Bailey & Love's SHORT PRACTICE of SURGERY

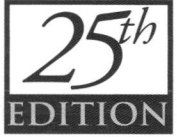

25th EDITION

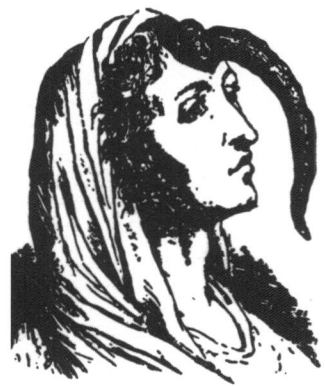

Sebaceous horn
(The owner, the widow Dimanche, sold water-cress in Paris)

A favourite illustration of Hamilton Bailey and McNeill Love,
and well known to readers of earlier editions of *Short Practice*.

Bailey & Love's
SHORT PRACTICE of SURGERY

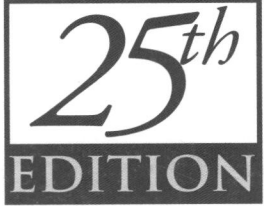

25th EDITION

Edited by

NORMAN S. WILLIAMS MS FRCS FMed Sci

Professor of Surgery and Centre Lead, Centre for Academic Surgery, Barts and the London School of Medicine and Dentistry, Queen Mary, University of London; Elected Member of the Council of the Royal College of Surgeons of England; President Elect of The Society of Academic and Research Surgery, UK

CHRISTOPHER J.K. BULSTRODE MCh FRCS(Orth)

Professor and Honorary Consultant Orthopaedic Surgeon, University of Oxford; Member of Council, Royal College of Surgeons of Edinburgh; Elected Member of the General Medical Council of the UK

P. RONAN O'CONNELL MD FRCSI FRCPS(Glas)

Professor of Surgery, University College Dublin, St Vincent's University Hospital, Dublin, Ireland

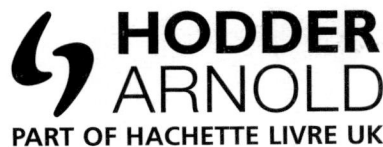

HODDER ARNOLD
PART OF HACHETTE LIVRE UK

First published in Great Britain in 1932
24th edition published in 2004
This 25th edition published in 2008 by Hodder Arnold, an imprint of
Hodder Education, part of Hachette Livre UK,
338 Euston Road, London NW1 3BH

http://www.hoddereducation.com

Whilst the advice and information in this book are believed to be true and
accurate at the date of going to press, neither the author[s] nor the
publisher can accept any legal responsibility or liability for any errors or
omissions that may be made. In particular (but without limiting the
generality of the preceding disclaimer) every effort has been made to
check drug dosages; however it is still possible that errors have been
missed. Furthermore, dosage schedules are constantly being revised and
new side-effects recognized. For these reasons the reader is strongly urged
to consult the drug companies' printed instructions before administering
any of the drugs recommended in this book.

British Library Cataloguing in Publication Data
A catalogue record for this book is available from the British Library

Library of Congress Cataloging-in-Publication Data
A catalog record for this book is available from the Library of Congress

ISBN 978 0 340 93932 1
ISBN [ISE] 978 0 340 93937 6
(International Students' Edition, restricted territorial availability)

1 2 3 4 5 6 7 8 9 10

Commissioning Editor: Joanna Koster
Project Editor: Clare Patterson
Production Controller: Andre Sim
Cover Designer: Helen Townson

Typeset in 9.5/11 pt Goudy by Phoenix Photosetting, Chatham, Kent
Printed and Bound in India

What do you think about this book? Or any other Hodder Arnold title?
Please visit our website: www.hoddereducation.com

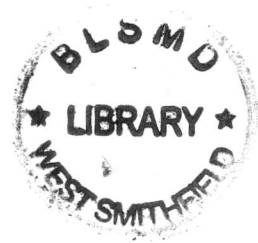

Contents

Editorial contributors

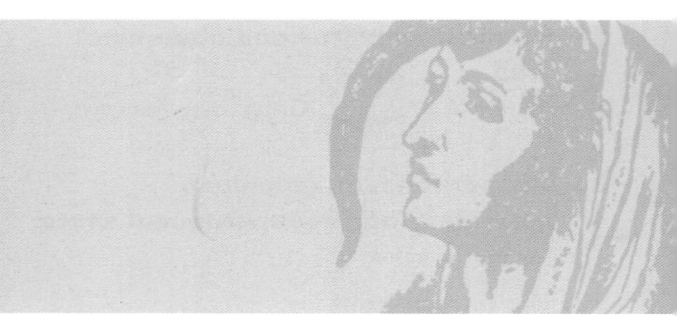

The editors would like to thank the following people who have made particular contributions to the 25th edition:

Section editor, Trauma

Robert Handley BSc MB ChB FRCS(Ed)
The Trauma Service, John Radcliffe Hospital, Oxford, UK

Editorial advisor, Paediatrics

Mark D. Stringer MS FRCS FRCP FRCS(Paed)
Department of Anatomy and Structural Biology, University of Otago, Dunedin, New Zealand; Formerly Professor of Paediatric Surgery, Leeds, UK

Imaging consultant

Stephen Eustace MB BCh MRCPI FRCR FFR RCSI
Consultant Radiologist, Mater Misericordiae University Hospital, Dublin, Ireland

Historical footnotes

John G. Fairer TD BA LLB MB BS FRCA
Formerly Anaesthetist, Charing Cross Hospital Medical School, London, UK

Andrew Wainwright BSc ChB FRCS(Tr and Orth)
Consultant Orthopaedic Surgeon, Nuffield Orthopaedic Centre NHS Trust, Oxford, UK

List of contributors

Derek Alderson MD FRCS
Barling Chair of Surgery, Queen Elizabeth Hospital,
Birmingham, UK

Gina M. Allen BM DCH MRCGP MRCP FRCR
Consultant Radiologist, Royal Orthopaedic Hospital and
Universities Hospitals, Birmingham, UK

Jonathan R. Anderson FRCS
Consultant in Cardiothoracic Surgery, Hammersmith Hospital,
London, UK

Nicholas C.M. Armitage DM FRCS
Consultant Colorectal and General Surgeon, Nottingham
University Hospitals Trust, Nottingham, UK

Shazad Ashraf BSc(Hons) MB ChB(Hons)
Bobby Moore Research Fellow, CRUK at the Weatherall
Institute of Molecular Medicine, Oxford, UK

D.L. Back BSc(Hons) MBBS FRCS(Ed)(Orth)
Consultant Orthopaedic Surgeon, Guy's and St Thomas'
Hospital, London, UK

Sarah J. Barton MBBS DMCC MRCS
Registrar, Trauma and Orthopaedics, Plymouth, UK

Grant J.E.M. Bates BSc BM BCh FRCS
Consultant ENT Surgeon, The Radcliffe Infirmary, and Senior
Clinical Lecturer, University of Oxford, Oxford, UK

David H. Bennett BSc DM FRCS
Department of Surgery, The Royal Bournemouth Hospital,
Bournemouth, UK

Satyajit Bhattacharya MS MPhil FRCS
Consultant Hepato-pancreato-biliary Surgeon, The Royal
London Hospital, London, UK

Kenneth D. Boffard BSc(Hons) MB BCh FRCS FRCS(Ed) FRCPS(Glas)
FCS(SA) FACS
Professor and Clinical Head, Department of Surgery,
Johannesburg Hospital and University of Witwatersrand,
Johannesburg, South Africa

Andrew W. Bradbury BSc MD FRCS(Ed)
Professor of Vascular Surgery, Birmingham Heartlands Hospital,
Birmingham, UK

J. Andrew Bradley PhD FRCS FMedSci
Professor of Surgery, University of Cambridge and Director of
Transplantation, Addenbrooke's Hospital, Cambridge, UK

Karim Brohi BSc FRCS FRCA
Consultant, Vascular and Trauma Section, The Royal London
Hospital, Whitechapel, London, UK

Kevin Burnand MB BS FRCS MS
Professor of Vascular Surgery, St Thomas' Hospital, London, UK

Christopher L.H. Chan BSc PhD FRCS
Senior Lecturer and Consultant Surgeon, Barts and the London
NHS Trust, London, UK

Sue Clark MD FRCS (Gen Surg)
Consultant Colorectal Surgeon, St Mark's Hospital, Harrow,
UK

Kevin Conlon MCh MBA FRCSI FACS FRCS
Chair of Surgery, Adelaide and Meath Hospital Dublin
incorporating The National Children's Hospital, Tallaght,
Dublin, Ireland

Paul Cool MD MedSc(Res) FRCS(Ed) FRCS(Orth)
Consultant Orthopaedic and Oncological Surgeon, Robert Jones
and Agnes Hunt Orthopaedic Hosptial, Oswestry, UK

Lord Darzi of Denham KBE HonFREng FMedSci
Paul Hamlyn Chair of Surgery, Professor of Surgery and Head of
Department, Department of Biosurgery and Surgical
Technology, Imperial College London, UK

Pradip K. Datta MS FRCS(Ed) FRCS(Eng) FRCSI FRCS(Glas)
Honorary Consultant Surgeon, Caithness General Hospital,
Wick, UK; and Member of Council and College Tutor, Royal
College of Surgeons of Edinburgh

Mark Davies FRCS FRCS(Tr & Orth)
Consultant Foot and Ankle Surgeon, The London Foot and
Ankle Centre, London, UK

Sanjay De Bakshi MS FRCS(Eng) FRCS(Ed)
Consultant Surgeon, Calcutta Medical Research Institute,
Kolkata, India

Brian R. Davidson MB ChB MD FRCPS(Glas) FRCS
Professor of HPB and Liver Transplant Surgery, Royal Free and University College School of Medicine, London, UK

Sunny Deo FRCS(Tr & Orth)
Consultant Orthopaedic Surgeon, Great Western Hospital, Swindon, UK

Len Doyal BA MSc
Emeritus Professor of Medical Ethics, St Bartholomew's and The Royal London School of Medicine and Dentistry, Queen Mary and Westfield College, University of London, UK

Michael J. Earley FRCSI FRCS(Plast) MCh
Consultant Plastic Surgeon, The Children's University Hospital, Dublin and the Mater Misericordiae Hospital, Dublin, Ireland; and Past President of the British Association of Plastic Reconstructive and Aesthetic Surgeons

Jonothan J. Earnshaw MB BS DM FRCS
Consultant Surgeon, Gloucestershire Royal Hospital, Gloucester, UK

Deborah M. Eastwood MB ChB FRCS
Great Ormond Street Hosptial for Children and the Royal National Orthopaedic Hospital, London, UK

Roger M. Feakins FRCPI FRCPath
Consultant Histopathologist, Barts and the London NHS Trust, London, and Professor of Gastrointestinal Pathology, Barts and the London, Queen Mary's School of Medicine and Dentistry, The University of London, UK

Kenneth C.H. Fearon MB ChB(Hons) MD FRCPS(Glas) FRCS(Ed) FRCS(Eng)
Professor of Surgical Oncology, University of Edinburgh, Royal Infirmary and Honorary Consultant Colorectal Surgeon, Western General Hospital, Edinburgh, UK

Christopher G. Fowler BSc MA MS FRCP FRCS(Urol) FEBU FHEA
Professor of Surgical Education, Barts and the London School of Medicine and Dentistry, Queen Mary, University of London, and Honorary Consultant Urologist, Barts and the London NHS Trust, London, UK

Brian J.C. Freeman MB BCh BAO DM FRCS(Tr & Oth)
Professor of Spinal Surgery, University of Nottingham and Consultant Spinal Surgeon, The Centre for Spinal Studies and Surgery, Nottingham University Hospitals NHS Trust, Nottingham, UK

O. James Garden BSc MB ChB MD FRCS(RCPSG) FRCS(Ed) FRCP(Ed) FRACS(Hon)
Regius Professor of Clinical Surgery and Honorary Consultant Hepatobiliary and Pancreatic Surgeon, Royal Infirmary, Edinburgh, UK

Peter V. Giannoudis BSc MB MD EEC(Ortho)
Professor of Trauma and Orthopaedic Surgery, University of Leeds, UK

Sudip Ghosh MBBS MS FRCS(Plast)(Eng)
Consultant in Plastic, Reconstructive and Cosmetic Surgery and Clinical Director of Burns, Stoke Mandeville Hospital, Aylesbury, UK

Giorgi Giorgobiani MD
Associate Professor of Surgery, Tbilisi State Medical University, Tbilisi, Georgia

Timothy Goodacre MBBS BSc FRCS
Senior Clinical Lecturer, Nuffield Department of Surgery, Oxford; Florey Lecturer in Clinical Medicine, Queen's College Oxford; Consultant Plastic and Reconstructive Surgeon, Oxford Radcliffe Hospitals, Oxford, UK

Adam R. Greenbaum MB BS MBA PhD FRCS(Plast) EBOPRAS
Consultant Plastic Surgeon, Guys and St. Thomas' NHS Foundation Trust and St John's Institute of Dermatology, St Thomas' Hospital, and Honorary Consultant Plastic Surgeon, King's College Hospital NHS Trust, London, UK

Robert Handley BSc MB ChB FRCS(Ed)
The Trauma Service, John Radcliffe Hospital, Oxford, UK

Hugo W.A. Henderson MA MB BS FRCOphth
Consultant Ophthalmologist and Ophthalmic Plastic Surgeon, The Royal Free Hampstead NHS Trust and The Royal National Throat Nose and Ear Hospital, London, UK

Joanna Hicks FRCS (Tr & Orth)
Consultant Paediatric Orthopaedic Surgeon, Stoke Mandeville Hospital, Aylesbury, UK

Shervanthi Homer-Vanniasinkam IBSc MD FRCSED FRCS
Consultant Vascular Surgeon, Leeds General Infirmary, Leeds, UK

David J. Howard FRCS FRCS(Ed)
Emeritus Senior Lecturer, University College London and Consultant Head and Neck Surgeon, Royal National Throat, Nose and Ear Hospital and Charing Cross Hospital, London, UK

Ian Hunt MB BS BSc(Hons) FRCS(C-Th)
Specialist Registrar Cardiothoracic Surgery, St George's Hospital, London, UK

Jonathan D. Jagger MB BS FRCS DO FRCS(Ophth)
Consultant Ophthalmic Surgeon, Royal Free Hosptial, London, UK

Srinath Kamineni BSc(Hons) MB BCh FRCS(Ed) FRCS(Orthopaedics and Trauma)
Consultant Elbow and Shoulder Surgeon, Cromwell Upper Limb Unit, Cromwell Hospital, London; Professor of Bioengineering, Brunel University, London; and Honorary Senior Clinical Lecturer, Imperial College London, UK

Stephen Kennedy MA(Oxon) MD MRCOG
Clinical Reader and Head of Department, Nuffield Department of Obstetrics and Gynaecology, University of Oxford, UK

Richard Kerr BSc MA MB BS MS FRCS
Consultant Neurological Surgeon, The Radcliffe Infirmary and Honorary Senior Lecturer, Nuffield Department of Surgery, Oxford, UK

Vikas Khanduja MB BS MRCS(G) MSc FRCS(Orth)
Consultant Orthopaedic Surgeon, Addenbrooke's, Cambridge University NHS Hospitals Trust, Cambridge, UK

Andrew N. Kingsnorth MS FRCS FACS
Professor of Surgery, Peninsula Medical School, Derriford Hospital, Plymouth, UK

Rohit Kotnis MB ChB BSc MRCS
Specialist Registrar in Trauma and Orthopaedics, Nuffield Orthopaedic Centre, Oxford, UK

Zygmunt H. Krukowski PhD FRCS(Ed) FRCP(Ed) Hon FRCS(Glas)
Consultant Surgeon, Aberdeen Royal Infirmary, Professor of Clinical Surgery, University of Aberdeen, Aberdeen, UK and Surgeon to the Queen in Scotland

Pawanindra Lal MS DNB MNAMS MNASc FRCS(Ed) FRCS(Glas)
Professor of Surgery, Maulana Azad Medical College, New Delhi, India

Ilana Langdon MB ChB MSc FRCS(Tr and Orth)
Consultant Orthopaedic Surgeon, Royal United Hospital, Bath, UK

Richard M. Langford FRCA
Senior Lecturer, St Bartholomew's and the Royal London School of Medicine at Queen Mary and Westfield College, London; Consultant Anaesthetist, St Bartholomew's Hospital, London, UK

John Leach MA BM BCh FRCS(Neuro.Surg)
Specialist Registrar in Neurosurgery, The John Radcliffe Hospital, Oxford, UK

David J. Leaper MD ChM FRCS FACS
Emeritus Professor of Surgery, University of Newcastle upon Tyne and Visiting Professor, Department of Wound Healing, Cardiff University, Cardiff, UK

Lisa Leonard BA MSc FRCS(T & O)
Consultant Orthopaedic Surgeon, Royal Sussex County Hospital, Brighton, UK

James Lindsay MA PhD BMBCh MRCP
Consultant Gastroenterologist, The Royal London Hospital, London, UK

Valerie J. Lund CBE MS FRCS FRCS(Ed)
Professor of Rhinology, The Ear Institute, University College London, London, UK

Peter J. Lunniss BSc MS FRCS
Senior Lecturer and Honorary Consultant Surgeon, Royal London and Homerton Hospitals, London, UK

John MacFie MD FRCS
Consultant Surgeon, Scarborough Hospital and Professor of Surgery, Postgraduate Medical Institute, University of Hull, UK

Pradeep Madhavan Dip NB(Surg) FRCS(Tr & Orth)
Consultant Spinal Surgeon, Taunton and Somerset NHS Foundation Trust, Taunton, UK

Vipul Mandalia MS
Specialist Registrar in Orthopaedics, Swindon and Marlborough NHS Trust, UK

Matthew Matson MRCP FRCR
Consultant Radiologist, Royal London Hospital, London, UK

Enda McVeigh MPhil FRCOG
Senior Fellow and Honorary Consultant Gynaecologist, John Radcliffe Hospital, Oxford, UK

Vivek Mehta MBBS FRCA
Consultant in Pain Medicine and Anaesthesia, St Bartholomew's Hospital, London, UK

Neil J.McC. Mortensen MD FRCS
Professor of Colorectal Surgery, John Radcliffe Hospital, Oxford, UK

Alastair J. Munro BSc FRCP(E) FRCR
Professor of Radiation Oncology, Ninewells Hospital & Medical School, Dundee, UK

John A. Murie MA BSc MD FRCS
Consultant Vascular Surgeon, The Royal Infirmary of Edinburgh, Edinburgh, UK

Ali Naraghi FRCR
Department of Medical Imaging, Mount Sinai Hospital and University Health Network, Toronto, Canada

Dinesh K. Nathwani MB ChB MSc FRCS(Tr & Orth)
Consultant and Honorary Senior Lecturer, Trauma and Orthopaedics, Charing Cross Hospital and Imperial College School of Medicine, London, UK

David E. Neal BSc FRCS FRCS(Ed) FMedSci
Professor of Surgical Oncology, Honorary Consultant Urological Surgeon, University of Cambridge, Cambridge, UK

P. Ronan O'Connell MB BCh BAO MD FRCSI FRCPS(Glas)
Professor of Surgery, University College Dublin, St Vincent's Hospital, Dublin, Ireland

Alistair Pace MD MRCS AFRCS MSc
Specialist Registrar in Trauma and Orthopaedics, Nottingham, UK

Simon Paterson-Brown MB BS MS MPhil FRCS(Ed) FRCS(Eng) MCS(Hong Kong)
Consultant General and Upper Gastrointestinal Surgeon and Honorary Senior Lecturer, Royal Infirmary Edinburgh, Edinburgh, UK

Rupert M. Pearse MB BS BSc MD FRCA DipICM(UK)
Consultant and Senior Lecturer in Intensive Care Medicine, Royal London Hospital, London, UK

Charles S. Perkins FDSRCS FFDRCSI FRCS
Consultant Oral and Maxillofacial Surgeon, Cheltenham General and Gloucestershire Royal Hospitals, Gloucestershire, UK

Ashley R. Poynton MD FRCSI FRCS(Tr & Orth)
Consultant Spinal Surgeon, National Spinal Injuries Unit, Mater Misericordiae University Hospital, Dublin, Ireland

John N. Primrose MD FRCS
Professor of Surgery, University of Southampton School of Medicine, Southampton General Hospital, Southampton, UK

Sanjay Purkayastha BSc(Hons) MBBS(Hons) MRCS(Eng)
Specialist Registrar and Clinical Lecturer in Surgery, Department of Biosurgery and Surgical Technology, Imperial College London, UK

Mamoon Rashid FRCS(Eng) FCPS(Pak)
Head of Department of Plastic Surgery, Combined Military Hospital Rawalpindi; Associate Professor of Surgery, Army Medical College Rawalpindi, Pakistan

Matthias Rothmund FACS FRCS(Hon)(Ed) FRCS ad eundem (Eng)
Professor and Chairman, Department of Surgery, Philipps University, Marburg, Germany

Robert W. Ruckley MB ChB FRCS FRCS(Ed)
Consultant Ear, Nose and Throat and Head and Neck Surgeon, Darlington Memorial Hospital, Darlington, UK

Richard Sainsbury MB BS MD FRCS
Consultant Surgeon, Southampton University Hospitals NHS Trust and Honorary Reader in Surgery, University College London, UK

Parminder Singh MB BS MRCS
Specialist Registrar in Trauma and Orthopaedics and Honorary Student Lecturer in the Nuffield Department of Orthopaedic Surgery, Nuffield Orthopaedic Centre, Oxford, UK

Jay Smith BSc MB BS MRCS(Eng) DipS&EMed GB&I
Specialist Registrar in Trauma and Orthopaedics, Guy's and St Thomas' Hospital, London, UK

William P. Smith FDSRCS FRCS
Consultant Maxillofacial Surgeon, Northampton General Hospital, Northampton, UK

Matthew C. Solan FRCS(Tr & Orth)
Consultant Trauma and Orthopaedic Surgeon, Royal Surrey County Hospital, Guildford, and London Foot and Ankle Centre, London, UK

Richard Stacey FRCS FRCS(SN)
Consultant Neurosurgeon, John Radcliffe Hospital, Oxford, and Lecturer in Clinical Medicine, Wadham College, Oxford, UK

Robert J.C. Steele MD FRCS(Ed) FRCS
Professor of Surgery, University of Dundee, UK

Mark D. Stringer MS FRCS FRCP FRCS(Paed)
Department of Anatomy and Structural Biology, University of Otago, Dunedin, New Zealand; Formerly Professor of Paediatric Surgery, Leeds, UK

Jeremy Thompson MChir FRCS
Consultant Gastrointestinal Surgeon, Chelsea and Westminster Hospital, London, UK

Tom Treasure MD MS FRCS
Professor of Cardiothoracic Surgery, Guy's Hospital, London, UK

Michael Tyler FRCS(Plast) MB ChM
Consultant Plastic Surgeon, Stoke Mandeville Hospital, Aylesbury, UK

Richard N. Villar MA MS FRCS
Consultant Orthopaedic Surgeon, The Wellington Hospital, London, UK

Birgit Whitman PhD
Research and Governance Manager, University of Bristol, UK

Marc Christopher Winslet MS FRCS
Professor of Surgery, Head of Department and Chairman of Division of Surgery and Interventional Sciences, University College London, Royal Free Hospital, London, UK

Preface

This is the 25th and hence Silver Jubilee edition of this world famous textbook. It has stood the test of time as evidenced by increasing sales, edition by edition, a tribute to the foresight of the original authors Hamilton Bailey and McNeill Love. Both set out to produce a high quality, comprehensive textbook to be enjoyed by both undergraduates and postgraduates. Part of their magic formula was to combine clear and concise text with numerous clinical photographs collected from their own archives. Most important was the frequent use of anecdote and aphorism to highlight points of clinical relevance, further enhanced by autobiographical notes beloved by all devotees of the book. We, the editors of this auspicious edition, therefore feel a particular responsibility following in the footsteps of the original authors and our colleague editors who continued this tradition over past editions. It is always difficult to blend the old with the new but this we have attempted to do. We present to the reader a comprehensive, modern surgical textbook which, we hope, retains the feel of the original. We have ensured that the text is liberally illustrated with high quality reproductions and line drawings. Some of Bailey and Love's original illustrations have been retained because they capture specific points so well that we have felt obliged to keep them. Similarly the autobiographical notes remain but have been updated. We have been particularly fortunate in this endeavour in retaining the services of Dr J.G. Fairer who, as a labour of love, has spent many hours ensuring the veracity of these notes. To help the budding young surgeon faced with that heart-sinking question from their boss, 'What instrument is that in your hand?' followed by 'And who was he?', we have started a new page in the appendix which gives answers to a few of the most common queries. Let us know if you think it is useful.

Despite the retention of some of the historical attributes that have made the book so popular over previous editions, the reader will find that the 25th edition is a book for our time. Whereas the past informs the present, it must never enslave the future. Thus each chapter starts with learning objectives and the text is liberally sprinkled with summary boxes that provide the busy student an easy aide memoire when revising for ubiquitous exams. We have given considerable thought to the order of the chapters and have grouped them into themed sections with the first concentrating on principles of surgery generic to all specialties. We believe this format provides a more logical sequence for the reader to that found in previous editions. We have also attempted to reduce repetition. For instance, most paediatric problems have been removed from the specialty chapters and are dealt with in a new chapter entitled 'Principles of paediatric surgery'. We are grateful to Mark Stringer, our paediatric advisor, who has masterminded this transition. Mark has also reviewed all the pertinent specialty chapters to ensure that where reference to paediatric conditions remains, it has been brought up to date. Other chapters have been merged to streamline the text. Where old chapters have been retained, they have been thoroughly revised and where appropriate new chapters have been introduced. The quality of diagnostic imaging reproduced has significantly benefited by review of our imaging advisor, Stephen Eustace, who has ensured a high standard of reproduction throughout.

Surgical textbooks need to be refreshed continually in order to keep up with ever-increasing developments. Continual renewal is an essential part of progress. Thus R.C.G. Russell, senior editor of four previous editions, has now stepped down. We thank Chris for his devotion to the book and his exemplary editorial skills that have undoubtedly contributed to its continued popularity. We welcome Ronan O'Connell to the editorial team. Ronan, as a past editor of the *British Journal of Surgery*, has brought new energy and strategic thinking into the organisation and content of the book. This, in turn, has invigorated the remaining two editors and hopefully enlivened the sections they are responsible for.

We have chosen our contributors carefully. Each was selected not only for surgical knowledge and expertise but also clarity in communication. Their instructions were to be ruthless in excising old material and to ensure current relevance of chapter content and that any recommendations for management were, as far as possible, evidence-based. We trust that this approach shines through. Without such a dedicated and meticulous group of contributors, this edition could never compete with the high quality of its predecessors. Their efforts are much appreciated. Our publishers have done sterling work to ensure that the production of the book is of the highest quality. They have striven for excellence including the elimination of typographical and grammatical errors. Nevertheless, in a volume of this size, some errors will inevitably have crept in. We have no doubt that these will, as in the past, be reported to us by our hawk-eyed readers, a valued Bailey and Love tradition.

Undergraduate and trainee curricula are continually changing as surgery evolves and becomes more specialised. There can be no doubt, however, that a house cannot be built on sand; a firm foundation is required. It is essential for all those who wish to pursue a career in surgery to have this firm base. They must be conversant with the general principles of surgery and have an appreciation of the basics of all specialties out with their own. Hence they need a reliable textbook that can provide this broad canvas. We very much hope that the Silver Jubilee Edition of this venerable textbook fulfils this requirement.

Norman S. Williams
Christopher J.K. Bulstrode
P. Ronan O'Connell
February 2008

Acknowledgements

Chapter 7, *Principles of oncology*, contains some material from 'Principles of oncology' by Robert J. Steele and Amy Leslie which appeared in the 24th edition. The material has been revised and updated by the current authors.

Chapter 8, *Surgical audit and research*, contains some material from 'An Approach to surgical audit and research' by Mark Emberton and Jan van der Meulen which appeared in the 24th edition. The material has been revised and updated by the current authors.

Chapter 10, *Diagnostic imaging*, contains some material from 'Diagnostic and interventional radiology' by Alison M. McLean and Matthew Matson and 'Musculoskeletal imaging' by David J. Wilson and Gina M. Allen which both appeared in the 24th edition. The material has been revised and updated by the current authors.

Chapter 13, *Preoperative preparation*, contains some material from 'Preparing a patient for surgery' by Peter Driscoll and Christopher J.K. Bulstrode which appeared in the 24th edition. The material has been revised and updated by the current authors.

Chapter 17, *Nutrition and fluid therapy*, contains some material from 'Nutrition' by Gordon L. Carlson and Edwin C. Clark which appeared in the 24th edition. The material has been revised and updated by the current author.

Chapter 24, *Neck and spine*, contains some material from 'The spine, vertebral column and spinal cord' by Richard C.S. Kerr and James Wilson-MacDonald which appeared in the 24th edition. The material has been revised and updated by the current author.

Chapter 25, *Trauma to the face and mouth*, contains some material from 'Maxillofacial injuries' by Charles S. Perkins and Richard P. Junpier which appeared in the 24th edition. The material has been revised and updated by the current author.

Chapter 32, *Sports medicine and sports injuries*, contains some material from 'Sports medicine and biomechanics' by Jonathan M. Webb and Christopher J.K. Bulstrode which appeared in the 24th edition. The material has been revised and updated by the current authors.

Chapter 34, *Upper limb – pathology, assessment and management*, contains some material from 'Problems in the shoulder and elbow' by Andrew J. Carr and Jon C. Clasper, and 'Wrist and hand' by David J. Warwick, both of which appeared in the 24th edition. The material has been revised and updated by the current author.

Chapter 35, *Hip and knee*, contains some material from 'Surgery for arthritis in the hip and knee' by Christopher J.K. Bulstrode and Ian K. Ritchie which appeared in the 24th edition. The material has been revised and updated by the current authors.

Chapter 46, *Oropharyngeal cancer*, contains material from 'Oral and oropharyngeal cancer' by John D. Langdon which appeared in the 24th edition. The material has been revised and updated by the current author.

Chapter 47, *Disorders of the salivary glands*, contains material from 'Disorders of the salivary glands' by William P. Smith and John D. Langdon which appeared in the 24th edition. The material has been revised and updated by the current author.

Chapter 49, *Adrenal glands and other endocrine disorders*, contains material from 'Parathyroid and adrenal glands' by Barnard Harrison which appeared in the 24th edition. The material has been revised and updated by the current author.

Chapter 54, *Venous disorders*, contains material from 'Venous disorders' by John H. Scurr which appeared in the 24th edition. The material has been revised and updated by the current author.

Chapter 59, *The oesophagus*, contains material from 'The oesophagus' by John Bancewicz which appeared in the 24th edition. The material has been revised and updated by the current author.

Chapter 63, *The gall bladder and bile ducts*, contains material from 'The gall bladder and bile ducts' by R.C.G. Russell which appeared in the 24th edition. The material has been revised and updated by the current author.

Chapter 64, *The pancreas*, contains material from 'The pancreas' by R.C.G. Russell which appeared in the 24th edition. The material has been revised and updated by the current author.

Chapter 65, *The small and large intestines*, contains material from 'The small and large intestines' by Neil J.McC. Mortensen and Oliver Jones which appeared in the 24th edition. The material has been revised and updated by the current authors.

Chapter 68, *The rectum*, contains material from 'The rectum' by Norman S. Williams which appeared in the 24th edition. The material has been revised and updated by the current author.

Chapter 69, *The anus and anal canal*, contains material from 'The anus and anal canal' by Norman S. Williams which appeared in the 24th edition. The material has been revised and updated by the current author.

Chapter 72, *The urinary bladder*, contains material from 'The urinary bladder' by David E. Neal and John D. Kelly which appeared in the 24th edition. The material has been revised and updated by the current author.

Chapter 73, *The prostate and seminal vesicles*, contains material from 'The prostate and seminal vesicles' by David E. Neal and John D. Kelly which appeared in the 24th edition. The material has been revised and updated by the current author.

Sayings of the great

Both Hamilton Bailey and McNeill Love, when medical students, served as clerks to Sir Robert Hutchison, 1871–1960, who was Consulting Physician to the London Hospital and President of the Royal College of Physicians. They never tired of quoting his 'medical litany', which is appropriate for all clinicians and, perhaps especially, for those who are surgically minded.

> From inability to leave well alone;
> From too much zeal for what is new and contempt for
>   what is old;
> From putting knowledge before wisdom,
>   science before art, cleverness before common sense;
> From treating patients as cases; and
> From making the cure of a disease more grievous than its
>   endurance,
> Good Lord, deliver.

To which may be added:

> The patient is the centre of the medical universe around which all our works revolve and towards which all our efforts trend.
>
> J.B. Murphy, 1857–1916, Professor of Surgery,
> Northwestern University, Chicago, IL, USA

> To study the phenomenon of disease without books is to sail an uncharted sea, while to study books without patients is not to go to sea at all.
>
> Sir William Osler, 1849–1919,
> Professor of Medicine, Oxford, UK

A knowledge of healthy and diseased actions is not less necessary to be understood than the principles of other sciences. By an acquaintance with principles we learn the cause of disease. Without this knowledge a man cannot be a surgeon. ... The last part of surgery, namely operations, is a reflection on the healing art; it is a tacit acknowledgement of the insufficiency of surgery. It is like an armed savage who attempts to get that by force which a civilised man would by stratagem.

> Hunter, 1728–1793, Surgeon, St George's Hospital,
> London, UK

Investigating Nature you will do well to bear ever in mind that in every question there is the truth, whatever our notions may be. This seems perhaps a very simple consideration; yet it is strange how often it seems to be disregarded. If we had nothing but pecuniary rewards and worldly honours to look to, our profession would not be one to be desired. But in its practice you will find it to be attended with peculiar privileges; second to none in intense interest and pure pleasures. It is our proud office to tend the fleshy tabernacle of the immortal spirit, and our path, if rightly followed, will be guided by unfettered truth and love unfeigned. In the pursuit of this noble and holy calling I wish you all God-speed.

> Promoter's address, Graduation in Medicine,
> University of Edinburgh, August, 1876, by Lord Lister,
> the Founder of Modern Surgery

PART
1 | Principles

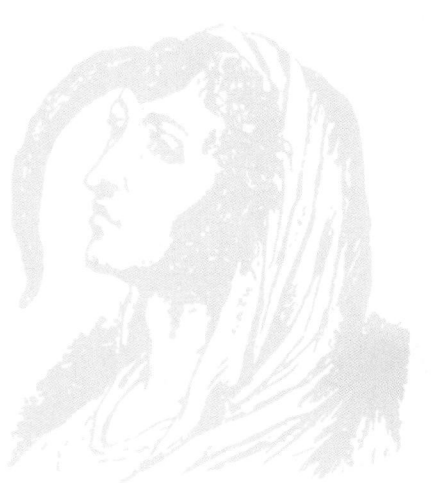

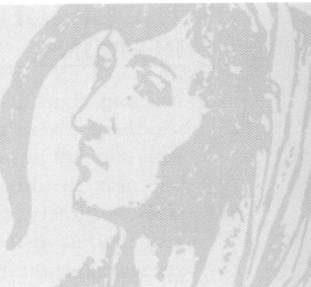

The metabolic response to injury

LEARNING OBJECTIVES

To understand:
- Classical concepts of homeostasis
- Mediators of the metabolic response to injury
- Physiochemical and biochemical changes that occur during injury and recovery

- Changes in body composition that accompany surgical injury
- Avoidable factors that compound the metabolic response to injury
- Concepts behind optimal perioperative care

BASIC CONCEPTS IN HOMEOSTASIS

In the eighteenth and nineteenth centuries, a series of eminent scientists laid the foundations of our understanding of homeostasis and the response to injury. The classical concepts of homeostasis and the response to injury are:

- 'The stability of the "milieu intérieur" is the primary condition for freedom and independence of existence.' (Claude Bernard)
  i.e. body systems act to maintain internal constancy
- 'Homeostasis: the co-ordinated physiological process which maintains most of the steady states of the organism.' (Walter Cannon)
  i.e. complex homeostatic responses involving the brain, nerves, heart, lungs, kidneys and spleen work to maintain body constancy
- 'There is a circumstance attending accidental injury which does not belong to the disease, namely that the injury done, has in all cases a tendency to produce both the deposition and means of cure.' (John Hunter)
  i.e. responses to injury are, in general, beneficial to the host and allow healing/survival

In essence, the concept evolved that the constancy of the 'milieu intérieur' allowed for the independence of organisms, that complex homeostatic responses sought to maintain this constancy, and that within this range of responses were the elements of healing and repair. These ideas pertained to normal physiology and mild/moderate injury. In the modern era, such concepts do not account for disease evolution following major injury/sepsis or the injured patient who would have died but for artificial organ support. Such patients exemplify less of the classical homeostatic control system (signal detector–processor–effector regulated by a negative feedback loop) and more of the 'open loop' system, whereby only with medical/surgical resolution of the primary abnormality is a return to classical homeostasis possible. Current understanding of such events as the response to major sepsis/injury relies on chaos theory and the use of a structured network knowledge-base approach.

As a consequence of modern understanding of the metabolic response to injury, elective surgical practice seeks to reduce the need for a homeostatic response by minimising the primary insult (minimal access surgery and 'stress-free' perioperative care). In emergency surgery, where the presence of tissue trauma/sepsis/hypovolaemia often compounds the primary problem, there is a requirement to augment artificially homeostatic responses (resuscitation) and to close the 'open' loop by intervening to resolve the primary insult (e.g. surgical treatment of major abdominal sepsis) and provide organ support (critical care) while the patient comes back to a situation in which homeostasis can achieve a return to normality (Summary box 1.1).

Summary box 1.1

Basic concepts

- **Homeostasis is the foundation of normal physiology**
- **'Stress-free' perioperative care helps to restore homeostasis following elective surgery**
- **Resuscitation, surgical intervention and critical care can return the severely injured patient to a situation in which homeostasis becomes possible once again**

This chapter aims to review the mediators of the stress response, the physiochemical and biochemical pathway changes associated with surgical injury and the changes in body composition that occur following surgical injury. Emphasis is laid on why knowledge of these events is important to understand the rationale for modern 'stress-free' perioperative and critical care.

Claude Bernard, 1813–1878, Professor of Physiology, The College de France, Paris, France.
Walter Bradford Cannon, 1871–1945, Professor of Physiology, Harvard University Medical School, Boston, MA, USA.
John Hunter, 1728–1793, Surgeon, St. George's Hospital, London, England. He is regarded as 'The Father of Scientific Surgery'.

THE GRADED NATURE OF THE INJURY RESPONSE

It is important to recognise that the response to injury is graded: the more severe the injury, the greater the response (Fig. 1.1). This concept not only applies to physiological/metabolic changes but also to immunological changes/sequelae. Thus, following elective surgery of intermediate severity, there may be a transient and modest rise in temperature, heart rate, respiratory rate, energy expenditure and peripheral white cell count. Following major trauma/sepsis, these changes are accentuated, resulting in a systemic inflammatory response syndrome (SIRS), hypermetabolism, marked catabolism, shock and even multiple organ dysfunction (MODS).

Not only is the metabolic response graded, but it also evolves with time. In particular, the immunological sequelae of major injury evolve from a pro-inflammatory state driven primarily by the innate immune system (macrophages, neutrophils, dendritic cells) into a compensatory anti-inflammatory response syndrome (CARS) characterised by suppressed immunity and diminished resistance to infection. In patients who develop infective complications, the latter will drive on-going systemic inflammation, the acute phase response and continued catabolism.

MEDIATORS OF THE METABOLIC RESPONSE TO INJURY

The classical neuroendocrine pathways of the stress response consist of afferent nociceptive neurones, the spinal cord,

thalamus, hypothalamus and pituitary (Fig. 1.2). Corticotrophin-releasing factor (CRF) released from the hypothalamus increases adrenocorticotrophic hormone (ACTH) release from the anterior pituitary. ACTH then acts on the adrenal to increase the secretion of cortisol. Hypothalamic activation of the sympathetic nervous system causes release of adrenalin and also stimulates release of glucagon. Intravenous infusion of a cocktail of these 'counter-regulatory' hormones (glucagon, glucocorticoids and catecholamines) reproduces many aspects of the metabolic response to injury. There are, however, many other players, including alterations in insulin release and sensitivity, hypersecretion of prolactin and growth hormone (GH) in the presence of low circulatory insulin-like growth factor-1 (IGF-1) and inactivation of peripheral thyroid hormones and gonadal function. Of note, GH has direct lipolytic, insulin-antagonising and pro-inflammatory properties (Summary box 1.2).

> **Summary box 1.2**
>
> **Neuroendocrine response to injury/critical illness**
>
> The neuroendocrine response to severe injury/critical illness is biphasic:
>
> - *Acute phase* characterised by an actively secreting pituitary and elevated counter-regulatory hormones (cortisol, glucagon, adrenaline). Changes are thought to be beneficial for short-term survival
> - *Chronic phase* associated with hypothalamic suppression and low serum levels of the respective target organ hormones. Changes contribute to chronic wasting

The innate immune system (principally macrophages) interacts in a complex manner with the adaptive immune system (T cells, B cells) in co-generating the metabolic response to injury (Fig. 1.2). Pro-inflammatory cytokines including interleukin-1 (IL-1), tumour necrosis factor alpha (TNFα), IL-6 and IL-8 are produced within the first 24 hours and act directly on the hypothalamus to cause pyrexia. Such cytokines also augment the hypothalamic stress response and act directly on skeletal muscle to induce proteolysis while inducing acute phase protein production in the liver. Pro-inflammatory cytokines also play a complex role in the development of peripheral insulin resistance. Other important pro-inflammatory mediators include nitric oxide [(NO) via inducible nitric oxide synthetase (iNOS)] and a variety of prostanoids [via cyclo-oxygenase-2 (Cox-2)].

Within hours of the upregulation of pro-inflammatory cytokines, endogenous cytokine antagonists enter the circulation [e.g. interleukin-1 receptor antagonist (IL-1Ra) and TNF-soluble receptors (TNF-sR-55 and 75)] and act to control the pro-inflammatory response. A complex further series of adaptive changes includes the development of a Th2-type counter-inflammatory response [regulated by IL-4, -5, -9 and -13 and transforming growth factor beta (TGFβ)] which, if accentuated and prolonged in critical illness, is characterised as the CARS and results in immunosuppression and an increased susceptibility to opportunistic (nosocomial) infection (Summary box 1.3).

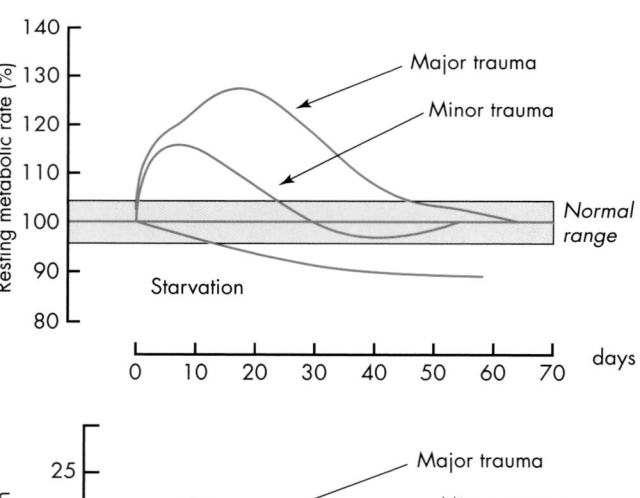

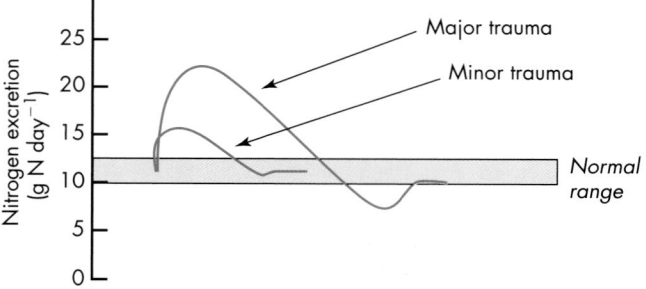

Figure 1.1 Hypermetabolism and increased nitrogen excretion are closely related to the magnitude of the initial injury and show a graded response.

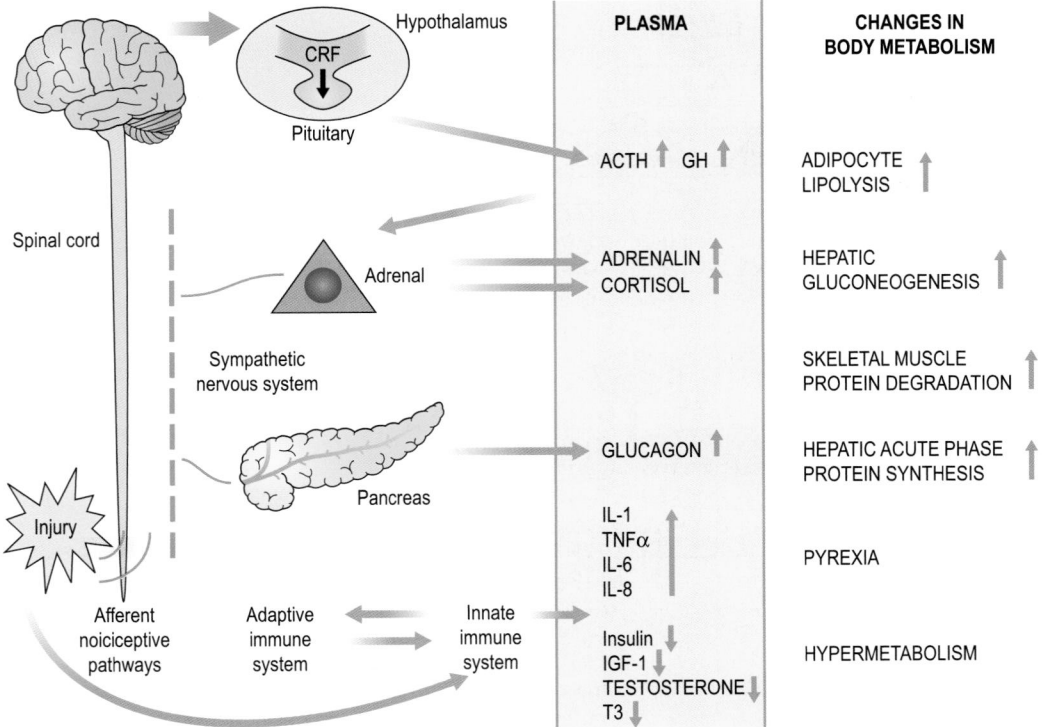

Figure 1.2 The integrated response to surgical injury (first 24–48 h): there is a complex interplay between the neuroendocrine stress response and the pro-inflammatory cytokine response of the innate immune system.

> **Summary box 1.3**
>
> **Systemic inflammatory response syndrome (SIRS) following major injury**
>
> - Is driven initially by pro-inflammatory cytokines (e.g. IL-1, IL-6 and TNFα)
> - Is followed rapidly by increased plasma levels of cytokine antagonists and soluble receptors (e.g. IL-1Ra, TNF-sR)
> - If prolonged or excessive may evolve into a counter-inflammatory response syndrome (CARS)

There are many complex interactions between the neuroendocrine, cytokine and metabolic axes. For example, although cortisol is immunosuppressive at high levels, it acts synergistically with IL-6 to promote the hepatic acute phase response. ACTH release is enhanced by pro-inflammatory cytokines and the noradrenergic system. The resulting rise in cortisol levels may form a weak feedback loop attempting to limit the pro-inflammatory stress response. Finally, hyperglycaemia may aggravate the inflammatory response via substrate overflow in the mitochondria, causing the formation of excess free oxygen radicals and also altering gene expression to enhance cytokine production.

At the molecular level, the changes that accompany systemic inflammation are extremely complex. In a recent study using network-based analysis of changes in mRNA expression in leucocytes following exposure to endotoxin, there were changes in the expression of more than 3700 genes with over half showing decreased expression and the remainder increased expression. The cell surface receptors, signalling mechanisms and transcription factors that initiate these events are also complex, but an early and important player involves the nuclear factor kappa B (NFκB)/*relA* family of transcription factors. A simplified model of current understanding of events within skeletal muscle is shown in Figure 1.3.

THE METABOLIC STRESS RESPONSE TO SURGERY AND TRAUMA: THE 'EBB AND FLOW' MODEL

In the natural world, if an animal is injured, it displays a characteristic response, which includes immobility, anorexia and catabolism (Summary box 1.4).

> **Summary box 1.4**
>
> **Physiological response to injury**
>
> The *natural* response to injury includes:
>
> - Immobility/rest
> - Anorexia
> - Catabolism
>
> The changes are designed to aid survival of moderate injury in the absence of medical intervention.

In 1930, Sir David Cuthbertson divided the metabolic response to injury in humans into 'ebb' and 'flow' phases (Fig. 1.4). The

Sir David Paton Cuthbertson, **1900–1989, Biochemist, Director of the Rowett Research Institute, Glasgow, Scotland.**

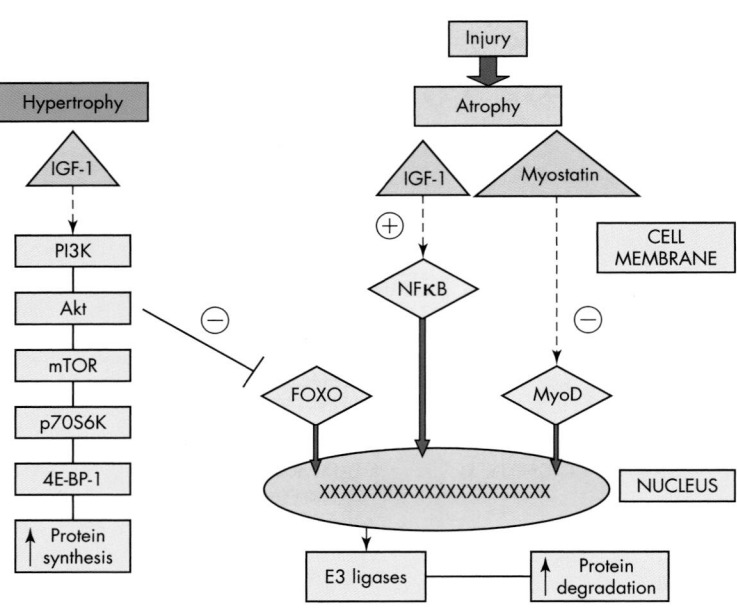

Figure 1.3 The major catabolic and anabolic signalling pathways involved in skeletal muscle homeostasis. FOXO, forkhead box sub-group O; IGF-1, insulin-like growth factor-1; mTOR, mammalian target of rapamycin; MyoD, myogenic differentiation factor D; NFκB, nuclear factor kappa B; PI3K, phosphatidylinositol 3-kinase; p70S6K, p70S6 kinase; 4E-BP-1, eukaryotic initiation translation factor 4E binding protein 1.

ebb phase begins at the time of injury and lasts for approximately 24–48 hours. It may be attenuated by proper resuscitation, but not completely abolished. The ebb phase is characterised by hypovolaemia, decreased basal metabolic rate, reduced cardiac output, hypothermia and lactic acidosis. The predominant hormones regulating the ebb phase are catecholamines, cortisol and aldosterone (following activation of the renin–angiotensin system). The magnitude of this neuroendocrine response depends on the degree of blood loss and the stimulation of somatic afferent nerves at the site of injury. The main physiological role of the ebb phase is to conserve both circulating volume and energy stores for recovery and repair.

Following resuscitation, the ebb phase evolves into a hypermetabolic flow phase, which corresponds to the SIRS. This phase involves the mobilisation of body energy stores for recovery and repair, and the subsequent replacement of lost or damaged tissue. It is characterised by tissue oedema (from vasodilatation and increased capillary leakage), increased basal metabolic rate (hypermetabolism), increased cardiac output, raised body temperature, leucocytosis, increased oxygen consumption and increased gluconeogenesis. The flow phase may be subdivided into an initial catabolic phase, lasting approximately 3–10 days, followed by an anabolic phase, which may last for weeks if extensive recovery and repair are required following serious injury. During the catabolic phase, the increased production of counter-regulatory hormones (including catecholamines, cortisol, insulin and glucagon) and inflammatory cytokines (e.g. IL-1, IL-6 and TNFα) results in significant fat and protein mobilisation, leading to significant weight loss and increased urinary nitrogen excretion. The increased production of insulin at this time is associated with significant *insulin resistance* and, therefore, injured patients often exhibit poor glycaemic control. The combination of pronounced or prolonged catabolism in association with insulin resistance places patients within this phase at increased risk of complications, particularly infectious and cardiovascular. Obviously, the development of complications will further aggravate the neuroendocrine and inflammatory stress responses, thus creating a vicious catabolic cycle (Summary box 1.5).

Summary box 1.5

Purpose of neuroendocrine changes following injury

The constellation of neuroendocrine changes following injury acts to:

- **Provide essential substrates for survival**
- **Postpone anabolism**
- **Optimise host defence**

These changes may be helpful in the short term, but may be harmful in the long term, especially to the severely injured patient who would otherwise not have survived without medical intervention.

KEY CATABOLIC ELEMENTS OF THE FLOW PHASE OF THE METABOLIC STRESS RESPONSE

There are several key elements of the flow phase that largely determine the extent of catabolism and thus govern the

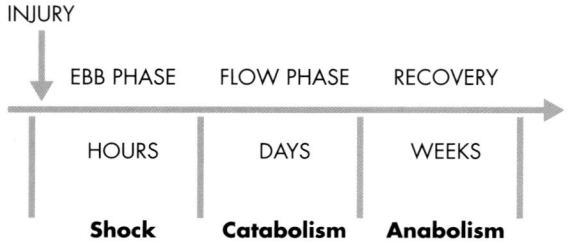

Figure 1.4 Phases of the physiological response to injury (after Cuthbertson 1930).

metabolic and nutritional care of the surgical patient. It must be remembered that, during the response to injury, not all tissues are catabolic. Indeed, the essence of this coordinated response is to allow the body to reprioritise limited resources away from peripheral tissues (muscle, adipose tissue, skin) and towards key viscera (liver, immune system) and the wound (Fig. 1.5).

Hypermetabolism

The majority of trauma patients (except possibly those with extensive burns) demonstrate energy expenditures approximately 15–25% above predicted healthy resting values. The predominant cause appears to be a complex interaction between the central control of metabolic rate and peripheral energy utilisation. In particular, central thermodysregulation (caused by the pro-inflammatory cytokine cascade), increased sympathetic activity, abnormalities in wound circulation [ischaemic areas produce lactate, which must be metabolised by the adenosine triphosphate (ATP)-consuming hepatic Cori cycle; hyperaemic areas cause an increase in cardiac output], increased protein turnover and nutritional support may all increase patient energy expenditure. Theoretically, patient energy expenditure could rise even higher than observed levels following surgery or trauma, but several features of standard intensive care (including bed rest, paralysis, ventilation and external temperature regulation) counteract the hypermetabolic driving forces of the stress response. Furthermore, the skeletal muscle wasting experienced by patients with prolonged catabolism actually limits the volume of metabolically active tissue (Summary box 1.6; see next section).

Summary box 1.6

Hypermetabolism

Hypermetabolism following injury:

- Is mainly caused by an acceleration of futile metabolic cycles
- Is limited in modern practice on account of elements of routine critical care

---

Alterations in skeletal muscle protein metabolism

Muscle protein is continually synthesised and broken down with a turnover rate in humans of 1–2% day^{-1}, and with a greater amplitude of changes in protein synthesis ($\pm$ twofold) than breakdown ($\pm$ 0.25-fold) during the diurnal cycle. Under normal circumstances, synthesis equals breakdown and muscle bulk remains constant. Physiological stimuli that promote net muscle protein accretion include feeding (especially extracellular amino acid concentration) and exercise. Paradoxically, during exercise, skeletal muscle protein synthesis is depressed, but it increases again during rest and feeding.

During the catabolic phase of the stress response, muscle wasting occurs as a result of an increase in muscle protein degradation (via enzymatic pathways), coupled with a decrease in muscle protein synthesis. The major site of protein loss is peripheral skeletal muscle, although nitrogen losses also occur in the respiratory muscles (predisposing the patient to hypoventilation and chest infections) and in the gut (reducing gut motility). Cardiac muscle appears to be mostly spared. Under extreme conditions of catabolism (e.g. major sepsis), urinary nitrogen losses can reach 14–20 g day^{-1}; this is equivalent to the loss of 500 g of skeletal muscle per day. It is remarkable that muscle catabolism cannot be inhibited fully by providing artificial nutritional support as long as the stress response continues. Indeed, in critical care, it is now recognised that 'hyperalimentation' represents a metabolic stress in itself, and that nutritional support should be at a modest level to attenuate rather than replace energy and protein losses.

The predominant mechanism involved in the wasting of skeletal muscle is the ATP-dependent ubiquitin–proteasome pathway (Fig. 1.6), although the lysosomal cathepsins and the calcium–calpain pathway play facilitatory and accessory roles.

Clinically, a patient with skeletal muscle wasting will experience asthenia, increased fatigue, reduced functional ability, decreased quality of life and an increased risk of morbidity and mortality. In critically ill patients, muscle weakness may be further worsened by the development of critical illness myopathy, a multifactorial condition that is associated with impaired excitation–contraction–coupling at the level of the sarcolemma and the sarcoplasmic reticulum membrane (Summary box 1.7).

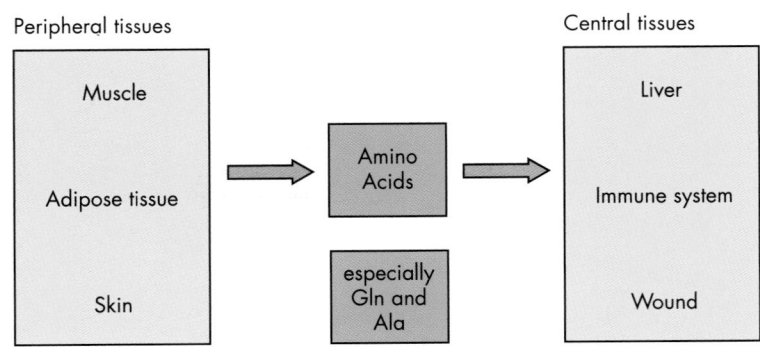

Peripheral tissues — Muscle, Adipose tissue, Skin → Amino Acids (especially Gln and Ala) → Central tissues — Liver, Immune system, Wound

Figure 1.5 During the metabolic response to injury, the body reprioritises protein metabolism away from peripheral tissues and towards key central tissues such as the liver, immune system and wound. One of the main reasons why the reutilisation of amino acids derived from muscle proteolysis leads to net catabolism is that the increased glutamine and alanine efflux from muscle is derived, in part, from the irreversible degradation of branched chain amino acids. Gln, glutamine; Ala, alanine.

Carl Ferdinand Cori, **1896–1984**, Professor of Pharmacology, and later of Biochemistry, Washington University Medical School, St. Louis, MI, USA and his wife Gerty Theresa Cori, **1896–1957**, who was also Professor of Biochemistry at the Washington University Medical School. In 1947 the Coris were awarded a share of the Nobel Prize for Physiology or Medicine 'for their discovery of how glycogen is catalytically converted'.

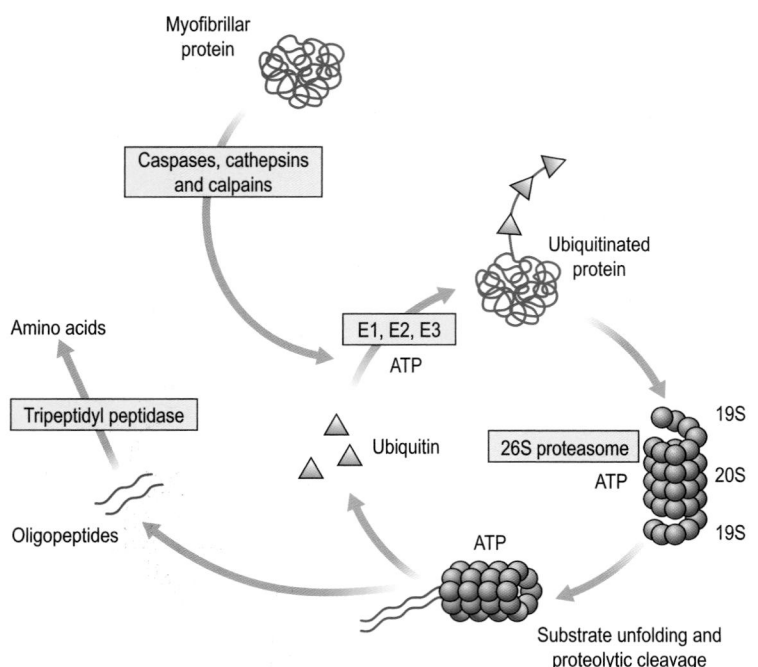

Figure 1.6 The intercellular effector mechanisms involved in degrading myofibrillar protein into free amino acids. The ubiquitin–proteasome pathway is a complex multistep process, which requires adenosine triphosphate (ATP) and results in the tagging of specific proteins with ubiquitin for degradation of proteasome. E1, ubiquitin-activating enzyme; E2, ubiquitin-conjugating enzyme; E3, ubiquitin ligase.

Summary box 1.7

Skeletal muscle wasting

- Provides amino acids for protein synthesis in central organs/tissues
- Is mediated at a molecular level mainly by activation of the ubiquitin–proteasome pathway
- Can result in immobility and contribute to hypostatic pneumonia and death if prolonged and excessive

---

Alterations in hepatic protein metabolism: the acute phase protein response (APPR)

The liver and skeletal muscle together account for > 50% of daily body protein turnover. Skeletal muscle has a large mass but a low turnover rate (1–2% day^{-1}), whereas the liver has a relatively small mass (1.5 kg) but a much higher protein turnover rate (10–20% day^{-1}). Hepatic protein synthesis is divided roughly 50:50 between renewal of structural proteins and synthesis of export proteins. Albumin is the major export protein produced by the liver and is renewed at the rate of about 10% day^{-1}. The transcapillary escape rate (TER) of albumin is about 10 times the rate of synthesis, and short-term changes in albumin concentration are most probably due to increased vascular permeability. Albumin TER may be increased threefold following major injury/sepsis.

In response to inflammatory conditions, including surgery, trauma, sepsis, cancer or autoimmune conditions, circulating peripheral blood mononuclear cells secrete a range of pro-inflammatory cytokines, including IL-1, IL-6 and TNFα. These cytokines, in particular IL-6, promote the hepatic synthesis of positive acute phase proteins, e.g. fibrinogen and C-reactive protein (CRP). The APPR represents a 'double-edged sword' for surgical patients as it provides proteins important for recovery and repair, but only at the expense of valuable lean tissue and energy reserves.

In contrast to the positive acute phase reactants, the plasma concentrations of other liver export proteins (the negative acute phase reactants) fall acutely following injury, e.g. albumin. However, rather than represent a reduced hepatic synthesis rate, the fall in plasma concentration of negative acute phase reactants is thought principally to reflect increased transcapillary escape, secondary to an increase in microvascular permeability (see above). Thus, increased hepatic synthesis of positive acute phase reactants is not compensated for by reduced synthesis of negative reactants (Summary box 1.8).

Summary box 1.8

Hepatic acute phase response

The hepatic acute phase response represents a reprioritisation of body protein metabolism towards the liver and is characterised by:

- *Positive* reactants (e.g. CRP): plasma concentration ↑
- *Negative* reactants (e.g. albumin): plasma concentration ↓

Insulin resistance

Following surgery or trauma, postoperative hyperglycaemia develops as a result of increased glucose production combined with decreased glucose uptake in peripheral tissues. Decreased glucose uptake is a result of insulin resistance which is transiently induced within the stressed patient. Suggested mechanisms for this phenomenon include the action of pro-inflammatory cytokines and the decreased responsiveness of insulin-regulated glucose transporter proteins. The degree of insulin resistance is proportional to the magnitude of the injurious process. Following routine upper abdominal surgery, insulin resistance may persist for approximately 2 weeks.

Postoperative patients with insulin resistance behave in a

similar manner to individuals with type II diabetes mellitus and are at increased risk of sepsis, deteriorating renal function, polyneuropathy and death.

The mainstay management of insulin resistance is intravenous insulin infusion. Insulin infusions may be used in either an *intensive* approach (i.e. sliding scales are manipulated to *normalise* the blood glucose level) or a *conservative* approach (i.e. insulin is administered when the blood glucose level exceeds a defined limit and discontinued when the level falls). Studies of postoperatively ventilated patients in the intensive care unit (ICU) have suggested that maintenance of normal glucose levels using intensive insulin therapy can significantly reduce both morbidity and mortality. Furthermore, intensive insulin therapy is superior to conservative insulin approaches in reducing morbidity rates. However, the mortality benefit of intensive insulin therapy over a more conservative approach has not been proven conclusively. The observed benefits of insulin therapy are probably simply as a result of maintenance of normoglycaemia, but the glycaemia-independent actions of insulin may also exert minor, organ-specific effects (e.g. promotion of myocardial systolic function).

CHANGES IN BODY COMPOSITION FOLLOWING INJURY

The average 70-kg male can be considered to consist of fat (13 kg) and fat-free mass (or lean body mass: 57 kg). In such an individual, the lean tissue is composed primarily of protein (12 kg), water (42 kg) and minerals (3 kg) (Fig. 1.7). The protein mass can be considered as two basic compartments, skeletal muscle (4 kg) and non-skeletal muscle (8 kg), which includes the visceral protein mass. The water mass (42 l) is divided into intercellular (28 l) and extracellular (14 l) spaces. Most of the mineral mass is contained in the bony skeleton.

The main labile energy reserve in the body is fat, and the main labile protein reserve is skeletal muscle. While fat mass can be reduced without major detriment to function, loss of protein mass results not only in skeletal muscle wasting, but also depletion of visceral protein status. Within lean tissue, each 1 g of nitrogen is contained within 6.25 g of protein, which is contained in approximately 36 g of wet weight tissue. Thus, the loss of 1 g of nitrogen

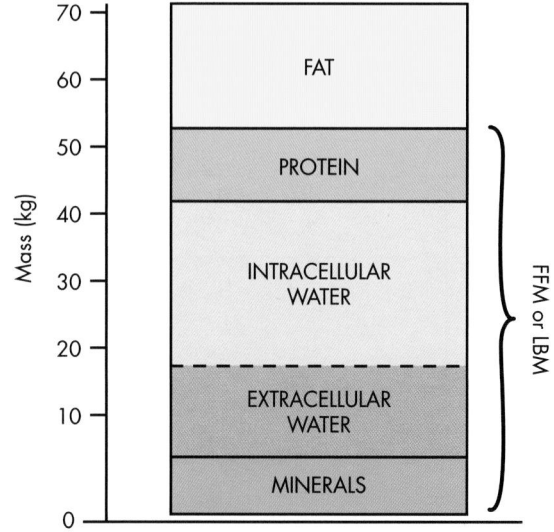

Figure 1.7 The chemical body composition of a normal 70-kg male. FFM, fat-free mass; LBM, lean body mass.

in urine is equivalent to the breakdown of 36 g of wet weight lean tissue. Protein turnover in the whole body is of the order of 150–200 g day⁻¹. A normal human ingests about 70–100 g protein day⁻¹, which is metabolised and excreted in urine as ammonia and urea (i.e. approximately 14 g N day⁻¹). During total starvation, urinary loss of nitrogen is rapidly attenuated by a series of adaptive changes. Loss of body weight follows a similar course (Fig. 1.8), thus accounting for the survival of hunger strikers for a period of 50–60 days. Following major injury, and particularly in the presence of on-going septic complications, this adaptive change fails to occur, and there is a state of 'autocannibalism', resulting in continuing urinary nitrogen losses of 10–20 g N day⁻¹ (equivalent to 500 g of wet weight lean tissue day⁻¹). As with total starvation, once loss of body protein mass has reached 30–40% of the total, survival is unlikely.

Critically ill patients admitted to the ICU with severe sepsis or major blunt trauma undergo massive changes in body composition (Fig. 1.8). Body weight increases immediately on

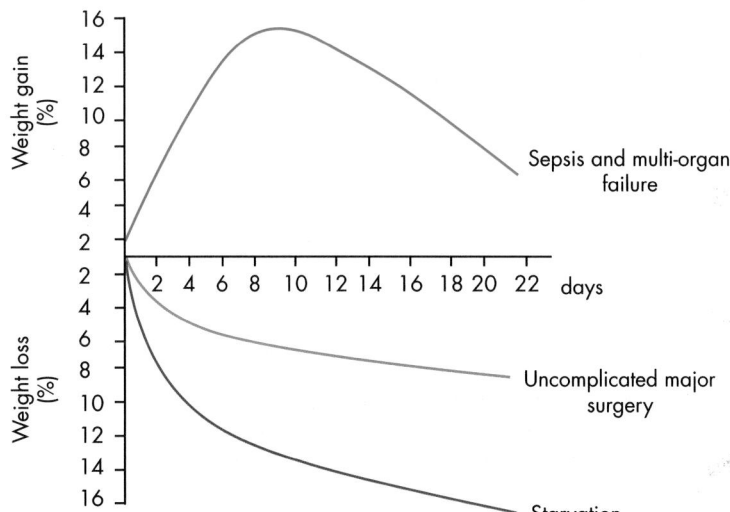

Figure 1.8 Changes in body weight that occur in serious sepsis, after uncomplicated surgery and in total starvation.

CHAPTER 1 | THE METABOLIC RESPONSE TO INJURY

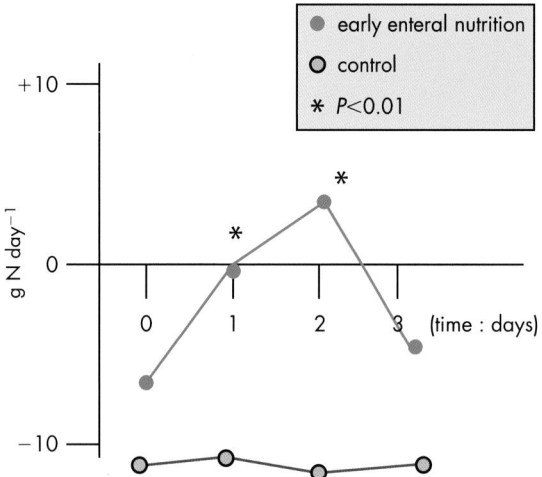

Figure 1.9 Effect of immediate enteral nutrition on nitrogen balance in patients managed with an enhanced recovery protocol following major colorectal surgery.

resuscitation with an expansion of extracellular water by 6–10 l within 24 hours. Thereafter, even with optimal metabolic care and nutritional support, total body protein will diminish by 15% in the next 10 days, and body weight will reach negative balance as the expansion of the extracellular space resolves. In marked contrast, it is now possible to maintain body weight and nitrogen equilibrium following major elective surgery (Fig. 1.9). This can be achieved by blocking the neuroendocrine stress response with epidural analgesia and providing early enteral feeding. Moreover, the early fluid retention phase can be avoided by careful intra-operative management of fluid balance, with avoidance of excessive administration of intravenous saline (Summary box 1.9).

Summary box 1.9

Changes in body composition following major surgery/critical illness

- Catabolism leads to a *decrease* in fat mass and skeletal muscle mass
- Body weight may paradoxically *increase* because of expansion of extracellular fluid space

---

AVOIDABLE FACTORS THAT COMPOUND THE RESPONSE TO INJURY

As noted previously, the main features of this metabolic response are initiated by the immune system, cardiovascular system, sympathetic nervous system, ascending reticular formation and limbic system. However, the metabolic stress response may be further exacerbated by anaesthesia, dehydration, starvation (including preoperative fasting), sepsis, acute medical illness or even severe psychological stress (Fig. 1.10). Thus, any attempt to limit or control these other factors is beneficial to the patient (Summary box 1.10).

Summary box 1.10

Avoidable factors that compound the response to injury

- Continuing haemorrhage
- Hypothermia
- Tissue oedema
- Tissue underperfusion
- Starvation
- Immobility

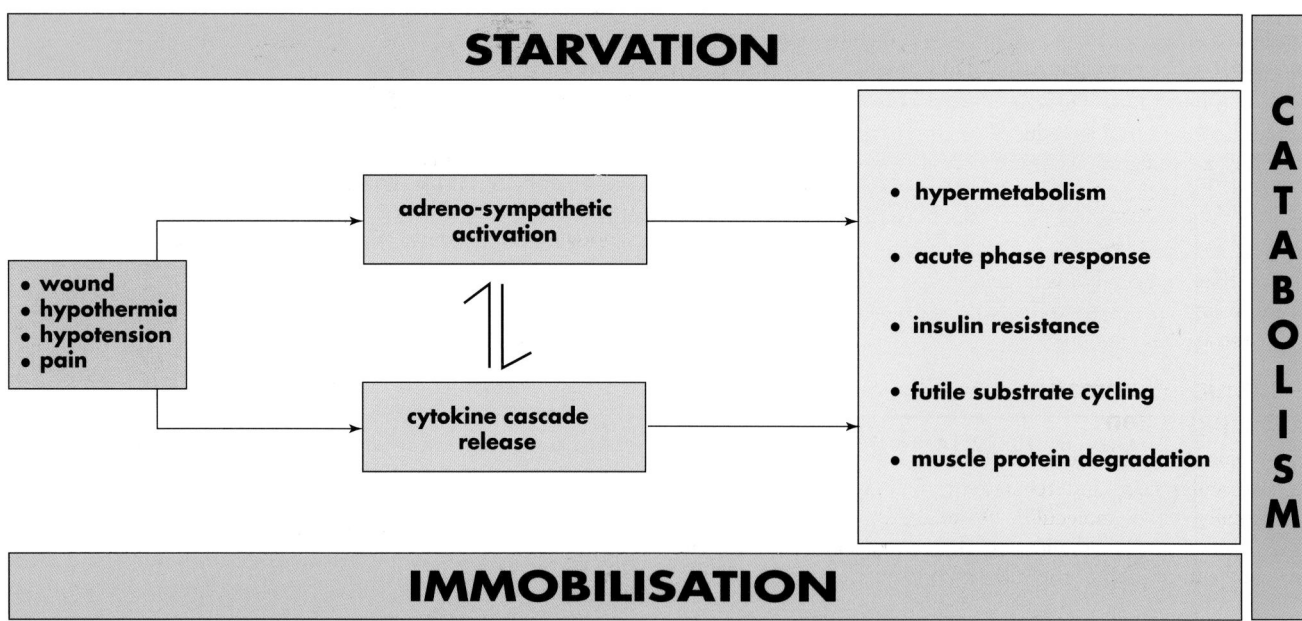

Figure 1.10 Factors that exacerbate the metabolic response to surgical injury include hypothermia, controlled pain, starvation, immobilisation, sepsis and medical complications.

Volume loss

During simple haemorrhage, pressor receptors in the carotid artery and aortic arch, and volume receptors in the wall of the left atrium, initiate afferent nerve input to the central nervous system (CNS), resulting in the release of both aldosterone and antidiuretic hormone (ADH). Pain can also stimulate ADH release. ADH acts directly on the kidney to cause fluid retention. Decreased pulse pressure stimulates the juxtaglomerular apparatus in the kidney and directly activates the renin–angiotensin system, which in turn increases aldosterone release.

Aldosterone causes the renal tubule to reabsorb sodium (and consequently also conserve water). ACTH release also augments the aldosterone response. The net effects of ADH and aldosterone result in the natural oliguria observed after surgery and conservation of sodium and water in the extracellular space. The tendency towards water and salt retention is exacerbated by resuscitation with saline-rich fluids. Salt and water retention can result in not only peripheral oedema, but also visceral oedema (e.g. stomach). Such visceral oedema has been associated with reduced gastric emptying, delayed resumption of food intake and prolonged hospital stay. Careful limitation of intraoperative administration of colloids and crystalloids (e.g. Hartmann's solution) so that there is no net weight gain following elective surgery has been proven to reduce postoperative complications and length of stay.

Hypothermia

Hypothermia results in increased elaboration of adrenal steroids and catecholamines. When compared with normothermic controls, even mild hypothermia results in a two- to threefold increase in postoperative cardiac arrhythmias and increased catabolism. Randomised trials have shown that maintaining normothermia by an upper body forced-air heating cover reduces wound infections, cardiac complications and bleeding and transfusion requirements.

Tissue oedema

During systemic inflammation, fluid, plasma proteins, leucocytes, macrophages and electrolytes leave the vascular space and accumulate in the tissues. This can diminish the alveolar diffusion of oxygen and may lead to reduced renal function. Increased capillary leak is mediated by a wide variety of mediators including cytokines, prostanoids, bradykinin and nitric oxide. Vasodilatation implies that intravascular volume decreases, which induces shock if inadequate resuscitation is not undertaken. Meanwhile, intracellular volume decreases, and this provides part of the volume necessary to replenish intravascular and extravascular extracellular volume.

Systemic inflammation and tissue underperfusion

The vascular endothelium controls vasomotor tone and microvascular flow, and regulates trafficking of nutrients and biologically active molecules. When endothelial activation is excessive, compromised microcirculation and subsequent cellular hypoxia contribute to the risk of organ failure. Maintaining

Alexis Frank Hartmann, **1898–1964, Paediatrician, St. Louis, MO, USA.**

normoglycaemia with insulin infusion during critical illness has been proposed to protect the endothelium, probably in part, via inhibition of excessive iNOS-induced NO release, and thereby contribute to the prevention of organ failure and death. Administration of activated protein C to critically ill patients has been shown to reduce organ failure and death and is thought to act, in part, via preservation of the microcirculation in vital organs.

Starvation

During starvation, the body is faced with an obligate need to generate glucose to sustain cerebral energy metabolism (100 g of glucose day^{-1}). This is achieved in the first 24 hours by mobilising glycogen stores and thereafter by hepatic gluconeogenesis from amino acids, glycerol and lactate. The energy metabolism of other tissues is sustained by mobilising fat from adipose tissue. Such fat mobilisation is mainly dependent on a fall in circulating insulin levels. Eventually, accelerated loss of lean tissue (the main source of amino acids for hepatic gluconeogenesis) is reduced as a result of the liver converting free fatty acids into ketone bodies, which can serve as a substitute for glucose for cerebral energy metabolism. Provision of at least 2 litres of intravenous 5% dextrose as intravenous fluids for surgical patients who are fasted provides 100 g of glucose day^{-1} and has a significant protein-sparing effect. Avoiding unnecessary fasting in the first instance and early oral/enteral/parenteral nutrition form the platform for avoiding loss of body mass as a result of the varying degrees of starvation observed in surgical patients.

Immobility

Immobility has long been recognised as a potent stimulus for inducing muscle wasting. Inactivity impairs the normal meal-derived amino acid stimulation of protein synthesis in skeletal muscle. Avoidance of unnecessary bed rest and active early mobilisation are essential measures to avoid muscle wasting as a consequence of immobility.

CONCEPTS BEHIND OPTIMAL PERIOPERATIVE CARE

Current understanding of the metabolic response to surgical injury and the mediators involved has led to a reappraisal of traditional perioperative care. There is now a strong scientific rationale for avoiding unmodulated exposure to stress, prolonged fasting and excessive administration of intravenous (saline) fluids. It is also important to realise that modulating the stress/inflammatory response at the time of surgery may have long-term sequelae over periods of months or longer. For example, β-blockers and statins have recently been shown to improve long-term survival after major surgery. It has been suggested that these effects may be due to suppression of innate immunity at the time of surgery. Equally, the use of epidural analgesia to reduce pain, block the cortisol stress response and attenuate postoperative insulin resistance may, via effects on the body's protein economy, favourably affects many of the patient-centred outcomes that are important to postoperative recovery but have largely been unmeasured to date, such as functional capacity, vitality and ability to return to work (Summary box 1.11).

Summary box 1.11

A proactive approach to prevent unnecessary aspects of the surgical stress response

- Minimal access techniques
- Blockade of afferent painful stimuli (e.g. epidural analgesia)
- Minimal periods of starvation
- Early mobilisation

FURTHER READING

Bessey, P.Q., Watters, J.M., Aoki, T.T. and Wilmore, D.W. (1984) Combined hormonal infusion simulates the metabolic response to injury. *Annals of Surgery* **200**: 264–81.

Calvano, S.E., Xioa, W., Richards, D.R. *et al.* (2005) A network-based analysis of systemic inflammation in humans. *Nature* **437**: 1032–7.

Cuthbertson, D.P. (1930) The disturbance of metabolism produced by bone and non-bony injury, with notes on certain abnormal conditions of bone. *Biochemistry Journal* **24**: 1244.

Fearon, K.C.H., Ljungqvist, O., von Meyenfeldt, M. *et al.* (2005) Enhanced recovery after surgery: a consensus review of clinical care for patients undergoing colonic resection. *Clinical Nutrition* **24**: 466–77.

Goldie, A.S., Fearon, K.C.H., Ross, J.A. *et al.* (1995) Natural crystokine antagonists and endogenous anti-endotoxin core antibodies in sepsis syndrome. *Journal of the American Medical Association* **274**: 172–7.

Lobo, D.N., Bostock, K.A., Neal, K.R. *et al.* (2002) Effect of salt and water balance on recovery of gastrointestinal function after elective colonic resection: a randomised controlled trial. *Lancet* **359**: 1812–18.

Moore, F.O. (1959) *Metabolic Care of the Surgical Patient.* W.B. Saunders Co., Philadelphia.

Van den Berghe, G., Wonters, P., Weckers, F. *et al.* (2001) Intensive insulin therapy in the critically ill patient. *New England Journal of Medicine* **345**: 1359–67.

Vanhorebeek, O., Langounche, L., Van den Berghe, G. (2006) Endocrine aspects of acute and prolonged critical illness. *Nature Clinical Practice: Endocrinology and Metabolism* **2**: 20–31.

Wilmore, D.W. (2002) From Cuthbertson to fast-track surgery: 70 years of progress in reducing stress in surgical patients. *Annals of Surgery* **236**: 643–8.

Shock and blood transfusion

INTRODUCTION

Shock is the most common and therefore the most important cause of death among surgical patients. Death may occur rapidly as a result of a profound state of shock or be delayed, resulting from the consequences of organ ischaemia and reperfusion injury. It is important, therefore, that every surgeon understands the pathophysiology and diagnosis of shock and haemorrhage, as well as the priorities for their management.

SHOCK

Shock is a systemic state of low tissue perfusion, which is inadequate for normal cellular respiration. With insufficient delivery of oxygen and glucose, cells switch from aerobic to anaerobic metabolism. If perfusion is not restored in a timely fashion, cell death ensues.

Pathophysiology

Cellular

As perfusion to the tissues is reduced, cells are deprived of oxygen and must switch from aerobic to anaerobic metabolism. The product of anaerobic respiration is not carbon dioxide but lactic acid. When enough tissue is underperfused, the accumulation of lactic acid in the blood produces systemic metabolic acidosis.

As glucose within cells is exhausted, anaerobic respiration ceases and there is failure of the sodium/potassium pumps in the cell membrane and intracellular organelles. Intracellular lysosomes release autodigestive enzymes and cell lysis ensues. Intracellular contents, including potassium, are released into the bloodstream.

Microvascular

As tissue ischaemia progresses, changes in the local milieu result in activation of the immune and coagulation systems. Hypoxia and acidosis activate complement and prime neutrophils, resulting in the generation of oxygen free radicals and cytokine release. These mechanisms lead to injury of the capillary endothelial cells.

These in turn further activate the immune and coagulation systems. Damaged endothelium loses its integrity and becomes 'leaky'. Spaces between endothelial cells allow fluid to leak out and tissue oedema ensues, exacerbating cellular hypoxia.

Systemic

Cardiovascular

As preload and afterload decrease there is a compensatory baroreceptor response resulting in increased sympathetic activity and release of catecholamines into the circulation. This results in tachycardia and systemic vasoconstriction (except in sepsis – see below).

Respiratory

The metabolic acidosis and increased sympathetic response result in an increased respiratory rate and minute ventilation to increase the excretion of carbon dioxide (and so produce a compensatory respiratory alkalosis).

Renal

Decreased perfusion pressure in the kidney leads to reduced filtration at the glomerulus and a decreased urine output. The renin–angiotensin–aldosterone axis is stimulated resulting in further vasoconstriction and increased sodium and water reabsorption by the kidney.

Endocrine

As well as activation of the adrenal and renin–angiotensin systems, vasopressin (antidiuretic hormone) is released from the hypothalamus in response to decreased preload and results in vasoconstriction and reabsorption of water in the renal collecting system. Cortisol is also released from the adrenal cortex, contributing to the sodium and water reabsorption and sensitising the cells to catecholamines.

Ischaemia–reperfusion syndrome

During the period of systemic hypoperfusion, cellular and organ damage progresses because of the direct effects of tissue hypoxia and local activation of inflammation. Further injury occurs once normal circulation is restored to these tissues. The acid and potassium load that has built up can lead to direct myocardial depression, vascular dilatation and further hypotension. The cellular and humoral elements activated by the hypoxia (complement, neutrophils, microvascular thrombi) are flushed back into the circulation where they cause further endothelial injury to organs such as the lungs and kidneys. This leads to acute lung injury, acute renal injury, multiple organ failure and death. Reperfusion injury can currently only be attenuated by reducing the extent and duration of tissue hypoperfusion.

Classification of shock

There are numerous ways to classify shock but the most common and clinically applicable way is that based on the initiating mechanism (Summary box 2.1).

All states are characterised by systemic tissue hypoperfusion and different states may coexist within the same patient.

Summary box 2.1

Classification of shock

- Hypovolaemic
- Cardiogenic
- Obstructive
- Distributive
- Endocrine

Hypovolaemic shock

Hypovolaemic shock is caused by a reduced circulating volume. Hypovolaemia may be due to haemorrhagic or non-haemorrhagic causes. Non-haemorrhagic causes include poor fluid intake (dehydration) and excessive fluid loss because of vomiting, diarrhoea, urinary loss (e.g. diabetes), evaporation and 'third-spacing', in which fluid is lost into the gastrointestinal tract and interstitial spaces, as for example in bowel obstruction or pancreatitis.

Hypovolaemia is probably the most common form of shock and is to some degree a component of all other forms of shock. Absolute or relative hypovolaemia must be excluded or treated in the management of the shocked state, regardless of cause.

Cardiogenic shock

Cardiogenic shock is due to primary failure of the heart to pump blood to the tissues. Causes of cardiogenic shock include myocardial infarction, cardiac dysrhythmias, valvular heart disease, blunt myocardial injury and cardiomyopathy. Cardiac insufficiency may also be caused by myocardial depression resulting from endogenous factors (e.g. bacterial and humoral agents released in sepsis) or exogenous factors, such as pharmaceutical agents or drug abuse. Evidence of venous hypertension with pulmonary or systemic oedema may coexist with the classic signs of shock.

Obstructive shock

In obstructive shock there is a reduction in preload because of mechanical obstruction of cardiac filling. Common causes of obstructive shock include cardiac tamponade, tension pneumothorax, massive pulmonary embolus and air embolus. In each case there is reduced filling of the left and/or right sides of the heart leading to reduced preload and a fall in cardiac output.

Distributive shock

Distributive shock describes the pattern of cardiovascular responses characterising a variety of conditions including septic shock, anaphylaxis and spinal cord injury. Inadequate organ perfusion is accompanied by vascular dilatation with hypotension, low systemic vascular resistance, inadequate afterload and a resulting abnormally high cardiac output.

In anaphylaxis, vasodilatation is caused by histamine release, whereas in high spinal cord injury there is failure of sympathetic outflow and adequate vascular tone (neurogenic shock). The cause in sepsis is less clear but is related to the release of bacterial products (endotoxins) and the activation of cellular and humoral components of the immune system. There is maldistribution of blood flow at a microvascular level with arteriovenous shunting and dysfunction of the cellular utilisation of oxygen.

In the later phases of septic shock there is hypovolaemia from fluid loss into the interstitial spaces and there may be concomitant myocardial depression, which complicates the clinical picture (Table 2.1).

Endocrine shock

Endocrine shock may present as a combination of hypovolaemic, cardiogenic and distributive shock. Causes of endocrine shock include hypo- and hyperthyroidism and adrenal insufficiency. Hypothyroidism causes a shock state similar to that of neurogenic shock as a result of disordered vascular and cardiac responsiveness to circulating catecholamines. Cardiac output falls because of low inotropy and bradycardia. There may also be an associated cardiomyopathy. Thyrotoxicosis may cause a high-output cardiac failure.

Adrenal insufficiency leads to shock as a result of hypovolaemia and a poor response to circulating and exogenous catecholamines. Adrenal insufficiency may result from pre-existing Addison's disease or it may be a relative insufficiency caused by a pathological disease state such as systemic sepsis.

Table 2.1 Cardiovascular and metabolic characteristics of shock

	Hypovolaemia	Cardiogenic	Obstructive	Distributive
Cardiac output	Low	Low	Low	High
Vascular resistance	High	High	High	Low
Venous pressure	Low	High	High	Low
Mixed venous saturation	Low	Low	Low	High
Base deficit	High	High	High	High

Thomas Addison, **1795–1860, Physician, Guy's Hospital, London, England, described the effects of disease of the suprarenal capsules in 1849.**

Severity of shock
Compensated shock

As shock progresses the body's cardiovascular and endocrine compensatory responses reduce flow to non-essential organs to preserve preload and flow to the lungs and brain. In compensated shock there is adequate compensation to maintain the central blood volume and preserve flow to the kidneys, lungs and brain. Apart from a tachycardia and cool peripheries (vasoconstriction, circulating catecholamines) there may be no other clinical signs of hypovolaemia.

However, this cardiovascular state is only maintained by reducing perfusion to the skin, muscle and gastrointestinal tract. There is a systemic metabolic acidosis and activation of humoral and cellular elements within the underperfused organs. Although clinically occult, this state will lead to multiple organ failure and death if prolonged because of the ischaemia–reperfusion effect described above. Patients with occult hypoperfusion (metabolic acidosis despite normal urine output and cardiorespiratory vital signs) for more than 12 hours have a significantly higher mortality rate, infection rate and incidence of multiple organ failure (see below).

Decompensation

Further loss of circulating volume overloads the body's compensatory mechanisms and there is progressive renal, respiratory and cardiovascular decompensation. In general, loss of around 15% of the circulating blood volume is within normal compensatory mechanisms. Blood pressure is usually well maintained and only falls after 30–40% of the circulating volume has been lost.

Mild shock

Initially there is tachycardia, tachypnoea and a mild reduction in urine output and the patient may exhibit mild anxiety. Blood pressure is maintained although there is a decrease in pulse pressure. The peripheries are cool and sweaty with prolonged capillary refill times (except in septic distributive shock).

Moderate shock

As shock progresses, renal compensatory mechanisms fail, renal perfusion falls and urine output dips below 0.5 ml kg^{-1}h^{-1}. There is further tachycardia and now the blood pressure starts to fall. Patients become drowsy and mildly confused.

Severe shock

In severe shock there is profound tachycardia and hypotension. Urine output falls to zero and patients are unconscious with laboured respiration.

Pitfalls

The classic cardiovascular responses described (Table 2.2) are not seen in every patient. It is important to recognise the limitations of the clinical examination and to recognise patients who are in shock despite the absence of classic signs.

Capillary refill

Most patients in hypovolaemic shock will have cool, pale peripheries with prolonged capillary refill times; however, the actual capillary refill time varies so much in adults that it is not a specific marker of whether a patient is shocked, and patients with short capillary refill times may be in the early stages of shock. In distributive (septic) shock the peripheries will be warm and capillary refill will be brisk despite profound shock.

Tachycardia

Tachycardia may not always accompany shock. Patients who are on β-blockers or who have implanted pacemakers are unable to mount a tachycardia. A pulse rate of 80 in a fit young adult who normally has a pulse rate of 50 is very abnormal. Furthermore, in some young patients with penetrating trauma, when there is haemorrhage but little tissue damage, there may be a paradoxical bradycardia rather than tachycardia accompanying the shocked state.

Blood pressure

It is important to recognise that hypotension is one of the last signs of shock. Children and fit young adults are able to maintain blood pressure until the final stages of shock by dramatic increases in stroke volume and peripheral vasoconstriction. These patients can be in profound shock with a normal blood pressure.

Elderly patients who are normally hypertensive may present with a 'normal' blood pressure for the general population but be hypovolaemic and hypotensive relative to their usual blood pressure. β-Blockers or other medications may prevent a tachycardic response. The diagnosis of shock may be difficult unless one is alert to these pitfalls.

Consequences
Unresuscitatable shock

Patients who are in profound shock for a prolonged period of time become 'unresuscitatable'. Cell death follows from cellular ischaemia, and the ability of the body to compensate is lost. There is myocardial depression and loss of responsiveness to fluid or inotropic therapy. Peripherally there is loss of the ability to maintain systemic vascular resistance and further hypotension ensues. The peripheries no longer respond appropriately to vasopressor agents. Death is the inevitable result.

Table 2.2 Clinical features of shock

	Compensated	Mild	Moderate	Severe
Lactic acidosis	+	++	++	+++
Urine output	Normal	Normal	Reduced	Anuric
Level of consciousness	Normal	Mild anxiety	Drowsy	Comatose
Respiratory rate	Normal	Increased	Increased	Laboured
Pulse rate	Mild increase	Increased	Increased	Increased
Blood pressure	Normal	Normal	Mild hypotension	Severe hypotension

CHAPTER 2 | SHOCK AND BLOOD TRANSFUSION

This stage of shock is the combined result of the severity of the insult and delayed, inadequate or inappropriate resuscitation in the earlier stages of shock. When patients present in this late stage and have minimal responses to maximal therapy it is important that the futility of treatment is recognised and that valuable resources are not wasted.

Multiple organ failure

As techniques of resuscitation have improved, more and more patients are surviving shock. When intervention is timely and the period of shock is limited, patients may make a rapid, uncomplicated recovery; however, the result of prolonged systemic ischaemia and reperfusion injury is end-organ damage and multiple organ failure.

Multiple organ failure is defined as two or more failed organ systems (Table 2.3). There is no specific treatment for multiple organ failure. Management is by supporting organ systems with ventilation, cardiovascular support and haemofiltration/dialysis until there is recovery of organ function. Multiple organ failure currently carries a mortality rate of 60%. Thus, prevention is vital by early aggressive identification and reversal of shock.

Table 2.3 Effects of organ failure

Lung	Acute respiratory distress syndrome
Kidney	Acute renal insufficiency
Liver	Acute liver insufficiency
Clotting	Coagulopathy
Cardiac	Cardiovascular failure

RESUSCITATION

Immediate resuscitation manoeuvres for patients presenting in shock are to ensure a patent airway and adequate oxygenation and ventilation. Once 'airway' and 'breathing' are assessed and controlled, attention is directed to cardiovascular resuscitation.

Conduct of resuscitation

Resuscitation should not be delayed in order to definitively diagnose the source of the shocked state; however, the timing and nature of resuscitation will depend on the type of shock and the timing and severity of the insult. Rapid clinical examination will provide adequate clues to make an appropriate first determination, even if a source of bleeding or sepsis is not immediately identifiable. If there is initial doubt about the cause of shock it is safer to assume the cause is hypovolaemia and begin with fluid resuscitation, followed by an assessment of the response.

In patients who are actively bleeding (major trauma, aortic aneurysm rupture, gastrointestinal haemorrhage) it is counterproductive to institute high-volume fluid therapy without controlling the site of haemorrhage. Increasing blood pressure merely increases bleeding from the site, and fluid therapy cools the patient and dilutes available coagulation factors. Thus, operative haemorrhage control should not be delayed and resuscitation should proceed in parallel with surgery.

Conversely, a patient with bowel obstruction and hypovolaemic shock must be adequately resuscitated before undergoing surgery otherwise the additional surgical injury and hypovolaemia induced during the procedure will exacerbate the inflammatory activation and increase the incidence and severity of end-organ insult.

Fluid therapy

In all cases of shock, regardless of classification, hypovolaemia and inadequate preload must be addressed before other therapy is instituted. Administration of inotropic or chronotropic agents to an empty heart will rapidly and permanently deplete the myocardium of oxygen stores and dramatically reduce diastolic filling and therefore coronary perfusion. Patients will enter the unresuscitatable stage of shock as the myocardium becomes progressively more ischaemic and unresponsive to resuscitative attempts.

First-line therapy, therefore, is intravenous access and administration of intravenous fluids. Access should be through short, wide-bore catheters that allow rapid infusion of fluids as necessary. Long, narrow lines such as central venous catheters have too high a resistance to allow rapid infusion and are more appropriate for monitoring than fluid replacement therapy.

Type of fluids

There is continuing debate over which resuscitation fluid is best for the management of shock. There is no ideal resuscitation fluid and it is more important to understand how and when to administer them. In most studies of shock resuscitation there is no overt difference in response or outcome between crystalloid solutions (normal saline, Hartmann's solution, Ringer's lactate) and colloids (albumin or commercially available products). Further, there is less volume benefit to the administration of colloids than had previously been thought, with only 1.3 times more crystalloid than colloid administered in blinded trials. On balance there is little evidence to support the administration of colloids, which are more expensive and have worse side-effect profiles.

Most importantly, the oxygen-carrying capacity of crystalloids and colloids is zero. If blood is being lost, the ideal replacement fluid is blood, although crystalloid therapy may be required while awaiting blood products.

Hypotonic solutions (e.g. dextrose) are poor volume expanders and should not be used in the treatment of shock unless the deficit is free water loss (e.g. diabetes insipidus) or patients are sodium overloaded (e.g. cirrhosis).

Dynamic fluid response

The shock status can be determined dynamically by the cardiovascular response to the rapid administration of a fluid bolus. In total, 250–500 ml of fluid is rapidly given (over 5–10 min) and the cardiovascular responses in terms of heart rate, blood pressure and central venous pressure (CVP) are observed. Patients can be divided into 'responders', 'transient responders' and 'non-responders'.

Responders show an improvement in their cardiovascular status, which is sustained. These patients are not actively losing fluid but require filling to a normal volume status.

Transient responders show an improvement but then revert to their previous state over the next 10–20 min. These patients either have moderate on-going fluid losses (either overt haemorrhage or further fluid shifts reducing intravascular volume).

Non-responders are severely volume depleted and are likely to have major on-going loss of intravascular volume, usually through persistent uncontrolled haemorrhage.

Alexis Frank Hartmann, 1898–1964, Paediatrician, St. Louis, MO, USA.
Sydney Ringer, 1835–1910, Professor of Clinical Medicine, University College Hospital, London, England.

Vasopressor and inotropic support

Vasopressor or inotropic therapy is not indicated as first-line therapy in hypovolaemia. As discussed above, administration of these agents in the absence of an adequate preload rapidly leads to decreased coronary perfusion and depletion of myocardial oxygen reserves.

Vasopressor agents (phenylephrine, noradrenaline) are indicated in distributive shock states (sepsis, neurogenic shock), in which there is peripheral vasodilatation and a low systemic vascular resistance, leading to hypotension despite a high cardiac output. When the vasodilatation is resistant to catecholamines (e.g. absolute or relative steroid deficiency), vasopressin may be used as an alternative vasopressor.

In cardiogenic shock or when myocardial depression complicates a shock state (e.g. severe septic shock with low cardiac output), inotropic therapy may be required to increase cardiac output and, therefore, oxygen delivery. The inodilator dobutamine is the agent of choice.

Monitoring

The *minimum* standard for monitoring of the patient in shock is continuous heart rate and oxygen saturation monitoring, frequent non-invasive blood pressure monitoring and hourly urine output measurements. Most patients will need more aggressive invasive monitoring including CVP and invasive blood pressure monitoring (Summary box 2.2).

Summary box 2.2

Monitoring for patients in shock

Minimum
- Electrocardiogram
- Pulse oximetry
- Blood pressure
- Urine output

Additional modalities
- Central venous pressure
- Invasive blood pressure
- Cardiac output
- Base deficit and serum lactate

Cardiovascular

As a minimum, cardiovascular monitoring should include continuous heart rate [electrocardiogram (ECG)], oxygen saturation and pulse waveform and non-invasive blood pressure. Patients whose state of shock is not rapidly corrected with a small amount of fluid should have CVP monitoring and continuous blood pressure monitoring through an arterial line.

Central venous pressure

There is no 'normal' CVP for a shocked patient, and reliance cannot be placed on an individual pressure measurement to assess volume status. Some patients may require a CVP of $5\,cmH_2O$, whereas others may require a CVP of $15\,cmH_2O$ or higher. Further, ventricular compliance can change from minute to minute in the shocked state, and CVP is a poor reflection of end-diastolic volume (preload).

CVP measurements should be assessed dynamically as the response to a fluid challenge (see above). A fluid bolus (250–500 ml) is infused rapidly over 5–10 min. The normal CVP response is a rise of $2-5\,cmH_2O$, which gradually drifts back to the original level over 10–20 min. Patients with no change in their CVP are empty and require further fluid resuscitation. Patients with a large, sustained rise in CVP have high preload and an element of cardiac insufficiency or volume overload.

Cardiac output

Cardiac output monitoring allows an assessment of not only the cardiac output but also the systemic vascular resistance and, depending on the technique used, end-diastolic volume (preload) and blood volume. Invasive cardiac monitoring using pulmonary artery catheters is becoming less frequent as new non-invasive monitoring techniques such as Doppler ultrasound, pulse waveform analysis and indicator dilution methods provide similar information without many of the drawbacks of more invasive techniques.

Measurement of cardiac output, systemic vascular resistance and preload can help distinguish the types of shock that are present (hypovolaemia, distributive, cardiogenic), especially when they coexist. The information provided guides fluid and vasopressor therapy by providing real-time monitoring of the cardiovascular response.

Measurement of cardiac output is desirable in patients who do not respond as expected to first-line therapy or who have evidence of cardiogenic shock or myocardial dysfunction. Early consideration should be given to instituting cardiac output monitoring in patients who require vasopressor or inotropic support.

Systemic and organ perfusion

Ultimately, the goal of treatment is to restore cellular and organ perfusion. Ideally, therefore, monitoring of organ perfusion should guide the management of shock (Table 2.4). The best measures of

Table 2.4 Monitors for organ/systemic perfusion

	Clinical	Investigational
Systemic perfusion	Base deficit; lactate; mixed venous oxygen saturation	
Organ perfusion		
Muscle	–	Near-infrared spectroscopy; tissue oxygen electrode
Gut	–	Sublingual capnometry; gut mucosal pH; laser Doppler flowmetry
Kidney	Urine output	–
Brain	Level of consciousness	Tissue oxygen electrode; near-infrared spectroscopy

---

Christian Johann Doppler, **1803–1853, Professor of Experimental Physics, Vienna, Austria, enunciated the 'Doppler Principle' in 1842.**

CHAPTER 2 | SHOCK AND BLOOD TRANSFUSION

organ perfusion and the best monitor of the adequacy of shock therapy remain the urine output; however, this is an hourly measure and does not give a minute-to-minute view of the shocked state. The level of consciousness is an important marker of cerebral perfusion, but brain perfusion is maintained until the very late stages of shock and, hence, is a poor marker of adequacy of resuscitation.

Currently, the only clinical indicators of perfusion of the gastrointestinal tract and muscular beds are the global measures of lactic acidosis (lactate and base deficit) and the mixed venous oxygen saturation.

Base deficit and lactate

Lactic acid is generated by cells undergoing anaerobic respiration. The degree of lactic acidosis, as measured by the serum lactate level and/or the base deficit, is a sensitive tool for both the diagnosis of shock and the monitoring of the response to therapy. Patients with a base deficit of over $6 \, mmol \, l^{-1}$ have much higher morbidity and mortality rates than those with no metabolic acidosis. Further, the duration of time in shock with an increased base deficit is important, even if all other vital signs have returned to normal (occult hypoperfusion – see below).

These parameters are measured from arterial blood gas analyses and, therefore, the frequency of measurements is limited and they do not provide minute-to-minute data on systemic perfusion or the response to therapy. Nevertheless, the base deficit and/or lactate should be measured routinely in these patients until they have returned to normal levels.

Mixed venous oxygen saturation

The percentage saturation of oxygen returning to the heart from the body is a measure of the oxygen delivery and extraction by the tissues. Accurate measurement is via analysis of blood drawn from a long central line placed in the right atrium. Estimations can be made from blood drawn from lines in the superior vena cava but these values will be slightly higher than those of a mixed venous sample (as there is relatively more oxygen extraction from the lower half of the body). Normal mixed venous oxygen saturation levels are 50–70%. Levels below 50% indicate inadequate oxygen delivery and increased oxygen extraction by the cells. This is consistent with hypovolaemic or cardiogenic shock.

High mixed venous saturation levels (> 70%) are seen in sepsis and some other forms of distributive shock. In sepsis there is disordered utilisation of oxygen at the cellular level and arteriovenous shunting of blood at the microvascular level. Thus, less oxygen is presented to the cells, cells cannot utilise what little oxygen is presented and venous blood has a higher oxygen concentration than normal.

Patients who are septic should, therefore, have mixed venous oxygen saturation levels of > 70%. Levels lower than this indicate that the patient is not only in septic shock but also in hypovolaemic or cardiogenic shock. Although the mixed venous oxygen saturation level is in the 'normal' range, it is low for the septic state and inadequate oxygen is being supplied to cells that cannot utilise oxygen appropriately. This must be corrected rapidly. Hypovolaemia should be corrected with fluid therapy and low cardiac output caused by myocardial depression or failure should be treated with inotropes (dobutamine) to achieve a mixed venous saturation level of > 70% (normal for the septic state).

New methods for monitoring regional tissue perfusion and oxygenation are becoming available, the most promising of which are muscle tissue oxygen probes, near-infrared spectroscopy and sublingual capnometry. Although these techniques provide information regarding perfusion of specific tissue beds, it is as yet unclear whether there are significant advantages over existing measurements of global hypoperfusion (base deficit, lactate).

Endpoints of resuscitation

It is much easier to know when to start resuscitation than when to stop. Traditionally patients have been resuscitated until they have a normal pulse, blood pressure and urine output; however, these parameters are monitoring organ systems whose blood flow is preserved until the late stages of shock. Therefore, a patient may be resuscitated to restore central perfusion to the brain, lungs and kidneys and yet the gut and muscle beds continue to be underperfused. Thus, activation of inflammation and coagulation may be on-going and, when these organs are finally perfused, it may lead to reperfusion injury and ultimately multiple organ failure.

This state of normal vital signs and continued underperfusion is termed occult hypoperfusion (OH). With current monitoring techniques it is manifested only by a persistent lactic acidosis and low mixed venous oxygen saturation level. The duration that patients spend in this hypoperfused state has a dramatic effect on outcome. Patients with OH for more than 12 hours have a two to three times higher mortality rate than that of patients with a limited duration of shock.

Resuscitation algorithms directed at correcting global perfusion endpoints (base deficit, lactate, mixed venous oxygen saturation) rather than traditional endpoints have been shown to improve mortality and morbidity in high-risk surgical patients; however, it is clear that, despite aggressive regimens, some patients cannot be resuscitated to normal parameters within 12 hours by fluid resuscitation alone. More research is under way to identify the pathophysiology behind this and investigate new therapeutic options.

HAEMORRHAGE

Haemorrhage must be recognised and managed aggressively to reduce the severity and duration of shock and avoid death and/or multiple organ failure. Haemorrhage is treated by arresting the bleeding, and not by fluid resuscitation or blood transfusion. Although necessary as supportive measures to maintain organ perfusion, attempting to resuscitate patients who have on-going haemorrhage will lead to physiological exhaustion (coagulopathy, acidosis and hypothermia) and subsequently death.

Pathophysiology

Haemorrhage leads to a state of hypovolaemic shock. As discussed above, this hypoperfused state results in cellular anaerobic metabolism and lactic acidosis. This acidosis leads to decreased function of the coagulation proteases, resulting in coagulopathy and further haemorrhage. This is exacerbated by ischaemic endothelial cells activating anti-coagulant pathways. Additionally, there is reduced perfusion to tissues, and the blood supply to the gut and muscle beds is reduced early in the compensatory process. Underperfused muscle is unable to generate heat and hypothermia ensues. Coagulation functions poorly at low temperatures and there is further haemorrhage, further hypoperfusion and worsening acidosis and hypothermia. These three factors result in a downward spiral leading to physiological exhaustion and death (Fig. 2.1).

Medical therapy has a tendency to worsen this effect. Intravenous blood and fluids are cold and exacerbate hypothermia. Further heat is lost by opening body cavities during surgery. Surgery usually leads to further bleeding and many crystalloid fluids are themselves acidic (e.g. normal saline has a pH of 6.7).

Every effort must therefore be made to rapidly identify and stop haemorrhage and to avoid (preferably) or limit physiological exhaustion from coagulopathy, acidosis and hypothermia.

Definitions

Revealed and concealed haemorrhage

Haemorrhage may be revealed or concealed. Revealed haemorrhage is obvious external haemorrhage, such as exsanguination from an open arterial wound or from massive haematemesis from a duodenal ulcer.

Concealed haemorrhage is contained within the body cavity and must be suspected, actively investigated and controlled. In trauma, haemorrhage may be concealed within the chest, abdomen, pelvis or retroperitoneum or in the limbs, with contained vascular injury or associated with long-bone fractures. Examples of non-traumatic concealed haemorrhage include occult gastrointestinal bleeding or ruptured aortic aneurysm.

Primary, reactionary and secondary haemorrhage

Primary haemorrhage is haemorrhage occurring immediately as a result of an injury (or surgery). Reactionary haemorrhage is delayed haemorrhage (within 24 hours) and is usually caused by dislodgement of clot by resuscitation, normalisation of blood pressure and vasodilatation. Reactionary haemorrhage may also result from technical failure such as slippage of a ligature.

Secondary haemorrhage is caused by sloughing of the wall of a vessel. It usually occurs 7–14 days after injury and is precipitated by factors such as infection, pressure necrosis (such as from a drain) or malignancy.

Surgical and non-surgical haemorrhage

Surgical haemorrhage is the result of a direct injury and is amenable to surgical control (or other techniques such as angioembolisation). Non-surgical haemorrhage is the general

ooze from all raw surfaces due to coagulopathy; it cannot be stopped by surgical means (except packing) but requires correction of the coagulation abnormalities.

Degree and classification

The adult human has approximately 5 litres of blood (70 ml kg^{-1} children and adults, 80 ml kg^{-1} neonates). Estimation of the amount of blood that has been lost is difficult and inaccurate and is usually an underestimation of the actual value.

External haemorrhage is obvious but it may be difficult to estimate the actual volume lost. In the operating room, blood collected in suction apparatus can be measured and swabs soaked in blood weighed.

The haemoglobin level is a poor indicator of the degree of haemorrhage as it represents a concentration and not an absolute amount. In the early stages of rapid haemorrhage, the haemoglobin concentration is unchanged (as whole blood is lost). Later, as fluid shifts from the intracellular and interstitial spaces into the vascular compartment, the haemoglobin and haematocrit levels will fall.

The degree of haemorrhage can be classified into classes 1–4 based on the estimated blood loss required to produce certain physiological compensatory changes (Table 2.5). Although conceptually useful there is variation across ages (the young compensate well, the old very poorly), between individuals (athletes vs. the obese) and because of confounding factors (e.g. concomitant medications, pain).

Treatment should therefore be based upon the degree of hypovolaemic shock according to vital signs, preload assessment, base deficit and, most importantly, the dynamic response to fluid therapy. Patients who are non-responders or transient responders are still bleeding and must have the site of haemorrhage identified and controlled.

Table 2.5 Traditional classification of haemorrhagic shock

	Class			
	1	**2**	**3**	**4**
Blood volume lost as percentage of total	<15%	15–30%	30–40%	>40%

Management

Identify haemorrhage

External haemorrhage may be obvious but the diagnosis of concealed haemorrhage may be more difficult. Any shock should be assumed to be hypovolaemic until proved otherwise and, similarly, hypovolaemia should be assumed to be due to haemorrhage until this has been excluded.

Immediate resuscitative manoeuvres

Direct pressure should be placed over the site of external haemorrhage. Airway and breathing should be assessed and controlled as necessary. Large-bore intravenous access should be instituted and blood drawn for cross-matching (see below). Emergency blood should be requested if the degree of shock and on-going haemorrhage warrants this.

Identify the site of haemorrhage

Once haemorrhage has been considered, the site of haemorrhage must be rapidly identified. Note that this is not to definitively

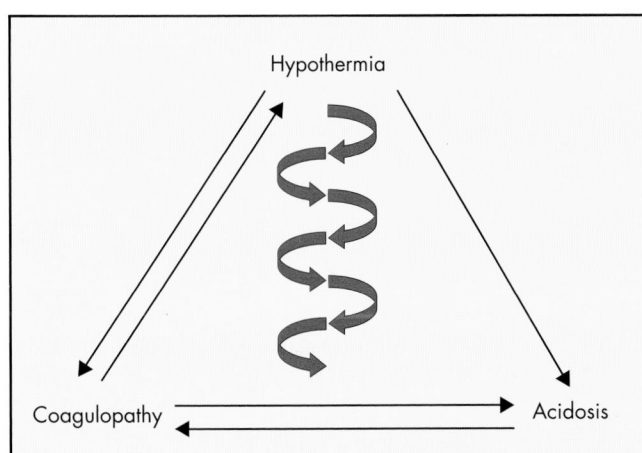

Figure 2.1 Physiological exhaustion: the triad of death.

identify the exact location but rather to define the next step in haemorrhage control (operation, angioembolisation, endoscopic control).

Clues may be in the history (previous episodes; known aneurysm; non-steroidal therapy for gastrointestinal bleeding) or examination (nature of blood: fresh, melaena; abdominal tenderness; etc.). For shocked trauma patients the external signs of injury may suggest internal haemorrhage, but cavitary haemorrhage must be excluded with rapid investigations (chest and pelvic radiography, abdominal ultrasound or diagnostic peritoneal aspiration).

Investigations for blood loss must be appropriate to the patient's physiological condition. Rapid bedside tests are more appropriate for profound shock and exsanguinating haemorrhage than investigations such as computerised tomography, which takes a long time and for which patient monitoring and treatment are difficult. Patients who are not actively bleeding can have a more methodical, definitive work-up.

Haemorrhage control

The bleeding, shocked patient must be moved rapidly to a place of haemorrhage control. This will usually be in the operating room but may be in other areas of the hospital such as the angiography or endoscopy suites. These patients require full surgical and anaesthetic support and full monitoring, and equipment must be available for their care.

Control must be achieved rapidly to prevent the patient entering the triad of coagulopathy–acidosis–hypothermia and becoming physiologically exhausted. There should be no unnecessary investigations or procedures before haemorrhage control, to minimise the duration and severity of shock. This includes prolonged attempts to volume-resuscitate the patient before surgery, which will result in further hypothermia and clotting factor dilution until the bleeding is stopped. Attention should be paid to correction of coagulopathy with blood component therapy to aid surgical haemorrhage control.

Surgery may need to be limited to the minimum necessary to stop bleeding and control sepsis. More definitive repairs can be delayed until the patient is physiologically capable of sustaining the procedure. This concept of tailoring the operation to match the patient's physiology and staged procedures to prevent physiological exhaustion is called 'damage control surgery'; this is a term borrowed from the military whereby the continued functioning of a damaged ship is ensured above conducting complete repairs, which would prevent a rapid return to battle.

Once haemorrhage is controlled, patients should be aggressively resuscitated and warmed and coagulopathy corrected. Attention should be paid to fluid responsiveness and the endpoints of resuscitation to ensure that patients are fully resuscitated and to reduce the incidence and severity of organ failure (Summary box 2.3).

Summary box 2.3

Damage control surgery

- **Arrest haemorrhage**
- **Control sepsis**
- **Protect from further injury**
- *Nothing else*

TRANSFUSION

The transfusion of blood and blood products has become commonplace since the first successful transfusion in 1829 (Table 2.6). Although the incidence of severe transfusion reactions and infections is now very low, in recent years it has become apparent that there is an immunological price to be paid for the transfusion of heterologous blood, which leads to increased morbidity and decreased survival in certain population groups (trauma, malignancy). Supplies are also limited and, therefore, the use of blood and blood products must always be judicious and justifiable in terms of clinical need.

Blood and blood products

Blood is collected from donors who have been previously screened to exclude any donor whose blood may have the potential to harm the patient or to prevent possible harm that donating a unit of blood may have on the donor. In the UK, up to 450 ml of blood is drawn, a maximum of three times a year. Each unit is tested for evidence of hepatitis B, hepatitis C, human immunodeficiency virus (HIV)-1, HIV-2 and syphilis. Donations are leucodepleted as a precaution against variant Creutzfeldt–Jakob disease (this may also reduce the immunogenicity of the transfusion). The ABO and Rhesus D blood group is determined, as well as the presence of irregular red cell antibodies. The blood is then processed into sub-components.

Whole blood

Whole blood is now rarely available in civilian practice as it is an ineffective use of the limited resource; however, whole blood

Table 2.6 History of blood transfusion

1492	Pope Innocent VIII suffers a stroke and is made to drink blood from three 10-year-old boys (paid a ducat each). All three boys died, as did the pope later that year
1665	Richard Lower in Oxford conducts the first successful canine transfusions
1667	Jean-Baptiste Denis reports successful sheep–human transfusions
1670	Animal–human transfusions are banned in France because of the poor results
1829	James Blundell performs the first successful documented human transfusion in a woman suffering post-partum haemorrhage.
1900	Karl Landsteiner discovers the ABO system
1914	The Belgian physician Albert Hustin performs the first non-direct transfusion, using sodium citrate as an anti-coagulant
1926	The British Red Cross institutes the first blood transfusion service in the world
1939	The Rhesus system is identified and recognised as the major cause of transfusion reactions

---

Hans Gerhard Creutzfeldt, **1885–1946, Neurologist, Kiel, Germany.**
Alfons Maria Jakob, **1884–1931, Neurologist, Hamburg, Germany.**

hand, benefit from early active mobilisation as this minimises adhesions between the tendon and the tendon sheath (see above for extrinsic tendon healing mechanism).

Skin cover by flap or graft may be required as skin closure should always be without tension and should allow for the oedema typically associated with injury and the inflammatory phase of healing. A flap brings in a new blood supply and can be used to cover tendon, nerve, bone and other structures that would not provide a suitable vascular base for a skin graft. A skin graft has no inherent blood supply and is dependent on the recipient site for nutrition.

SOME SPECIFIC WOUNDS

Bites

Most bites involve either puncture wounds or avulsions. Small animal bites are common in children (Fig. 3.4) and require cleansing and treatment according to the principles outlined in Summary box 3.4, usually under general anaesthetic.

Summary box 3.4

Managing the acute wound

- Cleansing
- Exploration and diagnosis
- Debridement
- Repair of structures
- Replacement of lost tissues where indicated
- Skin cover if required
- Skin closure without tension
- All of the above with careful tissue handling and meticulous technique

---

Ear, tip of nose and lower lip injuries are most usually seen in victims of human bites. A boxing-type injury of the metacarpo-phalangeal joint may result from a perforating contact with the teeth of a victim. Anaerobic and aerobic organism prophylaxis is required as bite wounds typically have high virulent bacterial counts.

Puncture wounds

Wounds caused by sharp objects should be explored to the limit of tissue blood staining. Needle-stick injuries should be treated according to the well-published protocols because of hepatitis and human immunodeficiency virus (HIV) risks. X-ray examination should be carried out in order to rule out retained foreign bodies in the depth of the wound.

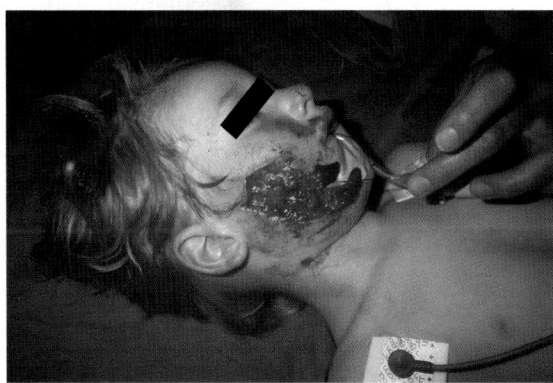

Figure 3.4 Dog bite in a child.

Haematomata

If large, painful or causing neural deficit, a haematoma may require release by incision or aspiration. In the gluteal or thigh region, there may be an associated disruption of fat in the form of a fat fracture, which results in an unsightly groove but intact skin. An untreated haematoma may also calcify and therefore require surgical exploration if symptomatic.

Degloving

Degloving occurs when the skin and subcutaneous fat are stripped by avulsion from its underlying fascia, leaving neurovascular structures, tendon or bone exposed. A degloving injury may be open or closed. An obvious example of an open degloving is a ring avulsion injury with loss of finger skin (Fig. 3.5). A closed degloving may be a rollover injury, typically caused by a motor vehicle over a limb. Such an injury will extend far further than expected, and much of the limb skin may be non-viable (Fig. 3.6). Examination under anaesthetic is required with a radical excision of all non-bleeding skin, as judged by bleeding dermis. Fluoroscein can be administered intravenously while the patient is anaesthetised. Under ultraviolet light, viable (perfused) skin will show up as a fluorescent yellowish green colour, and the non-viable skin for excision is clearly mapped out. However, the main objection to this method is that of possible anaphylactic shock due to fluoroscein sensitivity. Most surgeons therefore rely upon serial excision until punctate dermal bleeding is obvious. Split-skin grafts can be harvested from the degloved non-viable skin and meshed (Fig. 3.7) to cover the raw areas resulting from debridement.

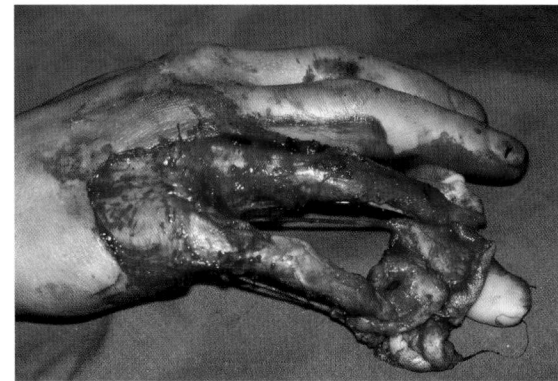

Figure 3.5 Degloving hand injury.

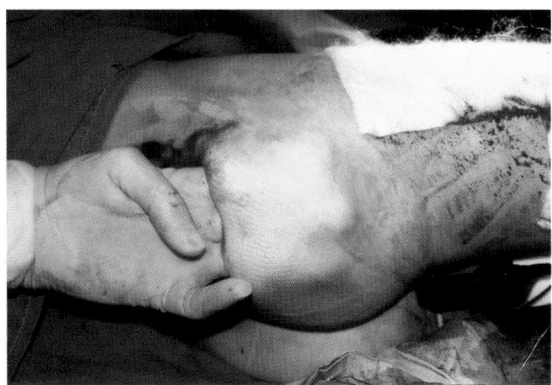

Figure 3.6 Degloving buttock injury.

CHAPTER 3 | WOUNDS, TISSUE REPAIR AND SCARS

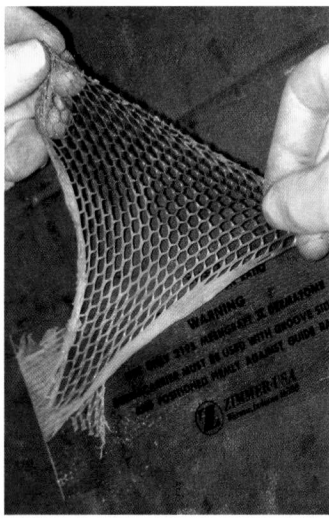

Figure 3.7 Meshed split-skin graft.

Compartment syndromes

Compartment syndromes typically occur in closed lower limb injuries. They are characterised by severe pain, pain on passive movement of the affected compartment muscles, distal sensory disturbance and, finally, by the absence of pulses distally (a late sign). They can occur in an open injury if the wound does not extend into the affected compartment.

Compartment pressures can be measured using a pressure monitor and a catheter placed in the muscle compartment. If pressures are constantly greater than 30 mmHg or if the above clinical signs are present, then fasciotomy should be performed. Fasciotomy involves incising the deep muscle fascia and is best carried out via longitudinal incisions of skin, fat and fascia (Fig. 3.8). The muscle will be then seen bulging out through the fasciotomy opening. The lower limb can be decompressed via two incisions, each being lateral to the subcutaneous border of the tibia. This gives access to the two posterior compartments and to the peroneal and anterior compartments of the leg. In crush injuries that present several days after the event, a late fasciotomy can be dangerous as dead muscle produces myoglobin which, if suddenly released into the bloodstream, causes myoglobinuria with glomerular blockage and renal failure. In the late treatment of lower limb injuries, therefore, it may be safer to amputate the limb.

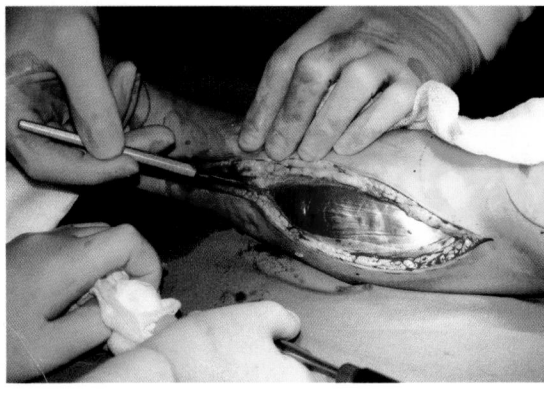

Figure 3.8 Fasciotomy of the lower leg.

High-pressure injection injuries

The use of high-pressure devices in cleaning, degreasing and painting can cause extensive closed injuries through small entry wounds. The liquid injected spreads along fascial planes, a common site being from finger to forearm. The tissue damage is dependent upon the toxicity of the substance and the injection pressure. Treatment is surgical with wide exposure, removal of the toxic substance and thorough debridement. Preoperative X-rays may be helpful where air or lead-based paints can be seen. It should be noted that amputation rates following high-pressure injection injuries are reported as being over 45%. Delayed or conservative treatment is therefore inappropriate.

CHRONIC WOUNDS

Leg ulcers

In developed countries, the commonest chronic wounds are leg ulcers. An ulcer can be defined as a break in the epithelial continuity. A prolonged inflammatory phase leads to overgrowth of granulation tissue, and attempts to heal by scarring leave a fibrotic margin. Necrotic tissue often at the ulcer centre is called slough. The more common aetiologies are listed in Summary box 3.5.

Summary box 3.5

Aetiology of leg ulcers

- Venous disease leading to local venous hypertension (e.g. varicose veins)
- Arterial disease, either large vessel (atherosclerosis) or small vessel (diabetes)
- Arteritis associated with autoimmune disease (rheumatoid arthritis, lupus, etc.)
- Trauma – could be self-inflicted
- Chronic infection – tuberculosis/syphilis
- Neoplastic – squamous or basal cell carcinoma, sarcoma

A chronic ulcer, unresponsive to dressings and simple treatments, should be biopsied to rule out neoplastic change, a squamous cell carcinoma known as a Marjolin's ulcer being the commonest. Effective treatment of any leg ulcer depends on treating the cause, and diagnosis is therefore vital. Arterial and venous circulation should be assessed, as should sensation throughout the lower limb. Surgical treatment is only indicated if non-operative treatment has failed or if the patient suffers from intractable pain. Meshed skin grafts (Fig. 3.7) are more successful than sheet grafts and have the advantage of allowing mobilisation, as any tissue exudate can escape through the mesh. It should be stressed that the recurrence rate is high in venous ulceration, and patient compliance with a regime of hygiene, elevation and elastic compression is essential.

Pressure sores

These can be defined as tissue necrosis with ulceration due to prolonged pressure. Less preferable terms are bed sores, pressure ulcers and decubitus ulcers. They should be regarded as preventable but

---

Jean-Nicholas Marjolin, **1780–1850, Surgeon, Paris, France, described the development of carcinomatous ulcers in scars in 1828.**

occur in approximately 5% of all hospitalised patients (range of 3% to 12% in published literature). There is a higher incidence in paraplegic patients, in the elderly and in the severely ill patient. The commonest sites are listed in Summary box 3.6.

Summary box 3.6

Pressure sore frequency in descending order

- Ischium
- Greater trochanter
- Sacrum
- Heel
- Malleolus (lateral then medial)
- Occiput

A staging system for description of pressure sores devised by the American National Pressure Ulcer Advisory Panel is shown in Summary box 3.7.

Summary box 3.7

Staging of pressure sores

Stage 1   Non-blanchable erythema without a breach in the epidermis

Stage 2   Partial-thickness skin loss involving the epidermis and dermis

Stage 3   Full-thickness skin loss extending into the subcutaneous tissue but not through underlying fascia

Stage 4   Full-thickness skin loss through fascia with extensive tissue destruction, maybe involving muscle, bone, tendon or joint

---

If external pressure exceeds the capillary occlusive pressure (over 30 mmHg), blood flow to the skin ceases leading to tissue anoxia, necrosis and ulceration (Fig. 3.9). Prevention is obviously the best treatment with good skin care, special pressure dispersion cushions or foams, the use of low air loss and air-fluidised beds and urinary or faecal diversion in selected cases. Pressure sore awareness is vital, and the bed-bound patient should be turned at least every 2 hours, with the wheelchair-bound patient being taught to lift themselves off their seat for 10 seconds every 10 minutes.

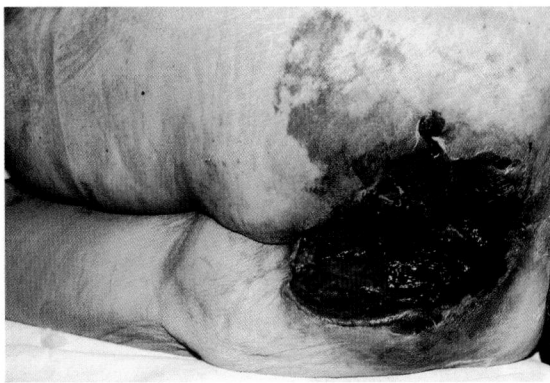

Figure 3.9 Pressure ulcer.

Surgical management of pressure sores follows the same principles involved in acute wound treatment (Summary box 3.4). The patient must be well motivated, clinically stable with good nutrition and adhere to the preventative measures advised postoperatively. Preoperative management of the pressure sore involves adequate debridement, and the use of vacuum-assisted closure (VAC) may help to provide a suitable wound for surgical closure (see below). The aim is to fill the dead space and to provide durable sensate skin. Large skin flaps that include muscle are best and, occasionally, an intact sensory innervated area can be included (e.g. extensor fascia lata flap with lateral cutaneous nerve of the thigh). If possible, use a flap that can be advanced further if there is recurrence and that does not interfere with the planning of neighbouring flaps that may be used in the future.

Vacuum-assisted closure

Applying intermittent negative pressure of approximately −125 mmHg appears to hasten debridement and the formation of granulation tissue in chronic wounds and ulcers. A foam dressing is cut to size to fit the wound. A perforated wound drain is placed over the foam, and the wound is sealed with a transparent adhesive film. A vacuum is then applied to the drain (Fig. 3.10). Negative pressure may act by decreasing oedema, by removing interstitial fluid and by increasing blood flow. As a result, bacterial counts decrease and cell proliferation increases, thereby creating a suitable bed for graft or flap cover.

NECROTISING SOFT-TISSUE INFECTIONS

These are rare but often fatal. They are most commonly polymicrobial infections with Gram-positive aerobes (*Staphylococcus aureus*, *Staphylococcus pyogenes*), Gram-negative aerobes (*Escherichia coli*, *Pseudomonas*, *Clostridium*, *Bacteroides*) and β-haemolytic *Streptococcus*. There is usually a history of trauma or surgery with wound contamination. Sometimes, the patient's own defence mechanism may be deficient. These infections are characterised by sudden presentation and rapid progression. The fact that deeper tissues are involved often leads to a late or missed diagnosis (Fig. 3.11). Clinical signs are shown in Summary box 3.8.

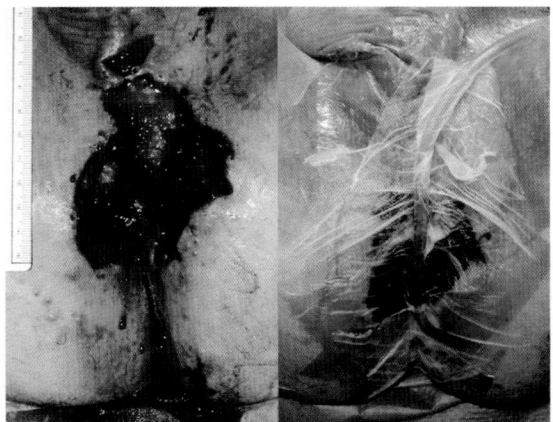

Figure 3.10 Vacuum-assisted closure (VAC) dressing of a large wound.

Hans Christian Joachim Gram, **1853–1938, Professor of Pharmacology (1891–1900) and of Medicine (1900–1923), Copenhagen, Denmark, described this method of staining bacteria in 1884.**

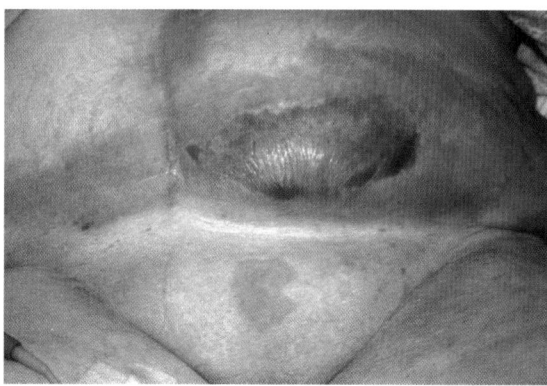

Figure 3.11 Necrotising fasciitis of the anterior abdominal wall.

Summary box 3.8

Sign of necrotising infections

- Oedema beyond area of erythema
- Crepitus
- Skin blistering
- Fever (often absent)
- Greyish drainage ('dishwater pus')
- Pink/orange skin staining
- Focal skin gangrene (late sign)
- Final shock, coagulopathy and multiorgan failure

There are two main types of necrotising infections: clostridial (gas gangrene) and non-clostridial (streptococcal gangrene and necrotising fasciitis). The variant of necrotising fasciitis with toxic shock syndrome results from *Streptococcus pyogenes* and is often called the 'flesh-eating bug' in this situation. Treatment is surgical excision with tissue biopsies being sent for culture and diagnosis. Wide raw areas requiring skin grafting often result.

SCARS

The maturation phase of wound healing has been discussed above and represents the formation of what is described as a scar. The immature scar becomes mature over a period lasting a year or more, but it is at first pink, hard, raised and often itchy. The disorganised collagen fibres become aligned along stress lines with their strength being in their weave rather than in their amount (this has been compared with steel wool being slowly woven into a cable). As the collagen matures and becomes denser, the scar becomes almost acellular as the fibroblasts and blood vessels reduce. The external appearance of the scar becomes paler, while the scar becomes softer, flattens and its itchiness diminishes. Most of these changes occur over the first 3 months but a scar will continue to mature for 1–2 years. Tensile strength will continue to increase but will never reach that of normal skin.

Scars are often described as being atrophic, hypertrophic and keloid. An atrophic scar is pale, flat and stretched in appearance, often appearing on the back and areas of tension. It is easily traumatised as the epidermis and dermis are thinned. Excision and resuturing may only rarely improve such a scar.

A hypertrophic scar is defined as excessive scar tissue that does not extend beyond the boundary of the original incision or wound. It results from a prolonged inflammatory phase of wound

healing and from unfavourable scar siting (i.e. across the lines of skin tension). In the face, these are known as the lines of facial expression.

A keloid scar is defined as excessive scar tissue that extends beyond the boundaries of the original incision or wound (Fig. 3.12). Its aetiology is unknown, but it is associated with elevated levels of growth factor, deeply pigmented skin, an inherited tendency and certain areas of the body (e.g. a triangle whose points are the xiphisternum and each shoulder tip).

The histology of both hypertrophic and keloid scars shows excess collagen with hypervascularity, but this is more marked in keloids where there is more type B collagen.

The treatment of both is difficult and is summarised in Summary box 3.9.

Summary Box 3.9

Treatment of hypertrophic and keloid scars

- Pressure – local moulds or elasticated garments
- Silicone gel sheeting (mechanism unknown)
- Intralesional steroid injection (triamcinolone)
- Excision and steroid injection[a]
- Excision and postoperative radiation (external beam or brachytherapy)[a]
- Intralesional excision (keloids only)
- Laser – to reduce redness (which may resolve in any event)
- Vitamin E or palm oil massage (unproven)

a. All excisions have high rates of recurrence.

Hypertrophic scars improve spontaneously with time, whereas keloids do not.

AVOIDABLE SCARRING

If the acute wound has been managed correctly (Summary box 3.4), most of the problems described here should not occur. However, the surgeon should always stress that there will be a scar of some description after wounding, be it planned or accidental. A dirt-ingrained (tattooed) scar is usually preventable by proper initial scrubbing and cleansing of the wound (Fig. 3.13). Late treatment may require excision of the scar or pigment destruction by laser.

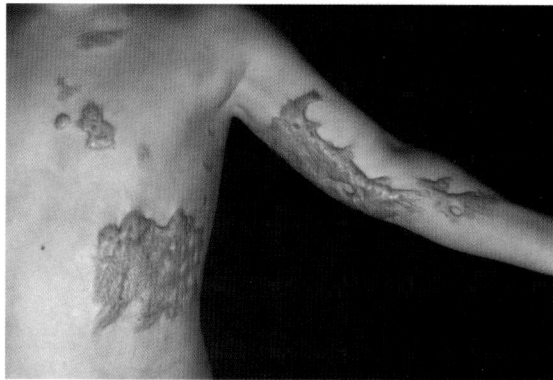

Figure 3.12 Multiple keloid scars.

Laser is an abbreviation for light amplification by stimulated emission of radiation. A laser is an intense beam of monochromatic light.

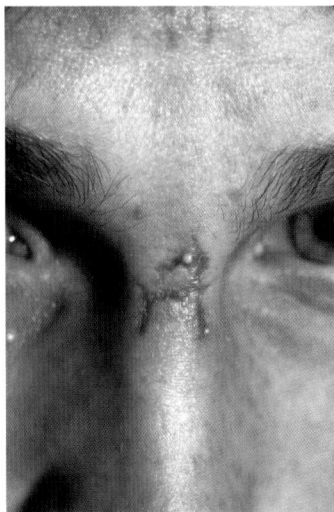

Figure 3.13 Dirt-ingrained scar.

Mismatched or misaligned scars result from a failure to recognise normal landmarks such as the lip vermilion/white roll interface, eyelid and nostril free margins and hair lines such as those relating to eyebrows and moustache. Treatment consists of excision and resuturing.

Poorly contoured scars can be stepped, grooved or pincushioned. Most are caused by poor alignment of deep structures such as muscle or fat, but trapdoor or pincushioned scars are often unavoidable unless the almost circumferential wound can be excised initially. Late treatment consists of scar excision and correct alignment of deeper structures or, as in the case of a trapdoor scar, an excision of the scar margins and repair using W- or Z-plasty techniques.

Suture marks may be minimised by using monofilament sutures that are removed early (3–5 days). Sutures inserted under tension will leave marks. The wound can be strengthened post suture removal by the use of sticky strips. Fine sutures (6/0 or smaller) placed close to the wound margins tend to leave less scarring. Subcuticular suturing avoids suture marks either side of the wound or incision.

CONTRACTURES

Where scars cross joints or flexion creases, a tight web may form restricting the range of movement at the joint. This may be referred to as a contracture and can cause hyperextension or hyperflexion deformity (Fig. 3.14). In the neck, it may interfere with head extension (Fig. 3.15). Treatment may be simple involving multiple Z-plasties (Fig. 3.16) or more complex requiring the inset of grafts or flaps. Splintage and intensive physiotherapy are often required postoperatively.

FURTHER READING

Brown, D.L. and Borschel, G.H. (2004) *Michigan Manual of Plastic Surgery*. Lippincott, Williams & Wilkins, Baltimore, MD, USA.

Georgiade, G.S., Riefkokl, R. and Levin, L.S. (1997) *Georgiade Plastic, Maxillofacial and Reconstructive Surgery*, 3rd edn. Williams & Wilkins, Baltimore, MD, USA.

McGregor, I.A. (1975) *Fundamental Techniques of Plastic Surgery*. Churchill Livingstone, Edinburgh.

Richards, A.M. (2002) *Key Notes on Plastic Surgery*. Blackwell Publishing, Oxford.

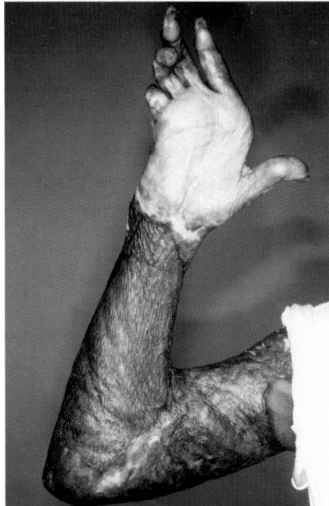

Figure 3.14 Burn contractures showing hyperextended fingers and hyperflexed elbow.

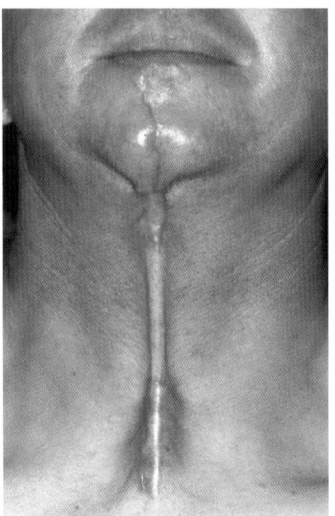

Figure 3.15 Post-traumatic (chainsaw) midline neck contracture.

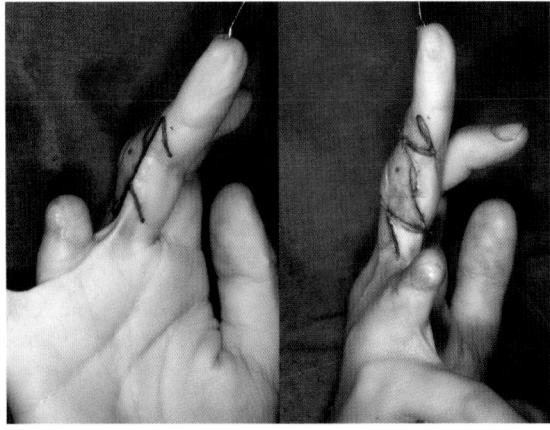

Figure 3.16 Multiple Z-plasty release of finger contracture.

Thomas, S. (2005) An introduction to the use of vacuum assisted closure. World wide wounds. Available online at: http://www.worldwide-wounds.com.

Westaby, S. (1985) *Wound Care*. William Heinemann Medical Books Ltd, London.

CHAPTER 3 | WOUNDS, TISSUE REPAIR AND SCARS

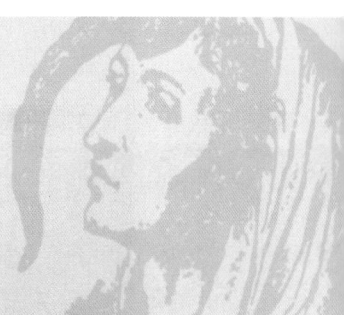

Surgical infection

LEARNING OBJECTIVES

To understand:
- The factors that determine whether a wound will become infected
- The classification of sources of infection and their severity
- The indications for and choice of prophylactic antibiotics
- The characteristics of the common surgical pathogens and their sensitivities
- The spectrum of commonly used antibiotics in surgery and the principles of therapy
- The misuse of antibiotic therapy with the risk of resistance [such as methicillin-resistant *Staphylococcus aureus* (MRSA)] and emergence (such as *Clostridium difficile* enteritis)

To learn:
- Koch's postulates
- The management of abscesses

To appreciate:
- The importance of aseptic and antiseptic techniques and delayed primary or secondary closure in contaminated wounds

To be aware of:
- The causes of reduced resistance to infection (host response)

To know:
- The definitions of infection, particularly at surgical sites
- What basic precautions to take to avoid surgically relevant health care-associated infections

PHYSIOLOGY AND PRESENTATION

Background

Surgical infection, particularly surgical site infection (SSI), has always been a major complication of surgery and trauma and has been documented for 4000–5000 years. The Egyptians had some concepts about infection as they were able to prevent putrefaction, testified by mummification skills. Their medical papyruses also describe the use of salves and antiseptics to prevent SSIs. This 'prophylaxis' had also been known earlier by the Assyrians, although less well documented. It was described again independently by the Greeks. The Hippocratic teachings described the use of anti-microbials, such as wine and vinegar, which were widely used to irrigate open, infected wounds before delayed primary or secondary wound closure. A belief common to all these civilisations, and indeed even later to the Romans, was that, whenever pus localised in an infected wound, it needed to be drained.

Galen recognised that this localisation of infection (suppuration) in wounds, inflicted in the gladiatorial arena, often heralded recovery, particularly after drainage (*pus bonum et laudabile*). Sadly, this dictum was misunderstood by many later healers, who thought that it was the production of pus that was desirable. Until well into the Middle Ages, some practitioners promoted suppuration in wounds by the application of noxious substances, including faeces, in the misguided belief that healing could not occur without pus formation. Theodoric of Cervia, Ambroise Paré and Guy de Chauliac observed that clean wounds, closed primarily, could heal without infection or suppuration.

The understanding of the causes of infection came in the nineteenth century. Microbes had been seen under the micro-

---

Hippocrates was a Greek Physician, and by common consent 'The Father of Medicine'. He was born on the Greek island of Cos off Turkey about 460 BC and probably died in 375 BC.

Galen, 130–200, a Roman Physician, who commenced practice as Surgeon to the Gladiators at Pergamum (now Bregama in Turkey) and later became personal Physician to the Emperor Marcus Aurelius and to two of his successors. He was a prolific writer on many subjects amongst them Anatomy, Medicine, Pathology and Philosophy. His work affected medical thinking for 15 centuries after his death. (Gladiator is Latin for 'Swordsman').

Theodoric of Cervia. Theodoric, 1210–1298, who was Bishop of Cervia published a book on Surgery ca. 1267.

Ambroise Paré, 1510–1590, a French Military Surgeon, who also worked at the Hotel Dieu, Paris, France.

Guy de Chauliac, ?1298–1368, was Physician and Chaplain to Pope Clement VI at Avignon, France. He was the author of 'Chirurgia Magna' which was published about 1363.

scope, but Koch laid down the first definition of infective disease (Koch's postulates; Summary box 4.1).

> **Summary box 4.1**
>
> **Koch's postulates proving the agency of an infective organism**
>
> - It must be found in considerable numbers in the septic focus
> - It should be possible to culture it in a pure form from that septic focus
> - It should be able to produce similar lesions when injected into another host

The Austrian obstetrician Ignac Semmelweis showed that puerperal sepsis could be reduced from over 10% to under 2% by the simple act of hand-washing between cases, particularly between post-mortem examinations and the delivery suite. He was ignored by his contemporaries.

Louis Pasteur recognised that micro-organisms were responsible for spoiling wine, turning it into vinegar. Joseph Lister applied this knowledge to the reduction of colonising organisms in compound fractures by using antiseptics. This allowed surgery without infection. However, his toxic phenol spray and principles of antiseptic surgery soon gave way to aseptic surgery at the turn of the century. Instead of killing the bacteria in the tissues (antiseptic technique), the conditions under which the operation was performed were kept free of bacteria (aseptic technique). This technique is still employed in modern operating theatres.

The concept of a 'magic bullet' (*Zauberkugel*) that could kill microbes but not their host became a reality with the discovery of sulphonamide chemotherapy in the mid-twentieth century. The discovery of the antibiotic penicillin is attributed to Alexander Fleming, but it was isolated by Florey and Chain. The first patient to receive penicillin was Police Constable Alexander in Oxford. He had a severe staphylococcal bacteraemia with metastatic abscesses. He responded to treatment, made a partial recovery before the penicillin ran out, then relapsed and died. Since then, there has been a proliferation of antibiotics with broad-spectrum activity.

However, most staphylococci are now resistant to penicillin, whereas streptococci remain sensitive, although they are now seen less commonly in surgical practice. Many bacteria develop resistance through the acquisition of β-lactamases, which break up the β-lactam ring in many antibiotics. The acquisition of extended spectrum β-lactamases (ESBLs) is an increasing concern in some Gram-negative organisms that cause urinary tract infections. In addition, there is increasing concern about the rising resistance of many other bacteria to antibiotics, in particular the emergence of methicillin-resistant *Staphylococcus aureus* (MRSA) and glycopeptide-resistant enterococci (GRE), which are also relevant in general surgical practice.

The synergy between aerobic Gram-negative bacilli and anaerobic *Bacteroides* spp. also presents a challenge to SSI prevention, especially abscesses after abdominal surgery. Broad-spectrum antibiotics can be given empirically to treat such infections but, if the organisms and their sensitivity are known, then more specific, narrow-range antibiotics can be given. The introduction of antibiotics for prophylaxis and for treatment, together with advances in anaesthesia and critical care medicine, has made possible surgery that would not previously have been considered. Faecal peritonitis is no longer inevitably fatal, and incisions made in the presence of such contamination can heal primarily without infection in 80–90% of patients with appropriate antibiotic therapy. Despite this, it is common practice in many countries to delay wound closure in patients in whom the wound is known to be contaminated or dirty. Waiting for the wound to granulate and then performing a delayed primary or secondary closure may be considered a better option (Summary box 4.2).

> **Summary box 4.2**
>
> **Advances in the control of infection in surgery**
>
> - Aseptic operating theatre techniques have replaced toxic antiseptic techniques
> - Antibiotics have reduced postoperative infection rates after elective and emergency surgery
> - Delayed primary, or secondary, closure remains useful in contaminated wounds

Surgical site infection in patients who have contaminated wounds, who are immunosuppressed or undergoing prosthetic surgery, is now the exception rather than the rule since the introduction of prophylactic antibiotics. The evidence for this is of the highest level. However, the value of prophylactic antibiotics in clean, non-prosthetic surgery remains controversial, although SSI rates after such surgery is high when judged by close, unbiased, post-discharge surveillance, using strict definitions.

PHYSIOLOGY

Micro-organisms are normally prevented from causing infection in tissues by intact epithelial surfaces. These are broken down in trauma and by surgery. In addition to these mechanical barriers, there are other protective mechanisms, which can be divided into:

- *chemical*: low gastric pH;
- *humoral*: antibodies, complement and opsonins;
- *cellular*: phagocytic cells, macrophages, polymorphonuclear cells and killer lymphocytes.

Robert Koch, 1843–1910, Professor of Hygiene and Bacteriology, Berlin, Germany, stated his 'Postulates' in 1882.
Ignac Semmelweis, 1818–1865, Professor of Obstetrics, Budapest, Hungary.
Louis Pasteur, 1822–1895, was a French Chemist, Bacteriologist and Immunologist who was Professor of Chemistry at the Sorbonne, Paris, France.
Joseph Lister, (Lord Lister), 1827–1912, Professor of Surgery, Glasgow, Scotland, (1860–1869), Edinburgh, Scotland, (1869–1877), and King's College Hospital, London, (1877–1892).
Sir Alexander Fleming, 1881–1955, Professor of Bacteriology, St Mary's Hospital, London, England, discovered Penicillium Notatum in 1928.
Howard Walter Florey, (Lord Florey of Adelaide), 1898–1968, Professor of Pathology, The University of Oxford, Oxford, England.
Sir Ernst Boris Chain, Professor of Biochemistry, Imperial College, London, England. Fleming, Florey and Chain shared the 1945 Nobel Prize for Physiology or Medicine for their work on Penicillin.

All these natural mechanisms may be compromised by surgical intervention and treatment.

Reduced resistance to infection has several causes (Summary box 4.3).

Summary box 4.3

Causes of reduced host resistance to infection

- Metabolic: malnutrition (including obesity), diabetes, uraemia, jaundice
- Disseminated disease: cancer and acquired immunodeficiency syndrome (AIDS)
- Iatrogenic: radiotherapy, chemotherapy, steroids

Host response is weakened by malnutrition, which can be recognised clinically, and most easily, as recent rapid weight loss that can be present even in the presence of obesity. Metabolic diseases such as diabetes mellitus, uraemia and jaundice, disseminated malignancy and AIDS are other contributors to infection and a poor healing response, as are iatrogenic causes including the immunosuppression caused by radiotherapy, chemotherapy or steroids (Summary box 4.4, and Figs 4.1 and 4.2).

Summary box 4.4

Risk factors for increased risk of wound infection

- Malnutrition (obesity, weight loss)
- Metabolic disease (diabetes, uraemia, jaundice)
- Immunosuppression (cancer, AIDS, steroids, chemotherapy and radiotherapy)
- Colonisation and translocation in the gastrointestinal tract
- Poor perfusion (systemic shock or local ischaemia)
- Foreign body material
- Poor surgical technique (dead space, haematoma)

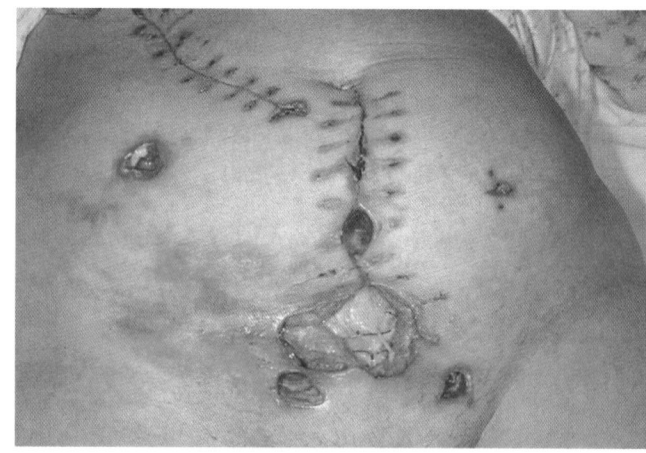

Figure 4.2 Delayed healing relating to infection in a patient on high-dose steroids.

When enteral feeding is suspended during the perioperative period, and particularly with underlying disease such as cancer, immunosuppression, shock or sepsis, bacteria (particularly aerobic Gram-negative bacilli) tend to colonise the normally sterile upper gastrointestinal tract. They may then translocate to the mesenteric nodes and cause the release of endotoxins (lipopolysaccharide in bacterial cell walls), which further increases susceptibility to infection and sepsis, through activation of macrophages and pro-inflammatory cytokine release (Fig. 4.3). The use of selective decontamination of the digestive tract (SDD) is based on the prevention of this colonisation. In the circumstances of reduced resistance, bacteria that are not normally pathogenic may start to behave as pathogens. This is known as opportunistic infection. Opportunistic infection with fungi is an example, particularly when prolonged and changing antibiotic regimens have been used.

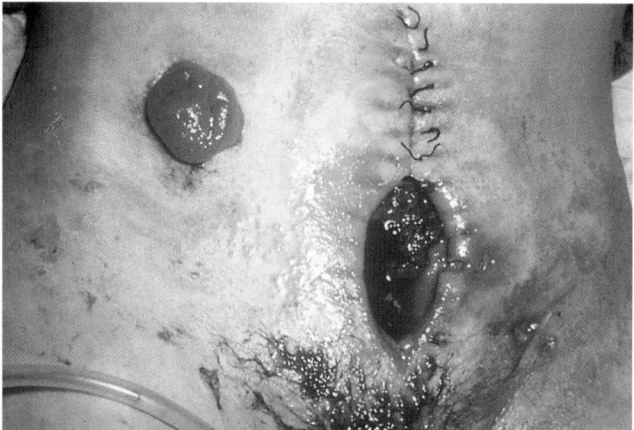

Figure 4.1 Major wound infection and delayed healing presenting as a faecal fistula in a patient with Crohn's disease.

Burrill Bernard Crohn, **1884–1983**, Gastroenterologist, Mount Sinai Hospital, New York, NY, USA, described regional ileitis in 1932.

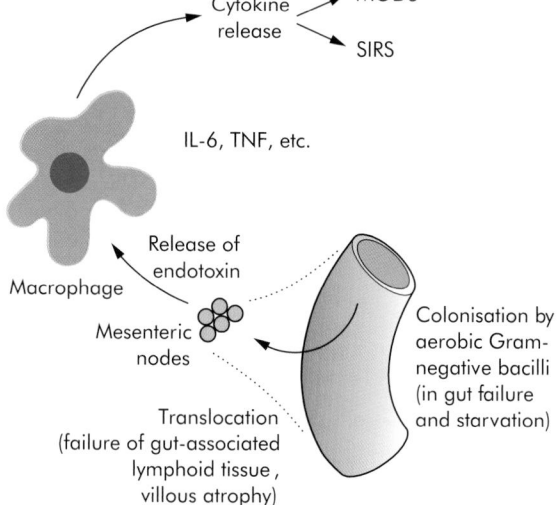

Figure 4.3 Gut failure, colonisation and translocation related to the development of multiple organ dysfunction syndrome (MODS) and systemic inflammatory response syndrome (SIRS). IL, interleukin; TNF, tumour necrosis factor.

The chance of developing an SSI after surgery is also determined by the pathogenicity of the organisms present and by the size of the bacterial inoculum. Devitalised tissue, excessive dead space or haematoma, all the results of poor surgical technique, increase the chances of infection. The same applies to foreign materials of any kind, including sutures and drains. If there is a silk suture in tissue, the critical number of organisms needed to start an infection is reduced logarithmically. Silk should not be used to close skin as it causes suture abscesses for this reason. These principles are important in prosthetic orthopaedic and vascular surgery, when large quantities of foreign material (prostheses and grafts) are deliberately left in the wound (Summary box 4.5)!

Summary box 4.5

Factors that determine whether a wound will become infected

- Host response
- Virulence and inoculum of infective agent
- Vascularity and health of tissue being invaded (including local ischaemia as well as systemic shock)
- Presence of dead or foreign tissue
- Presence of antibiotics during the 'decisive period'

There is a delay before host defences can become mobilised after a breach in an epithelial surface, whether caused by trauma or surgery. The acute inflammatory, humoral and cellular defences take up to 4 hours to be mobilised. This is called the 'decisive period', and it is the time when the invading bacteria may become established in the tissues. It is therefore logical that prophylactic antibiotics should be given to cover this period and that they could be decisive in preventing an infection from developing. The tissue levels of antibiotics should be above the minimum inhibitory concentration (MIC_{90}) for the pathogens likely to be encountered.

Local and systemic presentation

The infection of a wound can be defined as the invasion of organisms through tissues following a breakdown of local and systemic host defences, leading to cellulitis, lymphangitis, abscess and bacteraemia. The infection of most surgical wounds is referred to as superficial surgical site infection (SSSI). The other categories include deep SSI (infection in the deeper musculofascial layers) and organ space infection (such as an abdominal abscess after an anastomotic leak).

Pathogens resist host defences by releasing toxins, which favour their spread, and this is enhanced in anaerobic or frankly necrotic wound tissue. *Clostridium perfringens*, which is responsible for gas gangrene, releases proteases such as hyaluronidase, lecithinase and haemolysin, which allow it to spread through the tissues. Resistance to antibiotics can be acquired by previously sensitive bacteria by transfer through plasmids.

The human body harbours approximately 10^{14} organisms. They can be released into tissues by surgery, contamination being most severe when a hollow viscus perforates (e.g. faecal peritonitis following a diverticular perforation). Any infection that follows surgery may be termed primary or secondary (Summary box 4.6).

Summary box 4.6

Classification of sources of infection

- Primary: acquired from a community or endogenous source (such as that following a perforated peptic ulcer)
- Secondary or exogenous (HAI): acquired from the operating theatre (such as inadequate air filtration) or the ward (e.g. poor hand-washing compliance) or from contamination at or after surgery (such as an anastomotic leak)

Infection that follows surgery or admission to hospital is termed health care-associated infection (HAI). There are four main groups: respiratory infections (including ventilator-associated pneumonia), urinary tract infections (mostly related to urinary catheters), bacteraemia (mostly related to indwelling vascular catheters) and SSIs.

MAJOR AND MINOR SURGICAL SITE INFECTIONS

A major SSI is defined as a wound that either discharges significant quantities of pus spontaneously or needs a secondary procedure to drain it (Fig. 4.4). The patient may have systemic signs such as tachycardia, pyrexia and a raised white count [systemic inflammatory response syndrome (SIRS)] (Summary box 4.7).

Summary box 4.7

Major wound infections

- Significant quantity of pus
- Delayed return home
- Patients are systemically ill

Minor wound infections may discharge pus or infected serous fluid but should not be associated with excessive discomfort, systemic signs or delay in return home (Fig. 4.5). The differentiation between major and minor and the definition of SSI is important in audit or trials of antibiotic prophylaxis. There are scoring systems for the severity of wound infection, which are particularly useful in surveillance and research. Examples are the Southampton (Table 4.1) and ASEPSIS systems (Table 4.2).

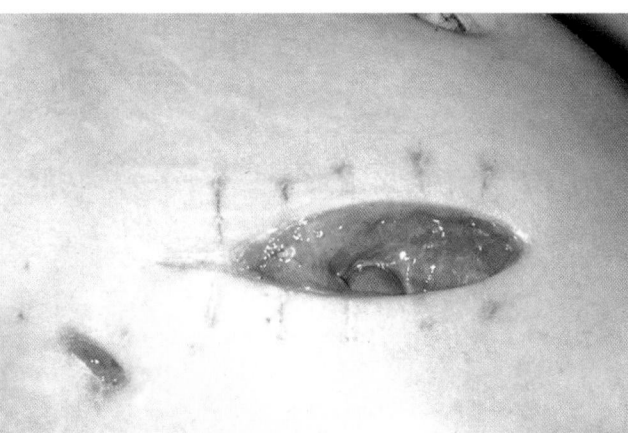

Figure 4.4 Major wound infection with superficial skin dehiscence.

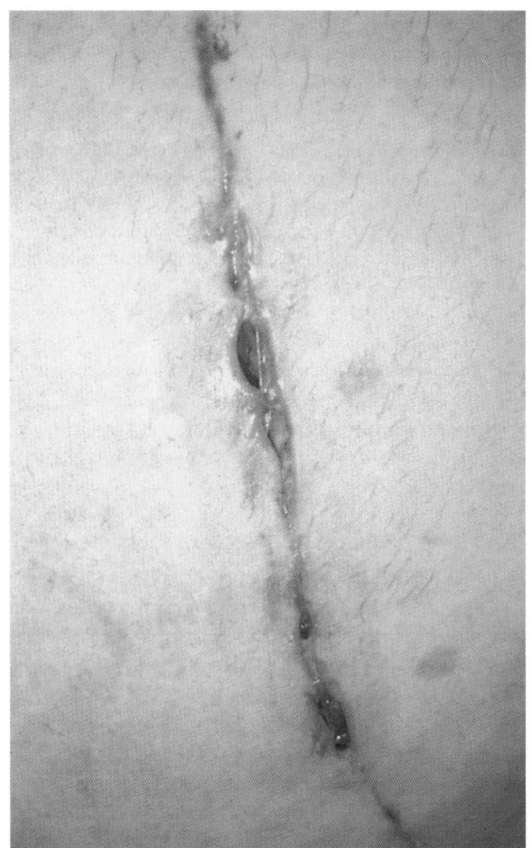

Figure 4.5 Minor wound infection that settled spontaneously without antibiotics.

Table 4.1 Southampton wound grading system

Grade	Appearance
0	Normal healing
I	Normal healing with mild bruising or erythema
Ia	Some bruising
Ib	Considerable bruising
Ic	Mild erythema
II	Erythema plus other signs of inflammation
IIa	At one point
IIb	Around sutures
IIc	Along wound
IId	Around wound
III	Clear or haemoserous discharge
IIIa	At one point only (≤ 2 cm)
IIIb	Along wound (> 2 cm)
IIIc	Large volume
IIId	Prolonged (> 3 days)
Major complication	
IV	Pus
IVa	At one point only (≤ 2 cm)
IVb	Along wound (> 2 cm)
V	Deep or severe wound infection with or without tissue breakdown; haematoma requiring aspiration

Table 4.2 The ASEPSIS wound score

Criterion	Points
Additional treatment	0
Antibiotics for wound infection	10
Drainage of pus under local anaesthesia	5
Debridement of wound under general anaesthesia	10
Serous discharge[a]	Daily 0–5
Erythema[a]	Daily 0–5
Purulent exudate[a]	Daily 0–10
Separation of deep tissues[a]	Daily 0–10
Isolation of bacteria from wound	10
Stay as in-patient prolonged over 14 days as result of wound infection	5

a. Scored for 5 of the first 7 days only, the remainder being scored if present in the first 2 months.

Accurate surveillance can only be achieved using trained, unbiased and blinded assessors. Most include surveillance for a 30-day postoperative period. The US Centers for Disease Control (CDC) definition insists on a 30-day follow-up period for non-prosthetic surgery and 1 year after implanted hip and knee surgery.

Types of localised infection

Abscess

An abscess presents all the clinical features of acute inflammation originally described by Celsus: *calor* (heat), *rubor* (redness), *dolour* (pain) and *tumour* (swelling). To these can be added *functio laesa* (loss of function: if it hurts, the infected part is not used). They usually follow a puncture wound of some kind, which may have been forgotten, as well as surgery, but can be metastatic in all tissues following bacteraemia.

Pyogenic organisms, predominantly *Staphylococcus aureus*, cause tissue necrosis and suppuration. Pus is composed of dead and dying white blood cells that release damaging cytokines, oxygen free radicals and other molecules. An abscess is surrounded by an acute inflammatory response and a pyogenic membrane composed of a fibrinous exudate and oedema and the cells of acute inflammation. Granulation tissue (macrophages, angiogenesis and fibroblasts) forms later around the suppurative process and leads to collagen deposition. If it is not drained or resorbed completely, a chronic abscess may result. If it is partly sterilised with antibiotics, an antibioma may form.

Abscesses contain hyperosmolar material that draws in fluid. This increases the pressure and causes pain. If they spread, they usually track along planes of least resistance and point towards the skin. Wound abscesses may discharge spontaneously by tracking to a surface, but may need drainage through a surgical incision. Most abscesses relating to surgical wounds take 7–10 days to form after surgery. As many as 75% of SSIs present after the patient has left hospital and may thus be overlooked by the surgical team. Their cost and management, which may be inadequate, is transferred to primary care (Summary box 4.8).

Aulus Aurelius Cornelius Celsus, **25 BC–50 AD, a Roman Surgeon. He was the author of 'De Re Medico Libri Octo'.**

> **Summary box 4.8**
>
> **Abscesses**
>
> - Abscesses need drainage with curettage
> - Modern imaging techniques may allow guided aspiration
> - Antibiotics are indicated if the abscess is not localised (e.g. evidence of cellulitis)
> - Healing by secondary intention is encouraged

Abscess cavities need cleaning out after incision and drainage and are encouraged to heal by secondary intention. All loculi need to be opened and curetted before resolution can occur. Persistent chronic abscesses may lead to sinus or fistula formation. In a chronic abscess, lymphocytes and plasma cells are seen. There is tissue sequestration and later calcification. Certain organisms are associated with chronicity, sinus and fistula formation. Common ones are *Mycobacterium* and *Actinomyces*. They should not be forgotten when these complications occur.

Perianastomotic contamination may be the cause of an abscess but, in the abdomen, abscesses are more usually the result of anastomotic leakage. An abscess in a deep cavity such as the pleura or peritoneum may be difficult to diagnose or locate even when there is strong clinical suspicion that it is present (Fig. 4.6). Plain or contrast radiographs may not be helpful, but ultrasonography, computerised tomography (CT), magnetic resonance imaging (MRI) and isotope scans are all useful and may allow guided aspiration without the need for surgical intervention.

The role of antibiotics in the treatment of wound abscesses is controversial unless there are signs of spreading infection such as cellulitis, lymphangitis or related sepsis. Surgical decompression and curettage of abscesses must be adequate whether antibiotics are used or not. Primary closure can be used, but delayed primary or secondary suture is safest once granulation tissue is mature and the wound is clean.

Cellulitis and lymphangitis

Cellulitis is the non-suppurative invasive infection of tissues. There is poor localisation in addition to the cardinal signs of inflammation. Spreading infection presenting in surgical practice is typically caused by organisms such as β-haemolytic streptococci (Fig. 4.7), staphylococci (Fig. 4.8) and *C. perfringens*. Tissue destruction, gangrene and ulceration may follow, which are caused by release of proteases.

Systemic signs (the old-fashioned term toxaemia) are common: SIRS, chills, fever and rigors. These follow the release of organisms, exotoxins and cytokines into the circulation. However, blood cultures are often negative.

Lymphangitis is part of a similar process and presents as painful red streaks in affected lymphatics. Cellulitis is usually located at the point of injury and subsequent tissue infection. Lymphangitis is often accompanied by painful lymph node groups in the related drainage area (Summary box 4.9).

> **Summary box 4.9**
>
> **Cellulitis and lymphangitis**
>
> - Non-suppurative, poorly localised
> - Commonly caused by streptococci, staphylococci or clostridia
> - SIRS is common
> - Blood cultures are often negative

SYSTEMIC INFLAMMATORY RESPONSE AND MULTIPLE ORGAN DYSFUNCTION SYNDROMES (MODS)

Sepsis is defined as the systemic manifestation of SIRS, with a documented infection, the signs and symptoms of which may

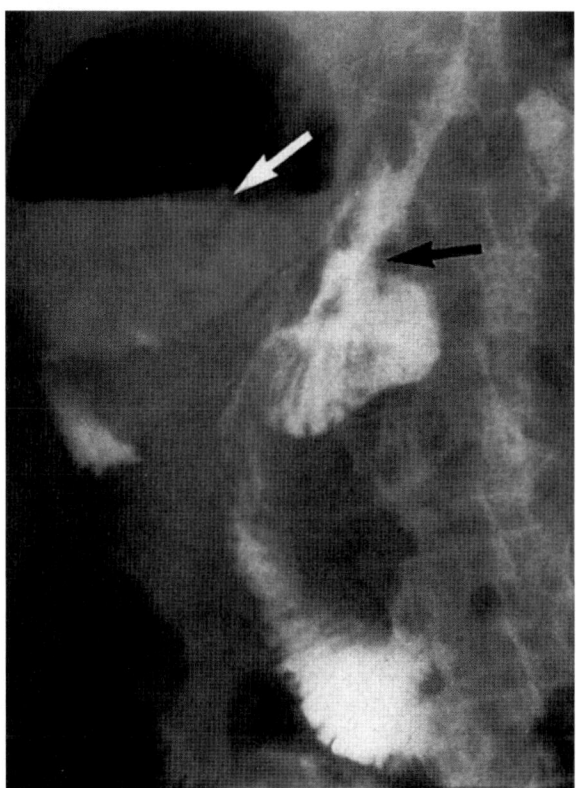

Figure 4.6 Plain radiograph showing a subphrenic abscess with a gas/fluid level (white arrow). Gastrografin is seen leaking from the oesophagojejunal anastomosis (after gastrectomy) towards the abscess (black arrow).

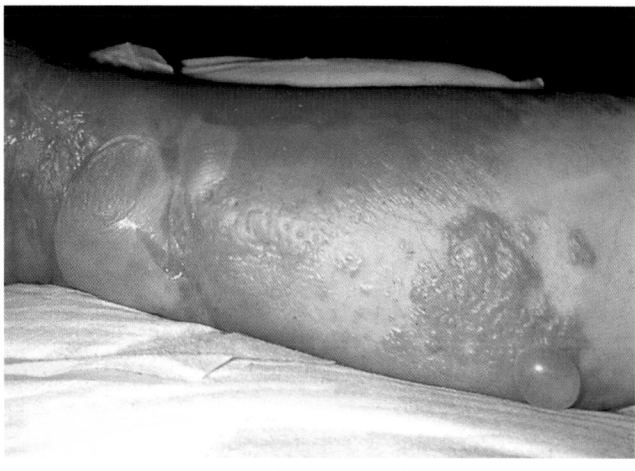

Figure 4.7 Streptococcal cellulitis of the leg following a minor puncture wound.

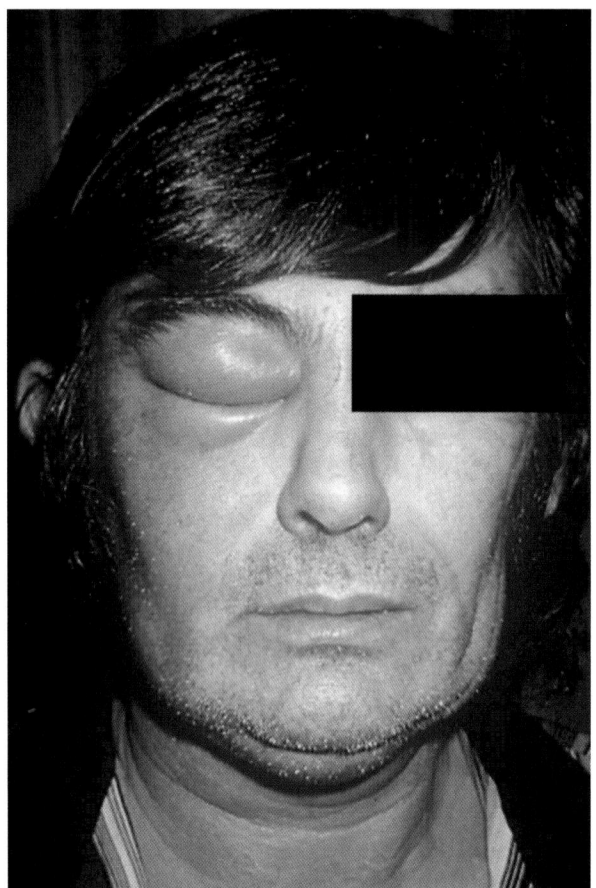

Figure 4.8 Staphylococcal cellulitis of the face and orbit following severe infection of an epidermoid cyst of the scalp.

also be caused by multiple trauma, burns or pancreatitis without infection. Serious infection, such as secondary peritonitis, may lead to SIRS through the release of lipopolysaccharide endotoxin from the walls of dying Gram-negative bacilli (mainly *Escherichia coli*) or other bacteria or fungi. This and other toxins cause the release of cytokines (Fig. 4.3, page 34). SIRS should not be confused with bacteraemia although the two may coexist (see Table 4.3).

Table 4.3 Definitions of systemic inflammatory response syndrome (SIRS) and sepsis

SIRS
Two of:
hyperthermia (> 38°C) or hypothermia (< 36°C)
tachycardia (> 90 min^{-1}, no β-blockers) or tachypnoea (> 20 min^{-1})
white cell count > 12×10^9 l^{-1} or < 4×10^9 l^{-1}
Sepsis is SIRS with a documented infection
Severe sepsis or sepsis syndrome is sepsis with evidence of one or more organ failures [respiratory (acute respiratory distress syndrome), cardiovascular (septic shock follows compromise of cardiac function and fall in peripheral vascular resistance), renal (usually acute tubular necrosis), hepatic, blood coagulation systems or central nervous system]

Theodor Escherich, 1857–1911, Professor of Paediatrics, Vienna, Austria, discovered the Bacterium Coli Commune in 1886.

Septic manifestations and multiple organ dysfunction syndrome (MODS) are mediated by the release of cytokines such as the interleukins (IL-6), tumour necrosis factor alpha (TNFα) and other substances released from polymorphonuclear and phagocytic cells. In its most severe form, MODS may progress into multiple system organ failure (MSOF). In this state, the body's resistance to infection is reduced (Summary box 4.10).

Summary box 4.10

Definitions of infected states

- SSI is an infected wound or deep organ space
- SIRS is the body's systemic response to an infected wound
- MODS is the effect that the infection produces systemically
- MSOF is the end-stage of uncontrolled MODS

Bacteraemia and sepsis

Bacteraemia is unusual following superficial SSIs but common after anastomotic breakdown (deep space SSI). It is usually transient and can follow procedures undertaken through infected tissues (particularly instrumentation in infected bile or urine). Bacteraemia is important when a prosthesis has been implanted, as infection of the prosthesis can occur. Sepsis accompanied by MODS may follow anastomotic breakdown. Aerobic Gram-negative bacilli are mainly responsible, but *Staphylococcus aureus* and fungi may be involved, particularly after the use of broad-spectrum antibiotics (Summary box 4.11).

Summary box 4.11

Bacteraemia and sepsis

- Sepsis is common after anastomotic breakdown
- Bacteraemia is dangerous if the patient has a prosthesis
- Sepsis may be associated with MODS

Specific wound infections

Gas gangrene

This is caused by *C. perfringens*. These Gram-positive, anaerobic, spore-bearing bacilli are widely found in nature, particularly in soil and faeces. This is relevant to military and traumatic surgery and colorectal operations. Patients who are immunocompromised, diabetic or have malignant disease are at greater risk, particularly if they have wounds containing necrotic or foreign material, resulting in anaerobic conditions. Military wounds provide an ideal environment as the kinetic energy of high-velocity missiles or shrapnel ($1/2 \cdot mv^2$; *m* is mass, *v* is velocity) causes extensive tissue damage. The cavitation which follows passage of a missile causes a 'sucking' entry wound, leaving clothing and environmental soiling in the wound in addition to devascularised tissue. Gas gangrene wound infections are associated with severe local wound pain and crepitus (gas in the tissues, which may also be noted on plain radiographs). The wound produces a thin, brown, sweet-smelling exudate, in which Gram staining will reveal bacteria. Oedema and spreading gangrene follow the release of collagenase, hyaluronidase, other proteases and alpha toxin. Early systemic complications with circulatory collapse and MSOF follow if prompt action is not taken (Summary box 4.12).

Summary box 4.12

Gas gangrene

■ Caused by *Clostridium perfringens*
■ Gas and smell are characteristic
■ Immunocompromised patients are most at risk
■ Antibiotic prophylaxis is essential when performing amputations to remove dead tissue

Antibiotic prophylaxis should always be considered in patients at risk, especially when amputations are performed for peripheral vascular disease with open necrotic ulceration. Once a gas gangrene infection is established, large doses of intravenous penicillin and aggressive debridement of affected tissues are required. The use of hyperbaric oxygen is controversial.

Clostridium tetani

This is another anaerobic, terminal spore-bearing, Gram-positive bacterium that can cause tetanus following implantation into tissues or a wound (which may have been trivial or unrecognised and forgotten). The spores are widespread in soil and manure, and so the infection is more common in traumatic civilian or military wounds. The signs and symptoms of tetanus are mediated by the release of the exotoxin tetanospasmin, which affects myoneural junctions and the motor neurones of the anterior horn of the spinal cord. A short prodromal period, which has a poor prognosis, leads to spasms in the distribution of the short motor nerves of the face followed by the development of severe generalised motor spasms including opsithotonus, respiratory arrest and death. A longer prodromal period of 4–5 weeks is associated with a milder form of the disease. The entry wound may show a localised small area of cellulitis; exudate or aspiration may give a sample that can be stained to show the presence of Gram-positive rods. Prophylaxis with tetanus toxoid is the best preventative treatment but, in an established infection, minor debridement of the wound may need to be performed and antibiotic treatment with benzylpenicillin provided in addition. Relaxants may also be required, and the patient may require ventilation in severe forms, which may be associated with a high mortality. The use of anti-toxin using human immunoglobulin ought to be considered for both at-risk wounds and established infection.

The toxoid is a formalin-attenuated vaccine and should be given in three separate doses to give protection for a 5-year period, after which a single 5-yearly booster confers immunity. It should be given to all patients with open traumatic wounds who are not immunised. At-risk wounds are those that present late, when there is devitalisation of tissue or when there is soiling. For these wounds, a booster of toxoid should be given or, if not immunised at all a three-dose course, together with prophylactic benzylpenicillin, but the use of anti-toxin is controversial because of the risk of toxicity and allergy.

Synergistic spreading gangrene (synonym: subdermal gangrene, necrotising fasciitis)

This is not caused by clostridia. A mixed pattern of organisms is responsible: coliforms, staphylococci, *Bacteroides* spp., anaerobic streptococci and peptostreptococci have all been implicated, acting in synergy. Abdominal wall infections are known as Meleney's synergistic hospital gangrene and scrotal infection as Fournier's gangrene (Fig. 4.9). Patients are almost always immunocompromised with conditions such as diabetes mellitus. The wound initiating the infection may have been minor, but severely contaminated wounds are more likely to be the cause. Severe wound pain, signs of spreading inflammation with crepitus and smell are all signs of the infection spreading. Untreated, it will lead to widespread gangrene and MSOF. The subdermal spread of gangrene is always much more extensive than appears from initial examination. Broad-spectrum antibiotic therapy must be combined with aggressive circulatory support. Locally, there should be wide excision of necrotic tissue and laying open of affected areas. The debridement may need to be extensive, and patients who survive may need large areas of skin grafting.

TREATMENT OF SURGICAL INFECTION

Now that patients are discharged more quickly after surgery and many procedures are performed as day cases, many SSIs are

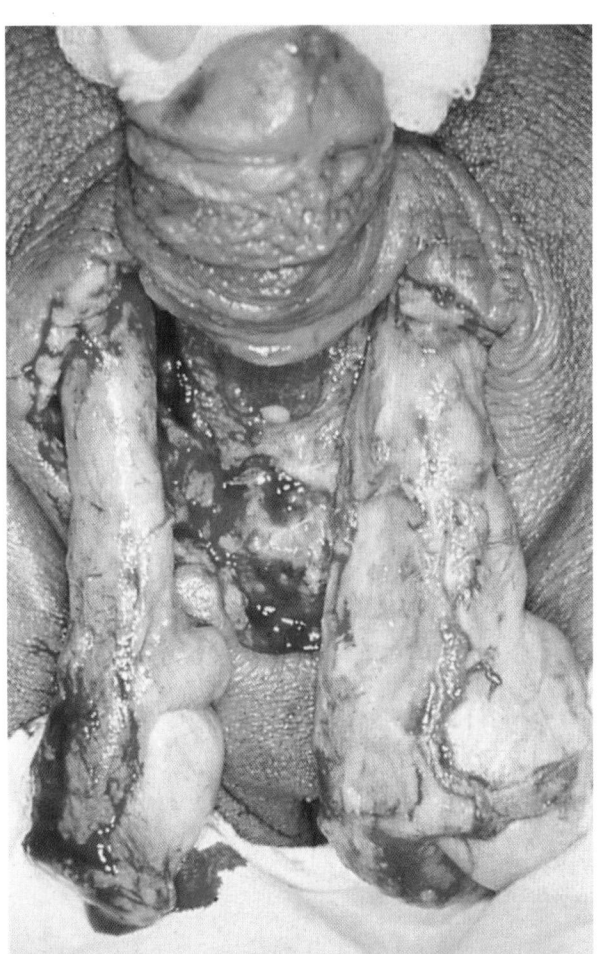

Figure 4.9 A classic presentation of Fournier's gangrene of the scrotum with 'shameful exposure of the testes' following excision of the gangrenous skin.

Frank Lamont Meleney, **1889–1963**, Professor of Clinical Surgery, Columbia University, New York, NY, USA.
Jean Alfred Fournier, **1832–1915**, Syphilologist, the Founder of the Venereal and Dermatological Clinic, Hôpital St. Louis, Paris, France.

missed by the surgical team unless they undertake a prolonged and carefully audited follow-up with primary care doctors. Suppurative wound infections take 7–10 days to develop, and even cellulitis around wounds caused by invasive organisms (such as the β-haemolytic *Streptococcus*) takes 3–4 days to develop. Major surgical infections with systemic signs (Fig. 4.10), evidence of spreading infection, cellulitis or bacteraemia need treatment with appropriate antibiotics. The choice may need to be empirical initially but is best based on culture and sensitivities of isolates harvested at surgery. Although the identification of organisms in surgical infections is necessary for audit and wound surveillance purposes, it is usually 2–3 days before sensitivities are known (Figs 4.11 and 4.12). It is illogical to withhold antibiotics until these are available but, if clinical response is poor by the time sensitivities are known, then antibiotics can be changed. This is unusual if the empirical choice of antibiotics is sensible; change of antibiotics promotes resistance and risks complications, such as *C. difficile* enteritis.

If an infected wound is under tension, or there is clear evidence of suppuration, sutures or clips need to be removed, with curettage if necessary, to allow pus to drain adequately. There is no evidence that subcuticular continuous skin closure contributes to or prevents suppuration. In severely contaminated

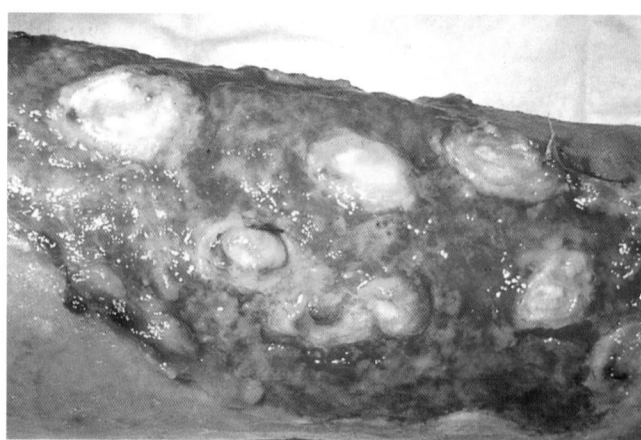

Figure 4.11 Mixed streptococcal infection of a skin graft with very poor 'take'.

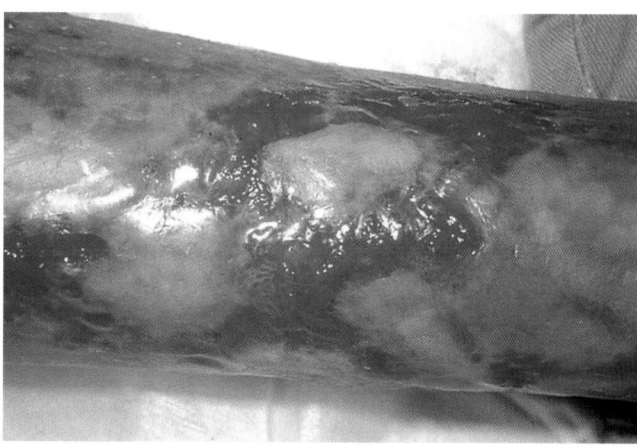

Figure 4.12 After 5–6 days of antibiotics, the infection shown in Fig. 4.11 is under control, and the skin grafts are clearly viable.

wounds, such as an incision made for drainage of an abscess, it is logical to leave the skin open. Delayed primary or secondary suture can be undertaken when the wound is clean and granulating (Figs 4.13 and 4.14). Leaving wounds open after a 'dirty' operation, such as laparotomy for faecal peritonitis, is not practised as widely in the UK as in the USA or mainland Europe (Summary box 4.13).

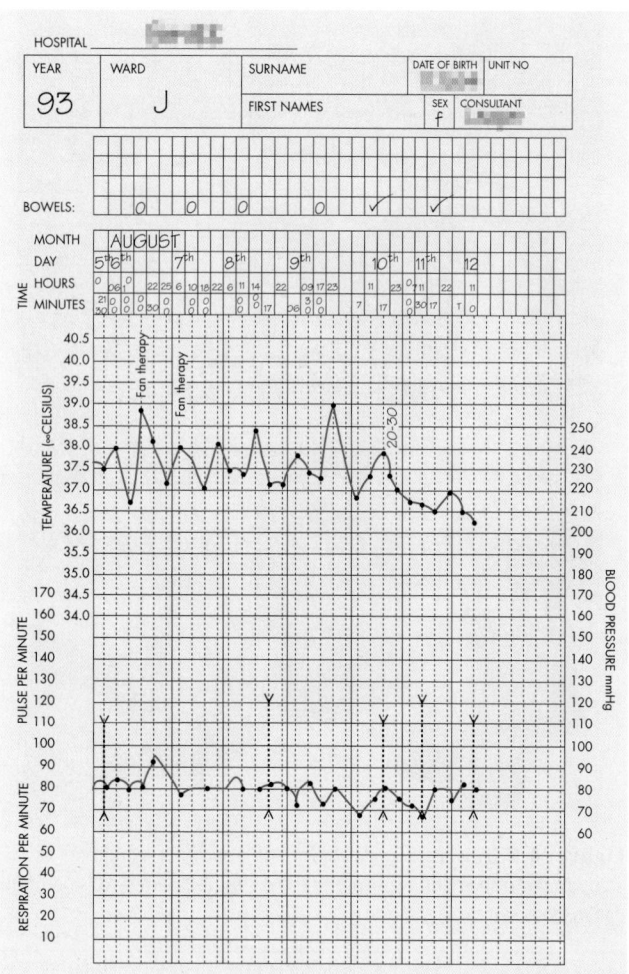

Figure 4.10 Classic swinging pyrexia related to a perianastomotic wound abscess that settled spontaneously on antibiotic therapy.

> **Summary box 4.13**
>
> **Surgical incisions through infected or contaminated tissues**
>
> - When possible, tissue or pus for culture should be taken before antibiotic cover is started
> - The choice of antibiotics is empirical until sensitivities are available
> - Wounds are best managed by delayed primary or secondary closure

When taking pus from infected wounds, specimens should be sent fresh for microbiological culture. Swabs should be placed in transport medium, but the larger the volume of pus sent, the more likely is the accurate identification of the organism

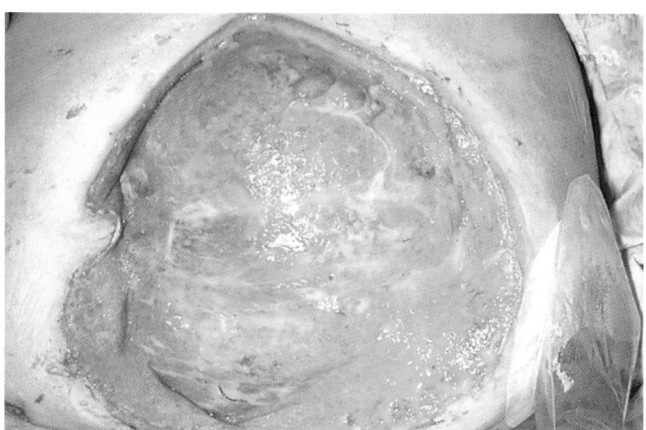

Figure 4.13 Skin layers left open to granulate after laparotomy for faecal peritonitis. The wound is clean and ready for closure.

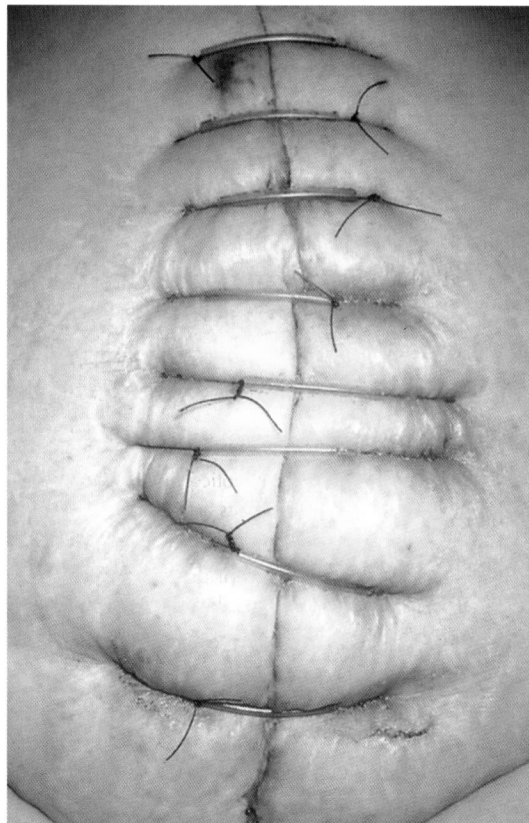

Figure 4.14 Secondary closure of wound.

involved. Providing the microbiologist with as much information as possible and discussing the results with him or her gives the best chance of the most appropriate antibiotic treatment. If bacteraemia is suspected, but results are negative, then repeat specimens for blood culture may need to be taken.

A rapid report on infective material can be based on an immediate Gram stain. Aerobic and anaerobic culture on conventional media allows sensitivities to be assessed by disc diffusion. Measurements of minimum inhibitory antibiotic concentrations (MIC_{90} in mg l^{-1}), together with measurements of endotoxin and cytokine levels, are usually only needed for research studies.

Many dressings are now available for use in wound care. These

are listed in Table 4.4. Polymeric films are used as incision drapes and also to cover sutured wounds, but are not indicated for use in wound infections. Agents that can be used to help debride open infected wounds and others to absorb excessive exudate or to encourage epithelialisation and the formation of granulation tissue are also listed (Fig. 4.15). Most contribute to the ideal moist wound environment, and there are others that provide an antibacterial to the wound. There is now a plethora of dressings containing silver or povidone iodine antiseptics, but the use of topical antibiotics should be avoided because of the risks of allergy and resistance.

Prophylaxis

Prophylactic antibiotics

If antibiotics are given empirically, they should be used when local wound defences are not established (the decisive period). Ideally, maximal blood and tissue levels should be present at the time at which the first incision is made and before contamination occurs. Intravenous administration at induction of anaesthesia is optimal. In long operations, those involving the insertion of a prosthesis, when there is excessive blood loss or when unexpected contamination occurs, antibiotics may be repeated 8 and 16 hours later. The choice of an antibiotic depends on the expected spectrum of organisms likely to be encountered, the cost and local hospital policies, which are based on experience of local resistance trends (Summary box 4.14).

Summary box 4.14

Choice of antibiotics for prophylaxis

- Empirical cover against expected pathogens with local hospital guidelines
- Single-shot intravenous administration at induction of anaesthesia
- Repeat only in prosthetic surgery, long operations or if there is excessive blood loss
- Continue as therapy if there is unexpected contamination
- Benzylpenicillin should be used if *Clostridium* gas gangrene infection is a possibility
- Patients with heart valve disease or a prosthesis should be protected from bacteraemia caused by dental work, urethral instrumentation or visceral surgery

---

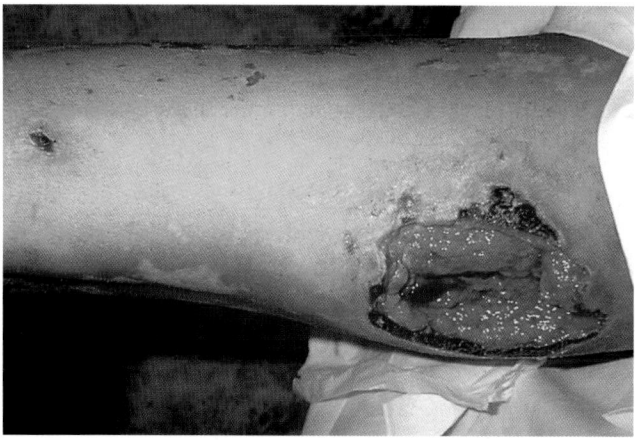

Figure 4.15 Infected animal bite/wound of the upper thigh, treated by open therapy following virulent staphylococcal infection. Deep cavity wounds such as this can be debrided and kept moist with many of the modern dressings listed in Table 4.4.

CHAPTER 4 | SURGICAL INFECTION

Table 4.4 Surgical dressings

Type	Name (example)	Indications and comments
Debriding agents	Benoxyl–benzoic acid Aserbine–benzoic acid Variclene–lactic acid	Used only in necrotic sloughing skin ulcers. Provide acidic environment. Claimed to enhance healing with debriding action
Enzymatic agents	Varidase–streptokinase/streptodornase	Activate fibrinolysis and liquefy pus on chronic skin ulcers
Bead dressings	Debrisan	Remove bacteria and excess moisture by capillary action in deep granulating wounds. Antimicrobials
	Iodosorb Other paste dressings	May be added but with questionable topical benefit
Polymeric films	Opsite Bioclusive Tegaderm	Primary adhesive transparent dressing for sutured wounds or donor sites
Foams	Silastic (elastomer)	Elastomeric dressing can be shaped to fit deep cavities and granulating wounds. Absorbent and non-adherent
	Lyofoam Allevyn	
Hydrogels	Geliperm Intrasite	Maintain moist environment. Polymers can absorb exudate or antiseptics (but adding antiseptics is of doubtful benefit). Semi-permeable, allow gas exchange
Hydrocolloids	Comfeel Granuflex	Complete occlusion. Promote epithelialisation and granulation tissue. Maintain moisture without gaseous exchange across them
Fibrous polymers	Kaltostat Sorbsan	Absorptive alginate dressings. Derived from natural (seaweed) source. Like polymeric hydrocolloids and hydrogels, they can be used to pack deep wounds
Biological membranes	Porcine skin, amnion	Used for superficial chronic skin ulcers. No proven advantage
Simple miscellaneous	Gauzes: viscose/cotton with non-adherent coating (Melolin) Tulles: non-adherent paraffin impregnation	Simple absorptive dressings only used as secondary dressings to absorb exudate. Added anti-microbials probably confer no benefit. Added charcoal absorbents may reduce swelling. Relatively cheap but of questionable effectiveness

The use of the newer, broad-spectrum antibiotics for prophylaxis should be avoided. Table 4.5 gives some examples of prophylaxis that can be used in elective surgical operations.

Lower limb amputation should be covered against C. *perfringens* using 1.2 g of benzylpenicillin intravenously at induction of anaesthesia and 6-hourly thereafter for 48 hours.

Patients with known valvular disease of the heart (or with any implanted vascular or orthopaedic prosthesis) should have prophylactic antibiotics during dental, urological or open viscus surgery. Single doses of broad-spectrum penicillin, for example amoxicillin, orally or intravenously administered, are sufficient for dental surgery. In urological instrumentation, a second-generation cephalosporin, such as cefuroxime, is sufficient, but in open viscus surgery, the addition of an imidazole such as metronidazole should be considered.

Preoperative preparation

Short preoperative hospital stay lowers the risk of acquiring MRSA, multiply resistant coagulase-negative staphylococci (MRCNS) and other organisms and the acquisition of HAIs. Medical staff should always wash their hands between patients, but compliance in some health-care working staff (particularly doctors!) is poor. Although the need for clean hospitals, emphasised by the media, is logical, the 'clean your hands campaign' is beginning to result in falls in the incidence of MRSA bacteraemias. The value of personal hygiene is obvious (to both patients and surgeons). Staff with open, infected skin lesions should not enter the operating theatres. Ideally, neither should patients, especially if they are having a prosthesis implanted. Antiseptic baths (usually chlorhexidine) are popular in Europe, but there is no hard evidence for their value in reducing wound infections. Preoperative shaving should be avoided except for aesthetic reasons or to prevent adherence of dressings. If it is to be undertaken, it should be undertaken immediately before surgery as the SSI rate after clean wound surgery may be doubled if it is performed the night before, because minor skin injury enhances superficial bacterial colonisation. Cream depilation is messy and hair clipping is best, with the lowest rate of infection (Summary box 4.15).

Table 4.5 Suggested prophylactic regimens for operations at risk

Type of surgery	Organisms encountered	Prophylactic regimen suggested
Vascular	*Staphylococcus epidermidis* (or MRCNS) *Staphylococcus aureus* (or MRSA) Aerobic Gram-negative bacilli (AGNB)	Three doses of flucloxacillin with or without gentamicin, vancomycin or rifampicin if MRCNS/MRSA a risk
Orthopaedic	*Staphylococcus epidermidis/aureus*	One to three doses of a broad-spectrum cephalosporin (with anti-staphylococcal action) or gentamicin beads
Oesophagogastric	Enterobacteriaceae Enterococci (including anaerobic/ viridans streptococci)	One to three doses of a second-generation cephalosporin and metronidazole in severe contamination
Biliary	Enterobacteriaceae (mainly *Escherichia coli*) Enterococci (including *Streptococcus faecalis*)	One dose of a second-generation cephalosporin
Small bowel	Enterobacteriaceae Anaerobes (mainly *Bacteroides*)	One to three doses of a second-generation cephalosporin with or without metronidazole
Appendix/colorectal	Enterobacteriaceae Anaerobes (mainly *Bacteroides*)	Three doses of a second-generation cephalosporin (or gentamicin) with metronidazole (the use of oral, poorly absorbed antibiotics is controversial)

MRCNS, multiply resistant coagulase-negative staphylococci; MRSA, methicillin-resistant *Staphylococcus aureus*.

Summary box 4.15

Avoiding surgical site infections

- Staff should always wash their hands between patients
- Length of patient stay should be kept to a minimum
- Preoperative shaving should be avoided if possible
- Antiseptic skin preparation should be standardised
- Attention to theatre technique and discipline
- Avoid hypothermia perioperatively and ensure supplemental oxygenation in recovery

Scrubbing and skin preparation

For the first operation of the day, aqueous antiseptics should be used, and the scrub should include the nails. Subsequent scrubbing should merely involve washing to the elbows, as repeated extensive scrubbing releases more organisms than it removes.

One application of an alcoholic antiseptic is adequate for skin preparation of the operative site. This leads to a more than 95% reduction in bacterial count. Antiseptics in common use are listed in Table 4.6.

Theatre technique and discipline also contribute to low infection rates. Numbers of staff in the theatre and movement in and out of theatre should be kept to a minimum. Careful and regular surveillance is needed to ensure the quality of theatre ventilation, instrument sterilisation and aseptic technique. Operator skill in gentle manipulation and dissection of tissues is much more difficult to audit, but dead spaces and haematomas should be avoided and the use of diathermy kept to a minimum. There is no evidence that drains, incision drapes or wound guards help to reduce wound infection.

There is the highest level of evidence-based medicine that the perioperative avoidance of hypothermia and supplemental oxygen during recovery can significantly reduce the rate of SSIs.

Postoperative care of wounds

Similar attention to standards is needed in the postoperative care of wounds. Secondary (exogenous) SSIs, as well as other HAIs, can be related to poor hospital standards. For example, outbreaks of MRSA infections are rare but serious, particularly with the advent of epidemic MRSA (E-MRSA) and new resistant strains that may express the Panton–Valentine leucocidin. The presence of this organism in wounds, and the number of MRSA bacteraemias, can be a marker of inadequate postoperative wound care, and it can be very difficult and expensive to screen for, identify and eradicate. Even in the community, new strains of MRSA (C-MRSA) are being recognised.

Careful audit should lead to changes in practice, and follow-up should ensure that audit loops are closed. It is critical that surgeons manage their own audit; league tables kept by non-medical or related personnel must be accurate. Scoring systems are useful in audit but, in general, have only been used in wound infection research (Tables 4.2 and 4.3, pages 36 and 38). Nevertheless, accurate audit ought to involve the use of trained, blinded observers in post-discharge surveillance of all HAIs, using validated and reproducible definitions.

CLASSIFICATION OF SURGICAL WOUNDS

Potential for infection

The best measure of wound contamination at the end of an operation is to sample tissue in the wound edge. The theoretical degree of contamination, proposed by the National Research Council (USA) over 40 years ago, relates well to infection rates (Table 4.7). When wounds are heavily contaminated or when an incision is made into an abscess, therapeutic antibiotics may be justified. In these cases, infection rates of more than 15% are expected. There is undisputed evidence that prophylactic antibiotics are effective in clean-contaminated and contaminated

Table 4.6 Classification of antiseptics commonly used in general surgical practice

Name	Presentation	Uses	Comments
Chlorhexidine (Hibiscrub)	Alcoholic 0.5% Aqueous 4%	Skin preparation Skin preparation. Surgical scrub in dilute solutions in open wounds	Has cumulative effect. Effective against Gram-positive organisms and relatively stable in the presence of pus and body fluids
Povidone–iodine (Betadine)	Alcoholic 10% Aqueous 7.5%	Skin preparation Skin preparation. Surgical scrub in dilute solutions in open wounds	Safe, fast-acting, broad spectrum. Some sporicidal activity. Anti-fungal Iodine is not free but combined with polyvinylpyrrolidone (povidone)
Cetrimide (Savlon)	Aqueous	Hand-washing Instrument and surface cleaning	*Pseudomonas* spp. may grow in stored contaminated solutions. Ammonium compounds have good detergent action (surface-active agent)
Alcohols	70% ethyl, isopropyl	Skin preparation	Should be reserved for use as disinfectants
Hypochlorites	Aqueous preparations (Eusol, Milton, Chloramine T)	Instrument and surface cleaning (debriding agent in open wounds?)	Toxic to tissues
Hexachlorophane	Aqueous bisphenol	Skin preparation Hand-washing	Has action against Gram-negative organisms

Table 4.7 SSI rates relating to wound contamination

Type of surgery	Infection rate (%)	Rate before prophylaxis
Clean (no viscus opened)	1–2	The same
Clean-contaminated (viscus opened, minimal spillage)	< 10	Gastric surgery up to 30% Biliary surgery up to 20%
Contaminated (open viscus with spillage or inflammatory disease)	15–20	Variable but up to 60%
Dirty (pus or perforation, or incision through an abscess)	< 40	Up to 60% or more

operations. Infection rates after non-prosthetic clean surgery may be higher than expected when carefully audited by post-discharge surveillance. Breast surgery, for example, is associated with a high risk of infection, or wound complications, which may be interpreted as a failure to heal and related to a high body mass index (BMI). The value of antibiotic prophylaxis is controversial in non-prosthetic clean surgery, with most trials showing no clear benefit.

BACTERIA INVOLVED IN SURGICAL INFECTION

Streptococci

Streptococci form chains and are Gram positive on staining (Fig. 4.16). The most important is the β-haemolytic *Streptococcus*, which resides in the pharynx of 5–10% of the population. In the Lancefield A–G carbohydrate antigens classification, it is the group A *Streptococcus*, also called *Streptococcus pyogenes*, that is

the most pathogenic. It has the ability to spread, causing cellulitis, and to cause tissue destruction through the release of enzymes such as streptolysin, streptokinase and streptodornase.

Streptococcus faecalis is an enterococcus in Lancefield group D. It is often found in synergy with other organisms, as is the γ-haemolytic *Streptococcus* and *Peptostreptococcus*, which is an anaerobe.

The name Eusol is derived from *E*dinburgh *U*niversity *S*olution *O*f *L*ime.
Rebecca Graighill Lancefield, 1895–1981, an American Bacteriologist, classified streptococci in 1933.

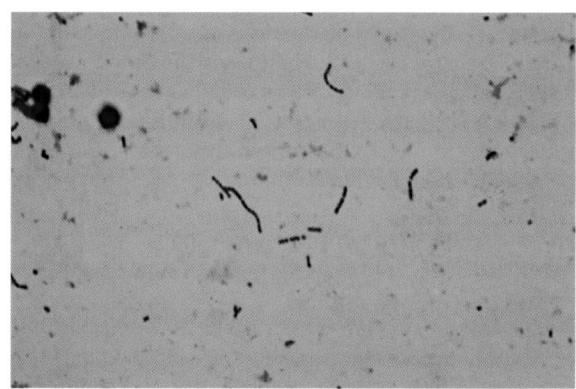

Figure 4.16 Streptococci.

Both *Streptococcus pyogenes* and *Streptococcus faecalis* may be involved in wound infection after large bowel surgery, but the α-haemolytic *Streptococcus viridans* is not associated with wound infections.

All the streptococci remain sensitive to penicillin and erythromycin. The cephalosporins are a suitable alternative in patients who are allergic to penicillin.

Staphylococci

Staphylococci form clumps and are Gram positive (Fig. 4.17). *Staphylococcus aureus* is the most important pathogen in this group and is found in the nasopharynx of up to 15% of the population. It can cause exogenous suppuration in wounds (and implanted prostheses). Strains resistant to antibiotics (e.g. MRSA) can cause epidemics and more severe infection. It is controversial but, if MRSA infection is found in a hospital, all doctors, nurses and patients may need to be swabbed so that carriers can be identified and treated. In parts of northern Europe, the prevalence of MRSA infections has been kept at very low levels using 'search and destroy' methods, which use these screening techniques and the isolation or treatment of carriers. Patients found to be positive on screening may be denied access to hospital. Some MRSA strains are now also resistant to vancomycin. Local policies on the management of MRSA depend on the prevalence of MRSA, the type of hospital or clinical specialty and the availability of facilities. Widespread swabbing, ward closures, isolation of patients and disinfection of wards all have to be carefully considered and involve all groups of practitioners. They may be expensive but necessary options.

Infections are usually suppurative and localised (see wound abscess, above). Most hospital *Staphylococcus aureus* strains are now β-lactamase producers and are resistant to penicillin, but most strains (MSSA) remain sensitive to flucloxacillin, vancomycin, aminoglycosides, some cephalosporins and fusidic acid (used in osteomyelitis). There are several novel and innovative antibiotics becoming available that have high activity against resistant strains. Some have the advantage of good oral activity (linezolid), some have a wide spectrum (tigecycline), have good activity in bacteraemia (daptomycin) but are relatively expensive, and some have side-effects involving marrow, hepatic and renal toxicity. Their use is justified but needs to be controlled by tight local policies and guidelines that involve clinical microbiologists.

Staphylococcus epidermidis (previously *Staphylococcus albus)*, also known as coagulase-negative staphylococci (CNS), was regarded as a commensal but is now recognised as a major threat in prosthetic (vascular and orthopaedic) surgery and in indwelling vascular catheters. They can be multiply resistant (MRCNS) to many antibiotics and represent an important cause of HAI.

Clostridia

Clostridial organisms are Gram-positive, obligate anaerobes, which produce resistant spores (Fig. 4.18). *Clostridium perfringens* is the cause of gas gangrene, and *C. tetani* causes tetanus after implantation into tissues or a wound (see specific wound infections, above).

Clostridium difficile is the cause of pseudomembranous colitis. This is another HAI, now more common than the incidence of MRSA bacteraemia, which is caused by the overuse of antibiotics. The cephalosporins and other anti-staphylococcal antibiotics seem to be the most implicated, but the inappropriate sequential use of several antibiotics puts patients most at risk. The key symptom of bloody diarrhoea can occur in small epidemics through poor hygiene. The elderly are particularly at risk and, in its most severe form, a severe colitis may lead to perforation and the need for emergency colectomy. There is a high mortality associated with this. Treatment involves resuscitation and antibiotic therapy with an imidazole or vancomycin. The fibrinous exudate is typical and differentiates the colitis from other inflammatory diseases; the recognition of the toxin is an early accurate diagnostic test.

Aerobic Gram-negative bacilli

These bacilli are normal inhabitants of the large bowel. *Escherichia coli* and *Klebsiella* spp. are lactose fermenting; *Proteus* is non-lactose fermenting. Most organisms in this group act in synergy with *Bacteroides* to cause SSIs after bowel operations (in particular, appendicitis, diverticulitis and peritonitis). *Escherichia coli* is a major cause of the HAI of urinary tract infection, although most aerobic Gram-negative bacilli (AGNB) may be involved, particularly in relation to urinary catheterisation. There is increasing concern about the development of ESBLs in many of this group of bacteria, which confer resistance to many antibiotics.

Pseudomonas spp. tend to colonise burns and tracheostomy wounds, as well as the urinary tract. Once *Pseudomonas* has colonised wards and intensive care units, it may be difficult to

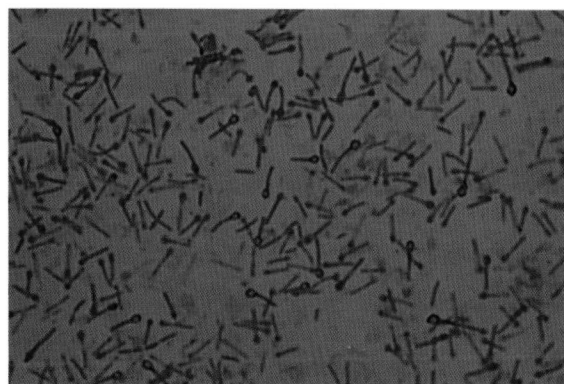

Figure 4.18 *Clostridium tetani* (drumstick spores).

Theodor Albrecht Edwin Klebs, 1834–1913, Professor of Bacteriology successively at Prague, Czechoslovakia; Zurich, Switzerland and The Rush Medical College, Chicago, IL, USA.

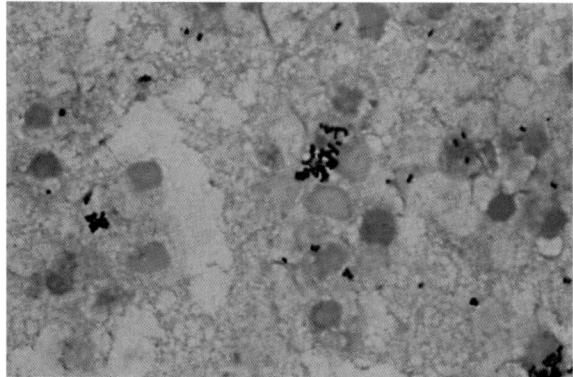

Figure 4.17 Staphylococcal pus.

CHAPTER 4 | SURGICAL INFECTION

eradicate. Surveillance of cross-infection is important in outbreaks. Hospital strains become resistant to β-lactamase as resistance can be transferred by plasmids. Wound infections need antibiotic therapy only when there is progressive or spreading infection with systemic signs. The aminoglycosides are effective, but some cephalosporins and penicillin may not be. Many of the carbapenems (e.g. meropenem) are useful in severe infections, whereas the quinolones have been made ineffective through their overuse and the development of ESBLs.

Bacteroides

Bacteroides are non-spore-bearing, strict anaerobes that colonise the large bowel, vagina and oropharynx. *Bacteroides fragilis* is the principal organism that acts in synergy with AGNB to cause SSIs, including intra-abdominal abscesses, after colorectal or gynaecological surgery. They are sensitive to the imidazoles (e.g. metronidazole) and some cephalosporins (e.g. cefotaxime).

PRINCIPLES OF ANTI-MICROBIAL TREATMENT

Anti-microbials may be used to prevent (see Prophylaxis, above) or treat established surgical infection (Summary box 4.16).

Summary box 4.16

Principles for the use of antibiotic therapy

- Antibiotics do not replace surgical drainage of infection
- Only spreading infection or signs of systemic infection justifies the use of antibiotics
- Whenever possible, the organism and sensitivity should be determined

---

The use of antibiotics for the treatment of established surgical infection ideally requires recognition and determination of the sensitivities of the causative organisms. Antibiotic therapy should not be held back if they are indicated, the choice being empirical and later modified depending on microbiological findings. However, once antibiotics have been administered, the clinical picture may become confused and, if a patient's condition does not rapidly improve, the opportunity to make a precise diagnosis may have been lost. It is unusual to have to treat SSIs with antibiotics, unless there is evidence of spreading infection, bacteraemia or systemic complications (SIRS and MODS). The appropriate treatment of localised SSIs is interventional radiological drainage of pus or open drainage and debridement.

There are two approaches to antibiotic treatment:

- A *narrow-spectrum antibiotic* may be used to treat a known sensitive infection; for example, MRSA (which may be isolated from pus) is usually sensitive to vancomycin or teicoplanin, but not flucloxacillin.
- *Combinations of broad-spectrum antibiotics* can be used when the organism is not known or when it is suspected that several bacteria, acting in synergy, may be responsible for the infection. For example, during and following emergency surgery requiring the opening of perforated or ischaemic bowel, any of the gut organisms may be responsible for subsequent peritoneal or bacteraemic infection. In this case, a triple-therapy combination of broad-spectrum penicillin, such as ampicillin

or mezlocillin, with an aminoglycoside, such as gentamicin, and metronidazole, may be used per- and postoperatively to support the patient's own body defences.

An alternative to the penicillins is a cephalosporin, e.g. cefuroxime. This has been a popular alternative as gentamicin toxicity and monitoring of levels are avoided, but the aminoglycosides remain inexpensive and effective. Other alternatives are piperocillin–tazobactam or monotherapy using a carbapenem.

In surgical units in which resistant *Pseudomonas* or other Gram-negative species (such as *Klebsiella*) have become 'resident opportunists', it may be necessary to rotate anti-pseudomonal and anti-Gram-negative antibiotic therapy (Summary box 4.17).

Summary box 4.17

Treatment of commensals that have become opportunist pathogens

- They are likely to have multiple antibiotic resistance
- It may be necessary to rotate antibiotics

The use of these routines, subsequent wound infection and the alternation of combinations of chemotherapy should be monitored by the infection control team and local hospital protocols. In treating patients who have surgical infection with systemic signs (SIRS and MODS), a failure to respond to antibiotics may indicate that there has been a failure of infection source control. If response is poor after 3–4 days, there should be a re-evaluation with a review of charts and further investigations requested to exclude the development or persistence of infection such as a collection of pus.

New antibiotics should be used with caution and, wherever possible, sensitivities should first be obtained. There are certain general rules on which the choice of antibiotics may be based. For example, it is unusual for *Pseudomonas aeruginosa* to be found as a primary infecting organism unless the patient has had surgical or hospital treatment. Local antibiotic sensitivity patterns vary from centre to centre and from country to country, and the sensitivity patterns of common pathogens should be known to the hospital microbiologist who should be involved.

ANTIBIOTICS USED IN TREATMENT AND PROPHYLAXIS OF SURGICAL INFECTION

Anti-microbials may be produced by living organisms (antibiotics) or by synthetic methods. Some are bactericidal, e.g. penicillins and aminoglycosides, and others are bacteriostatic, e.g. tetracycline and erythromycin. In general, penicillins act upon the bacterial cell wall and are most effective against bacteria that are multiplying and synthesising new cell wall materials. The aminoglycosides act at the ribosomal level, preventing or distorting the production of proteins required to maintain the integrity of the enzymes in the bacterial cell. Hospital and Formulary guidelines should be consulted for doses and monitoring of antibiotic therapy.

Penicillin

Benzylpenicillin has proved most effective against Gram-positive pathogens, including most streptococci, the clostridia and some of the staphylococci that do not produce β-lactamase. It is still effective against *Actinomyces*, which is a rare cause of chronic wound infection, and may be used specifically to treat spreading streptococcal infections. Penicillin is valuable even if other antibiotics are required as part of multiple therapy for a mixed infection. All serious infections, e.g. gas gangrene, require high-dose intravenous benzylpenicillin.

Flucloxacillin

This is a β-lactamase-resistant penicillin and is therefore of use in treating most community-acquired staphylococcal infections, but it has poor activity against other pathogens.

Ampicillin and amoxicillin

These β-lactam penicillins can be taken orally or may be given parenterally. Both are effective against Enterobacteriaceae, *Enterococcus faecalis* and the majority of group D streptococci, but not species of *Klebsiella* or pseudomonads. Their use is now rare as there are more effective alternatives.

Mezlocillin and azlocillin

These are ureidopenicillins with good activity against species of *Enterobacter* and *Klebsiella*. Azlocillin is effective against *Pseudomonas*. Each has some activity against *Bacteroides* and enterococci, but all are susceptible to β-lactamases. Combined with an aminoglycoside, mezlocillin is a valuable treatment for severe mixed infections, particularly those caused by Gram-negative organisms in immunocompromised patients. *There are more appropriate alternatives.*

Clavulanic acid is available combined with amoxicillin (Augmentin) and can be taken orally. This anti-β-lactamase protects amoxicillin from inactivation by β-lactamase-producing bacteria. It is of value in treating infections caused by *Klebsiella* strains and β-lactamase-producing *E. coli* but is not active against *Pseudomonas* spp. It can be used for localised cellulitis or superficial staphylococcal infections and infected human and animal bites. It is available for oral or intravenous therapy.

Cephalosporins

There are several β-lactamase-susceptible cephalosporins that are of value in surgical practice: cefuroxime, cefotaxime and ceftazidime are widely used. The first two are most effective in intra-abdominal skin and soft-tissue infections, being active against *Staphylococcus aureus* and most Enterobacteriaceae. As a group, the enterococci (*Streptococcus faecalis*) are not sensitive to the cephalosporins. Ceftazidime, although active against the Gram-negative organisms and *Staphylococcus aureus*, is also effective against *Pseudomonas aeruginosa*. These cephalosporins may be combined with an aminoglycoside, such as gentamicin, and an imidazole, such as metronidazole, if anaerobic cover is needed. Newer cephalosporins may be effective against organisms such as MRSA, but their spectra are usually limited.

Aminoglycosides

Gentamicin and tobramycin have similar activity and are effective against Gram-negative Enterobacteriaceae. Gentamicin is effective against many strains of *Pseudomonas*, although resistance has been recognised. All aminoglycosides are inactive against anaerobes and streptococci. Serum levels immediately before and 1 hour after intramuscular injection must be taken 48 hours after the start of therapy, and dosage should be modified to satisfy peak and trough levels. Ototoxicity and nephrotoxicity may follow sustained high toxic levels. These antibiotics have a marked post-antibiotic effect, and single, large doses are effective and may be

safer. Use needs to be discussed with the microbiologist, and local policies should be observed.

Vancomycin

This glycopeptide is most active against Gram-positive bacteria and has proved to be effective against MRSA, although vancomycin resistance (VRSA) is increasingly being reported. However, it is ototoxic and nephrotoxic, so serum levels should be monitored. It is effective against *C. difficile* in cases of pseudomembranous colitis.

Imidazoles

Metronidazole is the most widely used member of the imidazole group and is active against all anaerobic bacteria. It is particularly safe and may be administered orally, rectally or intravenously. Infections caused by anaerobic cocci and strains of *Bacteroides* and clostridia can be treated, or prevented, by its use. Metronidazole is useful for the prophylaxis and treatment of anaerobic infections after abdominal, colorectal and pelvic surgery.

Carbapenems

Meropenem, ertapenem and imipenem are members of the carbapenems. They are stable to β-lactamase, have useful broad-spectrum anaerobic as well as Gram-positive activity and are effective for the treatment of resistant organisms, such as ESBL-resistant urinary tract infections or serious mixed-spectrum abdominal infections (peritonitis).

Quinolones

Quinolones, such as ciprofloxacin, were active against a wide spectrum of organisms. Their widespread use has been related to the development of resistant organisms, and their role in treating surgical infection is limited.

HIV, AIDS AND THE SURGEON

The type I human immunodeficiency virus (HIV) is one of the viruses of surgical importance as it can be transmitted by body fluids, particularly blood. It is a retrovirus that has become increasingly prevalent through sexual transmission, both homo- and heterosexual, in intravenous drug addiction, through infected blood in treating haemophiliacs, in particular, and in sub-Saharan Africans. The risk in surgery is probably mostly through 'needlestick' injury during operations.

After exposure, the virus binds to CD4 receptors with a subsequent loss of CD4+ cells, T helper cells and other cells involved in cell-mediated immunity, antibody production and delayed hypersensitivity. Macrophages and gut-associated lymphoid tissue (GALT) are also affected. The risk of opportunistic infections (such as *Pneumocystis carinii* pneumonia, tuberculosis and cytomegalo virus) and neoplasms (such as Kaposi's sarcoma and lymphoma) is thereby increased.

In the early weeks after HIV infection, there may be a flu-like illness and, during the phase of seroconversion, patients present

---

Sub-Saharan Africans **come from that part of the African Continent which lies south of the Sahara Desert.**
Moritz Kaposi, **1837–1902, Professor of Dermatology, Vienna, Austria, described pigmented sarcoma of the skin in 1872.**

the greatest risk of HIV transmission. It is during these early phases that drug treatment, highly active anti-retroviral therapy (HAART), is most effective through the ability of these drugs to inhibit reverse transcriptase and protease synthesis, which are the principal mechanisms through which HIV can progress. Within 2 years, untreated HIV can progress to AIDS in 25–35% of patients, which is considered to be fatal.

Involvement of surgeons with HIV patients (universal precautions)

Patients may present to surgeons for operative treatment if they have a surgical disease and they are known to be infected or 'at risk', or because they need surgical intervention related to their illness for vascular access or a biopsy when they are known to have HIV infection or AIDS. Universal precautions have been drawn up by the CDC in the United States and largely adopted by the NHS in the UK (in summary):

- when there is a risk of splashing, particularly with power tools;
- use of a full face mask ideally, or protective spectacles;
- use of fully waterproof, disposable gowns and drapes, particularly during seroconversion;
- boots to be worn, not clogs, to avoid injury from dropped sharps;
- double gloving needed (a larger size on the inside is more comfortable);
- allow only essential personnel in theatre;
- avoid unnecessary movement in theatre;
- respect is required for sharps, with passage in a kidney dish;
- a slow meticulous operative technique is needed with minimised bleeding.

After contamination

Needle-stick injuries are commonest on the non-dominant index finger during operative surgery. Hollow needle injury carries the greatest risk of HIV transmission. The injured part should be washed under running water and the incident reported. Local policies dictate whether post-exposure HAART should be given. Occupational advice is required after high-risk exposure together with the need for HIV testing and the option for continuation in an operative specialty.

FURTHER READING

Cohen, I.K., Diegelmann, R.F. and Lindblad, W.J. (1992) *Wound Healing. Biochemical and Chemical Aspects*. W.B. Saunders, Philadelphia, PA.

Davis, J.M. and Shires, G.T. (1991) *Principles and Management of Surgical Infections*. J.B. Lippincott, Philadelphia, PA.

EWMA (2006) *Management of Wound Infection*. EWMA Position Document. Medical Education Partnership, London.

Grey, J.E. and Harding, K.G. (2006) *ABC of Wound Healing*. BMJ Books. Blackwell, Oxford.

Howard, R.J. and Simmons, R.L. (1988) *Surgical Infectious Diseases*, 2nd edn. Appleton and Lange, Norwalk, CT.

Leaper, D.J. and Harding, K.G. (1998) *Wounds: Biology and Management*. Oxford Medical, Oxford.

Leaper D.J., Harding, K.G. and Phillips, C.J. (2002) Management of wounds. In: Johnson. C. and Taylor, I. (eds) *Recent Advances in Surgery*, 25th edn. RSM Press, London, 13–24.

Majno, G. (1977) *The Healing Hand. Man and Wound in the Ancient World*. Harvard University Press, Cambridge, MA.

Schein, M. and Marshall, J.C. (2002) *Source Control*. Springer-Verlag, Berlin.

Taylor, E.W. (1992) *Infection in Surgical Practice*. Oxford Medical, Oxford.

Teot, L., Banwell, P.E. and Ziegler, U.E. (2004) *Surgery in Wounds*. Springer-Verlag, Berlin.

Williams, J.D. and Taylor, E.W. (2003) *Infection in Surgical Practice*. Arnold, London.

Surgery in the tropics

LEARNING OBJECTIVES

To be aware of:
- The common surgical conditions that occur in the tropics

To appreciate:
- That many patients do not seek medical help until late in the disease course

To know:
- The emergency presentations of the various conditions as patients in developing countries do not seek treatment until they are very ill

To be able to:
- Diagnose and treat these conditions, particularly as emergencies, in western hospitals because of the ease of global travel

To realise:
- That ideal management needs good teamwork between the surgeon, physician, radiologist, pathologist and microbiologist

INTRODUCTION

Most surgical conditions in the tropics are associated with parasitic infestations. With the ease of international travel, diseases that are common in the tropics and developing countries may be seen in the UK, especially presenting as emergencies.

This section deals with the conditions that a surgeon might occasionally encounter in a visitor to these shores. Details of the life cycles of the parasites will not be dealt with. Readers are, however, advised to refer to the 24th edition of this book should they wish details of the parasitology. The principles of surgical treatment are dealt with in the appropriate sections although, for operative details, the reader should refer to a relevant textbook.

AMOEBIASIS

Introduction

Amoebiasis is caused by *Entamoeba histolytica*. The disease is common in the Indian subcontinent, Africa and parts of Central and South America where almost half the population is infected. The majority remain asymptomatic carriers. The mode of infection is via the faeco-oral route, and the disease occurs as a result of substandard hygiene and sanitation. Amoebic liver abscess, the commonest extraintestinal manifestation, occurs in less than 10% of the infected population and, in endemic areas, is much more common than pyogenic abscess. Patients who are immunocompromised or alcoholic are more susceptible to infection.

Pathogenesis

The organism enters the gut through food or water contaminated with the cyst. In the small bowel, the cysts hatch, and a large number of trophozoites are released and carried to the colon where flask-shaped ulcers form in the submucosa. The trophozoites multiply, ultimately forming cysts, which enter the portal circulation or are passed in the faeces as an infective form that infects other humans as a result of insanitary conditions.

Having entered the portal circulation, the trophozoites are filtered and trapped in the interlobular veins of the liver. They multiply in the portal triads causing focal infarction of hepatocytes and liquefactive necrosis as a result of proteolytic enzymes produced by the trophozoites. The areas of necrosis eventually coalesce to form the abscess cavity. The term 'amoebic hepatitis' is used to describe the microscopic picture in the absence of macroscopic abscess. This is a differentiation in theory only as the medical treatment is the same.

The right lobe is involved in 80% of cases, the left in 10% and the rest are multiple. The right lobe of the liver is involved more often possibly because blood from the superior mesenteric vein runs on a straighter course through the portal vein into the larger lobe. The abscesses are most common high in the diaphragmatic surface of the right lobe. This may cause pulmonary symptoms and chest complications. The abscess cavity contains chocolate-coloured, odourless, 'anchovy sauce'-like fluid that is a mixture of necrotic liver tissue and blood. There may be secondary infection of the abscess. This causes the pus to be smelly. While pus in the abscess is sterile unless secondarily infected, trophozoites may be found in the abscess wall in a minority of cases. Untreated abscesses are likely to rupture.

Chronic infection of the large bowel may result in a granulomatous lesion along the large bowel, most commonly seen in the caecum, called an amoeboma (Summary box 5.1).

Summary box 5.1

Amoebiasis – pathology

- *Entamoeba histolytica* is the most common pathogenic amoeba in man
- The vast majority of carriers are asymptomatic
- Insanitary conditions and poor personal hygiene encourage transmission of the infection
- In the small intestine, the parasite hatches into trophozoites, which invade the submucosa producing ulcers
- In the portal circulation, the parasite causes liquefactive necrosis in the liver producing an abscess. This is the commonest extraintestinal manifestation
- The majority of abscesses occur in the right lobe
- A mass in the course of the large bowel may indicate an amoeboma

Clinical features

The typical patient with amoebic liver abscess is a young adult male with a history of pain and fever and insidious onset of non-specific symptoms such as anorexia, fever, night sweats, malaise, cough and weight loss, which gradually progress to more specific symptoms of pain in the right upper abdomen, shoulder tip pain, hiccoughs and a non-productive cough. A past history of bloody diarrhoea or travel to an endemic area raises the index of suspicion.

Examination reveals a patient who is toxic and anaemic. The patient will have upper abdominal rigidity, tender hepatomegaly, tender and bulging intercostal spaces, overlying skin oedema, a pleural effusion and basal pneumonitis – the last symptom is usually a late manifestation. Occasionally, a tinge of jaundice or ascites may be present. Rarely, the patient may present as an emergency due to the effects of rupture into the peritoneal, pleural or pericardial cavity.

Amoeboma

This is a chronic granuloma arising in the large bowel, most commonly seen in the caecum. It is prone to occur in longstanding amoebic infection that has been treated intermittently with drugs without completion of a full course, a situation that arises from indiscriminate self-medication, particularly in developing countries.

This can easily be mistaken for a carcinoma. An amoeboma should be suspected when a patient from an endemic area with generalised ill health and pyrexia has a mass in the right iliac fossa with a history of blood-stained mucoid diarrhoea. Such a patient is highly unlikely to have a carcinoma as altered bowel habit is not a feature of right-sided colonic carcinoma.

Investigations

The haematological and biochemical investigations reflect the presence of a chronic infective process: anaemia, leucocytosis, elevated erythrocyte sedimentation rate (ESR) and C-reactive protein (CRP), hypoalbuminaemia and deranged liver function tests, particularly elevated alkaline phosphatase.

Serological tests are more specific, with the majority of patients showing antibodies in serum. These can be detected by tests for complement fixation, indirect haemagglutination (IHA), indirect immunofluorescence and enzyme-linked immunosorbent assay (ELISA). They are extremely useful in detecting acute infection in non-endemic areas. IHA has a very high sensitivity rate in acute amoebic liver abscess in non-endemic regions and remains elevated for some time. The persistence of antibodies in a large majority of the population in endemic areas precludes its use there as a diagnostic investigation. In these cases, tests such as counter-immunoelectrophoresis are more useful for detecting acute infection.

An out-patient rigid sigmoidoscopy (using a disposable instrument) can be very useful particularly if the patient complains of bloody mucoid diarrhoea. Most amoebic ulcers occur in the rectosigmoid and are therefore within reach of the sigmoidoscope; shallow skip lesions and 'flask-shaped' or 'collar-stud' undermined ulcers may be seen, and can be biopsied or scrapings can be taken along with mucus for immediate microscopic examination. The presence of trophozoites distinguishes the condition from ulcerative colitis.

Imaging techniques

On ultrasound, an abscess cavity in the liver is seen as a hypoechoic or anechoic lesion with ill-defined borders; internal echoes suggest necrotic material or debris (Fig. 5.1). The investigation is very accurate and is used for aspiration, both diagnostic and therapeutic. Where there is doubt about the diagnosis, a computerised tomography (CT) scan may be helpful (Fig. 5.2).

Diagnostic aspiration is of limited value except for establishing the typical colour of the aspirate, which is sterile and odourless unless it is secondarily infected.

A CT scan may show a raised right diaphragm, a pleural effusion and evidence of pneumonitis (Fig. 5.3a and b).

An 'apple-core' deformity on barium enema would arouse suspicion of a carcinoma. A colonoscopy and biopsy are mandatory as the macroscopic appearance may be indistinguishable from carcinoma. In doubtful cases, vigorous medical treatment is given, and the patient's colon is imaged again in 3–4 weeks, as these masses are known to regress completely on a full course of drug therapy. However, it must be borne in mind that an amoeboma and carcinoma can coexist (Summary box 5.2).

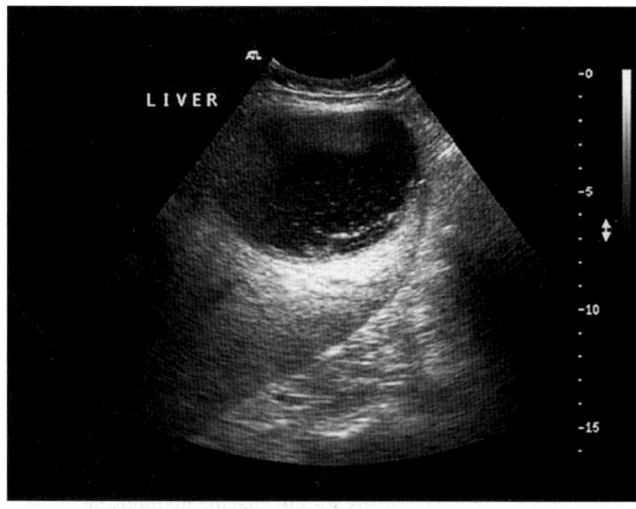

Figure 5.1 Ultrasound of the liver showing a large amoebic liver abscess with necrotic tissue in the right lobe.

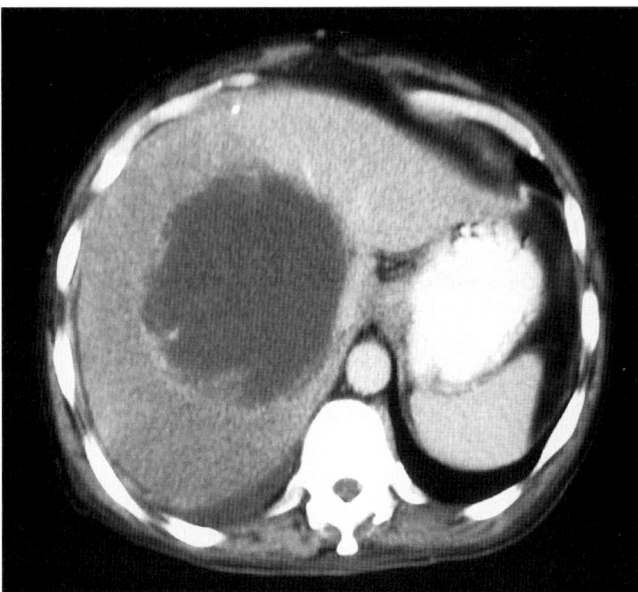

Figure 5.2 Computerised tomographic (CT) scan showing an amoebic liver abscess in the right lobe.

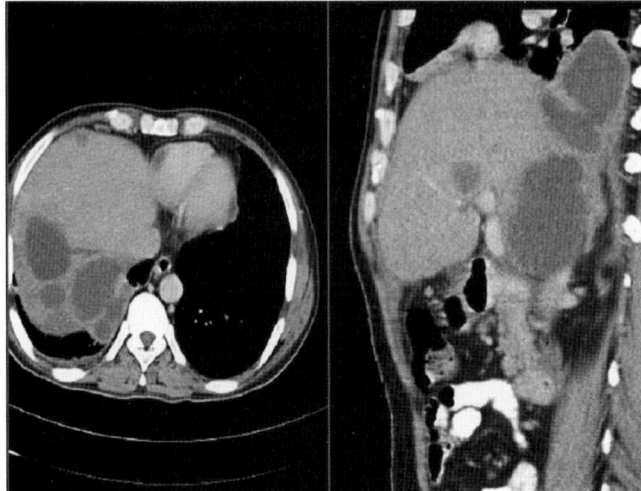

Figure 5.3 Computerised tomographic (CT) scans showing multiple amoebic liver abscesses with extension into the chest.

Summary box 5.2

Diagnostic pointers for infection with *Entamoeba histolytica*

- Bloody mucoid diarrhoea in a patient from an endemic area or following a recent visit to such a country
- Upper abdominal pain, fever, cough, malaise
- In chronic cases, a mass in the right iliac fossa = amoeboma
- Sigmoidoscopy shows typical ulcers – biopsy and scrapings may be diagnostic
- Serological tests are highly sensitive and specific outside endemic areas
- Ultrasound and CT scans are the imaging methods of choice

Treatment

Medical treatment is very effective and should be the first choice in the elective situation, with surgery being reserved for complications. Metronidazole and tinidazole are the effective drugs. After treatment with metronidazole and tinidazole, diloxanide furoate, which is not effective against hepatic infestation, is used for 10 days to destroy any intestinal amoebae.

Aspiration is carried out when imminent rupture of an abscess is expected. Aspiration also helps in the penetration of metronidazole, and so reduces the morbidity when carried out with drug treatment in a patient with a large abscess. If there is evidence of secondary infection, appropriate drug treatment is added. The threshold for aspirating an abscess in the left lobe is lower because of its predilection for rupturing into the pericardium.

Surgical treatment should be reserved for the complications of rupture into the pleural (usually the right side), peritoneal or pericardial cavities. Resuscitation, drainage and appropriate lavage with vigorous medical treatment are the key principles. In the large bowel, severe haemorrhage and toxic megacolon are rare complications. In these patients, the general principles of a surgical emergency apply. Resuscitation is followed by resection of bowel with exteriorisation. Then the patient is given vigorous supportive therapy. All such cases are managed in the intensive care unit.

An amoeboma that has not regressed after full medical treatment should be managed with a colonic resection, particularly if cancer cannot be excluded (Summary box 5.3).

Summary box 5.3

Amoebiasis – treatment

- Medical treatment is very effective
- In large abscesses, repeated aspiration is combined with drug treatment
- Surgical treatment is reserved for complications such as rupture into the pleural, peritoneal or pericardial cavities
- Acute toxic megacolon and severe haemorrhage are intestinal complications that are treated with intensive supportive therapy followed by resection and exteriorisation
- When an amoeboma is suspected in a colonic mass, cancer should be excluded by appropriate imaging

Further reading

Barnes, S.A. and Lillemore, K.D. (1997) Liver abscess and hydatid disease. In: Zinner, N.J., Schwartz, I. and Ellis, H. (eds). *Maingot's Abdominal Operations*, 10th edn, Vol. 2. Appleton and Lange, McGraw-Hill, 1527–45.

ASCARIS LUMBRICOIDES (ROUNDWORM)

Introduction

Ascaris lumbricoides, commonly called the roundworm, is the commonest intestinal nematode to infect the human and affects a quarter of the world's population. The parasite causes pulmonary symptoms as a larva and intestinal symptoms as an adult worm.

CHAPTER 5 | SURGERY IN THE TROPICS

Pathology and life cycle

The eggs can survive in a hostile environment for a long time. The hot and humid conditions in the tropics are ideally suited for the eggs to turn into embryos. The fertilised eggs are present in soil contaminated with infected faeces. Faeco-oral contamination causes human infection.

As the eggs are ingested, the released larvae travel to the liver via the portal system and then through the systemic circulation to reach the lung. The process of maturation takes up to 8 weeks. The developed larvae reach the alveoli, are coughed up, swallowed and continue their maturation in the small intestine. Sometimes, the young worm migrates from the tracheobronchial tree into the oesophagus, thus finding its way into the gastrointestinal tract, from where it can migrate to the common bile duct or pancreatic duct. The mature female, once in the small bowel, produces innumerable eggs that are fertilised and thereafter excreted in the stool to perpetuate the life cycle. Eggs in the biliary tract can form a nidus for a stone.

Clinical features

The larval stage in the lungs causes pulmonary symptoms – dry cough, chest pain, dyspnoea and fever – referred to as Loeffler's syndrome. The adult worm can grow up to 45 cm long. Its presence in the small intestine causes malnutrition, failure to thrive and abdominal pain. Worms that migrate into the common bile duct can produce ascending cholangitis and obstructive jaundice, while features of acute pancreatitis may be caused by a worm in the pancreatic duct.

Small intestinal obstruction can occur, particularly in children, due to a bolus of adult worms incarcerated in the terminal ileum. This is a surgical emergency. Rarely, perforation of the small bowel may occur from ischaemic pressure necrosis from the bolus of worms.

A high index of suspicion is necessary if one is not to miss the diagnosis. If a person from a tropical developing country, or one who has recently returned from an endemic area, presents with pulmonary, gastrointestinal, hepatobiliary and pancreatic symptoms, ascariasis infestation should be high on the list of possible diagnoses.

Investigations

Increase in the eosinophil count is common, in keeping with most other parasitic infestations. Stool examination may show ova. Sputum or bronchoscopic washings may show Charcot–Leyden crystals or the larvae.

Chest X-ray may show fluffy exudates in Loeffler's syndrome. A barium meal and follow-through may show a bolus of worms in the ileum (Fig. 5.4) or lying freely within the small bowel (Fig. 5.5). An ultrasound may show a worm in the common bile duct (Fig. 5.6) or pancreatic duct (Fig. 5.7). On magnetic resonance cholangiopancreatography (MRCP), an adult worm may be seen in the common bile duct in a patient presenting with features of obstructive jaundice (Fig. 5.8) (Summary box 5.4).

Summary box 5.4

Ascariasis – pathogenesis

- It is the commonest intestinal nematode affecting man
- Typically found in a humid atmosphere and poor sanitary conditions; hence is seen in the tropics and developing countries
- Larvae cause pulmonary symptoms; adult worms cause gastrointestinal, biliary and pancreatic symptoms
- Distal ileal obstruction due to bolus of worms; ascending cholangitis and obstructive jaundice from infestation of the common bile duct
- Acute pancreatitis when a worm is lodged in the pancreatic duct
- Perforation of the small bowel is rare

Treatment

The pulmonary phase of the disease is usually self-limiting and requires symptomatic treatment only. For intestinal disease, patients should ideally be under the care of a physician for treatment with anthelmintic drugs. Certain drugs may cause rapid death of the adult worms and, if there are many worms in the terminal ileum, the treatment may actually precipitate acute intestinal obstruction from a bolus of dead worms. Children who present with features of intermittent or subacute obstruction should be given a trial of conservative management in the form of intravenous fluids, nasogastric suction and hypertonic saline enemas. The last of these helps to disentangle the bolus of worms and also increases intestinal motility.

Surgery is reserved for complications such as intestinal obstruction that has not resolved on a conservative regimen, and when perforation is suspected. At laparotomy, the bolus of worms in the terminal ileum is milked through the ileocaecal valve into the colon for natural passage in the stool. Postoperatively,

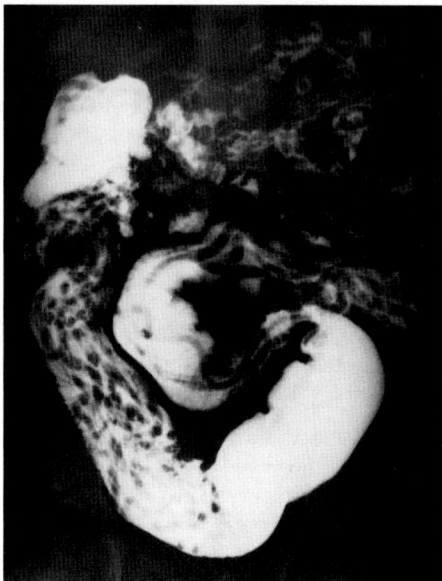

Figure 5.4 Barium meal and follow-through showing a bolus of roundworms in the ileum and multiple longitudinal filling defects in the small bowel from other worms. The patient presented with recurrent episodes of subacute intestinal obstruction (courtesy of Dr S.K. Agarwal, FRCR, New Delhi, India).

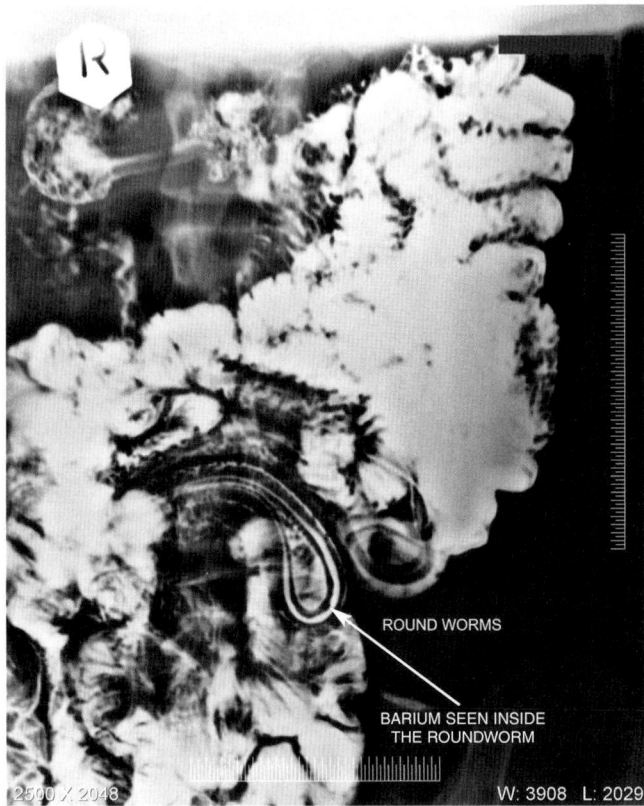

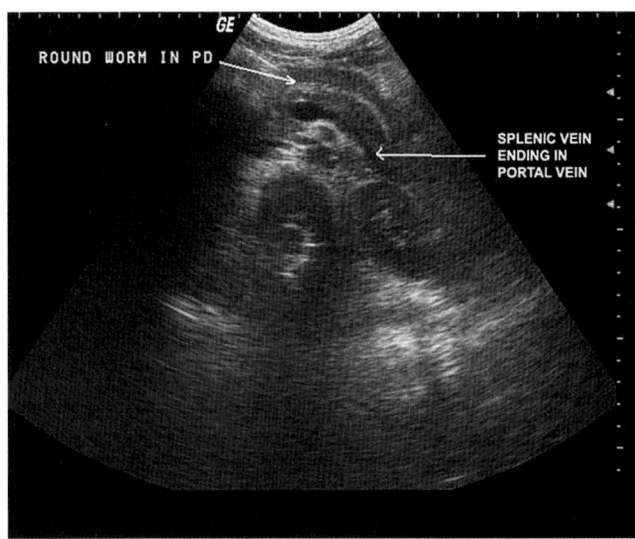

Figure 5.7 Ultrasound scan showing a roundworm in the pancreatic duct (PD). The patient presented with acute pancreatitis. The worm was seen to be moving in real time and was removed endoscopically (courtesy of Dr P. Bhattacharaya, Kolkata, India).

Figure 5.5 Barium meal and follow-through showing roundworms in the course of the small bowel with barium seen inside the worms in an 18-year-old patient who presented with bouts of colicky abdominal pain and bilious vomiting, which settled with conservative management (courtesy of Dr P. Bhattacharaya, Kolkata, India).

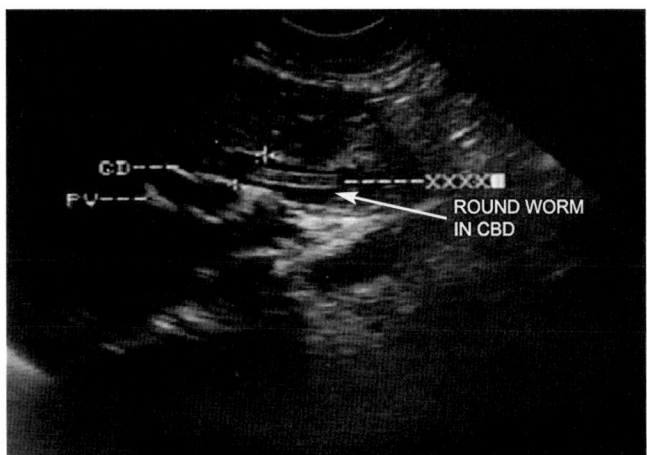

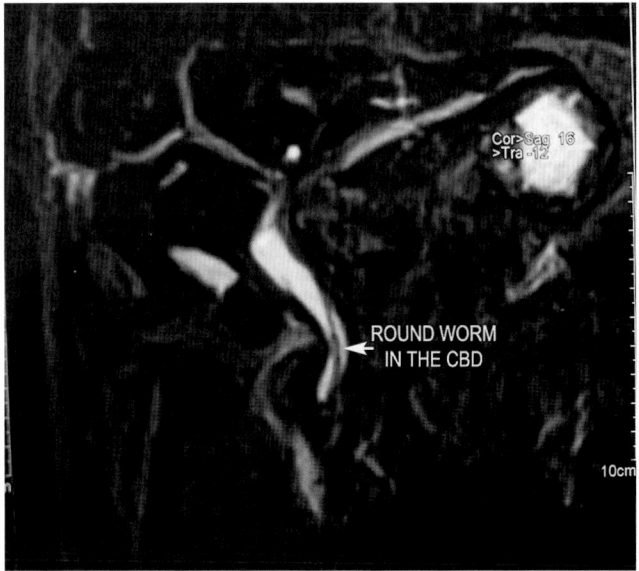

Figure 5.8 Magnetic resonance cholangiopancreatography (MRCP) showing a roundworm in the common bile duct (CBD). The worm could not be removed endoscopically. The patient underwent an open cholecystectomy and exploration of the CBD.

Figure 5.6 Ultrasound scan showing a roundworm in the common bile duct (CBD). The patient presented with obstructive jaundice and had asymptomatic gallstones. On endoscopic retrograde cholangiopancreatography (ERCP), part of the worm was seen outside the ampulla in the duodenum and was removed through the endoscope. Subsequent laparoscopic cholecystectomy was uneventful.

hypertonic saline enemas may help in the extrusion of the worms. Strictures, gangrenous areas or perforations need resection and anastomosis. If the bowel wall is healthy, enterotomy and removal of the worms may be performed (Fig. 5.9).

As a result of perforation due to roundworm, the parasites may be found lying free in the peritoneal cavity. The site of perforation may be brought out as an ileostomy because, in the presence of a large number of worms, closure or an anastomosis may be at risk of breakdown from the activity of the worms. Exteriorisation, although the ideal operation in severe sepsis, is unfortunately sometimes not done because of the reluctance on the part of the patient to accept such a procedure as good stoma care is not always available. In such circumstances, resection of the diseased ileum, closure of the distal bowel and end-to-side ileotransverse anastomosis is a good alternative.

When a patient is operated upon as an emergency for a

CHAPTER 5 | SURGERY IN THE TROPICS

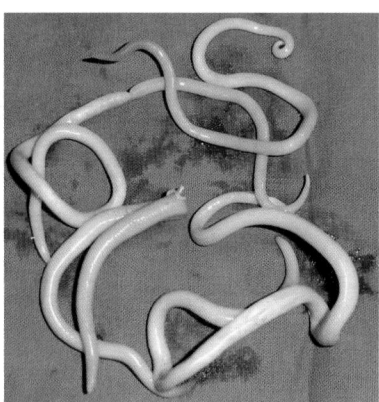

Figure 5.9 Roundworms removed at laparotomy in a 16-year-old patient who presented with acute intestinal obstruction (courtesy of the Pathology Museum, Calcutta Medical Research Institute, Kolkata, India).

suspected complication of roundworm infestation, the actual diagnosis at operation may turn out to be acute appendicitis, typhoid perforation or tuberculous stricture, and the presence of roundworms is an incidental finding. Such a patient requires the appropriate surgery depending upon the pathology.

Common bile duct or pancreatic duct obstruction from a roundworm can be treated by endoscopic removal, failing which open exploration of the common bile duct is necessary. Cholecystectomy is also carried out. A full course of anti-parasitic treatment must follow any surgical intervention (Summary box 5.5).

Summary box 5.5

Ascariasis – diagnosis and management

- Barium meal and follow-through will show worms scattered in the small bowel
- Ultrasound may show worms in the common bile duct and pancreatic duct
- Conservative management with anthelmintics is the first line of treatment even in obstruction
- Surgery is a last resort – various options are available

Further reading

Steinberg, R., Davies, J., Millar, A.J., Brown, R. and Rode, H. (2003) Unusual intestinal sequelae after operations for *Ascaris lumbricoides* infestation. *Paediatr Surg Int* **19(1–2)**: 85–7.

Wani, R.A., Parray, F.Q., Bhat, N.A., Wani, M.A., Bhat, T.H. and Farzana, F. (2006) Non-traumatic terminal ileal perforation. *World J Emerg Surg* **10**: 1–7.

ASIATIC CHOLANGIOHEPATITIS

Introduction

This disease, also called oriental cholangiohepatitis, is caused by infestation of the hepatobiliary system by *Clonorchis sinensis*. It has a high incidence in the tropical regions of South-east Asia, particularly among those living in the major sea ports and river estuaries. The organism, which is a type of liver fluke, resides in snails and fish that act as intermediate hosts. Ingestion of infected fish and snails when eaten raw or partly cooked causes the infection in humans and other fish-eating mammals, which are the definitive hosts.

Pathology

In humans, the parasite matures into the adult worm in the intrahepatic biliary radicles where they may reside for many years. The intrahepatic bile ducts are dilated with epithelial hyperplasia and periductal fibrosis. These changes may lead to dysplasia causing cholangiocarcinoma – the most serious complication of this parasitic infestation.

The eggs or dead worms may form a nidus for stone formation in the gall bladder or common bile duct, which becomes thickened and much dilated in the late stages. Intrahepatic bile duct stones are also caused by the parasite producing mucin-rich bile. The dilated intrahepatic bile ducts may lead to cholangitis, liver abscess and hepatitis.

Diagnosis

The disease may remain dormant for many years. Clinical features are non-specific, for example fever, malaise, anorexia and upper abdominal discomfort. The complete clinical picture can consist of fever with rigors due to ascending cholangitis, obstructive jaundice due to stones, biliary colic and pruritis. Acute pancreatitis may occur because of obstruction of the pancreatic duct by an adult worm. If any person or an emigrant to the west from an endemic area complains of symptoms of biliary tract disease, *Clonorchis* infestation should be considered in the differential diagnosis.

In advanced cases, liver function tests are abnormal. Confirmation of the condition is by examination of stool or duodenal aspirate, which may show the eggs or adult worms. Ultrasound scan findings can be characteristic showing the uniform dilatation of small peripheral intrahepatic bile ducts with only minimal dilatation of the common hepatic and common bile ducts, although the latter are dilated when the obstruction is caused by stones. The thickened duct walls show increased echogenicity and non-shadowing echogenic foci in the bile ducts representing the worms or eggs. Endoscopic retrograde cholangiopancreatography (ERCP) will confirm these findings (Summary box 5.6).

Summary box 5.6

Asiatic cholangiohepatitis – pathogenesis and diagnosis

- Occurs in the Far Eastern tropical zones
- Causative parasite is *Clonorchis sinensis*
- Produces bile duct hyperplasia, intrahepatic duct dilatation and stones
- Increases the risk of cholangiocarcinoma
- May remain dormant for many years
- When active, there are biliary tract symptoms in a generally unwell patient
- Stool examination for eggs or worms is diagnostic
- Ultrasound scan of hepatobiliary system and ERCP are also diagnostic

---

Treatment

Praziquantel and albendazole are the drugs of choice. However, the surgeon faces a challenge when there are stones not only in the gall bladder but also in the common bile duct. Cholecystectomy with exploration of the common bile duct is performed when indicated. Repeated washouts are necessary during the exploration, as the common bile duct is dilated and contains stones, biliary debris, sludge and mud. This should be followed by choledochoduodenostomy. As this is a disease with a prolonged and relapsing course, some surgeons prefer to do a choledochojejunostomy to a Roux loop. The Roux loop is brought up to the abdominal wall, referred to as 'an access loop', which allows the interventional radiologist to deal with any future stones.

As a public health measure, people who have emigrated to the west from an endemic area should be offered screening for *Clonorchis* infestation in the form of ultrasound of the hepatobiliary system. This condition can be diagnosed and treated and even cured when it is in its subclinical form. Most importantly, the risk of developing the dreadful disease of cholangiocarcinoma is eliminated (Summary box 5.7).

Summary box 5.7

Asiatic cholangiohepatitis – treatment

- Medical treatment can be curative
- Surgical treatment is cholecystectomy, exploration of the common bile duct and some form of biliary–enteric bypass
- Prevention – consider offering hepatobiliary ultrasound as a screening procedure to recently arrived migrants to the west from endemic areas

---

Further reading

Choi, B.I., Han, J.K., Hong, S.T. and Lee, K.H. (2004) Clonorchiasis and cholangiocarcinoma: etiologic relationship and imaging diagnosis. *Clin Microbiol Rev* **17**(3): 540–52.

FILARIASIS

Introduction

Filariasis is mainly caused by the parasite *Wuchereria bancrofti* carried by the mosquito. A variant of the parasite called *Brugia malayi* and *Brugia timori* is responsible for causing the disease in about 10% of sufferers. The condition affects more than 90 million people worldwide, two-thirds of whom live in India, China and Indonesia. According to the World Health Organization (WHO), filariasis is the second most common cause, after leprosy, of long-term disability.

Once bitten by the mosquito, the matured eggs enter the human circulation to hatch and grow into adult worms; the process of maturation takes about 1 year. The adult worms mainly colonise the lymphatic system.

Diagnosis

It is mainly males who are affected because females in general cover a greater part of their bodies, thus making them less prone to mosquito bites. In the acute presentation, there are episodic attacks of fever with lymphadenitis and lymphangitis.

Cesar Roux, **1857–1934**, Professor of Surgery and Gynaecology, Lausanne, Switzerland, described this method of forming a jejunal conduit in 1908.
Otto Eduard Heinrich Wucherer, **1820–1873**, a German Physician who practised in Brazil, South America.
Joseph Bancroft, **1836–1894**, an English Physician working in Australia.

Occasionally, adult worms may be felt subcutaneously. Chronic manifestations appear after repeated acute attacks over several years. The adult worms cause lymphatic obstruction resulting in massive lower limb oedema. Obstruction to the cutaneous lymphatics causes skin thickening, not unlike the 'peau d'orange' appearance in breast cancer, thus exacerbating the limb swelling. Secondary streptococcal infection is common (Fig. 5.10). Recurrent attacks of lymphangitis cause fibrosis of the lymph channels, resulting in a grossly swollen limb with thickened skin producing the condition of elephantiasis (Fig. 5.11). Bilateral lower limb filariasis is often associated with scrotal and penile elephantiasis. Early on, there may be a hydrocele underlying scrotal filariasis (Fig. 5.12).

Chyluria and chylous ascites may occur. A mild form of the disease can affect the respiratory tract, causing dry cough, and is

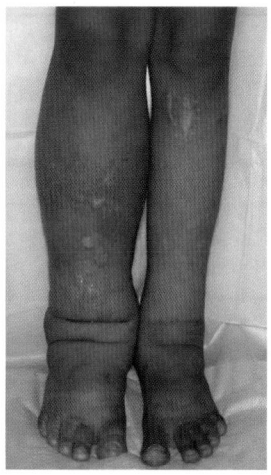

Figure 5.10 Bilateral lower limb filariasis with bacterial infection on the right side.

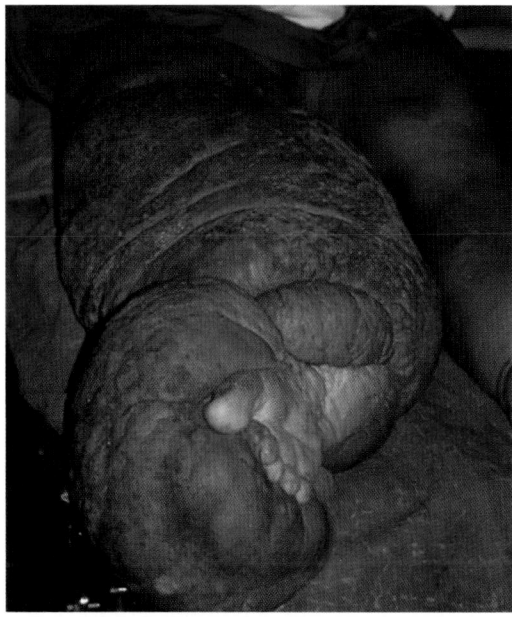

Figure 5.11 Elephantiasis of the lower limb (courtesy of Dr A. Golash, Kolkata, India).

---

peau d'orange **is French for 'orange skin'.**

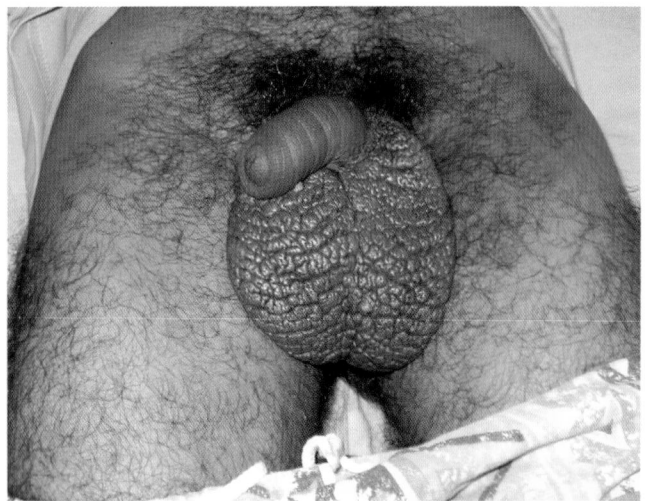

Figure 5.12 Filariasis of the scrotum with hydrocele.

referred to as tropical pulmonary eosinophilia. The condition of filariasis is clinically very obvious, and thus investigations in the full-blown case are superfluous. Eosinophilia is common, and a nocturnal peripheral blood smear may show the immature forms or microfilariae. The parasite may also be seen in chylous urine, ascites and hydrocele fluid.

Treatment

Medical treatment with diethylcarbamazine is very effective in the early stages before the gross deformities of elephantiasis have developed. In the early stages of limb swelling, intermittent pneumatic compression helps, but the treatment has to be repeated over a prolonged period.

A hydrocele is treated by the usual operation of excision and eversion of the sac with, if necessary, excision of redundant skin. Operations for reducing the size of the limb are hardly ever done these days because the procedures are so rarely successful (Summary box 5.8).

Summary box 5.8

Filariasis

- Caused by *Wuchereria bancrofti* that is carried by the mosquito
- Lymphatics are mainly affected, resulting in gross limb swelling
- Eosinophilia; immature worms seen in a nocturnal peripheral blood smear
- Gross forms of the disease cause a great deal of disability and misery
- Early cases are very amenable to medical treatment
- Intermittent pneumatic compression gives some relief
- The value of various surgical procedures is largely unproven

---

Further reading

Manjula, Y., Kate, V. and Ananthakrishnan, N. (2002) Evaluation of sequential intermittent pneumatic compression for filarial lymphoedema. *Natl Med J India* **15(4)**: 192–4.
World Health Organization (1995) The World Health Report – bridging the gaps. *World Health Forum* **16(4)**: 377–85.

HYDATID DISEASE

Introduction and pathology

Commonly called dog tape worm, hydatid disease is caused by *Ecchinococcus granulosus*. While it is common in the tropics, in the UK, the occasional patient may come from a rural sheep-farming community.

The dog is the definitive host and, as a pet, is the commonest source of infection transmitted to the intermediate hosts – humans, sheep and cattle. In the dog, the adult worm reaches the small intestine, and the eggs are passed in the faeces. These eggs are highly resistant to extremes of temperature and may survive for long periods. In the dog's intestine, the cyst wall is digested, allowing the protoscolices to develop into adult worms. Close contact with the infected dog causes contamination by the oral route, with the ovum thus gaining entry into the human gastro-intestinal tract.

The cyst is characterised by three layers, an outer *pericyst* derived from compressed host organ tissues, an intermediate hyaline *ectocyst* which is non-infective and an inner *endocyst* that is the germinal membrane and contains viable parasites which can separate forming daughter cysts. A variant of the disease occurs in colder climates caused by *Echinococcus multilocularis*, in which the cyst spreads from the outset by actual invasion rather than expansion.

Classification

In 2003, the WHO Informal Working Group on Echinococcosis (WHO-IWGE) proposed a standardised ultrasound classification based on the status of activity of the cyst. This is universally accepted, particularly because it helps to decide on the appropriate management. Three groups have been recognised:

Group 1: Active group – cysts larger than 2 cm and often fertile.
Group 2: Transition group – cysts starting to degenerate and entering a transitional stage because of host resistance or treatment, but may contain viable protoscolices.
Group 3: Inactive group – degenerated, partially or totally calcified cysts; unlikely to contain viable protoscolices.

Clinical features

As the parasite can colonise virtually every organ in the body, the condition can be protean in its presentation. When a sheep farmer, who is otherwise healthy, complains of a gradually enlarging painful mass in the right upper quadrant with the physical findings of a liver swelling, a hydatid liver cyst should be considered. The liver is the organ most often affected. The lung is the next most common. The parasite can affect any organ (Figs 5.13, 5.14a and b) or several organs in the same patient (Fig. 5.15a and b).

The disease may be asymptomatic and discovered coincidentally at post mortem or when an ultrasound or CT scan is done for some other condition. Symptomatic disease presents with a swelling causing pressure effects. Thus, a hepatic lesion causes dull pain from stretching of the liver capsule, and a pulmonary lesion, if large enough, causes dyspnoea. Daughter cysts may communicate with the biliary tree causing obstructive jaundice and all the usual clinical features associated with it in addition to symptoms attributable to a parasitic infestation (Fig. 5.16). Features of raised intracranial pressure or unexplained headaches in a patient from a sheep-rearing community should raise the suspicion of a cerebral hydatid cyst.

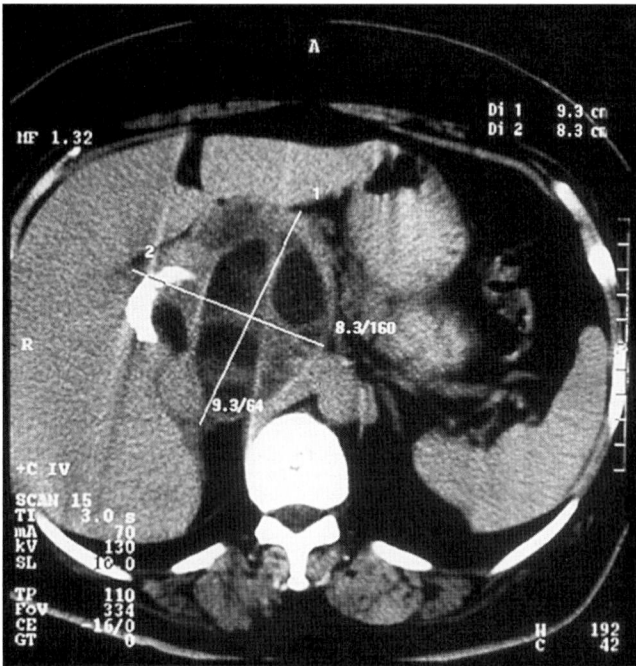

Figure 5.13 Computerised tomographic (CT) scan showing a hydatid cyst of the pancreas. A differential diagnosis of hydatid cyst or a tumour was considered. At exploration, the patient was found to have a hydatid cyst, which was excised followed by a 30-month treatment with albendazole, and remains free of disease.

The patient may present as an emergency with severe abdominal pain following minor trauma when the CT scan may be diagnostic (Fig. 5.17). Rarely, a patient may present as an emergency with features of anaphylactic shock without any obvious cause. Such a patient may subsequently cough up white material that contains scolices that have travelled into the tracheobronchial tree from rupture of a hepatic hydatid on the diaphragmatic surface of the liver.

Diagnosis

There should be a high index of suspicion. Investigations show a raised eosinophil count; serological tests such as ELISA and immunoelectrophoresis point towards the diagnosis. Ultrasound and CT scan are the investigations of choice. The CT scan shows a smooth space-occupying lesion with several septa (Fig. 5.18). An ultrasound of the biliary tract may show abnormality in the gall bladder and bile ducts. Hydatid infestation of the biliary system (Fig. 5.19) should then be suspected. Ultimately, the diagnosis is made by a combination of good history and clinical examination supplemented by serology and radiological imaging techniques (Summary box 5.9).

> **Summary box 5.9**
>
> ### Hydatid disease – diagnosis
>
> - In the UK, the usual sufferer is a sheep farmer
> - While any organ may be involved, the liver is by far the most commonly affected
> - Elective clinical presentation is usually in the form of a painful lump arising from the liver
> - Anaphylactic shock due to rupture of the hydatid cyst is the emergency presentation
> - CT scan is the best imaging modality – the diagnostic feature is a space-occupying lesion with a smooth outline with septa

Treatment

Here, the treatment of hepatic hydatid is outlined as the liver is most commonly affected, but the same general principles apply whichever organ is involved.

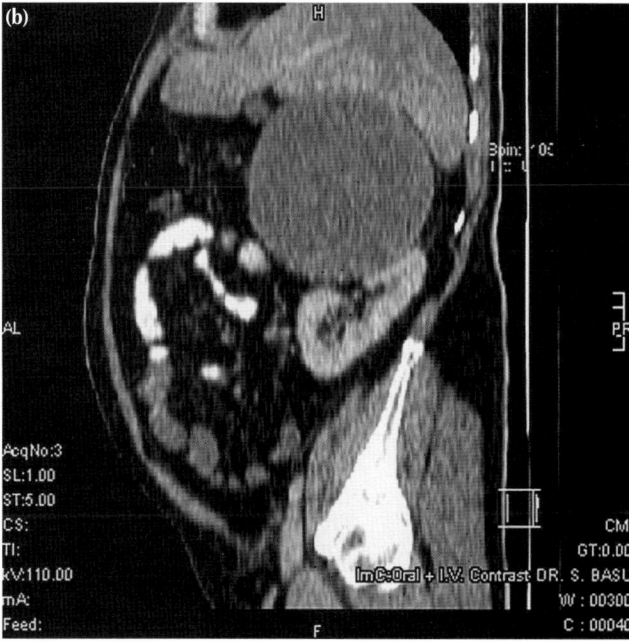

Figure 5.14 Anteroposterior (a) and lateral (b) views of computerised tomographic (CT) scans showing a large hydatid cyst of the right adrenal gland. The patient presented with a mass in the right loin and underwent an adrenalectomy (courtesy of Dr P. Bhattacharaya, Kolkata, India).

CHAPTER 5 | SURGERY IN THE TROPICS

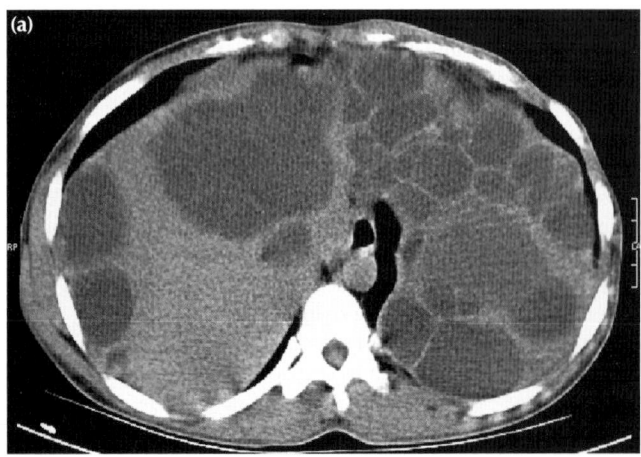

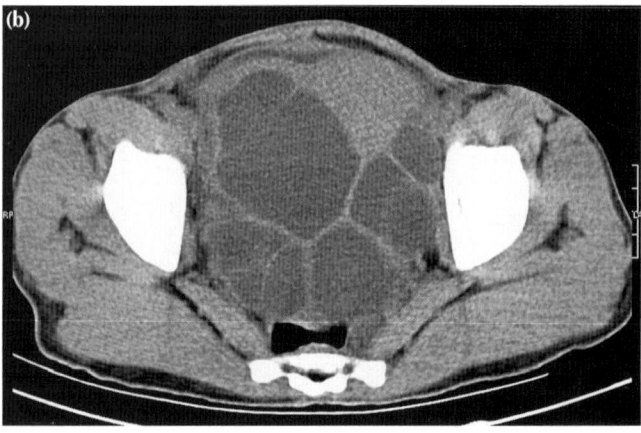

Figure 5.15 Computerised tomographic (CT) scan showing disseminated hydatid cysts of the abdomen (a) and pelvis (b). The patient was started on albendazole and lost to follow-up (courtesy of Dr P. Bhattacharaya, Kolkata, India).

These patients should be treated in a tertiary unit where good teamwork between an expert hepatobiliary surgeon, an experienced physician and an interventional radiologist is available. Surgical treatment by minimal access therapy is best summarised by the mnemonic PAIR – puncture, aspiration, injection and reaspiration. This is done after adequate drug treatment with albendazole, although praziquantel has also been used, both these drugs being available only on a 'named patient' basis.

Whether the patient is treated only medically or in combination with surgery will depend upon the clinical group (which gives an idea as to its activity), the number of cysts and their anatomical position. Radical total or partial pericystectomy with omentoplasty or hepatic segmentectomy (especially if the lesion is in a peripheral part of the liver) are some of the surgical options. During the operation, scolicidal agents are used, such as hypertonic saline (15–20%), ethanol (75–95%) or 1% povidone iodine, although some use a 10% solution. This may cause sclerosing cholangitis if biliary radicles are in communication with the cyst wall. A laparoscopic approach to these procedures is being tried.

Obviously, cysts in other organs need to be treated in accordance with the actual anatomical site along with the general principles described. An asymptomatic cyst which is inactive (group 3) may just be observed (Summary box 5.10).

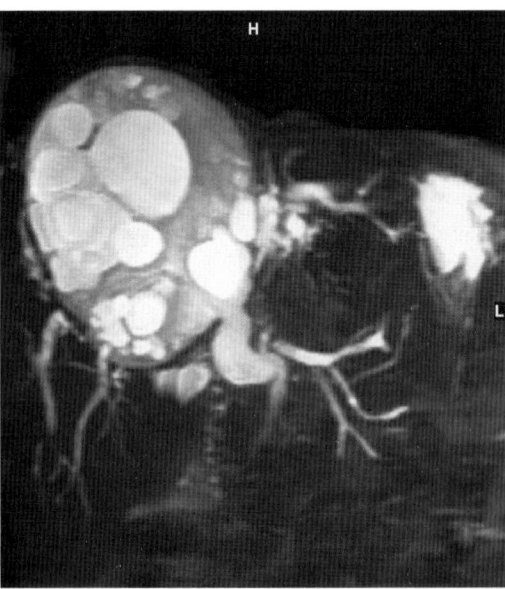

Figure 5.16 Magnetic resonance cholangiopancreatography (MRCP) showing a large hepatic hydatid cyst with daughter cysts communicating with the common bile duct causing obstruction and dilatation of the entire biliary tree (courtesy of Dr B. Agarwal, New Delhi, India).

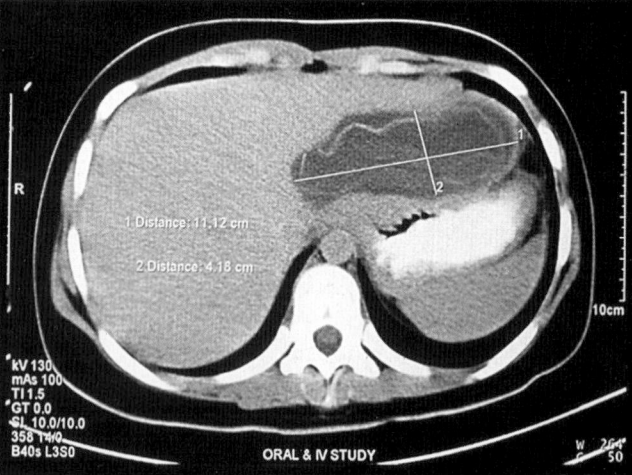

Figure 5.17 Computerised tomographic (CT) scan of the upper abdomen showing a hypodense lesion of the left lobe of the liver; the periphery of the lesion shows a double edge. This is the lamellar membrane of the hydatid cyst that separated after trivial injury. The patient was a 14-year-old girl who developed a rash and pain in the upper abdomen after dancing. The rash settled down after a course of anti-histamines. The CT scan was done 2 weeks later for persisting upper abdominal pain.

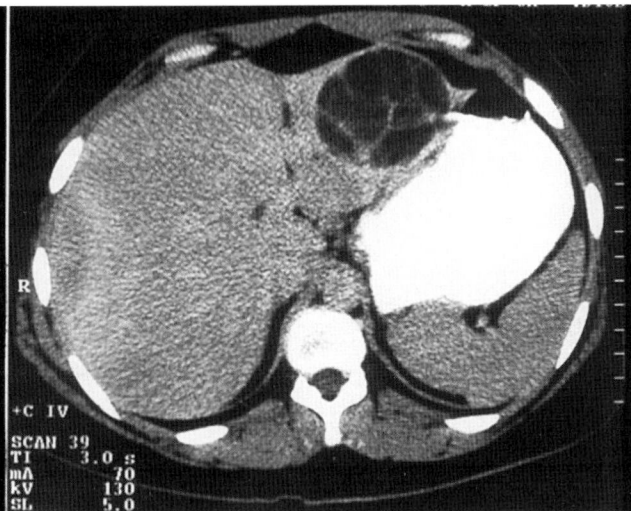

Figure 5.18 Computerised tomographic (CT) scan showing a hydatid cyst with septa in the left lobe of the liver.

Summary box 5.10

Hydatid cyst of the liver – treatment

- Ideally managed in a tertiary unit by a multidisciplinary team of hepatobiliary surgeon, physician and interventional radiologist
- Leave asymptomatic and inactive cysts alone – monitor size by ultrasound
- Active cysts should first be treated by a full course of albendazole
- Several procedures are available – PAIR, pericystectomy with omentoplasty and hepatic segmentectomy; it is important to choose the most appropriate option
- Increasingly, a laparoscopic approach is being tried

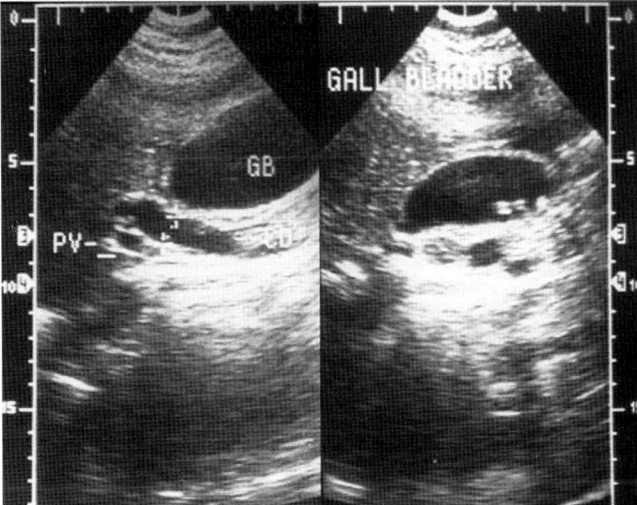

Figure 5.19 Ultrasound of the gall bladder (GB) and common bile duct (CBD) showing a dilated CBD. This is the same patient as in Fig. 5.18; the patient presented with jaundice from sludge in the CBD due to daughter cysts travelling down biliary channels in communication with the cyst.

Further reading

Barnes, S.A. and Lillemore, K.D. (1997) Liver abscess and hydatid disease. In: Zinner, N.J., Schwartz, I. and Ellis, H. (eds) *Maingot's Abdominal Operations*, 10th edn, Vol. 2. Appleton and Lange, McGraw Hill, 1527–45.

Chiodini, P. (2004) Parasitic infections. In: Russell, R.C.G., Williams, N.S. and Bulstrode, C.J.K. (ed.). *Bailey & Love's Short Practice of Surgery*, 24th edn. Arnold, London, 146–74.

WHO Informal Working Group (2003) International classification of ultrasound images in cystic echinococcosis for application in clinical and field epidemiological settings. *Acta Trop* 85(2): 253–61.

LEPROSY

Introduction

Leprosy, also called Hansen's disease, is a chronic infectious disease caused by the acid-fast bacillus, *Mycobacterium leprae*, that is widely prevalent in the tropics. Globally, India, Brazil, Nepal, Mozambique, Angola and Myanmar (Burma) account for 91% of all the cases; India alone accounts for 78% of the world's disease. Patients suffer not only from the primary effects of the disease but also from social discrimination, sadly compounded by the inappropriate term 'leper' for one afflicted with this disease. The use of the term 'leper', still used metaphorically to denote a social outcast, does not help to break down the social barriers that continue to exist against the sufferer.

Pathology

The disease is transmitted from the nasal secretions of a patient, the infection being contracted in childhood or early adolescence. After an incubation period of several years, the disease presents with skin, upper respiratory or neurological manifestations. The bacillus is acid fast but weakly so compared with *Mycobacterium tuberculosis*.

The disease is broadly classified into two groups – lepromatous and tuberculoid. In lepromatous leprosy, there is widespread dissemination of abundant bacilli in the tissues with macrophages and a few lymphocytes. This is a reflection of the poor immune response, resulting in depleted host resistance from the patient. In tuberculoid leprosy, on the other hand, the patient shows a strong immune response with scant bacilli in the tissues, epithelioid granulomas, numerous lymphocytes and giant cells. The tissue damage is proportional to the host's immune response. There are various grades of the disease between the two main spectra (Summary box 5.11).

Gerhard Henrik Armauer Hansen, **1841–1912, a Physician in charge of a Leper hospital near Bergen, Norway.**

Summary box 5.11

Mycobacterium leprae – pathology

- Leprosy is a chronic curable infection caused by *Mycobacterium leprae*
- It occurs mainly in tropical regions and developing countries
- The majority of cases are located in the Indian subcontinent
- Transmission is through nasal secretions
- It is attributed to poor hygiene and insanitary conditions
- The incubation period is several years
- The initial infection occurs in childhood
- Lepromatous leprosy denotes a poor host immune reaction
- Tuberculoid leprosy occurs when host resistance is stronger than virulence of the organism

Clinical features and diagnosis

The disease is slowly progressive and affects the skin, upper respiratory tract and peripheral nerves. In tuberculoid leprosy, the damage to tissues occurs early and is localised to one part of the body with limited deformity of that organ. Neural involvement is characterised by thickening of the nerves, which are tender. There may be asymmetrical well-defined anaesthetic hypopigmented or erythematous macules with elevated edges and a dry and rough surface – lesions called leprids. In lepromatous leprosy, the disease is symmetrical and extensive. Cutaneous involvement occurs in the form of several pale macules that form plaques and nodules called lepromas. The deformities produced are divided into primary, which are caused by leprosy or its reactions, and secondary, resulting from effects such as anaesthesia of the hands and feet.

Nodular lesions on the face in the acute phase of the lepromatous variety are known as 'leonine facies' (looking like a lion). Later, there is wrinkling of the skin giving an aged appearance to a young individual. There is loss of the eyebrows and destruction of the lateral cartilages and septum of the nose with collapse of the nasal bridge and lifting of the tip of the nose (Fig. 5.20). There may

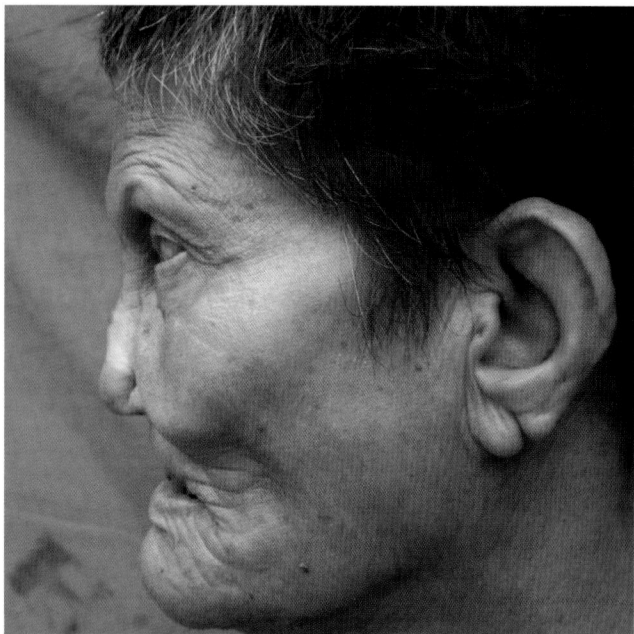

Figure 5.20 Lateral view of the face showing collapse of the nasal bridge due to destruction of nasal cartilage by leprosy.

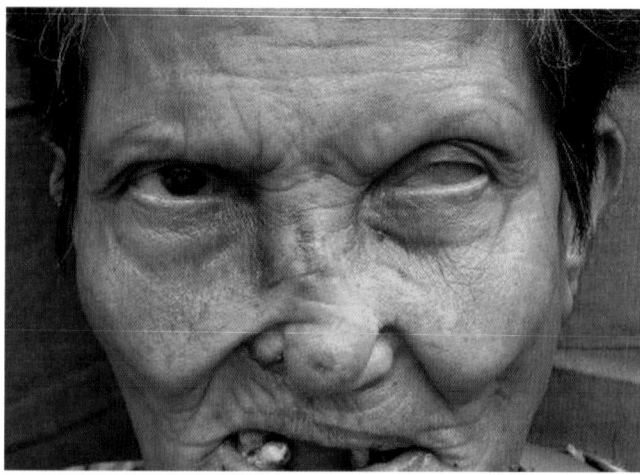

Figure 5.21 Frontal view of the face showing eye changes in leprosy – paralysis of orbicularis oculi and loss of eyebrows.

be paralysis of the branches of the facial nerve in the bony canal or of the zygomatic branch. Blindness may be attributed to exposure keratitis or iridocyclitis. Paralysis of the orbicularis oculi causes incomplete closure of the eye, epiphora and conjunctivitis (Fig. 5.21). The hands are typically clawed (Fig. 5.22a and b) because of involvement of the ulnar nerve at the elbow and the median nerve at the wrist. Anaesthesia of the hands makes these patients vulnerable to frequent burns and injuries. Similarly, clawing of the toes (Fig. 5.23) occurs as a result of involvement of the posterior tibial nerve. When the lateral popliteal nerve is affected, it leads to foot drop, and the nerve can be felt to be thickened behind the upper end of the fibula. Anaesthesia of the feet predisposes to trophic ulceration (Fig. 5.24), chronic infection, contraction and autoam-

(a)

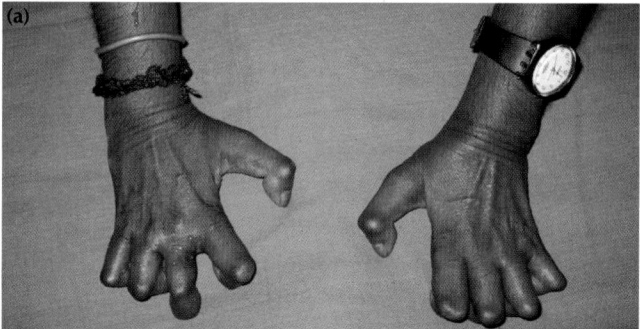

(b)

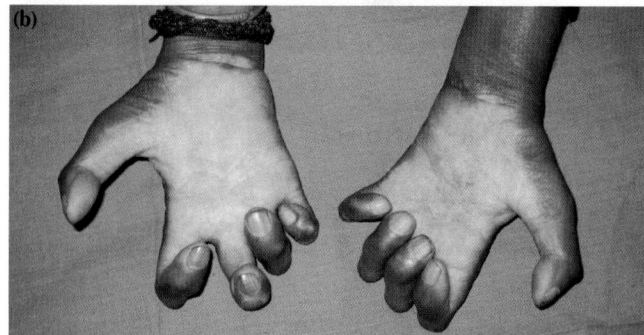

Figure 5.22 Typical bilateral claw hand from leprosy due to involvement of the ulnar and median nerves.

putation. Involvement of the testes causes atrophy, which in turn results in gynaecomastia (Fig. 5.25a and b). Confirmation of the diagnosis is obtained by a skin smear or skin biopsy, which shows the classical histological and microbiological features (Summary box 5.12).

Summary box 5.12

Leprosy – diagnosis

- Typical clinical features and awareness of the disease should help to make a diagnosis
- The face has an aged look about it with collapse of the nasal bridge and eye changes
- Thickened peripheral nerves, patches of anaesthetic skin, claw hands, foot drop and trophic ulcers are characteristic
- Microbiological examination of the acid-fast bacillus and typical histology on skin biopsy are confirmatory

---

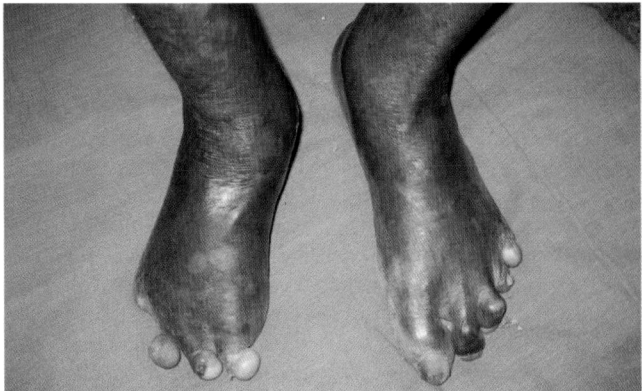

Figure 5.23 Claw toes from involvement of the posterior tibial nerve by leprosy; also note autoamputation of toes of the right foot.

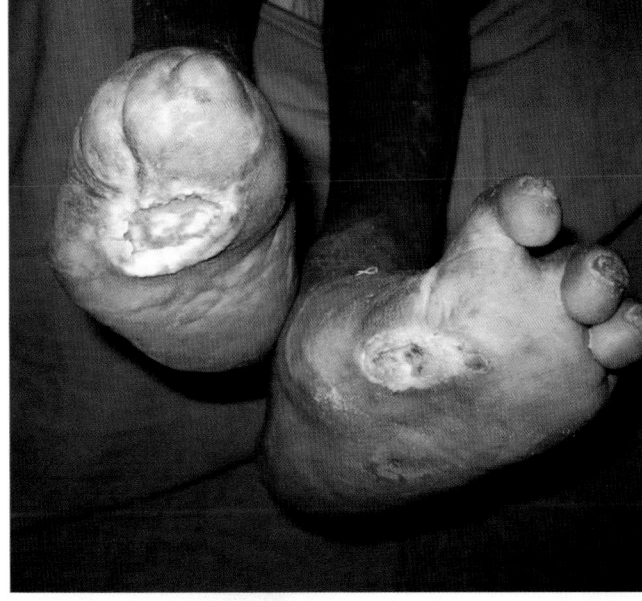

Figure 5.24 Bilateral trophic ulceration of the feet due to anaesthesia of the soles resulting from leprosy; also note claw toes on the left foot.

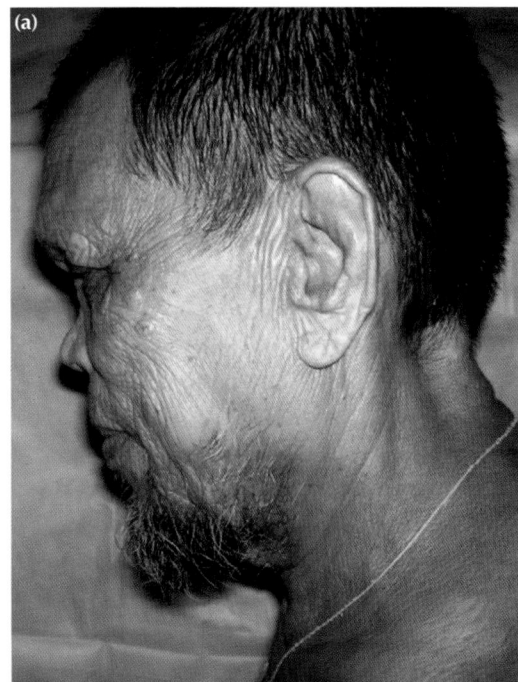

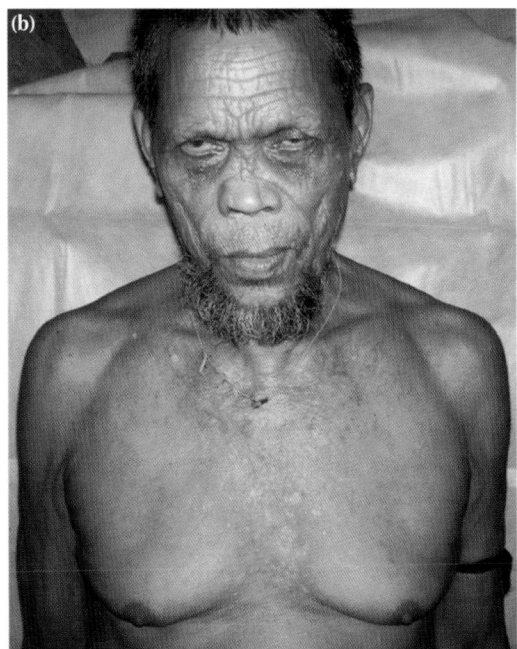

Figure 5.25 Typical leonine facies in leprosy (a) and gynaecomastia (b).

Treatment

A team approach between an infectious diseases specialist, plastic surgeon, ophthalmologist, hand and orthopaedic surgeon is important. Multiple drug therapy for 12 months is the key to treatment. This is carried out according to the WHO guidelines using rifampicin, dapsone and clofazimine. During treatment, the patient may develop acute manifestations. These are controlled with steroids.

Surgical treatment is indicated in advanced stages of the disease for functional disability of limbs, cosmetic disfigurement of

CHAPTER 5 | SURGERY IN THE TROPICS

the face and visual problems. These entail major reconstructive surgery, the domain of the plastic surgeon. Deformities of the hands and feet require various forms of tendon transfer, which need to be carried out by specialist hand or orthopaedic surgeons.

The general surgeon may be called upon to treat a patient when the deformity is so advanced that it requires amputation, or in an emergency situation when abscesses need to be drained.

All surgical procedures obviously need to be done under anti-leprosy drug treatment. This is best achieved by a team approach. Educating the patients about the dreadful sequelae of the disease so that they seek medical help early is important. It is also necessary to educate the general public that patients suffering from the disease should not be made social outcasts (Summary box 5.13).

Summary box 5.13

Leprosy – treatment

- **Multiple drug therapy for a year**
- **Team approach**
- **Surgical reconstruction requires the expertise of a hand surgeon, orthopaedic surgeon and plastic surgeon**
- **Education of the patient and general public should be the keystone in prevention**

Further reading

World Health Organization (2000) Leprosy – global situation. *Wkly Epidemiol Rec* **75**: 225–32.

POLIOMYELITIS

Introduction

Poliomyelitis is an enteroviral infection that sadly still affects children in developing countries – this is in spite of effective vaccination having been universally available for several decades. The virus enters the body by inhalation or ingestion. Clinically, the disease manifests itself in a wide spectrum of symptoms – from a few days of mild fever and headache to the extreme variety consisting of extensive paralysis of the bulbar form that may not be compatible with life because of involvement of the respiratory and pharyngeal muscles.

Diagnosis

The disease targets the anterior horn cells causing lower motor neurone paralysis. Muscles of the lower limb are affected twice as frequently as those of the upper limb (Fig. 5.26). Fortunately, only 1–2% of sufferers develop paralytic symptoms but, when they do occur, the disability causes much misery (Fig. 5.27). When a patient develops fever with muscle weakness, Guillain–Barré syndrome needs to be excluded. The latter has sensory symptoms and signs, and cerebrospinal fluid (CSF) analysis should help to differentiate the two conditions.

Georges Guillain, 1876–1961, Professor of Neurology, The Faculty of Medicine, Paris, France.
Jean Alexandre Barré, 1880–1967, Professor of Neurology, Strasbourg, France.

Guillain and Barré described this condition in a joint paper in 1916 whilst serving as Medical Officers in the French Army during the First World War.

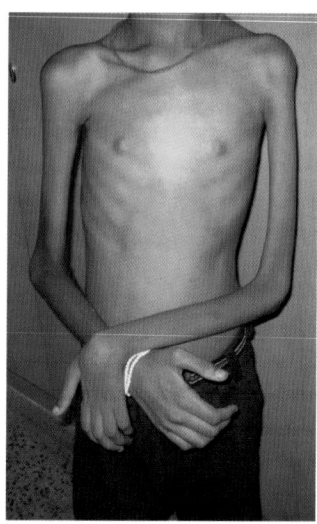

Figure 5.26 Polio affecting predominantly the upper limb muscles with wasting of the intercostal muscles.

Management

Surgical management is directed mainly towards the rehabilitation of the patient who has residual paralysis, the operations being tailored to that particular individual's disability. Children especially may show improvement in their muscle function for up to 2 years after the onset of the illness. Thereafter, many patients learn to manage their disability by incorporating various manoeuvres ('trick movements') into their daily life. The surgeon must be cautious in considering such a patient for any form of surgery.

Surgical treatment lies with the orthopaedic surgeon who needs to work very closely with the physiotherapist in both assessing and rehabilitating the patient. In the chronic form of the disease, operations are only considered after a very careful and detailed assessment of the patient's needs.

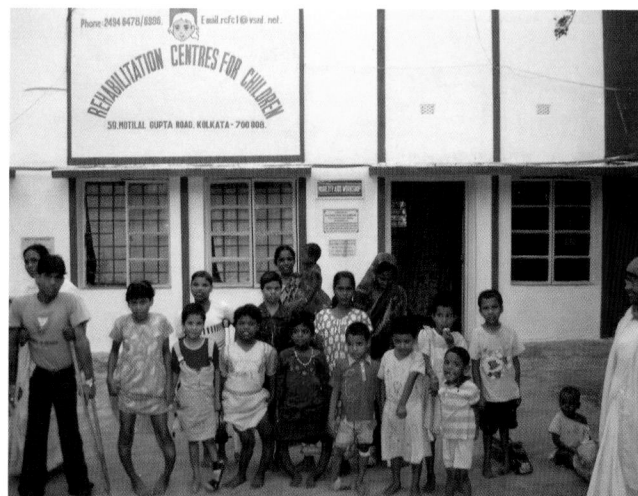

Figure 5.27 A group photograph at the Rehabilitation Centre for Children at Barisha, Kolkata, India. This centre used to treat exclusively children with polio deformities. As a result of a successful eradication programme, the centre now concentrates on deformities caused by other diseases. The patient on the extreme left had his knees arthrodesed as a young boy and now works for the centre (courtesy of Dr S.M. Lakhotia, MS, Dr P.K. Jain, MD, DA, Kolkata, India).

Surgical principles

(The following section has been contributed by Dr A. Golash, FRCSEd, Kolkata, India)

The goals of surgical treatment are to correct significant muscle imbalances and deformities of bones and soft tissues. The options are orthoses for static joint instabilities, operations such as tendon transfers for dynamic muscle imbalance and arthrodesis for permanent stabilisation of a flail joint.

The following are the common problems encountered and the suggested surgical solutions (Table 5.1).

Foot and ankle

The most common deformities are claw toes, cavovarus foot, dorsal bunion, talipes equinus, talipes equinovarus, talipes cavovarus, talipes equinovalgus and talipes calcaneus. Surgical intervention is only undertaken once the exact pattern of muscle paralysis and resultant deformity has been determined.

Knee

The common knee deformities are flexion contracture, quadriceps paralysis, genu recurvatum and flail knee. Flexion contracture of the knee is caused by a contracture of the iliotibial band (Fig. 5.28a and b) or isolated paralysis of the quadriceps muscle. Contractures of less than 20° can be treated by capsulotomy and hamstring lengthening. More severe contractures are corrected by supracondylar extension osteotomy of the femur. Quadriceps paralysis is treated by the transfer of one or more of the following tendons – biceps femoris, semitendinosus, sartorius and tensor fascia lata to quadriceps tendon and patella. Genu recurvatum is treated by tibial osteotomy and the transfer of one or more of the hamstring muscles to the patella. Flail knee is managed by the use of a long leg brace or knee arthrodesis.

Hip

Common problems are flexion and abduction contractures, hip instability due to paralysis of the gluteal muscles and paralytic hip dislocation. Flexion and abduction contracture of the hip is

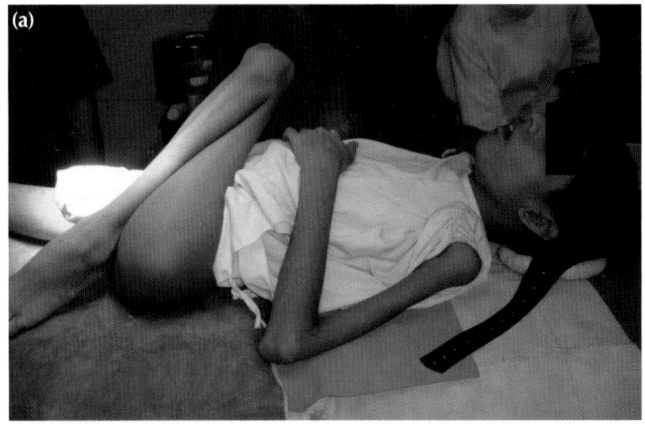

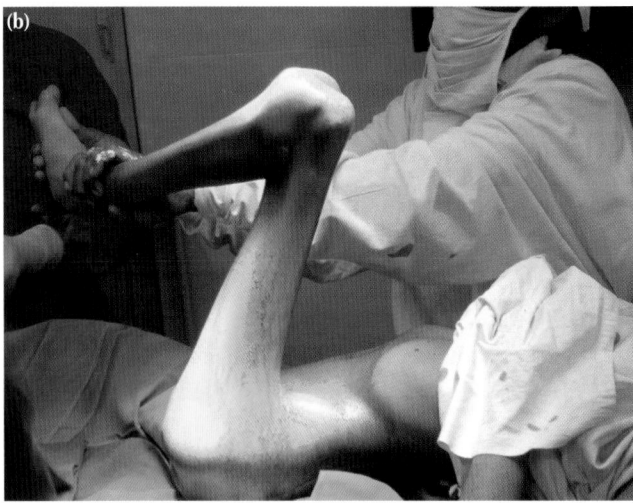

Figure 5.28 A 12-year-old patient with polio showing marked wasting of the left upper arm muscles with flexion contractures of the left knee and hip; there is equinus deformity of the foot (courtesy of Dr S.M. Lakhotia, MS, Dr P.K. Jain, MD, DA, Kolkata, India).

Table 5.1 Description and treatment of muscle imbalances in poliomyelitis

Paralysed muscle	Deformity	Treatment
Tibialis anterior	Equinus	Passive stretching and serial casting. Posterior capsulotomy and tendo achilles lengthening + anterior transfer of peroneus longus to the base of the second metatarsal
	Claw toes	Transfer of long toe extensors into the metatarsal neck + interphalangeal joint fusion
	Cavovarus	Plantar fasciotomy, release of intrinsic muscles + transfer of peroneus longus to the base of the second metatarsal, extensor hallucis longus to the neck of the first metatarsal
Tibialis anterior and tibialis posterior	Talipes equinovalgus	Serial casting followed by peroneus longus transfer to the base of the second metatarsal and one of the long toe flexors to the tibialis posterior
Tibialis anterior, toe extensors and peroneal muscles	Severe equinovarus deformity	Tendo achilles lengthening, anterior transfer of tibialis posterior to the base of the third metatarsal or middle cuneiform + anterior transfer of long toe flexors
Soleus/gastrocnemius	Talipes calcaneus	Tibialis anterior transfer to the calcaneal tuberosity and tendo achilles insertion

Achilles, the Greek Hero, was the son of Peleus and Thetis. When he was a child his mother dipped him in the Styx, one of the rivers of the Underworld, so that he should be invulnerable in battle. The heel by which she held him did not get wet, and was, therefore, not protected. Achilles died from a wound in the heel which he received at the siege of Troy.

usually accompanied by varying degrees of external rotation contracture; these can be corrected by complete release of the hip muscles. Very severe deformities need a complete release along with transfer of the crest of ilium.

Paralysis of the gluteus maximus and medius muscles results in an unstable hip that can prove very tiring along with an unsightly limp. Function can be improved by transferring muscles (external oblique, ilio-psoas) to replace gluteal muscles.

Trunk

Unbalanced paralysis causes scoliosis along with pelvic obliquity (Fig. 5.29). Complex bony procedures are needed to correct this deformity.

Shoulder

Disabilities caused by paralysis of the shoulder muscles can be corrected, to a certain extent, by tendon and muscle transfer (trapezius to deltoid) or by arthrodesis of the joint.

Elbow

Active elbow flexion and extension can be restored by muscle and tendon transfers. Elbow flexion can be restored by one of the following methods: flexorplasty, transfer of the pectoralis major muscle, transfer of the latissimus dorsi muscle or anterior transfer of the triceps tendon. Extension of the elbow can be restored by the posterior transfer of the deltoid muscle.

Wrist and hand

Treatment options are tendon transfer and wrist arthrodesis. Weakness of thumb opposition can be corrected by sublimis opponensplasty (Summary box 5.14).

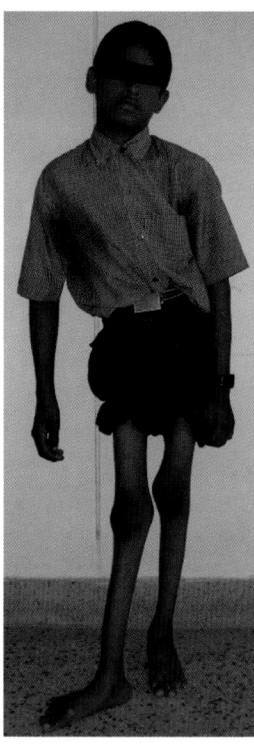

Figure 5.29 A young patient with polio showing paralysis of the lower limb and paraspinal muscles causing marked scoliosis and a deformed pelvis.

TROPICAL CHRONIC PANCREATITIS

Introduction

Tropical chronic pancreatitis is a disease affecting the younger generation from poor socio-economic strata in developing countries, seen mostly in southern India. The aetiology remains obscure with malnutrition, dietary, familial and genetic factors being possible causes. Alcohol ingestion does not play a part in the aetiology.

Aetiology and pathology

Cassava (tapioca) is a root vegetable that is readily available and inexpensive and is therefore consumed as a staple diet by people from a poor background. It contains derivatives of cyanide that are detoxified in the liver by sulphur-containing amino acids. The less well-off among the population lack such amino acids in the diet. This results in cyanogen toxicity causing the disease. Several members of the same family have been known to suffer from this condition; this strengthens the theory that cassava toxicity is an important cause because family members eat the same food.

Macroscopically, the pancreas is firm and nodular with extensive periductal fibrosis, with intraductal calcium carbonate stones of different sizes and shapes that may show branches and resemble a staghorn. The ducts are dilated. Microscopically, fibrosis is the predominant feature – intralobular, interlobular and periductal – with plasma cell and lymphocyte infiltration. There is a high incidence of pancreatic cancer in these patients (Summary box 5.15).

Diagnosis

The patient, usually male, is almost always below the age of 40 years and from a poor background. The clinical presentation is abdominal pain, thirst, polyuria and features of gross pancreatic insufficiency causing steatorrhoea and malnutrition. The patient looks ill and emaciated.

Initial routine blood and urine tests confirm that the patient has type 1 diabetes mellitus. This is known as fibrocalculous pancreatic diabetes, a label that is aptly descriptive of the typical pathological changes. Serum amylase is usually normal; in an acute exacerbation, it may be elevated. A plain abdominal X-ray shows typical pancreatic calcification in the form of discrete stones in the duct (Fig. 5.30). Ultrasound and CT scanning of the pancreas confirm the diagnosis. An ERCP as an investigation should only be done when the procedure is also being considered as a therapeutic manoeuvre for removal of ductal stones in the pancreatic head by papillotomy (Summary box 5.16).

Summary box 5.16

Diagnosis of tropical chronic pancreatitis

- The usual sufferer is a type 1 diabetic under 40 years of age
- Serum amylase may be elevated in an acute exacerbation
- Plain X-ray shows stones along the pancreatic duct
- Ultrasound and CT scan of the pancreas confirm the diagnosis
- ERCP may be used as a supplementary investigation and a therapeutic procedure

---

Treatment

The treatment is mainly medical with exocrine support using pancreatic enzymes, treatment of diabetes with insulin and the management of malnutrition. Treatment of pain should be along the lines of the usual analgesic ladder: non-opioids, followed by weak and then strong opioids and, finally, referral to a pain clinic.

Surgical treatment is necessary for intractable pain particularly when there are stones in a dilated duct. Removal of the stones, with a side-to-side pancreaticojejunostomy to a Roux loop, is the procedure of choice. As most patients are young, pancreatic resection is only very rarely considered, and then only as a last resort, when all available methods of pain relief have been exhausted (Summary box 5.17).

Summary box 5.17

Tropical chronic pancreatitis – treatment

- Mainly medical – pain relief, insulin for diabetes and pancreatic supplements for malnutrition
- Surgery is reserved for intractable pain
- Procedures are side-to-side pancreaticojejunostomy; resection in extreme cases

---

Further reading

Barman, K.K., Premlatha, G. and Mohan, V. (2003) Tropical chronic pancreatitis. *Postgrad Med J* **79**: 606–15.

TUBERCULOSIS OF SMALL INTESTINE

Introduction

Infection by *Mycobacterium tuberculosis* is common in the tropics. In these days of international travel and increased migration into the UK, tuberculosis in general and intestinal tuberculosis in particular are no longer clinical curiosities in the west. Any patient, particularly one who has recently arrived from an endemic area and who has features of generalised ill health and altered bowel habit, should arouse the suspicion of intestinal tuberculosis.

Pathology

When a patient with pulmonary tuberculosis swallows infected sputum, the organism colonises the lymphatics of the terminal ileum, causing transverse ulcers with typical undermined edges. The serosa is usually studded with tubercles. Histology shows caseating granuloma with giant cells (Fig. 5.31). This pathological entity, referred to as the ulcerative type, denotes a severe form of the disease in which the virulence of the organism outstrips the resistance of the host.

The other variety, called the hyperplastic type, occurs when host resistance is stronger than the virulence of the organism. It is caused by the drinking of infected milk. There is a marked inflammatory reaction causing hyperplasia and thickening of the terminal ileum because of its abundance of lymphoid follicles, thus causing narrowing of the lumen and obstruction. In both types, there may be marked mesenteric lymphadenopathy. Macroscopically, this type may be confused with Crohn's disease. The small intestine shows areas of stricture and fibrosis most pronounced at the terminal ileum (Fig. 5.32). As a result, there is shortening of the bowel with the caecum being pulled up into a subhepatic position (Summary box 5.18).

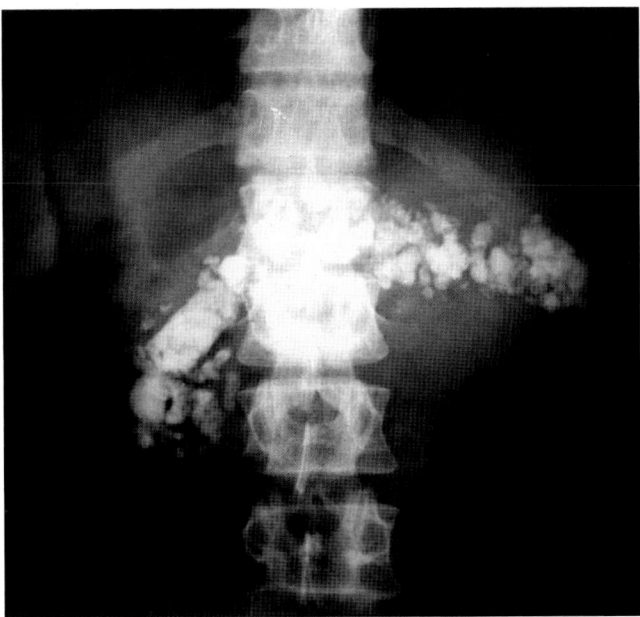

Figure 5.30 Plain X-ray of the abdomen showing large stones along the main pancreatic duct typical of tropical chronic pancreatitis (courtesy of Dr V. Mohan, Chennai, India).

Burrill Bernard Crohn, **1884–1983, Gastroenterologist, Mount Sinai Hospital, New York, NY, USA, described regional ileitis in 1932.**

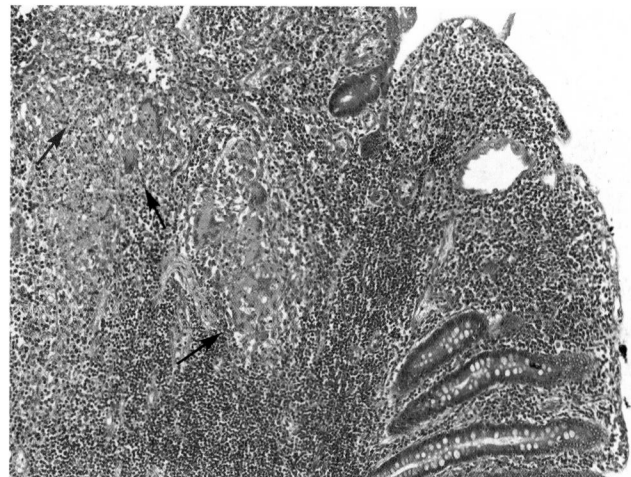

Figure 5.31 Histology of ileocaecal tuberculosis showing epithelioid cell granuloma (black arrows) with caseation (blue arrow) (courtesy of Dr A.K. Mandal, New Delhi, India).

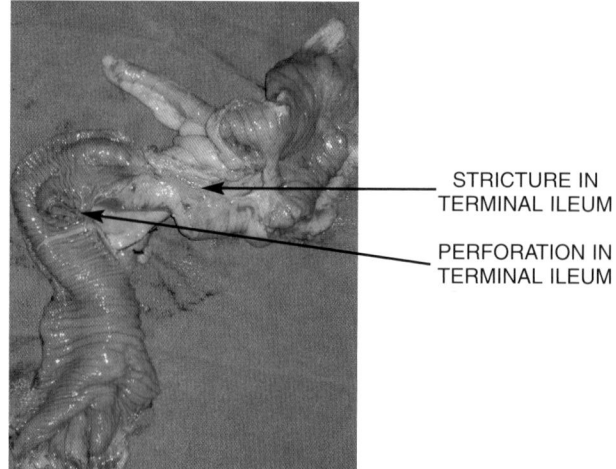

STRICTURE IN TERMINAL ILEUM

PERFORATION IN TERMINAL ILEUM

Figure 5.32 Emergency limited ileocolic resection: specimen showing tuberculous stricture in the terminal ileum and perforation of a transverse ulcer just proximal to the stricture.

Summary box 5.18

Tuberculosis – pathology

- Increasingly being seen in the UK, mostly among immigrants
- Two types are recognised – ulcerative and hyperplastic
- The ulcerative type occurs when the virulence of the organism is greater than the host defence
- The opposite occurs in the hyperplastic type
- Small bowel strictures are common in the hyperplastic type, mainly affecting the ileocaecal area
- In the ulcerative type, the bowel serosa is studded with tubercles
- Localised areas of ascites occur in the form of cocoons
- The lungs and other organs may also be involved simultaneously

Clinical features

Patients present electively with weight loss, chronic cough, malaise, evening rise in temperature with sweating, vague abdominal pain with distension and alternating constipation and diarrhoea. As an emergency, they present with features of distal small bowel obstruction from strictures of the small bowel, particularly the terminal ileum. Rarely, a patient may present with features of peritonitis from perforation of a tuberculous ulcer in the small bowel (Fig. 5.32).

Examination shows a chronically ill patient with a 'doughy' feel to the abdomen from areas of localised ascites. In the hyperplastic type, a mass may be felt in the right iliac fossa. In addition, some patients may present with fistula-in-ano, which is typically multiple with undermined edges and watery discharge.

As this is a disease mainly seen in developing countries, patients may present late as an emergency from intestinal obstruction. Abdominal pain and distension, constipation and bilious and faeculent vomiting are typical of such a patient who is in extremis.

There may be features of other system involvement such as the genitourinary tract, when the patient complains of frequency

of micturition. Clinical examination does not show any abnormality. The genitourinary tract should then be investigated (Summary box 5.19).

Summary box 5.19

Tuberculosis – clinical features

- Intestinal tuberculosis should be suspected in any patient from an endemic area who presents with weight loss, malaise, evening fever, cough, alternating constipation and diarrhoea and intermittent abdominal pain with distension
- The abdomen has a doughy feel; a mass may be found in the right iliac fossa
- The emergency patient presents with features of distal small bowel obstruction – abdominal pain, distension, bilious and faeculent vomiting
- Peritonitis from a perforated tuberculous ulcer in the small bowel can be another emergency presentation

Investigations

Raised ESR and CRP, low haemoglobin and a positive Mantoux test are usual, although the last is not significant in a patient from an endemic area.

Sputum for culture and sensitivity (the result may take several weeks) and staining by the Ziehl–Neelsen method for acid-fast bacilli (the result is obtained much earlier) should be done.

A barium meal and follow-through (or small bowel enema) shows strictures of the small bowel, particularly the ileum, typically with a high subhepatic caecum with the narrow ileum entering the caecum directly from below upwards in a straight line rather than at an angle (Figs 5.33a and b and 5.34a). Laparoscopy reveals the typical picture of tubercles on the bowel serosa,

Charles Mantoux, 1877–1947, Physician, Le Cannet, Alpes Maritimes, France, described the intra-dermal tuberculin skin test in 1908.
Franz Heinrich Paul Ziehl, 1859–1926, Neurologist, Lubeck, Germany.
Friedrich Carl Adolf Neelsen, 1854–1894, Pathologist, Prosector, the Stadt-Krankenhaus, Dresden, Germany.

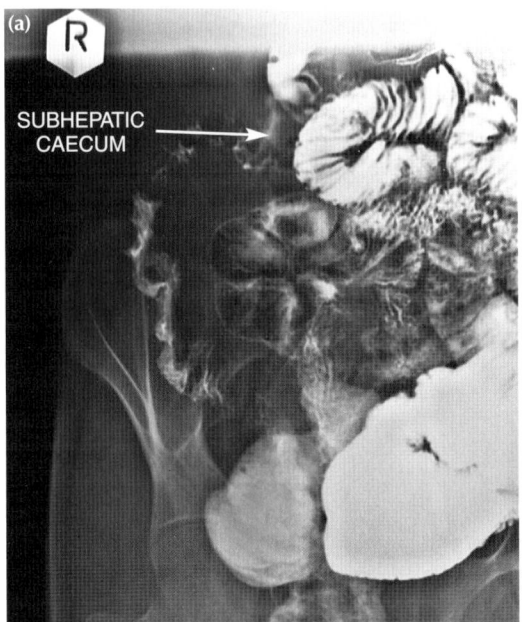

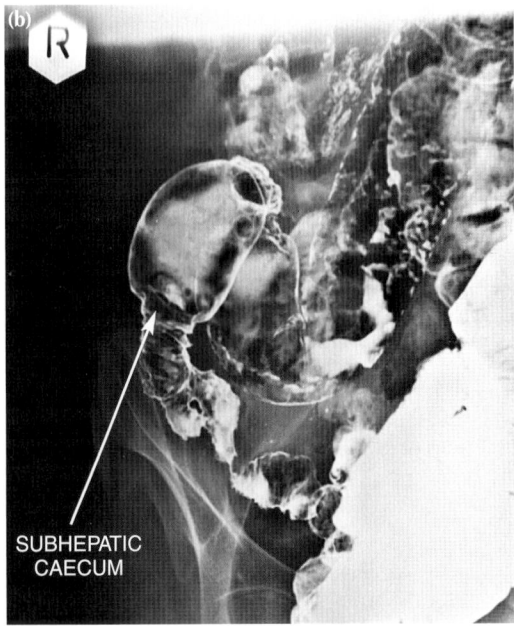

Figure 5.33 Series of a barium meal and follow-through showing strictures in the ileum with the caecum pulled up into a subhepatic position.

multiple strictures, a high caecum, enlarged lymph nodes, areas of caseation and ascites. Culture of the ascitic fluid may be helpful. A chest X-ray is essential (Fig. 5.34b).

If the patient complains of urinary symptoms, urine is sent for microscopy and culture, and the finding of sterile pyuria should alert the clinician to the possibility of tuberculosis of the urinary tract, when the appropriate investigations should be done.

In the patient presenting as an emergency, urea and electrolytes

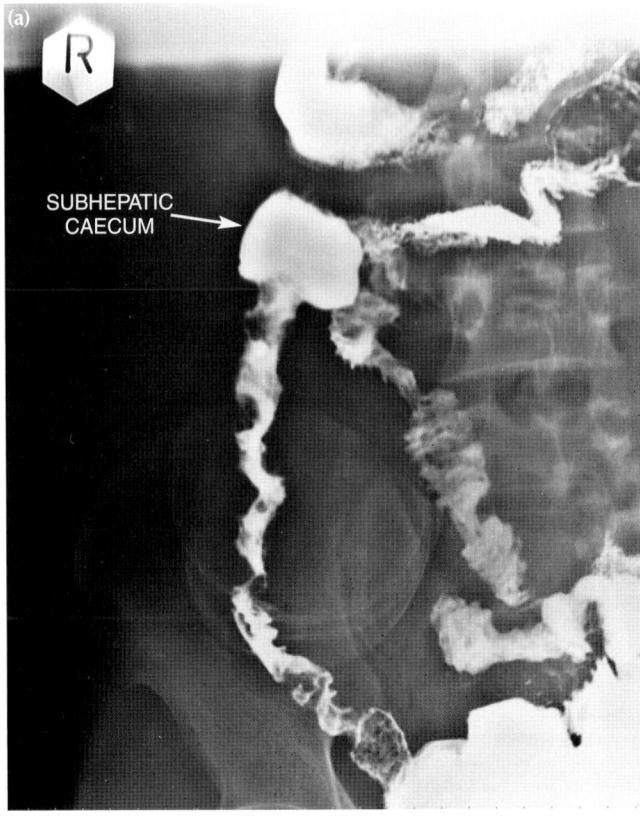

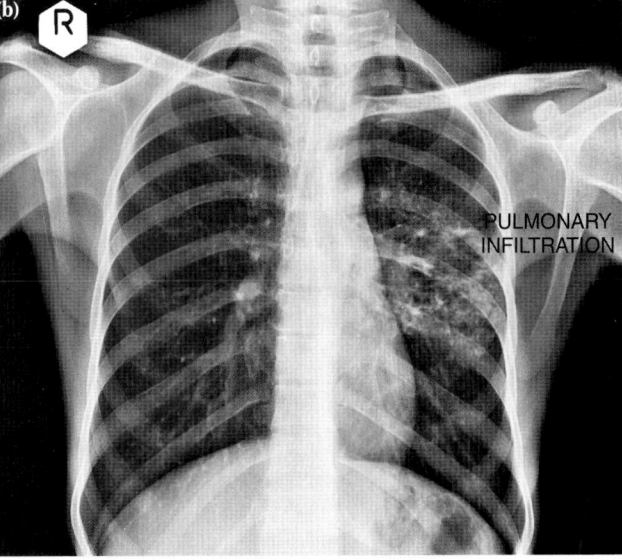

Figure 5.34 Barium meal and follow-through (a) and chest X-ray (b) in a patient with extensive intestinal and pulmonary tuberculosis, showing ileal strictures with high caecum and pulmonary infiltration.

show evidence of gross dehydration. Plain abdominal X-ray shows typical small bowel obstruction – valvulae conniventes of dilated jejunum and featureless ileum with evidence of fluid between the loops (Summary box 5.20).

Summary box 5.20

Intestinal tuberculosis – investigations

- Raised inflammatory markers, anaemia and positive sputum culture
- Ultrasound of the abdomen may show localised areas of ascites
- Chest X-ray shows pulmonary infiltration
- Barium meal and follow-through shows multiple small bowel strictures particularly in the ileum with a subhepatic caecum
- If symptoms warrant, the genitourinary tract is also investigated

---

Treatment

On completion of medical treatment, the patient's small bowel is reimaged to look for significant strictures. If the patient has features of subacute intermittent obstruction, bowel resection, in the form of limited ileocolic resection (Fig. 5.32) with anastomosis between the terminal ileum and ascending colon, strictureplasty or right hemicolectomy, is performed as deemed appropriate. The surgical principles and options in the elective patient are very similar to those for Crohn's disease.

The emergency patient presents a great challenge. Such a patient is usually from a poor socio-economic background, hence the late presentation of acute, distal, small bowel obstruction. The patient is extremely ill from dehydration, malnutrition, anaemia and probably active pulmonary tuberculosis. Vigorous resuscitation should precede the operation. At laparotomy, the minimum life-saving procedure is carried out, such as a side-to-side ileotransverse anastomosis for a terminal ileal stricture. If the general condition of the patient permits, a one-stage resection and anastomosis may be performed.

Thereafter, the patient should ideally be under the combined care of the physician and surgeon for a full course of anti-tuberculous chemotherapy and improvement in nutritional status; this may require 3–6 months of care. The patient who had a simple bypass procedure is reassessed and, when the disease is no longer active (as evidenced by return to normal of inflammatory markers, weight gain, negative sputum culture), an elective right hemicolectomy is done. This may be supplemented with strictureplasty for short strictures at intervals.

Perforation is treated by thorough resuscitation followed by resection of the affected segment. Anastomosis is performed provided it is regarded as safe to do so when peritoneal contamination is minimal and widespread disease is not encountered; otherwise, as a first stage, resection and exteriorisation is done followed by restoration of bowel continuity as a second stage later on after a full course of anti-tuberculous chemotherapy and improvement in nutritional status (Summary box 5.21).

Summary box 5.21

Tuberculosis – treatment

- Patients should ideally be under the combined care of a physician and surgeon
- Vigorous supportive and full drug treatment is mandatory in all cases
- Symptomatic strictures are treated by the appropriate resection, e.g. local ileocolic resection or strictureplasty as an elective procedure once the disease is completely under control
- Acute intestinal obstruction from distal ileal stricture is treated by thorough resuscitation followed by side-to-side ileotransverse bypass
- Once the patient has recovered with medical treatment, then the second-stage definitive procedure of right hemicolectomy is done
- One-stage resection and anastomosis can be considered if the patient's general condition permits
- Perforation is treated by appropriate local resection and anastomosis or exteriorisation if the condition of the patient is very poor; this is later followed by restoration of bowel continuity after the patient has fully recovered with anti-tuberculous chemotherapy

---

TYPHOID

Introduction

Typhoid fever is caused by *Salmonella typhi*, also called the typhoid bacillus. This is a Gram-negative organism. Like most infections occurring in developing countries in the tropics, the organism gains entry into the human gastrointestinal tract as a result of poor hygiene and inadequate sanitation. It is a disease normally managed by physicians, but the surgeon is called upon to treat the patient with typhoid fever because of perforation of a typhoid ulcer.

Pathology

Following ingestion of contaminated food or water, the organism colonises the Peyer's patches in the terminal ileum causing hyperplasia of the lymphoid follicles followed by necrosis and ulceration. The microscopic picture shows erythrophagocytosis with histiocytic proliferation (Fig. 5.35). If the patient is left untreated or inadequately treated, the ulcers may lead to perforation and bleeding. The bowel may perforate at several sites including the large bowel.

Diagnosis

A typical patient is from an endemic area or who has recently visited such a country and suffers from a high temperature for 2–3 weeks. The patient may be toxic with abdominal distension from paralytic ileus. The patient may have melaena due to haemorrhage from a typhoid ulcer; this can lead to hypovolaemia.

Blood and stool cultures confirm the nature of the infection and exclude malaria. Although obsolete in the UK, the Widal test

Daniel Elmer Salmon, 1850–1914, Veterinary Pathologist, Chief of the Bureau of Animal Industry, Washington DC, USA.
Johann Conrad Peyer, 1653–1712, Professor of Logic, Rhetoric and Medicine, Schaffhausen, Switzerland, described the lymph follicles in the intestine in 1677.
Georges Fernand Isidore Widal, 1862–1929, Professor of Internal Pathology, and later of Clinical Medicine, The Faculty of Medicine, Paris, France.

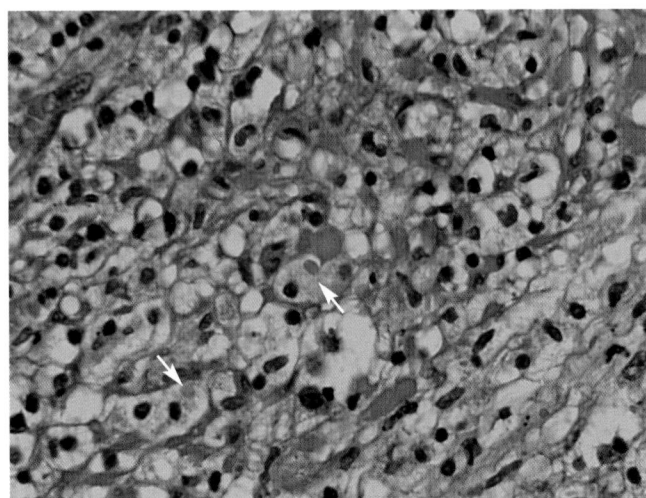

Figure 5.35 Histology of enteric perforation of the small intestine showing erythrophagocytosis (arrows) with predominantly histiocytic proliferation (courtesy of Dr A.K. Mandal, New Delhi, India).

is still done in the Indian subcontinent. The test looks for the presence of agglutinins to O and H antigens of *Salmonella typhi* and *paratyphi* in the patient's serum. In endemic areas, laboratory facilities may sometimes be limited. Certain other tests have been developed which identify sensitive and specific markers for typhoid fever. Practical and cheap kits are available for their rapid detection that need no special expertise and equipment. These are Multi-Test Dip-S-Ticks to detect immunoglobulin G (IgG), Tubex to detect immunoglobulin M (IgM) and TyphiDot to detect IgG and IgM. These tests are particularly valuable when blood cultures are negative (due to pre-hospital treatment or self-medication with antibiotics) or facilities for such an investigation are not available.

In the second or third week of the illness, if there is severe generalised abdominal pain, this heralds a perforated typhoid ulcer. The patient, who is already very ill, deteriorates further with classical features of peritonitis. An erect chest X-ray or a lateral decubitus film (in the very ill, as they usually are) will show free gas in the peritoneal cavity. In fact, any patient being treated for typhoid fever who shows a sudden deterioration accompanied by abdominal signs should be considered to have a typhoid perforation until proven otherwise (Summary 5.22).

Summary box 5.22

Diagnosis of bowel perforation secondary to typhoid

- The patient presents in, or has recently visited, an endemic area
- The patient has persistent high temperature and is very toxic
- Positive blood or stool cultures for *Salmonella typhi* and the patient is already on treatment for typhoid
- After the second week, signs of peritonitis usually denote perforation, which is confirmed by the presence of free gas seen on X-ray

---

Treatment

Vigorous resuscitation with intravenous fluids and antibiotics in an intensive care unit gives the best chance of stabilising the patient's condition. Metronidazole, cephalosporins and gentamicin are used in combination. Chloramphenicol, despite its potential side-effect of aplastic anaemia, is still used occasionally in developing countries. Laparotomy is then carried out.

Several surgical options are available, and the most appropriate operative procedure should be chosen judiciously depending upon the general condition of the patient, the site of perforation, the number of perforations and the degree of peritoneal soiling. The alternatives are closure of the perforation (Fig. 5.36a and b) after freshening the edges, wedge resection of the ulcer area and closure, resection of bowel with or without anastomosis (exteriorisation), closure of the perforation and side-to-side ileotransverse anastomosis, ileostomy or colostomy where the perforated bowel is exteriorised after refashioning the edges. After closing an ileal perforation, the surgeon should look for other sites of perforation or necrotic patches in the small or large bowel that might imminently perforate, and deal with them appropriately. Thorough peritoneal lavage is essential. The linea alba is closed leaving the rest of the abdominal wound open for delayed closure, as wound infection is almost inevitable and dehiscence not uncommon. In the presence of rampant infection, laparostomy may be a good alternative.

When a typhoid perforation occurs within the first week of illness, the prognosis is better than if it occurs after the second or third week because, in the early stages, the patient is less

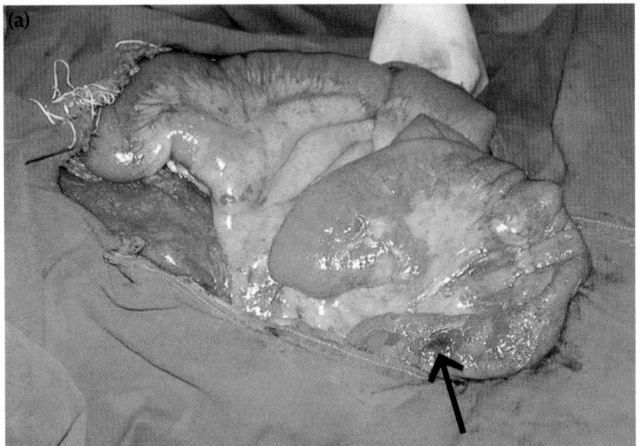

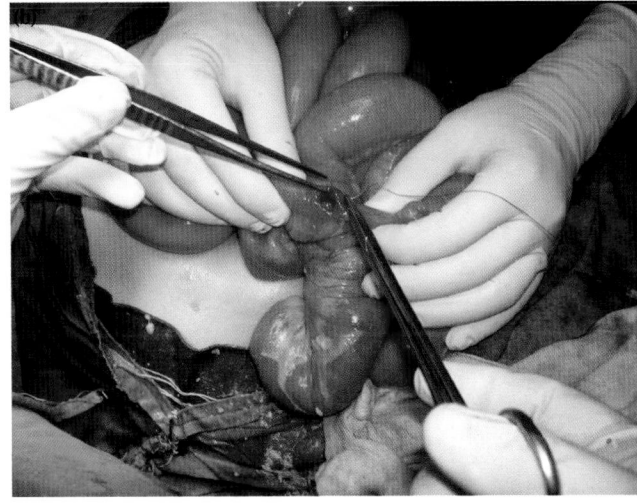

Figure 5.36 Typhoid perforation of the terminal ileum.

nutritionally compromised and the body's defences are more robust. Furthermore, the shorter the interval between diagnosis and operation, the better is the prognosis (Summary box 5.23).

Summary box 5.23

Treatment of bowel perforation from typhoid

- Manage in intensive care
- Resuscitate and give intravenous antibiotics
- Laparotomy – choice of various procedures
- Commonest site of perforation is the terminal ileum
- Having found a perforation, always look for others
- In the very ill patient, consider some form of exteriorisation
- Close the peritoneum and leave the wound open for secondary closure

---

Further reading

Adeniran, J.O., Taiwo, J.O. and Abdur-Raham, L.O. (2005) Salmonella intestinal perforation (27 perforations in one patient, 14 perforations in another): are the goal posts changing? *J Indian Assoc Pediatr Surg* **10**: 248–51.

Aziz, M., Qadir, A., Aziz, M. and Faizullah (2005) Prognostic factors in typhoid perforation. *J Coll Phys Surg Pakistan* **15(11)**: 704–7.

Olsen, S.J., Pruckler, J., Bibb, W. *et al.* (2004) Evaluation of rapid diagnostic tests for typhoid fever. *J Clin Microbiol* **42(5)**: 1885–9.

CHAPTER

6

LEARNING OBJECTIVES

To recognise and understand:
- The important anatomical, physiological and psychological differences between adults and children
- The structured approach to managing children with major trauma

- The pathology and the principles of management of common paediatric surgical conditions
- The spectrum of congenital malformations relevant to general surgery

INTRODUCTION

Children are not small adults. They suffer from different disorders and their physical and psychological responses are different. Their capacity for adaptation is greater but they must endure any consequences of disease and its management for longer. In contrast to adults they rarely have comorbidity from degenerative diseases or lifestyle problems but they can suffer the unique consequences of congenital malformations. Children must be treated within the context of their families. This chapter focuses on aspects of paediatric surgery relevant to general surgery.

ANATOMY AND PHYSIOLOGY

Anatomical differences between adults and children are important in surgery. Infants and small children (Table 6.1) have a wider abdomen, a broader costal margin and a shallower pelvis. Thus, the edge of the liver is more easily palpable below the costal margin and the bladder is an intra-abdominal organ. The ribs are more horizontal and respiratory function is more dependent on diaphragmatic movement. The umbilicus is relatively low lying. In the small child, transverse supraumbilical incisions are preferred to vertical midline ones for laparotomy. Abdominal scars grow with the child and may migrate – a gastrostomy sited in the epigastrium of the infant may end up as a scar over the costal margin (Summary box 6.1).

Table 6.1 Common terms

Preterm	< 37 completed weeks of gestation
Full term	Between 37 and 42 completed weeks of gestation
Neonate	Newborn baby up to 28 days of age
Infant	Up to 1 year of age
Child	All ages up to 16 years but often divided into preschool child (usually < 5 years), child and adolescent (puberty up to 16 years)

Summary box 6.1

Anatomy of the paediatric abdomen

- The abdomen is wider and the bladder intra-abdominal
- Transverse supraumbilical incisions are preferred to vertical midline ones
- Scars may migrate during growth

Thermoregulation is important in children undergoing surgery. The body surface area to weight ratio decreases with age and small children therefore lose heat more rapidly. Babies have less subcutaneous fat and immature peripheral vasomotor control mechanisms. The operating theatre must be warm and the infant's head (which may account for up to 20% of the body surface area compared with 9% in an adult) should be insulated. Infusions and respiratory gases may need to be warmed. The central temperature should be monitored and a warm air blanket is advisable during lengthy operations.

Infants undergoing surgery are vulnerable in other ways. Impaired gluconeogenesis renders them more susceptible to hypoglycaemia; blood glucose must be monitored and maintained above 2.6 mmol l^{-1}. Newborns are at risk of clotting deficiencies and should be given intramuscular vitamin K before major surgery. They are less able to concentrate urine or conserve sodium and have a greater obligatory water loss to excrete a given solute load. Fluid and sodium requirements are relatively high. Infants are prone to gastro-oesophageal reflux and have less well-developed protective reflexes, rendering them more at risk of pulmonary aspiration; adequate nasogastric aspiration is essential in those with gastrointestinal obstruction. Immaturity of the immune system increases the risk of infection, which can present with non-specific features such as poor feeding, vomiting and listlessness (Summary box 6.2).

Summary box 6.2

Special features that must be considered in children when preparing for surgery

Problem	Action
Thermoregulation	Warm fluids, warm theatre, insulate child
Hypoglycaemia	Maintain glucose above 2.6 mmol l^{-1}
Clotting	Give intramuscular vitamin K preoperatively to neonates
Fluid and electrolyte balance	Allow for higher sodium and fluid needs
Less postoperative catabolism	Relatively lower postoperative energy requirements
Gastro-oesophageal reflux	Use a nasogastric tube to prevent aspiration
Atypical presentations of infection	High index of suspicion
Psychology	Trained staff, day surgery for minor operations

Table 6.2 Basic paediatric data

(a) Weight

Age	Weight (kg)
Term neonate	3.5
1 year	10
5 years	20
10 years	30

Approximate guide: weight (kg) = 2 × (age in years + 4).

(b) Vital signs

Age (years)	Heart rate (beats min^{-1})	Systolic blood pressure (mmHg)	Respiratory rate (breaths min^{-1})
< 1	110–160	70–90	30–40
2–5	90–140	80–100	25–30
5–12	80–120	90–110	20–25

Systolic blood pressure ≈ 80 + (age in years × 2) mmHg.
Circulating blood volume ≈ 80 ml kg^{-1} (90 ml kg^{-1} in infants).

(c) Maintenance fluid requirements

Weight	Daily fluid requirement (ml kg^{-1} day^{-1})
Neonate	120–150
First 10 kg	100
Second 10 kg	50
Subsequent kg	20

(d) Maintenance electrolyte requirements

Weight	Sodium (mmol kg^{-1} 1 day^{-1})	Potassium (mmol kg^{-1} 1 day^{-1})	Energy (kcal kg^{-1} day^{-1})
< 10 kg	2–4	1.5–2.5	110
> 10 kg	1–2	0.5–1.0	40–75

Small bowel length in a term infant (duodenojejunal flexure to ileocaecal valve) ≈ 275 cm (adult length is almost 6 m).

The surgical management of children requires a working knowledge of normal weights, vital signs and fluid and electrolyte requirements at different ages (Table 6.2). Moderate (5–10%) dehydration is manifest by a decreased urine output, dry mouth, and sunken eyes and fontanelle. Severe dehydration (> 10%) causes decreased skin turgor, drowsiness, tachycardia and signs of hypovolaemia. Body weight is a critical measurement in children, not least because this is a major determinant of drug doses and fluid balance. Serial measures of weight and height provide a valuable index of general growth and nutrition (Fig. 6.1). Impaired growth is an important sign of disease in children and may be the dominant presenting feature in an adolescent with Crohn's disease. Delay in achieving normal developmental milestones can also be an indicator of ill health in children.

HISTORY AND EXAMINATION

The history should include details of any prenatal or neonatal problems as well as the relevant family medical and social background. Time, patience and a genuine interest are required to gain a rapport with the child and his/her parents or carers. Children should be told what to expect from an examination, investigation or surgical procedure in terms that they can understand. Fear, anxiety and pain can be reduced by involving parents and carers and by looking after the child in an appropriate environment with play facilities. Nursing and medical staff must be attuned to the needs of children. General health concerns are best discussed with a paediatrician, as is any concern about child abuse or neglect.

PRINCIPLES OF OPERATIVE SURGERY

Operative paediatric surgery demands meticulous and gentle technique, strict haemostasis, fine suture materials (with or without magnification aids) and attention to surgical principles,

Burrill Bernard Crohn, **1884–1983**, Gastroenterologist, Mount Sinai Hospital, New York, NY, USA, described regional ileitis in 1932.

e.g. maintaining well-vascularised tissues, avoiding tension and minimising tissue necrosis and contamination. Bipolar diathermy is particularly useful. Anatomy in children is clearer than in adults because there is less fat and the tissues are better demarcated.

Postoperatively, children often recover more quickly than adults. Postoperative analgesia must be adequate and appropriate, recognising the potential for respiratory depression with opioids. Nursing care by appropriately trained staff involves monitoring the airway and vital signs together with arterial oxygen saturation, fluid balance, temperature, pain control and glucose homeostasis. Maintenance intravenous fluids, e.g. 0.45% saline with 2.5% dextrose or isotonic saline, are being increasingly used instead of more hypotonic saline solutions to reduce the risk of iatrogenic hyponatraemia. Neonates require intravenous fluids with higher concentrations of glucose.

Abdominal wounds in infants and children can be safely closed with absorbable sutures using either a layered or mass closure technique. Non-absorbable sutures may occasionally be necessary, such as in the malnourished adolescent on steroids for inflammatory bowel disease. Wound dehiscence is rare and

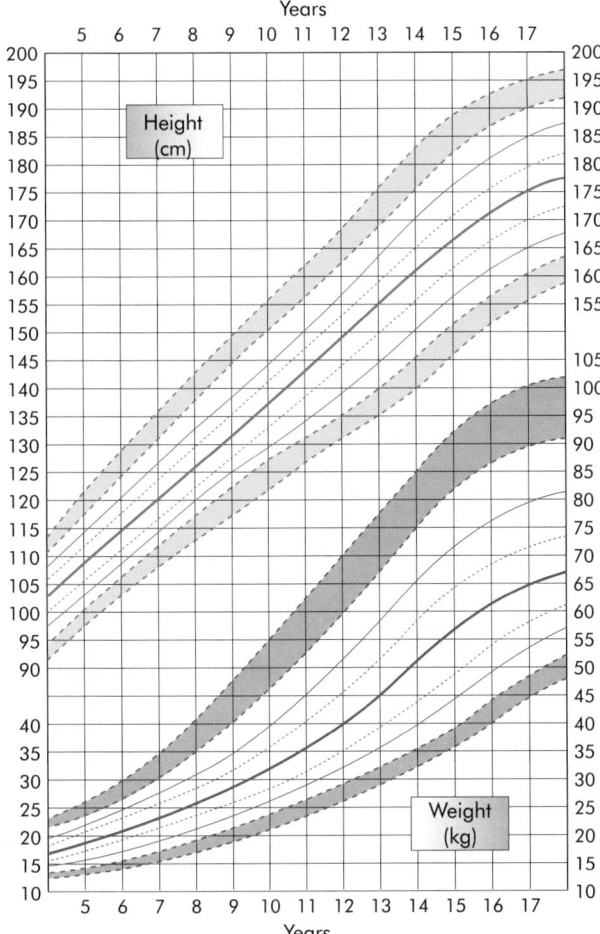

Figure 6.1 Growth chart for boys aged 5–18 years using the nine centile UK chart (Chart © Child Growth Foundation, reproduced with permission).

almost always the result of poor surgical technique. The use of single-layer interrupted extramucosal sutures for intestinal anastomosis is safe and effective. Clean skin incisions are best closed with absorbable subcuticular sutures. Surgical stapling devices are frequently used in paediatric gastrointestinal and thoracic surgery but staple lines should be oversewn. Endoscopic minimally invasive approaches can be used at all ages to achieve the same advantages as in adults, but instruments and insufflation pressures must be tailored to the size of the child (Summary box 6.3).

Summary box 6.3

Special features of surgical technique in children

- Gentle tissue handling
- Bipolar diathermy is preferred to unipolar during dissection
- Abdominal incisions can be closed with absorbable sutures
- Bowel can be anastomosed with interrupted single-layer extramucosal sutures
- Skin can be closed with absorbable subcuticular sutures

Stomas are necessary in some children. A gastrostomy may be required for nutritional support, particularly in the neurologically disabled child. Temporary intestinal stomas are used in the management of anorectal malformations, necrotising enterocolitis and Hirschsprung's disease; infants with a proximal colostomy or ileostomy frequently require salt supplements to avoid sodium deficiency, which causes poor weight gain.

Surgeons who operate on children should consider the long-term outcomes, i.e. the effects of surgical disease and its treatment during maturation and adult life. For example, ileal resection in the neonate may later be complicated by vitamin B12 deficiency, malabsorption of fat-soluble vitamins, gallstones, renal oxalate stones and, rarely, perianastomotic ulceration. Long-term concerns include the potential impact of surgical conditions and their treatment on future function (e.g. continence); fertility and sexuality; inheritance risks; psychosocial adaptation; and the potential risk of late malignancy (e.g. undescended testis, choledochal cyst, duplication cyst).

PAEDIATRIC TRAUMA

Trauma is a leading cause of death in children and adolescents in western countries. Many of these deaths are avoidable if prompt and effective treatment is given.

Primary survey

The structured approach to the child with major injuries advocated by the Advanced Trauma Life Support (ATLS) programmes is essential. The focus of the primary survey is on the *a*irway and cervical spine, *b*reathing, circulation and the control of bleeding, the assessment of conscious level, pupil size and reactivity and a rapid overview of all injuries. The shorter neck and relatively larger tongue of the child mean that respiratory obstruction will occur if the neck is overextended during maintenance of the airway. The assessment of breathing includes respiratory rate, signs of distress and the adequacy of chest expansion. The circulation is evaluated from vital signs, capillary refill time (normally ≤ 2 s), skin colour and temperature, and mental status. Normal ranges for heart rate, systolic blood pressure and respiratory rate are age-dependent (Table 6.2). Systolic blood pressure is often normal until at least 25% of the circulating blood volume has been lost.

Resuscitation

Life-threatening problems are treated as they are identified during the primary survey. High-flow oxygen should be provided in any patient with cardiorespiratory compromise. Endotracheal intubation and ventilation are required if oxygenation is inadequate, to control a flail chest or in children with a serious head injury (Glasgow Coma Score ≤ 8). Pneumothorax and haemothorax are treated by chest tube drainage. Seriously injured children require two large peripheral intravenous cannulae; additional sites of venous access include the long saphenous vein at the ankle, the femoral vein, the external jugular vein and, in babies, the scalp veins. Central venous access should only be attempted by an expert. Intraosseous infusion is particularly useful in small children (Fig. 6.2) (Summary box 6.4).

The Glasgow Coma Score was introduced in 1977 by William Bryan Jennet, Professor of Neurosurgery and Graham Michael Teasdale, a Neurosurgeon of the University Department of Neurosurgery, at the Institute of Neurological Sciences, The Southern General Hospital, Glasgow, Scotland.

Summary box 6.4

Fluid resuscitation of the hypovolaemic child after trauma

- Infuse 10 ml kg^{-1} of normal saline or colloid
  ⇓
- Assess cardiovascular response
  ⇓
- Infuse 10 ml kg^{-1} of normal saline or colloid
  ⇓
- Assess cardiovascular response
  ⇓
- Repeat if necessary
  ⇓
- If still hypovolaemic after a total of 40 ml kg^{-1} of crystalloid, transfuse packed red cells and consider urgent surgery

---

During resuscitation, details of the injury and past medical history are sought. Baseline blood tests and radiographs of the cervical spine (lateral), chest and pelvis are obtained. A major spinal cord injury can be present in a child without radiographic abnormalities and, after major trauma, a cervical spine injury should be assumed until it can be excluded by full neurological assessment; the neck must be immobilised. Other considerations include use of intravenous analgesia and, in the unconscious or ventilated child or those with major abdominal injuries, a nasogastric tube (orogastric if suspicion of a basal frontal skull fracture) and urethral catheter (if no evidence of urethral injury).

Secondary survey and emergency management

In a stable patient, the secondary survey attempts to identify all injuries in a systematic way by detailed clinical examination and appropriate investigations. Emergency treatment of chest and abdominal injuries is as follows:

- *Chest.* Children have relatively elastic ribs that rarely fracture. Lung contusion is common. A major thoracic injury may exist despite a normal chest radiograph. In all cases the airway is secured, oxygen is given and hypovolaemia is corrected with intravenous fluids. Tension pneumothorax requires prompt clinical diagnosis and immediate needle thoracocentesis (second intercostal space, mid-clavicular line) followed by chest tube drainage. Massive haemothorax is treated by chest tube drainage (fifth intercostal space, mid-axillary line). Cardiac tamponade may follow blunt or penetrating injury and requires emergency needle pericardiocentesis. Diaphragmatic rupture after blunt abdominal trauma is detected by chest radiography or computerised tomography (CT) scan; surgical repair is undertaken once the patient is stable.

- *Abdomen.* Blunt trauma is generally more common than penetrating injuries. The liver and spleen are more vulnerable in children because they are less well protected by the pliable rib cage. The abdomen must be carefully inspected for signs of patterned bruising, which indicates forceful compression against a rigid skeleton. Intra-abdominal or intrathoracic bleeding is likely in the shocked child with no obvious source of haemorrhage. Plasma amylase levels should be measured but may be normal despite pancreatic injury. The definitive radiological investigation of major abdominal trauma in the haemodynamically stable child is a CT scan with intravenous contrast (Fig. 6.3). When expert ultrasound scanning is readily available it can demonstrate free intra-abdominal fluid and solid organ injuries but it is not as sensitive and specific as CT. Diagnostic peritoneal lavage is obsolete in children because modern imaging is superior and the presence of intraperitoneal blood is not by itself a reason for laparotomy. Bowel perforation or deep penetrating trauma are indications for laparotomy.

Isolated splenic and/or liver injury can be safely and effectively managed non-operatively in the majority of children with blunt abdominal trauma; haemorrhage is frequently self-limiting. Unnecessary surgery and the long-term risks of splenectomy can be avoided.

Successful non-operative management of isolated blunt liver or spleen trauma requires:

- haemodynamic stability after resuscitation with no more than 40–60 ml kg^{-1} of fluid;
- a good-quality CT scan;
- no evidence of hollow visceral injury;
- frequent, careful monitoring and immediate availability of necessary surgical expertise/facilities.

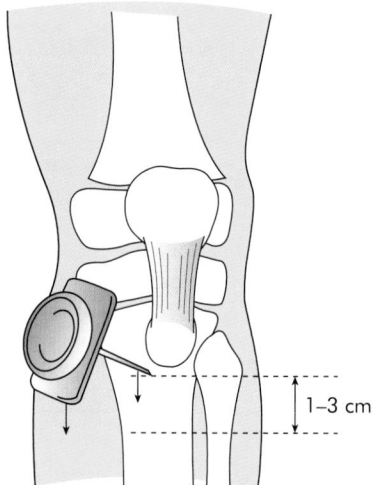

Figure 6.2 The intraosseous needle is inserted into the medullary cavity of the proximal tibia about 1–3 cm below the tibial tuberosity.

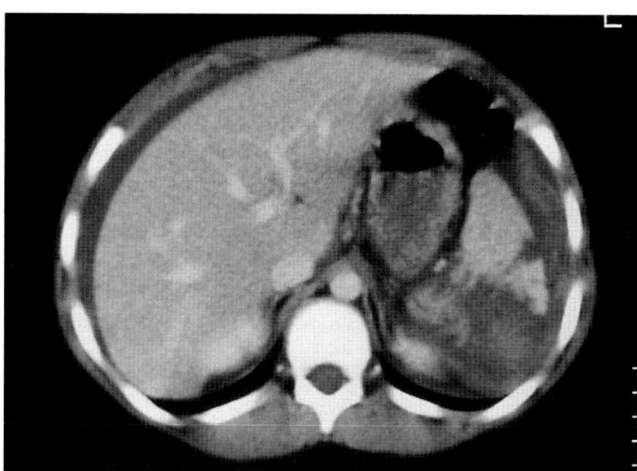

Figure 6.3 Abdominal computerised tomography scan after intravenous contrast in an 11-year-old boy showing a ruptured spleen (successfully managed non-operatively).

Children with ongoing intra-abdominal bleeding require laparotomy, but preliminary angiography and arterial embolisation can be useful in some cases of hepatic trauma. Bile leaks are uncommon and can usually be managed with radiological techniques. Uncomplicated non-operative cases of liver/spleen trauma can be discharged home after 5 days but activity should be restricted for 3–6 weeks and contact sports avoided for 2–3 months. Blunt renal trauma is also generally managed conservatively but an acutely non-functioning kidney following abdominal trauma may need urgent exploration with a view to revascularisation.

Patterns of injury

Patterns of injury often reflect the mechanism. For example, lap belt trauma from a motor vehicle crash may cause injury to the duodenum or jejunum and lumbar spine, bicycle handlebar injuries are associated with pancreatic or liver trauma (Fig. 6.4), straddle injuries may damage the urethra and pelvis, and run-over injuries may cause severe crushing of the chest and/or abdomen. Non-accidental injury must be considered if any of the following are present: multiple injuries at different stages of healing; different types of injury (e.g. soft tissue, fractures, burns or scalds, cuts and bruises); significant delay between the injury and seeking medical advice; an inconsistent or vague history; or inappropriate parental behaviour. Liaison with a paediatrician is essential in such cases (Summary box 6.5).

Summary box 6.5

Paediatric trauma

- Use ATLS principles
- Overextension of the neck will compromise the airway
- Cervical spine injury can be present without radiographic signs
- Intraosseous vascular access is helpful in small children
- Lung contusion can occur without rib fractures
- Patterned skin bruising suggests underlying organ injury
- In a stable child, abdominal injuries are best assessed by CT
- Isolated liver or splenic injury can usually be managed non-operatively

---

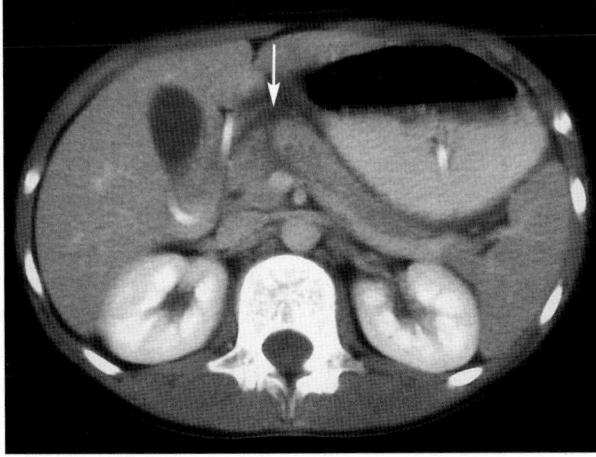

Figure 6.4 Abdominal computerised tomography scan showing a transection through the neck of the pancreas (arrow) from a bicycle handlebar injury.

COMMON PAEDIATRIC SURGICAL CONDITIONS

Inguinoscrotal disorders

Embryology

Most genital abnormalities in boys are the result of abnormal development. The testis develops from the urogenital ridge on the posterior abdominal wall. Gonadal induction to form a testis is regulated by genes on the Y chromosome. During gestation, the testis migrates down towards the internal ring, guided by mesenchymal tissue (gubernaculum). Inguinoscrotal descent of the testis is mediated by testosterone from the fetal testis. A tongue of peritoneum precedes the migrating testis through the inguinal canal (the processus vaginalis). This peritoneal pouch normally becomes obliterated after birth but failure of this process can lead to the development of an inguinal hernia or hydrocele (Fig. 6.5).

Inguinal hernia

Inguinal hernias in children are almost always indirect and due to a patent processus vaginalis. They are much more frequent in boys, especially if born prematurely. An inguinal hernia will develop in at least one in 50 boys and about 15% are bilateral. Rarely, bilateral inguinal hernias in a phenotypic girl may be the presenting feature of androgen insensitivity syndrome (testicular feminisation) and the hernia sac may then contain a testis.

An inguinal hernia typically causes an intermittent swelling in the groin or scrotum on crying or straining (Fig. 6.6). Unless an inguinal swelling is observed, diagnosis relies on the history and the presence of palpable thickening of the spermatic cord (or round ligament in girls). Some inguinal hernias present as a firm, tender, irreducible lump in the groin or scrotum as a result of obstruction by the external ring. The infant may be vomiting and irritable. Most incarcerated hernias in children can be successfully reduced by sustained gentle compression ('taxis') aided by cautious analgesia. Surgery is delayed for 24 hours to allow resolution of oedema. If reduction is impossible, emergency surgery is required because of the risk of strangulation of bowel (or ovary) and/or damage to the testis.

Inguinal herniotomy is performed via an inguinal skin crease incision and involves dissection, division and proximal ligation of the hernial sac. This is not a minor procedure in a neonate. In older infants, inguinal herniotomy is usually undertaken as a day-case operation provided that there is appropriate anaesthetic expertise (Summary box 6.6).

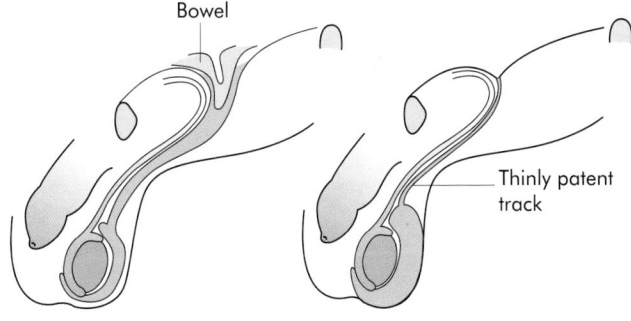

(a) Inguinal hernia   (b) Hydrocele

Figure 6.5 Inguinal hernia (a) and hydrocele (b) in children are the result of incomplete obliteration of the processus vaginalis.

CHAPTER 6 | PRINCIPLES OF PAEDIATRIC SURGERY

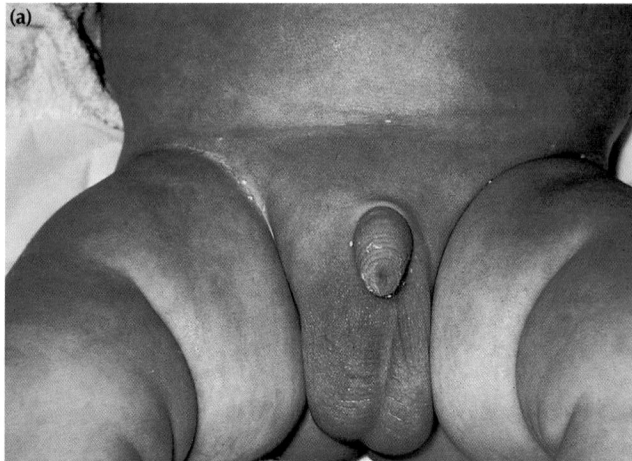

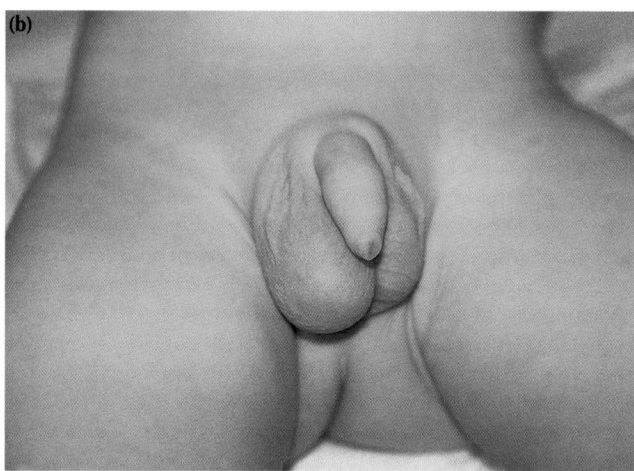

Figure 6.6 (a) An infant with a right inguinal hernia (the swelling is partially obscured by suprapubic fat) and (b) a boy with a right hydrocele.

Summary box 6.6

Inguinal hernias

- More common in premature boys
- 15% are bilateral
- Almost always indirect with a patent processus vaginalis
- Present with a groin lump that appears on straining or crying
- Incarcerated hernias can usually be reduced with gentle pressure
- If reduction is impossible emergency surgery is needed
- In infants, they must be repaired promptly to prevent the risk of strangulation
- The hernial sac is isolated then ligated and divided proximally

---

Hydrocele

A patent processus vaginalis that is too narrow to prevent the development of an inguinal hernia may nevertheless allow peritoneal fluid to track down around the testis to form a hydrocele. Hydroceles are unilateral or bilateral, asymptomatic, non-tender scrotal swellings. They may be tense or lax but typically transilluminate. The majority resolve spontaneously as the processus

continues to obliterate but surgical ligation is recommended in boys older than 2 years.

Undescended testis

This occurs when the testis is arrested along its normal pathway of descent. At birth, about 4% of full-term boys have unilateral or bilateral undescended testes (cryptorchidism), but by 3 months of age this figure is 1.5% and it changes little thereafter. The incidence is higher in preterm infants because the testis descends through the inguinal canal during the third trimester of pregnancy. Examination of the testes should be performed with warm hands once the boy has relaxed. The testis is usually palpable after gently massaging the contents of the inguinal canal towards the scrotum.

A *retractile* testis is typically present in the scrotum in early infancy; it can be manipulated into the bottom of the scrotum without tension but tends to be pulled up by the cremaster muscle. With time, the testis resides permanently in the scrotum; however, follow-up is advisable as, rarely, the testis subsequently ascends into the inguinal canal. An *ectopic* testis lies outside its normal line of descent, most often in the perineum or femoral triangle. An *undescended* testis may be palpable in the groin or at the neck of the scrotum or it may be impalpable if absent or located in the abdomen or inguinal canal.

Useful investigations include:

- *laparoscopy* – the optimum method of visualising the anatomy (Fig. 6.7);
- *ultrasound scan* – this has a limited role in detecting an inguinal testis in an obese boy;
- *hormonal* – in cases of bilateral impalpable testes, the presence of testicular tissue can be confirmed by recording a rise in serum testosterone in response to intramuscular injections of human chorionic gonadotrophin; these boys require specialist endocrine review.

Orchidopexy is usually undertaken as a day-case procedure. The testis is mobilised through an inguinal incision, preserving the vas deferens and testicular vessels. The associated patent processus vaginalis is ligated and divided and the testis is placed in a subdartos scrotal pouch. Orchidectomy is often advised for the

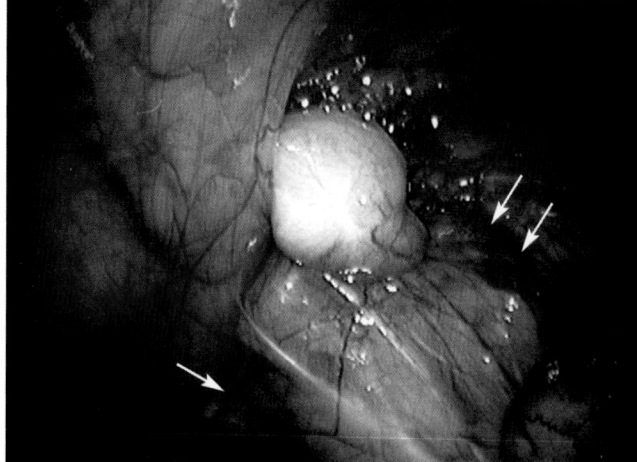

Figure 6.7 Laparoscopic view of a right-sided intra-abdominal testis visible at the internal ring. Vas (single arrow) and testicular vessels (double arrow).

unilateral intra-abdominal testis, which cannot be corrected by orchidopexy because of the future risk of malignancy. In cases of bilateral intra-abdominal testes, microvascular transfer and staged orchidopexy are two options available to preserve the testes if the testicular vessels are too short to permit a single-stage orchidopexy. The benefits of orchidopexy include:

- *Fertility.* To optimise spermatogenesis the testis needs to be in the scrotum below body temperature at a young age. Orchidopexy during the second year of life is currently recommended by paediatric surgeons. Fertility after orchidopexy for a unilateral undescended testis is near normal. Men with a history of bilateral intra-abdominal testes are usually sterile.
- *Malignancy.* Undescended testes are histologically abnormal and at an increased risk of malignancy. The greatest risk is for bilateral intra-abdominal testes. Early orchidopexy for a unilateral undescended testis may reduce the risk but this is not proven.
- *Cosmetic and psychological.* In an older boy a prosthetic testis can be inserted to replace an absent one (Summary box 6.7).

Summary box 6.7

The undescended testis

- A retractile testis can be drawn down into the bottom of the scrotum
- An undescended testis may be in the groin or impalpable in the abdomen
- An ectopic testis lies outside the normal line of descent
- Orchidopexy involves mobilising the testis and placing it in a subdartos pouch
- Orchidopexy before 2 years of age improves fertility, may reduce the risk of malignancy and has psychological benefits

---

The acute scrotum

Testicular torsion is most common in adolescents but may occur at any age, including in the perinatal period. The pain is not always centred on the scrotum but may be felt in the groin or lower abdomen. Oedema and erythema of the scrotal skin can be absent. Sometimes there is a history of previous transient episodes. Torsion of the testis must be relieved within 6–8 hours of the onset of symptoms for there to be a good chance of testicular salvage. At operation, viability of the testis is assessed after derotation. Three-point fixation of the contralateral testis with non-absorbable sutures corrects any anatomical predisposition to torsion (e.g. the bell-clapper testis). Expert assessment of testicular blood flow by colour Doppler ultrasound may help in the differential diagnosis but the scrotum must be explored urgently if torsion cannot be excluded.

A hydatid of Morgagni is an embryological remnant found on the upper pole of the testis. *Torsion of a testicular appendage* characteristically affects boys just before puberty (Fig. 6.8), possibly because of enlargement of the hydatid in response to gonadotrophins. The pain often increases over a day or two. Occasionally, the torted hydatid can be felt or seen (blue dot sign). Excision of the appendage leads to rapid resolution of

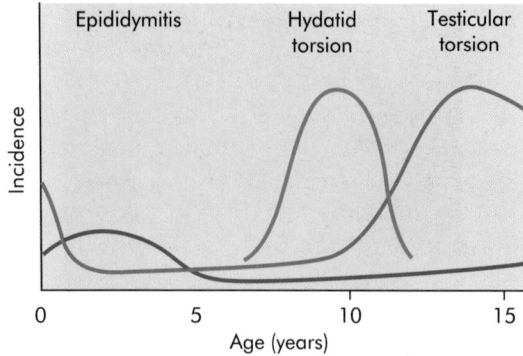

Figure 6.8 Acute scrotal pathology at different ages.

symptoms. Viral or bacterial *epididymo-orchitis* may cause an acute scrotum in infants and toddlers but the diagnosis is often only made after scrotal exploration. Other conditions that rarely cause acute scrotal symptoms and signs include idiopathic scrotal oedema (typically painless, bilateral inguinoscrotal redness and swelling in a young boy), an incarcerated inguinal hernia, vasculitis or a scrotal haematoma (Summary box 6.8).

Summary box 6.8

Diagnosis and treatment of the acute scrotum

- Torsion of the testis must be assumed until proven otherwise
- Testicular torsion can present with acute inguinal or abdominal pain
- Urgent surgical exploration is crucial if testicular torsion cannot be excluded
- Torsion of a testicular appendage usually occurs just before puberty
- An incarcerated inguinal hernia must be considered in the differential diagnosis

---

Abnormalities of the penis

Hypospadias

Failure of complete urethral tubularisation in the male fetus results in hypospadias, a common congenital anomaly affecting about one in every 200–300 boys. In most cases the urethra opens just proximal to the glans penis but in severe cases the meatus may be on the penile shaft or in the perineum. The dorsal foreskin is hooded and there is a variable degree of chordee (a ventral curvature of the penis most apparent on erection) (Fig. 6.9). Glanular hypospadias may be a solely cosmetic concern but more proximal varieties interfere with micturition and erection. In severe forms of hypospadias, additional genitourinary anomalies and intersex disorders should be excluded. Surgical correction of distal hypospadias is frequently undertaken before 2 years of age, often as a single-stage operation. Proximal varieties may require complex staged procedures. Surgery aims to achieve a terminal urethral meatus so that the boy can stand to micturate with a normal stream, a straight erection and a penis that looks normal.

Ritual circumcision must be avoided in infants with hypospadias because the foreskin is often required for later reconstructive surgery.

Giovanni Battista Morgagni, **1682–1771, Professor of Anatomy, Padua, Italy for 59 years. He is regarded as 'The Founder of Morbid Anatomy'.**

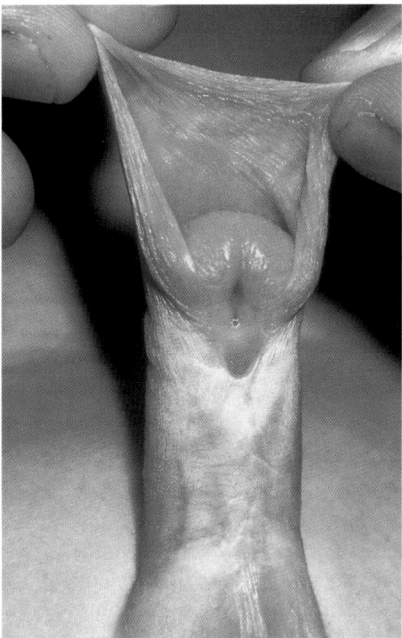

Figure 6.9 Hypospadias – note the hooded foreskin and the ventral meatus.

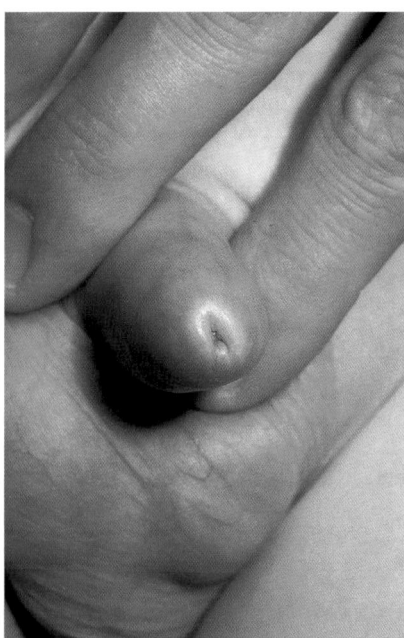

Figure 6.10 True phimosis from balanitis xerotica obliterans.

Circumcision

At birth, the foreskin is adherent to the glans penis. These adhesions separate spontaneously with time, allowing the foreskin to become retractile. At 1 year of age, about 50% of boys have a non-retractile foreskin. By 4 years this has declined to 10% and by 16 years to just 1%. Ballooning of the normal non-retractile foreskin may occur with micturition. Gentle retraction of the foreskin at bath times helps to maintain hygiene but forcible retraction should never be attempted. The presence of preputial adhesions, when the foreskin remains partially adherent to the glans, is normal and resolves spontaneously.

Circumcision is one of the earliest recorded operations and remains an important tradition in some cultures. Routine neonatal circumcision is performed in some western societies but the practice has been increasingly criticised. Proponents point out that circumcision reduces the incidence of urinary tract infection in infant boys; however, circumcision is not without risk of significant morbidity. The medical indications for circumcision are:

- *Phimosis.* This term is often wrongly applied to describe a normal, non-retractile foreskin. True phimosis is seen as a whitish scarring of the foreskin and is rare before 5 years of age (Fig. 6.10). It is caused by a localised skin disease known as balanitis xerotica obliterans, which also affects the glans penis and can cause urethral meatal stenosis.
- *Recurrent balanoposthitis.* A single episode of inflammation of the foreskin, sometimes with a purulent discharge, is not uncommon and usually resolves spontaneously; antibiotics are sometimes needed. Recurrent attacks are unusual but may be an indication for circumcision.
- *Recurrent urinary tract infection.* Circumcision is occasionally justified in boys with an abnormal upper urinary tract and recurrent urinary infection. It may also help boys with spina bifida who need to perform clean intermittent urethral catheterisation.

An emerging and still controversial indication for circumcision is in the prevention of sexually acquired human immunodeficiency virus (HIV) infection in communities where this disease is common; large clinical trials have recently shown that circumcision reduces the risk of HIV transmission.

Circumcision for medical reasons is best performed under general anaesthesia. A long-acting local anaesthetic regional block can be given to reduce postoperative pain. Circumcision is not a trivial operation; bleeding and infection are well-recognised complications and more serious hazards, such as injury to the glans, may occur if the procedure is not carried out by adequately trained personnel (Summary box 6.9).

Summary box 6.9

Circumcision

- Medical indications are phimosis and recurrent balanoposthitis
- Circumcision is not indicated for an otherwise healthy non-retractile foreskin
- Complications include bleeding and damage to the glans

Umbilical hernia

In the embryo the umbilical ring is a relatively large defect in the ventral abdominal wall transmitting several structures that subsequently connect the fetus to the placenta (Fig. 6.11). An umbilical hernia is common and caused by incomplete closure of the umbilical ring. Most resolve spontaneously within a year or two of birth and surgical repair is rarely necessary. Incarceration in an umbilical hernia is rare.

Infantile hypertrophic pyloric stenosis

In this acquired disorder, hypertrophy of the circular muscle layer increases the length and diameter of the pylorus. Boys are

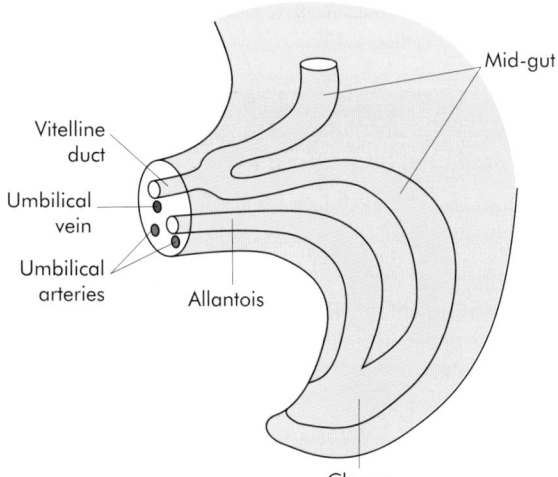

Figure 6.11 The embryonic umbilical ring; both the vitelline duct and the allantois can leave remnants (Meckel's diverticulum and urachus respectively).

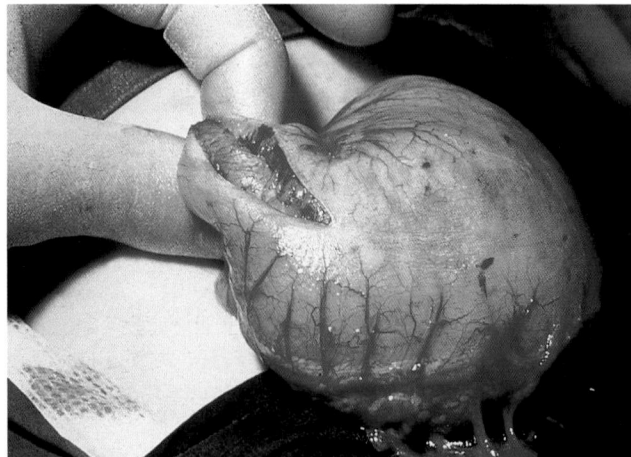

Figure 6.12 Pyloromyotomy for infantile hypertrophic pyloric stenosis.

affected four times more commonly than girls. The incidence is variable but in the UK it affects about three in every 1000 live-born infants. The aetiology is unknown but in some families there is a strong genetic predisposition. Infantile hypertrophic pyloric stenosis (IHPS) is classically associated with projectile vomiting between 2 and 8 weeks of age; it is rare after 3 months of age. Typically, the baby feeds hungrily and vomits non-bilious milk curds towards the end of a feed.

In most cases, IHPS can be diagnosed clinically. During a test feed there is visible gastric peristalsis passing from left to right across the upper abdomen and in a relaxed baby the pyloric 'tumour' is palpable as an 'olive' in the epigastrium or right upper quadrant. The diagnosis can be confirmed by an ultrasound scan, which shows the thickened pyloric muscle. IHPS is readily treated by surgery but the infant must first be adequately rehydrated and electrolyte/acid–base disturbances corrected; this may take 48 hours or more. IHPS classically causes a hypo-chloraemic alkalosis, the severity of which is related to the length of the history. Mild dehydration and alkalosis can be corrected by giving maintenance fluids (120–150 ml kg⁻¹ day⁻¹) of 0.45% saline with 5% dextrose containing 20 mmol of potassium chloride per litre. Extra fluid is needed to correct more severe dehydration. Oral feeding is discontinued and the stomach emptied with an 8–10 Fr nasogastric tube; on-going gastric losses should be replaced with normal saline containing potassium chloride. Blood glucose must be monitored and maintained.

Ramstedt's pyloromyotomy is performed under general anaes-thesia with endotracheal intubation and muscle relaxation. Via a transverse right upper quadrant muscle cutting incision, the pyloric tumour is delivered by gentle traction on the stomach. A serosal incision is made anterosuperiorly from the pyloroduodenal junction, where the muscle layer is thin, to the gastric antrum (Fig. 6.12). This region is relatively avascular. The pyloric muscle, which has a gritty consistency, is then separated widely down to the submucosa using artery forceps. The end result should be an

Wilhelm Conrad Ramstedt, **1867–1963, Surgeon, The Rafaelklinik, Münster, Germany, performed his first pyloromyotomy in 1911.**

intact bulging submucosa from duodenal fornix to gastric antrum. Perforation of the duodenal fornix is uncommon and not serious provided that it is recognised and repaired immediately. Minor bleeding as a result of venous congestion stops spontaneously but occasionally a larger gastric serosal vessel needs cautious diathermy coagulation. With experience, pyloromyotomy can be safely performed through a circumumbilical incision or laparo-scope with superior cosmesis.

Postoperatively, intravenous fluids are continued until oral feeding is re-established within 24 hours. Minor, transient vomit-ing is common and self-limiting. Surgical complications such as duodenal perforation, haemorrhage, wound infection and wound dehiscence are uncommon and avoidable. Pyloromyotomy has no significant long-term sequelae (Summary box 6.10).

Summary box 6.10

Infantile hypertrophic pyloric stenosis

- Most commonly affects boys aged 2–8 weeks
- Characterised by projectile vomiting after feeds
- Gastric peristalsis can be seen and a lump felt
- Fluid and electrolyte disturbances must be corrected before surgery
- Pyloromyotomy splits the hypertrophied muscle leaving the mucosa intact

Other common or serious causes of vomiting in infancy are shown in Table 6.3. Gastro-oesophageal reflux is common and tends to resolve spontaneously with maturity. Persistent symptoms require treatment with thickened feeds and anti-reflux medication. Complications such as failure to thrive or respiratory problems demand further investigation and, in some cases, fundoplication.

Intussusception

Intussusception, the invagination of one portion of the intestine into an adjacent segment, is uncommon but may be life-threaten-ing. Intussusception typically causes a strangulating bowel obstruction, which can progress to gangrene and perforation (Fig. 6.13). Intussusception is classified according to the site of the inner intussusceptum and outer intussuscipiens. In children,

Table 6.3 Vomiting in infancy

Bile-stained		
Neonate	Intestinal malrotation with volvulus	
	Duodenal/intestinal atresia/stenosis	
	Hirschsprung's disease	
	Necrotising enterocolitis	
	Incarcerated inguinal hernia	
	Meconium ileus	
Older infant	Intestinal malrotation with volvulus	
	Intussusception (often non-bilious initially)	
	Incarcerated inguinal hernia	
Non-bilious	Infantile hypertrophic pyloric stenosis	
	Gastro-oesophageal reflux	
	Feeding difficulties (technique/volume)	
	Non-specific marker of illness, e.g. infection (urinary tract infection, meningitis, gastroenteritis, respiratory), metabolic disorder, raised intracranial pressure, congenital adrenal hyperplasia, etc.	

more than 80% are ileocolic, beginning several centimetres proximal to the ileocaecal valve with their apex in the ascending or transverse colon.

In the majority of affected infants, intussusception is caused by hyperplasia of gut lymphoid tissue, which may in turn be secondary to viral infection. In 10% of children, intussusception is secondary to a pathological lead point such as a Meckel's diverticulum, enteric duplication cyst or even small bowel lymphoma. Such cases are more likely in children over the age of 2 years and in those with recurrent intussusception.

Intussusception can develop at any age and affect either sex but the peak incidence is between 5 and 10 months of age. Classically, a previously healthy infant presents with colicky pain and vomiting (milk then bile). Between episodes the child initially appears well. Later, they may pass a 'redcurrant jelly' stool. Clinical signs include dehydration, abdominal distension and a palpable sausage-shaped mass in the right upper quadrant. Rectal

examination may reveal blood or rarely the apex of an intussusceptum (Summary box 6.11).

Summary box 6.11

Presentation of intussusception

- Bilious vomiting in an infant is a sign of intestinal obstruction until proved otherwise
- Intussusception classically presents with colicky pain and vomiting
- Intussusception should be considered in any infant with bloody stools
- Peak incidence is between 5 and 10 months of age

A plain radiograph commonly shows signs of small bowel obstruction and a soft-tissue opacity. Diagnosis can be confirmed by an abdominal ultrasound scan or contrast enema. After resuscitation with intravenous fluids, broad-spectrum antibiotics and nasogastric drainage, non-operative reduction of the intussusception can be attempted using an air or barium enema (Fig. 6.14). Successful reduction can only be accepted if there is free reflux of barium or air into the small bowel, together with resolution of symptoms and signs in the patient. Non-operative reduction is contraindicated if there are signs of peritonitis or perforation, with a known pathological lead point or in the presence of profound shock. In experienced units, more than 70% of intussusceptions can be reduced non-operatively. Strangulated bowel and pathological lead points are unlikely to reduce. Perforation of the colon during pneumatic or hydrostatic reduction is a recognised hazard but is rare. Recurrent intussusception

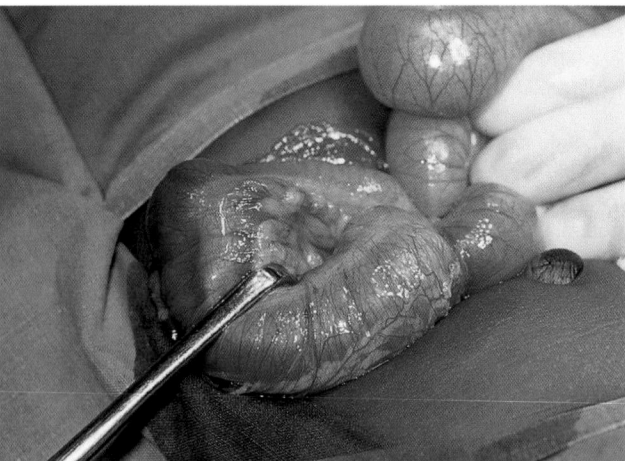

Figure 6.13 Operative appearances of an ileocolic intussusception causing small bowel obstruction.

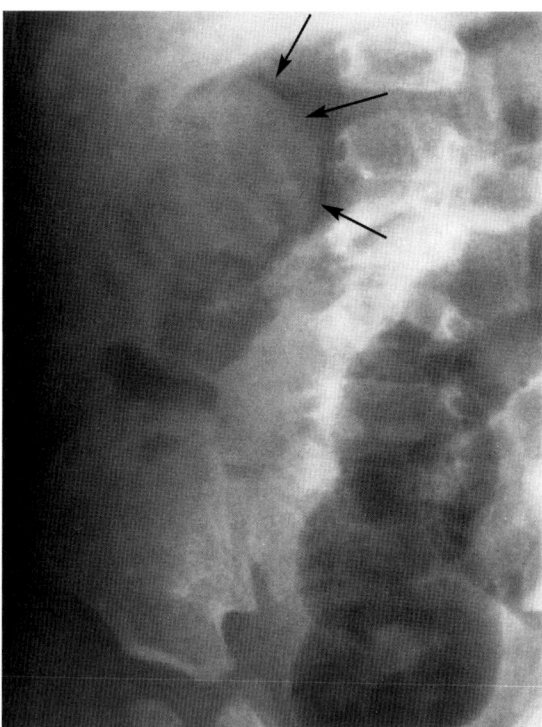

Figure 6.14 Air enema reduction of an intussusception (the arrows mark the soft tissue shadow of the intussusceptum).

occurs in up to 10% of patients after non-operative reduction (Summary box 6.12).

If non-operative reduction is contraindicated or unsuccessful, or if a pathological lead point is suspected, surgery is necessary. Via a right-sided transverse abdominal incision the intussusception is milked back by gentle compression from its apex. Both the intussusceptum and the intussuscipiens must be carefully inspected for areas of non-viability. An irreducible intussusception or one complicated by infarction or a pathological lead point requires resection and primary anastomosis.

Acute abdominal pain

Between one-third and one-half of children admitted to hospital with acute abdominal pain have non-specific abdominal pain. Another one-third have acute appendicitis. Relatively benign conditions such as constipation and urinary tract infection account for most of the remainder. A small proportion of children have more serious pathology.

History and examination

Time and patience are required to accurately evaluate the child with acute abdominal pain. The child is frightened and the parents are worried. Young children find it difficult to accurately describe or localise abdominal pain. The abdomen must be thoroughly inspected and, if necessary, repeatedly reassessed after analgesia. The genitalia, chest and neck must also be examined. A gentle abdominal examination of the sleeping toddler, before removing their clothes, may reveal tenderness, guarding or a mass. Rectal examination is not routinely necessary except if pelvic appendicitis is suspected. *Active observation* (Jones) is a valuable concept that acknowledges that a definitive diagnosis is not always possible when the patient is first seen. The surgeon reassesses the child after a few hours rather than waiting for any deterioration. Clear fluids and simple analgesics are allowed. This policy reduces the need for investigations and results in the removal of fewer innocent appendices (Summary box 6.13).

Peter Ferry Jones. **Formerly Professor of Clinical Surgery, The University of Aberdeen, Aberdeen, Scotland.**

Acute non-specific abdominal pain

The clinical features of non-specific abdominal pain are similar to acute appendicitis but the pain is poorly localised, not aggravated by movement and rarely accompanied by guarding. The site and severity of maximum tenderness often vary during the course of repeated examinations. Symptoms are typically self-limiting within 48 hours. The aetiology of non-specific abdominal pain in children is obscure but viral infections and transient intussusception account for some cases. Mesenteric adenitis, a viral infection causing widespread reactive lymphadenopathy, fever and diffuse abdominal pain is another cause. In some children, recurrent acute abdominal pain can be an expression of underlying psychosocial problems.

Acute appendicitis

Classical features are abdominal pain with localised tenderness and guarding in the right iliac fossa. Vomiting is common. Loose stools may occur with pelvic appendicitis. Some children complain of pain on micturition but this is abdominal pain rather than true dysuria; urine microscopy may show a sterile pyuria. The pulse rate and temperature tend to be normal or slightly elevated early on but a pyrexia of 39°C or greater accompanied by lower abdominal tenderness and guarding suggests a perforated appendix. The chest must always be examined because of the possibility of referred pain from a right lower lobe pneumonia. Most children with acute appendicitis prefer to lie still but there is the occasional stoic who remains active. Bowel sounds can still be audible in the child with peritonitis.

Acute appendicitis can be a difficult diagnosis in the preschool child who is more likely to present with peritonitis or an appendix mass: symptoms are poorly communicated, often nonspecific and easily confused with gastroenteritis or urinary infection; abdominal signs may be modified by antibiotics given for a presumed throat or ear infection; obstructing faecoliths are more common; and the greater omentum is poorly developed.

The treatment of acute appendicitis in children is surgical but only after adequate resuscitation with intravenous fluids, analgesia and broad-spectrum antibiotics. Appendicectomy can be performed laparoscopically or through a small muscle-splitting right iliac fossa incision. Peritoneal lavage with warm saline is essential with perforated appendicitis but a drain is only necessary in some cases of appendix abscess. An appendix mass usually responds to conservative management with antibiotics followed by interval appendicectomy 4–6 weeks later but some surgeons advocate early appendicectomy (Summary box 6.14).

Summary box 6.14

Acute appendicitis

- Vomiting and loose stools may be present
- Tenderness and guarding in the right iliac fossa is characteristic
- Exclude referred pain from right lower lobe pneumonia
- Take special care in diagnosing appendicitis in the preschool child
- Surgery is the treatment of choice but only after fluid resuscitation and antibiotics

---

Other causes of acute abdominal pain in children

- *Intestinal obstruction.* Consider intussusception, inguinal hernia, adhesions and Meckel's diverticulum.
- *Constipation.* Often overdiagnosed as a cause of acute abdominal pain, particularly as the plain abdominal radiograph of a dehydrated ill child frequently shows faecal loading. Constipation is more often a cause of acute abdominal pain in a child who has been treated for Hirschsprung's disease or an anorectal malformation.
- *Urinary tract disorders.* Urinary tract infection is an uncommon cause of acute abdominal pain. Urinary symptoms, fever and vomiting tend to predominate. Urinalysis, microscopy and culture are useful but a sterile pyuria may accompany acute appendicitis. Boys with pelviureteric junction obstruction can present with acute or recurrent abdominal pain and no urinary symptoms.
- *Gastroenteritis.* May cause colicky abdominal pain. Onset of pain before the diarrhoea and the presence of lower abdominal tenderness should raise suspicion of appendicitis. Pelvic tenderness on rectal examination may be a useful pointer to appendicitis.
- *Tropical diseases.* Ascariasis, typhoid and amoebiasis cause acute abdominal pain.

There are numerous rarer causes of acute abdominal pain in children including Henoch–Schönlein purpura, sickle cell disease, primary peritonitis, acute pancreatitis, biliary colic, testicular torsion, gynaecological pathology (e.g. ovarian cysts and tumours, pelvic inflammatory disease, haematometrocolpos) and urinary stone disease (Summary box 6.15).

Summary box 6.15

Rarer causes of acute abdominal pain in children

- Obstruction from intussusception, adhesions, Meckel's diverticulum or a hernia
- Constipation
- Urinary tract disorders
- Gastroenteritis
- Ascariasis
- Typhoid

Eduard Heinrich Henoch, 1820–1910, Professor of Diseases of Children, Berlin, Germany, described this form of purpura in 1868.
Johann Lucas Schönlein, 1793–1864, Professor of Medicine, Berlin, Germany, published his description of this form of purpura in 1837.

Urinary tract infection

Urinary tract infection in children should be diagnosed, investigated and treated promptly. Unlike adults, children often have an underlying urinary tract abnormality and they are at risk of developing renal scarring from ascending infection. Infection and obstruction is a particularly hazardous combination. Older children often complain of dysuria and frequency whereas infants with a urinary tract infection may simply present with vomiting, fever and/or poor feeding. Definite infection is confirmed by urine microscopy and culture showing a pure growth of a urinary pathogen with a colony count of $> 10^5$ organisms per ml and an associated pyuria. However, urine specimens from children are easily contaminated during collection and results must be interpreted with care.

A proven urinary tract infection should initially be investigated by ultrasound scan. Micturating cystography and radioisotope renography are helpful in excluding vesicoureteric reflux and renal scarring. Treatment is aimed at relieving symptoms, correcting an underlying cause and preventing renal scarring.

Vesicoureteric reflux is a common cause of urinary tract infection in children and is graded according to severity. Milder grades of reflux often improve with age but spontaneous resolution is less likely with more severe grades. Vesicoureteric reflux is initially treated with antibiotic prophylaxis. Surgical reimplantation of the ureter or endoscopic treatment to prevent ureteric reflux are reserved for children with symptomatic breakthrough infections, severe reflux, progressive renal scarring or associated urinary tract anomalies.

Children with *neuropathic bladders* (e.g. spina bifida) are at risk of secondary upper renal tract complications. Management of these children must take into account their dexterity and motivation. An adequate capacity, low-pressure bladder can frequently be managed by clean intermittent catheterisation but a high pressure bladder is hazardous and other strategies such as bladder augmentation may be necessary. Some of these children empty their bladder via a non-refluxing catheterisable channel fashioned from the appendix, the bowel or a redundant ureter interposed between the abdominal wall and bladder (Mitrofanoff) (Summary box 6.16).

Summary box 6.16

Urinary tract infection in children

- Needs prompt diagnosis, investigation and treatment to avoid permanent damage to kidneys
- Children often have an underlying urinary tract anomaly
- Symptoms are non-specific in infants
- Urine can be contaminated during collection
- The urinary tract should be checked with ultrasound in a confirmed urinary tract infection

---

Constipation

The passage of hard or infrequent stools is common in children. Severe constipation may be secondary to an anal fissure, Hirschsprung's disease, an anorectal malformation or a neuropathic bowel. A detailed history and examination of the abdomen, anus and spine will identify most causes. Rectal

---

Paul Mitrofanoff, B. 1934, Professor of Paediatric Surgery, Rouen, France.

examination and plain abdominal radiography may be helpful in severe cases. In the absence of specific underlying pathology, the child is best managed jointly with a paediatrician using a combination of diet, extra fluids, reward systems, laxatives and, in some cases, psychological intervention.

Rectal prolapse

Mucosal rectal prolapse can occur in toddlers and is exacerbated by straining or squatting on a potty. It is typically intermittent and frequently self-limiting. Rarely, it may be secondary to cystic fibrosis or spinal dysraphism. The differential diagnosis includes a prolapsing rectal polyp. Underlying factors such as constipation should be treated. Recurrent prolapse usually responds to injection sclerotherapy. Strapping the buttocks is ineffective.

Rectal bleeding

The aetiology and management of rectal bleeding depends on the age of the child, the type and quantity of bleeding and the associated symptoms. Unlike adults, malignancy is exceptionally rare. In infants, an anal fissure, necrotising enterocolitis, intussusception and allergic enterocolitis are possible causes. In older children, more common causes include an anal fissure, a juvenile polyp (Fig. 6.15) and certain gastroenteritides (e.g. *Campylobacter* infection); Meckel's diverticulum, duplication cyst and inflammatory bowel disease are less common. A careful history and examination together with stool microscopy and culture and a full blood count help to select those children who require further investigation by endoscopy, isotope scans, etc.

A Meckel's diverticulum (see Chapter 65) is a remnant of the vitelline duct that connected the embryonic mid-gut to the yolk sac. It is usually located about 60 cm proximal to the ileocaecal valve and is present in about 2% of individuals. Most Meckel's diverticula are clinically silent but if they contain ectopic gastric mucosa this can cause peptic ulceration and profuse (relatively painless) dark red rectal bleeding (Fig. 6.16). This complication occurs most often in young children. A technetium scan may confirm the presence of ectopic gastric mucosa. A Meckel's diverticulum may also be complicated by an obstructing band between the diverticulum and the umbilicus, diverticulitis, intussusception, intestinal volvulus, perforation or neoplasia. A pathological diverticulum should be completely excised (Summary box 6.17).

Summary box 6.17

Rectal problems in children

- *Constipation*: in severe cases exclude Hirschsprung's disease and an anorectal malformation
- *Rectal bleeding*: consider anal fissure, intussusception, colitis and Meckel's diverticulum

---

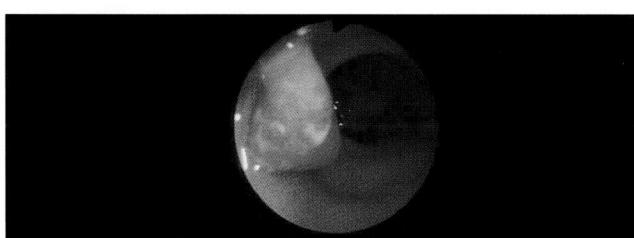

Figure 6.15 Colonic juvenile polyp – these are typically pedunculated.

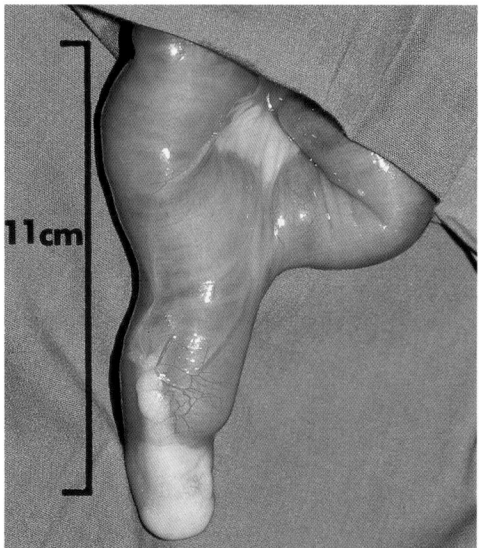

Figure 6.16 Meckel's diverticulum containing ectopic gastric mucosa.

Swallowed or inhaled foreign bodies

Coins are the most frequently swallowed foreign bodies in children. Once beyond the cardia, they almost never cause complications in a normal gastrointestinal tract. A plain radiograph of the chest and neck should establish if the coin is lodged in the oesophagus, in which case it should be removed endoscopically under general anaesthesia. Button batteries must be removed urgently if they remain in the oesophagus or stomach because they can cause gastrointestinal perforation or poisoning. The need to remove sharp objects depends on their size, the age of the child and their position in the gut.

An inhaled foreign body in a small child typically causes sudden-onset coughing and stridor. If there is worsening dyspnoea or signs of hypoxia then the infant should be given back blows in a head-down position. A Heimlich manoeuvre should be used in an older child. In a symptomatic but stable child, a unilateral wheeze or decreased air entry strongly suggests a residual foreign body. If the object is radiolucent, inspiratory and expiratory chest radiographs may show a hyperinflated lung from air trapping (Fig. 6.17). Such cases require bronchoscopy (Summary box 6.18).

Summary box 6.18

Swallowed or inhaled objects

- Most swallowed objects pass spontaneously
- Batteries need watching - they must pass quickly if their contents are not to leak
- Objects jammed in the airways or oesophagus need removing

Henry Jay Heimlich, **B. 1920, Thoracic Surgeon, Xavier University, Cincinnati, OH, USA.**

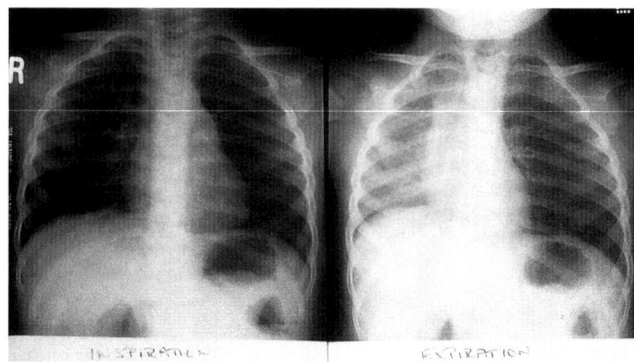

Figure 6.17 An inspiratory (left) and expiratory (right) chest radiograph demonstrating left-sided pulmonary air trapping after inhalation of a radiolucent foreign body.

Table 6.4 Incidence of selected congenital malformations in live-born infants

Malformation	Incidence
Thoracic	
Congenital diaphragmatic hernia	1:3000
Oesophageal atresia/tracheo-oesophageal fistula	1:3500
Cardiac	
Congenital heart disease	1:150
Gastrointestinal	
Gastroschisis	1:7500
Hirschsprung's disease	1:5000
Anorectal malformations	1:4–5000
Hepatobiliary	
Biliary atresia	1:17 000
Choledochal cyst	1:50 000
Urogenital	
Hypospadias	1:250
Pelviureteric junction obstruction	1:1000

CONGENITAL MALFORMATIONS

Excluding cutaneous haemangiomas and birthmarks, approximately 2% of babies are born with a major structural malformation. These may be isolated or multiple. Many are the result of genetic or teratogenic effects. There is an expanding cohort of adults who have sequelae from a congenital malformation or its treatment. Occasionally, a congenital abnormality presents for the first time in adulthood.

Most congenital malformations develop during embryonic life between the third and eighth weeks of gestation. During this phase the three germ layers (endoderm, mesoderm, ectoderm) give rise to rudimentary organ systems. Some malformations are caused by incomplete morphogenesis (e.g. oesophageal atresia) whereas others arise from redundant morphogenesis (e.g. Meckel's diverticulum).

Many major structural malformations can be detected and monitored before birth by prenatal ultrasound scan. Termination of pregnancy or planned delivery in a specialist centre can be considered for severe malformations. Prenatal diagnosis not only detects anatomical defects such as congenital diaphragmatic hernia and urinary tract anomalies but can also identify chromosomal abnormalities such as Down's syndrome and genetic disorders such as cystic fibrosis.

The incidence of congenital malformations is variable (Table 6.4). Some examples relevant to the general surgeon are briefly outlined in the following sections.

Oesophageal atresia

A blind proximal pouch with a distal tracheo-oesophageal fistula is the most common type (Fig. 6.18). Affected infants typically present soon after birth with frothy saliva and cyanotic episodes, exacerbated by any attempt to feed. The preceding pregnancy may have been complicated by maternal polyhydramnios. The diagnosis is confirmed by failure to pass a 10 Fr orogastric tube into the stomach; the tube is visible within an upper oesophageal pouch on the chest radiograph. The presence of abdominal gas signifies the tracheo-oesophageal fistula. Associated anomalies are common and include cardiac, renal and skeletal defects.

> John Langdon Haydon Down (sometimes given as Langdon-Down), **1838–1896,** Physician, The London Hospital, London, England, published 'Observations on an ethnic classification of idiots' in 1866.

The standard method of surgical repair is via a right-sided extrapleural thoracotomy within a day or two of birth. The fistula is divided and the tracheal side oversewn. The oesophageal ends are then anastomosed. Potential postoperative complications include anastomotic leak, stricture, recurrent fistula formation and gastro-oesophageal reflux. Infants with pure oesophageal atresia and no tracheo-oesophageal fistula are usually best managed by a temporary gastrostomy and delayed primary repair. Except for very-low-birthweight babies and those with major congenital heart disease, most infants with repaired oesophageal atresia have a good prognosis.

Congenital diaphragmatic hernia

Typically, there is a left-sided posterolateral diaphragmatic defect associated with herniation of abdominal viscera into the chest

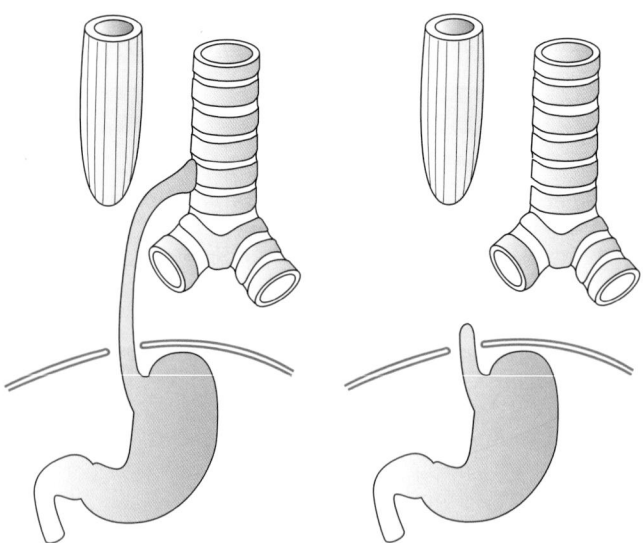

Figure 6.18 The two main varieties of oesophageal atresia. Atresia with a distal tracheo-oesophageal fistula, shown on the left, is the most common (about 85% of cases).

and pulmonary hypoplasia. Many cases are now detected by prenatal ultrasound scan. Prognosis is related to the severity of pulmonary hypoplasia. Despite intensive respiratory support, up to 30% of babies born with this condition die from neonatal respiratory failure. If the infant can be adequately oxygenated and stabilised, the diaphragmatic defect can be repaired. Attempts to salvage severely affected infants by fetal surgery (Harrison) have not yet improved overall survival rates. Small diaphragmatic hernias may present with respiratory or gastrointestinal symptoms in later childhood.

Intestinal atresia

Duodenal atresia (atresia = no lumen) may take the form of a completely obstructing membrane (Fig. 6.19) or the proximal and distal duodenum may be completely separated. The condition may be suspected from prenatal ultrasound scan findings of a 'double bubble' in the fetal abdomen together with maternal polyhydramnios. There is an association with Down's syndrome. Postnatally, the infant develops bilious vomiting if the atresia is distal to the ampulla. A plain abdominal radiograph is usually diagnostic (Fig. 6.20). Repair is by duodenoduodenostomy. Occasionally, there is a duodenal membrane with a small central perforation (duodenal stenosis), which may delay the onset of obstructive symptoms until later childhood.

The anatomy of jejunal/ileal atresia varies from an obstructing membrane through to widely separated blind-ended bowel ends associated with a mesenteric defect. Atresias may be single or multiple and are probably secondary to a prenatal vascular or mechanical insult causing sterile infarction of a segment of gut. They present with intestinal obstruction soon after birth. The proximal bowel is often extremely dilated and needs to be tapered prior to anastomosis to the distal bowel.

Intestinal obstruction and atresia may also occur in neonates with cystic fibrosis who develop inspissated meconium in the terminal ileum (meconium ileus). Meconium is a sterile mixture of epithelial cells, mucin and bile, formed as the fetus starts to swallow amniotic fluid. Any congenital intestinal obstruction may be complicated by meconium peritonitis, an aseptic peri-

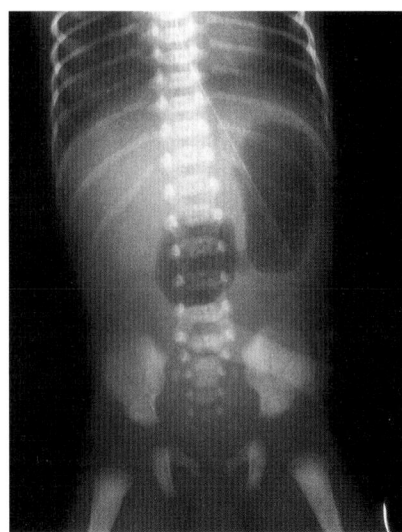

Figure 6.20 Neonatal radiograph showing the 'double bubble' of duodenal atresia.

tonitis developing late in intrauterine life or immediately after birth as a result of intestinal perforation. Typically, the baby is born with a firm, distended, discoloured abdomen and signs of intestinal obstruction. A plain abdominal radiograph may show dilated intestinal loops and areas of calcification. Occasionally, the cause of the intestinal perforation resolves spontaneously before birth but most neonates with meconium peritonitis will need surgery. Babies with uncomplicated meconium ileus (no associated atresia, volvulus or perforation) can sometimes be successfully treated by hyperosmolar contrast enemas to clear the inspissated meconium.

Intestinal malrotation

By the 12th week of gestation, the mid-gut has returned to the fetal abdomen from the extra-embryonic coelom and has begun rotating counterclockwise around the superior mesenteric artery axis. In classical intestinal malrotation, this process fails; the duodenojejunal flexure lies to the right of the midline and the caecum is central, creating a narrow base for the small bowel mesentery, which predisposes to mid-gut volvulus (Fig. 6.21). Malrotation with volvulus is life-threatening and typically presents with bilious vomiting. Bile-stained vomiting in the infant is a sign of intestinal obstruction until proved otherwise.

As the gut strangulates, the baby may pass bloodstained stools and becomes progressively sicker. An upper gastrointestinal contrast study confirms the malrotation (Fig. 6.21). Resuscitation and urgent surgery are needed to untwist the volvulus, widen the base of the small bowel mesentery, straighten the duodenum and position the bowel in a non-rotated position (Ladd's procedure). The appendix is usually removed to avoid leaving it in an abnormal site within the abdomen.

Abdominal wall defects

In gastroschisis, the fetal gut is extruded through a defect in the abdominal wall just to the right of the umbilicus. At birth, the

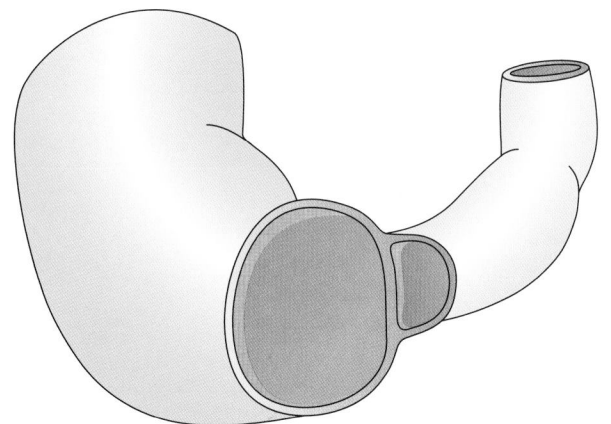

Figure 6.19 Congenital septum of duodenal obstruction at the commencement of the third part of the duodenum. The proximal gut is enormously dilated.

Michael R. Harrison, **B. 1943, Chief of Paediatric Surgery, San Francisco, CA, USA. A pioneer of foetal surgery.**

William Edwards Ladd, **Professor of Child Surgery, The University of Harvard, Boston, MA, USA.**

(a)

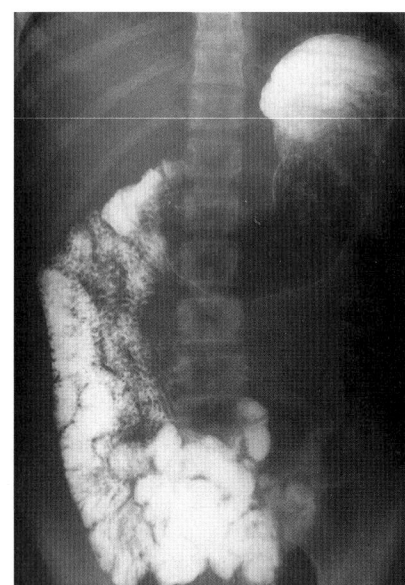

(b)

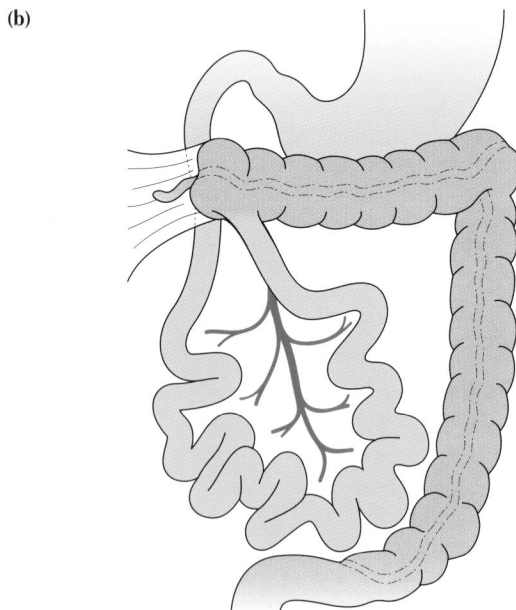

Figure 6.21 (a) Classical intestinal malrotation with a high central caecum and a duodenojejunal flexure to the right of the midline. (b) The narrow origin of the small bowel mesentery predisposes to mid-gut volvulus.

bowel is non-rotated, foreshortened and covered by a fibrinous peel (Fig. 6.22). After reduction of the bowel and closure of the defect, gastroschisis has a good prognosis although gut dysmotility delays recovery. Some infants have an intestinal atresia, which must also be repaired.

Exomphalos is a different type of anterior abdominal wall defect in which the fetal liver and gut are covered with a membranous sac from which the umbilical cord arises. It may be associated with chromosomal or cardiac anomalies.

Biliary atresia

The extrahepatic bile ducts are occluded causing obstructive jaundice and progressive liver fibrosis in early infancy. Biliary

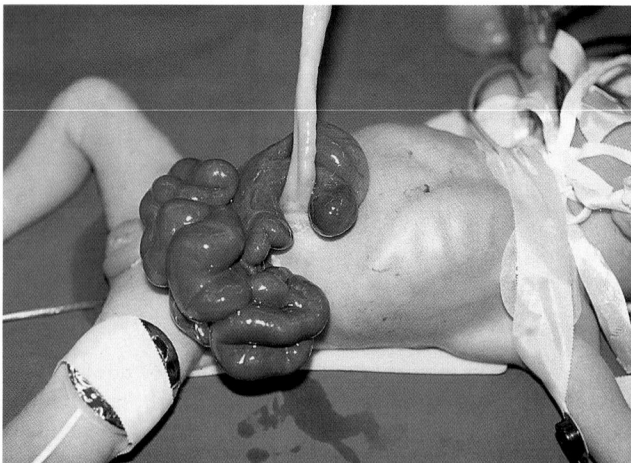

Figure 6.22 A newborn infant with gastroschisis.

atresia should be considered in any infant who remains jaundiced after 2 weeks of age. Affected infants have conjugated hyperbilirubinaemia and are at risk of a coagulopathy, which can be corrected by vitamin K. After excluding infective and metabolic causes of neonatal jaundice, the most useful investigations are an abdominal ultrasound scan (small irregular gall bladder and no visible bile ducts), a biliary radionucleide scan (no excretion) and a needle liver biopsy. Biliary atresia is treated by a Kasai portoenterostomy in which the occluded extrahepatic bile ducts are excised and a jejunal Roux loop is anastomosed to the hepatic hilum. Effective bile drainage is more likely if the operation is performed before 8 weeks of age and may obviate the subsequent need for liver transplantation.

Alimentary tract duplications

Alimentary tract duplications are rare. They are usually single, variable in size, and spherical or tubular. Most are located on the mesenteric border of the intestine. Typically, they are lined by alimentary tract mucosa and share a common smooth muscle wall and blood supply with the adjacent bowel, with which they may communicate. Duplications can contain heterotopic gastric mucosa and be associated with spinal anomalies. Most duplications present in infancy or early childhood with intestinal obstruction, haemorrhage, intussusception or perforation (Fig. 6.23). Presentation in adult life is also described. Rarely, this is because of malignant degeneration, which has been reported more often with rectal duplication cysts.

Complete excision is the treatment of choice.

Hirschsprung's disease

Hirschsprung's disease is characterised by the congenital absence of intramural ganglion cells (aganglionosis) and the presence of hypertrophic nerves in the distal large bowel. The absence of ganglion cells is due to a failure of migration of vagal neural crest cells into the developing gut. The affected gut is tonically contracted causing functional bowel obstruction. The aganglionosis is restricted to the rectum and sigmoid colon in 75% of patients (short segment), involves the proximal colon in 15% (long segment) and affects the entire colon

Mario Kasai, **Formerly Professor of Surgery, the University of Tokyo, Tokyo, Japan.**
Cesar Roux, 1857–1934, Professor of Surgery and Gynaecology, Lausanne, Switzerland described this method of forming a jejunal conduit in 1908.
Harald Hirschsprung, 1830–1916, Physician, The Queen Louise Hospital for Children, Copenhagen, Denmark, described congenital megacolon in 1887.

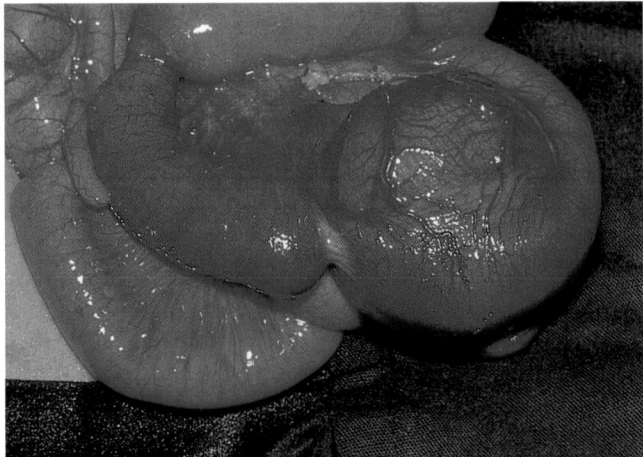

Figure 6.23 An ileal duplication cyst after derotating a localised intestinal volvulus.

and a portion of terminal ileum in 10% (total colonic aganglionosis). A transition zone exists between the dilated, proximal, normally innervated bowel and the narrow, distal aganglionic segment.

Hirschsprung's disease may be familial or associated with Down's syndrome or other genetic disorders. Gene mutations have been identified on chromosome 10 (involving the *RET* proto-oncogene) and on chromosome 13 in some patients. Hirschsprung's disease typically presents in the neonatal period with delayed passage of meconium, abdominal distension and bilious vomiting but it may not be diagnosed until later in childhood or even adult life, when it manifests as severe chronic constipation. Enterocolitis is a potentially fatal complication of the disease.

Definitive diagnosis of Hirschsprung's disease depends on histological examination of an adequate rectal biopsy by an experienced pathologist. A contrast enema may show the extent of the aganglionic segment (Fig. 6.24). Surgery aims to remove the aganglionic segment and bring down healthy ganglionic bowel to the anus; these 'pull-through' operations (e.g. Swenson, Duhamel, Soave and transanal procedures) can be done in a single stage or in several stages after first establishing a proximal stoma in normally innervated bowel. Most patients achieve good bowel control but a significant minority experience residual constipation and/or faecal incontinence.

Anorectal malformations

The anus is either imperforate or abnormally sited. Associated malformations of the sacrum and genitourinary tract are common. In boys, a perineal fistula (a 'low' defect) or an imperforate anus with a rectourethral fistula (Fig. 6.25) is most commonly seen. In girls, an anterior anus (low defect) or an imperforate anus with a fistula opening in the posterior vestibule (not vagina) is most common. Cloacal malformations, in which the rectum and genitourinary tract share a common outflow channel, are also seen in girls.

Diagnosis of a low malformation is usually possible by inspection of the infant's perineum alone. A lateral prone radiograph at about 24 hours of age can help by showing the distance between the rectal gas bubble and the anal skin. Most low malformations are treated by an anoplasty soon after birth. Higher, more com-

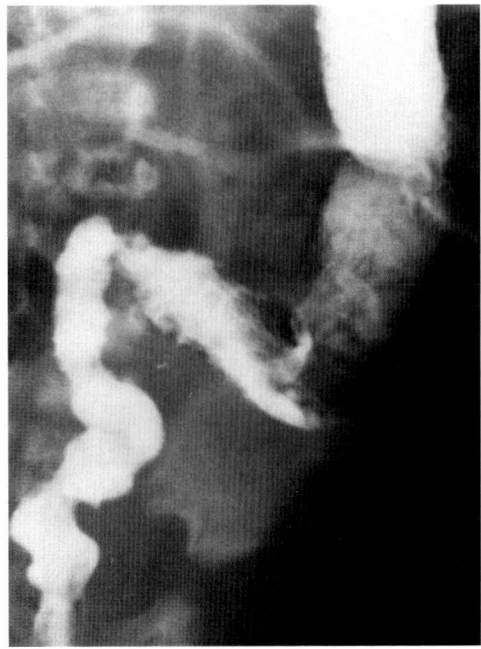

Figure 6.24 Barium enema in an infant showing a 'transition zone' in the proximal sigmoid colon between the dilated proximal normally innervated bowel and the contracted aganglionic rectum.

plex defects need a temporary colostomy; after detailed investigations, reconstructive surgery is undertaken at a few months of age. In the posterior sagittal anorectoplasty developed by Pena, dissection and reconstruction are performed through a midline sacroperineal incision. Any fistula is divided, the distal rectal pouch is mobilised and placed within the pelvic muscles of continence, and an inversion anoplasty is fashioned. Functional outcome is related to the type of anorectal malformation (low defects are associated with constipation, higher defects with faecal incontinence) and the integrity of the sacrum and pelvic muscles. For children with residual intractable faecal incontinence, antegrade colonic enemas administered via a catheterisable appendicostomy (Fig. 6.26) (the Malone procedure) enable the child to achieve social continence (Summary box 6.19).

Summary box 6.19

Congenital causes of intestinal obstruction

- *Intestinal atresia*: may be multiple
- *Cystic fibrosis*: can present with intestinal obstruction from inspissated meconium
- *Intestinal malrotation*: predisposes to potentially lethal midgut volvulus
- *Alimentary tract duplications*: may present with obstruction, haemorrhage or intussusception
- *Hirschsprung's disease*: typically presents with delay in passing meconium after birth
- *Anorectal malformations*: check the anus in babies with intestinal obstruction

---

Orvar Swenson, B. 1909, Professor of Surgery, Northern University, Chicago, IL, USA.
Bernard Georges Duhamel, 1917–1996, Professor of Sugery, Hôpital St. Denis, Paris, France.
F. Soave, 20th century Italian Paediatric Surgeon.

Alberto Pena, B. 1938, Professor of Pediatric Surgery, The Schneider Children's Hospital, New Heyde, NY, USA.
Padraig Seamus Malone, Contemporary, Paediatric Urologist, Southampton General Hospital, Southampton, England.

CHAPTER 6 | PRINCIPLES OF PAEDIATRIC SURGERY

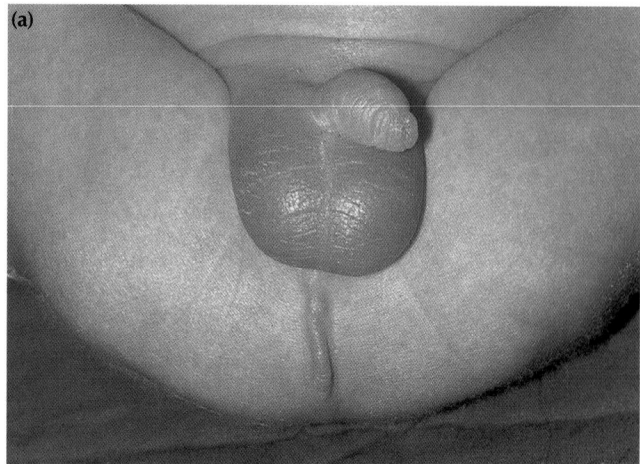

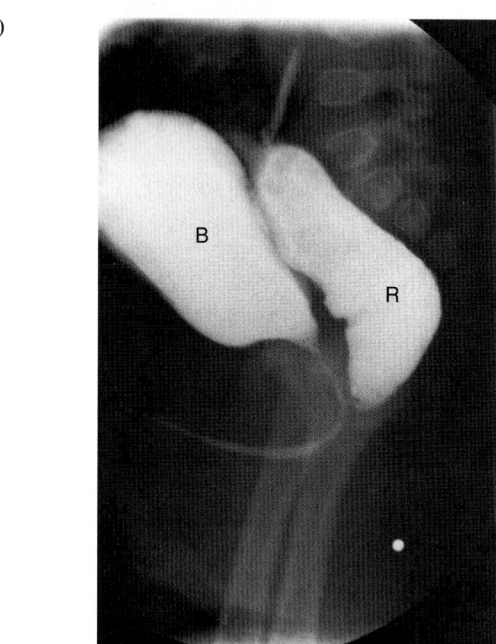

Figure 6.25 (a) An imperforate anus in a neonate associated with (b) a rectourethral fistula, visible on a contrast study performed via a sigmoid colostomy. The bladder is filled with contrast via the fistula and the radio-paque dot has been placed on the infant's perineum over the normal site of the anus. B, bladder; R, rectum.

Urinary tract malformations

Many of these malformations are now detected by prenatal ultrasound scan. Others present in childhood with urinary infection, obstruction or an abdominal mass. Urinary tract disorders in children are investigated by urine microscopy and culture, ultrasound scan, assessment of renal function and a combination of radioisotope renography (uptake and excretion), contrast radiology and endoscopy.

In many infants, prenatally diagnosed mild to moderate hydronephrosis resolves spontaneously. Those with more significant pelviureteric junction obstruction may be asymptomatic or present in later childhood with urinary tract infection or loin pain. Pyeloplasty is indicated for symptoms or impaired renal function. In boys, partial membranous obstruction in the poste-

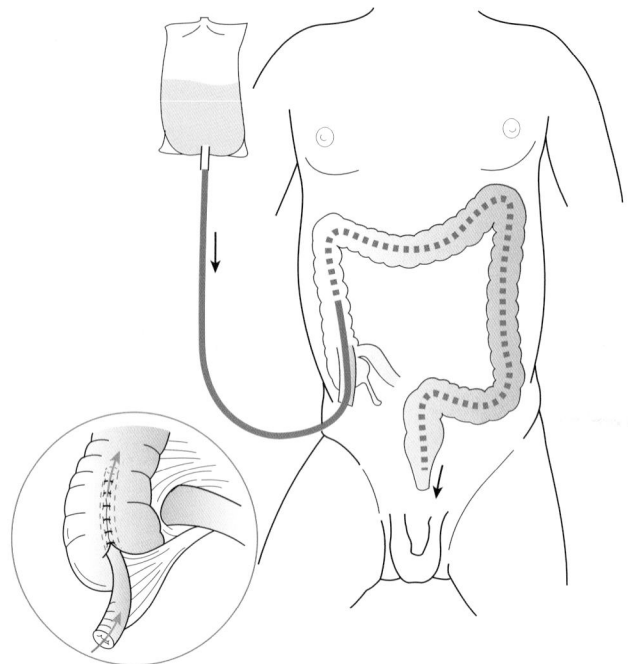

Figure 6.26 Appendicostomy for the delivery of antegrade colonic enemas.

rior urethra (valves) can cause a severe prenatal obstructive uropathy. This condition demands urgent investigation and treatment soon after birth to preserve bladder and kidney function. Renal failure develops in about one-third of affected boys despite early endoscopic ablation of the obstructing valves. Other congenital urinary tract malformations include ureteric abnormalities (e.g. duplex, ureterocoele, vesicoureteric reflux), multicystic dysplastic kidney and bladder exstrophy.

Necrotising enterocolitis

This is an acquired inflammatory condition of the neonatal gut, mostly affecting premature infants. It is not congenital. Immaturity, formula feeds (breast milk is protective), bacterial infection and impaired gut blood flow have been implicated in the pathogenesis. The neonate typically develops abdominal distension, bloody stools and bilious aspirates with signs of systemic sepsis. Patchy or extensive pneumatosis intestinalis progresses to necrosis and perforation of the gut (Fig. 6.27). A variable length of small and large bowel may be affected and the colon is frequently involved. Milder cases respond to antibiotics, gut rest and parenteral nutrition whereas more severe cases need urgent intestinal resection of infarcted bowel. A primary anastomosis is possible if the disease is reasonably localised.

PAEDIATRIC SURGICAL ONCOLOGY

Neoplasms are less common in children than adults but they are a leading cause of death (along with trauma) in children over 1 year of age. In western countries, leukaemia, central nervous system tumours, lymphomas and neuroblastoma account for most paediatric malignancies. The outlook for most childhood cancers has improved dramatically as a result of effective chemotherapy and collaborative multicentre clinical trials. Neuroblastoma and

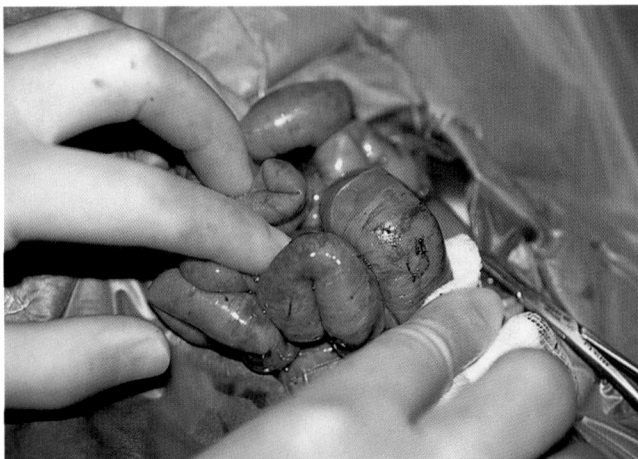

Figure 6.27 Operative appearances of neonatal necrotising entero-colitis. Note the intramural gas characteristic of this condition.

nephroblastoma are among the more common solid abdominal tumours.

Neuroblastoma is a malignancy of neuroblasts in the adrenal medulla or sympathetic ganglia and typically presents as an abdominal or paravertebral mass. It metastasises to lymph nodes, bones and liver and causes elevated urinary catecholamines. Small localised tumours are excised. More advanced tumours are treated by chemotherapy and surgery. Survival is related to tumour biology and stage (> 90% for small localised tumours, < 50% for advanced tumours).

Wilms' tumour (nephroblastoma) is a malignant renal tumour derived from embryonal cells; it typically affects children aged from 1 to 4 years. A mutation in the Wilms' tumour suppressor gene (*WT1*) is responsible for some cases. It usually presents as an abdominal mass. The tumour extends into the renal vein and vena cava and metastasises to lymph nodes and lungs. Treatment is with chemotherapy and surgery. Survival depends on tumour spread, completeness of surgical excision and histology but exceeds 70% even among patients with advanced tumours.

The maintenance of chronic central venous access is a critical part of the management of many children with cancer. A wide variety of access devices exist: external catheters and totally implantable ports with single or multiple lumens inserted via peripheral or central veins. External catheters made of silicone elastomer and commonly known as Broviac or Hickman catheters are inserted percutaneously or surgically into a central vein. A cuff around the extravascular subcutaneous portion of the line allows tissue ingrowth and subsequent catheter fixation. The internal jugular vein is often used for operative insertion and

Max Wilms, **1867–1918, Professor of Surgery, Heidelberg, Germany.**
John W. Broviac, **Formerly Nephrologist, University of Washington, Washington, DC, USA.**
Robert O. Hickman, **Formerly Nephrologist, University of Washington, Washington, DC, USA.**

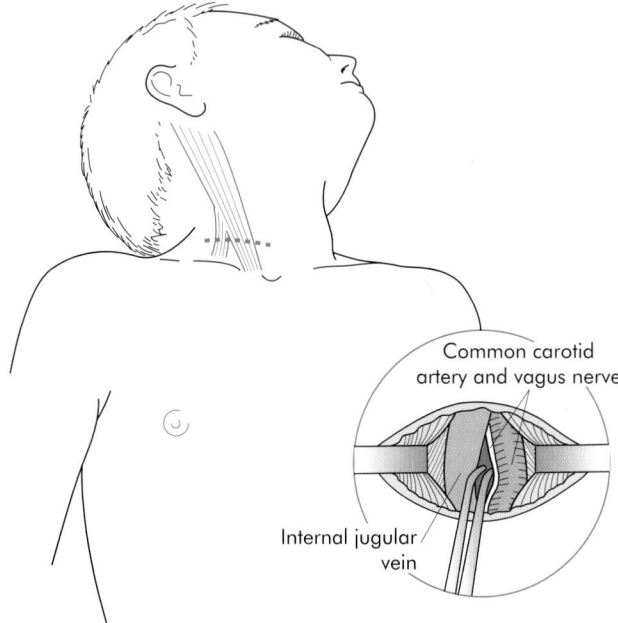

Figure 6.28 Exposure of the internal jugular vein for insertion of a tunnelled cuffed central venous catheter.

is exposed through a short transverse cervical incision above the medial end of the clavicle between the heads of sternomastoid (Fig. 6.28). Meticulous catheter placement and postoperative care are important in minimising complications.

FURTHER READING

Burge, D.M., Griffiths, D.M., Steinbrecher, H.A. and Wheeler, R.A. (eds) (2005) *Paediatric Surgery*, 2nd edn. Hodder Arnold, London.

Gearhart, J.P., Rink, R.C. and Mouriquand, P.D.E. (eds) (2007) *Pediatric Urology*. W.B. Saunders, Philadelphia, PA (in press).

Najmaldin, A.S., Rothenberg, S., Crabbe, D.C.G. and Beasley, S. (eds) (2005) *Operative Endoscopy and Endoscopic Surgery in Infants and Children*. Hodder Arnold, London.

Oldham, K.T., Colombani, P.M., Foglia, R.P. and Skinner, M.A. (eds) (2005) *Principles and Practice of Pediatric Surgery*. Lippincott Williams & Wilkins, Philadelphia, PA.

Puri, P. and Hollwarth, M.E. (eds) (2006) *Pediatric Surgery* (Springer Surgery Atlas Series). Springer-Verlag, Berlin.

Spitz, L. and Coran, A.G. (eds) (2006) *Rob and Smith's Operative Surgery. Pediatric Surgery*. 6th edn. Hodder Arnold, London.

Stringer, M.D., Oldham, K.T. and Mouriquand, P.D.E. (eds) (2006) *Pediatric Surgery and Urology: Long-Term Outcomes*, 2nd edn. Cambridge University Press, New York.

Wieteska, S., Mackway-Jones, K. and Phillips, B. (eds) (2005) *Advanced Paediatric Life Support. The Practical Approach*, 4th edn. Blackwell Publishing, Oxford.

CHAPTER 6 | PRINCIPLES OF PAEDIATRIC SURGERY

Principles of oncology

LEARNING OBJECTIVES

To understand:
- The biological nature of cancer
- The principles of cancer prevention and early detection

To appreciate:
- The principles of cancer aetiology and the major known causative factors

- The likely shape of future developments in cancer management
- The multidisciplinary management of cancer
- The principles of palliative care

WHAT IS CANCER?

History

Cancer has always been with us: dinosaur fossils from over 60 million years ago show evidence of malignancy; Egyptian mummies had cancer. The name itself comes to us through Greek and Latin words for a crab, from the Greek καρκινoς to the Latin *cancer*, and refers to the claw-like blood vessels extending over the surface of an advanced breast cancer. It is possible that cancer appeared on earth with the first vertebrates and that the earliest known tumour occurred in the jaw of an armoured fish about 350 million years ago. Given this history, we have to accept that cancer, at least for the higher vertebrates, is part of life itself.

The study of cancer has always been part of clinical medicine: theories have moved from divine intervention, through the humours, and are now firmly based on the cellular origin of cancer. Rudolf Virchow has the credit for being the first to demonstrate that cancer is a disease of cells and that the disease progressed as a result of abnormal proliferation. His views were encapsulated by his famous dictum 'omnes cellula e cellula' (every cell from a cell). In 1914, Theodor Boveri drew attention to the importance of chromosomal abnormalities in cancer cells and, by the 1940s, thanks to the work of Oswald Avery, we knew that DNA was the genetic material within the chromosomes. The key discovery came in 1953 when Watson and Crick described the structure of DNA and, as they put it themselves, 'It has not escaped our notice that the specific pairing we have postulated immediately suggests a possible copying mechanism for the genetic material'. This discovery paved the way for the study of what has become known as the molecular biology of cancer. We can now investigate, and sometimes even understand, the biochemical mechanisms whereby cancer cells are formed and which mediate their abnormal behaviour.

The psychopath within

Cancer cells are psychopaths. They have no respect for the rights of other cells. They violate the democratic principles of normal cellular organisation. Their proliferation is uncontrolled; their ability to spread is unbounded. Their inexorable, relentless progress destroys first the tissue and then the host.

In order to behave in such an unprincipled fashion, cells have to acquire a number of characteristics before they are fully malignant. No one characteristic is sufficient, and not all characteristics are necessary. These features, based on an article by Hanahan and Weinberg, are given in Summary box 7.1.

Rudolf Ludwig Carl Virchow, 1821–1902, Professor of Pathology, Berlin, Germany.
Theodor Heinrich Boveri, 1862–1913, Professor of Zoology and Comparative Anatomy, Wurzburg, Germany.
Oswald Theodore Avery, 1877–1955, a Bacteriologist at the Rockefeller Institute, New York, NY, USA.
James Dewey Watson, B. 1928, an American Biologist who worked at Cambridge, England, and later became Director of the Cold Spring Harbor Laboratory, New York, NY, USA.

Francis Harry Compton Crick, 1916–2004, a British Molecular Biologist who worked at the Cavendish Laboratory, Cambridge, England and later at the Salk Institute, San Diego, CA, USA. Watson and Crick shared the 1962 Nobel Prize for Physiology or Medicine with Maurice Hugh Frederick Wilkins, 1916–2004, of King's College, London.
Douglas Hanahan, The Department of Biochemistry and Biophysics and Hormone Research Institute, The University of California, San Francisco, CA, USA.
Robert A. Weinburg, The Whitehead Institute of Biomedical Research and Department of Biology, The Massachusetts Institute of Technology, Cambridge, MA, USA.

Malignant transformation

- Establish an autonomous lineage
  Resist signals that inhibit growth
  Acquire independence from signals stimulating growth
- Obtain immortality
- Evade apoptosis
- Acquire angiogenic competence
- Acquire the ability to invade
- Acquire the ability to disseminate and implant
- Evade detection/elimination
- Genomic instability
- Jettison excess baggage
- Subvert communication to and from the environment/milieu

Establish an autonomous lineage

This involves developing independence from the normal signals that control supply and demand. The healing of a wound is a physiological process; the cellular response is exquisitely coordinated so that proliferation occurs when it is needed and ceases when it is no longer required. The whole process is controlled by a series of signals telling cells when to divide and when not to divide. Cancer cells escape from this normal system of checks and balances: they grow and proliferate in the absence of external stimuli; they proliferate and grow despite signals telling them not to. Their division is inappropriate and remorseless. Oncogenes are a key factor in this process. An oncogene is an aberrant form of a normal cellular gene. Oncogenes were originally identified as sequences within the genome of viruses that could cause cancer. Initially, they were thought to be of viral origin but, surprisingly, turned out to be parts of the normal genome that were hitch-hiking between cells, using the virus as a vector. Viral oncogenes (v-*onc*) had sequence homology with normal cellular genes (c-*onc*) and are now presumed to be mutated versions of genes concerned with normal cellular husbandry. The implication of this is that we all carry within us the seeds of our own destruction: genetic sequences that, through mutation, can turn into active oncogenes and thereby cause malignant transformation.

Obtain immortality

According to the Hayflick hypothesis, normal cells are permitted to undergo only a finite number of divisions. For humans, this number is between 40 and 60. The limitation is imposed by the progressive shortening of the end of the chromosome, the telomere, that occurs each time a cell divides. Telomeric shortening is like a molecular clock and, when its time is up, it is time for that lineage to die out. Cancer cells can use the enzyme telomerase to rebuild the telomere at each cell division, so there is no telomeric shortening; it is as if the clock had never ticked, and the lineage will never die out. The cancer cell has achieved immortality.

Evade apoptosis

Apoptosis is a form of programmed cell death. Death occurs, not as the direct result of external events beyond the control of the

Leonard Hayflick, **B. 1928. In 1962,** whilst working at the Wistar Institute in Philadelphia, he noted that normal mammalian cells growing in culture had a limited, rather than an indefinite, capacity for self-replication.

cell, but as the direct result of internal cellular events instructing the cell to die. Unlike necrosis, apoptosis is an orderly process. The cell dismantles itself and packages itself up neatly for disposal (Fig. 7.1). There is a minimal inflammatory response. Apoptosis is a physiological process: cells in the web space of the embryo die by apoptosis; lymphocytes that could react to self also die by apoptosis. The process was rediscovered in 1972 and named apoptosis from the Greek απoπτωσıς, meaning the act of falling (as a dead leaf from a tree). Cells that should not be where they find themselves to be should, normally, die by apoptosis: death by apoptosis is an important self-regulatory mechanism in growth and development. Genes, such as *p53*, that can activate apoptosis function as tumour suppressor genes. Loss of function in a tumour suppressor gene will contribute to malignant transformation. Cancer cells will be able to evade apoptosis, which means that the wrong cells can be in the wrong places at the wrong times.

Acquire angiogenic competence

A mass of tumour cells cannot, in the absence of a blood supply, grow beyond a diameter of about 1 mm. This places a severe restriction on the capabilities of the tumour: it cannot grow much larger and it cannot spread widely within the body. However, if the mass of tumour cells is able to attract or to construct a blood supply, then it is able to quit its dormant state and behave in a far more aggressive fashion. The ability of a tumour to form blood vessels is termed angiogenic competence and is a key feature of malignant transformation.

Acquire the ability to invade

Cancer cells have no respect for the structure of normal tissues. They can, like tanks crossing farmland, demolish fences and boundaries. Cancer cells acquire the ability to breach the basement membrane and thus gain direct access to blood and lymph vessels. Cancer cells use three main mechanisms to facilitate invasion: they cause a rise in the interstitial pressure within a tissue; they secrete enzymes that dissolve extracellular matrix; and they acquire motility. Unrestrained proliferation and a lack of contact inhibition mean that cancer cells can directly exert pressure on the surrounding tissue and literally push themselves beyond the normal limits. Cancer cells secrete collagenases and

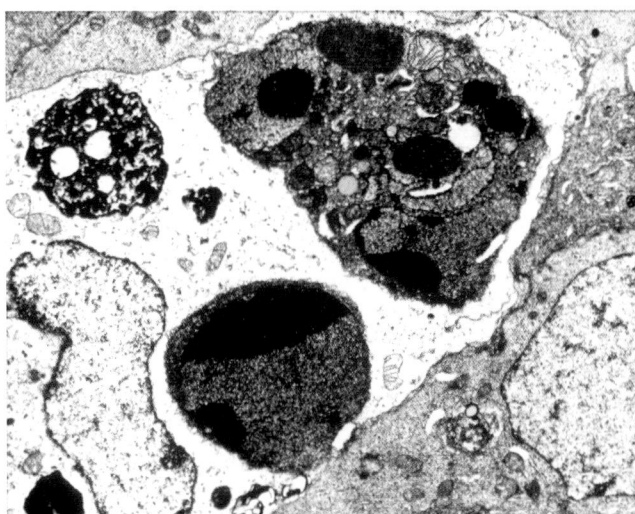

Figure 7.1 Electron micrograph of apoptotic bodies engulfed by a macrophage.

proteases that chemically dissolve any extracellular boundaries that would otherwise limit their spread through tissues. Cancer cells, by modulating the expression of cell surface molecules called integrins, are able to detach themselves from the extracellular matrix. The abnormal integrins associated with malignancy can also transmit signals from the environment to the cytoplasm and nucleus of the cancer cells ('outside-in signalling'), and these signals can induce increased motility.

Acquire the ability to disseminate and implant

As soon as motile cancer cells gain access to vascular and lymphovascular spaces, they have acquired the potential to use the body's natural transport mechanisms to distribute themselves throughout the body. Distribution is not, of itself, sufficient to cause tumours to develop at distant sites. The cells also need to acquire the ability to implant. As Paget pointed out over a century ago, there is a crucial relationship here between the seed (the tumour cell) and the soil (the distant tissue). Most of the cancer cells discharged into the circulation probably do not form viable metastases: circulating cancer cells can be identified in patients who never develop clinical evidence of metastatic disease. Clumping may be important in permitting metastases: outer cells protecting inner cells from immunological attack [like the testudo (tortoise) used by Roman legionnaires]. These outer protective cells may, on occasion, be normal lymphocytes.

Cancer can spread in this embolic fashion, but can also spread when individual cells migrate and implant. Whether spread occurs in groups or as individual cells, there is still the problem of crossing the vascular endothelium (and basement membrane) to gain access to the tissue itself. Cancer cells probably implant themselves in distant tissues by exploiting, and subverting, the normal inflammatory response. By expressing inflammatory cytokines, the cancer cells can fool the endothelium of the host tissue into becoming activated and allowing cancer cells access to the extravascular space. Activated endothelium expresses receptors that bind to integrins and selectins on the surface of leucocytes, and this binding allows the leucocytes to move across the endothelial barrier. Cancer cells simply subvert this physiological mechanism.

Evade detection/elimination

Cancer cells are simultaneously both 'self' and 'not self'. Although derived from normal cells ('self'), they are, in terms of their genetic make-up, behaviour and characteristics, foreign ('not self'). They are more like alien predators. As such, cancer cells ought to provoke an immune response and be eliminated. It is often hard to prove that something never happened. It is hard to prove that cancer cells are often eliminated by the body's own defence mechanisms, but it is entirely possible that malignant transformation is a more frequent event than the emergence of clinical cancer. The possible role of the immune system in eliminating nascent cancers was proposed by Paul Ehrlich in 1909 and revisited by both Sir Frank McFarlane Burnet and Lewis Thomas in the late 1950s. Cancer cells, or at least those that give rise to clinical disease, appear to gain the ability to escape detection by the immune system. This may be through suppressing the expression of tumour-associated antigens, a stealth approach, or it may be through actively coopting one part of the immune system to connive in helping the tumour to escape detection by other parts of the immune surveillance system – bribing a guard to distract his colleagues.

Genomic instability

A cancer is a genetic ferment. Cells are dividing without proper checks and balances. DNA is being copied, and the proofreaders have been retired or ignored. Mutations are arising all the time within tumours, and some of these mutations, particularly those in tumour suppressor genes, may have the ability to encourage the development and persistence of further mutations ('the mutator that mutates the mutator'). This gives rise to the phenomenon of genomic instability – as it evolves, a cancer contains an increasing variety and number of genetic aberrations: the greater the number of such abnormalities, the greater the chance of increasingly deviant behaviour.

Jettison excess baggage

Cancer cells are geared to excessive and remorseless proliferation. They do not need to develop or retain those specialised functions that make them good cellular citizens. They can therefore afford to repress or permanently lose those genes that control such functions. They become leaner and meaner. This may bring some short-term advantages. The longer term disadvantage is that what is today superfluous may, tomorrow, be essential. This can leave cancer cells vulnerable to external stress and may, in part, explain why some treatments for cancer work.

Subvert communication to and from the environment/milieu

Providing false information is a classic military strategy. Degrading the command and control systems of the enemy is an essential component of modern warfare. Cancer cells almost certainly use similar tactics in their battle for control over their host. Given the complexity of communication between and within cells, this is not an easy statement either to disprove or to prove. Nor does it offer any easy targets for therapeutic manipulation.

Malignant transformation

The characteristics of the cancer cell arise as a result of mutation. Only very rarely is a single mutation sufficient to cause cancer; multiple mutations are usually required. Colorectal cancer provides the classical example of how multiple mutations are necessary for the complete transformation from normal cell to malignant cell. Vogelstein and his colleagues identified the genes required and also postulated not only that it is necessary to have mutations in all the

---

Stephen Paget, 1855–1926, Surgeon, The West London Hospital, London, England. Paget's 'seed and soil' hypothesis is contained in his paper 'The Distribution of Secondary Growths in Cancer of the Breast', in the Lancet, 1889.
Paul Ehrlich, 1854–1915, Professor of Hygiene, The University of Berlin, and later Director of The Institute for Infectious Diseases, Berlin, Germany. In 1908 he shared the Nobel Prize for Physiology or Medicine with Elie Metchnikoff, 1845–1916, 'In recognition of his work on immunity'. Metchnikoff was Professor of Zoology at Odessa in Russia, and later worked at the Pasteur Institute in Paris, France.

Sir Frank McFarlane Burnett, 1899–1985, an Australian Virologist, at the Walter and Eliza Hall Institute, Melbourne, WA, Australia. Burnett shared the 1960 Nobel Prize for Physiology or Medicine with Sir Peter Brian Medawar, 1915–1987, Jodrell Professor of Zoology, University College, London, England, 'for their discovery of acquired immunological tolerance'.
Lewis Thomas, 1913–1993, an American Pathologist and Immunologist, who became President to the Sloan Kettering Memorial Institute, New York, NY, USA.
Bert Vogelstein, B. 1949, Molecular Biologist, Johns Hopkins Hospital, Baltimore, MD, USA.

relevant genes, but also that these mutations must be acquired in a specific sequence. This could be regarded as the poker hand view of the problem of transformation: not only do you need the right cards, but you need them in the right order. An alternative view is that malignant transformation involves the acquisition of mutations within a set of distinct regulatory pathways; within each pathway transforming mutations are mutually exclusive.

Cancer is usually regarded as a clonal disease. Once a cell has arisen with all the mutations necessary to make it fully malignant, it is capable of giving rise to an infinite number of identical cells, each of which is fully malignant. These cells divide, invade, metastasise and destroy but, ultimately, each is the direct descendant of that original, primordial, transformed cell. There is certainly evidence, mostly from haematological malignancies, to support the view that tumours are monoclonal in origin, but recent evidence challenges the universality of this assumption. Some cancers may arise from more than one clone of cells. Epigenetic modification refers to hereditable changes in DNA that are not related to the nucleotide sequence of the molecule. Epigenetic modification may give rise to distinct cancer cell lineages with differing biological properties. The interactions between cells from each lineage and the tissue within which such cells find themselves may determine the overall clinical behaviour of a tumour – and we return to Stephen Paget's seed and soil hypothesis from the late nineteenth century.

It takes a tissue to make a tumour. This provocative sentence encapsulates a more general approach to the problem of malignant transformation than the traditional, cell-based, reductionist view. 'No man is an island unto himself', and no cancer cell exists in isolation, uninfluenced by its physical and biochemical environment. This view applies the principles of systems biology to cancer and stimulates attempts to understand the role of the exchange of information between a cancer cell and its milieu in sustaining the malignant process.

The growth of a tumour

If it is accepted that a cancer starts from a single transformed cell, then it is possible, using straightforward arithmetic, to describe the progression from a single cell to a mass of cells large enough to kill the host. The division of a cell produces two daughter cells. The relationship 2^n will describe the number of cells produced after n generations of division. There are between 10^{13} and 10^{14} cells in a typical human being. A tumour 10 mm in diameter will contain about 10^9 cells. As $2^{30} = 10^9$, this implies that it would take 30 generations to reach the threshold of clinical detectability and, as $2^{45} = 3 \times 10^{13}$, fewer than 15 subsequent generations to produce a tumour that, through sheer bulk alone, would be fatal. This is an oversimplification because cell loss is a feature of many tumours and, for squamous cancers, as many as 99% of the cells produced may be lost, mainly by exfoliation. It will, in the presence of cell loss, take many cellular divisions to produce a clinically evident tumour – abundant opportunity for further mutations to occur during the preclinical phase of tumour growth. The growth of a

typical human tumour can be described by an exponential relationship, the doubling time of which increases exponentially – so called Gompertzian growth (see Fig. 7.2). This Gompertzian pattern has several important implications for the diagnosis and treatment of cancer (Summary box 7.2).

Summary box 7.2

Clinical implications of Gompertzian growth

- The majority of the growth of a tumour occurs before it is clinically detectable
- By the time they are detected, tumours have passed the period of most rapid growth, that period when they might be most sensitive to anti-proliferative drugs
- There has been plenty of time, before diagnosis, for individual cells to detach, invade, implant and form distant metastases
- 'Early tumours' are genetically old: plenty of time for mutations to have occurred, mutations that might confer spontaneous drug resistance (a probability greatly increased by the existence of cell loss)
- The rate of regression of a tumour will depend upon its age (the Norton–Simon hypothesis extends this: the rate of regression of a tumour will depend upon its growth rate at the time of treatment)

THE CAUSES OF CANCER

The interplay between nature and nurture

Both inheritance and environment are important determinants of whether or not an individual develops cancer. Although environ-

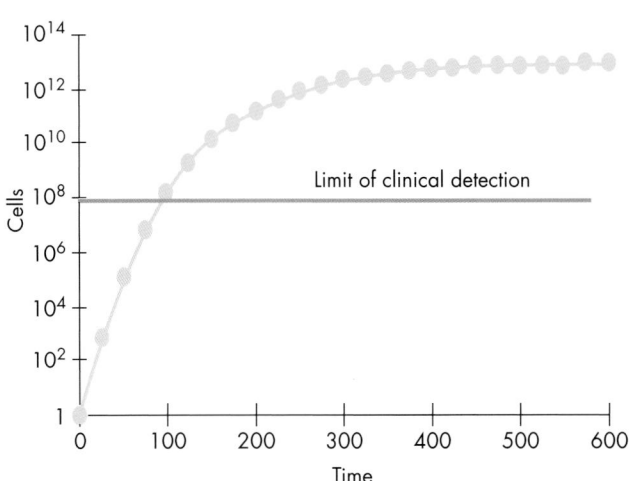

Figure 7.2 The Gompertzian curve describing the growth of a typical tumour. In its early stages, growth is exponential but, as the tumour grows, the growth rate slows. This decrease in growth rate probably arises because of difficulties with nutrition and oxygenation. The tumour cells are in competition: not only with the tissues of the host, but also with each other.

John Donne, 1573–1631, Metaphysical poet, and Dean of St. Paul's Cathedral, London, England. The quotation is from Donne's 'Meditation XVII'.
System Biology: a discipline in which a living entity is viewed as an integrated network in which the study of the interactions between genes, molecules and chemical reactions is as important as the study of the individual components of the network. The approach is synthetic rather than reductionist and embraces, rather than ignores, the inconvenient complexity of living organisms.

Benjamin Gompertz, 1779–1865. An insurance actuary who was interested in calculating annuities. To do this he needed to describe mathematically the relationship between life-expectancy and age. He was able to do this using the function (the Gompertzian Function) that bears his name. The Gompertzian function provides an excellent fit to data points plotting tumour size against time.

mental factors have been implicated in more than 80% of cases of cancer, this would still leave plenty of scope for the role of genetic inheritance: not just the 20% of tumours for which there is no clear environmental contribution but also, as environment alone can rarely cause cancer, the genetic contribution to the 80% of tumours to whose occurrence environmental factors contribute. As a plain example: not all smokers develop lung cancer; lung cancer can occur in people who have never smoked.

The knowledge we have concerning the causes of cancer can be used to design appropriate strategies for prevention or earlier diagnosis. As we find out more about the genes associated with cancer, genetic testing and counselling will play an increasing role in the prevention of cancer. These considerations are incorporated into Table 7.1 on the inherited cancer syndromes, and Table 7.2 on the environmental contribution to cancer.

Table 7.1 Inherited syndromes associated with cancer

Syndrome	Gene(s) implicated	Inheritance	Associated tumours and abnormalities	Strategies for prevention/early diagnosis
Familial adenomatous polyposis (FAP)/Gardner syndrome	*APC* gene	D	Colorectal cancer under the age of 25 years Papillary carcinoma of the thyroid Cancer of the ampulla of Vater Hepatoblastomas Primary brain tumours (Turcot's syndrome) Osteomas of the jaw CHRPE (congenital hypertrophy of the retinal pigment epithelium)	Prophylactic panproctocolectomy
Hereditary non-polyposis colorectal cancer (HNPCC)	DNA mismatch repair genes (*MLH1, MSH2, MSH6*)	D	Colorectal cancer (typically in the 40s and 50s)	Surveillance colonoscopies/polypectomies Non-steroidal anti-inflammatory drugs
HNPCC1	*MSH2*		Endometrium, stomach, hepatobiliary (Lynch's syndrome 1)	
HNPCC2	*MLH1*			
HNPCC3	*PMS1*			
Peutz–Jeghers syndrome	*STK11*	D	Bowel cancer, breast cancer, freckles round the mouth	Surveillance colonoscopy, mammography
Cowden's syndrome	*PTEN*	D	Multiple hamartomas of skin, breast and mucus membranes Breast cancer Neuroendocrine tumours Endometrial cancer, thyroid cancer	Active surveillance
Retinoblastoma	*RB*	D	Retinoblastoma Pinealoma Osteosarcoma	Surveillance of the uninvolved eye
Multiple endocrine neoplasia (MEN) type 1	*Menin*	D	Parathyroid tumours Islet cell tumours Pituitary tumours	Awareness of associations and paying attention to relevant symptoms
MEN type 2A	*RET*	D	Medullary carcinoma of the thyroid Phaeochromocytoma Parathyroid tumours	Regular screening of blood pressure, serum calcitonin and urinary catecholamines Prophylactic thyroidectomy

Eldon J. Gardner, **B. 1909**, Professor of Zoology, Utah State University, Salt Lake City, UT, USA.
Abraham Vater, **1684–1751**, Professor of Anatomy and Botany, and later of Pathology and Therapeutics, Wittenburg, Germany.
Jacques Turcot, **B. 1914**, Surgeon, Hôtel Dieu de Quebec Hospital, Quebec, Canada.
Henry T. Lynch, **B. 1928**, Oncologist, Chairman of the Department of Preventive Medicine, Creighton School of Medicine, California, USA.
John Law Augustine Peutz, **1886–1968**, Chief Specialist for Internal Medicine, St. John's Hospital, The Hague, The Netherlands.
Harold Joseph Jeghers, **1904–1990**, Professor of Internal Medicine, The New Jersey College of Medicine and Dentistry, Jersey City, NJ, USA.
One of the few clinical syndromes **named for the patient rather than the clinician**. Rachel Cowden was, in 1963, the first patient described with the syndrome. She died from **breast cancer at the age of 20.**

Table 7.1 Inherited syndromes associated with cancer – *continued*

Syndrome	Gene(s) implicated	Inheritance	Associated tumours and abnormalities	Strategies for prevention/early diagnosis
MEN type 2b	*RET*	D	Medullary carcinoma of the thyroid Phaeochromocytoma Mucosal neuromas Ganglioneuromas of the gut	Regular screening of blood pressure, serum calcitonin and urinary catecholamines Prophylactic thyroidectomy
Li–Fraumeni syndrome	*p53*	D	Sarcomas Leukaemia Osteosarcomas Brain tumours Adrenocortical carcinomas	Very difficult, as the pattern of tumours is so heterogeneous and varies from patient to patient
Familial breast cancer	*BRCA1, BRCA2*	D	Breast cancer Ovarian cancer Papillary serous carcinoma of the peritoneum Prostate cancer	Screening mammography Pelvic ultrasound Prostate-specific antigen in males Prophylactic mastectomy Prophylactic oophorectomy
Familial cutaneous malignant melanoma	*CDNK2A, CDK4*	D	Cutaneous malignant melanoma	Avoid exposure to sunlight, careful surveillance
Basal cell naevus syndrome (Gorlin)	*PTCH*	D	Basal cell carcinomas Medulloblastoma Bifid ribs	Careful surveillance, awareness of diagnosis (look for bifid ribs on X-ray)
Von Hippel–Lindau syndrome	*VHL*	D	Renal cancer Phaeochromocytoma Haemangiomas of the cerebellum and retina	Urinary catecholamines
Neurofibromatosis type 1	*NF1*	D	Astrocytomas Primitive neuroectodermal tumours Optic gliomas Multiple neurofibromas	A difficult problem; maintain a high index of suspicion concerning any rapid changes in the growth or character of any nodule
Neurofibromatosis type 2	*NF2*	D	Acoustic neuromas Spinal tumours Meningiomas Multiple neurofibromas	
Xeroderma pigmentosum	Deficient nucleotide excision repair (*XPA, B, C*)	R	Skin sensitive to sunlight; early onset of cutaneous carcinomas (SCCs, BCCs)	Avoidance of sun exposure Active surveillance and early treatment Retinoids for chemoprevention
Ataxia telangiectasia	*AT*	R	Progressive cerebellar ataxia Leukaemia Lymphoma Breast Melanoma Upper gastrointestinal	Active surveillance
Bloom's syndrome	*BLM helicase*	R	Sensitivity to UV light Leukaemia Lymphoma	Active surveillance

BCC, basal cell carcinoma; D, dominant; R, recessive; SCC, squamous cell carcinoma; UV, ultraviolet.

Frederick P. Li, **B.** 1940, Professor of Medicine, Harvard University Medical School, Boston, MA, USA.
Joseph F. Fraumeni, **B.** 1933, Director of Cancer Epidemiology and Genetics, The National Cancer Institute, Bethesda, MD, USA.
Robert Gorlin, **1923–2006**, Professor of Dentistry, The University of Minnesota, Minneapolis, MN, USA.
Eugen von Hippel, **1867–1939**, Professor of Ophthalmology, Göttingen, Germany.
Arvid Lindau, **1892–1958**, Professor of Pathology, Lund, Sweden.
David Bloom, **B.** 1892, a Dermatologist at the Skin and Cancer Clinic, New York University, New York, NY, USA.

Table 7.2 Environmental causes of cancer (and suggested measures for reducing their impact)

Environmental/ behavioural factor			Associated tumours	Strategy for prevention/ early diagnosis
Tobacco			Lung cancer Head and neck cancer	Ban tobacco Ban smoking in public places Punitive taxes on tobacco
Alcohol			Head and neck cancer Oesophageal cancer Hepatoma	Avoid excess alcohol Surveillance of high-risk individuals
UV exposure			Melanoma Non-melanoma skin cancer	Avoid excessive sun exposure, avoid sunbeds
Ionising radiation			Leukaemia Breast Lymphoma Thyroid	Limit medical exposures to the absolute minimum; safety precautions at nuclear facilities; monitor radiation workers
Viral infections	HPV		Cervix Penis	Avoid unprotected sex Vaccination
	HIV		Kaposi's sarcoma Lymphomas Germ cell tumours Anal cancer	Avoid unprotected sex Anti-retroviral therapy
	Hepatitis B		Hepatoma	Avoid contaminated injections/infusions Vaccination
Other infections	Bilharzia		Bladder cancer	Treatment of infection Cystoscopic surveillance
	Helicobacter pylori		Stomach cancer	Eradication therapy
Inhaled particles	Asbestos Wood dust		Mesothelioma Paranasal sinus cancers	Protect workers from inhaled dusts and fibres
Chemicals	Environmental pollutants/chemicals used in industry		Angiosarcoma (vinyl chloride) Bladder cancer (aniline dyes, vulcanisation of rubber) Lung, nasal cavity (nickel) Skin (arsenic) Lung (beryllium, cadmium, chromium) All sites (dioxins)	Protection of exposed workers; avoid chemical discharge and spillages
	Medical	Alkylating agents used in cytotoxic chemotherapy	Leukaemia Lymphoma Lung cancer	Avoid overtreatment; only combine drugs with ionising radiation when absolutely necessary
		Immunosuppressive treatment	Kaposi's sarcoma	As low a dose as possible, for as short a period as possible
		Stilbestrol	Adenocarcinoma of the vagina in daughters of treated mothers	Use of stilbestrol curtailed
		Tamoxifen	Endometrial cancer	Biopsy if patient on tamoxifen develops uterine bleeding
Fungal and plant toxins	Aflatoxins		Hepatoma	Appropriate food storage, screen for fungal contamination of foodstuffs

Table 7.2 Environmental causes of cancer (and suggested measures for reducing their impact)– *continued*

Environmental/ behavioural factor	Associated tumours	Strategy for prevention/ early diagnosis
Obesity/lack of physical exercise	Breast Endometrium Kidney Colon Oesophagus	Maintain ideal body weight, regular exercise

HIV, human immunodeficiency virus; HPV, human papillomavirus; UV, ultraviolet.

THE MANAGEMENT OF CANCER

Management is more than treatment

The traditional approach to cancer concentrates on diagnosis and active treatment. This is a very limited view and one that, in terms of the public health, may not have served society particularly well. It implies an attitude to the occurrence of cancer that is too fatalistic and an assumption that, once active treatment is complete, there is little more do be done. Prevention is forgotten and rehabilitation is ignored. The management of cancer can be considered as taking place along two axes: one is an axis of scale, from the individual to the world population; the other is an axis based on the unnatural history of the disease, from prevention through to rehabilitation or palliative care (see Fig. 7.3).

Prevention

Table 7.2 summarises the approaches that can be used in the prevention of cancer. In 1998, Sir Richard Doll estimated that 30% of cancer deaths were due to tobacco use and that up to 50% of cancer deaths were related to diet. Even allowing for overlap (smokers often have a poor diet), these are impressive figures and add some perspective to the often inflated claims made for the achievements of cancer treatment. Doll estimated that cancers related to occupation accounted for less than 4% of cancer deaths, and that environmental pollution accounted for less than 5% of deaths. Public attitudes to risk are not always logically consistent, and many well-intentioned attempts at cancer prevention fall foul of this simple fact.

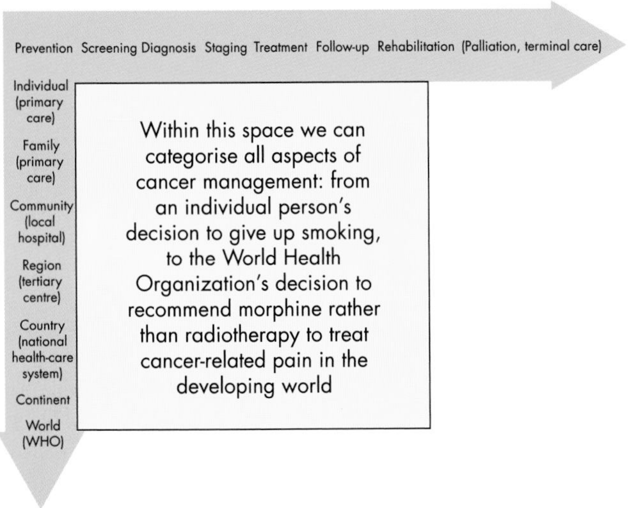

Screening

Screening involves the detection of disease in an asymptomatic population in order to improve outcomes by early diagnosis. It follows that a successful screening programme must achieve early diagnosis, and that the disease in question has a better outcome when treated at an early stage. The criteria that must be fulfilled for the disease, screening test and the screening programme itself are given in Summary box 7.3.

Figure 7.3 The management of cancer spans the natural history of the disease and all humankind, from the individual to the population of the world. WHO, World Health Organization.

Sir William Richard Shaboe Doll, **1912–2005, Regius Professor of Medicine, Oxford University, Oxford, England, and Sir Austin Bradford Hill, Professor of Medical Statistics, The London School of Hygiene and Tropical Medicine, London, England** published one of the definitive reports linking smoking to lung cancer in 1950.

> **Summary box 7.3**
>
> **Criteria for screening**
>
> ***The disease***
> - Recognisable early stage
> - Treatment at an early stage more effective than at a later stage
> - Sufficiently common to warrant screening
>
> ***The test***
> - Sensitive and specific
> - Acceptable to the screened population
> - Safe
> - Inexpensive
>
> ***The programme***
> - Adequate diagnostic facilities for those with a positive test
> - High-quality treatment for screen-detected disease to minimise morbidity and mortality
> - Screening repeated at intervals if the disease is of insidious onset
> - Benefit must outweigh physical and psychological harm

Merely to prove that screening picks up disease at an early stage, and that the outcome is better for patients with screen-detected disease than for those who present with symptoms, is an insufficient criterion for the success of a screening programme. This is because of inherent biases in screening, which make screen-detected disease appear to be associated with better outcomes than symptomatic disease. These biases are lead time bias, selection bias and length bias. Lead time bias describes the phenomenon whereby early detection of a disease will always prolong survival from the time of diagnosis when compared with disease picked up at a later stage in its development whether or not the screening process has altered the progression of the tumour (Fig. 7.4). Selection bias describes the finding that individuals who accept an invitation for screening are, in general, healthier than those who do not. It follows that individuals with screen-detected disease will tend, independently of the condition for which screening is being performed, to live longer. Length bias is brought about by the fact that slow-growing tumours are likely to be picked up by screening, whereas fast-growing tumours are likely to arise and produce symptoms in between screening rounds. Thus, screen-detected tumours will tend to be less aggressive than symptomatic tumours. Because of these biases, it is essential to carry out population-based randomised controlled trials and to compare a whole population offered screening (including those who refuse to be screened and those who develop cancer after a negative test) with a population that has not been offered screening. This research design has been applied to both breast cancer and colorectal cancer: in both cases, there was reduction in disease-specific mortality.

Diagnosis and classification

Accurate diagnosis is the key to the successful management of cancer. Diagnosis lies at the heart of the epidemiology of

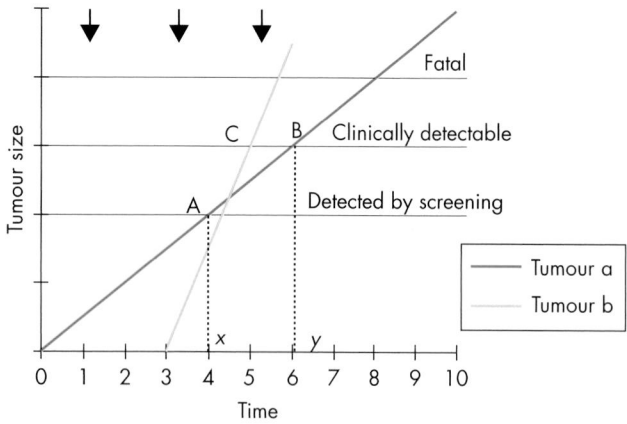

Figure 7.4 Lead time and length bias. Tumour a is a steadily growing tumour; its progress is uninfluenced by any treatment. The arrows indicate the timing of tests in a screening programme. The horizontal lines indicate three thresholds: detectability by screening; clinical detectability; and death due to tumour progression. Point A indicates the time at which the tumour would be diagnosed in a screening programme, and point B indicates the time at which the tumour would be diagnosed clinically, that is in the absence of any screening programme. If the date of diagnosis is used as the start time for measuring survival, then it is clear that, in the absence of any effect from treatment, the screening programme will, artefactually, add to the survival time. The amount of 'increased' survival is equal to $y - x$ years, in this example, just over 2 years. This artefactual inflation of survival time is referred to as lead time bias. Tumour b is a rapidly growing tumour; again, its progress is uninfluenced by treatment. It grows so rapidly that, in the interval between two screening tests, it can cross both the threshold for detectability by screening and that of clinical detectability. It will continue to progress rapidly after diagnosis, and the measured survival time will be short. This phenomenon, whereby those tumours that are 'missed' by the screening programme are associated with decreased survival, is called length bias.

cancer; if there is an inaccurate picture of the pattern of a disease, reliable inferences about its distribution and causes cannot be drawn. Precise diagnosis is crucial to the choice of correct therapy; the wrong operation or cytotoxic therapy, no matter how superbly carried out or how ingeniously designed, is useless. An unequivocal diagnosis is the key to an accurate prognosis; the answer to the question 'Doctor, how long have I got…?' is dependent upon knowing precisely what it is that is wrong. Only rarely can a diagnosis of cancer confidently be made in the absence of tissue for pathological or cytological examination. Cancer is a disease of cells and, for accurate diagnosis, the abnormal cells need to be seen. Different tumours are classified in different ways: most squamous epithelial tumours are simply classed as well (G1), moderate (G2) or poorly (G3) differentiated (Fig. 7.5). Adenocarcinomas are also often classified as G1, 2 or 3, but prostate cancer is an exception with widespread use of the Gleason system. The Gleason system grades prostate cancer according to the degree of differentiation of the two most prevalent architectural patterns. The final score is the sum of the two grades and can vary from 2 (1 + 1) to 10 (5 + 5), with the higher scores indicating poorer prognosis. The management of malignant lymphomas is based firmly upon histopathological classification: the first distinction is between Hodgkin's lymphoma (HL) and the non-Hodgkin's lymphoma (NHL). Each of these main types of lymphoma is then subclassified according to a different scheme. The World Health Organization/Revised European–American lymphoma (WHO/REAL) system classifies Hodgkin's lymphoma into classical HL (nodular sclerosis HL; mixed cellularity HL; lymphocyte depletion HL; lymphocyte-rich classical HL) and nodular lymphocyte-predominant HL. The WHO/REAL classification of NHL is considerably more complex and recognises 27 distinct pathological subtypes. It is perhaps no coincidence that the non-surgical treatment of lymphomas is, by and large, more successful than the non-surgical treatment of solid tumours. This suggests that precise and accurate subtyping of tumours enables appropriate selection of treatment and, in turn, this is associated with better outcome.

Investigation and staging

It is not sufficient simply to know what a cancer is; it is imperative to know its site and extent. If it is localised, then locoregional treatments such as surgery and radiation therapy may be curative. If the disease is widespread, then, although such local interventions may contribute to cure, they will be insufficient, and systemic treatment, for example with drugs or hormones, will be required. Staging is the process whereby the extent of disease is mapped out. Formerly, staging was a fairly crude process based on clinical examination and chest X-ray and the occasional ultrasound; nowadays, it is a highly sophisticated process, heavily reliant on the technology of modern imaging. These technological advances bring with them the implication that patients staged as having localised disease in 2007 are not comparable to patients described in 1985 as having localised disease. Many of these latter patients would, had they been imaged using the

Donald F. Gleason, **B. 1920, Pathologist, The University of Minnesota, Minneapolis, MN, USA.**
Thomas Hodgkin, **1798–1866, Curator of the Museum and Demonstrator of Morbid Anatomy, Guy's Hospital, London, England, described lymphadenoma in 1832.**

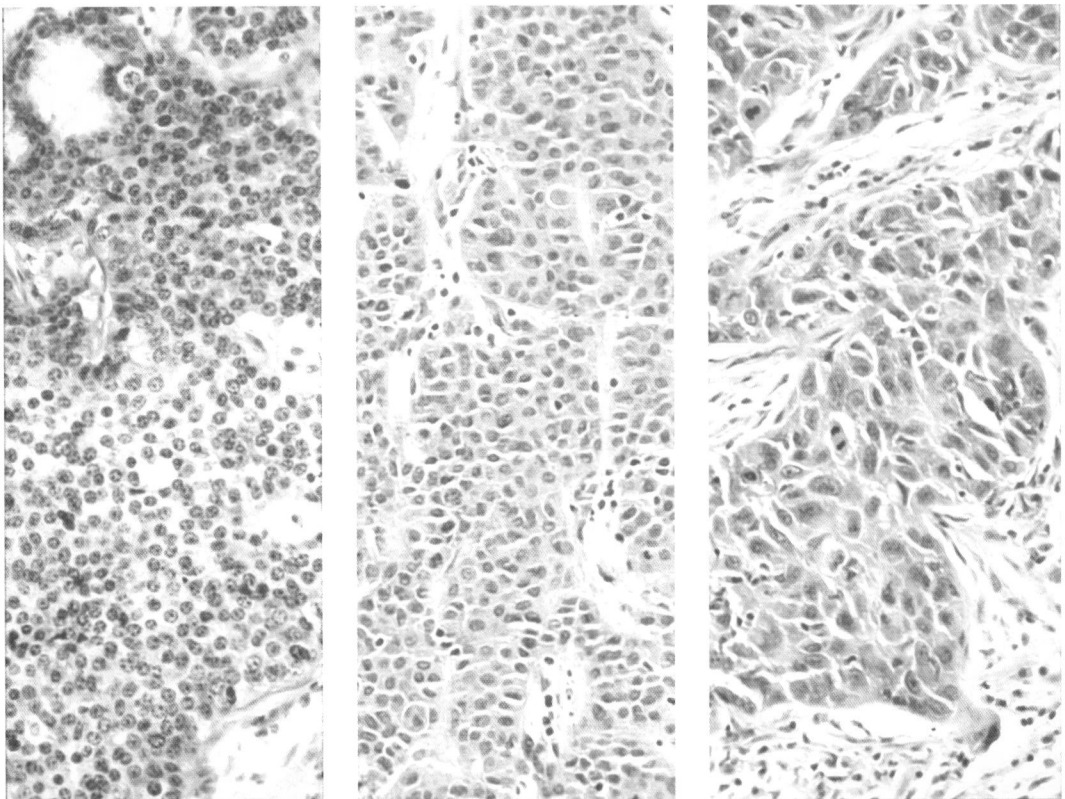

Figure 7.5 Three carcinomas showing different degrees of differentiation. Left to right: well differentiated, moderately differentiated and poorly differentiated.

technology of 2007, have had occult metastatic disease detected. This leads to the paradox of stage shift, also named, by Alvan Feinstein, the Will Rogers phenomenon. A change in staging system, or in the techniques used to provide baseline information concerning staging, can produce 'benefits' to patients at all stages of the disease. These benefits are, however, entirely artefactual and depend simply upon patients in each stage being enriched by patients with improved prognosis. The important cross-check to protect against being misled by stage shift is that the prognosis for the entire group (i.e. all stages pooled) has not been changed. Table 7.3 shows a worked example of stage shift.

The International Union against Cancer (UICC) is responsible for the TNM (tumour, nodes, metastases) staging system for cancer. This system is compatible with, and relates to, the American Cancer Society (AJCC) system for stage grouping of cancer. Examples of clinico-pathological staging systems for colon cancer are shown in Tables 7.4 and 7.5.

Therapeutic decision making and the multidisciplinary team

As the management of cancer becomes more complex, it becomes impossible for any individual clinician to have the intel-

CHAPTER 7 | PRINCIPLES OF ONCOLOGY

Table 7.3 Stage shift

Before new staging test				After new staging test				
Stage	Distribution (%)	Cure rate (%)	Number cured	Stage	Distribution (%)	Cure rate (%)	Number cured	'Improvement' in cure rate (%)
I	70	90	63	I	50	94	47	4
II	10	80	8	II	10	80	8	0
III	10	80	8	III	10	80	8	0
IV	10	50	5	IV	30	70	21	20
All	100		84	All	100		84	0

The cure rate improves in both stage I and stage IV, and there is no change in cure rates for stage II and stage III, after the introduction of a new staging investigation. The overall cure rate is, however, unchanged.

Alvan Feinstein, **1926–2001, American Clinician and Epidemiologist.**
Will Rogers (properly William Penn Adair Rogers), **1879–1935, American Actor, Humorist and Wit.**
There is much confusion **about the use of the terms 'multidisciplinary' and 'multiprofessional':** we use 'multidisciplinary' to imply the presence of various medically-qualified specialists (pathologists, radiologists etc.) and 'multiprofessional' implies the presence of specialists from non-medical backgrounds (nurses, social workers, radiographers).

Table 7.4 Staging of colorectal cancer

TNM	
TX	Primary tumour cannot be assessed
T0	No evidence of primary tumour
Tis	Intraepithelial or intramucosal carcinoma
T1	Tumour invades submucosa
T2	Tumour invades muscularis propria
T3	Tumour invades through the muscularis propria into the subserosa or into retroperitoneal (pericolic or perirectal) tissues

	a	Minimal invasion: < 1 mm beyond muscularis
	b	Slight invasion: 1–5 mm beyond muscularis
	c	Moderate invasion: 5–15 mm beyond muscularis
	d	Extensive invasion: > 15 mm beyond muscularis

T4	Tumour directly invades beyond bowel	
	a	Direct invasion into other organs or structures
	b	Perforates visceral peritoneum

NX	Regional lymph nodes cannot be assessed
N0	No metastases in regional nodes
N1	Metastases in 1–3 regional lymph nodes
N2	Metastases in ≥ 4 regional lymph nodes
MX	Not possible to assess the presence of distant metastases
M0	No distant metastases
M1	Distant metastases present

lectual and technical competence that is necessary to manage all the patients presenting with a particular type of tumour. The era of feigned omniscience is past. The formation of multidisciplinary teams represents an attempt to make certain that each and every patient with a particular type of cancer is managed appropriately. Teams should not only be multidisciplinary, they should be multiprofessional (Summary box 7.4).

Summary box 7.4

Members of the multiprofessional team

- Site-specialist surgeon
- Surgical oncologist
- Plastic and reconstructive surgeon
- Clinical oncologist/radiotherapist
- Medical oncologist
- Diagnostic radiologist
- Pathologist
- Speech therapist
- Physiotherapist
- Prosthetist
- Clinical nurse specialist (rehabilitation, supportive care)
- Palliative care nurse (symptom control, palliation)
- Social worker/counsellor
- Medical secretary/administrator
- Audit and information coordinator

There is widespread agreement, on the basis of remarkably little evidence, that multidisciplinary teams are essential for high-quality care. This gives rise to a belief, both quaint and naïve, that simply forming the team is sufficient and that the calibre and personal skills of the team members are of little consequence. There is remarkably little agreement, either in theory or in practice, as

Table 7.5 Relationships between staging systems for colorectal cancer

TNM	AJCC	Dukes	Modified Astler–Coller
TisN0M0	0	–	–
T1N0M0	I	A	A
T2N0M0	I	A	B1
T3N0M0	IIA	B	B2
T4N0M0	IIB	B	B3
T1 or T2 N1M0	IIIA	C	C1
T3 or T4 N1M0	IIIB	C	C2, C3
Any T N2M0	IIIC	C	C1, C2, C3
Any T Any N M1	IV	D	–

to the decision-making processes that are employed within the context of the multidisciplinary teams. There is a danger that the imprimatur of the team may be used to provide legitimacy for the opinions and prejudices of the dominant members of the team. The decision of the team should reflect an informed judgement made after discussion among equals, not the unqualified dogma espoused by the loudest voice. The advantages and disadvantages of multidisciplinary teams are summarised in Table 7.6. The challenge for the future is to reconcile a corporate approach to decision making with a respect for the individuality of each individual patient: their tumour, their circumstances, and their informed choices. There should be no class solutions in oncology.

Vernon B. Astler, **Surgeon, The Medical School of the University of Michigan, Ann Arbor, MI, USA.**
Frederick A. Coller, **Pathologist, The Medical School of the University of Michigan, Ann Arbor, MI, USA.**
Cuthbert Esquire Dukes, **1890–1977, Pathologist, St. Mark's Hospital, London, England.**

Table 7.6 The advantages and disadvantages of the multidisciplinary team

Advantages	Disadvantages
Open debate concerning management	An opportunity for rampant egotism and showing off
Patient has the advantage of many simultaneous opinions from many different specialties	Less confident and less articulate members of the team may not be able to express their views, even though their views may be extremely important
Decision making is open, transparent and explicit	May degenerate into a rubber-stamping exercise in which the class solutions implied by guidelines are unthinkingly applied to disparate individuals
Team members educate each other	Decisions are made in the absence of patients and their carers: the commodification of the person
A useful educational experience for trainees and students	Clinicians are able to avoid having to take responsibility for their decisions and their actions: the fig-leaf of 'corporate responsibility'
	Time-consuming and resource intensive: takes busy clinicians away from clinical practice for hours at a time

Principles of cancer surgery

For most solid tumours, surgery remains the definitive treatment and the only realistic hope of cure. However, surgery has several roles in cancer treatment including diagnosis, removal of primary disease, removal of metastatic disease, palliation, prevention and reconstruction.

Diagnosis and staging

In most cases, the diagnosis of cancer has been made before definitive surgery is carried out but, occasionally, a surgical procedure is required to make the diagnosis. This is particularly true of patients with malignant ascites where laparoscopy has an important role in obtaining tissue for diagnosis. Laparoscopy is also widely used for the staging of intra-abdominal malignancy, particularly oesophageal and gastric cancer. By this means, it is often possible to diagnose widespread peritoneal disease and small liver metastases that may have been missed on cross-sectional imaging. Laparoscopic ultrasound is a particularly useful adjunct for the diagnosis of intrahepatic metastases. Other examples in which surgery is central to the diagnosis of cancer include orchidectomy where a patient is suspected of having testicular cancer and lymph node biopsy in a patient with lymphoma. Recently, sentinel node biopsy in melanoma and breast cancer has attracted a great deal of interest. Here, a radiolabelled colloid is injected into or around the primary tumour, and the regional lymph node tumour is then scanned with a gamma camera that will pinpoint the lymph node nearest to the tumour. This lymph node can then be removed for histological diagnosis. Until recently, staging laparotomy was an important aspect of the staging of lymphomas but, with more accurate cross-sectional imaging and the much more widespread use of chemotherapy, this practice is now largely redundant.

Removal of primary disease

Radical surgery for cancer involves removal of the primary tumour and as much of the surrounding tissue and lymph node drainage as possible in order not only to ensure local control but also to prevent spread of the tumour through the lymphatics. Although the principle of local control is still extremely important, it is now recognised that ultraradical surgery probably has little effect on the development of metastatic disease, as evidenced by the randomised trials of radical vs. simple mastectomy for breast cancer. It is important, however, to appreciate that high-quality, meticulous surgery taking care not to disrupt the primary tumour at the time of excision is of the utmost importance in obtaining a cure in localised disease and preventing local recurrence.

Removal of metastatic disease

In certain circumstances, surgery for metastatic disease may be appropriate. This is particularly true for liver metastases arising from colorectal cancer where successful resection of all detectable disease can lead to long-term survival in about one-third of patients. With multiple liver metastases, it may still be possible to take a surgical approach by using *in situ* ablation with cryotherapy or radiofrequency energy. Another situation where surgery may be of value is pulmonary resection for isolated lung metastases, particularly from renal cell carcinoma.

Palliation

In many cases, surgery is not appropriate for cure but may be extremely valuable for palliation. A good example of this is the patient with a symptomatic primary tumour who also has distant metastases. In this case, removal of the primary may increase the patient's quality of life but will have little effect on the ultimate outcome. Other examples include bypass procedures such as an ileotransverse anastomosis to alleviate symptoms of obstruction caused by an inoperable caecal cancer or bypassing an unresectable carcinoma at the head of the pancreas by cholecysto- or choledochojejunostomy to alleviate jaundice.

Principles underlying the non-surgical treatment of cancer

The relationship between dose and response and the principle of selective toxicity

Non-surgical treatments, in common with surgery, have the potential to cause harm as well as benefit. Surgery is difficult to

---

in situ **is Latin for 'in the place'.**

quantify; it is hard to describe a mastectomy in units of measure. Both drugs and radiation can be expressed in reproducible units: milligrams in the case of drugs; Grays (Gy) in the case of radiation. Thus, in contrast to surgery, it is possible to construct dose–response relationships for both the benefits (such as tumour cure rate) and harms (such as tissue damage that is both severe and permanent) associated with non-surgical interventions. These curves (see Fig. 7.6) have the same general shape: they are sigmoidal. The practical consequence of this is that, over a relatively narrow dose range, we move from failure to success, from tolerability to disaster. It is possible, in theory, using dose–response curves to calculate an optimal dose for treating each tumour: the dose is that which is associated with the maximal probability of an uncomplicated cure. Lying behind the concept of the probability of an uncomplicated cure is the principle of selective toxicity: treatment must be delivered in such a way as to ensure that the damage done to the tumour is more than the damage done to the normal tissues. The treatment should be selectively toxic to the tumour and, as far as possible, should spare the normal tissues from damage. It is this simple principle that underpins both the selection of agents used to treat cancer and the schedules employed to deliver them. Although the graphical representations of the relationships between dose, response and the probability of uncomplicated cure are conceptually simple and intuitively appealing, they are, in clinical practice, completely impractical. The construction of full dose–response curves for all possible combinations of tumours and normal tissues is neither feasible nor ethical (you cannot knowingly

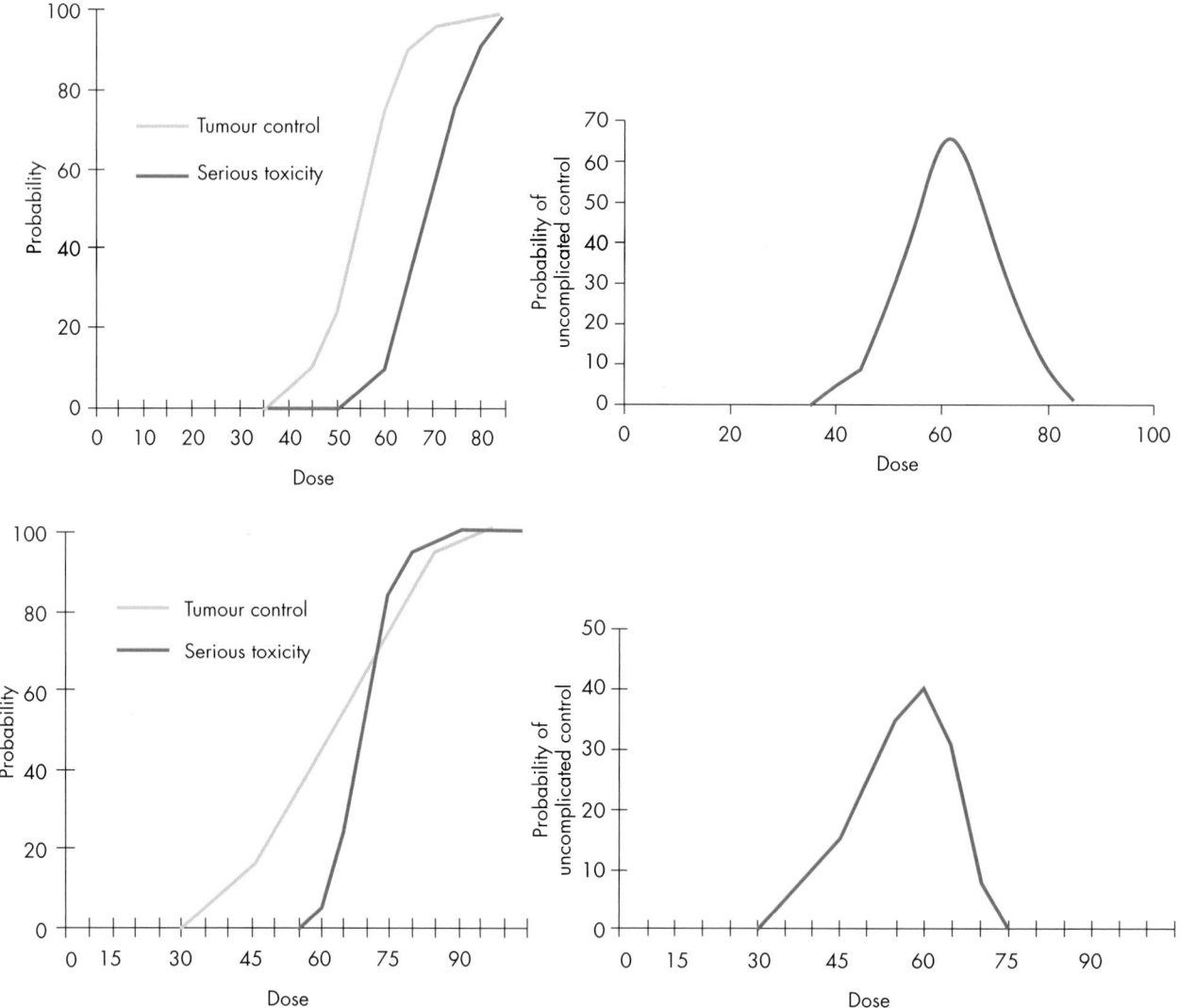

Figure 7.6 A schematic illustration of the relationship between dose, response and the probability of uncomplicated cure. The upper figures show ideal circumstances with steep dose–response relationships for both normal tissue damage and tumour control. The lower figures show something more like the real world. The dose–response relationship for tumour control is flatter, because tumours are heterogeneous and, consequently, the probability of uncomplicated cure is lower – even for the optimal dose (40% in the lower figure compared with 70% in the upper figure).

Louis Harold Gray, **1905–1965, Director, The British Empire Cancer Campaign Research Unit in Radiobiology, Mount Vernon Hospital, Northwood, Middlesex, England. A Gray (Gy) is the SI unit for the absorbed dose of ionizing radiation.**

expose a patient to a high risk of suffering harm, simply to provide another data point). Reliance, when it comes to defining optimal doses and schedules, must be on incomplete clinical data and a knowledge of the general shape of the relationship between dose and response.

General strategies in the non-surgical management of cancer

Curative surgery for cancer is guided by one simple principle: the physical removal of all identifiable disease. The principles underlying the non-surgical management of cancer are more complex. First, we have to consider the spatial distribution of the effects of our therapies: surgery and radiotherapy are local or, at best, locoregional treatments; drugs offer a therapy that is systemic (Fig. 7.7). Second, there is the question of the intent underlying the treatment. Occasionally, radiotherapy, chemotherapy or the combination of the two may be used with curative intent (Table 7.7). More usually, chemotherapy or radiotherapy is used to lower the risk of recurrence after primary treatment with surgery, so called adjuvant therapy. Implicit within the concept of adjuvant therapy is the realisation that much of what is done is unnecessary or futile, or both. The need for adjuvant therapy, to treat the risk that residual disease might be present after apparently curative surgery, is an acknowledgement of the current inability to detect or predict, with sufficient precision, the presence of residual disease. It also explains why the incremental benefits from adjuvant treatments are so small and why the existence of these benefits can only be proven using randomised controlled trials including many thousands of patients. As illustrated in Figures 7.8 and 7.9, our current approach to the selection of patients for post-surgical adjuvant treatment is both intellectually impoverished and inefficient. Patients would be far better off if, rather than so much time and effort having been invested in attempting to discover new 'cures' for cancer, equivalent resources had been devoted to devising clinically useful tests to detect residual cancer cells persisting after apparently successful initial therapy.

Radiotherapy

Within a month of their discovery in 1895, X-rays were being used to treat cancer. Despite over 100 years of use, and despite

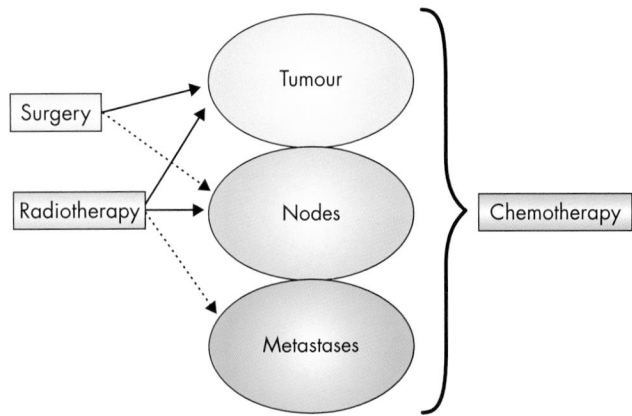

Figure 7.7 Schematic diagram to show the spatial scope of cancer treatments. Chemotherapy is systemic; surgery is mainly a local treatment. Radiotherapy is usually local or locoregional, but can, as in radio-iodine therapy for thyroid cancer, be systemic.

some outstanding clinical achievements, it is still not known how best to use radiation to treat cancer. Part of the difficulty arises because it is not known precisely how radiation treatment affects tumours or normal tissues. Up until about 20 years ago, it was assumed that the biological effects of radiation resulted from radiation-induced damage to the DNA of dividing cells. Nowadays, it is known that, although this undoubtedly explains some of the biological effects of radiation, it does not provide a full explanation. Radiation can, both directly and indirectly, influence gene expression: over 100 radiation-inducible effects on gene expression have now been described. These changes in gene expression are responsible for a considerable proportion of the biological effects of radiation upon tumours and normal tissues. It is pretentious, but true, to state that radiotherapy is a precisely targeted form of gene therapy for cancer.

The practicalities of radiation therapy are reasonably straightforward: define the target to treat; design the optimal technical set-up to provide uniform irradiation of that target; and choose that schedule of treatment that delivers radiation to that target in such a way as to maximise the therapeutic ratio (Fig. 7.10). One

Table 7.7 Examples of malignancies that may be cured without the need for surgical excision

Malignancy	Potentially curative treatment
Leukaemia	Chemotherapy (± radiotherapy)
Lymphoma	Chemotherapy (± radiotherapy)
Small cell lung cancer	Chemotherapy (± radiotherapy)
Tumours of childhood (rhabdomyosarcoma, Wilms' tumour)	Chemotherapy (± radiotherapy)
Early laryngeal cancer	Radiotherapy
Advanced head and neck cancer	Chemoradiation (synchronous chemotherapy and radiotherapy)
Oesophageal cancer	Chemoradiation (synchronous chemotherapy and radiotherapy)
Squamous cell cancer of the anus	Chemoradiation (synchronous chemotherapy and radiotherapy)
Advanced cancer of the cervix	Radiotherapy (± chemotherapy)
Medulloblastoma	Radiotherapy (± chemotherapy)
Skin tumours (BCC, SCC)	Radiotherapy

BCC, basal cell carcinoma; SCC, squamous cell carcinoma.

Max Wilms, **1867–1918**, Professor of Surgery, Heidelberg, Germany.

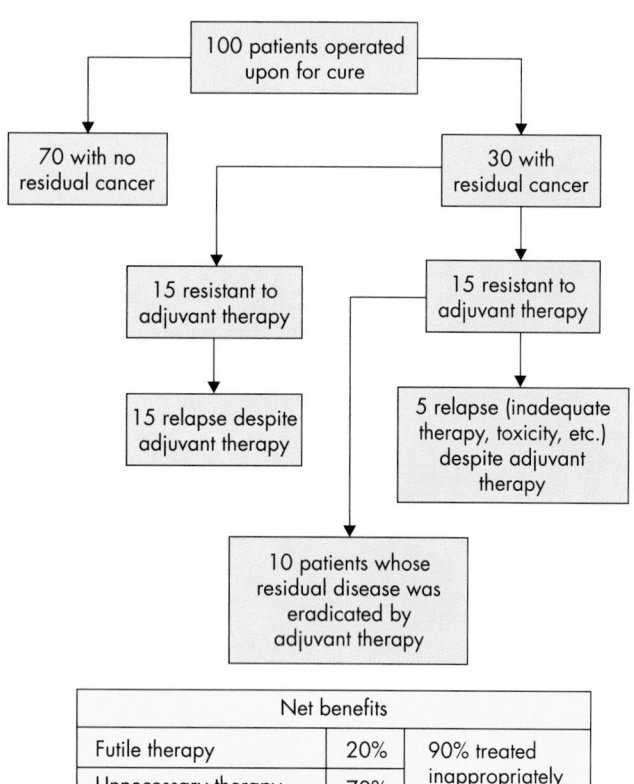

Figure 7.8 The concept of adjuvant therapy.

of the main problems with assessing a therapeutic ratio for a given schedule of radiation is that there is a dissociation between the acute effects on normal tissues and the late damage. The acute reaction is not a reliable guide to the adverse consequences of treatment in the longer term. As the late effects following irradiation can take over 20 years to develop, this poses an obvious difficulty: if the radiation schedule is changed, it will be known within 2 or 3 years whether or not the new schedule has improved tumour control; it may, however, be two decades before it is known, with any degree of certainty, whether the new technique is safe. Fractionated radiotherapy selectively spares late, as opposed to immediate, effects. For any given total dose, the smaller the dose per treatment (the larger the number of fractions), the less severe the late effects will be. The problem is that the greater the number of fractions of daily treatment, the longer the overall treatment time will be and the greater the opportunity will be for the tumour to proliferate during treatment. All fractionation is a compromise and, as a recent systematic review has shown, the evidence base for many widely accepted treatment schedules is remarkably slight. Thirty years ago, Withers defined the four Rs of radiotherapy (see Summary box 7.5); subsequently, we have added a fifth 'R' – intrinsic radiosensitivity. The clinical practice of radiation oncology operates within the limits defined by these five Rs.

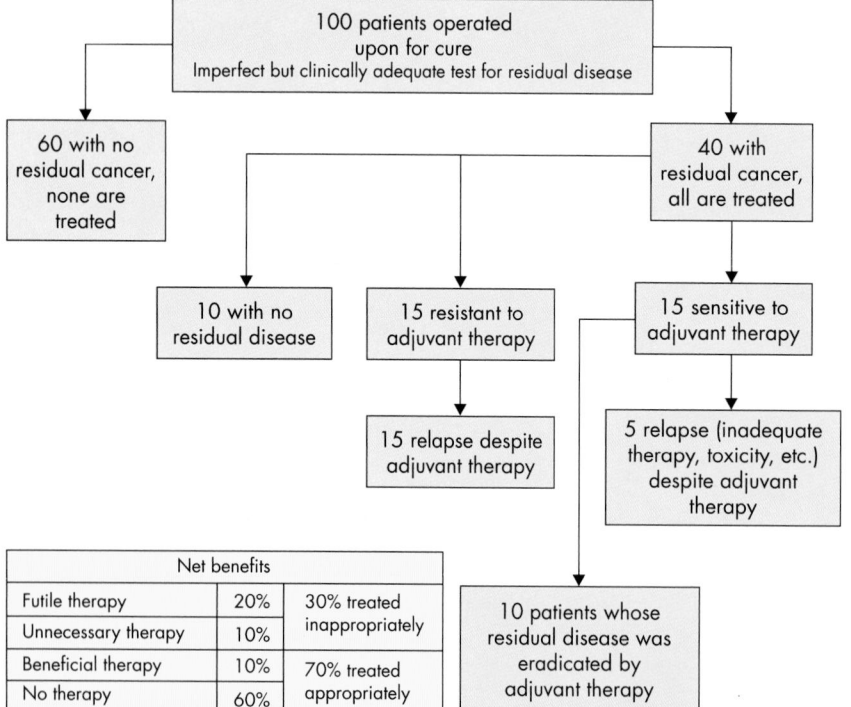

Figure 7.9 The concept of adjuvant therapy and testing for minimal residual disease.

H. R. Withers, **Professor of Radiation Oncology at the University of California, Los Angeles.**

Summary box 7.5

The five Rs of radiotherapy

- *Repair.* If given sufficient time between fractional doses of radiation, cells will repair the radiation-induced damage. Repair half-times are typically 3–6 hours. Fractionation offers a means whereby any differentials in repair capacity between tumour and normal cells may be exploited.
- *Reoxygenation.* Hypoxic cells are relatively radioresistant compared with well-oxygenated cells. Normal tissues are well oxygenated; tumours are often hypoxic. This is an obvious therapeutic disadvantage.
- *Repopulation.* As radiotherapy kills cancer cells, rapid proliferation of tumour cells is stimulated. Thus, during protracted treatment, production of cells by the tumour may equal, or even exceed, radiation-induced cell loss. It is thus better that the overall treatment time is as short as possible.
- *Redistribution.* The sensitivity of cells to radiation varies according to their position within the cell cycle. This may lead to a degree of synchronisation of cellular division within the tumour: ideally, fractions of radiotherapy should be timed to coincide with vulnerable phases of the cell cycle (late G2 and M).
- *Radiosensitivity.* Low dose rate irradiation experiments demonstrate that cells derived from tumours differ in their intrinsic sensitivity to radiation. Some cells are so intrinsically resistant to treatment that no clinically viable schedule of radiation therapy would eliminate them. Conversely, some cells may be so sensitive that virtually any schedule would be successful – the majority of cells will lie somewhere between these extremes.

Chemotherapy and biological therapies

As with radiotherapy, so with chemotherapy: selective toxicity is the fundamental principle underlying the use of chemotherapy in clinical practice. The importance of the principle is further emphasised by the fact that, by itself, chemotherapy is rarely sufficient to cure cancer. Chemotherapy is often (in effect if not in intent) a palliative rather than a curative intervention. As such, its use should be influenced by the cardinal principle of palliative treatment: treatment aimed at relieving symptoms should not, itself, produce unacceptable symptoms. To use the language of another era: we should not be 'making the cure of a disease more grievous than its endurance'. There are now over 95 different drugs licensed by the US Food and Drug Administration (FDA) for the treatment of cancer. Of these, over 65% are cytotoxic drugs, 15% are hormonal therapies and 15% are designed to interact with specific molecular targets – so called targeted therapies. Over 50% of these agents have been licensed since 1990: in terms of potential progress, achievement over the past 15 years has been equivalent to that in the previous 40 years. There are now many more options than there were 20 years ago and, perhaps more importantly, lessons have been learnt about how better to deploy resources. The classes of cytotoxic drugs, their mode of action and clinical indications are summarised in Table 7.8.

The newer 'targeted' therapies available for treating cancer present particular dilemmas. They offer modest prolongation of survival, often with minimal toxicity, but at considerable financial cost. When compared with conventional therapies, these drugs typically cost over £50 000 (US$94 000) per quality-adjusted life-year gained and, when overall resources are limited, they may be considered unaffordable: Table 7.9 (page 109) puts into context the cost-effectiveness of various clinical interventions. The current cost of targeted therapies should not obscure their importance: they represent the first attempts to translate advances in molecular biology into clinical practice. The discoveries of the mid-twentieth century are finally bearing fruit.

Principles of combined treatment

Cytotoxic drugs are rarely used as single agents; radiotherapy and chemotherapy are often given together. The rationale behind combination, as opposed to single-agent, drug therapy is straightforward and is somewhat analogous to that for combined antibiotic therapy: it is a strategy designed to combat drug resistance. By the time of diagnosis, many tumours will contain cancer cells that, through spontaneous mutation, have acquired resistance to cytotoxic drugs. Unlike antibiotic resistance, there is no need for previous exposure to the drug. Spontaneous mutation rates are high enough to allow the play of chance to permit the development, and subsequent expansion, of clones of cells resistant to drugs to which they have never been exposed. If drugs were used as single agents, then the further expansion of these *de novo* resistant subclones would limit cure. The problem can be mitigated by combining drugs together from the outset.

There are three main principles upon which the choice of drugs for combination therapy is based, the first of which should be self-evident: use drugs active against the diseases in question; use drugs with distinct modes of action; use drugs with non-overlapping toxicities. By using drugs with different biological effects, for example by combining an anti-metabolite with an agent that actively damages DNA, it may be possible to obtain a truly synergistic effect. It is inadvisable to combine drugs with similar adverse effects: combining two highly myelosuppressive drugs may produce an unacceptably high risk of neutropenic sepsis. Where possible, combinations should be based upon a consideration of the toxicity profiles of the drugs concerned (Summary box 7.6).

Summary box 7.6

Basic principles of combined therapy

- Use effective agents
- Use agents with different modes of action (synergy)
- Use agents with non-overlapping toxicities
- Consider spatial cooperation

In considering the combination of radiotherapy and chemotherapy, radiation could be considered as just another drug. There is, in addition to synergy and toxicity, another factor to consider in the combination of drugs and radiation – the concept of spatial cooperation. Chemotherapy is a systemic treatment; radiotherapy is not. Radiotherapy is, however, able to reach sites, such as the central nervous system and testis, that drugs may not reach effectively. This is why, for example in patients treated primarily with chemotherapy for leukaemias, lymphomas and small cell lung cancer, prophylactic cranial irradiation is part of the treatment protocol.

A synergistic effect is one in which the damage caused by giving the agents together is greater than the damage caused when the drugs are given separately.

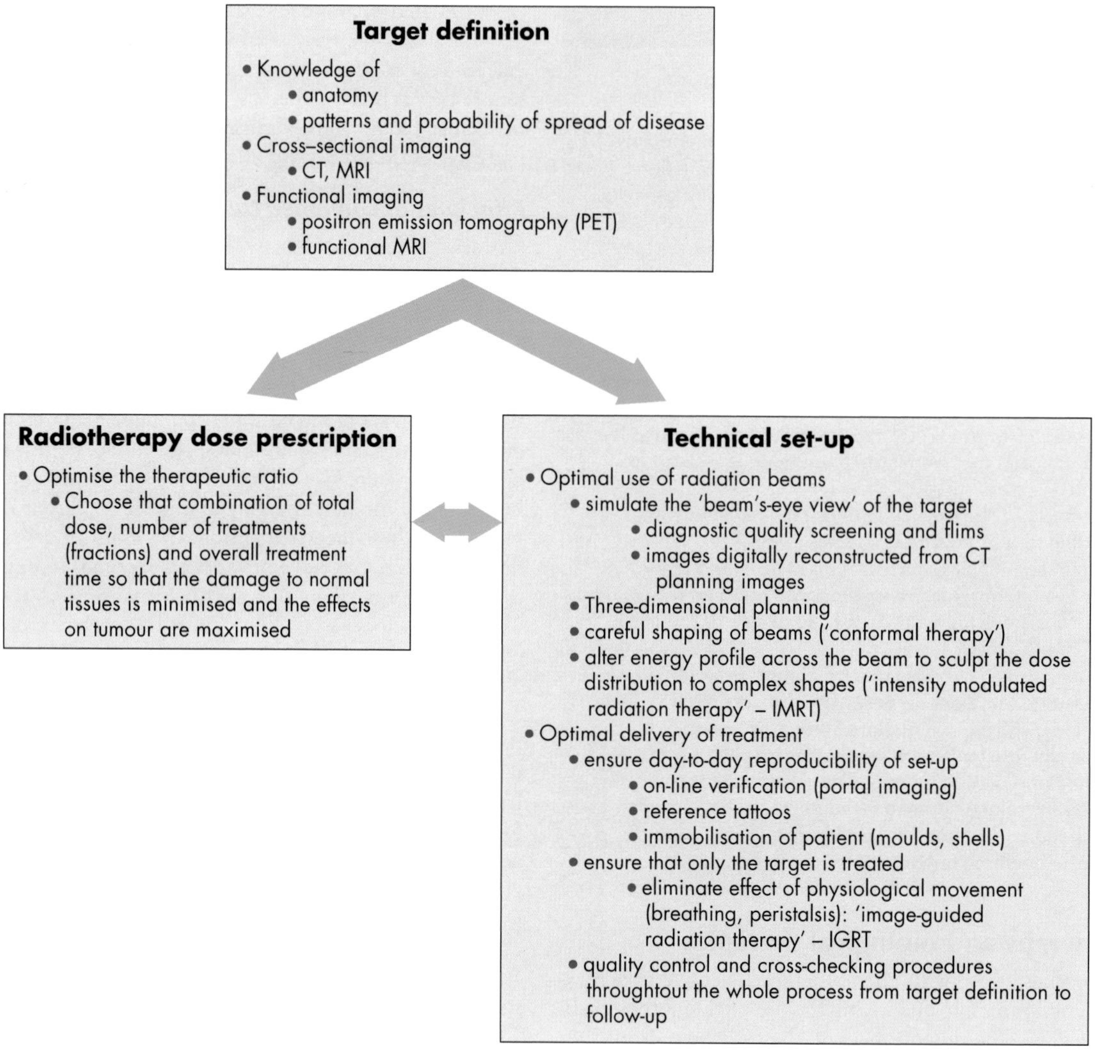

Figure 7.10 The processes involved in clinical radiotherapy. CT, computerised tomography; MRI, magnetic resonance imaging.

Palliative therapy

The distinction between palliative and curative treatment is not always clear cut. The distinction will become increasingly blurred as professional and public attitudes towards the management of cancer change. Ten years ago, cancer was perceived as a disease that was either cured or it was not; patients either lived or died. There was little appreciation that, for many patients, cancer might be a chronic disease. Nowadays, we are increasingly aware that many of the so called curative treatments are simply elegant exercises in growth delay. Five-year survival is not necessarily tantamount to cure. With the development of targeted therapies that regulate, rather than eradicate, cancer, this state of affairs is likely to continue. The aim of treatment will be growth control rather than the extirpation of every last cancer cell. Patients will live with their cancers, perhaps for years. They will die *with* cancer, but not necessarily *of* cancer. Against this background, the distinction between curative and palliative therapy seems somewhat arbitrary. The distinction may be arbitrary, but the control and relief of symptoms is crucial to the successful management of patients with cancer. Much of the fear associated with cancer is due to past failures to control patients' symptoms: there are folk memories of indignity and distress that affect peoples' current attitudes. Reluctance to attend for screening tests may be profoundly influenced by fears based on the past experiences of relatives and friends.

Patients fear the symptoms, distress and disruption associated with cancer almost as much as they fear the disease itself. Palliative treatment has as its goal the relief of symptoms. Sometimes, this will involve treating the underlying problem, as with palliative radiotherapy for bone metastases; sometimes it will not. Sometimes, it may be inappropriate to treat the cancer itself, but that does not imply that there is nothing more to be done; it simply means that there may be better ways to assuage the distress and discomfort caused by the tumour. Palliative medicine in the twenty-first century is about far more than optimal control of pain: its scope is wide, its impact immense (Table 7.10). The most important factor in the successful palliative management of a patient with cancer is that referral is made early enough in the course of the disease. There should be no abrupt change between curative and palliative modes of management; any such transition should be seamless.

Table 7.8 A summary of chemotherapeutic and biological agents currently used in cancer treatment

Class	Examples	Putative mode of action	Tumour types that may be sensitive to drug
Drugs that interfere with mitosis	Vincristine, vinblastine	Interfere with the formation of microtubules: 'spindle poisons'	Lymphomas Leukaemias Brain tumours Sarcomas
	Taxanes: Taxol, paclitaxel	Stabilise microtubules	Breast cancer Non-small cell lung cancer Ovarian cancer Prostate cancer Head and neck cancer
Drugs that interfere with DNA synthesis (anti-metabolites)	5-Fluorouracil (5-FU)	Inhibition of thymidylate synthase, false substrate for both DNA and RNA synthesis	Breast cancer Gastrointestinal cancer
	Capecitabine	Orally active prodrug that is metabolised to 5-FU. Inhibition of thymidylate synthase, false substrate for both DNA and RNA synthesis	Breast cancer Gastrointestinal cancer
	Methotrexate	Inhibition of dihydrofolate reductase	Breast cancer Bladder cancer Lymphomas Cervix cancer
	6-Mercaptopurine	Inhibits *de novo* purine synthesis	Leukaemias
	6-Thioguanine	Inhibits *de novo* purine synthesis	Leukaemias
	Cytosine arabinoside	False substrate in DNA synthesis	Leukaemias Lymphomas
	Gemcitabine	Inhibits ribonucleotide reductase	Non-small cell lung cancer Pancreatic cancer
Drugs that directly damage DNA or interfere with its function	Mitomycin C	DNA cross-linking, preferentially active at sites of low oxygen tension (a bioreductive drug)	Anal cancer Bladder cancer Gastric cancer Head and neck cancer Rectal cancer
	Cis-platinum	Forms adducts between DNA strands and interferes with replication	Germ cell tumours Ovarian cancer Non-small cell lung cancer Head and neck cancer Oesophageal cancer
	Carboplatin	Forms adducts between DNA strands and interferes with replication	Germ cell tumours Ovarian cancer Non-small cell lung cancer Head and neck cancer
	Oxaliplatin	Forms adducts between DNA strands and interferes with replication	Colorectal cancer
	Doxorubicin	Intercalates between DNA strands and interferes with replication	Breast cancer Lymphomas Sarcomas Kaposi's sarcoma
	Cyclophosphamide	A prodrug converted via hepatic cytochrome p450 to phosphoramide mustard; causes DNA cross-links	Breast cancer Lymphomas Sarcomas
	Ifosfamide	Related to cyclophosphamide, causes DNA cross-links	Small cell lung cancer Sarcomas
	Bleomycin	DNA strand breakage via formation of metal complex	Germ cell tumours Lymphomas

CHAPTER 7 | PRINCIPLES OF ONCOLOGY

Table 7.8 A summary of chemotherapeutic and biological agents currently used in cancer treatment – *continued*

Class	Examples	Putative mode of action	Tumour types that may be sensitive to drug
Drugs that directly damage DNA or interfere with its function – *continued*	Irinotecan	Inhibits topoisomerase 1 and thereby prevents the DNA from unwinding and repairing during replication	Colorectal cancer
	Etoposide	Inhibits topoisomerase 2; prevents the DNA from unwinding and repairing during replication	Small cell lung cancer Germ cell tumours Lymphomas
	Dacarbazine	A nitrosourea that requires activation by hepatic cytochrome p450. Methylates guanine residues in DNA	Brain tumours Sarcoma Melanoma
	Temozolomide	A nitrosourea but, unlike dacarbazine, does not require activation by hepatic cytochrome p450. Methylates guanine residues in DNA	Glioblastoma multiforme Melanoma
	Actinomycin D	Intercalation between DNA strands, DNA strand breaks	Rhabdomyosarcoma Wilms' tumour
Hormones	Tamoxifen	Blocks oestrogen receptors	Breast cancer
	Anastrazole	An aromatase inhibitor that blocks post-menopausal (non-ovarian) oestrogen production	Breast cancer
	Exemestane	An aromatase inhibitor that blocks post-menopausal (non-ovarian) oestrogen production	Breast cancer
	Letrozole	An aromatase inhibitor that blocks post-menopausal (non-ovarian) oestrogen production	Breast cancer
	Leuprolide	Analogue of gonadotrophin-releasing hormone; continued use produces downregulation of the anterior pituitary with a consequent fall in testosterone levels	Prostate cancer
	Goserelin	Analogue of gonadotrophin-releasing hormone; continued use produces downregulation of the anterior pituitary with a consequent fall in testosterone levels	Prostate cancer
	Buserelin	Analogue of gonadotrophin-releasing hormone; continued use produces downregulation of the anterior pituitary with a consequent fall in testosterone levels	Prostate cancer
	Cabergoline	Blocks prolactin release, a long-acting dopamine agonist	Prolactin-secreting pituitary tumours
	Bromocriptine	Dopamine agonist, blocks stimulation of the anterior pituitary	Pituitary tumours
	Cyproterone acetate	Blocks the effect of androgens	Prostate cancer
	Flutamide	Blocks the effect of androgens	Prostate cancer
	Nilutamide	Blocks the effect of androgens	Prostate cancer
	Bicalutamide	Blocks the effect of androgens	Prostate cancer
Inhibitors of receptor tyrosine kinases	Gefitinib	Inhibits EGFR tyrosine kinase	Non-small cell lung cancer
	Imatinib	Blocks the ability of mutant BCR-ABL fusion protein to bind ATP Inhibition of mutant c-KIT	Chronic myeloid leukaemia Gastrointestinal stromal tumours (GIST)
	Erlotinib	Inhibits EGFR tyrosine kinase	Non-small cell lung cancer Pancreatic cancer
	Sunitinib	Promiscuous tyrosine kinase inhibitor (PDGFR, VEGFR, KIT, FLT)	Renal cancer GIST refractory to Imatinib

Table 7.8 A summary of chemotherapeutic and biological agents currently used in cancer treatment – *continued*

Class	Examples	Putative mode of action	Tumour types that may be sensitive to drug
Inhibitors of receptor tyrosine kinases – *continued*	Lapatinib	Inhibits tyrosine kinases associated with EGFR and HER2	
Protease inhibitors	Bortezomib	Interferes with proteasomal degradation of regulatory proteins; in particular, prevents NF kappa B from preventing apoptosis	Multiple myeloma
Differentiating agents	All *trans*-retinoic acid	Induces terminal differentiation	Acute promyelocytic leukaemia
Farnesyl transferase inhibitors	Lonafarnib	Inhibition of farnesyl transferase and consequent inactivation of *ras*-dependent signal transduction	Leukaemia
	Tipifarnib	Inhibition of farnesyl transferase and consequent inactivation of *ras*-dependent signal transduction	Acute leukaemia Myelodysplastic syndrome
Antibodies directed to cell surface antigens	Trastuzumab	Antibody directed against HER2 receptor	Breast cancer
	Cetuximab	Antibody directed against EGFR receptor	Colorectal cancer Head and neck cancer
	Bevacizumab	Antibody directed against VEGFR	Colorectal cancer
	Rituximab	Antibody against CD20 antigen	Lymphomas
	Alemtuzumab	Antibody against CD52 antigen	Lymphomas
Inducers of apoptosis	Arsenic trioxide	Induces apoptosis by caspase inhibition Inhibition of nitric oxide	Acute promyelocytic leukaemia
Immunological mediators	Interferon alpha-2b	Activates macrophages, increases the cytotoxicity of T lymphocytes, inhibits cell division (and viral replication)	Renal carcinoma Melanoma Hairy cell leukaemia
	Thalidomide	Anti-inflammatory, stimulates T cells, anti-angiogenic	Myeloma

EGFR, epidermal growth factor receptor; NF, nuclear factor; PDGFR, platelet-derived growth factor receptor; VEGFR, vascular endothelial growth factor receptor.

Table 7.9 Comparison of various estimates of cost-effectiveness for selected clinical interventions

Intervention	Cost (in 2002 US dollars) per quality-adjusted life-year (QALY)
Annual CT chest screening for lung cancer in a 60-year-old male ex-smoker vs. no screening	$2.4 million
Laparoscopic inguinal hernia repair vs. expectant management in adults with inguinal hernia	$610
Stroke unit care vs. usual care in survivors of acute stroke	$1600
Lifetime vitamin D + calcium supplements vs. no supplements to prevent/treat osteoporosis in 70-year-old women	$8500
Letrozole vs. tamoxifen in the first-line management of post-menopausal women with advanced breast cancer	$120 000
Erlotinib vs. usual care in the treatment of relapsed non-small cell lung cancer	$104 000

CT, computerised tomography
Data from CEA (Tufts New England Medical Center) register (accessed via http://www.tufts-nemc.org/cearegistry/ on 15 November 2006) and the UK National Institute for Health and Clinical Excellence (accessed via http://www.nice.org.uk/page.aspx?c=153 on 15 November 2006).
Currently, in the UK, interventions costing less than US$60 000 (2002) are considered 'affordable', that is they fall below the WTP ('willingness to pay') threshold.

End-of-life care

End-of-life care is distinct from palliative care. Patients treated palliatively may survive for many years; end-of-life care concerns the last few months of a patient's life. Many issues, such as symptom control, are common to both palliative care and to end-of-life care, but there are also problems that are specific to the sense of approaching death. These may include a heightened sense of spiritual need, profound fear and the specific needs of those who are facing bereavement. 'I don't mind dying, I just don't want to be there when it happens' is a statement that expresses both the acceptance and the fear of death. We all live our own lives and

Table 7.10 An outline of the domains and interventions included within palliative and supportive care

Symptom assessment
    Pain, anorexia, fatigue, dyspnoea, etc.
    Treatment-related toxicity

Quality of life assessment

Symptom relief
    Drugs
    Surgery
    Radiotherapy
    Complementary therapies
        Acupuncture
        Homeopathy
        Aromatherapy, etc.

Psychosocial interventions
    Psychological support
    Relaxation techniques
    Cognitive behavioural therapy
    Counselling
    Group therapy
    Music therapy
    Emotional support

Physical and practical support
    Physiotherapy
    Occupational therapy
    Speech therapy

Information and knowledge
    Cancer back-up
    Maggie's centres

Nutritional support
    Dietary advice
    Nutritional supplements

Social support
    Patients
    Relatives and carers

Financial support
    Ensure uptake of entitlements
    Grants from charities, e.g. Macmillan Cancer Relief

Spiritual support

we all die our own deaths. The concept of the 'good death' has been embedded in many cultures over many centuries. As healthcare professionals, we deal with many deaths and sometimes forget that, for someone who wishes to die a 'good death', there are no replays: we only have one chance to get it right. This is why end-of-life care is worth considering in its own right and not as something synonymous with, or a mere appendage to, palliative care. Some of the issues unique to end-of-life care are summarised in Summary box 7.7.

Woody Allen, B. 1935, American Screen-writer, Director and Actor who, in his film 'Death', uses this version of a remark originally made by Mark Twain, (Samuel Langhorne Clemens), 1835–1910, the American Author.

Summary box 7.7

Issues at the end of life

- **Appropriateness of active intervention**
- **Euthanasia**
- **Physician-assisted suicide**
- **Living wills**
- **Bereavement**
- **Spirituality**
- **Support to allow death at home**
- **The problem of the medicalisation of death**

FUTURE DEVELOPMENTS IN THE MANAGEMENT OF CANCER

Developed world

Over the next 10 years, the cost of health care in general, and of cancer care in particular, will rise faster than our ability to afford it. The stark implication is that inequalities in care will increase, rather than decrease. Those who can afford expensive new treatments will be able to obtain them; those who are less well-off will have to do without. As cancer becomes a chronic disease, the duration of therapy will increase: instead of 3–6 months of relatively inexpensive chemotherapy, 3–4 years of extremely expensive biological therapy may be the norm. This compounds the problem of the unaffordability of treatment. There are some tough decisions to be made. One solution to this apparent dilemma is obvious but, politically, difficult to grasp: more effort needs to be put into the prevention and early detection of cancer. This makes sense in terms of both economics and social justice. Unfortunately, preventative and screening technologies lack the backing of the medico-industrial complex: there is more money to be made from treating with drugs than in attempting to persuade people to take exercise and eat a healthy diet or, for that matter, to send a sample of their faeces to a laboratory for faecal occult blood testing.

Developing world

Just as modern technology will increase the inequality in cancer services within the developed world so, for similar reasons, it will widen the gulf in cancer services between the developed world and the developing world. In many African countries, the annual per capita spending on health is less than US$50. Given this lack of resources, it is barely possible to diagnose, let alone treat, cancer. The problem is compounded by the high rate of human immunodeficiency virus (HIV) infection in the developing world. In southern Africa, over 50% of patients with cancer of the cervix are HIV positive. Both the HIV infection and the cancer are potentially preventable, by the use of condoms and human papillomavirus vaccination respectively. In addition, there are the other tumours related to acquired immunodeficiency syndrome (AIDS) to consider: Kaposi's sarcoma, lymphomas, squamous carcinomas of the conjunctiva. All cause morbidity, some are fatal and, in an impoverished country in the developing world, are fundamentally untreatable. The high prevalence of smoking among young people in China presages an epidemic of

---

Moritz Kaposi, 1837–1902, Professor of Dermatology, Vienna, Austria, described pigmented sarcoma of the skin in 1872.

lung cancer in that enormous population within the next 25 years.

A HEALTH WARNING

This has been a relatively simple account of a complex group of diseases. If cancer were simple, it would already have been cured. Investigating, understanding and treating cancer is fraught with ambiguities. However, we have deliberately tried to avoid ambiguity and have presented a series of gross oversimplifications: for every argument presented as fact, there are several counterarguments. We have, for example, stated that mutations are the driving force in forming tumours: one contrary view is that all tumours originate from gross rearrangements of chromosomes, and that mutations occur as secondary events. Another contrary view is that epigenetic events, such as global hypomethylation of genomic DNA, precede the acquisition of mutations and that, in order to flourish, a transforming event must occur within an epigenetic environment that is favourable. In this, as in many other instances, the conventional wisdom has been provided. The challenge for the future is to find out how much of conventional wisdom is true, and how much is not.

FURTHER READING

Bailar, J.C. and Gornik, H.L. (1997) Cancer undefeated. *N Engl J Med* **336(22)**: 1569–74.

Barcellos-Hoff, M.H. (2001) It takes a tissue to make a tumor: epigenetics, cancer and the microenvironment. *J Mammary Gland Biol Neoplasia* **6(2)**: 213–21.

Capasso, L.L. (2005) Antiquity of cancer. *Int J Cancer* **113(1)**: 2–13.

Doll, R. (1998) Epidemiological evidence of the effects of behaviour and the environment on the risk of human cancer. *Recent Results Cancer Res* **154**: 3–21.

Feinberg, A.P., Ohlsson, R. and Henikoff S. (2006) The epigenetic progenitor origin of human cancer. *Nature Rev Genet* **7(1)**: 21–33.

Feinstein, A.R., Sosin, D.M. and Well C.K. (1985) The Will Rogers phenomenon. Stage migration and new diagnostic techniques as a source of misleading statistics for survival in cancer. *N Engl J Med* **312(25)**: 1604–8.

Hanahan, D. and Weinberg, R.A. (2000) The hallmarks of cancer. *Cell* **100(1)**: 57–70.

Kerr, J.F., Wyllie, A.H. and Currie A.R. (1972) Apoptosis: a basic biological phenomenon with wide-ranging implications in tissue kinetics. *Br J Cancer* **26(4)**: 239–57.

Vogelstein, B. and Kinzler, K.W. (2004) Cancer genes and the pathways they control. *Nature Med* **10(8)**: 789–99.

Surgical audit and research

LEARNING OBJECTIVES

To understand:
- The planning and conduct of audit and research
- How to write up a project
- How to review a journal article and determine its value

INTRODUCTION

It is essential for a surgeon to understand the educational and legal framework in which he or she works. The agenda for medical education and clinical governance requires surgeons to expand their skills to encompass audit and research capabilities as useful tools for continued outcome measurement, service improvement and innovations for the benefit of patient care. The aim of this chapter is to enable improvements in patient experience as a result of a successful audit cycle or by recognising the need for research to determine a new and innovative way of treatment. It will also show how to keep track of personal clinical results. In addition, much clinical work is tedious and repetitive. Rigorous evaluation of even the most simple techniques and conditions can help to keep a surgeon stimulated throughout a long career and ensure good outcomes for patients, with benefits to society as a whole.

Large numbers of clinical papers appear in the surgical literature every year. Many are flawed, and it is important that a surgeon has the skills to examine publications critically. The best way to develop a critical understanding of the research and audit undertaken by others is to perform studies of one's own. The hardest part of audit and research is writing it up, and the hardest article to write is the first. This chapter also contains the information required to write a surgical paper and to evaluate the publications of others.

AUDIT OR RESEARCH?

It is important to determine at an early stage whether a project is audit or research, and sometimes that is not as easy as it seems. The decision will determine the framework in which the study is undertaken. Table 8.1 contains the information needed to make the decision and the formal processes that should be used for each.

AUDIT AND SERVICE EVALUATION

Clinical audit is a process used by clinicians who seek to improve patient care. The process involves comparing aspects of care (structure, process and outcome) against explicit criteria. Keeping track of personal outcome data and contributing to a clinical database ensures that a surgeon's own performance is monitored continuously and can be compared with a national data set to ensure compliance with agreed standards. If the care falls short of the criteria chosen, some change in the way that care is organised should be proposed. This change may be required at one of many levels. It might be an individual who needs training or an instrument that needs replacing. At times, the change may need to take place at the team level. Sometimes, the only appropriate action is change at an institutional level (e.g. a new antibiotic policy), regional level (provision of a tertiary referral centre) or, indeed, national level (screening programmes and health education campaigns).

Essentially two types of audits may be encountered: national audits (e.g. in the UK, the National Institute for Health and Clinical Excellence – NICE) and local/hospital audits. Both are designed to improve the quality of care. In an ideal world, national audits should be driven by needs identified in local and hospital-based audits that are closest to the patient. For example, hospital topics are often identified at the departmental morbidity and mortality meetings, where issues related to patient care are discussed. The reporting process might identify a possible national issue, and a national audit could be designed to be completed by the local audit department and surgical teams. The Vascular Society of Great Britain and Ireland is currently involving all its members in an evaluation of process and outcomes during carotid surgery. Issues that are of local importance are addressed within the local hospital, region or hospital trust (in the UK).

Audits are formal processes that require a structure. The following steps are essential to establish an audit cycle:

1. Define the audit question in a multidisciplinary team.
2. Identify the body of evidence and current standards.
3. Design the audit to measure performance against agreed standards based on strong evidence. Seek appropriate advice (local audit department in UK).
4. Measure over an agreed interval.
5. Analyse results and compare performance against agreed standards.

Table 8.1 Research, audit or service evaluation?

Research	Clinical audit	Service evaluation
The attempt to derive generalisable new knowledge including studies that aim to generate hypotheses as well as studies that aim to test them	Designed and conducted to produce information to inform the delivery of best care	Designed and conducted solely to define or judge current care
Quantitative research – designed to test a hypothesis Qualitative research – identifies/explores themes following established methodology	Designed to answer the question: 'Does this service reach a predetermined standard?'	Designed to answer the question: 'What standard does this service achieve?'
Addresses clearly defined questions, aims and objectives	Measures against a standard	Measures current service without reference to a standard
Quantitative research – may involve evaluating or comparing interventions, particularly new ones Qualitative research – usually involves studying how interventions and relationships are experienced	Involves an intervention in use ONLY. (The choice of treatment is that of the clinician and patient according to guidance, professional standards and/or patient preference)	Involves an intervention in use ONLY. (The choice of treatment is that of the clinician and patient according to guidance, professional standards and/or patient preference)
Usually involves collecting data that are additional to those for routine care but may include data collected routinely. May involve treatments, samples or investigations additional to routine care	Usually involves analysis of existing data but may include administration of simple interviews or questionnaires	Usually involves analysis of existing data but may include administration of simple interviews or questionnaires
Quantitative research – study design may involve allocating patients to intervention groups Qualitative research uses a clearly defined sampling framework underpinned by conceptual or theoretical justifications	No allocation to intervention groups: the health-care professional and patient have chosen intervention before clinical audit	No allocation to intervention groups: the health-care professional and patient have chosen intervention before service evaluation
May involve randomisation	No randomisation	No randomisation

Although any of the above may raise ethical issues, under current guidance, research requires ethics committee review, whereas audit and service evaluation do not.
Advice (in UK) from National Research Ethics Service (http://www.nres.npsa.nhs.uk/recs)

6 Undertake gap analysis:
   • If all standards are reached, reaudit after an agreed interval.
   • If there is a need for improvement, identify possible interventions such as training, and agree with the involved parties.
7 Reaudit.

Research study

During the design of the audit project, it might become apparent that there is a limited body of evidence available. In this case, the study should be structured as a research proposal. Research is designed to generate new knowledge and might involve testing a new treatment or regimen.

IDENTIFYING A RESEARCH TOPIC

The hardest part of research is to come up with a good idea. Once an idea has been formed, or a question asked, it needs to be transformed into a hypothesis. It is helpful to approach surgeons who regularly publish articles and who have a special interest in the surgical area being considered. As ideas are suggested, keep thinking whether the question posed really matters. Spend some time refining the question because this is probably the most important part of the study. Choosing the wrong topic at this stage can lead to many wasted hours. Once a topic has been identified, do not rush into the study. It is worth spending a considerable time investigating the subject in question. The worst possible thing is to find at the end of a long arduous study that the research or audit has already been done.

First port of call for information is the medical library. Look for current articles about the proposed research; review articles and meta-analyses can be particularly helpful. At this stage, most clinicians go to an electronic library and perform a database search. It is very important to learn how to do an accurate and efficient search as early as possible. Details are beyond the scope of this chapter, but most librarians will help out if a little interest and enthusiasm is shown. Current techniques involve searching on Medline or other collected databases but, as electronic information advances and the worldwide web becomes more user friendly, new search strategies may emerge. Collections of reviews are becoming available – the Cochrane Collaboration brings together evidence-based medical information and is available in most libraries (Table 8.2).

Once a stack of articles on the subject has been obtained, it is important that these are carefully perused. If the proposed project is still looking good after some thorough reading, it is worth further discussion with authors who have written a paper on a similar subject. All scientists are flattered by interest in their work. Now it should be possible to start to plan the research project.

PROJECT DESIGN

During the first phase, it is very important to keep in the mind some important questions (Summary box 8.1).

Summary box 8.1

Questions to answer before undertaking research

- Why do the study?
- Will it answer a useful question?
- Is it practical?
- Can it be accomplished in the available time and with the available resources?
- What findings are expected?
- What impact will it have?

Next to choosing the subject for study, time spent carefully designing a project is never wasted. There are many different types of scientific study. The design used totally depends on the study. Beloved of present scientists, the randomised controlled trial (RCT) is regarded as the best method of scientific research. It must not be forgotten that much surgical practice has been advanced by other different types of study such as those listed in Table 8.3. For example, testing a new type of operation often requires a pilot study to assess feasibility followed by a formal RCT.

Research can be qualitative or quantitative. Quantitative research allows hard facts to speak for themselves. A medical condition is analysed systematically using hard, objective endpoints such as death or amputation. In qualitative research, data often come from patient narratives, and the psychosocial impact of the disease and its treatment are analysed, for example narratives from patients with breast cancer. These sorts of data are often collected using quality-of-life measurements. A variety of different quality-of-life questionnaires exist to suit several different clinical situations. Much of the best research is both quantitative and qualitative.

As finances for health care are always limited, it is also important to include a cost–benefit analysis in any major area of research so that the value of the proposed intervention or change in treatment can be assessed.

Research should also be focused according to national (and international) strategies. Best Research for Best Health is the

Table 8.2 Electronic information sites

Database	Producer	Coverage	Availability[a]
Medline, including Pubmed (www.ncbi.nlm.nih.gov/pubmed/) and Biomed Central (www.pubmedcentral.nih.gov/)	US National Library of Medicine (NLM)	Worldwide journals; 9 million records since 1966	Subscription: CD-ROM, Internet
EMBASE (not free on-line)	Electronic version of *Excerpta Medica*	Good European drug/ pharmacology coverage; 6 million records since 1980	Subscription: CD-ROM, Internet
CINAHL (not free on-line)	Cumulated index to nursing and allied health literature	Worldwide journals and books, 95% English language; multidisciplinary: health psychology, community care, clinical guidelines and protocols, since 1982	Subscription: CD-ROM, Internet
ERIC (http://www.askeric.org)	Educational Resources Information Center, US Department of Education	Theory and practice of education; multidisciplinary; 1 million records since 1966	Free of charge: Internet Subscription: CD-ROM, Internet
Cochrane Collaboration (http://www.cochrane.co.uk)	BMJ Publishing Group	Evidence-based health care, systematic reviews, methodology, trials register, since 1995	Free of charge: Internet Subscription: CD-ROM, floppy disk, Internet
Omni (http://omni.ac.uk)	UK health-care libraries	Review websites on the Internet	Free of charge: Internet

a. Licensed to many organisations who provide their own interface. Main providers offering a pay-as-you-go service can be found: http://www.ovid.com or http://www.silverplatter.com

The Cochrane Collaboration **was formed in 1993 and named after Archibald Leman Cochrane, 1909–1988, Director of the Medical Research Council Epidemiology Unit, Cardiff, Wales, and later the first President of the Faculty of Community Medicine (now the Faculty of Public Health) of the Royal College of Physicians of London, England**

Table 8.3 Types of study

Type of study	Definition
Observational	Evaluation of condition or treatment in a defined population Retrospective: analysing past events Prospective: collecting data contemporaneously
Case–control	Series of patients with a particular disease or condition compared with matched control patients
Cross-sectional	Measurements made on a single occasion, not looking at the whole population but selecting a small similar group and expanding results
Longitudinal	Measurements are taken over a period of time, not looking at the whole population but selecting a small similar group and expanding results
Experimental	Two or more treatments are compared. Allocation to treatment groups is under the control of the researcher
Randomised	Two randomly allocated treatments
Randomised controlled	Includes a control group with standard treatment

current NHS research strategy for England and Wales. The aim is to support outstanding individuals, working in world-class facilities, conducting leading-edge research that is focused on the needs of patients and the public (http://www.dh.gov.uk/en/Policyandguidance/Researchanddevelopment/index.htm).

Sample size

Calculating the number of patients required to perform a satisfactory investigation is a very important prerequisite to the study. An incorrect sample size is probably the most frequent reason for research being invalid. Often, surgical trials are marred by the possibility of error caused by the inadequate number of patients investigated.

- *Type I error.* Benefit is perceived when really there is none (false positive)
- *Type II error.* Benefit is missed when it was there to be found (false negative)

Calculating the number of patients required in the study can overcome this bias. Unfortunately, it very often reveals that a larger number of patients is needed for the study than can possibly be obtained from available resources. This often means expanding enrolment by using a multicentre study. There is no point in embarking on a trial if it will never be possible to recruit an adequate population to answer the research question. Never forget that more patients will need to be randomised than the final sample size to take into account patients who die, drop out or are lost to follow-up.

The following is an example calculation for a study to recruit patients into two groups. In order to calculate a sample size, it is common practice to set the level of power for the study at 80% with a 5% significance level. This means that, if there is a difference between study groups, there is an 80% chance of detecting it. Based on previous studies, realistic expectations of differences between groups should be used to calculate the sample size. The formula below uses the figures of a reduction in event rate from 30% to 10% (e.g. a new treatment expected to reduce the complication rate such as wound infection from 30% = r to 10% = s).

$$8 \times [r(100-r) + s(100-s)]/(r-s)^2 \tag{8.1}$$

e.g. $8 \times [30(100-30) + 10(100-10)]/(30-10)^2 =$ 60 needed in each group

Eliminating bias

It is important to imagine how a study could be invalidated by thinking of things that could go wrong. One way to eliminate any bias inherent in the data collection is to have observers or recorders who do not know which treatment has been used (blinded observer). It might also be possible to ensure that the patient is unaware of the treatment allocation (single blind). In the best randomised studies, neither patient nor researcher is aware of which therapy has been used until after the study has finished (double blind). Randomised trials are essential for testing new drugs. In practice, however, in some surgical trials, randomisation may not be possible or ethical.

Study protocol

Now that the question to pose has been decided, and it has been checked that sufficient patients will be available to enrol into the study, it is time to prepare the detail of the trial. At this stage, a study protocol should be constructed to define the research strategy. It should contain a paragraph on the background of the proposed study, the aims and objectives, a clear methodology, definitions of population and sample sizes and methods of proposed analysis. It should include the patient numbers, inclusion and exclusion criteria and the timescale for the work. At this stage, it is useful to construct a flow diagram giving a clear summary of the research protocol and its requirements (Fig. 8.1). It is helpful to imagine the paper that will be written about the study, before it is performed. This may prevent errors in data collection.

When a study is planned, sufficient time should be reserved at the beginning for fund-raising and obtaining ethical and hospital approval, if required, and afterwards for collecting and writing up the data. A data collection form should be designed or a computer collection package developed. Do not forget that, if data are collected on computer, appropriate safeguards for privacy and confidentiality will be necessary to comply with legislation on data protection. It is important to ensure the cooperation of any other specialties or clinicians who will be involved in the study and to agree on the sharing of responsibility for the trial. This will also help to prevent disagreement about who takes the credit once a study is ready for presentation and publication.

Regulatory framework

In the UK, the implementation of the research governance framework by the Department of Health requires that independent ethical review is undertaken of all health and social care research (http://www.dh.gov.uk/assetRoot/04/12/24/27/04122427.pdf).

This is done by contacting the local ethics committee and following the guidance from the National Research Ethics Service

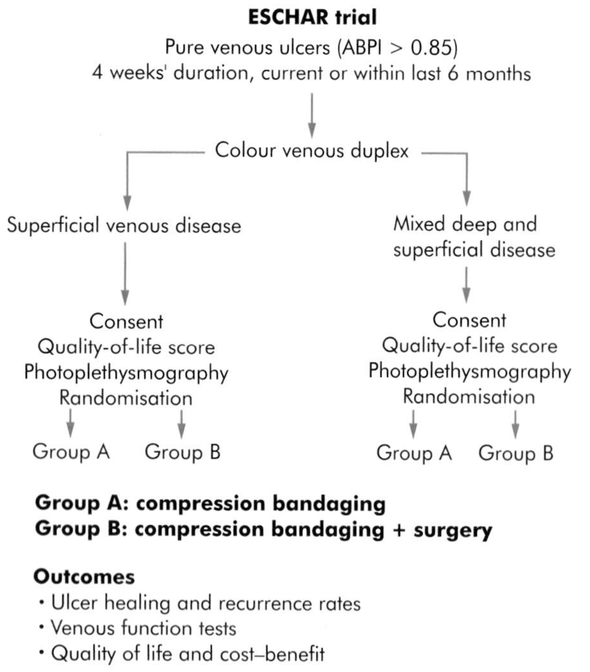

ESCHAR trial
Pure venous ulcers (ABPI > 0.85)
4 weeks' duration, current or within last 6 months

Colour venous duplex

Superficial venous disease

Mixed deep and
superficial disease

Consent
Quality-of-life score
Photoplethysmography
Randomisation

Consent
Quality-of-life score
Photoplethysmography
Randomisation

Group A   Group B

Group A   Group B

Group A: compression bandaging
Group B: compression bandaging + surgery

Outcomes
• Ulcer healing and recurrence rates
• Venous function tests
• Quality of life and cost–benefit

Figure 8.1 ESCHAR trial: completed in Gloucestershire, UK [Gohel, M.S. *et al.* (2005) *British Journal of Surgery* **92**: 291–297. Copyright British Journal of Surgery Society Ltd. Permission is granted by John Wiley & Sons Ltd on behalf of the BJSS Ltd.] ABPI, ankle–brachial pressure index.

(NRES). In addition, all studies should receive hospital trust approval, which ensures that the study complies with the legal framework for research. In the case of clinical trials, the European Union Clinical Trial Directive applies and is regulated by the Medicines and Health Care products Regulatory Agency (MHRA). A clinical trial should be registered with the European Clinical Trials Database (www.eudract.emea.europa.eu) or one of the other free databases (www.clinicaltrials.gov) before applying to NRES. It is then possible to apply to the MHRA for a Clinical Trial Authorisation in parallel to the NRES application. This can be a complicated and trying process, but most hospitals have research support units that will help if any problems are encountered. Editors of the major surgical journals now agree that all clinical trials should have been registered before an article relating to a trial can be published.

Peer review

Once your protocol is finalised, formal peer review is needed. In the UK, you will need to have evidence of peer review before submitting an application to the ethics committee and for hospital trust approval.

• If the research is part of a university course, the university should undertake this review.
• Surgeons working for the NHS can arrange their own peer review by experts who are not connected with the study. Alternatively, most Research and Development Support Units (NHS) will give guidance through the review process.
• Funders of research will usually undertake their own independent peer review. There is usually feedback from this process that often gives valuable advice about the study.

Ethics

In the first instance, common sense is the best guide to whether or not a study is ethical. It is still important to seek advice from an ethics committee whenever research is contemplated.

All studies involving animals require approval from statutory licensing authorities.

In the UK, and also in Australia, new therapeutic procedures and devices were registered and regulated through a body set up by the Surgical Royal Colleges: SERNIP (Safety and Efficacy Register of New Interventional Procedures). This process has now been subsumed by NICE who undertake a similar role.

Ethics committees prefer to see fully developed trial protocols, but it is often possible to get some preliminary advice from the committee chairman. Ethics committee forms may seem long and detailed, and it is important that these are filled in correctly. All dealings with ethics committees should be intelligent and courteous. Do attend the meeting at which your study will be discussed as it provides a forum for direct communication in relation to the study. It can save time as any possible concerns of the ethics committee can be addressed immediately, avoiding lengthy correspondence.

Do not embark on the study until the right approval has been granted. Ensure that a project does not incur hidden expenses to a hospital. The cost of non-routine investigations and extra treatments should be identified and covered by a grant application, or at least underwritten by a hospital finance department.

STATISTICAL ANALYSIS

Both audit and research commonly require statistical analysis. Many surgeons find the statistical analysis of a project the most difficult part. It is also the most commonly criticised part of papers written by other clinicians.

There are many useful books about statistics which can be consulted (see Further reading); if in any doubt, a statistician will be pleased to give assistance. Statisticians like to be consulted before research or audit has been conducted rather than being presented with the data at the end; they often give helpful advice over study design.

The following terms are frequently used when summarising statistical data:

• *Mean*: the result of dividing the total by the number of observations (the average).
• *Median*: the middle value with equal numbers of observations above and below – used for numerical or ranked data.
• *Mode*: the value with the highest frequency observed – used for nominal data collection.
• *Range*: the largest to the smallest value.

The most important decision for analysis is whether the distribution of results is normal, i.e. parametric or non-parametric. Normally distributed results have a symmetrical, bell-shaped curve, and the mean, median and mode all lie at the same value. The type of data collected determines which statistical test should be used.

1 Numerical and normally distributed (e.g. blood pressure) – use unpaired *t*-test to compare two groups, or paired *t*-test to assess whether a variable has changed between two time points.

2 Numerical but not normally distributed (e.g. tumour size) – use Mann–Whitney U-test to compare two groups, or a Wilcoxon signed rank test to assess whether a variable has increased/stayed the same/decreased between two time points.

3 Categorical (e.g. admitted to intensive care unit) – can use chi-squared test to compare two groups

(Please note: the use of any other test may benefit from professional advice.)

Confidence intervals are the best guide to the possible range in which the true differences are likely to lie. A confidence interval that includes zero usually implies a lack of statistical significance.

Scientists usually employ P-values to describe statistical chance. A P-value < 0.05 is commonly taken to imply a true difference. It is important not to forget that $P = 0.05$ simply means there is only a 1:20 chance that the differences between the variables would have happened by chance when there was no real difference. If enough variables are examined in any study, significant differences will occur simply by chance. Trials with multiple endpoints or variables require more sophisticated analysis to determine the significance of individual risk factors. Univariable or multivariable logistic regression analysis techniques may be appropriate.

Statistics simply deal with the chance that observations between populations are different, and should be treated with caution. Clinical results should show clear differences. If statistics are required to demonstrate differences between results, it is possible that they are unlikely to have major clinical significance.

Computer software packages available

Statistical computer packages offer a quick way of analysing descriptive statistics such as mean, median and range, as well as the most commonly used statistical tests such as the chi-squared test. Various packages are available commercially and are useful tools in data analysis.

ANALYSING A SCIENTIFIC ARTICLE

The simplest way to analyse an article from a scientific journal is to look at the check-list of requirements for good scientific research. A group of scientists and editors developed the CONSORT (Consolidated Standards of Reporting Trials) statement to improve the quality of reporting of RCTs. Looking in detail at the study design is often the best way of deciding whether a trial is any good. The CONSORT document includes a check-list for the conduct of good randomised trials (Table 8.4). Often clinicians overlook biases that others find obvious to detect, which can have a profound influence on the outcome of any study. Several scientists have tried to use scoring systems to grade clinical trials, as the label 'randomised clinical trial' does not always guarantee quality.

PRESENTING AND PUBLISHING AN ARTICLE

There is no point in conducting a research or audit project and then leaving the results unreported. Even when results are negative, they are worth distributing; no project is worthless. Most studies do not provide dramatic results, and few surgeons publish seminal articles.

The key to both presentation and publication is to decide on the message, and then aim for an appropriate forum. Big important randomised studies or national audits merit presentation at national meetings and publication in international journals. Small observational studies and audits are more often accepted for presentation at regional or hospital meetings and for publication in smaller specialist journals. Help and advice from clinicians familiar with presentation and publication are invaluable at this stage. The most important piece of advice is to follow accurately the instructions for journal submission. Most international meet-

Table 8.4 Check-list for authors

Heading	Sub-heading	Descriptor
Title		Identify as randomised trial
Abstract		Structured format
Introduction		Prospectively defined hypotheses, clinical objective
Methods	Protocol	Study population
		Intervention, timing
		Primary and secondary outcome
		Statistical rationale
		Stopping rules
	Assignment	Unit of randomisation
		Method: allocation schedule
	Masking (blinding)	
Results	Participant flow and follow-up	Trial profile, flow diagram
	Analysis	Estimated effect of intervention
		Summary data with appropriate inferential statistics
		Protocol deviation
Comment		Specific interpretation of study
		Sources of bias
		External validity
		General interpretation

From the CONSORT statement: *Journal of the American Medical Association* (1996) **276**: 637–639.

ings will accept presentations eagerly (especially by poster) as this increases the attendance at a conference.

Most surgeons publish research in peer-reviewed journals. The work that is submitted is checked anonymously by other surgeons before publication. If in doubt about whether to submit to a journal, many editors will give advice about the suitability of an article by letter or telephone.

Convention dictates that articles are submitted in IMRAD form – introduction, methods, results and discussion. Increasingly, electronic publication and the Internet may change the face of scientific publication and, in the next decade, these restrictions on style may disappear. For now, the IMRAD format remains inviolable. The length of an article is important: a paper should be as long as the size of the message. Readers of big randomised multicentre trials wish to know as much detail about the study as possible; reports on small negative trials should be brief.

Introduction

This should always be short. A brief background of the study should be presented and then the aims of the trial or audit outlined.

Methods

The methodology and study design should be given in detail. It is important to own up to any biases. Any new techniques or investigations should be detailed in full; if they are common practice or have been described elsewhere, this should be referenced instead of described.

Results

Results are almost always best shown diagrammatically using tables and figures if possible. Results shown in the form of a diagram need not then be duplicated in the text.

Discussion

It is important not to repeat the introduction or reiterate the results in this section. The study should be interpreted intelligently, and any suggestions for future studies or changes in management should be made. It is important not to indulge in flights of fantasy or wild imagination about future possibilities; most journal editors will delete these. Recently, a standard format for the discussion section has been promoted, and journals such as the *British Medical Journal* are keen that authors use it.

References

This section should include all relevant papers recording previous studies on the subject in question. The number should reflect the size of the message and the importance of the work. The reference section does not usually have to be exhaustive, but should include up-to-date articles. Remember to present the references in the style of the journal of submission.

EVIDENCE-BASED SURGERY

Surgical practice has been considered an art: ask 50 surgeons how to manage a patient and one will probably get 50 different answers. There is so much clinical information available that no surgeon can know it all. Evidence-based surgery is a move to find the best ways of managing patients using clinical evidence from collected studies. It was estimated that sufficient evidence to justify routine myocardial thrombolysis for heart attacks was available years before the randomised clinical studies that finally made it clinically accept-

able. No-one had gathered all the available information together. Centres such as the Cochrane Collaboration have been collecting randomised trials and reviews to provide up-to-date information for clinicians. The Cochrane Library presently includes a database of systematic reviews, reviews of surgical effectiveness and a register of controlled trials. The *British Journal of Surgery* has been collecting surgical randomised trials on its website archive for 10 years (www.bjs.co.uk). There are now almost 1000 annotated references that can be a valuable resource for scientific authors. As evidence accumulates, it is expected that this will gradually smooth out the differences between clinicians as the best way of managing patients becomes more obvious. Collecting published evidence together and analysing it often requires reviews of multiple randomised trials. These meta-analyses involve complex statistical analyses designed to interpret multiple findings and synthesise the results of multiple studies. There exist standard formats for the presentation of meta-analyses described in the QUORUM statement (a statement produced after a conference that was convened to address standards for improving the quality of reporting of meta-analysis of clinical RCTs).

FURTHER READING

Altman, D.G. (1991) *Practical Statistics for Medical Research*. Chapman & Hall, London.

Brown, R.A. and Swanson Beck, J. (1994) *Medical Statistics on Personal Computers*. BMJ Publishing Group, Plymouth.

Greenhalgh, T. (1997) *How to Read a Paper*. BMJ Publishing Group, London.

Guidelines for Clinical Practice: From Development to Use (1992) National Academic Press, Washington, DC.

Kelson, M. (1998) *Promoting Patient Involvement in Clinical Audit*. London College of Health and the Clinical Outcomes Group, London.

Kirkwood, B.R. (2003) *Essentials of Medical Statistics*, 2nd edn. Blackwell Publishing, Oxford.

Moher, D., Cooke, D.J., Eastwood, S. *et al.* (1999) Improving the quality of reports of meta-analyses of randomised controlled trials: the QUORUM statement. *Lancet* 354: 1896–900.

Morrell, C. and Harvey, G. (1999) *The Clinical Audit Handbook*. Baillière Tindall, London.

Schein, M., Farndon, J.R. and Fingerhut, A. (2001) *A Surgeon's Guide to Writing and Publishing*. Tfm Publishing, Kemberton, Shropshire.

Smith, R. (2006) *The Trouble with Medical Journals*. RSM Press Ltd, London.

Swinscow, T.D.V. (1996) *Statistics at Square One*, 9th edn. BMJ Publishing Group, London.

Walshe, K. (2000) Adverse events in health care: issues in measurement. *Quality in Health Care* 9: 47–52.

ON-LINE RESOURCES

Clinical Evidence: www.clinicalevidence.com

Cochrane Library: www.cochrane.org/index.htm

Consolidated Standards of Reporting Trials: www.consort-statement.org/Statement/revisedstatement.htm

National Institute for Health and Clinical Excellence (NICE): www.nice.org.uk

National Research Ethics Service: www.nres.npsa.nhs.uk/recs

Scottish Intercollegiate Guideline Network (SIGN): www.sign.ac.uk

Best Research for Best Health (Department of Health): www.dh.gov.uk/policyandguidance/researchanddevelopment

Surgical ethics

To understand:
- The importance of autonomy in good surgical practice
- The moral and legal boundaries and practical difficulties of informed consent
- Good practice in making decisions about the withdrawal of life-sustaining treatment

- The importance and boundaries of confidentiality in surgical practice
- The importance of appropriate regulation in surgical research
- The importance of rigorous training and maintenance of good practice standards

INTRODUCTION

Ethics and surgical intervention must go hand in hand. In any other arena of public or private life, if someone deliberately cuts another person, draws blood, causes pain, leaves scars and disrupts everyday activity, then the likely result will be a criminal charge. If the person dies as a result, the charge could be manslaughter or even murder. Of course, it will be correctly argued that the difference between the criminal and the surgeon is that the latter causes harm only incidentally. The surgeon's intention is to cure or manage illness, and any bodily invasion that it incurs is only with the permission of the patient.

Patients consent to surgery because they trust their surgeons. Yet what should such consent entail in practice and what should surgeons do when patients need help but are unable or unwilling to agree to it? When patients do consent to treatment, surgeons wield enormous power over them, the power not just to cure, but to maim, disable and kill. How should such power be regulated to reinforce the trust of patients and to ensure that surgeons practise to an acceptable professional standard? Are there circumstances, in the public interest, in which it is acceptable to sacrifice the trust of individual patients through revealing information that was communicated in what patients believed to be conditions of strict privacy?

These questions about what constitutes good professional practice concern ethics rather than surgical technique. Surgeons may be expert in the management of specific diseases but may have little understanding of how much and what sort of information is required for patients to give valid consent to treatment. Surgeons can understand the delicate techniques associated with specific types of procedures without necessarily knowing when these should be administered to patients who are unable to consent at all. Surgeons can recognise their own mistakes and those of colleagues without knowing how much should be said about them to others. And so it goes on.

Traditional surgical training offers little help in the resolution of such ethical dilemmas. This chapter provides guidance which is morally coherent, widely endorsed and legally justifiable. Our focus will be the practice of surgery within the UK, although much of the analysis will also apply to surgical work elsewhere.

RESPECT FOR AUTONOMY

Surgeons have a duty of care towards their human patients which goes beyond just protecting their life and health. Their additional duty of care is to respect the autonomy of their patients and their ability to make choices about their treatments, and to evaluate potential outcomes in light of other life plans. Such respect is particularly important for surgeons because, without it, the trust between them and their patients may be compromised, along with the success of the surgical care provided. We are careful enough at the best of times about whom we allow to touch us and to see us unclothed. It is hardly surprising that many people feel strongly about exercising the same discretion in circumstances in which someone is not only going to do these things but to inflict what may be very serious wounds on them as well.

For all these reasons, there is a wide moral and legal consensus that patients have the right to exercise choice over their surgical care. In this context, a right should be interpreted as a claim that can be made on others and that they believe that they have a strict duty to respect, regardless of their own preferences. Thus, to the degree that patients have a right to make choices about proposed surgical treatment, it then follows that they should be allowed to refuse treatments that they do not want, even when surgeons think that they are wrong. For example, patients can even refuse surgical treatment that will save their lives, either at present or in the future, through the formulation of advance directives specifying the types of life-saving treatments that they do not wish to have if they become incompetent to refuse them.

INFORMED CONSENT

In surgical practice, respect for autonomy translates into the clinical duty to obtain informed consent before the commencement of treatment. The word 'informed' is important here. Because of the extremity of their clinical need, patients might agree to surgery on the basis of no information at all. Agreement of this kind, however, does not constitute a form of consent that is morally or legally acceptable. Unless such patients have some understanding of what they are agreeing to, their choices may have nothing to do with planning their lives and thus do not count as expressions of their autonomy. Worse still, if patients are given no information, their subsequent choices may be based on misunderstanding and lead to plans and further decisions that they would not otherwise have made.

For agreement to count as consent to treatment, patients need to be given appropriate and accurate information. Such information should include:

- the condition and the reasons why it warrants surgery;
- the type of surgery proposed and how it might correct the condition;
- the anticipated prognosis and expected side-effects of the proposed surgery;
- the unexpected hazards of the proposed surgery;
- any alternative and potentially successful treatments other than the proposed surgery;
- the consequences of no treatment at all.

With such information, patients can link their clinical prospects with the management of other aspects of their life and the lives of others for whom they may be morally and/or professionally responsible. Good professional practice dictates that obtaining informed consent should occur in circumstances that are designed to maximise the chances of patients understanding what is said about their condition and proposed treatment, as well as giving them an opportunity to ask questions and express anxieties.

Where possible:

- a quiet venue for discussion should be found;
- written material in the patient's preferred language should be provided to supplement verbal communication;
- patients should be given time and help to come to their own decision;
- the person obtaining the consent should ideally be the surgeon who will carry out the treatment. It should not be – as is sometimes the case – a junior member of staff who has never conducted such a procedure and thus may not have enough understanding to counsel the patient properly.

Good communication skills go hand in hand with properly obtaining informed consent for surgery. It is not good enough just to go through the motions of providing patients with the information required for considered choice. Attention must be paid to:

- whether or not the patient has understood what has been stated;
- avoiding overly technical language in descriptions and explanations;
- the provision of translators for patients whose first language is not English;
- asking patients if they have further questions.

When there is any doubt about their understanding, surgeons should ask patients questions about what has supposedly been communicated to see if they can explain the information in question for themselves.

Surgeons have a legal, as well as a moral, obligation to obtain consent for treatment based on appropriate levels of information. Failure to do so could result in one of two civil proceedings, assuming the absence of criminal intent. First, in law, intentionally to touch another person without their consent is a battery, remembering that we are usually touched by strangers as a consequence of accidental contact. Surgeons have a legal obligation to give the conscious and competent patient sufficient information 'in broad terms' about the surgical treatment being proposed and why. If the patient agrees to proceed, no other treatment should ordinarily be administered without further explicit consent.

Negligence is the second legal action that might be brought against a surgeon for not obtaining appropriate consent to treatment. Patients may have been given enough information about what is surgically proposed to agree to be touched in the ways suggested. However, surgeons may still be in breach of their professional duty if they do not provide sufficient information about the risks that patients will encounter through such treatment. Although standards of how much information should be provided about risks vary between nations, as a matter of good practice, surgeons should inform patients of the hazards that in their view any reasonable person in the position of the patient would wish to know. In practice, surgeons should ask themselves what they or a close relative or friend should be entitled to know in similar circumstances.

Finally, surgeons now understand that, when they obtain consent to proceed with treatment, then patients are expected to sign a consent form of some kind. The detail of such forms can differ, but they often contain very little of the information supposedly communicated to the patient who signed it. Partly for this reason, the process of formally obtaining consent can become overly focused on obtaining the signature of patients rather than ensuring that appropriate types and amounts of information have been provided, and have been understood.

Both professionally and legally, it is important for surgeons to understand that a signed consent form is not proof that valid consent has been properly obtained. It is simply a piece of evidence that consent may have been attempted. Even when they have provided their signature, patients can and do deny that appropriate information has been communicated or that the communication was effective. Surgeons are therefore well advised to make brief notes of what they have said to patients about their proposed treatments, especially information about significant risks. These notes should be placed in the patient's clinical record.

PRACTICAL DIFFICULTIES

Thus far, we have examined the moral and legal reasons why the duty of surgeons to respect the autonomy of patients translates into the specific responsibility to obtain informed consent to treatment. For consent to be valid, patients must:

- be competent to give it – be able to understand, remember and deliberate about whatever information is provided to them about treatment choices, and to communicate those choices;

- not be coerced into decisions that reflect the preferences of others rather than themselves;
- be given sufficient information for these choices to be based on an accurate understanding of reasons for and against proceeding with specific treatments.

Surgeons will face four key practical difficulties in aspiring to these goals.

First, surgical care will grind to a halt if it is always necessary to obtain explicit informed consent every time a patient is touched in the context of their care. Fortunately, such consent is unnecessary because patients will already have given their implied consent to whatever bodily contact is required in order to fulfil the therapeutic goals when they gave their explicit consent to treatment. Yet the fact that this is so underlines the importance of obtaining proper and explicit consent in the first place, along with taking care to note any sign of the patient withdrawing that consent or placing restrictions on it – for example, through verbally refusing or physically resisting specific aspects of care.

Second, some patients will not be able to give consent because of temporary unconsciousness. This might be a by-product of their illness or injury, or it could simply be the result of the administration of general anaesthetic. The moral and legal rules that govern such situations are clear. Patients may be at risk of death or of serious and permanent disability if surgery is not immediately performed. The situation is then one of medical necessity, and intervention can occur in their best interests without consent. The exception is when it is known that patients have made a legally valid advance decision refusing treatment of the specific kind required. In any case, surgery that is not immediately necessary because of such risks should be postponed until patients regain consciousness and are able to give informed consent or refusal for themselves.

Surgeons must take care to respect this distinction between procedures that are therapeutically necessary and those that are done merely out of convenience, even when, in the course of one operation, they discover problems unknown to the patient that they believe to require further surgical work. For example, a surgeon was successfully sued for battery by a female patient for performing a hysterectomy thought to be in her best interests when all that she had explicitly consented to was a dilatation and curettage.

Third, informed consent may be made impossible by incompetence of other kinds. In the case of children, parents or someone with parental responsibility are ordinarily required to give explicit written consent on their behalf. This said, surgeons should:

- take care to explain to children what is being surgically proposed and why;
- always consult with children about their response;
- where possible, take the child's views into account and note that even young children can be competent to consent to treatment provided that they too can understand, remember, deliberate about and believe information relevant to their clinical condition.

When such competence is present, under English law, children can provide their own consent to surgical care, although they cannot unconditionally refuse it until they are 18 years old. With the exception of the latter, these provisions illustrate the importance of respecting as much autonomy as is present among child patients and remembering that, for the purposes of consent to medical treatment, they may be just as autonomous as adults.

If competence is severely compromised by psychiatric illness or mental handicap, other moral and legal provisions hold. If patients lack the autonomy to choose how to protect themselves as regards the consequences of their illness then others charged with protecting them must assume the responsibility. Yet care must be taken not to abuse this duty. Even when such patients have been legally detained for compulsory psychiatric care, it does not follow that such patients are unable to provide consent for surgical care. Their competence should be assumed and consent should be sought. If it is established with the help of their carers that such patients are also incompetent to provide consent for surgery and that they are at risk of death or serious and permanent disability, then therapy can proceed in their best interests. However, if treatment can be postponed, then this should be done until, as a result of their psychiatric care, patients become able either to consent or to refuse. As with children, respect should always be shown for as much autonomy as is present.

If, for whatever clinical reason, adult patients are permanently incompetent to consent to surgery, therapy can again proceed if it is necessary to save life, to prevent serious and permanent injury or, more electively, to alleviate discomfort and optimise care. The only exception is, again, when the patient has already formulated a legally valid advance decision refusing the specific treatments on offer and someone has been appropriately appointed by the patient as having appropriate power of lasting attorney (or possesses such power for any other judicial reason).

Otherwise, it is always a futile exercise to ask the relatives of incompetent patients to sign consent forms for surgery on adults who cannot do so for themselves. Indeed, to make such requests can be a disservice to relatives, who may feel an unjustified sense of responsibility if the surgery fails. This said, relatives should be treated with politeness and consulted about issues that pertain to determining the best interests of patients.

MATTERS OF LIFE AND DEATH

It has been noted that the right of a competent adult to consent to and refuse treatment is unlimited, including the refusal of life-sustaining treatment. Probably the example of this most familiar to surgeons is Jehovah's Witnesses, who refuse blood transfusions at the risk of their own lives. There can be no more dramatic example of the potential tension between the duties of care to protect life and health and to respect autonomy.

The tension does not stop here, however. For there will be some circumstances in which the protection of the life and health of patients is judged to be inappropriate; in which they are no longer able to be consulted; and in which they have not expressed a view about what their wishes would be in such circumstances. Here, if possible after discussion and consensus with the next of kin, a decision may be made to withhold or to withdraw life-sustaining treatment on behalf of the incompetent patient. The fact that such decisions can be seen as omissions to act does not excuse surgeons from morally and legally having to reconcile them with their ordinary duty of care. Ultimately, this can only be done through arguing that such omissions to sustain life are in the patient's best interests.

A Jehovah's Witness **is a member of a millenarian fundamentalist Christian sect founded in America in 1884. They have their own translation of the Bible which they interpret literally.**

CHAPTER 9 | SURGICAL ETHICS

The determination of best interests in these circumstances will rely on one of three objective criteria, over and above the subjective perception by the surgeon that the quality of life of the patient is poor. There is no obligation to provide or to continue life-sustaining treatment:

- If doing so is futile – when clinical consensus dictates that it will not achieve the goal of extending life. Thought of in this way, judgements about futility should not be linked to evaluations of a patient's quality of life and thus can be difficult to justify as long as treatment might stand even a very small chance of success.
- If patients are imminently and irreversibly close to death – in such circumstances, it would not be in the patient's best interests to prolong life slightly (e.g. through the application of intensive care) when, again, there is no hope of any sustained success. Not needlessly interfering with the process of a dignified death can be just as caring as the provision of curative therapy.
- If patients are so permanently and seriously brain damaged that, lacking awareness of themselves or others, they will never be able to engage in any form of self-directed activity. The argument here is backed up by morally and legally reasoning that further treatment other than effective palliation cannot be in the best interests of patients as it will provide them with no benefit.

When any of these principles are employed to justify an omission to provide or to continue life-sustaining treatment, the circumstances should be carefully recorded in the patient's medical record, along with a note of another senior clinician's agreement.

Finally, surgeons will sometimes find themselves in charge of the palliative care of patients whose pain is increasingly difficult to control. There may come a point in the management of such pain when effective palliation is possible at the risk of life because of the respiratory effects of the palliative drugs. In such circumstances, surgeons can with legal justification administer a dose that might be dangerous, although experts in palliative care are sceptical that this is ever necessary with appropriate training. In any case, the argument employed to justify such action refers to its 'double effect': that both the relief of pain and death might follow from such an action. As intentional killing (active euthanasia) is rejected as professional and legal medical practice throughout most of the world, a potentially lethal dose is regarded as appropriate only when it is motivated by palliative intent and this motivation can be documented.

CONFIDENTIALITY

Respect for autonomy does not entail only the right of competent patients to consent to treatment. Their entitlement to exercise control over their life and future corresponds to the duty of surgeons to respect their privacy – not to communicate information revealed in the course of treatment to anyone else without consent. Generally speaking, such respect means that surgeons must not discuss clinical matters with relatives, friends, employers and others unless the patient explicitly agrees. To do otherwise is regarded by all the regulatory bodies of medicine and surgery as a grave offence, incurring harsh penalties. For breaches of confidentiality are not only abuses of human dignity; they again undermine the trust between surgeon and patient on which successful surgery and the professional reputations of surgeons depend.

Important as respect for confidentiality is, however, it is not absolute. Surgeons are allowed to communicate private information to other professionals who are part of the health-care team – provided that the information has a direct bearing on treatment. Here, the argument is that patients have given their implied consent to such communication when they explicitly consent to a treatment plan. Certainly, patients cannot expect strict adherence to the principle of confidentiality if it poses a serious threat to the health and safety of others. There will be some circumstances in which confidentiality either must or may be breached in the public interest. For example, it must be breached as a result of court orders or in relation to the requirements of public health legislation. It may be ignored in attempts to prevent serious crime or to protect the safety of other known individuals who are at risk of serious harm.

RESEARCH

As part of their duty to protect life and health to an acceptable professional standard, surgeons have a subsidiary responsibility to strive to improve operative techniques through research, to assure themselves and their patients that the care proposed is the best that is currently possible. Yet, there is moral tension between the duty to act in the best interests of individual patients and the duty to improve surgical standards through exposing patients to the unknown risks that any form of research inevitably entails.

The willingness to expose patients to such risks may be further increased by the professional and academic pressures on many surgeons to maintain a high research profile in their work. For this reason, surgeons (and physicians, who face the same dilemmas) now accept that their research must be externally regulated to ensure that patients give their informed consent, that any known risks to patients are far outweighed by the potential benefits, and that other forms of protection for the patient are in place (e.g. proper indemnity) in case they are unexpectedly harmed. The administration of such regulation is through research ethics committees, and surgeons should not participate in research that has not been approved by such bodies. Equally, special provisions will apply to research involving incompetent patients who cannot provide consent to participate and research ethics committees will evaluate specific proposals with great care.

In practice, it is not always clear what is to count as surgical research that should be subjected to regulation and what constitutes a minor innovation dictated by the contingencies of a particular clinical situation. Surgeons must always ask themselves in such circumstances whether or not the innovation in question falls within the boundaries of standard procedures in which they are trained. If so, what may be a new technique for them will count not as research but as an incremental improvement in personal practice.

Yet, if the improvement is to be thought of in this way, no conclusions can be drawn from it to alterations in standard practice or to an evaluation of their efficacy. Equally, there will be no consequences for surgical training, as the innovation in question should only have been attempted against the background of the already existing training and experience of the surgeon in question. If a proposed innovation exceeds these conditions, then it does count as research and should be approved by a research ethics committee. Such surgical research should also be subject to a clinical trial designed to ensure that findings about outcomes are systematically compared with the best available treatment and that favourable results are not the result of arbitrary factors (e.g. unusual surgical skill among researchers) that cannot be replicated.

MAINTAINING STANDARDS OF EXCELLENCE

To optimise success in protecting life and health to an acceptable standard, surgeons must only offer specialised treatment in which they have been properly trained. To do so will entail sustained further education throughout a surgeon's career in the wake of new surgical procedures. While training, surgery should be practised only under appropriate supervision by someone who has appropriate levels of skill. Such skill can be demonstrated only through appropriate clinical audit, to which all surgeons should regularly submit their results. When these reveal unacceptable levels of success, no further surgical work of that kind should continue unless further training is undergone under the supervision of someone whose success rates are satisfactory. To do otherwise would be to place the interest of the surgeon above that of their patient, an imbalance that is never morally or professionally appropriate.

Surgeons also have a duty to monitor the performance of their colleagues. To know that a fellow surgeon is exposing patients to unacceptable levels of potential harm and to do nothing about it is to incur partial responsibility for such harm when it occurs. Surgical teams and the institutions in which they function should have clear protocols for exposing unacceptable professional performance and helping colleagues to understand the danger to which they may expose patients. If necessary, offending surgeons must be stopped from practising until they can undergo further appropriate training and counselling. Too often, such danger has had to be reported by individuals whose anxieties have not been properly heeded and who have been professionally pilloried rather than congratulated for their pains. Surgeons and anyone else discovered to have been participating in such 'cover up' and ostracism should share the blame and punishment for any resulting harm to patients.

CONCLUSION

The two general duties of surgical care are to protect life and health and to respect autonomy, both to an acceptable profes-

sional standard. The specific duties of surgeons are shown to follow from these: acceptable practice concerning informed consent, confidentiality, decisions not to provide, or to omit, life-sustaining care, surgical research and the maintenance of good professional standards. The final duty of surgical care is to exercise all these general and specific responsibilities with fairness and justice, and without arbitrary prejudice. The conduct of ethical surgery illustrates good citizenship: protecting the vulnerable and respecting human dignity and equality. To the extent that the practice of individual surgeons is a reflection of such sustained conduct, they deserve the civil respect which they often receive. To the extent that it is not, they should not practise the honourable profession of surgery.

FURTHER READING

Beauchamp, T. and Childress, J. (2001) *Principles of Biomedical Ethics.* Oxford University Press, London.

British Medical Association (2004) *Medical Ethics Today*, 2nd edn. BMJ Books, London.

British Medical Association, Law Society (2004) *Assessment of Mental Capacity: Guidance for Doctors and Lawyers.* BMJ Books, London.

British Medical Association (2007) *The Mental Capacity Act 2005 – Guidance for Health Professionals.* BMA, London.

General Medical Council (1998) *Seeking Patients' Consent: The Ethical Considerations.* GMC, London.

General Medical Council (2002) *Withholding and Withdrawing Life Prolonging Treatments: Good Practice in Decision Making.* GMC, London.

General Medical Council (2004) *Confidentiality: Protecting and Providing Information.* http://gmc-uk.org/guidance/current/library/confidentiality.asp

General Medical Council (2006) *Good Medical Practice.* GMC, London.

McCullough, L.B., Jones, J.W. and Brody, B.A. (eds) (1998) *Surgical Ethics.* Oxford University Press, New York.

Royal College of Paediatrics and Child Health (2002) *Good Medical Practice in Paediatrics and Child Health: Duties and Responsibilities of Paediatricians.* RCPCH, London.

Royal College of Surgeons (2002) *Good Surgical Practice.* RCS, London.

Senate of Surgery of Great Britain and Ireland (1997) *The Surgeon's Duty of Care: Guidance for Surgeons on Ethical and Legal Issues.* Royal College of Surgeons, London.

World Medical Association (2005) *Medical Ethics Manual.* WMA, Gerney-Voltaire.

For general information on medical ethics, see:
http://www.bma.org.uk/ap.nsf/content/splashpage
http://www.gmc-uk.org/
http://www.rcseng.ac.uk/
http://www.wma.net/e/ethicsunit/policies.htm

CHAPTER 9 | SURGICAL ETHICS

PART 2 | Investigation and diagnosis

Diagnostic imaging

LEARNING OBJECTIVES

To understand:

- The advantages of good working relationships and close collaboration with the imaging department in planning appropriate investigations

- The basic principles of radiation protection and know the law in relation to the use of ionising radiation
- The principles of different imaging techniques and their advantages and disadvantages in different clinical scenarios

INTRODUCTION

Appropriate surgical management of the patient relies on correct diagnosis. While clinical symptoms and signs may provide a firm diagnosis in some cases, other conditions will require the use of supplementary investigations including imaging techniques. The number and scope of imaging techniques available to the surgeon have dramatically increased within a generation from a time when radiographs alone were the mainstay of investigation. The development of ultrasound and colour Doppler, computerised tomography (CT) and magnetic resonance imaging (MRI) has enabled the surgeon to make increasingly confident diagnoses and has reduced the need for diagnostic surgical techniques such as explorative laparotomy. Faced with such a plethora of imaging to choose from, it is important that the patient is not sent on a journey through multiple unnecessary examinations.

As a basic principle, the simplest, cheapest test should be chosen that it is hoped will answer the clinical question. This necessitates knowledge of the potential complications and diagnostic limitations of the various methods. For example, in a patient presenting with the clinical features of biliary colic, an ultrasound examination alone may give enough information to enable appropriate surgical management. In more complex cases, it may be more efficient to opt for a single, more expensive investigation such as CT rather than embarking on multiple simpler and cheaper investigations that may not yield the answer. The choice of technique is often dictated by equipment availability, expertise and cost as well as the clinical presentation. However, it must be emphasised that, not infrequently, the most valuable investigation is a prior radiograph; this not only reduces the cost and the amount of radiation a patient receives but very often improves patient care.

HOW TO REQUEST IMAGING

Best practice depends on close collaboration between the radiologist and the referrer and must take into account local expertise

and access to facilities. The start of this important communication is most often the 'request card' (Summary box 10.1).

Summary box 10.1

Imaging request card

The important details are:

- name
- date of birth
- hospital number or other unique identifier code
- address and post code – the post code is often the key to patient administration system (PAS) databases
- patient's telephone number (enables quick contact)
- weight (obese patients may not be safe in a scanner or the table may not be able to accommodate their weight)
- in the case of female patients, the date of the last menses if the woman has not been sterilised (important for all radiation procedures and MRI to exclude the possibility of pregnancy)
- other relevant past medical history, i.e. diabetes, epilepsy, renal failure, allergies and anticoagulation, all of which can affect which contrast agent can be given safely
- the name of the clinician who is in charge of care and of the requesting clinician, with a legible contact number
- the most recent creatinine result if contrast agents are to be employed

---

Fortunately, electronic requesting via a radiology information system (RIS) allows the demographic data for a patient to be stored electronically and should make the requesting process easier.

When requesting imaging, consider what it is that you want to know from the investigation. Give a provisional diagnosis or state the clinical problem. For plain film radiography, it is best to allow the radiographer to decide on the best views. For more complex investigations, such as multidetector CT or MRI, the radiologist will protocol the examination in order to optimise the chance of a useful answer from the test. If you are unsure of the best method to answer the clinical problem, discuss with a radiologist.

INTERPRETING IMAGES

Highly complex imaging should be left to radiologists to interpret, but the clinician should be able to examine radiographs to exclude major abnormalities. The plain radiograph can be systematically examined using the system in Summary box 10.2.

Summary box 10.2
A simple system for checking radiographs

Label	Name of patient
Site	Date of examination
	Side (check marker)
	What part is the film centred on?
	Does the film cover the whole area required?
	Is there more than one view?
Quality	Is the penetration appropriate?
Compare	How have the appearances changed from previous images?
Conclude	Is the diagnosis clear?
	Is further imaging needed?

The systematic approach to examining a radiograph varies according to the part of the body being imaged. For instance, for a radiograph of an extremity, the alignment, the cortices and the medullary cavity of the individual bones, the joints and the soft tissues all need to be assessed on each view. You should develop, learn and practise your own method for ensuring that you study all of these in each case. This will take a long time when you start, but speed comes with practice.

Some abnormalities on the radiograph may prompt you to look at other areas of the film or may require an additional view to be taken. This knowledge can only be attained by reading and experience! Do not forget that radiologists are always delighted to help you with interpreting a film; they are not so happy when they have to report that an incorrect conclusion has been drawn.

HAZARDS OF IMAGING

Contrast media

There has been a dramatic increase in the use of contrast agents in recent years, mainly related to the increasing use of CT. Potential problems include allergic reaction and nephrotoxicity. The newer low-osmolality contrast media (LOCM) are 5–10 times safer than the older higher-osmolality agents. Reactions are rare: serious reactions occur in about 1:2500 cases and life-threatening reactions in about 1:25 000 cases. The risk of sudden death, however, has not changed with the new agents. Local policies for dealing with patients at increased risk vary between departments and, indeed, between countries. A recent publication from the Royal College of Radiologists (RCR) in the UK does not recommend routine steroid prophylaxis for patients at increased risk of allergic reaction, but rather the use of a LOCM and observation of the patient for 30 min after injection with the intravenous cannula still *in situ*, as most serious reactions occur

shortly after injection. Guidelines from the European Society of Uroradiology (ESUR), however, continue to advocate the use of steroids.

In patients with diabetes or renal impairment, a recent creatinine level should be available. The radiologist should be informed of any history of renal impairment, as all contrast media are nephrotoxic in patients with impaired renal function. The risks and benefits of contrast administration need to be carefully assessed in these patients and, if contrast is given, the lowest dose of a LOCM should be given. The British RCR does not recommend the routine use of *N*-acetylcysteine for renal protection.

Concerns about lactic acidosis in patients on metformin receiving contrast led to various recommendations for stopping the metformin. The latest RCR recommendations are that it can be continued in patients receiving 100 ml or less of intravenous contrast who are thought to have normal renal function. Other patients, including those who have intra-arterial contrast for angiography, should be discussed with the radiologist.

Allergic reactions to gadolinium diethyltriaminepentaacetic acid (DTPA) injection are rare, and gadolinium DTPA has been used as an alternative contrast agent in patients with iodine allergy. Mild reactions may occur in around 1:200 patients, with severe reactions in around 1:10 000 patients. Gadolinium DTPA has also been found to be nephrotoxic in patients with pre-existing renal failure. In addition, there have been some worrying reports of an association between gadolinium DTPA injection and the development of nephrogenic fibrosing dermopathy in patients with renal impairment.

HAZARDS OF IONISING RADIATION

The majority of ionising radiation comes from natural sources on the earth and cosmic rays, and this makes up the background radiation. However, medical exposure accounts for 12% of the total received by humans. The effects of ionising radiation can be broadly divided into two groups. The first group comprises predictable, dose-dependent (termed deterministic or non-stochastic) effects and includes, for example, the development of cataracts in the lens of the eye. These effects are important for those chronically exposed to radiation, including those using image intensifiers regularly. The second group comprises the all or nothing effects such as the development of cancer (termed stochastic). These effects are not dose dependent, but increase in likelihood with increased radiation dose.

The risk of radiation-induced cancer for plain films of the chest or extremities is very small, of the order of 1:1 000 000. However, that risk rises considerably for high-dose examinations such as CT of the abdomen or pelvis, where the lifetime excess risk of cancer increases to the order of 1:1000. Obviously, the risk of such examinations has to be balanced against the benefit to the patient in terms of increased diagnostic yield, and must also be viewed in the context that the lifetime risk of cancer for people generally is about 1:3. Nevertheless, techniques that do not use ionising radiation, such as ultrasound and MRI, should be carefully considered as alternatives, particularly in children and young people.

CURRENT LEGISLATION

In the UK, the Ionising Radiation (Medical Exposure) Regulations (IRMER) introduced in 2000 impose on the radiologist the duty to the patient to make sure that all studies involving radiation (plain radiographs, CT and nuclear medicine) are performed appropriately and to the highest standards. Inappropriate use of radiation is a criminal offence, so investigations involving radiation need careful consideration in order to prevent wasteful use of radiology (Summary box 10.3).

Summary box 10.3

Wasteful use of radiology

Results unlikely to affect patient management
  Positive finding unlikely
  Anticipated finding   Do I need it?
    probably irrelevant
    for management

Investigating too often
  Before disease could be   Do I need it now?
    expected to have
    progressed or resolved

Repeating investigations done previously
  Other hospital (?)
  GP (?)   Has it been done already?

Failing to provide adequate information
  Therefore wrong test   Have I explained the
    performed or   problem?
    essential view omitted

Requesting wrong investigation
  Discuss with radiologist   Is this the best test?

Overinvestigating   Are too many investigations
                                 being performed?

After: *Making the Best Use of a Department of Clinical Radiology*, 5th edn. Royal College of Radiologists, 2003.

Summary box 10.4 gives a summary of the responsibilities of both the radiologist and the referrer.

Summary box 10.4

Responsibilities

- Radiologists have a legal responsibility to keep imaging as safe as possible
- The referrer has a duty to balance risk against benefit
- The referrer must provide adequate clinical details to allow justification of the examination
- Avoid using portable (mobile) X-ray machines whenever practical
- Take all precautions when using an image intensifier
- The gonads, eyes and thyroid are especially vulnerable to radiation and should be protected

---

The Royal College of Radiologists has published a book, *Making the Best Use of a Department of Clinical Radiology* (5th edition, 2003), which has been adopted in many European countries. Local rules and guidelines are in place to deal with particular circumstances. Table 10.1, showing the radiation doses for common procedures, is taken from this publication.

There are special considerations for portable and fluoroscopy units. The longer an operator keeps the fluoroscopy unit running,

the higher the dose of radiation to all in the vicinity. Portable X-ray machines and fluoroscopic imaging equipment use much more radiation to achieve the same result. The staff, and patients in the next bed, are at risk when portable equipment is used. The result is also of lower quality, so portable X-ray machines should not be used unless absolutely necessary.

When using the image intensifier, lead aprons, thyroid shields, lead glasses and radiation badges should always be worn. Pregnancy in the female patient or staff must be excluded.

DIAGNOSTIC IMAGING

Basic principles of imaging methods

Conventional radiography

Despite the fact that it is over a hundred years since the discovery of X-rays by Roentgen in 1895, conventional radiography continues to play a central role in the diagnostic pathway of many acute surgical problems and particularly in chest disease, trauma and orthopaedics.

X-rays emitted from an X-ray source are absorbed to varying degrees by different materials and tissues and therefore cause different degrees of blackening of radiographic film, resulting in a radiographic image. This differential absorption is dependent partly on the density and the atomic number of different substances. In general, higher-density tissues result in a greater reduction in the number of X-ray photons and reduce the amount of blackening caused by those photons. In terms of conventional radiographs, a large difference in tissue structure and density is required before an appreciable difference is manifested radiographically. The different densities visible consist of air, fat, soft tissue, bone and mineralisation, and metal. Different soft tissues cannot be reliably distinguished as, in broad terms, they possess similar quantities of water (Fig. 10.1). Manipulation of X-ray systems and X-ray energies, as used in circumstances such as

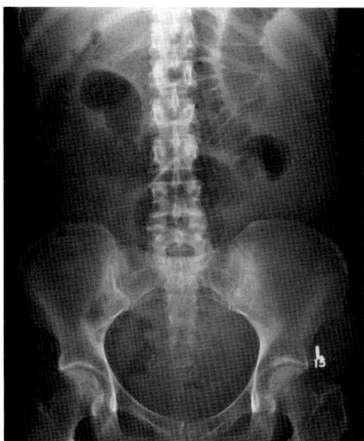

Figure 10.1 Supine abdominal radiograph of a patient with small bowel obstruction demonstrating multiple dilated small bowel loops. The different densities visible are air (within the bowel), bones, soft tissues and fat. The different soft tissues, subcutaneous and intra-abdominal, cannot be differentiated.

Wilhelm Conrad Roentgen, **1845–1923**, Professor of Physics, Wurtzburg, **(1888–1900),** and then at Munich, Germany. He was awarded the Nobel Prize for Physics in 1901 for his work on X-rays.

Table 10.1 Typical effective doses from diagnostic medical exposure in the 2000s

Diagnostic procedure	Typical effective dose (mSv)	Equivalent no. of chest radiographs	Approximately equivalent period of natural background radiation[a]
Radiographic examinations			
Limbs and joints (except hip)	< 0.01	< 0.5	< 1.5 days
Chest (single posteroanterior film)	0.02	1	3 days
Skull	0.07	3.5	11 days
Thoracic spine	0.7	35	4 months
Lumbar spine	1.3	65	7 months
Hip	0.3	15	7 weeks
Pelvis	0.7	35	4 months
Abdomen	1.0	50	6 months
Intravenous urography (IVU)	2.5	125	14 months
Barium swallow	1.5	75	8 months
Barium meal	3	150	16 months
Barium follow-through	3	150	16 months
Barium enema	7	350	3.2 years
CT head	2.3	115	1 year
CT chest	8	400	3.6 years
CT abdomen or pelvis	10	500	4.5 years
Radionuclide studies			
Lung ventilation (^{133}Xe)	0.3	15	7 weeks
Lung perfusion (^{99m}Tc)	1	50	6 months
Kidney (^{99m}Tc)	1	50	6 months
Thyroid (^{99m}Tc)	1	50	6 months
Bone (^{99m}Tc)	4	200	1.8 years
Dynamic cardiac (^{99m}Tc)	6	300	2.7 years
PET head (18F-FDG)	5	250	2.3 years

[a] UK average background radiation = 2.2 mSv per year; regional averages range from 1.5 to 7.5 mSv.
18F-FDG, 18F-2-fluoro-2-deoxy-D-glucose; CT, computerised tomography; ^{99m}Tc, ^{99m}technetium; PET, positron emission tomography.
From: *Making the Best Use of a Department of Clinical Radiology*, 5th edn. Royal College of Radiologists, 2003. By kind permission.

mammography, may allow better differentiation between some soft-tissue structures.

Despite this inherent lack of soft-tissue contrast, conventional radiography has many advantages. It is cheap, universally available, easily reproducible and comparable with prior examinations and, in many instances, has a relatively low dose of ionising radiation in contrast to more complex examinations. However, injudicious repeat radiography, particularly of the abdomen, pelvis and spine, can easily result in doses similar to CT.

The lack of soft-tissue contrast allows little assessment of the internal architecture of many abdominal organs. To obviate this problem, techniques employing the administration of contrast material combined with radiography have long been used. These techniques include intravenous urography and barium examinations (Fig. 10.2). In intravenous urography (IVU), intravenous administration of iodinated contrast material initially results in opacification of the renal parenchyma, followed by opacification of the pelvicalyceal system, ureters and bladder, allowing identification of pelvicalyceal morphology and filling defects (Fig. 10.3). Iodinated contrast material may even be instilled retrogradely into the bladder per urethra and combined with radiographs obtained during micturition to allow the assessment of the lower urinary tract.

A further modification of conventional X-rays uses fluorescent screens to allow real-time monitoring of organs and structures as opposed to the 'snapshot' images obtained with radiographs. This is used to follow the passage of barium through the bowel, obtaining dedicated images at specific points of interest only. Motility of the bowel can also be assessed in this way. Fluoroscopy is used extensively in interventional radiology and, in particular, in vascular intervention by allowing real-time assessment of the passage of intravascular iodinated contrast and the acquisition of multiple images per second to diagnose intravascular lesions and to guide treatment. Naturally, with the more sustained use of

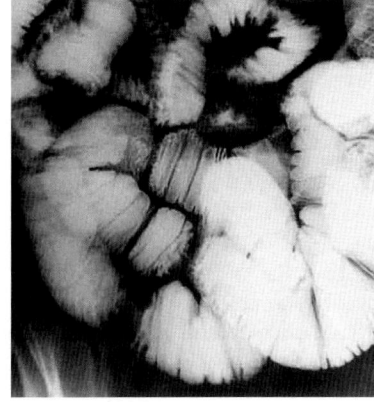

Figure 10.2 Barium examination of the small bowel demonstrates a focal short segment stricture of the distal ileum in a patient with Crohn's disease.

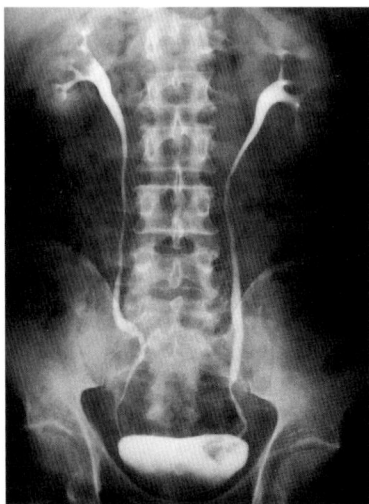

Figure 10.3 Intravenous urogram in a patient with macroscopic haematuria. There are focal irregular filling defects in the left side of the bladder and the right renal pelvis, consistent with multifocal transitional cell carcinomas.

ionising radiation, the cumulative doses tend to be greater than obtaining a conventional radiograph.

Ultrasound

Ultrasound is the second commonest method of imaging. It relies on high-frequency sound waves generated by a transducer containing piezoelectric material. The generated sound waves are reflected by tissue interfaces and, by ascertaining the time taken for a pulse to return and the direction of a pulse, it is possible to form an image. Medical ultrasound uses frequencies in the range 3–20 MHz. The higher the frequency of the ultrasound wave, the greater the resolution of the image, but the less depth of view from the skin. Consequently, abdominal imaging uses transducers with a frequency of 3–7 MHz, while higher-frequency transducers are used for superficial structures, such as musculoskeletal and breast ultrasound. Dedicated transducers have also been developed for endocavitary ultrasound such as transvaginal scan-

ning and transrectal ultrasound of the prostate, allowing high-frequency scanning of organs by reducing the distance between the probe and the organ of interest (Fig. 10.4). A further application of dedicated probes has been in the field of endoscopic ultrasound, allowing exquisite imaging of the wall of a hollow viscus and the adjacent organs such as the gastric wall and the pancreas.

Reflection of an ultrasound wave from moving objects such as red blood cells causes a change in the frequency of the ultrasound wave. By measuring this frequency change, it is possible to calculate the speed and direction of the movement. This principle forms the basis of Doppler ultrasound, whereby velocities within major vessels as well as smaller vessels in organs such as the liver and the kidneys can be measured. Doppler imaging is widely used in the assessment of arterial and venous disease, in which stenotic lesions cause an alteration in the normal velocity. Furthermore, diffuse parenchymal diseases such as cirrhosis may cause an alteration in the normal Doppler signal of the affected organ.

The advantages of ultrasound are that it is cheap and easily available. It is the first-line investigation of choice for assessment of the liver, the biliary tree and the renal tract (Figs 10.5 and 10.6). Ultrasound is also the imaging method of choice in obstetric assessment and gynaecological disease. High-frequency transducers have made ultrasound the best imaging technique for the evaluation of thyroid and testicular disorders in terms of both diffuse disease and focal mass lesions. It is also an invaluable tool for guiding needle placement in interventional procedures such as biopsies and drainages, allowing direct real-time visualisation of the needle during the procedure.

Ligament, tendon and muscle injuries are also probably best imaged in the first instance by ultrasound (Fig. 10.7). The ability to stress ligaments and to allow tendons to move during the investigation gives an extra dimension, which greatly improves its diagnostic value. The use of 'panoramic' or 'extended field of view' ultrasound (Fig. 10.8) provides images that are more easily interpreted by an observer not performing the examination, and are of particular assistance to surgeons planning a procedure.

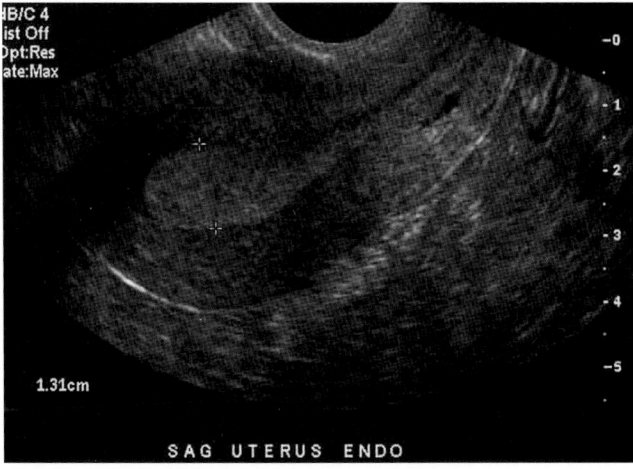

Figure 10.4 Longitudinal transvaginal ultrasound scan of the uterus demonstrating thickening of the endometrium in a patient during the secretory phase of the menstrual cycle.

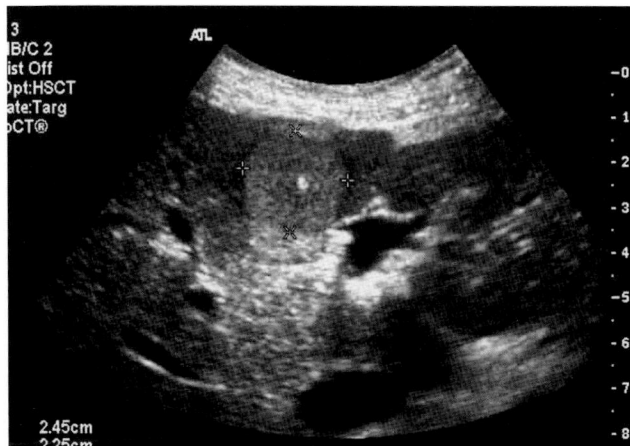

Figure 10.5 Transverse ultrasound image of the liver in a patient with colorectal cancer shows a solitary liver metastasis.

Christian Johann Doppler, **1803–1853, Professor of Experimental Physics, Vienna, Austria, enunciated the 'Doppler Principle' in 1842.**

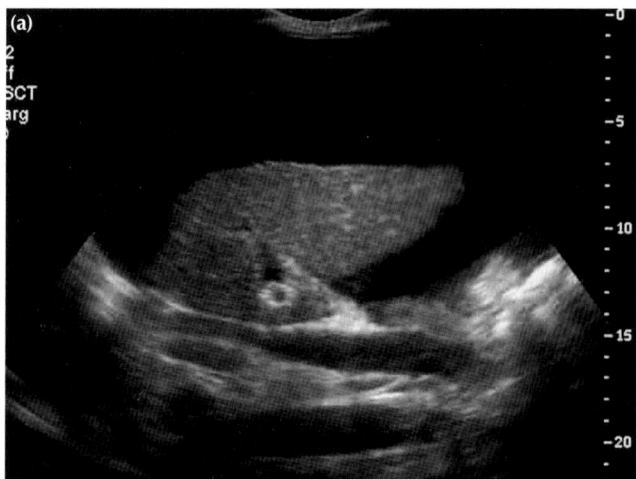

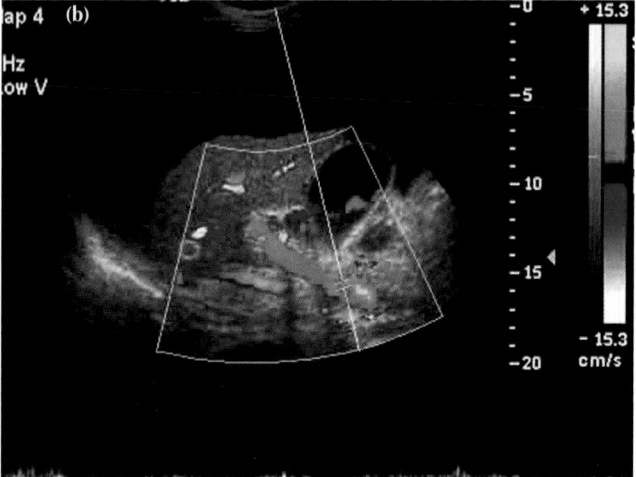

Figure 10.6 Sagittal ultrasound image of the liver (a) in a patient with cirrhosis demonstrates nodularity of the liver surface and extensive ascites. Doppler ultrasound (b) illustrates portal vein flow with a normal direction.

Ultrasound will demonstrate most foreign bodies in soft tissues, including those that are not radio-opaque.

The disadvantages of ultrasound are that it is highly operator dependent, and most of the information is gained during the actual process of scanning as opposed to reviewing the static images. Another drawback is that the ultrasound wave is highly attenuated by air and bone and, thus, little information is gained with regard to tissues beyond bony or air-filled structures; alternative techniques may be required to image these areas (Summary box 10.5).

Summary box 10.5

Ultrasound

Strengths
- No radiation
- Inexpensive
- Allows interaction with patients
- Superb soft-tissue resolution in the near field
- Dynamic studies can be performed
- First-line investigation for hepatic, biliary and renal disease
- Endocavitary ultrasound for gynaecological and prostate disorders
- Excellent resolution for breast, thyroid and testis imaging
- Good for soft tissue, including tendons and ligaments
- Excellent for cysts and foreign bodies
- Doppler studies allow assessment of blood flow

Weaknesses
- Interpretation only possible during the examination
- Long learning curve for some areas of expertise
- Resolution dependent on the machine available
- Images cannot be reliably reviewed away from the patient

Computerised tomography

There has been a great deal of development in CT technology over the last 30 years from the initial conventional CT scanners through to helical or spiral scanners and the current multi-detector machines. CT scanners consist of a gantry containing the X-ray tube, filters and detectors, which revolve around the patient, acquiring information at different angles and projections. This information is then mathematically reconstructed to produce a two-dimensional grey-scale image of a slice through the body. This technique overcomes the problem of superimposition

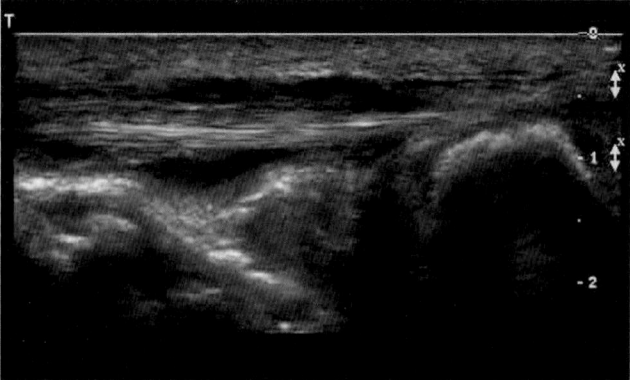

Figure 10.7 Ultrasound of the dorsal surface of the wrist shows the normal fibrillar pattern of the extensor tendons. There is increased fluid within the tendon sheath in this patient with extensor tenosynovitis.

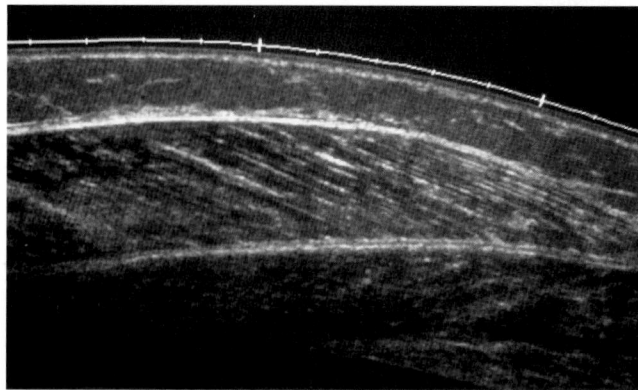

Figure 10.8 Panoramic ultrasound of the calf. The normal muscle fibres and the fascia can be identified over an area measuring approximately 12 cm.

of different structures, which is inherent in conventional radiography. Improvements in gantry design, advances in detector technology using more sensitive detectors and an increase in the number of detectors have resulted in an increase in spatial resolution as well as the speed at which the images are acquired. In early CT scanners, the table on which the patient was positioned moved in between the gantry revolution to allow imaging of an adjacent slice. Modern scanners allow for continuous movement of the table and the patient during the gantry revolution, thus greatly reducing the scan time. With modern equipment, it is now not only possible to obtain images of the chest, abdomen and pelvis in under 20 s, but these axial images can be reformatted in multiple planes with practically no degradation in image quality.

In addition, CT has a far higher contrast resolution than plain radiographs, allowing the assessment of tissues with similar attenuation characteristics. As with radiographs, the natural contrast of tissues is further augmented by the use of intravenous contrast medium. Rapid scanning of a volume of tissue also allows the scans to be performed at different phases of enhancement, which is advantageous in identifying different diseases. For instance, very early scanning during the arterial phase is ideally suited to the examination of the arterial tree and hypervascular liver lesions, whereas scanning performed after a delay may be better suited to the identification of other solid organ pathology such as renal masses. Furthermore, it is possible to obtain scans during several phases including the arterial and venous phases in the same patient, which may aid in the identification and characterisation of lesions.

CT is widely used in thoracic, abdominal (Fig. 10.9), neurological (Fig. 10.10), musculoskeletal (Fig. 10.11) and trauma imaging. The thinner collimation and improved spatial resolution have also resulted in the development of newer techniques such as CT angiography, virtual colonoscopy and virtual bronchoscopy. Furthermore, three-dimensional images can be reconstructed from the raw data to aid in surgical planning. The disadvantage of CT compared with ultrasound and conventional radiography lies largely in the increased costs and the far higher doses of ionising radiation. For instance, a CT scan of the abdomen and pelvis has a radiation dose equivalent to approximately 500 chest radiographs (Summary box 10.6).

Summary box 10.6

Computerised tomography

Strengths
- High spatial and contrast resolution
- Contrast resolution enhanced by imaging in arterial and/or venous phases
- Rapid acquisition of images in one breath-hold
- Imaging of choice for the detection of pulmonary masses
- Allows global assessment of the abdomen and pelvis
- Excellent for liver, pancreatic, renal and bowel pathology
- Three-dimensional reconstruction allows complex fracture imaging
- Multiplanar reconstruction and three-dimensional imaging, e.g. CT angiography and colonoscopy

Weaknesses
- High radiation dose
- Poor soft-tissue resolution of the peripheries and superficial structures
- Patient needs to be able to lie flat and still

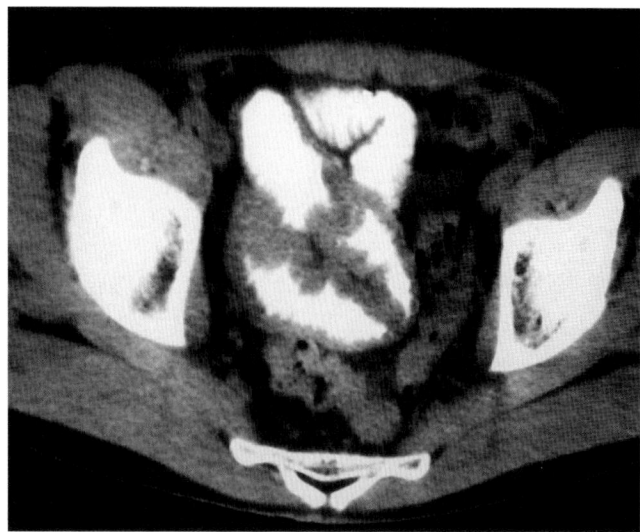

Figure 10.9 Axial computerised tomography scan through the pelvis with oral contrast administration illustrates loops of distal ileum with mural thickening in a patient with Crohn's disease.

Magnetic resonance imaging

Over the last 20 years, MRI has become an integral part of the imaging arsenal with ever-expanding indications. MRI relies on the fact that nuclei containing an odd number of protons or electrons have a characteristic motion in a magnetic field (precession) and produce a magnetic moment as a result of this motion. In a strong uniform magnetic field such as a MRI scanner, these nuclei align themselves with the main magnetic field and result in a net magnetic moment. A brief radiofrequency pulse is then applied to alter the motion of the nuclei. Once the radiofrequency pulse is removed, the nuclei realign themselves with the main magnetic field (relaxation) and in the process emit a radiofrequency signal that can be recorded, spatially encoded and used to construct a grey-scale image. The specific tissue characteristics define the manner and rate at which the nuclei relax. This relaxation is measured in two ways, referred to as the T1 and T2 relaxation times. The relaxation times and the proton density determine the signal from a specific tissue.

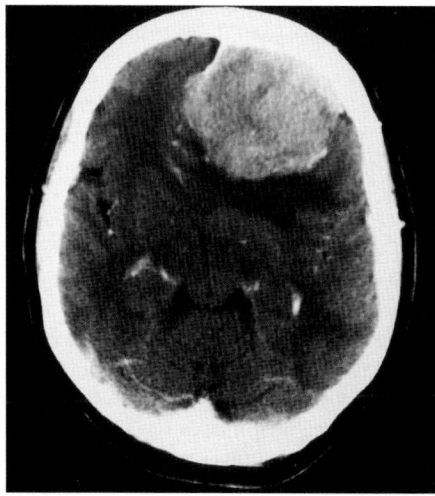

Figure 10.10 Axial computerised tomography scan of the head following intravenous contrast demonstrates a large mass lesion in the left frontal region in a patient with a large left frontal meningioma.

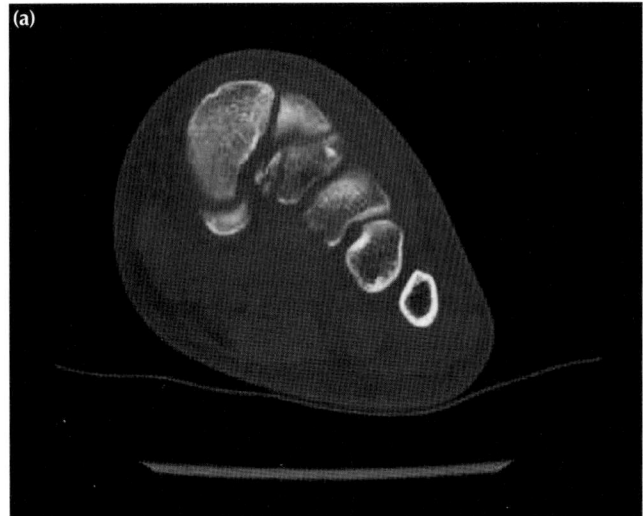

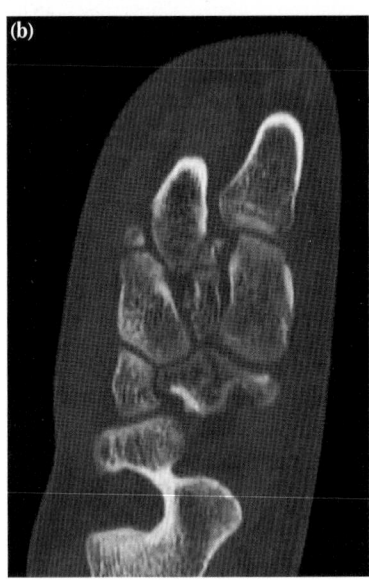

Figure 10.11 Coronal computerised tomography (a) and axial reformats (b) of the foot in a patient involved in a road traffic accident demonstrates Lisfranc fracture dislocation with a comminuted fracture of the base of the second metatarsal.

There are a large number of imaging sequences that can be used by applying radiofrequency pulses of different strengths and durations. The image characteristic and signal intensity from different tissues is governed by the pulse sequence employed and whether it is T1 weighted or T2 weighted. For instance, fat, methaemoglobin and mucinous fluid are bright on T1-weighted images, whereas water and thus most pathological processes, which tend to increase tissue water content, are bright on T2-weighted images. Cortical bone, air, haemosiderin and ferromagnetic materials are of very low signal on all pulse sequences. In general, T1-weighted images are superior in the delineation of anatomy, while T2-weighted images tend to highlight pathology better. For added tissue contrast, intravenous gadolinium may be

Jacques Lisfranc de St. Martin, **1790–1847, Professor of Surgery and Operative Medicine, Paris, France.**

administered. Other more specific contrast media are also available for liver, bowel and lymph node imaging.

MRI's exquisite contrast resolution, coupled with a lack of ionising radiation, is very attractive in imaging, particularly of tissues that have relatively little natural contrast. MRI also has the advantage of multiplanar imaging, as images can be acquired in any plane prescribed. It has traditionally been used extensively in the assessment of intracranial, spinal and musculoskeletal disorders (Figs 10.12–10.14), allowing a global assessment of bony and soft-tissue structures. More recent developments have resulted in new indications and applications. Today, MRI is commonly used in oncological imaging such as staging of rectal carcinoma and gynaecological malignancies, characterisation and identification of hepatic masses, assessment of the biliary tree [magnetic resonance

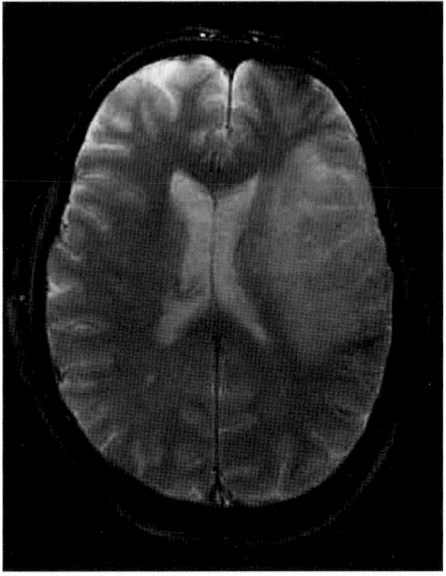

Figure 10.12 T2-weighted axial magnetic resonance imaging scan of the head in a patient with a large left-sided oligodendroglioma.

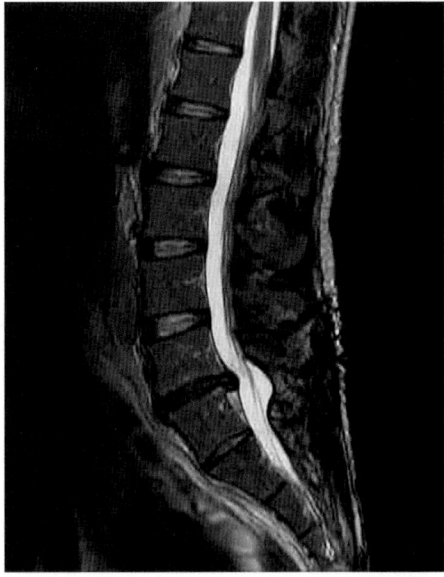

Figure 10.13 Sagittal T2-weighted magnetic resonance imaging scan of the lumbar spine demonstrates disc herniation in a patient with acute back pain.

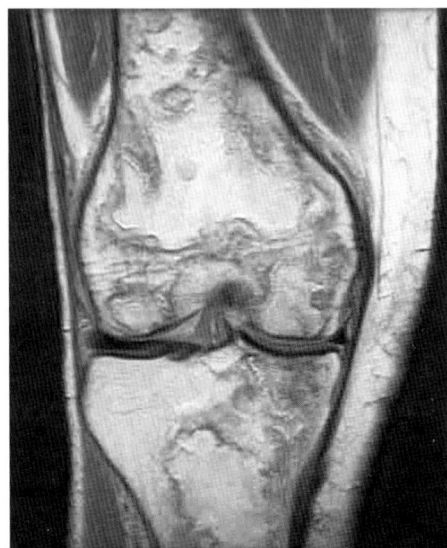

Figure 10.14 Coronal magnetic resonance imaging scan of the knee demonstrating extensive serpiginous areas of altered signal intensity in the distal femur and proximal tibia in a patient with bone infarcts secondary to oral corticosteroids.

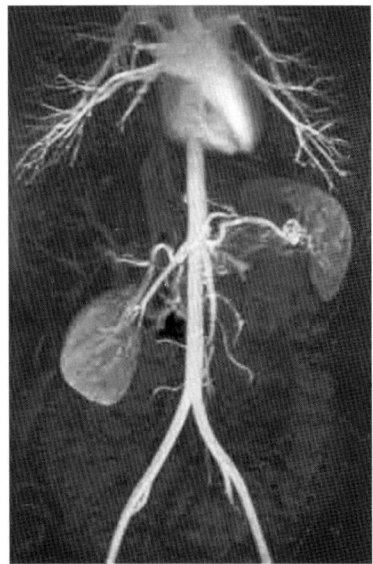

Figure 10.16 Maximum intensity projection image from a magnetic resonance angiogram demonstrating the abdominal aorta, common and external iliac arteries as well as parts of the pulmonary, mesenteric and renal vasculature.

cholangiopancreatography (MRCP) (Fig. 10.15)] and cardiac imaging. Techniques have also been developed which allow non-invasive angiography of the cranial and peripheral circulation (MR angiography) (Fig. 10.16).

However, the availability of MRI is still relatively limited in comparison with other imaging techniques, and it is time-consuming with respect to image acquisition and interpretation. Images are easily degraded by motion, including respiratory and cardiac motion. The use of respiratory and cardiac gating can minimise this, although bowel peristalsis can still be a problem. The long acquisition times require a cooperative patient who can lie very still, which can be difficult especially in claustrophobic individuals or those in pain. Furthermore, because of the use of high-strength magnetic fields, patients with some metallic implants, such as some aneurysm clips and prosthetic heart

valves, and those with implanted electronic devices such as pacemakers and defibrillators, cannot be examined. Some newer implants may, however, be MRI compatible, and patients with joint replacements can be studied safely (Summary box 10.7).

Summary box 10.7

Magnetic resonance imaging

Strengths
- No ionising radiation
- Excellent soft-tissue contrast
- Best imaging technique for
    Intracranial lesions
    Spine
    Bone marrow and joint lesions

Evolving use
- Staging
- MRCP
- MR angiography
- Breast malignancy
- Pelvic malignancy
- Cardiac imaging

Weaknesses
- Absolute contraindications
    Ocular metallic foreign bodies
    Pacemakers
    Cochlear implants
    Cranial aneurysm clips
- Relative contraindications
    First trimester of pregnancy
    Claustrophobia

Long scan times so patients may not be able to keep still, especially if in pain

Limited availability

Expensive

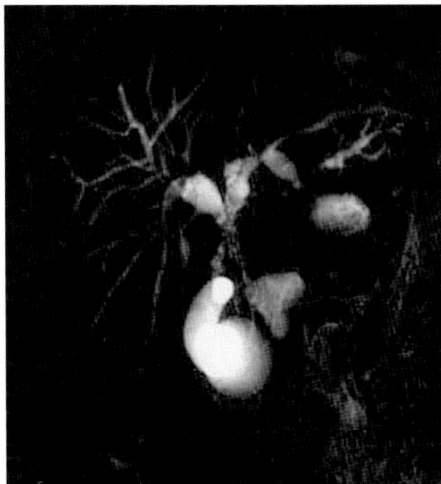

Figure 10.15 Magnetic resonance cholangiopancreatography demonstrating dilated central intrahepatic bile ducts and a stricture of the common bile duct in a patient with obstructive jaundice and cholangiocarcinoma.

CHAPTER 10 | DIAGNOSTIC IMAGING

Nuclear medicine

In other imaging techniques using ionising radiation such as CT and conventional radiography, the individual is exposed to ionising radiation from an external source and the radiation transmitted through the patient is recorded. In nuclear medicine, however, a radioactive element or radionuclide such as technetium, gallium, thallium or iodine is administered to the patient as part of a radiopharmaceutical agent, and a detector such as a gamma camera is then used to record and localise the emission from the patient, thus forming the image. The radionuclide is chosen and coupled with other compounds such that it is distributed and taken up in the tissues of interest. Therefore, a variety of radionuclides are required for imaging of different tissues. Nuclear medicine also differs from other means of imaging, which are largely anatomically based, as it also provides functional information.

Radionuclide imaging is widely used in bone imaging with very high sensitivity for assessing metastatic disease, metabolic bone disease, established arthropathies and occult infection and traumatic injuries (Fig. 10.17), although many of these applications are being replaced by MRI. In genitourinary disease, dynamic imaging can be performed to assess renal perfusion and function including obstruction, investigate renovascular hypertension and evaluate renal transplants. Radionuclide imaging is also commonly used in thyroid and parathyroid disorders, ischaemic cardiac disease, detection of pulmonary emboli and assessment of occult infection and inflammatory bowel disease.

Positron emission tomography (PET) is an extension of nuclear medicine, in which a positron-emitting substance such as ^{18}F is tagged and used to assess tissue metabolic characteristics. The most commonly used radiolabelled tracer is 18F-2-fluoro-2-deoxy-D-glucose (FDG), although other tracers can also be used in order to assess metabolic functions such as oxygen and glucose consumption and blood flow. Radioisotope decay

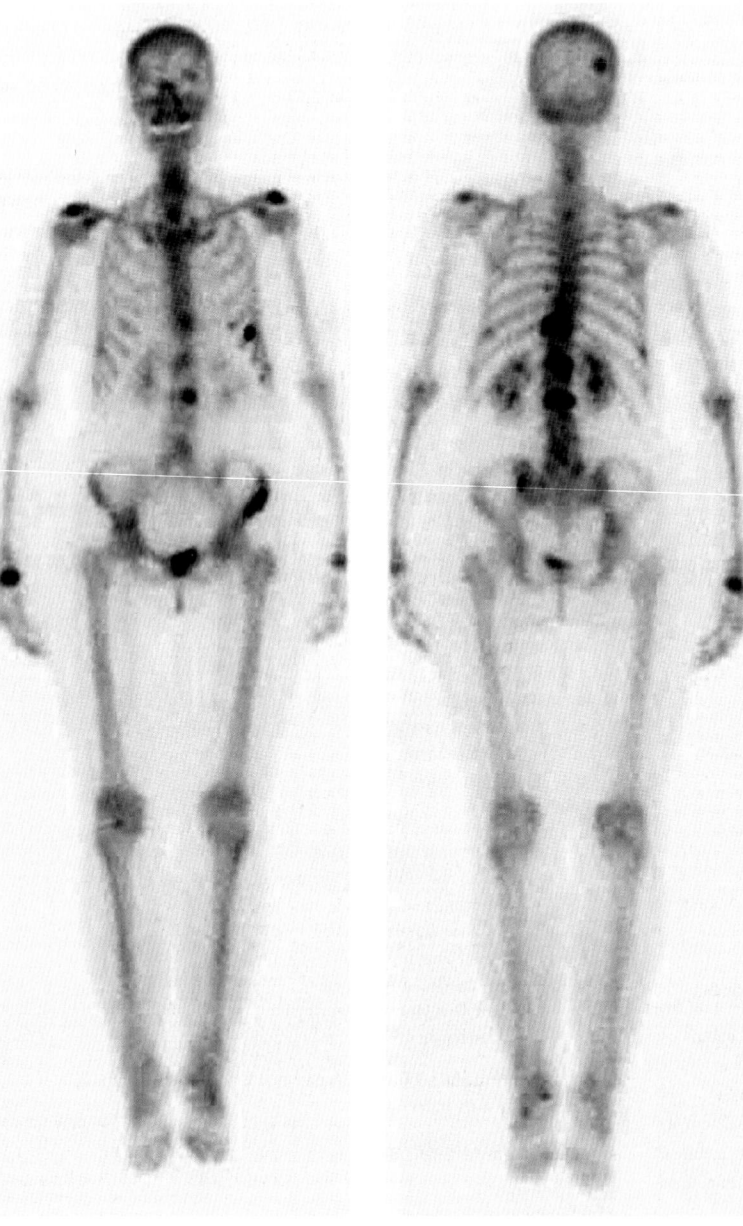

Figure 10.17 Bone scintigraphy in a patient with carcinoma of the breast illustrating bony metastatic deposits involving multiple vertebrae, the skull, pelvis and ribs.

causes the emission of a positron, which subsequently, within a few millimetres, collides with and annihilates an electron to produce a pair of annihilation photons. The drawbacks have been high cost, very limited availability and relatively low spatial resolution. The last of these has been addressed by PET/CT systems combining simultaneous PET imaging and CT, allowing the two sets of images to be registered so that the anatomical location of the abnormality can be localised more precisely (Summary box 10.8).

IMAGING IN ORTHOPAEDIC SURGERY

Introduction

Imaging is an intricate part of musculoskeletal diagnosis, and image-guided, minimally invasive techniques also play a major role in treatment. In broad terms, radiographs are the best method of looking for bony lesions or injuries, MRI shows bone marrow disease, muscle tendon and soft-tissue disorders, and ultrasound has better resolution than MRI for small structures, with the added advantage of showing dynamic changes. CT enables visualisation of the fine detail of bony structures, clarifying abnormalities seen on plain radiographs (Summary box 10.9).

There are occasions when a combination of techniques will be important, and due consideration should be given to reducing the ionising radiation burden to the patient, using ultrasound and MRI as primary investigations whenever appropriate.

Skeletal trauma

Musculoskeletal trauma is best imaged by an initial plain radiograph. All skeletal radiographs should be taken from two different angles, usually at right angles to each other. This is important in trauma because a fracture or dislocation may not be visible on a single view (Fig. 10.18). Occasionally, and in specific locations such as the scaphoid, more than two views are routinely performed. If this fails to make a clear diagnosis, or if there is suspicion of soft-tissue injuries, then cross-sectional studies are indicated.

In the spine, CT is a normal second-line investigation, but this is best performed with reference to good-quality radiographs, including oblique views if necessary (Summary box 10.10).

(a)

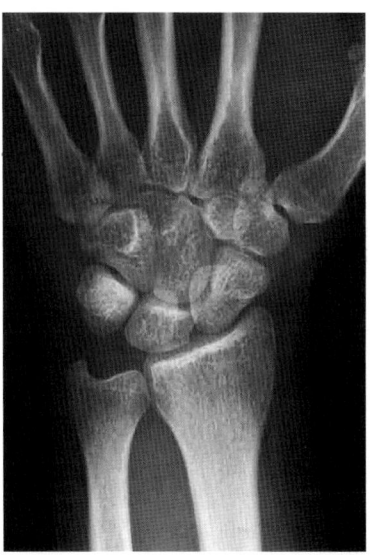

(b)

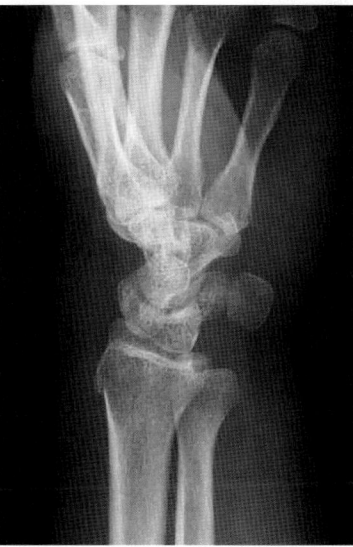

Figure 10.18 Anteroposterior radiograph of the wrist (a) in a patient following a fall does not show an acute bony injury. It is only on the second view (b) that a fracture of the dorsal cortex of the distal radius is visualised.

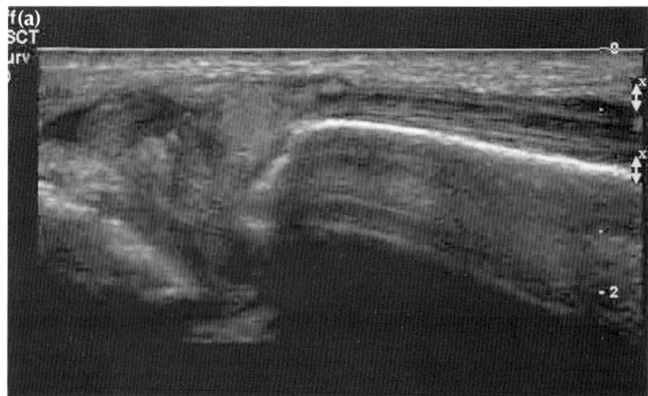

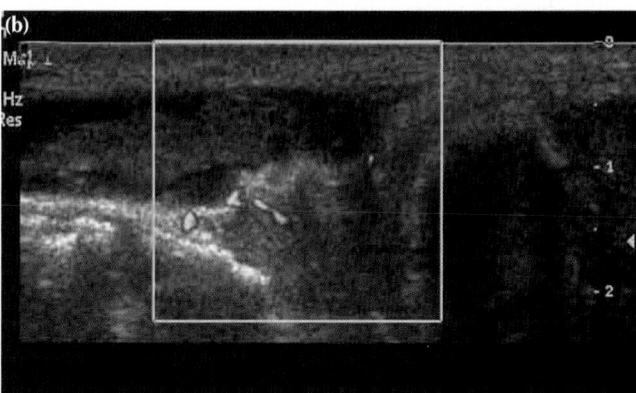

Summary box 10.10

Trauma imaging
- Initial imaging is radiography
- At least two views are needed
- Use CT for spine, intra-articular or occult fractures

Axial CT images alone may fail to diagnose some fractures, so three-dimensional reformatting is important to prevent errors. Sections should be thin, but care must be taken not to cover too wide an area, as the radiation burden may be excessive, particularly with multislice CT.

Degenerative disease

Synovitis

Radiographs are usually the first-line imaging investigation performed for the examination of joints. Typical changes of a degenerative or an erosive arthropathy are well known and understood. However, early arthropathy will be missed on radiographs and, with the advent of disease-modifying drugs, it is important to detect early synovitis before it is even apparent on clinical examination. Gadolinium DTPA-enhanced MRI is the most sensitive method for detecting synovial thickening of numerous joints, but ultrasound is also sensitive, albeit more laborious to perform. Ultrasound shows effusions and synovial thickening clearly, and shows the increased blood flow around the affected joints without the use of contrast agents (Figs 10.19 and 10.20).

Articular cartilage damage

Articular surface disease is difficult to detect using non-invasive techniques. MRI is probably the best method, although it is not sensitive to early chondral changes (Fig. 10.21) Higher field strength magnets (3 Tesla and above) with dedicated surface coils provide more precise assessment; however, MR arthrography is currently the imaging 'gold standard'. Saline mixed with a dilute

Figure 10.20 Ultrasound of the wrist (a) shows thickening of tissues on the dorsal aspect of the radiocarpal joint. (b) There is increased flow on power Doppler ultrasound in this patient with wrist synovitis and rheumatoid arthritis.

quantity of gadolinium DTPA is introduced into the joint by needle puncture, which is followed by an MRI examination. Using this technique, more subtle changes in the articular surface can be seen, including thinning, fissuring and ulceration. However, early softening of articular cartilage will not be visible. MR

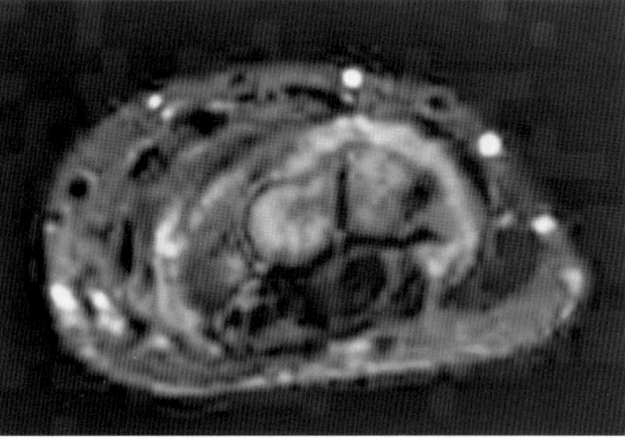

Figure 10.19 Axial T2-weighted fat-suppressed image of the wrist in a patient with rheumatoid arthritis demonstrating synovitis manifested as increased signal dorsal to the carpal bones.

Nikola Tesla, **1856–1943**, an American Physicist and Electrical Engineer who worked for the Westinghouse Company. A Tesla is the SI unit of magnetic flux density

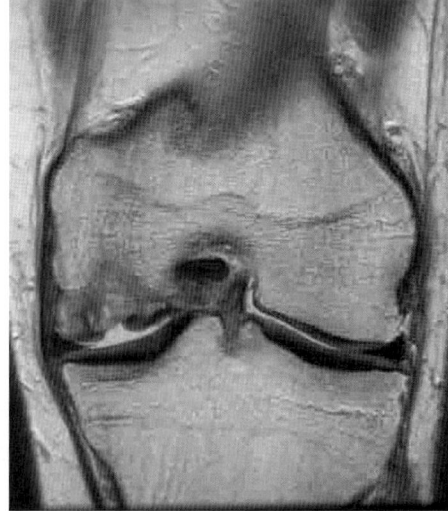

Figure 10.21 Coronal magnetic resonance imaging of the knee demonstrates a focal osteochondral abnormality of the medial femoral condyle with full-thickness loss of the articular cartilage and abnormality of the subchondral bone.

arthrography is also useful for detecting labral tears in the shoulder or hip (Fig. 10.22), and in the assessment of patients who have undergone a previous meniscectomy. The triangular fibrocartilage of the wrist is also difficult to assess fully without arthrography (Fig. 10.23).

In the shoulder, rotator cuff trauma and degenerative changes can be studied using ultrasound or MRI. In experienced hands, ultrasound has a higher accuracy rate, because image resolution is better and because the mechanical integrity of the cuff can be tested by dynamically stressing it (Fig. 10.24). MRI has the advantage of being able to show abnormalities in the subcortical bone.

In the majority of arthropathies and degenerative disorders, serial imaging is useful. Changes in films taken weeks or months apart are far easier to see and interpret than from a single snapshot study (Summary box 10.11).

Summary box 10.11

Imaging techniques for joint disease

- Radiographs are good for assessing established articular disease
- Synovitis can be detected using ultrasound or contrast-enhanced MRI
- Early damage to articular cartilage is difficult to image by conventional methods
- Rotator cuff lesions are best studied using ultrasound or MRI
- Destructive lesions are best studied first on plain radiographs
- MRI is best for staging tumours
- Biopsy can be guided by fluoroscopy, CT or ultrasound

Aggressive bone disease

The radiograph is the first imaging technique for destructive lesions in bones. There is considerable experience in the interpretation of these films, especially with regard to whether the lesion is benign or malignant (Fig. 10.25).

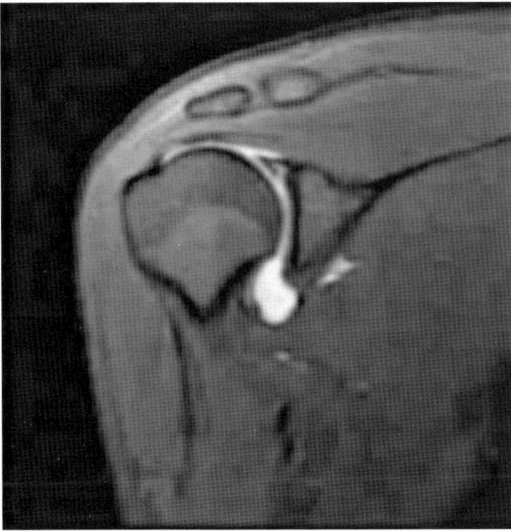

Figure 10.22 Coronal oblique T1-weighted fat-suppressed image of the right shoulder following intra-articular injection of diluted gadolinium demonstrates imbibition of the gadolinium mixture into the superior labrum in a patient with superior labrum anterior posterior (SLAP) tear.

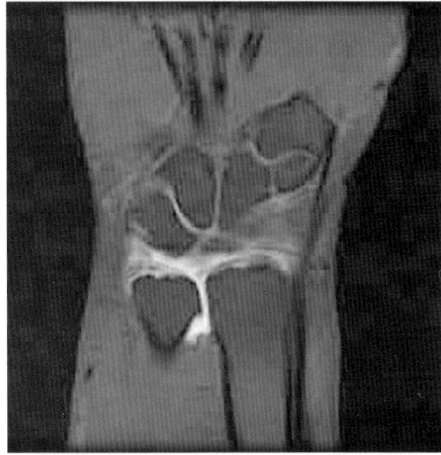

Figure 10.23 Coronal T1-weighted fat-suppressed image following injection of diluted gadolinium mixture into the radiocarpal joint shows extension of gadolinium into the distal radioulnar joint through a tear in the triangular fibrocartilage.

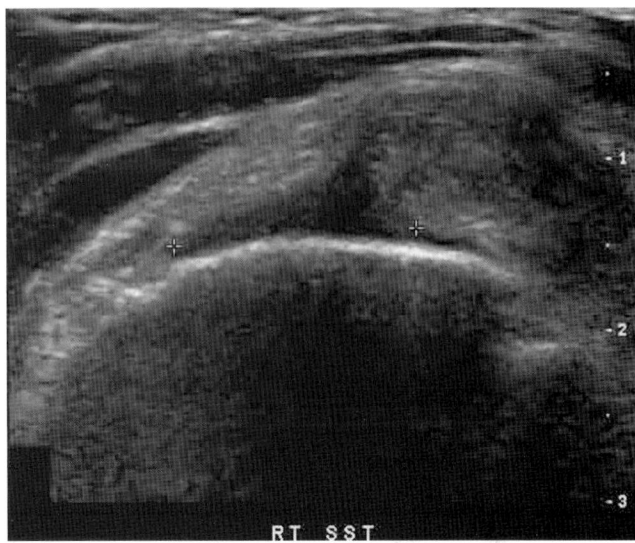

Figure 10.24 Ultrasound of the supraspinatus tendon identifies a partial tear of the tendon, which is predominantly articular sided but with a component that is nearly full thickness.

Radiographs are also vital in the assessment of soft-tissue calcification in tumours of muscle, tendon and subcutaneous fat. When a lesion is detected, there needs to be an early decision as to whether this is benign or malignant. If there is a suspicion of malignancy on the radiograph, or any uncertainty, then local staging is indicated. This is best performed by MRI for both bone and soft-tissue lesions (Fig. 10.26). At this stage, it is likely that a biopsy will be indicated, and preferably under image guidance. Soft-tissue and bone biopsy needles may be guided by CT, ultrasound or interventional MRI systems. The route of puncture should avoid vital structures and must be agreed with the surgeon, who will perform local excision if the lesion proves to be malignant. Care should be taken to avoid contaminating other compartments. In all circumstances, samples are best sent for both histopathological and microbiological examination. It may be difficult to tell on imaging whether or not a lesion is infected, and histology often provides a clear diagnosis in inflammatory

(a)

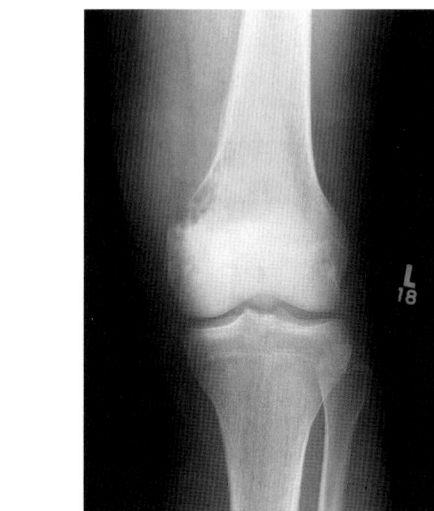

(b)

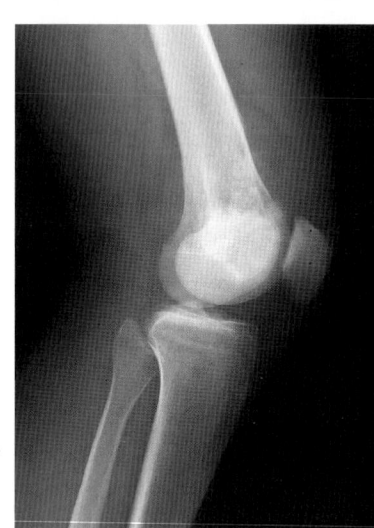

Figure 10.25 Anteroposterior (a) and lateral (b) radiographs of the left knee in a young patient with knee pain. There is a mixed lucent and sclerotic lesion of the distal femur with breach of the cortex medially and soft-tissue extension seen anteriorly and posteriorly. The location and appearances are consistent with osteosarcoma.

conditions. Bone scintigraphy is useful in detecting whether a lesion is solitary or multiple, although whole-body MRI is becoming available (Summary box 10.12).

> **Summary box 10.12**
>
> **Imaging of aggressive lesions in bone**
>
> - Plain radiographs are important as a first investigation
> - MRI is best for local staging
> - Bone scintigraphy or whole-body MRI for solitary or multiple lesion determination
> - CT detects lung metastases
> - Fluoroscopy, CT, MRI or ultrasound can be used to guide the biopsy

Mass lesions

Mass lesions in muscle and soft tissue are examined by ultrasound, which can be diagnostic in the majority of cases, thereby

(a)

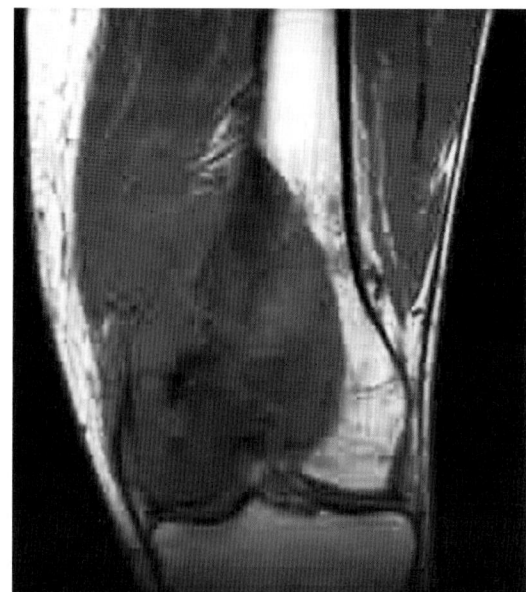

(b)

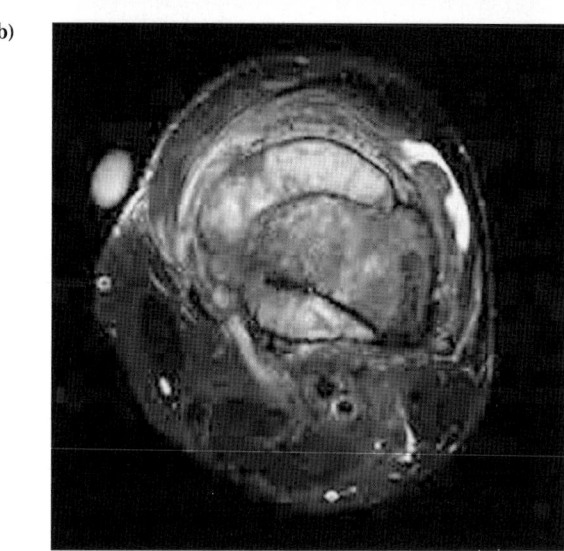

Figure 10.26 Coronal T1- (a) and axial T2-weighted fat-suppressed (b) images through the distal femur of the patient in Figure 10.25 illustrates the bony area involved, the soft-tissue extent of the tumour and the relationship of the neurovascular structures to the mass.

avoiding the need for further imaging. This is most often the case when a lesion is purely cystic and, as most soft-tissue masses are cysts, ultrasound is a very effective screening test. There are occasions when no mass lesion is found at the site of concern, and then reassurance can be offered. If the ultrasound examination is normal, this effectively excludes soft-tissue neoplasia. A reasonable protocol is to perform ultrasound on all palpable 'lesions' to exclude cysts, and on patients without any identifiable mass, and to proceed to MRI only when there is a solid or partly solid element to an unidentifiable lesion. Tumour vascularity is best assessed by Doppler ultrasound. It can be studied by intravenous gadolinium DTPA-enhanced MRI; however, this is a more expensive and invasive technique, providing no more information than Doppler ultrasound (Summary box 10.13).

Imaging of soft-tissue lesions

- Ultrasound is the best for screening; it is often the only imaging required
- MRI is best for local staging and follow-up
- Doppler ultrasound can assess vascularity cheaply and effectively
- Ultrasound is useful for biopsy

Infection

In the early stages of joint infection, the plain films may be normal, but they should still be performed to exclude bony erosions, in case a painful joint is the first sign of an arthropathy. Ultrasound examination is the easiest and most accurate method of assessing joint effusions, although, when an effusion is identified, it is not possible to discriminate between blood and pus. Aspiration guided by ultrasound is the best method of making this distinction. MRI may be required to assess early articular cartilage and bone involvement.

Radiographs should also be used to examine patients with suspected osteomyelitis. Although they may not detect early infection, they will demonstrate or exclude bony destruction, calcification and sequestrum formation. CT may be needed to give a cross-sectional view, in order to assess the extent of bony sequestrum.

MRI is perhaps the most sensitive method for detecting early disease and is the preferred technique to define the activity and extent of infection, as it shows not only the bony involvement but also the extent of oedema and soft-tissue involvement (Fig. 10.27). Abscesses may be detected or excluded, and subperiosteal oedema is readily visible. MRI can be used as a staging procedure to plan treatment, including surgical intervention.

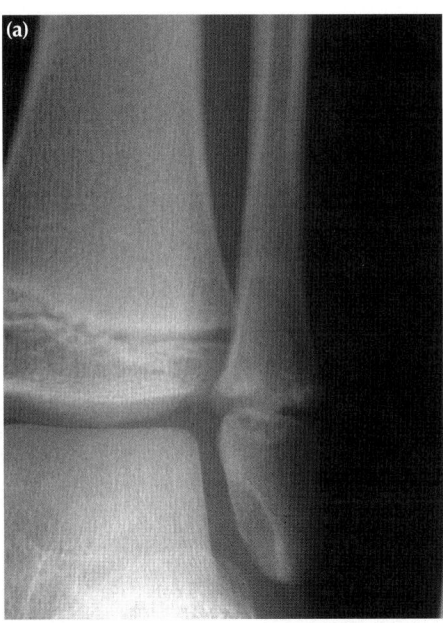
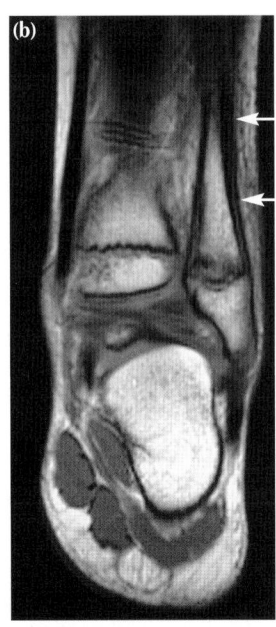
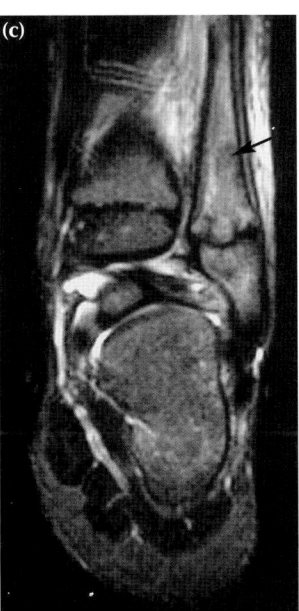
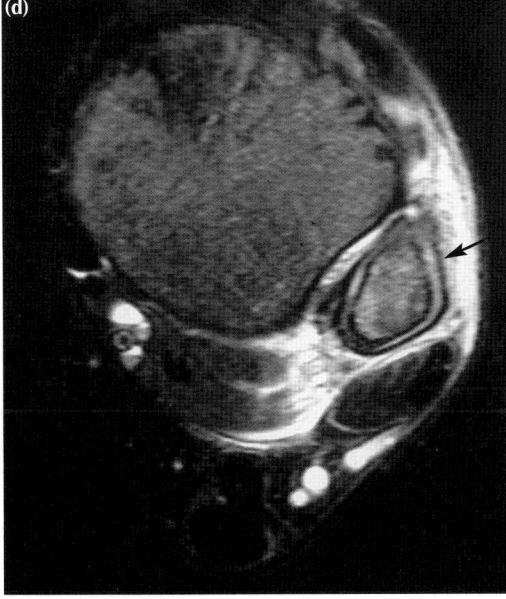

Figure 10.27 (a) The plain films of this 13-year-old are close to normal. On close inspection, there is a fine periosteal reaction on the fibula. (b) The coronal T1-weighted magnetic resonance image shows little more, but (c) the coronal fast STIR (short tau inversion recovery) images and (d) axial T2 fast spin echo with fat suppression show the oedema in bone as white and the extensive periosteal fluid with soft-tissue inflammation. The diagnosis is acute osteomyelitis.

CHAPTER 10 | DIAGNOSTIC IMAGING

Serial examinations can be used to follow the response to intravenous antibiotics and are very useful in the management of complex osteomyelitis. In cases of negative or equivocal MRI, nuclear medicine techniques such as bone scintigraphy can be very sensitive, and specialised studies using tracers such as gallium citrate or indium-labelled white cells increase specificity (Summary box 10.14).

Summary box 10.14

Imaging of potentially infected bone and joint

- Plain radiographs may be needed to exclude bone erosion
- Ultrasound is sensitive for an effusion, periosteal collections and superficial abscesses and can be used for guided aspiration
- CT is useful in established infection to look for sequestrum
- MRI is useful to define the activity of osteomyelitis, early infection and soft-tissue collections
- Bone scans are sensitive but of low specificity
- Complex nuclear medicine studies are useful in negative MR examinations or equivocal cases

---

Metabolic bone disease

Plain radiographs should be the first images of patients with metabolic bone disease. They may detect the subperiosteal erosions in hyperparathyroidism or, more commonly, the osteopenia in osteoporosis, but they cannot be used to quantify osteoporosis. The apparent density of the bone on the film is linked to the penetration of the rays, among other variables, as well as to the bone density. If a quantitative method is needed, however, bone mineral density using dual X-ray absorptiometry (DEXA) is the most accurate and practical. However, fractures will cause erroneously high readings, and they tend to occur in the vertebrae used for DEXA measurements. Quantitative CT is an alternative technique, although this is less readily available. Ultrasound transmission measurement in the extremities has its advocates, as it arguably measures factors that better represent the strength of bone rather than its density. Its limitations are that it cannot be used to study the vertebrae or hip, and these are the sites where osteoporotic fractures occur most frequently. MRI may be useful in detecting fractures and is an essential prerequisite to percutaneous vertebroplasty.

IMAGING IN MAJOR TRAUMA

Introduction

Trauma remains a major cause of mortality and morbidity in all age groups. Presented with a multiply injured patient, rapid and effective investigation and treatment are required to maximise the chances of survival and to reduce morbidity. Imaging plays a major role in this assessment and in guiding treatment. As with the clinical assessment, imaging is carried out according to the principles of primary and secondary surveys, identifying major life-threatening injuries of the airway, respiratory system and circulation before a more detailed and typically time-consuming assessment of other injures. At no point should imaging delay the treatment of immediately life-threatening injuries. As in other settings, the quickest and least invasive examinations should be performed first. A radiologist present in the trauma room at the time of patient assessment is able to rapidly evaluate the radiographs, relay this information back to the team and guide further imaging, which may include further plain films, CT, ultrasound and MRI.

Plain radiographs

Conventional radiography allows rapid assessment of the major injuries and can be carried out in the trauma room while the patient is clinically assessed and treated. Despite the time constraints, the number of staff involved and the restricted mobility of the patient, high-quality images can be routinely obtained with due care and attention.

There is no routine set of radiographs to be obtained, and the decision is based on the mechanism of injury, the stability of the patient's condition and whether the patient is intubated. The most commonly performed initial radiographs are a chest radiograph, a single anteroposterior view of the pelvis and a cervical spine series.

The supine chest radiograph should encompass an area from the lung apices to the costophrenic recesses and include the ribs laterally. Chest radiographs give valuable information in both blunt and penetrating trauma. Evaluation of the radiograph should be undertaken in a systematic manner to minimise the chances of missing an injury. In the first instance, the position of line and tubes including the endotracheal tube should be assessed followed by assessment of the central airways. Following this, the lungs should be evaluated for abnormal focal areas of opacification, which may represent aspiration, haemorrhage, haematoma or oedema as well as more diffuse opacification reflecting a pleural collection. Alternatively, relative focal or unilateral lucency may reflect a pneumothorax in the supine position. Evaluation of the mediastinum should include its position, which may be altered by tension pneumothoraces or large collections, as well as its contour, an alteration of which may reflect a mediastinal haematoma due to aortic or spinal injury. Finally, the skeleton and the soft tissue should be carefully examined for rib, vertebral, scapular and limb fractures as well as evidence of surgical emphysema and paraspinal haematomas (Fig. 10.28).

Pelvic radiographs are also commonly performed to screen for and assess fractures of the bony pelvis. The image should include the iliac crests in their totality and extend inferiorly to below the lesser trochanters. When assessing the film, the alignment of the sacroiliac joints and the symphysis pubis should be carefully examined, as some fractures, especially those of the sacral arcades, can be very subtle on the pelvic radiograph. The presence of pubic fractures raises the possibility of urethral injury and should alert clinicians to exercise caution with bladder catheterisation (Fig. 10.29).

The utility of cervical spine X-rays depends on the conscious level of the patient and the presence of distracting injuries. In fully conscious patients with an isolated neck injury, clinical assessment can be used to guide the need for X-rays. In patients with distracting injuries and/or altered consciousness, including intubated patients, radiography is required. Typically, in patients who are not intubated, at least three views are performed including an anteroposterior view, an open mouth odontoid peg view and a lateral view extending down to the cervicothoracic junction. These may be supplemented with trauma oblique views in which the tube is rotated rather than the patient. In intubated individuals, open mouth views cannot be performed, and soft-tissue assessment is impaired by the presence of the endotracheal tube, so CT should be used to supplement an initial lateral

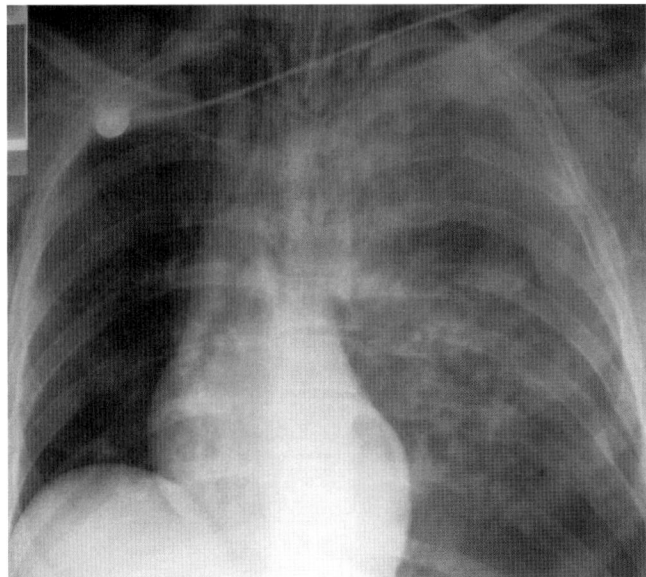

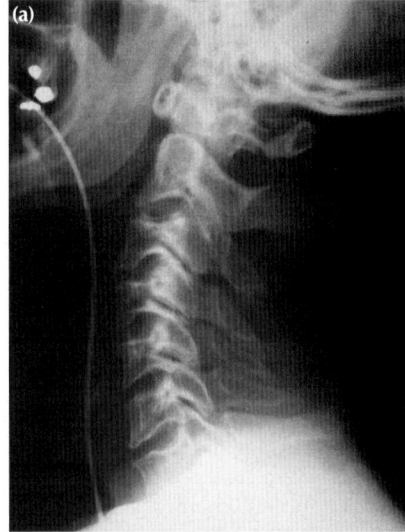

Figure 10.28 Supine chest radiograph of a patient involved in a road traffic accident. The patient is intubated. There are multiple left-sided rib fractures and extensive surgical emphysema. Depression of the left hemidiaphragm and mediastinal shift to the right suggest that there is a tension pneumothorax present.

radiograph (Fig. 10.30). When fractures are identified or when the radiographs do not fully examine the cervicothoracic junction, CT is indicated. If the patient is to undergo emergency CT examination for head or chest indications, a good-quality multi-detector CT study using thin sections and both coronal and sagittal reconstructions may be used to replace radiographs. CT may also be indicated when the radiographs appear normal but the nature of the injury or the clinical circumstances strongly suggest that the cervical spine may be injured.

Further radiographs of the thoracic and lumbar spine and the peripheral skeleton may be required depending on the clinical

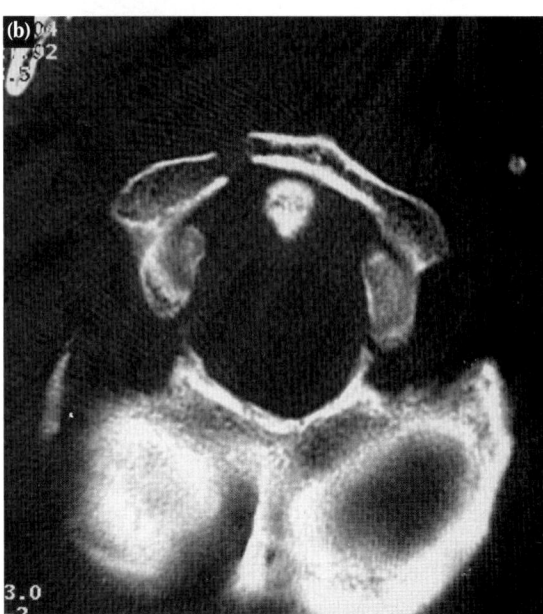

Figure 10.30 Lateral view of the cervical spine (a) fails to demonstrate the cervicothoracic junction. In addition, there appears to be a break in the posterior arch of C1. Computerised tomography of the cervical spine (b) demonstrated a fracture of the anterior arch as well as the posterior arch of C1.

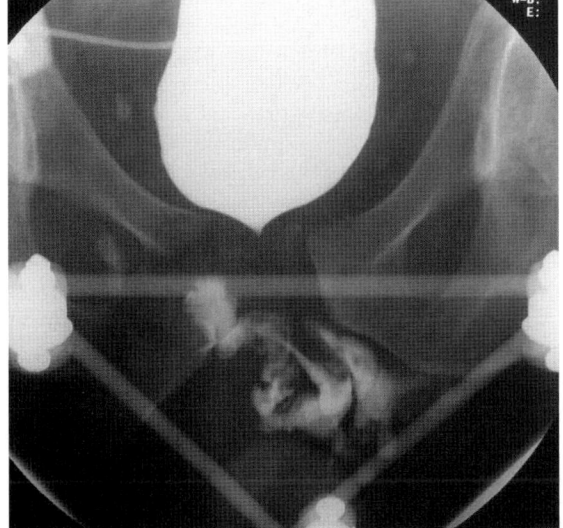

Figure 10.29 Retrograde urethrogram in a patient who sustained extensive pelvic fractures following a fall. The pelvic injuries have been stabilised using an external fixation device. The urethrogram identifies extensive injury to the urethra with extravasation of contrast.

setting. As with all skeletal radiographs, two perpendicular views are required for adequate assessment. Radiographs of the skull or facial bones have no role in the immediate assessment of the multitrauma individual except for immediate localisation of a penetrating object.

Ultrasound

Ultrasound has an evolving role in the assessment of acutely traumatised patients. The main current roles of ultrasound include the assessment of intraperitoneal fluid and haemopericardium (focused assessment with sonography for trauma, FAST), the evaluation of pneumothoraces in supine patients and in guiding intervention.

FAST ultrasound is a limited examination directed to look for intraperitoneal fluid or pericardial injury as a marker of underlying injury. This avoids the invasiveness of diagnostic peritoneal lavage. In the presence of free intraperitoneal fluid and an unstable patient, the ultrasound allows the trauma surgeon to explore the abdomen as a cause of blood loss. In the presence of fluid and a haemodynamically stable individual, further assessment by way of CT can be performed. However, it is important to realise that ultrasound has limitations in the identification of free fluid. This includes obscuration of fluid by bowel gas or extensive surgical emphysema. More organised haematoma may be more difficult to visualise. It must also be emphasised that the principal role of ultrasound is not to identify the primary solid organ injury, although this may be visualised. Occasionally, a second ultrasound scan may show free fluid in the presence of an initially negative FAST scan.

The detection of a pneumothorax on a supine radiograph can be very difficult. Ultrasound examination may be used to identify a radiographically occult pneumothorax. With a high-resolution linear probe, the pleura can be visualised as an echogenic stripe, and its motion with respiration can also be assessed. In the presence of a pneumothorax, the sliding motion of the pleura is lost. Ultrasound may also be used to detect a haemothorax or haemopericardium.

Finally, ultrasound may be of value in guiding the placement of an intravascular line by direct visualisation of the vessels. This can be especially advantageous in shocked patients.

Computerised tomography

CT is the main imaging method for the investigation of intracranial and intra-abdominal injuries and vertebral fractures. With current multidetector scanners a comprehensive examination of the head, spine, chest, abdomen and pelvis can be completed in less than 5 min. However, much more time is taken up in transferring the patient and the associated monitoring equipment onto the scanner. Therefore, the total time can be in excess of 30 min, and CT should be reserved for individuals whose condition is stable.

CT examination of the head is accurate in identifying treatable intracranial injuries (Figs 10.31 and 10.32) and should not

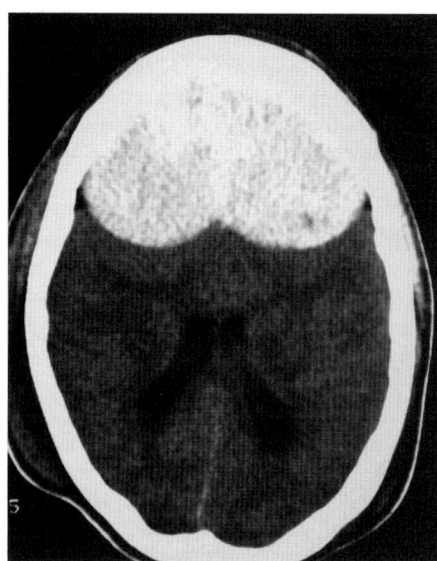

Figure 10.31 Computerised tomography of the head in a patient with head injury shows bilateral large frontal extradural collections.

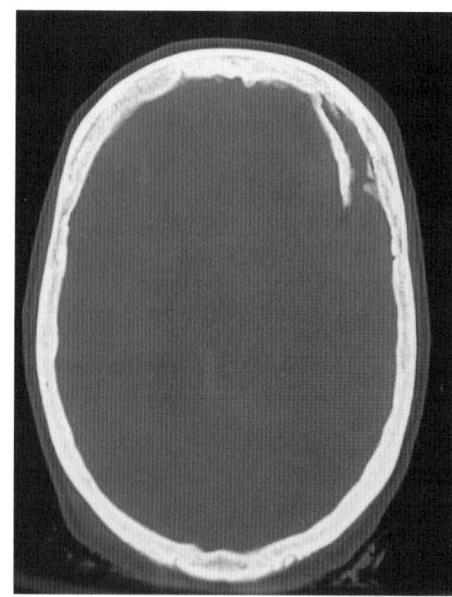

Figure 10.32 Computerised tomography of the head following head trauma shows a skull fracture with a large depressed component.

be delayed by radiography of peripheral injuries, as there is declining success in cases of intracranial collection when treated after the initial 3–4 hours. In comparison, identification of more widespread injuries such as diffuse axonal injury is relatively poor. Examination of facial injuries and cervical spine fractures can also be carried out at the same time as this only adds seconds to the examination. There is evidence that CT of the abdomen and pelvis is of benefit in multiple trauma when there is a head injury, as it often shows unexpected abnormalities, and this may affect the immediate management, especially if the patient deteriorates.

Chest CT with intravenous contrast agent is valuable in identifying vascular and lung injuries and is the most accurate way of demonstrating haemothorax and pneumothorax. The position of chest drains can be identified, allowing adjustment of position if necessary. Abdominal and pelvic CT is usually undertaken as an extension to the chest CT. If an abdominal examination is performed, the pelvis should be included to avoid missing pelvic injuries and free pelvic fluid. CT is an excellent means of identifying hepatic, splenic (Fig. 10.33) and renal injuries. Delayed examination after the administration of intravenous contrast agents allows assessment of the pelvicalyceal system in cases of renal trauma. Pancreatic and duodenal injuries may also be identified, but detection of these injuries may be more problematic. Using CT, the accuracy of detection of bowel or mesenteric injuries is less than it is for solid organ injury, and these injuries should be suspected when there is free intraperitoneal fluid without an identifiable cause (Fig. 10.34).

The image data may be reconstructed into thinner slices for the diagnosis of injuries to the thoracic and lumbar spine and for the better delineation of pelvic and acetabular fractures. Multidetector machines will be optimum for this purpose but, with older CT scanners, additional dedicated thin sections may be required for adequate examination. Complex intra-articular fractures of the peripheral skeleton such as calcaneal and tibial plateau fractures may be usefully examined by dedicated thin-section studies provided this does not delay the treatment of other more serious injuries (Fig. 10.35). CT angiography may be

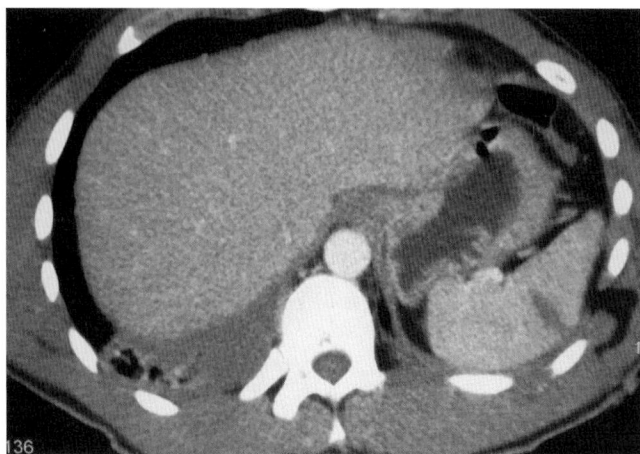

Figure 10.33 Post-contrast abdominal computerised tomography of a patient following blunt abdominal trauma shows a splenic laceration with herniation of mesenteric fat. A right-sided pleural collection is also evident.

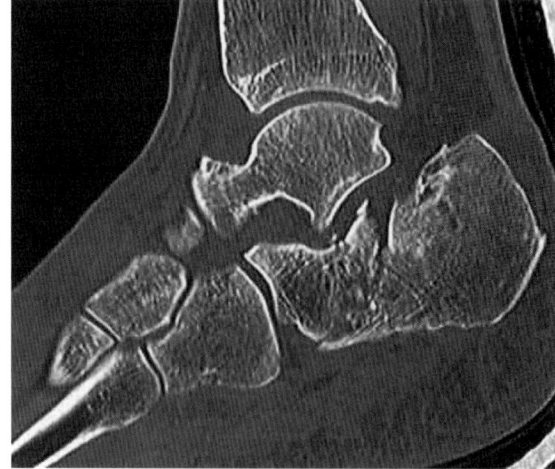

Figure 10.35 Sagittal reformats of computerised tomography of the calcaneus in a patient following a fall illustrate a comminuted calcaneal fracture with intra-articular extension into the posterior facet of the sub-talar joint.

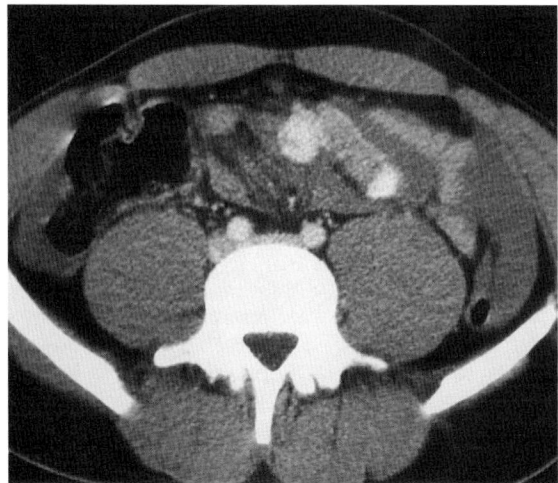

Figure 10.34 Post-intravenous contrast computerised tomography examination in a patient with a penetrating abdominal injury and mesenteric tear shows free fluid in the flanks and active extravasation of contrast centrally.

used to demonstrate vascular injuries in the limbs in those with penetrating injuries or complex displaced fractures.

Magnetic resonance imaging

The value of immediate MRI in trauma is relatively limited and is largely confined to the imaging of spinal injuries (Fig. 10.36). Access to urgent MRI is not widely available, and there are major practical problems in imaging patients who require ventilation or monitoring. MRI is therefore only practical in stable patients. All monitoring equipment must be MRI compatible, and ventilation support should be undertaken by staff skilled and experienced in these techniques as applied to the MRI environment. MRI may be used to stage injuries of the spinal cord and associated perispinal haematomas in patients with neurological signs or symptoms. MRI can supplement CT in spinal injuries by imaging soft-tissue injuries to the longitudinal and interspinous ligaments.

MRI is mandatory in patients in whom there is facetal dislocation if surgical reduction is being considered to minimise the risk of displacing soft-tissue or disc material into the spinal canal during reduction procedures. Subtle fractures may be difficult to identify, particularly if they are old, but an acute injury is normally identified by the surrounding oedema. Bony abnormities should be reviewed using CT, as fracture lines are hard to identify with MRI and unstable injuries may be overlooked. In the less acute setting, MRI may also be used to assess diffuse axonal injuries, with an accuracy exceeding CT.

Vascular interventional radiology

Angiography has been used for both the diagnosis and treatment of vascular injuries in the trauma patient. With the development and refinement of CT angiography techniques, the diagnostic role of interventional radiology may become more limited. Already, CT has a diagnostic accuracy similar to that of formal angiograms in patients with suspected aortic injuries, with the latter reserved for cases where CT has been suboptimal, doubt exists about the diagnosis or stent grafting is being considered. At present, peripheral angiograms are still performed, particularly in cases of penetrating injury, but as experience grows with CT peripheral angiography, this will probably become the preferred technique.

Endovascular techniques play an important role in the treatment of acute solid organ injuries, and the interventional radiologist should be consulted early in the decision-making process. Using coaxial catheter systems and a variety of available embolic agents such as soluble gelatine sponge and microcoils, selective embolisation and reduction of blood flow to the injured segment can be achieved without causing infarction. Selective embolisation techniques are also suitable for the treatment of patients with pelvic fractures with ongoing blood loss and volume issues. With penetrating and non-penetrating extremity trauma, balloon occlusion and embolisation may be employed to control haemorrhage, while the application of stent grafts can aid in re-establishing the circulation to the affected extremity.

CHAPTER 10 | DIAGNOSTIC IMAGING

(a)

(b)

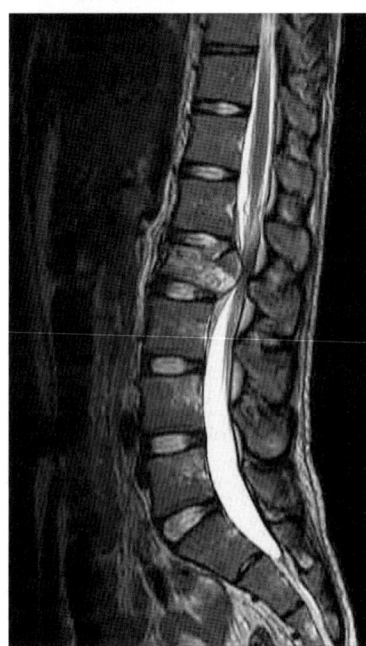

Figure 10.36 Sagittal T1-weighted (a) and T2-weighted (b) magnetic resonance imaging of the spine demonstrates a burst fracture of L2 causing neural compression.

Summary box 10.15

The investigation of the acute abdomen

Imaging tests	Indications/signs
Chest radiography (erect)	Free gas under the diaphragm
Anterior radiograph (supine)	Dilated bowel/gas pattern Gas inside/outside bowel Obstruction Closed loop Bowel wall oedema
IVU	Renal colic Ureteric obstruction by stone
Ultrasound	Ascites Cholecystitis/biliary colic Renal colic and bladder stones Abscess Obstruction – dilated fluid-filled bowel
Focused high-resolution ultrasound	Diverticulitis Appendicitis Bowel wall thickening/abscess
CT scan	Severe pancreatitis Diverticulitis Abscess Small bowel obstruction (high grade) Bowel infarction
Focused CT scan	Appendicitis Ureteric colic

Erect chest and supine abdomen radiographs remain the investigations of choice when perforation or intestinal obstruction is suspected (Figs 10.37 and 10.38). In many patients, these will provide sufficient information to determine further management. When the diagnosis is less clear, new imaging techniques are challenging the traditional approach. Both ultrasound and CT may contribute valuable information in inflammatory disease within the abdomen, notably in cholecystitis, diverticulitis, appendicitis and inflammatory bowel disease. CT is particularly useful in patients in whom there is a strong clinical suspicion of a collection, but the ultrasound examination is negative, as some collections may be overlooked using ultrasound. In some centres, the use of spiral CT as a first-line investigation is being promoted as a cost-effective alternative to increase the specificity of primary diagnosis.

In acute right upper quadrant pain, ultrasound is the best investigation for the gall bladder and biliary system and the best first-line test for liver disease. The pancreas is often well seen, dependent upon both the assiduousness of the scanning technique and the extent of upper abdominal gas.

Ultrasound can be a good first-line investigation for suspected appendicitis in patients in whom the diagnosis is not clinically obvious. It is especially useful in children and young adults and, in females, it will allow exclusion of a gynaecological cause. Thickened loops of terminal ileum or mesenteric abscess may be

IMAGING IN ABDOMINAL SURGERY

The acute abdomen

The term 'acute abdomen' encompasses many diverse entities. Imaging tests are selected based on the likely diagnosis, and the use of imaging early in the assessment process is highly desirable (Summary box 10.15).

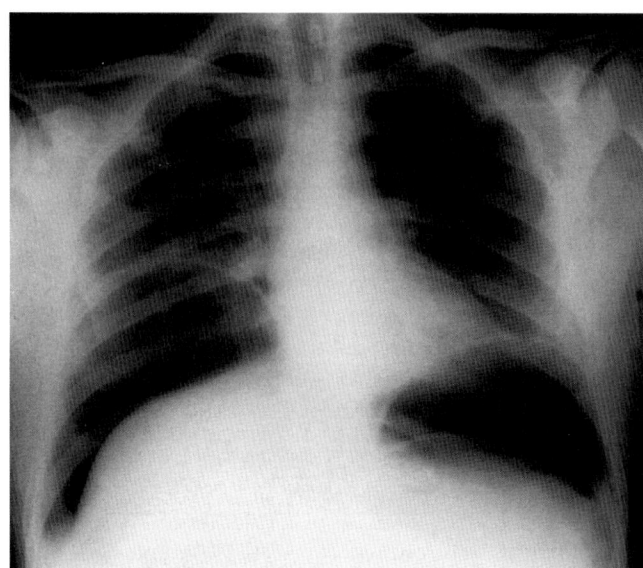

Figure 10.37 Erect chest radiograph showing marked bilateral elevation of the hemidiaphragms with a large volume of subdiaphragmatic free gas.

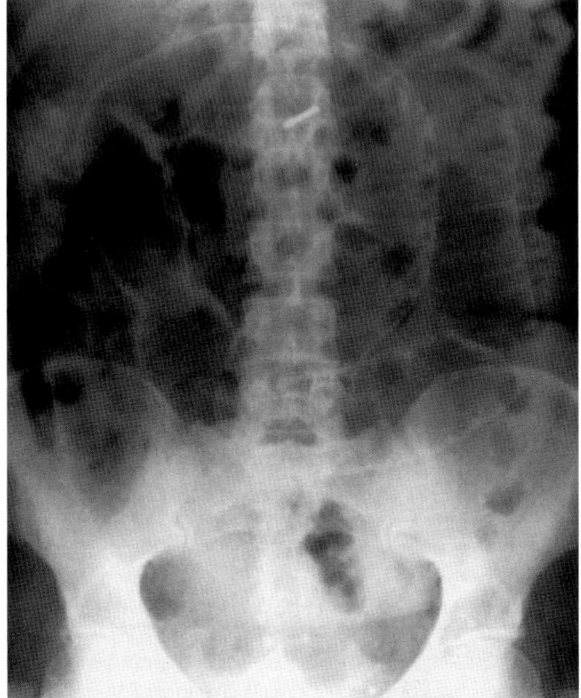

Figure 10.38 Pneumoperitoneum. The presence of free intraperitoneal air outlines the bowel so that both sides of the bowel wall can be seen (Rigler's sign).

identified in patients presenting with acute Crohn's disease. If there is remaining clinical doubt, then this may be resolved by a CT scan, which can be limited to the region of interest (Fig. 10.39).

In patients presenting with left iliac fossa pain and point tenderness, ultrasound may identify focal diverticulitis by the demonstration of bowel wall thickening and a paracolic or mesenteric collection. However, in most cases, CT is the best investigation for suspected diverticulitis and will allow staging of the disease to determine management. Barium enema is of limited value in this situation as the disease process is predominantly extraluminal (Fig. 10.40).

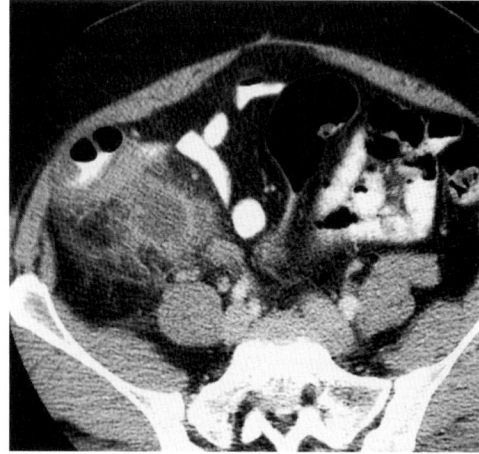

Figure 10.39 Computerised tomography (CT) scan. Acute appendicitis. Note the thickening of the caecal wall with a periappendiceal fluid collection indicating an appendix abscess.

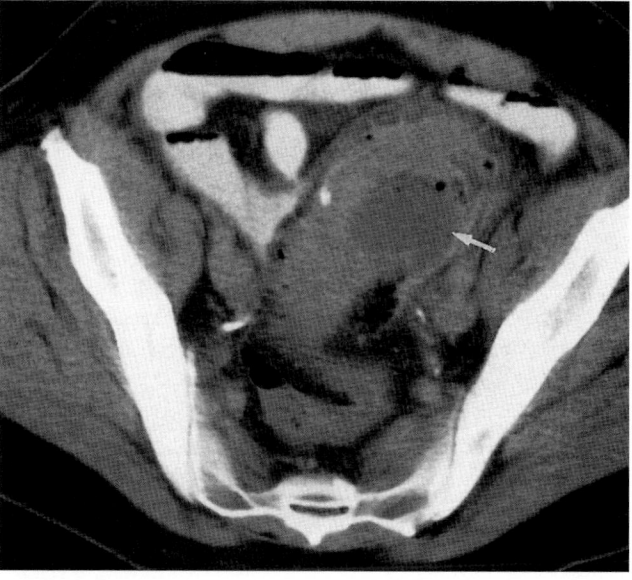

Figure 10.40 Computerised tomography scan showing a segment of thickened sigmoid colon with a paracolic abscess (arrow) in a patient with diverticulitis.

Bowel obstruction

Colonic obstruction is usually evident on the abdominal radiograph and, if this is equivocal, a limited unprepared contrast enema may confirm.

Although the abdominal radiograph is often diagnostic, small bowel obstruction can be more difficult to diagnose with confidence. Both ultrasound and CT are useful in demonstrating the presence of fluid-filled dilated small bowel loops in high-grade obstruction, and can identify the site and often the cause of the obstruction (Fig. 10.41). The use of CT, particularly in small bowel obstruction, has been widely advocated, although caution must be exercised in view of the radiation burden.

In subacute or low-grade obstruction, CT is very much less accurate and, in such cases, a small bowel enema (enteroclysis) is the investigation of choice.

IMAGING IN HEPATOBILIARY SURGERY

The techniques for imaging the liver, spleen, biliary tree and pancreas are discussed in Chapters 61, 62, 63 and 64 respectively.

IMAGING IN UROLOGY (SEE ALSO CHAPTER 70)

Renal colic

An initial abdominal radiograph and ultrasound will detect renal tract calculi in a proportion of patients and may reveal other causes for abdominal pain such as constipation. These techniques do not detect all calculi or causes of obstruction and, when negative, unenhanced helical CT is the most sensitive technique for the detection of ureteric calculi in renal colic and haematuria. Secondary signs of ureteric obstruction may also be appreciated, such as ureteric dilatation and stranding in the perinephric fat.

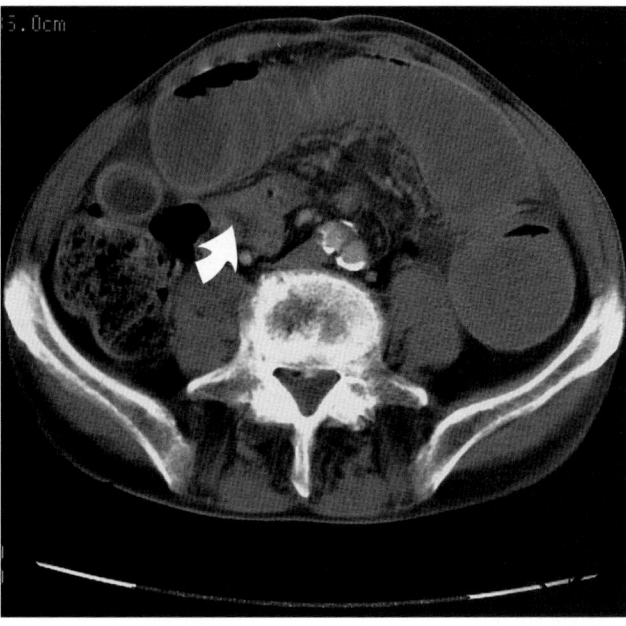

Figure 10.41 High-grade small bowel obstruction due to adhesions. Computerised tomography scan showing multiple, dilated, fluid-filled loops of small bowel with collapsed distal ileal loops beyond the point of obstruction (arrow).

A limited intravenous urogram remains a satisfactory alternative diagnostic test and has a lower radiation dose. Ultrasound may show a dilated collecting system, and the use of colour Doppler may demonstrate the absence of a ureteric jet into the bladder on the obstructed side or a twinkling artefact at the site of a calculus. However, in acute colic, the intrarenal collecting system may not be dilated and may result in a false-negative examination.

Haematuria

Analysis of the urine, including urine microscopy, will distinguish glomerular causes of haematuria such as immunoglobulin (Ig)A nephropathy from non-glomerular causes. The former will require renal ultrasound and chest radiography and further evaluation by nephrologists. The latter will require investigation of the entire urinary tract. Imaging should be accompanied by direct cystoscopy, as no imaging technique has sufficient sensitivity to exclude small bladder lesions. The initial investigation of haematuria varies between centres, but usually relies on IVU, ultrasound or both. Both have good sensitivity for detecting clinically important abnormalities, and there is little good evidence comparing the techniques upon which to base practice. Each technique has relative blind areas where sensitivity is reduced. Ultrasound is good for the detection of renal mass lesions but relatively less sensitive for urothelial lesions such as transitional cell carcinoma. Small non-obstructing calculi are also difficult to see, and combining ultrasound with plain film radiography improves their detection. Conversely, the IVU is sensitive for urothelial lesions and calculi, but may miss small renal mass lesions, particularly anteriorly or posteriorly projecting exophytic tumours.

CT is an extremely useful tool in the investigation of haematuria, but cost and radiation dose (see Table 10.1, p. 130) need to be considered against clinical benefit. As stated above, unenhanced CT is very sensitive in the detection of renal tract calculi. CT is more sensitive than ultrasound in the detection of renal mass lesions and is valuable in characterising solid tumours and in differentiating complex, potentially malignant cystic tumours from benign cystic lesions. With multidetector helical CT, the standard technique of contrast-enhanced CT may be modified to give reconstructed coronal images, sometimes with the use of abdominal compression. This technique, termed CT urography, can give excellent demonstration of the pelvicalyceal systems and ureters, equal or superior to standard IVU. Similar techniques have been developed for MR urography, with heavily T2-weighted coronal sequences depicting urine as a high signal.

IMAGING IN ONCOLOGY

Modern surgical treatment of cancer requires an understanding of tumour staging systems, as in many instances the tumour stage will define appropriate management. The development of stage-dependent treatment protocols involving neoadjuvant chemotherapy and preoperative radiotherapy relies on the ability of imaging to determine stage accurately before surgical and pathological staging. Once a diagnosis of cancer has been established, often by percutaneous or endoscopic biopsy, new imaging techniques can considerably improve the ability to define the extent of tumour, although the pathological specimen remains the 'gold standard'. Many staging systems are based on the tumour–node–metastasis (TNM) classification.

Tumour

In most published studies, cross-sectional imaging techniques (CT, ultrasound, MRI) are more accurate in staging advanced (T3, T4) than early (T1, T2) diseases, and the staging of early disease remains a challenge. In gut tumours, endoscopic ultrasound is more accurate than CT or MRI in the local staging of early disease (T1 and T2) by virtue of its ability to demonstrate the layered structure of the bowel wall and the depth of tumour penetration (Fig. 10.42). Developments in MRI may also improve the staging accuracy of early disease. MRI is extremely valuable in bone and soft-tissue tumour staging and in intracranial and spinal disease.

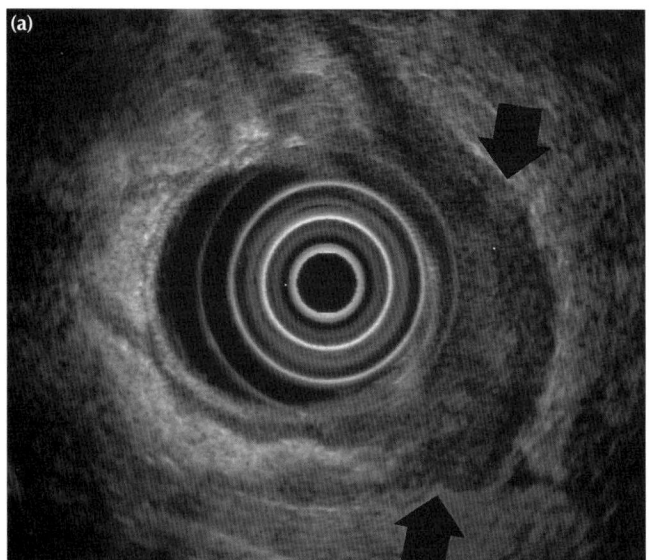

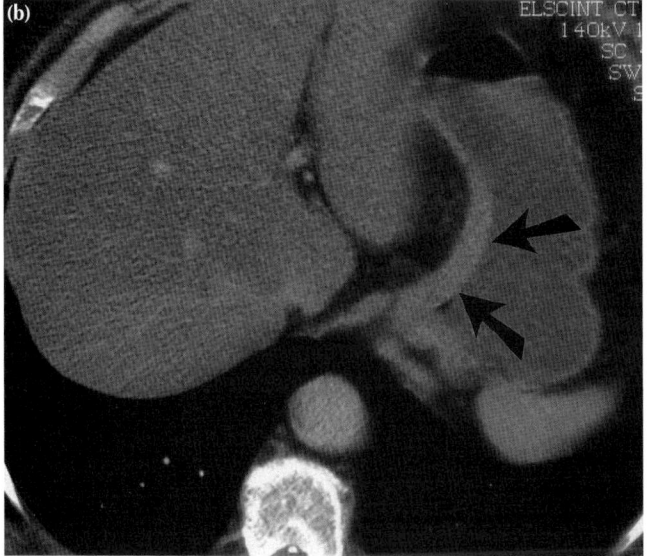

Figure 10.42 (a) Echo endoscopy in gastric cancer. The hypoechoic tumour (arrows) is destroying the layered structure of the gastric wall and extending out beyond the serosa. (b) Computerised tomography scan demonstrates thickening and enhancement of the gastric wall in the same area (arrows). The stomach is distended with water to provide low-density contrast.

Nodes

Accurate assessment of nodal involvement remains a challenge for imaging. Most imaging techniques rely purely on size criteria to demonstrate lymph node involvement, with no possibility of identifying micrometastases in normal-sized nodes. A size criterion of 8–10 mm is often adopted, but it is not usually possible to distinguish benign reactive nodes from infiltrated nodes. This is a particular problem in patients with intrathoracic neoplasms, in whom enlarged benign reactive mediastinal nodes are common. The echo characteristics of nodes at endoscopic ultrasound have been used in many centres to increase the accuracy of nodal staging, and nodal sampling is possible via either mediastinoscopy or transoesophageal biopsy under endoscopic ultrasound control. New radioisotope techniques are being developed using radiolabelled monoclonal antibodies against tumour antigens, which may increase the detection of nodal involvement by demonstrating micrometastases in non-enlarged nodes. There are current clinical studies of new MRI contrast agents that can identify tumour-infiltrated nodes.

Metastases

The demonstration of metastatic disease will usually significantly affect surgical management. Modern cross-sectional imaging has greatly improved the detection of metastases, but occult lesions will be overlooked in between 10% and 30% of patients. CT is the most sensitive technique for the detection of lung deposits, although the decision to perform CT will depend on the site of the primary tumour, its likelihood of intrapulmonary spread and the effect on staging and subsequent therapy of the demonstration of intrapulmonary deposits.

Ultrasound and CT are most frequently used to detect liver metastases. Contrast-enhanced CT can detect most lesions greater than 1 cm, although accuracy rates vary with the technique used and range from 70% to 90%. Recent studies suggest that MRI may be more accurate than CT in demonstrating metastatic disease. Although enhanced CT is used in most centres for screening for liver deposits, CT-AP (CT with arterial portography), which requires contrast injection via the superior mesenteric artery, is considered by many to be the most accurate technique for staging liver metastases if surgical resection is being considered. However, thin-section multislice CT with arterial and portal venous phase scanning is likely to replace this. Preoperative identification of the segment of the liver involved can be determined by translation of the segmental surgical anatomy, as defined by Couinaud, to the cross-sectional CT images (Fig. 10.43).

The technique of PET/CT is becoming a powerful tool in oncological imaging. This functional and anatomical imaging technique reflects tumour metabolism and allows the detection of otherwise occult metastases. The most common indications for PET/CT have been staging of lymphoma, lung cancer, particularly non-small cell lung cancer, and preoperative assessment of potentially resectable liver metastases such as colorectal carcinoma metastases.

Intraoperative ultrasound is an additional method of staging that provides superb high-resolution imaging of subcentimetre liver nodules that may not be palpable at surgery. This is often used immediately prior to resection of liver metastases.

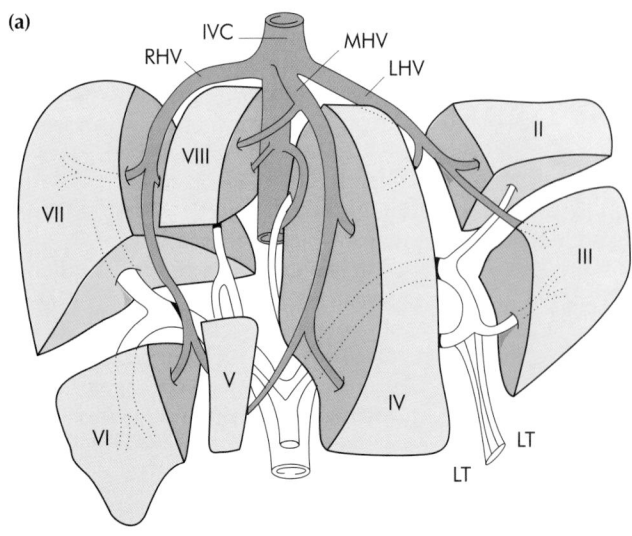

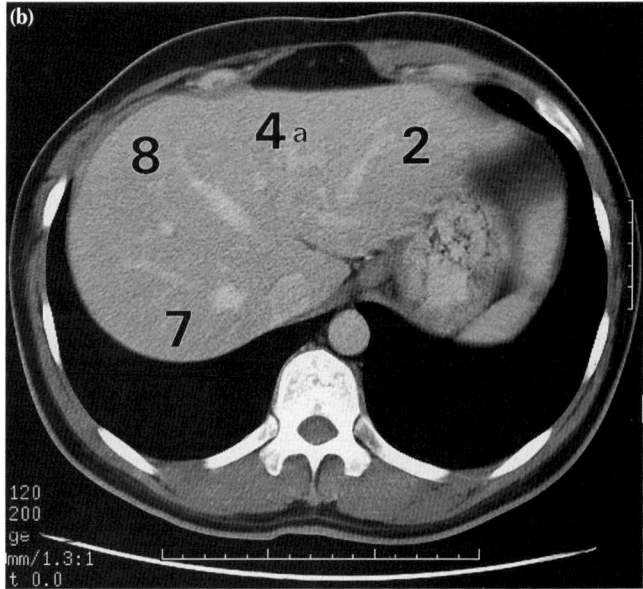

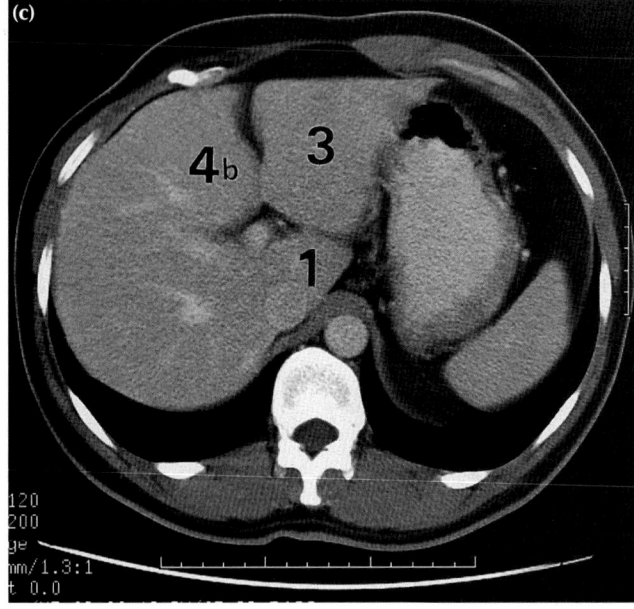

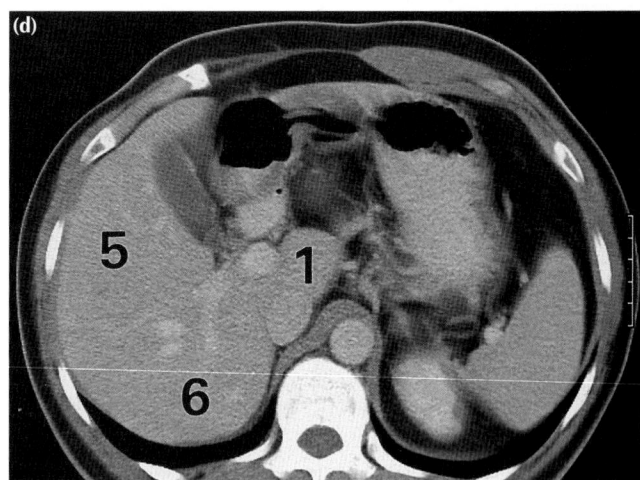

Figure 10.43 (a) Surgical lobes of the liver (after Couinaud). IVC, inferior vena cava; LHV, left hepatic vein; LT, ligamentum teres; MHV, middle hepatic vein; RHV, right hepatic vein. (b) Segmental anatomy on computerised tomography scan at the level of the hepatic veins. (c) Segmental anatomy at the level of the portal veins. (d) Segmental anatomy below the level of the portal veins.

FURTHER READING

Armstrong, P. and Wastie, M. (eds) (2001) *A Concise Textbook of Radiology*. Arnold, London.

Grainger, R.G., Allison, D.J. and Dixon, A.K. (eds) (2001) *Grainger & Allison's Diagnostic Radiology: A Textbook of Medical Imaging*, 4th edn. Harcourt Publishers, London.

Royal College of Radiologists (2003) *Making the Best Use of a Department of Clinical Radiology: Guidelines for Doctors*, 5th edn. Royal College of Radiologists, London.

Shuman, W.P. (1997) CT of blunt abdominal trauma in adults. *Radiology* **205:** 297–306.

Gastrointestinal endoscopy

CHAPTER 11

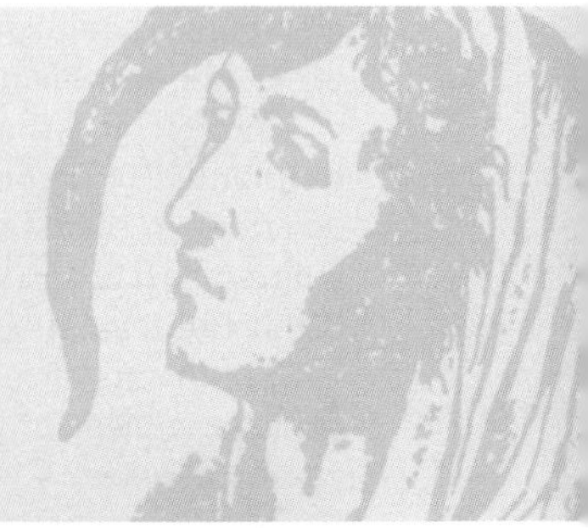

LEARNING OBJECTIVES

To gain an understanding of:

- The position of endoscopy as a therapeutic and diagnostic tool
- The basic organisation of an endoscopy unit and its equipment
- Consent and safe sedation
- The key points in managing endoscopy in diabetic patients and those on anticoagulants, as well as when to use antibiotic prophylaxis
- The indications for diagnostic and therapeutic endoscopy/colonoscopy/endoscopic retrograde cholangiopancreatography
- The recognition and management of complications
- Novel techniques for endoscoping the small bowel
- Advances in diagnostic ability

INTRODUCTION

The gastrointestinal tract has a myriad of functions such as digestion, absorption and excretion as well as the synthesis of a vast array of hormones, growth factors and cytokines. In addition, a complex enteric nervous system has evolved to control its function and communicate with the central and peripheral nervous systems. Finally, as the gastrointestinal tract contains the largest sources of foreign antigens to which the body is exposed, it houses well-developed arms of both the innate and acquired immune system. Therefore, it is not surprising that malfunction or infection of this complex organ results in a wide spectrum of pathology. However, its importance in disease pathogenesis is matched only by its inaccessibility to traditional examination.

Few discoveries in medicine have contributed more to the practice of gastroenterology than the development of diagnostic and therapeutic endoscopy. Although spectacular advances in radiology have occurred recently with the introduction of spiral computerised tomography (CT) and the increasing use of magnetic resonance imaging (MRI), the ability to take targeted mucosal biopsies remains a unique strength of endoscopy. Historically, radiological techniques were required to image areas of jejunum and ileum inaccessible to the standard endoscope; however the introduction of both capsule endoscopy and single/double-balloon enteroscopy allows both diagnostic and therapeutic access to the entire gastrointestinal tract. Image enhancement with techniques such as chromoendoscopy, magnification endoscopy and narrow band imaging allow increased resolution and near histological accuracy in lesion discrimination. The advances in the diagnostic accuracy of endoscopy lend themselves to disease surveillance for specific patient groups as well as population screening for gastrointestinal malignancy. Likewise there has been a rapid expansion in the therapeutic capability of endoscopy with both luminal and extraintestinal surgery being performed via endoscopic access.

As in all areas of interventional practice, a competent endoscopist must match a thorough grounding in anatomy and physiology with a clear understanding of the capabilities and limitations of the rapidly advancing techniques available. Perhaps most importantly they must also appreciate all aspects of patient care including pre-procedural management, communication before and during the procedure and the management of endoscopic complications. This chapter aims to guide the reader through these areas in addition to providing an introduction to the breadth of procedures that are currently performed.

HISTORY OF ENDOSCOPY

Over the last 50 years, endoscopy has become a most powerful diagnostic and therapeutic tool. However, its development required two obvious but formidable barriers to be overcome. First, the gastrointestinal tract is rather long and tortuous and, second, no natural light shines through the available orifices! Therefore, successful visualisation of anything beyond the distal extremities requires a flexible instrument with an intrinsic light source that can transmit images to the operator. The illumination issue was solved in 1879 by Thomas Edison, but 25 years elapsed before a light source was incorporated into the primitive rigid endoscopes available at that time. The first approach to gastrointestinal tortuosity was an instrument with articulated lenses and prisms, proposed by Hoffmann in 1911. Again, approximately two decades elapsed before this concept was

Thomas Alva Edison, **1847–1931, American Physicist and Inventor of Menlo Park, New Jersey, NJ, USA produced the first carbon filament electric light bulb in 1879.**

incorporated into a semiflexible gastroscope by Wolf, a fabricator of medical instruments, and Schindler, a physician.

The real breakthrough was the discovery that images could be transmitted using flexible quartz fibres. Although this was first described in the late 1920s, it was not until 1954 that Hopkins built a model of a flexible fibre imaging device. The availability of highly transparent optical quality glass led to the development in 1958 of the first flexible fibreoptic gastroscope by Larry Curtiss, a graduate student in physics, and Basil Hirschowitz, a trainee in gastroenterology. Over the next 30 years, the fibrescope evolved to allow examination of the upper gastrointestinal tract, the biliary system and the colon. In parallel with advances in diagnostic ability, a range of therapeutic procedures was developed (Table 11.1). Although the fibreoptic endoscope has been the workhorse of many endoscopy units over the last three decades, its obsolescence was guaranteed by the invention of the charge coupled device (CCD) in the 1960s, which allowed the creation of a digital electronic image, permitting endoscopic images to be processed by a computer and transmitted to television screens. Thus the modern endoscope was born (Fig. 11.1).

History does not sit still, and endoscopic evolution will continue with the replacement of much diagnostic endoscopy with cap-

Table 11.1 Historical landmarks of gastrointestinal endoscopy

1958	Development of fibreoptic gastroscope
1968	Endoscopic retrograde pancreatography
1969	Colonoscopic polypectomy
1970	Endoscopic retrograde cholangiography
1974	Endoscopic sphincterotomy (with bile duct stone extraction)
1979	Percutaneous endoscopic gastrostomy
1980	Endoscopic injection sclerotherapy
1980	Endoscopic ultrasonography
1983	Electronic (charge coupled device) endoscope
1985	Endoscopic control of upper gastrointestinal bleeding
1990	Endoscopic variceal ligation

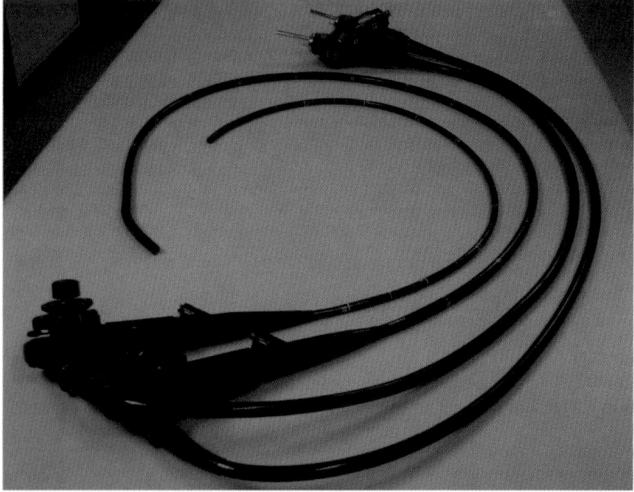

Figure 11.1 Photograph of standard gastroscope and colonoscope.

Harold Horace Hopkins, **1918–1994, Professor of Applied Optics, The University of Reading, Reading, England.**
Basil I. Hirschowitz, **Professor of Medicine, Birmingham, AL, USA.**

sule endoscopy and virtual imaging. Traditional endoscopy will therefore become increasingly therapeutic and historical divisions between medicine and surgery will become progressively blurred. As the complexity of the procedures increase, the distinction between specialist and general endoscopists will become more definite. This reinforces the need for all endoscopic practitioners to have a detailed understanding of the units in which they work and the instruments that they use.

THE MODERN ENDOSCOPY UNIT

Organisation

A well-designed endoscopy unit staffed by trained endoscopy nurses and dedicated administrative staff is essential to support good endoscopic practice and training. Clinical governance with regular appraisal and assessment of performance should be a routine process embedded within the unit philosophy. Endoscopist training demands particular attention, with a transparent process of skills- and theory-based education centred on practical experience and dedicated training courses. Experienced supervision of all trainee endoscopists is essential until competency has been obtained and assessed by an appropriately validated technique such as direct observation of practical skills (DOPS) and review of procedure logbooks. However, all endoscopists should keep an on-going log to record diagnostic and therapeutic procedure numbers and markers of competency such as colonoscopy completion rates, polyp detection rates, mean sedation use and complication rates. Central to this is an efficient data management system that provides outcome analysis for all aspects of endoscopy including adherence to guidelines, near misses, patient satisfaction, decontamination processes and scope tracking as well as the more obvious completion and complication rates.

Equipment

A full description of all available endoscopic equipment is beyond the scope of this chapter. However, each unit should have a sufficient range of endoscopes, processors and accessories as dictated by the local case mix and sufficient scope numbers to ensure smooth service provision. These should include both forward- and lateral-viewing gastroscopes, an enteroscope for proximal small bowel visualisation and a range of adult and paediatric colonoscopes to aid examination of both redundant and fixed colons. Dedicated small bowel centres require capsule endoscopy and a single/double-balloon enteroscope for ileojejunal therapeutics. An electrosurgical unit is the cornerstone of many therapeutic procedures and this may be supplemented by an argon plasma coagulation unit and laser units for advanced therapeutics in specialised centres.

Instrument decontamination

Endoscopes will not withstand steam-based autoclaving and therefore require high-level disinfection between cases to prevent transmission of infection. Although accessories may be autoclaved, best practice requires the use of disposable single use items whenever possible. All equipment should be decontaminated to an identical standard whether for use on immunocompromised/infected patients or not. This process involves two equally important stages: first, removal of physical debris from the internal and external surfaces of the instrument and, second, chemical neutralisation of all microbiological agents. A variety of agents are available and endoscopists should familiarise themselves with the agent in use in their department. Key points in endoscope decontamination are shown in Summary box 11.1.

Summary box 11.1

Disinfection of endoscopes

- All channels must be brushed and irrigated throughout the disinfection process
- All instruments and accessories should be traceable to each use, patient and cleaning cycle
- All staff should be trained and protected (particularly if glutaraldehyde is used in view of its immune-sensitising properties)
- Regular monitoring of disinfectant power and microbiological contamination should be performed

---

There are currently no reliable means of decontaminating scopes from contact with prion-associated conditions such as new variant Creutzfeldt–Jakob disease (nvCJD). Endoscopy should be avoided in patients thought to be at risk of this condition, as instruments require quarantine until the diagnosis can be excluded (which is often only possible post mortem). In many countries, previously exposed endoscopes are available if a patient with suspected nvCJD requires endoscopy.

CONSENT IN ENDOSCOPY

Approximately 1% of medical negligence claims in the USA relate to the practice of endoscopy. Many of these could have been avoided by a careful explanation of the procedure including an honest discussion of the risks and benefits. Therefore, obtaining informed consent is a cornerstone of good endoscopic practice. It preserves a patient's autonomy, facilitates communication and acts as a shield against future complaints and claims of malpractice.

The most important aspect of the consent procedure is that a patient understands the nature, purpose and risk of a particular procedure. Current guidelines would suggest that a patient should be informed of minor adverse events with a risk of more than 10% and serious events with an incidence of more than 0.5%. The key risks of endoscopy are summarised in Summary box 11.2.

Summary box 11.2

The risks of endoscopy

- Sedation
- Damage to dentition
- Aspiration
- Perforation or haemorrhage after endoscopic dilatation
- Perforation, infection and aspiration after percutaneous endoscopic gastrostomy insertion
- Perforation or haemorrhage after flexible sigmoidoscopy/colonoscopy with polypectomy
- Pancreatitis, cholangitis, perforation or bleeding after endoscopic retrograde cholangiopancreatography

---

Hans Gerhard Creutzfeldt, **1885–1964, a Neurologist, of Kiel, Germany.**
Alfons Marie Jakob, **1884–1931, a Neurologist of Hamburg, Germany.**

SAFE SEDATION

If performed competently the majority of diagnostic endoscopy and colonoscopy can be performed without sedation or with pharyngeal anaesthesia alone. However, therapeutic procedures may cause pain and patients are often anxious; thus in most countries sedation and analgesia are offered to achieve a state of conscious sedation (*not* anaesthesia). Medication-induced respiratory depression in elderly patients or those with comorbidities is the greatest cause of endoscopy-related mortality and, therefore, safe sedation practices are essential. The involvement of anaesthetists to advise on appropriate protocols is recommended (Summary box 11.3).

Summary box 11.3

Sedation in endoscopy

- Pharyngeal anaesthesia may increase the risk of aspiration in sedated patients
- Comorbidities must be identified so that sedation can be individualised
- All sedated patients require secure intravenous access
- Benzodiazepines reach their maximum effect 15–20 min after administration – doses should be titrated carefully, particularly in the elderly or those with comorbidities
- Co-administration of opiates and benzodiazepines has a synergistic effect – opiates should be given first and doses need to be reduced
- The use of supplementary oxygen is essential in all sedated patients
- Sedated patients require pulse oximetry to monitor oxygen saturation; high-risk patients or those undergoing high-risk procedures also require electrocardiogram monitoring
- A trained assistant should be responsible for patient monitoring throughout the procedure
- Resuscitation equipment and sedation reversal agents must be readily available
- The use of anaesthetic agents such as propofol for complex procedures requires specialist training
- The half-life of benzodiazepines is 4–24 hours – appropriate recovery and monitoring is essential. Post-procedural consultations may not be remembered, and patients must be advised not to drink alcohol or drive for 24 hours

---

ENDOSCOPY IN DIABETIC PATIENTS

As approximately 2% of the population is diabetic, managing glycaemic control before and after endoscopy is an essential aspect of endoscopic practice. Factors influencing management include the type of diabetes, the procedure that is planned, the preparation and recovery time, and the history of diabetic control in the individual patient. Thus, a poorly controlled insulin-dependant diabetic undergoing colonoscopy will require more input than a type 2 diabetic on oral hypoglycaemic medication undergoing upper gastrointestinal endoscopy. All patients should bring their own medication to the unit and should be advised not to drive in case there is an alteration in their glycaemic control. The majority of patients can be managed using clear protocols on an outpatient basis; however, elderly patients and those with brittle control should be admitted. In general, diabetic patients should be endoscoped first on the morning list. In complex cases the diabetic team should be involved.

ANTIBIOTIC PROPHYLAXIS

The majority of endoscopy can be performed safely without the need for routine antibiotic prophylaxis. However, given that certain endoscopic procedures are associated with a significant bacteraemia (Table 11.2), there are several specific situations where antibiotic cover is essential to prevent either bacterial endocarditis or infection of surgical prostheses. In general, the risk of infection relates to the level of bacteraemia and the risk of the underlying medical condition. Thus, patients with high-risk conditions such as prosthetic heart valves or a previous history of infective endocarditis should have prophylaxis for all endoscopic procedures, whereas those with moderate-risk conditions such as mitral valve prolapse with leaflet pathology or regurgitation only require antibiotics for procedures resulting in significant bacteraemia. Individual endoscopy societies have their own guidelines, which are widely available on the internet (e.g. the British Society of Gastroenterology guidelines are shown in Table 11.3; http://www.bsg.org.uk/pdf_word_docs/prophylaxis2001.pdf). Patients with severe neutropenia may also require antibiotic prophylaxis for endoscopy. The antibiotic regime used will depend on local guidelines. A standard protocol to prevent infective endocarditis is 1 g of amoxicillin and 120 mg of gentamicin intravenously 5–10 min before the procedure. Teicoplanin 400 mg intravenously can be used in patients who are allergic to penicillin.

In addition, procedures such as endoscopic percutaneous gastrostomy are associated with a significant incidence of wound or stoma infection, particularly if inserted for malignant disease. There is excellent evidence that antibiotic prophylaxis reduces this complication and a single intravenous injection of co-amoxiclav should be administered before the procedure. Ciprofloxacin is routinely used before endoscopic manipulation of an obstructed biliary tree to prevent sepsis. Finally, patients with

Table 11.2 Approximate incidence of bacteraemia in immunocompetent individuals following various procedures involving the gastrointestinal tract

Procedure	Incidence of bacteraemia (%)[a]
Rectal digital examination	4
Proctoscopy	5
Barium enema	11
Tooth brushing	25
Dental extraction	30–60
Colonoscopy	2–4
Diagnostic upper gastrointestinal endoscopy	4
Sigmoidoscopy	6–9
ERCP (no duct occlusion)	6
ERCP (duct occluded)	11
Oesophageal varices band ligation	6
Oesophageal varices sclerotherapy	10–50[b]
Oesophageal dilatation/prosthesis	34–54
Oesophageal laser therapy	35

[a]   Summary of published data.
[b]   Higher after emergency than after elective management.
ERCP, endoscopic retrograde cholangiopancreatography.

Table 11.3 Summary of consensus recommendations for endocarditis prophylaxis

Procedure	High-risk patient[a]	Moderate-risk patient[b]
OGD (+/– biopsy, banding)	+[c]	–
Colonoscopy (+/– polyp)	+	–
Flexible sigmoidoscopy	+	–
Oesophageal dilatation	+	+
Variceal sclerotherapy	+	+
ERCP (straightforward)	+	–
ERCP (obstructed system or pseudocyst)	+	+
Percutaneous endoscopic gastrostomy	+	+
Thermal procedure	+	+

[a]   Prosthetic valve, previous infective endocarditis, surgical conduit, complex congenital heart disease.
[b]   Complex left ventricular outflow including aortic stenosis, bicuspid valve; acquired valvulopathy, e.g. mitral valve prolapse with echo demonstration of substantial leaflet pathology and regurgitation.
[c]   +, antibiotic cover is indicated.
ERCP, endoscopic retrograde cholangiopancreatography; OGD, oesophagogastroduodenoscopy.

chronic liver disease and ascites undergoing variceal sclerotherapy should receive antibiotic prophylaxis to prevent bacterial peritonitis.

ANTICOAGULATION IN PATIENTS UNDERGOING ENDOSCOPY

Many patients undergoing endoscopy may be taking medication that interferes with normal haemostasis, such as warfarin, heparin, clopidogrel or aspirin. The key points to remember when managing anticoagulants in patients undergoing endoscopy are given in Summary box 11.4.

Summary box 11.4

Managing anticoagulants in patients undergoing endoscopy

It is important to recognise and understand:

- **The risk of complications related to the underlying gastrointestinal disease from anticoagulant therapy**
- **The risk of haemorrhage related to an endoscopic procedure in the setting of anticoagulant therapy**
- **The risk of a thromboembolic/ischaemic event related to interruptions of anticoagulant therapy**

Gastrointestinal bleeding in the anticoagulated patient

The risk of clinically significant gastrointestinal bleeding in patients on warfarin is increased, particularly in patients with a past history of similar events, if the international normalised ratio (INR) is above the therapeutic range or if they are taking concomitant aspirin/non-steroidal anti-inflammatory drugs (NSAIDs). In this situation the risk of reversing the anticoagulation must be weighed against the risk of on-going haemorrhage. If complete reversal is not appropriate, correction of the INR to approximately 1.5 is usually sufficient to allow endoscopic diagnosis and therapy. Anticoagulation can be resumed 24 hours after successful endoscopic therapy. If rapid resumption of anticoagulation is required, intravenous heparin should be used.

Elective endoscopy in the anticoagulated patient

Endoscopic procedures vary in their potential to produce significant or uncontrolled bleeding. Diagnostic oesophagogastroduodenoscopy (OGD), colonoscopy, enteroscopy and endoscopic retrograde cholangiopancreatography (ERCP) without sphincterotomy are considered low risk, as is mucosal biopsy. High-risk procedures include colonoscopic polypectomy (1–2.5%), gastric polypectomy (4%), laser ablation of tumour (6%), endoscopic sphincterotomy (2.5–5%) and procedures with the potential to produce bleeding that is inaccessible or uncontrollable by endoscopic means, such as dilatation of benign or malignant strictures, percutaneous gastrostomy insertion and endoscopic ultrasound (EUS)-guided fine-needle aspiration. Likewise, the probability of a thromboembolic complication during temporary cessation of anticoagulant therapy depends on the underlying medical condition (see Table 11.4) (Summary box 11.5).

Summary box 11.5

Recommendations concerning anticoagulant management

Low-risk procedures
- No adjustment to anticoagulation required
- Avoid elective procedures when anticoagulation is above the therapeutic range

High-risk procedure in a patient with a low-risk condition
- Discontinue warfarin 3–5 days before the procedure
- Consider checking the international normalised ratio on the day of the procedure

High-risk procedure in a patient with a high-risk condition
- Discontinue warfarin 3–5 days before the procedure
- Warfarin may be resumed the night of the procedure
- The decision to administer intravenous heparin should be individualised
- Intravenous heparin should be discontinued 4–6 hours before the procedure and may be resumed 2–6 hours after the procedure
- Heparin and warfarin should overlap until the international normalised ratio has stabilised within the therapeutic range
- The use of ambulatory low molecular weight heparin should be considered

---

Table 11.4 The risk of a thromboembolic event varies according to the underlying medical condition

Condition	Risk
Atrial fibrillation with valvular heart disease	High
Mechanical mitral valve	High
Mechanical valve and previous thromboembolic event	High
Deep vein thrombosis	Low
Uncomplicated atrial fibrillation	Low
Bioprosthetic valve	Low
Mechanical aortic valve	Low

Aspirin, non-steroidal anti-inflammatory drugs and anti-platelet therapies

Aspirin and NSAIDs inhibit platelet cyclo-oxygenase resulting in suppression of thromboxane A_2-induced platelet aggregation. Limited published data do not suggest an increased bleeding risk in patients taking standard doses and, therefore, there is no need to discontinue therapy before endoscopic procedures. Anecdotal evidence suggests an increased risk of bleeding after high-risk endoscopic procedures in patients taking clopidogrel and ticlodipine, although there are no clear data on which to base recommendations. Decisions to withhold therapy to prevent post-endoscopy haemorrhage must be weighed against the risk of an adverse coronary event. It would seem prudent to withhold therapy for 1 week before high-risk endoscopic therapy, particularly in patients taking concomitant aspirin.

UPPER GASTROINTESTINAL ENDOSCOPY

OGD is the most commonly performed endoscopic procedure in the world. Excellent visualisation of the oesophagus, gastro-oesophageal junction, stomach, duodenal bulb and second part of the duodenum can be obtained (Fig. 11.2). Retroversion of the gastroscope in the stomach is essential to obtain complete views of the gastric cardia and fundus (Fig. 11.2). Traditional forward-viewing endoscopes do not adequately visualise the ampulla, and a side-viewing scope should be used if this is essential. Likewise, although it is possible to reach the third part of the duodenum with a standard 120 cm instrument, a longer enteroscope is required if views beyond the ligament of Treitz are required. In addition to clear mucosal views, diagnostic endoscopy allows mucosal biopsies to be taken, which may either undergo processing for histological examination or be used for near-patient detection of *Helicobacter pylori* infection using a commercial urease-based kit. In addition, brushings may be taken for cytology and aspirates for microbiological culture.

Indications for oesophagogastroduodenoscopy

A full assessment of the role of OGD is outside the scope of this chapter. It will vary with local circumstances and the availability of alternative diagnostic techniques. OGD is usually appropriate when a patient's symptoms are persistent despite appropriate empirical therapy or are associated with warning signs such as intractable vomiting, anaemia, weight loss, dysphagia or bleeding. It is also part of the diagnostic work-up for patients with symptoms of malabsorption and chronic diarrhoea. However, increasing ease of access to OGD with the availability of 'open access' endoscopy has resulted in a significant number of unnecessary procedures being performed in young patients with dyspepsia or gastro-oesophageal reflux disease (GORD). This has led to a number of international gastroenterology societies proposing guidelines for the management of dyspepsia/GORD, including the empirical use of acid suppression and non-invasive *H. pylori* tests, such as urease breath tests and serology (e.g. the National Institute for Health and Clinical Excellence guidelines on dyspepsia; http://guidance.nice.org.uk/CG17/guidance/pdf/English/download.dsp). In addition to the role of OGD in diagnosis, it is also commonly used in the surveillance of neoplasia

---

Wenzel Treitz, **1819–1872, Professor of Pathology, Prague, The Czech Republic.**

(a)

(b)

(c)

(d)

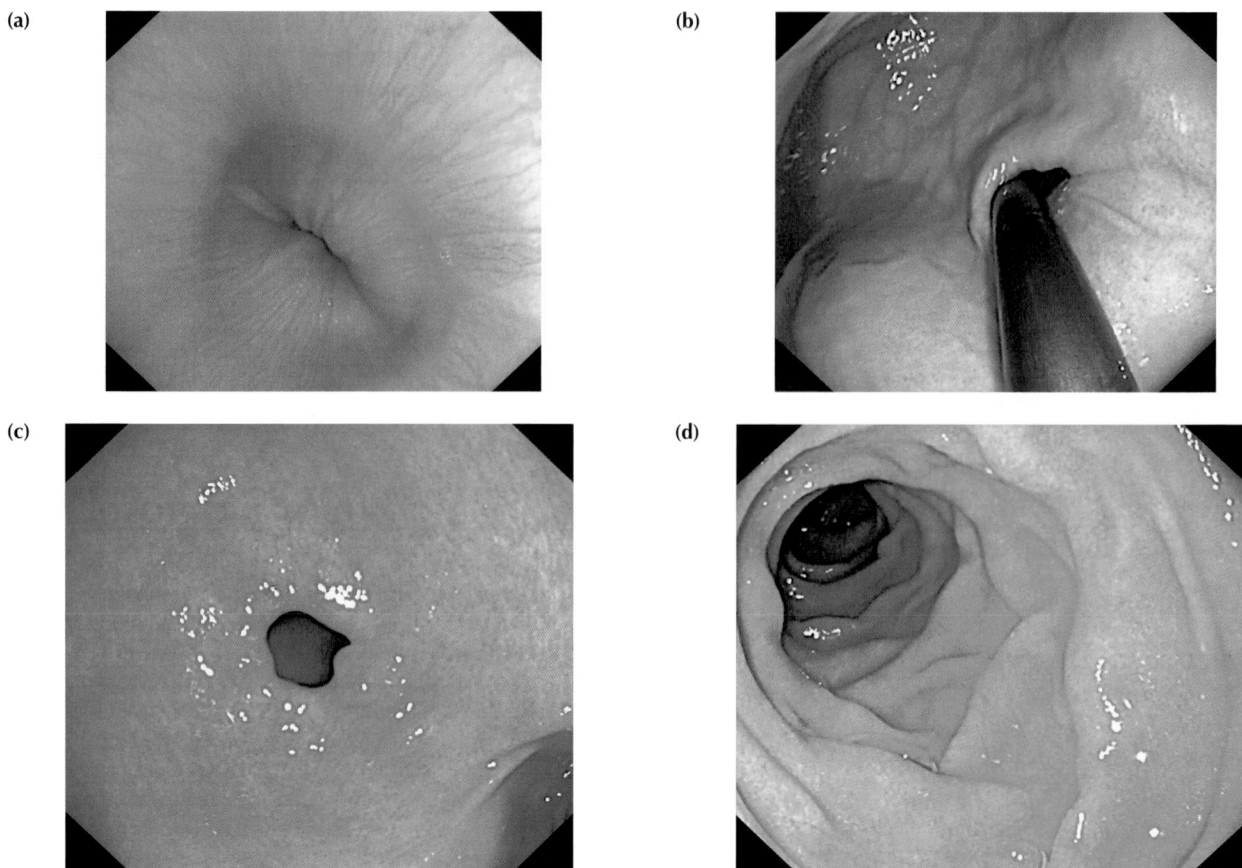

Figure 11.2 A normal upper gastrointestinal endoscopy showing the gastro-oesophageal junction (a), the gastric fundus in the 'J' position (b), the gastric antrum (c) and the second part of the duodenum (d).

development in high-risk patient groups. Whereas there is consensus about its role in genetic conditions such as familial adenomatous polyposis and Peutz–Jegher syndrome, controversy remains about the role and frequency of endoscopic surveillance in pre-malignant conditions such as Barrett's oesophagus and gastric intestinal metaplasia.

Therapeutic oesophagogastroduodenoscopy

Increasing technological advances have revolutionised the therapeutic applications of upper gastrointestinal endoscopy. However, appropriate patient selection and monitoring is essential to minimise complications. The most common therapeutic endoscopic procedure performed as an emergency is the control of upper gastrointestinal haemorrhage of any aetiology. Band ligation has replaced sclerotherapy in the management of oesophageal varices (Fig. 11.3) whereas sclerotherapy using thrombin-based glues can be used to control blood loss from gastric varices. Injection sclerotherapy with adrenaline coupled with a second haemostatic technique such as heater probe vessel obliteration or haemoclip application remains the technique of choice for a peptic ulcer

John Law Augustine Peutz, **1886–1968, Chief Specialist for Internal Medicine, St. John's Hospital, The Hague, The Netherlands.**
Harold Joseph Jeghers, **1904–1990, Professor of Internal Medicine, New Jersey College of Medicine and Dentistry, Jersey City, NJ, USA.**
Norman Rupert Barrett, **1903–1979, Surgeon, St. Thomas's Hospital, London, England.**

with an active arterial spurt or stigmata of recent haemorrhage (Fig. 11.4). This should be followed by 72 hours of intravenous proton pump inhibition in all cases. Chronic blood loss from angioectasia is most safely treated with argon plasma coagulation because of the controlled depth of burn compared with alternative thermal techniques (Fig. 11.5).

Therapeutic OGD is a cornerstone in the management of both benign and malignant upper gastrointestinal disease. Benign oesophageal and pyloric strictures may be dilated under direct vision with 'through the scope' (TTS) balloon dilators or the more traditional guidewire-based systems such as Savary–Guillard bougie dilators (Fig. 11.6). Intractable disease can be treated by the insertion of a removable stent. Likewise, the lower oesophageal sphincter hypertension associated with achalasia can be reduced by pneumatic balloon dilatation, although the procedure may need to be repeated every few years and the large (2–3 cm) balloons required are associated with a significantly increased risk of perforation. An alternative is the injection of botulinum toxin, which has a considerably more favourable side-effect profile but a shorter duration of benefit.

There are an increasing number of endoscopic techniques available to reduce gastro-oesophageal reflux, which rely on tightening the loose gastro-oesophageal junction by plication, the application of radial thermal energy or injection of a bulking agent. Although many of these techniques deliver short-term clinical benefits and a reduction in 24-hour oesophageal acid exposure, none has demonstrated long-term benefits in a group of

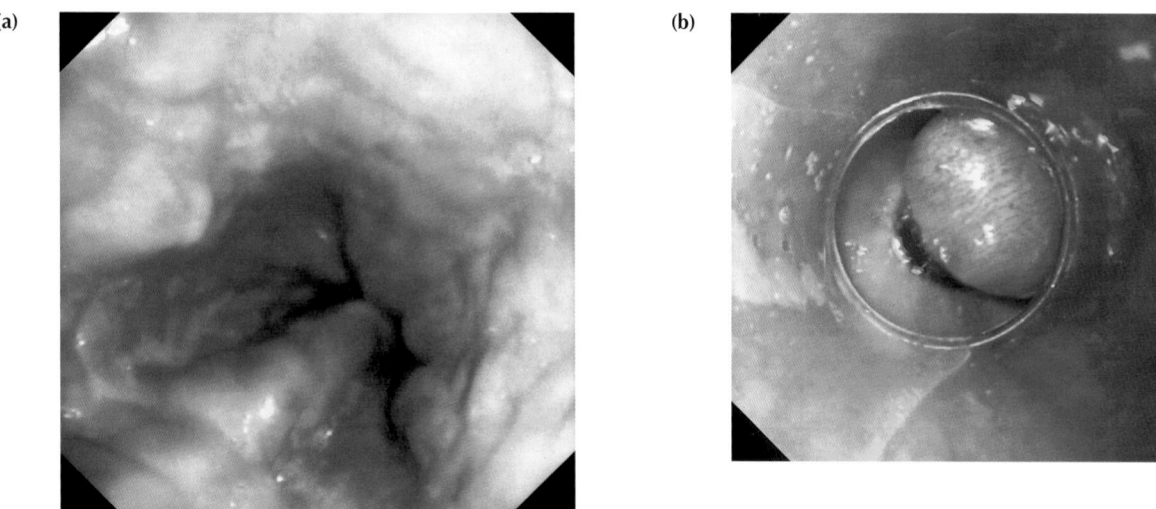

Figure 11.3 Grade 2 oesophageal varices (a), which can be treated by the application of bands to ligate the vessel and reduce blood flow (b).

patients resistant to proton pump inhibitors. Likewise, endoscopic techniques to tackle obesity, such as gastric balloon insertion, have not been associated with evidence of long-lasting benefit. In contrast, there is clear evidence that the insertion of a percutaneous endoscopic gastrostomy (PEG) tube enhances nutritional and functional outcome in patients unable to maintain oral nutritional intake (Fig. 11.7). PEG insertion is often a prelude to treatment of complex orofacial malignancy, and may be used to support nutrition in patients with alternative malignant, degenerative or inflammatory diseases.

The deployment of 'memory metal' self-expanding stents with or without a covering sheath inserted over a stiff guidewire leads to a significant improvement in symptomatic dysphagia and quality of life in patients with malignant oesophageal and gastric outlet obstruction (Fig. 11.8). Covered stents are the mainstay of treatment for benign or malignant tracheo-oesophageal fistulae. However, the area of greatest progress over the last few years has been in the endoscopic management of early oesophageal and gastric neoplasia with endoscopic mucosal resection (EMR) and the destruction of areas of high-grade dysplasia (HGD) using

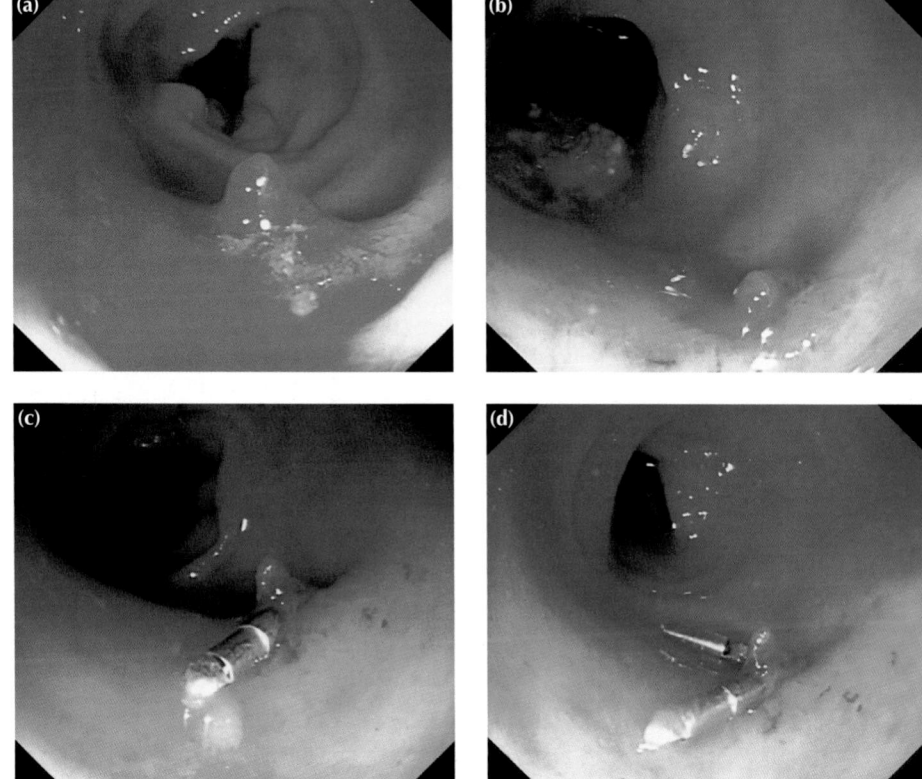

Figure 11.4 A gastric ulcer with active bleeding (a) is initially treated with adrenaline injection to achieve haemostasis (b). Two haemoclips are then applied to prevent rebleeding (c and d).

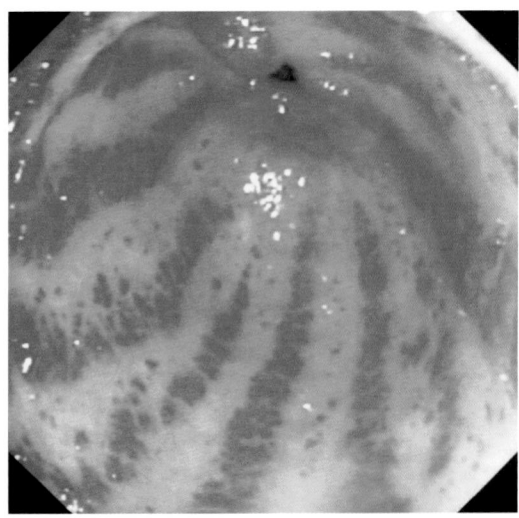

Figure 11.5 The classic appearance of gastric antral vascular ectasia (GAVE), which is often treated with argon plasma coagulation.

(a)

(b)

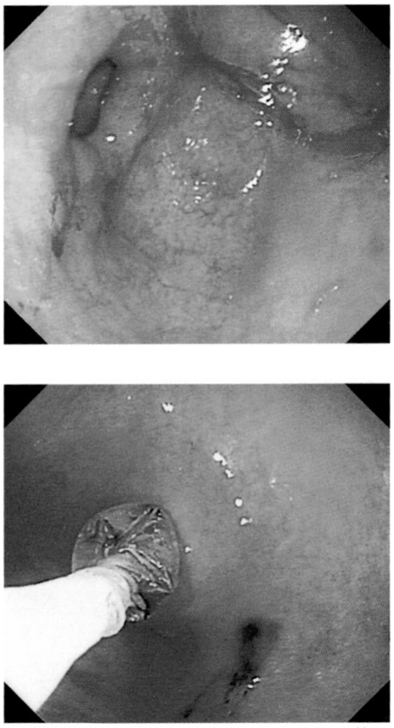

Figure 11.6 A pyloric stricture (a) can be dilated using a 'through the scope' balloon under direct vision to minimise complications (b).

either EMR (Fig. 11.9) or photodynamic therapy. However, long-term follow-up studies are required to ensure that the endoscopic ablation of areas of HGD has an impact on the progression to cancer.

Complications of diagnostic and therapeutic oesophagogastroduodenoscopy

Diagnostic upper gastrointestinal endoscopy is a safe procedure with minimal morbidity as long as appropriate patient selection and safe sedation practices are embedded in the unit policy. The mortality rate is estimated to be less than 1:10 000, with a complication rate of approximately 1:1000. As mentioned above, the

majority of adverse events relate to sedation and patient comorbidity. Particular caution should be exercised in patients with recent unstable cardiac ischaemia and respiratory compromise. Perforation can occur at any point in the upper gastrointestinal tract including the oropharynx. It is rare during diagnostic procedures and is often associated with inexperience. Perforation is more common in therapeutic endoscopy, particularly oesophageal dilatation and EMR for early malignancy. Early diagnosis significantly improves outcome and thus all staff must be alert to the symptoms (Summary box 11.6).

Summary box 11.6

Symptoms of endoscopic oesophageal perforation

- Neck/chest pain
- Abdominal pain
- Increasing tachycardia
- Hypotension
- Surgical emphysema

Prompt management includes radiological assessment using CT/water-soluble contrast studies, strict nil by mouth, intravenous fluids and antibiotics, and early review by an experienced upper gastrointestinal surgeon.

ENDOSCOPIC ASSESSMENT OF THE SMALL BOWEL

Introduction and indications

The requirement to visualise, biopsy and treat the small bowel is far less than in the stomach, biliary tree or colon, which has resulted in a time lag in technological advances. The most frequent indication is the investigation of gastrointestinal blood loss, which may present with either recurrent iron deficiency anaemia (occult haemorrhage) or recurrent overt blood loss per rectum (cryptic haemorrhage) in a patient with normal OGD (with duodenal biopsies) and colonoscopy. Other indications include the investigation of malabsorption; the exclusion of cryptic small bowel inflammation such as Crohn's disease in patients with diarrhoea/abdominal pain and evidence of an inflammatory response; targeting lesions seen on radiological images; and surveillance for neoplasia in patients with inherited polyposis syndromes.

A standard enteroscope is able to reach and biopsy lesions detected in the proximal small bowel; however, even in the most experienced hands this is limited to approximately 100 cm distal to the pylorus, although the use of a stiffening overtube may increase this somewhat. The procedure takes approximately 45 min and may be exceedingly uncomfortable, requiring high doses of sedation with the attendant increased risk of perforation and sedation-related morbidity. Sonde endoscopy, in theory, has the potential to examine the entire small bowel. In this procedure a long thin endoscope is inserted transnasally into the stomach and pushed through the pylorus with a gastroscope passed through the mouth. It is carried distally by peristalsis, which propels a balloon inflated at the tip. The technique has several limitations including a long examination time (6–8 hours), patient

Burrill Bernard Crohn, 1884–1983, Gastroenterologist, Mount Sinai Hospital, New York, NY, USA, described regional ileitis in 1932.

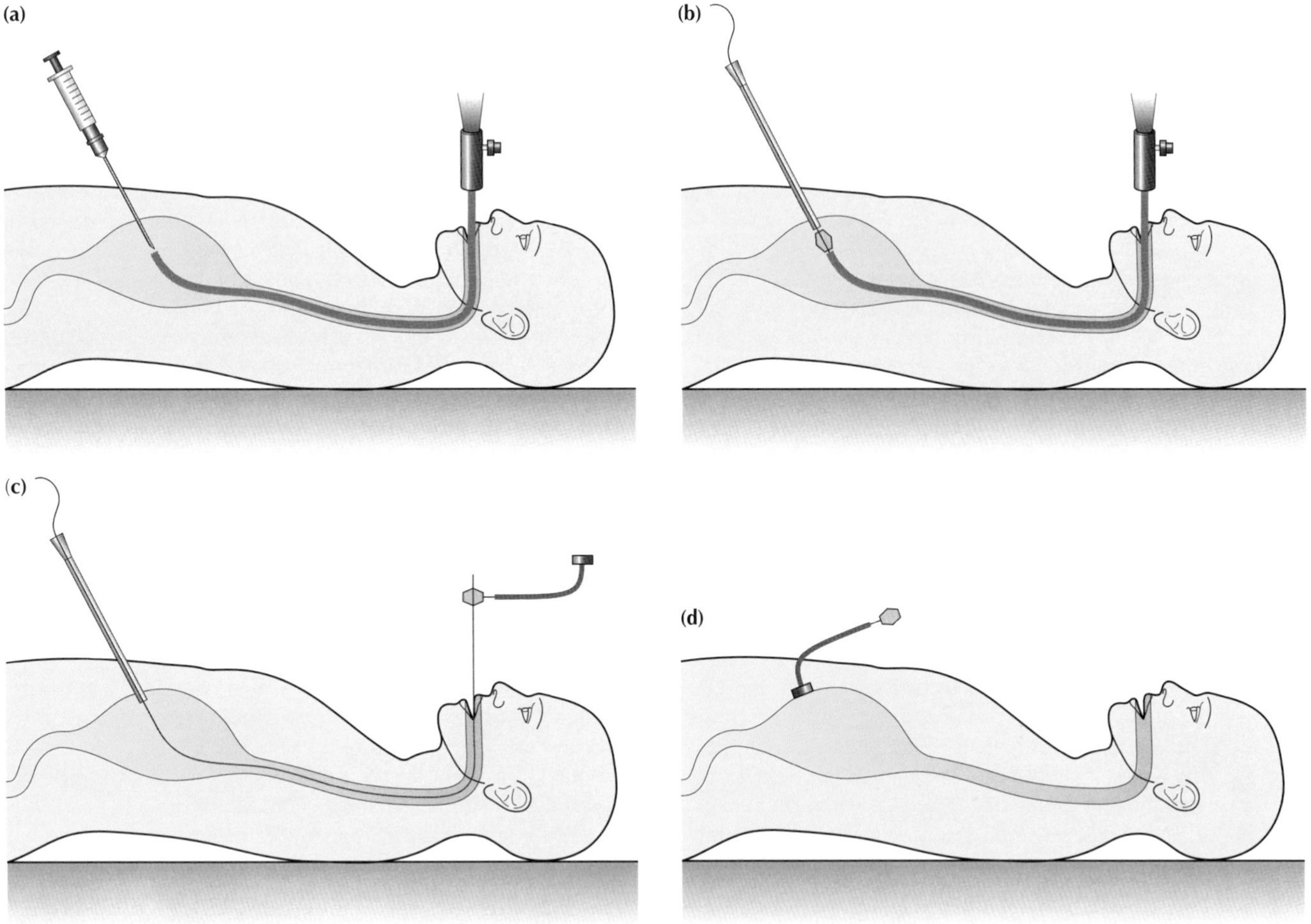

(a)

(b)

(c)

(d)

Figure 11.7 A schematic diagram of percutaneous endoscopic gastrostomy insertion. A standard endoscopy is performed to ensure that there are no contraindications to gastrostomy insertion. The stomach is insufflated with air and a direct percutaneous needle puncture made at a point where the stomach abuts the abdominal wall. Lignocaine is infused on withdrawal (a). A trochar is inserted and a wire passed into the stomach, which can be caught with a snare (b). The scope is withdrawn, pulling the wire out through the mouth, at which point it is attached to the gastrostomy tube (c). The gastrostomy is pulled through into the stomach and out through the track created by the trochar insertion (d).

discomfort, the danger of perforation and the inability to perform therapeutic procedures. For these reasons it is not widely performed and will soon become obsolete.

Therefore, until recently, barium follow-through or enteroclysis were the most effective imaging modalities to visualise the distal duodenum, jejunum and ileum. Obviously these techniques do not give true mucosal views, and outside specialist centres their decreasing use has led to diminished expertise and a

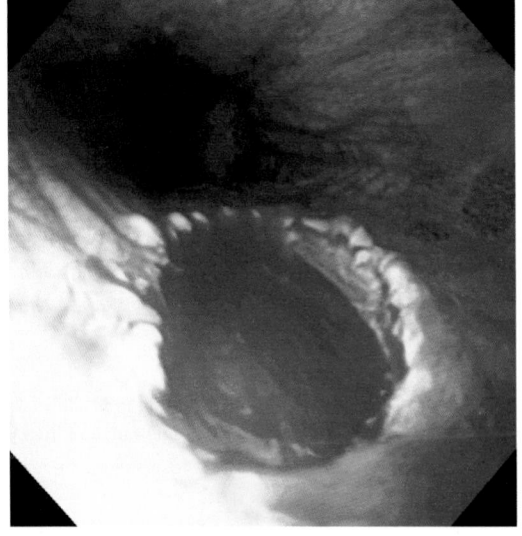

Figure 11.9 Novel upper gastrointestinal therapeutic uses of oesophagogastroduodenoscopy include the use of endoscopic mucosal resection to remove early gastric cancer leaving a clean base.

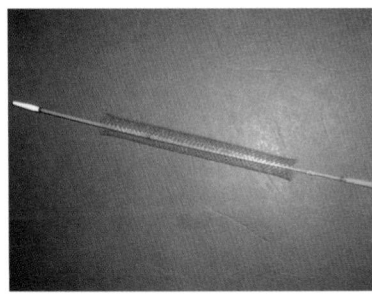

Figure 11.8 A self-expanding metal stent may be used to alleviate symptoms relating to malignant oesophageal strictures.

CHAPTER 11 | GASTROINTESTINAL ENDOSCOPY

reduced diagnostic yield. There have been rapid advances in axial radiological techniques such as MRI and CT enteroclysis, which demonstrate excellent diagnostic accuracy in this area (see Chapter 10). However, although these techniques may yield information about vascularity and bowel wall thickening, they do not allow direct mucosal views, have no biopsy capability and have limited scope in terms of therapeutics. Until recently, if an area of interest was outside the reach of a standard enteroscope, direct access via enterotomy under either laparoscopic or open surgery was required. Two major clinical advances over the last 2–3 years have revolutionised small bowel diagnosis and therapeutics. First, the development of the capsule endoscope allows diagnostic mucosal views of the entire small bowel to be obtained with minimal discomfort in unsedated patients. Second, the novel technique of single/double-balloon enteroscopy allows endoscopic access to the entire small bowel for biopsy and therapeutics (Table 11.5).

Capsule endoscopy

The prototype capsule endoscope was developed at the Royal London Hospital in the UK by Professor Paul Swain. Several companies have developed different systems for routine clinical use, but the basic principles remain identical. The technique requires three main components: an ingestible capsule, a portable data recorder and a workstation equipped with image-processing software. The capsule consists of an optical dome and lens, two light-emitting diodes, a processor, a battery, a transmitter and an antenna encased in a resistant coat the size of a large vitamin pill (Fig. 11.10). It acquires video images during natural propulsion through the digestive system that it transmits via a digital radio-frequency communication channel to the recorder unit worn outside the body; this also contains sensors which allow basic localisation of the site of image capture within the abdomen. Upon completion of the examination, the physician transfers the accumulated data to the workstation for interpretation via a high-capacity digital link. The workstation is a modified personal computer required for off-line data storage, interpretation and analysis of the acquired images, and report generation.

Clinical trials have been performed to evaluate the safety and efficacy of the system as a tool in the detection of small bowel diseases. Preliminary results show that the small bowel capsule provides good visualisation from mouth to colon with a high diagnostic yield. It compares favourably with the 'gold standard' techniques for the localisation of cryptic and occult gastrointestinal bleeding and the diagnosis of small bowel Crohn's disease. Use of the capsule endoscope is contraindicated in patients with known small bowel strictures in which it may impact, resulting in acute obstruction requiring retrieval at laparotomy or via laparoscopy. Severe gastroparesis and pseudo-obstruction are also relative contraindications to its use. Some units advocate a barium follow-through to exclude stricturing disease in all patients before capsule endoscopy. An alternative is to use a 'dummy' patency capsule that can be tracked via a hand-held device or conventional radiology as it passes through the intestine; it dissolves after 40 hours if it becomes impacted. Technology in this field is rapidly advancing with capsule systems designed to image the oesophagus and colon nearing the market. Prototype capsules that can be directed and deliver thermal therapy to angioectasia are in development.

Single/double-balloon enteroscopy

This technique allows the direct visualisation of and therapeutic intervention for the entire small bowel and may be attempted via either the oral or rectal route. Double-balloon enteroscopy was developed in 2001 in Japan; it involves the use of a thin enteroscope and an overtube, which are both fitted with a balloon. The procedure is usually carried out under general anaesthesia, but may be carried out with the use of conscious sedation. The enteroscope and overtube are inserted through either the mouth or anus and steered to the proximal duodenum/terminal ileum in the conventional manner. Following this the endoscope is advanced a small distance in front of the overtube and the balloon at the end is inflated. Using the assistance of friction at the interface between the enteroscope and intestinal wall, the small bowel is accordioned back to the overtube. The overtube balloon is then deployed and the enteroscope balloon is deflated.

Table 11.5 Comparison of the advantages and disadvantages of the currently available modalities to endoscope the small intestine

Technique	Advantages	Disadvantages
Traditional enteroscopy	Simple technique with wide availability Full range of therapeutics available Performed under sedation	Some discomfort Can only access proximal small bowel
Capsule endoscopy	Able to visualise the entire small bowel Preferable for patients No sedation Painless	No biopsies Not controllable and no accurate localisation Variable transit Incomplete studies due to battery life Not suitable for patients with strictures Large capsule to swallow
Double/single-balloon enteroscopy	Able to visualise the entire small bowel Full range of therapeutics	Requires sedation/general anaesthesia Patient discomfort May take 3–4 hours; may require admission Specialist centres only Complications include perforation

Christopher Paul Swain, **Contemporary**, Professor of Gastroenterology, The Royal London Hospital, London, England.

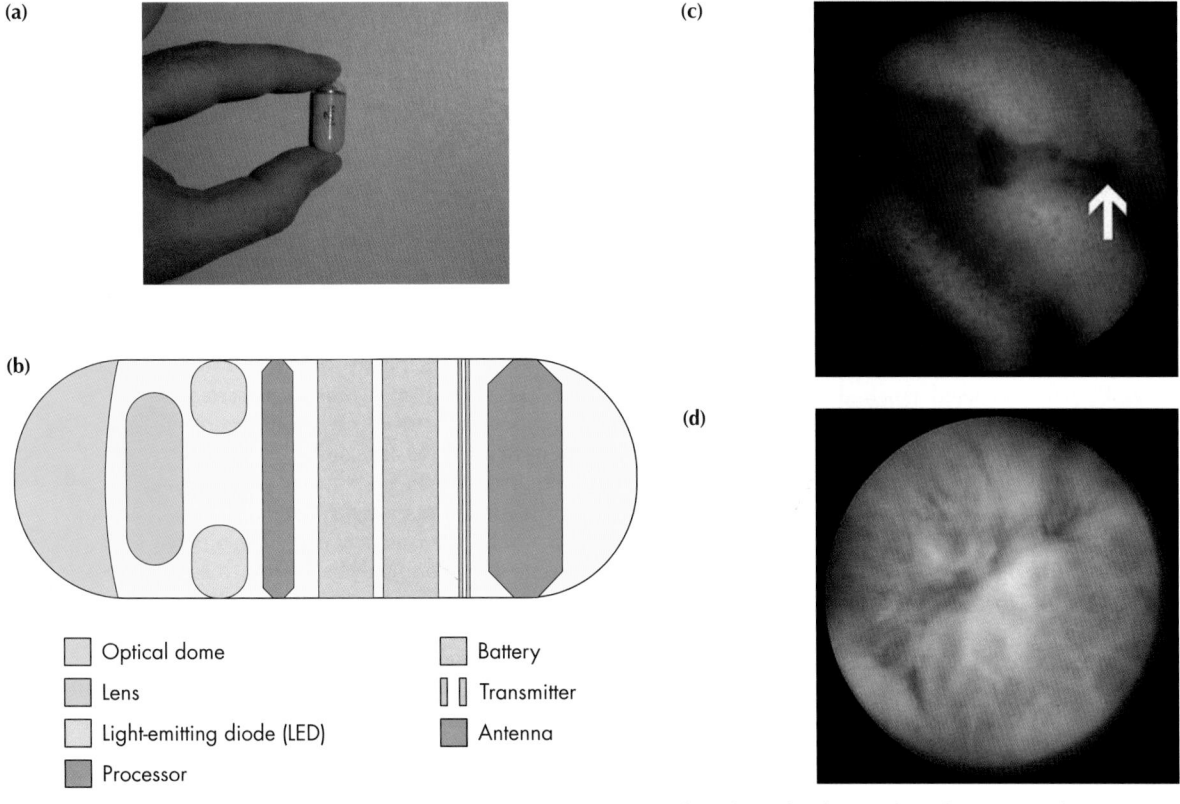

Figure 11.10 Complete diagnostic visualisation of the small bowel can be achieved with capsule endoscopy (a). The structure of the capsule is shown in (b). Clear mucosal pictures can be achieved here showing angioectasias (arrow) (c) and small bowel Crohn's disease (d).

The process is then continued until the entire small bowel is visualised (Fig. 11.11). In single-balloon enteroscopy, developed more recently, an enteroscope and overtube are used, but only the overtube has a balloon attached. A full range of therapeutics including diagnostic biopsy, polypectomy, argon plasma coagulation and stent insertion are available for balloon enteroscopy. Some experts advocate routine capsule endoscopy before balloon enteroscopy in an attempt to localise any lesions and plan whether oral or rectal access is more appropriate. The indications for single/double-balloon endoscopy are given in Summary box 11.7.

Summary box 11.7

Current established indications for single/double-balloon endoscopy

- Bleeding from the gastrointestinal tract of obscure cause
- Iron deficiency anaemia with normal colonoscopy and gastroscopy
- Visualisation of and therapeutic intervention for abnormalities seen on traditional small bowel imaging/capsule endoscopy

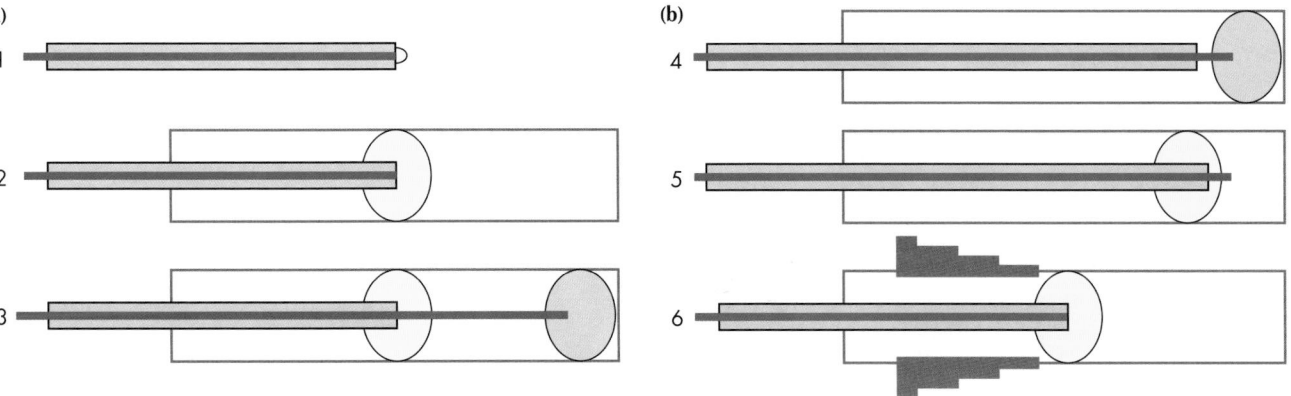

Figure 11.11 The technique of double-balloon enteroscopy is performed with an adapted enteroscope and overtube, both of which have inflatable balloons at their tip.

CHAPTER 11 | GASTROINTESTINAL ENDOSCOPY

ENDOSCOPIC RETROGRADE CHOLANGIOPANCREATOGRAPHY

This procedure involves the use of a side-viewing duodenoscope, which is passed through the pylorus and into the second part of the duodenum to visualise the papilla. This is then cannulated, either directly with a catheter or with the help of a guidewire (Fig. 11.12). Occasionally a small pre-cut is required to gain access. By altering the angle of approach one can selectively cannulate the pancreatic duct or biliary tree, which is then visualised under fluoroscopy after contrast injection. The significant range of complications associated with this procedure and improvements in radiological imaging using magnetic resonance cholangiopancreatography (MRCP) have rendered much diagnostic ERCP obsolete, and thus most procedures are currently performed for therapeutic purposes. There is still a role for accessing cytology/biopsy specimens.

Therapeutic endoscopic retrograde cholangiopancreatography

It is essential to ensure that patients have appropriate assessment prior to therapeutic ERCP, which is associated with a significant morbidity and occasional mortality. All patients require routine blood screening including a clotting screen. Assessment of respiratory and cardiovascular comorbidity is essential. Patients with an obstructed biliary system require antibiotic prophylaxis. The use of supplementary oxygen and both cardiac and oxygen saturation monitoring during the procedure are essential because of the high levels of sedation that are often required. The most common indication for therapeutic ERCP is the relief of biliary obstruction due to gallstone disease and benign or malignant biliary strictures. The pre-procedural diagnosis can be confirmed by contrast injection, which will clearly differentiate the filling defects associated with gallstones and the luminal narrowing of a stricture. If there is likely to be a delay in relieving an obstructed system, percutaneous drainage may be required.

The cornerstone of gallstone retrieval is an adequate biliary sphincterotomy, which is normally performed over a well-positioned guidewire using a sphincterotome connected to an electrosurgical unit. Most gallstones less than 1 cm in diameter will pass spontaneously in the days and weeks following a sphincterotomy, but most endoscopists prefer to ensure duct clearance

at the initial procedure to reduce the risk of impaction, cholangitis or pancreatitis. This can be achieved by trawling the duct using a balloon catheter or by extraction using a wire basket. If standard techniques fail, large or awkwardly placed stones can be crushed using mechanical lithotripsy. If adequate stone extraction cannot be achieved at the initial ERCP it is imperative to ensure biliary drainage with the placement of a removable plastic stent while alternative options are considered. These include surgery, endoscopically directed shockwaves under direct choledochoscopic vision using a mother and baby scope, and extracorporeal shockwave lithotripsy with subsequent ERCP to remove stone fragments.

Dilation of benign biliary strictures uses balloon catheters similar to those used in angioplasty inserted over a guidewire under fluoroscopic control. It is traditional to insert a temporary plastic stent to maintain drainage as several attempts at dilatation may be required. Self-expanding metal stents are most commonly used for the palliation of malignant biliary obstruction and are also normally inserted after a modest sphincterotomy. Correct stent placement can normally be confirmed by a flow of bile after release and by the presence of air in the biliary tree on follow-up plain abdominal radiographs. Stent malfunction, associated with recurrent or persistent biochemical cholestasis, may be due to poor initial stent position, stent migration, blockage with blood clot or debris, or tumour ingrowth. A repeat procedure is required to assess the cause, which can usually be remedied by the insertion of a second stent through the original one.

In addition to the standard techniques discussed above, ERCP is also used for pancreatic disease and the assessment of biliary dysmotility (sphincter of Oddi dysfunction) using manometry in specialist centres. Indications include pancreatic stone extraction, the dilatation of pancreatic duct strictures and the transgastric drainage of pancreatic pseudocysts. To minimise the risks of subsequent pancreatitis, pancreatic sphincterotomy is most safely performed after the placement of a temporary pancreatic stent to prevent stasis within the pancreatic duct.

Complications associated with endoscopic retrograde cholangiopancreatography

The same risks associated with other endoscopic procedures also apply to patients undergoing ERCP, but risks may be increased because of the increased patient frailty and high sedation levels

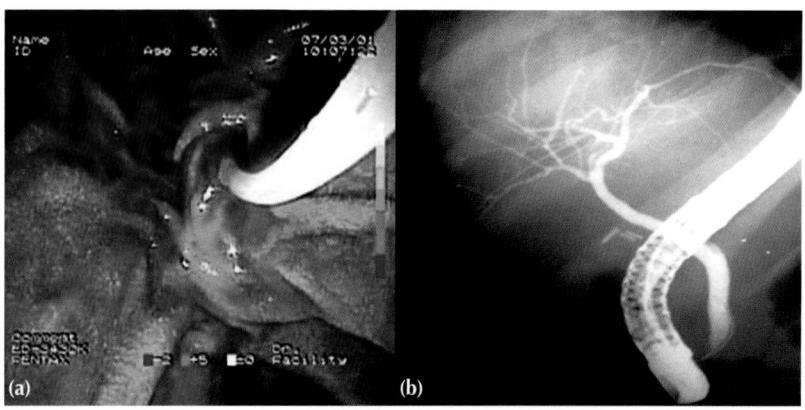

(a)　　　　　　　　　　　　(b)

Figure 11.12 During endoscopic retrograde cholangiopancreatography a side-viewing duodenoscope is positioned opposite the papilla, which can then be cannulated using either a catheter or a guidewire (a). Contrast is injected to achieve a cholangiogram (b).

Ruggero Oddi, **1845–1906**, Physiologist, Perugia, who later worked in Rome, Italy.

required. Complications specific to ERCP include duodenal perforation (1.3%)/haemorrhage (1.4%) after scope insertion or sphincterotomy, pancreatitis (4.3%) and sepsis (3–30%); the mortality rate approaches 1%. It is important to remember that post-sphincterotomy complications may be retroperitoneal and, therefore, CT scanning is essential in patients with pain, tachycardia or hypotension post-procedure. Although normally mild, post-ERCP pancreatitis can be severe with extensive pancreatic necrosis and a significant mortality rate. Many trials have assessed pharmacological strategies to reduce the incidence of pancreatitis, particularly in high-risk patients (Table 11.6). There is some evidence for the use of periprocedural nitroglycerine or rectal NSAIDs after a high-risk procedure.

COLONOSCOPY

Early attempts at colonoscopy were hindered by poor technique and the limitations of the available instruments. The ability to steer an endoscope around the entire colon and into the terminal ileum was made possible by the development of fully flexible colonoscopes with greater than 90° angulation of the tip. Advances in bowel preparation have enhanced mucosal visualisation during the examination. Two key revelations about the practical performance of colonoscopy have allowed skilled operatives to achieve a greater than 95% caecal intubation rate and frequent ileal intubation with minimal discomfort using light sedation. The first is that continued inward pressure of the endoscope results in the formation of loops within the mobile sigmoid and transverse colon, decreasing angulation control at the tip and removing the beneficial effect of shaft torque to aid steering around acute bends. The second is that pulling back the scope regularly with appropriate torque to ensure a straight passage through the sigmoid colon and around the splenic flexure greatly aids the completion of right-sided examination. Targeted abdominal hand pressure to prevent loops in a mobile colon and regular patient position change to enhance mucosal views and remove residual bowel content are also important aids to successful colonoscopy. It is essential that caecal intubation is confirmed to avoid missing pathology by incorrectly assuming that the caecal pole has been reached. The landmarks may not be clear and, therefore, visualisation of the appendix orifice or preferably terminal ileal intubation is necessary to confirm a complete colonoscopy (Fig. 11.13).

Mucosal biopsies may either be targeted to areas of abnormality

Table 11.6 Risk factors for post-ERCP pancreatitis

Definite	Suspected SOD
	Young age
	Normal bilirubin
	Prior ERCP-related pancreatitis
	Difficult cannulation
	Pancreatic duct contrast injection
	Pancreatic sphincterotomy
	Balloon dilatation of biliary sphincter
Possible	Female sex
	Low volume of ERCPs performed
	Absent CBD stone

CBD, common bile duct; ERCP, endoscopic retrograde cholangiopancreatography; SOD, sphincter of Oddi dysfunction.

(a)

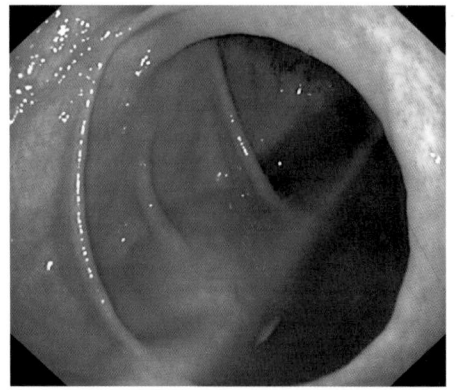

(b)

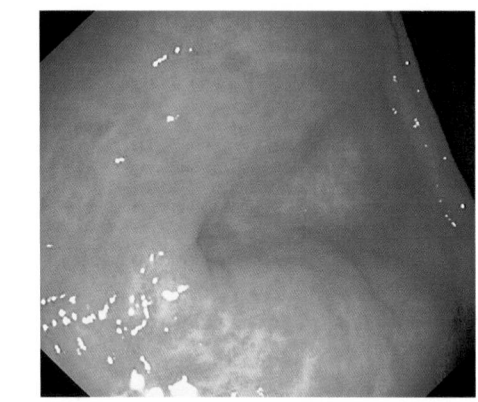

(c)

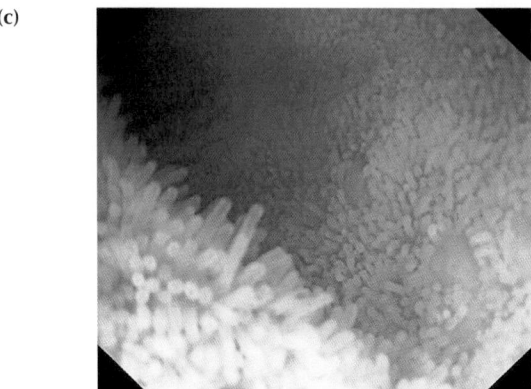

Figure 11.13 The caecal pole may not be easy to identify (a) and, therefore, the endoscopist should confirm complete colonoscopy by visualising the appendix orifice (b) or preferably intubating the terminal ileum (c), which demonstrates villi and Peyer's patches.

or random to exclude microscopic colitis in a patient with chronic diarrhoea but a macroscopically normal mucosa. Despite the increasing sophistication of radiological techniques to assess the colon such as CT colonography, the ability to biopsy areas of abnormality and resect polyps will ensure that colonoscopy remains the most appropriate investigation for the majority of patients (Summary box 11.8). Several countries including the USA and the UK have recently introduced colorectal cancer (CRC) screening programmes in the asymptomatic population once they reach a

Johann Conrad Peyer, 1653–1712, Professor of Logic, Rhetoric and Medicine, Schaffhausen, Switzerland, described the lymph follicles in the intestine in 1677.

predetermined age. The goal is to increase the number of early-stage CRCs detected and hence decrease mortality, as well as to identify and remove adenomatous polyps and prevent the onset of disease. There is on-going debate about the relevant benefits of different screening modalities including colonoscopy, CT colonography, flexible sigmoidoscopy and biannual/one-off faecal occult blood testing with colonoscopy only in positive patients. Whichever modality is used, colonoscopy is essential to resect any polyps identified and biopsy unresectable lesions.

Summary box 11.8

Indications for colonoscopy

- Rectal bleeding with looser or more frequent stools +/− abdominal pain related to bowel actions
- Iron deficiency anaemia (after biochemical confirmation +/− negative coeliac serology): oesophagogastroduodenoscopy and colonoscopy together
- Right iliac fossa mass if ultrasound is suggestive of colonic origin
- Change in bowel habit associated with fever/elevated inflammatory response
- Chronic diarrhoea (> 6 weeks) after sigmoidoscopy/rectal biopsy and negative coeliac serology
- Follow-up of colorectal cancer and polyps
- Screening of patients with a family history of colorectal cancer
- Assessment/removal of a lesion seen on radiological examination
- Assessment of ulcerative colitis/Crohn's extent and activity
- Surveillance of inflammatory bowel disease
- Surveillance of acromegaly/ureterosigmoidostomy

Therapeutic colonoscopy

The most common therapeutic procedure performed at colonoscopy is the resection of colonic polyps (Fig. 11.14). Retrieved specimens can be assessed for risk factors for neoplastic progression and an appropriate surveillance strategy determined. Small polyps up to 5 mm are removed by either cheese-wiring with a 'cold' snare or hot biopsy, during which the tip of a pedunculated polyp is grasped between biopsy forceps and tented away from the bowel wall. A brief burst of monopolar current is used to coagulate the stalk, allowing the polyp to be removed. Larger polyps with a defined stalk can be resected via snare polypectomy using coagulating current either *en bloc* or piecemeal depending on their size (Fig. 11.14). Post-polypectomy bleeding can be prevented by the application of haemoclips or an endoloop to the polyp stalk. Sessile polyps extending over several centimetres can be removed by endoscopic mucosal resection, which involves lifting the polyp away from the muscularis propria with a submucosal injection of saline to prevent iatrogenic perforation (Fig. 11.15). Any residual polyp is obliterated with argon plasma coapulation. Care should be taken with all polypectomies in the right colon where the wall may only be 2–3 mm thick.

APC and alternative thermal therapies such as heater probes are also used in the treatment of symptomatic angioectasias of the colon (Fig. 11.16). Laser photocoagulation may be used to debulk colonic tumours not suitable for resection. As with benign oesophageal strictures TTS balloons can be used to dilate short (less than 5 cm) colonic strictures. The dilatation of surgical anastomoses gives the most durable benefit as inflammatory strictures tend to recur even if intramucosal steroids are injected at the time of the dilatation. Finally, the colonoscopic placement of self-expanding metal stents may provide excellent palliation of inoperable malignant strictures (Fig. 11.17) and may also play an

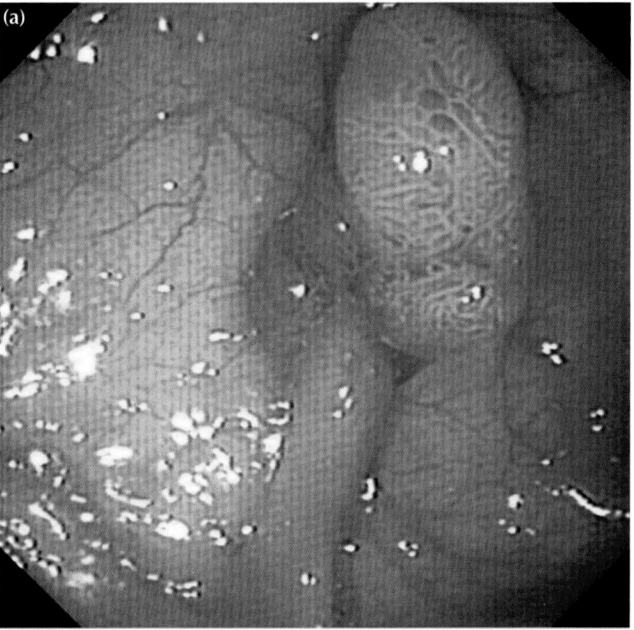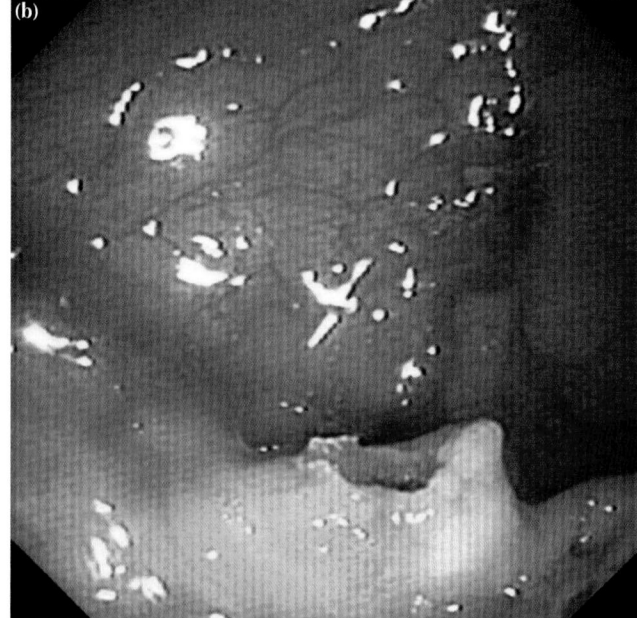

Figure 11.14 Colonoscopy is the most appropriate investigation to detect colonic polyps (a), which can be removed by snare polypectomy during the same procedure leaving a clean polyp base (b).

---

en bloc **is French for 'in a block'.**

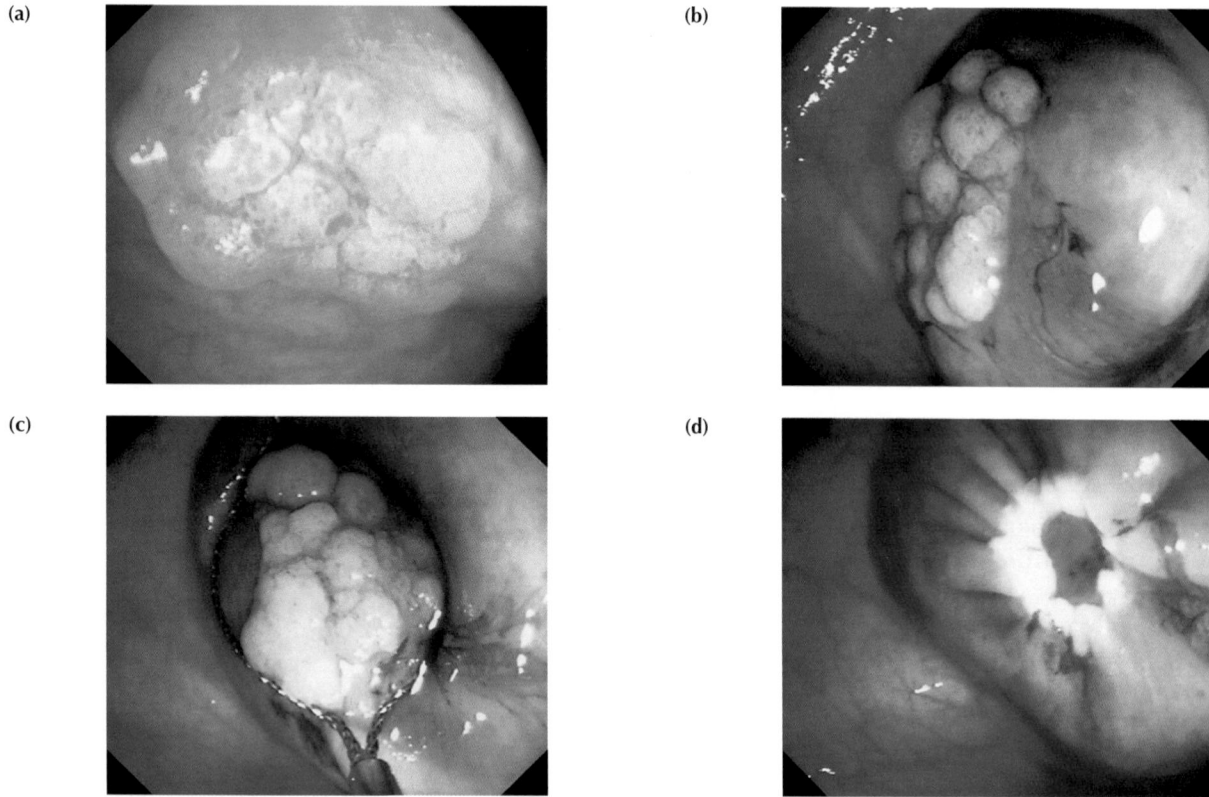

Figure 11.15 Large sessile polyps (a) can be removed by endoscopic mucosal resection. First the polyp is raised on a bed of injected saline containing dye (b). This ensures that there is no submucosal invasion and protects from transmural perforation. A snare is closed around the polyp (c), which is then resected leaving a clean excision base (d).

invaluable role in decompressing an obstructed colon to allow planned as opposed to emergency surgery.

Complications of colonoscopy

A competent endoscopist should cause few complications during routine diagnostic colonoscopy, although perforations have been reported as a result of excessive shaft tip pressure and with excessive air insufflation in severe diverticular disease. Total colonoscopy is contraindicated in the presence of severe colitis; a limited examination and careful mucosal biopsy only should be performed. Polypectomy is associated with a well-documented

rate of perforation (approximately 1%) and haemorrhage (1–2%). Immediate haemorrhage should be managed by re-snaring the polyp stalk where possible and applying tamponade for several minutes followed by careful coagulation if this is unsuccessful. Submucosal adrenaline injection and the deployment of haemo-clips are alternatives if this is not possible. Delayed haemorrhage

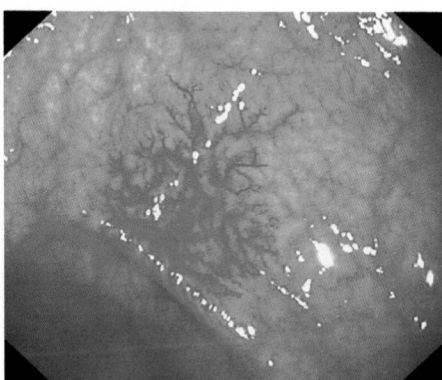

Figure 11.16 A large angioectasia of the colon. If this results in symptomatic anaemia, it should be obliterated with argon plasma coagulation.

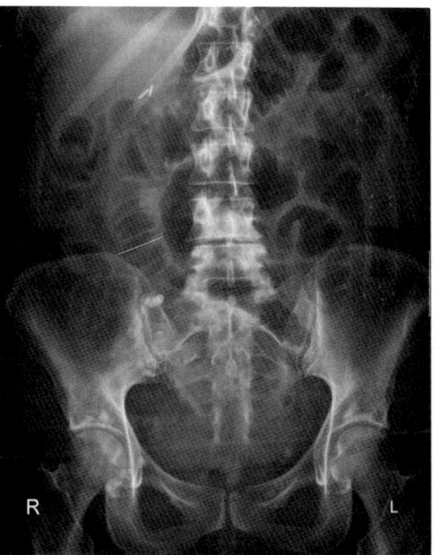

Figure 11.17 Malignant colonic obstruction can be palliated or temporarily relieved by insertion of a self-expanding metal stent.

CHAPTER 11 | GASTROINTESTINAL ENDOSCOPY

may occur 1–14 days post-polypectomy and can normally be managed by conservative observation. Transfusion may occasionally be required, but repeat colonoscopy is rarely necessary. If recognised at the time of polypectomy small perforations should be closed using clips and the patient admitted for observation. Symptoms of abdominal pain and cardiovascular compromise after a polypectomy should alert one to the risk of delayed perforation. Patients should be kept nil by mouth and receive intravenous resuscitation and antibiotics. Prompt assessment with plain radiography and a CT scan will often distinguish between a frank perforation and a transmural burn with associated localised peritonitis (the post-polypectomy syndrome). Assessment by an experienced colorectal surgeon is essential, as surgery is often the most appropriate course of action.

FUTURE DIRECTIONS IN ENDOSCOPY

Chromoendoscopy, narrow band imaging and high resolution magnification endoscopy

The ability to enhance lesion detection and achieve near-patient discrimination of pathology without the need for histology is a common theme of several active areas of endoscopic development. The goal is to allow accurate discrimination of dysplasia grade in areas of Barrett's oesophagus or quiescent ulcerative colitis and to aid polyp detection and the recognition of early gastric and colorectal cancer. The most widely available technique is chromoendoscopy, which involves the topical application of stains or pigments to improve tissue localisation, characterisation or diagnosis. Several agents have been described, which can broadly be categorised as absorptive (vital) stains such as methylene blue, contrast (reactive) stains such as indigo carmine, and those used for tattooing such as India ink. Narrow band imaging (NBI) relies on an optical filter technology that radically improves the visibility of capillaries, veins and other subtle tissue structures by optimising the absorbance and scattering characteristics of light. NBI uses two discrete bands of light: one blue at 415 nm and one green at 540 nm. Narrow band blue light displays superficial capillary networks whereas green light displays subepithelial vessels; when combined they offer an extremely high contrast image of the tissue surface. Finally, high-resolution magnifying endoscopy may be used alone or in combination with one of the above techniques to achieve near-cellular definition of the mucosa (Fig. 11.18).

CONCLUSIONS

Over the last 30 years endoscopy has become an integral part of the diagnostic work-up of patients with gastrointestinal disease. Whereas advances in radiology may obviate the need for some diagnostic procedures (routine OGD and ERCP), the ability to take mucosal biopsies will ensure that it retains a vital role. Moreover, on-going advances in technology such as magnifying endoscopy and chromoendoscopy are able to give near-histological quality definition to allow near-patient diagnosis. There have also been major advances in the range of conditions that are amenable to endoscopic therapy; such therapy may have substantially lower associated morbidity rates than traditional surgical approaches. However, as the scope of procedures widens and the age range/comorbidities of the patients increases it is beholden to the endoscopist to ensure that he or she adheres to

(a)

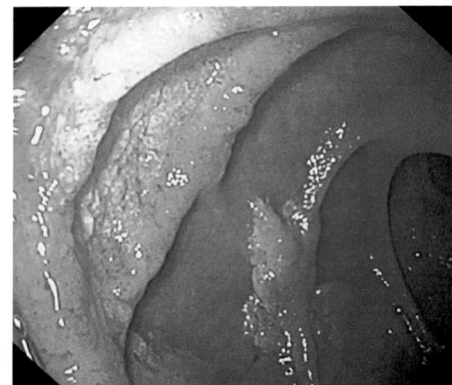

(b)

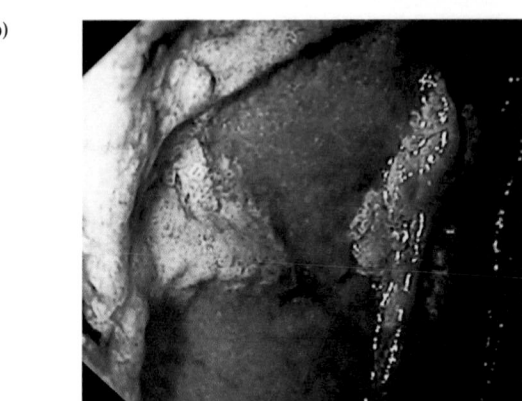

(c)

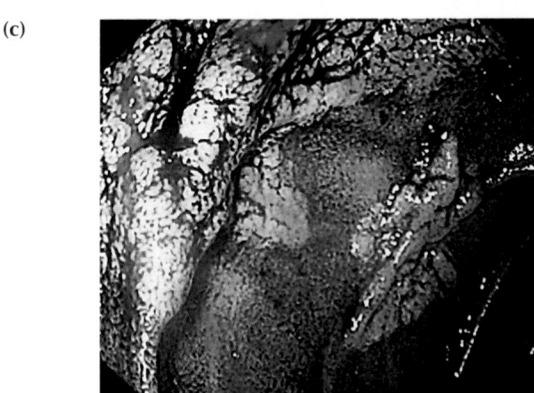

Figure 11.18 Endoscopic diagnostic accuracy can be improved by novel endoscopic techniques. This duodenal adenoma can be seen with conventional white light (a), but its full extent is more clearly delineated using narrow band imaging (b) or chromoendoscopy with indigo carmine (c).

appropriate governance/consent and sedation practice to minimise complications.

FURTHER READING

Cotton, P. and Williams, C. (2003) *Practical Gastrointestinal Endoscopy*, 5th edn. Blackwell Science, Oxford.

Saunders, B.P. (2005). Polyp management. In: Phillips, R.K.S. and Clark, S. (eds). *Frontiers in Colorectal Surgery*. tfm, Shrewsbury.

Tytgat, G., Classen, M., Waye, J. and Nakazawa, S. (2000) *Practice of Therapeutic Endoscopy*, 2nd edn. W.B. Saunders, London.

Weitz, J., Koch, M., Debus, J., Hohler, T., Galle, P.R. and Buchler, M.W. (2005) Colorectal cancer. *Lancet* **365**: 153–65.

Tissue diagnosis

INTRODUCTION

For centuries, macroscopic examination of autopsy material was the main form of tissue diagnosis. Microscopic examination of human tissue from autopsies and surgical procedures was introduced in the nineteenth century. Analysis of tissue samples is now an integral part of clinical management. Most tissue diagnosis is the responsibility of a histopathologist (or 'pathologist'), a medically qualified practitioner. The specialty now known as histopathology encompasses histopathology, cytopathology and autopsy (postmortem) work, and is heavily dependent on microscopy.

In the UK, the nature of the histopathologist's work has changed since the 1960s. There has been a steady increase in biopsy numbers, partly as a result of flexible endoscopy. Many resection specimens are assessed with management and prognosis in mind, the diagnosis having been made preoperatively. Screening programmes have had a major impact. New techniques have improved the quality and value of histopathological assessment, while autopsies have steadily decreased in number.

A modern histopathology department is usually located in a large hospital. Typically, more than 80% of specimens are from the gastrointestinal tract, gynaecological tract or skin. Highly specialised work, e.g. neuropathology, is confined to regional centres.

REASONS FOR ASSESSMENT OF TISSUE

There are several reasons for tissue analysis (Summary box 12.1). A new diagnosis may be made, e.g. squamous cell carcinoma, or a known diagnosis confirmed. Clues to a diagnosis may be found, e.g. granulomatous inflammation. Additional diagnoses may be excluded. For example, biopsies from Barrett's oesophagus may

Norman Rupert Barrett, **1903–1979, Surgeon, St Thomas's Hospital, London, England.**

confirm the diagnosis and also exclude pre-malignant change. Tissue analysis also helps to determine treatment and prognosis. For example, a liver biopsy from a patient with chronic hepatitis helps to determine therapy, exclude other diseases (e.g. steatohepatitis) and exclude complications (e.g. neoplasia). Tissue analysis, particularly assessment of resections, also helps surgeons to audit their performance.

A tissue sample does not always represent the entire patient. The interpretation of microscopic changes is enhanced by correlation with the macroscopic findings and the clinical picture. Accordingly, a request form with adequate clinical details should accompany all specimens. Useful details include site of biopsy, date of birth, gender, ethnicity, medications, relevant risk factors and past medical history.

Summary box 12.1

Reasons for tissue analysis

- To make new diagnoses
- To confirm suspected clinical diagnoses
- To exclude other diagnoses
- To assist with prognosis
- To help plan treatment
- Audit

TISSUE SPECIMENS

Routine tissue specimens received by a histopathology department include those intended for histopathological and cytopathological assessment (Summary box 12.2). Sometimes these two areas overlap.

Summary box 12.2

Common types of tissue sample

- Histology
    - Formalin-fixed tissue
        - Biopsy
            - Mucosal
            - Punch
            - Needle
            - Excision
            - Resection
        - Fresh tissue (usually for frozen section)
- Cytology
    - Cervical
    - Washings, brushings
    - Fine-needle aspirate (FNA)
    - Fluids

Histology

Specimens for histology are arbitrarily classified as biopsies and resections, although the word 'biopsy' means any tissue sample. Types of biopsy include punch biopsy, needle core biopsy and mucosal biopsy. An excision biopsy serves as both a diagnostic biopsy and a small resection. Samples for routine histology are placed in a fixative, almost always formalin (10% formaldehyde), so as to preserve morphology.

Cytology

Cytological specimens can be obtained from many sites using a variety of approaches. Some are easy to obtain, e.g. urine and sputum, whereas others require more intervention.

A conventional cervical smear is obtained by sampling the ectocervix with a spatula. Bronchial aspirates, washings and brushings, and gastrointestinal and biliary brushings sample a relatively wide area and may therefore be useful for the diagnosis of neoplasia. Fine-needle aspiration (FNA) cytology may be of accessible sites such as the breast, thyroid and superficial lymph nodes, while FNA from deeper structures, e.g. liver, pancreas, kidney and lung, is usually assisted by ultrasound or computerised tomography (CT) guidance. Transbronchial FNA may be used for mediastinal masses and transmucosal FNA for submucosal gastrointestinal lesions. Fluids may be submitted directly to the laboratory for cytological assessment.

Fresh tissue

The most common indication for submission of a fresh tissue sample (i.e. without fixative) is rapid frozen section diagnosis, but other indications are microbiological assessment, electron microscopy and various types of molecular pathological analysis. Before fixing a histology or cytology specimen, the operator should ask whether any of these investigations might be useful, e.g. microbiology if tuberculosis is suspected.

Risk management

Safety and risk management are priorities in the laboratory. Any risk of transmissible infection, e.g. hepatitis B, must be minimised by the use of warning labels, especially when fresh tissue is being submitted. Formalin kills most micro-organisms, but any risk of infection should still be notified. Formalin itself is toxic to the eyes and skin. Accordingly, leaking or faulty specimen containers should be discarded. Containers must be labelled with the patient's details and the sample site to minimise errors of identity (Fig. 12.1).

SPECIMEN PROCESSING

Histology specimen

On arrival in the histopathology department, specimens are given a unique number and submitted for macroscopic assessment and sampling ('cut up'). The largest specimens are opened (e.g. bowel) or sliced (e.g. uterus) and left to fix in formalin for at least 1 day (Fig. 12.2a–c). A written description is made. Representative samples ('blocks') are taken from any specimen too large to be processed whole (Fig. 12.3). This is usually done by a pathologist, especially if a case is complex. A local or national protocol is often followed. Samples from a cancer will include resection margins, tumour, lymph nodes, non-neoplastic tissue and other abnormal areas. Coloured inks may be used to identify resection margins and surfaces (Fig. 12.4a and b, page 170).

Specimens, or samples from specimens, are placed in plastic cassettes (Fig. 12.5, page 170), and then embedded in paraffin wax to make a block (Fig. 12.6, page 170). Sections with a thickness of 5 μm (microns) are cut from the block using a microtome (Fig. 12.7, page 171). The sections are placed on a glass slide and stained with haematoxylin and eosin (H&E) (Fig. 12.1). This work is done by trained staff, known in the UK as biomedical scientists (BMSs). High standards are necessary because a poorly cut section may have various artefacts, such as lines and folds, which impede accurate assessment. H&E staining has stood the test of time, probably because it is inexpensive, safe, fast, reliable and informative.

The stained sections are examined with a microscope (Fig. 12.8, page 171) by a histopathologist, who correlates the histological features with the clinical details and with the macroscopic description. After any appropriate further studies, the pathologist writes a report, which may be entered onto a computer system (Summary box 12.3).

Figure 12.1 Sections on glass slides stained with haematoxylin and eosin (H&E). Each slide has a unique specimen identifying number (06S022081), a letter corresponding to the biopsy site (A1–F1) and a site label (e.g. DUOBX for duodenal biopsy).

(a)

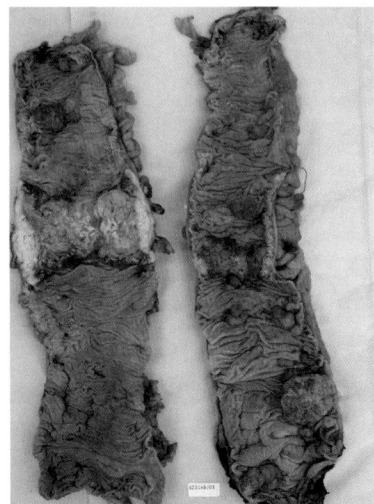

(b)

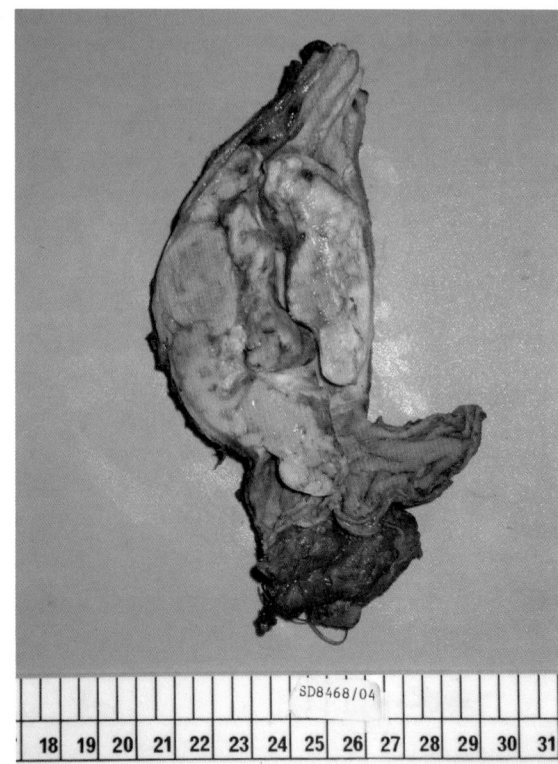

(c)

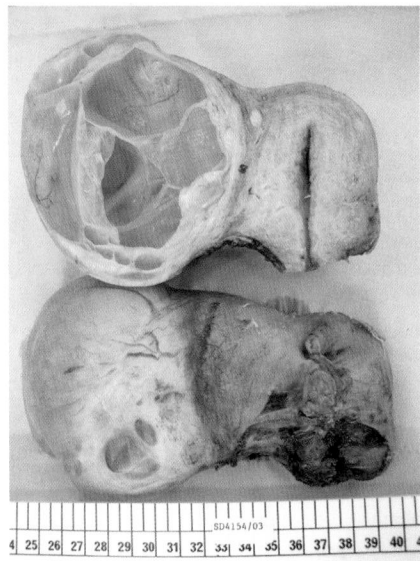

Figure 12.2 (a) A colon from a patient with familial adenomatous polyposis has been opened longitudinally to allow fixation. Multiple polyps and a carcinoma are seen. (b) An oesophagogastrectomy containing a distal oesophageal tumour has been opened and sliced to allow fixation. (c) A uterus and an adjacent cystic lesion have been bisected with a knife to allow fixation (all figures courtesy of Dr J. Chin Aleong, Barts and the London NHS Trust).

Summary box 12.3

Histological processing: sequence of events

- Biopsy or resection specimen received
- Description made
- Specimen sampled (if necessary)
- Specimen or samples from specimen placed in cassette(s)
- Paraffin wax block(s) made
- 5-μm sections cut
- Sections put on glass slides
- Sections stained with H&E
- Histopathologist examines slides
- Histology compared with clinical and macroscopic findings
- Further studies if necessary
- Report entered onto computer system

FROZEN SECTION SPECIMEN

Frozen section diagnosis is useful when a rapid answer is necessary. Surgeons are the main users of this service. A fresh (unfixed) tissue sample is frozen on a metal chuck, and sections are cut and stained within a few minutes. There are several disadvantages (Summary box 12.4). Fresh tissue carries a higher risk of infection than fixed tissue. The quality of a frozen section slide is inferior to that of routinely processed material, reducing the accuracy and precision of diagnosis. Small samples are required. Also, certain

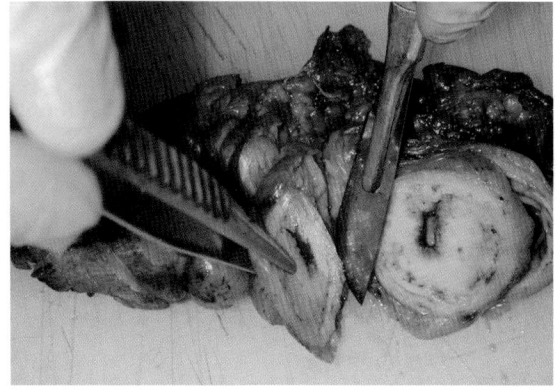

Figure 12.3 A sample is taken from a resection specimen with a scalpel.

(a)

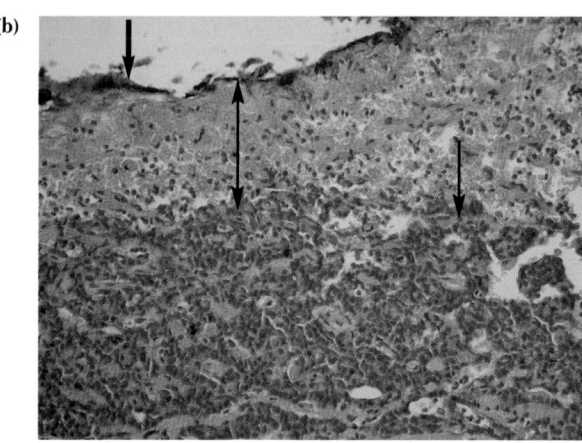

(b)

Figure 12.4 (a) An unopened pancreatoduodenectomy specimen (posterior view). Four inks of different colours have been painted onto various resection margins and external surfaces. (b) Yellow ink on the edge of a histology section (thick arrow). Tumour (thin arrow) lies close to the surface. The distance between the tumour and a surface or a resection margin can be measured (double-headed arrow).

types of tissue, e.g. fat, are difficult to process. Importantly, frozen sections are very time-consuming and disruptive for the histopathology department.

Summary box 12.4

Frozen section: advantages and disadvantages

Advantages:
- Quick diagnosis

Disadvantages:
- Labour intensive
- Disruptive
- Risk of infection
- Poorer quality sections
- Small sample required
- Some tissue types difficult to process

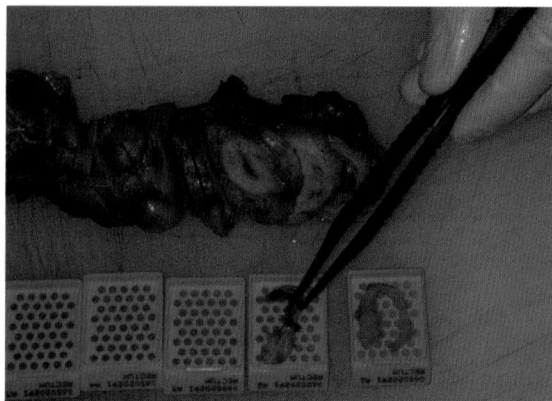

Figure 12.5 A sample from a resection specimen is placed in a cassette.

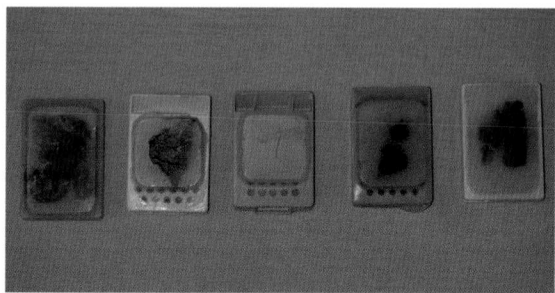

Figure 12.6 Paraffin wax blocks. Cassettes of different colours allow specimens to be organised into groups.

Cytology specimen

Many samples can be smeared immediately onto glass slides, fixed (usually in alcohol) or air dried, and stained immediately or later. Several slides are usually produced, some of which are stained with a Papanicolaou (Pap) stain and some with another method such as May–Grünwald–Giemsa (MGG) or Romanowsky. Cervical smears are usually stained with a Pap stain only (Fig. 12.9). For liquid-based cytology, the brushes used to obtain the sample are processed in the laboratory using purpose-built equipment.

Storage

Resection specimens are generally stored for about 4–6 weeks. Tissue blocks are retained for as long as space permits, typically for at least 30 years, while glass slides are typically retained for at least 10 years. Fresh tissue can be frozen and stored.

George Nicholas Papanicolaou, 1883–1962, Professor of Anatomy, Cornell University, New York, NY, USA, reported on the value of cervical smears in the diagnosis of carcinoma of the uterus in 1941.
Richard May, B. 1863, a Physician of Münich, Germany.
Ludwig Grunwald, B. 1863, an Otolaryngologist of Münich, Germany.
Gustav Giemsa, 1867–1948, a Bacteriologist who became Privatdozent in Chemotherapy, at The University of Hamburg, Hamburg, Germany.
Dimiti Leonidovich Romanovsky, 1861–1921, Professor of Medicine, St. Petersburg, Russia.

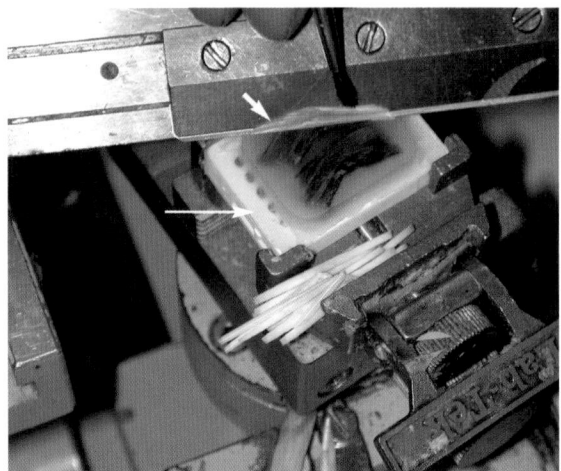

Figure 12.7 A section (thick arrow) being cut from a paraffin wax block (thin arrow) with a microtome.

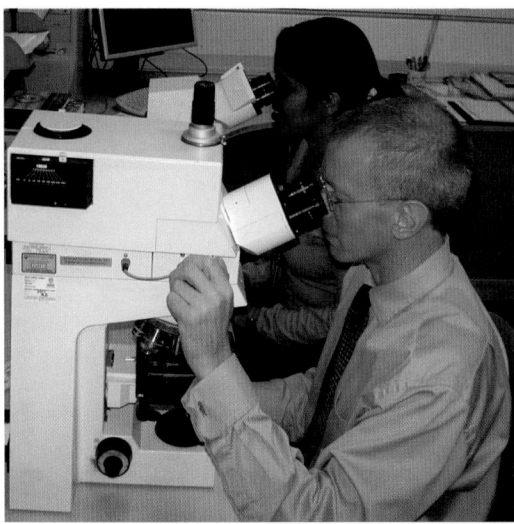

Figure 12.8 A double-headed microscope allows a histopathologist and a trainee to view a slide simultaneously.

PRINCIPLES OF MICROSCOPIC DIAGNOSIS

Diagnosis of malignancy

The main histological criteria for malignancy are metastasis, invasion, architectural changes and cytological features (Summary box 12.5).

Summary box 12.5

Microscopic features of malignancy

- Metastasis
- Invasion
    - Of surrounding tissue
    - Vascular
    - Perineurial
- Architectural abnormalities
- Necrosis
- Numerous mitotic figures
- Atypical mitotic figures
- Nuclear abnormalities
    - Pleomorphism
    - Enlargement
    - Hyperchromaticity
    - Chromatin clumping
- Nucleolar enlargement and multiplicity

Metastasis is diagnostic of malignancy. Invasion of surrounding structures suggests malignancy, while perineurial (Fig. 12.10) and vascular invasion (Fig. 12.11) strongly suggest malignancy. Other microscopic features of malignancy include architectural derangement, an increased number of mitotic figures, atypical mitoses and necrosis (tissue death) (Fig. 12.12). Cytological changes include nuclear enlargement, an increased nuclear:cytoplasmic ratio, nuclear pleomorphism (variation in shape) and nuclear hyperchromasia (dark colour) (Fig. 12.13). Multiplicity, irregularity and enlargement of nucleoli may also be seen (Fig. 12.13).

The diagnosis of malignancy depends on the site and type of tissue. In general, epithelial cells must invade beyond

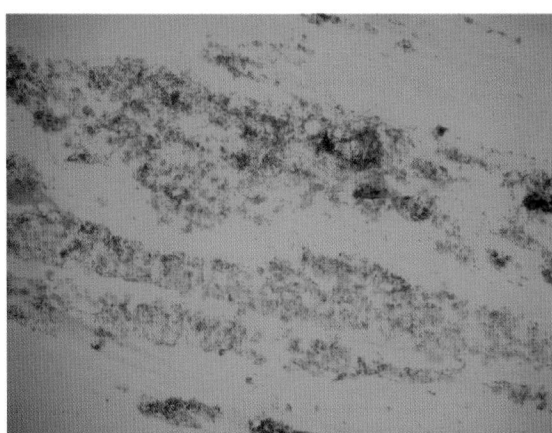

Figure 12.9 A cervical smear stained with a Papanicolaou stain. Numerous cells are present.

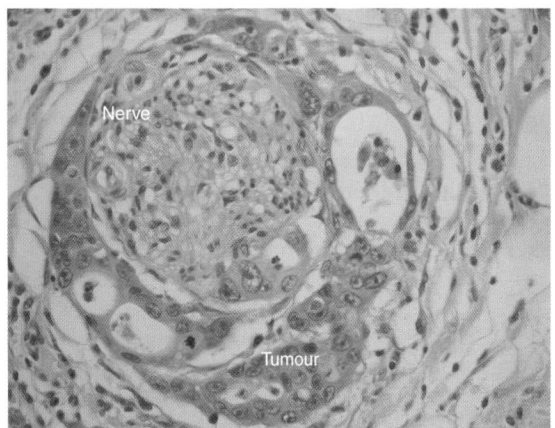

Figure 12.10 Perineurial invasion. A nerve is largely surrounded by tumour.

CHAPTER 12 | TISSUE DIAGNOSIS

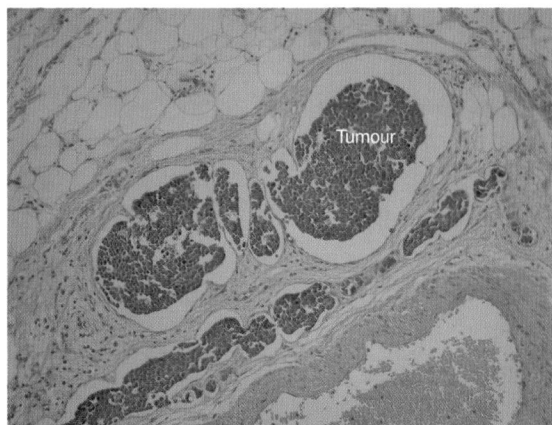

Figure 12.11 Vascular invasion. Aggregates of carcinoma cells are present within vessels.

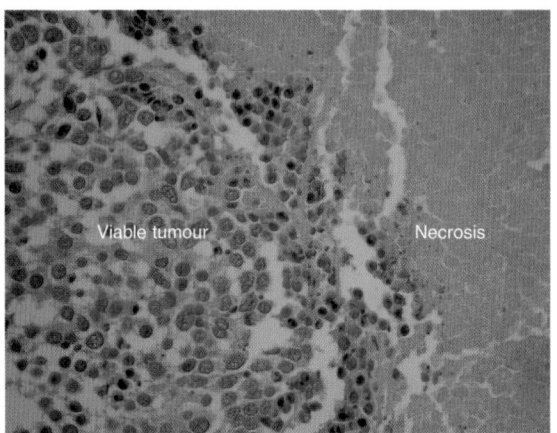

Figure 12.12 A poorly differentiated carcinoma. There is an area of necrosis.

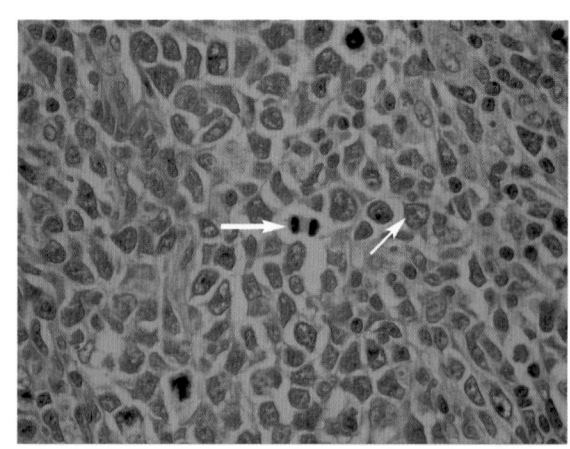

(a)

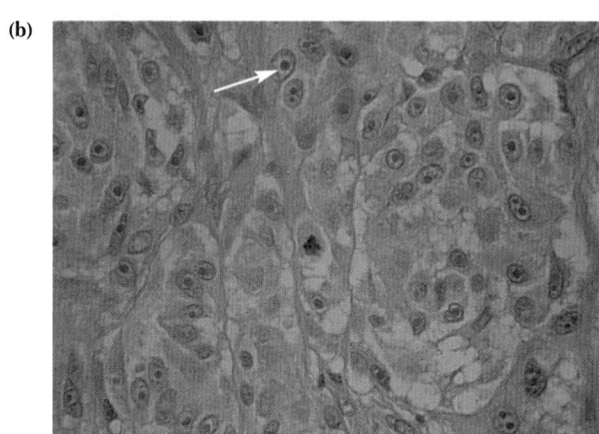

(b)

Figure 12.13 (a) A lymphoma showing cytological features of malignancy. There is nuclear pleomorphism (variation in appearance). Mitotic figures (thick arrow) are frequent. Many nuclei contain a prominent nucleolus (thin arrow). (b) A malignant melanoma showing nuclear pleomorphism and prominent nucleoli (arrow) (courtesy of Dr E. Husain, Barts and the London NHS Trust).

normal boundaries for malignancy to be diagnosed. The term 'dysplasia' indicates that microscopic features of carcinoma are present, but invasion has not occurred, e.g. cervical intraepithelial neoplasia (CIN), colorectal dysplasia (Fig. 12.14). However, in many types of non-epithelial tumour, the cytoarchitectural features, rather than invasiveness, are used to diagnose malignancy. In some cases, e.g. endocrine tumours, histological distinction between benign and malignant is impossible.

There are various causes of a false-positive diagnosis of malignancy. These include contamination of a specimen with tumour from elsewhere and interchanging of specimens. There are also numerous potential interpretative pitfalls for the histopathologist, the risk of which is reduced by thorough training, regular updating, discussion of difficult cases and avoidance of excessive workloads. The surgeon can also help to minimise interpretative errors by supplying adequate clinical details. For example, a history of radiotherapy is essential because radiation effects can mimic neoplasia. The histological changes in regenerating tissue, e.g. next to an ulcer, may also resemble malignancy (Summary box 12.6).

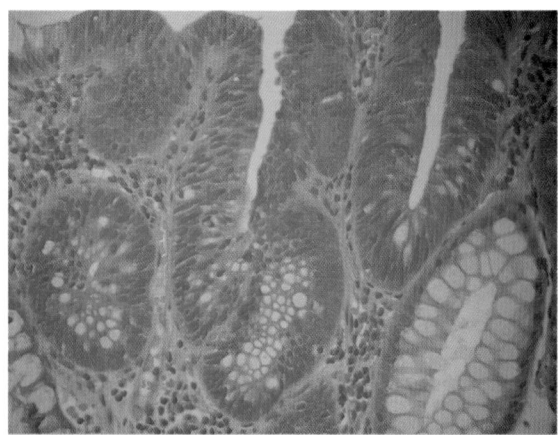

Figure 12.14 A colonic biopsy from a tubular adenoma with low-grade dysplasia. There is one non-dysplastic crypt (lower right corner). The remaining crypts show features of dysplasia, including nuclear stratification (multilayering) and nuclear hyperchromaticity (dark colour).

Histological types of malignancy

A malignant tumour showing features of epithelial differentiation, and typically arising in an epithelial layer, is a carcinoma. Other major types of malignancy include malignant melanoma (melanocytes), lymphoma (lymphoid cells) (Fig. 12.13a) and sarcoma (mesenchymal cells). In most cases, further subclassification is possible. For example, a carcinoma can be classified as squamous cell carcinoma (keratinisation) (Fig. 12.15), adenocarcinoma (tubule formation and mucin production) (Fig. 12.16), neuroendocrine carcinoma/small cell carcinoma (usually requiring immunohistochemical confirmation), clear cell carcinoma (Fig. 12.17), hepatocellular carcinoma or one of many other types.

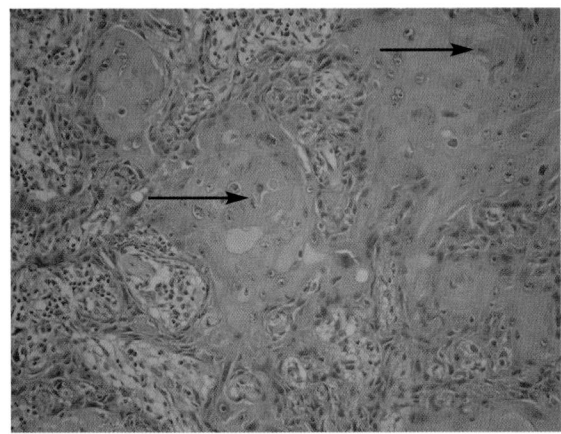

Figure 12.15 A squamous cell carcinoma. There are foci of keratinisation (arrows).

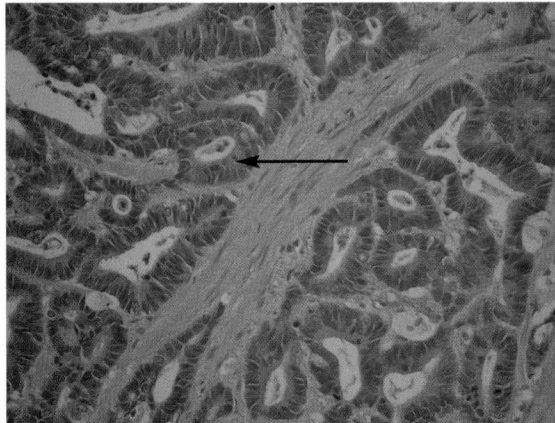

Figure 12.16 A well-differentiated adenocarcinoma. Gland formation (arrow) is obvious.

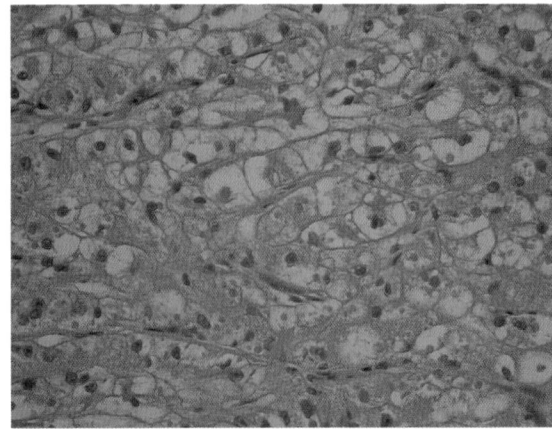

Figure 12.17 A metastatic clear cell carcinoma, composed of sheets of cells with clear cytoplasm. This is most likely to be of renal origin.

Prognostic factors for tumours

Tissue assessment is important for prognosis. Stage is the most important prognostic factor for most carcinomas, and the commonly used UICC (Union internationale contre le cancer) staging scheme depends heavily on the histopathological TNM category (pTpNpM), although the M(etastases) category is usually evaluated clinically. Grade may also be prognostic and is usually determined microscopically. Low-grade/well-differentiated tumours resemble their normal tissue counterparts (Fig. 12.16), whereas high-grade/poorly differentiated tumours do not (Figs 12.11 and 12.12). Other histological features associated with a poor prognosis include vascular invasion (Fig. 12.11), perineurial invasion (Fig. 12.10) and positive resection margins.

Inflammatory conditions

Acute inflammation is characterised by neutrophils (polymorphonuclear leucocytes) (Fig. 12.18), and chronic inflammation by lymphocytes and plasma cells. Other inflammatory cells include eosinophils (Fig. 12.19), mast cells and histiocytes. Granulomas (i.e. collections of epithelioid histiocytes) (Fig. 12.20a and b) raise the possibility of mycobacterial infection, fungal infection and a

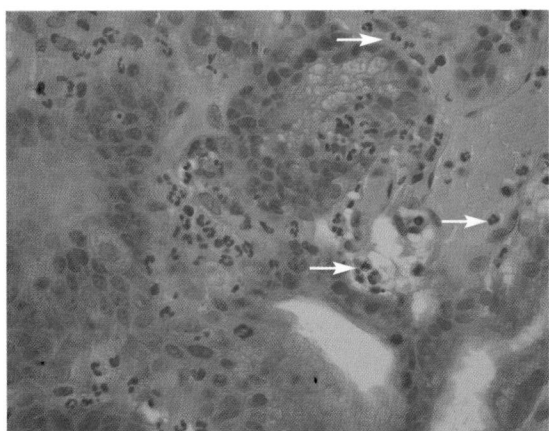

Figure 12.18 An acute inflammatory process characterised by neutrophils. Each arrow points to a neutrophil. Note the multilobated nuclei.

CHAPTER 12 | TISSUE DIAGNOSIS

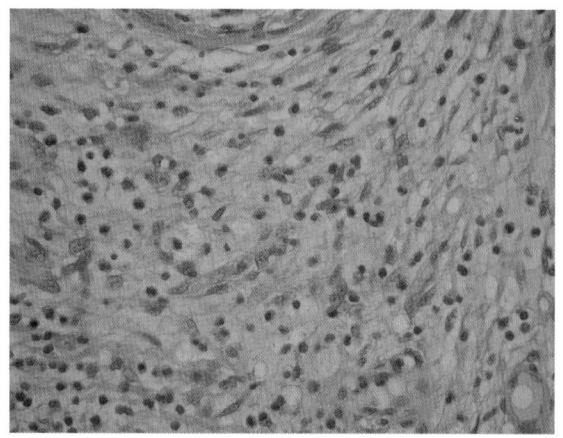

Figure 12.19 An inflammatory lesion in which eosinophils, characterised by bright red cytoplasm, are predominant.

(a)

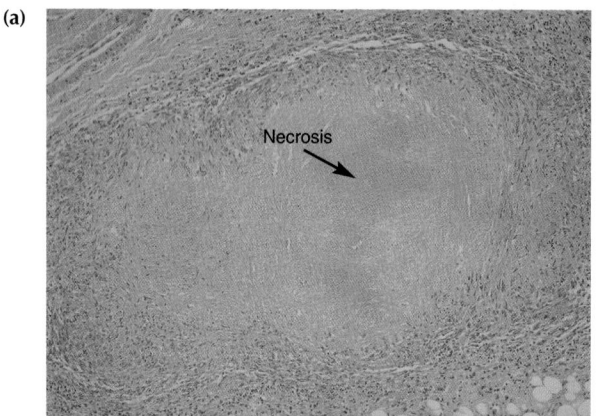

(b)

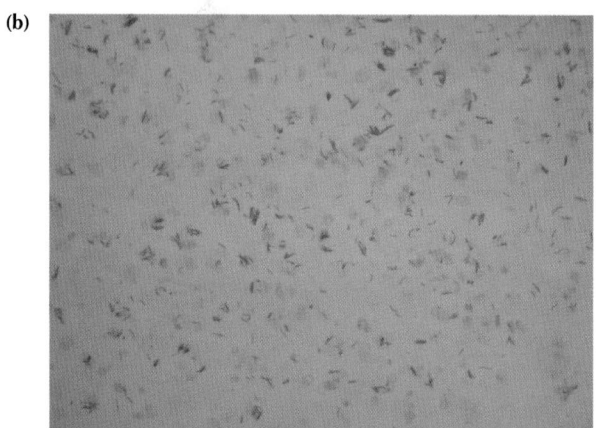

Figure 12.20 (a) A granuloma with central necrosis, suggesting tuberculosis. (b) A Ziehl–Neelsen stain (different case) shows numerous acid-fast bacilli.

reaction to foreign material, among numerous possible causes. Eosinophils in large numbers may reflect parasitic infection or allergy. Interpretation depends heavily on the site and clinical setting.

ASSESSMENT

Microscopy

Most tissue assessment depends on conventional light microscopy. Microscopes have several lenses with various powers of magnification, typically ranging from ×20 to ×400 or more. A low-power lens allows a sample to be scanned, and overall architecture to be assessed, while a high-power lens allows a closer more detailed view (Fig. 12.21a and b). A teaching arm and a digital camera can be attached to most microscopes (Fig. 12.8). Polarisation can be used to detect foreign material or to assess a special stain, e.g. Congo red.

Histological assessment

In a histological preparation, the microscopic structure of the tissue is preserved, allowing direct visualisation of architecture. Accordingly, the pathologist can see not only the characteristics of the cells that form the tissue, but also the way in which these cells are related to one another and the way in which different tissue compartments are arranged.

Cytological assessment

A cytological preparation consists of a sample of cells. Architecture cannot be determined, because intact tissue is absent or sparse (Figs 12.9 and 12.22a and b). Therefore, assess-

(a)

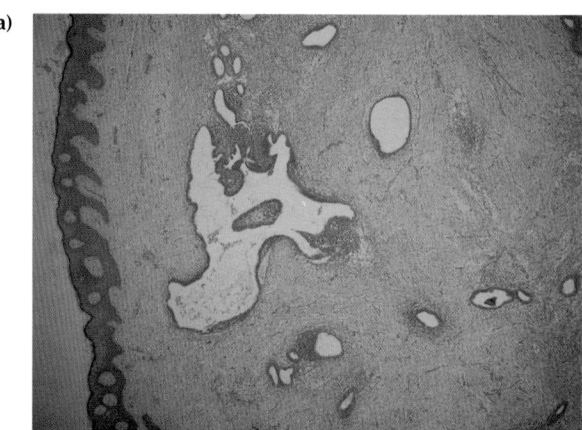

(b)

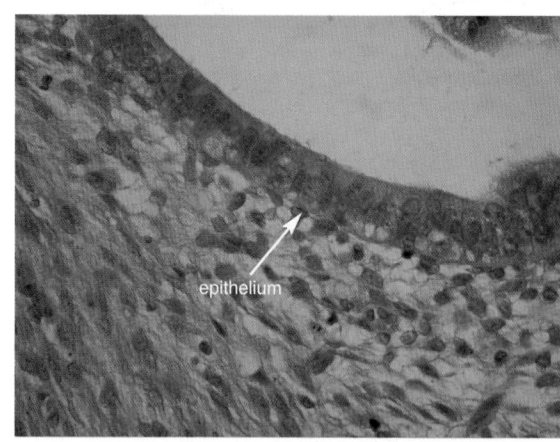

Figure 12.21 (a) Low-power view of an umbilical nodule. Glands are distributed irregularly through the stroma. (b) High-power view shows benign columnar epithelium lining the glands, favouring endometriosis over carcinoma.

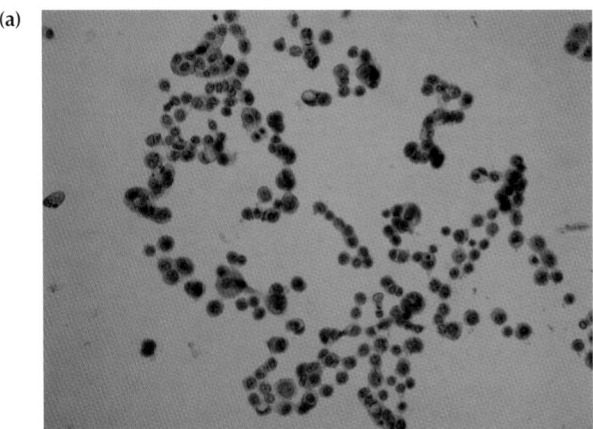

(a)

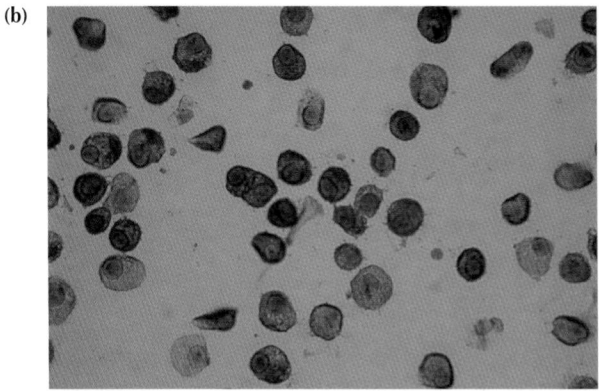

(b)

Figure 12.22 (a) A cytology preparation of a pleural effusion. Numerous cells with atypical features are present. (b) Immuno-histochemistry shows positive staining for carcinoembryonic antigen (CEA), favouring carcinoma over mesothelioma

ment relies mainly on the characteristics of the cells themselves. Accordingly, it may be difficult to diagnose malignancy, because many of the criteria, particularly invasiveness, cannot be assessed. However, cytology has several potential advantages over histology (Summary box 12.7). A wider area may be sampled, and obtaining a specimen may be easier and less traumatic. Processing times are usually shorter and costs lower. Also, non-medical staff can be trained to report, particularly cervical smears (Fig. 12.9).

Summary box 12.7

Cytology compared with histology

Advantages:
- Wider area may be sampled
- Sampling may be less invasive
- Fast
- Cheap
- Can be interpreted by non-medical staff

Disadvantages:
- Cannot assess tissue architecture
- Less amenable to further studies

Screening

Screening programmes aim to detect and treat pre-malignant tissue changes. They may rely on cytology, histology or both. The largest is the cervical cancer programme, which uses cytology initially, with biopsy and histology follow-up if appropriate. The breast cancer screening programme uses cytology and histology, while screening for cancer in ulcerative colitis relies entirely on histology.

Specimen adequacy

There are several possible reasons for an inadequate specimen (Summary box 12.8). The operator may fail to sample the intended organ or lesion, or may take too few samples to detect a heterogeneous abnormality. A sample from the centre of a necrotic or ulcerated lesion may not include viable tissue. Superficial biopsies from a carcinoma may fail to distinguish dysplasia (Fig. 12.14) from invasive carcinoma. Cautery and crush artefact may be severe enough to impede assessment. Cytology samples which have been spread too thickly may not be interpretable.

Summary box 12.8

Reasons for an inadequate sample

Histology and cytology:
- Failure to sample the intended organ or lesion
- Sample too limited
- Non-viable tissue

Histology:
- Sample too superficial
- Cautery artefact
- Crush artefact

Cytology:
- Thick smear

Further work

Further work is performed on a minority of histology specimens, and includes deeper levels, extra blocks, special stains and immunohistochemistry. *In situ* hybridisation, electron microscopy and polymerase chain reaction (PCR)-based methods may also be used. Some techniques can also be applied to cytology specimens (Summary box 12.9, Fig. 12.22a and b).

Summary box 12.9

Additional techniques

- Deeper levels
- Extra blocks
- Special stains
- Immunohistochemistry
- *In situ* hybridisation
- Electron microscopy
- PCR-based techniques
- Fluorescence *in situ* hybridisation (FISH)

DEEPER LEVELS AND EXTRA BLOCKS

The pathologist may request 'deeper levels', whereby the BMS cuts further into the paraffin block to obtain further sections. For example, deeper levels of an atypical but non-invasive epithelial lesion might show foci of invasion, allowing carcinoma to be diagnosed. Extra samples may be taken if a specimen has been sampled inadequately, e.g. if insufficient lymph nodes have been retrieved from a resection specimen.

SPECIAL STAINS

A 'special stain' is a stain that is not routine. Immunohisto-chemical stains are conventionally excluded from this category. Some special stains demonstrate normal substances in increased quantities or abnormal locations. The periodic acid–Schiff (PAS) stain demonstrates both glycogen and mucin, whereas a diastase PAS (D-PAS) stain demonstrates mucin, e.g. in an adenocarcinoma. Perls Prussian blue stain demonstrates iron accumulation (Fig. 12.23a and b), e.g. in haemochromatosis. A reticulin stain helps to demonstrate fibrosis (Fig. 12.24a and b). Elastic stains also show fibrosis and can highlight blood vessels by outlining their elastic laminae. Special stains can also reveal the accumulation of abnormal substances, e.g. a Congo red stain for amyloid (Summary box 12.10).

(a)

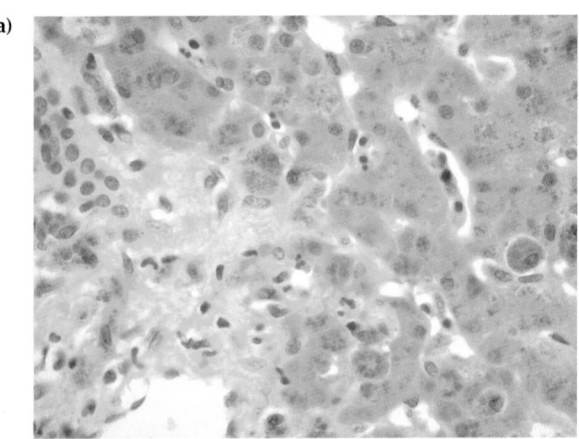

(b)

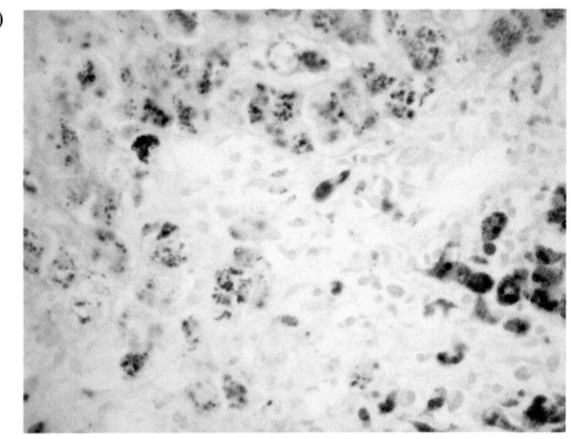

Figure 12.23 (a) Brown pigment in a biopsy. (b) A Perls stain is positive, indicating that the pigment is iron.

Hugo Schiff, **1834–1915, a German Biochemist who worked at Florence, Italy.**
Max Perls, **1843–1881, A Pathologist of Giesen, Germany.**
Congo Red **is Sodium diphenylbisazobisnaphthylamine sulphonate.**

(a)

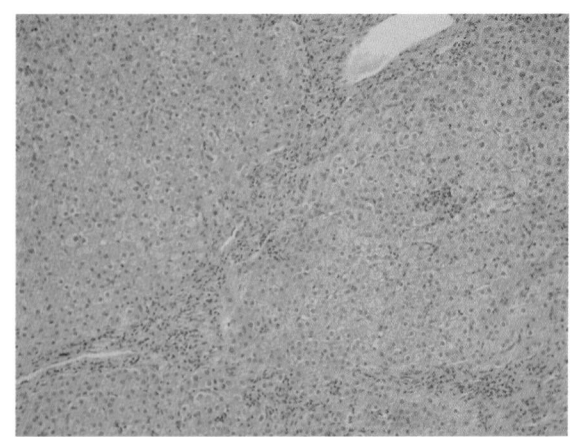

(b)

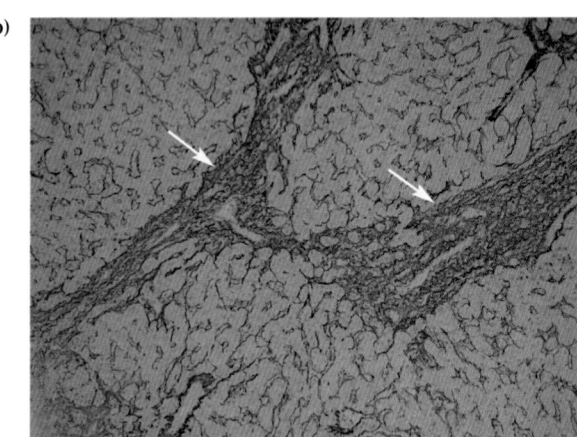

Figure 12.24 (a) A liver biopsy stained with haematoxylin and eosin (H&E) in which the severity of fibrosis cannot be determined. (b) A reticulin stain demonstrates fibrous bridges (arrows).

Summary box 12.10

Common special stains

- PAS: glycogen, fungi
- D-PAS: mucin
- Perls Prussian blue: iron
- Reticulin: reticulin fibres
- van Gieson: collagen
- Congo red: amyloid
- Ziehl–Neelsen: mycobacteria

Special stains are also useful for the diagnosis of infection. For example, a Ziehl–Neelsen stain demonstrates acid-fast bacilli, particularly mycobacteria, by staining them bright red in a blue background (Fig. 12.20a and b). Mycobacteria cannot be seen on H&E slides. Other micro-organisms that may be detectable on H&E but are easier to see with a special stain include fungi (PAS or Grocott stain), protozoa (Giemsa stain) and spirochaetes (Warthin–Starry stain).

Ira Thompson van Gieson, **1866–1913, an American Neuropathologist, described this stain in 1889.**
Franz Heinrich Paul Ziehl, **1859–1926, Neurologist, Lübeck, Germany.**
Friedrich Carl Adolf Neelsen, **1854–1894, Pathologist, Prosector, the Stadt-Krankenhaus, Dresden, Germany.**
Aldred Scott Warthin, **1866–1931, Professor of Pathology, The University of Michigan, Ann Arbor, MI, USA.**

IMMUNOHISTOCHEMISTRY

Immunohistochemistry, which was introduced in the 1970s, has had a major impact on histopathological diagnosis. This technique detects a specific antigen using an antibody. Numerous antibodies are now commercially available. The antibody is labelled with a dye and, when bound to its target antigen, is seen in the tissue section as a coloured stain, often brown (Fig. 12.25), allowing the presence of an antigen and its tissue distribution to be determined. Immunohistochemistry can be applied to fixed, fresh and frozen tissue and to cytological preparations (Fig. 12.22b). It is specific, safe, quick and relatively inexpensive. False-positive results can result from non-specific staining or cross-reaction with similar antigens.

Immunohistochemistry: tumour pathology

Immunohistochemistry has numerous applications in tumour pathology, including determination of cell type/direction of differentiation and elucidation of site of origin. Immunohistochemistry may also help to confirm neoplasia, determine the selection of treatment and refine prognostic predictions (Summary box 12.11).

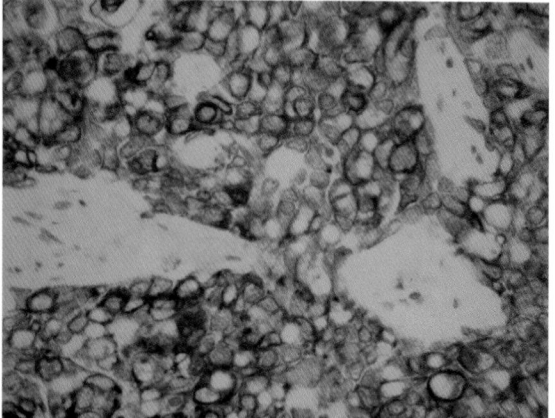

Figure 12.25 Diffuse immunohistochemical staining (brown) for a pancytokeratin marker in a malignancy, suggesting carcinoma.

Summary box 12.11

Some immunohistochemical stains used for tumours

- Cell type/site of origin:
  - Epithelial (carcinoma): cytokeratins
  - Lymphoid (lymphoma): CD3, CD20
  - Melanocytic (melanoma): S100
  - Neuroendocrine: CD56, chromogranin
  - Vascular: CD31, CD34
  - Myoid: desmin, actin

- Site of origin/cell type:
  - Prostate: prostate-specific antigen (PSA)
  - Lung: thyroid transcription factor-1 (TTF-1)
  - Thyroid: thyroglobulin
  - Colorectum: cytokeratin 20 (CK20)
  - Stomach, gynaecological, lung: cytokeratin 7 (CK7)
  - Liver: HepPar
  - Ovary: CA125

- Prognosis and treatment:
  - Breast carcinoma: receptors (ER, PR, HER2)
  - Endocrine tumours: Ki67 proliferative index
  - GIST: CD117

Various immunohistochemical stains are used to detect cell type. Cytokeratins are expressed by epithelial cells. Cytokeratin positivity suggests carcinoma (Fig. 12.25), but can also occur in other malignancies. Endothelial cell markers include CD31 and CD34, which may highlight vascular invasion or confirm a diagnosis of vascular neoplasia. Lymphoid markers include the pan-lymphoid marker CD45, the T-cell marker CD3 and the B-cell marker CD20. Markers of melanocytic differentiation include S100 and HMB45. Neuroendocrine/endocrine markers such as chromogranin and CD56 stain all neuroendocrine tumours including carcinoid, neuroendocrine carcinoma and small cell carcinoma.

The site of origin of a metastatic tumour may be suggested by H&E appearances. For example, a clear cell carcinoma (Fig. 12.17) is most likely to be of renal origin. In more difficult cases, markers of cell type (see above) provide clues. Other immunostains may provide further information. Some are highly specific, e.g. prostate-specific antigen (PSA) and thyroglobulin. Others are slightly less specific, e.g. thyroid transcription factor-1 (TTF-1), which favours bronchogenic origin, and HepPar, which favours hepatocellular origin. Individual cytokeratins include cytokeratin 7 (CK7), expressed by upper gastrointestinal, breast, lung and gynaecological malignancies, and CK20, expressed by colorectal carcinoma. Carcinoembryonic antigen (CEA) is seen in gastrointestinal and lung carcinomas (Fig. 12.22a and b), while CA125 is a marker for ovarian and other gynaecological tumours. However, a significant minority of tumours, especially if poorly differentiated, do not conform to these typical patterns. Therefore, the clinical picture, imaging results and H&E appearances must always be taken into account.

Immunohistochemistry may help to confirm malignancy. In lymphoid proliferations, light chain restriction (expression of only one immunoglobulin light chain) suggests clonality and favours neoplasia. S100 and actin stains can be used to identify the myoepithelial cell layer in a duct or gland; the absence of this layer around a neoplastic proliferation suggests invasiveness and favours malignancy.

Immunohistochemistry may play a role in the selection of treatment and prognostic predictions. Carcinomas of the breast are assessed for oestrogen receptor, progesterone receptor and HER2 status, while lymphomas are subjected to a comprehensive array of stains. Metastases from gastrointestinal stromal tumours (GIST) can be treated with the chemotherapeutic agent imatinib if they express CD117 (Fig. 12.26a and b). The management of endocrine tumours is influenced by the Ki67 proliferative index (Fig. 12.27).

Immunohistochemistry: infections

There are antibodies to many infective agents, including cytomegalovirus (CMV), Epstein–Barr virus (EBV), herpes simplex

Michael Anthony Epstein, **B. 1921, formerly Professor of Pathology, The University of Bristol, Bristol, England.**
Yvonne Barr, **B. 1931, a Virologist who emigrated to Australia. Epstein and Barr discovered this virus in 1964.**

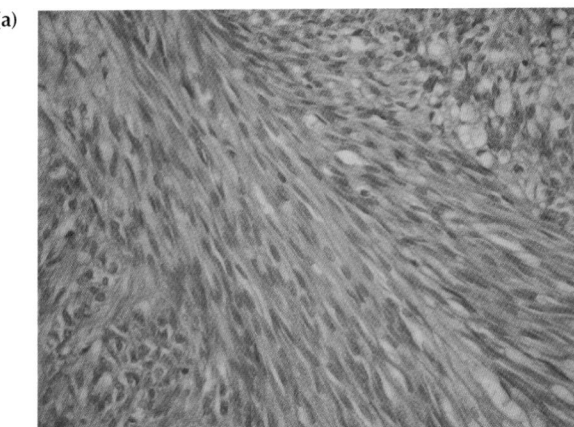

(a)

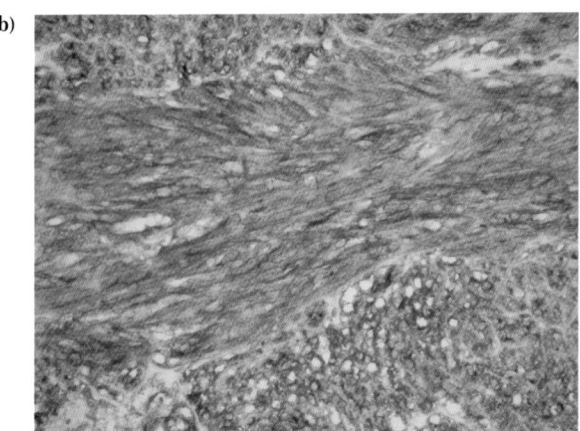

(b)

Figure 12.26 (a) A metastatic tumour composed of spindle cells. Gastrointestinal stromal tumour (GIST) was suspected. (b) Positive immunohistochemistry for CD117, confirming GIST, and indicating suitability for imatinib treatment.

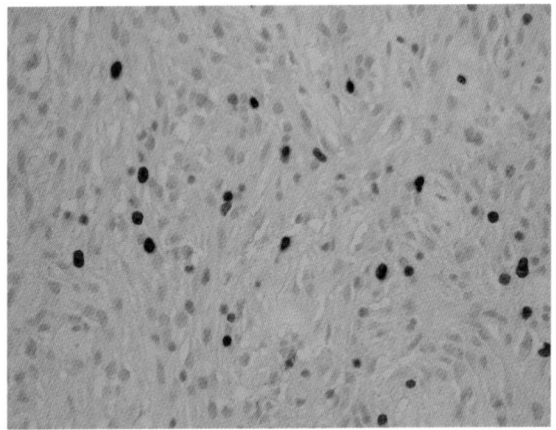

Figure 12.27 Immunohistochemistry for Ki67. The proliferative index is approximately 10%.

virus, human herpes virus 8 (HHV8) and hepatitis B. Some of these, e.g. EBV and HHV8, cannot be demonstrated by H&E and require immunohistochemistry or other techniques for their detection.

Immunohistochemistry: other applications

Immunoglobulin expression can be studied, and the abnormal accumulation of various proteins such as alpha-1-antitrypsin (A1AT) can be assessed. Amyloid can be characterised. Screening for mutations is another application (Summary box 12.12, see below).

Summary box 12.12

Uses of immunohistochemistry

- Cell type
- Neoplasia:
    Differentiation
    Metastasis: site of origin
    Confirmation of neoplasia
    Selection of treatment
    Prognosis
- Micro-organisms
- Other:
    Amyloid
    Immunoglobulins
    Other proteins

IN SITU HYBRIDISATION

This technique uses an oligonucleotide probe targeted at a specific RNA or DNA sequence and can be performed on fixed or fresh tissue sections. The presence or absence of a particular gene, and also its location, can be determined. Micro-organisms, including EBV (Fig. 12.28), CMV and human papillomavirus, can be detected.

ELECTRON MICROSCOPY

Electron microscopy allows tissue to be visualised at very high magnification, e.g. × 1000 to × 500 000. It may help to decide the lineage of a non-neoplastic or neoplastic cell in difficult cases, and may help to determine the nature of abnormal deposits, e.g. in renal disease. Unfortunately, it is time-consuming, labour intensive and expensive, and is now used selectively.

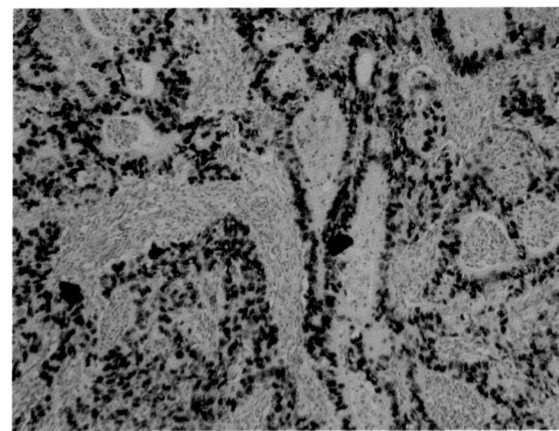

Figure 12.28 *In situ* hybridisation for Epstein–Barr virus (EBV) showing extensive nuclear positivity (black nuclei) in a gastric adenocarcinoma.

POLYMERASE CHAIN REACTION-BASED AND RELATED TECHNIQUES

The PCR amplifies DNA, yielding millions of copies from a single copy of a selected target. The amplified DNA is detected using various techniques, e.g. electrophoresis. RNA can also be amplified, using the technique of reverse transcriptase PCR (RT PCR). PCR is highly sensitive, fast and safe. However, it is expensive and has a high risk of contamination with DNA from outside sources. PCR can be performed on non-tissue samples (e.g. peripheral blood) and on homogenised tissue. PCR has an increasing number of clinical applications, including detection of mutations, confirmation of clonality and detection of infective agents (Summary box 12.13).

Summary box 12.13

Clinical applications of PCR to tissue samples

- Mutational analysis
- Clonality
- Loss of heterozygosity
- Chromosomal abnormalities
- Detection of micro-organisms

Detection of mutations

Mutational analysis comprises screening methods and direct sequencing. A germline mutation may predispose a patient to a specific disease or tumour. If the mutation is known, a sample of blood or tissue can be used to test patients and screen their families. For example, most patients with hereditary haemochromatosis are homozygous for a mutation of the *HFE* gene, while von Hippel–Lindau disease is caused by a mutation in the *vHL* gene. Mutations in colorectal carcinoma, whether sporadic or familial, include *APC* gene mutations (Fig. 12.29) and DNA

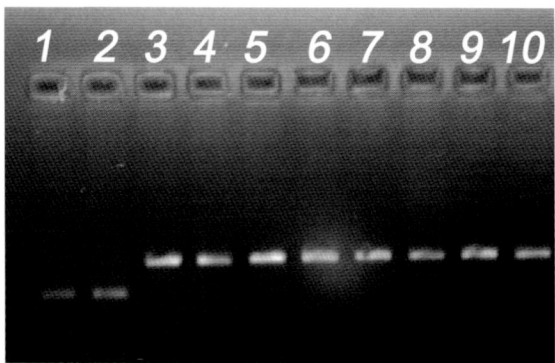

Figure 12.29 Mutation analysis of the *APC* gene. A variety of different tumours have been tested for mutation of the *APC* gene by polymerase chain reaction (PCR). Samples 1 and 2 (colorectal cancers) show loss of part of the *APC* gene resulting in smaller sized PCR products. All samples underwent sequence analysis, and point mutations (resulting in sequence change without loss of DNA) were identified in samples 5 and 7 (also colorectal cancers) (courtesy of Professor M. Ilyas, Nottingham University).

Eugen von Hippel, **1867–1939**, Professor of Ophthalmology, Göttingen, Germany. Arvid Lindau, **1892–1958**, Professor of Pathology, Lund, Sweden.

mismatch repair gene abnormalities with associated microsatellite instability (MSI). Screening methods for the latter include immunohistochemistry (Fig. 12.30) and DNA amplification of specific microsatellites. Screening results indicate whether direct sequencing for mutations is justified.

Clonality

Clonal immunoglobulin heavy chain (IgH) gene rearrangements in B-cell proliferations and clonal T-cell receptor gene rearrangements in T-cell proliferations favour neoplasia over reactive proliferations. These rearrangements can be detected using PCR and specific primers.

Loss of heterozygosity

In some centres, loss of heterozygosity (LOH) assessment is performed routinely on certain tumours, e.g. resected oligodendrogliomas (for which LOH at 1p and 19q is prognostic). PCR-based methods are the most reliable, but FISH has the potential to yield similar information and is quicker and cheaper.

(a)

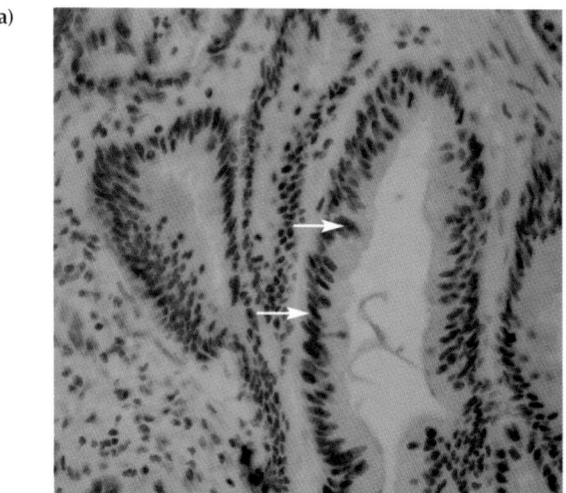

(b)

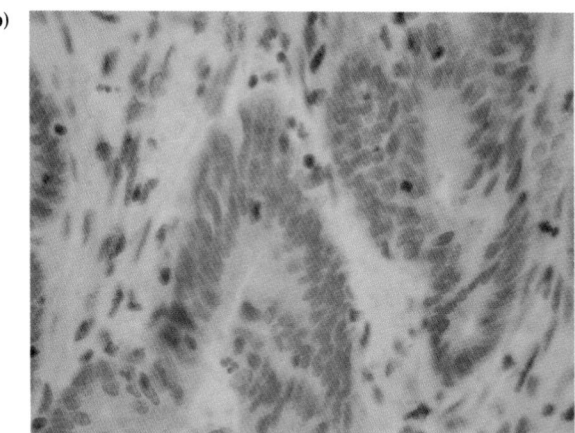

Figure 12.30 Immunohistochemical screening for microsatellite instability in a carcinoma. (a) Nuclear MLH1 expression is retained (arrows showing positively staining brown neoplastic nuclei). (b) In contrast, MSH2 expression is lost, suggesting microsatellite instability and mismatch repair gene abnormality.

CHAPTER 12 | TISSUE DIAGNOSIS

Micro-organisms

Conventional diagnosis of infection relies on microscopy, culture or serology. PCR can be used to amplify DNA from micro-organisms. This is often done on peripheral blood and other fluids, but can be performed on tissue.

CYTOGENETICS AND FISH

Cytogenetics is the study of chromosomes. Chromosomal abnormalities may be numerical, structural (e.g. translocations) or of other types. Conventional cytogenetics is time-consuming and requires fresh tissue. Interphase cytogenetics relies on the FISH technique, which is safe and fast and can be applied to fresh or fixed tissue. Interphase FISH is used for the analysis of chromosomal abnormalities, e.g. in haematological malignancies and genetic conditions such as trisomy 23. Immunohistochemistry and FISH are used to assess HER2 amplification in breast cancer. Translocations, amplifications and other changes can also be detected using PCR.

AUTOPSY

In the past, major advances in medical knowledge were sometimes based on autopsy findings. Autopsies remain very useful for medical education and audit. In the UK, there are two types of autopsy. The first is the coroner's post-mortem, where there is a legal need to establish the cause of death. The second is the hospital autopsy, which requires relatives' consent. In most cases, all organs are examined. Tissue may be retained for further examination if appropriate.

FURTHER READING

Kumar, V., Abbas, A.K. and Fausto, N. (2004) *Robbins and Cotran. Pathologic Basis of Disease*, 7th edn. Elsevier Saunders, Philadelphia.

Rosai, J. (ed.) (2004) *Rosai and Ackerman's Surgical Pathology*, 9th edn. Mosby, Philadelphia.

PART 3 | Perioperative care

Preoperative preparation

To understand:
- The tasks involved in preparing a patient for theatre
- The common problems affecting a patient's fitness for operation

- How to optimise a patient's medical state prior to anaesthesia/surgery
- How to take informed consent
- The organisation of an operating list

INTRODUCTION

A consultant surgeon leads a large team of people involved in safely seeing a patient through their individual operative experience. Even at an early stage in surgical training a trainee is a key member of that team.

Important aspects of the trainee's role in this process are:

1 *Gathering and recording* concisely all relevant information. Notes on the history, examination, investigation, conclusions and treatment plan should be clearly written, concise and yet comprehensive. The same applies to subsequent notes. They should allow other members of the team to familiarise themselves rapidly with the management plan and its rationale. It should be easy to check objective observations for any change in the patient's condition. If the notes are needed in court they should be a credit to the team, recording accurately the high level of care that has been given.
2 *Planning* to minimise risk and maximise benefit for the patient. Patients do not have to be medically fit before surgery is undertaken. This is simply not possible in many cases, especially when surgery is being undertaken as an emergency or when elective surgery is undertaken in the elderly. However, every effort should be made to find out what medical problems the patient has and how bad these are. Any problems should be treated if possible so that the risk to the patient is minimised. This will also involve balancing the potential harm caused by the delays involved in diagnosing and treating comorbidity with the benefits of taking time to bring problems under control. Elective patients should have all medical problems identified, assessed and addressed before being put onto an operative list; however, critically ill patients may only be able to receive rapid, continuous resuscitation on the way to theatre if they are to be treated in a timely manner.
3 *Being prepared* for adverse events and how to deal with them. Anticipating possible adverse events allows many of them to be avoided (e.g. making sure that the appropriate implant is available). Inevitably, things sometimes do not turn out as expected; comprehensive planning will have allowed contingency plans to

be made, ready for immediate implementation. One characteristic of an experienced surgeon is that there are rarely any surprises.
4 *Communicating* with the patient and all other members of the team. Communication errors are the source of many problems in patient care. Everyone, including the patient, should understand the surgical plan (Summary box 13.1).

Summary box 13.1

Preoperative patient preparation

- Gather and record concisely all relevant information
- Devise a plan to minimise risk and maximise benefit for the patient
- Consider possible adverse events and plan how to deal with them
- Communicate to ensure that everyone (including the patient) understands the surgical plan

---

PATIENT ASSESSMENT

Introduction

In the last 10 years there has been a major shift from in-patient to out-patient surgery. Alongside this, many patients requiring major in-patient elective surgery now arrive in hospital on the day of surgery. Preoperative assessment and optimisation have therefore become an increasingly important part of modern surgical practice.

At the start of each consultation the surgeon should introduce him/herself to the patient, explaining who he/she is. Patient details should be confirmed.

History

Do not assume that the history has already been adequately covered previously. Important points may have been overlooked in a busy out-patient clinic. In addition, there may have been a substantial delay between the clinic appointment and the admission for surgery, during which time symptoms and signs may have changed considerably.

There are a number of useful principles to adhere to when taking a history:

- *Listen.* What does the patient see as the problem? (Open questions.) Patients are allowed to describe their symptoms in their own words (try not to interrupt at this stage).
- *Clarify.* What does the patient expect? (Closed questions.) Clarify details in the history and explore the patient's hopes, fears and expectations of surgery. What outcome is the patient looking for?
- *Narrow the differential diagnosis.* (Focused questions.) Formulate a list of differential diagnoses as the story unfolds, with the most likely first. The order may change as the history progresses. Focused questions may help to exclude any outstanding differential diagnoses or highlight any ancillary problems that may need addressing.
- *Fitness.* What other comorbidities exist? (Fixed questions.) Some aspects of the history are not directly relevant to the diagnosis in hand but will be vital if anaesthesia and surgery are eventually necessary. Other conditions could alter the surgical plan or adversely affect the outcome unless they are identified and optimised. These factors all need to be considered before formulating the definitive management plan. Important negative findings must also be noted when they are important for the care plan, e.g. 'no problems with previous anaesthetics' (Summary box 13.2).

Summary box 13.2

Principles of history-taking

- *Listen*: what does the patient see as the problem? (Open questions)
- *Clarify*: what does the patient expect? (Closed questions)
- *Narrow* the differential diagnosis. (Focused questions)
- *Fitness*: what other comorbidities exist? (Fixed questions)

Layout of a standard history

Presenting complaint

The first few lines of the history should include the age and sex of the patient and, ideally, one sentence summarising the immediate problem(s) that the patient wants to resolve.

History of the presenting complaint

This section should describe the time course and severity of the patient's symptoms. Some assessment of the extent to which the problem is interfering with the patient's life should be made. What has the patient already tried to relieve the symptoms and what does the patient hope to achieve from any possible surgery? A useful mnemonic to help remember which of the basic features of the presenting complaint to explore is SORE POPE (Summary box 13.3).

Summary box 13.3

Features of the history of the presenting complaint to explore

- *Symptoms*, including features *not* present
- *Onset*
- *Relieving factors*
- *Exacerbating factors*
- *Pain*, nature of the pain, any radiation, etc.
- *Other therapies*
- *Planned surgery*
- *Expectations*

Past medical history

There will frequently be many negative responses in this section but any positive findings need to be recorded in some detail, including dates, causes, treatment and subsequent control of symptoms (Summary box 13.4).

Summary box 13.4

Key topics to review when taking the past medical history

Cardiovascular
- Ischaemic heart disease – angina, myocardial infarction[a]
- Hypertension[a]
- Heart failure
- Dysrhythmias
- Peripheral vascular disease
- Deep vein thrombosis and pulmonary embolism[a]
- Anaemia

Respiratory
- Chronic obstructive pulmonary disease
- Asthma[a]
- Fibrotic lung conditions
- Respiratory infections
- Malignancy

Gastrointestinal
- Peptic ulcer disease and gastro-oesophageal reflux
- Bowel habit – bleeding per rectum, obstruction
- Malignancy
- Liver disease – jaundice, alcohol, coagulopathy

Genitourinary tract
- Urinary tract infection
- Prostatism[a]
- Renal dysfunction

Neurological
- Epilepsy
- Cerebrovascular accidents and transient ischaemic attacks
- Psychiatric disorders
- Cognitive function

Endocrine/metabolic
- Diabetes
- Thyroid dysfunction
- Phaeochromocytoma
- Porphyria

Locomotor system
- Osteoarthritis
- Inflammatory arthropathy such as rheumatoid arthritis, including neck instability

Infectious diseases
- Human immunodeficiency virus
- Hepatitis
- Tuberculosis

Previous surgery
- Types of anaesthetic and any problems encountered[a]
- Have any members of the patient's family had particular problems with anaesthesia?

[a] These probably need recording even when negative as they are so important.

Drug history

Many patients also take alternative therapies such as herbal remedies or Chinese traditional medicine. It is important to list these as some therapies can interfere with the action of drugs such as warfarin. Enquiries should also be made about illegal drug use and any rehabilitation programme being followed. Ask about any allergic reactions, including their severity.

Social history

This should include a smoking and alcohol history as well as the patient's occupation and social circumstances. Social support is particularly important for the frail, elderly and disabled. Homeless patients and intravenous drug abusers present different challenges, as do those who are sole carers for disabled relatives. Identify problems early to formulate a sensible postoperative plan and prevent delays in discharge.

Examination

Keep patients warm and comfortable while they are being examined and always treat them with respect. Only expose parts of the body as they are required. Ideally a chaperone should always be present but this should certainly be the case for intimate examinations such as a vaginal or rectal examination. A full explanation of what is being done and why should be provided throughout. Painful areas should be approached with special caution and the patient's face watched throughout to check for signs of discomfort.

First, possible differential diagnoses should be actively excluded and any new complications that might make surgery more difficult highlighted, e.g. an inguinal hernia developing signs of bowel obstruction. Second, a general medical examination should be performed to identify the presence and severity of any comorbidities. If an operation has known complications (e.g. sciatic nerve damage in a patient receiving a total hip replacement) it is important to record the situation preoperatively, in case the problem pre-dates the surgery.

Summary box 13.5 highlights some important points to be noted in a general medical examination. The patient's nutritional status deserves special mention. This is an important determinant of surgical outcome. Patients with pre-existing nutritional impairment who are likely to be denied nutrition for a significant length of time because of the nature of their surgery or who have been septic or significantly injured are all at special risk. The body mass index (BMI) should be estimated for all patients if possible (body weight in kilograms divided by height in metres squared). A BMI of less than 18.5 indicates nutritional impairment and a BMI of less than 15 is associated with significant hospital mortality. Ask about recent weight loss and look for muscle wasting, loss of subcutaneous fat (the skin hanging in loose folds), oedema and alopecia (see Fig. 13.1) (Summary box 13.5).

Summary box 13.5

Key topics in the general medical examination

General
- Anaemia, jaundice, cyanosis, nutritional status, teeth, feet, leg ulcers (sources of infection)

Cardiovascular
- Pulse, blood pressure, heart sounds, bruits, peripheral pulses, peripheral oedema

Respiratory
- Respiratory rate and effort, chest expansion and percussion note, breath sounds, oxygen saturation

Gastrointestinal
- Abdominal masses, ascites, bowel sounds, bruits, herniae, genitalia

Neurological
- Conscious level, any pre-existing cognitive impairment or confusion, deafness, neurological status of limbs

Explaining to the patient

When the examination is complete the patient should be covered and made comfortable before discussing the proposed management plan. Allow the patient to ask questions.

Investigations

These should be ordered only when clinically indicated. Most hospitals have protocols to guide preoperative investigation requests. These are helpful but should not be followed blindly, as supplementary investigations are often required to aid surgical or anaesthetic planning. Request forms should be filled in clearly, including an explanation for why the request has been made. Record test results clearly in the notes, as well as the action taken to resolve any problems identified. Investigations that are commonly needed are described in the following sections.

Full blood count

This will be necessary in young women with menorrhagia or in any patient whose surgery may involve significant blood loss. It is usually necessary in older patients who may have undiagnosed

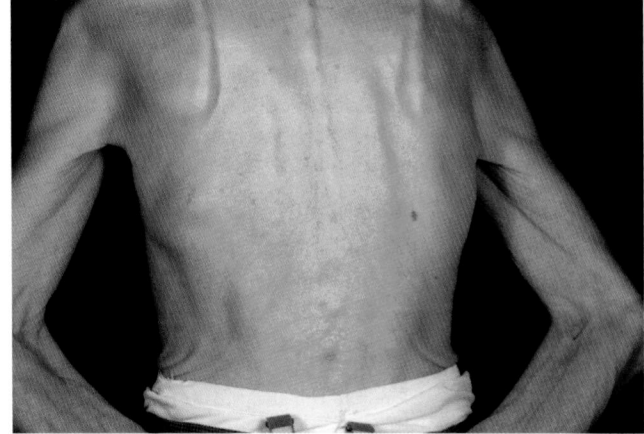

Figure 13.1 Cachectic male patient – mesothelioma of the left posterior chest wall.

CHAPTER 13 | PREOPERATIVE PREPARATION

anaemia. An abnormal white cell count will need further investigation to discover its cause.

Urea and electrolytes

This is normally necessary in patients over the age of 65, in patients who may lose a significant amount of blood in theatre or those with a history of cardiovascular, pulmonary or renal problems. It is also helpful in those taking regular diuretics.

Liver function tests

These are indicated in patients with jaundice, known or suspected hepatitis, cirrhosis, malignancy, portal hypertension, poor nutritional reserves or clotting problems.

Clotting screen

This is indicated for any patient on anticoagulants, with compromised liver function tests or evidence of a bleeding diathesis. It may also be advisable if the surgery may involve heavy blood loss.

Arterial blood gases

These are occasionally required for detailed assessment of some respiratory conditions, particularly if improvements might be achievable preoperatively. They are also useful if a significant acid–base disturbance is anticipated.

Electrocardiography

All departments will have guidelines on who should undergo electrocardiography (ECG). It is usually required in anyone over the age of 65, in all patients in whom significant blood loss is possible and in all those with a history of cardiovascular, pulmonary or anaesthetic problems.

Chest radiography

This is not usually required unless the patient has a significant cardiac history (including hypertension) or respiratory problems.

Further cardiac evaluation

Previous discussion with the anaesthetist and/or a cardiologist is advisable if there are cardiac problems. A resting ECG does not reliably predict ischaemic peroperative events. A ventricular ejection fraction of less than 35%, however, indicates a high risk of cardiac complications.

Further respiratory evaluation

Thoracic surgery usually requires a thorough respiratory work-up preoperatively. Otherwise, this is only indicated in patients with severe chronic obstructive airways disease [forced expiratory volume in 1 s (FEV_1) of < 40%] or poorly controlled asthma in which preoperative optimisation might be possible.

Temperature

Patients with a pyrexia should not be operated on until the cause has been identified and corrected if possible.

Urinalysis

Dipstick testing of urine is usually carried out preoperatively. It can detect urinary infection, biliuria, glycosuria and inappropriate osmolality. More detailed microscopic or biochemical analysis is indicated if the patient has a history of urinary tract problems or the urinalysis tests are abnormal.

β-Human chorionic gonadotrophin

This may be tested in blood or urine and used to confirm pregnancy. It is essential in all female patients of childbearing age with abdominal pain to exclude an ectopic pregnancy and in any unconscious female patient of childbearing age.

Sickle cell test

Usually the patient with sickle cell disease will know that they have this and inform the surgical team but it is important to exclude it in any unconscious patient from an affected part of the world. Sickle cell trait is less serious but should be tested for if a prolonged tourniquet time is anticipated.

Hepatitis/human immunodeficiency virus serology

Testing should be undertaken in any patient with a past history of high-risk exposure to infected body fluids, hepatitis or disorders associated with acquired immunodeficiency syndrome. Patient consent must usually be obtained before undertaking these tests, unless it is deemed that the patient lacks competence (see Obtaining consent, p. 192). In this situation the doctor must act in the patient's best interests.

Other radiological investigations

Patients with rheumatoid arthritis may have an unstable cervical spine, in which case the spinal cord can be injured during intubation. Flexion and extension lateral cervical spine radiographs should be obtained preoperatively to check for instability.

Orthopaedic surgery often requires careful planning on the basis of recent radiographs. Specialist views and imaging are sometimes required. It is important to check the requirements of the consultant concerned and make sure that the imaging (and not just the reports) is available at the time of surgery.

MANAGEMENT

Once the assessment process is completed a management plan can be drawn up in discussion with the patient. This should be carried out using language that the patient will understand. Often there will be two interdependent parts to this discussion.

First, the specific surgical diagnosis or diagnoses should be discussed. This discussion should include a systematic and logical presentation of any further investigations planned and treatment proposed. The possibility of not intervening should always be offered and the patient should be given ample time to voice their own concerns.

Second, confounding issues, such as medical comorbidities, may have been identified that will complicate the management plan. The risk of even a simple surgical procedure can be significantly increased by such comorbidities and this needs to be frankly discussed with the patient to allow truly informed consent to be given. It is not unusual for a patient in this situation to want time to think things over. If the patient is unsure it may be best to defer a final decision. Invite the patient to come back on another day with a prepared list of questions and suggest that they may wish to bring along a 'best friend' to help them at this important meeting. Inform the surgeon, the anaesthetist and any other relevant member of the team if you feel that you have identified a patient whose care may need to be out of the ordinary (Summary box 13.6).

SPECIFIC PREOPERATIVE PROBLEMS

Cardiovascular disease

Hypertension

The number of operations cancelled because of uncontrolled hypertension has been substantially reduced by preoperative assessment clinics. Patients with systolic pressures of 160 mmHg or above and diastolic pressures of 95 mmHg or above should have elective surgery deferred until their blood pressure is under control. Newly diagnosed hypertension may need further investigation to look for an underlying cause; the medical team may need to be involved.

For an acute admission requiring urgent surgery the blood pressure may need to be controlled more rapidly. It can be dangerous for a patient's blood pressure to drop precipitously and this should be carried out with the assistance of the medical team.

Ischaemic heart disease, including recent myocardial infarction

Recent myocardial infarction is a strong contraindication to elective anaesthesia. There is a significant mortality rate from anaesthesia within 3 months of infarction and elective procedures should ideally be delayed until at least 6 months have elapsed.

Significant or worsening angina needs investigation by a cardiologist before elective surgery (Fig. 13.2). If urgent surgery is required, aggressive medical therapy is indicated and meticulous optimisation of oxygenation and fluid balance throughout the perioperative period must be obtained.

Dysrhythmias

Fast atrial fibrillation must be controlled before surgery. The intervention necessary depends on the physiological state of the patient and the urgency of the surgery required. Regular measurement of serum potassium is essential, particularly if digoxin is being used.

Some conduction disorders may require pacing preoperatively, in particular second- or third-degree heart block. If a pacemaker is already fitted it is important to check whether it is programmable, as it will need to be switched to 'rate' or 'demand' mode preoperatively; expert cardiology support should be obtained for this. Most standard pacemakers are stable during anaesthesia but only bipolar diathermy should be used whenever possible. Figures 13.3 and 13.4 illustrate two cases requiring preoperative optimisation.

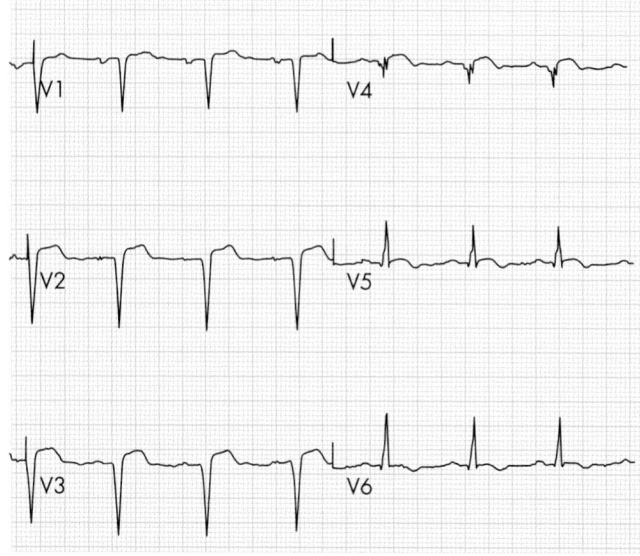

Figure 13.2 Preoperative electrocardiogram of a patient who complained of chest pain the previous day showing recent transmural anterior myocardial infarction with Q waves and ST elevation.

Cardiac failure

This needs careful work-up preoperatively and will require specialist medical input. Oxygenation and fluid balance are of critical importance in these patients and must be meticulously monitored and documented.

Anaemia and blood transfusion

Preoperative anaemia may result from bleeding or as a result of a chronic disease state. Preoperative transfusion should be considered if the preoperative haemoglobin concentration is below 8 g dl^{-1} or if the patient is symptomatic or actively losing blood.

In stable patients a small dose of a loop diuretic should be given with each alternate bag of blood. Each unit should be given over a sensible time period (usually 4 hours) and transfusion at night should be avoided. If possible, the transfusion should be given a day or so before the surgery to allow time for the

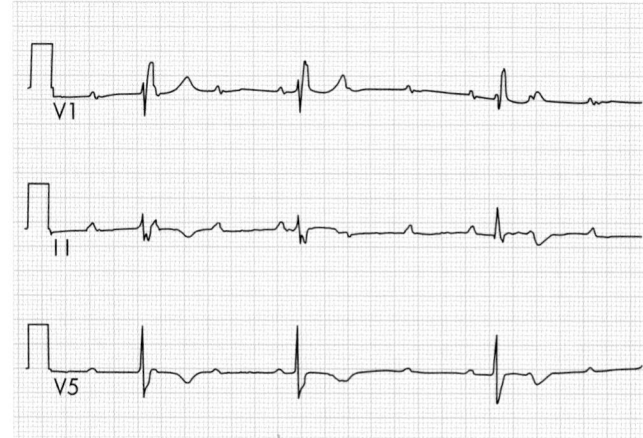

Figure 13.3 Routine preoperative electrocardiogram in an 83-year-old patient with no symptoms other than lethargy for the last 3 months. This shows complete heart block with dissociated P waves and QRS complexes, requiring preoperative pacing.

CHAPTER 13 | PREOPERATIVE PREPARATION

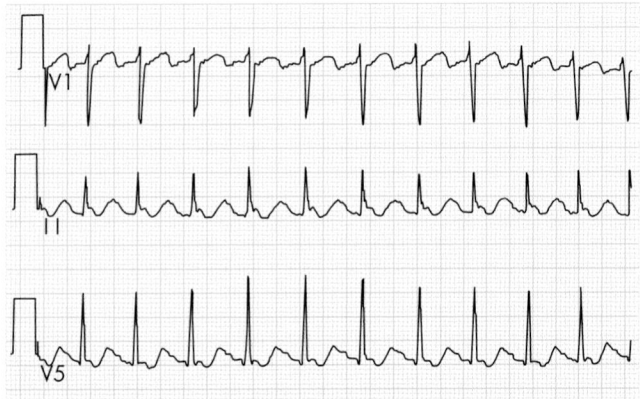

Figure 13.4 Atrial flutter with 2:1 block. Note the characteristic 'sawtooth' baseline, best seen in lead II. The cause should be treated and the rate controlled.

2,3-diphosphoglycerate levels to recover, so improving the oxygen-carrying capability of the cells. It is important to avoid rapidly transfusing patients with chronic macrocytic anaemia as heart failure can result. Other blood products such as platelets may also be required and may need to be requested well in advance if they are to be available on time.

Requests for blood must be carefully and clearly written to avoid the catastrophic complication of mis-transfusion. Mild febrile and allergic reactions are common with transfusion but high fevers and rigors require immediate cessation of the infusion and aggressive treatment for possible septic shock (Summary box 13.7).

Summary box 13.7

Preoperative transfusions

- Consider transfusion if haemoglobin level is less than 8 g dl⁻¹
- Consider carefully which products to use
- Order and write up blood products clearly
- Give the blood at a sensible time of day
- Consider co-administration of a loop diuretic
- Be prepared to treat any reactions rapidly

For major procedures a preoperative 'group and save' should be performed and blood cross-matched if necessary. Some units now use blood recycling systems in theatre, although paradoxically this does not seem to reduce the need for cross-matched blood.

Some patients will refuse blood transfusion (e.g. Jehovah's Witnesses). They should be asked to sign an extra consent form preoperatively making this explicit and accepting the consequences.

Prosthetic or leaking cardiac valves

Prophylactic antibiotic cover is usually necessary in these patients, especially if turbulent flow is likely to occur or the surgery may produce a bacteraemia.

A Jehovah's Witness **is a member of a millenarian fundamentalist Christian sect founded in America in 1884. They have their own translation of the Bible which they interpret literally.**

Respiratory disease

Infection

Significant lower respiratory tract infections should be treated before surgery except when the surgery is life-saving. Hospital protocols should be followed. The initial choice of antibiotic will depend on whether the infection was acquired at home or from hospital, and on the severity of the infection.

Patients with bronchiectasis and chronically infected sputum may need appropriate antibiotics combined with intensive physiotherapy. This may best be organised by admission to hospital several days before the surgery.

Asthma

The patient's usual inhalers should be continued. Brittle asthmatics may need oral steroid cover. The care plan will need to be discussed with the anaesthetist.

Chronic obstructive pulmonary disease

The anaesthetist must be informed if the chronic obstructive pulmonary disease (COPD) is significant, as regional anaesthetic techniques may need to be considered. Appropriate postoperative care will also need to be arranged and discussed with the patient and other members of the team. This may include booking an intensive therapy unit (ITU) bed.

Pulmonary fibrosis

There is no evidence that any treatment alters the course of this group of diseases but the anaesthetist will appreciate being warned about any cases in which gaseous exchange is significantly impaired.

Most respiratory conditions significantly increase postoperative morbidity and this should be made clear to the patient and mentioned in the consent. If the patient smokes they should be asked to stop at least 4 weeks before the surgery and the reasons be explained.

Gastrointestinal disease

Malnutrition

In the malnourished patient, treatment with nutritional support for a minimum of 2 weeks before surgery is required to have any impact on subsequent morbidity. If it is clear that the patient will not be able to eat for a significant time postoperatively, arrangements should be made to start nutritional support in the immediate postoperative phase. Chapter 17 covers this important topic in detail.

Obesity

Obesity is defined as a BMI of more than 30. These patients are at an increased risk of a number of postoperative complications. In some cases it might be better for the patient to delay surgery until they have lost weight. In others, extra prophylactic measures may need to be taken and the risks incorporated into the consent form (Summary box 13.8).

Summary box 13.8

Problems of surgery in the obese

Increased risk of:
- Difficulty intubating
- Aspiration
- Myocardial infarction
- Cerebrovascular accident
- Deep vein thrombosis and pulmonary embolism
- Respiratory compromise
- Poor wound healing/infection
- Pressure sores
- Mechanical problems – lifting, transferring, operating table weight limits

Regurgitation risk

Pulmonary aspiration can lead to acid pneumonitis, severe bronchospasm, pneumonia and death. Patients with a hiatus hernia, bowel obstruction or paralytic ileus, as well as emergency patients, are at a particularly high risk, even if they have been nil by mouth for an appropriate period.

A frequently used regime is 'no solids for 6 hours' and 'no clear fluids for 4 hours' before surgery. Some units now allow clear fluids up to 2 hours before surgery and the rules may be different again for infants.

Other management strategies may include the preoperative use of H2-receptor blockade, a nasogastric tube to empty a significantly distended stomach and specific anaesthetic techniques.

Jaundice

If the cause of jaundice is obstruction to the biliary tree it is important to ascertain whether there is associated sepsis (cholangitis). Infective causes may represent an increased risk to members of staff potentially exposed to body fluids and this should be highlighted to those concerned.

Jaundiced patients are also at risk of significant secondary complications. Impaired clotting occurs because of vitamin K deficiency and this should be corrected. There is also an increased risk of renal failure (hepatorenal syndrome) and so patients must be kept well hydrated, as well as a risk of other infections, so that prophylactic antibiotics will also be needed (Summary box 13.9).

Summary box 13.9

Surgery in the jaundiced patient

Causes of jaundice:
- Pre-hepatic – haemolysis
- Hepatic – hepatitis, cholangitis, alcohol
- Post-hepatic – biliary obstruction, drugs

Secondary complications of surgery:
- Clotting disorders
- Hepatorenal syndrome
- Infection

Genitourinary disease

Renal impairment

Prerenal

If the renal impairment appears to be a new finding, suspect a prerenal cause such as volume depletion. If previous tests of renal function are available for comparison, a disproportionate rise in urea concentrations compared with those of creatinine is diagnostic. Consider other causes of poor perfusion, particularly impairment of cardiac output.

Renal

A 'renal' cause for low urine output may arise following prolonged dehydration or the administration of certain nephrotoxic drugs [non-steroidal anti-inflammatory drugs (NSAIDs) and aminoglycoside antibiotics] or in the presence of several medical conditions. The cause of the problem should be removed and the advice of a physician sought. Prolonged dehydration may also affect platelet function and cause immunosuppression. Patients with chronic renal failure who do not require dialysis may easily be precipitated into end-stage failure by an episode of intraoperative hypotension or inadequate fluid management. Those already receiving dialysis will need to be treated 24 hours before surgery to ensure optimal fluid balance and electrolyte correction and to allow the necessary heparinisation to wear off. Further dialysis should be delayed for 24 hours after surgery if possible. Transplant patients should continue their immunosuppression and be covered with prophylactic antibiotics if necessary.

Postrenal

'Postrenal' causes of renal impairment include obstruction from any cause, e.g. renal calculi and prostate enlargement, or even a blocked catheter (Summary box 13.10).

Summary box 13.10

Renal impairment

- **Prerenal:**
  Dehydration
  Poor perfusion

- **Renal:**
  Acute – volume depletion, platelet function, immunosuppression
  Chronic – fluid balance, ?dialysis, ?transplantation

- **Postrenal:**
  Obstruction – calculi, prostate, blocked catheter

Urinary tract infection

Uncomplicated urine infections are seen most commonly, but not exclusively, in female patients. A male patient with outflow uropathy will almost invariably have chronically infected urine. Most centres treat such infections before high-risk elective surgery (such as joint replacement surgery) and wait for a negative result before proceeding. Urgent procedures rarely need delaying because of a urinary tract infection but antibiotics should be started and care taken to ensure that the patient maintains a good urine output.

In the systemically compromised patient, renal tract obstruction and pyelonephritis should be excluded.

Metabolic disorders

Diabetes

These patients are at high risk of complications. A careful preoperative assessment of their cardiovascular, peripheral vascular and neurological status should always be made. Possible preoperative risk-reduction strategies may include (but are not limited to) introducing lipid-lowering medication, improving diabetic control and treating significant vascular stenoses (Summary box 13.11).

Summary box 13.11

Surgical risks for the diabetic patient

- Increased risk of sepsis – local and general
- Neuropathic complications – pressure care
- Vascular complications – cardiovascular, cerebrovascular, peripheral
- Renal complications
- Fluid and electrolyte disturbances

Minor surgery in the non-insulin-dependent diabetic can be managed by simply omitting their morning dose of medication, listing them for early surgery and restarting treatment when they start eating postoperatively. For more significant surgery, and in the insulin-dependent diabetic, an intravenous insulin infusion will be required. This should be started when the patient first omits a meal and continued until they have recovered from the surgery. The plasma potassium level must be closely monitored.

There is a risk of life-threatening lactic acidosis in patients taking metformin who are to have contrast angiography. This drug should be discontinued 24 hours before the test and restarted 24–48 hours afterwards.

Adrenocortical suppression

Patients receiving oral adrenocortical steroids regularly (including up to 2 months before surgery) will have a degree of adrenocortical suppression. They will require extra doses of steroids around the time of surgery to avoid an addisonian crisis.

Other (rare) metabolic disorders

Familial porphyria, malignant hyperpyrexia and phaeochromocytoma are all rare conditions with specific, significant anaesthetic risks. The anaesthetist should be informed if these conditions are identified.

Coagulation disorders

Patients taking drugs that interfere with the clotting cascades

Warfarin is the commonest drug in this category. The reasons for the therapy should be established and the associated risks of stopping the treatment assessed.

For simple atrial fibrillation, warfarin can usually be stopped 3–4 days before surgery and then restarted at the normal dosage level on the evening after surgery. Check that the international normalised ratio (INR) has dropped to 1.5 or lower before surgery. Alternative perioperative anticoagulation is not required.

When the risk of thrombosis is significant, for instance with a mechanical heart valve, the warfarin should be replaced with an infusion of heparin, which is stopped 2 hours before surgery and restarted immediately afterwards. This will need close monitoring with sequential blood tests of the activated partial thromboplastin time (APTT).

Thomas Addison, **1795–1860**, Physician, Guy's Hospital, London, England, described the effects of disease of the suprarenal capsules in 1849.

For intermediate risk patients, a low molecular weight heparin may provide sufficient cover.

In some centres warfarin is not stopped for minor surgery, such as carpal tunnel release, and, if necessary, the effects of warfarin can be reversed using blood products and/or vitamin K. Vitamin K administration may cause prolonged resistance to warfarin and so should be used judiciously. The administration of low molecular weight heparin for any cause may preclude certain regional anaesthetic techniques, especially an epidural (because of the risk of a bleed in the spinal canal).

Anti-platelet agents such as aspirin and clopidogrel do not affect the INR or APTT but may affect bleeding times. The effects of these drugs cannot easily be acutely reversed, except with an infusion of new platelets. After these drugs are discontinued the effects are not reversed until the body manufactures new platelets; this commonly takes about a week. Most minor surgery can be safely undertaken without waiting this length of time but some anaesthetists are reluctant to use certain regional techniques if clopidogrel has been recently taken. For extensive surgery, or when considerable bleeding is anticipated, the safest policy is to wait if possible.

Acquired coagulopathy

For complex disorders, such as disseminated intravascular coagulation (DIC) and haemophilia, the treatment should be discussed with the haematologist.

Hypothermic patients bleed more than normal and they should be actively warmed before surgery. All patients should be kept warm in theatre, particularly during prolonged procedures.

Thrombophilia

An increased tendency to thrombosis is associated with a number of risk factors. Patients with a strong family history or previous personal history of thrombosis may have one of a number of genetic mutations. These include deficiencies in antithrombin III, protein S and C and anticardiolipin antibodies. Routine screening for these conditions is not recommended but if they are identified preoperatively management should be discussed with the haematology team (Summary box 13.12).

Summary box 13.12

Risk factors for thrombosis

- Increasing age
- Significant medical comorbidities (particularly malignancy)
- Trauma or surgery (especially of the abdomen, pelvis and lower limbs)
- Pregnancy/puerperium
- Immobility (including a lower limb plaster)
- Obesity
- Family/personal history of thrombosis
- Drugs, e.g. oestrogen, smoking

Reversible risk factors for thrombosis should be addressed before elective surgery if possible. After this has been carried out, individual risk factors should be taken into account to allow patients to be stratified into low-, moderate- or high-risk groups (Summary box 13.13).

Summary box 13.13

Risk groups for thrombosis

Low risk
- Minor surgery (less than 30 min), no risk factors, any age
- Major surgery (more than 30 min), no risk factors, less than age 40
- Minor trauma or medical illness

Moderate risk
- Major surgery (not orthopaedic or abdominal cancer), age 40+ or other risk factor
- Major medical illness, trauma or burns
- Minor surgery, trauma or illness in patient with a family/personal history

High risk
- Major surgery (elective or trauma orthopaedic, cancer) of the pelvis, hip or lower limb
- Major surgery, trauma or illness in a patient with a family/personal history
- Lower limb paralysis/amputation

Some routine prophylaxis is recommended for moderate- and high-risk groups but the exact regime will be dictated by the risk–benefit ratio in each patient. Mechanical and/or pharmacological prophylaxis may be used. Pharmacological prophylaxis carries a variable risk of undesirable bleeding (gastrointestinal, intracranial, intraoperative and postoperative haematoma) (Summary box 13.14).

Summary box 13.14

Prophylaxis against thrombosis

Mechanical
- Early mobilisation
- Neuraxial anaesthesia
- Leg compression stockings
- Calf and foot pumps

Pharmacological
- Heparin and low molecular weight heparin
- Warfarin
- Aspirin
- Pentasaccharides (e.g. fondaparinux – inhibits activated factor X)
- Direct thrombin inhibitors (e.g. melagatran and ximelagatran)

Neurological and psychiatric disorders

Peripheral neuropathies and myopathies may require prolonged ventilation postoperatively and this should be anticipated.

Anticonvulsants need to be continued perioperatively and may need to be changed to intravenous forms if starvation is prolonged.

Psychiatrically disturbed patients may require general rather than regional anaesthesia.

Certain psychiatric medications (particularly tricyclic antidepressants and monoamine oxidase inhibitors) may have unwanted interactions with anaesthetic and narcotic drugs. Ideally, monoamine oxidase inhibitors should be discontinued preoperatively.

Locomotor disorders

Specific complications of the inflammatory arthropathies should be identified preoperatively. The commonest, and potentially most catastrophic, of these is the unstable cervical spine in the patient with rheumatoid arthritis (Figs 13.5 and 13.6). If not handled carefully during intubation these patients can sustain significant spinal cord damage.

Most centres no longer stop disease-modifying drugs before surgery as this results in a flare-up of the disease that can take months to control and delays rehabilitation. Many of the disease-modifying drugs do increase the risk of wound-healing difficulties and infection but these effects are often longstanding and cannot be simply reversed by stopping the medication for a few weeks in isolation.

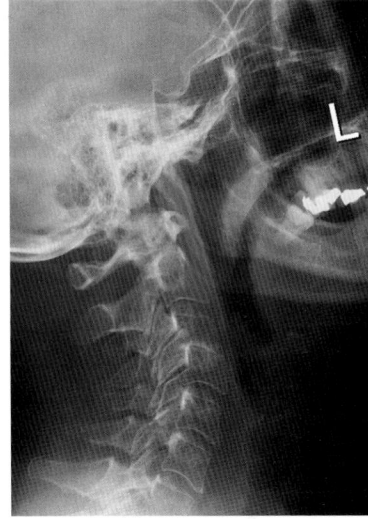

Figure 13.5 Extension view of cervical spine in patient with rheumatoid arthritis.

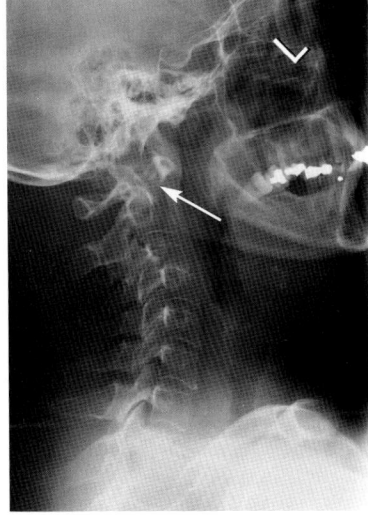

Figure 13.6 Flexion view in the same patient as in Figure 13.5. Note the huge increase in the atlantodens interval, implying significant instability at this level.

Remote site infection

Sources of potential bacteraemia, other than those already discussed, can compromise surgical results. Particularly significant is the risk of colonisation of any artificial material implanted at the time of surgery, such as in joint replacement surgery or arterial grafting. Sources of infection include infected toes and teeth. These should be treated preoperatively if possible. Appropriate antibiotic prophylaxis should be given if time does not permit complete eradication of the source of infection.

DOCUMENTATION

Clinical notes should be presented in a logical and economical manner. Investigations and a management plan should be clearly listed for action.

A drug chart should be completed including all of the patient's routine medication. Extra medications required perioperatively should be included, such as increased doses of corticosteroids, analgesia, antiemetics and thrombosis prophylaxis. Although the mainstay of infection prevention in the surgical patient is meticulous surgical technique, there is good evidence that prophylactic antibiotics can help reduce the incidence of this complication. The antibiotics prescribed should reflect the likely organisms involved. Most hospitals follow specific protocols for this. The drugs should be prescribed to allow peak serum concentrations to occur as the surgery starts. Only three doses (8-hourly) of prophylactic antibiotics should be given. Continuing antibiotics beyond the first 24 hours carries the risk that antibiotic resistance may develop, and there is no evidence of any benefit to the patient.

Certain procedures require bowel preparation to be given in advance and this should also be prescribed. Fluid charts and infusion pumps may also need to be organised.

OBTAINING CONSENT

The person obtaining consent should be fully conversant with the planned surgery, including all of the possible complications and alternatives.

Competence

To give informed consent adults (over 16 years) must be deemed competent. This requires that they can comprehend and retain the information discussed with them, believe it, and weigh up and choose from an array of treatment options. Children under 16 years of age can only give consent if they truly understand the nature, purpose and hazards of the relative treatment options. Although it is common to allow children to countersign the consent as they get older, it is still usually a parent who gives formal consent. A social worker can give consent for treatment for a child under a care order but if the child is in voluntary care the parent must still sign. For adults who are not deemed competent to give consent, treatment can still proceed if it is believed that it is in their best interests. It is usual to obtain two consultants' signatures in such cases and the reasons for the actions taken must be fully documented.

Stages in the consent process

The sections of most consent forms allow a structured approach to obtaining consent.

First, the patient's demographic details should be checked with the patient and the person obtaining consent should make it clear who they are and what their role is in the planned surgical episode.

Second, the planned operation should be outlined and confirmed with the patient. Alternatives to the proposed plan and the likely complications/outcomes of each choice (including doing nothing) should be discussed. All life- or limb-threatening complications and all minor complications with an incidence of 1% or more should be discussed. At this stage any risks specific to the patient should be discussed and recorded on the consent form (e.g. the extra risks arising from obesity). Steps that will be taken to minimise the risks and what will happen if complications do occur will also need to be discussed. Finally, it is important to check that the patient has understood what has been discussed and has no more questions.

If the preoperative preparation has been adequate the patient will be clear about the proposed plan and be happy to consent. Occasionally, new information may have been presented or the situation may have changed. The final decision is entirely the patient's and they must be given time and space to be completely comfortable with their choice (Summary box 13.15).

Summary box 13.15

Stages in the consent process

- Ensure competence (ensure that the patient can take in, analyse and express their view)
- Check details (correct patient)
- Make sure that the patient understands who you are and what your role is
- Discuss the treatment plan and sensible alternatives
- Discuss possible risks and complications (especially those specific to the patient)
- Discuss the type of anaesthetic proposed
- Give the patient time and space to make the final decision
- Check that the patient understands and has no more questions
- Record clearly and comprehensively what has been agreed

Marking

If the patient is to proceed directly to surgery this is a good time to mark the relevant side/limb if necessary.

MULTIPROFESSIONAL TEAM INVOLVEMENT

Organising an episode of surgical patient care involves a huge number of people and good communication is vital at all stages. The surgeon plays a key role in this team. A list of other people who may need to be involved is provided in Summary box 13.16.

Summary box 13.16

Multiprofessional team members

For theatre
- Ward staff
- List organiser and circulator
- Theatre nursing staff
- Anaesthetic staff, including operating department practitioners (ODPs)
- Other members of the surgical team
- Radiology department
- Pathology department

For postoperative recovery
- Rehabilitation staff
- Social care workers
- Children's ward staff
- ITU/high-dependency unit staff
- Specialist nurse counsellor (stoma/amputation)

The person responsible for organising the order and circulation of the operating list must be provided with essential information such as who has diabetes (to list them early) and which cases are 'dirty' (to list them last/later). High-risk cases, such as patients infected with human immunodeficiency virus or those with a latex allergy, must also be clearly documented.

Theatre scrub staff will need to be informed if any special equipment is required.

Postoperative recovery and discharge may be hastened by pre-operative planning with rehabilitation staff.

Children and parents may value a visit to the ward where they will be staying and a chance to meet staff there, including the play specialist if available. Patients who may spend some time on the intensive care ward or a similar unit may appreciate familiarising themselves with this daunting environment before they are admitted as a completely dependent patient.

Preoperative counselling with a specialist nurse can lessen the psychological impact of some types of surgery (e.g. limb amputation surgery or stoma formation).

FURTHER READING

General Medical Council (1998) *Seeking Patients' Consent: The Ethical Considerations*. GMC, London.

Kirk, R.M. and Ribbans, W.J. (2004) *Clinical Surgery in General*, 4th edn. RCS Course Manual. Churchill Livingstone, Edinburgh.

CHAPTER 13 | PREOPERATIVE PREPARATION

Anaesthesia and pain relief

LEARNING OBJECTIVES

To gain an understanding of:

- Anaesthetic duties preoperatively, peroperatively and postoperatively
- The techniques for maintaining an airway
- The special problems of day surgery
- The methods of providing pain relief – advantages and dangers

- The principles underlying the provision of postoperative analgesia
- The management of chronic pain and pain arising from malignant disease

HISTORY

The first successful demonstration of general anaesthesia took place at the Massachusetts General Hospital in Boston, USA on 16 October 1846 when Morton, a local dentist, administered ether to Gilbert Abbot so that John Collins Warren could operate upon a vascular tumour on the patient's neck. News of the operation reached England later that year and on the 21 December Liston, at University College Hospital, London, amputated a leg through the thigh under ether anaesthesia. In 1847, Simpson of Edinburgh introduced chloroform as an alternative to ether, and this was used extensively for general surgery, and also to relieve the pain of labour. This latter use was opposed by some members of the public who felt that relieving labour pains was contrary to the teaching of the Bible. Public recognition of the benefits of anaesthesia for childbirth was attained when Queen Victoria accepted chloroform from John Snow during the birth of Prince Leopold, in April 1853 (chloroform a la reine).

PRINCIPLES

Many advances in anaesthesia have facilitated or been driven by changes in surgical practice. Optimal patient care is dependent on good anaesthetic and surgical teamwork, with a joint approach to risk benefit assessment and preoperative optimisation of the patient's medical condition.

The importance of multidisciplinary collaborations at national level has been clearly demonstrated by the Confidential Enquiries into Maternal Deaths (triennial reports) and into Perioperative Deaths (CEPOD). These audits have enabled UK surgical and anaesthetic joint working parties to produce practice recommendations, which have resulted in influential documents such as *Pain after Surgery*.

Throughout, the anaesthetist's prime duty is to maintain the patient's safety and welfare, but it is also important to optimise the operative conditions. A collective duty of care exists to prevent injuries such as cutaneous burns or those to vulnerable structures such as nerves and eyes.

An anaesthetist's care extends into the postoperative period, at least until it has been clearly delegated to another person on the surgical ward or intensive care unit. Indeed, the modern anaesthetist is developing a more defined role as 'perioperative physician', with recognition of the continuing care beyond the immediate recovery period (Summary box 14.1).

William Thomas Green Morton, **1819–1868**, a dentist who practised in Boston, MA, USA.

John Collins Warren, **1778–1856**, Professor of Anatomy and Surgery, The Harvard Medical School, Boston, MA, USA.

Robert Liston, **1794–1847**, Surgeon, University College Hospital, London, England.

Sir James Young Simpson, **1811–1870**, Professor of Midwifery, Edinburgh, Scotland.

Alexandrina Victoria, **1819–1901**, Queen of the United Kingdom of Great Britain and Ireland, (**1837–1901**).

John Snow, **1813–1858**, a General Practitioner of London, England, who was one of the pioneers of anaesthesia.

Prince Leopold, **1853–1884**, who later became Duke of the Albany, was the eighth of Queen Victoria's nine children, and her fourth son.

Summary box 14.1

Responsibilities of an anaesthetist: patient's safety and welfare

- Make sure the patient's condition is optimal before surgery
- Ensure that the patient knows what is going to happen
- Coordinate the team during surgery
- Participate in the collective duty of the team to protect the patient from harm
- Supervise the safe recovery of the patient from anaesthesia and into the recovery period

PREPARATION FOR ANAESTHESIA

Recognition of general medical and specific anaesthetic risk factors facilitates the implementation of pre-emptive measures and improves patient safety. Early assessment, liaison with the anaesthetist and appropriate investigations avoid unnecessary delays. The anaesthetist who is to administer the anaesthetic during the operation should assess the patient preoperatively and participate in the preparation for surgery. The various aspects of postoperative pain relief, nutrition and rehabilitation should all be discussed with the patient preoperatively to make sure that they understand and can help with what is happening.

GENERAL ANAESTHESIA

Intraoperatively, the anaesthetist should provide the general anaesthetic triad of unconsciousness, pain relief and muscular relaxation, while ensuring maintenance of tissue perfusion and oxygenation.

General anaesthesia is most frequently induced intravenously and maintained by inhaled vapour such as halothane, enflurane or the more recent desflurane or sevoflurane. Propofol has replaced thiopentone as the commonest intravenous agent. It can also be used for maintenance in total intravenous anaesthesia (TIVA), by choice or when inhalational anaesthesia may be impractical such as during airway laser surgery, endoscopy or cardiopulmonary bypass. TIVA usually comprises propofol, combined with a short-acting opioid analgesic agent such as alfentanil or ultra-short-acting remifentanil, and neuromuscular blockade and pulmonary ventilation with a mixture of air and oxygen. The introduction of non-pungent sevoflurane has led to the renewed use of inhalational induction, particularly for children or 'needle-phobic' adults. It may also be used in patients who are at higher risk of developing airway obstruction.

Analgesic agents are also frequently injected at the time of anaesthetic induction, to reduce the cardiovascular response to tracheal intubation and to be effective by the time of surgical incision.

Although the use of nitrous oxide contributes analgesic and weak anaesthetic effects, its use is slowly declining as oxygen-enriched air mixtures become more popular, especially for longer cases. To provide a safety margin, at least 30% oxygen is added to the inspired mixture. Although still employed in some parts of the world, ether has generally been replaced by halothane, enflurane and isoflurane. The most recently introduced agents desflurane and sevoflurane have the advantages of fewer side-effects and more rapid recovery.

If compressed sources of oxygen, nitrous oxide or air are scarce, then air may drawn into the anaesthetic circuit either by the (unparalysed) patient's own respiratory effort or by a mechanical ventilator (Fig. 14.1) (Summary box 14.2).

Summary box 14.2

The general anaesthetic triad

- Unconsciousness
- Pain relief
- Muscle relaxation

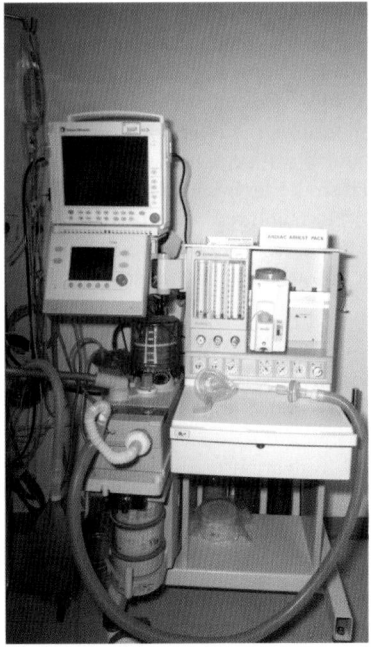

Figure 14.1 A continuous flow anaesthetic machine.

Management of the airway during anaesthesia

Loss of muscle tone as a result of general anaesthesia jeopardises airway patency and, hence, there is a requirement for methods to maintain the airway. These include manual techniques (e.g. jaw thrust) or the use of devices such as the Guedel or laryngeal mask airway or an endotracheal tube.

Sir Ivan Magill developed the endotracheal tube during the First World War to facilitate plastic surgery around the mouth without a face mask. The addition of a cuff to the tube allowed a seal of the trachea to protect the lungs from aspiration of blood or secretions and, later, to facilitate mechanical positive-pressure pulmonary ventilation.

The following means of airway control in the anaesthetised or unconscious patient are used:

- *Positioning of the tongue and jaw.* During a short procedure or before a definitive airway is inserted the anaesthetist thrusts the jaw forward from behind the temporomandibular joints, thereby lifting the tongue off the posterior pharyngeal wall. This may also be achieved by inserting an artificial oropharyngeal airway such as the Guedel airway. In these cases the anaesthetic gases are given through a face mask.
- *Laryngeal mask airway (LMA).* This was developed in the 1980s by Archie Brain, a UK anaesthetist. It is also inserted via the mouth and is positioned so that the mask covers the laryngeal inlet, which is sealed by an inflatable cuff. It provides a reliable means of maintaining the airway and frees the anaesthetist's hands from holding the patient's jaw or face mask. Its placement is less irritating to the patient's airway than

Arthur Ernest Guedel, **1883–1956**, Clinical Professor of Anesthesiology, The **University of Southern California, Los Angeles, CA, USA.**
Sir Ivan Whiteside Magill, **1888–1986**, Anaesthetist, The Westminster Hospital, **London, England.**
Archibald Ian Jeremy Brain, **Formerly Anaesthetist, The Royal Berkshire Hospital, Reading, Berkshire, England.**

endotracheal intubation. The technique is readily taught to non-anaesthetists for emergency airway management before endotracheal intubation (Fig. 14.2).

- *Endotracheal tube.* This may be passed into the trachea via either the mouth or the nose and is usually placed by direct laryngoscopy using a laryngoscope. Occasionally it is impossible to visualise the larynx in this way and a fibreoptic technique may be employed in which the tracheal tube is 'railroaded' over the flexible laryngoscope once the tip has been steered into the trachea (Figs 14.3–14.5).

Both the LMA and cuffed endotracheal tube facilitate artificial ventilation, but the cuffed endotracheal tube more reliably protects the lungs if there is a risk of pulmonary aspiration. If fluid or debris is likely to collect in the mouth from above (as in nasal surgery), an absorbent throat pack is placed in the oropharynx.

Endotracheal intubation is possible on most patients even in an emergency. However, on occasions it is impossible or airway control may be lost. There may even be accidental intubation of the oesophagus, which may initially go unrecognised.

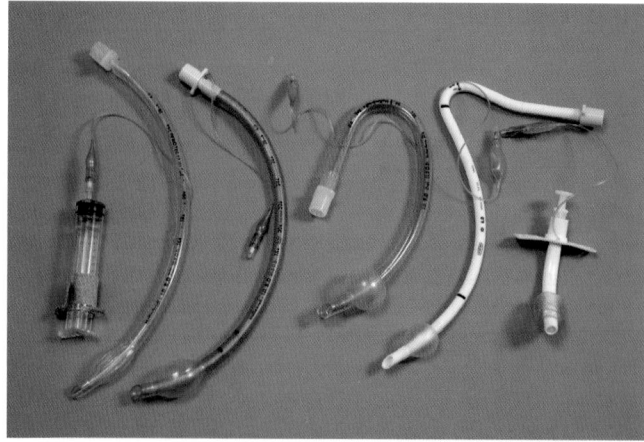

Figure 14.4 Endotracheal devices. From left to right: an uncut orotracheal tube; reinforced orotracheal tube; oral version of an RAE (Ring, Adair and Elwyn) preformed tube; nasal version of an RAE preformed tube; tracheostomy tube.

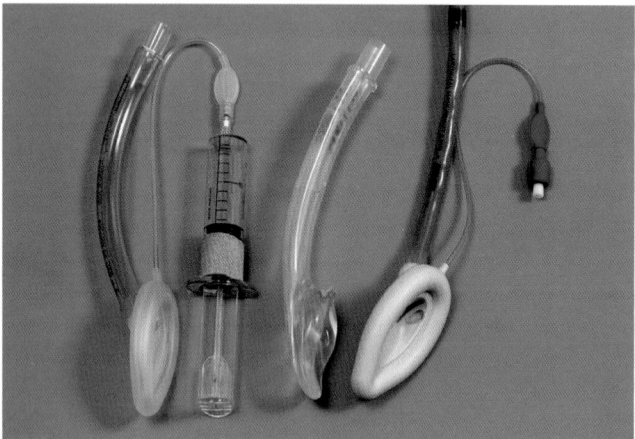

Figure 14.2 The laryngeal mask airway. The laryngeal mask airway (left), I-gel airway (centre) and reinforced laryngeal mask airway (right).

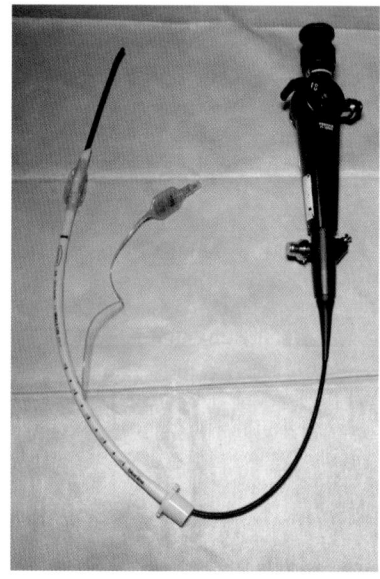

Figure 14.5 A fibreoptic intubating laryngoscope.

Other complications include:

- accidental intubation of a main bronchus;
- trauma to the larynx, trachea or teeth;
- aspiration of vomitus during neuromuscular blockade for intubation;
- disconnection or blockage of the tube;
- delayed tracheal stenosis – in children or after prolonged intubation.

Careful technique, vigilance and patient monitoring minimise these risks.

There are many modified tracheal tube designs including armouring to avoid kinking and the use of non-combustible materials (metal or Teflon) for laser surgery in the airway to avoid potentially fatal fires in the patient's airway.

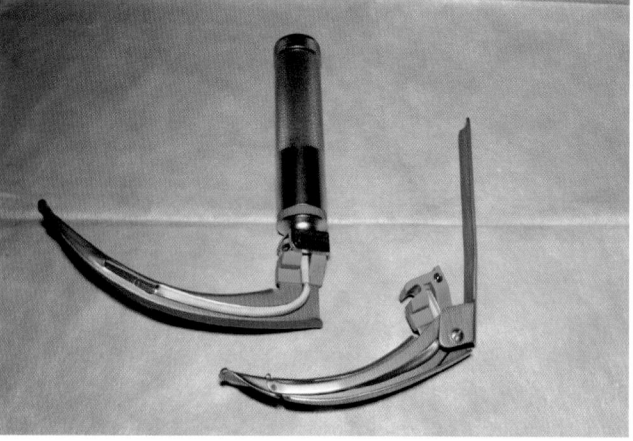

Figure 14.3 The Macintosh laryngoscope with a standard blade (left) and McCoy's modification of the Macintosh blade (right).

Sir Robert Reynolds Macintosh, **1897–1989,** Nuffield Professor of Anaesthetics, The University of Oxford, Oxford, England.

The RAE tube takes it name from the initials of the surnames of the people who introduced it, Wallace Harold Ring, John Adair and Richard Elwyn.

- *Tracheostomy tube.* Anaesthesia and pulmonary ventilation can be safely conducted through a tracheostomy tube using an inflatable cuff for airway control in place of an indwelling silver or fenestrated tracheostomy.
- *Endobronchial tube.* In open thoracic procedures such as pulmonary and oesophageal surgery, selective intubation of a main bronchus facilitates deflation of the lung on the operated side. Its use is also essential to protect the normal lung in the presence of a bronchopleural fistula.
- *Ventilation through a bronchoscope or endotracheal catheter.* The lungs can be ventilated during laryngotracheal surgery or bronchoscopy by intermittent jets of oxygen, which entrain air by the Venturi effect to generate enough pressure and flow to inflate the lungs (Summary box 14.3).

Summary box 14.3

Techniques for maintaining an airway

- Jaw thrust – only suitable for short term
- Guedel airway – holds tongue forwards but does not prevent aspiration
- Laryngeal mask – simple to insert, allows ventilation
- Endotracheal intubation – very secure protection of the airway
- Tracheostomy – used when airway needs protecting for prolonged periods

---

Neuromuscular blockade during surgery

The advent of neuromuscular blockade in the 1940s facilitated many advances in abdominal and thoracic surgery. Pharmacological blockade of neuromuscular transmission provides relaxation of muscles to facilitate surgery and mechanical positive pressure ventilation.

The depolarising muscle relaxant suxamethonium rapidly provides excellent intubating conditions of brief duration; however, it commonly causes postoperative diffuse muscle pains and, rarely, may cause a prolonged muscular block if the patient is deficient in plasma pseudocholinesterase.

The competitive neuromuscular blocking agents such as curare and its modern successors atracurium, cisatracurium, vecuronium and rocuronium share more predictable activity profiles and are less dependent on hepatorenal function for termination of action; however, they produce prolonged effects and, hence, require careful timing of doses so that the patient's muscle power is restored by the end of surgery. A peripheral nerve stimulator is also used to check for adequate depth of blockade during surgery and to confirm satisfactory recovery of neuromuscular function before resumption of spontaneous respiration and extubation of the trachea. It is essential to understand that these drugs are not hypnotic agents and are used as an adjunct to general anaesthesia, which is maintained by intravenous or inhalational anaesthetic agents to avoid any risk of accidental patient awareness.

Haemostasis and blood pressure control

Although the dangers of profound hypotension are well known nowadays, a 20–30% reduction of mean arterial blood pressure

Giovanni Battista Venturi, **1746–1822, Professor of Physics, The University of Modena, Modena, Italy.**

from the awake preoperative level in fit patients is still deemed acceptable, greatly improving the quality of the operative field and reducing total blood loss. Reduction of venous pressure at the wound by correct patient positioning and avoidance of any causes of venous obstruction will prevent excessive bleeding, as will maintenance of satisfactorily deep anaesthesia with slightly reduced arterial carbon dioxide tension.

Hypotensive drugs may be used to produce deliberate controlled hypotension if there is a clear surgical benefit to be obtained. However, preservation of cerebral perfusion and oxygenation must take priority over any other considerations.

Management of temperature during anaesthesia

Vasodilatation, cold infusions of fluid and loss of body heat by radiation and fluid evaporation from open body cavities results in hypothermia under anaesthesia. It is a particular hazard in children because of the high ratio of body surface area to body mass. The elderly are also at particular risk as hypothermia and shivering increase oxygen consumption and vascular resistance, predisposing to myocardial infarction. Careful intraoperative temperature control using warm air blowers and warming blankets and maintenance of fluids for intravenous infusion or irrigation of body cavities or organs (such as the bladder and renal pelvis) to body temperature greatly reduce postoperative morbidity.

Monitoring during anaesthesia

Safety is optimised by the mandatory continuous presence of an adequately trained anaesthetist and equipment for patient monitoring during anaesthesia and cardiopulmonary resuscitation. The basic parameters monitored are inspiratory oxygen concentration, oxygen saturation by pulse oximetry, expiratory carbon dioxide tension, blood pressure and the electrocardiogram. For major surgery, hourly urine volumes and invasive, direct monitoring of the circulation are also used. Ventilators and breathing circuits should all have airway pressure monitors, disconnection alarms and continuous analysis of the oxygen content (with oxygen supply failure alarms). There should also be a measure of anaesthetic concentration in the inspiratory gas mixture (Summary box 14.4).

Summary box 14.4

Tasks of the anaesthetist during anaesthesia

- Muscle relaxation – to allow ventilation and opening of wounds
- Pain control and unconsciousness – to minimise distress to patient
- Minimise blood loss – careful control of blood pressure
- Temperature – avoid hypothermia
- Monitoring – patient safety

Recovery from general anaesthesia

Recovery from general anaesthesia should be closely supervised by trained nursing staff skilled in airway management in an area equipped with the means for resuscitation and adequate monitoring devices. Inadequate breathing after general anaesthesia may result from:

- obstruction of the airway;
- central sedation from opioid drugs or anaesthetic agents;

- hypoxia or hypercarbia of any cause;
- hypocarbia from mechanical overventilation;
- persistent neuromuscular blockade.

An anaesthetist should be readily available to respond to any problem. For the seriously ill patient, a high-dependency unit or intensive care unit may be necessary until the patient's condition is satisfactory and stable.

General anaesthesia for day-case surgery

Driven by financial need and patient preference, day-case management is increasing worldwide, accounting for 70% of procedures in some countries. Although the principles remain the same, day-case patients have to recover rapidly from general anaesthesia and mobilise with the minimum of side-effects. Both longer and more complex operations are now conducted as day cases. Careful selection of patients is important. Coexisting diseases, the nature of the proposed surgery, the availability of a suitable escort and transport home, and domiciliary care all influence the decision as to whether day surgery is appropriate. Well-controlled non-debilitating chronic diseases do not preclude day care. Anaesthetics that promote rapid recovery such as propofol, sevoflurane and desflurane are preferred. Drugs with prolonged depressant central action, including pre-medicant drugs, are avoided. When possible, patients are managed with a laryngeal mask or face mask.

Postoperative analgesia must be given regularly to prevent breakthrough pain and should be strong enough to cope with the pain once the local anaesthetic has worn off. This is especially true in painful procedures such as hernia repair, haemorrhoidectomy, tubal surgery and meniscectomy (Summary box 14.5).

Summary box 14.5

Day or ambulatory surgery

- Being used more and more commonly even for major operations
- Preoperative assessment of social, medical and surgical needs is important
- Anaesthesia needs to be modified for rapid recovery
- Appropriate and regular postoperative analgesia will prevent breakthrough

---

General anaesthesia and cardiopulmonary bypass

The technique is discussed in Chapter 52.

LOCAL ANAESTHESIA

Local anaesthetic drugs may be used to provide anaesthesia on their own by local infiltration, by the use of regional anaesthetic techniques or by providing neuraxial blockade (intrathecal or epidural anaesthesia), or as an adjunct to general anaesthesia by providing pain relief extending to the postoperative period. The choice of local anaesthetic technique depends upon its feasibility for a particular procedure and the patient's willingness and ability to cooperate, as well the surgeon's and anaesthetist's preference. Local anaesthesia may be the reliable and traditional method for some minor surgical procedures but it is not infallible and may be contraindicated by allergy or local infection. Epidural and intrathecal (spinal) anaesthesia are ideal for some operations but may cause vasodilatation and systemic hypotension because they also block the sympathetic nerves.

Complications may be local, such as infection or haematoma, or systemic, if overdosage or accidental intravascular injection leads to toxic blood levels. The latter may manifest as depressed conscious level, convulsions and/or cardiac arrest (particularly bupivacaine), and may be heralded by circumoral paraesthesia and light-headedness. Prilocaine overdosage causes methaemoglobinaemia. Recently introduced local anaesthetics such as ropivacaine and levobupivacaine are claimed to have enhanced cardiovascular safety profiles.

The addition of adrenaline (commonly at a concentration of 1:200 000–1:125 000) to the local anaesthetic solution hastens the onset and prolongs the duration of action and permits a higher dose of drug to be used as it is more slowly absorbed into the circulation. Adrenaline should not be used in hypertensive patients or for patients taking either monoamine oxidase inhibitors or tricyclic antidepressant drugs, as its cardiovascular effects may be potentiated. It is contraindicated in end-arterial locations where there is no collateral circulation, such as fingers and toes or around the retinal artery.

Appropriately skilled personnel and resuscitation and oxygen equipment should always be available when local anaesthetic is being used because of the potential risk of life-threatening complications.

The sensible upper dose limits for the common local anaesthetic agents are given below (Table 14.1):

- *Lignocaine* 3 mg kg^{-1} or lignocaine with adrenaline (1:200 000) 7 mg kg^{-1}. Lignocaine 1% is effective for most sensory blocks. Thus, around 50 ml of lignocaine 1% (10 mg ml^{-1}) with adrenaline can be infiltrated into the tissues of a 70 kg patient.
- *Bupivacaine* 2 mg kg^{-1} (30 ml of 0.5% bupivacaine is more cardiotoxic than lignocaine but has a longer-lasting effect).

Table 14.1 Summary of drugs used for local anaesthesia

Name	Dose limit	Concentration	Comments
Lignocaine	3 mg kg^{-1} 7 mg kg^{-1a}	1%, 2%	Early onset, short acting, good for sensory blocks
Bupivacaine	2 mg kg^{-1}	0.25%, 0.5%	Longer lasting than lignocaine but more cardiotoxic; must never be injected into a vein
Ropivacaine	225 mg	0.2%, 1%	Less cardiotoxic; greater sensory than motor block
Prilocaine	400 mg	1%	Blue-brown skin colour indicates methaemoglobin toxicity
Levobupivacaine	150 mg	0.25%, 0.5%, 0.75%	An isomer of bupivacaine, less cardiotoxic

a   With adrenaline. Adrenaline enhances the effect of the local anaesthetic, prolongs its effect and allows larger doses to be used, but must not be given near end-arteries.

Bupivacaine 0.25% is effective for sensory block against a moderate stimulus. Bupivacaine must never be injected into a vein and is absolutely contraindicated for use in intravenous regional anaesthesia or Bier's block.

- *Ropivacaine* 225 mg. A recent addition, it is claimed to have an improved cardiovascular safety profile while providing relatively greater sensory than motor blockade.
- *Prilocaine* 400 mg. The presence of a blue-brown skin colour indicates methaemoglobin toxicity.
- *Levobupivacaine.* Recently introduced, the levobupivacaine stereoisomer potentially has an improved cardiovascular safety profile while maintaining equivalent potency (Summary box 14.6).

Summary box 14.6

Types of anaesthesia

- Local anaesthetic – suitable for day cases; contraindicated in infection
- Regional block – useful in an emergency when the patient is not starved; gives good postoperative pain relief
- Spinal and epidural anaesthetic – only to be used by an anaesthetist under full sterile conditions; allows on-going postoperative pain relief
- General anaesthetics are now safer and more controllable so still have an important role to play

---

Topical anaesthesia

Topical anaesthetic agents are used on the skin, the urethral mucosa, the nasal mucosa and the cornea. These agents include amethocaine, because it is well absorbed by mucosa; cocaine, for its vasoconstrictive properties; lignocaine; and prilocaine. A lignocaine and prilocaine eutectic mixture (EMLA cream) is commonly used on the skin of children before venepuncture.

Local infiltration

Infiltration of a local anaesthetic drug may be into or around a wound, ideally paying particular attention to neuroanatomical territories and boundaries. It is not necessary to starve the patient preoperatively unless the procedure carries a high risk of intravascular or intrathecal injection. Local infiltration is contraindicated near infection because it not only spreads the infection but is also ineffective, as the acidity produced by infection blocks the action of the drugs. It is also contraindicated in the presence of a clotting disorder as it may result in haemorrhage.

Regional anaesthesia

Regional anaesthesia involves the blockade of major nerve trunks innervating the site of surgery. It is most commonly used for limb, abdominal and thoracic surgery and obstetric analgesia and surgery. It may also be safer to use regional anaesthesia in an emergency when a patient has not been starved as the risk of aspiration of gastric contents is marginally reduced.

Spinal and epidural anaesthesia should only be conducted by anaesthetists using full aseptic techniques in a safe environment. Preoperative patient preparation for elective regional anaesthesia includes that required for general anaesthesia, with

---

August Karl Gustav Bier, 1861–1949, Professor of Surgery, Bonn, (1903–1907), and Berlin, Germany (1907–1932).

---

explanation of the local anaesthetic procedure. The recently introduced subcutaneous low molecular weight heparins (LMWH) for prophylaxis for deep venous thrombosis are longer acting than heparin and appear to have increased the risk of intraspinal haematoma. Epidural and spinal injections (and catheter insertion or removal) should only be performed at least 12 hours after a LMWH dose, and the next LMWH dose should be delayed by at least 2 hours. As with many perioperative management issues, optimal care depends upon close liaison between anaesthetist and surgeon.

Electrocardiogram, pulse oximetry and blood pressure measurements should be performed during regional anaesthesia. Oxygen by face mask should be given to frail or sedated patients during surgery.

If regional anaesthesia fails, general anaesthesia may be necessary. Compensation for an inadequate regional block by heavy sedation carries great dangers including airway obstruction and pulmonary aspiration of gastric contents. These may easily go unrecognised by a single operator; hence it is essential that a doctor other than the operator is present to continuously monitor and resuscitate the patient as necessary. In emergency surgery, regional anaesthesia carries the advantage of preserving the protective laryngeal reflexes, particularly in emergency obstetric anaesthesia, for which epidural or spinal regional anaesthesia is commonly the method of choice. The reduction in blood pressure with spinal and epidural anaesthesia can be advantageous in reducing intraoperative blood loss; however, it is essential to achieve haemostasis before wound closure and restoration of normal blood pressure.

Regional anaesthesia had very clear advantages over general anaesthesia when general anaesthetic agents carried high morbidity and mortality rates. In contemporary practice this advantage is less pronounced or even reversed. Regional anaesthesia does provide excellent analgesia into the postoperative period, reducing the need for centrally acting analgesic agents. In cardiovascular disease, although general anaesthesia with support of the circulation and pulmonary ventilation may confer less hypotension and tachyarrhythmias, exacerbating ischaemic heart disease and resultant angina. However, regional anaesthesia still remains advantageous for patients who have debilitating respiratory disease. The most clear indications for spinal and epidural anaesthesia are in obstetric practice to spare the mother from the risk of pulmonary aspiration because of the full stomach usually present in labour, and also to spare the newborn from the depressant action of the general anaesthetic and analgesic drugs.

Common local anaesthetic techniques

In awake patients the nerve blocks must provide comprehensive numbness throughout the surgical field. The following field blocks are commonly used:

- *Brachial plexus* block for surgery on the upper limb.
- *Field block* for inguinal hernia repair. The iliohypogastric and ilioinguinal nerves are blocked immediately inferomedial to the anterior superior iliac spine. The genitofemoral nerve is infiltrated at the mid-inguinal point and at the pubic tubercle. If a large volume of local anaesthetic is used, the peritoneal sac can be anaesthetised before the incision, but care must be taken to avoid drug toxicity. The line of the skin incision should also be infiltrated with the mixture.
- *Regional block* of the ankle. This can be used for surgery on the toes and minor surgery of the foot.

Intravenous regional anaesthesia (Bier's block)

The arm to be operated on is exsanguinated by elevation and/or compression, and then isolated from the general circulation by the application of a tourniquet inflated to a pressure well in excess of the systolic arterial pressure. The venous system is then filled with local anaesthetic agent, injected via a previously placed indwelling venous cannula. The drug diffuses from the bloodstream into the nerves to produce an effective block. The arm is more suitable for this procedure than the leg because the large volume of drug required for the latter can easily lead to toxicity. The tourniquet must only be deflated after adequate time has elapsed (at least 20 min) to allow for the residual venous drug load to fall to a safe level before it is washed back into the general circulation. Cardiac arrest or convulsions may well occur if the tourniquet is accidentally released before the drug is fixed. This is a particular risk with bupivacaine, which has been banned from use in this procedure. Up to 50 ml of prilocaine 0.5% is recommended as the safest agent to use. A separate medical practitioner should supervise the block and monitor the patient while the surgeon operates (Summary box 14.7).

Summary box 14.7

Bier's block

- Only safe in the upper limb
- Prilocaine is best – bupivacaine must *not* be used
- A second practitioner must be present to oversee the block
- The cuff must not be deflated for 20 min to prevent systemic toxicity

---

Spinal anaesthesia

Spinal anaesthesia in the awake patient is useful for some forms of surgery in the pelvis or lower limbs. Hyperbaric solutions of bupivacaine are injected as a 'single shot' into the cerebrospinal fluid to rapidly produce an intense blockade, usually within 5 min. Autonomic sympathetic blockade results in hypotension, so the patient should be preloaded with intravenous fluids and vasoconstrictor drugs may need to be given. If the hyperbaric solution is allowed to ascend too high, severe hypotension and ventilatory failure occur. This factor limits the use of spinal anaesthesia to surgery below the segmental level of T10. Intrathecal opioid drugs used in combination with local anaesthetics provide better postoperative analgesia but carry a significant risk of respiratory depression.

The incidence of postoperative headache as a result of cerebrospinal fluid leakage through the dural perforation is decreasing with the increasing use of modern needles (very fine with a round or pencil point tip and side aperture) designed to split rather than cut the dural fibres.

Epidural anaesthesia

Epidural anaesthesia is slower in onset than spinal anaesthesia but has the advantage of multiple dosing and prolonged use in the postoperative period as an indwelling catheter may be threaded into the epidural space. Urinary retention is common, necessitating catheterisation of the bladder. Epidural anaesthesia also includes sympathetic blockade but, being slower in onset, the resulting hypotension may be easier to control and can be advantageous for the surgery by reducing blood loss. Epidural anaesthesia used alone does not produce adequate analgesia for surgical intervention but, using a weak solution of bupivacaine or the newer ropivacaine, this technique produces a predominantly sensory block for analgesia after upper abdominal or thoracic surgery. The contemporary trend is to combine weak solutions of local anaesthetic with opioid agents such as the lipid-soluble diamorphine or fentanyl, the latter producing analgesia by their action on the opioid receptors in the spinal cord. However, the potential complication of epidural opioid analgesia is delayed respiratory arrest from rostral spread and central depression, as late as 24 hours after the last dose. Hence, regular monitoring of conscious level and respiratory rate, as well as the facility to immediately reverse the opioid with intravenous naloxone or to resuscitate, are essential prerequisites.

Caudal epidural anaesthesia is produced by injection of the local anaesthetic agent through the sacrococcygeal membrane. Used to supplement general anaesthesia, it provides very effective postoperative pain relief. This analgesic technique is much used in paediatric surgery (Fig. 14.6) (Summary box 14.8).

Summary box 14.8

Epidural block

- Slower action than spinal
- Blood loss in surgery is less
- Allows top-ups and is ideal for postoperative pain
- Epidurals containing opioids need careful monitoring for 24 hours

---

PERIOPERATIVE PAIN RELIEF (ACUTE PAIN MANAGEMENT)

Optimal management of acute postoperative pain requires planning, patient and staff education and tailoring of the regimen to the type of surgery and the needs of the individual patient. Of

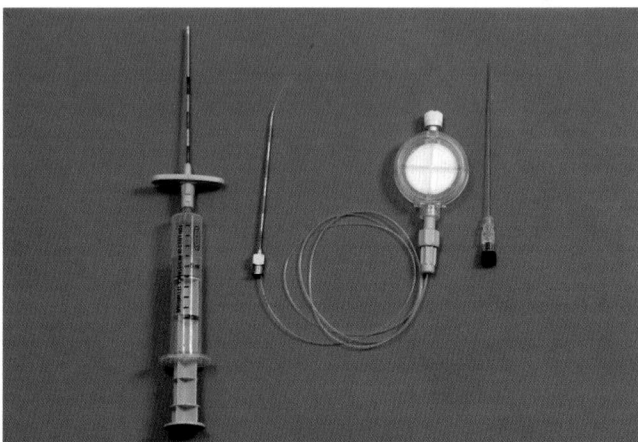

Figure 14.6 Equipment for epidural/spinal anaesthesia. A Touhy needle (curved tip Huber point) for epidural anaesthesia (left), an epidural catheter through a Touhy needle attached to a filter system (centre) and a spinal needle (right).

Edward Boyce Tuohy, **1908–1959, Professor of Anesthesiology, Georgetown Medical Center, Washington, DC (1947–1952), and later at the University of Southern California Medical School, Los Angeles, CA, USA.**
Ralph L. Huber, **1890–1953, a Dentist of Seattle, WA, USA.**

late, pain management has had to adapt to newer less invasive or destructive surgical techniques.

Patients vary greatly (up to eightfold) in their requirement for analgesia, even after identical surgical procedures. Undertreatment results in unacceptable levels of pain with tachycardia, hypertension, vasoconstriction and 'splinting' of the affected part. Painful abdominal and thoracic wounds restrict inspiration, leading to tachypnoea, small tidal volumes and inhibition of effective coughing and mobilisation. This predisposes to chest infection, delayed mobilisation, deep venous thrombosis, muscle wasting and pressure sores.

However, too much analgesic drug increases the risks of side-effects such as nausea, vomiting, somnolence and dizziness or, if greatly in excess, severe central effects including depressed consciousness and respiration. This can be avoided by sensible initial dosing, followed by titration until the patient is comfortable. Exaggerated fears of opioid-induced central depression and addiction have led all too commonly to the reluctance of staff to prescribe and administer adequate doses of opioids. Intermittent intramuscular dosing also leads to delays in administration of the 'controlled' opioids. The failure of pain relief is compounded by the slow time to onset of action.

A joint working party report of the Royal Colleges of Anaesthetists and Surgeons, *Pain after Surgery*, recommended the establishment of acute pain services comprising medical and nursing specialists to oversee the implementation of guidelines for practice, including the routine recording of pain levels and the education of both staff and patients. In hospital practice in the USA, a recent national initiative called 'Pain, the fifth vital sign' requires regular pain measurement, with staff to be alerted in the event of high scores. The joint working party report also encouraged the use of combined 'multimodal' analgesia comprising local anaesthesia and simple analgesics such as paracetamol (acetaminophen) and non-steroidal anti-inflammatory drugs (NSAIDs) with opioid drugs (Summary box 14.9).

Summary box 14.9

Acute postoperative pain relief

- Requires an expert team approach
- Pain levels must be measured regularly
- Analgesia is best given before pain breaks through
- A combination of analgesics gives best results
- Opioids should not be withheld
- The dose of analgesia used must be adequate to control the pain

---

Simple analgesic agents

In minor surgery and when the patient is able to eat after surgery, NSAIDs and paracetamol may be sufficient. Reye's syndrome, metabolic acidosis and hepatotoxicity in children have made paracetamol a preferable drug to aspirin in the younger age group. Within its dose recommendations paracetamol is a very safe and effective analgesic and is now widely available in intravenous formulation. Codeine phosphate is commonly favoured after intracranial surgery because of its intermediate respiratory depressant effect; however, it should not be given intravenously as it can then cause profound hypotension. Constipation is also not uncommon with codeine.

Ralph Douglas Kenneth Reye, 1912–1977, Director of Pathology, The Royal Alexandra Hospital for Children, Sydney, NSW, Australia, described this syndrome in 1963.

NSAIDs are useful as the main analgesic for moderate pain or as adjuvant therapy with opioids for severe pain. They cause non-specific cyclo-oxygenase (COX) inhibition, which results in side-effects including loss of gastric cytoprotection, renal homeostasis and platelet function. Rectal and intravenous diclofenac or intravenous ketorolac are commonly used NSAIDs in the perioperative period. Patients with a tendency towards peptic ulceration may need cover with proton pump inhibitors or misoprostol during analgesic treatment with anti-inflammatory agents.

Specific COX-2 inhibitor anti-inflammatory analgesics have the particular advantage in perioperative use of maintained platelet function but they may be contraindicated in some conditions such as ischaemic heart disease.

Stronger analgesic agents

With adjuvant analgesics in combination, regular intramuscular morphine injection can provide effective treatment for the majority of surgical patients. However, there are more sophisticated methods of pain management:

- *Patient-controlled analgesia (PCA)*. Opioid analgesia is injected intravenously or through an epidural cannula. The patient is trained to give a bolus dose of drug by pressing a button on a machine. The medical staff preset the strength, frequency and total dose of drug, which can be administered by the PCA machine over a given time. This method is popular with patients as they have control over their pain, while delays in administration of doses are avoided.
- *Local anaesthetic blocks*. These give excellent short-term analgesia but they require skill and have a small failure rate. Continuous catheter techniques provide prolonged pain relief but are generally only appropriate for in-patients.

Special methods of pain relief used under close supervision are:

- continuous epidural anaesthesia with opiate or local anaesthetic drugs;
- spinal opioids – generally very useful for appropriate types of surgery but again they require skill and are limited by concerns over severe respiratory depression.

Continuous intravenous or subcutaneous infusions of opioid analgesia carry the risk of overdosage in the more sensitive patient but are safe in the context of a continuously monitored high-dependency environment and careful dose titration.

Effective postoperative pain relief encourages early mobilisation and hospital discharge.

The methods described above can also be used for managing the pain of acute trauma (Summary box 14.10).

Summary box 14.10

Techniques for postoperative pain relief

- Regular intramuscular injections – may get pain breakthrough
- Local anaesthetic block – ideal if it works
- Indwelling epidural – good pain control; opioids may depress respiration
- Continuous infusions – reduce oscillations in pain relief but risk overdose
- Patient-controlled analgesia – pain relief titrated to patient's needs

---

CHAPTER 14 | ANAESTHESIA AND PAIN RELIEF

Chronic pain management

In surgical practice, the patient with chronic pain may present for treatment of the cause (e.g. pancreatitis) or have concomitant pathology. Surgery itself may have been the cause of the now chronic symptom, as acute pain may progress to chronic pain. There is a developing belief that inadequate treatment of acute pain may make this situation more likely.

Chronic, intractable pain may be of malignant or non-malignant origin and of several types:

- *Nociceptive pain.* Pain may result from musculoskeletal disorders or cancer activating cutaneous nociceptors. Prolonged ischaemic or inflammatory processes result in sensitisation of peripheral nociceptors and altered activity in the central nervous system leading to exaggerated responses in the dorsal horn of the spinal cord. The widened area of hyperalgesia and increased sensitivity (allodynia) has been attributed to increased transmission of afferent pain impulses consequent upon this spinal cord dynamic plasticity.
- *Neuropathic (or neurogenic) pain.* Pain is caused by the dysfunction of peripheral or central nerves (excluding the 'physiological' pain due to noxious stimulation of the nerve terminals). Neuropathic pain is classically 'burning', 'shooting' or 'stabbing' and may be associated with allodynia, numbness and diminished thermal sensation. It is poorly responsive to opioids. Examples include trigeminal neuralgia, metatarsalgia and postherpetic and diabetic neuropathy. Monoaminergic, tricyclic and anticonvulsant drugs are the mainstay of treatment.
- *Psychogenic pain.* Psychological factors play a greater or lesser role in many chronic pain syndromes. Whatever the primary cause may have been, depressive illness and chronic pain may exacerbate each other.

The treatment of pain of malignant origin differs from that of pain of a benign cause, which may be the more difficult to overcome. Drugs should preferably be taken by mouth, but the patient must be regularly reassessed to ensure that analgesia remains adequate as the disease process changes (Summary box 14.11).

Summary box 14.11

Chronic pain

- Inadequate control of acute pain may lead to chronic pain
- Chronic stimulation of nociceptors appears to produce sensitisation
- Dysfunction in nerves produces neuropathic pain
- Psychogenic pain – depression causes and is caused by chronic pain

---

Pain control in malignant disease

In intractable pain, the underlying principle of treatment is to encourage independence of the patient and an active life in spite of the symptom. The main guide to the management of cancer pain is provided by the World Health Organization, which portrays three levels of treatment – the 'pain stepladder':

- first rung: *simple analgesics* – aspirin, paracetamol, NSAIDs, tricyclic drugs or anticonvulsant drugs;
- second rung: *intermediate strength opioids* – codeine, tramadol or dextropropoxyphene;
- third rung: *strong opioids* – morphine (pethidine has been withdrawn from the second edition of the World Health Organization guide).

Oral opiate analgesia is necessary when the less powerful analgesic agents no longer control pain on movement or prevent the patient from sleeping. Fear that the patient may develop an addiction to opiates is usually not justified in malignant disease.

Oral morphine can be prescribed in short-acting liquid or tablet form and should be administered regularly every 4 hours until an adequate dose of drug has been titrated to control the pain over 24 hours. Once this is established, the daily dose can be divided into two separate administrations of enteric-coated, slow-release morphine tablets (MST morphine) every 12 hours. Additional short-acting morphine can then be used to cover episodes of 'breakthrough pain'. Nausea is a problem that is encountered early in the use of morphine treatment and it may need to be controlled with antiemetic agents, e.g. haloperidol, methotrimeprazine, metoclopramide or ondansetron. Nausea does not usually persist, but constipation is frequently a persistent complication requiring regular prevention by laxatives.

The infusion of *subcutaneous, intravenous, intrathecal or epidural opiate drugs* is necessary if a patient is unable to take oral drugs. Subcutaneous infusion of diamorphine is simple and effective to administer. Epidural infusions of diamorphine can be used in mobile patients with the aid of an external pump. Intrathecal infusions are prone to infection, but implantable reservoirs with pumps programmed by external computers are being used for long-term intrathecal analgesia. Intravenous narcotic agents may then be reserved for acute crises, such as pathological fractures.

Neurolytic techniques in cancer pain should only be used if the life expectancy is limited and the diagnosis is certain. The useful procedures are:

- subcostal phenol injection for a rib metastasis;
- coeliac plexus neurolytic block with alcohol for pain of pancreatic, gastric or hepatic cancer – image intensifier control is essential;
- intrathecal neurolytic injection of hyperbaric phenol – this technique is useful only if facilities for percutaneous cordotomy are not available because it can damage motor pathways;
- percutaneous anterolateral cordotomy to divide the spinothalamic ascending pain pathway – it is a highly effective technique in experienced hands, selectively eliminating pain and temperature sensation in a specific limited area.

Alternative strategies include:

- the use of anti-pituitary hormone drugs such as tamoxifen and cyproterone, which enables effective pharmacological therapy for the pain of widespread metastases instead of pituitary ablation surgery;
- palliative radiotherapy, which can be most beneficial for the relief of pain in metastatic disease;
- adjuvant drugs such as corticosteroids, which reduce cerebral oedema or inflammation around a tumour and may be useful in symptom control; tricyclic antidepressants, anticonvulsants and occasionally flecainide are also used to reduce the pain of nerve injury (Summary box 14.12).

Summary box 14.12

Techniques for managing chronic pain

- Oral opioids – initial nausea, long-term constipation
- Opioid infusions – useful if the patient cannot take drugs orally
- Neurolysis – only in limited life expectancy

Pain control in benign disease

Surgical patients may have persistent pain from a variety of disorders including chronic inflammatory disease, recurrent infection, degenerative bone or joint disease, nerve injury and sympathetic dystrophy. Chronic pain may result from persistent excitation of the nociceptive pathways in the central nervous system, invoking mechanisms such as spontaneous firing of pain signals at N-methyl-D-aspartate receptors in the ascending pathways. Such activity responds poorly to opiates; neuroablative surgery is unlikely to produce prolonged benefit and may make the pain worse.

As is well known, amputation of limbs may result in phantom limb pain, the likelihood being further increased if the limb was painful before surgery. Continuous regional local anaesthetic blockade (epidural or brachial plexus), established before operation and continued postoperatively for a few days, is believed to effectively reduce the establishment of phantom pain.

The following are treatments for chronic pain of benign origin:

- *Local anaesthetic and steroid injections.* These can be effective around an inflamed nerve and they reduce the cycle of constant pain transmission with consequent muscle spasm. Epidural injections are used for the pain of nerve root irritation associated with minor disc prolapse. This treatment should be in association with active physiotherapy to promote mobility.
- *Nerve stimulation procedures.* Acupuncture, transcutaneous nerve stimulation and the neurosurgical implantation of dorsal column electrodes aim to increase endorphin production in the central nervous system altering pain transmission.
- *Nerve decompression.* In patients who are fit for craniotomy, decompression of the trigeminal nerve at craniotomy is now performed for trigeminal neuralgia rather than percutaneous coagulation of the trigeminal ganglion.
- *Treatment of pain dependent on sympathetic nervous system activity.* Even minor trauma and surgery (often of a limb) can provoke chronic burning pain, allodynia, trophic changes and resultant disuse. The syndrome has been attributed to excessive sympathetic adrenergic activity inducing vasoconstriction and abnormal nociceptive transmission. Management may include:
  - a test response to systemic α-adrenergic blockade using intravenous phentolamine;
  - local anaesthetic injection of the stellate ganglion or lumbar sympathetic chain;
  - intravenous regional sympathetic blockade using guanethidine under tourniquet – this is now controversial as consistent evidence to confirm efficacy has not emerged, and some centres have abandoned this method.

- *Percutaneous chemical lumbar sympathectomy with phenol under radiographic control.* This is practised by both surgeons and anaesthetists for relief of rest pain in advanced ischaemic disease of the legs. It can also promote the healing of ischaemic ulcers by improving peripheral blood flow.
- *Drugs in chronic non-malignant pain.* Paracetamol and NSAIDs are the mainstay of musculoskeletal pain treatment, but NSAIDs are handicapped by gastrointestinal intolerance and peptic ulceration. These carry significant levels of non-compliance, contraindication and morbidity. Specific COX-2 inhibition, with preservation of protective COX-1 activity, promises to improve tolerability and safety in NSAID treatment. The tricyclic antidepressant drugs and anticonvulsant agents are often useful for diminishing the pain of nerve injury, although side-effects can prove troublesome and reduce compliance. Opioid analgesic drugs have been more commonly prescribed in more severe and debilitating non-malignant chronic pain with the advent of slow-release oral preparations of morphine and oxycodone and the development of transcutaneous patches delivering fentanyl and buprenorphine. Combinations of drugs often prove useful to achieve the optimum efficacy with minimal side-effects.

In the management of chronic pain of benign cause, a multidisciplinary approach by a team of medical and nursing staff working with pain specialists, psychologists, physiotherapists and occupational therapists can often achieve much more benefit than the use of powerful drugs. Multidisciplinary pain management programmes have been devised to help the chronic benign pain patients who do not respond to conventional means. They can help a number of patients to cope with the pain and maintain a higher quality of life (Summary box 14.13).

Summary box 14.13

Techniques for managing chronic pain in benign disease

- Local blocks
- Transcutaneous nerve stimulators
- Nerve decompression
- Amputation – only with good pain control before and after surgery
- Encourage activity
- Antidepressants
- A team approach is important

FURTHER READING

Australian and New Zealand College of Anaesthetists and Faculty of Pain Medicine (2005) *Acute Pain Management: Scientific Evidence*, 2nd edn. ANZCA, Melbourne.

Rawal, N. (ed.) (1998) *Management of Acute and Chronic Pain*. BMJ Books, London.

Wildsmith, I. and Armitage, E.N. (eds) (1990) *Principles and Practice of Regional Anaesthesia*. Churchill Livingstone, Edinburgh.

CHAPTER 14 | ANAESTHESIA AND PAIN RELIEF

Care in the operating room

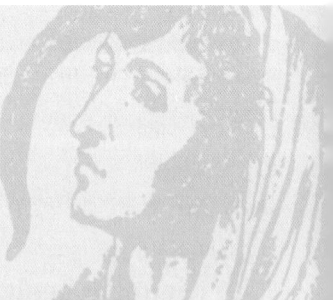

LEARNING OBJECTIVES

To understand:
- How to prepare a patient for theatre
- The process of gloving and gowning
- The process of preparation and draping the patient

- Behaviour in the operating room
- The process of writing an operative note

First do no harm

Hippocrates

PREOPERATIVE PREPARATION IMMEDIATELY BEFORE SURGERY

The patient should be seen by both the surgeon and the anaesthetist before any pre-medication is given.

1 The patient's identity should be confirmed and the patient should be asked to confirm what surgery is being carried out. The case notes should agree with this and with what is written on the operating schedule.
2 A check should be made that there has been no change in the patient's condition since they were last seen and, if the patient's condition has changed, this needs to be recorded.
3 Consent. The patient should be asked if they want the consent process to be repeated and, even if not, they should be asked whether they have any questions and whether they are happy to proceed with surgery. This should be recorded in the notes.
4 All relevant results, investigations and imaging must be available.
5 Adequate preoperative planning should have been undertaken and preferably recorded in the notes.
6 A check should be made for any sepsis (skin, teeth, urine and chest).
7 If there is the possibility of any neurovascular complications, the neurovascular status should also be recorded at this stage.
8 The side to be operated on should be marked with indelible pen.
9 The surgical area should be shaved either at this time or immediately before the incision is made (Summary box 15.1).

Hippocrates, c460–c375 BC, was a Greek Physician and Surgeon who is regarded by common consent to be 'The Father of Medicine'. He was born on the island of Cos off Turkey, and probably died about 375 BC.

Summary box 15.1

Preoperative checks with the patient

- Patient's name
- Condition
- Consent – mark side
- All investigations available
- Sepsis
- Pre-existing complications

Surgeon's preparation for the operation

All surgeons will have an envelope or ceiling to their surgical abilities, which is unique to them. A surgeon should only operate if he/she is capable of performing the surgery safely in the circumstances.

The surgeon must aim to optimise the patient's procedure by adequate preparation. This is highlighted in the traditional military saying: 'the seven "Ps" – prior preparation and planning prevents profoundly poor performance'. A simple measure of how well the preparation has been for an operation is the number of times that a runner needs to be sent out of the operating room to fetch another implant or piece of equipment during the actual operation.

Preoperative planning

Preoperative planning should cover all of the aspects of the surgical process. The preoperative planning process may be very brief and require minimal time in the case of routine, frequently undertaken and minor procedures, or it can be complex and prolonged with templating of radiographs and a pre-written surgical contingency plan for each phase of the surgical process.

Theatre team's preparation for the operation

The theatre team should be given as much notice as possible for the proposed operation. Every hospital and operating department will have a policy for the booking and scheduling of theatre cases, both for elective and emergency cases. Clearly, elective cases will be relatively easier to prepare for because the theatre team have more notice. Children are usually put first on operating lists to reduce the anxiety created by waiting. Diabetics and other patients whose conditions are potentially labile should also be put early on the list. Otherwise, the order of the list needs to be balanced carefully between the wishes of the surgeon, the anaesthetist and the operating and ward staff, as well as the patient.

Pre- and perioperative communication

Communication is one of the keys to good leadership and teamwork. The whole surgical team should be aware of the surgical plan on a 'need to know basis'. This includes the patient, ward staff, porters and the anaesthetic, surgical and recovery teams.

The theatre list

The theatre list should have as a header the date and the details of the theatre, surgeon and anaesthetist. For each operation the patient's name and number, the ward that they will be coming from, the operation title and the side of surgery, if appropriate, should be given. If a specific implant or equipment is required this must be specified. The need for other special equipment such as image intensification, a cell saver or a specific operating table should also be recorded. It is also helpful to note whether blood is available. It is a good idea to go over the list face-to-face with the theatre staff at least a day before surgery to make sure that nothing has been forgotten and that there are no further questions. This will be especially important for a complex or rare procedure, in which there may need to be a great deal of verbal communication of every aspect of the procedure, for example patient positioning, the position of the table in the room, which instrument sets are required and what type of dressing will be applied.

The anaesthetist should be aware of the operative procedure to estimate the effect on the physiology of the patient. This may affect the type of anaesthetic chosen. The need for preoperative prophylactic antibiotics should be discussed well in advance so that any antibiotic can be administered at an appropriate time. Any other possible requirements such as blood transfusion, platelet infusion or anti-haemophiliac fraction administration should be discussed with the anaesthetist before starting the operative procedure.

Supporting services, such as pathology for frozen sections or radiology for intraoperative imaging, will all appreciate as much notice as possible so that they can respond without delay (Summary box 15.2).

Summary box 15.2

Theatre staff preparation

- Operating list (order of patients)
- Special needs (implants and equipment)
- Cross-matched blood, imaging and investigations
- Extra staff (radiology, pathology)

Induction of anaesthesia

Before the patient is anaesthetised it is important that the patient is once again checked with regard to the following:

- the patient's name and identity label should be checked and confirmed;
- the nature of the operation should be confirmed with the patient;
- any dentures should be removed and any rings taped;

- the marking on the limb to be operated on should be confirmed;
- the appropriate consent form should be checked;
- preoperative antibiotics should be given.

Once the patient is anaesthetised the following can be undertaken:

- the patient is catheterised if indicated;
- the surgical site and monopolar diathermy site may require shaving in the hirsute patient; this is best carried out at this time rather than hours or the day before to prevent skin colonisation;
- a monopolar diathermy pad is applied if necessary (see below);
- a tourniquet is applied if appropriate (see Tourniquets);
- in some operating departments a 'pre-prep' or 'pre-scrub' using either soapy disinfectant or standard surgical skin preparation fluid may be undertaken.

The following general measures should be taken for the safe and effective use of diathermy:

- shave excess hair before applying the diathermy plate;
- make sure that the patient is not touching any earthed metal objects;
- ensure good contact between the patient and the plate, over an area of good muscle mass;
- check the plate if the patient is moved during surgery;
- place the plate as close as possible to the operative site;
- ensure that all connections to the generator are made before switching it on; always check the patient's skin at the site of the return electrode for signs of damage (Summary box 15.3).

Summary box 15.3

Positioning on the table

- The diathermy plate must be secure and well positioned
- The patient must be securely held on the table in the correct position
- There should be no contact between the patient and any metal surface
- All pressure areas should be protected

Tourniquets

The majority of limb tourniquets in use in contemporary practice are pneumatic tourniquets.

A tourniquet can and should be sized for the surgery to be undertaken. Small tourniquets can be used for digits, the simplest being either a rubber Penrose drain or the finger of a surgical glove with a small cut made in the tip; the finger of the glove is rolled down to exsanguinate the digit and then act as the tourniquet.

The skin underlying the tourniquet should be protected by either a specific tourniquet protector or some form of wool bandage as shown in Fig. 15.1a–c.

Most limb tourniquets are non-sterile, but sterile limb tourniquets are available and the smaller digit tourniquets are applied in the sterile field.

Charles Bingham Penrose, **1862–1925, Professor of Gynaecology, The University of Pennsylvania, Philadelphia, PA, USA, described this type of drain in 1890.**

Tourniquet application

An appropriately applied tourniquet, as shown in Fig. 15.1b, will minimise complications.

- Distal neurovascular status must be checked before inflation. If there is any sign of distal neuropathy or peripheral vascular disease (especially calcification of arteries) a tourniquet must not be used.
- The tourniquet must be placed as proximally as possible.
- The underbandaging or cover should be applied to the skin without creases.
- The tourniquet must be placed snugly enough so as not to slide down the limb but not so tight that it impedes exsanguination.
- An additional broad tape can be used to prevent surgical preparation solution from running under the tourniquet and causing skin damage.
- The distal limb can be exsanguinated before inflating the tourniquet if a completely blood-free field is needed (Fig. 15.1c). Care should be taken not to damage the skin with an Esmarch bandage wound on too tightly.

- As soon as the tourniquet is inflated then the time should be noted and arrangements made for a warning to be given to the surgeon as soon as that time exceeds 1 hour.
- Application of a safe tourniquet is a skilled process and is ultimately the surgeon's responsibility.
- It is also the responsibility of the surgeon to ensure that the tourniquet has been removed and that distal sensation and circulation has returned. This must be recorded in the notes (Summary box 15.4).

Summary box 15.4

Tourniquet

- ■ Note the distal neurovascular status before application
- ■ Care with position and padding
- ■ Exsanguinate the limb before inflation
- ■ Note the time of inflation
- ■ Deflate after 1 hour
- ■ Check return of circulation and sensation after deflation

---

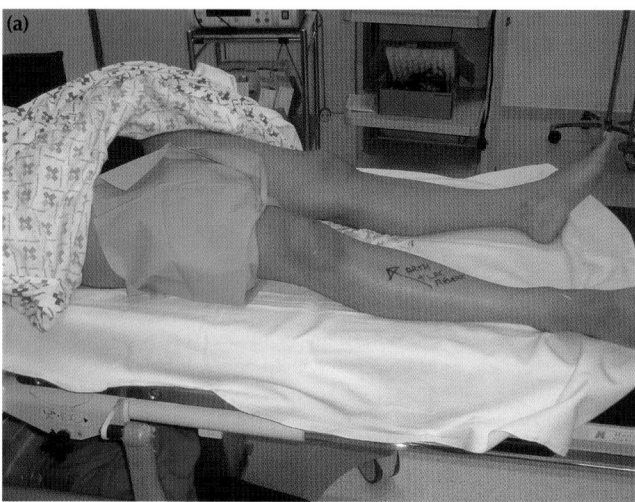

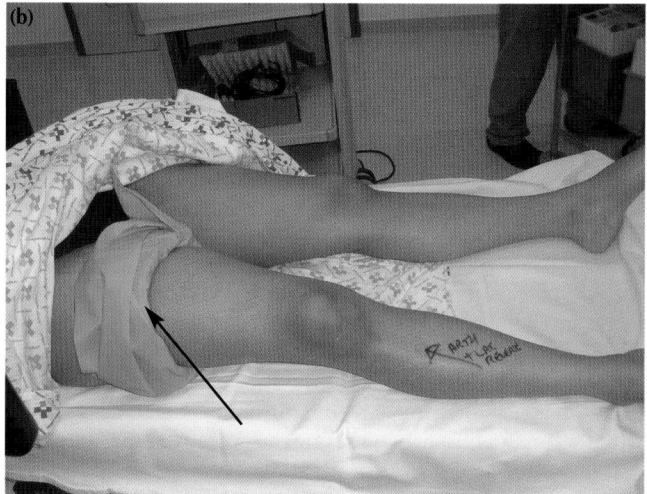

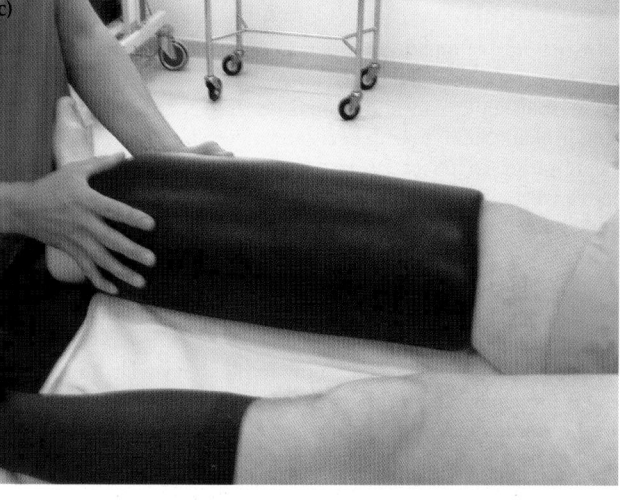

Figure 15.1 Tourniquet and tourniquet dressing. (a) Poor placement, too low – interfering with operative field. (b) Optimal placement of the tourniquet using a single-use tourniquet cover, which protects the skin under the tourniquet and has an adhesive strip to prevent ingress of preparation solution (arrow). This tourniquet is less likely to slip and provides a much larger skin preparation field, important as the patient is undergoing knee surgery. (c) Rhys-Davies exsanguinator.

Johann Friedrich August von Esmarch, **1823–1908, Professor of Clinical Surgery, Kiel, Germany,** devised this type of bandage whilst working as a military surgeon during the Franco–Prussian war (1870–71), and described its use in 1873.

Tourniquet complications

- Excessive tourniquet time causes both local pressure and distal ischaemic effects, with nerve damage and even compartment syndrome. Tourniquets should usually be let down after 1 hour unless close to the end of a procedure. They can then be reinflated after 5–10 min for a further hour.
- If the tourniquet pressure is inadvertently set too high, nerve and muscle damage beneath the cuff itself will occur. The generally recommended pressure level in adults is 200–250 mmHg for the upper limb (or 100 over systolic blood pressure) and 300–350 mmHg for the lower limb (or 150–200 over systolic blood pressure).
- Chemical burn or blistering from skin preparation leaking under the tourniquet.
- Tourniquet failure. This is generally the result of inadequate application of the tourniquet itself and is rarely caused by failure of the cuff or machine (which should be checked regularly). Failure may lead to some arterial inflow but with blocked venous outflow; this causes venous engorgement of the surgical field. The cuff will need removing at once and then reapplying if necessary.

THE OPERATION

Transfer and patient set-up

Transfer of patient from bed to operating table should be slow and smooth, ideally under the joint supervision of the anaesthetist and the surgeon as shown in Fig. 15.2. Protective gloves should be worn throughout the handling of the patient. This process can be assisted by the use of sliding boards or rollers carefully placed under the patient at the time of transfer, which are then removed until the end of surgery.

The patient should be firmly held on the table especially if the lateral position is needed for the operative procedure. All of the pressure areas should be well covered and protected, and limbs should be positioned to ensure that no bony prominence, vessels or nerves are compressed. Extra precautions should be taken with high-risk patients such as the elderly, as well as with excessively thin and obese patients.

No part of the skin surface should be in contact with any metal if diathermy is to be used.

Patients and theatre staff will need gonad and thyroid protection with lead shields if imaging is to be performed during the surgery.

Extensions of the operating table, e.g. arm board or leg holder, should be positioned either by the surgeon or by one of the team under appropriate supervision (see Fig. 15.3). The patient is then 'hooked-up' to the monitoring, intravenous infusion, diathermy and tourniquet apparatus as appropriate prior to skin preparation and draping of the operation site. A final check should now be made to ensure that the patient is safe on the table, as he/she will need to keep still for a given time period and may not be able to communicate or even feel developing problems because of the anaesthesia. This protection relates to the following:

- *Skin.* The operating table will be padded but additional soft padding under the back, buttocks, elbows and heels may be required, dependent on the patient's position for surgery.
- *Limbs* that are uninvolved in surgery, e.g. the arms, should be protected by arm boards with padding to further protect the ulnar nerve at the elbow. Legs in the lithotomy holders may need additional padding and bandaging to prevent movement of the limbs or pressure effects, both of which may cause tissue damage.
- *Side supports* may be needed to stop the patient sliding off the table if the patient is to be placed into a semi-decubitus lateral position.
- *Eyelids* may be taped to protect the corneas.

Asepsis

No operating room can be kept completely free of bacteria and, therefore, the risk of a wound becoming infected from contamination is always present. However, the risk can be minimised by strict theatre discipline.

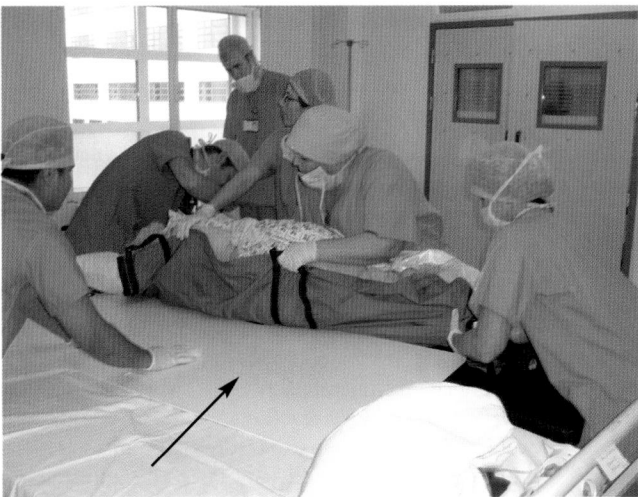

Figure 15.2 Patient transfer. Enough personnel are available to undertake the transfer. The anaesthetist supervises and protects the head, neck and airway. The patient is rolled and a sliding board (arrow) is placed under the patient and undersheet or canvas, which will allow the patient to slide across to the bed in a controlled fashion. Care is being taken by all of the team members to protect the whole patient.

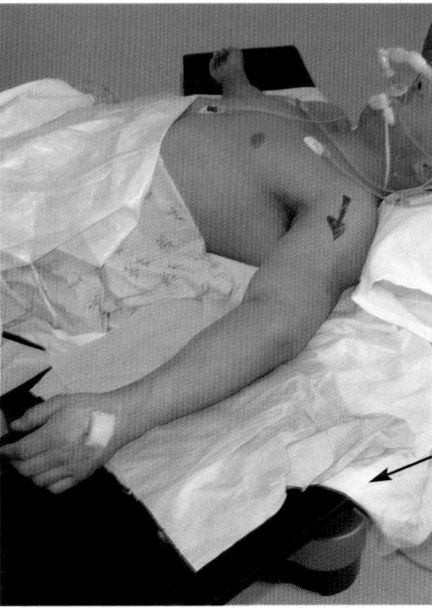

Figure 15.3 An example of an additional table attachment. The patient on an operating table with an arm board attached (arrow).

CHAPTER 15 | CARE IN THE OPERATING ROOM

Scrubbing

'Scrubbing up' is the process of washing the hands and arms prior to donning a gown and gloves, to minimise the microbial loads on parts of the surgical staff that might come into contact with the patient. Time spent scrubbing varies from unit to unit but as a general rule surgeons in training should usually start scrubbing before, and finish after, the senior surgeon. The commonest solutions used for hand-washing in the UK are 2% chlorhexidine gluconate or 7.5% povidone-iodine.

Excessive time or vigour in scrubbing may cause breakdown of the skin with an increased risk of infection. As a result, some centres are now adopting the use of water-free, spirit-based antiseptic solutions.

Scrub technique

1 Preparation before scrubbing:
   * You should not scrub if you have an open wound or an infection. (Uninfected cuts or abrasions can be covered after a routine scrub-up process by applying a sterile clear dressing before gloving.)
   * All jewellery on the hands should be removed.
2 A theatre hat, mask and eye protection should be fitted so that no hair is exposed and you are protected from splashback.
3 A sterile scrubbing brush and nail cleaner are used for 1–2 min to remove dirt from under the nails and from deep creases in the skin.
4 The hands are then washed systematically, paying special attention to the clefts between the fingers. This should be carried out on at least two further occasions, extending up the forearms to just below the elbows (see Fig. 15.4a). After applying disinfectant, the arms are washed from distal to proximal, with hands up and elbows flexed to avoid/minimise any contamination from the more proximal 'unclean' areas. The scrubbing surgeon in Fig. 15.4 demonstrates the correct position for scrubbing.
5 Following the final rinse the hands and arms should be raised to face level, away from the body. This allows water to drop from the elbows.
6 The hands and arms should be dried using a sterile towel for each side. Drying with each towel should start with the fingers and work across the hand and up the arm. The towel should then be discarded (see Fig. 15.4b).
7 The first scrub up of the day, therefore, should take about 5 min from start to drying.
8 If the surgeon stays within the theatre suite and there are no significant external contacts or contamination, subsequent scrub up will be shorter, with no need for the use of the nail cleaner or brush.

If the scrubbing procedure is interrupted, e.g. by touching the tap, the scrubbing procedure should be restarted. This is a common problem, particularly for those unused to the technique (Summary box 15.5).

Summary box 15.5

Scrubbing

■ Do not scrub if you have an infection
■ Make sure all hair is covered and that you are protected from splashes
■ Start scrubbing before, and finish after, the senior surgeon
■ Dry hands from distal to proximal

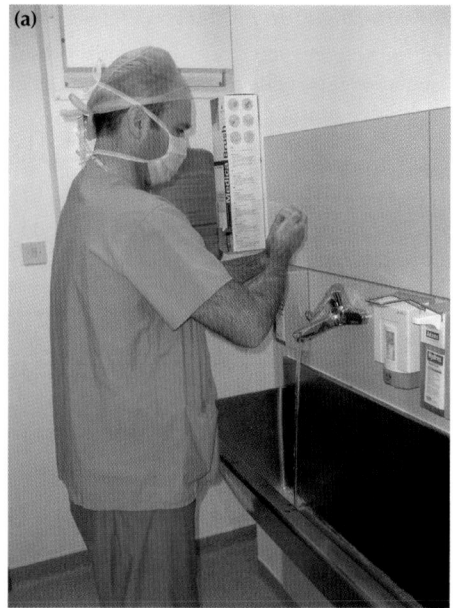

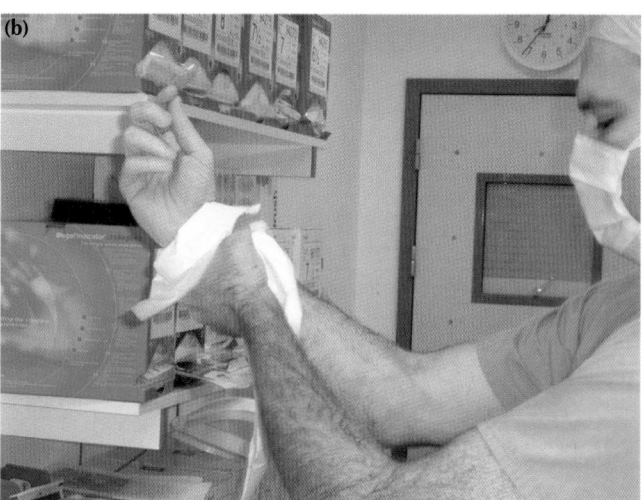

Figure 15.4 (a and b) Scrubbing up.

Types of scrub disinfectant solutions

Chlorhexidine gluconate has a residual effect and is effective for more than 4 hours. It has potent antiseptic activity against Gram-positive and Gram-negative organisms and some viruses but only moderate activity against the tubercle bacillus.

Iodine has some residual effects but these are not sustained for more than 4 hours. It is highly bactericidal, fungicidal and viricidal. There is some activity against bacterial spores and good activity against the tubercle bacillus. The iodine agents penetrate cell walls to produce anti-microbial effects. They may be irritating to the skin or cause allergic reactions.

The alcohols are highly effective, rapidly acting anti-microbial agents with broad-spectrum activity. They are effective in destroying Gram-positive and Gram-negative bacteria, fungi, viruses and tubercle bacilli, but are not sporicidal. Alcohol is an

---

Hans Christian Joachim Gram, **1853–1938, Professor of Pharmacology (1891–1900) and of Medicine (1900–1923),** Copenhagen, Denmark, described this method of staining bacteria in 1884.

inexpensive anti-microbial agent and one of the most widely used skin antiseptics, especially preceding subcutaneous and intramuscular injections and venepunctures; a 10-s drying after application enhances its effectiveness. Some alcohol scrub preparations will therefore avoid the use of water washing altogether, using a similar sequence of repeated hand and forearm washes.

Gowning

- The folded gown is lifted away from the surrounding wrapping and kept away from the trolley.
- The gown is grasped firmly at the neckline and allowed to unfold completely, with the inside facing the wearer.
- The arms are inserted into the armholes simultaneously (the front of the gown is not be touched with ungloved hands).
- Hands should stay inside the cuffs while gloving.
- The circulating theatre nurse should secure the gown at the neck and waist.
- If a wrap-around type of gown is worn, these ties are secured with the help of the circulating nurse once gloves are on.

Gloving

Gloves have two important functions. They prevent contamination of the surgical wound and they also protect the scrub team from the blood and body fluids of the patient. Double gloving

reduces the chance of a breach in this protection and allows the outer gloves to be changed if damaged. Double gloving is now a standard part of 'universal precautions' for minimising the transmission of human immunodeficiency virus (HIV) and hepatitis B and C (Fig. 15.5).

Once gowned and gloved, the hands must remain above waist level at all times, and when not involved in a sterile procedure the hands should be held together at chest height (do not tuck them into the armpits or dangle them!). Gloves are frequently perforated during surgical procedures, thus increasing the risk for surgical site infections. They should be changed if there is any suspicion of perforation (Summary box 15.6).

Summary box 15.6

Precautions when gloving/degloving

- Do not allow your skin to touch the outer surface of the glove
- Keep your fingers inside the sleeve of the gown until the glove is on
- If contamination occurs, both gown and gloves must be replaced
- Gloves are removed after the gown using a glove-to-glove, then skin-to-skin technique

---

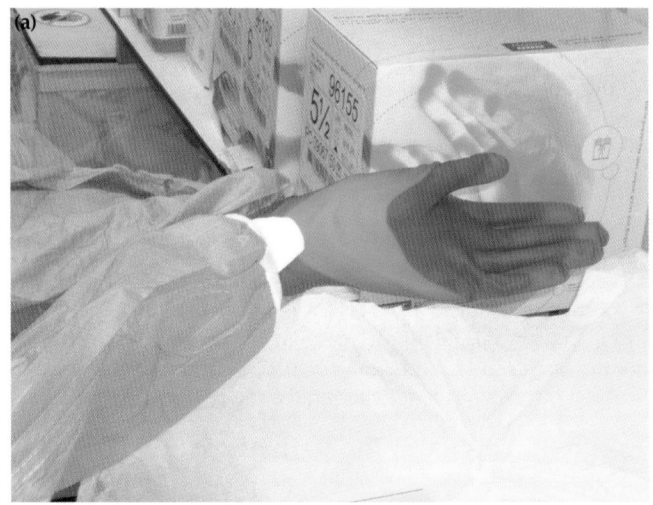

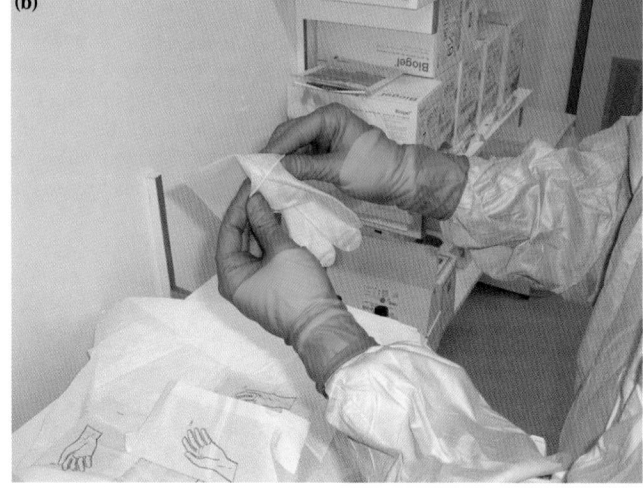

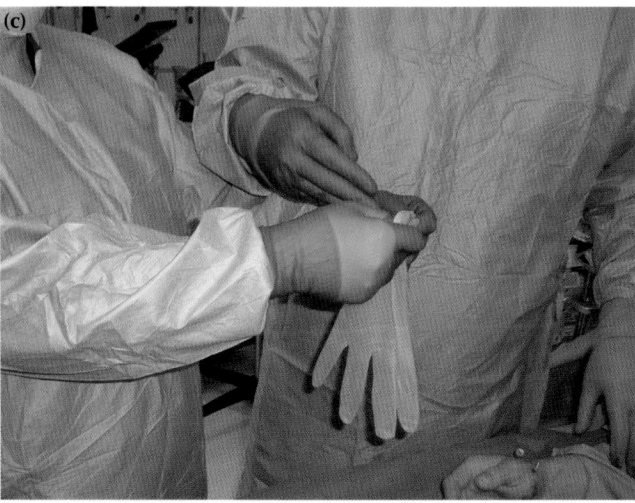

Figure 15.5 Gloving techniques. (a) The initial gloving occurs with the hands covered by the gown. The first glove is then placed onto the palmar surface and pulled into position. (b) The double gloving technique, with minimal touch technique. (c) The closed two-person gloving technique; the glove being held open by one person for the second to insert their hand into the glove.

The operating room/theatre

Temperature and humidity

Patients are at risk of becoming hypothermic during prolonged operations. Paralysis, cool intravenous fluid and large exposed wounds all add to this potential problem. To prevent such hypothermia ambient temperatures of between 24 and 26°C are recommended. However, most surgeons find such temperatures uncomfortable and fatigue quickly. Ideal working temperatures for surgeons are between 19 and 20°C. For prolonged operations a compromise often has to be made or a patient-warming blanket should be used. This is especially important in small children.

Relative humidity in theatres should be capable of adjustment in the range 40–60%.

Illumination

The light source in theatre should not produce shadow. It should be capable of producing a minimum of 40 000 lux at the incision site. Satellite lights can be employed; however, these create heat and subsequent convection currents and may therefore alter local airflow patterns, increasing the risk of wound contamination from airborne bacteria.

Ventilatory system

The aim of the airflow system is to keep air fresh, and this is measured by air changes per hour. The minimum standard number of airflow changes allowed in operating rooms in the UK is 17 per hour. Laminar flow will generally provide 100–300 air changes per hour and is used in operations in which airborne infection must be avoided at all costs (operations involving implants).

Movement

All staff should enter the theatre through the entry zone, which is used for scrubbing and gowning. The amount of movement in and around the operating room and table itself should be kept to a minimum. There should be doors clearly marked for entry and exit, as one-way traffic will minimise the risk of contamination.

Airborne contamination

Airborne bacteria in the theatre originate almost exclusively from personnel within the theatre. It has been shown that a person may shed from 3000 to 50 000 micro-organisms per minute depending on activity and clothing. The major source of these bacteria is the skin, which is often contaminated with *Staphylococcus aureus* and other benign coagulase-negative staphylococcal species. Bacteria also disperse from the upper respiratory tract.

Excessive or unnecessary movements, operating room/theatre overcrowding, poor scrubbing up, gowning and gloving technique, poor airflow and inappropriate temperatures and humidity can all conspire to increase the bacterial load within an operating room and the operating table zone, with potentially catastrophic infective sequelae (Summary box 15.7).

Summary box 15.7

External sources of contamination in the operating theatre

- Poor scrubbing up, gowning and gloving technique
- Excessive inappropriate movement into and out of the operating room
- Too many people in the operating room – excessive movement
- Unnoticed perforation of a glove
- Contamination of instruments by an unscrubbed person

THE PATIENT ON THE OPERATING TABLE

Hypothermia

Heat loss generally occurs through four main mechanisms:

- conduction – the transfer of body heat directly to colder objects;
- convection – through moving air currents;
- radiation – the transfer of heat to colder objects nearby;
- evaporation – the heat utilised during conversion of water to vapour.

Factors that predispose a patient to hypothermia include:

- long preoperative fasting (lowered patient metabolism);
- prolonged immobility on the operating table;
- the effects of anaesthetic agents, e.g. peripheral vasodilatation;
- evaporative heat loss from exposed viscera;
- emergency surgery on shocked patients who are already hypothermic;
- in children, the large surface area-to-weight ratio means that they lose heat quickly.

Hypothermia is associated with poor clotting (disseminated intravascular coagulation), cardiac arrhythmias, respiratory failure, sepsis and ultimately death. Warming blankets and warmed intravenous fluids can reduce the risk of hypothermia.

Accidental injury to the patient

- Tired assistants may lean on the patient. This may compromise the patient's ability to breathe.
- Retractors must be placed carefully, and then minimum pressure applied to avoid damaging soft tissues, especially nerves.
- Diathermy should be used sparingly to avoid excessive burning.
- Clips should not be applied blind when trying to control bleeding in case nerves are crushed too.

SKIN PREPARATION – 'PREPPING' AND DRAPING

The aim of skin preparation before surgery (often shortened to 'prepping') is to reduce the microbial count on the patient's skin to the minimal level possible, to inhibit microbial regrowth and contamination of the wound itself during surgery.

Cleaning removes all debris and the material on which micro-organisms exist. It is achieved with soaps or detergents and water in the 'pre-prep' phase.

Disinfection destroys micro-organisms provided that it comes into contact with them for long enough.

Sterilisation brings about the complete destruction of pathogenic micro-organisms and their spores. This process is used to ensure that drapes, instruments and implants are completely free of infective organisms.

Skin preparation

'Pre-prep'

The skin of the patient must be prepared before formal surgical skin preparation to remove soil and debris. If a plaster of Paris cast has just been removed, the skin should be washed with soapy disinfectant and then washed down with water or saline followed by application of surgical disinfectant ('prep') prior to the main prep. This pre-prep process is therefore not used for all patients and can be undertaken in the anaesthetic room. For patients undergoing elective surgery, a shower on the day of surgery with a soapy disinfectant should suffice.

Skin preparation solution – 'prep'

The solution used may have an aqueous or alcohol base. The agents commonly used are similar to those used in the surgical scrub solutions described in the section above. Care must be taken that the solution does not pool under the patient, as pooling can cause a chemical burn. In general, alcohol or spirit-based solutions are used when the skin is intact and aqueous solutions when there is an open wound.

Method of preparing the skin

The prep area should include the surgical site and a substantial area surrounding it, to minimise the possibility of micro-organism migration from unclean to clean areas during the surgical procedure. When the surgical site is part of a limb, it may be best practice to prep the entire limb. The cleansing of the skin should start at the incision site, working outwards in continually expanding circles away from the surgical site. The prep sponge/swab on a stick should then be discarded and a new clean swab taken.

Contaminated areas, e.g. axilla, groin or perineum, must be prepped last, and once the prep sponge has been used in this area it must be again be discarded. Two separate coats of prep are generally used, and some surgeons will then remove excess prep solution with a dry swab (see Fig. 15.6) (Summary box 15.8).

Summary box 15.8

Preparing the patient's skin ('prepping')

- Performed by staff who are scrubbed up
- Use aqueous solutions for open wounds, alcohol for intact skin
- Work from the incision site outwards
- Repeat at least twice
- Clean heavily contaminated areas last and then discard the prep sponge
- Remove excessive prep solution with a dry swab

Plaster of Paris **is a white powder, calcium sulphate hemi-hydrate (CaSO½H 0) which sets hard when water is added to it.**

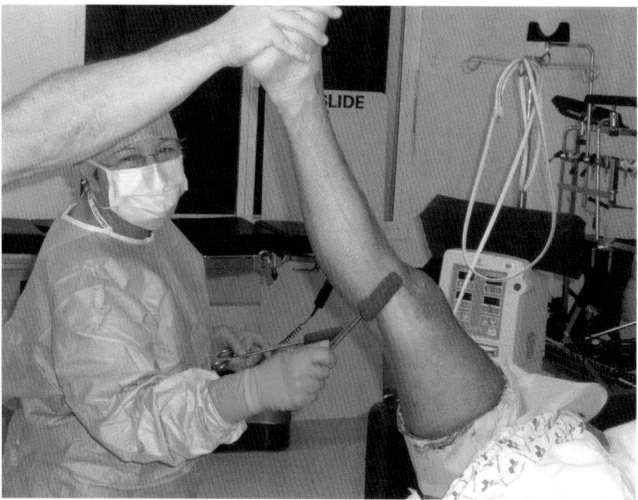

Figure 15.6 Prepping (skin preparation) and draping. Application of skin disinfectant solution to skin. Note that this is the second coat being applied to the posterior aspect of the leg. The leg holder is standing away from the scrub nurse and should be gloved. For this operation the foot is not being prepped.

Draping of the operative area

Surgical draping involves covering with sterile barrier material, 'drapes', the area immediately surrounding the operative site. Drape materials should resist penetration of microscopic particles and moisture, limiting the migration of micro-organisms into the surgical wound.

The purpose of surgical draping is to create and maintain a protective zone of asepsis, called a 'sterile field', so that all sterile items for the surgical procedure avoid touching any unclean surface (see Fig. 15.7a–c). Drapes should be handled only by personnel wearing sterile gloves and should be placed carefully and not disturbed once placed.

Both re-usable and disposable drapes and gowns are in use today. Disposable drapes are a more effective barrier to fluid penetration ('strike-through') and therefore prevent secondary ingress of micro-organisms. Re-usable drapes will lose their barrier quality if not properly laundered and must be routinely inspected for holes and tears.

Draping should allow access to the whole surgical incision and allow for extensile exposure if this is possibly going to be needed. The drapes should also be applied to allow the free movement of a limb if this is going to be necessary during the operation. When possible the edge of the drape nearest the incision should be stuck down onto the patient's skin, while the outer edge should be allowed to drop away off the edge of the operating table. The exposed skin around the incision area itself may be covered with a self-adhesive transparent drape, which should reduce wound contamination from the skin at the edge of the wound. The diathermy and sucker must be firmly attached to the drapes with enough slack to allow free movement. The outer ends of each are then passed off the operating table and from this point are regarded as unsterile.

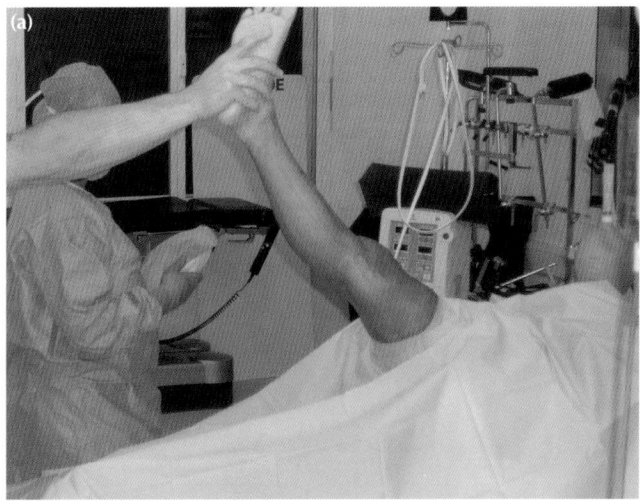

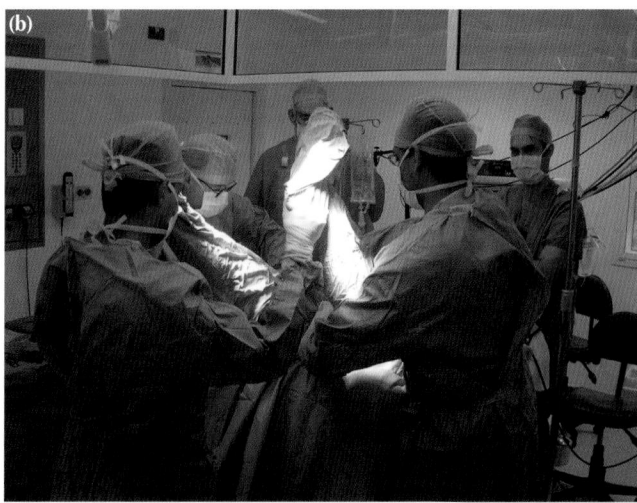

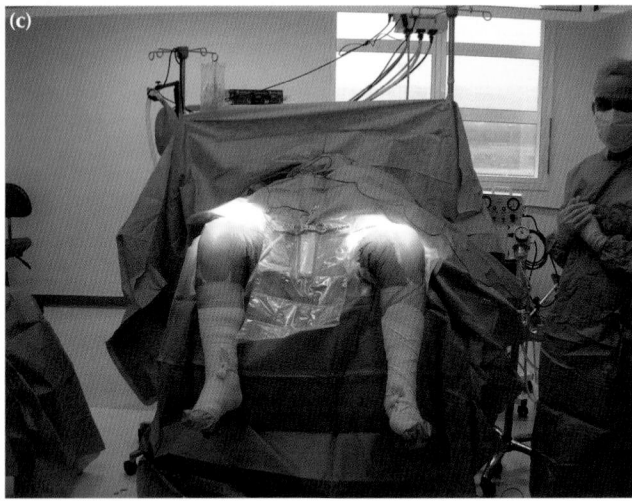

Figure 15.7 (a) A waterproof underdrape is applied with adhesive edges. A sterile waterproof stockingette is about to be applied by the scrub nurse, initially onto the forefoot with the unscrubbed assistant supporting the heel. The unsterile assistant will then move away carefully from the operating table. All of these drapes are disposable. (b) The stockingettes applied. (c) The final drapes are placed over the stockingettes, the operation sites are covered with clear adhesive and a sterile bandage is used to secure the stockingettes. In our department some of the surgeons will prep the feet entirely before draping. Note also the hand position of the surgeon.

GENERAL PRECAUTIONS FOR ESTABLISHING AND MAINTAINING ASEPTIC TECHNIQUE

Scrubbed personnel movements

Once the patient is draped the surgeon and assistant should keep their hands and arms on the table within the sterile field whenever possible. Their hands should not come near to their faces and should remain still when not actively involved in the surgery. Surgeons should only sit down if this is to be for the entire procedure. The seat should be covered with a sterile drape so that the surgeon's back stays sterile. Only sterile equipment can be used within the sterile field.

Instrument tables and/or trolleys and instruments

These are sterile only at table level. Anything extending over the edge of the table must be considered unsterile unless the sterile end is clipped to the drapes.

Behaviour of theatre personnel

Staff who are 'scrubbed up' only touch sterile items or areas. Staff who are not 'scrubbed up' only touch unsterile items or areas.

- Supplies are brought to the sterile team members by the circulator, who opens the outside wrappers on sterile packages. They pass the sterile contents to the scrub nurse by holding onto the object by the outer wrapper. The circulator ensures a sterile transfer to the sterile field.
- Staff who are not scrubbed avoid reaching over the sterile field. Staff who are scrubbed avoid leaning over the unsterile area.

Staff who are scrubbed up always:

- watch the sterile fields to guard against contamination;
- pass each other back to back or front to front;
- stay within the sterile field, facing the sterile area; they do not walk around or go outside the room;
- keep movement to a minimum to avoid contamination of sterile items or persons.

Staff who are not scrubbed up always:

- maintain a distance of at least 50 cm from the sterile field;
- face and observe a sterile area when passing it to be sure that they do not touch it;
- avoid walking through a sterile field (i.e. between the patient and the trays);
- keep all activity near the sterile field to a minimum.

Surgical assistants

Surgical assistants are frequently surgeons in training. They are therefore in theatre to help the senior surgeon and to learn as much as possible.

- *Preparation.* Assistants should review the anatomy before surgery and read up on the operation so that they can anticipate the actions of the senior surgeon and understand what she/he is trying to achieve. They should arrive at the operating theatre before the operating surgeon and should start scrubbing first, having first checked that the patient is ready for theatre.
- *At surgery.* The assistant should at all times try to provide the surgeon with the best access possible by placing and holding retractors and showing the surgeon the field where she/he will next be working, hence the need to know the anatomy and the operation in advance. Instruments and retractors should always be asked for by name.
- *After surgery.* The assistant should help transfer the patient safely off the table and may be allowed to write the operative note. Assistants should always keep an audit of all operations attended and what they have learnt from each case.

Universal precautions

Universal precautions are based on the concept that blood, blood products and body fluids of all persons are potential sources of infection, independent of diagnosis or perceived risk. Therefore, all staff must adhere rigorously to protective measures, which minimise exposure to these agents. The use of universal precautions involves placing barriers between staff and all blood and body fluids. The use and uptake of universal precautions has been patchy.

Universal precautions include:

- wearing of protective gloves, ideally with double layers;
- wearing of protective eyewear and mask;
- wearing of protective apron and gown;
- using safe sharp instrument handling techniques (as described below);
- undertaking hepatitis B vaccination for staff;
- covering open wounds that are clean;
- staff with infected wounds or active dermatitis should stay off work.

The following rules are important when handling sharp instruments:

- Sharp instruments should not be passed between surgeons and their assistants;
- Surgeons should be responsible for the safe placement of sharp instruments, usually into a bowl or tray, which can then be used to transfer them;
- Only one sharp instrument should be placed in the dish at a time;

- When two surgeons are operating simultaneously, each must have their own sharps dish;
- Used needles and other disposable sharp instruments must be discarded into an approved sharps container as soon as practicable.

POSTOPERATIVE CARE OF THE PATIENT

After the operation the patient should be safely transferred to the bed from the operating table, under the supervision of the anaesthetist and surgeon.

A clear operative note should be written immediately. This should include instructions on the postoperative care, including the thresholds for calling back the surgeon.

The following details should be included in the operative note:

1   Patient's details – full name, date of birth, hospital number, address, ward.
2   Date (and start/finish time) of operation.
3   Operating room.
4   Name of operation.
5   Surgeon, assistant, anaesthetist.
6   Anaesthetic type.
7   Patient positioning and set-up.
8   Was a tourniquet used, were antibiotics given, was the patient catheterised, type of skin preparation, method of draping.
9   Tourniquet time, if applicable.
10 Operative details including:
    - incision;
    - approach;
    - findings;
    - procedure (appropriate illustration, if appropriate);
    - complications, untoward events;
    - implants used;
    - closure, including suture material used;
    - dressing;
    - postoperative state (e.g. distal neurovascular status);
    - type of dressing used.
11 Postoperative instructions relevant to surgery:
    - observations required and frequency, e.g. 4-hourly pulse and blood pressure measurements for 24 hours;
    - possible complications and action to be taken if complications occur, e.g. if blood loss exceeds 500 ml in a drain call the surgeon;
    - treatment, e.g. intravenous fluids;
    - time lines for patient recovery, e.g. when to mobilise, when to resume normal oral intake, the need for physiotherapy, allowable movements, dressing changes.
12 Discharge and follow-up details; instruction for sutures, splints, casts, etc.

FURTHER READING

Garner, J.S. and Simmons, B.P. (1983) Guideline for isolation precautions in hospitals. *Infect Control* **4**: 245–325.

Hammond, J.S., Eckes, J.M., Gomez, G.A. and Cunningham, D.N. (1990) HIV, trauma, and infection control: universal precautions are universally ignored. *J Trauma* **30**: 555–61.

Odinsson, A. and Finsen, V. (2006) Tourniquet use and complications in Norway. *J Bone Joint Surg Br* **88-B**: 1090–2.

Osterman, J.W. (1995) Beyond universal precautions. *Can Med Assoc J* **152**: 1051–5.

Webb, J.B., Balaratnam, S. and Park, A.J. (2003) Flame burns: a forgotton danger of diathermy? *Surgeon* **1(2)**: 111–13.

Perioperative management of the high-risk surgical patient

LEARNING OBJECTIVES

To understand:

- The factors that put a patient at high risk from surgery and anaesthesia
- The problems of patients being treated as an emergency

- Classification and optimisation of high-risk patients
- The value of the critical care unit in the perioperative period

INTRODUCTION

Every surgical procedure involves some risk of significant postoperative complications or death. Whereas in most cases, this risk is well below 1%, a surgical population can easily be identified in which serious complications and death are much more frequent. Between 10% and 15% of in-patient surgical procedures appear to fall into this high-risk category and therefore represent an important cause of death and disability (Fig. 16.1). In the UK, 1.3 million hospital in-patients undergo general surgical procedures each year, of whom 166 000 can be identified as being at high risk of complications or death. The high-risk surgical population accounts for over 80% of surgical deaths but less than 15% of in-patient surgical procedures (Fig. 16.2). Of these high-risk surgical patients in the UK, 25 000 die postoperatively each year in hospital, and a further 115 000 patients who suffered complications will not survive in the long term.

The high-risk surgical population typically consists of elderly patients with coexisting medical conditions undergoing complex or major surgery, often as an emergency. Early identification and

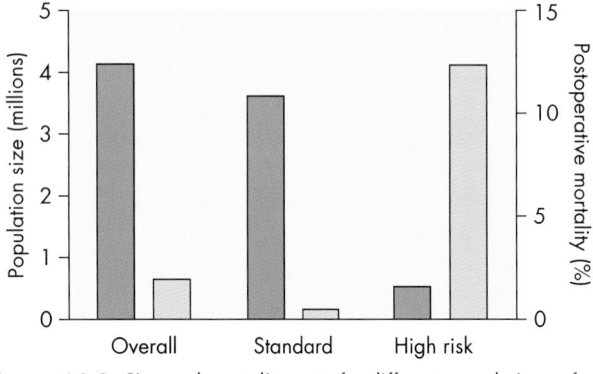

Figure 16.2 Size and mortality rates for different populations of surgical patients.

optimal care of the high-risk surgical patient will result in a substantial reduction in risk. The aim of this chapter is to describe the basic approach to the perioperative care of such patients (Summary box 16.1).

Summary box 16.1

Characteristics of the high-risk population

- Elderly
- Comorbid conditions
- Needing emergency surgery (no time for optimisation)

WHY ARE COMPLICATIONS SO FREQUENT IN THIS POPULATION?

Technical complications relating to specific anaesthetic and surgical procedures are well recognised and discussed elsewhere in this book. In this chapter, we are concerned with a range of more general factors which place the surgical patient at additional risk. The nature of risk varies widely with different surgical procedures and does not bear a simple relationship to the extent of tissue

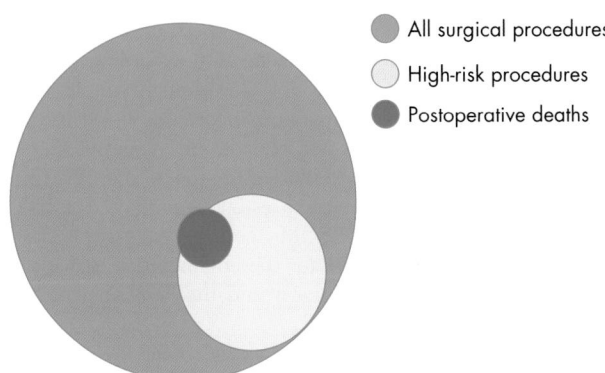

Figure 16.1 Distribution of postoperative deaths within the surgical population.

injury during surgery. In most cases, the overall risk of complications and death is a function of a range of patient- and surgery-related factors.

- Patient factors:
  - ischaemic heart disease;
  - chronic obstructive pulmonary disease;
  - diabetes;
  - advanced age;
  - poor exercise tolerance;
  - poor nutritional status.
- Surgical factors:
  - emergency surgery;
  - major or complex surgery;
  - body cavity surgery;
  - large anticipated blood loss;
  - large insensible fluid loss;
  - prolonged duration of surgery.
- Perioperative care factors:
  - inadequate critical care facilities;
  - insufficient patient monitoring;
  - lack of early intervention as complications develop.

Patient-related factors

In most cases, the underlying condition indicating surgical intervention will itself be associated with an increased risk of complications. For example, a patient who has developed severe peripheral vascular disease as a result of heavy smoking can be expected to suffer from significant ischaemic heart disease as well as chronic obstructive pulmonary disease. Other examples include poor nutritional status in a patient requiring cancer surgery and poor mobility in a patient requiring a major joint replacement. Comorbid diseases unrelated to the indication for surgery are also commonplace, with those affecting the respiratory and cardiovascular systems being most important.

The need for emergency treatment is perhaps the single most important factor raising the level of perioperative risk. This results from more serious and deteriorating acute pathology, the lack of opportunity to optimise medical management of comorbid illnesses, the presence of hypovolaemia which may be severe and dependence on junior medical staff often working outside office hours with minimal support or supervision.

Surgery- and anaesthesia-related factors

Tissue injury may result in a systemic inflammatory reaction leading to increased capillary permeability and insensible water losses from the intravascular compartment into the extracellular space. These 'third space' fluid losses tend to be most severe during and after procedures involving bowel resection. They may also be compounded by other forms of fluid loss such as prolonged preoperative fasting and insensible losses during surgery. Accurate estimation of these additional fluid requirements is a challenging but necessary aspect of perioperative care, as either inadequate or excessive perioperative replacement fluid may result in serious complications. Impaired coagulation may also increase the likelihood of haemorrhage.

Quite aside from psychological distress, pain is an important cause of postoperative complications. Excessive pain will result in poor mobility, deteriorating respiratory function (particularly following abdominal surgery), increased arterial pressure and myocardial work. Pain will therefore exacerbate the deteriorations in both cardiac and respiratory function that occur following major surgery. Optimal postoperative analgesia is therefore essential to ensure that the risk of cardiorespiratory complications is minimised.

Postoperative hypothermia is common in high-risk patients, particularly following prolonged or complex procedures, especially body cavity surgery. Hypothermia may result in shivering, confusion and delayed recovery from anaesthesia. These in turn lead to increased oxygen consumption, poor respiratory function and more frequent cardiorespiratory complications. High-risk patients have a higher likelihood of poor nutritional status as a result of their underlying pathology, compounded by ileus/being denied postoperative nutritional intake, poor appetite or simply experiencing difficulty feeding themselves (Summary box 16.2).

Summary box 16.2

Surgical and anaesthetic factors creating high risk

- Dehydration (shock before surgery, loss of fluids during surgery, inability to tolerate fluids postoperatively)
- Pain (reduces mobility, affects breathing and ability to take food and fluids)
- Hypothermia

IDENTIFICATION OF THE HIGH-RISK PATIENT

The previous section lists the common risk factors leading to a patient being high risk.

For example, an elderly patient with severe heart disease undergoing emergency surgery for a perforation of the large bowel will have a risk of complications in excess of 95%, and the risk of death may be higher than 50%. However, the difficulty with this approach is that perioperative risk is cumulative and depends on a complex interplay between different factors. Experience suggests that many high-risk patients are not identified, despite awareness of those factors that increase the incidence of postoperative complications and death. Consequently, there is continued interest in improving our methods of screening surgical patients and stratifying risk, in order to select the patients who require additional perioperative care. In some cases, this process may indicate a patient in whom the risks of surgery are not justified by the potential benefits.

One approach to this problem is the use of risk scoring systems to classify patients. The simplest and most commonly used system is the American Society of Anesthesiologists (ASA) score, which provides a basic classification according to subjective perception of risk (Table 16.1). Although simple to use, clinicians frequently classify patients incorrectly using the ASA score, and the system does not provide any objective estimate of the risk of death. An alternative approach is to use physiological and surgical variables to estimate predicted mortality. Examples include the POSSUM scoring system (Physiologic and Operative Severity Score for the enUmeration of Mortality and Morbidity) for general surgery and the Parsonnet score for

---

PARSONNET was developed by V. Parsonnet, and others, at the Newark Beth Israel Medical Center, New Jersey, NJ, USA, and is based on the publication 'A Method of Uniform Stratification of Risk for Evaluating the Results of Surgery in Aquired Adult Heart Disease' (1989).

Table 16.1 American Society of Anesthesiologists (ASA) score

ASA class	Description
Class I	A normal healthy patient
Class II	A patient with mild systemic disease that does not limit functional activity
Class III	A patient with severe systemic disease that limits functional activity
Class IV	A patient with severe systemic disease that poses a constant threat to life
Class V	A moribund patient who is not expected to survive for longer than 24 h, either with or without surgery

The addition of an 'E' denotes emergency surgery.

cardiac surgery. However, these systems were designed to describe populations of patients and are much less reliable when used to assess the individual. Consequently, scoring systems should not be used in isolation to assess perioperative risk.

The American College of Cardiology/American Heart Association (ACA/AHA) Task Force have issued detailed guidelines which help to stratify patients according to metabolic reserve. An important aspect of these guidelines is the use of metabolic equivalents (METs) to help to standardise the assessment of exercise tolerance based on activities of daily living. By stratifying patients in this way, it is possible to focus the use of preoperative investigations on those patients most in need. Although the MET is a useful concept, these guidelines are intended only for the identification and management of cardiac disease in patients undergoing elective surgery, and are not designed for the multifactorial situation of the high-risk surgical patient.

In contrast, anaerobic threshold testing is an increasingly popular method of preoperative assessment for elective surgery, although it requires resources and is still of limited availability. This technique involves the use of an exercise bike and continuous measurement of oxygen consumption to identify the threshold at which anaerobic respiration commences. A low anaerobic threshold appears to be associated with increased postoperative mortality rates and assists in determining appropriate levels of postoperative care. The difficulty with this approach is that the assessment is time-consuming and must be performed several days before surgery. Thus, we still need methods of evaluation to identify those patients in need of detailed risk assessment, and that are feasible for the emergency situation (Summary box 16.3).

Summary box 16.3

Surgical and anaesthetic risk scores

- ASA is frequently incorrectly applied
- POSSUM works best for populations not individuals
- MET measures exercise tolerance
- Anaerobic threshold needs measuring in advance of surgery
- No risk score is reliable in isolation

GENERAL ASPECTS OF PERIOPERATIVE CARE

Preoperative assessment

In addition to identifying the patient at increased risk, preoperative assessment should identify potentially reversible comorbid illness so that every effort can be made to optimise the patient's condition.

Preoperative assessment should be performed by both the anaesthetist and the surgeon and, when appropriate, by specialist physicians. A general assessment should always include an evaluation of respiratory and cardiac function. Other important factors to consider include are age, weight (ideally body mass index and girth measurements), smoking and alcohol intake, and general medical history and status (e.g. diabetes).

Careful evaluation of exercise tolerance will provide an indication of cardiorespiratory reserve. This is usually possible by asking the patient about common activities of daily living, for example the ability to climb a flight of stairs and the symptoms this provokes. Poor exercise tolerance generally reflects limitation in cardiorespiratory reserve. Objective assessments such as anaerobic threshold testing and METs help to identify the need for additional intraoperative monitoring and support and postoperative critical care admission. It may prove difficult to assess exercise tolerance in patients with poor mobility. Clinical examination should focus on the cardiac and respiratory systems (Summary box 16.4).

Summary box 16.4

Preoperative assessment for risk

- The history should focus on cardiac and respiratory problems
- Exercise tolerance gives a good guide to cardiac reserve
- Age and body mass index are useful indicators
- Check alcohol and tobacco intake
- Check medications

Preoperative medical therapy

Where significant comorbid disease has been identified, medical management should be reviewed according to current standards particularly for cardiorespiratory disease. The ACA/AHA Task Force guidelines discussed above form the basis of cardiac assessment in many centres. In some cases, patients may require percutaneous coronary intervention (angioplasty or stenting) or coronary artery bypass grafting prior to surgery. Preoperative bronchodilator therapy will be required in patients with reversible airflow limitation [e.g. asthma or chronic obstructive airways disease (COAD)]. A course of oral corticosteroids prior to surgery may also be necessary in such patients. The use of antibiotic therapy in patients with significant sputum production is tempting, but should be given careful consideration. Indiscriminate antibiotic use may simply result in the selection of resistant bacteria without any therapeutic benefit and, worse still, may greatly complicate the treatment of subsequent postoperative pneumonia. Preoperative physiotherapy is helpful for patients with chronic sputum production. Smoking cessation should be encouraged wherever possible with the offer of counselling and other practical support where available. In patients with chronic or end-stage renal failure, careful discussion with a nephrologist is needed to ensure optimal perioperative care and/or timing of haemodialysis prior to surgery (Summary box 16.5).

Summary box 16.5

Review medical treatment before surgery

- Coronary angiography may be indicated for patients with ischaemic heart disease
- Asthma and COAD may require bronchodilators and steroids
- Antibiotic therapy is not necessarily indicated for patients with chronic sputum production
- Patients should stop smoking
- Patients with renal failure need their surgery planned around dialysis
- Oral medication can be given with water even when a patient is 'nil by mouth'
- When possible, postpone surgery until the patient is optimised

---

Regular cardiovascular medications should usually be continued in the perioperative period, as omission of such medicines will increase the risk of perioperative hypertension and myocardial ischaemia. Oral medications may be administered prior to surgery with a small volume of water (perhaps 10 ml) without any increased risk of pulmonary aspiration. On a similar basis, most patients may be allowed oral medications after surgery, provided a common sense evaluation is performed.

Clinical management will often be influenced by the nature, indication and urgency of surgery. Ideally, surgery will be postponed until medical management has been optimised and a robust plan for perioperative care put in place. In practice, it is often not possible to achieve this and, clearly, this will not be possible where emergency surgery is required. In this situation, fluid resuscitation should be initiated and other aspects of care addressed as early as possible. Regardless of urgency, the early input of experienced colleagues should be considered, including the physicians, surgeons, anaesthetists and critical care specialists.

Critical care

The high-risk surgical patient may require admission to a critical care unit either before or after surgery.

Assessment of the surgical patient in critical care

Basic clinical assessment

Perioperative critical illness often conforms to a pattern. Simple and versatile clinical parameters may be used to establish the status of the patient. These generally include pulse rate, respiratory rate, arterial pressure, urine output, conscious level (Glasgow Coma Score), capillary refill time and the presence of peripheral cyanosis. The primary aim of perioperative critical care is to ensure adequate tissue perfusion and oxygenation. Measures of end-organ function and tissue perfusion such as urine output and Glasgow Coma Score should therefore be carefully assessed. Core–peripheral temperature gradient may also provide an

---

Glasgow Coma Score **was introduced in 1977 by William Bryan Jennet, Professor of Neurosurgery and Graham Michael Teasdale, a Neurosurgeon of the University Department of Neurosurgery, at the Institute of Neurological Sciences, Southern General Hospital, Glasgow, Scotland.**

---

indication of reduced tissue perfusion in circulatory shock. Basic non-invasive monitoring will include continuous electrocardiography (ECG) and pulse oximetry (SaO_2). Combined with close observation by specially trained medical and nursing staff, these simple techniques allow the prompt identification of any deterioration in clinical status (Summary box 16.6).

Summary box 16.6

Value of admission to critical care unit for perioperative care

- Enables optimal maintenance of tissue perfusion and oxygenation
- Allows close monitoring and rapid response to any instability

---

Invasive arterial pressure monitoring

Invasive arterial pressure monitoring is used to facilitate the immediate recognition of haemodynamic changes, especially in an unstable patient, as well as enabling repeated blood sampling for arterial blood gas analysis. Despite the benefits perceived for this form of monitoring, arterial blood pressure does not actually have a linear relationship with cardiac output or tissue perfusion and should be interpreted with caution. Nevertheless, invasive arterial pressure monitoring generally provides accurate and reliable data, although a damped waveform may occur with kinking of the cannula or thrombus formation.

Central venous pressure monitoring (CVP)

CVP is usually measured in the superior vena cava with a catheter inserted from either the internal jugular or the subclavian veins. The placement of these catheters may be extremely difficult in the hypovolaemic patient, and the inexperienced practitioner should seek advice and supervision. CVP is determined either through the use of a water manometer or, nowadays more commonly, via an electronic transducer attached to a monitor to give a continuous graphical display. The purpose of CVP measurement is to provide an estimate of intravascular volume status, sometimes termed preload. Invasive pressure measurement is frequently relied upon to assess volume status in the critically ill. However, venous pressure has a complex relationship with intravascular volume and may not provide a reliable indication of the need for intravenous fluid administration. The CVP *trend* in response to a fluid challenge (e.g. 200–500 ml given over 30 min) is considered to be more helpful than the absolute value when attempting to identify the hypovolaemic patient.

Arterial blood gas analysis

Arterial blood gas analysis will allow detailed assessment of both respiratory and metabolic status. Interpretation of blood gas data is straightforward and should be regarded as an essential skill for clinical staff involved in the care of the high-risk surgical patient. Reliable interpretation of blood gas data is dependent on a clear understanding of the recent clinical history, and it is vital to know the inspired (and hence alveolar) oxygen concentration when evaluating the arterial oxygen tension and saturation. Subsequent clinical decisions should be based on all the data available and not individual variables. This is particularly true when considering the administration of intravenous fluids to a patient with a significant base deficit or elevated serum lactate.

Cardiac output monitoring

Cardiac output monitoring may be desirable in critically ill patients who require intravenous fluid replacement or vasoactive infusions to stabilise their circulatory status. There are now a variety of commercially available invasive or non-invasive monitors that allow cardiac output measurement.

The pulmonary artery (or 'Swan–Ganz') catheter (PAC) is traditionally regarded as the gold standard method of cardiac output measurement at the bedside. The PAC is a balloon-tipped catheter, which is 'floated' through the great veins, right atrium and right ventricle until the tip lies in the pulmonary artery. Cardiac output is measured intermittently by the thermal indicator dilution technique, in which a bolus of cold fluid is injected proximal to the temperature sensor. Direct measurements include cardiac output, pulmonary artery pressure, central venous pressure, pulmonary artery occlusion pressure and mixed venous oxygen saturation. Derived data include systemic vascular resistance, oxygen delivery and oxygen consumption.

In recent years, the PAC has become less popular because it is perceived to be associated with an excessive complication rate. Although large trials refute this, the use of less invasive cardiac output monitoring is increasingly popular. The oesophageal Doppler technique involves the use of a probe placed in the oesophagus to measure blood velocity in the descending aorta by applying the Doppler shift principle. Aortic cross-sectional area is either estimated with a nomogram or measured directly, thus allowing the estimation of cardiac output. For the experienced operator, this is a quick and simple device to use. The probe is not well tolerated by conscious subjects, and use is therefore confined to the sedated or anaesthetised patient. The principal complication of its use is trauma to the pharynx and oesophagus, and this technique is contraindicated during or after pharyngeal and oesophageal surgery.

Transpulmonary lithium indicator dilution and arterial waveform analysis involves the use of an initial cardiac output measurement by the indicator dilution technique to calibrate arterial waveform analysis software and provide a continuous measurement of cardiac output. Lithium chloride indicator is injected as a bolus into a central vein; a lithium ion-sensitive electrode measures the indicator concentration in blood drawn from an arterial line by a small pump. This provides a calibration factor for continuous analysis of the arterial pressure waveform. Transpulmonary thermal indicator dilution and arterial waveform analysis is a very similar technique. In this case, cold saline is injected into a central vein, and the temperature change is measured using a thermistor-tipped arterial catheter sited in either the femoral or the axillary artery. Once calibrated, pulse contour analysis software is used to provide a continuous measurement of cardiac output (Summary box 16.7).

Summary box 16.7

Special monitoring techniques available in the critical care unit

- Oxygenation – invasive arterial gas with inspired oxygen monitoring
- Perfusion – cardiac output monitors – Swan–Ganz catheter, oesophageal Doppler probe, transpulmonary lithium and thermal sensors

---

General aspects of critical care

It is now routine practice in critical care to employ a 'bundle' of therapeutic strategies in all patients. Tight control of the patient's blood sugar involves the use of a sliding scale insulin infusion to achieve a blood glucose concentration between 4 and 8 mmol l^{-1}. This approach appears to be of particular benefit to patients who require prolonged postoperative critical care support. With the transfusion of stored red blood cells being associated with various complications including transfusion mismatch, infection and transfusion-related acute lung injury, the use of a more cautious haemoglobin concentration of 8 g dl^{-1} to trigger the transfusion of red blood cells may result in an improvement in outcome. Acquired adrenocortical depression is common in patients who develop septic shock. In such cases, the use of low-dose corticosteroids may reduce vasopressor requirements and improve mortality rates.

It has been traditional to withhold enteral nutrition from patients for several days following surgery, as a result of concerns that early enteral diet may jeopardise bowel anastomoses, exacerbate postoperative ileus and delay recovery. Some authorities have suggested that this approach may in itself be harmful as enterocytes may extract nutritional substrate directly from the gut lumen. Prolonged fasting could therefore result in atrophy of the intestinal mucosa with consequent translocation of bacteria across the bowel wall and an increase in infective complications. While this theory is unproven, it is, in carefully selected cases, usually possible to commence a liquid enteral feed immediately after surgery without any adverse effects. The increasing use of jejunostomy feeding tubes has facilitated this approach.

The importance of deep vein thrombosis prophylaxis should be emphasised as a vital aspect of the care of any surgical patient. The high-risk patient may present with a number of predisposing factors for thromboembolism, including smoking, obesity, malignancy and immobility (Summary box 16.8).

Summary box 16.8

General critical care

- Blood glucose – tight control using an insulin sliding scale
- Blood transfusion reaction – harden threshold for transfusion to 8 g dl^{-1}
- Steroids if there are signs of adrenocortical depression
- Start enteral feeding early (jejunal feeding tubes)
- Protect against deep vein thrombosis

Postoperative respiratory management

Major surgery under general anaesthesia will result in a number of physiological changes to the respiratory system, perhaps the most important of which is a reduction in functional residual

---

Harold James Charles Swan, **1922–2005**, Professor of Medicine, UCLA School of Medicine, Los Angeles, and Director of Cardiology, Cedars Sinai Medical Center, Los Angeles, CA, USA.
William Ganz, **b. 1919**, Cardiologist, Cedars Sinai Medical Center, Los Angeles, CA, USA. Swan and Ganz published the results of the use of their catheter in 1970.
Christian Johann Doppler, **1803–1853**, Professor of Experimental Physics, Vienna, Austria, enunciated the 'Doppler Principle' in 1842.

capacity (FRC). These changes will be further compounded by postoperative pain and the residual effects of anaesthesia to cause pulmonary atelectasis predisposing the patient to respiratory infection. Meanwhile, agitation, pain and shivering as a result of hypothermia may all result in an increase in oxygen consumption. The reduction in oxygen delivery at a time of increased demand in part explains the high incidence of postoperative respiratory failure among high-risk surgical patients with reduced respiratory reserve.

It is not necessarily advisable for the high-risk surgical patient to follow the routine of abrupt cessation of anaesthesia at the end of surgery, removal of the tracheal tube and a brief period of care in a postoperative recovery unit before discharge to a standard ward. Although this course of treatment will not necessarily result in complications, inadequate respiratory support in the hours immediately following surgery may lead to hypoxaemia, carbon dioxide retention, acidosis and deterioration in clinical status, precipitating the need for reintubation and ventilation.

Where available, the use of postoperative invasive ventilation will allow staff to discontinue sedation once the patient is cardiovascularly stable, normothermic and well hydrated with optimal analgesia. The amount of time required to achieve this may vary widely. Consequently, it may be necessary to continue invasive ventilation overnight and extubate the patient on the first postoperative day. In some institutions, the provision of extended postoperative recovery facilities or high-dependency units allows overnight invasive ventilation without the expense and complexity of full-scale intensive care (Summary box 16.9).

Summary box 16.9

Potential problems of early extubation vs. extended ventilation overnight

- Sudden extubation may lead to hypoxia from poor respiratory effort
- Atelectasis may prejudice oxygen transfer
- Carbon dioxide levels may rise, leading to acidosis
- Shivering, pain and shock lead to high oxygen demand

Mechanical (invasive) ventilation

The underlying management principles of postoperative mechanical (invasive) ventilation are the same for all critically ill patients. Recent research has emphasised the potential complications of excessive tidal volumes causing overdistension of alveoli termed *volutrauma*, while excessive airways pressure may result in *barotrauma*. It has now emerged that many cases of postoperative acute respiratory distress syndrome arise not as a result of surgery or associated sepsis, but from overly 'aggressive' postoperative invasive ventilation. Evidence suggests that tidal volumes should be maintained between 5 and 7 ml kg^{-1} wherever possible with a plateau pressure of 30 cmH$_2$O or less. In many patients, the resulting respiratory minute volume (MV) will be insufficient to maintain PaCO$_2$ at normal values. However, the mild degree of 'permissive' hypercapnia that results does not appear to be harmful as long as the arterial pH is maintained above 7.20. In practice, this is easily achieved in the absence of severe metabolic acidosis. This approach to ventilation is now often used during surgery as well.

Non-invasive ventilation (NIV)

Non-invasive ventilation via a tight-fitting face mask may prove a useful approach to postoperative respiratory management. This equipment is similar to that used for invasive ventilation (via a tracheal tube), and some modern ventilators may be used for both NIV and invasive ventilation. The chief benefit of NIV is that short periods of respiratory support may be provided without the need for general anaesthesia and tracheal intubation. Continuous positive airways pressure (CPAP) is a similar technique, which involves the application of a constant airways pressure (usually between 5 and 10 cmH$_2$O) via a tight-fitting face mask without cycling to a higher airways pressure during inspiration. The use of CPAP or NIV according to standardised protocols may facilitate early intervention for patients at risk, with subsequent reduction in the incidence of complications and a more rapid postoperative recovery. These non-invasive techniques of ventilation have also been shown to improve outcome in patients who develop postoperative respiratory failure unexpectedly. These techniques may obviate the need for initial invasive ventilation, or avoid respiratory deterioration and reintubation which risks significant morbidity for the patient.

Postoperative cardiovascular management

Most high-risk surgical patients will develop a degree of postoperative circulatory dysfunction. This may result from hypovolaemia, cardiac failure, haemorrhage, sepsis or a combination of these factors. In severe cases, these may result in circulatory shock, a state in which the perfusion of the tissues is insufficient to meet metabolic requirements.

General approach to treatment of circulatory shock

The **A**irway, **B**reathing, **C**irculation approach to assessment and management should be applied in every acutely ill patient. The purpose of this pragmatic approach to resuscitation is to ensure appropriate prioritisation, assessment and management of life-threatening disease. Circulatory shock is frequently associated with an inadequate airway due to reduced conscious level as well as impaired respiratory function. The resulting hypoxaemia will accelerate the deterioration in cardiac function. Airway and respiratory management should not be delayed to allow haemodynamic resuscitation, although such measures may be instituted simultaneously.

Hypovolaemia is commonplace following major surgery. Even a comparatively stable patient may have a degree of fluid depletion resulting from inadequate intake, haemorrhage and insensible losses. When a high-risk surgical patient develops signs of circulatory shock, it is, regardless of cause, appropriate to administer a 'fluid challenge'. Assessment of any response to fluid administration may provide more reliable evidence of hypovolaemia. This approach is unlikely to cause harm provided small volumes of fluid are administered and followed by careful and regular assessment. A 250-ml bolus of either intravenous crystalloid or colloid solution is generally considered appropriate. Where significant haemorrhage has occurred, the administration of packed red blood cells and other blood products will also be required. Improvement in pulse rate, urine output and conscious level are the most helpful indicators of fluid responsiveness. Arterial pressure may be misleading in the presence of circulatory shock and should be interpreted with caution (Summary box 16.10).

> **Summary box 16.10**
>
> **Diagnosis of perioperative hypovolaemia**
>
> - Many patients are hypovolaemic at or after surgery
> - A small fluid challenge will improve blood pressure, conscious state and urine output in a hypovolaemic patient
> - Vasopressor drugs and inotropics may be needed to improve tissue perfusion

Replacement of intravascular volume may not in itself be sufficient to restore haemodynamic stability. Vasopressor drugs may be required to increase systemic vascular resistance (i.e. by vasoconstriction), and inotropic support may be required to increase cardiac output. Once these interventions are required, admission to a critical care unit is usually required. This will also allow the use of cardiac output monitoring. In selecting an inotrope or adjusting existing therapy, the two most important variables are the mean arterial pressure and the cardiac output. Various inotropic drugs are available, each with a specific pattern of cardiac and peripheral vascular effects. The input of an experienced critical care specialist is necessary to ensure the appropriate management of such patients.

Specific measures in the treatment of circulatory shock

While the approach described above may be sufficient to restore circulatory status, in some situations, more specific interventions may be required. These may include surgery in a patient with sepsis, radiological drainage of a collection, surgery to control haemorrhage, and percutaneous coronary intervention. The use of these approaches in the critically ill patient is self-evident and emphasises the importance of the involvement of all appropriate senior specialists at an early stage.

Critical care outreach

In recent years, the role of critical care has been expanded to the concept of 'critical care without walls'. This term describes the delivery of critical care to the patient, regardless of location within the hospital, ensuring high standards of care and optimal outcome. Frequent reports of persistent failures in the care of critically ill patients on standard wards have resulted in the widespread introduction of mainly nurse-led critical care outreach teams to achieve this aim. It would seem obvious that a service that allows early assessment and intervention by experienced critical care practitioners would improve clinical outcomes. However, there is at present no convincing evidence of improved patient outcomes associated with the introduction of critical care outreach teams.

SPECIFIC MANAGEMENT STRATEGIES FOR THE HIGH-RISK SURGICAL PATIENT

Prophylactic perioperative β-blockade

Where significant cardiac disease is identified prior to surgery, medical management should be optimised in consultation with a cardiologist. The high mortality rates associated with postoperative myocardial infarction have led to the prophylactic use of nitrates, calcium channel antagonists and β-receptor antagonists in patients considered to be at risk of perioperative myocardial ischaemia. With the exception of β-receptor antagonists, none of these therapies has resulted in documented improvement in outcome.

The considerable metabolic and physiological demands of surgery may result in increased myocardial work and inadequate myocardial oxygen supply. The successful use of β-receptor antagonists in the management of ischaemic heart disease has suggested an indication for the use of these agents in perioperative care. A number of studies suggest that the prophylactic use of atenolol or bisoprolol may result in significant reductions in the incidence of perioperative myocardial ischaemic events. The results of an ongoing, large, multicentre trial may further confirm the value of this approach.

Goal-directed therapy

Perioperative management of the cardiovascular system will always involve predefined treatment limits or targets. These targets may be very basic, such as heart rate and blood pressure, or more sophisticated. Goal-directed therapy (GDT) is a term used to describe the perioperative administration of intravenous fluids and inotropic agents to achieve a predefined 'optimal' goal for oxygen delivery to the tissues. Oxygen delivery is a parameter that is calculated from measurements of cardiac output, haemoglobin concentration, SaO_2 and PaO_2. This approach was developed following the observation that, when routine parameters such as blood pressure and urine output were stabilised in all surgical patients, survivors had consistently higher cardiac output, oxygen delivery and oxygen consumption than those who subsequently died. The median values attained by the surviving patients in these observational studies were subsequently incorporated into GDT protocols as haemodynamic goals (Summary box 16.11).

> **Summary box 16.11**
>
> **Goal-directed therapy**
>
> - Treatment aimed at achieving predefined levels of oxygen delivery to tissues
> - Uses a multitude of treatment modalities depending on the patient's problem
> - Improves cardiac output, renal output, complication rates and patient survival

A number of studies have suggested that GDT may significantly reduce postoperative complication rates. Originally, GDT required the insertion of a pulmonary artery catheter and was continued throughout the perioperative period. However, more recent evidence suggests that this technique is most beneficial when applied for short periods during and after surgery. Significant reductions in complication rates may be achieved with up to 8 hours of postoperative GDT using a minimally invasive cardiac output monitoring technique. It is important to note that the sustained use of GDT in patients with established critical illness is not beneficial and may in fact be harmful.

The simultaneous recommendations for the use of perioperative GDT and β-receptor antagonists in the high-risk population have caused some confusion. While indications for the two therapeutic approaches may seem to be mutually exclusive, this is not the case. The use of prophylactic β-blockade in patients considered at high risk of perioperative myocardial ischaemia will not negate the benefits of goal-directed resuscitation during periods of hypovolaemia.

Intraoperative oesophageal Doppler-guided fluid therapy

The use of oesophageal Doppler cardiac output measurement to guide intravenous fluid therapy is related to the technique of GDT described above. This use of this monitor has proved popular, in part because of the simplicity of the technique, but also because the anaesthetist will generally be able to gain access to the head during surgery. On average, the use of oesophageal Doppler-derived cardiac output measurement does seem to be associated with a larger volume of fluid administration. However, it is important to note the wide variation in the volume of fluid required. This variability in estimated fluid requirements would suggest that the benefit of this approach does not relate to the administration of extra fluid but to the use of an accurate estimate of fluid volume requirements in each individual patient (Summary box 16.12).

Summary box 16.12

Oesophageal Doppler-guided fluid therapy

- Appears to allow more accurate estimation of a patient's fluid needs
- Improves outcome following major surgery
- Reduces the incidence and length of ileus

Oesophageal Doppler-guided fluid management has been shown to improve outcome following cardiac, orthopaedic and abdominal surgery. There is some evidence to believe that this approach to fluid management results in improved mesenteric perfusion and therefore less postoperative ileus. Three separate studies have shown an earlier return to enteral feeding and an associated reduction in duration of hospital stay.

SUMMARY

The majority of postoperative complications and deaths arise in a high-risk population of surgical patients. Increased awareness of this population with improved systems for the identification and treatment of the high-risk surgical patient is now increasingly important, as novel treatment strategies offer the prospect of significant improvements in outcome. However, a detailed multidisciplinary approach to perioperative care remains essential if the potential of these new approaches is to be realised.

FURTHER READING

Bersten, A., Soni, N. and Oh, T. (2003) *Oh's Intensive Care Manual*, 5th edn. Butterworth-Heinemann, London.

Cullinane, M., Gray, A.J., Hargraves, C.M., Lansdown, M., Martin, I.C. and Schubert, M. (2003) *The 2003 Report of the National Confidential Enquiry into Peri-operative Deaths*. NCEPOD, London.

Eagle, K.A., Berger, P.B., Calkins, H. *et al.* (2002) ACC/AHA guideline update for perioperative cardiovascular evaluation for noncardiac surgery – executive summary: a report of the American College of Cardiology/American Heart Association Task Force on Practice Guidelines. *J Am Coll Cardiol* **39**: 542–53.

Pearse, R.M., Harrison, D.A., James, P. *et al.* (2006) Identification and characterisation of the high-risk surgical population in the United Kingdom. *Crit Care* **10**: R81.

Nutrition and fluid therapy

LEARNING OBJECTIVES

To understand:

- The causes and consequences of malnutrition in the surgical patient
- Fluid and electrolyte requirements in the pre- and postoperative patient

- The nutritional requirements of surgical patients and the nutritional consequences of intestinal resection
- The different methods of providing nutritional support and their complications

INTRODUCTION

Malnutrition is common. It occurs in about 30% of surgical patients with gastrointestinal disease and in up to 60% of those in whom hospital stay has been prolonged because of postoperative complications. It is frequently unrecognised and consequently patients often do not receive appropriate support. There is a substantial body of evidence to show that patients who suffer starvation or have signs of malnutrition have a higher risk of complications and an increased risk of death in comparison with patients who have adequate nutritional reserves.

Long-standing protein–calorie malnutrition is easy to recognise (Fig. 17.1). Short-term undernutrition, which has similar adverse consequences, is an inevitable outcome of critical illness, major trauma, burns or surgery and impacts on patient recovery.

The aim of nutritional support is to identify those patients at risk of malnutrition and to ensure that their nutritional requirements are met by the most appropriate route and in a way that minimises complications.

PHYSIOLOGY

Metabolic response to starvation

After a short fast lasting 12 hours or less, most food from the last meal will have been absorbed. Plasma insulin levels fall and glucagon levels rise, which facilitates the conversion of 200 g of liver glycogen into glucose. The liver, therefore, becomes an organ of glucose production under fasting conditions. Many organs, including brain tissue, red and white blood cells and the renal medulla, can initially utilise only glucose for their metabolic needs. Additional stores of glycogen exist in muscle (500 g) but these cannot be utilised directly. Muscle glycogen is broken down

(glycogenolysis) and converted to lactate, which is then exported to the liver where it is converted to glucose (Cori cycle). With increasing duration of fasting (> 24 hours), glycogen stores are depleted and *de novo* glucose production from non-carbohydrate

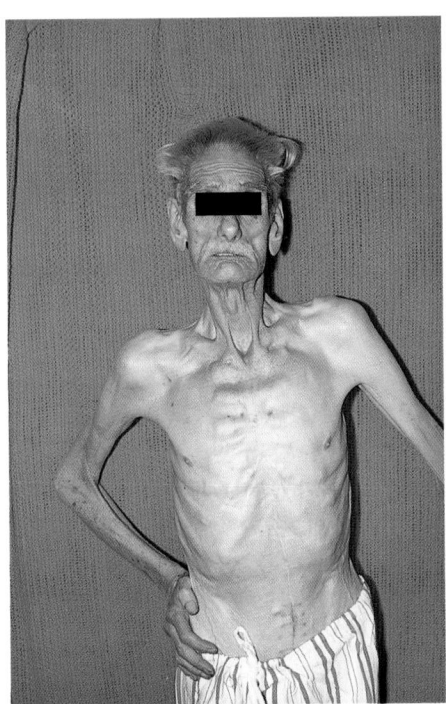

Figure 17.1 Severely malnourished patient with wasting of fat and muscle.

Carl Ferdinand Cori, 1896–1984, Professor of Pharmacology, and later of Biochemistry, Washington University Medical School, St, Louis, MO, USA, and his wife Gerty Theresa Cori, 1896–1957 who was also Professor of Biochemistry at the Washington University Medical School. In 1947 the Coris shared the Nobel Prize for Physiology or Medicine with Bernado Alberto Houssay, 'For their discovery of how glycogen is catalytically converted'.
de novo is Latin for 'from the beginning'.

precursors (gluconeogenesis) takes place, predominantly in the liver. Most of this glucose is derived from the breakdown of amino acids, particularly glutamine and alanine as a result of catabolism of skeletal muscle (up to 75 g per day). This protein catabolism in simple starvation is readily reversed with the provision of exogenous glucose (Fig. 17.2).

With more prolonged fasting there is an increased reliance on fat oxidation to meet energy requirements. Increased breakdown of fat stores occurs, providing glycerol, which can be converted to glucose, and fatty acids, which can be used as a tissue fuel by almost all of the body's tissues. Hepatic production of ketones from fatty acids is facilitated by low insulin levels and after 2–3 weeks of fasting the central nervous system may adapt to using ketone bodies as their primary fuel source. This conversion to a 'fat fuel economy' reduces the need for muscle breakdown by up to 55 g per day. Another important adaptive response to starvation is a significant reduction in the resting energy expenditure, possibly mediated by a decline in the conversion of inactive thyroxine (T_4) to active tri-iodothyronine (T_3). Despite these adaptive responses there remains an obligatory glucose requirement of about 200 g per day, even under conditions of prolonged fasting (Summary box 17.1).

Summary box 17.1

Metabolic response to starvation

- Low plasma insulin
- High plasma glucagon
- Hepatic glycogenolysis
- Protein catabolism
- Hepatic gluconeogenesis
- Lipolysis: mobilisation of fat stores
- Adaptive ketogenesis
- Reduction in resting energy expenditure (15–20 kcal kg^{-1} day^{-1})

Metabolic response to trauma and sepsis

This is described in full in Chapter 1 and summarised in Summary box 17.2.

Summary box 17.2

Metabolic response to trauma and sepsis

- Increased counter-regulatory hormones: adrenaline, noradrenaline, cortisol, glucagon and growth hormone
- Increased energy requirements (up to 40 kcal kg^{-1} day^{-1})
- Increased nitrogen requirements
- Insulin resistance and glucose intolerance
- Preferential oxidation of lipids
- Increased gluconeogenesis and protein catabolism
- Loss of adaptive ketogenesis
- Fluid retention with associated hypoalbuminaemia

From a nutritional point of view two factors deserve emphasis. First, in contrast to simple starvation, patients with trauma have impaired formation of ketones and *the breakdown of protein cannot be prevented by the administration of glucose* (Fig. 17.3). Second, although it is generally accepted that the metabolic response to trauma and sepsis is always associated with 'hypermetabolism' or

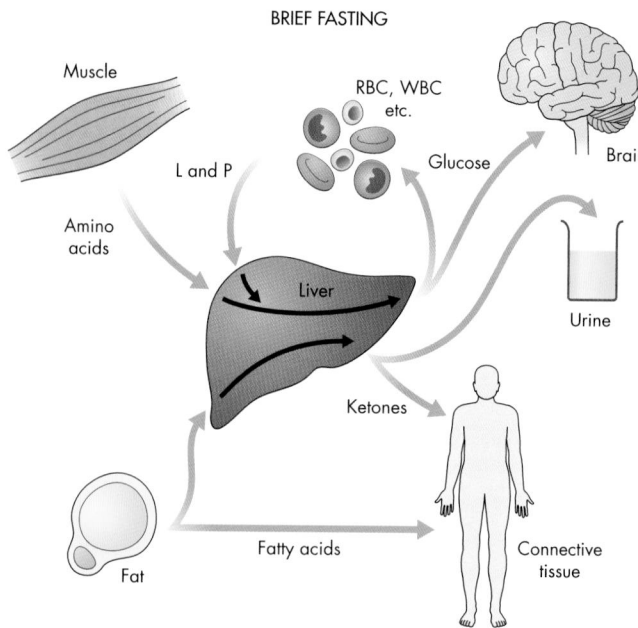

Figure 17.2 Schematic diagram to show metabolic response to fasting. L, lactate; P, pyruvate; RBC, red blood cells; WBC, white blood cells.

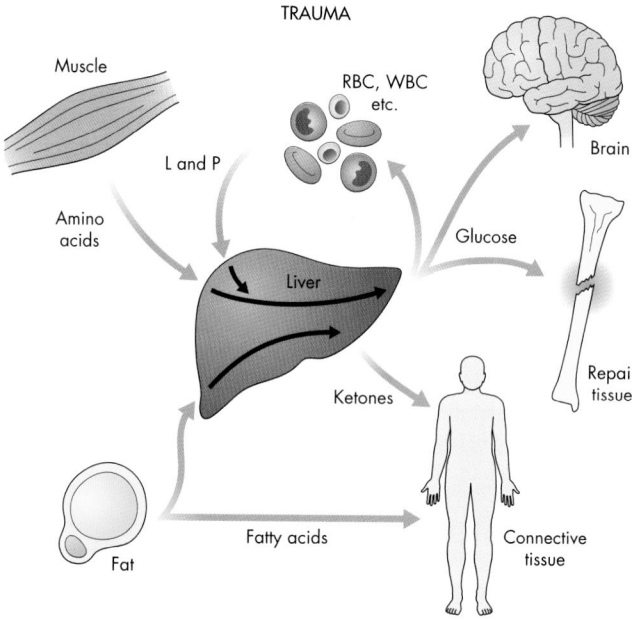

Figure 17.3 Schematic diagram showing metabolic response to trauma or sepsis. For abbreviations, see Fig. 17.2.

'hypercatabolism', these terms are ill defined and do not indicate the need for very high-energy intakes. There is no evidence to show that the provision of high-energy intakes is associated with an amelioration of the catabolic process and it may indeed be harmful.

NUTRITIONAL ASSESSMENT

Laboratory techniques

There is no single biochemical measurement that reliably identifies malnutrition. Albumin is not a measure of nutritional status. Although a low serum albumin level (< 30 g l^{-1}) is an indicator of poor prognosis, hypoalbuminaemia invariably occurs because of alterations in body fluid composition and because of increased capillary permeability related to on-going sepsis. Malnutrition is associated with defective immune function, and measurement of lymphocyte count and skin testing for delayed hypersensitivity frequently reveal abnormalities in malnourished patients. Immunity is not, however, a precise or reliable indicator of nutritional status, nor is it a practical method in routine clinical practice.

Body weight and anthropometry

A simple method of assessing nutritional status is to estimate weight loss. Measured body weight is compared with ideal body weight obtained from tables or from the patient's usual or pre-morbid weight. Unintentional weight loss of more than 10% of a patient's weight in the preceding 6 months is a good prognostic indicator of poor outcome. Body weight is frequently corrected for height, allowing calculation of the body mass index (BMI – defined as body weight in kilograms divided by height in metres squared). A BMI of less than 18.5 indicates nutritional impairment and a BMI below 15 is associated with significant hospital mortality. Major changes in fluid balance, which are common in critically ill patients, may make body weight and BMI unreliable indicators of nutritional status.

Anthropometric techniques incorporating measurements of skinfold thicknesses and mid-arm circumference permit estimations of body fat and muscle mass, and these are indirect measures of energy and protein stores. These measurements are, however, insufficiently accurate in individual patients to permit planning of nutritional support regimens. Similarly, use of bioelectrical impedence analysis (BIA) permits estimation of intra- and extracellular fluid volumes. These techniques are only useful if performed frequently on a sequential basis in individual patients. All of these techniques are significantly impaired by the presence of oedema.

Clinical

The possibility of malnutrition should form part of the work-up of all patients. A clinical assessment of nutritional status involves a focused history and physical examination, an assessment of risk of malabsorption or inadequate dietary intake and selected laboratory tests aimed at detecting specific nutrient deficiencies. This is termed 'subjective global assessment' and encompasses historical, symptomatic and physical parameters. Recently, the British Association of Parenteral and Enteral Nutrition introduced a Malnutrition Universal Screening Tool (MUST), which is a five-step screening tool to identify adults who are malnourished or at risk of undernutrition (Fig. 17.4).

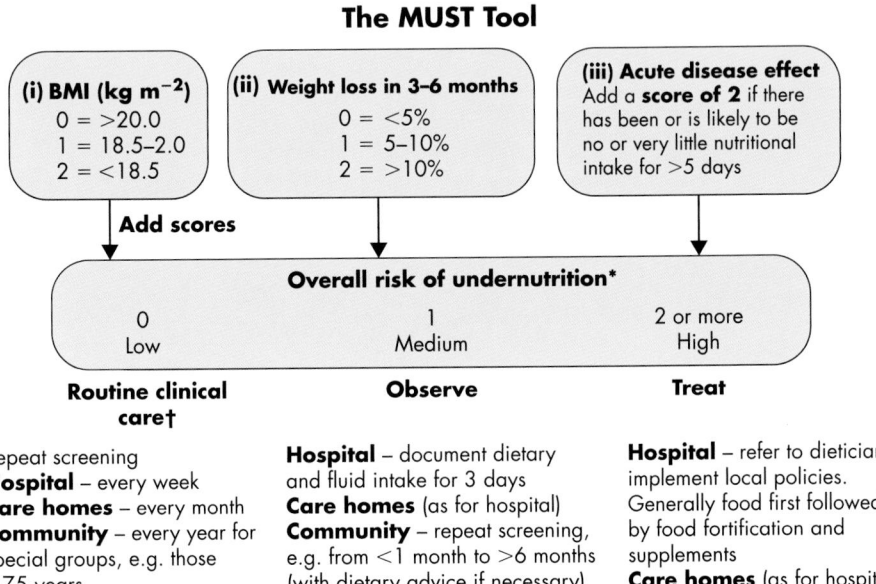

The MUST Tool

(i) BMI (kg m⁻²)
0 = >20.0
1 = 18.5-2.0
2 = <18.5

(ii) Weight loss in 3–6 months
0 = <5%
1 = 5–10%
2 = >10%

(iii) Acute disease effect
Add a **score of 2** if there has been or is likely to be no or very little nutritional intake for >5 days

Add scores

Overall risk of undernutrition*

| 0 | 1 | 2 or more |
| Low | Medium | High |

Routine clinical care†

Repeat screening
Hospital – every week
Care homes – every month
Community – every year for special groups, e.g. those >75 years

Observe

Hospital – document dietary and fluid intake for 3 days
Care homes (as for hospital)
Community – repeat screening, e.g. from <1 month to >6 months (with dietary advice if necessary)

Treat

Hospital – refer to dietician or implement local policies. Generally food first followed by food fortification and supplements
Care homes (as for hospital)
Community (as for hospital)

***If height, weight or weight loss cannot be established,** use documented or recalled values (if considered reliable). When measured or recalled height cannot be obtained, use knee height as surrogate measure.
If neither can be calculated, obtain an overall impression of malnutrition risk (low, medium, high) using the following:
(i) Clinical impression (very thin, thin, average, overweight);
(iia) Clothes and/or jewellery have become loose fitting;
(iib) History of decreased food intake, loss of appetite or dysphagia up to 3–6 months;
(iic) Disease (underlying cause) and psychosocial/physical disabilities likely to cause weight loss.

† Involves treatment of underlying condition, and help with food choice and eating when necessary (also applies to other categories).

Figure 17.4 The Malnutrition Universal Screening Tool (MUST) for adults [adapted from Elia, M. (ed.) (2003) *The MUST Report. Development and Use of the 'Malnutrition Universal Screening Tool' (MUST) for Adults*. A report by the Malnutrition Advisory Group of the British Association for Parenteral and Enteral Nutrition. Report No. ISBN 1 899467 70X, 152, with kind permission].

Marinos Elia, **Contemporary, Head of the Adult Clinical Nutrition Group, The Medical Research Council, Cambridge, England.**

FLUID AND ELECTROLYTES

Fluid intake is derived from both exogenous (consumed liquids) and endogenous (released during oxidation of solid foodstuffs) fluids. The average daily water balance of a healthy adult is shown in Table 17.1.

Fluid losses occur by four routes:

- *Lungs.* About 400 ml of water is lost in expired air each 24 hours. This is increased in dry atmospheres or in patients with a tracheostomy, emphasising the importance of humidification of inspired air.
- *Skin.* In a temperate climate, skin (i.e. sweat) losses are between 600 and 1000 ml day^{-1}.
- *Faeces.* Between 60 and 150 ml of water are lost daily in patients with normal bowel function.
- *Urine.* The normal urine output is approximately 1500 ml day^{-1} and, provided that the kidneys are healthy, the specific gravity of urine bears a direct relationship to volume. A minimum urine output of 400 ml day^{-1} is required to excrete the end products of protein metabolism.

Maintenance fluid requirements are calculated approximately from an estimation of insensible and obligatory losses. Various formulae are available for calculating fluid replacement based on a patient's weight or surface area. For example, 30–40 ml kg^{-1} gives an estimate of daily requirements.

The following are the approximate daily requirements of some electrolytes in adults:

- sodium: 50–90 mM day^{-1};
- potassium: 50 mM day^{-1};
- calcium: 5 mM day^{-1};
- magnesium: 1 mM day^{-1}.

The nature and type of fluid replacement therapy will be determined by individual patient needs. The composition of some commonly used solutions is shown in Table 17.2.

Note that Hartmann's solution also contains lactate (28 mM l^{-1}). Dextrose solutions are also commonly employed. These provide water replacement without any electrolytes and with modest calorie supplements (1 litre of 5% dextrose contains 400 kcal). A typical daily maintenance fluid regimen would consist of a combination of 5% dextrose with either Hartmann's or normal saline to a volume of 2 litres.

There has been much controversy in the literature regarding the respective merits of crystalloid versus colloid replacement. There is no consensus on this topic and the usual advice is to replace like with like. If the haematocrit is below 30%, blood transfusion may be required. There is increasing recognition, however, that albumin infusions are of little value.

In addition to maintenance requirements, 'replacement' fluids are required to correct pre-existing deficiencies and 'supplemental' fluids are required to compensate for anticipated additional intestinal or other losses. The nature and volumes of these fluids are determined by:

- A careful assessment of the patient including pulse, blood pressure and central venous pressure if available. Clinical examination to assess hydration status (peripheries, skin turgor, urine output and specific gravity of urine), urine and serum electrolytes and haematocrit.
- Estimation of losses already incurred and their nature: for example, vomiting, ileus, diarrhoea, excessive sweating or fluid losses from burns or other serious inflammatory conditions.
- Estimation of supplemental fluids likely to be required in view of anticipated future losses from drains, fistulae, nasogastric tubes or abnormal urine or faecal losses.
- When an estimate of the volumes required has been made, the appropriate replacement fluid can be determined from a consideration of the electrolyte composition of gastrointestinal secretions. Most intestinal losses are adequately replaced with normal saline containing supplemental potassium (Table 17.3).

NUTRITIONAL REQUIREMENTS

Total enteral or parenteral nutrition necessitates the provision of the macronutrients, carbohydrate, fat and protein, together with vitamins, trace elements, electrolytes and water. When planning a feeding regimen the patient should be weighed and an assessment made of daily energy and protein requirements. Standard tables are available to permit these calculations.

Daily needs may change depending on the patient's condition. Overfeeding is the most common cause of complications, regardless of whether nutrition is provided enterally or parenterally. It is

Table 17.1 Average daily water balance of a healthy adult in a temperate climate (70 kg)

Output	Volume (ml)	Intake	Volume (ml)
Urine	1500	Water from beverage	200
Insensible losses	900	Water from food	1000
Faeces	100	Water from oxidation	300

Table 17.2 Composition of crystalloid and colloid solutions (mM l^{-1})

Solution	Na	K	Ca	Cl	Lactate	Colloid
Hartmann's	130	4	2.7	109	28	
Normal saline (0.9% NaCl)	154			154		
Dextrose saline (4% dextrose in 0.18% saline)	30			30		
Gelofusine	150		< 1	150		Gelatin 4%
Haemacel	145	5.1	6.26	145		Polygelin 75 g l^{-1}
Hetastarch						Hydroxyethyl starch 6%

Alexis Frank Hartmann, **1898–1964, Paediatrician, St. Louis, MO, USA.**

Table 17.3 Composition of gastrointestinal secretions (mM l^{-1})

	Na	K	Cl	HCO$_3$
Saliva	10	25	10	30
Stomach	50	15	110	–
Duodenum	140	5	100	–
Ileum	140	5	100	30
Pancreas	140	5	75	115
Bile	140	5	100	35

essential to monitor daily intake to provide an assessment of tolerance. Failure to do so is the most common reason for inadequate nutrition. In addition, regular biochemical monitoring is mandatory (Table 17.4).

Macronutrient requirements

Energy

The total energy requirement of a stable patient with a normal or moderately increased need is approximately 20–30 kcal kg^{-1} day^{-1}. Very few patients require energy intakes in excess of 2000 kcal day^{-1}. Thus, in the majority of hospitalised patients in whom energy demands from activity are minimal, total energy requirements are approximately 1300–1800 kcal day^{-1}.

Carbohydrate

There is an obligatory glucose requirement to meet the needs of the central nervous system and certain haematopoietic cells, which is equivalent to about 2 g kg^{-1} day^{-1}. In addition, there is a physiological maximum amount of glucose that can be oxidised, which is approximately 4 mg kg^{-1} min, with the non-oxidised glucose being primarily converted to fat. Optimal utilisation of energy during nutritional support is ensured by avoiding the infusion of glucose at rates approximating physiological maximums and providing energy as a mixture of glucose and fat. Glucose is the preferred carbohydrate source.

Fat

Dietary fat is composed of triglycerides of predominantly four long-chain fatty acids. There are two saturated fatty acids – palmitic (C16) and stearic (C18) – and two unsaturated fatty acids – oleic (C18 with one double bond) and linoleic (C18 with two double bonds). In addition, smaller amounts of linolenic acid (C18 with three double bonds) and medium-chain fatty acids (C6–C10) are contained in the diet.

The unsaturated fatty acids linoleic and linolenic acid are considered essential because they cannot be synthesised *in vivo* from non-dietary sources. Both soybean and sunflower oil emulsions are rich sources of linoleic acid and provision of only 1 litre of emulsion per week avoids deficiency. Soybean emulsions contain approximately 7% alpha-linolenic acid (an omega-3 fatty acid). The provision of fat as a soybean oil-based emulsion on a regular basis will obviate the risk of essential fatty acid deficiency.

Safe and non-toxic fat emulsions based upon long-chain triglycerides (LCTs) have been commercially available for over 30 years. These emulsions provide a calorically dense product (9 kcal g^{-1}) and are now routinely used to supplement the provision of non-protein calories during parenteral nutrition. Energy during parenteral nutrition should be given as a mixture of fat together with glucose. There is no evidence to suggest that any particular ratio of glucose to fat is optimal as long as under all conditions the basal requirements for glucose (100–200 g day^{-1}) and essential fatty acids (100–200 g week^{-1}) are met. This 'dual energy' supply minimises metabolic complications during parenteral nutrition, reduces fluid retention, enhances substrate utilisation, particularly in the septic patient, and is associated with reduced carbon dioxide production.

Concerns have been expressed about the possible immunosuppressive effects of LCT emulsions. These are more likely to occur if the recommended infusion rates (0.15 g kg^{-1} hour^{-1}) are exceeded. Nonetheless, these concerns have prompted the development of newer emulsions based upon medium-chain triglycerides, omega-3 fatty acids and, most recently, structured

Table 17.4 Monitoring feeding regimens

Daily	Body weight
	Fluid balance
	Full blood count, urea and electrolytes
	Blood glucose
	Electrolyte content and volume of urine and/or urine and intestinal losses
	Temperature
Weekly (or more frequently if clinically indicated)	Urine and plasma osmolality
	Calcium, magnesium, zinc and phosphate
	Plasma proteins including albumin
	Liver function tests including clotting factors
	Thiamine
	Acid–base status
	Triglycerides
Fortnightly	Serum vitamin B12
	Folate
	Iron
	Lactate
	Trace elements (zinc, copper, manganese)

in vivo **is Latin for 'in a living thing'.**

triglycerides, which combine long- and medium-chain triglycerides in the same emulsion. The evidence of clinical benefit for these emulsions compared with conventional LCTs is tenuous, particularly if infusion rates are appropriate and hypertriglyceridaemia is avoided.

Protein

The basic requirement for nitrogen in patients without pre-existing malnutrition and without metabolic stress is 0.10–0.15 g kg^{-1} day^{-1}. In hypermetabolic patients the nitrogen requirements increase to 0.20–0.25 g kg^{-1} day^{-1}. Although there may be a minority of patients in whom the requirements are higher, such as after acute weight loss when the objective of therapy is long-term repletion of lean body mass, there is little evidence that the provision of nitrogen in excess of 14 g day^{-1} is beneficial.

Vitamins, minerals and trace elements

Whatever the method of feeding these are all essential components of nutritional regimens. The water-soluble vitamins B and C act as coenzymes in collagen formation and wound healing. Postoperatively, the vitamin C requirement increases to 60–80 mg day^{-1}. Supplemental vitamin B12 is often indicated in patients who have undergone intestinal resection or gastric surgery and in those with a history of alcohol dependence. Absorption of the fat-soluble vitamins A, D, E and K is reduced in steatorrhea and the absence of bile.

Sodium, potassium and phosphate are all subject to significant losses, particularly in patients with diarrhoeal illness. Their levels need daily monitoring and appropriate replacement.

Trace elements may also act as cofactors for metabolic processes. Normally, trace element requirements are met by the delivery of food to the gut and so patients on long-term parenteral nutrition are at particular risk of depletion. Magnesium, zinc and iron levels may all be decreased as part of the inflammatory response. Supplementation is necessary to optimise the utilisation of amino acids and to avoid refeeding syndrome.

FLUID AND NUTRITIONAL CONSEQUENCES OF INTESTINAL RESECTION

Up to 50% of the small intestine can be surgically removed or bypassed without permanent deleterious effects. With extensive resection (< 150 cm of remaining small intestine) metabolic and nutritional consequences arise, resulting in the disease entity known as short bowel syndrome. The clinical presentation of patients with short bowel syndrome is dependent upon the nature and extent of intestinal resection.

Small bowel motility

Small bowel motility is three times slower in the ileum than in the jejunum. In addition, the ileocaecal valve may slow transit. The adult small bowel receives 5–6 litres of endogenous secretions and 2–3 litres of exogenous fluids per day. Most of this is reabsorbed in the small bowel. In the jejunum the cellular junctions are leaky and jejunal contents are always isotonic. Fluid absorption in this region of bowel is inefficient compared with the ileum. It has been estimated that the efficiency of water absorption is 44% and 70% of the ingested load in the jejunum and ileum respectively. The corresponding figures for sodium are 13%

and 72% respectively. It can be seen, therefore, that the ileum is critical in the conservation of fluid and electrolytes (Table 17.5).

Ileum

The ileum is the only site of absorption of vitamin B12 and bile salts. Bile salts are essential for the absorption of fats and fat-soluble vitamins. The enterohepatic circulation of bile salts is critical to maintain the bile salt pool. Following resection of the ileum the loss of bile salts increases and is not met by an increase in synthesis. Depletion of the bile salt pool results in fat malabsorption. In addition, loss of bile salts into the colon affects colonic mucosa, causing a reduction in salt and water absorption, which increases stool losses.

Colon

Transit times in the colon vary between 24 and 150 hours. The efficiency of water and salt absorption in the colon exceeds 90%. Another important colonic function is the fermentation of carbohydrates to produce short-chain fatty acids. These have two important functions: first, they enhance water and salt absorption from the colon and, second, they are trophic to the colonocyte.

Effects of resection

Resection of proximal jejunum results in no significant alterations in fluid and electrolyte levels as the ileum and colon can adapt to absorb the increased fluid and electrolyte load. Absorption of nutrients occurs throughout the small bowel and resection of jejunum alone results in the ileum taking over this lost function. In this situation there is no malabsorption.

Resection of ileum results in a significant enhancement of gastric motility and acceleration of intestinal transit. Following ileal resection the colon receives a much larger volume of fluid and electrolytes and it also receives bile salts, which reduce its ability to absorb salt and water, resulting in diarrhoea. Even the loss of 100 cm of ileum causes steathorrea, which may necessitate the administration of oral cholestyramine to bind bile salts. With larger resections (> 100 cm) dietary fat restriction may be necessary. Regular parenteral vitamin B12 is required.

The most challenging patients are those with short bowel syndrome who have had in excess of 200 cm of small bowel resected together with colectomy. These patients will usually have a jejunostomy. They are conveniently divided into two groups termed 'net absorbers' and 'net secretors'. Absorbers characteristically have more than 100 cm of residual jejunum and they absorb more water and sodium from the diet than passes through the stoma. These patients can be managed without parenteral fluids.

Secretors usually have less than 100 cm of residual jejunum

Table 17.5 Intestinal luminal volume and absorption

	Volume (ml 24 h^{-1})	Sodium (mmol l^{-1})	Efficiency of water absorption (%)	Efficiency of sodium absorption (%)
Duodenum	9000	800	–	–
Jejunum	5000	700	44	13
Ileum	1500	200	70	72
Colon	100	3	93	99

and lose more water and sodium from their stoma than they take by mouth. These patients require supplements. Their usual daily jejunostomy output may exceed 4 kg per 24 hours. The sodium content of jejunostomy losses or other high-output fistulas is about 90 mmol l^{-1}. Jejunal mucosa is leaky and rapid sodium fluxes occur across it. If water or any solution with a sodium concentration of less than 90 mmol l^{-1} is consumed there is a net efflux of sodium from the plasma into the bowel lumen. It is therefore inappropriate to encourage patients with high-output jejunostomies (secretors) to drink large amounts of oral hypotonic solutions. Treatment begins with restricting the total amount of hypotonic fluids (water, tea, juices, etc.) consumed to less than a litre a day. Patients should be encouraged to take glucose and saline replacement solutions, which have a sodium concentration of at least 90 mmol l^{-1}. The World Health Organization (WHO) cholera solution has a sodium concentration of 90 mmol l^{-1} and is commonly used.

Complications of short bowel syndrome include peptic ulceration related to gastric hypersecretion, cholelithiasis because of interruption of the enterohepatic cycle of bile salts, and hyperoxaluria as a result of the increased absorption of oxalate in the colon predisposing to renal stones. Some patients with short bowel syndrome develop a syndrome of slurred speech, ataxia and altered affect. The cause of this syndrome is fermentation of malabsorbed carbohydrates in the colon to D-lactate and absorption of this metabolite. Treatment necessitates the use of a low carbohydrate diet.

Anti-secretory drugs reduce the amount of fluid secreted from the stomach, liver and pancreas. These include H2-receptor antagonists, proton pump inhibitors and the somatostatin analogue octreotide. Octreotide also reduces gastrointestinal motility. Anti-motility drugs include loperamide and codeine phosphate, which also decrease water and sodium output from the stoma by about 20%.

ARTIFICIAL NUTRITIONAL SUPPORT

The indications for nutritional support are simple (Fig. 17.5). Any patient who has sustained 5–7 days of inadequate intake or who is anticipated to have no intake for this period should be considered for nutritional support. The periods may be less in patients with pre-existing malnutrition. This concept is important because it emphasises that the provision of nutritional support is not specific to certain conditions or diseases. Although patients with Crohn's disease or pancreatitis, or those who have undergone gastrointestinal resections, may frequently require nutritional support, it is the fact that they have had inadequate intakes for defined periods that is the indication rather than the specific disease process.

Enteral nutrition

The term 'enteral feeding' means delivery of nutrients into the gastrointestinal tract. The alimentary tract should be used whenever possible. This can be achieved with oral supplements (sip feeding) or with a variety of tube-feeding techniques delivering food into the stomach, duodenum or jejunum.

A variety of nutrient formulations are available for enteral

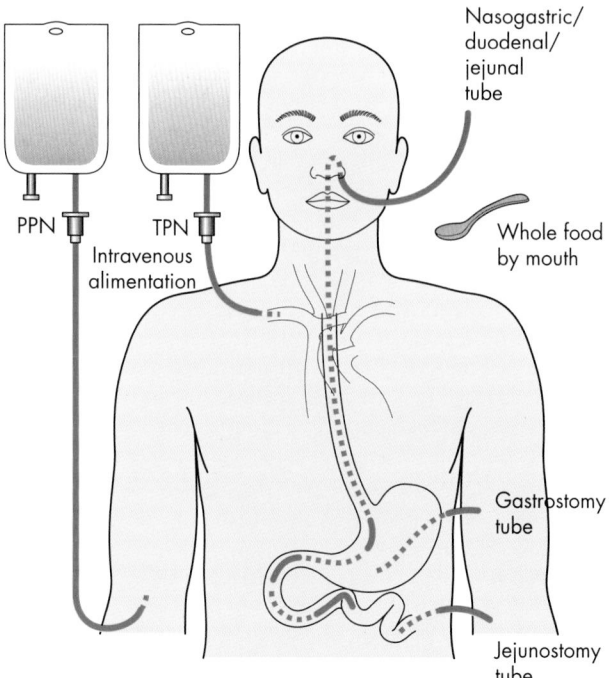

Figure 17.5 Techniques used for adjuvant nutritional support. PPN, partial parenteral nutrition; TPN, total parenteral nutrition. Redrawn with permission from Rick Tharp, rxkinetics.com.

feeding. These vary with respect to energy content, osmolarity, fat and nitrogen content and nutrient complexity. Most contain up to 1–2 kcal ml^{-1} and up to 0.6 g ml^{-1} of protein. Polymeric feeds contain intact protein and hence require digestion whereas monomeric/elemental feeds contain nitrogen in the form of either free amino acids or, in some cases, peptides. These are less palatable and are used much less frequently than in previous years. Newer feeding formulations are available that include glutamine and fibre to optimise intestinal nutrition or immunonutrients such as arginine and fish oils but these are expensive and their use is controversial.

Sip feeding

Commercially available supplementary sip feeds are used in patients who can drink but whose appetites are impaired or in whom adequate intakes cannot be maintained with *ad libitum* intakes. These feeds typically provide 200 kcal and 2 g of nitrogen per 200 ml carton. There is good evidence to demonstrate that these sip-feeding techniques are associated with a significant overall increase in calorie and nitrogen intakes without detriment to spontaneous nutrition. The evidence that these techniques improve patient outcomes is less convincing.

Tube-feeding techniques

Enteral nutrition can be achieved using conventional nasogastric tubes (Ryle's), fine-bore feeding tubes inserted into the stomach, surgical or percutaneous endoscopic gastrostomy (PEG) or, finally, post-pyloric feeding utilising nasojejunal tubes or various types of jejunostomy. The choice of method will be determined by local

Burrill Bernard Crohn, **1884–1983, Gastroenterologist, Mount Sinai Hospital, New York, NY, USA, described regional ileitis in 1932.**

ad libidum is Latin for 'at pleasure'.
John Alfred Ryle, **1889–1950, Regius Professor of Medicine, Cambridge University, and later Professor of Social Medicine, Oxford University, Oxford, England, introduced the Ryle's tube in 1921.**

circumstances and preference in many patients. Whichever method is adopted it is important that tube feeding is supervised by an experienced dietician who will calculate the patient's requirements and aim to achieve these within 2–3 days of the instigation of feeds. Conventionally, 20–30 ml are administered per hour initially, gradually increasing to goal rates within 48–72 hours. In most units feeding is discontinued for 4–5 hours overnight to allow gastric pH to return to normal. There is some evidence that this might reduce the incidence of nosocomial pneumonia and aspiration. There is good evidence to confirm that feeding protocols optimise the tolerance of enteral nutrition. In these, aspirates are performed on a regular basis and if they exceed 200 ml in any 2-hour period then feeding is temporarily discontinued.

Tube blockage is common. All tubes should be flushed with water at least twice daily. If a build-up of solidified diet occurs, instillation into the tube of agents such as chymotrypsin or papain may salvage a partially obstructed tube. Guidewires should not be used to clear blockages as these may perforate the tube and cause contiguous damage.

Nasogastric tubes are appropriate in a majority of patients. If feeding is maintained for more than a week or so a fine-bore feeding tube is preferable and is likely to cause fewer gastric and oesophageal erosions. These are usually made from soft polyurethane or silicone elastomer and have an internal diameter of < 3 mm.

Fine-bore tube insertion

The patient should be semirecumbent. The introducer wire is lubricated and inserted into the fine-bore tube (Fig. 17.6). The tube is passed through the nose and into the stomach via the nasopharynx and oesophagus. The wire is withdrawn and the tube is taped to the patient. There is a small risk of malposition into a bronchus or of causing pneumothorax. The position of the tube should be checked using plain abdominal radiography (Fig. 17.7). Alternatively, 5 ml of air can be injected and a stethoscope used to confirm bubbling from the stomach. Confirmation of position by pH testing is possible but limited by the difficulty of obtaining a fluid aspirate with narrow lumen tubes.

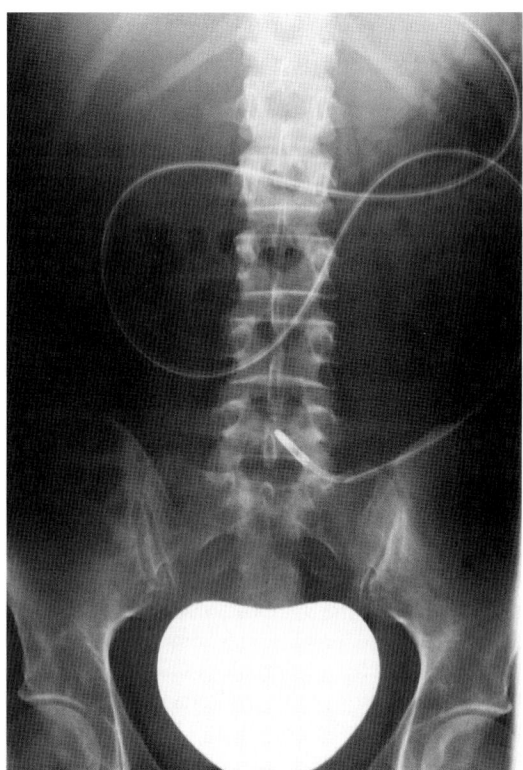

Figure 17.7 Radiograph of a tube similar to that in Figure 17.6 inserted beyond the duodenojejunal flexure.

Gastrostomy

The placement of a tube through the abdominal wall directly into the stomach is termed 'gastrostomy'. Historically, these were created surgically at the time of laparotomy. Today, the majority are performed by percutaneous insertion under endoscopic control using local anaesthesia (PEG) (Fig. 17.8).

Two methods of PEG are commonly used. The first is called the 'direct-stab' technique in which the endoscope is passed and the stomach filled with air. The endoscopist then watches a cannula entering the stomach having been inserted directly through the anterior abdominal wall. A guidewire is then passed through the cannula into the stomach. A gastrostomy tube (commercially available) may then be introduced into the stomach through a 'peel away' sheath. The alternative technique is the transoral or push-through technique whereby a guidewire or

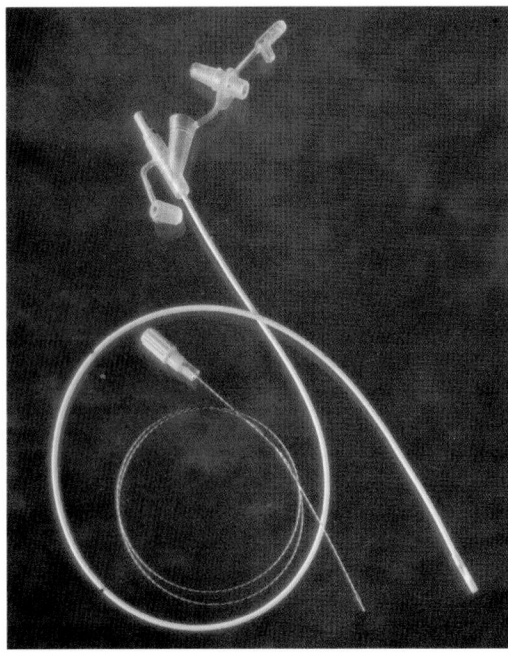

Figure 17.6 A fine-bore feeding tube with its guidewire.

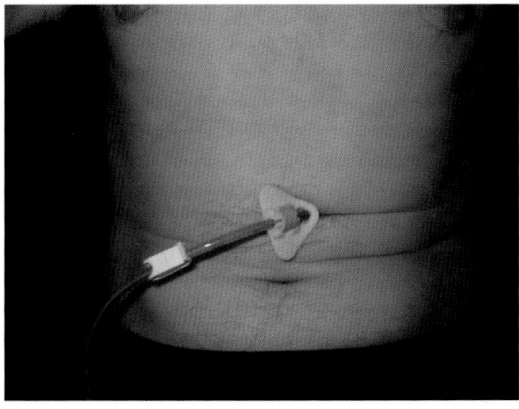

Figure 17.8 Percutaneous endoscopic gastrostomy tube.

suture is brought out of the stomach by the endoscope after trans-abdominal percutaneous insertion and is either attached to a gastrostomy tube or the tube is pushed over a guidewire. The abdominal end of the wire is then pulled, advancing the gastrostomy tube through the oesophagus and into the stomach. Continued pulling abuts it up against the abdominal wall.

If patients require enteral nutrition for prolonged periods (4–6 weeks) then PEG is preferable to an indwelling nasogastric tube; this minimises the traumatic complications related to indwelling tubes. PEG does have procedure-specific complications although these are uncommon. Necrotising fasciitis and intra-abdominal wall abscesses have been recorded. Sepsis around the PEG site is more common and may necessitate systemic antibiotics or repositioning. A persistent gastric fistula can occur on removal of a PEG if it has been in place for prolonged periods and epithelialisation of the tract has occurred. This necessitates surgical closure.

Jejunostomy

In recent years the use of jejunal feeding has become increasingly popular. This can be achieved using nasojejunal tubes or by placement of needle jejunostomy at the time of laparotomy. Some authorities advocate the use of jejunostomies on the basis that post-pyloric feeding may be associated with a reduction in aspiration or enhanced tolerance of enteral nutrition. In particular, there are many advocates of jejunostomies in patients with severe pancreatitis, in whom a degree of gastric outlet obstruction may be present, related to the oedematous head of pancreas. In most patients it is appropriate to commence with conventional nasogastric feeding and progress to post-pyloric feeding if the former is unsuccessful.

Nasojejunal tubes often necessitate the use of fluoroscopy or endoscopy to achieve placement, which may delay commencement of feeding. Surgical jejunostomies, even using commercially available needle-insertion techniques, do involve creating a defect in the jejunum, which can leak or be associated with tube displacement; both of these complications result in peritonitis.

Complications

Most complications of enteral nutrition can be avoided with careful attention to detail and appropriate infusion rates. Patients should be nursed semirecumbent to reduce the possibility of aspiration. Complications can be divided into those resulting from intubation of the gastrointestinal tract and those related to nutrient delivery. The former are more frequent with more invasive means of gaining access to the intestinal tract (see above). The latter include diarrhoea, bloating and vomiting. Diarrhoea occurs in more than 30% of patients receiving enteral nutrition and is particularly common in the critically ill. Up to 60% of patients in intensive care units may fail to receive their targeted intakes. There is no evidence that the incidence of diarrhoea and bloating is reduced by the use of half-strength feeds. It is important to introduce normal feeds at a reduced rate according to patient tolerance. Metabolic complications associated with excessive feeding are uncommon in enterally fed patients. There have been reports of nosocomial enteric infections associated with contamination of feeds, which should be kept in sealed containers at 4°C and discarded once opened.

In all patients it is essential to monitor intakes accurately as target intakes are often not achieved with enteral nutrition.

The complications of enteral nutrition are summarised in Summary box 17.3.

> **Summary box 17.3**
>
> ## Complications of enteral nutrition
>
> ### Tube-related
> - Malposition
> - Displacement
> - Blockage
> - Breakage/leakage
> - Local complications (e.g. erosion of skin/mucosa)
>
> ### Gastrointestinal
> - Diarrhoea
> - Bloating, nausea, vomiting
> - Abdominal cramps
> - Aspiration
> - Constipation
>
> ### Metabolic/biochemical
> - Electrolyte disorders
> - Vitamin, mineral, trace element deficiencies
> - Drug interactions
>
> ### Infective
> - Exogenous (handling contamination)
> - Endogenous (patient)

Parenteral nutrition

Total parenteral nutrition (TPN) is defined as the provision of all nutritional requirements by means of the intravenous route and without the use of the gastrointestinal tract.

Parenteral nutrition is indicated when energy and protein needs cannot be met by the enteral administration of these substrates. The most frequent clinical indications relate to those patients who have undergone massive resection of the small intestine, who have intestinal fistula or who have prolonged intestinal failure for other reasons.

Route of delivery: peripheral or central venous access

TPN can be administered either by a catheter inserted in the central vein or via a peripheral line. In the early days of parenteral nutrition the only energy source available was hypertonic glucose, which, being hypertonic, had to be given into a central vein to avoid thrombophlebitis. In the second half of the last century there were a number of important developments that have influenced the administration of parenteral nutrition. These include the identification of safe and non-toxic fat emulsions that are isotonic; pharmaceutical developments that permit carbohydrates, fats and amino acids to be mixed in single containers; and a recognition that the provision of energy during parenteral nutrition should be a mixture of glucose and fat and that energy requirement are rarely in excess of 2000 kcal day^{-1} (25–30 kcal kg^{-1} day^{-1}). These changes enabled the development of peripheral parenteral nutrition.

Peripheral

Peripheral feeding is appropriate for short-term feeding of up to 2 weeks. Access can be achieved either by means of a dedicated catheter inserted into a peripheral vein and manoeuvred into the central venous system [peripherally inserted central venous catheter (PICC) line] or by using a conventional short cannula in the wrist veins. The former method has the advantage of minimising inconvenience to the patient and clinician. These PICC lines have a mean duration of survival of 7 days. Their disadvantage is that when thrombophlebitis occurs the vein is irrevocably destroyed. In the alternative approach, intravenous nutrients are administered through a short cannula in wrist veins, infusing the patient's nutritional requirements on a cyclical basis over 12 hours. The cannula is then removed and re-sited in the contralateral arm. Peripheral parenteral nutrition has the advantage that it avoids the complications associated with central venous administration but suffers the disadvantage that it is limited by the development of thrombophlebitis (Fig. 17.9) Peripheral feeding is not indicated if patients already have an indwelling central venous line or in those in whom long-term feeding is anticipated.

Central

When the central venous route is chosen, the catheter can be inserted via the subclavian or internal or external jugular vein. There is good evidence to show that the safest means of establishing central venous access is by insertion of lines under ultrasound guidance; however, this will not be practicable for all cases. Most intensive care physicians and anaesthetists favour cannulation of internal or external jugular veins as these vessels are easily accessible. They suffer the disadvantage that the exit site is situated inconveniently on the side of the neck, where repeated movements result in disruption of the dressing with the attendant risk of sepsis. The infraclavicular subclavian approach is more suitable for feeding as the catheter then lies flat on the chest wall, which optimises nursing care (Fig. 17.10). For longer term parenteral nutrition Hickman lines are preferable. These are often inserted by a radiologist with fluoroscopic guidance or ultrasound. They incorporate a small cuff, which sits at the exit site of a subcutaneous tunnel. This is

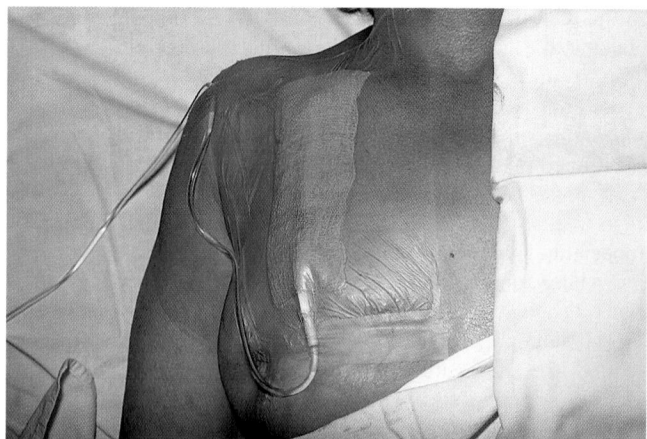

Figure 17.10 Infraclavicular subclavian line.

thought to minimise the possibility of line dislodgement and reduce the possibility of line sepsis. Whichever technique is employed, a post-insertion chest radiograph is essential before feeding is commenced to confirm the absence of pneumothorax and that the catheter tip lies in the distal superior vena cava to minimise the risk of central venous or cardiac thrombosis. Multilumen catheters can be used for the administration of TPN; one port should be employed for that sole purpose and strict protocols of care employed.

Complications of parenteral nutrition

The commencement of TPN may precipitate or accentuate underlying nutrient deficiency by encouraging anabolism. Common metabolic complications include fluid overload, hyperglycaemia, abnormalities of liver function and vitamin deficiencies. Fluid overload can be avoided by daily weighing of the patient. A weight change of $> 1\,\mathrm{kg\,day^{-1}}$ normally indicates fluid retention. Hyperglycaemia is common because of insulin resistance in critically ill patients. Even modest rates of glucose administration may be associated with hyperglycaemia. Hyperglycaemic patients undergoing surgery are known to run a substantially higher risk of infectious complications.

Abnormalities of liver enzymes are common in patients receiving TPN. Although the precise mechanisms are unclear, intrahepatic cholestasis may occur and hepatic steatosis and hepatomegaly have been reported. Reducing the fat content or infusion of fat-free TPN may be required. If liver enzymes continue to deteriorate TPN should be temporarily discontinued. In addition, overfeeding is a major factor in hepatic and other metabolic complications associated with TPN. Supplemental parenteral glutamine during parental nutrition should be considered, particularly in the critically ill patient.

Catheter-related sepsis occurs in 3–14% of patients. It may occur at the time of line insertion or afterwards by migration of skin bacteria along the external catheter surface. Some studies suggest that manoeuvring of the catheter hub due to frequent manipulations is a common cause. Contamination of the infusate is rare. Seeding on the catheter at the time of bacteraemia from a remote source may also cause catheter infection.

Diagnosis of catheter-related sepsis requires that the same organism is grown from the catheter tip as is recovered from blood and that the clinical features of infection resolve on removal of the catheter. Traditional methods of confirming line

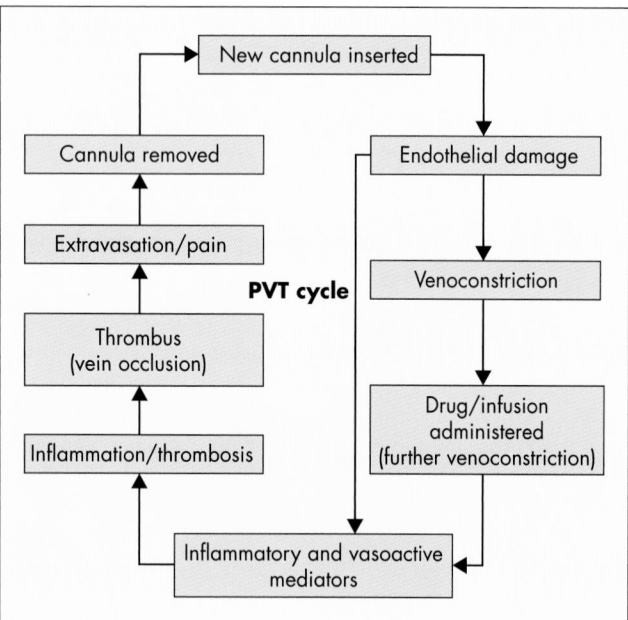

Figure 17.9 Cycle of causes of peripheral vein thrombophlebitis (PVT) [after Payne-James *et al.* (2001).

John Jason Payne-James, **Contemporary, Forensic Physician and Medical Writer,** Leigh-on-Sea, Essex, England.
Robert O. Hickman, **Formerly Nephrologist, The University of Washington, WA,** USA.

sepsis have necessitated removal of the line with subsequent bacteriological assessment. An alternative approach is to use an endoluminal brush passed down the catheter and withdrawn into a polythene sheath. The brush tip is cultured at the same time as performing blood cultures. Catheter sepsis is confirmed if identical organisms are cultured from brush and blood. A second alternative is to culture blood withdrawn through the catheter and compare this with peripheral blood cultures. If the colony count from the catheter sample is five or more times higher than that from peripheral blood then line sepsis is probable.

The complications of parenteral nutrition are summarised in Summary box 17.4.

Summary box 17.4

Complications of parenteral nutrition

Related to nutrient deficiency
- Hypoglycaemia/hypocalcaemia/hypophosphataemia/ hypomagnesaemia (refeeding syndrome)
- Chronic deficiency syndromes (essential fatty acids, zinc, mineral and trace elements)

Related to overfeeding
- Excess glucose: hyperglycaemia, hyperosmolar dehydration, hepatic steatosis, hypercapnia, increased sympathetic activity, fluid retention, electrolyte abnormalities
- Excess fat: hypercholesterolaemia and formation of lipoprotein X, hypertriglyceridaemia, hypersensitivity reactions
- Excess amino acids: hyperchloraemic metabolic acidosis, hypercalcaemia, aminoacidaemia, uraemia

Related to sepsis
- Catheter-related sepsis
- Possible increased predisposition to systemic sepsis

Related to line
- On insertion: pneumothorax, damage to adjacent artery, air embolism, thoracic duct damage, cardiac perforation or tamponade, pleural effusion, hydromediastinum
- Long-term use: occlusion, venous thrombosis

Refeeding syndrome

This syndrome is characterised by severe fluid and electrolyte shifts in malnourished patients undergoing refeeding. It can occur with either enteral or parenteral nutrition but is more common with the latter. It results in hypophosphataemia, hypocalcaemia and hypomagnesaemia. These electrolyte disorders can result in altered myocardial function, arrhythmias, deteriorating respiratory function, liver dysfunction, seizures, confusion, coma, tetany and death. Patients at risk include those with alcohol dependency, those suffering severe malnutrition, anorexics and those who have undergone prolonged periods of fasting. Treatment involves matching intakes with requirements and assiduously avoiding overfeeding. Calorie delivery should be increased slowly and vitamins administered regularly. Hypophosphataemia and hypomagnesaemia require treatment.

Nutrition support teams

Multidisciplinary nutrition teams ensure cost-effective and safe nutritional support, irrespective of how this is administered. The incidence of catheter-related sepsis is significantly reduced.

SUMMARY

Fluid therapy and nutritional support are fundamental to good surgical practice. Accurate fluid administration demands an understanding of maintenance requirements and an appreciation of the consequences of surgical disease on fluid losses. This requires knowledge of the consequences of surgical intervention and, in particular, intestinal resection.

Malnutrition is common in hospital patients. All patients who have sustained or who are likely to sustain 7 days of inadequate oral intake should be considered for nutritional support. This may be dietetic advice alone, sip feeding or enteral or parenteral nutrition. These are not mutually exclusive. The success or otherwise of nutritional support should be determined by tolerance to nutrients provided and nutritional endpoints such as weight. It is unrealistic to expect nutritional support to alter the natural history of disease. It is imperative that nutrition-related morbidity is kept to a minimum. This necessitates the appropriate selection of feeding method, careful assessment of fluid, energy and protein requirements, which are regularly monitored, and the avoidance of overfeeding.

ACKNOWLEDGEMENT

With thanks to Marcel Gatt, FRCS, who provided some illustrations and helped with proofreading the text.

FURTHER READING

Gibney, M., Elia, M., Ljungqvist, O. and Dowsett, J. (eds) (2005) *Clinical Nutrition* (The Nutrition Society Textbook Series). Blackwell Sciences, Oxford.

Payne-James, J., Grimble, G. and Silk, D. (eds) (2001) *Artificial Nutrition Support in Clinical Practice*, 2nd edn. Greenwich Medical Media, London.

Stroud, M., Duncan, H. and Nightingale, J. (2003) Guidelines for enteral feeding in adult hospital patients. *Gut* **52**: vii1–12.

CHAPTER 17 | NUTRITION AND FLUID THERAPY

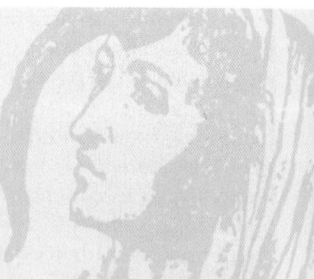

Basic surgical skills and anastomoses

CHAPTER

18

LEARNING OBJECTIVES

To understand:
- Surgical approaches, incisions and the use of appropriate instruments in surgery in general
- The indications for alternative technologies (glues and staples)

To know:
- The materials and methods used for surgical wound closure and anastomosis (sutures, knots and needles)

- The techniques for skin closure, artery and bowel anastomosis

To be aware of:
- The whole operative surgical team and the responsibility of each member in the care of sharps and perioperative care of instruments

INCISION OF SKIN

Skin and tissue incisions are usually made using scalpels with disposable blades. All sharp instruments, including needles, pose a risk of 'needle-stick' type injury and need to be passed within the operative team with great care using a kidney dish or similar. Attaching a blade to a scalpel handle, and its subsequent removal, is another simple skill that nevertheless needs to be learnt. This should be done using another instrument, such as a haemostat, and never using fingers. The blade shape and size is chosen for its purpose (Fig. 18.1). Blades for skin incisions usually have a curved margin; those used to make a passage for a drain through the skin or abdominal wall, or for an arteriotomy (which can be enlarged using arteriotomy scissors), have a sharp tip. When making an incision through skin and deeper layers for access, the knife should be pressed down firmly at right angles to the skin and then drawn across it. At the same time, tension should be applied across the line of the incision so that the skin springs apart cleanly (Fig. 18.2). It is important that the skin is not incised obliquely, as necrosis of the 'undercut' edge (not made at 90°) may occur. In long incisions of the lower limb, for vascular access, ischaemia of a skin edge risks infection, which can be disastrous because of the added risk of secondary haemorrhage from the anastomotic suture line. Diathermy, laser and harmonic scalpels can be used instead of blades when opening deeper tissues, as it is felt that they can reduce blood loss and save operating time, and may reduce postoperative pain.

SUTURE OF SKIN

Wounds should be closed with a minimum of tension. The edges of skin should gape slightly to allow swelling as the inflammation of healing occurs over the following few days. If a wound is closed tightly, swelling may cause wound edge necrosis and add to the risk of exogenous infection (Summary box 18.1).

Summary box 18.1

Closure of wounds

- Wound edges should be left slightly gaping to allow swelling
- Edges should be everted
- The knot should be placed to one side of the wound
- Knots must be secure, with the ends long enough to grasp when removing the suture

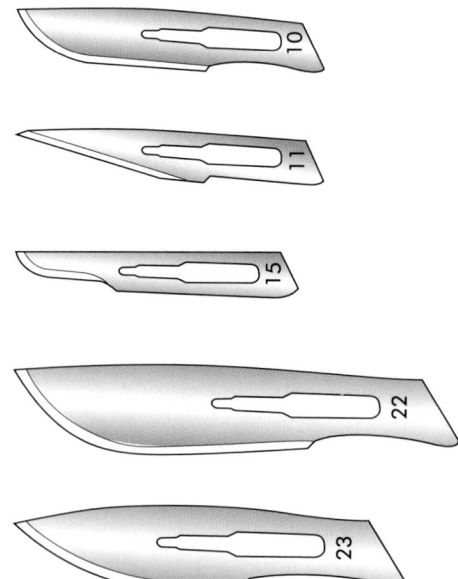

Figure 18.1 Scalpel blade sizes and shapes. The 11 blade is useful for arteriotomy, the 15 for minor operations and the rest for general use in incisions.

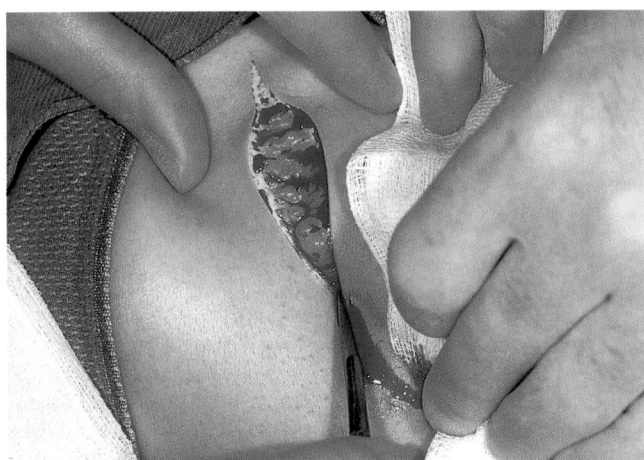

Figure 18.2 Skin incision. The skin is held taut between finger and thumb, and the incision is made with a clean sweep of the knife.

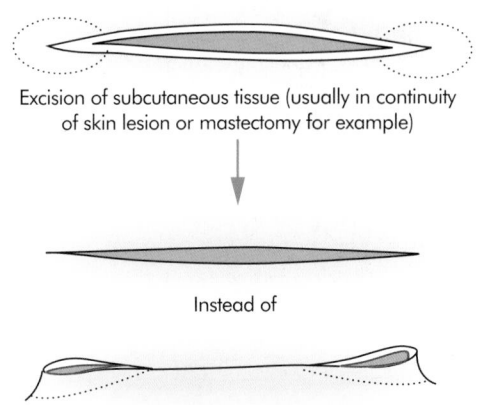

Figure 18.3 Avoidance of lateral incisional 'dog-ears'. The excision of subcutaneous tissue at the ends of a long incision can prevent 'dog-ears' at closure.

Needles are inserted at right angles to the skin for simple suture, using a supination/pronation movement of the wrist ('forehand' or 'backhand' suturing). Entry and exit points should be approximately the same distance from the wound edge as the thickness of the skin being closed. If the edge of the wound is gently everted with toothed forceps (the teeth can be used as a hook without grasping and injuring tissue) while the needle is inserted, a wider bite of the deeper tissue can be taken than the skin. The same can be done as the needle exits from the other side of the wound, ensuring that the suture takes a deep oval course through the tissues. When the suture is tightened, the wound edges should evert slightly (the best conditions for primary healing). If the suture enters and exits from the skin at an acute angle, the wound may become inverted with poor healing, and a poor cosmetic result needing revision.

As the suture is tightened, the knot should be drawn to one side to facilitate suture removal. When a non-absorbable suture is later removed, it needs to be cut immediately beneath the knot, and pulled out by the knot. The result is that the suture material contaminated by lying on the skin is lifted away without being drawn through the wound.

The final throw of the knot should be 'snugged' down, so that the knot cannot slip. The ends of the knot should be left long enough to be easy to grasp when they are being removed later, but not so long that they are tangled in adjacent sutures, or hair if the operative area has not been shaved.

As a general rule, each suture should be separated by a gap that is twice the thickness of the skin. If a wound is difficult to close, particularly after a large ellipse of skin has been removed, sutures can be placed alternately at each end of the wound, working towards the centre. If the wound has curves or zigzags, then 'stay sutures' at the tip of each corner make sure that the wound edges come together in the correct orientation, to avoid 'dog-ears' (Fig. 18.3). If a skin lesion is excised with overlying or surrounding skin, the wound length should be approximately three times the maximum width of the skin excised to allow closure with minimum distortion. If a wound is too short for the width of the excision, subcutaneous tissue can be excised under each end to prevent dog-ears. When a defect is large, and this technique cannot be used, several layers of side-to-side, from deep to superficial, continuous sutures can be placed in line with the incision.

The suture ends of each layer are brought out at the wound ends with the deepest layer the most distant from the wound end and the most superficial, in effect, being a subcuticular closure (see later). When the several strands are pulled, the wound comes together with no tension in any of the layers and leaving no dead space.

TYPES OF SKIN CLOSURE

Skin closure may be interrupted or continuous; or simple (Fig. 18.4a), mattress (Fig. 18.4b) or subcuticular (Fig. 18.4c). Interrupted sutures have the advantage that they can be removed individually, if a haematoma or infection forms locally, to help drain blood, or pus if a wound abscess develops later, without disruption of the whole suture line. They are disadvantaged by being slower to insert than continuous sutures. Mattress sutures appose skin edges tidily, ensure eversion and help to close the dead space in the subcutaneous fat layer. They are slower to insert than simple sutures but may avoid the need for a 'fat stitch' before closing skin. This 'fat stitch' may leave a poor cosmetic result; for example, after excision of a breast lump (when placed to close dead space and theoretically reduce the risk of haematoma), it may, through attachment to a breast compartment ligament, cause a permanent dimpling effect in the skin. Subcuticular sutures are cosmetically appealing but are more difficult to place in a wound that is curved. Any dead space in the subcutaneous fat layer may also need to be closed separately (but see the caution above in breast skin closure). Nevertheless, subcuticular closure is the most widely practised skin closure in virtually all specialties, although skin clips have their advocates.

Non-absorbable skin sutures are removed when the wound has healed to avoid scarring, infection and irritation. As a general rule, they are removed from the face in 2–3 days, the scalp in 5 days, the upper limb and groin in 7 days, the abdomen in 10 days, and the dorsum and lower trunk within 10–14 days. Although these timings are conventional, there is evidence that early removal may be followed by the 'spreading' of skin scars, particularly when there is tension. Prolonged wound support using adhesive paper strips (Steristrips), or the potential use of anti-scarring agents, may help to prevent this.

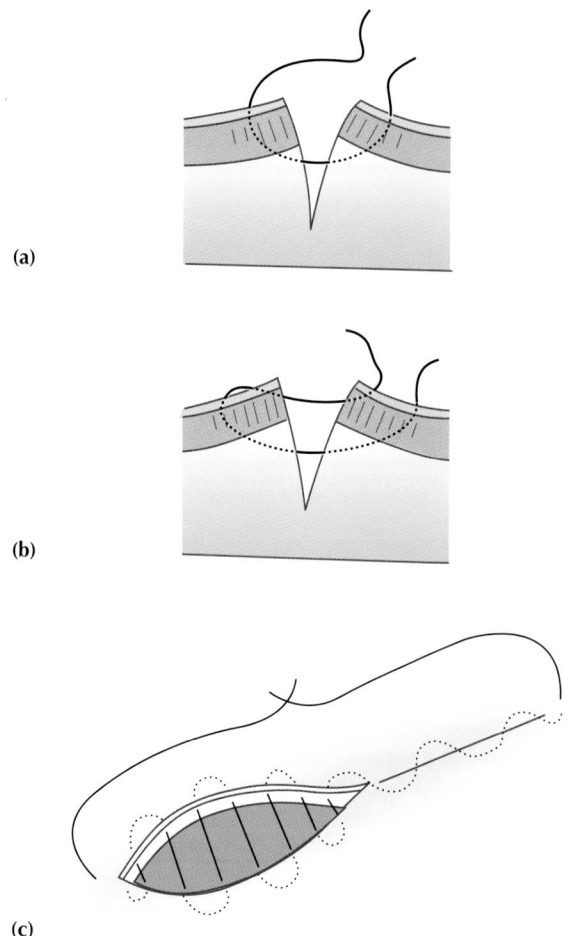

(a)

(b)

(c)

Figure 18.4 Types of skin closure. (a) Simple. (b) Mattress. (c) Subcuticular. Ends can be buried (absorbable) or left open (non-absorbable), with or without being secured by beads, until removal. Beads should be avoided in easily irritated areas such as the axilla.

No-touch technique

Suturing should be undertaken using a no-touch technique to reduce the risk of a needle-stick injury. Obviously, this is not possible when performing a subcuticular closure using a straight needle, still used by many for this type of closure (Summary box 18.2).

Summary box 18.2

No-touch technique

- Used whenever possible
- Needle holders should be suitable for the needle
- Avoids the risk of needle-stick injury

Needle holders should be appropriate for the job. Short-handled holders are used for skin closure, but long-handled holders are needed for sutures placed deep inside the body. They have hardened jaws, usually made of titanium, to hold needles securely, but they can damage or weaken suture material if used for making knots, or placed on the swage that holds the suture in the hollow needle. Needle holders are precision instruments that should be

checked pre- and postoperatively. Experienced surgeons know which type suits them best for different functions. Suturing deep in the pelvis needs a long needle holder and requires practice. The shorter needle holders used in skin closure can be mastered more quickly. Tissue forceps also have many styles, which need to be explored during operative surgical training. Atraumatic forceps are used for delicate tissues, but a toothed forceps can be used as a hook and can be helpful in skin closure without having to grasp tissue.

The needle should be held in the tip of the holder and placed about two-thirds of the way back from its tip, where there is usually a designed, flattened part to allow a secure grip that prevents rotation. If the needle is held too far back, the swage may be crushed and the needle could break or come apart from the suture material. If the needle is grasped by its tip it may bend or break and be lost in the incision, which will disconcert the 'scrub nurse'. Needles can be placed in their holders to be used forehand or backhand. This depends on the most convenient way that a suture line can be performed. Surgeons in training should become adept at both.

Suture materials (Tables 18.1 and 18.2)

There is evidence that traumatic and surgical wounds were closed in 3000 BC by the Egyptians using thorns and needles. They also used adhesive linen strips, similar to modern-day Steristrips. By 1000 BC, Indian surgeons were using horsehair, cotton and leather sutures. In Roman times, linen and silk and metal clips called fibulae were commonly used to close gladiatorial wounds. By the end of the nineteenth century, developments in the textile industry led to major advances, and both silk and catgut became popular as suture materials. Lister believed that catgut soaked in chromic acid (a form of tanning) prevented early dissolution in body fluids and tissues. Moynihan felt that chromic catgut was ideal as it could be sterilised, was non-irritant to tissues, kept its strength until its work was done and then disappeared. How wrong he turned out to be. Catgut does not have any of these desirable properties, apart from being sterilisable, and it certainly causes an inflammatory cellular reaction with release of proteases. It may also carry the risk of prion transmission if of bovine origin.

All the natural sutures, silk, cotton, linen and catgut, are being replaced by polymeric synthetic materials that cause minimal inflammatory reactions, are of predictable strength and absorb at an appropriate rate. They can be manufactured as monofilaments or braids, and can be coated with wax, silicone or polybutyrate to allow them to run smoothly through tissues and to knot securely. The absorbables cause a minimal tissue reaction as they are resorbed. To aid in the prevention of postoperative infection, particularly after prosthetic surgery, absorbable synthetic sutures may be impregnated with an antiseptic (Vicryl Plus, a polyglactin, is impregnated with triclosan). The integrity of some synthetic non-absorbables in holding healing tissues

---

Gladiators were so called because they fought with a Roman sword called a Gladius.
Joseph Lister (Lord Lister), 1827–1912, Professor of Surgery, Glasgow, Scotland (1860–1869), Edinburgh, Scotland (1869–1877) and King's College Hospital, London, England (1877–1892).
Berkeley George Andrew Moynihan, (Lord Moynihan of Leeds), 1865–1936, Professor of Clinical Surgery, The University of Leeds, Leeds, England.

Table 18.1 Suture materials in common use in surgery: non-absorbable

Suture	Types	Raw material	Tensile strength	Absorption rate	Tissue reaction	Contraindications	Frequent uses	How supplied
Silk	Braided or twisted multifilament. Dyed or undyed. Coated (with wax or silicone) or uncoated	Natural protein Raw silk from silkworm	Loses 20% when wet; 80–100% lost by 6 months. Because of tissue reactions and unpredictability, silk is increasingly not recommended	Fibrous encapsulation in body at 2–3 weeks Absorbed slowly over 1–2 years	Moderate to high Not recommended Consider suitable absorbable or non-absorbable	Not for use with vascular prostheses or in tissues requiring prolonged approximation under stress Risk of infection and tissue reaction makes silk unsuitable for routine skin closure	Ligation and suturing when long-term tissue support is necessary	10/0–2 with needles, 4/0–1 without needles
Linen	Twisted	Long staple flax fibres	Stronger when wet Loses 50% at 6 months; 30% remains at 2 years	Non-absorbable Remains encapsulated in body tissues	Moderate	Not advised for use with vascular prostheses	Ligation and suturing in gastrointestinal surgery. No longer in common use in most centres	3/0–1 with needles, 3/0–1 without needles
Surgical steel	Monofilament or multifilament	An alloy of iron, nickel and chromium	Infinite (> 1 year)	Non-absorbable Remains encapsulated in body tissues	Minimal	Should not be used in conjunction with prosthesis of different metal	Closure of sternotomy wounds Previously found favour for tendon and hernia repairs	Monofilament: 5/0–5 with needles; multifilament: 5/0–3/0 with needles
Nylon	Monofilament or braided multifilament Dyed or undyed	Polyamide polymer	Loses 15–20% per year	Degrades at approximately 15–20% per year	Low	None	General surgical use, e.g. skin closure, abdominal wall mass closure, hernia repair, plastic surgery, neurosurgery, microsurgery, ophthalmic surgery	Monofilament: 11/0–2 with needles (including loops in some sizes), 4/0–2 without needles; multifilament: 6/0–2 with needles, 3/0–1 without needles
Polyester	Monofilament or braided multifilament Dyed or undyed Coated (polybutylate or silicone) or uncoated	Polyester (polyethylene terephthalate)	Infinite (> 1 year)	Non-absorbable: remains encapsulated in body tissues	Low	None	Cardiovascular, ophthalmic, plastic and general surgery	Monofilament: (ophthalmic) 11/10; 10/0 with needles; multifilament: 5/0–1 with needles Ethibond 7/0–5 with needles
Polybutester	Monofilament. Dyed or undyed	Polybutylene terephthalate and polytetramethylene ether glycol	Infinite (> 1 year)	Non-absorbable: remains encapsulated in body tissues	Low	None	Exhibits a degree of elasticity. Particularly favoured for use in plastic surgery	7/0–1 with needles
Polypropylene	Monofilament. Dyed or undyed	Polymer of propylene	Infinite (> 1 year)	Non-absorbable: remains encapsulated in body tissues	Low	None	Cardiovascular surgery, plastic surgery, ophthalmic surgery, general surgical subcuticular skin closure	10/0–1 with needles

CHAPTER 18 | BASIC SURGICAL SKILLS AND ANASTOMOSES

Table 18.2 Suture materials in common use in surgery: absorbable

Suture	Types	Raw material	Tensile strength retention *in vivo*	Absorption rate	Tissue reaction	Contraindications	Frequent uses	How supplied
Catgut	Plain	Collagen derived from healthy sheep or cattle	Lost within 7–10 days. Marked patient variability. Unpredictable and not recommended	Phagocytosis and enzymatic degradation within 7–10 days	High	Not for use in tissues which heal slowly and require prolonged support. Synthetic absorbables are superior	Ligate superficial vessels, suture subcutaneous tissues. Stomas and other tissues that heal rapidly	6/0–1 with needles; 4/0–3 without needles
Catgut	Chromic	Collagen derived from healthy sheep or cattle. Tanned with chromium salts to improve handling and to resist degradation in tissue	Lost within 21–28 days. Marked patient variability. Unpredictable and not recommended	Phagocytosis and enzymatic degradation within 90 days	Moderate	As for plain catgut. Synthetic absorbables superior	As for plain catgut	6/0–3 with needles; 5/0–3 without needles
Polyglactin	Braided multifilament	Copolymer of lactide and glycolide in a ratio of 90:10, coated with polyglactin and calcium stearate	Approximately 60% remains at 2 weeks. Approximately 30% remains at 3 weeks	Hydrolysis minimal until 5–6 weeks. Complete absorption 60–90 days	Mild	Not advised for use in tissues which require prolonged approximation under stress	General surgical use where absorbable sutures required, e.g. gut anastomoses, vascular ligatures. Has become the 'workhorse' suture for many applications in most general surgical practices, including undyed for subcuticular wound closures. Ophthalmic surgery	8/0–2 with needles; 5/0–2 without needles
Polyglyconate	Monofilament. Dyed or undyed	Copolymer of glycolic acid and trimethylene carbonate	Approximately 70% remains at 2 weeks. Approximately 55% remains at 3 weeks	Hydrolysis minimal until 8–9 weeks. Complete absorption by 180 days	Mild	Not advised for use in tissues which require prolonged approximation under stress	Popular in some centres as an alternative to Vicryl and PDS	7/0–2 with needles
Polyglycolic acid	Braided multifilament. Dyed or undyed. Coated or uncoated	Polymer of polyglycolic acid. Available with coating of inert, absorbable surfactant poloxamer 188 to enhance surface smoothness. 87% excreted in urine within 3 days	Approximately 40% remains at 1 week. Approximately 20% remains at 3 weeks	Hydrolysis minimal at 2 weeks, significant at 4 weeks. Complete absorption 60–90 days	Minimal	Not advised for use in tissues which require prolonged approximation under stress	Uses as for other absorbable sutures, in particular where slightly longer wound support is required	9/0–2 with needles; 9/0–2 without needles
Polydioxanone (PDS)	Monofilament. Dyed or undyed	Polyester polymer	Approximately 70% remains at 2 weeks. Approximately 50% remains at 4 weeks. Approximately 14% remains at 8 weeks	Hydrolysis minimal at 90 days. Complete absorption at 180 days	Mild	Not for use in association with heart valves or synthetic grafts, or in situations in which prolonged tissue approximation under stress is required	Uses as for other absorbable sutures, in particular where slightly longer wound support is required	Polydioxanone suture (PDS) 10/0–2 with needles
Polyglycaprone	Monofilament	Copolymer of glycolite and caprolactone	21 days maximum	90–120 days		No use for extended support	Subcuticular in skin, ligation, gastrointestinal and muscle surgery	8/0–2 with needles

together can last indefinitely, such as the use of polypropylene in arterial anastomosis. Polyamide (nylon) is slowly biodegradable and therefore not suitable for this purpose. Many non-absorbables are presented as monofilaments, which eliminates interstices in the thread and makes knots less likely to be a nidus for infection by reducing the risk of bacterial biofilms and adherence, but requires more skill in tying secure knots (Summary box 18.3).

Summary box 18.3

Modern synthetic polymeric suture materials

- Inflammatory reaction is reduced
- Strength predictable (particularly with non-absorbables)
- Absorption more complete and predictable (with absorbables)
- Synthetic polymers can be monofilament or braided

Suture diameters vary from 0.02 to 0.8 mm. This corresponds to 0.2 to 8 on the metric system (millimetres times 10) and 10/0 to 5 on the British Pharmacopoeia (BP) system. The finest suture that will hold the wound secure, without it breaking or 'cheese-wiring' through the tissues, should be chosen. The amount of suture material used should be kept to a minimum, particularly when braided, to reduce bacterial colonisation. Suture material can be a nidus for infection, and knots can be the focus of a persistent and chronic inflammatory reaction (suture knot sinus).

Metal sutures, clips and staples

Mechanical stapling devices were first used successfully by Hümer Hültl, in Hungary, to close the stomach after resection. There is now a wide choice of linear, side-by-side and end-to-end stapling devices that give strong predictable suture lines, with minimal tissue necrosis. The staplers also allow access to difficult areas. For example, an oesophagogastric anastomosis can be performed without opening the chest. In an anterior resection, a staple gun may allow a low anastomosis to be performed quickly and without a colostomy, although a temporary loop ileostomy needs to be considered. The specific uses of stapling devices in surgery are described in the appropriate sections of this book. Most stapling devices are entirely disposable, relatively expensive, and now also available for minimally invasive surgery. Their cost is offset by the saving of operative time and increased range of surgery made possible. There are three basic types of gastrointestinal stapling device:

1 *Linear stapler* (Fig. 18.5a). A linear everting staple line is fashioned: used for closure of a viscus (e.g. duodenal stump closure after Pólya gastrectomy).
2 *Side-to-side stapler*, with or without a knife blade, for transection of a viscus between staple rows (Fig. 18.5b):
   a linear inverting anastomosis with transection: used for side-to-side intestinal anastomoses (e.g. gastroenterostomy);
   b linear staple line without transection: used for fashioning enteric reservoirs (e.g. ileal pouch);
   c linear staple line with transection: used for closure of a viscus (e.g. small bowel resection).
3 *End-to-end stapler* (Fig. 18.5c). Circular inverting anastomosis: used for end-to-end gastrointestinal anastomoses (e.g. closure of colostomy following Hartmann's procedure). These incorporate a circular knife blade.

Advances in laparoscopic surgery in recent years also owe much to the continuous refinement of clip and stapling devices designed to be used as laparoscopic instruments.

Metal clips for skin allow quick, accurate closure. Disposable units are more expensive than resterilisable Michel clips but save operating time. Skin clips are easy to remove with an appropriate, supplied device and give acceptable scars with a low infection rate. Inexpert placement can cause clips to drop out early, and cause skin edge overlap with a poor cosmetic result.

Stainless steel wire sutures have their place for the closure of the sternum after cardiac operations and in orthopaedic surgery. Their use in laparotomy closure has been superseded by modern synthetic non-absorbables.

Steristrips can be used to buttress a skin closure and can prevent 'spreading' of a scar. This can be useful, for example after a wide lump excision of the breast. Adhesive polyurethane films, such as Opsite, Tegaderm or Bioclusive, may have a similar property. Transparent dressings also allow wound inspection and may protect against cross-infection.

Needles

The choice of surgical needle (Fig. 18.6) is as important as the choice of suture. The needle holder chosen also needs to be appropriate; a large needle holder damages a small needle, and a large needle is unmanageable in a small needle holder. The passage of a needle through tissue should follow its curvature. This minimises tissue damage. The appropriate size and shape of cutting, or round-bodied atraumatic needle, needs to be chosen for the least traumatic passage through tissue. Shaped needles allow easier access for suturing. Examples are the J-shaped needle useful in low-approach femoral hernia repair, or the compound curve needle used in ophthalmic surgery. Hand needles should be avoided because of the risk of needle-stick injury. The tips of laparotomy closure needles are deliberately blunted by some of the manufacturers to reduce the risk of needle-stick injury. Needles may come with a loop suture (to avoid a knot at the end of a laparotomy) or as double-ended sutures (to facilitate arterial closure: see anastomoses).

Tissue glues

Cyanoacrylates

The use of tissue glues is not widespread despite much published work. The cyanoacrylates have been used for skin closure but require near perfect haemostasis if they are to work well. Some specific uses have been described such as the use in closure of a laceration on the forehead of a fractious child in Accident and Emergency (thereby dispensing with local anaesthetic and

---

Hümer Hültl, **Surgeon, St. Stephen's Hospital, Budapest, Hungary, described his gastric stapler in 1908.**
Eugen (Janö) Alexander Pólya, **1876–1944, Surgeon, St. Stephen's Hospital, Budapest, Hungary.**

Henri Albert Charles Antoine Hartmann, **1860–1952, Professor of Clinical Surgery, The Faculty of Medicine, The University of Paris, France.**
Gaston Michel, **1874–1937, French Surgeon.**

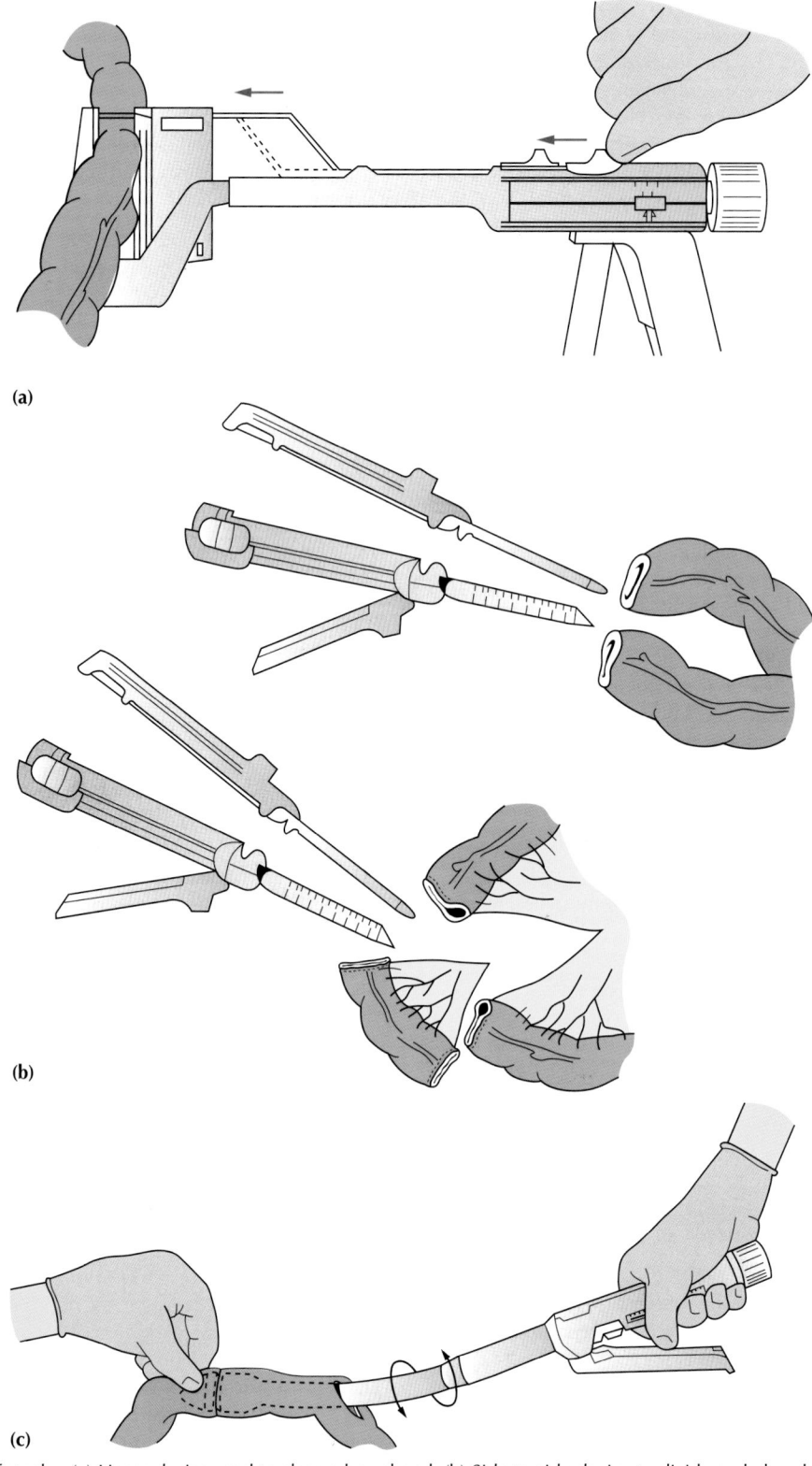

(a)

(b)

(c)

Figure 18.5 Types of stapler. (a) Linear device used to close a bowel end. (b) Side-to-side device to divide and close bowel or to allow side-to-side anastomosis. (c) End-to-end device used to anastomose bowel.

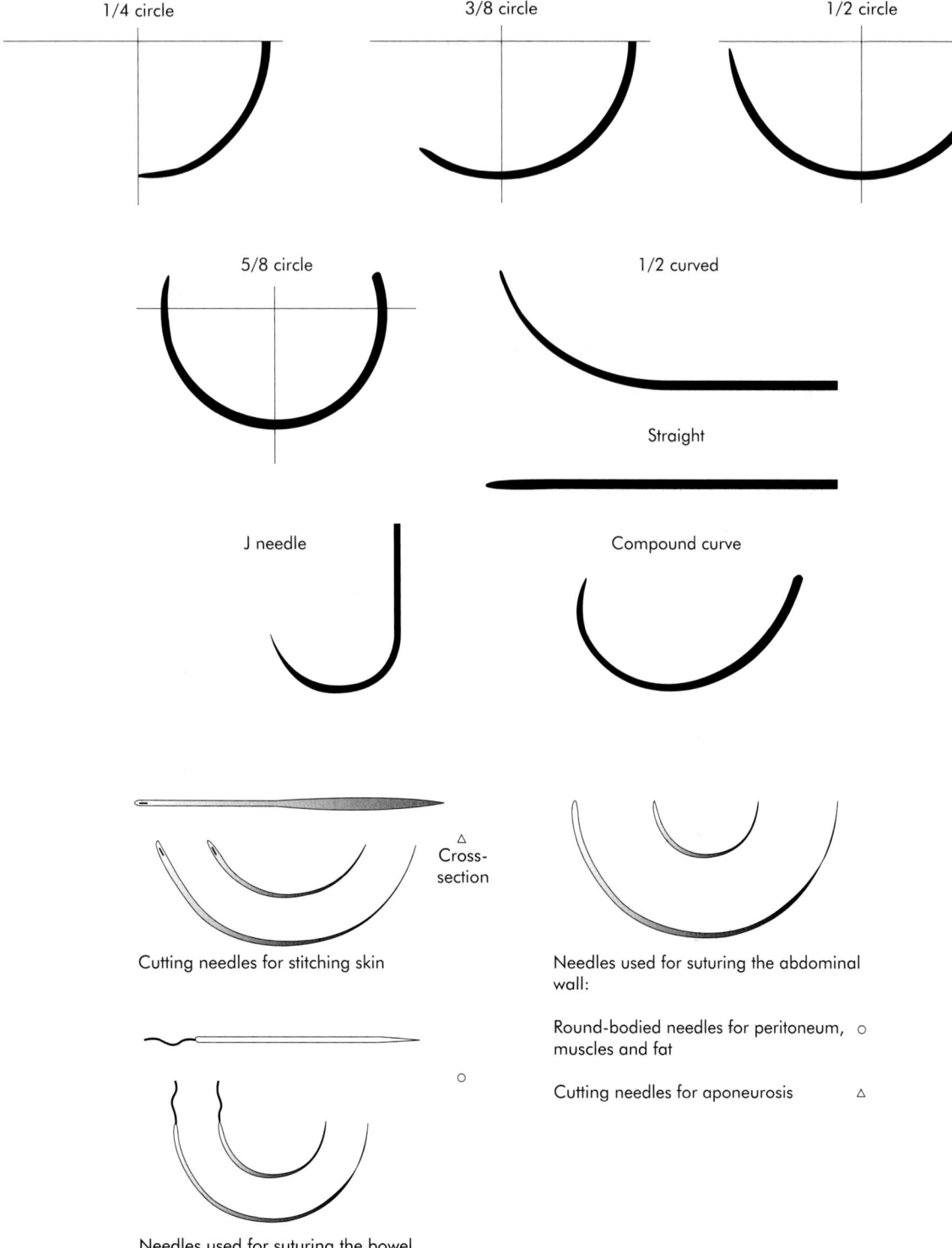

1/4 circle

3/8 circle

1/2 circle

5/8 circle

1/2 curved

Straight

J needle

Compound curve

△ Cross-section

Cutting needles for stitching skin

Needles used for suturing the abdominal wall:

Round-bodied needles for peritoneum, ○ muscles and fat

Cutting needles for aponeurosis   △

○

Needles used for suturing the bowel
The threads are swaged into the needles

Figure 18.6 Types of needles used for sutures. The sutures are swaged on to prevent a 'shoulder' and allow easy passage through tissues.

sutures). They are relatively expensive but quick to use, do not delay wound healing and are associated with an allegedly low infection rate.

Fibrin tissue glues

Tissue glues, involving fibrin, work on the conversion of fibrinogen by thrombin to fibrin with cross-linking by factor XIII; the addition of aprotinin retards break-up of the fibrin network by plasmin. The fibrinous network produced has good adhesive properties and has been used for haemostasis in the liver and spleen. It has also been used in neurosurgery for dural tears; in ear, nose and throat (ENT) and ophthalmic surgery; to attach skin grafts and prevent haemoserous collections under flaps; and in cardiac and general surgery for the prevention of postoperative adhesions in the pericardium and the peritoneum. Fibrin glues have been used to control gastrointestinal haemorrhage, using endoscopic injection, but do not work when bleeding is brisk. They are more effective in haemostasis when combined with collagen.

Knot tying

Secure knots are crucial in operative surgery. Most should be performed using an instrument such as a needle holder, with care being taken not to crush or damage the suture material incorporated into the knot.

Tying knots with the fingertips is useful when ligating at depth. Surgeons in training should practise these on the jigs devised for use in basic skill courses.

All knots should be square, but the two-throw reef (surgeon's) knot does not slip (Fig. 18.7). A granny knot is a two-throw knot using the same type of throw; its ability to slip is useful in produc-

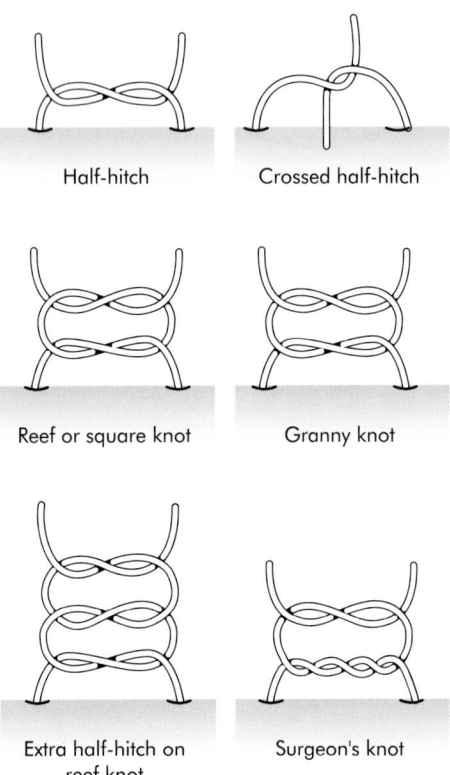

Half-hitch   Crossed half-hitch

Reef or square knot   Granny knot

Extra half-hitch on   Surgeon's knot
reef knot

Figure 18.7 Types of knot used in surgery.

ing the right tension (Fig. 18.7) prior to ensuring security with a third, double-throw knot (Fig. 18.7). In vascular surgery, some surgeons prefer the security of five or six throws, but a three-throw reef knot is probably as secure as the integrity of the suture being used. The Aberdeen knot can be used with a continuous suture to make a final knot. The free end of the suture is pulled through the final loop several times before being pulled through a final time prior to cutting. It gives a less bulky knot, useful at the end of closure of the deep layers of a laparotomy incision.

When knots are cut short, the free ends or 'ears' should be left at least 1–2 mm long. This is particularly important with monofilament non-absorbables. However, if the ends are left too long, they can cause wound irritation and add to the complications of wound pain and wound sinuses. If knots are not 'snugged down' tightly, a suture cut too short may slide and become undone. When tying, the throw should be taken to the tissue using an instrument or an index fingertip. If this is not done, the vessel being ligated bowstrings, and the ligature may dislodge or cut out; this is important for example when ligating the saphenofemoral junction during varicose vein surgery.

Ligatures can be tied using instruments or by hand when tissues are divided between forceps. The security of a ligature depends on good communication between surgeon and assistant as the tissue forceps is released and tissue tied without slippage. This needs practice.

Secure wound closure is crucial. Technical wound failure follows knots slipping, tissues tearing or breakage of sutures. When this occurs after laparotomy closure, the result is a burst abdomen, a disaster for the patient and a technical failure for the surgeon. This complication is avoided by the use of an appropriate material, polypropylene (Prolene) or polydioxanone suture (PDS), secure knots and appropriate tissue bites. It has been suggested by Jenkins that a suture length to wound length ratio of 4:1 indicates the optimum size of tissue bites and of suture spacing. The use of looped sutures, one starting from each end of the wound, requires only one knot, which also minimises the risk of a knot sinus or of wound pain (Summary box 18.4).

Summary box 18.4

Secure wound closure

- **Correct suture material**
- **Appropriate bites of tissue and suture spacing**
- **Secure knots**

ANASTOMOSIS

The word anastomosis comes from the Greek 'ανα', without, and 'στομα', a mouth, i.e. when a tubular viscus (bowel) or vessel (mostly arteries) is joined after resection or bypass without exteriorisation with a stoma. Anastomoses in the bowel were not undertaken successfully until the nineteenth century. Before that, experience was limited to exteriorisation or closure of simple lacerations. Lembert described his seromuscular suture technique for bowel anastomosis in 1826. Senn advocated a two-layer

---

Antoine Lembert, 1802–1851, Surgeon, Hôtel Dieu, Paris, France.
Nicolas Senn, 1844–1908, Professor of Surgery, Rush Medical College, Chicago, IL, USA.

technique for closure; Halsted favoured a one-layer extramucosal closure. Connell used a single layer of interrupted sutures incorporating all layers of the bowel. Kocher's method, a two-layer anastomosis, first a continuous all-layer suture using catgut, then an inverting continuous (or interrupted) seromuscular layer suture using silk, became the standard. There is evidence that inversion is safest in bowel (least likely to leak), although end-to-end staplers give an everted anastomosis without complication.

The single-layer extramucosal anastomosis, advocated by Matheson, causes the least tissue necrosis or luminal narrowing. There is probably little to choose between these techniques, provided basic essentials are observed. However, catgut and silk have been replaced by synthetic, usually absorbable, polymers.

Anastomosis of vessels was pioneered by Carrel. He advocated an everting anastomosis, with accurate opposition, to provide an intact endothelium that prevented platelet and thrombus deposition. The technique involved three stay sutures, which could be used to rotate the vessels and facilitate a continuous suture. The development of polymers, such as polypropylene which is not biodegradable, has made vascular anastomoses both safe and enduring.

Anastomosis of bowel

With good bowel preparation or an empty bowel, it is probably not necessary to apply clamps (even of the soft occlusion type), which are likely to cause some degree of tissue damage. If there is any risk of intestinal spillage during anastomosis, when bowel is unprepared or obstructed for example, atraumatic intestinal clamps should be used. Clamps must not impinge on the mesentery or its vasculature for fear of necrosis. Ideally, the bowel edges should be pink and bleeding prior to anastomosis. Excessive bleeding from the bowel wall may need oversewing if natural haemostasis is inadequate (Summary box 18.5).

Summary box 18.5

Essentials for safe bowel anastomosis

Local
- Good blood supply (no tension)
- Inverting anastomosis with appropriate suture
- Accurate apposition and suture technique (or stapling)
- Avoidance of tissue damage by clamps

Systemic
- Bowel preparation (and avoidance of spillage)
- Antibiotic prophylaxis
- Maintenance of good perfusion and tissue oxygenation during anaesthesia (correction of shock)
- Adequate nutritional attention
- Adequate resectional margins (cancer or inflammatory bowel disease) and avoidance of chemotherapy/radiotherapy

---

William Stewart Halsted, 1852–1922, Professor of Surgery, Johns Hopkins Hospital Medical School, Baltimore, MD, USA, described this suture in 1887.
Frank Gregory Connell, 1875–1968, Professor of Surgery, Rush Medical College, Chicago, IL, USA.
Emil Theodor Kocher, 1841–1917, Professor of Surgery, Berne, Switzerland.
Norman Alistair Matheson, Formerly Surgeon, Aberdeen Royal Infirmary, Aberdeen, Scotland.
Alexis Carrel, 1873–1944, was a Surgeon from Lyons in France who worked at the Rockefeller Institute for Medical Research in New York, NY, USA. He received the Nobel Prize for Physiology or Medicine in 1912 'In recognition for his works on vascular suture and the transplantation of blood vessels and organs.'

End-to-end two-layer technique

This technique (Fig. 18.8) can be practised on basic skills jigs. The bowel ends must be brought together without tension. Stay sutures, which avoid the need for tissue forceps, may help with the placement of the posterior, continuous, seromuscular layer and allow rotation of the anastomosis. The all-layers continuous inner suture can be undertaken with a double-ended suture to help to keep the anastomosis even, going from the middle posteriorly to the lateral edge on each side. At the corners, one or two Connell 'loop-on-the-mucosa' sutures help to invert the mucosa (Fig. 18.8a). The double-ended suture can then be tied in the middle (on the anti-mesenteric side of the bowel). Finally, the anastomosis is inverted using a seromuscular, anterior, continuous Lembert suture. The apposition of bowel edges should, in each layer, be as accurate as possible. Bites should be approximately 5 mm deep and 5 mm apart. Suture materials should be of 2/0–3/0 size and made of an absorbable polymer, which can be braided (e.g. polyglactin), or a monofilament (e.g. polydioxanone), mounted on an atraumatic round-bodied needle. Braided, coated sutures are the easiest to handle and knot.

Alternatively, the inner continuous all-layers suture can be undertaken first. An inverting seromuscular Lembert layer is then applied second. This risks mesenteric vascular damage and is not recommended. It is crucial to make sure that only bowel of similar diameter is brought together to form an end-to-end anastomosis. 'Parachuting' or 'purse-stringing' a proximal dilated bowel lumen into narrower distal bowel risks a poor anastomosis and subsequent leakage. In such a case, a side-to-side or end-to-side anastomosis may be safer. The Cheatle split (making a cut into the anti-mesenteric border) may help to enlarge the lumen of distal, collapsed bowel. The mesentery should always be closed to avoid the later risk of an internal hernia through a persistent mesenteric defect. Care must be taken in preventing mesenteric vessel damage as the anastomosis may need to be revised.

End-to-end one-layer technique; end-to-side anastomosis

These anastomoses (Fig. 18.9) can be undertaken using open, avoiding the use of occlusion clamps, or closed techniques. They are useful in the following circumstances:

- when access is not easy, as in transabdominal oesophagogastric anastomoses or after low anterior resection;
- when there is disparity in the bowel lumen;
- when the bowel serosa is lacking.

When interrupted sutures are required, a wide choice is available (Tables 18.1 and 18.2 above). There is no evidence that one technique is significantly superior to another (Fig. 18.10), but the interrupted single-layer extramucosal (seromuscular) suture is probably the most widely practised (Summary box 18.6).

Sir George Lenthal Cheatle, 1865–1951, Surgeon, King's College Hospital, London, England.

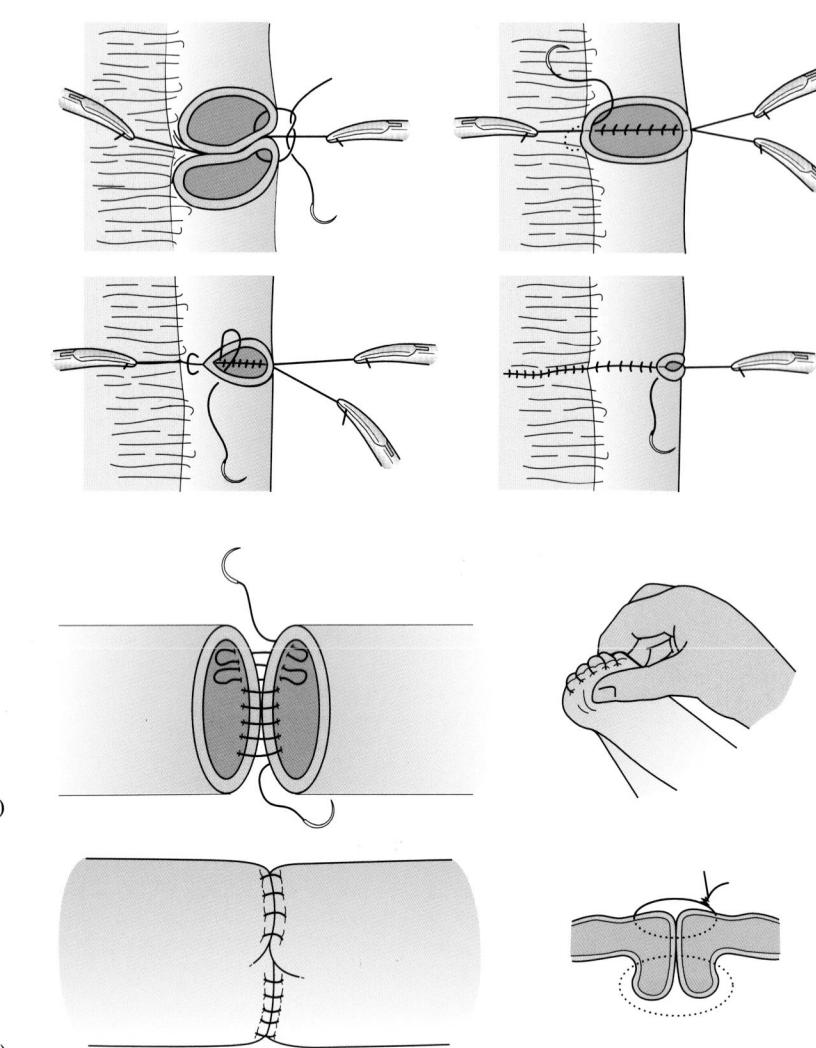

(a)

(b)

Figure 18.8 End-to-end, two-layer anastomosis in bowel (open). (a) The 'loop-on-the-mucosa' Connell stitch, which inverts the corners but is not haemostatic. (b) The second seromuscular outside layer that ensures mucosal inversion and can be performed as a single layer without the internal all-layers suture. The effect on a transverse section can be seen in the insert.

Summary box 18.6

Intestinal anastomosis

- Ensure viable bowel ends before and after anastomosis
- Use atraumatic clamps if soiling is a risk
- Avoid risk to mesenteric vessels by clamps or sutures
- Synthetic polymers are the most conventional sutures for hand-sewn inverting anastomoses
- Interrupted and continuous suture techniques are comparably safe
- Disposable staple units are an alternative with safe inverting or everting anastomoses

Anastomosis of vessels

Vascular anastomoses require more precision than bowel anastomoses as they must be immediately watertight at the end of the operation when the clamps are removed. The integrity of the suture also needs to be permanent. For this reason, polypropylene is one of the best sutures as it is not biodegradable. It should be used in its monofilament form, mounted on an atraumatic, curved, round-bodied needle. Knot security is important. The intimal suture line must be as smooth as possible to minimise the

risk of thrombosis and embolus, and regular to avoid leak. Suture size depends on vessel calibre: 2/0 is suitable for the aorta, 4/0 for the femoral artery and 6/0 for the popliteal to distal arteries. Microvascular anastomoses are made using a loupe and an interrupted suture down to 10/0 size (Summary box 18.7).

Summary box 18.7

Anastomosis of vessels

- Polypropylene-like sutures with indefinite integrity give the best results
- Intimal suture line must be smooth
- Knots must be secure
- Needle must pass from within outwards

Closure of an arteriotomy

The vessel walls must be treated with care, particularly the intima, and if manipulation is necessary, atraumatic forceps (such as DeBakey's) are needed. Vascular clamps should also be applied

Michael Ellis DeBakey, **B. 1908, Professor of Surgery, Baylor University, Houston, TX, USA.**

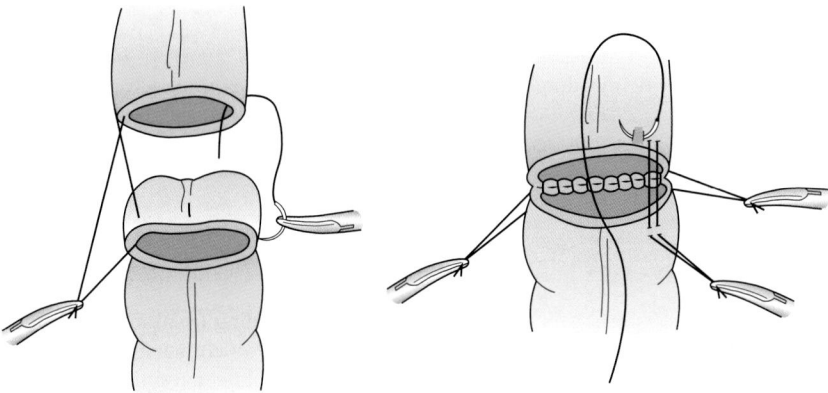

Figure 18.9 End-to-end, one-layer anastomosis in bowel (open).

with similar care. For the best exposure, the arterial wall can be retracted using a temporary looped suture, placed through all layers of the vessel at the midpoint of the proposed suture line and held on a haemostat. This exposure makes the first suture bite easier to place. Two single-ended sutures allow a knot to be placed externally at each end of the arteriotomy and a final knot to be easily placed in the middle at the end of each side of the arterial closure. Vessels should always be sewn with the needle moving from within to without the lumen to avoid creating an intimal flap and to fix any atherosclerotic plaque. The final closure is made easily at the middle of the arteriotomy where the

superior and inferior suture lines meet with the knot tied externally. This technique also simplifies the expulsion of air and any thrombus. The distal clamp is released before the final watertight knot is made. The proximal clamp can then be released without risk of distal embolus. Suture bites should be placed an equal distance apart, with the bite size dependent on the vessel diameter. Care needs to be taken to avoid damaging the suture, which can be torn by the instruments. The tip of the needle should be inserted at right angles to the surface of the intima and the curve of the needle followed to prevent vessel trauma. If the assistant follows by keeping the suture tight, the arteriotomy will be held up and open. This makes the next suture simple to place.

Closure of an arteriotomy with a vein patch

A transverse arteriotomy (Fig. 18.11) is less likely to stenose following closure than a longitudinal arteriotomy. However, a

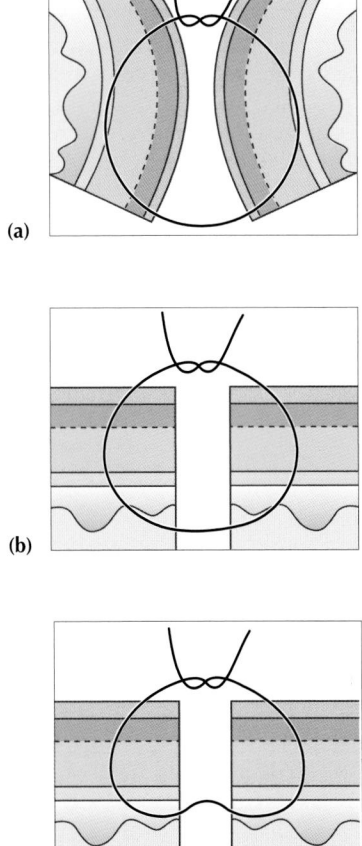

Figure 18.10 Different types of single-row sutures. (a) Lembert. (b) All-layer. (c) Extramucosal.

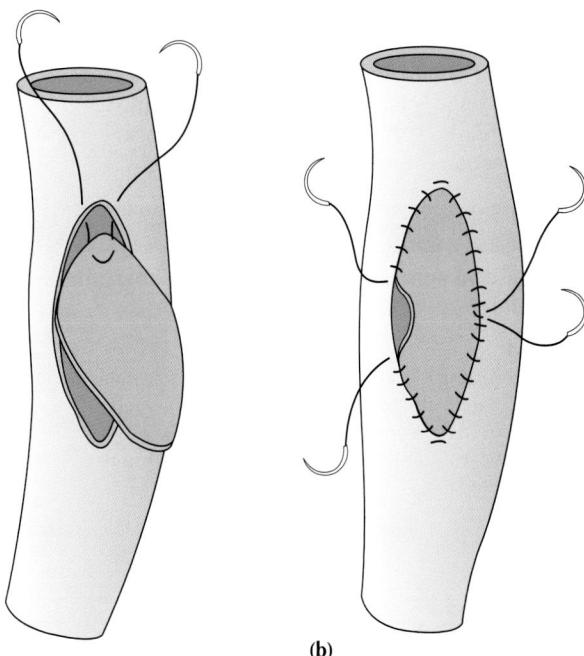

Figure 18.11 Closure of arteriotomy with a vein patch. This prevents stenosis. The use of double-ended sutures and an in–out technique from each end of the patch (a) allows final knots to be placed easily half-way down the patch and fixes the atherosclerotic plaque (b).

longitudinal arteriotomy is easier to make, and a vein patch graft can be used if there is any doubt about the size of the lumen. Once again, the suture line can be started at the top and bottom with a double-ended suture. The first knot is then placed half-way along the edge of the suture line. The closure is completed with a final knot on each side at the midpoint of the vein patch graft, using the in–out technique with fixation of plaque and avoidance of damage to the intima using atraumatic forceps.

End-to-end or side-to-side anastomoses

Most anastomoses involve the use of prosthetic material or vein grafts to bypass arterial disease. Continuous non-absorbable monomer sutures are used with the same in–out technique to ensure eversion. Double-ended sutures make the procedures easier. Gentle traction of the suture by the assistant keeps the lumen open as the suture line is completed. By leaving a tied suture long, the anastomosis can also be rotated to give better access to the suture line.

Complications after anastomoses

Difficult or poor exposure may lead to complications (Summary box 18.8).

Summary box 18.8

Complications after anastomosis

Leakage
- Bowel – peritonitis
- Vessel – haematoma, haemorrhagic shock (early), pseudoaneurysm (late)

Stenosis
- Bowel – obstruction after fibrous stricture or disease recurrence
- Vessel (early and late) – thrombosis, occlusion, gangrene

Inadequate mobilisation may leave an anastomosis under tension. A gentle respect for tissues is associated with fewer complications, although systemic factors need equal skill in recognition and correction (Summary box 18.9).

Summary box 18.9

Local and systemic adverse factors in anastomotic healing

Local
- Persisting disease process: cancer, chronic inflammation
- Distal obstruction
- Poor blood supply: rectum, oesophagus
- Poor technical aspects: haematoma, dead space, poor perfusion
- Presence of foreign body
- Gross contamination/infection

Systemic
- Shock of any cause
- Metabolic diseases: diabetes, uraemia, jaundice
- Immunosuppression: cancer, acquired immunodeficiency syndrome (AIDS), steroids
- Malnutrition: cancer

Complications include:

1 *Leakage*, which can occur early (vascular) or late (bowel), leading to haemorrhagic shock and peritonitis respectively.
2 *Bleeding* may need attention to a bowel edge prior to an anastomosis, by simple oversewing rather than diathermy, and revision if the anastomosis is complete. If overlooked, there may be the formation of a large haematoma (with risk of subsequent abscess if contaminated). The absence of bleeding at a bowel edge may indicate ischaemia; a bowel anastomosis that looks cyanosed needs serious consideration for refashioning. Urgent attention to persistent bleeding from an anastomotic edge is needed in vascular surgery, which may be arrested by: patience, gentle pressure and topical haemostatic agents such as Surgicel or Oxycel; an oversew at the bleeding anastomotic edge, which is undesirable as it may compromise the lumen; or the need for refashioning, which can be difficult, for example in an aortic neck. A pseudoaneurysm may result following revascularisation of a communicating haematoma.
3 Stenosis in bowel, which may be due to:
   a fibrosis following a leak;
   b inexpert technique;
   c recurrent tumour in a suture line.
4 Stenosis in arteries, which may be due to:
   a technical errors;
   b myo-intimal hyperplasia;
   c recurrent atherosclerosis.

CONCLUSION

Two of the most basic skills in surgery are suturing and knot tying. These techniques ought to be mastered before the surgeon in training enters the operating theatre. The surgical skills laboratory is the place to practise and master the techniques. Without practice, that skill will not develop.

FURTHER READING

Intercollegiate Basic Surgical Skills (2002) *Faculty and Participant Handbooks*, 3rd edn. Royal College of Surgeons of England, London.

Principles of laparoscopic and robotic surgery

LEARNING OBJECTIVES

To understand:
- The principles of laparoscopic and robotic surgery
- The advantages and disadvantages of such surgery

- The safety issues and indications for laparoscopic and robotic surgery
- The principles of postoperative care

DEFINITION

Minimal access surgery is a marriage of modern technology and surgical innovation that aims to accomplish surgical therapeutic goals with minimal somatic and psychological trauma. This type of surgery has reduced wound access trauma as well as being less disfiguring than conventional techniques. With increasing experience it offers cost-effectiveness both to health services and to employers by shortening operating times, shortening hospital stays and allowing faster recuperation.

EXTENT OF MINIMAL ACCESS SURGERY

Minimal access surgery has crossed all traditional boundaries of specialties and disciplines. Shared, borrowed and overlapping technologies and information are encouraging a multidisciplinary approach that serves the whole patient rather than a specific organ system. Broadly speaking, minimal access techniques can be categorised as follows.

Laparoscopy

A rigid endoscope is introduced through a sleeve into the peritoneal cavity. This is inflated with carbon dioxide to produce a pneumoperitoneum. Further sleeves or ports are inserted to enable instrument access and their use for dissection (Fig. 19.1). There is little doubt that laparoscopic cholecystectomy has revolutionised the surgical management of cholelithiasis and has become the mainstay of management of uncomplicated gallstone disease. With improved instruments and more experience it is likely that other advanced procedures, such as laparoscopic colectomies for malignancy, previously regarded as controversial, will also become fully accepted.

Thoracoscopy

A rigid endoscope is introduced through an incision in the chest to gain access to the thoracic contents. Usually there is no requirement for gas insufflation as the operating space is held open by the rigidity of the thoracic cavity.

Endoluminal endoscopy

Flexible or rigid endoscopes are introduced into hollow organs or systems, such as the urinary tract, upper or lower gastrointestinal tract, and respiratory and vascular systems (see Chapter 11).

Perivisceral endoscopy

Body planes can be accessed even in the absence of a natural cavity. Examples are mediastinoscopy, retroperitoneoscopy and retroperitoneal approaches to the kidney, aorta and lumbar sympathetic chain. Extraperitoneal approaches to the retroperitoneal organs, as well as hernia repair, are now becoming increasingly commonplace, further decreasing morbidity associated with visceral peritoneal manipulation. Other, more recent, examples include subfascial ligation of incompetent perforating veins in varicose vein surgery.

Arthroscopy and intra-articular joint surgery

Orthopaedic surgeons have long used arthroscopic access to the knee and have now moved their attention to other joints, including the shoulder, wrist, elbow and hip.

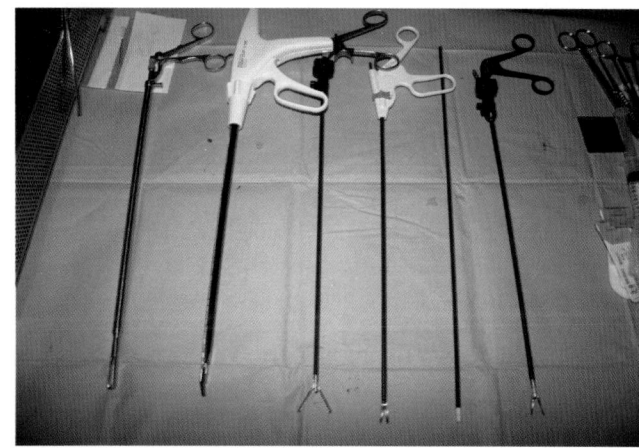

Figure 19.1 Basic laparoscopic instruments (photo courtesy of Daniel Leff).

Combined approach

The diseased organ is visualised and treated by an assortment of endoluminal and extraluminal endoscopes and other imaging devices.

SURGICAL TRAUMA IN OPEN, LAPAROSCOPIC AND ROBOTIC SURGERY

Most of the trauma of an open procedure is inflicted because the surgeon must have a wound that is large enough to give adequate exposure for safe dissection at the target site. The wound is often the cause of morbidity, including infection, dehiscence, bleeding, herniation and nerve entrapment. Wound pain prolongs recovery time and, by reducing mobility, contributes to an increased incidence of pulmonary atelectasis, chest infection, paralytic ileus and deep venous thrombosis.

Mechanical and human retractors cause additional trauma. Body wall retractors tend to inflict localised damage that may be as painful as the wound itself. In contrast, during laparoscopy, the retraction is provided by the low-pressure pneumoperitoneum, giving a diffuse force applied gently and evenly over the whole body wall, causing minimal trauma.

Exposure of any body cavity to the atmosphere also causes morbidity through cooling and fluid loss by evaporation. There is also evidence to suggest that the incidence of post-surgical adhesions has been reduced by the use of the laparoscope because there is less damage to delicate serosal coverings. In handling intestinal loops, the surgeon and assistant disturb the peristaltic activity of the gut and provoke adynamic ileus.

Minimal access surgery has many advantages, such as a reduction in the trauma of access and exposure and an improvement in visualisation (Summary box 19.1).

Summary box 19.1

Advantages of minimal access surgery

- Decrease in wound size
- Reduction in wound infection, dehiscence, bleeding, herniation and nerve entrapment
- Decrease in wound pain
- Improved mobility
- Decreased wound trauma
- Decreased heat loss
- Improved vision

LIMITATIONS OF MINIMAL ACCESS SURGERY

Despite its many advantages, minimal access surgery has its limitations. To perform minimal access surgery with safety, the surgeon must operate remote from the surgical field, using an imaging system that provides a two-dimensional representation of the operative site. The endoscope offers a whole new anatomical landscape, which the surgeon must learn to navigate without the usual clues that make it easy to judge depth. The instruments are longer and sometimes more complex to use than those commonly used in open surgery. This results in the novice being faced with significant problems of hand–eye coordination.

Some of the procedures performed by these new approaches are more technically demanding and are slower to perform. Indeed, on occasion, a minimally invasive operation is so technically demanding that both patient and surgeon are better served by conversion to an open procedure. Unfortunately, there seems to be a sense of shame associated with conversion, which is quite unjustified. It is vital for surgeons and patients to appreciate that the decision to close or convert to an open operation is not a complication but, instead, usually implies sound surgical judgement.

Another problem occurs when there is intraoperative arterial bleeding. Haemostasis may be very difficult to achieve endoscopically because blood obscures the field of vision and there is a significant reduction of the image quality owing to light absorption.

Another disadvantage of laparoscopic surgery is the loss of tactile feedback; this is an area of on-going research in haptics and biofeedback systems. Early work suggested that laparoscopic ultrasonography might be a substitute for the need to 'feel' in intraoperative decision-making. The rapid progress in advanced laparoscopic techniques, including biliary tract exploration and surgery for malignancies, has provided a strong impetus for the development of laparoscopic ultrasound. Although incompletely developed, this technique already has advantages that far outweigh its disadvantages.

In more advanced techniques, large pieces of resected tissue, such as the lung or colon, may have to be extracted from the body cavity. Occasionally, the extirpated tissue may be removed through a nearby natural orifice, such as the rectum or the mouth. At other times, a novel route may be employed. For instance, a benign colonic specimen may be extracted through an incision in the vault of the vagina. Several innovative tube systems have been shown to facilitate this extraction. Although tissue 'morcellators, mincers and liquidisers' can be used in some circumstances, they have the disadvantage of reducing the amount of information available to the pathologist. Recent reports of tumour implantation in the locations of port sites have raised important questions about the future of the laparoscopic treatment of malignancy. Although emerging evidence from large-scale UK and US prospective trials implicate surgical skill as an important aetiological factor, it is important to consider the biological implications of minimally invasive strategies on the tumours. The use of carbon dioxide and helium as insufflants causes locoregional hypoxia and may also change pH. The resultant modulation of spilled tumour cell behaviour is only now being elucidated.

Hand-assisted laparoscopic surgery is a well-developed technique. It involves the intra-abdominal placement of a hand or forearm through a minilaparotomy incision while pneumoperitoneum is maintained. In this way, the surgeon's hand can be used as in an open procedure. It can be used to palpate organs or tumours, reflect organs atraumatically, retract structures, identify vessels, dissect bluntly along a tissue plane and provide finger pressure to bleeding points while proximal control is achieved. In addition, several reports have suggested that this approach is more economical than a totally laparoscopic approach, reducing both the number of laparoscopic ports and the number of instruments required. Some advocates of the technique claim that it is also easier to learn and perform than totally laparoscopic approaches, and that there may be increased patient safety.

There is a growing need for improvement in dissection techniques in laparoscopic surgery and, specifically, for improving the safe use of electrosurgery and lasers. Ultrasonic dissection and tissue removal have been utilised by a growing number of specialties for several years. The adaptation of the technology to laparoscopic surgery grew out of the search for alternative, possibly safer, methods of dissection. The current units combine the functions of three or four separate instruments, reducing the need for instrument exchanges during a procedure. This flexibility, combined with the ability to provide a clean, smoke-free field, improves safety while shortening operating times.

Although dramatic cost savings are possible with laparoscopic cholecystectomy, the position is less clear-cut with other procedures. There is another factor that may complicate the computation of the cost–benefit ratio. A significant rise in the rate of cholecystectomy followed the introduction of the laparoscopic approach as the threshold for referring patients for surgery lowered. The increase in the number of procedures performed has led to an overall increase in the cost of treating symptomatic gallstones.

Three-dimensional systems are available but remain expensive and currently are not commonplace. Stereoscopic imaging for laparoscopy is still progressing. Future improvements in these systems will greatly enhance manipulative ability in critical procedures such as knot tying and dissection of closely underlying tissues. There are, however, some drawbacks, such as reduced display brightness and interference with normal vision because of the need to wear specially designed glasses for some systems. It is likely that brighter projection displays will be developed, at increased cost. However, the need to wear glasses will not be easily overcome.

Looking further to the future it is evident that the continuing reductions in the costs of elaborate image-processing techniques will result in a wide range of transformed presentations becoming available. It will ultimately be possible for a surgeon to call up any view of the operative region that is accessible to a camera and present it stereoscopically in any size or orientation, superimposed on past images taken in other modalities. Such augmented reality systems are being developed at present but are currently in relative infancy. It is for the medical community to decide which of these many potential imaginative techniques will contribute most to effective surgical procedures (Summary box 19.2).

Summary box 19.2

Limitations of minimal access surgery

- Reliance on remote vision and operating
- Loss of tactile feedback
- Dependence on hand–eye coordination
- Difficulty with haemostasis
- Reliance on new techniques
- Extraction of large specimens

ROBOTIC SURGERY

A robot is a mechanical device that performs automated physical tasks according to direct human supervision, a predefined program or a set of general guidelines using artificial intelligence techniques. In terms of surgery, robots have been used to assist surgeons during procedures. This has been primarily in the form of automated camera systems and telemanipulator systems, thus resulting in the creation of a human–machine interface.

Even though laparoscopic surgery has progressed greatly over the last two decades there are limitations. These include the restriction to two-dimensional views, reduced degrees of freedom, little or no tactile feedback and ergonomically difficult positions for the surgeon. Such problems undoubtedly affect surgical precision. This has led to interest in robotic master–slave systems (where the surgeon is the master, i.e. the operator, and the robot is the slave). Such devices have been under trial during the last 10 years. They offer many benefits, which have arisen as a result of new technology in lenses, cameras and computer software. The advantages are twofold: first for the patient (as per laparoscopic surgery, Summary box 19.1) and second for the surgeon. The advantages for the surgeon include better visualisation (higher magnification) with stereoscopic views; elimination of hand tremor allowing greater precision; improved manoeuvring as a result of the 'robotic wrist', which allows seven degrees of freedom; and the fact that large external movements of the surgical hands can be scaled down and transformed to limited internal movements of the 'robotic hands', extending the surgical ability to perform complex technical tasks in a limited space. Also, the surgeon is able to work in an ergonomic environment with less stress and achieve higher levels of concentration. The computer may also be able to compensate for the beating movement of the heart, making it unnecessary to stop the heart during cardiothoracic surgery. There may also be less need for assistance once surgery is under way.

Many surgical specialties have embraced the progression of robot-assisted techniques, including general surgery, cardiothoracic surgery, urology, orthopaedics, ear, nose and throat surgery and paediatric surgery. Specialities that use microsurgical techniques will particularly benefit in the future.

There are different robotic systems available (see Figs 19.2–19.5). Robotic camera systems include AESOP (Computer Motion, Goleta, California, USA) and EndoAssist (Armstrong

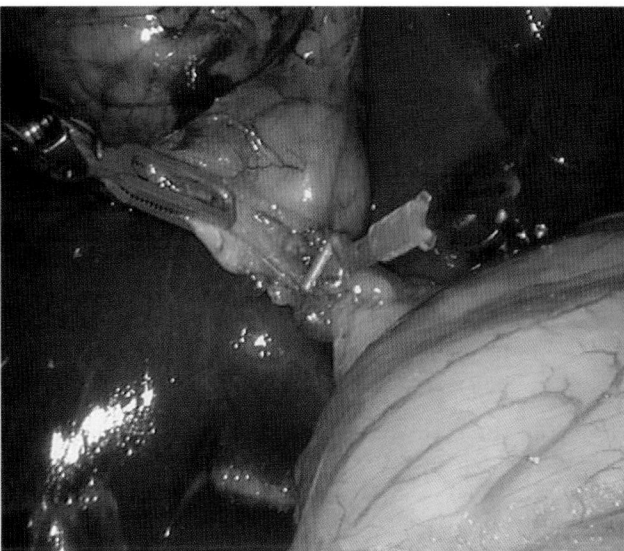

Figure 19.2 da Vinci manipulators used during robotic laparoscopic cholecystectomy. This demonstrates the robotic grasper holding and retracting the gall bladder neck while the robotic hook is used to free the overlying omentum on the gall bladder and cystic duct (courtesy of the Department of Biosurgery and Surgical Technology, Imperial College, London).

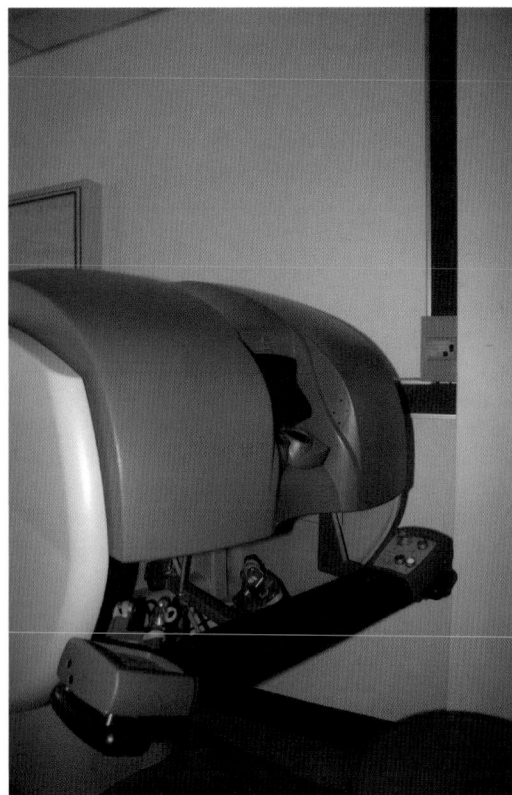

Figure 19.3 da Vinci console (photo courtesy of Daniel Leff).

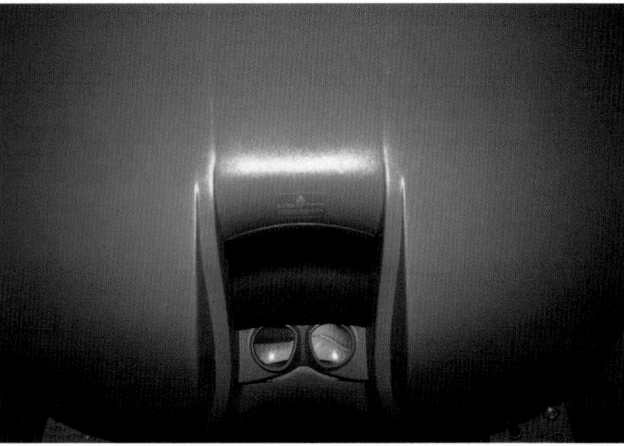

Figure 19.4 da Vinci console – binocular viewer (photo courtesy of Daniel Leff).

Healthcare Ltd, High Wycombe, UK). Telerobotic manipulators include the da Vinci (Intuitive Surgical, Inc., Menlo Park, California, USA) and ZEUS (Computer Motion, Goleta, California, USA) manipulators. Finally, telerobotics and tele-mentoring has been combined in systems such as SOCRATES (Computer Motion, Goleta, California, USA). All of these systems offer different advantages to the operating surgeon, ranging from reducing the need for assistants and providing better ergonomic operating positions to providing experienced guidance from surgeons not physically present in the operating theatre.

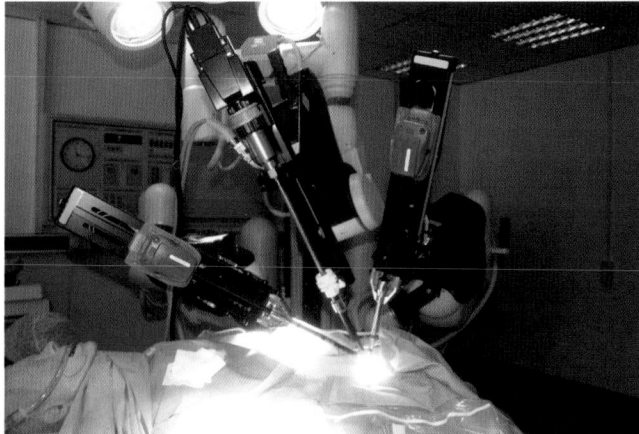

Figure 19.5 Slave unit: da Vinci arms set-up in a virtual operating theatre (photo courtesy of Daniel Leff).

PREOPERATIVE EVALUATION

Preparation of the patient undergoing laparoscopic or robotic surgery

Although the patient may be in hospital for a shorter period, careful preoperative management is essential to minimise morbidity.

History

Patients must be fit for general anaesthesia and open operation if necessary. Potential coagulation disorders (e.g. associated with cirrhosis) are particularly dangerous in laparoscopic surgery. As adhesions may cause problems, previous abdominal operations or peritonitis should be documented.

Examination

Routine preoperative physical examination is required as for any major operation. Although, in general, laparoscopic surgery allows quicker recovery, it may involve longer operating times and the establishment of the pneumoperitoneum may provoke cardiac arrhythmias. Severe chronic obstructive airways disease and ischaemic heart disease may be contraindications to the laparoscopic approach.

Particular attention should be paid to the presence or absence of jaundice, abdominal scars, palpable masses or tenderness.

Moderate obesity does not increase operative difficulty significantly, but massive obesity may make pneumoperitoneum difficult and standard instrumentation may be too short. Access may prove difficult in very thin patients, especially those with severe kyphosis.

Pre-medication

Pre-medication is the responsibility of the anaesthetist, with whom coexisting medical problems should be discussed.

Prophylaxis against thromboembolism

Venous stasis induced by the reverse Trendelenburg position during laparoscopic surgery may be a particular risk factor for deep vein thrombosis, as is a lengthy operation and the obesity of many patients. Subcutaneous fractionated heparin and anti-thromboembolic stockings should be used routinely in addition to pneumatic leggings during the operation. Patients already taking warfarin for other reasons should have this stopped temporarily or converted to intravenous heparin, depending on the underlying condition, as it is not safe to perform laparoscopic surgery in the presence of a significant coagulation deficit.

Urinary catheters and nasogastric tubes

In the early days of laparoscopic surgery, routine bladder catheterisation and nasogastric intubation were advised. Most surgeons now omit these but it remains essential to check that the patient is fasted and has recently emptied the bladder, particularly before the blind insertion of a Verres needle. However, currently, most general surgeons prefer the direct cut-down technique into the abdomen for the introduction of the first port for the establishment of the pneumoperitoneum (Hasson technique).

Informed consent

The basis of many complaints and much litigation in surgery, especially laparoscopic surgery, relates to the issue of informed consent. It is essential that the patient understands the nature of the procedure, the risks involved and, when appropriate, the alternatives that are available. A locally prepared explanatory booklet concerning the laparoscopic procedure to be undertaken is extremely useful.

In an elective case, a full discussion of the proposed operation should take place in the out-patient department with a surgeon of appropriate seniority, preferably the operating surgeon, before the decision is made to operate. On admission it is the responsibility of the operating surgeon and anaesthetist to ensure that the patient has been fully counselled, although the actual witnessing of the consent form may have been delegated. The patient should understand what laparoscopic surgery involves and that there is a risk of conversion to open operation. If known, this risk should be quantified, for example the increased risk with acute cholecystitis or in the presence of extensive upper abdominal adhesions. The conversion rate will also vary with the experience and practice of the surgeon. Common complications should be mentioned, such as shoulder tip pain and minor surgical emphysema, as well as rare but serious complications including injury to the bile ducts and visceral injury from trocar insertion or diathermy.

A few patients may insist on having an open procedure (probably influenced by accounts of mishaps) and the surgeon should be prepared to offer this, although most will opt for laparoscopy if the surgeon has extensive experience and an impressive safety record.

When obtaining consent for robotic surgery patients should be offered appropriate literature so that they are able to provide fully informed consent. As these procedures are still not routine, this should be carried out by the operating surgeon and, if the procedure is in the context of a clinical trial, the appropriate ethical approval and subsequent paperwork should be available to the patient before signing the consent form (Summary box 19.3).

Janos Verres, **1903–1979**, Chest Physician, and Chief of the Department of Internal Medicine, The Regional Hospital, Kapuvar, Hungary.
Harrith Hasson, **Professor of Gynecology, Chicago, IL, USA.**

Summary box 19.3

Preparation for laparoscopic or robotic surgery

- Overall fitness: cardiac arrhythmia, emphysema
- Previous surgery: scars, adhesions
- Body habitus: obesity, skeletal deformity
- Normal coagulation
- Thromboprophylaxis
- Informed consent

Preparation is very similar to that for open surgery and aims to ensure that:

- The patient is fit for the procedure
- The patient is fully informed and has consented
- Operative difficulty is predicted when possible
- Appropriate theatre time and facilities are available (especially important for robotic cases)

THEATRE SET-UP AND TOOLS

Operating theatre design, construction and layout is key to its smooth running on a daily basis. Originally, the video and diathermy equipment and other key tools used in laparoscopic surgery were moved around on stacks, taking up valuable floor space and cluttering up the theatre environment, which was not always ergonomic for the operating team. New theatres are designed with movable booms that come down from the ceiling; these are easy to place and do not have long leads or wires trailing behind them (Fig. 19.6). The equipment consists of at least two high-resolution LCD monitors, the laparoscopic kit for maintaining pneumoperitoneum and the audiovisual kit. The advent of DVD and other digital recording equipment has also led to these being incorporated into the rigs so that cases can be recorded with ease. This is further facilitated by cameras being inserted into the light handles of the main overhead lights so that open surgery can also be recorded without distracting the surgeons.

Image quality is vital to the success of laparoscopic surgery. New camera and lens technology allows the use of smaller cameras. Many centres now use 5 mm cameras routinely. Automatic focusing and charge-coupled devices (CCDs) are used to detect different levels of brightness and adjust for the best

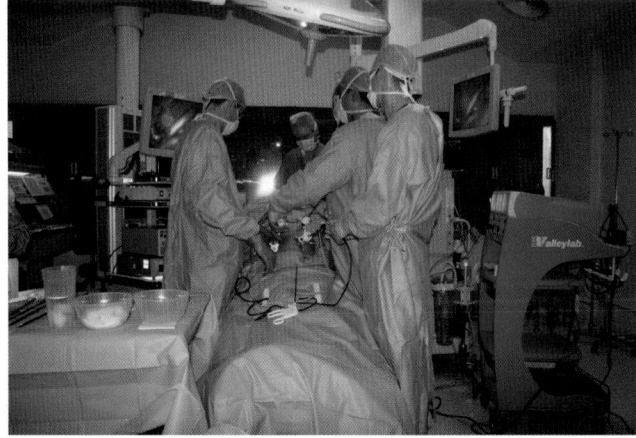

Figure 19.6 Modern laparoscopic theatre set-up (photo courtesy of Daniel Leff).

image possible. Flat panel monitors with high definition images are used to give the surgeon the best views possible. The usability of the kit has also improved; touch screen panels and even voice-activated systems are now available on the market.

As minimally invasive and robotic procedures have become routine in some institutions, the dedicated theatre team for such procedures has also evolved. Surgeons and anaesthetists, as well as scrub and circulating nurses, have become familiar with working with the equipment and each other. The efficient working of the team is crucial to high-quality surgery and quick yet safe turnover times. Laparoscopic tools have also changed. Disposable equipment is more readily available, which does unfortunately increase the cost of the surgery. However, easy to use, ergonomically designed and reliable surgical tools are essential for laparoscopic and robotic surgery. Simple designs for new laparoscopic ports are now being studied, with the aim of reducing the incidence of port-site hernias; see-through ports that allow the surgeon to cut down through the abdomen while observing the layers through the cameras and new light sources within the abdomen may be simple ideas that affect surgical technique in the near future.

GENERAL INTRAOPERATIVE PRINCIPLES

Laparoscopic cholecystectomy is now the 'gold standard' for operative treatment of symptomatic gallstone disease. The main negative aspect of the technique is the increased incidence of bile duct injury compared with open cholecystectomy. Better understanding of the mechanisms of injury, coupled with proper training, will avoid most of these errors. The following sections highlight the important technical steps that should be taken during any form of laparoscopic surgery to avoid complications.

Creating a pneumoperitoneum

There are two methods for creation of a pneumoperitoneum: open and closed. The closed method involves blind puncture using a Verres needle. Although this method is fast and relatively safe, there is a small but significant potential for intestinal or vascular injury on introduction of the needle or first trocar. The routine use of the open technique for creating a pneumoperitoneum avoids the morbidity related to a blind puncture. To achieve this, a 1-cm vertical or transverse incision is made at the level of the umbilicus. Two small retractors are used to dissect bluntly the subcutaneous fat and expose the midline fascia. Two sutures are inserted each side of the midline incision, followed by the creation of a 1-cm opening in the fascia. Free penetration into the abdominal cavity is confirmed by the gentle introduction of a finger. Finally, a Hasson trocar (or other blunt-tip trocar) is inserted and anchored with the fascial sutures (Fig. 19.7). The open technique may initially appear time-consuming and even cumbersome; however, with practice, it is more efficient overall.

Preoperative problems

Previous abdominal surgery

Previous abdominal surgery is no longer a contraindication to laparoscopic surgery, but preoperative evaluation is necessary to assess the type and location of surgical scars. As mentioned earlier, the open technique for insertion of the first trocar is safer. Before trocar insertion, the introduction of a fingertip helps to ascertain penetration into the peritoneal cavity and also allows

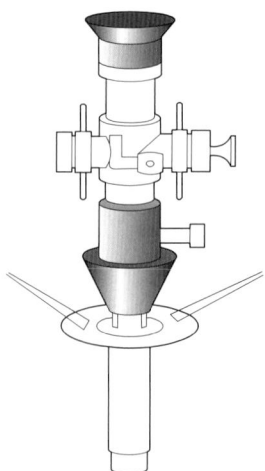

Figure 19.7 Open technique with Hasson port. Apply safe principles of closed technique.

adhesions to be gently removed from the entry site. After the tip of the cannula has been introduced, a 0° laparoscope is used as a blunt dissector to tease adhesions gently away and form a tunnel towards the quadrant where the operation is to take place. This step is accomplished by a careful pushing and twisting motion under direct vision. With experience, the surgeon learns to differentiate visually between thick adhesions that may contain bowel and should be avoided and thin adhesions that would lead to a window into a free area of the peritoneal cavity (Fig. 19.8).

Obesity

Laparoscopic and robotic surgery have proved to be safe and effective procedures in the obese population. In fact, some procedures are less difficult than their open counterparts for the morbidly obese patient. Technical difficulties occur, however, in obtaining pneumoperitoneum, reaching the operative region adequately and achieving adequate exposure in the presence of an obese colon. Increased thickness of the subcutaneous fat makes insufflation of the abdominal cavity more difficult. With the closed technique, a larger Verres needle is often required for morbidly obese patients. Pulling the skin up for fixation of the soft tissues is better accomplished with towel clamps. Only moderate

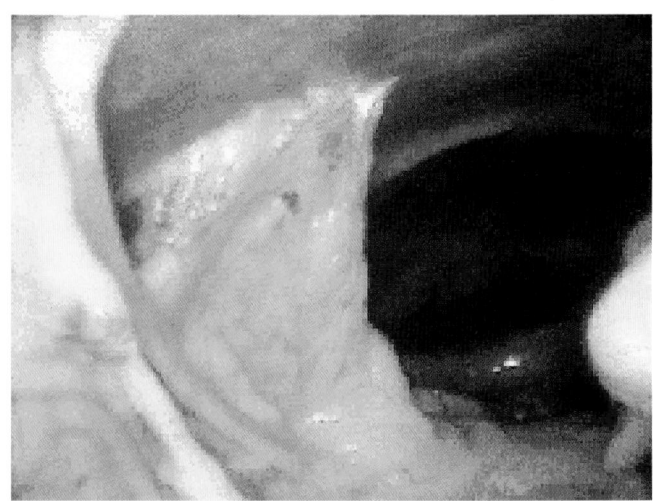

Figure 19.8 Intra-abdominal adhesion.

force should be used to avoid separating the skin farther away from the fascia. The needle should be passed at nearly a right angle to the skin and preferably above the umbilicus where the peritoneum is more firmly fixed to the midline. The open technique of inserting a Hasson trocar is easier and safer for obese patients. The main difficulty is reaching the fascia. A larger skin incision (1–3 cm), starting at the umbilicus and extending superiorly, may facilitate this. To reach the operative area adequately, the location of some of the ports has to be modified and, in some instances, larger instruments are necessary. When the length of the laparoscope appears to be insufficient to reach the operative area adequately, the initial midline port should be placed nearer to the operative field.

Operative problems

Perforation of the gall bladder (see also Chapter 63)

Perforation of the gall bladder is more common with the laparoscopic technique than with the open technique. Some authors have reported an incidence of up to 30% but it does not appear to be a factor in increasing the early postoperative morbidity. However, it is well known that bile is not a sterile fluid and bacteria can be present in the absence of cholecystitis. Unless the perforation is small, closure with endoloops should be attempted to avoid contamination.

Bleeding

In some of the larger series, bleeding has been the most common cause for conversion to an open procedure. Bleeding plays a more important role in laparoscopic surgery because of factors inherent to the technique. These include a limited field that can easily be obscured by relatively small amounts of blood, magnification that makes small arterial bleeding appear to be a significant haemorrhage and light absorption that obscures the visual field.

How to avoid bleeding

As in any surgical procedure the best way to handle intraoperative bleeding is to prevent it from happening. This can usually be accomplished by identifying patients at high risk of bleeding, having a clear understanding of the laparoscopic anatomy and employing careful surgical technique.

Risk factors that predispose to increased bleeding include:

- cirrhosis;
- inflammatory conditions (acute cholecystitis, diverticulitis);
- coagulation defects: these are contraindications to a laparoscopic procedure.

Bleeding from a major vessel

Damage to a large vessel requires immediate assessment of the magnitude and type of bleeding. When the bleeding vessel is identified, a fine-tip grasper can be used to grasp it and apply either electrocautery or a clip, depending on its size. When the vessel is not identified early and a pool of blood forms, compression should be applied immediately with a blunt instrument, a cotton swab or with the adjacent organ. Good suction and irrigation are of utmost importance. Once the area has been cleaned, pressure should be released gradually to identify the site of bleeding. Insertion of an extra cannula may be required to achieve adequate exposure and at the same time to enable the concomitant use of a suction device and an insulated grasper. Although most of the bleeding vessels can be controlled laparoscopically,

judgement should be used in deciding when not to prolong bleeding but to convert to an open procedure at an early stage.

Bleeding from the gall bladder bed

Bleeding from the gall bladder bed can usually be prevented by performing the dissection in the correct plane. When a bleeding site appears during detachment of the gall bladder, the dissection should be carried a little farther to adequately expose the bleeding point. Once this step has been performed, direct application of electrocautery usually controls the bleeding. If bleeding persists, indirect application of electrocautery is useful because it avoids detachment of the formed crust. This procedure is accomplished by applying pressure to the bleeding point with a blunt, insulated grasper and then applying electrocoagulation by touching this grasper with a second insulated grasper that is connected to the electrocautery device. One must be careful to keep all conducting surfaces of the graspers within the visual field while applying the electrocautery current.

Bleeding from a trocar site

Bleeding from the trocar sites is usually controlled by applying upwards and lateral pressure with the trocar itself. Considerable bleeding may occur if the falciform ligament is impaled with the substernal trocar or if one of the epigastric vessels is injured. If significant continuous bleeding from the falciform ligament occurs, haemostasis is achieved by percutaneously inserting a large, straight needle at one side of the ligament. A monofilament suture attached to the needle is passed into the abdominal cavity and the needle is exited at the other side of the ligament using a grasper (Fig. 19.9). The loop is suspended and compression is achieved. Maintaining compression throughout the procedure usually suffices. After the procedure has been completed, the loop is removed under direct laparoscopic visualisation to ensure complete haemostasis. When significant continuous bleeding from the abdominal wall occurs, haemostasis can be accomplished either by pressure or by suturing the bleeding site. Pressure can be applied using a Foley balloon catheter. The catheter is introduced into the abdominal cavity through the bleeding trocar site wound, the balloon is inflated and traction is placed on the catheter, which is bolstered in place to keep it under tension. The catheter is left *in situ* for 24 hours and then removed. Although

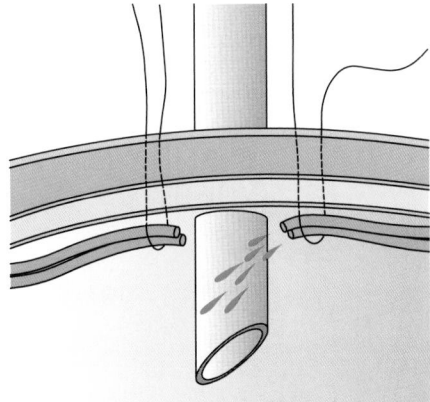

Figure 19.9 Port-side bleeding controlled with sutures.

Frederic Eugene Basil Foley, **1891–1966, Urologist, Ankher Hospital, St. Paul, MN, USA.**

this method is successful in achieving haemostasis, the author favours direct suturing of the bleeding vessel. This manoeuvre is accomplished by extending the skin incision by 3 mm at both ends of the bleeding trocar site wound. Two figure-of-eight sutures are placed in the path of the vessel at both ends of the wound.

Evacuation of blood clots

The best way of dealing with blood clots is to avoid them. As mentioned, careful dissection and identification of the cystic artery and its branches, as well as identifying and carrying out dissection of the gall bladder in the correct plane, help to prevent bleeding from the cystic vessels and the hepatic bed. Nevertheless, clot formation takes place when unsuspected bleeding occurs or when inflammation is severe and a clear plane is not present between the gall bladder and the hepatic bed. The routine use of 5000–7000 units of heparin per litre of irrigation fluid helps to avoid the formation of clots. When extra bleeding is foreseen, a small pool of irrigation fluid can be kept in the operative field to prevent clot formation. After clots have formed, a large-bore suction device should be used for their retrieval. Care should be taken to avoid suctioning in proximity to placed clips.

Principles of electrosurgery during laparoscopic surgery

Electrosurgical injuries during laparoscopy are potentially serious. The vast majority occur following the use of monopolar diathermy. The overall incidence is between one and two cases per 1000 operations. Electrical injuries are usually unrecognised at the time that they occur, with patients commonly presenting 3–7 days after injury with complaints of fever and abdominal pain. As these injuries usually present late, the reasons for their occurrence are largely speculative. The main theories are: (1) inadvertent touching or grasping of tissue during current application; (2) direct coupling between a portion of bowel and a metal instrument that is touching the activated probe (Fig. 19.10); (3) insulation breaks in the electrodes; (4) direct sparking to bowel from the diathermy probe; and (5) current passage to the bowel from recently coagulated, electrically isolated tissue. Bipolar diathermy is safer and should be used in preference to monopolar diathermy, especially in anatomically crowded areas. If monopolar diathermy is to be used, important safety measures include attainment of a perfect visual image, avoiding excessive current

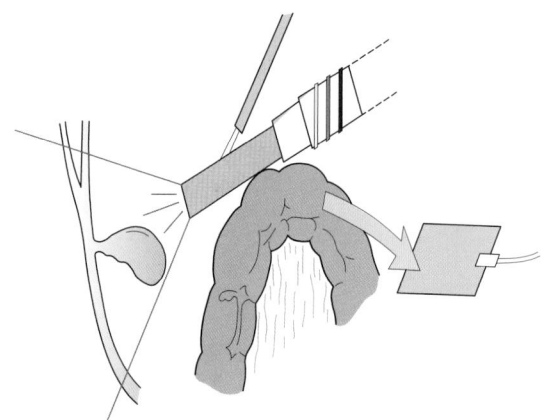

Figure 19.10 Direct coupling between bowel and laparoscope, which is touching the activated probe.

application and meticulous attention to insulation. Alternative methods of performing dissection, such as the use of ultrasonic devices, may improve safety.

Postoperative care

The postoperative care of patients after laparoscopic surgery is generally straightforward with a low incidence of pain or other problems. The most common routine postoperative symptoms are a dull upper abdominal pain, nausea and pain around the shoulders (referred from the diaphragm). There has been some suggestion that the instillation of local anaesthetic to the operating site and into the suprahepatic space, or even leaving 1 litre of normal saline in the peritoneum, serves to further decrease postoperative pain. It is a good general rule that if the patient develops a fever or tachycardia or complains of severe pain at the operation site, something is wrong and close observation is necessary. In this case routine investigation should include a full blood count, liver function tests, an amylase test and, probably, an ultrasound scan of the upper abdomen to detect fluid collections. If bile duct leakage is suspected, endoscopic retrograde cholangiopancreatography (ERCP) may be needed. If in doubt, re-laparoscopy or laparotomy should be performed earlier rather than later. Death following technical errors in laparoscopic cholecystectomy has often been associated with a long delay in deciding to re-explore the abdomen.

In the absence of problems, patients should be fit for discharge within 24 hours. They should be given instructions to telephone the unit or their general practitioner and to return to the hospital if they are not making satisfactory progress.

Nausea

About half of patients experience some degree of nausea after laparoscopic surgery and rarely this is severe. It usually responds to an antiemetic such as ondansetron and settles within 12–24 hours. It is made worse by opiate analgesics and these should be avoided.

Shoulder tip pain

The patient should be warned about this preoperatively and told that the pain is referred from the diaphragm and not due to a local problem in the shoulders. It can be at its worst 24 hours after the operation. It usually settles within 2–3 days and is relieved by simple analgesics such as paracetamol.

Abdominal pain

Pain in one or other of the port site wounds is not uncommon and is worse if there is haematoma formation. It usually settles very rapidly. Increasing pain after 2–3 days may be a sign of infection and, with concomitant signs, antibiotic therapy is occasionally required.

Analgesia

A 100-mg diclofenac suppository should be given at the time of the operation. It is important that the patient provides separate consent for this if the suppository is to be administered peroperatively. Suppositories may be administered a further two or three times postoperatively for relief of more severe pain. Otherwise 500–1000 mg of paracetamol 4-hourly usually suffices. Opiate analgesics cause nausea and should be avoided unless the pain is very severe. In this case, suspect a postoperative complication (as above). The majority of patients require between one and four doses of 1 g of paracetamol postoperatively.

Orogastric tube

An orogastric tube may be placed during the operation if the stomach is distended and obscuring the view. It is not necessary in all cases. It should be removed as soon as the operation is over and before the patient regains consciousness.

Oral fluids

There is no significant ileus after laparoscopic surgery except in resectional procedures such as colectomy or small bowel resection. Patients can start taking oral fluids as soon as they are conscious; they usually do so 4–6 hours after the end of the operation.

Oral feeding

Provided that the patient has an appetite, a light meal can be taken 4–6 hours after the operation. Some patients remain slightly nauseated at this stage but almost all eat a normal breakfast on the morning after the operation.

Patients will require advice about what they can eat at home. They should be told that they can eat a normal diet but should avoid excess. It seems sensible to avoid high-fat meals for the first week although there is no clear evidence that this is necessary.

Urinary catheter

If a urinary catheter has been placed in the bladder during the operation it should be removed before the patient regains consciousness. The patient should be warned of the possibility and symptoms of postoperative cystitis and told to seek advice in the unlikely event of this occurring.

Drains

Some surgeons drain the abdomen at the end of laparoscopic cholecystectomy although this is controversial. If a drain is placed to vent the remaining gas and peritoneal fluid it should be removed within 1 hour of the operation. If it has been placed because of excessive hepatic bleeding or bile leakage it should be removed when that problem has resolved, usually after 12–24 hours. Continued blood loss from a drain is an indication for re-exploration of the abdomen (Summary box 19.4).

Summary box 19.4

Surgical principles

- Meticulous care in the creation of a pneumoperitoneum
- Controlled dissection of adhesions
- Adequate exposure of operative field
- Avoidance and control of bleeding
- Avoidance of organ injury
- Avoidance of diathermy damage
- Vigilance in the postoperative period

DISCHARGE FROM HOSPITAL

Some surgeons discharge a proportion of their patients on the day of surgery but most are kept in overnight and discharged the following morning. Patients should not be discharged until they are seen to be comfortable and eating and drinking satisfactorily. They should be told that if they develop abdominal pain or other severe symptoms then they should return to the hospital or to their general practitioner.

Skin sutures

If non-absorbable sutures or skin staples have been used they can be removed from the port sites after 48 hours.

Mobility and convalescence

Patients can get out of bed to go to the toilet as soon as they have recovered from the anaesthetic and they should be encouraged to do so. Such movements are remarkably pain free when compared with the mobility achieved after an open operation. Similarly, patients can cough actively and clear bronchial secretions, and this helps to diminish the incidence of chest infections. Many patients are able to walk out of hospital on the evening of their operation and almost all are fully mobile by the following morning. Thereafter, the postoperative recovery is variable. Some patients prefer to take things quietly for the first 2–3 days, interspersing increasing exercise with rest. After the third day, patients will have undertaken increasing amounts of activity. The average return to work is about 10 days.

THE PRINCIPLES OF COMMON LAPAROSCOPIC PROCEDURES

The principles of common laparoscopic procedures are described in the appropriate chapters:

- laparoscopic cholecystectomy (Chapter 63);
- laparoscopic inguinal hernia repair (Chapter 57);
- laparoscopic anti-reflux surgery (Chapter 59);
- laparoscopic appendicectomy (Chapter 67).

Other elective laparoscopic or minimally invasive procedures that are becoming more widely utilised in certain specialist centres include:

- colectomy;
- splenectomy;
- nephrectomy;
- adrenalectomy;
- prostatectomy;
- thyroid and parathyroid surgery;
- aortic aneurysm surgery;
- single-vessel coronary artery bypass surgery;
- video-assisted thorascopic surgery (VATS).

Laparoscopy has also been used in certain emergency situations (in stable patients) in the hands of experienced laparoscopic surgeons. These may include diagnostic laparoscopy, repair of a perforated duodenal ulcer, laparoscopic appendicectomy, treatment of intestinal obstruction secondary to adhesions and, also, the laparoscopic evaluation of stable trauma patients.

Procedures that have been carried out using robotically assisted minimally invasive surgery include all of those listed above. Currently, robotic surgery still has certain disadvantages:

- increased cost;
- increased set-up of the system and operating time;
- socio-economic implications;
- significant risk of conversion to conventional techniques;
- prolonged learning curve;
- multiple repositioning of the arms can cause trauma;
- haemostasis;
- collision of the robotic arms in extreme positions.

Until these are overcome, by continued development of the technology and the drive of surgeons to progress in the field, robotically assisted surgery will not be commonplace. However, the potential for such systems is immense and continued research and clinical trials will pave the way for future generations of surgeons and patients alike.

THE FUTURE

Although there is no doubt that minimal access surgery has changed the practice of surgeons, it has not changed the nature of disease. The basic principles of good surgery still apply, including appropriate case selection, excellent exposure, adequate retraction and a high level of technical expertise. If a procedure makes no sense with conventional access, it will make no sense with a laparoscopic approach. Laparoscopic and robotic surgery training is key to allow the specialty to progress. The pioneers of yesterday have to teach the surgeons of tomorrow not only the technical and dextrous skills required but also the decision-making and innovative skills necessary for the field to continue to evolve. Training is often perceived as difficult as trainers have less control over the trainees at the time of surgery and caseloads may be smaller, especially in centres where laparoscopic and robotic procedures are not common. However, trainees now rightly expect exposure to these procedures and training systems should be adaptable for international exposure so that these techniques can be disseminated worldwide.

Improvements in instrumentation, the continued progress of robotic surgery and the development of structured training programmes are the key to the future of minimal access surgery. The use of robots in surgery has increased dramatically in the last decade. Indeed, robots are now available not only for assisting in surgery but also for aiding in the perioperative management of surgical patients. The remote presence systems (In Touch Health, Santa Barbara, California, USA; Figs 19.11 and 19.12) allow clinicians to assess patients in real time and interact with them while they are not on site or even if in a different continent. Continued advances in related technologies such as computer science will allow the incorporation of augmented reality systems alongside robotic systems to enhance surgical precision in image-guided surgery. Endoluminal robotic surgery is in its infancy but systems are being developed that will enable navigation within the colon to allow surgery on lesions in spaces that are accessible from the outside without an exterior incision being made. The advent of nanotechnology will also bring about much change in surgery. Miniaturisation will be possible, potentially allowing surgery at a cellular level to be carried out.

At present work has already started on single-port laparoscopy, in which a single port may act as a camera and have unfolding instruments open up once they are inside the peritoneum to perform the surgery, therefore reducing the number of port sites needed. Extensive research is also being carried out in the field of NOTES (natural orifice transluminal surgery). This is a technique whereby the peritoneal cavity is entered endoscopically, via a natural orifice (mouth, rectum, vagina) and the surgery is carried out using specialised endoscopic technology and techniques. Currently this has just started on a few human subjects, but most of the research is from animal models. NOTES cholecystectomy and appendicectomy have been successfully

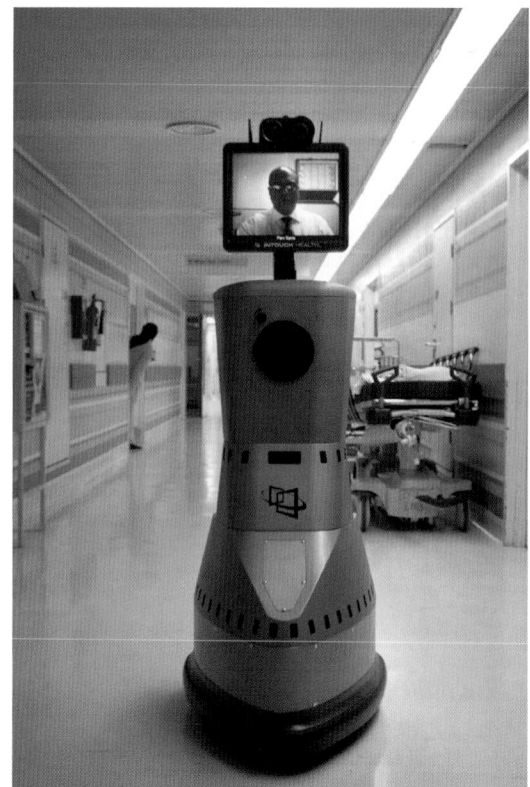

Figure 19.11 Remote presence robot (courtesy of the Department of Biosurgery and Surgical Technology, Imperial College, London).

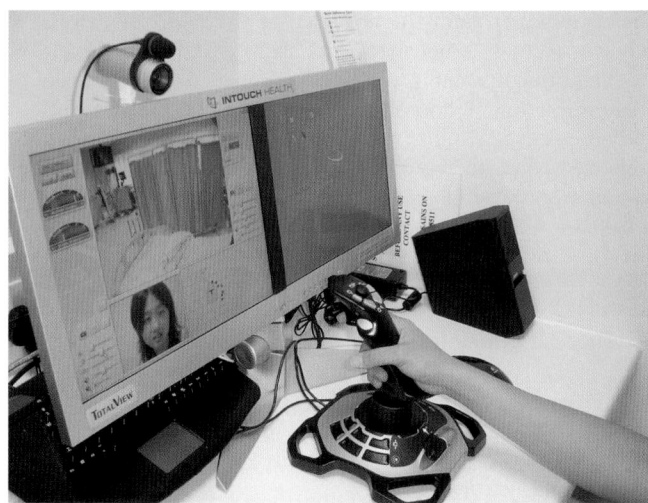

Figure 19.12 Remote presence console (courtesy of the Department of Biosurgery and Surgical Technology, Imperial College, London).

carried out in humans. Minimising the potential contamination of the peritoneum and the ability to carry out a safe closure of the peritoneal entry site are the main technical challenges of this type of minimally invasive and essentially 'scarless' or 'incisionless' surgery.

It is certain that there is much that is new in minimal access surgery. Only time will tell how much of what is new is truly better.

The cleaner and gentler the act of operation, the less the patient suffers, the smoother and quicker his convalescence, the more exquisite his healed wound.

Berkeley George Andrew Moynihan (1920)

Berkeley George Andrew Moynihan, (Lord Moynihan of Leeds), **1865–1936,** **Professor of Clinical Surgery, The University of Leeds, Leeds, England.**

FURTHER READING

Ballantyne, G.H., Marescaux, J. and Giulianotti, P.C. (eds) (2004) *Primer of Robotic and Telerobotic Surgery.* Lippincott Williams & Wilkins, Philadelphia, PA.

Cadiere, G.B., Houben, J.J., Bruyns, J., Himpens, J., Panzer, J.M. and Gelin, M. (1994) Laparoscopic Nissen fundoplication: technique and preliminary results. *Br J Surg* **81**: 400–3.

Cuschieri, A. (1992) A rose by any other name: minimal access or minimally invasive surgery. *Surg Endosc* **6**: 214.

Cuschieri, A. (1993) Laparoscopic anti-reflux surgery and repair of hiatal hernia. *World J Surg* **17**: 40–5.

Gill I.S., Sung, G.T. and Ballantyne, G.H. (eds) (2003) *Robotics in Surgery. Surg Clin N Am* **83(6)**.

McKernan, J.B. and Laws, H.L. (1994) Laparoscopic Nissen fundoplication for the treatment of gastroesophageal reflux disease. *Am Surg* **60**: 87–93.

Mouiel, J. and Katkhouda, N. (1994) Laparoscopic Rossetti fundoplication. In: Patterson-Brown, S. and Garden, J. (eds). *Principles and Practice of Laparoscopic Surgery.* W.B. Saunders, London, 262–76.

Nduka, C., Super, P., Monson, J.R.T. and Darzi, A. (1994) Cause and prevention of electrosurgical injury in laparoscopic surgery. *J Am Coll Surg* **179**: 161–79.

Purkayastha, S., Athanasiou, T., Casula, R. and Darzi, A. (2004) Robotic surgery: a review. *Hosp Med* **65**: 153–9.

CHAPTER 19 | PRINCIPLES OF LAPAROSCOPIC AND ROBOTIC SURGERY

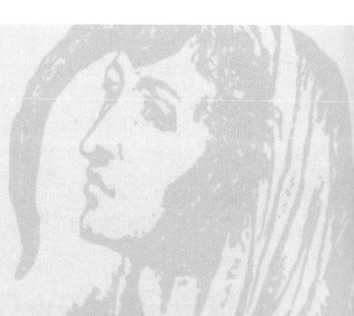

Postoperative care

LEARNING OBJECTIVES

To understand:
- The system of postoperative care
- The common and serious postoperative complications, their recognition, avoidance and treatment

- The system of daily entries in patients' records
- The system for discharging patients

INTRODUCTION

The aim of postoperative care is to provide the patient with as quick, painless and safe a recovery from surgery as possible.

GENERAL MANAGEMENT

The immediate postoperative period

In the immediate postoperative period the patient is nursed in a recovery area using one-to-one nursing and continuous monitoring. The role of the recovery nurse is to ensure that the patient is protecting their airway, breathing freely and perfusing adequately (*airway*, *breathing* and *circulation*). The recovery nurse should also monitor the patient's pain as the anaesthetic wears off and ensure that there are no early complications developing, such as bleeding from the wound or loss of distal circulation and/or sensation. Blood pressure, pulse and oxygen saturation are therefore monitored regularly and the results charted. Trends seen on these charts reassure the recovery nurse that the patient is recovering well or warn that a complication is developing (Summary box 20.1).

Summary box 20.1

Postoperative period

- Ensure airway, *breathing* and circulation are satisfactory
- Monitor pain
- Watch for complications
- Monitor blood pressure, pulse and oxygen saturation

If there are any special aspects that need monitoring (e.g. return of sensation) then instructions on how they are to be monitored should be written clearly in the postoperative care section of the operative notes as well as given verbally to the recovery nursing staff at handover of the patient.

Patient recovery

Once patients are fully conscious and comfortable and their vital functions are stable they are transferred to the general ward; however, patients who are at high risk may be transferred to a high-dependency or intensive care unit.

While on the ward patients should be visited at least morning and evening by medical staff to ensure that there is steady progress. All staff on these rounds must wash their hands between every patient.

A simple system for ensuring that everything is checked and recorded is represented by the acronym SOAP (*subjective*, *objective*, *assessment*, *plan*).

Subjective

Ask the patient how they are. Specifically, ask about pain, nausea and mobility. Anxiety, disorientation or a change in behaviour are often the first signs that complications are setting in.

Objective

Check the patient's charts for temperature, pulse and respiration (TPR), fluid balance and any special observations recorded by the nurses (such as colour of graft) (Fig. 20.1). The patient's pressure areas should be checked but, if the wound is to be inspected, proper sterile precautions must be observed. If possible, wounds should be left undisturbed for 48 hours after surgery to prevent contamination but the skin around the edge of the dressing should be checked for redness or blistering. The nursing staff therefore need to be warned so that the appropriate trolley is ready. Specific examinations also need to be recorded, such as bowel sounds after abdominal surgery or distal neurovascular status after orthopaedic procedures.

Regularly review nutritional status in those patients who may be in negative nitrogen balance. Deterioration can be gradual but nevertheless serious. Review all laboratory results and investigations. Review the drug chart to ensure that drugs are not being continued unnecessarily. Record all relevant findings (both negative and positive) clearly in the notes.

OBSERVATION AND PAIN ASSESSMENT

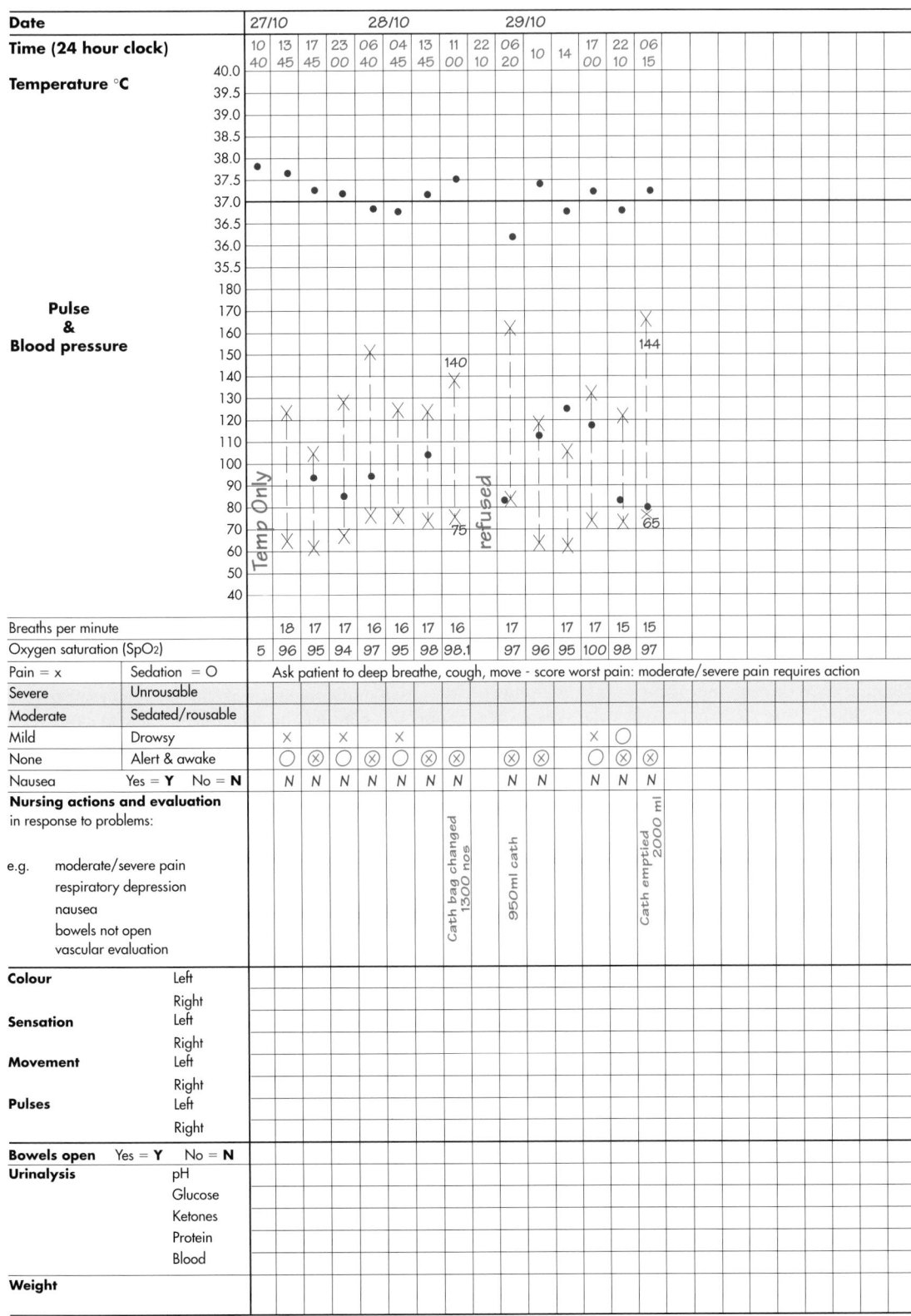

Figure 20.1 Postoperative nursing chart showing various monitoring parameters.

1996/Queen's Medical Centre/Acute Pain Service

Assessment

Review all of the information obtained under S and O and list the problems that the patient is now facing which need addressing.

Plan

Formulate and agree a plan with the patient and the staff and record that plan in the notes. This includes anticipating when discharge from hospital might occur and ensuring that everything is in place (e.g. social services) to prevent any unnecessary delay.

This is the minimum set of notes required on each patient every day. These notes should be dated, signed and legible.

Pain management

This is discussed in Chapter 14.

Fluid management

This is covered in Chapter 16.

COMPLICATIONS ASSOCIATED WITH THE INTRODUCTION OF INFUSION/ MONITORING SYSTEMS

Air embolism

This may occur when more than 15 ml of air is accidentally introduced during or after insertion of a venous catheter. The air enters the right atrium preventing adequate right heart filling and causing a drop in the blood pressure, a rise in the pulse rate and distension of the jugular venous pressure (JVP). It can be avoided by running fluids through the giving sets before connecting them to the patient. Patients should also be head-down when catheters are inserted into veins likely to be at a negative pressure (e.g. the jugular).

Phlebitis

A needle or catheter inserted into a vein will eventually result in inflammation around the area (phlebitis). The degree of phlebitis is related to not only the time of application but also the nature of the fluid being infused and the amount of bacterial contamination. Phlebitis may cause postoperative pyrexia and it is important that intravenous cannulae are regularly inspected for evidence of induration, oedema and tenderness and immediately removed if any of these signs are present. It is recommended that cannulae are marked with the date of insertion and changed at 72 hours. Cannulae that are carefully placed using full sterile precautions last longer than those which are not.

Finger necrosis

Arterial lines are usually inserted in patients who require continuous monitoring of pulse, blood pressure and arterial blood gases. They are usually inserted into the radial or femoral arteries. In some patients the blood supply to the hand arises predominantly from the radial artery, with little contribution from the ulnar artery. In these cases cannulation of the radial artery may disrupt the blood supply to the hand causing ischaemic necrosis of the fingers. In view of this it is important to check the patency of both arteries (using Allen's test) before inserting an arterial line (Summary box 20.2).

Edgar Van Nuys Allen, **1900–1961, Professor of Medicine, The Mayo Clinic, Rochester, MN, USA.**

> **Summary box 20.2**
>
> **Complications associated with monitoring systems**
> - Air embolism
> - Phlebitis
> - Finger necrosis

SPECIFIC POSTOPERATIVE COMPLICATIONS

Respiratory complications

Respiratory complications may be reduced by:

- using adequate analgesia, including epidurals, and using analgesia that depresses respiration carefully (e.g. opioids);
- administering oxygen using face masks or nasal prongs;
- arranging regular physiotherapy in patients with asthma and chronic obstructive airway disease;
- postponing surgery in patients with upper respiratory tract infections.

Shortness of breath

The commonest cause of postoperative dyspnoea (shortness of breath) and rapid shallow breathing is alveolar collapse or atelectasis. The diagnosis is confirmed by clinical examination and radiography (Fig. 20.2). Atelectasis usually responds to chest physiotherapy.

Abdominal surgical wounds may compromise respiratory function by splinting the diaphragm. Sudden onset of shortness of breath and tachypnoea (increased respiratory rate) may be caused by pulmonary embolism (Fig. 20.3), myocardial infarction/cardiac failure (Fig. 20.4), chest infection (Figs 20.5 and 20.6), pneumothorax (Fig. 20.7), acute bronchospasm or bronchopneumonia. These require immediate diagnosis and aggressive treatment.

A further cause of more gradual-onset postoperative shortness of breath is acute respiratory distress syndrome (ARDS). This may follow chest trauma, acute pancreatitis or sepsis, and results in poor oxygen transfer in the lungs even when the patient is given supplementary oxygen and is well perfused (Summary box 20.3).

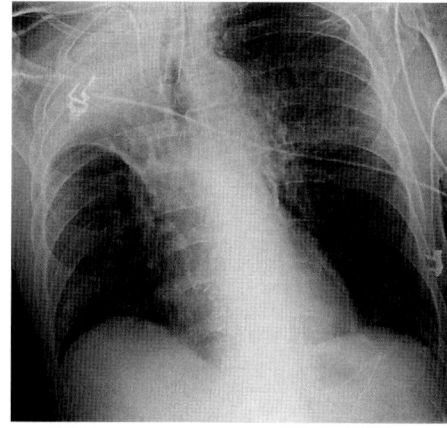

Figure 20.2 Radiograph showing right upper lobe atelectasis (courtesy of Prof. Stephen Eustace, Dublin).

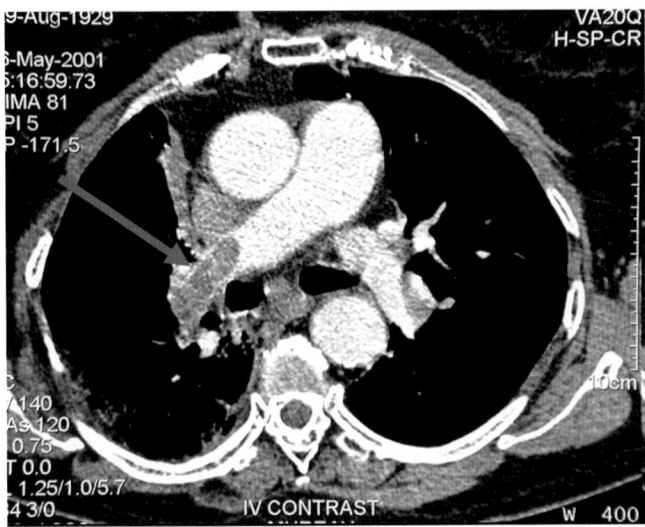

Figure 20.3 Computerised tomography (CT) scan showing pulmonary artery blood embolism (arrow) (courtesy of Prof. Stephen Eustace, Dublin).

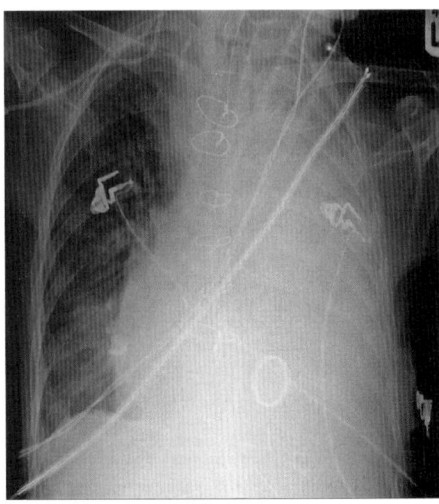

Figure 20.5 Radiograph showing lower left lobe consolidation (courtesy of Prof. Stephen Eustace, Dublin).

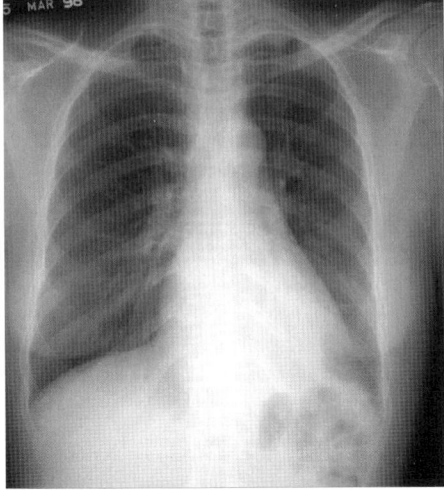

Figure 20.4 Radiograph showing a bilateral pleural effusion (courtesy of Prof. Stephen Eustace, Dublin).

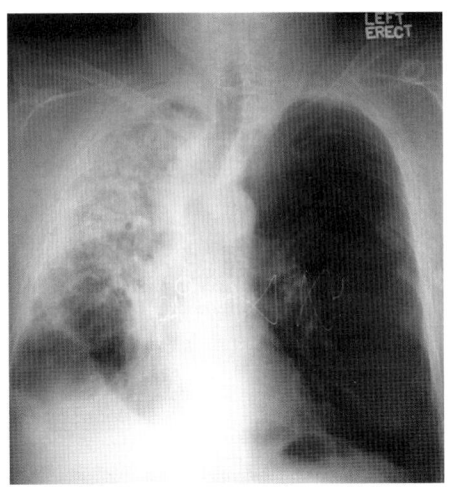

Figure 20.6 Radiograph showing classical *Staphylococcus aureus* pneumonia (courtesy of Prof. Stephen Eustace, Dublin).

Summary box 20.3

Causes of acute postoperative shortness of breath

- Myocardial infarction and heart failure
- Pulmonary embolism
- Chest infection
- Exacerbation of asthma or chronic obstructive airway disease

---

When the doctor is called to see a patient who has become short of breath, oxygen should be started immediately while taking a history and performing an examination. Intravenous access is needed and bloods should be taken for a full blood count and determination of electrolytes and cardiac enzymes, if appropriate. Arterial blood gases (ABGs) may also be needed. If chest infection is suspected the sputum should be sent for microbiology and

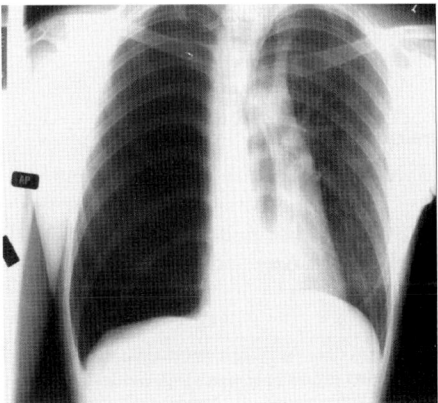

Figure 20.7 Radiograph showing a right tension pneumothorax with tracheal deviation to the left (courtesy of Prof. Stephen Eustace, Dublin).

CHAPTER 20 | POSTOPERATIVE CARE

Gram staining; blood culture and a chest radiograph may also be required and antibiotics should be given. Physiotherapy and appropriate drugs will be required if there is chronic obstructive airway disease (COAD) or asthma. An electrocardiogram will also be needed to exclude cardiac causes.

Any foreign bodies in the mouth, including dentures and vomitus, should be removed. The neck should be extended and the jaw pulled forward to allow the tongue to come forward, freeing the airway. The oral airway should be maintained and protected by an airway, e.g. Geudel's airway. In patients who have had mouth, throat or neck surgery, a cricothyroidotomy may be required or the neck wound may need to be opened up to release the haematoma causing pressure on the airway.

Cyanosis

In patients whose airway is clear but who develop cyanosis the problem may be in the lungs or in the circulation.

Common problems in the lung may be acute bronchospasm as a result of an asthmatic attack or there may be a pneumothorax detected by loss of air entry into the upper chest. Circulatory problems include sudden blood loss causing a decreased venous return, myocardial infarction or a massive pulmonary embolism.

Cardiovascular complications

Hypotension

The commonest cause of low blood pressure postoperatively is hypovolaemia, as a result of either bleeding or insufficient fluid replacement; however, a myocardial infarction may also present with hypotension, as can an overdose of analgesics, especially opioids. Specifically, epidural anaesthesia may be complicated by hypotension because of the vasodilatation of veins. Septic shock may also present in this way.

Whatever the cause of hypotension, the emergency treatment requires an increase in the fluid input with administration of high-flow oxygen. The patient should also be tilted head-down to maintain cerebral perfusion. A thorough examination should then be performed to determine the cause of the collapse (Summary box 20.4).

Summary box 20.4

Low blood pressure postoperatively

- Is the patient dehydrated?
- Has the patient had an epidural anaesthetic?
- Is the patient losing blood?
- Is the patient on too much morphine?
- Has the patient had a myocardial infarct?

Hypertension

High blood pressure may be dangerous in patients with ischaemic heart disease or cerebrovascular disease as it may precipitate infarction or stroke. Most causes of hypertension relate to inadequate pain relief or anxiety and usually settle with appropriate analgesia.

Hans Christian Joachim Gram, 1853–1938, Professor of Pharmacology, (1891–1900), and of Medicine, (1900–1923), Copenhagen, Denmark, described this method of staining bacteria in 1884.
Arthur Ernest Guedel, 1883–1956, Clinical Professor of Anesthesiology, The University of Southern California, Pasadena, CA, USA.

Deep vein thrombosis

There are several risk factors for deep vein thrombosis (DVT). Most patients with postoperative DVT show no physical signs; however, they may present with calf pain, swelling, warmth, redness and engorged veins. On palpation the muscle may be tender and there is a positive Homans' sign (calf pain on dorsiflexion of the foot); however, it must be emphasised that this sign is neither specific nor sensitive (Summary box 20.5).

Summary box 20.5

Risk factors for DVT

- Age > 60 years
- Recent surgery, particularly pelvic and lower limb surgery
- Immobilisation
- Trauma
- Oral contraceptive pill
- Obesity
- Heart failure
- Cancer
- Arteriopathy

Venography has been the standard diagnostic technique when DVT is suspected. It involves cannulation of a small vein in the foot and injection of contrast material to obtain a venogram. However, the deep veins of the lower limb may be scanned using duplex Doppler ultrasound to assess flow and thromboses. If a significant DVT is found (one that extends above the knee), treatment with intravenous heparin initially, followed by longer-term warfarin, should be started immediately. If untreated, DVT may result in chronic venous insufficiency, as a result of venous valvular damage, or pulmonary embolism, which may be fatal. In some patients with DVT, a caval filter may be required to decrease the possibility of pulmonary embolism.

Most hospitals have a DVT prophylaxis protocol. This may include the use of stockings, calf pumps and pharmacological agents such as low molecular weight heparin. No method of prophylaxis is foolproof and they all have their own complications, and so an optimal strategy needs to be developed, individualised to the patient and the operation that they are receiving (Summary boxes 6 and 7).

Summary box 20.6

Stratification of risk of DVT

Low
- Maxillofacial surgery
- Neurosurgery
- Cardiothoracic surgery

Medium
- Inguinal hernia repair
- Abdominal surgery
- Gynaecological surgery
- Urological surgery

High
- Pelvic elective and trauma surgery
- Total knee and hip replacement

John Homans, 1877–1954, Professor of Clinical Surgery, Harvard Medical School, Boston, MA, USA.
Christian Johann Doppler, 1803–1853, Professor of Experimental Physics, Vienna, Austria, enunciated the 'Doppler Principle' in 1842.

Prevention of DVT

- Early mobilisation
- Hydration
- Compression stockings
- Low molecular weight heparin as prophylaxis
- Calf pumps
- Minimise use of tourniquets

Gastrointestinal complications

Postoperative nausea and vomiting

This is a common problem and results in patient weakness and demoralisation. It may have an adverse effect on the outcome of surgery including wound dehiscence and pulmonary aspiration if the patient's airway is unprotected. Prolonged nausea and vomiting results in increased pain levels and a prolonged hospital stay. The following are predisposing factors for nausea and vomiting in postoperative patients:

- poorly controlled pain;
- use of opioids;
- surgery on the gastrointestinal tract, orthopaedic surgery or ear, nose and throat (ENT) surgery;
- female sex;
- young adult;
- history of preoperative vomiting;
- history of motion sickness or migraine;
- acute gastric dilatation.

In those patients who do not respond to antiemetics, nasogastric tubes should be inserted and the stomach should be adequately decompressed to prevent aspiration (Table 20.1).

Urinary complications

Urine output (oliguria/anuria)

Oliguria may be defined as urine output less than the minimum obligatory volume ($0.5\,\mathrm{ml\,kg^{-1}\,h^{-1}}$).

The commonest cause of oliguria postoperatively is reduced renal perfusion resulting from perioperative hypotension or inadequate fluid replacement. If untreated, acute renal failure may develop. To ensure that fluid management is adequate, daily input/output charting should be maintained. The urine output should be measured on an hourly basis after major surgery to detect early changes in renal function. The serum levels of urea and creatinine should be measured daily until the patient is fully recovered (see Chapter 17). The fluid chart must be checked daily by the medical staff and the fluid balance calculations checked, otherwise this important form of monitoring will be neglected and become unreliable. Patients who are left hypovolaemic or, hence, oliguric for any length of time will go into acute renal failure (Table 20.2).

If a postoperative patient develops a drop in the urine output it is sensible to first check whether the catheter is blocked. If hypovolaemia is suspected, a fluid challenge of 250 ml of intravenous fluid should be given over 1 hour. The urine output and JVP are then measured. If these parameters improve transiently then the patient is probably still underfilled and requires further fluid treatment. A central venous catheter may be considered to monitor intravascular volume. Once the patient has sufficient intravascular volume the urine output must be reassessed. If the urine output is still low then other causes must be sought. Sepsis needs to be aggressively treated and the opinion of critical care specialists may be sought. An abdominal ultrasound may be considered to exclude hydronephrosis resulting from blocked ureters. Nephrotoxic drugs should be stopped. If acute renal failure occurs or is imminent than the expertise of a nephrologist should be sought (Table 20.3).

Table 20.1 Treatment of postoperative nausea and vomiting

General measures	Adequate pain control
	Avoid opiates
	Keep stomach empty by aspirating (consider nasogastric tubes)
	Start oral feeding slowly
	Maintain hydration and blood pressure
	Epidural analgesia
Drugs	Dopamine receptor antagonists, e.g. prochlorperazine
	Metoclopramide
	H1 receptor antagonists, e.g. cyclizine
	5HT receptor antagonists, e.g. ondansetron

Table 20.2 Common causes of acute renal failure

Prerenal	Hypotension
	Hypovolaemia
Renal	Nephrotoxic drugs
	Gentamicin
	Steroids
	Myoglobinuria
	Sepsis
Postrenal	Ureteric injury
	Blocked urethral catheter

Table 20.3 Prevention of postoperative renal failure

Monitor renal function	Serum urea, creatinine and electrolytes
	Urine output monitoring
Assess volume status	Pulse and blood pressure
	Serial body weight
	Central venous pressure
	Pulmonary capillary wedge pressure
Optimise cardiac function	Monitor cardiac output
	Consider inotropic support
Relieve urinary obstruction	Prompt diagnosis
	Catheter drainage
	Surgical correction
Avoid nephrotoxins	Limit toxins
	Avoid aminoglycosides
	Adjust drug doses
Prevent sepsis	Catheter care
	Drain abscesses
	Give antibiotics
Consider diuretics	Mannitol and frusemide (furosemide)

CHAPTER 20 | POSTOPERATIVE CARE

Urinary retention

This is frequently seen in postoperative patients, particularly men who are bed-bound postoperatively. The inability to void after surgery is particularly common with pelvic and perineal operations or after procedures performed under spinal anaesthesia.

The causes of retention are related to the interference of neural mechanisms that are usually responsible for normal bladder emptying and over-distension of the bladder. Pain, fluid deficiency and accessibility of urinals and bed pans, as well as noisy overcrowded wards, may contribute to the problem. Retention may be confirmed by ultrasound and may require catheterisation.

Catheterisation should be performed prophylactically when an operation is expected to last 3 hours or longer or when large volumes of fluid are administered.

Urinary infection

This is the one of the most commonly acquired infections in the postoperative period. Patients who are immunocompromised or diabetic, or who have pre-existing urinary tract contamination, urinary retention or a history or presence of catheterisation, are known to be at higher risk. In those patients who are catheterised for less then 48 hours, the risk of bacteriuria is about 5%. Symptoms of urinary tract infection and cystitis include dysuria and mild pyrexia; however, pyelonephritis may cause severe flank tenderness in addition to high temperatures. Urinary tract infections should always be considered in the differential diagnosis of a patient with a temperature postoperatively. The diagnosis is confirmed by dipsticking the urine and sending samples for culture and sensitivity. Treatment involves adequate hydration and proper bladder drainage together with the use of relevant antibiotics in the light of laboratory sensitivities.

COMPLICATIONS RELATED TO SPECIFIC SURGICAL SPECIALTIES

Abdominal surgery

The abdomen should be examined daily for evidence of excessive distension, tenderness or drainage from wounds or drain sites. Patients undergoing abdominal surgery should be warned that they will have some discomfort on movement and coughing despite analgesia. Oral fluids may be reintroduced in most patients early on and there is a trend towards earlier feeding.

In certain operations, such as those for intestinal obstruction, a nasogastric tube may be used. It is useful after oesophageal and gastric procedures but of less use in lower colonic operations. It is of particular use in those patients suffering from ileus or a marked level of altered consciousness who are therefore liable to aspirate. The nasogastric tube should be allowed to drain into a small plastic bag. Free drainage may be supplemented by continuous suction.

The main complications to look out for in a postoperative abdominal surgical patient are:

- anastomotic leakage;
- bleeding or abscess;
- slow recovery of intestinal motor function (ileus).

Localised infection

An abscess may present with persistent abdominal pain, focal tenderness and a spiking fever. The patient may have prolonged ileus. If the abscess is deep-seated these symptoms may be absent. The patient will have a neutrophilic leucocytosis and may have positive blood cultures. An ultrasound or computerised tomography (CT) scan of the abdomen should identify any suspicious collection.

Paralytic ileus

Paralytic ileus may present with nausea, vomiting, refusal to eat, bowel distension and absence of flatus or bowel movements. Abdominal radiography reveals a dilated bowel.

Following laparotomy, gastrointestinal motility temporarily decreases. Treatment is usually supportive with maintenance of adequate hydration and electrolyte levels. However, intestinal complications may prolong ileus and so should be actively sought and treated whenever ileus persists. The return of function of the intestine occurs in the following order: small bowel, large bowel, stomach. This pattern allows the passage of faeces despite continuing lack of stomach emptying and, therefore, vomiting may continue even when the lower bowel has already started functioning normally.

Orthopaedic surgery

In patients having any limb surgery, including hip or knee arthroplasty, the distal neurovascular status of the limb needs to be reviewed regularly. In postoperative trauma cases, evidence of compartment syndrome should be actively sought for and treated by fasciotomy if suspected, especially if there has been significant soft-tissue injury or prolonged use of the tourniquet.

Patients with compartment syndrome complain of unremitting pain out of proportion to that expected. The pain is unrelieved by simple analgesia and requires increasing amounts of pain relief. Clinical examination reveals excessive pain on passively stretching the muscles in the affected compartment. The compartment is usually swollen and tense. In later stages there may be altered sensation. Pallor, pulselessness and paralysis are late signs. Plasters should always be split for the first 24 hours and the nurses given instructions to watch and record distal circulation every 4 hours. Check radiographs are only taken if there is a suggestion that the fracture has moved and/or when there is still time to remanipulate if necessary. If the patient has an external fixator, the pin sites should be regularly inspected for signs of infection. In patients who have undergone open reduction and internal fixation of fractures, the neurovascular status of the limb must be checked every half an hour initially by the nurses in recovery and then on the ward as dictated by the postoperative instructions. Radiographs of the limb concerned are required on a regular basis postoperatively to ensure that the fracture is healing.

Most orthopaedic procedures are carried out under tourniquet control. These are associated with ischaemia of limbs if applied for an excessive period of time. In view of this, patients who have had tourniquets applied in theatre should have the vascular supply to the limb carefully monitored in the immediate postoperative period (Summary box 20.8).

Neck surgery

Patients having neck surgery, e.g. thyroid surgery, must be observed for accumulation of blood in the wound, which may cause rapid asphyxia. A check also needs to be made pre- and postoperatively for damage to the recurrent laryngeal nerve. The findings must be recorded in the medical notes.

Thoracic surgery

Patients who have undergone a lobectomy or pneumonectomy are susceptible to fluid overload in the first 24–48 hours postoperatively. Hence, fluid intake should be restricted in such patients during this time period. Moreover, chest drains require regular review, noting whether they continue to swing, bubble or produce excess fluid. If the fluid in a chest drain swings then the drain has been inserted correctly in the pleural cavity; changes in pressure during inspiration and expiration cause the fluid to swing. If the chest drain continues to bubble then a bronchopleural fistula probably exists. A haemothorax or pleural effusion will reveal itself as a prolonged loss of blood or fluid, respectively, into the drain. Cardiac patients require continuous electrocardiography monitoring.

Neurosurgery

The intracranial pressure should be monitored closely postoperatively. A rise may be signalled by a deterioration in the state of consciousness as well as by neurological signs including pupil reflexes. Some patients may have an intracranial monitoring device to allow for more sensitive monitoring.

Vascular surgery

The patency of grafts and anastomoses in patients with femoropopliteal bypasses and abdominal aneurysmal repairs needs to be checked by regular clinical assessment of the limbs and by Doppler ultrasound.

Plastic surgery

The viability of flaps is crucial and the perfusion needs to be monitored regularly. The blood supply may be compromised by position, dressings or collection of fluids or blood beneath the flap.

Urology

Catheter patency must be ensured following urological surgery. In patients who have undergone transurethral resection of the prostate (TURP), continuous bladder irrigation may be used, and pulmonary oedema may develop if excess glycine from the irrigation fluid is absorbed into the circulation.

Diabetic patients

Whenever possible, diabetic patients should be put first on the operating list to avoid keeping them starved for longer than necessary as well as to provide adequate time for diabetic control to be stabilised during daylight hours. Diabetic patients undergoing surgery are usually commenced on a glucose–insulin infusion, and this should be continued until the patient is eating. If the patient is administered a long-acting insulin dose just before surgery or if too much insulin is given then there is the risk of hypoglycaemia. The maximum rate of infusion of insulin should rarely exceed $1.5\,U\,h^{-1}$ when using 5% dextrose. The patient should be started on an insulin sliding scale and the blood glucose level should be measured regularly. If the patient develops symptoms and signs of hypoglycaemia, the insulin infusion should be decreased and the rate of glucose infusion increased. Erratic and high glucose levels postoperatively may be caused by occult infection. Measures taken to check for, assess and treat known complications of surgery must be recorded in the medical notes. If a patient comes to harm as a result of developing a postoperative complication, the monitoring will only be assumed to be as good as what has been recorded in the notes.

GENERAL COMPLICATIONS

Fever

In total, 40% of patients develop pyrexia after major surgery; however, in 80% of cases no particular cause is found. Pyrexia does not necessarily imply sepsis. The inflammatory response to surgical trauma may manifest as temperature. In spite of this, a focus of infection must always be sought if a patient develops anything more than a slight pyrexia.

The causes of raised temperature postoperatively include:

- days 2–5: atelectasis of the lung;
- days 3–5: superficial and deep wound infection;
- day 5: chest infection including viral respiratory tract infection, urinary tract infection and thrombophlebitis;
- > 5 days: wound infection, anastomotic leakage, intracavitary collections and abscesses;
- infected intravenous cannula sites, DVTs, transfusion reactions, wound haematomas, atelectasis and drug reactions, which may also cause pyrexia of non-infective origin.

Patients with persistent pyrexia need a thorough review. Relevant investigations include full blood count, urine culture if urinary tract infection is suspected, sputum microscopy, chest radiography if indicated and blood cultures (Summary box 20.9).

Prophylaxis against infection

In patients who have had foreign material inserted operatively, including a hip or knee prosthesis in orthopaedic surgery or aortic valves in cardiovascular surgery, up to three doses of a prophylactic antibiotic should be administered, usually one dose preoperatively and two postoperatively. Bacteria can be incorporated into the biofilm that forms on the surface of the implant, where they are protected from antibiotics and from the natural defences of the body; prophylactic antibiotics appear to reduce the risk of any contamination developing into infection by destroying bacteria before they are incorporated into the biofilm.

Pressure sores

These occur as a result of friction or persisting pressure on soft tissues. They particularly affect the pressure points of a recumbent patient, including the sacrum, greater trochanter and heels. Risk factors are poor nutritional status, dehydration and lack of mobility. Those who are unconscious or who are unable to turn in bed should have their position in bed changed every 30 min to prevent pressure sores. High-risk patients may be nursed on an air filter mattress, which automatically alters the pressure areas. Early mobilisation prevents pressure sores and reduces respiratory complications (Summary box 20.10).

Summary box 20.10

Preventing pressure sores

- Address nutritional status
- Keep patients mobile or regularly turned if bed-bound

Confusional state

This develops in 10% of postoperative patients, especially elderly patients (Table 20.4). It is associated with increased morbidity and mortality as well as prolonged length of hospital stay.

Confusion may present with anxiety, incoherent speech,

Table 20.4 Causes of confusion

Renal	Renal failure/uraemia
	Hyponatraemia and electrolyte disorders
	Urinary tract infection
	Urinary retention
Respiratory	Hypoxia, e.g. chest infection
	Atelectasis
Cardiovascular	Pulmonary embolism
	Dehydration
	Septic shock
	Myocardial infarction
	Chronic heart failure
	Arrhythmia
Drugs	Opiates including heroin
	Hypnotics
	Cocaine
	Alcohol withdrawal
	Hypoglycaemia
Neurological	Epilepsy
	Encephalopathy
	Head injury
	Cerebrovascular accident
Idiopathic (rare)	Hypothyroid
	Hyperthyroidism
	Addison's disease

Thomas Addison, **1795–1860**, Physician, Guy's Hospital, London, England, described the effects of disease of the suprarenal capsules in 1849.

---

clouding of consciousness and destructive behaviour, e.g. pulling out of cannulae. Disorientation and change of environment, particularly in patients with a history of dementia, may precipitate confusion. These patients may present with sleep deprivation, anxiety, impaired thinking and memory, and disturbed emotions.

Drains

Drains are used to drain purulent collections, to prevent accumulation of blood or to indicate the possibility of leaking surgical anastomoses. In clean surgery, such as joint replacement, blood collected in drains can be transfused back into the patient provided that an adequate volume (>150 ml) is collected rapidly (<12 hours) and that a specifically designed drain and filter system is used.

The use of surgical drains has decreased in recent years as the evidence for their benefits has been questioned. They can result in complications and so should be used carefully. The complications associated with abdominal drains include:

- trauma during insertion;
- failure to drain because of incorrect placement or blockage;
- complications caused by disconnection;
- sepsis at drain sites;
- drain site metastases;
- erosion by the drain of adjacent tissue and perforation of abdominal viscera.

The quantity and character of drain fluid can be used to identify any abdominal complication resulting in fluid leakage (e.g. bile or pancreatic fluid) or bleeding. The excess loss of body fluids through the drain should be replaced by additional intravenous fluids. Blood loss through the drain should be investigated for the source. Any underlying coagulopathy should be excluded by checking the coagulation profile and platelet count. Angiography may be useful to identify the source of blood loss.

The absence of blood in the drain does not exclude heavy postoperative bleeding. If the patient's blood pressure and urine output are lower than expected the wound needs checking for a collection. Inspection, palpation and ultrasound can all help identify a developing haematoma.

Drains should be removed once the drainage has stopped or become less than 25 ml day^{-1}, as they are a potential track for contamination and infection into a wound. Drainage of bile or faecal matter indicates disruption of a biliary or intestinal anastomosis.

Nutrition

This is discussed in Chapter 17.

Blood transfusion

Most hospitals have a protocol for determining the number of units of blood that should be cross-matched before any given operation. Patients who are anaemic should have elective surgery postponed while the anaemia is investigated and, if possible, treated. During the first 24 hours after surgery, plasma or extracellular fluid loss may result in an artificially high measurement of haemoglobin. In a stable patient a top-up transfusion is indicated if the haemoglobin level falls below 8 g dl^{-1} or if the patient becomes short of breath. An unstable patient or one who may rebleed requires a higher threshold for transfusion. It is important that regular monitoring of pulse, blood pressure and temperature is carried out during transfusion to enable any transfusion reaction to be detected.

Complications of blood transfusion

Major/minor ABO incompatibility causes tachycardia, pyrexia, rash and pruritus in minor cases, and flushing, urticaria, bronchospasm and hypotension in severe reactions. The transfusion should be stopped at once if the patient develops these symptoms. A sample of the blood from the donor and recipient should be sent for culture and the remainder of the blood in the bag sent back to the transfusion department for recross-matching. In severe reactions, steroids and anti-histamines may be required.

Transmission of infection, including hepatitis, human immunodeficiency virus and Creutzfeldt–Jakob disease (CJD), and immunodeficiency in the recipient are all risks of transfusion and are increasingly becoming issues that cause a patient great anxiety (Summary box 20.11).

Summary box 20.11

Complications of blood transfusion

- Allergy
- Transmission of infection

Mobilisation

Immobilisation increases the risk of DVT, urinary retention, atelectasis, pressure sores and faecal impaction, so patients are now mobilised as soon as possible after surgery.

After a laparotomy patients are encouraged to sit out in a chair, even on the first postoperative day. This helps improve ventilation and reduces subsequent pulmonary complications by reducing the pressure on the diaphragm.

Wound care

Within hours of the wound being closed the dead space fills up with an inflammatory exudate. Within 48 hours of closure a layer of epidermal cells from the wound edge covers the bridge and hence sterile dressings applied in theatre should not be removed before this time. Wounds should be inspected only if there is any concern about their condition or the dressing needs changing. Inspection of the wound should be performed under sterile conditions. The wound may be red or discoloured with evidence of discharge, which may be serosanguinous or purulent in nature. If the wound looks inflamed, a wound swab may need to be taken and sent for Gram staining and culture. Infected wounds may need treatment with antibiotics or wound washout. This is especially important if a large haematoma is suspected that has started to drain. An infected haematoma can only be treated by returning the patient to theatre and washing out the infected material. Samples should be sent for bacteriology (before any antibiotics are given), any dead tissue excised and bleeding vessels identified and closed off. If there is any suspicion that contaminated or non-viable tissue remains then the wound should not be closed. It should be packed and then reviewed daily until it is clean, otherwise infection, especially synergistic gangrene, may develop.

Wound dressings should also be removed if they are wet as soaked dressings increase the bacterial contamination of the wound. Skin sutures or clips are usually removed between 6 and 10 days after surgery. They should remain for a shorter period when applied to the face or neck and should be left in longer where incisions go across creases, e.g. in the groin or in incisions closed under tension. If the wound is healing satisfactorily then the patient may be allowed to shower 1 week after surgery.

Wound healing is delayed in patients who are malnourished. Vitamin C deficiency interferes with collagen synthesis and vitamin A deficiency affects the rate of epithelisation. Deficiency of copper and other trace elements affects scar formation. In patients who lack these trace elements, supplements should be administered to aid healing. Steroids also inhibit the adequate healing of wounds as they inhibit the inflammatory response as well as protein synthesis and fibroblast proliferation. Diabetes, particularly if uncontrolled, also has a deleterious effect on wound healing.

Wound dehiscence

This is the partial or complete disruption of any or all of the layers in a wound. If it occurs in the abdomen it may be very distressing to the patient, causing extrusion of the bowel and other organs. Dehiscence may occur in up to 3% of abdominal wounds.

Wound dehiscence most commonly occurs from the fifth to the eight postoperative day when the strength of the wound is at its weakest. It most commonly occurs in abdominal wounds where it may herald an underlying intra-abdominal abscess. However, it may also occur in thoracotomy wounds, in particular sternal wounds.

Wound dehiscence usually presents with a serosanguinous discharge. The patient may have felt a popping sensation during straining or coughing. Most patients will need to return to the operating theatre for resuturing. In some patients it may be appropriate to leave the wound open and treat with dressings or vacuum-assisted closure (VAC) pumps (Summary box 20.12).

Summary box 20.12

Risk factors in wound dehiscence

General
- Malnourishment
- Diabetes
- Obesity
- Renal failure
- Jaundice
- Sepsis
- Cancer
- Patients on steroids

Local
- Inadequate or poor closure of wound
- Poor local wound healing, e.g. because of infection, haematoma or seroma
- Increased intra-abdominal pressure, e.g. in postoperative patients suffering from chronic obstructive airway disease, during excessive coughing

---

DISCHARGE OF PATIENTS

Following treatment in hospital patients are discharged home where they will continue to recover. Postoperative orthopaedic patients may be transferred to a rehabilitation centre where adequate supervision can be given and there is access to physiotherapy. Patients discharged home need a discharge letter detailing the postoperative plan for the patient. The 'immediate' discharge letter should leave the hospital with the patient. This is usually completed by the house surgeon and details the final diagnosis, the treatment and any complications that may have occurred. There should be advice for referring the patient back to hospital and indications for readmission if specific problems do occur. The GP should be informed of the subsequent care plan including follow-up arrangements. The formal discharge letter should be dictated as soon as possible after the discharge of the patient. It should detail preoperative findings, their management (operative or non-operative) and subsequent complications. Pathology results should be included if available and the basis of these in the subsequent care plan should be described along with the prognosis if appropriate.

Follow-up in clinic

Patients should only be reviewed in clinic when a key decision on management needs to be made. The findings and the care plan agreed with the patient at the clinic appointment should be included in a letter to the patient's GP as well as in a clear handwritten entry in the notes. This should include advice on how to recognise the onset of complications and what to do if there is concern. Patients should be discharged from clinic as soon as their GPs or they themselves can manage their care.

Day-case and fast-track surgery

There is a strong drive to do more surgery on a day-surgery basis; however, before patients are discharged home a check must be made that they are safe and that the discharge is appropriate to their best interests. Appropriate pain relief must be given and the patient must be able to call or return to a predetermined place if complications or problems occur.

Fast-track surgery or enhanced recovery after surgery (ERAS) is a multimodal comprehensive programme aimed at enhancing postoperative recovery and outcome. It has been pioneered in abdominal surgery but plans are being made to introduce the protocol into other specialties. The planned discharge after 48 hours in patients undertaking even major surgery has demonstrated a reduction in potential complications and enhanced recovery. The main thrust is to reduce the psychological and physiological stresses associated with operations, hence reducing tissue catabolism and organ dysfunction. Published evidence confirms the benefits of fast-track surgery including reduced hospitalisation, lower morbidity, cost-effectiveness, patient satisfaction and safety, and a low readmission rate. The concept encompasses the essence of optimum postoperative care including preoperative patient education, improved anaesthesia and use of epidural analgesia, adoption of modern surgical principles, optimised dynamic pain relief, early ambulation and early oral nutritional supplementation.

FURTHER READING

Burkitt, G., Quick, C. and Gatt, D. (1995) *Essential Surgery*, 2nd edn. Churchill Livingstone, UK.

Cuschieri, A. and Grace, P.A. (2003) *Clinical Surgery*. Blackwell, Oxford.

Ellis, H., Calne, R. and Watson, C.J.E. (1998) *Lecture Notes on General Surgery*, 9th edn. Blackwell, Oxford.

Forrest, A.P.M. and Carter, D.C. (1990) *Principles and Practice of Surgery*, 3rd edn. Churchill Livingstone, Edinburgh.

Grace, P.A. and Borley, N. (2006) *Surgery at a Glance*. Blackwell, Oxford.

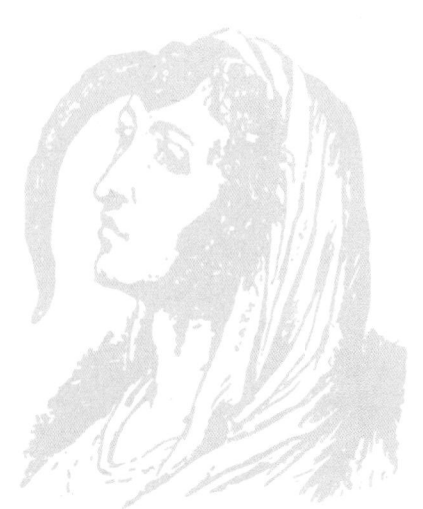

Introduction to trauma

LEARNING OBJECTIVES

To gain an understanding of:
- The importance of time in trauma management
- How to assess a trauma problem
- How to respond to a trauma problem
- The value of planning

WHAT IS TRAUMA?

Trauma is the study of medical problems associated with physical injury. The injury is the adverse effect of a physical force upon a person. There are a variety of forces that can lead to injury, including thermal, ionising radiation and chemical; these are discussed in Chapter 28. However, the force involved in most injuries is mechanical. The subject of trauma therefore centres upon the deleterious effects of kinetic energy on the human frame. In the next group of chapters we will explore trauma from a variety of perspectives related to different specialities. In this introduction we will look at the aspects that bind the whole topic together.

THE SCALE OF THE PROBLEM

Trauma is recognised as a serious public health problem. In fact, it is the leading cause of death and disability in the first four decades of life and is the third most common cause of death overall.

Millions of people are killed or disabled by injury each year. Of the 5 million people killed as a result of injuries in 2000, approximately 1.2 million people died of road traffic injuries, 815 000 from suicide and 520 000 from homicides. In the UK the accidental and deliberate injury standardised death rate (SDR) is 27.28 deaths of all ages per 100 000 inhabitants per year. Hundreds of thousands who survive their injuries experience long-term or permanent disabilities, time lost from work or family responsibilities, costly medical expenses, profound change in lifestyle, pain and suffering, regardless of gender, race or economic status. An injury affects more than just the injured person; it affects everyone who is involved in the injured person's life. The consequences of the modern chimaera of the motor vehicle accident (MVA) added to the global epidemic of violence can not be overstated.

Trauma is not just related to high-energy transfer in road accidents or violence. The elderly fall victim makes up the most common group to be admitted to hospital following injury in the UK. Fragility fractures represent an increasing load on health services. About 50 000 patients suffer a proximal femoral fracture each year in the UK, which is about 10 times the number of poly-trauma victims. About 30% of those over the age of 65 who suffer a proximal femoral fracture will die within a year of the incident, and most of the others will have diminished independence and mobility. It can be appreciated that this represents a huge burden on the health services and society in general.

The great majority of injuries are not life- or limb-threatening. Here the challenge is not only to treat the minor injuries but also to differentiate between those injuries that have some important aspects and those that are genuinely straightforward. For instance, in children, one must always be alert to the potential for non-accidental injury (NAI). There is a chilling statistic that in 66% of cases when children die as the result of abuse there has been some previous relevant contact with a health professional or social services. Again in children we also have to be alert to those injuries that represent a threat to future growth, thus having an effect disproportionate to their initial appearance. In all age groups we need to be wary of pathological fractures; here the more important problem may not be the injury itself but the underlying disease process (Summary box 21.1).

Summary box 21.1

Trauma: the scale of the problem

- Trauma is the major cause of death in the young
- Fragility fractures are an increasing burden
- Look beyond the obvious in trauma management

THE IMPORTANCE OF TIME

An identifying feature in the study of trauma is time. At time zero the person/patient is at their normal baseline. There is then some interaction with an external force leading to injury. The subsequent development of pathology, the response of the body by way of compensation and healing, and the external responses by health professionals all have a timeline; that timeline originates at time zero, the moment of injury. The timeline may be used to compare and consider the progress from time zero to other significant events or deadlines that follow.

Figure 21.1 depicts an estimate of the periods of time that may elapse from time zero to death or irretrievable damage for various injuries. It reflects the fact that some problems tend to lead to earlier death than others. An obstructed airway, a tension pneumothorax, an extradural haematoma or an ischaemic limb will all tend to progress along a characteristic time-line after the moment of initial injury. This creates an 'imperative of time' that shapes and provides a basis for the hierarchy of our initial medical response to the injured patient. Thus, an obstructed airway will need emergency initial management at the scene of the accident. An ischaemic limb may be dealt with urgently once the patient has reached a definitive treatment centre. The order ABCD, that is *airway*, *breathing*, *circulation* and *disability* (neurology), of the ATLS (Advanced Trauma Life Support) system is founded upon this time dependence.

To the raw diagram of the time from injury to death or irretrievable damage may be added other components. These are the time to understand or assess the nature of the problem and the time to respond effectively to that which has been discovered. Each of these will take a finite length of time and this is shown schematically for a generic condition in Fig. 21.2. It can be seen that in this example there is adequate time for an orderly process of all the stages of assessment followed by a response before irretrievable damage or death.

The block of time for assessment may be broken down further. Understanding and assessing the nature of the problem usually hinges on diagnosing the injury. An injury may be discoverable by special investigation or careful physical examination, or be very

obvious at different points on its timeline. An example is an evolving extradural haematoma: the initial skull fracture may be visible on radiography or computerised tomography (CT); as the haematoma develops it will first be visible on CT; later, it will be suspected on careful clinical examination; and, finally, it will become clinically very obvious. This is represented in Fig. 21.3a.

The next feature to add to the timeline is the response time. Once an obstructed airway is identified the response time to carry out a life-saving simple airway manoeuvre may be a matter of seconds. Thus, even at the stage when the diagnosis is clinically obvious there may still be time to resolve the problem before irretrievable damage occurs. However, when the diagnosis is an extradural haemorrhage, the average response time from identification of the problem to surgical resolution may be measured in hours. This may seem an unduly long time, but bringing the patient to an operating theatre with a neurosurgeon takes time to arrange as seen in Fig. 21.3b. If we now combine the various features of a timeline for the single condition of extradural haematoma, difficulties become apparent. In Fig. 21.3c it is seen that if the response is only initiated once the diagnosis is very obvious there may be insufficient time left to resolve the problem before death. This seems to suggest that we need to initiate a response to a problem before we are sure of its existence. This apparent paradox will be explored further. However, for the moment it can be likened to the need to identify a cancer at an early stage to give the best chance of successful treatment. A common approach to such a problem is to screen the at-risk population, and the same principle applies in trauma.

As we will see, much of the medical preparation and planning related to trauma is aimed at reducing the diagnosis time and the response time so that they will fit into the time available before death or irretrievable damage. To revise the meanings of these terms, the diagnosis time is the time between injury and recognition of the problem and the response time is the time that elapses between identifying the problem and the intervention required to deal with it being completed. We can reduce these times by using a practised approach to the initial stages of the

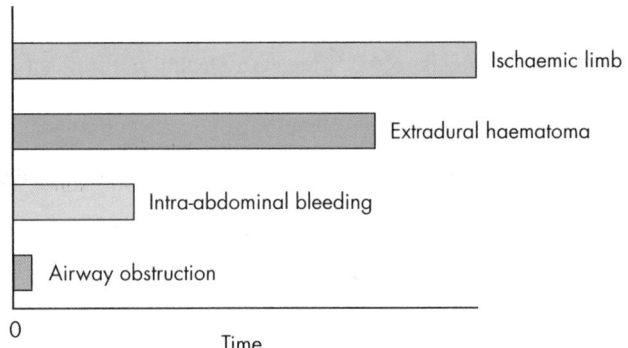

Figure 21.1 Estimated time from incident to death or irretrievable damage for various conditions.

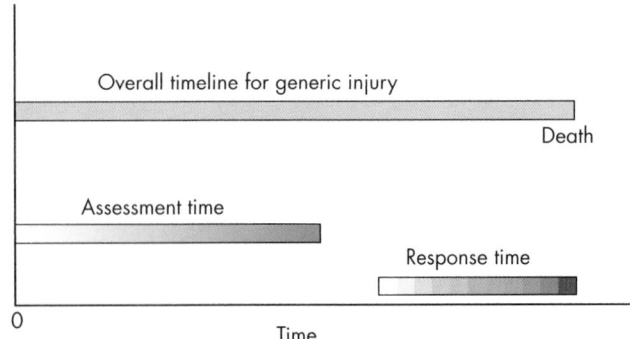

Figure 21.2 Diagrammatic representation of the relationship between assessment and response times. In this example there is time to assess and respond effectively before death.

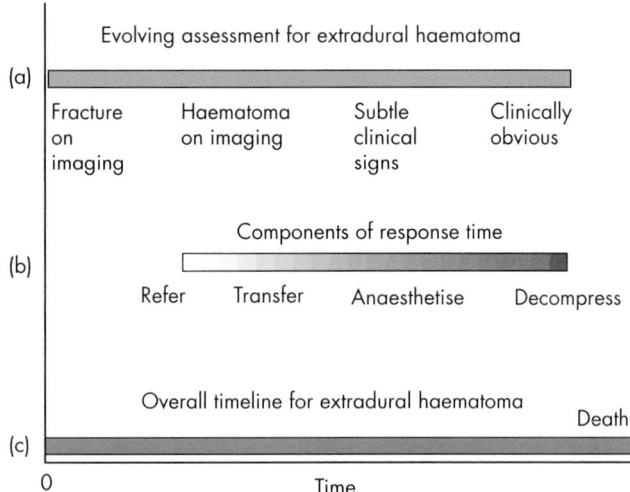

Figure 21.3 Diagrammatic representation of the relationship between assessment and response times for extradural haematoma. (a) The stages of assessment, (b) the components of the response, and (c) the overall time from incident to death. It can be seen that relying on obvious clinical signs gives insufficient time to respond effectively.

management of a polytrauma patient. This does not absolve us from thinking but it does mean that we can have a pre-existing structure upon which to build. This allows us to move forward more rapidly. This structured initial approach allows for more straightforward teamwork and standardisation of the equipment required. This practised familiarity brings confidence to a difficult situation.

The pressure of time determines the manner in which we deal with the multiply injured patient. The normal sequence of history, examination, provisional diagnosis, special investigations, diagnosis and management plan is not appropriate. When dealing with the multiply injured a quite different approach is needed. As will be seen, the primary survey used in ATLS combines the identification of life-threatening problems with their management. It has evolved to improve the chances of the necessary actions being taken within the available time to save life and limb. The system has to allow diagnosis and response within the timeline for the injuries sustained.

The model of a timeline need not be restricted to the multiply injured. The role of time when dealing with an elderly person who has been injured is still present but is frequently ignored. There may be hidden urgent issues. Thus, when dealing with the elderly we too readily label a patient with the most obvious problem (such as a hip fracture) without performing the vital initial physiological triage. They may have a primary cardiac, respiratory or neurological problem that has resulted in a fall and the response to this may be the most urgent issue. Therefore, the timeline is not only relevant to the acute and obviously urgent clinical issues. As noted at the beginning of this chapter a timeline may be used to compare and consider the progress from time zero to other significant events or deadlines that follow. The response time to arrange a discharge from hospital for the elderly patient may be protracted. Figure 21.4 demonstrates that, with such a long response time, to allow for discharge at the appropriate clinical time the social planning needs to commence almost at the time of admission. This is well before it would seem clinically reasonable but to achieve an efficient system it is quite necessary. This approach allows an emergency unit to get as close as is possible to the practice of effective elective units where discharge plans are made before the patient is admitted.

Time also plays a part in how we deal with more minor injuries. There is a need and expectation that these patients will be dealt with rapidly; however, there is then a danger, especially with inexperienced doctors, that corners will be cut and key problems missed. Focusing on the important issues without risking missing problems is a difficult skill. However, the risks can be reduced. Although not all patients will be seen by more than one doctor, another health professional, usually a nurse, will see them and their insights should not be ignored. A common safety net for the front-line medical staff is that all radiographs of patients discharged are independently reviewed by a radiologist. Should their findings differ from those in the clinical record the patient can be recalled and reassessed.

Timelines reveal that things change. As a consequence, reassessment can be of vital importance. An observation, a radiograph or a blood test are only snapshots in time. Repeated observation will reveal trends that may make a diagnosis more straightforward. Modern monitoring allows this continuing vigilance to be carried out more straightforwardly. Graphical recording of results in a single place makes trends easier to follow.

Although the pressure and relevance of time shapes our response to the injured it should not be allowed to degrade it (Summary box 21.2).

> **Summary box 21.2**
>
> **The importance of time**
>
> - Time pressure shapes our management of trauma
> - There is a finite time to assess
> - There is a finite time to respond
> - For success these must fit into the available time before irretrievable damage or death

ASSESSMENT AND RESPONSE

The breakdown of our approach to the injured into two components of assessment and response has been introduced. Although the two concepts overlap and intertwine it is helpful to explore them separately.

The assessment of trauma

At time zero, a person in their baseline condition comes together with an external force to produce injury. Understanding this relationship between the patient, the mechanism of injury and the injury produced is the key to understanding the problem that has to be solved. It is helpful both when making a diagnosis and a treatment plan for an individual and also for structuring the thinking of the management of trauma in general. The relationship can be expressed simply as: *mechanism + patient = injury*.

The initial nature of these variables may be quite obvious (overt) or hidden (covert). As clinicians we need to convert everything to the overt so that appropriate clinical responses can be made. We can only treat what we have found; we can only resolve the problems that we have identified.

A tidy relationship between the mechanism, the patient and the resulting injury is often obvious. Thus, a previously healthy 40-year-old man falling vertically 2 metres and landing on his feet may sustain an os calcis fracture. From this position of understanding we can move swiftly forward to investigate and treat.

In cases in which the mechanism is not known reliably the

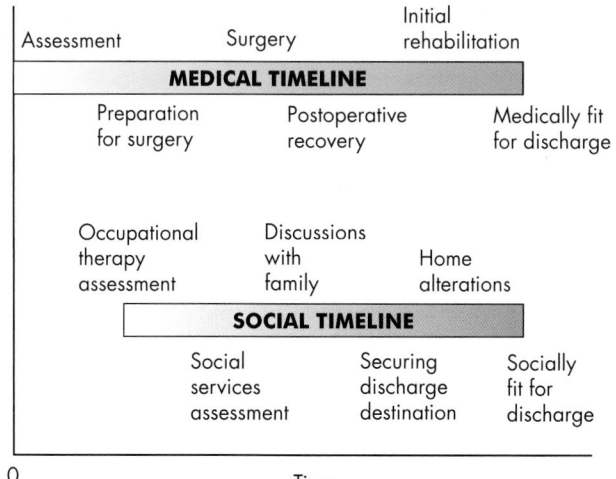

Figure 21.4 Social and medical timelines for an elderly patient with a proximal femoral fracture. Discharge can only occur when both are complete.

other variables may be clearer and the equation can be rewritten as: *injury − patient = mechanism*. So, if we can see an obvious injury and we know that the patient was previously fit and well we may well be able to work out the likely mechanism of injury. This approach can be useful when assessing the unconscious patient. By using a presumptive mechanism of injury deduced from obvious clinical findings we can begin to search for covert injuries. For example, when an obtunded patient is brought in from a car crash and has facial and chest injuries, we can deduce that the impact was head-on and that we need to check particularly carefully for other injuries associated with such a mechanism, such as to the feet (around the pedals) and the knees (dashboard injuries). Thus, the real value of an equation is not in describing or demonstrating the overt or obvious but rather guiding the search for the covert or hidden.

On some occasions the equation appears not to apply at first sight and can be expressed as: *mechanism + patient ≠ injury*. This failure of the relationship is not real but apparent. If the three variables do not fit together something has probably been misjudged, and the factor that is causing the failure of the clinical picture to 'add up' must be sought. It may be that some aspect of the injury has not yet been discovered, the mechanism suggested may not be genuine or there may be some aspect of the patient before the injury of which one is unaware. To expand on this theme we will explore overt and covert examples of each of the variables in the equation (Summary box 21.3).

Overt mechanisms

Overt mechanisms of injury are the most common. The patient presents with a history that includes a mechanism. The broad groups of mechanisms described are blunt, penetrating, thermal and blast. We will concentrate on the first two groups as in civilian practice these are the most frequent. Usually the distinction between blunt and penetrating is quite clear, but even at this simple level some injuries with wounds are poorly served by this terminology. In orthopaedic trauma the distinction is best made by use of the terms open and closed. An open tibial fracture caused by a gunshot is accepted as a penetrating wound, whereas an open tibial fracture following a tackle at football would generally be considered as a blunt trauma with an open wound. Many penetrating injuries involve the use of weapons, whereas many blunt injuries are the result of acceleration/deceleration such as falls or road accidents. Although the precision in the use of words is helpful it is more important to understand the principles involved. In these circumstances it is important to understand the patterns of injury that may be associated with a particular mechanism and that when the skin is breached infection is more likely.

Penetrating mechanisms

The easiest of these to understand is the incision caused by a knife. We are used to knives both at home when we eat and as surgeons when we operate. A knife has a sharp edge that may cut tissues with which it makes contact; these effects are easily appreciated because they happen in a timescale that we understand. A knife damages only what it can reach. A good history of the length of blade coupled with an entry point allows for a potential pattern of injury to be imagined and then individual components to be confirmed or excluded by examination, special investigation or wound exploration.

Thus, an incisional injury over an extremity is readily evaluated as long as the relevant anatomy is known. The distal perfusion, peripheral nerve function and tendon and muscle function can all be assessed by clinical examination. Should penetration of a joint be suspected then the problem is different. This is an example of a situation in which understanding the timeline is of value. The consequences of a septic arthritis are severe and if treatment is delayed until the condition is clinically obvious then it may be too late to remedy. Therefore the diagnosis of joint penetration needs to be excluded by screening the at-risk group. This exclusion can be achieved by exploration and washing out of the at-risk joint, which will normally require operating theatre time and an anaesthetic. If a large joint is involved, for example the knee, an algorithm such as that in Fig. 21.5 can help identify those joints that need formal exploration. One component of this algorithm is to fill the joint until tense with sterile saline and watch whether fluid leaks through the traumatic wound. This will indicate whether the joint has been penetrated. If the joint has been breached a formal procedure in an operating theatre is required, but this is now therapeutic and not exploratory. It is a sound general principle that operating theatre time should be for therapy and not diagnosis whenever possible.

In assessing the effects of an incisional mechanism over the torso the first step is again to decide which structures are at risk. This may seem simple but it is not always easy to determine the direction that a blade has entered. The anatomy can also be confusing; it is worth recalling that the abdominal contents extend

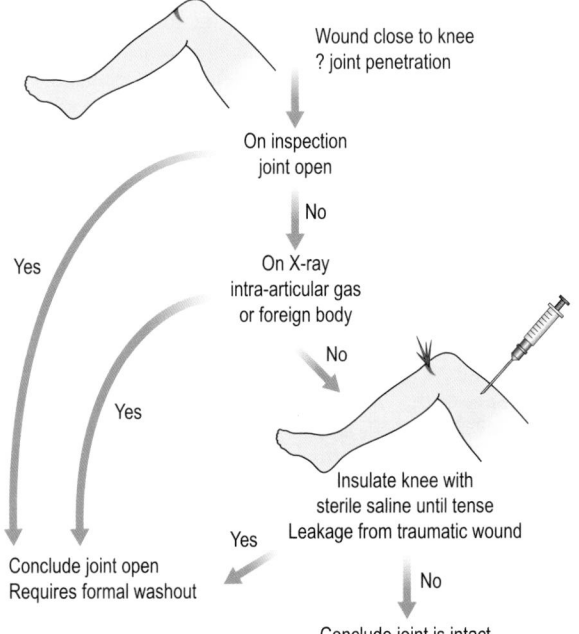

Figure 21.5 Algorithm for assessing a wound that has potentially entered a joint.

higher than normally expected, up to the level of the fifth rib in expiration. A notable feature of stab injuries is that they are often eminently treatable; even cardiac injuries can be treated with a realistic chance of success if identified early (Summary box 21.4).

Summary box 21.4

Incisional injuries

- Require knowledge of anatomy
- The abdominal contents extend high into the chest
- Even cardiac injuries are treatable if recognised early and treated quickly

---

Penetrating injuries caused by firearms are not so intuitively understood as incisional injuries. A low-velocity projectile behaves more or less like a stabbing injury. However, as the velocity increases, the energy increases in line with $E = \frac{1}{2}mv^2$; as the amount of energy increases, the ability of the system to dissipate that introduced energy in a simple way is overcome. In the case of high-velocity projectiles the result is not like anything we are familiar with in day-to-day life. Furthermore, these projectiles are deliberately designed to produce particular results: some are designed to kill whereas others are designed to maim but not kill. In a military conflict it is more disabling and demoralising to your opponent's forces if individuals do not die but consume resources in their treatment and protection.

The high-velocity bullet crushes particles of the human body in its pathway and produces lateral acceleration away from the point of impact. This motion of the tissue particles away from their original position produces a cavity. Two types of cavity are produced: (1) permanent cavity – one that remains after the initial impact; (2) temporary cavity – one that lasts for milliseconds, and may no longer be apparent during the physical examination of the wounded. This temporary cavitation can extend well beyond the boundaries of the apparent injury (Fig. 21.6). High-speed photography shows the dramatic nature of the temporary deformation, which happens on a timescale with which we are not generally familiar. Awareness of this phenomenon will lead the treating surgeon to perform an adequate exploration and, if appropriate, a more radical wound excision than would otherwise be used (Summary box 21.5).

Summary box 21.5

Firearm injuries

- Low-velocity bullets behave like knife injuries
- High-velocity bullets cause cavitation
- The temporary cavity is large and draws in foreign materials
- The permanent cavity is smaller and gives no clue to the extent of damage

---

Blunt mechanisms

The blunt mechanism can be considered as direct or indirect. A direct mechanism is when the damage occurs at or close to the site of impact. An indirect mechanism is when the damage occurs at a distant site after transmission of that force. The following examples, in which two different mechanisms leading to fracture of the ulna are considered, may help to understand this. Should an

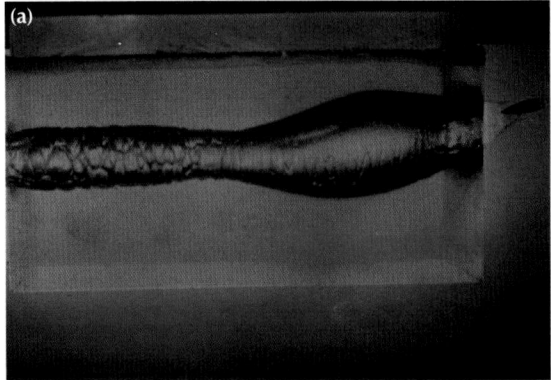

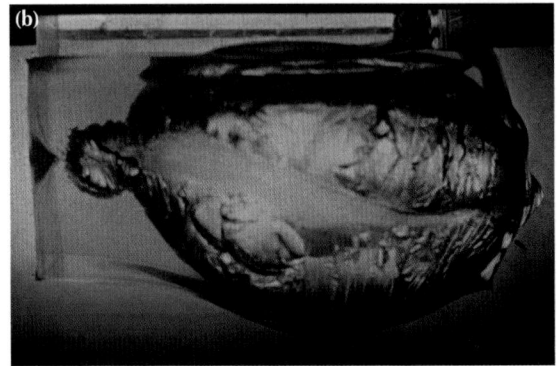

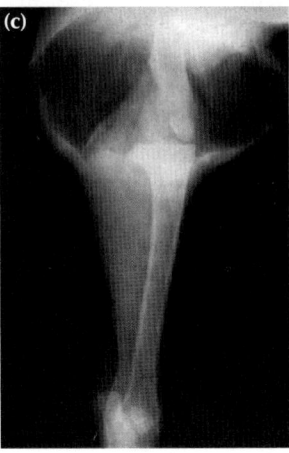

Figure 21.6 (a) and (b) show a projectile passing through a gelatin block. In (a) there is low energy transfer and in (b) there is high energy transfer. (c) Shows the effect of high energy transfer on tissues. Photo courtesy of Prof J Ryan.

attacker strike with a strong stick the victim may protect their head by raising their arm. The blow will then fall on the ulna. This may cause an isolated fracture of that bone generally called a 'nightstick fracture' (a nightstick being a weapon of enforcement carried by the police). This is clearly a direct injury. All of the injury is concentrated at the site of application of the force; the soft tissues may be bruised, contused or lacerated at the site. A different situation occurs if a person falls on an outstretched hand. This may lead to a fracture of the ulna but here the mechanism is indirect. The force has been transmitted through the body's tissues to a site at some distance from its application. It is unlikely that an ulnar fracture would occur in isolation in such circumstances and the 'associated injuries' should be sought. In this instance, the associated injury is often a dislocation of the radial head, the whole injury complex being called a Monteggia fracture dislocation. These injuries are demonstrated diagrammatically in Fig. 21.7. The injury is often missed and the consequences are severe in the growing child. Thus, we should always evaluate the elbow fully (radiologically and clinically) in an apparently 'isolated' ulnar fracture, especially if the mechanism was indirect, usually a fall onto the hand. The timeline in these circumstances is not pressing. The injury can be adequately treated for some weeks after it occurs, but once the diagnosis has been missed and the wrong label applied it becomes progressively more difficult to rectify.

An analogous situation occurs in the paired bones of the lower leg. A footballer may fracture the shaft of the fibula as the result of a direct blow; however, the fracture may be the consequence of an indirect twisting injury at the ankle. The direct injury is often a trivial injury requiring little or no treatment. The indirectly sustained high fibular fracture associated with an ankle injury is often quite unstable and requires operative treatment. A useful history of the mechanism is often very difficult to obtain in such circumstances. However, the history immediately after the injury may be helpful: a player who can continue to play or walk demonstrates some stability, whereas the person who cannot weight bear at all may have instability. Once again, as with the ulnar fracture, the associated injuries should be sought by clinical (tenderness away from the site of the obvious injury suggesting an indirect mechanism) and radiological assessment. Figure 21.8 shows how inferred instability of the ankle in an indirect injury is demonstrated by stress views taken under anaesthesia. This is another example of screening the at-risk population so that an appropriate treatment response can be made. If the initial opportunity of diagnosis is missed the condition may become clinically apparent only once united in a poor position and it is then difficult to resolve.

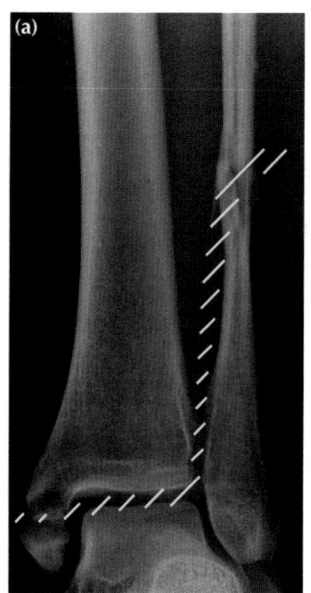
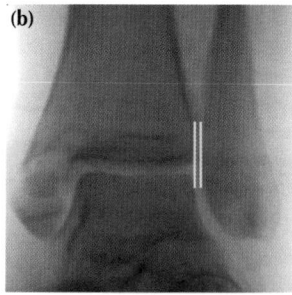
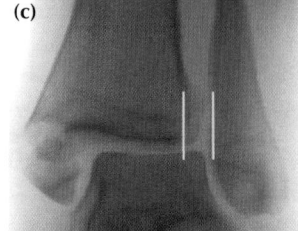

Figure 21.8 Ankle fracture. (a) The potential line of injury is shown by the hatching. (b) Neutral view under anaesthesia. (c) The instability is confirmed by the stress view, which shows the opening of the inferior tibiofibular syndesmosis.

The energy transmission in an indirect mechanism may be via a solid structure such as a bone, as in the examples above, or it may be via the soft tissues or fluid. Some of the resulting injuries can be quite unexpected. A compressive force to the abdomen will cause a rise in pressure that may be transmitted by the vascular system. A sudden back pressure at the heart can lead to damage to the valves. The results of direct mechanisms are easier to understand as the damaging effects are often more localised.

Even when the patient was alert before and after the event, it can be surprisingly difficult to be sure of the mechanism as it affected the injured part. The rapidity and unexpectedness of accidents means that precision in history is often hard to obtain.

Overt patients

The nature of some patients as a substrate for injury is obvious. Individuals with different physical characteristics will respond differently to mechanical insult. In the standard history taken, a quick categorisation of a patient is normally carried out.

As we take a history we intuitively group patients to assess the nature of their likely injuries. Children, adults and the elderly are three obvious separate groups. We anticipate different injuries in these different groups even if the mechanism is the same. For instance, if three people – a child, a young adult and an elderly person – fall together on an icy path, what might happen to them? The child will bounce, get up and do it again because it was fun. The adult will sprain or break their wrist. The elderly person breaks their hip.

Why the differences? With a low centre of gravity and less mass the child will have much less energy to dissipate in a simple fall. Their tissues are generally strong and more elastic and so do not break with trivial injury. Minor injuries in children are very common because they do a lot of silly things. However, there are times when their physical structure makes them vulnerable. As is discussed in Chapter 27, the growth plate of a bone can be a point

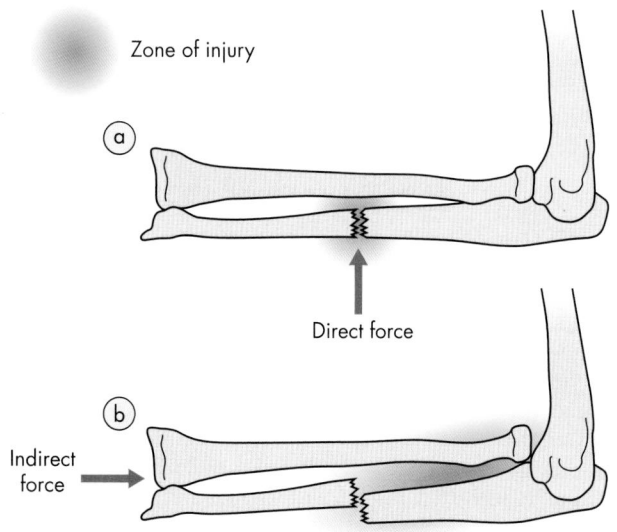

Figure 21.7 Two examples of a fracture of the ulna. (a) A nightstick fracture from a direct blow. (b) A Monteggia fracture from an indirect force.

Giovanni Battista Monteggia, **1762–1815, Professor of Anatomy and Surgery, Ospedale Maggiore, Milan Italy.**

of relative weakness, particularly as the child approaches puberty.

The adult reacts quickly to the fall and so is able to dissipate energy using the hand and arm as a shock absorber. This may prevent injury but should this protective mechanism be overwhelmed a wrist injury may result.

The elderly person does not react as rapidly and so they fall further before their deceleration mechanisms come into play. They have more energy to dissipate and yet their tissues are less able to cope. They are therefore more vulnerable to a serious fracture.

Overt injuries

Some injuries are so obvious that they may present before any mechanism or patient details are known. It may therefore be the presence of one overt injury that leads to the search for another; the obvious injury is being used just as a history would in other circumstances. The most obvious injuries will be those that are visible externally. It is for this reason that there is an E at the end of ABCDE in the ATLS system: E is for *exposure* – look for the clues.

A wound suggests a penetrating injury and thought should be given to the underlying structures at risk. A contusion over the knee of a driver suggests a dashboard injury. Finger-shaped bruises on a child's arms suggest NAI.

A good example of a minor but obvious injury helping in a timeline is singed facial hair. Singed facial hair often associated with carbonaceous sputum suggests inhalational burns. Calling an anaesthetic colleague when singed nasal hair is first noted is far better than a crash call 15 min later when laryngeal oedema obstructs the airway of a patient with an inhalational burn.

Exposing the patient comes readily to those dealing with trauma. The perils of not exposing the patient were demonstrated in an infamous case in the UK. A patient already in hospital for another problem had 'collapsed' by the phone within the hospital and was dealt with by the cardiac arrest team. The patient responded poorly to treatment and it was only some time later that the bullet on their chest radiograph was noticed. Following this the bullet wound on their back was found. A helpful adage borrowed from radiology is that 'unless you are very lucky you only find what you look for'.

Covert mechanisms

Sometimes, when the normal relationship of *mechanism + patient = injury* does not seem to hold, the hidden information may be in the mechanism. The most obvious examples are in situations in which there has been a deliberate attempt to mislead.

Conscious sensible patients reporting their own injuries will generally tell the truth; however, sometimes to protect themselves or others they may fabricate a mechanism. The risk here is that if the mechanism is incorrect the wrong pattern of injuries may be anticipated. Potentially this could lead to an important injury being overlooked or diagnosed late. Thus, the man who fell from 6 metres when jumping from his lover's window does not help achieve an accurate diagnosis if he reports the mechanism as a twist to his ankle from a stumble. Similarly, if it is not admitted that an injury results from an assault then no action can reasonably be taken to help protect that person from further aggression. This situation is most commonly encountered when the patient is the victim of abuse within a relationship. The patient should be given the opportunity to tell their story, but it should not always be believed.

More commonly, the problem of a hidden mechanism arises when the patient is unable to give their own history. A very young child or an elderly person is both physically and mentally vulnerable. They may have been physically abused but be unable to report it. In these circumstances the mechanism of injury may have been criminal. A list of some of the factors that should make one suspicious of the history and suspect that NAI has occurred is given below:

- history clearly inconsistent with the injuries sustained;
- changing history;
- aggressive behaviour of carers at interview;
- injuries of different ages;
- posterior rib injuries;
- long bone fractures in a pre-ambulatory child.

The interests of the patient are paramount and so we need to not only identify injuries that need treatment but also protect patients from further harm. The timeline of importance here is that which has shown that 66% of children who die as the result of abuse have been in contact with a health or social work professional before the fatal episode. We have already accepted that to adequately treat an extradural haematoma we must respond to subtle indicators in the history and physical examination to allow our response to begin early enough to be effective. An analogous situation applies with child abuse – if we ignore the early signs we may be too late to prevent the later episode in which real harm is done. NAI is a very difficult problem to deal with. As clinicians we are more comfortable trying to help everyone; acting to police a situation does not come naturally. The simple early response is to admit the at-risk person on clinical grounds. This allows time for a considered response. Who provides this will depend on the situation where we work.

In some criminal situations the nature of any overt injuries may provide important evidence of the mechanism. Such evidence may be affected by our medical assessment and treatment. Although we should not compromise the medical management of an injured person, it is folly not to bear in mind at every stage that the victim of an assault may need good forensic evidence at some later date to convict their assailant. Indeed, the injured victim of an assault may later become a murder victim (Summary box 21.6).

Summary box 21.6

Covert mechanisms

- Patients usually tell the truth but may not if criminal activity is involved
- Fear of abuse may prevent vulnerable patients telling the truth
- If NAI is suspected you have a responsibility to take action
- Patients likely to have covert medical problems need careful checking even if their injury appears to have a simple mechanical cause

---

Covert patients

When the mechanism and the injury are obvious but inconsistent, it may be that there is something previously unknown about the patient to discover. Most commonly this is a pre-existing pathology. Thus, a healthy adult who breaks their femur following a trivial insult may well have had a pathological weakness of the bone, such as a neoplasm. Thoughtless treatment of this as a simple fracture, without tissue diagnosis, staging, etc., may result in entirely inappropriate treatment with unnecessary loss of limb or life.

Injury in the older patient may be the manifestation of general health problems. Falls in the elderly can be divided into those caused by mechanical factors and those caused by medical problems. The division into these two categories is difficult in practice. However, it is true to say that, although the obvious injury may be the fractured proximal femur, the hidden patient factor may be the transient ischaemic attack or abnormal cardiac rhythm that caused the fall. Rather like the practice of the secondary survey looking for covert injury in the polytraumatised patient, a medical secondary survey is required as a screen in the elderly.

A hidden problem with the patient should also be sought in some potential child abuse cases. The defence in a court case may suggest that repeated injury was not the result of repeated abusive mechanisms but rather an undue propensity to injury. It may be claimed that the allegedly abused child has osteogenesis imperfecta and that the explanation of the multiple fractures is weak bones. The arguments here are a specialist area. Our role is more straightforward in providing a record of the initial evidence in an unbiased, professional and thorough manner.

Covert injuries

Looking for the hidden injury can follow three methods:

1 the deductive approach;
2 the look everywhere approach;
3 the focused exclusion approach.

The deductive approach – patterns of injury

One can apply common sense and experience to the search for hidden injuries. Injuries occur in patterns along the lines of energy transmission. Finding an obvious injury may therefore lead to one that is hidden. A good example is the child restrained by a lap seatbelt in the rear of a car involved in a frontal collision. There may be an obvious flexion spinal injury, e.g. a Chance fracture. What may be less obvious but should be sought is damage to the immobile retroperitoneal structures, the pancreas or duodenum.

Certain mechanisms are associated with particular patterns of injury. Thus, if the mechanism and perhaps some of the obvious injuries are known, one can seek the less obvious injury. An unrestrained passenger in a head-on car crash will hit their knee on the dashboard. If the tibia is the site of impact the patient has to

be evaluated for a potential rupture of the posterior cruciate ligament and a posterior hip dislocation. A dislocation of the knee should immediately raise concerns about damage to the popliteal artery and injury to it should be excluded. Table 21.1 gives some examples of patterns of associated injuries.

The look everywhere approach

One of the mainstays of trauma evaluation is the secondary survey. The essence is that once the initial life-saving manoeuvres have been completed you look everywhere for further injury. This detailed examination may take place shortly after admission, the following morning on the ward round or sometimes a week later when the patient first regains consciousness. A foot injury, a scaphoid fracture, a ruptured diaphragm and a peripheral nerve injury are all injuries that can be overlooked and cause long-term morbidity.

As its name suggests, the look everywhere secondary survey comes later in the sequence of the ATLS approach. However, the emphasis placed on the timeline at the beginning of this chapter and the need for early diagnosis is leading to a different look everywhere approach. The ATLS system has included a plain pelvic and a chest radiograph as part of the primary survey. This may confirm a clinical diagnosis but is also a screening tool to identify injuries that may progress to a clinical problem; the response to that injury can then be initiated earlier. The threshold for using more generalised investigations such as CT scanning, ultrasound, cardiac echo and magnetic resonance imaging (MRI) to check for these covert injuries is progressively being lowered. Some emergency departments now have CT scanners in their resuscitation rooms. A head-to-pelvis CT scan is being used to replace the early plain radiographs of the chest and the pelvis. A CT scan is more sensitive and specific and its use to identify injury before the clinical signs present is certain to increase.

The focused exclusion approach

Some injuries or conditions are for some reason missed on a surprisingly regular basis. This suggests that a normal deductive approach is not always adequate. When there is any suggestion of the presence of these injuries they should be actively sought and excluded. The evolution of head injury assessment in the UK illustrates this point very well. The National Institute for Health and Clinical Excellence (NICE) issues guidelines for clinical practice. The NICE guidelines for the investigation of head injury have lowered the threshold for a head CT, the objective being to

Table 21.1 Examples of patterns of injury

Mechanism	Obvious features	Covert injuries
Left-sided impact from road traffic accident	Lateral compression of the pelvis Left-sided pneumothorax	Splenic rupture Extradural haematoma
Flexion distraction (lap belt)	Chance fracture of the lumbar spine Dislocated knee Head injury	Duodenal rupture Popliteal artery disruption Cervical spine fracture
Electrocution	Burn on hand and collapse	Posterior dislocation of the shoulder
Dashboard impact	Knee wound	Posterior dislocation of the hip

George Quentin Chance, **Formerly Director of Diagnostic Radiology, The Derby Group of Hospitals, Derbyshire, England.**

avoid intracranial injuries being misdiagnosed and, more fundamentally, to demonstrate the problem at an early enough stage in the timeline for a medical response to be mounted. A consequence of very early imaging is that the findings, even on investigation, may not be well developed. As the guidelines suggest there needs to be a willingness to repeat investigations if indicated to detect evolving problems.

Other injuries that can cause disability but are easily missed are listed in Chapter 27. They are overlooked regularly so one must presume that the normal deductive processes for identifying them do not work. Therefore, if such injuries are suspected they should be positively excluded by focused history, examination and investigation (Summary box 21.7).

Summary box 21.7

Trauma assessment

- Know the timelines for important diagnoses
- Prioritise the assessment accordingly
- Positively exclude critical diagnoses
- If required, screen at-risk patients before clinical signs are apparent

---

The response to trauma

Once an assessment has been made based on the factors of mechanism, patient and injury discussed above, the response must be planned and executed. At the same time the patient will have an evolving response to injury. On the positive side, physiological compensatory and reserve mechanisms will be recruited and healing processes will be initiated. Countering this there may be progressive pathophysiological responses, the consumption of resources and decompensation.

The patient's response to injury

The patient's own homeostatic mechanisms will respond to the injury and there will be physiological and pathophysiological changes. In the light of this evolution of responses we may alter the nature or the timing of our interventions.

A simple example is body temperature. A drop in body temperature is common after injury; this may be due to exposure, inactivity, damp, blood loss or loss of vasomotor control. The body's own thermoregulatory mechanisms may not be able to resolve the problem and so we must be prepared to support that role – body temperature should be monitored and heat loss prevented as required. It may not be possible to do this adequately in an operating theatre during a surgical procedure.

Similarly, oxygenation can be monitored and support may be given by way of increased inspired oxygen or different modes of ventilation. However, it is often the case that the ventilators available in an operating theatre are not as sophisticated and flexible as those in an intensive care unit.

The response to blood loss is not only an evolving situation for an individual patient but our response to it also changes. The patient calls on compensatory mechanisms when blood is lost. As long as organ perfusion is adequate, low blood pressure is not a problem in its own right. The body has a finite resource of clotting factors and the injured lung does not tolerate excess fluid. These factors combined have led to a tendency to draw back from large-scale early fluid replacement. Instead, the emphasis is placed on identifying and stopping the source of bleeding. The evolution of permissive hypotensive resuscitation will no doubt continue in parallel with the more liberal use of investigations such as CT, which allow early therapeutic treatment and not just supportive treatment.

The patient also mounts a generalised immunological response to trauma. This has an impact on their ability to tolerate surgical interventions. There is growing evidence that procedures should be timed and staged to better fit the conditions created by the patient's systemic immune response.

The medical response to injury

Initial management

The structure of ATLS is discussed in Chapter 22. For some patients reducing the elapsed time from injury to useful intervention is critical. Preparation can aid this process. When a department is made aware of the impending arrival of a seriously injured patient a decision is made as to whether to call the 'trauma team'; if appropriate, this will allow a trained team of nurses and doctors to be waiting to meet the patient. While waiting, equipment is made ready, a leader is identified and each team member is given a role. Protective clothing will be needed: gloves to protect from fluids and lead aprons to protect from X-rays.

For the medical and nursing staff the beginning of the patient's pathway can become familiar just like any routine journey and, thus, planning becomes less complex. However, if wasteful delays are to be avoided, alternatives need to be available if for some reason the routine cannot be followed. Anticipating and dealing with potential rate-limiting steps in the patient's journey will allow delays to be avoided and reduce the response time. The component of the response that will be the rate-limiting step will depend on local as well as general circumstances. Examples of causes of delay are obtaining a CT scan, getting the patient into an operating theatre or obtaining a necessary specialist opinion. Such steps that can potentially bring the progress of the patient to a halt need to be addressed early and sometimes in a way that may seem out of the normal sequence. This is one of the major roles of the team leader who should have an overview and be able to foresee and pre-empt problems. Whenever a system is protocol driven someone should be in a position to take the responsibility to break protocol if required to keep the overall process flowing.

Having a practised common pathway can be disadvantageous; a patient with the wrong 'label' may go along the wrong pathway. We all have to be wary of labelling. When a patient has sustained obvious polytrauma and arrives on a stretcher with a cervical collar in place it is initially straightforward and appropriate to label them as an emergency. Should two patients with identical histories and injuries arrive in an emergency department with one on a spine board and the other in a chair, the former will be treated as if more severely injured when in fact that may not be the case. We must make our own judgements on reasonable evidence and not rely on the labels (in this case the cervical collars) applied by others.

Labelling is most frequently a dangerous problem in the elderly. A patient with an obviously short externally rotated leg may be quickly given the label '#NOF' (fracture neck of femur). There are a number of problems with this practice. The notation itself is misleading as the fracture is often intertrochanteric; thus, PFF for proximal femoral fracture is a better term. However, even this is inappropriate as it concentrates on the orthopaedic label rather than the whole patient. The incorrect label may mask the fact that the patient could be dying. The patient may have fallen as a consequence of a cardiac arrhythmia or other comorbidity; the early labelling as #NOF or PFF may therefore send the patient off on entirely the wrong pathway. All vulnerable patients should have a physiological triage to avoid such problems. This means assessing the airway, respiratory rate, blood pressure, pulse rate and consciousness. All of these assessments are more important, even in the elderly, than the presence of a fractured hip.

Beyond the first hour

The primary survey of ATLS encourages the identification and treatment of life-threatening problems. Once these have been addressed there may be other problems that require intervention. The timing and order of these interventions is a matter of judgement. There has been an evolution in the approach to the management of polytrauma. It has been variously said that a patient may be 'too sick to operate on' or that they may be 'too sick *not* to operate on'. The work of Bone in particular has promoted the concept of early definitive stabilisation of long bone fractures to allow better control of the pathophysiology of trauma. Others have highlighted the need in some circumstances for limited early intervention, sometimes called 'damage control surgery'. This is followed by definitive treatment when the patient is better able to tolerate it. In orthopaedic trauma the debate has focused on whether long bone fractures should be fixed temporarily or definitively. In general surgery the question is whether the abdomen should be definitively treated or packed. Any patient needing a sequence of interventions, e.g. laparotomy, femoral nailing, tibial nailing, should have the most important done first. Thus, if there needs to be a break in the procedures for any reason the most important interventions will have been completed. As each component of a sequence of procedures nears its

end, a decision needs to be made whether it is safe or appropriate to proceed to the next stage. Monitoring of core temperature, coagulation, base excess, etc., will help this decision to be made on rational grounds. If the patient's pathophysiology is deteriorating it may be decided to halt the surgery after life-saving or damage control surgery. An abdomen may be packed rather than subjected to a definitive procedure and the femoral fracture may be held with an external fixator rather than an intramedullary nail. The patient can then be transferred to the more controlled environment of an intensive care unit and return for definitive surgery when physiologically and immunologically better able to tolerate it; this may be hours or days later.

The evolving surgical plan can be crystallised into the patient's records as a written note. However, a very useful adjunct is to record it on a whiteboard in the operating theatre. This informs others of the intended pathway of treatment so that preparations can be made. An example of such a tactic is shown in Fig. 21.9. Note the alternative pathway that exists should the patient's general condition require a shorter procedure, when the femur can be temporarily stabilised with an external fixator rather than definitively fixed with a nail.

Local protocols and guidelines

A general guideline such as ATLS deals with some aspects of patient management and is used in many institutions. However, hospitals generally have individual policies to guide or direct decision making in smaller areas of practice. Examples are prophylaxis against infection and thromboembolism, the use of steroids in spinal injury and clearance of the cervical spine. These represent the efforts of individuals within an institution to plan for common and foreseeable circumstances. These protocols allow for easier and quicker decision making. Their application should protect the patient and, in an increasingly litigious world, the doctor as well.

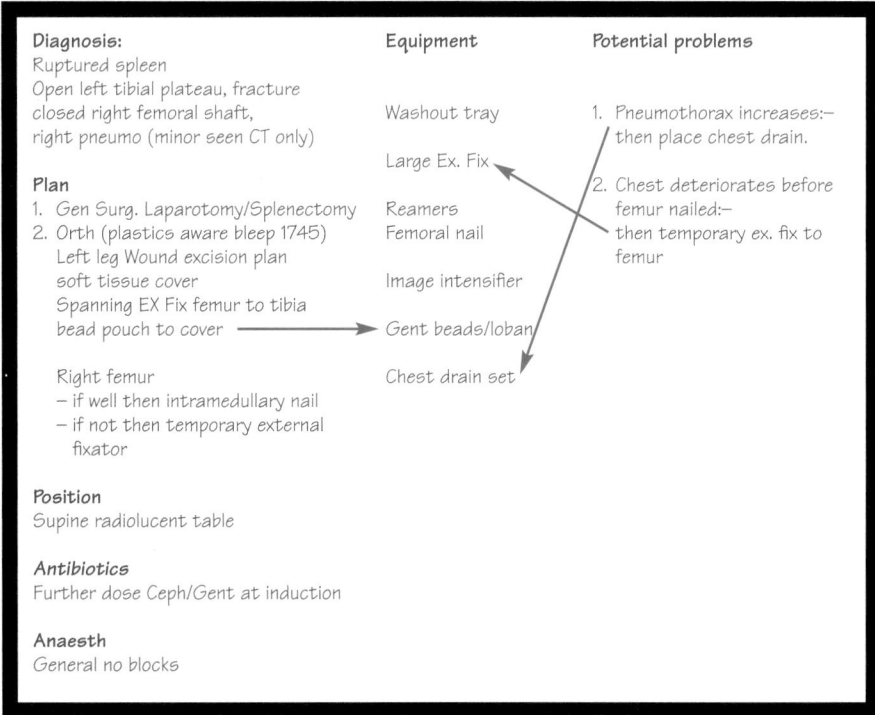

Figure 21.9 An example of a surgical tactic on a whiteboard in the operating theatre.

'Clearing' of the spine is a practice that has particular relevance to trauma. The early policy for managing the spine in polytrauma patients is straightforward; it can be summarised as 'suspect and protect'. This approach is widely employed and so in emergency departments very many patients have their spine protected. However, this is a precautionary protective approach and at some stage one has to have a strategy for discontinuing protection or 'clearing' the spine in those patients in whom it is not required. The 'gold standard' is clinical examination of the fully conscious, undistracted patient combined with any necessary investigations. The problem arises if a patient is not going to be fully conscious for some time. Maintaining spinal precautions for such a patient is costly, time-consuming and prone to complications. Pressure sores may develop under a collar, neck lines are less accessible and more nurses are needed for turning. However, the patients involved are likely to be those with higher-energy injury mechanisms in which spinal injury is more likely. Hospitals should have policies in place for such a situation. If no such policy exists and spinal precautions are withdrawn randomly it degrades the initial care that has been given. In the event that it is not possible to exclude spinal injury on clinical grounds the managing clinicians may request clearance on radiological grounds. The images should be assessed by an experienced radiologist and it must be recorded in the patient's records and signed that the spine has been cleared. An example of such a policy for clearing the spine is given in Table 21.2.

Record-keeping for the injured patient is both important and difficult. It is often said that trends in a patient's condition are more important than isolated observations. Because an injured patient may be cared for by a large number of individuals, trends can only become apparent by reference to the sequential recorded notes. If each individual clinician records their observations in an 'individual' manner it becomes very difficult to identify trends. Adoption of the Glasgow coma scale to monitor the level of consciousness demonstrates the advantage of using a consistent system of recording observations. Such sequential observations, especially when displayed on a single chart, demonstrate trends. The clinical evolution of a problem such as raised intracranial pressure secondary to an extradural haematoma is then easier to identify (Summary box 21.8).

Summary box 21.8

The response to trauma

- Guidelines and protocols speed and streamline management
- Pre-empt time-limiting steps to avoid delay
- Respond to the evolving condition of the patient

Responding to a local complex injury

Responding to a local complex injury, e.g. a fracture with a vascular injury, provides a good example of the difficulties that are encountered when planning and executing a multispecialty procedure. A fracture with a vascular injury may be open or closed. The first imperative is to recognise that the vascular injury exists. The clock for the warm ischaemic time starts running at the time that the circulation is occluded; this may be the time of injury or later. Management plans and interventions can only make progress once the injury is noticed. It is clearly important to make the diagnosis as soon as possible. The presence of an occluded or divided artery should be detectable clinically. However, sometimes the initial vascular injury may lead to only a partial interruption of blood flow. With vigilance and a high level of suspicion, the correct diagnosis may be reached before complete occlusion. An example is with a penetrating injury to the thigh or a dislocated knee. Both injuries can be associated with vessel damage. An ankle–brachial index of less than 0.9 suggests arterial injury even in the presence of palpable pulses. This will prompt early arteriography, which may allow the surgical response to be prepared earlier and with more chance of success. This is another example of screening an at-risk group to reduce the assessment time and allow more time for a clinical response.

Once the vascular deficit is apparent the question that needs to be answered is at what level the injury is situated. If the level of injury is obvious, time expended in arteriography is not profitable.

Managing the injury usually requires the cooperation of at least two surgical disciplines. The first step is to agree on a working diagnosis. Both parties should be happy with the structure of the surgical plan. The surgical approach, that is the anatomical route for dissection, will need discussion. An example of how conflict may occur is given by the case of surgery in the vicinity of the knee: the 'vascular approach' may damage some of the medial hamstring structures that might be needed later in an orthopaedic reconstructive procedure. It is generally preferable to avoid multiple approaches, so a compromise should be considered.

The teams should then agree on the sequence of events. Management of the injury will require the completion of a number of steps; these may include restoration of perfusion, definitive vascular anastomoses, wound excision and exploration (if an open fracture), provisional fracture stabilisation, definitive fracture fixation and fasciotomies. If the vascular anastomosis is the first step to be completed, this may then discourage the thorough wound excision of an open fracture or hinder fracture fixation, and the anastomosis may itself be damaged. If the progress to theatre has been rapid it may be possible to carry out a rapid wound excision and fracture fixation and still leave time for an anastomosis before the safe warm ischaemia time of about 4 hours has been exceeded. The advantage of avoiding unnecessary angiography is apparent when working against the clock. If it is clear that there is not sufficient time for this sequence of definitive procedures to be followed it may be possible to place a temporary shunt in the vessels to allow perfusion so that fracture fixation may be completed before the definitive anastomosis is performed.

Table 21.2 An example of a policy for clearing the spine in the obtunded patient

Cervical spine	Fine-quality CT scans of C0–T4, reformatted and assessed in the axial, sagittal and coronal planes. Powers ratio to assess the atlanto-occipital junction
Thoracolumbar spine (T4 distally)	Either good-quality anteroposterior and lateral plain films or CT scans reformatted and assessed in the anteroposterior, lateral and axial planes

CHAPTER 21 | INTRODUCTION TO TRAUMA

Planning an individual operation

The central part of a surgeon's work is operating. Dealing with injuries is not repetitive and so thought and planning are required. Even when an individual surgeon is involved in performing the surgery, care is delivered as part of a team. It is good practice to think through the plan for the operating theatre. Mental rehearsal of a procedure may allow potential hazards to be predicted and avoided. For example:

- As the procedure is planned it may become apparent that the proposed surgical approach will not allow the access required. In a whiteboard exercise this can readily be altered. This cannot be done if the first time this problem is appreciated is after the skin has been cut.
- It may be decided in planning that another surgeon is better suited to perform a particular procedure.

The use of the whiteboard in theatre, discussed earlier in the context of multiple injuries, is equally applicable for the isolated injury. An example of a surgical tactic for a segmental tibial fracture is given in Fig. 21.10. This not only helps the surgeon to be clear about the procedure in his or her own mind but also informs others. The position of the patient, the surgical approach, position of the image intensifier, method of fracture reduction and instruments required, and method of fixation and implants required are all noted. Theatre staff, anaesthetic staff, radiographers, etc. can all see what is intended and it can also act as a teaching aid. A trainee may be asked to complete the whiteboard plan; they then have to commit to a plan of action and not just drift along. An important addition to the planned progress of the procedure is a list of potential problems or hazards. The strategies that will be used to deal with these problems should they arise can then be considered and prepared for (Summary box 21.9).

Summary box 21.9

Planning an individual operation

- Plan procedures before performing them
- Commit a plan to paper
- Share a surgical plan by use of a whiteboard

(a)

Diagnosis	Equipment	Problems/solutions

Open segmental fracture left tibia
 	
Procedure
– Excise wound with plastics
– Plan soft tissue cover
– Secure nail entry point
– Ream segment through traumatic wound
– Statically lock nail
– Dress wound with a bead pouch
– Continue antibiotics until definitive soft-
   tissue cover
	– Radiolucent table
	– Tourniquet (during wound excision)
	– Soft tissue tray
	– Washout tray
	   9 litres washout
	– Reamers
	– Cannulated tibial IM nail
	
	In reserve
	external fixator/long plates
		– Segment viable but too narrow to
		   nail/proceed to bridge plate or ex. fix
		   depending on soft tissue
		– Segment non-viable/remove segment
		   place temp ex. fix with view to
		   subsequent Illizarov transport
		– On passing nail malalignment of
		   proximal fragment/remove nail and
		   place blocking screw

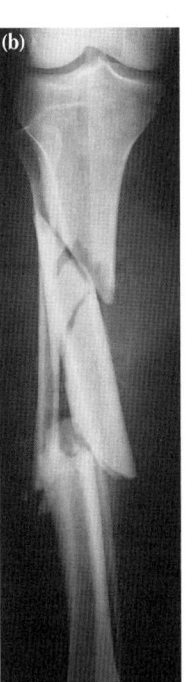
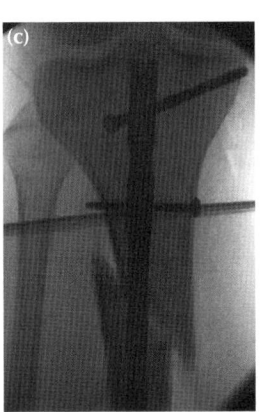
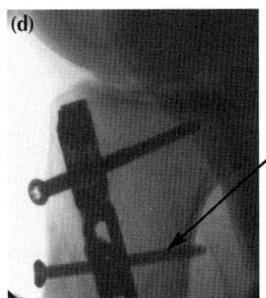
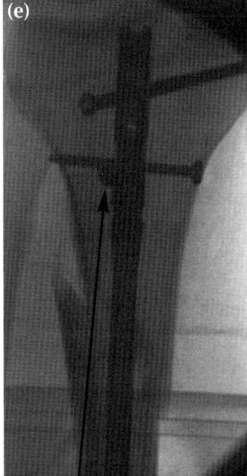

Blocking screw

Figure 21.10 (a) Theatre whiteboard with surgical tactic and (b) radiograph for a complex grade IIIb open segmental tibial fracture. One of the foreseen problems has occurred as the proximal fragment is malreduced (c). The nail was removed and an anteroposterior blocking screw was placed (highlighted) (d and e). The fracture is then well reduced.

The response to the mechanism of injury (injury prevention)

When assessing the *mechanism + patient = injury* relationship it is easy for the doctor to focus on managing the injury; however, the mechanism of injury can also be addressed, that is we should aim to prevent rather than just treat injury.

When a mechanism of injury becomes particularly prevalent or has serious consequences it is prudent to take steps to either remove the mechanism or reduce the consequences.

Accidents occur in a variety of places: the home, the workplace and the roads are the most common. The strategy and motivation for prevention varies from place to place. Within the workplace there is legislation to protect employees and a tendency for an injured employee to sue the employer. Thus, although some work environments are naturally dangerous, many advances in safety have been made. Within the home, legislation has little effect on behaviour. The safety of the structure of a home may be influenced by building regulations but the thrust is on education of the individual. It is difficult to educate adults to behave more safely and so accidents in the home remain very common. Simple measures such as avoiding loose rugs or cables, polished floors and unnecessary steps are common sense. There is evidence to suggest that incorporating accident prevention education into the appropriate parts of the school curriculum is more likely to be successful.

Road safety is a contentious issue. The safe management of the kinetic energy of travel would seem to be a straightforward physical problem. Great advances have been made in the technology of motor vehicles to protect drivers. Restricting speed, separating vehicles travelling in different directions and segregating motor vehicles from vulnerable road users such as pedestrians are not popular measures. The political power of the motorist tends to obstruct progress in this area.

The response to the potential NAI is to involve the appropriate agencies in an attempt to prevent further problems. This is a difficult role for doctors as it involves having a quite different relationship with the patient and the family to that which is normally adopted. In general, our training is to be empathetic and trusting; however, we have to be alert, professional and act in the best interests of the child or other vulnerable person (Summary box 21.10).

Summary box 21.10

Response to the mechanism of injury

- The saying that 'prevention is better than cure' is true
- Legislation and education are required
- Prevent further abuse by responding to the initial clues

The response to patient factors

Another approach to injury prevention is to alter the patient. This particularly applies to the epidemic of injuries in the elderly. Falls are the commonest mechanism of injury, so one can try to address the cause or the effects of falls. Fall prevention clinics are now common. The at-risk patients are assessed and remediable causes of falls are addressed. Postural hypotension, transient ischaemic attacks, arrhythmias, etc. can be identified and treated. Unfortunately, the number of patients considered to be at risk is so large that the coverage of such clinics is as yet quite inadequate.

Elderly people will continue to fall, so we can try to minimise the effect of the fall. Schemes such as using hip protector pads to cushion a fall have been tried with limited success. The area most likely to expand and give results is that of strengthening the skeleton. Identifying those at risk of osteoporosis, screening them and then treating appropriately offers a hope of reducing the incidence of low energy fractures. There was initial scepticism about the expense of such treatments and the potentially huge number of people who would require them. It is now accepted that treatment targeted appropriately will be cost-effective by reducing later fractures with the consequent costs of hospitalisation, morbidity and mortality.

Another of the patient factors discussed earlier is when injury occurs in pathological tissues, the common example being a fracture of a bone with a neoplastic deposit. This should influence management in one of two ways. When there is a doubt as to whether the tumour is a primary or secondary it is important to think before treatment. Injudicious operative management of a fracture associated with a primary deposit may prejudice proper tumour management; when the situation allows a proper opinion should be obtained. When dealing with obvious secondary deposits the situation is quite different. Aggressive surgical management is often justified to allow an early return to function. A person with a limited life expectancy should not spend long periods of time rehabilitating (Summary box 21.11).

Summary box 21.11

Response to patient factors

- Pre-empt injury with the use of fall prevention clinics
- Carry out targeted osteoporosis treatment
- Do not treat thoughtlessly an injury that is possibly secondary to a primary neoplasm

---

CONCLUSION

Trauma is usually the adverse consequence of a mechanical force on a patient. The prime importance of time in trauma care needs to be appreciated. At time zero there is a relationship between the mechanism, the patient and the injury. The components of this relationship should fit together in a rational manner. When this rational fit is not apparent, great care should be taken to look for hidden injuries, pre-existing pathology or some deliberate deception in the given history.

There is a timeline that progresses from the moment of injury. Prompt understanding of the problems is key in allowing an early reaction. It may not be possible to wait for overt clinical signs and so diagnoses should be positively sought and in some circumstances patients screened. There is a minimum response time to initiate and complete the interventions to deal with the problems. Preparation can reduce this response time. Knowledge of realistic response times is important, because only then does the clinician know the real urgency of initiating action.

When presented with an injured patient the early management is largely protocol driven. As more details become known and the patient moves towards definitive care a more individual plan is made. This plan coordinates the different specialities and should be flexible to allow for evolving pathology. Someone should be responsible for the patient.

CHAPTER 21 | INTRODUCTION TO TRAUMA

Trauma does not just consist of care of the young injured. Increasingly the injured patient will be elderly. The team involved needs to reflect the needs of these elderly patients.

Trauma need not only be addressed by tackling the injury itself. Preventative measures should be employed when particular mechanisms can be identified as being common or important causes of injury. For example, prophylactic measures may reduce the propensity for individuals to fall or reduce the consequences of those falls when they occur.

The following chapters in this section will look further at these principles as applied to specific regions or surgical disciplines (Summary box 21.12).

Summary box 21.12

Conclusion

- The management of trauma is dependent upon time
- Multiple specialties may be involved but do not lose sight of the overall problem
- Planning increases the chances of success

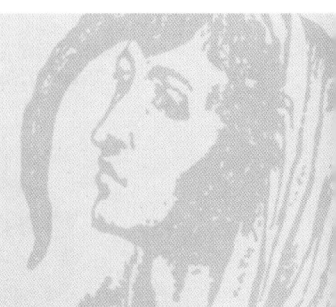

Early assessment and management of trauma

LEARNING OBJECTIVES

To identify:
- The sequence of priorities in the early assessment of the injured patient

To learn:
- The principle of triage in immediate management of the injured patient
- The concepts of injury recognition prediction based on the mechanism and energy of injury

To apply:
- The principles of primary and secondary surveys in the assessment and management of trauma

- Techniques for the initial resuscitative and definitive care aspects of trauma

To perform:
- The necessary protocols to allow early stabilisation of the patient leading on to definitive care

To recognise:
- Certain important groups of patients and their differing management

EPIDEMIOLOGY

Trauma is the commonest cause of death in the population between the ages of 1 and 40 years worldwide. It is a huge drain on health resources in both the developed and the developing world. By 2020, it is estimated that injuries will be the third leading cause of death and disability worldwide. In addition to killing people, injuries cause lifelong disabilities and many other health problems with serious consequences for individuals, families, communities and health-care systems.

The World Health Organization data published in 2002 revealed the following points worthy of consideration:

- An estimated 5 million people worldwide died from injuries in 2000 – a mortality rate of 83.7 per 100 000 population.
- Injuries accounted for 9% of the world's deaths in 2000 and 12% of the world's burden of disease.
- Road traffic injuries are the leading cause of injury-related deaths worldwide. More than 90% of the world's deaths from injuries occur in low- and middle-income countries.
- The low- and middle-income countries of Europe have the highest injury mortality rates.
- The South-east Asia and Western Pacific regions account for the highest number of injury deaths worldwide.
- Globally, injury mortality among men is twice that among women.
- Males in Africa and Europe have the highest injury-related mortality rates.
- Young people between the ages of 15 and 44 years account for almost 50% of the world's injury-related mortality.
- Mortality from road traffic injuries and interpersonal violence in males is almost three times higher than that in females.

- Injury profiles including morbidity and mortality statistics differ between Third and First World countries largely on account of the availability of health-care resources being significantly diminished in the Third World. Road traffic injuries in the developing world are now the third highest cause of death. Probable factors include the large numbers of pedestrians and cyclists (many living below the poverty line) involved in these injuries; overcrowding of public transport; poor road maintenance and few speed restrictions (Fig. 22.1).

Falls

Globally, an estimated 391 000 people died as a result of falls in 2002, making it the second leading cause of unintentional injury death worldwide after road traffic injuries. A quarter of all fatal falls occurred in the high-income countries. Europe and the Western Pacific region combined account for nearly 60% of the total number of fall-related deaths worldwide.

Males in the low- and middle-income countries of Europe have by far the highest fall-related mortality rates worldwide.

In all regions of the world, adults over the age of 70 years, particularly females, have significantly higher fall-related mortality rates than younger people. However, children account for the largest morbidity – almost 50% of the total number of disability-adjusted life-years (DALYs) lost globally to falls occur in children under 15 years of age.

With ever increasing population growth and increased life expectancy, the injury mortality and morbidity statistics are likely to be skewed towards the two ends of the age spectrum, making the paediatric and the elderly populations very important with respect to global health care and economics.

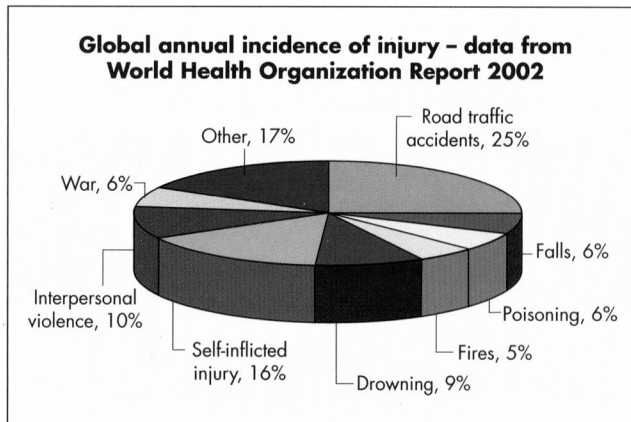

Figure 22.1 Worldwide annual incidence of injury.

INTRODUCTION

Modern trauma care is increasing in its complexity and management and, despite measures to reduce the incidence of trauma worldwide, it looks likely to remain the 'unsolved epidemic' of the future. The economic impact of trauma and injury is huge globally. Lost wages, medical expenses, administration costs, property damage and indirect costs contribute to the annual cost of over $400 billion in the USA alone.

Many significant changes have improved trauma care, and many have concentrated on a systematic focused methodology for the management of trauma, particularly in the initial stages. In fact, one can argue that it is the initial assessment that is probably the most important factor in the subsequent outcome of the trauma patient, as it is at this stage that a subsequent care pathway and protocol is formed for definitive treatment.

In essence, trauma can be divided into two basic types:

- Serious and life-threatening injury;
- Significant trauma requiring treatment but not immediately life threatening.

While it is acknowledged that the two can and often do overlap, it is important for the initial assessment to efficiently and carefully distinguish between the two.

The approach to the traumatised patient is very different from that of a patient with an undiagnosed medical condition as, in the latter, an extensive history, past medical history, physical examination from head to toe, differential diagnosis and investigations ordered to confirm or refute this diagnosis are undertaken. In the trauma setting, it is often not possible to obtain such information immediately; hence, a standardised protocol of management is required. The Advanced Trauma Life Support (ATLS) system was therefore created initially in the USA and rapidly taken up globally. At present, over 40 countries worldwide are actively providing the ATLS course to their physicians. In the UK, it is a prerequisite qualification for higher surgical training, and the surgeon cannot be fully accredited unless he or she has successfully completed an ATLS provider course (Summary box 22.1).

Summary box 22.1

The steps in the ATLS philosophy

- Primary survey with simultaneous resuscitation – identify and treat what is killing the patient
- Secondary survey – proceed to identify all other injuries
- Definitive care – develop a definitive management plan

Although it has been acknowledged in recent literature that the ATLS philosophy has its limitations, it still remains probably the most significant advance in trauma care and management in the last three decades. In fact, once the attending clinician is versed in the structure and protocol of the philosophy, it becomes very easy to apply this to any trauma event whether large or small, hence the importance of its emphasis throughout this chapter. Later chapters will deal with the specifics of injury management by region but, before the clinician even gets to the definitive management, it is important that an initial assessment protocol is followed.

There are important considerations when managing paediatric trauma and trauma in the elderly population, which will be discussed later in this chapter.

Triage

Triage is an important concept in modern health-care systems, and three essential phases have developed:

1 pre-hospital triage – in order to despatch ambulance and pre-hospital care resources;
2 at the scene of trauma;
3 on arrival at the receiving hospital.

The brief behind establishing these systems focused on the identification of those immediately at risk of loss of life, then moving to the management of urgent cases and prioritising these into clinically stable but seriously ill and into the most appropriate order for evacuation, and identifying the most appropriate receiving unit. In many western countries, subspecialisation is becoming more and more common, and there are discrepancies in the local availability of services such as neurosurgery, vascular surgery, plastic surgery, orthopaedic surgery and even intensive care facilities in all district admitting units and, as in the US model, many places are giving consideration to the establishment of specialised trauma units that cater for those seriously injured. However, at present, the logistical systems and financial resources that have to be put in place make this an idealistic rather than a realistic goal. Nevertheless, the concept of triage is an important one and should be understood, and it remains the entry point to an organised system of care to maximise outcome in any medical framework.

In trauma, two types of triage situation usually exist:

1 *Multiple casualties.* Here, the number and severity of injuries do not exceed the ability of the facility to render care. Priority is given to the life-threatening injuries followed by those with polytrauma.
2 *Mass casualties.* The number and severity of the injuries exceed the capability and facilities available to the staff. In this situation, those with the greatest chance of survival and the least expenditure of time, equipment and supplies are prioritised (see Chapter 30).

MECHANISMS OF TRAUMA

Blunt trauma: patterns of injury

The most common cause of blunt trauma is the motor vehicle. Injuries related to motor vehicles are related to several key factors: the mass and speed of the vehicle at the moment of impact; whether the occupants of the vehicle were restrained; whether the occupant was ejected; and the interaction of the occupant or pedestrian with vehicle parts. Speed is a critical factor: a 10% increase in impact speed translates into a 40% rise in the case fatality risk for both restrained and unrestrained occupants. Ejection from a vehicle is associated with a significantly greater incidence of severe injury. Use of seatbelts is thought to reduce the risk of death or serious injury for front-seat occupants by approximately 45% (Fig. 22.2). Unbelted rear-seat occupants are also at increased risk of serious injury in motor vehicle accidents (MVAs); they may be ejected or thrown forward into the back of the front seat; the impact from unbelted rear-seat passengers on front-seat occupants can be a major determinant of injury. It is estimated that, when rear seatbelts are worn, the risk of death for belted front-seat occupants is reduced by 80%. Although seatbelts reduce mortality overall, they cause a specific pattern of internal injuries. Patients with seatbelt marks have been found to have a fourfold increase in thoracic trauma and an eightfold increase in intra-abdominal trauma compared with those without seatbelt marks (Fig. 22.3) (Summary box 22.2).

Summary box 22.2

Energy and injury prevention

- A 10% increase in speed of impact increases pedestrian fatality risk by 40%
- Seatbelts reduce the risk of injury in a vehicle by 45%

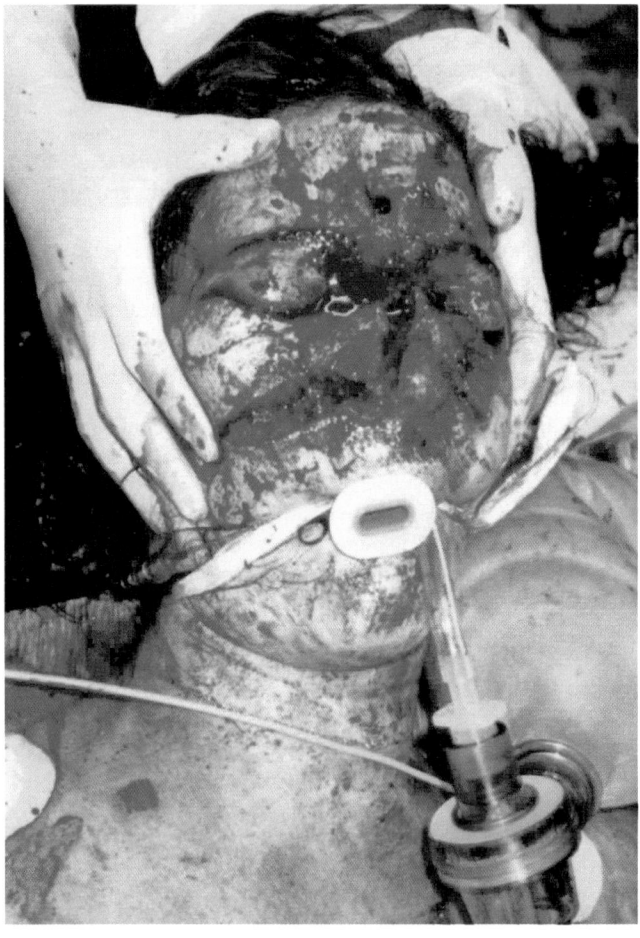

Figure 22.2 Unrestrained driver with severe craniofacial injury (courtesy of Johannesburg Hospital Trauma Unit).

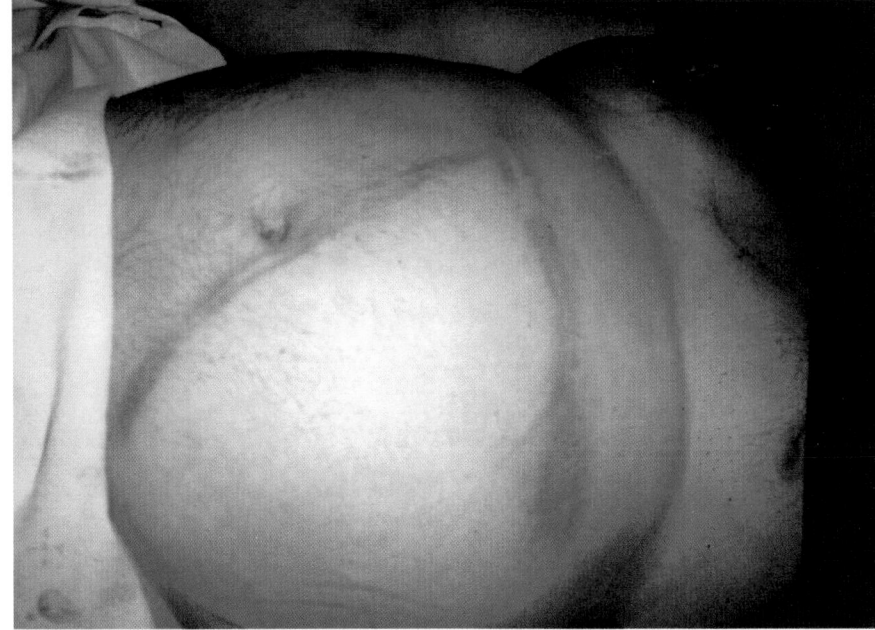

Figure 22.3 Seatbelt mark after motor vehicle accident (courtesy of Johannesburg Hospital Trauma Unit).

In direct frontal MVAs, airbags provide a reduced risk of fatality of approximately 30%. In all crashes, the reduction in risk of death has been estimated at 11%. However, airbags may also cause specific patterns of injury. Three separate at-risk groups have been identified: adult drivers, school-aged children riding in the front passenger seat and infants installed in rear-facing infant car seats placed in the front passenger seat. Adults tend to have severe chest injuries; the infants usually sustain neck or head injury and are unrestrained. Children in the front seat have also died as a result of airbag deployment despite the use of lap and shoulder restraints. In order to reduce the risk of airbag-induced injury, children younger than 12 years should be properly restrained in the back seat. Infants (aged < 1 year) in rear-facing child safety seats should never ride in the front seat of a vehicle fitted with a passenger-side airbag. All vehicle occupants should wear seatbelts, and the seat should be moved as far back as possible from the steering wheel or dashboard.

Motorcyclists experience a death rate 35 times greater than the occupants of cars. Helmets reduce the risk of fatal head injury by about one-third and reduce the risk of facial injury by two-thirds. Fractures of the lower extremities are also common in motorcyclists, occurring in approximately 40% of motorcyclists hospitalised for non-fatal injuries. Injuries due to bicycles account for 800 deaths and approximately 500 000 injuries treated at hospitals every year in the US. Children aged 5–14 years have the highest rates of injury, and head injury accounts for 75% of the deaths. Helmets have been shown to reduce the risk of brain injury for bicyclists by nearly 90%.

Injuries to pedestrians occur disproportionately among school-aged children, the elderly and the intoxicated. Children are most at risk when they live in areas of high traffic density where kerbside parking is prevalent, traffic speed is high and few alternative play areas are available. Poverty, household crowding and poor parental supervision are compounding factors (Summary box 22.3).

Summary box 22.3

Types of injury

- Blunt, e.g. car bonnet
- Penetrating, e.g. knife
- Blast, e.g. bomb
- Crush, e.g. building collapse
- Thermal

Penetrating trauma

Although the incidence of penetrating injuries is increasing, such injuries are uncommon in the UK compared with other countries. Factors include the proximity of the underlying viscera to the path of the penetrating object and the velocity of the missile. The distance from the weapon to the wound may give important information regarding the energy of the injury and therefore predict internal damage.

Blast injury

Terrorism is now a global phenomenon. It is conceivable that civilian, as well as military, surgeons will be exposed to patients injured in explosions. (See Chapter 30).

Crush injury

The association between crush injury, rhabdomyolysis and acute renal failure was first reported during the Second World War in victims trapped during the 'London Blitz'. It has been reported in earthquake and mining accident survivors, after excessive exercise and when limbs have been forced into abnormal postures for prolonged periods, such as during general anaesthesia or coma induced by alcohol or drugs. Prolonged crushing of a muscle mass causes death of the muscle cells, with release of myoglobin and

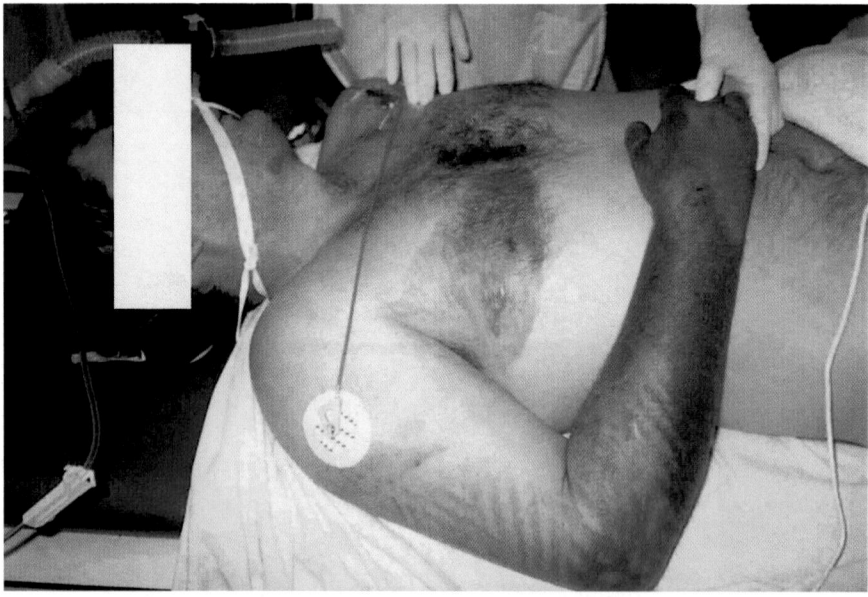

Figure 22.4 Crush injury to the arm and chest due to prolonged entrapment in a motor vehicle accident (courtesy of Johannesburg Hospital Trauma Unit).

The London Blitz. This is the name given to the German air raids on London between the 7th of September 1940 and the 11th of May 1941, during which it is estimated that more than 15,000 people were killed. Blitz is short for Blitzkrieg, the German for 'lightning war'.

vasoactive mediators into the circulation. Injured muscle also sequesters many litres of fluid, reducing the effective intravascular volume, which results in renal vasoconstriction and ischaemia. Myoglobin is concentrated in the tubules, and precipitates, leading to tubular obstruction.

Early and aggressive volume loading of patients, preferably prior to extrication, is the best treatment. Intensive care is required with close attention to fluid balance and renal replacement therapy if required. Compartment syndrome of a limb may occur (Fig. 22.4) (Summary box 22.4).

Summary box 22.4

Crush injury

- Muscle cells die. If reperfused, they release myoglobin
- Injured tissue sequesters fluid
- Renal shutdown results
- Treatment is fluid loading with monitoring of renal output to maintain diuresis

---

Thermal injury

See Chapter 28 on Burns.

Alcohol and drugs

Alcohol and other forms of substance abuse are major associated factors in all forms of trauma. Drivers with illegal blood alcohol levels account for nearly one-third of non-fatal injuries, and half of driver deaths. Injury to drunken pedestrians shows even greater alcohol relatedness, as pedestrian accidents account for nearly three-quarters of adult traffic deaths. There is a strong association between problem drinking and high-risk behaviour, such as dangerous driving and violent, aggressive behaviour. Illicit drug use often leads to interpersonal violence as a consequence of the effects of the drugs and the crime required to fund the habit.

ASSESSMENT AND MANAGEMENT OF THE SERIOUSLY INJURED

It is important to remember the trimodal distribution of deaths from trauma with regard to time, first described by Trunkey in the 1980s. There are three 'peaks' as follows:

- Immediate – 50% of all deaths, not possible to save. Usually as a result of massive head injury/brainstem injury/major cardiovascular event.
- Early – within the first few hours, often death from torso trauma.
- Late – 20% of deaths. Usually from organ failure and sepsis, influenced by inadequate early resuscitation and care.

From this emerged the concept of the 'golden hour' to describe the urgent need for treatment of trauma victims within the first hour after injury.

Importance of the multidisciplinary team approach

The team approach to trauma is essential to achieve the best possible outcomes. It is, however, resource intensive. The available personnel and resources can become overwhelmed quickly in non-hospital settings, smaller institutions in underdeveloped countries and mass casualty situations. Regardless of this, it is essential that the care team is organised prior to patient arrival. Leadership and unity of command are essential, as is communication, with rapid identification of the individual team members. A trauma team leader should be identified prior to patient arrival, who will direct the evaluation and initial resuscitation. By definition, therefore, the person responsible for this role should ideally not have an active hands-on role, but be more a 'traffic controller and information collator'. Additional physicians and midlevel providers are responsible for airway management, conducting primary and secondary surveys and other procedures as necessary. Radiographers should be immediately available and properly trained in the imaging required. Early consultation with senior neurosurgeons, general/vascular surgeons and orthopaedists will be needed. The changing modern media world requires that media involvement is usually immediate, and it is important that there is a spokesperson who acts as a mode of communication between the team caring for the individual(s) and the outside world. This is particularly important in the mass casualty situation where hospitals should have systems in place specifically for communication purposes. Of even more importance is the communication with the patient and members of their immediate family, who must not be neglected even in the seriously injured (Summary box 22.5).

Summary box 22.5

Managing a major trauma situation

- Plan for this eventuality
- Set up the team before the patients arrive
- Organise lines of communication and command

Preparation

- Pre-hospital phase – there must be good coordination and communication pathways set up prior to transfer of the injured from the scene of injury. This will allow time for mobilisation of the team and resources at the receiving hospital (Fig. 22.5).
- In-hospital phase – a resuscitation area should be available

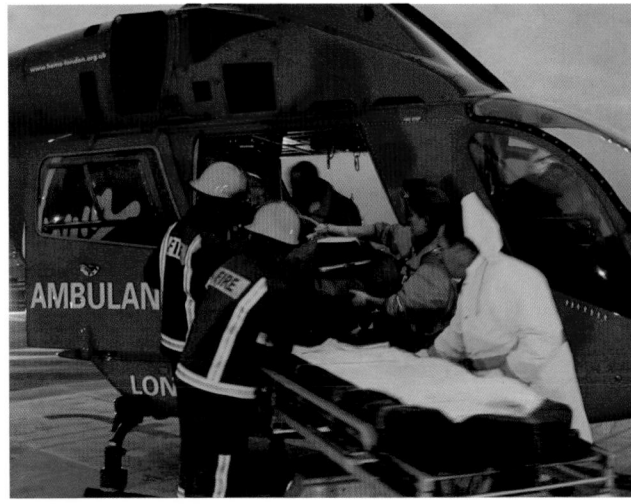

Figure 22.5 The importance of teamwork in pre-hospital care (courtesy of the London Helicopter Emergency Service).

and secured. Equipment in this area should be checked daily and placed where it is immediately accessible. Warmed intravenous crystalloid solutions should be prepared and ready for immediate attachment on arrival. The laboratory team should be warned that blood may be urgently needed. The team should be prepared, ideally with specialty name badges, and standard disease prevention protocols should be put in place, e.g. masks, eye protection, water-impervious aprons, X-ray gowns, gloves, etc. Handover from pre-hospital personnel should be succinct and standardised: **M**echanism of injury, **I**njuries identified including information on injuries to other casualties involved in the same event, vital **S**igns at the scene and any **T**reatment administered (MIST) is one such example.

PRIMARY SURVEY AND RESUSCITATION

This includes early triage, and many centres in the USA, UK and Europe have scoring systems to help to identify treatment priorities. The process is based on the energy of trauma, the vital signs and injuries sustained. Patient management must consist of a rapid primary evaluation, resuscitation of vital functions, a more detailed secondary assessment and, finally, the initiation of definitive care. This is the heartbeat core of the ATLS system and constitutes the ABCDE of trauma care (Summary box 22.6).

Summary box 22.6

ABCDE of trauma care

- A – Airway maintenance and cervical spine protection
- B – Breathing and ventilation
- C – Circulation with haemorrhage control
- D – Disability: neurological status
- E – Exposure: completely undress the patient and assess for other injuries

---

Airway with cervical spine protection

The airway must be evaluated first. If there is vocal response from the patient, then the patient's airway is not immediately at risk, but repeated assessment is prudent. If there is no or limited response, then a rapid investigation and assessment for signs of airway obstruction should be undertaken. This includes inspection for foreign bodies, maxillofacial or mandibular fractures, tracheal or laryngeal injury or oedema (see Fig. 22.2, p. 287).

The Glasgow Coma Score (GCS) is routinely used in head trauma, and further details can be found in Chapter 23. Patients with a significant head injury, where there is an altered level of consciousness or a GCS of 8 or less, usually require placement of a definitive airway. Special considerations must be given to the paediatric airway because of its unique anatomical laryngeal features (see the later section on paediatric trauma).

Measures to ensure a patent airway should be instituted while protecting the cervical spine. Initially, the chin lift or jaw thrust manoeuvres are recommended to achieve this task. A normal neurological examination should not exclude a cervical spine injury. Protection of the cervical spine should be maintained throughout either by stabilisation equipment or by a member of

---

The Glasgow Coma Source **was introduced in 1977 by William Bryan Jennet and Graham Michael Teasdale of The Southern General Hospital, Glasgow, Scotland.**

---

the trauma team when it is required that the patient be moved or turned (Summary box 22.7).

Summary box 22.7

Airway assessment

- Check verbal response
- Clear mouth and airway with large-bore sucker
- If GCS ≤ 8, consider a definitive airway; otherwise use jaw thrust or chin lift

---

Breathing and ventilation

Oxygen must be administered to all trauma patients, usually at high flow and via a reservoir mask. Ventilation requires an adequately functioning chest wall, lungs and diaphragm, and each must be systematically evaluated. Signs of surgical emphysema, dilatation of the neck veins, symmetry of the chest wall, respiratory effort and rate should be evaluated and recorded. Percussion and auscultation should be performed both front and back after log rolling.

Acute tension pneumothorax, flail chest with contusion, massive haemothorax and open pneumothorax are examples of life-threatening injuries that must be identified in the primary survey, i.e. they are *not* radiological diagnoses. Critical findings include the absence of or asymmetry of breath sounds, tracheal deviation, hyperresonance (consistent with tension pneumothorax) or dullness to percussion (haemothorax). Treat pneumothorax, haemothorax and tension pneumothorax with a tube thoracostomy. As an emergency measure in tension pneumothorax, immediately decompress with the insertion of a needle into the pleural space in the mid-clavicular line two fingerbreadths below the clavicle, followed by chest drain insertion. Furthermore, it should be noted that, when intubation and ventilation have been necessary in the unconscious patient, a re-evaluation should occur, as intubation and securing of the airway itself may unmask an underlying chest injury. Open chest wounds ('sucking') should be occluded with a three-sided dressing followed by intercostal drain placement through a separate incision. If there is evidence of massive haemothorax (> 1.5 litres of blood), it may lead to severe respiratory compromise, cardiac tamponade and compression of the affected lung; in this situation, operative control of the bleeding is likely to be required immediately (Summary box 22.8).

Summary box 22.8

Breathing

- Give 100% oxygen at high flow
- Check for tension pneumothorax
- Decompress at once if tension pneumothorax is suspected (needle in the second intercostal space)

Circulation and control of bleeding

Assessment here centres on three critical clinical observations:

1 *Conscious level.* If this is impaired or altered, one must assume that the patient has lost a significant amount of blood as cerebral perfusion has become compromised.

2 *Skin colour.* A patient with pink skin and warm peripheries is rarely critically hypovolaemic, and the converse is true for a pale, ashen, grey-looking patient with ominous signs of hypovolaemia.

3 *Pulse.* Full, slow, regular peripheral pulses are usual signs of relative normovolaemia, whereas a rapid, thready pulse or, worse still, one that is not peripherally palpable is a grave sign of hypovolaemic shock, and blood volume must be rapidly restored. Pulse rate changes occur as a rule prior to any shift in the blood pressure.

Recent emphasis has been given to the over-riding priority being primary haemorrhage control and timely surgical intervention rather than overaggressive fluid resuscitation ('permissive hypotension'), but one should guard against complacency, particularly in the at-risk groups, i.e. the elderly, children, patients with head injuries and those in whom the pre-hospital phase has been longer than normal. The elderly and the paediatric population will be discussed as special groups later in the chapter; they have very different physiological responses to volume loss (Summary box 22.9).

> **Summary box 22.9**
>
> **Circulation (assessment and warning signs)**
>
> ■ Deteriorating conscious state
> ■ Pallor
> ■ Rapid thready pulse is a more reliable and earlier warning sign than a fall in blood pressure

Disability

The GCS allows for a very rapid assessment of the patient's level of consciousness, pupillary size and reaction, motor function and, therefore, injury level and is also a good prognostic indicator. Further details can be found in Chapter 23.

It should be noted, however, that hypoglycaemia, alcohol and drug abuse may also alter the level of consciousness and should also be excluded. As always throughout the assessment, one must evaluate and re-evaluate constantly to ensure that evolving problems are identified, especially after head injury.

Exposure

The patient must be fully exposed and examined front and back using a carefully controlled log roll. Spinal alignment must be maintained during this procedure with in-line traction. Hypothermia can be rapid following trauma, and warming air blankets are vitally important in the resuscitative phase.

Adjuncts to the primary survey

These include blood samples for full blood count (FBC), coagulation studies, plasma chemistry (urea and electrolytes and, sometimes, toxicology or other case-specific indices), transfusion screening (group and cross-match, etc.), 12-lead electrocardiography (ECG) monitoring and pulse oximetry, if available. The blood can be taken at the same time as securing intravenous access with two large-bore cannulae (14–16G). Other adjuncts are urinary and gastric catheters. Care should be taken when passing gastric catheters nasally in the presence of maxillofacial injury or suspected base of skull fracture. If urethral injury is suspected, as in the case of pelvic diastasis, one should obtain an emergency room urethrogram prior to catheterisation. Rectal and external genital examination is necessary before catheterisation to rule out serious retroperitoneal injury. Signs include blood at the meatus, scrotal or labial ecchymosis and a high riding prostate in males. Perform a dipstick urinalysis to rule out occult haematuria (Summary box 22.10).

> **Summary box 22.10**
>
> **Adjuncts to the primary survey**
>
> ■ Blood – FBC, urea and electrolytes, clotting screen, glucose, toxicology, cross-match
> ■ ECG
> ■ Two wide-bore cannulae for intravenous fluids
> ■ Urinary and gastric catheters
> ■ Radiographs of the cervical spine and chest

Radiographs that are routinely requested and should be available as portable images in the resuscitation room are:

• *Lateral cervical spine.* Note that a normal lateral cervical spine does *not* rule out injury to the cervical spine; once the patient has been successfully stabilised, it is essential that further X-rays are taken, i.e. anteroposterior view and peg/open mouth view. These views should then be correlated with the clinical cervical spine examination prior to announcing that the patient is cleared of cervical spine injury (Fig. 22.6).

• *Anteroposterior chest.* Look at mediastinal size and shift, evidence of pneumothorax/haemothorax (Figs 22.7 and 22.8), fractures of the ribs, surgical emphysema, diaphragmatic shape and position and evidence of pulmonary contusion. A widened mediastinal shadow may represent an aortic rupture.

• *Anteroposterior pelvis.* Looking essentially for fractures and pelvic discontinuity that have the potential for massive blood loss and fatality (Fig. 22.9).

Other more specialised forms of imaging, such as ultrasound, computerised tomography, angiography and diagnostic peritoneal

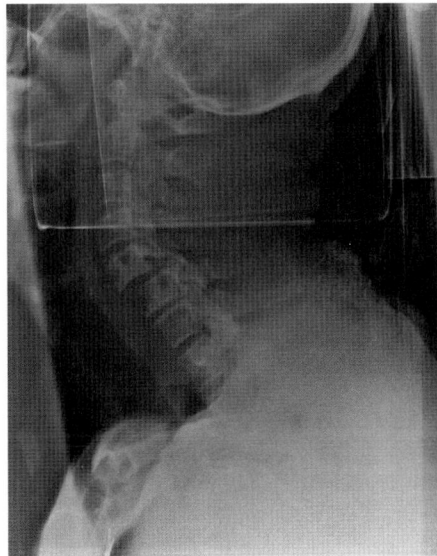

Figure 22.6 Lateral emergency room cervical spine X-ray showing complete subluxation of cervical vertebrae C5 and C6.

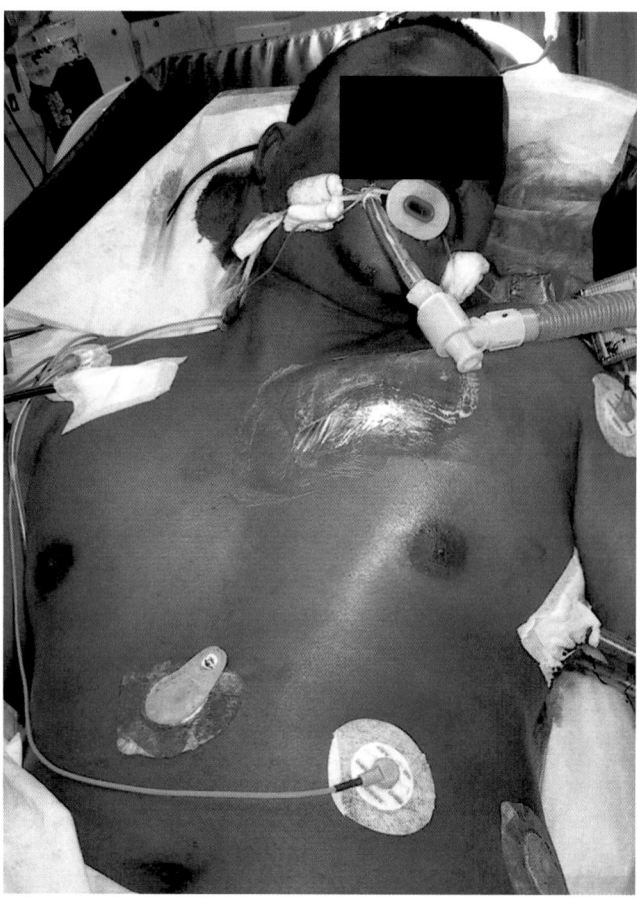

Figure 22.7 Gunshot to the chest (courtesy of Johannesburg Hospital Trauma Unit).

lavage, should be considered after the secondary survey and only when the patient is stable after initial resuscitation.

SECONDARY SURVEY

This starts *after* completion of the primary survey and once initial resuscitative measures have commenced. The purpose of the secondary survey is to identify all injuries and perform a more thorough 'head to toe' examination. If possible, it is here that the patient's history is reviewed. Again, the AMPLE mnemonic from the ATLS group is helpful here (Summary box 22.11).

Summary box 22.11

Review of patient's history (AMPLE)

- Allergy
- Medication including tetanus status
- Past medical history
- Last meal
- Events of the incident

Subsequent physical examination

Examine each region of the body for signs of injury, bony instability and tenderness to palpation.

- *Head and face*. Evaluate the head and face for maxillofacial fractures, ocular injury, open head injury and any evidence of bleeding or discharge from the ears suggestive of a basal skull fracture. Inspect the mouth, mandible, zygoma, nose and ears. This excludes midfacial injury and potential airway compromise.
- *Neck*. Inspect and palpate the cervical spine anteriorly and posteriorly for haematomas, crepitus, tenderness and evidence

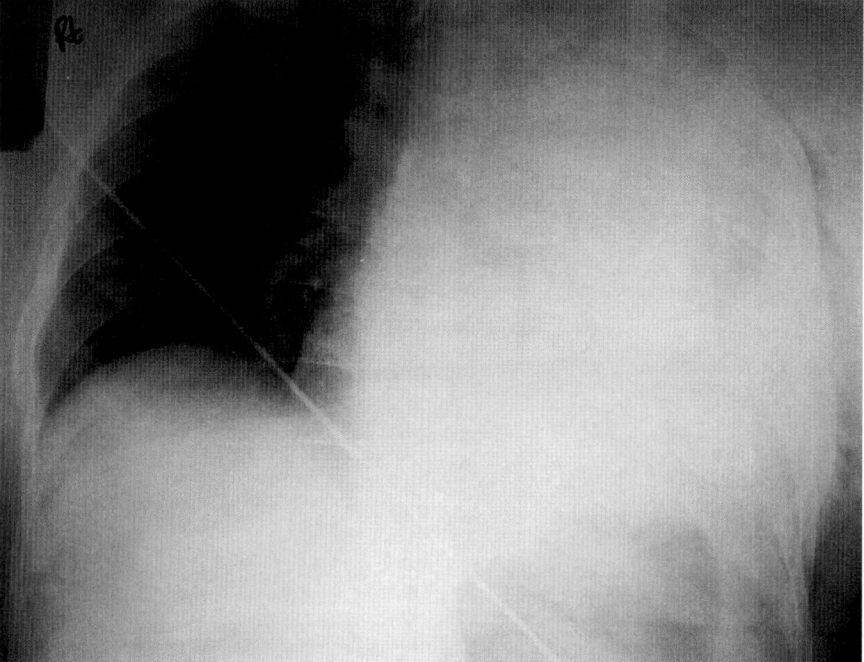

Figure 22.8 Chest radiograph in the same patient as in Fig. 22.7, demonstrating a massive haemothorax (courtesy of Johannesburg Hospital Trauma Unit).

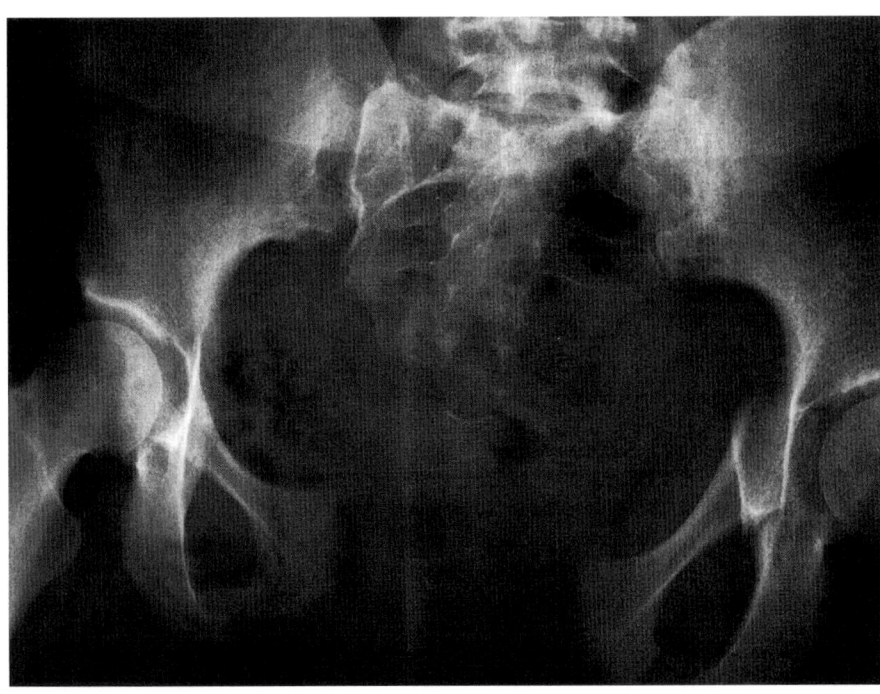

Figure 22.9 Open book pelvic fracture with haemodynamic instability requiring urgent stabilisation (courtesy of Johannesburg Hospital Trauma Unit).

of steps on palpation. In trauma where the cause and energy of injury is uncertain and where there has been a significant maxillofacial or head injury, assume a cervical spine injury until definitively excluded with radiology and clinical evaluation. The spine is held immobilised with a hard collar, sandbag and tape across the forehead. Wounds should be fully evaluated and formally explored in theatre if deeper than the platysma muscle layer.

- *Chest.* Review the primary survey and perform full palpation and auscultation of the chest wall front and (once log rolled) back. Palpate the entire chest wall including the clavicle, sternum and ribs. Sternal fractures have a high incidence of damage to the underlying cardiovascular structures, and monitoring must be present for 24–48 hours after injury. Distended neck veins, distant heart sounds and narrow pulse pressure may suggest cardiac tamponade.
- *Neurological.* Examine the GCS repeatedly (at least every 15 min). Perform a full neurological examination if the patient's condition allows. Any evidence of sensory and motor disturbance requires full spinal immobilisation and urgent review by the neurosurgeons or spinal orthopaedic surgeons with imaging as appropriate.
- *Abdomen and pelvis.* Inspect for distension, explore low-velocity local wounds to assess the depth of involvement; high-velocity injuries should be urgently evaluated in the operating room. Palpate the iliac crests for instability to detect significant fractures. Inspect the perineum for evidence of ecchymosis or bleeding. A rectal examination is needed to assess tone, prostate level and to look for bleeding. A high index of suspicion is often required with abdominal injuries, so frequent re-evaluation is important as injuries may not manifest themselves in the early stages.
- *Extremities.* It is often here that attention is diverted immediately when a dramatic injury to the limbs presents itself (Fig. 22.10). It is important to note that, unless there is severe

haemorrhage, the injury to the limb is not immediately life threatening and focus *must* be maintained on the primary survey and sequence as above. Obviously deformed limbs should be manipulated into as near anatomical alignment as possible, remembering to document neurovascular status before and after the intervention. Palpate the upper and lower limbs meticulously and systematically and document all findings. Remember to move the relevant joints to exclude dislocations. Neurovascular status must be recorded for each limb especially if a fracture is identified proximally.

- *Log roll.* Once the patient has been evaluated anteriorly, it is imperative that a log roll is performed to inspect the back. One member of the team is responsible for maintaining in-line spinal stabilisation (usually the anaesthetist when the patient is intubated), and it is on this person's orders that a gentle log roll is performed. Remember that at least four people are required for a safe log roll procedure: one for the spinal in-line traction, one for the torso and one for the pelvis and lower limbs (which ideally should be strapped together). The fourth person removes the spinal board and performs a detailed assessment of the back. Inspect the entire spine from occiput to sacrum for bony abnormalities. Identify any penetrating injuries or exit wounds from gunshot injuries and dress accordingly. Percuss, palpate and auscultate the posterior chest wall.

Re-evaluation

This cannot be stressed enough. It is an integral process in the initial assessment of major trauma and should not stop once the patient leaves the emergency room. It is often some hours or days before injuries to the hands, carpus, feet and ankles are picked up, and this is usually once the patient has stabilised and regained a level of consciousness. It is here that the initial triage of the patient can be assessed and modified accordingly, as minor trauma may evolve into major trauma as time passes.

Continuous monitoring is invaluable here, especially of the

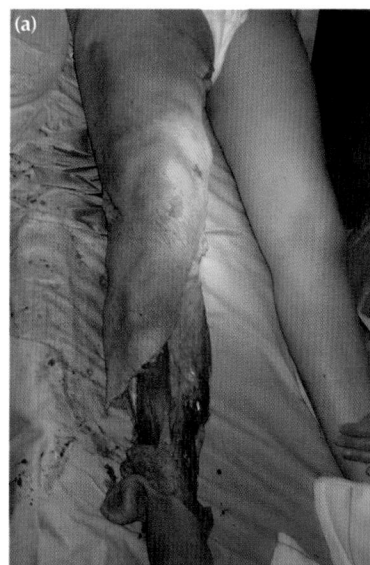

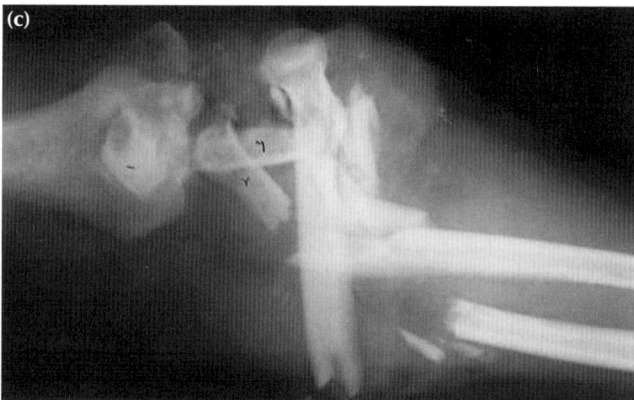

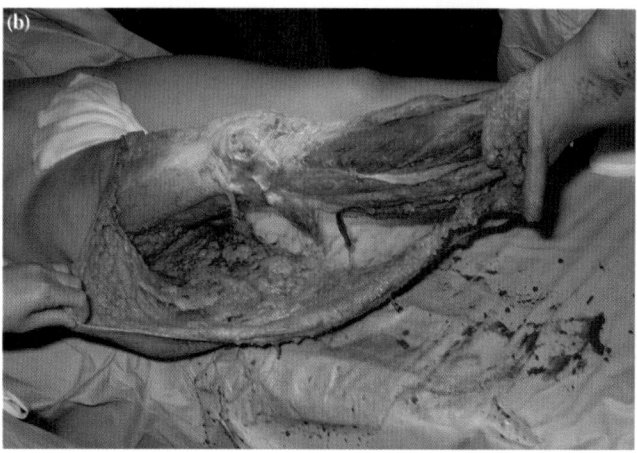

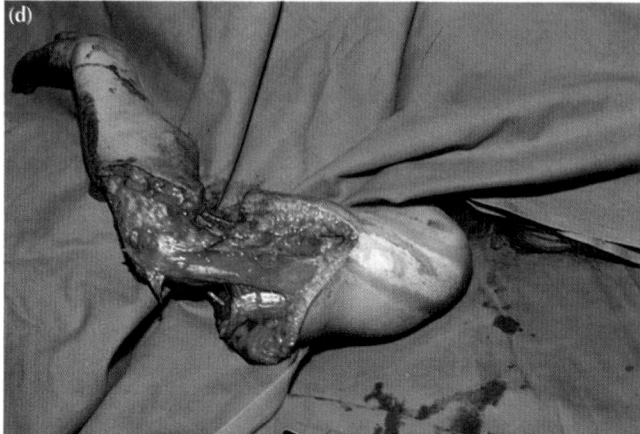

Figure 22.10 (a–d) Severe degloving injuries to the upper and lower limbs following a high-speed road traffic accident. The initial appearance and severity of the injury should not detract from following the important ATLS sequence in evaluating and treating immediate life-threatening injuries.

vital signs and urinary output. In the adult, an output of $0.5\,\mathrm{ml\,kg^{-1}\,h^{-1}}$ should be adequate, whereas in the paediatric patient, one should expect twice this rate. Pulse oximetry is a useful real-time measure of oxygenation and is sensitive to sudden changes in the patient's ventilation and airway.

Analgesia

Often neglected, it is very important to provide relief of pain in the initial management. Pain and anxiety can produce changes to the vital signs, and it is important that adequate relief is provided. This is usually by a titrated intravenous dose of opiate. The dose must be administered judiciously to avoid respiratory depression and also masking important changes in the patient's status.

Documentation and legal considerations

It is very important to keep meticulous records. Time should be documented for all entries as, in the trauma setting, changes can be rapid. Accurate record-keeping can be facilitated by having a member of the nursing staff whose sole job is to collate and record the information – of course, this is resource dependent. Consent should be sought before treatment if possible; however, in cases where the patient has life-threatening

injury and consent is not possible, it makes sense to treat first and obtain formal consent retrospectively. Forensic evidence must be kept in cases admitted as a result of criminal activity; bullets, clothing, etc. must not be discarded but should be kept for the police. Blood alcohol concentrations and those of other drugs can be very important evidence and have substantial legal implications.

Definitive care and transfer

Definitive care will be discussed in subsequent chapters, but it is important to recognise that there should be as little delay as possible in reaching this stage. Much has been made of the 'golden hour' concept, and one often finds that the majority of patients spend this hour at the scene of injury. Increasingly, it is recognised that early transfer to an appropriate care facility is the most important contributor to successful outcome. When it becomes mandatory to transfer the patient from the initial receiving hospital, the patient must be haemodynamically and cardiovascularly stable. An experienced anaesthetist should be sent with the patient, the airway should be secured and the patient intubated if necessary. Life-saving surgery, e.g. splenectomy, may need to be performed prior to transfer for other injuries.

SPECIAL SUB-GROUP CONSIDERATIONS

Essentially, initial trauma assessment and management in those without serious life-threatening injury is very similar to the guidelines indicated previously. Obviously, a good triage system needs to be in place locally to give first priority to those seriously ill. The assessment philosophy above is a very simple and reproducible one, and there is no reason why similar guidelines and protocols should not be followed when managing those who are not seriously traumatised.

However, there remain two very important groups worthy of separate consideration in the initial management and assessment of trauma, and these are the paediatric and elderly populations. Trauma receiving centres are likely to admit a large proportion of these two population sub-groups in future purely as a result of the rising global population and the increased survival of paediatric numbers worldwide. Each will be considered separately highlighting the differences in initial trauma assessment and management from the adult population.

PAEDIATRIC TRAUMA

Injury is the leading cause of mortality among children and adolescents. Road traffic accidents are the leading cause followed by drowning, house fires, homicides and falls. In fact, falls represent the leading cause of injury in children below the age of 10 years. The sequence of assessment, i.e. ABCDE, resuscitation, secondary survey and definitive care, is the same for adults and children but, in children, the signs of severe injury may be delayed on account of their greater physiological capacity to respond to the injury initially. However, once the physiology decompensates, the rapid deterioration can be devastating. Most serious paediatric trauma is blunt head injury. As a result, it is respiratory distress that occurs more frequently than cardiovascular compromise. The treating physician must be aware of the anatomical and physiological characteristics that make children unique. Children have a smaller body mass and, therefore, there is a greater force applied per unit surface area. The energy is transmitted to a body with less fat, less connective tissue and an immature skeleton; therefore, injuries to multiple organs are more frequent. As the surface area to body volume ratio is high, thermal energy loss is higher and one must guard against hypothermia.

Airway and cervical spine control

Control of the airway is the first priority. Unlike adults, the cause of arrest is not usually cardiac, but respiratory. Anatomically, children differ from adults in that they have a smaller and anterior larynx, floppy epiglottis, short trachea and large tongue. As in the adult, the airway can be opened via the chin lift or jaw thrust manoeuvres. The mouth and oropharynx are cleared of secretions and debris and, prior to inserting mechanical methods of airway maintenance, the child must be pre-oxygenated. The oral

airway should only be inserted in the unconscious child or else gagging and vomiting are likely. The airway should be carefully inserted directly into the oropharynx rather than passing it backwards and rotating 180° as in the adult. This is to minimise iatrogenic injury to the soft palate in children. The size of the endotracheal tube is estimated by the diameter of the child's fifth digit or, more accurately, by the use of the Broselow tapes. Cuffed endotracheal tubes are rarely needed for children under 9 years of age because of the delicate structures within the airway and the fact that the cricoid ring provides an adequate seal. Children can have a more pronounced vagal response to intubation, and this can be minimised by atropine pretreatment, which also reduces the secretions, permitting easier visualisation. Nasotracheal intubation in children younger than 9 years should not be performed because of the possibility of damage to the cranial vault and to the fragile soft tissues causing bleeding. Once past the glottis, the tube should be advanced only 2–3 cm below the vocal cords as the trachea is shorter in infants, and there is a very real risk of intubating the right mainstem bronchus, compromising gaseous exchange. First auscultation and then chest X-ray should be performed to confirm the position of the tube, remembering to re-evaluate regularly to ensure that the tube has not dislodged. Surgical cricothyroidectomy is rarely indicated in the infant or small child, but can be performed in the older child (usually 12 years of age) when the cricothyroid membrane is easily palpable.

Cervical spine control is similar in the child and, again, injury must be assumed, particularly when there has been serious, significant, high-energy trauma.

Breathing and ventilatory control

The respiratory rate in the child decreases with age. Infants require 40–60 breaths per minute, whereas the older child breathes 20 times per minute (Table 22.1). Hypoxia is a common cause of cardiorespiratory arrest; however, before this, hypoventilation causes a respiratory acidosis, which is the commonest acid–base disturbance in the injured child. Correction must be through adequate and controlled ventilation. Flail chest and aortic rupture are uncommon in children due to the elastic nature and resilience of the underlying structures. Pulmonary contusions are not evident in the early chest X-ray but, as before, re-evaluation is necessary for the following 24–48 hours.

Circulation with haemorrhage control

Vital signs vary with age (Table 22.1). Hypotension is a late and ominous sign of hypovolaemic shock. A 30% reduction in circulatory volume is required to manifest a change in the vital signs. Tachycardia is the primary response to circulatory compromise in children but, as in adults, may well be anxiety induced. More subtle signs are loss of peripheral pulse, skin mottling, cooled extremities and reduced pulse pressure. If intravenous access has failed after two attempts, consideration should be given to intraosseous access, especially in children younger than 6 years of

Table 22.1 Paediatric vital signs

Normal vital signs by age	Pulse (beats per min)	Systolic blood pressure (mmHg)	Respiratory rate (breaths per min)
Infant (< 1 year)	160	80	40
Preschool (< 5 years)	140	90	30
Adolescent (> 10 years)	120	100	20

age. The uninjured proximal tibia is the ideal route or, alternatively, the distal femur. The infusion should be discontinued once suitable peripheral access has been acquired. Other options are percutaneous femoral vein access or saphenous vein cutdown at the ankle. Urinary output monitoring should take into account the differences in urinary output with age (Table 22.2).

Disability

Head injury is the commonest cause of disability and death among children in trauma. The principles of assessment and management are similar to those in the adult population with strict avoidance of hypoxia and hypovolaemia. Diffuse axonal injury is more common in children than in adults, who have a higher incidence of intracranial mass lesions.

Exposure

As mentioned above, surface area to volume ratios make children particularly vulnerable to environmental changes, hypothermia in particular. Precautions must be taken in the emergency setting to prevent this occurrence. Overhead lamps or heaters, warming blankets and warmed intravenous fluids and blood are often necessary (Fig. 22.11).

Paediatric secondary survey

This is essentially similar to the head to toe examination described earlier. Consideration must be given to the fact that the liver and spleen are the commonest organs to be injured, and many of these injuries can be managed non-operatively but, as usual, extreme vigilance in monitoring and re-evaluation is mandatory. A number of visceral injuries are more common in children:

- duodenal haematoma or pancreatic injury – secondary to a handlebar striking the right upper quadrant in under-developed anterior abdominal musculature;
- small bowel perforation and mesenteric injuries;
- bladder injury is more common due to pelvic shallowness;
- restraint from a lap belt (less common now) results in enteric disruption, especially if there is an associated 'chance' fracture of the lumbar spine.

Child abuse

Intentional harm to a child is a sad and distressing part of dealing with childhood injury. There are certain markers to look for, and early identification and alerting of child protection authorities may be the single most important intervention for the child involved and prevent a potential future fatality (Summary box 22.12).

Summary box 22.12

Markers for non-accidental injury

- Repeated hospital visits for minor injuries
- Late presentations and multiple visits to different hospitals
- Vague or inconsistent history from the child's parent or guardian and the child
- Withdrawn behaviour of the child with resistance to examination
- History of abuse in a sibling
- Bite marks, finger marks, belt marks or cigarette burns
- Multiple fractures of different ages
- Perineal injury
- Intracranial haemorrhage without a history of MVA

Table 22.2 Urine output by age in the paediatric population

Age	Optimal urine output
Infant (< 1 year)	2 ml kg^{-1} h^{-1}
Preschool (1–5 years)	1.5 ml kg^{-1} h^{-1}
Child–adolescent (6–16 years)	1 ml kg^{-1} h^{-1}

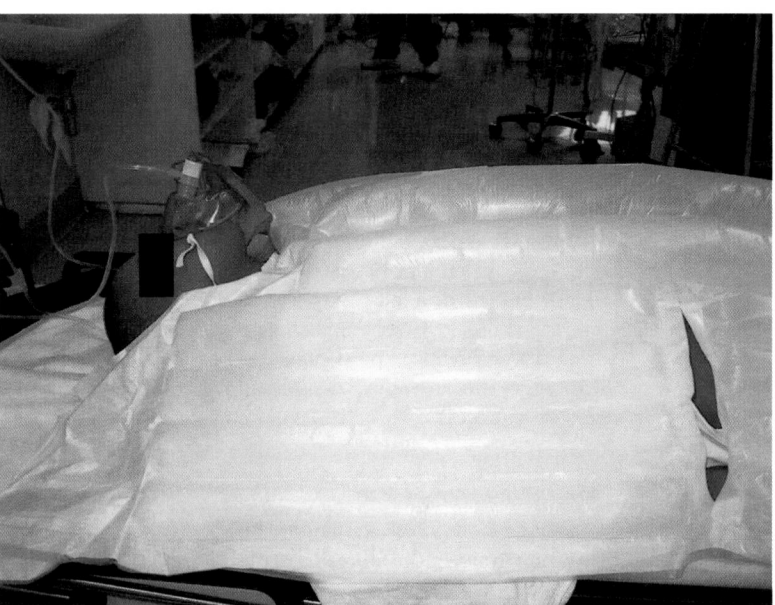

Figure 22.11 External warming blanket (courtesy of Johannesburg Hospital Trauma Unit).

George Quentin Chance, **Formerly Director of Diagnostic Radiology, The Derby Group of Hospitals, Derbyshire, England.**

TRAUMA IN THE ELDERLY POPULATION

There has been recent exposure in the literature with regard to injury in this group of patients, and trauma in the elderly population presents many challenges for the treating physicians. Some of these are not easily overcome due to the fragility of the patient's physiological status and comorbid medical conditions. Despite these poor outcomes, several reviews have advocated an aggressive approach to management because as many as 85% of elderly people return to independent function after significant trauma. It has been documented that trauma care of the injured elderly in a recognised trauma centre resulted in a sevenfold increase in survival compared with a standard receiving unit. This implies that, if one applies careful and considerate management to this fragile group of individuals, good outcome is possible. Unfortunately, despite this, it is often this very group of individuals that is neglected and triaged to low-priority treatment when compared with the younger generation. A study by Velmahos et al. in the USA revealed that mortality was significantly reduced when trauma teams were activated purely on the criteria of age alone (70 years or above) rather than waiting for changes in vital parameters. In the USA, the three leading causes of mortality from injury are falls, road traffic accidents and burns. As many as 40% of elderly people who fall will die, but the majority survive resulting in increased hospital stay and repeated visits.

Once the problems have been identified, it is very important for the attending physician to take into consideration the physiological and biological fragility of the elderly trauma patient. It does not require high-velocity or high-energy trauma to put the elderly life at risk following injury. An elderly patient may only be surviving with just enough physiological reserve, and any injury no matter how insignificant may prove fatal (Fig. 22.12). Initial assessment and, more importantly, management has to be even more meticulous in this sub-group of patients. Iatrogenic fluid overload is common, as the newly qualified resident, well versed in the management of normal adult trauma, applies the same principles of resuscitation to the elderly patient. This is a fundamental error of judgement and can have devastating consequences.

The initial assessment, however, does follow the same basic rules of primary survey, resuscitation and secondary survey followed by definitive care or transfer.

Airway and cervical spine control

This is the same for the elderly as it is in the normal population. However, one should watch for dentition status, nasopharyngeal fragility as in children, macroglossia and cervical spine and temporomandibular joint arthritis. Stiffness in the cervical spine may make the usual airway clearing measures difficult.

Breathing and ventilation

In patients with a known history of chronic obstructive airways disease, it may be prudent to consider early intubation and ventilation because of their instability in maintaining respiratory drive. Mortality rates following chest injuries in the elderly are higher; rib fractures and pulmonary contusion are not well tolerated. Pulmonary complications such as atelectasis, pneumonia and pulmonary oedema occur with great frequency and are not helped, as mentioned, by overzealous fluid prescription.

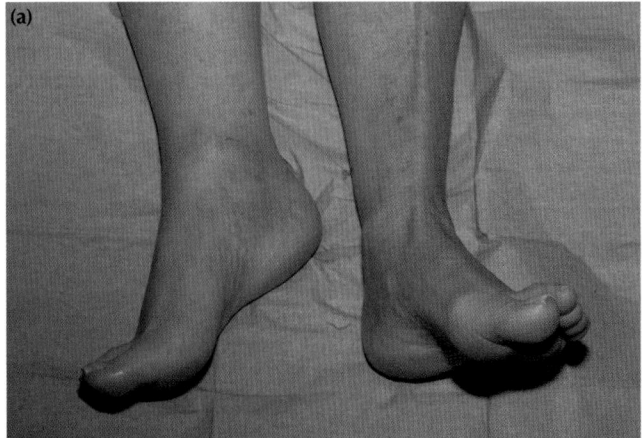

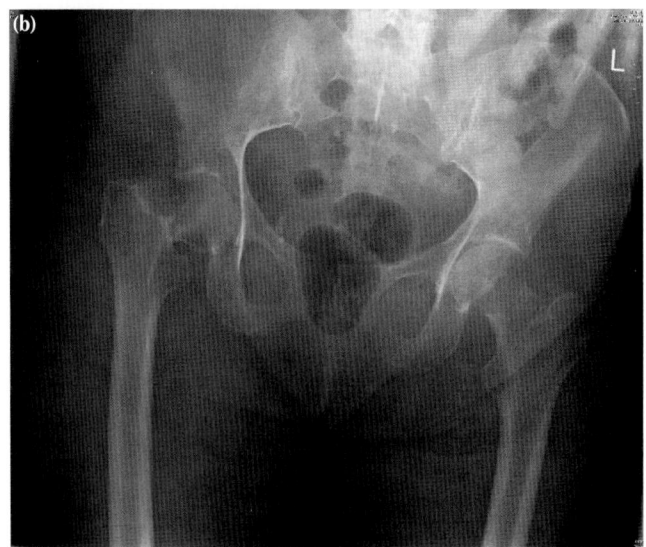

Figure 22.12 Classical shortened externally rotated right lower limb of a subcapital fractured neck of femur – it should be emphasised that this represents a significant major trauma in this vulnerable group of elderly individuals.

Circulation

By the age of 65 years, nearly 50% of the population has coronary artery stenosis. The maximum heart rate decreases with age and, therefore, it may be difficult to detect ongoing hypovolaemic shock just from the pulse rate. Urinary response changes with age; the elderly kidney is more susceptible to damage from hypovolaemia, medications and other nephrotoxins. When assessing the cardiovascular status, it is important to try and establish what the normal systolic blood pressure (SBP) is for that particular patient. An SBP of 120 mmHg may be reassuring in the young but, in the elderly, the level may indicate severe and significant life-threatening shock. Because of this limited cardiac reserve, it is essential that diagnosis of haemorrhage is rapid with early adjuncts used to assist in the diagnosis. Retroperitoneal haemorrhage may occur from relatively minor pelvic or hip fractures, and a patient who fails to stabilise after fluid resuscitation may require prompt angiography and embolisation. Prompt treatment or transfer to an appropriate facility may be life saving.

Disability

Cerebral atrophy is common with increasing age. This leads to increased space within the cranium and therefore some protection from contusion. It is surprising how much blood can collect around the brain before there are overt symptoms. Pre-existing medical conditions may be a cause of confusion in the elderly, making assessment of head injury difficult. Osteoporosis can lead to increased risk of spinal fractures after even very minor injury. Spinal injury may be more common because of pre-existing stiffness and spinal stenosis, thus predisposing to central and anterior cord syndromes.

Exposure and environment

Reduced thermoregulatory ability is well documented in the elderly. Skin vascularity and dermal thickness reduce with age, making wound healing potentially hazardous. It is essential that, as in children, the elderly patient is protected from the effects of hypothermia during the initial assessment and management.

Secondary survey in the elderly

Again, a full head to toe examination must be undertaken after careful 'AMPLE' history-taking. Owing to the friable skin condition, spinal injury should be ruled out quickly, and prolonged use of the spinal board should be avoided, reducing the risk of pressure sores developing. It is commonly a musculoskeletal injury that the patient presents with after a fall, and this is largely as a consequence of pre-existing osteoporosis and osteopenia. Muscle mass decreases with age and, at the age of 50 years, the decline is as high as 10% per decade. The result of this is that the underlying bones and joints are less protected. The commonest fracture is in the proximal femur followed by the humerus and wrist. Isolated hip fractures do not generally cause shock, but the patient has sustained a serious injury to the body and general metabolism. Often, patients are dehydrated and have been lying on the floor for several hours before being discovered. Recent literature suggests that careful resuscitation in these patients followed by early surgical stabilisation improves survival significantly. Analgesia is important in the elderly. Morphine can be titrated and given in small intravenous doses (0.5–1 mg) until adequate pain relief is achieved. A comprehensive medication history allows careful planning of treatment and can serve as warning signs for potential problems. Above all, a multidisciplinary approach must be adopted including the patient and their relatives if the definitive treatment plans are to be successful.

SUMMARY

Trauma is a massive and growing worldwide health burden. Despite injury prevention strategies, a significant number of the world's population will be exposed to or involved in trauma. In the initial assessment and management of these patients, it is demonstrated that the ATLS approach is still the most reproducible protocol for successful outcome. A team approach must be utilised, and good organisation of the system leads to very real reductions in mortality and morbidity globally. The paediatric and elderly are special groups of individuals who have unique inherent differences that must be recognised but, essentially, the framework for assessment remains the same. It is only through education and training that truly significant inroads can be made into this hugely debilitating and resource-intensive 'disease'.

FURTHER READING

Jacobs, D. (2003) Special considerations in geriatric injury. *Curr Opin Crit Care* **9**: 535–9.

Jacobs, D., Plaisier, B., Barie, P. and Hammond, J. (2003) Practice management guidelines for geriatric trauma: the EAST Practice Management Guidelines Work Group. *J Trauma* **54**: 391–416.

Peden, M., McGee, K. and Sharma, G. (2002) *The Injury Chart Book: A Graphical Overview of the Global Burden of Injuries*. World Health Organization, Geneva.

The American College of Surgeons' Committee on Trauma (2004) *Advanced Trauma Life Support Course*. American College of Surgeons, Chicago, IL.

Velmahos, G.C., Jindal, A., Chan, L.S. *et al.* (2001) Insignificant mechanism of injury: not to be taken lightly. *J Am Coll Surg* **192**: 147–52.

WEBSITE ADDRESSES

American Association for the Surgery of Trauma: www.aast.org
Eastern Association for the Surgery of Trauma: www.east.org
Trauma.org: www.trauma.org
American Orthopaedic Trauma Association: www.ota.org

Head injury

LEARNING OBJECTIVES

To understand:
- The anatomy and physiology of the skull and brain
- The classification of head injuries
- Secondary brain injury and its avoidance
- The safe treatment of head injuries

EPIDEMIOLOGY

Head injury is a frequent cause of emergency department attendance, accounting for approximately 3.4% of all presentations, with an incidence of around 450 cases per 100 000 population per year. In the UK, around 500 000 children with head injury attend hospital every year and head injury admissions account for nearly 10% of all paediatric hospital admissions.

Head injury associated with traumatic brain injury (TBI) occurs with an incidence of 20–40 cases per 100 000 population per year. It is the most common cause of death in young adults (age 15–24 years) and is more common in males than females. Road traffic accidents (RTAs) are the most common cause of TBI in the UK, followed by falls and assaults.

The cost of a poor outcome from TBI is measured not only in personal terms but also in the socio-economic costs of neuro-rehabilitation, long-term nursing and supportive care, and lost income generation.

PATHOPHYSIOLOGY

Brain metabolism

Brain oxygen consumption ($CMRO_2$, cerebral metabolic rate for oxygen) is about 3.5 ml $100\,g^{-1}\,min^{-1}$. The brain relies on blood-borne glucose for 90% of its energy requirements.

Cerebral blood flow and autoregulation

Normal cerebral blood flow is approximately 55 ml $100\,g^{-1}\,min^{-1}$ and is usually maintained at a constant level via mechanisms termed cerebral autoregulation. This is despite variations in mean arterial pressure (MAP) of between 50 and 150 mmHg.

In TBI, mechanisms of cerebral autoregulation become disordered. Cerebral blood flow then fluctuates with MAP and the brain is more vulnerable to hypotension.

Intracranial pressure and brain herniation

The brain is confined by a rigid container, the skull. The addition of a mass lesion can initially be compensated for by the displacement of cerebrospinal fluid (CSF) and venous blood out of the intracranial cavity. During this period the intracranial pressure (ICP) will remain at normal levels (Fig. 23.1). As further expansion of the mass lesion occurs, quite small increases in volume result in relatively large increases in ICP, brain herniation and rapid clinical deterioration (Figs 23.2 and 23.3).

Primary vs. secondary brain injury

Primary brain injury occurs at the time of impact and includes injuries such as brainstem and hemispheric contusions, diffuse axonal injury and cortical lacerations.

Secondary brain injury occurs at some time after the moment of impact and is often preventable. The principle causes of secondary brain injury are hypoxia, hypotension, raised ICP, reduced cerebral perfusion pressure and pyrexia (Summary box 23.1). Prevention of secondary brain injury results in improved neurological outcome after head injury and may make the difference between independent survival and dependent survival/death.

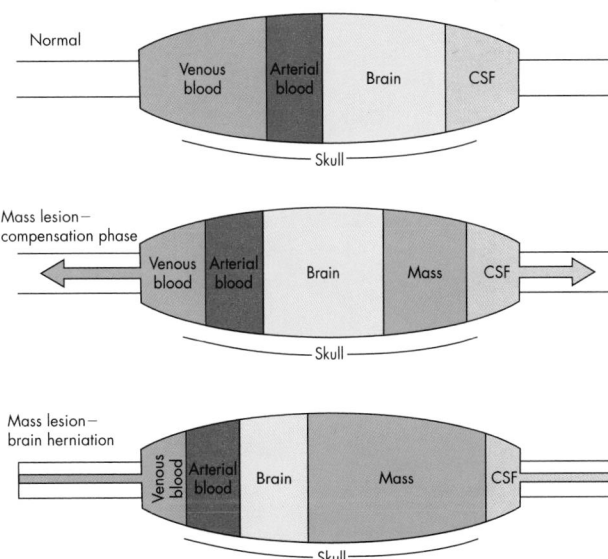

Figure 23.1 As a mass lesion increases in size there is initially a compensation during which the intracranial pressure remains normal. After the point of decompensation, very small increases in size of the mass lesion cause marked increases in intracranial pressure.

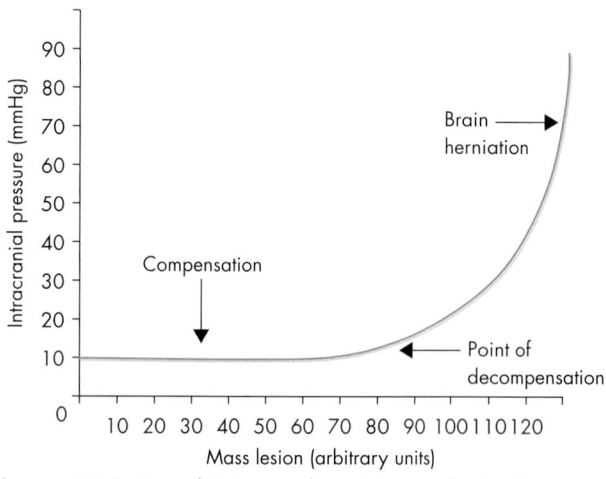

Figure 23.2 Normal intracranial contents are brain tissue, cerebrospinal fluid (CSF) and arterial and venous blood. During the compensation phase, CSF and venous blood volumes are reduced. When this egress of CSF and venous blood is maximal, further increases in the size of the mass lesion will cause brain herniation.

Summary box 23.1

Causes of secondary brain injury

- Hypoxia: $Po_2 < 8$ kPa
- Hypotension: systolic blood pressure (SBP) < 90 mmHg
- Raised intracranial pressure (ICP): ICP > 20 mmHg
- Low cerebral perfusion pressure (CPP): CPP < 65 mmHg
- Pyrexia
- Seizures
- Metabolic disturbance

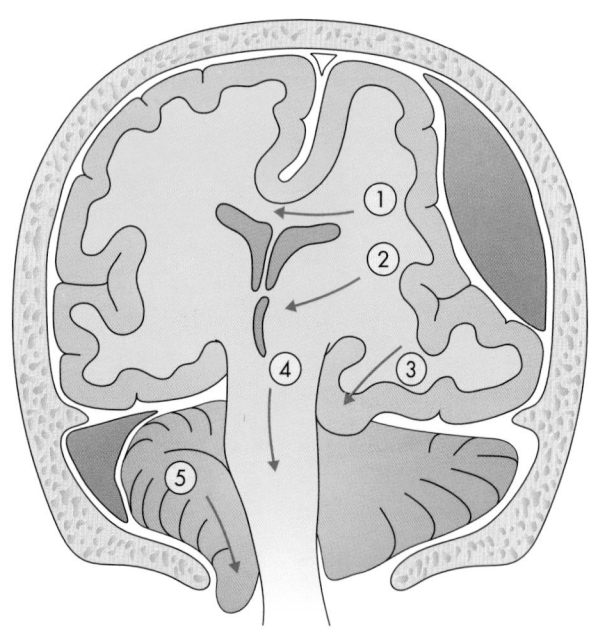

Figure 23.3 Brain herniation. Herniation of the cingulate gyrus under the falx cerebri is called subfalcine herniation (1). Herniation is associated with midline shift (2). Herniation of the uncus of the temporal lobe (3) is associated with compression of the ipsilateral third nerve. Central herniation (4) and tonsillar herniation (5) are associated with compression of brainstem structures.

CLASSIFICATION OF HEAD INJURY

Glasgow Coma Score

Severity of head injury is classified according to the Glasgow Coma Score (GCS) (Table 23.1), as the GCS – and in particular the motor score – is the best predictor of neurological outcome:

- minor head injury: GCS 15 with no loss of consciousness (LOC);
- mild head injury: GCS 14 or 15 with LOC;
- moderate head injury: GCS 9–13;
- severe head injury: GCS 3–8.

Blunt vs. penetrating

Head injury may be classified as blunt or penetrating. Penetrating head injuries are further divided into low-velocity injuries such as those caused by stabbing and high-velocity injuries such as gunshot injuries (Figs 23.4 and 23.5).

Morphological

A head injury may be classified according to the type of injury that has occurred.

Skull fractures may be divided into vault or base of skull fractures. Vault fractures may be open or closed, linear or comminuted, depressed or non-depressed. Base of skull fractures may or may not be associated with CSF rhinorrhoea and otorrhoea or cranial nerve palsy.

Intracranial haematomas may be extradural, subdural, subarachnoid or intracerebral. Areas of mixed-density intracerebral haematoma in head injury are termed contusions.

CLINICAL FEATURES

History

A history (Summary box 23.2) should begin with the mechanism of injury. A dangerous mechanism of injury such as a fall from a

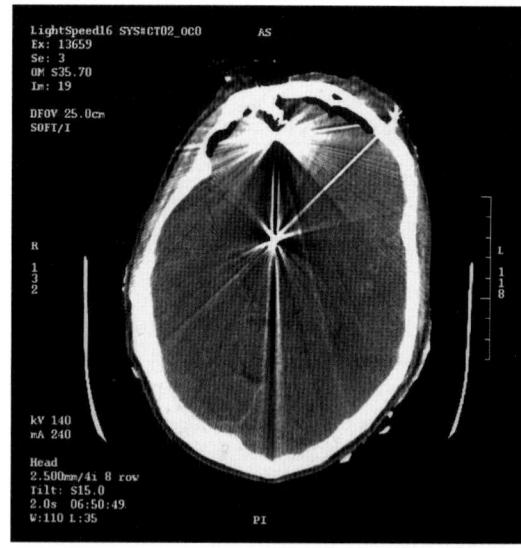

Figure 23.4 High-velocity penetrating head injury. This axial computerised tomography (CT) scan of the head was performed for a patient with a shotgun injury. Note the frontal soft tissue swelling, skull fracture and intracranial air (black). The shotgun pellets cause large CT artefacts: one pellet is lodged in the frontal lobe, the other sits just in front of the brainstem in the prepontine cistern.

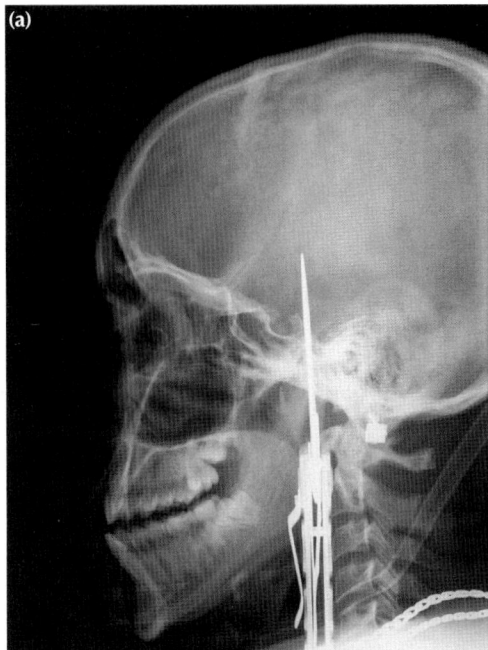

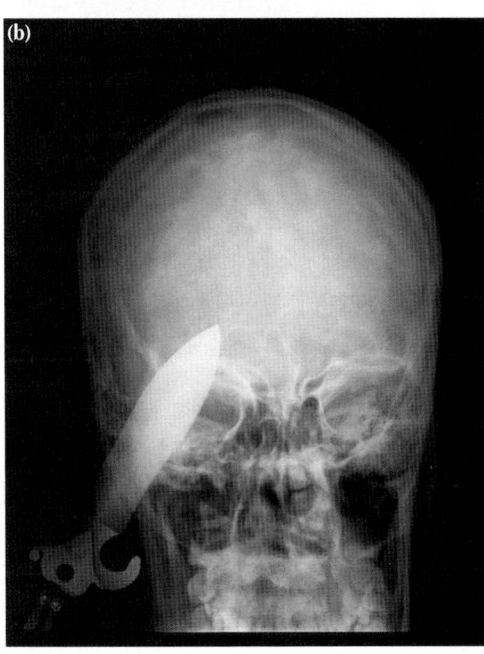

Figure 23.5 Low-velocity penetrating head injury. Lateral (a) and anteroposterior (b) skull radiographs of a patient who has sustained a stab wound to the head.

height or a high-speed motor vehicle accident should make you suspicious of multisystem injury, including spinal injury. A head injury with LOC when there is no clear accidental mechanism of injury should prompt you to think of non-accidental causes of collapse, such as syncope or aneurysmal subarachnoid haemorrhage, or medical conditions, such as hypoglycaemia.

Try to establish the neurological status of the patient at the time of the injury and soon afterwards. Is there a history of LOC or amnesia? Amnesia may be antegrade (for events after the injury) or retrograde (for events preceding the injury). Was the

patient responding, moving and talking appropriately after the incident? Was there evidence of seizure activity?

In the severely head-injured patient, what was the GCS at the scene, prior to intubation or on arrival at hospital? Have there been any abnormalities of pupillary responses? Is there a history of possible hypoxia or cardiovascular instability?

As with all trauma patients, any available history regarding pre-existing medical conditions, medication and drug allergies will be useful. In particular, the use of medications such as anticoagulants or anti-platelet drugs will be relevant to a patient with an intracranial haematoma. Is there a history of alcohol or illicit drug use? Is the patient on insulin?

Summary box 23.2

Taking a history in head injury

- **Mechanism of injury**
- **Loss of consciousness or amnesia**
- **Level of consciousness at scene and on transfer**
- **Evidence of seizures**
- **Probable hypoxia or hypotension**
- **Pre-existing medical conditions**
- **Medications (especially anticoagulants)**
- **Illicit drugs and alcohol**

Examination

Examination (Summary box 23.3) should begin with resuscitation and a primary survey. The cervical spine should be immobilised with three-point fixation. 'D' in the ABCDE approach to a primary survey stands for disability and should include assessment of pupillary size and reactivity, GCS and the presence of focal neurological signs. A full head, neck and peripheral nerve examination is performed as part of the secondary survey. Neurological examination should be repeated frequently and recorded, as changes in neurological status imply alterations in ICP and changes in the GCS (especially deterioration) are much more important indicators of the need for treatment than any absolute level.

The GCS is composed of eye (E), verbal (V) and motor (M) responses (see Table 23.1). The best possible score is 15/15 and

Table 23.1 Glasgow Coma Score (GCS)

Eyes open	Spontaneously	4
	To verbal command	3
	To painful stimulus	2
	Do not open	1
Verbal	Normal oriented conversation	5
	Confused	4
	Inappropriate/words only	3
	Sounds only	2
	No sounds	1
	Intubated patient	T
Motor	Obeys commands	6
	Localises to pain	5
	Withdrawal/flexion	4
	Abnormal flexion (decorticate)	3
	Extension (decerebrate)	2
	No motor response	1

the worst possible score is 3/15. For each category, the score given is the best score obtained during the examination. For example, if a patient localises to pain on one side and extends to pain on the other then the motor score is 5/6. If the patient is not eye opening or obeying commands in response to verbal stimuli, then a painful stimulus must be applied. This stimulus should ideally be applied in the region of trigeminal nerve innervation, such as the supraorbital ridge, but it is commonly accepted practice to use a sternal rub or trapezius squeeze. A patient who is eye opening to painful stimuli, saying occasional words and flexing to pain has a GCS of 9/15 (E2, V3, M4). Always record the three components of the GCS and use this when communicating with other doctors. If a patient is intubated then the verbal score is 'T'. For example, a patient who opens eyes to speech (E2), is intubated (VT) and localises to pain (M5) has a GCS of 7T/15.

The pupillary light response should be recorded. The pupillary size is recorded in millimetres and the light response as present, sluggish or absent. Anisocoria or an asymmetrical sluggish response may suggest partial third nerve dysfunction on the side with the larger or sluggish pupil, implying uncal herniation as a result of a mass on the ipsilateral side. As the third nerve becomes increasingly compromised the ipsilateral pupil will become fixed and dilated. There are several pitfalls in the examination of pupillary responses in a head-injured patient. It may be difficult or impossible to expose the cornea because of periorbital bruising. Direct ocular trauma may cause a traumatic mydriasis that can be confused with a third nerve palsy. Traumatic mydriasis is suspected if there is evidence of ocular trauma and if the pupillary dilatation has been present since the time of injury. The patient may have cataracts or other pre-existing causes of anisocoria such as a Holmes–Adie pupil.

Secondary survey in a head-injured patient also includes a detailed examination of the head, face and neck. First, look and feel the scalp. There may be evidence of external head injury such as subgaleal haematoma or scalp laceration, which may be a cause of significant external blood loss. Palpation of a scalp laceration may reveal an underlying skull fracture with or without a CSF leak. Look for clinical evidence of skull base fracture: bilateral periorbital bruising (raccoon eyes), Battle's sign (bruising over the mastoid, see Fig. 23.6), CSF rhinorrhea or otorrhea, or haemotympanum. Bleeding from an ear may result from local trauma or from a skull base fracture with a perforated tympanum. A skull base fracture may be associated with a facial or vestibulo-cochlear cranial nerve injury. Examine the eyes. Look for evidence of injury to the conjunctiva or cornea. Re-examine the pupils. Using an ophthalmoscope, look for major hyphaema or retinal detachment. Examine eye movements: gaze paresis, dysconjugate gaze or roving eye movements suggest midbrain or brainstem dysfunction. Assess the facial skeleton for evidence of orbital ridge, zygomatic or maxillary fractures.

A peripheral nerve examination should record limb tone, evidence of motor weakness or sensory loss, and reflexes. In those patients with an associated spine injury it is important to document neurological deficits, particularly if the patient is likely to be

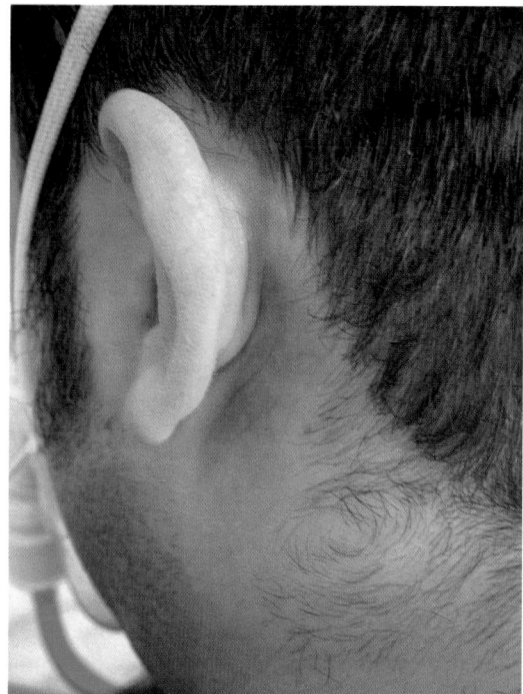

Figure 23.6 Battle's sign. A skull base fracture may be associated with bruising over the mastoid process.

moved to the operating theatre or to intensive care where such an assessment will not be possible for some time afterwards.

The neurological examination must be recorded and repeated in a patient admitted with head injury. A change in neurological status that is picked up early will result in timely investigation and treatment of emergent problems and will help prevent secondary brain injury.

Summary box 23.3

Examination in head injury

- Glasgow Coma Score
- Pupil size and response
- Lateralising signs
- Signs of base of skull fracture
  - Bilateral periorbital oedaema (raccoon eyes)
  - Battle's sign (bruising over mastoid)
  - Cerebrospinal fluid rhinorrhoea or otorrhoea
  - Haemotympanum or bleeding from ear
- Full neurological examination: tone, power, sensation, reflexes

---

MANAGEMENT OF MILD HEAD INJURY (GCS 14–15)

The majority of patients presenting to hospital with a mild head injury are discharged from the emergency department after history, examination and a period of observation. The following criteria must be met before discharge: the patient must have a

A raccoon is a small mammal native to North and Central America which has a pale face with dark rings round its eyes.

GCS of 15/15 with no focal neurological deficit; the patient must be accompanied by a responsible adult and should not be under the influence of alcohol or other drugs; verbal and written head injury advice must be given to the patient and their accompanying adult.

Written head injury advice describes to patients the symptoms that should prompt them to obtain further medical advice, which usually involves a return to the emergency department. These include persistent or worsening headache despite analgesia, persistent vomiting, drowsiness, visual disturbance such as double or blurred vision, and development of weakness or numbness in the limbs.

Some patients with mild head injury are at significant risk of intracranial haematoma and require a computerised tomography (CT) scan. Selecting which patients should have a CT scan is not always easy. On the one hand, scanning all patients with minor head injury would be expensive, time-consuming and would unnecessarily expose thousands of patients to ionising radiation. On the other hand, a missed intracranial haematoma is a potentially life-threatening medical error. The National Institute for Health and Clinical Excellence (NICE) has published some guidelines for when to carry out a CT scan in a patient with mild head injury (Summary box 23.4). If a patient fulfils the criteria for a CT scan according to these guidelines, then the decision to discharge the patient without a scan should only be made by a senior clinician experienced in the management of head injury.

Summary box 23.4

NICE guidelines for computerised tomography (CT) in head injury

- Glasgow Coma Score (GCS) < 13 at any point
- GCS 13 or 14 at 2 hours
- Focal neurological deficit
- Suspected open, depressed or basal skull fracture
- Seizure
- Vomiting > one episode

Urgent CT head scan if none of the above but:
- Age > 65
- Coagulopathy (e.g. on warfarin)
- Dangerous mechanism of injury (CT within 8 hours)
- Antegrade amnesia > 30 min (CT within 8 hours)

MANAGEMENT OF MODERATE TO SEVERE HEAD INJURY

Management of a patient with a moderate to severe head injury begins with resuscitation and a primary survey. The principle aim of treatment is the prevention of secondary brain injury and this is best achieved by the avoidance of hypoxia and hypotension. It follows that investigations such as a CT scan of the head are of secondary importance to restoring normal oxygenation and blood pressure, even if that means going to the operating theatre to prevent on-going abdominal or pelvic blood loss. The cervical spine must be immobilised with three-point fixation until such time as an appropriate radiological investigation can be performed.

Having completed the primary survey and established the presence of a moderate to severe head injury, the next appropriate step is a CT scan of the head. This investigation is aimed

at identifying an intracranial haematoma, the evacuation of which will reduce intracerebral pressure and reduce the likelihood of secondary brain injury. The CT scan will also provide information about scalp soft tissue injury, skull fracture, including base of skull fracture, and lesions not requiring immediate surgery, such as small intracerebral contusions. In the case of an intubated patient, it is useful at this point to request, in addition to a CT scan of the head, a CT scan of the entire cervical spine with three-dimensional reformatting to expedite radiological cervical spine clearance.

Early consultation with the local neurosurgical service is advised. Simple measures to reduce ICP include positioning the patient with the head up 20–30° [reverse Trendelenburg (head up) when the spine has not been cleared] and making sure that the cervical immobilisation collar is not so tight as to restrict venous return from the head. In patients with pupillary dilatation suggesting acutely raised ICP, the administration of 0.5 mg kg^{-1} of 20% mannitol will temporarily reduce ICP during interhospital transfer or on the way to theatre. Excessive use of this osmotic diuretic can lead to hypovolaemia and hypotension.

SURGICAL MANAGEMENT OF HEAD INJURY

Extradural haematoma

An extradural haematoma (EDH) is a neurosurgical emergency. An EDH is nearly always associated with a skull fracture and is more common in young male patients. The skull fracture is associated with tearing of a meningeal artery and a haematoma accumulates in the space between bone and dura. The most common site is temporal, as the pterion is not only the thinnest part of the skull but also overlies the largest meningeal artery – the middle meningeal. An EDH may also occur in other regions such as frontal as well as in the posterior fossa. They are not always arterial: disruption of a major dural venous sinus can result in an EDH. The force required to sustain a skull fracture can be surprisingly small – a fall from standing or a single blow to the head.

The classical presentation of an EDH, occurring in less than one-third of cases, is initial injury followed by a lucid interval when the patient complains of a headache but is fully alert and orientated with no focal deficit. After minutes or hours a rapid deterioration occurs, with contralateral hemiparesis, reduced conscious level and ipsilateral pupillary dilatation as a result of brain compression and herniation. This type of presentation reinforces the important point that there may be no primary brain injury with an EDH. Early recognition and treatment of the condition is likely to result in full recovery whereas delays in diagnosis and treatment can result in death from secondary brain injury. Of course, a patient with an EDH may also sustain a primary brain injury and have a reduced conscious level from the time of injury.

The features of an EDH on a CT scan are a lentiform (lens-shaped or biconvex) hyperdense lesion between the skull and brain (Fig. 23.7). There may be an associated mass effect on the underlying brain, with or without a midline shift. Areas of mixed density may be seen in a lesion that is actively bleeding.

The treatment of an EDH is immediate surgical evacuation

Friedrich Trendelenburg, **1844–1924, Professor of Surgery successively at Rostock (1875–1882), Bonn (1882–1895) and Leipzig (1895–1911), Germany. The Trendelenburg position was first described in 1885.**

(a)

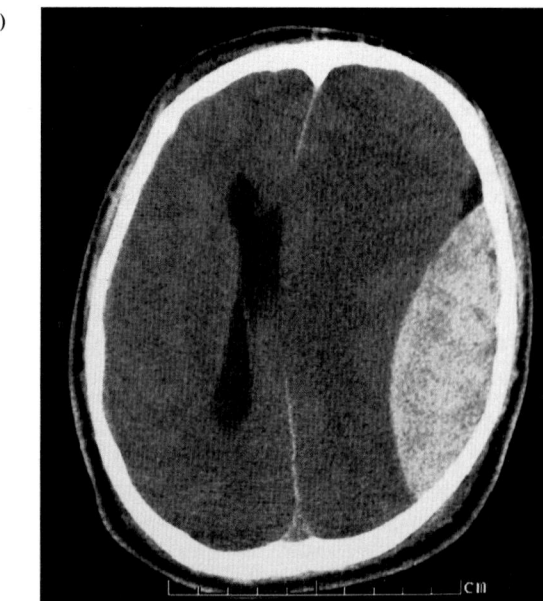

(b)

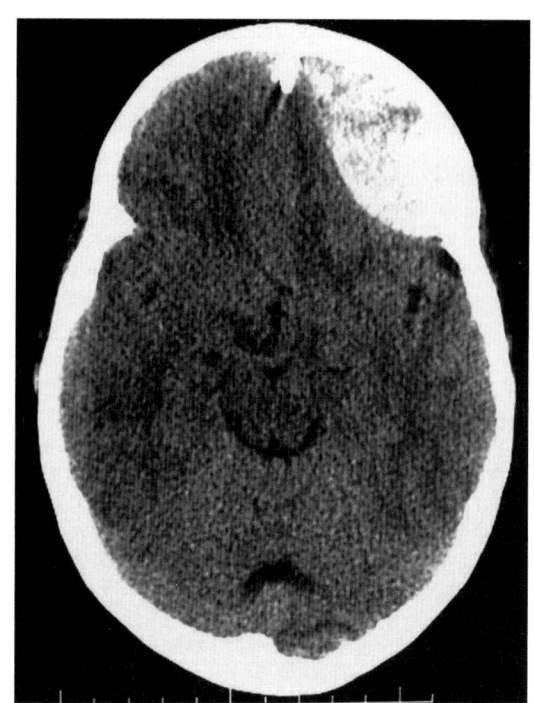

(c)

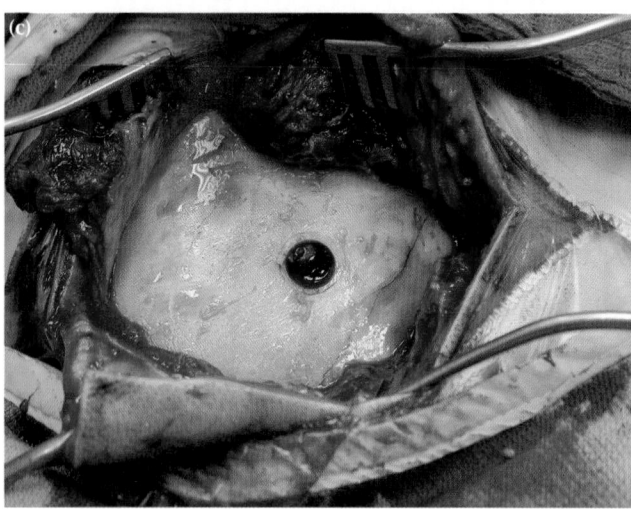

Figure 23.7 (a) An axial computerised tomography (CT) scan of a large left-sided extradural haematoma with mass effect and midline shift. (b) An axial CT scan of a left frontal extradural haematoma. Note the biconvex shape of the haematomas. (c) A surgical temporal bone exposure showing a linear skull fracture with underlying extradural haematoma visible through a burr hole.

via a craniotomy. Access to neurosurgical services often requires an interhospital transfer and delays in time to theatre have a direct impact on patient outcome. Expedited transfer and good communication between medical teams is the key to good results. The overall mortality for all cases of EDH is about 18% but for isolated EDH it is about 2%.

Acute subdural haematoma

Acute subdural haematoma (ASDH) differs from EDH in terms of pathophysiology, presentation and prognosis.

An ASDH accumulates in the space between the dura and the arachnoid. To produce a subdural haematoma there has usually been some disruption of a cortical vessel or brain laceration, and ASDH is nearly always associated with a significant primary brain injury. Patients with ASDH usually present with an impaired conscious level from the time of injury, but further deterioration can occur as the haematoma expands.

The CT appearance of an ASDH is also hyperdense (acute blood) but the haematoma spreads across the surface of the brain giving it a rather diffuse and concave appearance (Fig. 23.8). This occurs because there is less resistance to blood moving through the subdural space than through the extradural space.

The treatment of an ASDH is usually evacuation via a craniotomy. Small haematomas with little mass effect may be managed conservatively in neurosurgical centres. It may be inappropriate to perform surgery on cases with a very poor prognosis: factors such as best GCS, pupillary reactivity, age and presence of anticoagulants must be taken into account. Early consultation with neurosurgery is advised.

The mortality rate from ASDH is much higher than for EDH and is as high as 40% in some series.

Subarachnoid haemorrhage

Although aneurysms are the most common cause of spontaneous subarachnoid haemorrhage, trauma is by far the commonest cause of subarachnoid haemorrhage overall. In rare cases, a spontaneous aneurysmal haemorrhage immediately precedes a head injury. Traumatic subarachnoid haemorrhage is managed conservatively.

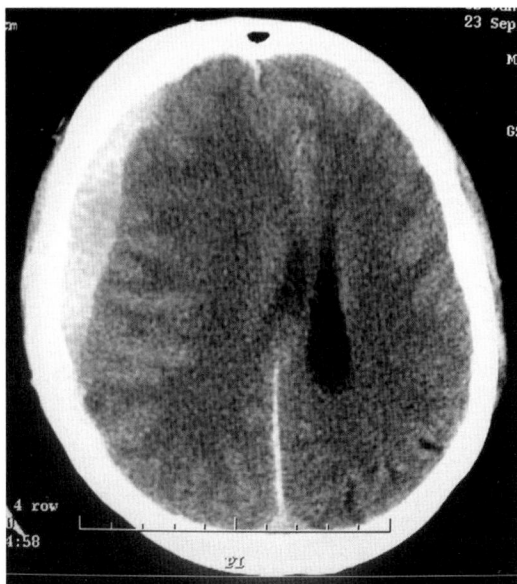

Figure 23.8 An axial computerised tomography (CT) scan of a right-sided acute subdural haematoma. Note the midline shift to the left. The right hemisphere is swollen relative to the left, reflecting an underlying primary brain injury on the right.

Chronic subdural haematoma

Chronic subdural haematomas (CSDH) usually occur in the elderly and are more common in those on anti-coagulant or anti-platelet agents. There is usually but not always a history of minor head injury in the weeks or months prior to presentation. It is thought that small bridging veins tear and cause a small ASDH which is clinically silent. As the haematoma breaks down it increases in volume, leading to a mass effect on the underlying brain.

Clinical features of CSDH include headache, cognitive decline, focal neurological deficits and seizures. It is important to exclude hypoxic, metabolic and endocrine disorders in this group of patients.

The CT appearance of a CSDH is variable. Acute blood (0–10 days) is hyperdense whereas subacute blood (10 days to 2 weeks) is isodense relative to brain; chronic blood (> 2 weeks) is hypo-dense. A CSDH will often have areas of more recent haemor-rhage in more dependent (posterior) areas and is then termed an acute-on-chronic subdural haematoma. The extent of acute ver-sus chronic blood is important as it affects the method of haematoma evacuation.

Treatment of a CSDH and most acute-on-chronic subdural haematomas is evacuation via burr hole(s) rather than cranio-tomy. This is an important distinction as burr holes can be easily performed under local anaesthetic in an elderly patient with extensive comorbidity.

Cerebral contusions

Cerebral contusions are common in head injury and result from the brain being damaged by impacting against the skull either at the point of impact (the 'coup') or on the other side of the head ('contre-coup') or as the brain slides forwards and backwards over the ridged cranial fossa floor (most often affecting the inferior frontal lobes and temporal poles).

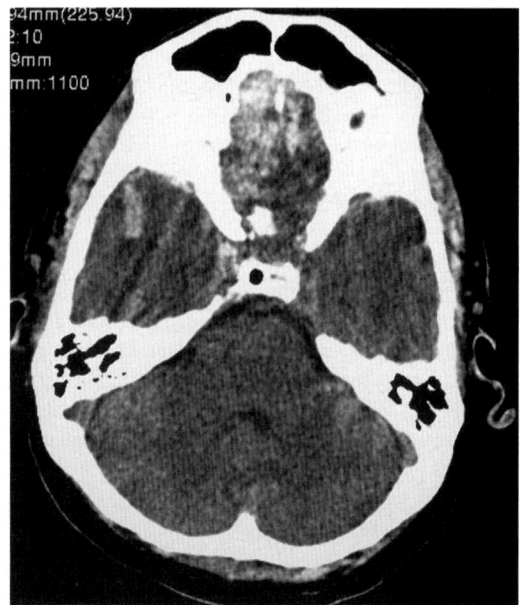

(a)

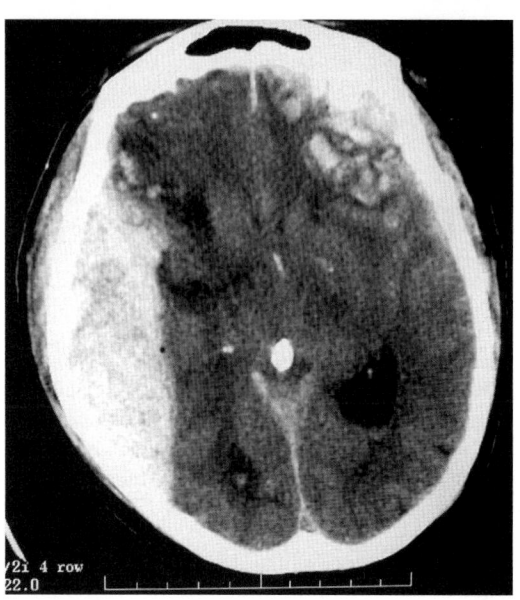

(b)

Figure 23.9 (a) An axial computerised tomography (CT) scan show-ing cerebral contusions at the base of the frontal lobe bilaterally and in the right temporal pole. (b) An axial CT scan showing a right extradural haematoma as well as widespread cerebral contusions, which are worse in the left frontal lobe, and traumatic subarachnoid blood in the third and lateral ventricles.

Cerebral contusions on CT appear heterogeneous with mixed areas of high and low density (Fig. 23.9). There may be an asso-ciated mass effect. A contusion may be described as an intracere-bral haematoma if the lesion contains a large amount of fresh haemorrhage and therefore appears uniformly hyperdense.

Cerebral contusions rarely require immediate surgical treat-ment. A head-injured patient with cerebral contusions must be admitted for observation as these lesions will tend to mature and expand for 48–72 hours following injury. A small proportion of cerebral contusions will require delayed surgical evacuation to reduce the mass effect.

CHAPTER 23 | HEAD INJURY

Intracranial pressure monitoring

ICP monitoring is a useful adjunct in the management of unconscious patients with head injury. A sustained ICP of > 20 mmHg is associated with a worse outcome. The ICP can also be used to calculate the cerebral perfusion pressure (see Circulation and cerebral perfusion pressure, below). An ICP monitor may be parenchymal or ventricular (Fig. 23.10).

Decompressive craniectomy

Controversy still surrounds the use of decompressive craniectomy. The purpose of a decompressive craniectomy is to control the ICP in patients without a focal intracerebral haematoma in whom the ICP is refractory to maximal medical therapy. The operation involves removing a large section of skull and opening the dura, allowing the swollen brain to expand underneath the scalp (Fig. 23.11). The bone flap is stored and can be replaced 3–6 months later when the patient has made a good neurological recovery and the brain swelling has resolved.

Summary box 23.5

Surgical management of raised intracranial pressure

- Early evacuation of focal haematomas: EDH, ASDH
- Cerebrospinal fluid drainage via ventriculostomy
- Delayed evacuation of swelling contusions
- Decompressive craniectomy

MEDICAL MANAGEMENT OF SEVERE HEAD INJURY

Environment

Severe head injury is best managed in a neurointensive care setting and mortality is reduced compared with general units even if no neurosurgery is performed (Fig. 23.12). The patient should be positioned with the head up 30° if spinal clearance allows. It is important to ensure that the cervical immobilisation collar does not obstruct venous return from the head.

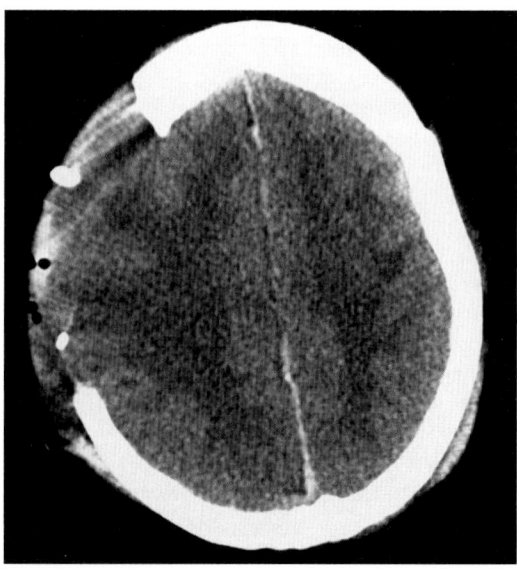

Figure 23.11 Decompressive craniectomy. A right-sided decompressive craniectomy has been performed allowing the swollen right hemisphere to herniate through the skull defect. This procedure can help to control raised intracranial pressure. The bone flap can be stored and replaced at a later date.

Airway and ventilation

A definitive airway is required in cases of severe head injury for several reasons: the patient in traumatic coma is unable to protect their airway and is at risk of aspiration; gas exchange may be impaired; the safe interhospital transfer of a patient with an impaired conscious level and who is at risk of further neurological deterioration en route requires intubation.

Normal gas exchange in the head-injured patient must be confirmed and maintained. Hypoxia and hypercapnia will result in increased brain ischaemia and secondary brain injury. A single episode of hypoxia with a $PO_2 < 8$ kPa is associated with a worse outcome in traumatic coma.

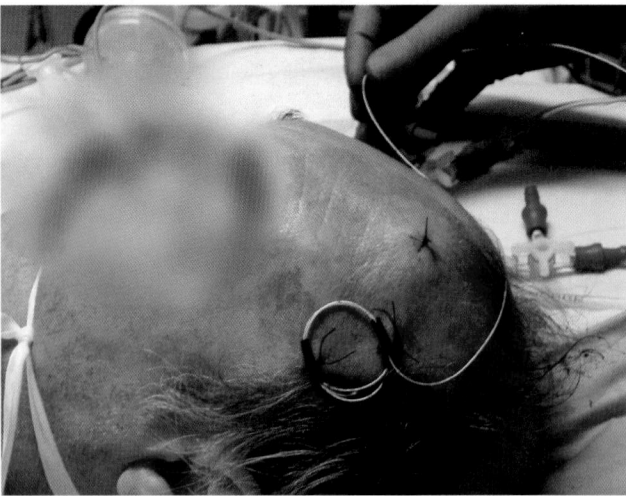

Figure 23.10 Intracranial pressure (ICP) monitoring. A tunnelled parenchymal ICP monitor can be inserted through a twist drill burr hole, in this case into the left frontal lobe.

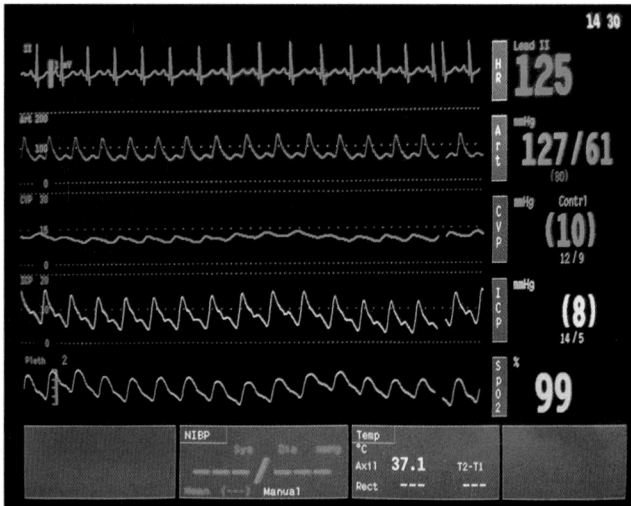

Figure 23.12 Monitoring in neurointensive care. The traces from top to bottom display electrocardiogram (ECG), continuous arterial blood pressure, central venous pressure, intracranial pressure and oxygen saturation.

In the intubated patient, normocapnia is maintained: PCO_2 4.5–5.0 kPa. The cerebral vasculature is reactive to CO_2 levels. A rise in PCO_2 in a head-injured patient with an abnormally high ICP will result in generalised cerebral vasodilatation, an increase in cerebral blood volume, further raised ICP and reduced cerebral perfusion. Conversely, a fall in PCO_2 will result in generalised vasoconstriction, a fall in cerebral blood volume and a drop in ICP. Although this global effect on ICP may seem beneficial it occurs at the expense of perfusion of ischaemic areas of the brain and therefore will result in a higher likelihood of cerebral infarction than recovery from ischaemia. It is for this reason that hyperventilation to induce hypocapnia is used only by anaesthetists experienced in the care of head-injured patients as an emergency measure, to temporarily reduce ICP while definitive care or urgent investigation is being organised.

Circulation and cerebral perfusion pressure

Hypotension sits alongside hypoxia as a major cause of secondary brain injury. A single episode of hypotension with a systolic blood pressure of < 90 mmHg is associated with a worse outcome in traumatic coma. Cerebral perfusion pressure should be maintained at > 65 mmHg in severely head-injured patients. This is an independent prognostic factor in neurological outcome. Global cerebral perfusion can be estimated by the equation:

$$\text{Cerebral perfusion pressure} = \text{mean arterial pressure} - \text{intracranial pressure} \tag{23.1}$$

$$CPP = MAP - ICP$$

If the ICP is 20 mmHg, it follows that the MAP should be ≥ 85 mmHg.

Control of intracranial pressure

Normal ICP is 8–12 mmHg. A sustained ICP of > 20 mmHg is associated with poor outcome. As well as the environmental, respiratory and circulation measures outlined above, measures to reduce ICP include:

- *Sedation*, with or without muscle relaxants.
- *Use of diuretics*. Judicious use of diuretics such as furosemide and mannitol will temporarily reduce cerebral swelling and ICP.
- *Thermoregulation*. Pyrexia will increase the brain metabolic rate and should be avoided. Active cooling to reduce the metabolic rate is of questionable overall benefit but is used in some centres.
- *Use of barbiturates*. The use of agents such as thiopentone reduces the brain metabolic rate and helps reduce ICP. Barbiturates are associated with respiratory and metabolic complications and can take days to clear from the body. Dosage is guided by burst suppression on electroencephalogram (EEG) monitoring.
- *Maintaining fluid and electrolyte balance*. Severely brain-injured patients are susceptible to disturbances of sodium haemostasis such as diabetes insipidus and syndrome of inappropriate antidiuretic hormone (SIADH).
- *Seizure control*. Seizures increase the brain metabolic rate and should be controlled. Prophylactic anticonvulsants may reduce seizures in the first week.

Steroids in severe head injury are associated with increased mortality and should not be used.

Summary box 23.6

Medical management of raised intracranial pressure

- Position head up 30°
- Avoid obstruction of venous drainage from head
- Sedation +/– muscle relaxant
- Normocapnia 4.5–5.0 kPa
- Diuretics: furosemide, mannitol
- Seizure control
- Normothermia
- Sodium balance
- Barbiturates

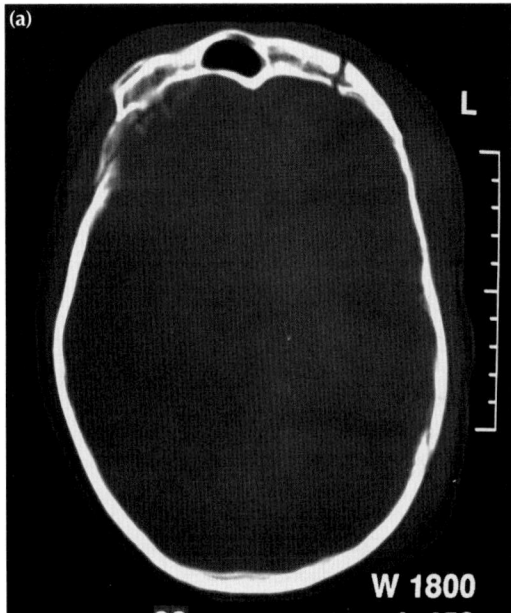

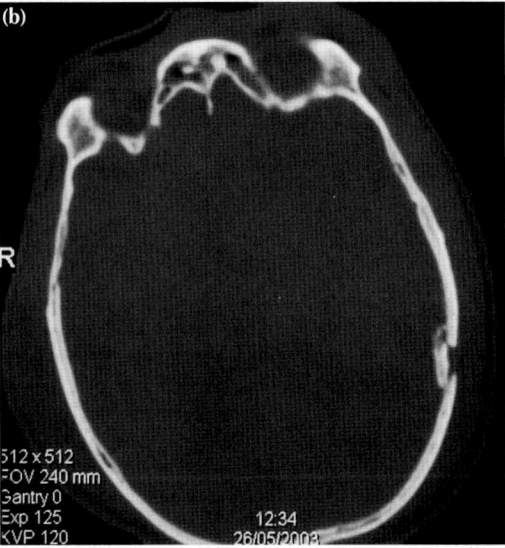

Figure 23.13 Axial computerised tomography (CT) scans with bone windowing showing and minimally displaced right fronto-orbital, left frontal and left parietal fractures (a) and a displaced left parietal skull fracture (b).

CHAPTER 23 | HEAD INJURY

SKULL FRACTURES

Skull vault fractures

Indications for surgery for skull fracture include elevation of significantly depressed fragments and wound debridement for compound fractures, particularly if there is evidence of underlying dural injury such as contusion or CSF leak. Fracture elevation is rarely needed for cosmesis alone (Fig. 23.13 on the previous page).

Base of skull fractures

Base of skull fractures may be associated with seventh or eighth nerve palsies. CSF otorrhoea or rhinorrhoea often resolves spontaneously. Antibiotics are not required prophylactically unless for concomitant facial fractures. A delayed craniotomy and anterior fossa dural repair is occasionally required for persistent CSF leak to prevent meningitis.

LONG-TERM SEQUELAE OF HEAD INJURY

Neurorehabilitation

Long-term management of the brain-injured patient requires the concerted efforts of medical, nursing, physiotherapy and speech and occupational therapy teams.

Neuropsychology

Neuropsychological sequalae are common after head injury and sometimes occur after relatively minor head injury. Post-concussional symptoms include headache, dizziness, impaired short-term memory and concentration, easy fatigability, emotional disinhibition and depression.

Seizures

Long-term epilepsy affects < 5% of patients admitted with head injury. The use of prophylactic anticonvulsants does not seem to change the long-term incidence of epilepsy.

Delayed CSF leak

Patients with delayed or on-going CSF leak should be investigated with CT cisternography or CSF isotope studies prior to surgical repair.

OUTCOMES AFTER HEAD INJURY

Outcome scores

The Glasgow Outcome Score (GOS) is shown in Table 23.2. A good recovery (GOS 5) does not mean that there is no deficit but implies independent functioning and the possibility of returning to work. Patients with GOS 4 remain independent though with a disabling deficit. Patients with severe disability (GOS 3) are dependent on others for at least some of their care. Patients in a vegetative state (GOS 2) show no awareness of themselves or their environment. This state is not considered permanent until at least 1 year after traumatic brain injury.

Table 23.2 Glasgow Outcome Score (GOS)

Good recovery	5
Moderate disability	4
Severe disability	3
Persistent vegetative state	2
Dead	1

FURTHER READING

Advanced textbooks

Ganong, W.F. (2003) Circulation through special regions. In: Ganong, W.F. (ed.). *Review of Medical Physiology*, 21st edn. McGraw Hill, New York.

Marshall, L.F. and Grady, M.S. (2004) Trauma. In: Winn, H.R. (ed.). *Youman's Neurological Surgery*, 5th edn. Saunders, Philadelphia, PA.

Rengachary, S. and Ellenbogen, R. (2004) *Principles of Neurosurgery*, 2nd edn. Mosby, Philadelphia, PA.

Neck and spine

LEARNING OBJECTIVES

To be familiar with:
- The accurate assessment of spinal cord injuries
- The mechanisms of spinal injuries and the pathophysiology of spinal cord trauma
- The basic management of spinal trauma and the major pitfalls

- The prognosis of the various types of spinal cord injury, factors affecting functional outcome and common associated complications

EPIDEMIOLOGY OF SPINAL CORD INJURY

The incidence of spinal cord injury ranges from 27 to 47 cases per million population per year. Road traffic accidents remain the leading cause of spinal cord injuries worldwide. Pre-hospital survival and life expectancy of spinal cord injury victims have improved significantly.

EVOLUTION OF THE MANAGEMENT OF SPINAL CORD INJURY

There is clear evidence to show that fewer complications, a decreased length of stay and improved patient outcome occur when patients with spinal cord injury are treated in a specialised unit (Summary box 24.1).

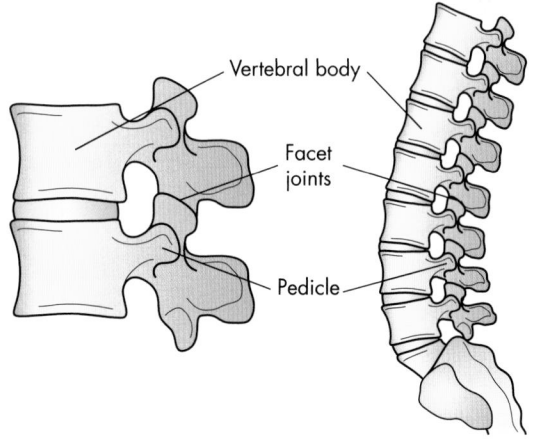

Figure 24.1 The spinal motion segment.

Summary box 24.1

Spinal cord injury

- The incidence of spinal cord injury remains constant
- Pre-hospital and post-injury survival have increased significantly
- Outcome is improved in regional/national spinal cord injury centres

---

ANATOMY OF THE SPINE AND SPINAL CORD

Spinal column anatomy

The vertebral column is composed of a series of motion segments (Fig. 24.1). A motion segment consists of two adjacent vertebrae, intervertebral disc and ligamentous restraints (Fig. 24.2). The neural elements are contained within the spinal canal.

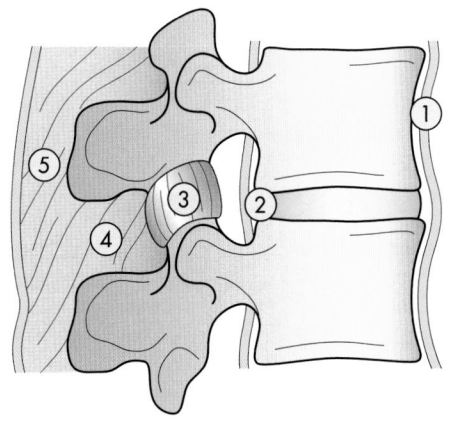

Figure 24.2 Ligamentous spinal restraints. (1) Anterior longitudinal ligament; (2) intervertebral disc and posterior longitudinal ligament; (3) facet joint capsule; (4) interspinous ligament; (5) supraspinous ligament.

Regional variations

Upper cervical spine anatomy is designed to facilitate motion (Fig. 24.3), and stability in this region is dependent on ligamentous restraints (Fig. 24.4). Upper cervical spinal cord injury is uncommon as the canal is capacious. The anatomy of each vertebra from C3–C7 is similar.

The cervicothoracic junction is a transitional zone, going from mobile to fixed, and is thus prone to injury. It may be difficult to visualise this area on radiography (Fig. 24.5).

The thoracic spine is relatively rigid because of the stabilising influence of the thorax. Significant disruption of the thoracic spine requires major energy transfer and associated visceral and vascular injuries are common.

The thoracolumbar junction is another transitional zone that is prone to injury; this is the most common area of injury outside the cervical spine (Fig. 24.6).

The three-column concept of spinal stability

The spinal column can be divided into three columns: anterior, middle and posterior (Fig. 24.7). When all three columns are injured the spine is unstable. Instability may also exist in some two-column injuries (Summary box 24.2).

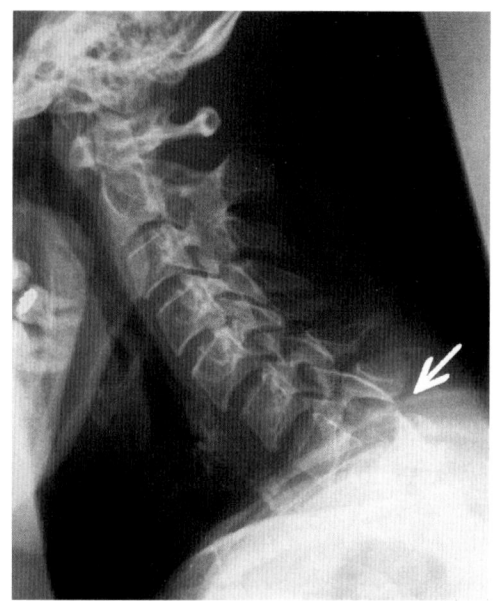

Figure 24.5 Cervicothoracic facet subluxation (easily missed with inadequate radiography).

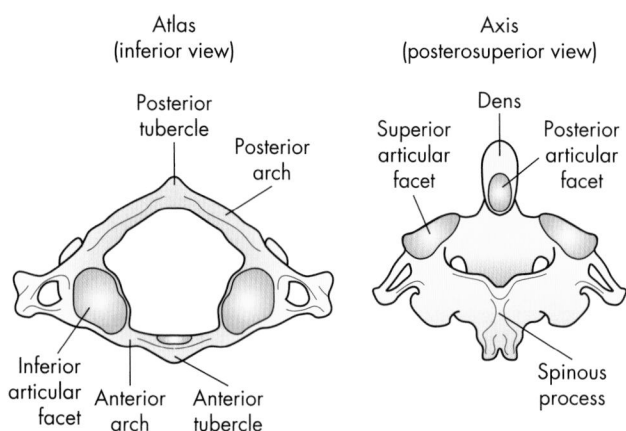

Figure 24.3 Atlantoaxial bony anatomy.

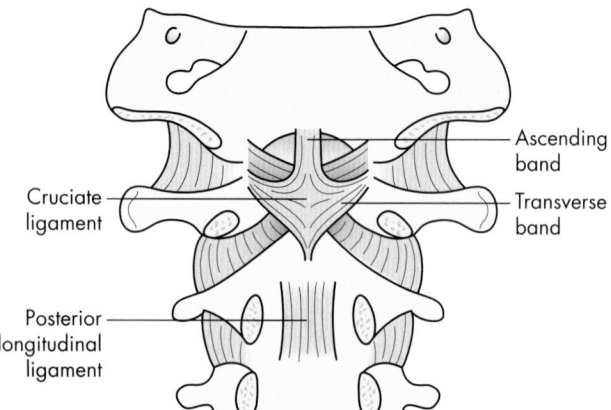

Figure 24.4 Atlantoaxial ligaments.

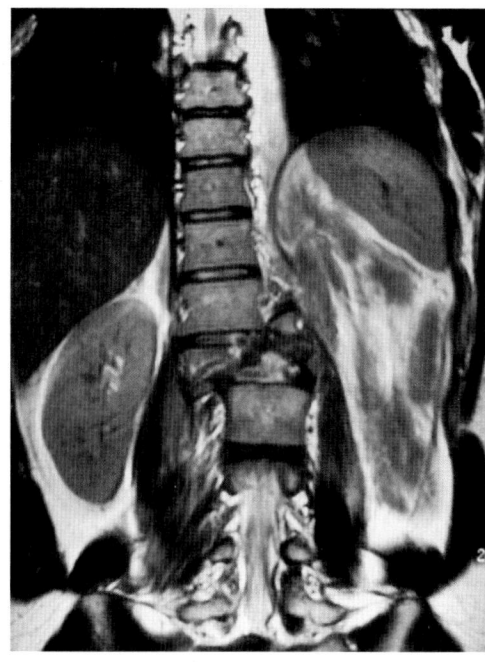

Figure 24.6 Coronal T2-weighted magnetic resonance imaging scan demonstrating a fracture dislocation at the thoracolumbar junction.

Summary box 24.2

Spinal column anatomy

- Upper cervical spine stability is dependent on ligamentous restraints
- Major energy transfer is required to significantly disrupt the thoracic spine
- The cervicothoracic and thoracolumbar junction are transitional zones and are therefore prone to injury
- The need for surgical fixation of a spine fracture depends upon the stability of the fracture type

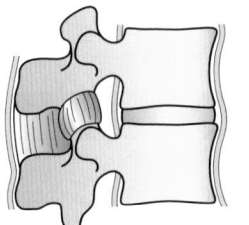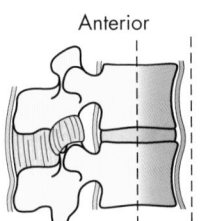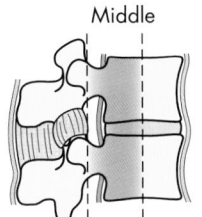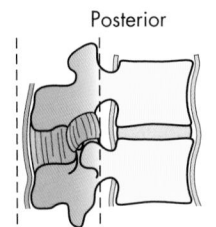

Anterior Middle Posterior

Figure 24.7 The three-column model of spinal stability.

Spinal neuroanatomy

The spinal cord extends from the foramen magnum to the T12/L1 junction where it ends as the conus medullaris (Fig. 24.8). Below this level lies the cauda equina. Figure 24.9 illustrates a cross-section of the spinal cord. It consists of central grey matter (neuronal cell bodies) surrounded by white matter (axons). The lateral spinothalamic tracts transmit pain and temperature sensation, the lateral corticospinal tracts are responsible for motor function and the posterior columns transmit position, vibration and deep pressure sensation.

A spinal nerve root exits on both sides of the spinal cord at each level. There are eight cervical roots. The C1 root exits above the C1 body, the C2 root exits between C1 and C2 and the C8 root exits below C7. All thoracic and lumbar nerve roots exit below the pedicle of the same number.

PATHOPHYSIOLOGY OF SPINAL CORD INJURY

The primary injury

This injury occurs when the skeletal structures fail to dissipate the energy of the primary mechanical insult, resulting in direct energy transfer to the neural elements. The injury may occur directly by flexion, extension, axial loading, rotation or traction, or by compression of the cord by a fragment of bone and/or disc material.

The secondary injury

Haemorrhage, oedema and ischaemia result in a biochemical cascade that causes the secondary injury. This may result in further loss of neurological function. Prolonged hypotension and poor oxygenation compound the situation so it is important that the patient is adequately resuscitated. The spinal column should be realigned as soon as possible in cases of cord injury in which dislocation or subluxation is present. Ongoing spinal cord compression from disc material and/or bony fragments may require surgical intervention (Summary box 24.3).

Summary box 24.3

Pathophysiology of spinal cord injury

- The spinal cord contains tracts that are topographically arranged
- Spinal cord injury involves both primary and secondary phases
- Therapeutic strategies are directed at reducing the secondary injury

---

PATIENT ASSESSMENT

Basic points

Approach every trauma patient in the same manner using Advanced Trauma Life Support (ATLS) principles. Assume that

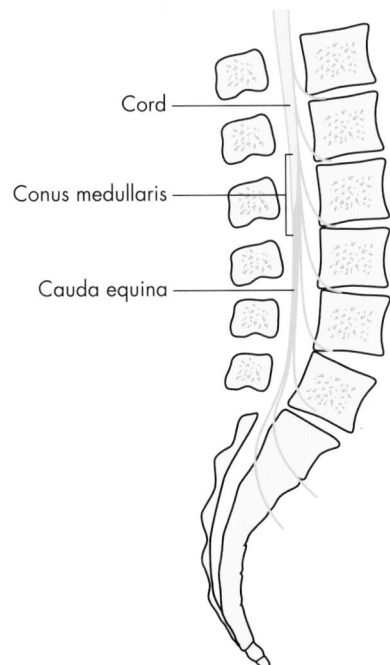

Cord

Conus medullaris

Cauda equina

Figure 24.8 The spinal cord ends at T12/L1 as the conus medullaris, which gives rise to the cauda equina.

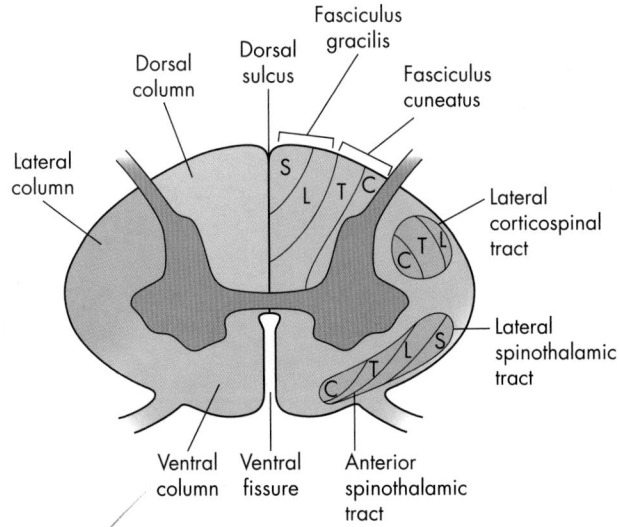

Dorsal column · Dorsal sulcus · Fasciculus gracilis · Fasciculus cuneatus · Lateral column · Lateral corticospinal tract · Lateral spinothalamic tract · Ventral column · Ventral fissure · Anterior spinothalamic tract

Figure 24.9 A cross-section of the spinal cord. C, cervical; L, lumbar; S, sacral; T, thoracic.

CHAPTER 24 | NECK AND SPINE

every trauma patient has a spinal injury until proven otherwise; all assessment, resuscitation and life-saving procedures must be performed with full spinal immobilisation (Fig. 24.10). However, patients must be removed from spinal boards as soon as possible to avoid skin breakdown, particularly in cases of spinal cord injury and unconsciousness.

There should be a high index of suspicion of spinal injury if any of the following are evident:

- neurological deficit;
- multiple injuries;
- head injury;
- facial injury;
- high-energy injury (e.g. fall from a height);
- abdominal bruising from a seatbelt, suggestive of a possible lumbar spine injury.

The polytrauma patient

Spinal injuries often result from high-velocity trauma and associated injuries are common:

- spinal injury at another level: 10–15% of cases;
- head and facial injury: 26% of cases;
- major chest injury: 16% of cases;
- major abdominal injury: 10% of cases;
- long bone/pelvic fracture: 8% of cases.

The unconscious patient

Full assessment of the spine in this situation is difficult. Definitive clearance of the spine may not be possible in the initial stages. Spinal immobilisation should be maintained until magnetic resonance imaging (MRI) of the entire spine has been used to rule out injury or the cervical spine has been screened while being flexed and extended under image intensifier control.

The pain-free patient

In a conscious patient spinal injury can be excluded if:

- there is no pain;
- palpation of the spine is non-tender;
- neurological examination is normal;
- there is a pain-free range of movement;

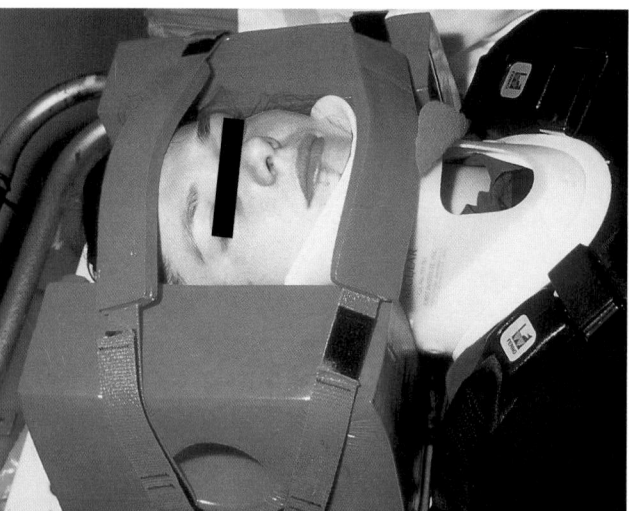

Figure 24.10 Spinal immobilisation.

- there are no other serious injuries that may mask spinal symptoms (Summary box 24.4).

Summary box 24.4

Patient assessment

- Use ATLS principles in all cases of spinal injury
- In polytrauma cases suspect a spinal injury
- A second spinal injury at a remote level may be present in 10% of cases
- Spinal boards cause pressure sores

PERTINENT HISTORY

The mechanism and velocity of injury should be determined at an early stage.

PHYSICAL EXAMINATION

Initial assessment

It is important to be aware that spinal cord injury may mask signs of intra-abdominal injury.

Identification of shock

Three categories of shock may occur in spinal trauma:

- *Hypovolaemic shock.* This presents with hypotension, tachycardia and cold clammy peripheries. It is most often caused by haemorrhage and is treated with appropriate fluid replacement.
- *Neurogenic shock.* Hypotension occurs with a normal heart rate or bradycardia and warm peripheries. It is caused by unopposed vagal tone resulting from cervical spinal cord injury above the level of sympathetic outflow (C7/T1). Care must be taken to avoid fluid overload.
- *Spinal shock.* This is characterised by paralysis, hypotonia and areflexia. It usually lasts for only 24 hours. When it starts to resolve the bulbocavernosus reflex (Fig. 24.11) returns. The patient should be regularly reassessed neurologically to determine the true extent of neurological injury.

Spinal examination

The entire spine must be palpated and the overlying skin inspected. A formal spinal log roll must be performed to achieve this (Fig. 24.12). Significant swelling, tenderness or palpable steps or gaps suggest a spinal injury. Note the presence of any wounds that might suggest penetrating trauma and document the condition of the skin, particularly over the pressure areas.

Neurological examination

The American Spinal Injury Association (ASIA) neurological evaluation system (Fig. 24.13) is internationally accepted and has low inter- and intraobserver variability.

Motor function is assessed using the Medical Research Council (MRC) grading system (0–5) and is confined to key muscle groups. Sensory function is assessed using the dermatomal map (Fig. 24.13). Pinprick and light touch sensation are assessed at key dermatomal points and scored from 0 to 2. A rectal examination is performed to assess anal tone, voluntary anal contraction and perianal sensation. Preservation of perianal sensation

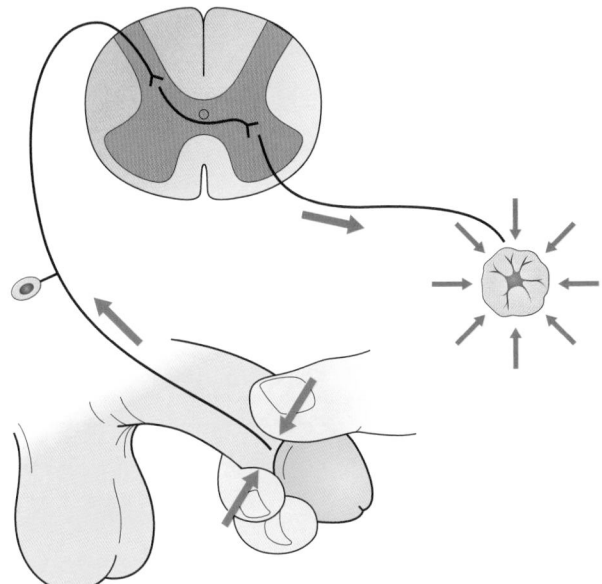

Figure 24.11 The bulbocavernosus reflex (this can be elicited in female patients by traction on the Foley catheter).

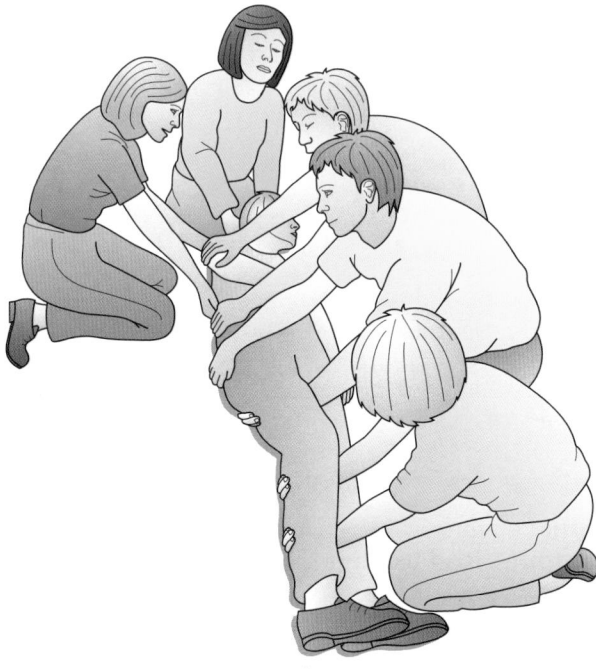

Figure 24.12 Spinal log roll.

indicates an incomplete cord injury and suggests that there should at least be some recovery.

On completion of the neurological assessment the following should be known:

- the presence or absence of a neurological injury;
- the probable level of injury;
- whether the injury is complete or incomplete;
- the type of spinal cord injury;
- the level of impairment.

Level of neurological injury

This is simply the most caudal (lowest) neurological level with normal neurological function.

Complete versus incomplete spinal cord injury

A spinal cord injury is incomplete when there is preservation of perianal sensation.

Types of incomplete spinal cord injury

Central cord syndrome This results from injury to the central portions of the spinal cord. This can occur when hyperextension results in the cord being pinched by pre-existing degenerative narrowing of the spinal canal. Distal motor function in the legs is typically spared whereas the upper limbs and hands may be profoundly affected. This reflects the topographical arrangement of the cord. Younger patients often recover substantially but may be left with a permanent loss of fine motor hand function.

Brown-Séquard syndrome This is typically seen in cord hemisection caused by penetrating trauma. This results in ipsilateral loss of power, proprioception and vibration sense with a contralateral loss of pain and temperature sensation below the level of injury because of the arrangement of the various spinal cord tracts (Fig. 24.9). This type of spinal cord injury carries a good prognosis.

Anterior spinal syndrome Flexion–compression injuries to the cervical spine may damage the anterior spinal artery, cutting off the blood supply to the anterior two-thirds of the spinal cord. Posterior column function is preserved but the prognosis is poor.

Posterior cord syndrome This rare injury results from isolated posterior column injury. Motor function is preserved but joint position sense is lost.

Cauda equina syndrome This is most frequently associated with large central disc herniations at L4/5 and L5/S1. Patients typically describe numbness around the perineum and down the inside of the thighs (saddle paraesthesia). They may also be unable to pass urine and have loss of anal tone. If possible, imaging and surgery should be undertaken within hours of the onset of symptoms as the prognosis deteriorates rapidly over time.

Level of neurological impairment

The ASIA neurological impairment scale is based on the Frankel classification of spinal cord injury:

- A: absent motor and sensory function;
- B: sensory function present, motor function absent;
- C: sensory function present, motor function present but not useful (MRC grade < 3/5);
- D: sensory function present, motor function useful (MRC grade ≥ 3/5);
- E: normal function (Summary box 24.5).

CHAPTER 24 | NECK AND SPINE

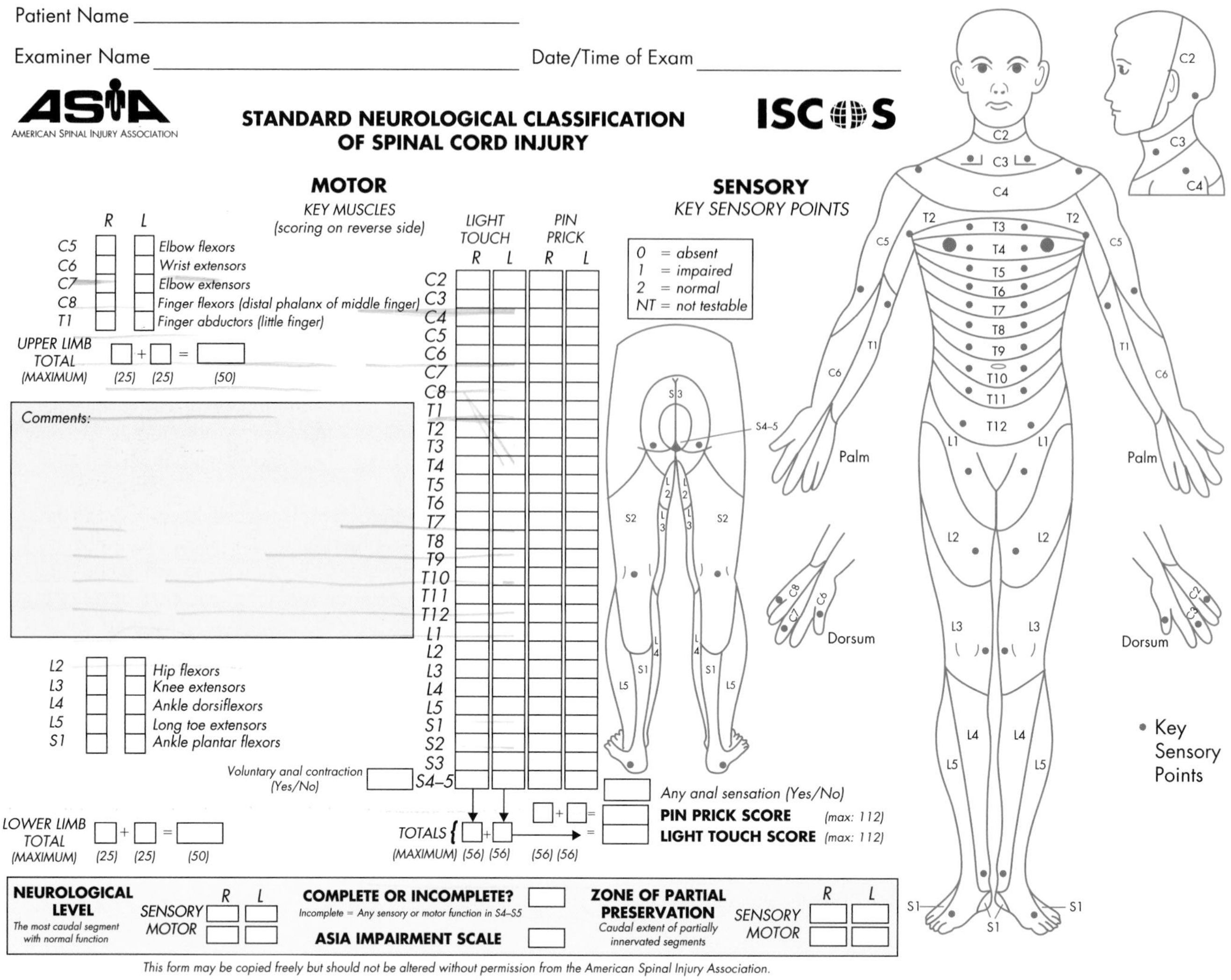

Patient Name _____

Examiner Name _____   Date/Time of Exam _____

Figure 24.13 American Spinal Injury Association neurological evaluation.

Summary box 24.5

Physical examination

- Shock after spinal injury can be hypovolaemic, neurogenic or spinal
- The ASIA scoring system should be used to evaluate patients with spinal cord injury
- Prognoses of spinal injury depends on the type of injury

DIAGNOSTIC IMAGING

Plain radiographs

In total, 85% of significant spinal injuries will be seen on the standard lateral cervical spine radiograph recommended at the resuscitation of polytraumatised patients. If the thoracocervical junction cannot be visualised, even with a swimmer's view, a computerised tomography (CT) scan should be obtained.

Significant loss of vertebral body height, sagittal deformity and widening of the interpedicular distance (on the anteroposterior view) may signify an unstable injury of a vertebra (Figs 24.14–24.16).

Computerised tomography

CT scanning remains the most sensitive imaging modality in spinal trauma. Complex fracture patterns can be understood and an accurate assessment of spinal canal compromise by bony fragments can be made (Fig. 24.17). Sagittal reconstruction is an important modality in assessing posterior column stability.

Magnetic resonance imaging

MRI is best at visualising the soft-tissue elements of the spine (Fig. 24.18). It is possible to see spinal cord haemorrhage and epidural and prevertebral haematomas. Spinal cord haemorrhage carries a poor prognosis. MRI is not good at assessing bony structures and has a relatively low sensitivity in identifying fractures (particularly those in the posterior element).

In cases of spinal trauma without neurological injury, plain radiographs and CT usually give sufficient information, unless it is particularly important to exclude disrupted ligaments (Summary box 24.6).

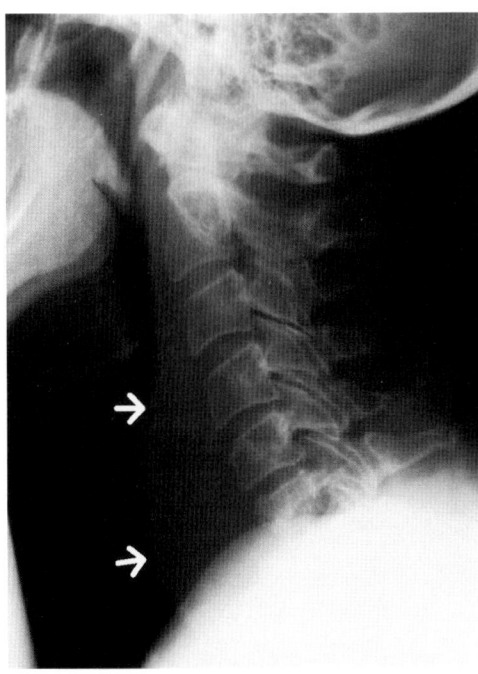

Figure 24.14 Large prevertebral haematoma.

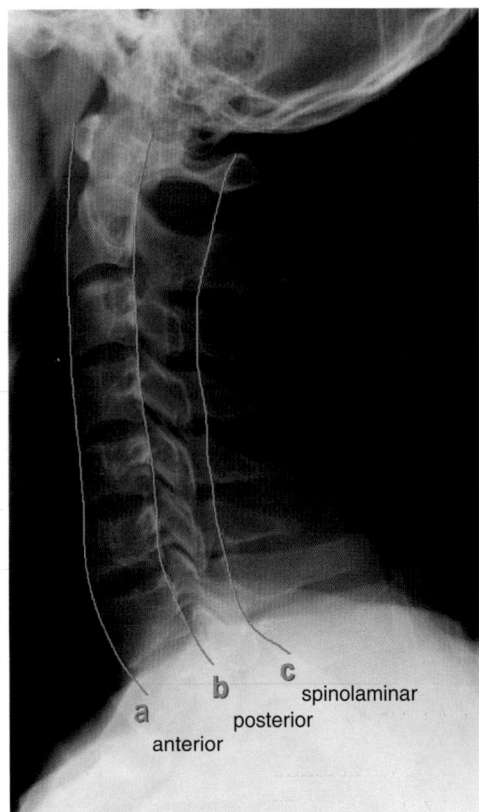

Figure 24.15 The anterior, posterior and spinolaminar lines are useful for identifying anterior translation on lateral radiographs of the neck. a, anterior; b, posterior; c, spinolaminar.

CLASSIFICATION AND MANAGEMENT OF SPINAL AND SPINAL CORD INJURIES

General points

In cases of neurological injury, initial intervention is aimed at reducing the secondary injury, preventing further deterioration and allowing return of neurological function in some cases. Most spinal trauma centres no longer use steroids in cases of spinal cord injury as there is no evidence that they work.

Basic management principles

Spinal realignment

In cases of cervical spine subluxation or dislocation, skull tongs (Fig. 24.19) are used to apply traction. The alternative is open reduction and operative realignment using internal fixation (Fig. 24.20). A halo brace can be used to perform a closed realignment of cervical fractures (Fig. 24.21).

Stabilisation

If a spinal fracture or dislocation is unstable (moves abnormally when stressed) there is a risk of new or further neurological injury as well as painful post-traumatic deformity. Many spinal injuries can be managed non-operatively with external support but, when possible, internal fixation should be used. The only absolute

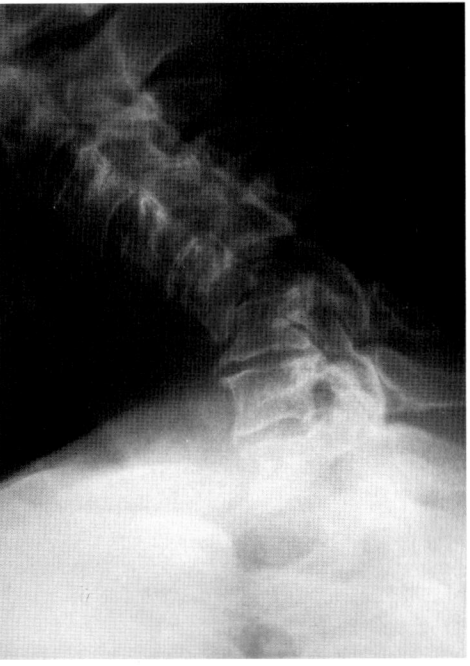

Figure 24.16 Lateral cervical spine radiograph showing obvious spinal instability with marked sagittal angulation and translation. This patient walked into the out-patient department.

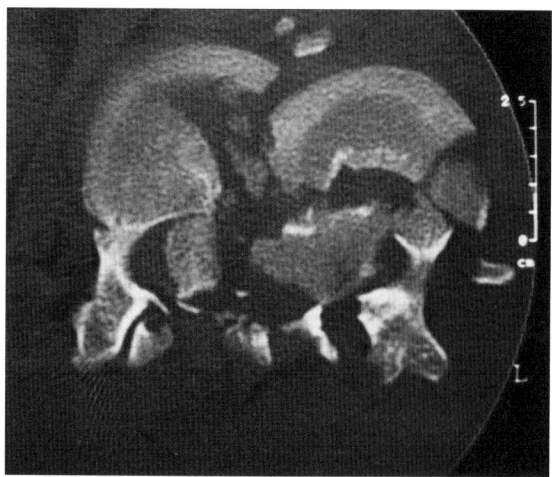

Figure 24.17 Axial computerised tomography demonstrating a double vertebral body and high-grade spinal canal compromise consistent with a thoracolumbar fracture–dislocation.

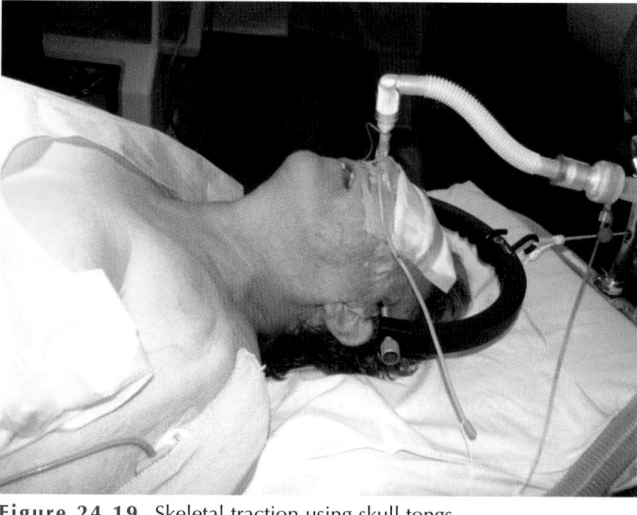

Figure 24.19 Skeletal traction using skull tongs.

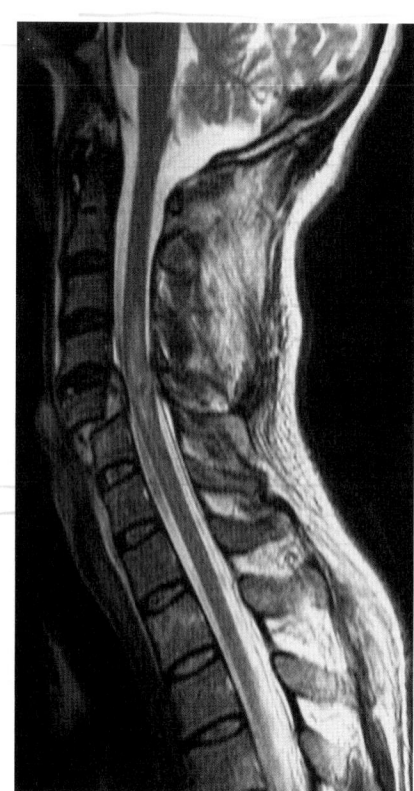

Figure 24.18 Sagittal T2-weighted magnetic resonance imaging demonstrating a cervical spine subluxation and spinal cord contusion.

indication for surgery in spinal trauma is deteriorating neurological function. All other indications are relative.

Early stabilisation has the advantage that it allows early mobilisation of the patient.

Decompression of the neural elements

Spinal realignment is important in this regard. Compression of the cord by bone and/or disc material requires surgical removal

(Fig. 24.22). Most spinal surgeons agree that, in cases of incomplete cord injury and progressive neurology, expeditious surgery is appropriate.

In cases of complete cord injury timing of surgery is less important as the prognosis neurologically is unlikely to be affected; however, relatively early surgery with realignment and stabilisation may facilitate early mobilisation and reduce in-patient complications. Decompression of the spinal cord may also reduce the risk of post-traumatic syrinx formation (Summary box 24.7).

Summary box 24.7

Management of spinal trauma

- The management of spinal trauma depends on the presence or absence of neurological deficit
- Deteriorating neurological status is an absolute indication for surgical intervention
- Many spinal cord injury units no longer advocate the use of high-dose corticosteroids

---

SPECIFIC SPINAL INJURIES

Upper cervical spine (skull to C2)

Craniocervical dislocation

This injury is the consequence of high-energy trauma and is usually fatal. It may be anterior, posterior or vertical (Fig. 24.23). Power's ratio (Fig. 24.24) is used to assess skull translation. In survivors, careful occipitocervical fusion is required. A halo brace should be applied before surgery to prevent intraoperative dislocation.

Atlantoaxial instability

The most common form is a rotatory subluxation in children. This is usually of spontaneous onset but can be traumatic. The

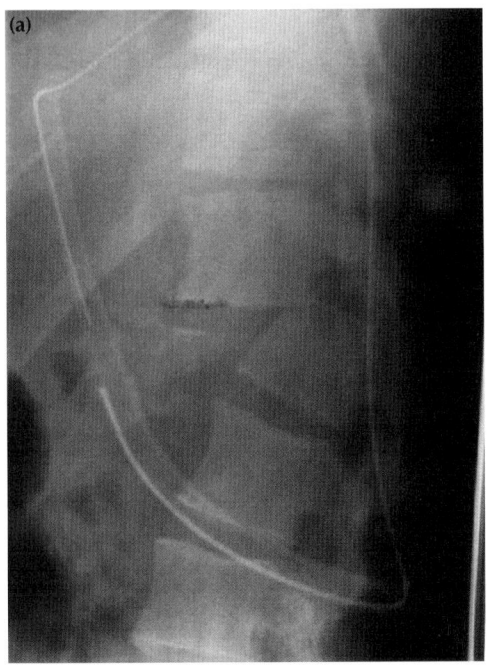

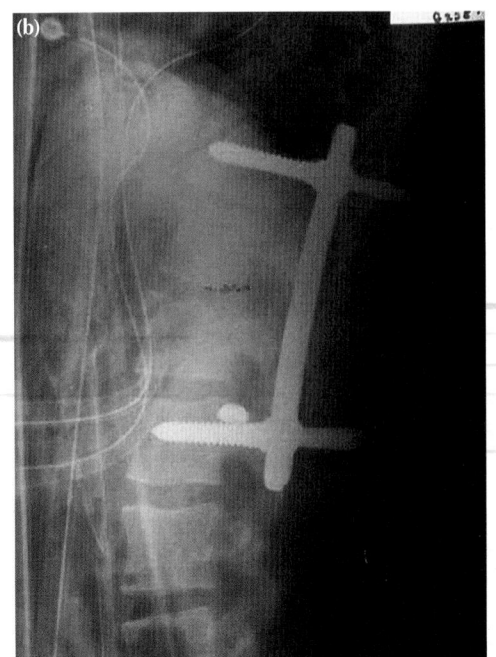

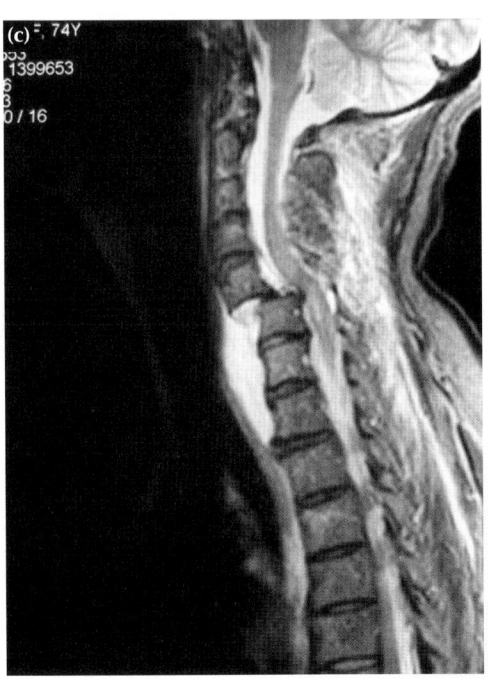

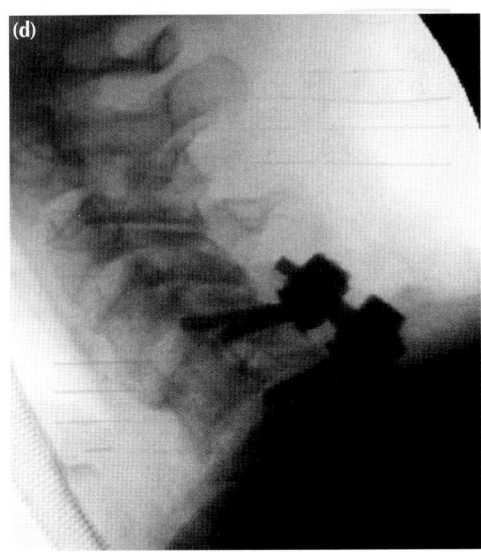

Figure 24.20 (a) Thoracolumbar fracture–dislocation; (b) treated with open reduction and posterior fixation. (c) Bifacetal cervical spine dislocation; (d) posterior stabilisation following closed reduction.

child presents with a cock-robin appearance. Halter traction results in realignment in the majority of cases.

Isolated, traumatic transverse ligament rupture leading to C1/2 instability is uncommon and is treated with posterior C1/2 fusion (Fig. 24.25).

Occipital condyle fracture

This is an uncommon injury that is usually associated with head

injuries and identified on CT. The majority of fractures are stable and can be treated in a hard collar for 8 weeks.

Jefferson fractures (C1 ring)

These injuries are associated with axial loading of the cervical spine, which can be stable or unstable (Fig. 24.26a and b). Associated transverse ligament rupture may occur (Fig. 24.26c). Unstable Jefferson fractures should be treated in a halo jacket for

A robin **is a small red-breasted bird of the thrush family which carries its head on one side.**

Sir Geoffrey Jefferson, **1886–1961, Professor of Neurosurgery, University of Manchester, England.**

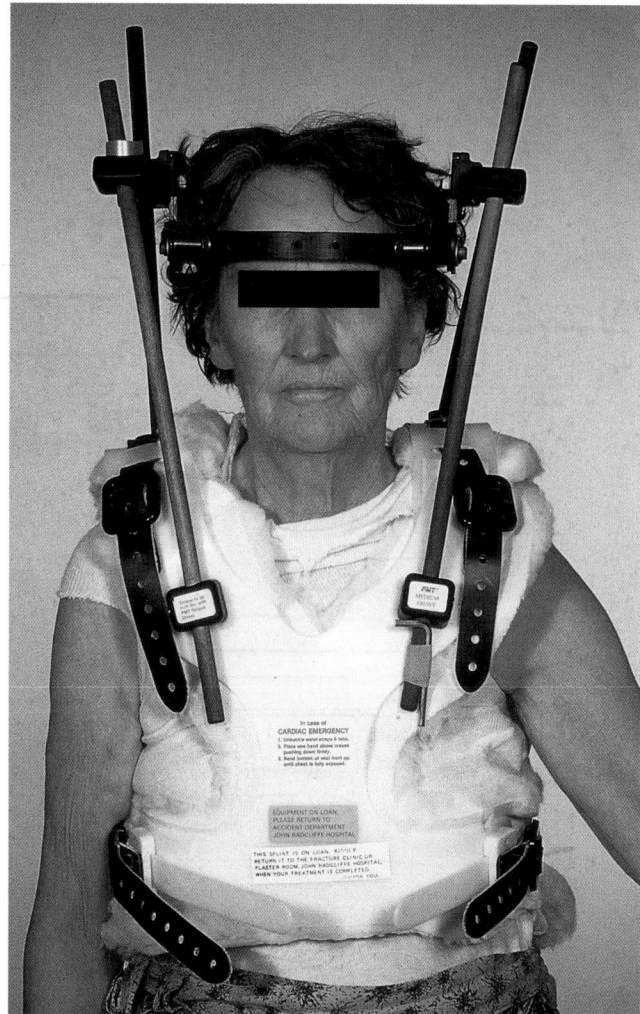

Figure 24.21 External immobilisation using a halo jacket.

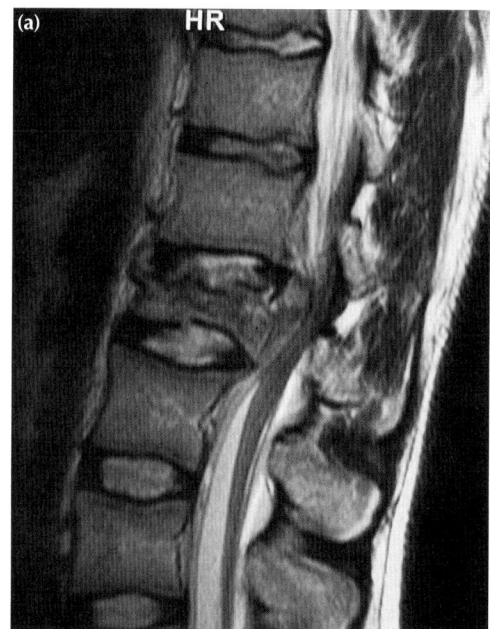

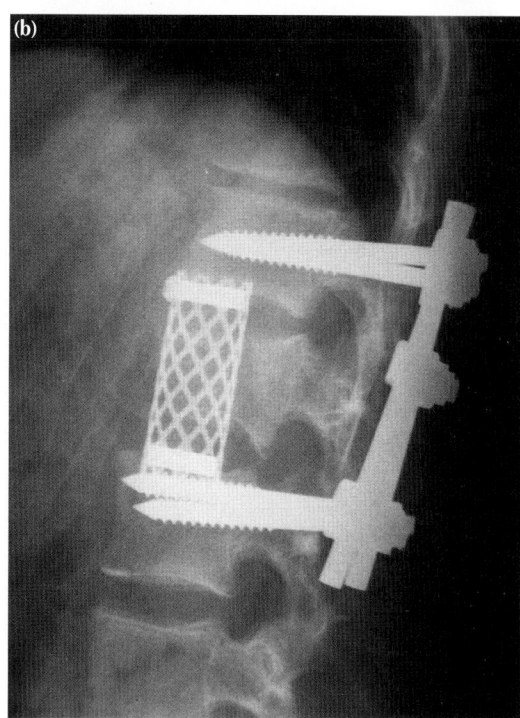

Figure 24.22 (a) Sagittal T2-weighted magnetic resonance imaging showing an L1 burst fracture and neural compression; (b) treated with combined anterior and posterior surgery.

3 months followed by flexion–extension stress radiography to check stability. Persistent C1/2 instability will need C1/2 or occiput–C2 fusion.

Odontoid fractures

There are three types of odontoid fracture (Fig. 24.27). Type I fractures are uncommon and are usually stable, requiring no immobilisation. Type II fractures may fail to unite, particularly those with significant displacement on presentation and those in the elderly. Type III fractures extend into the C2 vertebral body and usually readily unite. Neurological injury is rare. The majority of acute injuries are treated non-operatively in a halo jacket for 3 months. Internal fixation with an anterior compression screw is indicated in displaced fractures in younger patients with good bone quality (Fig. 24.28).

Posterior C1/2 fusion is required in cases of non-union. Elderly patients often develop a fibrous pseudoarthrosis that is relatively stable and does not require surgery.

Hangman's fracture

This injury can be considered as a traumatic spondylolisthesis of C2/3 resulting from bilateral C2 pedicle fractures secondary to hyperextension (Fig. 24.29). The majority can be treated non-operatively in a halo jacket or brace. Those with significant

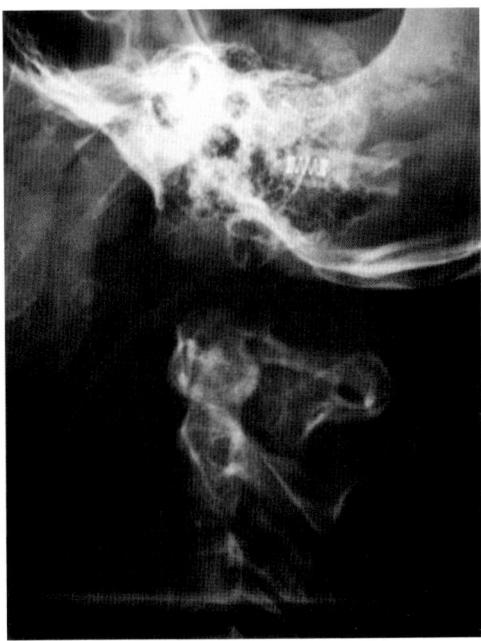

Figure 24.23 Vertical occipitocervical dislocation.

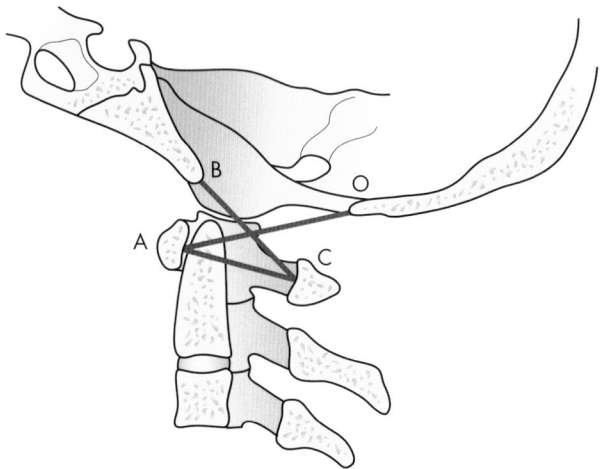

Figure 24.24 Power's ratio. BC/OA A ≥ 1 indicates anterior translation, ≤ 0.75 indicates posterior translation. B, anterior margin of the foramen magnum; C, anterior margin of the C1 posterior arch; O, posterior margin of the foramen magnum; A, posterior margin of the C1 anterior arch.

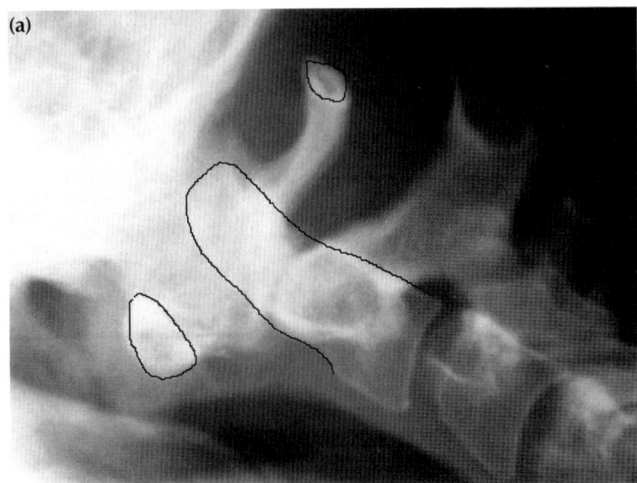

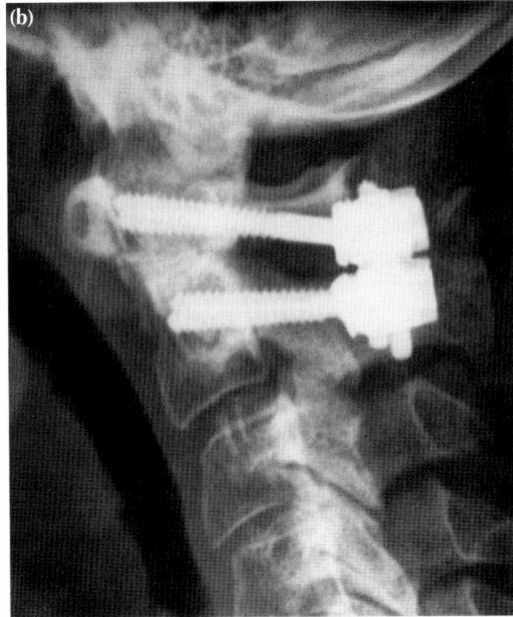

Figure 24.25 (a) Atlantoaxial subluxation. (b) C1/2 posterior fusion using C1 lateral mass and C2 pedicle screws.

displacement or associated facet dislocation are treated operatively, usually with posterior stabilisation.

Subaxial cervical spine (C3–C7)

The pattern of lower cervical spine injury depends on the mechanism of trauma. Many of the more severe injuries are associated with spinal cord injury.

Wedge fracture

This results from hyperflexion and is usually stable without neurological injury. It is treated in a brace or halo for 3 months.

Burst fracture

This occurs secondary to axial loading of the cervical spine. Bony fragments may explode into the spinal canal and cause neurological injury (Fig. 24.30a). Surgical intervention may be required to remove the fractured vertebral body, decompress the spinal cord and then stabilise with internal fixation (Fig. 24.30b).

Burst fractures without neurological deficit can be treated non-operatively in a halo jacket.

Tear-drop fracture

The mechanism of injury is hyperextension. Unstable fractures require operative treatment.

Facet subluxation/dislocation

The pattern of injury ranges from facet subluxation, through unifacetal dislocation to bifacetal dislocation (Fig. 24.31). Bifacetal

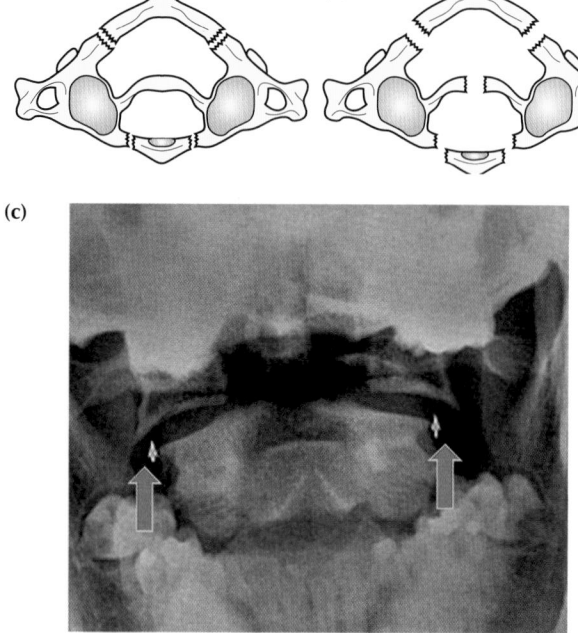

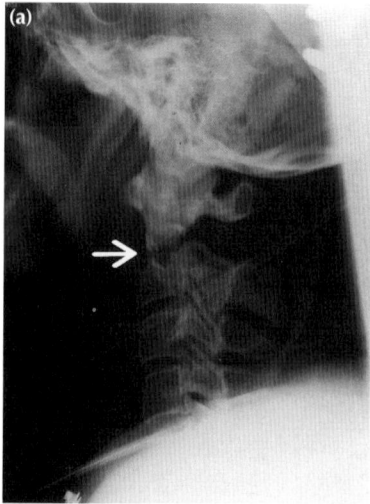

Figure 24.26 Stable (a) versus unstable (b) Jefferson's fracture of C1. (c) Open mouth view of C1/2 demonstrating C1 lateral mass deviation. Rupture of the transverse ligament is present when the combined lateral mass deviation exceeds 6.9 mm.

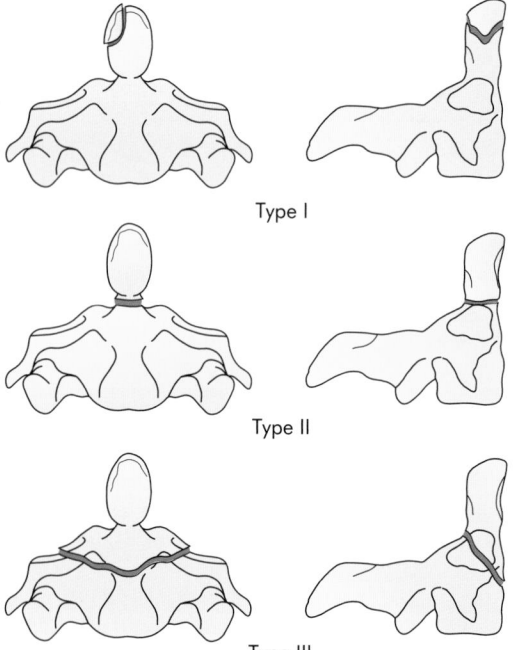

Type I

Type II

Type III

Figure 24.27 Types of odontoid fracture.

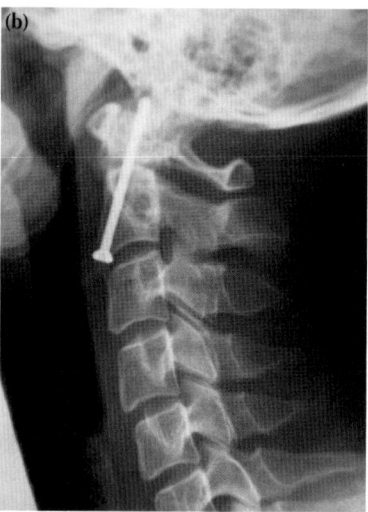

Figure 24.28 (a) Type II odontoid fracture; (b) treated with an anterior compression screw.

dislocation is associated with spinal cord injury in the majority of cases. The mechanism of injury is a combination of axial loading and flexion leading to compression at the anterior aspect of the spine and distraction of the posterior elements. The majority are pure ligamentous injuries with associated disruption of the inter-

vertebral disc. Surgical stabilisation is required in most cases; awake, closed reduction with skeletal traction is recommended when possible. In cases of incomplete paralysis or normal neurology, a pre-traction MRI should be considered to identify disc herniations that may then press on the cord and damage it during reduction (Summary box 24.8).

Summary box 24.8

Cervical spine injuries

- The majority of upper cervical spinal injuries are treated non-operatively
- Spinal cord injury is more commonly associated with subaxial cervical spinal injuries
- In cases of facet dislocation a pre-traction MRI should be considered

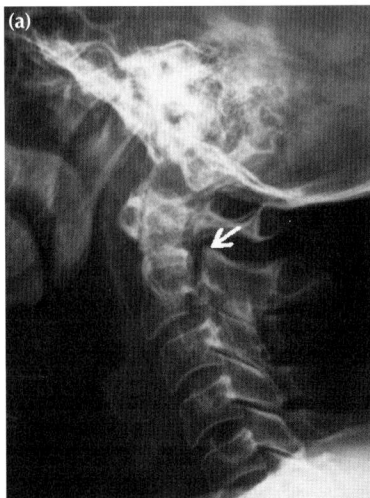

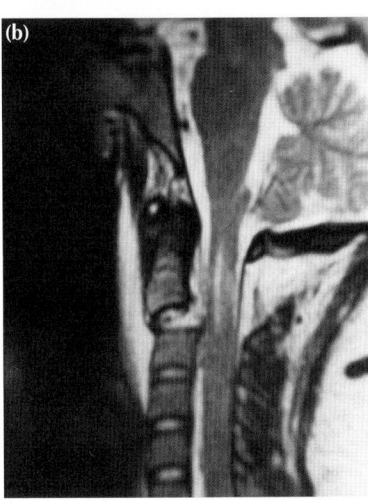

Figure 24.29 (a) Hangman's fracture of C2 with minimal forward translation. (b) C2/3 subluxation with spinal cord contusion.

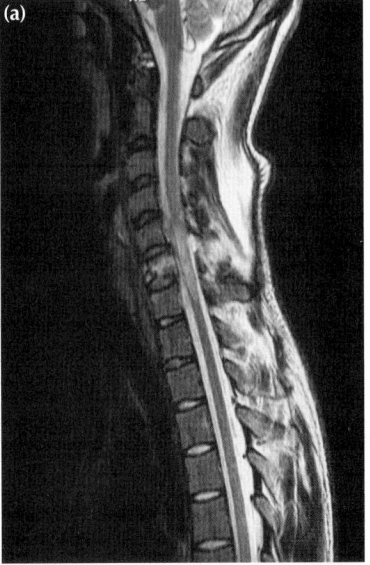

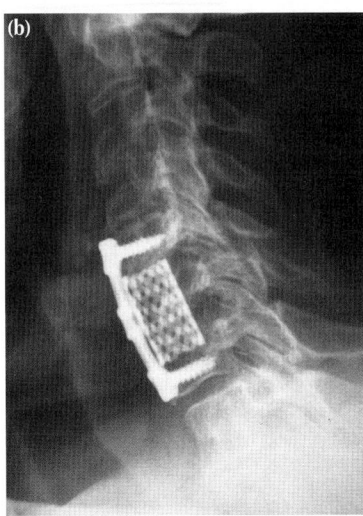

Figure 24.30 (a) Cervical burst fracture with spinal cord contusion; (b) treated by anterior decompression and reconstruction.

Thoracic and thoracolumbar fractures

Fractures that are highly unstable with an associated risk of neurological deficit should be fixed surgically. The AO (Arbeitsgemeinschaft für Osteosynthesefragen) classifies fractures into three main types, A, B and C, with injuries becoming progressively more unstable from A to C. There is also an increasing risk of associated neurological injury.

Type A fractures primarily involve the vertebral body. Type B injuries have additional distraction/disruption of the posterior elements and type C injuries are rotational. The majority of type B and type C injuries require surgical stabilisation. Burst fractures are included in type A.

Thoracic spine (T1–T10)

Osteoporotic wedge compression fractures in the elderly are the most common injury in this group. These are stable so can be treated symptomatically. Fractures that remain sympto-

> AO, Arbeitsgemeinschaft für Osteosynthesefragen which may be translated from the German as 'Working Party on Problems of Bone Repair'.

matic for more than 6 weeks can be treated with percutaneous bone cement augmentation, known as vertebroplasty. Specialised balloons can also be inserted and inflated in an attempt to restore vertebral height (kyphoplasty) and relieve pain (Fig. 24.32).

The combination of thoracic spine disruption and a sternal fracture (Fig. 24.33) carries a significant risk of aortic rupture. Multiple posterior rib fractures and rib dislocations above and below a thoracic spinal injury signify a major rotational injury to the chest and are associated with vascular injury and significant pulmonary contusion (Fig. 24.34).

Upper thoracic spinal column injuries can be difficult to diagnose with plain radiography. High-quality CT sagittal reformats are best.

Posterior instrumentation is indicated in almost all unstable thoracic spinal injuries as braces do not provide adequate stability and the risk of neurological deterioration can be considerable.

CHAPTER 24 | NECK AND SPINE

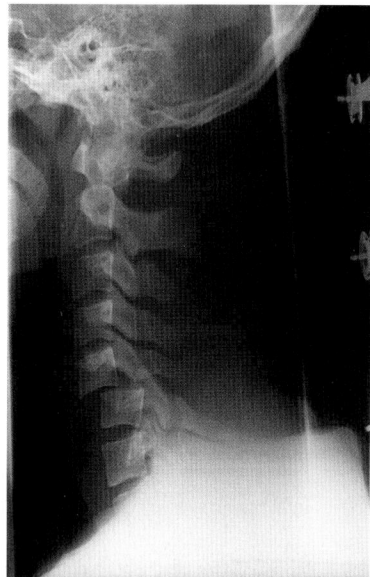

Figure 24.31 C5/6 bifacetal dislocation.

Thoracolumbar spinal fractures (T11–S1)

The thoracolumbar junction is prone to injury as it represents a transition zone from fixed to mobile segments. There is a wide spectrum of possible injuries, ranging from minor wedge fractures to spinal dislocation (Fig. 24.35).

Burst fractures

These are comminuted fractures of the vertebral body. The distance between the pedicles is widened and bone is retropulsed into the spinal canal (Fig. 24.36). Many of these fractures can be treated non-operatively. Surgical intervention is indicated when there is neurological compromise or the fracture is unstable. Instability is determined by loss of anterior vertebral body height of > 50%, sagittal plane angulation of > 30° and spinal canal compromise of > 50%. An anterior approach with vertebral corpectomy, canal clearance and anterior reconstruction (Fig. 24.37) is the treatment of choice for a burst fracture with neurological compromise.

Chance fractures

These are flexion–distraction injuries and are classically associated with the use of lap belts (Fig. 24.38). They may be bony or soft tissue in nature and predominantly occur at the thoracolumbar junction. Duodenal, pancreatic and/or aortic rupture can occur in these injuries and there must be a high index of suspicion (Summary box 24.9).

Summary box 24.9

Thoracic and thoracolumbar fractures

- Unstable thoracic spine fractures are commonly associated with vascular and/or visceral injuries
- Thoracolumbar flexion–distraction injuries may result in duodenal, pancreatic and/or aortic rupture

---

George Quentin Chance, **Formerly Director of Diagnostic Radiology, The Derby Group of Hospitals, Derbyshire, England.**

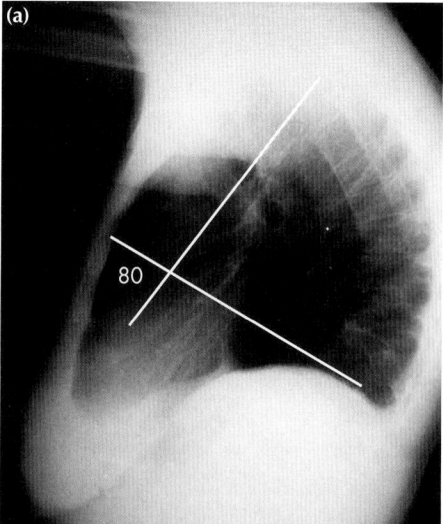
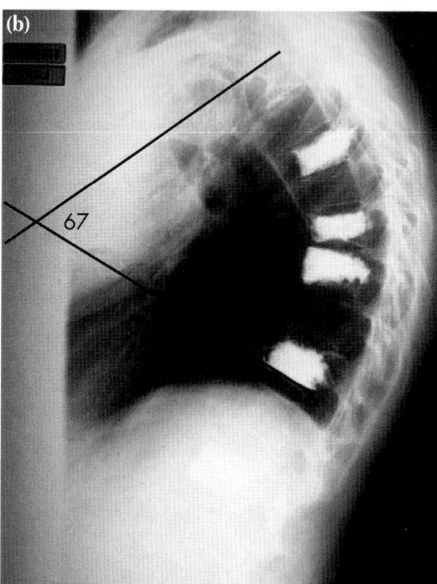

Figure 24.32 (a) Lateral radiograph showing multiple osteoporotic compression fractures. (b) Reduction in thoracic kyphotic deformity following four-level kyphoplasty.

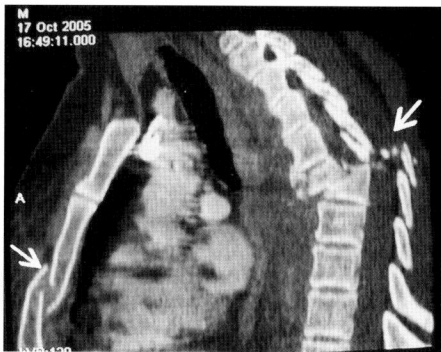

Figure 24.33 Sagittal computerised tomography reconstruction showing an upper thoracic spine fracture–dislocation and associated sternal fracture.

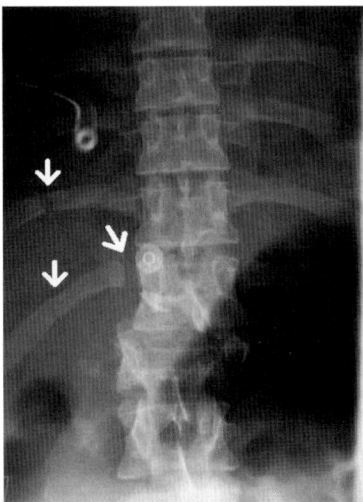

Figure 24.34 Rotational (type C) injury at the thoracolumbar junction. Note the rib fractures and dislocation (arrows) and the presence of a chest tube.

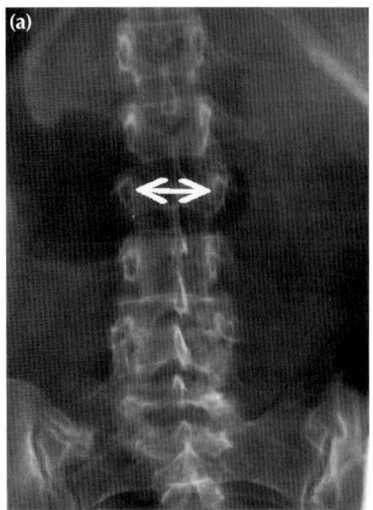

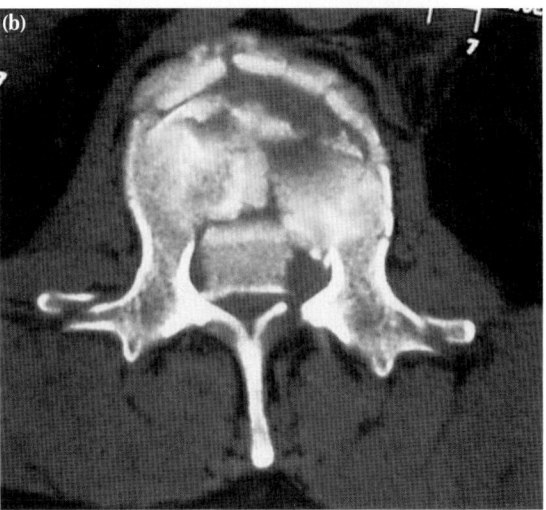

Figure 24.36 Lumbar burst fracture with increase in interpedicular distance (a) and spinal canal compromise (b).

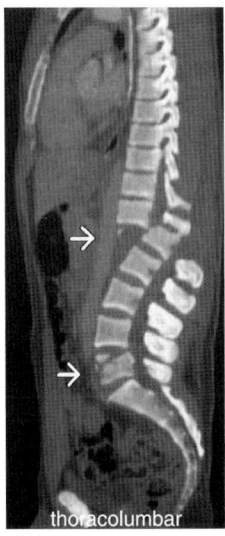

Figure 24.35 Total spinal sagittal computerised tomography reconstruction demonstrating a thoracolumbar fracture–dislocation and fracture of L5.

SCIWORA (SPINAL CORD INJURY WITHOUT OBJECTIVE RADIOLOGICAL ABNORMALITY)

This phenomenon occurs in children and is related to hyperelasticity of the vertebral column. In most cases spinal cord traction is the mechanism of neurological injury.

MRI scanning may demonstrate the level of cord injury and is useful in demonstrating compressive lesions, e.g. epidural haematoma.

REHABILITATION AND PATIENT OUTCOME

The goal of spinal cord injury rehabilitation is to maximise remaining neurological function. The functional ability that may be achieved is dependent on the level of neurological impairment and this is outlined in Table 24.1.

Prognosis of spinal cord injury

Life expectancy following spinal cord injury

Despite continuing improvements in survival following spinal cord injury, life expectancy remains reduced (Table 24.2). Pneumonia, pulmonary emboli and septicaemia are the most frequent causes of premature death in this population group. Renal failure is no longer the leading cause of death because of advances in urological management. Age at injury and level of injury are the most important prognostic factors.

Prognosis for neurological recovery

The prognosis of incomplete cord injury is highly variable and is influenced by the type of cord injury (syndromes), age of the patient and associated injuries.

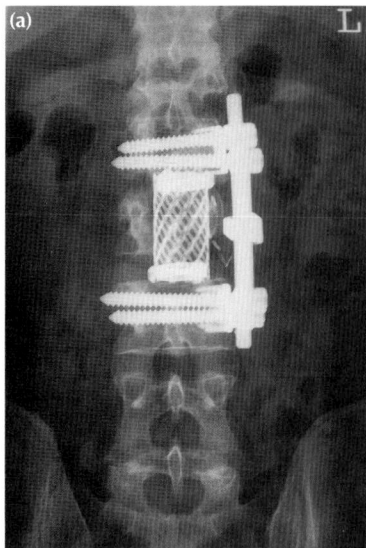

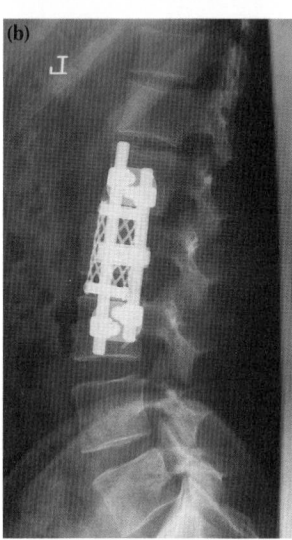

Figure 24.37 Anterior spinal reconstruction for a lumbar burst fracture.

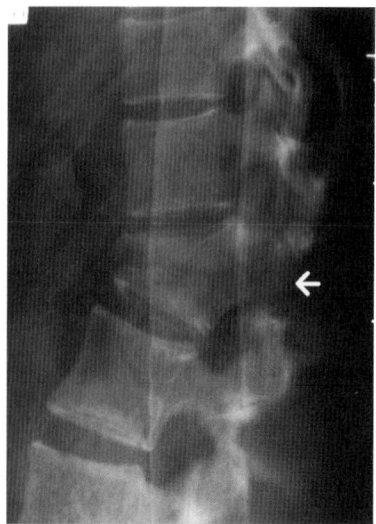

Figure 24.38 A bony Chance fracture at the thoracolumbar junction secondary to a lap belt injury.

Complications associated with spinal cord injury

Pain and spasticity

Neurogenic pain is extremely common following spinal cord injury and in some cases may be difficult to control. Once reflex activity returns spasticity can be problematic. Intrathecal infusion of baclofen may be required in resistant cases.

Autonomic dysreflexia

This is a paroxysmal syndrome of hypertension, hypohydrosis (above level of injury), bradycardia, flushing and headache in response to noxious visceral and other stimuli. It is most commonly triggered by bladder distension or rectal loading from faecal impaction.

Neurological deterioration

Post-traumatic syringomyelia may cause late (> 3 months post-injury) neurological deterioration and occurs in 3–5% of spinal cord injury cases. Increase in pain and/or spasticity, ascending loss of pain and temperature sensation, and ascending loss of deep tendon reflexes are some of the features associated with this

Table 24.1 Expected functional outcome versus level of cervical spinal cord injury

Level of injury	Functional goal
C3–C4	Power wheelchair with mouth or chin control; verbalise care, communicate through adaptive equipment; may be ventilator dependent
C5	Power wheelchair; dress upper body; self-feed with aids; wash face with assistance
C6	Propel power wheelchair, possibly push manual wheelchair; transfer with assistance; dress upper body (lower body with assistance); self-groom with aids; bladder/bowel care with assistance; self-feed with splints; able to drive
C7	Manual wheelchair; independent transfer; dress (with aids), feed, bath and self-care; bladder and bowel care with assistance
C8–T4	Independent with most activities of daily living, transfers, manual wheelchair and bowel and bladder care
T5–T12	As above but with more ease; independent with all self-care activities. T12: possible to walk with walker and long leg braces (difficult and highly demanding)
L1–L5	Independent; walk with short or long leg braces
S1–S5	Independent; able to walk if capable of pushing off (S1) (may need brace); bladder, bowel and sexual function may remain compromised

Table 24.2 Life expectancy (years) post-injury according to severity of injury and age at injury

(a) For persons who survive the first 24 hours

Age at injury (years)	No SCI	Motor functional at any level	Paraplegic	Low tetraplegic (C5–C8)	High tetraplegic (C1–C4)	Ventilator dependent at any level
20	58.4	52.8	45.6	40.6	36.1	16.6
40	39.5	34.3	28.0	23.8	20.2	7.1
60	22.2	17.9	13.1	10.2	7.9	1.4

(b) For persons surviving at least 1 year post-injury

Age at injury (years)	No SCI	Motor functional at any level	Paraplegic	Low tetraplegic (C5–C8)	High tetraplegic (C1–C4)	Ventilator dependent at any level
20	58.4	53.3	46.3	41.7	37.9	23.3
40	39.5	34.8	28.6	24.7	21.6	11.1
60	22.2	18.3	13.5	10.8	8.8	3.1

SCI, spinal cord injury.

condition, which warrant early MRI assessment of the cord. Expanding cavities require neurosurgical intervention.

Thromboembolic events

Approximately 30% of spinal cord-injured patients develop a clinically significant deep vein thrombosis. Fatal pulmonary embolus is reported in 1–2% of all spinal cord injury deaths within the first 3 months of injury, with the highest risks within the first 3 weeks. Prophylactic intervention is therefore important in this patient group.

Heterotopic ossification and contractures

The most frequent areas affected by heterotopic ossification are hips, knees, shoulders and elbows. It occurs in 25% of spinal cord-injured patients. Patients should receive prophylactic sodium etidronate or indomethacin. Surgery for joint ankylosis should only be considered when the process becomes dormant (normal alkaline phosphatase level, negative isotope bone scan).

Soft tissue contractures around joints may occur where opposing muscle groups have unequal power. These are avoided by appropriate physical therapy, positioning and splinting. Surgical release may be required in certain cases.

FURTHER READING

Aebi, M., Thalgott, J.S. and Webb, J.K. (1998) *AO ASIF Principles in Spine Surgery*. Springer-Verlag, Berlin.

Bridwell, K.H. and DeWald, R.L. (eds) (1997) *The Textbook of Spinal Surgery*. Lippincott-Raven, Philadelphia, PA.

British Orthopaedic Association (2006) *The Initial Care and Transfer of Patients With Spinal Cord Injuries*. British Orthopaedic Association, London.

Cotler, J.M., Simson, M.J., An, H.S. and Silveri, C.P. (eds) (2000) *Surgery of Spinal Trauma*. Lippincott, Williams & Wilkins, Philadelphia, PA.

Fardon, D.F., Garfin, S.R., Abitbol, J.J., Boden, S.D., Herkowitz, H.H. and Mayer, T.G. (eds) *Orthopaedic Knowledge Update: Spine 2*. American Academy of Orthopaedic Surgeons, Rosemont, IL.

Weinstein, J.N. (ed.) (2006) Spinal trauma focus issue. *Spine* **31(11S)**: S1–104.

CHAPTER 24 | NECK AND SPINE

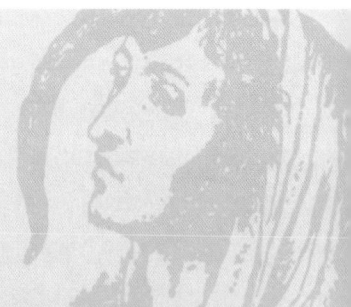

Trauma to the face and mouth

CHAPTER

25

INTRODUCTION

Injuries to the orofacial region are common, but the majority are relatively minor in nature. A few are major and complex, requiring exacting technique and meticulous care in management. It must always be remembered that an intact and unscarred face is important to the well-being of the individual, and thus all injuries, however trivial, should be treated thoughtfully and sympathetically, with every effort made to produce an optimal outcome. In addition, even trivial blows to the face may:

- cause injuries that compromise the airway;
- directly or indirectly cause a head injury;
- cause injuries to the cervical spine.

EPIDEMIOLOGY

Injuries to the orofacial soft tissues, dentition and facial skeleton result from sporting activities, accidents and intentional violence. Formerly, road traffic accidents were the commonest cause of maxillofacial injuries in the UK. However, the compulsory wearing of seatbelts and the use of car air bags and laminated windscreens have reduced the incidence of such injuries as a result of road traffic accidents. However, the decrease in injuries from this source has been almost matched by the increase in deliberate injury from civil assault where 'putting the boot in' has become a fashion, with often appalling results.

Many studies have demonstrated significant variation in the aetiological causes of orofacial injuries in different parts of the world, and even within the same continent. This can perhaps be accounted for by both variation in data collection and also the classification of such injuries, which may vary significantly between researchers. In addition, many factors affect the causes of orofacial injuries, and these may also explain the varying epidemiological and incidence figures seen in differing geographical regions:

- *Social factors.* Interpersonal violence has steadily increased and, in many countries, is now the commonest cause of orofacial injuries. This increase is noticed to a greater extent in conurbations and urban areas, often fuelled by alcohol excess and 'binge' drinking.
- *Climatic factors.* Countries lying within temperate latitudes often demonstrate variations in weather that may be associated with an increased incidence of injuries. The arrival of snow and freezing weather during the winter and increased traffic volumes and interpersonal violence during the warmer months of the year often produce seasonal variations in the incidence of injuries.
- *Road traffic accidents.* Legislation and improved vehicular design have lessened the number of injuries presenting as a result of road traffic accidents. Air bag provision, seatbelts, laminated windscreens and drink/drive laws have all helped in reducing orofacial injuries. The enforcement of lower speed limits has not, as yet, been shown to reduce injuries.

CLINICAL EFFECTS

The mouth and nasal passages form part of the upper aerodigestive tract, and lacerations and fractures of the facial skeleton may give rise to immediate or delayed respiratory obstruction. Immediate obstruction may arise from inhalation of tooth fragments, accumulation of blood and secretions, and loss of control of the tongue in the unconscious or semiconscious patient. To avoid this, the patient should always be nursed in the semiprone position (Fig. 25.1) with the head supported on the bent arm, and never lying on their back. Damaged teeth, blood and secretions can then fall out of the mouth, and gravity pulls the tongue

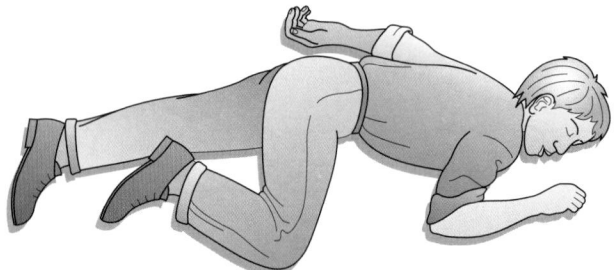

Figure 25.1 The patient should be nursed in the semiprone position to allow secretions, blood and foreign bodies to fall from the mouth.

forward. As the patient is manoeuvred into the correct nursing position, the neck should be supported and held in a neutral position – a protective collar is advisable until a fracture of the cervical spine has been excluded. An intracranial injury should always be considered as a possibility, however minor the injury to the face.

Initial haemorrhage after a facial injury can be dramatic. Sustained bleeding is unusual, but emergency measures to stabilise the facial fractures and control bleeding may be required. The most likely causes of circulatory failure in a facial injury are accompanying skeletal fractures or a ruptured viscus, and these should always be actively sought in the shocked patient.

Oedema is a particular feature of all fractures of the facial skeleton and tends to develop within 60–90 minutes. Thus, a patient with a shattered face may appear to have a good airway immediately after the blow, but the airway may change rapidly and become occluded by swelling of the tongue or facial and pharyngeal tissues. This problem must always be borne in mind when the middle third of the face is involved. In Le Fort III fractures (see below), the maxilla may be thrust downwards and backwards along the base of the skull. As it does so, the posterior teeth of the upper and lower jaws contact prematurely and the mouth is held open (Fig. 25.2), giving the impression of a good airway. As oedema develops, the soft palate and tongue may swell to meet, so closing the pharyngeal airway and leading to respiratory distress and even obstruction (Fig. 25.3). Whenever this is suspected, the 'golden hour' must be used to insert an oropharyngeal airway, even though the patient may appear conscious and the airway not obstructed. If this is not done, an emergency tracheostomy may have to be undertaken later with potential risk to the patient (Summary box 25.1).

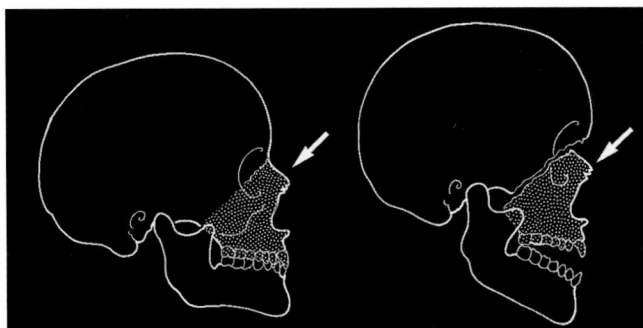

Figure 25.2 A blow from the front of the face may separate the facial skeleton from the base of the skull and thrust it downwards and backwards.

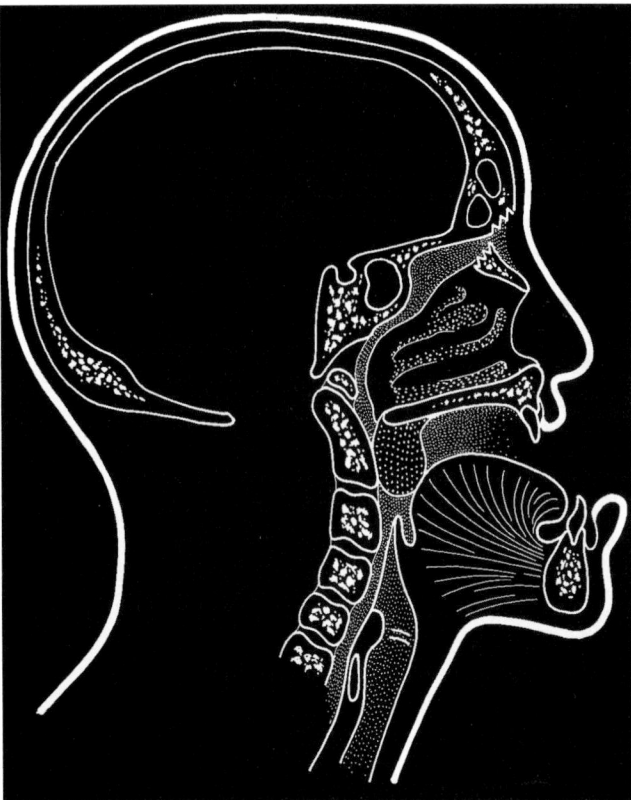

Figure 25.3 Loss of nasopharyngeal space and oedema of the soft palate and tongue may close off the airway in severe maxillofacial injuries, 2–3 hours after the injury.

Summary box 25.1

Facial injuries

- Are potentially life-threatening (can compromise the airway)
- Can distract the clinician from other injuries
- May be associated with injuries to the brain and cervical spine
- Are cosmetically very important

EXAMINATION OF THE PATIENT

The examination of the patient should be under a good light with consideration of the airway and other collateral injuries in mind. It is easy to be distracted from examining the whole patient by the dramatic effects of the facial injury. The rapid onset of oedema may make examination of the face and routine head injury observations difficult – occasionally, it is impossible to prise the eyelids apart to examine the pupils, for instance. Lacerations should be explored first and, if necessary, cleaned using sterile saline or aqueous antiseptic solution.

Once the pattern and extent of soft-tissue injury has been established and recorded, attention should be directed towards the hard tissues. Regardless of the apparent site of the injury, the whole head should be examined visually and by palpation starting with the vault of the skull. A blow to the face may result in the head being thrown back against a hard object, and a bruise or laceration on the occiput can be missed. Bruising over the mastoid process, or Battle's sign, may be indicative of a middle cranial fossa fracture. The face should be examined from the front. Any asymmetry and displacements should be noted, although oedema may make this difficult. Gentle palpation, using both hands and wearing surgical gloves, gives the most information in searching for step deformities. Tenderness over sites of known weakness and potential for fracture (see below) is a very good guide to the possibility of there being an underlying fracture. A suitable system is to examine from above downwards – the supraorbital and infraorbital ridges, the nasal bridge and the zygomas, including the arches. The mandible should then be examined starting at the condyles bilaterally and then following the posterior and lower border of the mandible as far as the midline. The majority of middle third injuries are accompanied by some degree of epistaxis (except isolated zygomatic arch fractures), and Le Fort II and III injuries frequently have a cerebrospinal fluid (CSF) leak with anterior or posterior CSF rhinorrhoea. A particularly useful sign in the fractured zygoma is the frequent subconjunctival haemorrhage, which will often be found to have no posterior limit when the patient is asked to look to the other side (Fig. 25.4). This may be suggestive of a fracture of the associated zygomatic complex.

The patient should then be examined intraorally with good illumination. The lips should be parted and the occlusion of the teeth examined. The maxillary and mandibular dentition normally 'fit' together even if the occlusion is naturally irregular – if they do not, a fracture of the jaws may be suspected. All fractures involving the alveolus (the tooth-bearing portion of the jaw in the dentate patient) tear the gingivae and are compound into the mouth (Fig. 25.5): the examiner should look for signs of bleeding. A haematoma in the floor of the mouth is a good indication of a fracture of the mandible, particularly in edentulous cases. Alignment of the teeth should be noted, and any missing or broken teeth and dental restorations/prostheses should be carefully recorded. The occlusal plane must be examined for the presence of step defects, often indicative of a fracture of the underlying bone. The patient should be asked to bring the teeth together, so

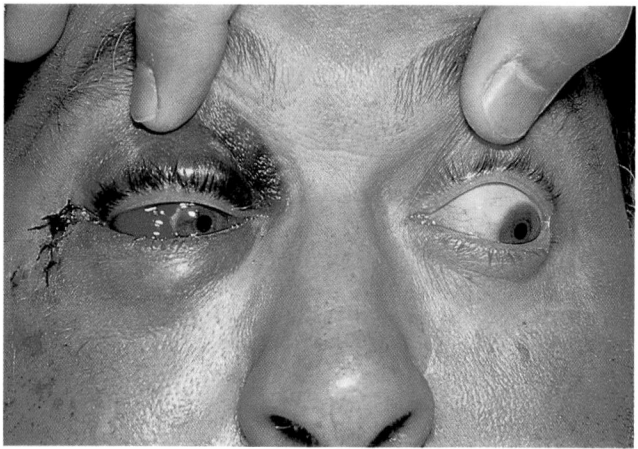

Figure 25.4 Fractures of the zygoma may often be associated with subconjunctival haemorrhage. This example shows no posterior border to the haemorrhage as the patient looks away from the side of the fracture.

William Henry Battle, 1855–1936, Surgeon, St Thomas' Hospital, London, England.

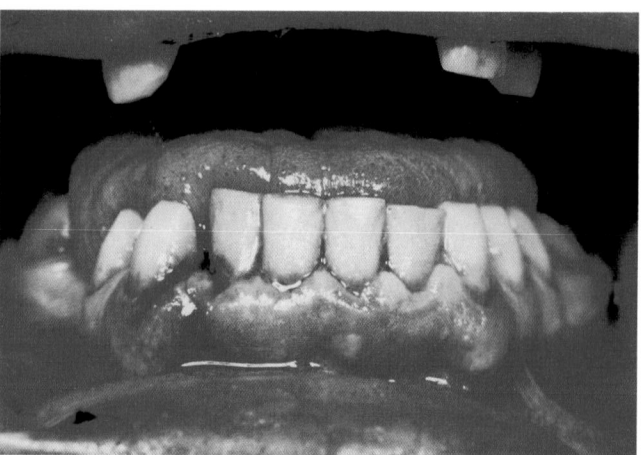

Figure 25.5 A fracture of the right parasymphysis of the mandible, demonstrating a tear of the gingivae in the lower right lateral incisor/canine region.

that any occlusal anomalies may be observed and, in some cases, independent movement of the fragments may then be detected. Movement of the jaw should be tested – deviation from the midline at rest or on opening suggests a fracture of the side to which the jaw is deviating.

If a fracture of the maxilla is suspected, the maxillary dental arch should be grasped between the index finger, middle finger and thumb of one hand in the incisor region, while the other is placed on the forehead. If the maxilla is fractured, gentle movement forward and backward, or side to side, will reveal movement between the examining hands. With the mandible, gentle manipulation across the suspected site of a fracture will confirm the presence of a fracture if 'springing' is felt and seen. Confirmation of a fractured zygoma may be made by palpating the fractured antral wall above the upper molar teeth in the buccal sulcus.

Soft-tissue injuries within the oral cavity should be identified and recorded. Lacerations of the oral mucosa may occur independently of hard-tissue injuries, and can often involve the buccal mucous membrane and tongue. Degloving lacerations most commonly involve the labial sulcus and the body of the mandible. Tongue injuries demand careful assessment as lacerations are often underestimated in terms of their depth and potential for dehiscence. Furthermore, tongue lacerations may be a source of potential haemorrhage, which may be delayed on occasion. Palatal lacerations tend to occur in young children who fall onto objects held in the oral cavity, especially pens and pencils. With such a history, the suspicion of retained foreign bodies must be considered.

The maxillofacial examination is then turned to the relevant cranial nerves. Anaesthesia or paraesthesia indicates a fracture proximally along the course of the nerve. Thus, anaesthesia/paraesthesia of the cheek and upper lip suggests a fracture involving the infraorbital foramen or floor of the orbit, while anaesthesia/paraesthesia of the lower lip suggests a fracture of the mandibular body. Facial palsy may indicate severance of branches of the facial nerve that are involved in facial lacerations, particularly penetrating wounds of the parotid gland. In the absence of lacerations, facial palsy may be suggestive of a fractured temporal bone.

It is important to confirm that the patient has sight in both eyes. This may be difficult in the very oedematous patient with marked periorbital oedema, but a pen torch shone directly through the lids will confirm gross optic nerve function. Where possible, pupil size and reflexes to light should be observed and recorded, as should eye movements. Diplopia should be checked for by asking the patient to follow the light of a pen torch in both central and extremes of gaze. Diplopia may be indicative of damage to the III, IV or VI cranial nerves or, more commonly, damage to the thin orbital plates of bone, particularly the floor of the orbit.

All findings should be recorded accurately, preferably with diagrams to include measurements of lacerations, abrasions and areas of tissue loss. Photographs of the initial injury can be very helpful if litigation is likely to follow (Summary box 25.2).

Summary box 25.2

Examination of facial injuries

- Commence with lacerations and soft-tissue injuries
- Systematically examine bones including the occiput and cranial vault
- Check dental occlusion and palpate the mouth
- Check cranial nerves
- Photographs are useful

ADDITIONAL INVESTIGATIONS

Blood tests

Baseline full blood count and biochemistry should be obtained. Blood should be grouped when it is thought that significant bleeding has occurred and more bleeding is likely.

Radiological investigations

Table 25.1 demonstrates the radiographic views utilised in the diagnosis of maxillofacial injuries. Coronal computerised tomography (CT) scanning has superseded tomographic views in the diagnosis of orbital floor fractures, and coronal and axial CT scanning is often the choice of radiographic investigation in the more complex middle third fractures (Fig. 25.6). A chest radiograph is indicated if there is any suggestion of inhalation of dental fragments or dental prostheses. It should be remembered, however, that polymethylmethacrylate used in the construction of dentures may not appear radiopaque on plain radiographs.

Table 25.1 Radiological views for specific fractures

Site of fracture	Radiographs
Mandible: body and ramus	OPT, lateral obliques, lower occlusal, PA mandible
Mandible: condyles	OPT, PA mandible with mouth open, Toller transpharyngeal views
Maxilla	OM 15° and 30°, lateral facial bones
Zygomatic complex	OM 15° and 30°, submentovertex
Orbital blow-outs	OM 15° and 30° and tomograms
Nasal bones	Lateral nasal bones, occipitofrontal
Frontal bones	Lateral skull, occipitofrontal

OPT, orthopantomogram; PA, posteroanterior; OM, posteroanterior occipitomental.

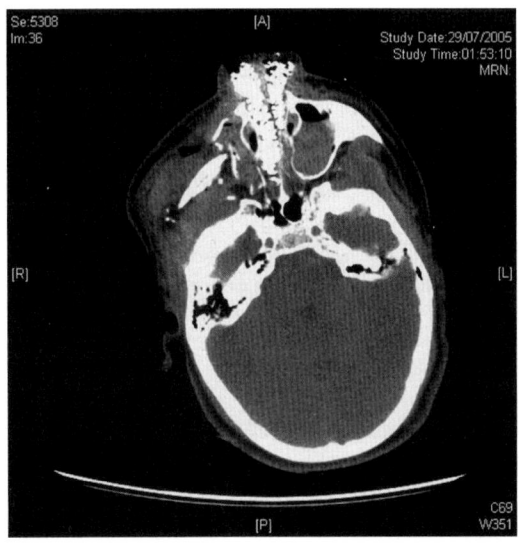

Figure 25.6 Computerised tomographic (CT) scan showing a comminuted fracture of the right maxilla and zygomatic complex (nasal pack in place).

Posteroanterior occipitomental radiographs taken at 15° and 30° are the optimum initial radiographs to illustrate the site and displacement of a middle third fracture. A panoramic oral radiograph, or orthopantomogram (Fig. 25.7), is the radiograph of choice for the mandible as it shows the whole bone from condyle to condyle. If the patient cannot be positioned in the machines to achieve these views, radiographs should wait until the patient is fit enough. Poor radiographs can be misleading, and treatment can only be based on adequate radiographs or scans.

FRACTURES OF THE FACIAL SKELETON

Fractures of the facial skeleton may be divided into those of the upper third (above the eyebrows), the middle third (above the mouth) and the lower third (the mandible). Fractures tend to occur through points of weakness – the sutures and foramina – and in thin unsupported bone.

The upper third

The patterns of fracture of the skull tend to be random, but there are points of weakness, mainly involving the frontal sinuses and the supraorbital ridges.

The middle third

In 1911, René Le Fort classified fractures according to patterns which he created on cadavers using varying degrees of force. The Le Fort classification is used extensively today throughout the world. While Le Fort classified the fractures from superior to inferior, the custom today is that the classification runs inferiorly to superiorly (Fig. 25.8).

The Le Fort I fracture effectively separates the alveolus and palate from the facial skeleton above. The fracture line runs through points of weakness from the nasal piriform aperture

---

René Le Fort, 1869–1951, was a French Surgeon who classified facial fractures after macabre research in which he dropped rocks and other heavy objects on the faces of cadavers.

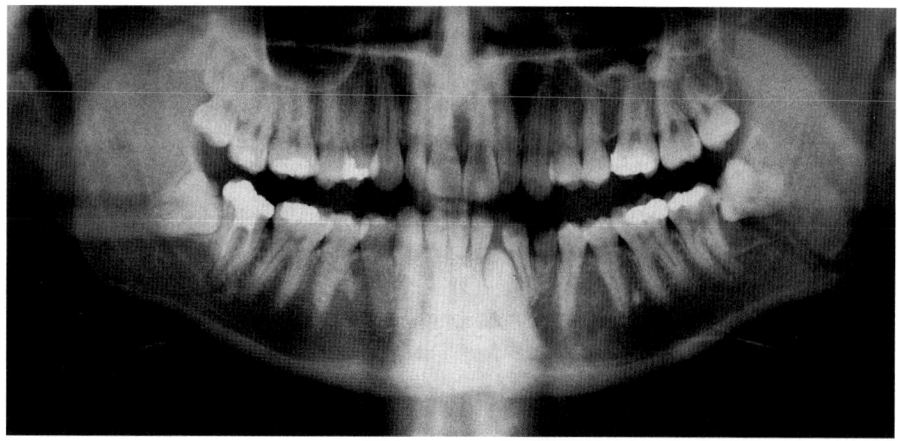

Figure 25.7 An orthopantomogram demonstrating a fracture of the left angle of the mandible.

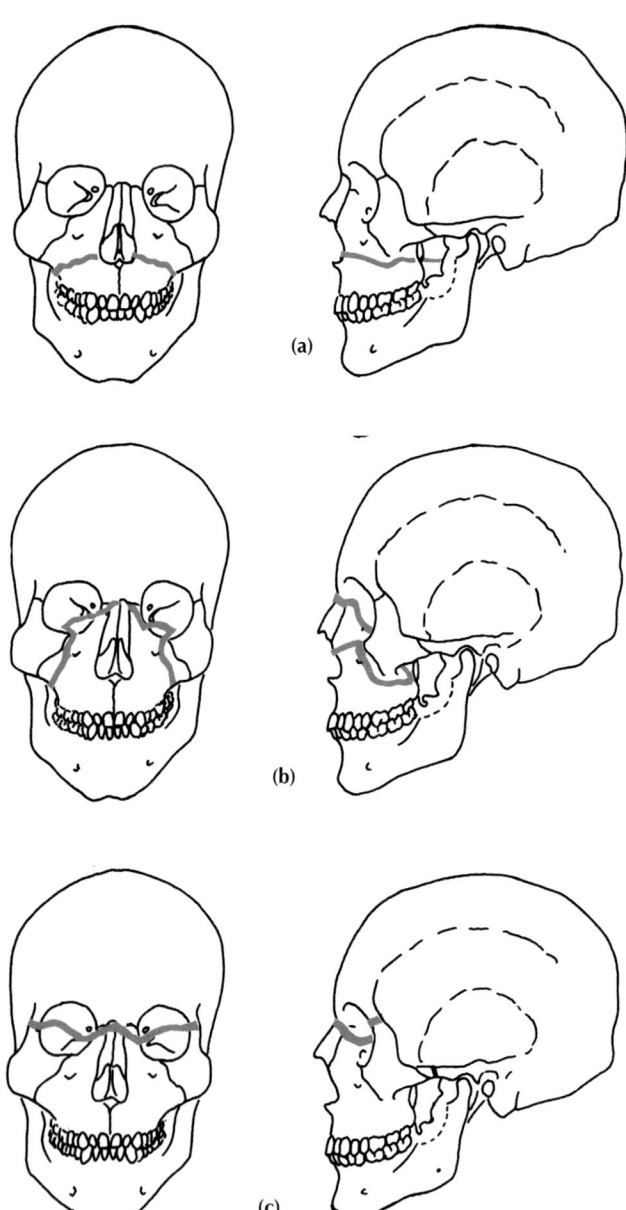

Figure 25.8 Maxillary fractures as classified by Le Fort. (a) Le Fort I; (b) Le Fort II; (c) Le Fort III.

through the lateral and medial walls of the maxillary sinus, running posteriorly to include the lower part of the pterygoid plates.

The Le Fort II fracture is pyramidal in shape. The fracture involves the orbit, running through the bridge of the nose and the ethmoids, whose cribriform plate may be fractured, leading to a dural tear and CSF rhinorrhoea. It continues to the medial part of the infraorbital rim and often through the infraorbital foramen. By definition, the orbital floor is always involved. It continues posteriorly through the lateral wall of the maxillary antrum at a higher level than the Le Fort I fracture to the pterygoid plates at the back.

The Le Fort III fracture effectively separates the facial skeleton from the base of the skull – the fracture lines run high through the nasal bridge, septum and ethmoids, again with the potential for dural tear and CSF leak, and irregularly through the bones of the orbit to the frontozygomatic suture. The zygomatic arch fractures, and the facial skeleton is separated from the bones above at a high level through the lateral wall of the maxillary sinus and the pterygoid plates.

The Le Fort fractures are seldom confined exactly to the original classification, and combinations of any of the above fractures may occur.

The zygomatic complex

This is the most common fracture of the middle third of the face, apart from the nose. The fractures occur through points of weakness – the infraorbital margin, the frontozygomatic suture, the zygomatic arch and the anterior and lateral wall of the maxillary sinus. Tears of the antral mucosa may lead to epistaxis on the affected side, and damage to the infraorbital nerve may cause paraesthesia in its sensory distribution (Summary box 25.3).

Summary box 25.3

Fractures of the zygomatic complex

- Damage to the infraorbital nerve is common, causing numbness on the cheek

---

Blow-out fractures of the orbit

Direct trauma to the globe of the eye may push it back within the orbit. The globe is a fairly robust structure and, as it is thrust backwards, the pressure increases within the orbit, and the weaker plates of bone may fracture, without necessarily fracturing the bones of the orbital rim. Such injuries can occur when a blunt object strikes the globe. The weakest plate of bone, most commonly the orbital floor, fractures, and the orbital contents herniate down into the maxillary antrum. This soft-tissue herniation may lead to muscular dysfunction, particularly the inferior oblique and inferior rectus, leading to failure of the eye to rotate upwards. Enophthalmos and diplopia can follow, although both may initially be concealed by oedema. Paraesthesia in the distribution of the infraorbital nerve may be an important clue to the blow-out fracture. Any fracture that involves the orbital floor (Le Fort II and zygomatic complex) must be considered to have the potential for orbital content entrapment too.

There should be a high index of suspicion of any possible orbital blow-out fracture. The signs and symptoms of such injuries are often masked in the early stages, with enophthalmos and ocular problems becoming apparent later. Significant delay in treatment may be associated with less success than early diagnosis and planned treatment (Fig. 25.9). It is wise to assume that, if any signs or symptoms are suggestive of a possible orbital floor injury, such an injury exists, until proven otherwise with coronal CT scans (Summary box 25.4).

Summary box 25.4

Blow-out fractures of the orbit

- Damage to the infraorbital nerve is common, causing numbness of the cheek
- Any fracture that involves the orbital floor (Le Fort II and zygomatic complex) has the potential for orbital content entrapment

Naso-ethmoidal complex fractures

Fractures of the naso-ethmoidal complex, as opposed to isolated nasal bone fractures, are usually comminuted fractures involving the nasal bones, frontal processes of the maxilla, medial and sometimes infraorbital rims and the maxillary processes/anterior sinus wall of the frontal bones. Such injuries can cause significant deformity (Fig. 25.10) and, because of disruption of the medial canthal ligaments, may cause traumatic telecanthus.

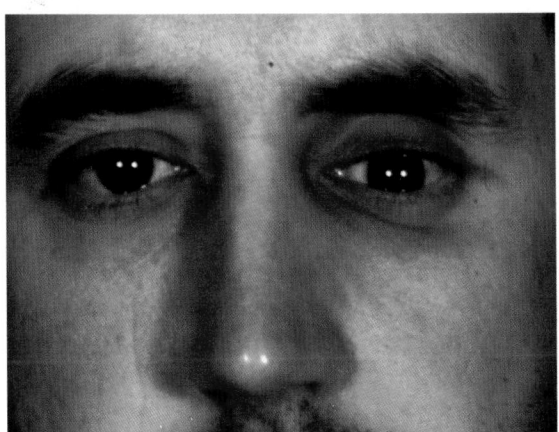

Figure 25.9 Previously undiagnosed left orbital blow-out fracture, presenting 3 months after the initial injury. Enophthalmos and lowered pupillary level are evident.

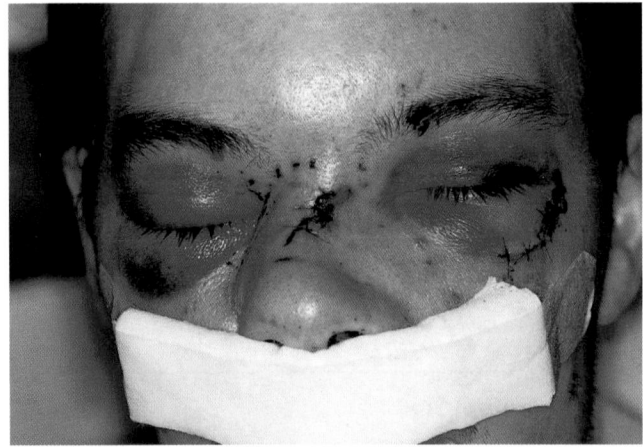

Figure 25.10 Naso-ethmoidal complex fracture, demonstrating gross nasal deformity and traumatic telecanthus.

Fractures of the mandible

The condylar neck is the weakest part of the mandible and is the most frequent site of fracture (Fig. 25.11), while other fractures tend to occur through unerupted teeth (the impacted wisdom tooth) or where the roots are long (the canine tooth). The mandible may fracture directly at the point of the blow, or indirectly where the force from the blow is transmitted and the mandible fractures at a point of weakness distant from the original blow. The latter is characteristically seen in the so called 'guardsman' fracture, where a blow to the chin point may cause a fracture of the symphysis or parasymphysis of the lower jaw, and indirect transmission of the kinetic energy causes a unilateral or bilateral fracture of the mandibular condyles. Individual sharp blows with a blunt instrument may fracture a segment away from the mandible. Blows from below may cause the mandible to be thrust upwards, fracturing the alveolus and teeth as they strike the maxillary dentition.

Much has been made in the past of the 'butterfly' fracture of the mandible. Here, a segment of mandible is detached from the rest of the mandible in the canine regions. The segment of bone may include the anterior insertion of the tongue (genioglossus and geniohyoid). Theoretically, the tongue may fall back and occlude the airway. First, the fracture is exceedingly rare and,

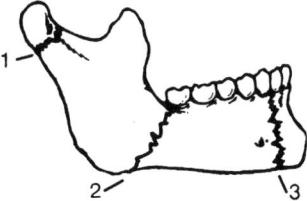

Figure 25.11 The patterns of fracture of the mandible. (1) The neck of the condyle is the most common site, followed by (2) the angle of the mandible through the last tooth. (3) The third point of weakness is in the region of the canine tooth.

A 'guardsman' fracture is so called because it refers to the Queen's Guards who, when they fainted on parade, still held themselves in a position of attention. As a consequence, if they fell forward, the first point of contact with the ground would be the point of the chin. This resulted in a direct fracture of the symphysis/parasymphysis of the mandible, and indirect fractures of both mandibular condyles.

CHAPTER 25 | TRAUMA TO THE FACE AND MOUTH

second, the patient can still control the tongue, if nursed in the correct position (see earlier) (Summary box 25.5).

> **Summary box 25.5**
>
> **Fractures of the mandible**
>
> ■ The condylar neck is the weakest and most common site
> ■ Indirect transmission of energy may fracture the mandibular condyle(s)

TREATMENT

Soft-tissue injuries

Facial soft tissues have an excellent blood supply and heal well. They should be sutured as soon as possible following the injury after careful exploration, debridement and cleaning, particularly where foreign bodies may be embedded. Many lacerations may be closed using local anaesthesia, injecting into the edges of the wound. If the patient is due to have a general anaesthetic and there is a delay, the wounds should be temporarily closed in advance, using local anaesthesia. Tissue sufficiently traumatised to have lost its blood supply should be removed with a sharp scalpel, and the edge to which it is to be apposed trimmed to fit as appropriate.

Great care should be taken to replace tissues accurately, particularly in cosmetically important landmarks such as the vermilion border of the lips, the eyelids and nasal contours. Haemostasis is important. Muscle and underlying tissues should be brought together with absorbable sutures so that the edges of the wound lie passively within 2 mm of their final position. Then fine monofilament sutures (5/0 or 6/0) are used to bring the wound edges together (Fig. 25.12). Sutures should be placed so as to avoid compromising the blood supply of the apices of small flaps. Vacuum drains are used where there is concern over dead space beneath the wounds. The lacerations should be covered with antibiotic ointment two or three times per day, and broad-spectrum antibiotics should be prescribed. Ideally, alternate sutures should be removed from the third day with the remaining sutures removed on the fifth day.

Intraoral lacerations require careful debridement, and closure in layers with resorbable suture materials. Lacerations to mobile structures such as the tongue and soft palate can often be underestimated in terms of their depth. Failure to close the deeper layers of intraoral lacerations may predispose to later dehiscence,

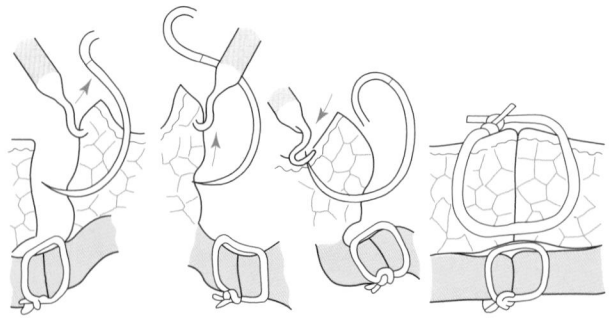

Figure 25.12 Facial wound. The method of skin closure avoiding inversion of the wound edges. The skin suture has a greater bite of deep tissue than at the surface.

with resultant scars that are thickened and uncomfortable to the patient (Summary box 25.6).

> **Summary box 25.6**
>
> **Facial lacerations**
>
> ■ Wounds must be cleaned to avoid tattooing
> ■ Replace tissues accurately, especially the vermilion border

Skin loss

Loss of facial skin in any significant amount is a relatively rare occurrence in all but the more severe maxillofacial injuries. However, substantial skin and deeper tissue loss does occur as a result of human bite injuries (Fig. 25.13), most commonly the nose and ear. Small areas of tissue loss can be dealt with by careful undermining of the surrounding soft tissues, with the defect being closed primarily, providing there is no significant tension on the wound edges and no resulting distortion of the surrounding tissues or structures. Larger areas of skin loss require careful assessment and planned reconstruction with grafts and local tissue flaps.

Facial nerve injury

The branches of the facial nerve may be severed in the depths of a lateral facial wound. If this is suspected, primary repair should be attempted, particularly where clinical signs suggest that a major division is involved. Locating the divided branches in oedematous and damaged tissue can prove extremely difficult. Proximal and distal flaps in relatively normal adjacent tissue may have to be raised to identify the nerve on each side of the laceration. The severed nerve ends may then be approximated using

(a)

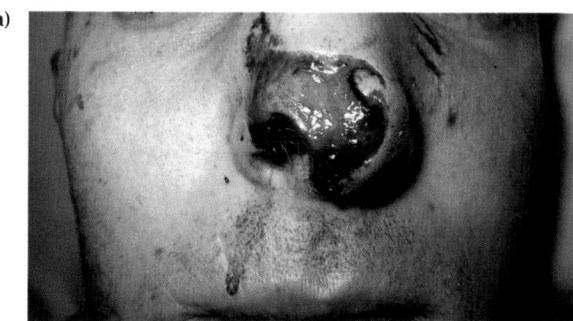

(b)

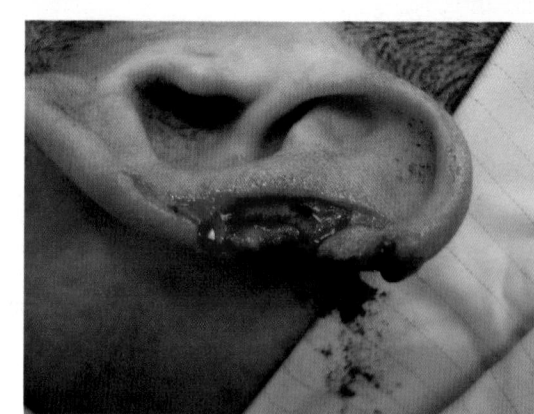

Figure 25.13 Skin and cartilage loss sustained as a result of human bite injuries. (a) Nose; (b) ear.

an operating microscope, and the nerve and laceration sutured. Attempts at primary repair should always be undertaken, as secondary repair is generally unsatisfactory (Summary box 25.7).

Summary box 25.7

Facial nerve injury

- Primary repair is the most appropriate treatment

Parotid duct

Lacerations in the same vicinity as those that transect the facial nerve may also transect the parotid duct. The suggested management is to insert a fine cannula in the parotid duct from within the mouth and pass it posteriorly until it appears in the wound. The position of the proximal duct should then be identified and this portion passed over the cannula, so approximating the severed portions of the duct. The two portions of the duct are then anastomosed, and the cannula left in position for several days in an attempt to prevent post-anastomotic stricture (Summary box 25.8).

Summary box 25.8

Parotid duct transection

- Cannulate from the mouth and anastomose over the stent

The lacrimal apparatus

The nasolacrimal apparatus may be involved in damage to the eyelids and skeletal facial injuries involving the naso-orbital region. The tissues are generally grossly oedematous, and the manipulation required to reduce the fractures adds to the difficulty of identifying the cannaliculae. Most surgeons do not attempt repair primarily but refer to an ophthalmic surgeon if epiphora becomes a problem later. Surprisingly, few patients suffer epiphora after a year has elapsed from the injury.

Fractured nasal bones

The nasal bones are the most commonly fractured bones of the facial skeleton. Best results are obtained when soft-tissue oedema has been allowed to settle so that accurate reduction can be achieved. Surgery should ideally be carried out within a week of the injury as, if left any longer, reduction may become difficult or impossible. Reduction should be directed first to repositioning the nasal bones, disimpacting with Walsham's forceps with the external blade covered with rubber tubing, so as to avoid damage to the skin. The nasal bones are first moved laterally to disimpact them and then medially to reposition them. The septum is then grasped with Asch's forceps, manipulated until it is straight and then positioned in the groove of the nasal crest and vomer. It should be remembered, however, that the nasal septum often cannot be adequately manipulated into position and may require formal septoplasty at a later date. Asch's forceps may also be used to pull the disimpacted nasal bones forward to their previous position.

William Johnson Walsham, 1847–1903, Surgeon, St Bartholomew's Hospital, London, England.
Morris Joseph Asch, 1833–1902, Surgeon, New York Eye and Ear Hospital, New York, NY, USA.

Fractures involving the naso-ethmoidal complex require open reduction and fixation, and any disruption of the medial canthal attachments demands replacement of these structures in their correct anatomical position. The nasal bones may need supporting by a pack within the nasal bridge. Variations on nasal packing exist, but most packs should be removed at 2–3 days following the nasal bone reduction. A protective nasal plaster may be placed and should be removed at 5–7 days (Summary box 25.9).

Summary box 25.9

Nasal fractures

- Treatment is best undertaken within 1 week, once the swelling has settled

---

Frontal bone fractures

The presence of depressed frontal bone fractures and fractures of the posterior wall of the frontal sinus demands that neurosurgical collaboration should be sought. However, fractures of the anterior wall of the sinus are amenable to maxillofacial techniques for reduction and fixation. Access may be through pre-existing lacerations overlying the area, but excellent access with minimal morbidity is achieved using the bicoronal scalp flap (see later). Bone fragments may then be reduced and fixed using small titanium bone plates and screws (Fig. 25.14). Any missing bone should be replaced with bone grafts, thereby avoiding any cosmetic forehead depression postoperatively.

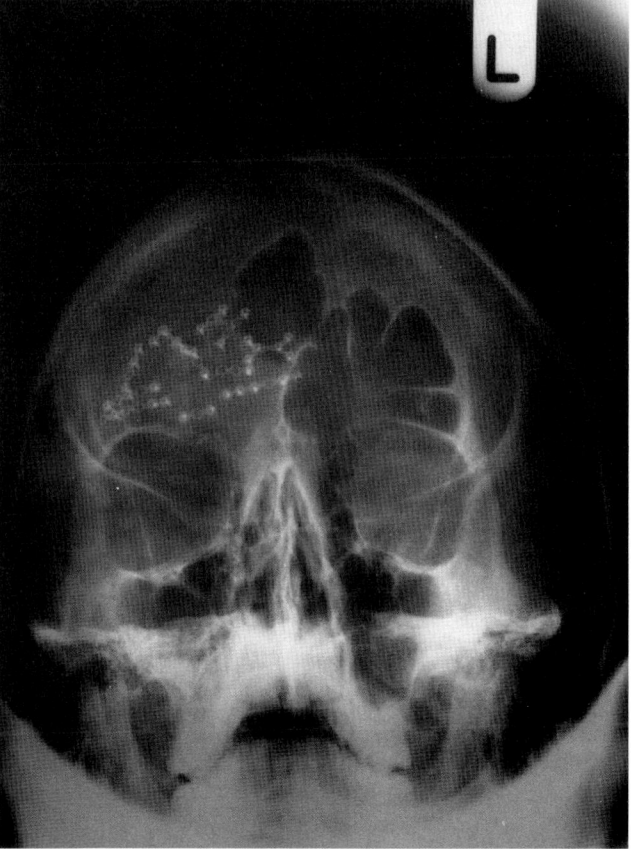

Figure 25.14 Radiograph demonstrating multiple plate fixation of an anterior wall in a frontal sinus fracture.

Fractures of the maxilla

The principle of reducing and stabilising fractures of the frontal and facial bones is that the surgeon starts at the top and works down. Where there are extensive lacerations, these may be used, perhaps with small extensions, to approach the fracture sites. Where no convenient lacerations exist, fractures of the frontal bone, supraorbital ridge and nasal root may be approached through a bicoronal incision at the vault of the skull, high in the hair line. The incision is taken from just in front of each ear across the vault of the skull and reflected forwards until the supraorbital ridges are exposed. The supraorbital nerves are identified and freed, and the flap extended as required. The nasal bones, lateral orbital rim, frontal bones and zygomatic arches may all be exposed through this approach. All the fractured bones may be reduced and fixed by stainless steel wire or titanium mini/microplates under direct vision. Bone deficiencies in this area may be made up with free, outer cortical cranial bone grafts, with the donor sites available through the bicoronal incision. Where there has been disruption of the medial canthal ligaments, these may be identified and sutured/wired to the opposite side to restore canthal width.

When the stabilisation of the upper part of the face is complete, attention may be turned to the midface. Incisions in the lower eyelid (blepharoplasty incision), lower conjunctival sac or infraorbital region are used to explore fractures of the infraorbital rim. These also give access to the orbital floor and are used to treat orbital blow-out fractures. The fractured rim may be fixed using mini/microplates or wires as above, and the floor of the orbit reconstructed with bone, titanium mesh or alloplastic material according to choice, often held by wires or screws.

The lower part of the maxilla is approached through a gingival sulcus incision above the maxillary teeth as far back as the second molar. Fractures may be identified with ease through this route and fixed with plates or wires. The dental arch is restored to its original shape as far as possible so that it matches the pre-morbid occlusion with the mandibular arch. To achieve accurate location, dental arch bars or eyelet wires (see below) may need to be applied. Where this is anticipated, the necessary wiring is undertaken before the main part of the operation is commenced.

The principle of treatment is to restore the fragments to their original position. To achieve this, it is usually necessary to reduce the maxilla first with Rowe's disimpaction forceps, which grasp the palate between the nasal and palatal mucosa. Considerable force is sometimes required in a series of downwards, forwards and sideways movements to mobilise it. After 2–3 weeks, full disimpaction is often impossible.

With the advent of maxillofacial plating systems, indirect or external fixation with pins, fames and haloes is seldom used. If the fragments are multiple and the whole restored maxilla remains unstable, external fixation may be the only answer. Then the principle is that the mandible is fixed to the cranium, with the maxilla as a 'sandwich' between the two. Cranial fixation is by means of a halo or supraorbital pins, and mandibular fixation is by pins inserted into the body of the mandible on each side. All the pins are connected together with connecting bars secured by universal joints. When the teeth of each jaw are fixed together with intermaxillary fixation, the anteroposterior position of the facial bones is likely to be correct. The vertical dimension is adjusted through the connecting bars fixed by universal joints onto the pins. This means that the jaws are fixed together during recovery, and careful attention should be given to advising the recovery staff on how to release the apparatus in an emergency (Summary box 25.10).

Summary box 25.10

Fixation of maxillary fractures

- Orbital floor deficiencies can be made up with grafts, alloplasts or titanium mesh
- Dental wiring may be needed to stabilise the dental arch and achieve the correct occlusion
- External fixation is only rarely used

Fractures of the mandible

Fractures of the mandible were frequently reduced indirectly and then fixed with intermaxillary fixation (IMF). IMF is simply a means of splinting the upper and lower arches of teeth together (Fig. 25.15). However, the introduction of maxillofacial plating systems using initially stainless steel and latterly titanium has significantly altered the management of patients sustaining fracture of the mandible. Prior to the introduction of these plating systems, patients would often have their jaws 'wired together' for a period of up to 6 weeks. Now, although patients may be placed in temporary IMF during their operative procedure, it is more often than not released at the end of the procedure when the rigid plate fixation has been applied (Fig. 25.16).

The majority of fractures of the mandible require reduction and fixation under general anaesthetic. The fractures may be explored through intraoral or extraoral incisions according to the access required. Pre-existing lacerations overlying the mandible may be used to gain access to the fracture (Fig. 25.17). Any fractured teeth should be removed, as should those previously compromised by extensive caries or infection. It is unnecessary to remove healthy teeth in the fracture line. To be sure of achieving a correct dental occlusion, it is wise to use temporary intraoperative IMF. There are occasions where, in spite of rigid fixation with titanium miniplates, IMF or elastic traction is still required in the

Norman Lester Rowe, 1915–1991, Maxillofacial Surgeon, Queen Mary's University Hospital, Roehampton, London, England.

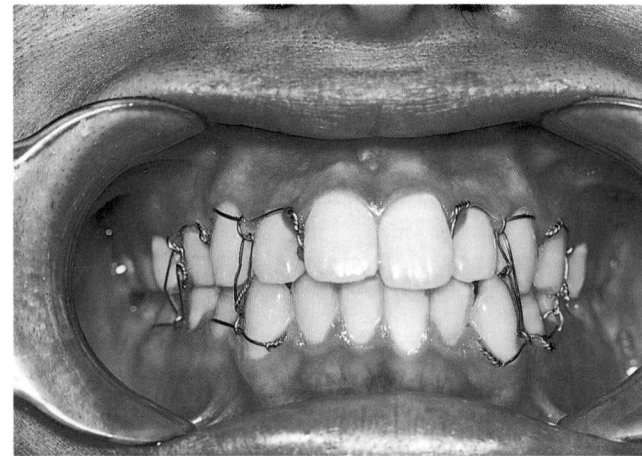

Figure 25.15 Intermaxillary fixation using eyelet wires.

(a)

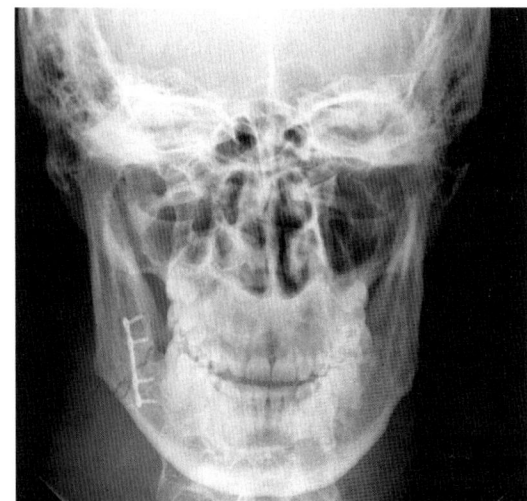

(b)

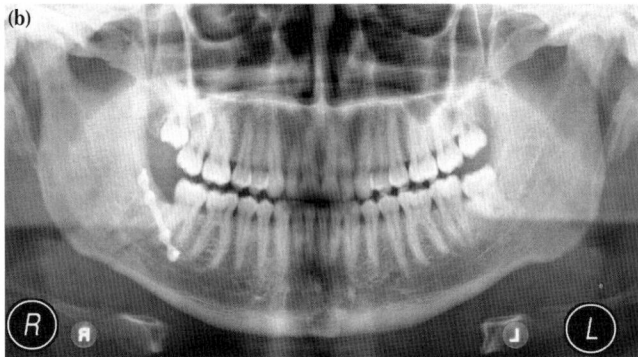

Figure 25.16 A fractured mandible treated by open reduction and fixation using a titanium miniplate. No postoperative intermaxillary fixation (IMF) has been used. (a) Posteroanterior view; (b) orthopantomogram.

postoperative period. In this event, the IMF is removed during the recovery from anaesthesia, so as not to risk complications involving the airway. The IMF may then be reapplied when the patient has fully recovered from the general anaesthetic.

Fractures of the edentulous (non-tooth-bearing) mandible are generally reduced and then fixed using titanium plates. In the very atrophic mandible, the raising of the periosteum should be kept to a minimum as the blood supply to the jaw may be compromised.

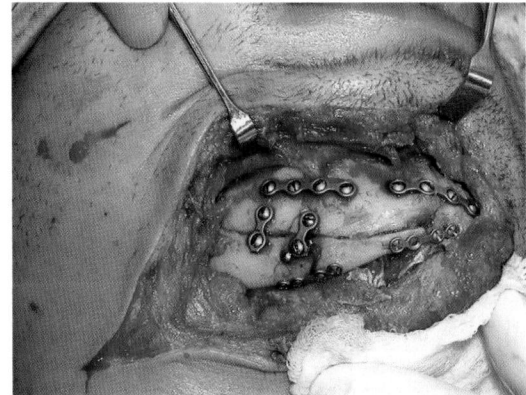

Figure 25.17 Comminuted fracture of the mandible approached through a pre-existing laceration.

Where there is concern that the blood supply may be seriously disadvantaged by the insertion of plates, Gunning's splints may be constructed. These require dental impressions to be taken, and the splints are then constructed by the maxillofacial technician in the laboratory. In effect, they are like upper and lower dentures, but with the teeth replaced with plastic in which hooks are placed. Each splint is wired to the respective jaw – the mandible, with wires going around the mandible (circum-mandibular wires) and the maxilla by a choice of wiring techniques supporting the splint from a stable point in the middle third of the facial skeleton. When the fracture has been reduced and the splints wired in place, the hooks placed on the buccal surfaces of the splints are used to apply IMF and hence fixation for the reduced fracture (Summary box 25.11).

> **Summary box 25.11**
>
> **Fixation of the mandible**
>
> ■ Plating has made long-term jaw wiring almost redundant

Fractures of the mandibular condyle may cause disturbance of the occlusion with deviation of the mandible to the side of the fracture. In unilateral fractures, which are minimally displaced, this disturbance may not be evident. However, displaced unilateral fractures and bilateral condylar fractures often present with such a disturbance and, as such, constitute an indication for open reduction and fixation of one of the condylar fractures to prevent the formation of an anterior open bite. This open bite develops due to the vertical pull of the muscles of mastication shortening the ramus height. The posterior teeth contact first and the anterior teeth remain apart. Functionally and cosmetically, this is very undesirable and is almost impossible to counteract by secondary procedures. Simply to fix the mandible in IMF, with or without a posterior bite block to overcome the tendency to open bite, is insufficient. Open reduction and fixation of the fractured mandibular condyle within 7–10 days of the original injury is indicated if such an anterior open bite is evident in a unilateral condylar fracture with significant displacement, or in a bilateral condylar fracture (Summary box 25.12).

> **Summary box 25.12**
>
> **Fixation of mandibular condyles**
>
> ■ If displaced or bilateral, with significant occlusal disturbance, surgical intervention will be required
> ■ Reduction and plating prevents anterior open bite

Fractures of the zygomatic complex

Second to the fractured nasal bone, this is the most common fracture of the middle third of the facial skeleton. Displacement is usually posteriorly, although it is important to assess the actual displacement by studying the occipitomental radiographs. Most fractures may be reduced by the Gillies temporal approach. This entails an incision in the hair line, superficial to the temporal

Thomas Brian Gunning, 1813–1889, American dentist.
Sir Harold Delf Gillies, 1882–1960, Plastic Surgeon, St Bartholomew's Hospital, London, England.

fossa, about 15 mm long, at 45° to the vertical. It is deepened down to and through the temporalis fascia. A channel is prepared behind the fascia and down to the body of the zygoma and arch. A Bristow's or Rowe's elevator is then inserted beneath the body of the zygoma or arch, according to the site of the fracture. Force is then applied in the opposite direction to the displacement of the fracture. After reduction, the position of the zygoma can be checked by palpating the bony prominences of the zygomatic arch, and the lateral and inferior orbital rims. As all fractures of the zygoma, other than those solely of the arch, involve the orbital floor, it is essential to apply a forced duction test to ensure no limitation of movement of the inferior oblique and inferior rectus muscles. For this to be done, the lower eyelid is retracted and the inferior rectus grabbed in the lower fornix. The globe can then be rotated upwards and should move freely. Any restriction in movement suggests entrapment of the infraorbital soft tissues, and the floor of the orbit should be explored as for a blow-out fracture (see below).

Should the fracture be unstable, open reduction and fixation of the fracture may be necessary. The frontozygomatic suture may be exposed by a small incision just behind the lateral part of the eyebrow and visualised. Displacements may be reduced and fixed with intraosseous wires or bone plates. Occasionally, it is necessary to explore and fix fractures at the infraorbital rim (see above) (Summary box 25.13).

Summary box 25.13

Fixation of fractures of the zygomatic complex

- The arch is elevated
- Ocular tethering should be checked if the fracture involves the orbital floor
- Regular postoperative observations must be made for retrobulbar haematoma

---

All patients who have had operations involving the orbit should have formal eye observations in the postoperative period. The condition of the eye, pupil size and light reaction should be recorded. Occasional complications occur, the most serious of which is a developing retrobulbar haematoma. Increasing proptosis and loss of vision constitute a postoperative emergency requiring immediate action to reduce the pressure of the haematoma.

Orbital blow-out fractures

The mechanism has been explained above. These fractures are ideally treated within 10–14 days of the original injury. The aim of treatment is to reduce any soft-tissue herniation of the periorbita (Fig. 25.18), restore the continuity of the orbital floor and restore any functional deficit of ocular function caused by extraocular muscle dysfunction. The floor of the orbit is approached either through a blepharoplasty incision in the lower eyelid or through the inferior fornix. Keeping superficial to the tarsal plate of the lower lid, the infraorbital margin is identified and the periosteum raised, attempting to avoid displacement of the delicate fragments of bone constituting the fracture. The periorbital soft tissues are gently separated from the bone of the

Walter Rowley Bristow, **1882–1947**, Orthopaedic Surgeon, St Thomas' Hospital, London, England.

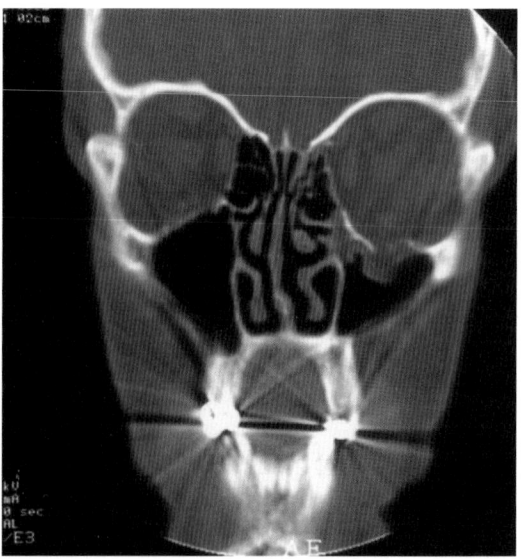

Figure 25.18 Coronal computerised tomographic (CT) scan showing a left orbital blow-out fracture, with evident soft-tissue herniation into the maxillary antrum.

fracture and freed so that no trapping or soft-tissue herniation into the antrum remains. Defects of the orbital floor may be made up with bone grafts from a variety of sources, titanium mesh or other suitably rigid materials. Many surgeons use reinforced silastic or resorbable materials. These materials may be fixed in place with wires, screws or plates. If the fragments are very unstable owing to comminution or the size of the blow-out is excessively large, packing the antrum via a Caldwell–Luc approach may be necessary. When the orbital floor has been adequately reduced and periorbital soft tissue freed from the fracture, the antrum may be packed from above downwards with ribbon gauze soaked in Whitehead's varnish, taking care not to overpack the antrum and so displace the orbital contents. The pack should be removed at 3 weeks (Summary box 25.14).

Summary box 25.14

Orbital blow-out fractures

- Defects of the orbital floor can be made up with bone graft or with synthetic materials

---

Intraoral injuries

Intraoral injuries will often occur in coexistence with facial and jaw injuries. However, oral injuries to the dentition, the dentoalveolar bone and the oral mucosa or combinations of these commonly occur in isolation and, in many cases, present to accident and emergency departments of general hospitals.

George Walter Caldwell, **1866–1946**, Otolaryngologist, who practised successively in New York, NY, San Francisco, CA, and Los Angeles, CA, USA. He described his operation for treating suppuration in the maxillary antrum in 1893.
Henri Luc, **1855–1925**, Otolaryngologist, Paris, France, described his operation in 1889.
Walter Whitehead, **1840–1913**, Surgeon, the Royal Infirmary, Manchester, England. Whitehead's varnish consists of iodoform, benzoin, storax and Tolu balsam in ether.

Dental injuries

Isolated injury to the dentition is extremely common. Several studies have reported that up to one-third of 11-year-old children in the UK will have sustained some type of injury to their dentition.

Treatment of such dental injuries lies within the remit of the dental surgeon, but many of these patients may initially present to accident and emergency departments of general hospitals. Occasionally, urgent treatment may be necessitated, especially in respect of avulsed teeth.

Patterns of dental injury depend on several factors. The site of the blow, the resilience of the supporting structures of the teeth and the direction and energy of the impact all have an effect in determining the type of injury sustained. The possibility of underlying injury to the jaw and temporomandibular joint (TMJ) should always be considered and, as with maxillofacial injuries in general, the possibility of cervical spine and cerebral injuries should never be overlooked.

Dental injuries may be classified as crown fractures, root fractures or luxation injuries, with the last including avulsion injury. Combinations of the three main groups may also occur. Any missing fragment of tooth should be accounted for. Implantation of dental fragments into the perioral soft tissues and the possibility of inhalation must be excluded.

Loss of dental enamel may result in the exposure of dentine or the dental pulp (Fig. 25.19). Such injury will expose dentinal tubules, which allow bacterial, thermal and chemical irritants to attack the dental pulp. Whether such injury is symptomatic or not, referral to the patient's dental surgeon as soon as possible is necessitated as possible pulpal necrosis will complicate the chances of successful dental reconstruction of the damaged dentition.

Avulsed teeth

When teeth are completely avulsed, the periodontal ligament and cemental layers are ruptured. In addition, the periapical nerves and apical vessels are severed. Such teeth can be reimplanted, but the success of such reimplantation depends on several factors. The stage of root development, the length of time the tooth is in either dry or wet storage, the type of media used for wet storage, correct handling of the tooth and appropriate splinting are all factors affecting the overall prognosis in dental reimplantation.

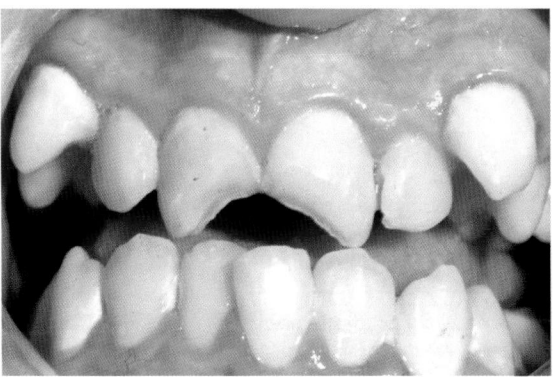

Figure 25.19 Fractured upper central incisors, involving enamel and dentine.

Ideally, immediate reimplantation is the treatment of choice, but this is seldom feasible at the scene of the accident. Once out of the socket, periodontal ligament cells can survive a dry period of up to 30 minutes without significant harm. After 60 minutes of dry storage, few periodontal cells will retain their viability, and the chances of successful reimplantation decrease significantly. Wet storage can increase periodontal ligament cell vitality, and such storage may increase the chances of successful reimplantation. The patient's own saliva or fresh milk is the best transport medium available to the lay person. Water should not be used because of its osmotic effects on the periodontal ligament cells. The aim of delayed reimplantation should be to reimplant the tooth as soon as possible, once local anaesthetic has been administered. The socket should be gently irrigated with normal saline to remove any clot/debris. The tooth should be held by the crown, and the root gently irrigated with saline to remove debris before the tooth is firmly reimplanted in the socket. Referral to the patient's dental surgeon for semirigid fixation for a period of 7–10 days is necessary, and oral antibiotics are required for a period of 5–7 days following reimplantation (Summary box 25.15).

Summary box 25.15

Dental injuries

- Avulsed teeth should ideally be implanted within 60 minutes of the injury
- The best transport medium for avulsed teeth is the patient's own saliva or fresh milk

---

General

Fractures of the facial skeleton are almost always compound, and prophylactic antibiotics are important. Penicillin/amoxicillin and metronidazole singly or in combination are ideal for those patients who are not allergic. The cephalosporins are an alternative.

All patients with fractures of the facial skeleton benefit from intraoperative and postoperative dexamethasone to reduce facial oedema (Summary box 25.16).

Summary box 25.16

General principles in facial fractures

- Prophylactic antibiotics should be given
- Dexamethasone may reduce facial oedema

FURTHER READING

Andreasen, J.O., Andreasen, F. and Anderrson, L. (eds) (2007) *Textbook and Color Atlas of Traumatic Injuries to the Teeth*, 4th edn. Blackwell Munksgaard, Oxford.

Ward-Booth, P., Eppley, B. and Schmelzeisen, R. (2003) *Maxillofacial Trauma and Esthetic Reconstruction*. Churchill Livingstone, Edinburgh.

Williams, J.Ll. (ed.) (1994) *Rowe and Williams' Maxillofacial Injuries*, 2nd edn. Churchill Livingstone, Edinburgh.

Chest and abdomen

CHAPTER
26

LEARNING OBJECTIVES

To understand:
- That the management of injury is based on physiology rather than anatomy
- The gross and surgical anatomy of the chest and abdomen
- The pathophysiology of torso injury
- The limitations of clinical assessment in the injured patient

- The special investigations and their limitations
- The operative approaches to the thoracic cavity
- The special features of an emergency room thoracotomy for haemorrhage control
- The indications for and techniques of the trauma laparotomy
- The philosophy of damage control surgery

INTRODUCTION

The torso is generally regarded as the area between the neck and the groin, made up of the thorax and abdomen. This is the largest area of the body and is commonly injured following both blunt and penetrating trauma. Because injury does not respect anatomical boundaries, division of the body into abdomen and thorax is artificial, and injury to the torso, with its associated physiological consequences, is more appropriate.

Traditionally, death from trauma has had a 'trimodal' distribution, with 50% of deaths occurring in the pre-hospital environment, 30% during the first few hours and the remaining 20% occurring later. With better pre-hospital care, patients are reaching hospital earlier, and now some 50% of deaths occur in the early in-hospital environment (Fig. 26.1).

About 42% of deaths are the result of brain injury, but some

39% of all trauma deaths are caused by major haemorrhage, usually from torso injury. Many of these are the result of a failure to appreciate the magnitude of the bleeding (Fig. 26.2).

Although initially, injury was treated on an anatomical basis, it has become clear that physiology should be the over-riding consideration, and the driver of successful resuscitation is therefore the restoration of normal physiology. Techniques such as 'damage control resuscitation' and 'damage control surgery' have dramatically improved survival through an understanding of the best techniques required to restore physiological stability.

The Advanced Trauma Life Support (ATLS) course of the American College of Surgeons was developed in 1977 and is the cornerstone of advanced resuscitation. The principles include:

- early assessment and primary survey;
- simultaneous aggressive resuscitation;

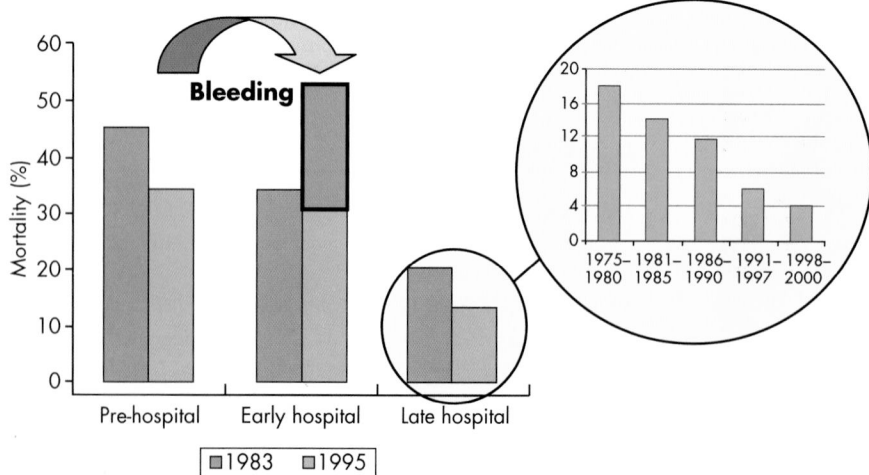

Figure 26.1 Changes in the trimodal distribution of trauma death. More efficacious emergency medical services has shifted pre-hospital to early hospital death. Today most deaths occur within 12 hours of arrival at hospital. Late deaths due to post-surgical complications are declining [from Turnkey, D.D. (1983) *Scientific American* **149**: 28–35; Sauaia, A. (1995) *Journal of Trauma* **38**: 185–93, Annual Report Klinik für unfallschirugie, Univärsitsklinikum Essen].

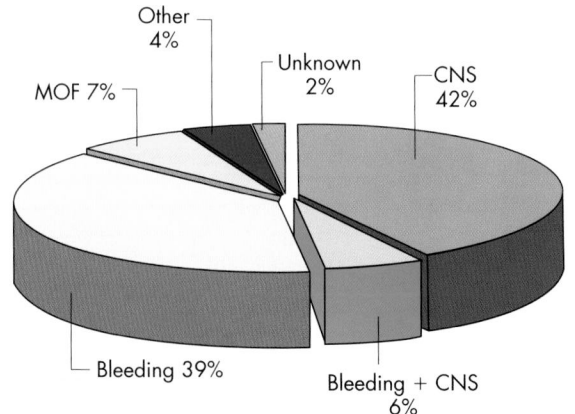

Figure 26.2 Causes of death in trauma. CNS, central nervous system; MOF, multiple organ failure.

- a careful secondary survey with full examination:
  - front to back;
  - top to toe;
- transfer to a definitive site of care.

The concept of the trauma team – with each person having designated responsibilities – was developed to enable a careful assessment to be made in patients with multiple injuries and a treatment plan to be developed that recognises the need to treat the greatest threats to life first and ensure the early control of major bleeding and contamination. The philosophy also includes the concept of triage:

- the sorting of patients, with the most severely injured patients being treated first;
- the sorting of injuries, so that the most compelling threats to life, e.g. bleeding sites, receive priority (Summary box 26.1).

Summary box 26.1

Trauma to the abdomen

- The proportion of patients surviving severe torso injury until arrival at hospital is increasing
- 40% of all trauma deaths are a result of torso injury
- Rapid assessment and resuscitation will improve survival rates

---

INJURY MECHANISMS ASSOCIATED WITH TORSO TRAUMA

With a careful history and an understanding of the injury mechanism it is often possible to predict the type of injury that might occur. For example, in motor vehicle accidents:

- motor vehicle occupants, if unrestrained, suffer a classic 'triad' of injury to the face, chest and knees;
- pedestrians suffer injury to the lower legs and pelvis from the vehicle, with an associated head injury from the impact with the ground;
- lap belts can result in acute flexion over the belt with corresponding vertebral injury;
- injuries to the duodenum and/or pancreas can occur as a result of compression between, for example, the steering wheel or a seatbelt and the vertebral column.

For specific anatomy, refer also to the chapters on individual organ injury (Chapters 21–30).

- general surgery requires a knowledge of anatomy and pathology;
- trauma surgery requires a knowledge of physiology and anatomy.

Injury often traverses different anatomical zones of the body, affecting anatomical structures on both sides of traditional anatomical zones. These zones are known as junctional zones.

Junctional zones

The key junctional zones are:

- between the neck and the thorax;
- between the thorax and the abdomen;
- between the abdomen, the pelvic structures and the groin.

These zones represent surgical challenges in terms of both the diagnosis of the area of injury and the surgical approach, which have to be balanced against the physiological stability of the patient.

Root of the neck

Most injuries affecting the base of the neck (junctional zone 1) also affect the upper mediastinum and thoracic inlet. Choice of access is determined by the need for surgical control of the vascular structures contained within.

The mediastinum

The zone overlying the mediastinum with its major vessels and the heart is also an extremely high-risk area for penetrating wounds. Any wound in this region should immediately raise the suspicion of an associated cardiac or major vascular injury even in the absence of initial gross physical signs.

Diaphragm

The thorax and abdomen are separated by the diaphragm. The diaphragm is mainly responsible for breathing, and moves with breathing from the fourth to the eighth interspace. Any penetrating injury of the lower half of the chest may therefore have penetrated the diaphragm and entered the abdomen. Injuries in this junctional zone, therefore, should be evaluated as if both cavities had been penetrated (Fig. 26.3).

Pelvic structures and groin

The pelvis contains a large plexus of vessels, both venous and arterial. Should injury occur, control of haemorrhage can prove to be exceptionally difficult and may require control of both inflow and outflow. This may involve surgical control at the groin of the external iliac and femoral vessels, as well as at the aortic and cava level.

Retroperitoneum

Injury to the retroperitoneum is often difficult to diagnose, especially in the presence of other injury, and the signs may be masked. Intraperitoneal diagnostic tests (ultrasound and diagnostic peritoneal lavage) may be negative. The best diagnostic modality is the computerised tomography (CT) scan, but this requires a physiologically stable patient. The retroperitoneum is divided into three zones (Fig. 26.4):

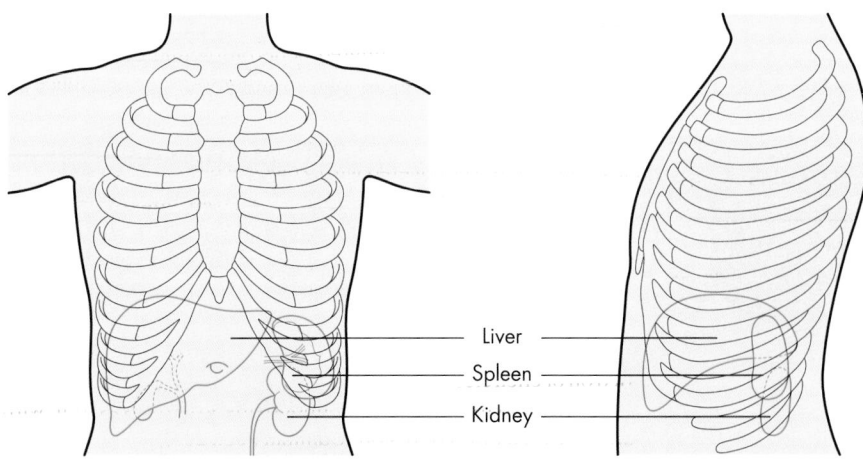

Figure 26.3 The extent of the abdomen.

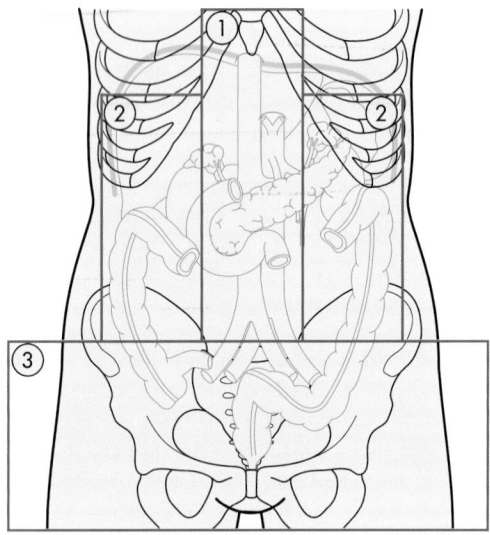

Figure 26.4 The zones of the retroperitoneum. Zone 1: central; zone 2: lateral; zone 3: pelvic.

- zone 1 (central): central haematomas should always be explored, with proximal and distal vascular control;
- zone 2 (lateral): lateral haematomas are usually renal in origin and can be managed non-operatively, sometimes with angioembolisation;
- zone 3 (pelvic): pelvic haematomas are exceptionally difficult to control and should, whenever possible, not be opened; they should be controlled with packing (intra- or extrapelvic) and angioembolisation (Summary box 26.2).

Summary box 26.2

Junctional zones

- ■ Neck
- ■ Mediastinum
- ■ Diaphragm
- ■ Groin
- ■ Retroperitoneum

Injuries in these large zones pose diagnostic and treatment problems

---

CRITICAL PHYSIOLOGY

Resuscitation of all injuries to the chest and abdomen should follow traditional ATLS principles (Table 26.1).

Bleeding is the major problem with torso trauma. This may be obvious at the time of evaluation; however, in the young fit individual, bleeding into the chest and abdomen may be subtle and difficult to assess (Table 26.2). Bleeding occurs from five major sites – 'one on the floor and four more':

- external (i.e. skin);
- chest;
- abdomen;
- pelvis;
- extremities (e.g. fractures).

Although obvious injury may be present, traditional indicators are unreliable in young patients. As always, the physiology should be assessed, especially in the light of the history of the injury. Another reason why traditional indicators (such as pulse rate) may be unreliable is because the patient is 'unseen' before arrival in the resuscitation room and the previous physiological state is unknown – a fit individual may have a very low pulse rate

Table 26.1 ATLS principles of resuscitation

A	Airway
B	Breathing
C	Circulation
D	Disability (neurology)
E	Environment and Exposure

Table 26.2 Clinical indicators of potential on-going bleeding in torso trauma

Physiological	Increasing respiratory rate
	Increasing pulse rate
	Falling blood pressure
	Rising serum lactate
Anatomical	Visible bleeding
	Injury in close proximity to major vessels
	Penetrating injury with a retained weapon

normally and so a raised rate for that individual may still appear as low.

THORACIC INJURY

Thoracic injury accounts for 25% of all injuries. In a further 25%, it may be a significant contributor to the subsequent death of the patient. In most of these patients, the cause of death is haemorrhage.

Chest injuries are often life-threatening, either in their own right or in conjunction with other system injuries. About 80% of patients with chest injury can be managed non-operatively, and the key is early physiological resuscitation followed by diagnosis. A reproducible and safe approach to the diagnosis and management of chest injury is taught by the ATLS course of the American College of Surgeons.

Investigation

Routine investigation in the emergency department of injury to the chest is based on clinical examination, supplemented by chest radiography. In the unstable patient, chest radiography is the investigation of first choice, provided that it does not interfere with resuscitation. Ultrasound can be used to differentiate between contusion and the actual presence of blood. A chest tube can be a diagnostic procedure as well as a therapeutic one, and the benefits of insertion often outweigh the risks.

The pitfalls of investigation are:

- failure to auscultate both front and back (an inflated lung will 'float' on a haemothorax, so auscultation from the front may sound normal);
- failure to check whether the trachea is central;
- failure to pass a nasogastric tube if rupture of the diaphragm is suspected;
- pursuing radiological investigation (radiography or CT scan) before, or instead of, resuscitation if the patient is haemodynamically unstable.

Computerised tomography scan

The CT scan, especially using the newer multislice scanning technology, has become the principal and most reliable examination for major injury in thoracic trauma. Scanning with contrast allows for three-dimensional reconstruction of the chest and abdomen, as well as of the bony skeleton. In blunt chest trauma the CT scan will allow the definition of rib and vertebral fractures, as well as showing haematomas, pneumothoraces and pulmonary contusion. In penetrating trauma the scan may show the track of the missile and allow the planning of definitive surgery.

CT scanning has replaced angiography as the diagnostic modality of choice for the assessment of the thoracic aorta (Summary box 26.3).

> **Summary box 26.3**
>
> **Investigation of chest injuries**
>
> - Directly or indirectly involved in 50% of trauma deaths in the USA
> - 80% can be managed non-operatively
> - A chest radiograph is the investigation of first choice
> - A spiral CT scan provides rapid diagnoses in the chest and abdomen
> - A chest drain can be diagnostic as well as therapeutic

Management

Most patients who have suffered penetrating injury to the chest can be managed with appropriate resuscitation and drainage of haematoma.

If a sucking chest wound is present, this should not be fully closed but should be covered with a piece of plastic, closed on three sides, to form a one-way valve, and then an underwater drain should be placed. No attempt should be made to close a sucking chest wound until controlled chest drainage has been achieved.

In blunt injury most bleeding occurs from the intercostal or internal mammary vessels and it is relatively rare for these to require surgery. If bleeding does not stop spontaneously the vessels can be tied off or encircled. In blunt chest compressive injury there is injury to the ribs and frequently to the underlying structures as well, with an associated lung contusion (Summary box 26.4).

> **Summary box 26.4**
>
> **Closed management of chest injuries**
>
> - About 80% of chest injuries can be managed closed
> - If there is an open wound insert a chest drain
> - Do not close a sucking chest wound until a drain is in place
> - If bleeding persists, the chest will need to be opened

The patient *in extremis* with exsanguinating chest haemorrhage will be discussed in the section on Emergency room thoracotomy (ERT; p. 345).

Life-threatening injuries can be remembered as the *deadly dozen*. Six are immediately life-threatening and should be sought during the primary survey and six are potentially life-threatening and should be detected during the secondary survey (Table 26.3).

Efficient initial assessment should focus on identifying and correcting the immediate threats to life. A high index of suspicion must be maintained thereafter to diagnose the potential threats to life as their symptoms and signs can be very subtle. Early consultation and referral to a trauma centre is advised in cases of doubt.

Immediate life-threatening injuries

Airway obstruction

Early preventable trauma deaths are often due to lack of or delay in airway control. Dentures, teeth, secretions and blood can

Table 26.3 The 'deadly dozen' threats to life from chest injury

Immediately life threatening	Airway obstruction
	Tension pneumothorax
	Pericardial tamponade
	Open pneumothorax
	Massive haemothorax
	Flail chest
Potentially life threatening	Aortic injuries
	Tracheobronchial injuries
	Myocardial contusion
	Rupture of diaphragm
	Oesophageal injuries
	Pulmonary contusion

contribute to airway obstruction in trauma. Bilateral mandibular fracture, expanding neck haematomas producing deviation of the pharynx and mechanical compression of the trachea, laryngeal trauma such as thyroid or cricoid fractures and tracheal injury are other causes of airway obstruction.

These patients need intubation (with simultaneous protection of the cervical spine). Early intubation is very important, particularly in cases of neck haematoma or possible airway oedema. Airway distortion can be insidious and progressive and can make delayed intubation more difficult if not impossible.

Tension pneumothorax

A tension pneumothorax develops when a 'one-way valve' air leak occurs either from the lung or through the chest wall. Air is forced into the thoracic cavity without any means of escape, completely collapsing the affected lung. The mediastinum is displaced to the opposite side, decreasing venous return and compressing the opposite lung.

The most common causes are penetrating chest trauma, blunt chest trauma with parenchymal lung injury and air leak that did not spontaneously close, iatrogenic lung punctures (e.g. due to subclavian central venepuncture) and mechanical positive-pressure ventilation.

The clinical presentation is dramatic. The patient is panicky with tachypnoea, dyspnoea and distended neck veins (similar to pericardial tamponade). Clinical examination can reveal tracheal deviation (a late finding – not necessary to clinically confirm diagnosis), hyperresonance and absent breath sounds over the affected hemithorax. Tension pneumothorax is a clinical diagnosis and treatment should not be delayed by waiting for radiological confirmation (Fig. 26.5).

Treatment consists of immediate decompression and is managed initially by rapid insertion of a large-bore needle into the second intercostal space in the mid-clavicular line of the affected hemithorax. This is immediately followed by insertion of a chest tube through the fifth intercostal space in the anterior axillary line.

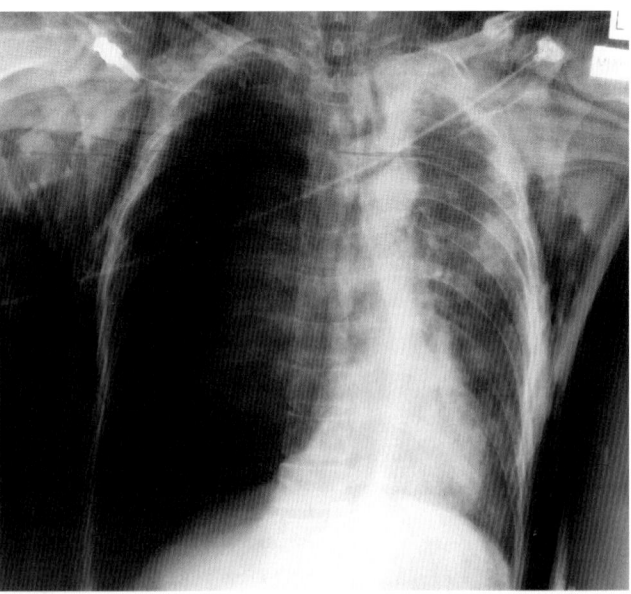

Figure 26.5 Radiological appearance of a tension pneumothorax.

Pericardial tamponade

Pericardial tamponade must be differentiated from tension pneumothorax in the shocked patient with distended neck veins. It is most commonly the result of penetrating trauma. Accumulation of a relatively small amount of blood into the non-distensible pericardial sac can produce physiological obstruction of the heart. All patients with penetrating injury anywhere near the heart plus shock must be considered to have cardiac injury until proven otherwise. Classically the presentation consists of venous pressure elevation, decline in arterial pressure with tachycardia, and muffled heart sounds (note that this can mimic tension pneumothorax). A high index of suspicion and further diagnostic investigations (e.g. chest radiography showing an enlarged heart shadow or a cardiac echo showing fluid in the pericardial sac, and insertion of a central line with a rising central venous pressure) are required for the subclinical case. In cases in which major bleeding from other sites has taken place, the neck veins may be flat.

Needle pericardiocentesis may allow the aspiration of a few millilitres of blood, and this, along with rapid volume resuscitation to increase preload, can buy enough time to move to the operating room. However, in penetrating injury to the heart there is usually a substantial clot in the pericardium, which may prevent aspiration. Pericardiocentesis has a high potential for iatrogenic injury to the heart and it should at the most be regarded as a desperate temporising measure in a transport situation [under electrocardiogram (ECG) control]. The correct immediate treatment of tamponade is operative (sternotomy or left thoracotomy), with repair of the heart in the operating theatre if time allows or otherwise in the emergency room.

To summarise, the pitfalls of pericardial tamponade are:

- neck veins may be flat if the patient has bled substantially from elsewhere and is therefore in volume collapse;
- the central venous pressure may not be elevated if the circulating volume is depleted, e.g. because of other injuries;
- pericardiocentesis is a temporising measure only with a high complication rate and is not a substitute for immediate operative intervention – it proves only that there is a 'clot' on both ends of the needle!

Open pneumothorax ('sucking chest wound')

This is due to a large open defect in the chest (> 3 cm), leading to equilibration between intrathoracic and atmospheric pressure. Air accumulates in the hemithorax (rather than in the lung) with each inspiration, leading to profound hypoventilation on the affected side and hypoxia. Signs and symptoms are usually proportionate to the size of the defect. If there is a valvular effect, increasing amounts of air will result in a tension pneumothorax (see above).

Initial management consists of promptly closing the defect with a sterile occlusive plastic dressing (e.g. Opsite), taped on three sides to act as a flutter-type valve. A chest tube is inserted as soon as possible in a site remote from the injury site. Definitive treatment may warrant formal debridement and closure, preferably in the operating room, and all such patients should be referred early.

The following points are important in the management of an open pneumothorax:

- a common problem is using too small a tube – a 28FG or larger tube should be used in an adult;

- if the lung does not reinflate, the drain should be placed on low-pressure (5 cm water) suction;
- a second drain is sometimes necessary (but see Tracheo-bronchial injuries);
- physiotherapy and active mobilisation should begin as soon as possible.

Massive haemothorax

The most common cause of massive haemothorax in blunt injury is continuing bleeding from torn intercostal vessels or occasionally the internal mammary artery.

Accumulation of blood in a hemithorax can significantly compromise respiratory efforts by compressing the lung and preventing adequate ventilation. Such massive accumulation of blood presents as haemorrhagic shock with flat neck veins, unilateral absence of breath sounds and dullness to percussion. The treatment consists of correcting the hypovolaemic shock, insertion of an intercostal drain and, in some cases, intubation.

Blood in the pleural space should be removed as completely and rapidly as possible to prevent on-going bleeding, empyema or a late fibrothorax. Clamping a chest drain to tamponade a massive haemothorax is usually not helpful.

Initial drainage of more than 1500 ml of blood or on-going haemorrhage of more than 200 ml h⁻¹ over 3–4 hours is generally considered an indication for urgent thoracotomy.

The following points are important in the management of massive haemothorax:

- clinical examination may be misleading if only done from the supine position, as the lung may 'float' on the haemothorax and breath sounds anteriorly may be normal;
- caution is required in a case that drains more than 500 ml into the drainage bottle but has persistent dullness or radiographic opacification.

Flail chest

A flail chest occurs when a segment of the chest wall does not have bony continuity with the rest of the thoracic cage. This condition usually results from blunt trauma associated with multiple rib fractures, i.e. three or more ribs fractured in two or more places. The blunt force required to disrupt the integrity of the thoracic cage typically produces an underlying pulmonary contusion as well. The diagnosis is made clinically, not by radiography. On inspiration the loose segment of the chest wall is displaced inwards and less air therefore moves into the lungs. To confirm the diagnosis the chest wall can be observed for paradoxical motion of a chest wall segment for several respiratory cycles and during coughing. Voluntary splinting as a result of pain, mechanically impaired chest wall movement and the associated lung contusion are all causes of the hypoxia. The patient is also at high risk of developing a pneumothorax or haemothorax.

Traditionally, treatment consisted of mechanical ventilation to 'internally splint' the chest until fibrous union of the broken ribs occurred. The price for this was considerable in terms of intensive care unit resources and ventilation-dependent morbidity. Currently, treatment consists of oxygen administration, adequate analgesia (including opiates) and physiotherapy. If a chest tube is *in situ*, intrapleural local analgesia can be used as well. Ventilation

in situ is Latin for 'in place'.

is reserved for cases developing respiratory failure despite adequate analgesia and oxygen. Surgery to stabilise the flail chest is currently in use again; it may be useful in a selected group with isolated or severe chest injury and pulmonary contusion who have been shown to benefit from internal operative fixation of the flail segment.

Potentially life-threatening injuries

Thoracic aortic disruption

Traumatic aortic rupture is a common cause of sudden death after an automobile collision or fall from a great height. The vessel is relatively fixed distal to the ligamentum arteriosum, just distal to the origin of the left subclavian artery. The shear forces from a sudden impact disrupt the intima and media. If the adventitia is intact, the patient may remain stable. For the subgroup of immediate survivors, salvage is frequently possible if aortic rupture is identified and treated early. It should be clinically suspected in patients with asymmetry of upper or upper and lower extremity blood pressure, widened pulse pressure and chest wall contusion. Erect chest radiography can also suggest thoracic aortic disruption, the most common radiological finding being a widened mediastinum (Fig. 26.6). The diagnosis is confirmed by aortography or a contrast spiral CT scan of the mediastinum (Fig. 26.7) and to a lesser extent by transoesophageal echocardiography.

Initially, management consists of control of the systolic arterial blood pressure (to less than 100 mmHg). Thereafter, an endovascular intra-aortic stent can be placed or the tear can be operatively repaired by direct repair or excision and grafting using a Dacron graft.

The following points are important in the management of thoracic aortic disruption:

- in the presence of competing chest and abdominal injury, treat the abdominal injury first;
- look for a difference in the measured pressures between the arms and legs and for a radiofemoral delay;
- if the mediastinum is widened on the supine film, repeat the X-ray in the erect position if possible;
- the 'gold standard' for diagnosis in aortic rupture is the aortogram, but a multislice CT scan with contrast yields similar results.

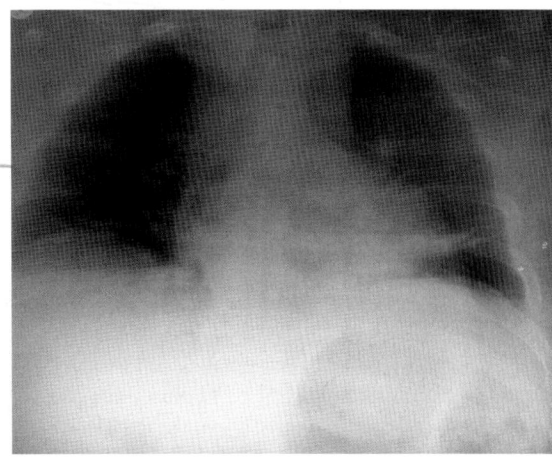

Figure 26.6 Chest radiograph showing a widened mediastinum.

CHAPTER 26 | CHEST AND ABDOMEN

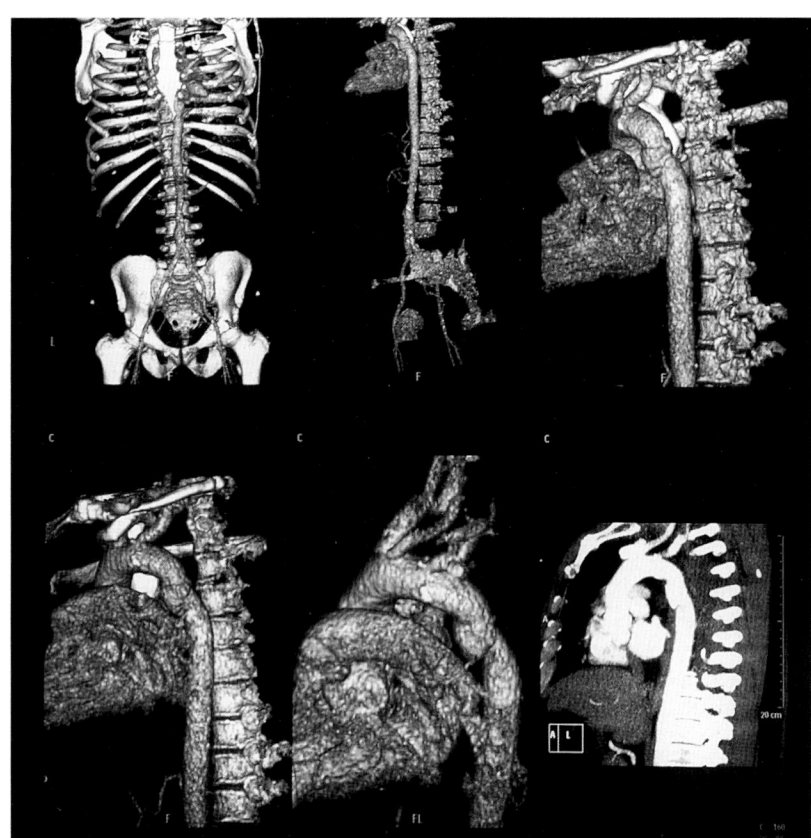

Figure 26.7 Computerised tomography scan showing aortic disruption.

Tracheobronchial injuries

Severe subcutaneous emphysema with respiratory compromise can suggest tracheobronchial disruption. A chest drain placed on the affected side will reveal a large air leak and the collapsed lung may fail to re-expand. If after insertion of two drains the lung fails to re-expand, referral to a trauma centre is advised.

Bronchoscopy is diagnostic. Treatment involves intubation of the unaffected bronchus followed by operative repair.

Blunt myocardial injury

Significant blunt cardiac injury that causes haemodynamic instability is rare. Blunt myocardial injury should be suspected in any patient sustaining blunt trauma who develops ECG abnormalities in the resuscitation room.

Although a good deal has been written regarding diagnosis, the most reliable sign of significant injury to the myocardium is an abnormal 12-lead ECG. Two-dimensional echocardiography may show wall motion abnormalities. A transoesophageal echocardiogram may also be helpful. There is very little evidence that enzyme estimations have any place in diagnosis; a rise in troponin I may be a useful adjunct but is not of primary value in making the diagnosis.

All patients with myocardial contusion diagnosed by conduction abnormalities are at risk of developing sudden dysrhythmias and should be monitored for the first 24 hours. After this interval the risk for sudden onset of dysrhythmias decreases substantially, unless the patient comes under significant extra stress such as that produced by a general anaesthetic.

Diaphragmatic injuries

Any penetrating injury to or below the fifth intercostal space should raise the suspicion of diaphragmatic penetration and, therefore, injury to abdominal contents. Diagnostic laparoscopy may have a role in this situation.

Blunt injury to the diaphragm is usually caused by a compressive force applied to the pelvis and abdomen. The diaphragmatic rupture is usually large, with herniation of the abdominal contents into the chest. Diagnosis of blunt diaphragmatic rupture is missed even more often than penetrating injuries in the acute phase.

Most diaphragmatic injuries are silent and the presenting features are those of injury to the surrounding organs. There is no single standard investigation. Chest radiography after placement of a nasogastric tube may be helpful (as this may show the stomach herniated into the chest). Contrast studies of the upper or lower gastrointestinal tract, CT scan and diagnostic peritoneal lavage all lack positive or negative predictive value. The most accurate evaluation is by video-assisted thoracoscopy (VATS) or laparoscopy, the latter offering the advantage of allowing the surgeon to proceed to a repair and additional evaluation of the abdominal organs.

Operative repair is recommended in all cases. All penetrating diaphragmatic injury must be repaired via the abdomen and not the chest, to rule out penetrating hollow viscus injury.

The thorax is at negative pressure and the abdomen is at positive pressure. The late complication of rupture of the diaphragm is herniation of abdominal contents into the chest. These include stomach, small bowel, large bowel and spleen. Strangulation of any of the contents can occur, which has a high mortality rate.

Oesophageal injury

Most injuries to the oesophagus result from penetrating trauma; blunt injury is rare. A high index of suspicion is required if the diagnosis is to be made in a timely manner. The patient can present with odynophagia (pain on swallowing foods or fluids), subcutaneous or mediastinal emphysema, pleural effusion, air in the retro-oesophageal space and unexplained fever within 24 hours of injury. Mediastinal and deep cervical emphysema must be seen as evidence of an aerodigestive injury until proven otherwise.

The mortality rate rises exponentially if treatment is delayed for more than 12–24 hours. A combination of oesophagogram in the decubitus position and oesophagoscopy confirm the diagnosis in the great majority of cases. The treatment is operative repair and drainage.

Pulmonary contusion

Pulmonary contusion is caused by haemorrhage into the lung parenchyma, usually underneath a flail segment or fractured ribs. This is a very common, potentially lethal chest injury and the major cause of hypoxaemia after blunt trauma. It is an independent risk factor for pneumonia and adult respiratory distress syndrome (ARDS).

The natural progression of pulmonary contusion is worsening hypoxemia for the first 24–48 hours. The chest radiography findings are typically delayed and non-segmental. Contrast CT scanning can be confirmatory. If abnormalities are seen on the admission chest radiograph, the pulmonary contusion is severe. Haemoptysis or blood in the endotracheal tube is a sign of pulmonary contusion.

In mild contusion the treatment is oxygen administration, aggressive pulmonary toilet and adequate analgesia. In more severe cases mechanical ventilation is necessary. Although one should be careful not to overload these patients with fluid to avoid pulmonary oedema, establishment of normovolaemia is critical for adequate tissue perfusion and fluid restriction is not advised.

EMERGENCY THORACOTOMY

Emergency thoracic surgery is an essential part of the armamentarium of any surgeon dealing with major trauma. A timely thoracotomy for the correct indications can be the key step in saving an injured patient's life.

Indications for thoracotomy include:

- internal cardiac massage;
- control of haemorrhage from injury to the heart;
- control of haemorrhage from injury to the lung;
- control of intrathoracic haemorrhage from other causes;
- control of massive air leak.

Thoracotomy can be broadly divided into the following:

- emergency (resuscitative) thoracotomy for control of life-threatening bleeding;
- planned thoracotomy for repair of specific injury.

The clinical decision as to whether a casualty requires an ERT can be transferred to the operating room or whether further investigations are required can be more complex than it initially

sounds. It is far better to perform a thoracotomy in the operating room, either through an anterolateral approach or a median sternotomy, with good light and assistance and the potential for autotransfusion and potential bypass, than it is to attempt heroic emergency surgery in the resuscitation suite. However, if the patient is *in extremis* with a falling systolic blood pressure, despite volume resuscitation, there is no choice but to proceed immediately with a left anterolateral thoracotomy in an attempt to relieve the situation. In certain circumstances, when care is futile, it may not need to be performed at all. A resuscitation room thoracotomy following blunt trauma has limited indications and is rarely successful.

Emergency room thoracotomy

ERT should be reserved for those patients suffering penetrating injury *in whom signs of life are still present*. Patients who have received cardiopulmonary resuscitation (CPR) in the pre-hospital phase of their care are unlikely to survive, and electrical activity must be present. The survival rates for ERT in patients with penetrating trauma in whom the blood pressure is falling despite adequate resuscitation are shown in Table 26.4.

It is important to make a distinction between:

- ERT for the control of haemorrhage or tamponade or, in some situations, for internal cardiac massage;
- urgent planned thoracotomy for definitive correction of the problem – this usually takes place preferably in the more controlled environment of the operating theatre.

In certain situations, ERT is considered futile:

- CPR in the absence of endotracheal intubation for more than 5 min;
- CPR for more than 10 min (with or without endotracheal intubation);
- blunt trauma when there have been no signs of life at scene (see above).

Planned emergency thoracotomy

Planned emergency thoracotomy implies an emergency thoracotomy performed as a planned procedure in the operating room, directed at the management of a specific injury. As such, the approach chosen is dependent on the indication for surgery and the organ injured (Table 26.5). The thoracotomy may be right- or left-sided, and these may be joined, resulting in the so called 'clamshell incision'. Alternatively, certain organs are best approached through a median sternotomy.

Posterolateral thoracotomy is not generally used in the emergency situation because of the difficulties in positioning of the patient.

Continuing blood loss

The first principle of all care is to assess and treat the patient according to the physiology. Initial blood loss of more than

Table 26.4 Survival rates for thoracotomy in patients with penetrating trauma

Blood pressure despite resuscitation	Survival (%)
> 60 mmHg	60%
> 40 mmHg	30%
< 40 mmHg	3%

Table 26.5 Different approaches to the contents of the chest cavity

Approach	Best for
Left anterolateral thoracotomy	Left lung and lung hilum
	Thoracic aorta
	Origin of left subclavian artery
	Left side of heart
	Lower oesophagus
Right anterolateral thoracotomy	Right lung and lung hilum
	Azygos veins
	Superior vena cava
	Infracardiac inferior vena cava
	Upper oesophagus
	Thoracic trachea
Median sternotomy	Anterior aspect of heart
	Anterior mediastinum
	Ascending aorta and arch of aorta
	Pulmonary arteries
	Carina of the trachea

1500 ml indicates the potential for class III shock, and any on-going bleeding must be dealt with surgically, as soon as possible. Similarly, an on-going blood loss of more than 200 ml h^{-1} for 3 consecutive hours requires resuscitative surgery to stop the bleeding.

ABDOMINAL INJURY

Patients who have suffered abdominal trauma can generally be classified into the following categories based on their physiological condition after initial resuscitation:

- haemodynamically 'normal' – investigation can be full and treatment planned;
- haemodynamically 'stable' – investigation is more limited and is aimed at establishing whether the patient can be managed non-operatively, whether angioembolisation can be used or whether surgery is required (and, if so, which cavity);
- haemodynamically 'unstable' – immediate surgical correction of the bleeding is required.

A trauma laparotomy is the final step in the pathway to delineate intra-abdominal injury. Occasionally it is difficult to determine where the compelling source of bleeding is in the shocked multiply injured patient and, if doubt still exists, especially in the presence of other injuries, a laparotomy may still be the safest option.

Investigation

Investigations are driven by the cardiovascular status of the patient. A patient's physiology is the key to the value of radiological imaging, as stable patients will generally be able to have a CT scan. Radiography for the evaluation of torso trauma is only of limited value in stable trauma patients, as CT will provide greater and more anatomically accurate information. This applies to the chest, abdominal cavity and pelvis.

In patients with penetrating injury, metal markers (e.g. bent paper clips) should be placed on all external wounds before plain films are taken, irrespective of the area being radiographed, as this allows an assessment of the trajectory and helps to correlate

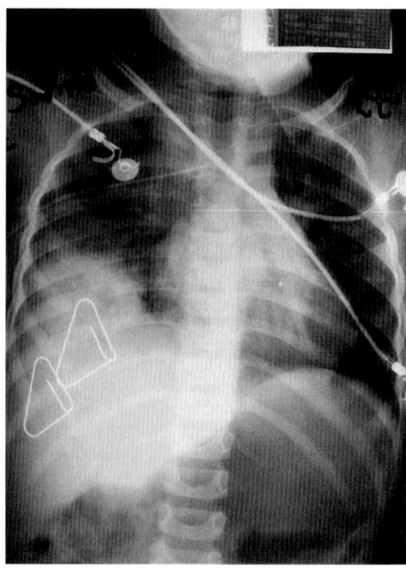

Figure 26.8 Abdominal radiograph of a gunshot wound showing bullet markers.

the number of holes and the number of missiles (i.e. whether two holes are indicative of one missile passing through or two missiles, both retained internally) (Fig. 26.8).

The patient's physiology must be assessed and, if there as an indication that the patient is bleeding, then the source must be found. Blood loss into the abdomen can be subtle and there may be no clinical signs (blood is not an irritant and may not initially cause any abdominal pain). Distension may be subjective. If stable, the best and most sensitive modality is a CT scan with intravenous contrast; however, in the unstable patient, this is generally not possible. Examination in unstable patients should take place in the emergency department or operating theatre.

Diagnostic peritoneal lavage

Diagnostic peritoneal lavage (DPL) is a test used to assess the presence of blood in the abdomen. A gastric tube is placed to empty the stomach and a urinary catheter is inserted to drain the bladder.

A cannula is inserted below the umbilicus, directed caudally and posteriorly. The cannula is aspirated for blood (> 10 ml is deemed as positive) and, following this, 1000 ml of warmed Ringer's lactate solution is allowed to run into the abdomen and is then drained out. The presence of > 100 000 red cells μl^{-1} or > 500 white cells μl^{-1} is deemed positive (this is equivalent to 20 ml of free blood in the abdominal cavity). Drainage of lavage fluid via a chest drain indicates penetration of the diaphragm.

Although DPL has largely been replaced by focused abdominal sonar for trauma (FAST; see below), it remains the standard in many institutions where FAST is not available or is unreliable. DPL is especially useful in the hypotensive, unstable patient with multiple injuries as a means of excluding intra-abdominal bleeding.

DPL has a 97–98% sensitivity rate for blood and a 1% complication rate. In total, 10–15% of laparotomies performed on the

Sydney Ringer, 1835–1910, Professor of Clinical Medicine, University College Hospital, London, England.

basis of a 'positive' DPL do not require active intervention. In principle, therefore, a negative DPL is often more helpful than a positive one, because the presence of blood in the abdomen does not necessarily require surgery.

Focused abdominal sonar for trauma

FAST is a technique whereby ultrasound imaging is used to assess the torso for the presence of blood, either in the abdominal cavity or in the pericardium. The purpose of the ultrasound evaluation of the injured casualty is to determine the presence of free intra-abdominal or pericardial fluid. The technique therefore focuses only on four areas:

- pericardial;
- splenic;
- hepatic;
- pelvic.

There is no attempt to determine specific injury. Repeated studies have shown that FAST is a rapid, reproducible, portable and non-invasive bedside test that is equally of use in the hospital resuscitation room or on military deployment. FAST can be performed simultaneously with resuscitation and it has been unequivocally demonstrated that trained operators can perform FAST accurately. It is commonly used as the bedside investigation of choice for detection of intra-abdominal blood in abdominal trauma. Extensions of the FAST technique to include assessment of the chest for haemothorax and pneumothorax, as well as assessment of the extremities, depend on the experience of the operator and are not yet widely accepted.

FAST is accurate for the detection of > 100 ml of free blood; however, it is very operator and experience dependent and, especially if the patient is very obese or the bowel is full of gas, it may be unreliable. Hollow viscus injury is difficult to diagnose, even in experienced hands, with a low sensitivity (29–35%) for organ injury without haemoperitoneum. FAST is unreliable for excluding injury in penetrating trauma. If there is doubt, the FAST examination should be repeated (Summary box 26.5).

Summary box 26.5

FAST

- It detects free fluid in the abdomen or pericardium
- It will not reliably detect less than 100 ml of free blood
- It does not identify injury to hollow viscus
- It cannot reliably exclude injury in penetrating trauma
- It may need repeating or supplementing with other investigations

---

Computerised tomography

CT has become the 'gold standard' for the intra-abdominal diagnosis of injury in the stable patient. The scan is performed using intravenous contrast and often oral contrast as well. CT is sensitive for blood and has the added advantage of sensitivity for the diagnosis of retroperitoneal injury. An entirely normal abdominal CT is usually sufficient to exclude injury.

The following points are important when performing CT:

- despite its tremendous value, it remains an inappropriate investigation for unstable patients who have a risk of rapid decompensation while in the scanner;

- if duodenal injury is suspected from the mechanism of injury, oral contrast may be helpful;
- if rectal and distal colonic injury is suspected in the absence of blood on rectal examination, rectal contrast may be helpful;
- in multislice CT examinations, fat may erroneously appear to be 'free air'.

Diagnostic laparoscopy

Diagnostic laparoscopy (DL) is a valuable screening investigation in penetrating trauma to detect or exclude peritoneal penetration and/or diaphragmatic injury in stable patients following an abdominal or thoracoabdominal stab wound. DL is not appropriate for use in the unstable patient.

In most institutions, evidence of penetration requires a laparotomy to evaluate organ injury, as it is difficult to exclude all intra-abdominal injuries laparoscopically. When used in this role DL reduces the non-therapeutic laparotomy rate. DL is not a substitute for open laparotomy, especially in the presence of haemoperitoneum or contamination.

INDIVIDUAL ORGAN INJURY

Liver

The majority of injuries to the liver occur as a result of blunt injury. Most are relatively minor in severity and can be managed non-operatively. Many are not even suspected at the time. With the widespread use of CT for the evaluation of trauma patients, minor solid organ injury (liver, spleen, kidneys) is being diagnosed more frequently. Many of these injuries were not even recognised before the use of CT scanning.

Blunt liver trauma occurs as a result of direct injury. The liver is a solid organ and compressive forces can easily burst the liver substance. The liver is compressed between the force and the rib cage or vertebral column.

Penetrating trauma to the liver is relatively common, primarily related to the size of the liver in the abdominal cavity and, therefore, its vulnerability to injury. Bullets have a shock wave and when they pass through a solid structure such as the liver they cause significant damage some distance from the actual track of the bullet. Not all penetrating wounds require operative management and a number may stop bleeding spontaneously.

In the stable patient, CT is the investigation of choice. It provides information on the liver injury itself, as well as on injuries to the adjoining major vascular and biliary structures. Close proximity injury and injury in which there is a suggestion of a vascular component should be reimaged, as there is a significant risk of the development of subsequent ischaemia.

Liver injury can be graded using the American Association for the Surgery of Trauma (AAST) Organ Injury Scale (OIS) (www.aast.org/injury). These are useful as research and audit tools and can be used to help drive management decisions.

Management

With liver injury it is the cardiovascular status of the patient that ultimately drives the patient towards either the operative or the non-operative approach. The CT images and volume of blood in the abdomen can be assessed to give an idea of the severity of the liver injury; however, even high-grade injuries may be managed non-operatively in the stable patient. Surgery is required only in the presence of other organ injury, increasing instability or failure of non-operative management.

The management of liver injuries can be summarised as 'the four Ps':

- push;
- Pringle;
- plug;
- pack.

At laparotomy the liver is reconstituted as best as possible in its normal position and bleeding is controlled by direct compression (push). The inflow from the portal triad is controlled by a Pringle's manoeuvre, with direct compression of the portal triad, either digitally or using a soft clamp (Fig. 26.9). This has the effect of reducing arterial and portal venous inflow into the liver although it does not control the backflow from the inferior vena cava and hepatic veins. Any holes due to penetrating injury can be plugged directly and, after controlling any arterial bleeding, the liver can then be packed (see Damage control surgery, p. 350).

Bleeding points should be controlled locally when possible and, after packing, such patients should undergo angiography; any vessels that are still bleeding can be embolised. It is not usually necessary to suture penetrating injuries of the liver. If there has been direct damage to the hepatic artery it can be tied off. Damage to the portal vein must be repaired, as tying off the portal vein carries a greater than 50% mortality rate. If it is not technically feasible to repair the vein at the time of surgery, it should be shunted and the patient referred to a specialist centre (see Damage control, p. 350). A closed suction drainage system must be left *in situ* following hepatic surgery.

Penetrating injuries and deep tracts can be plugged using silicone tubing or a Sengstaken–Blakemore tube.

Finally, the liver can be definitively packed, restoring the anatomy as closely as possible (see Damage control surgery). Placing omentum into cracks in the liver is not recommended (Summary box 26.6).

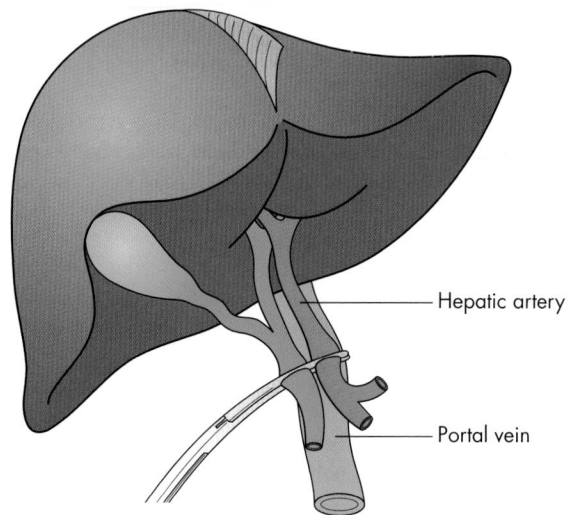

Figure 26.9 The Pringle manoeuvre.

James Hogarth Pringle, **1863–1941**, Surgeon, The Royal Infirmary, Glasgow, Scotland.
Robert William Sengstaken, **b.1923**, Surgeon, Garden City, NY, USA.
Arthur Hendley Blakemore, **1897–1970**, Associate Professor of Surgery, The College of Physicians and Surgeons, Columbia University, New York, NY, USA.

Summary box 26.6

Liver trauma

- Blunt trauma occurs as the result of direct compression
- Penetrating trauma of the upper abdomen or lower thorax can damage the liver
- CT scanning is the investigation of choice
- Surgical management consists of push, Pringle, plug and pack
- The hepatic artery can be tied off but not the portal vein (stent)
- Closed suction should always be used

Biliary injuries

Isolated traumatic biliary injuries are rare and occur mainly from penetrating trauma. They often occur in association with injuries to other structures that lie in close proximity, e.g. common bile duct injuries are often associated with portal vein injuries. The common bile duct can be repaired over a T-tube or drained and referred to appropriate care as part of damage control.

Spleen

Splenic injury occurs from direct blunt trauma; the spleen is often injured by direct energy applied to the overlying ribs (ninth to 11th ribs). Most isolated splenic injuries, especially in children, can be managed non-operatively. However, in adults, especially in the presence of other injury, physiological instability, coagulopathies, etc., laparotomy and direct splenorrhaphy should be considered. The spleen can be packed, repaired or placed in a mesh bag. Splenectomy may be a safer option, especially in the unstable patient with multiple potential sites of bleeding. In certain situations, selective angioembolisation of the spleen can play a role.

Following splenectomy there are significant though transient changes to blood physiology. The platelet count rises and may reach $10^7\,\mu l^{-1}$. The white cell count rises and may mimic sepsis.

Pancreas

Most pancreatic injury occurs as a result of blunt trauma. The major problem is that of diagnosis, because the pancreas is a retroperitoneal organ and, therefore, examinations such as DPL, FAST, etc. are non-specific. CT remains the mainstay of accurate diagnosis. Amylase estimation is only relatively helpful because a low amylase (present in up to 50% of injury) does not exclude pancreatic injury.

Classically the pancreas should be treated with conservative surgery and closed suction drainage. Injuries are treated according to the OIS system of the AAST. Injuries to the tail are treated by closed suction drainage, with distal pancreatectomy if the duct is involved. Proximal injuries (to the right of the superior mesenteric artery) are treated as conservatively as possible, although partial pancreatectomy may be necessary. The pylorus can be temporarily closed (pyloric exclusion) in association with a gastric drainage procedure. A Whipple's procedure (pancreaticoduodenectomy) is rarely needed and should not be performed in the emergency situation because of the very high associated

Allen Oldfather Whipple, **1881–1963**, Valentine Mott Professor of Surgery, The College of Physicians and Surgeons, Columbia University, New York, NY, USA.

mortality rate. A damage control procedure with packing and drainage should be performed and the patient referred for definitive surgery once stabilised.

Stomach

Most stomach injuries are caused by penetrating trauma. Blood may be present and is diagnostic if found in the nasogastric tube.

Surgical repair is performed but great care must be taken to examine the stomach fully, as an injury to the front of the stomach can be expected to have an 'exit' wound elsewhere on the organ.

Duodenum

Duodenal injury is frequently associated with injuries to the adjoining pancreas. Like the pancreas the duodenum lies retroperitoneally and so injuries are hidden and only discovered late or at laparotomy performed for other reasons. The only sign may be gas in the periduodenal tissue seen at CT.

Smaller injuries can be repaired primarily. Major injuries and those also involving the head of the pancreas should undergo initial damage control surgery and be referred for definitive care.

Small bowel

The small bowel is frequently injured as a result of blunt trauma. The individual loops may be trapped, causing high-pressure rupture of a loop or tearing of the mesentery. In penetrating injury, wounds may be multiple.

Small bowel injuries need urgent repair at laparotomy. Haemorrhage control as always takes priority and these wounds can be temporarily controlled with simple sutures. The small bowel can be temporarily occluded until haemorrhage control has been achieved. In blunt trauma the mesenteric vessels can be torn and bleeding actively – this may dictate the extent of a resection (see Damage control surgery). Resections should be carefully planned to limit the loss of viable small bowel but should be weighed against an excessive number of repairs or anastomoses. A combination of resection and repair should be used to avoid loss of significant lengths of bowel. Haematomas in the small bowel mesenteric border need to be explored to rule out perforation. With low-energy wounds, primary repair can be performed after debridement of any dead tissue, whereas more destructive wounds associated with military type weapons require resection and anastomosis.

Colon

Injuries to the colon from blunt injury are relatively infrequent. However, in penetrating injury, colonic injuries are not uncommon. If relatively little contamination is present and the viability of the colon is satisfactory, such wounds can be repaired primarily. If, however, there is extensive contamination, the patient is physiologically unstable or the bowel is of doubtful viability, then the colon can be closed off or a subsequent defunctioning colostomy formed.

Rectum

Only 5% of colon injuries involve the rectum. The majority are caused by penetrating injury, although occasionally the rectum may be damaged following fracture of the pelvis. Digital rectal examination to assess for the presence of blood is part of the examination of the trauma patient and, especially with an abdominal penetrating injury, the presence of blood is evidence of colorectal injury. These injuries are often associated with bladder and proximal urethral injury.

The location of the injury determines the management strategy. With intraperitoneal injuries, the rectum is managed as for colonic injuries. Full-thickness extraperitoneal rectal injuries should be managed with either a diverting end-colostomy and closure of the distal end (Hartmann's procedure) or a loop colostomy. Presacral drainage is generally no longer used.

In penetrating trauma it is important that the number of small bowel holes and missiles, e.g. bullets, add up to an even number, because although occasionally wounds may be tangential, this is the exception rather than the rule. For every 'entrance' wound there should either be an 'exit' wound or a residual missile.

Renal and urological tract injury

In the stable patient CT scanning with contrast is the investigation of choice. CT will enable the assessment of renal injury and, with delayed films, will enable the assessment of more distal injury.

For assessment of bladder injury a cystogram should be performed. A minimum of 400 ml of contrast is instilled into the bladder via a urethral catheter. The volume is essential because a small volume may not leak from a small bladder injury once the cystic muscle has contracted. It is important to assess the films as follows:

- with two views – anteroposterior and lateral;
- on two occasions – full and post-micturition.

Generally, renal injury is managed non-operatively unless the patient is unstable. The kidney can be angioembolised if required.

Ureteric injury is rare and is generally due to penetrating injury. Most ureters can be repaired or diverted if necessary.

Intraperitoneal ruptures of the bladder, usually from direct blunt injury, will require surgical repair. Extraperitoneal ruptures are usually associated with a fracture of the pelvis and will heal with adequate urine drainage (Summary box 26.7).

Summary box 26.7

Injuries to structures in the abdomen

- In children splenic injury can be managed non-operatively
- Duodenal injuries are associated with pancreatic damage
- Small bowel injuries need urgent repair
- Large bowel injuries can be resected and stapled off in damage limitation surgery
- Rectal injuries may be best managed initially with a defunctioning colostomy
- Kidney and urinary tract damage is best diagnosed with enhanced CT scanning
- Intra-abdominal bladder tears need formal repair and drainage

---

ABDOMINAL COMPARTMENT SYNDROME AND THE OPEN ABDOMEN

Raised intra-abdominal pressure has far-reaching consequences for the patient; the syndrome that results is known as abdominal

---

Henri Albert Charles Antoine Hartmann, **1860–1952, Professor of Clinical Surgery, The Faculty of Medicine, The University of Paris, Paris, France.**

compartment syndrome (ACS). ACS is a major cause of morbidity and mortality in the critically ill patient and its early recognition is essential (Table 26.6).

In all cases of abdominal trauma in which the development of ACS in the immediate postoperative phase is considered a risk, the abdomen should be left open and managed as for damage control surgery.

DAMAGE CONTROL

Following major injury, protracted surgery in the physiologically unstable patient with the 'deadly triad' – the combination of hypothermia, acidosis and coagulopathy – carries a very high mortality rate. 'Damage control' or 'damage limitation surgery' is a concept that originated from naval architecture, whereby a ship was designed to have areas sealed off in the case of damage, to limit flooding.

The application of damage control to the trauma patient has come from the realisation that minimising surgery until the physiological derangement can be corrected is the best way of improving outcome. The surgery is restricted to only two goals:

- stopping any active surgical bleeding;
- controlling any contamination.

The operation is then suspended and the abdomen temporarily closed. The patient's resuscitation continues in the intensive care unit. Once the physiology has been corrected, the patient warmed and the coagulopathy corrected, the patient is returned to the operating theatre for any definitive surgery.

The key philosophy of damage control can be summarised as follows:

- to keep the patient alive at any cost, utilising an unconventional approach and abbreviated surgical technique to limit the depletion of physiological reserve;
- to be part of the resuscitation process, in which there is initial surgical control of haemorrhage and contamination followed by rapid closure, assisting in the restoration of normal physiology.

Table 26.6 Effect of raised intra-abdominal pressure on individual organ function

Organ	Effect
Renal	Increase in renal vascular resistance leading to a reduction in glomerular filtration rate and impaired renal function
Cardiovascular	Decrease in venous return resulting in decreased cardiac output because of both a reduction in preload and an increase in afterload
Respiratory	Increased ventilation pressures because of splinting of the diaphragm, decreased lung compliance and increased airway pressures
Visceral perfusion	Reduction in visceral perfusion
Intracranial effects	Severe rises in intracranial pressures

Damage control resuscitation

This is a new concept that has evolved following recent military experience, in which the concept of damage control has been broadened to include the techniques used in resuscitation as well as in surgery. In the group of unstable trauma patients who are candidates for damage control surgery the time in the emergency department is minimised and the resuscitation of the patient is carried out in the operating room and not in the resuscitation bay. The resuscitation is individualised through repeated point of care testing in the operating room of haemoglobin level, acidosis (pH and lactate) and clotting, and is therefore directed towards the early delivery of biologically active colloids, clotting products, recombinant factor VIIa and whole blood in order to buy time. The physiological disturbances that are associated with the downward spiral of acidosis, coagulopathy and hypothermia in these serious injuries are predicted and attempts are made to avoid them rather than react to them.

Damage control surgery

The decision that damage control surgery is required should be made at the earliest opportunity, preferably in the emergency department or at the beginning of the operation. An early decision improves communication of the strategy with the whole surgical and anaesthetic team, expedites time to the operating room, limits time in surgery and allows earlier admission thereafter to the intensive care unit where the resuscitation can be best completed. Damage control is a staged process (Table 26.7).

Patient selection is the key to appropriate damage control. This is summarised in Table 26.8.

The initial surgical focus is haemorrhage control, which is followed by control and limitation of contamination. This is achieved using a range of abbreviated techniques including simple ligation of bleeding vessels, shunting of major arteries and veins, drainage, temporary stapling off of bowel, and therapeutic packing.

Following the above the abdomen is closed in a temporary fashion using a sheet of plastic (e.g. Opsite) over the bowel, an intermediate pack to allow suction, and a further sheet of adherent plastic drape to the skin to form a watertight and airtight seal. Suction is applied to the intermediate pack area to collect abdominal fluid. This technique is known as the 'Vacpac' or 'Opsite sandwich' (Fig. 26.10).

The closure is not without its own significant morbidity including atmospheric enteric fistula formation, heat loss and excessive fluid loss and, therefore, attempts to close the abdomen should be proactive. Successful closure may require aggressive off-loading of fluid and even haemofiltration to achieve this if the patient will tolerate it. The best situation is closure of the abdominal fascia, or, if this cannot be achieved, then skin closure only. Occasionally, mesh closure can be used, with skin grafting over the mesh and subsequent abdominal wall reconstruction.

Table 26.7 The stages of damage control surgery

Stage	
I	Patient selection
II	Control of haemorrhage and control of contamination
III	Resuscitation continued in the intensive care unit
IV	Definitive surgery
V	Abdominal closure

Table 26.8 Indications for damage control surgery

Anatomical	Inability to achieve haemostasis
	Complex abdominal injury, e.g. liver and pancreas
	Combined vascular, solid and hollow organ injury, e.g. aortic or caval injury
	Inaccessible major venous injury, e.g. retrohepatic vena cava
	Demand for non-operative control of other injuries, e.g. fractured pelvis
	Anticipated need for a time-consuming procedure
Physiological (decline of physiological reserve)	Temperature < 34°C
	pH < 7.2
	Serum lactate > 5 mmol l⁻¹ [N (Normal) < 2.5 mmol l⁻¹]
	Prothrombin time (PT) > 16 s
	Partial thromboplastin time (PTT) > 60 s
	> 10 units blood transfused
	Systolic blood pressure < 90 mmHg for > 60 min
Environmental	Operating time > 60 min
	Inability to approximate the abdominal incision
	Desire to reassess the intra-abdominal contents (directed relook)

As soon as control has been achieved the patient is transferred from the operating theatre to the intensive care unit where resuscitation is continued; the aim of this is the correction of hypothermia, acidosis and coagulopathy. Following this, further physiological investigation or radiological intervention can be carried out.

The next stage of damage control is definitive surgery. The team should aim to perform definitive anastomoses, vascular reconstruction and closure of the body cavity within 24–72 hours of injury; however, this must be individualised to the patient, the response to critical care resuscitation and the injury complexes, and must be judged on its own merits. Undue haste and a premature return to theatre will convert a definitive second operation into a second damage control procedure and result in further physiological insult for the patient; however, undue delay may increase the risk of intra-abdominal sepsis and the progression of previously unrecognised injuries.

The abdomen is closed as soon as possible, bearing in mind the risks of ACS.

Thoracic damage control is conceptually based on the same philosophy, i.e. that haemorrhage control and focused surgical procedures minimise further surgical insult and lead to improved survival in the unstable trauma patient. The focus of thoracic damage control is to rapidly control bleeding and limit air leaks using the fastest procedures available to minimise the operative time.

In abdominal damage control, abbreviated surgical techniques are performed that will require secondary procedures. The physiological impact of injuries to the thorax dictate that the thoracic techniques utilised are more single-stage definitive techniques. These are often performed in an abbreviated and occasionally more radical fashion, e.g. using staplers to resect injured lung, the lung twist to temporarily control lung parenchymal bleeding, *en masse* pneumonectomy and, more rarely, thoracic packing for diffuse bleeding and rapid techniques for the temporary closure of the chest.

The indications and techniques for emergency thoracotomy have already been described.

Damage control applies equally to the extremities, with shunting of blood vessels, fasciotomy and removal of contaminated tissue. Subsequent definitive management can be carried out at a later stage (Summary box 26.8).

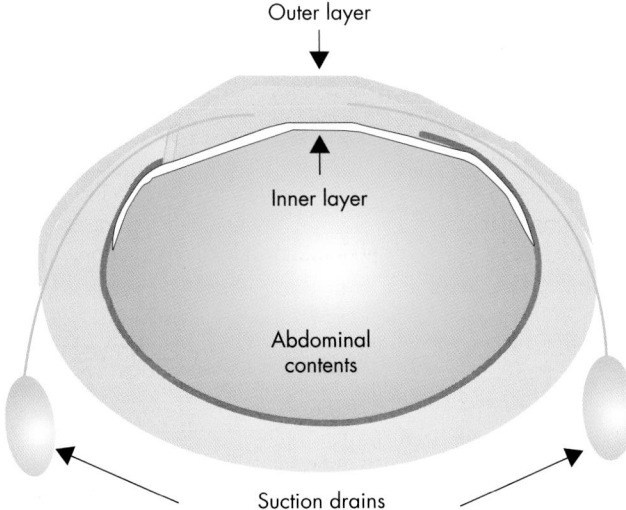

Outer layer

Inner layer

Abdominal contents

Suction drains

Figure 26.10 Abdominal closure following damage control surgery.

Summary box 26.8

Damage control

- **Resuscitation is carried out in the operating room using biologically active fluids**
- **Surgery is the minimum needed to stabilise the patient**
- **The aim of surgery is control of haemorrhage and limitation of contamination**
- **Secondary surgery is aimed at definitive repair**

---

en masse is French for 'in a body'.

INTERVENTIONAL RADIOLOGY

Interventional radiology can be useful in the management of torso trauma as both an investigative and a therapeutic tool for patients with vascular injury. Angioembolisation following demonstration of on-going bleeding in splenic and renal injury is a valuable technique. Interventional radiology is also widely used to evaluate for and control pelvic bleeding when clinically appropriate. Significant liver injuries that require therapeutic packing at laparotomy are at risk of on-going bleeding. Arteriography can be used to define and embolise bleeding vessels before a planned return to the operating room. In penetrating trauma, interventional radiology can be used to identify pseudoaneurysms and arteriovenous fistulae, which can be stented if required.

NON-OPERATIVE MANAGEMENT

Universally preferred for the management of solid organ injury in haemodynamically stable children, non-operative management of solid abdominal organ injury has rapidly gained acceptance in the management of adults as well. A stable patient and accurate imaging by CT are prerequisites for this approach. More widespread CT now accurately diagnoses many low-grade organ injuries to the liver, spleen and kidneys, which are frequently self-limiting with minimal intra-abdominal blood loss. Close observation for any signs of deterioration or bleeding is important as 2–15% will have concomitant hollow viscus injuries. Failure of non-operative management is uncommon and typically occurs within the first 12 hours after injury. Therefore, if correctly selected, the vast majority of these patients will avoid surgery, requiring less blood transfusion and sustaining fewer complications than operated patients.

Antibiotics in torso trauma

There is no level 1 evidence to recommend the use of antibiotics for the insertion of chest drains. However, they should be used in all cases of penetrating abdominal trauma.

FURTHER READING

American Association for the Surgery of Trauma. Organ Injury Scaling System. Available online at: http://www.aast.org (accessed 2007).

American College of Surgeons (2003) *Advanced Trauma Life Support Course Manual*. American College of Surgeons, Chicago.

Boffard, K.D. (ed) (2007) *Definitive Surgery of Trauma Care*, 2nd edn. Hodder Arnold, London.

Eastern Association for the Surgery of Trauma. Guidelines for practice management: evidence-based guidelines. 4a: Blunt aortic injury; 4b: Blunt myocardial injury; 4c: Evaluation of blunt abdominal trauma; 4d: Non-operative management of liver and spleen; 4e: Penetrating intraperitoneal colon injuries; 4f: Pain management in blunt thoracic trauma; 4g: Prophylactic antibiotics in penetrating abdominal trauma; 4h: Prophylactic antibiotics in tube thoracostomy. Available online at: http//:www.east.org (accessed 2007).

Moore, E.E., Feliciano, D.V. and Mattox, L.K. (eds) (2004) *Trauma*, 5th edn. McGraw Hill, New York.

World Society for Abdominal Compartment Syndrome. Abdominal compartment syndrome. Available online at: http//:www.wsacs.org (accessed 2007).

Extremity trauma

To gain an understanding of:
- How to identify whether an injury exists
- The important injuries not to miss

- The principles of the description and classification of fractures
- The range of available treatments
- How to select an appropriate treatment

INTRODUCTION

The objective when managing any injured person is to restore maximum function with minimum risk. The first duty is to identify and treat any immediate threats to life. The management of skeletal injuries has to take its rightful place in the overall care of the patient. For the multiply injured, following the Advanced Trauma Life Support (ATLS) system, this rightful place is usually when the primary survey and initial resuscitation have been completed. Very occasionally the haemorrhage associated with a fracture may be life-threatening; thus a pelvic injury may require urgent stabilisation or a major open fracture direct pressure to control blood loss. Most often, extremity injuries are encountered in the secondary survey. The relevant history, including the mechanism of the incident, a top-to-toe clinical examination and appropriate special investigations can be taken into account. Extremity injuries are identified and diagnosed, and their treatment is then planned and executed according to priority.

DIAGNOSIS, DESCRIPTION AND CLASSIFICATION OF INJURY

The first step is to establish the existence of an injury; it can then be described, classified and treated. Missing an injury can be serious, both medically and legally. It is usually easy to diagnose a musculoskeletal injury and so we become complacent. However, Table 27.1 contains a list of injuries for which it is known from the mistakes of others that the diagnosis is easily missed and that this error may have adverse consequences. We may each have only one chance in our career to make some of these diagnoses, so we must be prepared for the first case. We cannot just learn constructively from our own experience.

Assessment – history and examination

A relevant history should be taken. This will provide symptoms, a mechanism and general information about the patient. From the symptoms and mechanism likely injuries can be considered, sought and excluded. The general history should include factors that may affect diagnosis, treatment and objective. Known metastatic disease or generalised bone pathology will contribute to the diagnosis and affect the management plan. Diabetes and the use of anticoagulants are two common factors affecting management. Because the aim of treatment is restoration of function it is necessary to be clear as to the level of pre-injury function. This is gauged from occupation, hobbies, handedness and responsibilities. A mother with young children may need rapid restoration of function; a sportsperson or musician may not accept what would normally be considered a good result.

In isolated injuries, examination should focus on the history and symptoms. Local features of tenderness, deformity, abnormal movement and loss of function will then guide the use of investigations. In many respects the most important part of the clinical examination is of those areas adjacent to the area to be investigated, for it is here that many injuries are missed. For instance, in the case of injuries to the lower extremity, many hindfoot, midfoot and Achilles tendon injuries are missed as the investigation chosen is often an ankle radiograph, and when this is normal the patient is falsely reassured.

In the multiply injured or obtunded patient, the absence of

Table 27.1 Extremity injuries not to miss

Posterior dislocation of the shoulder
Lateral condylar mass fracture of the distal humerus
Peri-lunate dislocation
Scaphoid fracture
Tarsometatarsal fracture dislocation
Compartment syndrome
Vascular injury with knee dislocation
Talar neck fracture
Slipped upper femoral epiphysis
Achilles tendon rupture

Achilles, the Greek Hero, was the son of Peleus and Thetis. When he was a child his mother dipped him in the Styx, one of the rivers of the Underworld, so that he should be invulnerable in battle. The heel by which she held him did not get wet, and was, therefore, not protected. Achilles died from a wound in the heel which he received at the siege of Troy.

history and symptoms is compensated for by performing a top-to-toe clinical examination as part of the secondary survey.

The discovery of one injury is not the conclusion of the search but a prompt to look for associated injuries. This search is guided by the knowledge that injuries occur in patterns, e.g. a dislocated knee is often associated with a vascular injury, a head injury may mask a fractured cervical spine. In 15% of cases in which a spinal fracture has been identified there is another spinal injury at a separate site. An important discipline, particularly when managing the multiply injured patient, is the repeat examination; the 'morning after' ward round is a time for a further secondary survey to search for occult injuries. Once the information has been gathered there should be a rational relationship such that *patient + mechanism = injury.*

Principles of investigation

Imaging is performed to confirm or exclude possible injury guided by the history and examination. It adds precision to the diagnosis, which aids in planning treatment. A summary of the available methods is given in Table 27.2.

For almost 100 years the mainstay of the orthopaedic surgeon's investigation has been the plain radiograph. Radiographs should include orthogonal views (two views at 90° separation) and, for long bones, should show the joints above and below the injury. Other imaging modalities are now being used more frequently. Computerised tomography (CT) scans are invaluable for defining more complex patterns of a fracture, particularly adjacent to a joint. They are now also being used for the global assessment of the multiply injured person. As scan acquisition times decrease and physiological monitoring improves, the dangers for the multiply injured patient of being isolated in a scanner are reduced and the benefits of accurate diagnosis increased. Ultrasound is used to assess soft-tissue structures, e.g. Achilles tendon or rotator cuff injuries. Magnetic resonance (MR) scanning is used primarily to show soft-tissue injury, particularly around the knee. Imaging needs to be used intelligently; there is an adage in radiology that 'unless you are very lucky you only find what you look for'. Injuries with a reputation for being missed, such as a posterior dislocation of the shoulder, should be actively sought whenever there is any chance that they may be present (Fig. 27.1) (Summary box 27.1).

> **Summary box 27.1**
>
> **Finding an injury**
>
> - Relate all of the information gathered in the equation patient + mechanism = injury
> - Look specifically for 'easily missed injuries'
> - Re-examine the multiply injured patient

DESCRIPTION AND CLASSIFICATION OF MUSCULOSKELETAL INJURY

Description of injury

An injury needs to be described in plain language. This initial act of description is for the benefit of the diagnosing doctor, *not* for someone else. It begins to translate the information that has been gathered into a rational entity, which can then guide management. This act of description naturally leads to classification. Classification encourages precision in assessment and again aids management decisions; however, the limitations of classification should be recognised. Even the common systems are interpreted by individuals in a surprisingly wide variety of ways. Effective communication depends on a sensible blend of description and classification.

The soft-tissue injury

There are two components of soft-tissue injury that need to be identified: the degree of damage to the soft-tissue envelope around the fracture and the integrity of the important structures passing through the area, primarily the arteries and nerves. The state of the soft-tissue envelope over a fracture is an indicator of the degree of compromise of the local blood supply and resistance to infection. Open and closed fractures are the most easily recognised group. An open fracture is present when the fracture haematoma is exposed by a breach in an epithelial surface; this is usually skin but is sometimes mucous membrane of the bowel or vagina. When present a wound should initially be described in plain terms, e.g. 'a ragged 6-cm laceration over the anterior aspect of the midshaft of the left tibia with contused skin edges but no gross contamination'. A photograph, including a scale, should be obtained. The wound

Table 27.2 Investigation modalities

Modality	Good for	Problems
Plain radiographs	Fractures and dislocations. Easily available	Radiation. Not good for soft tissues
Computerised tomography	Bony spinal injury Global view in polytrauma Planning treatment of complex fractures	Radiation dose. Availability. Safety in severe injuries
Ultrasound scan	Soft-tissue injuries	Operator dependency
Magnetic resonance imaging	Soft-tissue problems and fractures	Availability and expensive Difficult to use in the ventilated patient
Bone scan	Stress fractures and tumours	Radiation dose
Fluoroscopy	Checking progress of surgery	Small field of view Quality Image distortion

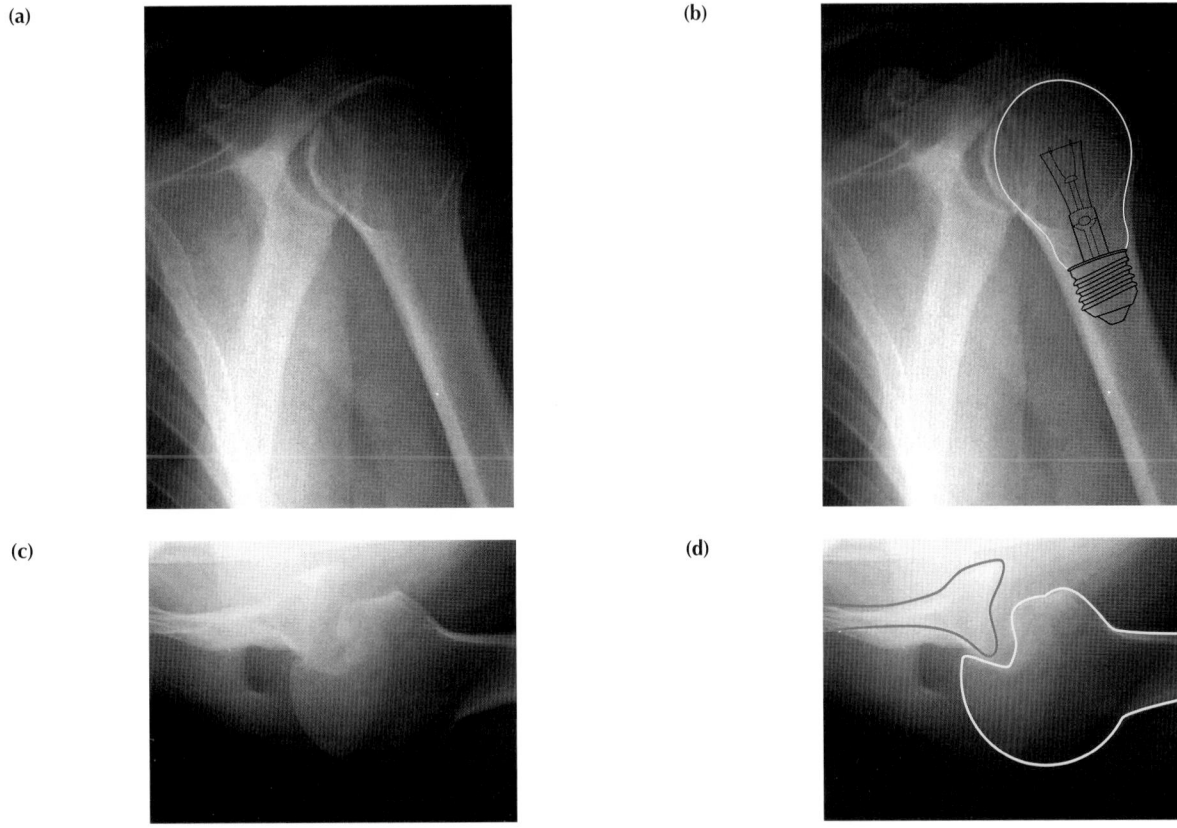

Figure 27.1 Posterior dislocation of the shoulder. (a) Anteroposterior view; (b) origin of the light bulb sign; (c) axial projection demonstrating how much easier it is to visualise the injury on this view; (d) axial projection highlighting this point and further demonstrating the impacted fracture in the humeral head, or Hill–Sachs lesion.

should then be covered and not be disturbed again until definitive treatment is given in an operating theatre.

Just because a fracture is closed does not mean that the injury to the soft-tissue envelope cannot be described. There may still be bruising, swelling, contusion, tissue shearing or crushing. The closed soft-tissue injury may have characteristics that will affect the timing of interventions and the likely outcome.

Injuries to arteries and nerves

Major arterial injuries may be limb- or life-threatening and require early recognition. Suspicion will be raised by a history of penetrating trauma or of displaced injuries at particular sites, e.g. the knee. It should be routine to record the circulation distal to a fracture or dislocation. This record should be specific, e.g. 'dorsalis pedis present' or 'capillary refill < 2 s', not just 'neuro-vascularly intact'. The role and timing of diagnostic imaging techniques is debatable because although they aid diagnosis, they also delay treatment. The warm ischaemia time should be kept to below 4 hours. If the level of the injury is clinically obvious it is best to proceed to treatment; on-table arteriography can then be obtained if required.

Nerve injuries should be identified by clinical examination and recorded. It is important that if operative treatment of a fracture is planned the preoperative neurological status is recorded. As with the vascular examination, the findings should be recorded in such a way that they can be interpreted without ambiguity. This should not be taken as an invitation to be precise beyond knowledge. For instance, if the examiner does not know the function of the axillary nerve it is misleading to record that it has been tested. A diagram recording findings is often the simplest method of record.

Compartment syndrome

When the hydrostatic pressure within a fascial compartment increases sufficiently it will compromise the effective circulation within the compartment leading to tissue ischaemia and necrosis. The most reliable clinical symptom is disproportionately severe pain, and the most useful sign is pain on passive stretching of the involved compartment. It is not an easy diagnosis to make as patients are expected to have pain after a fracture; the symptoms may be masked by analgesics. Additionally, examination may be difficult because of the placement of splints and dressings. Of note is that peripheral pulses are generally not affected and alteration in sensation is a late sign. The nature of the fracture is not a good guide to development of the syndrome. It can occur with low-energy and high-energy injuries, closed or open. Compartment syndromes are most frequently recognised in the lower leg, but they can occur wherever there is a closed compartment. Some injuries require particular vigilance, including crush injuries to the foot and hand, and displaced humeral supracondylar fractures in children.

The reliance on pain to achieve a diagnosis is clearly a problem in the obtunded patient. Here there is a good argument for measurement of compartment pressures. There is some evidence that it may be wise to monitor the compartment pressure in all tibial fractures.

The bony injury

To the soft-tissue injury is added a description of the bony injury. The terminology used in this description is illustrated in Fig. 27.2. Now look at Fig. 27.3 and describe what you see. Plain language should be used to describe the injury: thus, a '45° oblique fracture at the junction of the proximal and middle thirds of the right tibia with an associated fibular fracture' gives a clear unambiguous picture (this example is used again later). A satisfactory description generally needs the following components:

- which bone is injured;
- the region of the bone injured;
- whether the fracture is simple or multifragmentary;

- the direction of the fracture line – transverse, oblique or spiral;
- whether the fragment is displaced or undisplaced;
- if displaced, the alignment, length and rotation;
- any evidence of pre-existing pathology;
- any associated joint dislocation.

Although in adults the fracture line is generally complete, i.e. it extends through both cortices, in children the different mechanical qualities of the bone may lead to other patterns in which the fracture line is incomplete. These are termed torus and greenstick fractures (Fig. 27.4). Compression fractures occur when cancellous bone is crumpled; an example is a wedge compression fracture of a vertebral body. A similar injury is an impacted fracture; here the fracture occurs at the metaphyseal/diaphyseal junction. The hard cortical bone is driven into the cancellous bone, analogous to a cone being driven into an ice-cream; this pattern commonly occurs at the humeral neck. Some injuries are hard to describe in plain language, for example physeal injuries in children. Almost all communication utilises the Salter–Harris classification, which is described later (Summary box 27.2).

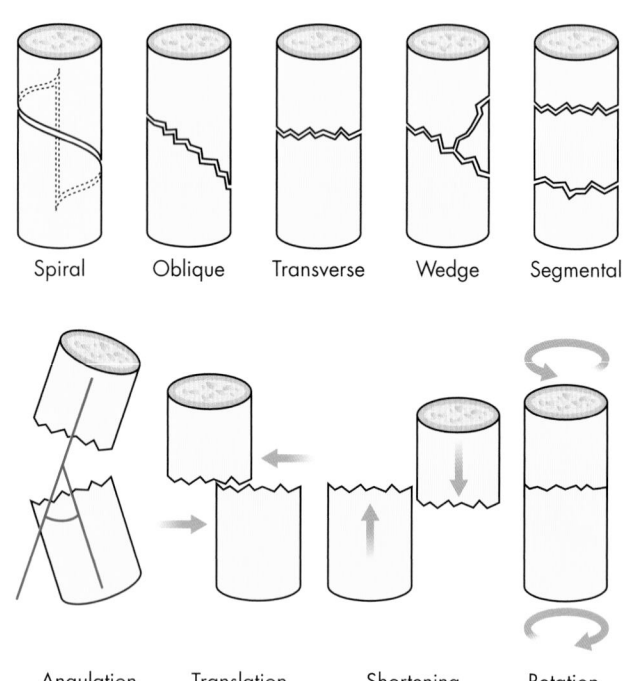

Spiral   Oblique   Transverse   Wedge   Segmental

Angulation   Translation   Shortening   Rotation

Figure 27.2 Descriptive terms for fractures.

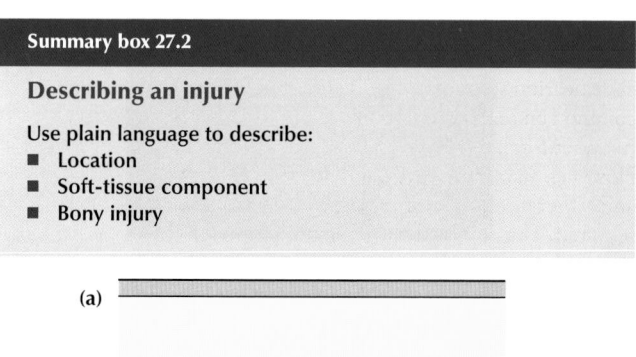

Summary box 27.2

Describing an injury

Use plain language to describe:
- **Location**
- **Soft-tissue component**
- **Bony injury**

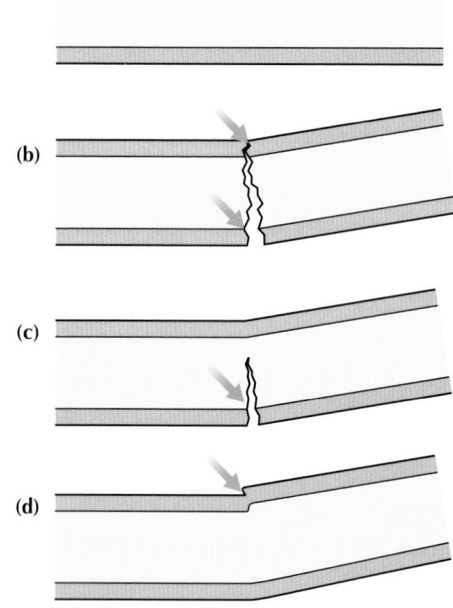

Figure 27.4 Types of bony injury. (a) Uninjured bone; (b) adult transverse fracture failure across the whole bone; (c) greenstick fracture; the bone has failed on the tension side; (d) torus or buckle fracture; the bone has failed on the compression side.

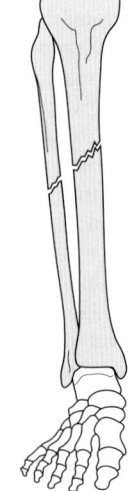

Robert Bruce Salter, **formerly Professor of Orthopaedic Surgery, The University of Toronto, Ontario, Canada.**
W. R. Harris, **formerly Professor of Orthopaedic Surgery, The University of Toronto, Ontario, Canada.**

Figure 27.3 Fracture of the shaft of the tibia.

Classification of injury

To formalise the description of the injury, use a classification. This encourages precision in the assessment and may enhance communication and management decisions.

Soft-tissue injury

Despite the emphasis placed upon management of the soft tissues, it remains common practice that unless it is an open injury the soft-tissue component of an injury is described and not classified. There are classification systems available for closed soft-tissue injuries when required.

Open injuries are generally classified; the system most commonly used is that of Gustillo and Anderson. This classification is based on a study of a large group of open tibial fractures. Of note is that the grade of the injury is not determined by the size of the wound alone: thus, a high-energy fracture with a < 1 cm wound is a grade III fracture. The injury cannot be finally classified until its full extent is appreciated on completion of the initial wound excision. The classification is summarised in Table 27.3.

Bony injury in adults

There are many eponymous and anatomically localised fracture classification systems; some are referred to later. Some fractures are common enough and sufficiently well studied that evidence-based treatment related to such a local system can be carried out. However, many fractures are treated on the basis of 'principles' and, therefore, a principle-based system of classification is required. The AO (Arbeitsgemeinschaft für Osteosynthesefragen)

Table 27.3 Gustillo and Anderson open fracture classification

Type I	A low energy open fracture with a wound less than 1 cm long and clean
Type II	An open fracture with a laceration more than 1 cm long without extensive soft tissue damage, flaps or avulsion
Type III	Characterised by high energy injury irrespective of the size of the wound. Extensive damage to soft tissues, including muscles, skin, and neurovascular structures, and a high degree of contamination. Multifragmentary and unstable fractures

Sub-groups of type III

A	Adequate soft tissue cover of a fractured bone after stabilisation
B	Inadequate soft tissue cover of a fractured bone after stabilisation ie flap coverage required
C	Open fracture associated with an arterial injury requiring repair

Source: Gustillo et al., 1984

Ramon Balgoa Gustilo, **Surgeon, Hennepin County Medical Center, Minneapolis, MN, USA.**
John T. Anderson, **Surgeon, Hennepin County Medical Center, Minneapolis, MN, USA.**
AO is short for Arbeitsgemeinschaft für Osteosynthesefragen which may be translated from the German as 'Working Party on Problems of Bone Repair'.

system provides such a principle-based comprehensive classification of fractures. It allows and encourages a comparison of fractures of similar types from different body regions. Principle-based treatment can flow from this principle-based classification. Thus, it can easily be seen that a partial articular fracture of the distal radius is very similar to that of a tibial plateau. The system is organised to identify the site and nature of a fracture. Initially, the site is identified by two numbers: the first records which bone is involved and the second which segment of that bone (Fig. 27.5). The classified fracture is recorded as an alphanumeric; for instance, the tibial fracture described at the beginning of this section is a 42A2. The '4' and the '2' are simply shorthand for the tibial shaft. The letter begins to define the nature of the fracture as shown in Fig. 27.6; in this case it is a simple or 'A-type' diaphyseal fracture. The final number given refines the record of the fracture pattern; for a simple diaphyseal fracture '1' represents a spiral, '2' an oblique and '3' a transverse fracture. The system goes into further detail but this requires reference to the AO classification book (see Further reading).

Thus, although the alphanumeric is not what one would use for verbal communication with a colleague, it does have advantages. It requires clear consideration of the fracture pattern to reach a conclusion, i.e. it directs the assessment. It allows succinct recording in a database, which is then easily searched. Thus, the principle-based classification system guides principle-based treatment.

Growth plate injuries

In children some fractures are similar to those seen in adults, but there are also specific injuries to the growth plate region. The physis contains cells that are responsible for longitudinal bone growth. Trauma is the most common cause of physeal arrest, which may be partial or complete. A bridge of bone (bony bar) forms between the epiphysis and metaphysis. From then on growth will be altered leading to relative shortening or angulation.

The classification of Salter and Harris is used to describe the nature of the epiphyseal injury. These patterns of injury are shown in Fig. 27.7 and a description of the types and their characteristics is given below:

- Type I – a transverse fracture along the line of the physis; the growing zone is not usually injured so there is no growth disturbance. This fracture is common.
- Type II – similar to a type 1 injury but the fracture line deviates off into the metaphysis at one end, producing a metaphyseal fragment; seldom affects growth. This fracture is common.
- Type III – passes along the physis and then deviates into the epiphysis (intra-articular); rarely results in significant deformity but can lead to joint incongruity. This fracture is not common.
- Type IV – crosses the physis passing from the epiphysis into the metaphysis; interferes with the growing layer of cartilage cells so can cause premature focal fusion of the physis followed by deformity. This fracture is not common.
- Type V – a crush injury of the physis; associated with growth disturbances at the physis. Diagnosis may be difficult as the radiograph may look normal; however, premature closure of the physis reveals the diagnosis. This fracture is rare.
- Type VI – rare injury consisting of an injury to the perichondral structures by direct trauma, e.g. heat or chemical (Summary box 27.3).

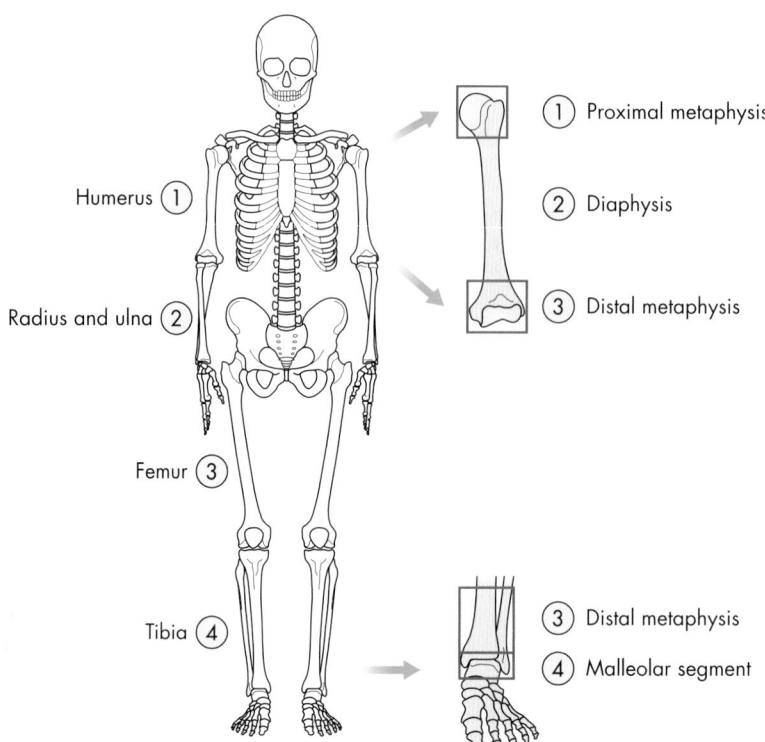

Figure 27.5 The AO classification system: the first two numbers specify the site of the fracture.

Summary box 27.3

The value of classification

- Encourages and directs evaluation of the injury
- Assists planning of treatment
- Guides prognosis
- Results in easier data retrieval
- Allows comparison with the results of other surgeons

THE RESPONSE TO INJURY

The natural response to a fracture, that is the natural history of a fracture, is that the broken bone will heal. It may well heal in a satisfactory position and have a satisfactory functional outcome. However, it may fail to unite, be slow to unite, unite in a poor position, become infected or have a combination of these problems. Consideration of these possible outcomes and how we might influence them is at the heart of making management decisions.

Bone healing

Fractures naturally tend to heal and may do so by indirect or direct mechanisms:

- *Indirect (secondary) bone healing.* Indirect (secondary) bone healing occurs with a callus precursor and is referred to as enchondral ossification. This tends to occur when the bone ends are not perfectly aligned and when there is some movement at the fracture site during the healing process. Such secondary bone healing is broadly characterised by three main phases: inflammation, repair with callus formation and remodelling of immature woven bone to mature lamellar bone. It may be thought of as the natural way for a bone to heal.

- *Direct (primary) bone healing.* This occurs without callus formation. It is like the normal process of remodelling with cutting cones crossing the fracture and new lamellar bone being laid down. It tends to occur when the fracture ends are closely opposed and there is no relative movement between them.

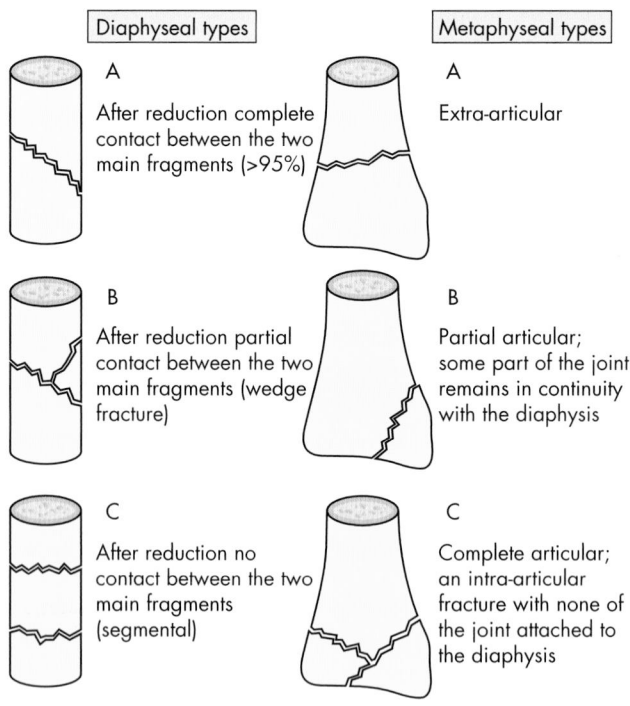

Figure 27.6 The AO classification system: the letter defines the nature of the fracture.

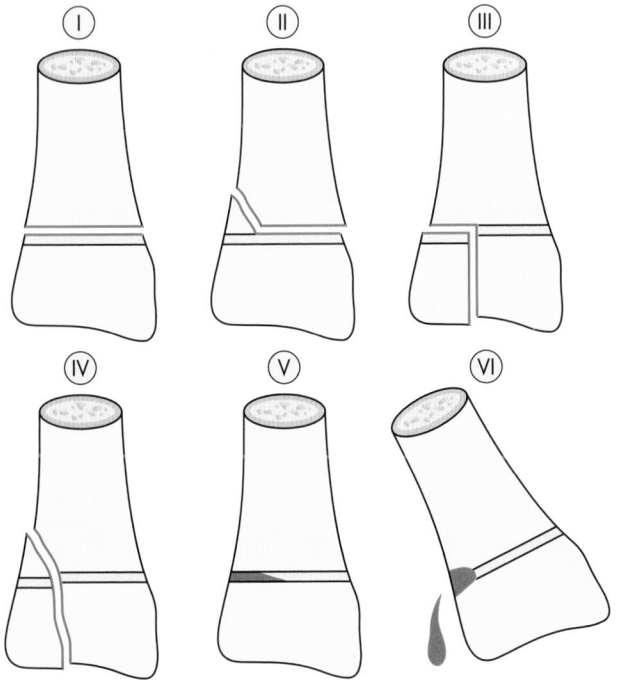

Figure 27.7 The Salter–Harris classification of growth plate injuries.

Thus, one of the components of a successful outcome in fracture healing is for the healing tissues to differentiate into bone. For this to occur the appropriate mechanical and biological conditions have to be met. Perren and Cordey in 1980 proposed the 'interfragmentary strain theory'. They suggested that loading that leads to an increase in the length of the bone (strain) of less than 2% is advantageous to fracture union. Applying this theory has led to two approaches to fracture fixation. One may try to achieve absolute stability between fragments when bone is fixed so that the broken surfaces do not move relative to each other. This leads to direct healing. It is achievable in simple fracture patterns when they are reduced precisely and compressed together. Relative stability is when the fracture fragments can move relative to each other. The amount of movement between the fracture fragments does not only depend upon the surgical construct but also on the applied loads. Therefore, before commencing definitive treatment it is important to consider what one is trying to achieve. Does the patient need to weight-bear, does the joint need to be mobilised early and are there multiple injuries to consider? Unsurprisingly, this means considering the whole patient and not just the broken bone.

Bone union is not just dependent upon mechanical factors. The healing tissues require an adequate blood supply. Therefore, when the injury has led to significant soft-tissue damage, union is likely to be slow. At the time of surgery, care must be taken to minimise disruption to the blood supply of the healing tissues. Smoking has been shown to delay fracture healing. Non-steroidal anti-inflammatory medications also seem to delay fracture healing; they are therefore best avoided in situations in which union is likely to be slow.

Adverse outcomes

Malunion

Malunion is when the bone unites in an incorrect position. What constitutes an incorrect position is debatable and varies from

bone to bone. As a guide, an articular step should not be greater than the thickness of the articular cartilage. In the lower limb angulation or rotation should not exceed 5°. Visible deformity is seldom acceptable.

Non-union

Non-union of a fracture may be defined as failure to show progressive clinical or radiographic signs of healing. The principle types of non-union are atrophic, hypertrophic and infected. These can be secondary to failure of biology and/or mechanical environment and patient factors (smoking). In atrophic non-union, the fracture gap is filled by fibrous tissue and the bone fragments remain mobile. Hypertrophic union occurs when there is excessive movement at the fracture site, leading to abundant periosteal bone formation. Union fails because stability is insufficient to allow bridging of the fracture gap. If stability is provided, union is likely.

Infected non-union

Infected non-union merits a separate mention as it is a potentially catastrophic complication. Its treatment is often prolonged, multistaged and can result in loss of the limb. Open fractures are therefore treated with minimisation of infection as the main priority. The risk–benefit balance should always be considered before embarking on treatment.

Delayed union

Delayed union is the term used to describe a fracture that has not healed in the expected time. Fractures in children tend to heal more rapidly than fractures in adults, and upper limb fractures can heal more quickly than lower limb fractures. Fractures in children may unite (the bone ends stick together) within 2–3 weeks and consolidate in 4–6. Femoral fractures in adults may take 12 weeks to unite and 24 weeks until they are as strong as they were before (consolidation) (Summary box 27.4).

> **Summary box 27.4**
>
> **Fracture healing**
>
> - *Mechanics* – the strain theory – determine whether healing is indirect or direct
> - *Biology* – the blood supply needs to be intact; avoid smoking and non-steroidal anti-inflammatory drugs
> - *Infection* – must be guarded against

Understanding outcome

Estimating the potential benefits and disadvantages of treatment interventions can be difficult. Table 27.4 lists the potential advantages and disadvantages of treatment. A key factor is to have some knowledge of the natural history of the injury, i.e. what will happen if nothing is done. When this is known some estimate can be made of the potential for improvement or the risk of doing harm.

It can help to look at outcome in a graphical manner; such a picture can help to conceptualise when and how vigorously to intervene. In Fig. 27.8a the blue line shows what the progress of the patient would have been if the injury had not occurred: the general quality of life is plotted against the passage of time. Even had the injury not occurred at some stage the quality of life would deteriorate and the patient would eventually die. The red line

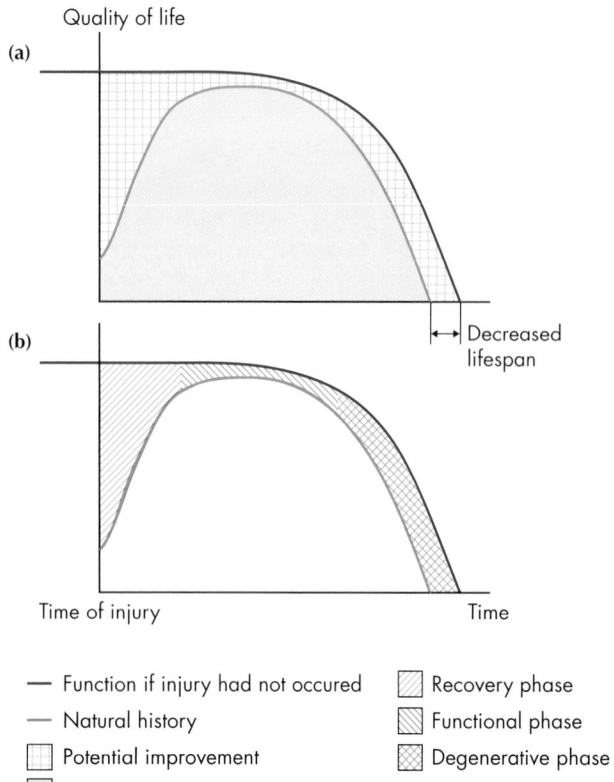

— Function if injury had not occured

— Natural history

▢ Potential improvement

▢ Potential harm

▨ Recovery phase

▧ Functional phase

▩ Degenerative phase

Figure 27.8 Graphical representation of the potential benefits and disadvantages of treatment interventions. (a) The hatched area between the two curves represents the potential for beneficial therapeutic intervention. The beige area beneath the natural history curve represents the potential for detrimental effects of intervention. (b) The area of potential benefit can be divided into three phases: recovery, functional and degenerative.

Table 27.4 Risks and benefits of fracture treatment

Benefits	Risks
Pain relief	Anaesthesia
Prevention of infection	Introduction of infection
Restoration of anatomy	Damage to soft tissues and
Early movement of the limb	neurovascular structures
Early movement of the patient	Devitalising bone
Improved function	Need for implant removal
Reduced risk of secondary	Financial cost (cost of
arthritis	treatment)
Financial cost (time off work)	

shows the natural history of an imagined injury, that is the effect of the injury on the patient's quality of life without any treatment being given. Thus the area between these curves represents the opportunity for treatment to provide some improvement on the natural history, presuming that the best we can hope for is to get the patient's condition back to what it would have been had the injury not occurred.

Figure 27.8b shows how the possible clinical benefit can be divided into an early, plateau and late phase. The early phase equates to improved function during recovery or while healing is

taking place, e.g. an intramedullary nail for a femoral shaft fracture. The plateau (functional) phase equates to better function after healing, e.g. ensuring leg length equality, stable joints and decreased pain. The late phase relates to the avoidance of secondary complications such as degenerative arthritis. If the patient's outcome dips below the natural history curve at any stage then it can be seen that treatment has actually caused a poorer outcome than if none had been offered. Thus the area below the natural history curve represents the potential for treatment to be disadvantageous and cause harm.

Such a graphical approach can be used to illustrate whether or not treatment interventions are rational. This can be seen with the examples given later for the treatment of pathological and paediatric injuries. What is clear is that unless the natural history of an injury is known then rational treatment decisions are not possible.

PRINCIPLES OF FRACTURE MANAGEMENT

As noted above the aims of treatment are to restore function safely with minimal complications. The first principle is to consider whether any intervention is necessary; many fractures require no or just symptomatic treatment. The interventional management of the bony injury has two components: reduction and stabilisation. They can each be achieved by a variety of methods and these methods will have mechanical and biological consequences.

Reduction

A fracture can be reduced by closed or open means. Each method has the same components, being some way of moving the fragments and some way of judging whether the desired position has been achieved. The accuracy of reduction required varies from site to site, with the nature of the planned stabilisation and with the anticipated mode of healing.

The assessment of the adequacy of fracture reduction may be made within the zone of injury or outside of it. Direct viewing of the fracture ends may be with the naked eye at open operation or by using imaging or arthroscopy. Outside of the zone of injury the adequacy may be assessed with reference to the other limb, again by just looking or by imaging. Generally, a combination of methods is used. Reference to Fig. 27.2 (see p. 356) demonstrates that the fracture with rotational deformity is difficult to depict graphically and for the same reason is often not noticed on radiography or at open surgery. However, merely looking at the whole limb and comparing it with the normal side generally reveals whether the rotational reduction is adequate.

The other component of reduction is moving or manipulating the fragments. Manipulating a fracture by a closed technique, i.e. without surgically exposing the bone, is an art. The key is to utilise the remaining soft tissues; they will tend to guide the bony fragments. The most elegant way is to reverse the mechanism of the injury. Charnley in 1950 demonstrated this with a simple model; it is easy to make a similar model using a broken pencil and some sellotape. The sequence of injury and reversal is illustrated in Fig. 27.9.

At open operation the bony fragments can be manipulated just as in a closed reduction; it is easier because the bony

Sir John Charnley, **1911–1982, Professor of Orthopaedic Surgery, The University of Manchester, Manchester, England.**

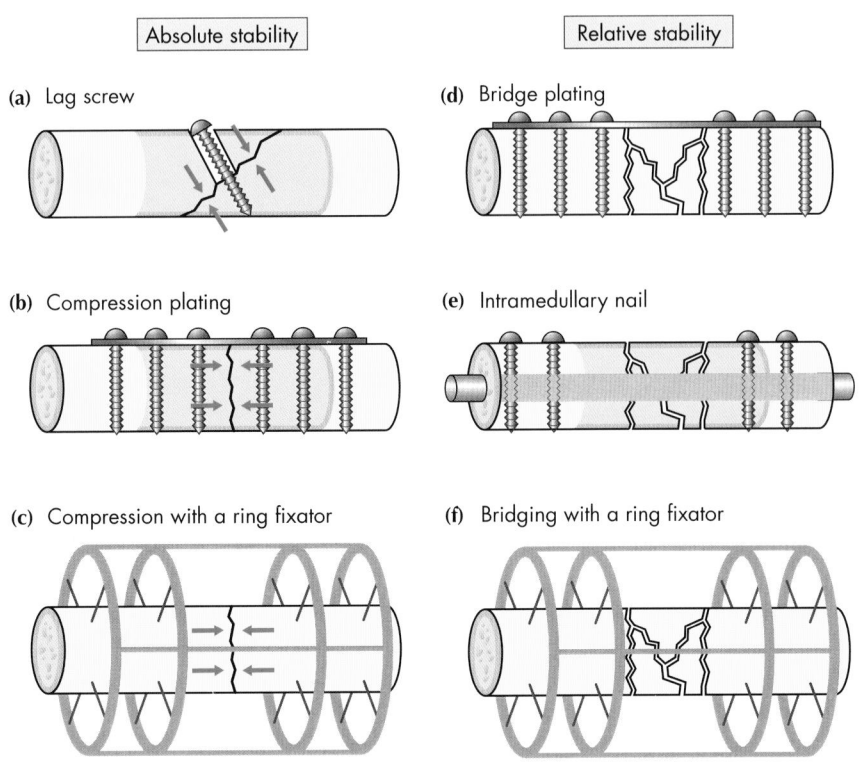

Figure 27.9 How absolute and relative stability can be achieved. The same implants may be used to achieve different mechanical effects.

fragments can be watched. The fragments can also be moved by applying clamps directly to the bone. The adequacy of the reduction with a simple fracture pattern can be judged by direct reference to the fracture fragments themselves, just as when making a simple jigsaw. With more complex fracture patterns exposure of all of the individual fragments may devitalise them and so reduction is assessed indirectly by restoring the overall position of the limb (Summary box 27.5).

Summary box 27.5

Reduction

- **Reduction has two components – moving the fragments and assessing adequacy**
- **Each component can be carried out within the zone of injury or beyond the zone of injury**

Stabilisation

Most often when a fracture has been reduced it needs to be held or stabilised while healing progresses.

When choosing a technique of stabilisation the aim is to:

1 optimise the biological and mechanical environment to create conditions favourable for fracture healing;
2 reduce the period of disability by speeding healing or allowing function during the healing process.

The mechanical environment can be altered to achieve the desired stability, either absolute or relative. *Absolute stability* is when the bone behaves as if it is not fractured. This is generally achieved by precise reduction and compression of the fracture ends. No displacement should occur during the loading permitted

in the postoperative period. This provides the environment for direct bone healing. In contrast, *relative stability* will produce a situation that allows some movement in proportion to the load applied. This stimulates callus formation and secondary bone healing. Fig. 27.9 shows some of the configurations that can be used to achieve relative and absolute stability. Simple fracture patterns allow absolute stability to be obtained; in the more complex fracture patterns the biological cost of achieving precise reduction (soft-tissue stripping, etc.) may outweigh the advantages.

Methods used for stabilising a fracture

Casting and splinting

A cast is a moulded orthopaedic appliance that may be composed of plaster of Paris or fibreglass; it is useful in the stabilisation of a fracture, either as a temporary or a definitive treatment.

When a cast is applied it should be remembered that, following a fracture, there may be significant soft-tissue swelling which may increase before it subsides. By applying a full (circumferential) cast, the increasing swelling will lead to tightness of the limb within the cast. There is then a risk of neurovascular damage, skin damage and compartment syndrome. A plaster slab may be used instead, in which the plaster material is not circumferential but the securing bandages are, and, as a consequence, tightness can still occur. The best way to avoid tightness is to apply a full cast and then split it through all of the layers down to the skin once it has set. Whichever method is used for treatment the surgeon should assess the risk of cast tightness and take appropriate

---

Plaster of Paris **is a white chrystalline powder, Calcium Sulphate Hemihydrate, CaSO ½HO, which sets hard when water is added to it.**

precautions. This may involve admitting a patient for a period of observation or providing instructions for the patient and family to follow in the event of problems.

When a cast has been applied as a first aid measure to provide stability and comfort, no particular moulding is required. However, when the fracture has been manipulated and reduced as described in Fig. 27.10 the cast needs to be applied in such a way as to prevent redisplacement. This requires the use of the available intact structures. The soft-tissue hinge is placed in tension and the reduced bone is placed in compression. The cast is then applied and moulded to stabilise the fracture using a so called 'three-point fixation'. Once moulded, plaster providing such three-point fixation appears bent; this leads to the adage that 'if you want a straight bone then you need a bent plaster' (Fig. 27.11).

The advantages and disadvantages of casting and splinting are described in Table 27.5.

Traction

Traction is pulling to change or hold the position of fracture fragments. The advantages and disadvantages of traction are given in Table 27.6. The technique works because of the integrity of the

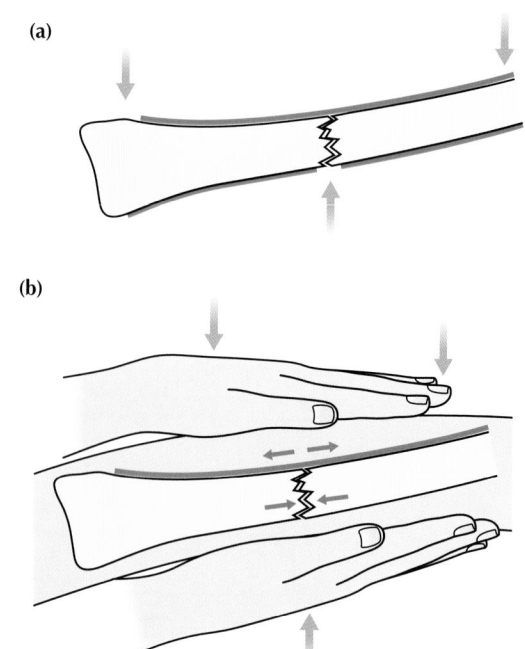

Figure 27.11 (a) The position achieved at the end of the manipulation described in Figure 27.11. (b) Demonstration of how by moulding the cast the intact periosteum is kept under tension and the bone under compression; thus, the remaining mechanical properties are used to achieve stability.

surrounding soft tissues (otherwise, on pulling, the fragments would just get further apart). Traction can be used both as a temporary and as a definitive treatment. Traction splints are often used for temporary stabilization of a fracture. So long as the patient is not moving, for Newton's law to be satisfied, there must be equal opposing forces. Static traction, that is between two fixed points, is well illustrated by a Thomas-type splint (Fig. 27.12a). This gives pain relief and stability, allowing the patient to be transported. In dynamic traction the pull is exerted by a system of weights, balanced with the patient's own body weight, which provides the opposing force (Fig. 27.12b).

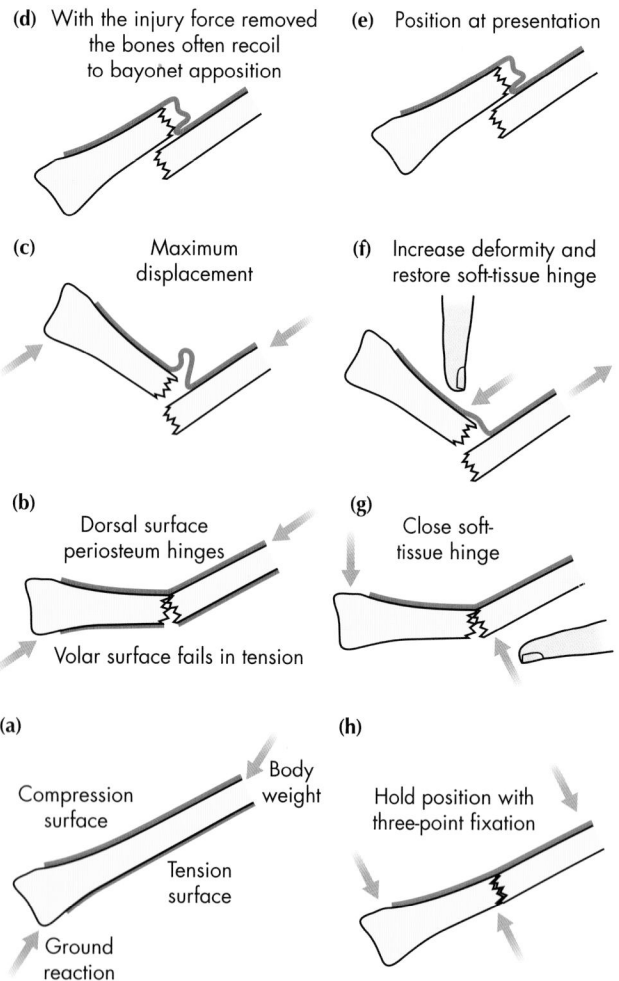

Figure 27.10 (a–d) Representation of how the mechanism of injury causes the bony and soft-tissue injury. (e–h) Representation of how the residual mechanical properties of the tissues may be used to effect and hold a reduction.

Table 27.5 Advantages and disadvantages of casting and splinting

Advantages	No wound
	No interference with fracture site
	Cheap
	Adjustable
	No implants to remove
Disadvantages	Limited access to the soft tissues
	Cumbersome (particularly in the elderly)
	Interferes with function
	Poor mechanical stability
	'Plaster disease'

Sir Isaac Newton, 1642–1727, Lucasian Professor of Mathematics, Cambridge University, Cambridge, England.
Hugh Owen Thomas, 1834–1891, A General Practitioner of Liverpool, England. He is regarded as 'The Founder of Orthopaedic Surgery' although never holding a hospital appointment preferring to treat patients in their own homes. He introduced the Thomas splint in 1875.

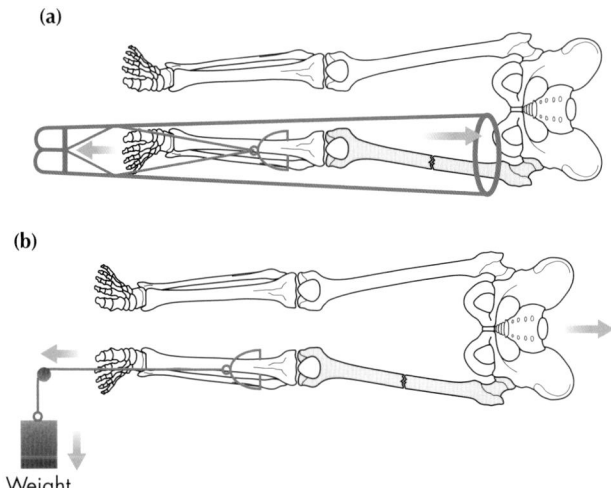

(a)

(b)

Weight

Figure 27.12 (a) Static traction with a Thomas splint. The force and counterforce are contained within a static system. The load is applied to the patient through the tibial traction pin via a cord tightened with a Spanish windlass. The counterforce is applied through pressure by the splint on the ischial tuberosity. (b) A dynamic system in which the load is applied by weights suspended from the tibial pin and the counterforce is the patient's own weight.

Table 27.6 Advantages and disadvantages of traction

Advantages	No wound in zone of injury
	No interference with fracture site
	Materials cheap
	Adjustable
Disadvantages	Restricts mobility of patient
	Expensive in hospital time
	Skin pressure complications
	Pin site infection
	Thromboembolic complications

Traction can be applied either using the skin (skin traction) or by direct coupling to the bone with pins or wires (skeletal traction). It can be simple or complicated. The simplest practical example of traction is the use of a collar and cuff to treat a proximal humeral fracture. As long as the patient is upright, gravity provides the traction. The role of the doctor is simply to advise the patient to sleep in a chair instead of a bed to maintain the dependency of the arm. More complex systems of weights, counterweights and pulleys can be used to provide the appropriate force required to maintain alignment of a lower limb fracture. The concept of a controlled and uncontrolled fragment is helpful; failure to understand this can lead to failure of traction. As the terms suggest, a controlled fragment is one that the surgeon can manoeuvre into the position that he or she wishes; an uncontrolled fragment is one over which the surgeon has no control. Thus, in the proximal femoral fracture the proximal fragment tends to remain flexed and abducted however great the traction, i.e. it is uncontrolled. The key is to move the controlled distal fragment into line with the uncontrollable proximal fragment.

In the UK traction is rarely used for definitive treatment in adults. Although the equipment for traction is inexpensive, the technique is costly in terms of the length of hospital stay. Public opinion has also changed and there is an unwillingness to remain in hospital for prolonged periods. Nursing a patient on traction can be difficult once the familiarity with the system is lost. Prolonged bed rest may lead to pressure sores, thromboembolism, pneumonia and atelectasis.

Plates and screws

A screw is normally used to join two things together. Instinctively we expect a screw to squeeze these things together when tightened. This is achieved because the hole under the screw head is greater in diameter than the threads of the screw, which allows the screw to glide in this hole. Thus, further tightening after the head impacts will cause compression. This method can be used to compress two bony fragments (the technique is then called a lag screw) or a plate to the bone. When a fracture can be reduced precisely a lag screw may be used to compress the fragments together to provide absolute stability. This single vulnerable lag screw will provide absolute stability but will not provide a strong durable fixation. It may be protected by a plate, termed a neutralisation plate. This is a classic method of stable internal fixation and is ideal for fractures such as those of the radial and ulnar shafts. The same plate and screws may be used in different ways, to provide different sorts of fixation. Table 27.7 shows the advantages and disadvantages of plate fixation.

Open reduction and internal fixation (ORIF) is the term generally associated with the use of such implants in the fashion described above. However, as with other branches of surgery, fracture fixation has become less invasive. With better intraoperative imaging, minimally invasive osteosynthesis (MIO) has evolved in which fractures are reduced and fixed though smaller incisions. It is presumed that this will reduce morbidity and speed recovery.

A recent development is the locking plate. Here the screw has a threaded head that tightens into the plate. The screws are not floppy within the plate but 'lock' when tightened. This gives angular stability similar to that of an external fixator and seems particularly advantageous in elderly bone and at metaphyseal/diaphyseal junctions.

Intramedullary nailing

The diaphysis of a long bone with its medullary canal is essentially a tube. It has long been realised that there are advantages to placing the stabilisation device inside the canal. The technique has evolved alongside improvements in intraoperative radiographic imaging. In this situation the surgeon's eyes are the image

Table 27.7 Advantages and disadvantages of plate and screw fixation

Advantages	Can be used when anatomical reduction is required
	Allows early mobilisation
	Can provide absolute or relative stability
Disadvantages	May interfere with fracture site
	Periosteal/soft-tissue damage
	Does not normally allow for immediate load-bearing
	Potential for infection
	Metalwork complications
	?Need for plate removal

intensifier. An intramedullary nail is usually made of steel or titanium. It may be solid, hollow or slotted in cross-section. An intramedullary nail will by its nature protect against angulatory displacement and translation. To extend the range of fractures suitable for stabilisation with a nail the implant normally has transverse holes at either end; this allows locking of the nail to the bone with further screws to control rotation and length.

Modern nailing is a minimally invasive technique. The nail is introduced in a series of planned steps, aided by specific instrumentation. After fracture reduction a guidewire is placed down the medulla, which then guides reamers. These enlarge or make uniform the canal until finally the nail itself can be introduced. Nails can be placed with or without reaming and much (probably too much) has been made of the comparison. Table 27.8 summarises this debate.

Because standard nails are introduced at the ends of a bone they are not suitable for the growing bone where they would transgress a growth plate. Elastic nails have been developed that can be placed without disrupting the physis. By using opposing pre-bent elastic nails, sufficient stability can be gained to control a paediatric fracture. They have revolutionised the treatment of children's femoral fractures in the same way that standard nails have for adult fractures. They allow for early mobilisation and a much earlier discharge from hospital.

The advantages and disadvantages of intramedullary nailing are described in Table 27.9.

External fixation

External fixation is a mechanical construction to hold a fracture. Each side of the fracture is coupled to the fixator and the major part of the device is external to the skin. The couple to the bone is via either half-pins (that is stiff metal rods typically 5–6 mm in diameter) or tensioned wires (typically 1.8 mm in diameter), which are then secured to the frame by clamps.

A great advantage of external fixation is that the immediate environment of the fracture may be left intact with the frame bridging the zone of injury (Table 27.10). This facility to bridge an injured area is commonly used as a temporary measure. For a complex fracture this can provide safe stability while the condition of the soft tissue improves or further imaging is obtained, or the patient's general condition improves before other definitive fixation. When used for definitive treatment external fixation also has the advantage over internal fixation in that the mechanical properties of the frame can be adjusted to suit the changing mechanical needs of the healing bone. This concept is most simply applied when a frame is destabilised as a fracture heals so that progressively more load is taken through the bone. It may be that the fracture is thought to require more stability in which case the frame may be adjusted to apply continuous compression. The mechanical environment may be manipulated in more complex ways. Callus may be distracted to allow for correction of a deformity, lengthening of a limb or transport of a bone segment to fill a defect. These advanced uses of external fixation were to a large extent developed by Ilizarov using tensioned wire circular frames.

The prime disadvantage is that an external fixator always has 'pin sites', i.e. the point where the pins or wires penetrate the skin. The pin sites require care as they may become infected or tether soft tissues, thereby interfering with function, and may generally irritate the patient. An infected pin site may compromise a later planned change to another technique for definitive fixation; however, it is usually safe to leave a frame in place for up to 10 days. A poorly placed temporary fixator may compromise the later definitive treatment and so a plan is always helpful.

Specific indications for external fixators include:

- emergency stabilisation of a long bone fracture in the polytrauma patient thought too unwell to have other interventions – 'damage control orthopaedics';
- stabilisation of a dislocated joint after reduction, e.g. a spanning fixator across the knee joint while the vascular surgeons repair an arterial injury with a knee dislocation;
- complex periarticular fractures – temporary stabilisation to allow the soft tissues to settle before definitive fixation, e.g. a distal tibial (pilon) fracture;
- fractures associated with infection;
- treating fractures with a bone loss.

Table 27.8 A comparison of reamed vs. unreamed nailing (an assumption is that nails used unreamed are usually thinner than those used reamed)

	Reamed IMN	Unreamed IMN
Insertion time	Longer	Quicker
Time to union	Shorter	Longer
Size of implant	Larger	Smaller
Reduction of distal fractures	Easier	More difficult
Strength of construct	More	Less

IMN, intramedullary nail.

Table 27.9 Advantages and disadvantages of intramedullary nailing

Advantages	Minimally invasive
	Early weight-bearing
	Less periosteal damage than open reduction and internal fixation
	Seldom need removal
Disadvantages	Increased risk of fat emboli/chest complications
	Infection difficult to treat
	Difficult to remove if broken

Table 27.10 Advantages and disadvantages of external fixation

Advantages	No interference with fracture site
	Adjustable after application: alignment; biomechanics
	Soft tissues accessible for plastic surgery
	Rapid stabilisation of fracture
	Hardware easy to remove
Disadvantages	Pin site infection
	Interferes with plastic surgical procedures
	Soft-tissue tethering
	Cumbersome for the patient

Gavriil Abramovich Ilizarov, **1921–1993, Orthopaedic Surgeon, Kurgan, Western Siberia, Russia.**

Wires

A Kirschner wire (also called a K-wire) is a thin, flexible wire made of stainless steel, available in various diameters. The wires can be smooth or threaded (the latter are used in situations in which backing out of the pin is undesirable). They have multiple uses as shown in Table 27.11. Transfixing wires can be passed percutaneously to keep fracture fragments reduced. They are cheap and often quick and simple to use. They have been used extensively around the hand and wrist as definitive fixation. Another common use of wires is for temporary fixation intraoperatively. Thus, a provisional reduction can be held with wires while the more definitive and robust fixation is applied.

Flexible wires are also used in fracture fixation. In situations in which the mechanical loads on the fracture are predictable a technique called tension band wiring is popular. Thus, at the patella and the olecranon a 'figure-of-eight' tension band wire can provide reliable stability. This is a dynamic fixation such that, when a predictable load is applied to the bone, compression across the fracture site is actually increased.

Complications of K-wires are pin track infection, wire breakage, loss of fixation and migration of the wire. Migration of a wire is a potentially serious problem and, as a consequence, their use in some areas is ill-advised. K-wires placed around the clavicle have been known to migrate, penetrating the thoracic cavity and even the heart.

Arthroplasty

Arthroplasty surgery for degenerative change has the objective of relieving pain and restoring function. Similar objectives apply in the treatment of the injured. It is thus strange that replacing the damaged surfaces of a joint is seen by some as a failure of fracture surgery. This is quite illogical as there are clearly situations when this is the best treatment. Prosthetic replacements, manufactured from metal alloys, may be used for treating articular fractures affecting a variety of joints. The implants used can be seen in Chapters 31–38 on elective orthopaedics, in which joint replacement is a mainstay of treatment. The indications in trauma may be fracture or patient related. In general, the problems of late loosening or wear mean that their use is confined to the older patient. The principles are discussed in the section on hip fractures (intracapsular fractures), but replacement surgery can be indicated in proximal humeral, elbow and occasionally knee injuries. In the proximal humerus, a multi-fragmentary fracture that is considered unsalvageable by internal fixation methods can be treated with a shoulder hemiarthroplasty.

The advantages of prosthetic replacement over internal fixation are earlier full weight-bearing and the elimination of non-union, avascular necrosis and failure of fixation. The disadvantages include a more extensive procedure, increased blood loss and the risk of prosthetic dislocation.

Table 27.11 Indications for K-wire insertion

Temporary fixation
Definitive fixation – with small fracture fragments (e.g. wrist fractures and hand injuries)
Tension band wiring (fractures of the patella and olecranon)
Temporary immobilisation of a small joint

Martin Kirschner, **1879–1942, Professor of Surgery, Heidelberg, Germany, introduced the use of skeletal traction wires in 1909.**

MANAGEMENT BY TYPE AND REGION

Having discussed the principles of assessment and the principles of the available treatments for extremity injury the two can now be amalgamated. The motive for treatment is to restore function, to reduce the area on the graph between the curve of the natural history of the injury and that of the uninjured person. The AO classification distinguishes between diaphyseal and metaphyseal fractures and they are approached differently. Many fractures can be managed without operation. Table 27.12 gives some of the general indications for operative stabilisation. Two simple questions to ask of a fracture are: 'Does it need to be reduced?' and 'Does it need to be held?'

Diaphyseal fractures

The diaphysis is composed predominantly of a tube of dense cortical bone. Fracture treatment is aimed at restoring function by achieving bony union with correction of the length, alignment and rotation. In many diaphyseal fractures, if the bone heals with the adjacent joints in their normal relationship, the anatomical reduction of the fracture fragments at the fracture site is of secondary importance. This is demonstrated in Fig. 27.13 which shows C-type fractures treated in this way.

Femoral shaft fractures

The anatomy of the proximal femur allows easy access to the medullary canal for inserting an intramedullary device nail. A statically locked intramedullary nail is suitable for the vast majority of adult femoral shaft fractures irrespective of their pattern. With an isolated femoral shaft fracture the patient can be expected to mobilise rapidly postoperatively and may only be hospitalised for a few days.

Traction was traditionally used as definitive treatment for these fractures but it is now most commonly used as a first aid measure to provide pain relief and maintain length while transferring a patient or before operative fixation. Both methods of treatment can have satisfactory outcomes but the earlier return to function favours surgery.

Tibial shaft fractures

When the fracture is sufficiently stable, generally an A-type pattern, casting is the safest and cheapest choice. A full-leg cast is

Table 27.12 Indications for surgery in limb trauma (the main indication is that operation will produce a better outcome; the principles are given below)

A fracture requiring treatment that is unsuitable for non-operative measures
Open fractures
Failed non-operative management
Multiple injuries
Pathological or impending pathological fractures
Displaced intra-articular fractures
Fractures through the growth plate, where arrest is possible (Salter–Harris type III–V)
Avulsion fractures that compromise the functional integrity of a ligament/tendon around a joint (e.g. olecranon fracture)
Established non-unions or malunions

CHAPTER 27 | EXTREMITY TRAUMA

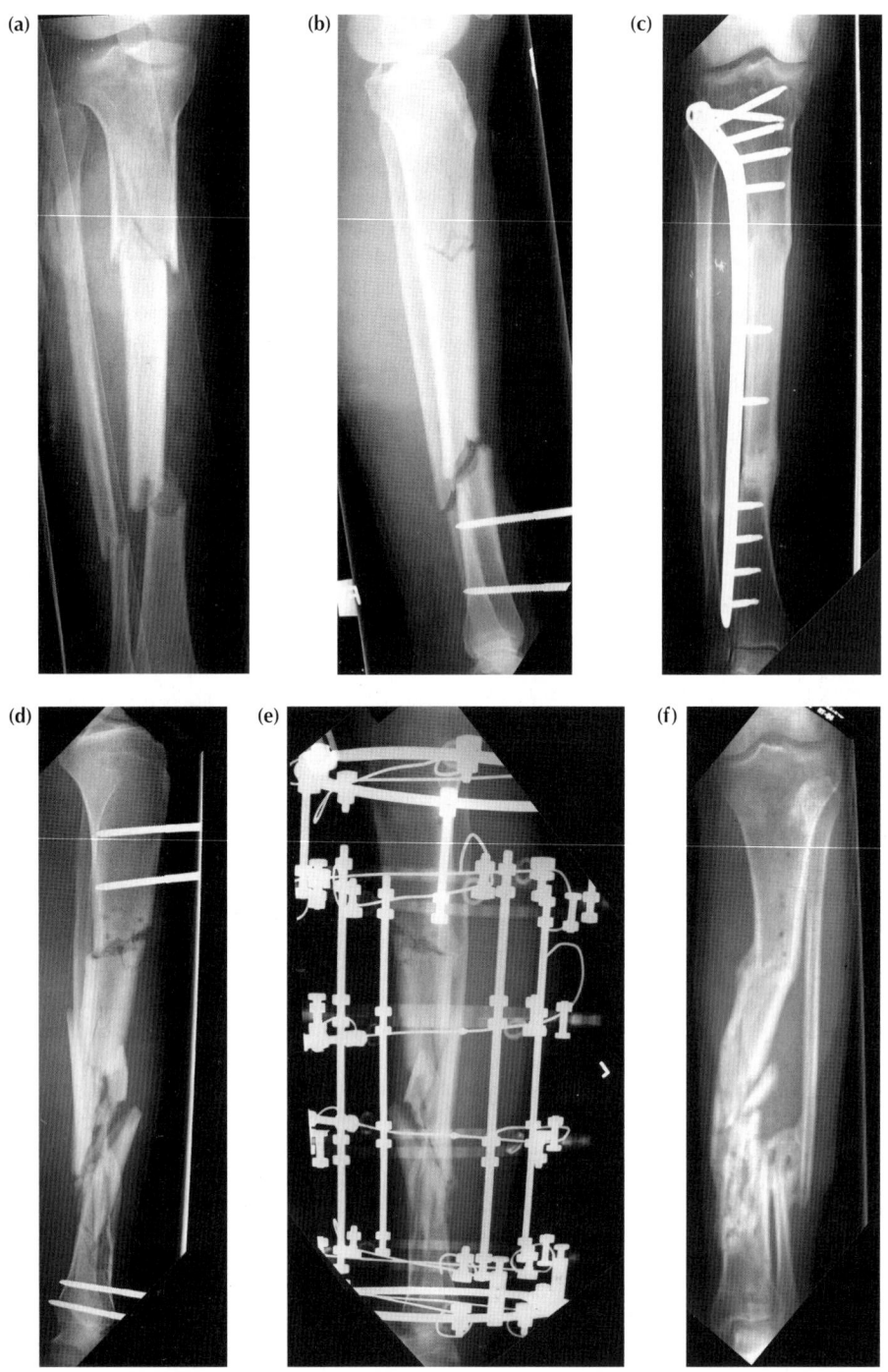

Figure 27.13 (a) and (d) are C-type or segmental tibial fractures. Each was a high-energy injury. (b) and (e) show a temporary spanning external fixator applied in each case. (c) and (f) show definitive relative stability was achieved with different methods of bridging fixation. Healing was by indirect means in both cases. Despite irregularities at the fracture sites the overall position was satisfactory and function was good.

applied and split to the skin. Once the risk of compartment syndrome has passed the cast is completed. By 4 weeks it can generally be changed to a moulded, patella tendon-bearing, below-knee cast. This allows the knee to move. Cast treatment requires frequent and careful monitoring and there should be no hesitation in changing the cast should the reduction be deteriorating. To correct minor deformity in a controlled and comfortable manner the cast may be wedged.

Surgery to a tibial shaft fracture is often indicated either as a result of instability (B- or C-type fractures) or other injuries. Currently, when surgery is required, intramedullary nailing is the most frequent choice. There is a high incidence of anterior knee pain following this and so it should be used with caution in those patients who have to kneel. Malunion is common in nailed fractures of the proximal tibial shaft; thus, plating fractures closer to the metaphysis is a good option, provided that the soft tissues are satisfactory. External fixation remains a good option for a wide range of shaft fractures. The subcutaneous position of the tibia makes pin placement and pin site care relatively straightforward. The tibia is the most common of the major bones to be involved in an open fracture. When soft-tissue procedures will be necessary, intramedullary nailing gives the plastic surgeons the best access for soft-tissue reconstruction and is generally the stabilisation method of choice.

Humeral shaft fractures

In humeral shaft fractures the maintenance of limb length and alignment is nowhere near as important as in the leg. The majority of humeral shaft fractures can be treated non-operatively with a simple protective functional brace and a collar and cuff. This is the safest and cheapest option. The indications for operative management include an open fracture, the presence of other injuries such as head injury, multiple injuries, ipsilateral arm fractures and failed non-operative management. In these circumstances, fixation and stability can be achieved by either plating or intramedullary nailing. The rate of non-union is significantly higher when nailing the humerus than when nailing the femur or tibia; thus, plating is generally the treatment of choice. Figure 27.14 shows a plated B-type diaphyseal fracture. Should the need for fixation be combined with signs of radial

nerve damage, plating has the advantage of allowing exploration of the nerve.

Radius and ulna

Although the radius and ulna appear outwardly similar to other long bones, they can best be visualised as the two components of a large joint. Their relationship requires precise anatomical restoration if they are to function normally in supination and pronation. This precision is best and most easily achieved by open reduction and plate fixation (Summary box 27.6).

> **Summary box 27.6**
>
> **Diaphyseal fractures**
>
> - Restore length, alignment and rotation
> - Consider whether primary or secondary bone healing is the objective
> - Radius and ulna need precise reduction to function

Metaphyseal fractures

Fractures in the metaphyseal region are classified as A type if they are extra-articular, B type if they are partial articular and C type if they are complete articular.

In an A-type fracture the joint surfaces remains intact so congruity is not an issue. Therefore, the problem may be thought of as being similar to that of treating a diaphyseal fracture; however, there are two differences that need attention. First, the injury and the subsequent treatment, being close to a joint, are more liable to cause joint stiffness. Second, the bone on either side of the fracture is not of a similar type or quality. It is generally easier to obtain a mechanical hold on the diaphyseal bone of the shaft than on the spongy bone of the metaphysis; thus the quality of fixation may be imbalanced. This imbalance in fixation is even more apparent when dealing with osteoporotic bone.

With B- and C-type fractures the joint surfaces themselves are involved. Thus, in addition to providing stability and overall alignment, the congruity of the joint surface is also important.

The management of metaphyseal injuries to the distal humerus, distal radius, distal femur, proximal tibia and distal tibia is very similar and is principle based with some regional influences. The main difference between the various sites is the scale of the metalware employed.

In an A-type metaphyseal fracture the emphasis is on maintaining length, alignment and rotation while allowing continued function. This requires sound fixation as demonstrated in Fig. 27.15. In this instance the fixation has been achieved with a plate and screws but it could equally have been carried out with an external fixator.

In a B-type partial articular fracture joint congruity is the prime objective. This can often be maintained with relatively lightweight fixation as the load borne by the metalware itself is less (Fig. 27.16). B-type fractures when they require surgery are nearly always treated with screws, or screws and plates.

The C-type or complete articular fracture combines both of these features, having the need for joint congruity and alignment, and is demonstrated in the tibial plateau in Fig. 27.17. The articular component of the fracture is generally held with screws, allowing for interfragmental compression. The metaphyseal component of the fracture may be held as in the A-type fracture, with plates and screws or an external fixator.

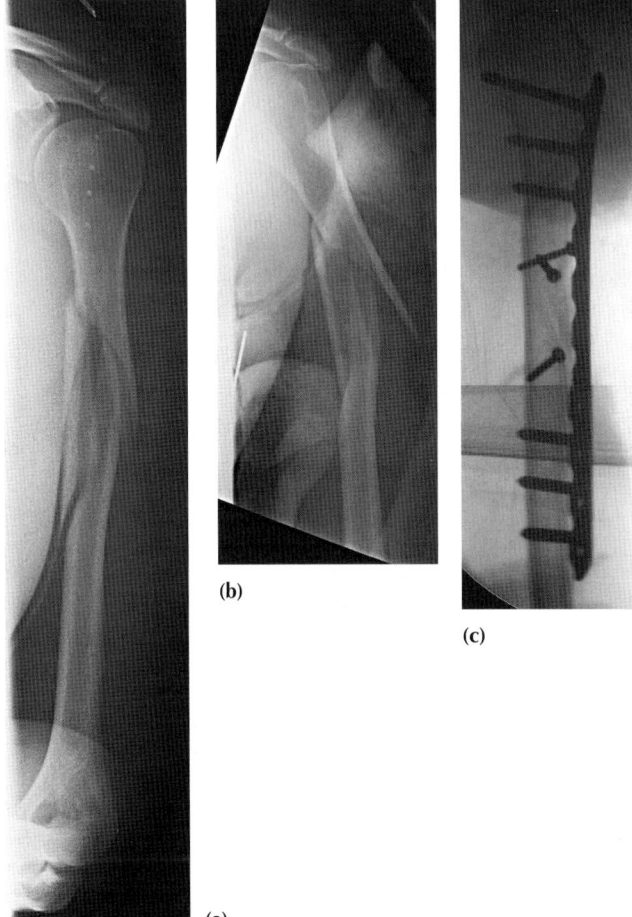

(b)

(c)

(a)

Figure 27.14 A B-type humeral shaft fracture. This fracture could not be controlled by non-operative means and was treated with lag screws protected by a plate.

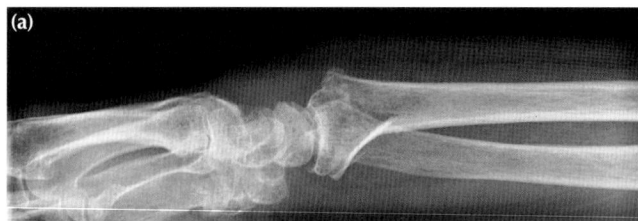

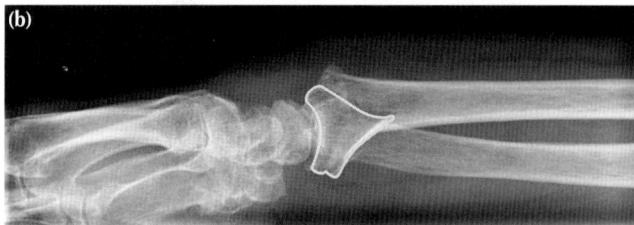

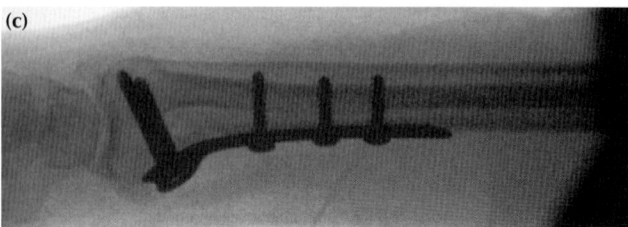

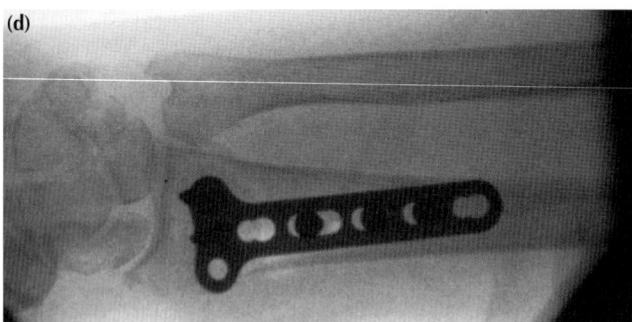

Figure 27.15 An A-type or extra-articular metaphyseal fracture. A plain lateral radiograph of this Smith-type fracture (a and b). Fracture fixed to a plate. There is *no* interfragmental compression. The plate is pushing against or buttressing the distal fragment (c and d).

Achieving the final definitive fixation for an articular fracture may be the final step in the procedure. A good example is a pilon fracture. The soft tissue surrounding the ankle is particularly vulnerable following injury. It is therefore common practice to place a spanning external fixator across the joint until such time as appropriate investigations are available and the soft tissues are ready for definitive surgery.

Distal radial fractures

Because of the frequency of their occurrence distal radial fractures deserve separate mention. The common fractures in this area are A type, i.e. extra-articular. The Colles' fracture with dorsal and radial angulation can generally be treated by manipulation and casting. When this does not provide sufficient stability

a useful technique to have available is intrafocal wiring, popularised by Kapandji. In this technique, the wires are placed through the fracture site, then angled to stabilise the distal fragment and secured through the opposite cortex of the proximal fragment (Fig. 27.18).

When the displacement is in the opposite direction, i.e. volar, the so called Smith's fracture stability is difficult to achieve by casting. Access for wiring is awkward and so plating is generally employed.

The management of intra-articular distal radial fractures, particularly in the young adult, is evolving rapidly. The advent of CT has allowed for a better understanding of the patterns of injury. When there is significant articular displacement, formal open reduction and fixation with plates and screws is being performed in a very similar fashion to dealing with a tibial plateau fracture but with smaller implants. Customised locking plates are being used more frequently. Despite the popularity of these approaches the strength of the supporting evidence is not great.

Ankle fractures

The eventual functional outcome of ankle fractures depends upon the position of union. Thus, if the fracture is stable it requires only symptomatic treatment. An unstable ankle fracture requires reduction and maintenance of reduction until bony union. This can be achieved operatively or non-operatively. The important step is therefore to assess the stability. This may be inferred by the clinical history (a dislocated ankle) or the pattern of bony injury (e.g. both medial and lateral bony injury) or it may be assessed directly by an examination under anaesthesia. The maintenance of reduction is more reliable with operation and so in the younger patient this is generally the preferred option. In the elderly there is no clear evidence for choosing between operative and non-operative management.

Managing fractures in the skeletally immature

Many injuries are dealt with in an analogous way in the child and the adult; however, there are naturally differences. As discussed in Chapter 21 there needs to be constant vigilance for evidence of non-accidental injury.

Children's fractures heal more rapidly than adults'. The acceptable reduction may differ because of the extent of remodelling that is possible. This remodelling potential is dependent upon the growth remaining and the location of the fracture. The nearer the fracture is to the growth plate, the greater the remodelling capacity. Deformity is more acceptable in the plane of motion of the adjacent joint. Remodelling is greatest at the ends of the bone that contribute most to longitudinal growth. For example, fractures at the distal femur have more potential to remodel than proximal femoral fractures. Significant remodelling is also expected at the proximal humerus (70% of longitudinal growth). Children younger than 10 years of age have a greater potential capacity to remodel than children older than 10 years of age.

Repeated attempts to reduce a physeal fracture may injure the physis leading to growth arrest. Internal fixation should not cross the physis. When this is absolutely necessary, the smallest and smoothest pin should be used.

Trauma is the commonest cause of physeal arrest, and occurs

Abraham Colles, 1773–1843, Professor of Surgery, The Royal College of Surgeons in Ireland, and Surgeon, Dr. Steven's Hospital, Dublin, Ireland.

Robert William Smith, 1807–1873, Professor of Surgery, Trinity College, Dublin, Ireland, described the reverse Colles' fracture in 1847.

(a)

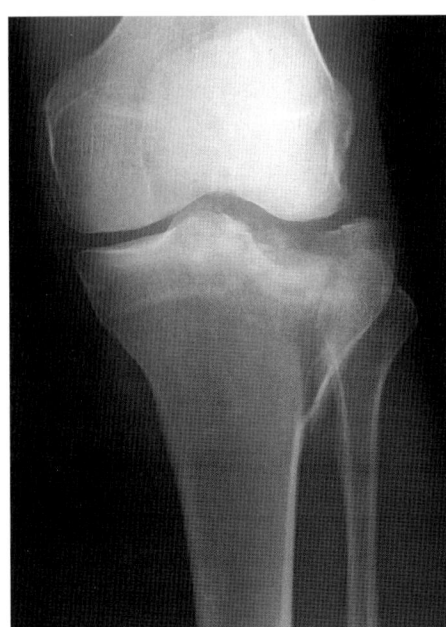

(b)

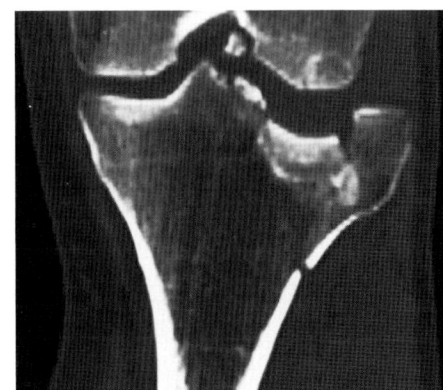

(c)

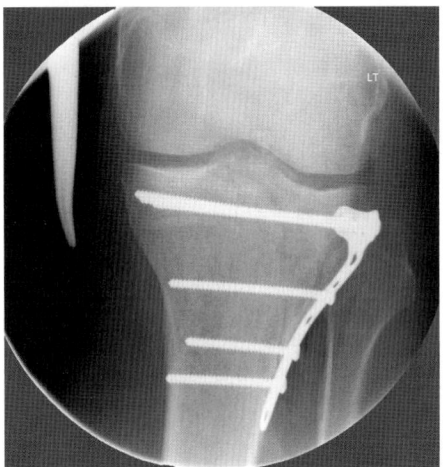

Figure 27.16 A B-type or partial articular fracture. (a) Plain radiograph; (b) computerised tomography clarifies the injury; (c) fixation with plate and screws achieving compression across a previously reduced fracture.

when a bony bridge forms between the metaphysis and epiphysis. Complete arrest is most commonly seen after a crush injury to the growth plate (Salter–Harris type V). The commonest area for growth arrest is the distal femur, proximal and distal tibia and the distal radius. Injured physeal plates tend to close prematurely before the normal contralateral side, despite the successful restoration of growth.

The thicker and stronger periosteum contributes both to fracture stability and to fracture reduction if some of it (known as the 'periosteal hinge') remains intact on the compression side of the fracture. The physis is weaker than bone in torsion, shear and bending, and so fractures easily.

Children rarely experience non-union and frequently heal their fractures more rapidly than adults. In general, the rate of healing is inversely proportional to age.

Complications unique to childhood include growth arrest, progressive angular or rotational deformity and overgrowth of a long bone (post-femoral fracture).

The indications for operative intervention are fewer in children than adults (see Pathological failure, p. 376; Fig. 27.27c). The generally benign natural history of children's fractures means that the risk of complications often does not balance favourably against a small potential advantage.

Specific injuries

Distal radial fracture

The commonest area of fracture in children is the distal radius. Fractures proximal to the growth plate may be treated

symptomatically or by manipulation under anaesthesia (MUA). There is no clear rule as to the amount of deformity that can be accepted. Clinically obvious deformity should probably be corrected at any age; otherwise, a maximum radiological deformity of 20° is acceptable in the plane of movement of the adjacent joint. As puberty approaches, fractures should be treated as for the adult.

A special case is when the distal radial fracture is sufficiently displaced to require manipulation that the ulna itself is intact. Secondary redisplacement is common under these circumstances and it is advisable to hold the radius with primary K-wiring. When the growth plate is involved in a distal radial fracture it is generally a Salter–Harris type I or II injury. MUA and casting is usually adequate and growth disturbance is uncommon after primary treatment; however, should the fracture reduction be lost, one should seldom proceed to a second manipulation. The second manipulation is much more likely to cause damage to the physis and subsequent growth problems.

Distal humeral (supracondylar) fracture

The markedly displaced supracondylar fracture is associated with two main complications. Neurovascular compromise may arise early and residual deformity is a late complication. The treatment of the former is early reduction, as the bone spike protruding from the proximal fragment may actually be pressing on the structures. Should the problem be with the circulation it will generally be resolved once reduction is carried out. Even when the brachial artery itself is involved there is usually adequate distal flow from

(a)

(b)

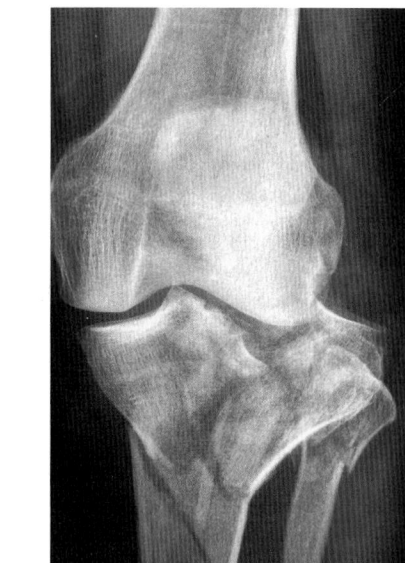

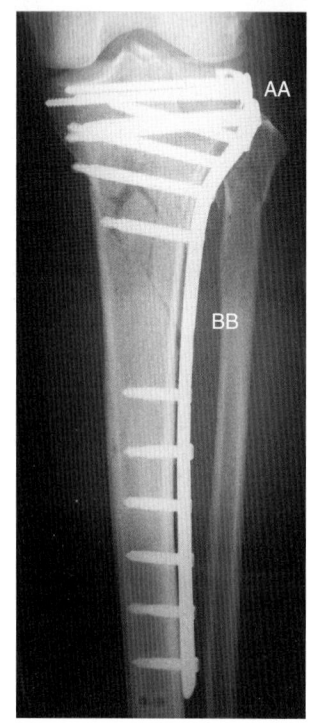

Figure 27.17 (a) A C-type proximal tibial articular fracture, i.e. none of the joint remains attached to the diaphysis. (b) The small plate and screws (AA) are used to compress the joint fragments, aiming for absolute stability. The heavy duty fixed angled device (BB) spans the fracture and provides relative stability.

the collateral vessels provided as a sonata me is carried out. Arterial repair is seldom necessary.

The late complication of a supracondylar fracture is deformity. This is due not to an interference with growth (the fracture is proximal to the growth plate) but to poor initial reduction or loss of reduction. As noted above, deformity in the plane of the adjacent joint tends to correct satisfactorily. It is the varus/valgus angulatory deformity that is critical at the elbow. This is very difficult to assess initially as the deformity only

(a)

(b)

(c)

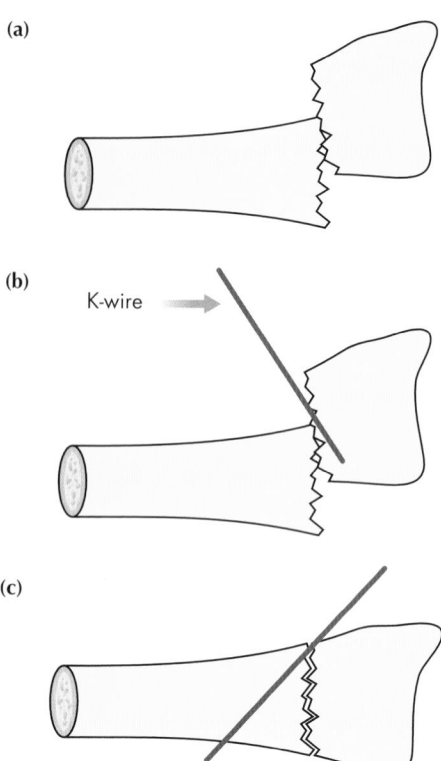

Figure 27.18 (a) A displaced distal radial fracture. (b) A wire is introduced percutaneously by hand through the fracture site. (c) The fracture is manipulated into a reduced position (*not* levered using the wire). Once reduced the wire is advanced under power into the opposite cortex, securing the reduction.

becomes obvious once full extension is regained, which may be many months later.

A minimally displaced supracondylar fracture is a benign injury and can be treated symptomatically. When a displaced fracture can be manipulated into a satisfactory position it sometimes appears stable as soon as the elbow is put in flexion. It is tempting to leave this injury in a flexed cast for stability. The authors' opinion is that if a supracondylar fracture needs to be reduced it should then be held with K-wires.

Lateral condylar mass fracture

This injury is easily missed and is an example of the apparently benign injury that may have significant morbidity if it goes unrecognised. Clinically the clue is localised lateral tenderness. The radiograph may show just a flake off the distal humeral metaphysis above the capitellum (Fig. 27.19). This is an intra-articular fracture that crosses the growth plate. If it is displaced or unstable it should be primarily fixed. A injury of this nature that is missed can progress to non-union or malunion with growth arrest, or, if an attempt is made to reduce the fracture late under direct vision, it may develop avascular necrosis.

Slipped upper femoral epiphysis

This injury is readily missed. A painful hip in a child approaching puberty should arouse suspicion. The injury can be diagnosed on plain radiography as seen in Fig. 27.20. When treated in its early stages the outcome is excellent; if it progresses to a more severe slip then the outcome is poor.

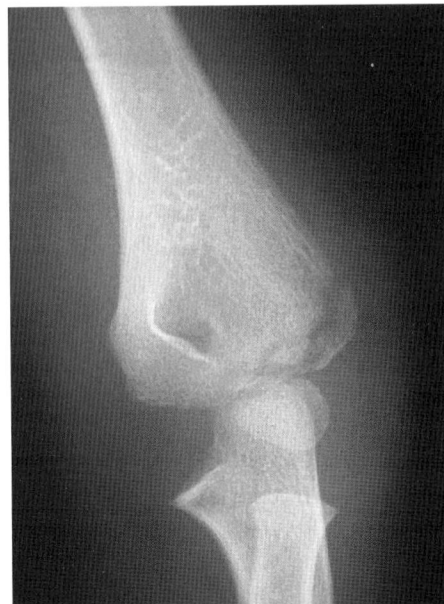

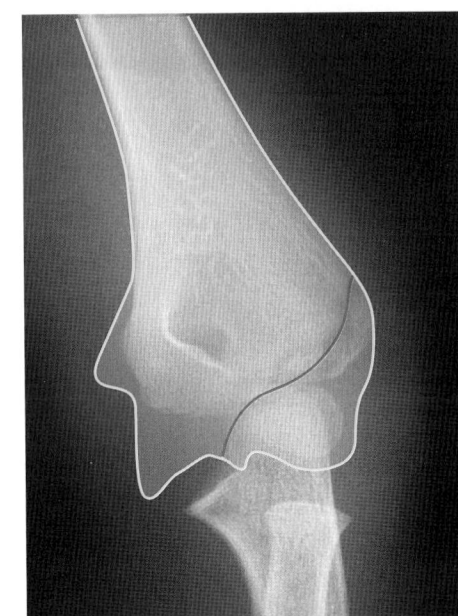

Figure 27.19 Lateral condylar mass fracture. (a) Plain radiograph showing the metaphyseal fracture. (b) The yellow shows the shape of the distal humerus including the cartilaginous analogue, and the red shows the true extent of the injury, i.e. a significant intra-articular fracture.

Femoral shaft fracture

The management of femoral shaft fractures in children is evolving in a similar way to how the management of the adult fracture evolved, albeit 20 years later. These fractures can be managed with traction and the shorter time to union makes this more acceptable. Until recently, unless there was another indication for surgical fixation such as a head injury or other long bone fracture, most were managed non-operatively; now, only in the very young is this the case. With children under 12–15 kg, simple gallows traction is appropriate. Here the legs are suspended vertically with the buttocks just off the bed. This maintains an adequate position and nappy changes are straightforward. With older

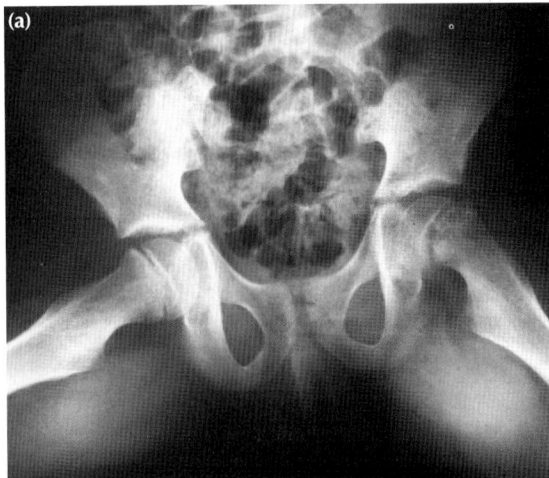

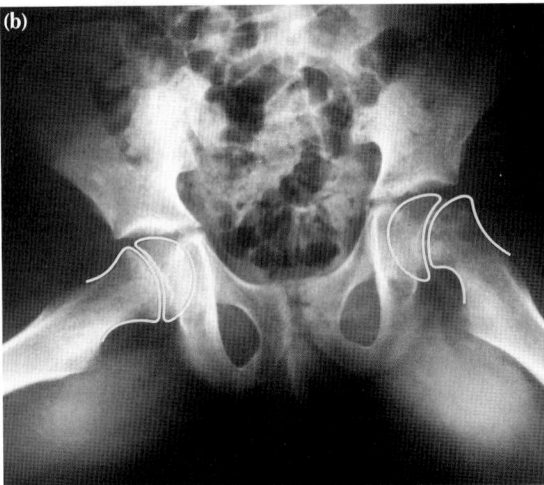

Figure 27.20 Slipped left upper femoral epiphysis. (a) Plain radiograph; (b) the injury highlighted.

children, as the necessary period of traction increases, so does the tendency for operative fixation. Standard intramedullary nailing poses a risk to the proximal growth plate and should be avoided in girls below 12 years and boys below 14 years. As previously mentioned, flexible intramedullary nails may be placed to avoid the growth plate (Fig. 27.21).

Tibial shaft fracture

In a child with an unstable tibial fracture that is not amenable to cast management, external fixation, elastic nailing and plating are all reasonable options (Summary box 27.7).

Summary box 27.7

Fractures in the skeletally immature

- Do not forget non-accidental injury
- Be reluctant to re-manipulate a physeal injury
- Elastic nails are a significant step forward in fracture treatment in children
- Not many fractures require operative intervention in children

CHAPTER 27 | EXTREMITY TRAUMA

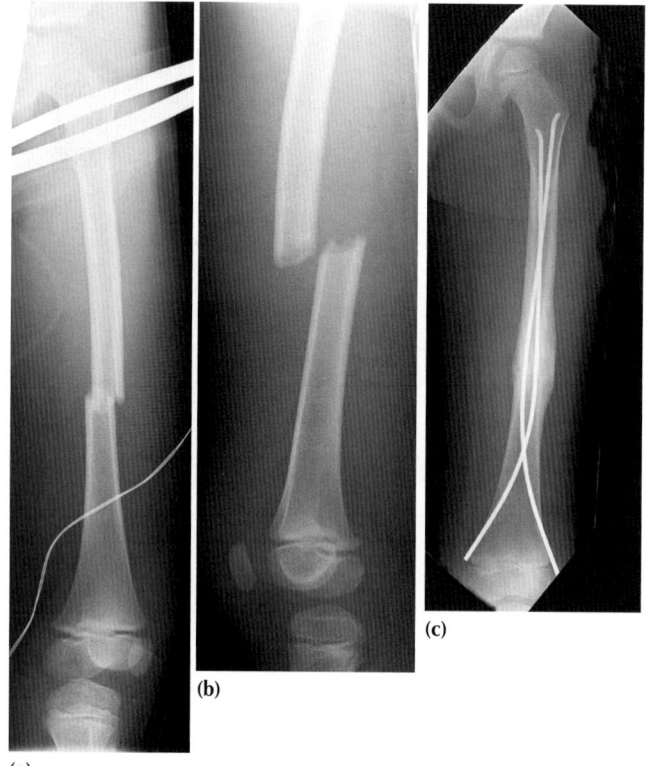

(a)

Figure 27.21 Femoral shaft fracture in a child, which has been stabilised with elastic nails.

Osteoporotic fractures

In osteoporosis there is a decrease in bone mass and strength. Eventually, a relatively minor strain can cause a fracture (fragility fracture). These fractures, occurring mainly in the elderly, constitute the bulk of the orthopaedic trauma workload of a UK hospital. They can sometimes be treated in just the same way as injuries in younger stronger bone. However, there are other considerations. The elderly have less capacity to tolerate an injured limb and, thus, it is often not possible for them to partially weight-bear. Therefore, if treatment is to allow them to function, fixation must be able to tolerate full weight-bearing. If this cannot be achieved then it is frequently necessary for the patient to have a prolonged period of hospitalisation. For general management it is important to follow local guidelines for osteoporosis management and falls prevention.

Internal fixation in osteoporotic bone remains a challenge. The hold of screws inserted into the bone is often suboptimal. This leads to 'backing out' of the screws and subsequent loss of fracture reduction. Locking plates may help to overcome this problem. In a locking plate and construction the integrity of the structure depends upon the tightness of the screw in the plate rather than the tightness of the screw in the bone (Fig. 27.22b).

The need for early restoration of function would seem to guide the surgeon towards more intervention. However, this has to be balanced against the poorer quality of the soft tissues and, therefore, the greater likelihood of wound problems. However, on balance, the treatment of fractures in the elderly is generally more aggressive to try to achieve earlier function as depicted in the outcome curves discussed earlier.

(a)

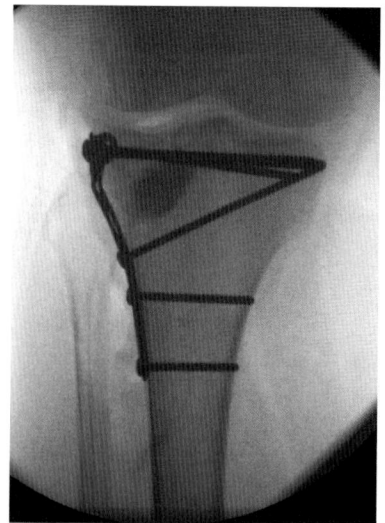

(b)

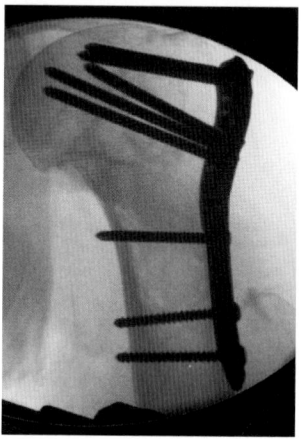

Figure 27.22 Variations in fixation technique suited to osteoporotic bone. (a) Norian bone substitute has been injected to support the lateral tibial plateau in the partial articular fracture. (b) A locking plate in a proximal humerus. The screws are threaded into the plate to make a fixed-angle device.

Intra-articular fractures

It is not always necessary to obtain a perfect anatomical reduction of an intra-articular fracture in an elderly osteoporotic patient, and it is even more difficult to hold it. The long-term complication of degenerative change is of relatively less importance in the elderly. Thus, in dealing with a tibial plateau fracture in an older person the object of operative fixation is different from that in the younger person – it is primarily stability and not congruity that is required. The first stage of an operation to treat a tibial plateau fracture in the elderly is an examination under anaesthesia. If the joint is stable then there is no indication for operative treatment. When operation is required it can be helpful to augment the bone. Figure 27.23a shows a case in which the bone substitute Norian has been used to help support the reduced joint surface.

Proximal femoral fractures

Proximal femoral fractures fall into two groups: extracapsular and intracapsular. The blood supply to the femoral head and neck travels down through the hip capsule and then back up the femoral neck. Fractures of the femoral neck inside the capsule

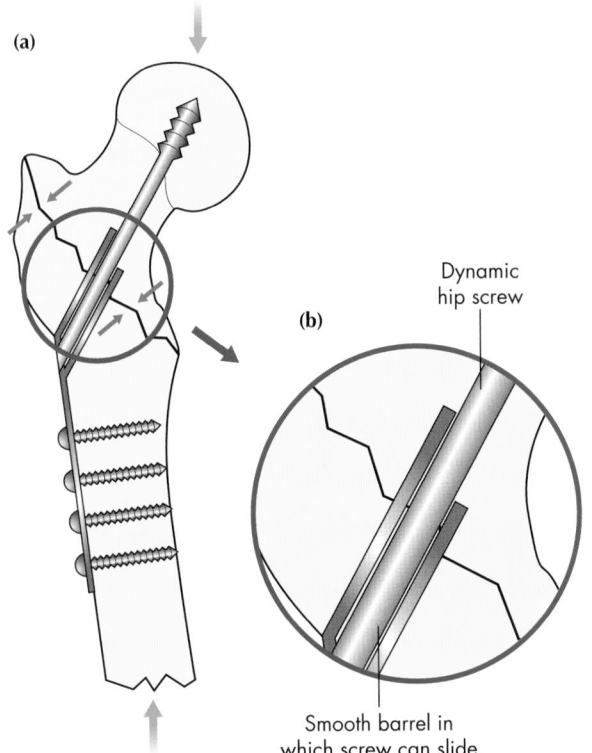

(a)

(b)

Dynamic hip screw

Smooth barrel in which screw can slide

Figure 27.23 (a) A dynamic hip screw for fixing a trochanteric proximal femoral fracture. This allows for compression at the fracture site on load-bearing and protects the femoral head from penetration by the screw when the osteoporotic bone settles. (b) Insert to show the sliding screw in the barrel.

(intracapsular or subcapital) are liable to sever the blood supply to the head of the femur and so need to be treated differently to those outside the capsule.

Extracapsular fracture

Biological fixation principles are used to fix this type of fracture. Indirect reduction using a traction table is followed by fixation with a dynamic hip screw (DHS) placed using an image intensifier. The dynamic nature of the implant allows the fragments to impact together when the patient walks, as shown in Fig. 27.23. This stimulates healing while improving stability and protects the femoral head from penetration by the implant.

Intracapsular fracture

Most patients presenting with an intracapsular (subcapital) fractured neck of femur are elderly and osteoporotic. Early mobilisation offers their best chance of sustaining such independence as they have. If the fracture has displaced, then the probability is that fixation of the articular fragment will be tenuous and prone to failure, coupled with the knowledge that the femoral head may have lost its blood supply. An elderly patient will have difficulty protecting a delicate fixation. Therefore, often the treatment of choice is to simply replace the compromised femoral head with an artificial head (a hemi-arthroplasty). This treatment is not ideal in younger patients, but what then what constitutes a 'younger' patient is open to debate. The alternatives for the younger patient are:
(a) to make an attempt to reduce and fix the fracture generally holding it reduced with screws placed under image intensifier

control, in the knowledge that a proportion of these fixations will fail but that if successful the patient has their own hip.
Or:
(b) to perform a total hip replacement, which is mechanically sounder but a more extensive procedure and more expensive.

This question of fixing or replacing in relation to articular fractures has analogies in other joints (Summary box 27.8).

Summary box 27.8

Osteoporotic fractures

- Fragility fractures are the commonest cause of trauma admission
- The elderly do not tolerate immobility
- Fixation techniques are extended with fixed-angle devices and bone augmentation
- Manage osteoporosis
- Manage falls

Injuries to the foot and hand

Foot injuries

Severe injuries to the foot are surprisingly disabling. They have a greater tendency to impact on the ability to work than long bone fractures.

Foot injuries are frequently missed, especially in the polytrauma setting. Even when injury is suspected the clinical localisation of an injury and the interpretation of radiographs can be difficult.

Calcaneal fractures

The os calcis is the largest and most frequently fractured hindfoot bone. The commonest cause of injury is a fall from a height. Associated injuries include lumbar spine and lower extremity fractures, occurring in 10–20% of cases. Plain radiographs often do not demonstrate the scale of destruction and CT is necessary for evaluation. Figure 27.24 shows an intra-articular fracture of the os calcis. When accurate reduction and fixation is achievable it would seem to be beneficial. When a good reduction is not achievable the benefit of operation is less clear.

Talus fractures and dislocations

The talus consists of three parts (head, neck and body) and articulates superiorly with the distal tibia and inferiorly with the calcaneus and navicular. The talus has no muscular or tendinous attachments and therefore its blood supply is tenuous. The blood supply comes from two sources: extraosseous and intraosseous. Talar neck fractures are the commonest injury and are usually high energy (historically termed 'aviator's astragalus'). A significant complication is avascular necrosis of the talus. The goal of treatment is anatomical reduction and stable fixation, which helps reduce the risk of osteonecrosis. Hawkins' sign can be seen approximately 6–8 weeks after injury on plain radiographs. This appears as subchondral lucency of the talar dome, which signifies bony reabsorption, i.e. a viable bone.

Tarsometatarsal (Lisfranc) joint injuries

The tarsometatarsal joint is a very strong weight-bearing structure. It requires significant force to injure it. Poorly treated

Jacques Lisfranc de St. Martin, **1790–1847, Professor of Surgery and Operative Medicine, Paris, France.**

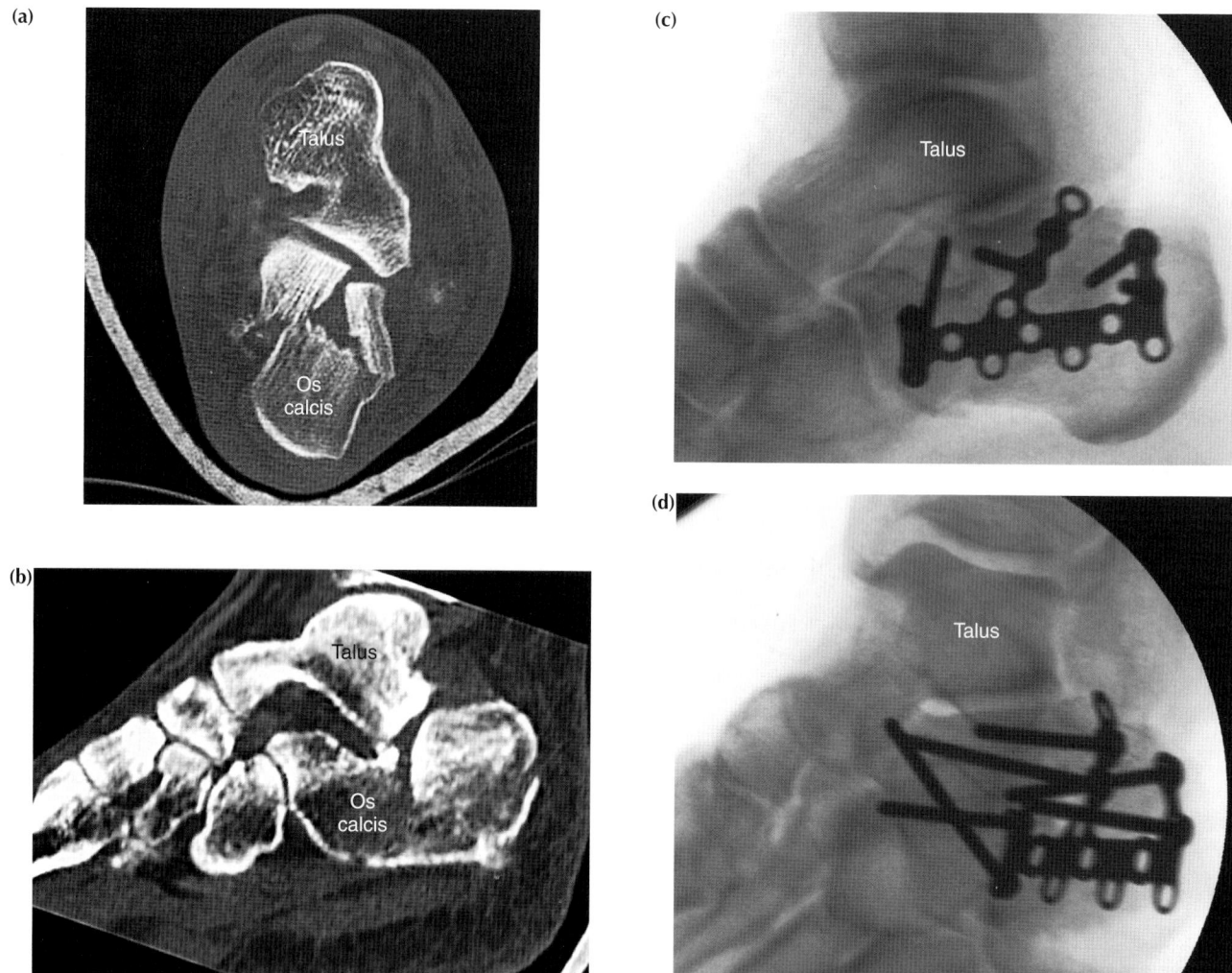

Figure 27.24 Axial (a) and sagittal (b) views of a displaced intra-articular fracture of the os calcis. (c and d) Intraoperative views of the reconstruction. Both the overall shape and the articular surface have been restored.

injuries of this joint can give rise to long-term debilitating symptoms. It is therefore surprising that these injuries are frequently missed. The key to diagnosis is careful localisation of symptoms and signs, which when looked for are usually significant. Once suspected the injury is then confirmed on plain radiography and delineated further with CT. The treatment of the displaced injury is open reduction and internal fixation.

Achilles tendon rupture

Up to 20% of these injuries are missed at initial presentation. The typical history of a sensation of being kicked behind the ankle whilst playing sport is frequently given. Sometimes there is a palpable gap. Simmonds' test – squeezing the calf to produce passive plantarflexion of the ankle – is usually positive. Many regimes for treatment exist. A logical progression is to confirm the diagnosis on ultrasound, proceeding to percutaneous repair of those tendons with a gap of > 5 mm in plantarflexion, and treating those with a smaller gap non-operatively.

Franklin Adin Simmonds, **1911–1983, Orthopaedic Surgeon, The Rowley Bristow Hospital, Pyrford, Surrey, England.**

Hand injuries

Some injuries to the hand are easily missed and are therefore worth discussing further.

Scaphoid fracture

The scaphoid is the most commonly injured carpal bone. The scaphoid is made up of the proximal and distal poles, a tubercle and the waist. The proximal pole is completely intra-articular and receives all of its blood supply from the distal branches of the radial artery. This enters the scaphoid in a retrograde fashion (distal to proximal). Therefore, fractures in the proximal pole are most at risk of non-union or avascular necrosis. In contrast, distal pole fractures tend to heal without problems. Figure 27.25 shows a scaphoid fracture and demonstrates how awkward it can be to make the diagnosis on standard anteroposterior and lateral views of the wrist.

The mechanism of injury is typically a fall onto the outstretched hand with the wrist in radial deviation and dorsiflexed. Fractures of the scaphoid waist occur most frequently. Examination usually reveals tenderness in the anatomical snuffbox. The suspected diagnosis is initially based on clinical findings. Plain radiographs may not show a fracture line for up to 10 days.

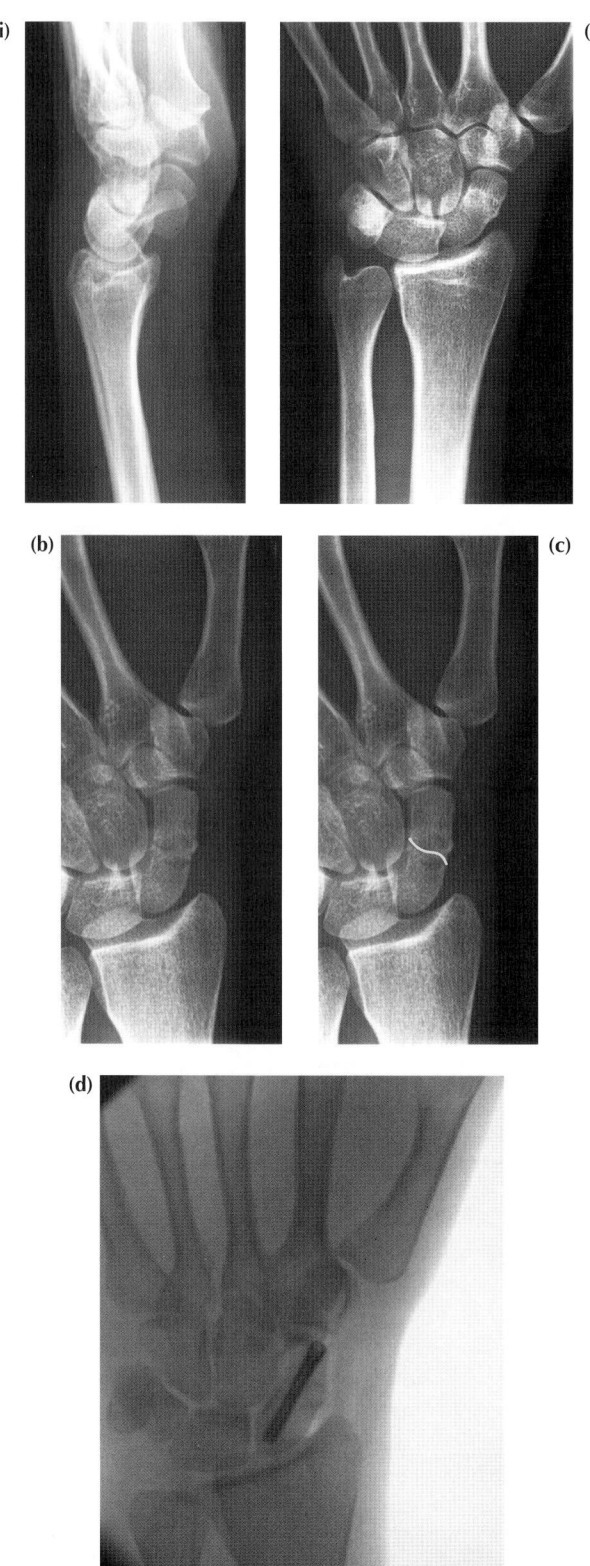

Therefore, a patient with an equivocal examination is treated in a cast. Immobilisation is implemented empirically to reduce the risk of non-union and subsequent avascular necrosis. A repeat clinical and radiographic assessment should be performed between 10 and 14 days post-injury. In the presence of a fracture line the cast is reapplied. If the radiographs are normal but clinical suspicion remains, further imaging using a bone scan or MRI scan can be helpful. Open reduction (using a compression screw) is required for unstable fractures (> 1 mm displacement or angulation). Complications of scaphoid fractures include non-union, avascular necrosis, malunion and carpal instability.

Lunate dislocation

The lunate forms a part of the proximal row of the carpus with the scaphoid and triquetrum. Articulating with the radius, this row forms the radiocarpal joint.

The lunate resides in the concavity of the lunate fossa of the distal radius. Interosseus ligaments hold it to the adjacent scaphoid and triquetrum.

Perilunate dislocations are often unrecognised. Clinical examination reveals significant swelling of the entire carpus. The diagnosis is made with plain radiographs (Fig. 27.26); the lateral view demonstrates the 'spilled tea cup sign' with volar tilt of the lunate. Acute injuries may be initially treated with closed reduction and casting. Irreducible or unstable injuries require open reduction and stabilisation with K-wires. Note that associated injuries such

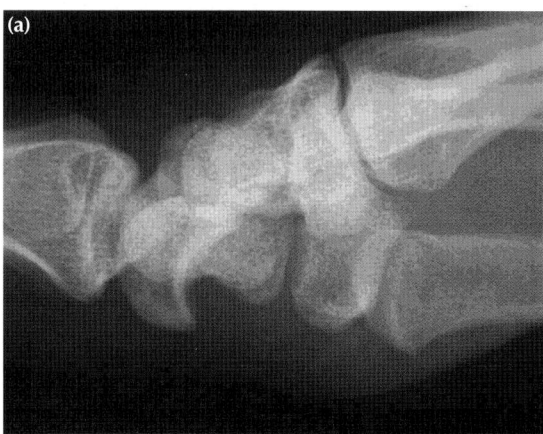

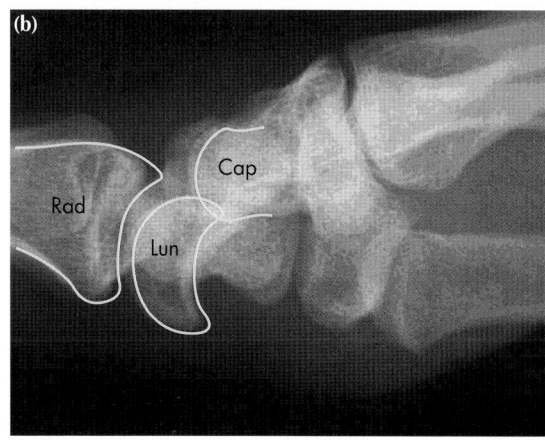

Figure 27.25 Scaphoid fracture. (a) Anteroposterior and lateral views in which the injury is difficult to see. (b and c) Oblique views with the fracture line highlighted. (d) In this case of a young patient the fracture was treated with early fixation.

Figure 27.26 Perilunate dislocation. (a) A plain lateral radiograph of the wrist. (b) The outline of the perilunate dislocation is highlighted. Cap, capitate; Lun, lunate; Rad, radius.

CHAPTER 27 | EXTREMITY TRAUMA

as scaphoid and radial styloid fractures, as well as median nerve injury, should be excluded.

Thumb metacarpophalangeal ulnar collateral ligament

The integrity of this ligament is important for effective lateral key pinch. Injury to the ulnar collateral ligament is commonly referred to as 'gamekeeper's thumb' or 'skier's thumb', and is caused by the thumb being forced laterally away from the rest of the hand. Tenderness is located on the ulnar aspect of the metacarpophalangeal joint. To assess the integrity of the ligament, perform a stress test.

Cast immobilisation can be used in the treatment of partial tears with a good endpoint. A complete tear with instability (excessive opening of the joint when compared with the other side) or a displaced fracture requires open repair.

Pathological failure

When abnormal bone gives way, this is referred to as a pathological fracture. Examples include primary bone tumours and bony metastases, osteomyelitis, metabolic bone disease (osteomalacia, Paget's disease, osteoporosis) and haematopoietic disease (myeloma, lymphoma, leukaemia). Up to 80% of metastatic disease arises from the breast, thyroid, lungs, kidneys and prostate. The most common locations include the ribs, spine, pelvis, humerus and femur.

The typical history is of a minor trauma. This aspect of the history should alert the surgeon to the possibility of an underlying bony pathology. Physical examination should be directed to identifying the primary cause of the lesion. When suspected, investigations should be performed to ascertain the underlying pathology before definitive treatment. Blood tests, a chest radiograph and full-length views of the fractured bone are essential. A bone scan is the most sensitive indicator of skeletal disease.

If it is possible that the bony deposit is a primary tumour then operative treatment should not be commenced without careful thought. Many primary tumours can be treated constructively; however, this treatment may be compromised if tissue planes are disrupted by ill-considered operative management.

The common situation is a fracture through a metastasis and the presumption is that the patient has a limited life expectancy. Treatment is therefore aimed at regaining immediate mobility and relief of pain. As can be seen in Fig. 27.27 there is a clear rationale for aggressive treatment to restore function despite the risks. A patient with a limited life expectancy does have the time to invest in prolonged treatment and rehabilitation. Adjuvant radiotherapy or chemotherapy should be considered in consultation with an oncologist.

The goals of surgical treatment are to reduce pain and to splint the bone so that the patient can use it. Femoral, tibial and humeral fractures are nailed where possible. Some juxta-articular fractures that would require protection if treated with ORIF and bone grafting may be mobilised earlier if bone cement is substituted for the graft. Prophylactic stabilisation should be considered in patients with metastases where there has been cortical bone destruction of ≥ 50% or a femoral lesion longer than 2.5 cm, pathological fracture of the lesser trochanter and persistent pain after irradiation (Summary box 27.9).

Sir James Paget, **1814–1899, Surgeon, St. Bartholomew's Hospital, London, England.**

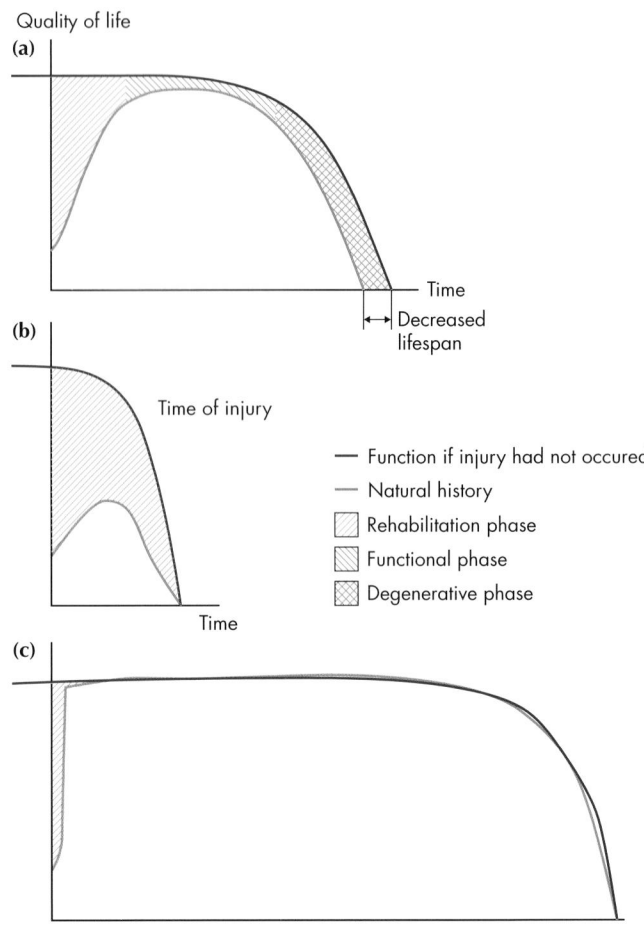

Figure 27.27 Comparative outcome curves for a normal adult (a), pathological fracture (b) and paediatric fracture (c). (a) The generic outcome curve as shown in Figure 27.8 for a patient with a life expectancy of > 20 years. There is a rehabilitation, functional and degenerative phase to consider. (b) It is seen that the short life expectancy of a patient with a pathological fracture secondary to metastases means that only the rehabilitation phase is relevant. The patient must be able to function before bone healing. This justifies aggressive treatment. (c) The paediatric fracture with benign natural history. Any marginal early gain has to be considered in the light of great potential for long-term detriment should there be complications.

Summary box 27.9
Pathological failure
■ **Do not operate on what might be a primary tumour without careful thought**
■ **Fractures through secondary tumours are treated aggressively to optimise early function**

CONCLUSION

The management of extremity trauma is in theory quite straightforward. The first step is to realise that an injury exists as a missed injury cannot be treated. The injury then needs to be understood – this generally involves description and classification. When there is clear evidence as to the best method of treatment for a particular injury this should be followed. When such evidence is lacking, as is generally the case, the treatment of fractures is generally principle based (Summary box 27.10).

Summary box 27.10
Summary of extremity trauma
■ Realise that an injury exists
■ Find the characteristics of the injury, describe and classify it
■ Consider the natural history of the injury
■ Treatment is guided by outcome if known or by principle if not
■ Beware of injuries that are 'easily missed'

FURTHER

Bone, L.R, Johnson, K. versus delayed stabilizat **71A(3)**: 336–40.

Charnley, J. (1950) *The Closed Treat* Livingstone, Edinburgh.

Gustillo, R.B. and Anderson, J.T. (1976) Prevent treatment of 1025 open fractures of long bones. **58A(4)**: 453–8.

Mast, J., Jakob, R. and Ganz, R. (1989) *Planning and Reduction Te in Fracture Surgery.* Springer-Verlag, Berlin.

Muller, M.E., Nazarian, S. and Koch, P. (1988) *The AO Classification of Fractures.* Translated by J. Schatzker. Springer-Verlag, Berlin.

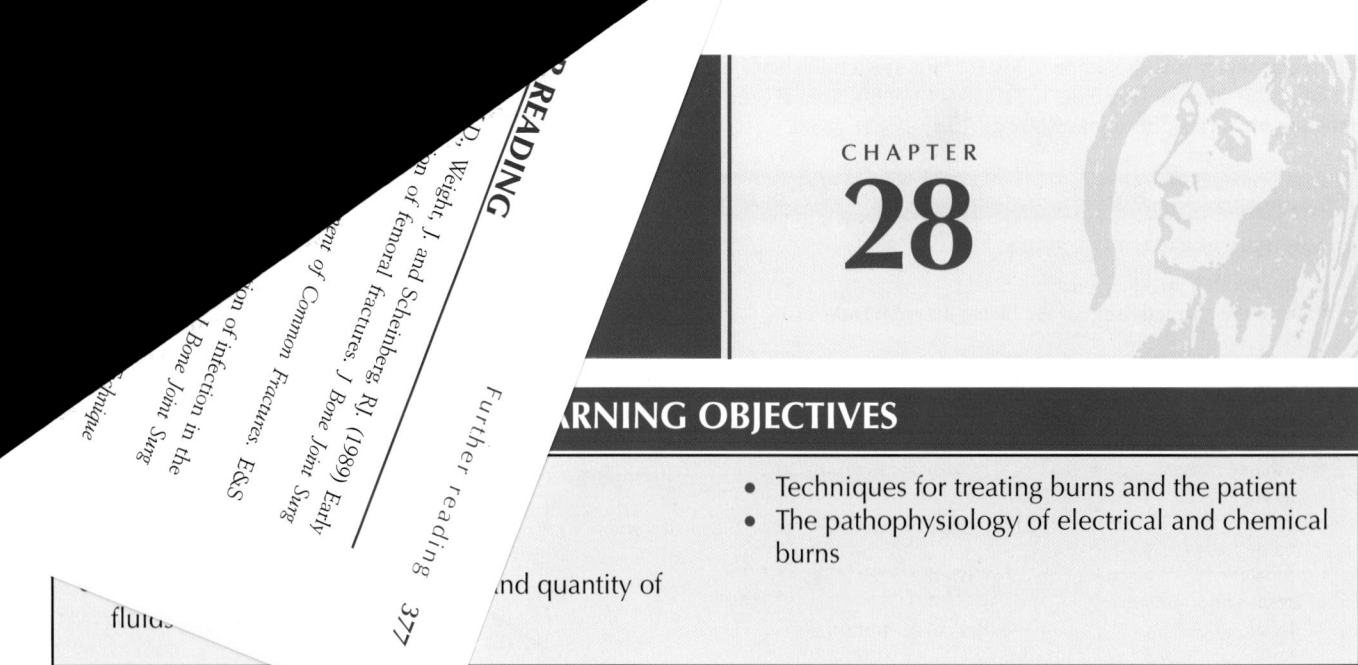

D. Weight, J and Schenberg, RJ (1989) Early
...on of femoral fractures. J Bone Joint Surg

...nt of Common Fractures. J Bone Joint Surg

...ion of infection in the
...I Bone Joint Surg
...chnique

Further reading 377

CHAPTER

28

LEARNING OBJECTIVES

- Techniques for treating burns and the patient
- The pathophysiology of electrical and chemical burns

...nd quantity of

fluids

INTRODUCTION

The incidence of burn injury varies greatly between cultures. In the UK (population 65 million), each year around 175 000 people visit accident and emergency (A&E) departments suffering burns, of whom about 13 000 need to be admitted. About 1000 have severe burns requiring fluid resuscitation, and half of the victims are under 16 years of age.

The majority of burns in children are scalds caused by accidents with kettles, pans, hot drinks and bath water. Among adolescent patients, the burns are usually caused by young males experimenting with matches and flammable liquids. In adults, scalds are not uncommon but are less frequent than flame burns. Most electrical and chemical injuries occur in adults. Cold and radiation are very rare causes of burns. Associated conditions in adults, such as mental disease (attempted suicide or assault), epilepsy and alcohol or drug abuse, are underlying factors in as many as 80% of patients with burns admitted to hospital in some populations.

Legislation, health promotion and appliance design have reduced the incidence of burns, with regulations regarding flame-retardant clothes and furniture, the promotion of smoke alarms, the design of cookers and gas fires, the almost universal use of cordless kettles and the education of parents to keep their hot water thermostat to 60°C all playing their part (Summary box 28.1).

Summary box 28.1

Prevention of burns

A significant proportion of burns can be prevented by:

- Implementing good health and safety regulations
- Educating the public
- Introducing of effective legislation

The last 50 years have seen great strides made to reduce both morbidity and mortality from burn injuries. The coming years will see a better understanding of the control of physiology along with improvements in reconstruction and rehabilitation.

A vast spectrum of injuries can arise from a burning accident, from the trivial to some of the most dramatic injuries that humans survive. The management of the major burn injury represents a significant challenge to every member of the burns team – burns doctors, surgeons, anaesthetists, ward and theatre nurses, physiotherapists, occupational therapists, dietitians, bacteriologists, physicians, psychiatrists, psychologists and the many ancillary staff whose cleaning and supply services are vital to the successful running of a burns unit. A large burn injury will have a significant effect on the patient's family and friends and the patient's future.

The importance of multidisciplinary care needs to be stressed for the adequate and effective care of the burn patient.

THE PATHOPHYSIOLOGY OF BURN INJURY

Burns cause damage in a number of different ways, but by far the most common organ affected is the skin. However, burns can also damage the airway and lungs, with life-threatening consequences. Airway injuries occur when the face and neck are burned. Respiratory system injuries usually occur if a person is trapped in a burning vehicle, house, car or aeroplane and is forced to inhale the hot and poisonous gases (Summary box 28.2).

Summary box 28.2

Warning signs of burns to the respiratory system

- Burns around the face and neck
- A history of being trapped in a burning room
- Change in voice
- Stridor

INJURY TO THE AIRWAY AND LUNGS

Physical burn injury to the airway above the larynx

The hot gases can physically burn the nose, mouth, tongue, palate and larynx. Once burned, the linings of these structures will start to swell. After a few hours, they may start to interfere with the larynx and may completely block the airway if action is not taken to secure an airway (Summary box 28.3).

Summary box 28.3

Dangers of smoke, hot gas or steam inhalation

- Inhaled hot gases can cause supraglottic airway burns and laryngeal oedema
- Inhaled steam can cause subglottic burns and loss of respiratory epithelium
- Inhaled smoke particles can cause chemical alveolitis and respiratory failure
- Inhaled poisons, such as carbon monoxide, can cause metabolic poisoning
- Full-thickness burns to the chest can cause mechanical blockage to rib movement

---

Physical burn injury to the airway below the larynx

This is a rare injury as the heat exchange mechanisms in the supraglottic airway are usually able safely to absorb the heat from hot air. However, steam has a large latent heat of evaporation and can cause thermal damage to the lower airway. In such injuries, the respiratory epithelium rapidly swells and detaches from the bronchial tree. This creates casts, which can block the main upper airway.

Metabolic poisoning

There are many poisonous gases that can be given off in a fire, the most common being carbon monoxide, a product of incomplete combustion that is often produced by fires in enclosed spaces. This is the usual cause of a person being found with altered consciousness at the scene of a fire. Carbon monoxide binds to haemoglobin with an affinity 240 times greater than that of oxygen and therefore blocks the transport of oxygen. Levels of carboxyhaemoglobin in the bloodstream can be measured. Concentrations above 10% are dangerous and need treatment with pure oxygen for more than 24 hours. Death occurs with concentrations around 60%.

Another metabolic toxin produced in house fires is hydrogen cyanide, which causes a metabolic acidosis by interfering with mitochondrial respiration.

Inhalational injury

Inhalational injury is caused by the minute particles within thick smoke, which, because of their small size, are not filtered by the upper airway, but are carried down to the lung parenchyma. They stick to the moist lining, causing an intense reaction in the alveoli. This chemical pneumonitis causes oedema within the alveolar sacs and decreasing gaseous exchange over the ensuing 24 hours, and often gives rise to a bacterial pneumonia. Its presence or absence has a very significant effect on the mortality of any burn patient.

Mechanical block on rib movement

Burned skin is very thick and stiff, and this can physically stop the ribs moving if there is a large full-thickness burn across the chest.

INFLAMMATION AND CIRCULATORY CHANGES

The dangers to the airway and respiration described above are readily apparent, but the cause of circulatory changes following a burn are more complex. The changes occur because burned skin activates a web of inflammatory cascades. The release of neuropeptides and the activation of complement are initiated by the stimulation of pain fibres and the alteration of proteins by heat. The activation of Hageman factor initiates a number of protease-driven cascades, altering the arachidonic acid, thrombin and kallikrein pathways.

At a cellular level, complement causes the degranulation of mast cells and coats the proteins altered by the burn. This attracts neutrophils, which also degranulate, with the release of large quantities of free radicals and proteases. These can, in turn, cause further damage to the tissue. Mast cells also release primary cytokines such as tumour necrosis factor alpha (TNF-α). These act as chemotactic agents to inflammatory cells and cause the subsequent release of many secondary cytokines. These inflammatory factors alter the permeability of blood vessels such that intravascular fluid escapes. The increase in permeability is such that large protein molecules can also now escape with ease. The damaged collagen and these extravasated proteins increase the oncotic pressure within the burned tissue, further increasing the flow of water from the intravascular to the extravascular space.

The overall effect of these changes is to produce a net flow of water, solutes and proteins from the intravascular to the extravascular space. This flow occurs over the first 36 hours after the injury but does not include red blood cells. In a small burn, this reaction is small and localised but, as the burn size approaches 10–15% of total body surface area (TBSA), the loss of intravascular fluid can cause a level of circulatory shock. Furthermore, once the area increases to 25% of TBSA, the inflammatory reaction causes fluid loss in vessels remote from the burn injury. This is why such importance is attached to measuring the TBSA involved in any burn. It dictates the size of inflammatory reaction and therefore the amount of fluid needed to control shock (Summary box 28.4).

Summary box 28.4

The shock reaction after burns

- Burns produce an inflammatory reaction
- This leads to vastly increased vascular permeability
- Water, solutes and proteins move from the intra- to the extravascular space
- The volume of fluid lost is directly proportional to the area of the burn
- Above 15% of surface area, the loss of fluid produces shock

---

Hageman **is the surname of the individual in whom the deficiency of the factor was first discovered.**

CHAPTER 28 | BURNS

OTHER LIFE-THREATENING EVENTS WITH MAJOR BURNS

The immune system and infection

The inflammatory changes caused by the burn have an effect on the patient's immune system. Cell-mediated immunity is significantly reduced in large burns, leaving them more susceptible to bacterial and fungal infections. There are many potential sources of infection, especially from the burn wound and from the lung if this is injured, but also from any central venous lines, tracheostomies or urinary catheters present.

Changes to the intestine

The inflammatory stimulus and shock can cause microvascular damage and ischaemia to the gut mucosa. This reduces gut motility and can prevent the absorption of food. Failure of enteral feeding in a patient with a large burn is a life-threatening complication. This process also increases the translocation of gut bacteria, which can become an important source of infection in large burns. Gut mucosal swelling, gastric stasis and peritoneal oedema can also cause abdominal compartment syndrome, which splints the diaphragm and increases the airway pressures needed for respiration.

Danger to peripheral circulation

In full-thickness burns, the collagen fibres are coagulated. The normal elasticity of the skin is lost. A circumferential full-thickness burn to a limb acts as a tourniquet as the limb swells. If untreated, this will progress to limb-threatening ischaemia (Summary box 28.5).

Summary box 28.5

Other complications of burns

- Infection from the burn site, lungs, gut, lines and catheters
- Malabsorption from the gut
- Circumferential burns may compromise circulation to a limb

IMMEDIATE CARE OF THE BURN PATIENT

Pre-hospital care

The principles of pre-hospital care are:

- *Ensure rescuer safety.* This is particularly important in house fires and in the case of electrical and chemical injuries.
- *Stop the burning process.* Stop, drop and roll is a good method of extinguishing fire burning on a person.
- *Check for other injuries.* A standard ABC (airway, breathing, circulation) check followed by a rapid secondary survey will ensure that no other significant injuries are missed. Patients burned in explosions or even escaping from fires may have head or spine injuries and other life-threatening problems.
- *Cool the burn wound.* This provides analgesia and slows the delayed microvascular damage that can occur after a burn injury. Cooling should occur for a minimum of 10 min and is effective up to 1 hour after the burn injury. It is a particularly important first aid step in partial-thickness burns, especially scalds. In temperate climates, cooling should be at about 15°C, and hypothermia must be avoided.

- *Give oxygen.* Anyone involved in a fire in an enclosed space should receive oxygen, especially if there is an altered consciousness level.
- *Elevate.* Sitting a patient up with a burned airway may prove life-saving in the event of a delay in transfer to hospital care. Elevation of burned limbs will reduce swelling and discomfort.

Hospital care

The principles of managing an acute burn injury are the same as in any acute trauma case:

A Airway control.
B Breathing and ventilation.
C Circulation.
D Disability – neurological status.
E Exposure with environmental control.
F Fluid resuscitation.

The possibility of injury additional to the burn must be sought both clinically and from the history, and treated appropriately. The major determinants of severity of any burn injury are the percentage of TBSA that is burned, the presence of an inhalation injury and the depth of the burn (Summary box 28.6).

Summary box 28.6

Major determinants of the outcome of a burn

- Percentage surface area involved
- Depth of burns
- Presence of an inhalational injury

These aspects are therefore some of the primary diagnostic aims of the acute admission and, although there is this vast spectrum of burns severity, most of the principles covered below will apply to all patients. Not all burned patients will need to be admitted to a burns unit (Summary box 28.7).

Summary box 28.7

The criteria for acute admission to a burns unit

- Suspected airway or inhalational injury
- Any burn likely to require fluid resuscitation
- Any burn likely to require surgery
- Patients with burns of any significance to the hands, face, feet or perineum
- Patients whose psychiatric or social background makes it inadvisable to send them home
- Any suspicion of non-accidental injury
- Any burn in a patient at the extremes of age
- Any burn with associated potentially serious sequelae including high-tension electrical burns and concentrated hydrofluoric acid burns

---

Airway

The burned airway creates symptoms by swelling and, if not managed proactively, can completely occlude the upper airway. The treatment is to secure the airway with an endotracheal tube until the swelling has subsided, which is usually after about 48 hours. The symptoms of laryngeal oedema, such as change in voice, stridor, anxiety and respiratory difficulty, are very late symptoms. Intubation at this point is often difficult or impossible owing to swelling, so acute cricothyroidotomy equipment must be at hand when intubating patients with a delayed diagnosis of airway burn. Because of this, early intubation of suspected airway burn is the treatment of choice in such patients. The time-frame from burn to airway occlusion is usually between 4 and 24 hours, so there is time to make a sensible decision with senior staff and allow an experienced anaesthetist to intubate the patient (Summary box 28.8).

Summary box 28.8

Initial management of the burned airway

- Early elective intubation is safest
- Delay can make intubation very difficult because of swelling
- Be ready to perform an emergency cricothyroidotomy if intubation is delayed

---

Thus, the key in the management of airway burn is the history and early signs, rather than the symptoms. The history is that of obligatory inhalation of hot gases such as in a house or car fire. Clues include blisters on the hard palate, burned nasal mucosa and loss of all the hair in the nose (the anterior hairs are often burned), but perhaps the most valuable signs are the presence of deep burns around the mouth and in the neck (Summary box 28.9).

Summary box 28.9

Recognition of the potentially burned airway

- A history of being trapped in the presence of smoke or hot gases
- Burns on the palate or nasal mucosa, or loss of all the hairs in the nose
- Deep burns around the mouth and neck

Breathing

Inhalational injury

Time is a factor; anyone trapped in a fire for more than a couple of minutes must be observed for signs of smoke inhalation. Other signs that raise suspicion are the presence of soot in the nose and the oropharynx and a chest radiograph showing patchy consolidation.

The clinical features are a progressive increase in respiratory effort and rate, rising pulse, anxiety and confusion and decreasing oxygen saturation. These symptoms may not be apparent immediately and can take 24 hours to 5 days to develop.

Treatment starts as soon as this injury is suspected and the airway is secure. Physiotherapy, nebulisers and warm humidified oxygen are all useful. The patient's progress should be monitored using respiratory rate, together with blood gas measurements. If the situation deteriorates, continuous or intermittent positive pressure may be used with a mask or T-piece. In the severest cases, intubation and management in an intensive care unit will be needed.

The key, therefore, in the management of inhalational injury is to suspect it from the history, institute early management and observe carefully for deterioration.

Thermal burn injury to the lower airway

These rare injuries can occur with steam injuries. Their management is supportive and the same as that for an inhalational injury.

Metabolic poisoning

Any history of a fire within an enclosed space and any history of altered consciousness are important clues to metabolic poisoning. Blood gases must be measured immediately if poisoning is a possibility. Carboxyhaemoglobin levels raised above 10% must be treated with high inspired oxygen for 24 hours to speed its displacement from haemoglobin. Metabolic acidosis is a feature of this and other forms of poisoning.

Once again, the key to diagnosing these injuries is suspicion from the history. Blood gas measurement will confirm the diagnosis. The treatment is oxygen.

Mechanical block to breathing

Any mechanical block to breathing from the eschar of a significant full-thickness burn on the chest wall is obvious from the examination. There will also be carbon dioxide retention and high inspiratory pressures if the patient is ventilated. The treatment is to make some scoring cuts through the burned skin to allow the chest to expand (escharotomy). The nerves have been destroyed in the skin, and this procedure is not painful for the patient.

ASSESSMENT OF THE BURN WOUND

Assessing size

Burn size needs to be formally assessed in a controlled environment. This allows the area to be exposed and any soot or debris washed off. Care should be taken not to cause hypothermia during this stage. In the case of smaller burns or patches of burn, the best measurement is to cut a piece of clean paper the size of the patient's whole hand (digits and palm), which represents 1% TBSA, and match this to the area. Another accurate way of measuring the size of burns is to draw the burn on a Lund and Browder chart (Fig. 28.1), which maps out the percentage TBSA of sections of our anatomy. It also takes into account different proportional body surface area in children according to age. The rule of nines, which states that each upper limb is 9% TBSA, each lower limb 18%, the torso 18% each side and the head and neck 9%, can be used as a rough guide to TBSA outside the hospital environment (Summary box 28.10).

Summary box 28.10

Assessing the area of a burn

- The patient's whole hand is 1% TBSA, and is a useful guide in small burns
- The Lund and Browder chart is useful in larger burns
- The rule of nines is adequate for a first approximation only

---

Assessing depth from the history

The first indication of burn depth comes from the history (Table 28.1). The burning of human skin is temperature and time dependent. It takes 6 hours for skin maintained at 44°C to suffer irreversible changes, but a surface temperature of 70°C for 1 s is all that is needed to produce epidermal destruction. Taking an

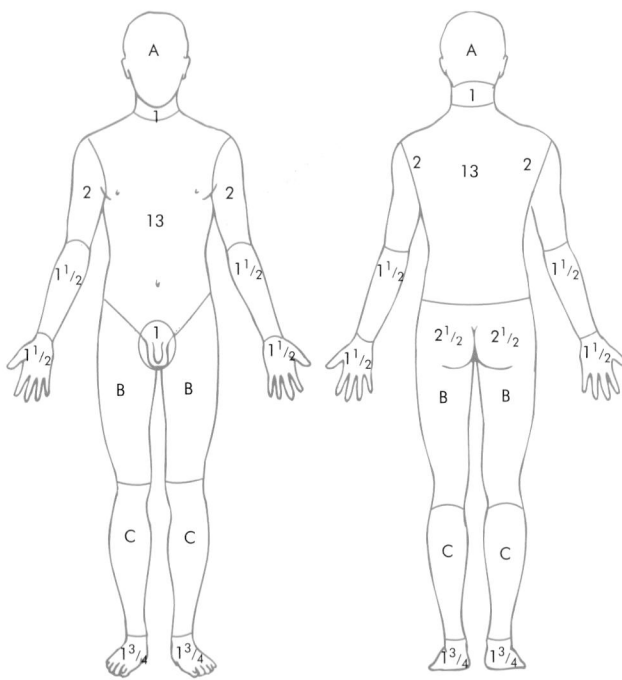

Relative percentage of area affected by growth

Age in years	0	1	5	10	15	Adult
A Head	9	8	6	5	4	3
B Thigh	2	3	4	4	4	4
C leg	2	2	3	3	3	3

Figure 28.1 The Lund and Browder chart.

Table 28.1 Causes of burns and their likely depth

Cause of burn	Probable depth of burn
Scald	Superficial, but with deep dermal patches in the absence of good first aid. Will be deep in a young infant
Fat burns	Deep dermal
Flame burns	Mixed deep dermal and full thickness
Alkali burns including cement	Often deep dermal or full thickness
Acid burns	Weak concentrations superficial, strong concentrations deep dermal
Electrical contact burn	Full thickness

example of hot water at 65°C: exposure for 45 s will produce a full-thickness burn, for 15 s a deep partial-thickness burn and for 7 s a superficial partial-thickness burn (Summary box 28.11).

Summary box 28.11

Assessing the depth of a burn

■ The history is important – temperature, time and burning material
■ Superficial burns have capillary filling
■ Deep partial-thickness burns do not blanch but have some sensation
■ Full-thickness burns feel leathery and have no sensation

Superficial partial-thickness burns

The damage in these burns goes no deeper than the papillary dermis. The clinical features are blistering and/or loss of the epidermis. The underlying dermis is pink and moist. The capillary return is clearly visible when blanched. There is little or no fixed capillary staining. Pinprick sensation is normal. Superficial partial-thickness burns heal without residual scarring in 2 weeks. The treatment is non-surgical (Fig. 28.2).

Deep partial-thickness burn

These burns involve damage to the deeper parts of the reticular dermis (Fig. 28.3). Clinically, the epidermis is usually lost. The exposed dermis is not as moist as that in a superficial burn. There is often abundant fixed capillary staining, especially if examined after 48 hours. The colour does not blanch with pressure under the examiner's finger. Sensation is reduced, and the patient is unable to distinguish sharp from blunt pressure when examined with a needle. Deep dermal burns take 3 or more weeks to heal without surgery and usually lead to hypertrophic scarring (Fig. 28.4, see page 384).

Full-thickness burns

The whole of the dermis is destroyed in these burns (Fig. 28.5, see page 384). Clinically, they have a hard, leathery feel. The appearance can vary from that similar to the patient's normal skin to charred black, depending upon the intensity of the heat. There is no capillary return. Often, thrombosed vessels can be seen under the skin. These burns are completely anaesthetised: a needle can be stuck deep into the dermis without any pain or bleeding.

FLUID RESUSCITATION

The principle of fluid resuscitation is that the intravascular volume must be maintained following a burn in order to provide sufficient circulation to perfuse not only the essential visceral organs such as the brain, kidneys and gut, but also the peripheral tissues, especially the damaged skin (Summary box 28.12).

Summary box 28.12

Fluids for resuscitation

■ In children with burns over 10% TBSA and adults with burns over 15% TBSA, consider the need for intravenous fluid resuscitation
■ If oral fluids are to be used, salt must be added
■ Fluids needed can be calculated from a standard formula
■ The key is to monitor urine output

Intravenous resuscitation is appropriate for any child with a burn greater than 10% TBSA. The figure is 15% TBSA for adults. In some parts of the world, intravenous resuscitation is commenced only with burns that approach 30% TBSA. If oral resuscitation is to be commenced, it is important that the water given is not salt free. It is rarely possible to undergo significant diuresis in the first 24 hours in view of the stress hormones that are present. Hyponatraemia and water intoxication can be fatal. It is therefore appropriate to give oral rehydration with a solution such as Dioralyte.

The resuscitation volume is relatively constant in proportion

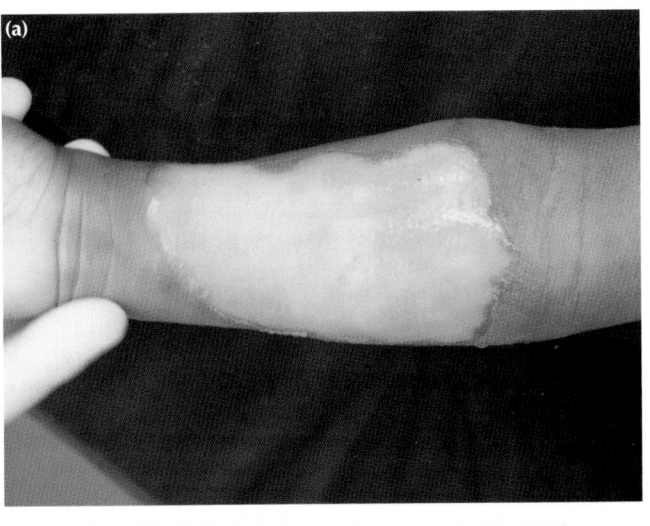

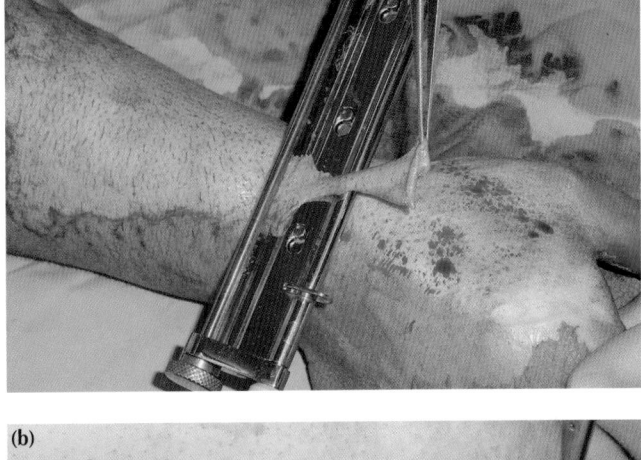

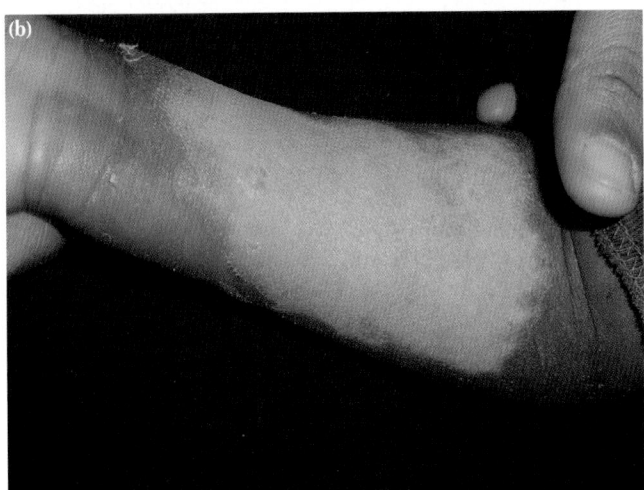

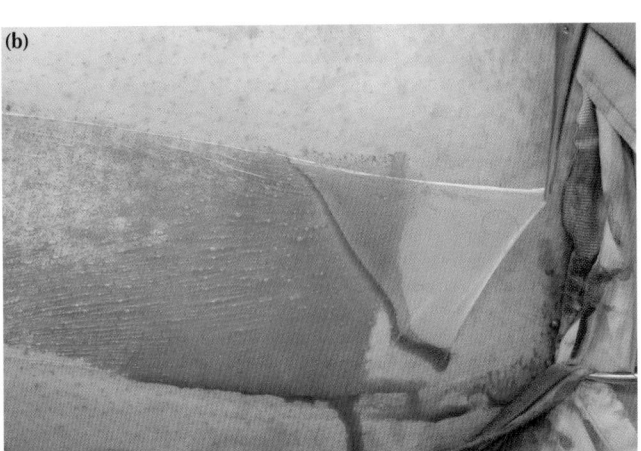

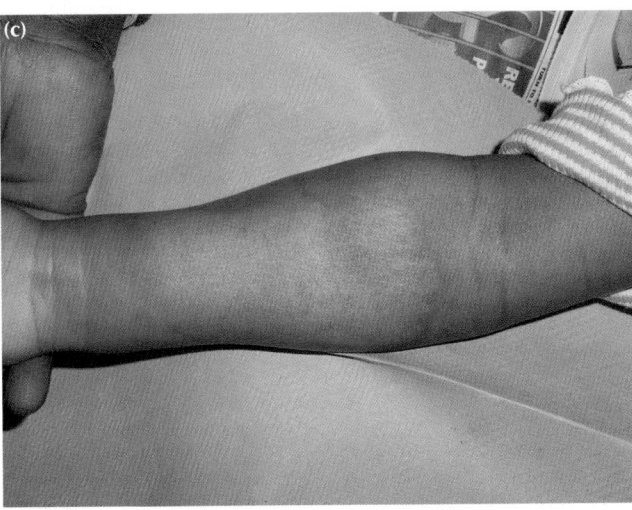

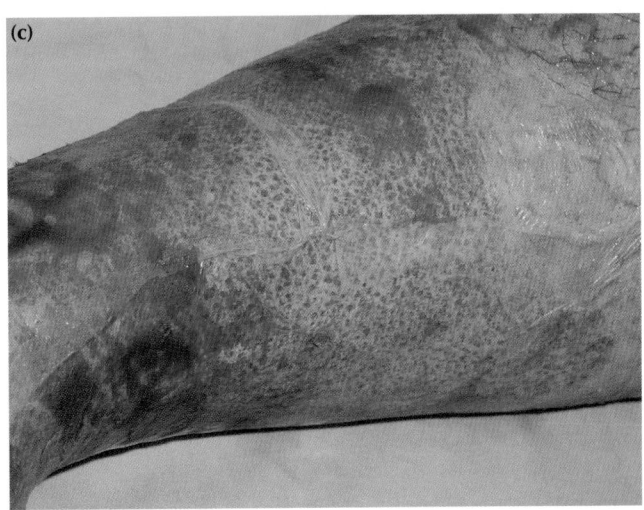

Figure 28.2 (a) A superficial partial-thickness scald 24 hours after injury. The dermis is pink and blanches to pressure. (b) At 2 weeks, the wound is healed but lacks pigment. (c) At 3 months, the pigment is returning.

Figure 28.3 (a) A deep dermal burn undergoing tangential shaving. The dead dermis is removed layer by layer until healthy bleeding is seen. The burn is pale because it was dressed with silver sulphadiazine cream, but no blanching was visible under this layer. The patient was unable to differentiate between pressure from the sharp and blunt ends of a needle. (b) A thin, split-thickness graft harvested from the thigh. (c) The thin graft is placed in the dermal remnants. The rete pegs can be seen between the remnants of the dermis through the graft.

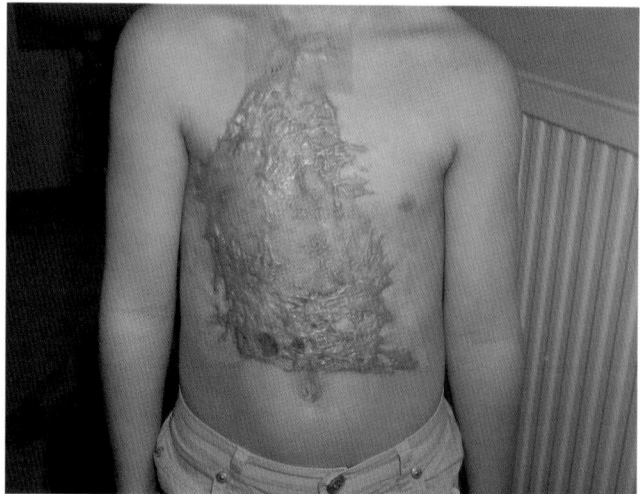

Figure 28.4 Hypertrophic scarring following a deep dermal burn.

to the area of the body burned and, therefore, there are formulae that calculate the approximate volume of fluid needed for the resuscitation of a patient of a given body weight with a given percentage of the body burned. These regimens follow the fluid loss, which is at its maximum in the first 8 hours and slows, such that, by 24–36 hours, the patient can be maintained on his or her normal daily requirements.

There are three types of fluid used. The most common is Ringer's lactate or Hartmann's solution; some centres use human albumin solution or fresh-frozen plasma, and some centres use hypertonic saline.

Perhaps the simplest and most widely used formula is the Parkland formula. This calculates the fluid to be replaced in the first 24 hours by the following formula:

$$\text{Total percentage body surface area} \times \text{weight (kg)} \times 4 = \text{volume (ml)} \quad (28.1)$$

Half this volume is given in the first 8 hours, and the second half is given in the subsequent 16 hours.

Crystalloid resuscitation

Ringer's lactate is the most commonly used crystalloid. Crystalloids are said to be as effective as colloids for maintaining intravascular volume. They are also significantly less expensive. Another reason for the use of crystalloids is that even large protein molecules leak out of capillaries following burn injury; however, non-burnt capillaries continue to sieve proteins virtually normally.

In children, maintenance fluid must also be given. This is normally dextrose–saline given as follows:

- 100 ml kg^{-1} for 24 hours for the first 10 kg;
- 50 ml kg^{-1} for the next 10 kg;
- 20 ml kg^{-1} for 24 hours for each kilogram over 20 kg body weight.

Hypertonic saline

Human albumin solution (HAS) is a commonly used colloid.

Hypertonic saline has been effective in treating burns shock for many years. It produces hyperosmolarity and hypernatraemia. This reduces the shift of intracellular water to the extracellular space. Advantages include less tissue oedema and a resultant decrease in escharotomies and intubations.

Colloid resuscitation

Plasma proteins are responsible for the inward oncotic pressure that counteracts the outward capillary hydrostatic pressure. Without proteins, plasma volumes would not be maintained as there would be oedema. Proteins should be given after the first 12 hours of burn because, before this time, the massive fluid shifts cause proteins to leak out of the cells.

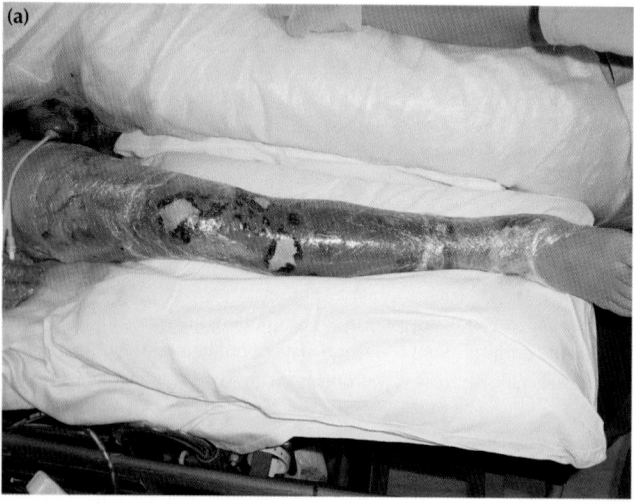
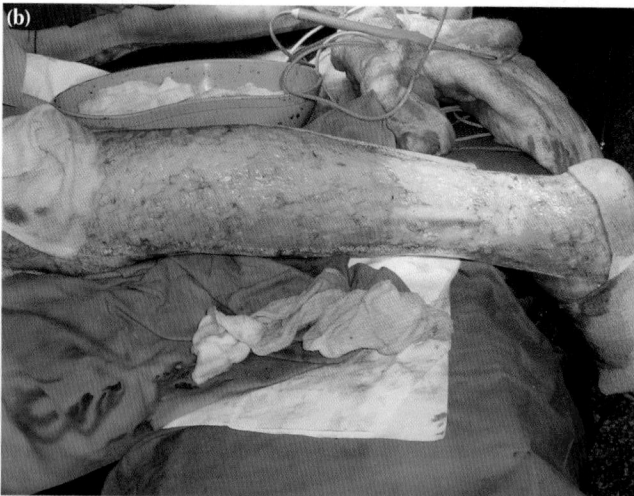

Figure 28.5 (a) A full-thickness burn on admission just prior to escharotomy. The wound is wrapped in cling film while in transit. The patient's facial burn is shown in Figure 28.8. (b) Excision of the same full-thickness burn, down to healthy fat.

Sydney Ringer, 1835–1910, Professor of Clinical Medicine, University College Hospital, London, England.
Alexis Frank Hartmann, 1898–1964, Paediatrician, St. Louis, MO, USA.

The commonest colloid-based formula is the Muir and Barclay formula:

- 0.5 × percentage body surface area burnt × weight = one portion;
- periods of 4/4/4, 6/6 and 12 hours respectively;
- one portion to be given in each period.

Monitoring of resuscitation

The key to monitoring of resuscitation is urine output. Urine output should be between 0.5 and 1.0 ml kg^{-1} body weight per hour. If the urine output is below this, the infusion rate should be increased by 50%. If the urine output is inadequate and the patient is showing signs of hypoperfusion (restlessness with tachycardia, cool peripheries and a high haematocrit), then a bolus of 10 ml kg^{-1} body weight should be given. It is important that patients are not over-resuscitated, and urine output in excess of 2 ml kg^{-1} body weight per hour should signal a decrease in the rate of infusion.

Other measures of tissue perfusion such as acid–base balance are appropriate in larger, more complex burns, and a haematocrit measurement is a useful tool in confirming suspected under- or overhydration. Those with cardiac dysfunction, acute or chronic, may well need more exact measurement of filling pressure, preferably by transoesophageal ultrasound or with the more invasive central line.

TREATING THE BURN WOUND

Escharotomy

Circumferential full-thickness burns to the limbs require emergency surgery (Fig. 28.6). The tourniquet effect of this injury is easily treated by incising the whole length of full-thickness burns. This should be done in the mid-axial line, avoiding major nerves (Table 28.2). One should remember that an escharotomy can cause a large amount of blood loss; therefore, adequate blood should be available for transfusion if required.

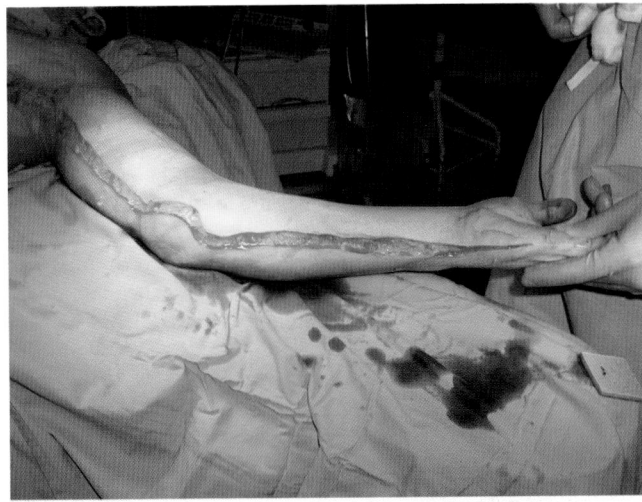

Figure 28.6 A full-thickness burn to the upper limb with a mid-axial escharotomy. The soot and debris have been washed off.

Ian Fraser Kerr Muir, **formerly Plastic Surgeon, The Aberdeen Royal Infirmary, Aberdeen, Scotland.**

Thomas Laird Barclay, **D. 2007, formerly Plastic Surgeon, The Royal Infirmary, Bradford, England.**

Table 28.2 Key features of escharotomy placement

Upper limb	Mid-axial, anterior to the elbow medially to avoid the ulnar nerve
Hand	Midline in the digits. Release muscle compartments if tight. Best done in theatre and with an experienced surgeon
Lower limb	Mid-axial. Posterior to the ankle medially to avoid the saphenous vein
Chest	Down the chest lateral to the nipples, across the chest below the clavicle and across the chest at the level of the xiphisternum
General rules	Extend the wound beyond the deep burn. Diathermy any significant bleeding vessels. Apply haemostatic dressing and elevate the limb postoperatively

Thereafter, the management of the burn wound remains the same irrespective of the size of the injury. The burn needs to be cleaned, and the size and depth need to be assessed. Full-thickness burns and deep partial-thickness burns that will require operative treatment will need to be dressed with an antibacterial dressing to delay the onset of colonisation of the wound.

Full-thickness burns and obvious deep dermal wounds

The four most common dressings for full-thickness and contaminated wounds are listed in Summary box 28.13.

Summary box 28.13

Options for topical treatment of deep burns

- 1% silver sulphadiazine cream
- 0.5% silver nitrate solution
- Mafenide acetate cream
- Serum nitrate, silver sulphadiazine and cerium nitrate

Dressings with nanocrystalline silver

- *Silver sulphadiazine cream (1%).* This gives broad-spectrum prophylaxis against bacterial colonisation and is particularly effective against *Pseudomonas aeruginosa* and also methicillin-resistant *Staphylococcus aureus*.
- *Silver nitrate solution (0.5%).* Again, this is highly effective as a prophylaxis against *Pseudomonas* colonisation, but it is not as active as silver sulphadiazine cream against some of the Gram-negative aerobes. The other disadvantage of this solution is that it needs to be changed or the wounds resoaked every 2–4 hours. It also produces black staining of all the furniture surrounding the patient.
- *Mafenide acetate cream.* This is popular, especially in the USA, but is painful to apply. It is usually used as a 5% topical solution but has been associated with metabolic acidosis.

Hans Christian Joachim Gram, **1853–1938, Professor of Pharmacology (1891–1900) and of Medicine (1900–1923), Copenhagen, Denmark, described this method of staining bacteria in 1884.**

CHAPTER 28 | BURNS

- *Silver sulphadiazine* and *cerium nitrate*. This is also a very useful burn dressing, especially for full-thickness burns. It induces a hard effect on the burned skin and has been shown in certain instances, especially in elderly patients, to reduce some of the cell-mediated immunosuppression that occurs in burns. Cerium nitrate forms a sterile eschar and is specially useful in treating burns when a conservative treatment option has been chosen. Cerium nitrate has also been shown to boost cell-mediated immunity in these patients.

Superficial partial-thickness wounds and mixed-depth wounds

Around the world, a wide variety of substances are used to treat these wounds, from honey or boiled potato peel to synthetic biological dressings with live cultured fibroblasts within the matrix. This is testament to the fact that superficial partial-thickness burns will heal almost irrespective of the dressing. Thus, the key lies with dressings that are easy to apply, non-painful, reduce pain, simple to manage and locally available. The choice of dressings does, however, become crucial in the case of burns that border on being deep dermal (Fig. 28.7). Here, the choice of dressing can make the difference between scar and no scar and/or operation and no operation. Some of the options for dressing choice are described below.

If the wound is heavily contaminated as a result of the accident, then it is prudent to clean the wound formally under a general anaesthetic. With more chronic contamination, silver sulphadiazine cream dressing for 2 or 3 days is very effective and can be changed to a dressing that is more efficient at promoting healing after this period.

The simplest method of treating a superficial wound is by exposure. The initial exudate needs to be managed by frequent changes of clean linen around the patient but, after a few days, a dry eschar forms, which then separates as the wound epithelialises. This is often used in hot climates and for small burns on the face. However, this method is painful and requires an intensive amount of nursing support. A variation on this theme is to cover the wound with a permeable wound dressing such as Mefix or Fixamol. This allows the wounds to dry but, because it is a covering, it avoids the problems of the wound adhering to the sheets and clothes. A similar method of managing these types of burn is to place a Vaseline-impregnated gauze (with or without an antiseptic such as chlorhexidine) over the wound. An alternative is a fenestrated silicone sheet (e.g. Mepitel). These can then be backed with swabs to absorb the exudate. The Vaseline gauze or silicone layer is used to prevent the swabs adhering to the wound and reduces the stiffness of the dry eschar, preventing it from cracking so easily. The swabs need to be changed after the first 48 hours as they are often soaked. After that, they can be left for longer.

More interactive dressings include hydrocolloids and biological dressings. Hydrocolloid dressings need to be changed every 3–5 days. They are particularly useful in mixed-depth burns as the high protease levels under the occlusive dressings aid with the debridement of the deeper areas of burn. They also provide a moist environment, which is good for epithelialisation. Duoderm is a hydrocolloid dressing. There is good evidence for its value in burns.

Biological, synthetic (e.g. Biobrane) and natural (e.g. amniotic membranes) dressings also provide good healing environments

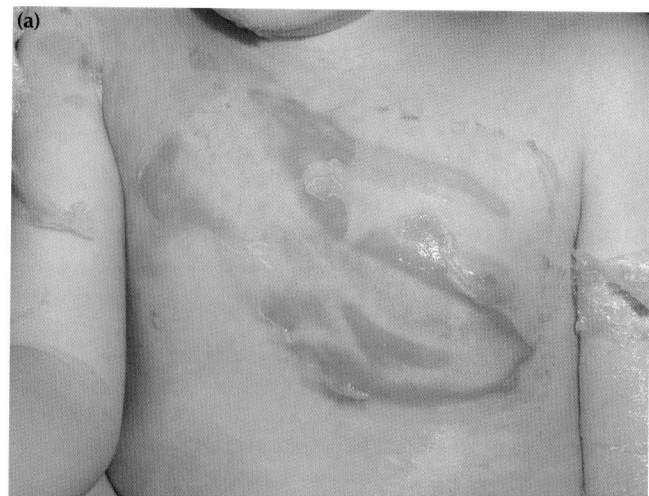

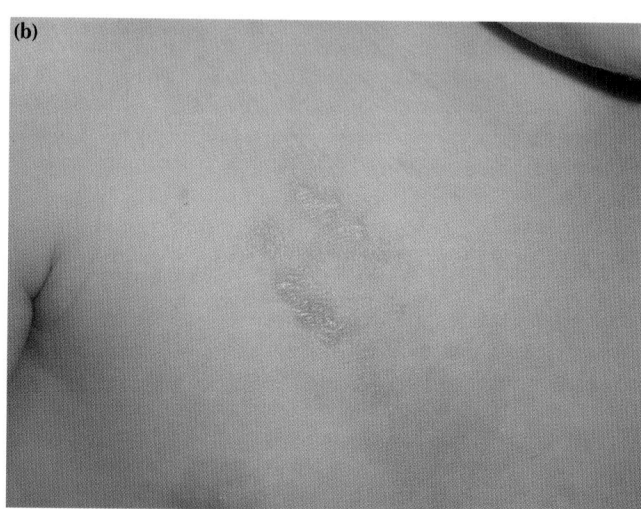

Figure 28.7 (a) A scald to the chest from boiling water, mainly superficial but in some areas close to being deep dermal. This was treated with a hydrocolloid dressing. (b) There are two tiny areas of hypertrophy indicating how close the burn was to being deep dermal. The good first aid this patient received probably made a difference to the outcome.

and do not need to be changed. They are ideal for one-stop management of superficial burns, being easy to apply and comfortable. However, they will become detached if applied to deep dermal wounds as the eschar needs to separate. They are therefore not as useful in mixed-depth wounds (Summary box 28.14).

> **Summary box 28.14**
>
> **Principles of dressings for burns**
>
> - Full-thickness and deep dermal burns need antibacterial dressings to delay colonisation prior to surgery
> - Superficial burns will heal and need simple dressings
> - An optimal healing environment can make a difference to outcome in borderline depth burns

Early debridement and grafting is the key to effectively treating deep partial- and full-thickness burns in a majority of cases.

ADDITIONAL ASPECTS OF TREATING THE BURNED PATIENT

Analgesia

Acute

Analgesia is a vital part of burns management. Small burns, especially superficial burns, respond well to simple oral analgesia, paracetamol and non-steroidal anti-inflammatory drugs. Topical cooling is especially soothing. Large burns require intravenous opiates. Intramuscular injections should not be given in acute burns over 10% of TBSA, as absorption is unpredictable and dangerous.

Subacute

In patients with large burns, continuous analgesia is required, beginning with infusions and continuing with oral tablets such as slow-release morphine. Powerful, short-acting analgesia should be administered before dressing changes. Administration may require an anaesthetist, as in the case of general anaesthesia or midazolam and ketamine, or less intensive supervision, as in the case of morphine and nitrous oxide.

Energy balance and nutrition

One of the most important aspects in treating burns patients is nutrition. Any adult with a burn greater than 15% (10% in children) of TBSA has an increased nutritional requirement. All patients with burns of 20% of TBSA or greater should receive a nasogastric tube. (Feeding should start within 6 hours of the injury to reduce gut mucosal damage.) A number of different formulae are available to calculate the energy requirements of patients (Summary box 28.15).

Summary box 28.15

Nutrition in burns patients

- Burns patients need extra feeding
- A nasogastric tube should be used in all patients with burns over 15% of TBSA
- Removing the burn and achieving healing stops the catabolic drive

Burn injuries are catabolic in the acute episode. Successful management of the patient's energy balance involves a number of strategies. The catabolic drive continues while the wound remains unhealed and, therefore, rapid excision of the burn and stable coverage of the wound are the most significant factors in reversing this. Obligatory energy utilisation must be reduced to a minimum by keeping the patient warm with good environmental control. The excess energy requirements must be provided for and the nutritional balance monitored by measuring weight and nitrogen balance.

Commonly used feeding formulae

Curreri formula
Age 16–59 years: $(25)W + (40)TBSA$
Age 60+ years: $(20)W + (65)TBSA$

Sutherland formula
Children: $60\,kcal\,kg^{-1} + 35\,kcal\%TBSA$
Adults: $20\,kcal\,kg^{-1} + 70\,kcal\%TBSA$

Protein needs
Greatest nitrogen losses between days 5 and 10
20% of kilocalories should be provided by proteins

Davies formula
Children: $3\%\,kg^{-1} + 1\,g\%TBSA$
Adults: $1\,g\,kg^{-1} + 3\,g\%TBSA$

Monitoring and control of infection

Patients with major burns are immunocompromised, having large portals of entry to pathogenic and opportunistic bacteria and fungi via the burn wound (Summary box 28.16). They have compromised local defences in the lungs and gut due to oedema, and usually have monitoring lines and catheters, which themselves represent portals for infection.

Summary box 28.16

Infection control in burns patients

- Burns patients are immunocompromised
- They are susceptible to infection from many routes
- Sterile precautions must be rigorous
- Swabs should be taken regularly
- A rise in white blood cell count, thrombocytosis and increased catabolism are warnings of infection

Control of infection begins with policies on hand-washing and other cross-contamination prevention measures. Bacteriological surveillance of the wound, catheter tips and sputum helps to build a picture of the patient's flora. If there are signs of infection, then further cultures need to be taken and antibiotics started. This is often initially on a best guess basis, hence the usefulness of prior surveillance; close liaison with a bacteriologist is essential. In patients with large burns that remain catabolic, the core temperature is usually reset by the hypothalamus above 37°C. Significant temperatures are those above 38.5°C, but often other signs of infection are more useful to the clinician. These include significant rise or fall in the white cell count, thrombocytosis, increasing signs of catabolism and decreasing clinical status of the patient.

Nursing care

Burns patients require particularly intensive nursing care. Nurses are the primary effectors of many decisions that directly affect healing. Bandaged hands and joints, stiff and painful, need careful coaxing. Personal hygiene, baths and showers all become time-consuming and painful but are vital parts of the patient's physiotherapy. Their success or failure has a powerful psychological impact on the patient and his or her family.

Physiotherapy

All burns cause swelling, especially burns to the hands. Elevation, splintage and exercise reduce swelling and improve the final outcome. The physiotherapy needs to be started on day 1, so that the message can be reinforced on a daily basis.

Psychological

A major burn is an overwhelming event, outside the normal experience, which overwhelms the patient's coping ability, suspends the patient's sense of safety and causes post-traumatic reactions. These are normal and usually self-limiting, receding as the patient heals. The features of this intensity of experience are of intrusive reactions, arousal reactions and avoidance reactions.

The intrusive reactions include flashbacks and other intrusive experiences. Arousal reactions include sleep disturbance, anger and panic attacks. Avoidance reactions include avoidance behaviour and emotional numbness. Patients also often have a sense of grief, guilt and self-blame. Psychological help and support for the patient and family is an important part of treating a severely burned patient. Vigilance for post-traumatic stress disorder is also important.

SURGERY FOR THE ACUTE BURN WOUND

Any deep partial-thickness and full-thickness burns, except those that are less than about 4 cm^2, need surgery. Any burn of indeterminate depth should be reassessed after 48 hours. This is because burns that initially appear superficial may well deepen over that time. Delayed microvascular injury is especially common in scalds (Summary box 28.17).

Summary box 28.17

Surgical treatment of deep burns

- Deep dermal burns need tangential shaving and split-skin grafting
- All but the smallest full-thickness burns need surgery
- The anaesthetist needs to be ready for significant blood loss
- Topical adrenaline reduces bleeding
- All burnt tissue needs to be excised
- Stable cover, permanent or temporary, should be applied at once to reduce burn load

---

The essence of burns surgery is control. First and foremost, the anaesthetist needs good control of the patient. A wide-bore cannula should be used, and the patient's blood pressure must be monitored adequately. If a large excision is considered, then an arterial line (to monitor blood pressure) and a central venous pressure monitor are needed. The anaesthetist also needs measurements and control of the acid–base balance, clotting time and haemoglobin levels. The core temperature of the patient must not drop below 36°C otherwise clotting irregularities will be compounded, so the temperature in the operating environment must be kept warm.

For most burn excisions, subcutaneous injection of a dilute solution of adrenaline 1:1 000 000 or 1:500 000 and tourniquet control are essential for controlling blood loss.

In deep dermal burns, the top layer of dead dermis is shaved off until punctate bleeding is observed and the dermis can be seen to be free of any small thrombosed vessels (Fig. 28.3a, see page 383). A topical solution of 1:500 000 adrenaline also helps to reduce bleeding, as does the application of the skin graft. The use of a tourniquet during burn excisions in the limbs helps to decrease blood loss and maintain control.

Full-thickness burns require full-thickness excision of the skin (Fig. 28.5b, see page 384). In certain circumstances, it is appropriate to go down to the fascia but, in most cases, the burn excision is down to viable fat. Wherever possible, a skin graft should be applied immediately. With very large burns, the use of

synthetic dermis or homografts provides temporary stable coverage and will allow complete excision of the wound and thus reduce the burn load on the patient.

Postoperative management of these patients obviously requires careful evaluation of fluid balance and levels of haemoglobin. The outer dressings will quickly be soaked through with serum and will need to be changed on a regular basis to reduce the bacterial load within the dressing.

Physiotherapy and splints are important in maintaining range of movement and reducing joint contracture. Elevation of the appropriate limbs is important. The hand must be splinted in a position of function after grafting, although the graft needs to be applied in the position of maximal stretch. Knees are best splinted in extension, axillae in abduction. Supervised movement by the physiotherapists, usually under direct vision of any affected joints, should begin after about 5 days.

Delayed reconstruction and scar management

Delayed reconstruction of burn injuries is common for large full-thickness burns. In the early healing period, acute contractures around the eye need particular attention. Eyelids must be grafted at the first sign of difficulty in closing the eyelids, and this must be done before the patient has any symptoms of exposure keratitis (Fig. 28.8). Other areas that require early intervention are any contracture causing significant loss of range of movement of a joint. This is particularly important in the hand and axilla (Summary box 28.18).

Summary box 28.18

Delayed reconstruction of burns

- Eyelids must be treated before exposure keratitis arises
- Transposition flaps and Z-plasties with or without tissue expansion are useful
- Full-thickness grafts and free flaps may be needed for large or difficult areas
- Hypertrophy is treated with pressure garments
- Pharmacological treatment of itch is important

Established contracture can be treated in a number of ways. Burn alopecia is best treated with tissue expansion of the unburned hair-bearing skin. Tissue expansion is also a useful technique for isolated burns and other areas with adjacent normal skin. Z-plasty is useful in the situation in which there is a single band and a transposition flap is useful in wider bands of scarring (Fig. 28.9). In areas of circumferential or very broad areas of scarring, the only real treatment is incision and replacement with tissue. By far the best tissue for replacement is from either a full-thickness graft or vascularised tissue as in a free flap. Occasionally, the situation requires the less ideal covering of split skin, possibly with an artificial dermis such as Integra (Fig. 28.10). These last two options require prolonged scar management after their use.

Hypertrophy of many scars will respond to pressure garments. These need to be worn for a period of 6–18 months. Where it is difficult to apply pressure with pressure garments, or with smaller areas of hypertrophy, silicone patches will speed scar maturation, as will intralesional injection of steroid. Itching and dermatitis in burn scar areas are common. Pharmacological treatment of itch is an essential adjunct to therapy.

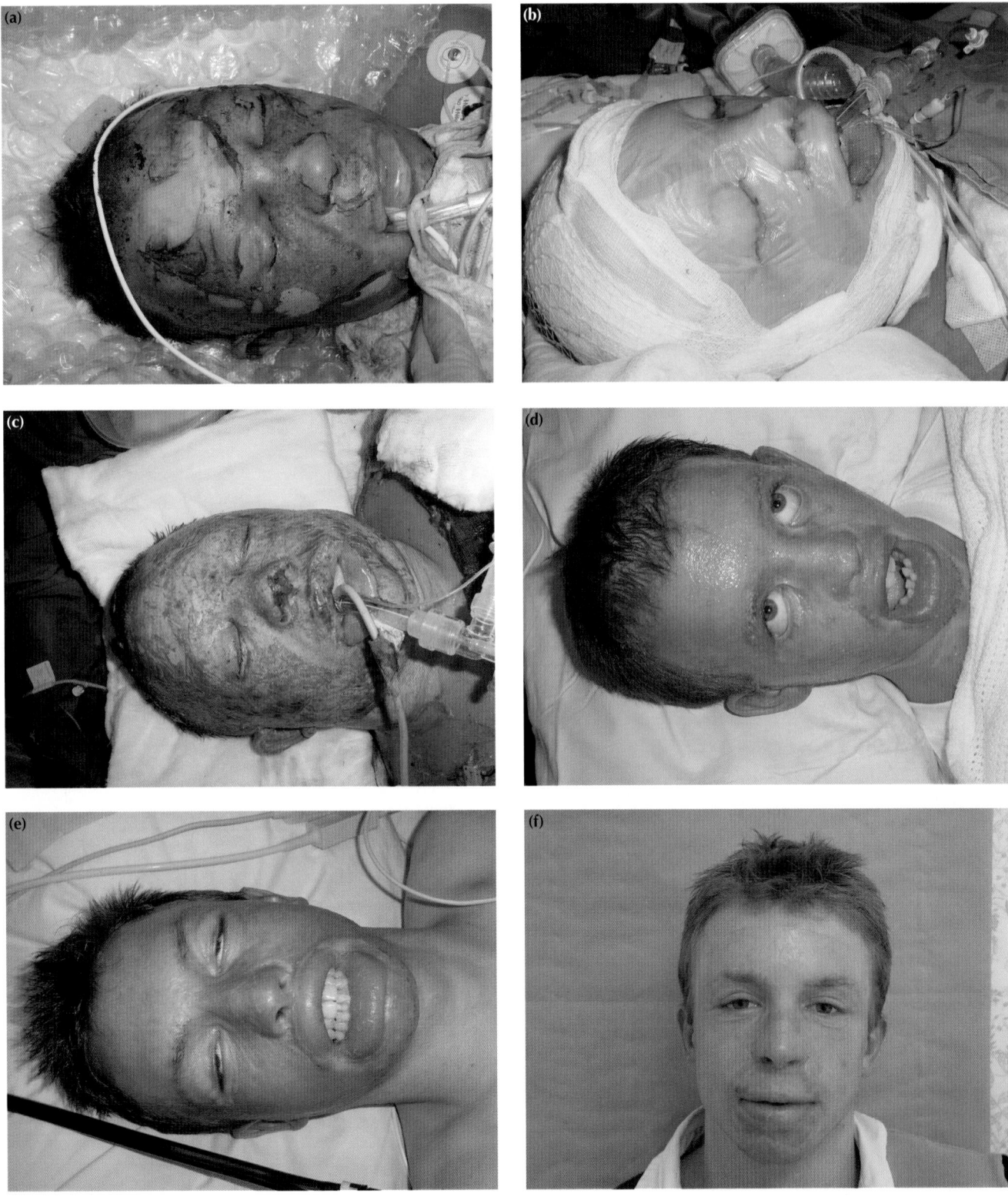

Figure 28.8 (a) A mixed superficial and deep burn to the face after a petrol explosion. The patient's airway was protected prior to transfer. He has an orogastric tube and feeding has commenced. (b) The face dressed with a hydrocolloid dressing. The endotracheal tube is wired to the teeth. (c) Day 6: the swelling is still present. (d) Six weeks after injury. With the mouth wide open, the lower eyelids are pulled down, demonstrating the intrinsic and extrinsic shortening of the eyelids. (e) Three months after injury. The eyelids have been grafted but note the contracture of the lips. (f) Six months after injury. The patient has had grafts to the upper and lower lips.

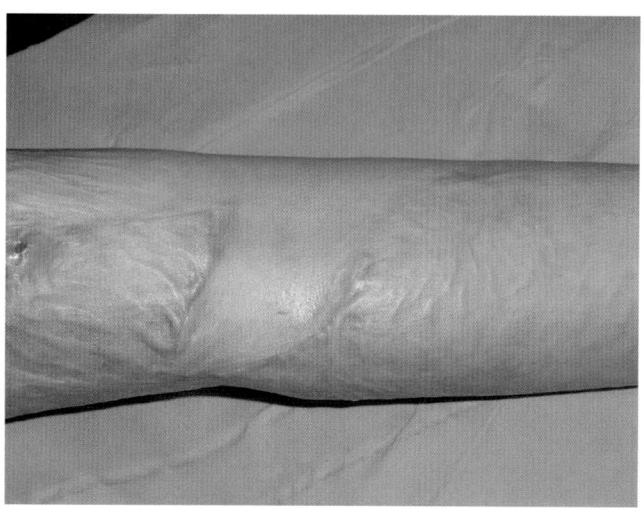

Figure 28.9 A transposition flap bringing normal skin across a scarred elbow.

MINOR BURNS/OUT-PATIENT BURNS

Local burn wound care

Blisters

Whether to remove blisters or leave them intact has been the subject of much debate. Proponents of blister removal quote laboratory studies which show that blister fluid depresses immune function, slowing down chemotaxis and intracellular killing and also acting as a medium for bacterial growth.

Conversely, other authors advocate leaving blisters intact as they form a sterile stratum spongiosum. Leaving a ruptured blister is not advised.

Initial cleaning of the burn wound

Washing the burn wound with chlorhexidine solution is ideal for this purpose.

Topical agents

For initial management of minor burns that are superficial or partial thickness, dressings with a non-adherent material such as Vaseline-impregnated gauze or Mepitel are often sufficient. These dressings are left in place for 5 days. These burns, by definition, should be healed after 7–10 days. Various topical creams and

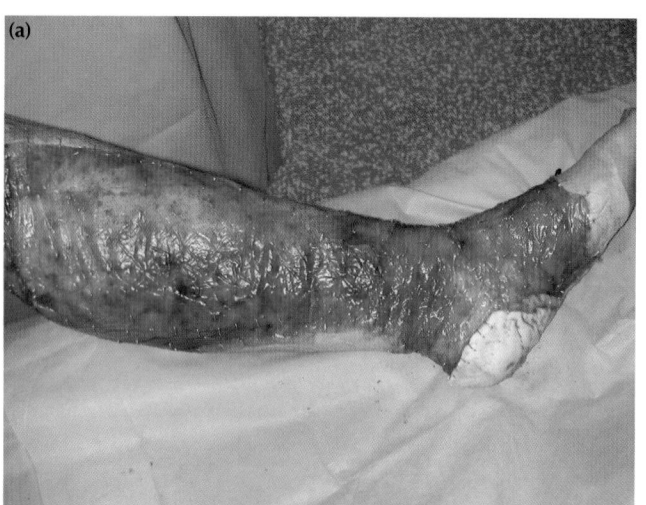

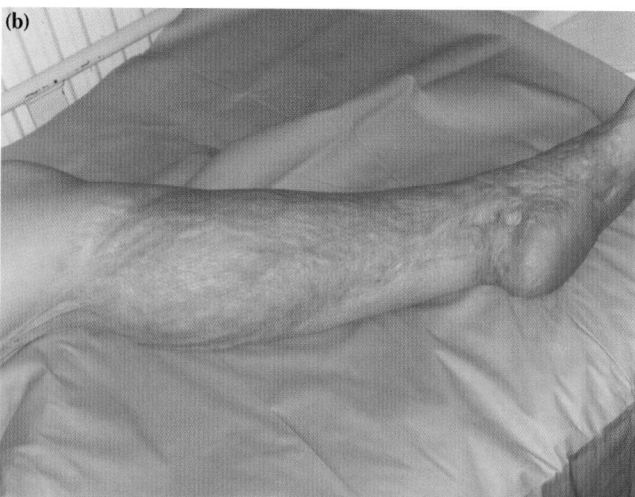

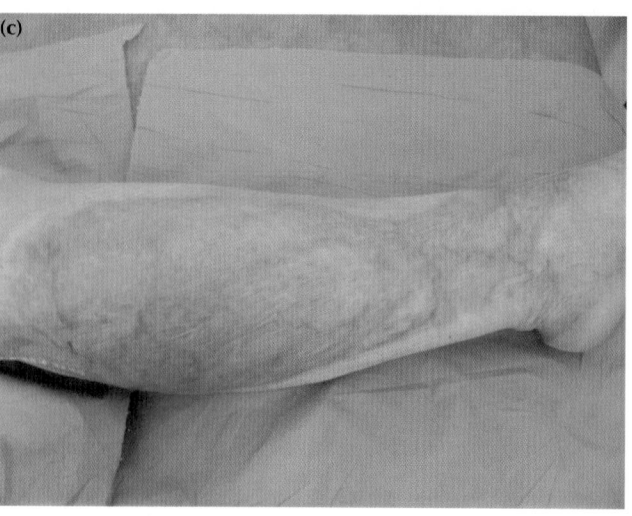

Figure 28.10 (a) A healed full-thickness leg burn prior to resurfacing with Integra. (b) The burn scar has been excised, and the raw surface of the artificial dermis is shown prior to split-skin grafting. (c) The rest after resurfacing with the artificial dermis Integra. The skin is smoother but remains scarred and still has no skin appendages such as hair or sweat glands.

ointments have been used for the treatment of minor burns. All published comparative data show no advantage of these agents over petroleum gauze.

Silver sulphadiazine (1%) or Flamazine is the most commonly used topical agent. However, it should be avoided in pregnant women, nursing mothers and infants less than 2 months of age because of the increased possibility of kernicterus in these patients.

Dressing the minor burn wound

This very important facet of burn care has unfortunately had virtually no objective studies. The aims of dressing are to decrease wound pain and to protect and isolate the burn wound. The small superficial burn requires Vaseline gauze or another non-adherent dressing such as Mepitel as the first layer. Following this, gauze or Kerlix is wrapped around with sufficient tightness to keep the dressing intact but not to impede the circulation. This is further wrapped with bandage. It is important to realise that bulkiness of dressings in the minor burn wound depends upon the amount of wound discharge. A special case is burns of the hands where dressings should be minimised so as not to impede mobilisation and physiotherapy.

Synthetic burn wound dressings are popular as they:

* decrease pain associated with dressings;
* improve healing times;
* decrease out-patient appointments;
* lower overall costs.

Biobrane is a bilaminar dressing made up of an inner layer of knitted nylon threads coated with porcine collagen and an outer layer of rubberised silicone impervious to gases but not to fluids and bacteria. Wounds to be dressed with Biobrane should be carefully selected. Burn wounds should be fresh (less than 24 hours), sensate, show capillary blanching and refill. Biobrane should be applied to the wound after removal of all blisters. It should be checked at 48 hours for adherence and any signs of infection. It should be removed if any sign of infection is found.

Duoderm or hydrocolloid dressings are not bulky, help in healing and can be kept in place for 48–72 hours. They provide a moist environment, which helps in re-epithelialisation of the burn wound.

Healing of burn wounds

Burns that are being managed conservatively should be healed within 3 weeks. If there are no signs of re-epithelialisation in this time, the wound requires debridement and grafting.

Infection

Infection in the minor burn should be tackled very aggressively as it is known to convert a superficial burn to a partial-thickness burn and a partial- to a deep partial-thickness burn respectively. It should be managed using a combination of topical and systemic agents. Debridement and skin grafting should also be considered.

Itching

Most burn patients have itchy wounds. Histamine and various endopeptides are said to be the causative factors of itching. This is another area that lacks controlled trials; therefore, management varies greatly. Anti-histamines, analgesics, moisturising creams, aloe vera and antibiotics have all been tried with varying degrees of success.

Traumatic blisters

The healed burn wound is prone to getting traumatic blisters because the new epithelium is very fragile. Non-adherent dressings usually suffice; regular moisturisation is also useful in this condition.

NON-THERMAL BURN INJURY

Electrical injuries

Electrical injuries are usually divided into low- and high-voltage injuries, the threshold being 1000 V (Summary box 28.19).

Summary box 28.19
Electrical burns
■ Low-voltage injuries cause small, localised, deep burns
■ They can cause cardiac arrest through pacing interruption without significant direct myocardial damage
■ High-voltage injuries damage by flash (external burn) and conduction (internal burn)
■ Myocardium may be directly damaged without pacing interruption
■ Limbs may need fasciotomies or amputation
■ Look for and treat acidosis and myoglobinuria

Low-tension injuries

Low-tension, or domestic appliance, injuries do not have enough energy to cause destruction to significant amounts of subcutaneous tissues when the current passes through the body. The resistance is too great. The entry and exit points, normally in the fingers, suffer small deep burns; these may cause underlying tendon and nerve damage, but there will be little damage between. The alternating current creates a tetany within the muscles, and thus patients often describe how they were unable to release the device until the power was turned off. The main danger with these injuries is from the alternating current interfering with normal cardiac pacing. This can cause cardiac arrest. The electricity itself does not usually cause significant underlying myocardial damage, so resuscitation, if successful, should be lasting.

High-tension injuries

High-tension electrical injuries can be caused by one of three sources of damage: the flash, the flame and the current itself.

When a high-tension line is earthed, enormous energy is released as the current travels from the line to the earth. It can arc over the patient, causing a flash burn. The extremely rapid heating of the air causes an explosion that often propels the victim backwards. The key here is that the current travelled from the line to the earth directly and not through the patient. The flash, however, can go on to ignite the patient's clothes and so cause a normal flame burn.

In accidents with overhead lines, the patient often acts as the conduction rod to earth. In these injuries, there is enough current to cause damage to the subcutaneous tissues and muscles. The entry and exit points are damaged but, importantly, the current can cause huge amounts of subcutaneous damage between these two points. These can be extremely serious injuries.

The damage to the underlying muscles in the affected limb can cause the rapid onset of compartment syndrome. The release of the myoglobins will cause myoglobinuria and subsequent renal dysfunction. Therefore, during the resuscitation of these patients,

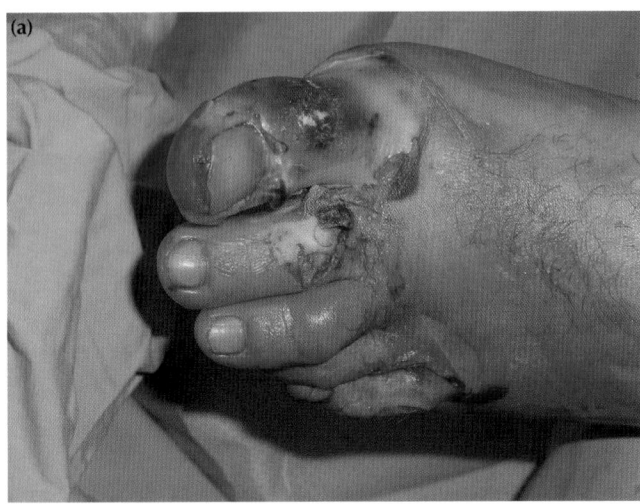
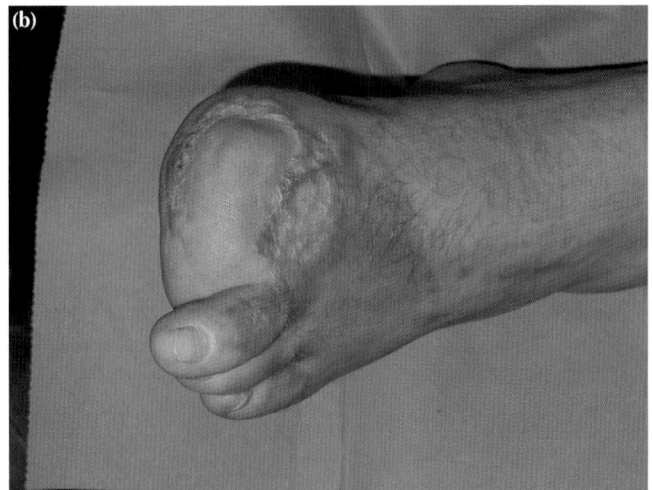

Figure 28.11 (a) An exit wound of a high-tension injury, with a dead big toe and significant damage to the medial portion of the second toe. (b) Amputation and cover with the lateral portion of the second toe.

efforts must be made to maintain a high urine output of up to 2 ml kg^{-1} body weight per hour. Severe acidosis is common in large electrical burns and may require boluses of bicarbonate. These patients are also at risk of myocardial damage as a result of direct muscle damage rather than by interference with cardiac pacing. This gives rise to significant electrocardiogram changes, with raised cardiac enzymes. If there is significant damage, there is rapid onset of heart failure. In the case of a severe injury through a limb, primary amputation is sometimes the most effective management (Fig. 28.11).

Chemical injuries

There are over 70 000 different chemicals in regular use within industry. Occasionally, these cause burns. Ultimately, there are two aspects to a chemical injury. The first is the physical destruction of the skin, and the second is any poisoning caused by systemic absorption (Summary box 28.20).

Summary box 28.20

Chemical burns

- Damage is from corrosion and poisoning
- Copious lavage with water helps in most cases
- Then identify the chemical and assess the risks of absorption

---

The initial management of any chemical injury is copious lavage with water. There are only a handful of chemicals for which water is not helpful, for example phosphorus, which is a component of some military devices, and elemental sodium, which is occasionally present in laboratory explosions. These substances need to be physically removed with forceps; however, it is extremely rare that any medical practitioner will encounter these in his or her lifetime. The more common injuries are caused by either acids or alkalis. Alkalis are usually the more destructive and are especially dangerous if they have come into contact with the eyes. After copious lavage, the next step in the management of any chemical injury is to identify the chemical and its concentration and to elucidate whether there is any underlying threat to the patient's life if absorbed systemically.

One acid that is a common cause of acid burns is hydrofluoric acid. Burns affecting the fingers and caused by dilute acid are relatively common. The initial management is with calcium gluconate gel topically; however, severe burns or burns to large areas of the hand can be subsequently treated with Bier's blocks containing calcium gluconate 10% gel. If the patient has been burnt with a concentration greater than 50%, the threat of hypocalcaemia and subsequent arrhythmias then becomes high, and this is an indication for acute early excision. It is best not to split-skin graft these hydrofluoric acid wounds initially, but to do this at a delayed stage.

Ionising radiation injury

These injuries can be divided into groups depending on whether radiation exposure was to the whole body or localised. The management of localised radiation damage is usually conservative until the true extent of the tissue injury is apparent. Should this damage have caused an ulcer, then excision and coverage with vascularised tissue is required.

Whole-body radiation causes a large number of symptoms. The dose of radiation either is or is not lethal. A patient who has suffered whole-body irradiation and is suffering from acute desquamation of the skin has received a lethal dose of radiation, which can cause a particularly slow and unpleasant death. Non-lethal radiation has a number of systemic effects related to the gut mucosa and immune system dysfunction. Other than giving iodine tablets, the management of these injuries is supportive (Summary box 28.21).

Summary box 28.21

Radiation burns

- Local burns causing ulceration need excision and vascularised flap cover – usually with free flaps
- Systemic overdose needs supportive treatment

August Karl Gustav Bier, **1861–1949**, Professor of Surgery, Berlin, Germany.

Cold injuries

Cold injuries are principally divided into two types: acute cold injuries from industrial accidents and frostbite (Summary box 28.22).

Summary box 28.22

Cold injuries

- The damage is more difficult to define and slower to develop than burns
- Acute frostbite needs rapid rewarming, then observation
- Delay surgery until demarcation is clear

Exposure to liquid nitrogen and other such liquids will cause epidermal and dermal destruction. The tissue is more resistant to cold injury than to heat injury, and the inflammatory reaction is not as marked. The assessment of depth of injury is more difficult, so it is rare to make the decision for surgery early.

Frostbite injuries affect the peripheries in cold climates. The initial treatment is with rapid rewarming in a bath at 42°C. The cold injury produces delayed microvascular damage similar to that of cardiac reperfusion injury. The level of damage is difficult to assess, and surgery usually does not play a role in its management, which is conservative, until there is absolute demarcation of the level of injury.

FURTHER READING

British Burns Association (2004) *Emergency Management of Burns*, 8th edn. UK Course Pre-reading. British Burns Association.

Herndon, D. (ed.) (2007) *Total Burn Care*, 3rd edn. Saunders and Elsevier, Philadelphia, PA.

Pape, S., Judkins, K. and Settle, J. (2000) *Burns: The First Five Days*, 2nd edn. Smith and Nephew, Romford.

Plastic and reconstructive surgery

CHAPTER
29

LEARNING OBJECTIVES

To understand:
- The spectrum of plastic surgical techniques used to restore bodily form and function
- The relevant anatomy and physiology of tissues used in reconstruction
- The various skin grafts and how to use them appropriately
- The principles and use of flaps
- How to use plastic surgery to manage difficult and complex tissue loss

HISTORICAL CONTEXT

Reconstructive plastic (from the ancient Greek *plassein*, to mould or shape – also the stem for our modern use of the materials termed plastics) surgery involves using various techniques to restore form and function to the body when tissues have been damaged by injury, cancer or congenital loss. Its origins can be traced back to ancient Egypt, with wound care depicted in hieroglyphs on papyrus, to India in the sixth century BC, where Sushruta described using the forehead flap to reconstruct a nose, and to Al-Zahrawi, the tenth-century Islamic surgical scholar from Cordoba. Modern techniques were developed after the First World War, especially with Sir Harold Gillies' work on reconstructing facial injuries (Fig. 29.1), which was enabled by new safe anaesthetic intubation (Sir Ivan Magill). Later in the twentieth century, renewed understanding of detailed soft tissue anatomy led to an explosion in the use of new flaps, which with microsurgical methods, craniofacial surgery and tissue expansion resulted in an entirely new set of techniques becoming available to surgeons for reconstructing parts.

Today, the need for reconstructive plastic surgery, especially in developing nations, has never been greater. Road, war and domestic injury inflict life-diminishing effects, which plastic surgery can reduce. The reconstructive surgeon's 'toolbox' is now very diverse and will continue to grow in order to address problem wounds and tissue defects, which arise as modern medical care is more successful in treating cancer, preserving life into old age and salvaging victims of trauma.

ANATOMY RELATED TO RECONSTRUCTIVE SURGERY

Skin

The surface of the skin is important as a biological layer for homeostasis. Restoring the skin surface is therefore critical even if the underlying structures can await later reconstruction. Epidermis regenerates from deeper follicular elements, with the most superficial layer losing vascularity and acting as a barrier to fluid loss and providing important protection against invasion by micro-

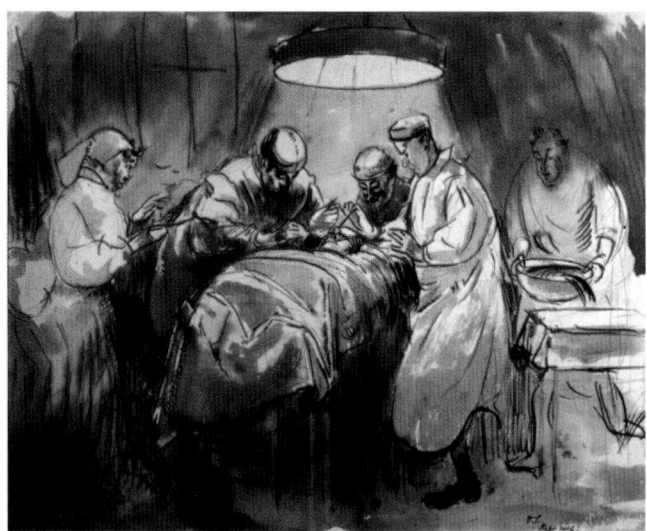

Figure 29.1 Sir Harold Gillies operating during the First World War – 'the birth of plastic surgery'. Picture by Henry Tonks (by kind permission of the Royal College of Surgeons of England).

Sir Harold Delf Gillies, **1882–1960**, Plastic Surgeon, St. Bartholomew's Hospital, London, England.
Sir Ivan Whiteside Magill, **1888–1986**, Anaesthetist, Westminster Hospital, London, England.

Henry Tonks, **1862–1937**, commenced a career in surgery, but abandoned it for art, and became, from 1917 to 1930, Slade Professor at the Westminster School of Art, London, England.

organisms. (Epidermal keratinocytes can be artificially cultured *in vitro* and are used in some wound management systems.)

The depth of the dermis and the amounts of elastin and skin adnexal elements such as sweat glands and hair follicles vary depending on the functional requirements of the area concerned. This means that some areas are much more vulnerable to injury than others, e.g. the fine flexible elastic skin of the eyelid rapidly suffers a full-thickness burn after a flash burn, whereas thick back skin suffers only a partial loss after the same flash burn.

Skin vascularity is derived from fine perforating vessels that run through underlying muscles or through fascial septal layers, and then horizontally in a subcutaneous plane from which capillaries branch (Fig. 29.2). Nerves run axially out from major trunks and are less well defined than most perforating blood vessels.

When local, random-pattern skin flaps are raised, they are lifted at the subcutaneous level and are nourished by the subdermal plexus of blood vessels. However, this plexus can only survive a limited distance from the more substantial arterial branches running in the fascial, septal or muscle-perforating planes. Understanding the anatomy of different parts of the skin and tissues to be moved is a key element of successful plastic surgery.

Without skin, wounds heal by *secondary intention* with fibrosis and contracture (Fig. 29.3), and underlying structures are vulnerable to necrosis, chronic infection and dysfunction.

Graft anatomy

Split-thickness skin grafts

Split-thickness skin grafts are harvested by taking all of the epidermis together with some dermis, leaving the remaining dermis behind to heal the donor site. The thicker the dermis that is taken (seen by more brisk punctate bleeding at the donor site; Fig. 29.4), the more durable will be the graft once healed (although it might take longer and require more care), but also the more difficult will be donor site healing (Summary box 29.1).

Summary box 29.1

Split-thickness skin grafts

- Thicker knife-gap settings recognised give rise to fewer but brisker bleeding points on the donor site
- Thicker grafts heal with less contracture and are more durable
- Thinner donor sites heal better
- Grafts are hairless and do not sweat (these structures are not transferred)

Full-thickness skin grafts

Full-thickness grafts are harvested to incorporate the whole dermis, with the underlying fat trimmed away – unless elements of fat (or even cartilage as well) are deliberately left attached to form a *composite graft*. Full-thickness and composite grafts require the best handling and postoperative nursing to help ensure that they 'take' in their transplanted site.

How does a skin graft survive?

Split-thickness skin grafts survive initially by *imbibition* of plasma from the wound bed; after 48 hours fine anastomotic connections

In vitro **is Latin for 'in the glass'.**

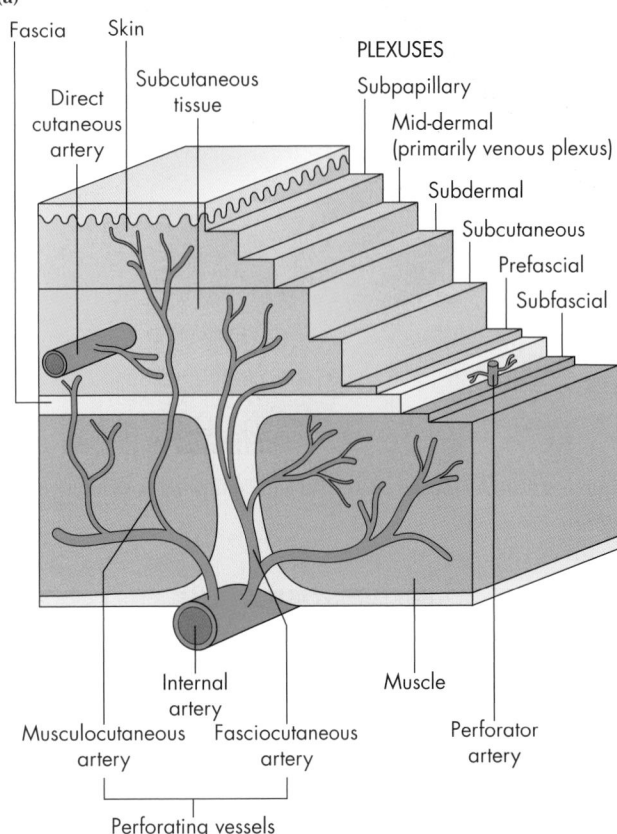

(a)

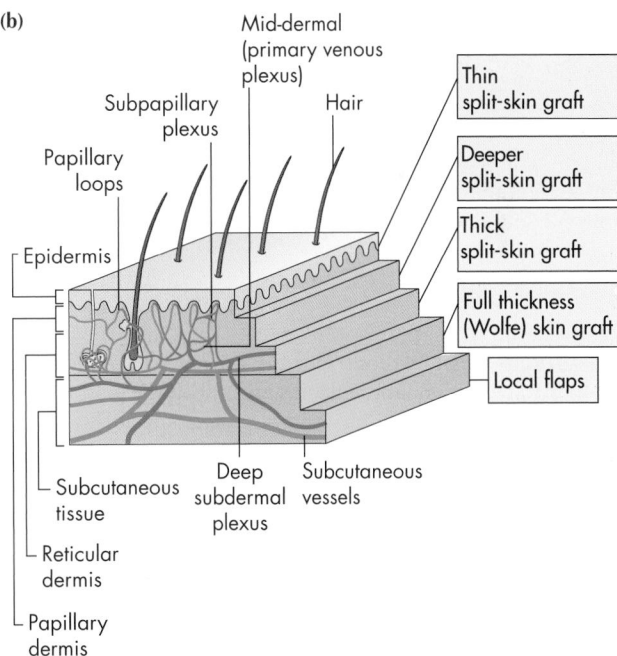

(b)

Figure 29.2 Diagram of skin anatomy with vascular plexus.

are made, which lead to *inosculation* of blood. Capillary ingrowth then completes the healing process with fibroblast maturation. Because only tissues that produce granulation will support a graft, it is usually *contraindicated* to use grafts to cover exposed tendons, cartilage or cortical bone.

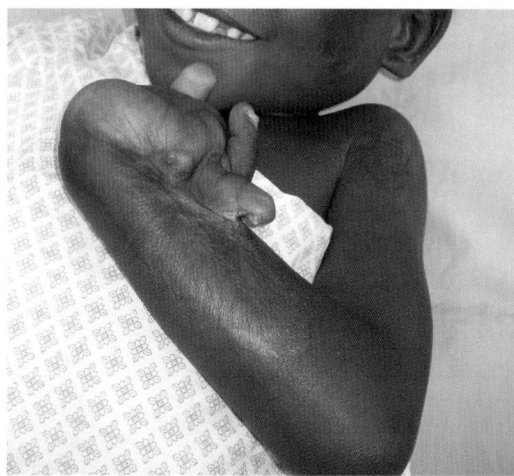

Figure 29.3 A severely contracted hand following burn to the dorsal aspect.

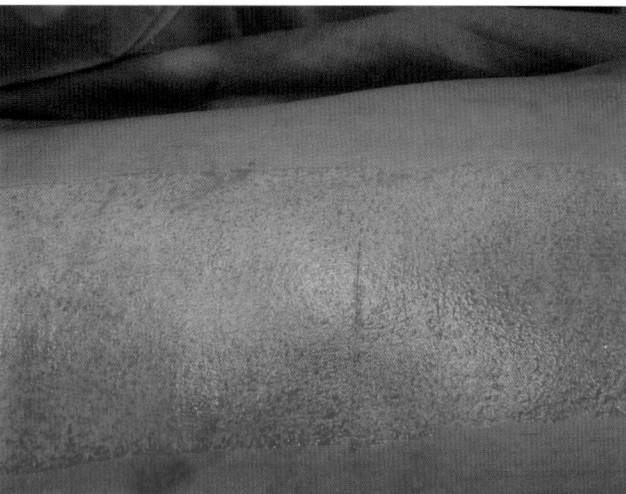

Figure 29.4 Fine punctate bleeding from a split-thickness skin graft donor site.

Skin grafts inevitably contract, with the extent of contracture determined by the amount of dermis taken with the graft and the level of postoperative splintage and physiotherapy applied to the grafted site.

CLASSIFICATION

The reconstructive 'toolbox'

Plastic surgery has a number of means available for managing a given problem. Sometimes, a problem is managed using a 'ladder' approach, with the simplest methods being used first and only moving to more complex methods when absolutely necessary. However, this is not always the best way to proceed. If resources permit, it is often more cost-effective and better functionally for the patient to begin with a more complex treatment, with other easier managements held in reserve as 'lifeboats'. Plastic surgeons now prefer to think of the range of options available as a 'toolbox' from which they can take the most appropriate method to solve

a problem, taking into account available skill, resources and the consequences of failure.

The scope of plastic surgery

The tools of reconstruction are used for a wide range of conditions:

- trauma:
  - soft-tissue loss (skin, tendons, nerves, muscle);
  - hand and lower limb injury;
  - faciomaxillary;
  - burns;
- cancer:
  - skin, head and neck, breast, soft tissue sarcoma;
- congenital:
  - clefts and craniofacial malformations;
  - skin, giant naevi, vascular malformations;
  - urogenital;
  - hand and limb malformations;
- miscellaneous:
  - Bell's (facial) palsy;
  - pressure sores;
  - aesthetic surgery;
  - chest wall reconstruction.

A few key principles that can also be applied to other surgical specialties should be observed. In many reconstructions, success depends upon good rapid wound healing, which itself depends upon attention to detail from the surgeon. Adequate debridement, careful technique, gentle handling of tissues and consideration of blood supply are all key factors that influence outcome (Table 29.1).

The placement of incisions can be critical, especially in reducing the appearance of scars on the face and in areas of tension. When possible, incisions should lie in the lines of minimal tension (described by Langer but frequently different from those originally noted) (Fig. 29.5).

Grafts

Grafts are tissues that are transferred without their blood supply, which therefore have to revascularise once they are in a new site. They include the following:

- *Split-thickness skin grafts* (of varying thickness). These are sometimes called Thiersch grafts. They are used to cover all sizes of

Table 29.1 Plastic surgery principles

Optimise wound by adequate debridement or resection
Wound or flap must have a good blood supply to heal
Place scars carefully – 'lines of election'[a]
Replace defect with similar tissue – 'like with like'[b]
Observe meticulous surgical technique
Remember donor site 'cost'

[a] Lines of election – analogous to Langer's lines of minimal skin tension.
[b] Millard, D.R. (1986) *Principalization of Plastic Surgery*. Little & Brown, Boston.

Sir Charles Bell, **1774–1842**, Surgeon, The Middlesex Hospital, London, England, and from 1835 until his death, Professor of Surgery, The University of Edinburgh, Scotland.
Karl Ritter von Edenberg Langer, **1819–1887**, Professor of Anatomy, Vienna, Austria, described these lines in 1862.

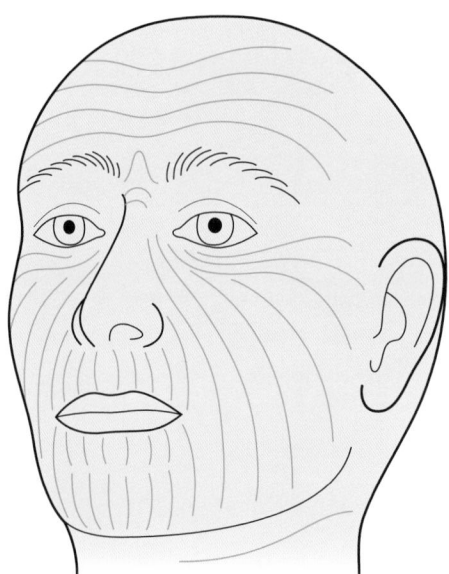

Figure 29.5 Lines of relaxed skin tension.

wound, are of limited durability and will contract. They may be used to provide valuable temporary wound closure before better cosmetic secondary correction after rehabilitation.
- *Full-thickness skin grafts* (Wolfe grafts). Used for smaller areas of skin replacement where good elastic skin that will not contract is required (such as fingers, eyelids, facial parts).
- *Composite skin grafts* (usually skin and fat, or skin and carti-

lage). Often taken from the ear margin and useful for rebuilding missing elements of nose, eyelids and fingertips.
- *Nerve grafts.* Usually taken from the sural nerve but smaller cutaneous nerves may be used.
- *Tendon grafts.* Usually taken from the palmaris longus or plantaris tendon (runs just anteromedial to the Achilles tendon) and used for injury loss or nerve damage correction.

Flaps

Flaps are tissues that are transferred with a blood supply. They therefore have the advantage of bringing vascularity to the new area. Flaps can be raised to consist of any specific tissue; for skin flaps the following will illustrate the types that exist (Fig. 29.6):

- *Random flaps.* Three sides of a rectangle, bearing no specific relationship to where the blood supply enters; the length to breadth ratio is no more than 1.5:1. This pattern can be lengthened by 'delaying' the flap, a process in which the cuts are partially made and the flap is part lifted at a first operation; it is then replaced, thus 'training' the blood supply from a single border of the rectangle. At a second procedure it is raised further and finally transferred.
- *Axial flaps.* Much longer flaps, based on known blood vessels supplying the skin. This technique was rediscovered in the 1960s/70s and enables many long thin flaps to be safely moved across large distances.
- *Pedicled/islanded flaps.* The axial blood supply of these flaps means that they can be swung round on a stalk or even fully 'islanded' so that the business end of the skin being transferred can have the pedicle buried (Fig 29.7).

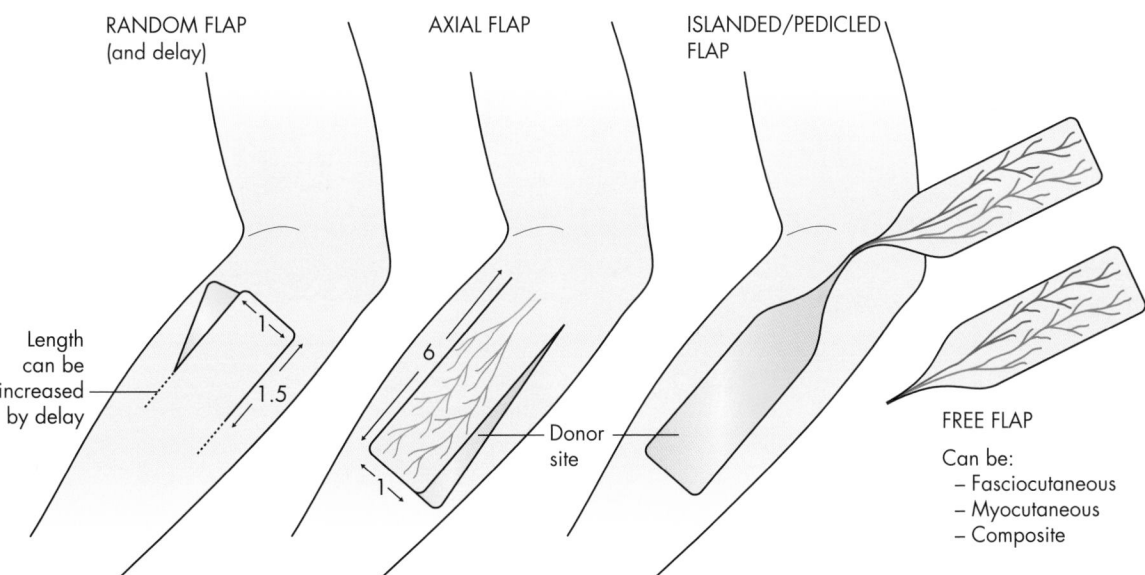

Figure 29.6 Skin flaps, from simple to complex.

Karl Thiersch, 1822–1895, Professor of Surgery, Leipzig, Germany. He was a pioneer of free skin grafts, and described his method of skin grafting in 1874.
John Reissburg Wolfe, 1824–1904, Ophthalmic Surgeon, Glasgow, Scotland, described full thickness skin grafts in 1875, and in the same year used forearm skin to construct an eyelid.
Achilles, the Greek Hero, was the son of Peleus and Thetis. When he was a child his mother dipped him in the Styx, one of the rivers of the Underworld, so that he should be invulnerable in battle. The heel by which she held him did not get wet, and was, therefore, not protected. Achilles died from a wound in the heel which he received at the siege of Troy.

CHAPTER 29 | PLASTIC AND RECONSTRUCTIVE SURGERY

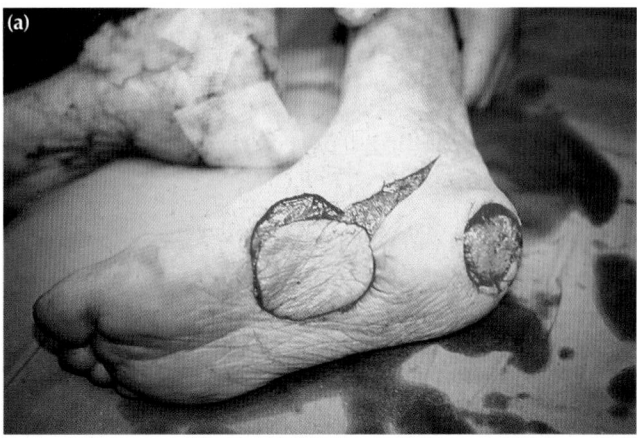

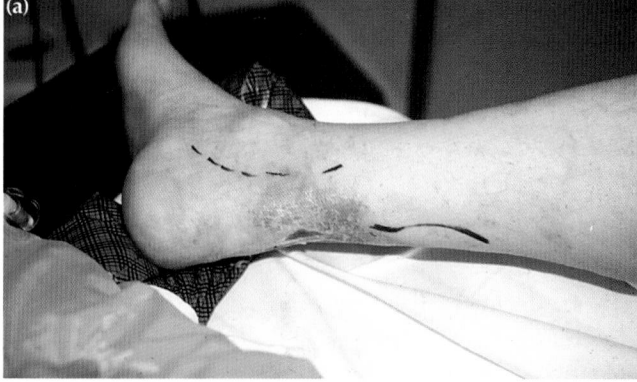

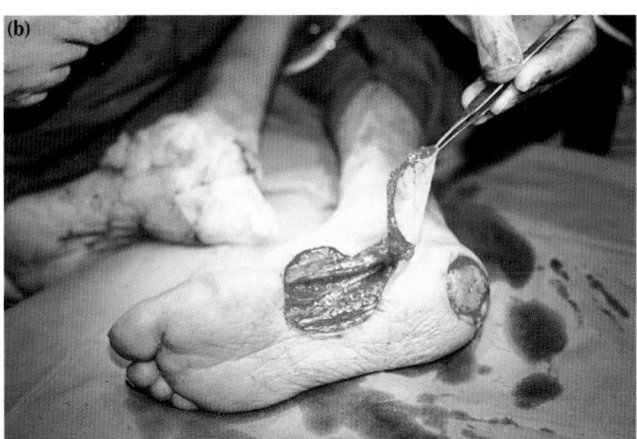

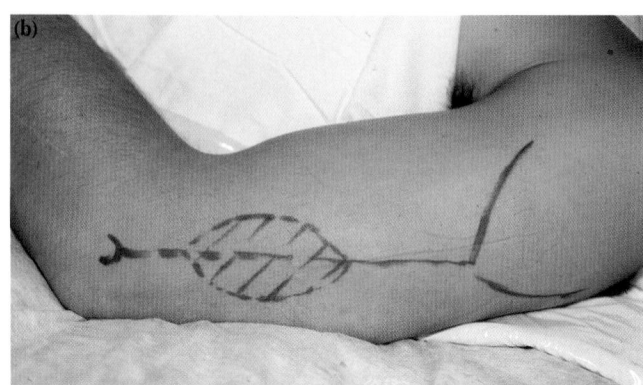

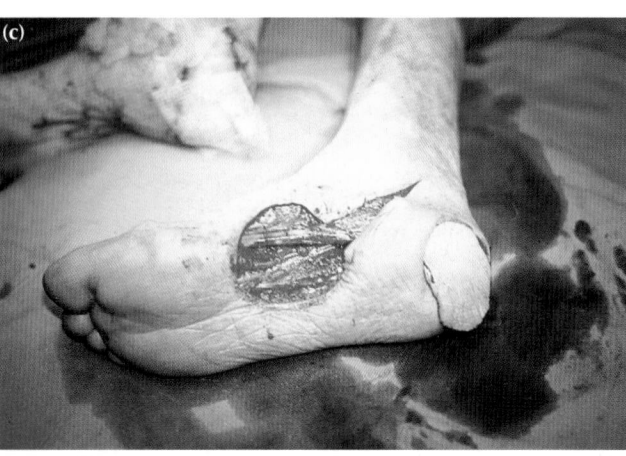

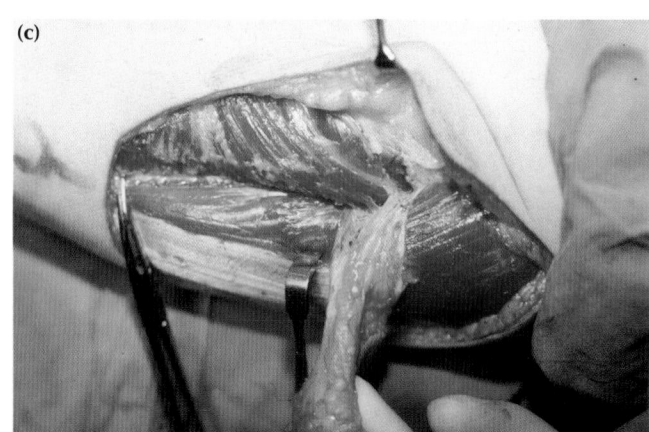

Figure 29.7 (a–c) Islanded pedicled flap used from instep to resurface heel defect.

- *Free flaps.* The blood supply has been isolated, disconnected and then reconnected using microsurgery at the new site (Fig. 29.8).
- *Composite flaps.* Various tissues are transferred together, often skin with bone or muscle (osseocutaneous or myocutaneous flaps respectively).
- *Perforator flaps.* This description refers to a whole new subgroup of axial flaps in which tissues are isolated on small perforating vessels that run from more major blood vessels to supply the surface.

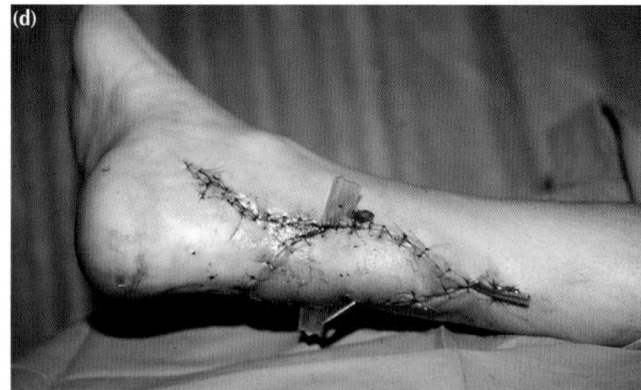

Figure 29.8 (a–d) Free lateral arm fasciocutaneous flap used to resurface a tendo Achilles defect.

Skin substitutes

One solution to the problem presented by major skin loss with inadequate skin donor sites has been to use artificially engineered skin substitutes. These vary from thin sheets of autologous keratinocytes, to artificial collagen matrices with embedded fibroblasts and a keratinocyte sheet covering. They are costly but are becoming widely used, and it is likely that tissue-engineered products will continue to be developed in an attempt to solve difficult reconstructive problems.

Tissue expansion

This technique is valuable in using 'local' tissue for reconstruction. The natural ability of tissue to expand has been harnessed clinically since the experiments of Austad and the clinical work of Radovan in the 1970s. It is a technique borrowed from nature, and it is observed during pregnancy when skin expands over the underlying mass. It involves placing a device – usually an expandable balloon constructed from silicone – beneath the tissue to be expanded and progressively enlarging the volume with fluid while the overlying tissue accommodates to the changed vascular pressure (Fig. 29.9). The fluid (usually sterile saline) is introduced via a self-sealing port attached to a filling tube that enters the balloon. It may be introduced as frequently as can be tolerated by the patient until the tissues are stretched enough to be used for reconstruction. The tissues expanded do not hypertrophy but there are major changes in the collagen structure.

The process is time-consuming although it can be very valuable in problematic cases. It is invaluable for sharing remaining areas of scalp hair after severe burns, removing major congenital skin naevi and restoring full-thickness skin over previously grafted limb wounds.

It must *never* be used under irradiated tissues (such as mastectomy sites), which will not expand but necrose (Summary box 29.2).

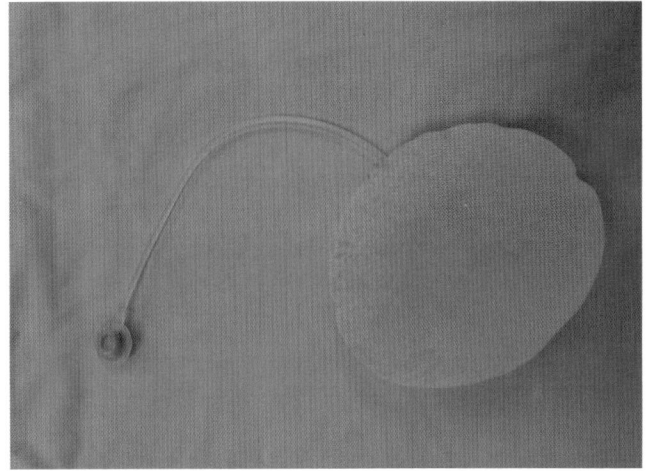

Figure 29.9 Tissue expander.

Implants and prosthetics

Many tissue deficiencies cannot be adequately reconstructed with autologous tissue, however sophisticated the technique used. In such circumstances, implants are part of the reconstructive surgical 'toolbox'; they include solid and soft silicone materials, many forms of filler including collagen and polymers, and osseointegratable anchor points for prosthesis fixation.

> **Summary box 29.2**
>
> **Tissue expansion**
>
> **Advantages**
> - Well-vascularised tissue
> - Tissue next to defect so likely to be of similar consistency
> - Good colour match
>
> **Disadvantages**
> - Multiple expansion episodes (sometimes painful)
> - Cost of device
> - High incidence of infection and extrusion (especially limbs)

Vacuum-assisted closure

The use of negative pressure applied to a tissue defect has positive effects on wound closure, as well as making difficult and complex wounds more manageable during the early stages of granulation. Exudate is removed and the suction pressure affects angiogenesis and tissue regeneration. The technique can be applied as part of early wound management before definitive surgical closure has been planned, or in some cases to avoid the need for surgery altogether. The foam sponge dressing is connected by a tube to a negative pressure pump that can be controlled to give intermittent suction.

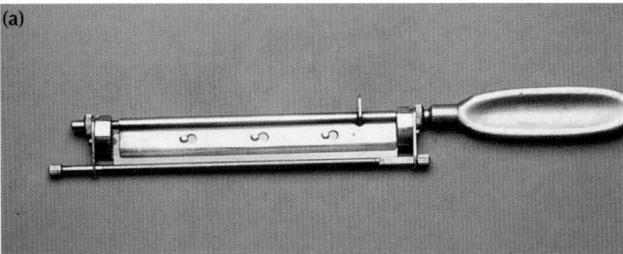
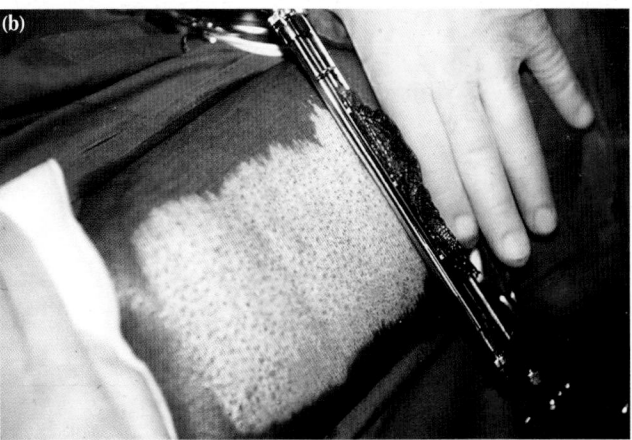

Figure 29.10 Hand-held skin knife (a) and harvesting skin with hand-held knife (b).

ASSESSMENT AND DIAGNOSTIC PLANNING

Formation of a definitive treatment plan, carefully considering all available options for care with the whole of the patient's needs in mind, is a vital component of wise plastic surgical practice. This is never more so than when managing major trauma cases in the acute setting or when planning major cancer man-agement, which might be staged over a period of treatments and procedures. If the reconstructive surgeon can be involved in early wound debridement and incisions, vital flap pedicles can be protected and the functional and cosmetic outcome made optimal. This pattern of shared team care has become the norm in many units demonstrating good outcomes from major trauma salvage.

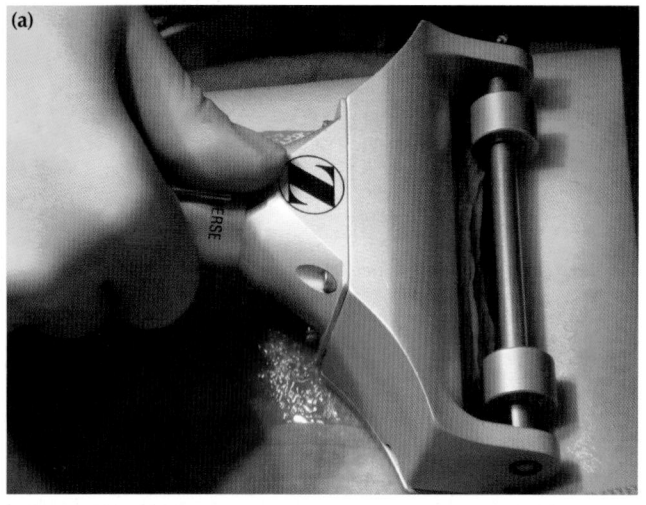
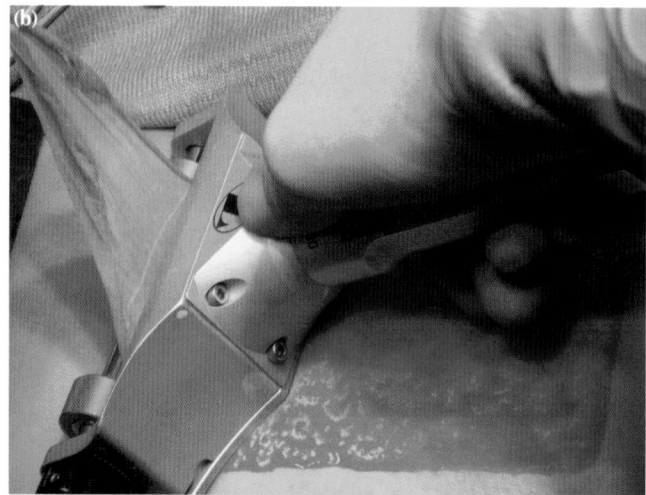
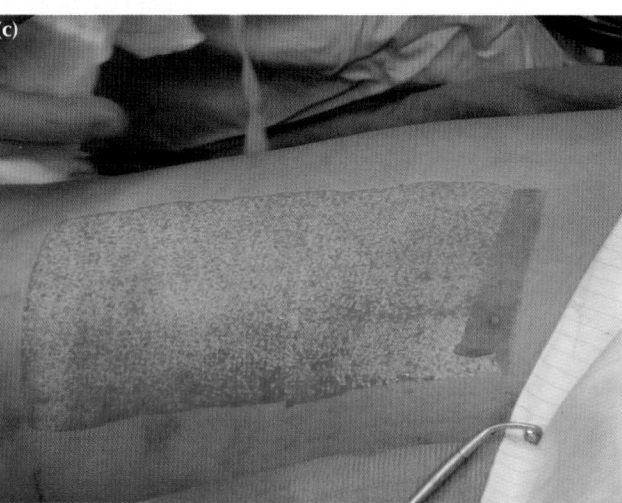
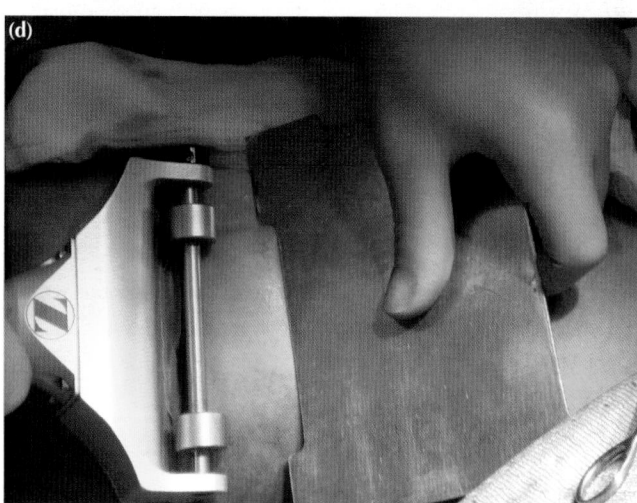
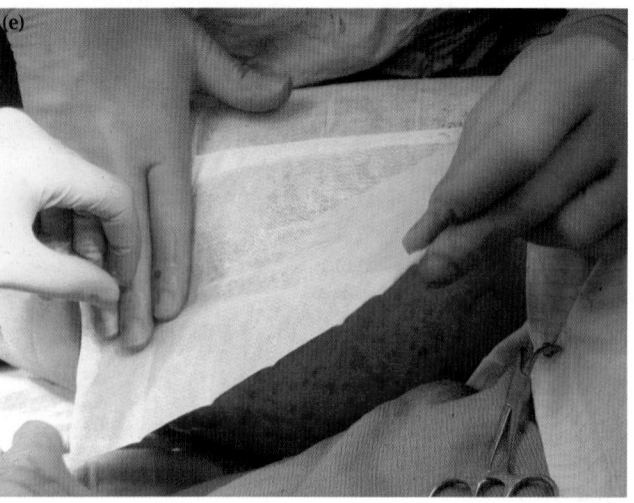

Figure 29.11 Power dermatome harvest of a split-thickness skin graft, with the correct method of providing skin tension (a–d), and dressing of donor site with adhesive material (e).

The initial assessment of wounds involves adequate removal of devitalised tissue, assessment of which vital structures will need reconstruction immediately and which might be better reconstructed later, and assessment of the degree of contamination involved, which will require further cleaning. Further planning will include the definitive soft-tissue cover of the wound and functional rehabilitation with full psychosocial rehabilitation.

TREATMENT AND COMPLICATIONS

Split-thickness skin grafts

Split-thickness skin grafts are taken with either hand-held (Fig. 29.10) or powered skin knives (Fig. 29.11). The most used donor site is the thigh, with the buttock preferable in children and cosmetically sensitive individuals. For larger grafts almost any flat surface can be harvested, including the scalp if shaved (a very good and useful donor site). The thickness of the graft harvested, ease of graft 'take' and donor site healing must be weighed against the lack of durability of thin split-thickness skin grafts.

Split grafts can be perforated to allow exudates to escape and improve 'take'; they can be further meshed to allow expansion (Fig. 29.12). This is carried out on a device that cuts a series of slits along the skin, allowing it to expand from a ratio of anything from 1:1.5 to about 1:6.

Grafts will only take on a bed on which they can become vascularised. Preparation of the wound bed is therefore an essential part of a successful graft (Figs 29.13 and 29.14). Graft failure is commonly caused by pus, exudate or residual dead tissue beneath the skin, haematoma or shearing forces. A clean healthy wound bed with a meshed graft tied in place to stop movement will encourage success. The group A β-haemolytic *Streptococcus* can destroy split grafts completely (and also convert a donor site to a full-thickness defect) and so the presence of this micro-organism is a *contraindication* to grafting.

Full-thickness skin grafts

Small dermal grafts (Wolfe grafts) can be taken from behind the ear, the groin creases and the neck, with easy direct closure of the donor site. Older people can sustain larger harvests because of skin laxity. Large full-thickness skin graft use is uncommon and requires great care to obtain a good take. Large donor sites

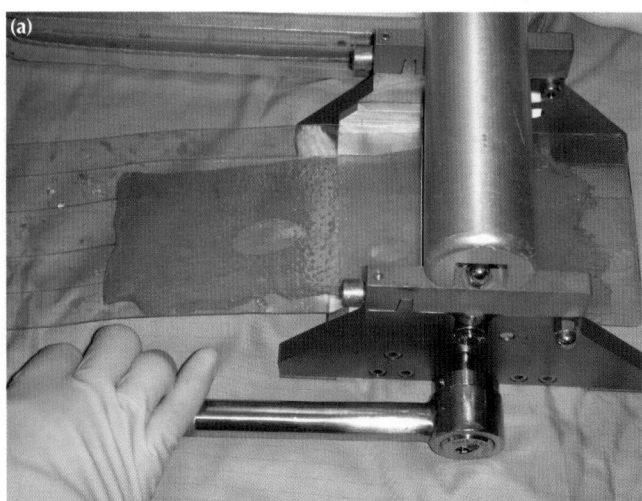

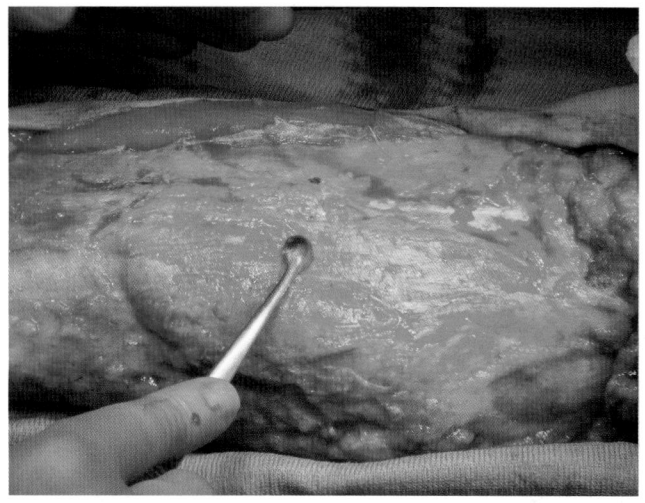

Figure 29.13 Cleaning a wound of excessive granulation tissue before grafting.

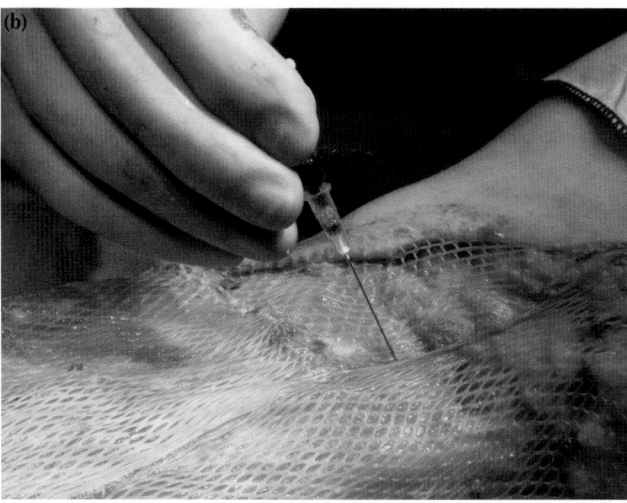

Figure 29.12 Split-thickness skin graft mesher (a) and meshed skin applied to wound (b).

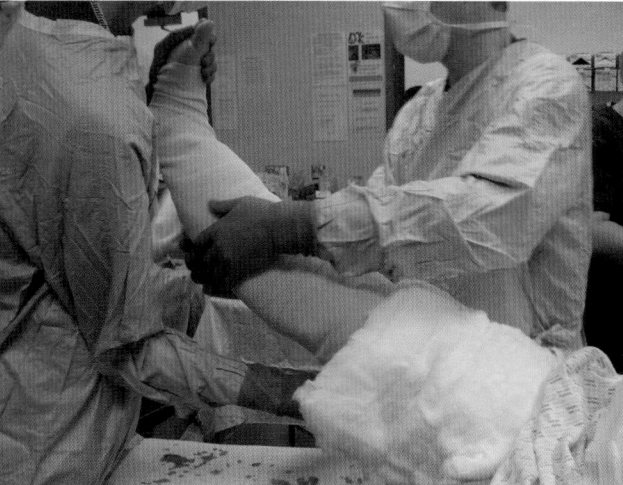

Figure 29.14 Application of a firm pressure dressing to ensure stability of the graft.

CHAPTER 29 | PLASTIC AND RECONSTRUCTIVE SURGERY

require secondary split-thickness skin grafting. Major secondary burn contractures of the face and flexion creases can achieve remarkable functional and cosmetic improvement using such large grafts, particularly as the remaining facial muscle function can still produce a more natural appearance than when covered by a bulky full-thickness skin flap. Smaller full-thickness grafts are useful for contracture release around sensitive facial and extremity structures.

Technique

The shape of the graft needed is drawn and copied onto a small template (paper or cloth), which is used to transfer the same shape to the donor site. Full-thickness skin is cut; grafts take best if additional underlying fat is removed, after which the graft is applied with normal skin tension and tied down with a pressure dressing. The graft will remain vulnerable to shearing forces for several weeks after application.

Flaps

Local flaps

A local flap is raised next to a tissue defect in order to reconstruct it. Basic patterns include (Fig. 29.15):

- *transposition flap*: the most basic design, leaving a graftable donor site (Fig. 29.16);
- *Z-plasty*: for lengthening scars or tissues;

TRANSPOSITION FLAP

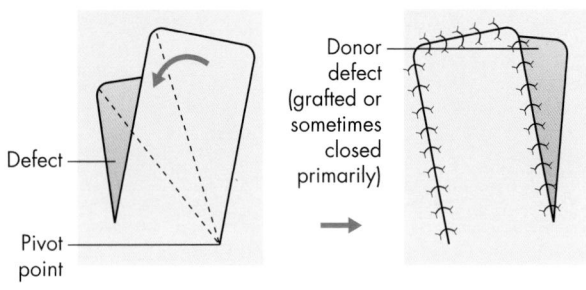

Z-PLASTY

Two triangular transposition flaps interposed

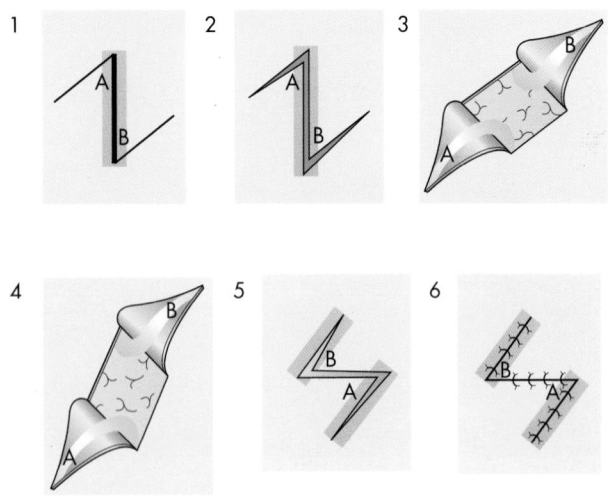

(a)

BILOBED FLAP

Uses a flap to close a convex defect, and a second smaller flap to close the donor site

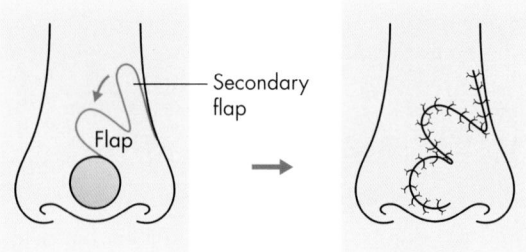

BIPEDICLE FLAP

A 'bucket-handle' flap supplied from both ends. Useful to rebuild the lower eyelid

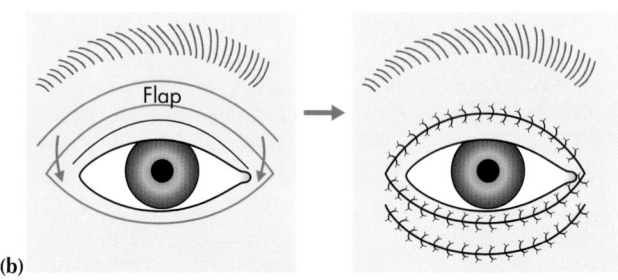

(b)

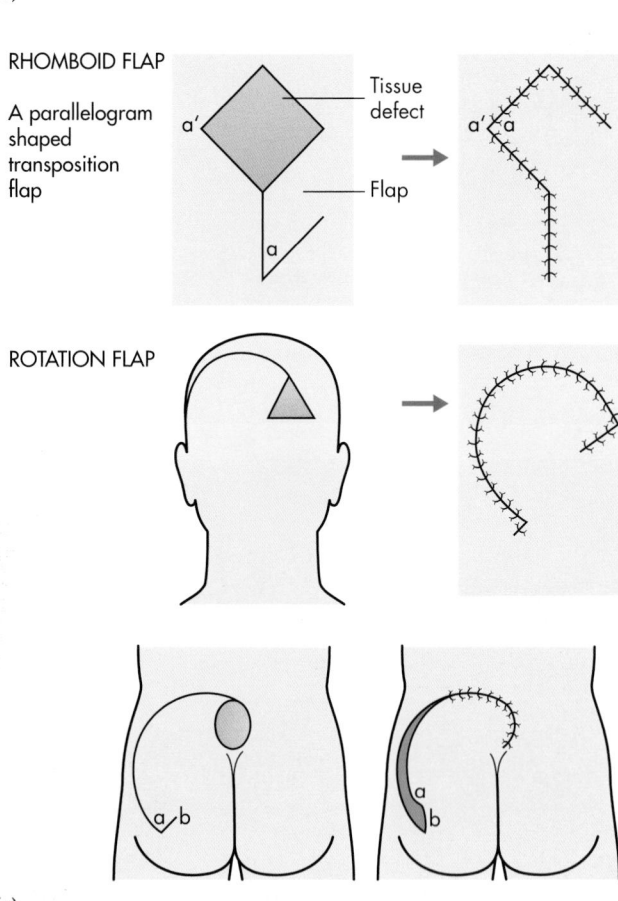

RHOMBOID FLAP

A parallelogram shaped transposition flap

ROTATION FLAP

(c)

Figure 29.15 Local flap diagrams. (a) Transposition and Z-plasty flaps; (b) bilobed and bipedicled flaps; (c) rhomboid and rotation flaps. (*continued opposite*)

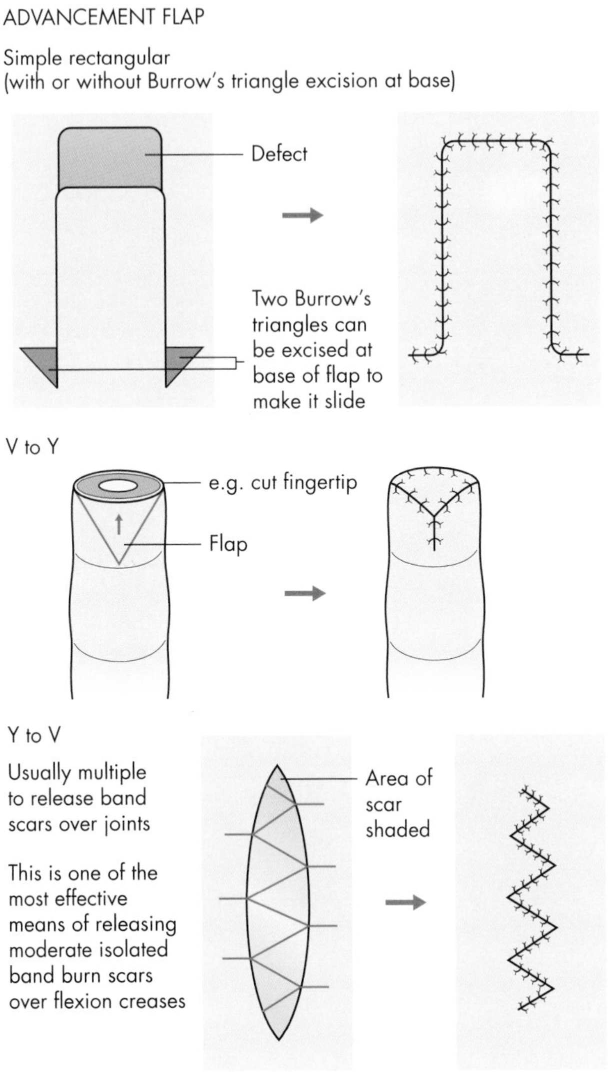

ADVANCEMENT FLAP

Simple rectangular
(with or without Burrow's triangle excision at base)

Defect

Two Burrow's triangles can be excised at base of flap to make it slide

V to Y

e.g. cut fingertip

Flap

Y to V

Usually multiple to release band scars over joints

This is one of the most effective means of releasing moderate isolated band burn scars over flexion creases

Area of scar shaded

(d)

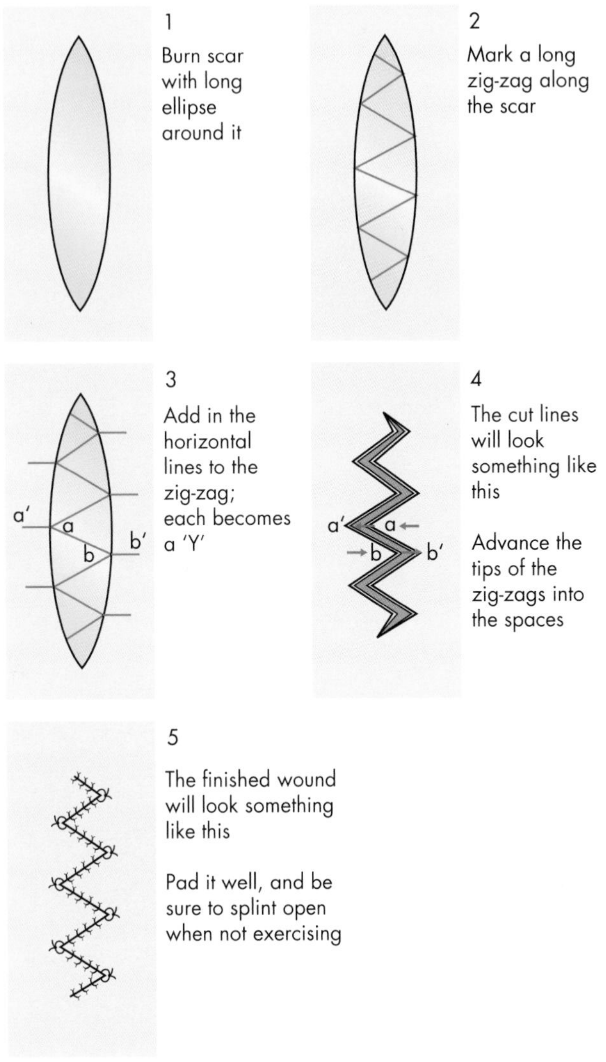

1
Burn scar with long ellipse around it

2
Mark a long zig-zag along the scar

3
Add in the horizontal lines to the zig-zag; each becomes a 'Y'

a' a b' b

4
The cut lines will look something like this

a' a b' b

Advance the tips of the zig-zags into the spaces

5
The finished wound will look something like this

Pad it well, and be sure to splint open when not exercising

(e)

Figure 29.15 (*continued*) Local flap diagrams. (d) Advancement flaps; (e) multiple Y-to-V plasty for burn scar.

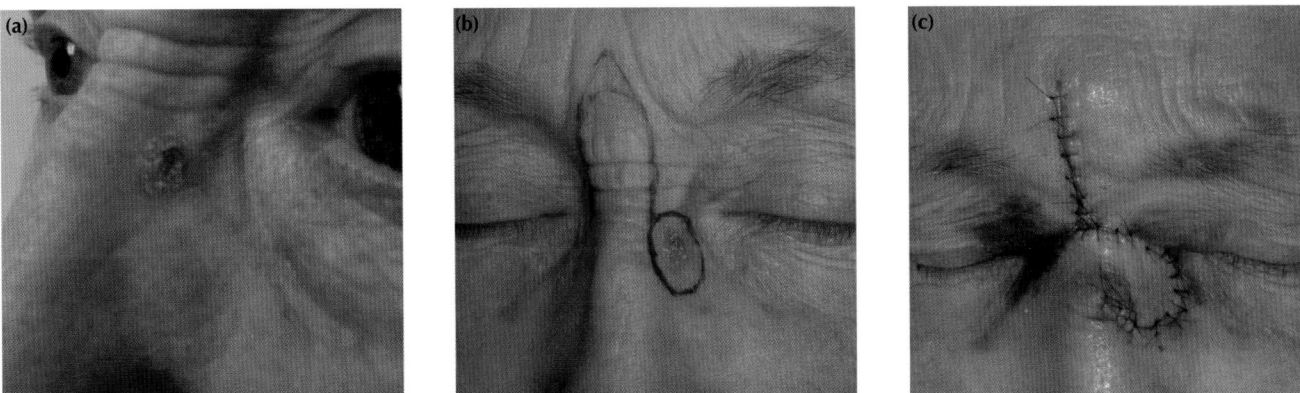

Figure 29.16 (a–c) Example of transposition flap (in this case from glabellar area to inner canthal defect). (*continued overleaf*)

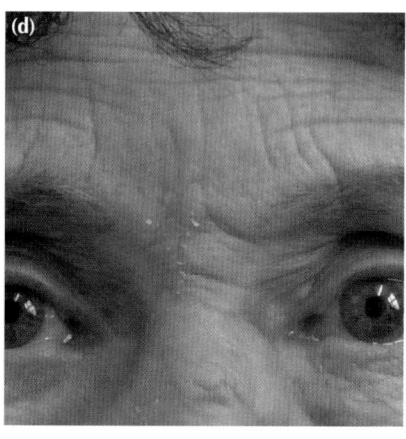

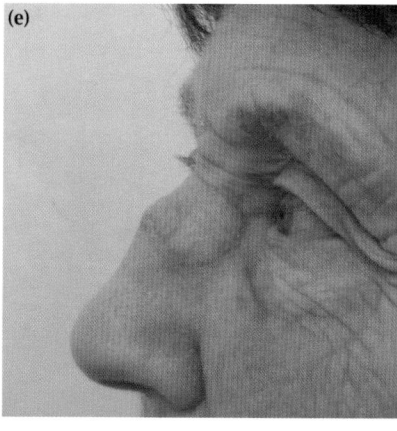

Figure 29.16 (*continued*) (d and e) Appearance at 1 month post-transfer.

- *rhomboid flap*: for cheek, temple, back and flat surface defects;
- *rotation flap*: for convex surfaces;
- *advancement flap*: for flexor surfaces; may need triangles excised at the base to make it work (commonly called Burrow's triangles);
- *V-to-Y advancement*: commonly used for fingertips and extremities;

- *bilobed flap*: for convex surfaces, especially the nose (Fig. 29.17);
- *bipedicle flap*: for eyelids, rarely elsewhere.

All flaps must be raised in the subcutaneous plane. Gentle undercutting of margins helps to close the donor site. The art of making local flaps work is to pull available local spare lax skin into the defect, so that the scar when closed sits in a good 'line of

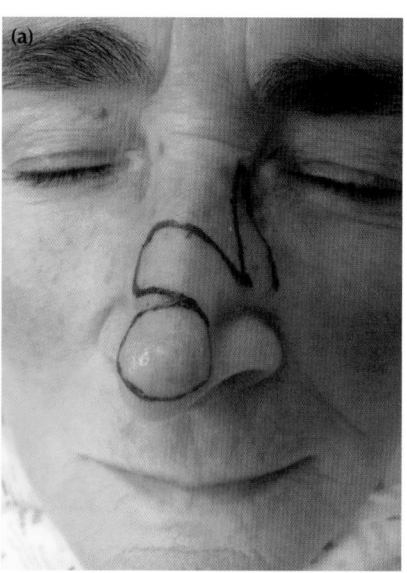

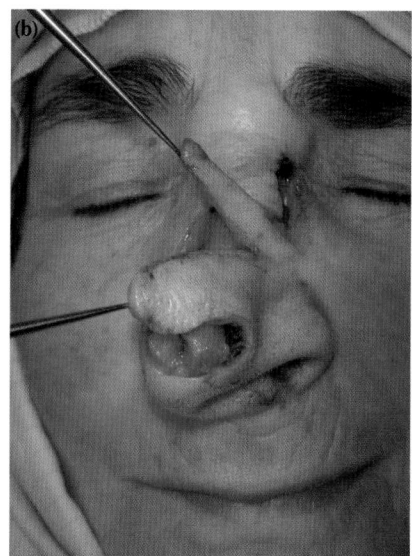

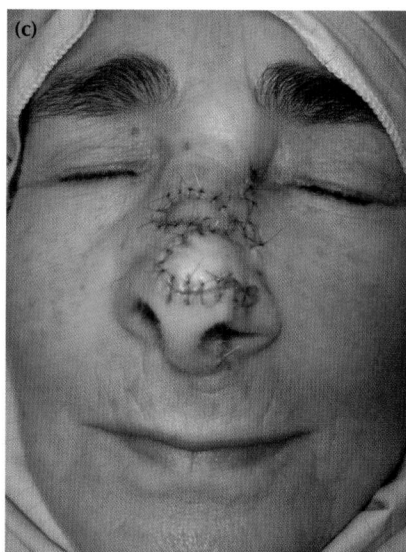

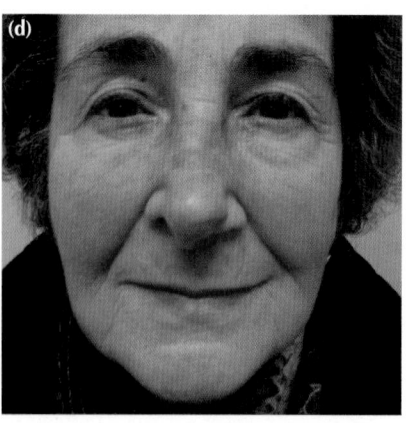

Figure 29.17 (a–c) Example of a bilobed flap (in this case from nose to defect on tip following excision of a basal cell carcinoma). (d) Appearance at 6 weeks post-transfer.

Karl August von Burrow, **1809–1974, Surgeon, Konigsberg, Germany.**

election'. Local flaps are usually not based on specific blood vessels but are very useful in head and neck and smaller defect reconstructions. Good planning is essential to gain the best result from these flaps (Summary box 29.3).

Combined local flaps

In some circumstances, such as burn contracture release, local flaps can usefully be combined to import surplus tissue from a wide area adjacent to a scar or defect that needs removal. Examples are the W-plasty and the multiple Y-to-V plasty, which is a very versatile means of releasing an isolated band scar contracture over a flexion crease (Fig. 29.18).

Distant flaps

To repair defects in which local tissue is inadequate, distant flaps can be moved on long pedicles that contain the blood supply. The pedicle may be buried beneath the skin to create an island flap or left above the skin and formed into a tube.

The most common means of moving flaps long distances while still attached are with a long muscular pedicle that contains a dominant blood supply (a *myocutaneous flap*) (Fig. 29.19) or with a long fascial layer that likewise contains a major septal blood supply (a *fasciocutaneous flap*) (Fig. 29.20). These flaps can carry large composite skin parts for reconstruction very great distances, e.g. from the abdomen to the chest (for breast reconstruction),

from the chest to the face (for oral cancer reconstruction) and from the calf to the knee.

There are a vast number of carefully described myocutaneous and fasciocutaneous flaps throughout the body, all of which are based on known blood vessels. They are reliable when the anatomy of the blood supply is known by the surgeon and the skin is raised carefully in continuity with the underlying fascia or muscle, through which the small perforating vessels run to supply the piece of skin that is being transferred. They are the 'workhorse' of plastic surgery worldwide because they do not require complex equipment to raise and they can solve the majority of reconstructive problems.

Microsurgery and perforator flaps

With fine instruments and materials it has become commonplace to be able to disconnect the blood supply of the flap from its donor site and reconnect it in a distant place using the operating microscope.

The free tissue transfer is now the best means of reconstructing major composite loss of tissue in the face, jaws, lower limb and many other body sites, as long as resources allow it (Fig. 29.21). The operative procedure is similar whether the defect is newly produced from a recent injury or cancer resection or whether it is to be used for the secondary correction of a deformity such as rebuilding a mastectomy deformity. At the site of the defect the surgeon must be sure that all contaminated and dead tissue has been thoroughly cleared and cleaned, a process commonly described as debridement, although that term strictly refers to the release of constricting tissue. If this removal of poorly viable tissue is in doubt, then consideration should be given to delaying the reconstruction.

The surgeon must then find a suitable blood supply for the tissue transfer at the site to be reconstructed. A good arterial flow in and venous return out, without external tissue pressure (such as from surrounding wound induration), is of paramount importance in achieving a successful transfer. The flap is then raised (Table 29.2) and transferred using magnification (Fig. 29.22). Free muscle transfers should be reanastomosed within 1–2 hours if possible; fasciocutanous flaps are more robust and can survive slightly greater ischaemic times (Summary box 29.4).

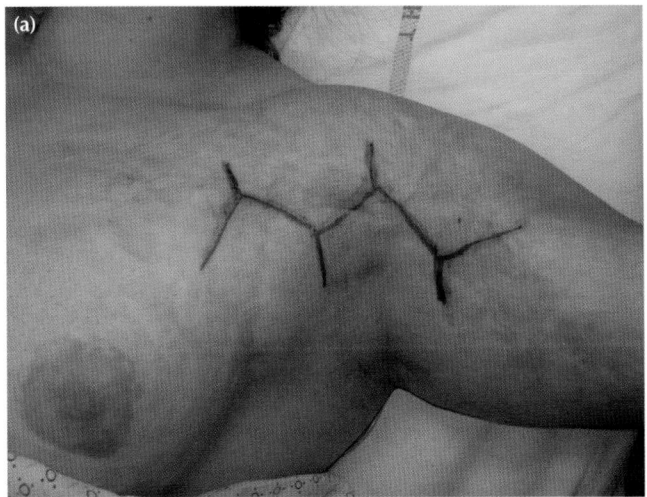 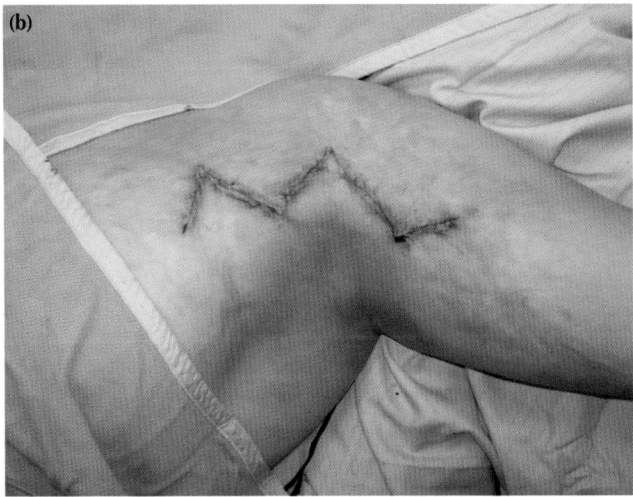

Figure 29.18 (a and b) Y-to-V flap to release axillary contracture.

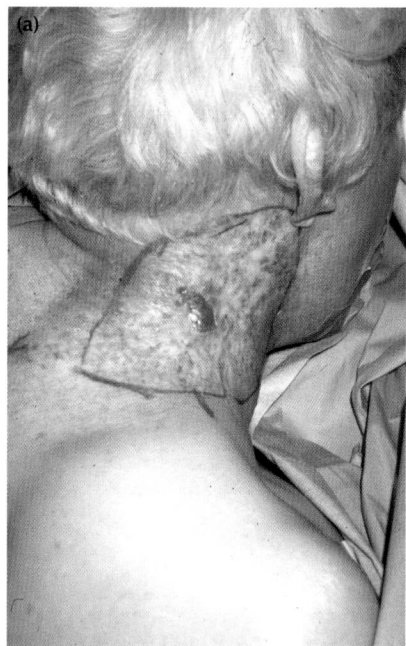

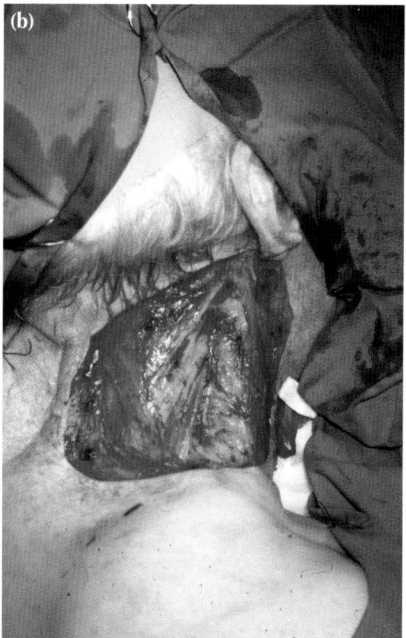

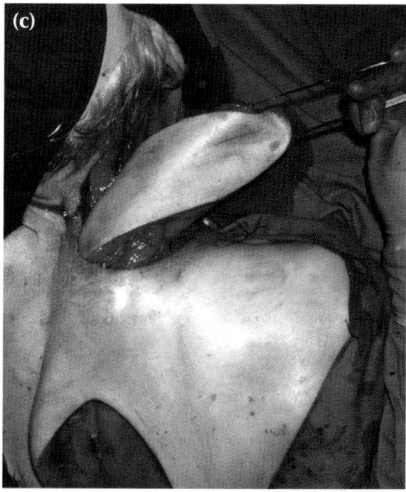

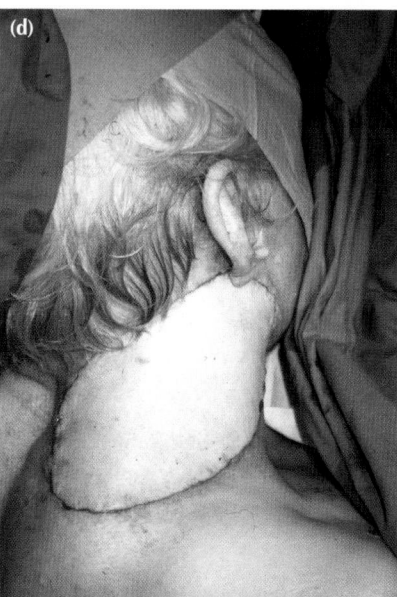

Figure 29.19 Trapezius pedicled myocutaneous flap to an area of recurrent squamous carcinoma in neck.

Table 29.2 Common free tissue transfer donor sites

Muscle only	Latissimus dorsi
	Rectus abdominis
	Gracilis
Myocutaneous	Latissimus dorsi
	Transverse rectus abdominis
Fasciocutaneous	Radial forearm flap
	Scapular
	Lateral arm
	Groin
Osseous	Fibula (may be cutaneous as well)
	Forearm
	Iliac crest
Fascial	Temporoparietal
Miscellaneous	Jejunum – for oesophageal reconstruction
	Pectoralis minor – for facial reanimation
	Omentum – for chest wall and limb defects

Summary box 29.4

Free tissue transfer (or free flap)

Advantages
- Being able to select exactly the best tissue to move
- Only takes what is necessary
- Minimises donor site morbidity

Disadvantages
- More complex surgical technique
- Failure involves total loss of all transferred tissue
- Usually takes more time unless the surgeon is experienced

Recent developments have led to surgeons dissecting distant flaps free from the carrier muscle or fascia, to reduce further the donor morbidity. These distant 'perforator' flaps increase the flexibility of the use of the flap tissue while reducing donor site problems. Future flap design is moving towards individualised flaps

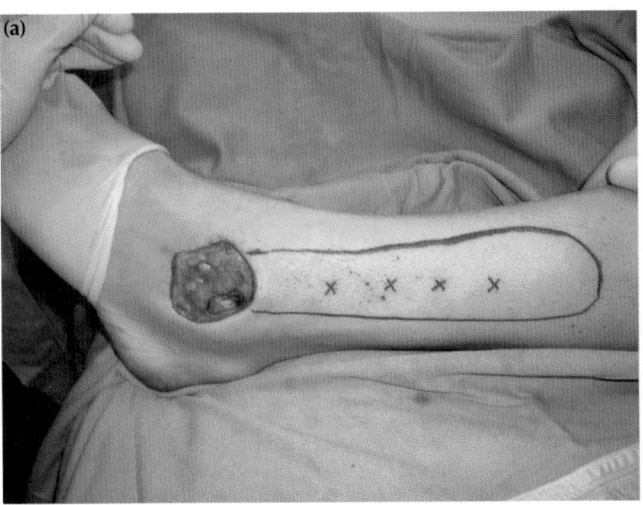

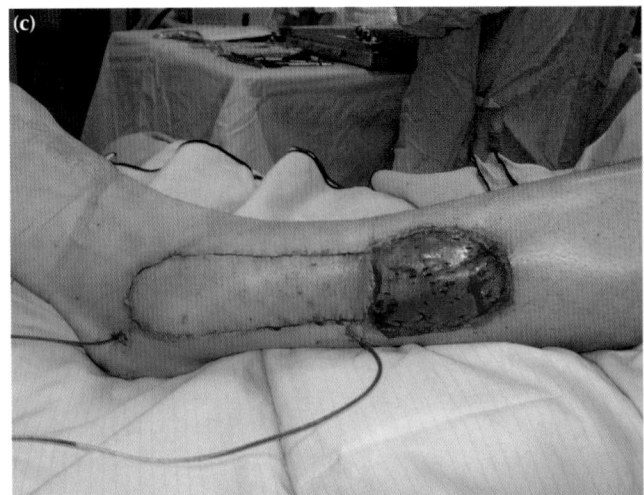

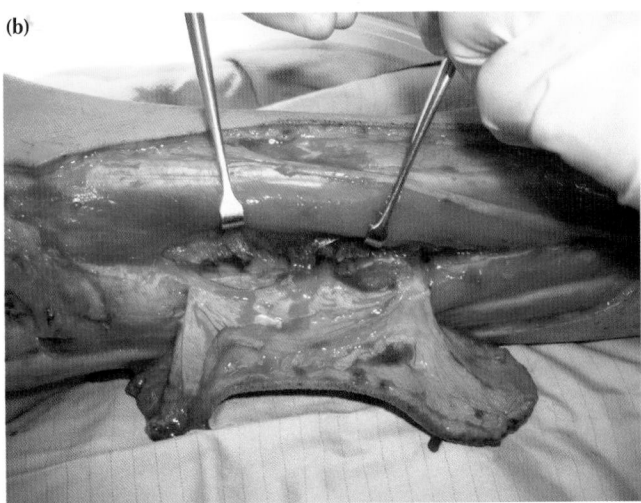

Figure 29.20 (a) Defect at ankle with the flap to be transferred outlined and the position of the perforating vessels (identified with hand-held Doppler device) marked with crosses; (b) flap raised with preserved septal perforators to skin paddle clearly visible; (c) flap rotated into position to cover the defect; proximal donor defect covered with a split-thickness skin graft [case courtesy of Mr David Johnson FRCS(Plast)].

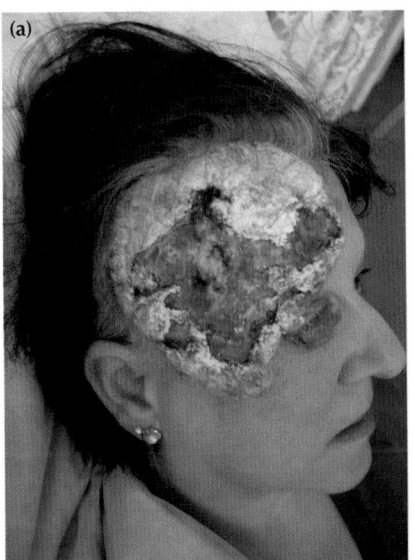

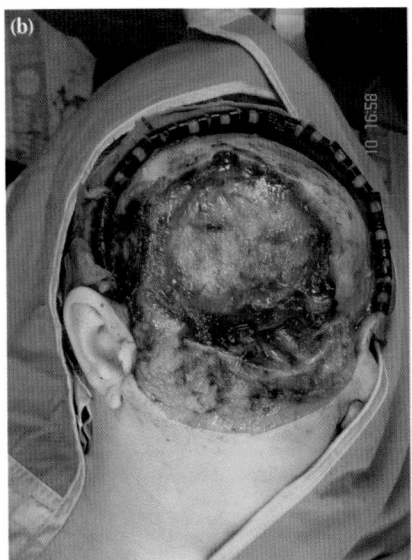

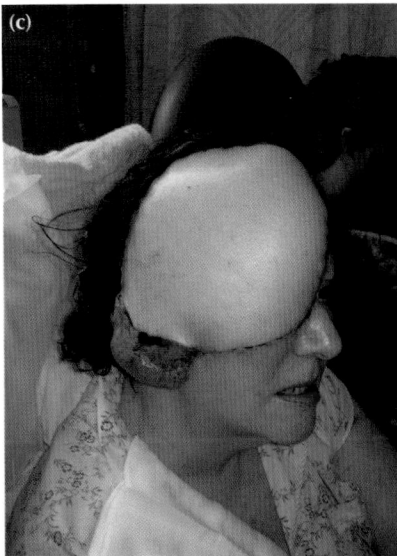

Figure 29.21 (a–c) Large myocutaneous free flap (latissimus dorsi) to cover an exposed cranial defect following the excision of advanced basal cell carcinoma [case courtesy of Mr David Johnson FRCS(Plast)].

CHAPTER 29 | PLASTIC AND RECONSTRUCTIVE SURGERY

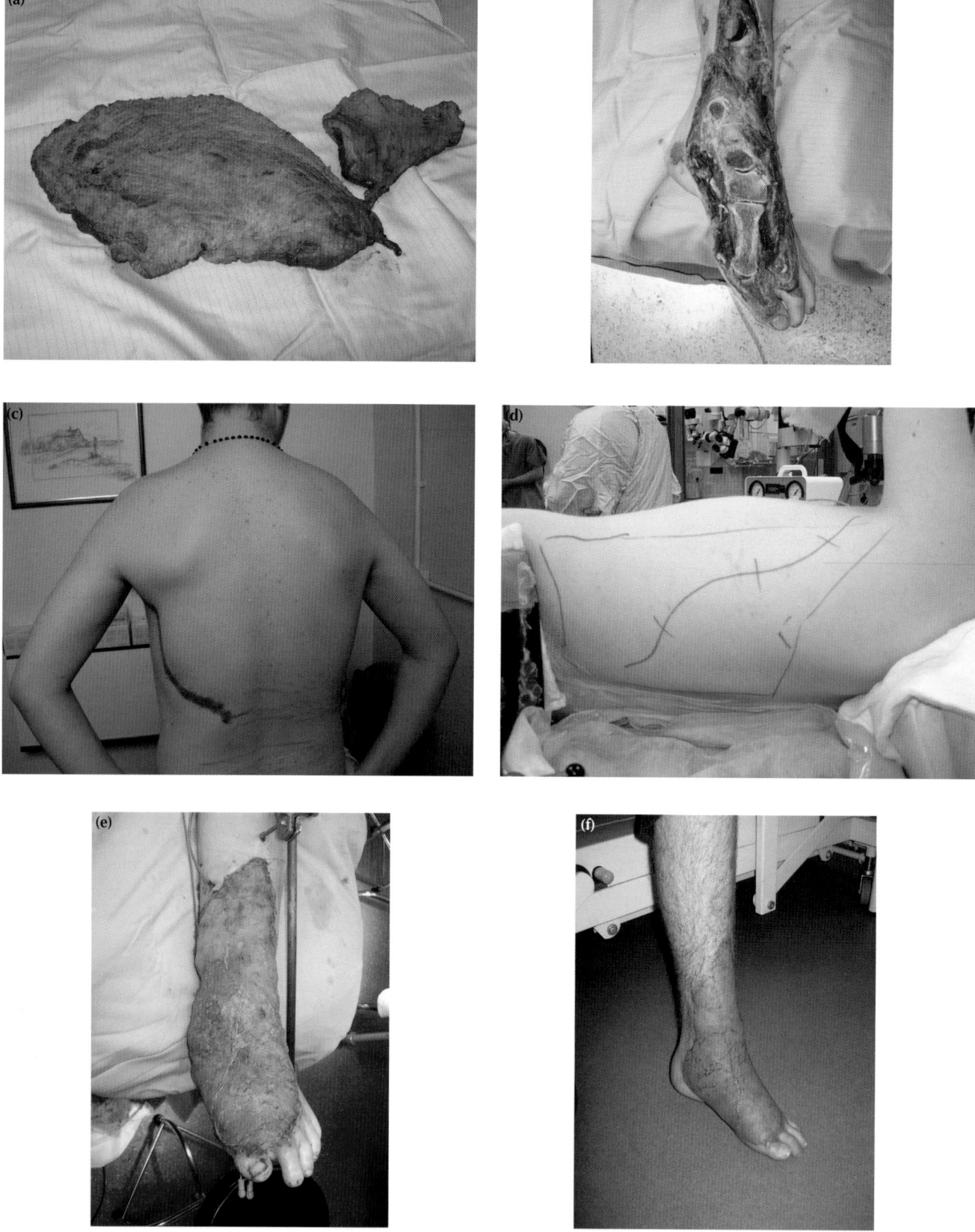

Figure 29.22 Large 'chimeric flap' of latissimus dorsi and serratus anterior muscles (a) to cover a complex open wound of the foot and ankle (b), illustrating the donor site (c and d) and fully covered defect (e and f) [case courtesy of Mr David Johnson FRCS(Plast)].

customised in freestyle fashion for the specific reconstructive requirement demanded.

Care of flaps and monitoring

After a flap has been moved it should be observed for tissue colour, warmth and turgor, and be pressed to assess blanching and capillary refill time. Loss of arterial inflow results in pale, cold, flaccid tissue; loss of venous outflow results in blue congestion, increased turgor, rapid capillary refill and initially a warm flap. In a pedicled flap, such venous congestion may be relieved by releasing suture tension; applying leeches to suck out excess venous blood is a last resort when no other means of restoring venous drainage can be obtained.

The most common causes of flap failure are:

- poor anatomical knowledge when raising the flap (such that the blood supply is deficient from the start);
- flap inset with too much tension;
- local sepsis or a septicaemic patient;
- the dressing applied too tightly around the pedicle;
- microsurgical failure in free flap surgery (usually caused by problems with surgical technique).

'Wet, warm and comfortable'

The best advice for postoperative flap care for major tissue transfers is to keep the patient 'wet, warm and comfortable'. This means that the patient should be well hydrated with a hyperdynamic circulation, a very warm body temperature and well-controlled analgesia to reduce catecholamine output.

Reconstructing complex areas

Certain areas such as the eyelids, nose, lips, ears, genitalia, fingers, breast and intraoral structures often require a combination of methods to produce the most functional and acceptable outcome for the patient. Planning such reconstruction involves considering each cosmetic subunit involved in the defect and bringing the best tissue to rebuild it. An example is the Indian forehead rhinoplasty of Sushruta, which involves transposition of a pedicled fasciocutaneous flap from forehead to nose, with the donor site usually thin skin grafted but occasionally closed primarily in small flaps. It remains the finest means of transporting cosmetically correct tissue to the nose.

FURTHER READING

Achauer, B.M., Erikson, E., Guruyon, R., Coleman, J.J., Russell, R.C. and Vander Kolk, C.A. (eds) (2000) *Plastic Surgery Indications, Operations and Outcomes*, Vols 1–5. Mosby, St Louis.

Cormack, G.C. and Lamberty, B.G.H. (1986) *The Arterial Anatomy of Skin Flaps*. Churchill Livingstone, Edinburgh.

Geddes, C.R., Morris, S.F. and Neligan, P.C. (2003) Perforator flaps: evolution, classification, and applications. *Ann Plastic Surg* **50**: 90–9.

Koshima, I. and Soeda, S. (1989) Inferior epigastric artery skin flaps without rectus abdominis muscle. *Br J Plastic Surg* **42**: 645–8.

MacGregor, A.D. and MacGregor, I.A. (2000) *Fundamental Techniques in Plastic Surgery*, 10th edn. Churchill Livingstone, Edinburgh.

Mathes, S.J. (2006) *Plastic Surgery*, Vols 1–8. W.B. Saunders, Philadelphia.

Mustarde, J.C. and Jackson, I.T. (1988) *Plastic Surgery in Infancy and Childhood*. Churchill Livingstone, Edinburgh.

Nabri, I.A. (1983) El Zahrawi (936–1013 AD), the father of operative surgery. *Ann R Coll Surg Engl* **65**: 132–4.

Serafin, D. (1996) *Atlas of Microsurgical Composite Tissue Transplantation*. W.B. Saunders, Philadelphia.

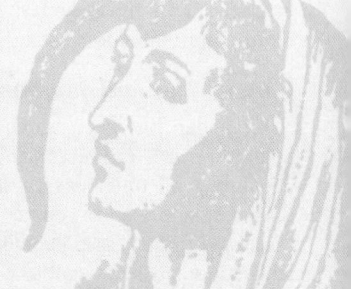

Disaster surgery

'At all defining moments in history, either the man defines the moment or the moment defines the man.'

Ron Shelton, from the film 'Tin Cup'

LEARNING OBJECTIVES

To recognise and understand:
- The common features of various disasters
- The principles behind the organisation of the relief effort and of triage in treatment and evacuation

- The role and limitations of field hospitals
- The features of conditions peculiar to disaster situations and their treatment

INTRODUCTION

Natural disasters such as floods and earthquakes provide a constant reminder of the awesome power and capricious nature of our planet. The depletion of the ozone layer and global warming mean that the future may hold in store natural events that will be even greater in magnitude than the ones experienced before. Alongside the ravages of nature is our own propensity to damage our fellow man. National conflicts and ideological differences have not lessened over the millennia and the resultant 'unnatural disasters' have the potential to rival the natural ones in enormity and the impact on human life. The spectre of terrorist attacks on major world cities constantly haunts security organisations and health-care providers.

COMMON FEATURES OF MAJOR DISASTERS

Any event that results in the loss of human life is disastrous, but most accidents, such as aeroplane and train crashes, are limited in the number of people involved. Conversely, tsunamis and nuclear explosions leave in their wake massive destruction over large areas, which may transcend national boundaries. All the apparatus of a society that respond to such disasters (the civil administration, emergency services, fire brigades and hospitals) may themselves be rendered non-functional (Fig. 30.1). Large numbers of people may require immediate shelter and food in addition to their requirements for medical care.

A breakdown of communication is inevitable and is accompanied by widespread panic and a disruption of civil order. Access to the disaster area may be limited because of the destruction of bridges, road and rail links. In the face of such extensive damage to the infrastructure of society, the armed forces are usually called upon to help restore civil order and initiate the reconstructive effort (Summary box 30.1).

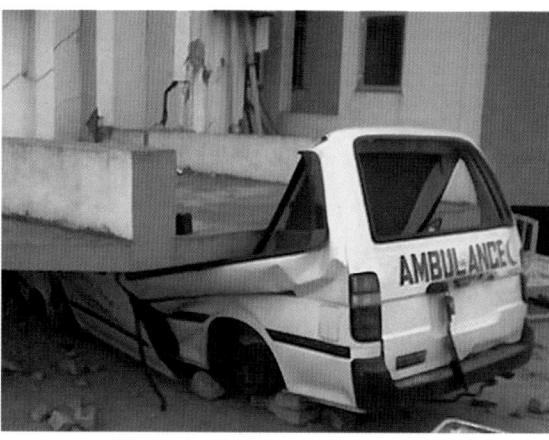

Figure 30.1 Damage to emergency medical services.

Summary box 30.1

Common features of major disasters

- Massive casualties
- Damage to infrastructure
- A large number of people requiring shelter
- Panic and uncertainty among the population
- Limited access to the area
- Breakdown of communication

FACTORS INFLUENCING RELIEF EFFORTS AND PROVISION OF MEDICAL AID

Communication is the critical factor that determines the response from the authorities. Its restoration is a priority so that first-hand information about the magnitude of the disaster can be obtained as quickly as possible. Wireless technology and satellite imagery have revolutionised the way in which real-time information can be obtained (Fig. 30.2). Even so, there is a lag period between the occurrence of the disaster and the response from the establishment.

The location of the disaster area, whether rural or urban, has a significant bearing on relief efforts. Terrorist attacks and nuclear events are more likely to be targeted towards large population centres where emergency services are better developed and high-standard hospital facilities are available. On the other hand they are also densely populated, cramped with high-rise buildings and may have limited access by road and air. Natural disasters can strike anywhere but can be particularly difficult to manage if they occur in remote areas as relief efforts are hampered by geographical isolation and the lack of a suitable infrastructure for dealing with a major calamity.

The time-frame in which a disaster occurs also has an impact on the relief efforts. Earthquakes and blasts unleash havoc in fractions of a second but floods and hurricanes may continue for several days and nuclear fallout can damage the ecosystem for years to come. Another noteworthy aspect is the state of development of the country; disasters in the developing world can seldom be managed without significant outside assistance (Summary box 30.2).

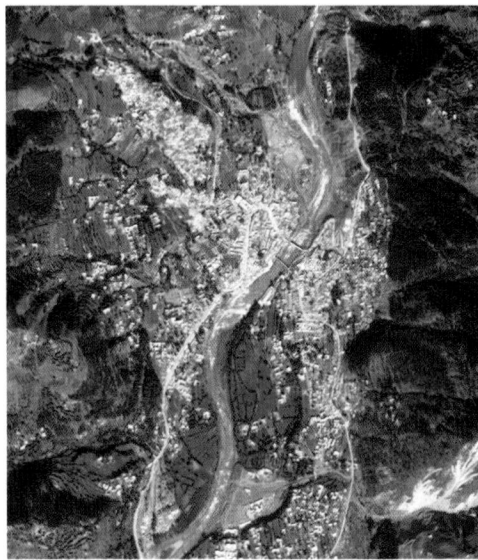

Figure 30.2 Satellite image showing destruction of a bridge as a result of flood.

Summary box. 30.2

Factors influencing rescue and relief efforts

- Status of communications
- Location, whether rural or urban
- Accessibility of the location
- Time-frame in which disaster occurs
- Economic state of development of the area

SEQUENCE OF RELIEF EFFORTS AFTER A DISASTER

Establishing a chain of command

In many countries there are organisations that deal with disasters, such as the Federal Emergency Management Authority (FEMA) in the USA. In others, an ad-hoc administrative hierarchy is established to coordinate the efforts of the teams participating in relief efforts. The actual organisation that deals with a particular disaster will depend upon the circumstances but the principles of each organisation remain the same (Fig. 30.3).

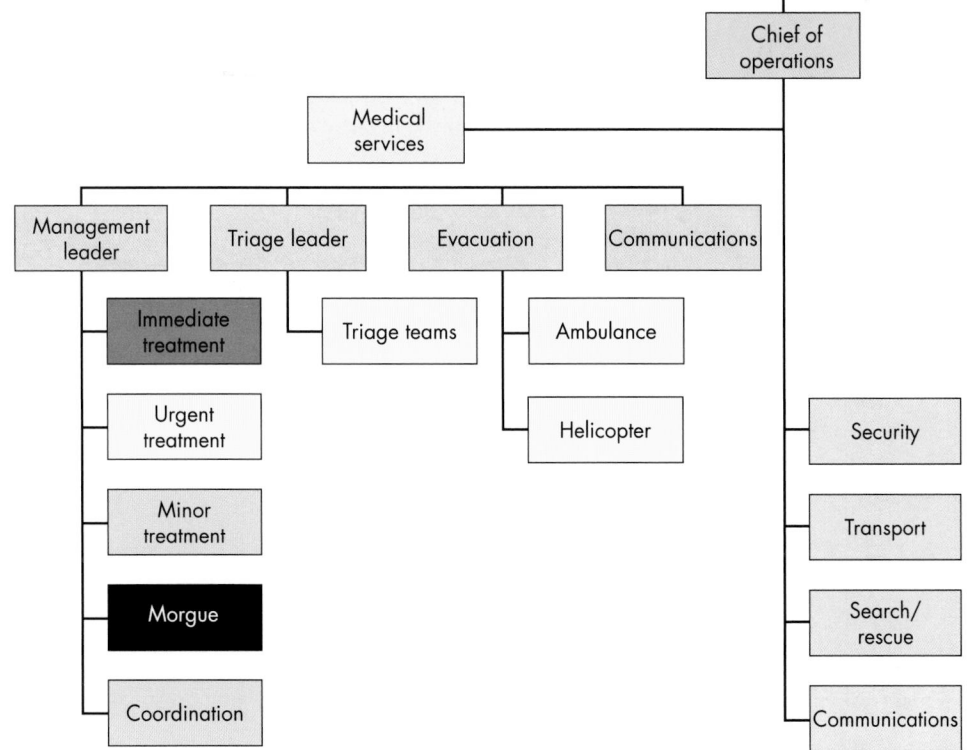

Figure 30.3 Organisation chart for disaster management.

Damage assessment

The first and often the most difficult objective in disaster management is an accurate assessment of the damage and the number of casualties. All sources of information must be employed, not just the official channels. Given the public's morbid fascination with such events, the 24-hour news services are frequently the first on the scene and can be an important source of information.

Mobilising resources

The next step is mobilisation of human and material resources appropriate to the size and nature of the disaster. Although all modes of transport available need to be considered, helicopters are the quickest way in for the first responders (Fig. 30.4).

The initial groups of personnel to respond must include experienced senior staff who can quickly assess the situation, make immediate decisions and organise further assistance.

Rescue operation

Early coordination of the rescue effort will allow optimal use of limited resources. Self-help will already be under way in the form of the less injured helping the more gravely hurt. Rescue teams

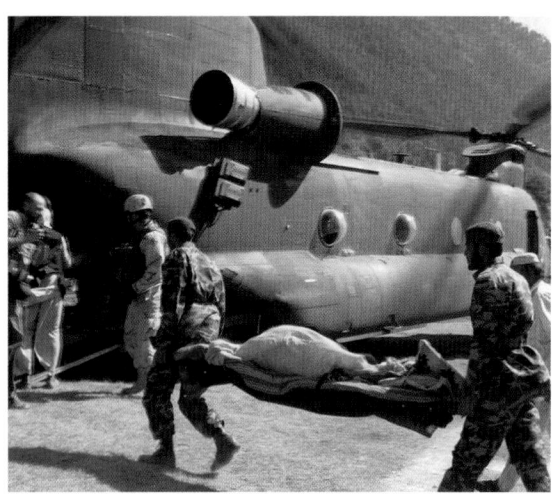

Figure 30.4 Heli-evacuation.

from the outside must work with local volunteers who are familiar with the area.

The first priority is to prevent further damage from occurring, both to people and to the infrastructure. Fires should be put out, people moved away from falling debris and well-meaning non-professionals stopped from embarking on hazardous rescue efforts.

The types of injuries that will be encountered by rescue workers will depend upon the delay between the start of the disaster and the arrival of rescue workers. Patients with head injuries and abdominal and thoracic trauma will either have been treated or have succumbed to their injuries within 48–72 hours of a disaster. After the first 2 weeks, the only casualties requiring treatment are those with complex limb trauma (Fig. 30.5).

Coordination with relief agencies

A laudable aspect of globalisation is the immediate outpouring of help from governments and various non-government organisations that occurs in response to a disaster on the other side of the world. Some organisations, for example Rescue and Preparedness in Disasters (RAPID), deal with search and rescue whereas others, such as the International Committee of the Red Cross (ICRC) and Oxfam, provide general disaster-related relief (Fig. 30.6). United Nations (UN) agencies such as the World Health Organization (WHO), the World Food Programme (WFP) and the UN High Commissioner for Refugees (UNHCR) deal with medical care, food provision and refugees respectively. The authorities need to coordinate the efforts of these organisations for optimal results, as medical aid in isolation is inadequate without the simultaneous provision of safe drinking water, food, clothing and shelter. The scale of the disaster and the immediate and long-term requirements should be clearly communicated so that appropriate and timely help is received. Rescue teams should be prepared to be self-sufficient and not rely on the local infrastructure, which may have been destroyed.

Safety of the helpers

Rescue and relief workers are a diverse group of individuals and, whereas policemen and members of rescue organisations are trained to deal with the breakdown in civil order that occurs in

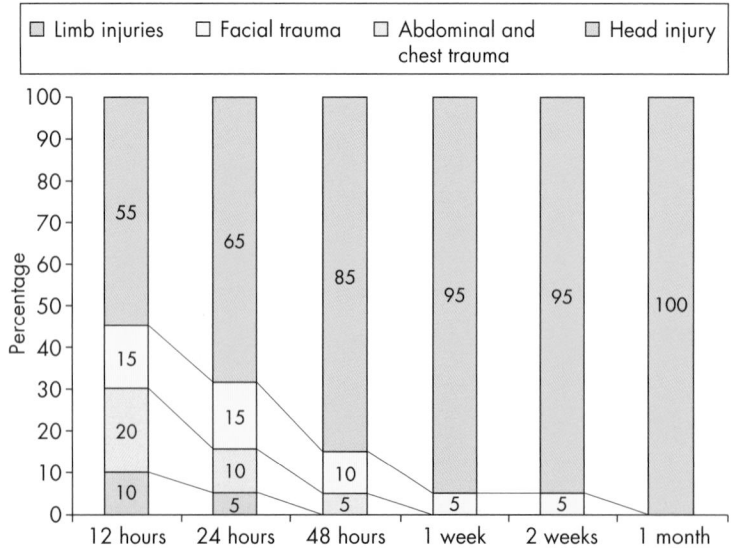

Figure 30.5 Time line showing the type of injuries encountered at different times in a disaster.

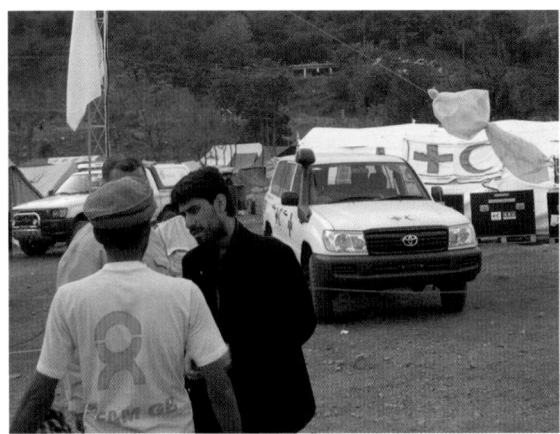

Figure 30.6 Oxfam and the International Committee of the Red Cross provide generalised relief.

the wake of disasters, volunteer workers may have little experience of such situations. It is not uncommon for mobs to loot stores of food and other essentials in a disaster, especially if help has arrived late. This results in injuries, occasionally serious, to personnel trying to provide an equitable distribution of goods. During armed conflicts and civil wars, rival groups have prevented humanitarian assistance reaching the neediest, and even structures bearing the Red Cross and Red Crescent have been targeted. It is therefore imperative that the local authorities make it a point to safeguard the lives and property of aid workers to allow them to work without duress and fear.

Dealing with the media

Disasters act like a magnet to the media and, in today's world of 24-hour news coverage, the media exert a powerful influence in shaping public opinion. They are frequently accused of dramatising the situation and only emphasising the inadequacies of the relief effort. Aid workers may find dealing with the media difficult as their priorities are rightly different. Nevertheless it is essential to establish a working relationship between the two groups. To prevent conflicting statements a spokesperson should be appointed, who must be kept informed of the latest situation. With careful handling the media can become a powerful ally and play a constructive role in identifying problems, galvanising aid and keeping the public informed.

Triage

Derived from the French verb 'trier', triage means 'to sort' and is the cornerstone of the management of mass casualties. It aims to identify the patients who will benefit the most by being treated the earliest, ensuring *the greatest good for the greatest number*. Its value has been proved in battlefields since the Napoleonic wars and it is still practised in hospital emergency departments. In a broader sense it determines who will be treated first, what mode of evacuation is best and which medical facility is optimal for the management of the patient. Numerous studies show that only 10–15% of disaster casualties are serious enough to require hospitalisation. By sorting out the minor injuries, triage lessens the immediate burden on medical facilities. Deciding who should receive priority when faced with hundreds of seriously injured

victims is a daunting prospect. There is a tendency for senior doctors to believe that their services are better utilised in the actual management of patients rather than in triage. This is a mistake and it is crucial that this task be undertaken by someone senior, who has the training and experience to make these crucial decisions. It is important to remember the changing clinical picture of an injured person. To keep pace, triage needs to be undertaken at various levels, i.e. in the field, before evacuation and at the hospital.

Triage areas

For efficient triage the injured need to be brought together at one location. Any undamaged structures that can accommodate and shelter a large number of wounded, such as school buildings and stadia, are suitable. A good water supply and ease of access are useful. Areas should then be reserved for patient holding, emergency treatment and decontamination (in the event of discharge of hazardous materials). An area should also be designated to serve as a morgue, preferably a little removed from the holding and treatment areas.

Practical triage

Emergency life-saving measures should proceed alongside triage and actually help the decision-making process. The assessment and restoration of airway, breathing and circulation are critical and are discussed in Chapter 22. A simple visual check of the injuries is notoriously unreliable. Vital signs and a general physical examination should be combined with a brief history taken by a paramedic or volunteer worker if it is available.

Documentation for triage

Accurate documentation is an inseparable part of triage and should include basic patient data, vital signs with timing, brief details of injuries (preferably on a diagram) and treatment given. In addition, a system of colour-coded tags attached to the patient's wrist or around the neck is employed by emergency medical services. The colour denotes the degree of urgency with which a patient requires treatment (Fig. 30.7).

Triage categories

There is no universally accepted method of triage. Nevertheless, all methods use simple criteria based on vital signs and a rapid clinical assessment, taking into account the patient's ability to walk, the mental status and the presence or absence of ventilation or capillary perfusion. A commonly used four-tier system is presented in Table 30.1. Triage carries serious consequences, especially for patients who are consigned to the unsalvageable category. It should be carried out with compassion but also be clear and decisive.

Evacuation of casualties

This is a major logistics exercise especially in a 'diffuse' catastrophe such as an earthquake or a tornado. It is good practice to carry out a quick re-triage before deciding on the sequence of transport and destination of the injured. Decisions regarding the best destination for each patient need to be based on how far it is safe for them to travel and whether the facilities that they need for definitive treatment will be available. If decisions are not made carefully some hospitals may be swamped with patients whereas others with

FRONT   **BACK**

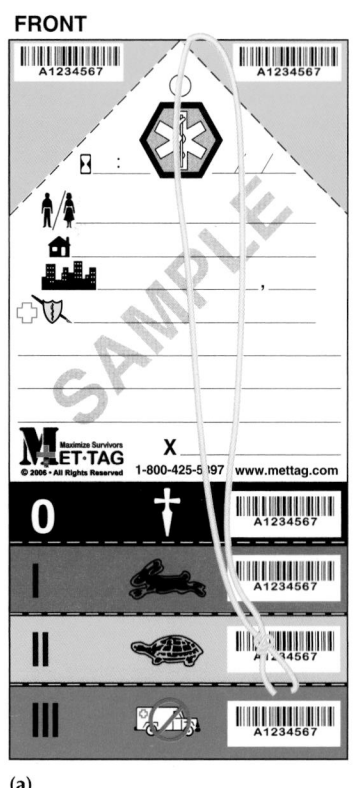

(a)

FRONT   **BACK**

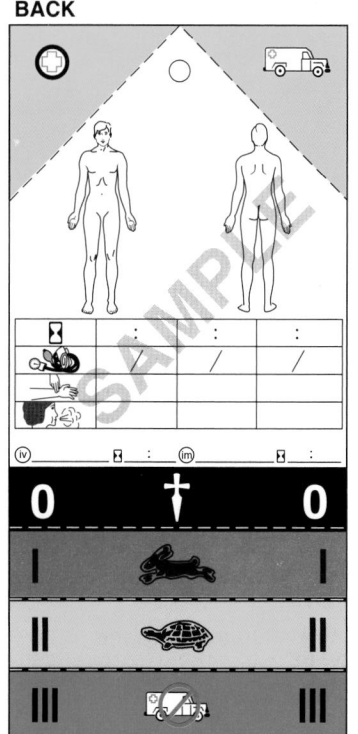

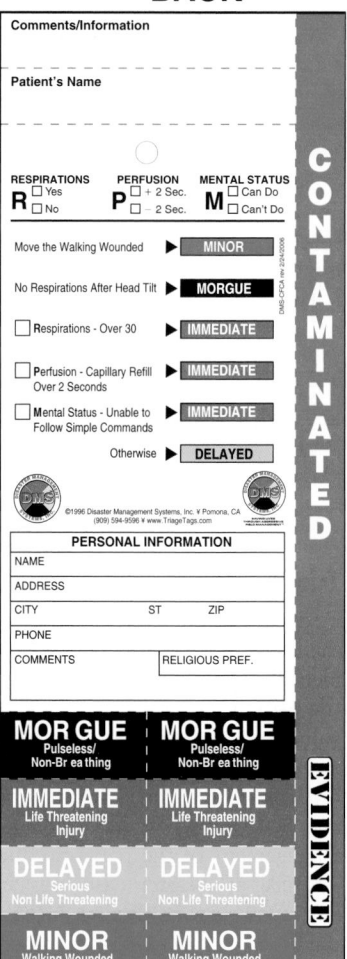

Figure 30.7 Triage tags. (a) Courtesy of TACDA & METTAG products, American Civil Defense Association. (b) Courtesy of Disaster Management Systems.

(b)

Table 30.1 Triage categories

Priority	Colour	Medical need	Clinical status	Examples
First (I)	Red	Immediate	Critical but likely to survive if treatment given early	Severe facial trauma, tension pneumothorax, profuse external bleeding, haemothorax, flail chest, major intra-abdominal bleed, extradural haematomas
Second (II)	Yellow	Urgent	Critical, likely to survive if treatment given within hours	Compound fractures, degloving injuries, ruptured abdominal viscus, pelvic fractures, spinal injuries
Third (III)	Green	Non-urgent	Stable, likely to survive even if treatment is delayed for hours to days	Simple fractures, sprains, minor lacerations
Last (0)	Black	Unsalvageable	Not breathing, pulseless, so severely injured that no medical care is likely to help	Severe brain damage, very extensive burns, major disruption/loss of chest or abdominal wall structures

better facilities receive only a small number. The paramedics accompanying the casualties should be familiar with safe transport techniques. A patient with a spinal injury should be strapped to the spine board, the hard collar adjusted and the head fixed to the board with tape. Chest tubes, urinary catheters, endotracheal tubes, tracheotomy tubes and intravenous lines must be properly secured. These measures will help prevent the 'second accident' that plagues casualty transportation. For patients obliged to travel for a long time, an adequate supply of essentials such as intravenous fluids, dressings, pain medication and oxygen must be arranged. Care must be exercised in the case of unaccompanied minor children; cases must be clearly documented and social services informed (Summary box 30.3).

Summary box 30.3

Essentials of casualty evacuation

- Re-triage to prioritise the injured
- Select appropriate medical facilities
- Select appropriate means of transport
- Prevent the 'second accident'
- Ensure an adequate supply of materials

Field hospitals

The decision to set up field hospitals will depend upon the location of the disaster, the number of casualties and the speed with which evacuation can be affected. The two basic types of field hospitals are the traditional tented structure and the modular type housed in containers (Fig. 30.8).

The modular type is self-contained and can be operational as soon as it reaches the disaster area but the containers are heavy and require an intact road or rail link to be transported. The tented structures require an initial period of setting up before they can be functional but they are very portable and components can be carried in small vehicles or air dropped. Whichever type is chosen, it must be equipped with an X-ray plant, operating rooms, vital signs monitors, sterilising equipment, a blood bank, ventilators and basic laboratory facilities.

Management in the field

Field hospitals principally function in three main areas (Table 30.2).

First aid

Care for patients with minor injuries involves suturing of lacerations, splinting simple fractures and sprains and applying bandages

Table 30.2 Type of treatment given in field hospitals

	Examples	Further
First aid	Suturing cuts and lacerations, splinting simple fractures	Review at local hospital
Emergency care for life-threatening injuries	Endotracheal intubation, tracheotomy, relieving tension pneumothorax, stopping external haemorrhage, relieving an extradural haematoma, emergency thoracotomy/laparotomy for internal haemorrhage	After damage control surgery, transfer patients to base hospitals once stable
Initial care for non-life-threatening injuries	Debridement of contaminated wounds, reduction of fractures and dislocations, application of external fixators, vascular repairs	Transfer patients to base hospitals for definitive management

CHAPTER 30 | DISASTER SURGERY

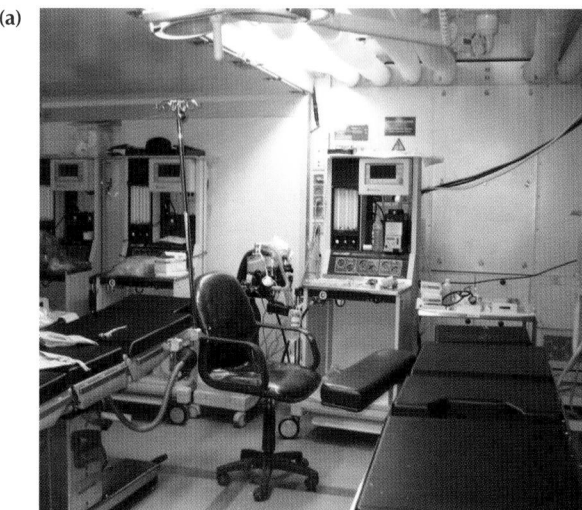

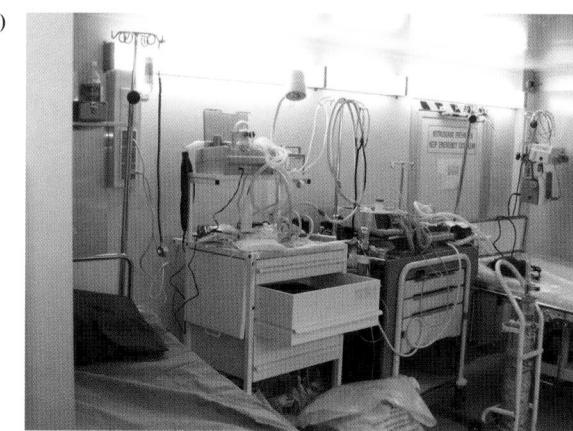

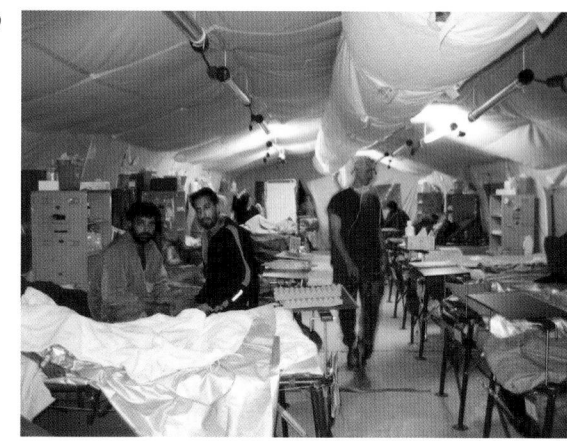

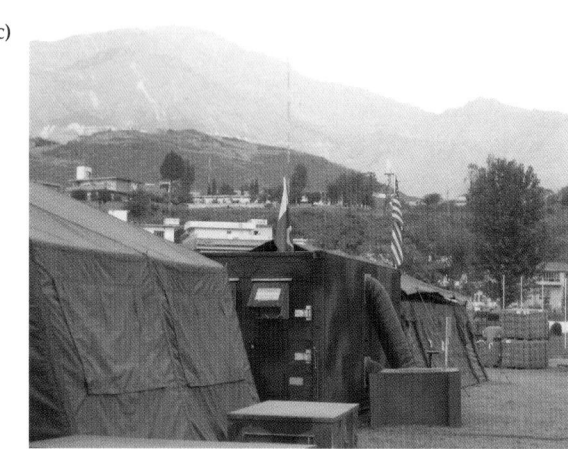

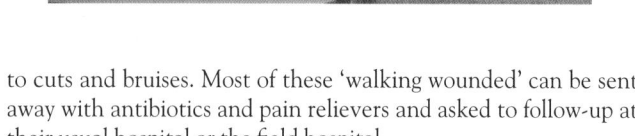

Figure 30.8 Field hospitals: (a) and (b) modular type; (c) tented structure; (d) interior of a tented field hospital.

to cuts and bruises. Most of these 'walking wounded' can be sent away with antibiotics and pain relievers and asked to follow-up at their usual hospital or the field hospital.

Emergency care for immediate life-threatening injuries

There are many patients who may be saved by relatively simple measures provided that they are taken urgently. Endotracheal intubation, tracheotomy, relieving a tension pneumothorax, closing an open pneumothorax and stopping profuse external haemorrhage fall into this category. Major procedures may include an emergency thoracotomy or laparotomy to stop massive or persistent internal bleeding and evacuation of an extradural haematoma. These procedures are indicated in the field only if the patient is unlikely to survive an attempt at transfer to a base hospital. Amputation for clearly devitalised limbs and gas gangrene should be undertaken at field hospitals.

Initial care for non-life-threatening injuries

Many patients will present with serious injuries that require complex, prolonged care. Compound limb fractures, degloving injuries, dislocations of major joints, major facial injuries and complex hand injuries all fall into this category. These patients will need specialised orthopaedic and plastic surgical care requiring transfer to the appropriate facility. Replantations of totally amputated limbs and other extensive reconstructive procedures should not be attempted in field hospitals as they are very time

consuming and divert resources and personnel to the treatment of a few patients.

Debridement

Taken from the French meaning to 'unleash or cut open', debridement has come to mean more than simply the laying open of tissues. It plays a crucial part in the management of trauma. Wounds sustained in disasters are often heavily contaminated, containing foreign bodies and non-viable tissues (Fig. 30.9). Debridement reduces the chances of anaerobic and necrotising infections and can prevent systemic sepsis. The following principles of debridement apply to all contaminated wounds, including gunshot and shrapnel injuries:

- It should be undertaken by surgeons who are well versed in trauma surgery, in a sterile environment with good lighting.
- After the administration of anaesthesia, the first step is a thorough cleansing of the injured area by copious irrigation with normal saline, preferably carried out under tourniquet to reduce blood loss. Pulse lavage, if available, is ideal for this but a large syringe can also be used (Fig. 30.10). Next, the wound is palpated and all foreign matter is removed using forceps. In-driven dirt is best removed using a nail brush as even small particles of retained dirt result in permanent tattooing. Dirt intimately enmeshed in the soft tissues can only be removed by excision. Open joints should be thoroughly irrigated and all foreign material removed.

(a)

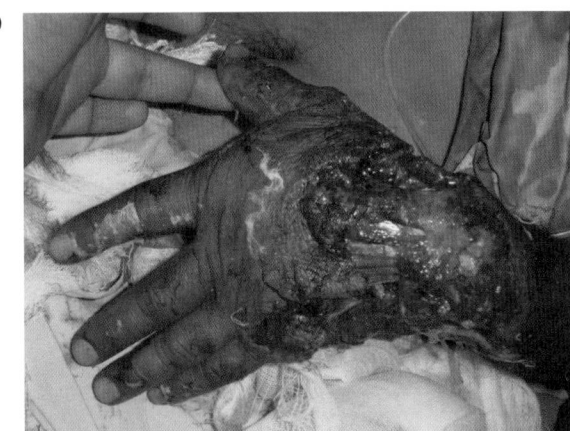

(b)

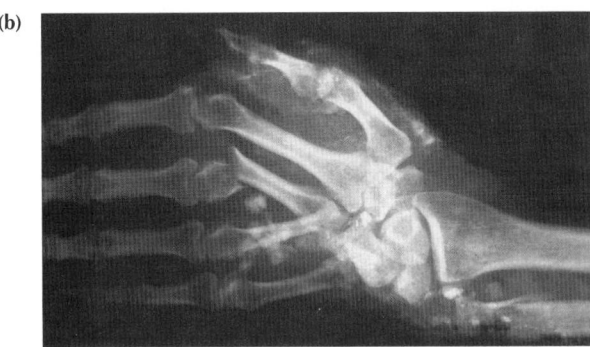

Figure 30.9 Gross contamination typically seen in wounds sustained in disasters. The radiograph shows numerous radio-opaque foreign bodies in the soft tissues.

- Wounds with a small external opening but more extensive cavitation (firearm injuries, high-impact injuries) should be generously enlarged in a longitudinal direction along with the deep fascia to gain better access and decompress the underlying muscles. This helps to visualise the damaged structures, gain proximal and distal control for vascular injuries and identify severed ends of major nerves and tendons.
- The next step is excision of all dead and devitalised tissue. It is advisable at this stage to let down the tourniquet to check the vascularity of the tissues. Skin excision should be kept to a minimum as it is quite resistant to trauma and only the margins of the wound need to be trimmed back to healthy bleeding edges. Removal of devitalised muscle is essential and should be undertaken generously. Muscle that is pale or dark in colour, has a soft consistency, does not contract on pinching and does not bleed on cutting is definitely non-viable. Small pieces of crushed bone lying free should be removed. Large segments of bone that retain some soft-tissue attachment should be left undisturbed. In patients with traumatic amputations, the bone ends are tidied, the skin and muscle edges trimmed to the lowest level possible and the wound left open.
- In patients with associated fractures, skeletal stabilisation should be obtained before embarking on any repairs. External fixators are invaluable for this and make wound management easier (Fig. 30.11).
- In major trauma in the acute setting, only vascular repairs are justified. For lacerated vessels the ends are trimmed and anastomosis performed. In case of loss of substance of the vessel wall a vein patch or reversed vein graft may be used. Silicone tubing may be used as a temporary bypass (stent) while vascular repair is being carried out in patients with critically compromised distal circulation.
- Nerves and tendons should not be dissected out nor any attempt made at definitive repair in wounds with tissue devitalisation and gross oedema, as it leads to poor results. The key structures should simply be identified and the edges trimmed and tagged with non-absorbable sutures to facilitate repair during subsequent exploration.
- Wounds sustained in disasters are heavily contaminated and not suitable for primary closure. However, blood vessels (whether repaired or simply exposed) and exposed joint surfaces need to be covered. This can be achieved by using adjoining muscle or skin loosely tacked with a few sutures. The wound is then covered with fluffed gauze and sterile cotton and the extremity splinted with a plaster of Paris slab, even if there is no fracture. For the upper extremity, elevation with a drip stand and, for the lower limb, elevation on a couple of pillows are important to reduce oedema.
- Broad-spectrum antibiotics, such as third-generation cephalosporins, are started prophylactically and continued for 5–7 days.
- The wound should be reinspected at 24–48 hours to assess the viability of the tissues and the distal circulation. The wounds are closed between the fourth and sixth day if there is no infection. Tension should be avoided and liberal use of partial-thickness skin grafts to achieve wound closure is

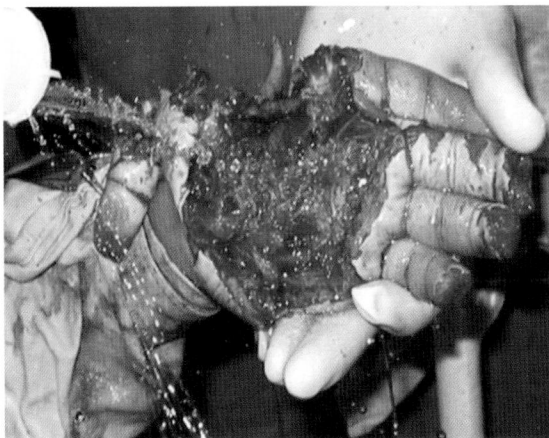

Figure 30.10 Lavage with normal saline to decontaminate a wound.

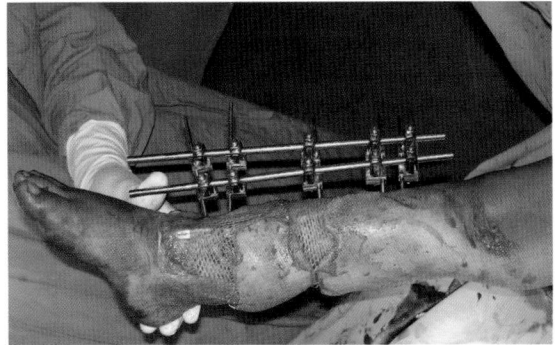

Figure 30.11 External fixators provide skeletal stabilisation and allow easy management of the soft tissues.

CHAPTER 30 | DISASTER SURGERY

recommended. Skin staplers are particularly useful and time saving when dealing with large numbers of casualties.

- In wounds with gross infection no attempt at closure is made until infection is eradicated. These wounds are re-explored to make sure that there are no residual foreign bodies or devitalised tissue. Surface swabs are not useful but tissue should be taken for microbiological culture. Vacuum-assisted closure (Vac-Pac) has emerged as a very useful tool for irregular and deeply cavitating wounds. It utilises low-pressure suction to evacuate exudate, promote sprouting of granulation tissue and reduce the size of the wound (Fig. 30.12). Once the wounds are free from infection secondary closure can be undertaken (Summary box 30.4).

Summary box 30.4

Principles of debridement and initial wound care

- Obtain generous exposure through skin and fascia
- Identify neurovascular bundles
- Excise devitalised tissue
- Remove foreign bodies
- Repair major vessels
- Obtain skeletal stabilisation with external fixators
- Only tag cut tendons and nerves
- Leave wound open and delay primary closure
- Avoid tight dressings
- Elevate injured limb

DEFINITIVE MANAGEMENT

This is undertaken at major hospitals. Hospitals should be alerted to the expected number of casualties so that the staff are prepared. Hospitals are selected on the basis of the facilities available and the number of injured that they can handle. The number of beds available is seldom a good guide to capacity as the ancillary resources required for trauma patients are more than for the typical case mix of a hospital. It is estimated that only half the bed strength of a hospital should be utilised to provide optimum care.

(a)

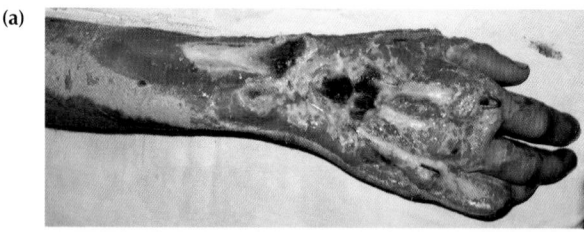

(b)

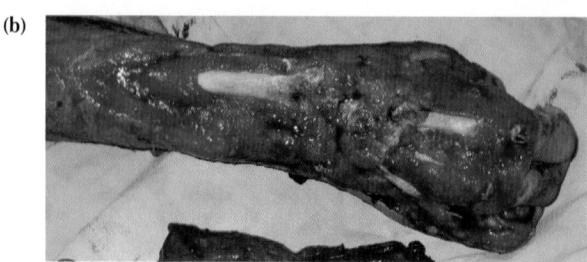

Figure 30.12 Use of low-pressure vacuum therapy in preparing a wound for secondary closure.

Hospital reorganisation

Hospitals are organised according to the type of patients treated and the facilities that they offer, but reorganisation of services is unavoidable during disasters. This includes transferring patients with non-urgent conditions to other facilities, augmenting surgical services, reorganising the specialist rota and redesignating medical wards as surgical care areas to accommodate the patient load. A quick check of hospital inventories should be undertaken to ensure availability of essential equipment and medicines and an appeal for blood donations should be broadcast (Summary box 30.5).

Summary box 30.5

Sequence of the relief effort in major disasters

- Establish chain of command
- Establish communication
- Damage assessment
- Mobilise resources
- Rescue operation
- Triage
- Emergency treatment
- Evacuation
- Definitive management

SPECIFIC ISSUES

There is no injury that is peculiar to disasters. Destruction of buildings and explosions can produce the whole spectrum of external injuries from minor cuts to extensive degloving, compound fractures and amputations. Internal organ damage is frequent and, unless immediate help is available, accounts for the major share of early mortality figures. People trapped under fallen buildings may suffer crush injuries and crush syndrome if the duration is prolonged. Those near an explosion can suffer injury to the lungs and abdominal viscera, as well as burns because of the heat of the blast.

Crush injuries and missile injuries cause extensive tissue damage and gross contamination, both favourable conditions for anaerobic and micro-aerophillic infections.

Limb salvage

The Mangled Extremity Severity Score (MESS) and its modifications are useful in making a judgement about limb salvage. In the past, extensive tissue loss, neurovascular damage and loss of long fragments of bone were all considered indications for amputation. Currently, with the use of microvascular flaps, wounds of any dimension can be covered with healthy tissue in a single stage. If performed in time, vascular repairs can salvage most acutely ischaemic limbs. Distraction osteogenesis and vascularised bone transfers can restore bony continuity in all but the most massive bone losses. In view of these developments the indications for amputation in trauma have undergone a paradigm shift and the majority of patients who reach a tertiary-care facility within 24 hours are candidates for limb salvage (Fig. 30.13). This assumes that debridement and, if required, vascular repairs have been performed in a field medical facility. Restoration of vascular continuity is the critical issue and a limb is unlikely to survive if vascular repairs of major limb vessels are delayed for more than 4–6 hours.

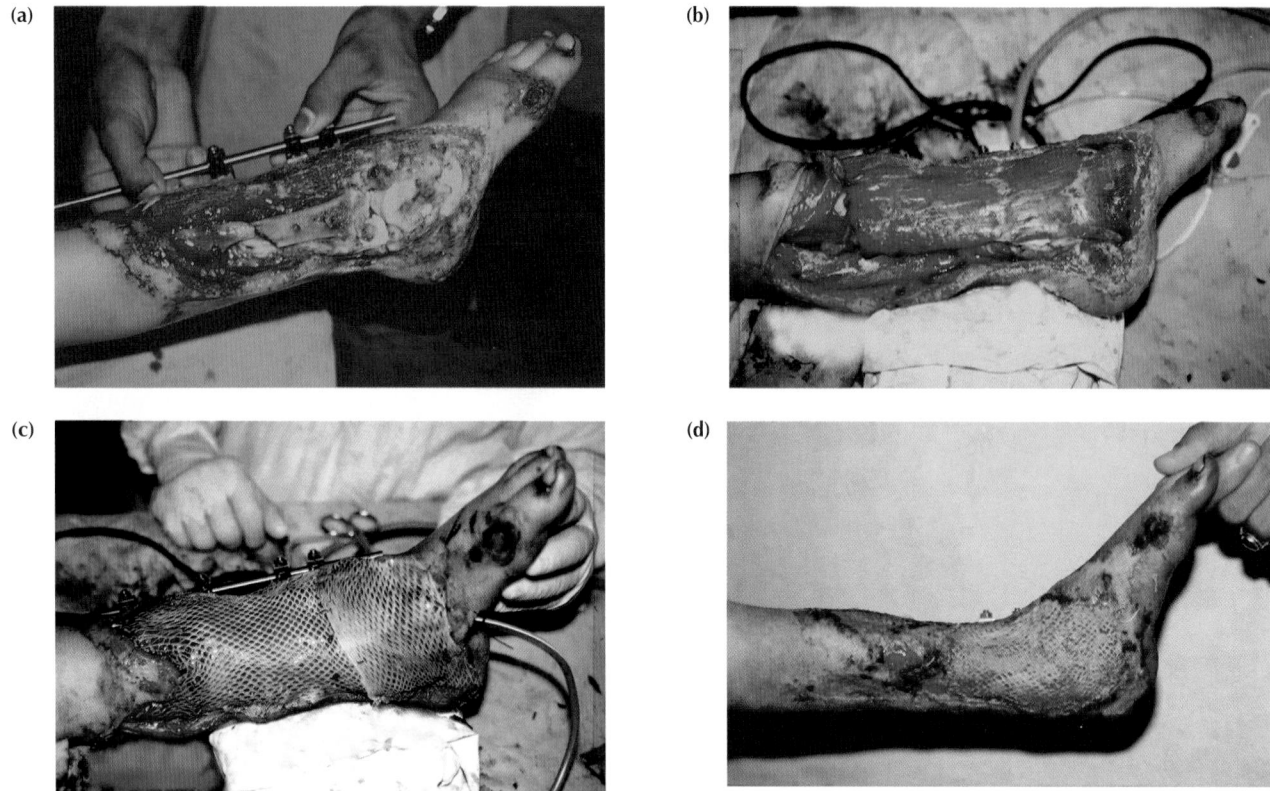

Figure 30.13 Badly traumatised lower limb. Reconstruction has been performed using a microvascular rectus abdominis flap covered with a skin graft.

Facial injuries

The management of facial injuries follows the same general principles of debridement and delayed closure as already outlined. Because of the functional and cosmetic importance of facial structures, skin and soft-tissue excisions are kept to a minimum. There is a robust blood supply to the face and the ability to counter infection is therefore very high. Even in patients who present late with gross contamination, a careful debridement followed by delayed primary closure can lead to good results (Fig. 30.14).

Tetanus

This potentially fatal condition, also called 'lockjaw', is caused by *Clostridium tetani*, a Gram-positive spore-forming bacillus occurring naturally in the intestines of humans and animals and in the soil. It enters the body through a wound and replicates, thriving on the anaerobic conditions present in devitalised tissues. It produces tetanospasmin, a potent exotoxin that binds to the neuromuscular junctions of the central nervous system neurones, rendering them incapable of neurotransmitter release. This leads to failure of inhibition of motor reflex responses to sensory stimulation. The result is generalised contractions of agonist and antagonist muscles causing tetanic spasms. The median incubation period is 7 days, ranging from 4–14 days.

Early symptoms are painful spasms of the masseter and facial muscles resulting in the classical risus sardonicus (Fig. 30.15). The spasms spread to involve the muscles of respiration and the laryngeal musculature. Spasms of the paravertebral and extensor limb musculature produce opisthotonus, an arching of the whole body. Laryngeal muscle spasm leads to apnoea and, if prolonged, to asphyxia and respiratory arrest. The spasms can be brought on by the slightest of sensory stimuli. They may be sustained and severe enough to produce long-bone fractures and joint dislocations.

The diagnosis is obvious once it is fully manifest. There are three aspects of management:

- *Prevention*. Wounds contaminated with soil are likely to harbour the organism and active immunisation is indicated by administering 0.5 ml of tetanus toxoid intramuscularly. Patients with gross contamination of deeply cavitating wounds should also receive 250–500 U of human anti-tetanus globulin (ATG) intramuscularly to provide passive immunisation and neutralise the circulating toxin (in clinical tetanus, 3000–10 000 U of ATG should be administered). Wound manipulation should be avoided for 2–3 hours after ATG administration to minimise tetanospasmin release.
- *Local wound care*. This includes a thorough wound debridement to eliminate the anaerobic environment. Intravenous administration of $10–24 \times 10^6$ U day^{-1} of penicillin G is effective and should be continued for 10–14 days. The wound should be closed using the delayed primary or secondary closure techniques (see above).
- *Supportive care for established disease*. These patients are nursed in an intensive care unit (ICU) environment, free from strong sensory stimuli. Unnecessary manipulations are avoided. Diazepam is useful in preventing the onset of spasms but if spasms become frequent and sustained the patient should be paralysed, intubated and placed on a ventilator. The patient is

CHAPTER 30 | DISASTER SURGERY

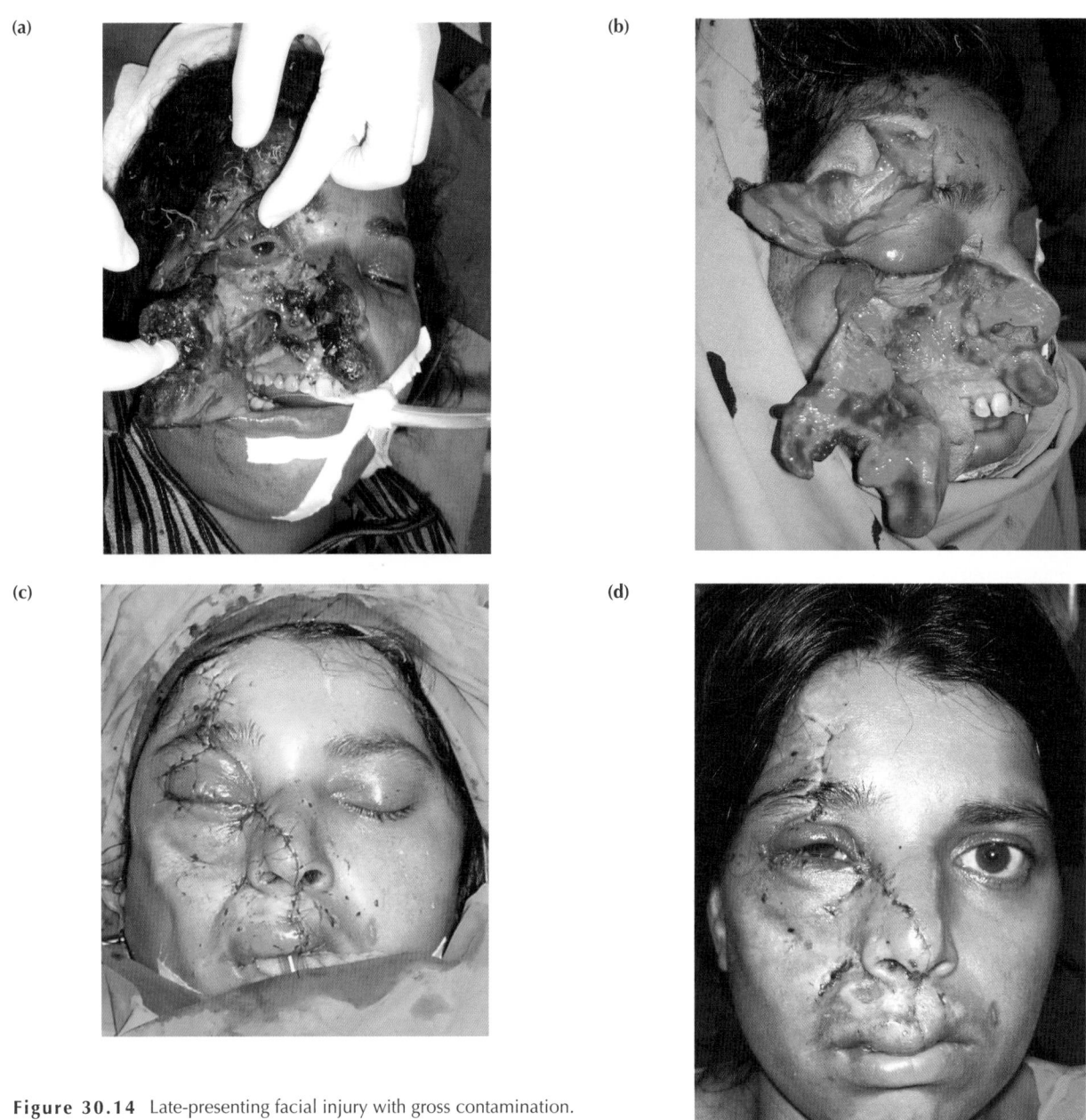

Figure 30.14 Late-presenting facial injury with gross contamination. A thorough debridement followed by delayed primary closure has yielded good results.

then gradually weaned off the ventilator under cover of anticonvulsants. The overall mortality rate is around 45%, prognosis being determined by the incubation period and the time from the first symptom to the first tetanic spasm. In general, shorter intervals indicate a poorer prognosis. Clinical tetanus does not result in immunity and so survivors should receive active immunisation with toxoid to prevent recurrence.

Necrotising fasciitis

This is a dangerous and rapidly spreading infection of the fascial planes leading to necrosis of the subcutaneous tissues and overlying skin. It is caused by β-haemolytic streptococci and, occasionally, *Staphylococcus aureus* but may take the form of a polymicrobial infection associated with other aerobic and anaerobic pathogens, including *Bacteroides, Clostridium, Proteus, Pseudomonas* and *Klebsiella*. It is termed Fournier's gangrene when it affects the perineal area and Meleney's synergistic gangrene when it involves the abdominal wall. The underlying pathology is identical and includes acute inflammatory infiltrate, extensive necrosis, oedema and thrombosis of the microvasculature. The area becomes

Theodor Albrecht Edwin Klebs, 1834–1913, **Professor of Bacteriology successively at Prague, Czechoslovakia, Zurich, Switzerland and the Rush Medical College, Chicago, IL, USA.**
Jean Alfred Fournier, 1832–1915, **the founder of the Venereal and Dermatological Clinic, Hôpital St Louis, Paris, France.**
Frank Lamont Meleney, 1889–1963, **Professor of Clinical Surgery, Columbia University, New York, NY, USA.**

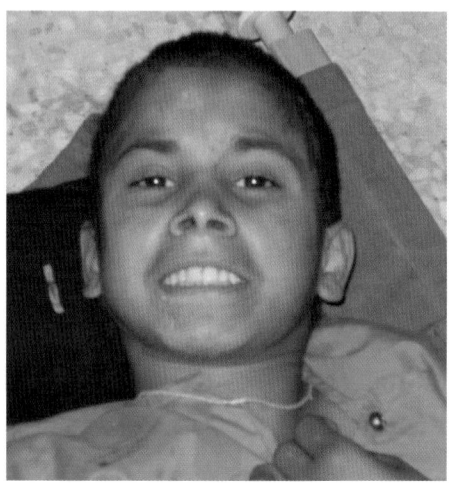

Figure 30.15 Risus sardonicus of 'lockjaw' (courtesy of Dr Samira Ajmal FRCS).

oedematous, painful and very tender. The skin turns dusky blue and black secondary to the progressive underlying thrombosis and necrosis (Fig. 30.16). The area may develop bullae and progress to overt cutaneous gangrene with subcutaneous emphysema. It spreads to contiguous areas but occasionally also produces skip lesions that later coalesce. It is accompanied by fever and severe generalised toxicity. Renal failure as a result of hypovolaemia and cardiovascular collapse caused by septic shock may occur. The rate of progression can catch the unwary by surprise and unless aggressively treated it leads to serious consequences with a mortality rate approaching 70%.

The diagnosis is usually made on clinical grounds. Creatinine kinase levels may show enormous elevation and biopsy of the fascial layers can confirm the diagnosis. Patients are admitted to ICU and treated aggressively with careful monitoring of volume derangements and cardiac status. Oxygen supplementation is advantageous and endotracheal intubation is required in patients unable to maintain their airway.

High-dose penicillin G along with broad-spectrum antibiotics such as third-generation cephalosporins and metronidazole should be given intravenously until the patient's toxicity abates. The cornerstone of management is surgical excision of the necrotic tissue. The fascial planes are opened with ease as the infection produces inflammatory degloving and the yellowish-green necrotic fascia is visible. Devitalised tissue should be removed generously, preferably going beyond the area of induration. This can lead to profuse bleeding and it is wise to have blood already cross-matched. The wound is lightly packed with fluffed gauze and dressed. This process should be continued on a daily basis as the necrosis is prone to spread beyond the edges of the excised wound. In patients who survive, this results in a large wound, which will require skin grafting or flap coverage.

Recently, the role of hyperbaric oxygen (HBO) has become more established. It is claimed that it is bactericidal, improves neutrophil function and promotes wound healing. The patient is placed in a high-pressure chamber and 100% oxygen administered at a pressure of 2–3 atmospheres. Studies have shown a

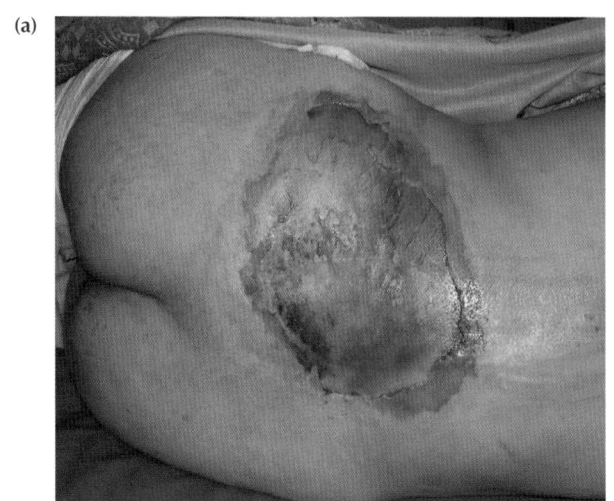

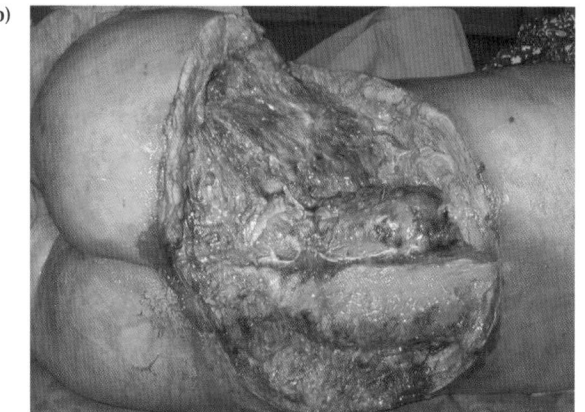

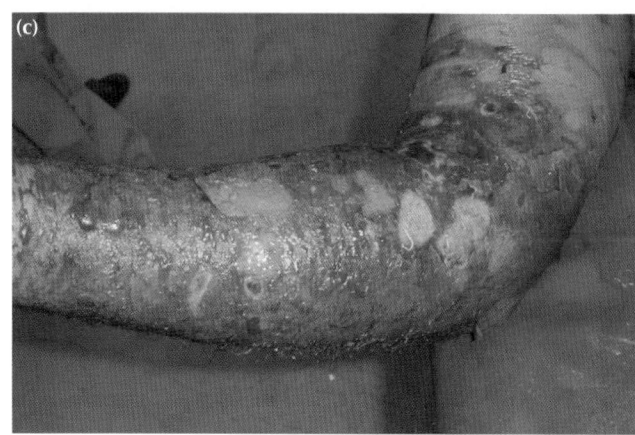

Figure 30.16 (a) Necrotising fasciitis at presentation and (b) rapid progression seen after 24 hours. (c) Typical bullae and induration.

CHAPTER 30 | DISASTER SURGERY

reduction in mortality rate in patients treated with HBO (9–20%) compared with patients who did not receive HBO (30–50%). The main limitation to its use is availability of the pressure chamber.

Gas gangrene

This is a dreaded consequence of inadequately treated missile wounds, crushing injuries and high-voltage electrical injuries. It is a rapidly progressive, potentially fatal condition characterised by widespread necrosis of the muscles and subsequent soft-tissue destruction. The common causative organism is *Clostridium perfringens*, a spore-forming, Gram-positive saprophyte that flourishes in anaerobic conditions. Other organisms implicated in gas gangrene include *C. bifermentans*, *C. septicum* and *C. sporogenes*. They are present in the soil and have also been isolated from the human gastrointestinal tract and female genital tract. Non-clostridial gas-producing organisms such as coliforms have also been isolated in 60–85% of cases of gas gangrene.

Clostridium perfringens produces many exotoxins but their exact role is unclear. Alpha-toxin, the most important, is a lecithinase, which destroys red and white blood cells, platelets, fibroblasts and muscle cells. The phi-toxin produces myocardial suppression whereas the kappa-toxin is responsible for the destruction of connective tissue and blood vessels.

Wounds become contaminated with clostridial spores and the devitalised tissue, foreign bodies and premature wound closure provide the anaerobic conditions necessary for spore germination. The usual incubation period is < 24 hours but it can range from 1 hour to 6 weeks. A vicious cycle of tissue destruction is initiated by rapidly multiplying bacteria and locally and systemically acting exotoxins. Locally, this results in spreading necrosis of muscle and thrombosis of blood vessels while progressive oedema further compromises the blood supply. The typical feature of this condition is the production of gas (composed of nitrogen, hydrogen sulphide and carbon dioxide) that spreads along the muscle planes. Systemically, the exotoxins cause severe haemolysis and, combined with the local effects, this leads to rapid progression of the disease, hypotension, shock, renal failure and acute respiratory distress syndrome (ARDS).

The earliest symptom is acute onset of pain that increases in severity as the myo-necrosis progresses. The limb swells up and the wound exudes a serosanguinous discharge. The skin is involved secondary to underlying muscle necrosis, turning brown and progressing to a blue-black colour with the appearance of haemorrhagic bullae (Fig. 30.17). The characteristic sickly sweet odour and soft tissue crepitus caused by gas production appear with established infection but the absence of either does not exclude the diagnosis. These local signs are accompanied by pyrexia, tachycardia disproportionate to body temperature, tachypnoea and alteration in mental status.

The diagnosis is made on the basis of history and clinical features: a peripheral blood smear may suggest haemolysis; a Gram stain of the exudate reveals large Gram-positive bacilli without neutrophils; and the biochemical profile may show metabolic acidosis and renal failure. Radiography can visualise gas in the soft tissues and computerised tomography (CT) scans are useful in patients with chest and abdominal involvement.

Hans Christian Joachim Gram, **1853–1938, Professor of Pharmacology (1891–1900) and Medicine (1900–1923), Copenhagen, Denmark, described this method of staining bacteria in 1884.**

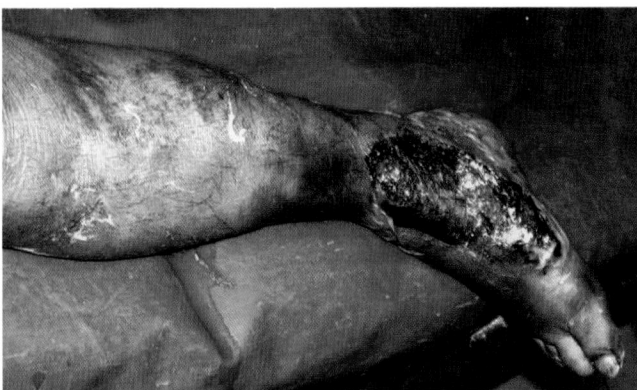

Figure 30.17 Typical picture of spreading gas gangrene caused by crush injury.

Patients should be admitted to ICU and treated aggressively with careful monitoring. High-dose penicillin G and clindamycin, along with third-generation cephalosporins, should be given intravenously until the patient's toxicity abates. The mainstay of management is early surgical excision of the necrotic tissue. The muscle planes are opened through generous longitudinal incisions and all devitalised tissue is removed, going beyond the area of induration. Abdominal involvement may necessitate excision of the wall musculature. Excision should be continued daily until the process of necrosis has stopped spreading. In established gas gangrene with systemic toxicity, amputation of the involved extremity is life saving and should not be delayed. No attempt is made at closure, amputation stumps are left open and the wound is lightly packed with saline-soaked gauze and dressed.

The role of HBO is not as clear as in necrotising fasciitis but it is recommended in severe cases if the facilities are available.

Blast injuries

Mechanism of explosive blast injury

The explosive pressure accompanying the bursting of bombs or shells ruptures their casing and imparts a high velocity to the fragments. These can cause even more devastating injury to the tissues than bullets. In addition, all explosions are accompanied by a complex blast wave composed of a blast pressure wave (dynamic overpressure) and the mass movement of air (blast wind). Like sound waves, blast pressure waves flow over and around an obstruction and affect anyone sheltering behind a wall or in a trench. A mass movement of air from the rapid expansion of gases at the centre of the explosion displaces air at supersonic speed. This results in injury patterns ranging from traumatic amputation to total body disruption. When a blast pressure wave hits the body, the force of the impact sets up a series of stress waves that are capable of internal injury, particularly at air–fluid interfaces. Thus, injury to the ear, lungs, heart and, to a lesser extent, the gastrointestinal tract is notable.

General management of blast injuries

The structures injured by the primary blast wave, in order of prevalence, are the middle ear, the lungs and the bowel. However, the commonest urgent clinical problem in survivors is penetrating injury caused by blast-energised debris and fragments of the exploding device. Many of those exposed will have blunt, blast and thermal injuries in addition to more obvious penetrating wounds. The deafness of blast victims caused by tympanic membrane rupture makes communication difficult and may complicate early assessment. Here, the primary survey and resuscitation phases of a system such as Advanced Trauma and Life Support (ATLS) are particularly apt. The management of penetrating wounds differs little from that of missile wounds referred to earlier. The soft-tissue wounds are usually heavily contaminated with dirt, clothing and secondary missiles such as wood, masonry and other materials from the environment. Such contaminants may be driven deeply into adjacent tissue planes opened up by the force of the explosion. In blast injuries, one cannot be sure of complete wound excision and it is imperative that wounds should be left open at the end of the initial operation and delayed primary closure performed.

Crush injury and syndrome

A crush injury occurs when a body part is subjected to a high degree of force or pressure, usually after being squeezed between two heavy or immobile objects. Damage related to crush injury includes lacerations, fractures, bleeding, bruising, compartment syndrome and crush syndrome. It can have disastrous consequences on local tissues with extensive destruction and devitalisation (Fig. 30.18).

Crush syndrome

The association between crush injury, rhabdomyolysis and acute renal failure was first reported in victims trapped during the 'London Blitz'. It is seen in earthquake and mining accident survivors and in battlefield casualties. Prolonged crushing of muscle releases myoglobin and vasoactive mediators into the circulation. It also sequesters many litres of fluid, reducing the effective intravascular volume and resulting in renal vasoconstriction and ischaemia. The myoglobinuria leads to tubular obstruction.

The treatment of crushed casualties should begin as soon as they are discovered. Rescuers must be alert to the presence of associated injuries (Fig. 30.19). Aggressive volume-loading of patients, preferably before extrication, is the best treatment. After provision of first aid and starting intravenous fluids the patient should be catheterised to measure output. In adults, a saline infusion of $1000\text{--}1500\,\mathrm{ml\,h^{-1}}$ should be initiated. Alkalinisation increases the solubility of acid haematin in urine and aids its excretion and should be continued until myoglobin is no longer detectable in the urine. Mannitol administration can reduce the reperfusion component of this injury. Once a flow of urine is observed, a mannitol–alkaline diuresis of up to $8\,\mathrm{l\,day^{-1}}$ should be maintained, keeping the urinary pH greater than 6.5.

Intensive care is required with close attention to fluid balance and renal replacement therapy if required.

(a)

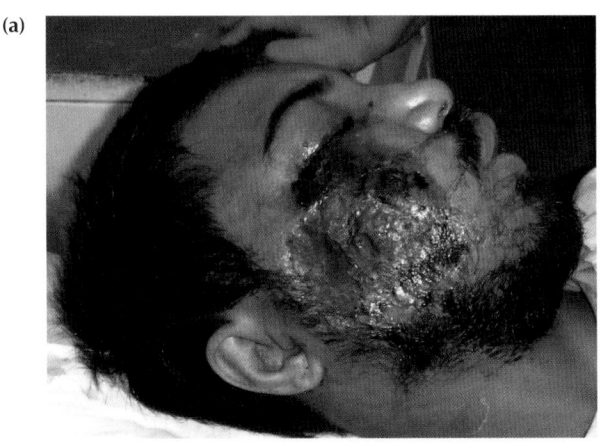

(c)

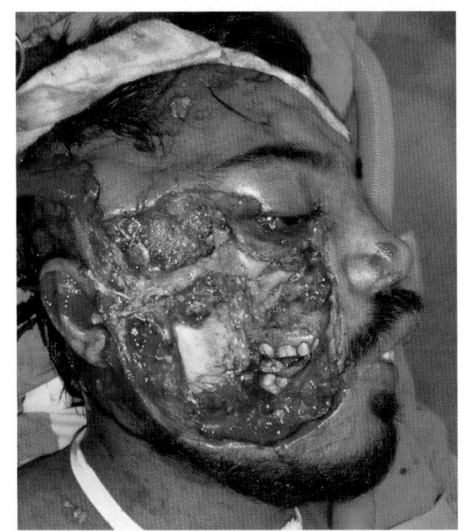

(b)

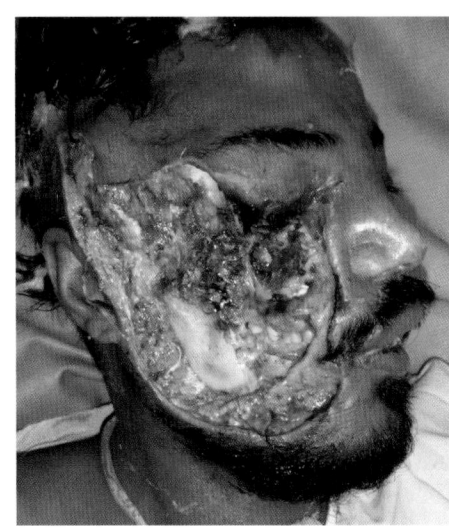

Figure 30.18 Extensive crush injury in a man trapped in a fallen house. The depth to which the soft tissues have been devitalised is seen clearly.

The London Blitz. This is the name given to the German air raids on London between 7 September 1940 and 11 May 1941, during which it is estimated that over 15 000 people were killed. Blitz is short for Blitzkrieg, the German for 'lightning war'.

CHAPTER 30 | DISASTER SURGERY

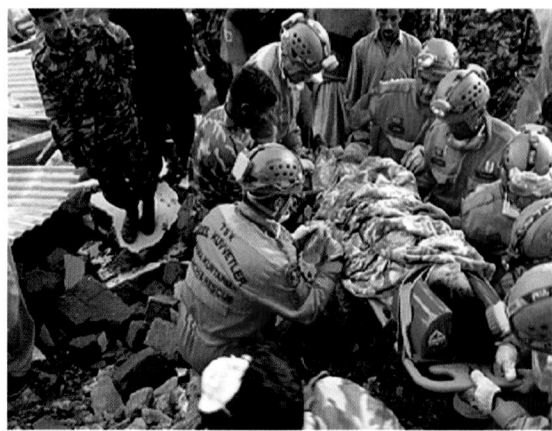

Figure 30.19 Rescuers must be prepared for injuries to the spine. Treatment of crush syndrome should start before extrication.

Compartment syndrome

For further details see Chapter 27.

Hypothermia

Hypothermia is a major cause of morbidity and mortality during disasters in cold regions and at high altitudes. It develops rapidly if the individual is immersed in water, covered with wet clothing or exposed to windy conditions. The body responds to cold temperatures by peripheral vasoconstriction as a result of catecholamine release and shivering caused by increased tone of the musculature. If the hypothermia continues unabated, the body's metabolism declines, with bradycardia and hypoventilation. The risk of ventricular fibrillation increases at temperatures below 28°C (82.4°F) and cerebral metabolism is decreased by 6–7% per 1°C drop in temperature.

In mild hypothermia symptoms are vague, including dizziness, lethargy, joint stiffness and nausea. The skin becomes pale and cold and the patient may exhibit confusion and impaired judgement, which progresses to uncoordinated movements and slurred speech. In severe hypothermia the mental status is further impaired, leading to hallucinations, stupor, and coma. Cardiac arrest usually occurs at 20°C (68°F).

The diagnosis is based on a history of exposure and is confirmed by rectal temperatures of 35°C (95°F) or less. The principles of treatment in the field include preventing further heat loss, restoring the core temperature and avoiding ventricular fibrillation.

The patient should be moved into dry shelter and wet clothing removed. A fire should be built or a stove lit to increase the temperature of the surroundings. No fluids should be given by mouth and the patient should be warmed passively. This is a safe and simple method of treating mild hypothermia and often the only choice in the field. The patient is covered with blankets or a sleeping bag and rewarmed for 24 hours at a room temperature of 25–33°C (77–91.4°F). Blood volume should be expanded using crystalloid solutions (warmed to 45°C/111°F). In adults, 300–500 ml should be administered rapidly, with the subsequent rate of infusion adjusted according to the blood pressure.

Severe hypothermia (< 28°C/82.4°F) should be treated as a life-threatening emergency. If the patient is breathing, humidified oxygen (10 l min⁻¹) should be administered using a non-rebreathing mask. If the patient is not breathing, ventilation should be initiated with an Ambu(RT) bag connected to a humidified, heated oxygen delivery system. Supplemental oxygen is necessary to prevent hypoxia, reduce the risk of ventricular fibrillation and treat pulmonary oedema.

Even after prolonged cardiac arrest, resuscitation is possible, and patients should not be declared dead until they are first rewarmed. If the patient is still not breathing, endotracheal intubation should be undertaken to maintain the airway. External cardiac compression must be continued in pulseless patients for some time. A central line or a venous cut-down should be established to administer warm fluids and for pressure measurements. A Foley catheter is passed to monitor urine output. Cardiac arrhythmias represent an immediate threat to life, but most revert spontaneously with rewarming. At core body temperatures below 30°C (86°F), the heart is usually unresponsive to defibrillation and inotropic agents, so medications are best withheld until rewarming has been achieved.

In severe hypothermia, active rewarming is required, which involves the internal or external addition of heat to the body: externally by heating blankets and warm water immersion; internally by heated humidified inhalation, peritoneal dialysis, haemodialysis or extracorporeal bypass.

Frost bite and immersion injuries

For further details see Chapter 28.

HANDING OVER

Follow-up and secondary problems

The medical aspect of disaster management does not involve a single short-term effort. It requires a long-term commitment and involvement of various disciplines. Because of the large numbers of casualties, the initial treatment received by patients is directed towards the anatomical restoration of damaged structures. This does not always translate into good functional results. There are therefore numerous patients who will need secondary procedures such as nerve, tendon and bone grafts, release of contractures and treatment of chronic infection (osteomyelitis). This second wave of patients is encountered 3–6 months following a major catastrophe and appropriate arrangements should be made to deal with this.

Designated centres

Initially, the casualties seen in major disasters are scattered amongst many hospitals. After the first few weeks most of the acute problems have been dealt with and only those patients who require longer-term treatment remain. At this point it is advisable to designate a particular hospital as a centre for patients with spinal cord injuries and complex limb trauma, who require combined orthopaedic and plastic surgical care along with rehabilitation. It concentrates resources and expertise and makes it easier to follow up these patients. This may not always be possible because of logistic reasons, as many patients prefer to be treated near their places of residence.

DISASTER PLANS

Disasters are by their very nature unforeseen events and planning for them may seem paradoxical. It has, however, been shown that

Frederic Eugene Basil Foley, **1891–1966, Urologist, Ankher Hospital, St Paul, MN, USA.**

disaster planning not only works but also saves lives. Unfortunately, the message only seems to register in the aftermath of a real disaster. Disaster planning is a wide field but a résumé of the important aspects follows.

Establishment of a national level disaster management organisation

This is the first step in the planning for disasters. Most developed countries already have such an agency, which can formulate policy at the national level and has the infrastructure to react quickly when the need arises.

Anticipating disasters

Areas close to active volcanoes and geological fault lines are at risk from seismic disturbances whereas regions along major rivers are liable to flood. The urban centres of all countries are now potential targets for terrorist attacks. It is important to not only carry out threat assessments but also, if possible, set up an early warning system. This allows information to be relayed to the population at risk, hopefully before a calamity occurs. For this to work there has to be close liaison with the meteorological services, seismology experts and intelligence agencies.

Evacuation planning

Evacuation of large population centres as a prelude to or in the wake of an impending disaster is a complex exercise. Yet it may be the most prudent course of action to remove as many people as possible from harm's way. Clear identification of exit routes for different areas must be determined and communicated to the populations at risk. Evacuation drills are very useful in areas that are at high risk of natural calamities and for high-rise buildings in urban areas.

Organisation of emergency services

Emergency services such as the fire brigade, police and ambulance service must have definite roles and areas of responsibility assigned to them to ensure a smooth and coordinated response during a crisis. Members of these teams must be included in the planning phase to ensure that the final plan is practicable and reflects the situation on the ground.

Medical planning

The role of medical services has been discussed in detail in the preceding sections. Identification of hospitals able to take large numbers of casualties and the location of areas that can be used for patient holding and triage in case of mass casualties is very important. Planners should estimate realistically the number of acute patients that each hospital in a region can treat optimally. Hospitals that offer specialised services, e.g. trauma and burns centres, intensive care facilities and neurosurgical services, should be identified and their role during a major crisis made clear. Ambulance services and search and rescue organisations must be kept fully informed of the situation at all times because they will be responsible for patients reaching the appropriate destinations. Suitable hospitals in the surrounding areas must be designated as overflow hospitals in the eventuality of a very large volume of patients.

FURTHER READING

Burkle, F.M., Jr, Sanner, P.H. and Wolcott, B.W. (1984) *Disaster Medicine: Application for the Immediate Management and Triage of Civilian and Military Disaster Victims.* Medical Examination Publishing, New York.

der Heide, E.A. (1989) *Disaster Response: Principles of Preparedness and Coordination.* Mosby, St Louis, MO.

Husum, H., Gilbert, M. and Wisborg, T. (2000) *Save Lives Save Limbs – Life Support for Victims of Mines, Wars and Accidents.* Third World Network, Malaysia.

Mattox, K., Feliciano, D.V. and Moore, E.E. (eds) (2000) *Trauma,* 4th edn. McGraw Hill, New York.

CHAPTER 30 | DISASTER SURGERY

PART 5 | Elective orthopaedics

Clinical examination

To understand how to:
- Take a general orthopaedic history

- Perform a systematic examination of each region of the musculoskeletal system

INTRODUCTION

The components of the musculoskeletal system include the bones, joints, ligaments, muscles and tendons as well as the neurological and vascular structures. A simple system allows a concise yet comprehensive history to be taken and a reliable examination to be performed, which will reveal all of the common as well as the more rare but dangerous musculoskeletal problems that are likely to be encountered in clinical practice.

HISTORY

Introduction

- Introduce yourself and check the patient's name.
- Explain what you are going to do, obtain verbal consent and ensure that the patient is comfortable.

Take a history

- *Presenting complaint.* Start with an open-ended question. Ask the patient to 'explain what the problem is' in their own words. Ask the patient what their hopes and expectations are from the interview.
- *History of the presenting complaint* ('the three Ws'). When did you first notice the problem? What were you doing when it started? Was is sudden or did it develop gradually?
- *Associated symptoms.* Ask about the following: pain; swelling; instability – 'giving way'; mechanical symptoms (e.g. locking, clicking, clunking); loss of power; altered sensation.
- *Functional impairment.* Ask whether the patient is having difficulties performing activities of daily living: upper limb, e.g. personal hygiene, feeding; lower limb, e.g. putting on shoes and socks, standing.
- *Past medical history (PMH).* Comorbidities may affect the patient's fitness for an anaesthetic, e.g. diabetes, asthma, previous heart attack or stroke. Check for any previous problems with anaesthetics.
- *Past relevant surgical procedures.*
- *Drug history.* Ask about the following in particular: anticoagulants, steroids, aspirin, immunosuppressants, oral contraceptive pill and hormone replacement therapy.
- *Social history.* Tailor questions to the patient's condition:

patient's age; hand dominance; employment status; dependents; alcohol; smoking and hobbies; home help; accommodation – own house, residential or nursing home; use of walking aids; mental test score assessment (Summary box 31.1).

Summary box 31.1

Taking a history

- Introduce yourself and put the patient at ease
- Explain what you are doing and ensure that the patient agrees
- Presenting complaint – ask an open question
- History of presenting complaint and associated symptoms
- Functional impairment
- Past medical history and relevant surgical history
- Drug and social history

MUSCULOSKELETAL EXAMINATION

General principles

Apley described a useful and systematic approach to clinical examination. This approach is divided into three parts:

- look;
- feel;
- move.

Look

The inspection begins as soon as you enter the examination room. Look around the room for any walking aids. Remember to look at the whole patient and not just at the joint of interest. For example:

- look at the hands for rheumatoid arthritis;
- look at the eyes for Horner's syndrome;
- look for any obvious upper or lower limb or spinal deformity.

Alan Graham Apley, **1914–1996, Director of Orthopaedic Surgery, St. Thomas' Hospital, London, England.**
Johann Friedrich Horner, **1831–1886, Professor of Ophthalmology, Zurich, Switzerland, described this syndrome in 1869.**

Gait

The gait cycle is all of the activity between the initial contact of the foot with the ground and the succeeding initial contact of the same limb. There are two main stages: the stance phase (60%) and the swing phase (40%). Ask the patient to stand, and inspect from the front, side and back. Then, ask the patient to walk using any walking aids. Some of the types of limp that might be present are described in Table 31.1.

Focused inspection

Adequately expose the joint above and below. Expose the opposite limb for comparison. Make sure that the patient is comfortable. It may be easier for you and the patient if they remain standing for the first part of the examination. When a couch is used, make sure that it is in the centre of the room (not against the wall) so that you can work on both sides of the patient.

Remember that all joints are covered by an envelope of soft tissues and skin. Look at the *skin* for:

- surgical scars;
- bruising (may indicate recent injury or a bleeding disorder);
- erythema (e.g. cellulitis);
- ulcers (e.g. arterial, vascular or neuropathic);
- rashes;
- sinuses (e.g. secondary to osteomyelitis);
- hair loss and the presence or absence of sweating;
- pigmentations or raised lesion (e.g. café au lait spots or neuro-fibromas).

Look at the *soft tissues* for:

- swelling (e.g. may indicate a joint effusion);
- lumps (consider which tissue layer they are arising from);
- muscle wasting (e.g. may be secondary to disuse atrophy, neuropathy);
- muscle fasciculation (lower motor neurone pathology).

Look at the *bones* for:

- abnormal limb alignment – comparison with the other side may be helpful;
- deformity.

Feel

Ask the patient if they have any areas of tenderness. Ensure that you do not cause the patient pain – watch their face as you feel. It may be easier (especially with children) to feel the normal side first.

Skin

The aim of sensory testing is to establish a pattern of sensory loss. Look for a dermatomal (may indicate spinal root or peripheral nerve pathology) or glove and stocking distribution (may indicate a neuropathy, e.g. diabetes).

Perform a screening test by lightly stroking both limbs. Record whether the patient feels a difference. If none is noticed there is no need to spend more time on the neurological examination. If there is a difference then a full neurological examination should now be performed.

Soft tissues

- *Tenderness.* Try to determine the actual anatomical structure from which the pain arises (e.g. subcutaneous fat, bursae, nerves, arteries).
- *Lumps and effusions.* Determine the characteristics of any lump or effusion using Table 31.2 as a guide.
- *Pulses.* Palpate the distal pulses (or capillary return) of the limb. Recording distal neurovascular status before and after surgery is essential. Acute loss of circulation to a limb is a surgical emergency. Absence of distal pulses is an absolute contraindication to elective surgery in that limb.

Bone

Palpate the contours of the joint and assess for tenderness. For superficial joints, such as the knee, the joint line can be felt and checked for lumps and tenderness.

Move

There are three stages to assessing movement. The words used to describe a particular movement are shown in Table 31.3.

- *Active.* Ask the patient to move the joint within the limits of their pain.
- *Passive.* Move the joint yourself. Record the range of movement in 'degrees' (a goniometer may be helpful).
- *Stability.* Stability has a *static* and a *dynamic* component: static tests assess the integrity of the ligaments and joint (bone) surfaces; dynamic tests assess the integrity and functions of the muscles and tendons. Ask the patient to actively move the joint through its range of motion while you try to stop the movement. Record power using the Medical Research Council (MRC) grading system as illustrated in Table 31.4. Consider the muscles that drive each movement, the

Table 31.1 Types of limp

Type of limp	Pathology
Antalgic	Hip joint arthritis
Trendelenburg	Weakness of hip abductors
High-stepping gait	Foot drop secondary to common peroneal nerve palsy
Spastic	Cerebral palsy
Ataxic	Cerebellar pathology

Friedrich Trendelenburg, **1844–1924, Professor of Surgery, Rostock (1875–82), Bonn (1882–95), and Leipzig, Germany (1895–1911). The Trendelenburg position was first described in 1885.**

Table 31.2 Swelling – an acronym for history and examination of a lump

Start	Did it appear after trauma or gradually on its own?
Where	Anatomical site and layer (skin, fat, muscle); does it move in relation to these?
External features	Size, surface and definition of margins
Lymph nodes	Are the local ones enlarged?
Liquid	Is it fluctuant? Can it be transilluminated?
Internal features	Is it hard? Is it tender?
Noise	Is there a thrill? Is there a bruit?
General	Examination of the whole patient for general lumps

Table 31.3 Terminology used to describe the direction of movement

Flexion	Forward or anterior movement of the trunk or limb
Lateral flexion	Bending of the forward-facing head and trunk to either side
Extension	Backward or posterior movement
Abduction	A movement away from the midline of the body
Adduction	A movement towards the midline of the body
Internal rotation	Rotation towards the midline of the body
External rotation	Rotation away from the midline
Supination	Movement of the forearm so that the palm faces anteriorly
Pronation	Movement of the forearm so that the palm faces posteriorly
Circumduction	A combination of flexion, abduction, extension and adduction without rotation
Inversion	Movement of the foot that directs the sole of the foot medially
Eversion	Movement of the foot that directs the sole of the foot laterally
Retraction	Backwards movement of the head, jaw or shoulders

peripheral nerves that supply them and the nerve root values (Table 31.5).

In the following sections, in addition to the approach of 'Look, Feel, Move', we have included details of special tests for each joint as well as neurological examination of the limb. The peripheral nerve examination comprises sensory and motor testing, reflexes, tone and coordination and proprioception (Summary box 31.2).

Summary box 31.2

Musculoskeletal examination

- Introduce yourself and put the patient at ease
- Assess the gait
- Look
- Feel
- Move
- Special tests
- Neurological examination
- Pulses

Table 31.4 The Medical Research Council grading system of muscle power

Grade	Description
0	No movement
1	Flicker of movement
2	Active movement with gravity elimination
3	Active movement against gravity
4	Active movement against resistance but power less than full
5	Normal power

CLINICAL EXAMINATION OF THE SPINE

The spinal column consists of 33 vertebrae with 23 intervertebral discs. This is supported by numerous ligaments and para-spinal muscles.

When observed from the front (coronal plane) with the patient standing and the hips and knees fully extended, the head should be centred over the sacrum. A 'plumb line' dropped from the spinous process of C7 should fall through the gluteal crease (Fig. 31.1). If it falls to either side of the cleft, lateral tilt of the spine is present. The ear, shoulder and greater trochanter of the hip should lie in the same vertical plane. When the patient is observed from the side, assess the four physiological sagittal plane curves (cervical and lumbar lordosis, and the thoracic and sacral kyphosis) (Fig. 31.2).

Cervical spine

Look

Ensure that the shoulders, back muscles and scapulae can be seen. Look for muscle wasting and asymmetry of the neck creases and check that the shoulders are level and that there is a normal cervical lordosis (range 20–40°).

Feel

Stand behind the patient and support the patient's chin:

- *Soft tissues.* Feel for spasm of the para-spinal muscles.
- *Bone.* Palpate the spinous processes (tenderness and alignment); the spinous processes of C7 (vertebra prominens) and T1 are usually large and are easily palpable at the base of the neck.

Move

Motion occurs in three planes: flexion/extension, bending and rotation (Fig. 31.3):

- *Flexion* (45°)/*extension* (55°). Ask the patient to bend their neck forwards – place the chin on the chest. Measure the

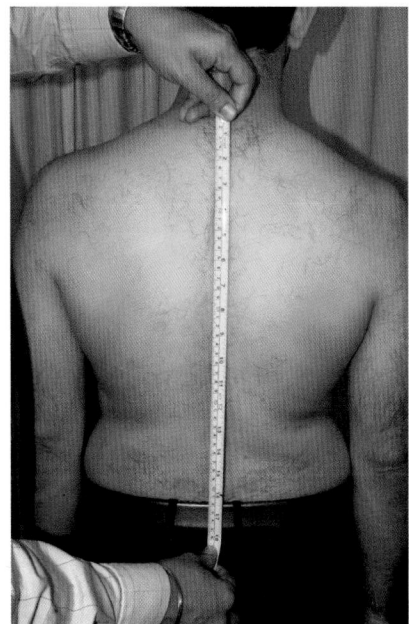

Figure 31.1 Plumb line.

Table 31.5 Peripheral nerves

Root level	Sensation	Motor	Reflex
C5	Lateral upper arm	Deltoid	Biceps
C6	Lateral forearm	Wrist extension	Brachioradialis
C7	Middle finger	Triceps	Triceps
C8	Little finger	Finger flexors	–
T1	Medial forearm	Interossei	–
L1	Anterior thigh	Psoas	–
L2	Anterior thigh/groin	Quadriceps	–
L3	Anterior and lateral thigh	Quadriceps	–
L4	Medial leg and foot	Tibialis anterior	Knee jerk
L5	Lateral leg and first dorsal web space	Extensor hallucis longus	–
S1	Lateral and plantar foot	Gastrocnemius/perineals	Achilles
S2–S4	Perianal	Bladder and foot intrinsics	–

(a)

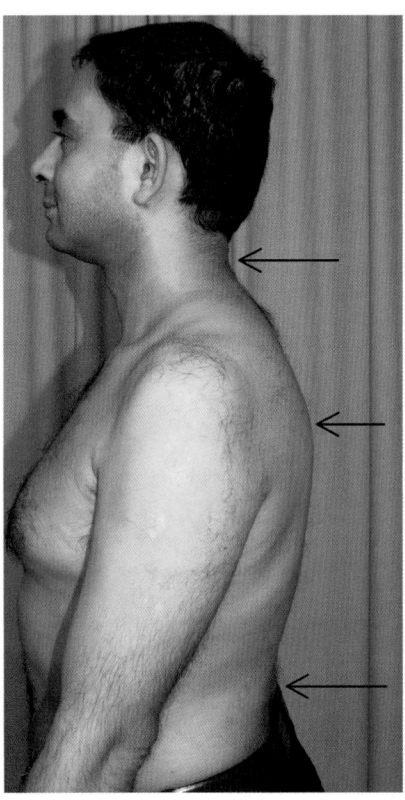

(b)

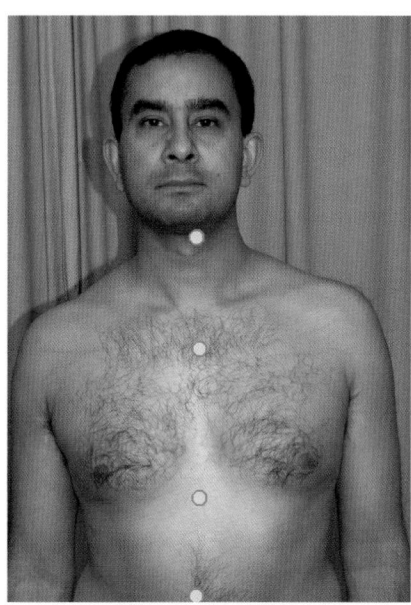

(c)

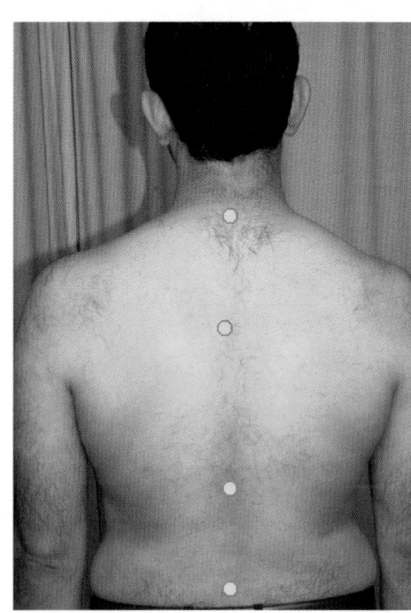

Figure 31.2 Standing sagittal profile of cervical and lumbar lordosis (a), and thoracic (b) and sacral (c) kyphosis.

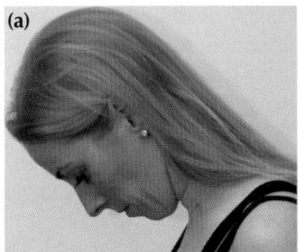
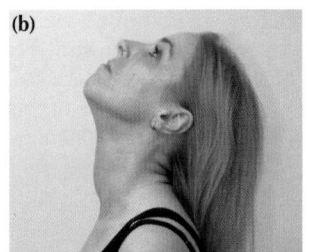
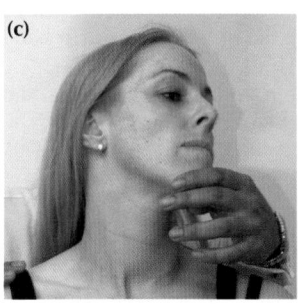
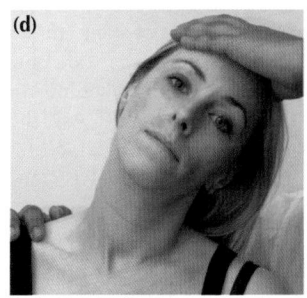

Figure 31.3 Cervical spine flexion/extension (a and b), rotation (c) and bending (d).

distance from the chin to the sternum. Ask the patient to extend their neck by looking up at the ceiling.
- *Right/left bending* (40°). Ask the patient to lay their ear on their ipsilateral shoulder.
- *Right/left rotation* (70°). Ask the patient to look over each shoulder while not moving the chest wall.

Neurological

Focus your examination on the C5 to T1 nerve roots. These supply the upper extremities (Fig. 31.4).

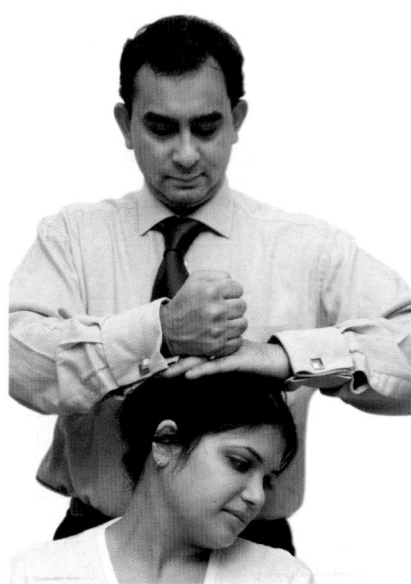

Figure 31.4 Spurling's test for cervical spine nerve root entrapment. Extend the cervical spine and rotate the head to each shoulder in turn. The presence of a shooting pain down the arm may indicate cervical nerve root compression.

Thoracic spine

Pathology commonly presents with pain and deformity. The thoracic spine is normally convex with a gentle kyphosis (normal range 20–45°).

Look

Ensure that the front and the back from the neck to the gluteal cleft can be visualised. Note skin markings (e.g. café au lait spots, hairy patches). These may suggest occult neurology or bony pathology.

- *Front.* Asymmetry of the shoulder and rib cage suggests scoliosis.
- *Back.* Look for a difference in the height of the iliac crests (pelvic tilt). Assess for coronal plane deformity such as scoliosis (lateral curvature of the thoracic spine with rotation). A rib hump suggesting a structural scoliosis may be visible.
- *Side.* Assess for sagittal plane deformity such as an increased kyphosis.

Feel

Palpate with one hand supporting the patient's pelvis.

Move

Range of motion is limited in the thoracic spine:

- *'Forward bending test'* (Fig. 31.5). Ask the patient to bend forwards to touch their toes:
  - *structural scoliosis*: a rib hump will increase in size (bulge posteriorly on the thoracic convex side) as the patient bends forwards; this is diagnostic of idiopathic thoracic scoliosis (rotatory deformity);
  - *functional scoliosis*: the spine straightens as the patient bends forwards and no rib hump is visible; this flexible deformity is

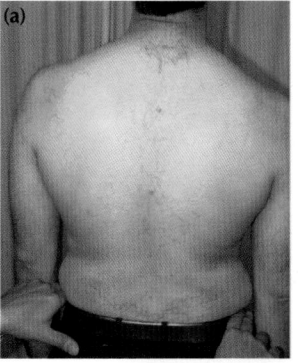
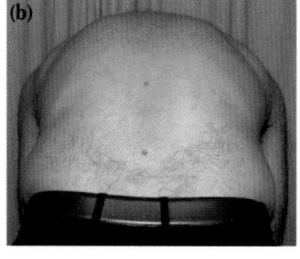
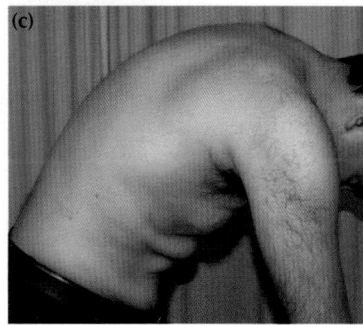

Figure 31.5 Forward bending test.

secondary to other abnormalities such as abnormal leg lengths and muscle spasm in the lumbar region.

- *Lateral bending* can be used to assess the flexibility of a scoliosis. Radiographs are taken in this position to supplement the assessment.

Lumbar spine

Examination should include the pelvis, hips, lower limbs, gait and peripheral vascular system as well as the lumbar region. Irritation of nerves in the lumbar spine can mimic problems in the lower limb. Always consider referred pain.

Look

- *Back.* Check the skin at the base of the spine for hairy tufts and dimples (underlying spina bifida). Prominence of the spinal muscles on one side may be the result of muscle spasm secondary to pain.
- *Side.* The lumbar spine has a smooth concavity known as the lumbar lordosis (normal range is 40–60°). Muscle spasm is a cause of loss of the normal lordosis.

Feel

Feel for any 'step-off' in the spinous processes. This may indicate forward slippage of one of the vertebrae on another.

Move

Movement occurs in flexion, extension, lateral bending and rotation (Fig. 31.6). Record the motion in each plane in degrees. Remember that a significant portion of lumbar flexion is achieved through the hip joint.

- *Forward flexion* is a measure of lumbar flexibility. The skin of the lumbar spine stretches as the patient bends forwards. To measure flexion, place the tip of your thumb over the T12–L1 junction and the tip of your index finger of the same hand over the lumbosacral junction. Ask the patient to bend forwards and touch the toes (normal range 40–60°). Measure the distance by which your thumb and the tip of your index finger separate.
- *Lateral bending.* Ask the patient to slide their right hand down the outer side of their right leg and then their left hand down the outside of their left leg. Note the distance that each hand moves down that side of the thigh.
- *Rotation.* Stand behind the patient and hold their pelvis still with both hands. Ask the patient to twist around and look over their shoulder. Note the angle that the shoulder girdle forms with the pelvis (range 3–18°).

Special tests

- *Lasègue's straight leg raise test* (Fig. 31.7). This test increases tension along the sciatic nerve (L5 and S1 nerve roots). With the patient supine, elevate the leg with the knee bent to check pain-free movement of the hip. Then, the knee is straightened, allowing the hip to extend until tension is removed from the hamstring muscles. Finally, the ankle is dorsiflexed firmly, tugging on the sciatic nerve. If the patient experiences pain running down the leg the test is positive.
- *Contralateral stretch test.* Elevate the asymptomatic leg; if pain is reproduced in the other leg the test is considered positive (Summary box 31.3).

(a)

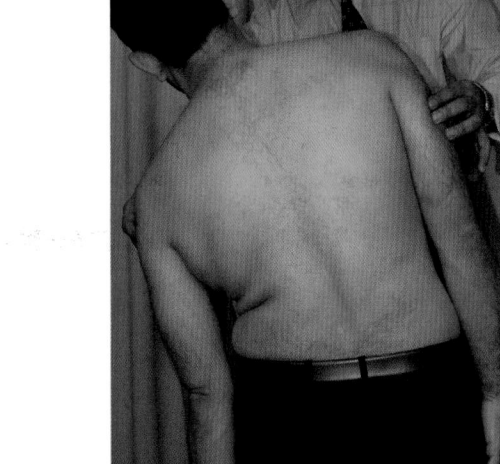

(b)

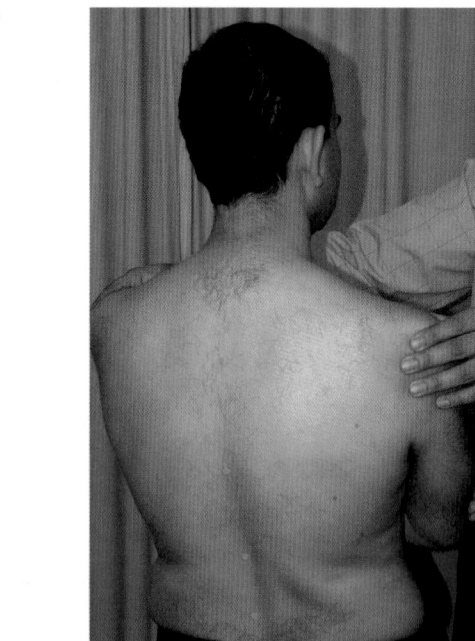

Figure 31.6 Lumbar flexion/extension, lateral bending (a) and rotation (b).

Charles Ernest Lasègue, **1816–1863, Professor of Medicine, The Univesity of Paris, and Physician, La Salpêtrière, Paris, France.**

(a)

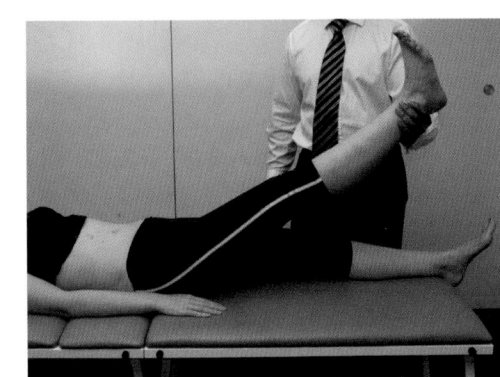

(b)

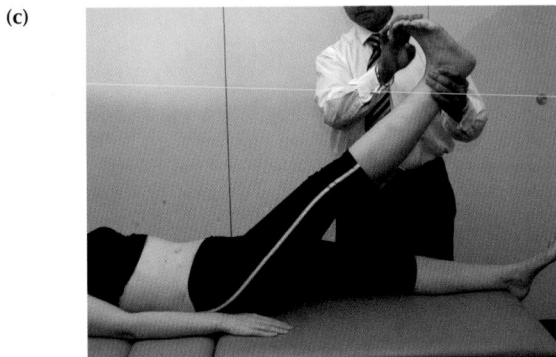

(c)

Figure 31.7 Lasègue's straight leg test.

Summary box 31.3

Spine examination

Inspection of the standing patient
■ From the front and back (coronal plane)
■ From the side (saggittal plane)

Palpation
■ Palpation of the posterior bony elements and the para-spinal muscles

Move
■ Assess flexion, extension, lateral rotation and bending

Neurological
■ Assess sensation, tone, power, reflexes, proprioception and coordination

Special tests
■ Spurling's test
■ Forward bending test
■ Lasègue's straight leg test
■ Contralateral stretch test

CLINICAL EXAMINATION OF THE HAND AND WRIST

The hand and wrist should be thought of as one functional unit. The muscles may be divided into extrinsic (the muscle bellies in the forearm) and intrinsic (origins and insertions within the hand alone). The 'flexors' (volar side) flex the wrist and fingers and the 'extensors' (dorsal surface) extend the digits and fingers.

Look

Inspect the posture of both hands. A nerve lesion will produce a specific resting position (e.g. an ulnar nerve lesion will produce clawing of the little and ring fingers).

- *Skin*. Assess for scars, discolouration (café au lait spots, erythema) and loss of hair. The nails may reveal systemic disease (e.g. psoriatic pitting). Look for tight bands in the palm (Dupuytren's contracture). Loss of sweating is seen in complex regional pain syndrome.
- *Soft tissue*. Centrally located swellings at the wrist may indicate a ganglion arising from the wrist joint itself; de Quervain's tenosynovitis may present with a swelling around the radial styloid.
- Check for thenar, hypothenar (Fig. 31.8) and intrinsic muscle wasting. To assess thenar eminence wasting, place the hands side by side with the thumbs upwards and look down and

(a)

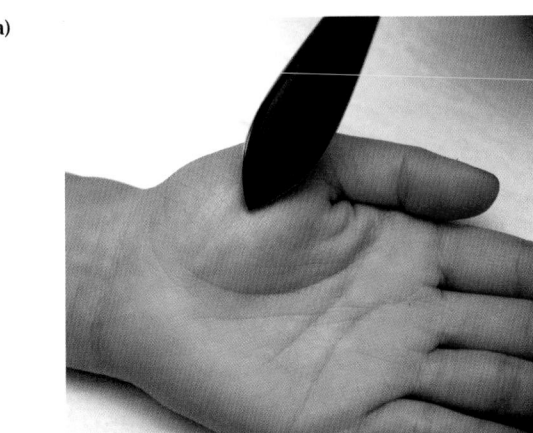

(b)

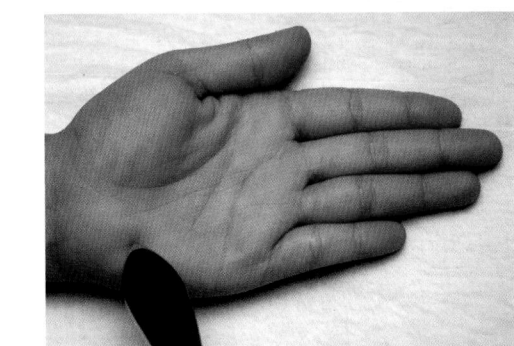

Figure 31.8 Thenar (a) and hypothenar (b) wasting.

Baron Guillaume Dupuytren, **1777–1835, Surgeon, Hôtel Dieu, Paris, France,** described this condition in 1831.
Friedrich Joseph de Quervain, **1868–1940, Professor of Surgery, Berne, Switzerland,** described this form of tenosynovitis in 1895.

CHAPTER 31 | CLINICAL EXAMINATION

compare the thenar regions. Patterns of muscle wasting are shown in Table 31.6.

- *Bones.* Look for bony deformity (dinner fork deformity, Colles' fracture). Typical bony deformities are described in Table 31.7.

Feel

- *Skin.* If there is any question of abnormal sensation on a simple stroke test comparing both sides, proceed to the two-point discrimination test using the sharp ends of a paper clip. Record the minimum distance between the tips of the paper clip at which the patient is able to recognise two points. Table 31.8 describes the anatomical region supplied by the median, ulnar and radial nerves.
- *Pen sliding test.* To assess the absence or presence of sweating, slide a pen along the radial border of the index finger. If the pen slides smoothly, this may indicate loss of sweating.
- *Soft tissue*:
  - *blood vessels*: check the radial and ulnar artery pulses; assess the capillary refill time, which is normally less than 2 s; Allen's test should be performed before surgery (Table 31.9 and Fig. 31.9);
  - *nerves*: compressive neuropathies are most commonly seen affecting the median nerve [see Tinel's (Fig. 31.10a) and Phalen's (Fig. 31.10b) test in Table 31.9];
  - *palmar fascia*: feel for palmar thickening and skin pits; long finger-like structures (cords), most commonly affecting the ring and little fingers, are suggestive of Dupuytren's disease.
- *Bones.* Palpate from the radial to the ulnar side of the wrist joint. In the trauma setting, palpate the anatomical snuff box (Fig. 31.11). A fracture of the scaphoid may cause tenderness.

The scaphoid tubercle, pisiform and the hook of hamate are all palpable on the volar aspect of the wrist.

Move

The wrist can be moved into flexion and extension, and ulnar and radial deviation.

- *Wrist.* Extension is tested by asking the patient to push the hands together into a 'prayer' position (Fig. 31.12a). If there is loss of extension, the palms will not meet and/or one forearm will be dropped. It is essential that the elbows remain at the same level. Palmar flexion is tested in a similar fashion but with the hands pointing down and the back of the hands in contact (Fig. 31.12b). Ulnar and radial deviation are tested by taking the patient's hand in your own and moving the hand into these directions.
- *Hand.* A general screening assessment is to ask the patient to roll up their fingers from full extension to full flexion. This will reveal a trigger finger.

Extensors and flexors

Asking the patient to grip two of your fingers in their fist tests the power of the extensors of the wrist (radial nerve) because they are needed to brace the wrist. It also tests the power of the flexors in the forearm (median nerve). Asking the patient then to extend and spread their fingers apart against resistance tests the intrinsic muscles of the hand (mainly the ulnar nerve).

Finger flexors

- *Superficialis tendon test.* The flexor digitorum profundus (FDP) usually has one muscle belly from which tendons to all of the fingers arise. The FDP can be immobilised by holding all of the fingers in extension; this allows the superficialis tendon to be tested in isolation. Hold all of the fingers in full extension except the finger to be tested. Ask the patient to actively flex that finger. If the test finger is able to flex, the superficialis tendon to that finger is working. Repeat for the other fingers individually (Fig. 31.13).

Table 31.6 Patterns of muscle wasting in the hand

Thenar wasting	Median nerve palsy (C8)
Hypothenar wasting	Ulnar nerve palsy (T1)
Intrinsic wasting	Ulnar nerve palsy (T1)

Table 31.7 Bony deformities of the hand

Anatomical site	Name	Association
Distal interphalangeal joint (DIPJ)	Heberden's nodes	Osteoarthritis
Proximal interphalangeal joint (PIPJ)	Buchard's node	Osteoarthritis
Hyperextension of the metacarpo-phalangeal joint (MCPJ), flexion of the PIPJ and hyperextension of the DIPJ	Boutonnière deformity	Rheumatoid arthritis
Hyperextension of the MCPJ and PIPJ and flexion of the DIPJ	Swan neck deformity	Rheumatoid arthritis
Flexion of the MCPJ with hyperextension of the interphalangeal joint	Z deformity of the thumb	Rheumatoid arthritis
Subluxation of the MCPJ	Ulnar drift	Rheumatoid arthritis

Abraham Colles, **1773–1843**, Professor of Surgery, The Royal College of Surgeons in Ireland, and Surgeon, Dr. Steven's Hospital, Dublin, Ireland.
Edgar van Nuys Allen, **1900–1961**, Professor of Medicine, The Mayo Clinic, Rochester, MN, USA.
Jules Tinel, **1879–1952**, Physician, Hôpital Beaujon, Paris, France.
George S. Phalen, **Contemporary**, Orthopaedic Surgeon, The Cleveland Clinic, Cleveland, OH, USA.
William Heberden (Snr), **1710–1801**, a Physician who practised first in Cambridge, and later in London, England.
Charles Jacques Bouchard, **1837–1915**, Physician, Dean of the Faculty of Medicine, Paris, France.
Boutonnière **is French for 'button-hole'.**

(a)

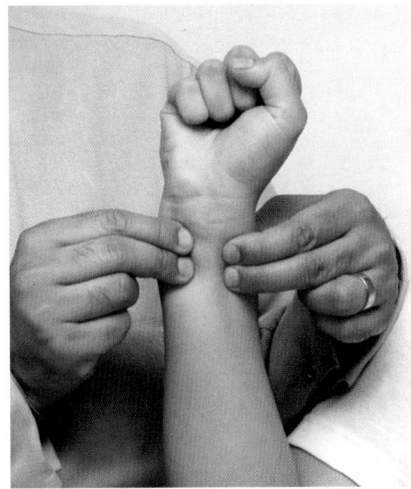

(b)

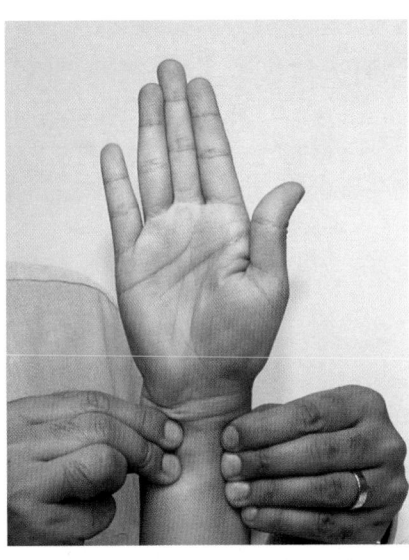

(c)

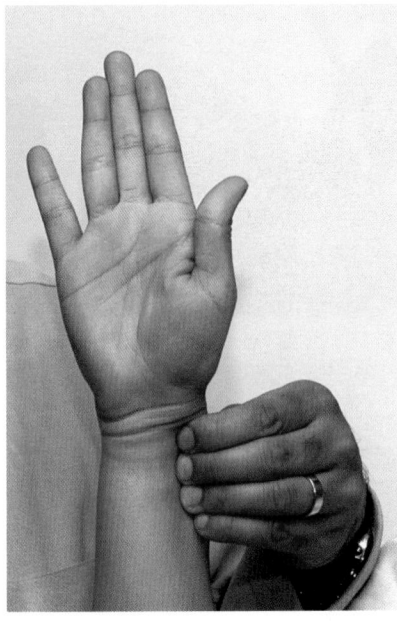

Figure 31.9 (a–c) Performing Allen's test.

Table 31.8 Sensory distribution of the nerve supply to the hand

Nerve	Sensory distribution
Ulnar	Little finger and ulnar half of the ring finger
Median	Thumb, index, middle and radial half of the ring finger
Radial	Base of the thumb on the dorsum of the hand

Table 31.9 Special hand tests

Test	Technique	Significance
Allen's test	Elevate the hand and apply digital pressure on the radial and ulnar arteries to occlude them. Ask the patient to make a fist several times. The tips of the finger should go pale. Release each artery in turn and observe the return of colour	Tests the adequacy of the blood supply to the hand from the radial and ulnar arteries and the arcade between them
Tinel's test	Tap over the nerve of interest. Tingling may indicate nerve compression	Identifies compression of a peripheral nerve
Phalen's test	Place the wrist in maximum flexion with the elbows extended	Compression of the medial nerve causes paraesthesia
Froment's sign	Ask the patient to grip a sheet of paper between the index finger and thumb of both hands. Grip the paper yourself similarly. Ask the patient to resist as you attempt to pull the paper away.	A positive test indicated by flexion of the thumb interphalangeal joint suggests weakness of the adductor pollicis muscle supplied by the ulnar nerve. Recruitment of the median nerve-innervated flexor pollici brevis explains the thumb posture

CHAPTER 31 | CLINICAL EXAMINATION

(a)

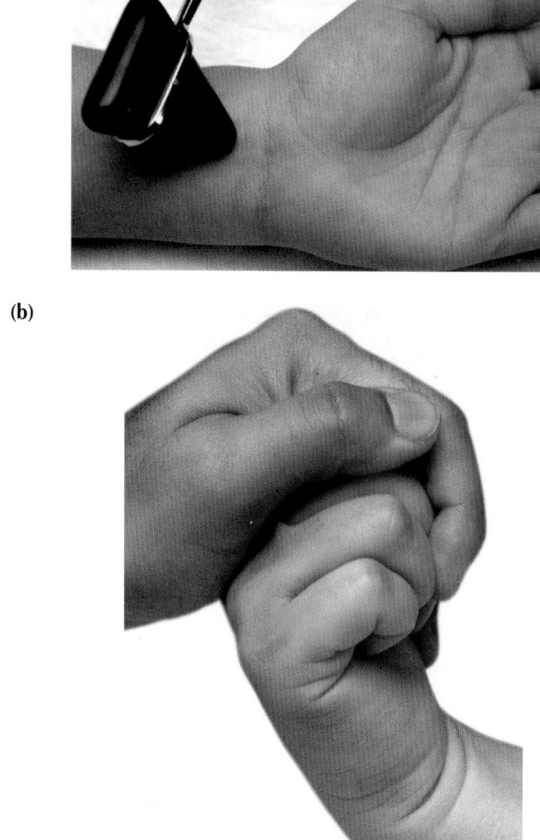

(b)

Figure 31.10 (a) Tinel's test; (b) Phalen's test.

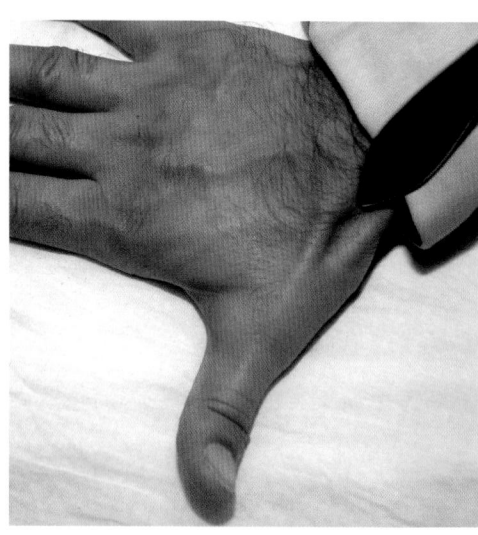

Figure 31.11 Palpating the anatomical snuff box between the tendons of extensor pollicis longus and abductor pollicis brevis.

(a)

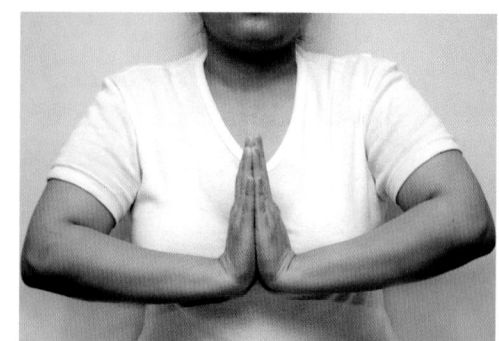

(b)

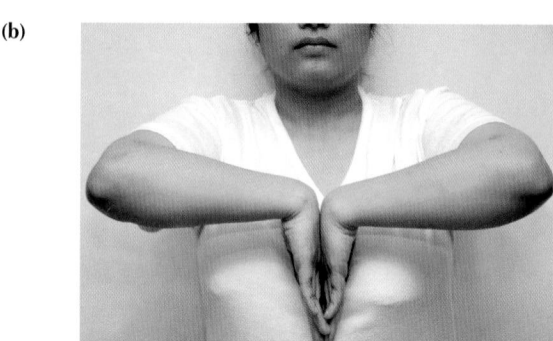

Figure 31.12 Testing the range of (a) wrist extension; (b) wrist flexion.

(a)

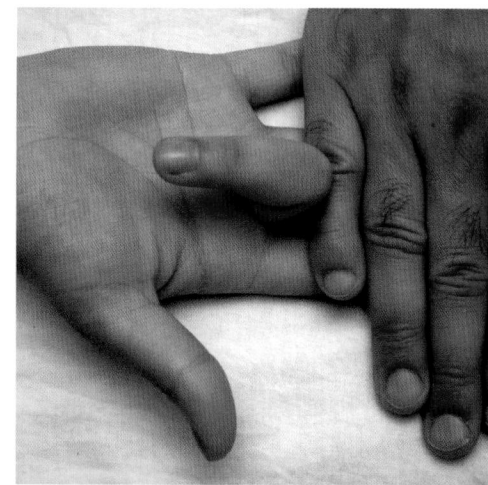

(b)

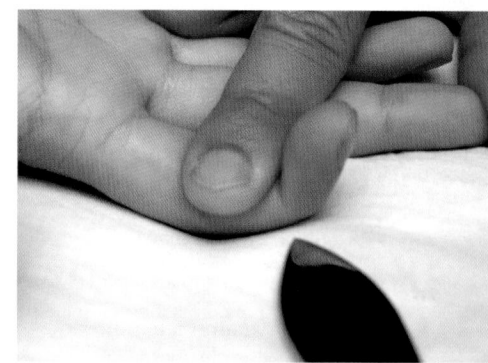

Figure 31.13 Testing the (a) flexor digitorum superficialis; (b) flexor digitorum profundus.

Other muscles

- *Thenar eminence:*
  - The abductor pollicis brevis, opponens pollicis and flexor pollicis brevis can be tested together by opposing the thumb to the little finger.
  - The flexor pollicis longus supplied by the anterior interosseus nerve (branch of the median nerve) can be tested by asking the patient to bring the tips of the thumb and index finger together (the 'OK' sign – Fig. 31.14).
  - The integrity of the extensor pollicis longus tendon is tested by asking the patient to lift the thumb off a table with the palm flat on the table (Fig. 31.15).
- *Adductor pollicis.* Test using Froment's sign (see Table 31.9 and Fig. 31.16).

Thumb abductor pollicis brevis

This muscle is supplied by the median nerve. With the hand lying flat on a table with the palm facing upwards, ask the patient to raise the thumb towards the ceiling. Ask the patient to resist as you push the thumb back towards the palm (Fig. 31.17) (Summary box 31.4).

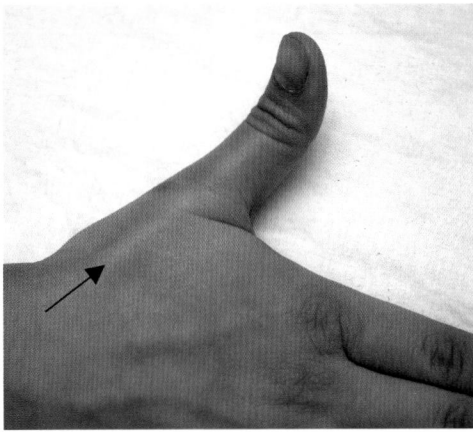

Figure 31.15 Testing the integrity of extensor pollicis longus.

Summary box 31.4

Hand and wrist examination

Inspection of the standing patient
- Dorsum and palm – asymmetry, deformity, muscle wasting

Inspection of the supine patient
- Skin, scars, soft tissues
- Palpation of bony structures and joints of the hand

Movements
- Wrist – flexion and extension, ulnar and radial deviation
- Hand – thumb movements, metatarsophalangeal joints and small joints of the hand

Special tests
- Allen's test
- Tinel's and Phalen's test for the median nerve
- Froment's sign
- Finkelstein's test

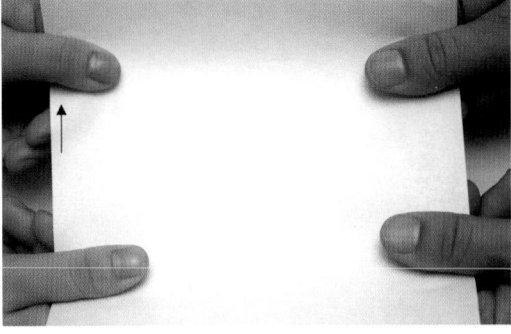

Figure 31.16 Froment's sign; the arrow illustrates the flexed posture of the thumb interphalangeal joint, indicating weakness of the ulnar nerve-innervated adductor pollicis muscle.

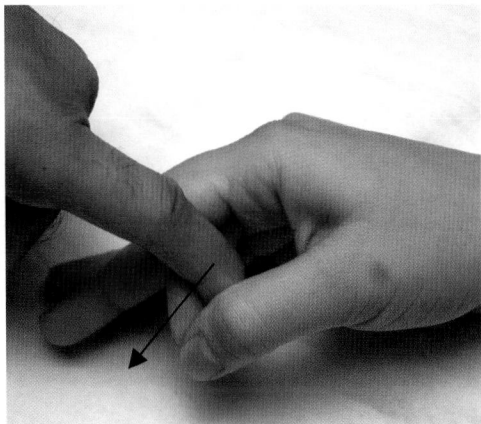

Figure 31.14 Test for flexor pollicis longus supplied by the anterior interosseus nerve.

Jules Froment, **1878–1946, Professor of Clinical Medicine, Lyons, France.**

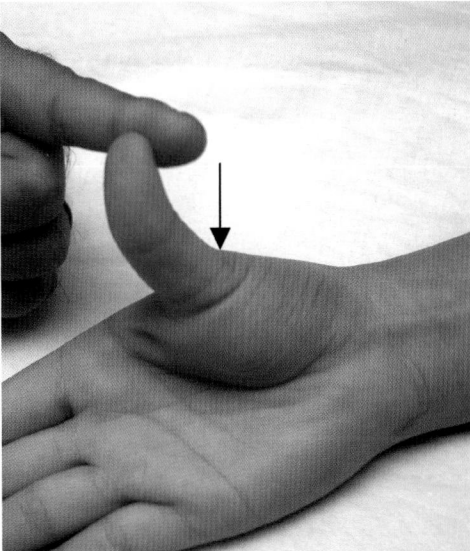

Figure 31.17 Testing the power of the abductor pollicis brevis supplied by the median nerve.

CLINICAL EXAMINATION OF THE ELBOW

The elbow is a hinge joint formed by the articulation of the ulna and radius with the humerus.

Look

Look for obvious asymmetry, abnormal posture and deformity (cubitus varus or valgus).

- *Skin.*
- *Soft tissues.* Look for any swellings, e.g. olecranon bursa, rheumatoid nodules, gouty tophi.
- *Muscle wasting.* Examine the biceps and triceps muscle bulk. Note that compression of the ulnar nerve at the elbow leads to wasting distally in the hypothenar eminence and intrinsic muscles of the hand – assess the hand for the presence of clawing and wasting.
- *Bone.* With the elbow in extension, look at the axis between the upper arm and forearm. There is a physiological valgus ('carrying angle') of 9–14° (2–3° greater in women) (Fig. 31.18). This angle allows the elbow to be tucked into the waist depression above the iliac crest:
    - cubitus varus (gun-stock deformity): the carrying angle is reversed, secondary to a supracondylar fracture;
    - cubitus valgus: the carrying angle is increased, caused by malunion of a distal humeral fracture;
    - there is normally a physiological hyperextension of the elbow (5°).

Feel

- *Soft tissues.* An effusion may be elicited by performing a cross-fluctuation test. The ulnar nerve can be rolled under your fingers placed between the medial epicondyle and the olecranon. Test the distal sensation in the hand and assess the vascular status.
- *Bones.* The three palpation landmarks are the medial and lateral epicondyles and the apex of the olecranon. These form an equilateral triangle when the elbow is flexed to 90°. The radial head is palpated with the examiner's thumb while the other hand pronates and supinates the forearm. On the medial side, palpate the medial epicondyle. Posteriorly, palpate the olecranon fossa.

Move

- *Flexion–extension.* The normal range is from –5° (slight hyperextension) to 150°. Ask the patient to bend the elbow from the fully straight position (Fig. 31.19).
- *Pronation and supination.* With the elbows at 90° and the palms facing upwards (full supination), ask the patient to turn the forearm so that the dorsum of the hand faces upwards (full

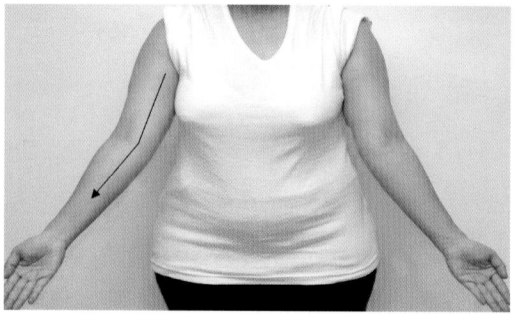

Figure 31.18 Carrying angle of the elbow illustrating the normal cubitus valgus.

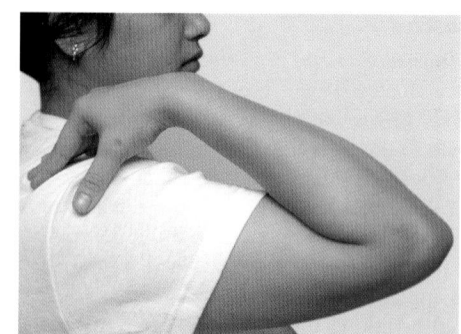

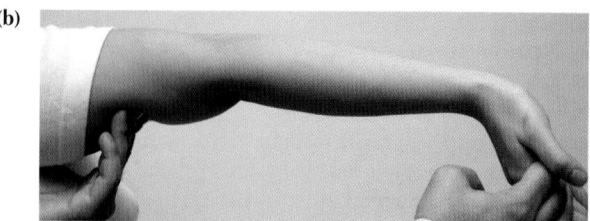

Figure 31.19 (a) Elbow flexion; (b) elbow extension.

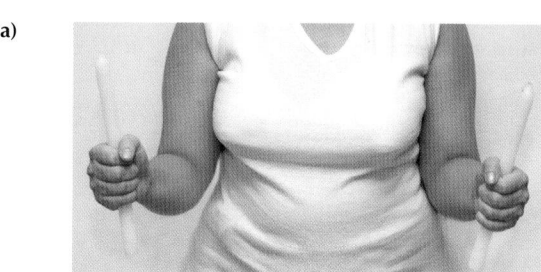

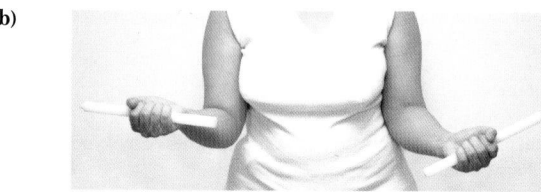

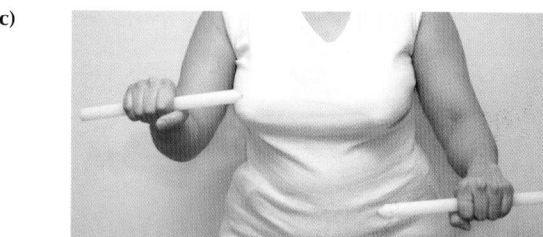

Figure 31.20 Testing forearm rotation: (a) mid-prone position; (b) full supination; (c) full pronation.

pronation) (Fig. 31.20). The normal values are 70° pronation and 90° supination.

Special tests and diagnoses

Tennis elbow and golfer's elbow

These are inflammatory processes of the tendons that attach the large muscle mass of the forearm to the lateral or medial epicondyle.

- *Medial epicondylitis (synonym = golfer's elbow).* The medial epicondyle is the common origin of the forearm flexors and the pronator muscle. Palpate the medial epicondyle for tenderness. The diagnostic test is resisted wrist flexion, which reproduces the pain over the medial epicondyle.

- *Lateral epicondylitis (synonym = tennis elbow)*. The lateral epicondyle is the common origin of the forearm extensors. Palpate for tenderness – usually just distal (5–10 mm) to the epicondyle near the origin of the extensor carpi radialis brevis muscle. Wrist extension against resistance with the elbow extended should provoke the patient's symptoms (Summary box 31.5).

Summary box 31.5

Elbow examination

Inspection of the standing patient
- Front – asymmetry, carrying angle, deformity
- Back – olecranon fossa

Inspection of the supine patient
- Skin, scars, soft tissues, deformity
- Palpation of bony structures

Movements
- Flexion and extension, pronation and supination

Special tests
- Tennis and golfer's elbow
- Stability testing
- Ulnar nerve compression
- Biceps tendon

CLINICAL EXAMINATION OF THE SHOULDER

Pain arising from the shoulder joint may be felt anterolaterally. Referred pain may present from the cervical spine, heart, mediastinum and the diaphragm.

Look

Assess the attitude of the limb.

- *Skin*. Check for surgical scars. An anterior scar is used for the deltopectoral approach. At the side, the deltoid splitting approach and lateral arthroscopic portals may be seen. Posteriorly, arthroscopic portal sites can be seen.
- *Soft tissues*. Wasting of the deltoid muscle is commonly seen after shoulder dislocation when there is a temporary loss of function of the axillary nerve that supplies it.
- *The rotator cuff* comprises four muscles: supraspinatus, infraspinatus, subscapularis and teres minor. Wasting of these muscles may occur following a rotator cuff injury.
- *Bone*. Look for any obvious deformity or prominence. A fracture of the middle third clavicle is the commonest cause. A dislocation may be suspected by a loss of normal shoulder contour. The more common anterior dislocation often presents with an anterior bulge and a squared-off shoulder.

Feel

Generalised pain in the shoulder may arise from the neck or the shoulder joint itself. More localised pain is often indicative of acromioclavicular joint pathology.

- *Skin*. Test sensation in the upper part of the lateral aspect of the arm ('regimental badge area') (Fig. 31.21). Loss may

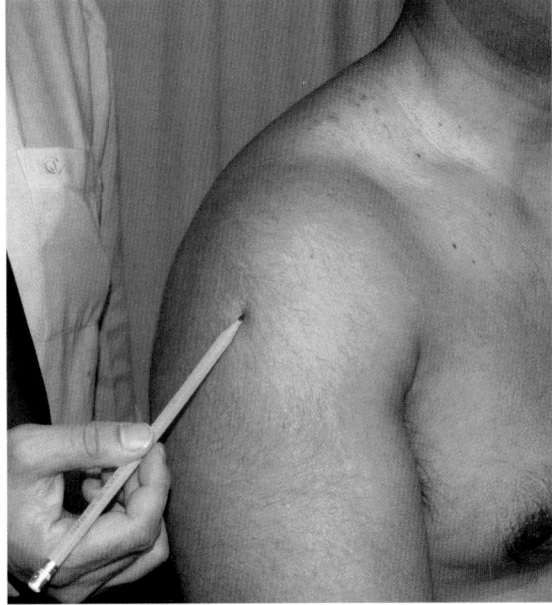

Figure 31.21 The area of skin supplied by the axillary nerve – the 'regimental badge area'.

indicate damage to the axillary nerve (following shoulder dislocation).

- *Bones*. Palpate the acromioclavicular and sternoclavicular joints and the clavicle.

Move

Differentiate between movements of the shoulder joint and scapulothoracic movement of the scapula on the chest wall. Patients with a painful shoulder will commonly move from the scapulothoracic joint. Stabilise the scapula by placing the thumb over the coracoid process and the fingers of the same hand over the spine of the scapula. Start in the 'neutral position' with the arms by the side, elbows extended and the palm facing forwards. Note any pain throughout the range of movement (Fig. 31.22).

- *Forward flexion*. Ask the patient to raise their hands in front to touch the ceiling while keeping the elbows extended (0–180°).
- *Extension*. Ask the patient to extend both arms behind (0–30°).
- *Abduction*. Shoulder abduction involves the glenohumeral joint and scapulothoracic movement. The first 60° of movement is mainly at the glenohumeral joint. Beyond this the scapula begins to rotate on the thorax and final movements are almost entirely scapulothoracic. Raise the arms sideways until the fingers point to the ceiling (180°).
- *Adduction*. Ask the patient to touch their other shoulder tip.
- *Internal rotation*. Ask the patient to touch their back with the dorsum of the hand and to raise their hand up the back as high as possible (normal range is thoracic spine level T7–9).
- *External rotation*. With the arms by the sides, bend the elbow to 90° and rotate the forearms to the mid-prone position. Ask the patient to separate their hands as much as possible (0–40°).

Special tests and diagnoses

Impingement syndrome

This is impairment of rotator cuff function within the subacromial bursa. It may lead to inflammation (tendinitis) or a partial or

(a)

(b)

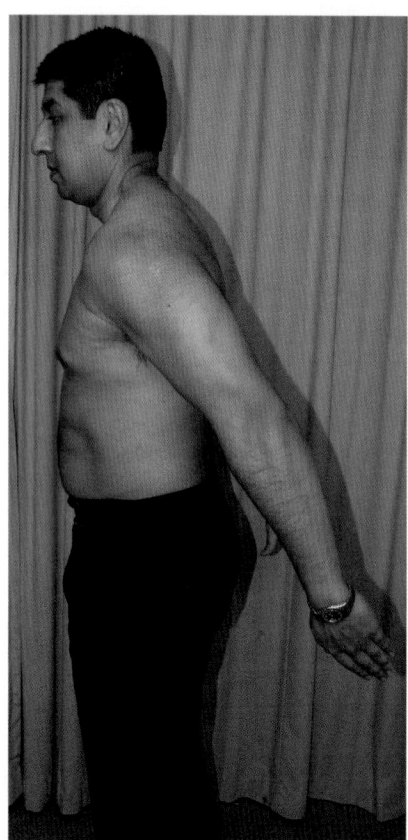

(c)

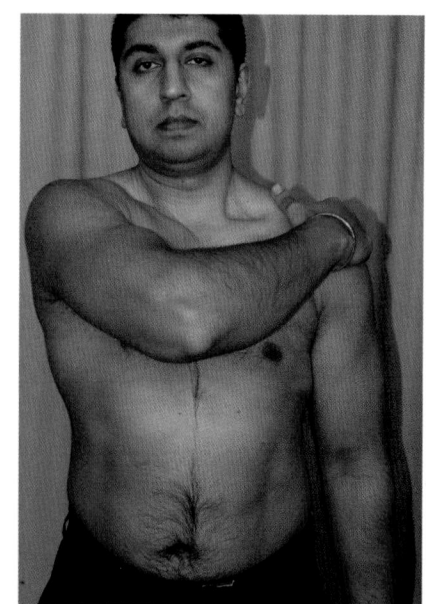

(d)

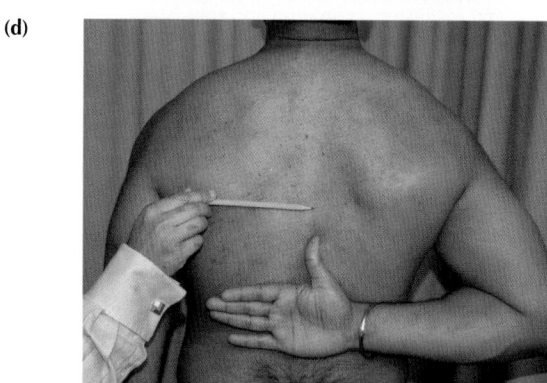

(e)

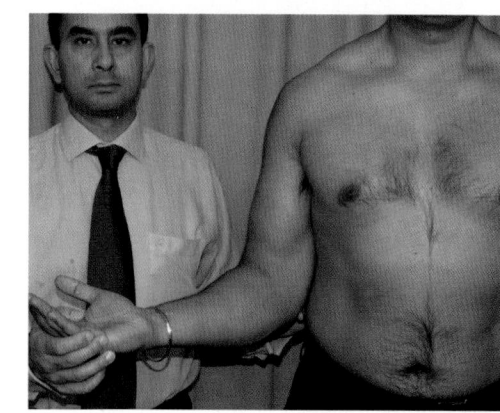

Figure 31.22 Movements of the shoulder: (a) forward flexion; (b) extension; (c) adduction; (d) internal rotation; (e) external rotation.

full-thickness tear. Impingement is characterised by pain and weakness on abduction and internal rotation.

- *Painful arc test* (Fig. 31.23). Ask the patient to abduct their arms from their sides. The presence of pain from 60° to 120° is positive.
- *Jobe's test (empty can)* (Fig. 31.24). Ask the patient to abduct the arm to 90° elevation in the scapula plane with full internal rotation (empty can position). Ask the patient to resist downward pressure. The presence of pain is a positive test.

Shoulder instability

Instability may be defined as a shoulder that slips in and out of joint (dislocation) more than once or twice, or frequently slips partially out of joint and then returns on its own. Instability can be anterior, posterior, inferior or multidirectional.

- *Apprehension test* (Fig. 31.25). With the patient supine or standing, flex the elbow to 90° and abduct the shoulder to 90°. Now externally rotate the shoulder. Apprehension indicates anterior instability (Summary box 31.6).

Summary box 31.6

Shoulder examination

Inspection of the standing patient
- Front – asymmetry, deformity
- Side – muscle wasting
- Back – muscle wasting, scapula

Inspection of the supine patient
- Skin, scars, soft tissues, deformity
- Palpation of shoulder girdle (sternum to scapula)

Movements
- Flexion and extension, abduction and adduction, internal and external rotation

Special tests
- Impingement syndrome – painful arc, Jobe's test, Hawkins' test
- Shoulder instability – apprehension, relocation test, sulcus sign
- Rotator cuff assessment
- Acromioclavicular joint pathology
- Frozen shoulder vs. glenohumeral osteoarthritis

(a)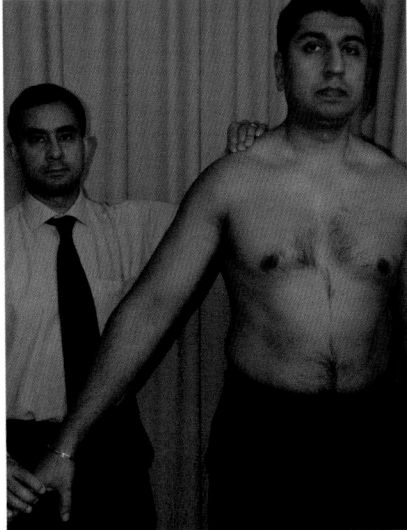

(b)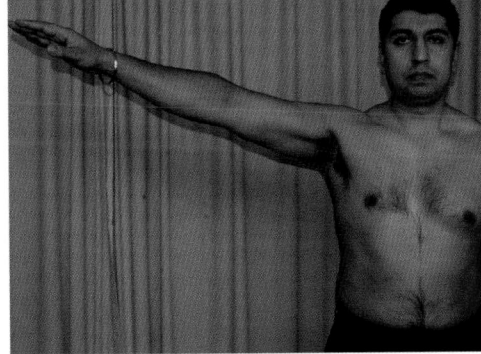

(c)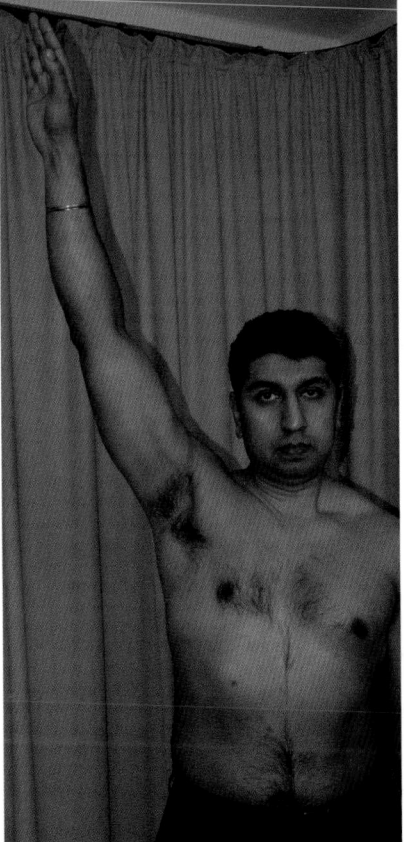

Figure 31.23 Painful arc test for rotator cuff impingement.

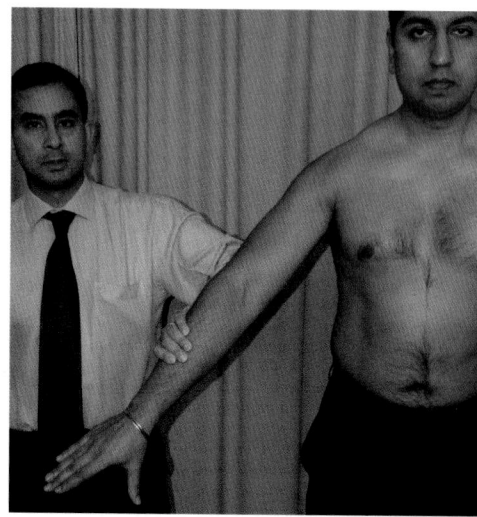

Figure 31.24 Jobe's test for rotator cuff impingement.

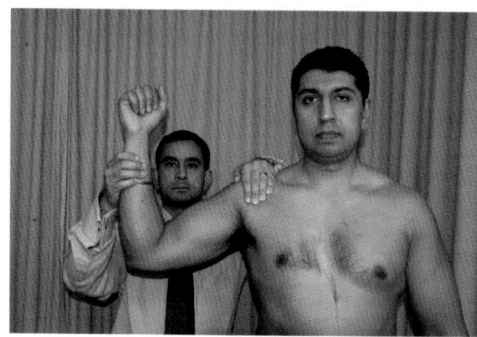

Figure 31.25 Anterior apprehension test for anterior shoulder instability.

CLINICAL EXAMINATION OF THE HIP JOINT

The hip is a synovium-lined ball and socket joint. Typical clinical diseases of the hip that may be encountered in children and adults are shown in Table 31.10.

A patient complaining of hip pain should undergo a careful examination of the spine, abdomen, pelvis, groin and thigh. In addition, consider a gynaecological examination in women.

Look

With the patient standing, look at the front, side and back of the hip. Look around the room for walking aids and heel raises in the shoes.

- *Skin.* Look for scars and sinuses.
- *Soft tissues.* Muscle wasting may be present as a consequence of hip arthritis or primary muscle or neurological disease.
- *Bone.* Look at the posture of the limb and assess for adduction deformity; fixed adduction may be present in severe osteoarthritis and cerebral palsy, and makes the leg appear short because the pelvis is tilted (apparent shortening).

Feel

- *Soft tissues.* Tenderness overlying the greater trochanter may suggest trochanteric bursitis or an abductor enthesopathy.

Table 31.10 Common clinical diseases of the hip in children and adults

Children	Adults
Developmental dysplasia of the hip	Primary osteoarthritis
Transient synovitis of the hip	Secondary osteoarthritis
Perthe's disease	Inflammatory arthritis
Septic arthritis and osteomyelitis	Avascular necrosis
Slipped capital femoral epiphysis	Labral tears
Juvenile idiopathic arthritis	Referred pain

Move

The hip joint can be moved into flexion, extension, abduction and adduction and internal and external rotation (Fig. 31.26). True hip movement ends when the pelvis begins to move. To detect true hip movement simultaneously place a finger/hand on the anterior superior iliac spine (ASIS) contralateral to the hip being examined. Remember to compare both sides.

Passive movement

Hip flexion and extension (120–0°)

The patient is asked to lie on their back and then roll themselves into a ball, flexing the hips and the spine fully. A comparison of the flexion of the two hips can be made in this position. The patient is then asked to hold onto one knee with both hands (thereby fixing the pelvis in flexion) and the other leg is allowed to extend down onto the couch. A note is made of any fixed flexion deformity (inability of the thigh to come down onto the couch). This hip is then returned to full flexion and the patient grasps that knee while dropping the other hip into extension. This modified Thomas's test is the most comfortable and accurate way of measuring flexion and extension of the hip (Fig. 31.27).

Rotation

- *Internal rotation (45°).* With the hip flexed to 45° and the knee in 90° of flexion, hold the front of the knee with one hand and the foot with the other. Internally rotate the hip (the foot goes outwards), then externally rotate the hip (the foot goes in). The angle that the tibia makes with the vertical indicates the range of movement. Pain at the extremes of movement suggest inflammation in the hip.
- *Abduction (40°).* The hip should be abducted by moving the leg away from the midline with the other hand on the patient's pelvis to detect any tilt in the pelvis.

Special tests

- *Trendelenburg test* (Fig. 31.28). Face the patient and ask them to place their hands on the palm of your hands for support. Then ask them to stand first on one leg, then the other. Increased pressure from the opposite hand as they take weight through the weak hip indicates a positive Trendelenburg test.
- *Leg length discrepancy (LLD).* The inequality may be in the hip joint, femur, tibia, ankle or foot or a combination of these. The pathology may be from the bone being too short or too long (Summary box 31.7). When assessing LLD, place both legs in the same position. For example, if there is an adduction deformity

Hugh Owen Thomas, **1834–1891**, General Practitioner, Liverpool, England. He is regarded as the founder of Orthopaedic Surgery. He never held a hospital appointment preferring to treat patients in their own homes.

(a)
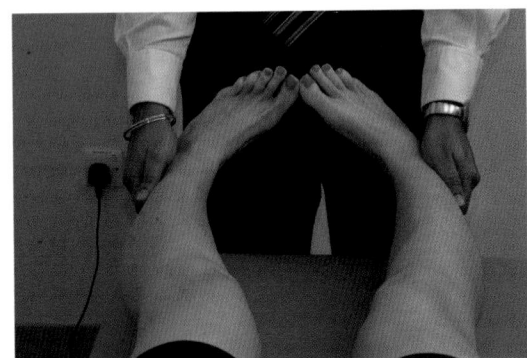

(b)
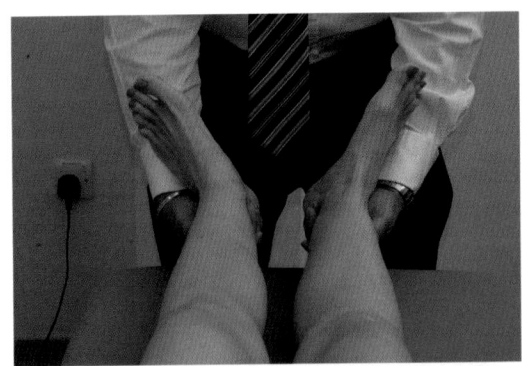

(c)
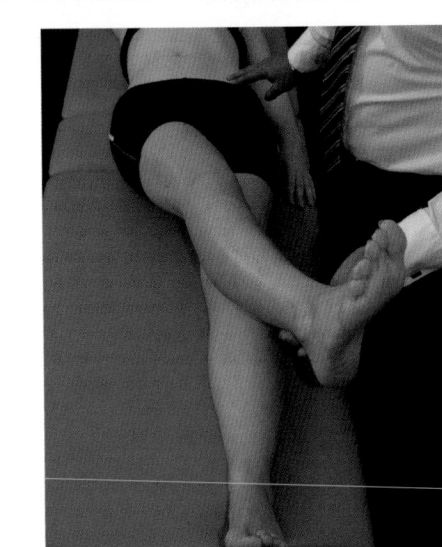

(d)
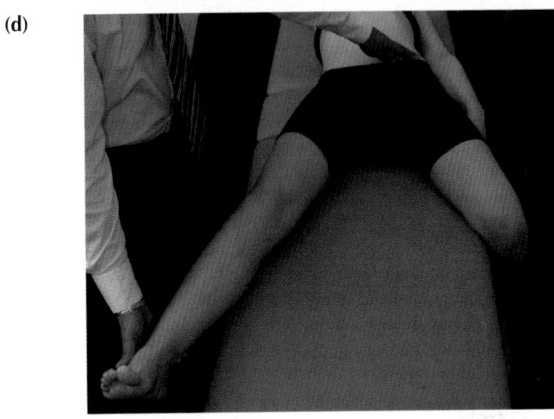

Figure 31.26 Hip movements: (a) internal rotation; (b) external rotation; (c) adduction; (d) abduction.

present in the affected leg, place the good leg in the same degree of adduction. LLD can be caused by a real difference in the leg lengths (the bones are different lengths) or by a deformity that makes the leg appear short because the pelvis must be tilted to get the leg onto the ground. The first is called 'real' LLD. The second is called 'apparent' LLD. Both are real to the patient but the cause and therefore the treatment are different.

- *Gait*. Hip disease can present with an altered gait pattern. The common types of abnormal gait are described in Table 31.11 (Summary box 31.8).

Summary box 31.7

Common causes of limb length inequality in the hip

- Osteoarthritis
- Hip fracture
- Hip dislocation
- Hip dysplasia
- Avascular necrosis
- Fixed flexion deformity

Table 31.11 Common limps observed in hip disease

Gait Pattern	Description
Weak: Trendelenburg	May lead to pelvic sway or tilt. The patient swings the body over the weak hip to stay in balance when it is weight bearing
Painful: antalgic	The rhythm is dot–dash, with a short period spent on the painful limb
Unbalanced: broad-based	May be caused by ataxia, e.g. cerebellar pathology. The rhythm also tends to be disordered
Loss of muscle control: high-stepping	May be due to loss of proprioception or a drop foot. This leads to difficulty in clearing the toes during the swing phase and the patient compensates by externally rotating the leg and flexing the hip and knee
Deformity: in-toeing	Can be caused by persistent femoral anteversion. The foot may catch on the back of the calf of the weight-bearing leg, tripping the patient

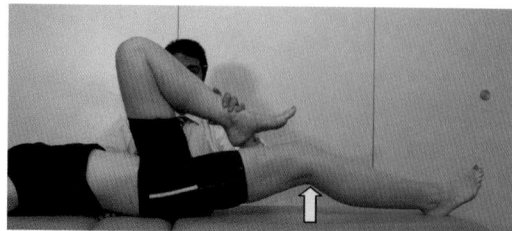

Figure 31.27 Modified Thomas's test for assessing a fixed flexion deformity. A fixed flexion deformity of the right hip is indicated by an inability to fully straighten the right leg (arrow).

(a)

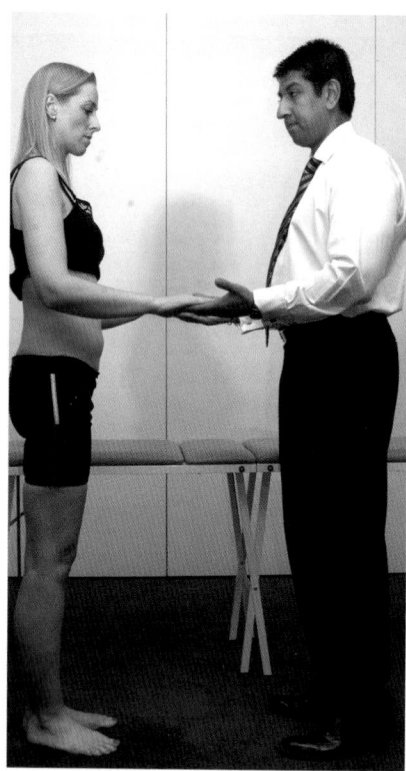

(b)

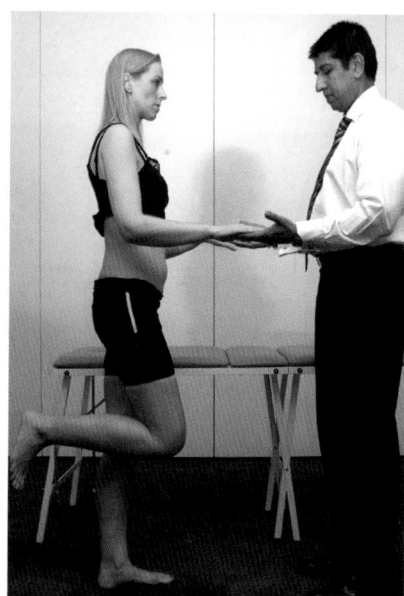

Figure 31.28 Trendelenburg test.

> **Summary box 31.8**
>
> **Hip examination**
>
> *Inspection of the standing patient*
> - Front – pelvic tilt, rotational deformity
> - Side – lumbar lordosis
> - Back – pelvic tilt, scoliosis, gluteal wasting
> - Gait – Trendelenburg, antalgic
>
> *Inspection of the supine patient*
> - Skin, scars, soft tissues, deformity
> - Palpation of the anterior joint line, adductor origin, greater trochanter, ischial tuberosity
>
> *Movements*
> - Flexion and extension
> - Abduction and adduction
> - Internal and external rotation
>
> *Special tests*
> - Thomas's test
> - Leg length assessment – real/apparent
> - Trendelenburg test
> - Snapping hip
> - Impingement tests

CLINICAL EXAMINATION OF THE KNEE

The knee is a synovial hinged joint. There are three compartments: medial, lateral and patellofemoral. The quadriceps, quadriceps tendon, patella, patella tendon and tibial tuberosity comprise the extensor mechanism of the knee.

The anterior cruciate ligament (ACL) provides primary restraint to anterior displacement of the tibia. The posterior cruciate ligament (PCL) provides posterior restraint of the tibia. The medial collateral ligament (MCL) resists valgus and external rotation forces whereas the lateral collateral ligament (LCL) resists varus forces.

Look

Look at the front, sides and back of both knees and for any walking or mobility aids or external appliances.

- *Skin.* Check for scars.
- *Soft tissues.* Look for wasting of the quadriceps and swelling in front of and behind the knee.
- *Bone.* Look for overall alignment (varus or valgus deformity). Measure the intermalleolar distance if a valgus deformity is present. With varus deformity, measure the distance between the medial aspect of both knees. From the side of the knee look for fixed flexion or recurvatum (hyperextension).

Gait

Look for antalgic gait (osteoarthritis) and varus thrust (collapse of the knee into more varus as weight is taken on that leg).

Feel

- *Soft tissue.* Feel the tendons for quadriceps and patellar tendon rupture.
- *Fluid displacement test.* Place your hand on the superior aspect of the suprapatellar pouch and move it inferiorly, attempting to displace any fluid into the knee joint. Maintain your hand at the

level of the superior pole of the patella. Now look to see if the normal gutters on either side of the knee are less noticeable because of fluid distension. Stroke the back of your hand over either gutter in turn. Look at the opposite gutter to see if there is filling.

- *Patellar tap test.* This test is used when a large effusion is present. Place one hand on either side of the patella and, with the other hand, push down on the patella. With an effusion, fluctuance is present as the patella moves towards the joint.
- *Bone.* Feel the tibial tuberosity, inferior pole of the patella, patella facets, origin and insertion of the knee ligaments and joint line (medial and lateral). Remember to palpate for any popliteal swellings. Note the height of the patella.

Move

The knee moves principally in flexion (0–135°) and extension (from 0 to –10°) (Fig. 31.29). Assess hyperextension by placing one of your hands on the anterior aspect of the distal femur. Now lift the distal tibia with the other hand. Measure the angle or the height that the heel can be lifted off the couch before the knee starts to move.

Perform a lag test to assess the integrity of the extensor mechanism. The patient is asked to lift the leg up off the bed (10°) with the knee straight. They are then asked to bend the knee and then straighten it again with the leg still held in the air. If they are unable to re-straighten the knee they have a positive lag. This indicates significant weakness of the quadriceps mechanism.

In the presence of an apparent fixed flexion deformity of the knee (seen in osteoarthritis), decide if this is arising from the knee or hip joint. To differentiate, sit the patient up with the knees hanging over the edge of the couch; this obliterates the effect of any hip flexion deformity. Passively try to extend the knee fully. With a flexion deformity of the knee, this is not possible.

Special tests

Collateral ligaments

To assess the ligaments, place the leg under your arm. Flex the knee to 10° to relax the posterior capsule (the MCL and LCL are taut in full extension and lax in flexion). Stress each ligament in turn by applying a valgus or varus force. With your index fingers simultaneously palpate over the collateral ligaments. Assess for signs of instability (excessive opening of the joint). The quality of the endpoint should be noted. Compare both sides (Fig. 31.30).

- *Medial collateral ligament.* A lax MCL or deficient lateral compartment may cause knee instability when applying a valgus stress. It is important to note that the valgus stress test should be applied with the knee in 30° of flexion. Valgus instability in full extension (0°) should alert you to a possible posterior structure injury (e.g. posterior capsule, posterior cruciate ligament).
- *Lateral collateral ligament.* A lax LCL or deficient medial compartment may cause knee instability when applying a varus stress in 10° of flexion. Instability in full extension (0°) suggests injury to the medial structures. In a suspected lateral injury, evaluation of the peroneal nerve must be performed.

Anterior cruciate ligament

The most sensitive test for evaluation of the ACL is the Lachmann test.

- *The Lachmann test* (Fig. 31.31). Flex the knee to 15–30° and pull the proximal tibia forwards. Excessive laxity may indicate rupture of the ACL. Anterior translation of the tibia associated with a soft or no endpoint is a positive test. The test may be negative in chronic ruptures as the ACL stump can scar to the PCL.
- *Anterior draw test* (Fig. 31.32a). Flex both knees to 90° and look for a posterior sag (compare the height of the tibial tuberosities). This may indicate an injury to the PCL. Stabilise the feet by sitting on them. Now place your hands around the proximal and posterior aspect of the tibia. With your index fingers, push up the hamstrings to remove their effect. Now pull the tibia forwards and measure any laxity; any laxity must be compared with the other knee. The degree of laxity can be graded: grade I (0–5 mm), grade II (5–10 mm) and grade III (> 10 mm).

Posterior cruciate ligament

The PCL is the primary restraint to posterior tibial translation between 30° and 90° of knee flexion. At 90°, the PCL accepts 95% of the posterior translational forces. Isolated PCL injuries are graded by the degree of posterior translation of the tibia with the knee in 90° of flexion. Look for a posterior sag with the knees flexed to 90°. The posterior draw test is the most reliable clinical test for a PCL injury.

- *Posterior draw test* (Fig. 31.32b). Perform the test with the knee flexed to 90°. Push the anterior aspect of the proximal tibia posteriorly and compare any laxity with the other side. If more than 10 mm of posterior tibial translation is noted at 30° and/or 90° of knee flexion, a combined PCL and posterolateral corner injury may be present. An evaluation of the competency of the posterolateral corner is necessary.

(a)

(b)

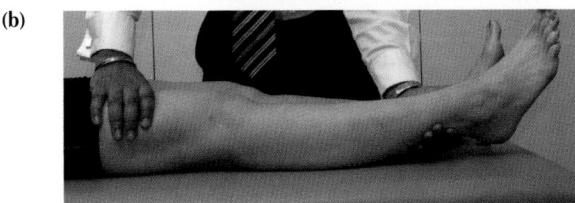

Figure 31.29 Knee flexion and extension.

(a)
(b)
(c)
(d)

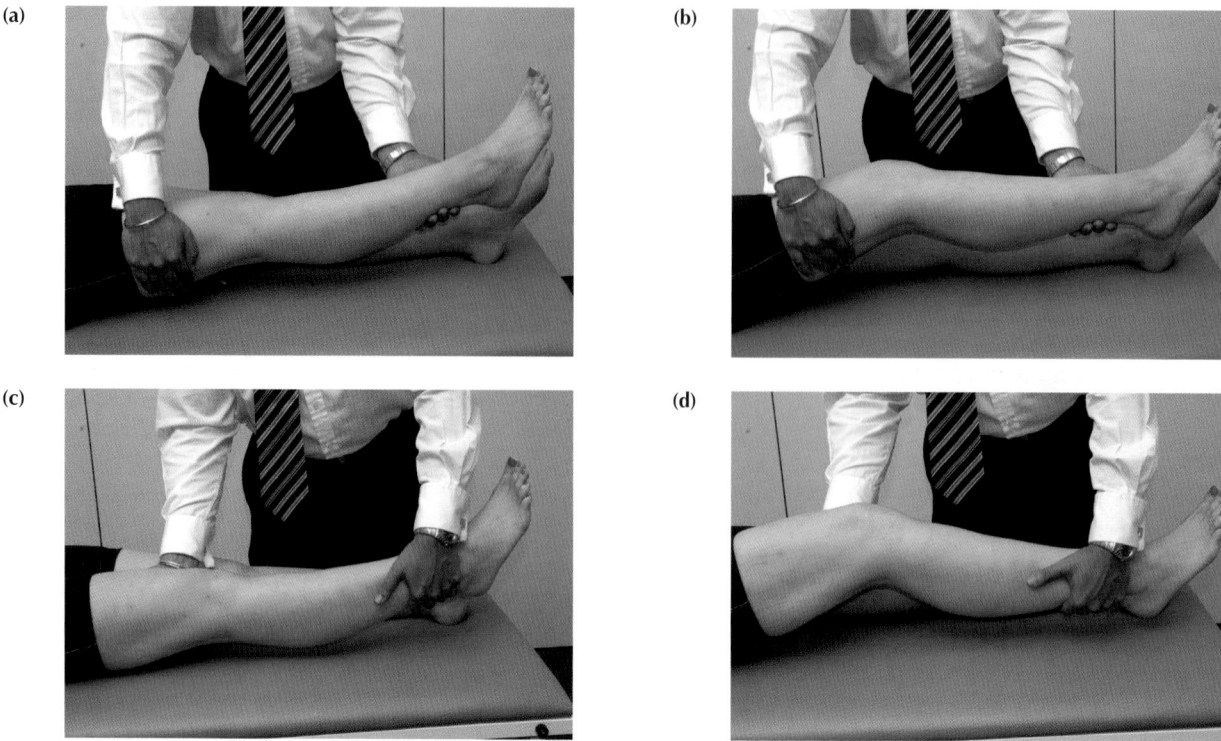

Figure 31.30 Assessing the medial and lateral collateral ligaments.

Menisci

The presence of palpable joint line tenderness is the most sensitive clinical examination test for a meniscal tear. Flex the knee to 90° and palpate the joint line using your thumb and index finger. Note any areas of tenderness. The well-known tests for meniscal tears (McMurray's test and Apley's grind test) are unreliable and so are not described here.

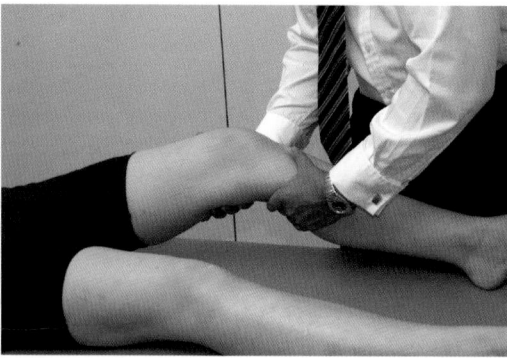

Figure 31.31 Lachmann's test: flex the knee to 15–30° and pull the proximal tibia forwards.

Thomas Porter McMurray, **1887–1949, Professor of Orthopaedic Surgery, Liverpool University, Liverpool, England.**

(a)

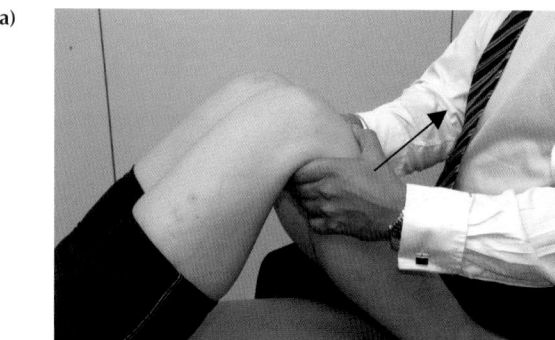

(b)

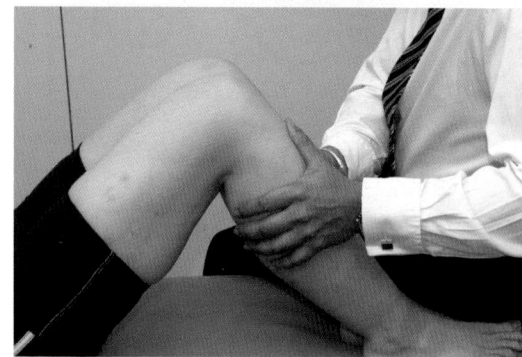

Figure 31.32 (a) Anterior draw test for anterior cruciate ligament stability; (b) posterior draw test for posterior cruciate ligament stability.

Patellofemoral joint

The patella normally enters the trochlea from a lateral position and becomes centralised with increasing knee flexion, travelling in a 'J' pattern. Measure the 'Q' angle.

- *Patellar tracking* (Fig. 31.33). Sit the patient and ask them to let their legs hang off the end of the couch with the knees flexed to 90°. Ask the patient to slowly extend the knee to full extension. Toward the end of extension, look for lateral subluxation of the patella ('J' sign). This indicates maltracking.
- *Patellar apprehension (Fairbank's) test (for instability).* Attempt

(a)

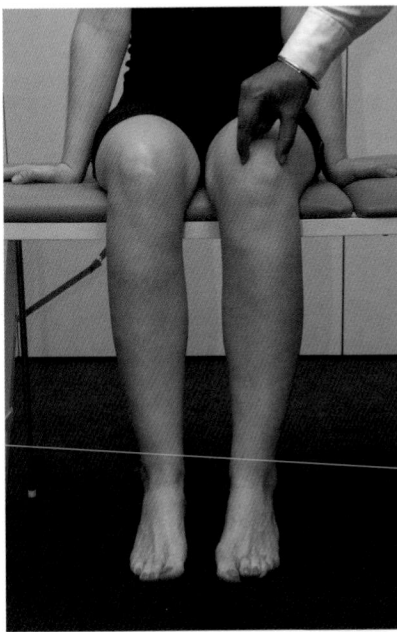

(b)

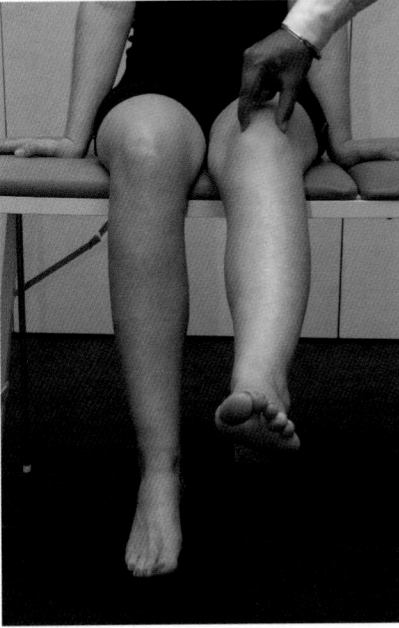

Figure 31.33 Patellar tracking.

Sir Harold Arthur Thomas Fairbank, **1876–1961**, Orthopaedic Surgeon, King's College Hospital, London, England.

to laterally displace the patella with the knee in extension. Patients with instability contract their quadriceps muscle or complain of pain. With the patient supine and the quadriceps relaxed, flex the knee to 30° whilst trying to push the patella laterally. With instability the patient may react with apprehension. In addition, the quadriceps muscle may contract in an attempt to realign the patella.

Patellar tendon

The patellar tendon serves as the distal extent of the extensor mechanism. Rupture usually occurs at the osseotendinous junction. This results in an inability to actively perform and maintain full knee extension. A rupture presents with diffuse swelling in the anterior knee. A high-riding patella (patella alta) is present secondary to the unopposed pull of the quadriceps muscle. A defect in the tendon is usually palpable. When the rupture extends through the medial and lateral retinaculae, active extension is lost.

Quadriceps tendon rupture

Rupture of the quadriceps tendon occurs relatively infrequently and usually in patients older than 40 years of age. The patient presents with swelling, tenderness and a palpable defect in the tendon (Summary box 31.9).

Summary box 31.9

Knee examination

Inspection of the standing patient
- Front – alignment (varus/valgus/rotational deformity), muscle bulk
- Side – fixed flexion deformity
- Back – popliteal swellings, hamstrings
- Gait – antalgic, high stepping gait (foot drop), varus thrust

Inspection of the supine patient
- Skin, scars, soft tissues, deformity
- Palpation of the extensor mechanism, medial and lateral joint lines and collateral ligaments, hamstrings, tibial tuberosity, fibular head

Movements
- Flexion and extension

Special tests
- Patellar apprehension test and extensor mechanism
- Cruciate ligaments
- Collateral ligaments
- Menisci

CLINICAL EXAMINATION OF THE FOOT AND ANKLE

The foot can be divided into three parts – the hindfoot (calcaneus, talus), the midfoot (navicular, cuboids, cuneiforms) and the forefoot (metatarsals and phalanges).

Look

Ask the patient to stand and assess the overall limb alignment. Assess pelvic obliquity, limb length discrepancy (and its level), valgus/varus deformities of the knee and rotational alignment. Check for contractures of the hips and knees, Now focus your attention on the foot itself:

- *Foot shape.* Assess the overall shape of the forefoot from the front. From the side, look for the normal medial arch (Fig. 31.34a). The hindfoot is best appreciated from behind. Now look at the vertical relationship between the Achilles tendon and the calcaneus (normal heel valgus of 5–7°). Look from behind and count the number of toes that can be seen. The 'too many toes' sign demonstrates increased forefoot abduction [pes planus (flat foot)] and a splayed forefoot. Foot shapes that may be encountered include neutral foot (no overall deformity), skew foot (hindfoot valgus and forefoot adduction), metatarsus adductus (neutral hindfoot and adduction of the metatarsus), pes planus (collapse of the medial arch) and pes cavus or high arch (increased medial arch). The possible causes of pes planus and pes cavus are shown in Summary boxes 31.10 and 31.11 respectively.

(a)

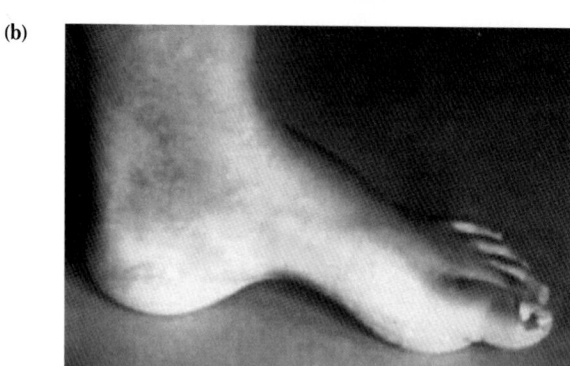

(b)

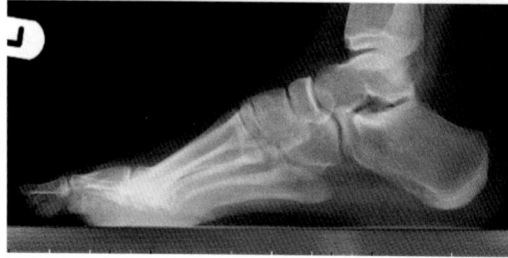

Figure 31.34   (a) Normal medial longitudinal arch of the foot. (b) Clinical and radiological appearance of pes cavus.

Summary box 31.10

Causes of pes planus

- Normal variant
- Hyperlaxity syndrome, e.g. Marfan's syndrome
- Tarsal coalition – rigid and painful flat foot (Fig. 31.39a, p. 453)
- Tibial posterior dysfunction

Summary box 31.11

Causes of pes cavus (Fig. 31.34b)

- Spinal anomalies, e.g. spina bifida
- Hereditary sensorimotor neuropathies such as Charcot–Marie–Tooth disease
- Charcot foot (e.g. neuropathic foot)
- Post-compartment syndrome (e.g. Volkmann's ischaemic contracture)

- *Skin.* A bunion or red swelling on the medial aspect of the metatarsophalangeal joint (MTPJ) is common. This is an area of inflamed skin with an underlying subcutaneous bursa and a joint osteophyte. Systemic manifestations include gouty tophi and thin fat pads under the metatarsal heads as seen in rheumatoid arthritis. Remember to assess the appearance of the nails.
- *Soft tissues.* Swelling may indicate soft tissue or joint pathology. Muscle wasting is most commonly seen on the dorsum of the foot and in the clefts between the metatarsals. If present, a full neurological examination of the upper and lower limbs should be performed including the spine.
- *Bones.* Look for any bony prominences or exostoses. Common forefoot deformities are shown in Table 31.12.

Table 31.12 Common forefoot deformities

Deformity	Metatarsophalangeal joint	Proximal interphalangeal joint	Distal interphalangeal joint
Claw toe	Hyperextension	Flexion	Flexion
Hammer toe	Normal	Flexion	Flexion
Mallet toe	Normal	Normal	Flexion
Hallux valgus or varus	Valgus or varus position	Normal	–

Gait

Ask the patient to walk up and down the room. Look for a high stepping gait (foot drop), painful (antalgic) gait (ankle and foot joint pain) and a short propulsive phase (forefoot pain).

Footwear

Inspect the footwear. This may reveal areas of abnormal weight bearing. With normal wear of the sole a corner is typically worn off the posterolateral aspect of the heel (heel strike). In addition, there may be a circular wear pattern under the ball of the big toe (toe-off phase).

- External appearance. Look at the materials used, the metal supports and heel raise, depth and width.
- Internal appearance. Look at the insoles, arch supports and heel cups.

Feel

- Skin. Reduced sensation in a glove and stocking distribution is seen with diabetes.
- Soft tissues. The posterior tibial and the dorsal pedis pulses should be identified (Fig. 31.35). Palpate the tibialis anterior tendon and the long extensor tendons on the dorsum of the foot. From the back, palpate the Achilles tendon. Palpate the peroneal tendons from the lateral side and the tibialis posterior tendon from the medial side. The sinus tarsi can be assessed. This is an anatomical space bounded by the talus and calcaneus and is recognisable as a soft-tissue depression

(a)

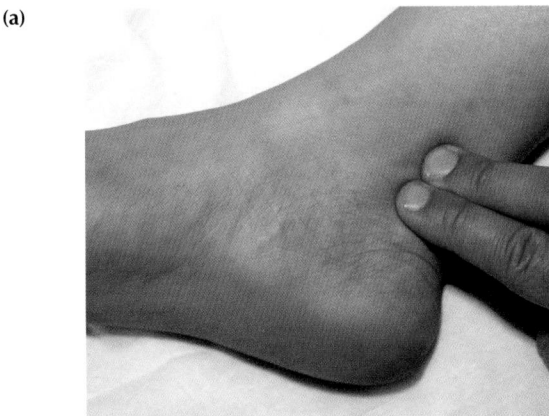

(b)

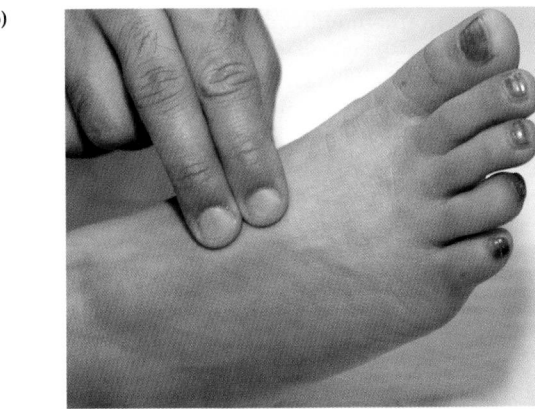

Figure 31.35 (a) Palpation of the posterior tibial pulse; (b) palpation of the dorsalis pedis pulse.

anterior to the lateral malleolus. It is filled with fat and the extensor digitorum brevis muscle. Sinus tarsi syndrome may occur. This may be caused by injury to the interosseous talocalcaneal ligament or the subtalar joint. There is pain and tenderness over the sinus tarsi with subjective hindfoot instability. The pain is characteristically relieved by local anaesthetic injection.

- Bones. Feel for deformity, bony prominences and loose bodies:
  - ankle joint: the medial and lateral malleoli, anterior and posterior joint line, lateral gutter and ligament complex, the syndesmosis (front of the ankle), medial gutter and medial ligament complex;
  - subtalar joint: palpate each facet;
  - midtarsal joints: the talonavicular and calcaneocuboid joints;
  - tarsometatarsal joints (TMTJ): note that the second TMTJ is several millimetres proximal to the others; movement is minimal in the second ray, limited in the third ray, moderate in the fourth and fifth rays and very variable in the first ray.
- Specific structures to palpate:
  - calcaneus (heel bone): the commonest cause of pain is plantar fasciitis; this may present with numbness, burning and electric shock sensations, which are worse in the morning and improve as the day goes on; identify the exact point of tenderness;
  - tendons: examine for contracture of the Achilles tendon insertion and the peroneal or tibialis posterior tendons;
  - head of talus: invert and evert the patient's foot;
  - sustentaculum tali: palpate one fingerbreadth below the medial malleolus; this important structure serves as an attachment for the spring ligament;
  - cuneiforms (medial, middle and lateral), MTPJs, web spaces and all the forefoot bones.

Move

The movements of the foot and ankle are linked via the ankle, subtalar and midfoot joints. Remember the acronyms PAED – pronation, abduction, eversion and dorsiflexion – and SAPI – supination, adduction, plantarflexion and inversion.

Ankle (Fig. 31.36)

- Dorsiflexion. Test dorsiflexion with the knee both flexed and extended. If restriction is greater with the knee extended than flexed, the contracture is principally in the gastrocnemius. Restriction that is equal in all knee positions is caused by a contracture principally of the soleus.
- Plantarflexion. Ask the patient to touch the floor with their foot (15°). Weakness suggests injury to the Achilles tendon or pathology affecting the S1 nerve root.

Subtalar joint (Figs 31.37 and 31.38)

Hold the talar neck and ask the patient to move their heel from side to side. Repeat using a hand on the heel to move the joint and apply a varus and valgus stress while feeling for movements of the talus. Holding the talus as opposed to the tibia isolates subtalar from ankle motion. (Normal range is 5° in each direction.)

- Inversion. Ask the patient to move their foot in towards them.
- Eversion. Ask the patient to move their foot out to the side.

(a)

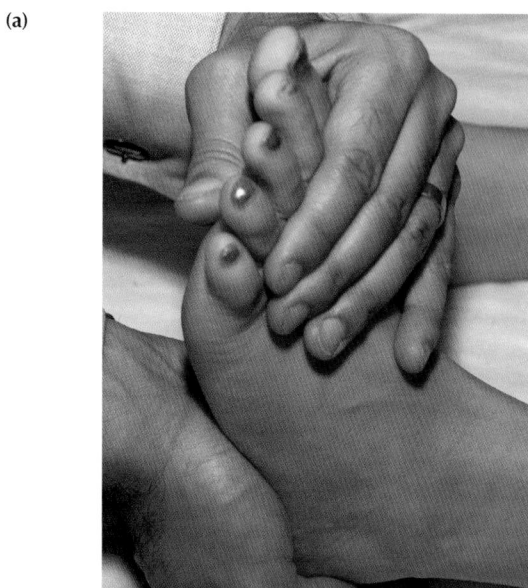

(b)

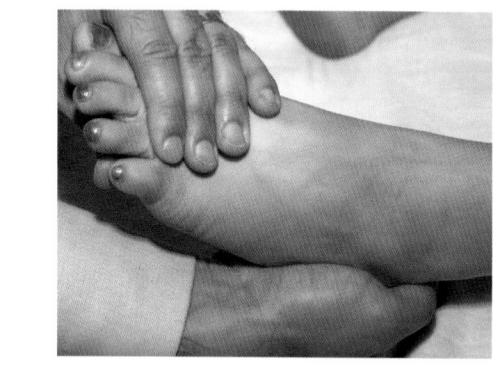

Figure 31.36 (a) Ankle dorsiflexion and (b) ankle plantarflexion.

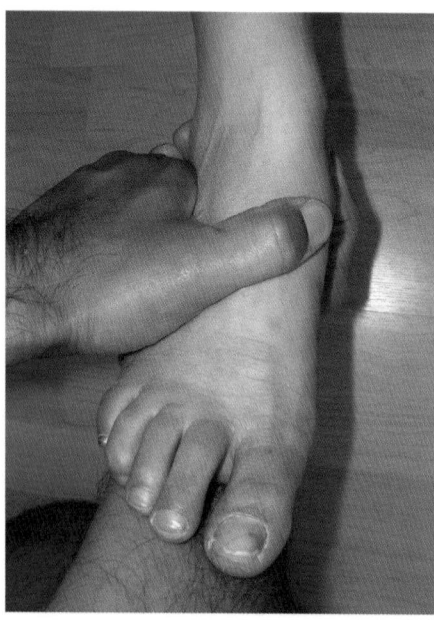

Figure 31.37 Testing subtalar joint motion.

(a)

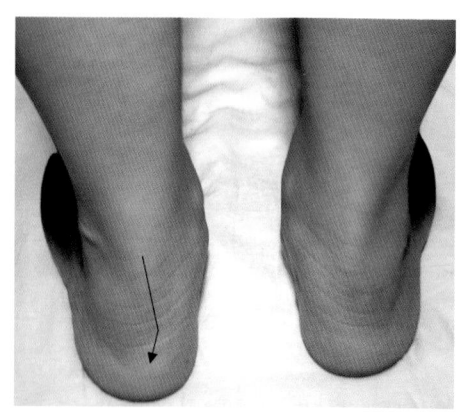

(b)

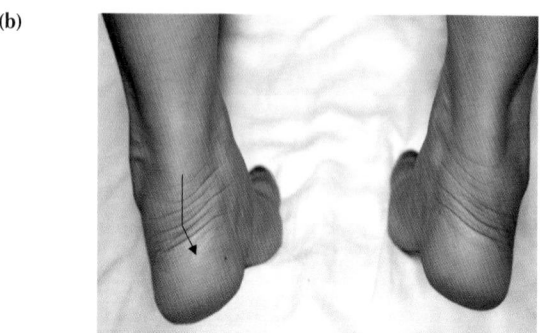

Figure 31.38 Testing subtalar joint flexibility.

Midtarsal joint

Hold the heel with one hand and move the forefoot medially (adduction = 20°) and laterally (abduction = 10°) with the other hand.

Tarsometatarsal joint

Hold the midfoot and manipulate each metatarsal up and down to estimate the passive range of movement.

Metatarso-phalangeal joint

Test extension (70–90°) by asking the patient to lift the toes to the ceiling and test flexion (45°) by pointing the toes to the floor. Normal toe-off requires 35–40° of dorsiflexion.

Special tests

Achilles tendon

Feel the gastrocnemius and soleus bellies and the whole length of the tendon for gaps (rupture), tenderness or swelling. Also identify the posterolateral (Haglund's) prominence of the calcaneus and palpate the retro-Achilles bursa.

The best test for integrity of the tendon is the *Thompson's or Simmonds' test*. Do not be misled by the patient's ability to stand on tiptoes – some people can do this using their long toe flexors alone. Lie the patient prone and allow the calves to rest on your

Achilles, the Greek Hero, was the son of Peleus and Thetis. When he was a child his mother dipped him in the Styx, one of the rivers of the underworld, so that he should be invulnerable in battle. The heel by which she held him did not get wet, and was, therefore, not protected. Achilles died from a wound in the heel which he received at the siege of Troy.
Patrik Haglund, 1870–1937, Swedish Orthopaedic Surgeon.
Franklin Adin Simmonds, 1911–1983, Orthopaedic Surgeon, The Rowley Bristow Hospital, Pyrford, Surrey, England.

forearms. Squeeze each calf in turn and watch for movement at the ankle joint. Lack of movement may indicate a rupture.

Subtalar joint flexibility

Ask the patient to stand on their toes and observe the heel from behind; the heel moves normally from valgus to varus indicating flexibility. The *Coleman's block test* is used to assess the flexibility of the subtalar joint. Ask the patient to stand on a 2-cm block with the great toe over the medial edge, resting on the floor. Now look from behind. If the hindfoot varus remains, the subtalar joint is fixed. If it corrects to valgus, the joint is mobile (Fig. 31.38).

Flat foot flexibility

Use the Windlass and Jack's test to distinguish a flexible from a fixed flat foot (Fig. 31.39):

- *Windlass test*. Ask the patient to stand on their toes and observe the arch of the foot on the medial aspect. As soon as the patient stands on their toes, the arch forms. Failure of this indicates a fixed flat foot.
- *Jack's test*. With the patient standing, lift up the great toe. The arch should form in the flexible flat foot.

(a)

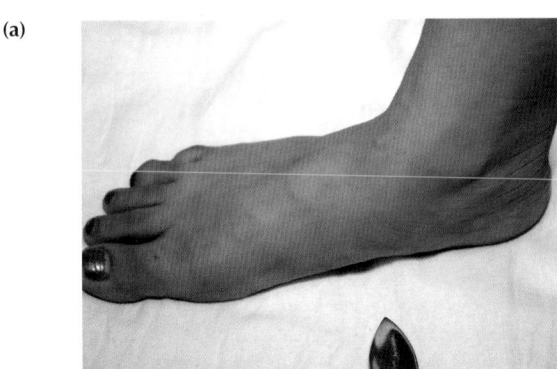

(b)

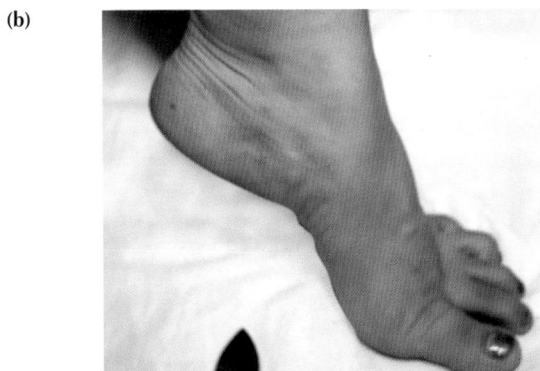

(c)

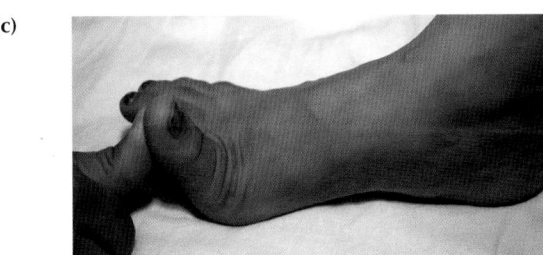

Figure 31.39 (a) Flat foot appearance with a reduced medial longitudinal arch; (b) Windlass test; (c) Jack's test.

Ankle stability

Trauma to the ankle is a common cause of instability. Accurate assessment may be difficult in the acute setting because of pain.

- *Anterior draw test*. With the foot resting over the bed, hold the heel with one hand and the front of the tibia with the other. Move the heel forwards on the fixed tibia. Compare with the other side. Instability of the syndesmosis may be palpable (Fig. 31.40).
- *Squeeze test for distal tibiofibular stability*. Compress the proximal calf. Pain at the ankle may indicate separation of the distal fibula from the tibia.
- *Tilt test*. Hold the talus at the neck rather than the heel so that you can be sure that any tilt is in the ankle and not the subtalar joint.

Tarsometatarsal joint stability

Stability can be assessed by pushing each joint up and down. Standing lateral radiographs may be used in addition.

Tibialis anterior

Ask the patient to walk on their heels with their feet inverted; the tibialis anterior tendon can be seen. With the patient's feet resting over the edge of the couch, ask the patient to actively dorsiflex and invert their foot to reach your hand. Palpate the tibialis anterior muscle.

Tibialis posterior

Pathology of the tibialis posterior typically presents with posteromedial ankle pain, swelling and gradual onset of a flat foot. When assessing the tendon, look for swelling along its course, a flat foot with heel valgus, the 'too many toes' sign and prominence of the talar head. Palpate for tenderness, swelling or gaps in the tendon. To test integrity:

- Ask the patient to perform a single foot tiptoe test on both sides. The inability to lift the affected heel off the ground is suggestive of a tibialis posterior tendon injury or insufficiency.
- To test strength, position the foot in the plantarflexed and inverted position. Ask the patient to hold this position while you push against their foot.

Dorsiflexors

Tendinitis of the long toe dorsiflexors usually presents in athletes. Pain affects gait in the early contact phase. Palpate for swelling,

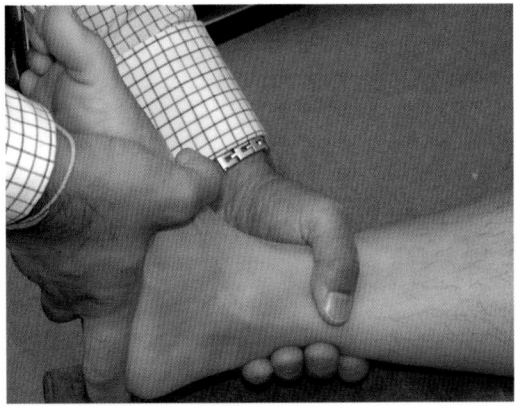

Figure 31.40 Anterior draw test.

gaps or any tenderness. Ask the patient to move the foot into dorsiflexion and to hold this position while you push the foot down.

Inability to dorsiflex the foot is referred to as foot drop. Causes include stroke, spinal injury, spinal stenosis or disc prolapse, peripheral nerve injury (e.g. sciatic, common and deep peroneal) or a peripheral neuropathy.

Peroneals

Peroneal tendon pathology presents with swelling and/or pain of the lateral hindfoot or midfoot. There may be a history of the ankle 'giving way'. Presentations of peroneal tendon pathology include:

- *'peroneal spasm'*: may be seen in tarsal coalition; here, the muscles are usually contracted secondary to the hindfoot valgus;
- *peroneal tendon dislocation*: attempt to dislocate the tendons by dorsiflexing and everting the foot.

The peroneus longus may be palpated just before it crosses under the foot to insert onto the base of the first metatarsal. Ask the patient to plantarflex the first metatarsal. Test strength and integrity by active and resisted eversion while you palpate the tendons for swelling, tenderness or gaps.

Morton's neuroma

This condition represents thickening of the tissue that surrounds the digital nerve leading to the toes as the nerve passes under the ligament connecting the metatarsals in the forefoot. It is most frequent between the third and fourth toes. A neuroma presents with burning pain in the ball of the foot that radiates to the involved toes. The condition is difficult to diagnose and requires a high index of suspicion. Palpate in the web space between the symptomatic toes for a mass. Compression of the metatarsals may

Thomas George Morton, **1835–1903, Surgeon, The Pennsylvania Hospital, Philadelphia, PA, USA, described this condition in 1876.**

elicit a 'click' between the bones (Molders' click) (Summary box 31.12).

> **Summary box 31.12**
>
> **Ankle and foot examination**
>
> ***Inspection of the standing patient***
> - Front – alignment, foot shape and deformity
> - Side – medial arch
> - Back – heel position
> - Gait – antalgic, high stepping gait (foot drop)
>
> ***Inspection of the supine patient***
> - Skin, scars, soft tissues, bony deformity
> - Palpation of the ankle, subtalar, midfoot and forefoot joints
>
> ***Movements***
> - Dorsiflexion, plantarflexion, inversion, eversion
>
> ***Special tests***
> - Flexibility of the subtalar joint and a flat foot
> - Joint stability, Morton's neuroma
> - Tendons – tibialis posterior and anterior, Achilles tendon, peroneals and dorsiflexors

FURTHER READING

Aitken, D. McCrae (1935) *Hugh Owen Thomas: His Principles and Practice*. Oxford University Press, London.

Ganz, R., Parvizi, J., Beck, M., Leunig, M., Nötzli, H. and Siebenrock, K.A. (2003) Femoroacetabular impingement: a cause for osteoarthritis of the hip. *Clin Orthop* **217**: 112–20.

Miller, M.D., Bergfeld, J.A., Fowler, P.J., Harner, C.D. and Noyes, F.R. (1999) The posterior cruciate ligament injured knee: principles of evaluation and treatment. *Instr Course Lect* **48**: 199–207.

Neer, C.S. (1983) Impingement lesions. *Clin Orthop* **173**: 70–7.

Rang, M. (1966) *Anthology of Orthopaedics*. E&S Livingstone, Edinburgh, 139–43.

Sports medicine and sports injuries

To understand:
- The common sports injuries
- The treatment and rehabilitation plans in sports medicine
- The common conditions associated with different joints
- The importance of rehabilitation

INTRODUCTION

When the normal physical limits of human tissues are exceeded, injury occurs. This is particularly associated with participation in any form of physical activity. Understanding how the injury occurred, the biomechanics of the forces involved, the relevant anatomy, the healing process and how to rehabilitate the injured joint are encompassed in the field of sports medicine.

The incidence of injuries differs between different sports. Although obviously aggressive physical contact sports, e.g. rugby, American football and wrestling, have a high incidence of major injuries, it is of note that sports such as cricket also have a high incidence of injuries (2.6–24.4 per 10 000 hours played). Many of these injuries are relatively minor injuries to the hand, but all need to be treated appropriately to prevent a chronic state occurring.

DIAGNOSIS OF SPORTS INJURIES

History

The incident leading to the injury can provide valuable information on the nature of the injury and also reveal occult injuries. For example, the direction of impact in a sliding football tackle should alert you to the nature of any knee or ankle injuries – damage to the medial collateral ligament (MCL) of the knee from a lateral impact, inversion injury of the ankle.

Injuries can be broadly classified as:

- acute extrinsic injuries, e.g. haematoma, cuts, grazes;
- acute intrinsic injuries – this is when a structure has been stressed beyond its limit, e.g. ligament sprains, dislocations and fractures;
- chronic injuries, which may be exacerbated by a new event.

Examination

Accurate diagnosis of the injury immediately after the incident is often difficult, with pain and muscle spasm masking signs. The principles of Advanced Trauma Life Support (ATLS) should also be considered before focusing on the more obvious injury.

Subsequent examination during the process of recovery may require you to watch the individual actually perform their sport, to enable an accurate assessment of the injury and how it might be prevented in the future.

PROTECTIVE EQUIPMENT AND ORTHOTICS

When correctly used, protective equipment can help prevent injuries occurring (Fig. 32.1); however, it can provide an athlete with a false sense of security that injuries may not happen; for example, protective head gear will not necessarily prevent concussion. Badly fitting protection may in itself cause injury, e.g. ulceration and infections.

The principles of protection may be achieved by:

- absorbing the energy of the impact;
- diffusing the impact over a larger area;
- limiting the movement of a joint;
- preventing infection.

REHABILITATION

Rehabilitation of the injured athlete is an essential part of the treatment plan. By dividing it into four stages an effective rehabilitation plan can be devised.

Stage one involves the immediate treatment of the injury. Use of the basic acronym PRICE will help reduce the length of the inflammatory process and promote quicker rehabilitation:

- *p*rotect;
- *r*est;
- *i*ce;
- *c*ompression;
- *e*levation.

Stage two involves restoring the movement of the injured joint. Pain and swelling have usually started to settle.

Drugs have a role to play in the treatment of most injuries and can help reduce the time needed before a return to sport is possible.

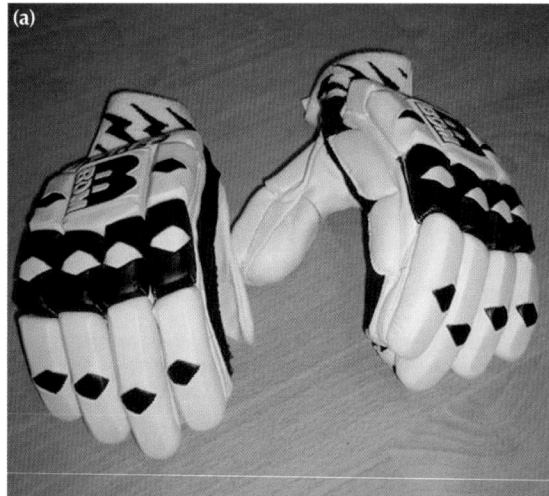

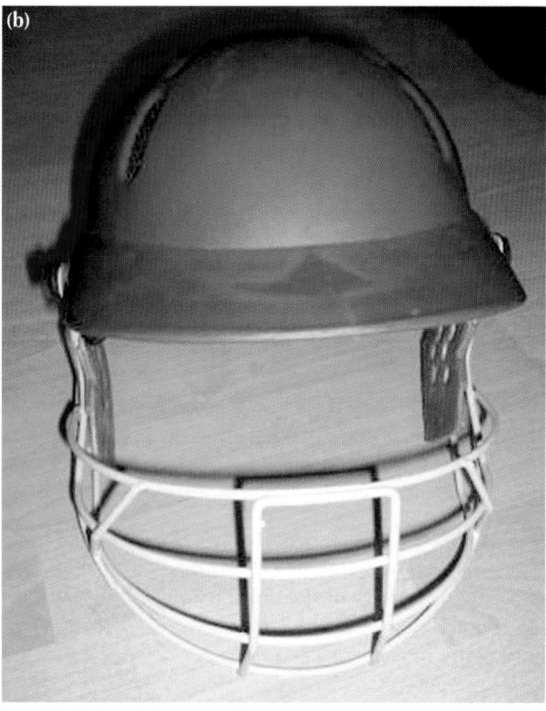

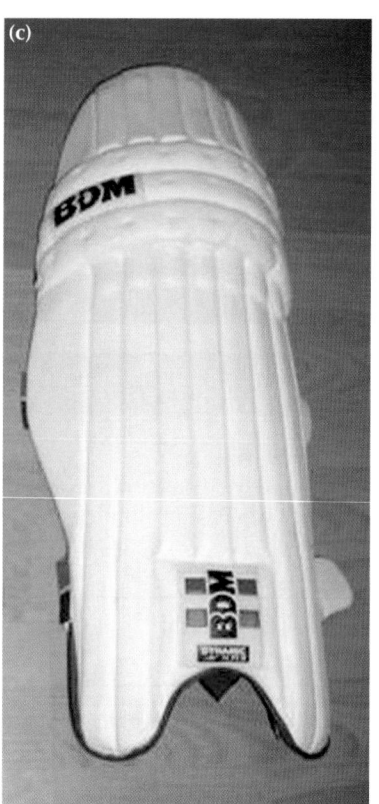

Figure 32.1 (a–c) Protective equipment.

Simple analgesics such as non-steroidal anti-inflammatory drugs (NSAIDs) are beneficial in reducing pain and oedema. Corticosteroids, e.g. cortisone and prednisolone, are also useful in reducing oedema and inflammation in chronic conditions; however, they are associated with re-rupture of tendons and long-term use is also associated with osteoporosis. Before prescribing any drugs it is important to be aware of the International Olympic Committee's guidelines on doping for athletes (Table 32.1), for example whether a given drug is banned. A positive drug test can have a devastating effect on an athlete's career and on your reputation.

Restoration of movement is an essential part of the rehabilitation process: the longer a structure is out of use the more atrophy there will be. In severe cases, contractures and osteoporosis may develop.

Initially, passive movements may be applicable, using continuous passive movement machines. As healing occurs, more active exercises can be undertaken. These include isometric exercises, in which the muscle is contracted but the joint controlled by it is not moved. Isotonic exercises are those in which the muscle contracts under a constant load and the joint is moved through a range of movement. A physiotherapist is an essential part of the rehabilitation team, to control and monitor progress.

GENERAL TISSUE INJURIES

Different types of tissue sustain different types of damage and heal at differing rates.

Muscles

Bleeding within any muscle may be extensive and it is essential to recognise whether this is intramuscular bleeding, and therefore more prone to compartment syndrome, or intermuscular bleeding.

Table 32.1 Classes of banned drugs

Class of drug	Mode of action	Examples
Stimulants	These cause the autonomic nervous system to speed up different parts of the brain, resulting in faster reflexes. This may help sprinters. Increased confidence and aggression may help boxers. The secondary weight loss may be desirable in dancers and gymnasts	Amphetamines, cocaine, ephedrine, caffeine, β_2-agonists, phenylpropanolamine
Anabolic steroids	These drugs can increase muscle bulk, strength, weight and acceleration. They improve injury repair, reduce recovery time and improve overall performance	Stanozolol, nandrolone, testosterone, oxandrolone, methanedione
β_2-Agonists	As well as acting as stimulants, when taken systemically they can have powerful anabolic effects. Clenbuterol has a marked stimulatory effect on fast-twitch muscle fibres and causes lipolysis	Clenbuterol, salbutamol, terbutaline, salmeterol
Narcotics	These can result in an increased pain threshold and a feeling of invincibility, which may be beneficial in sports in which aggression and physical contact are required, e.g. rugby	Morphine, pethidine, buprenorphine
Peptides and hormones	Actions are specific to the hormone. Erythopoietin can increase the number of circulating red blood cells, improving the oxygen-carrying capacity of the athlete. This is useful in distance and endurance sports	Human chorionic gonadotrophin, human growth hormone, erythropoietin
Diuretics	These can help induce rapid and temporary weight loss as well as masking the use of other banned substances. This can help in weight-category sports such as rowing and horse racing	Furosemide, bendroflumethiazide, mannitol, bumetanide

Intermuscular bleeding is more likely to be responsible for superficial bruising and is less prone to compartment syndrome.

The principles of treating any soft tissue injury are the same and the PRICE formula is again useful.

The patient requires rehabilitation and education to prevent the injury from recurring. Occasionally, the haematoma does not resolve and a cyst may develop. This may require surgical excision but there is an associated risk of infection. Deep bruising may produce osteoid – myositis ossificans traumatica – which is difficult and slow to treat.

Tendons

Tendons consist of dense type 1 collagen bundles that are attached to the bone by Sharpey's fibres. The bundles or fascicles are surrounded by a sheath of connective tissue called the epitendon, which is in turn enclosed within a paratendon (tendon sheath). The tendons transmit load from the muscles to the bone.

When tendons are damaged they repair themselves by fibroblasts laying new collagen and macrophages clearing the damaged tissue. This means that there is a period of weakness, approximately 7–10 days post injury, when care should be taken in the mobilisation protocol to avoid re-rupture. It may take 6 months for full strength to return.

Tendon pathology (apart from rupture) can be divided into three types:

- *paratendinitis* – this is inflammation of the paratendon and is very painful; it responds well to conservative therapies;

William Sharpey, **1802–1880, Professor of Anatomy and Physiology, University College, London, England, described these fibres in 1848.**

- *paratendinitis with tendinosis*;
- *pure tendinosis* – this is degeneration within the tendon and may only manifest itself when a rupture has occurred; pre-rupture prophylactic treatment is difficult and controversial.

Ligaments

Ligaments transmit tensile forces across joints and help stabilise them. They are similar in structure to tendons but have a higher elastin content and mechanoreceptors for proprioception.

Ligament injuries can be graded as follows:

- grade 0: normal ligament, normal joint stability;
- grade 1: tenderness of the injured ligament, no increase in joint laxity;
- grade 2: partial disruption – tenderness and increased joint laxity with an endpoint;
- grade 3: complete disruption – tenderness and marked increase in joint laxity with no endpoint.

When assessing the stability of joints it is essential to compare both sides. There is a great deal of variation in laxity between and among different groups, e.g. young vs. old, women vs. men, those with hypermobility disorders.

The principles of treatment are the same as for tendons, while remembering that prolonged immobilisation can cause stiffness and reduce the strength of the repair. There is, therefore, a fine balancing act between early mobilisation with reduced swelling and stiffness and mobilisation too early, resulting in re-injury and delayed healing.

Bursae

Between most joints and the overlying tissues there are small

CHAPTER 32 | SPORTS MEDICINE AND SPORTS INJURIES

fluid-filled endothelium-lined sacs, which decrease the frictional forces. These sacs can become inflamed, swollen and acutely painful. Common sites are the:

- olecranon;
- psoas tendon;
- greater trochanter;
- pre-patellar;
- infrapatellar;
- retrocalcaneal.

The symptoms are usually self-limiting and settle without intervention. Occasionally, aspiration, steroid injections or excision may be required.

Bone

Bone is a unique dynamic structure that is continuously adapting throughout life and which heals itself depending on the stresses placed on it (Wolff's law). Fractures heal best when the broken ends of the bone are opposed. Healing occurs in three recognised phases:

- *inflammation*: immediate haematoma formation followed by granulation tissue formation over the next few days;
- *repair*: immature callus forms over weeks and more mature bone over the following months;
- *remodel*: remodelling of the bone occurs according to Wolff's law.

Stress fractures

Any repetitive activity may cause a stress fracture in virtually any bone (Fig. 32.2). They are common and characterised by poorly localised pain that is worse on exercise. Confirming the diagnosis in the early stages can be difficult as plain radiographs will appear normal. Technetium bone scans or magnetic resonance imaging (MRI) will often clarify the diagnosis.

Stress fractures are more common in endurance athletes and women. Other pathologies or contributing factors need to considered, including osteosarcoma and chronic compartment syndrome.

Treatment involves resting from the exacerbating activity; this often requires long periods without undergoing training. Psychological support and alternative forms of exercise will need to be organised to help the athlete through this depressing time (Summary box 32.1).

Summary box 32.1

General tissue injuries

- ■ **Define tendon pathology**
- ■ **Classify ligament injuries**
- ■ **Name the common bursa sites**
- ■ **Three phases of bone repair**

PELVIS, HIP AND THIGH INJURIES

Massive trauma to this area produces fractures and dislocations that can be life-threatening (see Chapter 27). Soft-tissue injuries

---

Julius Wolff, **1836–1902**, Professor of Orthopaedic Surgery, Berlin, Germany, enunciated 'Wolff's Law' in 1892.

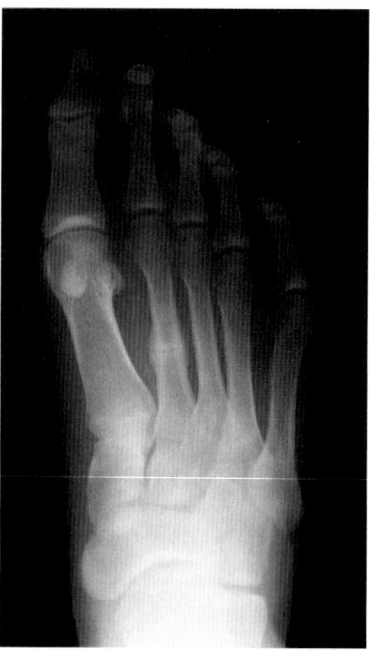

Figure 32.2 Radiograph of a metatarsal stress fracture.

in this area may be subtle and easily missed as attention is focused on the larger fractures and dislocations.

Quadriceps contusion (cork thigh, charley horse)

This is usually the result of a direct blow. A haematoma develops in the rectus femoris with pain, swelling and stiffness. Compartment syndrome needs to be excluded. Initially, the knee should be immobilised in extension; then the muscle is gradually returned to pain-free movement.

Quadriceps rupture

This may occur when kicking balls, especially in football and rugby. Classically, the patient cannot perform a straight leg raise. The torn tendon ends need to be brought together and held as securely as possible so that gentle mobilisation (low load) can be started as soon as possible and stiffness avoided.

Hamstring strain

This is common and usually occurs after a quick muscle contraction. It is usually the short head of the biceps that tears. It should respond to the standard PRICE formula.

Groin strain

This is a difficult area to diagnose and treat. The differential diagnosis includes:

- herniae;
- fractures;
- tumours;
- gynaecological and urinary problems;
- sexually transmitted diseases, e.g. *Chlamydia*;
- stress fractures;
- osteitis pubis.

All athletes are prone to groin strains and they can quickly become an acute-on-chronic injury. Treatment is conservative whenever possible and surgery should not be considered before 6–12 months of treatment.

Bony injuries

Besides the usual fractures and dislocations that may be seen, the pelvis is susceptible to a number of other injuries:

- *Avulsion of the iliac spine.* This is seen in adolescent footballers following a sudden contraction of the rectus femoris or after the leg is brought rapidly to a standstill (such as kicking a wet football) (Figs 32.3 and 32.4).
- *Ischial apophysitis.* This inflammation of the ischial tuberosity is seen in adolescent runners. Occasionally, the hamstring may actually avulse.
- *Osteitis pubis.* This is a self-limiting condition with tenderness of the symphysis pubis and is common in cricketers (Fig. 32.5).

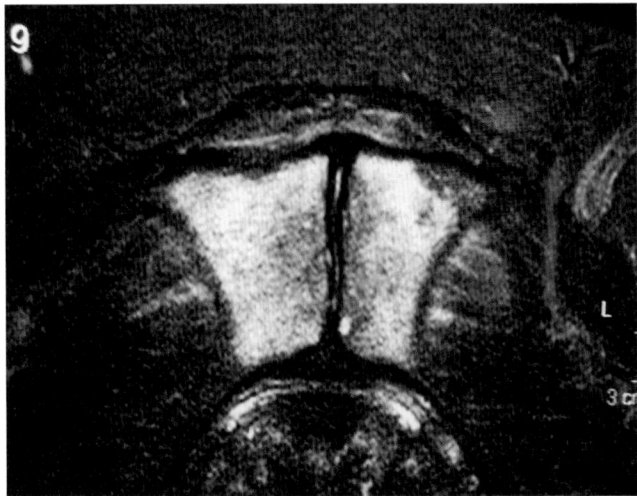

Figure 32.5 Computerised tomography scan of osteitis pubis with cyst formation.

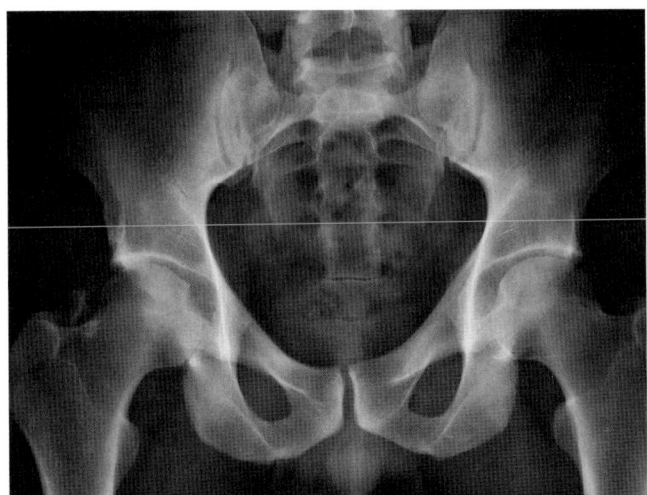

Figure 32.3 Radiograph of a ruptured rectus femoris.

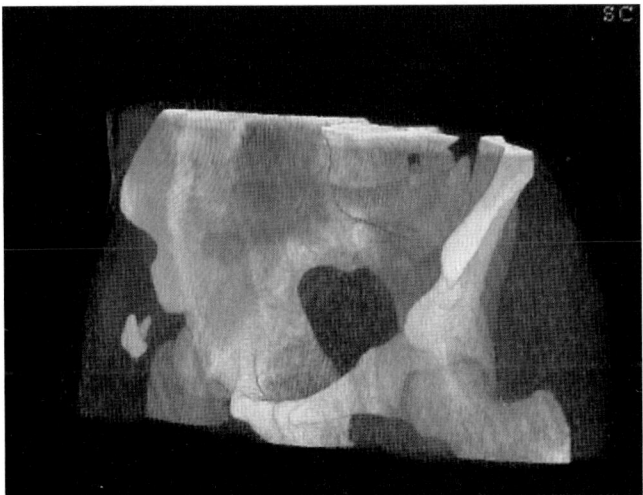

Figure 32.4 Computerised tomography scan demonstrating a ruptured rectus femoris.

KNEE AND KNEE INJURIES

The knee is a complex hinge joint that also allows some rotational movement. It is highly susceptible to injury from most sports, in particular contact sports. Pain felt in the knee area may be referred from the hip, spine or ankle.

Ligamentous injuries

The knee has four main ligaments.

Medial collateral ligament

When a lateral (valgus) force is applied to the knee, the MCL is susceptible to damage, particularly at the femoral insertion, resulting in pain and valgus instability. Grade 1 and 2 tears are usually partial, whereas grade 3 injuries are characterised by > 1 cm of joint opening and other associated ligament injuries. Treatment involves bracing, early weight-bearing and quadriceps exercises.

Lateral collateral ligament

When a medial (varus) force is applied to the knee, the lateral collateral ligament (LCL) is susceptible to damage. Isolated injuries to this ligament are rare because of the presence of other reinforcing structures, e.g., the biceps femoris, iliotibial band and popliteus. However, damage to the LCL is often associated with more extensive disruption of the posterolateral corner, which is a far more significant injury often requiring surgical intervention.

Cruciate ligaments

There are two cruciate ligaments in the knee, which are intracapsular and extrasynovial. They prevent anterior and posterior translation of the tibia on the femur.

Anterior cruciate ligament

Anterior cruciate ligament (ACL) injuries are the most common knee ligament injuries seen in all forms of sport. They are more common in women, jumpers and footballers. An ACL injury is a classic twisting injury with internal rotation and anterior translation of the tibia. In the acute injury there is pain and often a large haemarthrosis, making assessment of the ligament difficult.

CHAPTER 32 | SPORTS MEDICINE AND SPORTS INJURIES

Diagnosis of an ACL injury can be made using a number of diagnostic tests, including the anterior draw test and Lachman's test (see Figs 32.6–32.8). Once the haemarthrosis has resolved, examination is easier and a positive pivot shift, anterior draw test or Lachman's test are usually conclusive. It is associated with other injuries, such as an MCL sprain and meniscal tear, so these need to be excluded.

Rehabilitation of the quadriceps and hamstrings may stop many athletes requiring surgical intervention; however, if instability of the knee continues, surgical reconstruction may be appropriate (Fig. 32.9).

Posterior cruciate ligament

Posterior cruciate ligament (PCL) injuries are less common and are frequently misdiagnosed. The severity of the damage can easily be underestimated. They usually result from a direct blow to the tibia. The 'dashboard injury' is a PCL rupture caused by a motor vehicle accident (MVA). An unrestrained person in the front seat is thrown forwards onto the dashboard. The knee takes the brunt of the force and the tibia is driven backwards. When

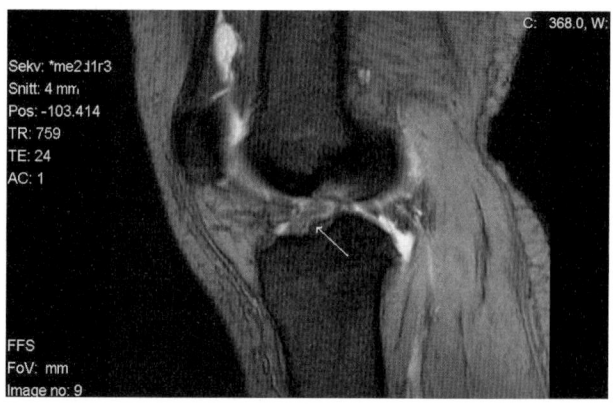

Figure 32.8 Magnetic resonance imaging of a ruptured anterior cruciate ligament.

the mobility of the injured knee is compared with that of the other side, a posterior sag can be clearly seen (Fig. 32.10).

Often the posterolateral corner complex is also damaged and acute reconstruction is now advocated. The surgery is complex and the results are variable.

Meniscal injuries

Menisci are avascular semilunar structures made from fibrocartilage. They help transmit load and act as shock absorbers in the knee. When a rotatory force is applied between the femur and the tibia, i.e. twisting to change direction, then a tear can occur in the meniscus.

There is usually pain and a small effusion may develop over a few days. There is not usually any blood in this as menisci have no blood supply. If a bucket-handle tear results then the patient

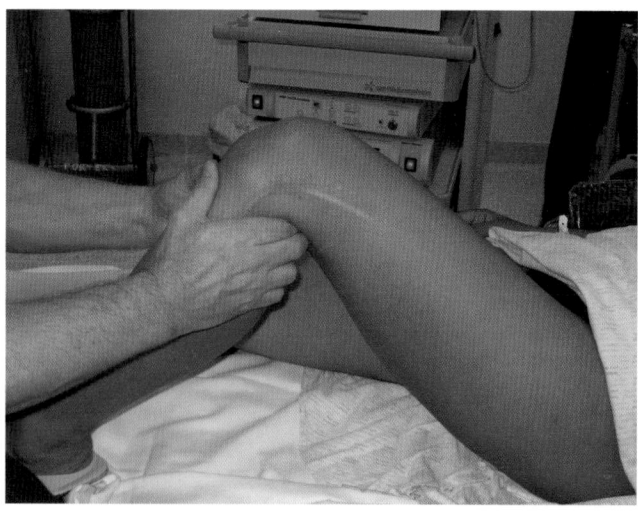

Figure 32.6 Anterior draw test.

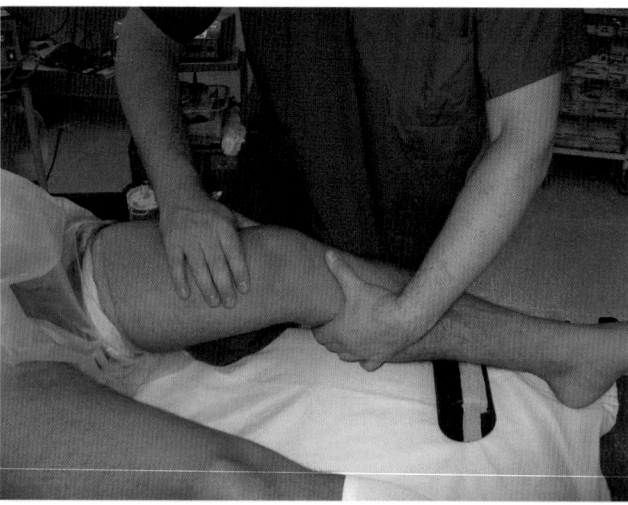

Figure 32.7 Lachman's test.

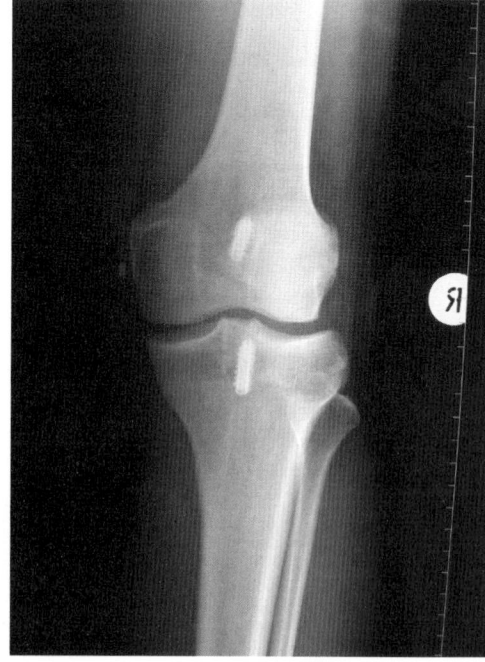

Figure 32.9 Radiograph of a postoperative anterior cruciate ligament repair.

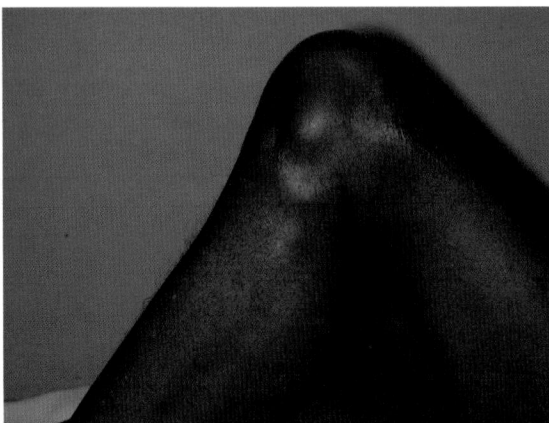

Figure 32.10 Posterior sag of the knee.

may find that the knee locks. The McMurray and Apley grind tests are sometimes positive. An MRI scan may help if the diagnosis is unclear but, ultimately, arthroscopic resection of the tear may be required (Fig. 32.11). In adolescents, meniscal repair is encouraged, especially if the tear is in the periphery where there is a blood supply.

Patellofemoral injuries

This joint is subject to numerous problems such as tracking disorders, instability, chondromalacia patellae and bursitis. The most common symptom is anterior knee pain.

Chondromalacia patellae

This is said to be softening of the patellar articular cartilage although the true aetiology is not known. It is particularly common in female adolescents although the cartilage may appear normal on arthroscopy. Treatment should be centred around quadriceps strengthening and taping exercises, to improve the strength and coordination of the muscle that controls tracking of the patella.

Patellar instability

Dislocation and subluxation may be the result of significant trauma but are frequently chronic conditions, made worse by poor musculature and a shallow femoral trochlea (Fig. 32.12).

Immediate management should be to reduce the patella and sometimes aspirate the haemarthrosis (if large) for pain relief. Immobilisation in extension for 2 weeks combined with isometric quadriceps exercises should be started. When the quadriceps bulk has returned and stability of the knee improved then a graduated return to activity can be undertaken.

Recurrent dislocation and subluxation may require a surgical procedure to overcome the problem, but there is no ideal solution.

Patellar tendinitis (jumper's knee)

This is an apophysitis (inflammation) of the patellar tendon as it inserts into the patella. It is associated with pain, swelling and

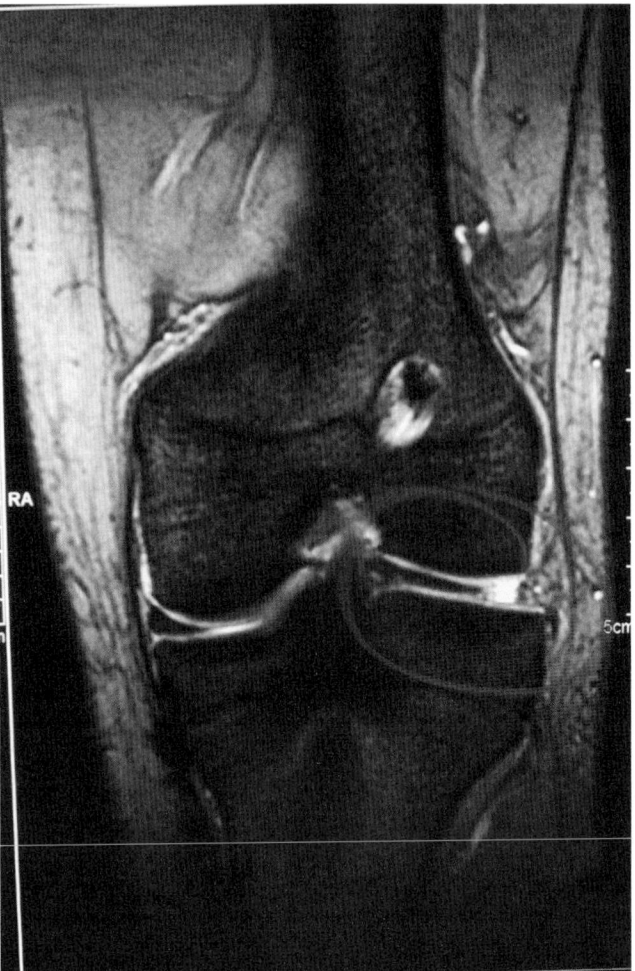

Figure 32.11 *In situ* meniscal tear as seen on a magnetic resonance imaging scan.

crepitus. Conservative management with physiotherapy is the mainstay of treatment. Surgery is rarely required.

Hoffa's disease

Bleeding into the anterior fat pad can cause anterior knee pain. It is most common in adolescents and those with hypermobility and may start with a hyperextension injury. Gymnasts and those practising sports requiring flexibility are more at risk. Treatment should start with modifying activities and occasionally arthroscopic resection.

Plica syndrome

Plica are folds of synovial membrane within the knee. If they become scarred or thickened from trauma or overuse, pain and clicking may result. This can occur in any sport but is more common in football, skiing and rugby. It is often an incidental finding in a normal arthroscopic examination. Surgical resection may relieve the problem.

Thomas Porter McMurray, **1887–1949, Professor of Orthopaedic Surgery, the University of Liverpool, Liverpool, England.**
Alan Graham Apley, **1914–1996, Director of Orthopaedic Surgery, St. Thomas' Hospital, London, England.**

Albert Hoffa, **1859–1907, Orthopaedic Surgeon, Berlin, Germany, described chronic synovitis of the knee in 1904.**

CHAPTER 32 | SPORTS MEDICINE AND SPORTS INJURIES

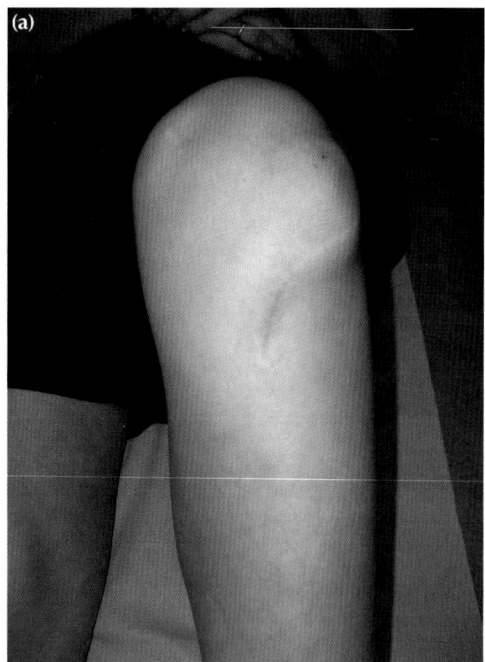

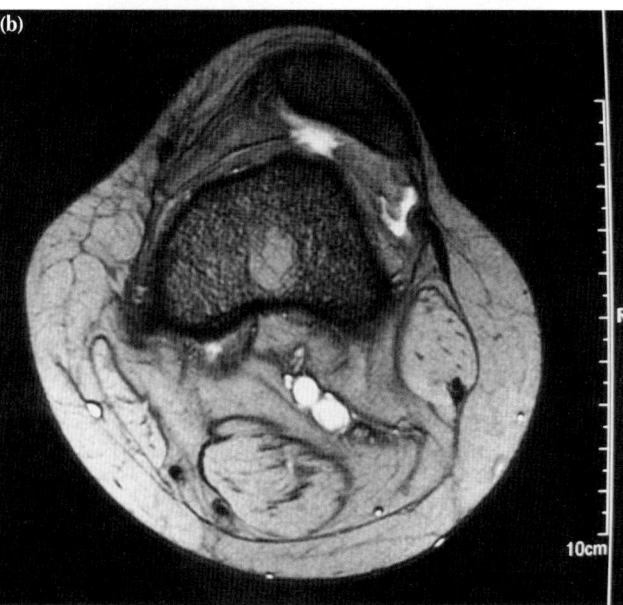

Figure 32.12 Dislocated patella.

Iliotibial band syndrome

The insertion of the iliotibial band into the lateral epicondyle may become inflamed. This is particularly common in runners. Stretching, rest and, if necessary, steroid injections should resolve it (Summary box 32.2).

Summary box 32.2

Knee injuries

- The knee is a hinge joint allowing flexion, extension and some rotation
- There are four main knee ligaments, all susceptible to injury
- The menisci act as shock absorbers and assist in reducing friction
- Pain in the knee may be referred – look for other causes

ANKLE INJURIES

Ankle sprains

Soft-tissue injuries around the ankle joint are common and usually involve the anterior talofibular ligament and the calcaneofibular ligament. Eversion/abduction forces cause trauma to the medial ligament complex, whereas inversion/adduction forces lead to injury of the lateral complex.

Type I sprains involve minor ligamentous injury, type II sprains occur with incomplete ligamentous injury and type III sprains involve complete disruption of a ligament or multiple ligaments.

Ankle sprain diagnosis can be difficult in the acutely painful, post-traumatic ankle joint. Immediate treatment should involve the PRICE routine, which will assist in the recovery; the ankle joint should then be reassessed after 4–7 days. Routine anteroposterior and lateral radiographs should be taken when indicated to exclude a bony injury. Stress views may be indicated but often require an general anaesthetic. MRI imaging of the ankle joint has been shown to be 90% accurate in diagnosing lateral ligament injuries.

Complete rupture of the medial ligament rarely occurs in isolation and is often associated with disruption of the syndesmosis. Damage to either of these structures leads to lateral shift of the talus on everting the ankle (Fig. 32.13). This can predispose to prolonged instability because of failure of the ligament to heal and osteoarthritis as the talus repeatedly impinges on the tibia.

Treatment of an ankle sprain aims to provide a stable ankle with good anatomical alignment and function. Type I and II sprains (incomplete ligament rupture) require protection with an ankle brace or strapping, with early mobilisation and functional

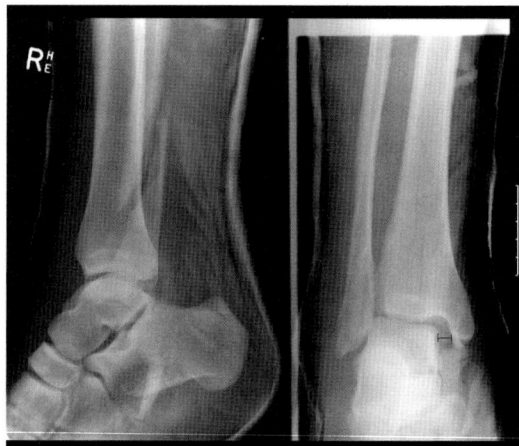

Figure 32.13 Ankle showing a talar shift (bar).

range of motion exercises. It is essential for patients to undergo neuromuscular retraining exercises directed by a physiotherapist to help provide a stable ankle with a good range of movement. The treatment of type III sprains is controversial. Some advocate early surgical repair; however, secondary repair of ruptured ligaments, even years later, has produced comparable results.

Peroneal tendon injuries

Injuries to the peroneal tendons are relatively rare and often misdiagnosed but they can be serious as the peroneal tendons are the dynamic stabilisers of the hindfoot in inversion. They are more prevalent in patients with cavus feet or feet with high medial longitudinal arches. If the sheath is damaged they may sublux anteriorly, giving a snapping sensation. This will require surgical repair. Plain radiography, computerised tomography (CT) or MRI may be helpful in confirming the diagnosis.

Low-grade sprains should respond to bracing and physiotherapy. Complete rupture of the peroneal tendons requires surgical exploration and repair.

Tibialis posterior injuries

Disorders of the tibialis posterior lead to unilateral flat foot deformity. It is more common in women and in the middle-aged athlete and is often a chronic injury. It is characterised by hindfoot valgus along with pronation and abduction of the fore- and midfoot respectively. The deformity is easily identified in the weight-bearing patient; however, it is not always apparent on the lateral X-ray.

Pain around the medial ankle and hindfoot is common, exacerbated by exercise. If it is untreated the foot remains in a chronically pronated position and the pain shifts laterally.

Treatment consists of orthotic shoe implants or splinting to improve the foot position, thereby relieving the pain caused by the foot deformity. This can be combined with NSAIDs and localised steroid injections if indicated. Surgical repair in severe cases may be warranted.

Tibialis anterior injuries

Acute inflammation within the tendon sheath of the tibialis anterior tendon is common in long-distance runners. There is pain, swelling and crepitus over the tendon. It usually resolves with a period of rest and rehabilitation.

Achilles tendon injuries

Tendinitis

This is pain and/or swelling of the Achilles tendon. If the inflammation of the tendon becomes chronic then the tendon develops multiple microtears and loses its organised structure; this is called Achilles' tendonosis. Achilles' tendinitis is caused by a sudden increase in activity that involves the Achilles tendon, i.e. plantarflexion. It is common in athletes and those who participate in sports on an infrequent basis. Patients with pes

> Achilles, the Greek hero, was the son of Peleus and Thetis. When he was a child his mother dipped him in the Styx, one of the rivers of the Underworld, so that he should be invulnerable in battle. The heel by which she held him did not get wet, and was, therefore, not protected. Achilles died from a wound in the heel that he received at the siege of Troy.

planus (flat feet) are more susceptible to develop Achilles' tendinitis as their flat, over-pronated foot places greater demands on the tendon.

Ultrasound or MRI is helpful to confirm the diagnosis.

Initially, the condition should be treated by immobilisation in a cast or boot to rest the tendon combined with NSAIDs and PRICE. Physiotherapy with stretching and strengthening exercises is often beneficial. Cases that fail to respond to conservative measures may require surgical repair.

Rupture

The feeling of a sharp blow to the back of the ankle and an inability to dorsiflex the foot are characteristic of an Achilles tendon rupture. It is classically seen in middle-aged squash and badminton players. Clinically, it can be confirmed using Simmonds' test; this involves squeezing the calf muscles and seeing the foot plantarflex if the tendon is intact.

Tears at the musculotendinous junction can be treated conservatively using a plantarflexed cast or boot for 6–9 weeks. Midsubstance tendon tears can be treated conservatively or by surgical repair. Re-rupture in the first year following injury can occur with either treatment method: there is a 6–10% risk after treatment with conservative methods vs. 3–4% after operative repair. In the long term the re-rupture rate is the same but the risk of nerve damage and skin necrosis is solely associated with operative repair (Summary box 32.3).

Summary box 32.3

Ankle injuries

■ Ankle sprains are graded from I to III, depending on the structures that are injured
■ Common tendon injuries are to the Achilles tendon, tibialis posterior and peroneal tendons

---

FOOT INJURIES

Plantar fasciitis

Typically, this may occur in a middle-aged active patient with a unilateral painful heel. Pain is worse in the morning and on getting out of bed or up from a chair. The pain becomes a dull ache increasing in severity.

Clinically, there may be an area of tenderness around the calcaneal tuberosity on the inferomedial aspect of the calcaneum. A calcaneal spur is present in 50% of cases, which is of unknown significance.

Treatment is varied and includes shoe inserts/heel cups, NSAIDs and local steroid injections. Success with each modality is variable but, as the condition is usually self-limiting over a period of 18 months, one will probably be associated with curing the condition. In cases that are resistant to conservative management, surgical release of the origin of the plantar fascia may be indicated.

Retrocalcaneal bursitis

The calcaneal insertion of the Achilles tendon has a superficial bursa that can become irritated; an associated Haglund's (bony lump) deformity may also be present. It responds well to footwear modification. Occasionally, surgical resection of the calcaneal tuberosity may be attempted but the lump often recurs.

Nerves

Sural nerve entrapment

This commonly occurs in runners and presents with pain along the lateral aspect of the foot. It is often associated with chronic ankle sprains due to the presence of scar tissue. Nerve conduction studies show slow conduction. Initial treatment with manipulation/massage of soft tissues to break down adhesions should help. In resistant cases surgical release is required.

Morton's neuroma

There are many theories regarding the aetiology of Morton's neuroma but it is widely accepted that it occurs in the post-traumatic foot, especially with associated metatarsal fractures.

Patients complain of pain or aching around the metatarsal heads that is exacerbated by walking and relieved by rest or massaging the affected area. Ultrasound or MRI confirms the diagnosis. Lifestyle and footwear modification with or without injection of steroids into the affected web space have limited success. Surgical resection of the neuroma forms the mainstay of treatment.

Bones

Turf toe (plantar capsular ligament sprain)

Pain at the metatarsophalangeal joint (MTPJ) of the big toe may be caused by repetitive jamming of the big toe or pushing off while running and jumping. It is a classic cricketing injury. Hyperextension of the first MTPJ tears the MTPJ capsule and causes pain, swelling and stiffness. Joint instability and even dislocation at the MTPJ can occur in severe cases.

Diagnosis is by clinical means with radiography being performed to exclude any fractures. Treatment consists of avoiding the activity for 3–4 weeks with elevation and ice, to allow the capsule to heal. Orthotic shoe inserts that limit movement at the MTPJ can help to prevent recurrence.

Metatarsalgia

Pain felt in the ball of the foot around the metatarsal heads is called metatarsalgia. It commonly occurs at the heads of the second, third and fourth metatarsals. It is caused by excessive pressure being exerted on the metatarsal heads because of poor footwear, participating in high-impact activities without proper footwear, pes cavus, a tight Achilles tendon, first ray instability, hammer toe or claw toe.

The pain is under one or more of the metatarsal heads and the patient may describe it as a feeling of walking on pebbles.

Treatment is by adaptation of footwear and use of an orthotic metatarsal insole, which offloads the metatarsal heads.

Freiberg's disease

Avascular necrosis of the second metarsal head is called Freiberg's disease (Fig. 32.14). It is most commonly seen in ado-

lescents before epiphyseal closure. Pain is diffusely spread in the forefoot. Treatment consists of activity modification with or without orthotic insoles or metatarsal bars. Surgical resection will leave a short toe.

Sever's disease (calcaneal apophysitis)

Sever's disease is heel pain developing in the teenager and is associated with a growth spurt. The hindfoot has poor flexibility and altered biomechanics. The vertical orientation of the apophyseal plate where the Achilles tendon inserts into the calcaneum makes it prone to shearing forces. It is common in soccer players and gymnasts who perform frequent running or jumping movements. Treatment consists of activity modification and stretching exercises and may be coupled with heel cushion inserts. Once the growth plate fuses the symptoms should resolve.

Stress fractures

Stress fractures are classically associated with constant impact sports, such as running or jumping on hard surfaces. Common sites for fractures are the neck of the second metatarsal (March fractures), the sesamoids of the great toe and the navicular in dancers and horse riders. It is caused by repetitive loading of the bone leading to microfractures across the bone. If the rate of formation of microfractures exceeds the reparative ability of the bone, a stress fracture forms and causes pain.

They are more common in women and this may be associated with the 'female athlete triad' of bulimia/anorexia, amenorrhoea and osteoporosis.

The treatment of stress fractures is rest from the causative activity, usually for 6–8 weeks. This does not mean a cessation of all sport but rather adapting and using other training modalities to maintain fitness, muscle strength and flexibility. A premature return to sport may result in a chronic injury developing (Summary box 32.4).

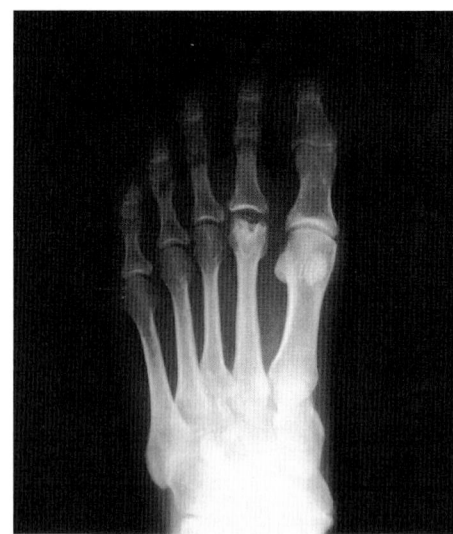

Figure 32.14 Radiograph of Freiberg's disease.

Thomas George Morton, 1835–1903, Surgeon, the Pennsylvania Hospital, Philadelphia, PA, USA, described this condition in 1876.
Albert Henry Freiburg, 1869–1940, Professor of Orthopaedic Surgery, the University of Cincinnati, OH, USA, described this condition in 1926.

James Warren Sever, 1878–1964, Orthopaedic Surgeon, the Children's Hospital, Boston, MA, USA, described apophysitis of the os calcis in 1912.
March fractures are so called because they commonly occur in troops who have marched long distances.

SHOULDER AND UPPER LIMB INJURIES

The shoulder consists of three joints, all of which can be injured. The glenohumeral joint is inherently unstable and is therefore prone to injury, particularly in sports that rely on throwing.

Instability

Shoulder instability is extremely common and can range from dislocations through to subluxations. Eventually, it may require a minimal external force for such events to occur. Males under the age of 25 years with a first-time dislocation have a 60% chance of recurrence, a 10% chance of contralateral instability and a 20% chance of developing arthritis.

Dislocations should be reduced as quickly as possible and, after a short period of immobilisation, intensive rehabilitation should be started to build strength and coordination around the shoulder.

Tendinitis and tears of the rotator cuff

Damage to the rotator cuff is particularly common in bowlers and the older athlete. Overload and impingement as a result of abnormal acromial anatomy may be at fault. It is characterised by pain over the anterior shoulder that radiates down the arm, is worse at night and which presents difficulties in raising the arm above the head. Speed's and Yergason's tests are usually positive. Treatment includes modifying activities and cortisone injections. Arthroscopic debridement can also be considered.

Rotator cuff tears are more common in the elderly athlete and are rarely amenable to surgery. In the younger athlete a significant force must have been applied for a tear to occur; repair offers a good chance of success.

Acromioclavicular joint dislocation

This is common in cyclists, wrestlers and after a fall onto the shoulder. Unless the clavicle buttonholes through the muscle, treatment is usually conservative.

Occasionally, a direct blow to the lateral end of the clavicle may result in osteolysis of the end of the clavicle. This is usually self-limiting but does leave a noticeable gap.

Sternoclavicular joint dislocation

Again, this is associated with falls onto the shoulder, resulting in dislocation of the joint anteriorly. It can be treated conservatively. Urgent reduction is needed if the displaced bone is compromising the thoracic outlet.

Muscles

Rupture of the pectoralis major, long head of the biceps and subscapularis are the most common muscle injuries around the shoulder. They are particularly common in weightlifters and wrestlers, in which case an association with performance-enhancing drugs should be considered. Biceps ruptures can be treated conservatively but the other two injuries may require surgical repair (Summary box 32.5).

THE ELBOW

Injuries to the elbow are less common than injuries to other joints and are generally caused by overuse. This occurs in golf, tennis, baseball and events involving throwing.

Lateral and medial epicondylitis

Lateral epicondylitis (tennis elbow)

This is tendinitis of the origin of the extensor carpi radialis brevis and is a problem in older athletes. Pain is localised to the insertion of the extensor muscles on the lateral side of the elbow and is typically made worse by shaking hands or opening doors. It is self-limiting over a year; treatment with NSAIDs, acupuncture and injections have all proved to be effective.

Medial epicondylitis (golfer's elbow)

This is inflammation of the flexor tendon origin on the medial side of the elbow and is caused by exercise involving repetitive throwing. Pain radiates from the medial epicondyle down the forearm and is exacerbated by pronation. There may be associated ulnar nerve symptoms. Treatment is the same as for lateral epicondylitis.

Osteochondritis dissecans of the elbow

Although this condition can affect any joint, gymnasts and cricketers are particularly at risk. It involves spontaneous necrosis of the capitellum, resulting in bony fragments that cause crepitus, pain and locking of the joint. Arthroscopic removal is advised.

THE HAND AND WRIST

Injuries to the hand and wrist are very common in all forms of sport. They can terminate a sporting career and can have a devastating effect on everyday life.

The anatomy of the hand is highly complex, with tendons, muscles, nerves and synovial sheaths all working closely together to allow fine, complex movements. Even relatively minor damage to any of these structures can affect the whole function of the hand.

Careful assessment of the injured hand is essential. Each individual nerve and tendon should be examined. A small puncture wound can suggest that there is only minimal damage

CHAPTER 32 | SPORTS MEDICINE AND SPORTS INJURIES

internally; however, a missed severed tendon or index finger lateral digital nerve can have long-term major consequences.

Compression of the nerves

The median nerve

Repetitive weight training can cause compression of the median nerve in a number of areas: the ligament of Struthers, pronator teres, carpal tunnel and the origin of the flexor digitorum superficialis.

Symptoms of parasthesiae and a positive Tinel's sign are diagnostic. Treatment by activity modification should relieve the symptoms although, occasionally, surgical release is required.

The ulnar nerve

As the ulnar nerve traverses Guyon's canal it may be compressed. This can occur in cyclists who hyperextend their wrists and press down on the handlebars. Again, activity modification and splinting should relieve the symptoms.

The radial nerve

Compression of the radial nerve can be hard to differentiate from lateral epicondylitis. If the radial nerve is compressed, stressing the extensor carpi radialis brevis should reproduce the symptoms. Again, activity modification and forearm splinting should resolve this.

The carpus

Fractures and dislocations of the carpus are discussed in Chapter 27. The scaphoid bone is particularly vulnerable in gymnasts and weightlifters who dorsiflex their wrists under extreme loads. This causes the scaphoid to impact against the radius and gives wrist pain. An osteophyte develops causing impingement; this usually needs excision.

Sir John Struthers, **1823–1899, Professor of Anatomy, the University of Aberdeen, Scotland.**
Jules Tinel, **1879–1952, Physician, Hôpital Beaujon, Paris, France.**
Jean Casimir Felix Guyon, **1831–1920, Professor of Surgical Pathology, Paris, France.**

Fingers

Dislocations of the joints and injuries to the collateral ligaments and tendons are very common injuries. For example, gamekeeper's/skier's thumb is caused by marked radial deviation of the proximal phalanx on the metacarpal, causing the ulnar collateral ligament to stretch and ultimately rupture. Partial tears can be treated in a splint but complete ruptures will need surgical intervention. Mallet/baseball finger is a rupture of the distal insertion of the extensor tendon and can be treated conservatively. The more subtle ruptured middle slip of the extensor mechanism at the proximal interphalangeal joint is often missed, resulting in a boutonnière deformity, which will often need surgical intervention.

Flexor tendons may also rupture at the distal interphalangeal joint. This is commonly seen in rugby and wrestling as the athlete attempts to grab the opponent's jersey, hence the name jersey finger; it requires early surgical intervention.

ACKNOWLEDGEMENTS

M.J.K. Bankes FRCS Orth, Consultant Orthopaedic Surgeon, Guy's and St Thomas' Hospital NHS Trust.
A.J. Davies FRCS Orth, Consultant Orthopaedic Surgeon, Guy's and St Thomas' Hospital NHS Trust.

FURTHER READING

Anderson, M.K. and Hall, S.J. (1997) *Fundamentals of Sports Injury Management.* Williams & Wilkins, Baltimore, MD.
Martin, M. and Yates, W.N. (1998) *Therapeutic Medications in Sports Medicine.* Williams & Wilkins, Baltimore, MD.
Sherry, E. and Wilson, S. (1998) *Oxford Handbook of Sports Medicine.* Oxford University Press, Oxford.

Boutonnière, **French for button-hole.**

The spine

EPIDEMIOLOGY

The lifetime prevalence of low back pain has been reported at between 60 and 80%. By comparison, the lifetime prevalence of true sciatica has been reported at 5.3% in men and 3.7% in women. It is generally accepted that 90% of acute episodes of low back pain settle, allowing return to work within 6 weeks. However, some 3–4% of the population aged between 16 and 44 years and 5–7% of the population aged between 45 and 64 years will report back problems as a 'chronic sickness'.

The lifetime prevalence of neck pain reported in the literature varies from 66% to 71%. A higher prevalence is noted in females, those of advanced years, those with previous injury and those with perceived high job demands. The true incidence of brachalgia has not been reported in the literature.

CLINICAL ANATOMY

The normal thoracic kyphosis is between 20° and 50° (mean 35°) and increases with age. The normal lumbar lordosis is between 40° and 80° (mean 60°). Most lumbar lordosis occurs between L4 and S1, and decreases with age. When standing, the normal sagittal vertical axis (sagittal plumb-line) falls from the odontoid process through the C7–T1 disc space and crosses the spinal column at the T12–L1 disc space, before reaching the posterior superior corner of the S1 vertebral body.

The spinal nerve roots include 8 cervical, 12 thoracic, 5 lumbar, 5 sacral and 1 coccygeal. Dorsal and ventral roots join to form spinal nerves. The ventral root and the dorsal root ganglion lie within the intervertebral foramen. The neural foramen is bounded superiorly and inferiorly by pedicles, anteriorly by the disc and posteriorly by the facet joint. Degenerative changes in these structures may lead to neural compromise. Disruption of the medial or inferior pedicle cortex with pedicle instrumentation should be avoided to minimise the risk of injury to the nerve root or dura. When considering the spinal canal, it is helpful to describe parasagittal subdivisions including the central canal, lateral recess, foraminal and extraforaminal zones to assist when correlating radiological findings with operative findings. Laminar overlap within the lumbar spine decreases from L1 to S1 so that, at the L5–S1 level, discectomy requires *less* bone removal than a more proximal discectomy (Summary box 33.1).

The blood supply of the spinal cord is derived from the vertebral, deep cervical, intercostal and lumbar arteries. The arteries of the spinal cord include the anterior spinal artery and two posterior spinal arteries. In the cervical spine, the anterior spinal artery arises from the vertebral artery. The vertebral artery enters the transverse foramen of C7 and travels cephalad to pass through the foramen magnum. Radicular arteries enter the vertebral canal through the intervertebral foramen and divide into anterior and posterior radicular arteries, which in turn supply the anterior and posterior spinal arteries. The most significant radicular artery to the cervical cord arises from the deep cervical artery and travels with the left C6 spinal nerve. The radicular artery of Adamkiewicz makes a major contribution to the anterior spinal artery, supplying the lower spinal cord. It originates on the left in 80% of people, usually accompanying the ventral root of T9, T10 or T11, but can originate anywhere from T5 to L5. Ligation of segmental vessels over the midpoint of the vertebral body will minimise the risk of injury to this important artery.

Albert Adamkiewicz, **1850–1921, Professor of Pathology, The University of Krakow, (Cracow), Poland, described the arterial supply of the spinal cord in 1882.**

Injury to the superior gluteal artery and cluneal nerves can occur during bone graft harvest from the posterior iliac crest. The incision should, therefore, stay within 70 mm of the posterior iliac crest. An incision made parallel to the cluneal nerves and perpendicular to the posterior iliac crest decreases the morbidity. The lateral femoral cutaneous nerve may be injured when harvesting bone from the anterior iliac crest. By operating at least 2 cm posterior to the anterior superior iliac crest and harvesting from the outer cortex of the ilium, the risk is reduced.

HISTORY AND PHYSICAL EXAMINATION

History taken from a patient with back pain should include questions on age, history of malignant disease, unexplained weight loss, intake of immunosuppressive drugs, duration of symptoms, responsiveness to previous treatment, pain that is worse at rest and urinary or other infections. In cauda equina syndromes, there will usually be a history of difficulty with micturition, loss of anal sphincter tone and faecal incontinence, saddle anaesthesia around the anus, perineum and genitals, and widespread progressive motor weakness in the legs and gait disturbance (Summary box 33.2).

Summary box 33.2

Cauda equina syndrome

A spectrum of:

- Low back pain
- Uni- or bilateral sciatica
- Saddle anaesthesia
- Motor weakness in the lower extremities
- With variable rectal and urinary symptoms

For patients with neck pain, sensory disturbance, widespread motor weakness and long tract signs, the possibility of cervical myelopathy should be considered. For the diagnosis of spinal stenosis, the most commonly found symptom from the history is reduced walking distance. Other specific causes of back pain such as infections, benign tumours and inflammatory disease are found in fewer than 1% of patients seen in general practice. Summary box 33.3 lists the commonly accepted 'red flags' that allow diagnostic triage into those with serious pathology of the spine (such as fractures, tumours or cauda equina syndrome) and those *without* serious pathology.

Summary box 33.3

'Red flags' according to the evidence-based guidelines (the most common indications from history and examination for pathological findings requiring special attention)

- Back pain in children <18 years with considerable pain or onset >55 years
- History of violent trauma
- Constant progressive pain at night
- History of cancer
- Systemic steroids
- Drug abuse, human immunodeficiency virus infection
- Weight loss
- Systemic illness
- Persisting severe restriction of motion
- Intense pain or minimal motion
- Structural deformity
- Difficulty with micturition
- Loss of anal sphincter tone or faecal incontinence; saddle anaesthesia
- Widespread progressive motor weakness or gait disturbance
- Inflammatory disorders (ankylosing spondylitis) suspected
- Gradual onset <40 years
- Marked morning stiffness
- Persisting limitation of motion
- Peripheral joint involvement
- Iritis, skin rashes, colitis, urethral discharge
- Family history

The psychosocial history helps to estimate prognosis and to plan therapy. The New Zealand guidelines introduced the concept of 'yellow flags'. The most useful items are a history of failed previous treatment, substance abuse and disability compensation. Brief screening questionnaires for depression and psychosocial problems offer important therapeutic opportunities.

The examination should exclude pathology of the shoulder, hip, knee, sacroiliac joint and vascular system. The normal range of motion in the cervical spine is 45° of flexion, 55° of extension, 70° of rotation and 40° lateral bend. Spurling's test for radiculopathy is a reproduction of arm pain by hyperextension and lateral rotation towards the symptomatic side. This manoeuvre decreases the size of the intervertebral foramen. Tone, power, coordination, reflexes and sensation should be checked on both upper and lower limbs (Tables 33.1 and 33.2). Myelopathy or upper motor neurone (UMN) lesions are suggested by hyperreflexia, a positive Hoffmann's sign (if the middle finger is flicked

Table 33.1 Neurological evaluation of the upper limb

Neurological level	Motor	Sensation	Reflex
C5	Deltoid	Lateral arm	Biceps
C6	Wrist extensors and extensor carpi radialis longus	Lateral forearm	Brachioradialis
C7	Triceps	Middle finger	Triceps
C8	Long finger flexors	Medial forearm	No reflex
T1	Interosseus muscles	Medial arm	No reflex

Johann Hoffmann, **1857–1919, Professor of Neurology, Heidelberg, Germany.**

Table 33.2 Neurological evaluation of the lower limb

Neurological level	Motor	Sensation	Reflex
L2	Hip flexion	Anterior thigh, groin	No reflex
L3	Knee extension	Anterior and lateral thigh	Patellar (L3, 4)
L4	Ankle dorsiflexion	Medial leg and foot	Patellar (L3, 4)
L5	Extensor hallucis longus	Lateral leg and foot	No reflex
S1	Ankle plantarflexion	Lateral foot and little toe	Achilles

into extension, the thumb and other fingers flex briskly), upgoing plantar responses and, in the case of a high cervical myelopathy, a positive scapulohumeral reflex (tapping on the spine of the scapula or tip of the acromion in the caudal direction leads to elevation of the scapula or abduction of the humerus). Other manifestations of hyperreflexia include ankle and patellar clonus. Typical signs of radiculopathy [lower motor neurone (LMN) lesion] include flaccid paralysis, muscle atrophy, loss of reflexes and muscle fasciculation.

Schober's test determines the degree of actual excursion in flexion and extension, which is decreased in ankylosing spondylitis. Functional testing by observation of heel walking (ankle dorsiflexion L4 myotome), toe walking (ankle plantarflexion S1 myotome) and deep knee bend (quadriceps L3 and L4 myotomes) can give a quick assessment of lower limb power. However, formal testing of all five myotomes should be performed (Table 33.2). The knee, ankle and Babinski reflexes should also be assessed. A positive passive straight leg raise test produces radicular pain distal to the knee at less than 70° of elevation. If the contralateral straight leg raise is positive for radicular pain in the symptomatic leg, this is strongly suggestive of nerve root compression. Lasègue's sign denotes straight leg raise radiculopathy aggravated by ankle dorsiflexion, while the bowstring sign denotes straight leg raise radiculopathy aggravated by applying pressure over the popliteal fossa. The femoral stretch test is less specific than the sciatic straight leg raise. When positive, it produces anterior thigh symptoms and indicates an L3 or L4 radiculopathy. The patient is examined in the prone position with the knee flexed, and the hip is then passively extended.

The sacroiliac joints can be assessed by applying manual compression across the iliac wings or by performing the FABER (flexion, abduction, external rotation, figure-of-four test) test of the hip to rule out sacroiliac instability and pain.

Examination for scoliosis involves inspection of the patient standing and in forward flexion (Adams' test) to assess rib or loin prominence. Relative shoulder heights and waist asymmetry should be noted. The skin should be examined for cutaneous neurofibromata, café au lait patches or axillary freckles commonly present in neurofibromatosis. Neurological examination should include abdominal reflexes. Leg lengths should be measured. In the case of kyphosis, the sagittal alignment and forward gaze should be assessed.

Waddell *et al.* (1979) developed and validated a series of signs and tests that have proved helpful in identifying individuals who are magnifying or exaggerating symptoms. The signs include three observations of pain behaviour (pain in a non-anatomical distribution, pain out of proportion to the stimulus, exaggerated pain behaviour such as grimacing) and four tests (skin roll produces 'radicular' symptoms, pain on simulated spinal rotation, back pain on axial compression of the head, and variable straight leg raise in the supine and sitting positions). Waddell's signs of incongruency do not explain why a patient is exaggerating. A patient may be seeking some secondary gain. Patients with three or more of these signs typically respond poorly to either surgery or physiotherapy unless the underlying cause of the abnormal behaviour is corrected (Summary box 33.4).

> **Summary box 33.4**
>
> **Non-organic physical signs in low back pain**
>
> - *Tenderness*: superficial or non-anatomical
> - *Simulation tests*: axial loading or rotation
> - *Distraction tests*: variable straight leg raises
> - *Regional disturbances*: non-anatomical sensory or motor loss
> - *Over-reaction*: grimacing, muscle tremor, etc.

INVESTIGATIONS

The most common diagnostic imaging tests used to evaluate spinal disorders include plain radiographs, magnetic resonance imaging (MRI), computerised tomography (CT), CT myelography and isotope bone scanning. These investigations are extremely sensitive but relatively non-specific. For example, at least one-third of asymptomatic patients have been noted to have 'abnormalities' on MRI scans. All investigations must therefore be carefully correlated with the clinical findings.

Plain radiographs

It is not necessary to order spine radiographs for every patient presenting with neck or low back pain. Plain radiographs of a patient with cervical, thoracic or lumbar pain may be indicated for those patients less than 20 years of age or over 50 years of age, for patients who have failed to respond to conservative treatment, for patients who have sustained trauma or suffered night pain or with a history of carcinoma, fever or weight loss. Standing radiographs of the whole spine are important for the full assessment of scoliosis. Radiographs cannot diagnose early-stage tumour or infection, because significant bone destruction (between 40% and 60% of bone mass) must occur before a radiographic abnormality is detected (Summary box 33.5).

Joseph Francois Felix Babinski, **1857–1932, Neurologist, Hôpital de la Pitie, Paris, France.**
Charles Ernest Lasègue, **1816–1863, Professor of Medicine, The University of Paris, and Physician, La Salpêtrière, Paris, France.**

Summary box 33.5

Need for plain radiography

Plain radiographs of the lumbar, thoracic or cervical spine may be indicated for:

- Patients under 20 years of age
- Patients over 50 years of age
- History of trauma
- History of carcinoma
- History of night pain, fever or weight loss

Magnetic resonance imaging

This allows detailed visualisation of the disc, thecal sac, epidural space, neural elements, paraspinal soft tissues and bone marrow, while avoiding the use of ionising radiation. It is contraindicated for patients with pacemakers, drug pumps or spinal cord stimulators.

Computerised tomography

This investigation is the best test for bone anatomy. Three-dimensional reconstructions are often useful for the assessment of congenital spinal deformity. CT myelography is now rarely used, but does have utility in revision cases or for those patients unable to have MRI.

Bone scintigraphy

Isotope bone scanning is a highly sensitive, but non-specific test useful for screening of the skeletal system for metastatic disease, discitis or vertebral body osteomyelitis, or to assess the relative activity of bone lesions such as pars interarticulares defects or a pseudarthrosis. When investigating spondylolysis, a single-photon emission CT (SPECT) scan will provide both planar and cross-sectional images. ^{99m}Technetium hydroxymethylene diphosphonate is administered intravenously. The technetium is adsorbed into the hydroxyapatite matrix of bone, and the activity is recorded with a gamma camera. In the case of multiple myeloma or purely lytic metastases, the bone scan may not show increased activity as these tumours may not stimulate a significant *osteoblastic* response. The use of a mobile gamma probe can assist in the perioperative localisation and excision of both osteoid osteoma and osteoblastomas.

Bone densitometry

Bone density can be measured using dual-energy X-ray absorptiometry (DEXA). It is widely used to assess bone mass and is necessary to confirm the diagnosis of osteoporosis. The bone density is usually checked at three sites: the spine, the hip and the distal radius.

Discography

This involves the injection of a radio-opaque contrast agent into a presumed degenerated and painful disc as a preoperative test for performing spinal fusion or as a method of choosing the level of fusion (Fig. 33.1). It is commonly used in the lumbar spine, and less commonly in the cervical spine. It is possible to assess disc morphology and to confirm whether or not the intervertebral disc is the pain generator. Although controversial, there are reports in the literature demonstrating improved outcome following lumbar fusion in patients who were selected by positive lumbar discography.

Facet joint injections

For patients who predominantly have facet joint arthropathy, X-ray-guided facet joint injections may be both diagnostic and

(a)

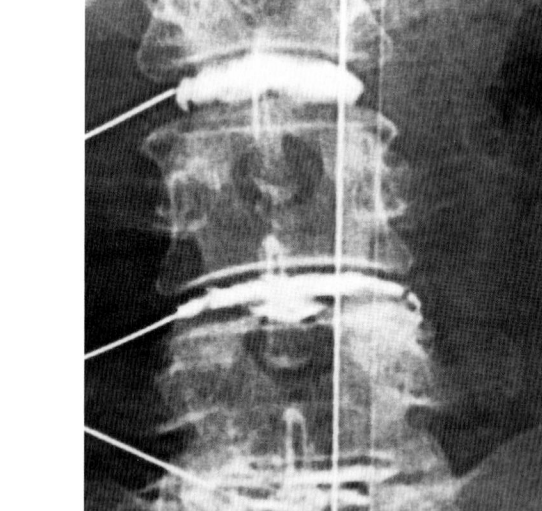

(b)

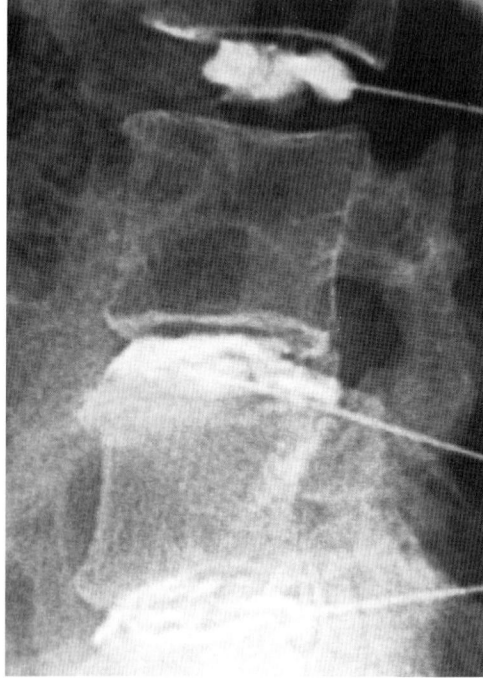

Figure 33.1 Lumbar discography. Anteroposterior (a) and lateral (b) radiographs following injection of contrast media into the lower three lumbar discs. Typical low back pain was reproduced when injecting the L4/5 and L5/S1 disc. The patient experienced no pain when the L3/4 disc was injected.

therapeutic. Local anaesthetic combined with steroid is injected in the region of the facet.

Foraminal epidural steroid injections

For patients with radiculopathy due to a prolapsed intervertebral disc or lateral recess stenosis, a targeted foraminal epidural steroid injection of local anaesthetic and steroid may provide important diagnostic information and have a lasting therapeutic effect. The introduction of these techniques has been shown to significantly reduce the number of patients required to undergo traditional lumbar microdiscectomy.

Spinal biopsy

CT-guided or open biopsy is often performed to obtain tissue for diagnostic study in cases of suspected tumour and/or infection.

CLASSIFICATION

It is useful to classify low back pain into three main groups: mechanical, non-mechanical and miscellaneous (Table 33.3).

TUMOURS OF THE SPINE

Metastatic tumours

These are the most common tumours of the spine, accounting for 98% of all spine lesions. The commonest malignancies that metastasise to the spine include breast (21%), lung (14%), prostate (7.5%), renal (5%), gastrointestinal (5%) and thyroid (2.5%). The most frequent pathway for spread of metastatic deposits is through the venous system. Batson's plexus of veins extends along the entire spinal column, providing a connection with the major organ systems most commonly involved in metastatic spinal disease. Other methods by which metastatic disease spreads to the spine are listed in Table 33.4 (Summary box 33.6).

Summary box 33.6

Commonest malignancies that metastasise to the spine (in order of frequency)

- Breast
- Lung
- Prostate
- Renal
- Gastrointestinal
- Thyroid

Over 80% of patients with spinal metastases present with progressive unrelenting *pain*, and only 20% present with spinal cord compression. Plain radiographs may show an absent pedicle (see Fig. 33.3a) ('winking owl' sign), vertebral cortical erosion and/or vertebral collapse. Investigations should include a full blood count (FBC), erythrocyte sedimentation rate (ESR), calcium, phosphate, alkaline phosphatase, prostate-specific antigen, serum protein electrophoresis, thyroid function tests, nutritional indices and either a CT-guided or open biopsy. Most metastases are *osteoblastic* and will show up on bone scintigraphy; however, osteolytic lesions such as multiple myeloma and hypernephroma may not show up on an isotope bone scan.

Treatment options include orthotic treatment, steroids (dexamethasone), radiotherapy, chemotherapy, hormonal therapy, surgery or a combination of any of the above. Radiotherapy promotes re-ossification of the vertebral body and reduces tumour load. It can be very effective for reducing 'bone pain'. Breast, lung and prostate metastases and lymphoma are highly radiosensitive. Gastrointestinal adenocarcinoma, metastatic melanoma, thyroid and renal carcinoma are radioresistant. Small cell carcinoma of the lung, Ewing's sarcoma, thyroid carcinoma, breast carcinoma and neuroblastoma are usually sensitive to chemotherapy and should have chemotherapy as the first line of management. Adenocarcinoma of the lung is resistant to chemotherapy.

Surgery should be reserved for those patients whose life expectancy exceeds 3 months. Indications for surgery include a lack of definitive diagnosis, progressive neurological deficit despite the administration of steroids and/or radiotherapy, spinal instability, incapacitating pain or radioresistant tumours. Relative contraindications to surgery include multiple spinal metastases, widespread visceral or brain metastases or an expected survival of less than 3 months. Preoperative embolisation of spinal tumours can dramatically reduce perioperative blood loss, which is particularly useful for vascular tumours such as renal cell carcinoma, thyroid carcinoma and Ewing's sarcoma.

Surgical approaches usually involve spinal decompression and stabilisation with instrumentation over multiple segments. The anterior column may be reconstructed with allograft, methylmethacrylate, titanium mesh or carbon fibre cages.

Primary spine tumours

These may be benign, intermediate or malignant. They include the *bone-forming tumours* such as osteoid osteoma, osteoblastoma (Fig. 33.2) and osteosarcoma, the *cartilage-forming tumours* such as chondroma, osteochondroma and chondrosarcoma, the *giant cell tumours* such as osteoclastoma, the *round cell tumours* such as Ewing's sarcoma, malignant lymphoma and myeloma, the *vascular tumours* such as haemangioma and haemangioendothelioma (Fig. 33.3) and a number of *tumour-like lesions* such as the aneurysmal bone cyst or eosinophilic granuloma. These are discussed further in Chapter 37.

Benign tumours tend to occur in the posterior elements; malignant tumours tend to involve the vertebral body. Osteoblastoma, aneurysmal bone cyst and giant cell tumour all

Table 33.3 Classification of low back pain (Carragee and Hannibal 2004)

I	Mechanical	e.g. spondylolysis, spondylolisthesis, facet joint arthropathy, discogenic low back pain, spinal stenosis
II	Non-mechanical	e.g. tumour, infection, inflammatory spondyloarthopathy
III	Miscellaneous	e.g. osteoporosis, viscerogenic referred pain, psychogenic pain

---

Oscar V. Batson, 1894–1979, an American Otolaryngologist.
James Ewing, 1866–1943, Professor of Pathology, Cornell University Medical College, New York, NY, USA, described this type of sarcoma in 1921.

(a)

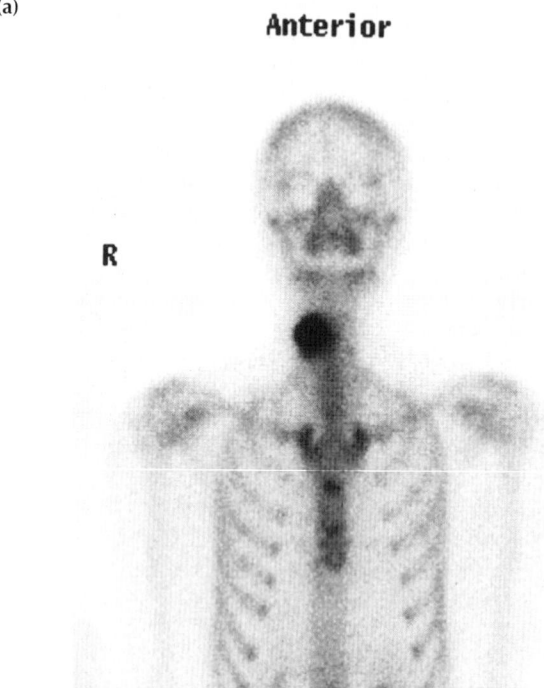

(b)

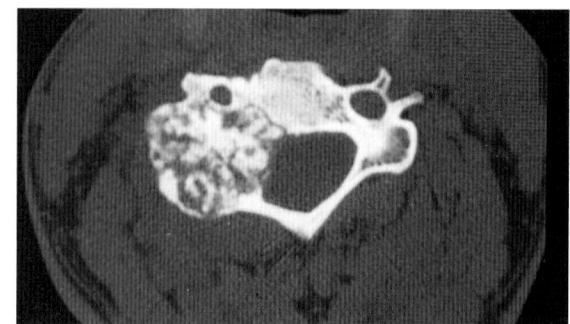

(d)

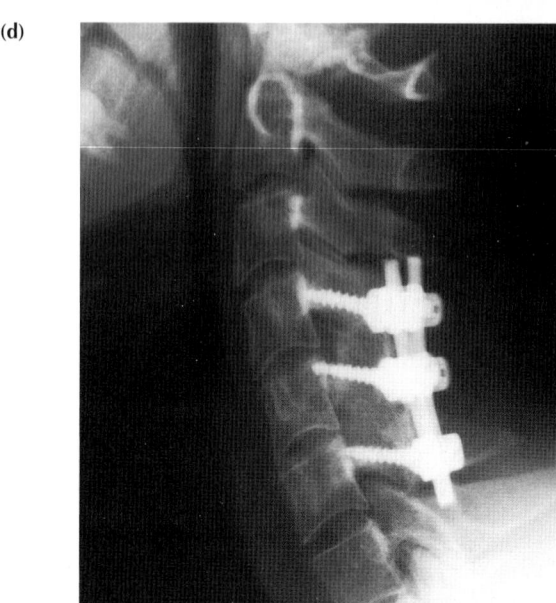

(c)

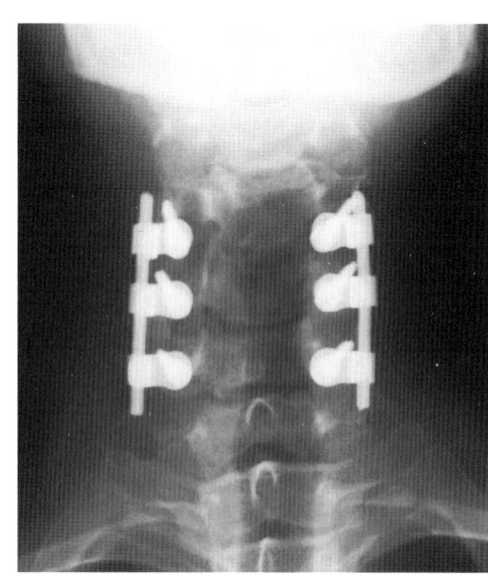

Figure 33.2 Osteoblastoma arising from the posterior elements of the fifth cervical vertebra. This 21-year-old man presented with severe unremitting neck pain. An isotope bone scan (a) demonstrated increased uptake in C5. An axial computerised tomography scan (b) further delineated the expansive lesion. The tumour was successfully removed with the aid of an intraoperative gamma probe to confirm complete excision. (c) and (d) show the postoperative anteroposterior and lateral radiographs, respectively, following reconstruction with a tricortical bone graft, lateral mass screws and rods.

have a relatively high rate of local recurrence. These tumours may present with pain or neurological deficit. The WBB (Weinstein, Boriani, Biagini) surgical staging system divides the vertebra into 12 radiating zones in clockwise order and allows an assessment of the extent of the tumour and assists in planning whether *en bloc* tumour excision is feasible.

Table 33.4 Methods by which metastatic disease spreads to the spine

1	Embolisation through the venous system (Batson's plexus)
2	Embolisation through the arterial system
3	Direct extension
4	Lymphatic spread

Osteoid osteoma was first described by Jaffe in 1935. The tumour consists of a small nidus of highly vascularised osteoblasts producing osteoid surrounded by dense sclerotic bone. Patients usually present between the ages of 10 and 25 years and complain of night pain that is not relieved by non-steroidal anti-inflammatory drugs or salicylates. The typical pain is related to prostaglandin production by the nidus.

Osteoblastomas are histologically very similar to osteoid osteomas, but are larger, with a nidus greater than 15 mm in diameter, and they behave in a more aggressive way (Fig. 33.2). Curative treatment of these lesions involves complete surgical excision of

Henry Lewis Jaffe, **1896–1979, American Pathologist.**

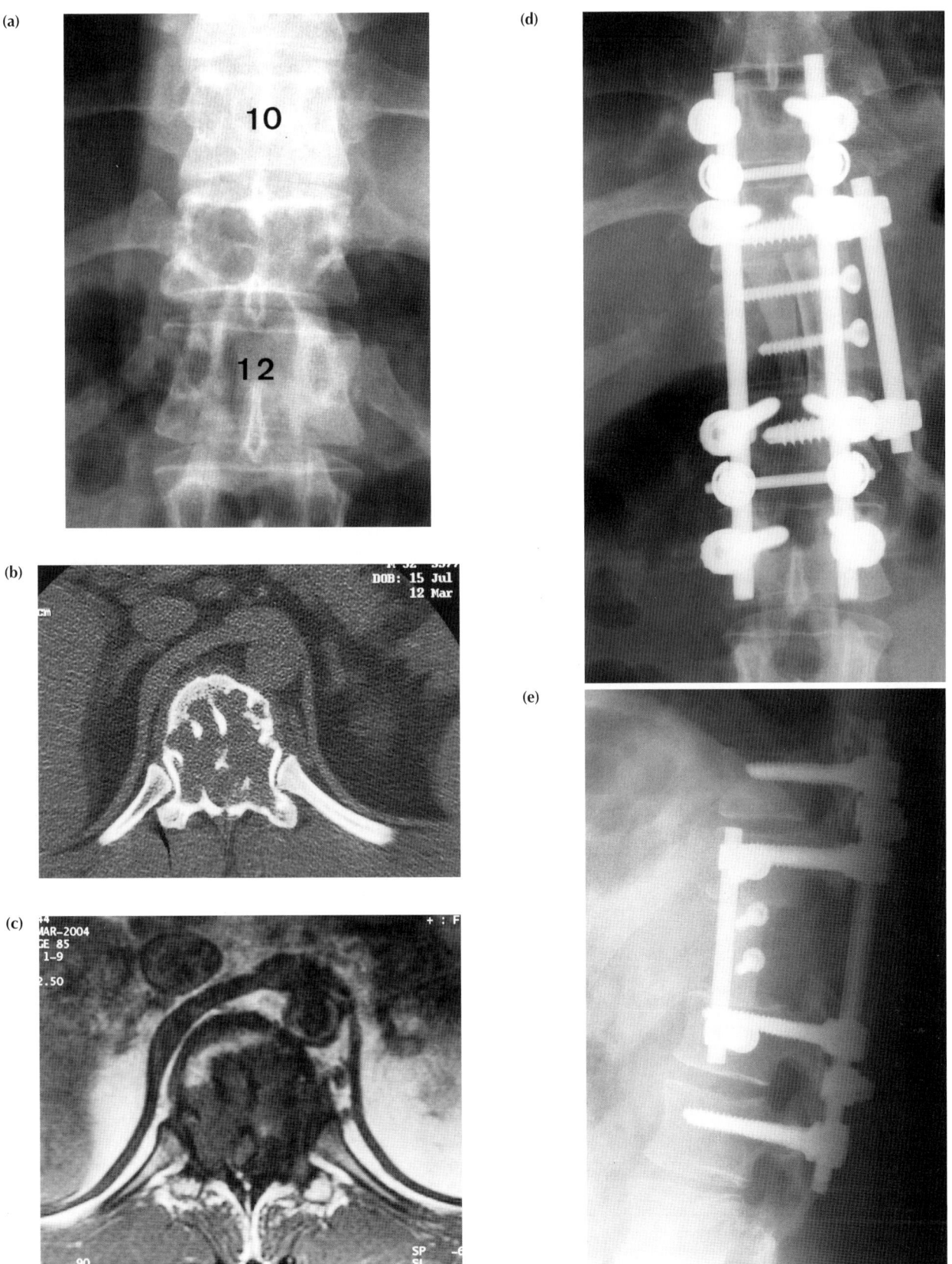

Figure 33.3 Haemangioendothelioma arising from the body of the 11th thoracic vertebra. This 34-year-old man presented with signs of spinal cord compression and severe pain in the lower thoracic region. The anteroposterior radiograph (a) demonstrated loss of both pedicles at T11. Axial computerised tomography (b) confirmed a lytic lesion. Magnetic resonance imaging (c) demonstrated spinal cord compression on the axial T1-weighted scan. The patient underwent a staged posterior stabilisation, total *en bloc* spondylectomy and anterior column reconstruction. (d) and (e) show the postoperative anteroposterior and lateral radiographs respectively.

the nidus. The preoperative administration of radiopharmaceuticals and a sterile gamma probe intraoperatively can help to localise these bony tumours and confirm complete excision at the conclusion of surgery.

Intradural tumours

These are rare. They may be intramedullary (within the substance of the cord) or extramedullary (outside the cord). Most are extramedullary and benign; the commonest are meningiomas and neurofibromas. Intramedullary tumours include ependymomas and astrocytomas.

Intradural tumours can be multiple, occurring as part of a systemic syndrome (e.g. von Recklinghausen syndrome, neurofibromatosis type I and von Hippel–Lindau syndrome, multiple haemangiomablastomas). Any malignant tumour can metastasise via the normal cerebrospinal fluid pathways. Patients usually show progressive neurological deficits with little pain.

Ependymomas are treated by surgical resection, with radiotherapy reserved for malignant or incompletely resected lesions. Astrocytomas are often infiltrative, with variable histology. They may be treated surgically using the carbon dioxide laser or ultrasonic aspirator, whereas others believe radiation therapy to be the treatment of choice.

INFECTIONS OF THE SPINE

Pyogenic infections

Pyogenic vertebral osteomyelitis is primarily a lesion of the disc and its osseous margins (Fig. 33.4). The most common method by which an organism spreads to the spine is via the haematogenous route (either by lodging in the end-arteriolar network in the vertebral end-plate or via retrograde flow from the pelvic venous plexus to the perivertebral venous plexus of Batson). Alternative routes include contiguous spread from adjacent soft tissue infection or direct implantation, e.g. traumatic penetration. The disc is nearly always involved in pyogenic vertebral infection. In contrast, granulomatous infection typically does *not* involve the disc space.

Risk factors for pyogenic vertebral osteomyelitis include advancing age, intravenous drug abuse, diabetes, renal failure, recent infections and trauma. *Staphylococcus aureus* accounts for 30–55% of infections. Gram-negative organisms such as *Escherichia coli*, *Pseudomonas* species and *Proteus* species are associated with recent genitourinary infections or procedures and intravenous drug abuse. Anaerobic infections are uncommon, but may be seen in diabetic patients and after penetrating trauma.

The principles of treatment of bone infection are discussed in Chapter 37.

Operative intervention should be considered for:

- an open biopsy (when a closed biopsy has failed);
- failure of medical management (persistent pain, elevated ESR);
- drainage of abscesses;
- decompression of spinal cord compression;
- correction of progressive spinal deformity;
- correction of progressive spinal instability.

The surgical approach should include radical anterior debridement with reconstruction followed by staged or simultaneous posterior spinal stabilisation.

Epidural abscess

This condition is often a surgical emergency. The majority of cases occur within the thoracic spine. The patient presents with increasing pain, fevers, raised ESR and raised white cell count. Without treatment, significant neurological deficit occurs and, eventually, paralysis may develop.

Tuberculosis

This is discussed in Chapter 5.

DEGENERATIVE CONDITIONS OF THE SPINE

Cervical radiculopathy

Patients present with neck and arm pain (brachalgia), paraesthesia and motor weakness in the distribution of the compromised nerve root (radiculopathy). A disc herniation at the C5–C6 level causes compromise of the C6 nerve root, resulting in weakness of the biceps and wrist extensors, loss of the brachioradialis reflex and diminished sensation of the radial forearm into the thumb and index finger. Foraminal stenosis caused by degenerative changes may also lead to radiculopathy.

Symptoms often settle with conservative treatment including physiotherapy to restore lordosis and range of motion, medication for neuropathic pain (amitriptyline, gabapentin or pregabalin) or fluoroscopically guided foraminal epidural steroid injections of local anaesthetic and steroid. Intractable pain or functional neurological deficit is an indication for surgical intervention. Surgical options include anterior cervical discectomy (with or without the application of a cervical spine locking plate), posterior lamino-foraminotomy or cervical total disc replacement.

Cervical myelopathy

Degenerative change in the cervical spine leading to spinal cord compression is the commonest cause of cervical myelopathy in patients over 55 years of age (Fig. 33.5). LMN changes occur at the level of the lesion, with atrophy of the upper extremity muscles, particularly the intrinsic muscles of the hands. UMN findings are noted *below* the level of the lesion and may involve both upper and lower extremities. Typically, spasticity and hyperreflexia are noted in the legs. There may be neck pain, stiffness, spastic gait, loss of manual dexterity or problems with sphincter control.

The method of surgical decompression depends on where the pathology is located. For multilevel disease, a cervical laminectomy from C3 to C6 is commonly performed. If the cervical spine is kyphotic, additional instrumentation (lateral mass screws and posterior rods) should be added to restore cervical lordosis and assist in achieving a fusion. An alternative to laminectomy is canal-expansive laminoplasty. This procedure gained popularity in Japan, where the incidence of ossification of the posterior

(a)

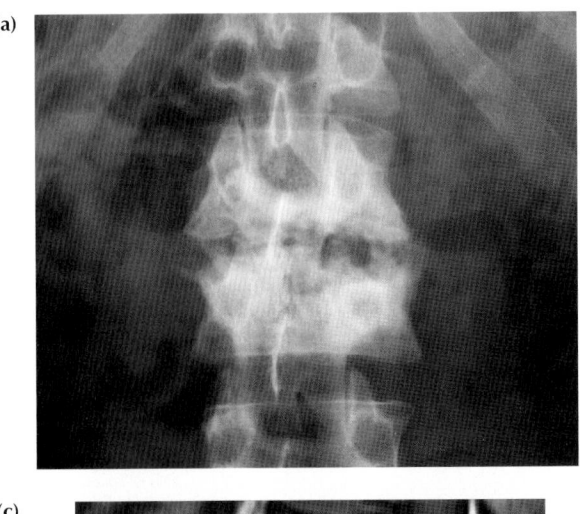

(b)

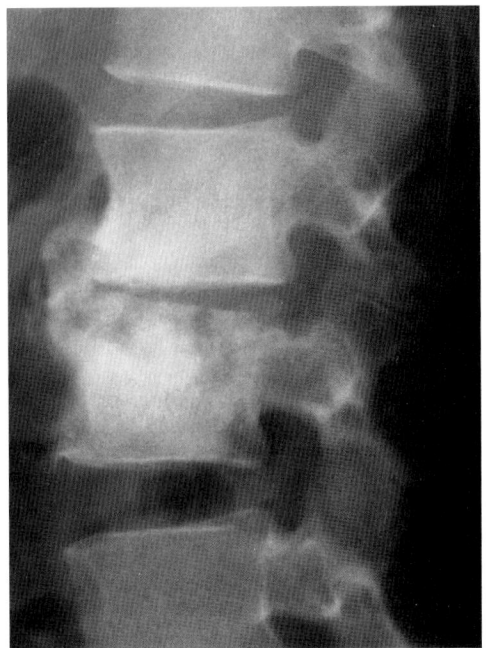

(c)

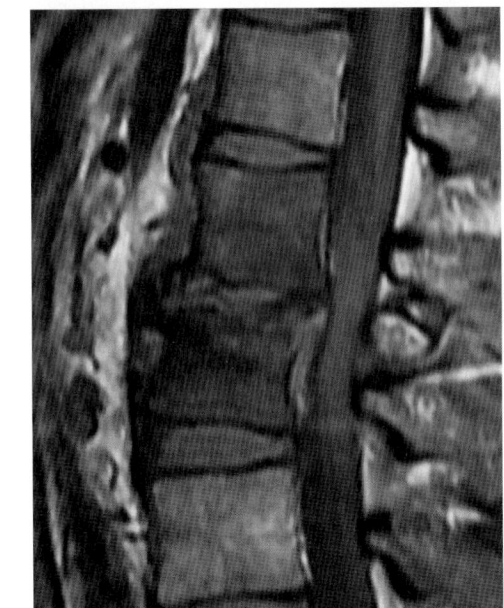

(d)

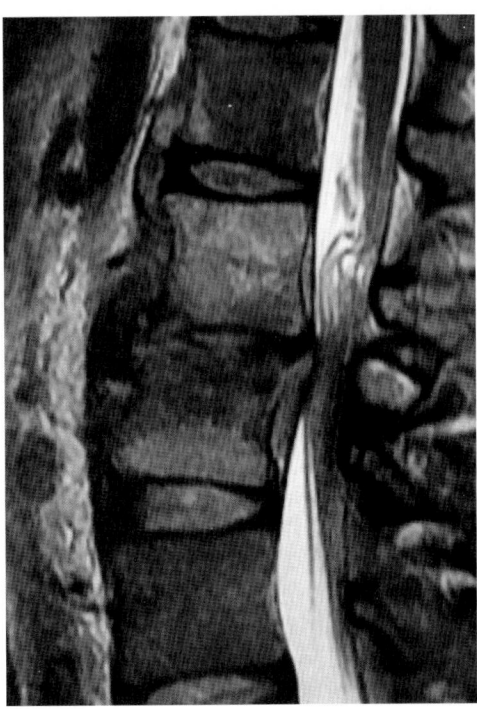

Figure 33.4 Discitis and vertebral body osteomyelitis arising from the lumbar L2/3 disc. This 46-year-old man presented with back pain, fever, malaise and night sweats. Anteroposterior (a) and lateral (b) radiographs revealed loss of disc space and sclerosis. Magnetic resonance imaging revealed *decreased* signal in the vertebral body and disc on T1-weighted scan (c) and *increased* signal in the vertebral body and disc on T2-weighted scan (d). The man underwent a Harlow Wood biopsy under general anaesthetic. The causative organism was identified as *Staphylococcus aureus*. He was successfully treated with intravenous antibiotics and an orthosis.

longitudinal ligament remains high. Anterior surgical options include anterior corpectomy and strut grafting.

Axial neck pain

Surgery for pure axial neck pain is controversial. Many authors have used cervical discography in an attempt to isolate the pain source before proceeding with anterior cervical discectomy and fusion. However, reviewing the literature, there is *no* evidence of benefit for this type of surgery for this indication.

Thoracic disc herniation

Thoracic disc herniations are rare, accounting for less than 2% of all discectomy procedures. Disc protrusions occur predominantly in the distal thoracic segments between T8 and T12. Herniations may be soft or calcified. Typically, the patient presents with axial pain, radiculopathy or myelopathy. MRI is invariably required to demonstrate protrusions and the degree of neural compromise. Thoracic disc protrusions identified on MRI may be *asymptomatic*. Conservative treatment including

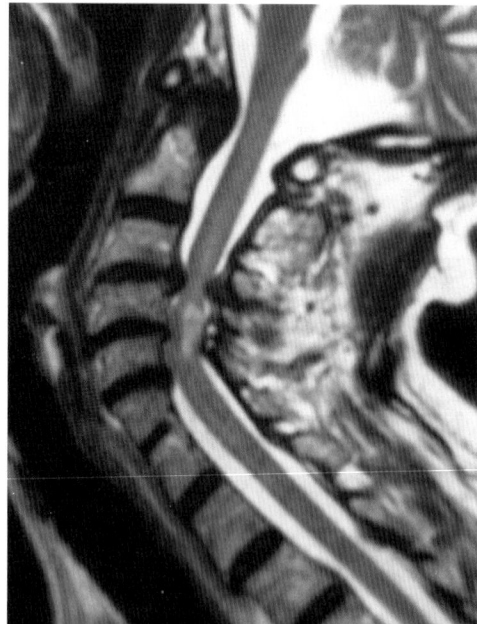

Figure 33.5 Cervical myelopathy. Magnetic resonance image showing a block fusion at C6/7 with adjacent level degenerative changes and compromise of the spinal cord at C3/4, C4/5 and C5/6. Signal change was noted within the cord, particularly at the C4/5 level.

non-steroidal anti-inflammatory drugs, physiotherapy and general fitness should be tried initially. Discectomy and interbody fusion is an appropriate surgical treatment for progressive spinal cord compression or unremitting radicular pain. Surgery may be performed via a thoracotomy or, for a soft disc prolapse, via a thoracoscopic approach. Surgery for pure axial pain is *not* recommended.

Lumbar disc herniation

A symptomatic lumbar disc herniation occurs during the lifetime of approximately 2% of the population. Risk factors include male gender, age (30–50 years), heavy lifting or twisting, stressful occupation, lower income and cigarette smoking.

Herniations may be described as a *protrusion* (displaced disc material remains in continuity with the disc of origin and contained by the annulus fibrosus), an *extrusion* (disc material migrating through the annulus fibrosus but contained by the posterior longitudinal ligament) or *sequestered* (disc material lying free in the spinal canal). This material may be *central*, *posterolateral*, *foraminal* or *extraforaminal*. Over 90% of lumbar disc herniations occur at the L4–5 or L5–S1 levels. A posterolateral disc protrusion will affect the *traversing* root, e.g. an L5–S1 disc protrusion affects the S1 nerve root. A far-lateral disc protrusion (extraforaminal) will affect the *exiting* nerve root, e.g. far-lateral L5–S1 disc protrusion affecting the L5 nerve root (Fig. 33.6). Symptoms typically commence with a period of back pain followed by sciatica. There may be paraesthesia, motor weakness, loss of reflexes and a reduction in straight leg raise.

A large midline disc herniation may compress the cauda equina, leading to a syndrome defined by bowel and/or bladder difficulties, saddle anaesthesia and lower limb sensory and motor deficits. Surgery for cauda equina syndrome should be performed

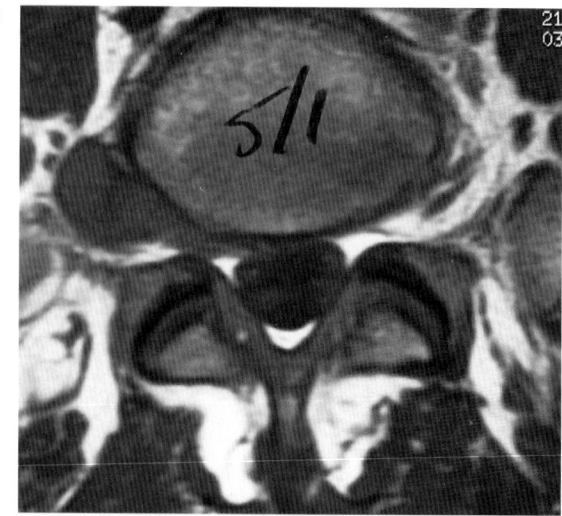

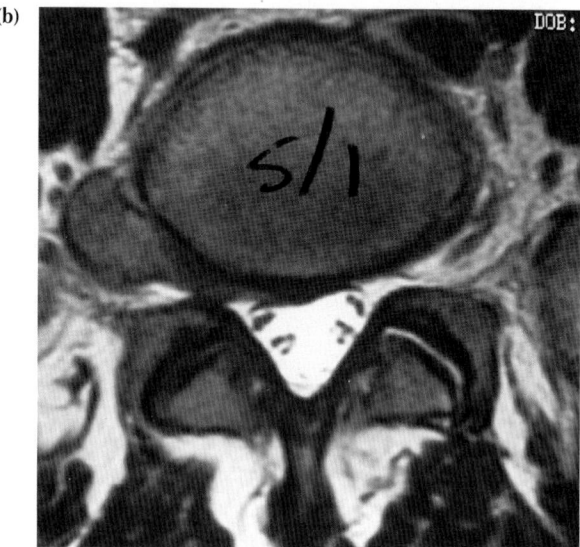

Figure 33.6 Far-lateral disc prolapse at L5/S1. A right-sided far-lateral disc protrusion is noted at L5/S1 on the T1-weighted (a) and the T2-weighted (b) magnetic resonance imaging scan. The patient presented with an L5 radiculopathy.

within 24 hours of the onset of symptoms to allow the optimum recovery of neural elements.

For simple sciatica, a period of 6–12 weeks of conservative treatment is advised. Up to 70% of patients will settle within this period. Epidural steroid injections may be helpful. Microdiscectomy is the standard surgical intervention for those in whom conservative treatment has failed. Surgical excision removes both the source of the pressure and the initiator of the inflammatory response.

Spinal stenosis

Spinal stenosis is characterised by back, buttock or leg pain. Symptoms are often provoked by exercise. Symptoms of spinal claudication can be distinguished from vascular claudication because they are frequently associated with neurological symptoms, are often worse in extension, and pedal pulses are present on clinical examination.

Plain radiographs may show degenerative changes with or without degenerative spondylolisthesis. MRI scans will reveal neural compromise. Stenosis is caused by a combination of facet joint hypertrophy, disc bulge and ligamentum flavum thickening.

Symptoms progress in approximately 20% of patients who receive no treatment. The condition may be treated successfully by surgical intervention. Laminectomy with preservation of the facet joints is a reasonable option, particularly when normal lumbar lordosis is preserved. Others prefer multilevel laminotomies with undercutting of the facet joints, trimming of the ligamentum flavum and removal of disc bulges. Such a segmental procedure is considered to be less destabilising than laminectomy. Preservation of the midline structures via a spinous process osteotomy is an alternative approach. Recently, an interspinous process decompression system (X-stop) has been found to be effective for patients suffering from lumbar spinal stenosis when compared with non-operative therapy.

Discogenic low back pain

Discogenic low back pain has been defined as a continuum of diagnostic categories (internal disc disruption, degenerative disc disease, segmental instability) reflecting various stages of degenerative pathology affecting the intervertebral disc. Patients typically present with chronic relapsing episodes of low back pain. MRI studies may show decreased signal intensity within the disc, high-intensity zones in the posterior annulus (suggestive of an annular tear) and surrounding Modic changes in the adjacent end-plates. A recent study has compared rehabilitation with spinal fusion for such candidates. The authors concluded that both groups reported reductions in disability during the 2 years of follow-up and recommended that patients should be offered rehabilitation prior to surgical intervention.

For those patients who fail to improve with conservative measures, provocative lumbar discography may help to confirm the pain generator. Intradiscal electrothermal therapy (IDET) was heralded as a new treatment for patients with discographically proven discogenic low back pain. There are two randomised controlled trials assessing the efficacy of IDET. The first showed modest overall benefit, and the second showed IDET to be no more effective than placebo for the treatment of chronic discogenic low back pain.

Lumbar fusion may be considered for treatment of low back pain of discogenic origin in patients who fail to improve after a minimum of 6 months of appropriate non-surgical care. In one randomised study, lumbar fusion diminished pain and decreased disability more efficiently than commonly used non-surgical treatment. Many techniques including non-instrumented posterolateral fusion, instrumented posterolateral fusion, anterior lumbar interbody fusion (Fig. 33.7), posterior lumbar interbody fusion and combined anterior and posterior (circumferential) fusion have been used. The literature remains unclear as to the best method; however, it seems apparent that lumbar interbody fusion, i.e. the anterior or posterior techniques, provides a higher fusion rate when compared with posterolateral fusion, although this does not necessarily translate to a superior clinical outcome.

A recent study has compared a total disc replacement (Fig. 33.8) with an anterior lumbar interbody fusion for the treatment of mechanical low back pain caused by one-level degenerative disc disease. The authors found the clinical outcomes in both groups to be *equivalent* at 2 years, suggesting that total disc replacement remained a viable option for this condition.

(a)

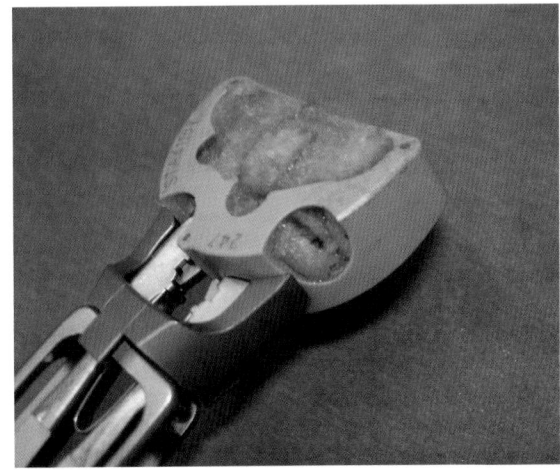

(b)

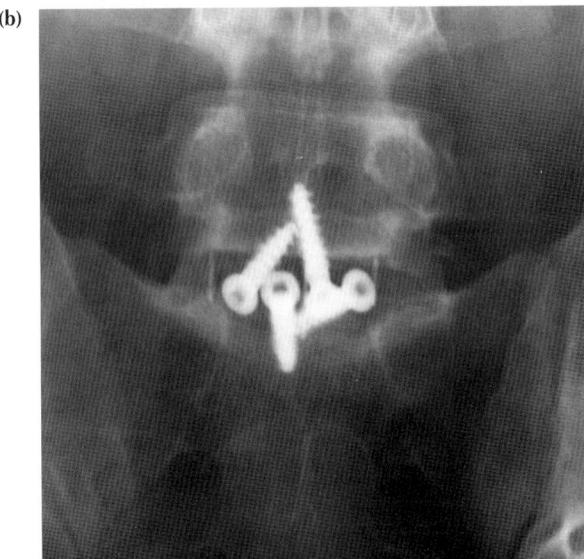

(c)

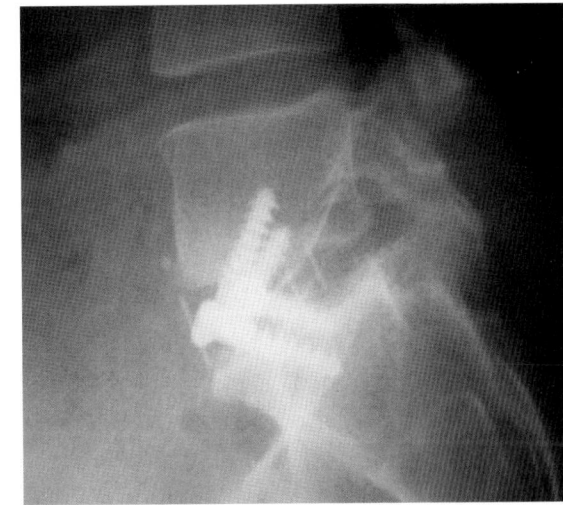

Figure 33.7 Anterior lumbar interbody fusion. The PEEK (polyethylethylketone) cage has been packed with bone graft prior to insertion (a); (b) and (c) show the anteroposterior and lateral postoperative radiographs respectively.

CHAPTER 33 | THE SPINE

(a)

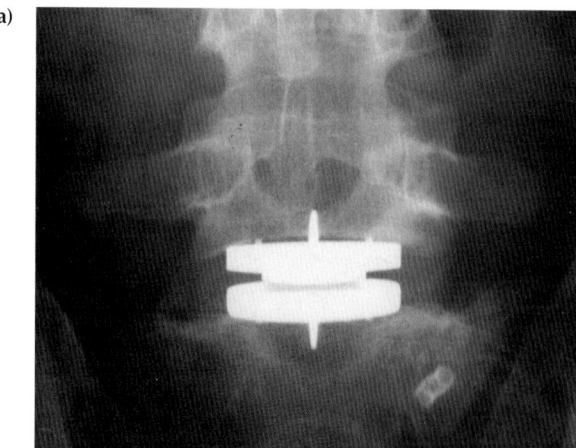

(b)

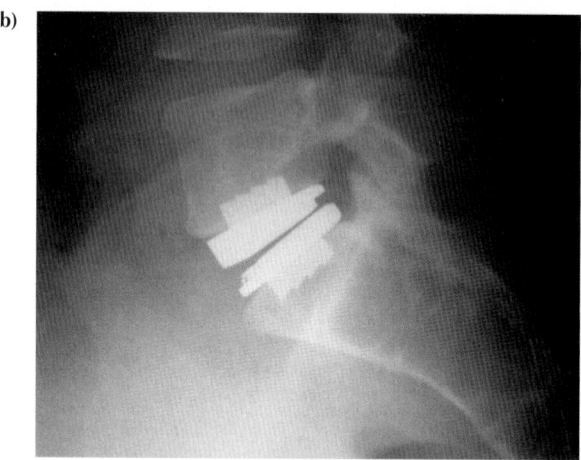

Figure 33.8 Lumbar total disc replacement. (a) Anteroposterior radiograph with 30° of cranial inclination. (b) Lateral radiograph with the implant appropriately positioned.

SPONDYLOLYSIS AND SPONDYLOLISTHESIS

Spondylolysis

This is a unilateral or bilateral defect in the region of the pars interarticularis without vertebral slippage. Persistent motion through the fracture may result in a pseudarthrosis. The incidence is reported at approximately 4% by the age of 6 years and 6% by the age of 14 years. Many cases remain asymptomatic. The incidence in the young athletic population varies between 15% and 47%.

The diagnosis may be made with standing anteroposterior and lateral X-rays of the lumbosacral spine. Oblique radiographs are no longer acceptable because of the high radiation dose. SPECT scanning and a reverse-gantry CT scan are usually used to make the diagnosis, although MRI is increasingly being used as a first-line investigation.

Treatment involves rest, non-steroidal anti-inflammatory medication, activity modification and a lumbosacral orthosis that reduces lumbar lordosis. For patients who remain symptomatic despite an adequate trial of non-operative care, surgery in the form of a direct repair (modified Buck's fusion) may be indicated. Patients under 25 years of age without evidence of disc or facet

pathology and with a pars defect of less than 3–4 mm have favourable outcomes following such a direct repair. If disc degeneration is established, then an alar transverse or intertransverse lumbar fusion is recommended.

Spondylolisthesis

Spondylolisthesis is a forward slippage of the vertebral body engendered by a break in the continuity or elongation of the pars interarticularis (Fig. 33.9). Wiltse *et al.* (1976) classified spondylolisthesis into six types (Table 33.5).

The Meyerding classification describes the degree of slip and refers to the amount of translation of the superior vertebra relative to the inferior vertebra (Table 33.6). One vertebra may sublux completely on the underlying vertebra, a condition called spondyloptosis.

Patients may present with back pain, an associated L5 nerve root pain and/or hamstring spasm. For patients past the third decade of life, it is unusual for spondylolisthesis to produce pain and, more commonly, the pain results from secondary degenerative changes in the disc and facet joints.

(a)

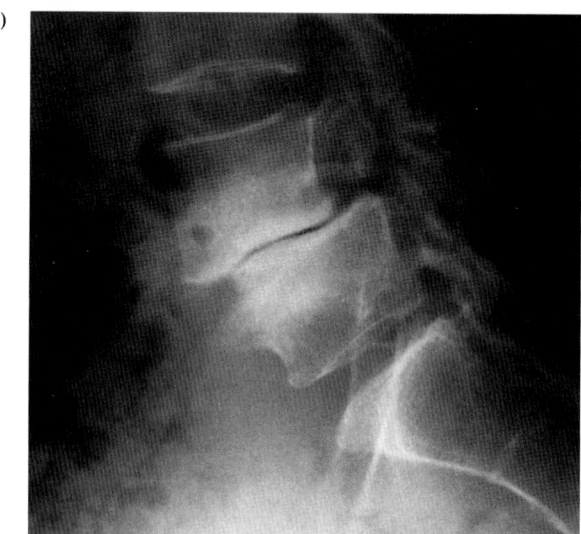

(b)

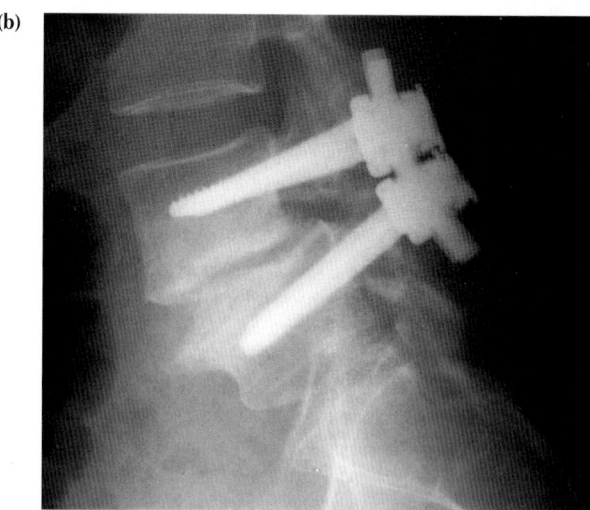

Figure 33.9 Lytic spondylolisthesis L4/L5. (a) Lateral radiograph showing a Meyerding grade I spondylolisthesis. The patient underwent a decompression and instrumented fusion *in situ* (b).

Table 33.5 The Wiltse classification of spondylolisthesis

Type 1	Dysplastic	Associated with congenital deficiency of the L5–S1 articulation
Type 2	Isthmic	Associated with a lesion of the pars interarticulares. Three subtypes: 2A: lytic defect of the pars 2B: elongated or attenuated pars 2C: acute pars fracture
Type 3	Degenerative spondylolisthesis	Segmental instability due to disc degeneration and facet arthrosis
Type 4	Traumatic	Acute fracture in the region of the posterior elements, other than the pars interarticulares
Type 5	Pathological	Generalised bone disease resulting in attenuation of the pars (e.g. metabolic, neoplastic)
Type 6	Post-surgical	After decompression of the lumbar spine

Table 33.6 The Meyerding classification for the degree of slip of spondylolisthesis

Grade I	1–25%
Grade II	26–50%
Grade III	51–75%
Grade IV	76–100%

For patients who have intractable low back or radicular pain, progressive slips in skeletally immature patients or neurological symptoms, surgery may be indicated. For low-grade slips (Meyerding grade I/II), an *in situ* posterolateral fusion is the procedure of choice. If there is *objective* evidence of neural compression (e.g. weakness of extensor hallucis longis), a spinal decompression should be performed at the same time.

For high-grade (Meyerding grade III/IV) slips, treatment is more controversial. Opinion is divided on whether to reduce the slip first and then fuse, or simply to fuse *in situ*. Problems with reduction include injury to the L5 nerve root, cauda equina nerve roots and sacral fixation failure. Neurological complications may be avoided by slow reduction with an external fixator followed by definitive fusion.

INFLAMMATORY SPONDYLOARTHROPATHY

Rheumatoid arthritis

Between 33% and 50% of patients develop atlanto-axial subluxation (AAS) within 5 years of diagnosis of rheumatoid arthritis. Some 2–10% of patients with AAS develop myelopathy over the next 10 years. Once diagnosed with myelopathy, 50% of patients die within 1 year. Approximately 20% of patients develop symptomatic subaxial disease. Neurological symptoms may occur as a result of direct compression by bone or soft tissue or from neural ischaemia.

The Ranawat classification of neurological function is useful for patients with rheumatoid arthritis (Table 33.7) (Summary box 33.7).

Chitranjan S. Ranawat, **Orthopaedic Surgeon, The Hospital for Special Surgery, New York, NY, USA.**

> **Summary box 33.7**
>
> **Recommendations for spinal surgery in rheumatoid arthritis**
>
> - AAS with a posterior atlanto-dental interval (PADI) of 14 mm or less
> - AAS with at least 5 mm of basilar invagination
> - Subaxial subluxation with a sagittal canal diameter of 14 mm or less

Table 33.7 Ranawat classification of neurological function

Grade	Description
I	No neurological deficit
II	Subjective weakness with hyperreflexia and dysaesthesia
III	Objective weakness with long tract signs Two subtypes: IIIa Ability to walk IIIb Quadriparetic/non-ambulatory

Rheumatoid patients with myelopathy often have a very poor prognosis. In one series, 100% became bedridden within 3 years of onset of myelopathy and one-third died suddenly. The morbidity is very high, with only 25% of patients (Ranawat IIIb) who underwent surgical decompression having a favourable outcome. Early surgical stabilisation is therefore recommended. Techniques of occipitocervical fixation now utilise bicortical screw fixation to the occiput, transarticular fixation across the C1–2 joint and lateral mass screws in the subaxial cervical spine.

Ankylosing spondylitis

This condition is discussed in Chapter 37.

Should a patient with ankylosing spondylitis (AS) present following trauma, a high index of suspicion for occult fractures should be present. It is common for AS patients to develop epidural haematomas with subtle neurological deficit.

Patients with a significant fixed flexion deformity at the cervicothoracic junction ('chin-on-chest' deformity), limited forward gaze, eating and swallowing difficulties may be treated with an extension osteotomy of the cervical spine (Fig. 33.10). Surgery

CHAPTER 33 | THE SPINE

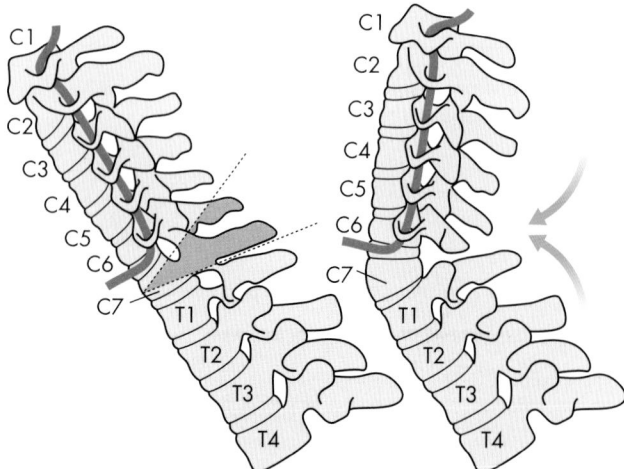

Figure 33.10 Cervical osteotomy for correction of cervico-thoracic kyphosis. Planned resection lateral view for closing wedge osteotomy (left) and lateral view after closure of the osteotomy (right).

is performed under general anaesthesia after an awake fibreoptic intubation. The spinal cord is monitored with somatosensory and motor-evoked potentials. A halo is applied and the osteotomy carried out at the C7–T1 level. The osteotomy is closed under precise control and stabilised with instrumentation and a posterior fusion.

Primary thoracic kyphosis can be corrected by multiple thoracic osteotomies, or the overall spinal deformity can be corrected by a compensatory osteotomy in the lumbar spine. Lumbar osteotomy is best performed by a transpedicular closing wedge osteotomy at the second or third lumbar vertebra, i.e. below the conus and held in place by rigid posterior instrumentation and fusion.

SPINAL DEFORMITY

Spinal deformity may be categorised into a coronal plane deformity (scoliosis) or a sagittal plane deformity (kyphosis). Further classification may be made on the basis of aetiology into congenital, neuromuscular, syndrome-related and idiopathic. The appropriate radiograph for scoliosis is a standing posteroanterior projection of the whole spine. When surgery is contemplated, supine lateral bending radiographs are performed to assess the flexibility of the curve. Curve magnitude is assessed using the Cobb method. This involves identifying the superior end-plate of the most cranial vertebra pointing in towards the concavity, and the inferior end-plate of the most caudal end-plate pointing in towards the concavity, and measuring the angle subtended by these two lines. The criterion for diagnosis of scoliosis is a Cobb angle of 10° or more. Curves of less than 10° are referred to as spinal asymmetry (Summary box 33.8).

Summary box 33.8
Aetiology of scoliosis
■ Congenital
■ Neuromuscular
■ Syndrome-related
■ Idiopathic

Skeletal maturity may be assessed radiographically using the Risser sign, which describes the ossification of the iliac apophysis. The status of the triradiate cartilage of the acetabulum may also be useful to assess remaining growth potential. The triradiate cartilage closes before the iliac apophysis appears (Risser 0) at about the time of peak growth velocity. Patients with abnormal neurological examination, e.g. asymmetrical abdominal reflexes, or patients for whom surgical correction is planned should have an MRI examination of the *whole* spine to look for intraspinal pathology (e.g. syringomyelia, low-lying conus, diastematomyelia or a tethered cord). These findings may well result in a change in the operative strategy.

Congenital scoliosis

This is caused by vertebral anomalies that produce a frontal plane growth asymmetry. The anomalies are present at birth, but the curvature may take years to be clinically evident. These deficiencies occur in the embryonic period of intrauterine development (before 48 days' gestation) and are commonly associated with cardiac and urological abnormalities. It is thought that the *Homeobox* genes of the Hox class are responsible for congenital spinal malformations. Hemivertebrae can readily be detected on antenatal ultrasound at 20 weeks.

Congenital spinal anomalies can be classified into defects of *segmentation*, defects of *formation* or a combination of the two (mixed). Radiographs may show asymmetry in the number of pedicles, absent ribs or rib fusions. An unsegmented bar is suggested when the corresponding ribs and/or pedicles are conjoined. Block or wedge vertebrae have a low chance of progression. Hemivertebrae have a risk of progression of between 1° and 2.5° per year. Unilateral unsegmented bars progress at the rate 6–9° per year, and unilateral unsegmented bars with contralateral hemivertebrae are at the greatest risk of progression, sometimes exceeding 10° per year.

Specific associations have been described in the VACTERLS syndrome including the following congenital anomalies: vertebral, anorectal, cardiac, tracheo-oesophageal fistula, radial limb dysplasia, lung abnormalities and single umbilical artery.

Close observation of spinal growth is required until skeletal maturity is reached. Brace treatment is ineffective for the primary structural curve, which is often short and rigid, but it may have a role in the control of compensatory curves. Investigations should include renal ultrasound, cardiac echo and MRI of the whole spine (intraspinal pathology is present in up to 30%).

For progressive curves, surgical options include posterior fusion *in situ*, hemivertebra excision with correction, convex hemiepiphysiodesis combined with a Luque trolley construct, or combined anterior and posterior fusion. Anomalous blood supply of the spinal cord is not uncommon, and great care must be taken when tying off segmental vessels on the front of the spine.

Neuromuscular scoliosis

This may be due to *neuropathic* disorders, such as cerebral palsy, spinocerebellar degeneration, syringomyelia, quadriplegia, spinal muscular atrophy and poliomyelitis, or *myopathic* disorders, such as Duchenne muscular dystrophy and myotonic dystrophy. A

Joseph Charles Risser, **Professor of Orthopaedic Surgery, Loma Linda University, Los Angeles, CC, USA.**
Guillaume Benjamin Amand Duchenne, **1806–1875, a neurologist who worked successively in Boulogne and Paris, France, but who never held a hospital appointment.**

progressive spinal deformity producing disturbance in quality of life or threatening compromise of cardiorespiratory function can be treated by correction and fusion using a posterior approach. There is good evidence that stabilisation of the spine in children with Duchenne muscular dystrophy who are able to walk, before the respiratory compromise is too severe to allow a general anaesthetic, may increase their lifespan by several years. Problems not uncommonly encountered during operations on children with neuromuscular scoliosis include excessive blood loss, malignant hyperthermia, latex allergy and difficulty with monitoring neurological function.

Idiopathic scoliosis

Idiopathic scoliosis can be divided into *early onset* (before 8 years of age) (Fig. 33.11) and *late onset* (after 8 years of age; typical adolescent idiopathic scoliosis) (Fig. 33.12). The distinction is important, as the number of alveoli in the lung does not increase after the age of 8 years. Patients with severe curves in

(a)

(b)

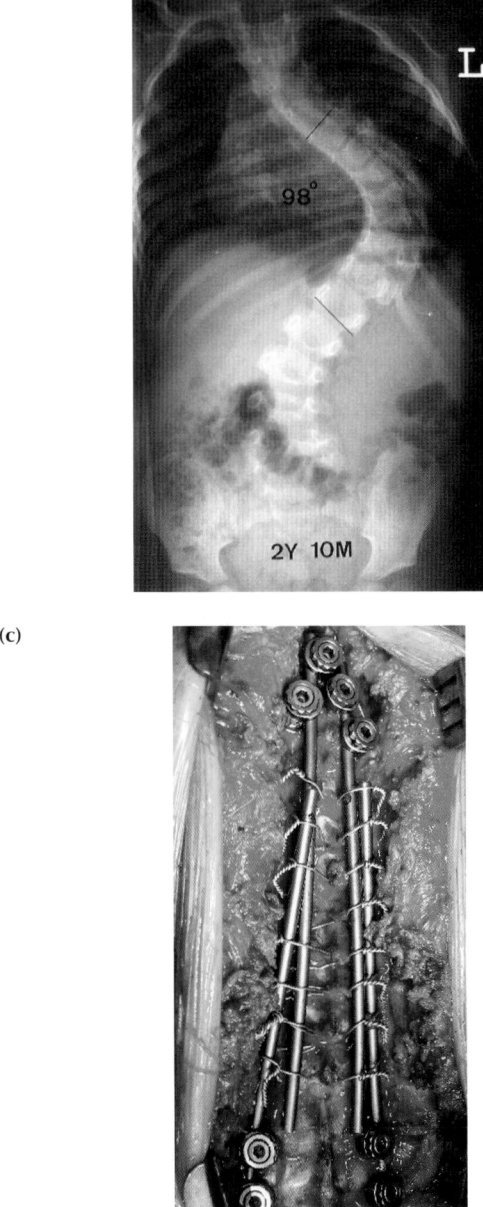

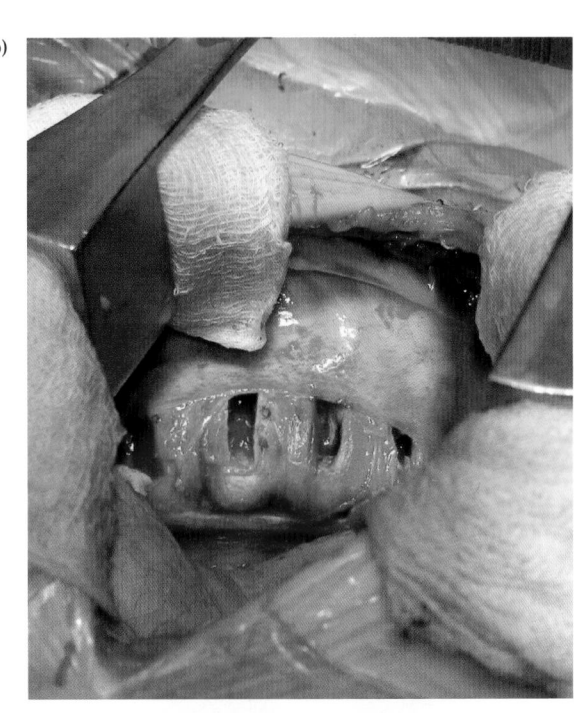

(c)

(d)

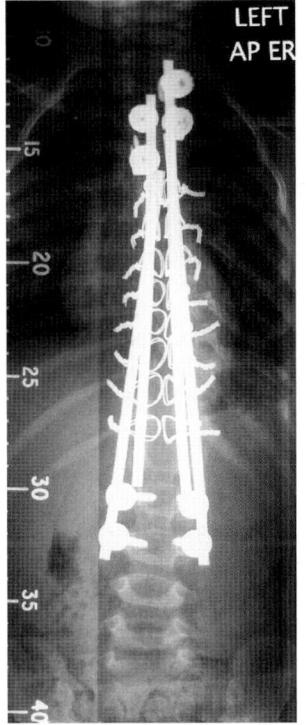

Figure 33.11 Early-onset idiopathic scoliosis. The anteroposterior standing radiograph (a) demonstrates a Cobb angle of 98° and dextrocardia. This 34-month-old boy underwent a convex hemiepiphysiodesis over the apical four discs (b), followed by posterior Luque trolley instrumentation *without* fusion to correct the spinal deformity and allow continued growth (c and d).

CHAPTER 33 | THE SPINE

(a)

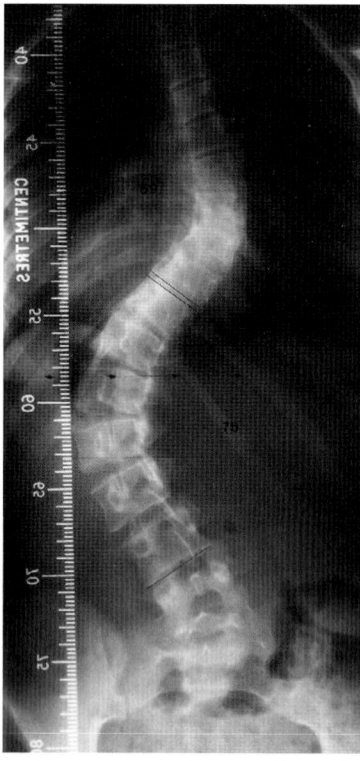

(b)

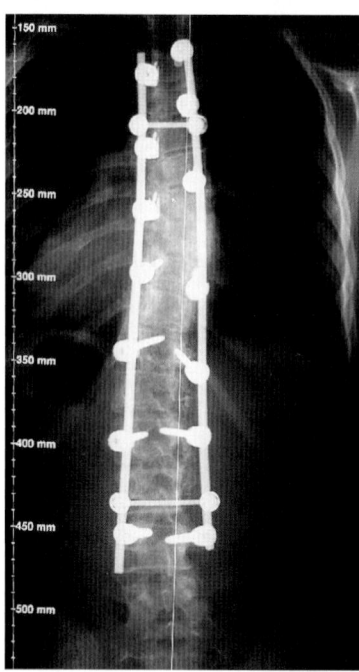

Figure 33.12 Late-onset idiopathic scoliosis. This 15-year-old girl had a progressive scoliosis with unacceptable cosmesis. The standing radiograph (a) demonstrated a right thoracic curve with a Cobb angle of 59° and a left thoracolumbar curve of 75°. Both curves were flexible on supine bending films. She underwent a posterior correction and instrumented fusion from T4 to L4 (b).

the early-onset group may develop cor pulmonale and right ventricular failure resulting in premature death. Adolescent idiopathic scoliosis is associated with a normal or near-normal life expectancy.

The prevalence of curves with a Cobb angle greater than 10° is between 0.5% and 3%. The prevalence of curves greater than 30° is between 1.5 and 3 per 1000. Risk factors for progression include female gender, remaining skeletal growth, curve location and curve magnitude. Not all curves stabilise when skeletal maturity is reached. In long-term studies, 68% experienced curve progression; the most marked progression of 1° per year was observed in thoracic curves between 50° and 75°.

Idiopathic curves of less than 25° are monitored with clinical and radiographic examination. In growing children (Risser 0–1, pre-menarche) with curves between 20° and 29°, a brace may be indicated. Bracing is used to prevent curve progression and generally does not lead to permanent curve improvement. Curves beyond 45° are not amenable to brace treatment.

Surgery in the form of corrective instrumentation and spinal fusion is indicated for curve progression beyond 40°, truncal imbalance and unacceptable cosmesis. Surgery may involve posterior surgery, anterior surgery or a combination of both. During surgery, continuous electrical spinal cord monitoring is used in the form of somatosensory evoked potentials and, more recently, motor-evoked potentials. The risk of permanent neurological injury for such patients is 0.02% (1:5000); the risk of incomplete neurological injury is 0.4% (1:250).

Scheuermann's kyphosis

This condition was initially described as a rigid kyphosis associated with wedged vertebral bodies usually involving the 7th to 10th thoracic vertebrae, presenting with backache. At least three adjacent vertebrae must be wedged by at least 5° each. Typically, a thoracic kyphosis of 50–90° may exist. The incidence has been estimated at 1–8% of the population. The condition is more common in males.

Physiotherapy directed at postural improvement and hamstring release may be useful. Bracing for skeletally immature patients with kyphosis up to 65° may be effective in arresting progression. Indications for surgery include pain, progressive deformity greater than 70°, unacceptable cosmesis, and neurological and cardiac pulmonary compromise. Neurological deficits have been reported relating to thoracic disc herniation, epidural cysts or hyperkyphosis.

If surgery is contemplated, a hyperextension lateral radiograph (over a bolster) is performed to assess flexibility. If the kyphosis fails to correct to less 50°, an anterior release and disc excision may be required. This may be carried out via a thoracotomy or an endoscopic approach, to be followed by a posterior correction and fusion, typically from T2 to L2. Alternatively, posterior chevron osteotomies may prevent the need for an anterior release. Care should be taken if the curve has a low apex (e.g. T10–11), when posterior instrumentation should be extended to the first lordotic disc.

DEVELOPMENTAL ABNORMALITIES

Developmental abnormalities of the spine and spinal cord can be divided into primary bony disorders (e.g. congenital scoliosis as

Holger Werfel Scheuermann, **1877–1960**, Radiologist, The Municipal Hospital, Sundby, Copenhagen, Denmark, described Juvenile Kyphosis in 1920.

discussed above) and primary neurological disorders (e.g. spina bifida, Arnold–Chiari malformation and spinal dysraphism).

Spina bifida

Spinal bifida is caused by a failure of fusion of the vertebral arches and possibly the underlying neural tube. Spina bifida cystica has an incidence of 1:300 live births. This is now decreasing as a consequence of folic acid supplementation, antenatal ultrasound and the measurement of alpha-fetoprotein levels. The condition is usually obvious at birth. A neurological examination of the structures *below* the defect should be carefully performed. The head should be examined for evidence of hydrocephalus (bulging fontanelle or excessive head circumference). There are two basic types:

- *Meningocele*: the meninges herniate through the bony defect and are covered by skin.
- *Myelomeningocele*: the roof of the defect is formed by exposed neural tissue with 75% of cases developing hydrocephalus.

A meningocele with good-quality skin over the defect may be treated conservatively. A meningocele with a more prominent sac can be excised at 3–6 months. The management of myelomeningocele is more controversial. Enthusiasm for closing all defects has been replaced by a more selective approach with the recognition that it was inappropriate to operate on children with severe hydrocephalus, a large open defect and no distal neurological function. The majority of these children die in their first year from hydrocephalus or from an infection if closure is not attempted. With antibiotics, early surgical closure and shunts to prevent hydrocephalus, half the children who survive the first 24 hours will reach school age.

The aims of surgery are to return the nervous tissue to the spinal canal, to preserve the cerebrospinal fluid absorption capacity and to cover the defect with fascia and skin. Following surgery, regular examinations are required to detect hydrocephalus. Long-term problems include skin, bone and joint deformity and the complications associated with a neuropathic bladder.

Arnold–Chiari malformation

Arnold–Chiari malformation occurs when the medulla oblongata and the cerebellar tonsils extend through the foramen magnum into the cervical spinal canal, causing pressure on the lower medulla. Hydrocephalus and impaired neurological function are common, and there is a strong association with spina bifida and syringomyelia. The presentation is variable because of its complex aetiology. Symptoms may include headache, vomiting, visual disturbance, diplopia, mental dullness, lack of coordination, paralysis of the extremities, cerebellar ataxia and sensory disorders. Plain radiographs may show a *small* posterior cranial fossa, but the condition is best demonstrated by MRI or CT myelography. Management consists of decompressing the foramen magnum and, usually, the posterior arch of the atlas to restore normal cerebrospinal fluid flow.

Spinal dysraphism

This is a group of disorders arising from abnormal embryological formation of tissues: all are associated with a progressive neurological deficit as the result of cord tethering and traction or cord compression. There is a strong association with spina bifida.

In diastematomyelia, there is an abnormal bony or cartilaginous spur projecting across the middle of the vertebral canal, dividing the dural tube and spinal cord in two. Between 50% and 70% of patients have a skin naevus, dimple or hairy patch when the spine is examined. Diastematomyelia is more common in females and most commonly occurs in the thoracolumbar region. It often presents during the growth spurt with upper limb weakness, abnormal gait, urinary incontinence or spinal deformity.

Syringomyelia

In 1824, Olivier d'Angers described a spinal cord cavity in continuity with the fourth ventricle, which he called syringomyelia. Patients may present with sensory disturbance, weakness of the hands, loss of pain and temperature sensation or progressive kyphoscoliosis. Hindbrain herniation can lead to headache, neck ache, ataxia, spasticity and lower cranial nerve palsies.

If associated with a type I Arnold–Chiari malformation (where cerebrospinal fluid outflow obstruction is implicated), then a posterior cranial fossa decompression is indicated to restore cerebral spinal fluid outflow through the foramen of Magendie. If the cause is an intramedullary spinal cord tumour, excision of the tumour should restore cerebrospinal fluid communication with the central canal. If the origin of the syrinx is post traumatic, the obstruction should be relieved by decompression. Fluid diversion should not be the primary or only treatment of syringomyelia. Notwithstanding this, diversion to the peritoneum (syringo-peritoneal) or pleural spaces (syringo-pleural) has been used with moderate success.

METABOLIC BONE DISEASES AFFECTING THE SPINE

Osteoporosis

This is characterised by a decreased amount of normally mineralised bone per unit volume, resulting in skeletal fragility and an increased risk of fracture. Osteoporosis may be classified into primary or secondary types.

Primary osteoporosis is further subdivided into type I or postmenopausal osteoporosis and type II or senile osteoporosis. Type I osteoporosis is due to oestrogen deficiency occurring in females, 5–10 years after the menopause. It is associated with vertebral body fractures, intertrochanteric hip fractures and distal radial fractures. Type II osteoporosis occurs as a result of ageing and calcium deficiency. It is associated with vertebral body fractures, femoral neck fractures and pelvic fractures. Secondary osteoporosis occurs as a result of endocrinopathies such as Cushing's disease.

Bone mineral density is measured with dual-energy X-ray absorptiometry (DEXA). Ideally, the bone density is measured in

Julius Arnold, 1835–1915, Professor of Pathological Anatomy, The University of Heidelberg, Heidelberg, Germany, described this condition in 1894.
Hans Chiari, 1851–1916, Professor of Pathological Anatomy, Strasbourg, Germany, (Strasbourg was returned to France in 1918 after the end of the First World War) gave his account of this condition in 1891.

Francois Magendie, 1783–1855, Professor Pathology and Physiology, The College of France, Paris, and Physician, Hôtel Dieu, Paris, France.
Harvey Williams Cushing, 1869–1939, Professor of Surgery, The Johns Hopkins University, Baltimore, MD (1903–1912), and at The Harvard University Medical School, Boston, MA, USA (1912–1932), described this syndrome in 1932.

the spine, distal radius and hip with bone mineral density reported in terms of two absolute values: T-score (units of standard deviation compared with the density of a healthy 30-year-old) and Z-score (units of standard deviation compared with age- and sex-matched control subjects). The World Health Organization has defined osteoporosis in terms of the T-score: osteoporosis is said to occur when the T-score is more than 2.5 standard deviations below the peak. A 1-point decrease in standard deviation in the T-score is associated with a 2.5-fold increased risk of a spine fracture.

Patients with osteoporosis may present with pain after minimal trauma or loss of height and an exaggerated thoracic kyphosis. Medications used to prevent and treat osteoporosis include the bisphosphonates (alendronate, risedronate), oestrogen or hormone replacement therapy and calcitonin.

Patients with painful thoracic fractures may be treated with short-term bed rest, analgesics and a spinal orthosis. If still painful 6 weeks after the injury, patients may be considered for vertebroplasty or kyphoplasty. Vertebroplasty involves the injection of polymethylmethacrylate bone cement (PMMA) under pressure into the vertebral body under fluoroscopic guidance. The goal of the procedure is to *stabilise* the spine and *decrease pain* associated with compression fractures.

Kyphoplasty, on the other hand, involves inserting bilateral bone tamps with balloons into the vertebral body. These are inflated under fluoroscopic control with the bone tamp re-expanding the body, elevating the end-plates to reduce the fracture deformity. The balloons are then deflated and removed, and PMMA is placed into the cavity created by the balloons. The goals of kyphoplasty are *spinal stabilisation*, *pain relief* and *restoration of vertebral body height*. Significant complications have been reported, including nerve root injury and spinal cord injury resulting from cement extravasation along with cement embolism, infection and hypotension.

Osteomalacia

This is characterised by delayed or impaired mineralisation of bone matrix resulting in bone fragility. Causes include nutritional deficiency, gastrointestinal malabsorption and renal tubular defects. Patients present with generalised bone pain and tenderness in the appendicular skeleton. Findings may include pseudofractures, Looser's zones and biconcave vertebra (cod-fish vertebra). Laboratory investigations may show a low or normal serum calcium, elevated parathyroid hormone, low serum phosphate, raised serum alkaline phosphatase and increased urine phosphate. A bone biopsy will show increased width and extent of osteoid seams. The disease is usually treated with vitamin D therapy with or without calcium supplementation.

FURTHER READING

Carragee, E.J. and Hannibal, M. (2004) Diagnostic evaluation of low back pain. *Orthop Clin North Am* **35**: 7–16.

Fairbank, J., Frost, H., Wilson-McDonald, J. *et al.* (2005) Randomised controlled trial to compare surgical stabilisation of the lumbar spine with an intensive rehabilitation programme for patients with chronic low back pain: The MRC spine stabilisation trial. *BMJ* **330**: 1233–8.

Freeman, B.J.C., Fraser, R.D., Cain, C.M.J., Hall, D.J. and Chapple, D.C.L. (2005) A randomised double-blind controlled trial: intradiscal electrothermal therapy versus placebo for the treatment of chronic discogenic low back pain. *Spine* **30**: 2369–77.

Fritzell, P., Hägg, O., Wessperg, P. and Nordwall, A. (2001) Volvo award in clinical science: lumbar fusion versus non-surgical treatment for chronic low back pain. A multi-centre randomised controlled trial from the Swedish lumbar spine study group. *Spine* **26**: 2521–34.

Nachemson, A. and Vingård, E. (2000) Assessment of patients with neck and back pain: a best-evidence synthesis. In: Nachemson, A. and Johnsson, E. (eds). *Neck and Back Pain: The Scientific Evidence of Causes, Diagnosis and Treatment*. Lippincott, Williams and Wilkins, Philadelphia, PA, Chapter 9, 189–236.

Waddell, G., McCulloch, J.A., Kummel, E.D. *et al.* (1979) Volvo award in clinical science: non organic physical signs in low-back pain. *Spine* **5**: 117–25.

Wiltse, L.L., Newman, P.H. and Macnab, I. (1976) Classification of spondylosis and spondylolisthesis. *Clin Orthop* **117**: 23–9.

Emil Looser, **1877–1936, Surgeon, Zurich, Switzerland, described this condition in 1920.**

Upper limb – pathology, assessment and management

34

To understand:
- Anatomy and physiology relevant to upper limb pathology

To be able to explain:
- The diagnosis and treatment of common upper limb problems

SHOULDER GIRDLE

Anatomy and function

The humerus, scapula, clavicle, manubrium sterni and chest wall are the osseous elements of the shoulder girdle. The main muscle groups are those that control the scapulothoracic and glenohumeral joints, in order that the hand may be placed in space, as defined by a sphere centred on the latter. The clavicle, through the medial sternoclavicular joint and the lateral acromioclavicular joints, acts as a load-transmitting bony strut between the upper limb and the axial skeleton. The whole shoulder girdle moves around the sternoclavicular joint, controlled and limited by those muscles between the thorax and scapula (e.g. trapezius, levator scapulae, rhomboids, serratus anterior and pectoralis minor) and thorax and humerus (e.g. pectoralis major and latissimus dorsi). The glenohumeral joint is controlled by the deltoid and the rotator cuff muscles, the latter composed of the anterior subscapularis, superior supraspinatus and superoposterior infraspinatus and teres minor. The scapula is integral to shoulder motion by moving around the posterior aspect of the thorax and, in combination, these joints comprising the shoulder girdle afford the greatest range of motion of all the joints of the body, with stability primarily the function of soft-tissue static and dynamic stabilisers (Fig. 34.1) (Summary box 34.1).

Summary box 34.1

Function of the shoulder

- To enable the hand to manipulate the environment as described by an arc centred on the shoulder joint
- The design is a compromise between mobility, stability and strength

---

Clinical history and physical examination

The clinical history and examination are detailed in Chapter 31, but the essential elements to clarify are those that commonly pertain to either loss of joint stability, e.g. anterior/posterior/multidirectional/habitual instability, or loss of joint motion, e.g. primary or secondary frozen shoulder, and pain sources around

the shoulder girdle, e.g. calcific tendinitis, rotator cuff disease, superior labrum anterior posterior (SLAP) tears, etc.

Congenital abnormalities

Sprengel's shoulder

This is the commonest congenital pathology around the shoulder, and is due to the abnormal descent of the scapula from its embryonic midcervical position. The clinical presentation is a high, small and rotated scapula with a connection to the cervical spine in 50% of cases, by a bony bar, fibrous band or an omovertebral body. Other congenital deformities may be associated, notably rib abnormalities, scoliosis of the thoracic spine or cervical spine

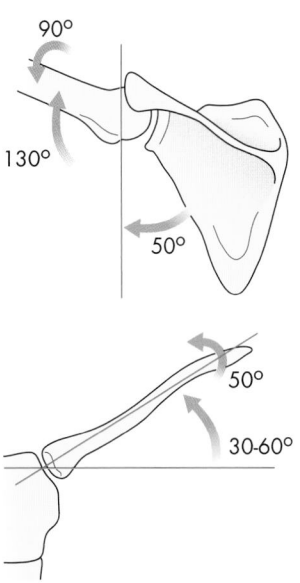

Figure 34.1 Relative motion of the elements of the shoulder girdle.

Otto Gerhard Karl Sprengel, **1852–1915, Surgeon, Grossherzogliches Krankenhaus (the Grand Ducal Hospital), Brunswick, Germany, described congenital high scapula in 1891.**

CHAPTER 34 | UPPER LIMB – PATHOLOGY, ASSESSMENT AND MANAGEMENT

anomalies including the Klippel–Feil syndrome (congenital fusion of the cervical vertebrae) (Fig. 34.2). The management is usually for cosmetic rather than functional reasons, especially in unilateral cases. Excision of the omovertebral body or superior angle has a satisfactory cosmetic effect. When functional improvement is the primary goal, complex reconstructive procedures are required.

Acquired abnormalities

The vast majority of acquired conditions present with some degree of pain in the shoulder region. The commonest of these acquired pathologies involve the rotator cuff musculature, especially the supraspinatus muscle–tendon unit. The spectrum of pathology that affects the rotator cuff presents, in order of severity, with painful arc syndrome, subacromial impingement, partial-thickness tears, full-thickness tears and cuff tear arthropathy. Calcific tendinitis, frozen shoulder and degenerative arthritis form the remainder of the common painful conditions of the shoulder (Summary box 34.2).

Summary box 34.2

Shoulder pain

- The second commonest musculoskeletal pain after back pain
- The supraspinatus muscle–tendon unit is most commonly diseased and painful

---

Rotator cuff disease

The rotator cuff musculature, in particular the supraspinatus tendon, has a relatively poor blood supply, and this predisposes it to degeneration and tearing. The anterolateral portion of the tendon is initially affected; the resultant swelling can lead to impingement on the undersurface of the anterior acromion with its attached coracoacromial (CA) ligament. This leads to pain, particularly on active abduction or flexion, and initially leads to a painful arc between 60° and 120° (Fig. 34.3).

It is believed that abnormalities of the bone occur, with hooking of the anterior acromion. These may be secondary changes, rather than the primary cause of the pain, but surgical treatment is often to remove part of the undersurface of the acromion and CA ligament (Fig. 34.4).

History and examination

The commonest patient characteristics are middle-age, a history of overuse or specific injury or a gradual onset of symptoms. The pain tends to be exacerbated with overhead activities and reaching across the body, e.g. putting washing on a line or grooming the opposite side of the head. Weakness is a feature in some patients that indicates a rotator cuff tear, as opposed to tendonosis.

Physical examination can rarely reveal local tenderness. Active movements may be limited and usually reproduce the symptoms, which occur between 60° and 120° of abduction and flexion (Fig. 34.3). There is usually much less pain on passive movement, and this confirms the mechanical and dynamic nature of the pain. Weakness of the supraspinatus and infraspinatus, when found, suggests the possibility of a tear in the muscles. Specific impingement tests have been described and help to confirm the diagnosis (Figs 34.5 and 34.6). Radiographs may be normal, but there are usually signs of subacromial sclerosis (Summary box 34.3).

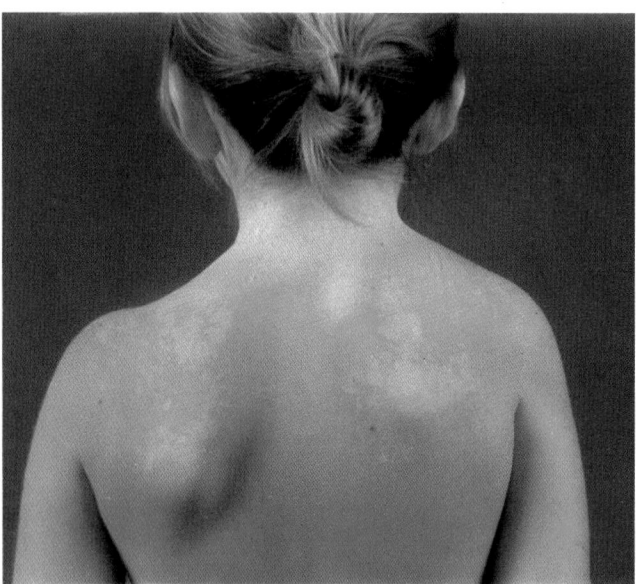

Figure 34.2 Sprengel's shoulder (right) of a 4-year-old girl.

Maurice Klippel, 1858–1942, Neurologist, Hôpital Tenon, Paris, France.
André Feil, 1889–?, Neurologist, Paris, France.
Klippel and Feil **described this condition in a joint paper in 1912.**

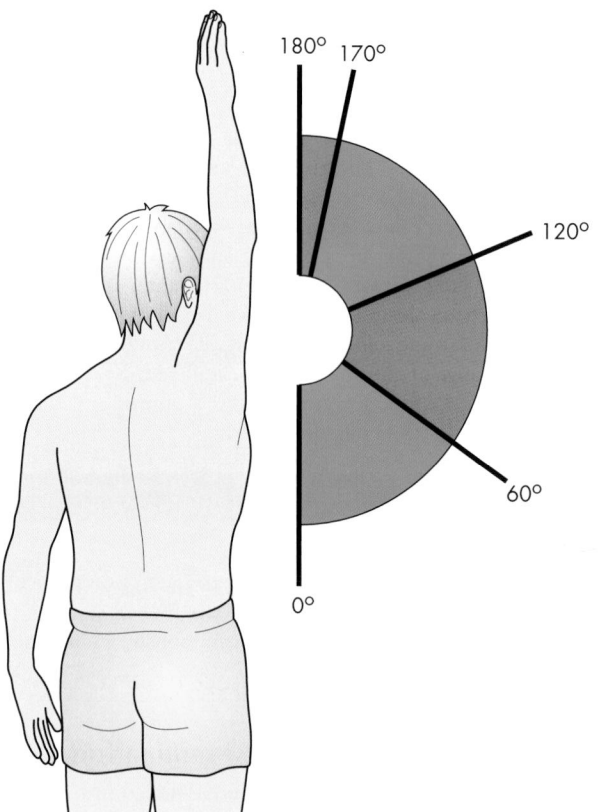

Figure 34.3 Arcs of shoulder girdle motion with subacromial impingement pain between 60° and 120° of abduction, and acromioclavicular joint pain between 170° and 180°.

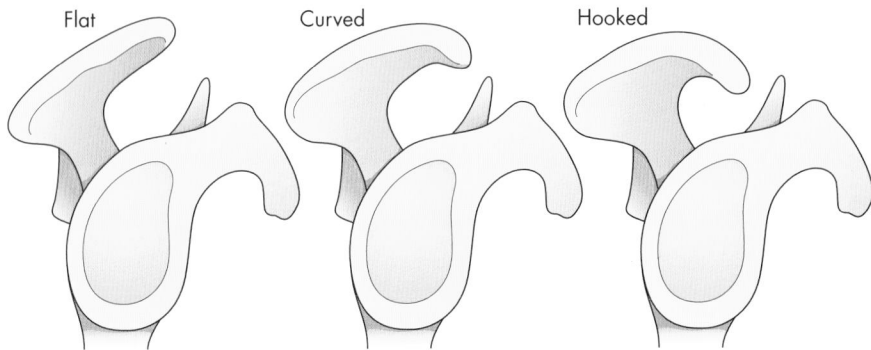

Flat   Curved   Hooked

Figure 34.4 The three commonest acromial morphologies.

Summary box 34.3

Supraspinatus problems

- Commonly in middle-age
- Activity related, especially the arm above the head
- No local tenderness
- Passive movement is less painful than active
- Local anaesthetic into the subacromial region is diagnostic
- Subacromial steroid is therapeutic in the early tendonosis stage
- Steroids should not be injected without knowledge of the presence of a tear

Subacromial injection of local anaesthetic can temporarily improve symptoms, if the diagnosis is correct, and is a valuable diagnostic tool. Steroid injections should only be used if the patient is not a surgical candidate, or if there is clinical and other diagnostic information to exclude the presence of a repairable tear. In such cases, the steroid, in the form of a depot, can lead to

symptom resolution, although this tends to be temporary. In cases of tendonosis, the anti-inflammatory steroid effect allows the rotator cuff the opportunity to be rehabilitated adequately.

Investigations

An out-patient clinic subacromial local anaesthetic injection is a useful confirmatory test. Imaging modalities include plain radiography, ultrasound and magnetic resonance imaging (MRI). The last two can determine the presence, size and location of a tear, and are useful preoperative planning tools (Fig. 34.7).

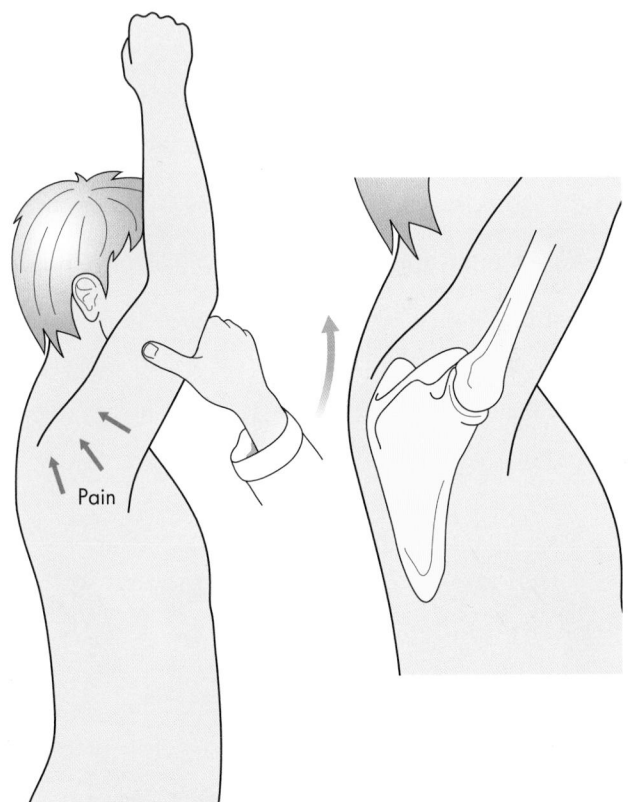

Figure 34.6 Neer's impingement test. Pain is reproduced with full forward flexion.

Charles Sumner Neer II, **Orthopaedic Surgeon, Columbia-Presbyterian Medical Center, New York, NY, USA.**

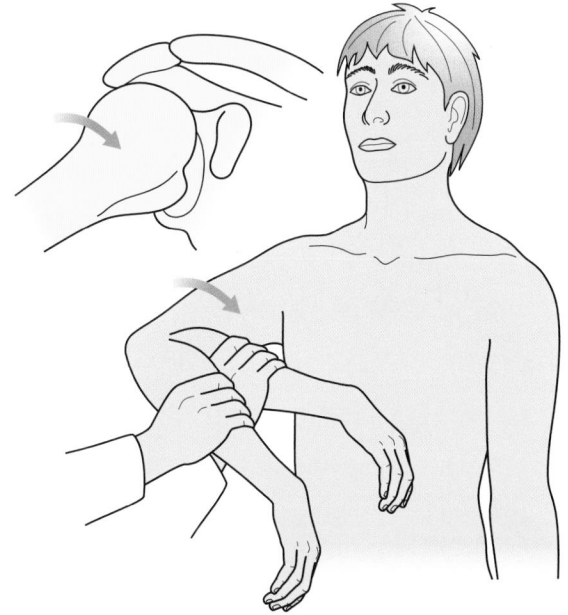

Figure 34.5 Hawkin's impingement test. Impingement pain is reproduced when the shoulder is internally rotated with 90° of forward flexion, thereby locating the greater tuberosity underneath the acromion.

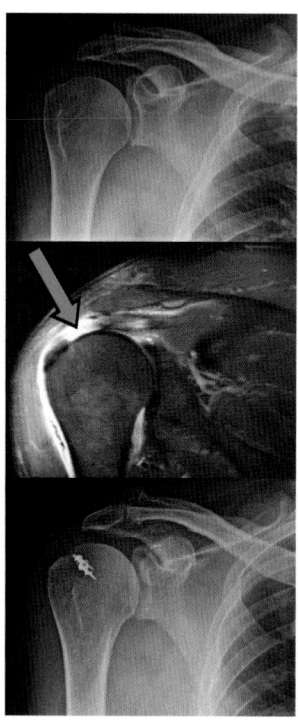

Figure 34.7 (Top) Plain anteroposterior (AP) radiograph demonstrating a roughened subacromion and greater tuberosity. (Middle) T2–weighted coronal magnetic resonance imaging scan demonstrating a retracted supraspinatus tear (red arrow). (Bottom) Postoperative AP radiograph demonstrating anchor fixation of the rotator cuff tear.

Treatment

It is likely that most early cuff disease, impingement and tendonosis, will settle with non-operative treatment. The initial treatment is by a maximum of three depot steroid injections over a 12-month period if each injection is demonstrated to give good symptomatic relief. Specific rehabilitation should aim to balance the whole rotator cuff, thereby resisting the proximal vector of the deltoid. Surgery is required in those who do not respond to this non-operative rehabilitation or if the symptoms persist beyond a reasonable period of time, as defined by the patient and surgeon, a minimum period of 6 months. Rotator cuff decompression (arthroscopic or open) is performed by removing the acromial overhang and dividing the CA ligament.

In addition, repair of a rotator cuff tear may be required. In the absence of a rotator cuff tear, the prognosis is good (Summary box 34.4).

Summary box 34.4

Treatment of subacromial irritation

- Non-operative treatment includes injections and cuff rehabilitation
- Surgery is indicated if symptoms fail to settle after a minimum of 6 months
- Surgery decompresses the rotator cuff

Rotator cuff tears

Patients with rotator cuff tears are generally older than patients with impingement, and it should be remembered that such tears form a spectrum of pathology from an early stage with small tears to the late stage of complete tear of all muscles. The supraspinatus muscle tears initially at the anterolateral edge of the tendon, progressing posteriorly to include the remainder of the supraspinatus, infraspinatus and teres minor, thereby creating, in the end-stage pathology, a bald greater tuberosity. The muscle–tendon unit retracts medially once detached. The patient is usually unaware of the rotator cuff tearing, and large tears of several years' duration may be present before the patient seeks medical attention (Fig. 34.8) (Summary box 34.5).

Summary box 34.5

Rotator cuff tears

- Occur in older age groups compared with impingement
- 4–20% of 40- to 50-year-olds have an asymptomatic tear
- > 50% of > 70-year-olds have an asymptomatic tear
- Treatment is required in symptomatic patients unresponsive to conservative management
- Outcomes are better following surgical repair of smaller than larger tears
- Subacromial decompression is important for pain relief following cuff repair
- Staged rehabilitation is crucial for good outcomes after surgical intervention

---

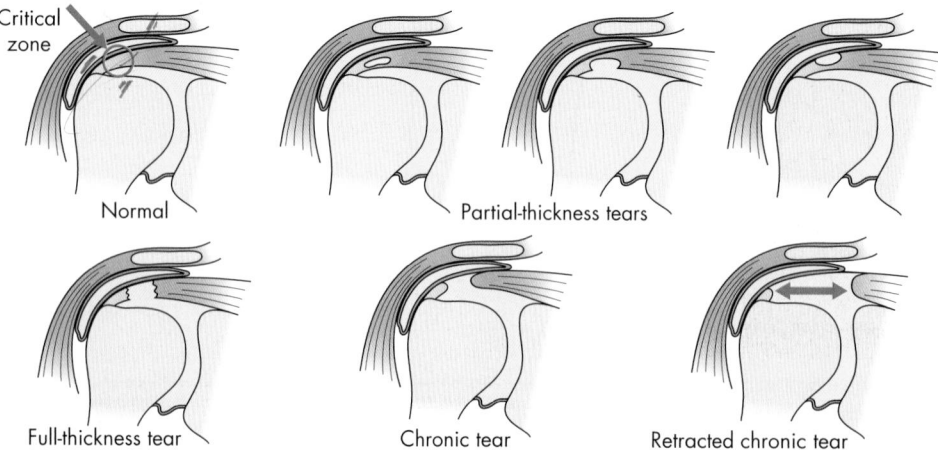

Critical zone

Normal

Partial-thickness tears

Full-thickness tear

Chronic tear

Retracted chronic tear

Figure 34.8 Various stages of rotator cuff tear. Initial partial-thickness tears have the potential to progress to full-thickness and retracted tears.

Small tears of the supraspinatus

These are very common and may be found in up to 50% of the normal population, according to MRI data, in the absence of any specific shoulder symptoms. The tear is usually less than 1 cm in length and, in the absence of pain, is insufficient to cause any observable weakness.

Treatment of small tears is dependent on the presence and severity of cuff symptoms. In the absence of symptoms, conservative cuff rehabilitation and regular review generally suffice. Symptom and/or tear progression are indicators for rotator cuff repair, with adjunctive decompression if impingement is defined to be a significant part of the pathology.

Intermediate tears

Tears of 2–4 cm are usually associated with symptoms of impingement and/or weakness of the shoulder, and frequently require decompression and repair of the supraspinatus. Arthroscopic or open approaches can be adequately utilised to perform the repair and decompression. The tendon is mobilised and then sutured into a bony trough created on the edge of the greater tuberosity, using suture anchors or osseous sutures. Results of repair are good for intermediate tears, but full recovery will take several months, with an emphasis placed on a graduated rehabilitation protocol.

Large rotator cuff tears

Tears greater than 5 cm (massive) may extend into the infraspinatus and teres minor and are usually associated with weakness of the shoulder. Abduction is typically limited to below 60°, often with a characteristic hunching of the shoulder (Fig. 34.9). With such massive tears, superior humeral head migration can occur, thereby further impairing function. A consequence of the resultant joint incongruity is secondary osteoarthritis of the glenohumeral joint, known as 'cuff tear arthropathy' (Fig. 34.10).

Large cuff tears that are significantly symptomatic and debilitating to the patient should be considered for repair and subacromial decompression. However, such chronic, degenerate tears are not always repairable, even after surgical mobilisation, because of

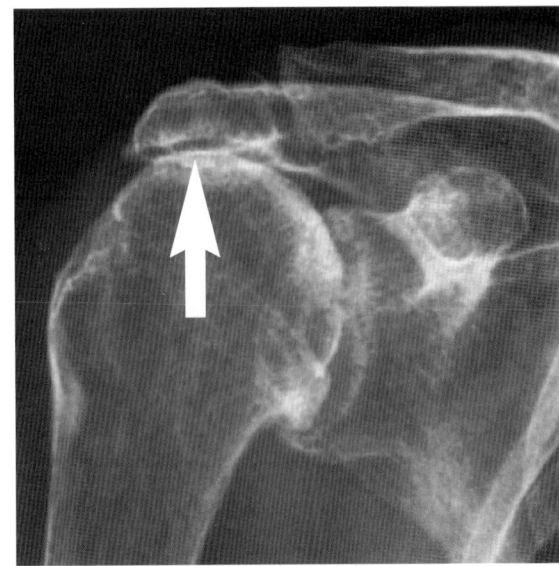

Figure 34.10 A massive rotator cuff tear that has led to proximal humeral head migration and secondary osteoarthritis of the glenohumeral joint, 'cuff tear arthropathy'.

medial muscle–tendon retraction and loss of elasticity of the structure. Options for defect closure include muscle tendon transfers and patch grafts (synthetic or xenografts), although the results of such procedures are less than satisfactory. A primary source of poor results, in this case, is the loss of contractility of the chronically retracted muscles, which undergo disuse atrophy and fatty infiltrative degeneration.

The majority of patients with massive irreparable tears complain of pain rather than loss of function. A successful treatment strategy is to repair, to the greater tuberosity, as much of the mobilised cuff that has retained adequate elasticity, which constitutes a partial repair, in combination with a minimal decompression. Good pain relief and some functional improvement are to be expected. A simple decompression without a partial repair may produce short-term pain relief, but has the potential for accelerated head migration and further erosion of the acromial bone stock.

Acute rotator cuff tears

Most tears of the supraspinatus result from degeneration and, as discussed above, will be associated with impingement symptoms. Occasionally, a large tear of the rotator cuff can result from trauma in the absence of any previous shoulder symptoms. These patients present soon after the event with profound weakness and loss of function but minimal pain. On examination, there is marked restriction of abduction, usually to less than 90°, with a characteristic hunching of the shoulder. This is due to elevation and rotation of the scapula to attempt to aid abduction. Diagnosis is confirmed by ultrasound or MRI, and early exploration and repair are indicated. Unlike the large degenerate cuff tears, the acute tear is usually repairable if surgery is carried out early. Often no decompression is necessary, as the front edge of the acromion is normal with no evidence of overhang. In middle-aged and elderly patients, an acute cuff tear can occur after shoulder dislocation, on the background of a pre-existent chronic degenerate tear (Summary box 34.6).

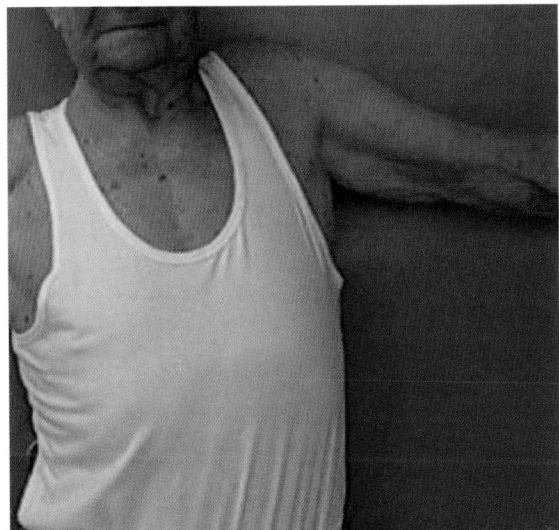

Figure 34.9 A 75-year-old patient with a > 5 cm retracted rotator cuff tear attempting to abduct the left shoulder, which is limited, by lack of balanced motor power, to below 60°.

Summary box 34.6

Acute rotator cuff tears

- Present with little pain but profound weakness
- Early repair gives good results

Frozen shoulder

This is a description of a painful and stiff shoulder condition of varying aetiologies, some of which remain poorly defined and termed 'idiopathic'. The rotator interval between supraspinatus and subscapularis is affected, as is the shoulder capsule. The disease most commonly affects females in their fifth decade, and is more common in diabetics and patients with heart or thyroid disease. Summary box 34.7 gives a brief summary of the condition.

Summary box 34.7

Frozen shoulder

- Idiopathic or secondary to other defined pathologies
- Symptoms – pain followed by reduced shoulder motion
- Idiopathic usually in females in the fifth decade
- Spontaneous resolution reported in between 1 and 3 years
- Differential diagnoses include calcific tendinitis and rotator cuff tear

History and examination

Idiopathic frozen shoulder is characterised by spontaneous, often severe pain of sudden onset, and may follow minor trauma. Sleep is often disturbed, and the differential diagnoses include infection, fractures and rotator cuff tears. In the early stages, the shoulder is difficult to examine owing to pain but, as the disease progresses, the range of motion reduces, both actively and passively. Local tenderness is often felt anteriorly over the rotator interval. The pathognomonic sign of frozen shoulder is loss of external rotation, and this differentiates it from rotator cuff disease. Plain radiographs exclude other intra-articular pathology.

Clinical course

The clinical course of frozen shoulder can be divided into three stages as follows:

Stage 1 – Painful phase. This can last for 2–9 months. The shoulder becomes increasingly painful, especially at night, and the patient uses the arm less and less. The pain is often very severe, and may be unrelieved by simple analgesics.
Stage 2 – Stiffening phase. This can last for 4–12 months and is associated with a gradual reduction in the range of movement of the shoulder. The pain usually resolves during this period, although there is commonly still an ache, especially at the extremes of the reduced range of movement.
Stage 3 – Thawing phase. This lasts for a further 4–12 months and is associated with a gradual improvement in the range of motion.

The clinical course runs over a period of 1–3 years, and the condition usually resolves without any long-term sequelae.

Treatment

Often no treatment is required, and the condition will resolve as described above. The range of motion may be slightly reduced compared with the unaffected side, but the vast majority of patients have no functional problems.

Treatment in the acute stage is pain relief. Corticosteroids may be tried but have variable effects, and should be avoided if imaging reveals a potentially repairable rotator cuff tear to be present. Active and passive mobilisation can be carried out if comfort allows, but aggressive/painful physiotherapy should be discouraged.

Surgery is usually reserved for prolonged stiffness affecting function, but can also produce good pain relief in the acute stage. Manipulation under anaesthetic may produce an increased range of motion. Arthroscopic distension of the joint with saline allows inspection of the shoulder before treatment. If these measures fail to produce any benefit, open release of the rotator interval can be carried out through an anterior approach, or preferably through an arthroscopic release.

Calcific tendinitis

This is a common disorder of unknown aetiology, which results in an acutely painful shoulder. Calcium is deposited within the supraspinatus, and it is thought that this may be part of a degenerative process or a consequence of a partial degenerative tear of the tendon. The differential diagnosis includes frozen shoulder, with both conditions occurring most commonly in middle-aged women.

History and examination

This pain is usually of rapid onset, often with no precipitating cause. In common with impingement, the pain is felt on the anterolateral aspect of the shoulder and is worse with activity, particularly overhead activities. The pain can be very severe and usually disturbs sleep. On examination, the shoulder is tender anterolaterally, and there is often some painful restriction of active, and sometimes passive, motion. External rotation will be possible, and this differentiates the condition from frozen shoulder.

The calcific deposits can be seen on plain radiographs (Fig. 34.11), lying within the supraspinatus tendon, inferior to the acromion and just medial to the tuberosity of the humerus. They can also be seen on ultrasound and MRI scans.

Treatment

Simple analgesia should be tried, together with rehabilitation. Calcific tendinitis usually responds to subacromial injection of corticosteroid, although a course of several injections may be necessary. The condition is often self-limiting, with resolution of the symptoms and resorption of the calcium.

Surgery

Resistant cases of calcific tendinitis are an indication for surgical treatment. Open excision of the calcific deposits can be carried out through a sabre incision, although arthroscopic subacromial decompression is a less invasive alternative. The calcific deposit can be debrided and removed and, if the remaining cavity is considerable, a simple closure can be performed.

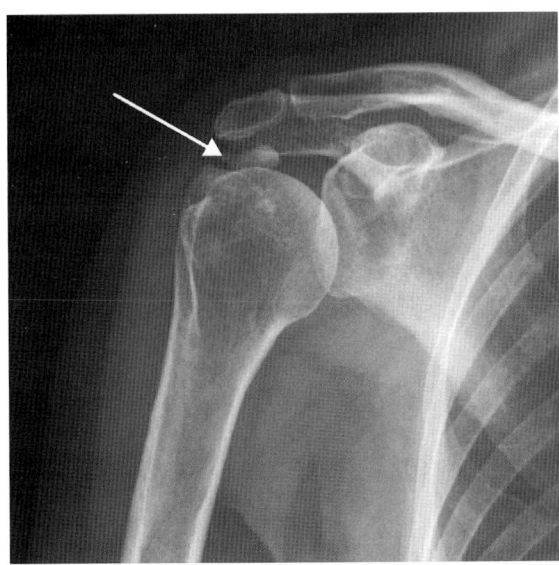

Figure 34.11 Radiograph demonstrating calcific tendinitis.

The prognosis for calcific tendinitis is generally good. Summary box 34.8 summarises the condition.

Summary box 34.8

Calcific tendinitis

- Commonly of unknown aetiology
- Rapid symptomatic onset, usually in middle-aged women
- Plain radiography often reveals the calcific deposits
- The majority of cases are self-limiting
- Resistant cases may be helped by subacromial decompression and deposit removal

---

Arthritis of the shoulder

Rheumatoid arthritis

The glenohumeral joint is commonly involved in inflammatory arthritides, particularly rheumatoid arthritis, with up to one-third of these patients developing severe problems, prior to the introduction of modern disease-modifying agents. Initially, pain is related to synovitis, and this responds to medical management, including intra-articular steroid injection.

Impingement symptoms can also occur, either with or without a rotator cuff tear. These will respond to subacromial injection, but decompression may be indicated. Arthroscopic synovectomy can be carried out at the same time but, in general, open synovectomy is not indicated in the management of rheumatoid arthritis of the shoulder. Chemical synovectomy may be indicated for symptoms that are resistant to medical treatment, but this is not commonly performed for rheumatoid arthritis.

For advanced disease, glenohumeral arthroplasty is indicated, with very good relief of pain, but there is often little improvement in the preoperative stiffness, as this is more a function of the peri-articular soft tissues (Summary box 34.9).

Summary box 34.9

Shoulder problems in rheumatoid arthritis

- One-third of cases have glenohumeral joint involvement
- Impingement can lead to rotator cuff tears
- Arthroscopic synovectomy is symptomatically effective
- Glenohumeral joint arthroplasty improves pain, but motion to a lesser degree

---

Osteoarthritis

Osteoarthritis of the glenohumeral joint is either primary or, more commonly, secondary. Secondary arthritis is commonly post-traumatic (Fig. 34.12) or a result of end-stage rotator cuff disease, in association with a massive tear of the cuff and superior migration of the humeral head (see Fig. 34.10, p. 489).

Treatment

Medical management is the first line of treatment but, if unsuccessful, surgical options are indicated. The two surgical avenues of management are debridement or joint arthroplasty; realigning osteotomies, akin to the knee, have no proven benefit in the shoulder. Whereas shoulder debridement is less predictable for long-term symptomatic relief, both total shoulder replacement (Fig. 34.13) and hemiarthroplasty (Fig. 34.14), without glenoid replacement, have good results in correctly indicated patients. A standard total shoulder arthroplasty should only be carried out if the rotator cuff is intact. In most rheumatoid patients and all patients with cuff tear arthropathy, the cuff is deficient, and the surgical options include hemiarthroplasty, hooded glenoid total shoulder arthroplasty (Fig. 34.15) or a reverse polarity total shoulder arthroplasty (Fig. 34.16). Shoulder arthroplasty is an effective pain-relieving procedure, but is less predictable in restoring motion, especially above shoulder level motion.

Arthrodesis of the joint is an alternative in younger patients, especially with a history of sepsis or any neurological problem that could destabilise a joint replacement. The peroperative morbidity is higher, and 3–4 months of immobilisation are required for union to occur. The patient retains a moderate range of movement at the shoulder, as a result of motion at the scapulothoracic articulation (Summary box 34.10).

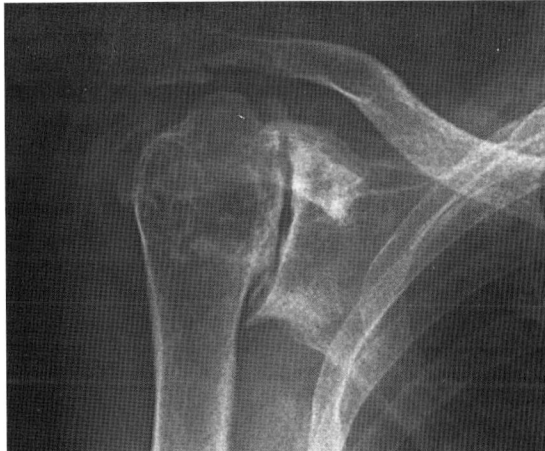

Figure 34.12 Post-traumatic arthritis with malunion of the proximal humerus, collapse of the humeral head and other features of osteoarthritis (subchondral sclerosis and osteophytes).

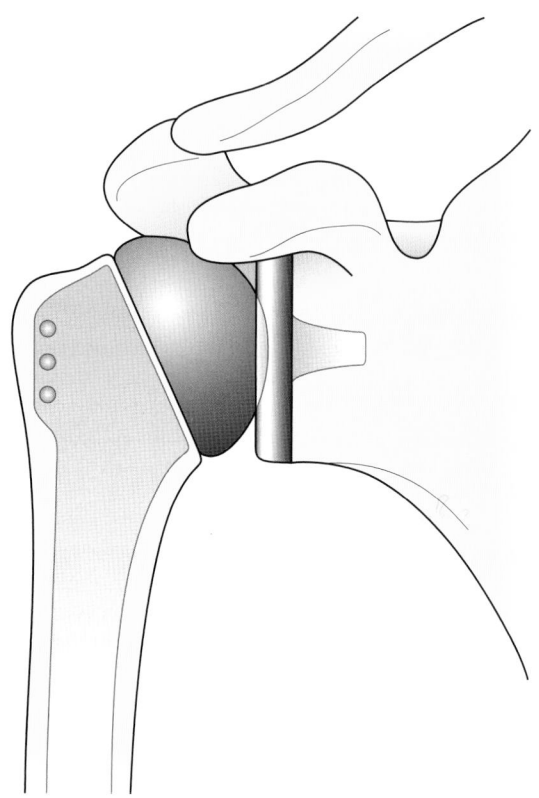

Figure 34.13 Total shoulder arthroplasty, for osteoarthritis, with an intact rotator cuff (from Kvitne, R.S. and Jobe, F.W. The diagnosis and treatment of anterior instability in the throwing athlete. *Clin Orthop* 1993, **291**: 107–23). With permission of the publisher.

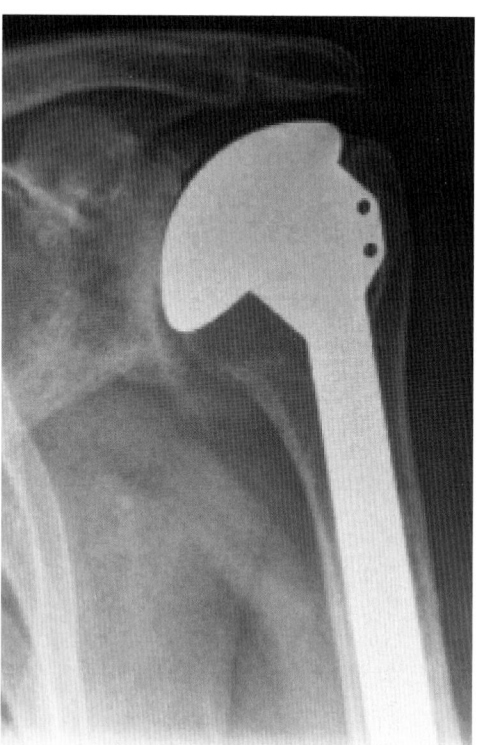

Figure 34.14 Hemiarthroplasty in a patient with an intact rotator cuff and reasonable chondral surface on the glenoid. An oversized hemiarthroplasty is an option in the presence of a massive rotator cuff tear.

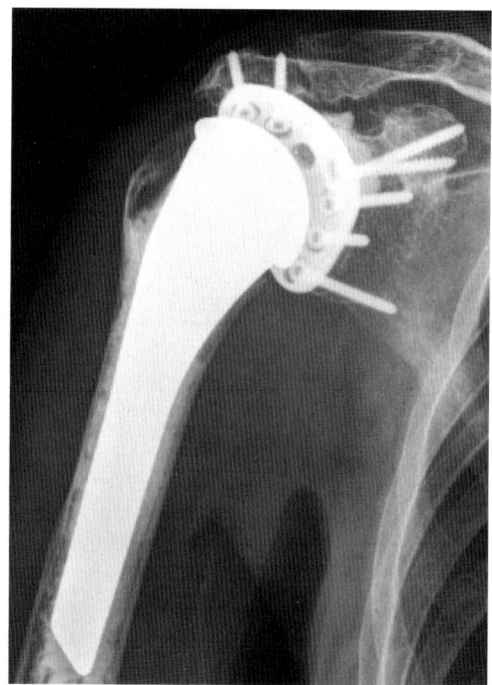

Figure 34.15 Hooded glenoid total shoulder arthroplasty for cuff-deficient arthropathy. The hooded glenoid resists superior migration of the humeral head, thereby allowing the deltoid to generate a centred rotatory torque and enabling the shoulder to be elevated and abducted.

Summary box 34.10

Shoulder osteoarthritis management

- Severe cases are treated by partial or total joint replacement
- If the rotator cuff is beyond repair, a standard total joint replacement is not an option
- Cuff tear arthropathy options are hemiarthroplasty, hooded glenoid or reverse polarity joint replacement
- Pain relief is predictably achieved, but range of motion improvement is less predictable
- Glenohumeral arthrodesis is an option in younger patients
- Post-arthrodesis motion is surprisingly good as a result of scapulothoracic motion

---

Acromioclavicular joint arthritis

Degenerative changes of the acromioclavicular joint are relatively common on plain radiographs and are often age related. Symptomatic disease usually manifests in males between 20 and 50 years of age and is frequently post-traumatic. Commonly, sports or manual occupations that load the upper limbs are implicated. The presence of inferior osteophytes implies the potential for impingement of the underlying rotator cuff.

History and examination

The pain is activity related and, unlike most causes of shoulder pain, is well localised, with the patient pointing to the acromioclavicular joint as the source of the pain. On examination, there is usually a bony abnormality, with prominence of the lateral end of the clavicle. This may be tender, and movement of the joint by depressing the clavicle while pushing up the humerus will

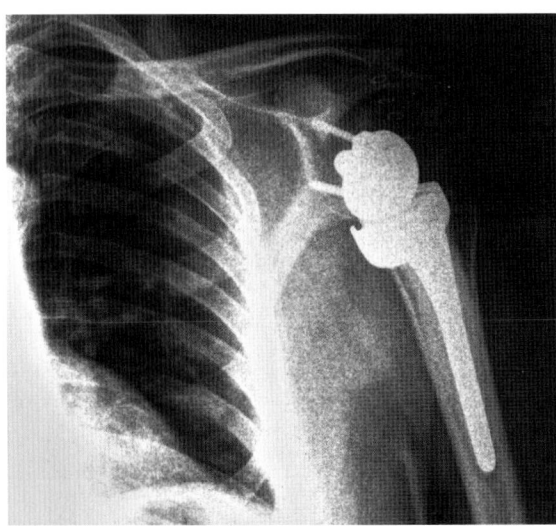

Figure 34.16 Reverse polarity total shoulder arthroplasty for cuff-deficient arthropathy. The glenosphere resists superior migration of the humerus, thereby allowing deltoid function.

reproduce the pain. Flexing and adducting the arm to place the hand behind the opposite shoulder will also produce pain. An intra-articular injection of local anaesthetic will confirm the joint as the site of the pain. If the symptoms are related to the inferior osteophytes, the pain is less localised, and impingement signs and symptoms are present.

Treatment

Intra-articular injection of corticosteroids usually produces some benefit, and a course of three injections is a standard course of treatment. If medical management fails, then surgery may be appropriate. The distal 0.5–1 cm of the clavicle is excised by an arthroscopic excision or open approach, with good relief of pain and no functional difficulties. In patients with predominantly impingement symptoms, arthroscopic debridement of the osteophytes can be carried out (Summary box 34.11).

Summary box 34.11

Acromioclavicular joint problems

- Usually secondary to either repetitive overload or trauma
- Inferior osteophytes can impinge on the underlying cuff
- Intra-articular local anaesthetic can aid diagnosis
- Intra-articular steroid injection is helpful in some cases
- Excision of the lateral end of the clavicle is curative if recalcitrant to conservative measures

---

Long head of biceps tendon rupture

A relatively common condition, predominantly in the middle to elderly age groups. The pathomechanics appears to involve abrasion of the tendon in the bicipital groove and is associated with rotator cuff tears. Most patients present with few symptoms, although they often seek advice acutely.

History and examination

Usually, the patient feels a sense of 'something giving way' in the front of the shoulder, and this sensation is often linked to a specific exertional event, e.g. lifting or pulling. The upper arm is

often bruised, and elbow flexion produces a swelling in the front and middle of the arm. The lump is initially tender and power is diminished (Fig. 34.17).

Treatment

In the vast majority of cases, the treatment is reassurance that the pain and bruising will resolve and that the power will improve over several months (Summary box 34.12).

Summary box 34.12

Proximal biceps tendon rupture

- Rupture of the long head is the commonest
- There is an association with rotator cuff pathology
- Surgery is rarely indicated
- A swelling remains but the power improves over several months

---

Instability of the glenohumeral joint

Traumatic dislocation of the shoulder is the commonest of all dislocations, with recurrent dislocations or instability being commoner age-related sequelae. A significant proportion (> 50%) of under 25-year-olds develop either recurrent subluxations or dislocations. A sub-group of shoulder instability patients dislocate their shoulders after relatively little force (atraumatic dislocation), while another sub-group is able to dislocate or sublux under their own volition (habitual dislocation). A careful clinical history, physical examination and plain radiographs (including lateral and axillary views) often accurately define the pathology in most cases.

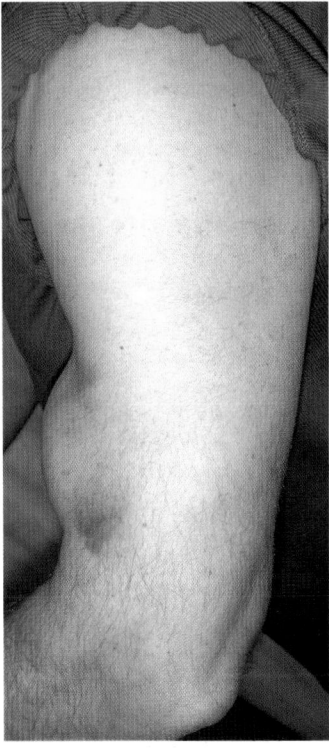

Figure 34.17 Long head of biceps tendon rupture – an obvious change in upper arm shape is evident along with acute bruising on the lateral aspect.

Classification

There are many ways of classifying shoulder instability, based on the direction and degree of traumatic energy, as well as differentiating between subluxations and dislocations. There is a spectrum of instability, but three broad groups of instability can be considered (Summary box 34.13).

Summary box 34.13

Classification of dislocations

- Traumatic – unidirectional; surgery usually successful
- Atraumatic – multidirectional, painful; responds to surgery
- Habitual – voluntary with ligament laxity, painless; surgery usually contraindicated
- Remember – patients may have a combination of the above aetiologies

---

Recurrent traumatic instability

Predominantly unidirectional and commonly anteroinferior. There is a notable traumatic event initially, although less energy is required on subsequent occasions. The patient experiences apprehension during activities that place the humeral head at risk of displacing towards the vulnerable direction. The shoulder may sublux or dislocate, which may or may not require medically supervised reduction. On examination, there is a full range of motion; with forced abduction and external rotation, apprehension is elicited (Fig. 34.18). Other joints are usually normal. As discussed in the section on trauma, there is usually a Bankart defect, with detachment of the anteroinferior glenoid labrum and damage to the humeral head (Figs 34.19 and 34.20) and, if the instability causes functional difficulties, surgery is indicated. For anterior instability, repair of the Bankart defect, in addition to some tightening of the capsule, will produce good results in 90–95% of patients. This is carried out either through an open anterior deltopectoral approach or arthroscopically (Fig. 34.21). For recurrent posterior instability (which is uncommon), tightening of the posterior capsule is curative, through either an open or an arthroscopic approach (Summary box 34.14).

Summary box 34.14

Recurrent traumatic shoulder instability

- A traumatic event is initially noted
- Subsequent dislocations/subluxations become easier
- Commonest direction of instability is anteroinferior
- Normal range of motion but positive apprehension sign
- Surgical treatment repairs the labral lesion and tightens the capsule

---

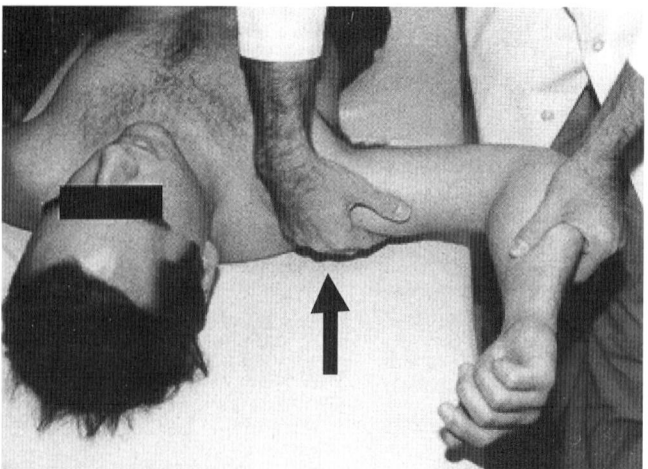

Figure 34.18 Shoulder instability can be clinically tested with an apprehension test; the photograph demonstrates the test while the patient is supine, but the same test can be performed with the patient sitting. The arrow indicates the direction of humeral head instability in common anteroinferior instability.

Atraumatic instability

Although there may be an initiating event, this is often less traumatic, for example a fall climbing stairs rather than a sporting injury. In many cases, there is no initial injury, and the instability may occur in more than one direction. The shoulder usually subluxes rather than dislocates, and the patient can often self-reduce the shoulder. The subluxation is painful, and the patient cannot dislocate the shoulder voluntarily. On examination, generalised ligament laxity is commonly present, and the shoulder can often be subluxed inferiorly to produce a sulcus sign, with a lateral sulcus appearing beneath the acromion as the arm is pulled down. Apprehension tests are again positive, but often in more than one direction. Anterior and posterior drawing of the humeral head often allows laxity to be appreciated (Fig. 34.22).

Physiotherapy, by an experienced therapist, should be tried first in these patients. As well as muscle strengthening, re-education of the patient, and of the shoulder, is necessary, and specific muscle groups may need to be targeted.

Approximately half of patients will require surgery, and a capsular tightening procedure is carried out either through an anterior approach or arthroscopically. This is a successful procedure, but there is a higher failure rate than with patients found to have a Bankart defect. Arthroscopic capsular shrinkage appears not to have an independent role in such patients, although it may have an, as yet incompletely defined, adjunctive role to capsular plication.

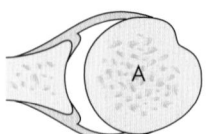 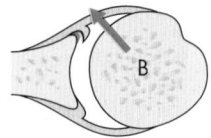 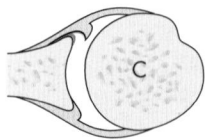 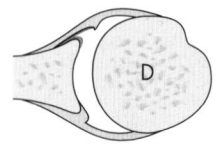 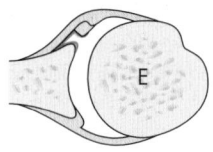

Figure 34.19 Schematic representation of Bankart's lesions, which form a spectrum of pathology from minor labral detachment (B) to large detachments with glenoid rim fractures (bony Bankart; E).

Arthur Sydney Blundell Bankart, 1879–1951, Orthopaedic Surgeon, the Middlesex Hospital, London, England.

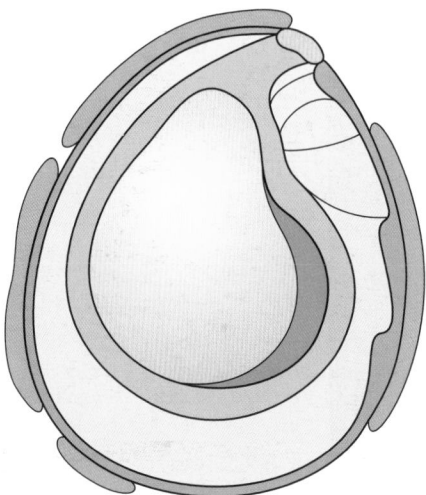

Figure 34.20 An end-on view of the glenoid labrum, demonstrating a labral detachment (red), with the rotator cuff muscles (brown), long head of biceps tendon and labrum (grey).

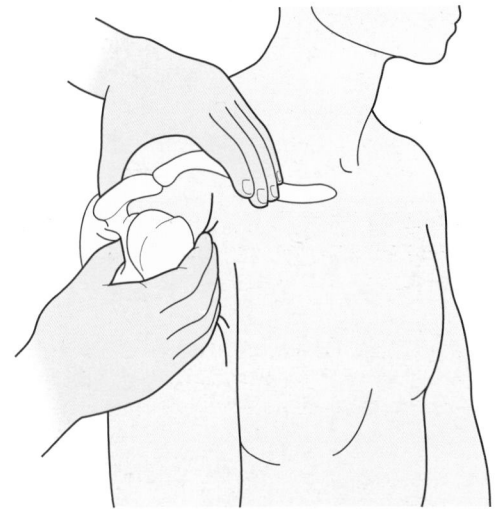

Figure 34.22 Generalised laxity can be appreciated by drawing the humeral head in anterior and posterior directions, and further confirmed by the sulcus sign.

Habitual dislocation

This is a much smaller group of patients, but one that does not respond well to surgical treatment. The patient is able to sublux the shoulder at will, either anteroinferiorly (Fig. 34.23) or posteriorly (Fig. 34.24), and this is usually not painful. There is underlying joint laxity, which is usually generalised, and there is rarely a significant traumatic event. The patient may sublux the shoulder as a 'party trick' or for emotional or psychological reasons.

It is vital that these patients are assessed and managed by an experienced therapist. The patient must be educated to avoid subluxing the shoulder and shown exercises as appropriate. Biofeedback re-education of muscles is important. Surgery is associated with a high failure rate and should be avoided in the vast majority of cases. However, recalcitrant cases can be treated by temporary paralysis of the dislocating muscle groups with botulinum toxin, while the stabilising muscle groups are re-educated.

DISORDERS OF THE ELBOW

Tennis elbow (lateral epicondylitis)

This is the most common cause of elbow pain excluding traumatic conditions, and usually occurs in patients in their 30s to 50s. The aetiology is unknown in the majority of cases, but the condition commonly follows a period of overactivity, particularly unaccustomed activity that involves active extension of the wrist. The tendon of extensor carpi radialis brevis is most commonly involved and, at exploration, a partial muscle tear and chronic inflammatory tissue may be evident (Summary box 34.15).

Summary box 34.15

Tennis elbow

- Strenuous or overactivity may precede symptoms
- Anterodistal lateral epicondyle tenderness
- Resisted wrist extension is a reliable diagnostic test
- Local anaesthetic injection is diagnostically helpful
- Vast majority improve with supervised conservative management
- Open or arthroscopic release yields good results in recalcitrant cases
- Arthroscopic release also identifies associated pathology

History and examination

The patient complains of pain around the lateral epicondyle and in the back of the forearm with certain activities. There is not usually

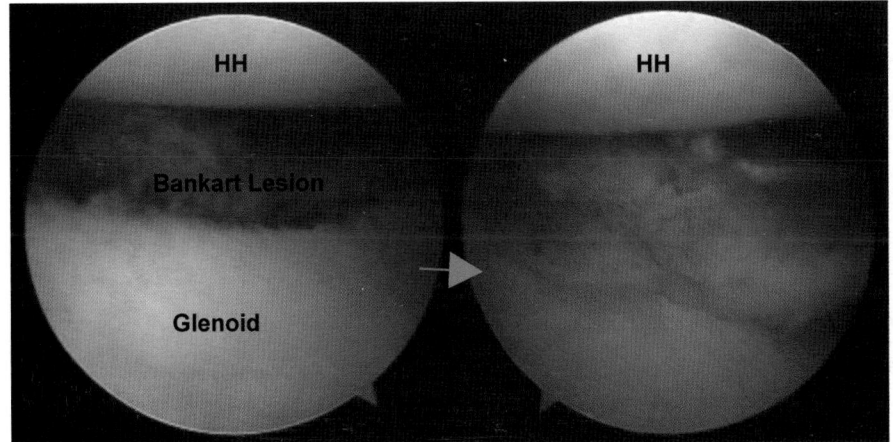

Figure 34.21 An arthroscopic view of a detached labrum (a) followed by an arthroscopic repair (b). The red arrow indicates where the labrum has been re-attached to the rim of the glenoid. HH, humeral head.

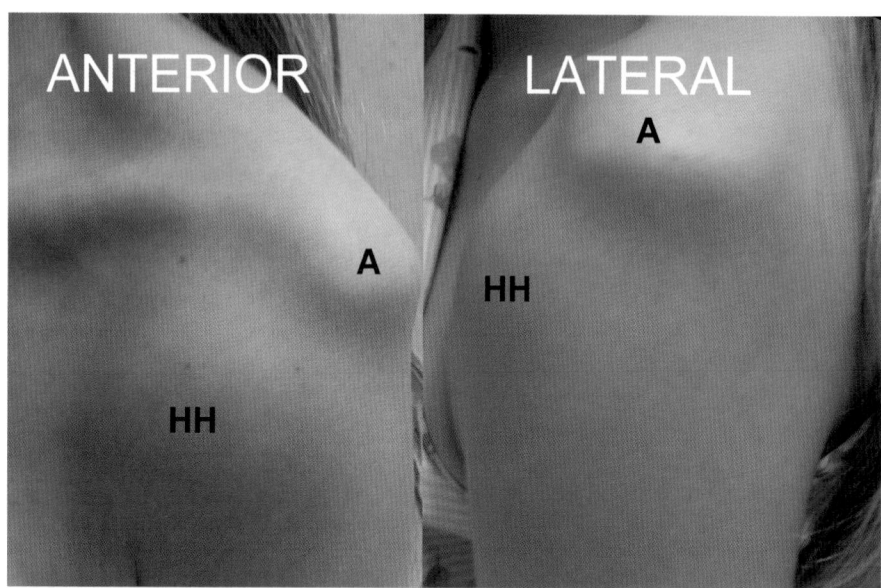

Figure 34.23 Anteroinferior habitual subluxation of the left shoulder in a 12-year-old girl. This was treated successfully with a combination of botulinum toxin to the pectoralis major muscle, biofeedback muscle re-education and a temporary anterior glenoid rim K-wire. A, acromion; HH, humeral head.

a history of trauma, but the patient may relate the onset to a period of unusual or strenuous activity. On examination, the patient is locally tender, which is commonly just distal and anterior to the lateral epicondyle rather than at the apex of the epicondyle itself. Forced palmar flexion and pronation (Fig. 34.25) or resisted wrist extension against resistance (Fig. 34.26) reproduces the pain. Pain with resisted middle finger metacarpophalangeal joint extension distinguishes the source as the extensor digitorum communis origin. The diagnosis is essentially a clinical one, aided by a local anaesthetic injection into the lateral epicondylar region. The need for ultrasound or MRI is minimal, as the vast majority are adequately diagnosed with clinical examination.

Treatment

The prognosis is generally good with most cases resolving without medical input, especially if the precipitating activity is avoided. Persistent cases can be aided with simple analgesia or a local injection of hydrocortisone, depending on severity, but repeated injections should be avoided. Other effective non-surgical measures include extensor mass stretching exercises and deep massage of the extensor mass, followed by cooling the elbow with ice packs. Open or arthroscopic surgery (Fig. 34.27) may be indicated occasionally, and local excision of the abnormal tissue will produce good results in 70–90% of patients.

(a)

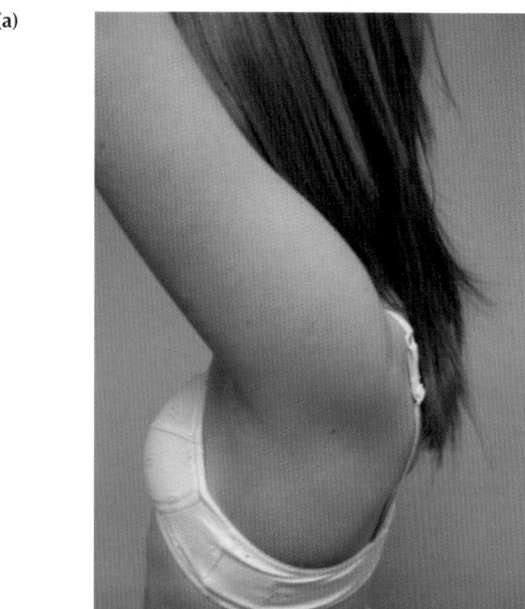

(b)

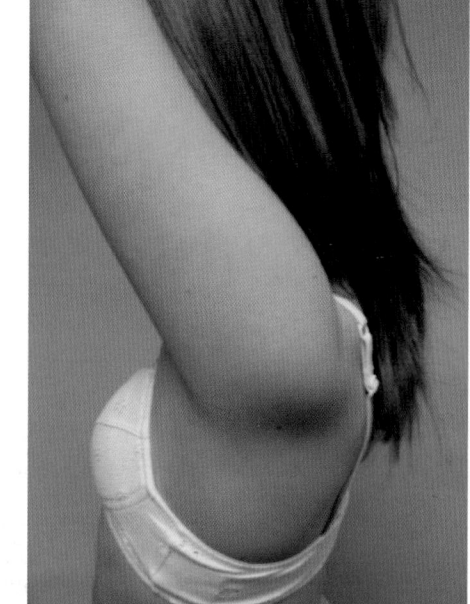

Figure 34.24 Posterior habitual instability of the shoulder in a 14-year-old girl that completely responded to biofeedback muscle re-education; (a) reduced, (b) posteriorly subluxed.

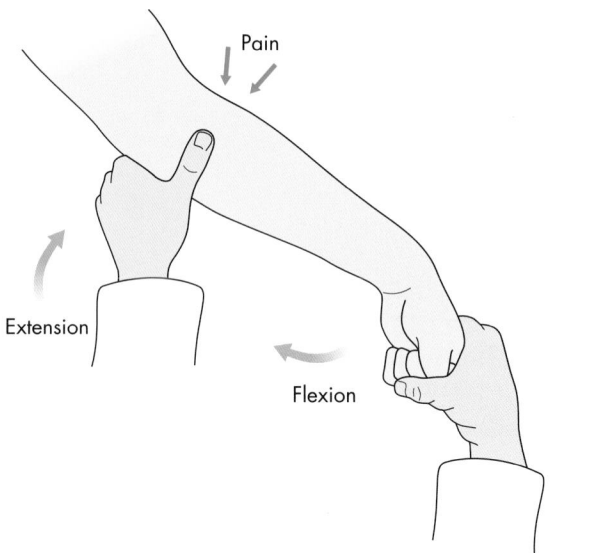

Figure 34.25 Tennis elbow test 1. Pain is reproduced with wrist flexion and forearm pronation against resistance.

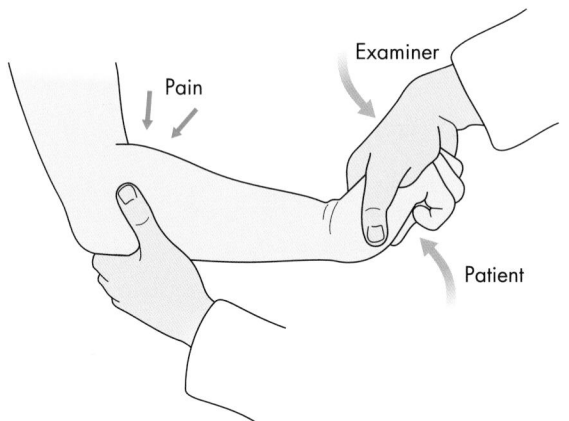

Figure 34.26 Tennis elbow test 2. Pain is reproduced with resisted wrist extension.

Golfer's elbow (medial epicondylitis)

This is less common and involves the flexor–pronator origin at the medial epicondyle. Ulnar nerve symptoms due to irritation or compression are part of the differential diagnosis, and treatment follows similar lines. If non-surgical management fails and surgical excision of the degenerate muscle origin is carried out, further imaging such as ultrasound or MRI is occasionally required, but this is essentially a clinical diagnosis.

Arthritis of the elbow

Rheumatoid arthritis

The elbow is commonly involved in rheumatoid arthritis, which can be a source of discomfort and functional limitation. Medical management is increasingly successful, but surgery is occasionally required. Radial head excision and synovectomy (open or arthroscopic) is effective for painful and restricted pro-supination, with good short-term results, although relapses are frequent. Elbow arthroplasty is a very effective modality for pain relief and functional restoration in end-stage disease (Fig. 34.28), with up to

(a)
(b)
(c)

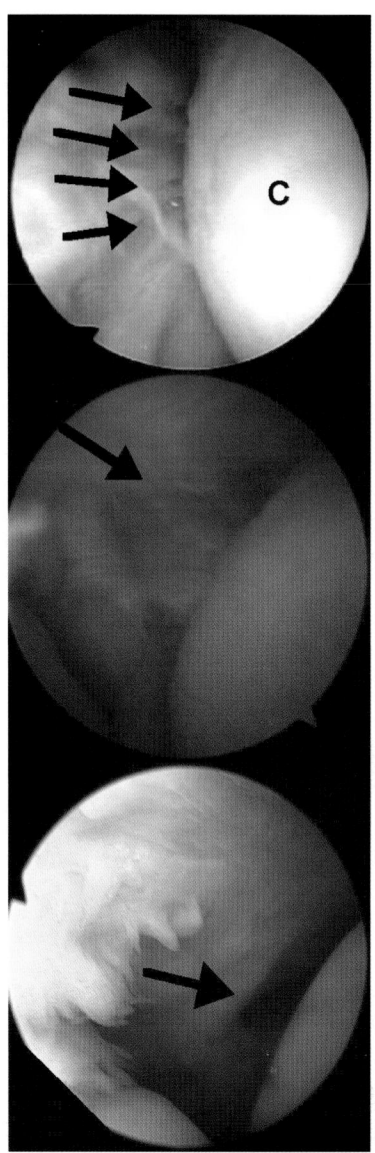

Figure 34.27 Arthroscopic view of tennis elbow. Arrows highlight the visible pathology. (a) Capsular splits; (b) capsular partial rupture; (c) complete capsular and extensor carpi radialis brevis rupture. C, capitellum.

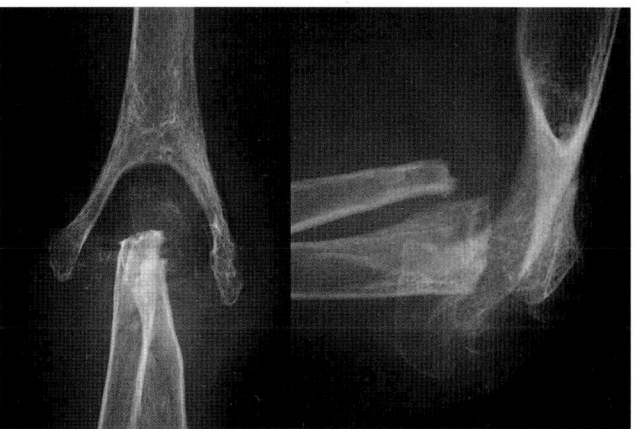

Figure 34.28 Typical end-stage rheumatoid arthritic destruction of the elbow joint, with characteristic erosion of the olecranon process and distal humeral columns.

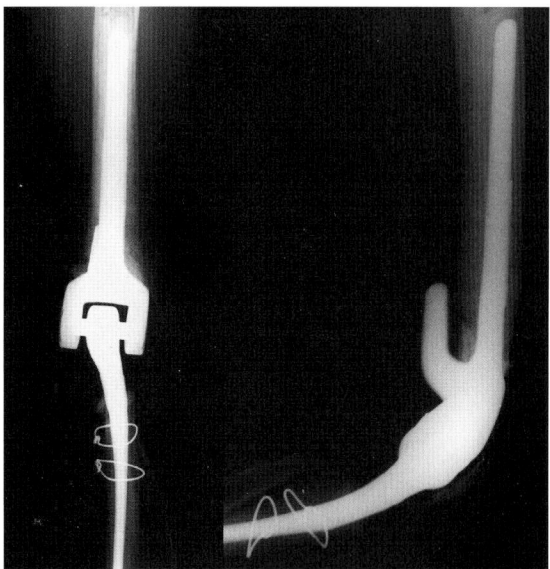

Figure 34.29 A linked total elbow arthroplasty (Coonrad–Morrey) of the patient from Fig. 34.28. Of note is the lack of olecranon process and columns.

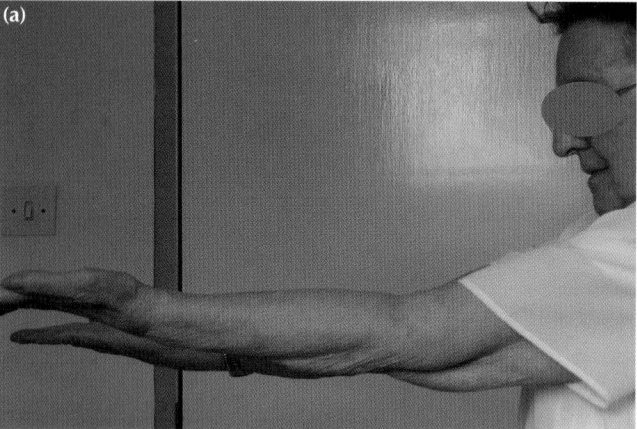

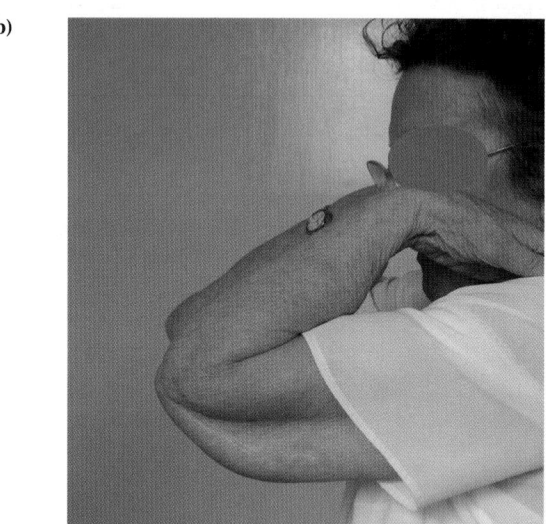

90% implant survival at 10 years (Fig. 34.29), with gross bony destruction. The functional outcomes are gratifying and of significant benefit to this group of debilitated patients (Fig. 34.30) (Summary box 34.16).

Figure 34.30 Final functional outcome of the patient in Fig. 34.28, 1 year after a Coonrad–Morrey linked total elbow arthroplasty.

Summary box 34.16

Rheumatoid arthritis of the elbow

- Surgical management is less frequently required due to the success of medical treatment
- A painful rheumatoid radial head can be excised to improve pain and pro-supination
- End-stage elbow disease is well treated with a total elbow arthroplasty
- Elbow replacement surgery is technically challenging if little bone stock is present

---

Osteoarthritis

Primary osteoarthritis of the elbow is increasing in frequency, but most cases of arthritis are secondary to previous trauma, osteochondritis dissecans or congenital problems. The typical patient demographic is a 40- to 60-year-old male, working in a heavy manual occupation (Fig. 34.31). Pain is the primary problem, along with locking although, on examination, there will usually be some crepitus, pain with motion and some degree of fixed flexion deformity. The history and examination should concentrate on differentiating the pain of a degenerate joint, which is activity related and predictable, from that of sudden unexpected pain and locking, which suggests loose bodies within the elbow (Figs 34.32 and 34.33). In addition, ulnar nerve symptoms are more common in the arthritic elbow.

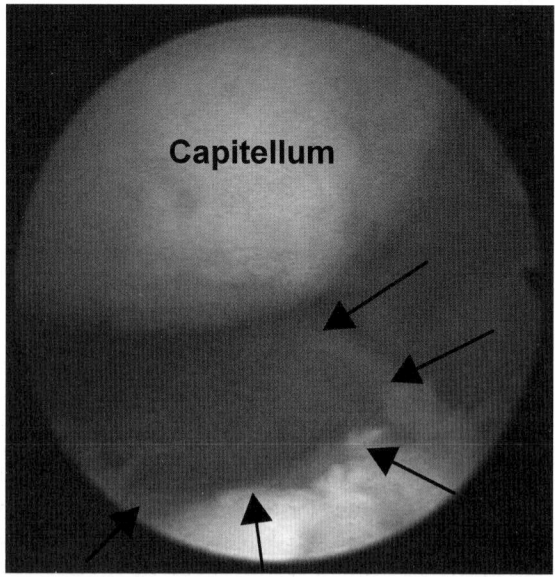

Figure 34.31 Arthroscopic view of primary osteoarthritis (arrows) of the radiocapitellar joint in a young male labourer.

(a)

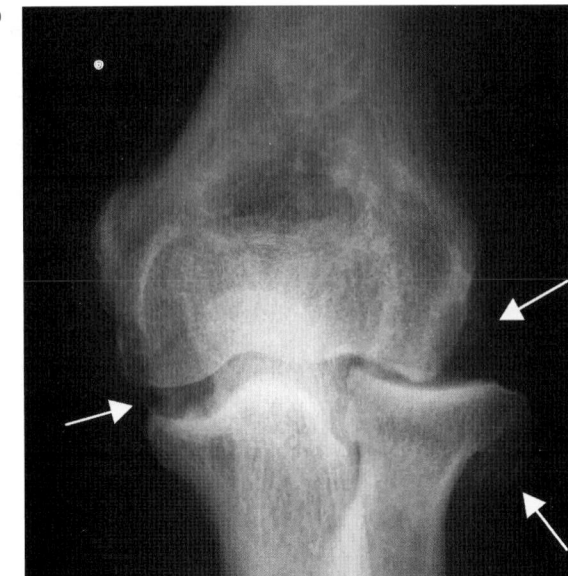

(b)

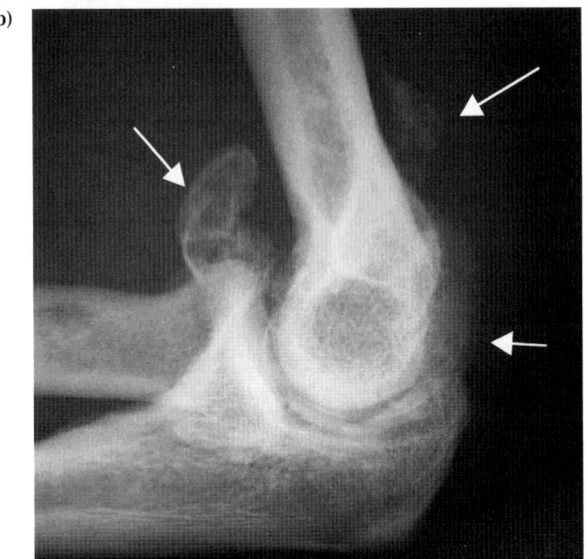

Figure 34.32 Plain radiographs of primary degenerative osteoarthritis of the elbow. White arrows, osteophytes.

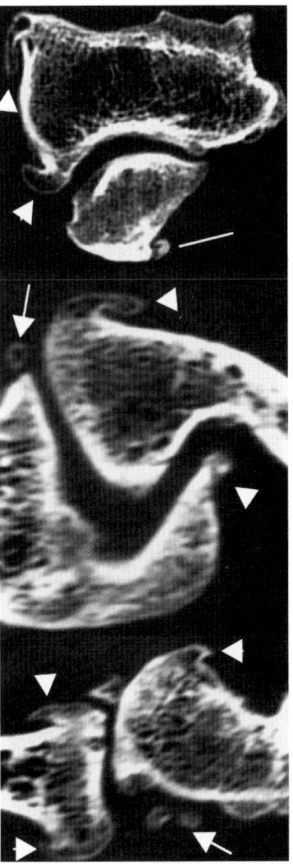

Figure 34.33 Computerised tomography scans of primary degenerative osteoarthritis of the elbow. Arrows, loose bodies; arrow heads, osteophytes; white line, broken osteophyte.

Treatment

No treatment is required in most cases other than reassurance about the nature of the condition. Osteoarthritic elbows seldom deteriorate rapidly, and the symptoms often improve after retirement. For the patient who is unable to carry out normal activities, there are surgical procedures that alleviate symptoms but may not guarantee a return to heavy manual work. Debridement, with or without augmentation with hyaluronic acid supplementation, will alleviate painful symptoms and increase the range of motion in the earlier stages; loss of motion is rarely a major complaint. Interposition arthroplasty using tendon, fascia or cutis is an option, although the outcomes are less predictable. Prosthetic joint arthroplasty is better for a more predictable symptomatic relief, but patients wishing to return to a heavy manual profession should be precluded. Other options that are less acceptable but should be considered in certain situations are resection arthroplasty and arthrodesis.

In general, the results of elbow replacement for osteoarthritis are not as good as for rheumatoid arthritis, probably as a consequence of different lifestyles of the patients (Summary box 34.17).

Summary box 34.17

Elbow osteoarthritis

- Initial management – decrease forces across elbow
- Decrease activities, change occupation
- Joint-preserving measures include arthroscopic/open debridement
- When conservative measures fail, consider prosthetic arthroplasty in low-demand patients

---

Loose bodies

After the knee, the elbow is the second commonest site of symptomatic loose bodies. The most common cause is osteoarthritis but, in younger patients, osteochondritis dissecans is the usual cause. Most patients complain of sudden unexpected pain and locking of the elbow, and often they have to shake or manipulate the elbow to relieve it. Plain radiographs will confirm the diagnosis in 90% of cases, and further investigation is not necessary (Fig. 34.34). Arthroscopic removal (Fig. 34.35) is effective and, in the presence of mechanical symptoms, good results can be expected. The removal of loose bodies from a degenerate elbow in isolation

(a)

(b)

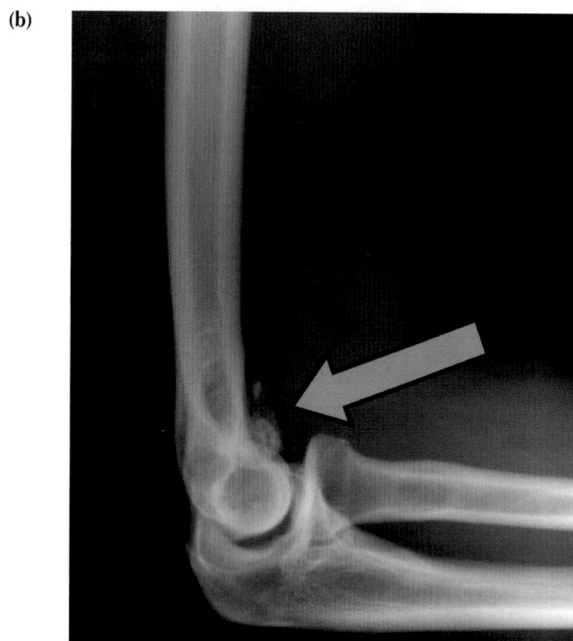

Figure 34.34 Radiograph of elbow loose bodies.

may not result in any lasting benefit, due to the degenerative symptomatology from the remainder of the joint (Summary box 34.18).

Summary box 34.18

Other common elbow problems

- Osteochondritis dissecans – occurs in teenage boys Detached fragments can be repaired or removed
- Olecranon bursitis – usually chemical not septic
- Ulnar nerve compression – may present with numbness in the hand. May need to be decompressed

---

Osteochondritis dissecans

Osteochondritis dissecans is much less common in the elbow than in the knee, and usually affects the capitellum. Teenage boys are usually affected, and the condition is often related to sporting activities. The main symptoms are pain and swelling and, on

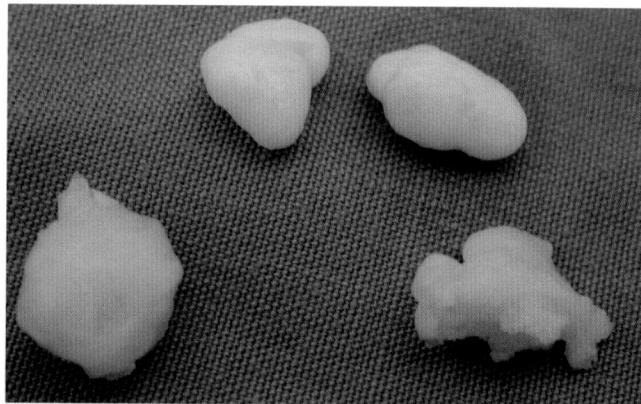

Figure 34.35 Loose bodies arthroscopically removed from the patient in Fig. 34.33.

examination, there is loss of full extension. Treatment is normally conservative, with a rest from sports, but arthroscopic removal may be required if the fragment detaches and the patient develops mechanical symptoms suggestive of a loose body.

Olecranon bursitis

Inflammation of the olecranon bursa is relatively common. The elbow is often very red, warm, swollen and painful, and a septic arthritis may initially be suspected. The signs and symptoms are, however, confined to the back of the elbow (Fig. 34.36), and movement within an arc of 30–130° is usually possible. The bursitis is usually chemical rather than infective, and management consists of rest, ice, anti-inflammatories and a compression dressing. If there is any suspicion of a penetrating wound, antibiotics should be administered, but formal drainage of the bursa should be avoided, unless purulent material is present.

Chronic bursitis can occur and may be associated with calcific nodules of the bursal lining (Fig. 34.37). When troublesome, surgical excision is beneficial.

Distal biceps tendon rupture

Rupture of the distal insertion of the biceps is an uncommon condition that usually occurs in younger patients, particularly after a

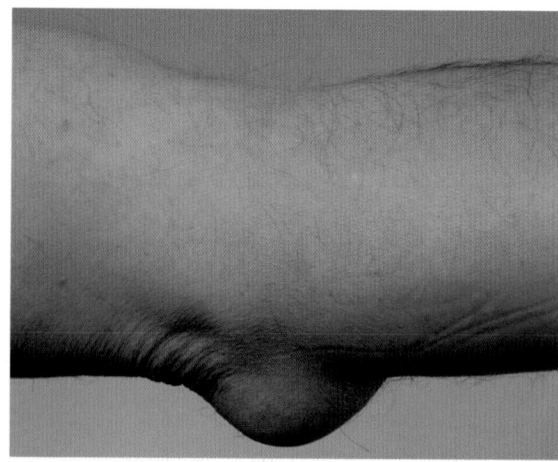

Figure 34.36 Olecranon bursa.

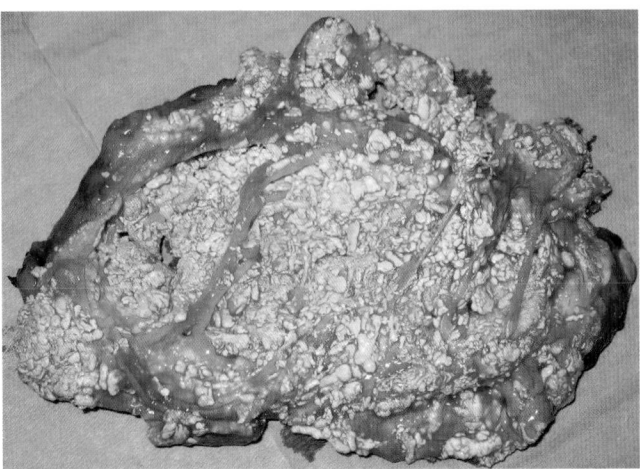

Figure 34.37 A very large chronic olecranon bursa, excised and its internal lining exposed, revealing a dense calcific component to the lining.

sporting injury. Again, pain and weakness are present but, unlike rupture of the long head, the weakness will not improve. Surgical repair is indicated in the demanding younger age groups, with good functional restoration (Fig. 34.38).

Ulnar nerve compression

This is the second commonest peripheral nerve entrapment after carpal tunnel syndrome. The most common sites of compression are around the elbow, especially if associated with a significant cubitus valgus angular deformity (Fig. 34.39): there are a number of other possible sites:

- the arcade of Struthers and the medial intermuscular septum – as the nerve passes into the posterior compartment of the distal humerus;
- medial epicondyle – particularly if osteophytes are present;
- cubital tunnel – as the nerve passes between the two heads of the flexor carpi ulnaris (Fig. 34.40).

A nerve palsy may also be due to a flexion or a valgus deformity of the elbow.

History and examination

Unlike carpal tunnel syndrome, compression of the ulnar nerve may not be painful, and the patient may present with weakness of the hand in association with paraesthesia. On examination, a positive Tinel's sign is usually present, particularly at the site of compression, and wasting (Fig. 34.41) and weakness of the intrinsic muscles of the hand are evident. Nerve conduction studies have an unpredictable diagnostic value in the earlier stages of the pathology, and are frequently no more informative than a good clinical examination. Plain radiographs are of value to screen for deformity, medial impinging osteophytes and medial epicondylar pathology.

Sir John Struthers, **1823–1899, Professor of Anatomy, the University of Aberdeen, Aberdeen, Scotland.**
Jules Tinel, **1879–1952, Physician, Hôpital Beaujon, Paris, France.**

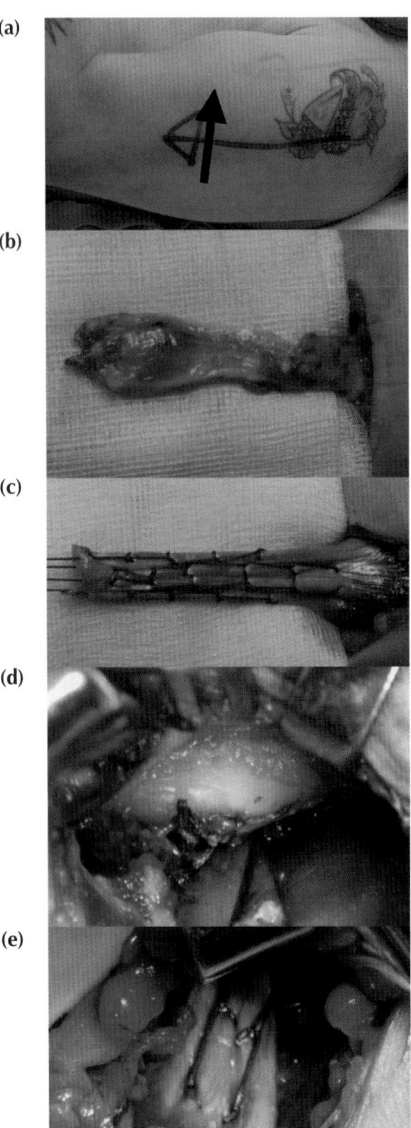

Figure 34.38 Rupture of the distal biceps tendon. (a) Change in contour of the distal arm (arrow), (b) ruptures the end of the distal tendon, (c) is secured with a non-absorbable suture, (d) reattached to the bicipital tuberosity of the radius, (e) and inspected to confirm an adequate tension.

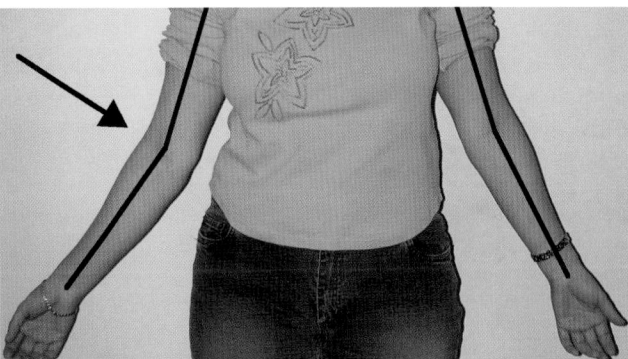

Figure 34.39 Significant cubitus valgus deformity of the right elbow in a 32-year-old female, following a malunited childhood supracondylar fracture.

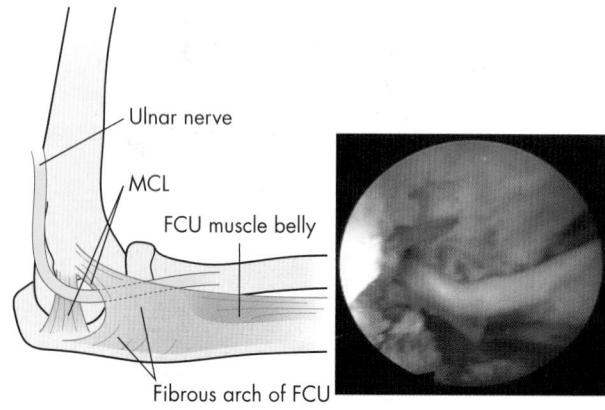

Figure 34.40 Anatomy of the cubital tunnel site of ulnar nerve compression, with a view of arthroscopic ulnar nerve decompression (inset). FCU, flexor carpi ulnaris; MCU, medial collateral ligament.

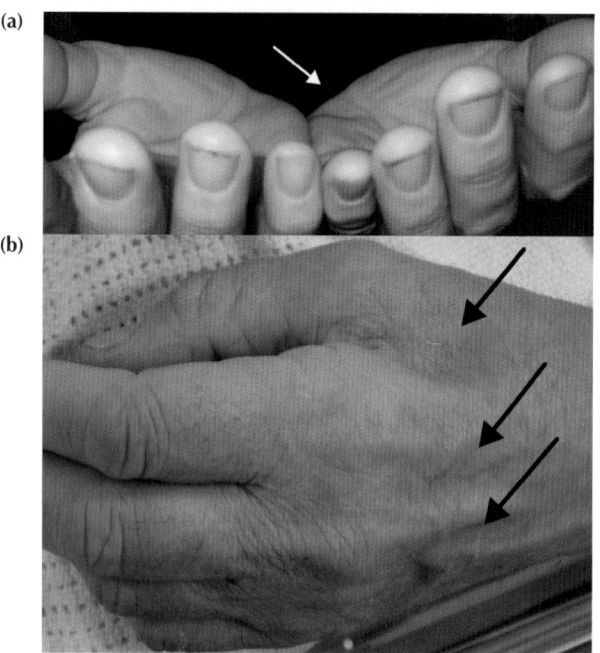

Figure 34.41 Clinical signs of ulnar neuropathy. (a) Hypothenar eminence wasting; (b) interosseous muscle wasting.

Treatment

Despite the absence of pain, decompression of the nerve should be carried out. The nerve can be explored through an open or arthroscopic approach. Surgical options include simple decompression, decompression with partial medial epicondylectomy and anterior transposition. Transposition is usually necessary in cases of deformity or if the nerve is unstable after decompression. For most other situations, decompression without transposition is sufficient, provided all sites of possible compression have been explored.

Any paraesthesia should resolve, but the prognosis for the return of hand power should be guarded as the recovery is unpredictable.

Compression of both radial and median nerves at the elbow occurs, but this is much less common than ulnar nerve compression.

INFECTIONS OF THE UPPER LIMB

Osteomyelitis

Osteomyelitis of the upper limb is very uncommon in adults, unless there are specific predisposing factors such as penetrating wounds. As with other sites, staphylococci and streptococci are commonly implicated, although other organisms may be encountered in the immunocompromised patient. The treatment of osteomyelitis of the upper limb does not differ from that in other sites.

In children, osteomyelitis of the proximal humeral metaphysis can occur, but this is much less common than osteomyelitis of the proximal femur or around the knee.

Septic arthritis

In both adults and children, septic arthritis of the shoulder or elbow is uncommon. Arthroscopy is preferred to formal arthrotomy for washing out the shoulder. The elbow may be washed out arthroscopically or via a lateral Kocher-type approach.

Tuberculosis

The shoulder and elbow are relatively uncommon sites for tuberculosis (TB), but the incidence appears to be increasing (Fig. 34.42), and treatment is along conventional lines. Secondary degeneration can occur and may be difficult to manage. A previously infected joint is one of the few indications for shoulder arthrodesis, but the elbow presents a dilemma. Arthrodesis of the elbow is not a good procedure, and there is little information on the outcome of other methods of treatment after previous TB (Summary box 34.19).

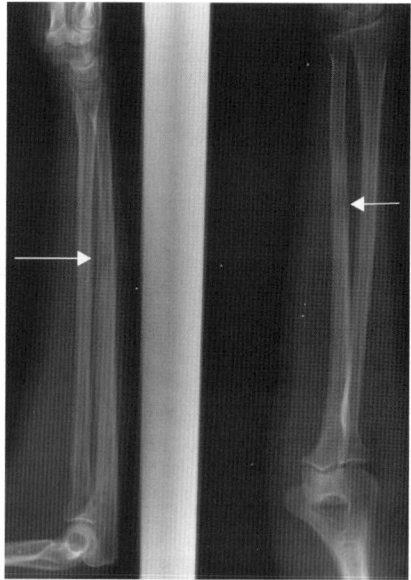

Figure 34.42 Tuberculosis of the ulnar shaft in an Indian female, revealing a bony erosive lesion, which responded to conventional antituberculous chemotherapy without surgery.

Emil Theodor Kocher, **1841–1917, Professor of Surgery, Berne, Switzerland.**

CHAPTER 34 | UPPER LIMB – PATHOLOGY, ASSESSMENT AND MANAGEMENT

Tumours of the upper limb

Tumours are unusual around the elbow, but the proximal humerus is a relatively common site. It is the third most common site for both osteosarcomas and fibrosarcomas after the distal femur and proximal tibia. Treatment is along conventional lines. The shoulder is the second most common peripheral site after the proximal femur for chondrosarcomas, and the scapula body is also a common site. The principal method of treatment for chondrosarcomas is surgical excision, and this may be technically difficult around the shoulder. Subtotal excision of the scapula can be carried out with good preservation of function if the glenoid can be left. The humerus is also a relatively common site for lymphomas and Ewing's tumour. Treatment is, again, along conventional lines (Summary box 34.20).

Benign and intermediate tumours such as osteochondromas, giant cell tumours and aneurysmal bone cysts are also relatively common. The proximal humerus is the most common site for unicameral bone cysts, which are thought to represent an abnormality of cells of the growth plate (Fig. 34.44). They commonly present as pathological fractures in children around the age of 10 years and affect boys more commonly than girls. The lesion may

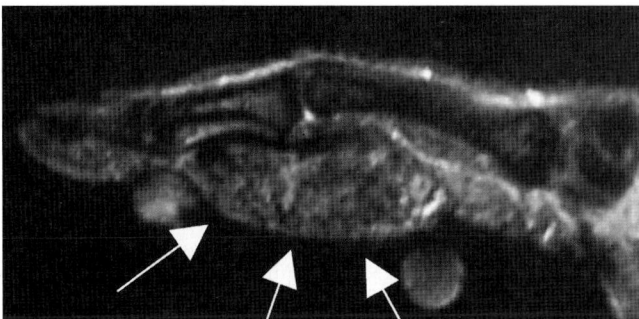

Figure 34.43 Giant cell tumour (arrows) of the tendon sheath (magnetic resonance imaging).

James Ewing, **1866–1943, Professor of Oncology, Cornell University Medical College, New York, NY, USA, described this type of sarcoma in 1921.**

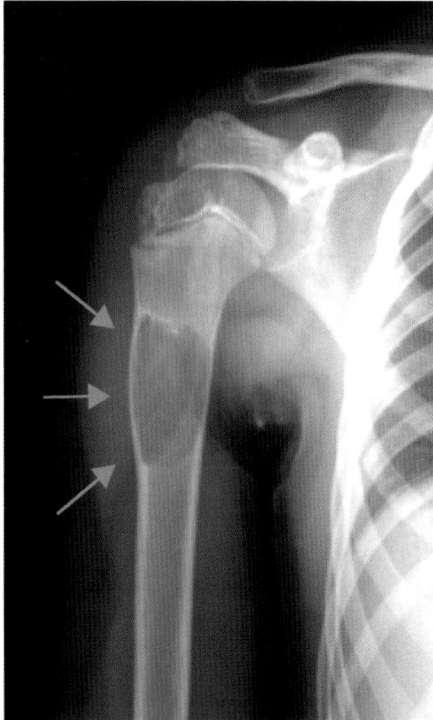

Figure 34.44 Unicameral bone cyst (arrows) of the proximal humerus in a 12-year-old boy.

resolve after fracturing, but local medical treatment is often required. Benign soft-tissue tumours that are common are lipomas (Fig. 34.45) and fibromas (Fig. 34.46), with ganglia (Fig. 34.47) sometimes posing diagnostic challenges.

The humeral shaft is a common site for secondary deposits (Fig. 34.48), and intramedullary nailing may be required for pathological fracture or impending fracture, if the patient is fit for surgery. In the majority of cases, primary tumours are found in the breast or prostate, but secondary spread from the thyroid, lung, kidney and bowel can also occur.

HAND

Function

The hand is a complicated and highly sensate organ that is designed to manipulate the environment, and therefore has some prerequisites to function effectively (Summary box 34.21).

The index finger works against the thumb, which acts as a post, in order to achieve a fine pinch grip, e.g. picking up a small object, whereas the little and ring fingers provide power grip, e.g. holding a hammer, and curl into the palm. The thumb presses against the side of the index finger for key grip and presses the tips of the index and middle fingers for chuck grip (holding a pen). All

(a)

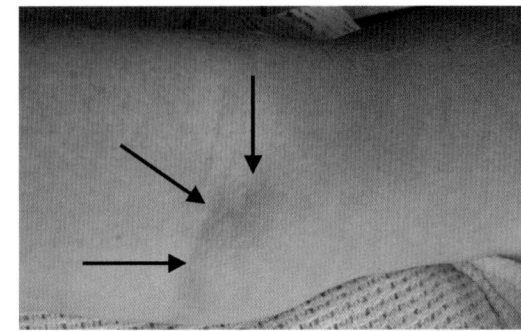

(b)

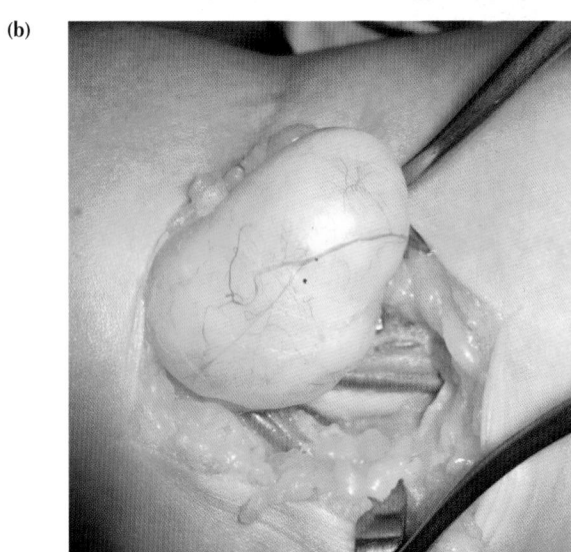

Figure 34.45 Antecubital lipoma (arrows), which presented with median nerve compression neuropathic symptoms. (a) Antecubital swelling; (b) lipoma defined with the underlying median nerve and brachial artery/vein.

(a)

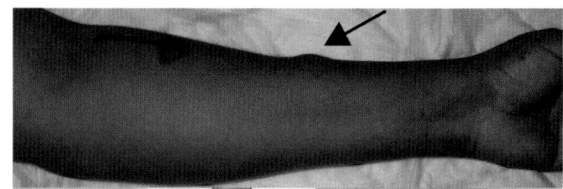

(b)

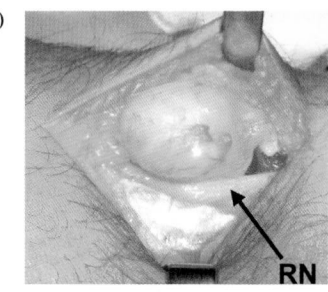

(c)

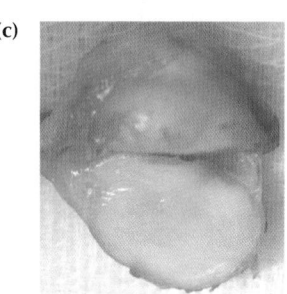

Figure 34.46 Fibroma of the forearm. (a) Swelling on the radial border of the mid-forearm, a firm but mobile swelling. (b) Fibroma defined with the underlying radial nerve, which was the source of the sensory neuropathy. (c) Fibroma bivalved revealing a dense fibrous interior.

the fingers curl for hook grip (holding a suitcase). A stable wrist is required to allow these hand functions (Summary box 34.22).

Summary box 34.22

The five functions of the hand

- Fine pinch, e.g. picking up a small object
- Power grip, e.g. holding a hammer
- Key grip, e.g. holding a key
- Chuck grip, e.g. holding a pen
- Hook grip, e.g. carrying a suitcase

Clinical history and physical examination

The initial clinical history should ascertain the patient's age, occupation and left or right handedness. An important aspect of assessment is the function and pain of the hand with a lesser importance placed on cosmesis, with care being taken to assess rotational malalignments of the digits (Fig. 34.49). Sensation and weakness are also specifically questioned.

Tendons

Examination should begin with inspection for deformity, scars, nodules, etc. Tendon function can be tested with the passive tenodesis method: the wrist is moved from flexion to extension passively, normal function is demonstrated by the fingers curling into flexion with wrist extension and should open with wrist flexion. This motion arc should be smooth and coordinated, thereby establishing the function of each tendon.

Nerves

The neurological status of the hand should be assessed by sensation on each side of the digits (light touch and two-point discrimination). Tinel's test (nerve percussion that produces tingling) allows the examination of a compressed nerve or a nerve tip that is regenerating and advancing following an injury. Sweat gland function in the hand, assessed by passing a pen across the surface of a digit, can assess whether a nerve is intact, in which case the pen sticks to the skin, or severed, if the pen glides smoothly over the skin without resistance.

Circulation

The capillary refill time can be examined with nailbed compression and observing the time taken to reperfuse. Arterial supply by the radial and ulnar arteries can be tested with the Allen test: the patient elevates and tightly clenches the fist. The Allen test can identify whether both radial and ulnar arteries are intact. In this

---

Edgar van Nuys Allen, **1900–1961, Professor of Medicine, the Mayo Clinic, Rochester, MN, USA.**

(a)

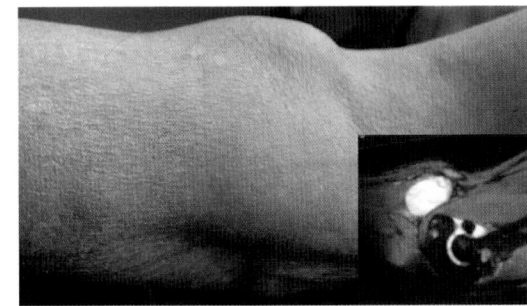

(b)

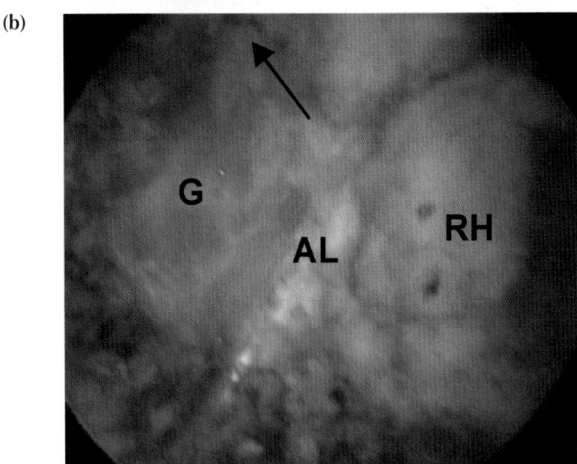

Figure 34.47 Antecubital ganglion (G) causing considerable elbow discomfort. (a) Antecubital soft and fluctuant swelling, with a magnetic resonance imaging inset revealing a fluid-filled mass. (b) Arthroscopic excision view revealing its close relationship to the annular ligament (AL) and radial nerve (arrow). RH, radial head.

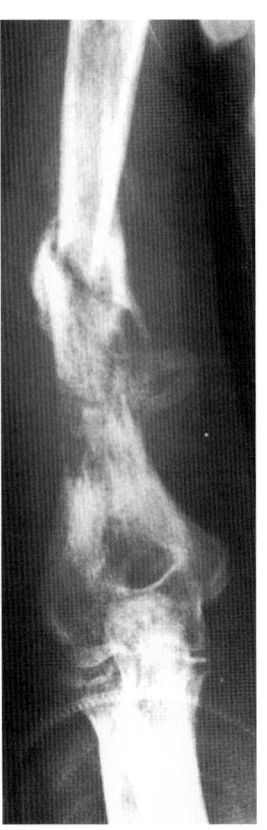

Figure 34.48 A pathological distal humeral shaft fracture through a secondary renal cell carcinoma deposit. This patient was not fit for surgery and hence was treated in a plaster cast.

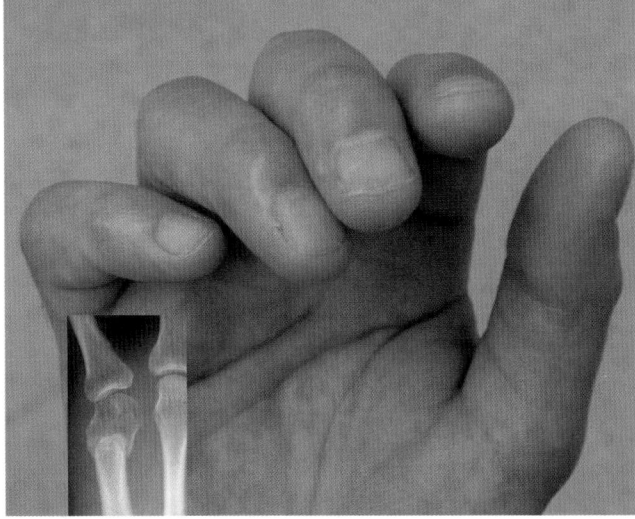

Figure 34.49 Rotational malalignment of the little finger.

test, the patient squeezes his or her hand to express the blood, and then both arteries are compressed by the examiner's fingers. The hand will be white. The examiner then releases one artery; if the hand does not 'pink up', that artery is occluded or divided. The test is repeated for the other artery. Compression of the fingernail will cause it to go white. On release of the examiner's finger, return of a normal pink colour within 2 s confirms a proper distal artery circulation (Fig. 34.50) (Summary box 34.23).

Summary box 34.23

Examination of the hand

- Tendons – passive tenodesis test for function
- Nerves – two-point discrimination for sensation
- Nerves – skin sweat test for autonomic nerve function
- Arteries – Allen's test for circulation

Investigations

The following are specific investigations for the hand and wrist: (1) electrophysiology provides data regarding nerve function and is helpful in carpal and Guyon's tunnel syndromes if the clinical picture is not conclusive; (2) MRI can be helpful to detect Kienböck's lunate and scaphoid fracture fragment vascularity; (3) radioisotope bone scans can be helpful in elusive cases of wrist pain for increased signals identifying areas of higher vascularity; (4) wrist arthroscopy can be a useful diagnostic aid for triangular fibrocartilage complex (TFCC) tears, carpal instabilities and arthritis.

(a)

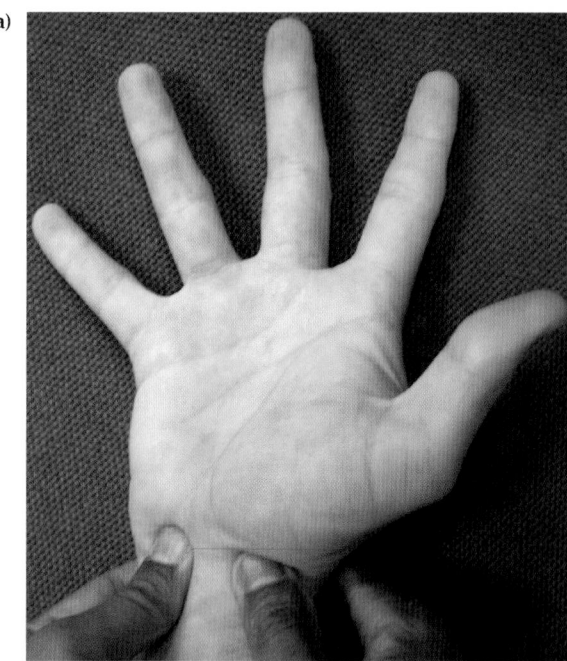

(b)

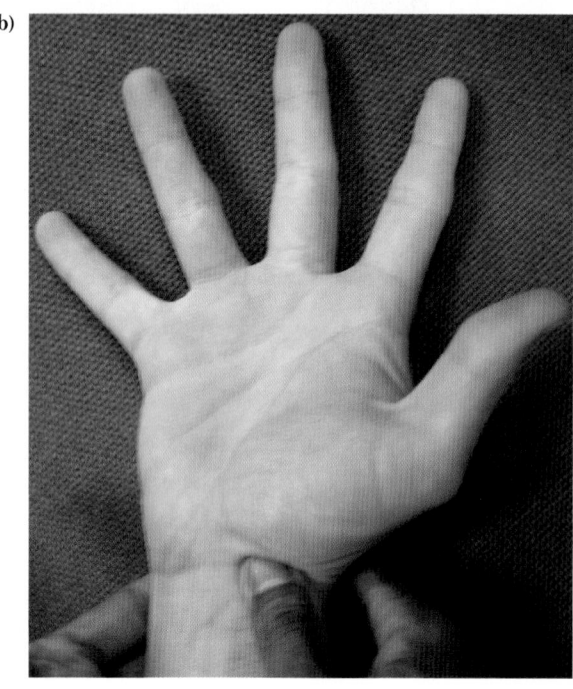

(c)

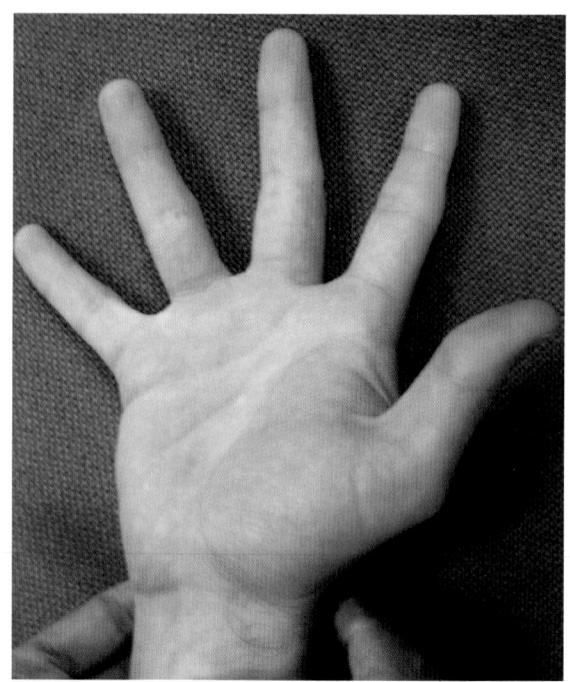

Figure 34.50 Allen's test.

Hand treatment – basic principles

Prevent swelling and stiffness

Following injury, surgery or infection, the hand swells (Fig. 34.51), leading to an extended metacarpophalangeal joint and flexed interphalangeal joint position. This position can, if prolonged, lead to collateral ligament shrinkage; as the wrist swells, it tends to fall into a position of flexion, the metacarpophalangeal joints extend and the interphalangeal joints flex. This position becomes permanent as the collateral ligaments shrink and the oedematous tissues fibrose. The hand cannot then function properly. To avoid this, the following three principles should be observed:

1 *Elevation* in a high sling, without excess elbow flexion, which impairs venous drainage.
2 *Splintage.* The wrist should be splinted initially in the position of safety – the 'Edinburgh' position described by James is designed to avoid fixed flexion contractures. Dressings must not be too tight.
3 *Movement.* Rehabilitation should be planned to mobilise all joints as early as possible (Summary box 34.24).

John Ivor Pulsford James, **1913–2001, Professor of Orthopaedic Surgery, the University of Edinburgh, Edinburgh, Scotland.**

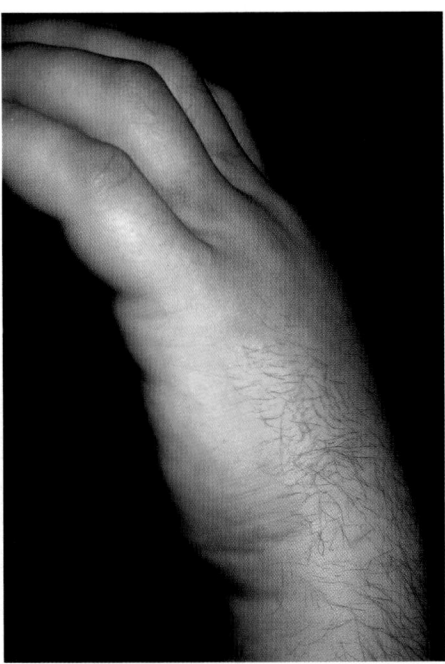

Figure 34.51 Hand swelling following surgery is to be avoided.

Many other basic principles apply to the surgical treatment of the hand and are listed in Summary box 34.25.

Thumb ulnar collateral ligament

Gamekeeper's thumb is a chronic overuse stretching of the ulnar collateral ligament of the thumb. An acute form of this injury is the skier's thumb, radial hyperabduction of the thumb. Patients present with pain and instability of the thumb when attempting to maintain a power pinch grip between the thumb and index finger. Most stable sprains can be managed conservatively with 3–4 weeks of splintage. When unstable, the ulnar collateral ligament should be either repaired, if possible, or reconstructed with a suitable graft.

Triangular fibrocartilage complex

This is a structure that is in continuity with the dorsal and volar wrist capsules and primarily serves to stabilise the distal radio-ulnar joint and acts as part of the proximal articulation of the triquetrum. It can undergo traumatic or degenerative tears, thereby presenting with ulna-sided wrist pain, and distal radio-ulnar instability. Diagnosis by magnetic resonance arthrography or diagnostic arthroscopy can effectively lead to repair of the traumatic tears and debridement of the ragged degenerative tears.

Infections

Most hand infections can be treated initially with elevation, static splintage and presumptive antibiosis. Surgical drainage may be necessary if pus is evident, and antibiosis should be altered in accordance with microbiological investigation of the pus. If swelling and inflammation settles, with or without surgical intervention, supervised motion is instigated to avoid stiffness (Summary box 34.26).

Paronychia

Acute paronychia is the commonest hand infection, often due to inappropriate nail trimming or skin picking around the nail fold (Fig. 34.52). After initial inflammation, pus accumulates beside the nail and needs to be surgically released, with or without the excision of the outer quarter of the nail. Chronic paronychia appears over several weeks and is usually a fungal infection, unrelated to the acute form. It commonly occurs in patients whose hands are frequently immersed, and microscopy of scrapings and fungal cultures reveals the diagnosis. Management ranges from advice to keep the hand dry and the use of anti-fungal creams to nail fold surgery.

Pulp space (felon)

Pus trapped between the specialised fingertip septae causes intense fingertip pain, and may lead to terminal phalangeal bone infection, erosion and sequestrum formation. The last of these

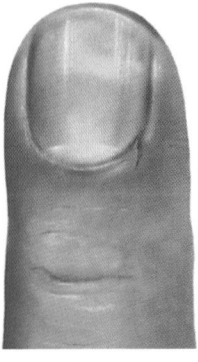

Figure 34.52 Acute paronychia.

will need to be drained and debrided. A common differential diagnosis with small vesicles and crusts is the self-resolving herpetic whitlow, especially in dental workers, caused by the herpes simplex virus.

Flexor tendon sheath infection

The clinical presentation is of a swollen flexed finger, which is painful with passive motion and tender on tendon sheath palpation. If the infection, commonly by *Staphylococcus* or *Streptococcus*, is untreated, adhesions between the tendon and its sheath lead to a stiff and useless finger. Management is by early saline irrigation of the sheath, with a catheter passed into the sheath, with early motion once signs of inflammation resolve.

Bites

Animal or human bites can lead to infection and consequent loss of function, commonly due to *Staphylococcus*. Broad-spectrum antibiotics are generally effective. Wounds should be explored thoroughly, excised, washed out, damaged tendons repaired and splinted, and appropriate antibiotics commenced.

Other infections

Mycobacterial infections

Tuberculosis in the hand may involve the tenosynovium, joints or bone. The most dramatic form is the compound palmar ganglion, with synovial swelling, proximal and distal to the transverse carpal ligament. The diagnosis is made with a biopsy, and synovectomy and prolonged chemotherapy are the basis of treatment.

Pilonidal sinus

A hair implanted in the palm or web space can cause a recurrently infected cyst (Fig. 34.53), which should be excised.

Palmar space infections

The whole hand becomes swollen and tender, as pus collects on either side of the septum. Treatment is by incision and drainage and thorough washout of the wound.

Web space infections

Pus can collect in the potential space surrounding the lumbricals, which pass from the palm, across the deep transverse metacarpal ligament into the extensor mechanism. The web space swells, and swelling tends to spread adjacent fingers apart. Pus is drained through a longitudinal incision over the web space.

Arthritis

Rheumatoid arthritis

Rheumatoid arthritis has many deforming and devastating effects and presents with the classic symptoms of morning stiffness, symmetrical arthritis, especially involving the hand, hand deformities and rheumatoid nodules. Further diagnostic criteria include seropositive rheumatoid factor and radiographic changes, e.g. erosive changes and periarticular decalcification (Table 34.1). Rheumatoid synovitis (pannus) destroys ligaments, tendons and joints, producing pain, deformity and loss of function. Zig-zag collapse is a typical rheumatoid feature, e.g. boutonnière (Fig. 34.54), swan neck (Fig. 34.55), and ulnar drift of the metacarpophalangeal joints with radial drift of the wrist. Simple activities of daily living, such as thumb pinch and opening jars, stress the weakened ligaments, thus producing greater deformities. Any treatment is primarily dictated by pain and disability, not deformity (Summary box 34.27).

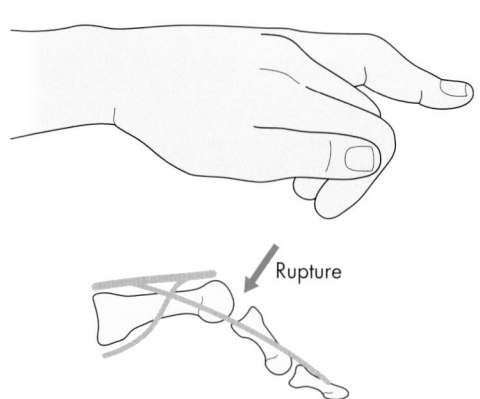

Figure 34.54 Boutonnière deformity.

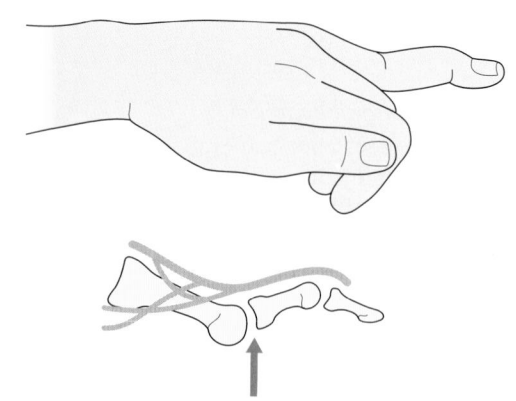

Figure 34.55 Swan neck deformity.

Boutonnière **is French for button-hole.**

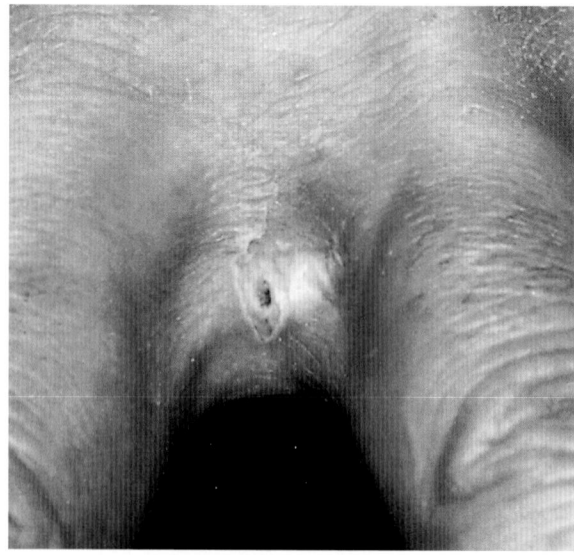

Figure 34.53 Pilonidal sinus in a barber.

Table 34.1 Radiographic differences between rheumatoid and osteoarthritis

Rheumatoid arthritis	Osteoarthritis
Periarticular osteoporosis/ subchondral erosions	Subchondral sclerosis and cysts
Periarticular soft-tissue swelling	Less pronounced swelling
Joint space narrowing	Joint space narrowing
Marginal erosions	Marginal osteophytes
Joint deformity/malalignment	Less pronounced deformities
Ankylosis	Less common ankylosis

Summary box 34.27

Deformities in rheumatoid arthritis

Fingers
- Swan neck deformity
- Boutonnière deformity
- Extensor tendon rupture
- Flexor tendon rupture
- Flexor synovitis

Metacarpophalangeal joints
- Flexion
- Ulnar deviation
- Subluxation, dislocation

Wrist
- Radial deviation
- Carpal supination
- Prominent ulnar head
- Extensor tenosynovitis

Management

Non-operative treatment is primarily directed at slowing progression and improving symptoms. Specific aids help patients to perform daily tasks, e.g. turning taps and opening jars, and splints improve symptoms during flare-ups, all of which serve to decrease further damage to weakened ligaments. The primary indications for operative treatment are: (1) pain relief; (2) functional improvement; (3) to prevent disease progression; and (4) cosmesis. In general, the hand and wrist should be treated after the shoulder and elbow, and the more reliable operations, e.g. wrist and thumb fusion, should be considered prior to less predictable operations, e.g. soft-tissue reconstructions, as discussed below.

1 Synovectomy can improve pain and increase function, even following tendon rupture, eliminate trigger finger and cure carpal tunnel syndrome in these patients.
2 Excision of the distal ulna may reduce the risk of extensor tendon rupture, protects the repair of ruptured extensor tendons and has a cosmetic benefit. Post-excision instability can be treated with soft-tissue stabilisation or ulna head arthroplasty.
3 Prosthetic arthroplasty of the wrist is relatively unpredictable, whereas metacarpophalangeal and interphalangeal joint replacement is more predictable for pain relief and functional improvement, with the proviso of functioning soft-tissue stabilisers, e.g. repairable/reconstructable collateral ligaments and tendons.
4 Arthrodesis of the wrist, thumb and some of the smaller joints provides good pain relief, and creates a stable axis against which other parts of the hand can function. For example, when the flexor pollicis longus tendon ruptures and is symptomatic, the most reliable solution is to arthrodese the interphalangeal joint of the thumb.
5 Tendon reconstructions. Some ruptured tendons cause significant morbidity, often solved by either a local joint fusion or tendon transfer, e.g. extensor indicis transfer for an extensor pollicis longus rupture. Multiple tendon ruptures can be treated by creating a mass tendon action, with side-to-side tendon suture or multiple tendon transfers.

Osteoarthritis

Wrist

The radiocarpal joint can develop primary or secondary osteoarthritis, e.g. after intra-articular trauma and infection (Fig. 34.56). Non-operative management begins with conservative measures, e.g. analgesia, splints, activity modification and activity aids. Operative management, following failed conservative treatment, includes wrist arthrodesis in 20° extension and radiocarpal arthroplasty, a much less predictable option than fusion. Specific and localised arthritis of the carpus, e.g. post-scaphoid fracture or scapholunate disruption, can be managed with either fragment excision or limited arthrodesis. Pisotriquetral arthritis, with clinical tenderness and confirmed by a 30° supinated lateral radiograph (Fig. 34.57), can be treated with rest, splintage, corticosteroid injection or pisiform excision as a last resort.

Hand

Commonly affected are the distal interphalangeal (Heberden's nodes), proximal interphalangeal (Bouchard's) and the thumb carpometacarpal joints (Fig. 34.58). Symptoms rarely correlate with appearance or radiographic appearances. Affected joint arthrodesis eliminates pain at the expense of motion, but function is often well tolerated. Joint arthroplasty (Fig. 34.59) is an option

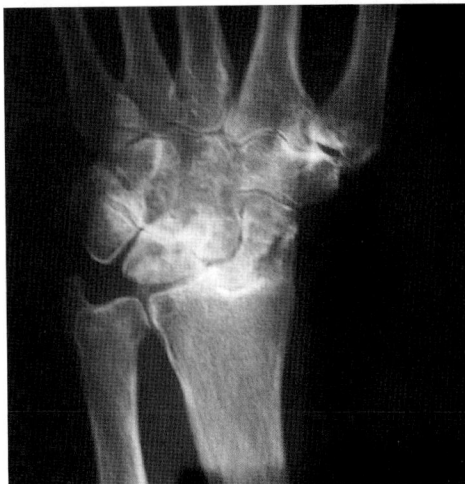

Figure 34.56 Radiocarpal osteoarthritis.

William Heberden (Snr), 1710–1801, a Physician who practised first in Cambridge, and from 1748 in London, England, described these nodes in 1802.
Charles Jacques Bouchard, 1837–1915, Physician, Dean of the Faculty of Medicine, Paris, France.

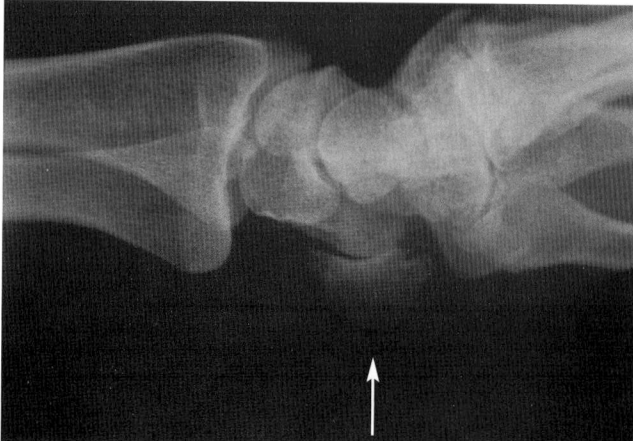

Figure 34.57 Pisotriquetral arthritis (arrow).

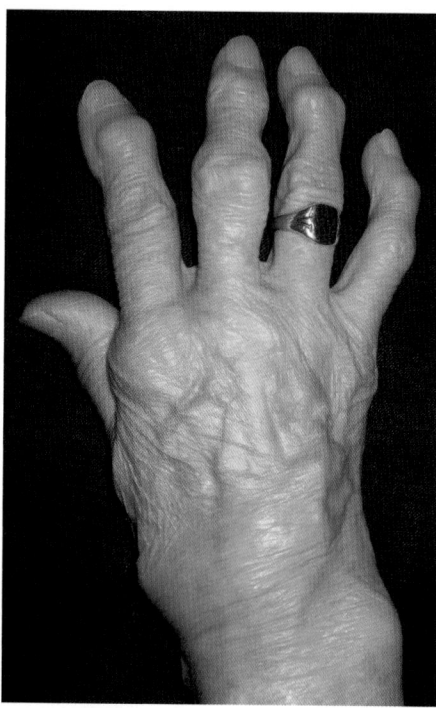

Figure 34.58 Osteoarthritis of the hand.

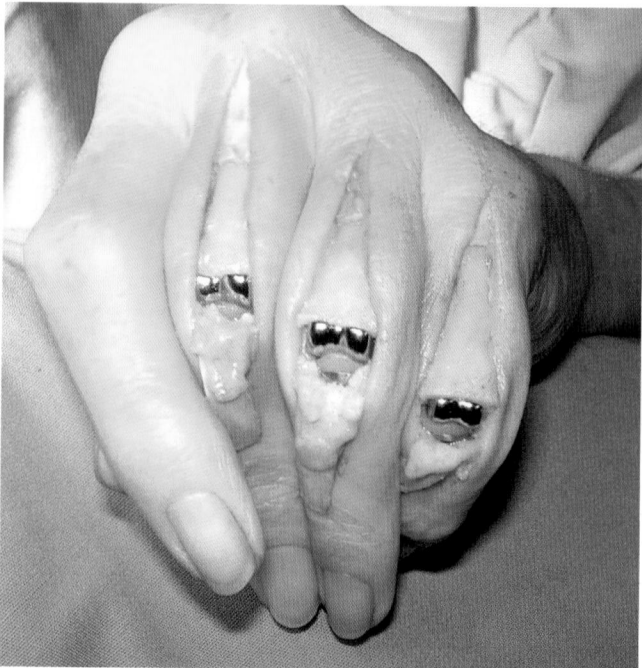

Figure 34.59 Proximal interphalangeal joint replacement.

Other arthritides

Gout

Gout commonly causes pain, joint redness and occasional tophi, and can be differentially diagnosed as septic arthritis. Serum urate and negative microscopic birefringence of joint aspirated sodium urate crystals are diagnostic.

Psoriasis

Psoriatic arthropathy of the hand and wrist is asymmetrical, with pitted nails and destructive radiographic features including a pencil in cup appearance.

Systemic lupus erythematosus

Systemic lupus erythematosus arthropathy is common in young females (15–25 years), with rheumatoid-like deformities, but without joint narrowing or erosions.

Dupuytren's contracture

An autosomal dominant trait with an association with Anglo-Saxon lineage, age, smoking, use of vibrating tools, pulmonary tuberculosis, epilepsy, acquired immunodeficiency syndrome (AIDS) and alcoholic cirrhosis. Clinical features include palmar nodules, skin puckering, cords of the palm and digits, flexion contractures of the digits, Garrod's knuckle pads [thickened skin on proximal interphalangeal joint (PIPJ) dorsum; Fig. 34.60]. Penile thickening and curvature (Peyronie's disease) and plantar

in some cases, as is trapezial excision for basal thumb arthritis (Summary box 34.28).

Summary box 34.28

Wrist and hand osteoarthritis (management)

■ Wrist arthrodesis – maintains acceptable function and improves pain
■ Distal interphalangeal joint fusion – maintains acceptable function
■ Excision of the trapezium – improves pain but decreases stability and reduces pinch strength

---

Baron Guillaume Dupuytren, **1777–1835**, Surgeon, Hôtel Dieu, Paris, France, described this condition in 1831.
Sir Archibald Edward Garrod, **1857–1936**, Regius Professor of Medicine, the University of Oxford, Oxford, England, described this condition in 1893.
Francois de la Peyronie, **1678–1747**, Surgeon to King Louis XIV of France, and Founder of the Royal Academy of Surgery, Paris, France.

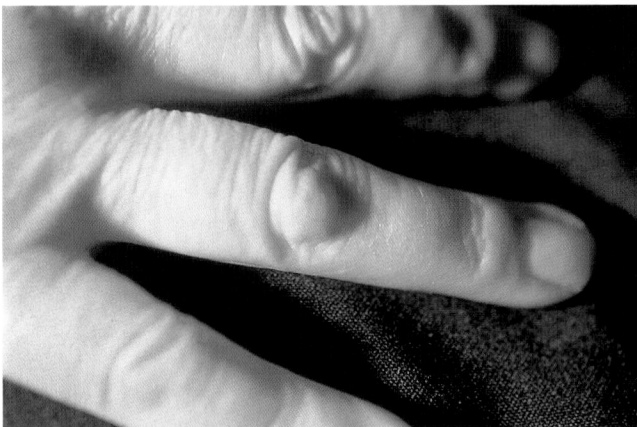

Figure 34.60 Garrod's knuckle pads.

thickening (Ledderhose's disease) are associations. Deformities that rapidly progress or are of functional consequence are indications for surgical correction. Surgical goals include deformity correction, protection of neurovascular bundles, which are often intricately entangled with the fibrous tissue, and skin coverage, often requiring Z-plasties (Fig. 34.61) (Summary box 34.29).

Summary box 34.29

Dupuytren's contracture

- Autosomal dominant inheritance (trait)
- Fibroblastic hyperplasia with resultant skin nodules, cords and deformities
- Management is surgical if rapidly progressive or functionally debilitating

---

Tendon disorders

Trigger finger

Triggering occurs in a finger or thumb when there is size disproportion between a flexor tendon and its sheath, often with a

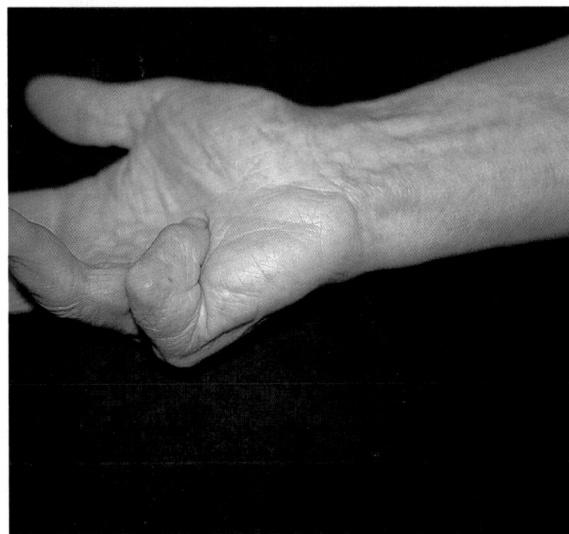

Figure 34.61 Dupuytren's disease.

Georg Ledderhose, **1855–1925, a German Surgeon, described this disease in 1894.**

nodule developing in the tendon (Fig. 34.62). Initial management is with a steroid injection into the sheath, followed by surgical tendon sheath release if non-responsive, with careful preservation of the digital nerves. Rheumatoid triggering may be due to synovitis or tendon nodules, and treatment is with synovectomy and excision of a slip of the flexor digitorum superficialis tendon without dividing the A1 pulley (Summary box 34.30).

Summary box 34.30

Trigger finger

- Flexor sheath thickening catches the flexor tendon/nodule
- Often painful with attempted straightening of the digit
- Initial management is with tendon sheath steroid injection
- Surgical release of the A1 pulley relieves the symptoms
- Paediatric trigger thumb and fingers frequently resolve spontaneously
- Rheumatoid triggering is treated by synovectomy, partial tendon excision, but sheath preservation

---

de Quervain's disease

This is believed to be an overuse pathology of the abductor pollicis longus and extensor pollicis brevis in the first dorsal wrist compartment, most common in middle-aged females, although pregnancy and inflammatory arthritides are also implicated. Dorsoradial wrist pain and tenderness, along with Finkelstein's test (pain with wrist and thumb ulnar deviation while the thumb is fully flexed), are diagnostic. Management ranges from non-steroidal anti-inflammatory analgesia, splintage and steroid injection to surgical release of the extensor retinaculum of the first compartment if the non-operative measures fail.

Neuropathies

Median nerve (carpal tunnel syndrome)

A common pathology presenting with painful wakening at night with tingling in the radial three and a half digits of the hand. There may also be weakness of the abductor pollicis brevis, leading to clumsiness with fine movements. Advanced cases may be observed to have thenar eminence wasting. Specific reliable clinical tests include: (1) Tinel's percussion over the carpal

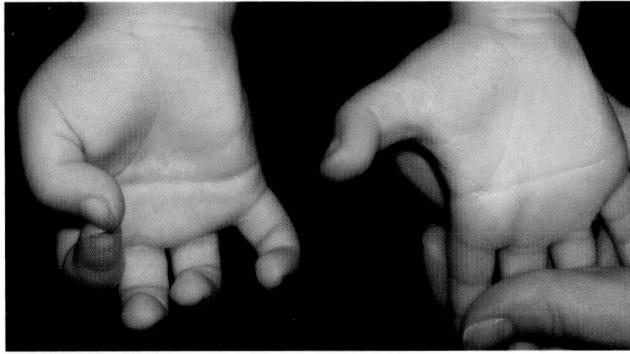

Figure 34.62 Trigger thumb in a child.

Fritz de Quervain, **1868–1940, Professor of Surgery, Berne, Switzerland, described this form of tenosynovitis in 1895.**

tunnel; (2) Phalen's test (reproduction of paraesthesia with full wrist flexion); and (3) carpal tunnel compression with full wrist flexion. Rarely does electrophysiological testing add to the clinical tests, but it is a good tool for tracking changes. Non-operative treatment modalities include night splintage of the wrist in extension and steroid injections into the carpal tunnel. Operative options serve to de-roof the carpal tunnel, thereby creating space for the nerve, without compression (Summary box 34.31).

Summary box 34.31

Carpal tunnel syndrome

- Night pain is common and relieved by shaking the hand
- Less common features are numbness and clumsiness
- Thenar wasting is an advanced sign
- Clinically, Tinel's and Phalen's tests are useful
- Electrophysiology is rarely useful beyond clinical tests
- Treatment options include splints, steroid injection and surgical decompression

---

Ulnar nerve (Guyon's tunnel syndrome)

Compression of the ulnar nerve due to ganglia, osteophytes or fractured hook of hamate can lead to hypothenar wasting (Fig. 34.63) and ulnar territory dysfunction, with preservation of dorsal sensation of the little finger and the ulnar half of the ring finger.

Kienböck's disease

Commonly thought to be an avascular phenomenon, the aetiology is unclear, but probably involves both ischaemia and microtrauma of the lunate. A possible correlation with a negative ulnar variance (relatively short ulna) has been suggested. The pathological stages progress from sclerosis to collapse and, finally, arthritis. Clinical presentation with wrist pain and weakness can be positively diagnosed with plain radiographs and MRI scans; the latter are able to detect very early lesions before they are visible on radiographs (Fig. 34.64). Early-stage treatment is with wrist splintage, with analgesia, or radial shortening to reduce compressive forces, thereby potentially decreasing the risk of disease progression. Advanced stage disease may require limited fusion to alleviate pain.

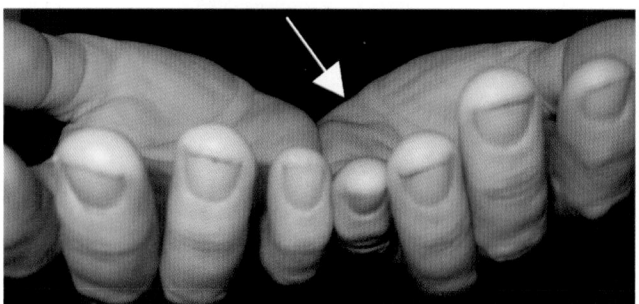

Figure 34.63 Ulnar nerve neuropathy with hypothenar wasting (arrow).

George S. Phalen, Orthopaedic Surgeon, the Cleveland Clinic, Cleveland, Ohio, OH, USA.

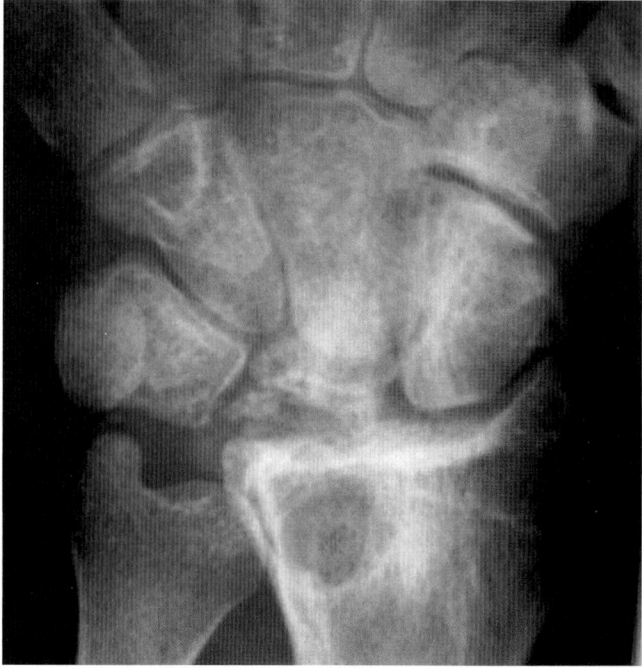

Figure 34.64 Kienböck's disease.

Ganglion cysts

These are the commonest hand swellings, causing patient concern and occasional discomfort. They are commonest on the wrist dorsum, but can be on the volar surface (Fig. 34.65). Physical examination reveals a smooth, fluctuant, transilluminable swelling, most which resolve following aspiration or being 'hit with a large book'. Surgical excision aims to remove the whole ganglion, including its connection to the underlying joint/sheath. Patients should be informed regarding the possibility of recurrence.

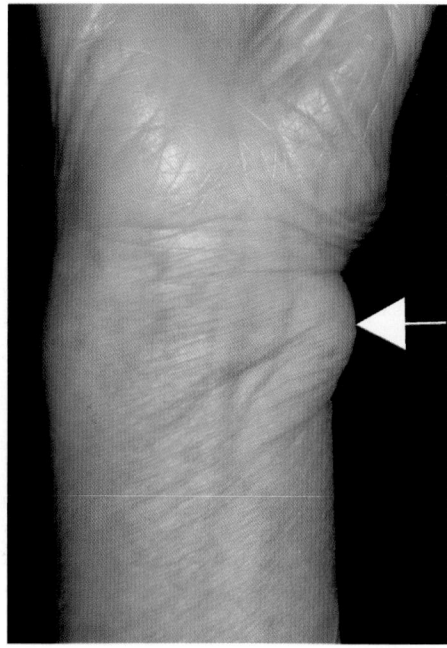

Figure 34.65 Volar wrist ganglion (arrow).

Congenital differences

The true rate of congenital malformations is difficult to assess, but a fundamental has to be correct identification (Fig. 34.66), communication of the findings to the parents and child, and management involving a multidisciplinary team. The classification by Swanson, later adopted by the International Federation of Societies of Surgeries of the Hand, is reproduced in Table 34.2.

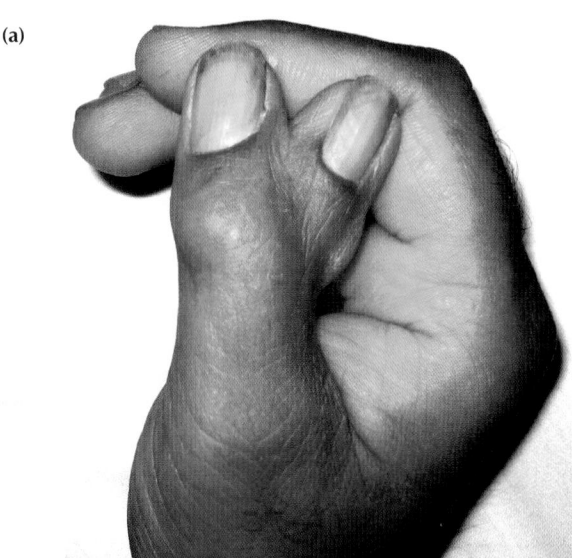

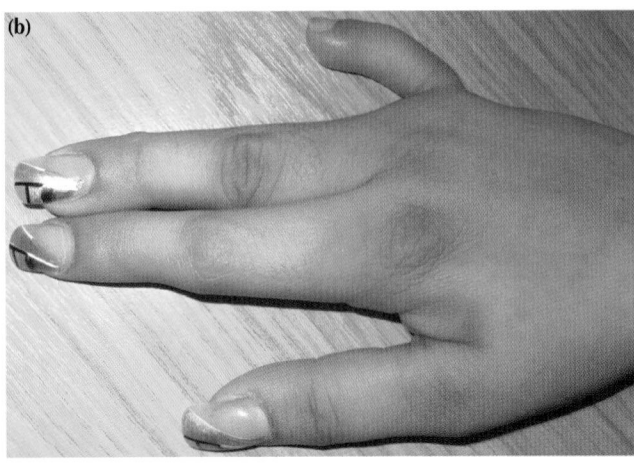

Figure 34.66 Congenital deformities in the hand. (a) Thumb duplication. (b) Absent fourth ray with constriction ring of the fifth digit.

Table 34.2 Congenital malformations (hand and wrist)

A	Defects in formation due to arrested development	(1) Transverse agenesis (2) Longitudinal agenesis (a) radial ray aplasia; (b) median ray aplasia; (c) ulnar ray aplasia (3) Thumb aplasia/hypoplasia
B	Defects in differentiation/separation	(1) Syndactyly (2) Camptodactyly (3) Clinodactyly (4) Kirner's deformity (5) Radioulnar synostosis
C	Duplications	(1) Supernumerary phalanges (2) Supernumerary digits (polydactyly) (Fig. 34.66)
D	Excess development/hyperplasia	Macrodactyly
E	Insufficient development/hypoplasia	Thumb hypoplasia
F	Constricting (amniotic) bands	Simple amniotic band syndrome
G	Generalised skeletal anomalies	Marfan's, Turner's and Down's syndromes

FURTHER READING

Lister, G. (1993) *The Hand* 3rd edn. Churchill Livingstone, Edinburgh.
Magee, D. (1997) *Orthopaedic Physical Assessment*, 3rd edn. W.B. Saunders, St. Louis.
Morrey, B. (2000) *The Elbow and its Disorders*, 3rd edn. W.B. Saunders, St Louis.
Nobuhara, K. (2003) *The Shoulder*, World Scientific, Singapore.

Antonin Bernard-Jean Marfan, **1858–1942, Physician, Hôpital des Enfants-Malades, Paris, France, described this syndrome in 1896.**
Henry Hubert Turner, **1892–1970, Professor of Medicine, the University of Oklahoma, OK, USA, described this syndrome in 1938.**
John Langdon Haydon Down (sometimes given as Langdon Down), **1828–1896, Physician, the London Hospital, London, UK, published his classification of aments in 1866.**

CHAPTER 34 | UPPER LIMB – PATHOLOGY, ASSESSMENT AND MANAGEMENT

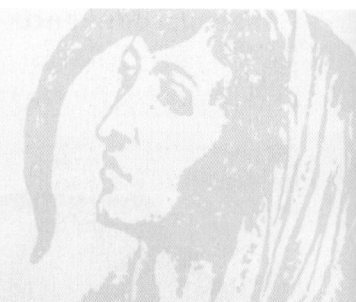

Hip and knee

THE HIP JOINT

Applied anatomy

The hip joint is a ball and socket joint formed by the head of the femur and the cup-shaped acetabulum. The femoral head and the acetabulum are covered with hyaline articular cartilage throughout, except at the fovea capitis on the femoral head and the base of the acetabulum (Fig. 35.1). The joint allows a considerable range of movement but is inherently stable because of its bony anatomy and the static and dynamic stabilisers. The static stabilisers are composed of the ligaments, the capsule and the labrum, whereas

the muscles running across the joint constitute the dynamic stabilisers. The joint is supported by the iliofemoral and pubofemoral ligaments anteriorly and the ischiofemoral ligament posteriorly. Another structure contributing to stability is the acetabular labrum, which is a triangular fibrocartilagenous structure attached to the rim of the acetabulum except at the base where it is replaced by the transverse ligament. The labrum helps in deepening the socket and also provides a negative suction effect in the joint, thereby enhancing stability. The ligamentum teres, which is attached to the acetabular notch and the transverse ligament and to the fovea capitis, may also have a role in providing stability to the joint. The short external rotator muscles posteriorly, the psoas muscle anteriorly and the abductors acting on the greater trochanter laterally are the dynamic stabilisers of the joint.

The femoral head derives its blood supply mainly from the retinacular branches of the medial circumflex femoral artery and there is a small contribution from the artery of the ligamentum teres (Summary box 35.1).

Summary box 35.1

Anatomy

- The hip joint is a ball and socket joint
- It is stabilised by static and dynamic stabilisers
- Static stabilisers include the capsule, ligaments and labrum
- Dynamic stabilisers comprise the muscles acting across the joint
- Blood supply to the femoral head is mainly derived from the medial circumflex femoral artery

---

Biomechanics of the hip joint

Biomechanics is the study of the forces acting on the living body and involves both kinetic and kinematic analysis. Kinematics is the study of motion without reference to forces whereas kinetics

Acetabulum   Capsule

Iliofemoral ligament

Capsule   Ligamentum teres

Interotrochanteric line

Figure 35.1 Anatomy of the hip joint.

relates to the effect of forces on bodies producing motion. Kinematic analysis of the hip joint shows that it allows a large range of movement; average degrees of movement in each direction are summarised in Summary box 35. 2.

Summary box 35.2

Range of movement in the hip joint

- Flexion – 115°
- Extension – 30°
- Abduction – 50°
- Adduction – 30°
- Internal rotation – 45°
- External rotation – 45°

Kinetic analysis reveals that forces as high as one and a half times body weight can be exerted across the hip joint during activities of daily living and this is primarily the result of contraction of muscles crossing the joint. The abductors, because of their insertion on the greater trochanter and the lateral side of the femur, help in supporting the pelvis when the patient stands on one leg and thereby form the basis of a Trendelenburg test (Fig. 35.2) (Summary box 35.3).

Summary box 35.3

Forces going through the hip joint

- Lifting leg from bed – one and a half times body weight
- Standing on one leg – three times body weight
- Running and jumping – 10 times body weight

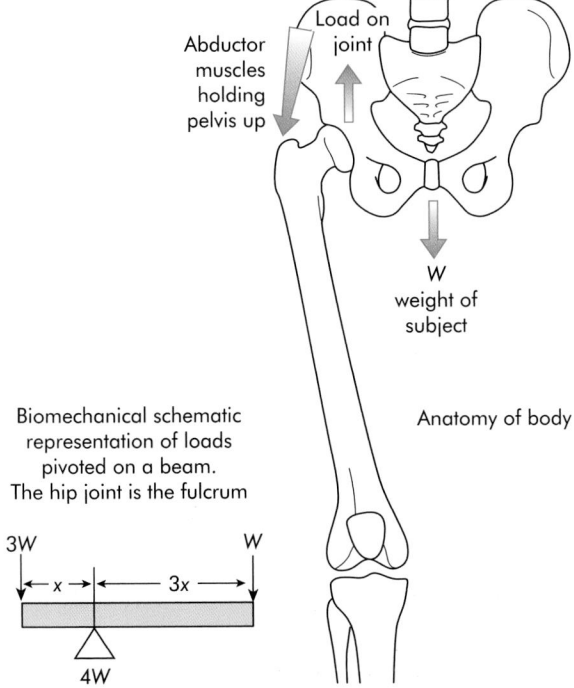

Figure 35.2 Load on the hip joint when subject (weighing W) stands on one leg. Hopping increases the load from 4 to 10W.

Friedrich Trendelenburg, **1844–1924, Professor of Surgery, Rostock (1875–1882), Bonn, (1882–1895) and Leipzig, Germany, (1895–1911).**

Conditions affecting the hip joint

The pathological state of the hip joint in the paediatric age group and secondary to trauma is covered in Chapters 38 and 27 respectively. This chapter focuses on the acquired pathological conditions in the adult.

Avascular necrosis

Introduction and aetiology

Avascular necrosis (AVN) or osteonecrosis of the femoral head occurs because of an interruption in the blood supply to the femoral head, which causes bone death. This leads to collapse of the femoral head with degenerative changes setting in the joint eventually. It can be idiopathic or secondary to other pathology. The most common cause is trauma and, of the non-traumatic causes, excessive alcohol intake and the use of systemic steroids are the most common (Summary box 35.4).

Summary box 35.4

Aetiology of AVN of the femoral head

- Sickle cell disease
- Haemoglobinopathies
- Caisson disease
- Hyperlipidaemia
- Systemic lupus erythematosus
- Gaucher's disease
- Chronic liver disease
- Antiphospholipid antibody syndrome
- Radiotherapy
- Chemotherapy
- Human immunodeficiency virus
- Hypercoagulable states (protein C and protein S deficiency)

Clinical features

AVN of the femoral head usually occurs in men aged from 35 to 45 and is bilateral in over 50% of patients. The patient is frequently asymptomatic in the early stages of the disease process and therefore a high index of suspicion is required for initial diagnosis. However, as the disease progresses the patient may complain of an ache in the groin and clinical examination may reveal an effusion, a limp and limitation of movement.

Investigations

A weight-bearing anteroposterior (AP) radiograph of the pelvis along with a lateral radiograph of the affected hip should be obtained. The classical features of AVN on radiography include increased sclerosis in the early stages, the crescent sign indicating subchondral bone resorption and, eventually, flattening in the later stages indicating a segmental head collapse (Fig. 35.3). However, radiographs may be normal in the early stages of the disease and, therefore, the most sensitive and specific way of investigating these patients is with magnetic resonance imaging (MRI). MRI allows the disease to be recognised before it is apparent on radiography as it enables bone oedema and marrow changes to be identified, as well

---

A caisson **is a watertight chamber used to protect construction workers during the building of underwater structures.**
Philippe Charles Ernest Gaucher, **1854–1918, Physician, Hôpital St. Louis, Paris, France, described familial splenic anaemia in 1882.**

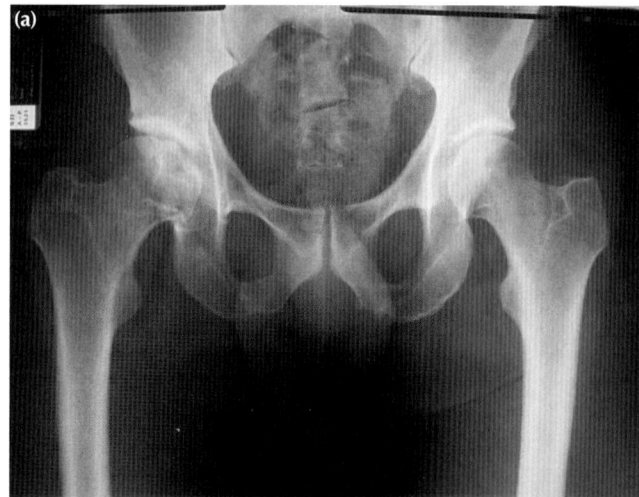

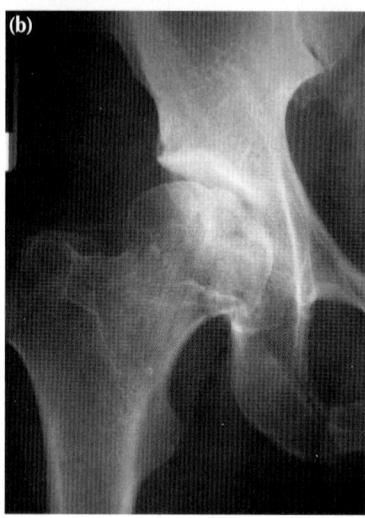

Figure 35.3 (a and b) Radiological appearance of avascular necrosis of the femoral head.

as accurately revealing the extent of involvement of the femoral head, thereby helping in prognosis (Fig. 35.4).

In 1985 Ficat classified the disease into five stages. In 1995 Steinberg modified this classification into seven stages based upon the type of radiological change on MRI and radiography (Table 35.1).

Table 35.1 Steinberg's classification of avascular necrosis of the femoral head

Stage	Description
0	Normal or non-diagnostic radiograph, bone scan or MRI
I	Normal radiograph, abnormal MRI or bone scan
II	Sclerosis and cysts
III	Subchondral collapse, crescent sign
IV	Flattening of the head, normal acetabulum
V	Acetabular involvement
VI	Obliteration of joint space

MRI, magnetic resonance imaging

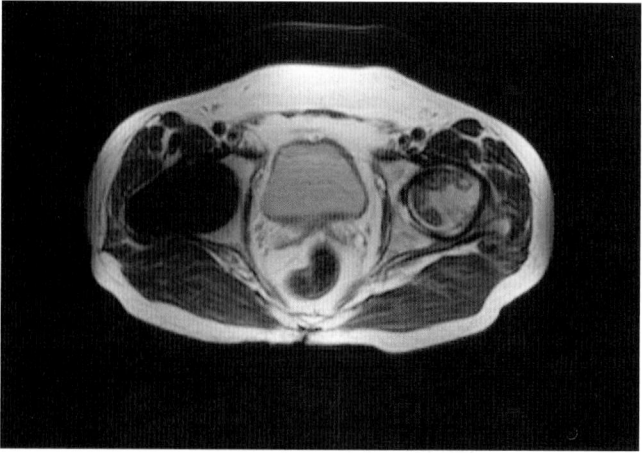

Figure 35.4 Magnetic resonance imaging scan of the hip joint showing avascular necrosis and the extent of involvement of the femoral head.

Stages I–IV are further divided into A, B or C depending upon the extent of involvement of the femoral head.

Treatment

The appropriate treatment of patients with AVN is dependent on the stage of the disease. Broadly, the seven stages can be divided into two groups: pre-collapse and collapse. In the pre-collapse group the principle is to preserve and preferably revascularise the femoral head, whereas in the collapse group the aim is to replace the femoral head. Conservative treatment in AVN usually leads to poor results and is therefore not recommended. The prognosis is largely dependent upon the extent of head involvement. Surgical treatment for the pre-collapse stage includes core decompression, which is aimed at relieving intravascular congestion in the femoral head and thereby pain. This can be achieved with or without bone grafting; a vascularised bone graft can also be used to enhance bone formation.

The post-collapse stage can be treated with a femoral osteotomy, which aims to transfer the weight-bearing area of the femoral head and thereby protect the collapsed segment; however, if degenerative change has set in, it is preferable to consider a replacement, either in the form of a resurfacing arthroplasty (Fig. 35.5) or a total joint replacement (Fig. 35.6) (Summary box 35.5).

Summary box 35.5

AVN of the femoral head

- Idiopathic AVN is the most common, followed by AVN secondary to trauma, alcohol abuse and the use of systemic steroids
- Patients are asymptomatic in the early stages and therefore a high index of suspicion is necessary for initial diagnosis
- MRI scans are essential for early diagnosis
- Treatment is based upon whether the patient presents in a pre-collapse or post-collapse stage
- The principle of treatment in the pre-collapse stage is to preserve the femoral head, whereas in the collapsed stage the aim is to replace it
- Prognosis is dependent upon the extent of head involvement

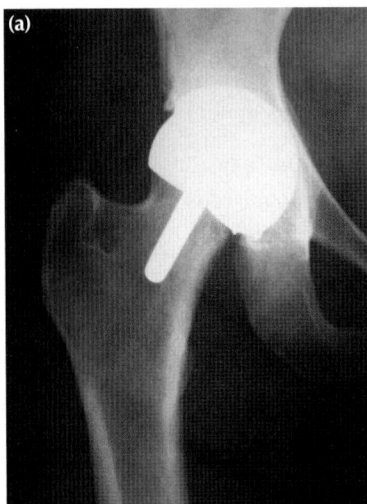

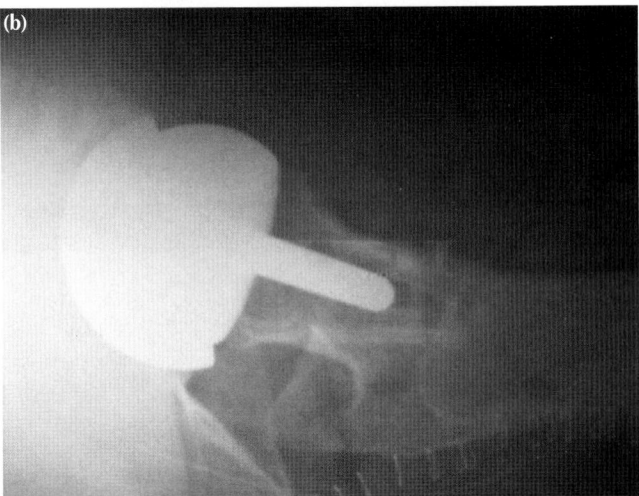

Figure 35.5 Anteroposterior (a) and lateral (b) radiographs of the hip showing a resurfacing arthroplasty.

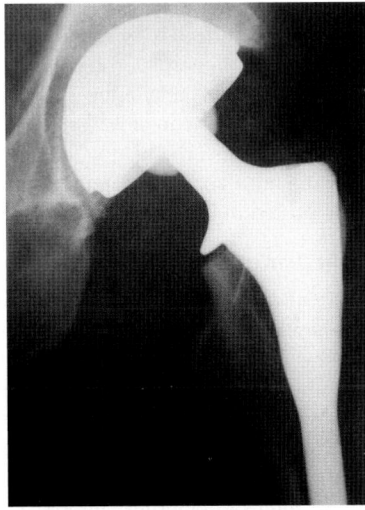

Figure 35.6 Radiograph showing an uncemented total hip replacement *in situ*.

Osteoarthritis

Introduction and aetiology

Osteoarthritis is a non-inflammatory condition that is characterised by progressive damage and loss of the articular cartilage. The progressive nature of the disease process is the result of the body's innate inability to regenerate hyaline articular cartilage. Osteoarthritis is termed as primary or secondary depending upon whether a predisposing cause can be identified for its development.

A multitude of factors including genetic, biochemical and mechanical influences have been implicated in the development of primary osteoarthritis. Despite these theories the exact mechanism for the development of primary osteoarthritis remains unknown and it is thereby termed idiopathic. However, recently, femoroacetabular impingement (FAI) has been proposed as an aetiological factor responsible for the development of primary osteoarthritis. The theory is based on the observation that, in certain hips with aberrant morphological features, an abnormal contact occurs between the proximal femur and the acetabular rim during the terminal range of movement, leading to lesions of the acetabular labrum and/or the adjacent acetabular cartilage. This type of repetitive abutment in due course leads to progressive loss of the articular cartilage and labral lesions because of a sheering stress, resulting in degenerative joint disease if the underlying cause is not addressed.

Secondary osteoarthritis usually develops following trauma, AVN of the femoral head, developmental dysplasia, slipped capital femoral epiphysis, Perthes' disease and enzymatic degradation of the articular cartilage in septic arthritis (Summary box 35.6).

Summary box 35.6

Aetiology of osteoarthritis

Primary
- Cause unknown, termed idiopathic
- Femoroacetabular impingement implicated as a possible cause

Secondary
- Trauma
- AVN
- Perthes' disease
- Developmental dysplasia of the hip
- Slipped capital femoral epiphysis
- Septic arthritis

Clinical features

The most consistent symptom is pain in the groin followed by limitation of movement. Groin pain occurs secondary to irritation of the obturator nerve, which crosses the hip joint. The pain may also radiate down to the knee joint and in some cases the only presenting feature may be a painful knee. In the early stages of the disease, pain is activity related but as the disease progresses the patient also complains of pain at rest. The patient frequently complains of night pain and may also find it difficult to get into a comfortable position while sleeping. Functionally, most have difficulty in putting on their shoes/socks and getting into and out of

Georg Clemens Perthes, **1869–1927**, Professor of Surgery, Tubingen, Germany, described osteochondritis of the femoral capital epiphysis in 1910.

a bath or a car. As the pain increases the joint gradually loses its movement because of muscle spasm, reluctance to move the joint and fibrosis of the capsule.

Clinical examination may reveal gluteal muscle wasting and an effusion with crepitus anteriorly. There may also be a limp with a positive Trendelenburg's sign. Shortening is a consistent feature and by the time that most patients present to the surgeon they are using a walking stick in the opposite hand for support. There is limitation of movement, particularly rotation in the earlier stages of the disease process; in the later stages of the disease the limb is in a position of fixed external rotation, adduction and flexion.

Investigations

Radiographs in the AP and lateral plane should be obtained (Fig. 35.7). The characteristic features include a reduction of joint space, which correlates to the loss of articular cartilage, sclerosis in the periarticular bone, which is a result of increased stresses on the surrounding bone, subchondral cyst and osteophyte formation. Eventually, a collapsed femoral head may also be evident. There may also be features suggesting previous trauma or surgical intervention, developmental dysplasia, Perthes' disease or slipped capital femoral epiphysis in cases of secondary osteoarthritis.

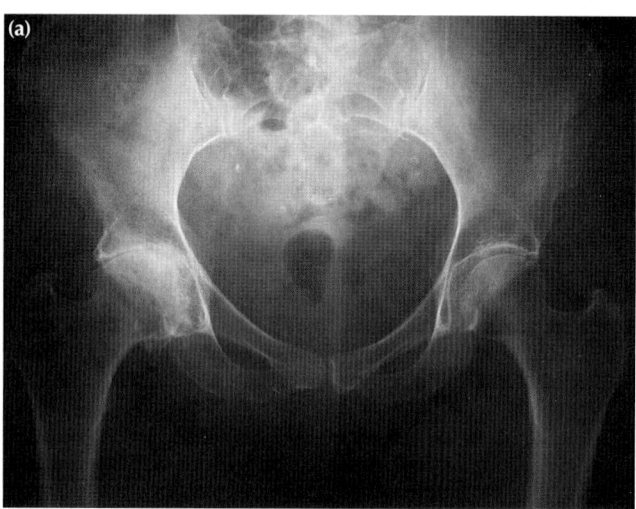

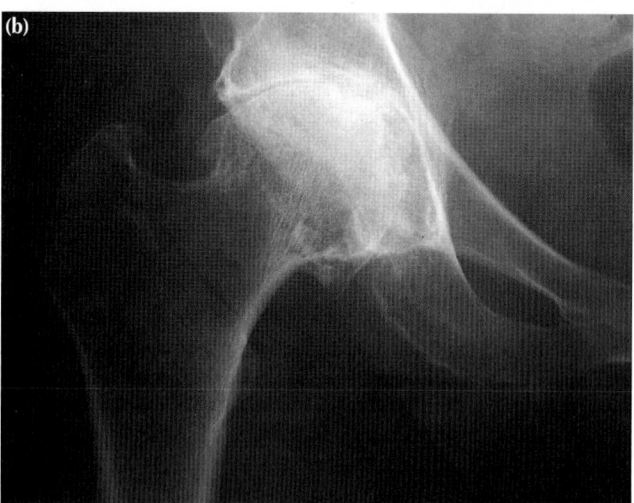

Figure 35.7 Anteroposterior (a) and enlarged anteroposterior (b) radiographs of the hip joint showing osteoarthritis.

Treatment

There is no specific pharmacological therapy for osteoarthritis; however, conservative treatment with non-steroidal anti-inflammatories, glucosamine sulphate, regular exercise and physiotherapy to improve muscle strength and range of movement, and modification of lifestyle with loss of weight does help. Also, patients are encouraged to use a walking stick in the opposite hand to offload the affected joint.

The indications for surgery are relentless pain, limitation of lifestyle and activities of daily living, and failure of conservative treatment. The surgical options include an arthrodesis, an osteotomy or a joint replacement in the form of a resurfacing arthroplasty or a total joint replacement. The choice of a particular procedure is based upon the age of the patient, the lifestyle and activity status and the stage of the disease. The principle behind each of these procedures is described in Surgical procedures of the hip.

The dictum that patients should receive a joint replacement only in the end stage of osteoarthritis when they are in severe pain and activities of daily living are markedly restricted has certainly evolved over the last decade. More and more joint replacements are now being performed based on limitation of lifestyle and individual needs, thereby making it a truly life-improving operation (Summary box 35.7).

> **Summary box 35.7**
>
> **Osteoarthritis of the hip**
>
> - Osteoarthritis is a non-inflammatory condition leading to progressive damage of the articular cartilage
> - The most consistent features are pain and limitation of movement
> - Characteristic radiological findings include reduction of joint space, joint-line sclerosis, subchondral cysts and osteophyte formation
> - Conservative treatment includes walking aids, non-steroidal analgesics, glucosamine and physiotherapy
> - Surgical options include an arthroscopy, an osteotomy, an arthrodesis and a joint replacement

Inflammatory arthritis

The hip joint can also be affected by inflammatory arthritides; however, this is not as common as osteoarthritis. This group includes rheumatoid arthritis, ankylosing spondylitis, gout and chondrocalcinosis, juvenile rheumatoid arthritis and systemic lupus erythematosus. Of these, rheumatoid arthritis and ankylosing spondylitis are the most common conditions affecting the hip joint. These are discussed in Chapter 37.

Labral tears, articular cartilage and soft tissue injury

The hip joint is frequently a source of pain following injury in sport. Most of these injuries went undiagnosed in the past because of the unavailability of appropriate imaging techniques and also a lack of interest in and knowledge of sports medicine. However, this trend has changed following the recognition of sports and exercise medicine as a specialty in itself and the introduction of contrast-enhanced MRI and arthrograms.

A spectrum of injuries including muscle contusions and strains, acetabular labrum and ligamentum teres tears, and articular cartilage injuries can now be diagnosed and managed effectively arthroscopically. A detailed account of these injuries is covered in Chapter 32.

Surgical procedures

Osteotomies around the hip

The goal of an osteotomy around the hip is to restore anatomy to as normal as possible and redistribute forces evenly across the joint, thereby eliminating excessive point loading. This can be achieved by performing an osteotomy on the femoral or the acetabular side, depending upon the desired goal, e.g. an excessive valgus neck–shaft angle and an uncovered femoral head on the lateral aspect can be corrected by carrying out a varus femoral osteotomy. Similarly, a redirection osteotomy on the acetabular side can also be performed to improve coverage of the femoral head. The common indications for an osteotomy around the hip include:

- developmental dysplasia of the hip;
- Perthes' disease;
- osteoarthritis in a young patient;
- slipped upper femoral epiphysis;
- AVN.

Ideally, an osteotomy should be considered in a young patient who maintains a good range of movement of the hip and has minimal symptoms. Radiographs should show a reasonable amount of joint space and thorough preoperative planning is essential to assess whether the desired position can be achieved postoperatively. Three-dimensional computerised tomography (CT) scans may be essential for appropriate preoperative planning. Osteotomies may also be performed when arthritic change has set in – these are termed salvage osteotomies.

Arthrodesis of the hip

Arthrodesis or fusion of the hip is an uncommon operation. It is generally reserved for young patients with severe osteoarthritis who have heavy manual jobs and in whom joint replacements would fail fairly quickly. The aim is to achieve a painless joint by fusing it in a functional position, which is about 30° of flexion, 15° of external rotation and 5° of abduction. This can be achieved by an intra-articular dynamic hip screw or by an extra-articular plate with screws.

Several problems can occur following an arthrodesis including excessive loading of the ipsilateral knee, the contralateral hip and the spine. In addition, degenerative change in these joints in the long term is the rule rather than the exception. Therefore, any pathology in these joints preoperatively does preclude an arthrodesis.

Joint replacement

Osteoarthritis of the hip affects 10–25% of those over the age of 65 years and over 50 000 total hip replacements are performed annually in the UK. The results of surgery are encouraging. In good hands, up to 95% of patients will have a well-functioning hip at 10 years. In the best series, 85% will still be functioning at 20 years, although many are still in place only because the patients are too old and infirm for them to be changed. Following surgery the quality of life approaches normal for a healthy individual. Pain is reduced, mobility increases and sleep as well as social and sexual function is improved. Nevertheless, with the ever-increasing number of patients with joint replacements, the number of patients whose replacement has failed or worn out and who now want a revision, or even a revision of a revision, is rising rapidly.

The ideal joint replacement – principles and design

The decision of which implant to use is a difficult one as there are over 100 available on the market. However, the decision process can be made easier by considering the elementary features of an ideal joint replacement. The main purpose of implanting a joint in the body is to allow a mechanical device to take over the function of the native joint effectively. Therefore, for any joint replacement to be successful it should be biocompatible and made of inert materials. It should be well fixed to the host tissue and the design should incorporate features to allow a good range of movement. The bearing surfaces should produce the least amount of friction and the material released from the bearing surface should be non-toxic and non-carcinogenic. Finally, any joint implanted should ideally outlive the patient (Summary box 35.8).

Summary box 35.8

Features of an ideal joint replacement

- Biocompatible
- Made of relatively inert materials
- Well fixed to the host tissue and allowing a good range of movement
- Bearing surfaces should be designed to minimise friction
- Material released from the bearings should be non-toxic
- Should ideally outlive the patient

Materials

Most of the implants available currently are made of metal. The metals commonly used are stainless steel, titanium and cobalt–chrome alloy; of these, cobalt–chrome alloy is the most common. The advantages of using a metal alloy are that the implants are able to withstand high loads, are relatively inert and can be manufactured easily. However, they do pose problems in terms of ion release if they are used as bearing surfaces. Also, corrosion can be a cause for concern if two dissimilar metals are used.

Bearing surface

The total hip replacement designed by Charnley uses a joint surface of metal on high-density polyethylene. This is described as a hard-on-soft bearing surface and has a high coefficient of friction. High-density polyethylene has good shock-absorbing properties but does wear slowly over the years, producing small particles that can stimulate an inflammatory response in the joint, which can ultimately be responsible for aseptic loosening of the joint. The stimulated macrophages resorb bone and may also stimulate osteoclasts to do the same. There has therefore been a move towards using bearing surfaces that do not produce wear particles and the concept of hard-on-hard bearing is quite popular currently.

Ceramic femoral heads bearing on polyethylene cups have far

Sir John Charnley, **1911–1982, Professor of Orthopaedic Surgery, University of Manchester, Manchester, England.**

lower friction, but ceramic femoral heads on ceramic acetabular cups have the lowest friction of all. They are, however, very difficult and very expensive to manufacture. Metal-on-metal bearings also have a low coefficient of friction and produce small-sized wear particles. These bearing surfaces were frequently used in the past but earned a bad reputation because of a high rate of loosening secondary to manufacturing problems. A summary of the advantages and disadvantages of each bearing surface is provided in Table 35.2.

Fixation

Artificial joints must bed securely into the bones each side of the joint so that the implant does not work loose. This can be achieved with the help of cement or biological interdigitation between the prosthesis and bone (Table 35.3).

Traditionally, hip replacements were fixed into a bed of polymethylmethacrylate (PMMA) cement (Fig. 35.8a). The cement acted as a grout (spacer) between the implant and the bone and provided a static form of fixation. Cement does not possess the ability to remodel and it therefore loosens in time as the bone continues to remodel. Also, as the cement sets, some of the monomer is released into the patient's bloodstream, which can cause a drop in blood pressure.

On the other hand, biological fixation can be achieved by providing a rough surface on the prosthesis for bone to grow into the prosthesis or by bone growing onto the prosthesis; this is a dynamic form of fixation (Fig. 35.8b). This type of biological fixation can also be enhanced by coating the surface of the prosthesis with hydroxyapatite. Hydroxyapatite is an osteoconductive agent and bone essentially binds to it.

Surgical approaches to the hip, postoperative course and complications

Once a decision has been made on which implant to use, the operation can be performed via a posterior approach, an anterolateral or Hardinge approach, a trochanteric osteotomy or an anterior approach (Table 35.4). Each approach has its own

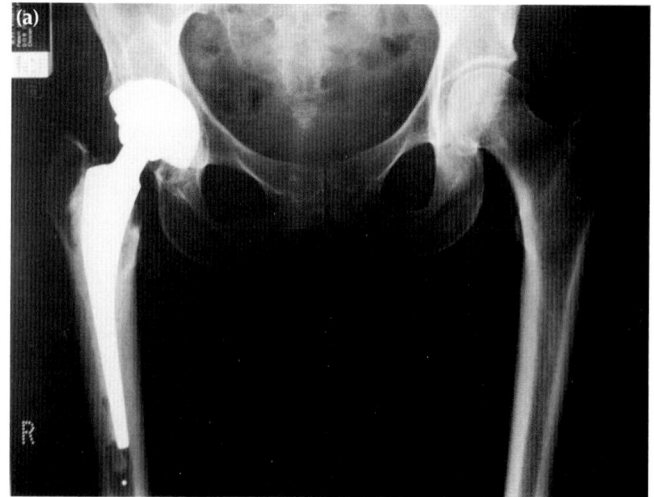

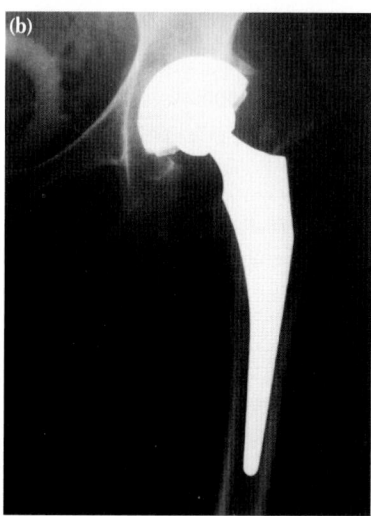

Figure 35.8 Radiographs of a cemented (a) and non-cemented (b) femoral component.

Table 35.2 Bearing surfaces

Type of bearing	Advantages	Disadvantages
Metal on polyethylene	Proven efficacy; easy to manufacture; cheap	High friction; high wear rates; wear particles excite an inflammatory response, which leads to osteolysis
Ceramic on polyethylene	Lower friction	Expensive; ceramic fracture can be a problem
Ceramic on ceramic	Low friction	Very expensive; ceramic can fracture
Metal on metal	Lowest friction	Bad reputation as has failed in the past; metal ion release is a problem; expensive

Table 35.3 Fixation of implants

Method of fixation	Advantages	Disadvantages
Cemented	Implant does not need to fit cavity exactly; well-proven results	Cement gets hot; fragments may cause third-body wear and stimulate aseptic loosening; difficult to remove at revision; non-biological and static fixation
Uncemented	No cement needed; fixation more secure; dynamic and biological fixation	Fit must be perfect; osseous integration does not always work; expensive

Table 35.4 Surgical approaches to the hip

Surgical approach	Anatomical interval and muscle
Posterior	Along the fibres of the gluteus maximus
Anterolateral/Hardinge	Parts of the gluteus medius and minimus are reflected off the greater trochanter
Anterior	Interval is developed between the sartorius and rectus femoris and the tensor fascia lata
Trochanteric	A trochanteric osteotomy is required

advantages and disadvantages and the description of each approach is beyond the scope of this chapter; however, the kind of approach used by any surgeon eventually depends on training and experience. There is also a move towards minimally invasive surgery and shortening the size of the incision. The proponents of this concept have described a two-incision approach wherein the femoral component is inserted via a small incision around the greater trochanter and the acetabular component via an incision in the groin. Although the concept is attractive no long-term benefits have been conclusively shown over the conventional technique. Eventually, whichever approach is taken, it is essential to be able to implant a prosthesis that has the correct offset, a correct centre of rotation, the correct component orientation and which equalises leg lengths and is able to relieve the patient's symptoms.

The preoperative preparation of the patient is covered in Chapter 13. The postoperative course involves a 5- to 7-day stay in hospital where the patient is encouraged to mobilise independently. Before discharge, the occupational therapist assesses the patient's home and arranges for any modifications that may be required to assist the patient, e.g. a raised toilet seat. Following discharge, physiotherapy is continued for a period of 6–8 weeks and the patient is advised to continue their own exercises subsequently. The clips/sutures are removed 2 weeks following discharge. The patient is advised to wear thromboembolic deterrent (TED) stockings and continue with oral anticoagulation for 6 weeks following surgery. Follow-up visits are arranged at 6 weeks, 3 months, 6 months and then yearly post-surgery. Although hip replacement is a fairly successful and safe procedure, it does have associated complications. A comprehensive list of complications is given in Summary box 35.9.

Summary box 35.9

Complications of total hip replacement

Intraoperative complications
- Nerve injury – sciatic, femoral and obturator
- Vascular injury – femoral vein and artery
- Femoral fracture

Postoperative complications
- Deep vein thrombosis and pulmonary embolism
- Infection
- Dislocation (Fig. 35.9)
- Leg length inequality
- Heterotopic ossification
- Implant loosening

Revision total hip replacement

Revision of a total hip replacement is required if the patient is symptomatic secondary to implant loosening (Fig. 35.10), recurrent dislocations or a periprosthetic fracture. Loosening of the implant can occur because of an infection or as a result of aseptic osteolysis caused by an inflammatory response secondary to particle wear.

In the initial stages of loosening the patient complains of pain, which is experienced mainly on weight-bearing. A history of infection in the immediate postoperative period may suggest infection as a cause of implant loosening. The patient should be investigated with a full blood count, an evaluation of erythrocyte sedimentation rate and C-reactive protein, appropriate radiography, a radioisotope scan and a synovial fluid and tissue biopsy to determine whether the loosening is secondary to an infection.

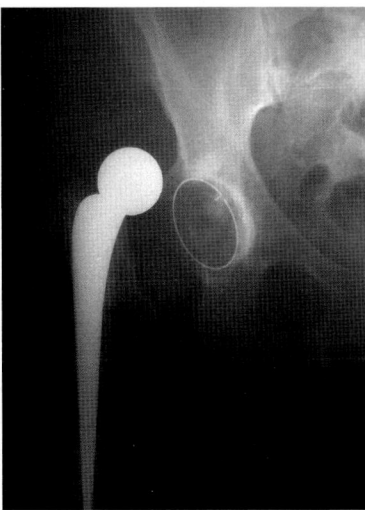

Figure 35.9 Dislocation of the hip.

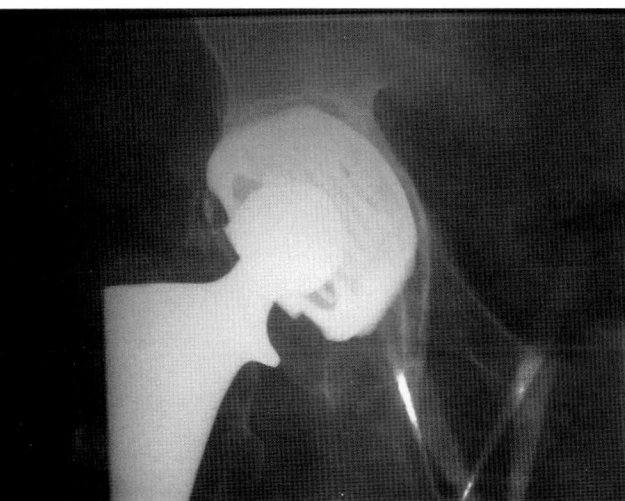

Figure 35.10 Acetabular loosening.

CHAPTER 35 | HIP AND KNEE

Once the definitive diagnosis has been made, a revision is planned. If the loosening is secondary to infection, a two-staged revision is usually preferred. The first stage consists of removal of the native implant, a thorough debridement and implantation of an antibiotic-loaded cement spacer with institution of appropriate antibiotics for a period of 6 weeks or more. Following this a second-stage procedure, which involves removal of the cement spacer and implantation of the new prosthesis, is performed.

In the case of aseptic loosening, revision is performed as a single-stage procedure. If there has been a significant amount of bone loss, bone grafting may be required and the patient should be advised of this preoperatively. The results following a revision hip replacement are not as good as those following a primary total hip replacement and the rate of complications, especially dislocation, is also higher.

THE KNEE

Applied anatomy

The knee joint is a complex hinge joint formerly described as *ginglymus* (meaning hinge). The joint is inherently unstable because of its articular morphology but stability is provided by a number of ligaments that hold the joint together and form the static stabilisers. The muscles acting across the joint form the dynamic stabilisers.

The medial and lateral menisci are fibrocartilagenous structures that help in deepening the joint surface and also aid shock absorption (Fig. 35.11).

The medial and the lateral collateral ligaments prevent trans-lation in the mediolateral plane. The medial collateral ligament is a broad, flat, membranous band situated near the posterior aspect, which is attached to the medial condyle of the femur superiorly and to the medial condyle and the medial surface of the tibia inferiorly. The ligament is composed of a superficial and a deep layer, the deep layer being intimately adherent to the medial meniscus. The fibular or the lateral collateral ligament, on the other hand, is a rounded, fibrous, cord-like structure, which is attached to the lateral femoral condyle superiorly and to the head of the fibula inferiorly.

The cruciate ligaments are situated in the centre of the joint, nearer to the posterior than the anterior surface. The anterior cruciate ligament is attached to the tibial spine and passes upwards, backwards and laterally to attach to the medial and posterior aspect of the lateral femoral condyle. Its primary function is to prevent anterior translation of the tibia on the femur. The posterior cruciate ligament arises from the posterior aspect of the tibia and passes upwards, forwards and medially to insert on the anterior aspect of the medial femoral condyle. Its main function is to prevent posterior translation of the femur on the tibia.

The joint is covered by a synovial membrane throughout and has a number of bursae surrounding it, which are frequently the focus of inflammation and infection.

The dynamic stabilisers of the knee joint consist of the quadriceps femoris crossing it anteriorly; the biceps femoris and popliteus laterally; the sartorius, gracilis, semitendinosus and semimembranosus medially; and the popliteus posteriorly (Summary box 35.10).

> **Summary box 35.10**
>
> **Anatomy of the knee joint**
>
> - The joint is a complex hinge joint
> - It is inherently unstable because of its articular and bony anatomy
> - Stability is provided by static and dynamic stabilisers
> - Static stabilisers include the capsule, the menisci, the collateral ligaments and the cruciate ligaments
> - Dynamic stabilisers consist of the muscles crossing the joint

Biomechanics

Axes of the lower limb

The anatomical axes of the femur and tibia are along their respective shafts. However, the mechanical axis of the lower limb runs from the centre of the femoral head to the centre of the ankle. It passes just medial to the medial tibial spine in the knee. The anatomical axis of the lower limb is in 6° valgus compared with the mechanical axis. It is important to understand this concept because, when replacing the knee, the aim is to recreate the correct mechanical axis and not the anatomical axis (Fig. 35.12).

Kinematics and kinetics

The knee joint allows movement mainly in one plane, i.e. sagittal with a limited amount of rotation, which varies with the degree of flexion. As the flexion increases, so does the range of rotation. Normal range of movement is between 10° of hyperextension and 130° of flexion. Kinematic studies reveal that movement about the knee joint is a complex combination of rolling and sliding; in

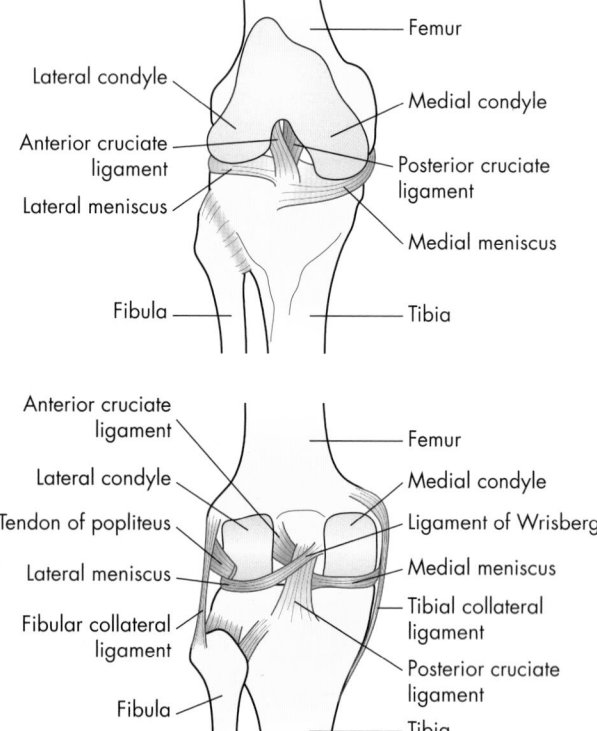

Figure 35.11 Anatomy of the knee joint.

Ginglymus **from the Greek** *gigglymos*, **a hinge.**

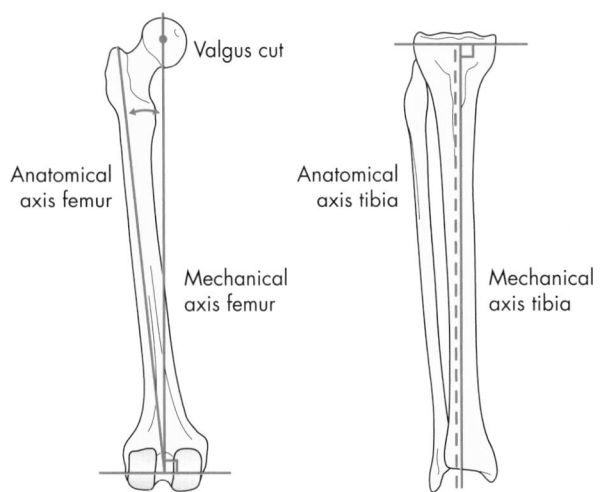

Figure 35.12 Axes of the lower limb. Anatomical and mechanical axes are coincident. Adapted from Miller, M. *Review of Orthopaedics, 4th edn.* 2004, Elsevier, Philadelphia. By kind permission of the publishers.

addition, the femur internally rotates around the larger medial femoral condyle during the last 15° of extension.

Kinetic analysis reveals that loads as high as three times body weight are transmitted while level walking, and up to four times body weight while climbing stairs. The patella, apart from protecting the knee joint during injury, also helps in extension; it increases the lever arm and aids in load distribution. It has a thick articular cartilage that is designed to bear loads of up to seven times body weight while squatting and jogging. While descending stairs the compressive forces between the patella and femur are in the range of two to three times body weight (Summary box 35.11).

Summary box 35.11

Biomechanics of the knee joint

- The anatomical axis of the lower limb is 6° valgus to the mechanical axis
- The main range of movement of the knee joint is in the sagittal plane with minimal rotation, which increases as the flexion increases
- Three to four times body weight is transmitted via the knee while level walking and climbing stairs
- The patella has the thickest articular cartilage and loads as high as seven times body weight are transmitted while squatting or jogging

---

Conditions affecting the knee joint

The pathology of the knee joint secondary to trauma, in sporting injuries and in the paediatric age group is covered in Chapters 27, 32 and 38 respectively. This section deals with acquired pathology in the adult.

Osteoarthritis of the knee

The knee is one of the most common joints to be affected by osteoarthritis and the incidence is higher in women than in men. At least 3% of women over the age of 75 years are affected by the

disease. Secondary osteoarthritis in the knee may occur because of a previous fracture, a neuropathic joint, osteonecrosis or a previous meniscectomy. Primary osteoarthritis of the knee, as in the hip, is due to a multitude of causes and is therefore termed idiopathic.

Clinical features and investigations

Most patients present with pain that is fairly well localised to the compartment involved. In the initial stages of the disease the pain is related to activity but as the disease progresses the pain changes to a constant ache that can disturb the patient's sleep as well. Pain also occurs on changing position, i.e. getting up from a sitting position, and can be severe on weight-bearing. The patient's walking speed and distance are markedly reduced and climbing stairs can be cumbersome.

Clinical examination reveals that the patient has an antalgic gait and uses a walking aid. Examination of the knee per se may reveal a varus or a valgus deformity with a swelling. A varus deformity seems to occur more frequently in the osteoarthritic knee whereas the valgus deformity is a constant feature of the rheumatoid knee. The range of movement, especially extension, is restricted and the knee may be unstable in the sagittal or coronal plane. Crepitus is felt throughout the range of movement. It is essential to assess the distal pulses in these patients because of the higher incidence of peripheral vascular disease in this age group.

Weight-bearing AP and lateral radiographs along with a view of the patellofemoral joint should be obtained. The radiographs reveal joint-space narrowing, subchondral sclerosis, subchondral cysts and osteophytes (Fig. 35.13). In advanced stages, lateral subluxation of the tibial plateau on the femur may also be seen.

Treatment

Conservative treatment is commenced with advice on modification of lifestyle, losing weight and exercising to improve the quadriceps. Protective weight-bearing (walking aids) and using knee braces can be beneficial in relieving pain. Non-steroidal anti-inflammatories are helpful in reducing inflammation in acute stages and glucosamine sulphate has also been found to be useful in improving symptoms.

If conservative treatment fails then surgery must be considered. Surgical options include an arthroscopy if the patient complains of pain in a specific compartment secondary to a degenerate meniscal tear, an osteotomy, an arthrodesis, or a total

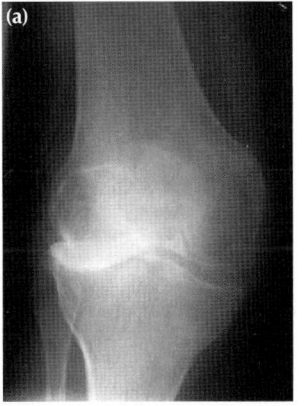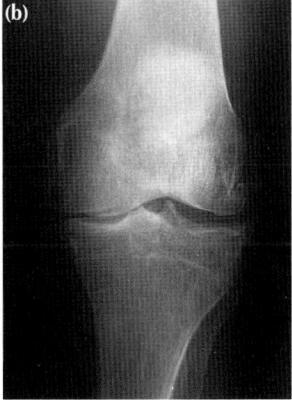

Figure 35.13 Osteoarthritis of the knee.

or unicompartmental knee replacement; the basis behind each of the above-mentioned surgical options is discussed in Surgical procedures, below (Summary box 35.12).

Summary box 35.12

Osteoarthritis of the knee

- More common in elderly women
- Activity-related pain is the initial symptom
- Clinical examination reveals a deformity with restriction in range of movement
- Radiographs show joint-space narrowing, subchondral cysts and sclerosis, and osteophytes
- Treatment is conservative in the initial stages followed by a joint replacement in the end-stage of the disease process

---

Surgical procedures

Arthroscopy of the knee

Arthroscopy of the knee has a well-established place in the diagnosis and treatment of cartilage, meniscal and ligament injuries. However, it should be noted that arthroscopy is not a substitute for a good clinical examination; the importance of getting a thorough history and eliciting appropriate clinical signs cannot be overemphasised.

The most common indications for performing an arthroscopy of the knee joint are summarised in Summary box 35.13.

Summary box 35.13

Indications for arthroscopy of the knee joint

- Meniscal tear – for repair or resection
- Anterior and posterior cruciate ligament tears – for reconstruction
- Loose bodies – for removal
- Osteochondritis dissecans
- Septic arthritis – for debridement and washout
- Inflammatory arthritis – for assessment of the joint and occasionally synovectomy
- Osteoarthritis – for assessment, resection of degenerate tears of the meniscus and a washout
- Diagnosis of unexplained knee pain; also offers the possibility of obtaining a synovial biopsy
- Tibial plateau fractures; allows intraoperative assessment of the articular surface while fixing these difficult fractures

---

Osteotomies about the knee

Degenerative arthritis can lead to varus or valgus deformities in the knee joint. This leads to an imbalance in the stresses exerted on the affected compartment, which further predisposes to acceleration of degenerative changes in that compartment. In this situation, the goal of an osteotomy is to redistribute the forces equally, thereby unloading the involved compartment by correcting the deformity.

The ideal patient for an osteotomy is a well-motivated young adult who is not overweight, who has disease limited to a single compartment and who has a good preoperative range of movement.

The osteotomies commonly performed are a closing-wedge high tibial osteotomy on the lateral side or an opening-wedge tibial osteotomy on the medial side for a varus knee. For the valgus knee, if the deformity is mild, correction can be achieved by a varus-producing osteotomy on the tibial side; if the deformity is larger, e.g. more than 12–15°, a supracondylar osteotomy is essential on the femoral side.

Arthrodesis of the knee

Arthrodesis of the knee is reserved for a neuropathic joint; as a salvage procedure for an infected joint following a total knee replacement or septic arthritis; for traumatic arthritis in a young patient; or for malignant lesions affecting the knee joint. However, in clinical practice the most common indication is a failed total knee replacement.

Arthrodesis can be achieved by the intramedullary method using a long intramedullary nail or via an extramedullary method using external fixation and compression. The final preferred position of an arthrodesed knee is about 5–8° of valgus, 0–10° of external rotation and 10–15° of flexion to allow clearance of the foot while walking.

Total knee replacement

The rapid rise in the number of total hip replacements has been followed by a similar rise in the number of total knee replacements as this operation is now found to have a similar success rate to that of a total hip replacement. In the knee, the medial compartment (the load-bearing part of the joint) seems to be particularly susceptible to osteoarthritis in old age. In rheumatoid arthritis the lateral compartment of the knee is more commonly affected. In all cases, the patellofemoral and the opposite tibiofemoral compartment eventually become involved, producing the end-stage of tricompartmental disease.

The goals of a total knee replacement are to alleviate pain and correct deformity. The principles of an ideal joint replacement remain the same as in the hip; however, the design features are significantly different in the knee compared with the hip.

In its simplest form, the knee replacement can be considered as a resurfacing procedure, in which the articular surfaces of the tibia and the femur are replaced with metal and the menisci are replaced by a polyethylene insert (Fig. 35.14). The natural knee joint is not congruent (one surface does not fit within the other). Therefore, to obtain stability the artificial knee joint needs to be restrained. If an artificial knee is completely restrained, e.g. a hinge knee, then the translational loads that occur within the knee on movement are transmitted directly to the implant–bone interface and this results in early loosening. On the other hand, if the artificial knee is only partially restrained by making the tibial component slightly concave, then the femoral component slides as well as rolls on the tibial component. This allows the normal movements to occur within the joint but creates point loading (high stresses at a specific point) at the tibiofemoral joint surface. Most of the condylar knee replacements on the market are currently of the latter design; however, it is a compromise in trying to create as much congruency as possible (to spread the load) with as much freedom of movement as possible (to minimise implant–bone interface loading).

Technically, the goals of a knee replacement are to achieve the correct mechanical alignment, a good balance of the collateral ligaments and the correct position of the joint line, and to ensure that the patella tracks appropriately over the femoral condyle. In the context of the balancing of the collateral ligaments it is essential to understand the concept behind the development of contractures and deformity. Degenerative changes in the knee joint lead to constant overloading of one compartment and this in turn

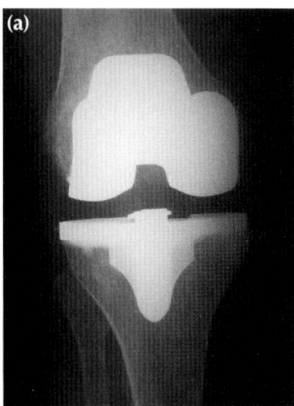

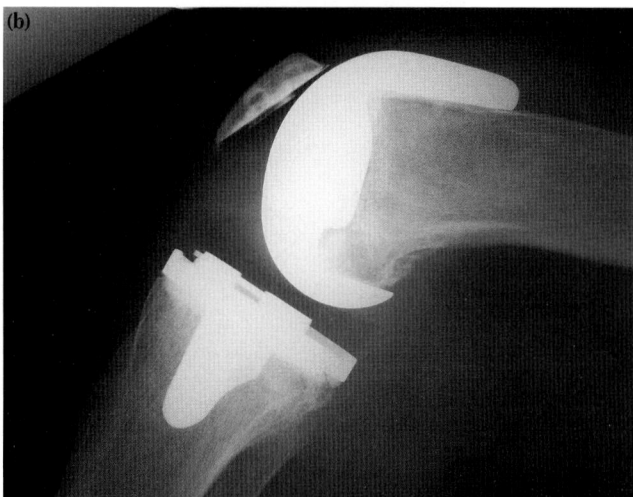

Figure 35.14 Total knee replacement.

causes the collateral ligament on that side to contract and on the other side to stretch. This eventually leads to the production of a varus or a valgus deformity. Therefore, the collateral ligaments need to be preserved and then released on the contracted side to allow balancing so that both the ligaments are in equal tension and length throughout the range of movement (Summary box 35.14).

Summary box 35.14

Technical goals of a total knee replacement

- Correct mechanical alignment
- Correct positioning of the joint line
- Accurate collateral ligament balancing
- Good patellar tracking over the femoral condyle

Surgical exposure involves a midline vertical incision centred over the knee and, subsequently, a medial parapatellar incision to expose the joint. Rarely, a subvastus approach is used because it offers the advantage of preserving the quadriceps and theoretically the possibility of a quicker recovery. However, as in the hip, whichever approach is used it is essential to be able to perform a knee replacement safely and achieve the technical goals of a well-positioned and a well-aligned knee.

The postoperative period is centred on building up the quadriceps and in the early phase the patient is encouraged to do an active straight leg raise. This is followed by an intensive course of physiotherapy for 6 weeks to 3 months to strengthen the quadriceps and achieve full extension. The patient should be assessed at 6 weeks, 3 months, 6 months, 1 year and yearly thereafter following surgery.

Complications

Complications following a total knee replacement can be related to the patient, the operation or the rehabilitation period. As in the hip they can be divided into intraoperative and postoperative complications (Summary box 35.15).

Summary box 35.15

Complications of total knee replacement

Intraoperative complications

- Neurovascular injury
- Tibial or femoral fracture
- Malalignment
- Tourniquet injury – neurovascular

Postoperative complications

- Infection
- Thromboembolism
- Osteolysis and loosening
- Instability due to inappropriate ligament balancing
- Stiffness
- Chronic pain – complex regional pain syndrome

Unicompartmental knee replacement

The natural history of osteoarthritis of the knee shows that the disease starts in the medial compartment in 92% of cases and then progresses into the other compartments. This was the basis for the development of the unicompartmental knee replacement. In its current form, both the fixed- and mobile-bearing options are available and the results reported in most series are good at 10 years (Fig. 35.15).

The ideal candidate for a unicompartmental knee replacement is a patient who is over 60 years of age, not physically active, not obese and who has disease limited to one compartment with not more than 15° of deformity (which is correctable) and no instability.

The operation is performed via a 5–7 cm incision and the quadriceps is preserved. The patient is usually discharged earlier than with a total knee replacement. It is a conservative procedure as it allows bone stock to be preserved and, should it fail, a total knee replacement can still be performed with good results.

Revision total knee replacement

The main causes for revision in the knee are implant loosening secondary to infection or polyethylene wear leading to osteolysis. Other causes include a periprosthetic fracture, maltracking of the patella, malalignment (Fig. 35.16a) and ligament instability. Tibial component loosening is more common than femoral component.

The patient should be assessed thoroughly for ligament instability as the choice of implant depends upon the integrity of the collateral ligaments. If the collateral ligaments are non-functional a constrained implant is necessary. Also, as in the hip, it is of paramount importance to investigate whether the loosening is secondary to infection because a two-staged approach may

CHAPTER 35 | HIP AND KNEE

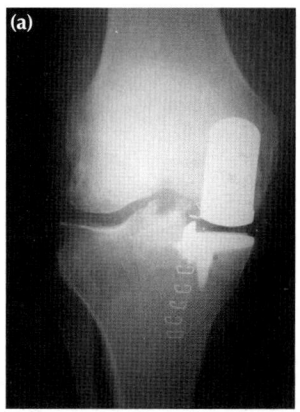

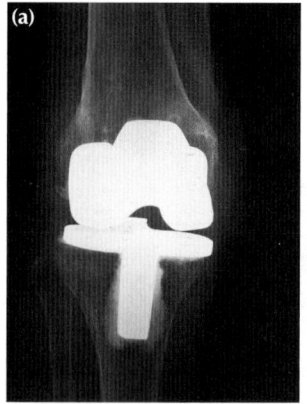

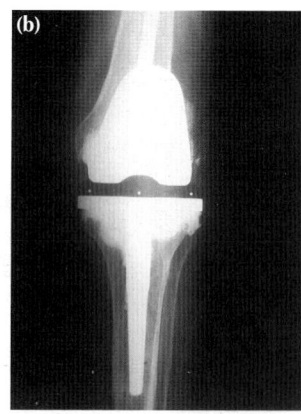

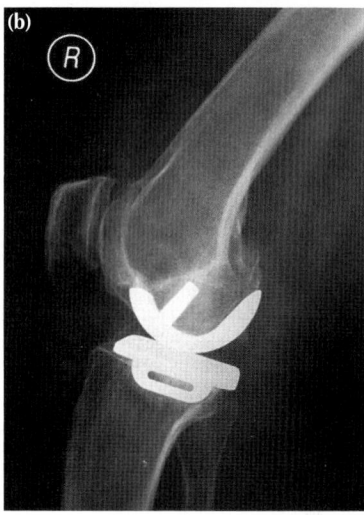

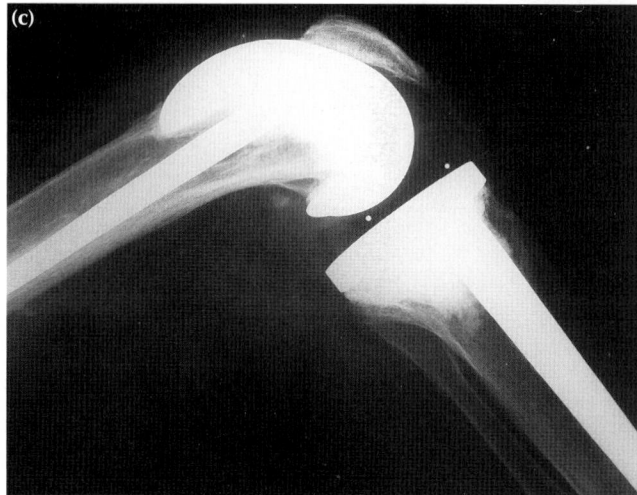

Figure 35.15 Unicompartmental knee replacement.

Figure 35.16 Radiographs of a malaligned knee (a) and a well-aligned revised knee (b and c).

be warranted in such cases. Finally, like the primary total knee replacement, the goals of a revision total knee replacement are to implant a well-aligned, well-balanced and stable knee (Fig. 35.16b and c).

FURTHER READING

Bulstrode, C., Buckwalter, J., Carr, A., Fairbank, J., Marsh, L., Wilson-MacDonald, J. and Bowden, G. (2002) *Oxford Textbook of Trauma and Orthopaedics*. Oxford University Press, Oxford.

Miller, M.D. (2004) *Review of Orthopaedics*, 4th edn. Saunders, Philadephia, PA.

Solomon, L., Warwick, D.J. and Nayagam, S. (2005) *Apley's Concise System of Orthopaedics and Fractures*, 3rd edn. Hodder Arnold, London.

Foot and ankle

To understand:

- The common problems affecting the foot and ankle in each age group
- The basic anatomy and biomechanics of the foot and ankle
- The principles behind the treatment of each condition, be it conservative or surgical

- The significance of progressive neurological diseases
- The advances in the management of disorders of the foot and ankle and that modern surgical practice is still evolving

INTRODUCTION

All foot conditions are congenital, developmental or acquired. Foot and ankle disorders fall into two broad categories: those that affect the paediatric population and those that affect adults.

ANATOMY

There are 26 main bones in the foot (seven tarsal bones, five metatarsals and 14 phalanges) plus the two sesamoids of the hallux and a variable number of other sesamoid and accessory bones.

Movements at the ankle joint are mainly dorsiflexion and plantarflexion but, because the talus is wider anteriorly than posteriorly, dorsiflexion of the ankle leads to external rotation of the fibula at the syndesmosis. This means that the foot externally rotates with dorsiflexion and internally rotates with plantarflexion.

Stability is conferred upon the ankle by the shape of the medial, lateral and posterior malleoli and the integrity of the medial and lateral ligaments and the inferior tibiofibular ligaments.

The subtalar joint is divided into anterior, middle and posterior facets and, along with the talonavicular and calcaneocuboid joints, makes up the triple joint complex. These joints are responsible for inversion and eversion of the hind and midfoot with most of the movement occurring at the talonavicular joint.

The second tarsometatarsal joint is recessed relative to the first and third and acts as a 'keystone'. Disruption of this joint (Lisfranc's injury) leads to loss of the transverse arch and an acquired flat foot.

Jacques Lisfranc, 1790–1847, Professor of Surgery and Operative Medicine, Paris, France.

The lower leg is divided into four compartments:

- the superficial posterior – gastrocnemius, soleus and plantaris;
- the deep posterior – tibialis posterior, flexor digitorum longus and flexor hallucis longus;
- the lateral – peroneus brevis and peroneus longus;
- the anterior – tibialis anterior, extensor hallucis longus, extensor digitorum longus and peroneus tertius.

There is only one muscle on the dorsum of the foot, the extensor digitorum brevis. The muscles on the plantar aspect of the foot are divided into four layers, the first being the most superficial. The plantar fascia is a very important structure that takes its origin from the heel and inserts into the bases of the proximal phalanges of the toes. At toe-off, the fascia tightens and accentuates the medial plantar arch and helps provide a rigid lever arm, the so-called 'windlass mechanism'.

The blood supply of the foot is from the anterior tibial, the posterior tibial and the peroneal arteries. The following nerves supply sensation to the foot: posterior tibial, saphenous, sural, superficial and deep peroneal (Fig. 36.1) (Summary box 36.1).

Summary box 36.1

Anatomy of the foot

- There are 26 major bones in the foot
- There are four layers of muscles in the sole of the foot
- The blood supply of the foot is from the anterior and posterior tibial arteries plus the peroneal artery

BIOMECHANICS

The human foot has evolved to allow orthograde bipedal locomotion (upright walking); it is adapted for walking, running and jumping as well as standing. During walking there are vertical,

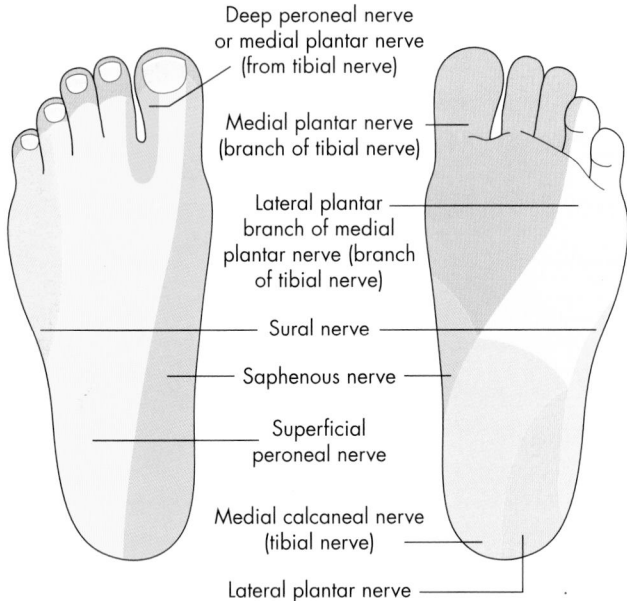

Deep peroneal nerve
or medial plantar nerve
(from tibial nerve)

Medial plantar nerve
(branch of tibial nerve)

Lateral plantar
branch of medial
plantar nerve (branch
of tibial nerve)

Sural nerve

Saphenous nerve

Superficial
peroneal nerve

Medial calcaneal nerve
(tibial nerve)

Lateral plantar nerve

Figure 36.1 Cutaneous nerve supply of the foot. Courtesy of Bartleby.com.

horizontal and lateral body displacements. The forces that act on the human body are those created by muscular activity and gravity.

During walking the centre of pressure moves from the heel to the metatarsal area and then the great toe and the pressure pattern can be measured using a force plate.

The walking cycle is divided into the stance (62%) and swing (38%) phases. The stance phase is divided into three intervals: (1) heel strike to foot flat; (2) foot flat until the body passes over the ankle; and (3) ankle joint plantarflexion to toe-off. During walking up to 12% of the gait cycle is spent with both feet in the stance phase but with running there is a period when neither foot is in contact with the ground, the 'float' phase. During running the cycle time is shortened but the forces generated are very much increased.

Some confusion surrounds the terminology used to describe foot motion. Plantar- and dorsiflexion are movements in the sagittal plane. Inversion is tilting of the plantar surface of the foot towards the midline and eversion is the opposite movement. Adduction is movement of the foot towards the midline in the transverse plane and abduction is away from the midline. Supination is a combination of adduction, inversion and plantarflexion and pronation is the opposite movement, i.e. abduction, eversion and dorsiflexion. The subtalar joint moves around a single inclined axis. The flatter the foot the more horizontal the axis and the greater the supinatory/pronatory forces applied to the foot. In such individuals the forces on the tibialis posterior tendon are increased and the tendon is prone to dysfunction. The transverse tarsal (talonavicular and calcaneocuboid) joints are parallel and therefore more flexible with the heel everted, and non-parallel and therefore 'locked' when inverted. At heel strike the heel is everted thus allowing the foot to accommodate to the terrain encountered but, at toe-off, the heel is inverted, thereby providing a rigid lever for propulsion. It is worth remembering that isolated fusion of the talonavicular joint leads to loss of 90% of motion in the triple joint complex whereas a calcaneocuboid joint fusion only abolishes 30% of inversion/eversion (Summary box 36.2).

Summary box 36.2

Biomechanics

- Human walking is known as orthograde bipedal locomotion
- The gait cycle is divided into swing and stance phases
- Running generates increased forces, shortens the gait cycle and has a float phase when neither foot touches the ground

PAEDIATRIC CONDITIONS

Congenital talipes equinovarus (Fig. 36.2)

This deformity (clubfoot), with characteristic equinus and varus positioning of the foot, is apparent at birth. Associated conditions (e.g. arthrogryposis, myelomeningocoele) must be excluded. The condition is more prevalent in boys and affects 1:1000 live births. Both limbs are affected in up to 50% of cases. The relationship of the talus to the calcaneus is abnormal and, in addition, the talus is smaller than usual.

It is essential that both treating physician and parents understand that the limb will never be normal – even after successful treatment the foot remains small with underdeveloped calf musculature. The aim of treatment is to achieve a plantigrade foot that is both stable and painless. Better understanding of the pathology has allowed manipulative techniques, combined with appropriate Achilles tendon lengthening, to achieve these goals

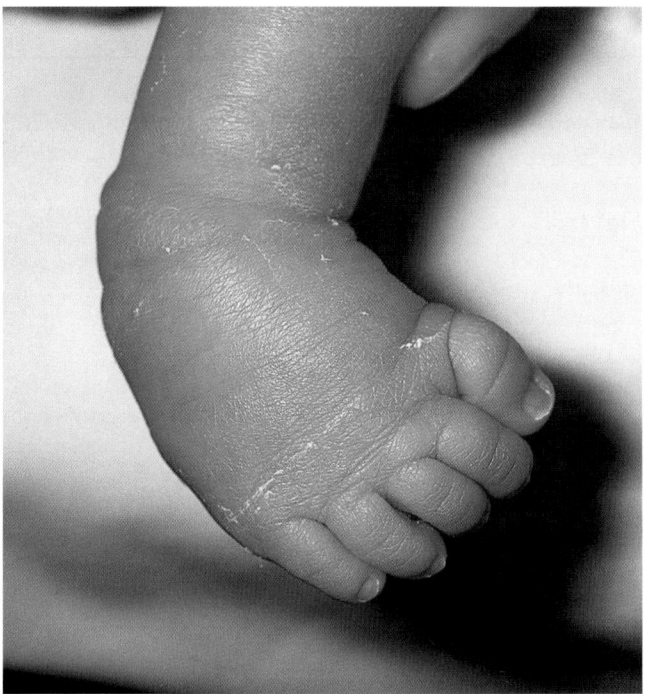

Figure 36.2 Clubfoot.

Achilles, the Greek hero, was the son of Peleus and Thetis. When he was a child his mother dipped him in the Styx, one of the rivers of the Underworld, so that he should be invulnerable in battle. The heel by which she held him did not get wet, and was, therefore, not protected. Achilles died from a wound in the heel, which he received at the siege of Troy.

without the need for major soft tissue release (the Ponseti technique). Surgery is best undertaken before 1 year of age. Sequential release of tendons, ligaments and joint capsules allows reduction of the deformity. A long posteromedial (Turco) or circumferential (Cincinnati) incision can be used. Talonavicular reduction is held with temporary K-wire fixation and serial below-knee casts.

Undercorrected residual or relapsed clubfoot

In older children who may or may not already have had surgery, a combination of osteotomies, tendon transfers and soft-tissue release is required. Some centres report encouraging results using circular external fixation.

Metatarsus adductus

The forefoot is medially deviated on the hindfoot. A variety of other terms (metatarsus varus, skewfoot) are used to describe the spectrum of this condition.

In most cases manipulative treatment taught to the parents is sufficient. Splintage at night with straight-last shoes aids the maintenance of correction. Only rarely is surgery required. Soft-tissue release of the abductor hallucis muscle and shortening osteotomy of the cuboid is one of several surgical techniques described.

Calcaneovalgus foot

This positional deformity in which the ankle joint is excessively dorsiflexed will correct with manipulative treatment. Splintage with serial casting may be required for more rigid cases, but consideration should first be given to alternative diagnoses, such as congenital vertical talus or a neurological abnormality.

Cavus foot

See Pes cavus.

Flat foot

The key to successful management is to differentiate between idiopathic flexible flat foot (requiring no treatment) and flat foot associated with an underlying abnormality.

Rigid flat foot

Congenital vertical talus gives the foot a characteristic rocker-bottom shape. The head of the talus is palpable in the sole of the foot. There is dorsolateral dislocation of the navicular. Treatment options include serial casting or surgery. The latter often needs to include more than a soft-tissue release to achieve reduction of the joint.

Tarsal coalition

In this condition there is incomplete separation of the developing bones in the hindfoot. The most common coalitions are talocalcaneal and calcaneonavicular (Fig. 36.3). The coalition may be bony, cartilaginous or fibrous. Pain with activity is the usual presenting complaint.

Martin Kirschner, **1879–1942, Professor of Surgery, Heidelberg, Germany** introduced the use of skeletal wires in 1909.

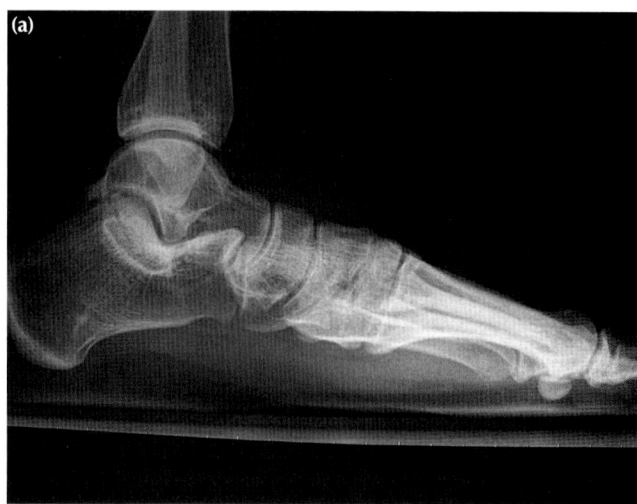

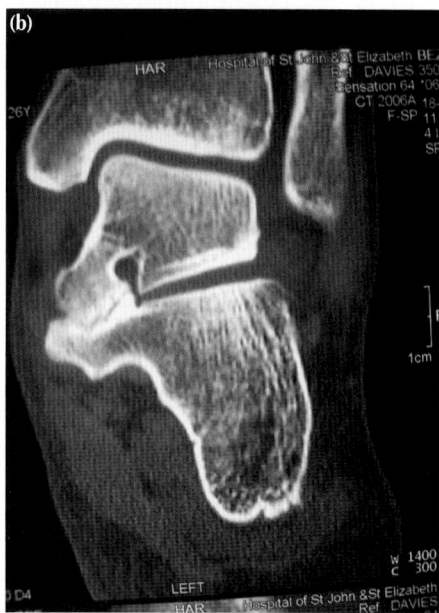

Figure 36.3 Tarsal coalition (talocalcaneal).

Commonly, the medial longitudinal arch is of low height and the heel is in valgus. If these features do not correct when the child stands on tiptoe then the deformity is not correctable (i.e. the Windlass test is negative). Plain radiographs and axial imaging determine the pathology.

Activity modification or casting may allow symptoms to settle. Surgery to excise the coalition has better results in children than in young adults. Fusion of the affected joint reliably relieves pain in older patients or if excision is not successful.

Other causes

The subtalar joint may be the first joint involved in rheumatoid arthritis (RA). Rare causes of hindfoot pain include osteomyelitis, fracture or bone tumour. All may present with pain and a flat foot deformity.

Flexible flat foot

Most flexible flat feet are painless and require no treatment. Orthotics have been shown to be of no long-term benefit. In rare painful cases the synchondrosis between the secondary ossification centre of the navicular and the main body of the bone may be the cause. Treatment should be symptomatic for as long as possible, in the expectation that the pain will resolve at skeletal maturity. Surgical treatment for recalcitrant cases aims to fuse the synchondrosis or remove the accessory ossicle.

Hallux valgus

Surgical treatment is best reserved until skeletal maturity. Congruent joints must be identified and the distal metatarsal articular angle corrected without producing joint subluxation (see Pathology in the adult, Hallux valgus, below).

Cerebral palsy

Ankle and foot disorders in patients with cerebral palsy evolve as the muscle balance changes, even though the central nervous system lesion is non-progressive. For non-ambulatory patients, splintage using an ankle/foot orthosis (AFO) to maintain the foot in a plantigrade position and stretch the tight calf is a safe and helpful treatment. In ambulatory patients, surgery to lengthen the Achilles tendon should not be undertaken in isolation without assessment of the knees and hips because of the possibility of causing a deterioration in the ability to walk.

Traumatic conditions

Transitional fractures of the ankle

Paediatric ankle fractures include a small sub-group that requires careful assessment and treatment. The distal tibial growth plate closes in a predictable pattern and children who injure their ankles during this period of maturation may have either a Tillaux fracture or a Triplane fracture (Fig. 36.4). In the former injury the anterior tibiofibular ligament causes avulsion of the anterolateral tibial epiphysis. The fracture is intra-articular. In a Triplane injury the fracture line forms a complex appearance, best appreciated with computerised tomography (CT). Treatment of displaced fractures is by accurate reduction and internal fixation.

PATHOLOGY IN THE ADULT

The forefoot

Hallux valgus

Hallux valgus is deviation of the big toe away from the midline, i.e. towards the lesser toes, and is usually associated with a bunion, an erythematous swelling on the medial aspect of the first metatarsal head (Fig. 36.5). It is a common condition that affects mainly shod populations, women more than men, and which is often bilateral. It is believed that the tendency to hallux valgus is inherited and that closed-in shoes accelerate the development of the condition. Other factors that predispose to the development of hallux valgus include:

- metatarsus primus varus;
- hypermobility of the first metatarsocuneiform joint (less common);
- a round metatarsal head as opposed to a flat head.

Paul Jules Tillaux, 1834–1904, Professor of Surgery, Paris. France.

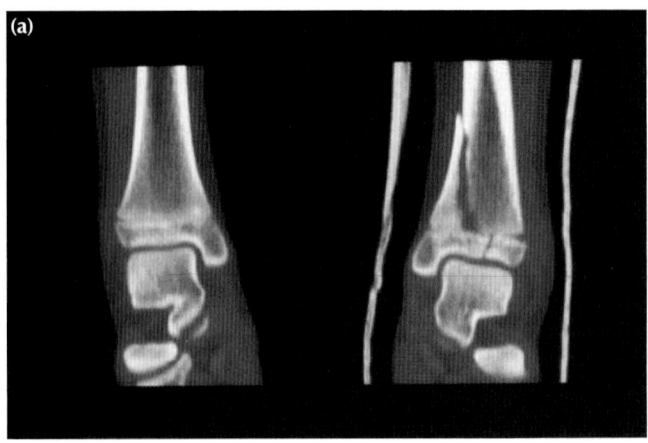

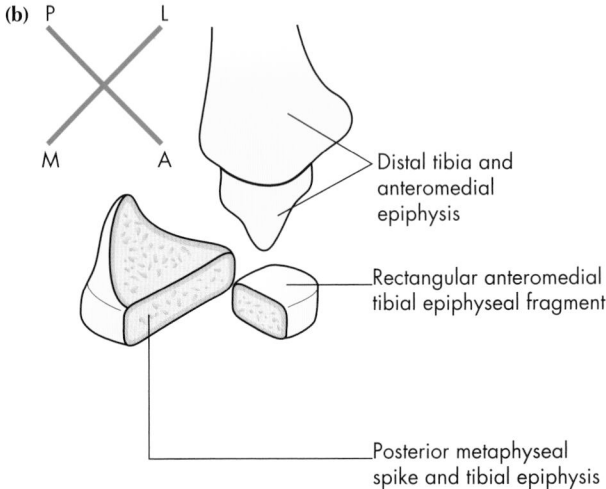

A, anterior; L, lateral
M, medial; P, posterior.

Distal tibia and anteromedial epiphysis

Rectangular anteromedial tibial epiphyseal fragment

Posterior metaphyseal spike and tibial epiphysis

Figure 36.4 Triplane fracture.

Hallux valgus can occur as a result of trauma and will often follow amputation of the second toe. Joint hyperelasticity (e.g. Ehlers–Danlos syndrome) and anything that leads to attenuation of the medial capsule can give rise to the deformity. With increasing deformity the first ray becomes defunctioned, and overload of the second metatarsophalangeal (MTP) joint results in pain and swelling and eventually hammering of the second toe.

When examining a patient the following should be documented:

- extent of valgus deformity;
- range of motion;
- pronation of hallux;
- second toe deformity/MTP joint tenderness;
- medial arch height;
- any other foot deformity.

Edvard Ehlers, 1863–1937, Professor of Clinical Dermatology, Copenhagen, Denmark, described this condition in 1901.
Henri Alexandre Danlos, 1844–1912, Dermatologist, Hôpital St. Louis, Paris, France, gave his account of this condition in 1908.

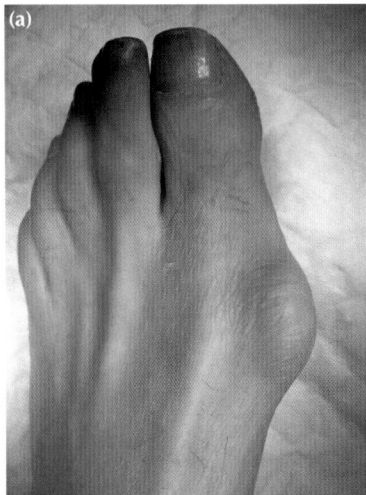

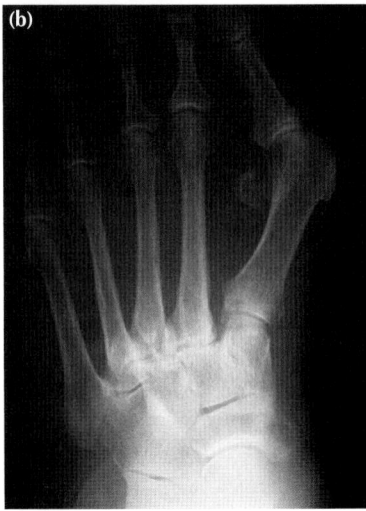

Figure 36.5 Hallux valgus and bunion.

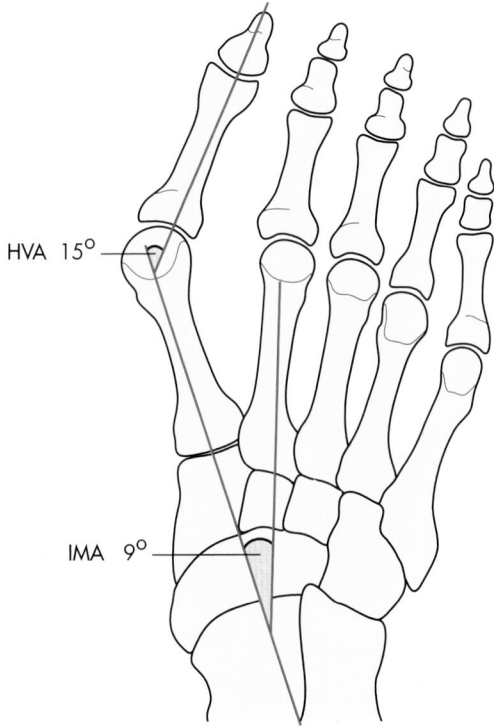

HVA, Hallux valgus angle
IMA, Intermetatarsal angle

Figure 36.6 Diagram of hallux valgus angles.

Hallux valgus is classified as follows:

- mild [hallux valgus angle (HVA) < 20°];
- moderate (HVA 20–40°);
- severe (HVA > 40°) (Fig. 36.6).

The only investigations required are weight-bearing anteroposterior and lateral radiographs of the foot and a non-weight-bearing oblique radiograph if there are lesser toe issues.

The decision-making process regarding management is not straightforward. The options are, however, simple: do nothing, modify footwear or carry out surgery. The problem with footwear modification is that it often involves providing a shoe with a wide and deep toe box, which is unacceptable to many. Operating for purely cosmetic reasons is difficult to justify but, if a young patient has a significant deformity, it is likely that the deformity will worsen. Surgery is therefore recommended for those patients with significant pain and/or significant deformity, providing that they understand the risks involved, the importance of following post-operative instructions and the fact that it takes 6–12 months to make a full recovery.

The more deformed the foot, the more technically demanding the surgery. For mild deformities a distal osteotomy (e.g. chevron) is usually adequate. For moderate deformities the surgeon is more likely to use a shaft (e.g. Scarf, Fig. 36.7) or a basal (proximal chevron or crescentic) osteotomy. Severe deformities can be corrected by shaft and basal osteotomies but sometimes a fusion of the first tarsometatarsal joint (modified Lapidus) or a first MTP joint fusion can be effective. Operations such as a Keller's excision arthroplasty should no longer be performed now that more 'anatomical' procedures are available.

The prognosis without surgery is usually a slow progression of the deformity over many years. Surgery should produce 90% satisfaction rates, especially if patients are properly informed as to what they might expect. The complications of surgery are infection, cutaneous nerve damage, recurrence/overcorrection of deformity, stiffness and overload of the second MTP joint (transfer lesion) (Summary box 36.3).

Summary box 36.3

Hallux valgus

- Bunions affect women more than men
- Patients with hallux valgus have inherited a tendency to develop the condition
- Not all patients need surgery
- The choice of operation is determined by the severity of the deformity

William Lordan Keller, **1874–1959**, Head of the Department of Surgery, the Walter Reed Hospital, Washington, DC, USA, described this operation in 1904.

CHAPTER 36 | FOOT AND ANKLE

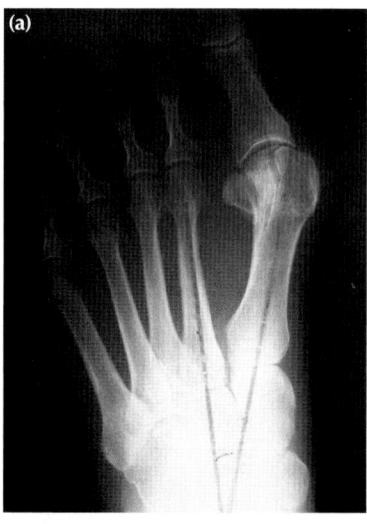

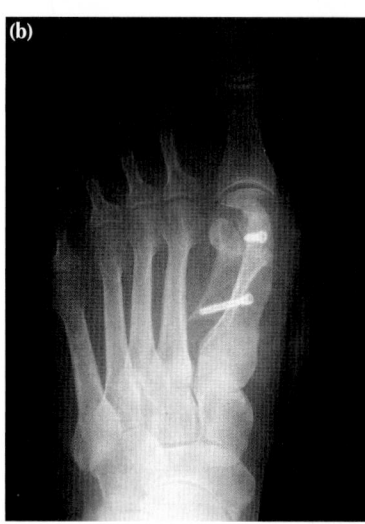

Figure 36.7 Pre- (a) and postoperative (b) radiographs of a Scarf osteotomy.

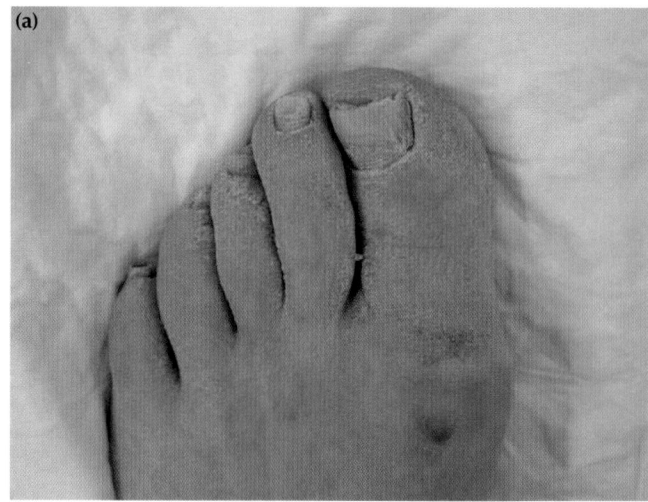

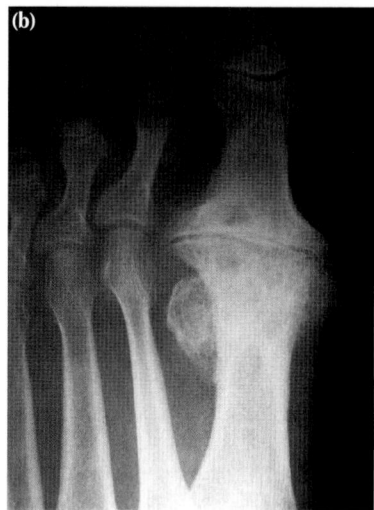

Figure 36.8 Clinical (a) and radiographic (b) appearances of hallux rigidus.

Hallux rigidus

Hallux rigidus is a painful condition of the hallux MTP joint characterised by loss of motion and osteophyte formation (Fig. 36.8). Hallux limitus is a term that is synonymous with this condition but which implies restriction in terms of movement. It is a common condition in adults. There is also a juvenile form that is associated with excessive length of the first metatarsal and/or an osteochondral lesion of the first metatarsal head and possibly elevation of the metatarsal head (metatarsus elevatus). In adults there is often a history of trauma or repetitive microtrauma (sport) but, occasionally, there is a strong family history of the condition. It is also said to be associated with a flat metatarsal head. Patients complain of stiffness and pain on weight-bearing and certain shoes will be a lot more uncomfortable than others. Clinical examination will often reveal a dorsal swelling (dorsal bunion), joint-line tenderness and a restricted range of motion. Pain at the extreme of dorsiflexion often implies impingement of the synovium between osteophytes.

There are three grades of hallux rigidus based on subjective, objective and radiological findings. Grade I is mild and there may only be some stiffness and some dorsal spurring. Grade II is moderate and is associated with significant pain, stiffness and moderate joint-space narrowing, whereas in Grade III there is severe pain, profound stiffness and almost complete obliteration of the joint space.

Non-operative treatment involves analgesics and/or non-steroidal anti-inflammatory drugs (NSAIDs), footwear and activity modification. A steroid injection may give short-term pain relief and physiotherapy may help a small percentage of sufferers. The most effective non-operative treatment is provision of a stiff-soled shoe with a deep toe box. This combination splints the joint and protects it from pressure.

The mainstays of surgical management are cheilectomy (from the Greek *cheilos*, for 'lip') and fusion. A cheilectomy is a radical joint debridement and resection of the dorsal 30% of the metatarsal head. It is the procedure of choice if pain is only at the extremes of motion and at least 50% of the articular cartilage remains. Fusion is for the severely affected and is an effective means of abolishing pain. It does, however, restrict the height of heel that can be worn. A fusion will still allow sports participation. Joint replacement has yet to be proven as a successful form of treatment (Summary box 36.4).

Lesser toe deformities

Lesser toes can be the source of great misery. There are four types of lesser toe deformity (Table 36.1). Hammer toes (Fig. 36.9) result from mechanical overload whereas mallet and curly toes occur as a result of soft-tissue/muscle imbalance of non-neurological origin. These three types often affect a single digit. The fourth type, clawing, has a neurological cause, often affects all the lesser toes and needs to be appropriately investigated (Fig. 36.10).

These deformities may be flexible or fixed and symptomatic or asymptomatic. For symptomatic flexible deformities soft-tissue surgery is usually adequate but for fixed deformities bony procedures are required. Non-operative treatment involves appropriate padding and footwear modification.

Freiberg's disease (Fig. 36.11)

This condition is uncommon but affects the second metatarsal head in teenagers (girls more than boys). It is thought that it is caused by ischaemic necrosis of the epiphysis, resulting in pain and swelling of the joint. It will often settle with rest but sometimes surgery is required to tidy up the joint. Rarely, a closing wedge osteotomy of the metatarsal head is required but excision of the whole head should never be performed.

Morton's neuroma and metatarsalgia

Metatarsalgia means 'pain in the region of the metatarsals' and is as non-specific a term as 'headache'. It usually occurs secondary to joint problems or irritation of a nerve. Morton's neuroma is a painful condition that arises from compression of the common digital nerve between the third and fourth metatarsal heads (90% of cases). In 10% of cases the nerve between the second and third metatarsal heads is affected. Characteristically, the patient will only experience pain when wearing shoes and the tighter the shoe the greater the problem. The affected toes often go numb and the patient will remove the shoe and rub the foot to gain relief. Non-

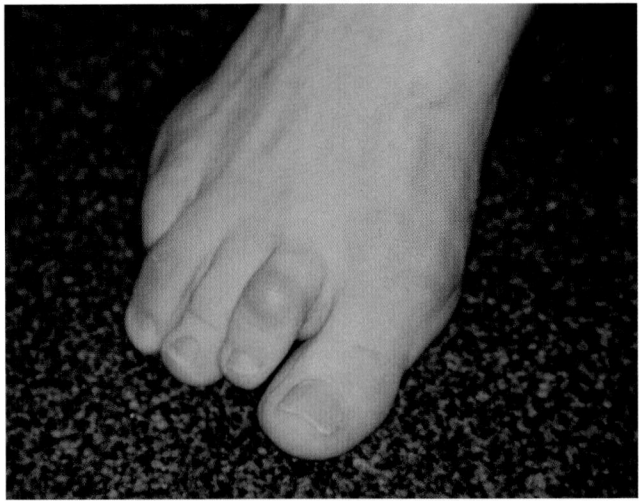

Figure 36.9 Hammer toe.

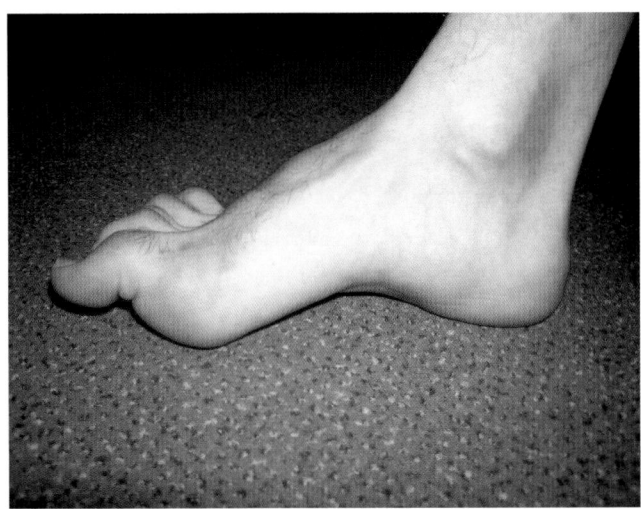

Figure 36.10 Claw toes.

operative treatments include advice about footwear, an orthosis (pre-metatarsal dome) to splay the metatarsal heads or an injection of steroids for short-term relief. Surgery involves resection or transposition of the neuroma and is usually highly successful; however, the neuroma can regrow and the affected toes will

Table 36.1 Types of lesser toe deformity

Deformity	MTPJ	PIPJ	DIPJ	Comments
Hammer toe	Extended	Flexed	Extended or flexed	Associated with hallux valgus. Second toe most common
Mallet toe	Normal	Normal	Flexed	
Curly toe	Medial deviation and rotated	Medial deviation and rotated	Medial deviation and rotated	Affects third, fourth or fifth toes
Claw toe	Extended	Flexed	Flexed	Look for underlying neurological diagnosis

DIPJ, distal interphalangeal joint; MTPJ, metatarsophalangeal joint; PIPJ, proximal interphalangeal joint.

Albert Henry Freiberg, **Professor of Orthopaedic Surgery, University of Cincinnati, Cincinnati, OH, USA, gave his account of this condition in 1926.**
Thomas George Morton, **1835–1903, Surgeon, the Pennsylvania Hospital, Philadelphia, PA, USA, described this condition in 1876.**

CHAPTER 36 | FOOT AND ANKLE

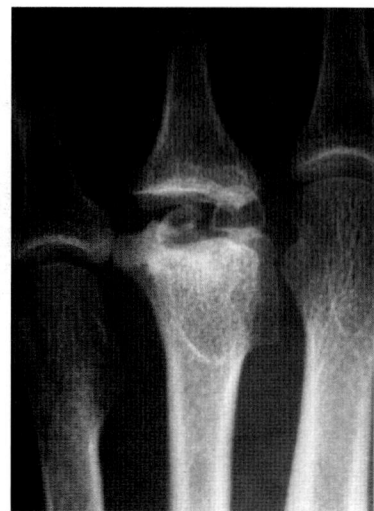

Figure 36.11 Freiberg's disease.

be permanently numb if the nerve is removed. It is essential to distinguish between a second MTP joint synovitis (often seen in hallux valgus) and a second space neuroma (Summary box 36.5).

Summary box 36.5

Morton's neuroma

- Morton's neuroma most commonly affects the third web space
- It is important to distinguish a second space neuroma from a second MTP synovitis
- Surgical excision of a neuroma is often successful

Midfoot and hindfoot

The hindfoot comprises the ankle joint and the calcaneus. The midfoot comprises the remaining tarsal bones as far as the tarsometatarsal joints. The majority of problems affecting this part of the body relate to joint and tendon disorders. These problems can be broadly divided into mechanical/degenerative disorders and inflammatory conditions. Osteoarthritis (OA) can affect any of the joints as can inflammatory arthritides such as RA.

Degenerative joint conditions

Degenerate joints may be asymptomatic but usually present with pain, swelling and/or deformity. There may or may not be a history of trauma or repeated microtrauma. If a foot is swollen and deformed but without pain there is likely to be an underlying neuropathy. In the majority of cases pain will be the reason for the patient seeking help. On examination there is usually joint-line tenderness and it is therefore very important to be familiar with the surface anatomy of the joints of the foot. The diagnosis and the extent of any deformity are usually confirmed by plain weight-bearing radiography. Before recommending treatment it is important to assess the level of a patient's symptoms.

Non-operative treatments include analgesics, non-steroidal medication, footwear modification (including bracing), activity modification, physiotherapy and judicious usage of intra-articular steroids. One should never forget that a walking stick can also be helpful. Surgery is reserved for those patients who fail non-operative treatment.

Operative treatment for OA will usually be in the form of arthrodesis (fusion). This is normally carried out via an open approach but arthroscopic ankle arthrodesis is now an established procedure. When there is significant osteophyte formation and impingement without significant OA, osteophyte removal can be extremely effective. Osteophytes that cause impingement tend to be anterior whereas posterior impingement tends to be caused by an os trigonum. In severe OA of the ankle debridement has no role but joint replacement of the ankle (Fig. 36.12) is finally becoming a viable alternative to fusion in selected cases (low-demand patients without significant deformity).

In the past it was felt that a triple fusion should be performed when any of the joints of the triple joint complex needed fusing but it is now deemed preferable to fuse only the affected symptomatic joints.

Inflammatory joint conditions

The treatment of conditions such as RA is very similar in principle to that outlined above for OA. In RA, however, it is essential that the medical management of the condition is optimised before considering surgery. It is also important to realise that these patients often have multiple joint involvement and the postoperative period can pose major problems in terms of

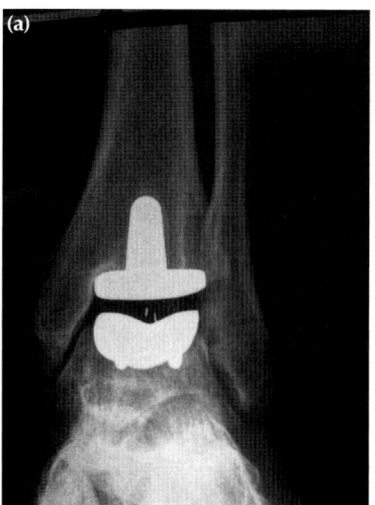

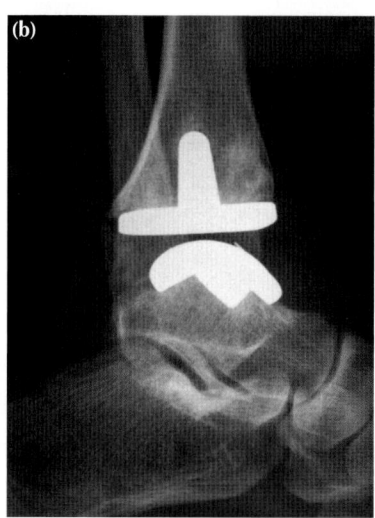

Figure 36.12 Total ankle arthroplasty.

mobility. It is essential to remember that knee deformity must be addressed before corrective hindfoot surgery is undertaken (Summary box 36.6).

Tendon disorders

Tenosynovitis occurs as a result of injury or overuse or is secondary to inflammatory joint conditions. Rest, anti-inflammatory medication and physiotherapy are often helpful but, in inflammatory conditions, tenosynovectomy may be required.

The tendons most commonly affected by degeneration are the Achilles, tibialis posterior and peroneii (brevis more than longus). Achilles 'tendinitis' is either mid-substance or insertional (Fig. 36.13). The former will often settle with non-operative strategies and time but the insertional type often requires debridement and resection of the prominent calcaneal tuberosity. The peroneus brevis is prone to longitudinal tears and splitting, particularly in patients with high-arched feet (Fig. 36.14). Surgical repair is often necessary and quite effective.

The tibialis posterior tendon tends to fail in overweight individuals and those who have flat feet. Often, after unaccustomed exercise, the tendon swells and is painful. The diagnosis is rarely made early. Rest, splinting and anti-inflammatory medication can help in the early stages but, with time, the foot becomes flatter and the tendon ceases to work. Many individuals will require surgical treatment in the form of a medial displacement calcaneal osteotomy, flexor digitorum longus or flexor hallucis longus tendon transfer and spring ligament repair. Failure to treat this condition can lead to spectacular deformity (Fig. 36.15).

Ankle instability

Most people who sustain an ankle sprain will recover, particularly if they receive prompt physiotherapy. However, some individuals

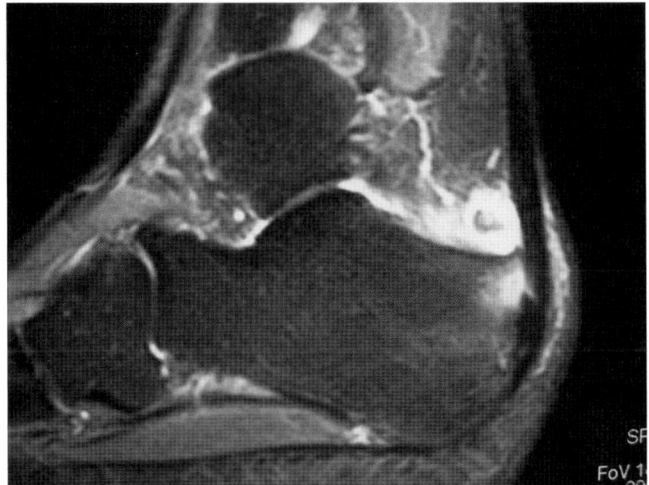

Figure 36.13 Insertional Achilles tendinitis.

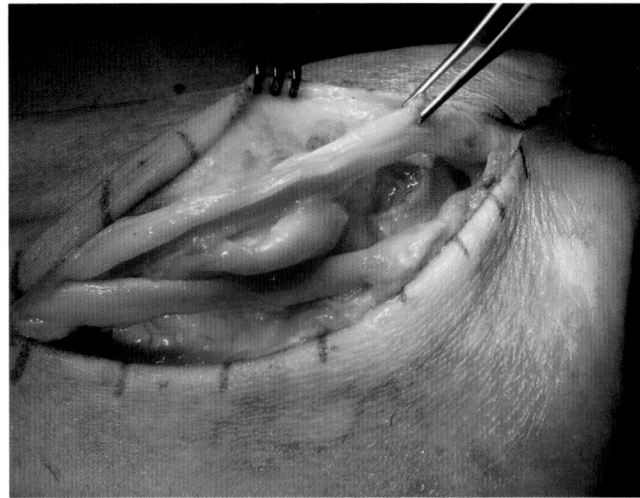

Figure 36.14 Split and degenerate peroneus brevis.

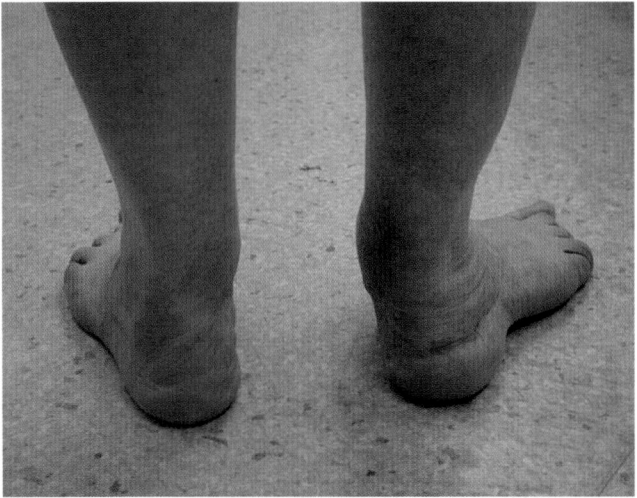

Figure 36.15 A tibialis posterior tendon-deficient foot.

develop significant instability. The frequency of episodes of giving way varies enormously with some patients suffering daily sprains. If physiotherapy is unsuccessful at resolving the problem, an anatomical reconstruction using the Brostrom method is usually curative.

Osteochondral lesions of the talus

Nearly all lateral and 70% of medial osteochondral lesions of the talus (OLTs) follow a traumatic episode. They can vary from a chondral flap to a large loose OLT (Fig. 36.16). If progress appears slow following an ankle sprain and the patient complains of a poorly localised ache within the ankle an OLT should be suspected. Diagnosis is confirmed on magnetic resonance imaging (MRI). Arthroscopic debridement is often required but is not always successful. Osteochondral autologous transplantation (OATS) from the knee, or cartilage culture and transplantation, may be considered for such cases.

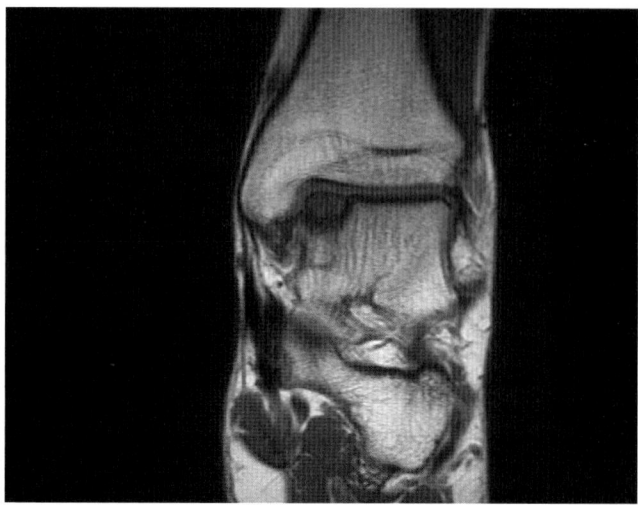

Figure 36.16 Magnetic resonance imaging of an osteochondral lesion of the talus.

Pes cavus

Pes cavus sometimes presents in adults (Fig. 36.17). It is usually bilateral and most cases will be associated with an underlying neurological condition, the most common being Charcot–Marie–Tooth disease. These patients may present with recurrent ankle sprains or fifth metatarsal stress fractures. Precise diagnosis is confirmed with nerve conduction studies. Surgical correction of deformity is often required but not curative in this progressive disease. If a teenager presents with a unilateral pes cavus an underlying tethering of the spinal cord (diastematomyelia) should be suspected (Summary box 36.7).

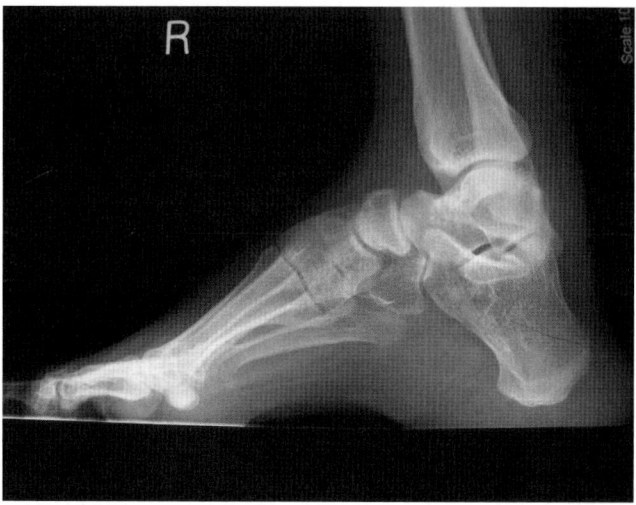

Figure 36.17 Pes cavus.

Jean Martin Charcot, **1825–1893**, Physician, La Salpêtrière, Paris, France.
Pierre Marie, **1853–1940**, Neurologist, Hospice de Bicêtre, Paris, France, later becoming Professor of Pathological Anatomy in the Faculty of Medicine, and finally, in 1918, Professor of Neurology.
Howard Henry Tooth, **1856–1925**, Physician, St Bartholomew's Hospital, and the National Hospital for Nervous Diseases, Queen Square, London, England, described peroneal muscular atrophy in 1886 independently of Charcot and Marie.

> **Summary box 36.7**
>
> **Pes cavus**
>
> - Pes cavus needs neurological investigation
> - About 80% of cases of pes cavus are associated with a neurological disease
> - The commonest cause is Charcot–Marie–Tooth disease
> - Unilateral pes cavus – think diastematomyelia

Acquired flat foot

In adults there are a number of conditions that should be considered when a foot becomes flat. Often, it is a flat foot that becomes even flatter. The causes are:

- tibialis posterior tendon dysfunction;
- tarsometatarsal arthritis/injury (Fig. 36.18);
- Charcot neuroarthropathy, e.g. diabetes;
- inflammatory/degenerative arthritis of the subtalar/talonavicular joints;
- spring ligament rupture.

Non-operative treatment is appropriate except in the acute trauma situation. Surgical intervention may be required in other cases but is rarely required in the Charcot foot unless unacceptable deformity or ulceration occurs. Patients with tibialis posterior tendon dysfunction have medial ankle pain and swelling and often have considerable difficulty performing a single heel raise (Summary box 36.8).

> **Summary box 36.8**
>
> **Acquired flat foot**
>
> - Tibialis posterior tendon dysfunction and tarsometatarsal OA are common causes of an acquired flat foot
> - Orthoses, rest and NSAIDs can help with symptomatic relief
> - Surgery is a major undertaking but often highly successful at achieving symptomatic relief

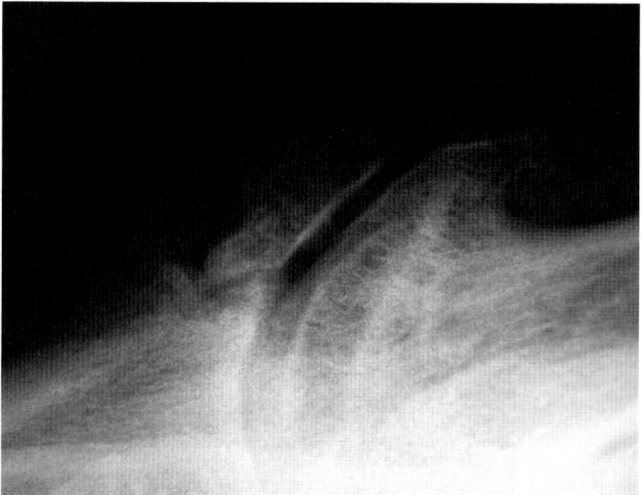

Figure 36.18 Tarsometatarsal arthritis.

Tumours

Tumours can be benign or malignant. Malignant tumours of the foot are vanishingly rare but do occur. The two most common benign tumours of the foot are ganglia and angioleiomyomas (Fig. 36.19); these tumours may need surgical excision.

Infection

Septic arthritis in the foot or ankle is rare; when it occurs it usually follows a surgical procedure but it can also arise as a result of haematogenous spread. Treatment is immediate surgical drainage and administration of appropriate high-dosage antibiotics. The most common causative organism is *Staphylococcus aureus* with methicillin-resistant *S. aureus* (MRSA) becoming more prevalent. Even with prompt treatment chondrolysis often occurs and subsequent degenerative changes develop rapidly.

Osteomyelitis can be equally devastating. Prompt and appropriate management with rest and high-dosage antibiotics can successfully treat the condition. Treatment continues until the patient is apyrexial, the foot quiescent and the inflammatory markers normal. Chronic osteomyelitis is treated using similar principles when a flare-up occurs but cure can only be achieved by surgical excision of the infected bone.

Foot infections are either acute or chronic and arise as a result of direct inoculation or haematogenous spread. Treatment is with rest, elevation and appropriate antibiotics but surgical debridement may be required, especially with conditions such as necrotising fasciitis (*Streptococcus pyogenes*).

In immunocompromised patients opportunistic infections can arise and, in diabetics, failure to treat with debridement can lead to amputation. It is important to realise that radiographs in the early stages of infection are usually normal and that diagnosis is made on clinical suspicion and with blood tests and more sophisticated imaging such as MRI or bone scanning.

Tuberculosis can affect the foot and is associated with major bony damage; it responds surprisingly well to debridement and appropriate anti-tuberculous therapy (Fig. 36.20).

Diabetes

Diabetics have foot problems secondary to neuropathy and microvascular changes. They are at increased risk of infection

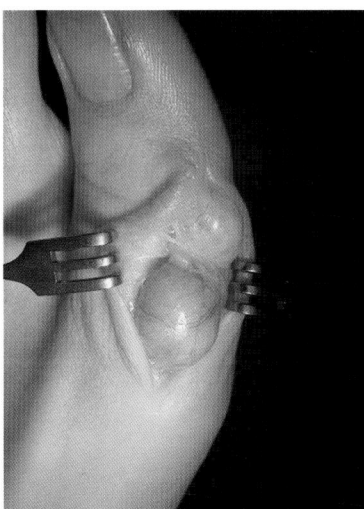

Figure 36.19 Angioleiomyoma of the hallux.

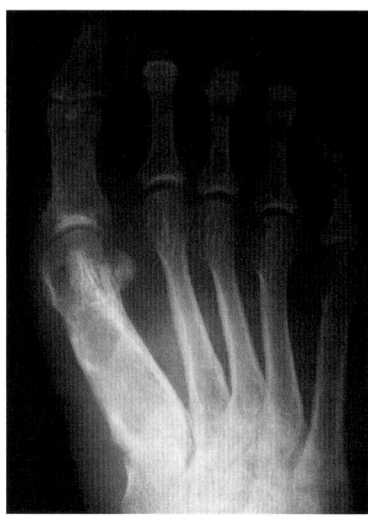

Figure 36.20 Tuberculosis of the foot.

and ulceration, and trauma (sometimes trivial) can lead to collapse of the foot, also known as Charcot neuroarthropathy (Fig. 36.21). There are three stages (Eichenholtz) to the process of Charcot neuroarthropathy, which takes up to 18 months to run its course: stage I, fragmentation; stage II, coalescence; and stage III, bone consolidation. It is essential to distinguish between infection and neuroarthropathy; however, in the acute situation this can be difficult. Infection requires appropriate antibiotic therapy and/or surgical debridement whereas the acute Charcot foot requires appropriate splintage in a Charcot retaining orthotic walker (CROW) or a total contact cast (TCC). If there is no history of skin damage, infection is unlikely, but inflammatory markers and MRI can help differentiate between the two conditions.

Ulceration can lead to major morbidity and amputation (Fig. 36.22). Ulcers need to be treated and when ulcer healing has occurred the aim should be to keep the foot ulcer free (Summary box 36.9).

> **Summary box 36.9**
>
> **Diabetes**
>
> Diabetics are prone to infection because of:
> - Peripheral neuropathy
> - Peripheral vascular disease
> - Impaired resistance to infection

Entrapment neuropathies

Any nerve supplying the foot can become entrapped and result in pain, and treatment often requires surgical decompression. Tarsal tunnel syndrome is much rarer than carpal tunnel syndrome in the hand.

Heel pain

The commonest cause of heel pain is plantar fasciitis. Pain is located inferomedially within the heel and is worst first thing in the morning and after periods of rest. It often, but not always, follows unaccustomed activity in a middle-aged overweight

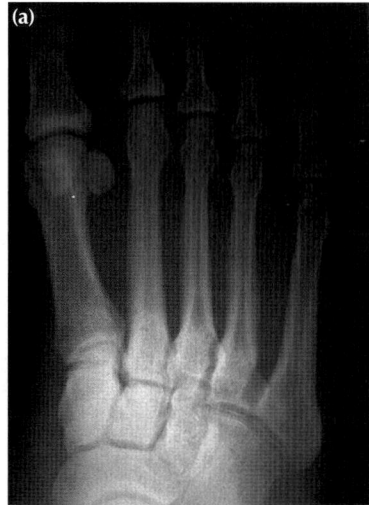

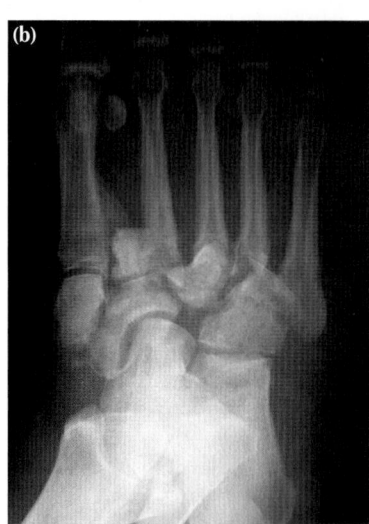

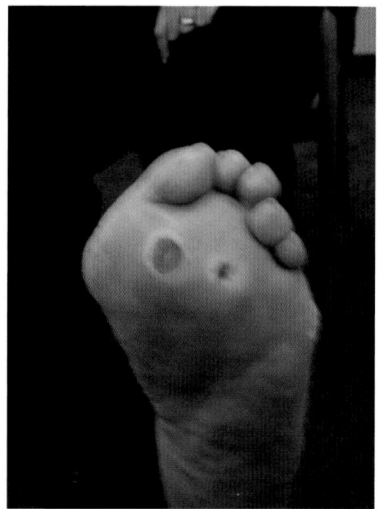

Figure 36.22 Diabetic foot ulcer.

Figure 36.21 Charcot foot. Radiographs taken at the time of a trivial injury (a) and 6 weeks later (b).

individual. Treatment includes cortisone injection, physiotherapy, analgesics and orthoses. The majority of cases settle within 18 months and surgery is rarely required or successful.

Amputation

In orthopaedics, amputation is usually carried out for uncontrolled infection, trauma or tumour. The level of amputation is chosen to allow optimal wound healing and prosthetic fitting. It is carried out when the patient is clearly going to be better off without the foot (or leg).

CONCLUSION

Major advances have occurred and will continue to emerge in the subspeciality of foot and ankle surgery. As a general rule, non-operative measures should be tried before surgery is considered. Modern foot and ankle surgery has a lot to offer sufferers and most patients will do well and be satisfied if treatment is tailored to their needs and they are informed about what to reasonably expect from the treatment.

FURTHER READING

Bulstrode, C., Buckwalter, J., Carr, A., Fairbank, J., Marsh, L., Wilson-MacDonald, J. and Bowden, G. (2002) *Oxford Textbook of Trauma and Orthopaedics*. Oxford University Press, Oxford.

Miller, M.D. (2004) *Review of Orthopaedics*, 4th edn. Saunders, Philadelphia, PA.

Solomon, L., Warwick, D.J. and Nayagam, S. (2005) *Apley's Concise System of Orthopaedics and Fractures*, 3rd edn. Hodder Arnold, London.

Inflammation and infection and musculoskeletal tumours

LEARNING OBJECTIVES

Inflammation and infection in bones and joints

To understand:

- Common diseases causing inflammation of the musculoskeletal system with their characteristic features in terms of history, examination, pathogenesis, investigation, treatment and prognosis
- Characteristic features in the history and examination of infection of bone and joint
- Treatment of infection of bone and joint

Musculoskeletal tumours

To understand:

- Symptoms and signs that suggest the presence of a benign or malignant musculoskeletal tumour
- Action to be taken with suspicious lesions
- Value of centres of excellence for staging, biopsy and multidisciplinary assessment
- Staging before biopsy
- Diagnosis before treatment
- Taking a biopsy
- Surgical treatment of musculoskeletal tumours
- Surgical treatment in metastatic disease, pathological fracture or impending fracture

INFLAMMATION AND INFECTION IN BONES AND JOINTS

RHEUMATOID ARTHRITIS

The commonest type of inflammatory arthritis is rheumatoid arthritis, which affects approximately 3% of women and 1% of men in Northern Europe. The prevalence is less in other areas of the world but tends to rise with urbanisation. Patients with rheumatoid arthritis are not seen represented in historical western art and literature. This suggests that it is a modern disease in Europe. However, changes characteristic of the disease are recognised in ancient Native American skeletons, leading to speculation that it originated in the New World. The disease appears to arise from a cell-mediated (T-cell) autoimmune response, but there may be an underlying infectious aetiology. Once the T-cell response is triggered, there is a release of cytokines, including interleukins IL-1 and IL-6, and tumour necrosis factor (TNF), which cause the inflammatory reaction. The disease has a predilection for small joints in the hands and feet and is usually symmetrical. However, it can involve any joint, and also affects tissues elsewhere in the body. There is inflammation of the soft tissues and synovial hyperplasia, containing lymphocytes and plasma cells. A layer of inflammatory tissue called a 'pannus' spreads over the joint surfaces and erodes the subchondral bone, denuding articular cartilage. There is chronic mononuclear cell infiltration and neovascularisation. Rheumatoid factor (RF) is found in approximately 80% of cases of the disease (and in 1–5% of the unaffected population). The extra-articular manifestations are found in the skin, eyes, lungs, heart and kidneys. Amyloid may also arise, as well as neuritis secondary to vasculitis (Summary boxes 37.1 and 37.2).

Summary box 37.1

Rheumatoid arthritis

- Occurs in around 3% of women and 1% of men
- Caused by a cell-mediated (T-cell) autoimmune response
- Rheumatoid factor positive in 80%
- Often starts with symmetrical disease affecting small joints of the hands and feet

---

Summary box 37.2

Extra-articular manifestations of rheumatoid arthritis

- Skin – subcutaneous nodules
- Eyes – scleritis, iritis
- Lungs – interstitial lung disease, pleural effusion
- Heart – myocarditis
- Kidneys – nephritis
- Amyloid – lungs, kidneys, heart, bowel
- Compression and vascular neuritis

The diagnostic criteria for rheumatoid arthritis were devised by the American College of Rheumatology (1987). This involves the patient having four of the seven criteria listed in Table 37.1.

The onset is often insidious with joint stiffness and polyarthritis but may be acute in approximately 30% of patients, presenting with malaise and low-grade fever. Hands and feet are commonly affected early in the disease. On examination there are joint effusions and synovitis. These cause swelling, warmth, erythema and stiffness of the affected joints with pain on movement.

There are very characteristic patterns of disease and deformity seen in the hand and wrist. Inflammation of the tendons (tenosynovitis) commonly affects flexor and extensor tendons of the hand and wrist, producing swelling and crepitus. Eventually tendons may rupture, so that passive range of movement exceeds active. Rupture is especially common in the extensor tendons of the little finger (Figs 37.1–37.3). It is usual for the erythrocyte sedimentation rate (ESR) and C-reactive protein (CRP) to be elevated (Summary box 37.3).

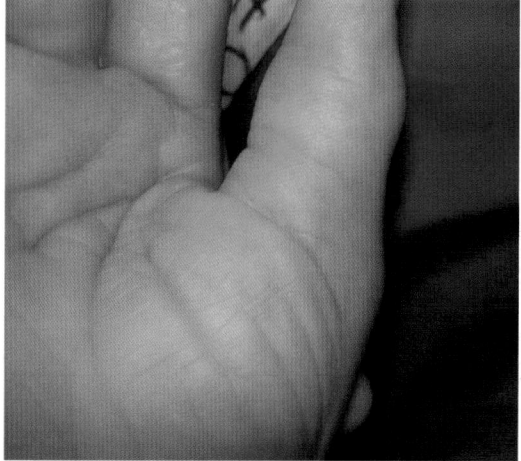

Figure 37.1 Flexor pollicis longus tenosynovitis.

Summary box 37.3

Problems in the hand and wrist caused by rheumatoid arthritis

- Radial deviation of the wrist
- Extensor tendon ruptures
- Ulnar deviation metacarpophalangeal joints
- Z-deformity of the thumb
- Boutonnière deformity of the fingers
- Swan neck deformities
- Carpal tunnel syndrome

Longstanding, stable, mild cases of rheumatoid arthritis can be treated with analgesics and non-steroidal anti-inflammatory drugs (NSAIDs). However, it is now believed that the disease is best treated aggressively in its early phase before erosions and extra-articular pathology can occur. This may prevent long-term recruitment of the autoimmune cascade. The treatment is with disease-modifying anti-rheumatic drugs (DMARDs) such as methotrexate, gold, sulphasalazine/Salazopyrin, leflunomide, penicillamine and ciclosporin. The most recent development of anti-TNF drugs such as etanercept and infliximab may revolutionise treatment. Corticosteroid therapy continues to be useful,

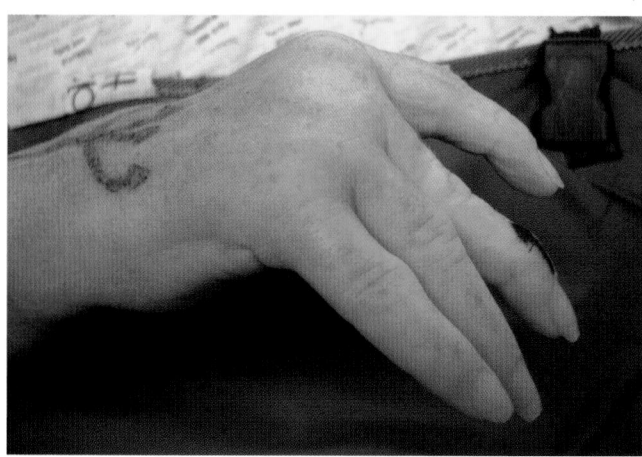

Figure 37.2 Swan neck deformity.

Table 37.1 American College of Rheumatology criteria for diagnosis of rheumatoid arthritis

Morning stiffness lasting at least 1 hour

Active arthritis of three or more joints simultaneously

Active arthritis of at least one hand joint (wrist, MCPJ or PIPJ)

Symmetrical arthritis

Subcutaneous rheumatoid nodules on extensor surfaces, juxta-articular or over bony prominences

Rheumatoid factor

Radiographic changes of periarticular erosions or osteopenia in affected joints, not osteoarthritis

MCPJ, metacarpophalangeal joint; PIPJ, proximal interphalangeal joint.

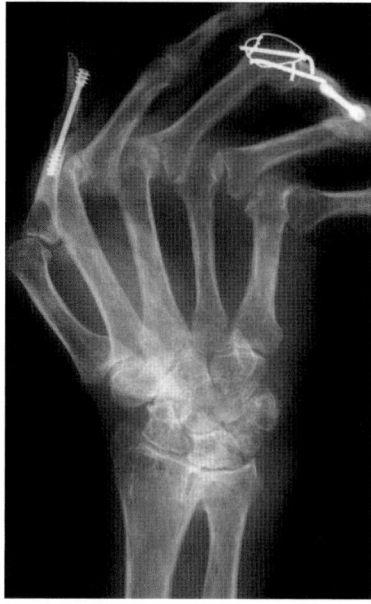

Figure 37.3 Rheumatoid wrist and hand radiograph, showing arthritis of the distal radioulnar joint, wrist with radial deviation, dislocated ulnar, deviated metacarpophalangeal joints, screw arthrodesis of the thumb interphalangeal joint and wired arthrodesis of the finger proximal interphalangeal joints.

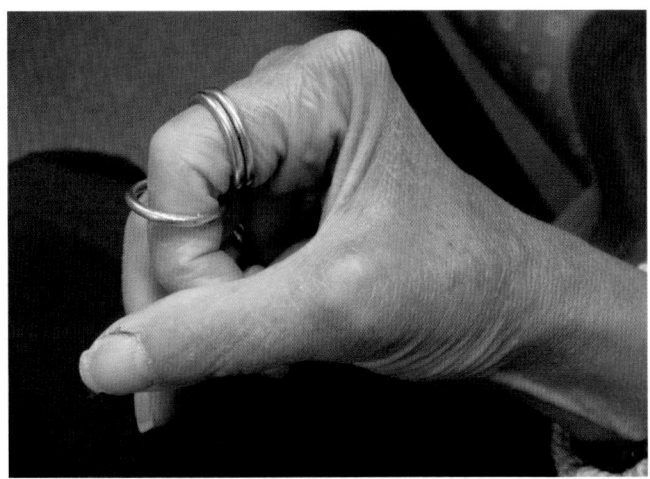

Figure 37.4 Silvis ring worn to prevent proximal interphalangeal joints hyperextension (swan neck deformity) but allow flexion.

systemically, topically and by local injection into joints or around tendons.

Splints can be helpful to reduce pain and improve function (e.g. unstable wrist, swan neck deformity (Fig. 37.4). They probably do not often prevent deformity. Orthotics are useful for the foot and ankle.

For the moment surgery is still very important for rheumatoid arthritis. Surgical options for joints include arthrodesis [especially for cervical spine, finger proximal interphalangeal joints (PIPJ), the wrist, ankle and hindfoot], and joint replacement (for major joints including the elbow, metacarpophalangeal joints and even the wrist). There are a few sites where excision arthroplasty is used such as the distal ulna and radial head (Figs 37.5 and 37.6).

If tenosynovitis is resistant to medical treatment, it should be treated with tenosynovectomy to prevent tendon rupture. If rupture occurs, it is treated with tendon transfer (e.g. extensor indicis proprius to ruptured extensor pollicis longus). An alternative is interposition grafting (often using palmaris longus) or arthrodesis in a functional position of the joint previously controlled by the tendon (e.g. of the thumb IPJ after flexor pollicis longus rupture; see Fig. 37.3) (Summary box 37.4).

Summary box 37.4

Surgery for rheumatoid arthritis

- Synovectomy – for inflamed joints
- Tenosynovectomy for inflamed tendon sheaths
- Arthrodesis (fusion) – finger joints (IPJs), wrist, spine, ankle and hindfoot
- Joint replacement (hip, knee, elbow, shoulder, metacarpophalangeal joints)

GOUT AND PSEUDOGOUT

Gout was first described in the fourth century by Hippocrates. Gout affects approximately 1% of the UK population, mostly men

---

Hippocrates **was a Greek Physician, and by common consent 'The Father of Medicine'. He was born on the Greek island of Cos off Turkey about 460 BC, and probably died in 375 BC.**

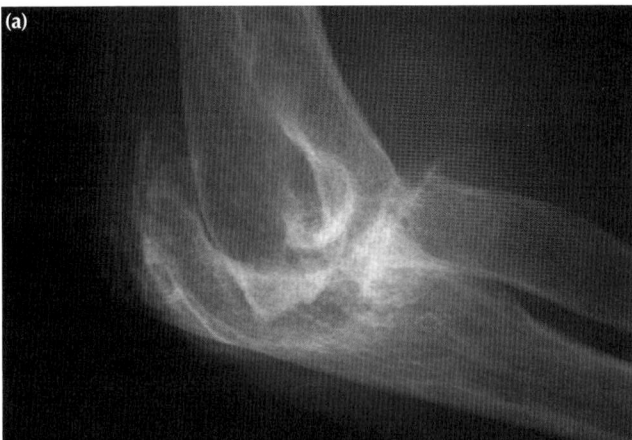

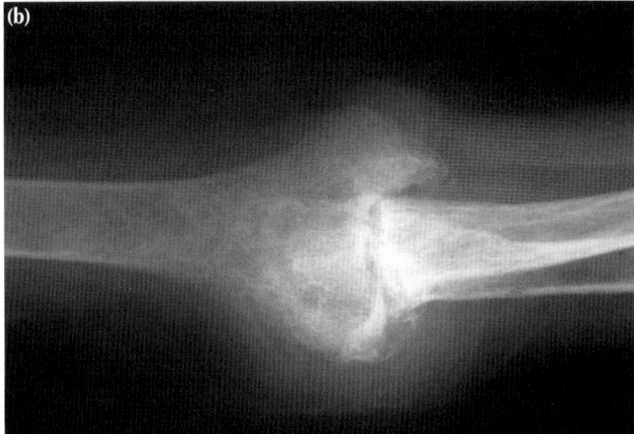

Figure 37.5 Anteroposterior and lateral radiographs of a rheumatoid elbow. There is significant erosion and bone loss of elbow with rheumatoid arthritis.

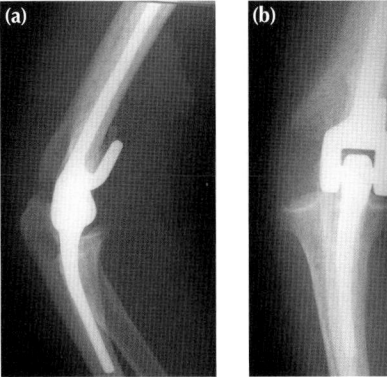

Figure 37.6 Radiograph of elbow with total elbow replacement.

over 40. Pseudogout affects the elderly, both men and women. There is excess urate in the blood and tissues. Over time, crystals of urate form in and around joints, causing inflammation (Fig 37.7). Renal calculi may also form.

The initial presentation is usually with a single joint affected in an acute attack. The first metatarsophalangeal joint is affected in half of first attacks. Other common sites are the small joints of the hand, wrist, elbow, mid-tarsal joints, ankle and knee. The

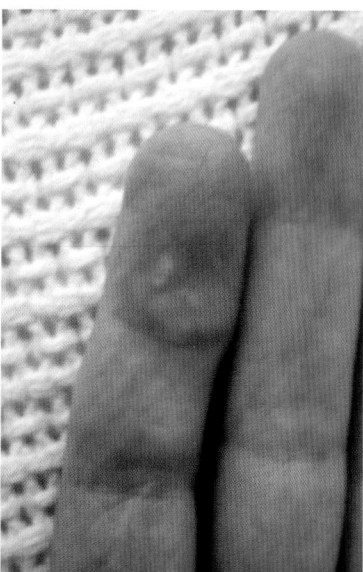

Figure 37.7 Gouty tophus.

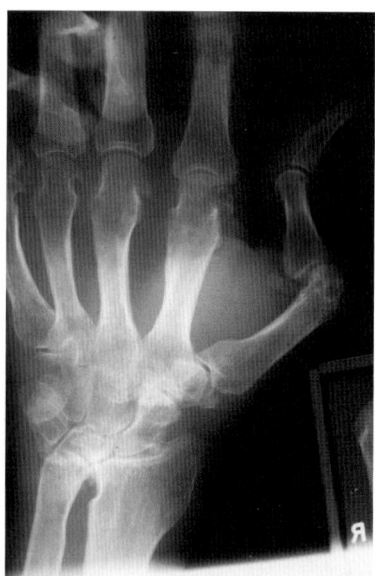

Figure 37.8 Radiograph of hand and wrist with changes characteristic of gout.

larger joints and axial skeleton are rarely affected, and certainly never in the first attack. The pain develops over a few hours, often overnight. There is intense inflammation of the affected joint, with erythema, swelling and extreme tenderness; even bedclothes touching the joint cannot be tolerated. There may be fever and malaise.

Investigations should include serum urate; however, this may be lowered during an acute attack and should be measured between attacks, using two separate fasting samples. There may be a neutrophilia, and raised CRP during an acute attack. Renal function should be checked.

Definitive diagnosis rests upon demonstration under polarised light of negatively birefringent monosodium urate monohydrate crystals within the synovial fluid, obtained by joint aspiration. The synovial fluid will be turbid with a high neutrophil count.

The main differential diagnoses of acute gout are pseudogout and septic arthritis. These may co-exist, so the aspirate should also be examined with a Gram stain and cultured for organisms.

A radiograph of the affected joint is usually normal during an initial attack, but may show punched-out eccentric, asymmetrical juxta-articular erosions after repeated attacks. (Fig. 37.8) These have normal bone density around the cysts, contrasting with the ill-defined, symmetrical, marginal erosions with osteopenia seen in rheumatoid arthritis. The higher the hyperuricaemia, the worse the destruction in most cases (Fig 37.9).

Treatment of the acute attack involves pain relief with anti-inflammatories, and/or aspiration. Attempting to lower the serum urate may conversely prolong the attack – and should be avoided.

Pseudogout [calcium pyrophosphate deposition disease – (CPPD)] leads to pyrophosphate deposition within the joints. It is the most common cause of acute mono-arthropathy in the elderly and is most likely to affect the knee, wrist, shoulder or ankle. Calcium pyrophosphate shows positively birefringent crystals under polarised light. The radiograph in pyrophosphate arthropathy may show changes of osteoarthritis and calcification within the meniscii of the knee, the triangular fibrocartilage on the ulnar side of the wrist, or the symphysis pubis. More rarely, there is calcification within hyaline cartilage.

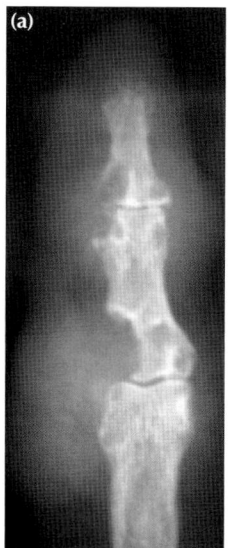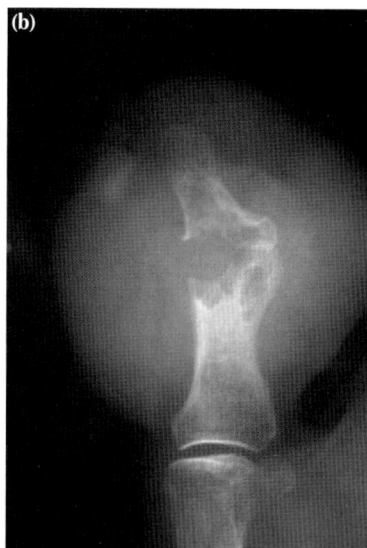

(a) (b)

Figure 37.9 Characteristic radiographic features of neglected gout in index finger (left) and thumb (right), same patient as in Fig 37.7.

THE SPONDYLOARTHROPATHIES

The spondyloarthropathies are a heterogeneous group or spectrum of disorders, including ankylosing spondylitis, reactive arthritis and psoriatic arthritis. They are associated with HLA-B27 and a negative rheumatoid factor.

Ankylosing spondylitis

Ankylosing spondylitis affects approximately 0.5% of men and 0.2% of women in the UK. This most commonly starts in the late teens, twenties or thirties. There is a strong genetic component, being associated with HLA-B27.

The disease principally affects the sacroiliac joints, axial skeleton and peripheral joints, starting with sacroiliitis. The sacroiliac

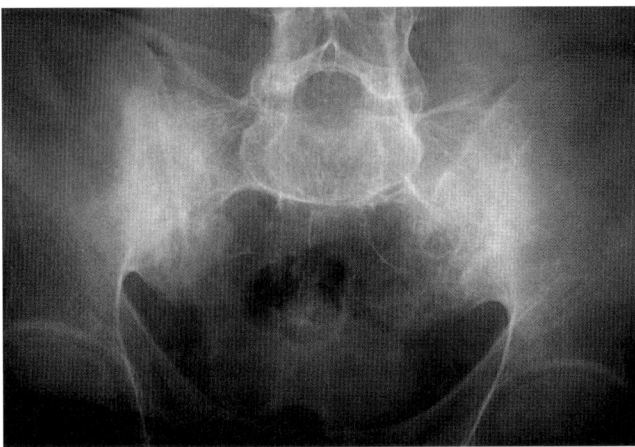

Figure 37.10 Radiograph showing sacroiliitis in ankylosing spondylitis.

Table 37.2 Radiological changes in the sacroiliac joint in ankylosing spondylitis

0	Normal
I	Minimal changes
II	Sclorosis, some erosions
III	Severe erosions, pseudodilatation of joint space, limited ankylosis
IV	Ankylosis

joint changes are classified on plain radiographs as shown in Table 37.2 and Fig. 37.10. Patients usually present with inflammatory low back and buttock pain. Over time, increasing stiffness of the spine is seen, with a flattening of the normal lumbar lordosis, and then a thoracic kyphosis. The rib cage stiffens and so lung capacity becomes limited (Figs 37.11 and 37.12). A fixed flexion deformity of the hips is common. This is compensated for by flexion of the knees, so that the patient adopts a 'question mark' posture. Enthesitis (inflammation at the insertion of tendon or ligament to bone) commonly occurs at the insertion of the Achilles tendon or the plantar fascia on the calcaneus.

Sacroiliitis can be seen very early in the disease process on magnetic resonance imaging (MRI). Ultrasound can be useful in the diagnosis of enthesitis. Plain radiography shows characteristic changes, as described above, commonly known as 'bamboo spine'.

Medical treatment with regular physiotherapy is important to maintain range of movement. Around 10% of patients require total hip replacement. Occasionally a corrective osteotomy of the kyphosis is needed to allow forward vision. The stiff spine makes patients susceptible to unstable spinal fractures.

REACTIVE ARTHRITIS (REITER'S DISEASE)

Stoll described this triad of urethritis, uveitis and arthritis in 1776, Reiter redescribing the condition much later. The condition starts

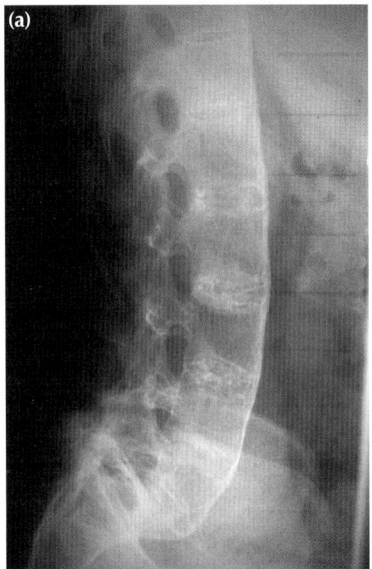

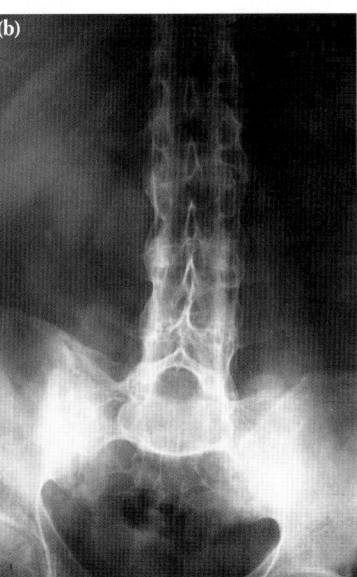

Figure 37.11 Lumbar spine radiographs showing 'bamboo spine' changes in ankylosing spondylitis.

with an infection as the gastrointestinal or genitourinary systems with a triggering organism, such as *Shigella* or *Chlamydia*. This is followed by a reactive synovitis and arthritis with effusion (Table 37.3). The precipitating infection may be asymptomatic, especially *Chlamydia* in women. *Yersinia* causes arthritis inversely proportional to the severity of the gastrointestinal symptoms. Patients have either an oligoarthritis or a monoarthritis, and the lower limb joints are most commonly affected. The joint is acutely inflamed with erythema, swelling/synovitis and effusion. Enthesitis is usually present in addition to the arthritis, affecting the Achilles tendon and plantar fascia insertions on the calcaneus. Sacroiliitis and dactylitis are also seen. Ocular manifestations include conjunctivitis (which has often settled

Hans Conrad Julius Reiter, **1881–1968, President if the Health Service, and Honorary Professor of Hygiene at the University of Berlin, Germany, described this disease in 1916.**
Maximilian Stoll, **1742–1787, Physician, Vienna, Austria.**

Kiyoshi Shiga, **1870–1957, a Japanese Bacteriologist, who was Dean of the Medical Faculty of the Keijo Imperial University, Chosen, Japan.**

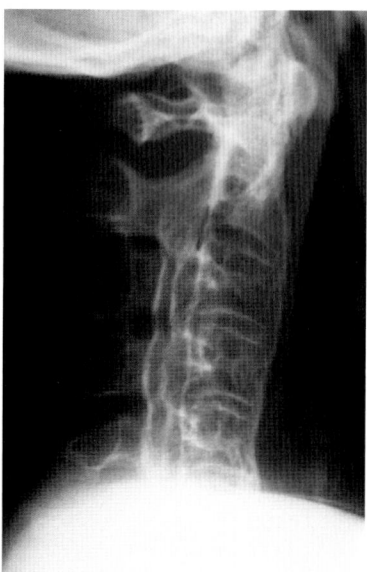

Figure 37.12 Radiograph of cervical spine in ankylosing spondylitis.

Table 37.3 Features and causes of reactive arthritis

Classic clinical features	Classic infective organisms
Asymmetrical oligoarthritis, especially lower limb	*Salmonella* *Campylobacter*
Enthesitis	*Yersinia*
Extra-articular signs, e.g. uveitis	*Shigella* *Chlamydia*

when the arthritis presents) or acute anterior uveitis. Abnormal investigations include raised ESR and particularly CRP (> 100 mg l^{-1}). Assays for antinuclear antibodies and RF are negative.

Affected joints require rest and occasionally splintage. Joint aspiration is also useful for symptomatic relief. This may be followed by corticosteroid injection once septic arthritis has been excluded.

ARTHRITIS ASSOCIATED WITH PSORIASIS OR COLITIS

Psoriatic arthritis affects 5–40% of the 1–3% of people with skin psoriasis. There is a similar association with ulcerative colitis and Crohn's disease in 10–20% of patients. Radiographs show an inflammatory type of arthritis, with 'whiskering': erosive changes at the margins of joints with adjacent new bone. When severe, erosion often produces a 'pencil-in-cup' radiographic appearance (Fig 37.13). Changes in the axial skeleton are similar to those seen in ankylosing spondylitits. Appearances may resemble

Daniel Elmer Salmon, **1840–1914**, Veterinary Pathologist, Chief of the Bureau of Animal Industry, Washington, DC, USA.
Alexandre Emile Jean Yersin, **1863–1943**, Bacteriologist, Institute Pasteur, Paris, France.
Burrill Bernard Crohn, **1884–1983**, Gastroenterologist, Mount Sinai Hospital, New York, NY, USA, described regional ileitis in 1932.

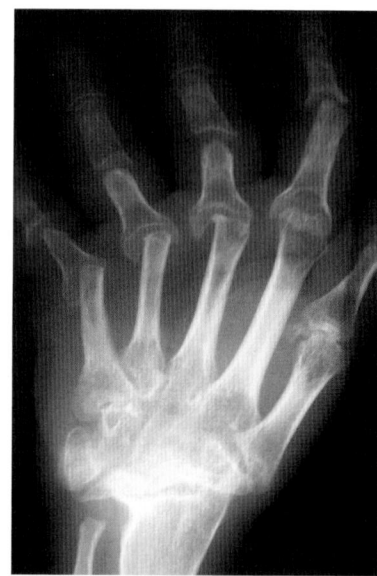

Figure 37.13 'Pencil-in-cup' appearance of metacarpophalangeal joints in psoriatic arthritis.

Forestier's disease (diffuse idiopathic spinal hyperostosis; Fig 37.14). Skin therapy has no effect on arthritis. Treatment options include NSAIDs, intra-articular or paratendinous steroid injection, DMARDs (sulphasalazine, methotrexate, ciclosporin). Surgical options are similar to those described for rheumatoid arthritis.

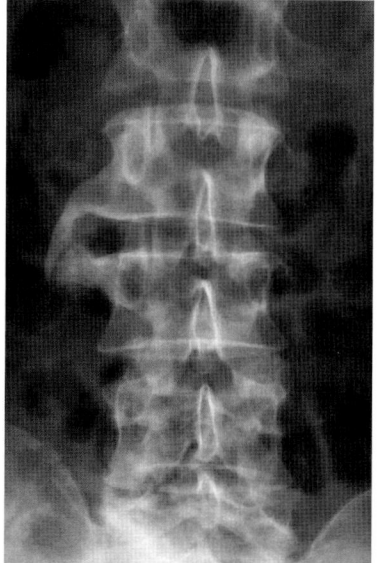

Figure 37.14 Lumbar spine radiograph showing changes of psoriatic arthropathy.

JUVENILE RHEUMATOID ARTHRITIS

This affects mostly girls under 5. The late-onset pauciarticular type affects more boys. The systemic type often starts in children

Jacques Forestier, **1890–1978**, a French Rheumatologist, described this condition in 1950.

under 5 and affects boys and girls equally. The pathophysiology is similar to that of rheumatoid arthritis but the effects are different because the bones and joints are growing. Hyperaemia can increase growth in the short term, but chronic disease may result in very small bones. Severe and longstanding disease may cause ankylosis and soft-tissue contractures. The most frequently affected joint is the knee. Other commonly affected joints are the ankle, wrist, hip and cervical spine. The pauciarticular type affects younger children. The polyarticular cases may involve several joints simultaneously or sequentially and also include tenosynovitis. While the arthritis is active, the child may feel unwell and have a low-grade pyrexia. The temporomandibular joints are very frequently extremely stiff, making anaesthesia difficult and fibreoptic intubation may be required. Surgery is generally restricted to soft-tissue releases and occasional synovectomy until cessation of growth, but joint replacement is increasingly indicated in early adult life as prostheses have become more reliable.

SYSTEMIC LUPUS ERYTHEMATOSUS

This is an autoimmune disorder that can present with symptoms and signs in almost any part of the body. The aetiology is multifactorial, including genetic, hormonal and environmental factors. There is often an effusion, but rarely synovitis. Hip pain raises suspicion of avascular necrosis (AVN) of the femoral head, a complication of systemic corticosteroid therapy. MRI gives early diagnosis. Investigations should include antinuclear antibody assay. An increase in anti-dsDNA antibody or anti-Sm antibody level is virtually specific for systemic lupus erythematosus (SLE). Surgery for SLE is less often indicated than for rheumatoid arthritis. Metacarpophalangeal joint subluxation is treated with silicone arthroplasty and soft-tissue reconstruction. Some patients benefit from interphalangeal joint arthrodesis in a functional position for severe deformities. Femoral head AVN may indicate total hip replacement (Summary box 37.5).

> **Summary box 37.5**
>
> **Other causes of inflammatory joint disease**
>
> - Gout – deposition of urate crystals – commonly affects big toe
> - Pseudo-gout – calcium pyrophosphate (birefringent crystals) – larger joints
> - Ankylosing spondylitis – HLA-B27-positive – sacroiliac joints affected first
> - Reactive arthritis – urethritis, uveitis and arthritis; triggered by bowel infection
> - Associated arthritis – psoriasis and ulcerative colitis
> - Juvenile rheumatoid arthritis – commonly starts in girls under 5
> - SLE – anti-Sm antibodies diagnostic

SEPTIC ARTHRITIS

Septic arthritis occurs at any age, most commonly at the extremes of age. In adults, the immunocompromised are most at risk, including intravenous drug abusers, diabetics and sufferers of rheumatoid arthritis. Infection can arise from contamination of the joint following trauma, but it also appears possible that

bacteria can settle in the joint from a transient bacteraemia in the blood (which occurs regularly in us all) as well as from a full-blown septicaemia (blood poisoning).

The most commonly affected joints are the hip in neonates and the knee in children and adults. In around 10% of cases more than one joint is involved. The patient with acute septic arthritis usually has a short history and is sometimes very unwell, with a high pyrexia (if septicaemic). However, septic arthritis may present only with severe joint pain, and the patient may be apyrexial much of the time, and then only develop a low-grade pyrexia from time to time. A high index of suspicion is required if the diagnosis is to be made quickly. One cardinal sign is that the joint is held immobile in the 'position of comfort', and there is severe pain if any attempt is made to move the affected joint actively or passively. Radiographs show no change for 7–10 days. Ultrasound scanning and guided aspiration is useful, especially for the hip in small children. Treatment of the septic joint consists of removal of pus and reduction of joint pressure as soon as possible. Intravenous antibiotics should be started immediately after samples and blood cultures have been taken. Cefuroxime is a good empirical choice until organism and/or sensitivities are identified, as it covers staphylococci and gram-negative organisms. Repeated aspiration may be needed, but if the effusion re-accumulates a safer option is to perform open arthrotomy and wash-out. The capsule is left open, and skin sutured. In the knee or shoulder an arthroscopic washout can be performed. Common infective organisms are shown in Table 37.4.

TUBERCULOUS ARTHRITIS

This had become uncommon in the UK, but was still prevalent in the developing world. There is now a resurgence in the developed world from travel, immigration, more immunocompromised/elderly patients and drug addicts. The usual organism is *Mycobacterium tuberculosis*, 3–5% of cases affect the skeleton, half in the spine. It presents with a chronic history, usually from haematogenous spread. Osseous tuberculosis affects the metaphysis or subchondral bone. If host resistance is poor, destruction extends along and out of the bone. A 'cold abscess' (not inflamed) or fistula may form. Spinal involvement is commonly paradiscal, but vertebral, anterior or posterior infections or 'skip

Table 37.4 Organisms most commonly involved in bone and joint infections

Staphylococcus aureus	Overall the commonest in all sites and age groups
ß-Haemolytic streptococci and anaerobes	Also cause acute infection
Escherichia coli, group B streptococci	Neonates
Haemophilus influenzae	Non-immunised toddlers
Aerobic gram-negative rods	Discitis in the elderly

Hans Christian Joachim Gram, **1853–1938, Professor of Pharmacology, (1891–1900), and of Medicine (1900–1923), Copenhagen, Denmark, described this method of staining bacteria in 1884.**

lesions' affecting non-adjacent vertebrae are seen. Diagnosis is based on joint aspirate or biopsy. MRI can delineate disease extent within bone and soft tissues, especially spine. Tuberculin skin testing and blood tests are usually unhelpful. Treatment is anti-tuberculous chemotherapy; early surgery is required only for cord compression with paraplegia. Debridement is occasionally indicated (Summary box 37.6).

Summary box 37.6

Septic arthritis

- Commonest in babies and the elderly
- Extreme pain on moving the joint
- Diagnosis by ultrasound-guided aspiration of effusion
- Commonest organism is *Staphylococcus aureus* but *Escherichia coli* and others can occur in neonates
- Needs early decompression and high-dose antibiotics
- Tuberculous arthritis often affects the spine

INFECTION IN JOINT REPLACEMENTS

In a prosthetic infection the ulcer is more indolent, and the patient is rarely unwell. Occasionally, acute infection can present in the early postoperative phase (less than 1% of cases in good units). Others develop later but most almost certainly began from contamination at the time of surgery. Low-virulence organisms, particularly skin commensals such as *Staphylococcus epidermidis* and also methicillin-resistant *Staphylococcus aureus* (MRSA) are frequently the cause. If bacteria introduced at the time of surgery survive, they appear to get buried in a protein layer (biofilm) associated with the interface between the healing bone and the implant. In this position they cannot replicate quickly but they are also immune to antibiotics. However, they produce a low-grade inflammatory response which causes pain and rapid loosening of the implant; CRP will rise rather than fall. If infection is suspected, treatment should be started as soon as possible if the implant is to be saved. A firm diagnosis is best made by opening the joint and taking multiple biopsy specimens of the synovium and membrane around the implant. If there is no sign of infection then nothing further need be done until the culture results return, but if there is felt to be excessive inflammation but no gross infection, an aggressive clearance of all soft tissues and a washout of the wound is performed. This is followed by high-dose intravenous antibiotics. If infection is obvious (frank pus in the joint), the joint replacement needs removing with all the cement as well. Some surgeons immediately replace the prosthesis with a new one (one-stage revision), others leave the patient without a joint for a minimum of 3 months and treat with high-dose antibiotics while they wait for the infection to clear. Then they put in a new implant (two-stage revision). If the infection does not settle, then the patient may need to be left without a joint. This is called the Girdlestone operation in the hip (Summary box 37.7).

Gathorne Robert Girdlestone, 1881–1950, Nuffield Professor of Orthopaedics, The University of Oxford, Oxford, England.

Summary box 37.7

Infected joint replacement

- Most are avoidable with good theatre technique and prophylactic antibiotics
- Indolent onset with pain, weakness and failure to improve after surgery
- Persistent raised ESR and CRP; positive culture at biopsy
- One- or two-stage revision needed with long-term antibiotics

---

OSTEOMYELITIS

This is commonest in children (decreasing), and the elderly or immunocompromised (increasing). The elderly most commonly have vertebral osteomyelitis, whereas children develop infection in a long bone metaphysis. The commonest organism is *Staphylococcus aureus*, despite the infrequency of staphylococcal bacteraemia, presumably because of that organism's particular ability to infect bone. Acute osteomyelitis is usually regarded as that which occurs before there is actual bone death, while chronic osteomyelitis involves infection both within and around bone that has died.

Osteomyelitis is classified according to cause:

- haematogenous;
- post-traumatic;
- contiguous (from neighbouring tissue – e.g. diabetic foot ulcer).

The history is usually short, 48 hours or less. Initially, there is bone pain and marked tenderness without visible inflammation. When infection spreads subperiosteally, local and systemic signs of infection appear. Pus then forms in bone and soft tissues. The appearance of the bone does not change for 10–14 days so radiographs are a baseline for future change and to exclude differential diagnoses (Ewing's sarcoma, leukaemia). Softening of soft-tissue planes may be seen. Ultrasound gives an early diagnosis and if fluid or oedema can be seen aspiration provides an organism in 70% of cases. MRI is useful for visualising deeper bones, e.g. pelvis. Full blood count (FBC), ESR, CRP and blood cultures are all useful indicators. When repeated they can give a guide to the success of treatment. Treatment with empirical intravenous antibiotics should start immediately after cultures have been taken. Likely organisms are those also listed for septic arthritis. A definitive choice is directed by sensitivities once available. Antibiotic treatment should be continued for several weeks. Surgery (or interventional radiology) is indicated to evacuate abscesses. Bone drilling is not routinely required. With modern antibiotic therapy, the high mortality and permanent disability caused by osteomyelitis have dramatically improved. Now, only 5% of cases develop long-term sequelae. Chronic osteomyelitis is typically seen in elderly patients who developed acute osteomyelitis in the pre-antibiotic era. This is rarely 'cured', and reactivates at times of poor health or trauma. Pathology shows necrotic bone, new bone formation and chronic inflammation. Antibiotics (or natural host defences) cannot reach organisms within dead tissues, and disease continues. Necrotic cortical bone is extruded. This is called a 'sequestrum'. The encasing live bone, the 'involucrum', may be perforated by openings which can lead to the skin as a sinus. Treatment combines clearance of all dead and contaminated tissues, bone de-roofing, intramedullary reaming and intravenous antibiotics. Wound closure, often with local or free flaps is preferred (Summary box 37.8).

INFECTIONS OF SOFT TISSUE

See the section on necrotising fasciitis in Chapter 30.

MUSCULOSKELETAL TUMOURS

The most common malignant bone tumours are metastases (Fig. 37.15). As a result of advances in oncological treatment, the number of patients presenting with skeletal failure due to metastatic disease is increasing. The most common tumours that metastasise to bone are breast, prostate, lung, kidney and thyroid carcinomas (Fig. 37.16).

Multiple myeloma (Fig. 37.17) is a malignant neoplasm arising from the plasma cells in the bone marrow. It is usually multicentric. If the condition is solitary it is called a plasmacytoma. Malignant primary sarcomas of bone are very rare. The most common of these is osteosarcoma (Fig. 37.18). Osteosarcoma has two peaks in incidence, one in adolescence, the other later in life, arising in patients with Paget's disease and those who have had previous radiotherapy (Fig. 37.19). Chondrosarcoma (Figs 37.20–37.22) and Ewing's sarcoma (Fig. 37.23, p. 550) make up most of the rest. Ewing's sarcoma occurs in adolescence, while the incidence of chondrosarcoma increases from middle age onwards. Some conditions are associated with an increased likelihood of developing malignant disease in bone and/or cartilage (Table 37.5). Soft-tissue tumours are also quite rare and most are benign, with only one in a hundred being malignant (Fig. 37.24, p. 551).

Malignant tumours usually metastasise to bone by means of haematogenous spread. The spine is the third most common site for metastases, after the lung and liver. Although most patients with systemic cancer will have metastatic disease in the spine before they die, only 10% are symptomatic. Tumour cells metastasise to the spine via Batson's venous plexus. These retroperitoneal veins have no valves and allow retrograde spread by embolisation to the spine and proximal long bones (Fig. 37.25,

Sir James Paget, 1814–1899, Surgeon, St. Bartholomew's Hospital, London, England, described osteitis deformans in 1877.
James Ewing, 1866–1943, Professor of Pathology, The Cornell University Medical College, New York, NY, USA, described this type of sarcoma in 1921.
Oscar V. Batson, 1894–1979, an American Otolaryngologist.

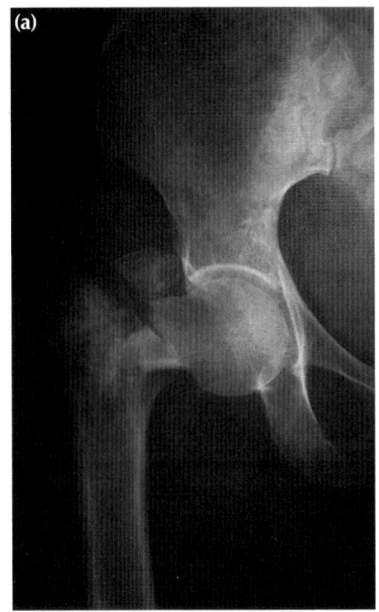

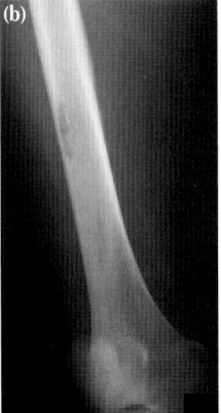

Figure 37.15 (a) Pathological fracture of the proximal femur through metastatic breast carcinoma. (b) Radiographs of the whole femur show a further, more distal metastatic deposit.

p. 551). Metastases can be lytic, sclerotic or mixed. Lytic metastases usually arise from tumours that are vascular. However, they can also occur in very aggressive, destructive tumours with no healing response from the bone. Sclerotic lesions are commonly from the prostate.

BONE TUMOURS

Bone tumours are classified according to the tissue of origin. These include:

- metastases – may show histological features of their tissue of origin;
- haematopoetic tumours – e.g. myeloma;
- osteogenic tumours – e.g. osteosarcoma;
- chondrogenic tumours – e.g. chondrosarcoma;
- others – e.g. Ewing's sarcoma.

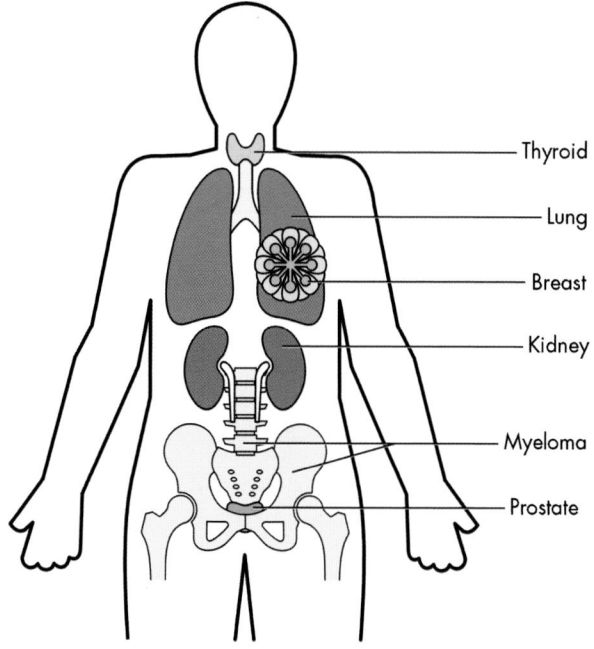

Figure 37.16 Malignant tumours commonly metastasising to bone.

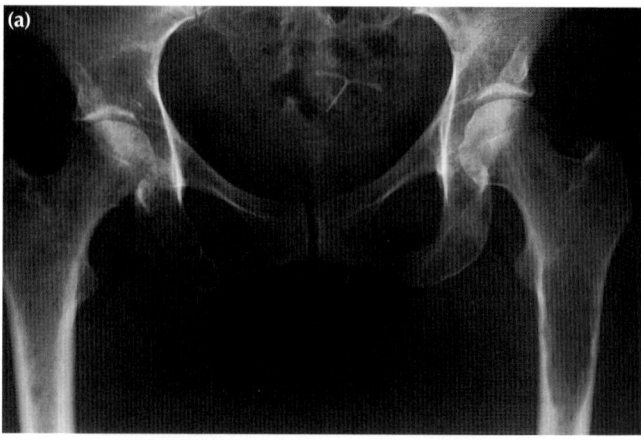

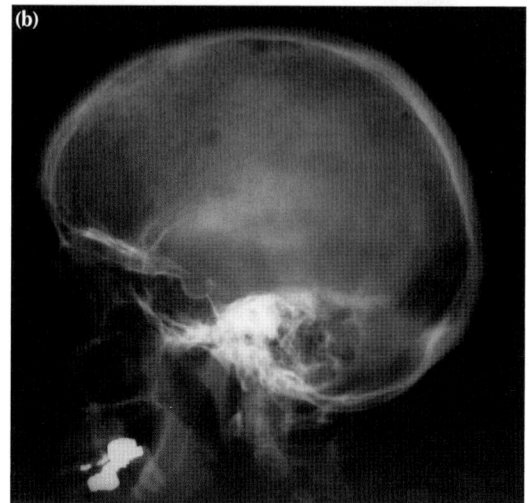

Figure 37.17 (a) Multiple myeloma with a large deposit in the left proximal femur. (b) Multiple myeloma with multiple deposits in the skull.

METASTASES

The vast majority of tumours spreading to the skeleton are carcinomas; but not infrequently the primary tumour is never found. Metastases are rare in children, but can occur from neuroblastoma, rhabdomyosarcoma and clear cell carcinoma of the kidney (Summary boxes 37.9 and 37.10).

Summary box 37.9

Most common bone metastases (93%)

- Breast
- Prostate
- Lung
- Renal
- Thyroid

Summary box 37.10

Commonest sites of bone metastases

- Spine
- Proximal femur
- Proximal humerus

Table 37.5 Conditions associated with an increased risk of malignant disease in bone and cartilage

High risk	Moderate risk	Low risk
Maffucci's syndrome (enchondromatosis and angiomas of soft tissue)	Diaphyseal aclasia (multiple osteochondromas)	Chronic osteomyelitis
Ollier's disease (enchondromatosis)	Polyostotic Paget's disease	Osteonecrosis
Familial retinoblastoma syndrome	Radiation osteitis	Fibrous dysplasia, osteogenesis imperfecta, osteoblastoma and chondroblastoma

---

Angelo Maffuci, **1845–1903, Professor of Pathological Anatomy, Pisa, Italy.**
Louis Xavier Eduard Leopold Ollier, **1830–1900, Professor of Surgery, Lyons, France, described enchondromatosis in 1899.**

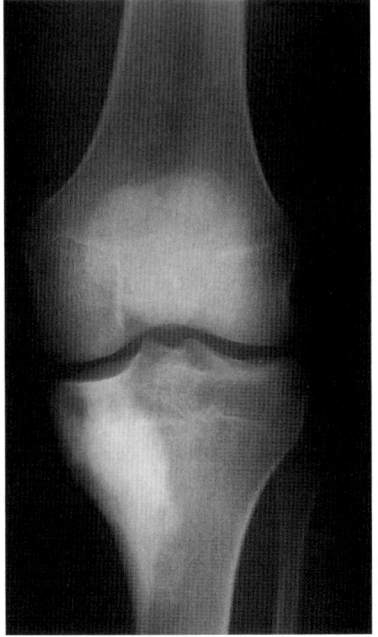

Figure 37.18 Sclerotic osteosarcoma of the proximal tibia.

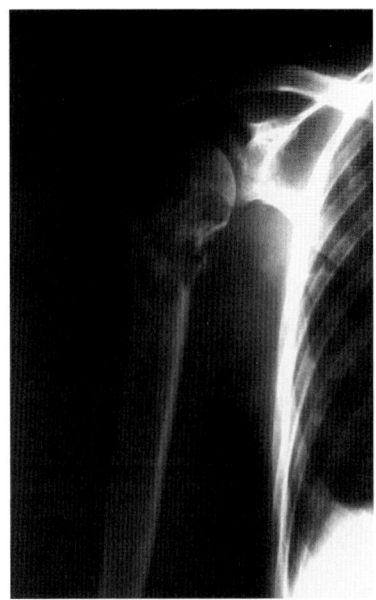

Figure 37.19 Radiation-induced osteosarcoma of the proximal humerus (following treatment for breast carcinoma).

HAEMATOPOETIC TUMOURS

There are no benign neoplasms of the haematopoetic system. Malignant tumours can be divided into two groups:

- solitary plasmacytoma/multiple myeloma (see Fig. 37.17 p. 548);
- lymphomas – malignant neoplasm of the lymphoid cells (Summary box 37.11).

Summary box 37.11

Malignant bone tumours

- ■ Plasmacytoma – solitary form of multiple myeloma
- ■ Osteosarcoma – could be secondary to Paget's disease and radiotherapy
- ■ Chondrosarcoma
- ■ Ewing's sarcoma

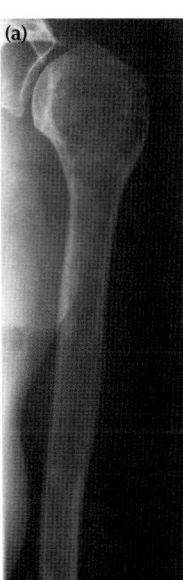

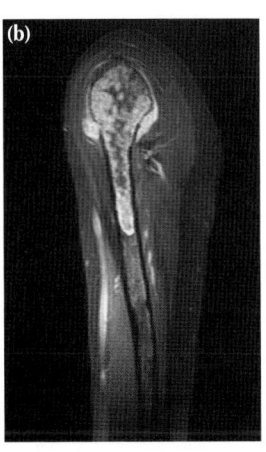

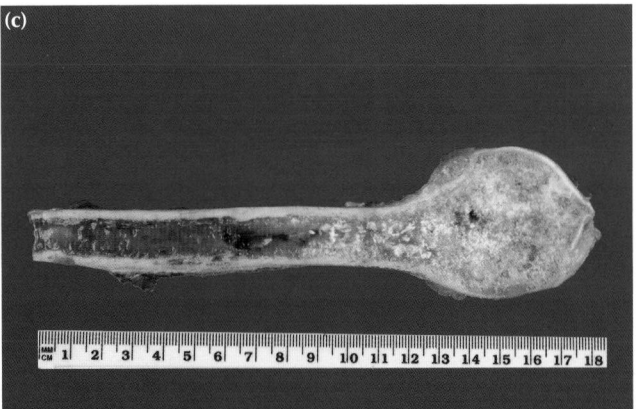

Figure 37.20 (a) Chondrosarcoma of the proximal humerus with multiple calcifications. (b) Magnetic resonance imaging scan showing extensive involvement. (c) Excised chondrosarcoma of the proximal humerus.

CHAPTER 37 | INFLAMMATION AND INFECTION AND MUSCULOSKELETAL TUMOURS

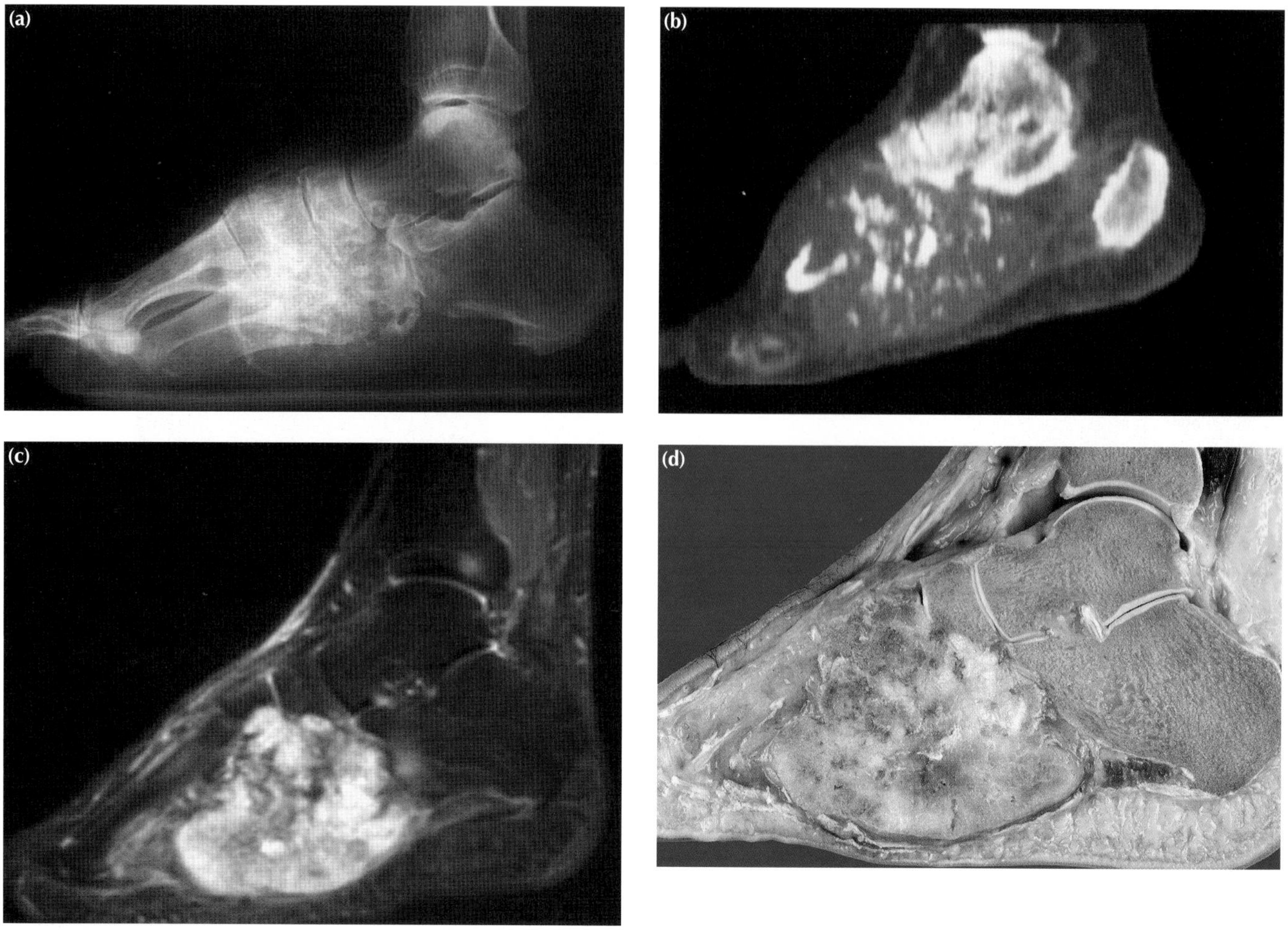

(a)

(b)

(c)

(d)

Figure 37.21 (a) Chondrosarcoma of the foot. (b) Computerised tomography scan reconstruction showing multiple calcifications. (c) T2-weighted magnetic resonance imaging scan shows high signal in chondrosarcoma. (d) Excised chondrosarcoma of the foot.

OSTEOGENIC TUMOURS

These tumours produce osteoid or bony matrix.

Osteoid osteoma (Figs 37.26 and 37.27) is a benign bone-forming lesion which is small but very painful. Usually, symptoms occur at night and are typically relieved by anti-inflammatories. Children and adolescents are frequently affected. Osteomas can occur in any bone but are common in the proximal femur.

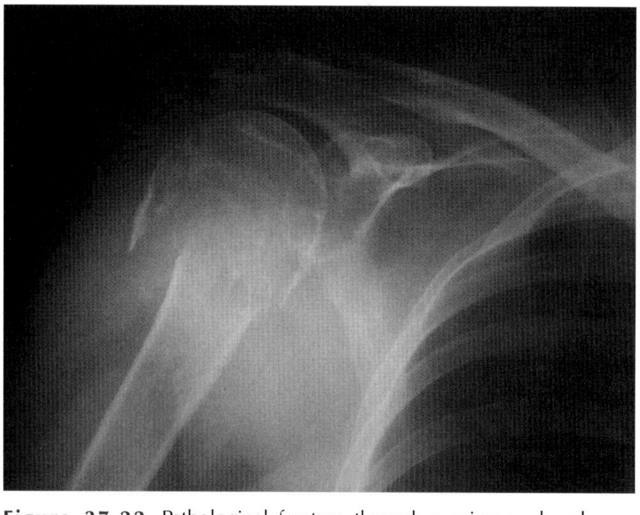

Figure 37.22 Pathological fracture through a primary chondrosarcoma of the proximal humerus.

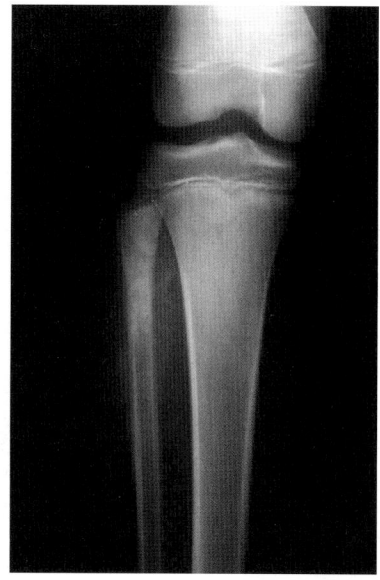

Figure 37.23 Ewing's sarcoma of the proximal fibula.

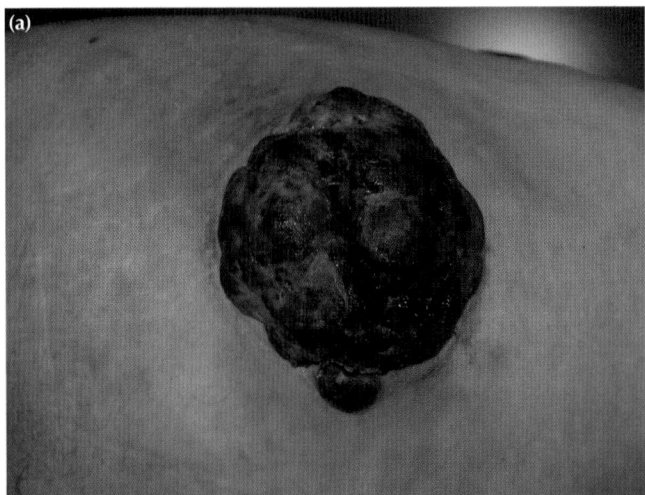

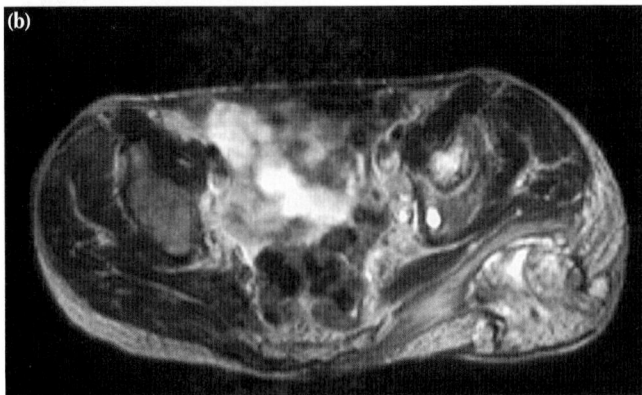

Figure 37.24 (a) Large, fungating soft-tissue sarcoma of the buttock. (b) Magnetic resonance imaging scan showing a large fungating sarcoma of the buttock.

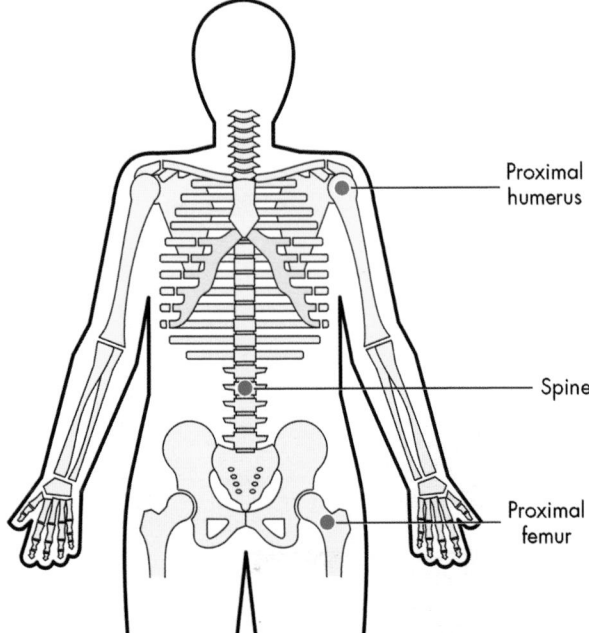

Figure 37.25 Common sites of metastatic bone disease.

Proximal humerus

Spine

Proximal femur

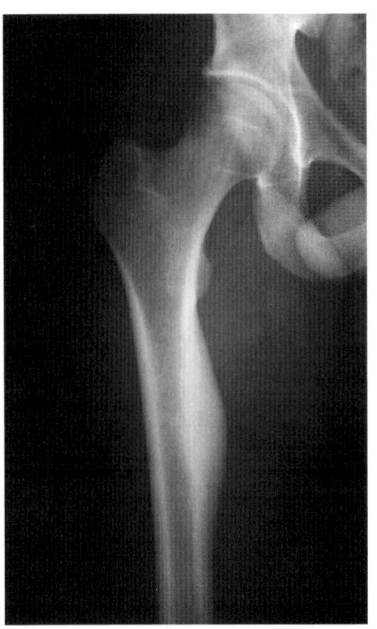

Figure 37.26 Radiograph showing osteoid osteoma of the proximal femur with reactive bone formation.

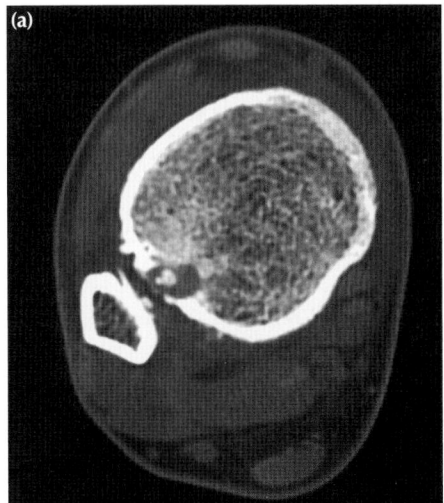

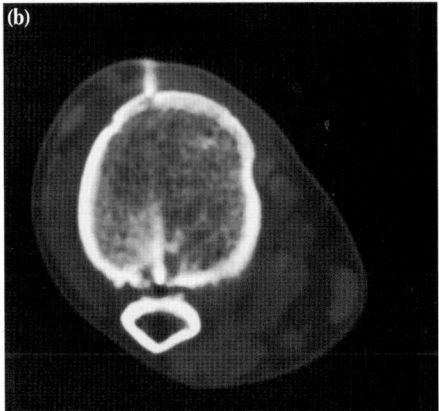

Figure 37.27 (a) Axial computerised tomography (CT) scan showing an osteoid osteoma nidus in the distal tibia. (b) CT-guided radio-frequency thermocoagulation of an osteoid osteoma of the distal tibia. The scan shows the electrode *in situ*.

Osteoid osteomas are usually diaphyseal in location and give rise to a dense cortical reaction (Fig. 37.26). Osteoblastoma is the larger more aggressive counterpart of osteoid osteoma that commonly occurs in the spine.

Osteosarcoma (see Figs 37.18 and 37.19, p. 549) is most common in the distal femur, followed by proximal tibia, proximal humerus and distal tibia. Radiologically and histologically the tumour can be sclerotic (Fig. 37.18), chondroblastic, teleangiectic and of other more unusual histological forms. Usually, osteosarcomas are intraosseous, but they can also arise from the surface of the bone. Paraosteal osteosarcoma (Fig. 37.28) is a low-grade osteosarcoma that arises from the surface of the bone. It frequently affects the distal femur and proximal tibia. The clinical symptoms are often mild and longstanding (Summary box 37.12).

Summary box 37.12

Tumours producing bone

- Osteoid osteoma – small and painful; produce a dense cortical reaction
- Osteoblastoma – larger and more aggressive than osteoid osteoma
- Osteosarcoma – malignant; commonest in lower femur and upper tibia

---

CHONDROGENIC TUMOURS

These tumours produce chondroid matrix. The biological spectrum of these tumours ranges from very benign to highly malignant.

Osteochondroma (Figs 37.29 and 37.30) is a benign cartilage-capped bony projection. It is thought to originate from the physis. The bony projection is always growing away from the joint towards the diaphyseal region of the bone. It has no structures attached to it. Osteochondromas can be pedunculated or sessile. The stalk or base is always continuous with the intramedullary cavity of the bone. They are usually solitary, but can be multiple (Fig. 37.31) in diaphyseal aclasia (autosomal dominant inheritance). Complications include mechanical symptoms, nerve impingement, vascular pseudo-aneurysm, fracture and infarction. Increasing size or pain, particularly after skeletal maturity, is concerning and may indicate malignant transformation. The incidence of malignant transformation is less than 1% in solitary osteochondromas and 1–3% in diaphyseal aclasia.

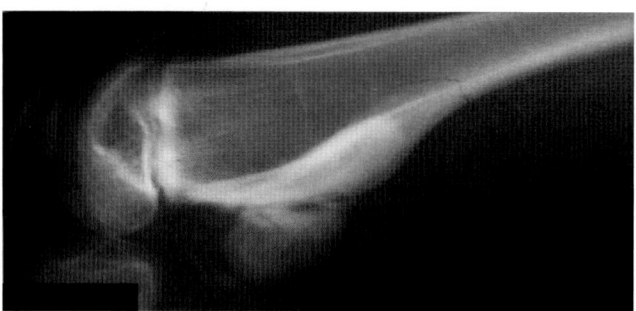

Figure 37.28 Paraosteal osteosarcoma of the distal femur in an unusually young patient. There is no continuity with the intramedullary cavity of the femur.

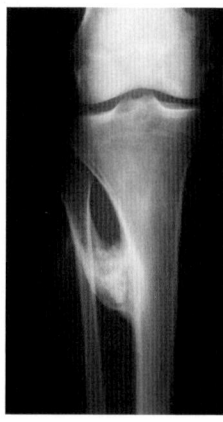

Figure 37.29 Pedunculated osteochondromas of the proximal fibula with pseudarthrosis. Osteochondromas always grow away from the physis.

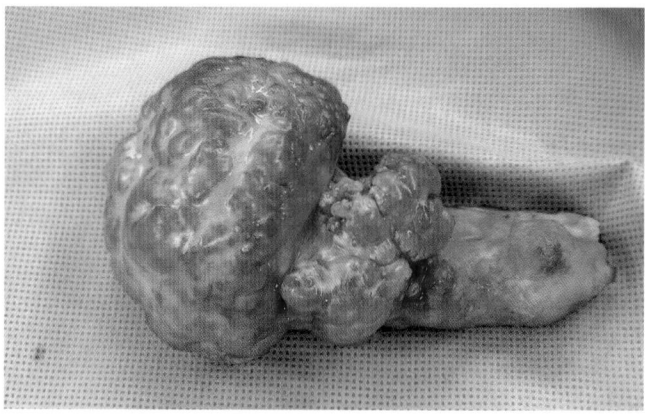

Figure 37.30 Excised pedunculated osteochondroma showing cartilage cap.

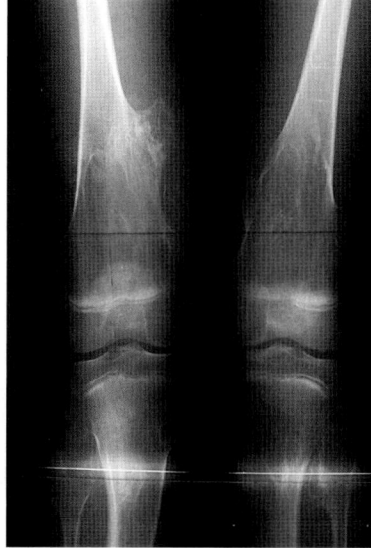

Figure 37.31 Multiple osteochondromas in diaphyseal aclasia.

Enchondroma (Fig. 37.32) is a benign cartilaginous neoplasm within the intramedullary cavity of bone. Approximately 50% are in the hands and feet. Enchondroma is the most common bone tumour in the hand. A large proportion of these tumours are entirely asymptomatic, and diagnosis is often incidental. They can present with pain, swelling or pathological fracture. Patchy calcification, expansion and scalloping can be visible on the radiographs, but some are only diagnosed on MRI scan. Ollier's disease is a developmental condition characterised by multiple enchondromas. In Maffucci syndrome, the multiple enchondromas are associated with multiple angiomas. Malignant transformation to chondrosarcoma can occur in approximately 20% of patients with Ollier's disease and is almost inevitable in patients with Maffucci syndrome.

Chondroblastoma (Fig. 37.33) is a benign cartilage-producing tumour that occurs in the epiphyses of children. It is most common around the knee. Pain is often severe with associated inflammation and possibly joint effusion. Radiologically, there is an often barely visible lytic lesion in the centre of the epiphysis. The diagnosis is often missed, and bone scan can aid in the localisation of the lesion.

Chondrosarcoma (see Figs 37.20–37.22, pp. 549–50) is a malignant tumour with cartilage differentiation. The biological spectrum is very wide; it ranges from very low-grade lesions to highly aggressive dedifferentiated tumours. Clinically, the presenting symptom is pain and or swelling. Symptoms are often longstanding. Radiological and pathological correlation is particularly important in the evaluation of this condition. Clear cell chondrosarcoma is a rare form of chondrosarcoma that occurs in the epiphysis (Fig. 37.34 and Summary box 37.13).

Summary box 37.13

Tumours producing cartilage

- Osteochondroma – cartilage capped; grows away from the physis
- Enchondroma – inside bone; commonest in the hands and feet
- Chondroblastoma – in the epiphyses of adolescents
- Chondrosarcoma – of varying malignancy

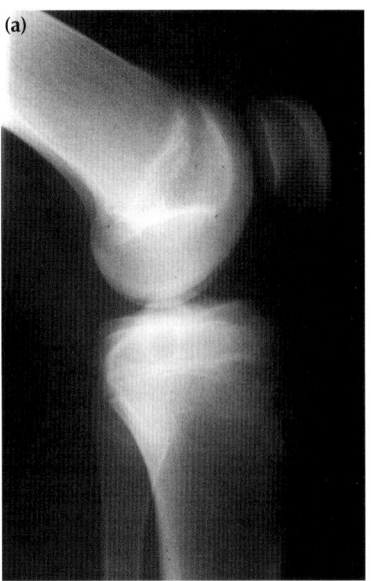

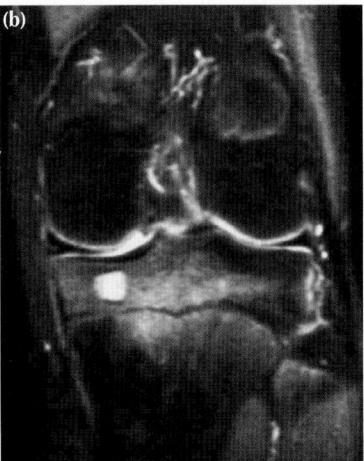

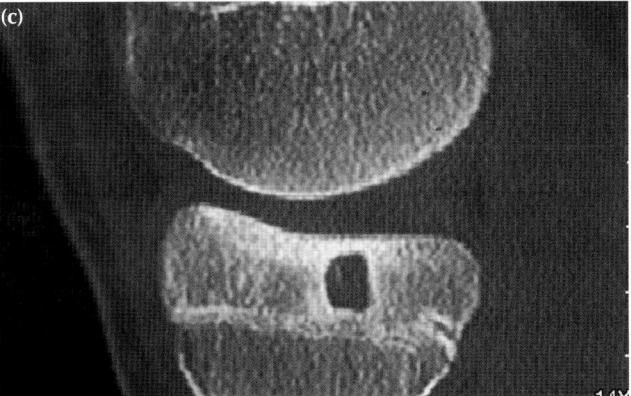

Figure 37.33 (a) Lateral radiograph with barely visible chondroblastoma in the epiphysis of the proximal tibia. (b) Coronal T2-weighted magnetic resonance imaging scan showing chondroblastoma in the epiphysis of the proximal tibia with surrounding oedema. (c) Sagittal computerised tomography reconstruction showing calcification within a chondroblastoma of the proximal tibial epiphysis.

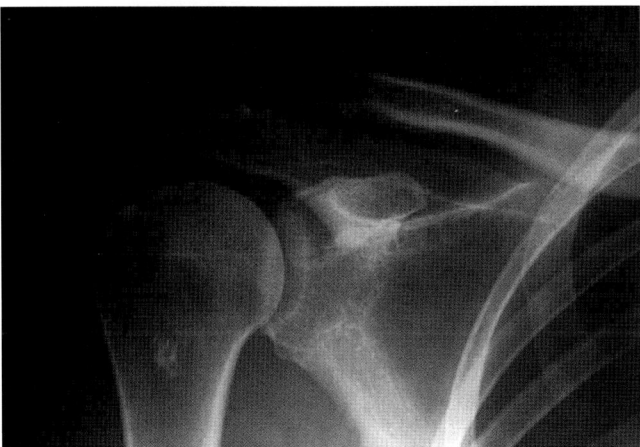

Figure 37.32 Calcification in benign enchondroma of the proximal humerus.

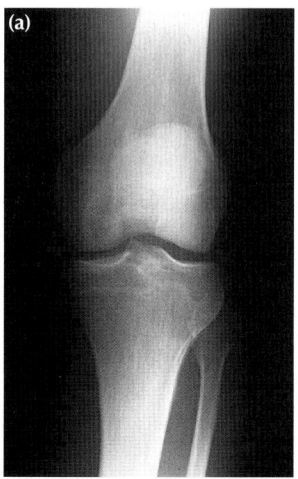

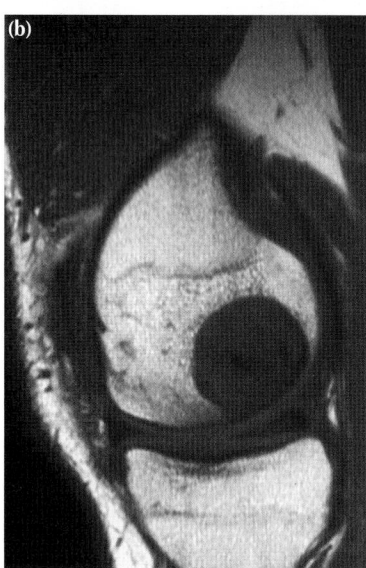

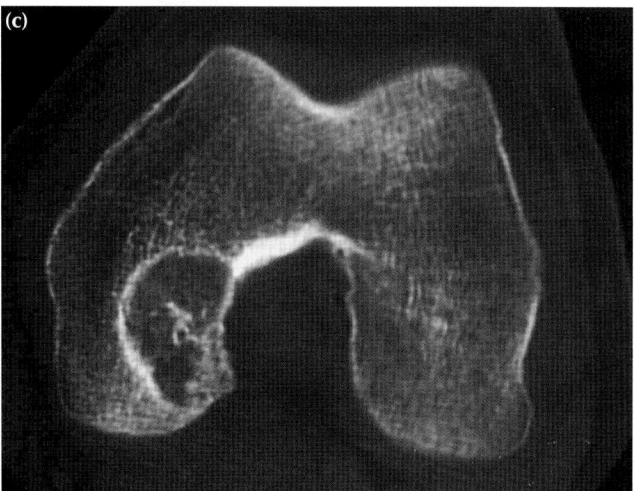

Figure 37.34 (a) Clear cell chondrosarcoma of the medial femoral condyle. (b) Sagittal T1-weighted magnetic resonance imaging scan showing clear cell chondrosarcoma in the medial femoral condyle. (c) Computerised tomography scan reconstruction shows calcification within the lesion.

OTHER BONE TUMOURS

Simple bone cyst, or unicameral bone cyst (Fig. 37.35), is a membrane-lined cavity filled with serous fluid. It usually occurs in the proximal long bones of children.

Aneurysmal bone cyst (Fig. 37.36a) is a benign cystic lesion of bone consisting of blood-filled spaces separated by fibrous septa. The lesion is much more aggressive than a simple bone cyst and often presents with pain and swelling. Plain radiographs show commonly aggressive features with eccentric expansion of the cortex and an open physis. Scans often show multiple fluid levels (Fig. 37.36b).

Giant cell tumour of bone (Fig. 37.37) is a benign aggressive tumour with large osteoclast-like giant cells. It usually occurs between ages 20 and 45, when the physes have closed. Giant cell tumour typically affects the epiphysis of long bones, especially around the knee, proximal humerus and distal radius.

Eosinophilic granuloma (Fig 37.38) is a rare neoplastic proliferation of Langerhans cells. It can be unifocal, multifocal or disseminated (respectively: eosinophilic granuloma, Hand–Schuller–Christian disease, Letterer–Siwe disease). There is a predilection for the skull and diaphyses of long bones. In the spine it can present with vertebral collapse (vertebra plana). Radiographs can appear aggressive with punched-out lesions and periosteal reaction.

Fibrous dysplasia (Fig. 37.39) is a benign fibro-osseous lesion that can be monostotic or polyostotic. It usually affects the long bones, ribs and skull. Patients can present with pain, swelling and/or fracture. Hip fractures can produce a shepherd's crook deformity. Radiologically there is often expansion and a ground glass appearance. Cysts may well be present.

Ewing's sarcoma (see Fig. 37.23, p. 550) is a round cell sarcoma of bone. It tends to arise in the diaphyses of long bones or the pelvis. Patients usually present with a painful mass and may have general symptoms with fever, anaemia and increased ESR. Radiologically the bone appears moth-eaten and may show an

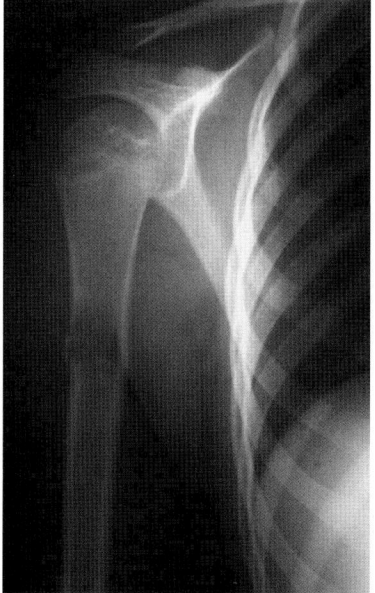

Figure 37.35 Pathological fracture through a simple bone cyst with the pathognomic fallen leaf sign. The fracture healed and the cyst consolidated without operative intervention.

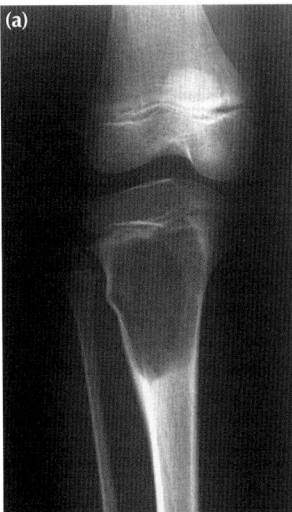

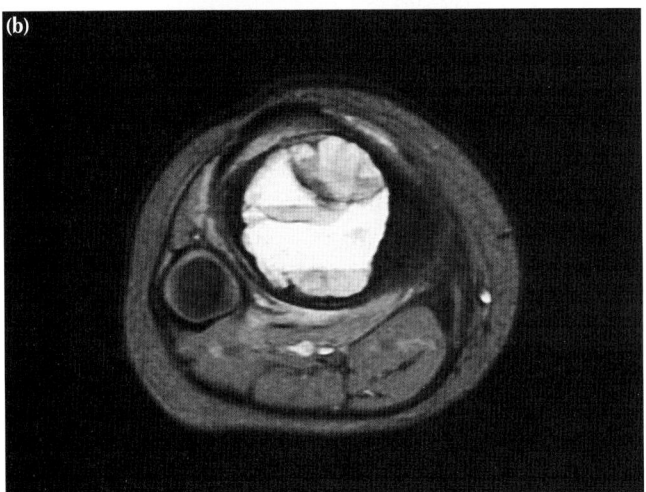

Figure 37.36 (a) Aneurysmal bone cyst with pathological fracture of the proximal tibia. (b) Magnetic resonance imaging scan shows multiple fluid levels.

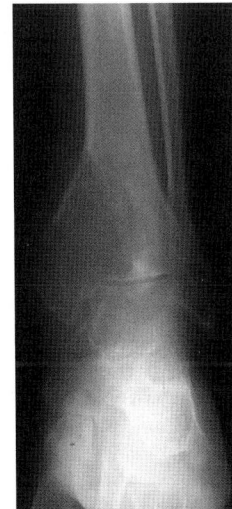

Figure 37.37 Giant cell tumour of the medial malleolus.

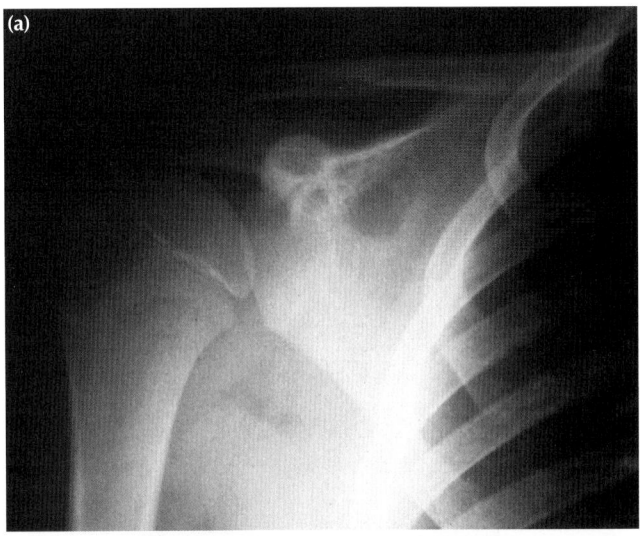

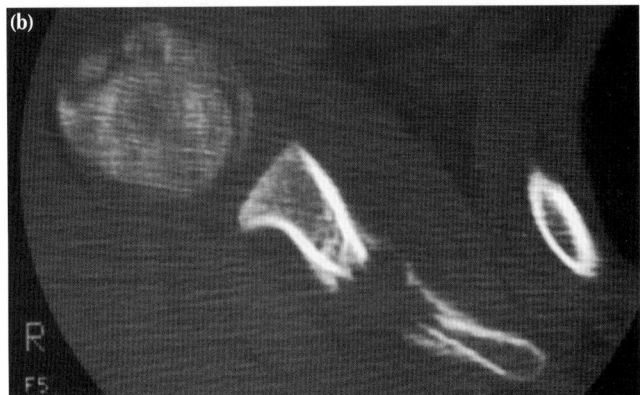

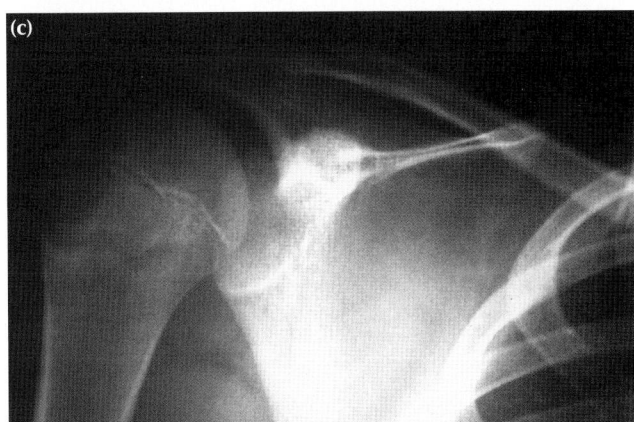

Figure 37.38 (a) Eosinophilic granuloma of the scapula. (b) Computerised tomography scan shows a 'punched-out' lesion. (c) Spontaneous resolution.

'onion-skin' periosteal reaction. There is often significant inflammation with oedema on the MRI scan.

Bone tumours can also be classified according to their site (Tables 37.6 and 37.7). Epiphyseal tumours are likely to be benign. Bone tumours are usually staged using the Enneking staging system.

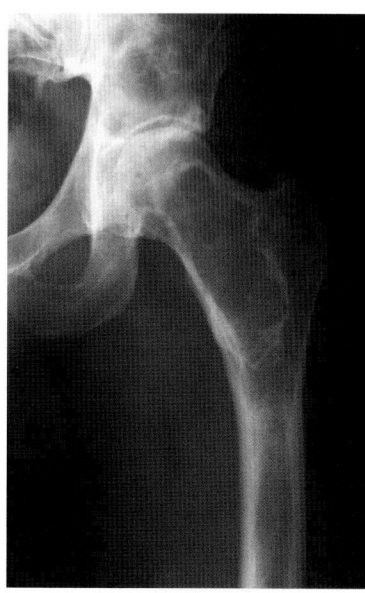

Figure 37.39 Fibrous dysplasia affecting the proximal femur.

Benign tumours are staged as:

- latent, i.e. osteochondroma;
- active, i.e. osteoid osteoma;
- aggressive, i.e. giant cell tumour.

Latent lesions are usually asymptomatic and often discovered incidentally. Active lesions, such as osteoid osteoma, do present with mild symptoms and continue to grow. A giant cell tumour is an example of an aggressive lesion. Aggressive lesions tend to grow rapidly. For malignant tumours, the Enneking system combines stage and grade of a tumour (Table 37.8). The compartment is the bone that is involved with the tumour. A tumour is extra-compartmental when the tumour has breached the cortex of the bone as visible on the plain radiographs. Most bone tumours are Enneking stage 2B at diagnosis (Summary boxes 37.14 and 37.15).

Table 37.6 Classification of bone tumours by site

Tumour and site Diaphyseal	Metaphyseal	Epiphyseal
Eosinophilic granuloma	Most	Chondroblastoma
Osteoid osteoma		Intra-articular osteoid osteoma
Fibrous dysplasia		Giant cell tumour (physis closed)
Adamantinoma		Clear cell chondrosarcoma
Ewing's sarcoma		

Table 37.7 Common diaphyseal bone tumours according to age

Age	Most common diaphyseal tumour
< 10	Eosinophil granuloma
Teenage	Ewing's sarcoma
Adult	Lymphoma
> 60	Metastasis? Myeloma?

Table 37.8 The Enneking staging system for bone tumours

Low-grade	Intracompartmental	1A
	Extracompartmental	1B
High-grade	Intracompartmental	2A
	Extracompartmental	2B
Any grade	Metastases	3

Summary box 37.14

Other bone tumours

- Simple bone cyst – proximal long bones of children
- Aneurysmal bone cyst – more aggressive, expanding
- Giant cell tumour – found in the epiphyses around the knee
- Fibrous dysplasia – may be multiple; found in long bones, ribs and skull
- Ewing's – round cell sarcoma; patients may have fever and anaemia

---

Summary box 37.15

Warning signs of bone tumour

- Non-mechanical bone pain
- Especially common around the knee in young adolescents
- Radiographs raise concern

SOFT-TISSUE TUMOURS

These tumours are also classified according to the cell of origin. Most types have a benign and a malignant counterpart [i.e. lipoma (Fig. 37.40) and liposarcoma]. The biological spectrum of these tumours is wide and full multidisciplinary assessment is essential to make a correct diagnosis. The Trojani system, based on tumour differentiation, mitotic count and tumour necrosis, is often used to grade soft tissue tumours. The tumour–node–metastasis (TNM) system is used for staging (Summary box 37.16).

Summary box 37.16

Warning signs of soft tissue tumour

- Larger than 5 cm
- Increasing in size
- Painful
- Deep to the fascia
- Recurrence after previous excision

HISTORY AND EXAMINATION, INVESTIGATION AND DIAGNOSIS

In the assessment of musculoskeletal tumours, a multidisciplinary approach that allows clinical, radiological and pathological correlation is essential to establish a correct diagnosis. Treatment of primary bone and soft-tissue tumours should only take place in an institution that has a full multidisciplinary team (centre of excellence).

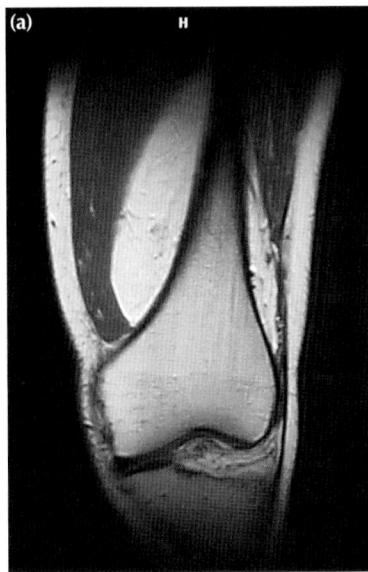

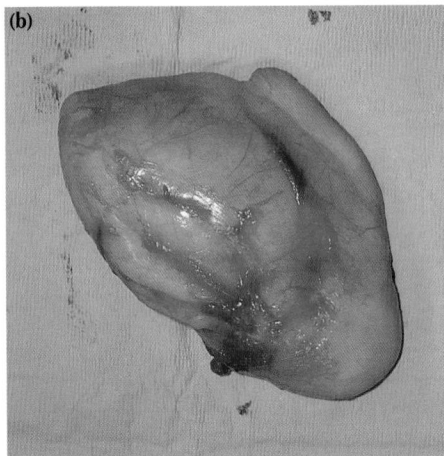

Figure 37.40 (a) Coronal T1-weighted magnetic resonance imaging scan showing a benign lipoma deep to the quadriceps muscle. (b) Excised benign lipoma.

When a musculoskeletal tumour is suspected:

- Stop
- Think
- Stage.

History and examination

Bone tumours

Non-mechanical and/or night pain, particularly in the young adolescent, is a concerning symptom and a primary bone tumour should be suspected. Symptoms that resolve with aspirin are suggestive of an osteoid osteoma.

The principles of management of primary bone tumours are:

- a high index of suspicion;
- early referral to a tumour centre;
- careful imaging studies;
- biopsy after completion of imaging investigations;
- minimally invasive technique for biopsy;
- a multidisciplinary approach to management.

Patients with a past medical history of malignancy who present with back pain should be considered to have metastatic disease until proved otherwise. Plain radiographs of the spine and routine blood tests are the minimum that is required. For metastatic disease of bone:

- the extent of metastases is best demonstrated on a bone scan;
- prophylactic treatment of any impending fracture should be considered;
- radiotherapy and internal fixation improve pain and quality of life;
- beware the 'solitary' metastasis (Fig. 37.41). This could be a primary bone tumour and *full staging, including biopsy*, is required.

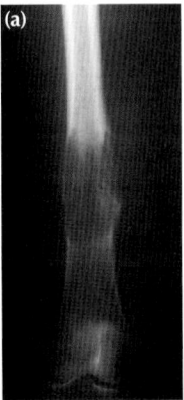

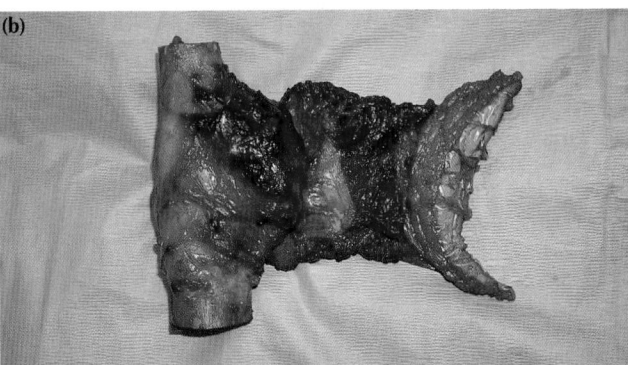

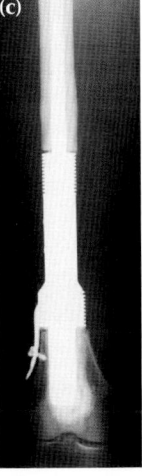

Figure 37.41 (a) A patient with a previous history of breast carcinoma presented with a solitary lesion in the femur. Biopsy showed primary bone sarcoma and the lesion was excised. (b) *En bloc* excision, including the biopsy track. (c) Reconstruction with endoprosthetic replacement.

CHAPTER 37 | INFLAMMATION AND INFECTION AND MUSCULOSKELETAL TUMOURS

Multiple myeloma (see Fig. 37.17, p. 548) is the most common primary malignancy of bone in adults:

- It should be considered in all patients with back pain over 65 years of age.
- Back pain with an ESR > 100 mm h^{-1} is multiple myeloma until proved otherwise.
- Monoclonal gammopathy is diagnostic.
- Elevated urinary and serum Bence Jones proteins are diagnostic.

Soft-tissue tumours

Soft-tissue swellings are common and the vast majority are benign. Symptoms and signs that suggest malignant disease are:

- *pain*;
- *size*: larger than 5 cm and/or increasing;
- *position*: deep to fascia;
- *behaviour*: recurrence after previous excision (whatever the pathology).

Each of these factors has a 25% risk of malignancy.

Staging

Primary musculoskeletal tumours should be staged according to local and distant features:

- Local
  - plain radiographs of the whole affected bone or soft tissue lesion (see Fig. 37.15, p. 547);
  - MRI of the whole affected bone or soft-tissue lesion;
  - computerised tomography (CT) scan;
  - ultrasound scan (for soft-tissue tumours only).
- Distant
  - blood tests; including FBC, ESR, profile, calcium and myeloma screen;
  - plain radiographs of the chest;
  - CT scan of the lungs;
  - bone scan (for bone tumours only);
  - ultrasound scan of the abdomen (if renal metastasis is a possibility).

For bone tumours, plain film radiographs are the most informative, but appropriate scans are required for further confirmation and staging. Imaging should always include the whole of the affected bone to look for satellite lesions and skip metastases. Satellite lesions occur within, whereas skip lesions occur beyond the reactive zone of the tumour. Both primary bone sarcomas and soft-tissue sarcomas commonly metastasise to the lungs and a CT scan is an essential part of the staging. Patients who present with a lytic bone lesion could have a renal primary and an ultrasound scan of the kidneys is advised. Biopsy without this could result in unexpected massive blood loss (Summary box 37.17).

Summary box 37.17

Staging

- Plain radiography is most informative for bone tumours
- Always image the whole bone in case of skip lesions
- CT of the lung detects lung metastases
- Lytic lesions require ultrasound of the abdomen to check for a renal primary

---

Henry Bence Jones, **1813–1873**, Physician, St. George's Hospital, London, England.

Biopsy

A biopsy is performed only when the staging process is completed. This should be done in the centre performing the definitive surgical procedure. Image-guided biopsies have a higher diagnostic accuracy as areas of radiological concern can be targeted. If image-guided biopsy is performed, close discussion between radiologist and surgeon is required to ascertain that the correct biopsy route is used. It is essential that the biopsy track is excised at the time of definitive surgery (Figs 37.41–37.43). Biopsies for bone tumours are usually taken using a Jamshidi needle (Fig. 37.44), whereas Trucut needles are preferred for soft-tissue tumours.

The principles of biopsy are as follows:

- A tourniquet can be used, but exsanguination should be avoided as this can release tumour cells in the circulation.
- Use longitudinal incisions that are part of an extensile approach.
- Do not cross compartments.
- The biopsy track will have to be excised at the time of definitive surgery (Summary box 37.18).

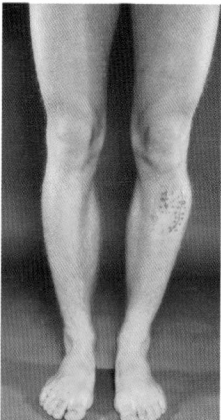

Figure 37.42 Poorly placed biopsies, making subsequent surgical excision of the track impossible.

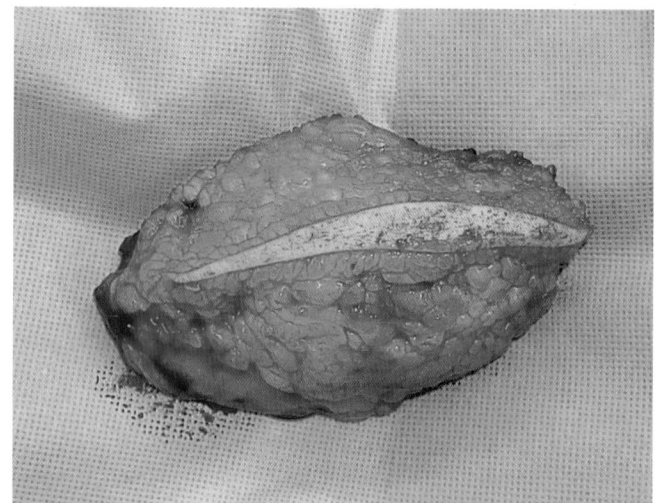

Figure 37.43 *En bloc* excised tumour and biopsy track.

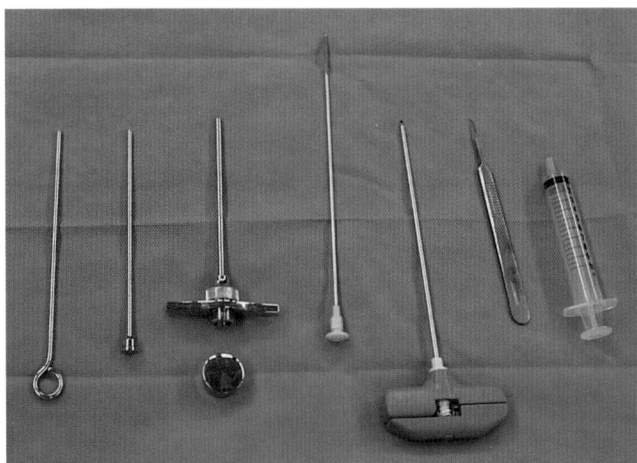

Figure 37.44 Bone biopsy instruments.

Summary box 37.18

Biopsy

- Only biopsy once staging is completed
- Biopsy should be performed at the centre undertaking the main surgery
- Image-guided biopsy is more reliable
- The biopsy track must be excised at definitive surgery
- Jamshidi needles for bone; Trucut needles for soft tissues

Assessment

The assessment of any bone or soft-tissue lesion can be divided into three phases. The first two phases can be performed in a district general hospital, but the third phase is best done in a tumour treatment centre (Table 37.9). Patients with metastatic disease often require resuscitation for electrolyte imbalance, anaemia, cardiorespiratory problems or hypercalcaemia before surgical treatment can be considered. Hypercalcaemia can be treated effectively with fluid resuscitation and pamidronates (Fig. 37.45). The risk of pathological fracture needs to be assessed. This is best assessed using the Mirels score (Table 37.10).

TREATMENT, PROGNOSIS AND COMPLICATIONS

Primary bone tumours

Most latent and active benign bone tumours are treated by intralesional curettage. Packing of the cavity with graft of bone

substitutes is usually not required. Simple bone cysts can heal following pathological fracture and an initial observant approach following fracture is best. If the cyst persists following union of the fracture, a variety of treatments, including injection with steroid or bone marrow and surgical curettage, have been described. Osteoid osteomas can resolve spontaneously. However, symptoms are often pronounced and most patients are treated by CT-guided thermocoagulation. Large or more rapidly growing benign bone tumours might require more extensive surgical excision and reconstruction. Malignant primary bone tumours require a more

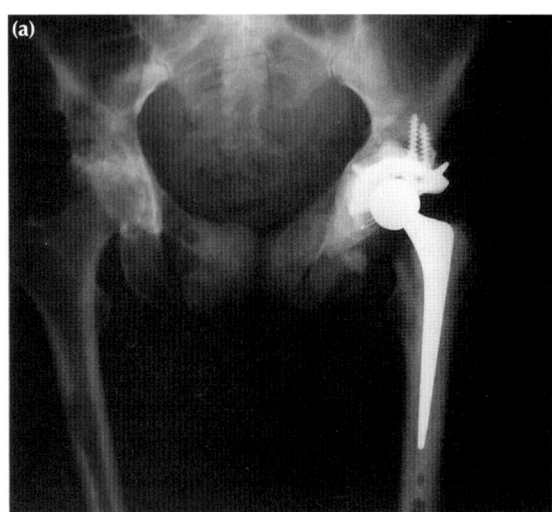

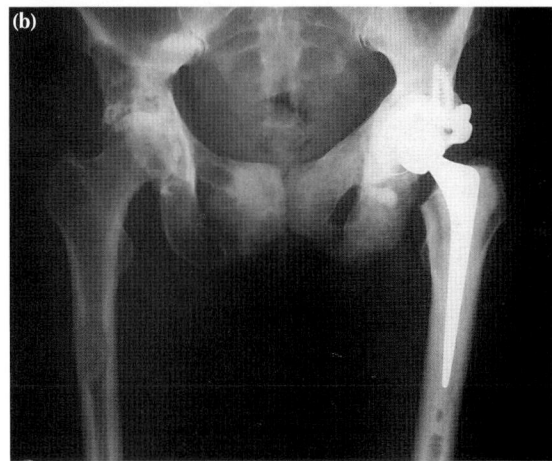

Figure 37.45 (a) Multiple deposits of metastatic breast carcinoma and lytic deposit in the right proximal femur. (b) Consolidation following treatment with pamidronate.

Table 37.9 The three phases of assessment of lesions

Phase 1 (within 24 hours)	Phase 2 (within first week)	Phase 3 (at tumour centre)
History and examination	Bone scan	CT scan of lesion
Blood assays	Ultrasound scan of the abdomen	MRI scan of lesion
Radiograph of whole bone	CT scan of chest	Biopsy
Chest radiograph		

CT, computerised tomography, MRI, magnetic resonance imaging.

Table 37.10 The Mirels scoring system for risk of pathological fracture

| | Score | | |
	1	2	3
Site	Upper limb	Lower limb	Peritrochanter
Pain	Mild	Moderate	Functional
Size	< 1/3	1/3–2/3	> 1/3
Lesion	Blastic	Mixed	Lytic

Score > 8, high risk of fracture – urgent prophylactic treatment needed; score < 7 low risk of fracture – stabilisation of the bone not immediately needed.

Table 37.11 Classification of surgical resection margins

Intralesional	Resection through the lesion
Marginal	Resection through the reactive zone of the tumour
Wide	Resection outside the reactive zone of the tumour
Radical	Excising the whole affected compartment

aggressive approach. Osteosarcoma and Ewing's sarcoma are treated with neoadjuvant chemotherapy and surgery. Chondrosarcomas are not sensitive to chemotherapy or radiotherapy and treatment is surgical.

The surgical options for malignant primary bone tumours are:

- amputation or van Ness rotationplasty;
- excision alone (for dispensable bones);
- excision and replacement with a graft or prosthesis.

If surgical excision is undertaken it is important for the biopsy track to be excised *en bloc* with the surgical specimen to avoid local recurrence through the biopsy track (see Figs 37.41 and 37.43, p. 557 and 558). Following excision the resection margins can be classed as shown in Table 37.11.

In most cases, limb salvage with excision and reconstruction is possible (Fig. 37.46). Only a minority of cases have neurovascular invasion and require amputation. Limb salvage, compared with amputation, has a slightly higher rate of local recurrence. However, no difference in overall survival has been demonstrated (Summary boxes 37.19 and 37.20).

Summary box 37.19

Treatment – benign bone tumours

- Benign lesions can be simply curetted
- CT-guided thermocoagulation is used for osteoid osteoma
- Large benign tumours may require reconstruction

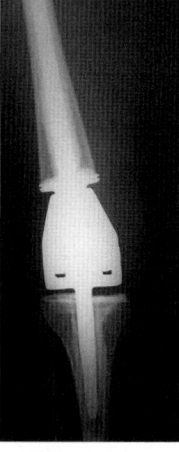

Figure 37.46 Endoprosthetic replacement of the distal femur.

en bloc **is French for 'in a block'.**

Summary box 37.20

Treatment of malignant bone tumours

- Osteosarcomas and Ewing's sarcoma require neoadjuvant chemotherapy
- Chondrosarcomas are insensitive to radiotherapy or chemotherapy
- Most malignant tumours can be treated with limb salvage.
- There is no difference in survival between amputation and limb salvage

---

Metastatic bone tumours

Surgical treatment in patients with metastatic bone disease is palliative. This should be kept in mind when planning treatment. Surgery is unable to lengthen life in patients with metastatic bone disease, but it can shorten it. Spinal surgery may be required for stabilisation of the spine and/or decompression in patients with (impending) cord compression. Surgery in the peripheral skeleton is mainly for treatment of (impending) pathological fracture.

Renal metastases tend to be very vascular and massive blood loss can be encountered during surgery. Therefore, preoperative embolisation should be considered just before surgery to prevent blood loss (Fig. 37.47). Treatment of myeloma is mainly haematological. Surgical treatment is only required for complications such as fracture and spinal cord compression. Solitary plasmacytoma is an exception and surgical excision is usually advised.

Patients with a previous history of malignancy may present with a (solitary) bony lesion or pathological fracture. It should not be assumed that this is a metastatic lesion (see Fig. 37.41, p. 557). Prior to planning surgical treatment it is important to ascertain that the diagnosis is correct. Staging including biopsy will be required to exclude a malignant primary bone tumour. Prior to planning surgical treatment for patients with metastatic bone disease it is important to have an assessment of:

- survival: prognosis of the primary tumour (Fig. 37.48);
- quality of life;
- medical fitness;
- biomechanical/risk of fracture;
- single or multiple bone lesions;
- response to adjuvant treatment such as radiotherapy and hormonal treatment;
- radiotherapy – before or after surgery?

It is difficult to give strict guidelines for the surgical management of patients with metastatic bone disease. However, when a prolonged disease-free interval is expected, prosthetic replacement is usually preferred to intramedullary nailing. A high failure rate is associated with internal fixation of pathological fractures (Fig. 37.49). Prior to surgical treatment it is essential to stabilise the patient's medical condition. Pamidronate can have a dramatic effect and might make surgery unnecessary (see Fig. 37.45, p. 559). Epiphyseal and metaphyseal lesions are best treated with

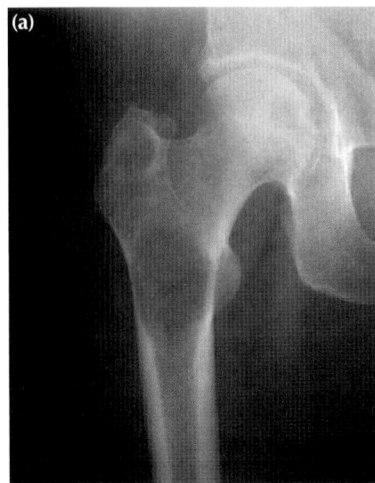

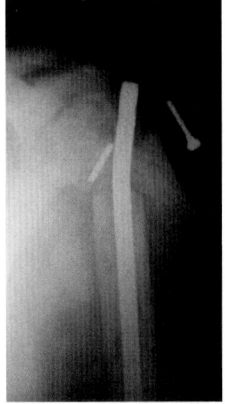

Figure 37.49 Failed metalwork following fixation of a metastatic fracture.

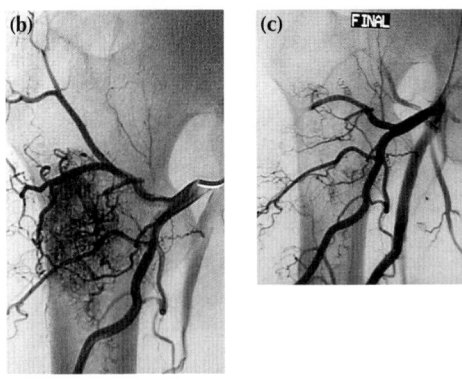

Figure 37.47 (a) Lytic metastasis of renal cell carcinoma. (b) Angiogram shows increased vascularity. (c) Following embolisation.

Summary box 37.21

Treatment of bone metastases

- Surgery cannot lengthen life but may shorten it
- Spines may need stabilising and nerves or the spinal cord decompressing
- Long bones will need stabilising if a pathological fracture is imminent
- Patients who have a possibility of long survival may need a prosthesis
- Radiotherapy relieves pain

---

prosthetic replacement, whereas diaphyseal lesions are usually best treated with an intramedullary nail. In the shoulder, prosthetic replacements have poor function and internal fixation usually gives the best results. However, in hip lesions the best treatment is joint replacement.

Solitary breast and renal metastases can have a prolonged disease-free survival so excision and replacement rather than fixation should be the treatment of choice (Summary box 37.21).

Soft-tissue tumours

Malignant soft-tissue tumours are preferably excised with as wide a margin as possible. As in bone tumours, it is important for the biopsy track to be excised *en bloc* with the surgical specimen (see Fig. 37.43, p. 558). The skin might require reconstruction with a split-skin graft (Fig. 37.50) or skin flap (Fig. 37.51). In general, skin flaps are preferred as they allow for early administration of radiotherapy. Following surgical excision of high-grade soft-tissue sarcomas, adjuvant radiotherapy should be considered. Preoperative radiotherapy can also have good results, but there is a risk of wound healing problems following surgery. Chemotherapy has a limited role in the treatment of soft tissue sarcomas.

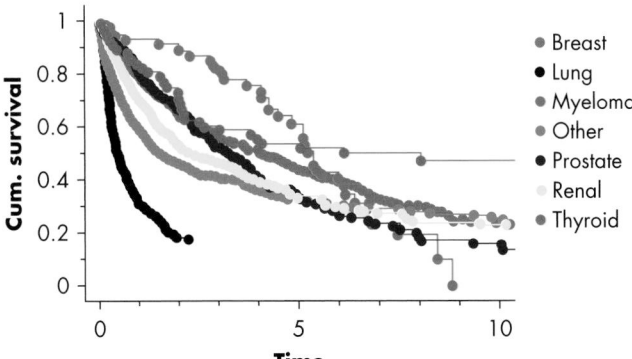

Figure 37.48 Survival curves of patients who present with bony metastasis.

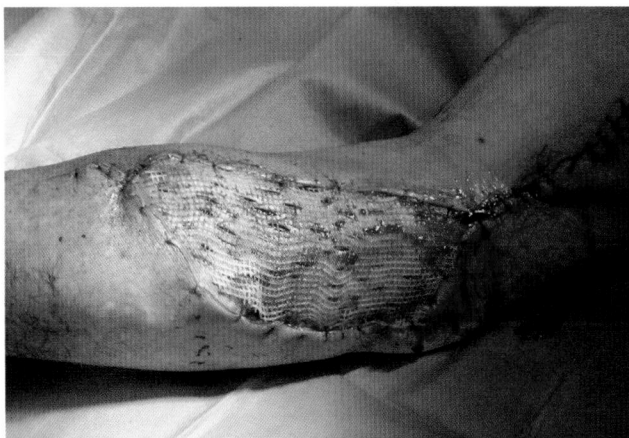

Figure 37.50 Excised soft tissue sarcoma and reconstruction with a split-skin graft.

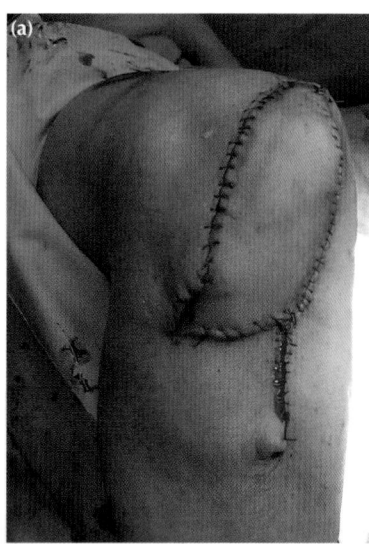

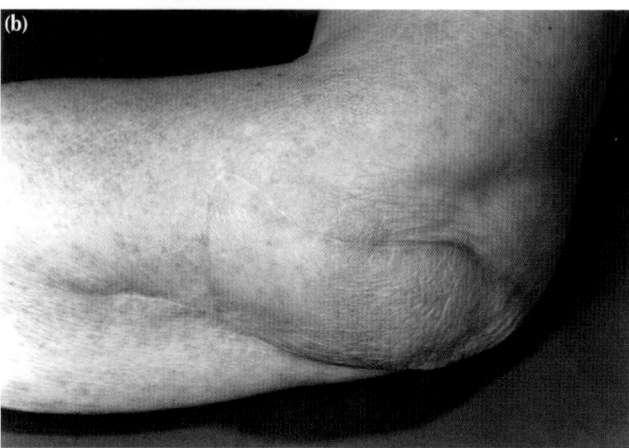

Figure 37.51 (a) Excised soft-tissue sarcoma and reconstruction with skin flap. (b) Final result following radiotherapy.

ACKNOWLEDGEMENTS

Parts of this chapter were previously published in the 24th edition of this volume under the title 'Diseases of bones and joints', authored by Tony Berendt and Martin McNally. Their material has been added to and updated by the current authors.

The original diagrams were prepared by Andy Biggs, Robert Jones and Agnes Hunt Orthopaedic Hospital, Oswestry, UK.

FURTHER READING

Inflammation and infection in bones and joints

Doherty, M., Hazleman, B., Hutton, C. *et al.* (1998) *Rheumatology Examination and Injection Techniques*, 2nd edn. Elsevier, London.

Hakim, A., Clunie, G.J.A. and Haq, I. (2002) *Oxford Handbook of Rheumatology*, 2nd edn. Oxford University Press, Oxford.

Snaith, M. (2004) *ABC of Rheumatology*, 3rd edn. Blackwell BMJ Books, Oxford.

Warwick, D.J., Solomon, L., Nayagam, S. and Apley, A.G. (2001) *Apley's System of Orthopaedics and Fractures*, 8th edn. Butterworth Heinemann, London.

Muskuloskeletal tumours

Cool, P. and Grimer, R. (2000) Pathological fractures of the extremities. *Trauma* **2**: 101–11.

Cool, P., Grimer, R. and Rees, R. (2005) Surveillance in patients with sarcoma of the extremities. *Eur J Surg Oncol* **31**: 1020–4.

Enneking, W.F., Spanier, S.S. and Goodman, M.A. (1980) A system for the surgical staging of musculoskeletal sarcoma. *Clin Orthop Relat Res* **153**: 106–20.

Fletcher, C.D.M., Unni, K.K. and Mertens, F, (eds) (2002) *World Health Organization Classification of Tumours. Pathology and Genetics Tumours of Soft Tissue and Bone*. IARC Press, Lyon.

Mankin, H.J., Lange, T.A. and Spanier, S.S. (1982) The hazards of biopsy in patients with malignant primary bone and soft tissue tumors. *J Bone Joint Surg* **64A**: 1121–7.

Mirels, H. (1989) Metastatic disease in long bones. *Clin Orthop* **249**: 256–64.

Wedin, R. and Bauer, H.C. (2005) Surgical treatment of skeletal metastatic lesions of the proximal femur: endoprosthesis or reconstruction nail? *J Bone Joint Surg* **87**: 1653–7.

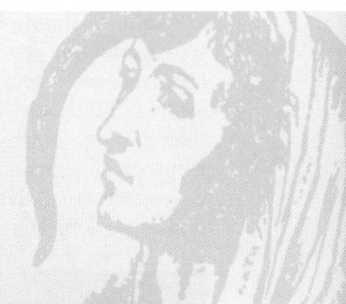

Paediatric orthopaedics

CHAPTER

38

LEARNING OBJECTIVES

To be familiar with:
- The normal development of the musculoskeletal system and understand how deformity can arise through failure of normal development
- The difference between normal variants and pathological deformity
- The diagnosis and treatment of developmental hip dysplasia

- The presentation and management of other conditions affecting the hip in childhood
- The management of clubfoot
- The need to consider, diagnose and treat appropriately musculoskeletal infection in childhood

INTRODUCTION

Young skeletons have the potential to heal rapidly and remodel but growth plate injury or muscle imbalance may lead to progressive deformity. The conservative treatment of common conditions, such as developmental dysplasia of the hip (DDH) and clubfoot, combines the remodelling ability of the growing skeleton with an understanding of the Heuter–Volkmann principle and Wolff's law (Summary box 38.1): by improving the biomechanical environment, abnormal growth patterns may be reversed. In contrast, in conditions such as Blount's disease and physeal trauma, growth plate damage leads to asymmetrical growth and deformity.

> **Summary box 38.1**
>
> **Laws governing the remodelling of bone**
>
> ***Heuter–Volkmann principle***
> - Compressive forces inhibit growth
> - Tensile forces stimulate growth
>
> ***Wolff's Law***
> - Bone is deposited and resorbed in accordance to the stresses placed upon it

Recently, the molecular and genetic bases of some congenital musculoskeletal conditions have been established, which may lead to new avenues of prevention and treatment. In other childhood conditions, such as Perthes' disease, the aetiology remains a matter of speculation, reflected in the variety of controversial treatment methods available.

DEVELOPMENT OF THE MUSCULOSKELETAL SYSTEM

Embryogenesis of the limbs starts with formation of the upper limb bud on the lateral wall of the embryo 4 weeks after fertilisation, followed promptly by the lower limb bud. By 2 months, differentiation of the limb elements is complete. The majority of congenital limb anomalies arise during this interim period.

Three intercoordinated signalling centres control different aspects of limb development. The *apical ectodermal ridge* (AER) is a thickened layer of ectoderm that condenses over the limb bud. It acts as a signalling centre to guide differentiation of the mesoderm into appropriate structures in a proximal-to-distal direction and is responsible for interdigital necrosis and, hence, separation of the webbed digits. The *zone of polarising activity* (ZPA), within the posterior margin of the limb bud, functions as a signalling centre for anterior-to-posterior limb development via the sonic hedgehog protein. The *wingless-type* (Wnt) signalling centre, in the dorsal ectoderm, secretes factors that induce the underlying mesoderm to adopt dorsal characteristics, developing dorsal-to-ventral axis configuration and alignment of the limb.

Certain limb anomalies are directly related to alterations in these centres. For example, removal of the AER during embryogenesis yields a truncated limb similar to a congenital amputation, and prohibits interdigital necrosis, causing syndactyly.

> Richard von Volkmann, 1830–1889, Professor of Surgery, Halle, Germany.
> Julius Wolff, 1836–1902, Professor of Orthopaedic Surgery, Berlin, Germany.
> Walter Putnam Blount, 1900–1992, Professor of Orthopaedic Surgery, Marquette University, Milwaukee, WI, USA, described this condition in 1937.

> Georg Clemens Perthes, 1869–1927, Professor of Surgery, Tübingen, Germany.

An error during limb development may disturb other organ systems that are developing simultaneously; therefore, some limb anomalies are associated with systemic disorders whereas others are not. Many of the systemic conditions are more important than the limb anomaly and accurate identification allows treatment of life-threatening problems, such as cardiac anomalies. Conversely, an extensive work-up for an isolated anomaly (e.g. a transverse deficiency) is unnecessary (Summary box 38.2).

Summary box 38.2

Development of the musculoskeletal system

- Occurs between 4 and 8 weeks after fertilisation
- AER controls proximal-to-distal differentiation and interdigital necrosis
- ZPA controls posterior-to-anterior differentiation
- Wnt controls dorsal-to-ventral differentiation

NORMAL VARIANTS

Normal variants require no intervention. The most common causes of concern are intoeing, bowlegs, knock-knees and flat foot. If the child fails to follow the normal development pattern or there are functional problems help may be required.

Normal variants are usually symmetrical, symptom free and without stiffness or systemic problems. There is often a family history of similar complaints. The child should have had no significant perinatal problems and should have achieved all developmental milestones normally.

Intoeing gait

Intoeing, defined as a negative foot progression angle, can originate from anywhere in the lower limb and may result from a combination of torsional components (Fig. 38.1 and Table 38.1).

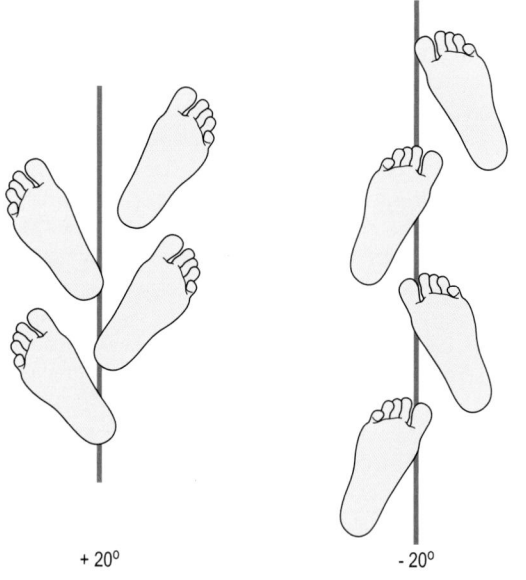

+ 20°   - 20°

Figure 38.1 Foot progression angle: a positive angle is caused by an extoeing gait, a negative angle by an intoeing gait.

Table 38.1 Common sites and causes of intoeing gait in childhood

Site	Cause
Femur/hip	Persistent femoral neck anteversion
Tibia	Internal tibial torsion
Foot	Metatarsus varus

Persistent femoral anteversion

All femurs have an anteverted neck at birth. As the femur lengthens it also rotates, reducing this anteversion to around 7° in the adult; however, if the anteversion persists, the child intoes. Clinically, there will be excessive internal rotation at the hip joint. Spontaneous correction usually occurs but if a significant deformity is still present by 12–13 years of age and function is impaired then a corrective osteotomy may be justified. Development of external tibial torsion (a normal process) may compensate for persistent femoral anteversion.

Internal tibial torsion

This is assessed by the foot/thigh angle and is commonly associated with physiological tibia vara in infants. Spontaneous correction can be expected by age 4.

Metatarsus varus

This foot deformity is often mobile and spontaneous correction occurs in 90% of patients by the age of 2–4 years. If the deformity is not easily correctable then stretching, corrective plasters or straight-last shoes may be helpful. Surgical release is rarely indicated.

Other abnormalities of gait

Toe walking

Toe walking is a phase in normal gait development. If the gait does not mature to a heel–toe pattern by the age of 3 years, conservative treatment with physiotherapy and casting may be used. Surgical lengthening of a contracted gastrocsoleus complex may become necessary in the older child. If toe walking starts after walking age a spinal or neuromuscular aetiology such as a tethered cord or a muscular dystrophy must be considered.

Extoeing

Extoeing is less common than intoeing but may result from relative femoral retroversion, external tibial torsion or flexible flat feet. The young child may be late walking because of poor balance associated with the externally rotated foot posture. This condition improves as the child grows.

Knock-knees and bowlegs

Normal children change their leg shape dramatically as they grow. All children start life with bowlegs, often accompanied by tibial torsion. By the age of 2–3 years they have developed knock-knees, which regress towards the normal adult tibiofemoral angle of 7° valgus by the age of 7 (Fig. 38.2).

Traditionally, deformity is quantified by measuring the intercondylar or intermalleolar distance although this is not very accurate. Further investigation is needed when the deformity is severe, asymmetrical or symptomatic. The most common pathological causes are previous trauma, rickets or a skeletal dysplasia.

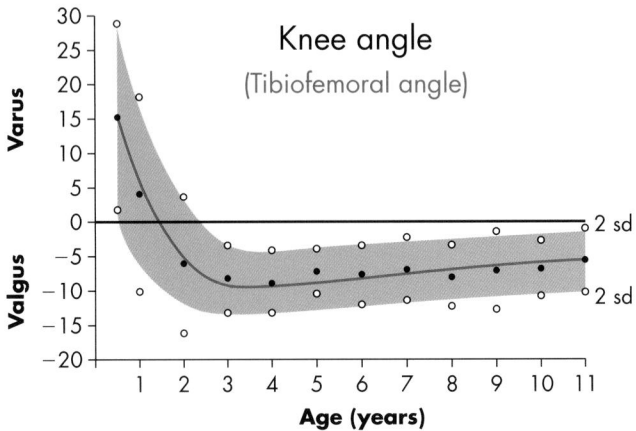

Figure 38.2 Graph to show the normal tendency of limb alignment to change from varus to valgus with growth.

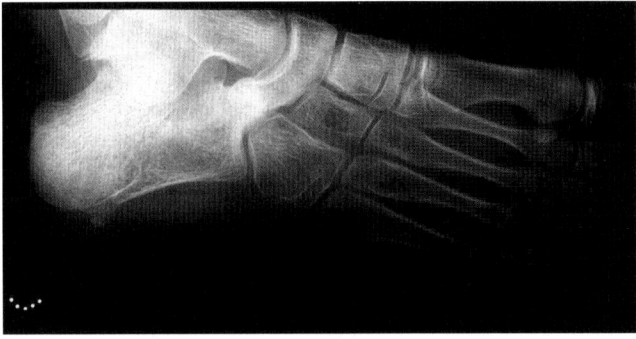

Figure 38.3 Oblique radiograph of the foot that shows the most common form of tarsal coalition, a calcaneonavicular bar.

Flat foot

All children under 3 years have flat feet because the medial longitudinal arch has not yet developed. Most adults do not have flat feet and, thus, the natural history of flat feet is for improvement, although genetic factors (both family and racial) may influence this.

The painless, flexible flat foot needs no treatment. Orthoses *do not* alter the natural history of the condition but can alleviate symptoms *if* they arise.

The symptomatic, rigid flat foot is usually the result of a tarsal coalition or inflammation and requires appropriate medical or surgical treatment (Fig. 38.3 and Table 38.2) (Summary box 38.3).

Summary box 38.3

Normal variants

- Intoeing or extoeing may be caused by extremes of femoral torsion, tibial torsion or foot deformity
- It is essential to look for neurological abnormalities in toe walkers
- Children's legs are often bowed until the age of 2 years and then knock-kneed until the age of 6 or 7
- Flat feet that are flexible and painless do not need treatment

---

Postural abnormalities

Many babies are subjected to moulding pressures while *in utero*. At birth they have 'postural abnormalities' such as torticollis, calcaneovalgus feet and plagiocephaly. A careful examination will exclude significant abnormalities and postural problems improve with time and some stretching exercises.

Table 38.2 All flat feet have a flattened medial arch with a valgus heel but the two major types of flat feet should be distinguished from each other

Type	Characteristics
Flexible	On tiptoe the arch is restored and the heel corrects into varus; subtalar joint movements are full and pain free
Rigid	On tiptoe the arch fails to return; subtalar joint movements are restricted and often painful

CONGENITAL AND DEVELOPMENTAL ABNORMALITIES OF THE SKELETON

Although many generalised or focal skeletal abnormalities are identified on antenatal ultrasound scans or at birth, others only become apparent with growth. Skeletal disorders are often linked to soft-tissue abnormalities; the presence of a skin dimple or vascular malformation should make the clinician look for a more generalised condition.

Congenital limb malformations usually arise from failure of differentiation but may result from inadequate or excessive growth of all or part of a limb. Most congenital malformations fit the classification shown in Table 38.3.

Many congenital anomalies require surprisingly little treatment and cause minimal functional disability whereas others, such as proximal femoral focal deficiency and radial club hand, pose considerable management challenges in which the functional and cosmetic needs of the child and the family must be balanced with the available resources and expertise. Despite advances in limb reconstruction techniques there is relatively little high-quality evidence-based data from skeletally mature patients to support their widespread use. In the meantime, considerable advances are also being made in the field of amputation prosthetics and rehabilitation.

Generalised skeletal dysplasias

This chapter cannot discuss all forms of skeletal dysplasia but the following more common conditions are representative of the challenges posed.

Table 38.3 Classification of congenital limb malformations

Category	Example
Failure of formation of parts	
Transverse	Congenital amputation
Longitudinal	Fibular hemimelia
Failure of differentiation	Vertebral body fusion; syndactyly
Duplication	Extra digits
Overgrowth	Gigantism; macrodactyly
Undergrowth	
Congenital constriction band syndrome	Often affects hands/feet with poor formation of the digits
Generalised skeletal abnormalities	Skeletal dysplasia, e.g. achondroplasia

Achondroplasia

This is the most common skeletal dysplasia that doctors see. The cause is a defect in the *FGFR3* gene on chromosome 4 that codes for fibroblast growth factor receptor 3. Enchondral bone formation is most affected and thus the patient presents with disproportionate short stature and classic clinical and radiographic features. The most characteristic feature is that the limbs are disproportionately short compared with the trunk (Fig. 38.4).

Relative underdevelopment of the foramen magnum and spinal stenosis can cause significant neurological difficulties.

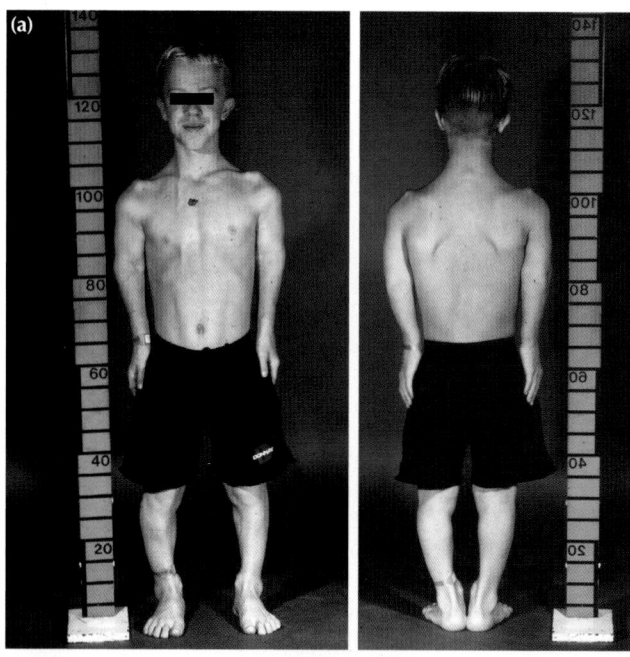

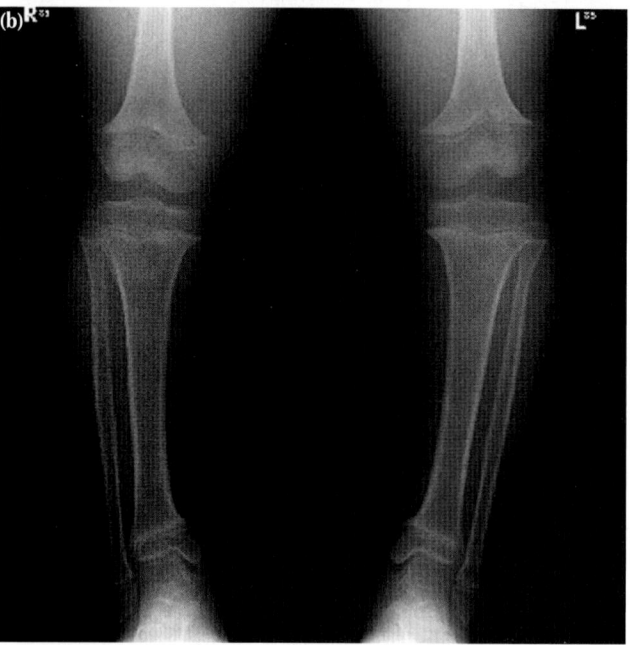

Figure 38.4 Achondroplasia. (a) Clinical photograph of a child with achondroplasia. (b) Radiograph of the lower limb of a child with achondroplasia showing short limbs, widened metaphyses and a varus deformity of the distal tibia.

Correction of limb alignment may be necessary and the use of limb lengthening techniques is popular in some countries.

Hereditary multiple exostoses – diaphyseal aclasis

Exostoses grow as the child grows and may cause cosmetic or functional difficulties that justify excision. The later the excision is performed, the less the risk of recurrence and/or physeal damage. Differential growth between the paired bones of the lower arm and leg can lead to joint deformity and loss of function. Distortion of the physis secondary to altered mechanical forces may exacerbate this problem. Growth abnormalities should be predicted and aggressive treatment designed to prevent deformity may be necessary (Fig. 38.5).

Enchondromas

An abnormality in the ossification of the cartilage columns of the physis may be the precursor of these cartilaginous masses. They are discussed in Chapter 37.

Fibrous dysplasia

This common disorder often presents as a chance finding on radiography and probably results from a somatic mutation causing defective bone formation (Fig. 38.6). This is discussed in Chapter 37 (Summary box 38.4).

Summary box 38.4

Congenital and developmental abnormalities of the skeleton

- Achondroplasia most affects endochondral ossification and presents with disproportionate dwarfism
- Exostoses may cause cosmetic or functional problems secondary to growth disturbance
- Enchondromas mostly occur in the hands and feet – multiple enchondromas occur in Ollier's disease and Maffucci's syndrome

---

METABOLIC BONE DISEASE

Rickets

There are various causes of the clinical condition described as rickets but in all cases the primary problem can be described as inadequate mineralisation of growing bone (Table 38.4).

In severe cases skeletal deformities along with classic radiographic features may surround every physis (Fig. 38.7).

The mainstay of treatment is medical to improve mineralisation. Deformity correction occurs with growth. Surgery may be necessary for the management of pathological fractures or to correct mechanical alignment associated with residual deformity *when* the medical condition has been controlled.

Osteogenesis imperfecta

Osteogenesis imperfecta (OI) or 'brittle bone disease' represents a spectrum of conditions linked by a qualitative and/or quantitative

---

Louis Xavier Edouard Léopold Ollier, 1830–1900, Professor of Surgery, Lyons, France, described enchondromatosis in 1899.
Angelo Maffucci, 1845–1903, Professor of Pathological Anatomy, Pisa, Italy, described this syndrome in 1881.

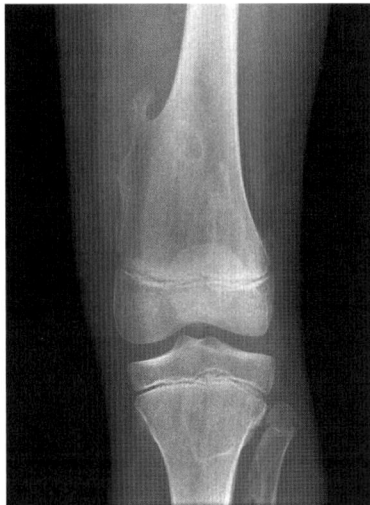

Figure 38.5 Radiograph of the knee showing multiple broad-based osteochondromas.

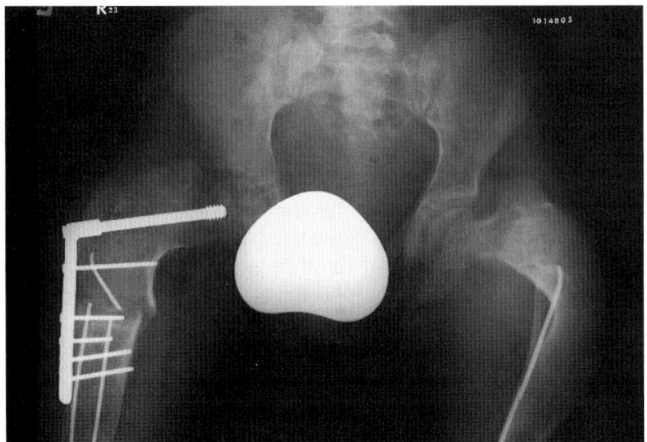

Figure 38.6 The diaphyseal lesions of fibrous dysplasia classically have a 'ground glass' appearance and, if extensive, may be associated with angular deformity or pathological fracture.

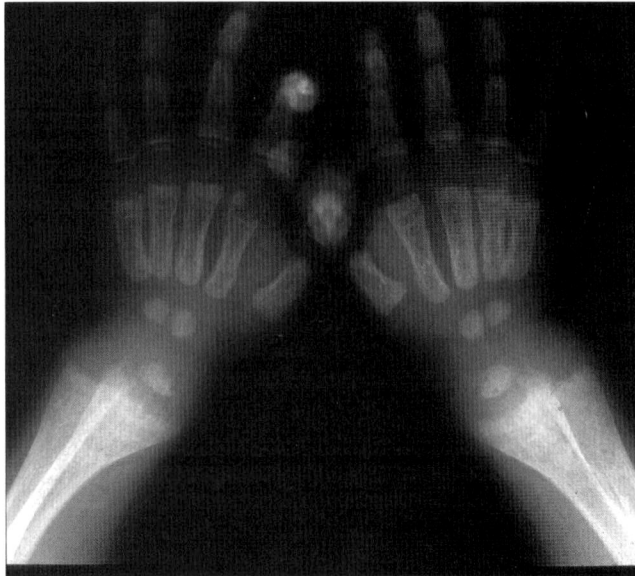

Figure 38.7 Radiographs demonstrate widened physes with cupped, flared metaphyses.

bone turnover. This reduces bone pain and fracture rate, which in turn improves weight-bearing mobility and, subsequently, bone strength (Fig. 38.8).

When a bone fractures care must be taken to minimise disuse osteoporosis and maintain normal bone alignment. Treatment options range from simple casting techniques to more specialised procedures that include intramedullary nailing to correct/maintain limb alignment while allowing growth (Fig. 38.9) (Summary box 38.5).

> **Summary box 38.5**
>
> **Metabolic bone disease**
>
> - Rickets, resulting from nutritional or other causes, is characterised by failure of bone mineralisation
> - In osteogenesis imperfecta there is a defect in type I collagen production
> - In severe forms of osteogenesis imperfecta, frequent fractures lead to progressive deformity and treatment with bisphosphonates may reduce the fracture rate

ABNORMALITIES OF THE HIP

Developmental dysplasia of the hip

This term describes the spectrum of hip instability ranging from the irreducibly dislocated hip to the hip that is correctly located but associated with a shallow ('dysplastic') acetabulum.

malfunction of collagen production. Many specific genetic defects have been identified; most are caused by mutations in the collagen *1A1* or *1A2* gene on chromosome 17q or 7q respectively. The bone may break easily but it usually heals promptly and well. All structures that contain collagen may be affected, which accounts for the ligamentous laxity, blue sclerae and poor teeth found in some forms of this disease.

Cyclical bisphosphonate treatment has become popular in the management of severe OI. Its use decreases bone resorption and

Table 38.4 Common causes of rickets

Nutritional	Reduced intake of vitamin D and calcium (high intake of phytates or oxalates may be contributory)
Environmental	Inadequate exposure to sunlight
Gastrointestinal disease	e.g. Crohn's disease, gluten-sensitive enteropathy
Genetic	e.g. X-linked hypophosphataemia
Renal disease	e.g. end-stage renal failure, renal tubular anomalies. Secondary hyperparathyroidism changes may be present

CHAPTER 38 | PAEDIATRIC ORTHOPAEDICS

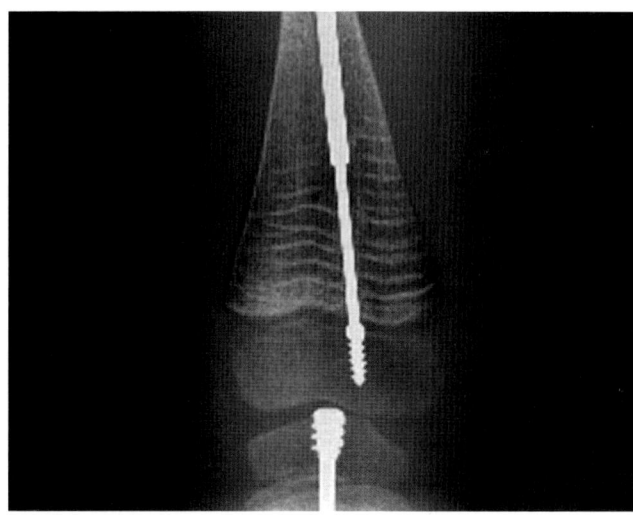

Figure 38.8 Radiograph of a child with osteogenesis imperfecta who has been treated with cyclical bisphosphonates. Multiple growth lines are visible in addition to an intramedullary device.

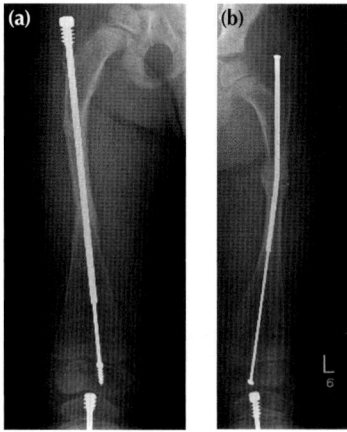

Figure 38.9 Radiograph of two adolescent femora showing different types of intramedullary alignment device *in situ*.

Reflecting the spectrum of pathology there is a spectrum of presentation of DDH from birth to adult life: in a neonate there may be instability, a toddler may limp, an adolescent may experience exercise-induced pain and, in an adult, there may be pain as a result of degenerative arthritis.

Incidence

The incidence of neonatal instability may be as high as 20 cases per 1000 births whereas the incidence of dislocated hips is about 2 cases per 1000 live births; this is because many hips that are unstable at birth will stabilise spontaneously.

Aetiology (Table 38.5)

- *Gender.* DDH is five times more common in girls than boys, possibly related to hormonal factors causing temporary joint laxity.
- *Breech presentation.* Up to 20% of breech babies, particularly with the extended breech (hips and knees extended), have DDH.

Table 38.5 Risk factors associated with an increased incidence of hip dislocation

DDH	Female gender
	Breech position
	Family history and/or ethnic origin
	Oligohydramnios and/or associated moulding abnormalities
Teratologic hip dislocation	Associated syndromic features
	Neuromuscular conditions

- *Birth order.* DDH is more common in firstborns because the primigravid uterus is tighter, restricting movement, and in the left hip, as a result of the common fetal position.
- *Oligohydramnios.* This restricts fetal movement and may also increase the risk of other postural deformities such as torticollis and metatarsus adductus; the presence of these factors raises the possibility of DDH.
- *Family history.* The incidence of DDH is increased significantly with a positive family history. This may reflect faulty acetabular development or excessive ligamentous laxity. When there is joint laxity the clinical diagnosis of DDH can be difficult as there may be no limitation of hip abduction.
- *Racial and seasonal variations.* DDH is more common in certain regions and in certain races. The incidence is low among African but high in Navaho Indian populations, perhaps because of a combination of genetic and environmental factors; swaddling the legs together will exacerbate an unstable hip whereas carrying the baby astride the carer's hip encourages a position of hip flexion and abduction that will help stability. DDH is more common in babies born in winter.

DDH is often found in association with generalised syndromes or neuromuscular conditions such as spina bifida and arthrogryposis. Sometimes these conditions are occult and can lead to unexplained problems during treatment. These teratologic hips are often resistant to surgical intervention and the results are poor. The overall condition and prognosis of the child must also be considered.

Diagnosis

Neonates

All newborn babies should be screened clinically for instability and limitation of hip abduction. The hips should be examined again at 6 weeks.

Clinical instability The knees and hips are flexed and the thigh held by the examiner with the thumb along the medial aspect and the ring or middle finger behind the greater trochanter. The hips are gently abducted while lifting the greater trochanter upwards with the finger. A dislocated hip may reduce during this manoeuvre with a soft clunk – the Ortolani test (Fig. 38.10a). The examiner should note if both hips abduct fully. If the hip does abduct fully, then, as a continuous movement, the hip is adducted while pressing gently downwards on the knee with the palm and inside of the thumb. An unstable hip may dislocate or

---

The Navaho Indians **are an American Indian people from New Mexico and Arizona, USA.**

(a) Ortolani

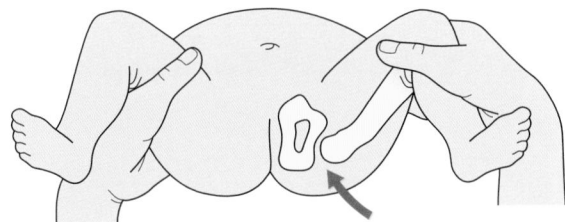

(b) Barlow

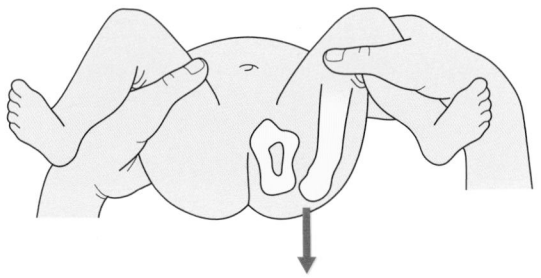

Figure 38.10 Line diagram illustrating the Ortolani and Barlow tests for developmental dysplasia of the hip.

sublux with a soft clunk – the Barlow test (Fig. 38.10b). With an irreducible hip there is no clunk of reduction but there will usually be limitation of abduction. Bilateral dislocation may be missed as abduction is symmetrical, and abduction may be normal when there is ligamentous laxity.

Ultrasound Ultrasound can confirm clinical suspicion of dislocation or instability and be used to monitor the early treatment (Fig. 38.11). It can also be used as a screening tool, either universally or in 'at-risk' groups. As the sonographic appearance of most hips matures (becomes less dysplastic) spontaneously there is a risk of overtreatment if scans are performed too early. If delayed, the best opportunity for acetabular remodelling may be lost. Ideally, therefore, screening scans should be performed between 4 and 6 weeks after birth and treatment instigated promptly.

X-ray Plain radiographs can also be used to evaluate dysplasia from about 12 weeks. The appearance of the femoral ossific nucleus is often delayed in the presence of dysplasia (Fig. 38.12).

Infant

The hips should be checked as part of routine developmental monitoring, looking in particular for limitation of abduction in flexion, limb asymmetry, such as an extra thigh crease, or limb shortening.

Marius Ortolani, **Orthopaedic Surgeon, Instituto Provinciale Per L'Infanzia di Ferrara, Italy, described this test in 1937.**
Thomas Geoffrey Barlow, **1915–1975, Orthopaedic Surgeon, The Salford Royal Hospital, Salford, England.**

Child

Children present with a limp. The affected leg tends to be short and externally rotated and there may be unilateral tiptoe walking. There is an extra thigh crease and limited abduction. However, the signs may be subtle and easily misinterpreted as normal development in an unsteady toddler. If both hips are affected there will be a waddling gait.

Adolescent

Discomfort after exercise is the usual feature but the pain may be in the knee. Typically, a radiograph shows dysplasia and possibly subluxation.

Adult

Pain is the usual complaint and radiographs may show degenerative change as well as dysplasia (Summary box 38.6).

Summary box 38.6

Diagnosis of DDH

- All neonates are screened clinically using the Barlow and Ortolani tests, at birth and then again at 6 weeks
- Ultrasound is used to confirm and monitor hip stability and as a screening test, particularly in 'at-risk' babies
- Radiography can be carried out from 3 months onwards
- Older children may present with a limp

Management

When diagnosed early, conservative treatment is likely to be successful, but after walking age, surgery is usually required. However, the principles are the same; the objective is to obtain a stable, congruous reduction and to avoid damage to the capital epiphysis [avascular necrosis (AVN)] or growth plate. Such damage is a major complication, causing stiffness, coxa vara and shortening.

Neonate

Some normal hips are unstable at first because of ligamentous laxity, but these stabilise within the first couple of weeks of life and do *not* need treatment. Ultrasound will confirm whether the acetabulum is normal.

Hips that remain unstable or are dislocated at rest are treated with harnesses or splints devised to maintain the hip safely in the reduced position of abduction and flexion. A harness (e.g. Pavlik harness) allows controlled movement and may be safer but it requires close supervision (Fig. 38.13). It is also possible to ultrasound hips in the harness to check on progress. A splint (e.g. von Rosen) holds the hips more rigidly but carries a greater risk of AVN. Excessive abduction should be avoided with either type of device. If the hips fail to relocate or stabilise or can only be held reduced in excessive abduction then treatment should be discontinued.

Infant

Successful treatment with a harness is unusual after 4–6 months of age. For the late-presenting hip or the hip that fails conservative treatment, an examination under anaesthetic may allow a

Sophus von Rosen, **Orthopaedic Surgeon, Malmo General Hospital, Malmo, Sweden.**

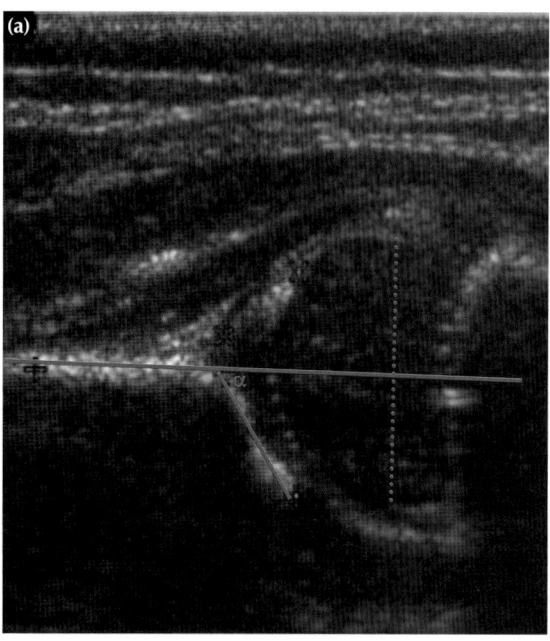

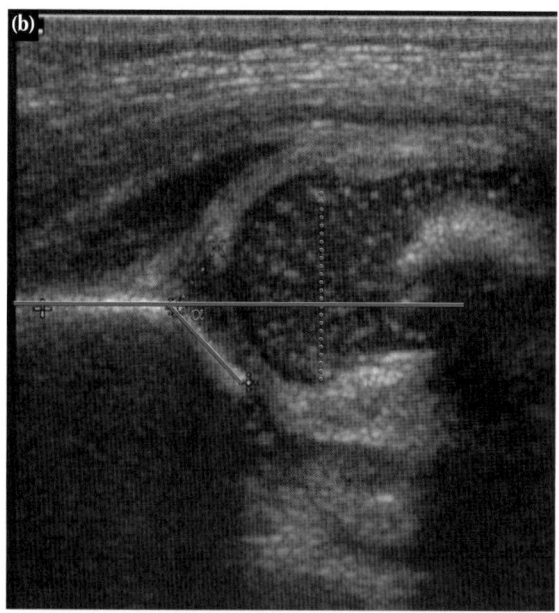

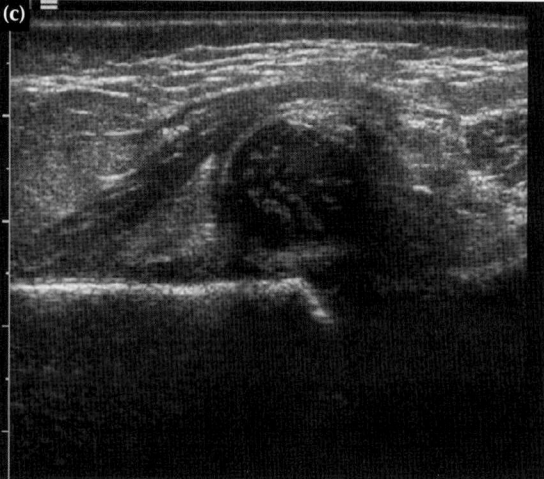

Figure 38.11 Ultrasound images of an infant hip. (a) Normal hip with a high α angle and a Morin index of 50% (defined as the percentage of the femoral head covered by the acetabulum, i.e. the portion lying below the horizontal red line). (b) Grossly dysplastic hip with a low α angle and a Morin index of < 50%. This hip is likely to be unstable on dynamic ultrasound scanning, i.e. Barlow positive. (c) A dislocated hip joint.

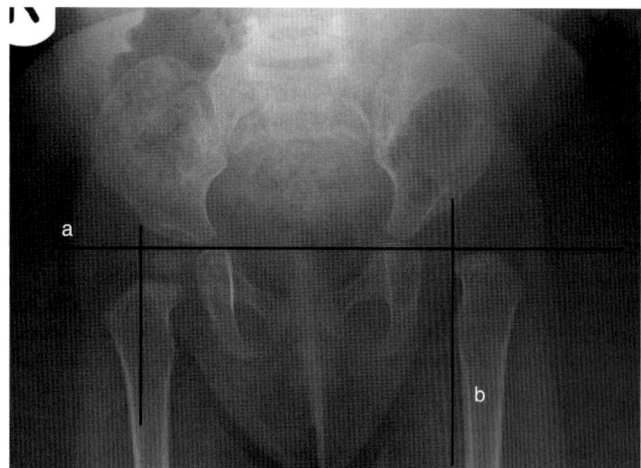

Figure 38.12 Anteroposterior pelvic radiograph showing Hilgenreiner's line (a) and Perkins' line (b). The femoral head (ossific nucleus) of a normal hip lies in the inner lower quadrant. The right hip is normal, the left hip has developmental dysplasia of the hip.

closed reduction to be attempted. The arthrogram shows whether a concentric reduction is present and, if not, it will indicate which structures are blocking reduction and a psoas/adductor release can be performed as necessary. A closed reduction must be held with a short- or long-leg hip spica cast for some months.

If the hip is irreducible or can only be held in an extreme position with a small safe zone then this treatment method must be abandoned and an open reduction considered via a medial approach or, in an older infant, via an anterior approach (Summary box 38.7).

Summary box 38.7

Management of early DDH

- Many hips that are unstable in the first few days of life do not need treatment
- Until the age of 4–6 months, a harness or splint is usually effective
- In older babies, closed reduction is still sometimes possible
- For failed closed treatment, open surgical reduction may be required

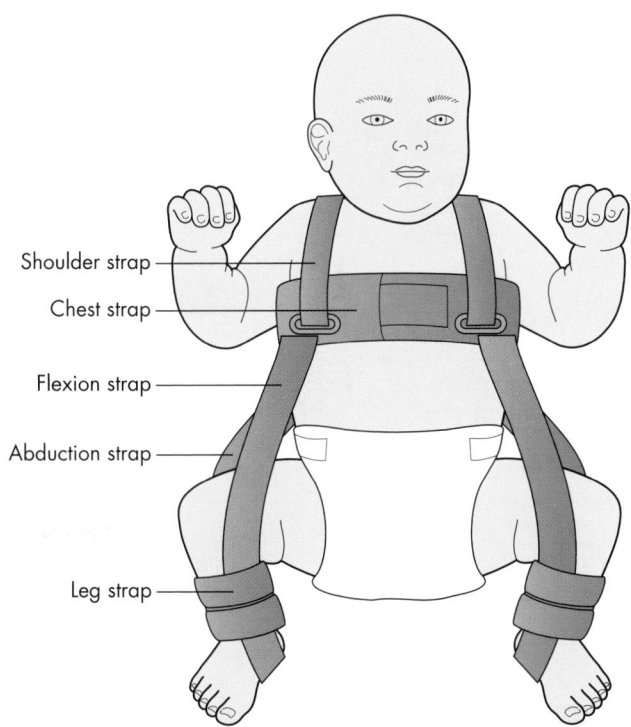

Shoulder strap

Chest strap

Flexion strap

Abduction strap

Leg strap

Figure 38.13 The anterior strap of the Pavlik harness controls hip flexion whereas the posterior strap limits adduction and encourages abduction.

Toddler and young child

The older the child, the less likely that reduction by closed methods will succeed (Fig. 38.14). Open reduction together with bony realignment is necessary. The traditional approach is to carry out open reduction via an anterior approach after the age of 1 year. Earlier surgery via the medial approach can be considered but access is limited and no additional surgery such as capsulorraphy or bony realignment can be performed through the same incision. The anterior approach offers excellent access. A pelvic osteotomy may be required to reorient or close down the acetabulum, and

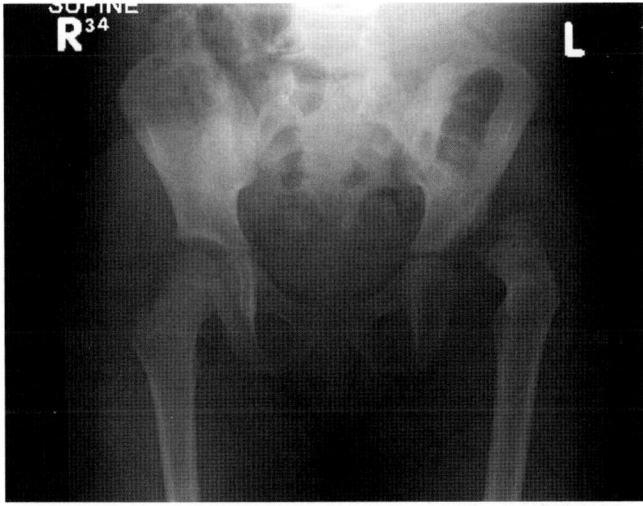

Figure 38.14 Anteroposterior pelvic radiograph showing acetabular dysplasia with subluxation (developmental dysplasia of the hip) of the left hip. This child presented at the age of 4.

femoral shortening or derotation osteotomies are often used to improve stability.

Older child

In the older child a similar approach can be used. Acetabuloplasty is frequently required. The older the child, the more difficult and unrewarding surgery becomes. In bilateral cases surgery is often not undertaken in children aged over 6–8 years and in unilateral cases over age 8–10 years.

Adolescent and young adult

These hips are often subluxed. Investigations are required to see if the hip can be reduced and, if so, if that position can be recreated with a combination of pelvic and femoral osteotomies. For the hip that cannot be reduced, some form of acetabular augmentation may reduce symptoms and delay the onset of degenerative change requiring hip arthroplasty (Summary box 38.8).

Summary box 38.8

Management of late-presenting DDH

- The older the child, the more likely it is that they will need surgery
- Femoral osteotomy can stabilise the hip and reduce pressure on the femoral head
- Pelvic osteotomy can redirect or reshape the acetabulum
- Acetabular remodelling ceases at the age of 6 years
- Avascular necrosis is a risk of treatment of DDH at any stage

---

Secondary procedures and complications

Regular follow-up is required to ensure that the hip remains concentrically reduced and that the acetabulum continues to develop. Acetabular remodelling continues up until the age of 6 years and may be assessed objectively by measuring the acetabular index or, in children over 5 years, the centre–edge angle (Fig. 38.15).

If the acetabulum does not improve then a variety of operations are available. For example, the innominate osteotomy or shelf procedures both improve cover. Significant AVN with relative overgrowth of the greater trochanter can cause a Trendelenburg limp and distal transfer of the trochanter may help. Occasionally, a leg length difference needs treatment. In the long term there is an increased risk of osteoarthritis necessitating hip replacement or resurfacing.

Legg–Calvé–Perthes' disease

This condition is characterised by the development of AVN of the proximal femoral epiphysis and is probably one of the most controversial topics in paediatric orthopaedics.

Incidence and aetiology

The condition is rare and affects boys predominantly, most commonly between the ages of 4 and 8 years. The aetiology is

---

Arthur Thornton Legg, 1874–1939, Orthopaedic Surgeon, The Children's Hospital, Boston, MA, USA.
Jacques Calvé, 1875–1927, Orthopaedic Surgeon, La Fondation Franco-Americaine, Berck Plage, Pas-de-Calais, France.
Legg, Calvé and Perthes all described osteochondritis of the head of the femur independently in 1910.

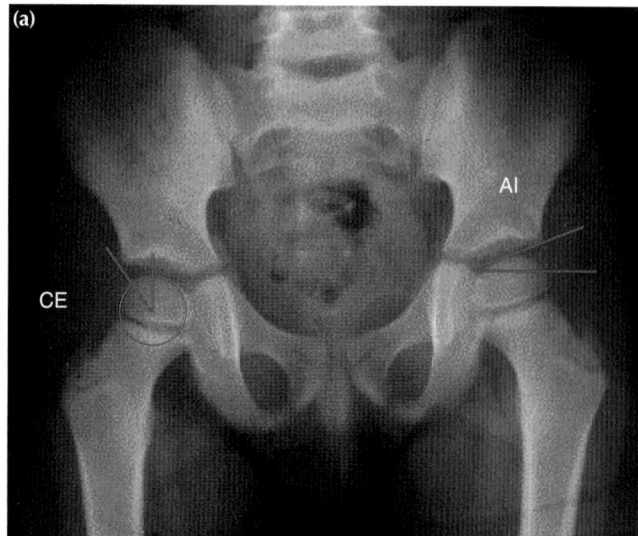

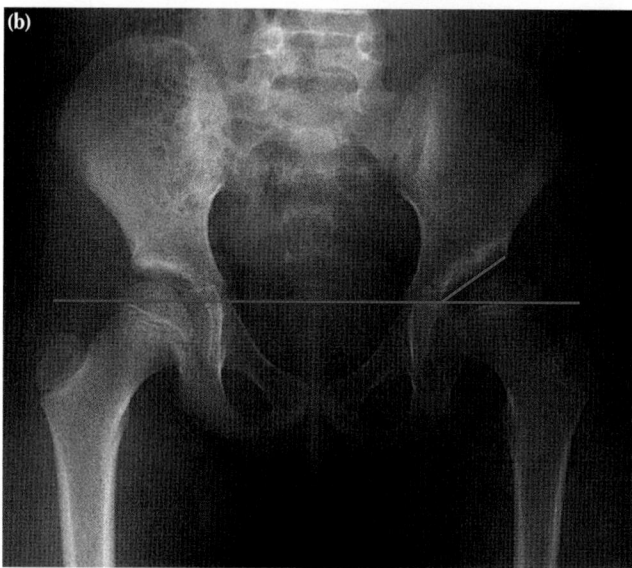

Figure 38.15 Anteroposterior pelvic radiographs demonstrating the acetabular index (AI) and the centre–edge (CE) angle. (a) Normal hips; (b) the left hip shows residual dysplasia. The AI is increased compared with the normal right hip. The left CE angle would be smaller than the right too but is has not been measured on this radiograph.

unknown although a variety of factors have been implicated. Up to 10% of patients may develop bilateral disease.

Recently, thrombophilia secondary to protein deficiencies has been cited as an aetiological factor but there is little supporting evidence for this (Summary box 38.9).

Summary box 38.9

Factors implicated in the pathogenesis of Perthes' disease

- Low birthweight
- High birth order
- Abnormalities in anthropometric measurements
- Delayed bone age
- Low socio-economic status

Pathology

Once established the process follows a relatively well-defined course. The avascular change may affect the whole of the femoral head or only part of it. The avascular bone may collapse and this is followed by fragmentation of the ossific nucleus and subsequent healing with revascularisation and regeneration of the bony epiphysis; in this respect Perthes' disease is a self-limiting condition but, during the collapse and fragmentation phases, femoral head deformity occurs.

Diagnosis

The history, clinical examination and anteroposterior and 'frog' lateral radiographs of the pelvis make the diagnosis. An intermittently painful hip (or knee) with a limp and restriction of hip movements requires investigation. The radiographic features will vary with the stage of the disease and may not correlate with the clinical condition (Fig. 38.16).

AVN of the femoral head may be due to other causes and a differential diagnosis should be considered, particularly if the radiographic changes are bilateral (Summary box 38.10).

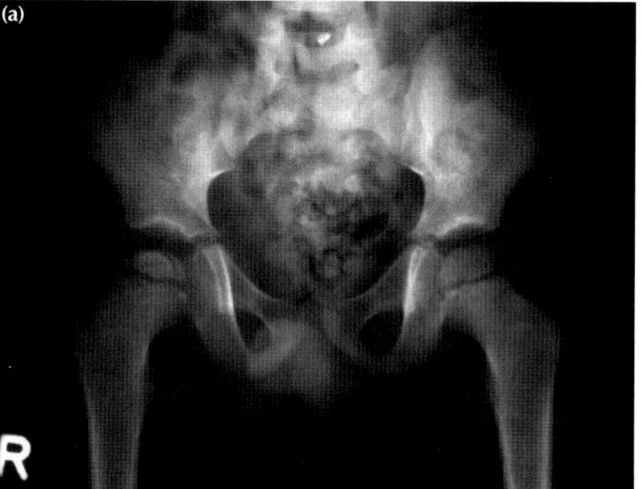

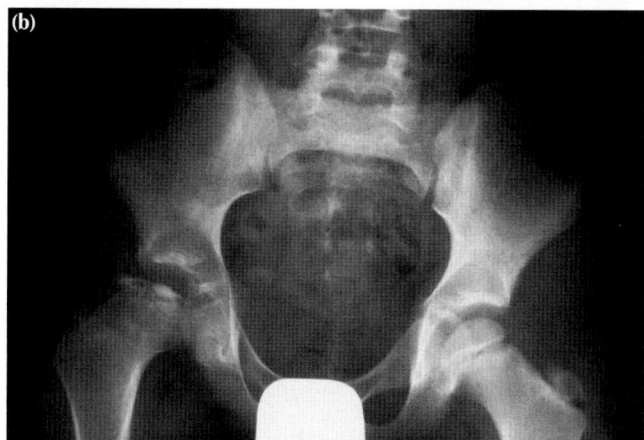

Figure 38.16 Anteroposterior pelvic radiographs of Perthes' disease demonstrating whole head involvement. (a) Right-sided disease; the process is in an early phase. The area of dense necrotic bone is visible (b). There has been collapse and fragmentation.

Management (Table 38.6)

The aim of treatment is to minimise femoral head deformity and, hence, reduce the likelihood of secondary acetabular dysplasia. To encourage sphericity of the head it is important to maintain a good range of movement with regular analgesia and physiotherapy and avoid joint contractures developing. Some restriction of sporting activity is advisable but the routine use of crutches and/or wheelchairs is to be discouraged because of the flexion/adduction posture that they promote. Brace management on its own seems ineffective in maintaining movement or head sphericity, perhaps because the 'good' hip moves more readily than the affected hip.

The role of operative treatment is controversial. Surgery can be performed early to prevent deformity secondary to femoral head collapse or late to 'salvage' a poor mechanical situation, such as hinge abduction occurring because of deformity. In this case the surgery must be performed after the stage of collapse when the head is no longer vulnerable to loading pressures, otherwise recurrent deformity develops.

Joint distraction (arthrodiastasis) via an articulated external fixator to preserve some joint movement may maintain femoral head height but there are no long-term results available yet.

Not all hips with deformity require 'salvage' surgery. With time, remodelling of deformity does occur, with secondary acetabular changes leaving an aspherical but congruent hip joint. Thus, young children, with more time to remodel, have a better prognosis. Long-term follow-up may be required to deal with sequelae such as mechanical symptoms caused by loose osteochondral fragments, a Trendelenburg gait secondary to trochanteric overgrowth or a short-leg gait. A leg length discrepancy may exacerbate the poor mechanical situation associated with coxa breva and trochanteric overgrowth. Degenerative change may occur in adult life.

There are other conditions (all eponymous) in which there are radiographic changes of AVN (Table 38.7). Again, the radiographic changes 'heal' but the change in shape of the affected bone may lead to secondary joint stiffness and loss of function (Summary box 38.11).

Slip of the upper (capital) femoral epiphysis

The physis links the proximal femoral epiphysis (the femoral head) to the metaphysis of the femoral neck. In certain physiological or pathological conditions a 'complete fracture' or a 'stress fracture' through the physis allows the epiphysis to displace on the femoral neck in a manner similar to that which occurs with an intracapsular femoral neck fracture. The leg comes to lie in a shortened, externally rotated position. There is usually painful limitation of hip joint movement. Hilton's law, which states that a joint is supplied by the same nerves as the muscles that move the joint, explains why so many children present with knee pain although the pathology is in the hip.

Table 38.6 A guide to some of the surgical options available for the management of Perthes' disease

Timing	Type of procedure	Comments	Aim
Early	Femoral osteotomy Innominate osteotomy Shelf acetabuloplasty	Varus and derotation	To cover ('contain') the vulnerable femoral head
Intermediate	Arthrodiastasis	Hinged distraction to allow movement	To reduce deforming pressures on the femoral head
Late	Femoral osteotomy Cheilectomy Arthrotomy Trochanteric epiphyseodesis	Valgus and extension; to remove osteochondral fragments	To improve joint congruity and hence function; to improve joint mechanics
Contralateral limb	Distal femoral epiphyseodesis		To improve leg length discrepancy and reduce effects on hip joint mechanics

John Hilton, **1805–1878, Surgeon, Guy's Hospital, London, England.**

Table 38.7 Other conditions (commonly classified as osteochondroses) in which the radiographic appearance is of avascular necrosis

Condition	Affected bone
Keinbock's disease	Lunate
Panner's disease	Capitellum of the humerus
Freiberg's disease	Metatarsal head – usually the second
Köhler's disease	Navicular

Incidence and aetiology

Slip of the upper (capital) femoral epiphysis (SUFE or SCFE) is rare, with an incidence of around 5 cases per 100 000 population. Boys are affected most commonly: the peak incidence is related to the start of puberty and, hence, is earlier in girls than in boys. At this stage, secondary to hormonal changes, the strength of the growth plate, its resistance to shear and its orientation are changing. The hip is therefore 'at risk' and normal forces, exacerbated by obesity and repetitive minor trauma, may precipitate a slip.

Other conditions such as hypothyroidism and renal failure also increase the risk of a slip. Patients who have undergone radiotherapy treatment may be at increased risk if the treatment has weakened the physis and/or been responsible for pituitary hormonal changes.

Diagnosis

The diagnosis is suggested by the history and examination and confirmed on plain radiography (Fig. 38.17). Displacement is

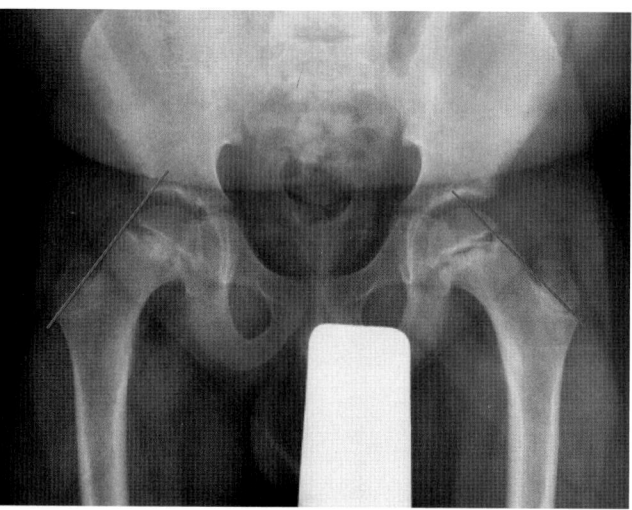

Figure 38.17 Anteroposterior pelvic radiograph demonstrating a mild slip of the upper (capital) femoral epiphysis on the right side. A line drawn along the upper margin of the femoral neck should transect the femoral head (left side) – if it does not do so (right side) a slip is present. There are many other radiographic features that help confirm the diagnosis but the changes are often subtle.

Robert Kienbock, 1871–1953, **Professor of Radiology, Vienna, Austria, described this condition in 1910.**
Hans Jessen Panner, 1871–1930, **Radiologist of Copenhagen, Denmark, described this condition in 1927.**
Albert Henry Freiberg, 1869–1940, **Professor of Orthopaedic Surgery, The University of Cincinnati, Cincinnati, OH, USA, described this disease in 1926.**
Alban Köhler, 1874–1947, **Radiologist of Wiesbaden, Germany, described this disease in 1908.**

sometimes difficult to identify on an anteroposterior radiograph but more obvious on a lateral view.

Classification

The severity of the slip can be graded on the lateral radiograph by how much of the metaphysis is uncovered (Table 38.8).

The condition can also be classified according to its timing. Epiphyseal displacement can occur slowly with the patient presenting with *chronic* symptoms or suddenly with an *acute* onset of symptoms or there may be an acute episode on the background of chronic symptoms (*acute-on-chronic*).

Management

Following an *acute* episode the patient is often unable to bear weight through the leg and the slip is considered to be *unstable* by the Loder classification. Displacement is often *moderate or severe*. This situation is very similar to a displaced intracapsular femoral neck fracture in a child or young adult. An acute severe unstable SUFE is an emergency: poor treatment will result in death of the femoral head. The risk of AVN is considerable and is reduced by prompt screw fixation to stabilise the 'fracture' (Fig. 38.18). A gentle repositioning of the femoral head may be acceptable and often occurs inadvertently with the reduction of muscle spasm that accompanies the general anaesthetic. Current evidence suggests that to be effective such treatment must take place within 24 hours of injury. If delayed the outcome of treatment may be worse than the natural history of the condition, and the rate of AVN increases.

With *chronic* slips the patient is usually able to weight bear, albeit with pain, and the slip is considered stable. Screw or pin fixation *in situ* will relieve pain and often improve the range of movement but permanent reduction in abduction, flexion and internal rotation will be present (Fig. 38.19). The leg is slightly short.

In the *acute-on-chronic* case, repositioning of the acute element of the slip may be feasible. Full correction is impossible and must not be attempted.

If the slip is severe it may be impossible to place a screw in a satisfactory position in the epiphysis, even by starting anteriorly on the metaphyseal neck. In addition, despite fixation *in situ*, there may be significant, persistent malalignment leading to restriction of joint movement. In such cases a realignment osteotomy must be considered. As with all osteotomies, the closer the correction is to the site of deformity, the better the outcome; however, in this situation, the risks of AVN or chondrolysis complicating correction at the level of the physis may be unacceptably high, in which case a more distal osteotomy, for example in the intertrochanteric region, could be considered.

Bilateral slips do occur and the reported incidence is variable.

Table 38.8 Grading of the severity of slip of the upper (capital) femoral epiphysis

Slip severity	Metaphysis uncovered (%)
Mild	< 33
Moderate	33–66
Severe	> 66

Randall Loder, **Professor of Orthopaedic Surgery, Philadelphia, PA, USA.**

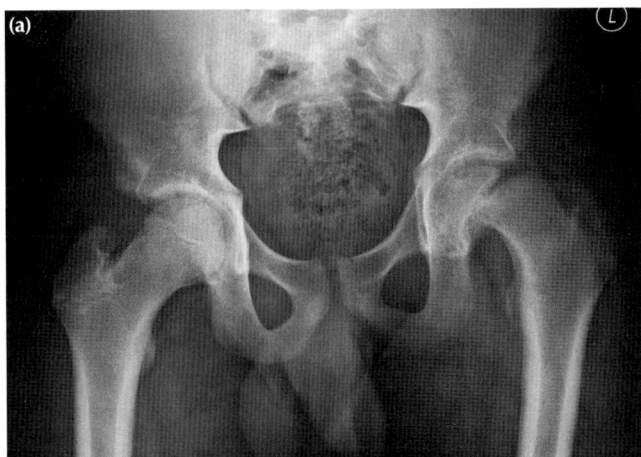

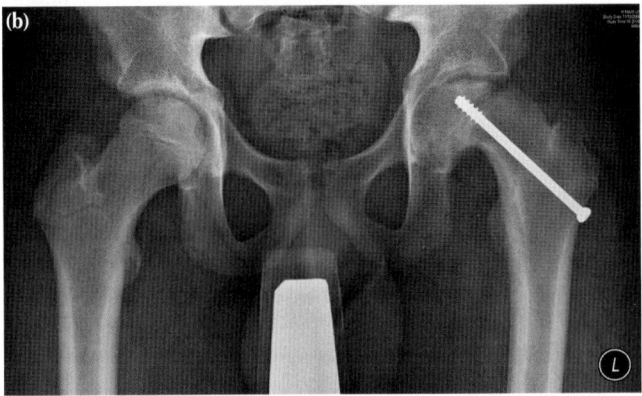

Figure 38.18 Anteroposterior pelvic radiograph showing a left-sided acute severe unstable slip of the upper (capital) femoral epiphysis. (a) At presentation; (b) following partial repositioning and fixation with a cannulated screw.

Prophylactic pinning of the normal but 'at-risk' hip may be considered (Summary box 38.12).

Summary box 38.12

Slip of the upper (capital) femoral epiphysis

- Occurs in prepubertal children, mainly boys
- Often presents with knee pain and the leg may be shortened and externally rotated
- Classification may be according to the severity of slip, whether acute or chronic, or whether stable or unstable – all may affect the prognosis
- Most slips are pinned *in situ* with a single screw in the centre of the epiphysis
- Avascular necrosis is the most feared complication of both the condition and its treatment

---

ABNORMALITIES OF THE KNEE AND LOWER LEG

Many knee problems are self-limiting. Others require surgical consideration to reduce the risk of degenerative change in the longer term.

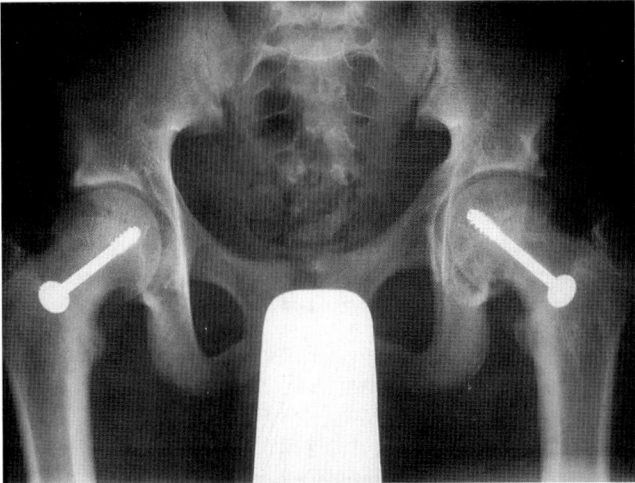

Figure 38.19 Anteroposterior radiograph showing screw fixation *in situ* of a case of bilateral chronic slip of the upper (capital) femoral epiphysis. Note the position of the screw entry point on the anterior femoral neck.

Osteochondritis dissecans

Osteochondritis dissecans (OCD) is found most commonly in the knee although it does affect other joints. An osteochondral fragment becomes partially or completely separated from the joint surface. Magnetic resonance imaging (MRI) is usually diagnostic. In mild cases, or those treated early with rest and activity modification, the fragment may remain attached and heal. If it detaches, partially or completely, mechanical symptoms may require treatment. Treatment aims to encourage bone healing via fixation of the fragment but, in certain cases, the loose body must simply be removed. Younger children have a better prognosis.

Discoid meniscus

This invariably affects the lateral meniscus, which is abnormally thick, covering much of the tibial surface. The knee may snap or clunk when extended and there is often pain, especially when the meniscofemoral ligament is torn. MRI is usually diagnostic. Surgery is only required for pain or mechanical symptoms.

Anterior knee pain

In children, the extensor mechanism is the commonest site of knee pain.

Osgood–Schlatter disease is a traction apophysitis of the patellar tendon insertion, probably caused by the high biomechanical strain as the mobile ligament inserts via a bone/cartilage 'sandwich' onto the apophysis. Pain, tenderness and swelling at the tibial tubercle, exacerbated by exercise, are diagnostic and radiographs are unnecessary. (The normal apophysis often appears fragmented.) Treatment is rest and analgesia, and the condition resolves once the apophysis has fused.

Patellofemoral pain is common in adolescents and often attributed to a degree of patellar maltracking. Treatment, as with

---

Robert Bailey Osgood, 1873–1956, Professor of Orthopaedic Surgery, Harvard University Medical School, Boston, MA, USA.
Carl Schlatter, 1864–1934, Professor of Surgery, Zurich Switzerland.
Osgood and Schlatter described osteochondritis of the tibial tubercle independently in 1903.

more extreme degrees of patellar instability, starts with physiotherapy to develop the quadriceps muscles, particularly vastus medialis. Surgery is rarely appropriate.

Fibular hemimelia

In this longitudinal deficiency there is failure of formation of the lateral 'column' of the lower leg (Fig. 38.20 and Table 38.9). Management varies with the severity of the deficiency and treatment options range from the use of a shoe raise, through multiple episodes of limb equalisation surgery to amputation. An early prediction of the leg length discrepancy at maturity allows a realistic treatment plan to be devised for the patient that includes an honest assessment of final outcome and the time required to achieve this.

Blount's disease

In this condition there is disordered growth in the posteromedial tibial physis. The aetiology is unknown but the infantile form is more common in those of Afro-Caribbean origin. The adolescent-onset disease affects all ethnic origins. Risk factors include early walking and obesity. The child presents with progressive and often severe tibia vara with significant intoeing. There are classical features on radiography (Fig. 38.21).

Treatment is surgical and, following correction of limb alignment via an osteotomy, an epiphyseodesis of the remaining physis may be necessary to prevent recurrence of deformity.

Congenital pseudarthrosis of the tibia

This rare condition presents clinically with an anterolateral bow of the tibia with or without a fracture. Classic radiographic

Table 38.9 Classical radiographic features of fibula hemimelia

Foot and ankle	Absent lateral rays; tarsal coalition; ball and socket ankle joint
Lower leg	Absent or deficient fibula; tibial bow
Knee	Absent cruciate ligaments; deficient lateral femoral condyle
Femur	Relative hypoplasia
Limb length and alignment	Short; external rotation ± valgus

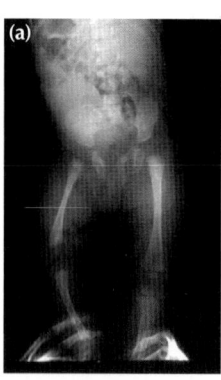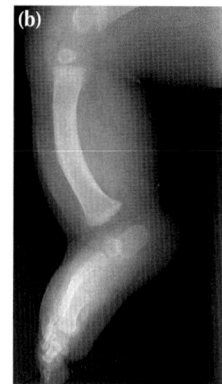

Figure 38.20 Anteroposterior (a) and lateral (b) radiographs of two lower limbs showing some of the features of a fibular hemimelia: absent 5th ray in the foot, absent fibula and deformed tibia.

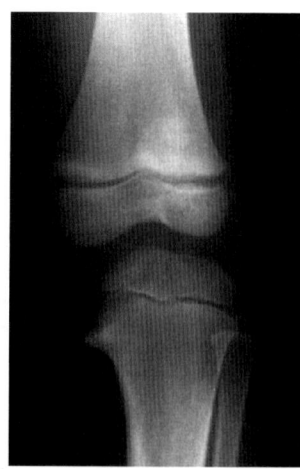

Figure 38.21 Anteroposterior radiograph of the left knee demonstrating changes compatible with Blount's disease affecting the posteromedial tibial physis with changes in both the epiphysis and the metaphysis.

changes are noted and up to 50% of cases are thought to be associated with neurofibromatosis. Once fractured the tibia is reluctant to heal and long-term orthotic treatment may be necessary, with subsequent surgical procedures designed to obtain bony union and restore leg length (Summary box 38.13).

Summary box 38.13

Abnormalities of the knee and lower leg

- *Osteochondritis dissecans* – better prognosis in children than adults
- *Discoid meniscus* – usually lateral, may require surgery
- *Anterior knee pain* – treatment almost always conservative
- *Fibular hemimelia* – associated with abnormality from the hip distally
- *Blount's disease* – clinically, a sharp proximal tibial angulation
- *Congenital pseudarthrosis* of the tibia – anterolateral bowing

---

ABNORMALITIES OF THE FOOT AND ANKLE

Parents are often concerned that minor foot abnormalities will cause their child to be clumsy or slow. This is rarely the case. A careful examination excludes significant pathology and explanation reassures parents.

Club foot

In this condition, more correctly called congenital talipes equinovarus (CTEV), the foot is deformed in three planes (Fig. 38.22). In true CTEV the deformity is fixed. Intrauterine moulding can cause an identical pattern of deformity that is postural and correctable.

Incidence and aetiology

The overall incidence varies from one to six cases per 1000 live births, depending on racial differences. It is more common in boys and bilateral in approximately 50% of cases. A family history is

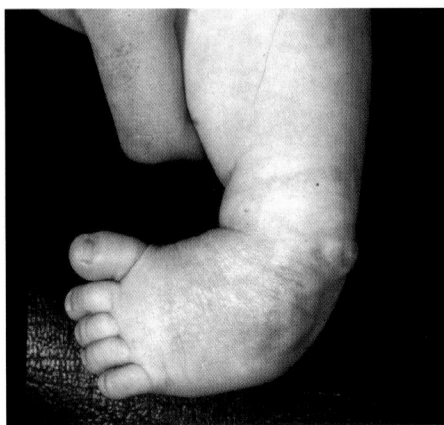

Figure 38.22 Anteroposterior photograph of a foot showing the classic deformities associated with a clubfoot. The hindfoot is in equinus and varus, there is midfoot cavus and the forefoot lies adducted and apparently supinated, although actually pronated relative to the hindfoot.

common but inheritance is likely to be multifactorial. Most cases are idiopathic but as the outcome varies with the aetiology it is important to consider the cause when planning treatment (Table 38.10).

Pathology

The talonavicular joint is subluxed with the navicular displaced medially and plantarwards with respect to a deformed talar head and neck. Ligaments, particularly the calcaneofibular ligament, and tendon sheaths, such as the posterior tibial tendon sheath, are shortened and thickened and have been shown to contain contractile myofibroblasts. Conversely, gastrocsoleus and posterior tibial muscles are smaller and thinner than normal, with reduced myofibrils and increased connective tissue, possibly because of a regional nerve abnormality. The vascular supply via the dorsalis pedis may be altered. Theories abound but it is not known which abnormalities are primary and which occur as the deformity develops.

Clinical assessment

It is usually possible to distinguish the postural clubfoot from the structural (rigid) foot, although not always immediately after birth.

The postural clubfoot may need some physiotherapist input via stretching or casting but can soon be manipulated into a 'normal' position of 45° of abduction and full dorsiflexion with the calcaneus well down in the heel pad. Medial creases are minimal and posterior creases shallow and multiple. Some studies suggest that

Table 38.10 Several different types of clubfoot are recognised

Type	Example
Postural	
Idiopathic	
Neuromuscular	Spina bifida; arthrogryposis; spinal cord anomalies – must be considered in feet that resist treatment or relapse
Syndromic	Trisomy 15

intrauterine moulding is important in the development of both DDH and the postural clubfoot and recommend neonatal hip screening for these 'at-risk' infants.

The structural clubfoot has fixed deformity with elements of equinus, varus and supination and cannot be corrected beyond neutral. Cavus is often marked. The heel feels 'empty' as the calcaneus is held up by the shortened tendo Achilles. There is a deep medial and single posterior crease.

All children with structural clubfoot deformity have an associated small calf and a small foot. Some tibial shortening may become apparent with growth. They should be examined carefully for abnormal neurological signs of intraspinal pathology.

Both Pirani and Dimeglio have developed scoring systems based on the appearance of the foot in the position of maximal correction. These can be used to predict response to treatment and to monitor progress (Summary box 38.14).

Summary box 38.14

Clubfoot

- Triplanar deformity, with hindfoot equinus and varus, midfoot cavus and forefoot adduction and supination
- Incidence is one to six cases per 1000 live births, more common in boys and with a familial tendency
- Most cases are idiopathic but neuromuscular causes include spina bifida and arthrogryposis
- Scoring systems, such as those of Pirani and Dimeglio, can be used to assess the severity

---

Family counselling

The diagnosis of CTEV may be made during an antenatal ultrasound, at which time counselling is limited by uncertainty as to the severity of the deformity. Antenatal counselling is a good opportunity to accustom the parents to the idea of a lengthy period of treatment. At the same time they can be reassured that the child with clubfoot will walk, run and play with his/her peers. The same advice applies if the first meeting is post-natally.

Treatment

Recently, there has been a major swing from operative to non-operative treatment of clubfoot.

Ponseti method

The method described by Ponseti is associated with successful correction of the foot deformity in 95% of cases without the need for a formal surgical release. The technique has been introduced successfully worldwide but a learning curve exists. Treatment commences within a few days of birth. A specific series of manoeuvres results in gradual correction of the deformity, using a series of well-moulded above-knee plaster casts (Fig. 38.23). The head of the talus is the fulcrum around which the rest of the foot swivels, using direct pressure on the first ray and counterpressure over the lateral aspect of the talar head with the distal femur supported. The first ray is elevated to remove the cavus by supinating the forefoot relative to the hindfoot. The varus, inversion and adduction are then gradually corrected by abducting the foot. The calcaneus rotates under the talus into a neutral position. After the forefoot has been corrected, most feet (about 80%)

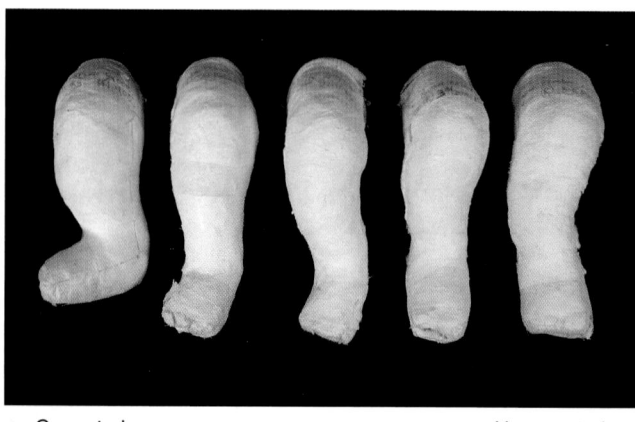

Corrected ←——————————————→ Uncorrected

Figure 38.23 A photograph of a series of casts documenting the stepwise correction of the foot deformity with the Ponseti method of serial manipulation and casting.

Table 38.11 The four stages of a peritalar release that might be required for the correction of a severe clubfoot deformity

Site	Structures requiring lengthening or release
Posterior	Tendo Achilles Ankle and subtalar joints Calcaneofibular ligament Posterior elements of the peroneal tendon sheaths
Medial	Abductor hallucis Tibialis posterior Talonavicular joint Toe flexors
Lateral	Calcaneocuboid joint
Plantar	Plantar ligaments Plantar fascia
Protect	*Neurovascular bundle* *Talocalcaneal interosseous ligament (if possible)*

require a percutaneous Achilles tenotomy in order to dorsiflex the foot satisfactorily.

Once corrected the foot position is maintained by a foot abduction orthosis (FAO) that holds the feet in external rotation and slight dorsiflexion. The FAO is worn full-time for 3 months and at 'night and nap-time' for at least 18 months. Compliance may be difficult to achieve as the child gets older but failure to do so is associated with a higher relapse rate. Recurrent deformity can be treated with further plasters, even in older children, but a tibialis anterior tendon transfer may be required around the age of 2½–4 years for dynamic supination.

There is evidence that feet treated with the Ponseti method are less stiff, less likely to be painful and less subject to overcorrection than those treated surgically. It has the advantage that it can be performed successfully even when surgical facilities are limited. Other conservative regimes have been reported; some are variations on the Ponseti method and others are more resource-intensive. Overall, the results are not as good as with the true Ponseti method.

Surgical treatment

When conservative treatment fails, surgical intervention is required, ideally before walking age.

Surgical release is generally performed 'à la carte', with sequential release of the pathologically tight structures via either a Turco incision on the medial side of the foot or the Cincinnati incision, which runs circumferentially from the naviculo-cuneiform joint medially to the sinus tarsi laterally (Table 38.11).

This approach allows reduction of the subluxed joints but stabilisation may require the use of temporary Kirschner wires. Deformity correction should not be compromised by wound closure and the Cincinnati incision particularly can be left open to heal by secondary intention to preserve ankle position.

Postoperative casting is followed by splinting and physiotherapy as required. Good or excellent results are reported in 60–80% of children treated surgically, but stiffness and over- or undercorrection are common complications.

Martin Kirschner, **1879–1942, Professor of Surgery, Heidelberg, Germany, introduced the use of skeletal traction wires in 1909.**

Secondary surgery for such complications is often difficult and requires a careful assessment of the residual deformity in both the forefoot and hindfoot. Growth disturbance of the distal tibial physis must be considered. Surgical procedures may involve further soft-tissue releases or tendon transfers but, in the presence of fixed deformity, bony correction is often necessary. The foot becomes progressively stiffer with each surgical intervention (Summary box 38.15).

Summary box 38.15

Treatment of clubfoot

- The Ponseti method of serial casting is successful in 95% of feet, avoiding formal surgical release although percutaneous tenotomy is usually required
- The standard sequence is elevation of the first ray, gradual abduction to 60° and, finally, dorsiflexion, usually following Achilles tenotomy
- Tibialis anterior transfer can be used to correct dynamic supination in toddlers and older children
- Surgical release may need to address posterior, medial, plantar and lateral structures, and may result in a stiffer foot than one treated conservatively

Other foot and ankle conditions

Most postural deformities of metatarsus adductus and calcaneo-valgus feet improve spontaneously although in a small proportion minor residual deformity persists.

Congenital vertical talus (CVT) is rare and often associated with neuromuscular conditions such as arthrogryposis and spinal dysraphism. Clinically, there is a stiff 'rocker-bottom' foot and the underlying abnormality is dorsal dislocation of the navicular on the talus (Fig. 38.24). Correction is surgical.

In *tarsal coalition* there is failure of segmentation of adjacent tarsal bones. Presentation is usually in children of school age (up to teens) with hindfoot pain and recurrent ankle sprains. The stiff subtalar joint cannot accommodate uneven ground. The most common coalitions are talocalcaneal and calcaneonavicular (see Fig. 38.3, p. 565). Radiography, computerised tomography (CT) or bone scan may be required to confirm the diagnosis. Treatment

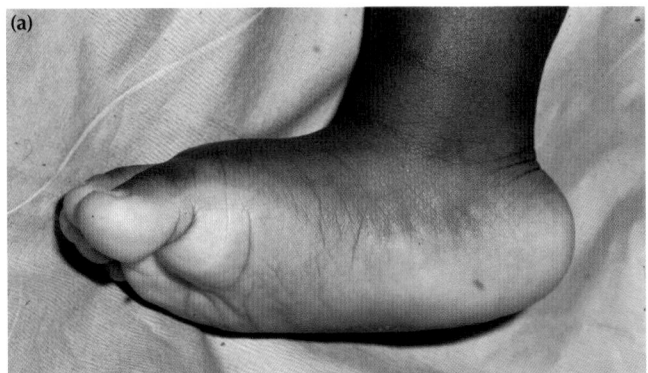

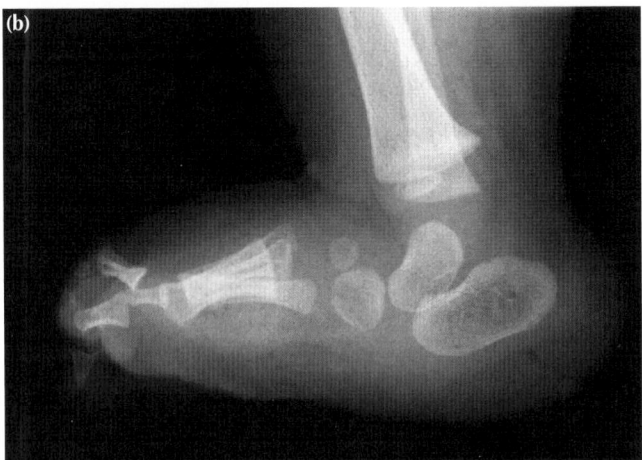

Figure 38.24 Congenital vertical talus. (a) Lateral photograph demonstrating a 'rocker-bottom foot'. (b) Lateral radiograph showing hindfoot equinus and suggesting dorsal subluxation of the non-ossified navicular and forefoot with respect to the head of the talus.

is initially conservative but, if the coalition requires surgical excision, this should be carried out before significant degenerative changes develop.

Curly toes that are flexed and medially deviated are common, often familial and rarely need treatment. They are caused by relative tightness of the toe flexors. Strapping is ineffective. Flexor tenotomy is used when there are symptoms such as rubbing, callosities and difficulty with shoe wear.

Other causes of foot pain in children include osteochondroses (see Table 38.7):

- *Köhler's disease*. This presents with dorsal forefoot pain and swelling in young children. The alarming radiological appearances resolve spontaneously and without sequelae.
- *Sever's disease* (enthesopathy of the calcaneal apophysis). This presents with heel pain related to activity. Tightness in the calf muscle complex may be a contributing factor.
- *Freiberg's osteochondrosis*. This presents with forefoot pain and avascular change in the second metatarsal head. It may be asymptomatic and can present at any age as an incidental finding on radiography. Occasionally it remains symptomatic because of changes within the joint. Bony spurs and osteochondral fragments may need excision (Summary box 38.16).

Summary box 38.16

Other foot and ankle conditions

- Congenital vertical talus – presents as 'rocker-bottom' foot
- Tarsal coalition – presents as a stiff, painful flat foot
- Curly toes are common – most do not need treatment
- Osteochondroses are almost always self-limiting

ABNORMALITIES OF THE UPPER LIMB

Minor abnormalities of the fingers are common (Table 38.12) and frequently require some surgical intervention; however, it must be remembered that, although hand appearance is important, comfort and function are more so.

Function must also be the most important consideration when managing other, more extensive, abnormalities of the upper limb. Treatment is delayed until hand dominance has been established and it is clear what problems a specific deformity are causing in a given child. Children are very adaptable and cope with certain disabilities much more readily than their parents or doctors expect.

Radial club hand

This longitudinal failure of formation is commonly associated with other malformations, for example as part of the VACTERL syndrome (abnormal *v*ertebrae, *a*nus, *c*ardiovascular system, *t*rachea, *r*enal system and *l*imb buds). The clinical presentation of

Table 38.12 Common minor congenital anomalies affecting the hand

Anomaly	Definition	Treatment
Extra/accessory digits		Excise/amputate when necessary
Syndactyly	Failure of separation of digits	Separation with/without skin grafting for functional or cosmetic reasons
Trigger thumb (digit)		Release of the A1 pulley of the flexor tendon sheath
Clinodactyly (usually the fifth digit)	Abnormal angulation of the digit in the radioulnar plane	Surgical treatment of the delta phalanx if deformity progressive or interfering with hand function
Camptodactyly (usually the fifth digit)	Fixed flexion deformity of proximal interphalangeal joint	Splinting/physiotherapy; surgery rarely indicated

---

James Warren Sever, **1878–1964, Orthopaedic Surgeon, The Children's Hospital, Boston, MA, USA, described apophysitis of the os calcis in 1912.**

the upper limb problem depends on the severity of the malformation and, most specifically, whether the thumb is present and functional (Fig. 38.25). Treatment is a balance of conservative measures including physiotherapy and splinting and the judicious use of surgery to centralise and stabilise the hand and wrist on what is essentially a single bone forearm. Thumb reconstruction may be technically challenging. In later childhood, forearm lengthening may be considered.

An ulnar club hand is less common.

Radioulnar synostosis

This is a rare condition in which failure of separation of the embryonic radius and ulna proximally results in no forearm rotation with the hand held in a fixed position. The condition often presents in childhood when the fixed position, for example of full pronation, may become a functional problem. If it is, osteotomy of the forearm bones can change the fixed position but no surgical procedure can restore the range of movement.

Congenital radial head dislocation

The dislocation is usually posterolateral compared with the classic anterior dislocation that accompanies a Monteggia fracture–dislocation (Fig. 38.26). Some restriction of elbow joint movement and forearm rotation is noted and there may be some pain on activity. Excision of the prominent radial head may be required (Summary box 38.17).

Summary box 38.17

Upper limb abnormalities

- Radial club hand is highly associated with other congenital anomalies, for example as part of the VACTERL syndrome
- Radioulnar synostosis usually presents some time after birth with fixed forearm rotation
- Congenital radial head dislocation is usually posterolateral

---

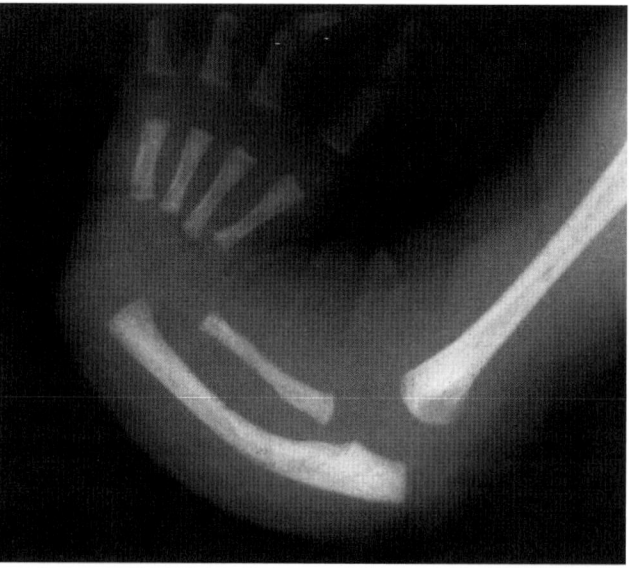

Figure 38.25 Anteroposterior radiograph of a radial club hand demonstrating a short radius, a deformed ulna and an absent thumb.

Giovanni Battista Monteggia, 1762–1815, Professor of Anatomy and Surgery, Ospedale Maggiore, Milan, Italy.

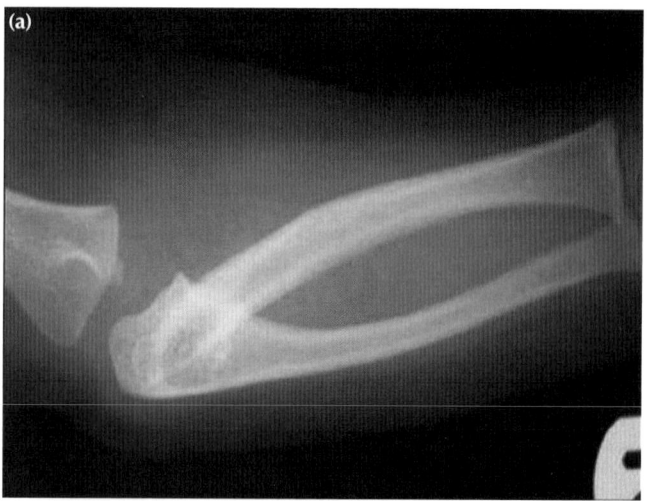

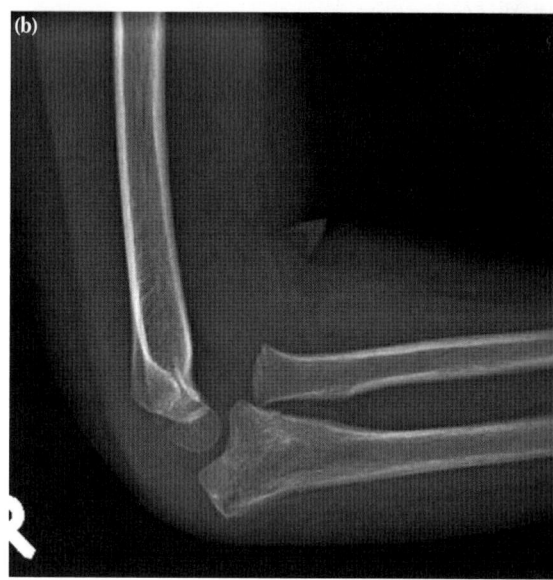

Figure 38.26 Radial head dislocation. (a) Lateral radiograph of a forearm showing a proximal radioulnar synostosis with a posterolateral dislocation of the radial head. Note the underdeveloped radial head and neck. (b) Lateral radiograph of a traumatic anterior dislocation of the radial head with a normal appearance to the head and neck and a deformity in the proximal ulna.

SPINAL DEFORMITIES AND BACK PAIN

Congenital deformities

By definition these problems are present at birth and are either failures of formation or of segmentation of vertebral bodies. Failure of formation may result in a hemivertebra. Failure of segmentation may produce a unilateral bar or bilateral bar (i.e. fusion).

The clinical result is usually a scoliosis (Fig. 38.27), and treatment is based on the potential for curve progression. When a kyphosis results, progressive neurological deficit is common. Bracing is ineffective for congenital vertebral deformities.

Scoliosis

The term 'scoliosis' describes deviation and rotation of the spine such that the most obvious deformity is lateral curvature; the

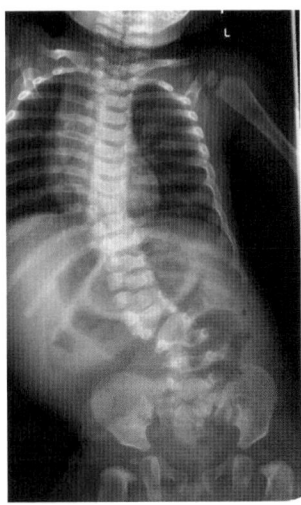

Figure 38.27 Anteroposterior radiograph of the spine demonstrating multiple congenital vertebral anomalies including hemivertebrae.

rotational component is often most apparent in forward flexion (the forward bend or Adams test), when the rib asymmetry creates a 'rib hump' (Fig. 38.28).

The aetiology may be idiopathic, neuromuscular, syndrome-related or congenital, and this, as well as the age of onset, affects the natural history.

Idiopathic scoliosis is common and may be classified according to the age of onset (Table 38.13). In general, the earlier the onset, the more likely the deformity is to be progressive.

The adolescent idiopathic curve is the most common, affecting girls more commonly than boys, but careful assessment must exclude other diagnoses. Full neurological examination and exclusion of leg length discrepancy are essential. Idiopathic scoliosis is generally not painful and so the presence of significant pain requires exclusion of infection and, in particular, tumour. Radiological assessment is by measurement of the Cobb angle (Fig. 38.29). Curves with a Cobb angle of < 20° do not need treatment, progressive curves of 25–40° are generally treated with bracing and those over 40° are considered for surgery (Summary box 38.18).

Table 38.13 Classification of idiopathic scoliosis

Type	Age of onset
Infantile	0–3 years
Juvenile	4–10 years
Adolescent	11–18 years
Adult	Onset at maturity

Summary box 38.18

Scoliosis

- Deformity is multiplanar and includes a rotational component
- Aetiology may be congenital (underlying bony malformation), neuromuscular, syndromic or idiopathic
- Adolescent idiopathic scoliosis is the most common type
- Back pain associated with scoliosis may be associated with an acquired cause such as infection or tumour
- Treatment depends on the severity and likelihood of curve progression – it varies from observation, through bracing to surgery

Kyphosis

Normal kyphosis is 20–50°. When it exceeds this the cause may be postural or structural. Structural kyphosis is most commonly

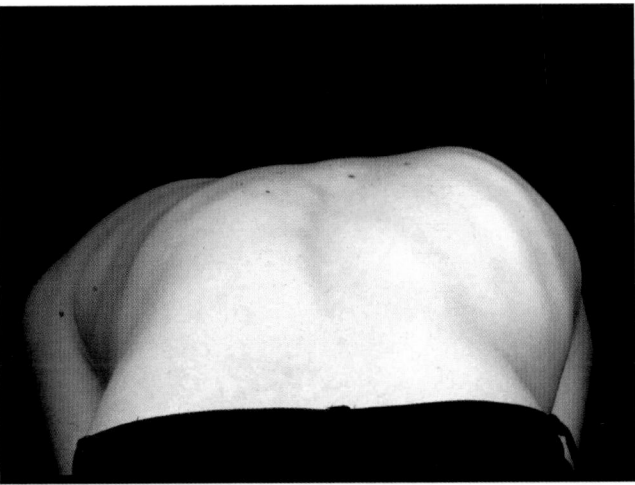

Figure 38.28 Clinical photograph of the Adams forward bend test that demonstrates the presence of a rib hump and the level of the curve.

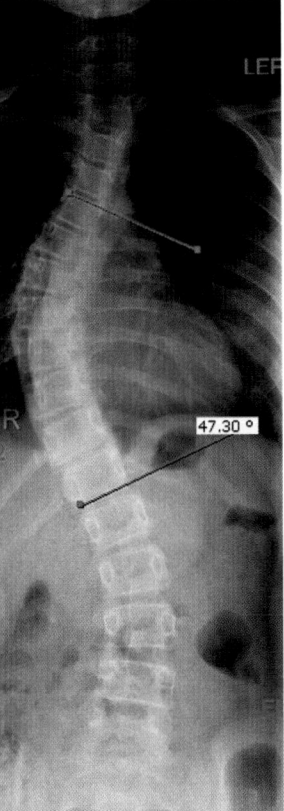

Figure 38.29 Anteroposterior radiograph of a spine with a scoliosis (right thoracic), with a Cobb angle of 47°.

CHAPTER 38 | PAEDIATRIC ORTHOPAEDICS

secondary to *Scheuermann's disease*, which presents as progressive kyphosis in adolescence and is characterised radiologically by vertebral wedging of 5° or more at three adjacent levels and vertebral end-plate changes. The aetiology is unknown. Treatment ranges from physiotherapy and bracing to surgery, depending on the degree of deformity, progression and symptoms.

Spondylolisthesis

Spondylolysis refers to a defect in the pars interarticularis of the vertebra. There are six types: congenital (dysplastic facet joints), isthmic (weak or elongated pars), degenerative, post-traumatic, pathological or post-surgical. *Spondylolisthesis* occurs when the upper vertebra slips forward on the lower; it is graded according to the percentage slip, measured by relating the slipped vertebra to the one below (Table 38.14).

Mild slips are often asymptomatic and do not require treatment. Treatment (physiotherapy, bracing and surgery) depends on the degree of slip and symptoms; mechanical back pain may respond to conservative methods but the development or threat of neurological involvement usually requires surgical intervention.

Torticollis

In torticollis the head is tilted toward and rotated away from the tight sternocleidomastoid muscle.

Congenital torticollis is usually secondary to intrauterine moulding but may present with fixed sternocleidomastoid contracture or with a palpable mass in the muscle. Plagiocephaly may develop and there is a strong correlation with DDH, requiring careful screening of the hips. Most cases resolve with stretching but, occasionally, surgical release of the sternocleidomastoid at one or both ends is needed.

Acquired torticollis is less common and may be caused by gastro-oesophageal reflux, posterior fossa tumour/other regional abnormality, inflammation/infection, ocular problems or atlanto-axial rotatory subluxation. A more comprehensive work-up is therefore required for torticollis presenting after the neonatal period.

Back pain

Children report back pain less frequently than adults although more than half will have had an episode by their late teenage years. Back pain that is mild, intermittent or occurs only on strenuous activity is usually self-limiting; however, back pain in a child is in itself a 'red flag' for serious spinal pathology (Summary box 38.19).

Table 38.14 Classification of spondylolisthesis according to severity of the slip

Grade	Percentage slip
0	No slip
1	< 25%
2	26–50%
3	51–75%
4	> 75%
Spondyloptosis	> 100% – complete translation

Holger Werfel Scheuermann, **1877–1960, Radiologist, The Municipal Hospital, Sundby, Copenhagen, Denmark, described juvenile kyphosis in 1920.**

Summary box 38.19

'Red flag' symptoms and signs for spinal pathology

- Systemic illness, fever or weight loss
- Progressive neurological deficit
- Unrelenting or night pain
- Spinal deformity

All of these require urgent further investigation with a full blood count (FBC), measurement of erythrocyte sedimentation rate (ESR) and C-reactive protein (CRP), plain radiography and MRI or other appropriate imaging. Other causes of back pain include intra-abdominal, renal and systemic pathology; all must be considered but, once excluded, physiotherapy should help improve symptoms (Summary box 38.20).

Summary box 38.20

Other spinal conditions

- Excessive kyphosis may be caused by Scheuermann's disease
- Spondylolisthesis is forward slip of one vertebra on another; it may cause mechanical and, rarely, neurological symptoms
- Torticollis may be congenital and usually responds to stretching of the fibrosed sternocleidomastoid muscle. Acquired torticollis requires elimination of a number of causes
- Back pain with red flag symptoms and signs requires urgent investigation

NEUROMUSCULAR CONDITIONS

Joint stability and limb function depend on the complex integration of a normal musculoskeletal system and a normal neurological system. Damage to either can lead to a variety of conditions linked only by the fact that they are never curable. Thus, management must be directed at helping the child cope with their disability, minimising further deterioration and maximising function. It is important to have an understanding of what the damage is and what the future holds. Several factors need to be considered (Summary box 38.21).

Summary box 38.21

Factors to be considered in the assessment of a neuromuscular disability

- Is the insult to the neurological system progressive or non-progressive?
- Is it located centrally or peripherally?
- Is it general or focal?
- Is it associated with other abnormalities or not?

Spina bifida and polio are classic lower motor neurone lesions whereas cerebral palsy and head injuries affect upper motor neurones and the higher centres and there may be other disabilities such as poor vision, epilepsy and intellectual difficulties to consider.

In children it must be remembered that, even if the initial insult to the neuromuscular system is not progressive, the effects of the insult will change with growth. Damage to any level of the neuromuscular system by whatever cause leads to an alteration in tone and muscle imbalance associated with decreased control of movement. Altered muscle pull, particularly in combination with the effects of gravity, alters bone growth leading to deformity and joint contracture. Muscles are almost always relatively weak and, thus, with body growth and an increase in weight, the muscle is no longer strong enough to control a heavier limb, particularly when deformity means it is working at a mechanical disadvantage.

A multidisciplinary approach to management is essential; therefore, although surgeons must have an understanding of both surgical and non-surgical options, they must *not* work alone. Good physiotherapists and orthotists will reduce the need for surgical intervention, and the results of surgery will be severely compromised if these practitioners are not available to help in the postoperative period.

In conditions such as Duchenne muscular dystrophy there is a substantial evidence base for the benefits of certain surgical procedures; however, in other conditions, such as cerebral palsy, there are fewer long-term validated studies that show significant benefits of surgery.

In general, it is important to maintain a full range of passive joint movement and thus maintain good muscle length and tendon excursion. This is easier to achieve in patients with a flaccid paralysis or low tone. The maintenance of muscle strength is also important. The use of splints, positioning techniques and seating and sleeping systems is essential in most cases. The aim is to prevent the development of a fixed contracture.

Surgery has a valuable role in the management of carefully selected patients (Table 38.15). The surgeon must anticipate the general effects of surgery on the patient, for example altering ankle posture may affect knee and hip posture/function, the patient must have the intellectual ability and motivation to recover from the surgical procedure (Summary box 38.22).

Summary box 38.22

Principles of treatment of neuromuscular conditions

- A neurological defect, whether progressive or not, may cause progressive deformity as the skeleton grows
- A multidisciplinary approach is essential
- Primary therapy aims to maintain range of movement and prevent fixed contractures, with an emphasis on managing tone and position
- Surgery has a limited role in the management of neuromuscular conditions

---

Cerebral palsy

Cerebral palsy is caused by a non-progressive insult to the developing brain in the perinatal period; in most cases only risk factors, such as prematurity, rather than specific causes, such as hypoxia, can be identified. The effects of cerebral palsy may only become apparent as the child grows and fails to reach the expected developmental milestones. Investigations at this stage may help with aetiology and may predict the pattern of the cerebral palsy, for example premature babies may show evidence of periventricular leucomalacia on a brain MRI, which is associated with the development of a spastic diplegia with relative preservation of intellectual function.

In general, the pattern of involvement can be classified according to the anatomical site involved and the effect on muscle tone (Table 38.16). The prognosis for walking can be predicted by identifying evidence of neurological development, i.e. the loss of primitive reflexes.

An important aspect of management is the control of high tone. Tone can be reduced with drugs such as diazepam and baclofen. Alternatively, neuromuscular blockers such as botulinum toxin can bring about a focal reduction in tone. This toxin prevents acetylcholine release at the neuromuscular junction and, hence, transmission at the motor end-plate. The effect is temporary, giving a window of opportunity in which the physiotherapists can work to stretch agonists and strengthen antagonists. It is important to differentiate between dynamic and fixed contractures; the latter will not respond to tone management or splinting.

Table 38.15 General types of surgical procedure that might be considered in the management of a patient with a neuromuscular condition

Surgical procedure	Aim of treatment
Lengthening of the muscle–tendon unit	Restore joint range (but results in relative muscle weakness)
Tendon transfer	Improve functional movement; rebalance muscle forces, after correction of the fixed deformity
Release of joint contracture; correction of bony deformity	Restore mechanical alignment, which may allow muscles to work in a more efficient manner
Fuse/stabilise/relocate joints	Improve posture/function
	Reduce pain
Neurological procedures, e.g. selective dorsal rhizotomy, intrathecal baclofen pumps	Reduce tone
Leg equalisation procedures	Improve lower limb mechanics

Guillaume Benjamin Amand Duchenne, (Duchenne de Boulogne), **1806–1875, a Neurologist who worked successively in Boulogne and Paris, France, but who never held a hospital appointment.**

CHAPTER 38 | PAEDIATRIC ORTHOPAEDICS

Table 38.16 Classification of cerebral palsy with respect to muscle tone and site of involvement

	Characteristics
Tone	
Low	
High	
Mixed	Often low tone in trunk with high tone in the limbs
Variable	High tone and low tone apparent in the same limb on different occasions
Site	
Hemiplegia	Arm more affected than leg
Diplegia	Legs more affected than arms
Total body involvement	Often significant intellectual impairment

The classic cerebral palsy gait patterns show spasticity with the flexors most obviously affected. The child with spastic diplegia has problems at all levels of the lower limb. Multilevel surgery is popular but knowing when to operate and what to operate on is difficult. Observational gait analysis is a skill that improves with practice; computerised gait analysis provides objective evidence of joint movement and mechanics in multiple planes (Fig. 38.30). Appropriate bone and soft-tissue procedures can then be planned. Botulinum toxin can help manage postoperative pain and spasm.

In the child with total body involvement (TBI) and high muscle tone, hip subluxation and eventual dislocation cause some ethical dilemmas (Fig. 38.31). How hard should you work to keep a hip in joint when the patient themselves may be unaware of any difficulty? Current thinking is that the hip should be kept in joint by the simplest means possible but surgical intervention should be performed early if necessary. Spinal involvement is also common and, again, aggressive

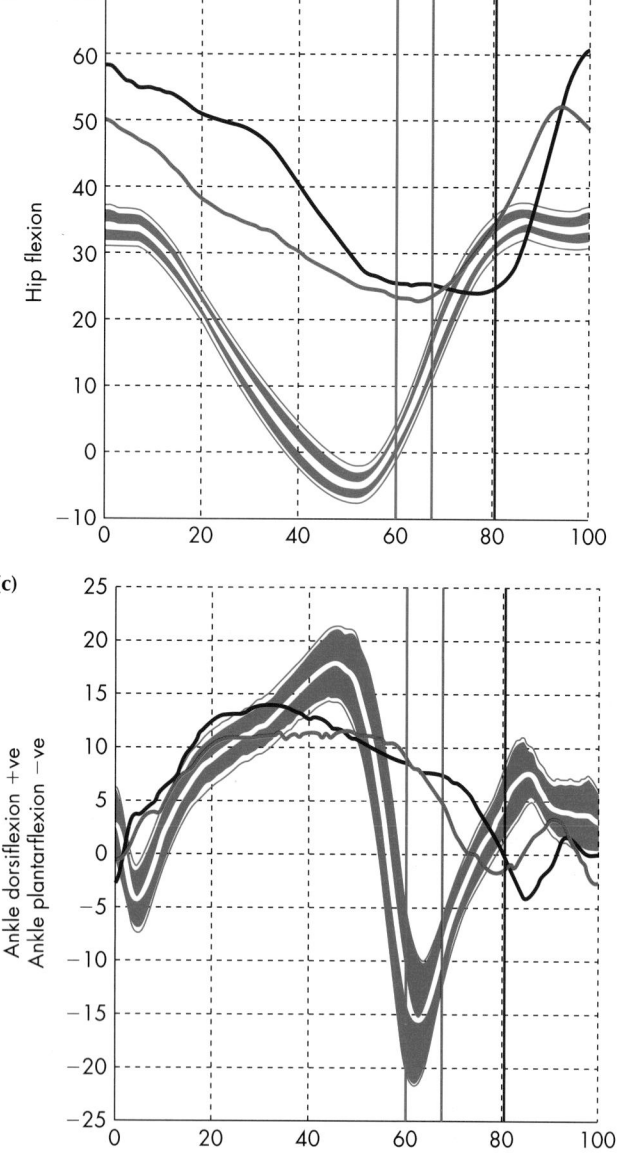

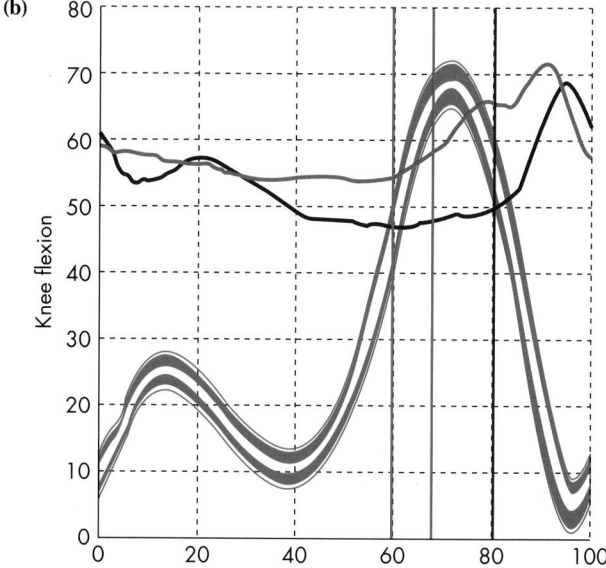

Figure 38.30 a–c Gait analysis graphs such as these demonstrate the normal range of joint movements (green band) at hip (a), knee (b) and ankle (c) during the stance and swing phases of gait. The abnormal joint ranges are shown in red (right leg) and blue (left leg) and demonstrate the excessive hip flexion and lack of knee extension and abnormal knee mechanics associated with the 'crouch' gait of a child with cerebral palsy.

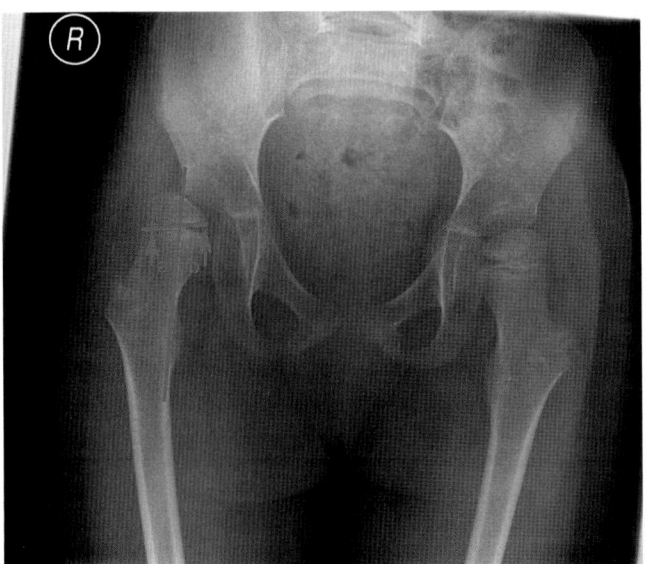

Figure 38.31 Anteroposterior pelvic radiograph of a child with spastic cerebral palsy. Both hips are subluxed. Reimer's migration percentage (a/a + b as a percentage) has been measured as approximately 60% on the right hip.

management may be required, with specific attention given initially to seating position and subsequently to spinal bracing or surgery.

Overall, it is important to remember what the child's needs will be once they reach adulthood. Independent mobility and effective means of communication are two of the most important requirements. Hence, it may not be appropriate to invest time and effort into gaining an upright posture if mobility will be achieved via an electric wheelchair and a hand-controlled car (Summary box 38.23).

Summary box 38.23

Cerebral palsy

- Brain injury is non-progressive
- Classified as hemiplegia, diplegia and TBI
- Tone may be high, low or variable but there is generalised, relative muscle weakness
- In ambulant children, gait analysis may be used to plan surgery or botulinum toxin injections given to improve gait
- In TBI, primary concerns are hip subluxation and spinal deformity

---

Polio

Although an effective polio vaccine has been available for many years the disease still occurs. About 1–2% of patients develop neurological problems when the virus affects the anterior horn cells. Muscle weakness is proportionate to the number of motor units destroyed. Patients often develop trick movements to cope with their muscle weakness and minor joint contractures might actually improve function. Careful assessment before surgery is essential and both the surgeon and the patient must understand the goals of treatment.

Spina bifida

The extent of the disability varies with the level of the lesion and there may be upper motor neurone involvement with spasticity as well as the more classic lower motor neurone lesion. Hydrocephalus may contribute to this. Muscle imbalance leads to secondary joint deformity but the accompanying sensory disturbance, which is often profound, may affect the choice of surgical and non-surgical options.

Muscular dystrophy

Many types of muscular dystrophy exist and the presentation in terms of severity and distribution of involvement is varied. Surgical intervention can be useful for improving quality of life. This is best achieved by operating early to release joint contractures and maintain walking ability and good spinal posture.

Brachial plexopathy

The obstetric brachial plexus injury is still common. It may have a devastating effect on upper limb function, particularly if anti-gravity motor activity has not recovered by the age of 6 months. Neural repair may be necessary in the first few months of life and, later, surgical interventions aim to prevent joint contractures and improve function.

INFECTION

Bone and joint infection remain frequent causes of significant morbidity throughout the world.

Septic arthritis

Joint infection is usually secondary to haematogenous spread but direct inoculation does occur, and sometimes surprisingly easily, for example during a neonatal venepuncture. Diagnosis can be difficult in the very young and in those presenting with overwhelming sepsis. Neonates, children who are immunocompromised and those with sickle cell disease are all at increased risk. At the other end of the clinical spectrum the differentiation between joint sepsis and transient synovitis of the hip can also cause concern.

Classically, the child presents with pain, fever and a reluctance to move or to use the joint; in the lower limb joints this translates to a reluctance to weight bear. On examination, local tenderness and painful restriction of movement are apparent and in superficial joints signs of inflammation may be obvious, with joint swelling and an effusion.

Investigations should include FBC, ESR, CRP and blood culture specimens. Plain radiographs help to exclude other diagnoses and may identify an area of osteomyelitis. Ultrasound scans of deep seated joints, such as the hip, are particularly useful to identify joint effusions (Fig. 38.32). Other investigations such as MRI may be useful on occasion but should not be regarded as a necessity. Good clinical skills, regular patient review and a high index of suspicion are more useful. Four clinical predictors have been identified that differentiate between septic arthritis and transient synovitis (Summary box 38.24 and Table 38.17).

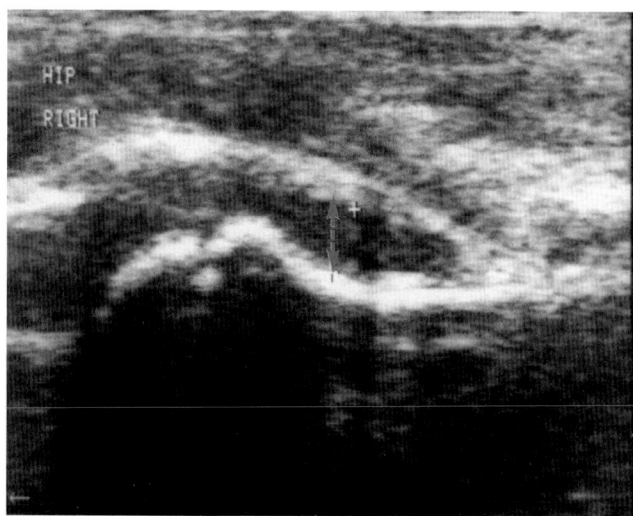

Figure 38.32 Ultrasound scan of a hip joint. A large effusion is distending the joint capsule. The dotted line represents the distance between the femoral neck and the joint capsule.

Summary box 38.24

The clinical predictors of Kocher *et al.* for the diagnosis of a septic joint

- History of fever
- Non weight-bearing
- Erythrocyte sedimentation rate > 40 mm h⁻¹
- White cell count > 12 × 10⁹ μl⁻¹

Pus in a joint is destructive because the proteases produced by leucocytes destroy both the collagen matrix of the articular cartilage and the bacteria. AVN may also occur secondary to pressure effects or ischaemic infarction. The treatment of a presumed septic arthritis is thus the prompt removal of pus from the joint and appropriate adequate antibiotic therapy. Pain relief and rest are also important. The general health and nutrition of the patient must also be considered and treated.

Joint fluid can be aspirated and if pus is confirmed then a formal washout must be performed; standard teaching states that the joint must be opened, irrigated thoroughly and free drainage encouraged via the capsulotomy (a section of joint capsule is often removed). Recently, some literature supports repeated aspiration/irrigation via a large-bore cannula or a small arthroscope. Antibiotic usage is guided by the local hospital policy, the source of the infection, the Gram stain and, in due course, the culture and sensitivity of the organism identified. The joint

Table 38.17 The value of the clinical predictors of Kocher *et al.* in determining the likelihood of the joint being septic

No of positive predictors	Predicted probability of joint sepsis
0	< 0.2%
1	3.0%
2	40.0%
3	93.1%
4	99.6%

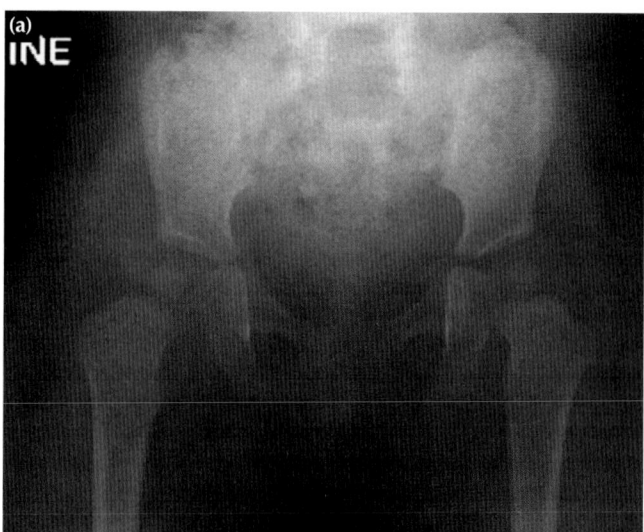

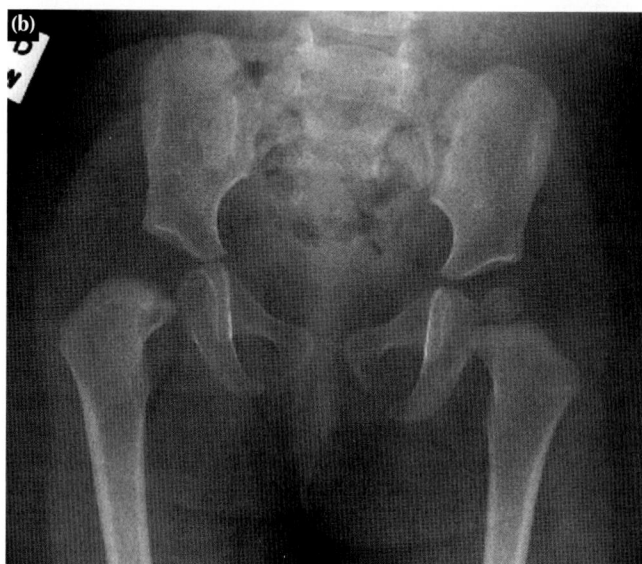

Figure 38.33 Septic arthritis of the right hip. (a) Anteroposterior pelvic radiograph with subtle signs of right hip subluxation. (b) Anteroposterior pelvic radiograph 6 months later showing destruction of the femoral head secondary to late treatment of a septic joint.

capsule may have been distended by the presence of fluid and softened by the inflammatory process and this can lead to joint instability with subluxation or even frank dislocation, particularly in the hip joint (Fig. 38.33a). In such cases the joint must be splinted in the reduced position whilst the inflammatory process settles.

The most frequently identified organism is *Staphylococcus aureus*. Streptococcal infection is also common and other organisms are more prevalent in certain age groups, e.g. the neonate, in certain conditions, e.g. sickle cell disease, or in certain countries. The *Haemophilus influenzae* type B (Hib) vaccine has essentially eliminated *Haemophilus influenzae* as a cause of infection.

Improvement is judged clinically and by monitoring the inflammatory markers. Reaccumulation of pus does occur and must be suspected and treated promptly if the child fails to improve (Summary box 38.25).

Summary box 38.25

Septic arthritis

■ Diagnosis is difficult in neonates and the immunocompromised
■ Typical presentation is pain, fever and a reluctance to move the joint or weight-bear
■ Investigations should include FBC, ESR, CRP, blood cultures and appropriate imaging studies, combined with astute clinical skills
■ Pus in a joint can destroy articular cartilage and cause avascular necrosis
■ Treatment is prompt removal of pus, appropriate antibiotic therapy, pain relief and splintage

Osteomyelitis

As with septic arthritis, bone infection is usually caused by haematogenous spread. Infection often occurs in long bones in which the slow vascular flow within the looped vessels of the metaphysis combined with microtrauma encourages seeding of infection during a bacteraemia (Fig. 38.34a).

Inflammation follows and, if purulent material develops, the pressure effects of the subsequent abscess will lead to progressive bony destruction. Pus can pass through cortical bone and will then elevate the strong periosteum, a process that may render the cortical bone avascular. As in cases of trauma or tumour, the periosteal elevation is a potent stimulus for new bone formation. In cases of untreated or chronic infection this new bone or involucrum may surround the dead bone, the sequestrum, leading to a 'bone-within-a-bone' appearance (Fig. 38.34b).

The presentation and investigation of osteomyelitis is similar to that for joint sepsis. The differentiation between the two may be difficult and a sympathetic joint effusion may occur with metaphyseal osteomyelitis. Thus, if there are no organisms seen on microscopy of a joint aspirate the possibility of a coexisting osteomyelitis must be considered. The metaphysis of a long bone may be intracapsular and infection may spread easily into the joint once the periosteum is breached. In the neonate, proximal femoral osteomyelitis and septic arthritis are essentially the same condition (Fig. 38.34c).

The general treatment principles for the management of infection must be adhered to. Pus needs to be drained but otherwise the treatment is medical. Debate continues over the duration of treatment and indeed whether antibiotics should be parenteral or oral during this time. Overtreatment probably does occur but each case deserves to be treated on its merits, remembering that the child may be immunocompromised and malnourished. The risks of undertreatment are considerable (Summary boxes 38.26 and 38.27).

Summary box 38.26

The general treatment principles for bone and soft tissue infection

■ Rest/splintage of affected limb
■ Analgesia
■ Surgical drainage of pus
■ Appropriate antibiotics via a suitable route and for the correct time
■ Treatment of the underlying condition, e.g. nutritional deficiency, sickle cell disease

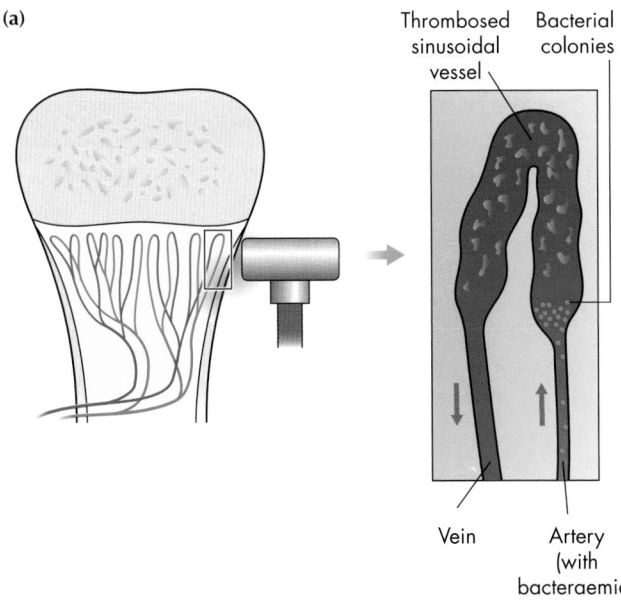

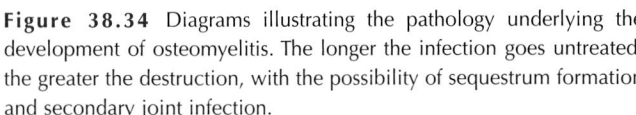

(a) Thrombosed sinusoidal vessel — Bacterial colonies — Vein — Artery (with bacteraemia)

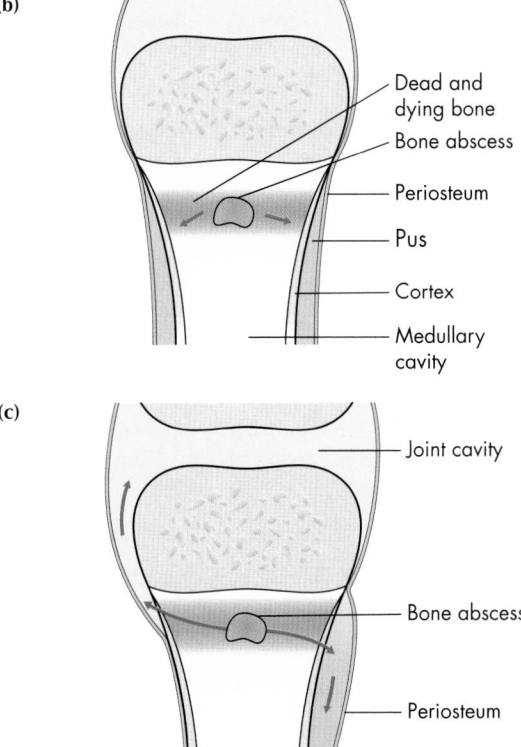

(b) Dead and dying bone — Bone abscess — Periosteum — Pus — Cortex — Medullary cavity

(c) Joint cavity — Bone abscess — Periosteum

Figure 38.34 Diagrams illustrating the pathology underlying the development of osteomyelitis. The longer the infection goes untreated, the greater the destruction, with the possibility of sequestrum formation and secondary joint infection.

> **Summary box 38.27**
>
> **Osteomyelitis**
>
> - Occurs by haematogenous spread, enhanced by microtrauma
> - If untreated, new involucrum envelops the dead sequestrum
> - A joint effusion may be sympathetic or caused by direct spread from the adjacent metaphysis
> - Treatment is drainage of pus when present, appropriate and often prolonged antibiotic therapy, pain relief and splintage

Complications of bone and joint sepsis

Most cases of bone and joint sepsis, if treated appropriately, resolve with no sequelae. However, significant complications can occur, particularly in terms of chronic infection and in cases in which there has been damage to the joint and/or the physis and the secondary growth centre in the epiphysis. In the neonate, vascular channels pass through the physis, connecting the metaphysis with the epiphysis, and a poorer outcome may ensue (see Fig. 38.33b, p. 586). Orthopaedic follow-up should be continued until normal growth patterns are documented.

Meningococcal sepsis

The often debilitating, late orthopaedic sequelae of meningococcal septicaemia are secondary to endotoxin-induced microvascular injury and subsequent ischaemic physeal damage.

Tuberculosis

Tuberculosis is still common. The clinical presentation is often more insidious, with general features such as malaise and weight loss combined with a boggy joint swelling, muscle wasting and joint contractures. Spinal deformity and neurological symptoms are particular problems.

Chronic relapsing/recurrent multifocal osteomyelitis

Although radiographic features suggest subacute or chronic osteomyelitis, laboratory and histopathological findings in chronic relapsing/recurrent multifocal osteomyelitis are usually non-specific and microbiological culture is negative. This is probably an inflammatory rather than an infective condition.

Discitis

Children who refuse to weight-bear may also complain of back pain and may have a discitis. There is continued debate regarding the aetiology of this condition, which may be infective or inflammatory. If the vertebral bodies are involved, infection is assumed.

Brodies's abscess

Subacute or chronic infections may present with radiographic features of a cyst with a sclerotic wall.

Sir Benjamin Collins Brodie, 1783–1862, Surgeon, St. George's Hospital, London, England, described 'Brodie's Abscess' in 1828.

CLINICAL DILEMMAS

The limping child

Children may limp because of pain, weakness, deformity or to gain attention, and the causes vary from sepsis to a spinal tumour and from a leg length discrepancy to a shoe that rubs. It is essential to exclude serious causes and the 'surgical sieve' helps to identify the most likely diagnoses (Summary box 38.28).

> **Summary box 38.28**
>
> **A guide to the clinical assessment of the limping child**
>
> - Symptom onset: sudden or gradual?
> - Symptom duration
> - Concurrent events: recent viral infection, trauma, new shoes, new sport?
> - General health: is the child well?

The examination must include all joints and soft tissues and, in addition, a brief neurological examination, measurement of leg length and an assessment of pain at rest or on weight bearing.

Many conditions, such as sepsis and juvenile arthritis, can present at any age but certain hip conditions are more likely in particular age groups (Table 38.18).

Plain radiographs should usually include both anteroposterior and 'frog' lateral views of the pelvis. Always bear in mind the possibility of a tumour; further imaging such as MRI may be required.

Non-accidental injury

No child is exempt but some children are at particular risk of non-accidental injury (NAI), including those under the age of 3 and those with disabilities. A careful clinical assessment is required (Fig. 38.35) (Summary boxes 38.29 and 38.30).

> **Summary box 38.29**
>
> **Factors that raise concern in the clinical assessment of suspected non-accidental injury**
>
> *History*
> - Delay in seeking medical advice
> - Inconsistent story
> - Mechanism of injury inconsistent with pattern of injury
>
> *Examination*
> - Unexpected bruising to the buttocks/back of legs
> - 'Finger-mark' bruises
> - Bruising of various ages
> - Burns, deep scratches, etc.

Table 38.18 Age at presentation of certain hip conditions

Age (years)	Diagnosis
1–3	Late presenting developmental dysplasia of the hip; sepsis
3–10	Transient synovitis; Perthes' disease
11–15	Slipped upper femoral epiphysis

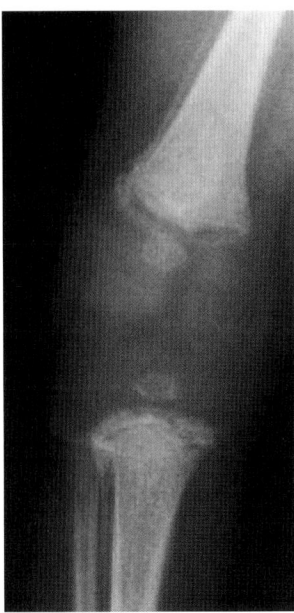

Figure 38.35 Anteroposterior radiograph of a knee showing metaphyseal corner fractures that are often considered to be pathognomonic of non-accidental injury. Non-accidental injury must also be considered in any fracture that presents late or without an adequate explanation.

> **Summary box 38.30**
>
> **Fracture patterns with a high specificity for non-accidental injury**
>
> - Corner or bucket-handle metaphyseal fractures
> - Multiple fractures at different stages of healing/old fractures
> - Scapular fractures
> - Posterior rib fractures
> - Any fracture in a child below walking age

Whenever there is suspicion of NAI, the case should be discussed with the relevant child protection team. All injuries should be documented carefully and photographed if appropriate. If there are concerns for the child's immediate safety it may be prudent to admit the child until further checks have been made. It is important to remember that child abuse occurs in different forms: emotional, physical, sexual and neglect.

FURTHER READING

Benson, M.K.D., Fixsen, J.A. and MacNicol, M.F. (eds) (2002) *Children's Orthopaedics and Fractures*, 2nd edn. Harcourt, London.

Kocher, M.S., Mandiga, R., Zurakowski, D., Barnewolt, C. and Kasser, J.R. (2004) Validation of a clinical prediction rule for the differentiation between septic arthritis and transient synovitis of the hip in children. *J Bone Joint Surg Am* **86–A**: 1629–35.

Loder, R.T., Richards, B.S., Shapiro, P.S., Reznick, L.R. and Aronson, D.D. (1993) Acute slipped capital femoral epiphysis: the importance of physeal stability. *J Bone Joint Surg Am* **75**: 1134–40.

Morrissy, R.T. and Weinstein, S.L. (eds) (2006) *Lovell and Winter's Pediatric Orthopaedics*, Vols 1 and 2, 6th edn. Lippincott, Williams and Wilkins, Philadelphia, PA.

PART 6 | Skin and subcutaneous tissue

Skin and subcutaneous tissue

FUNCTIONAL ANATOMY AND PHYSIOLOGY OF SKIN

Skin can be divided into an outer layer, the *epidermis* and an inner layer, the *dermis*. Deep to the dermis is the *hypodermis*, which is composed of subcutaneous fat and remnants of the *panniculus carnosus*.

Epidermis

The epidermis is composed of keratinised, stratified, squamous epithelium and can be subdivided further into five layers: the *stratum basale* (deepest), the *stratum spinosum*, the *stratum granulosum*, the *stratum lucidum* and the *stratum corneum* (superificial). It accounts for 5% of the total skin (Fig. 39.1).

The majority of epidermal cells are keratinocytes arranged in layers. The basal epidermis (stratum basale) also contains melanocytes. Keratinocytes are classified according to their depth in the epidermis and their degree of differentiation. Keratinocytes grow and are replaced via mitoses in the cells of the stratum granulosum. As they mature and die, they travel up and out from deep to superficial, losing their nuclei and organelles as they progress before forming the stratum corneum, which ultimately separates and sloughs off to form house dust! The other keratinocyte layers in the skin (the strata lucidum, granulosum and spinosum) are variably

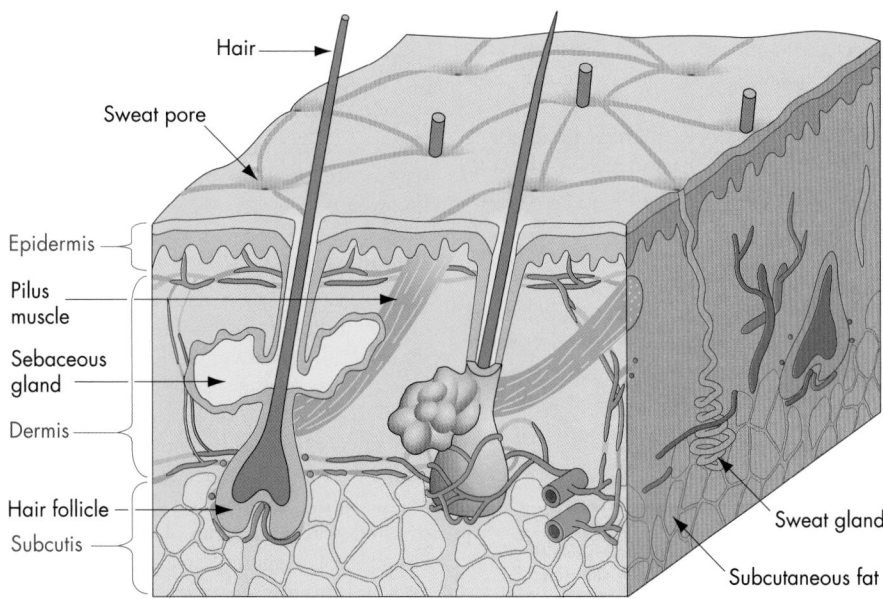

Figure 39.1 Three-dimensional diagram of the structural layers of the skin and its adnexal structures. (Reproduced from Simonsen T, Aarbakke J, Kay I, Coleman I, Sinnot P and Lysaa R, *Illustrated Pharmacology for Nurses*, London: Hodder Arnold, 2006 with kind permission of the illustrator Roy Lysaa.)

present according to body site – for instance, all three are present in the glabrous skin of the palms and soles of the feet (Summary box 39.1).

Summary box 39.1

Layers of the skin

Epidermis
- Stratum corneum
- Stratum lucidum
- Stratum granulosum
- Stratum spinosum
- Stratum basale

Dermis
- Papillary layer
- Reticular layer

Melanocytes are dendritic cells of neural crest origin, which are usually located in the basal epidermis. Each melanocyte synthesises the brown-black pigment melanin, which is transferred via membrane processes to the keratinocytes in the strata granulosum and spinosum. Melanin is positioned within keratinocytes to shield the nuclei from ultraviolet radiation (UVR). Ethnic differences in skin colour are determined by variations in the amount, combination and distribution of melanin within the keratinocytes, rather than differences in the number of melanocytes.

Dermis

The dermis constitutes 95% of the skin and is structurally divided into two layers. The superficial papillary layer is composed of delicate collagen and elastin fibres in ground substance, into which a capillary and lymphatic network ramifies. The deeper reticular layer is composed of coarse branching collagen, layered parallel to the skin surface.

The epidermis and dermis meet at the dermo-epidermal junction in a three-dimensional, wave-like arrangement, in which epidermal rete pegs project down and interdigitate with upward-pointing dermal papillary ridges containing vascular and lymphatic plexi.

The skin also contains specialised cells such as Langerhans cells, the role of which is to engulf antigens and present them to T cells. Merkel cells and Meissner and Pacinian corpuscles have a role in mechanosensation.

Skin adnexa

Adnexal structures such as hair follicles and sebaceous and sweat glands span both the epidermal and dermal layers and contain some keratinocytes in their ducts. In injuries in which epidermis is lost, re-epithelialisation occurs from these structures as well as from the wound margins.

Paul Langerhans, **1847–1888**, Professor of Pathological Anatomy, Freiberg, Germany.
Friedrich Sigmund Merkel, **1845–1919**, Professor of Anatomy successively at Rostock, Königsberg (now Kaliningrad in Russia) and Göttingen, Germany.
George Meissner, **1829–1905**, successively Professor of Anatomy and Physiology, Basle, Switzerland, Professor of Zoology and Physiology, Freiburg, Germany, and Professor of Physiology, Göttingen, Germany.
Filippo Pacini, **1812–1883**, Professor of Anatomy and Physiology, Florence, Italy.

Hair follicles

The human body has two types of hair: *vellus hairs* are a fine, downy, non-pigmented hair that covers the body for 3 months *in utero*, then is eventually shed before birth, apart from the face. *Terminal hairs* are thicker, pigmented and long and are usually found on the scalp, face, axillae, groins, arms and legs and then variably elsewhere according to ethnic, hormonal and genetic predisposition. Hairs are keratinised shafts of tissue that grow out from the bulb at the base of each hair follicle. Each hair follicle has a growth cycle of three phases: during anagen phase the hair grows, then it regresses during catagen phase (during which the hair is shed), and then the follicle remains quiescent for several months during telogen phase before entering a new anagen phase. Hair follicles can only be killed during the anagen (growth) phase. Strips of smooth muscle (erector pili) are inserted into the wall of the hair follicle and lead to hair elevation in times of stress and cold.

Sebaceous glands

Most are hair follicle appendages situated between each hair follicle and its erector pili muscle. When the erector pili muscle contracts to elevate the hair, it compresses the gland and sebum is released (an example of holocrine secretion). The function of the sebum is to act as a skin lubricant and physical protective barrier.

Sweat glands

Eccrine and apocrine glands are simple sweat glands that open into pores in hair follicles. Eccrine glands are distributed throughout the entire body surface except on the lips. These glands secrete sweat in response to emotion or during thermoregulation. Apocrine glands are found in the axillary and groin areas and become active at puberty. Their secretion, which becomes characteristically malodorous after degradation by bacteria, varies in response to emotion and hormone secretion.

Skin thickness

Skin thickness varies with age and body area. It is thinner in children than in adults in any given region. The dermis is between 15 and 40 times thicker than the epidermis, but starts to thin during the fourth decade as part of the ageing process. The epidermis is thickest on the palms, soles, back and buttocks, and is thinnest on the eyelids (0.5–1 mm on sole of the foot, 0.05–0.09 mm on the eyelid).

Blood supply of the skin

In the last 25 years, the 'angiosome model' has furthered our understanding of the anatomical blood supply of the skin and therefore the ability to reconstruct soft-tissue defects using vascularised flaps of various tissue compositions. With respect to its blood supply, the body can be envisaged as three-dimensional segments of tissue called angiosomes, each with an arterial supply and a venous drainage. Blood equilibrates and flows between neighbouring angiosomes via 'choke' vessels, which tend to be situated within muscles. Cutaneous arteries, which are direct branches of segmental arteries (concentrated at the dorsoventral axes and intermuscular septae), perforate the underlying muscles or run directly within fascial layers to the skin from the deep tissues (Fig. 39.2).

The blood supply to the skin anastomoses in subfascial, fascial,

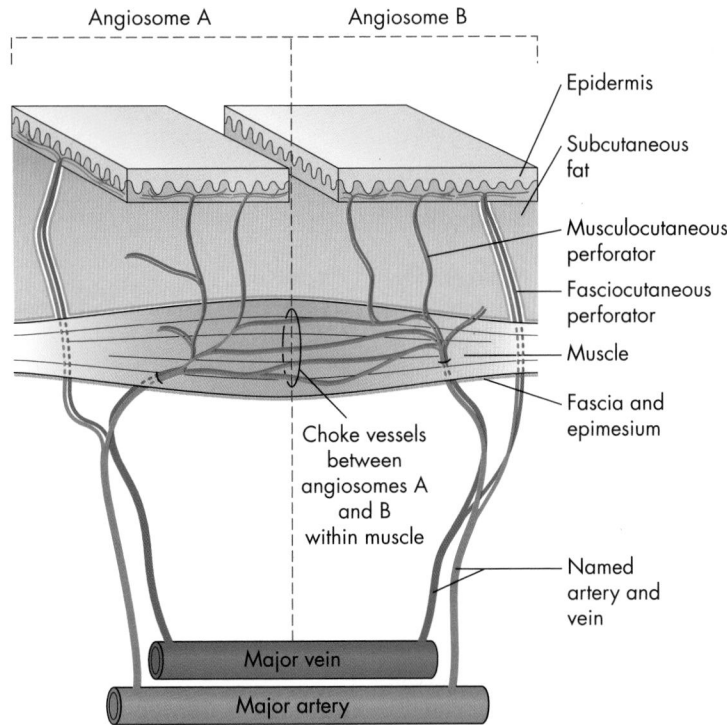

Figure 39.2 Schematic showing two neighbouring angiosomes. Note the choke vessels within the muscle spanning the two cutaneous territories of angiosome A and B – two common examples of myocutaneous flaps which utilise this physiology include the rectus abdominus and the latisimus dorsi flaps.

subdermal, dermal and subepidermal plexi. The epidermis contains no blood vessels so epidermal cells derive nourishment by diffusion.

The venous drainage of the skin is via both valved and unvalved veins. The unvalved veins allow an oscillating flow between cutaneous territories within the subdermal plexus, equilibrating flow and pressure. The valved cutaneous veins drain via plexi to the deep veins.

Anomalies of skin metabolism

Blood flow to the skin can vary between 5 and 100 ml $100\,g^{-1}$ min^{-1} in the temperature range 20–40°C. Therefore, the skin has a potential blood supply that is 20–100 times greater than its metabolic and thermoregulatory requirements. Despite this, the blood supply is inadequate to support wound healing alone, as evidenced by the fact that either primary closure or granulation tissue is required for healing to occur.

A teleological explanation for this apparent excess blood supply is in the restitution of mechanical integrity after the myriad of injuries (such as scratching, stretching, compressing, heating and cooling) to which our skin is constantly subjected.

Skin functions optimally at temperatures below body core temperature and can tolerate long periods of ischaemia (allowing it both to be grafted and to be expanded and used in reconstructive surgery – see Chapter 29).

FUNCTION OF THE SKIN

Human skin and subcutaneous tissue have several important functions:

- barrier to the environment: trauma, radiation, pathogens;
- temperature and water homeostasis;
- excretion (e.g. urea, sodium chloride, potassium, water);
- endocrine and metabolic functions;
- sensory organ for pain, pressure and movement.

Skin grafts

Grafts of the skin can be used to reconstruct wounds having been harvested as a split- (leaving some epidermal components) or full-thickness graft. The process by which a skin graft adheres to and heals a wound is a unique and unnatural process, in which normal wound healing at the recipient site is altered by the presence of the graft. The survival of a skin graft is largely dependent on how fast the graft derives a new blood supply from the wound on which it is placed. Until the graft establishes a new blood supply, nutrition is derived by diffusion through the fibrin layer formed between it and the wound bed. After 48–72 hours, a fine capillary network grows into the graft and anastomoses with the native vasculature of the graft. Factors that inhibit this process (formation of haematoma, seroma or bacterial exudate between graft and wound bed) will decrease the likelihood that the graft will 'take' successfully (see Chapter 29).

Ulcers

An ulcer is a discontinuity of an epithelial surface. It is characterised by progressive destruction of the surface epithelium and a base which may be necrotic granulating or malignant. Ulcers can be classified as non-specific, specific and malignant (Table 39.1 and Fig. 39.3).

Sinuses

A sinus is a blind-ending tract that connects a cavity lined with granulation tissue (often an abscess cavity) with an epithelial

Table 39.1 Classification of common types of ulcer

Ulcer	Type
Peptic	Non-specific
Pressure sores (decubitus ulcers) and ischaemic ulcers	Non-specific
Gravitational ulcers – venous insufficiency	Non-specific
Secondary infective – wound infection and abscess drainage	Non-specific
Traumatic ulcers	Non-specific
Neuropathic ulcers – diabetes, tabes dorsalis, leprosy	Non-specific
Iatrogenic – intravenous fluid extravasation	Non-specific
Dermatitis artefacta – self-mutilation	Non-specific
Aphthous	Non-specific
Primary infective – herpes simplex, tuberculosis, fungal, syphilis	Specific
Gastrointestinal tract and skin	Malignant

surface. Sinuses may be congenital or acquired. Congenital sinuses arise from the remnants of embryonic ducts that persist instead of being obliterated after involution during embryonic development. Acquired sinuses occur as result of the presence of a retained foreign body (e.g. suture material), specific chronic infection (e.g. tuberculosis, actinomycosis or a dental abscess), inflammation (e.g. Crohn's disease), malignancy or inadequate drainage of the cavity (Fig. 39.4).

Treatment of a sinus is directed at removing the underlying cause. Biopsies should always be taken from the wall of the sinus to exclude malignancy or specific infection. For specific management of the disease conditions, please refer to the appropriate chapter.

Fistulas

A fistula is an abnormal communication between two epithelially lined surfaces. This communication or tract may be lined by granulation tissue but may become epithelialised in chronic cases. Fistulas may be congenital or acquired. Examples of congenital fistulas include tracheo-oesophageal and branchial fistulas. Acquired fistulas include fistula-*in-ano*, enterocutaneous fistula following Crohn's disease or postoperative anastomotic

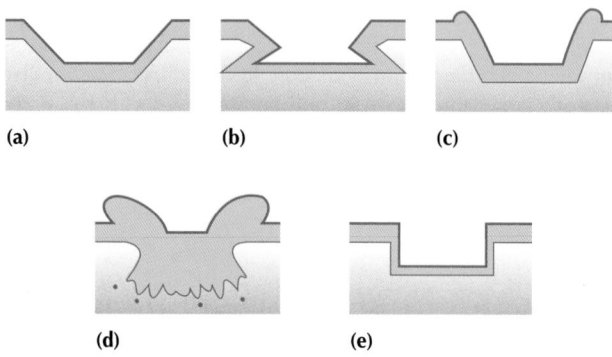

(a)   (b)   (c)

(d)   (e)

Figure 39.3 Some characteristic shapes of the edges of ulcers. (a) Non-specific ulcer: note the shelving edge. (b) Tuberculous ulcer: note the undermined edge. (c) Basal cell carcinoma (rodent ulcer): note the rolled edge, which may exhibit small blood vessels. (d) Epithelioma: note the heaped-up, everted edge and irregular thickened base. (e) Syphilis: note the punched-out edge and thin base, which may be covered with a 'wash-leather' slough.

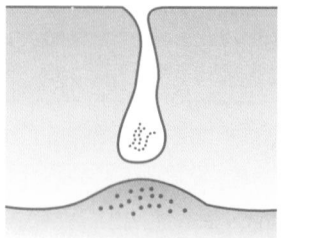
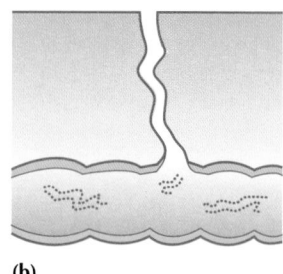

(a)   (b)

Figure 39.4 A sinus (a) and a fistula (b); both usually arise from a preceding abscess. (a) This is a blind track, in this case a pilonidal abscess. (b) This a track connecting two epithelium-lined surfaces, in this case a colocutaneous fistula from colon to skin.

complications and arteriovenous fistula, which may be traumatic or iatrogenic (for haemodialysis).

Again, management of the fistula is directed to treating the underlying aetiology (see appropriate chapter).

PATHOPHYSIOLOGY OF THE SKIN AND SUBCUTANEOUS TISSUES

Radiation damage

UVR and ionising radiation (IR) damage cellular DNA via the tumour suppressor gene *p53*, inhibiting cellular repair and apoptotic mechanisms. There is also evidence that efferent immune responses are impaired after skin exposure to UVR, so facilitating neoplasia.

Ultraviolet radiation

UVR is divisible into types A, B and C according to wavelength. UVR is the principal cause of all types of skin cancer. Its effects are attenuated by melanin and there is an inverse relationship between melanin content and skin susceptibility to UV-induced neoplasia. Some protection is afforded by the stratum corneum, which reflects and refracts UVR, and by clothing, protective creams, cloud cover and buildings.

Ionising radiation

The effects of IR are dose and time dependent. The skin with its rapid cellular turnover exhibits signs soon after exposure. High-frequency rays cause electron coupling at the molecular level damaging proteins, polysaccharides and lipids.

Infrared radiation

Infrared radiation generates heat with cumulative exposure posing the risk of thermal burns.

Cutaneous ageing

The natural process of cutaneous ageing is accelerated by exposure to UVR. The epidermis becomes thinner because and the dermo-epidermal papillae flatten. Numbers of melanocytes and Langerhans cells decrease.

In the dermis, the amount of glycosaminoglycans, proteoglycans and elastin decreases. Dermal collagen content decreases by 6% each decade and the proportion of type I collagen increases relative to that of type III. The rete pegs flatten and the dermis becomes less adherent to the hypodermis. Generally skin appendages decrease in number and function.

In total, these changes, in combination with gravity and life events, result in the characteristic sagging, stretched and wrinkled skin of the elderly and the prematurely aged skin characteristic of the sun exposed.

Congenital/genetic disorders

Neurofibromatosis (Fig. 39.5)

There are two distinct neurofibromatosis syndromes in which Schwann cells form tumours. Each is caused by different genes on different chromosomes; 70% are autosomal dominant and 30% arise from sporadic mutations. Neurofibromatosis (NF) 1 or von Recklinghausen's disease is the more common variant, affecting approximately 1:4000 births. It arises from a gene mutation on chromosome 17. Skin manifestations can appear in early life, with the development of more than five smooth-surfaced café au lait spots, subcutaneous neurofibromata, armpit or groin freckling, and Lisch nodules.

Naevoid basal cell carcinoma (Gorlin's) syndrome

This is an autosomal dominant inherited condition caused by an abnormality in the tumour suppressor gene on chromosome 9q22–31 that codes for the 'patched' protein; 90% of patients develop multiple basal cell carcinomas (BCCs). Patients may also exhibit specific phenotypical characteristics including overdeveloped supraorbital ridges, broad nasal roots, hyperteliorism, bifid ribs, scoliosis, brachymetacarpalism, palmar pits and molar odontogenic cysts.

Xeroderma pigmentosum

Described by Kaposi in 1874, this syndrome is caused by an abnormality on the 'patched' gene of chromosome 9q, resulting in aberrant nucleotide repair during cellular DNA maintenance. It has an autosomal recessive inheritance conferring an > 2000-fold increase in skin cancer risk. Sufferers have an intolerance of UVR, which is manifested as erythema, pigmentation and photophobia. This leads to premature skin ageing and the development of multiple neoplasms, with most affected individuals dying in early adulthood from metastatic disease (60% mortality by 20 years of age).

Gardner's syndrome

This is an autosomal dominant disease variant of familial adenomatous polyposis caused by an abnormal gene on chromosome 5. Gardner's syndrome can cause the development of cutaneous pathology, such as multiple epidermoid cysts and lipomata.

Ferguson–Smith's syndrome (Fig. 39.6)

A rare, autosomal dominant abnormality on chromosome 9q. This results in a syndrome that can be traced to a single familial line from western Scotland, with affected individuals developing multiple self-healing squamous cell carcinomas (SCCs).

Cutaneous manifestations of generalised disease

Many diseases have cutaneous manifestations that may present in surgical practice. These include necrobiosis lipoidica, granuloma annulare in diabetes mellitus and pyoderma gangrenosum in inflammatory bowel disease.

Hyperhidrosis

This condition involves excessive eccrine sweating of the palms, soles of the feet, axillae and groins. This can cause functional and social problems, but can be controlled, depending on severity, with anti-perspirants or periodic local injections with botulinum toxin A. More resistant cases are treated by endoscopic cervical sympathectomy.

Lipodystrophy

Lipodystrophy (lipoatrophy) is a localised or generalised loss of fatty tissue, which can have primary or secondary causes. It is most commonly seen as a complication of long-term administration of insulin, following treatment of HIV with protease inhibitors or in transplant recipients.

It can be treated in selected cases with local injections of poly-L-lactic acid, autologous fat grafting or free tissue transfer to fill out the contour defect that results.

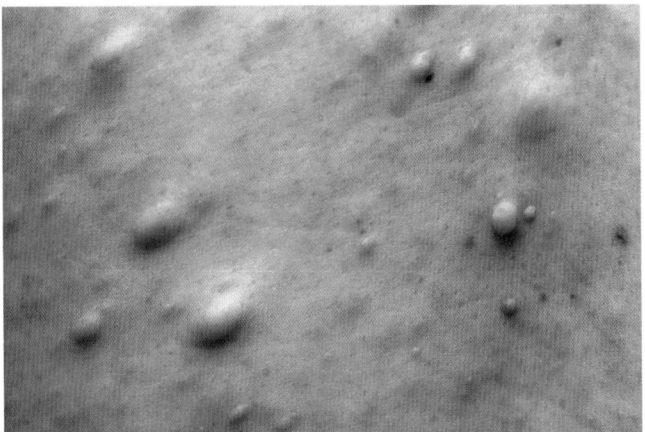

Figure 39.5 Neurofibromatosis (courtesy of St John's Institute for Dermatology, London, UK).

Theodor Schwann, **1810–1882, Professor of Anatomy successively at Louvain, (1839–1848), and Liege, Belgium (1849–1880).**
Friedrich Daniel von Recklinghausen, **1833–1910, Professor of Pathology, Strasbourg, France, described generalised neurofibromatosis in 1882.**
Karl Lisch, **B. 1907, Ophthalmologist, Wörgl, Austria.**
Robert J. Gorlin, **1923–2006, Professor of Oral Pathology, the University of Minnesota, Minneapolis, MN, USA.**
Moritz Kaposi, **1837–1902, Professor of Dermatology, Vienna, Austria.**

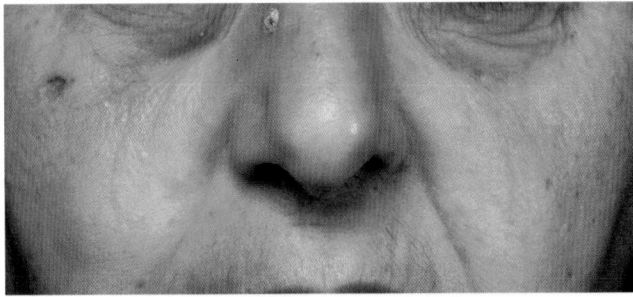

Figure 39.6 Mid-face of a patient with Ferguson–Smith's syndrome. Note the two tumours at different stages of development: on the nose and the right cheek (courtesy of St John's Institute for Dermatology, London, UK).

Eldon J. Gardner, **B. 1909, Professor of Zoology, Utah State University, Salt Lake City, UT, USA.**
John Francis Ferguson-Smith, **1888–1978, Dermatologist, The Victoria Infirmary, Glasgow, Scotland.**

CHAPTER 39 | SKIN AND SUBCUTANEOUS TISSUE

Inflammatory conditions

Hidradenitis suppurativa (Fig. 39.7)

This is a chronic inflammatory disease culminating in suppurative skin abscesses, sinus tracts and scarring. It most commonly occurs in the skin of the axillae and groins, which contains apocrine glands. Less common sites include the scalp, breast, chest and perineum.

Hidradenitis suppurativa appears to have a genetic predisposition with variable penetrance, and is strongly associated with obesity and smoking. Women are four times more likely to be affected than men.

The pathophysiology involves follicular occlusion followed by folliculitis and secondary infection with skin flora (usually *Staphylococcus aureus* and *Propionibacterium acnes*). Clinically, patients develop tender, subcutaneous nodules which may not point and discharge, but which usually progress to cause chronic inflammation and scarring.

This condition is managed by advising patients to stop smoking and lose weight where appropriate. Symptoms can be reduced by the use of antiseptic soaps, tea tree oil and non-compressive and aerated underwear. Medical treatments include topical and oral antibiotics and anti-androgen drugs.

In selected cases, patients may require radical excision of the affected skin and subcutaneous tissue with reconstruction. Healing by secondary intention more frequently leads to contracture and functional impairment than when plastic surgical techniques such as skin grafting or flap transposition are used.

Pyoderma gangrenosum (Fig. 39.8)

Pyoderma gangrenosum is characterised by cutaneous ulceration with purple undermined edges. It occurs secondary to heightened, immunological reactivity, usually from another

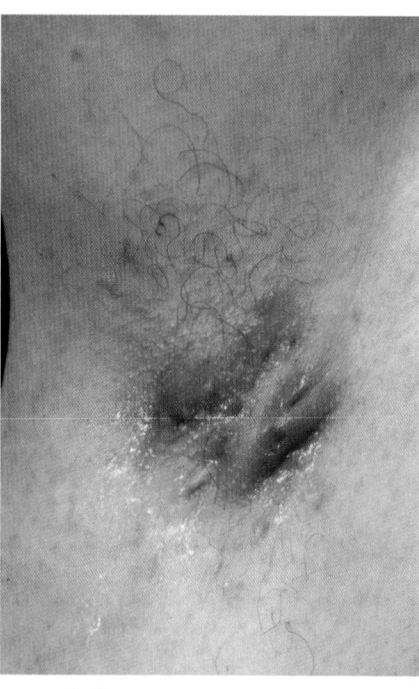

Figure 39.7 Hydradenitis suppurativa affecting the axilla (courtesy of St John's Institute for Dermatology, London, UK).

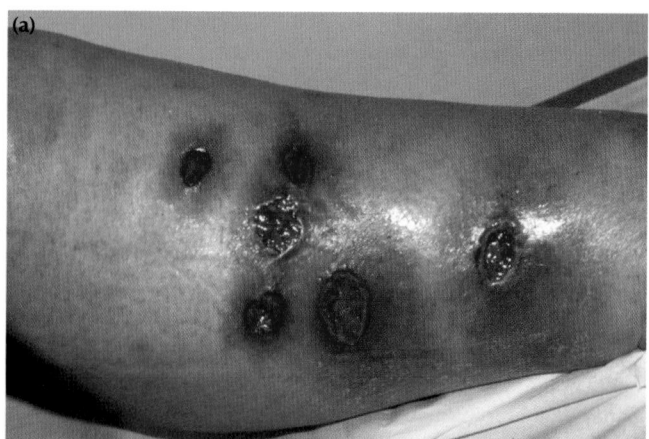

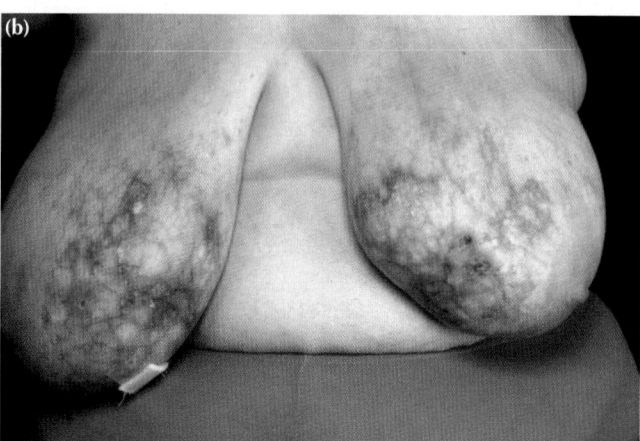

Figure 39.8 Pyoderma gangrenosum affecting the legs (a) and the breasts (b) (courtesy of St John's Institute for Dermatology, London, UK).

disease process such as inflammatory bowel disease, rheumatoid arthritis, non-Hodgkin's lymphoma or Wegener's granulomatosis.

Cultures from ulcers often grow Gram-negative streptococci. These skin lesions generally respond to steroids. Surgery is rarely indicated and may exacerbate the condition.

Inflammation and abnormal wounds after healing

Abnormal scars

Ideally, a scar after trauma, and especially after a surgical incision with primary closure, will be thin and pigmented similarly to the surrounding skin after healing and inflammation are complete.

Scars that heal under tension between the two apposed skin edges in the first 9 weeks (while maximum scar strength is being achieved) are prone to stretching.

Scars that result from healing by secondary intention, or which are subject to tension in two dimensions after primary closure, may become hypertrophic. Hypertrophic scars are elevated but confined within the boundary of the initial injury or incision. They tend to form soon after the causal injury, and affect the young, rather than the elderly, and females more than males. The anterior chest, shoulders and deltoid regions are particularly

Thomas Hodgkin, **1798–1866, Curator of the Museum and Demonstrator of Morbid Anatomy, Guy's Hospital, London, England.**

predisposed to hypertrophic scarring. They may regress spontaneously over several years (Fig. 39.9).

Keloid scars and hypertrophic scars are often confused, but it is important to be able to distinguish the two. Keloid scars resemble hypertrophic scars superficially in that they are elevated, but, unlike hypertrophic scars, they extend beyond the boundary of the original injury or incision. They can form, in some instances, within previously normal scars, months or years after injury – often apparently in response to hormonal stimuli at puberty or during pregnancy and diminishing sometimes after the menopause. Males and females are equally prone to keloid scars, but dark skin types, especially skins of African genetic origin, are 15 times more likely to form them. There is also a strong familial tendency, with both autosomal recessive and dominant inheritance described, and they are associated with Ehlers–Danlos syndrome and scleroderma. Wound tension does not play a role in their genesis and they have never been noted in albino skin.

There are some similarities between keloid and hypertrophic scars: both involve abnormal collagen metabolism resulting in a higher than usual proportion of type III collagen. They are more likely to form in wounds that undergo inflammation without resolution for more than 3 weeks, and both are associated with tissue hypoxia and sustained levels of transforming growth factor (TGF)β1 and -2 (rather than TGFβ3), within the wound. However, they differ histologically: keloid scars contain thick collagen and have increased levels of epidermal hyaluronic acid, whereas hypertrophic scars have a more nodular microscopic structure with fine collagen bundles and increased concentrations of α-actin.

Management of abnormal scars

Despite having different aetiologies, hypertrophic and keloid scars share several treatments in common, which only adds to the confusion that surrounds them.

Non-surgical treatments

Pressure from massage, compressive dressings or clip-on earrings increases collagenase activity and decreases collagen synthesis within either type of scar and, likewise, silicone applied as a dressing or oil diminishes both scars – possibly via an immune mechanism – with more effect on hypertrophic than keloid scars. Corticosteroids decrease collagen synthesis and so both types of scar may respond to intralesional injections, which should avoid the hypodermis so as not to cause hypodermal fat atrophy. Cryotherapy and intralesional steroids injections combined work well in treating keloid scars. Radiotherapy can be used for intractable keloid scars, but its use should be balanced against longer term side-effects as patients tend to be young and will live long enough to develop the long-term sequelae of radiation damage.

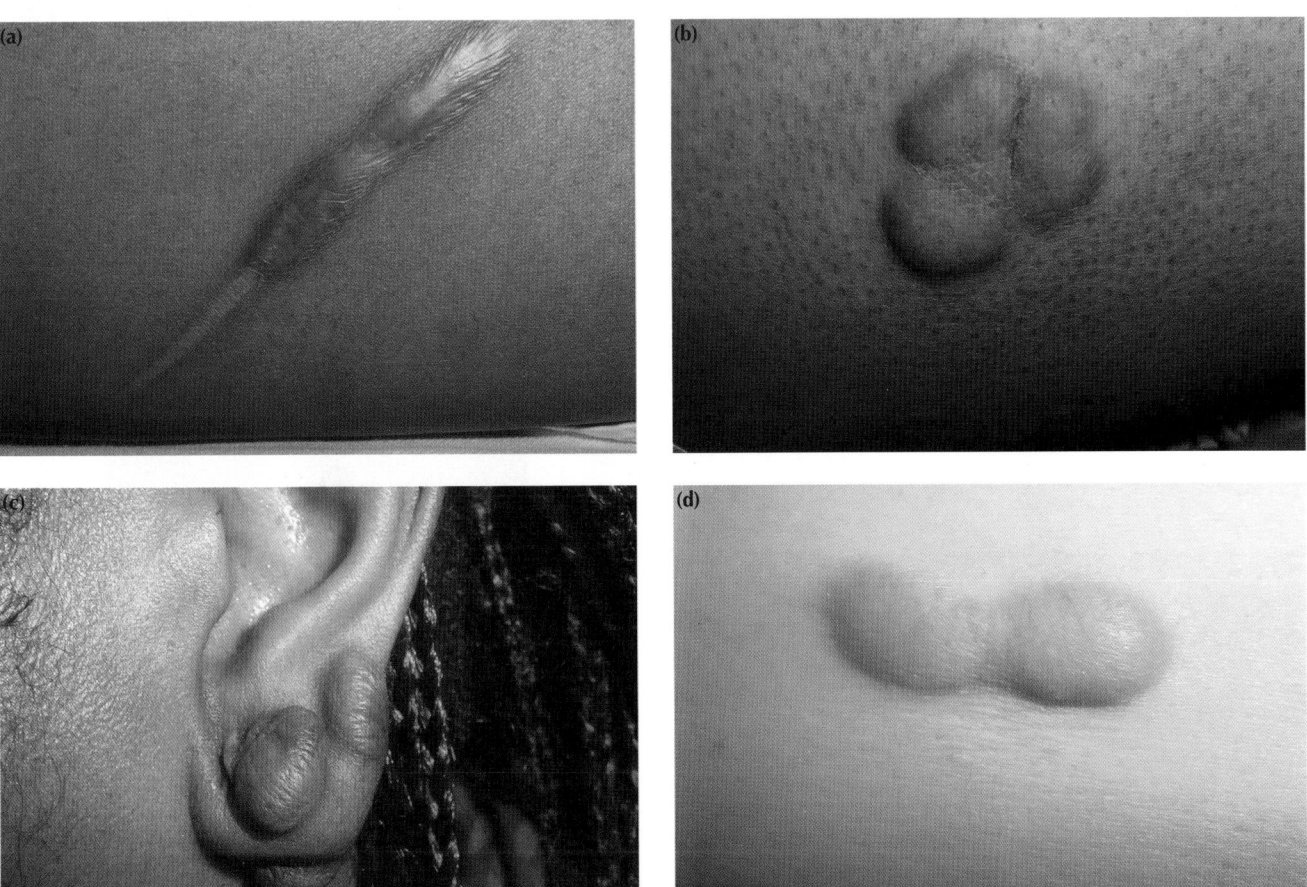

Figure 39.9 (a) Hypertrophic scar after a knife wound – it is raised and stretched, but confined to the boundary of the initial incision. (b) Keloid scar at the site of a bacille Calmette–Guérin vaccination: note how the scar has spread beyond the initial tiny puncture. (c) Keloid scar, following an ear piercing, which is dumbbell shaped, in three dimensions – this became keloid several years after the piercing. (d) Keloid scar in a white-skinned individual at the site of a mosquito bite (courtesy of Mr A.R. Greenbaum).

CHAPTER 39 | SKIN AND SUBCUTANEOUS TISSUE

Surgical treatments

Surgery alone for keloid scars that are resistant to non-surgical treatments carries a 50–80% recurrence rate – less so for hypertrophic scars, especially if the resulting defect can be closed without tension using a local flap. Surgery is usually combined with intralesional steroid administration per- and postoperatively and can also be combined with radiotherapy. Where possible, pressure should be applied postoperatively for 2 months. A very good compromise in treating keloid scars, which has a lower rate of recurrence but a suboptimal cosmetic result, is to perform an 'intralesional' excision, leaving the rim of the original scar behind – this seems to fool the scar into not realising it has been mostly removed.

Infections

Skin and soft-tissue infections can be localised or spreading and necrotising or non-necrotising. Localised or spreading non-necrotising infections usually respond to broad-spectrum antibiotics. Localised necrotising infections will need surgical debridement as well as antibiotic therapy. Spreading, necrotising soft-tissue infection constitutes a life-threatening surgical emergency, requiring immediate resuscitation, intravenous antibiotic therapy and urgent surgical intervention with radical debridement.

Impetigo (Fig. 39.10)

Impetigo is a superficial skin infection with staphylococci, streptococci or both. It is highly infectious and usually affects children. Impetigo is characterised by blisters that rupture and coalesce to become covered with a honey-coloured crust. Treatment is directed at washing the affected areas and applying topical antistaphylococcal treatments, and broad-spectrum oral antibiotics if streptococcal infection is implicated.

Erysipelas (Fig. 39.11)

This is a sharply demarcated streptococcal infection of the superficial lymphatic vessels, usually associated with broken skin on the face. The area affected is erythematous and oedematous. The patient may be febrile and have a leucocytosis. Prompt administration of broad-spectrum antibiotics after swabbing the area for culture and sensitivity is usually all that is necessary.

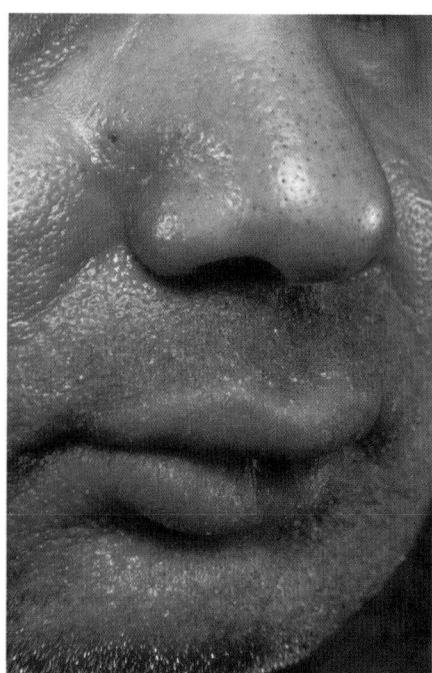

Figure 39.11 Erysipelas (courtesy of St John's Institute for Dermatology, London, UK).

Cellulitis/ lymphangitis (Fig. 39.12)

Cellulitis is a bacterial infection of the skin and subcutaneous tissue that is more generalised than erysipelas. It is usually associated with previous skin trauma or ulceration. Cellulitis is characterised by an expanding area of erythematous, oedematous tissue that is painful and associated with a fever, malaise and leucocytosis. Erythema tracking along lymphatics may be visible (lymphangitis). The commonest causative organism is *Streptococcus*. Blood and skin cultures for sensitivity should be taken

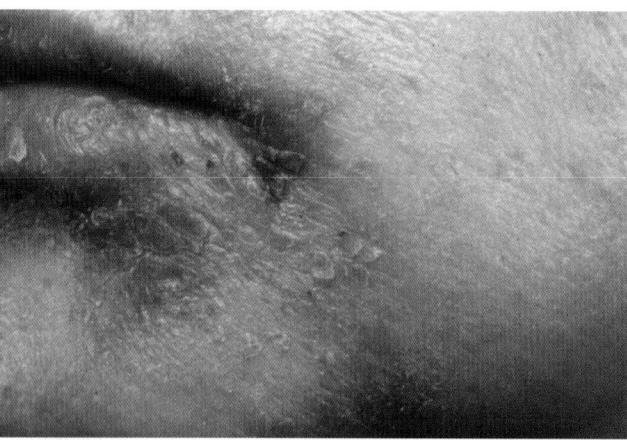

Figure 39.10 Impetigo. Note the honey-coloured crust (courtesy of St John's Institute for Dermatology, London, UK).

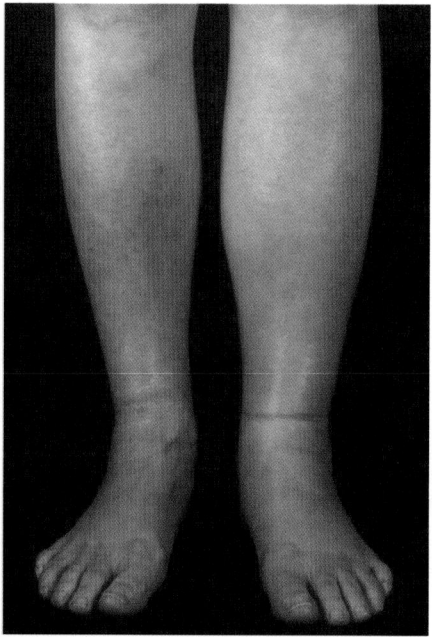

Figure 39.12 Cellulitis affecting the left leg (courtesy of St John's Institute for Dermatology, London, UK).

before prompt administration of broad-spectrum intravenous antibiotics and elevation of the affected extremity.

Necrotising fasciitis (Fig. 39.13)

Necrotising fasciitis was first described by Paré in the sixteenth century. Meleney's synergistic gangrene and Fournier's gangrene are all variants of a similar disease process (Summary box 39.2).

Summary box 39.2

Necrotising fasciitis

- Surgical emergency
- Polymicrobial synergistic infection
- 80% have a history of previous trauma or infection
- Rapid progression to septic shock
- Urgent resuscitation, antibiotics and surgical debridement
- Mortality 30–50%

Necrotising fasciitis results from a polymicrobial, synergistic infection – most commonly a streptococcal species (group Aβ haemolytic) in combination with *Staphylococcus*, *Escherichia coli*, *Pseudomonas*, *Proteus*, *Bacteroides* or *Clostridium*; 80% have a history of previous trauma/infection and over 60% commence in the lower extremities. Predisposing conditions include:

- diabetes;
- smoking;
- penetrating trauma;
- pressure sores;
- immunocompromised states;
- intravenous drug abuse;
- skin damage/infection (abrasions, bites and boils).

Classical clinical signs include: oedema stretching beyond visible skin erythema, a woody hard texture to the subcutaneous tissues, an inability to distinguish fascial planes and muscle groups on palpation, disproportionate pain in relation to the affected area with associated skin vesicles and soft-tissue crepitus. Lymphangitis tends to be absent. Early on patients may be febrile and tachycardic, with a very rapid progression to septic shock. If radiographs have been taken, they may demonstrate air in the tissues, but ideally, the diagnosis will have been made promptly on the basis of symptoms and signs without recourse to 'screening radiography' because unnecessary delay may be lethal.

Management should commence with urgent fluid resuscitation, monitoring of haemodynamic status and administration of high-dose broad-spectrum intravenous antibiotics. This is a surgical emergency and the diseased area should be debrided as soon as possible, until viable, healthy, bleeding tissue is reached. Early review in the operating theatre and further debridement is advisable, together with the use vacuum-assisted dressings. Early skin grafting in selected cases may minimise protein and fluid losses. Mortality of between 30% and 50% can be expected even with prompt operative intervention.

Purpura fulminans

This is a rare condition in which intravascular thrombosis produces haemorrhagic skin infarction. This progresses rapidly to septic shock and disseminated intravascular coagulation. It is usually seen in children, but can occur in adults. It may be subdivided into three types based on aetiological mechanism.

Acute infectious purpura fulminans (Fig. 39.14)

This is the commonest form of purpura fulminans and is caused by either an acute bacterial or viral infection. *Neisseria*

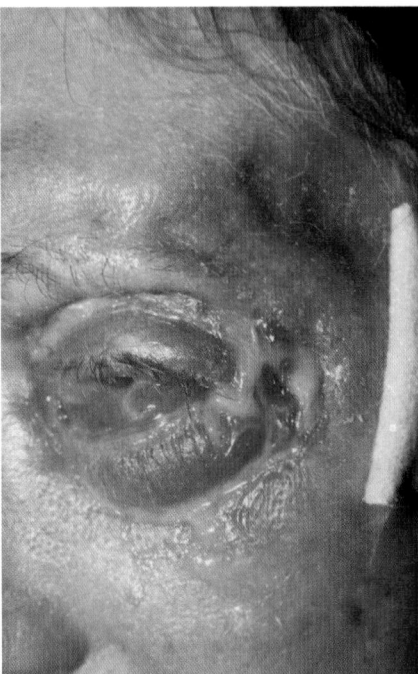

Figure 39.13 Necrotising fasciitis affecting the left orbit and facial skin (courtesy of St John's Institute for Dermatology, London, UK).

Ambroise Paré, 1510–1590, a French Military Surgeon, who also worked at the Hôtel Dieu, Paris, France.
Frank Lamont Meleney, 1889–1963, Professor of Clinical Surgery, Columbia University, New York, NY, USA.
Jean Alfred Fournier, 1832–1915, Syphilologist, Founder of the Venereal and Dermatological Clinic, Hôpital St Louis, Paris, France.

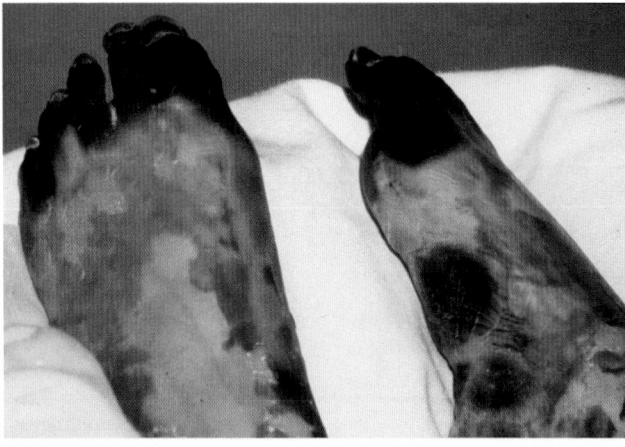

Figure 39.14 Menigococcal septicaemia. Note the sharply demarcated necrotic areas distal to the affected end or perforating arteries with surrounding normal skin (courtesy of St John's Institute for Dermatology, London, UK).

Albert Ludwig Siegmund Neisser, 1855–1916, Director of the Dermatological Institute, Breslau, Germany (now Wroclaw, Poland).

CHAPTER 39 | SKIN AND SUBCUTANEOUS TISSUE

meningitidis and varicella are the most common causal organisms. Acute infectious purpura fulminans causes an acquired protein C deficiency as endotoxins produce an imbalance in the procoagulant and anticoagulant endothelial activity. Acute infectious purpura fulminans is most common in children under 7 years, following an upper respiratory tract infection or in asplenia. Clinically, an initial petechial rash is observed, which develops into confluent echymoses and haemorrhagic bullae, which, in turn, necrose to form well-demarcated lesions that form hard eschars. Extensive tissue loss is common, which often culminates in limb amputation. Acute infectious pupura fulminans is associated with a mortality rate of 40–50% usually a result of multiorgan failure.

Neonatal purpura fulminans

This is an inherited deficiency of protein C and protein S, primarily affecting children, causing extensive venous thrombosis of the skin and viscera in the first days of life.

Idiopathic purpura fulminans

Usually follows a viral illness after a latent period before the development of the clinical picture of purpura fulminans.

Skin and soft-tissue cysts

Milia (Fig. 39.15)

These are tiny hard keratin retention cysts seen both in babies and also in the elderly after chronic sun exposure damage.

Epidermal cysts (Fig. 39.16)

These are cysts lined with true stratified squamous epithelium derived from the infundibulum of the hair follicle or traumatic inclusion. They are commonly known as sebaceous cysts and are often found on hairy areas of the body such as the scalp, trunk and face. They are fixed to the skin and usually have a central punctum and are often indentable with pressure.

Treatment depends on the clinical state of the cyst. When they are inflamed or infected, they should be incised and drained initially, and removed later once the inflammation and induration has subsided. It is important to excise the cyst in its entirety as failure to do so usually results in recurrence.

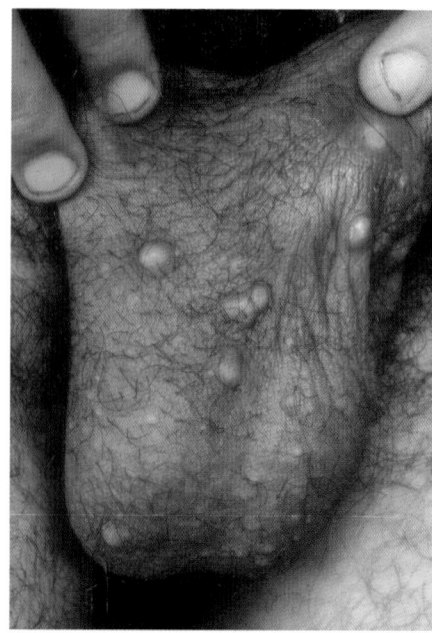

Figure 39.16 Multiple scrotal epidermal cysts (courtesy of St John's Institute for Dermatology, London, UK).

Meibomian cysts are epidermal cysts found on the free edge of the eyelid. A chronic Meibomian cyst is called a chalazion. Tricholemmal (pilar/pilosebaceous) cysts can be confused with epidermal cysts, except that they are derived from the epidermis of the external root sheath of the hair follicle; 90% are found in the scalp and 70% are multiple.

SKIN TUMOURS

Benign lesions

Basal cell papilloma (seborrhoeic keratosis, senile keratosis, verruca senilis) (Fig. 39.17)

These are soft warty lesions, which are often pigmented and hyperkeratotic. They are formed from the basal layer of epidermal

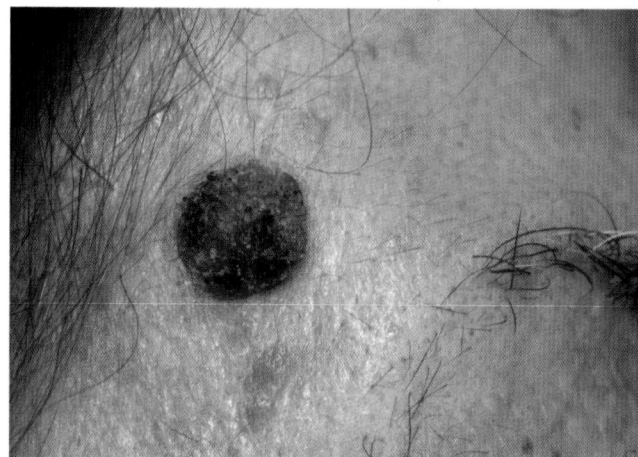

Figure 39.17 Basal cell papilloma (courtesy of St John's Institute for Dermatology, London, UK).

Heinrich Meibom, (Meibomius), **1638–1700, Professor of Medicine, History and Poetry, Helmstadt, Germany, described these glands in 1666.**

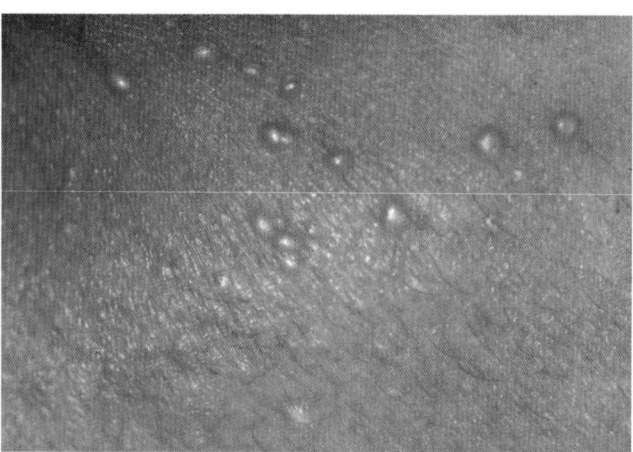

Figure 39.15 Milia (courtesy of St John's Institute for Dermatology, London, UK).

cells and contain melanocytes. They are one of commonest benign skin tumours in the elderly.

Papillary wart (verruca vulgaris)

This is a benign skin tumour arising from infection with the human papillomavirus (HPV), which is also responsible for plantar warts and condylomata acuminata.

Freckle (ephilis)

A freckle is an area of skin that contains a normal number of melanocytes, producing an abnormally large number of melanin granules.

Lentigo

Lentigenes are small, sharply circumscribed pigmented macules that are a marker for sun damage and some systemic syndromes. Solar lentigenes are commoner in fairer skins. An example of a systemic syndrome associated with lentigenes is Peutz–Jeghers syndrome.

Moles/naevi

Melanocytes migrate from the neural crest to the basal epidermis during embryogenesis. When these melanocytes layer in the epidermis they form a simple mole. Melanocytes that aggregate in the dermis or at the dermo-epidermal junction are called naevus cells.

Junctional naevus (Fig. 39.18)

A junctional naevus is a deeply pigmented macule or papule that occurs commonly in childhood or adolescence. It represents a dermo-epidermal proliferation of naevus cells, and usually progresses to form a compound or intradermal naevus with advancing age. It may be found on any part of the body but has no malignant potential. Benign mucosal lesions tend to be junctional naevi.

Compound naevus (Fig. 39.19)

This is a maculopapular, pigmented lesion that becomes most prominent during adolescence. It represents a junctional proliferation of naevus cells with nests and columns in the dermis.

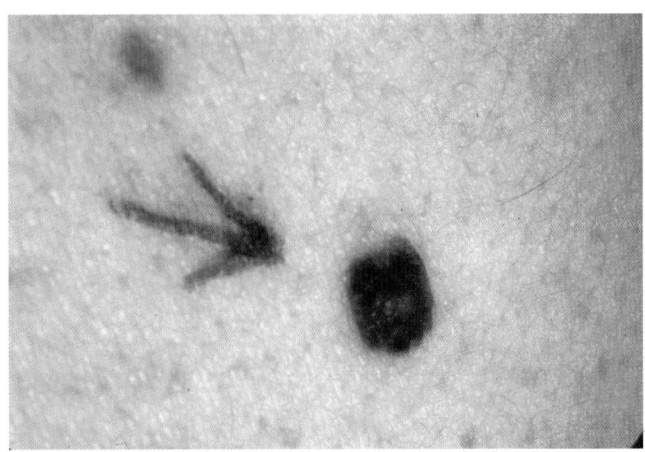

Figure 39.19 Compound naevus (courtesy of St John's Institute for Dermatology, London, UK).

Intradermal naevus (Fig. 39.20)

Intradermal naevi are faintly pigmented papules in adults showing no junctional proliferation but a cluster of dermal melanocytes. These commonly occur on the face.

Spitz naevus (Fig. 39.21)

These are reddish brown (occasionally deeply pigmented) nodules previously termed 'juvenile melanoma'. They most commonly occur on the face and legs, growing rapidly initially and then remaining static. The differential diagnosis is melanoma, and excision biopsy is warranted if there is doubt as to the diagnosis.

Spindle cell naevus

Spindle cell naevi are densely, black lesions that contain spindle cells and atypical melanocytes at the dermo-epidermal junction. They are commonly seen on the thighs and affect women more frequently. They may have malignant potential.

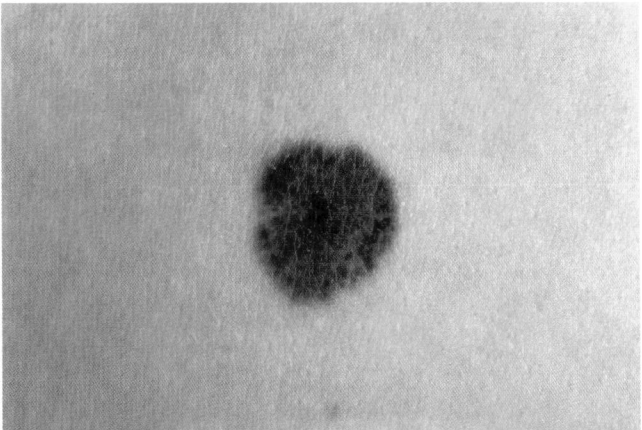

Figure 39.18 Junctional naevus (courtesy of St John's Institute for Dermatology, London, UK).

John Law Augustine Peutz, **1886–1968**, Chief Specialist for Internal Medicine, St John's Hospital, The Hague, The Netherlands.
Harold Joseph Jeghers, **1904–1990**, Professor of Internal Medicine, New Jersey College of Medicine and Dentistry, Jersey City, NJ, USA.

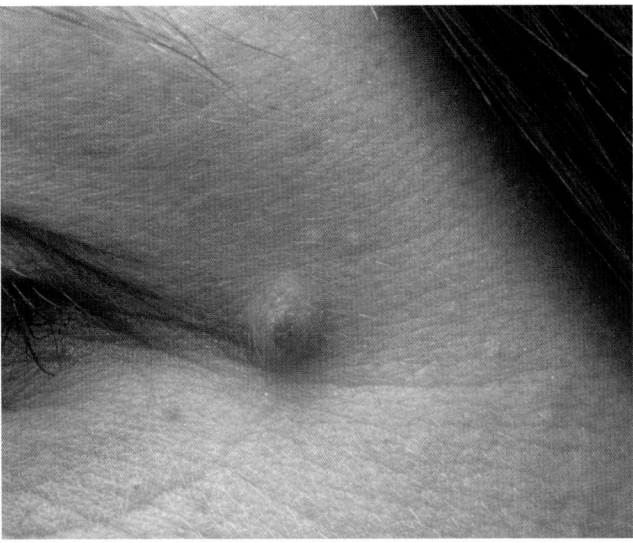

Figure 39.20 Intra-dermal naevus (courtesy of St John's Institute for Dermatology, London, UK).

CHAPTER 39 | SKIN AND SUBCUTANEOUS TISSUE

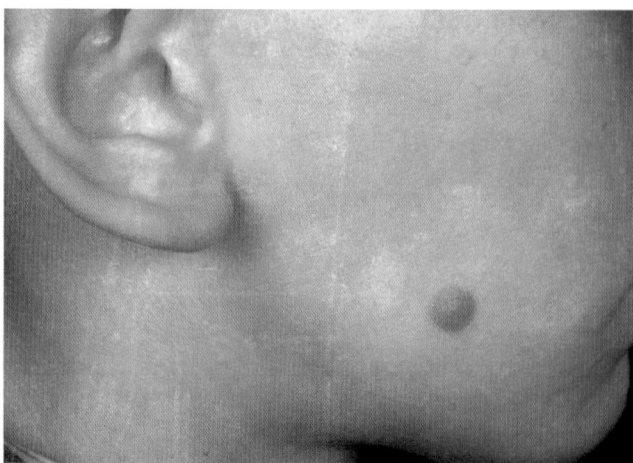

Figure 39.21 Spitz naevus (courtesy of St John's Institute for Dermatology, London, UK).

Halo naevus (Fig. 39.22)

The halo of depigmentation around any benign naevus represents an antibody response to melanocytes. The importance of this depigmentation is that it may also appear around a malignant melanoma (MM). Halo naevi are associated with vitiligo.

Café au lait spots (Fig. 39.23)

These are coffee-coloured macules of variable size (from a few millimetres up to 10 cm). Multiple, smooth-bordered lesions are associated with neurofibromatosis type 1 and McCune–Albright syndrome. They are more commoner in dark-skinned races.

Naevus spilus (Fig. 39.24)

This is also known as speckled lentiginous naevus. It is similar in appearance to a café au lait spot but with hyperpigmented speckles throughout. It is a benign lesion that is associated with various cutaneous diseases. The mainstay of management is observation and serial photography as malignant transformation is possible but rare.

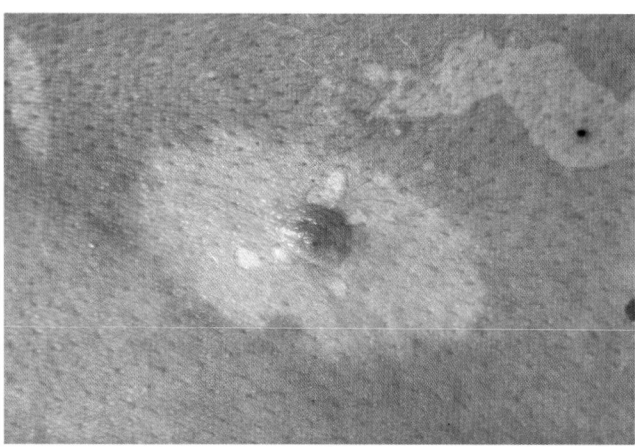

Figure 39.22 Halo naevus (courtesy of St John's Institute for Dermatology, London, UK).

Sophie Spitz, B. 1910, American Pathologist.
Donovan James McCune, 1902–1976, American Paediatrician.
Fuller Albright, 1900–1969, Physician, Massachusetts General Hospital, Boston, MA, USA.

(a)

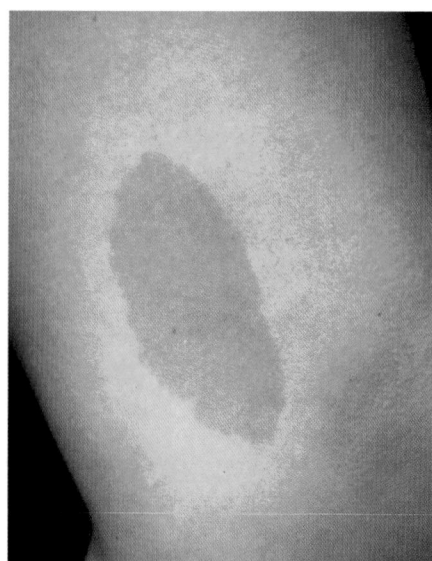

(b)

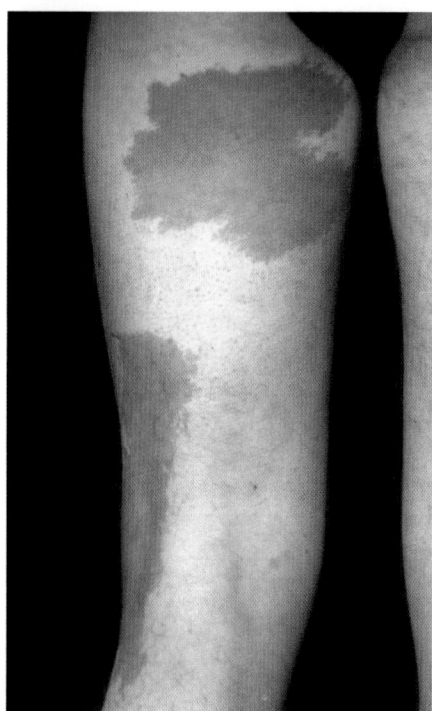

Figure 39.23 Café au lait spots. Note the two topographical variants: in (a) the spot has a smooth 'coast of California' border, whereas the upper spot in (b) has an irregular 'coast of Maine' border. Multiple smooth bordered lesions are commonly associated with syndromes (courtesy of St John's Institute for Dermatology, London, UK).

Mongolian spot (Fig. 39.25)

A Mongolian spot is a congenital, blue-grey macule found over the sacral skin area. Pigmentation initially deepens and then regresses completely by age 7 years.

Blue naevus (Fig. 39.26)

A blue naevus is a benign skin lesion that is four times commoner in children, typically affecting the extremities and face.

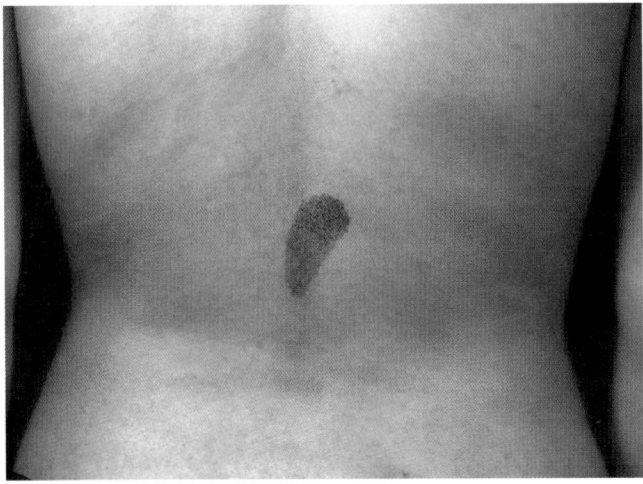

Figure 39.24 Naevus spilus (courtesy of St John's Institute for Dermatology, London, UK).

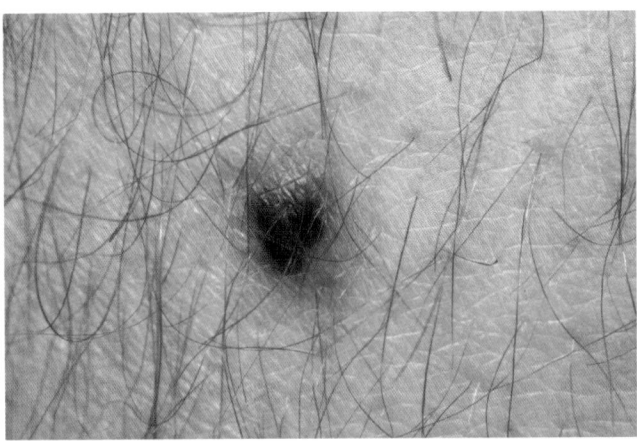

Figure 39.26 Blue naevus (courtesy of St John's Institute for Dermatology, London, UK).

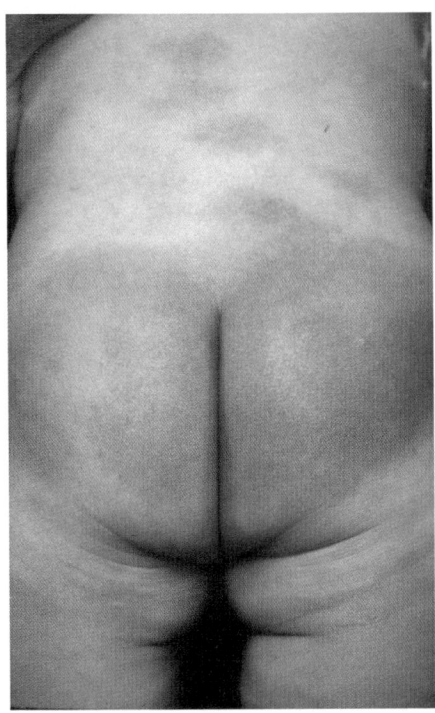

Figure 39.25 Mongolian spot (courtesy of St John's Institute for Dermatology, London, UK).

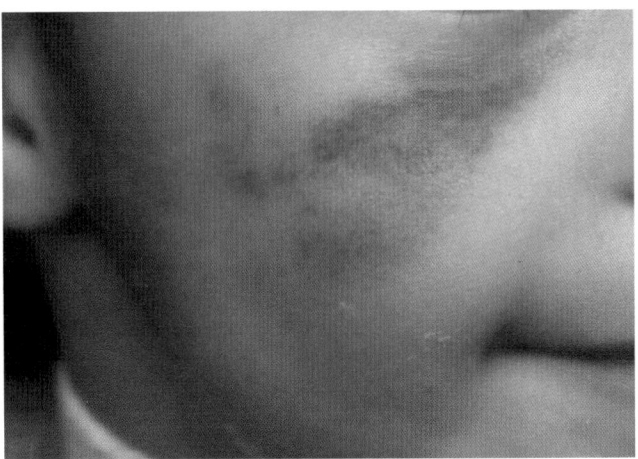

Figure 39.27 Naevus of Ota (courtesy of St John's Institute for Dermatology, London, UK).

Naevi of Ota and Ito (Figs 39.27 and 39.28)

The naevus of Ota is a dermal, melanocytic hamartoma presenting as a characteristically blue or grey macule in the ophthalmic and maxillary dermatomes of the trigeminal nerve. It is four times more common in women, with peaks of incidence in infancy and adolescence, suggesting a hormonal influence. It is most frequently seen in Oriental and African races.

Minoru Ito, 1892–1986, Professor of Dermatology, Tohoku University, Sendai, Honshu, Japan.

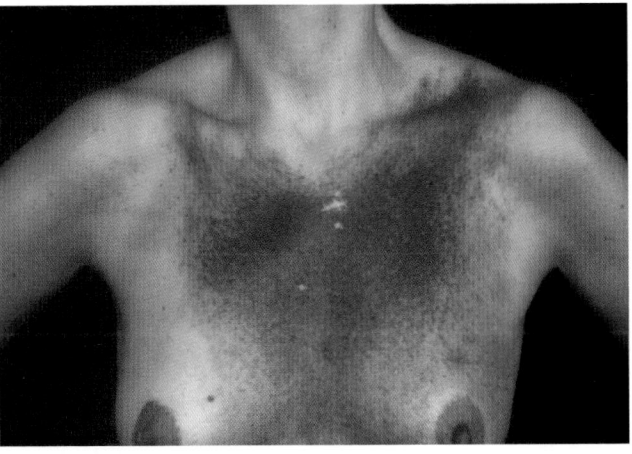

Figure 39.28 Naevus of Ito (courtesy of St John's Institute for Dermatology, London, UK).

The naevus of Ito is characterised by dermal melanocytosis in the shoulder region and can occur simultaneously in a patients with naevus of Ota. It is most frequently seen in Oriental and African races.

Hair follicles

Trichoepithelioma

Trichoepithiomas are small skin-coloured nodules most often found in the nasolabial fold. Clinically and histologically, they look similar to BCC.

Pilomatrixoma (calcifying epithelioma of Malherbe)

These are benign tumours of hair matrix cells characterised by basaloid and eosinophilic ghost cells. They commonly calcify and 40% are found in the under-10 age group.

Tricholemmoma (naevus sebaceous of Jadassohn) (Fig. 39.29)

Tricholemmoma is a congenital hamartoma with the appearance of a linear verrucous naevus. These were believed to form BCCs in up to 10% of cases after puberty, but reviewed histology casts doubt on the frequency with which this occurs, although it is recognised that they have an increased potential for malignant change.

Adenoma sebaceum (tuberous sclerosis, Bourneville's disease) (Fig. 39.30)

Typically these are red facial papules (angiofibromas) that are found usually on the nasolabial folds, cheek and chin. They form part of the disease process in tuberous sclerosis. Skin lesions

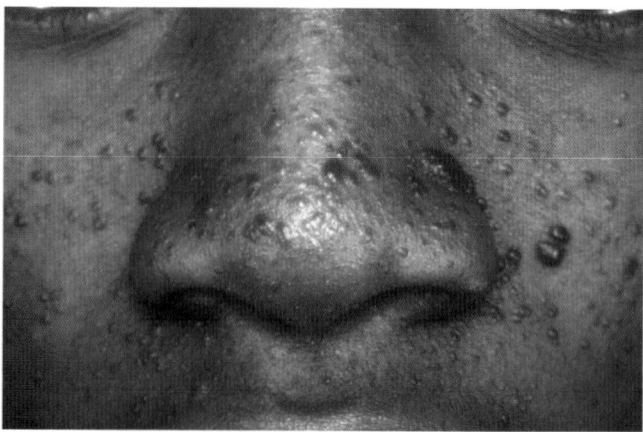

Figure 39.30 Adenoma sebaceum (courtesy of St John's Institute for Dermatology, London, UK).

usually appear in children under 10 years of age and increase in size and number until adolescence. Cosmetic removal with carbon dioxide or pulse–dye lasers or scalpel is possible.

Rhinophyma (Fig. 39.31)

Rhinophyma is an end-stage sequela of acne rosacea. It is hypertrophy and hyperplasia of the sebaceous glands and tends to affect elderly men (male to female ratio 12:1). Up to 3% of cases may have an occult BCC. Treatment by dermabrasion or laser resurfacing produces good results.

Sweat glands

Cystadenoma (hydrocystadenomas, hidradenomas)

These are 1- to 3-cm translucent blue cystic nodules.

Eccrine poroma (papillary syringoma)

These are single raised or pedicled lesions found most often on the palm or sole.

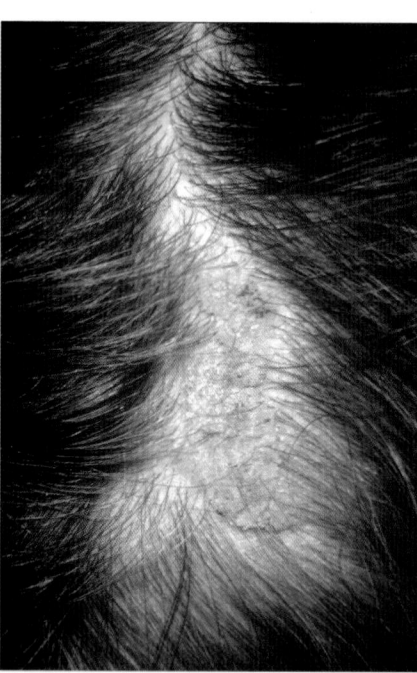

Figure 39.29 Naevus sebaceous of Jadassohn (courtesy of St John's Institute for Dermatology, London, UK).

Josef Jadassohn, **1863–1936**, a Dermatologist of Breslau, Germany (now Wroclaw, Poland).
Desire M. Bourneville, **1840–1909**, Physician, Le Bicêtre, Paris, France.

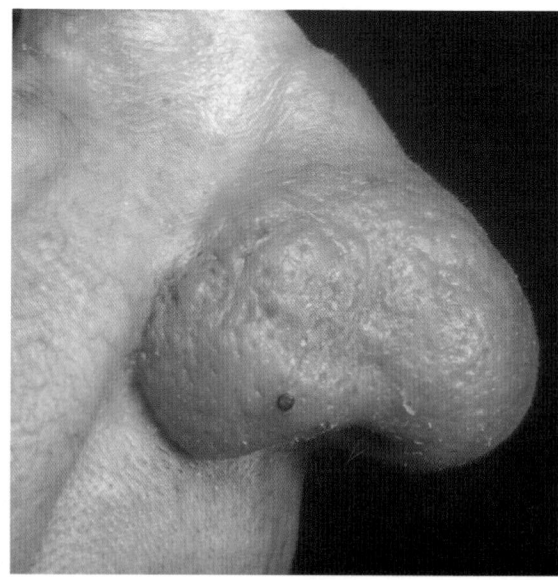

Figure 39.31 Rhinophyma (courtesy of St John's Institute for Dermatology, London, UK).

Cylindroma (turban tumour)

A variant of eccrine spiradenoma, which can be multiple on the scalp and can coalesce to form a 'turban tumour'.

Pre-malignant lesions

Actinic/solar keratoses (Fig. 39.32)

These are areas of dyskeratosis and cellular atypia, with sub-epidermal inflammation, but a normal dermo-epidermal junction. Up to 20% go on to form SCCs.

Cutaneous horn (Fig. 39.33)

A cutaneous, keratin accumulation, which, by definition, has a height greater than its base diameter; 10% will have an underlying SCC.

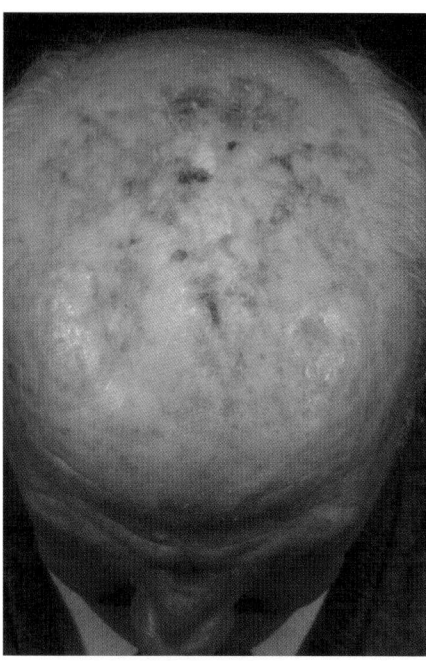

Figure 39.32 Actinic keratosis (courtesy of St John's Institute for Dermatology, London, UK).

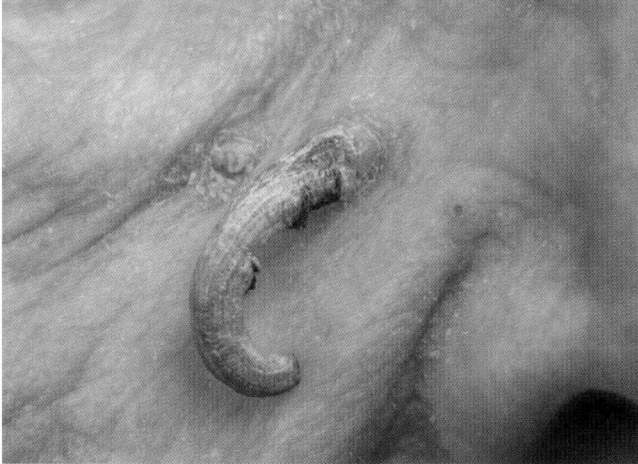

Figure 39.33 Cutaneous horn (courtesy of St John's Institute for Dermatology, London, UK).

Keratoacanthoma (Fig. 39.34)

Classically, this a cup-shaped growth that exhibits symmetry about its middle. The central crater is filled with a plug of keratin. It is twice as common in men and is usually found on the face of 50- to 70-year-olds. Keratoacanthoma has an unclear aetiology; it may be caused by papilloma virus infecting a hair follicle during the anagen phase of the growth cycle, but it has also been associated with smoking and chemical carcinogen exposure. Lesions can grow to between 1 and 3 cm over 6 weeks and then they typically resolve spontaneously over the subsequent 6 months. Removal of the central keratin plug may speed resolution. However, excision is recommended as the differential diagnosis includes anaplastic SCC and the excision scar is often better than that which remains after resolution.

Bowen's disease (Fig. 39.35)

This is an SCC *in situ*, of which 3–11% progress to SCC. It is currently not thought to be a paraneoplastic condition. Chronic solar damage and inorganic arsenic compounds have been implicated as aetiological factors in the development of Bowen's disease and HPV16 has also been documented as a cause.

Bowen's disease often presents as a slowly enlarging, erythematous, scaly patch or plaque. It may occur anywhere on the muco-cutaneous surface of the body. On the glans penis, it is often called erythroplasia of Queyrat, although somewhat unfairly because the condition was described 50 years earlier by Paget (Fig. 39.36).

Topical therapy with 5-fluorouracil or imiquimod is an effective treatment. Alternatives include surgical excision with a 4-mm margin or Mohs' micrographic surgery for larger or recurrent lesions.

Extramammary Paget's disease (Fig. 39.37)

This is a form of intra-epidermal adenocarcinoma, which may occur in the genital or perianal regions or in cutaneous sites that

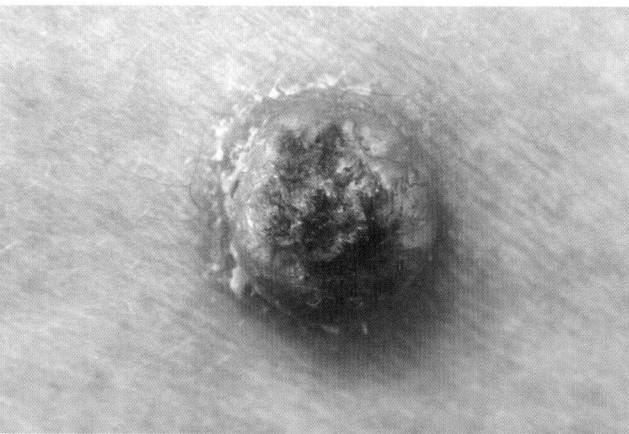

Figure 39.34 Keratoacanthoma (courtesy of St John's Institute for Dermatology, London, UK).

John Templeton Bowen, **1857–1941, Professor of Dermatology, Harvard University Medical School, Boston, MA, USA, described this intradermal precancerous skin lesion in 1912.**
Auguste Queyrat, **1856–1933, Dermatologist, Paris, France, described this condition in 1911.**
Frederic E. Mohs, **a twentieth century American Surgeon.**

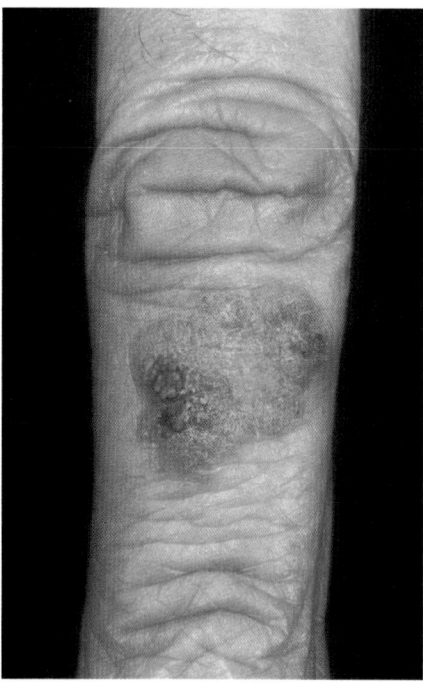

Figure 39.35 Bowen's disease – Squamous cell carcinoma *in situ* (courtesy of St John's Institute for Dermatology)

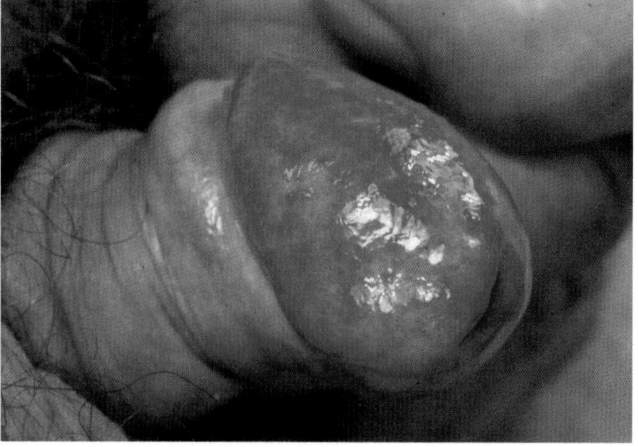

Figure 39.36 Erythroplasia of Queyrat – Squamous cell carcinoma *in situ* on the glans penis; also called Paget's disease of the penis (courtesy of St John's Institute for Dermatology, London, UK).

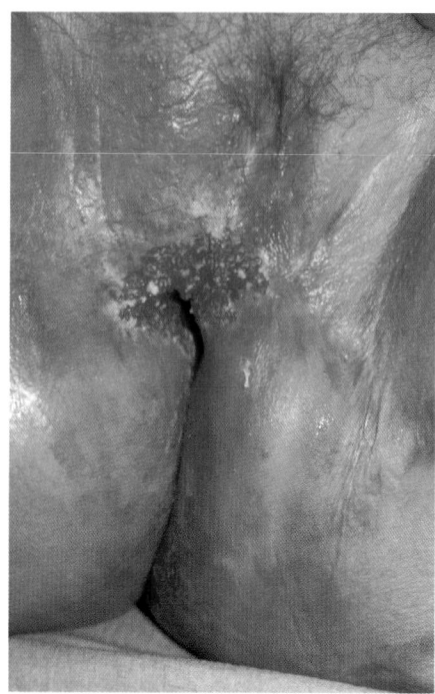

Figure 39.37 Extramammary Paget's disease (courtesy of St John's Institute for Dermatology, London, UK).

and into the subdermal fat and muscle. There is general agreement that GCPNs are precursors of MM but the magnitude of this risk is unclear, largely due to the lack of well-conducted studies and poor classification. A 3–5% lifetime risk of melanoma is quoted. In total, 1:3 childhood MM arise in patients with GCPN but the risk decreases with advancing age: 15% present at birth, 62% present by puberty and 99% by 45 years of age. MM arising

are rich in apocrine glands, such as the axilla. Approximately 25% of extramammary Paget's disease is associated with an underlying *in situ* or invasive neoplasm. The early skin changes are subtle and may mimic an eczematous lesion or intertrigo. Surgical excision forms the basis of treatment.

Giant congenital pigmented naevus (GCPN) or giant hairy naevus (Fig. 39.38)

This naevus causes a great deal of confusion as its definition and management are contentious. It is a hamartoma of naevo-melanocytes that has a tendency to dermatomal distribution. It has a similar histology to compound naevi, but the naevus cells are distributed variably from the epidermis throughout all layers

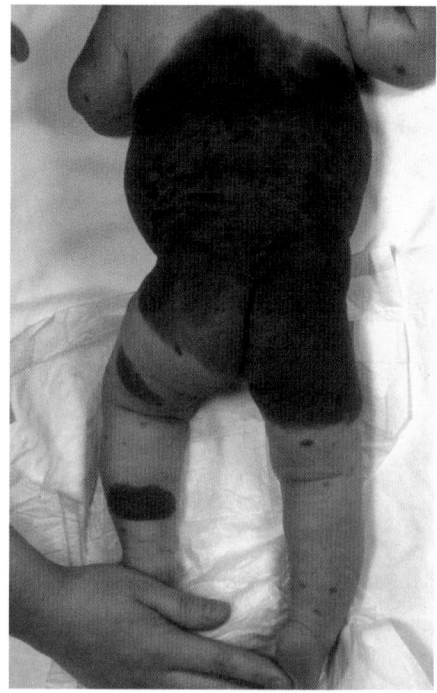

Figure 39.38 Giant congenital pigmented naevus (courtesy of St John's Institute for Dermatology, London, UK).

within GCPN is more likely in axial rather than extremity lesions. Retroperitoneal or intracranial melanosis in association with GCPN of the back or scalp respectively is associated with MM presenting before the age of 3 or in the third decade.

A multidisciplinary management approach is advocated for these birthmarks, with initial investigations directed towards discovering neurocutaneous melanosis, as leptomeningeal involvement may necessitate a shunt to avoid raised intracranial pressure.

Removal of GCPN can be considered for both aesthetic and oncological reasons but the evidence to support complete excision to avoid developing MM is poor. Various possibilities for partial or complete removal exist – none is completely successful. They include perinatal curettage, dermabrasion, laser resurfacing and surgical excision with reconstruction using a split-skin graft or after neighbouring skin has been expanded to allow coverage of the defect.

Dysplastic (atypical) naevus (Fig. 39.39)

Dysplastic naevi are irregular proliferations of atypical melanocytes at the basal layer of the epidermis. They have variegated pigmentation with irregular borders, measuring more than 5 mm in size. Dysplastic naevi can have a familial inheritance and carry a 5–10% risk of forming superficial spreading melanoma.

Malignant lesions

Basal cell carcinoma

Usually a slow-growing, locally invasive malignant tumour of pluripotential epithelial cells arising from basal epidermis and hair follicles, hence affecting the pilosebaceous skin (Summary box 39.3).

Summary box 39.3

BCC

- Slow growing
- Caused by UV light
- 90% nodular/nodular cystic
- High- and low-risk BCC

Epidemiology

The strongest predisposing factor to BCC is UVR. The incidence of BCC therefore increases with proximity to the equator,

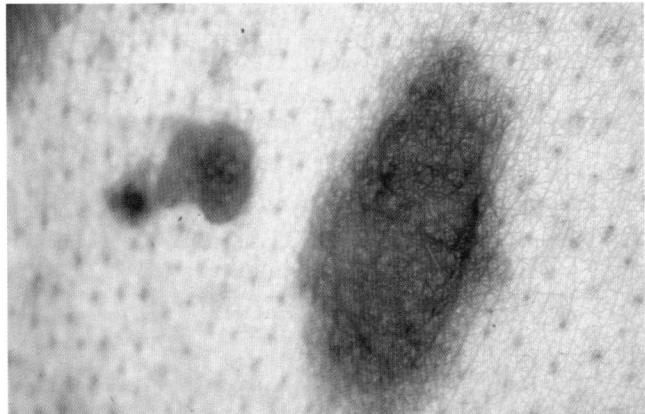

Figure 39.39 Dysplastic naevus (courtesy of St John's Institute for Dermatology, London, UK).

although, interestingly, 33% arise in parts of the body that are not typically sun exposed. It occurs in the middle-aged or elderly, with 90% of lesions found on the face above a line from the lobe of the ear to the corner of the mouth. Other predisposing factors include exposure to arsenical compounds, coal tar, aromatic hydrocarbons, IR and genetic skin cancer syndromes. White-skinned people are almost exclusively affected. Overall, 95% occur between the ages of 40 and 80 years and they are more common in men.

Pathogenesis

BCCs have no apparent precursor lesions and their development is proportional to the initial dose of the carcinogen, but not duration of exposure. BCCs rarely metastasise, are hard to culture and resist transplantation. All of this suggests that a multistep mechanism for their development is unlikely, and that mesodermal factors acting as intrinsic promoters coupled with an initiation step is the most likely explanation for their development.

Macroscopic appearance (Fig. 39.40)

BCC can be divided into localised (nodular, nodulocystic, cystic, pigmented and naevoid) and generalised lesions, which can be superficial (multifocal or superficial spreading) or infiltrative (morphoeic, ice pick and cicatrising). Nodular and nodulocystic variants account for 90% of BCCs.

Microscopic appearance (Fig. 39.41)

In total, 26 histological types have been described. The characteristic finding is of ovoid cells in nests with a single, outer 'palisading' layer. It is only the outer layer of cells that actively divide. This may explain why tumour growth rates are slower than the cell cycle speed would suggest, and why incompletely excised lesions are more aggressive. Morphoeic BCCs synthesise type IV collagenase and so spread rapidly.

Prognosis

There are 'high-risk' and 'low-risk' BCCs. High-risk BCCs are those which are large (> 2 cm), are located at specific sites (near the eye, nose, ear) or which have ill-defined margins. Recurrent tumours and those forming in the presence of immunosuppression are also higher risk.

Management

Treatment can be surgical or non-surgical. Margins should always be assessed and marked under loupe magnification and vary between 2 and 15 mm depending on the macroscopic variant. When margins are ill defined or tissue is at a premium (nose, eyes), either Mohs' micrographic surgery or a two-stage surgical approach with subsequent reconstruction after confirmation of clear margins is advisable. The histological sample must be orientated and marked for pathological examination.

Mohs' micrographic surgery is a method used by dermatological surgeons (dermatologists who have undergone extra training in techniques of cutaneous surgery and histopathology) to excise skin cancer under microscopic control. It has been demonstrated to minimise recurrence rates and maximise conservation of surrounding normal tissue when treating suitable skin tumours. The technique is, therefore, considered the optimal treatment for poorly demarcated, recurrent or incompletely excised BCCs (including BCCs around the nose, eyes and ears, where clearance may be uncertain, significant morbidity may be associated with

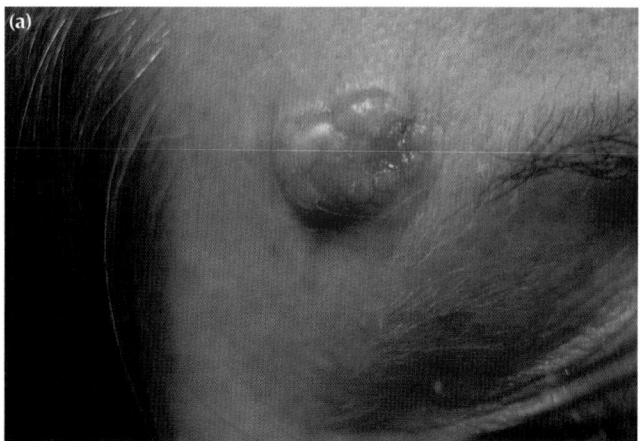

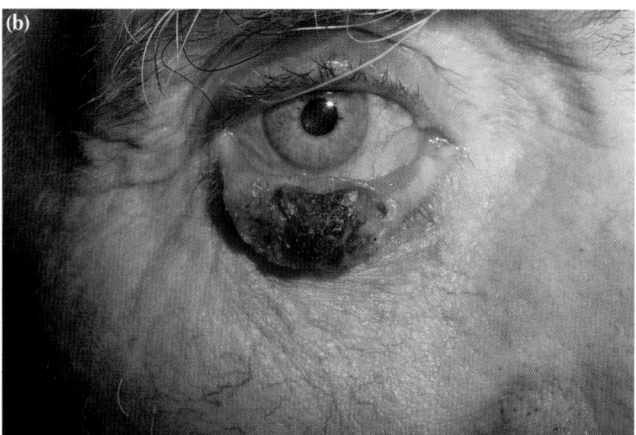

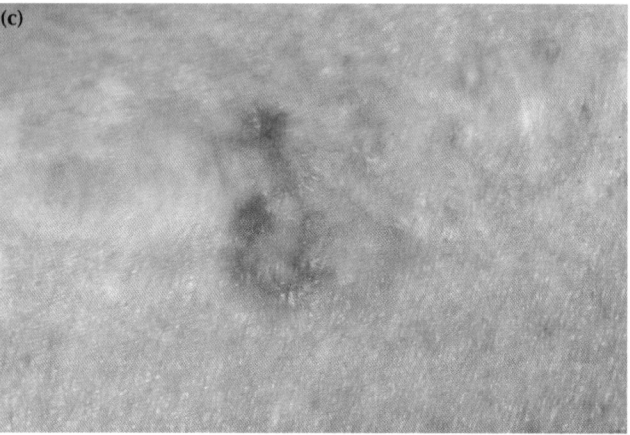

Figure 39.40 (a) A nodulocystic basal cell carcinoma (BCC). Note the characteristic pearly surface with telangectasia. (b) An ulcerating BCC on the lower eyelid. (c) A recurrent morphoeic BCC ((a) and (b) courtesy of Mr A.R. Greenbaum; (c) courtesy of St John's Institute for Dermatology, London, UK).

incomplete excision and where reconstruction with a flap is preferable cosmetically). It can also be used for excision of SCCs, dermatofibrosarcoma protuberans and lentigo maligna (using either frozen section and immunohistochemistry or horizontal paraffin-embedded sections).

Mohs' micrographic surgery is performed under local anaesthesia (which is one of its limitations) and involves an initial

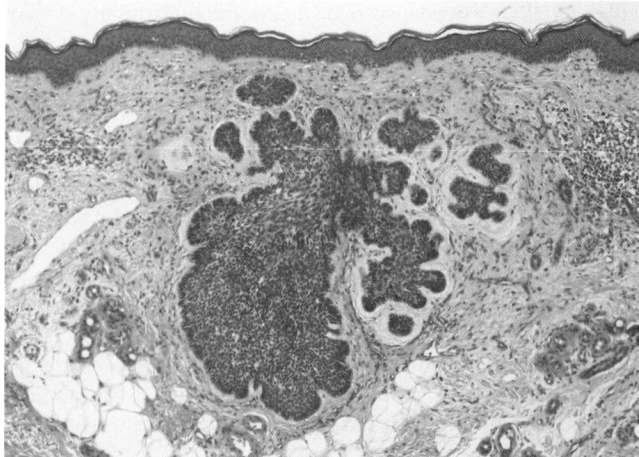

Figure 39.41 A basaloid, epithelial tumour with palisading cells on the periphery of the tumour that sits within a mucinous stroma (courtesy of Dr Catherine di Stefanato, Consultant Dermatopathologist, St John's Institute for Dermatology, London, UK).

'saucerising excision' of the primary tumour's visible extent. The sample and the defect are then marked and orientated. A map of the specimen is drawn and characterised using different coloured stains in different quadrants. A histotechnician and a Mohs' surgeon work together: the histotechnician receives a tissue sample from the Mohs' surgeon, which is then sectioned horizontally (including lateral and deep margins in the same slide) and stained with haematoxylin and eosin. The Mohs' surgeon then examines the slides for the presence of residual tumour and excises more tissue from the relevant parts of the mapped defect as necessary. In theory, the technique offers complete evaluation of the lateral and deep margins of tumour excision and so should be dependable. Complete excision rates exceeding 99% are the rule in trained and experienced hands.

In elderly or infirm patients, radiotherapy produces similar recurrence rates to surgery. Superficial tumours can also be treated with topical treatments (5-fluorouracil, imiquimod) or cryotherapy. Cosmetically, radiotherapy scars age badly so plastic surgery is always likely to be the better option if possible for patients who are likely to live longer than 10 years.

Excision must be complete as there is a 67% recurrence rate if margins are grossly involved and a 33% recurrence rate within 2 years with microscopic involvement or when reported 'close'. Patients with uncomplicated, completely excised lesions can be discharged, with follow-up reserved for patients with tumours in high-risk areas, globally sun-damaged skin, syndromes (e.g. naevoid BCC syndrome) and incompletely excised tumours if further surgery is declined.

Cutaneous squamous cell carcinoma

SCC is a malignant tumour of keratinising cells of the epidermis or its appendages. It also arises from the stratum basale of the epidermis but, unlike BCC, it expresses cytokeratins 1 and 10.

Epidemiology

SCC is the second most common form of skin cancer. It is four times less common than BCC and usually affects the elderly. It is strongly related to cumulative sun exposure and damage, and is twice as common in men and in white-skinned individuals living nearer the equator. SCC is also associated with chronic inflammation (chronic sinus tracts, pre-existing scars, osteomyelitis, burns, vaccination points) and immunosuppression (organ-transplant recipients). When a SCC appears in a scar it is known as a Marjolin's ulcer.

The time taken to develop a SCC after radiation exposure is proportional to the wavelength of the radiation. SCC is also caused by chemical carcinogens (arsenicals, tar) and infection with HPV5 and HPV16. There is also evidence that current and previous tobacco use doubles the relative risk of cutaneous SCC (Summary box 39.4).

Summary box 39.4

SCC

- Associated with UV light exposure, chronic inflammation and viral infection
- Ulcerated lesions
- Metastasis in 2% of cases

Macroscopic appearance (Fig. 39.42)

The early appearance of SCC may vary from smooth nodular to verrucous, papillomatous and ulcerating lesions. However, all variants will eventually ulcerate as they grow. The ulcers have a characteristically everted edge and are surrounded by inflamed, indurated skin. The main differential diagnoses of SCC are actinic keratosis, BCC, keratoacanthoma, pyoderma gangrenosum and warts.

Microscopic appearance (Fig. 39.43)

Characteristic irregular masses of squamous epithelium are noted to proliferate and invade the dermis from the germinal layer. This tumour stains positive for cytokeratins 1 and 10. SCC can be histologically graded according to Broder's histological grading. This system describes the proportion of de-differentiated cells (i.e. the ratio of pleomorphic and anaplastic to normal cells).

The histopathology report on an SCC should include information on the pathological pattern (e.g. adenoid), the cellular morphology (e.g. spindle), the Broder's grade, the depth of invasion,

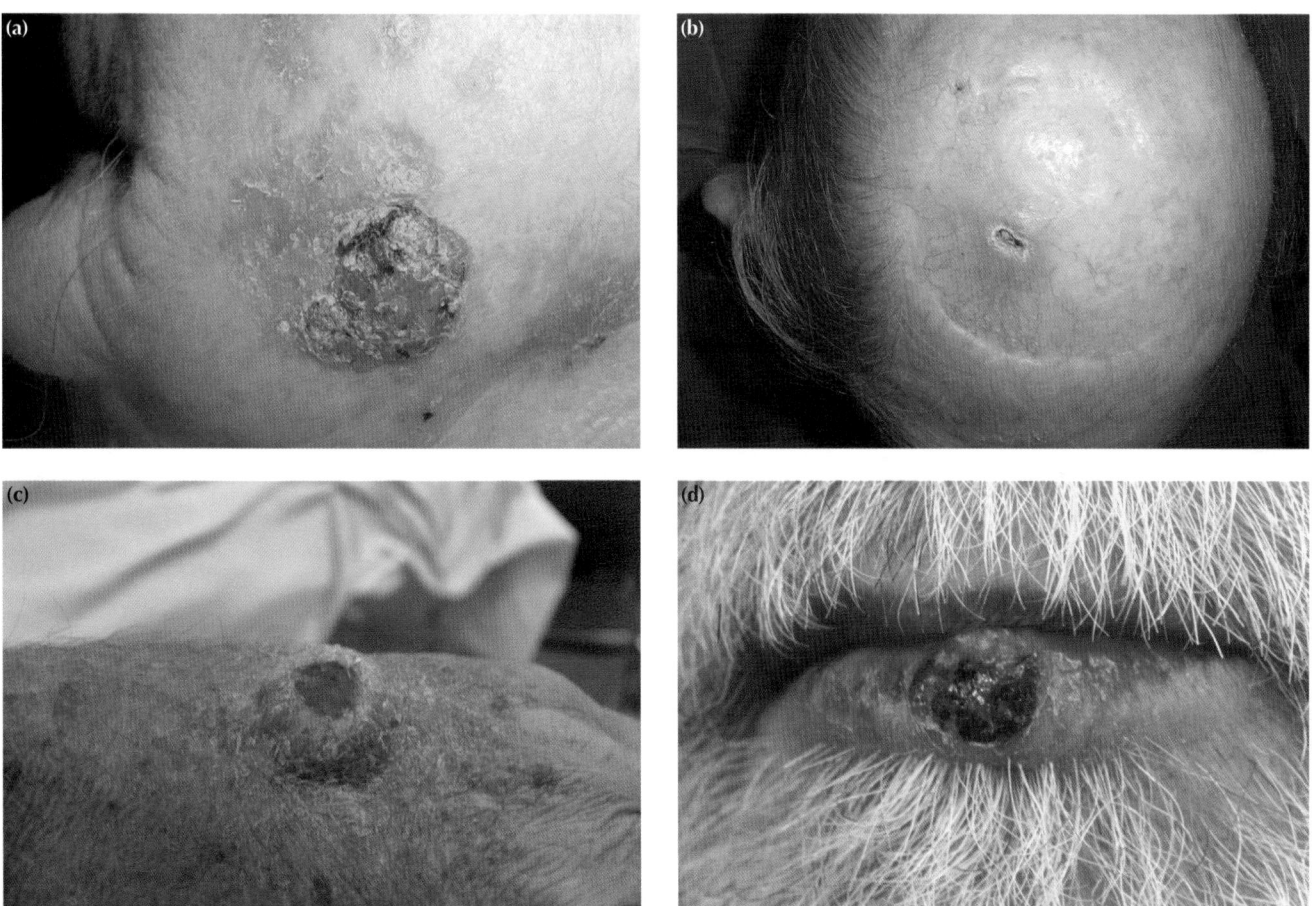

Figure 39.42 (a) A squamous cell carcinoma (SCC) on the face. (b) A recurrent SCC arising in a previously skin-grafted area of the scalp. (c) An SCC arising on the dorsum of the hand in a renal transplant recipient on immunosuppressive therapy. (d) An SCC arising on the lip of a smoker who worked outside on a farm ((a–c) courtesy of Mr A.R. Greenbaum; (d) courtesy of St John's Institute for Dermatology, London, UK).

Jean-Nicholas Marjolin, **1780–1850, Surgeon, Paris, France, described the development of carcinomatous ulcers in scars in 1828.**
Albert Compton Broders, **1885–1964, an American Pathologist of Minnesota, USA.**

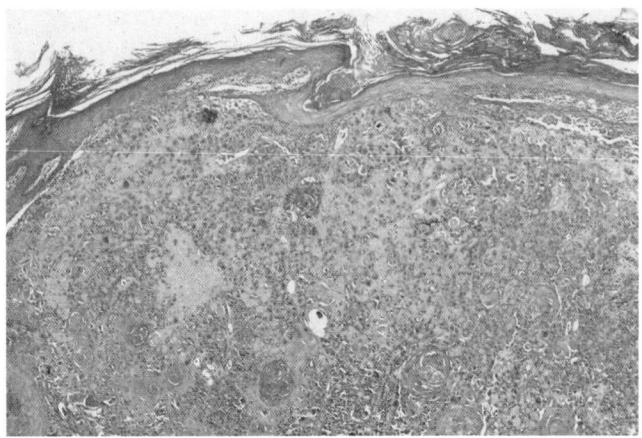

Figure 39.43 An invasive, epidermal keratinising tumour characterised by proliferation of atypical squamous cells with 'horn pearls' (courtesy of Dr Catherine di Stefanato, Consultant Dermatopathologist, St John's Institute for Dermatology, London, UK).

the presence of any perineural or vascular invasion and the deep and peripheral margin clearance (Table 39.2).

Prognosis

There are several independent prognostic variables for SCC:

1 *Invasion*:
   a *Depth*: the deeper the lesion, the worse the prognosis. For SCC < 2 mm, metastasis is highly unlikely, whereas if > 6 mm, 15% of SCCs will have metastasised;
   b *Surface size*: lesions > 2 cm have a worse prognosis than smaller ones.
2 *Histological grade*: the higher the Broder's grade, the worse the prognosis.
3 *Site*: SCCs on the lips and ears have higher local recurrence rates than lesions elsewhere, and tumours at the extremities fare worse than those on the trunk.
4 *Aetiology*: SCC that arises in burn scars, osteomyelitic skin sinuses, chronic ulcers and areas of skin that have been irradiated has a higher metastatic potential.
5 *Immunosuppression*: SCC will invade further in those with impaired immune response.
6 *Prognosis*: Tumours with perineural involvement have a worse prognosis and require a wider than usual clearance.

The overall rate of metastasis is 2% for SCC – usually to regional nodes – with a local recurrence rate of 20%.

Management

SCC is a heterogeneous tumour with a malignant behaviour that varies between subtypes. Management must therefore address the need for definitive treatment, the possibility of in-transit metastasis and the tumour's tendency for lymphatic metastasis.

Surgical excision is the only means of providing accurate histology. The margins for primary excision should be tailored to surface size in the first instance. This should ideally be assessed using surgical loupe magnification. A 4-mm clearance margin should be achieved if the SCC measures < 2 cm across, and a 1-cm clearance margin if it measures > 2 cm.

Overall, 95% of local recurrence and regional metastases occur within 5 years, so follow-up beyond this period is not indicated.

Cutaneous malignant melanoma

MM is a cancer of melanocytes. It usually arises in skin but can form anywhere that melanocytes exist, such as in the bowel mucosa, the retina and the leptomeninges.

Epidemiology
Cutaneous melanoma is caused largely by exposure to UVR. Its rise in incidence reflects social behaviour and increased recreational activity in the sun amongst white-skinned races that are not suited to sun exposure. Although it accounts for less than 5% of skin malignancy generally it is responsible for over 75% of deaths related to skin malignancy.

Worldwide, MM accounts for 3% of all malignancy. It is the commonest cancer in young adults (20–39 years) and is the most likely cause of cancer-related death.

Distribution between the sexes varies around the world and reflects occupational and recreational exposure to sunlight. Likewise, geographical distribution reflects exposure of white-skinned individuals to sunlight: Auckland, New Zealand, currently reports the highest incidence per capita, and before that Brisbane, Australia, held that distinction.

Of all patients with MM, 5% will develop a second primary melanoma. Overall, 7% of all MMs present as occult metastasis from an unknown primary.

Pathophysiology
Exposure to UVR is the major causal factor for developing MM. Cumulative exposure favours the development of lentigo maligna melanoma, whereas 'flash fry' exposure – typical of rapidly acquired holiday tans – favours the other morphological variants (Summary box 39.5).

Summary box 39.5
MM
■ **Rising incidence**
■ **Caused by UV exposure**
■ **Superficial spreading form is the most common**
■ **Breslow thickness is the most important prognostic indicator until there is lymph node involvement**
■ **Sentinel node biopsy is useful for staging disease**

Table 39.2 TNM classification and staging of squamous cell carcinoma

Size	Nodes	Metastases	Grade
T1 = < 2 cm	N0 = no regional nodes	M0 = no metastases	G1 = low grade
T2 = 2–5 cm	N1 = regional nodes	M1 = distant metastases	G2 = moderately differentiated
T3 > 5 cm			G3 = high grade or highly anaplastic
T4 = muscle or bony invasion			

Stage I = T1, N0, M0 ; stage II = T2–3, N0, M0; stage III = T4, N0, M0 and any T, N1, M0; stage IV = any T, any N1, M1(+).

A small proportion of MM is genetically mediated, as in xeroderma pigmentosum, which increases the relative risk of developing MM to 1000. Immunosuppression secondary to drugs or HIV infection will increase the incidence of MM by 20- to 30-fold.

The risk factors for developing MM are summarised below:

1 xeroderma pigmentosum (relative risk = 1000);
2 past medical or family history of MM with dysplastic naevi (relative risk = 33–1269);
3 previous melanoma (relative risk = 84);
4 high total number of naevi (relative risk = 3.4, if > 20 naevi);
5 dysplastic naevi (10% lifetime risk);
6 red hair (relative risk = 3);
7 tendency to freckle (relative risk = 1.9);
8 immune compromised conditions: HIV infection, Hodgkin's disease, ciclosporin A therapy;
9 GCPN (increased risk);
10 history of sunburn – especially in childhood.

Macroscopic appearance

Only 10–20% of MMs form in pre-existing naevi, with the remainder arising *de novo* in previously normally pigmented skin. The most likely naevi to form MMs are the junctional and compound types. Macroscopic features in a pre-existing naevus that suggest malignant change are listed in Summary box 39.6.

Summary box 39.6

Macroscopic features in naevi suggestive of MM

- **Change in *size* – any adult naevus > 6 mm is suspect (for reference a lead pencil diameter is 7 mm) and anything changing to > 10mm is more likely to be malignant than benign**
- **Shape**
- **Colour**
- **Surface (nodularity or ulceration)**
- **Satellite lesions (discrete pigmented areas spreading away from the primary)**
- **Tingling/itching/serosanguinous discharge (usually late signs)**
- **Blood supply: melanomas > 1 mm thick have a blood supply that can be found with a hand-held Doppler monitor, so 'Doppler-positive' pigmented lesions should be excised**

There are four common macroscopic variants of MM. In addition, there are several other notable, but rarer forms.

Superficial spreading melanoma (Fig. 39.44)

This is the commonest type (70%) and the most likely to arise in a pre-existing naevus; classically, after several years of slow change, there follows a rapid growth of a darker pigmented area in a junctional naevus in the preceding months before presentation. Nodularity within superficial spreading melanoma heralds the onset of the vertical growth phase.

Nodular melanoma (Fig. 39.45)

This accounts for 15% of all MMs and tends to be more aggressive than superficial spreading melanomas, with a shorter clinical onset. These lesions typically arise *de novo* in skin and are more

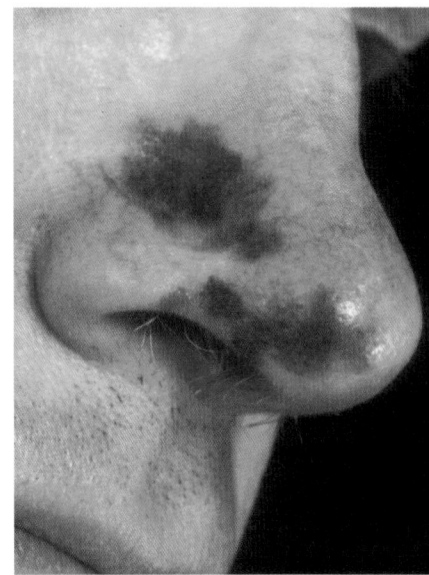

Figure 39.44 Superficial spreading melanoma (courtesy of St John's Institute for Dermatology, London, UK).

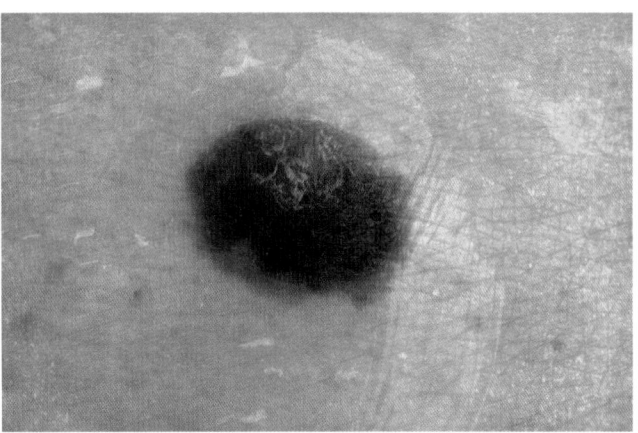

Figure 39.45 Nodular melanoma (courtesy of St John's Institute for Dermatology, London, UK).

common in men than women, often presenting in middle age and usually on the trunk, head or neck. They typically appear as blue-black papules, 1–2 cm in diameter and, because they lack the horizontal growth phase, they tend to be sharply demarcated. Up to 5% are amelanotic.

Lentigo maligna melanoma (Fig. 39.46)

This was previously also known as Hutchinson's melanotic freckle. This variant presents as a slow-growing, variegated, brown macule (a lentigo) on the face, neck or hands of the elderly. They are positively correlated with prolonged, intense sun exposure, affecting women more than men. They account for between 5% and 10% of MMs. *In situ* melanoma in this variant is called lentigo maligna.

Sir Jonathan Hutchinson, 1828–1913, Surgeon, St Bartholomew's Hospital, London, UK.

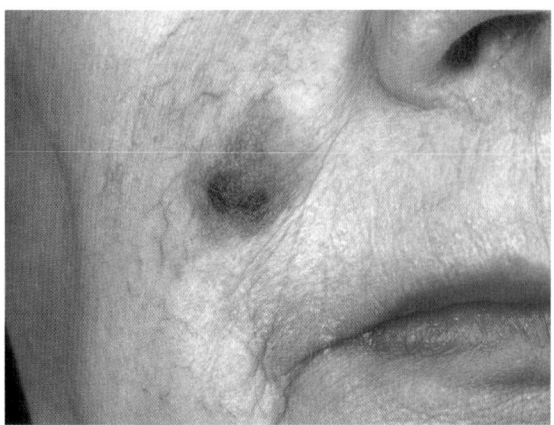

Figure 39.46 Lentigo maligna melanoma (courtesy of St John's Institute for Dermatology, London, UK).

Lentigo maligna melanomas are thought to have less metastatic potential than other variants as they take longer to enter a vertical growth phase. Nonetheless, when they have entered the vertical growth phase their metastatic potential is the same as any other melanoma.

Acral lentiginous melanoma (Fig. 39.47)

Acral lentiginous melanoma affects the soles of feet and palms of hands. It is rare in white-skinned individuals (2–8% of MMs) but more common in the Afro-Caribbean, Hispanic and Asian populations (35–60%). It usually presents as a flat, irregular macule in later life; 25% are amelanotic and may mimic a fungal infection or pyogenic granuloma.

MMs under the fingernail are usually superficial spreading melanomas rather than acral lentiginous melanomas. For finger- or toenail lesions it is vital to biopsy the nail matrix rather than just the pigment on the nail plate. A classical feature of a

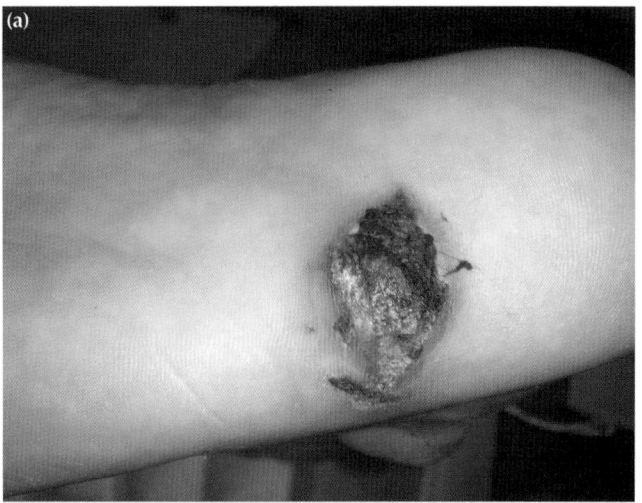

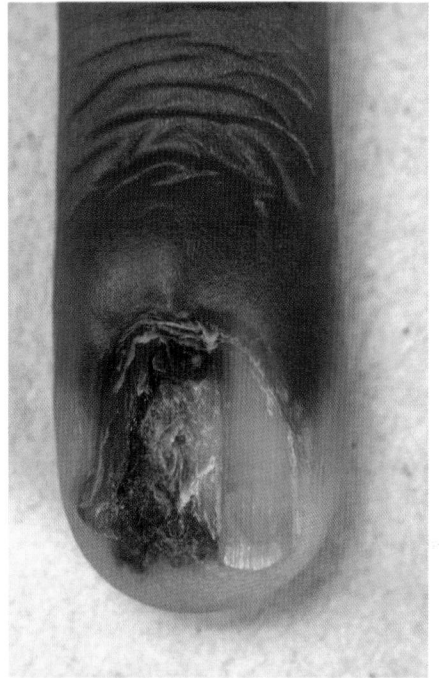

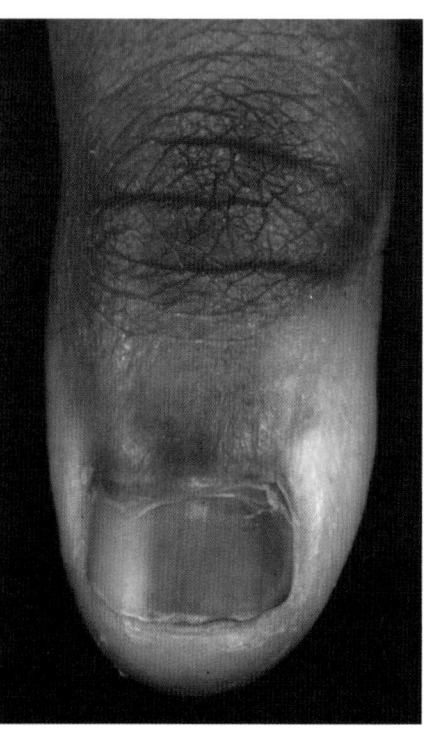

Figure 39.47 (a) Acral lentiginous melanoma on the sole of the foot (courtesy of Mr A.R. Greenbaum). (b) Subungual melanoma – probably a superficial spreading melanoma. Note the swelling proximal to the nail fold. (c) Benign racial melanonychia ((b) and (c) courtesy of St John's Institute for Dermatology, London, UK).

subungual melanoma is Hutchinson's sign: nail-fold pigmentation then widens progressively to produce a triangular pigmented macule with associated nail dystrophy. The differential diagnosis is 'benign racial melanonychia', which produces a linear dark streak under a nail in a dark-skinned individual. Malignancy is unlikely if the nail fold is uninvolved.

Miscellaneous

Amelanotic melanoma is, as the name suggests, not pigmented. It often arises in the gastrointestinal tract, presenting with obstruction or as a metastasis from an unknown primary.

Desmoplastic melanoma is mostly found on the head and neck region. It has a propensity for perineural infiltration and often recurs locally if not widely excised. It may be amelanotic clinically.

Microscopic appearance

Malignant change occurs in the melanocytes in the basal epidermis; while *in situ*, atypical melanocytes are limited to the dermo-epidermal junction and show no evidence of dermal involvement. During the horizontal growth phase, cells spread along the dermo-epidermal junction, and although they may breach the dermis their migration is predominantly radial. During the vertical growth phase, the dermis may be invaded; the greater the depth of invasion, the greater is the metastatic potential of the tumour.

Management

History and clinical examination should be directed at discovering the primary lesion and identifying local, regional or distant spread. Clinical photography is useful when choosing to observe a lesion rather than perform excision biopsy for definitive histo-pathological diagnosis. An excision biopsy with a 2-mm margin of skin and a cuff of subdermal fat is acceptable in the first instance. Incision biopsy is occasionally indicated – for instance, in large lesions on the face where an excision biopsy of the whole lesion would be disfiguring.

Biopsy and pathological examination provide the first step towards staging melanoma. The Breslow thickness of a melanoma (measured to nearest 0.1 mm from the granular layer to the base of the tumour) is the most important prognostic indicator in the absence of lymph node metastases. The American Joint Committee on Cancer (AJCC) staging system then takes lymph node and distant metastases into account (Table 39.3).

Investigations

Guidelines for staging are contentious – published UK guidelines for investigating MM seem currently to be aimed at detecting stage IV disease, whereas one could and arguably should, aim investigations towards detecting occult stage II disease in order to upstage patients and then treat them accurately and appropriately. Thus, offering sentinel node biopsy (SNB) to patients with clinical stage II disease seems prudent (and follows the AJCC staging system used in the USA and the UK guidelines), and investigations for stage III disease should be directed to individual clinical presentation.

Local treatment

The treatment for melanoma is surgery. Lentigo maligna (melanoma *in situ*) should be excised completely in most clinical situations because of the risk of it entering the vertical growth phase to become lentigo maligna melanoma. A complete excision with a clinical 5-mm margin requires no further treatment.

Table 39.3 American Joint Committee on Cancer 2001 staging for malignant melanoma

Stage	Primary tumour	Lymph node	Metastases
0	*In situ*	No nodal involvement	No distant metastases
IA	< 1 mm, no ulceration		
IB	< 1 mm, with ulceration > 1 but < 2 mm, no ulceration		
IIA	> 1 but < 2 mm, with ulceration > 2 but < 4 mm, no ulceration		
IIB	> 2 but < 4 mm, with ulceration > 4 mm, no ulceration		
IIC	> 4 mm, with ulceration		
IIIA	Any Breslow, no ulceration	Micrometastasis	
IIIB	Any Breslow, with ulceration Any Breslow, no ulceration Any Breslow, with or without ulceration	Micrometastasis ≤ 3 palpable nodes In transit metastases/satellites	
IIIC	Any Breslow, with ulceration Any Breslow, with or without ulceration	≤ 3 palpable nodes ≥ 4 palpable or matted nodes or nodes plus in transit metastases	
IV			M1: skin, subcutaneous or distant M2: lung M3 all other sites/ or any site plus ↑ [LDH]

[LDH], concentration of lactate dehydrogenase.

CHAPTER 39 | SKIN AND SUBCUTANEOUS TISSUE

For melanoma < 1 mm deep, wide local excision with a 1-cm margin is sufficient. For deeper lesions, a 2-cm margin is recommended, as there is no evidence that wider margins make a difference.

Regional lymph nodes

The likelihood of metastatic spread to regional lymph nodes is proportional to the Breslow thickness of the melanoma. The management of regional lymph nodes has been a contentious topic for well over a century. Historically, some advocated simultaneous elective lymph node clearance at the time of wide excision of the primary melanoma, whereas others favoured a later, therapeutic lymphadenectomy only if regional metastases became clinically evident.

Certainly evidence from retrospective studies suggested that patients with thick melanomas had better survival after elective lymphadenectomy, whereas data from prospective randomised studies were less convincing except in specific sub-groups. However, electively clearing regional nodes in those patients whose melanomas have not metastasised derives them no benefit and exposes them unnecessarily to the morbidity and complications of a major surgical procedure. Ideally, therefore, one would like to be able to select the group of patients in whom melanoma has spread to regional lymph nodes and treat only these patients. This goal underpins SNB, which is based on the hypothesis that lymphatic metastasis proceeds as an orderly process that can be predicted by mapping the lymphatic drainage from a primary tumour to the first or 'sentinel' node in the regional lymphatic basin, a hypothesis that has been borne out in both animal and human studies. When SNB is performed according to consensus standards, it is predictive of the regional nodal status in 99% of cases. There is negligible benefit in performing SNB in patients whose primary melanoma is thinner than 1 mm – only 4% of sentinel nodes would be expected to be positive for tumours with a Breslow thickness of < 1.25 mm. In practice, 70–80% of patients with metastases in the sentinel nodes will have no other involved regional nodes so, although the current standard approach is to proceed to completion lymphadenectomy, this will overtreat a significant number of sentinel node-positive patients, which appears to be a better option than potentially undertreating 20–30% of patients with positive sentinel nodes. Evidence of objective survival benefit from SNB is currently unavailable but several large prospective clinical trials are in progress to investigate this; meanwhile, SNB remains part of the AJCC staging system.

Current treatment for biopsy positive nodal disease is block dissection of the regional lymph nodes to remove all the lymph nodes in that regional basin.

Adjuvant therapy

None is of proven benefit, with clinical trials currently looking at vaccine and interferon treatments.

Prognosis

The Breslow thickness of the primary tumour offers the best correlation with survival in stage I disease. The higher the mitotic index, the poorer the prognosis of the primary tumour; this has greater significance than the presence or absence of ulceration.

Alexander Breslow, **1928–1980, American Pathologist.**

The presence of lymph node metastases is the single most important prognostic index in melanoma, outweighing both tumour and host factors. The number of affected nodes and the presence of extranodal extension are also significant outcome predictors. Once regional nodes are involved clinically, 70–85% of patients will have occult distant metastases.

Merkel cell (dermal mechanoreceptor) tumour (Fig. 39.48)

This is an aggressive malignant tumour of Merkel cells. It usually affects the elderly and is four times more common in women than men. Treatment is with wide local excision, aiming for a 25- to 30-mm margin, followed by radiotherapy.

VASCULAR LESIONS

Congenital: haemangiomata and vascular malformations

These can be subclassified *biologically* into vascular tumours or vascular malformations based on their endothelial characteristics or *radiologically* into haemangiomata and vascular and lymphatic malformations based on their vascular dynamics.

Haemangiomata

These are benign endothelial tumours that affect three girls for every boy. They may go unnoticed at birth or be evident as a faint 'herald' patch. Haemangiomata grow rapidly in the first year of life, then slowly involute over several years, with 70% having resolved by 7 years of age.

The clinical appearance of a haemangioma depends on its depth relative to the dermis and the growth phase in which it is observed. Early proliferating lesions are bright red, irregularly surfaced, papular lesions reminiscent of strawberries; deeper lesions may be blue or skin coloured. Involution typically begins with the

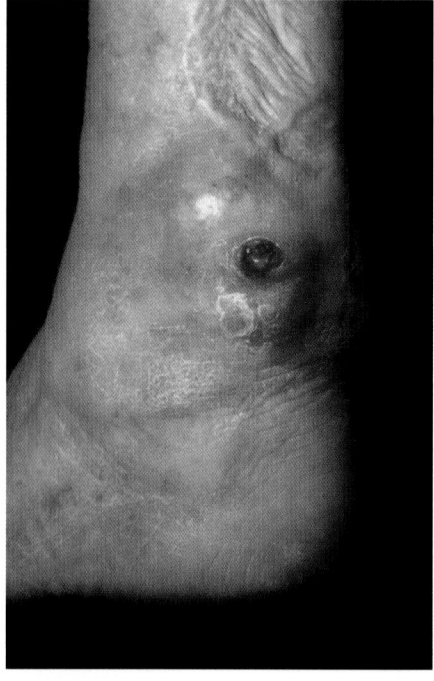

Figure 39.48 Merkel cell tumour (courtesy of St John's Institute for Dermatology, London, UK).

fading of colour, leaving greyish areas, and the lesion softens and shrinks at the same time. When involution is complete, often all that remains is the 'crêpe paper'-textured area of skin which may be redundant and stretched locally.

Haemangiomata may occur anywhere in the body, but the majority are central rather than peripheral and 60% are on the head. The majority of haemangiomata require no specific treatment. Most clinical problems needing intervention occur during the early proliferative growth phase. Periorbital lesions may obstruct the visual fields and cause deprivational amblyopia. Total obstruction of one visual field for more than a week during the first year of life may result in permanent visual impairment. Pressure on the globe from a large lesion near the eye can cause astigmatism and an ophthalmologist should be involved with all such patients immediately.

Neonates are obligate nasal breathers, so large haemangiomata that obstruct the nose pose a serious risk. Rarely, skin ulceration over a haemangioma can cause haemorrhage but this usually settles acutely with localised compression. Blood-borne bacteria can lodge in haemangiomata and produce a nidus for septicaemia and localised necrosis. Large haemangiomata can trap platelets leading to thrombocytopenia (Kasabach–Merritt syndrome) and large visceral or multiple lesions can cause congestive heart failure secondary to shunting of blood.

The management of most clinical problems is primarily nonsurgical. Systemic corticosteroids induce involution in up to 60% (2 mg kg^{-1} for 3 weeks, then a tapering dose). The primary role of surgery is in the management of abnormally textured or redundant skin left behind after involution.

Vascular malformations

Vascular malformations affect boys and girls equally. They arise secondary to errors in development of the vascular elements during the eighth week *in utero* and are associated with numerous congenital syndromes. They are invariably present at birth but may be missed if deep to the skin. Vascular malformations subsequently grow in proportion to a child's growth (other than in response to sepsis or hormonal stimulation). Stasis can lead to a localised, consumptive coagulopathy in large venous malformations. Low-flow malformations may cause skeletal hypoplasia, whereas high-flow malformations can cause hypertrophy.

Common vascular birthmarks

Salmon patch (Fig. 39.49)

A haemangioma that presents as a pink macule, usually at the nape of the neck, in 50% of infants. It is caused by an area of persistent fetal dermal circulation and usually disappears within a year.

Capillary haemangioma (strawberry naevus) (Fig. 39.50)

The commonest birthmark, which is found most commonly on the head and neck; 90% appear at birth and, as a consequence of intravascular thrombosis, fibrosis and mast cell infiltration, 10% resolve each subsequent year, with 70% resolved by the age of 7 years. White-skinned individuals are affected most commonly and girls are affected three times more than boys.

Haig H. Kasabach, **1898–1943, Radiologist, the Presbyterian Hospital, New York, NY, USA.**
Katharine K. Merritt, **B. 1886, American Paediatrician.**

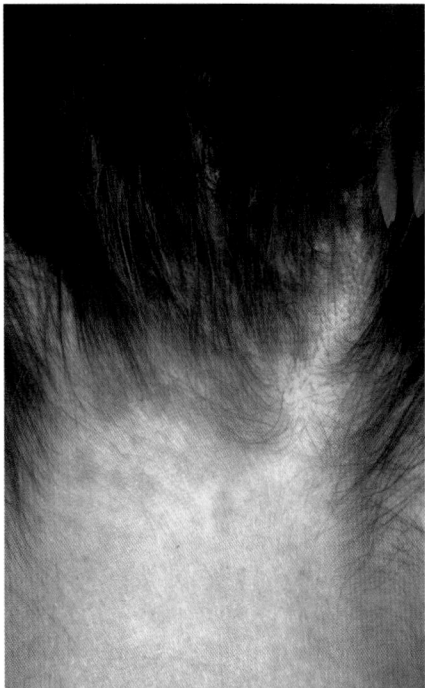

Figure 39.49 Salmon patch (courtesy of St John's Institute for Dermatology, London, UK).

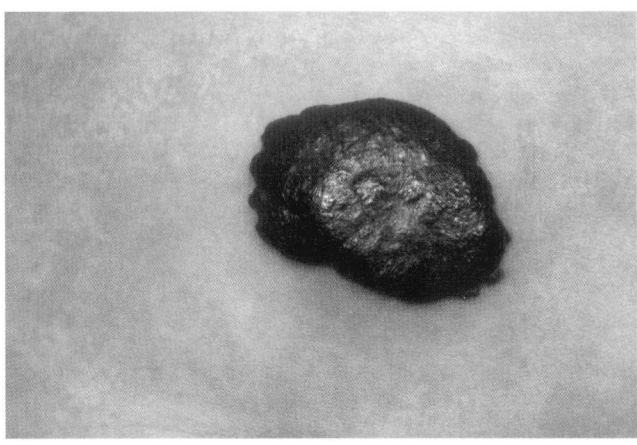

Figure 39.50 Capillary haemangioma (courtesy of St John's Institute for Dermatology, London, UK).

'Port-wine' stains (Fig. 39.51)

These arise from capillary malformations and are 20 times less common than capillary haemangiomata; they result from defective maturation of cutaneous sympathetic innervation during embryogenesis, leading to localised intradermal capillary vasodilatation. At birth, they appear as flat, smooth, intensely purplestained areas, most frequently on the head and neck, often within the maxillary and mandibular dermatomes of the trigeminal nerve; with age their surfaces become more keratotic and nodular.

Treatment with intense pulsed light and pulse–dye laser are

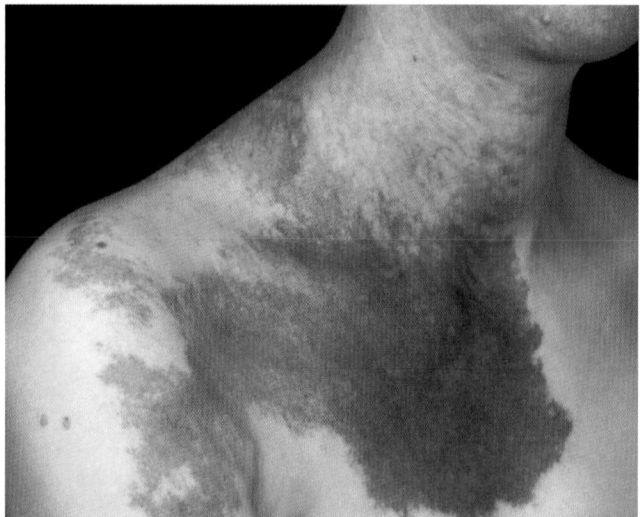

Figure 39.51 'Port-wine' stain (courtesy of St John's Institute for Dermatology, London, UK).

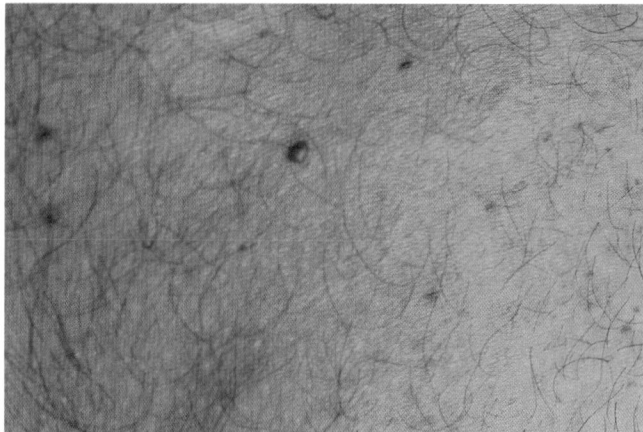

Figure 39.52 Campbell de Morgan spot (courtesy of Mr A.R. Greenbaum).

successful. Port-wine stain (PWS) is associated with several syndromes:

- *Sturge–Weber syndrome.* PWS affecting trigeminal dermatomes; associated with epilepsy and glaucoma (secondary to ipsilateral, leptomeningeal angiomatosis), cortical atrophy and visual field defects.
- *Klippel–Trenaunay–Weber syndrome.* PWS on a limb with associated bone and soft tissue hypertrophy and lateral varicose veins when the lower limb is involved. It is called Parkes–Weber syndrome if there is an associated arteriovenous malformation.
- *Proteus syndrome.* PWS and regional gigantism in association with lymphatic (lymphaticovenous) malformation. Hypertrophy is always asymmetrical.

Acquired

Campbell de Morgan spots (Fig. 39.52)

These are arteriovenous fistulae at the dermal capillary level that usually, although not exclusively, occur in skin on the trunk of older patients. Multiple lesions are associated with liver disease.

Spider naevi (Fig. 39.53)

These are angiomata that appear (and may disappear) spontaneously at puberty or in two-thirds of pregnant women, usually disappearing in the puerperium. Spider naevi are also associated with chronic liver disease. They can be treated with intense pulsed-light or pulse–dye laser.

William Allen Sturge, **1850–1919, Physician, the Royal Free Hospital, London, UK.**
Frederick Parkes Weber, **1863–1962, Physician, the German Hospital, Dalston, London, UK.**
Maurice Klippel, **1858–1942, Neurologist, La Salpêtrière, Paris, France.**
Paul Trenaunay, **B. 1875, a French Neurologist. Klippel and Trenaunay described this condition in a joint paper in 1900.**
Proteus **was a minor sea-god of Greek mythology, who had the power of prophesy and was able to assume different shapes in order to avoid answering questions.**
Campbell Greig de Morgan, **1811–1876, Surgeon, the Middlesex Hospital, London, UK.**

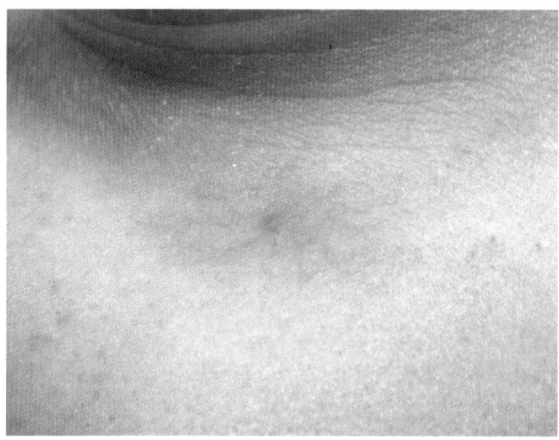

Figure 39.53 Spider naevus (courtesy of St John's Institute for Dermatology, London, UK).

Pyogenic granuloma (Fig. 39.54)

These share many histological characteristics of haemangiomata and are probably a subtype thereof. Most are small (0.5–1.5 cm), raised, pedunculated, soft, red nodular lesions showing superficial ulceration and a tendency to bleed after trivial trauma. They should be excised with a minimal margin.

Glomus tumour (Fig. 39.55)

These arise from subcutaneous arteriovenous shunts (Sucquet–Hoyer canals) especially in the corium of the nail bed. Typically, they are small, purple nodules measuring a few millimetres in size, which are disproportionately painful in response to insignificant stimuli (including cold exposure). Subungual varieties may be invisible causing paroxysmal digital pain.

Angiosarcoma ('malignant angioendothelioma') (Fig. 39.56)

Angiosarcoma is a rare, highly malignant tumour arising from vascular endothelial cells. The *lymphangiosarcoma* variant arises

J.P. Sucquet, **Fl 1840–1870, an Anatomist of Paris, France.**
Heinrich Hoyer, **1834–1907, Professor of Histology, Embryology and Anatomy, the Central Medical School, the Polish University, Warsaw, Poland.**

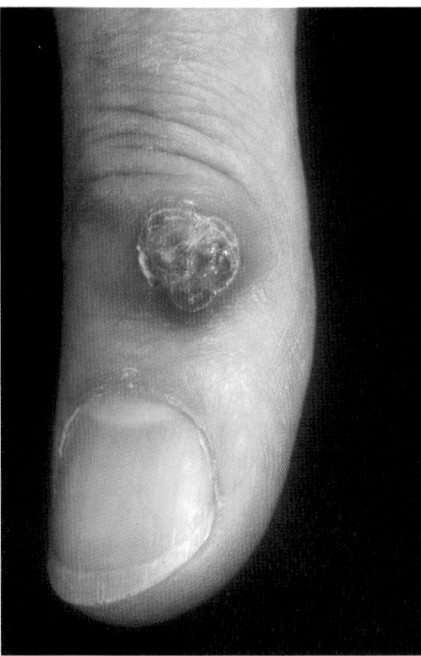

Figure 39.54 Pyogenic granuloma (courtesy of St John's Institute for Dermatology).

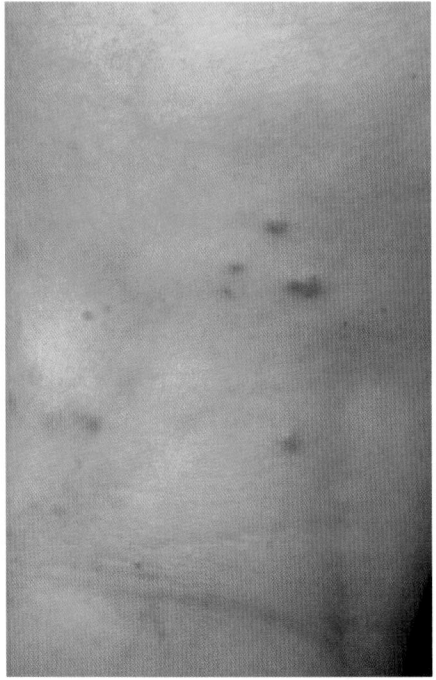

Figure 39.55 Glomus tumour (courtesy of St John's Institute for Dermatology).

from lymphatic endothelium and can develop in lymphoedematous tissue, particularly on an extremity. Proliferation is rapid, with early systemic spread.

Kaposi's sarcoma (Fig. 39.57)

This is a malignant, proliferative tumour of vascular endothelial cells, which was first described as a rare tumour in elderly Jewish men but is now usually associated with immune compromise after

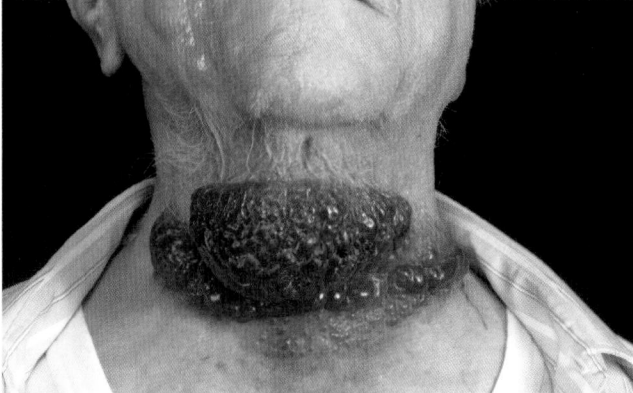

Figure 39.56 Angiosarcoma (courtesy of St John's Institute for Dermatology, London, UK).

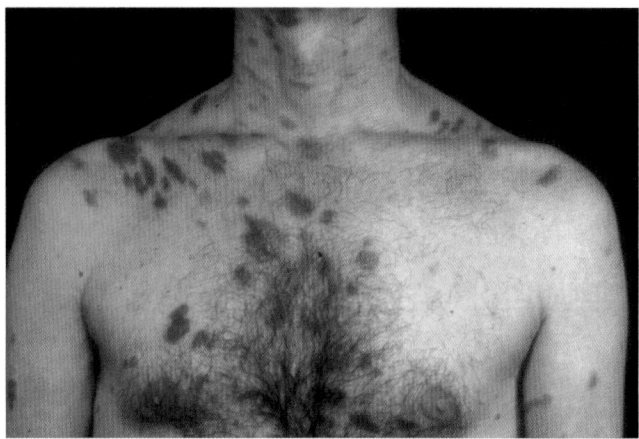

Figure 39.57 Kaposi's sarcoma (courtesy of St John's Institute for Dermatology, London, UK).

transplantation or human immunodeficiency virus (HIV) infection. There appears to be a causal link with infection by human herpesvirus 8 and immune dysfunction. Kaposi's sarcoma usually starts as a red-brown, indurated, plaque-like skin lesion that becomes nodular and then ulcerates. Treatment is with radiotherapy.

WOUNDS: CONGENITAL

Cutis aplasia congenita

This is a rare condition characterised by congenital absence of the epidermis, dermis and, in some cases, subcutaneous tissues, with underlying bony defects in 20%. Lesions may occur on any body surface, but localised scalp agenesis is most frequent. Treatment depends on the severity of the presentation but usually involves plastic surgery.

Parry–Romberg disease

This is an uncommon and poorly understood progressive, hemifacial atrophy of skin, soft tissue and bone. Its incidence is

Caleb Hillier Parry, 1755–1822, Physician, the General Hospital, Bath, UK.
Moritz Heinrich Romberg, 1795–1873, a German Neurologist who was Director of the University Hospital, Berlin, Germany.

unknown and its inheritance uncertain but it affects women more commonly than men.

It usually starts when a patient is in his or her late twenties but can present in childhood when the resulting deformity is worse because it is magnified by differential growth elsewhere. The commonest presentation is confined to lipodystrophy, but mixed atrophy of skin, fat, muscle, cartilage and bone combined result in the classic *coup de sabre* deformity.

The condition is self limiting, usually by 5–10 years after onset. Once the condition is stable, plastic surgical techniques can be employed alone or in combination to reconstruct an aesthetic contour.

Spina bifida

Failure of closure of the caudal neuropore during the fourth week *in utero* results in the incomplete development of some or all of the structural elements posterior to the spinal cord. This can occur anywhere, but is most common in lumbar vertebrae and presents as two gross variants: *spina bifida occulta*, in which there is a variable bony defect without neural protrusion (and which is, therefore, asymptomatic) and *spina bifida cystica*, in which there is herniation of the meninges (meningocele), spinal cord (myelocele) or, most commonly, both (meningomyelocele). Management ideally involves a multidisciplinary approach and is directed towards protecting the spinal cord, preventing cerebrospinal fluid contamination and secondary hydrocephalus and meningitis.

WOUNDS: ACQUIRED

Pressure sores

These begin with tissue necrosis at a pressure point (next to a bony prominence) and develop into a cone-shaped volume of

> Coup de Sabre **is French for 'a sabre cut', a vertical cut across the shoulder from the front to the back.**

necrotic loss (with the cone's tip superficial). As many as 10% of acute hospital in-patients will suffer some degree of pressure sore; the majority affect the elderly and patients with spinal injury or decreased sensibility. Overall, 80% of paraplegics will get a pressure sore and 8% will die as a result.

The pathogenesis of pressure sores revolves around unrelieved pressure: an increase in local tissue pressure above that of perfusion pressure produces ischaemic necrosis that is directly proportional to the duration and degree of pressure and inversely proportional to the area over which it is applied. Muscle and fat are more susceptible to pressure than skin.

In a patient who has no predisposing factors (who developed a sore while unable to move but who normally can move), management is aimed at debridement and repair of the defect as necessary on the assumption that recurrence will not occur once normal function and sensibility returns. In the paraplegic, recurrence is likely, so management should involve a multidisciplinary approach with surgery used sparingly once all other predisposing factors have been addressed. Primary treatment involves relieving pressure (special mattress, nursing care, relief of muscle spasm and contractures), optimising nutrition, correcting anaemia, preventing infection and using dressings. Surgery involves thorough debridement to promote healing and plastic surgery to reconstruct the defect if vacuum-assisted closure is unable to heal it.

FURTHER READING

Balch C.M., Buzaid A.C., Soong, S.J. *et al.* (2001) Final version of the American Joint Committee on Cancer staging system for cutaneous melanoma. *J Clin Oncol* **19**: 3635–48.

Du Vivier, A. (2002) *Atlas of Clinical Dermatology*, 3rd edn. Churchill Livingstone, London.

McKee, P.H., Calonje, E. and Granter, S. (2005) *Pathology of the Skin*, 3rd edn. Mosby, St Louis.

Weedon, D. (2002) *Skin Pathology*. Churchill Livingstone, London.

PART 7 | Head and neck

Elective neurosurgery

LEARNING OBJECTIVES

To understand and know:
- The pathophysiology of raised intracranial pressure and hydrocephalus
- The common causes, presentations, investigation and treatment options for intracranial infection

To be able to:
- Describe the presenting features, investigation and treatment of intracranial tumours

- Understand the diagnosis and management of intracranial haemorrhage
- Define the role of surgery in the management of epilepsy, pain and movement disorders
- Recognise the common compressive peripheral neuropathies
- Understand the principles involved in defining brain death

RAISED INTRACRANIAL PRESSURE

An understanding of raised intracranial pressure (ICP) pathophysiology is crucial to understanding the presentation and treatment of the common neurosurgical conditions (Summary box 40.1).

Summary box 40.1

Raised intracranial pressure

- Results in reduced cerebral perfusion and brain herniation
- The major causes of raised ICP are haematomas, tumours and hydrocephalus

---

Pathophysiology

Normal intracranial pressure

Normal ICP varies from 5 to 15 mmHg in the adult at rest. ICP varies with venous pressure and is thus affected by factors such as gravitational drainage and manoeuvres that raise intrathoracic pressure (coughing, Valsalva, positive pressure ventilation) or lower it (normal inspiration). Normal values in small children and infants are lower than for adults.

Aetiology of raised intracranial pressure

The principle causes of raised ICP are mass lesions, hydrocephalus and cerebral oedema.

The Monro–Kellie doctrine describes the skull as a rigid container that encloses the brain, cerebrospinal fluid (CSF) and

---

Alexander Monro, (Secundus), **1733–1817, Professor of Anatomy, Edinburgh, Scotland.**

---

arterial/venous blood. The addition of a new mass lesion such as a growing tumour or haematoma can initially be compensated for by the egress of CSF and venous blood from the skull. During this compensation phase, there is only a small increase in ICP. When compensation is maximal, there is then a rapid rise in ICP for relatively small increases in volume. This increased pressure causes compression and herniation of the brain (see figures in Chapter 23).

Cerebral oedema may be cytotoxic or vasogenic. Cytotoxic oedema refers to cerebral swelling as a result of cellular engorgement and can occur in both neurones and glia in response to insults such as ischaemia. Vasogenic oedema results from an accumulation of extracellular cerebral fluid, usually as a result of breakdown of the blood–brain barrier and leakage of fluid through 'leaky' capillaries. Vasogenic oedema is commonly seen with tumours such as metastases, malignant gliomas and meningiomas.

Hydrocephalus is discussed later in this chapter.

Raised intracranial pressure and cerebrovascular physiology

The brain does not store much energy and is unable to utilise anaerobic metabolism. The brain is therefore critically dependent on a constant flow of oxygen and glucose via the cerebral arterial vasculature. In the absence of arterial blood flow, brain tissue will be viable for only a few minutes.

In normal circumstances, cerebral blood flow is maintained at a constant rate despite fluctuations in mean arterial pressure (MAP) of between 50 and 150 mmHg via mechanisms termed cerebral autoregulation (Fig. 40.1). These mechanisms include neural regulation via aortic and carotid baroreceptors, and local factors such as arteriolar responsiveness to oxygen and carbon dioxide.

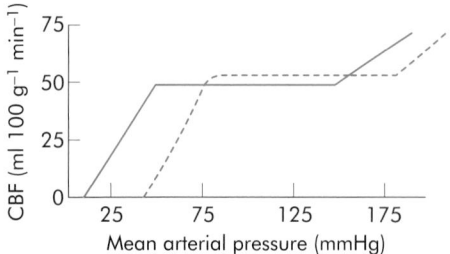

Figure 40.1 Autoregulation of cerebral blood flow (CBF): CBF remains constant over a wide range of mean arterial pressure. The curve is shifted to the right in patients with hypertension.

In the injured brain, cerebral autoregulation may be impaired either locally or globally. Cerebral blood flow is then dependent on MAP with a fall in MAP leaving the brain susceptible to ischaemia, and a rise in MAP resulting in hyperaemia, increased cerebral blood volume and thus raised ICP. Cerebral perfusion can be estimated by the following formula: cerebral perfusion pressure (CPP) = MAP – ICP. Studies of patients in traumatic coma have shown that poor prognostic factors include an ICP of > 20–25 mmHg or a CPP of < 60 mmHg.

Cerebral herniation

Sub-falcine herniation refers to shift of the cingulate gyrus of one hemisphere under the falx cerebri (a tough vertical dural fold between the two hemispheres) and across to the contralateral side. The thin wall dividing the lateral ventricles (septum pellucidum) may shift from the midline.

Uncal herniation refers to shift of the medial temporal lobe (uncus) medially towards the tentorial hiatus. As this occurs, the nearby oculomotor (third) nerve is stretched, causing dilatation and fixation of the ipsilateral pupil. This is usually accompanied by a rapidly progressive contralateral hemiparesis as pressure is exerted on the ipsilateral cerebral peduncle. Unusually, compression of the contralateral cerebral peduncle against the free edge of the tentorium (Kernohan's notch) causes an ipsilateral hemiparesis in association with an ipsilateral third nerve palsy.

Tentorial herniation refers to a downwards shift of midbrain structures through the tentorial hiatus. Tonsillar herniation refers to a downwards shift of the cerebellar tonsils and medulla through the foramen magnum. This type of herniation is associated with death due to compression and/or ischaemia of the cardiorespiratory centres.

Clinical features

Symptoms of raised ICP in a patient include headaches that tend to be worse in the early morning or on lying down and may improve with ambulation. Associated symptoms include nausea, vomiting or visual disturbance, particularly double vision or blurred vision. The headache may be exacerbated by coughing, straining or bending. In addition there may be symptoms relevant to the location of the pathology, for example, cognitive and personality change, unsteadiness of gait and incontinence of urine in frontal lobe pathology or right-sided weakness and garbled speech

James Watson Kernohan, **1896–1981**, Pathologist, the Mayo Clinic, Rochester, MN, USA.

in dominant temporal lobe pathology. As ICP increases further, relatives may report lethargy or drowsiness followed by unconsciousness and coma (Table 40.1).

Raised ICP may be associated with papilloedema on fundoscopy (Fig. 40.2). There may also be diplopia due to a sixth nerve palsy; this nerve is vulnerable to downwards cerebral shift of any cause due to its long intracranial course, sometimes called a *false localising sign*. There may be abnormalities of conjugate gaze. In particular, impaired upgaze or sun-setting may be seen as part of Parinaud's syndrome, caused by pressure on the dorsal midbrain (Fig. 40.3).

Raised ICP is associated with impaired consciousness and coma as measured by the Glasgow Coma Score (see Chapter 23).

Table 40.1 Symptoms of raised intracranial pressure

Headache	Early morning
	Worse on lying down
Nausea and vomiting	
Visual blurring or double vision	
Drowsiness	

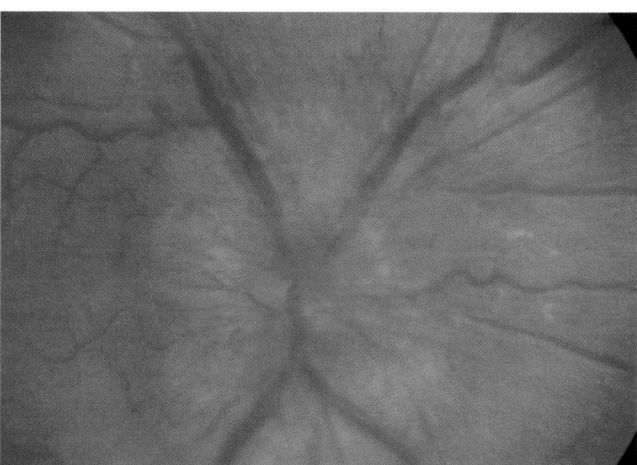

Figure 40.2 Papilloedema showing a swollen optic disc with blurred margins.

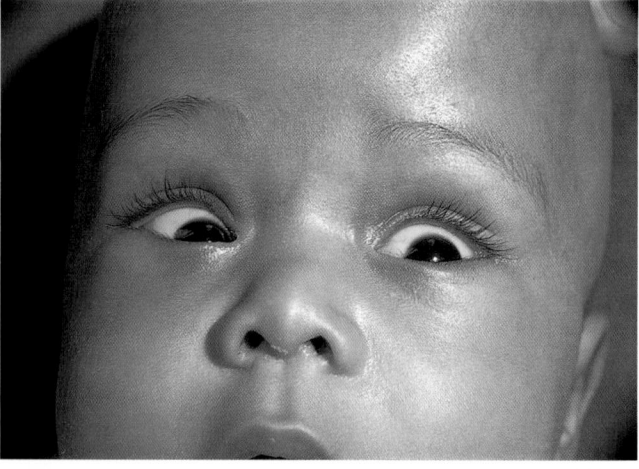

Figure 40.3 Child with 'sun-setting' eye sign due to hydrocephalus.

In infants, raised ICP causes a bulging fontanelle, progressive macrocephaly with sutural diastasis, and dilatation of scalp veins rather than papilloedema (Table 40.2).

Treatment

Appropriate treatment of raised ICP depends on identifying the cause.

Medical

For a review of the medical management of raised ICP in head injury, see Chapter 23.

Mannitol is an osmotic diuretic that can be used in emergency settings to reduce ICP: the dose is 0.5–1.0 g kg^{-1}.

Vasogenic oedema is often treated with the administration of high-dose steroids in the form of dexamethasone, for example 8 mg twice daily. Steroids reduce the permeability of the blood–brain barrier and are useful in reducing cerebral swelling prior to definitive treatment of the underlying cause of the vasogenic oedema.

A carbonic anhydrase inhibitor such as acetazolamide can play a role in control of raised ICP in idiopathic intracranial hypertension and acts by reducing CSF production.

Surgical

A variety of mass lesions can cause raised ICP and are amenable to surgical treatment via craniotomy: in trauma, acute extradural and subdural haematomas, intracerebral contusions and chronic subdural haematomas; in cerebrovascular pathology, superficial lobar haematomas, haematomas associated with ruptured aneurysms; in neuro-oncology, a variety of primary and secondary tumours. Occasionally, surgical control of ICP will involve a large bony decompression (craniectomy), such as in traumatic brain injury or extensive middle cerebral artery (MCA) infarction.

HYDROCEPHALUS

Hydrocephalus is a condition in which there is disequilibrium between CSF production and absorption, leading to raised ICP, and is often associated with dilated ventricles. Not all patients with ventriculomegaly have hydrocephalus and not all patients with hydrocephalus necessarily have enlarged ventricles (Summary box 40.2).

Summary box 40.2

Hydrocephalus

- Hydrocephalus may be obstructive or communicating
- Treatment is with removal of the causative lesion or by CSF diversion procedures

---

Table 40.2 Signs of raised intracranial pressure

Papilloedema
Sixth nerve palsy
Impaired upgaze
Focal neurological deficits
Impaired conscious level
In infants:
Progressive macrocephaly
Bulging anterior fontanelle
Dilated scalp veins
Sun-setting eyes

Cerebrospinal fluid physiology

The total CSF volume in an adult is about 150 ml and it is distributed between the cerebral ventricles (approximately 35 ml), the cerebral subarachnoid space and the spinal thecal sac. CSF production occurs at a rate of approximately 0.33 ml min^{-1} or 450 ml day^{-1}, resulting in a turnover of three volumes per day (Table 40.3).

CSF production is primarily by the choroid plexus of the ventricles and is an active process independent of ICP. Some CSF production occurs by transependymal spread through the ventricular walls from the cerebral extracellular fluid, and from the spinal dural nerve root sheaths. CSF flows from the lateral ventricles, through the foramen of Munro, into the third ventricle and then into the cerebral aqueduct and fourth ventricle before exiting into the subarachnoid space via the midline foramen of Magendie and lateral foramina of Lushka. CSF absorption is a pressure-dependent passive process involving filtration across the arachnoid villi, which are abundant along the superior sagittal sinus into which the CSF is absorbed.

Relative to plasma, CSF has a lower potassium and calcium content but is richer in chloride and magnesium. Normal protein content is 0.15–0.45 g l^{-1}. CSF is slightly acidic relative to plasma (pH 7.33–7.35).

Aetiology of hydrocephalus

Hydrocephalus can be obstructive or communicating (Table 40.4 and Fig. 40.4). *Obstructive hydrocephalus* can be caused by any lesion blocking the CSF pathways from the lateral ventricles to

Table 40.3 Cerebrospinal fluid physiology

Volume	150 ml
Production	20 ml h^{-1}
	80% by choroid plexus
	Active process
Absorption	At arachnoid villi
	Pressure dependent
Relative to plasma	Reduced K$^+$ and Ca^{2+}
	Increased Cl$^-$ and Mg^{2+}
	pH 7.33–7.35

Table 40.4 Aetiology of hydrocephalus

Obstructive hydrocephalus	Lesions within the ventricle
	Lesions in the ventricular wall
	Lesions distant from the ventricle but with a mass effect
Communicating hydrocephalus	Post haemorrhagic
	CSF infection
	Raised CSF protein
Excessive CSF production (rare)	Choroid plexus papilloma/carcinoma

CSF, cerebrospinal fluid.

Francois Magendie, **1783–1855, Professor of Pathology and Physiology, at the College of France, and Physician, Hôtel Dieu, Paris, France.**
Hubert von Luschka, **1820–1875, Professor of Anatomy, Tubingen, Germany.**

CHAPTER 40 | ELECTIVE NEUROSURGERY

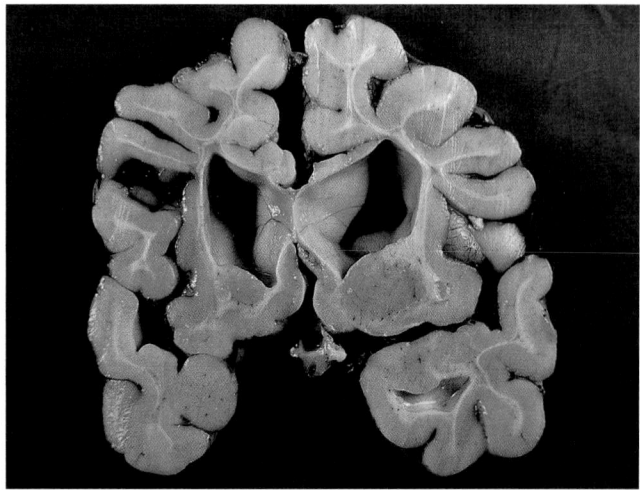

Figure 40.4 Pathological specimen of a hydrocephalic brain.

the fourth ventricle (Fig. 40.5). Susceptible sites include the foramen of Munro (colloid cyst of the third ventricle) and cerebral aqueduct (congenital aqueduct stenosis, tectal plate glioma). Lesions may be within the ventricle, in the ventricular wall or distant from the ventricle but exerting mass effect on it. Posterior fossa mass lesions are more likely than supratentorial lesions to present with obstructive hydrocephalus because the fourth ventricle is easily compressed within the relatively small posterior fossa. *Communicating hydrocephalus* refers to circumstances in which the intracerebral CSF pathways are patent but there is accumulation of CSF, usually due to impaired CSF absorption.

This may be because the CSF constituents have altered such as in cases of meningitis or subarachnoid haemorrhage (SAH).

Normal-pressure hydrocephalus is a specific form of communicating hydrocephalus that tends to affect the elderly. The clinical triad is ataxia, cognitive decline and urinary incontinence, and there is ventriculomegaly on imaging. Although one-off measurements of CSF pressure may be normal the syndrome is thought to arise from impaired CSF absorption, resulting in intermittent high pressure, and some patients respond clinically to CSF diversion with ventriculoperitoneal shunting.

Investigation

Lumbar puncture is contraindicated in *obstructive hydrocephalus* because of the risk of causing tonsillar herniation and death.

Ventricular size can be assessed with a computerised tomography (CT) scan of the brain (Fig. 40.6). The ventricles may be enlarged as a result of generalised cerebral atrophy or localised neuronal cell loss (*ex vacuo* dilatation) as well as by hydrocephalus. In children, chronic raised ICP can result in copper-beating of the skull (Fig. 40.7).

A magnetic resonance imaging (MRI) scan of the brain can provide better anatomical detail of lesions causing hydrocephalus and is particularly useful in the diagnosis of aqueduct stenosis. A midline T2-weighted MRI scan can be used to assess the suitability of a patient for a third ventriculostomy by identifying the relationships of the floor of the third ventricle, basilar artery and clivus.

ICP monitoring with a parenchymal probe placed into the frontal lobe via a twistdrill burrhole is a useful diagnostic tool for patients in whom hydrocephalus or CSF shunt dysfunction is suspected.

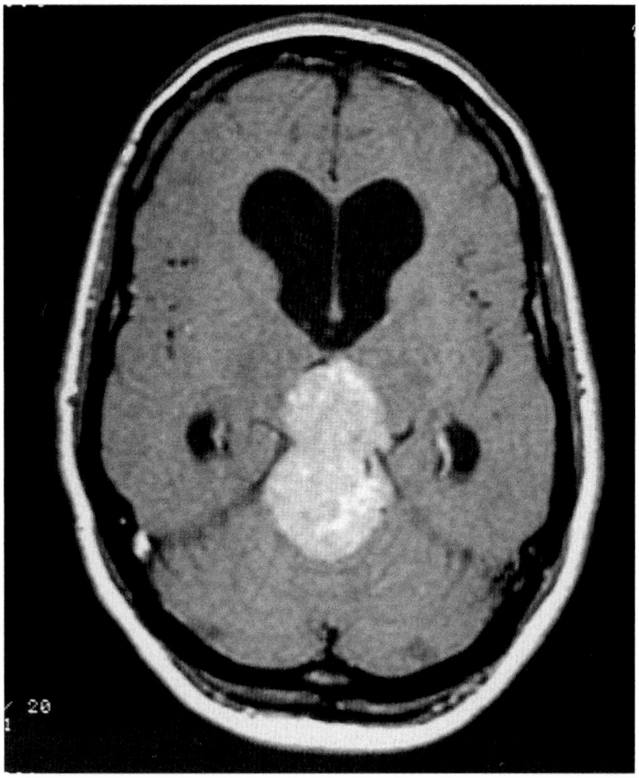

Figure 40.5 Pineal region tumour causing obstructive hydrocephalus.

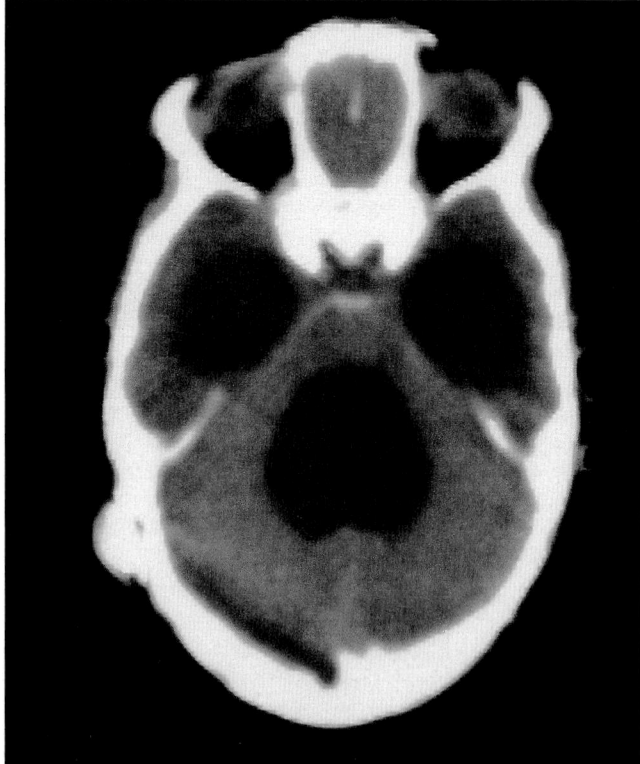

Figure 40.6 Axial computerised tomography scan, showing a neonate with hydrocephalus and markedly dilated ventricles. The temporal horns, normally just visible, are particularly enlarged.

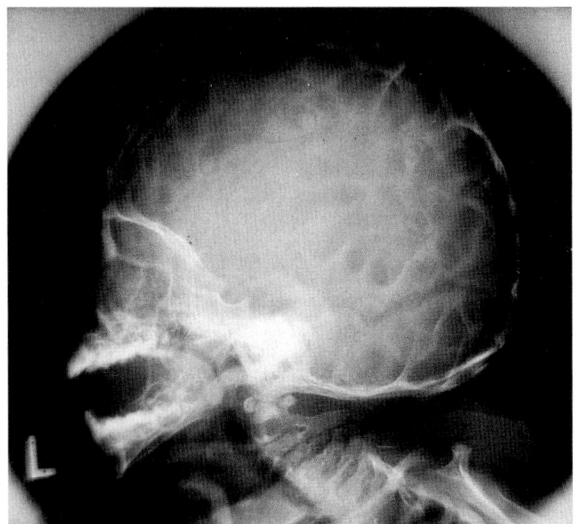

Figure 40.7 Lateral skull radiograph showing copper-beating, which is indicative of chronic raised intracranial pressure.

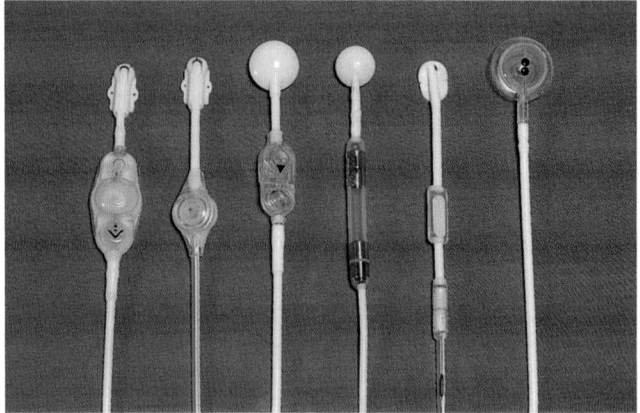

Figure 40.8 Various types of cerebrospinal fluid shunt.

In *communicating hydrocephalus*, a lumbar puncture may be both diagnostic, by measurement of opening pressure, and therapeutic, by draining a volume of CSF that allows the closing pressure to be within normal limits.

In the diagnosis of normal pressure hydrocephalus, other diagnostic procedures include the CSF tap test (clinical evaluation before and after withdrawal of 20–30 ml of CSF via lumbar puncture) and CSF infusion studies. These involve infusing saline into the thecal sac while measuring the pressure to obtain an estimate of resistance to CSF outflow. Values of CSF outflow of $> 14 \, \text{mmHg ml}^{-1} \text{min}^{-1}$ have a positive predictive value for responsiveness to ventriculoperitoneal shunt insertion.

Management

Management of hydrocephalus will depend on the underlying cause. Options include removing a causative mass lesion, ventricular shunting or third ventriculostomy.

Removing a causative mass lesion

Intracranial mass lesions may present with obstructive hydrocephalus. In some circumstances it may be appropriate to treat the hydrocephalus by tumour removal and decompression of the CSF pathways, perhaps with the insertion of an external ventricular drain (EVD) to cover the early postoperative period. In other cases, such as a patient who presents with an impaired conscious level secondary to obstructive hydrocephalus, it may be appropriate to treat the hydrocephalus with an EVD or ventriculoperitoneal shunt and allow the patient to recover before undertaking tumour surgery.

Ventriculoperitoneal shunt

A ventriculoperitoneal shunt involves the insertion of a catheter into the lateral ventricle (usually right frontal or occipital) (Fig. 40.8). The catheter is then connected to a shunt valve under the scalp and finally to a distal catheter, which is tunnelled subcutaneously down to the abdomen and inserted into the peritoneal cavity. If the CSF pressure exceeds the shunt valve pressure, then CSF will flow out of the distal catheter and be absorbed by the peritoneal lining.

Other options for distal catheter placement include the right atrium via the deep facial and jugular vein (ventriculo-atrial shunt) or the pleural cavity (ventriculopleural shunt).

Shunt valves have a variety of mechanisms of action, which include diaphragm and ball-in-cone systems. These valves are pressure regulated but others are flow regulated. Pressure-regulated valves are susceptible to *siphoning*, a term that describes increased shunt flow when gravity acts on a column of fluid such as the distal shunt tubing in an upright patient. Most shunt valves are available in two or three different performance settings (such as high, medium and low pressure). For patients in whom the correct valve setting is difficult to determine, a programmable valve can be inserted. This allows the valve pressure to be adjusted by the application of an external magnet without the need for surgery. Shunt valves usually have an in-built CSF reservoir on the ventricular side of the valve, which may be useful for shunt tapping to obtain a CSF sample.

Shunt complications

The most common complications include shunt blockage and infection. Approximately 15–20% of shunts are revised within the first 3 years.

Shunt blockage may affect the ventricular catheter, shunt valve or distal catheter. Causes of blockage include choroid plexus adhesion, blood, cellular debris or misplacement of the distal catheter in the pre-peritoneal space. More than one-half of cases of shunt blockage are subsequently shown to be infected.

Shunt infection affects between 1% and 7% of shunt insertions and is usually caused by skin commensals, such as *Staphylococcus epidermidis*. Neonates are susceptible to *Escherichia coli* and haemolytic streptococcal infections. Risk factors for infection include very young children, open myelomeningocele, longer operative time and excessive staff movement into and out of theatre. Most infections become apparent clinically by 6 weeks and over 90% are apparent within 6 months. Treatment is by removal of the shunt, external CSF drainage and treatment of infection prior to re-insertion of the shunt at a different site. The introduction of antibiotic-impregnated catheters has resulted in a reduction in shunt infection rates.

Shunt systems may overdrain leading to subdural haemorrhage or slit ventricle syndrome. Other complications are common to intracranial surgery and include seizures (5%), CSF leak, stroke and intracerebral haemorrhage (< 1%).

Endoscopic third ventriculostomy

An endoscopic third ventriculostomy (ETV) involves the insertion of a neuroendoscope into the frontal horn of the lateral ventricle and then into the third ventricle through the foramen of Munro. A stoma can be created in the floor of the third ventricle in between the mamillary bodies and infundibular (pituitary) recess. CSF can then communicate freely between the ventricular system and interpeduncular subarachnoid space. The technique is particularly useful when there is obstruction of the CSF pathways below the third ventricle such as with aqueduct stenosis or posterior fossa mass lesions.

It has an advantage over shunting in that no tubing is left in the patient and therefore infection rates are lower. ETVs may block off, however, with about one-half of these patients ending up with a shunt. Rare, but serious, complications include basilar artery rupture or memory impairment from injury to the fornix. The procedure is less useful for communicating types of hydrocephalus or in infants of less than 6 months of age, but has a success rate of over 70% for accepted indications.

External drains

External drains can be placed within the ventricle (EVD) or the lumbar thecal sac (lumbar drain). These are useful for temporary CSF drainage and can be used to administer intrathecal antibiotics to treat CSF infection.

INTRACRANIAL INFECTION (SUMMARY BOX 40.3 AND TABLE 40.5)

Summary box 40.3

Intracranial infection

- Cerebral abscess can be caused by local or haematogenous spread
- Subdural empyema can be difficult to diagnose and requires urgent surgical drainage
- Common cerebral mass lesions in human immunodeficiency virus – acquired immunodeficiency syndrome (HIV-AIDS) include toxoplasmosis and lymphoma

---

Meningitis

Meningitis is a life-threatening infection that, if left untreated, will progress through meningeal inflammation, subpial encephalopathy, cortical venous thrombosis, cerebral oedema and death. The causative pathogens are age dependent (Table 40.6). Presentation is with fever, neck stiffness, photophobia and altered conscious level. Investigation is via CT and lumbar puncture, and treatment is by prompt administration of intravenous antibiotics such as cefotaxime. Aciclovir is usually added empirically to cover herpes simplex virus infection. Neurosurgical

Table 40.5 Types of intracranial infection

Meningitis
Extradural empyema
Subdural empyema
Cerebral abscess

Table 40.6 Organisms causing meningitis

Neonate	Group B *Streptococcus* *Listeria* Enterobacteriae
Infant	*Streptococcus pneumoniae* *Neisseria meningitidis* *Haemophilus influenzae*
Young child/adult	*Streptococcus pneumoniae* *Neisseria meningitidis*
Immunocompromised patient	*Cryptococcus* *Mycobacterium tuberculosis* *Listeria*

intervention is seldom required but some patients require shunting for post-meningitic communicating hydrocephalus. Subdural effusions are common in infants with hydrocephalus but rarely need surgical intervention except to rule out subdural empyema.

Cerebral abscess

Pathology

Intracerebral abscess may occur as a result of direct spread from air sinus infection, following surgery or from haematogenous spread especially associated with respiratory infection, endocarditis or dental infection. In around 25% of cases no cause is found. Patients at increased risk of cerebral abscess formation include those with cyanotic heart disease and those who are immunocompromised: patients with diabetes, solid organ transplant, haematological malignancy or long-term steroids.

A 2- to 3-day period of early cerebritis with inflammatory cell inflammation is followed by late cerebritis over days 4–9, with the formation of a necrotic core and increasing numbers of macrophages and fibroblasts (Fig. 40.9). After 10 days, a capsule begins to form and is firm and mature by day 14 (Fig. 40.10).

In a non-compromised host the causative organisms include anaerobic and micro-aerophilic streptococci, staphylococci, enterobacteria and anaerobes. Immunocompromised hosts are also susceptible to other infections including *Nocardia*, *Listeria*, *Aspergillus*, *Candida*, *Cryptococcus* and *Toxoplasma*.

Diagnosis

Presentation is with focal signs, seizures and raised ICP, as with other mass lesions, but the time course is often short. Patients may be febrile or have a raised peripheral white cell count or inflammatory markers. However, many patients with cerebral abscess show no markers of systemic infection. An intracerebral abscess appears as a ring-enhancing mass lesion on CT (Fig. 40.10) or MRI and the lesions may be multiple in the case of haematogenous spread. Differential diagnosis includes primary brain tumour and cerebral metastasis. A diffusion-weighted MRI may help differentiate between a tumour and an abscess because the latter will show restricted diffusion, but false negatives and positives occur. Where there is doubt, a ring-enhancing lesion should be treated as a cerebral abscess until proven otherwise.

Treatment

Cerebral abscess is usually treated by surgical drainage followed by administration of intravenous antibiotics for at least 6 weeks.

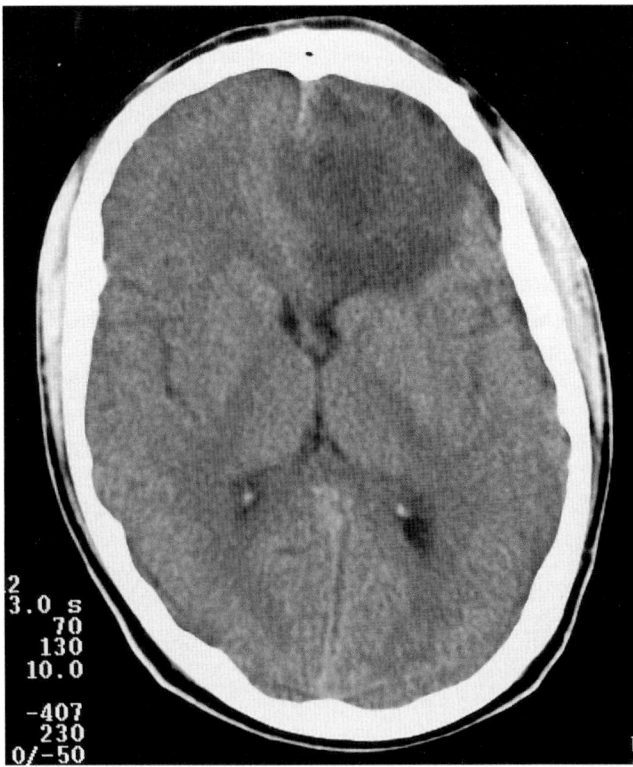

Figure 40.9 Axial computerised tomography scan with contrast of a patient with frontal sinusitis and epilepsy, showing a hypodense area of cerebritis in the left frontal region.

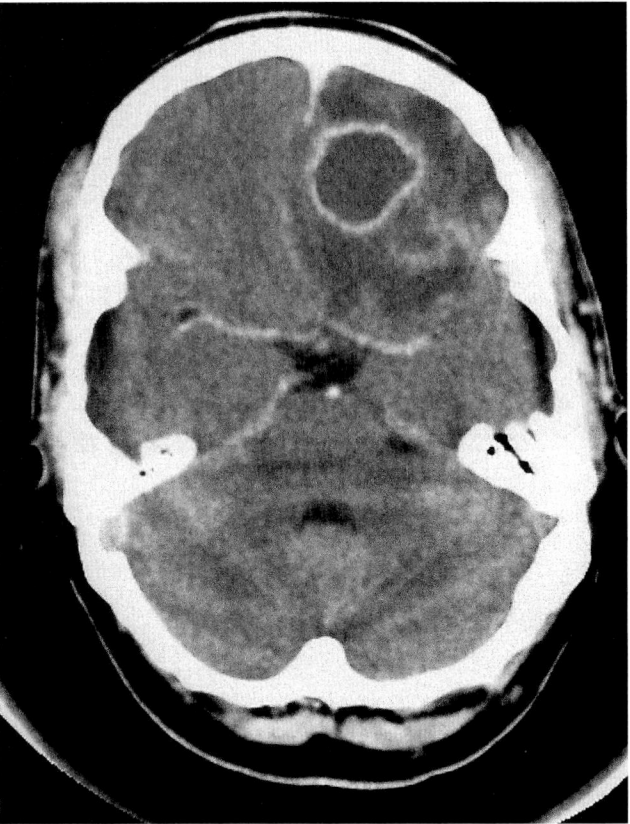

Figure 40.10 Axial computerised tomography scan with contrast of the same patient as in Fig. 40.9 but 2 weeks later. A ring-enhancing lesion has developed, typical of a pyogenic abscess.

Surgical drainage is often by image-guided aspiration, which may need to be repeated several times during the course of the illness. Excision of the abscess wall is an option and may be required for lesions that fail to resolve and multilocular or posterior fossa abscesses. Antibiotic therapy is rationalised according to microbiological culture and sensitivity, and regular surveillance scanning is recommended during therapy and for some months after therapy to pick up recurrences. Multiple small abscesses may be treated medically with antibiotics targeted against organisms isolated from systemic sources but rigorous surveillance is essential. Stereotactic aspiration of one of the lesions to confirm the organism is often desirable.

Steroids are reserved for cases with significant oedema or mass effect and their routine use is discouraged because of their negative impact on antibiotic therapy. Owing to the high risk of seizures, patients should also be treated with anticonvulsants.

Outcome

The overall mortality for cerebral abscess has fallen with the advent of CT and image-guided surgery to around 4% from 40% in earlier decades. It remains the case that a delay in diagnosis and treatment is highly dangerous. If a cerebral abscess is allowed to progress and ruptures into the ventricle, then the rate of mortality is over 80%.

Subdural empyema

Subdural empyema is less common than cerebral abscess but carries a high mortality (5–10%). Infection usually spreads locally from sinusitis and the pus collects over the cerebral convexity and in the parafalcine space (Fig. 40.11). Location in the subdural space encourages cortical venous thrombophlebitis with consequent venous infarction. Causative organisms are usually streptococci such as *Streptococcus viridans* or *Streptococcus milleri*.

Presentation is with headache, fever and meningism. Seizures are common and focal neurological deficits may progress quickly to altered mental state and coma. Diagnosis by non-contrast CT can be difficult and a high index of suspicion must be used – a small parafalcine collection of fluid may be all that is visible. MRI is useful when the diagnosis is doubtful.

Treatment is by craniotomy and thorough drainage of the pus, followed by intravenous antibiotic treatment, anticonvulsants and radiological surveillance as for cerebral abscess.

Tuberculosis

Tuberculosis may affect the central nervous system (CNS) by causing meningoencephalitis or small tumour-like masses of granulomatous tissue called tuberculomas that tend to appear at the base of the cerebral hemispheres. Tuberculoma is a very common cause of intracerebral mass lesion in India. True cerebral abscess in tuberculosis is rare except in patients with AIDS.

Diagnosis of tuberculosis is usually by lumbar puncture. There will be an increased opening pressure with increased CSF white cell count, mainly lymphocytes. Protein is elevated and glucose reduced but not as much as in bacterial meningitis. CSF culture may take several weeks but polymerase chain reaction (PCR) detection is more rapid.

The management of tuberculosis is with drug therapy except

CHAPTER 40 | ELECTIVE NEUROSURGERY

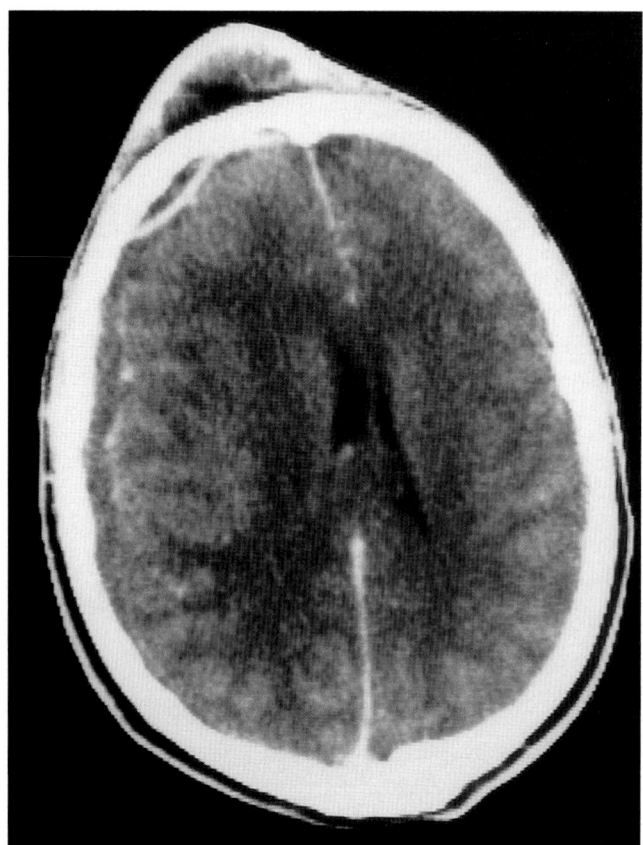

Figure 40.11 Axial computerised tomography scan with contrast showing a right hemisphere subdural empyema and a right frontal Pott's puffy tumour.

in cases when hydrocephalus requires shunt insertion or diagnostic doubt necessitates biopsy.

Parasitic central nervous system infections

Neurocysticercosis

Infection with the pork tapeworm is endemic in areas of Eastern Europe, Asia, South America and Africa. Ingestion of the larval form via contaminated human faeces results in cysticercosis. The larvae burrow through the duodenum and gain access to the systemic circulation, including to the brain. In the brain, larval infection stimulates cyst formation with intense inflammation. They show on CT as ring-enhancing cysts. Presentation may be with seizures, raised pressure or cranial nerve deficits from basal arachnoiditis.

Treatment is with anti-helminthic drugs such as praziquantel or albendazole. The only role for surgery is to treat hydrocephalus or when there is diagnostic doubt.

Toxoplasmosis

Toxoplasma species are obligate intracellular parasites that can be ingested from contact with raw beef, lamb or cat faeces. Infection is more common in the immunocompromised host, especially in the context of AIDS.

Percivall Pott, 1714–1788, Surgeon, St Bartholomew's Hospital, London, UK, described the 'Puffy Tumour' in 1760.

Neurosurgery and human immunodeficiency

Patients with HIV-AIDS may present with a variety of CNS manifestations including HIV-related meningitis and opportunistic infections. The most common focal brain lesions, in descending order of frequency, are: toxoplasmosis, primary CNS lymphoma, progressive multifocal leucencephalopathy and cryptococcal abscess. Surgical biopsy is reserved for cases of diagnostic doubt.

Toxoplasmosis

Toxoplasmosis occurs in 15–30% of patients with AIDS and usually occurs late in the course of the disease when the CD4 count is less than 400 cells/mm³. The resulting abscesses represent over 70% of the cerebral mass lesions in AIDS. They are usually multiple (> 5), prefer a basal ganglia or subcortical location and demonstrate ring enhancement. Treatment is with pyrimethamine and sulphadiazine.

Primary central nervous system lymphoma

Primary CNS lymphoma occurs in about 10% of AIDS patients, is associated with Epstein–Barr virus infection and carries a worse prognosis than in the normal population. Unlike in the normal population, ring enhancement on CT or MRI is common, thus sometimes making a differentiation from toxoplasmosis on imaging criteria difficult. CSF cytology may be positive on lumbar puncture. It may be reasonable to treat for toxoplasmosis and reserve biopsy for those patients who do not respond.

Progressive multifocal leucencephalopathy

This condition is caused by JC virus (a human polyoma virus) infection, with AIDS being the most common underlying disorder. The pathology is oligodendrocyte destruction and presentation is with progressive focal deficits and altered cognition. On imaging, the lesions are located in the white matter and may be multiple, but do not demonstrate enhancement or a mass effect. There is no specific treatment other than that of the underlying disorder and death usually occurs within a few months.

Cryptococcal abscess

Cryptococcus is a fungal infection that causes meningitis but also cerebral abscess in AIDS patients. The organism or its antigens may be detected in the CSF. Treatment is with amphotericin B and fluconazole.

Creutzfeldt–Jakob disease

Creutzfeldt–Jakob disease (CJD) is a transmissible spongiform encephalopathy caused by an abnormal prion protein. It has a variant form (vCJD), which was described in 1996 after an epidemic of bovine spongiform encephalopathy in the UK.

The neurosurgeon may become involved by performing a brain biopsy when diagnosis of CJD is suspected. CJD is transmissible and standard sterilisation methods are inadequate. Disposable instruments must be used in cases in the UK for which a diagnosis of CJD is a possibility. Any non-disposable equipment must be quarantined until a final diagnosis is known and is then destroyed if CJD is confirmed. Because of the risk of vCJD transmission, neuroendoscopes used on those patients born before 1 January 1997 must be kept separate from those used on other patients. All neuroendoscopy accessories must be single use and disposable.

INTRACRANIAL TUMOURS

Intracranial tumours is a term encompassing a great variety of pathological entities ranging from developmental to benign, low-grade and frankly malignant mass lesions. An abridged version of the World Health Organization (WHO) classification of intracranial tumours is shown in Table 40.7. The cells of origin that form the majority of intracranial tumours include meningothelial cells, glial cells, metastatic deposits and pituitary cells. Any mass lesion within the skull is a threat to the integrity of brain function and therefore even histologically benign tumours can threaten life (Summary box 40.4).

Summary box 40.4

Intracranial tumours

- Intracranial tumours may present with seizures, focal neurological deficit, raised ICP or endocrine disturbance
- Cerebral metastases are the most common intracranial tumours
- Benign tumours may cause life-threatening intracranial complications
- For aggressive tumours, management options include steroids, surgery, radiotherapy and chemotherapy

---

Aetiology

The majority of primary brain tumours are sporadic. Various possible environmental risk factors such as smoking, diet, occupation and mobile phone use have been studied with no causative link proven. Some brain tumours are linked with known genetic abnormalities and this list is enlarging on an annual basis. Neurofibromatosis type 1 is caused by a mutation on chromosome 17, which encodes the protein neurofibromin and is associated with astrocytomas as well as neurofibromas. Neurofibromatosis type 2 is caused by a mutation on chromosome 22, which encodes the protein schwannomin, and is characterised by bilateral vestibular Schwannomas (acoustic neuromas) as well as an increased incidence of meningiomas. Li–Fraumeni syndrome is caused a mutation of the gene encoding p53 protein on chromosome 17 and is associated with astrocytomas, as is the *PTEN* gene mutation of Cowden's disease and also hereditary non-polyposis colorectal cancer syndrome. Familial adenomatous polyposis syndrome (*APC* gene mutation) and basal cell naevus syndrome (*PTCH* gene mutation) are associated with medulloblastoma.

Clinical features

Intracranial tumours can present with seizures, focal neurological deficits, raised ICP, seizures or endocrine dysfunction, or can be incidental findings.

Focal deficits

The type of focal neurological deficit will depend on the location of the lesion. With regard to the time-course of neurological symptoms, a steady progression of symptoms over time suggests a structural lesion more than the acute deficit of vascular pathology. An exception to this may be the acute deficit produced by haemorrhage into a malignant glioma, a melanoma metastasis or pituitary apoplexy (see the section on pituitary tumours).

Frontal lobe lesions tend to present with personality change, gait ataxia and urinary incontinence, contralateral hemiparesis if posterior frontal and dysphasia if involving the left inferior frontal gyrus. Parietal lesions are associated with sensory inattention, dressing apraxia, astereognosis and, if on the dominant side, acalculia, agraphia, left–right disorientation and finger agnosia (Gerstmann's syndrome). Temporal lobe lesions may be associated with disturbance of memory, contralateral superior quadrantanopia or hemiparesis and, if on the dominant side, dysphasia. Occipital lesions are often associated with visual field deficits, most commonly an incomplete contralateral homonymous hemianopia.

Other classical focal deficits associated with tumours include: bitemporal hemianopia with a pituitary macroadenoma; anosmia, ipsilateral optic atrophy and contralateral papilloedema with an

Table 40.7 World Health Organization classification of brain tumours

Neuroepithelial tumours	Gliomas	Astrocytomas
		Oligodendrogliomas
		Ependymoma
		Choroid plexus tumour
	Pineal tumours	
	Neuronal tumours	Ganglioglioma
		Gangliocytoma
		Neuroblastoma
	Medulloblastoma	
Nerve sheath tumours	Vestibular Schwannoma	
Meningeal tumours	Meningioma	
Pituitary tumours		
Germ cell tumours	Germinoma	
Lymphomas	Teratoma	
Tumour-like malformations	Craniopharyngioma	
	Epidermoid tumour	
	Dermoid tumour	
	Colloid cyst	
Metastatic tumours		
Contiguous extension from regional tumours, e.g. glomus tumour		

CHAPTER 40 | ELECTIVE NEUROSURGERY

anterior skull base meningioma (Foster–Kennedy syndrome); and ipsilateral hearing loss, tinnitus and dysequilibrium with a vestibular Schwannoma.

Raised intracranial pressure

Intracranial tumours may be associated with raised ICP by a variety of mechanisms, including direct mass effect, vasogenic oedema and obstructive hydrocephalus.

Seizures

The type of seizure may give a clue as to the location of the tumour: for example, parietal lesions causing simple partial seizures, which may become secondarily generalised, medial temporal lesions causing complex partial seizures and so on.

Gliomas

Gliomas include astrocytomas, oligodendrogliomas and mixed tumours. They are graded according to the WHO classification from I to IV according to histological criteria including cellularity, nuclear pleomorphism, mitoses, vascular proliferation and necrosis. A grade I tumour, such as a pilocytic astrocytoma, is the least aggressive; a grade IV tumour, such as a glioblastoma multiforme, is the most aggressive (Fig. 40.12).

Pilocytic astrocytoma is most common in children and young adults, with a peak incidence at the age of 10 years. Common sites include the cerebellum, optic nerve and chiasma, hypothalamus and brainstem. It may be possible to cure posterior fossa tumours by complete surgical excision.

Diffuse astrocytomas (WHO grade II) are most common in the fourth decade of life and often present with seizures or are incidental findings. Optimum treatment remains controversial. Options include surveillance scanning only, biopsy to confirm diagnosis or maximal resection. Radiotherapy may be given early or, more usually, after clinical or radiological progression. Diffuse astrocytomas cannot be cured by any treatment modality and tumour progression is likely, often to a higher grade, within 3–5 years.

High-grade gliomas, including anaplastic astrocytomas (WHO grade III) and glioblastoma (WHO grade IV) are most common in the fifth and sixth decades of life respectively. Glioblastoma is the most common adult glial tumour. Treatment includes surgery to confirm the diagnosis and achieve a macroscopic excision when possible. Surgery is usually followed by high-dose (60 Gy) focused irradiation for those patients with a good performance status. Chemotherapy options include oral temozolomide, either concurrently or after radiotherapy. Chemotherapy wafers impregnated with carmustine may be inserted into the surgical cavity at the time of resection. Despite recent advances, the prognosis for a glioblastoma remains poor with a median survival of 12 months and 2-year survival of only 26% (Fig. 40.13).

The prognosis for a patient with a glioma depends on the histological grade, cell type, tumour size and patient factors such as age and performance status.

Cerebral metastases

Cerebral metastases are by far the most common intracranial tumours and will affect approximately one in every four cancer sufferers. They tend to occur in the fifth to seventh decades. The tumours of origin and their relative frequency are shown in Table 40.8.

The majority of patients with cerebral metastases have multiple lesions and are not suitable candidates for surgery. Palliation with steroids and whole-brain irradiation remain options. Occasionally, the diagnosis is unclear and a biopsy is required.

Patients with a solitary cerebral metastasis may be candidates for excision via a craniotomy if they are in good clinical condition and the primary disease is well controlled. In these circumstances surgery and radiotherapy prolongs life compared with radiotherapy

Table 40.8 Origin of cerebral metastases

Origin	Percentage
Lung	40
Breast	10–30
Melanoma	5–15
Colon, renal	–
Unknown	15

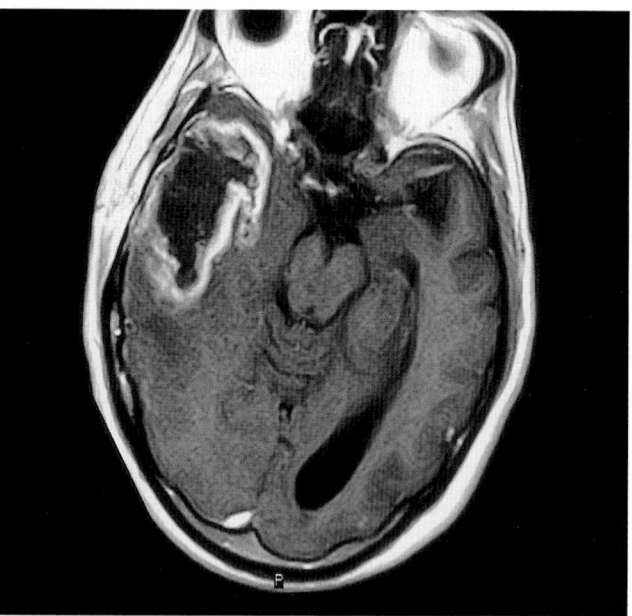

Figure 40.12 Axial T1-weighted magnetic resonance imaging scan with gadolinium, showing a glioblastoma multiforme.

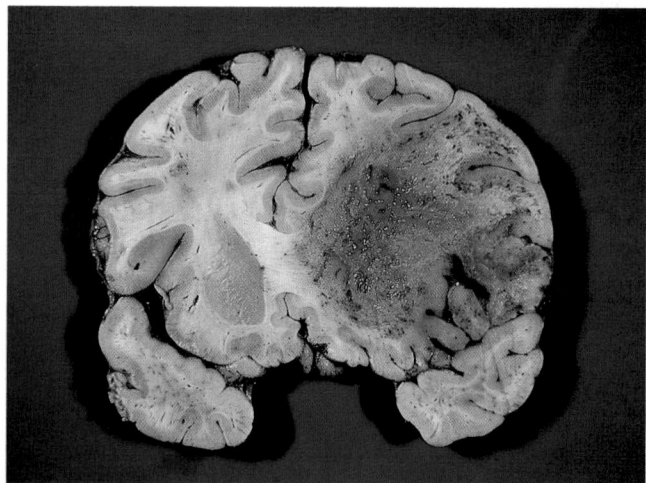

Figure 40.13 Pathological specimen of a glioblastoma multiforme.

alone. Some studies suggest that if two or even three metastases are present and all lesions can be safely removed, then the prognosis is similar to those with a solitary metastasis. Focused radiation therapy is an alternative to craniotomy.

Meningiomas

Meningiomas arise from meningothelial cells and represent around 15–20% of all intracranial tumours (Fig. 40.14). Meningiomas are usually benign although atypical and malignant forms can occur. Around 80% are supratentorial occurring in sites such as the convexity (20%), parafalcine area (20%), sphenoid ridge (10%), tuberculum sellae (10%) and olfactory groove (10%). They may occur within the ventricle (2–5%).

Meningiomas disturb brain function by mass effect, stimulation of vasogenic oedema, direct brain invasion or obstructive hydrocephalus. The tumours may grow slowly over many years and a decision to undertake surgery must consider the patient's neurological status, age and comorbidity. A course of steroids to reduce oedema preoperatively is often desirable.

The chance of recurrence of a benign meningioma depends on the extent of resection those that are completely excised have a 10-year recurrence rate of 10%, increasing to 20% if the dural origin is diathermied but not excised and 30% for subtotal excision.

Radiotherapy is reserved for more aggressive tumour types or difficult surgical locations such as the cavernous sinus.

Pituitary tumours

These account for 10–15% of all intracranial tumours. The majority are benign adenomas that are classified according to size, local invasiveness, the patient's endocrine status, ultrastructure and immunohistochemical staining. Metastases may occur, usually in elderly patients in the posterior pituitary. The differential diagnosis of a sellar region mass includes craniopharyngioma, meningioma, aneurysm and Rathke's cleft cyst.

The most common pituitary adenomas are prolactinoma (30%), non-functioning adenoma (20%), growth hormone-secreting adenoma (15%) and adrenocorticotrophic hormone (ACTH)-secreting adenoma (10%).

Clinical features

Pituitary adenomas may present with mass effect or endocrine disturbance. Mass effect may cause a bitemporal hemianopia due to pressure on the optic chiasma or cause dysfunction of cranial nerves III, IV and VI (Fig. 40.15). Endocrine dysfunction will depend on the secretory properties of the tumour if any: galactorrhoea and primary/secondary amenorrhoea in a prolactinoma, Cushing syndrome in an ACTH-producing tumour (Cushing's disease) and acromegaly or gigantism in a growth hormone-secreting tumour (Table 40.9).

Pituitary apoplexy results in the sudden onset of headache, visual loss, ophthalmoplegia and possibly altered conscious level. It is caused by haemorrhagic infarction of a pituitary tumour. The sudden headache and meningism is similar to the presentation of aneurysmal SAH. Preoperative resuscitation should include steroid cover, and urgent decompression is usually required.

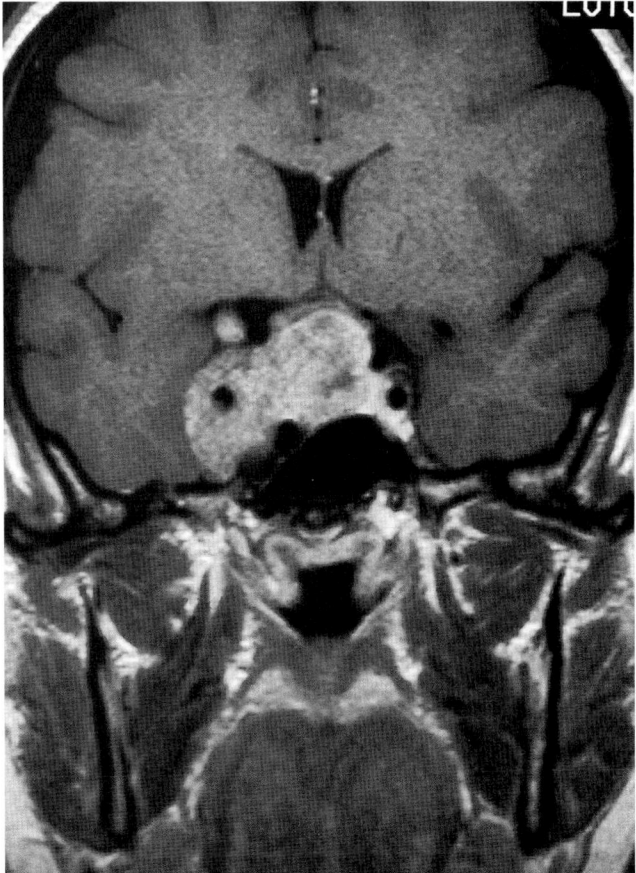

Figure 40.15 Pituitary non-functioning macroadenoma with suprasellar extension and right cavernous sinus invasion.

Harvey Williams Cushing, **1869–1939, Professor of Surgery, Harvard University Medical School, Boston, MA, USA.**

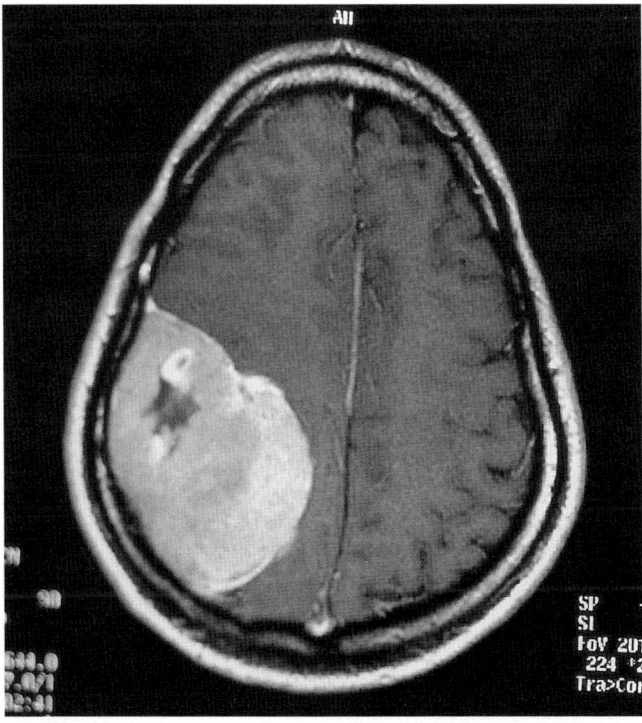

Figure 40.14 Axial T1-weighted magnetic resonance imaging scan with gadolinium, showing a large right parietal convexity meningioma.

CHAPTER 40 | ELECTIVE NEUROSURGERY

Table 40.9 Clinical syndromes for secretory pituitary tumours

Prolactin	Galactorrhoea
	Primary or secondary amenorrhoea
	Impotence
Growth hormone	Acromegaly
	Gigantism if prepubertal
Adrenocorticotrophic hormone	Cushing's disease

Investigation

A patient with a suspected pituitary tumour should undergo formal visual field and acuity testing, MRI scan of the pituitary region and baseline assessment of pituitary function including prolactin, fasting serum and urinary free cortisol, growth hormone and insulin-like growth factor-1, follicle-stimulating hormone, luteinising hormone and thyroid function.

It is essential that the patient's endocrine status is established particularly with regards to the ACTH–cortisol axis and prolactin. Cortisol deficiency must be corrected, especially in the perioperative period. A high prolactin level may indicate a prolactinoma and preclude the need for surgery (see below) but it is important to be aware that pituitary stalk compression from other tumours can moderately elevate the prolactin level. Diagnosis of an ACTH-secreting tumour can be difficult and will often involve the use of specialised tests such as petrosal sinus sampling as well as a dexamethasone suppression test.

Treatment

The aim of treatment of pituitary tumours is to alleviate mass effect, restore or replace normal endocrine function and prevent recurrence. Management requires close cooperation between neurosurgeon and endocrinologist.

Prolactinomas should be initially treated medically with dopamine agonists such as cabergoline or bromocryptine. Growth hormone-secreting tumours may be amenable to medical treatment with somatostatin analogues such as octreotide or dopamine agonists.

Surgical management of pituitary tumours requires transsphenoidal surgery either with an operating microscope or endoscope assisted. Large tumours with suprasellar extension may need to be managed by craniotomy as well. Surgical success as determined by normalisation of endocrine dysfunction and lack or recurrence varies according to the condition being treated and the size of the tumour. Complications of trans-sphenoidal surgery include CSF leak (3%), visual deterioration (1%), major vessel injury (1%) and panhypopituitarism (1%). Diabetes insipidus occurs following manipulation of the pituitary stalk and is usually transient.

Vestibular Schwannoma (acoustic neuroma)

Vestibular Schwannoma is the most common intracranial nerve sheath tumour and is benign. It may occur sporadically or in association with neurofibromatosis type 2 (bilateral vestibular Schwannomas being diagnostic of this condition).

Theodor Schwann, 1810–1882, Professor of Anatomy, successively at Louvain, (1839–1848), and Liege, Belgium (1849–1880).

Presentation is usually with a combination of hearing loss, tinnitus and dysequilibrium. Facial numbness and weakness are less common. Large tumours may present with symptoms of brainstem compression or hydrocephalus.

Imaging with MRI will demonstrate a tumour that may be in the internal auditory canal (intracanalicular) or extend through the meatus into the cerebellopontine angle (Fig. 40.16). Differential diagnosis includes meningioma, metastasis and epidermoid tumour.

Management depends on the size of the tumour and the presentation. Small intracanalicular tumours may be treated by radiological surveillance. Larger tumours could be considered for radiosurgery or craniotomy and excision. Open surgery is the favoured option for large tumours with brainstem compression. Hydrocephalus may need to be relieved via a ventriculoperitoneal shunt.

Preservation of facial nerve and hearing function will depend on preoperative function as well as the size of the tumour. Facial nerve preservation is possible in about 90% of tumours that are < 4 cm but in only 70% of those that are > 4 cm. Hearing preservation (retrosigmoid or middle fossa approach) is possible in around 50% of tumours that are < 1 cm but very unlikely in tumours that are > 2 cm.

Intracranial tumours in children

Intracranial tumours are the most common solid tumours in children.

In neonates, tumours tend to be of neuroectodermal origin and most are supratentorial. Tumour types include:

- teratoma;
- primitive neuroectodermal tumour;
- high-grade astrocytoma;
- choroid plexus papilloma/carcinoma.

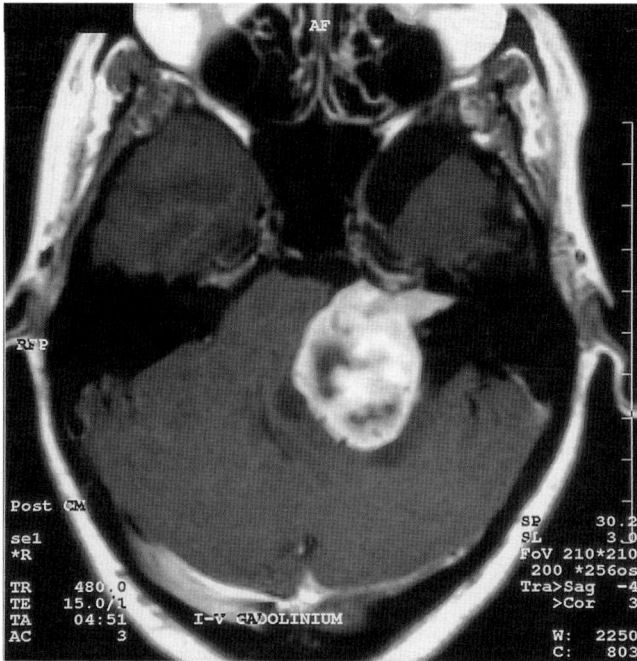

Figure 40.16 Axial T1-weighted magnetic resonance imaging scan with gadolinium, showing a left vestibular Schwannoma.

In older children, the majority of tumours are infratentorial and one of three types:

- medulloblastoma;
- ependymoma;
- pilocytic astrocytoma.

Other tumours include supratentorial low-grade gliomas, craniopharyngioma and brainstem gliomas.

VASCULAR NEUROSURGERY (SUMMARY BOX 40.5)

Summary box 40.5

Vascular neurosurgery

- Aneurysmal SAH should be suspected in a patient with a sudden, severe headache
- Complications of aneurysmal SAH include re-bleeding, delayed ischaemic neurological deficit and hydrocephalus
- Patients with symptomatic carotid stenosis may benefit from carotid endarterectomy
- Arteriovenous malformations may present with seizures, focal neurological deficit or haemorrhage

Aneurysmal subarachnoid haemorrhage

The most common cause of SAH by far is trauma. On the other hand, non-traumatic SAH is caused by:

- aneurysms (75%);
- arteriovenous malformations (AVMs; 10%);
- idiopathic causes (10%);
- tumours.

Epidemiology

Aneurysmal SAH most commonly occurs in the sixth decade of life and has an incidence of about 10–15:100 000 population per year (Fig. 40.17). Risk factors include hypertension, a positive family history of SAH and, particularly in younger patients, cocaine abuse. Those with two first-degree relatives who have had aneurysmal SAH have a 15% chance of harbouring an intracranial aneurysm themselves. Other associated conditions include polycystic kidney disease (15% chance of aneurysm, increased risk of aneurysm rupture), fibromuscular dysplasia (7–20%) and other connective tissue disorders.

Clinical features

SAH can be difficult to diagnose clinically and missing the diagnosis often ends in a disastrous outcome for the patient. A high index of suspicion is therefore required in patients with a normal physical examination.

The typical presentation is the sudden onset of an unusual headache. This is often described as the worst headache of a patient's life or like being struck forcefully on the back of the head. The location of the headache is often occipital or cervical. There may be associated nausea, vomiting and photophobia. It is not uncommon for patients to experience transient loss of consciousness and collapse. There may be a history of less severe headache some days prior to the ictus – the warning or sentinel headache. Post-coital SAH may occur. Differential diagnosis includes migraine and post-coital cephalgia.

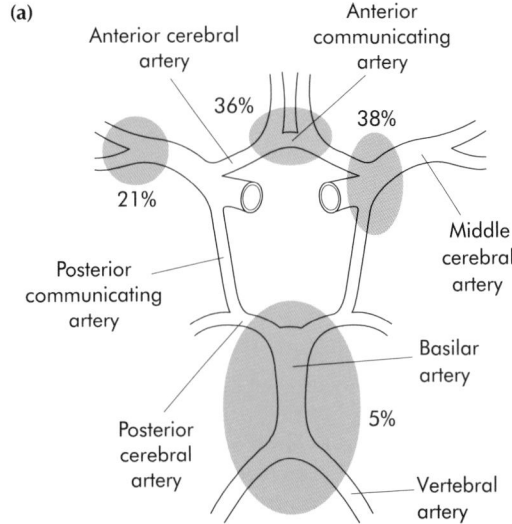

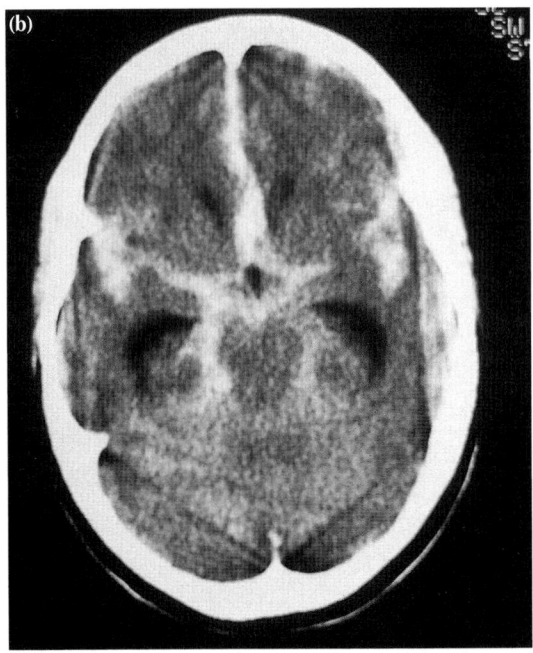

Figure 40.17 (a) Main sites of intracranial supraclinoid aneurysms. (b) Axial computerised tomography scan demonstrating a diffuse subarachnoid haemorrhage with hydrocephalus.

Physical examination may be entirely normal. Meningism with neck stiffness and photophobia should be sought. The development of a third nerve palsy in the context of a sudden severe headache should put in mind SAH from a ruptured posterior communicating artery aneurysm, because of the proximity of this nerve and artery. Patients may have an altered level of consciousness and clinically SAH is graded according the World Federation of Neurological Surgeons system (Table 40.10). Focal neurological deficits in the limbs at presentation suggest a focal intracerebral haematoma or vascular dissection. Patients in the more severe grades are more likely to exhibit the systemic complication of SAH: cardiac tachyarrhythmias and neurogenic pulmonary oedema. A Cushing's response (hypertension and bradycardia) may be seen in patients with altered consciousness secondary to raised ICP.

Table 40.10 World Federation of Neurological Surgeons Grading of subarachnoid haemorrhage

Grade	Glasgow Coma Scale	Focal deficits*
I	15	–
II	13–14	–
III	13–14	+
IV	7–12	±
V	3–9	±

*Focal deficit = dysphasia or limb weakness.

Investigation

CT scan is positive in aneurysmal SAH in 95% of cases if performed within 48 hours but the sensitivity falls off rapidly with increased time from ictus as blood is cleared from the subarachnoid space. A positive CT scan precludes a lumbar puncture.

A lumbar puncture is indicated in those patients with a suspicious history for SAH but a negative CT scan (Fig. 40.18). These patients are likely to be in a good clinical state with no neurological deficit. The CSF should be spun down and the supernatant analysed with a spectrophotometer between wavelengths of 350 and 650 nm. The first breakdown product in blood to be seen is oxyhaemoglobin (413–415 nm), which appears from around 2–12 hours. Bilirubin (450–460 nm) appears later and a bilirubin peak is diagnostic of SAH. False negatives may occur if the lumbar puncture is performed within 12 hours of the ictus. False positives may occur in the presence of a traumatic tap or increased serum bilirubin. Remember that a traumatic tap (fresh procedure-related blood in the sample) does not exclude an SAH – it merely means that the lumbar puncture may not give a useful result.

In patients with a highly suspicious history and an unrevealing lumbar puncture result, a CT angiogram or formal cerebral angiogram is required (Fig. 40.19).

Management

Once a diagnosis of SAH has been made, and the patient has been resuscitated, the management priorities are:

- confirm the presence or absence of an aneurysm;
- prevent the main complications of aneurysmal rupture:
  - rebleeding;
  - delayed ischaemic neurological deficit;
  - hydrocephalus;
  - hyponatraemia.

The presence of an aneurysm can be confirmed by diagnostic cerebral digital subtraction angiography (DSA) or CT angiogram. Treatment of a ruptured aneurysm to prevent rebleeding is either by endovascular coiling or surgical clipping via a craniotomy (Figs 40.20 and 40.21). There is evidence that for small anterior circulation aneurysms a poor outcome is less likely (relative risk reduction 23.9%) with endovascular coiling and this is one of the factors that has led to a dramatic increase in aneurysm coiling in

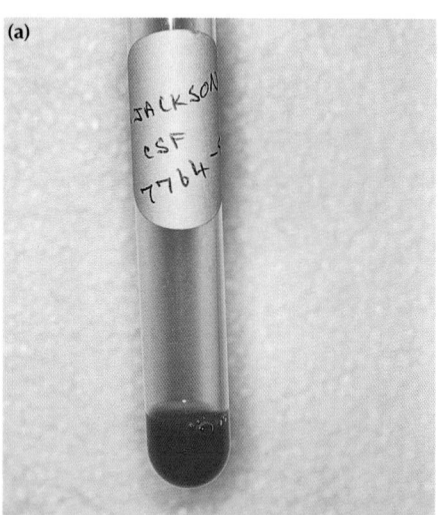

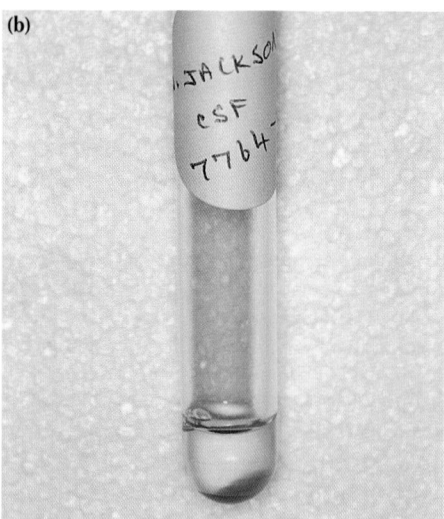

Figure 40.18 Cerebrospinal fluid (CSF) sample for a patient presenting with subarachnoid haemorrhage. (a) Test tube showing blood-stained CSF. (b) Test tube showing the sample after having been spun down and demonstrating xanthochromia in the supernatant. Spectrophotometry should be used to test for pigments.

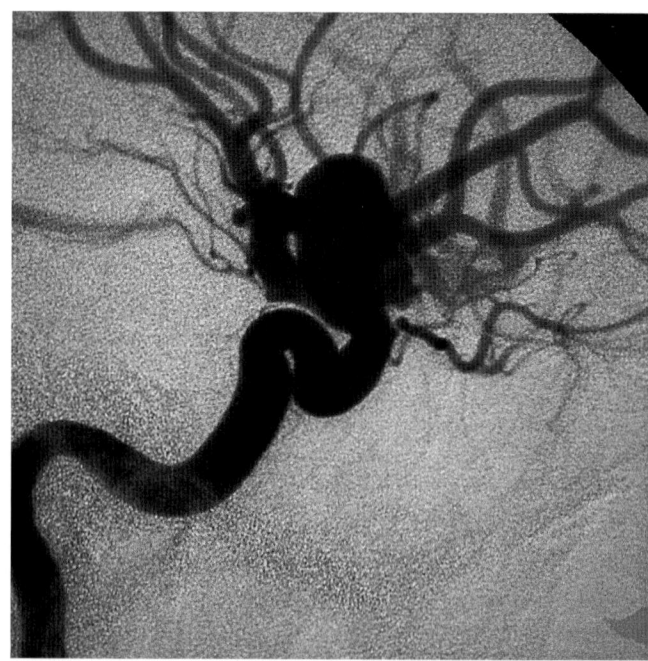

Figure 40.19 Cerebral angiogram demonstrating a middle cerebral artery aneurysm.

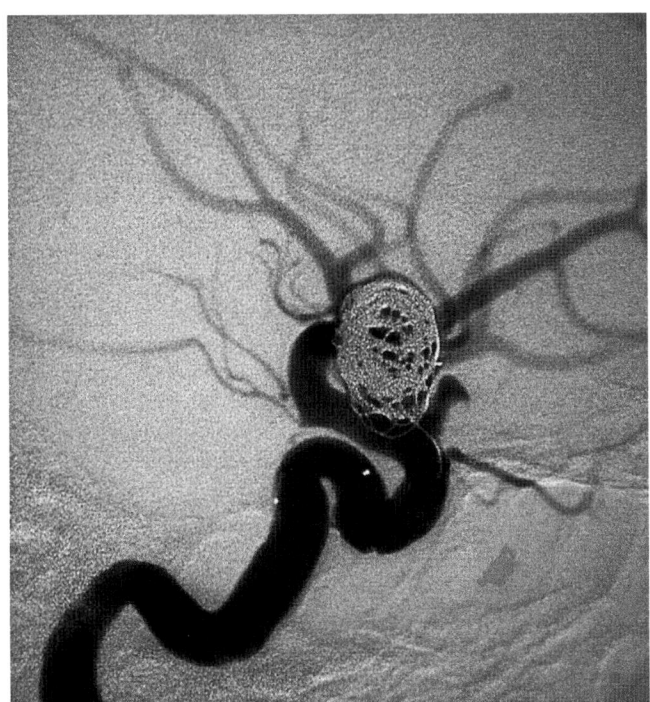

Figure 40.20 The middle cerebral artery aneurysm in Fig. 40.19 undergoing embolisation with Gugliemi detachable coils.

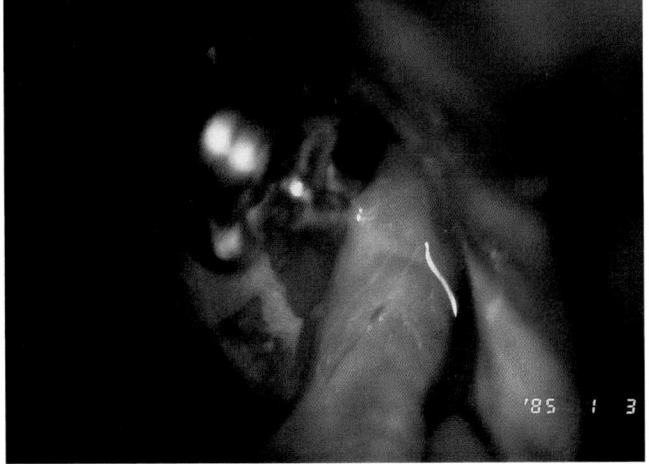

Figure 40.21 Microscope picture of a clipped aneurysm.

recent years. There is still a role for surgery, and the decision about best treatment modality is based on characteristics of the aneurysm (size, dome to neck ratio, incorporation of branching vessels), operator experience and patient preference.

Delayed ischaemic neurological deficit (DIND) is the occurrence of focal neurological deficits, usually between 4 and 10 days after the SAH and often attributed to cerebral 'vasospasm'. DIND is a major cause of morbidity and mortality following subarachnoid haemorrhage, resulting in death in 7% and permanent morbidity in another 7%. Cerebral vasospasm may affect any of the cerebral arteries and occurs in response to blood in the subarachnoid space via uncertain mechanisms. Patients with a larger blood load are at higher risk of vasospasm. The diagnosis of DIND is made after exclusion of other complications such as

rebleeding, hydrocephalus and electrolyte disturbance, particularly hyponatraemia. A cerebral angiogram if performed may demonstrate cerebral artery narrowing. Treatment is with hypertension (inotropes may be required), hypervolaemia and haemodilution. The deficits of DIND are often reversible if diagnosed and treated in a timely fashion. Angioplasty, either chemical or with a balloon, plays a role in the treatment of short-segment large artery spasm. The incidence of DIND can be lowered (30% fewer cerebral infarctions) by prophylaxis with nimodipine (60 mg, 4-hourly) and hypervolaemia (8-hourly normal saline).

Hydrocephalus affects about 20% of patients who have a SAH, and around one-half of those with hydrocephalus will go on to require a ventriculoperitoneal shunt. Hydrocephalus early in the course of the disease is often treated by external ventricular drainage: acute blood clot in the ventricles may act as an obstructive mass lesion rendering lumbar puncture unsafe. Continuous CSF drainage is desirable and an EVD can be used to monitor ICP in the comatose patient. A ventriculoperitoneal shunt can be inserted if the patient requires it, once the red blood cell count in the CSF has fallen to < 500 mm^{-3}.

Hyponatraemia is common after SAH and is often caused by cerebral salt wasting (CSW) rather than the syndrome of inappropriate antidiuretic hormone secretion (SIADH). The distinction is an important one as in CSW the problem is excessive salt loss, probably due to a natriuretic factor, with relative dehydration. The treatment is with volume loading and salt replacement. In SIADH the problem is retention of water and is treated by fluid restriction. In SAH, incorrectly diagnosing a patient with SIADH when in fact they have CSW is potentially dangerous, as inappropriate fluid restriction will lead to hypovolaemia and an increased incidence of DIND. Biochemical tests (plasma and urine sodium and osmolarity) do not help distinguish between the two conditions. Estimating the fluid status of the patient prior to treatment is the best way of distinguishing the two conditions, but in SAH the patients are usually already being filled with intravenous fluids as part of DIND prophylaxis. Expert endocrinological advice may be required.

Prognosis

Aneurysmal SAH is not a benign condition. If only the grade I patients are considered, approximately one-half will go back to equivalent full-time employment. Neuropsychological sequelae are common. One-year mortality rates are about 10% for grade I patients, rising to over 40% for patients in grades IV–V. Moderate to severe disability is likely to affect at least 30% of survivors.

Arteriovenous malformations

Cerebral AVMs are lesions containing abnormal vessels with arteries feeding directly into veins without the normal interposed capillary bed, resulting in a high-pressure and high-flow vascular shunt. They may be congenital or acquired.

AVMs may present with headache, seizures, focal deficits or bleeding. Once an AVM has bled, then it has an approximately 2–4% per year risk of rebleeding although this risk may be much higher in the first 6 weeks. Bleeding can occur from intranidal aneurysms or flow aneurysms on feeding arteries, in which case the urgency of treatment is greater.

The diagnosis, suspected by vessels and calcification within a lesion seen on CT or MRI can be confirmed by cerebral angiography (Figs 40.22 and 40.23). Treatment can be endovascular (often using tissue glue), by stereotactic radiosurgery or surgical via craniotomy with factors such as AVM nidal size, functional

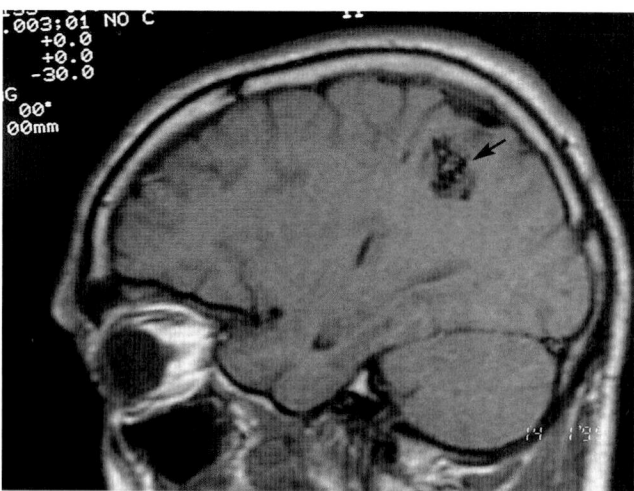

Figure 40.22 Sagittal T1-weighted magnetic resonance imaging scan of a young man presenting with a seizure. This demonstrates a serpiginous lesion (arrow) with low-signal flow voids that are typical of an arteriovenous malformation.

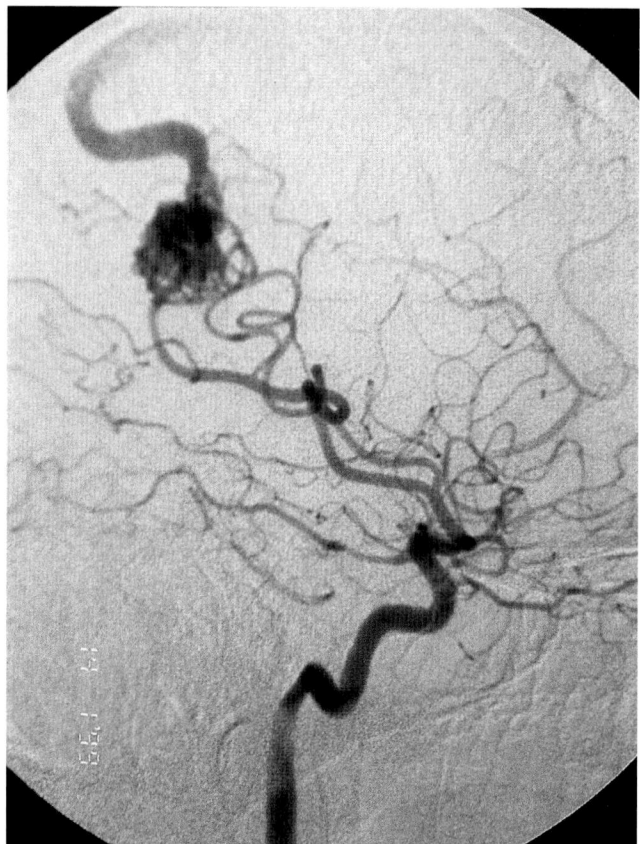

Figure 40.23 Lateral cerebral angiogram of the same patient as in Fig. 40.22. This demonstrates the arteriovenous malformation being filled by a branch of the middle cerebral artery and draining into the superior sagittal sinus.

importance of surrounding brain, number and type of feeding arteries, and superficial or deep venous drainage being taken into account (Fig. 40.24).

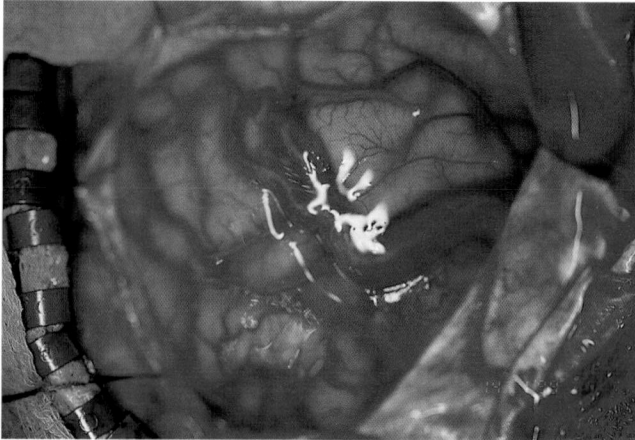

Figure 40.24 Intraoperative picture of the same patient as in Figs 40.22 and 40.23. The large superficial draining vein can be seen.

Cavernomas

A cavernoma is a benign angiographically occult cluster of abnormal sinusoidal blood vessels that may be associated with a developmental venous anomaly. They are more common in the supratentorial than infratentorial compartment and may be multiple. Cavernomas can present with seizures, focal signs and haemorrhage or they may be discovered incidentally. Surgery is recommended if seizures are refractory to medical therapy or to prevent rebleeding although the annual risk of haemorrhage is low.

Moyamoya disease

Moyamoya means 'puff of smoke' in Japanese. The condition, occurring in young patients, involves progressive occlusion of both internal carotid arteries in the region of the carotid siphon. The subsequent development of small capillary-like vessels followed by collateralisation from the external carotid artery underlies the angiographic findings. Presentation is with ischaemia or haemorrhage.

Surgical treatment options include:

- encephalosynangiosis (temporalis muscle to pia-arachnoid);
- superficial temporal artery (STA)–MCA bypass (STA to MCA);
- encephalodurarteriosynangiosis (STA to dura);
- omental pedicle transposition.

Surgery for stroke

Spontaneous intracerebral haemorrhage

When considering a patient for surgery for a spontaneous intracranial haemorrhage, one must always consider the possibility of an underlying lesion such as a tumour, vascular malformation or aneurysm.

In general terms, craniotomy and haematoma evacuation will do little to improve focal deficits from haemorrhagic cerebrovascular accidents. The role of surgery is to reduce raised ICP due to mass effect and therefore prevent brain herniation and perhaps improve the recovery of brain tissue in the surrounding ischaemic penumbra. A recent international trial centred in the UK (STICH), showed no benefit for surgery over conservative management in cases where the surgeon was uncertain whether or not to operate. Those likely to benefit from surgery are young patients with superficial haematomas and a falling Glasgow Coma Score.

Carotid endarterectomy

Carotid endarterectomy is indicated for symptomatic (recent transient ischaemic attack or stroke) patients with severe carotid artery stenosis. A North American trial demonstrated a 2-year ipsilateral stroke absolute risk reduction of 17% (26 vs. 9%) for surgery versus conservative management, with a number-needed-to-treat of six. These results were backed up by a similar European trial. The benefits of surgery for symptomatic patients with moderate stenosis or asymptomatic patients with severe stenosis are less clear-cut.

Posterior fossa infarction

Patients with posterior fossa infarction (haemorrhagic or ischaemic) are susceptible to brainstem compression and obstructive hydrocephalus from cerebral swelling. In selected patients, it is appropriate to offer decompressive craniectomy and infarct/clot evacuation.

Middle cerebral artery infarction

Infarction encompassing all or much of the MCA territory is associated with a high morbidity and mortality. In young patients in particular it is associated with malignant cerebral swelling. Recent trials have sought to address the question of whether there is overall benefit to a large decompressive craniectomy. As this operation will prevent herniation and coning, there was a concern that widespread use of the technique might result in a large increase in the number of survivors with severe disability. There is now evidence that surgery reduces mortality and increases those survivors with a modified Rankin score (mRS) of 1–4 but does not increase the number of patients with a mRS of 5 (bedbound).

EPILEPSY SURGERY

Epilepsy is the most common neurological disorder but only a small fraction of epilepsy patients are considered suitable candidates for epilepsy surgery. All cerebral mass lesions may present with seizures, but epilepsy surgery as a subspecialty deals primarily with non-lesional or at least non-tumour-related seizures (Summary box 40.6).

Summary box 40.6

Epilepsy surgery

- Epilepsy surgery candidates are identified through extensive preoperative work-up
- Epilepsy surgery procedures include invasive monitoring, resective operations and disconnection operations

---

History and examination

For a patient to be considered for resective epilepsy surgery there must be concordance between clinical, radiological and electrophysiogical data. In addition the patient should be under the care of a neurologist with a special interest in epilepsy and it should have been demonstrated that the seizures are refractory to best medical therapy. The seizures must adversely affect quality of life. Detailed information about seizure frequency, type, severity and location is required. Patients with mesial temporal sclerosis may give a history of complicated febrile seizures at a young age.

Electroencephalography

Scalp surface electrode recording can give valuable information about seizure localisation, particularly in the complex partial seizures of temporal epilepsy. Complex software analysis is used to compare ictal with interictal recordings. Video telemetry, accessed on an in-patient basis, is used to capture a run of seizures with synchronous clinical and electroencephalogram data collection.

Occasionally additional information about localisation is desirable. Surgical diagnostic procedures include the insertion of subdural grid or strip electrodes and, occasionally, depth electrodes.

Neuropsychology

Neuropsychological evaluation is important for two reasons: to assess the patient's baseline functional state and to evaluate the likely chance of postoperative language and memory deficits in temporal lobe epilepsy surgery. The latter assessment is made during the sodium amytal or Wada test.

Imaging

In mesial temporal sclerosis, an MRI scan will demonstrate loss of hippocampal volume and internal architecture and altered signal. MRI may also show lesions such as cortical dysplasia, low-grade tumours or gliosis.

An ictal SPECT (single-photon emission CT) scan can identify a seizure-onset zone by measurement of regional cerebral perfusion. A radioactive compound (^{99m}Tc HMPAO) is injected soon after seizure onset and is fixed in the brain for around 6 hours, during which time the scan is performed.

Interictal positron emission tomography (PET) scans using radiolabelled fluorodeoxyglucose (^{18}Fl FDG) may localise a seizure focus by demonstrating a region of hypometabolism.

Surgery: resective procedures

Surgery for mesial temporal sclerosis includes temporal lobectomy and selective amygdalo-hippocampectomy. With correct patient selection, seizure cure rates of 70% can be achieved. Anatomical or functional hemispherectomy is used for conditions such as Rasmussen's encephalitis (Fig. 40.25).

Surgery: disconnection and modulation procedures

Corpus callosotomy may improve quality of life for patients with drop attacks. Multiple subpial transactions may be used to disconnect a seizure focus from the surrounding cortex. The mode of action of a vagal nerve stimulator is uncertain but the device may improve seizures in idiopathic epilepsy.

FUNCTIONAL NEUROSURGERY (SUMMARY BOX 40.7)

Summary box 40.7

Functional neurosurgery

- Functional neurosurgery modulates the nervous system to alleviate symptoms from movement disorders, pain syndromes and spasticity

---

John A. Wada, **a twentieth century Japanese–Canadian Neurologist.**

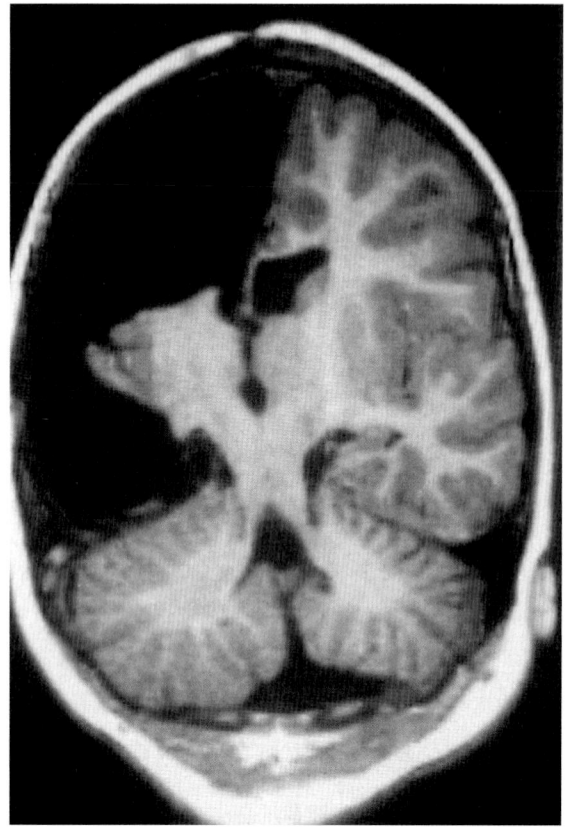

Figure 40.25 Coronal T2-weighted magnetic resonance imaging scan image following an anatomical hemispherectomy.

Movement disorder surgery

Deep brain stimulation (DBS) involves the stereotactic implantation of an electrode into the deep grey matter to alter brain function. The electrodes are connected to a pulse generator, the settings of which can be adjusted by an external programmer. DBS is generally preferred to lesion surgery as its effects are reversible and adjustable.

Parkinson's disease

DBS for Parkinson's disease targets either the subthalamic nucleus or globus pallidus interna. Surgery is reserved for those experiencing intolerable side-effects of medical therapy, such as dyskinesias. Tremor, rigidity and dyskinesia are the symptoms most likely to improve.

Dystonia

Options for focal dystonia include botulinum toxin injection and focal denervation surgery. Generalised dystonia may be treated with levodopa. For refractory cases, the target for DBS for dystonia is the globus pallidus interna bilaterally.

Tremor

The DBS target for tremor is the Vim nucleus of the thalamus.

James Parkinson, **1755–1824, a General Practitioner of Shoreditch, London, UK.**

Surgery for pain

Painful conditions can often be managed by treatment of the underlying cause, medication of escalating strength, physical therapy and local injections when appropriate. Some patients have pain syndromes that are severe and refractory to conventional management; for these, a variety of functional neurosurgical procedures can be considered.

Spinal cord stimulators

Spinal cord stimulation (SCS) involves the insertion of electrodes onto the dura of the spine either by open laminotomy or percutaneously (Fig. 40.26). The electrodes are connected to a pulse generator implanted subcutaneously. Candidates for SCS include those with chronic leg pain following failed spinal decompressive surgery or those with arachnoiditis, peripheral vascular disease or angina.

Deep brain stimulation

Some patients with chronic pain syndromes such as from thalamic stroke are candidates for DBS. Targets include periaqueductal grey and the sensory thalamic nuclei.

Cordotomy/rhizotomy

In selected pain syndromes symptomatic improvement may be gained by dorsal root rhizolysis or surgical interruption of the spinothalamic tract (cordotomy).

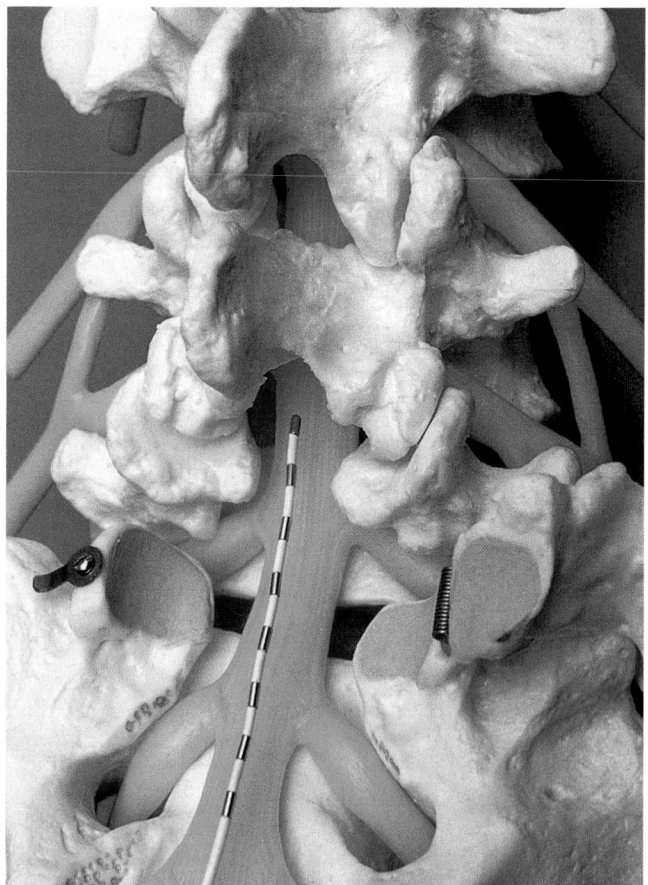

Figure 40.26 A spine model demonstrating the position of an epidural electrode.

Trigeminal neuralgia

Trigeminal neuralgia is a condition of severe episodic lancinating facial pain occurring in the distribution of the trigeminal nerve. The aetiology of the condition is unclear but vascular compression of the trigeminal nerve near the root entry zone seems to play a part. Bilateral trigeminal neuralgia should raise the suspicion of multiple sclerosis. Structural causes should be excluded by MRI.

Treatment is initially with medication such a carbamazepine or gabapentin. Refractory cases are considered for surgical treatments, which include:

- percutaneous treatments:
  - trigeminal ganglion techniques:
    - glycerol injection;
    - radiofrequency thermocoagulation;
    - balloon compression;
    - local nerve block;
- microvascular decompression via craniotomy;
- stereotactic radiosurgery.

Intrathecal drug delivery

An intrathecal catheter can be introduced into the lumbar spine region and connected to a subcutaneous pump containing either opiates for pain relief or baclofen to treat spasticity (Fig. 40.27).

DEVELOPMENTAL ABNORMALITIES (SUMMARY BOX 40.8 AND TABLE 40.11)

Summary box 40.8

Developmental abnormalities

- Spinal dysraphism is a term that encompasses a wide range of conditions resulting from abnormal CNS development
- Premature fusion of skull sutures causes abnormalities of skull shape

Arachnoid cysts

Arachnoid cysts are benign fluid-filled intracranial mass lesions, possibly formed by splitting of the arachnoid membrane. Around

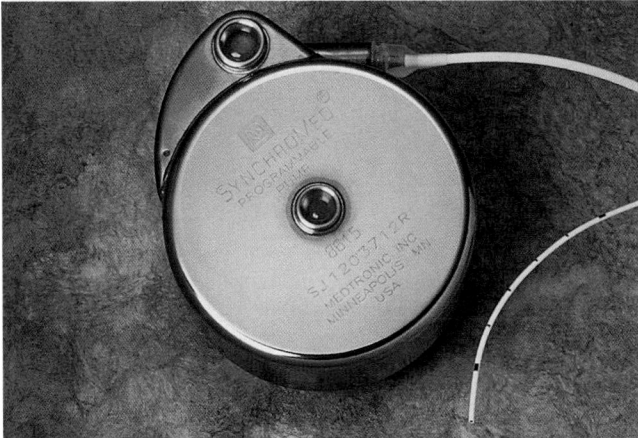

Figure 40.27 A Medtronic synchronised programmable intrathecal drug delivery system.

Table 40.11 Developmental abnormalities

Arachnoid cysts	
Spinal dysraphism	Spina bifida occulta
	Myelomeningocele
	Lipomyelomeningocele
	Tethered cord syndrome
Encephaloceles	
Chiari malformations	
Craniosynostosis	

one-half of them are located in the Sylvian fissure, whereas others occur in the cerebellopontine angle and the suprasellar and posterior fossa regions. They often present in the paediatric age group: some remain aymptomatic, others enlarge in size, causing a mass effect, and others may present with haemorrhage. Surgery is reserved only for symptomatic lesions and options include endoscopy and fenestration into a cistern or ventricle, or shunting.

Spinal dysraphism
Myelomeningocele

Myelomeningocele is a developmental abnormality of the caudal thoracodorsal spine and results from a failure of primary neuralation (neural tube defect). The incidence has decreased in recent times to about 0.5:1000 births. Aetiology is multifactorial but is associated with folate deficiency, some anticonvulsant medications and family history. Diagnosis may be made prenatally using ultrasound and predicted using maternal alpha-fetoprotein levels or amniocentesis.

Surgical repair of an open myelomeningocele is recommended within 72 hours of birth to prevent infection. The majority of patients have hydrocephalus and will require a ventriculoperitoneal shunt. All patients with a myelomeningocele will have a Chiari II malformation (see next page).

Tethered cord syndrome

Associated with myelomeningocele and spina bifida occulta, this condition involves a low-lying conus medullaris and thickened filum terminale. Presentation may be with progressive neurological deficit, spasticity, bladder dysfunction or scoliosis. Surgical treatment involves untethering of the cord to prevent further neurological deterioration.

Spinal lipoma and lipomomyelomeningocele

Lipomas may occur within the normally located conus (lower cord) or be associated with distraction of neural tissue out of the spinal canal. Presentation is with a back mass or lower limb and bladder dysfunction. Surgery aims to preserve neural function and prevent the development of a tethered cord.

Encephaloceles

Encephaloceles, the developmental herniation of cerebral tissue through a cranial defect, occur with a frequency of approximately 1–4:1000 births (Fig. 40.28). They may be occipital, nasofrontal (more common in South-east Asia), fronto-ethmoidal or basal. Surgical repair is required to prevent infection, especially if skin covering is absent, and to reconstruct the skull.

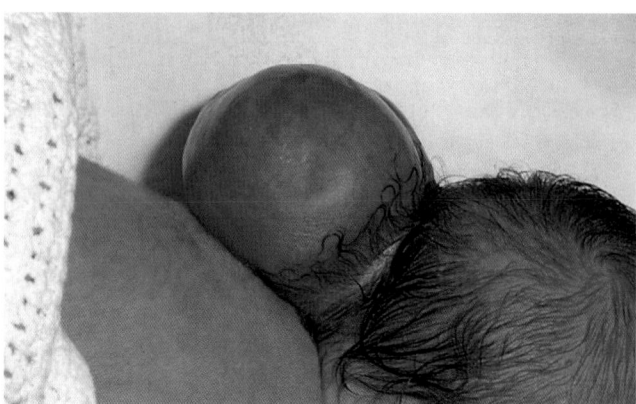

Figure 40.28 An occipital encephalocele.

Chiari malformation

Chiari malformation is used to describe herniation of the posterior fossa contents (e.g. cerebellar tonsils) through the foramen magnum:

- normal: up to 5 mm of tonsillar descent through the foramen magnum;
- Chiari I: > 5 mm of tonsillar descent;
- Chiari II: descent of the tonsils and cerebellar vermis.

Chiari I malformation tends to present in young adults, with headaches that are exacerbated by coughing and straining. There may be signs associated with brainstem compression or spinal cord fluid cavity (syrinx).

Chiari II malformations tend to present in infancy, with signs of brainstem compression such as poor feeding, stridor and apnoeic spells.

Treatment of Chiari malformations is directed first towards associated hydrocephalus followed by consideration of foramen magnum decompression.

Craniosynostosis

Craniosynostosis, or premature fusion of the cranial sutures, may affect single or multiple sutures. Premature fusion leads to restricted growth in a plane at 90° to the suture, resulting in presentation with an abnormal head shape (Figs 40.29 and 40.30). Sagittal synostosis causes a narrow boat-shaped head with frontal and occipital bossing (scaphocephaly); bicoronal synostosis causes a shortened forehead (brachycephaly); metopic synostosis causes trigonocephaly. Unicoronal and unilambdoid synostosis must be differentiated from the much more common anterior and posterior plagiocephaly (positional flattening of the head).

There are rare genetic conditions associated with craniosynostosis, some of which are caused by abnormalities of the fibroblast growth factor receptor genes, such as the following syndromes:

- Crouzon;
- Apert;
- Pfeiffer;
- Saethre–Chotzen.

Hans Chiari, **1851–1916**, Professor of Pathology, the German University, Prague, Czech Republic.
Octave Crouzon, **1874–1938**, Neurologist, La Salpêtrière, Paris, France.
Eugene Apert, **1868–1940**, Physician, L'Hôpital des Enfants-Malades, Paris, France.

Surgery aims to correct deformity and prevent the development of raised ICP.

PERIPHERAL NERVE DISORDERS

Carpal tunnel syndrome

This is entrapment of the median nerve at the wrist. Risk factors include diabetes, obesity, thyroid disorders and acromegaly. The patient complains of numbness and pins and needles in the median 3½ digits, worse at night and relieved by handshaking. Symptoms can progress to weakness and loss of hand function. Examination reveals altered sensation in the median 3½ digits (but not the palm), wasting of the thenar eminence and weakness of abductor policis brevis. Symptoms may be elicited by tapping over the carpal tunnel (Tinel's sign) or wrist flexion (Phalen's test).

The diagnosis can be confirmed by nerve conduction studies and treatment is with wrist splinting, steroid injection or carpal tunnel decompression.

Ulnar nerve entrapment at the elbow

Ulnar nerve entrapment at the elbow can cause pain, numbness and tingling in the ulnar 1½ digits of the hand, progressing to loss of hand function. Signs include wasting and weakness of the small muscles of the hand and the hypothenar eminence. Froment's sign, elicited by asking the patient to hold a piece of paper in the first web space while the examiner tries to slide it out, is flexion of the thumb on attempted thumb adduction. Nerve conduction studies confirm the diagnosis, which is treated by surgical decompression.

Meralgia parasthetica

Compression of the lateral nerve of the thigh as it passes beneath the inguinal ligament can cause pain, tingling and numbness in the lateral thigh. Treatment may be by weight loss if appropriate, steroid injection or surgical decompression.

Thoracic outlet syndrome

Thoracic outlet syndrome can be caused by a cervical rib or a fibrous band from the C7 transverse process to the first rib. Compression of the lower brachial plexus roots (C8, T1) and subclavian artery explains the symptoms and signs: neural compression causes radicular arm pain with wasting, weakness and numbness in a C8/T1 distribution.

Investigation may include plain cervical radiograph, nerve conduction studies and brachial plexus MRI. Treatment is by surgical decompression, dividing the fibrous band or removing the cervical rib.

BRAINSTEM DEATH

Brainstem death is defined by irreversible loss of consciousness, loss of brainstem reflexes and apnoea (absence of respiratory drive) and these patients are therefore mechanically ventilated in an intensive care setting. Brainstem death is equivalent to death and is one of the criteria for the harvesting of organs for transplant from a heart-beating donor.

George S. Phalen, **Orthopaedic Surgeon**, the Cleveland Clinic, Cleveland, OH, USA.
Jules Froment, **1878–1946**, Professor of Clinical Medicine, Lyons, France.

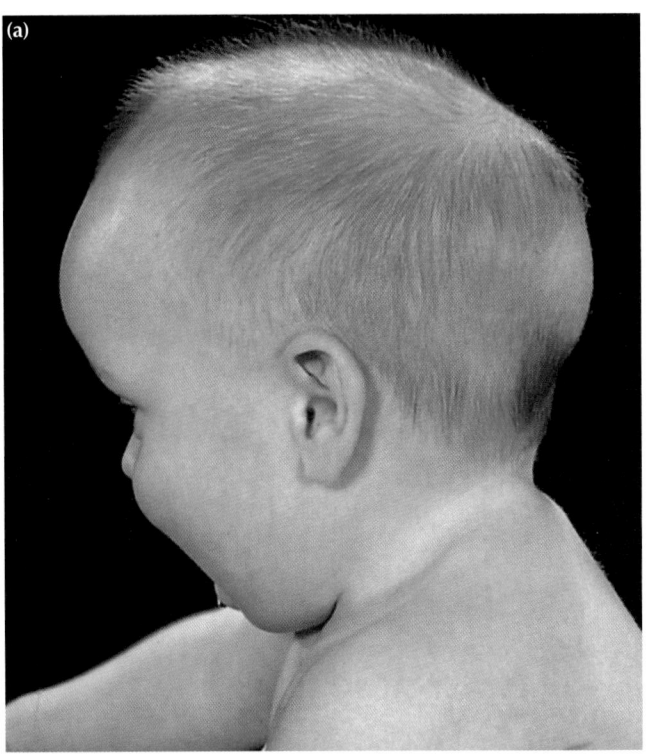

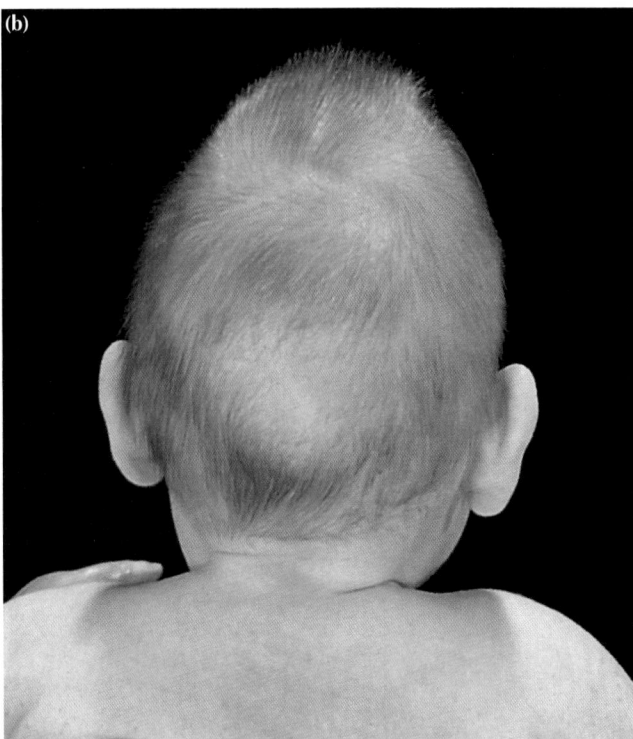

Figure 40.29 Characteristic appearance of scaphocephaly due to sagittal suture synostosis.

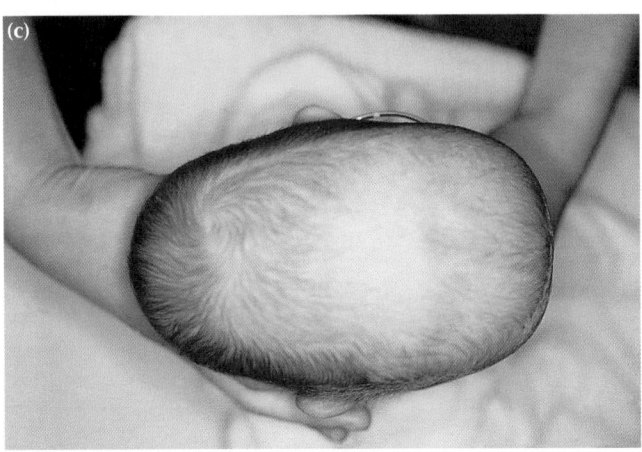

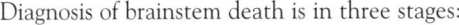

Diagnosis of brainstem death is in three stages:

- identification of the cause of irreversible coma (Fig. 40.31);
- exclusion of reversible causes of coma;
- clinical demonstration of absence of brainstem reflexes.

The brainstem reflexes tested for are:

- pupillary reaction to light;
- corneal reflex;
- vestibulo-ocular reflex;
- cough reflex;
- gag reflex;
- motor response to central pain;
- apnoea test: apnoea despite a carbon dioxide increase to > 6.65 kPa.

All reflexes must be absent and are tested for twice by two doctors.

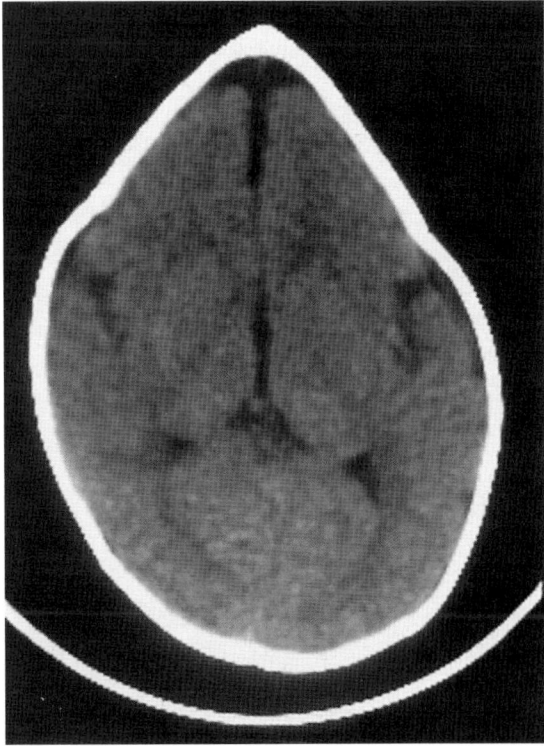

Figure 40.30 Axial computerised tomography scan showing severe trigonocephaly due to premature fusion of the metopic suture.

CHAPTER 40 | ELECTIVE NEUROSURGERY

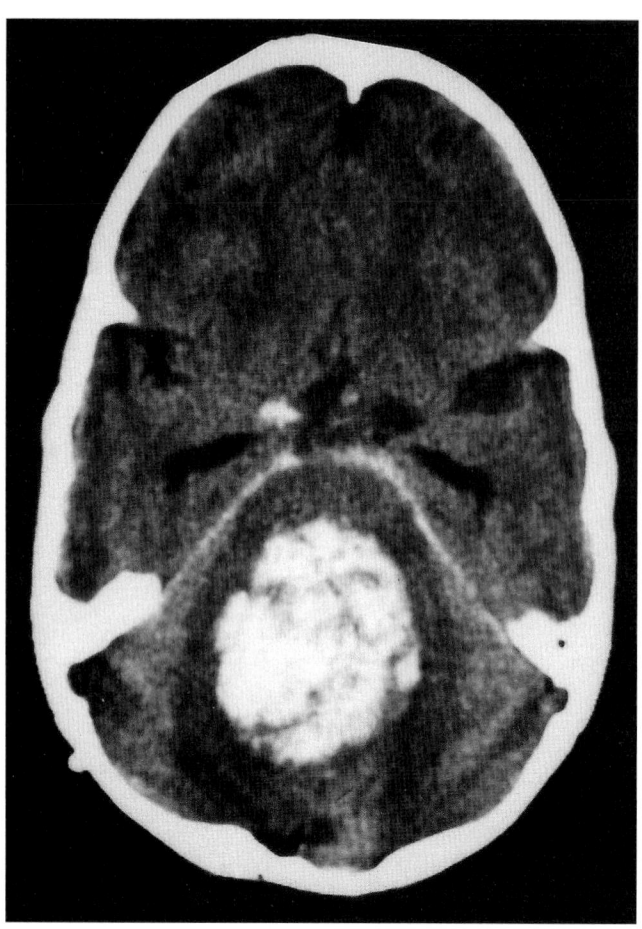

Figure 40.31 Axial computerised tomography scan showing a fatal posterior fossa haematoma.

FURTHER READING

Ganong, W.F. (2005) *Review of Medical Physiology*, 22nd edn. McGraw-Hill Medical: Maidenhead.

Kaye, A.H. (2005) *Essential Neurosurgery*, 3rd edn. Blackwell Publishing: Oxford.

Kiernan, J.A. (2005) *Barr's The Human Nervous System: An Anatomical Viewpoint*. Lippincott, Williams and Wilkins: Baltimore.

Lindsay, K.W. and Bone, I. (1999) *Neurology and Neurosurgery Illustrated*, 4th edn. Churchill Livingstone, London.

Winn, H.R. (2004) *Youman's Neurological Surgery*, 5th edn. Saunders: Philadelphia.

The eye and orbit

To understand and appreciate:
- The common ocular disorders and recognise ophthalmic symptoms and specific signs
- The value of special investigations
- When specialist referral is appropriate

OCULAR ANATOMY

Adnexae

The lids comprise skin, connective tissue, the orbicularis oculi (VIIth nerve) and the tarsal plate, with multiple meibomian glands opening posterior to the lashes and lined with conjunctiva, which is reflected onto the sclera. The upper lid is elevated by the levator muscle (IIIrd nerve) and has a horizontal strip of sympathetically innervated Müller's muscle, giving rise to 2 mm of ptosis in Horner's syndrome. Both lids are attached to the orbital rim by the medial and lateral canthal tendons. Both have a rich vascular supply and are innervated by V1 above and V2 below.

Lacrimal system

The almond-shaped lacrimal gland lies under the upper outer orbital rim and opens into the upper conjunctival fornix through 10–15 ducts. Tears are swept across the globe by the lids and evaporate or pass into the upper and lower lid puncta, and then into the canaliculi to join the common canaliculus, which passes into the lacrimal sac under the medial canthal tendon. The sac is drained by the nasolacrimal duct into the nose, opening in the inferior meatus under the inferior turbinate.

The globe (Fig. 41.1)

The cornea is the 12 mm-diameter window of the eye, 0.5 mm thick centrally; its clarity is due to the regular arrangement of collagen bundles and relative dehydration. It merges into the sclera at the corneoscleral junction (the limbus), the insertion of the bulbar conjunctiva. The sclera, which is 1 mm thick, comprises four-fifths of the wall of the eye, and gives attachment to the extraocular muscles. It is perforated by the long and short posterior ciliary arteries and the vortex veins and is contiguous with the optic nerve sheath. The uvea comprises iris, ciliary body and vascular choroid. The optic nerve is continuous with the retina and retinal pigment epithelium. The most sensitive part of the retina, the macula, lies

at the posterior pole within the vascular arcade. The biconvex lens and capsule are suspended by the suspensory ligament, over 300 tiny fibres attached to the ciliary muscle. Aqueous humour arises from the ciliary processes, hydrates the vitreous gel, passes through the pupil into the anterior chamber between the iris and the cornea and then drains out through Schlemm's canal in the drainage angle. The inner retina is supplied by the central retinal artery and drained by the central retinal vein.

Orbit

The orbit is four-sided and pyramidal in structure, housing the globe, optic nerve, the four rectus and two oblique muscles, the

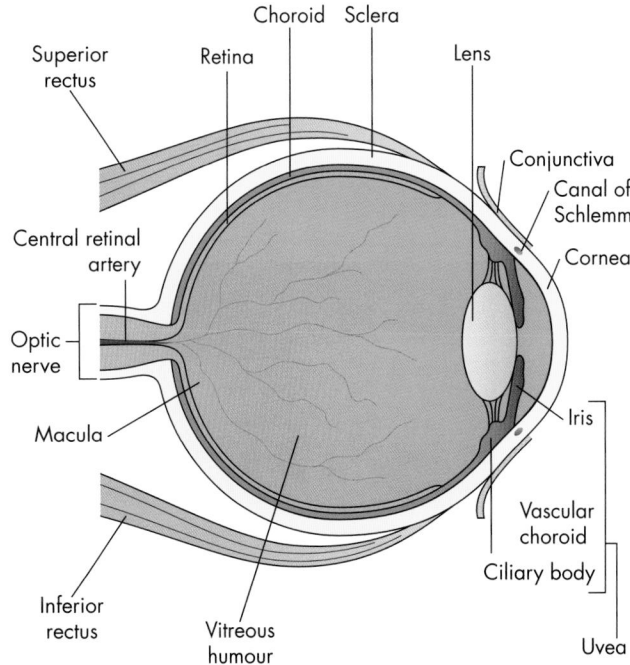

Figure 41.1 Anatomy of the eye.

Labels: Choroid Sclera Retina Lens Superior rectus Conjunctiva Canal of Schlemm Cornea Central retinal artery Optic nerve Iris Macula Vascular choroid Ciliary body Inferior rectus Vitreous humour Uvea

Johannes Peter Müller, **1801–1858, Professor of Anatomy and Physiology, Berlin, Germany.**
Johan Friedrich Horner, **1831–1886, Professor of Ophthalmology, Zurich, Switzerland, described this syndrome in 1869.**

Friedrich Schlemm, **1795–1858, Professor of Anatomy, Berlin, Germany.**

lacrimal gland, orbital fat, the IIIrd, IVth, Vth and VIth cranial nerves, the ophthalmic artery with its tributaries and the ophthalmic veins, which anastamose anteriorly with the face and posteriorly with the cranial cavity. Above is the frontal lobe of the brain, temporally the temporal fossa, inferiorly the maxillary sinus and nasally the lacrimal sac and ethmoidal and sphenoidal air sinuses. The optic nerve passes through the optic canal to the chiasm, with other nerves and vessels passing through the superior ophthalmic fissure.

PERIORBITAL AND ORBITAL SWELLINGS

Swellings related to the supraorbital margin

Dermoid cysts

Dermoid cysts are usually external angular cysts although they may occur medially (Fig. 41.2). They often cause a bony depression by their pressure and they may have a dumbbell extension into the orbit. They can also erode the orbital plate of the frontal bone to become attached to dura and for this reason it is important to image the area by computerised tomography (CT) before excision.

Neurofibromatosis

Neurofibromatosis may also produce swellings above the eye. The diagnosis can usually be confirmed by an examination of the whole body, as there are often multiple lesions. Proptosis can also result (Fig. 41.3). Other ophthalmic features may be present.

Swellings of the lids

Meibomian cysts (chalazion)

These are the most common lid swellings (Fig. 41.4). A meibomian cyst is a chronic granulomatous inflammation of a meibomian gland. It may occur on either upper or lower lids and presents as a smooth, painless swelling. It can be felt by rolling the cyst on the tarsal plate. It can be distinguished from a stye (hordeolum), which is an infection of a hair follicle and is usually painful. Persistent meibomian cysts are treated by incision and curettage from the conjunctival surface. Styes are treated by antibiotics and local heat.

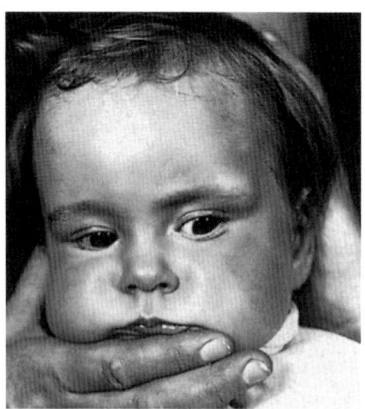

Figure 41.2 External angular dermoid.

Heinrich Meibom (Meibomius), **1638–1700, Professor of Medicine, History and Poetry, Helmstadt, Germany, described these glands in 1666.**

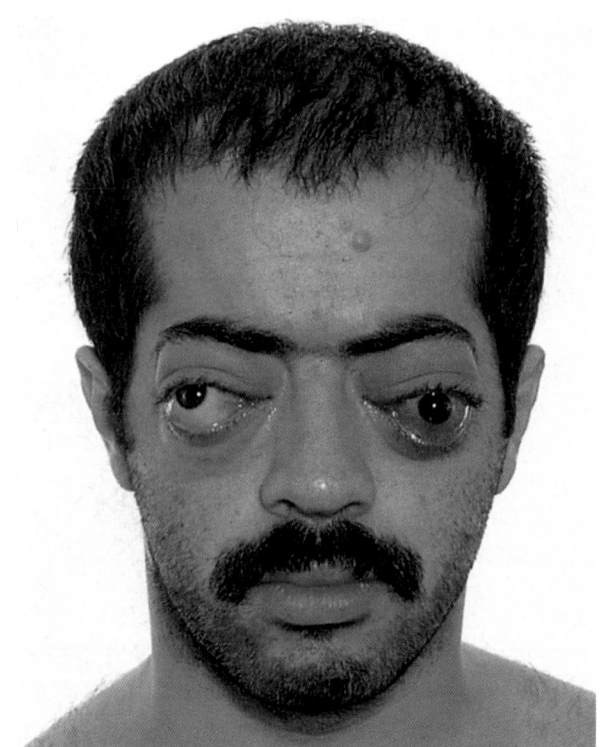

Figure 41.3 Neurofibroma in the orbit with proptosis, and also similar lesions in the forehead.

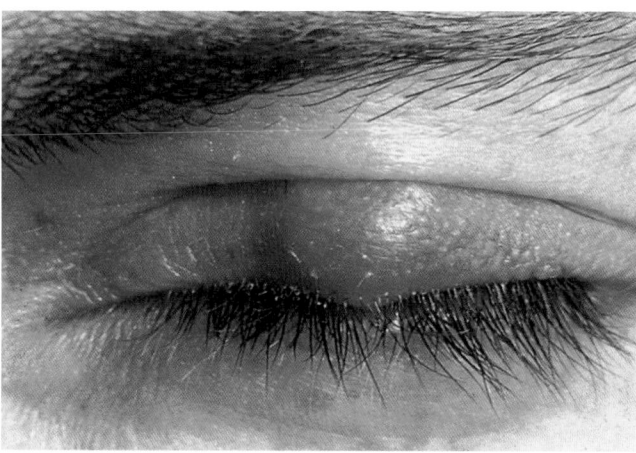

Figure 41.4 Meibomian cyst (courtesy of Mr D. Spalton, FRCS).

Basal cell carcinomas (rodent ulcers)

This is the most common malignant tumour of the eyelids (Fig. 41.5). It is locally malignant, is more common on the lower lids and usually starts as a small pimple that ulcerates and has raised edges. It is easily excised in the early stages. Histological confirmation that the excision is complete is required. More extensive lesions may require specialist techniques such as Mohs' micrographic surgical excision controlled by frozen section. Local radiotherapy or cryotherapy can be carried out; however, recurrence is more common, more aggressive and more difficult to detect (Summary box 41.1).

Frederic E. Mohs, **a 20th century American Surgeon.**

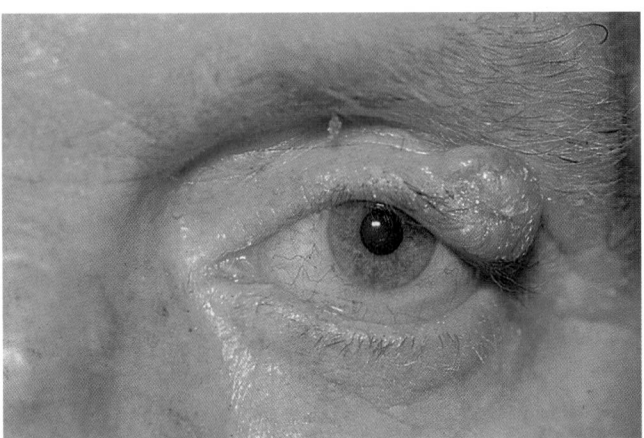

Figure 41.5 Rodent ulcers (courtesy of Mr J. Beare, FRCS).

Other lid swellings

Other types of lid swelling can occur but they are less common. They include sebaceous cysts, papillomas, keratoacanthomas, cysts of Moll (sweat glands) (Fig. 41.6) or Zeis (sebaceous glands) and molluscum contagiosum. When molluscum contagiosum occurs on the lid margin, it can give rise to a mild chronic kerato-conjunctivitis and should be curetted or excised.

Carcinoma of the meibomian glands and rhabdomyosarcomas are rare lesions; they need to be treated by radical excision. Atypical or meibomian cysts that recur should be biopsied.

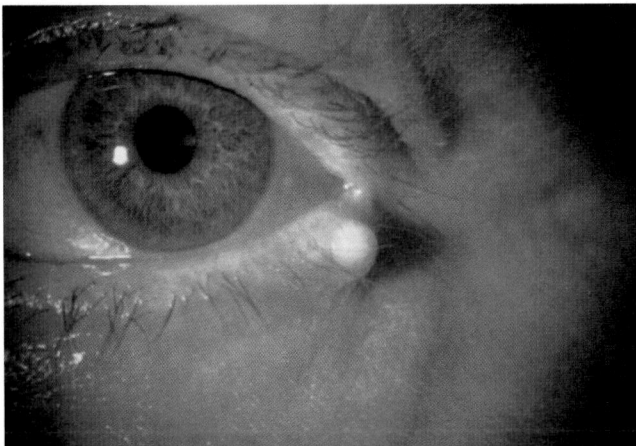

Figure 41.6 Cyst of Moll.

Jacob Antonius Moll, **1832–1913, Ophthalmologist of The Hague, The Netherlands.** Edward Zeis, **1807–1868, Professor of Surgery, Marburg, (1844–1850), who later worked at Dresden, Germany, described these glands in 1835.**

Swellings of the lacrimal system

Lacrimal sac mucocele

This occurs from obstruction of the lacrimal duct beyond the sac and results in a fluctuant swelling that bulges out just below the medial canthus. It can become infected to give rise to a painful tense swelling (acute dacryocystitis). If untreated it may give rise to a fistula. Treatment is by performing a bypass operation between the lacrimal sac and the nose [a dacryocystorrhinostomy (DCR)]. Watering of the eye can occur due to eversion of the lower lid (ectropion), which causes loss of contact between the lower punctum and the tear film, or from reflex hypersecretion as a result of irritation of inturning lashes in entropion, and these must be distinguished from a mucocele.

Lacrimal gland tumours

These are swellings of the lacrimal glands, which lie in the upper lateral aspect of the orbit. Eventually they lead to impairment of ocular movements and displacement of the globe forwards, downwards and inwards. Pathologically the tumours resemble parotid tumours and they can be pleomorphic adenomas with or without malignant change, carcinomas or muco-epidermoid tumours.

Orbital swellings

Orbital swellings result in displacement of the globe and limitation of movement. A full description of orbital swellings is outside the realm of this text but some of the most common causes include the following:

- *Pseudoproptosis.* This results from a large eyeball, as seen in congenital glaucoma or high myopia.
- *Orbital inflammatory conditions* that result in orbital cellulitis (Fig. 41.7).
- *Haemorrhage* after trauma or retrobulbar injection.
- *Neoplasia* affecting the lacrimal gland, the optic nerve, the orbital walls or the nasal sinuses, e.g. glioma (neurofibromatosis) (see Fig. 41.3, p. 646), meningioma and osteoma (Fig. 41.8).
- *Dysthyroid exophthalmos* (Figs 41.9–41.11). This may be unrelated to active thyroid disease but can start after thyroidectomy and may need urgent tarsorrhaphy, large doses of steroids or even orbital decompression if the eyeball is threatened by exposure or optic nerve compression. This is most easily done into the nasal sinuses. CT and magnetic resonance imaging (MRI) scans are useful in diagnosis.

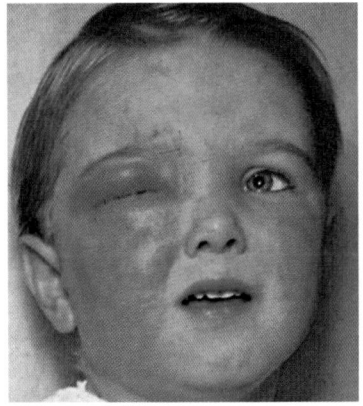

Figure 41.7 Orbital cellulitis.

CHAPTER 41 | THE EYE AND ORBIT

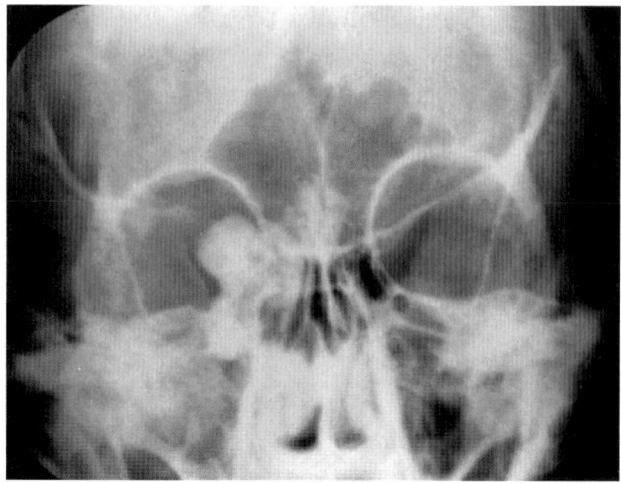

Figure 41.8 Radiograph showing an osteoma on the nasal side of the orbit giving rise to proptosis.

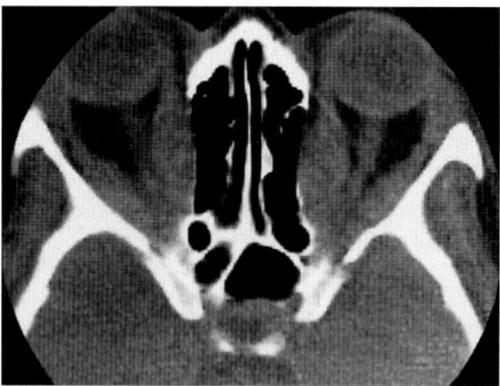

Figure 41.9 Computerised tomogram of the orbit in dysthyroid exophthalmos, showing swollen muscles (courtesy of Dr Glyn Lloyd).

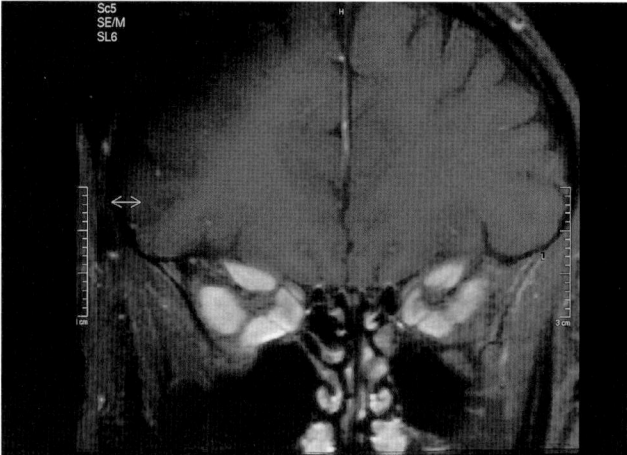

Figure 41.10 Magnetic resonance imaging scan of a coronal view of the orbit, showing enlarged muscles in thyroid disease (courtesy of Dr Juliette Britton).

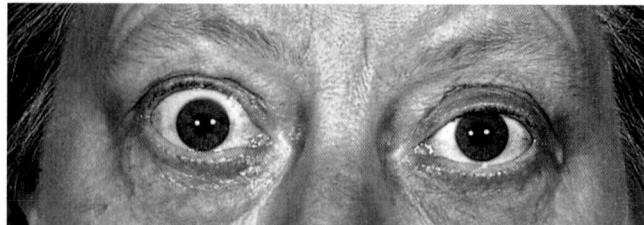

Figure 41.11 Exophthalmos in dysthyroid eye disease.

- *Pseudotumour,* or malignant lymphoma.
- *Haemangiomas* of the orbit (Fig. 41.12).
- *Tumour metastases.* These are rare. In children they usually arise from neuroblastomas of the adrenal gland, whereas in adults the oesophagus, stomach, breast and prostate can be sites of primary lesions.

Diagnostic aids

Diagnostic aids include radiography, CT, MRI, ultrasonography and, less commonly, tomography and orbital venography.

Treatment

Treatment is directed to the cause of the lesion if at all possible, taking care to prevent exposure of the eye, diplopia or visual impairment from optic nerve compression.

INTRAOCULAR TUMOURS

Children

Retinoblastoma is a multicentric malignant tumour of the retina, which can be bilateral. Some are sporadic but many are hereditary. Children with a family history should be carefully monitored from birth. It is often not spotted until the tumour fills the globe and presents as a white reflex in the pupil or as a squint (Fig. 41.13). The differential diagnosis includes retinopathy of prematurity, primary hyperplastic vitreous and intraocular infections. If the tumour is large, enucleation may be required, but radiotherapy, cryotherapy or laser treatment can cure small lesions. Liaison with a paediatric oncologist is essential (Summary box 41.2).

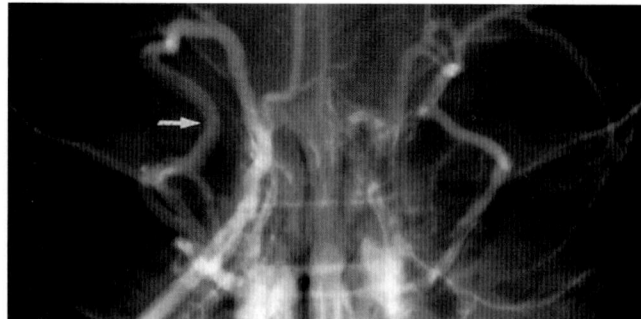

Figure 41.12 Capillary haemangioma in a child. An orbital venogram demonstrates displacement of the second part of the superior ophthalmic vein (arrow) (courtesy of Dr Glyn Lloyd).

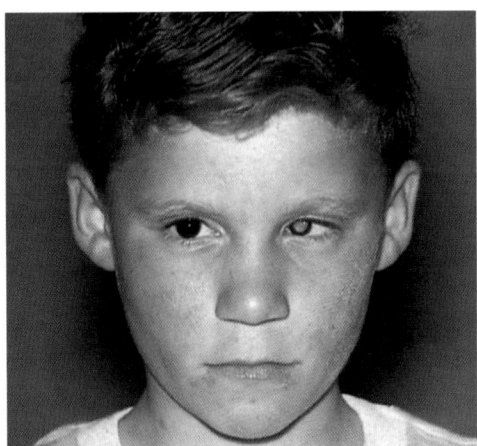

Figure 41.13 Retinoblastoma giving rise to a white pupillary reflex. This child was first seen with a convergent squint and discharged without a fundus examination. He was next seen many years later with a 'white reflex' and died soon after diagnosis (courtesy of M.A. Bedford, FRCS).

Summary box 41.2

Intraocular tumours

- All children with a squint should have a fundal examination to exclude a retinoblastoma
- A blind painful eye may hide a melanoma

Adults

Malignant melanoma is the most common tumour and it originates in the pigment cells of the choroid (Fig. 41.14), ciliary body or iris. It can present with a reduction in vision, a vitreous haemorrhage or by the chance finding of an elevated pigmented lesion in the eye. Tumour growth is variable but, as a general rule, the more posterior the lesion, the more rapidly progressive it is likely to be. Spread may be delayed for many years; however, the liver is frequently involved, hence the advice 'beware of the patient with a glass eye and an enlarged liver'. Treatment is by light or laser

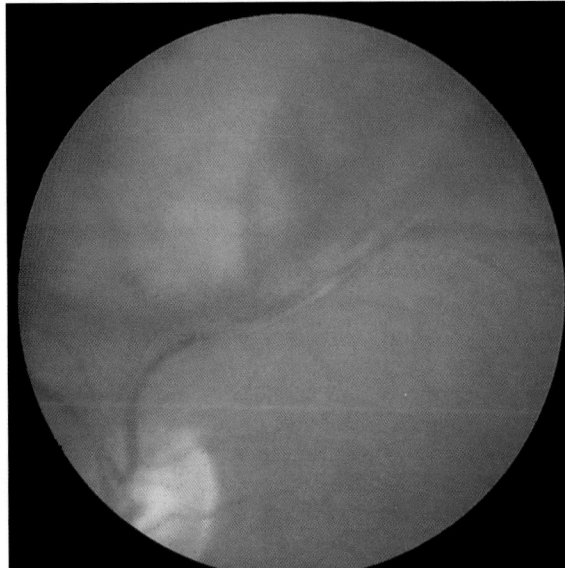

Figure 41.14 Choroidal melanoma.

coagulation, radioactive plaque, radiotherapy, enucleation and, in selected cases, local excision using hypotensive anaesthesia. Diagnosis is made by direct observation and/or ultrasound, which shows a solid tumour (Fig. 41.15).

INJURIES INVOLVING THE EYE AND ADJACENT STRUCTURES

Corneal abrasions and ulceration

The cornea is frequently damaged by direct trauma or by foreign bodies (Fig. 41.16). Ulceration can occur with infection or after damage to the facial nerve. Post-herpetic ulceration is common and serious if not treated. Fluorescein instillation illuminated by blue light shows up corneal ulceration at an early stage (Summary box 41.3).

Summary box 41.3

Corneal abrasions

- A drop of fluorescein dye illuminated by a blue light reveals even the smallest corneal abrasion

---

Treatment is by protection (eye pads, tarsorrhaphy or a bandage contact lens) and antibiotics topically and rarely systemically:

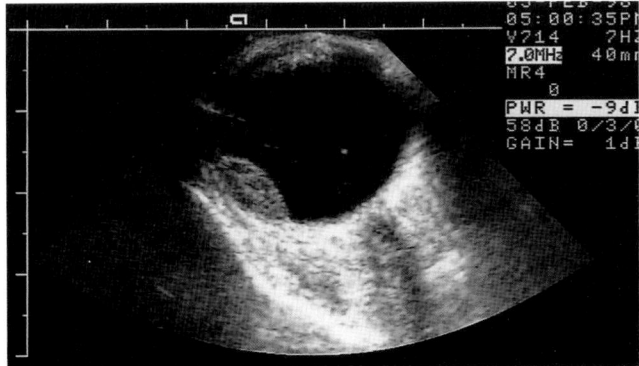

Figure 41.15 B-scan showing choroidal melanoma (courtesy of Dr Marie Reston).

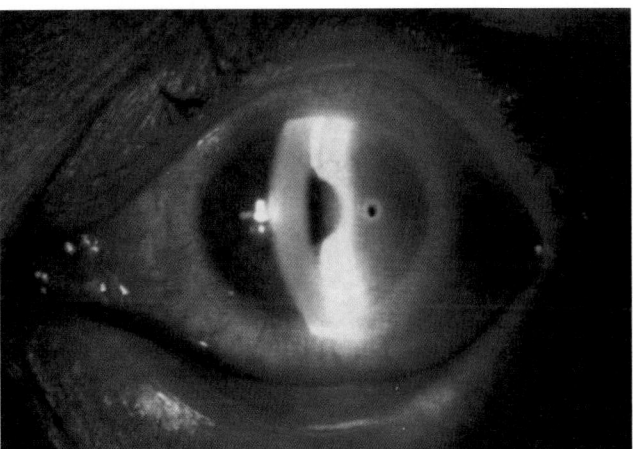

Figure 41.16 Corneal foreign body.

0.5% chloramphenicol or ofloxacin eye drops are commonly used. The eye is made more comfortable by the use of mydriatics such as homatropine or cyclopentolate. Herpes simplex ulcers are treated with aciclovir ointment. In countries in the Far and Middle East, chronic infection with trachoma can cause corneal opacification and blindness. Corneal grafting is the only cure for an opaque cornea. Rarely, osteo-odonto keratoprosthesis can be attempted in very severe cases of opaque corneas that are not suitable for grafting. Acanthamoeba is a rare serious cause of corneal infection. This infection usually follows the use of contact lenses. Specialist management and treatment is recommended.

Blunt injuries to the eye and orbit

The floor of the orbit is its weakest wall and in blunt trauma, such as a blow from a fist, it is often fractured without fractures of the other walls. This is called a blow-out fracture. Clinical signs are enophthalmos, bruising around the orbit, maxillary hypoaesthesia, limitation of upward gaze and diplopia. This occurs when the extraocular muscles or orbital septa become trapped in the fracture and can be identified as a soft-tissue mass in the antrum on a radiograph (Fig. 41.17), although CT scans or tomograms may be necessary. Surgical repair of the orbital floor with freeing of the trapped contents may be necessary if troublesome diplopia persists or enophthalmos is marked. A child with an orbital floor fracture requires urgent assessment as a 'greenstick' fracture can result in ischaemia of a trapped inferior rectus muscle and may require urgent surgery. If an orbital haemorrhage is too extensive to examine the eye, it may be necessary to examine the eye under anaesthesia because there may be a hidden perforation of the globe. Injuries to the lids and lid margins must be repaired, and if the lacrimal canaliculi are damaged they should be repaired if possible, especially the lower canaliculus as 75% of tear drainage goes through it.

Blunt injuries can also cause damage to the optic nerve, which can result in blindness and a total afferent nerve defect (Figs 41.18 and 41.19).

Concussion injuries

Concussion injuries of the eye can give rise to several problems, which include the following:

- *Iritis*. Inflammation, treated with topical steroids.
- *Hyphaema* (blood in the anterior chamber) (Fig. 41.20). Rest and sedation, particularly in children, are advised because the

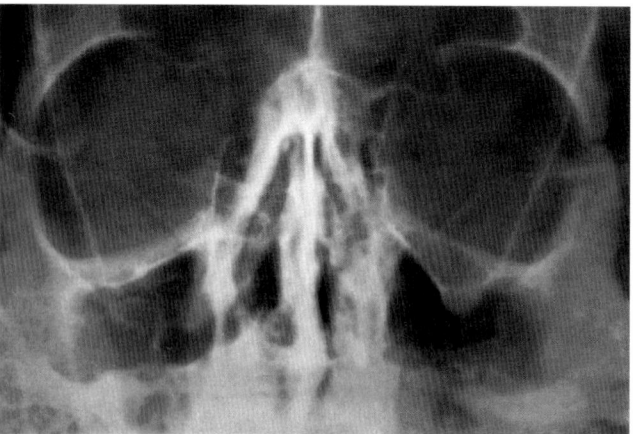

Figure 41.17 Radiograph showing a blow-out fracture of the orbit (left) with soft tissue in the antrum (courtesy of Dr Glyn Lloyd).

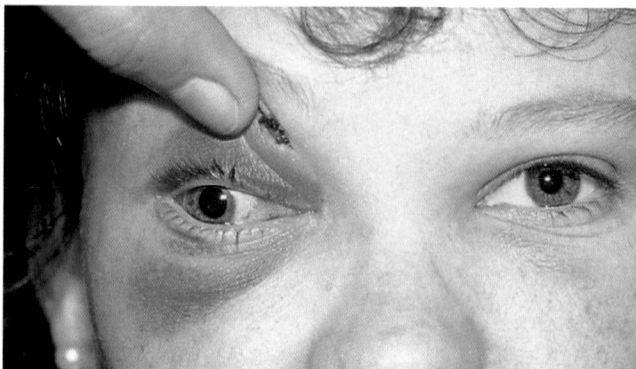

Figure 41.18 Injury from a ski stick into the right brow. Vision reduced to 'no perception of light' (courtesy of J. Beare, FRCS).

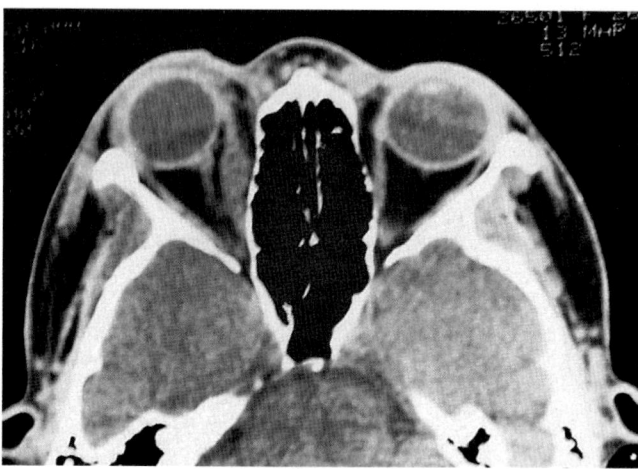

Figure 41.19 Scan of orbit from Fig. 41.18 showing a massive swelling of the medial rectus (courtesy of J. Beare, FRCS).

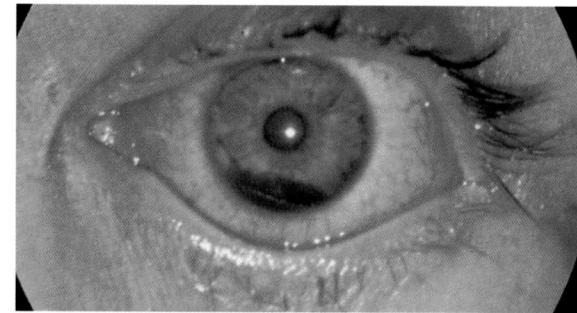

Figure 41.20 Hyphaema. Blood in the vitreous chamber after concussional injury.

main danger in this condition is secondary bleeding, resulting in an acute rise in intraocular pressure and blood staining of the cornea. The use of anti-fibrinolytic agents (ε-aminocaproic acid) has been advocated and, if the pressure rises, surgery to wash out the blood may be necessary.

- *Subluxation of the lens*. This is suspected if the iris, or part of the iris, 'wobbles' on movement (iridodonesis).
- *Secondary glaucoma*. This is often associated with recession of the drainage angle.
- *Retinal and macular haemorrhages and choroidal tears* (Fig. 41.21).

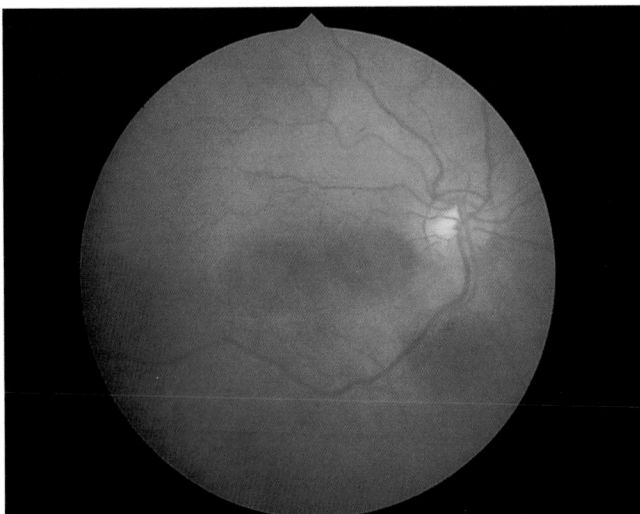

Figure 41.21 Retinal haemorrhage from a cricket bat injury (courtesy of J. Beare, FRCS).

- *Retinal dialysis.* This may lead to a retinal detachment and permanent damage to vision (Fig. 41.22).

Penetrating eye injuries

These occur when the globe is penetrated, often in road traffic and other major accidents (Fig. 41.23), and also in injuries from sharp instruments. The compulsory wearing of seatbelts in motor vehicles has substantially reduced the incidence of this type of eye injury, by up to 73% in the UK. The presence of an irregular pupil suggests prolapse of the iris and should arouse the suspicion of a penetrating injury. Treatment is prompt primary repair to restore the integrity of the globe. If a perforation is suspected, extensive eye examination should not be attempted before anaesthesia because this may lead to further extrusion of the intraocular contents. If the fundal view is poor, ultrasonography and orbital imaging are indicated. Secondary corneal grafting, lensectomy and vitrectomy have considerably improved the visual prognosis; these must be done by an experienced eye surgeon. Injuries to the optic nerves must also be excluded in severe accidents.

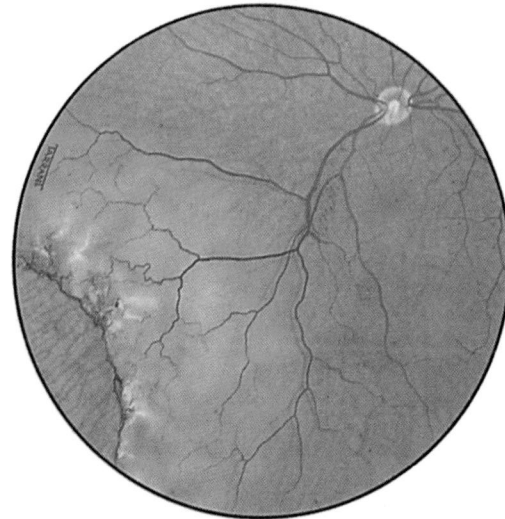

Figure 41.22 Retinal dialysis after concussional injury.

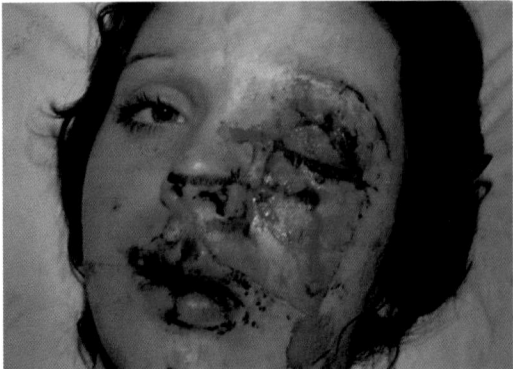

Figure 41.23 Facial lacerations from a windscreen injury. Beware of a perforating eye injury.

Intraocular foreign bodies

Intraocular foreign bodies must always be excluded when patients attend the accident and emergency department with an eye injury and a history of working with a hammer and chisel or a history of a potentially high-velocity injury. Radiography of the orbits should always be performed, and ferrous and copper foreign bodies should always be removed. B-scan ultrasonography can also assist in localising foreign bodies when a vitreous haemorrhage or cataract is present. CT can be used, but MRI is contraindicated (Summary box 41.4).

Summary box 41.4

Penetrating eye injuries

- A distorted and irregular pupil warrants the careful exclusion of a penetrating eye injury

---

Burns

Radiation burns

These occur after exposure to ultraviolet radiation after arc welding or excessive sunlight (snow blindness) and sun lamps. Such burns cause intense pain and photophobia as a result of keratitis, which starts some hours after exposure. Mydriatic and local steroids with antibiotic drops ease the condition, and healing usually occurs after 24 hours.

Thermal burns

If these involve the full thickness of the lids, corneal scarring may occur from exposure, and immediate corneal protection is necessary. A splash of molten metal may cause marked local necrosis and may lead to permanent corneal scarring. Treatment is to remove any debris by irrigation and to instill local atropine, antibiotics and steroids to prevent superadded infection and scarring. Lid reconstruction may be necessary.

Chemical burns

Chemical burns, and especially alkali burns, can be serious because ocular penetration occurs quickly and ischaemic necrosis can result (Fig. 41.24). Immediate irrigation until the pH is neutral will ensure that the chemical is diluted as much as possible, and all particles should be removed from the fornices. Treatment can then be continued as with thermal burns. Well-fitting goggles should prevent such injuries.

CHAPTER 41 | THE EYE AND ORBIT

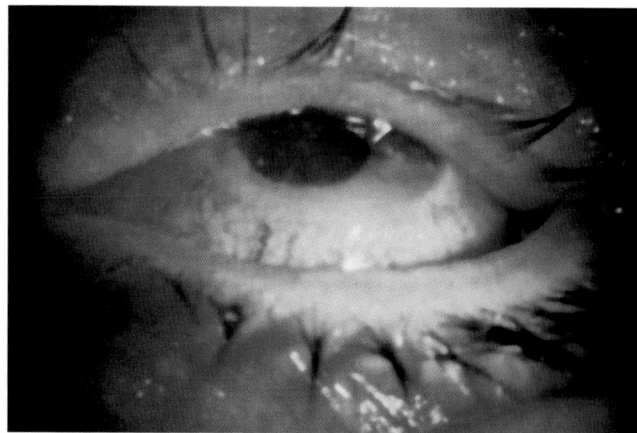

Figure 41.24 Chemical burn showing conjunctival necrosis.

DIFFERENTIAL DIAGNOSIS OF THE ACUTE RED EYE

This is important in the management of minor ocular complaints and the recognition of conditions that require expert attention. Possible causes of the acute red eye include:

- subconjunctival haemorrhage;
- conjunctivitis;
- keratitis;
- uveitis;
- episcleritis and scleritis;
- acute glaucoma.

Any condition with pain, visual impairment or a pupil abnormality suggests a more serious diagnosis.

Subconjunctival haemorrhage

This presents as a bright-red eye, often noticed incidentally with only minimal discomfort and normal vision. Causes include coughing, sneezing, minor trauma, hypertension and, rarely, a bleeding disorder. Reassurance and treatment of the underlying cause are required.

Conjunctivitis

Symptoms are grittiness, redness and discharge. Causes are infective, chemical, allergic or traumatic. In the newborn it can be serious; gonococcal and chlamydial infection must be excluded. Bacterial conjunctivitis is common, purulent, usually self-limiting and treated with topical broad-spectrum antibiotics. Chlamydial and adenovirus infections must be considered. Adenoviral infections usually affect one eye much more in severity and onset, tending to be more watery than sticky, and are often associated with a palpable preauricular gland.

Vernal conjunctivitis (Fig. 41.25) is a form of allergic conjunctivitis, usually worse in the spring and early summer and often associated with other allergic problems such as hay fever. Clinically, most signs are under the upper lid, which may have a cobblestone appearance instead of a smooth surface.

Giant pupillary conjunctivitis with large papillae under the upper lid may be seen in soft contact lens wearers. This is usually caused by an allergy to the sterilising solutions and may be helped by either using a preservative-free solution or using daily-wear disposable lenses.

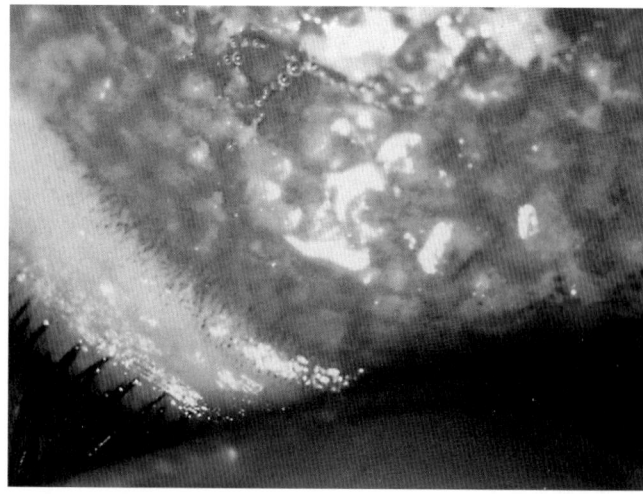

Figure 41.25 Vernal conjunctivitis (spring catarrh) showing cobblestone appearance under the upper lid.

Kaposi's sarcoma can rarely present like a subconjunctival haemorrhage (Fig. 41.26).

Considerable conjunctival irritation can be caused by the lids turning in (entropion) (Fig. 41.27) or turning out (ectropion)

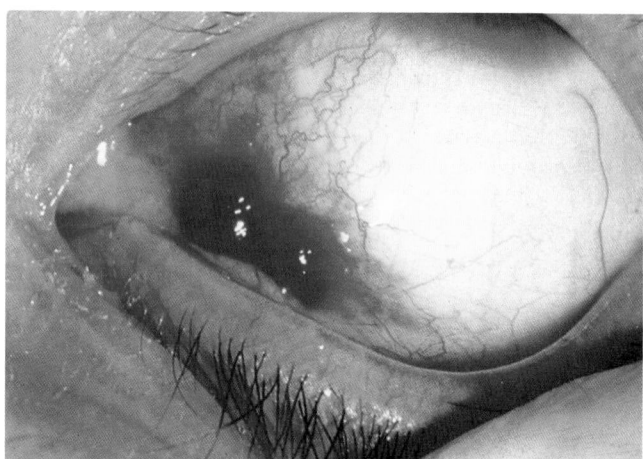

Figure 41.26 Kaposi's sarcoma of conjunctiva.

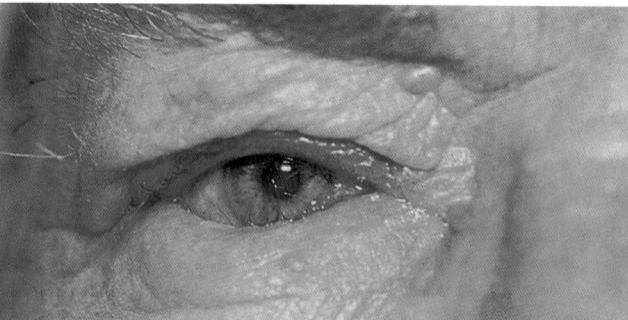

Figure 41.27 Entropion (courtesy of J. Beare, FRCS).

Moritz Kaposi, 1837–1902, Professor of Dermatology, Vienna, Austria, described pigmented sarcoma of the skin in 1872.

(Figs 41.28 and 41.29), and by ingrowing lashes. The lids should be repaired surgically to their normal position.

Vision is not commonly affected in conjunctivitis but, with some viral infections, a keratitis may be present and result in visual impairment and pain. All of the other conditions are painful and usually affect vision.

Keratitis (inflammation of the cornea)

Herpes simplex infection is the most serious cause of an acute red eye and presents as a dendritic (branching) ulcer, shown easily by staining with fluorescein or Bengal Rose. It is treated with aciclovir ointment five times per day. The use of steroid drops must be avoided as this can make the condition much worse (Fig. 41.30).

Corneal ulceration may occur as a result of ingrowing lashes or corneal foreign bodies, marginal ulceration and infected abrasions. Infected ulcers can occur in patients wearing soft contact lenses. Herpes zoster (shingles) may affect the ophthalmic division of the Vth nerve and can give rise to a keratitis and uveitis. It is important to avoid the use of steroid drops until a diagnosis has been made. Local anaesthetic drops should also not be given on a regular basis.

Uveitis

This can be anterior (iritis) or, more rarely, posterior. In anterior uveitis, the pupil will be small, sometimes irregular, there is

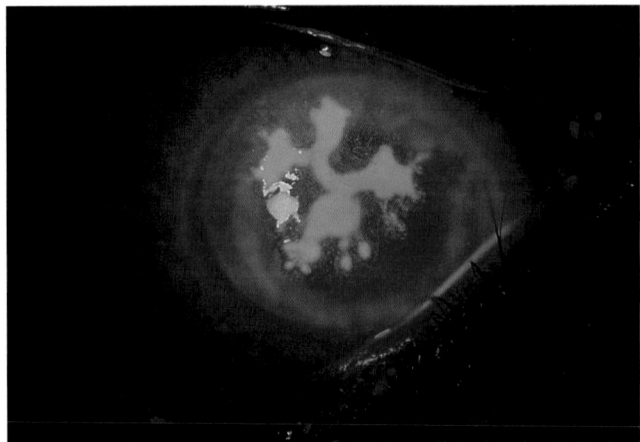

Figure 41.30 Dendritic staining caused by herpes keratitis.

circumcorneal injection and there may be keratic precipitates present on the posterior surface of the cornea. Pain, photophobia and some visual loss are usually present. Posterior uveitis can present with a white eye and blurred vision. It usually takes a chronic course. Granulomatous diseases, Behçet's disease, Reiter's syndrome, toxoplasmosis and cytomegalovirus infection should be excluded. Topical systemic steroids and, sometimes, immunosuppressive drugs are useful in treating these conditions.

Episcleritis and scleritis

Episcleritis or inflammation of the episcleral tissue often occurs as an idiopathic condition (Fig. 41.31).

Scleritis is a less common, more serious, condition in which the deeper sclera is involved. There is often an associated uveitis and severe pain. Thinning of the sclera may result. Systemic non-steroidal anti-inflammatory drugs (NSAIDs) or steroids may be required to treat the condition adequately.

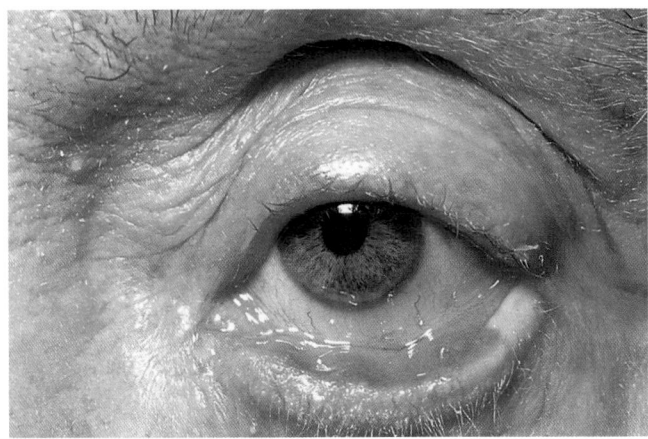

Figure 41.28 Ectropion, lower lid (courtesy of J. Beare, FRCS).

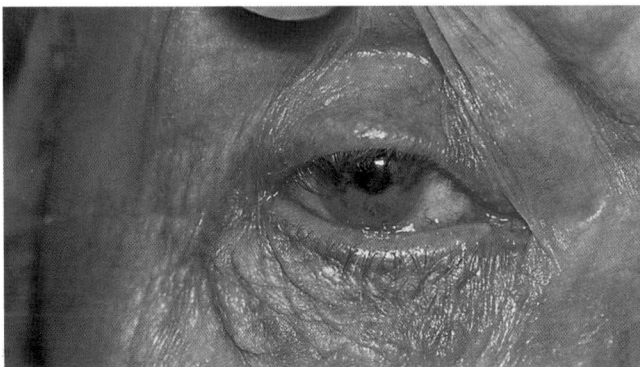

Figure 41.29 Ectropion, upper lid – chronic staphylococcal infection (courtesy of J. Beare, FRCS).

Bengal Rose, (or Rose Bengal) is Dichlortetraiodofluorescein.

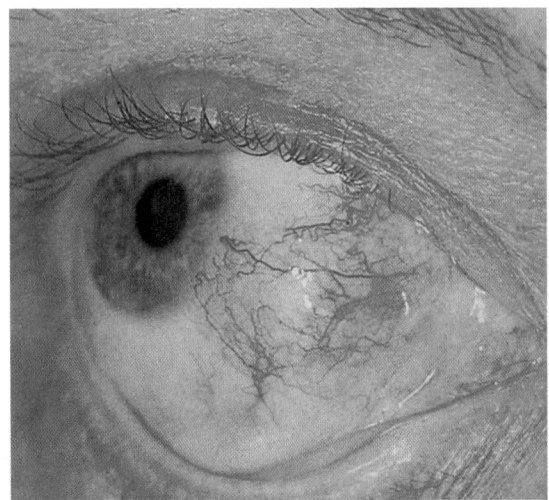

Figure 41.31 Episcleritis.

Hulusi Behçet, 1889–1948, Professor of Dermatology, Istanbul, Turkey, described this disease in 1937.
Hans Conrad Julius Reiter, 1881–1968, President of the Health Service, and Honorary Professor of Hygiene at the University of Berlin, Germany, described this disease in 1916.

Scleritis is often associated with severe rheumatoid conditions. The presence of scleritis suggests that there is active systemic disease and it requires systemic work-up including renal function tests.

Acute glaucoma

This usually occurs in older, often hypermetropic, patients. The cornea becomes hazy, the pupil oval and dilated, the vision poor and the eye feels hard. In severe cases pain may be accompanied by vomiting and the condition can be mistaken for an acute abdominal problem. Tonometry (intraocular measurement) is diagnostic. Urgent treatment to reduce the pressure with pilocarpine, acetazolamide and, if refractory, mannitol should be started, followed by a surgical iridectomy or laser iridotomy. The condition is usually bilateral and the second eye usually needs a prophylactic iridotomy at the same time.

Except for a simple conjunctivitis and subconjunctival haemorrhage, which are self-limiting, the management of an acute red eye requires expert treatment and a specialist opinion should be sought. A painful eye with a IIIrd nerve palsy often signifies an intracranial aneurysm and should be investigated immediately.

PAINLESS LOSS OF VISION

This may occur in one or both eyes, and the visual loss may be transient or permanent. Possible causes are:

- obstruction of the central retinal artery (Fig. 41.32);
- obstruction of the central retinal vein (Fig. 41.33);
- cranial arteritis;
- ischaemic optic neuropathy;
- migraine and other vascular causes;
- retrobulbar neuritis and papillitis;
- vitreous and retinal haemorrhages;
- retinal detachment (Fig. 41.34);
- macular hole, cyst or haemorrhage;
- cystoid macular oedema, often after surgery;
- hysterical blindness;
- cataract;
- glaucoma;
- macular degeneration.

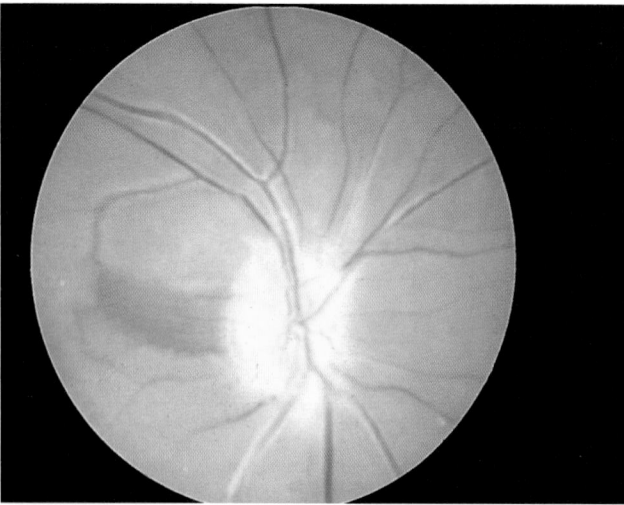

Figure 41.32 Retinal artery occlusion.

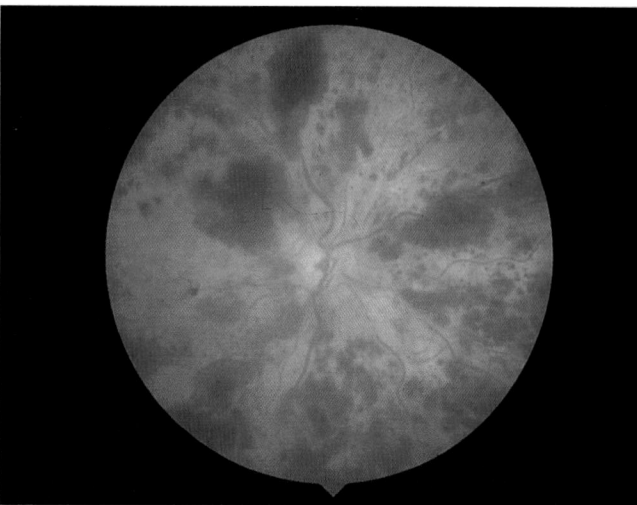

Figure 41.33 Central retinal vein occlusion.

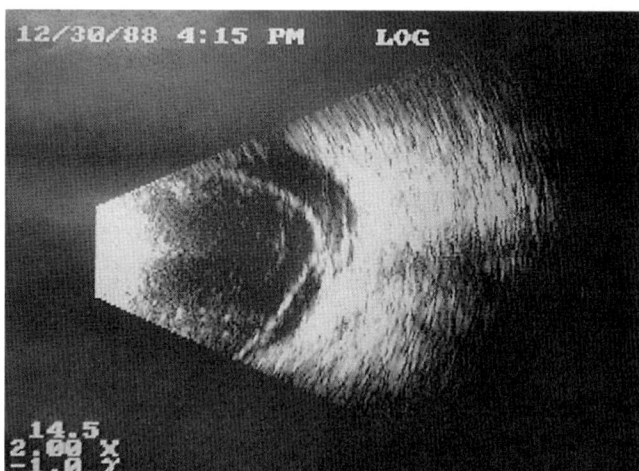

Figure 41.34 B-scan of a retinal detachment.

Specialist help should be sought in any case of loss of vision. The erythrocyte sedimentation rate and C-reactive protein should be measured immediately if cranial arteritis is suspected, and the carotid system should be examined for bruits and other signs of arteriosclerosis in cases of ischaemic optic neuropathy and central retinal artery occlusion. Glaucoma, hypertension, hyperviscosity syndromes and diabetes should be looked for in cases of central vein thrombosis.

RECENT DEVELOPMENTS IN EYE SURGERY

In the last two decades, eye surgery has become a microsurgical specialty. Cataract surgery has been transformed by changes in local anaesthesia, implants, phakoemulsification and small-incision surgery, which allows compressible silicone or acrylic implants to be inserted through a 3-mm incision. The implant power can be more accurately measured by new formulae and the use of A-scan ultrasonography or laser wavefront biometry, and multifocal and accommodative lenses are now available.

There are new treatments for eye disorders that involve abnormal growth of blood vessels in the back of the eye, such as the wet form of age-related macular degeneration. Photodynamic therapy involves the activation of the drug verteporfin in a localised area of the eye using a laser. Antivascular endothelial antibodies such as the drug ranibizumab may be injected directly into the vitreous cavity to reduce new vessel proliferation.

Developments in vitreous surgery have enabled membranes to be peeled off the retina and macular holes to be repaired, and have also increased the success rate in retinal detachment surgery with the additional use of gases and silicone oil or heavy liquid inserted into the vitreous cavity tamponading the retina.

Some paralytic squints can be helped by the use of adjustable sutures or injections of botulinum toxin into the overacting muscles. Refractive errors can be treated either by surgery (arcuate or radial keratotomy) or by the excimer laser. These can be combined with laser *in situ* keratomeilusis (LASIK) surgery, which involves cutting a corneal flap and performing the laser surgery at a deeper level. There have been some concerns about defective contrast sensitivity and problems with night vision after laser correction of myopia. Phakic implants have also been used to correct high refractive errors. Corneal topography aids the accuracy of corneal and refractive surgery and the increased use and quality of CT and MRI scans has revolutionised the diagnosis of orbital and intracranial lesions involving the optic pathways (Figs 41.35–41.37). Fluorescein angiography, indocyanine green angiography, and the scanning laser opthalmoscope (SLO) are invaluable in the diagnosis and treatment of macular conditions. The glaucoma detection (GDx) retinal nerve fibre analyser and Heidelberg retinal tomography (HRT) are increasingly used in the diagnosis and management of glaucoma.

LASERS IN OPHTHALMOLOGY

These were originally used for coagulation. The ruby laser was superseded by the argon blue–green laser and then the argon green-only laser, as the blue light was dangerous both to the operator and to the patient's macula. Yellow and red wavelengths are also used and the doubled-frequency doubled yttrium–aluminium–garnet (YAG) laser can be used as a coagulator with a wavelength of 533 nM. The photodisruptive YAG laser was developed together with extracapsular surgery and is used for

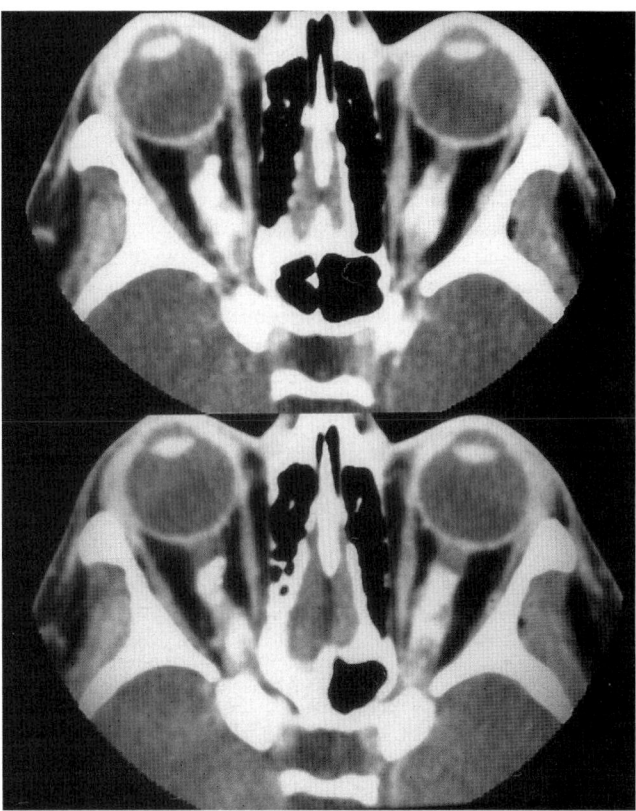

Figure 41.36 High-resolution computerised tomography through the orbits showing dense calcification of the optic nerve sheaths typical of optic nerve meningioma (courtesy of Dr Juliette Britton).

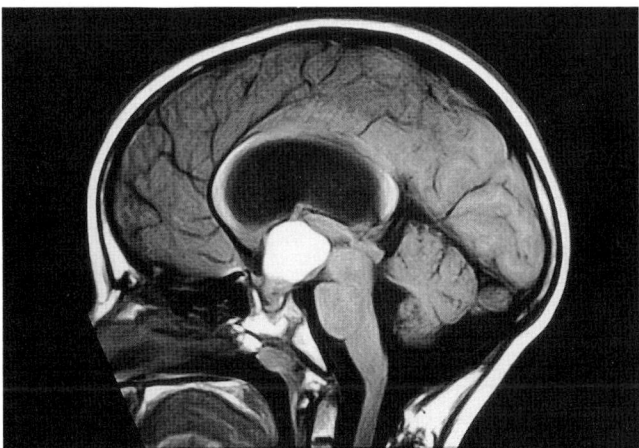

Figure 41.35 Magnetic resonance imaging scan, sagittal view. Craniopharyngioma. The mass in the suprasellar cistern is of high signal intensity because of the proteinaceous fluid that the cyst contains (courtesy of Dr Juliette Britton).

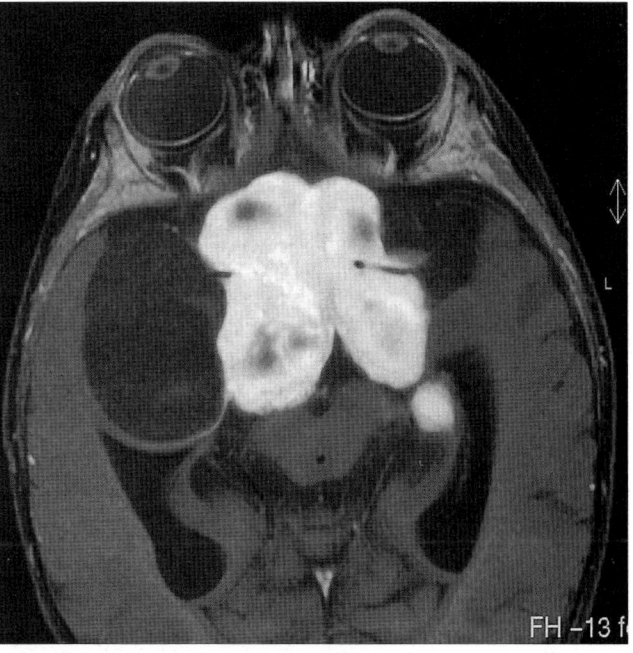

Figure 41.37 Axial enhanced magnetic resonance imaging scan showing a mass involving the optic chiasma and extending down the optic nerves and tracts.

CHAPTER 41 | THE EYE AND ORBIT

capsulotomies, iridotomies and cutting anterior vitreous bands. In continuous mode it can be used to treat severe glaucomas.

Holmium and erbium lasers have been used to create subconjunctival drainage in glaucoma; the potassium–titanyl–phosphate (KTP) and holmium lasers can also be used in lacrimal obstruction during endoscopic DCR operations. CO_2 lasers are used to remove external lesions of the eyelids, and photoablative excimer lasers are used for refractive surgery. The diode laser can be used both as a retinal photocoagulator and for treating the ciliary body in advanced cases of glaucoma. Lasers combined with phakoemulsification to liquefy the human lens are being developed. Laser technology is advancing and new forms of lasers will be developed for use in the assessment, diagnosis and management of eye disorders.

SURGICAL PROCEDURES

Excision of an eyeball

Indications include a blind, painful eye, a blind, cosmetically poor eye, intraocular neoplasm and, in cadavers, for use in corneal grafting.

The operation

The speculum is introduced between the lids and opened. The conjuctiva is picked up with toothed forceps and divided completely all round as near as possible to the cornea. Tenon's capsule is entered and each of the rectus tendons is hooked up on a strabismus hook and divided close to the sclera. The speculum is now pressed backwards and the eyeball projects forwards. Blunt scissors, curved on the flat, are insinuated on the inner side of the globe, and these are used to sever the optic nerve. The eyeball can now be drawn forwards with the forceps, and the oblique muscles, together with any other strands of tissue that are still attaching the globe to the orbit, are divided. A swab, moistened with hot water and pressed into the orbit, will control the haemorrhage. If an orbital implant is inserted to give better eye movement, the muscles are sutured to the implant at the appropriate sites. The subconjunctival tissues and conjunctiva are closed in layers.

Evisceration of an eyeball

Evisceration is preferred to excision in panophthalmitis, minimising the risk of orbital and intracranial spread with meningitis. The sclera is transfixed with a pointed knife a little behind the corneosclerotic junction, and the cornea is removed entirely by completing the encircling incision in the sclera. The contents of the globe are then removed with a curette, care being exercised to remove all of the uveal tract. At the end of the operation the interior must appear perfectly white. A ball orbital implant made of acrylic or hydroxyapatite is placed within the orbit behind the sclera to improve the appearance when the artificial eye is fitted.

Incision and curettage of chalazion (meibomian cyst)

The lid margin is everted to allow the application of a meibomian clamp. The ring of the clamp is placed on the palpebral conjunctiva with the granuloma in the centre. An incision is made with a small blade in the axis of the gland. The herniating granulomatous tissue is removed with a curette and the cavity is scraped clean. Recurrent cysts may have to have the cyst wall dissected away with scissors. A biopsy may be necessary in atypical or recurrent cysts to exclude malignant change.

ACQUIRED IMMUNODEFICIENCY SYNDROME AND THE EYE

Kaposi's sarcomas, purplish or brown non-pruritic nodules or macules, are a frequent early manifestation of acquired immunodeficiency syndrome (AIDS). Commonly affecting the face, especially the tip of the nose, the lesions may involve the eyelids and the conjunctiva. They respond to chemotherapy and so excision is not usually necessary.

Fundus lesions are 'non-infective' or 'infective'. The non-infective retinopathy is a microangiopathy consisting of cotton wool spots and blot haemorrhages. These fade over several weeks and do not affect vision. The most common infective retinitis is caused by cytomegalovirus (CMV). The retinal lesions are irregular areas of white necrosis and associated scattered haemorrhages. The appearance is likened to a 'pizza pie'. The borders of the lesions expand as a 'brushfire', leaving behind an atropic pigmented retina. CMV retinitis is progressive and the lesions expand over a few months so that the entire retina is involved over a period of about 6 months, causing absolute blindness.

Treatment is with a course of ganciclovir or foscarnet given intravenously. Both drugs can be injected directly into the vitreous. Long-term maintenance therapy is essential to prevent further progression. A Vitrasert is a ganciclovir slow-release implant that is surgically inserted into the vitreal cavity and anchored to the sclera. It is effective in preventing progression for 9 months.

The other retinal infections are rare and include toxoplasmosis, *Pneumocystis*, *Candida*, *Cryptococcus*, herpes zoster and syphilis.

The most effective treatment of CMV retinitis and all retinal infections is the recovery of the patient's immunocompetence. This can be achieved using anti-retroviral drug combinations against human immunodeficiency virus (HIV). When the patient's immunity is restored, the retinitis becomes atrophic. Reduced vision is permanent.

Neuro-ophthalmological complications in AIDS have been reported, most frequently as nerve palsies associated with intracranial infections with cryptococci and toxoplasmosis, or as a manifestation of an intracranial lymphoma.

FURTHER READING

Findlay, R.D. and Payne, P.A.G. (1997) *The Eye in General Practice*, 10th edn. Butterworth-Heinemann, Oxford.

Kanski, J. (2007) *Clinical Ophthalmology: A Systematic Approach*, 6th edn. Butterworth-Heinemann, Oxford.

Kline, L.B. and Bajandas, F.J. (2003) *Neuro-Ophthalmology Review Manual*, 5th edn. Slack Incorporated, NJ, USA.

Olver, J. and Cassidy, L. (2005) *Ophthalmology at a Glance*. Blackwell Publishing, Oxford.

Wills Eye Hospital (2004) *The Wills Eye Manual: Office and Emergency Room Diagnosis and Treatment of Eye Disease*, 4th edn. Lippincott Williams & Wilkins, Philadelphia, PA.

Jacques Rene Tenon, **1724–1816, Surgeon, La Salpêtrière, Paris, France.**

Cleft lip and palate: developmental abnormalities of the face, mouth and jaws

LEARNING OBJECTIVES

To understand:
- The aetiology and classification of cleft lip and palate
- The principles of reconstruction of cleft lip and palate

- The key features of the perioperative care of the child with cleft lip and palate
- The associated complications of cleft lip and palate and their management

INTRODUCTION

Clefts of the lip, alveolus and hard and soft palate are the most common congenital abnormalities of the orofacial structures. They frequently occur as isolated deformities but can be associated with other medical conditions, particularly congenital heart disease. They are also an associated feature in over 300 recognised syndromes.

All children born with a cleft lip and palate need a thorough paediatric assessment to exclude other congenital abnormalities. In certain circumstances genetic counselling must be sought if a syndrome is suspected.

INCIDENCE

The incidence of cleft lip and palate is 1:600 live births and of isolated cleft palate is 1:1000 live births. The incidence increases in Oriental groups (1:500) and decreases in the black population (1:2000). The highest incidence reported for cleft lip and palate occurs in the Indian tribes of Montana, USA (1:276).

Although cleft lip and palate is an extremely diverse and variable congenital abnormality, several distinct sub-groups exist, namely cleft lip with/without cleft palate (CL/P), cleft palate (CP) alone and submucous cleft palate (SMCP).

The typical distribution of cleft types is:

- cleft lip alone: 15%;
- cleft lip and palate: 45%;
- isolated cleft palate: 40%.

Cleft lip/palate predominates in males whereas cleft palate alone appears to be more common in females. In unilateral cleft lip the deformity affects the left side in 60% of cases.

AETIOLOGY

Contemporary opinion on the aetiology of cleft lip and palate is that cleft lip and palate and isolated cleft palate have a genetic predisposition and a contributory environmental component. A family history of cleft lip and palate in which the first-degree relative is affected increases the risk to 1:25 live births. Genetic influence is more significant in cleft lip/palate than cleft palate alone, in which environmental factors exert a greater influence.

Environmental factors implicated in clefting include maternal epilepsy and drugs, e.g. steroids, diazepam and phenytoin. The role of antenatal folic acid supplements in preventing cleft lip and palate remains equivocal.

Although most clefts of the lip and palate occur as an isolated deformity, Pierre Robin sequence remains the most common syndrome. This syndrome comprises isolated cleft palate, retrognathia and a posteriorly displaced tongue (glossoptosis), which is associated with early respiratory and feeding difficulties.

Isolated cleft palate is more commonly associated with a syndrome than cleft lip/palate and cleft lip alone. Over 150 syndromes are associated with cleft lip and palate, although Stickler's (ophthalmic and musculoskeletal abnormalities), Shprintzen's (cardiac anomalies), Down's, Apert's and Treacher–Collins' syndromes are most frequently encountered (Summary box 42.1).

Summary box 42.1

Cleft lip and palate

- Associated with other congenital abnormalities
- Incidence varies between races from 1:300 to 1:2000 live births
- Aetiology is both genetic and environmental

Pierre Robin, **1867–1950, Professor, The French School of Dentistry, Paris, France,** described this syndrome in 1929.
Gunnar B. Stickler, **B. 1925, Paediatrician, The Mayo Clinic, Rochester, MN, USA.**
John Langdon Haydon Down, (sometimes given as Langdon-Down), **1828–1896, Physician, The London Hospital, London, England, published his classification of** aments in 1866.
Eugene Apert, **1868–1940, Physician, L'Hopital des Infants-Malades, Paris, France,** described this syndrome in 1906.
Edward Treacher Collins, **1862–1932, Ophthalmic Surgeon, The Royal London Ophthalmic Hospital, and Charing Cross Hospital, London, England, described** this syndrome in 1900.

ANATOMY OF CLEFT LIP AND PALATE

Cleft lip

The abnormalities in cleft lip are the direct consequence of disruption of the muscles of the upper lip and nasolabial region. The facial muscles (Fig. 42.1) can be divided into three muscular rings of Delaire: the nasolabial muscle ring surrounds the nasal aperture; the bilabial muscle ring surrounds the oral aperture; and the labiomental muscle ring envelops the lower lip and chin regions.

Unilateral cleft lip

In the unilateral cleft lip, the nasolabial and bilabial muscle rings are disrupted on one side resulting in an asymmetrical deformity involving the external nasal cartilages, nasal septum and anterior maxilla (premaxilla) (Fig. 42.2a and b). These deformities influence the mucocutaneous tissues causing a displacement of nasal skin onto the lip and a retraction of labial skin, as well as changes to the vermilion and lip mucosa. All these changes need to be considered in planning the surgical repair of the unilateral cleft lip.

Bilateral cleft lip

In the bilateral cleft lip the deformity is more profound but symmetrical. The two superior muscular rings are disrupted on both sides producing a flaring of the nose (caused by lack of nasolabial muscle continuity), a protrusive premaxilla and an area of skin in front of the premaxilla devoid of muscle, known as the prolabium (Fig. 42.3a and b). As in the unilateral cleft lip, the muscular, cartilaginous and skeletal deformities influence the mucocutaneous tissues, which must be respected in planning the repair of the bilateral cleft lip.

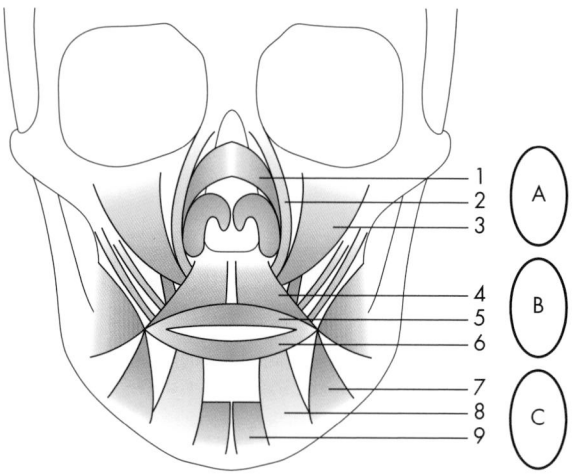

Figure 42.1 The muscle chains of the face: frontal view. The nasal cartilages are represented in blue. A, nasolabial (muscles 1–3); B, bilabial (muscles 4–6); C, labiomental (muscles 7–9); 1, transverse nasalis; 2, levator labii superioris alaeque nasi; 3, levator labii superioris; 4, orbicularis oris (oblique head) – upper lip; 5, orbicularis oris (horizontal head) – upper lip; 6, orbicularis oris – lower lip; 7, depressor anguli oris; 8, depressor labii inferioris; 9, mentalis.

Jean Delaire, **Professor of Stomatology and Maxillofacial Surgery, The Univesity of Nantes, Nantes, France from 1960 until 1991.**

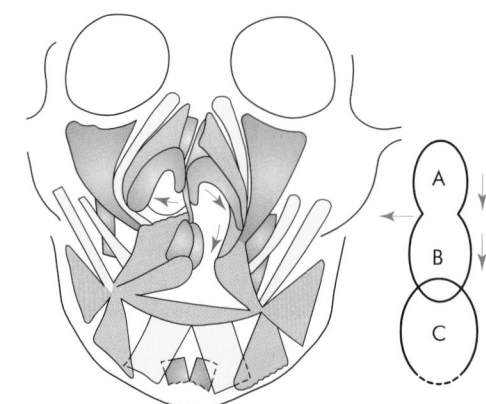

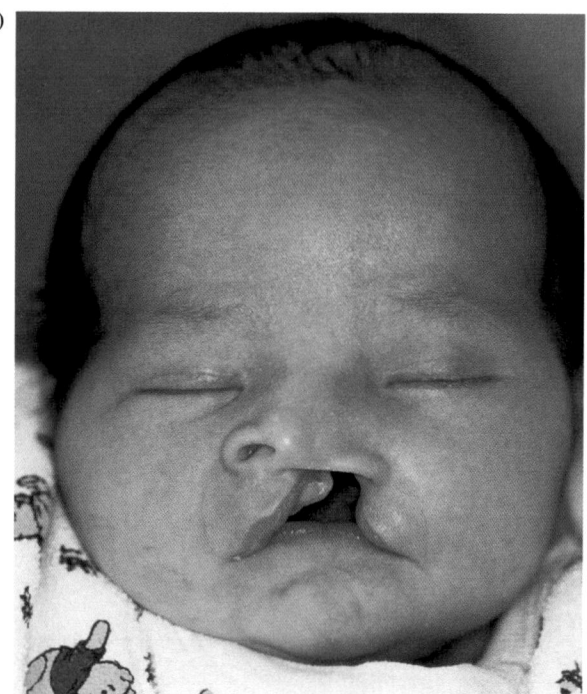

Figure 42.2 (a) Schematic representation of disruption of the nasolabial and bilabial muscle chains in unilateral (left) cleft lip. A, nasolabial; B, bilabial; C, labiomental. (b) Unilateral cleft lip before muscular reconstruction.

Cleft palate

Embryologically, the *primary* palate consists of all anatomical structures anterior to the incisive foramen, namely the alveolus and upper lip. The *secondary* palate is defined as the remainder of the palate behind the incisive foramen, divided into the hard palate and, more posteriorly, the soft palate.

Cleft palate results in failure of fusion of the two palatine shelves. This failure may be confined to the soft palate alone or involve both hard and soft palate. When the cleft of the hard palate remains attached to the nasal septum and vomer, the cleft is termed *incomplete*. When the nasal septum and vomer are completely separated from the palatine processes, the cleft palate is termed *complete* (Summary box 42.2).

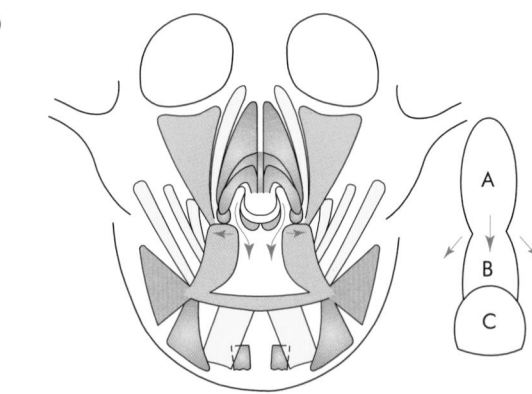

Soft palate

In the normal soft palate, closure of the velopharynx, which is essential for normal speech, is achieved by five different muscles functioning in a complete but coordinated fashion. In general, the muscle fibres of the soft palate are orientated transversely with no significant attachment to the hard palate.

In a cleft of the soft palate (Fig. 42.4a) the muscle fibres are orientated in an anteroposterior direction, inserting into the posterior edge of the hard palate (Fig. 42.4b).

Hard palate

The normal hard palate can be divided into three anatomical and physiological zones (Fig. 42.5). The central *palatal fibromucosa* is very thin and lies directly below the floor of nose. The *maxillary fibromucosa* is thick and contains the greater palatine neurovascular bundle. The *gingival fibromucosa* lies more lateral and adjacent to the teeth.

In performing surgical closure of cleft palate the changes associated with the cleft must be understood to obtain an anatomical and functional repair. In complete cleft palate the median part of the palatal vault is absent and the palatal fibromucosa is reduced in size. The maxillary and gingival fibromucosa are not modified in thickness, width or position.

CLASSIFICATION

Any classification for such a diverse and varied condition as cleft lip and palate needs to be simple, concise, flexible and exact but graphic. It must be suitable for computerisation but descriptive and morphological. An example of such a classification is the LAHSHAL system, which is able to describe site, size and extent, as well as type of cleft (Fig. 42.6).

Complete clefts of the lip, alveolus and hard and soft palate are designated as capitals L, A, H and S respectively. Incomplete clefts are recorded in lower case letters whereas microform clefts are documented with asterisks. Hence, LAHSHAL is the anatomical paraphrase of a complete bilateral cleft lip and palate. Another example, lahSh, represents an incomplete right unilateral cleft lip and alveolus with a complete cleft of soft palate extending partly onto the hard palate.

PRIMARY MANAGEMENT

Antenatal diagnosis

An antenatal diagnosis of cleft lip, whether unilateral or bilateral, is possible by ultrasound scan after 18 weeks of gestation. Isolated cleft palate cannot be diagnosed by antenatal scan. When an antenatal diagnosis is confirmed, referral to a cleft surgeon is appropriate for counselling to allay fears. Photographs of cleft lip shown to parents 'before and after' surgery are invaluable. Introduction to a parent support group and meeting parents

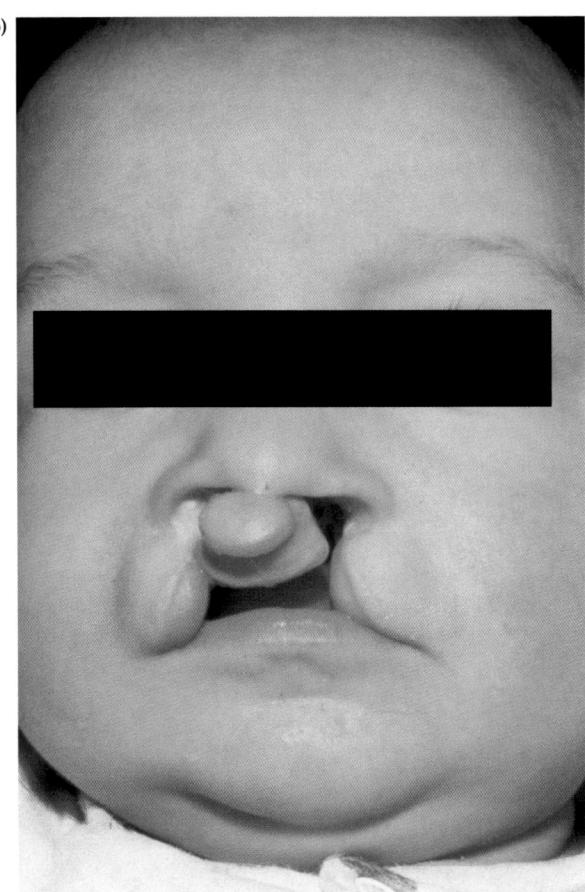

Figure 42.3 (a) Schematic representation of disruption of the nasolabial and bilabial muscle chains in bilateral cleft lip. A, nasolabial; B, bilabial; C, labiomental. (b) Bilateral cleft lip before muscular reconstruction.

of a child with a similar cleft who has undergone surgery may also be extremely helpful (Summary box 42.3).

CHAPTER 42 | CLEFT LIP AND PALATE

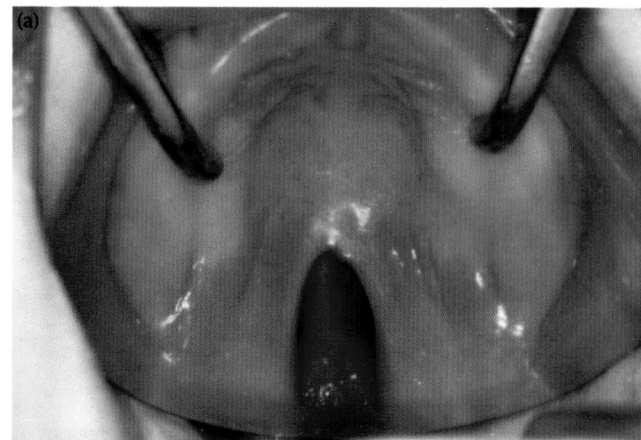

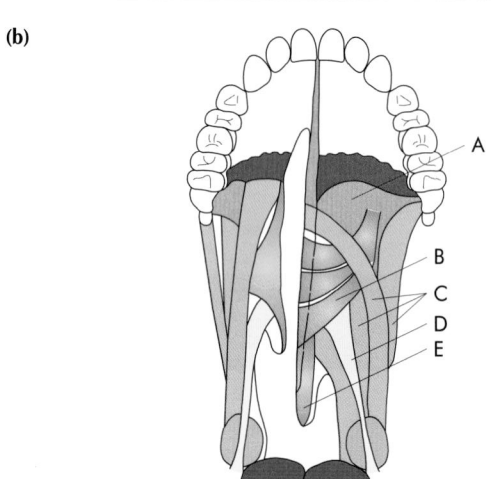

Figure 42.4 (a) Cleft of soft palate and incomplete cleft of hard palate. (b) Muscles of the soft palate: left, cleft palate; right, normal anatomy. A, tensor palati; B, levator palati; C, palatopharyngeus; D, palatoglossus; E, musculus uvulae.

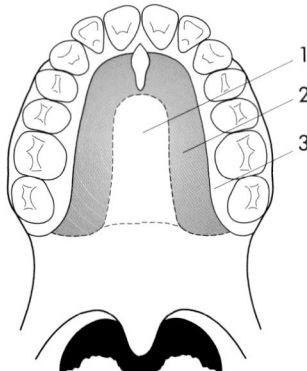

Figure 42.5 The three mucosal zones of the hard palate. 1, palatal fibromucosa; 2, maxillary fibromucosa; 3, gingival fibromucosa.

Feeding

Most babies born with cleft lip and palate feed well and thrive, provided that appropriate advice is given and support is available. Some mothers are successful in breast-feeding, particularly when the cleft is incomplete and confined to the lip. Good feeding patterns can be established with soft bottles (e.g. Mead Johnson)

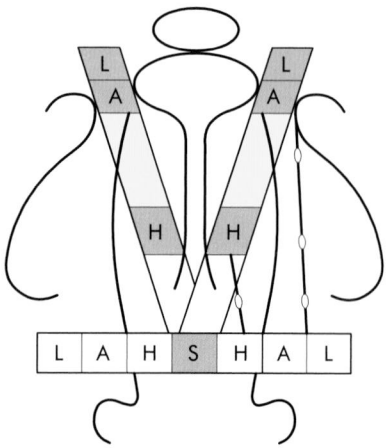

Figure 42.6 LAHSAL: an anatomical representation of cleft lip (L), alveolus (A) and hard (H) and soft palate (S).

and modified teats (orthodontic, Nuyk). Simple measures such as enlarging the hole in the teat often suffice. Feeding plates, constructed from a dental impression of the upper jaw, are rarely necessary to improve feeding. Some babies are provided with an active plate that aims not only to improve feeding but also reduce the width of the cleft lip and palate prior to surgery. The long-term benefit of such a regime remains unproven.

Airway

Major respiratory obstruction is uncommon and occurs exclusively in babies with Pierre Robin sequence. Hypoxic episodes during sleep and feeding can be life-threatening. Intermittent airway obstruction is more frequent and is managed by nursing the baby prone. More severe and persistent airway compromise can be managed by 'retained nasopharyngeal intubation' to maintain the airway. Surgical adhesion of the tongue to the lower lip (labio-glossopexy) in the first few days after birth is an alternative but less commonly practised method of management (Summary box 42.4).

Summary box 42.4

Problems immediately after birth

- Some babies are able to feed normally but some will need assistance
- Breathing problems in Pierre Robin sequence may be life-threatening

---

PRINCIPLES OF CLEFT SURGERY

The ultimate goal in cleft lip and palate management is a patient with a normal appearance of lip, nose and face, whose speech is normal and whose dentition and facial growth fall within the range of normal development.

Surgical techniques are aimed at restoring normal anatomy. With the exception of rare conditions such as holoprosencephaly, there is no true hypoplasia of the tissues involved on either side of the cleft. There is, however, displacement, deformation and underdevelopment of the muscles and facial skeleton. Emphasis is placed on muscular reconstruction of the lip, nose and face as well as muscles of the soft palate. Normal or near-normal anatomy promotes normal function, thereby encouraging normal growth and development of lip, nose, palate and facial skeleton. An in-depth understanding of the anatomy of the cleft is invaluable if the surgeon is to achieve normal, or near-normal, anatomical reconstruction (Summary box 42.5).

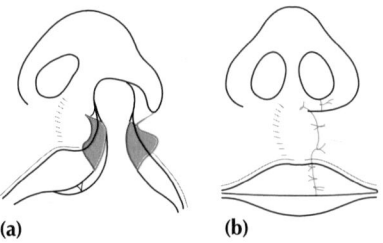

Figure 42.7 (a and b) Skin incisions (highlighted in red) for left unilateral complete cleft lip (after Delaire).

Summary box 42.5

Surgical anatomy

- Normal lip, face and nose
- There is underdevelopment and displacement of the muscles
- Restoration of normal anatomy encourages normal facial growth and function

---

Surgical techniques

There have been many different surgical techniques and sequences advocated in cleft lip and palate management. Cleft lip repair is commonly performed between 3 and 6 months of age whereas cleft palate repair is frequently performed between 6 and 18 months.

The Delaire technique and sequence (Table 42.1) is one of many regimes currently practised.

Cleft lip surgery

Skin incisions (Figs 42.7 and 42.8) are developed to restore displaced tissues, including skin and cartilage, to their normal position, while gaining access to the facial, nasal and lip musculature.

Table 42.1 Timing of primary cleft lip and palate procedures (after Delaire)

Cleft lip alone		
Unilateral (one side)	One operation at 5–6 months	
Bilateral (both sides)	One operation at 4–5 months	
Cleft palate alone		
Soft palate only	One operation at 6 months	
Soft and hard palate	Two operations	Soft palate at 6 months Hard palate at 15–18 months
Cleft lip and palate		
Unilateral	Two operations	Cleft lip and soft palate at 5–6 months Hard palate and gum pad with or without lip revision at 15–18 months
Bilateral	Two operations	Cleft lip and soft palate at 4–5 months Hard palate and gum pad with or without lip revision at 15–18 months

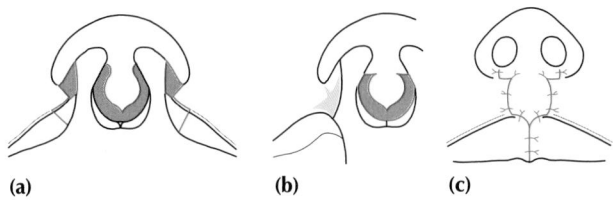

Figure 42.8 (a–c) Skin incisions for bilateral complete cleft lip, showing the shaded area from Fig. 42.7a. Areas for removal of excess mucosa (a) or skin (b) (after Delaire).

Muscular continuity is achieved by subperiosteal undermining over the anterior maxilla. Nasolabial muscles are anchored to the premaxilla with non-resorbable sutures. Oblique muscles of orbicularis oris are sutured to the base of the anterior nasal spine and cartilaginous nasal septum. Closure of the cleft lip is completed by suturing the horizontal fibres of orbicularis oris to achieve a functioning oral sphincter (Figs 42.9 and 42.10).

When the cleft lip is incomplete (Figs 42.11a and Fig. 42.12a), meticulous assessment of the cleft deformity is of paramount importance, as complete muscle disruption may be present leading to nasal and skeletal deformity. Full muscular exposure and reconstruction is imperative in many incomplete clefts if facial symmetry is to be achieved (Figs 42.11b and 42.12b).

Cleft palate surgery

Cleft palate closure can be achieved by one- or two-stage palatoplasty. The surgical principle is mobilisation and reconstruction of the aberrant soft palate musculature (Fig. 42.13a and b) together with closure of the residual hard palate cleft by minimal dissection and subsequent scar formation (Fig. 42.14a and b). Excess scar formation in the palate adversely affects growth and development of the maxilla. The philosophy of two-stage closure encourages a physiological narrowing of the hard palate cleft to minimise surgical dissection at the time of the second procedure (Summary box 42.6).

Summary box 42.6

Principles of surgery

- Cleft lip surgery attaches and reconnects the muscles around the oral sphincter
- Cleft palate surgery aims to bring together mucosa and muscles with minimal scarring
- Two-stage procedures attempt to minimise dissection

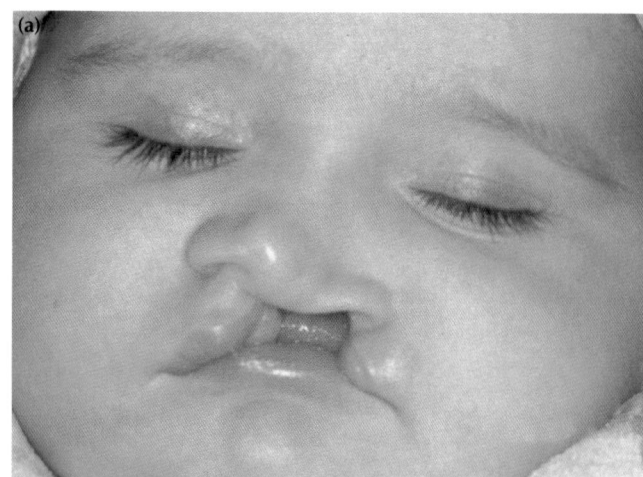

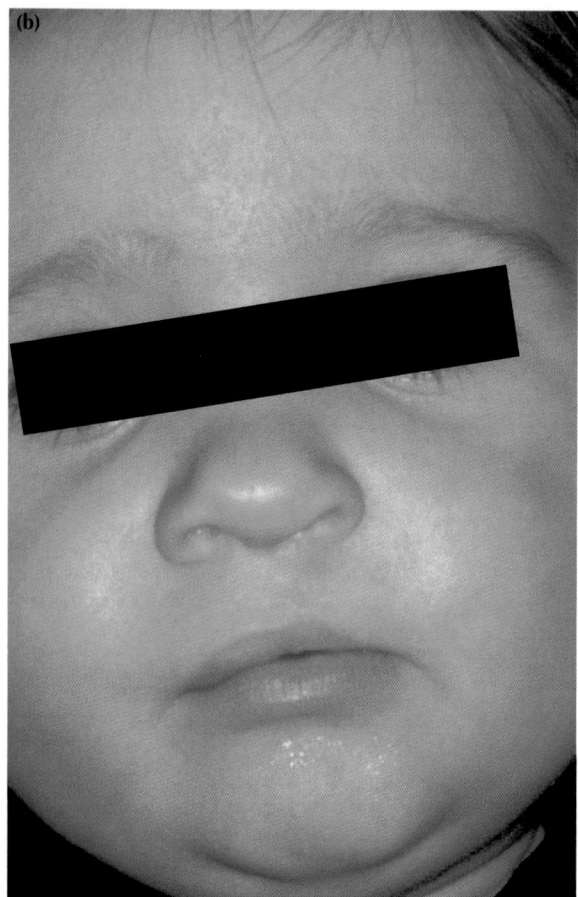

Figure 42.9 Unilateral complete cleft lip before (a) and after (b) muscular reconstruction.

SECONDARY MANAGEMENT

Following primary surgery, regular review by a multidisciplinary team is essential. Many aspects of cleft care require long-term review:

- hearing;
- speech;
- dental development;
- facial growth.

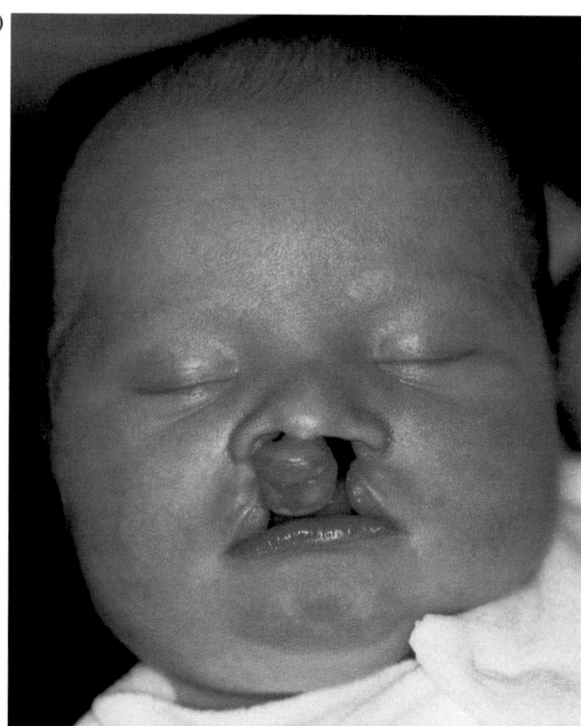

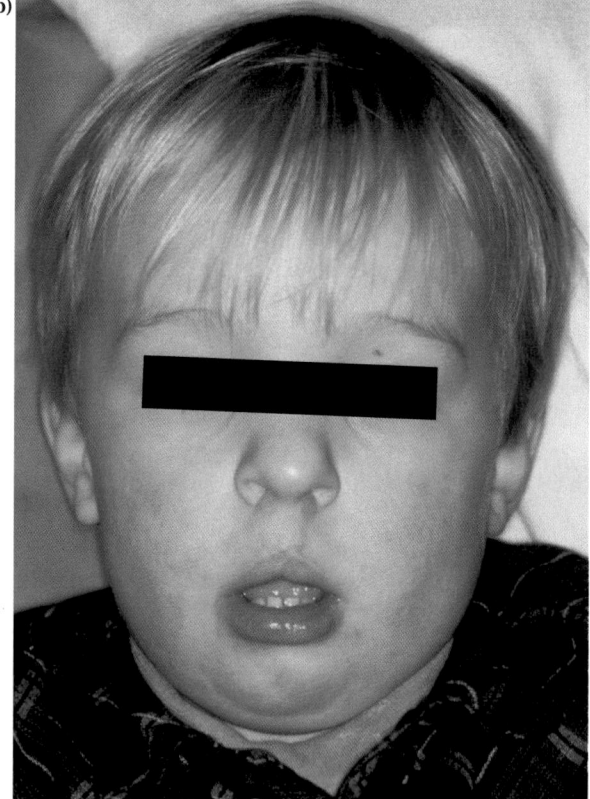

Figure 42.10 Bilateral cleft lip before (a) and after (b) muscular reconstruction.

Hearing

Eustachian tube dysfunction plays a central role in the pathogenesis of otitis media with effusion in babies and children born with a cleft palate. Children with a cleft lip alone exhibit the same

(a) 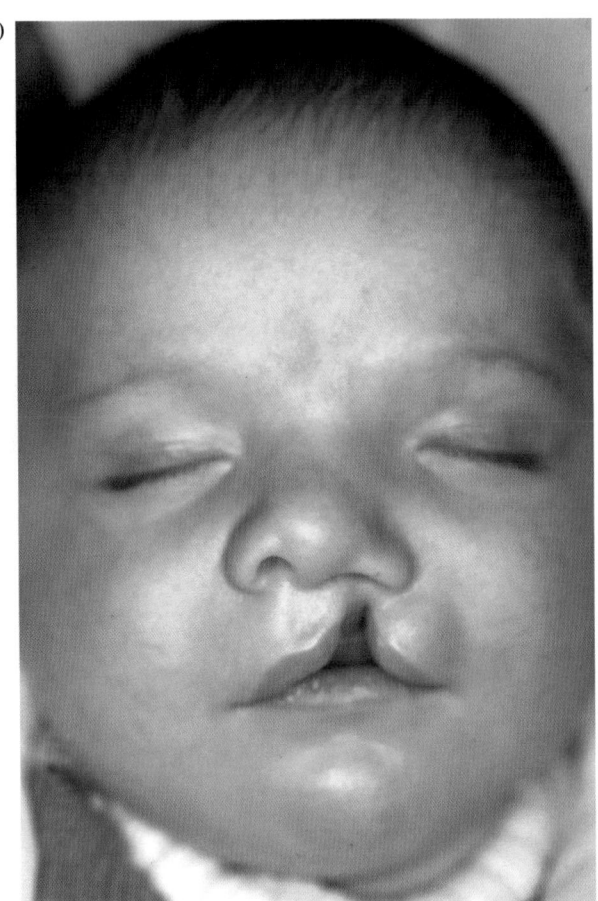 (b)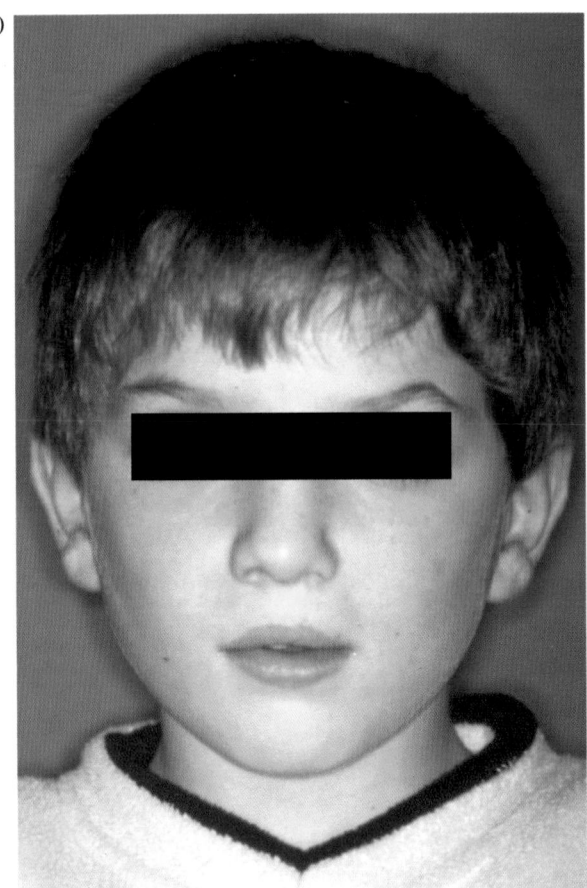

Figure 42.11 Unilateral incomplete cleft lip before (a) and after (b) muscle reconstruction.

frequency of otitis media as their age-matched non-cleft counterparts. It has been recently recognised that a child with a craniofacial anomaly including cleft lip and palate is at increased risk of a sensorineural hearing deficit. All children born with a cleft lip and palate should undergo assessment before 12 months of age for *sensorineural and conductive hearing loss* by auditory brainstem responses (ABR) and tympanometry respectively.

Sensorineural hearing loss is managed with a hearing aid whereas the management of secretory otitis media remains more controversial. Early (6–12 months) prophylactic myringotomy and grommet insertion temporarily eliminates middle ear effusion. Regular audiological testing may be as appropriate, reserving surgery for established secretory otitis media with infection. No firm evidence is available to support the interventional approach over the conservative regime. Nevertheless, the relationship between hearing loss and potential speech problems remains important. Regular audiological assessment during childhood is of utmost importance.

Speech

Initial speech assessment should be performed early (18 months) and repeated regularly to ensure that problems are identified early and managed appropriately.

Common speech problems associated with cleft lip and palate are:

- *Velopharyngeal incompetence.* This is associated with increased nasal airflow and resonance producing a nasal or 'hypernasal'

quality to speech. It frequently reflects poor function of the soft palate associated with inadequate muscle repair.
- *Articulation problems.* These arise either as a compensatory mechanism to overcome velopharyngeal incompetence or less commonly are caused by jaw/dental and occlusal abnormalities. Videofluoroscopy, nasal airflow studies (aerophonoscopy) and nasendoscopy are helpful in defining the exact mechanism of the problem, aiding management.
- *Speech problems.* These are managed by speech and language therapy; secondary palatal surgery, either intravelar veloplasty (muscular reconstruction of soft palate) or pharyngoplasty; and speech training devices (Summary box 42.7).

Summary box 42.7

Associated hearing and speech problems

- Higher incidence of sensorineural and conductive hearing loss
- Regular hearing tests are important if speech is to develop normally
- Speech problems may result from airflow problems

Dental

Dental anomalies are common findings in children with cleft lip and/or palate. Various phenomena including delayed tooth development, delayed eruption of teeth and morphological

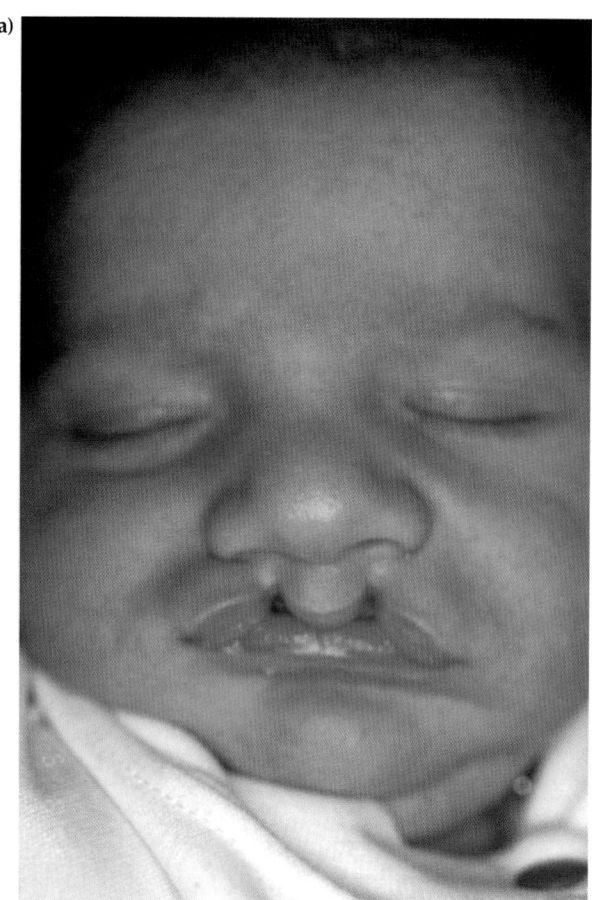

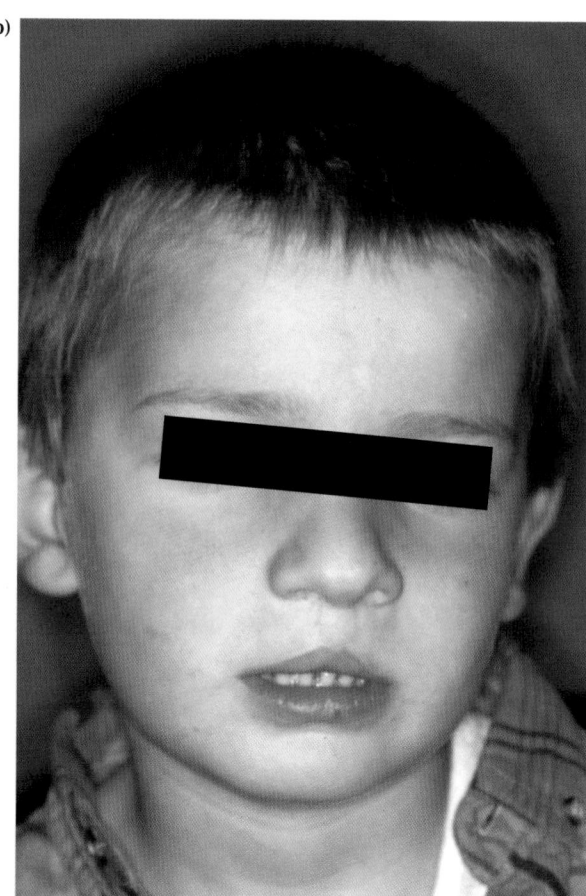

Figure 42.12 Bilateral incomplete cleft lip before (a) and after (b) muscular reconstruction.

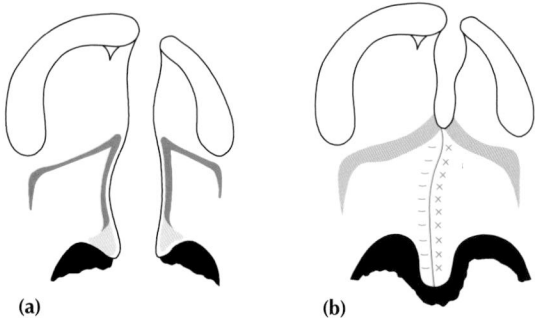

Figure 42.13 (a and b) Method of repair of cleft palate. First-stage palatoplasty to reconstruct muscles of the soft palate. Red lines represent incisions, and orange areas raw surfaces.

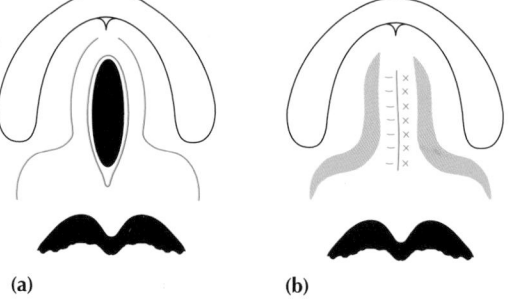

Figure 42.14 (a and b) Schematic representation of closure of the hard palate. Second-stage palatoplasty achieved with two-layered closure. Red lines represent incisions, and orange areas raw surfaces.

abnormalities are well documented. The number of teeth may be reduced (hypodontia) or increased (hyperdontia), occurring most commonly in the region of the cleft alveolus involving the maxillary lateral incisor tooth. These abnormalities can occur in both primary and secondary dentition.

All children with cleft lip and palate should undergo regular dental examination. Dental management should also include preventative measures such as dietary advice, fluoride supplements and fissure sealants.

A well-maintained and disease-free dentition in childhood is

an absolute prerequisite for orthodontic treatment (Summary box 42.8).

Summary box 42.8

Dental problems

- Too many/too few teeth or problems with eruption of teeth are common
- Good dentition is essential for successful reconstructive surgery

Orthodontic management

Many children with cleft lip and palate require orthodontic treatment. Orthodontic treatment is commonly carried out in two phases:

1 Mixed dentition (8–10 years) – to expand the maxillary arches as a prelude to alveolar bone graft.
2 Permanent dentition (14–18 years) – to align the dentition and provide a normal functioning occlusion. This phase of treatment may also include surgical correction of a malpositioned/retrusive maxilla by maxillary osteotomy (Fig. 42.15a and b).

Secondary surgery for cleft lip and palate

Good outcome in cleft lip and palate is directly attributable to the quality of the primary surgery. Secondary cleft procedures include:

- cleft lip revision (unilateral and bilateral);
- alveolar bone graft;
- simultaneous lip revision and alveolar bone graft;
- secondary palate procedures, e.g. veloplasty and pharyngoplasty, closure of a palatal fistula;
- dentoalveolar procedures, including transplantation of teeth/insertion of osseo-integrated dental implants;
- orthognathic surgery;
- rhinoplasty.

Cleft lip revision

Indications for revisional surgery to the previously repaired cleft lip are dependent on the site and severity of the residual deformity.

Revisional surgery should be delayed for 2 years after primary lip closure unless the surgeon is of the opinion that the initial procedure was inadequate, particularly with respect to muscular reconstruction.

Indications for revision include:

- lip deformity:
  - malaligned vermilion;
  - asymmetrical Cupid's bow;
  - muscle discontinuity or malalignment;
- nasal deformity:
  - lateral drift of alar base;
  - poor nasal tip projection;
  - deviation of cartilaginous nasal septum into the non-cleft nostril.

Residual nasal deformity is an external manifestation of incomplete reconstruction of the nasolabial muscle ring.

Examples of lip revision are shown in Figs 42.16–42.19 (Summary box 42.9).

Summary box 42.9

Cleft lip revision surgery

- Should be delayed for at least 2 years after primary surgery
- Aims to improve incomplete primary reconstruction

Cupid's Bow. **Cupid, the Roman God of Love,** is often depicted holding a double-curved bow which he uses to shoot arrows into his victims.

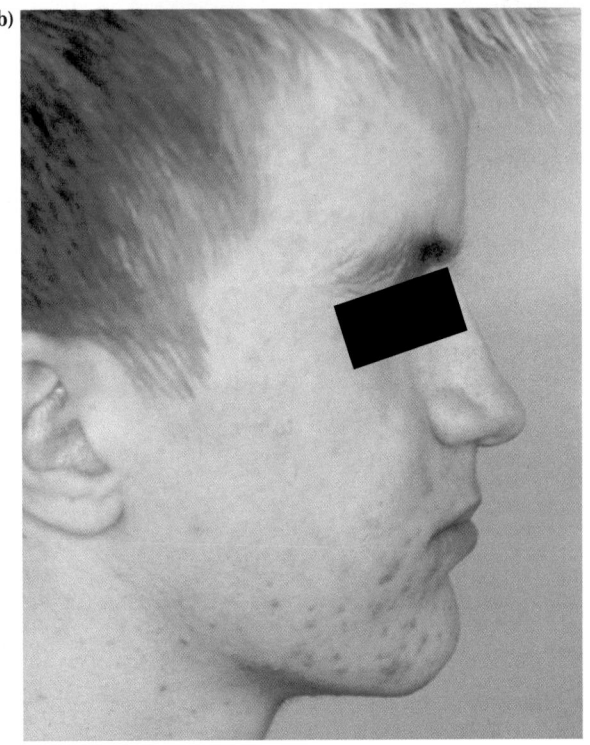

(a)

(b)

Figure 42.15 Correction of midface retrusion by maxillary advancement osteotomy, before (a) and after (b) surgery.

Alveolar bone grafting

Alveolar bone grafting in a mixed dentition is a well-established procedure for patients with a residual alveolar cleft associated

CHAPTER 42 | CLEFT LIP AND PALATE

(a)
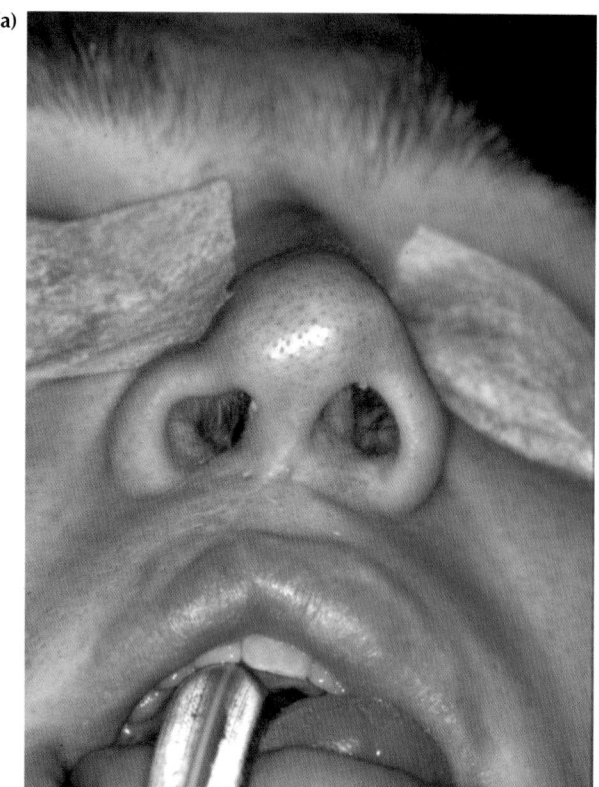

(b)
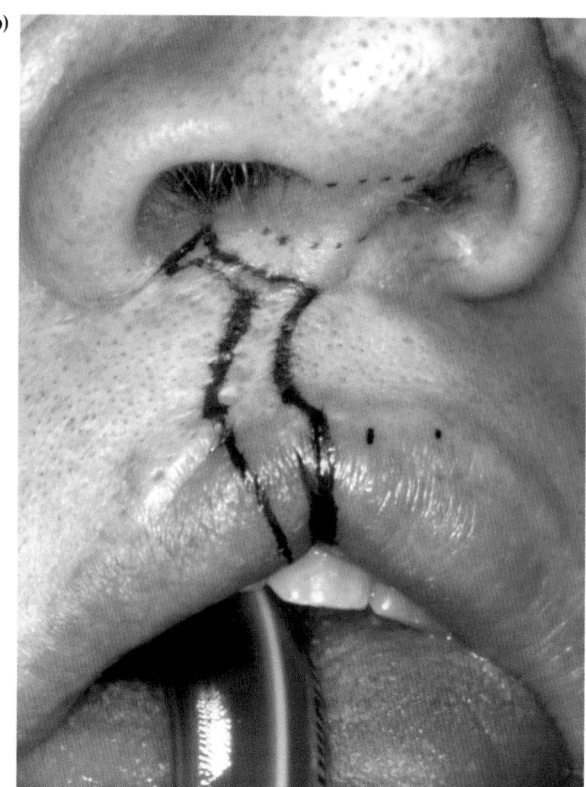

(c)
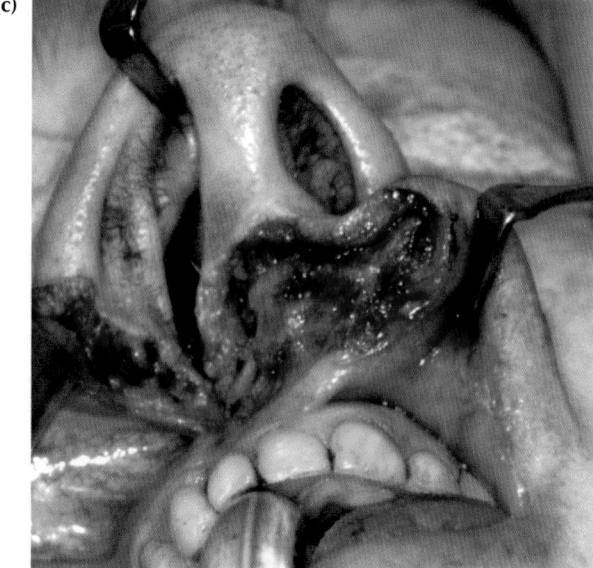

(d)
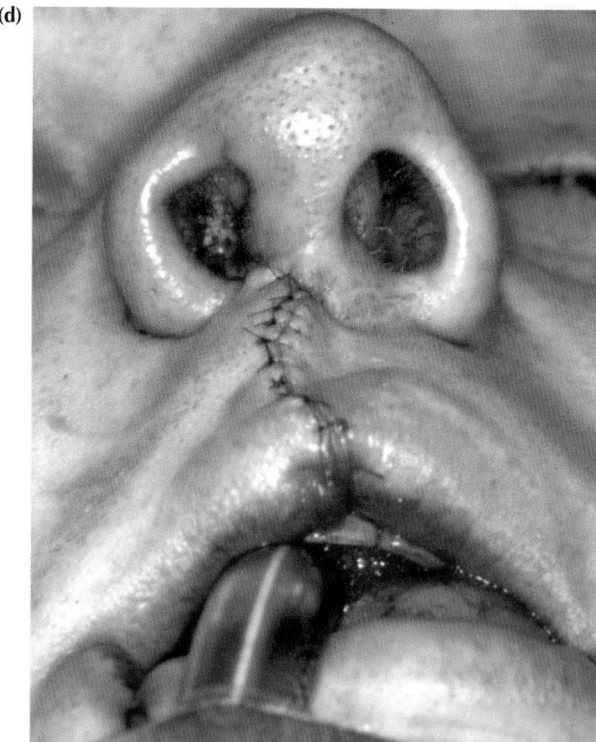

Figure 42.16 (a) Revision of unilateral complete cleft lip, seen from below. (b) Skin incisions. (c) Wide exposure of nasolabial and orbicularis oris muscle. (d) Lip closure highlighting improved nasal symmetry.

with cleft lip and palate. The rationale for performing alveolar bone grafting includes:

- stabilisation of maxillary segments;
- to promote eruption of the canine tooth into the cleft site;
- to enhance bony support of the teeth adjacent to the cleft alveolus;
- to promote closure of the oronasal fistula;
- to close residual fistula of the anterior palate;
- to provide adequate bone stock to receive an osseo-integrated dental implant where a tooth is congenitally absent.

Normally, but not universally, patients undergo a period of orthodontic treatment prior to bone grafting. The collapsed maxillary

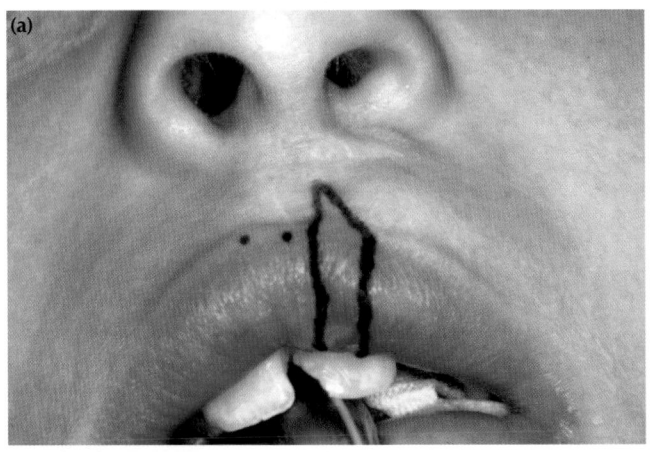

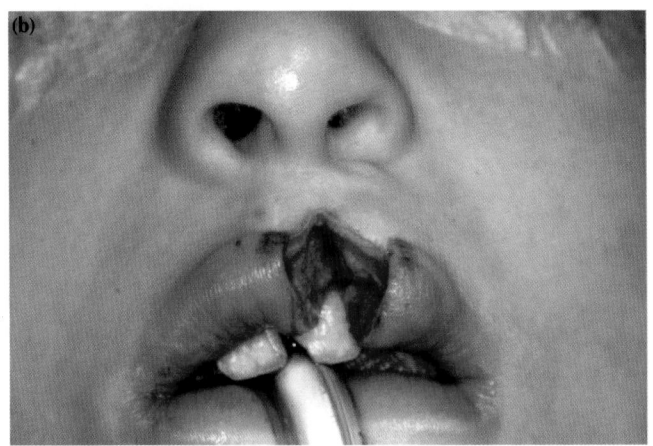

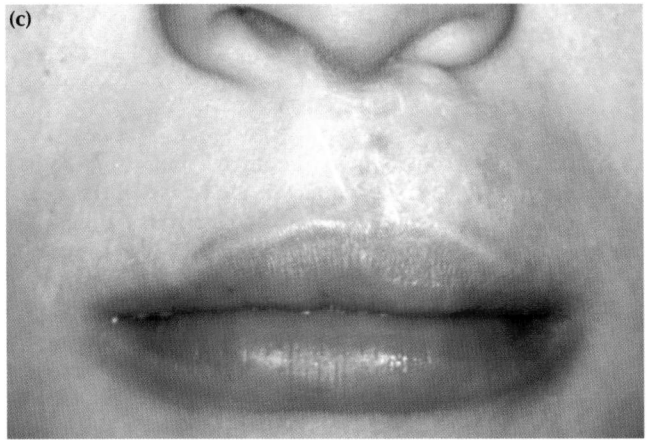

Figure 42.17 (a) Asymmetrical Cupid's bow. Revision of unilateral cleft lip – skin markings. (b) Identification and realignment of orbicularis oris muscle. (c) Postoperative appearance.

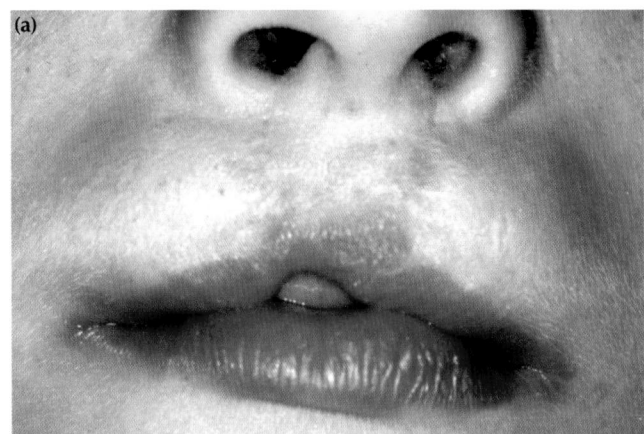

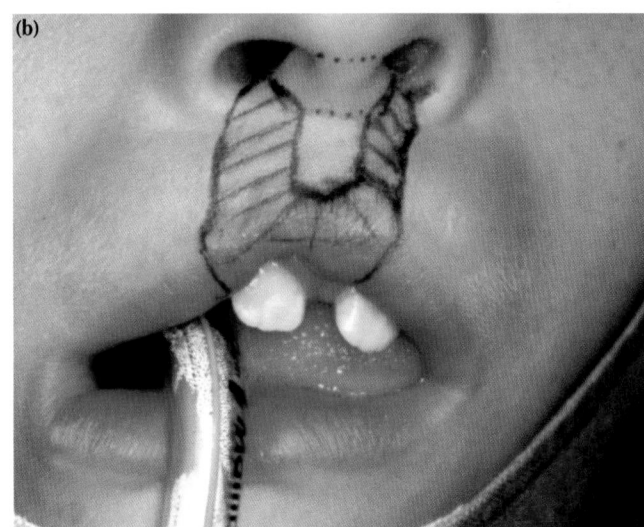

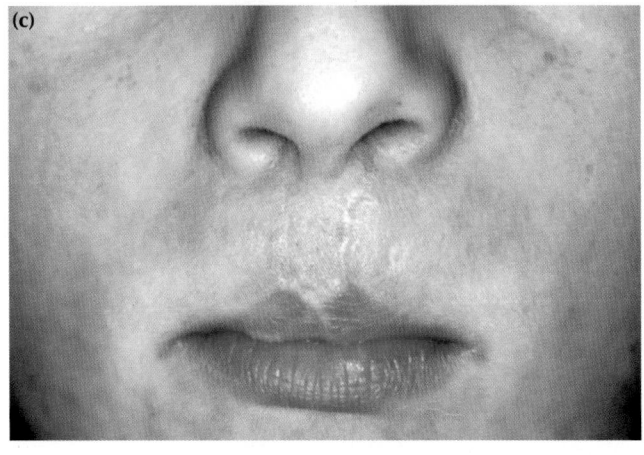

Figure 42.18 (a) Revision of bilateral cleft lip with reconstruction of nasolabial muscles. (b) Skin incisions and development of philtrum. (c) Postoperative view – improved nasal and lip symmetry.

segment is expanded orthodontically to widen the cleft alveolus. The surgery is best performed before the canine tooth erupts (between 8 and 11 years of age). There is a consensus that earlier bone grafting may be beneficial not only for the unerupted canine tooth but also to promote eruption and bony support to the adjacent central and lateral incisor when present. Alveolar bone grafting can also be performed simultaneously with secondary lip revision (Fig. 42.20).

Cancellous bone is harvested from either the iliac crest or

tibial plateau. This is achieved either through an open approach or preferably through a small incision utilising a trephine. When the defect is very small, alternative bone sites, e.g. mental symphysis, are sometimes advocated. Bone grafting is a highly successful procedure when carried out in experienced hands, with over 90% of patients achieving acceptable interdental alveolar

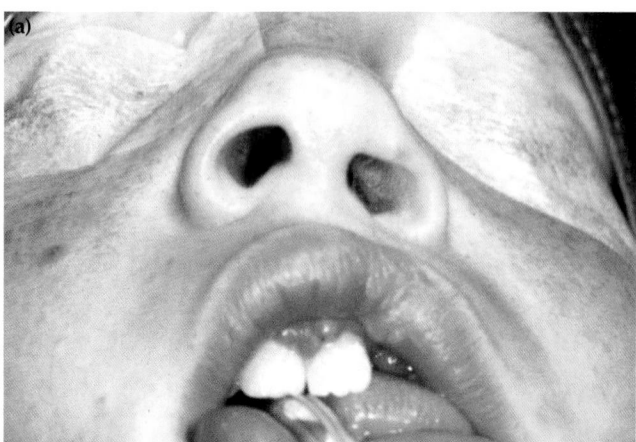

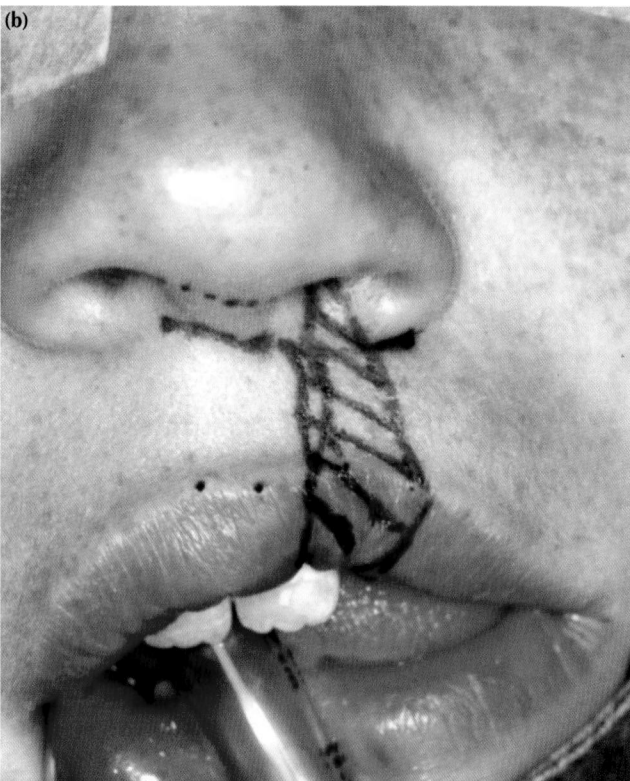

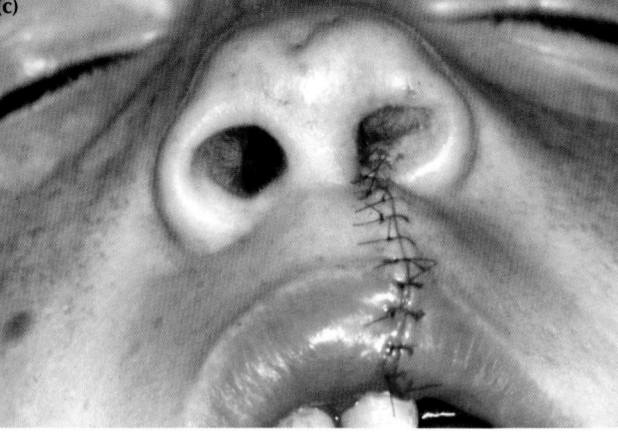

Figure 42.19 (a) Revision of left unilateral cleft lip to correct nasal deformity. (b) Skin incision. (c) Postoperative view.

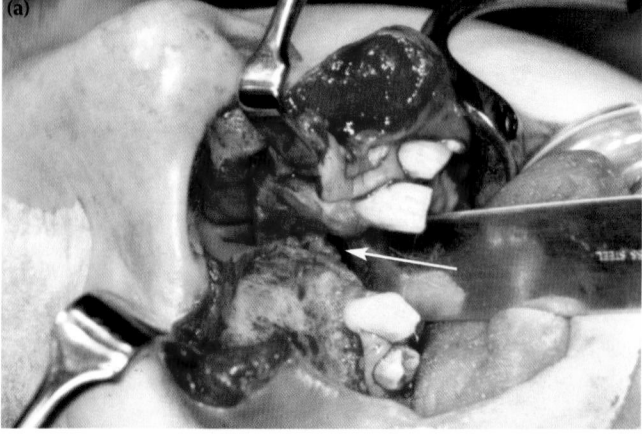

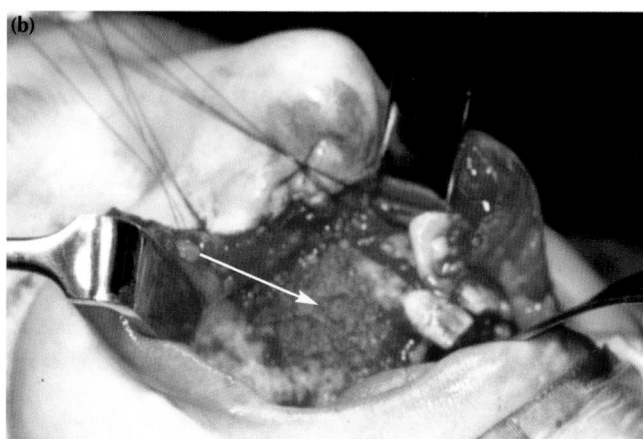

Figure 42.20 (a) Peroperative view of alveolar bone graft demonstrating defect in alveolus (arrow) (simultaneous lip revision). (b) Cancellous bone graft (arrow) packed into defect.

bone height, but it does require the interaction of surgeon and orthodontist. When the lateral incisor is absent and the canine tooth fails to erupt, surgical exposure of the canine tooth may be required to aid its eruption. It is a fundamental principle that, following alveolar bone grafting, efforts should be made to ensure that a tooth erupts into the alveolar bone graft site. Failure to provide a tooth in the alveolar bone graft site usually results in bony resorption in the long term. This can be overcome by the insertion of an osseo-integrated implant into the grafted site, thereby preserving bone stock (Fig. 42.21) (Summary box 42.10).

Summary box 42.10

Alveolar bone grafting

- Aimed at supplementing orthodontic treatment
- Promotes normal eruption of canine and other teeth

Orthognathic surgery

Impaired growth of the midface (maxilla) is now attributed to poor and traumatic primary surgery. Surgical techniques must endeavour to minimise scarring, although in many cases patients have a genetic predisposition to poor midfacial growth. Elective maxillary advancement or bimaxillary surgery is often indicated

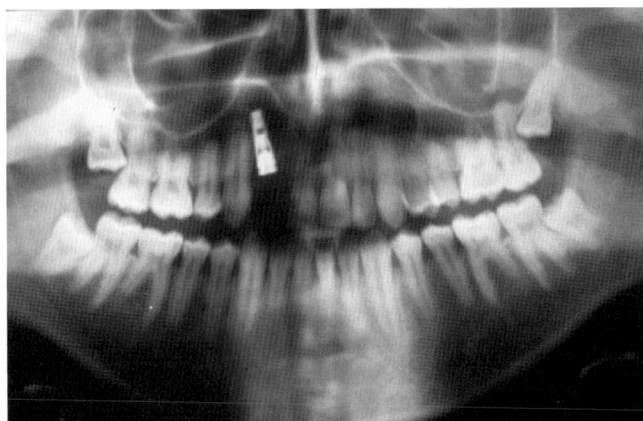

Figure 42.21 Radiographic appearance of an implant in an alveolar bone graft site.

to restore aesthetics and dental occlusal harmony. Orthognathic surgery is usually performed when facial growth is complete (16 years in female patients, 19 years in male patients).

The principal dentofacial deformity associated with cleft lip and palate is underdevelopment in both the horizontal and vertical direction of the maxilla. This leads to a pseudoprognathism in late adolescence, which is not correctable by orthodontic fixed-appliance therapy alone. Patients needing orthognathic surgery can be identified as early as 10 years old, although planning and treatment does not commence until 14–15 years of age. Treatment with fixed appliances to align teeth in each dental arch is carried out over a period of 18–24 months as a prelude to orthognathic surgery. Orthognathic surgery may require maxillary osteotomy advancement alone (Fig. 42.15a and b, see p. 665) or bimaxillary osteotomy and genioplasty (Fig. 42.22). Rigid fixation with or without bone grafting of the maxilla is essential as cleft lip and palate patients undergoing orthognathic surgery have a high risk of a skeletal relapse as a result of the scarring associated with primary cleft lip and palate surgery.

Open septorhinoplasty

Following revisional cleft lip and palate surgery, orthognathic surgery and alveolar bone grafting, many patients still require definitive surgical nasal correction. In patients with cleft lip and palate, open rhinoplasty is preferred to gain access to the external cartilaginous framework, which is frequently deformed (Fig. 42.23). The principal deformity is a collapse of the lower lateral cartilage on the cleft side together with a dislocation of the cartilaginous septum into the non-cleft nostril. The open method ensures adequate access and repositioning of the cartilaginous framework as a tertiary procedure to improve nasal tip projection, correct septal deformity and relocate alar cartilages. A postauricular onlay graft to the middle crus of the cleft nostril lower lateral cartilage may be required to enhance good nasal tip projection and symmetry (Summary box 42.11).

Summary box 42.11

Deformities requiring nasal reconstruction

- Collapse of the lower lateral cartilage on the cleft side
- Dislocation of cartilaginous septum into the non-cleft nostril

---

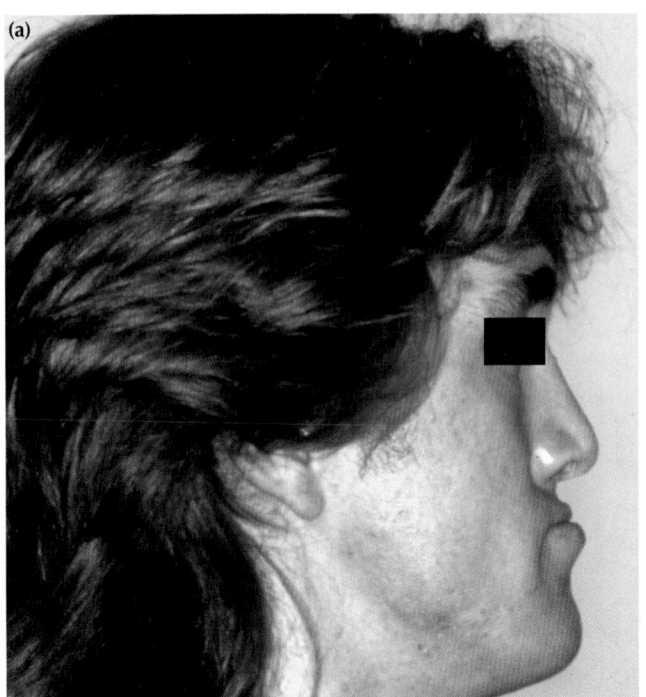

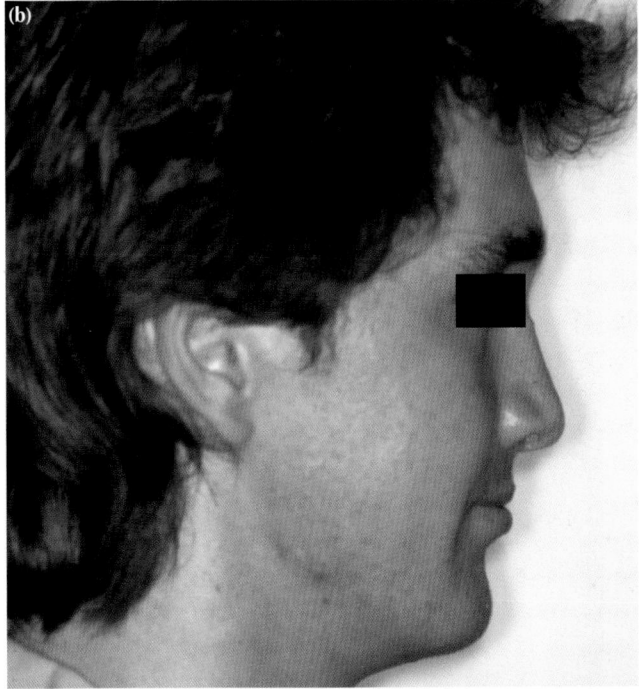

Figure 42.22 (a) Lateral view of an adult a with previously repaired cleft lip and palate demonstrating mandibular prognathism and maxillary retrusion. (b) Postoperative appearance following maxillary advancement and mandibular setback surgery.

Summary

The management of children with cleft lip and palate is complex, requiring the skill of a multidisciplinary team. Each team should include professionals who are appropriately qualified with specialist training, treating an adequate number of patients per year. Meticulous record keeping of photography, radiology, dental casts

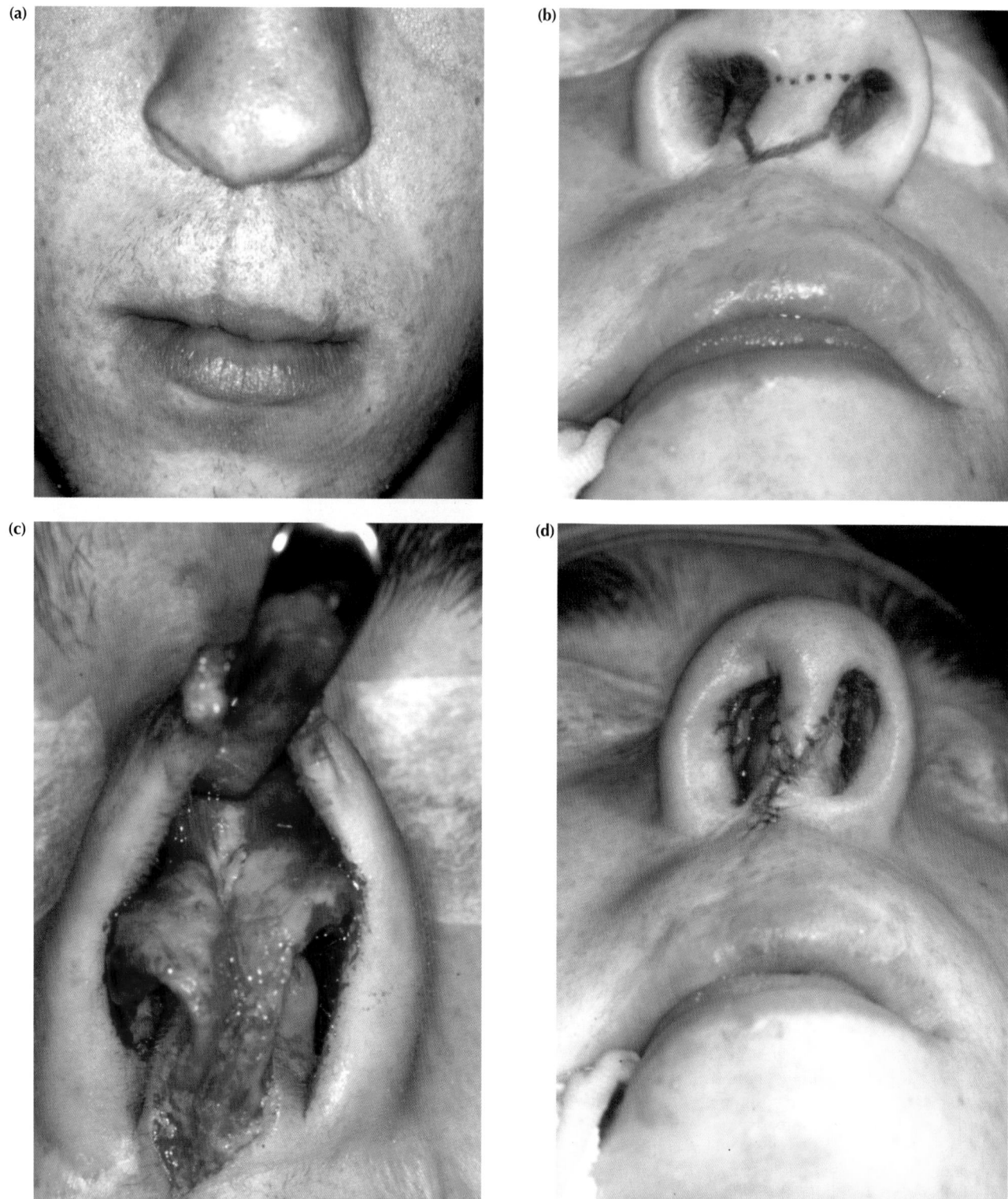

Figure 42.23 (a) Characteristic nasal deformity of a non-functional unilateral cleft lip repair. (b) Incisions for open rhinoplasty. (c) Exposure of the cartilaginous skeleton of the external nose. (d) Repositioning of external nasal cartilages to improve nasal tip projection.

and speech recordings are indispensable to permit regular audits and improve outcomes.

DEVELOPMENTAL ABNORMALITIES OF THE TEETH AND JAWS

Teeth

Developmental abnormalities of the teeth can be divided into:

- abnormality in number;
- defects of structure and size;
- disorders of eruption of teeth.

Number

Anodontia is the term that is strictly applied to congenital absence of all teeth, which may involve both deciduous and permanent dentition. This is a rare condition that is often hereditary.

Partial anodontia is a much more common disorder in which there is a failure of development of the primary or more commonly the secondary dentition. Teeth that are most frequently absent are the third molars (wisdom teeth), second premolars and maxillary lateral incisor teeth.

Partial anodontia is associated with certain systemic disorders:

- ectodermal dysplasia;
- Down's syndrome;
- cleft lip and palate.

Management of partial anodontia involves prosthetic replacement of the teeth, usually in combination with orthodontic treatment. Congenitally missing teeth can be replaced with removable prostheses, fixed prostheses or, more recently, the use of osseo-integrated dental implants.

Additional teeth (*hyperdontia*) can occur alone or in association with other syndromes. Additional teeth are termed *supernumerary* teeth and are often impacted in the jaw with abnormal morphology. The most common site for supernumerary teeth is the maxillary incisor region, particularly in the midline (mesiodens). When additional teeth are of a similar morphology to the normal dentition, the term supplemental is appropriate. Supplemental teeth are common in the maxillary incisor and premolar regions, and less common in the wisdom tooth region when they are termed the fourth molars. Most supernumerary teeth are removed to encourage the eruption of the permanent dentition (Summary box 42.12).

Summary box 42.12

Problems with numbers of teeth

- Absent teeth can be replaced with prosthetic teeth, which may involve osseo-integrated implants
- Supernumerary teeth are often impacted and are removed to allow eruption of secondary dentition

---

Defects of the structure of teeth

Structural changes of the teeth can occur as a consequence of genetic disorders or environmental factors.

Genetic disorders frequently include *amelogenesis imperfecta* and *dentinogenesis imperfecta,* which affect the enamel and dentine of the teeth respectively. Both of these conditions are characterised by defects in both dentitions, in which all teeth are affected. In amelogenesis imperfecta the defects are variable and may involve changes in structure (hypoplasia) or in mineralisation (hypocalcification). The loss of enamel leads to rapid attrition of the teeth to gum level in early adolescence. Dentinogenesis imperfecta results in soft dentine associated with short roots. Dentinogenesis imperfecta is strongly associated with osteogenesis imperfecta.

Acquired conditions producing changes in the structure of the teeth may be either local or systemic. Local causes are usually the consequence of trauma to the deciduous predecessor tooth, which interferes with enamel formation (amelogenesis). Common examples of systemic causes that produce tooth structure disruption are:

- measles;
- rickets;
- hypoparathyroidism;
- tetracycline;
- fluoride (Summary box 42.13).

Summary box 42.13

Causes of defects of the structure of teeth

Congenital
- Amelogenesis imperfecta
- Dentinogenesis imperfecta

Acquired local
- Trauma

Acquired systemic
- Disease – measles, rickets
- Drugs – fluoride, tetracycline

Disorders of eruption

Both primary and secondary dentition erupt in a specific sequence, although the timing of eruption does vary from child to child. Delayed eruption of teeth may involve a single tooth or may involve the entire dentition.

Local factors

There are numerous factors that impair the eruption of a single tooth. These include:

- loss of space/overcrowding;
- additional teeth;
- dentigerous cysts;
- retention of deciduous tooth.

Systemic factors

These can prevent the eruption of multiple teeth. Examples of such conditions include:

- metabolic diseases – cretinism and rickets;
- osteodystrophies – cleidocranial dysostosis and fibrous dysplasia;
- hereditary gingival fibromatosis.

Management of unerupted teeth involves the removal of the obstruction to eruption, including supernumerary teeth, as well as the relief of crowding. Patients with cleidocranial dysostosis should undergo long-term follow-up with regular radiographic assessment. Supernumerary teeth, as and when they appear,

CHAPTER 42 | CLEFT LIP AND PALATE

should be removed to encourage the eruption of permanent dentition in adolescence. Many patients with cleidocranial dysostosis require multiple operations to expose teeth and encourage eruption (Summary box 42.14).

Jaws

Disproportionate growth between the maxilla and mandible can occur, which results in derangement of the dental occlusion. The occlusion can be classified into three different subtypes:

- class I: a normal relationship of upper and lower incisors and molar dentition;
- class II: the mandibular teeth are placed posterior to the maxillary teeth;
- class III: the mandibular teeth are placed anterior to the maxillary teeth.

This classification is usually, but not invariably, the consequence of aberrant skeletal development of the maxilla and mandible, such that in a class II condition there is usually an underdevelopment of the mandible (mandibular retrognathia), whereas in a class III condition there may be simultaneous overgrowth of the mandible (mandibular prognathism) and underdevelopment of the maxilla (maxillary hypoplasia).

In the Caucasian population the commonest deformity of the facial skeleton is an underdevelopment of the mandible (retrognathia), producing a skeletal class II relationship often associated with excessive vertical growth of the maxilla. Bimaxillary protrusion is rare but is a characteristic of African races.

Condylar hyperplasia is an idiopathic condition seen in patients between 15 and 30 years of age, in which there is hyperplasia of the neck of the mandibular condyle. This gives an asymmetrical growth to the jaw in both a vertical and horizontal plane.

Facial disproportionate growth is also a characteristic of many syndromes. Such syndromes include:

- Treacher-Collins' syndrome;
- Crouzon's syndrome;
- Apert's syndrome;
- Pierre Robin sequence.

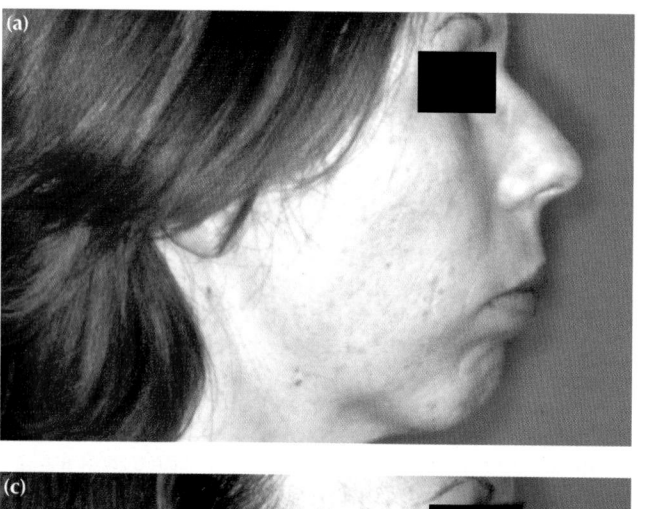
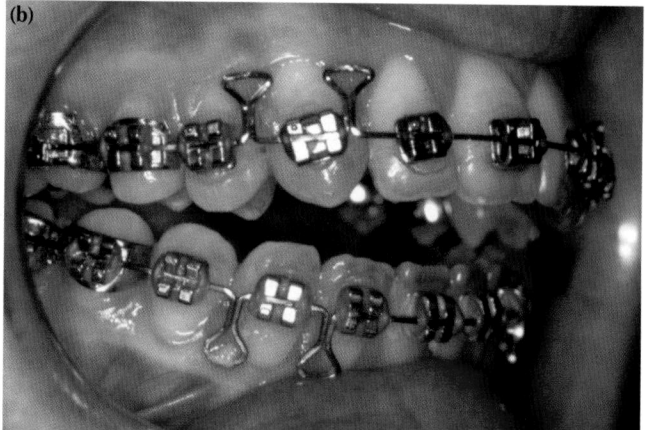
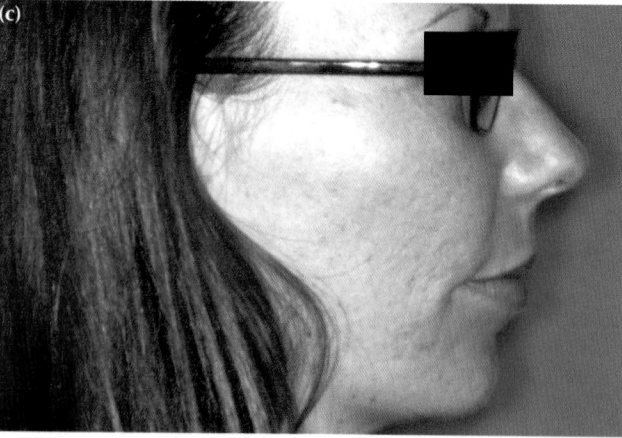
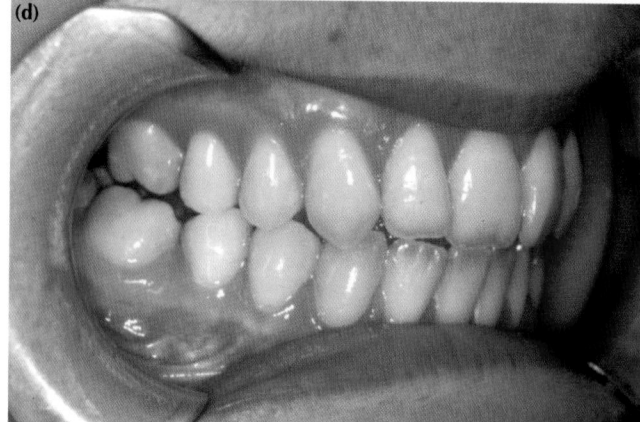

Figure 42.24   (a) Profile of class II relationship with vertical growth of maxilla and mandibular retrognathia. (b) Preoperative occlusion with anterior open bite. (c) Postoperative view following superior repositioning of maxilla, mandibular advancement and genioplasty. (d) Postoperative occlusion.

Octave Crouzon, 1874–1938, Physician, La Salpêtrière, Paris, France, described this condition in 1912.

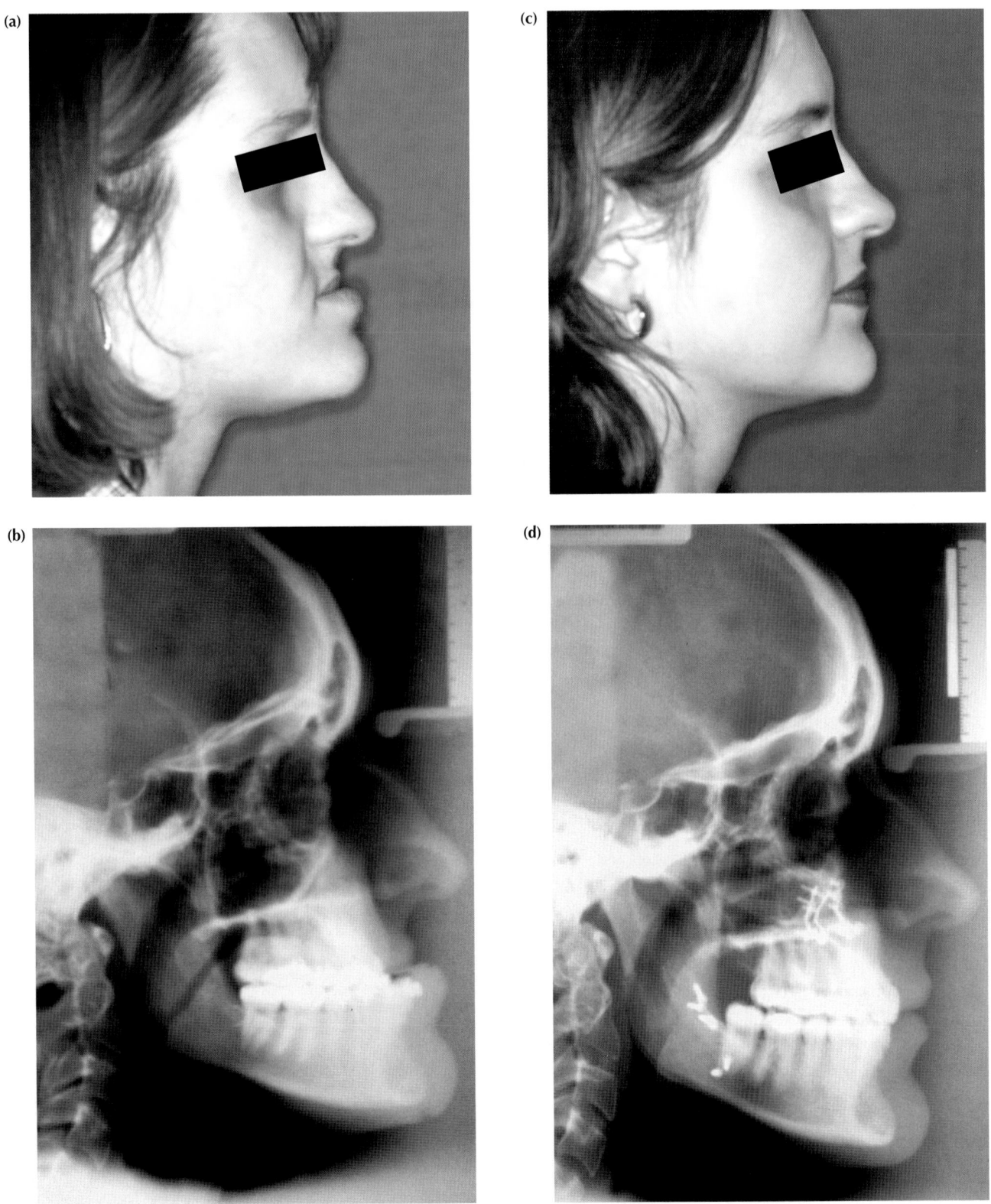

Figure 42.25 (a) Profile of class III skeletal relationship and maxillary hypoplasia and mandibular prognathism. (b) Lateral skull radiograph. (c) Profile following bimaxillary osteotomy. (d) Postoperative radiograph following bimaxillary osteotomy demonstrating internal fixation. (Part (e) overleaf).

(e)

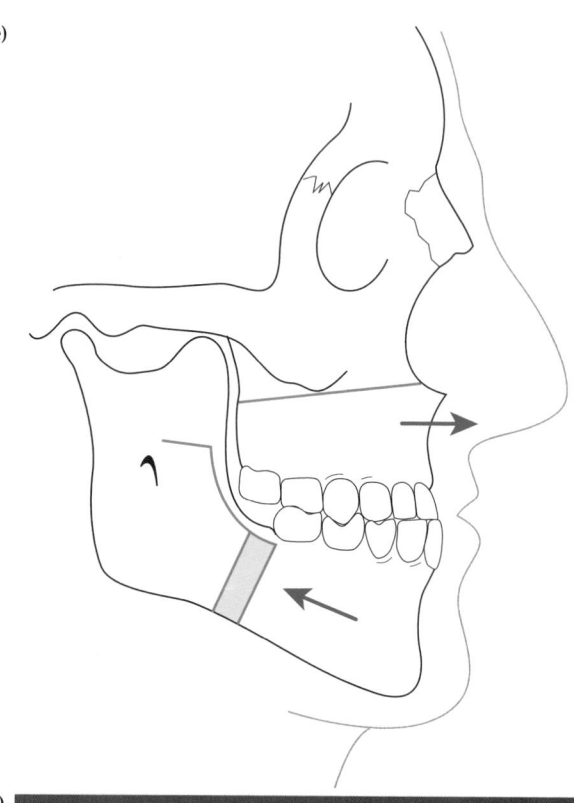

Figure 42.25 *continued* (e) Schematic representation of bimaxillary osteotomy with maxillary advancement and mandibular retrusion.

(a)

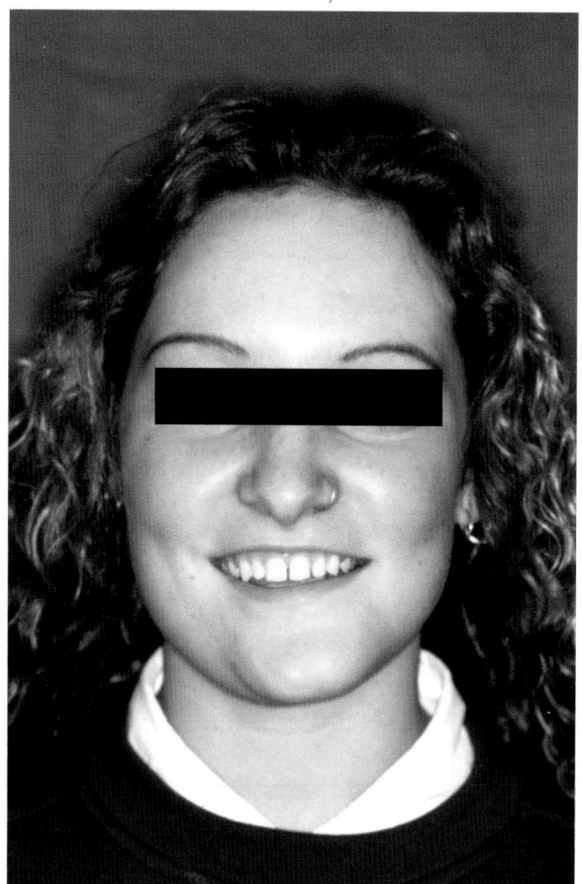

(b)   Right lateral   Anterior

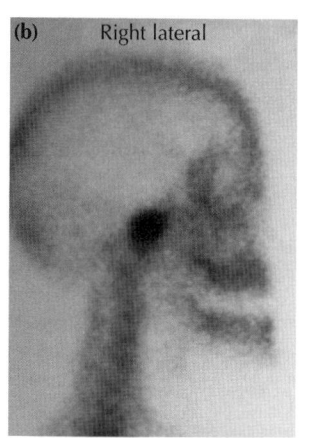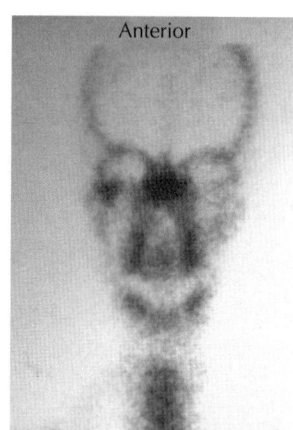

(c)

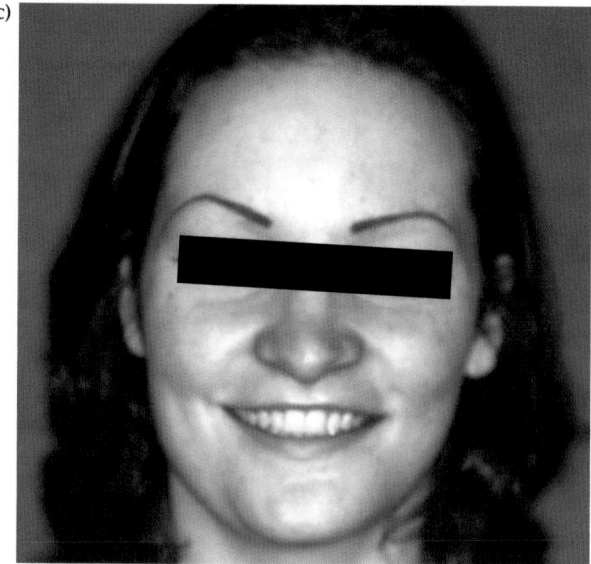

Figure 42.26 (a) Condylar hyperplasia with mandibular asymmetry. (b) Bone scan revealing increased bone activity in the right mandibular condyle. (c) Postoperative appearance following bimaxillary osteotomy to correct facial asymmetry.

Orthognathic surgery

Orthognathic surgery is the term given to the surgical correction of deformities of the jaw. It is usually undertaken in close cooperation between orthodontic and maxillofacial surgeons. Surgery is directed at simultaneously changing the position of both maxilla and mandible at the end of the growth period. This is termed bimaxillary osteotomy. Treatment planning usually commences at the age of 12–13 years, in which the orthodontist aligns the dental arches in correct relation for each jaw. This frequently results in an accentuation of the facial deformity at the end of the orthodontic phase of treatment. Treatment normally takes 2 years, in which orthognathic surgery is performed towards the end of orthodontic treatment, although orthodontic treatment in the form of fixed appliances usually continues postoperatively for up to 6 months after surgery. Surgical planning should be meticulous and involves clinical examination and cephalometric assessment in the form of radiograph analysis, as well as study model analysis, working in close cooperation with maxillofacial technologists.

Orthognathic surgery is generally carried out through intraoral incisions, in which the upper and lower jaws are mobilised by achieving osteotomy cuts with saws and drills (Fig. 42.24). Following mobilisation of the mandible and maxilla, the jaws are repositioned and held with titanium plates and screws placed through an intraoral approach. This frequently avoids the use of intermaxillary fixation and allows earlier function of the jaws as well as improved early dietary intake. Examples of orthognathic surgery are shown in Figs 24.25 and 42.26.

Patients with syndromic conditions such as hemifacial microsomia and Crouzon's and Treacher-Collins' syndromes require the services of a craniofacial surgeon. As these syndromes are extremely rare, management and surgery should only be carried out in designated centres. The principal treatment is to correct the deformity from the cranium downwards, with correction of the cranial deformity within the first 3 years of life and correction of the residual midfacial and lower facial deformity in childhood and adolescence.

A relatively new innovation is the introduction of distraction osteogenesis in the management of craniofacial deformity. This technique, in its infancy within maxillofacial surgery, may greatly change and reduce the requirements for major surgery in patients with severe facial deformity (Summary box 42.15).

Summary box 42.15

Principles of orthognathic surgery

- Orthodontist aligns the dental arches
- Surgery then corrects the jaw deformity

FURTHER READING

Markus, A.F. and Delaire, J. (1993) Functional primary closure of cleft lip. *Br J Oral Maxillofac Surg* **31**: 281–91.

Markus, A.F., Delaire, J. and Smith W.P. (1992) Facial balance in cleft lip and palate. I: Normal development and cleft palate. *Br J Oral Maxillofac Surg* **30**: 287.

Markus, A.F., Delaire, J. and Smith W.P. (1992) Facial balance in cleft lip and palate. II: Cleft lip and palate and secondary deformities. *Br J Oral Maxillofac Surg* **30**: 296.

Markus, A.F., Smith, W.P. and Delaire, J. (1993) Primary closure of cleft palate: a functional approach. *Br J Oral Maxillofac Surg* **31**: 71–7.

Smith, W.P., Markus, A.F. and Delaire, J. (1995) Primary closure of the cleft alveolus: a functional approach. *Br J Oral Maxillofac Surg* **33**: 156–65.

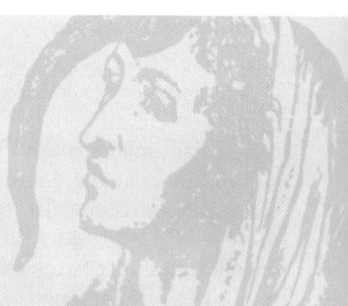

The nose and sinuses

To be familiar with:
- The basic anatomy of the nose and paranasal sinuses
- The principles of managing post-traumatic nasal and septal deformity
- The causes and management of epistaxis
- The diagnosis and management of nasal polyposis
- The clinical features of sinus infection and its treatment and potential complications
- The common sinonasal tumours, their presentation, investigation and principles of treatment

BASIC ANATOMY OF THE NOSE AND PARANASAL SINUSES

The supporting structures of the nose are shown in Fig. 43.1. The septum consists of the anterior quadrilateral cartilage, the perpendicular plate of the ethmoid and the vomer (Fig. 43.2). The lateral wall of the nasal cavity contains the superior, middle and inferior turbinates (Fig. 43.3). Opening onto the lateral nasal wall

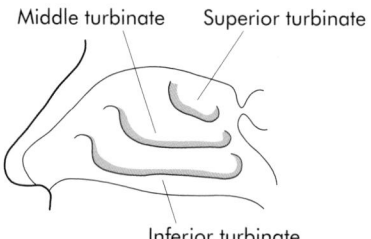

Figure 43.3 The right lateral nasal wall.

are the ostea of all of the nasal sinuses except the sphenoid sinus (Figs 43.4 and 43.5)

The nasal fossae and sinuses receive their blood supply via the external and internal carotid arteries. The external carotid artery supplies the interior of the nose via the maxillary and sphenopalatine arteries. The greater palatine artery supplies the anteroinferior septum via the incisive canal. The contribution from the internal carotid artery is via the anterior and posterior ethmoidal arteries,

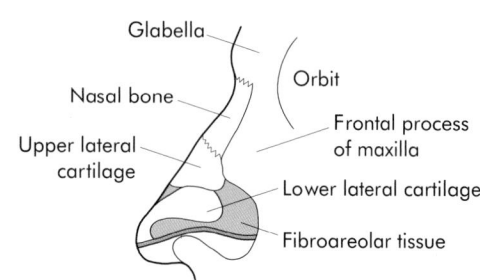

Figure 43.1 The nasal skeleton.

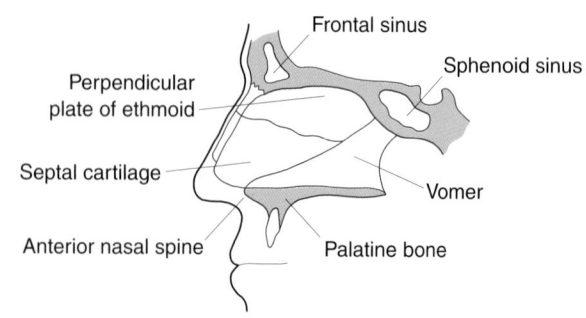

Figure 43.2 The left side of the nasal septum.

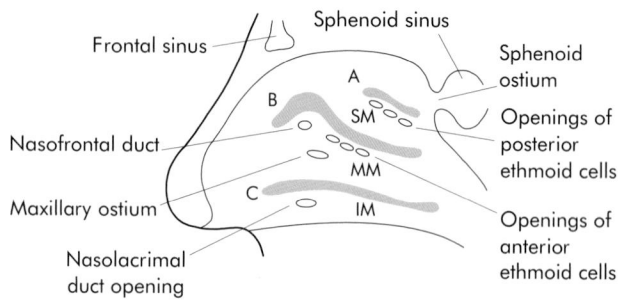

Figure 43.4 The right lateral nasal wall with turbinates removed to show the sinus ostia. A, insertion of superior turbinate; B, insertion of middle turbinate; C, insertion of inferior turbinate; SM, superior meatus; MM, middle meatus; IM, inferior meatus.

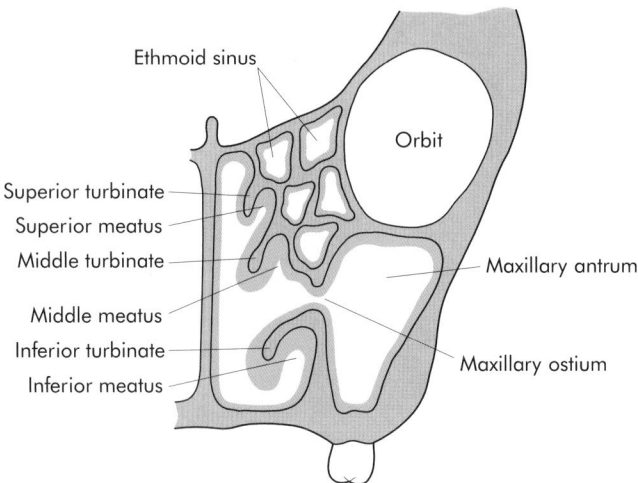

Figure 43.5 Coronal section through the left maxillary and ethmoid sinuses.

which are branches of the ophthalmic artery (Fig. 43.6). All of these arteries anastomose to form a plexus of vessels (Kiesselbach's plexus) on the anterior part of the nasal septum. Venous drainage is via the ophthalmic and facial veins and the pterygoid and pharyngeal plexuses. Intracranial drainage into the cavernous sinus via the ophthalmic vein is of particular clinical importance because of the potential for intracranial spread of nasal sepsis.

EXAMINATION OF THE NOSE AND PARANASAL SINUSES

Internal inspection of the nasal fossae can be achieved to a limited extent with the use of a Thudichum's speculum. A more thorough examination and assessment of the nose is possible with the use of either rigid or flexible endoscopes. Application of a vasoconstrictor/analgesic spray such as lidocaine hydrochloride 5% (w/v) with phenylephrine hydrochloride 0.5% (w/v) shrinks down the nasal mucosa and improves the view.

IMAGING OF PARANASAL SINUSES

Plain radiographs are of limited value in the assessment of sinus disease. A minimum of four views, namely occipitomental,

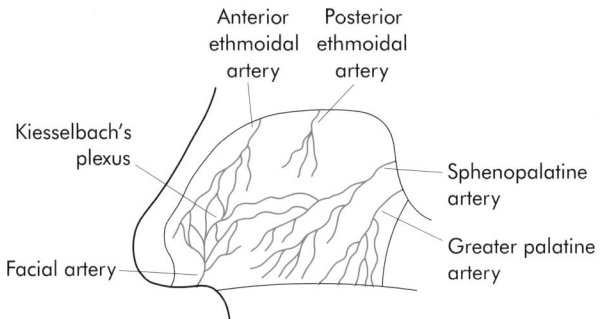

Figure 43.6 Arterial blood supply to the left side of the nasal septum.

Wilhelm Kiesselbach, **1839–1902, Professor of Otology, Erlangen, Germany.**
Johann Ludwig Wilhelm Thudichum, **1829–1901, Biochemist and General Practitioner, London, England.**

occipitofrontal, submentovertical and lateral, are required to demonstrate the paranasal sinuses adequately. Computerised tomography (CT) scanning is far superior in demonstrating sinus pathology. Coronal and axial scans are necessary for detailed assessment.

TRAUMA TO THE NOSE AND PARANASAL SINUSES

Fracture of the nasal bones

Blunt injury to the nose may fracture the nasal bones. This can be a simple crack of the nasal bones without displacement, but greater force may result in deviation of the bony nasal complex laterally (Fig. 43.7). A blow directly from the front may depress the bony pyramid or cause a comminuted fracture and widening of the bridge of the nose. The fracture line can extend into the lacrimal bone and tear the anterior ethmoidal artery producing catastrophic haemorrhage. This may be delayed, occurring only as the soft-tissue swelling subsides and the torn artery opens up.

Violent trauma to the frontal area of the nose can result in a fracture of the frontal and ethmoid sinuses extending into the anterior cranial fossa. Dural tears and brain injuries, which may be open or closed, are then at risk from ascending infection from the nose or sinuses. This may progress to meningitis or brain abscess.

Cerebrospinal fluid (CSF) rhinorrhoea is a certain sign of a dural tear. There may be associated surgical emphysema, proptosis with or without loss of vision, or a frontal pneumoencephalocoele. Anosmia occurs in 75% of patients with these injuries and cranial nerves II–VI may be injured. A clear discharge from the nose may be identified as CSF by a simple stix test confirming the presence of glucose, which is not present in nasal mucus. Such injuries are managed by neurosurgical exploration to remove bone fragments, close the dura and repair the skull base. Late complications of this injury include CSF fistula, recurrent late

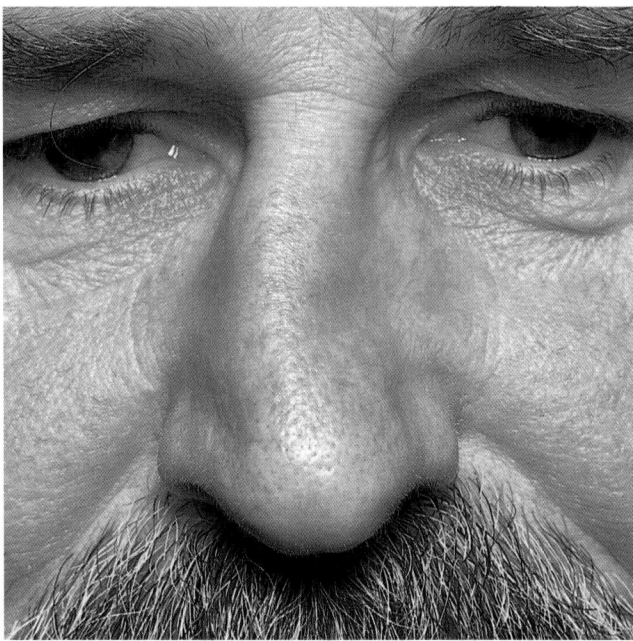

Figure 43.7 Fracture of the nasal bones with displacement of the bony nasal complex to the right side.

meningitis, brain abscess, osteomyelitis and the formation of mucopyocoeles.

Management of fractured nasal bones

Fractured nasal bones are often accompanied by extensive overlying soft tissue swelling and bruising, which may hinder the assessment of the underlying bony deformity. Reviewing the patient after 4–5 days when the soft tissue swelling has diminished will allow a better assessment of any deformity. If there is a significant degree of nasal deformity then this can be corrected by manipulation of the nasal bones under local or general anaesthesia. This should be carried out within 10–20 days of the injury while the bony fragments are still mobile. The deviated nasal bones are repositioned to restore the correct alignment of the nose or, in the case of a depressed fracture, the fragments are elevated and supported if necessary with anterior nasal packing. Often a satisfactory result can be obtained by manipulation alone but, should this fail, a rhinoplasty procedure may be necessary to obtain further improvement in the appearance of the nose.

Septal injury

A blunt injury of moderate force may lead to lateral displacement or deformity of the septal cartilage, restricting the nasal airway. A C-shaped fracture of the septal cartilage and the anterior portion of the perpendicular plate of the ethmoid bone is known as a Jarjavay fracture. Unlike the nasal bones the nasal septum cannot be manipulated back into position and requires a formal septoplasty procedure to restore the anatomy and the patency of the nasal airways.

Springing of the septal cartilage with separation of the overlying mucoperichondrium and subsequent bleeding into this potential space will cause a septal haematoma, which may be unilateral or bilateral. The haematoma will give rise to nasal obstruction and can easily be overlooked in the presence of extensive facial injuries. Untreated, a septal haematoma will progress to abscess formation and ultimately result in necrosis of the septal cartilage. Robbed of this support the tip of the nose will collapse. A septal haematoma should be treated by incision and evacuation of the blood clot. The insertion of a small silicone drain and packing of the nasal fossa will prevent reaccumulation and allow the mucoperichondrium to readhere to the septal cartilage. A broad-spectrum prophylactic antibiotic should be prescribed (Summary box 43.1).

Summary box 43.1

Nasal trauma

- Do not overlook a septal haematoma
- Displaced nasal bone fractures should be reduced within 10–20 days of injury
- Severe persistent epistaxis suggests lacrimal bone fracture and injury to the anterior ethmoid artery
- Cerebrospinal fluid rhinorrhoea indicates a fracture involving the frontal or ethmoid sinuses with a dural tear

---

THE NASAL SEPTUM

Septal deformity

In some individuals a naturally occurring deviated nasal septum may give rise to significant nasal obstruction. In others, minor nasal trauma is responsible for displacement of the septum and restriction of the nasal airway (Fig. 43.8). The physical obstruction of the nasal airway by a deviated septum is readily apparent on anterior rhinoscopy. Further encroachment of the anterior nasal airway can occur if the ventral edge of the septal cartilage is dislocated from the columella and projects into the nasal vestibule. Inferior turbinate hypertrophy is frequently seen on the concave side of a deviated nasal septum.

Septal deformity can be corrected by a septoplasty procedure or a submucous resection (SMR) of the septum. In the former procedure the septal cartilage is preserved but the anatomical abnormalities giving rise to its deformity, such as a twisted maxillary crest or inclination of the bony septum, are corrected. In the SMR procedure the deformed septal cartilage is excised while preserving the dorsal strut along with the anterior 5 mm of septal cartilage in order to support and maintain the normal shape of the nasal tip. Both operations are performed through a vertical incision of the septal mucosa with elevation of mucoperichondrial flaps.

Complications of septal surgery include septal perforation. If too much cartilage is excised in the SMR procedure, loss of support to the dorsum of the nose may result in a supra-tip depression or drooping of the tip of the nose.

Septal perforation

A hole in the nasal septum causes a turbulent airflow through the nose and a resulting sensation of nasal blockage. The causes of septal perforation are listed in Summary box 43.2. The most common cause is a complication of septal surgery when there is loss of cartilage and a bilateral breach in the mucoperichondrium.

Summary box 43.2

Causes of septal perforations

- Trauma
  - Surgical following septal surgery
  - Nose picking
- Infection
  - Syphilis
  - Tuberculosis
- Vasculitis
  - Wegener's granulomatosis
- Tumours
- Toxins
  - Chrome salts
  - Cocaine
- Idiopathic

Septal perforations seldom heal spontaneously. They give rise to extensive crusting at the margins of the perforation, often with mucosal bleeding. If situated to the front of the septum,

---

Jean Francois Jarjavay, **1815–1868, Professor of Anatomy and Surgery, The Faculty of Paris, Paris, France.**

Friedrich Wegener, **1907–1990, Professor of Pathology, Lübeck, Germany, described this form of granulomatosis in 1939.**

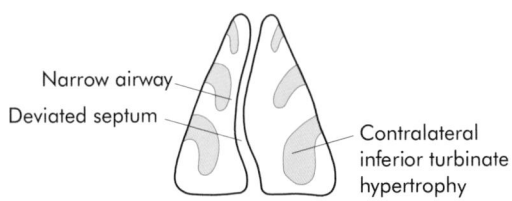

Figure 43.8 Coronal section through the anterior nasal fossae with deviated nasal septum to the right side.

embarrassing whistling can occur with nasal respiration. Crusting can be controlled to a degree with nasal douches or the use of topical antiseptic creams to minimise nasal drying. A great variety of operations have been described to close septal perforations but none has met with universal success. A more certain option is to occlude the perforation by inserting a Silastic biflanged prosthesis (Figs 43.9 and 43.10).

Wegener's granulomatosis is a systemic idiopathic autoimmune disease affecting the nose, lungs and kidneys. Mucosal granulations on the nasal septum destroy the cartilage, producing a septal perforation and a saddle deformity of the nose. Nasal symptoms include excessive crusting, blockage and serosanguinous discharge. Laboratory findings include a high erythrocyte sedimentation rate and may demonstrate impaired creatinine

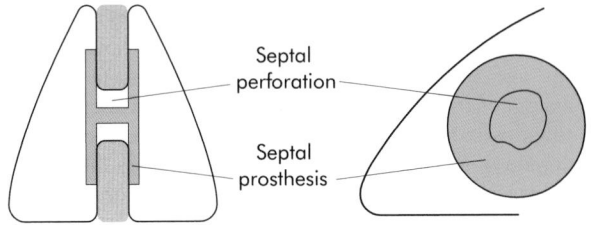

Figure 43.9 Anterior and lateral views of septal perforation occluded with prosthesis.

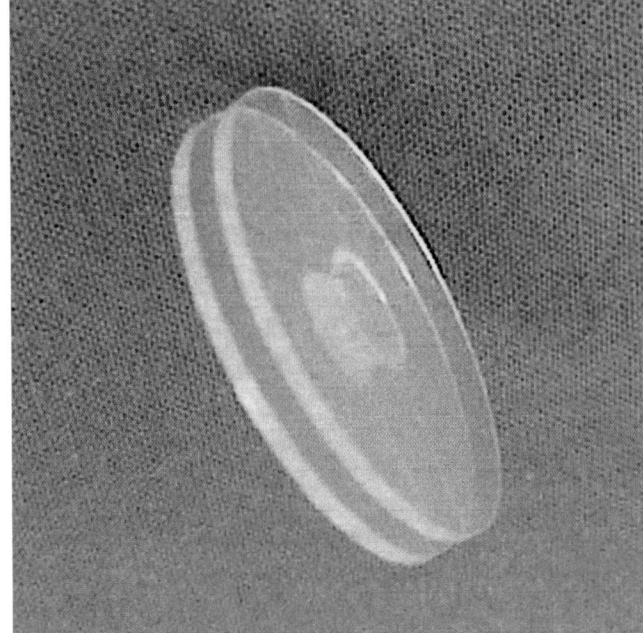

Figure 43.10 Silastic prosthesis for septal perforation.

clearance. The presence of antineutrophil cytoplasmic antibodies (ANCA) is 80–100% sensitive in disseminated disease and 60–70% sensitive in upper airway disease.

EPISTAXIS

The causes of epistaxis are listed in Summary box 43.3. The most common site of bleeding is from Kiesselbach's plexus in Little's area of the anterior portion of the septum (see Fig. 43.6). Less often bleeding is from the lateral nasal wall. Anterior bleeding is common in children and young adults as a result of nose blowing or picking. In the elderly, arteriosclerosis and hypertension are the underlying causes of arterial bleeding from the posterior part of the nose. Epistaxis commonly occurs in elderly patients on warfarin or aspirin. Less common causes are trauma, foreign bodies within the nose, blood diseases, disorders of coagulation and malignant tumours of the nose or sinuses. Hereditary haemorrhagic telangiectasia (Osler's disease) gives rise to recurrent multifocal bleeding from thin-walled vessels deficient in muscle and elastic tissue (Fig. 43.11).

Juvenile angiofibroma is an uncommon condition that affects adolescent boys and may lead to massive life-threatening episodes of bleeding. It has a peak incidence between 14 and 18 years and can very rarely occur in adult men. It is a benign tumour that arises from the sphenopalatine fossa and expands into the nasopharynx as a smooth, lobulated red mass. The tumour extends aggressively through foramina and fissures into the ethmoid and sphenoid sinuses, orbit and skull base and eventually enters the cranial cavity. Lateral growth can occur into the infratemporal fossa (Summary box 43.3).

Summary box 43.3

Causes of epistaxis

Local
- **Nose picking**
- **Nasal trauma**
- **Nasal foreign bodies**
- **Tumours**
- **Infection**
- **Granulomatous disorders**
- **Juvenile angiofibroma**

Systemic
- **Hypertension**
- **Warfarin therapy**
- **Aspirin therapy**
- **Haemophilia**
- **von Willebrand's disease**
- **Leukaemia**
- **Haemorrhagic telangiectasia**

James Laurence Little, **1836–1885**, Professor of Surgery, The University of Vermont, Montpelier, VT, USA.
Sir William Osler, **1849–1919**, Professor of Medicine successively at McGill University, Montreal, Canada; The University of Philadelphia, Pennsylvania, PA, and The Johns Hopkins University, Baltimore, MD, USA, finally becoming Regius Professor of Medicine at Oxford University, Oxford, England in 1904.
Erik Adolf von Willebrand, **1870–1949**, Physician, Diakonissanstaltens Hospital, Helsinki, (Helsingfors), Finland, described hereditary pseudohaemophilia in 1926.

CHAPTER 43 | THE NOSE AND SINUSES

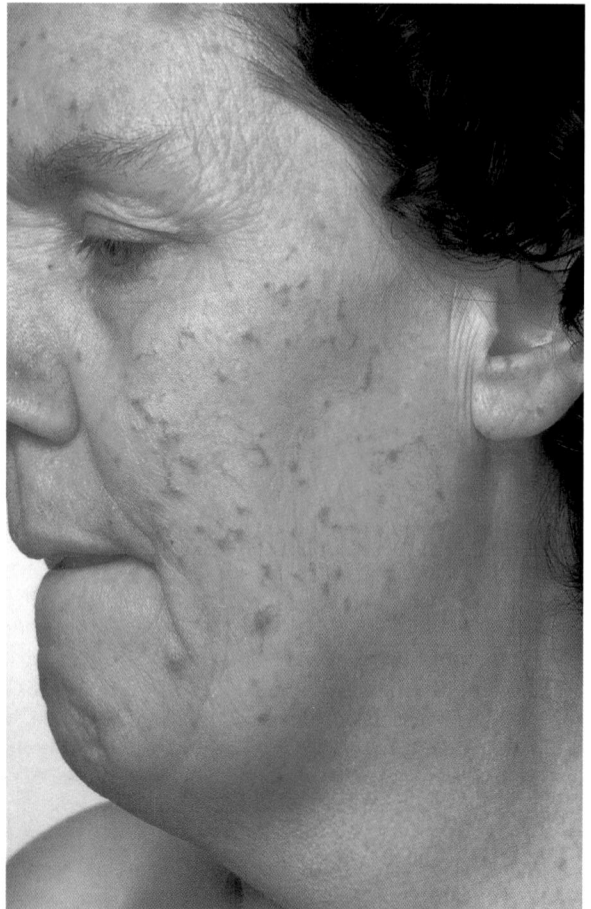

Figure 43.11 Osler's disease showing the multiple telangiectasia.

Diagnosis is made with contrast CT scanning or magnetic resonance imaging (MRI). Anterior bowing or indentation of the posterior antral wall (Holman–Miller or antral sign) is the classical finding but may be seen in other expansive lesions in this area. It is a very vascular tumour, which should not be biopsied because of the risk of uncontrollable haemorrhage. Excision is best carried out by a surgeon experienced in the management of the condition. Preoperative embolisation of the feeding blood vessels may help to reduce blood loss during surgery. Sometimes the tumour is managed with radiotherapy.

Management of epistaxis

Bleeding from Kiesselbach's plexus may be controlled by silver nitrate cautery under local anaesthesia. Posterior bleeding, as seen in the elderly, may require anterior nasal packing either with Vaseline-impregnated ribbon gauze or absorbable sponge. An alternative to anterior packing is the use of an inflatable epistaxis balloon catheter (Fig. 43.12). The catheter is passed into the nose and the distal balloon is inflated in the nasopharynx to secure it. The proximal balloon, which is sausage shaped, is then inflated within the nasal fossa to compress the bleeding point. Although usually effective they can be uncomfortable.

Sometimes anterior nasal packing alone is not sufficient to control haemorrhage and posterior nasal packing may be required. This is usually carried out under general anaesthesia by inserting a gauze pack into the nasopharynx, which is then secured by tapes passed through each side of the nose and tied

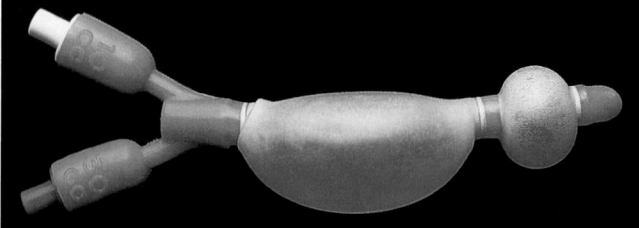

Figure 43.12 Epistaxis balloon catheter.

together across a protected columella. A third tape is brought out through the mouth and taped to the patient's cheek. The nasal fossae are then packed with anterior nasal packs. All packs are left in place for 48 hours and prophylactic antibiotics are given. The tape attached to the cheek is to facilitate removal of the pack, usually achieved without a general anaesthetic. Endoscopic-assisted cautery or clipping of a posterior bleeding point can be an effective alternative to nasal packing.

In uncontrolled life-threatening epistaxis in which the above methods have proved ineffective, haemostasis is secured by vascular ligation. Depending on the origin of bleeding it may be necessary to ligate the internal maxillary artery in the pterygopalatine fossa and the anterior and posterior ethmoidal arteries. An alternative measure is external carotid artery ligation above the origin of the lingual artery.

In Osler's disease, anterior nasal packing is best avoided if at all possible because it is most likely to lead to further mucosal trauma and bleeding. High-dose oestrogen induces squamous metaplasia of the nasal mucosa and has been used effectively in treating this condition. In some cases it may be necessary to resort to excision of the diseased nasal mucosa via a lateral rhinotomy and replacement with a split-skin graft, a procedure known as a septodermoplasty. It is not unknown, however, for the grafted skin to undergo similar abnormal vascular change over time (Summary box 43.4).

Summary box 43.4

Epistaxis

- The commonest causes are nose picking, hypertension and anticoagulant therapy
- Young people bleed from the anterior septum – Kiesselbach's plexus
- Elderly people bleed from the posterior part of the nose
- Silver nitrate cautery is used to control anterior bleeding
- Moderate bleeding may require anterior nasal packing
- Severe bleeding may require anterior and posterior nasal packing
- Persistent bleeding may require endoscopic cautery/ clipping or arterial ligation

---

NASAL POLYPS

Pathology

Nasal polyps are benign swellings of the ethmoid sinus mucosa of unknown origin. Histologically, the polyps contain a waterlogged stroma infiltrated with inflammatory cells and eosinophils. The majority of nasal polyps arise from the ethmoid sinuses, with each individual ethmoid air cell giving rise to a single polyp as its swollen mucosal lining prolapses out of the air cell to hang down inside the nasal cavity. Polyps can arise from the other nasal sinuses and a single large polyp arising from the maxillary antrum is referred to as an antrochoanal polyp (Fig. 43.13). This usually fills the nose and eventually prolapses posteriorly down into the nasopharynx.

There is a clear association between nasal polyps and three distinct clinical conditions: asthma, aspirin sensitivity and cystic fibrosis. Samter's triad of nasal polyps, aspirin allergy and asthma is not uncommon; however, there is no conclusive evidence that polyps are caused by allergy. Several inflammatory mediators have been isolated from nasal polyps including vascular cell adhesion molecule (VCAM)-1, nitric oxide synthase and cys-leukotrienes (Cys-LT) but their role in the aetiology of polyps is unclear. Fungal colonisation of nasal mucosa has been implicated as a possible aetiological factor. Leukotriene, chemical mediators and interleukin inhibitors may have a role in the future management of nasal polyposis.

Clinical features

Patients present with nasal obstruction, watery rhinorrhoea, sinus infection and often anosmia. Polyps are easily identifiable within the nose as pale semitransparent grey masses, which are mobile and insensitive when palpated with a fine probe. This allows them to be distinguished from hypertrophied turbinates. If left untreated, extensive nasal polyposis will eventually cause expansion of the nose and the polyps may prolapse out through the nasal vestibule (Fig. 43.14).

Malignancy should be considered in adults with unilateral nasal polyps whereas in children such polyps must be distinguished from a meningocoele or encephalocoele by high-resolution CT scanning of the anterior cranial fossa. Nasal polyps are unusual in children and, if multiple, they occur in conjunction with cystic fibrosis in 10% of cases.

Management of nasal polyps

Medical treatment with systemic steroids will often reduce the size of nasal polyps and give short-term relief of nasal blockage. Unfortunately the polyps tend to recur when the treatment stops. Polyps occurring in association with cystic fibrosis are usually more resistant to systemic steroid treatment. Low-dose topical corticosteroid nasal sprays may reduce the growth of nasal polyps

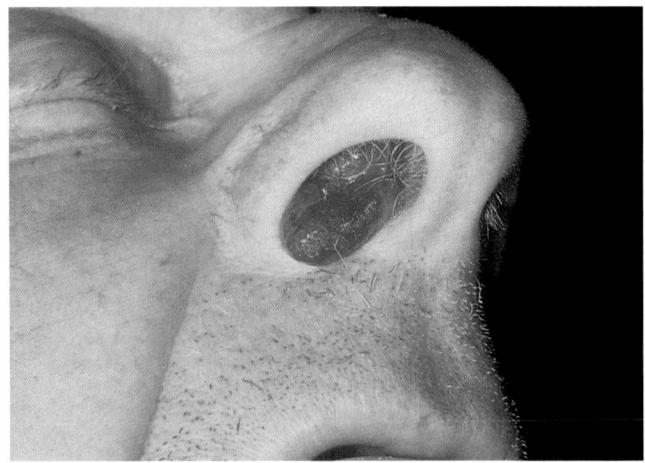

Figure 43.14 Nasal polyp in right nasal vestibule.

but are relatively ineffective in massive nasal polyposis. They can be useful in retarding the regrowth of polyps after surgical removal. If nasal steroid sprays are used in children, monitoring is required to avoid potential growth suppression.

Surgical treatment is required in patients with severe nasal obstruction and pansinusitis that is refractory to medical treatment. Polyps may be removed either by avulsion with a nasal snare or endoscopically with a powered nasal microresector. (Fig. 43.15). Antral lavage should be performed at the same time. Preoperative CT scans allow evaluation of any anatomical variations and changes caused by polyposis or previous surgery. The objective is to remove all of the polypoid disease and provide adequate sinus ventilation. All polyps should be submitted for histological examination.

Polyps often recur after surgery in a seemingly random and unpredictable way, sometimes within a few months or even after several years. Long-term treatment with a low-dose topical steroid nasal spray postoperatively lessens the tendency for polyps to recur. After multiple recurrences, external ethmoidectomy should be considered (Summary box 43.5).

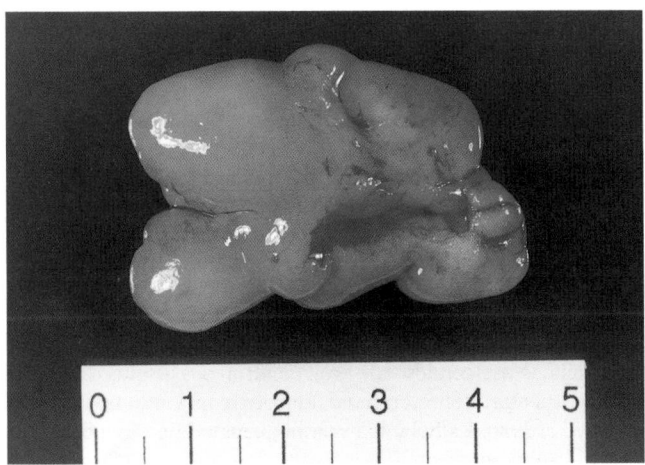

Figure 43.13 Antrochoanal polyp.

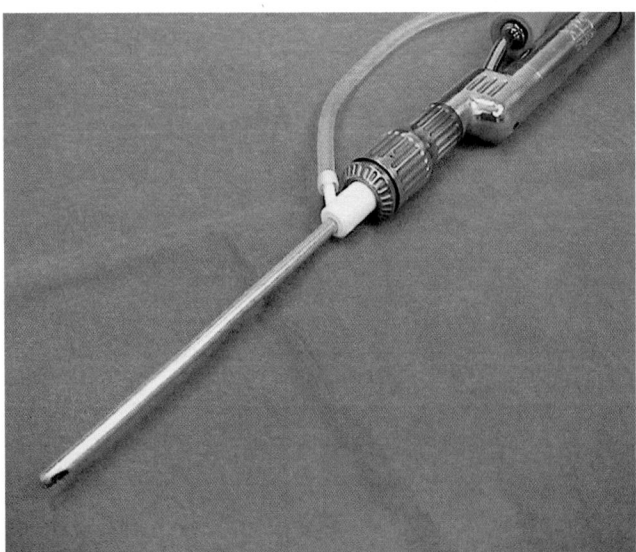

Figure 43.15 Powered nasal microresector.

CHAPTER 43 | THE NOSE AND SINUSES

Summary box 43.5

Nasal polyps

- Polyps are insensitive to touch and are mobile
- Simple polyps are bilateral
- Unilateral nasal polyps should be removed for histology
- Bleeding polyps may indicate malignancy
- Meningocoele and encephalocoele must be excluded in children with polyps
- Polyps can be removed with a snare or a powered microresector
- Recurrent polyps may require external ethmoidectomy
- Transitional papilloma may mimic simple nasal polyps
- All polyps should be submitted for histology

MAXILLARY SINUSITIS

Clinical features

Local disorders such as nasal polyps, deviated nasal septum or upper dental sepsis may predispose to sinus infection. Patients with persistent maxillary sinusitis have mucopurulent postnasal discharge, headache, which is variable in severity and location, facial pain and nasal obstruction. Irritation of the superior alveolar nerve may give rise to referred upper toothache. The nasal mucosa is swollen and bathed in mucopurulent secretions. Plain sinus radiographs may show a fluid level in the antrum or complete opacity (Fig. 43.16).

The most likely causative organisms are *Streptococcus pneumoniae* and *Haemophilus influenzae*. As the infection becomes chronic the likelihood of anaerobic infection increases. The consideration of *Branhamella catarrhalis* as a primary pathogen and the possible involvement of β-lactamase-producing strains of *H. influenzae* will influence the choice of antibiotic treatment. About 10% of infections of the maxillary antrum are caused by dental sepsis from anaerobic organisms. The resultant mucopurulent

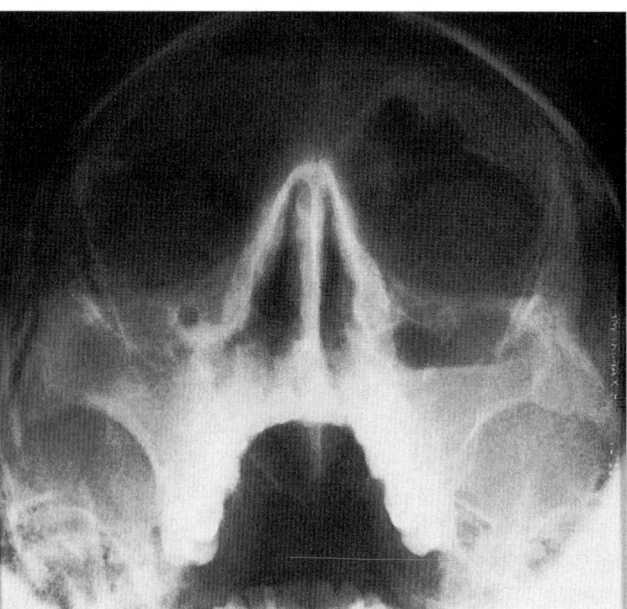

Figure 43.16 Plain radiograph showing the fluid level in the left maxillary antrum and total opacity of the right antrum.

nasal secretion has a foul taste and smell. Complications of maxillary sinusitis include acute cellulitis or osteitis.

Treatment

Adequate penetration of antibiotics into chronically inflamed sinus mucosa is doubtful and, therefore, treatment may need to be prolonged. Topical nasal decongestants such as ephedrine nasal drops will often encourage the sinus to drain.

Antral lavage under general anaesthesia allows confirmation of the diagnosis and provides the opportunity to obtain samples for bacteriology. The antrum is entered through the inferior meatus below the inferior turbinate where the bone separating the antrum from the nasal fossa is extremely thin and can be easily penetrated by a trocar and cannula (Fig. 43.17).

If infection has caused a significant degree of inflammation and fibrosis of the lining of the antrum then the natural ostium may be completely obstructed. In this situation an intranasal inferior meatal antrostomy may be fashioned to facilitate drainage from the antrum. Alternatively, intranasal endoscopic techniques may be employed to create a middle meatal antrostomy or enlarge the natural ostium. Endoscopic nasal surgery allows a more functional approach to diseases of the paranasal sinuses and the indications for radical antrostomy are on the decline. Areas of chronically diseased mucosa and infected granulation tissue hinder mucociliary transport and lymphatic drainage, leading to retained secretions and the perpetuation of infection. Endoscopic surgery directed towards the middle meatus and the ethmoid system allows precise removal of diseased mucosa with minimal trauma to adjacent tissues and leads to quicker healing with return to normal function. By removing fibrotic tissue from the narrow recesses within the nose, ventilation and internal drainage of the sinuses can be restored (Summary box 43.6).

Summary box 43.6

Maxillary sinusitis

- The most common causative organisms are *Streptococcus pneumoniae* and *Haemophilus influenzae*
- Anaerobic infection may result from dental sepsis
- Acute infection should be treated with antibiotics and topical decongestants
- Antral lavage is diagnostic and therapeutic
- Intranasal antrostomy or endoscopic middle meatal antrostomy may be required
- Complications of untreated infection include cellulitis, osteitis and involvement of the orbit

FRONTOETHMOIDAL SINUSITIS

When treated promptly with antibiotics and topical nasal decongestants this type of sinus infection is unlikely to be a long-term problem. If allowed to persist, chronic frontoethmoiditis gives rise to mucopurulent catarrh, frontal headache or a feeling of pressure between the eyes, nasal obstruction and hyposmia. Nasal endoscopy will confirm pus issuing from the middle meatus. The ethmoid sinuses can only be properly assessed radiologically by CT scanning, including coronal as well as axial sections.

If frontoethmoiditis fails to settle with conservative treatment

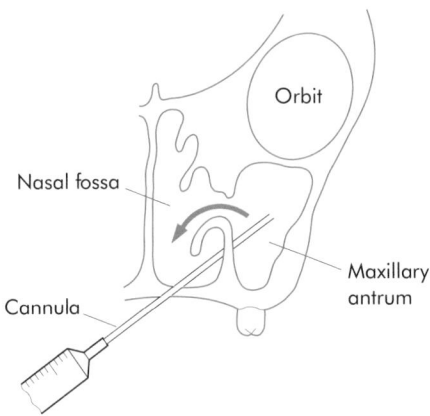

Figure 43.17 Diagram of left maxillary antral lavage.

then frontal sinus drainage may be required. Complications of frontoethmoiditis are potentially extremely serious. Orbital cellulitis (Fig. 43.18) may occur and can progress to an extraperiosteal abscess, which typically displaces the eyeball down, forwards and laterally. If unrecognised and untreated this can lead to blindness. Treatment consists of intravenous broad-spectrum antibiotics and orbital decompression by an external approach. Orbital cellulitis may also progress to cavernous sinus thrombosis and septicaemia. Spread of infection by direct bone penetration or via the diploic vein can give rise to extradural, subdural or frontal lobe abscess formation (Summary box 43.7).

Summary box 43.7

Frontoethmoiditis

- Assessment is best achieved by CT scanning
- It may require open surgical drainage
- Chronic infection may require an obliterative osteoplastic flap procedure
- Orbital infections may threaten sight
- Intracranial spread may cause meningitis, cerebral abscess or cavernous sinus thrombosis

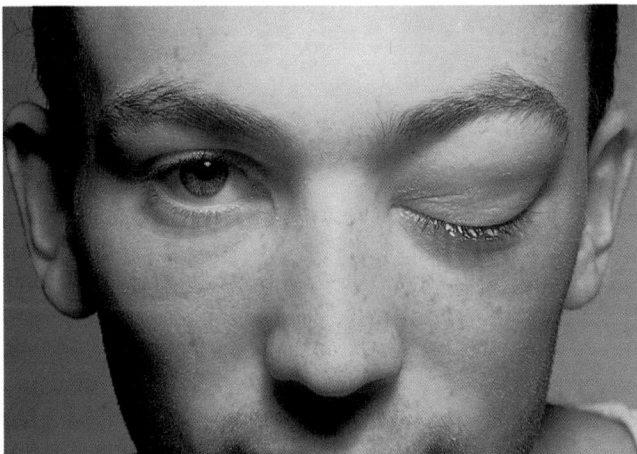

Figure 43.18 Left periorbital cellulitis complicating acute left ethmoiditis.

TUMOURS OF THE NOSE AND SINUSES

There are a wide variety of tumours that can occur in the nose or paranasal sinuses. Tumours arising in the nasal fossa may present with unilateral nasal obstruction, persistent unilateral anterior rhinorrhoea, postnasal catarrh or epistaxis. These are common, non-specific symptoms and a high index of suspicion is required to avoid missing such a diagnosis. Unfortunately, the diagnosis is often delayed. Symptoms that may suggest the possibility of sinonasal malignancy include unilateral blood-stained rhinorrhoea, facial swelling and proptosis.

Benign tumours

Simple papillomas or viral warts can grow inside the nasal vestibule. They can be confused with carcinomas and are best excised for histological diagnosis.

Osteomas of the nasal skeleton are not uncommon and are usually detected on radiography as an incidental finding (Fig. 43.19). In symptomatic individuals the osteoma can be removed via the frontal sinus or an external ethmoidectomy.

Transitional cell papillomas can occur both in the nasal cavity and the nasal sinuses. They are sometimes referred to as inverted papillomas because histologically the hyperplastic epithelium inverts into the underlying stroma. The papillomas are covered with transitional epithelium. They can be quite extensive and give rise to nasal obstruction and sometimes epistaxis. They may be mistaken for simple nasal polyps. In 25% of cases the diagnosis is made by the pathologist after a routine nasal polypectomy. When large they can erode the lateral nasal wall and infiltrate the antrum or ethmoid

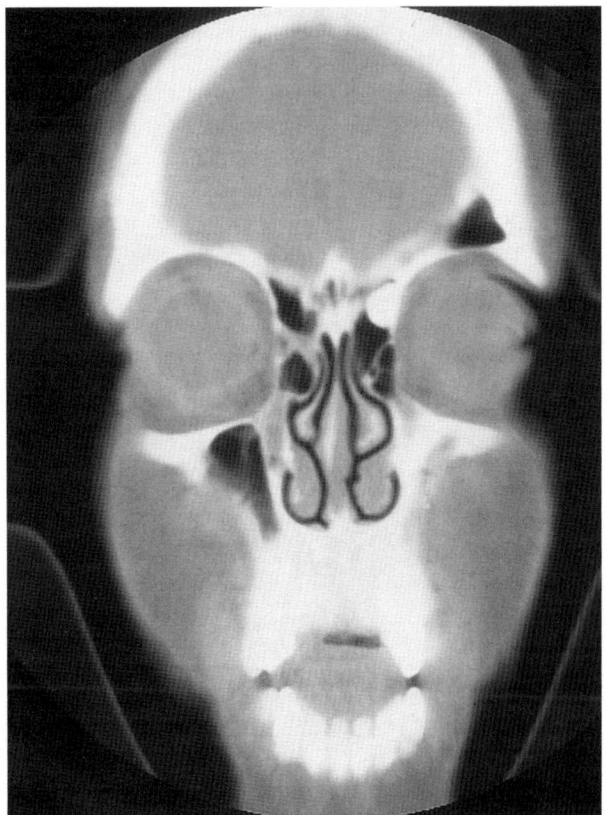

Figure 43.19 Coronal computerised tomography scan showing a small osteoma in the right ethmoid sinus adjacent to the orbit.

sinus. Calcification within the tumour may be seen on CT scanning along with sclerosis of bone at the margins of the growth (Fig. 43.20). Transitional cell papillomas can undergo malignant change; synchronous lesions occur in 5–10% of cases whereas metachronous lesions develop in 1%. For this reason more radical surgery is employed than for simple polyps to ensure complete removal of all papillomata; this will usually involve a partial maxillectomy.

Malignant tumours

The most common malignant tumours to occur within the nasal cavity and paranasal sinuses are squamous cell carcinoma (Fig. 43.21), adenoid cystic carcinoma and adenocarcinoma. Adenocarcinoma has been linked to exposure to hard wood dust in the furniture industry. Adenoid cystic carcinomas arise from minor salivary glands, which can be found in the nose. Almost 50% of sinonasal cancers originate on the lateral nasal wall and 33% arise from the maxillary antrum. The incidence of ethmoid cancers is 5% and frontal/sphenoid cancers 2.5%.

Presenting symptoms include unilateral nasal obstruction, chronic nasal discharge, which is often haemorrhagic and offensive, and loss of skin sensation on the face (trigeminal nerve). There may be swelling of the cheek, buccal sulcus or medial canthus of the eye and a feeling of fullness or pressure within the nose or face. Suspicious signs of invasion of neighbouring tissues include diplopia, proptosis, loosening of the teeth (Fig. 43.22), trismus, cranial nerve palsies and regional lymphadenopathy.

A biopsy can be taken at the time of nasal endoscopy to provide a tissue diagnosis whereas assessment of bone erosion and the extent of the disease can be determined by CT scanning (Fig. 43.23).

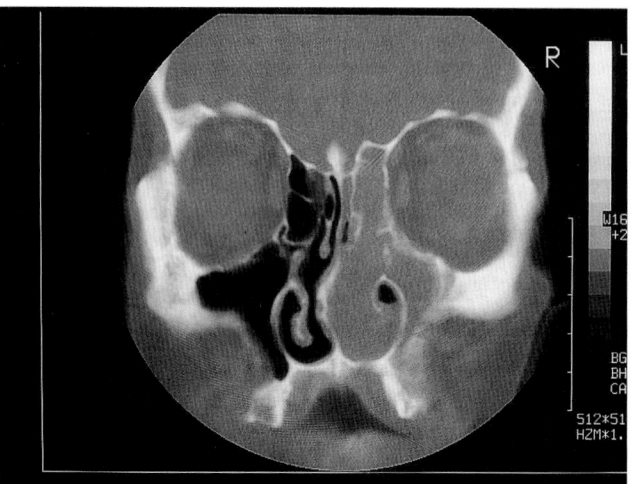

Figure 43.20 Coronal computerised tomography scan showing extensive transitional cell papilloma involving the right maxillary antrum and ethmoid sinuses.

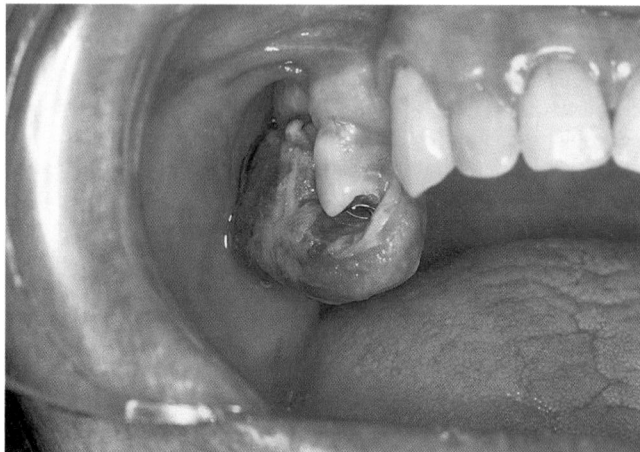

Figure 43.22 Maxillary antral carcinoma presenting through an oroantral fistula.

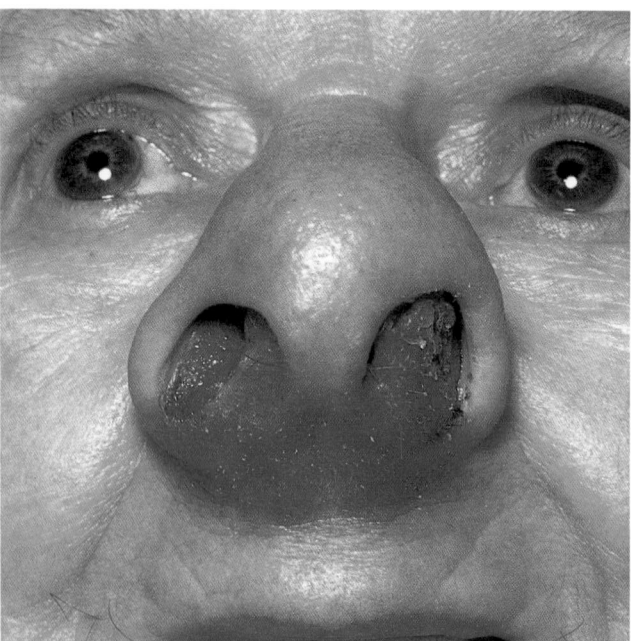

Figure 43.21 Squamous cell carcinoma of the nasal septum.

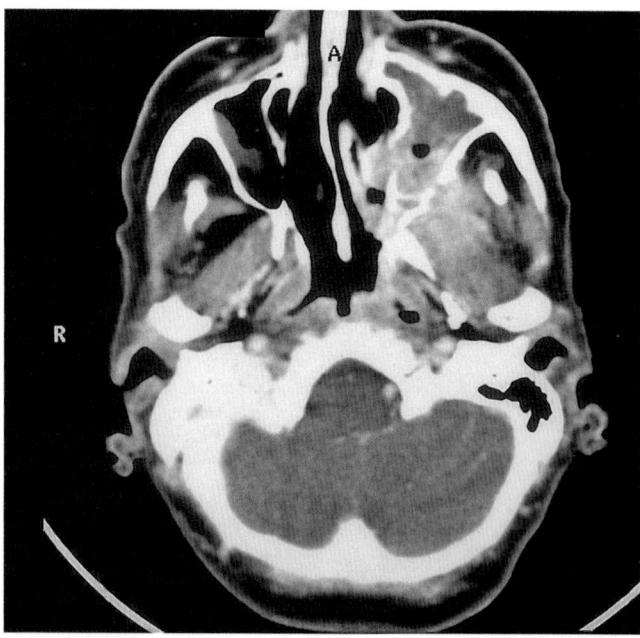

Figure 43.23 Axial computerised tomography scan of paranasal sinuses showing extensive maxillary antral carcinoma invading adjacent structures.

Patients with sinus or intranasal malignancy are best managed in a combined clinic where the expertise of ear, nose and throat (ENT) surgeons, maxillofacial surgeons and radiotherapists can be employed. Detailed surgical management is outside the scope of this book but the adequacy of any surgical resection will need to be confirmed by frozen section control of soft tissue margins. Surgery is followed by radiotherapy. At present, chemotherapy is reserved for possible palliation of inoperable tumours (Summary box 43.8).

Summary box 43.8

Tumours of the nose and sinuses

- A wide variety of tumour types can occur in the nose or sinuses
- Unilateral nasal blockage, discharge and bleeding are often presenting symptoms in nasal or sinus tumours
- Osteomas are often asymptomatic
- Transitional cell papilloma is the most common benign tumour – this tumour may undergo malignant change
- Squamous cell carcinoma is the most common malignant tumour
- Almost 50% of sinonasal cancers arise on the lateral nasal wall and 33% in the maxillary antrum
- Multidisciplinary management of malignant sinonasal tumours requires input from ENT surgeons, maxillofacial surgeons and radiotherapists

FURTHER READING

Mackay, I.S. and Bull, T.R. (1988) *Scott Brown's Otolaryngology.* Butterworths, London.

Maran, A.G.D. and Lund, V.J. (1990) *Clinical Rhinology.* Thieme, New York.

Wigand, M.E. (1990) *Endoscopic Surgery of the Paranasal Sinuses and Anterior Skull Base.* Thieme, New York.

CHAPTER 43 | THE NOSE AND SINUSES

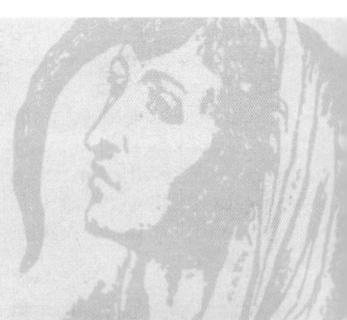

CHAPTER

44

The ear

LEARNING OBJECTIVES

To be familiar with:
- The anatomy of the ear
- The conditions of the outer, middle and inner ear
- The examination of the ear including hearing tests

To understand that:
- The outer layer of the tympanic membrane migrates outwards

- There are two types of chronic otitis media
- The facial nerve can be damaged by trauma and ear disease
- Chronic ear disease can lead to intracranial sepsis
- There are two types of hearing loss: conductive and senorineural

INTRODUCTION

The mammalian ear is an evolutionary masterpiece. Its highly complex 'three-dimensional anatomy' is best learnt by dissecting cadaver temporal bones. In this chapter the 'surgical anatomy' is described followed by the conditions that affect the outer, middle and inner ear.

SURGICAL ANATOMY OF THE EAR

The external ear

The external ear consists of the pinna and the ear canal. The pinna is made of yellow elastic cartilage covered by tightly adherent skin. The external and middle ear develop from the first two branchial arches. The external ear canal is 3 cm in length; the outer two-thirds is cartilage and the inner third is bony. The skin on the lateral surface of the tympanic membrane is highly specialised and migrates outwards along the ear canal. As a result of this migration most people's ears are self-cleaning. The external canal is richly innervated and the skin is tightly bound down to the perichondrium so that swelling in this region results in severe pain.

The lymphatics of the external ear drain to the retroauricular, parotid, retropharyngeal and deep upper cervical lymph nodes.

The tympanic membrane and middle ear

The tympanic membrane has three layers: an inner mucosal layer, a dense fibrous middle layer and the outer stratified squamous epithelium. The upper portion that lies above the lateral process of the malleus is called the pars flaccida. The lower portion is called the pars tensa (Fig. 44.1).

The middle ear contains the ossicles. It is bounded laterally by the tympanic membrane, medially by the cochlea and anteriorly

by the Eustachian tube, and posteriorly it communicates with the mastoid air cells (Fig. 44.2). Entwined in this tiny space is the facial nerve, which pursues a tortuous course through the middle ear and exits the skull base at the stylomastoid foramen. The middle ear is separated from the middle fossa by a thin sheet of bone known as the tegmen.

The tympanic membrane and ossicles act as a transformer system converting vibrations in the air to vibrations within the fluid-filled inner ear.

The inner ear

The inner ear comprises the cochlea and vestibular labyrinth (saccule, utricle and semicircular canals). These structures are embedded in dense bone called the otic capsule.

The cochlea is a minute spiral of two and three-quarter turns. Within this spiral, perilymph and endolymph are partitioned by the thin Reissner's membrane. The endolymph has a high concentration of potassium, similar to intracellular fluid, and the perilymph has a high sodium concentration and communicates with the cerebrospinal fluid (CSF). Maintenance of the ionic gradients is an active process and is essential for neuronal activity.

There are approximately 15 000 hair cells in the human cochlea. They are arranged in rows of inner and outer hair cells. The inner hair cells act as mechanicoelectric transducers, converting the acoustic signal into an electric impulse. The outer hair cells contain contractile proteins and serve to tune the basilar membrane on which they are positioned.

Bartolomeo Eustachio, (Eustachius), ?1513–1574, was appointed Physician to the Pope in 1547, and Professor of Anatomy at Rome, Italy, in 1549.
Ernst Reissner, 1824–1878, Professor of Anatomy at Dorpat, and later at Breslau, Germany, (now Wroclaw, Poland), described the vestibular membrane of the cochlea in 1851.

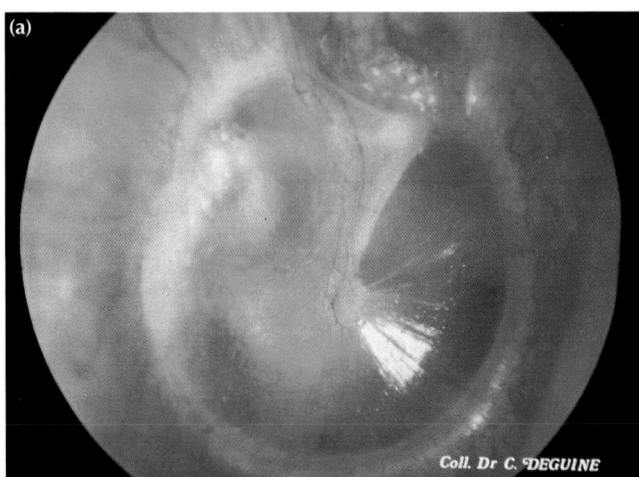

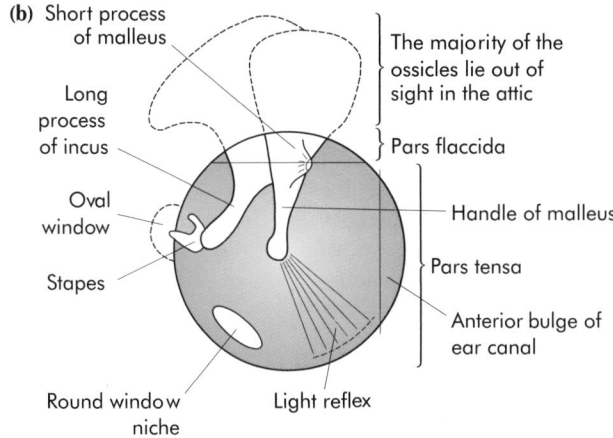

(b)

- Short process of malleus
- Long process of incus
- Oval window
- Stapes
- Round window niche
- The majority of the ossicles lie out of sight in the attic
- Pars flaccida
- Handle of malleus
- Pars tensa
- Anterior bulge of ear canal
- Light reflex

Figure 44.1 (a) Right tympanic membrane and (b) diagram to illustrate anatomy (courtesy of Dr Christian Deguine).

Each inner hair cell responds to a particular frequency of vibration. When stimulated, it depolarises and passes an impulse to the cochlear nuclei in the brainstem.

The vestibular labyrinth consists of the semicircular canals, utricle and saccule and their central connections. The three semicircular canals are arranged in the three planes of space at right angles to each other. Like the auditory system, hair cells are present. In the lateral canals, the hair cells are embedded in a gelatinous cupula. Shearing forces, caused by angular movements of the head, produce hair cell movements and generate action potentials. In the utricle and saccule the hair cells are embedded in an otoconial membrane that contains particles of calcium carbonate. These respond to changes in linear acceleration and the pull of gravity.

Impulses are carried centrally by the vestibular nerve and connections are made to the spinal cord, cerebellum and external ocular muscles.

The sensory nerve supply

The external ear is supplied by the auriculotemporal branch of the trigeminal nerve (Vth), which supplies most of the anterior half of the pinna and the external auditory meatus. The greater auricular nerve (C2/3), together with branches of the lesser occipital nerve (C2), supply the posterior part of the pinna. The VIIth, IXth and Xth cranial nerves also supply small sensory branches to the external ear; this explains why the vesicles of herpes zoster

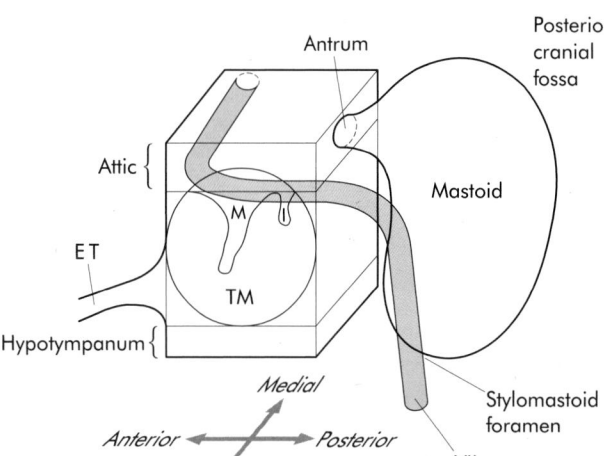

Figure 44.2 Diagram to show the relations of the middle ear (courtesy of Dr Christian Deguine). ET, Eustachian tube; M, malleus; TM, tympanic membrane; VII, facial nerve.

affecting the VIIth nerve appear in the concha (see Fig. 44.34, p. 701). The middle ear is supplied by the glossopharyngeal nerve (IXth).

This complicated and rich sensory innervation means that referred otalgia is common and may originate from the normal area of distribution of any of the above nerves. A classic example is the referred otalgia caused by cancer of the larynx (Summary box 44.1).

Summary box 44.1

Applied anatomy

- The skin on the outer surface of the eardrum migrates outwards so that the ear canal is 'self-cleaning'
- Infection of the middle ear and mastoid can easily spread to the cranial cavity
- The facial nerve pursues a tortuous course through the middle ear
- The ear has a rich sensory innervation so that 'referred otalgia' is common
- Cancer of the larynx can present with otalgia

Taking a thorough history is the most important part of the assessment; the symptoms that need to be enquired after are listed in the summary box below (Summary box 44.2).

Summary box 44.2

History taking

Ask about:
- Earache, pain and itch
- Hearing loss
- Discharge: type, quantity and smell
- Tinnitus
- Vertigo
- Facial movements
- Speech and development (in children)
- Past history: head injury, baro- or noise trauma, ototoxics, family history and previous ear surgery

---

CHAPTER 44 | THE EAR

EXAMINATION OF THE EAR

The tools of the trade are shown in Fig. 44.3. Examination of the ear is part of the general ear, nose and throat (ENT) examination. Make the patient comfortable and explain what you are going to do. Sit at the same height as the patient. Inspect the pinna and mastoid. The technique of otoscopy is shown in Fig. 44.4. Gently retract the pinna to straighten the ear canal. Systematically examine the canal, the pars tensa and pars flaccida. The mobility of the tympanic membrane can be tested with the pneumatic attachment. The Rinne and Weber tuning fork tests are used to

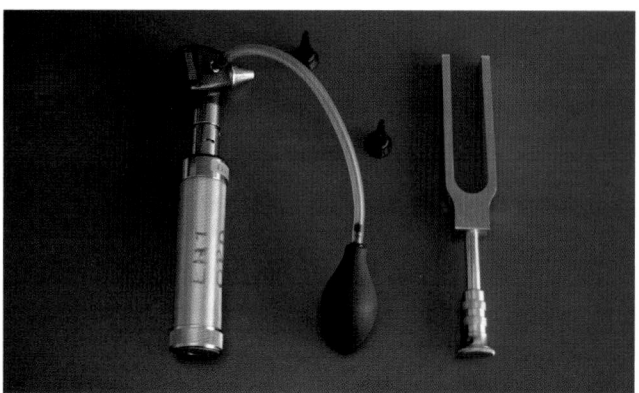

Figure 44.3 Tools of the trade: a fibreoptic otoscope, with pneumatic attachment and a selection of specula. Also a 512-Hz tuning fork.

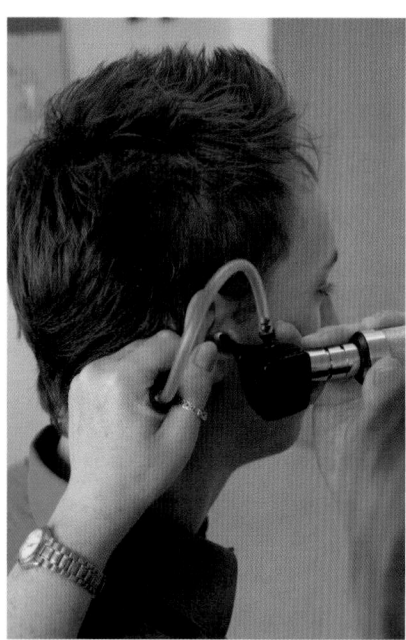

Figure 44.4 The correct method of holding the otoscope: note the pinna is retracted to straighten the ear canal. Hold the barrel of the otoscope so that the examiner's little finger is balanced on the patient's cheek; this prevents the speculum impinging on the tympanic membrane in case of sudden movement.

Friedrich Heinrich Adolf Rinne, **1819–1868, German Otologist.**
Friedrich E. Weber-Liel, **1832–1891, German Otologist.**

distinguish between a conductive and a sensorineural hearing loss.

The Rinne and Weber tuning fork tests

A 512-Hz fork is used. In the Rinne test the tuning fork is placed behind the ear and then in front and the patient is asked in which position the fork sounds loudest. In a normal test, air conduction (in front) is better than bone conduction. When the bone conduction is heard better than the air conduction the most common reason is a conductive hearing loss; however, occasionally this abnormal result can occur when there is a dead ear. In this scenario, sound is transmitted across the bony skull and heard in the other ear.

In the Weber test the vibrating fork is placed in the midline (forehead) and the patient is asked to indicate in which ear the sound is loudest. Normally the sound is heard in the middle but if a conductive hearing loss is present on one side the sound localises to that side. Alternatively, if one ear has a sensorineural hearing loss the sound lateralises to the better cochlea.

The cranial nerves and especially the function of the facial nerve should be examined.

Although conversational testing can give a useful guide to the level of hearing, pure tone audiometry in a soundproof booth is the best way of establishing the air and bone hearing levels (Fig. 44.5). Other common audiological tests include speech audiometry, tympanometry, stapedial reflexes, electric response audiometry, otoacoustic emissions, caloric testing and electronystagmography (see Further reading).

Radiological investigation

Computerised tomographic (CT) scanning of the temporal bones is routinely used preoperatively to show detailed individual anatomy, as well as alerting the surgeon to anatomical variants. Pus, bone and air are shown well on high-resolution CT and so this is the imaging method of choice for investigating cholesteatoma and bony abnormalities (Fig. 44.6).

Magnetic resonance imaging (MRI) is better than CT at imaging soft tissue (e.g. facial and auditory nerve) and is the best method for imaging tumours of the acoustic nerves (Fig. 44.7).

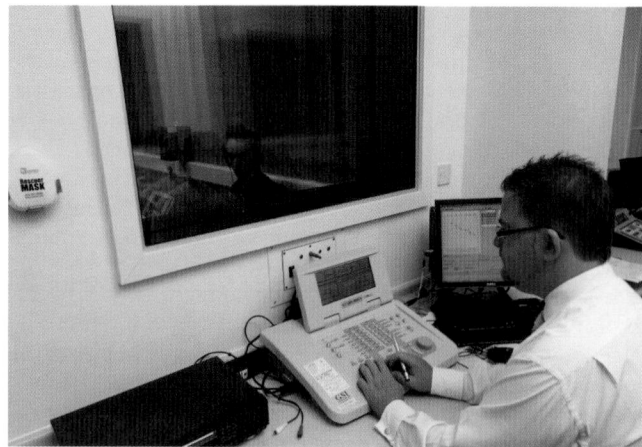

Figure 44.5 Audiometry: the patient sits in a soundproof room and the audiologist presents sounds at different thresholds and records the responses.

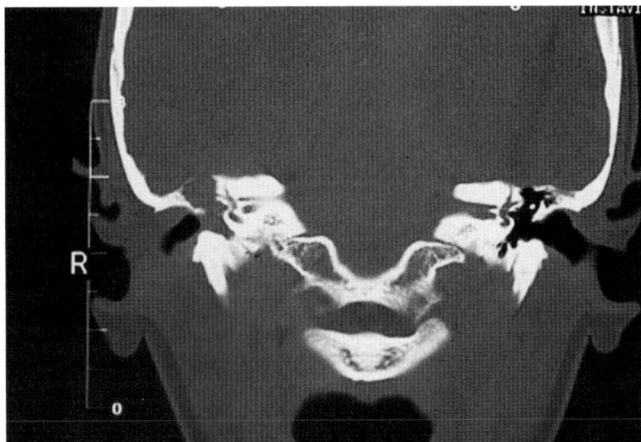

Figure 44.6 The CT scan shows a normal left ear; note the air filled middle ear and the incus and stapes and the lateral and semicircular canals and IAM can be seen. In the right ear the entire middle ear and mastoid is opaque and filled with soft tissue. This is the typical appearance of cholesteatoma.

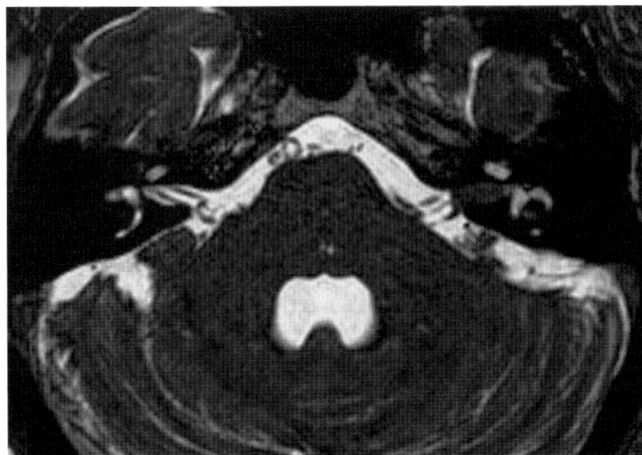

Figure 44.7 The MRI image is a high resolution T2-weighted image at the level of the IAMs showing an intra-cannalicular acoustic neuroma (AN) on the left and a normal IAM on the right (Courtesy of Dr Peiter Petorius).

CONDITIONS OF THE EXTERNAL EAR

Congenital anomalies

Congenital anomalies can range from total absence of the ear through to minor cosmetic deformities. The external and middle ear originate from the first and second branchial arches, whereas the cochlea is of neuroectodermal origin. This means that an individual may have a gross deformity of the external and/or middle ear but a normal cochlea. In these circumstances, sound can be transmitted from a hearing aid connected to an osseo-integrated peg that is screwed into the mastoid bone. This type of device is known as a bone-anchored hearing aid (BAHA).

Children who have a significant deformity of the pinna (microtia) can be helped with osseo-integrated implants to which a prosthetic ear is connected (Fig. 44.8). The prosthetic ear can be unclipped before playing violent sport, for example rugby, and this unsettles the opposition (Summary box 44.3)!

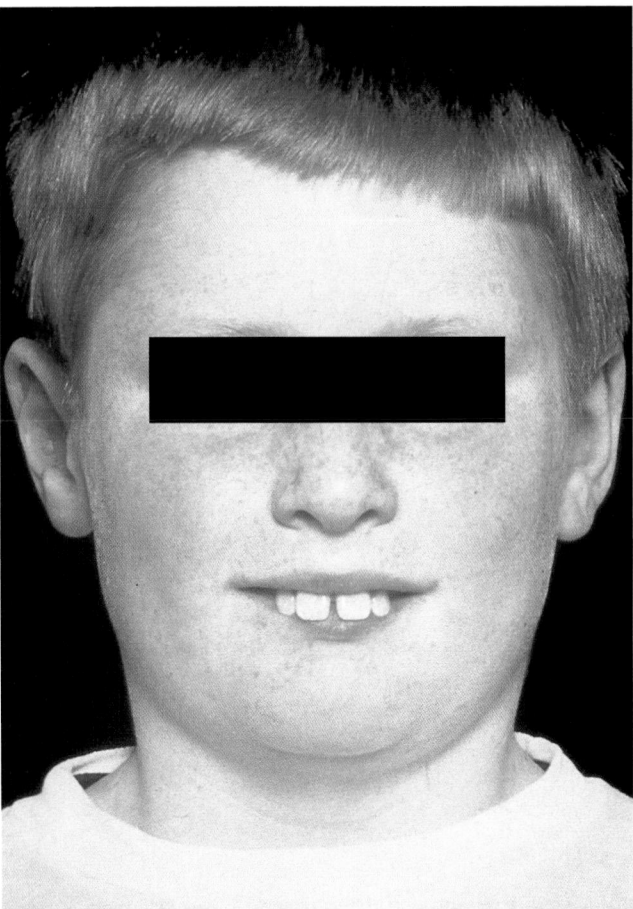

Figure 44.8 This young man can remove his prosthetic right ear, which is attached to an osseo-integrated stud, before playing rugby.

Summary box 44.3

Congenital anomalies of the external ear

- The external and middle ear originate from the first and second branchial arches but the cochlea is neuroectodermal in origin
- An individual can have a congenital abnormality of the pinna and middle ear with a normal cochlea and, therefore, the potential for normal hearing. Haematoma of the pinna needs draining and a pressure dressing
- Osseo-integration allows a prosthetic ear and hearing aid to be attached to the skull

---

Pre-auricular sinuses are a common congenital abnormality and occasionally need excising because of recurrent infections and discharge. Prominent ears can be corrected by scoring the cartilage to create a fold.

Trauma

A haematoma of the pinna occurs when blood collects under the perichondrium. The cartilage receives its blood supply from the perichondrial layer and will die if the haematoma is not evacuated, resulting in a cauliflower ear. A generous incision under general anaesthetic, with a pressure dressing or compressive sutures and antibiotic cover, is recommended (Fig. 44.9).

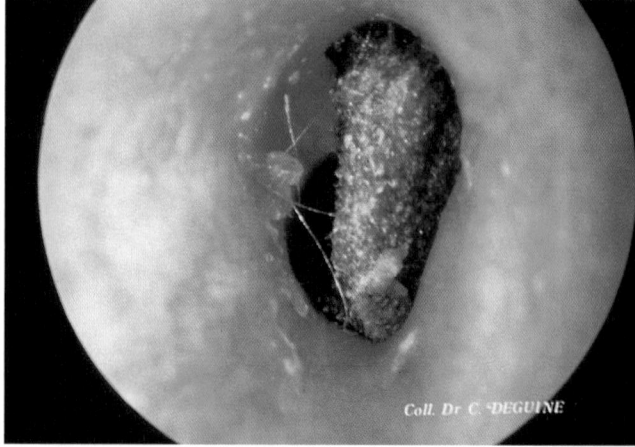

Figure 44.10 Removal of a foreign body from the ear canal can be a challenge (courtesy of Dr Christian Deguine).

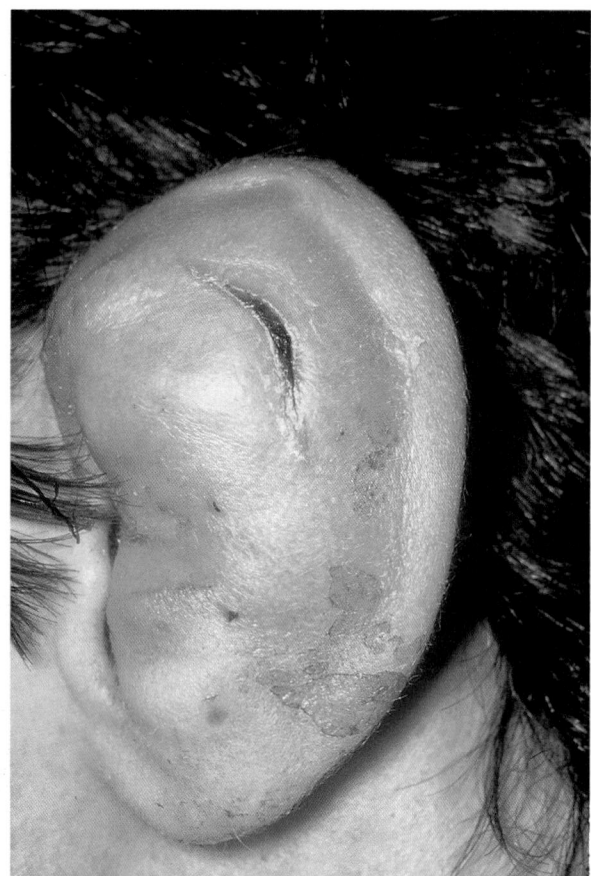

Figure 44.9 Haematoma of the pinna.

Foreign bodies in the ear canal need to be treated with the greatest respect. If an object is not easily removed at the first attempt it is better to do it with the aid of a microscope and general anaesthesia. An active 2-year-old with a bead in the ear can be a formidable opponent (Fig. 44.10) (Summary box 44.4).

> **Summary box 44.4**
>
> **Trauma of the external ear**
>
> - A haematoma of the pinna requires thorough drainage, antibiotics and a compressive dressing or sutures
> - A 2-year-old with a foreign body in the ear canal is a formidable opponent; consider general anaesthesia.

Inflammation

Otitis externa is common and consists of generalised inflammation of the skin of the external auditory meatus. The cause is often multifactorial but includes general skin disorders, such as psoriasis and eczema, and trauma. Common pathogens are *Pseudomonas* and *Staphylococcus* bacteria, *Candida* and *Aspergillus*. Once the skin of the ear canal becomes oedematous, skin migration stops and debris collects in the ear canal. This acts as a substrate for the pathogens. The hallmark of acute otitis externa is severe pain (apparently on a par with childbirth). Movement of the pinna elicits pain, which distinguishes it from otitis media.

The initial treatment is with topical antibiotics and steroid ear drops, together with analgesia. If this fails, meticulous removal of the debris with the aid of an operating microscope is required. Fungal infection can be recognised by the presence of hyphae within the canal (Fig. 44.11). Fungal infection causes irritation and itch. The treatment is meticulous removal of the fungus and any debris, as well as stopping any concurrent antibiotics.

Systemic antibiotics are rarely required for otitis externa but should be used if cellulitis of the pinna occurs (Fig. 44.12).

Necrotising otitis externa is a rare but important condition. It presents as a severe, persistent, unilateral otitis externa in an immunocompromised individual. It is important to think of the diagnosis in an elderly diabetic patient. Usually the infecting organism is *Pseudomonas aeruginosa*. Osteomyelitis of the skull base occurs and several cranial nerves (VII, IX, X) may be destroyed by the progressing infection. Intensive systemic antibiotics are required and the disease process should be monitored by high-resolution imaging (Summary box 44.5).

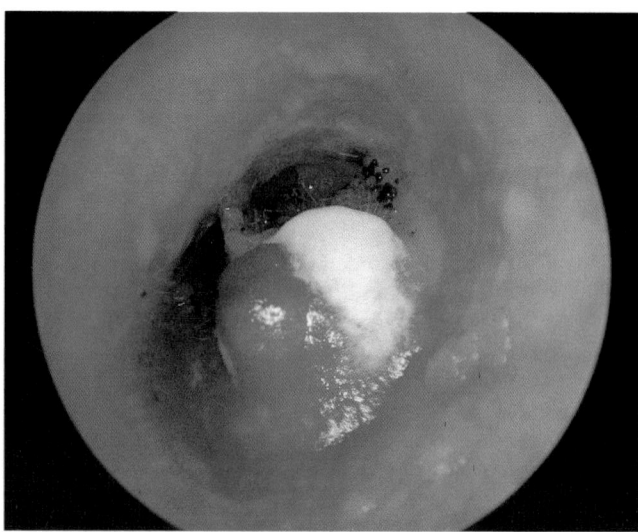

Figure 44.11 Fungal otitis externa; note the spores.

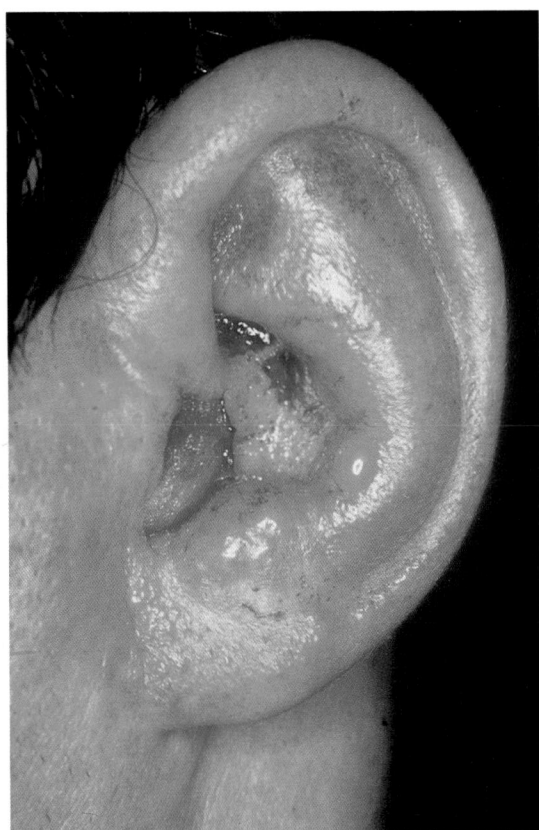

Figure 44.12 Cellulitis of the pinna.

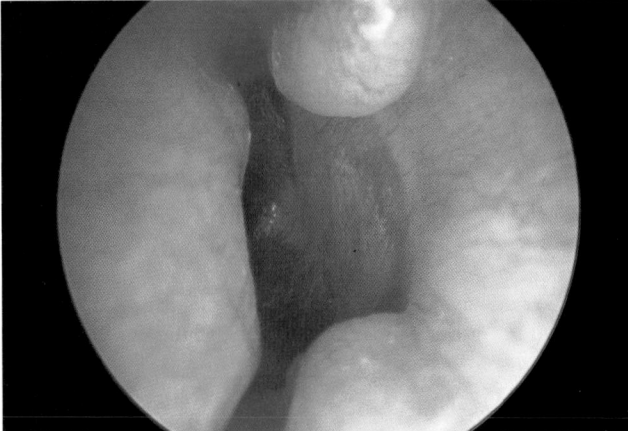

Figure 44.13 Osteomas grow from the bony part of the ear canal in response to cold and so are found in swimmers, surfers and divers. Treatment is only required if the osteomas occlude the ear canal.

Summary box 44.5

Types of otitis externa

- Acute bacterial otitis externa is very common and extremely painful; treat with topical steroids and topical antibiotics
- Systemic antibiotics should be reserved for cellulitis of the pinna
- Chronic otitis externa needs the underlying dermatitis to be treated; topical steroid in spirit applications is recommended
- Fungal otitis externa itches and can be diagnosed by the presence of hyphae and spores; treat with meticulous cleaning and stop antibiotics
- Necrotising otitis externa is a progressive skull base infection that occurs in immunocompromised individuals and can be life-threatening; intensive long-term antibiotic treatment is required

---

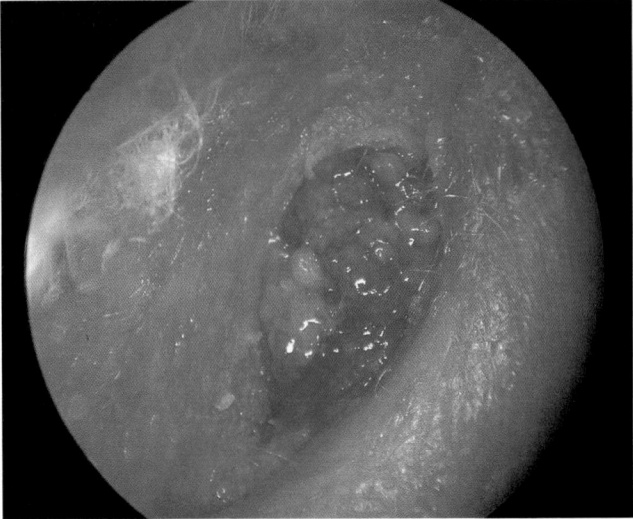

Figure 44.14 Squamous cell carcinomas of the external ear usually originate from the pinna; in this case the tumour is growing from the canal (courtesy of Mr P. Beasley).

Neoplasms

Benign osteomas arise from the bone of the ear canal in individuals who swim in cold water (Fig. 44.13). No treatment is required unless the osteomas obstruct the canal. Other benign tumours include papillomas and adenomas.

Malignant primary tumours of the external ear are either basal cell or squamous cell carcinomas (Fig. 44.14). Both may present as ulcerating or crusting lesions that grow slowly and may be ignored by elderly patients. Squamous cell carcinomas metastasise to the parotid and/or neck nodes. The ear canal may be invaded by tumours from the parotid gland and post-nasal space carcinomas, which 'creep' up the Eustachian tube. All resectable malignant tumours of the ear are treated primarily with surgery, with or without the addition of radiation therapy.

CONDITIONS OF THE MIDDLE EAR

Congenital anomalies

Congenital anomalies of the middle ear may be associated with other general congenital deformities. There are a number of branchial arch syndromes, e.g. Pierre Robin's, craniofacial dysostosis, Down's and Treacher Collins' syndromes. If there is an

Pierre Robin, **1867–1950, Professor, The French School of Dentistry, Paris, France, described this syndrome in 1929.**
John Langdon Haydon Down, (sometimes given as Langdon-Down), **1828–1896, Physician, The London Hospital, England, published his classification of aments in 1866.**
Edward Treacher Collins, **1862–1932, Ophthalmic Surgeon, The Royal London Ophthalmic Hospital, and Charing Cross Hospital, London, England, described this syndrome in 1900.**

external ear abnormality it should raise suspicion of an underlying middle ear deformity. Middle ear deformity can be assessed by high-resolution CT scanning and, if the inner ear is normal, reconstructive surgery of the middle ear can be successful.

Trauma

Trauma to the middle ear can result in a perforated tympanic membrane (Fig. 44.15a). Such perforations usually heal spontaneously (Fig. 44.15b). Trauma can also result in ossicular discontinuity and it is usually the incus that is displaced. Tympanoplasty operations are available to reconstruct the damaged ossicular chain and repair the tympanic membrane (Summary box 44.6)

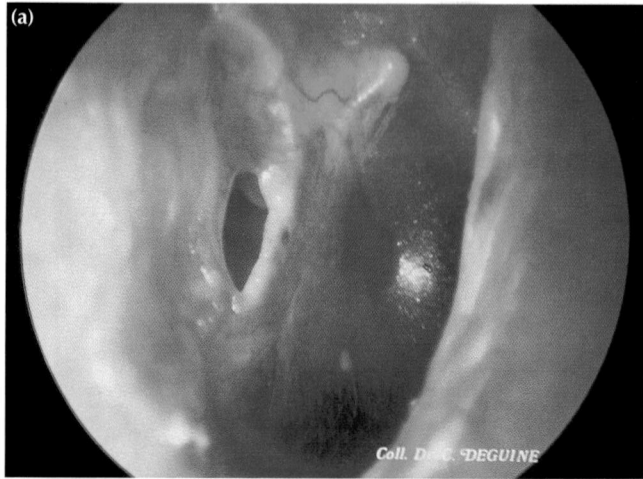

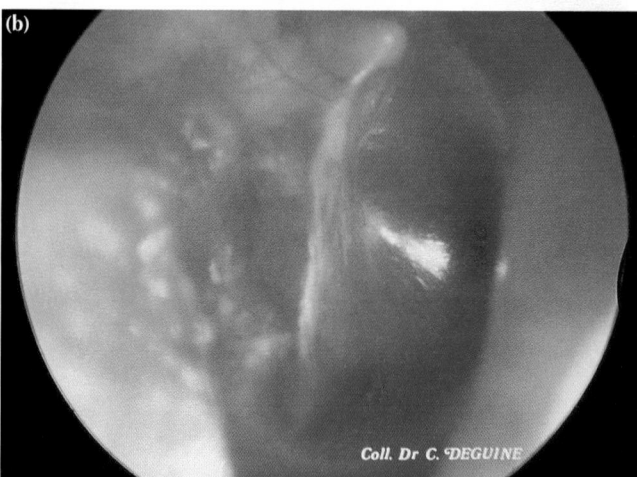

Figure 44.15 (a) Traumatically perforated tympanic membrane. (b) The same tympanic membrane 2 days later (courtesy of Dr Christian Deguine). [Reproduced from O'Donoghue, G.M., Bates, G.J. and Narula, A. (1991) *Clinical ENT*, with permission from Oxford University Press, Oxford.]

Summary box 44.6

Congenital anomalies and trauma of the middle ear

- Congenital anomalies may be isolated or associated with general congenital deformities
- CT can identify middle ear abnormalities that may be corrected by surgery
- Traumatic perforations of the tympanic membrane usually heal spontaneously but explosive and welding injuries do not
- A myringoplasty is an operation that repairs the tympanic membrane
- With severe head trauma the incus can be displaced, which leads to a conductive hearing loss

---

Suppurative otitis media

Suppurative otitis media is extremely common in childhood and is characterised by purulent fluid in the middle ear. Mastoiditis may be associated with otitis media because the mastoid air cells connect freely with the middle ear space. The tympanic membrane bulges because of pressure from the pus in the middle ear (Fig. 44.16). The child suffers extreme pain until the tympanic membrane bursts. The most common infecting organisms are *Streptococcus pneumoniae* and *Haemophilus influenzae*. Appropriate systemic antibiotics should be given for 10 days.

Mastoiditis (Fig 44.17) requires hospital admission and intravenous antibiotics. If the infection does not resolve quickly, a cortical mastoidectomy is required, together with a myringotomy.

Otitis media with effusion (glue ear)

The majority of children experience at least one episode of glue ear. It is primarily thought to be caused by poor Eustachian tube function. Oxygen is continually being absorbed by the middle ear mucosa and this results in a negative middle ear pressure unless the Eustachian tube opens to replenish the air. This negative middle ear pressure initially results in transudation of fluid into the middle ear space (Fig. 44.18). If the hypoxia continues, a mucoid exudate is produced by the glands within the middle ear mucosa. This sticky exudate is referred to as 'glue ear'.

The following symptoms may be associated with glue ear:

- hearing impairment, which often fluctuates;
- delayed speech;
- behavioural problems;
- recurrent ear infections, which occur because the exudate is an ideal culture medium for micro-organisms;
- reading and learning difficulties at school.

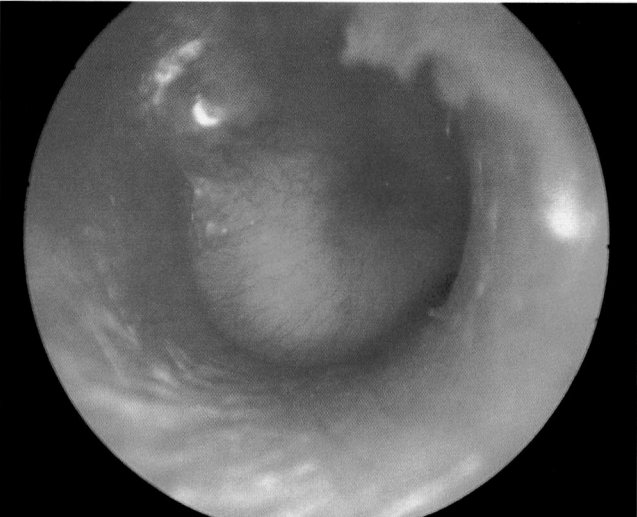

Figure 44.16 Acute otitis media of the left ear; note the bulging tympanic membrane.

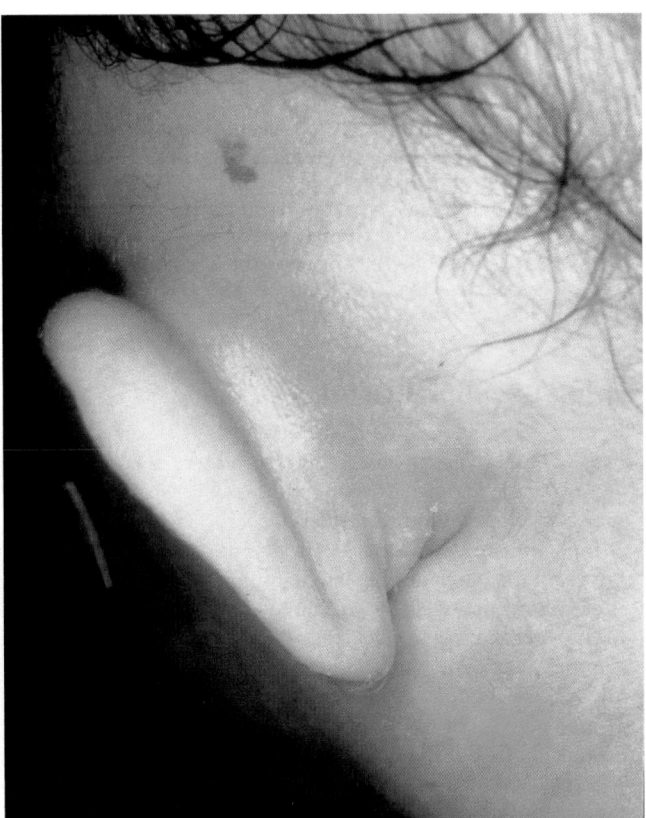

Figure 44.17 Child with acute mastoiditis whose tympanic membrane is shown in Fig. 44.16.

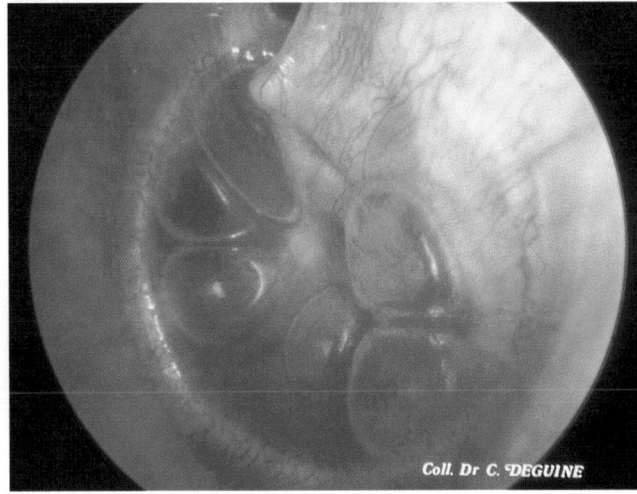

Figure 44.18 The initial serous transudate of glue ear, left ear (courtesy of Dr Christian Deguine). [Reproduced from O'Donoghue, G.M., Bates, G.J. and Narula, A. (1991) *Clinical ENT*, with permission from Oxford University Press, Oxford.]

The otoscopic findings with glue ear

The otoscopic findings of exudative glue ear are of a dull drum that is immobile on pneumatic otoscopy. The tympanic membrane is retracted and radial blood vessels may be present (Fig. 44.19).

In children first presenting with bilateral glue ear, 50% will be better within 6 weeks. Initially, a 'wait and watch' policy is

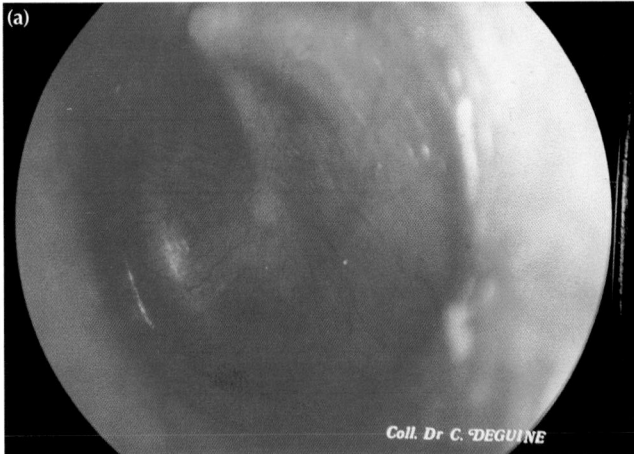

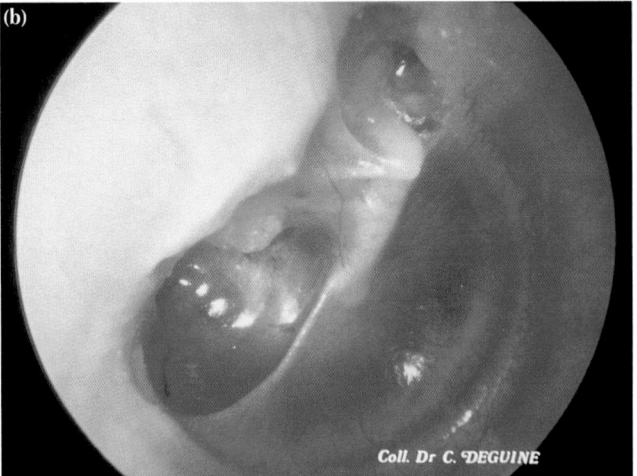

Figure 44.19 (a) Left exudative glue ear. The tympanic membrane is dull and retracted. The light reflex has gone and there are radial blood vessels. The drum does not move with pneumatic otoscopy. (b) Right ear. Advanced exudative glue ear with retraction pockets (courtesy of Dr Christian Deguine). [Reproduced from O'Donoghue, G.M., Bates, G.J. and Narula, A. (1991) *Clinical ENT*, with permission from Oxford University Press, Oxford.]

therefore appropriate. If a bilateral conductive hearing loss persists, the child will miss out on educational opportunities and may not fulfil his or her academic potential; in these circumstances treatment is required.

Medical treatment is of limited value. The Otovent device (Fig. 44.20) may improve Eustachian tube function and is worth trying. However, surgical intervention is the only effective way of curing glue ear. Both ventilation tubes (grommets) (Fig. 44.21) and adenoidectomy are effective. The controversy is not whether surgery works but when to intervene.

Insertion of ventilation tubes and/or an adenoidectomy requires a general anaesthetic. The ventilation tube is placed in the anterior inferior portion of the tympanic membrane. The ventilation tubes stay in position for approximately 6–18 months and are then extruded because of the migratory behaviour of the tympanic membrane. There is no reason why children with ventilation tubes should not be allowed to swim.

A middle ear effusion in adults is relatively rare and, when it occurs, it does not usually last long. The condition is often

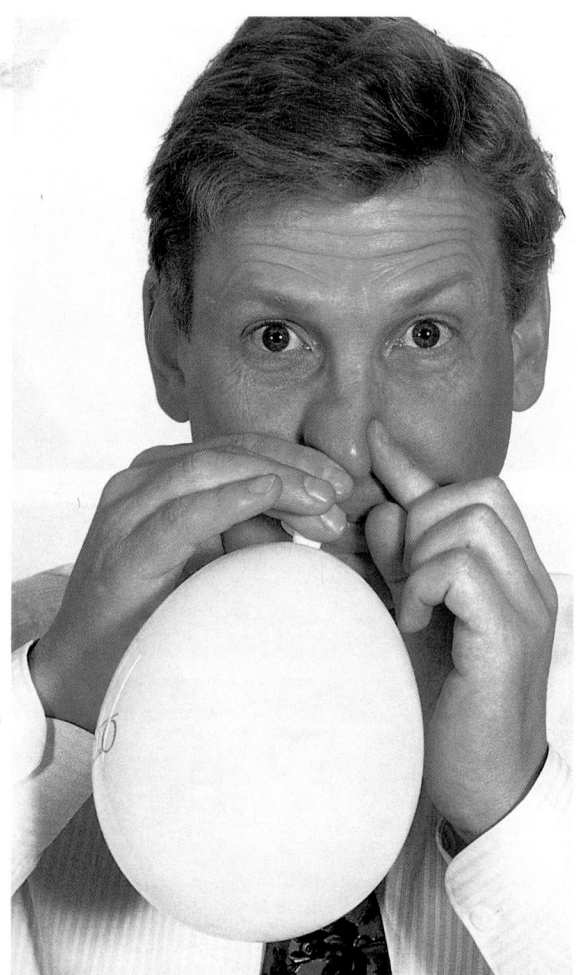

Figure 44.20 Otovent device demonstrated by the author.

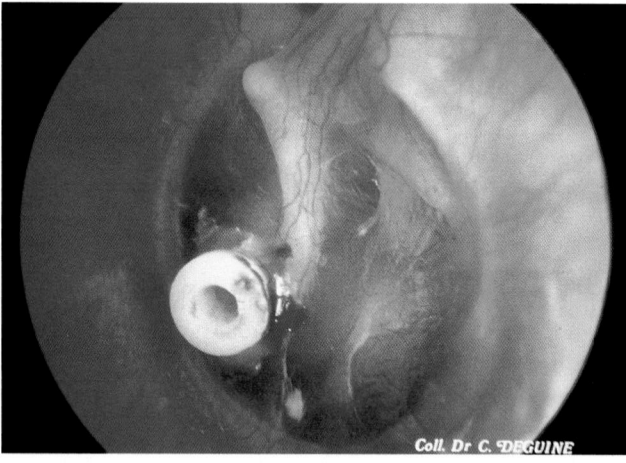

Figure 44.21 Ventilation tube in tympanic membrane, left ear (courtesy of Dr Christian Deguine).

associated with an upper respiratory tract infection. A persistent unilateral effusion in an adult should always be viewed with suspicion. A nasopharyngeal carcinoma may cause the effusion by blocking the opening of the Eustachian tube in the post-nasal space. This is the most common carcinoma in men in southern China (Summary box 44.7).

Summary box 44.7

Acute suppurative otitis media and glue ear

■ Acute suppurative otitis media can progress to mastoiditis
■ Glue ear is very common in children and usually resolves without treatment
■ Persistent hearing loss and/or recurrent acute otitis media is best treated with grommets and/or an adenoidectomy
■ A persistent middle ear effusion in an adult is rare and may be caused by a cancer of the post-nasal space, especially in Chinese and Asian races

---

Chronic suppurative otitis media

Chronic suppurative otitis media (CSOM) is classified into two types: (1) tubotympanic disease, in which there is a perforation of the pars tensa; and (2) atticoantral disease, in which a retraction pocket develops from the pars flaccida.

Tubotympanic CSOM results from trauma or infection. When perforated the tympanic membrane usually repairs itself but if the outer layer of the tympanic membrane fuses with inner mucosa a chronic perforation results (Fig. 44.22). The patient's main symptoms are of an intermittent mucoid discharge associated with a mild conductive hearing loss. It is rare for this type of disease to be associated with intracranial complications.

A diagnosis is made on otoscopy and the tuning forks usually suggest a conductive hearing impairment. The first-line treatment is topical antibiotics and steroid drops and, on occasion, microsuction. If medical treatment fails the patient may request

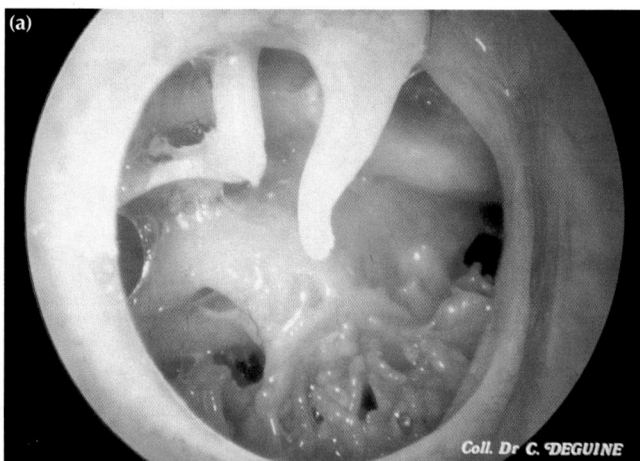

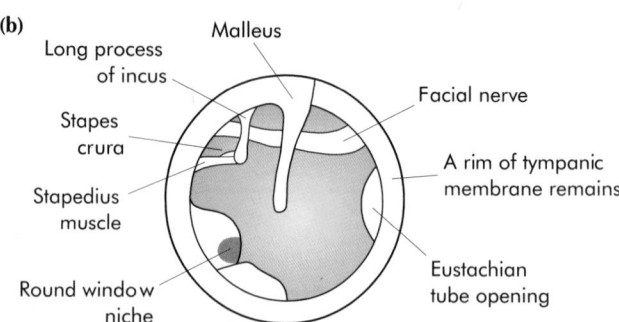

Figure 44.22 (a) Tubotympanic chronic suppurative otitis media showing central perforation, right ear. (b) Anatomy (courtesy of Dr Christian Deguine).

an operation to graft the tympanic membrane. This operation is termed a myringoplasty (type I tympanoplasty). The edges of the perforation are freshened and a small piece of temporalis fascia is inserted under the tympanic membrane to graft the drum. The raw epithelial edges then grow across the graft to repair the tympanic membrane.

Atticoantral CSOM (also known as cholesteatoma) is important because of the complications associated with it. The exact aetiology of cholesteatoma is not known although poor Eustachian tube function is implicated. Patients with cleft palates have relatively poor Eustachian tube function and have a higher incidence of cholesteatoma.

A retraction pocket develops in the pars flaccida and, if the squamous epithelium cannot migrate out of this pocket, a cholesteatoma results. A low-grade osteomyelitis results in the release of fatty acids from the bone, which gives the discharge its characteristic faecal smell. Invariably, the discharge is accompanied by hearing loss and mild discomfort. The patient may simply put up with these symptoms until a severe complication occurs.

The hearing loss that is caused by cholesteatoma may be conductive as a result of ossicular erosion or sensorineural as a result of cochlea damage. Vestibular symptoms may occur because of erosion of the semicircular canals or the migration of toxins into the vestibule. Erosion of the facial nerve is relatively unusual.

The close proximity of the middle ear and mastoid to the middle and posterior cranial fossae means that intracranial sepsis can result from chronic ear disease. The infection spreads to the dura via emissary veins, which connect the middle ear mucosa to the dura, or by direct extension of the disease through the bone. Meningitis, extradural, subdural or intracerebral abscess, or a combination of these may occur. Diagnosis should be suspected on otoscopy (Fig. 44.23). Pus, crusts, granulations or a whitish debris in the attic are hallmarks of the disease. Examination under the microscope, audiometry and, sometimes, CT scanning are indicated.

The treatment is surgical and follows the principle of exposing the disease, excising the disease and then exteriorising the affected area. Three commonly applied operations for this disease are an atticotomy, modified radical mastoidectomy or combined approach tympanoplasty (Summary box 44.8).

Summary box 44.8

Chronic suppurative middle ear disease

There are two main types of CSOM:
- Tubotympanic CSOM, in which there is a hole in the eardrum and frequently a mucoid discharge; this is seldom serious
- Atticoantral CSOM (cholesteatoma). In this condition, squamous epithelium has invaded a retraction pocket in the attic part of the eardrum and is known as a cholesteatoma. Presents with hearing loss and faecal smell from the ear. It is a common cause of intracranial sepsis

Tuberculous otitis media

This is an important cause of suppuration in many countries. The diagnosis should always be considered in any ear that fails to respond to standard therapy. A swab for appropriate culture studies, coupled with chest radiography, will usually confirm the diagnosis.

Otosclerosis

This is a condition in which new abnormal spongy bone is laid down in the temporal bone. Of particular importance is the bone that is laid down around the footplate of the stapes, which impedes the mobility of the stapes and results in a conductive hearing loss (Fig. 44.24). Toxins released from the new bone formation may also cause a gradual sensorineural hearing loss. Otosclerosis is more common in women and in 50% of patients

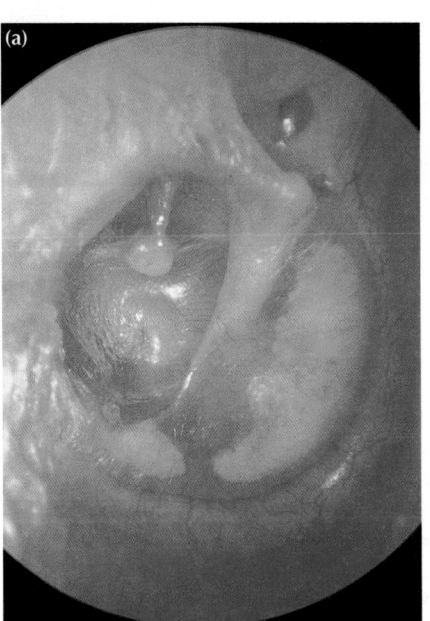 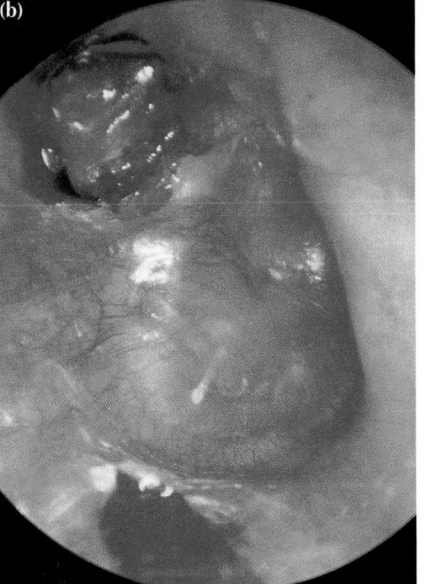 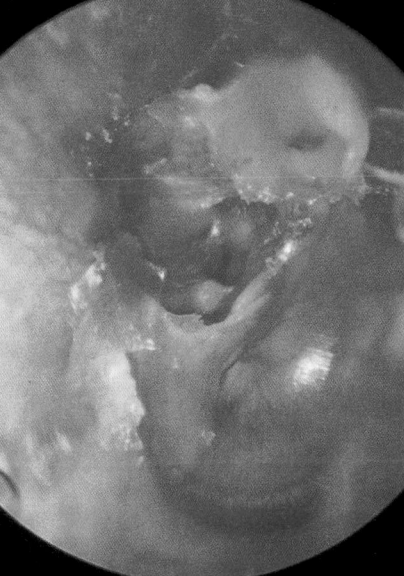

Figure 44.23 (a) Empty attic retraction pocket, right ear. (b) Attic crust covering cholesteatoma, right ear. (c) Attic erosion with cholesteatoma, right ear.

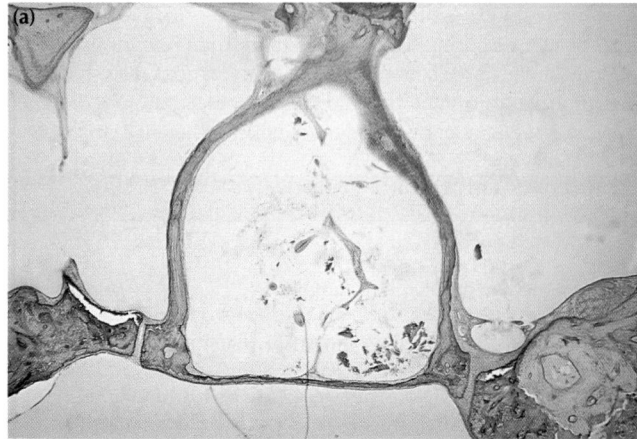

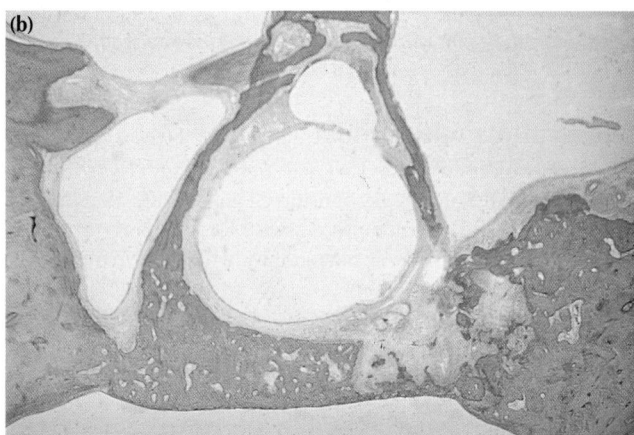

Figure 44.24 Section of normal stapes (a) and section of stapes affected by otosclerosis (b).

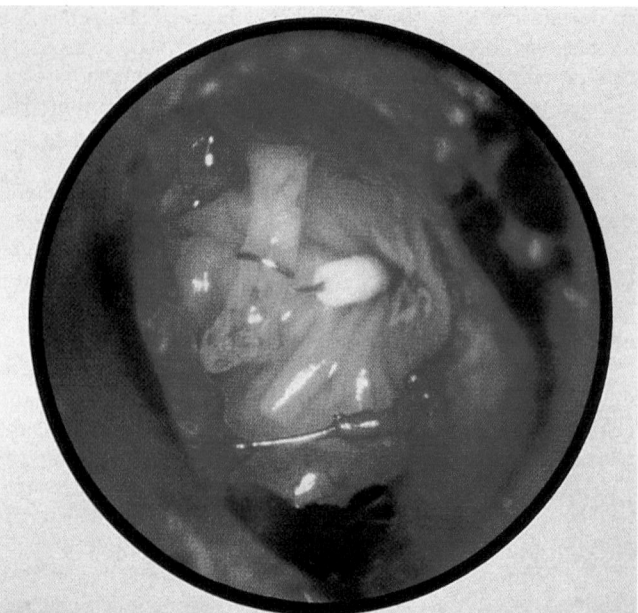

Figure 44.25 The stapedotomy operation showing the piston linking the incus to the vein graft, left ear.

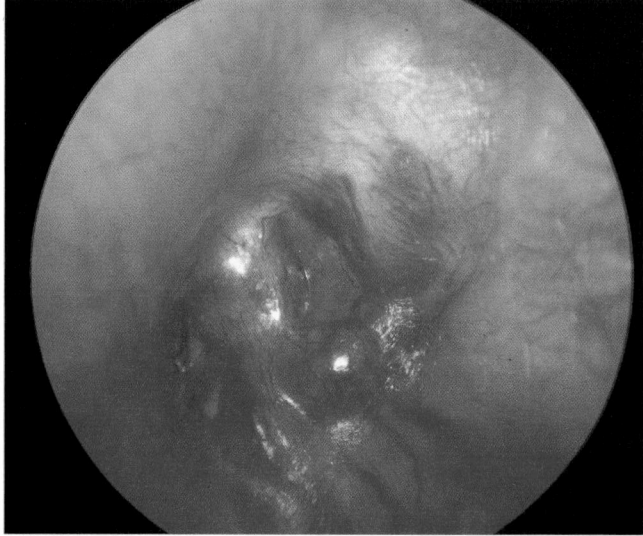

Figure 44.26 Glomus tumour in the middle ear, left ear.

there is a family history. The typical presentation is of a conductive hearing loss in a young woman, with the condition being exacerbated by the hormonal flux of pregnancy. A similar type of stapes fixation occurs in osteogenesis imperfecta and is known as van der Hoeve's syndrome. Otosclerosis is often bilateral. A diagnosis should be suspected in any patient with a conductive hearing loss and a normal tympanic membrane.

The treatment options are simple reassurance, a hearing aid or a stapedotomy operation. The stapes crura are removed and a small hole is drilled in the fixed stapes footplate. A vein graft is then inserted over the hole and a piston linking the incus to the vein graft is delicately placed in position (Fig. 44.25). In 90% of cases the operation is highly successful but rare complications include severe sensorineural hearing loss and balance disturbance.

Neoplasms

Middle ear tumours are rare with the most common being a glomus tumour (Fig. 44.26). Glomus tumours arise from non-chromaffin paraganglionic tissue. The carotid body tumour arising in the neck is an example of this type of tumour. In the temporal bone, three types of glomus tumour are recognised and classification depends on the location: glomus tympanicum

> J. van der Hoeve **described this syndrome in 1918.**

(arising in the middle ear), glomus jugularae (arising next to the jugular bulb) and glomus vagali (skull base).

Pulsatile tinnitus is a classic symptom and the hearing loss that occurs may be either conductive or sensorineural. Palsies of the VIIth, IXth, Xth, XIth and/or XIIth nerves may occur. The classic sign is a cherry-red mass lying behind the tympanic membrane. An audible bruit may be heard with a stethoscope over the temporal bone. The treatment of choice is preoperative embolisation followed by surgical excision. Radiotherapy is also effective.

Squamous cell carcinoma may also occur within the middle ear. It usually presents with deep-seated pain and a blood-stained discharge. Facial paralysis often occurs. Squamous carcinomas usually arise in a chronically discharging ear and can arise in a chronically infected mastoid cavity. Radical surgical excision with or without radiotherapy provides the only chance of cure (Summary box 44.9).

CONDITIONS OF THE INNER EAR

Congenital anomalies

Congenital inner ear disorders may be associated with external or middle ear abnormalities or exist on their own. The most common anomaly is dysplasia of the membranous labyrinth, although dysplasia of the bony labyrinth and even total aplasia of the ear may occur. Intrauterine infections, including rubella, toxoplasmosis and cytomegalovirus infection, can cause inner ear damage. Perinatal hypoxia, jaundice and prematurity are also risk factors for a hearing loss. After birth, meningitis may cause profound sensorineural hearing loss.

If a child's parents suspect a hearing impairment it is important to believe them, especially when glue ear has been excluded. In children in whom there is a suspicion of sensorineural hearing loss, brainstem-evoked audiometry is used to establish hearing thresholds (Fig. 44.27). If some hearing is present, the early fitment of hearing aids can maximise the neural plasticity that is present in the developing brain. If a child has a profound hearing loss, early intervention with a cochlear implant is the ideal solution (Fig. 44.28). Most cases of profound sensorineural hearing loss are due to loss of cochlear hair cells, so that an implant inserted through the round window can selectively stimulate the cochlear neurones, which usually remain intact. The results of cochlear implantation are miraculous but it is expensive technology.

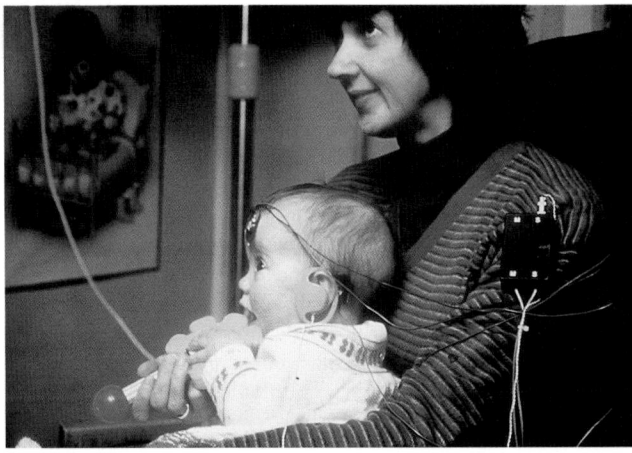

Figure 44.27 Evoked-response audiometry. A simple non-invasive objective test of hearing thresholds. [Reproduced from O'Donoghue, G.M., Bates, G.J. and Narula, A. (1991) *Clinical ENT*, with permission from Oxford University Press, Oxford.]

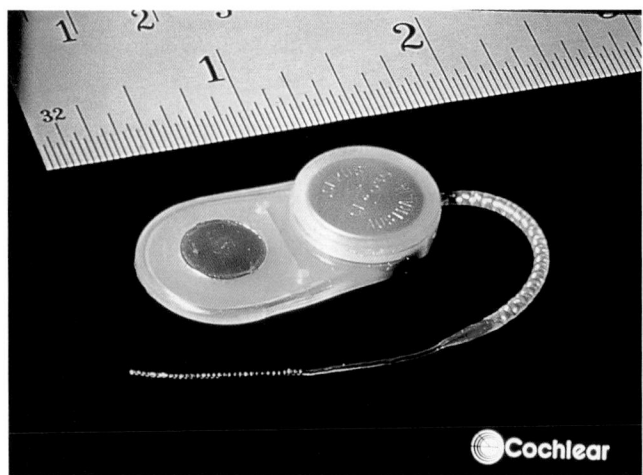

Figure 44.28 Multichannel cochlear implant (Cochlear Corporation).

Presbycusis

Presbycusis is characterised by a gradual loss of hearing in both ears, with or without tinnitus. The hearing loss usually affects the higher frequencies and a classical audiogram is shown in Fig. 44.29. The consonants of speech lie within the high-frequency range, which makes speech discrimination difficult. Examination of an elderly person's cochlea shows loss of hair cells, particularly at the basal turn of the cochlea. With ageing the dynamic range of hearing is also reduced so that elderly people often find loud noises uncomfortable. This phenomenon is known as 'recruitment'.

Many patients with presbycusis are concerned that they may lose their hearing completely and they need reassurance. Hearing aid technology has improved dramatically and most patients can benefit (Fig. 44.30). Care and attention to detail when fitting the hearing aid is essential, together with monitoring of the patient's progress. If this does not occur the hearing aid ends up in the bedroom drawer.

Tinnitus

Tinnitus is an abnormal noise that appears to come from the ear or within the head. It may have an extrinsic cause, for example the pulsatile tinnitus of a glomus tumour. Usually, however, the tinnitus is generated within the cochlea. Most people will experience tinnitus at some time in their lives. Tinnitus frequently accompanies presbycusis, as well as any other condition that damages the inner ear structures. Most individuals adapt to the presence of tinnitus but in some patients it proves intrusive. Reassurance and relaxation therapy are highly effective as are hearing aids for patients who also have presbycusis. An ENT surgeon who was a keen fisherman found that he could not hear his tinnitus when fishing next to a waterfall. From this observation, tinnitus maskers were developed (Fig. 44.31). A masker provides a similar noise to the tinnitus and 'blanks it out'.

Trauma

Noise exposure

Hair cells within the cochlea are damaged by sudden acoustic trauma (blast injury or gunfire) or prolonged exposure to excessive noise. The sensorineural hearing loss that results is greatest at high frequencies (particularly 4000 Hz) and is often accompanied by tinnitus (Fig. 44.32). The law in the UK requires that

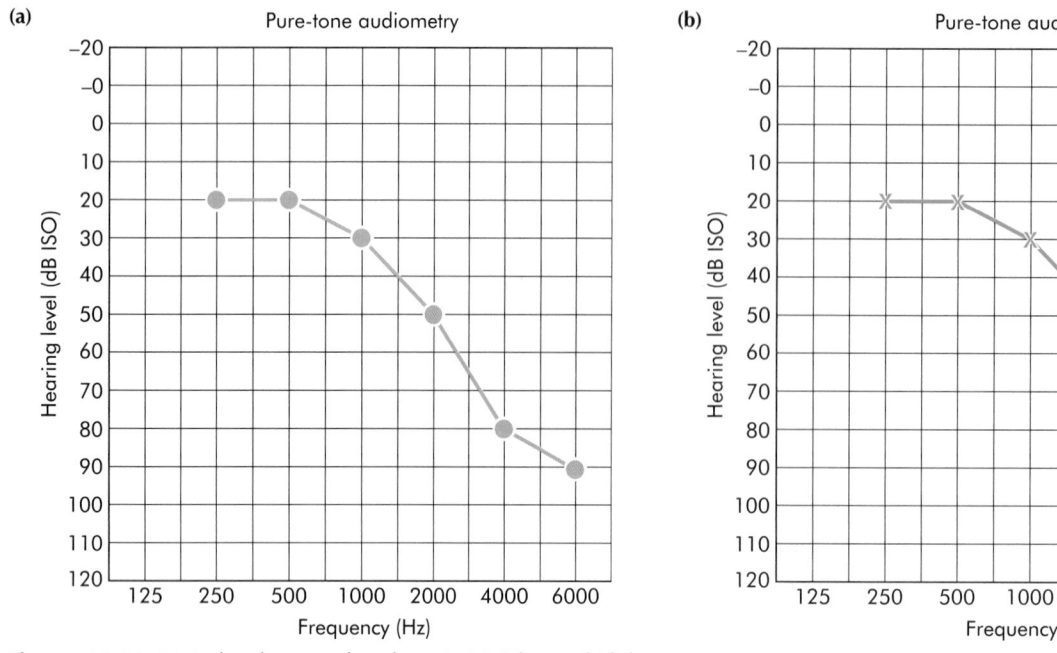

Figure 44.29 Typical audiogram of presbycusis: (a) right ear; (b) left ear.

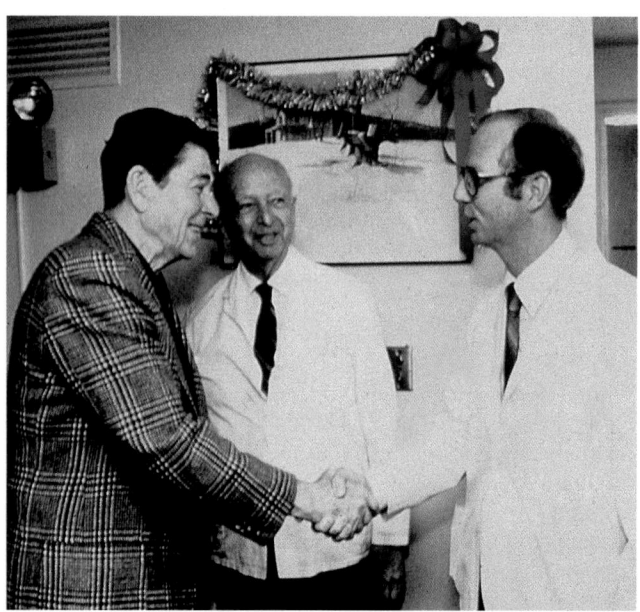

Figure 44.30 A well-known patient receives his hearing aid.

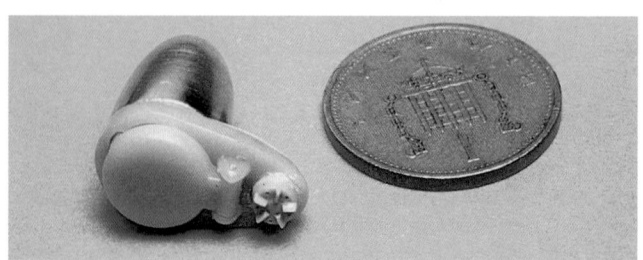

Figure 44.31 A tinnitus masker.

workers are protected from noise but in a disco an individual relies on common sense!

Head injury

The otic capsule is the hardest bone in the body but, if trauma to the head is severe, temporal bone fractures may occur. These tend to be either longitudinal (80%) or transverse (20%). Transverse fractures usually involve the labyrinth and lead to a sensorineural hearing loss that is permanent. Profound vertigo occurs initially, followed by gradual compensation. In about 50% of cases there is an associated facial nerve paralysis. When assessing a severely injured patient it is important to record the facial nerve function and, in particular, whether any facial weakness is partial or total. Important physical findings that may accompany a skull base fracture include a haematoma over the mastoid bone (Battle's sign), blood in the external ear or a laceration along the roof of the external canal. CSF otorrhoea or CSF rhinorrhoea (if the tympanic membrane is intact) may occur. A conductive hearing loss may be present because of fluid in the middle ear or disruption of the ossicular chair. A high-resolution CT scan is required to assess skull base fractures.

Barotrauma

Rapid changes in pressure across the labyrinthine membranes may occur with diving or flying and may allow air to be forced into the cochlea. Any individual with a sudden sensorineural hearing loss requires urgent hospital admission and, in those with a history of barotrauma, it may be appropriate to raise the tympanic membrane and to search for a leak of perilymph in the region of the oval or round window.

William Henry Battle, **1855–1936**, Surgeon, St. Thomas's Hospital, London, **England.**

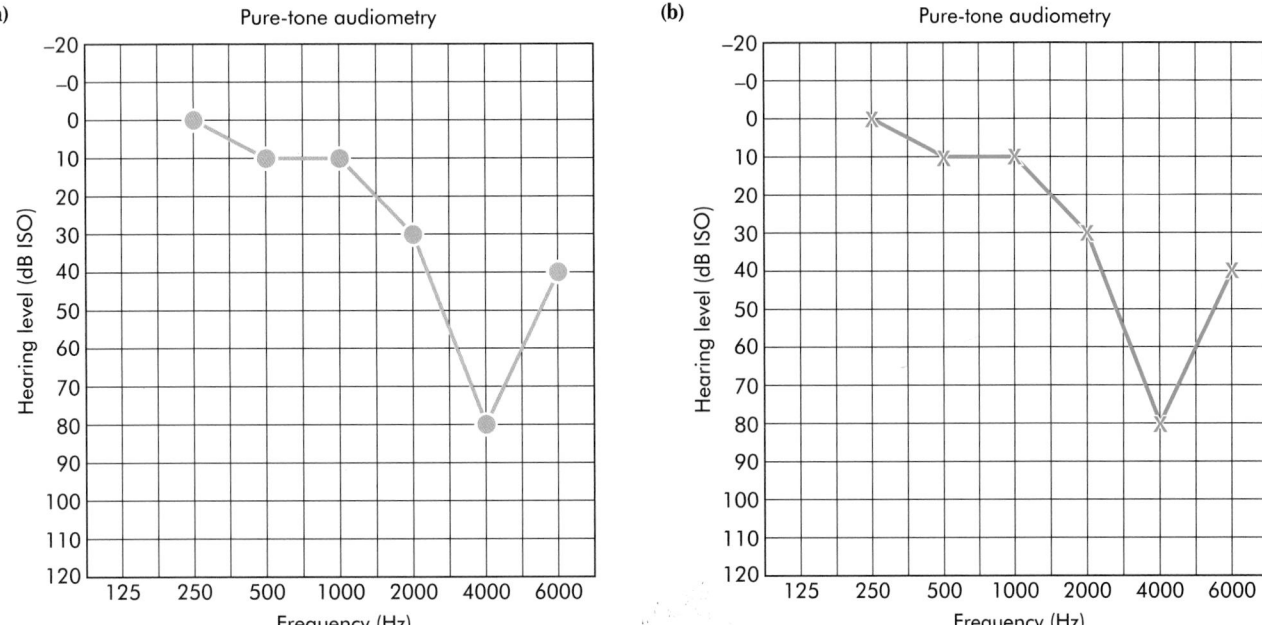

Figure 44.32 A typical audiogram of noise damage: (a) right ear; (b) left ear.

Drug ototoxicity

Certain drugs differentially affect the cochlea, causing hearing loss and tinnitus, whereas others affect the vestibular system, causing vertigo. Aminoglycosides are well known to be ototoxic, as is cis-platinum. Recognition of risk factors, such as poor renal function in patients being treated with aminoglycosides, is most important. Although many topical ear drops contain aminoglycosides there is little evidence that such topical treatment causes sensorineural hearing loss if used for short periods.

Benign paroxysmal positional vertigo

Benign paroxysmal positional vertigo (BPPV) may follow head or neck trauma. Vertigo is an illusion of movement and BPPV is characterised by intermittent attacks of vertigo that occur when the head is moved in a certain position. Typically, the vertigo only lasts for a few seconds and is not associated with other otological symptoms. Positional testing can evoke nystagmus and helps in the diagnosis of this condition. The condition is usually self-limiting, and special manoeuvres described by Epley help the majority of patients (Fig. 44.33).

Reduction in cochlear blood flow

This is the most likely cause for most cases of sudden onset of severe sensorineural hearing loss. All patients with a sudden sensorineural hearing loss should be referred immediately for specialist treatment. The treatment consists of bed rest, steroids and the administration of carbogen (an oxygen and carbon dioxide mixture). In total, 5% of patients with an acoustic neuroma present with sudden sensorineural hearing loss and, therefore, radiological investigation is required to exclude this diagnosis.

Inflammation

Viral infections are thought to account for acute vestibular failure. This condition is characterised by a sudden onset of

vertigo. The vertigo is so severe that the patient goes to bed for 5 days. Central compensation then occurs, although recurring episodes of vertigo can occur for up to 18 months.

Menière's disease

The aetiology is not known but the pathology is well documented. There is an excessive accumulation of endolymphatic fluid (hydrops) and it is thought that the distension of the endolymphatic compartment may rupture Reissner's membrane, which leads to mixing of endolymph and perilymph. The condition is characterised by a triad of symptoms: intermittent attacks of vertigo, a fluctuating sensorineural hearing loss and tinnitus. The patient often has a sensation of pressure in the affected ear before an attack. The hearing loss typically affects the lower frequencies. The vertigo characteristically lasts between 30 min and 6 hours and is often accompanied by nausea and vomiting. The investigations include pure tone audiometry, electrocochleography and an MRI scan to exclude an acoustic neuroma. Medical treatment with betahistadine and diuretics is effective, with selective destruction of the vestibular labyrinth by percolating gentamicin through a grommet being reserved for resistant cases.

Facial paralysis

Viral infections that involve the facial nerve are one of the most common causes of facial weakness (80%). Bell's palsy results from a viral infection of the facial nerve. The nerve swells and is compressed within the temporal bone. Early treatment with high-dose steroids is appropriate. Not all facial nerve palsies are due to viral infection and a thorough otoneurological examination is

John M. Epley, **20th century American Otologist.**

Prosper Menière, **1799–1862, Physician, The Institute for Deaf Mutes, Paris, France, described this condition in 1861.**
Sir Charles Bell, **1774–1842, Surgeon, The Middlesex Hospital, London, England (1812–1835), and later Professor of Surgery, The University of Edinburgh, Scotland (1836–1842).**

CHAPTER 44 | THE EAR

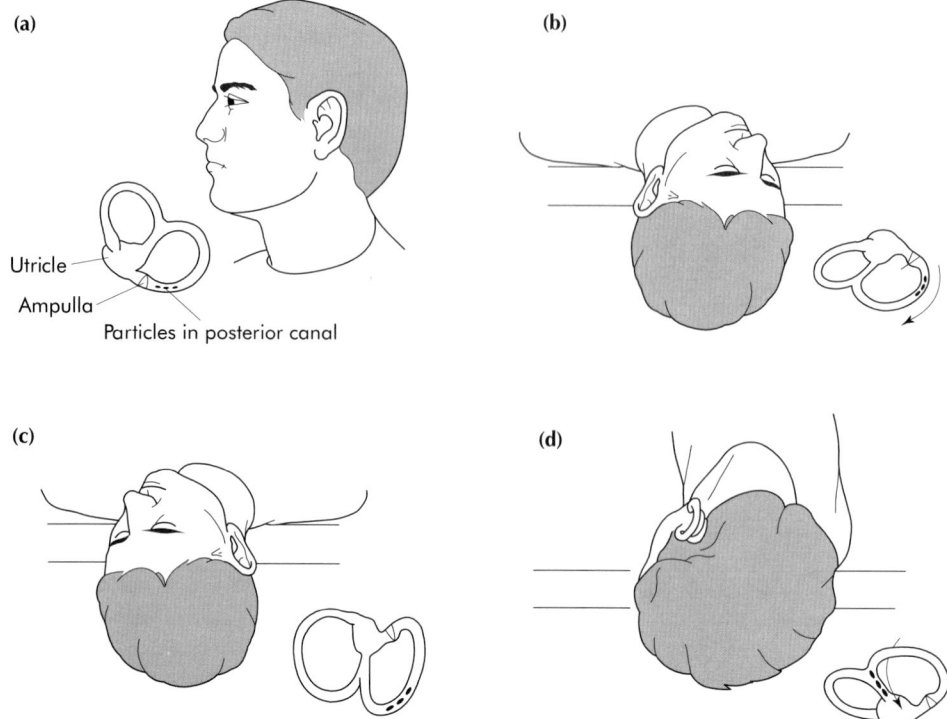

Figure 44.33 The Epley manoeuvre for benign paroxysmal positional vertigo.

required. The facial nerve can be damaged at the cerebello-pontine angle, within the internal auditory meatus, within the middle ear, at the skull base and within the parotid gland. It is essential to consider these potential sites of facial nerve damage in any patient with VIIth nerve paralysis (Summary box 44.10).

Summary box 44.10

Facial paralysis

- The facial nerve passes through the middle ear and mastoid
- When considering a paralysis, think 'complete' or 'partial'
- Protect the eye: carry out a full otoneurological examination to find the cause
- If acute consider steroids and anti-viral agents

Ramsay-Hunt syndrome

This is caused by herpes zoster and is characterised by facial paralysis, pain and the appearance of vesicles on the tympanic membrane, ear canal and pinna (Fig. 44.34). It is accompanied by vertigo and sensorineural hearing loss (VIIIth nerve). Treatment with aciclovir is effective if given early.

The metabolic causes of inner ear damage

These include diabetes mellitus and thyroid disease, both of which may cause sensorineural hearing loss.

James Ramsay Hunt, **1874–1937, Professor of Neurology, The Columbia College of Physicians and Surgeons, New York, NY, USA.**

Neoplasms

These are uncommon but can present with sensorineural hearing loss, tinnitus and vertigo. Acoustic neuromas, which are actually schwannomas of the vestibular division of the VIIIth nerve, are the most common, followed by meningiomas. Acoustic neuromas grow slowly and somewhat unpredictably and as they expand can cause cranial nerve palsies, brainstem compression and raised intracranial pressure. The early symptoms are a unilateral sensorineural hearing loss or unilateral tinnitus or both. It is important to diagnose these tumours early and remove them when they are small. The morbidity and mortality from surgery is directly related to tumour size. If the tumour is removed when it is small, there is an extremely good chance of preserving facial nerve function.

The investigation of choice for detecting acoustic neuromas is MRI (Fig. 44.35). The treatment options include a 'wait and see' policy, which may be appropriate for an elderly patient with minimal symptoms. MRI can be used to monitor the tumour.

In a small number of centres, stereotactic radiotherapy is used to treat small tumours; however, surgical resection is the most common treatment. There are three main approaches: a middle fossa approach, used for small tumours only; the translabyrinthine approach, entirely through the ear; and the suboccipital approach via a craniotomy. The physiological monitoring of the facial nerve and auditory nerve during surgery has improved acoustic nerve surgery results (Summary box 44.11).

Friedrich Theodor Schwann, **1810–1882, Professor of Anatomy and Physiology, successively at Louvain (1839–1848), and Liege (1848–1880), Belgium, described the neurilemma in 1839.**

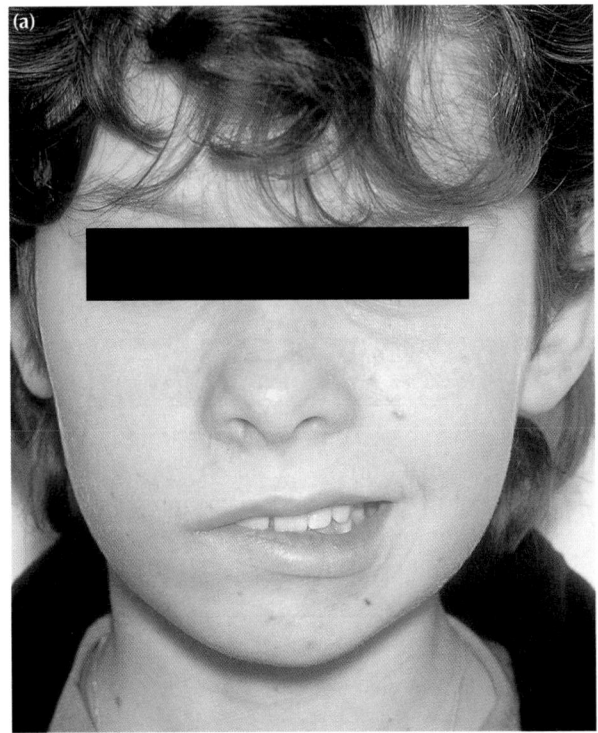

(a)

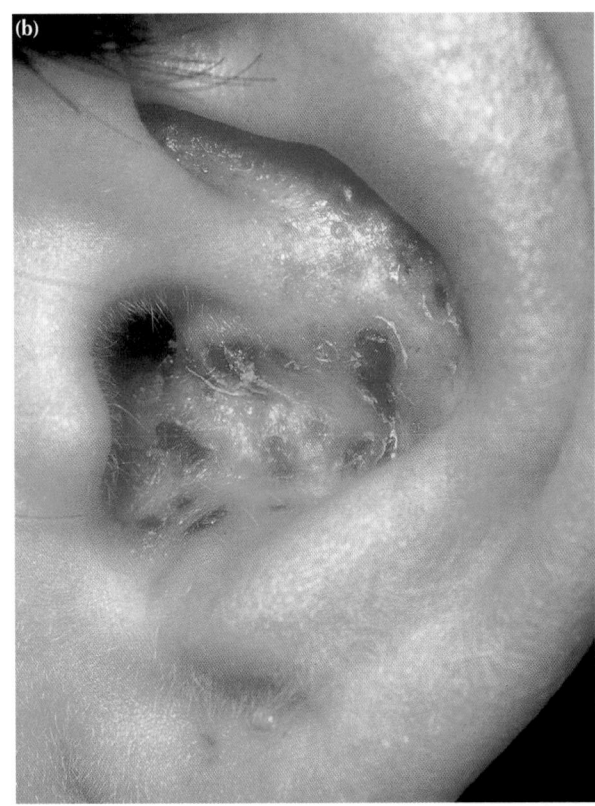

(b)

Figure 44.34 Herpes zoster infection of the VIIth (a) and VIIIth (b) nerves with vesicles on the pinna.

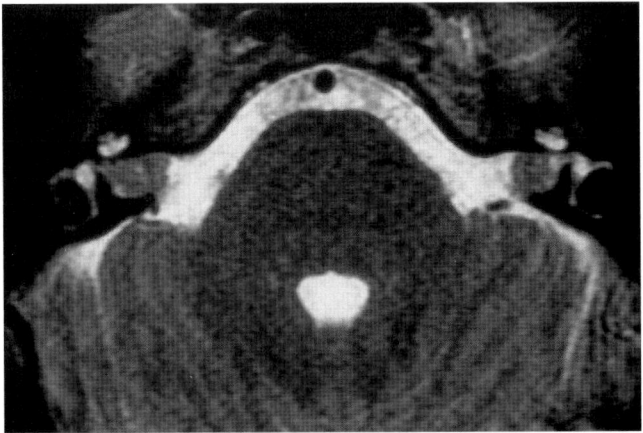

Figure 44.35 Magnetic resonance imaging scan of an acoustic neuroma, which presented with unilateral sensorineural hearing loss and tinnitus.

Summary box 44.11

Conditions of the inner ear

■ Presbycusis is the bilateral high-frequency loss associated with ageing
■ Unilateral tinnitus or sensorineural hearing loss needs to be investigated to exclude acoustic neuroma
■ Sudden sensorineural hearing loss needs immediate treatment, and radiological investigation in the case of acoustic neuroma
■ Menière's disease presents with the triad of sensorineural hearing loss, tinnitus and vertigo

FURTHER READING

Gleeson, M. (ed) (2008) *Scott-Brown's Otorhinolaryngology: Head and Neck Surgery*, 7th rev. edition. Hodder Arnold, London.

Mawson, S., Ludman, H. and Wright, T. (1998) *Diseases of the Ear*. Oxford University Press, Oxford.

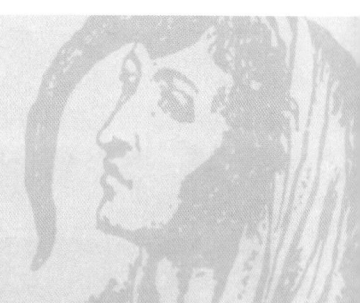

Pharynx, larynx and neck

CHAPTER 45

CLINICAL ANATOMY AND PHYSIOLOGY

The pharynx

The pharynx is a fibromuscular tube forming the upper part of the respiratory and digestive passages. It extends from the base of the skull to the level of the sixth cervical vertebra at the lower border of the cricoid cartilage where it becomes continuous with the oesophagus. It is divided into three parts: the nasopharynx, oropharynx and hypopharynx (Fig. 45.1).

Nasopharynx

The nasopharynx lies anterior to the first cervical vertebra and has the openings of the Eustachian tubes in its lateral wall,

behind which lie the pharyngeal recesses, the fossae of Rosenmüller. The adenoids are situated submucosally at the junction of the roof and posterior wall of the nasopharynx.

Oropharynx

This is bounded above by the soft palate, below by the upper surface of the epiglottis and anteriorly by the anterior faucial pillars. The oropharynx contains the palatine tonsils situated in the lateral wall between the anterior and posterior pillars of the fauces. They are part of the complete ring of lymphoid tissue (Waldeyer's ring) together with the adenoids and lingual tonsils on the posterior third of the tongue. This ring of lymphoid tissue occupying the entry to the air and food passages is constantly exposed to new antigenic stimuli and is an important part of the mucosa-associated lymphoid tissues (MALT), which process antigen and present it to T helper cells and B cells (Fig. 45.2).

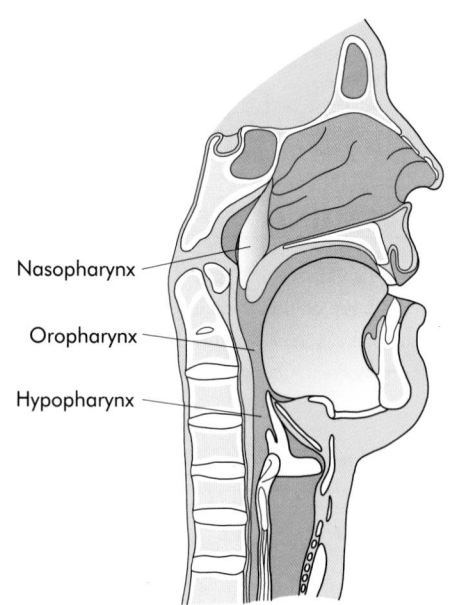

Figure 45.1 The component parts of the pharynx.

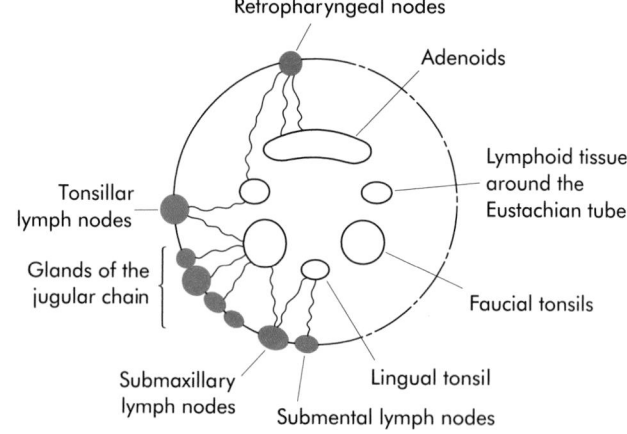

Figure 45.2 Waldeyer's ring.

The tissue of Waldeyer's ring undergoes physiological hypertrophy during early childhood as the child is exposed to increasing amounts of antigenic stimuli, and there is often a similar hypertrophy of the cervical lymph nodes.

It also has an exceptionally good blood supply from the facial artery, which may be closely related to the lower pole, and laterally a plexus of paratonsillar veins, which may be the source of serious venous bleeding following tonsillectomy.

Hypopharynx

The hypopharynx is bounded above and anteriorly by the sloping laryngeal inlet. Its inferior border is the lower border of the cricoid cartilage where it continues into the oesophagus. The hypopharynx is commonly divided into three areas: the pyriform fossae, the posterior pharyngeal wall and the post-cricoid area. The mucosa of these areas is, however, continuous so disease processes, such as squamous carcinoma, can easily involve more than one area and may also spread submucosally. The motor nerve supply of the pharynx and larynx is the vagus nerve.

Understanding of the physiology of normal swallowing and the problems caused by disease has been enhanced in the last two decades by the use of videofluoroscopy in which the passage of a bolus of radio-opaque liquid or solid from the point at which it enters the oral cavity down to its passage within the stomach is examined radiologically. It is considerably more accurate than a barium swallow.

Swallowing is mediated via efferent fibres passing to the medulla oblongata through the second division of the trigeminal nerve (V), glossopharyngeal nerve (IX) and vagus nerve (X) (Fig. 45.3). The afferent pathway is from the nucleus ambiguus and is mediated via the glossopharyngeal (IX), vagus (X) and hypoglossal (XII) nerves. Damage to these major cranial nerves at any point along their pathway, by trauma or disease, may cause dysphagia with or without aspiration.

The main function of the larynx is not the production of voice but the protection of the tracheobronchial airway and lungs; it closes completely during swallowing.

RELATIONS OF THE PHARYNX (FIG. 45.4)

Parapharyngeal space

This potential space lies lateral to the pharynx and extends from the base of the skull above to the superior mediastinum below. It is occupied by the carotid vessels, internal jugular vein, deep cervical lymph nodes, the last four cranial nerves and the cervical sympathetic trunk.

Infection and suppuration of the cervical lymph node in the parapharyngeal space most commonly occurs from infections of the tonsils or teeth (particularly the third lower molar tooth). It may then spread up to the skull base or down to the para-oesophageal region and superior mediastinum.

Retropharyngeal space

This potential space lies posterior to the pharynx, bounded anteriorly by the posterior pharyngeal wall and its covering buccopharyngeal fascia and posteriorly by the cervical vertebrae and their covering muscles and fascia. It contains the retropharyngeal lymph nodes, which are usually paired lateral nodes but which are separated by a tough median partition that connects the prevertebral with the buccopharyngeal fascia.

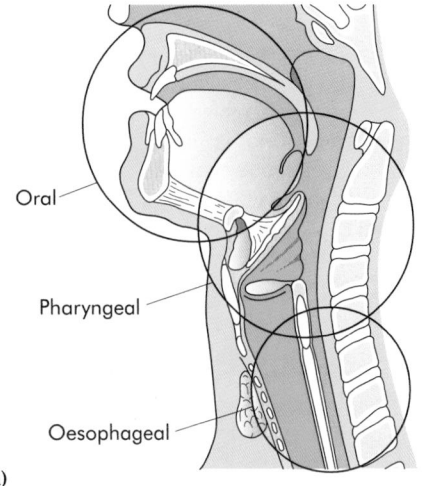

(a)

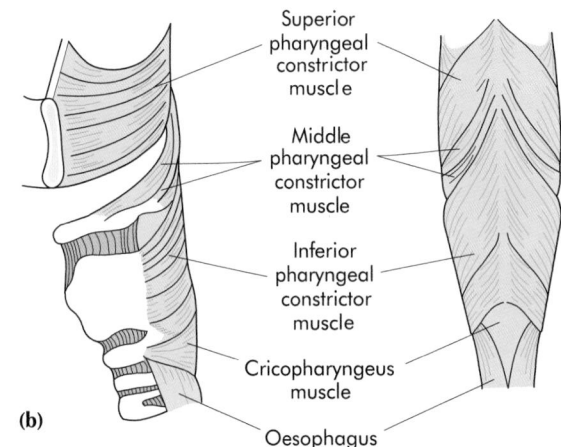

(b)

Figure 45.3 The three phases of swallowing (a) and the muscles involved (b).

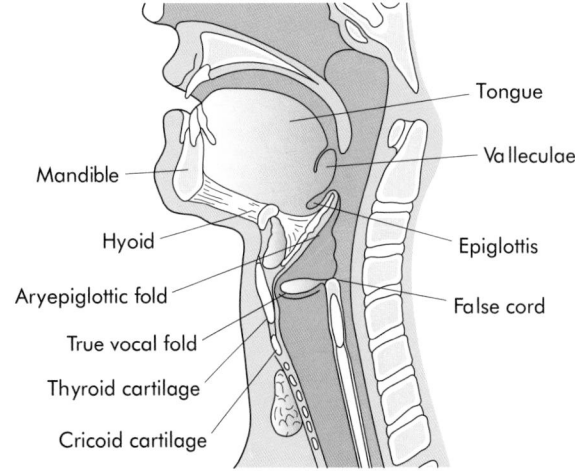

Figure 45.4 Sagittal diagram of upper aerodigestive tract.

These nodes are more developed in infancy and young children, and it is at this age that they are most likely to be involved in inflammatory processes, which, if severe, may affect swallowing and respiration as a consequence of gross swelling and suppuration of the retropharyngeal space.

CHAPTER 45 | PHARYNX, LARYNX AND NECK

Larynx

The larynx is the protective sphincter that closes off the airway during swallowing and, in humans and some other mammals, is responsible for the production of sound. The larynx has a mainly cartilaginous framework that may ossify in later life, and which consists of the hyoid bone above, the thyroid and cricoid cartilages and the intricate arytenoid cartilages posteriorly.

The cricoid cartilage is the only complete ring in the entire airway and bounds the subglottis, which is the narrowest point of the airway. This is the most common site for damage from an endotracheal tube used for intensive care unit ventilation in seriously ill patients.

An anatomical description of the larynx divides it into the supraglottis, glottis and subglottis (Fig. 45.5). The true vocal folds (often incorrectly called the vocal cords) are normally white in contrast to the pink mucosa of the rest of the larynx and airway. The true vocal folds meet anteriorly at the midlevel of the thyroid cartilage, whereas posteriorly they are separate and attached to an arytenoid cartilage. This arrangement produces the 'V' shape of the glottis (Fig. 45.6).

Nerve supply

The sensory nerve supply to the larynx above the vocal folds is from the superior laryngeal nerve and below the vocal folds is from the recurrent laryngeal nerve. Both these nerves are branches of the vagus nerve (X). The motor nerve supply to the larynx is from the recurrent laryngeal nerve, which is a branch of the vagus nerve and which supplies all intrinsic muscles. Only one of these intrinsic muscles, the posterior cricoarytenoid, abducts the vocal folds during respiration. All other intrinsic muscles adduct the cords. As all of the intrinsic muscles of the larynx are supplied by the recurrent laryngeal nerve, damage to this nerve or to the vagus nerve will cause paralysis of the vocal fold on the side of the damage.

Views on indirect laryngoscopy

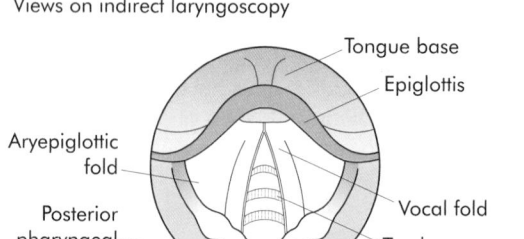
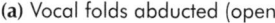
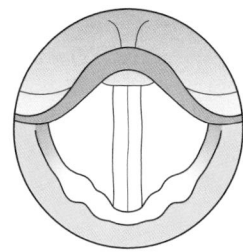

(a) Vocal folds abducted (open)

(b) Vocal folds adducted (closed)

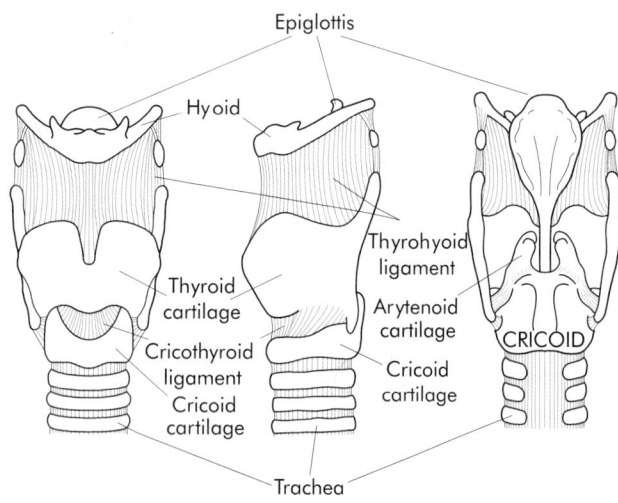

Figure 45.5 Anatomy of the larynx. [Reprinted from Aird's Companion in Surgical Studies, 2nd edn, Burnand, K.G. and Young, A.E. (eds), 1998, Fig. 20.37, with permission from Elsevier.]

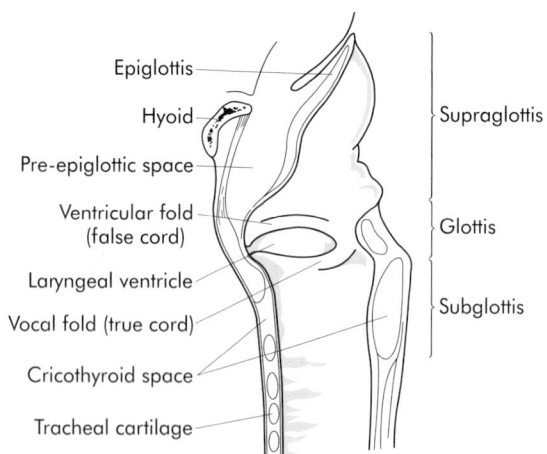

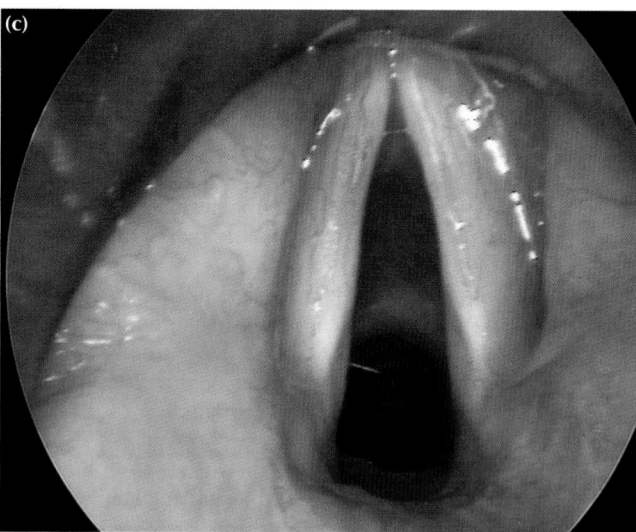

Figure 45.6 A view of the larynx on indirect laryngoscopy: (a) vocal folds abducted; (b) vocal folds adducted. (c) Photograph of normal larynx in abduction. [Adapted from Aird's Companion in Surgical Studies, 2nd edn, Burnand, K.G. and Young, A.E. (eds), 1998, Fig. 20.38, with permission from Elsevier.]

Phonation/speech

The larynx functions by closing the vocal fold against the air being exhaled from the lungs, but the rise in subglottic pressure forces the vocal folds apart slightly for an instant of time with accompanying vibration of the vocal fold epithelium. The opening and closing occurs in rapid sequence to produce a vibrating column of air, which is the source of sound.

Paralysis or disease of the vocal folds or closely associated laryngeal structures will give rise to disturbance of the sound, producing hoarseness.

The functions of the larynx are given in Summary box 45.1.

Summary box 45.1

Functions of the larynx

Protection of the lower respiratory tract by
- Closure of the laryngeal inlet
- Closure of the false cords
- Closure of the glottis
- Cessation of respiration
- Cough reflex

Phonation

Respiration
- Control of pressure

Fixation of chest
- Aids lifting, straining and climbing

The neck

The neck is divided into anterior and posterior triangles by the sternocleidomastoid muscle. The anterior triangle extends from the inferior border of the mandible to the sternum below, and is bounded by the midline and the sternocleidomastoid muscle. The posterior triangle extends backwards to the anterior border of the trapezius muscle and inferiorly to the clavicle. The upper part of the anterior triangle is commonly subdivided into the submandibular triangle above the digastric muscle and the submental triangle below. The lymphatic drainage of the head and neck is of considerable clinical importance (Fig. 45.7). The most important chain of nodes are the jugular nodes (also called cervical), which run adjacent to the internal jugular vein. The other main groups are the submental, submandibular, pre- and post-auricular, occipital and posterior triangle nodes.

A system of levels is used to describe the location of these neck nodes (Fig. 45.8). The upper jugular nodes, level II, which contain the large jugulodigastric node, drain the naso- and oropharynx, including the tonsils, posterolateral aspects of the oral cavity, and the superior aspects of the larynx and pyriform fossae. They are the most common site of enlargement and may be palpated along the anterior border of the sternocleidomastoid muscle.

Metastatic spread of squamous cell carcinoma (80% of head and neck cancer) most commonly occurs with tumours of the nasopharynx, tongue base, tonsil, pyriform fossae and supraglottic larynx. When an enlarged neck node is detected and malignant disease is suspected, these five primary sites must be carefully examined.

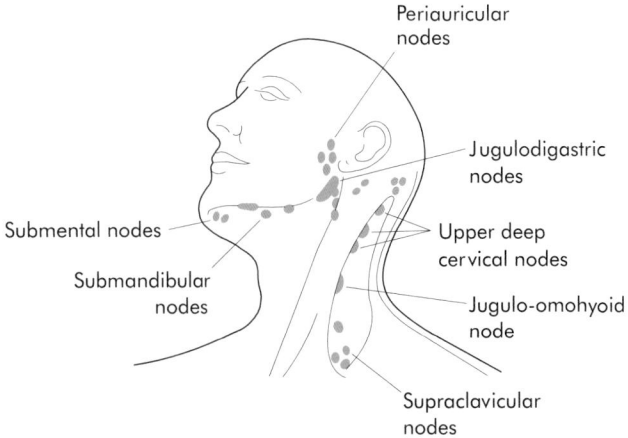

Figure 45.7 Distribution of cervical lymph nodes.

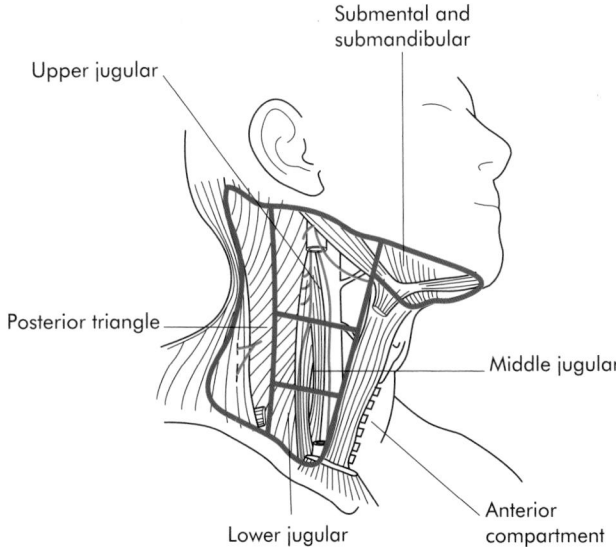

Figure 45.8 The level system for describing location of lymph nodes in the neck. Level 1, submental and submandibular group; level II, upper jugular group; level III, middle jugular group; level IV, lower jugular group; level V, posterior triangle group; level VI, anterior compartment group.

CLINICAL EXAMINATION

Pharynx and larynx

Before examination of the pharynx, the oral cavity should be examined with the aid of a good light and tongue depressors. A reflecting mirror on the head or a headband-mounted fibreoptic light source permits use of both hands to hold instruments. Inspection should include the buccal mucosa and lips, the palate, the tongue and floor of the mouth, all surfaces of the teeth and gums, opening and closing of the mouth and dental occlusion. Patients should be asked to elevate the tongue to the roof of the mouth and protrude the tongue to both the right and the left. Palpation may be required using one or two fingers gently intraorally to feel any swellings and this may be combined with extraoral palpation of the submental and submandibular lymph nodes and salivary glands.

Following examination of the oral cavity, the oropharynx is then inspected with the tongue depressor placed firmly onto the tongue base to depress it inferiorly. The anterior and posterior faucial pillars, the tonsil, retromolar trigone and posterior pharyngeal wall should all be inspected for colour changes, ulceration, pus, foreign bodies and swellings. Even with an experienced examiner, approximately one-third of patients cannot tolerate the depression of the posterior base of tongue without gagging. Pain and trismus as a consequence of pharyngolaryngeal or neck pathology may additionally add to the difficulty of the examination.

Fibreoptic nasendoscopes passed through the nose with or without topical anaesthesia allow high-quality examination of the entire nasopharynx, oropharynx and larynx in over 90% of patients.

The neck

The patient should be examined sitting with the whole neck exposed so that both clavicles are clearly seen. The neck is inspected from in front and the patient asked to swallow, preferably with the aid of a sip of water. Movements of the larynx and any swelling in the neck are noted. The patient should be asked to protrude the tongue if there is a midline neck swelling. A thyroglossal cyst will move upwards with the tongue protrusion. The patient is then examined from behind with the chin flexed slightly downwards to remove any undue tension in the strap muscles, platysma and sternocleidomastoids. The neck is palpated bilaterally in a sequential manner comparing the two sides of the neck.

On examining for a lump in the neck, it is often helpful to ask the patient to point to the lump first. Ask if the lump is tender. A swelling beneath the sternomastoid muscle may be considerably larger than thought on palpation. If malignancy is suspected (hard, irregular or fixed to overlying skin or to deep structures), inspection of the nasopharynx, tonsils, tongue base, pyriform fossae and supraglottic larynx is essential (Summary box 45.2).

Summary box 45.2

Key points of history and examination

Mouth
- Adequate light source and two spatulas to examine the mouth
- Examine
  - Teeth, gums, gingival sulci
  - Buccal mucosa, opening of parotid duct
  - Floor of mouth
  - Hard and soft palates
  - Retromolar trigone region ('coffin corner')
  - Anterior and posterior faucial pillars, tonsils
  - Posterior pharyngeal wall
  - Tongue (observe full movements)
- Palpate
  - Salivary glands/ducts

Larynx, oropharynx and hypopharynx
- Indirect laryngoscopy
  - Mirror and headlight
- Direct flexible fibreoptic pharyngolaryngoscopy

Nasopharynx
- Rigid Hopkins' rod endoscopy
- Flexible fibreoptic nasendoscopy

Neck
- Inspection
  - Tongue protrusion
  - Observe swallowing
- Palpation
  - If a mass is palpable, evaluate for size, site, shape, consistency, superficial and deep fixation, fluctuation, transillumination, auscultation

---

INVESTIGATIONS OF THE PHARYNX, LARYNX AND NECK

Plain lateral radiographs

Plain lateral radiographs of the neck and cervical spine may show soft tissue abnormalities; of particular importance is the depth and outline of the prevertebral soft tissue shadow. The outline of the laryngotracheal airway may be a useful guide to the presence of disease in the pharynx and larynx.

There should be no air within the upper oesophagus. If seen endoscopy is advised. Radio-opaque foreign bodies may be seen impacted in the pharynx, larynx or upper oesophagus on these radiographs.

Barium swallow

Barium liquid video fluoroscopic studies record the movement of a small quantity of radio-opaque liquid and allow detailed evaluation of the oral and pharyngeal phases of swallowing (Figs 45.9 and 45.10).

Computerised tomography scanning

Computerised tomography (CT) scanning provides much improved demonstration of disease in the pharynx, larynx and neck. Intravenous contrast given at the same time as the CT scan (dynamic scanning) further improves the demonstration of disease in these areas (Fig. 45.11).

Other techniques

Magnetic resonance imaging (MRI) is being increasingly used and may give better soft tissue definition of some diseases, but poorer definition of bony and cartilaginous structures (Fig. 45.12). Ultrasound scanning can be useful in differentiating solid

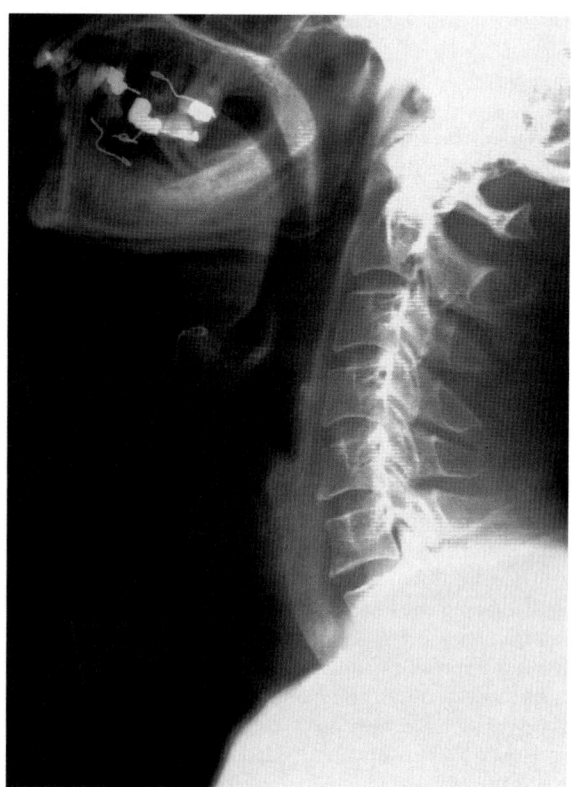

Figure 45.9 Plain lateral radiograph showing normal anatomy.

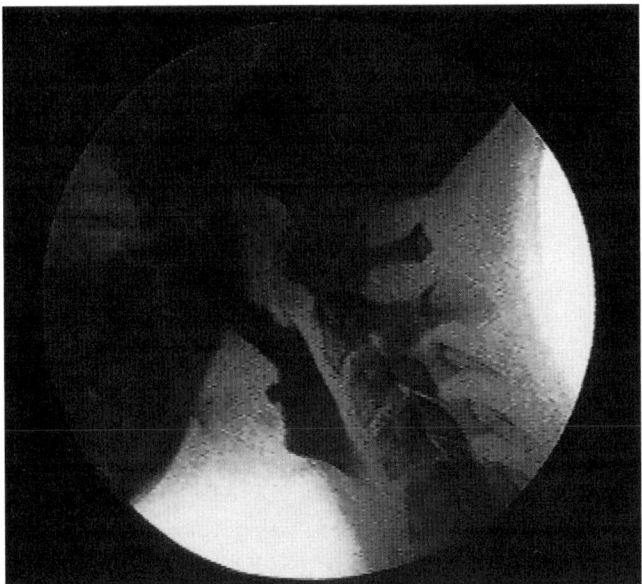

Figure 45.10 Videofluoroscopy image showing liquid barium in the upper pharynx in a normal swallow.

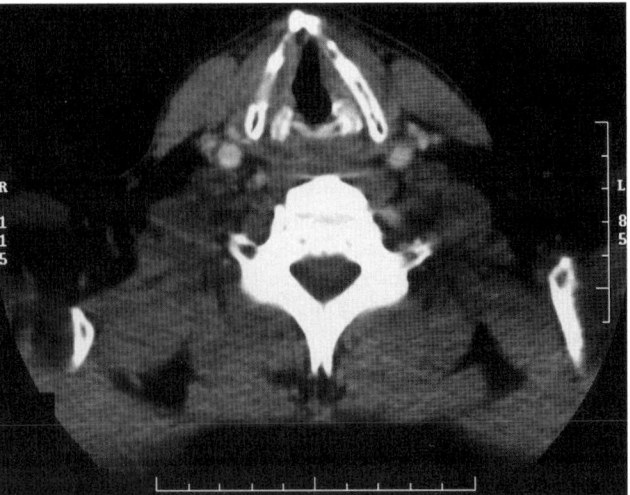

Figure 45.11 Axial computerised tomography scan through the larynx at the level of the glottis.

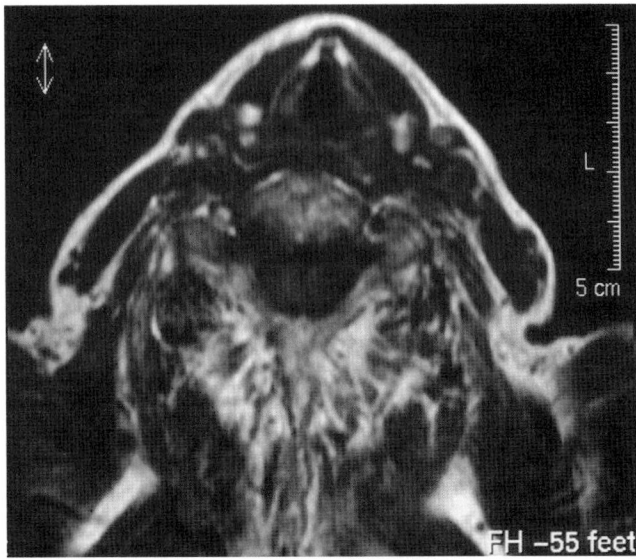

Figure 45.12 Axial magnetic resonance imaging scan at the same level as Fig. 45.11.

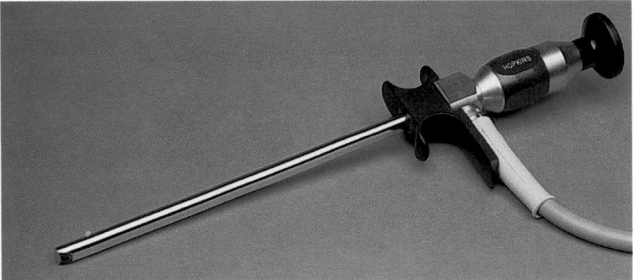

Figure 45.13 A rigid Hopkins' rod or endoscope.

lesions, e.g. malignant lymph nodes from cystic lesions such as a branchial cyst.

Fine-needle aspiration cytology

This technique can be performed under local anaesthesia. It is useful particularly if a neck lump is thought to be malignant. Increasingly high rates of accurate histological diagnosis are reported and there is no evidence of spread of tumour through the skin track caused by the fine hypodermic needle used with this technique. Fine-needle aspiration may be further aided by ultrasound or CT guidance.

Angiography or digital subtraction vascular imaging

These may be indicated if a vascular lesion such as a carotid body tumour is suspected. Angiography may have a therapeutic role to play by facilitating embolisation of the lesion.

Direct pharyngoscopy and laryngoscopy

Examination of the pharynx, larynx and neck under general anaesthesia may be required if there are problems with the routine examination of patients such as an inadequate view as a result of trismus from pain, poor patient compliance, or large obstructive pharyngeal or laryngeal pathology. These examinations may be further aided by the use of an operating microscope or rigid endoscope (Hopkins' rods) (Fig. 45.13).

DISEASES OF THE PHARYNX

Nasopharynx

Enlarged adenoid

The most common cause of an enlarged adenoid (there is only one nasopharyngeal adenoid, despite the common use of the term

Harold Horace Hopkins, 1918–1994, Professor of Applied Optics, The University of Reading, Reading, England. He invented the rigid rod endoscope (Hopkins' Rod, 1954), and contributed to the development of the fibres for flexible endoscopes.

'adenoids') is physiological hypertrophy. The size of the adenoid alone is not an indication for removal. It is often associated with hypertrophy of the other lymphoid tissues of Waldeyer's ring. If excessive hypertrophy causes blockage of the nasopharynx in association with tonsil hypertrophy, the upper airway may become compromised during sleep causing obstructive sleep apnoea.

Obstructive sleep apnoea

This condition is becoming increasingly diagnosed and is important because it can cause sleep deprivation and secondary cardiac complications. It has been implicated in some cases of sudden infant death syndrome. The most common symptom is snoring, which is typically irregular, with the child actually ceasing respiration (apnoea) and then restarting with a loud inspiratory snort. The child is often restless and may take up strange sleep positions as he or she tries to improve the pharyngeal airway. Surgical removal of the tonsils and adenoid is curative, but it is important to avoid sedative premedications and opiate analgesics postoperatively because they may further depress the child's respiratory drive.

Obstructive sleep apnoea may also occur in adults, where the obstruction may result from nasal deformity, a hypertrophic soft palate associated with an altered nasopharyngeal isthmus, obesity and general narrowing of the pharyngeal airway, or supraglottic laryngeal pathology. Surgery may be indicated following investigation by means of a sleep study, during which measurement of the patient's sleep pattern and arterial oxygenation are undertaken.

Hypertrophy of adenoid tissue most commonly occurs between the ages of 4 and 10, but the adenoid tissue usually undergoes spontaneous atrophy during puberty, although some remnants may persist into adult life (Fig. 45.14). The relationship of adenoid enlargement to recurrent secretory otitis media or recurrent acute otitis media is not entirely clear.

Adenoidectomy (Figs 45.15 and 45.16)

Adenoid tissue can be removed alone or in conjunction with a tonsillectomy. The indications for adenoidectomy are:

* obstructive sleep apnoea associated with post-nasal obstruction;

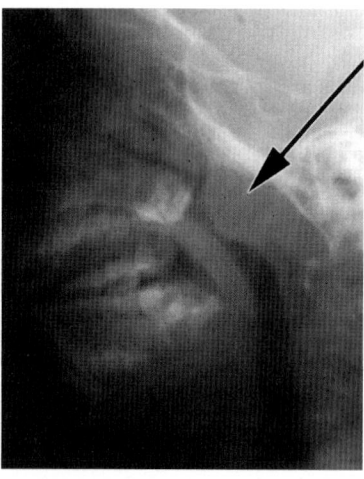

Figure 45.14 Plain lateral radiograph showing a large pad of adenoid tissue (arrow) in the post-nasal space.

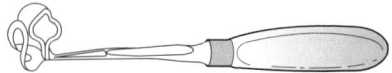

Figure 45.15 St Clair Thomson's adenoid curette.

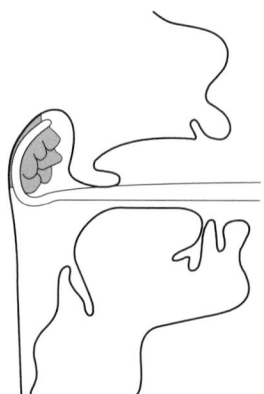

Figure 45.16 Curettage of the adenoid.

* post-nasal discharge;
* recurrent acute otitis media or prolonged serous otitis media, usually longer than 3 months' duration;
* recurrent rhinosinusitis.

Removal of the adenoid

Operative technique The adenoid tissue is removed with a guarded curette pressed against the roof of the nasopharynx and then carried downwards in a moderately firm sweeping movement bringing the excised adenoid into the oropharynx. The guard on the curette secures the adenoid and prevents it from dropping inferiorly into the airway. A post-nasal swab is placed into the nasopharynx until all haemorrhage has ceased.

Reactionary or secondary haemorrhage during the recovery period may require a nasopharyngeal pack under a further anaesthetic. This can occasionally cause respiratory depression in children and adults, and strict observation is required while the pack is in place.

TUMOURS OF THE NASOPHARYNX

Benign

There are two main types of benign tumour of the nasopharynx: the angiofibroma and the antrochoanal polyp. Both are rare.

Angiofibroma

This tumour is confined to young male patients most commonly between the ages of 8 and 20 years. It usually causes progressive nasal obstruction, recurrent severe epistaxis, purulent rhinorrhoea and occasionally loss of vision because of compression of the optic nerve. Although the tumour is rare, these symptoms in a young male patient should always arouse suspicion. The tumour is most common in northern India although the reasons for this are unknown. Clinical examination often shows a tumour in the nasal cavity or nasopharynx, but CT scanning best demonstrates the extent of the tumour and its accompanying bony erosion. MRI scanning defines the soft-tissue extent and, with these two modern investigations, angiography is rarely indicated. Biopsy should be avoided unless clinical and radiological examination are not diagnostic because of the risk of bleeding.

Surgical resection requires adequate exposure either through a midfacial approach or lateral rhinotomy (Figs 45.17 and 45.18). Both allow ligation of the feeding maxillary artery. Most recently, endoscopic resection has been used for smaller lesions.

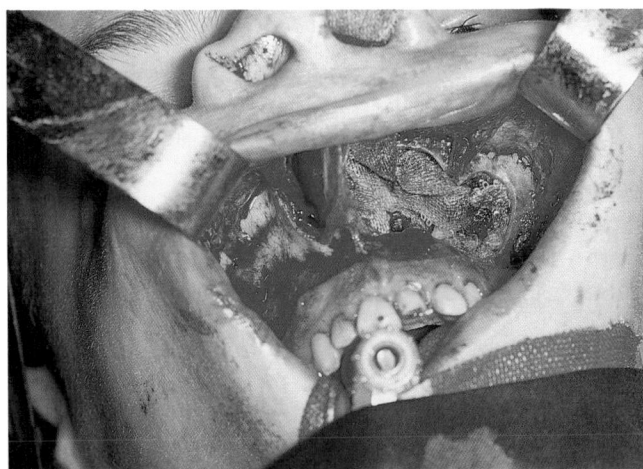

Figure 45.17 Intraoperative photograph showing exposure during a midfacial degloving approach.

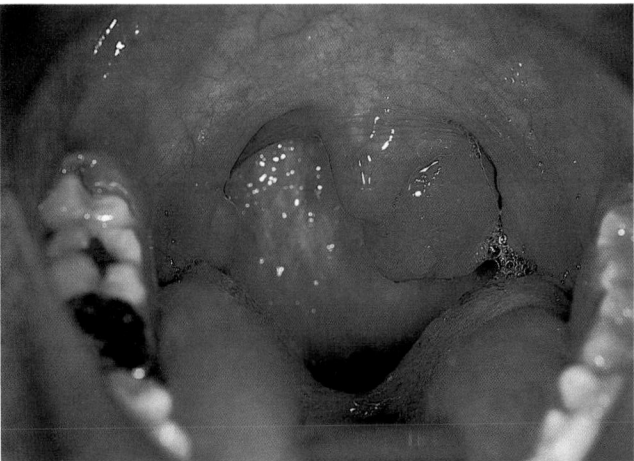

Figure 45.19 Intraoral view showing a fleshy polyp hanging in the oropharynx.

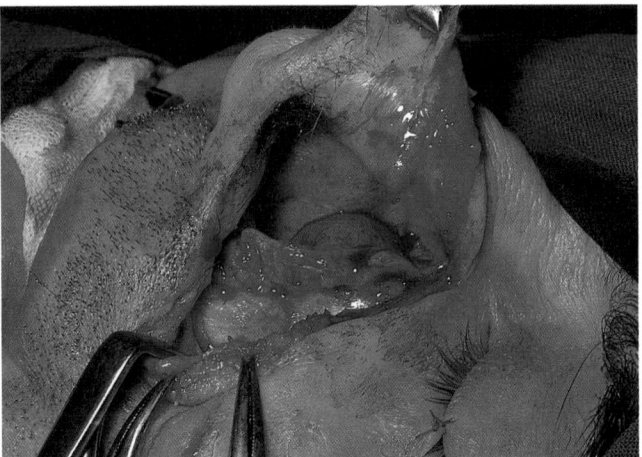

Figure 45.18 Intraoperative photograph showing an incision in lateral rhinotomy.

Antrochoanal polyp

This relatively uncommon lesion is a benign mucosal polyp that arises in the maxillary antrum and prolapses into the nasal cavity where it expands backwards into the nasopharynx and occasionally into the oropharynx (Figs 45.19 and 45.20). It may mimic an angiofibroma from which it is distinguished by its avascularity and pale colour, and its site of origin on endoscopic examination and imaging. It requires complete removal via an endoscopic approach through the middle meatus or, occasionally, a Caldwell–Luc procedure.

Malignant

Nasopharyngeal carcinoma

Nasopharyngeal carcinomas are usually squamous cell carcinoma and have a very variable incidence. In most parts of the world,

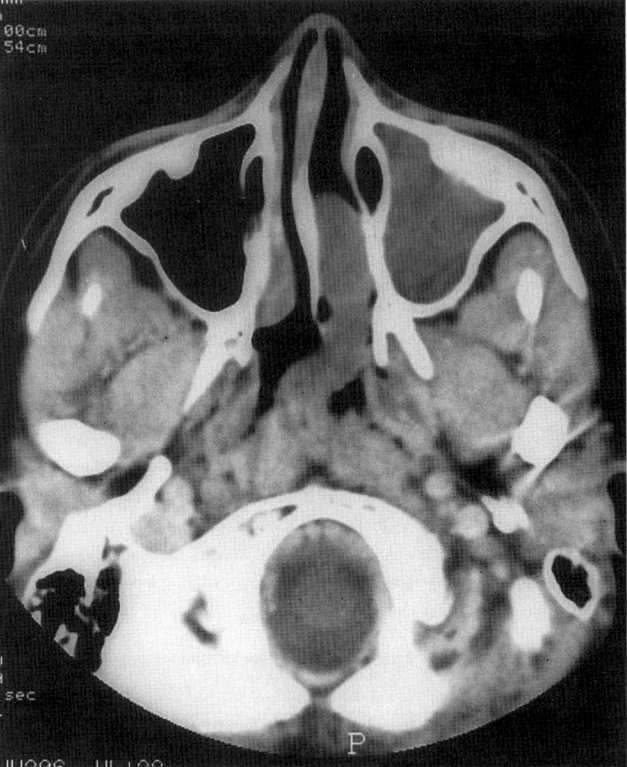

Figure 45.20 Axial computerised tomogram of an antrochoanal polyp (as seen in Fig. 45.19), with opaque maxillary antrum and a mass in the nasal cavity and nasopharynx.

the tumour is rare with an annual incidence of 1 case per 100 000 population; however, among southern Chinese populations the rate is 30–50 cases per 100 000 population. The aetiology of nasopharyngeal carcinoma is multifactorial. Genetic susceptibility, early infection by the Epstein–Barr virus and consumption of

George Walter Caldwell, **1834–1918**, Otolaryngologist, who practised successively in New York, San Francisco, and Los Angeles, USA, devised this operation for treating suppuration in the maxillary antrum in 1893.
Henri Luc, **1855–1925**, Otolaryngologist, Paris, France, described his operation in 1889.

Micheal Anthony Epstein, **B. 1921**, formerly Professor of Pathology, The University of Bristol, Bristol, England.
Yvonne Barr, **B. 1931**, a Virologist who emigrated to Australia. Epstein and Barr discovered this virus in 1964.

CHAPTER 45 | PHARYNX, LARYNX AND NECK

traditional diets, particularly salted fish, are known to contribute (Summary box 45.3).

Summary box 45.3

Aetiological factors in nasopharyngeal carcinoma

- Genetic, e.g. Cantonese
- Infective, e.g. Epstein–Barr virus
- Environmental, e.g. salted fish

The majority of tumours are undifferentiated with a characteristic morphology, comprising over 90% of nasopharyngeal malignancy in endemic areas. Rare epithelial tumours are adenocarcinoma and adenoid cystic carcinoma. B- and T-cell lymphomas also occur in this region and should not be confused with the more common undifferentiated carcinoma. Nasopharyngeal carcinoma has a bimodal distribution with an increased incidence in teenagers and young adults and then again in the 50–60 age group.

Clinical features

Symptoms are closely related to the position of the tumour in the nasopharynx and the degree of distant spread if any. Early symptoms are often minimal and may be ignored by both patient and doctor. Approximately 50% of patients will present with a mass of malignant nodes in the neck, indicating an advanced tumour. This percentage is even higher in patients under 21 years of age. Fine-needle aspiration or a biopsy of a neck node showing undifferentiated carcinoma requires immediate thorough examination of the nasopharynx. In about 5% of patients, the nasopharynx may look normal or minimally asymmetrical but contains submucosal nasopharyngeal carcinoma. A biopsy of the nasopharynx is essential if there is suspicion of nasopharyngeal malignancy. Nasal complaints occur in one-third of patients and aural symptoms of unilateral deafness as a consequence of Eustachian tube obstruction and secretory otitis media occur in approximately 20%. Neurological complications with cranial nerve palsies as a result of disease in the skull base occur relatively late in the disease, but are a poor prognostic factor (Summary box 45.4).

Summary box 45.4

Nasopharyngeal carcinoma: main presenting complaints

Systemic
- Cervical lymphadenopathy

Local
- Unilateral serous otitis media, otalgia
- Nasal obstruction, bloody discharge, epistaxis
- Cranial nerve palsies, especially III–VI then IX–XII

Investigation is by direct inspection with a flexible or rigid nasendoscope and biopsy under topical or general anaesthesia. Serological investigation for Epstein–Barr virus-associated antigenic markers in combination with the clinical and histological examination is valuable for the early detection of disease. Highly sensitive assays for anti-viral antibodies together with the newly discovered virus-associated serological markers are useful in early detection. Immunoglobulin (Ig)A anti-viral capsid antigen antibody has recently been evaluated in mass surveys in southern China and has been found to be an excellent screening method for the early detection of nasopharyngeal carcinoma in high-risk groups.

Imaging

Imaging is essential for staging and to determine the extent of disease. CT of the head, neck and chest has a major role in planning radiotherapy and assessing the response to treatment, diagnosing recurrence and detecting complications.

Treatment

The primary treatment of nasopharyngeal carcinoma is radiotherapy as the majority of the tumours are radiosensitive undifferentiated squamous cell carcinomas. Elective bilateral external radiotherapy is given to the skull base and neck in all patients, even when no neck nodes are apparent. Brachytherapy (intracavitary and interstitial radiotherapy) and chemotherapy are increasingly used. For early disease, 3-year disease-free survival rates of more than 75% are common; however, in advanced disease the results are less good, with 3-year disease-free survival rates of 30–50%.

OROPHARYNX

Acute tonsillitis

This common condition is characterised by a sore throat, fever, general malaise, dysphagia, enlarged upper cervical nodes and sometimes referred otalgia. Approximately half the cases are bacterial, the most common cause being a pyogenic group A streptococcus. The remainder are viral and a wide variety of viruses have been implicated, in particular infectious mononucleosis, which may be mistaken for bacterial tonsillitis.

On examination, the tonsils are swollen and erythematous, and yellow or white pustules may be seen on the palatine tonsils, hence the name 'follicular tonsillitis' (Fig. 45.21). A throat swab should be taken at the time of examination as well as blood for Paul–Bunnell testing.

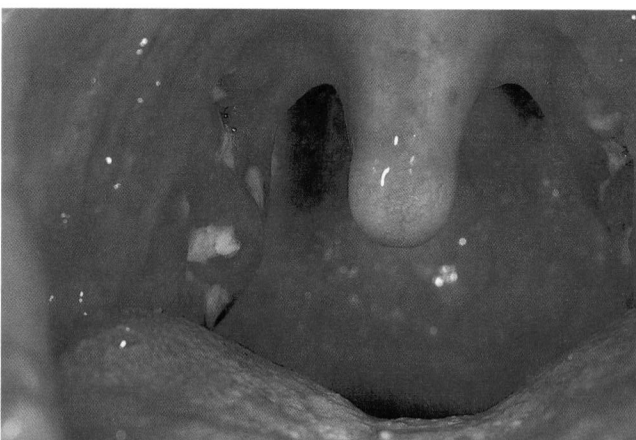

Figure 45.21 Acute follicular tonsillitis.

John Rodman Paul, 1893–1971, **Professor of Preventative Medicine, Yale University, New Haven, CT, USA.**
Walls Willard Bunnell, 1902–1966, **an American Physician. Paul and Bunnell described this test in 1932.**

Treatment

Paracetamol or similar analgesia may be administered to relieve pain and gargles of glycerol–thymol are soothing. The condition is frequently sensitive to benzyl- or phenyoxymethylpenicillin (penicillin V) and these are given until antibiotic sensitivities are established. Ampicillin is avoided as it may precipitate a rash in patients with infectious mononucleosis. Most cases resolve in a few days.

Quinsy

This is an abscess in the peritonsillar region that causes severe pain and trismus (Fig. 45.22). The trismus caused by spasm induced in the pterygoid muscles may make examination difficult but may be overcome by instillation of local anaesthesia into the posterior nasal cavity (anaesthetising the sphenopalatine ganglion) and the oropharynx. Inspection reveals a diffuse swelling of the soft palate just superior to the involved tonsil, displacing the uvula medially. In more advanced cases, pus may be seen pointing underneath the thin mucosa.

Treatment

In the early stages intravenous broad-spectrum antibiotics may produce resolution. However, if there is frank abscess formation, incision and drainage of the pus can be carried out under local anaesthesia. A small scalpel is best modified by winding a strip of adhesive tape around the blade so that only 1 cm of the blade projects. In teenagers and young adults, the patient sits upright and an incision is made approximately midway between the base of the uvula and the third upper molar tooth (Fig. 45.23). This may produce immediate release of pus, but, if not, a dressing forceps is pushed firmly through the incision and, on opening, pus may then be encountered. In small children, general anaesthesia is required.

Chronic tonsillitis

Chronic tonsillitis usually results from repeated attacks of acute tonsillitis in which the tonsils become progressively damaged and provide a reservoir for infective organisms.

Tonsillectomy

Recurrent acute tonsillitis is the most common relative indication for tonsillectomy in children and adolescents, although it is important that these attacks are well documented and do not

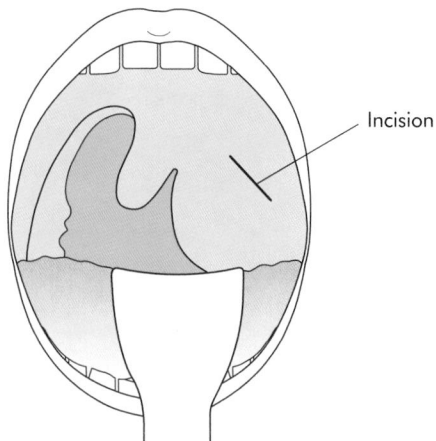

Figure 45.23 Site of incision in peritonsillar abscess.

simply constitute a minor viral sore throat. Chronic tonsillitis more frequently affects young adults in whom it is important to establish that chronic mouth breathing secondary to nasal obstruction is not the main problem rather than the tonsils themselves. Absolute indications for tonsillectomy are when the size of the tonsils is contributing to airway obstruction or a malignancy of the tonsils is suspected (Table 45.1).

Ideally, the procedure should be undertaken when the tonsils are not acutely infected, and it is important to discuss factors that may increase the tendency to bleed. Blood transfusion is rarely required, but it is normal practice to type and screen blood for cross-match in children under 15 kg in weight.

Dissection tonsillectomy is carried out under general anaesthesia. The mucosa of the anterior faucial pillar is incised and the tonsil capsule identified. Using blunt dissection, the tonsil is separated from its bed until only a small inferior pedicle is left (Fig. 45.24). Usually a snare is used to separate it from the lingual tonsil. A tonsil swab is placed in the tonsillar bed and pressure applied for some minutes, following which bleeding points may be controlled by ligature or by bipolar diathermy.

Following surgery, the patient is kept under close observation for any systemic or local evidence of bleeding, with regular pulse and blood pressure measurements and observation to see if the patient is swallowing excessively (Fig. 45.25). Postoperatively patients are encouraged to eat normally. Paracetamol is preferred to aspirin-containing analgesics. Patients are allowed home on the following day and are warned that they may experience otalgia as a result of referred pain from the glossopharyngeal

Table 45.1 Indications for tonsillectomy

Absolute	Sleep apnoea, chronic respiratory tract obstruction, cor pulmonale
	Suspected tonsillar malignancy
Relative	Documented recurrent acute tonsillitis
	Chronic tonsillitis
	Peritonsillar abscess (quinsy)
	Tonsillitis resulting in febrile convulsions
	Diphtheria carriers
	Systemic disease caused by β-haemolytic *Streptococcus* (nephritis, rheumatic fever)

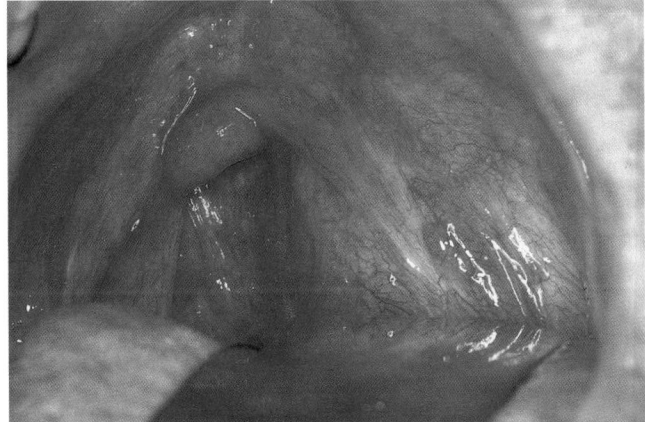

Figure 45.22 Quinsy (peritonsillar abscess).

CHAPTER 45 | PHARYNX, LARYNX AND NECK

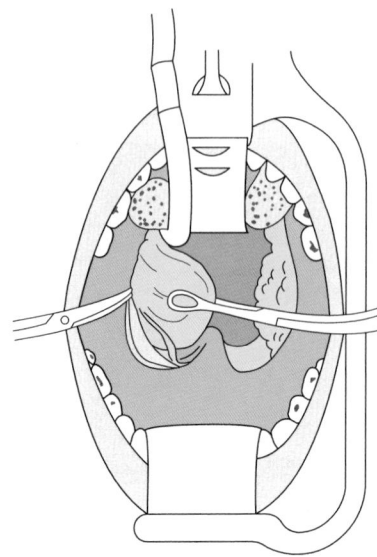

Figure 45.24 Removal of the tonsils.

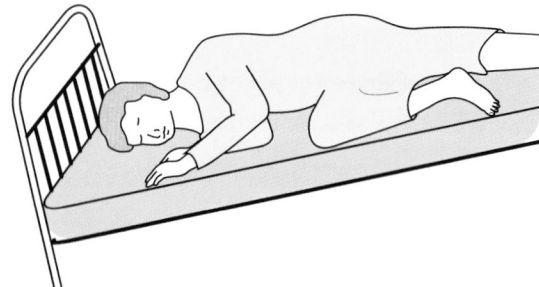

Figure 45.25 Positioning of the patient after tonsillectomy.

nerve and that secondary haemorrhage may occur up to 10 days following the surgery.

Haemorrhage is the most common complication in the immediate postoperative period. Local pressure may help in mild cases, but it is generally wisest to return to theatre for definitive treatment, particularly in younger patients. Under general anaesthesia, it may be possible to identify a bleeding spot, but often a more generalised ooze is observed and suturing of the tonsil bed combined with the application of Surgicel and bipolar diathermy is often more successful than attempted placement of ligatures.

Late haemorrhage is generally secondary to infection and patients should be commenced on intravenous antibiotics with aerobic and anaerobic cover. Significant or persistent bleeding may require a further general anaesthetic and undersewing of the surgical bed, which by this time will often be covered with slough and granulation tissue. Postoperative tonsillar haemorrhage is still a serious and life-threatening complication and should not be underestimated, particularly in the younger patient (Summary box 45.5).

Summary box 45.5

Complications of tonsillectomy

Anaesthetic
- Traumatic intubation
- Cardiopulmonary arrest
- Malignant hyperthermia

Surgical
- Haemorrhage (immediate or late)
- Infection
- Pain/otalgia
- Postoperative airway obstruction
- Velopharyngeal insufficiency

Parapharyngeal abscess

Parapharyngeal abscess may be confused with a peritonsillar abscess, but the maximal swelling is *behind* the posterior faucial pillar and there may be little oedema of the soft palate. The patient is usually a young child and there may be a severe general malaise. In early cases, admission to hospital and the institution of fluid replacements coupled with intravenous antibiotics may produce resolution. In advanced cases, drainage and intravenous antibiotics are required. With an obvious abscess pointing into the oropharynx, drainage may be carried out with a blunt instrument or the glove finger, but general anaesthesia is frequently required and the expertise of a senior anaesthetist, good illumination and good suction are absolutely essential. A large parapharyngeal abscess may compromise both the airway and swallowing.

Acute retropharyngeal abscess

This is the result of suppuration of the retropharyngeal lymph nodes and, again, is most commonly seen in children, with most cases occurring under 1 year of age. It is associated with infection of the tonsils, nasopharynx or oropharynx, and is frequently accompanied by severe general malaise, neck rigidity, dysphagia, drooling, a croupy cough, an altered cry and marked dyspnoea.

Dyspnoea may be the prominent symptom and may also be accompanied by febrile convulsions and vomiting. These children should always be carefully examined. Inspection of the posterior wall of the pharynx may show gross swelling and an abscess pointing beneath the thinned mucosa.

In countries where diphtheria still occurs, an acute retropharyngeal abscess may be confused with this, but the presence of the greyish green membrane aids differentiation. Occasionally, a foreign body, most commonly a fish bone which has perforated the posterior pharyngeal mucosa, will give rise to a retropharyngeal abscess in older children and young adults. Intravenous antibiotics are commenced immediately but surgical drainage of the abscess is often necessary. It requires experienced anaesthesia because, on induction, care must be taken to avoid rupturing the abscess. The airway is protected by placing the child in a head-down position while a pair of dressing forceps guided by the finger may be thrust into an obvious abscess in the posterior wall and the contents evacuated. On other occasions, an approach anterior and medial to the carotid sheath via a cervical incision may be required.

Chronic retropharyngeal abscess

This condition is now rare and is most commonly the result of an extension of tuberculosis of the cervical spine, which has spread through the anterior longitudinal ligament to reach the retropharyngeal space. In addition to the retropharyngeal swelling seen intraorally there may be fullness behind the sternocleidomastoid muscle on one side. In contrast to an acute retropharyngeal abscess, this condition occurs almost solely in adults.

Radiology usually shows evidence of bone destruction and loss of the normal curvature of the cervical spine. The spine may be quire unstable and undue manipulation may precipitate a neurological event.

A chronic retropharyngeal abscess must not be opened into the mouth, as such a procedure may lead to secondary infection. Drainage of the abscess may not be necessary if suitable treatment of the underlying tuberculosis disease is instituted. If it is necessary, drainage should be carried out through a cervical incision anterior to the sternocleidomastoid muscle with an approach anterior and medial to the carotid sheath to enter the retropharyngeal space. The cavity is opened and suctioned dry after taking biopsy material. Occasionally, surgery is required to decompress the spinal cord if there is a progressive neurological deficit.

Glandular fever (infectious mononucleosis)

This systemic condition is usually caused by the Epstein–Barr virus, but similar features can be caused by cytomegalovirus or toxoplasmosis. The tonsils are typically erythematous with a creamy grey exudate and appear almost confluent, usually symmetrical in contrast to a quinsy. In addition to the discomfort and dysphagia, patients may drool saliva and have respiratory difficulty, particularly on inspiration. They commonly have a high temperature and gross general malaise with other notable cervical or generalised lymphadenopathy. Occasionally, an enlarged spleen or liver may be detected. The condition is most frequent in teenagers and young adults. The diagnosis can be confirmed by serological testing showing a positive Paul–Bunnell test, an absolute and relative lymphocytosis, and the presence of atypical monocytes in the peripheral blood.

Treatment

Analgesia and maintenance of fluid intake are important. A small number of patients require admission to hospital if the airway is compromised and a short course of steroids may be helpful. Antibiotics are of little value and ampicillin is contraindicated because of the frequent appearance of a widespread skin rash. Rarely if the airway is severely compromised, an unhurried elective tracheostomy under local anaesthesia is safer and less traumatic than an emergency intubation. Emergency tonsillectomy is contraindicated because of the generalised pharyngeal oedema and compromised airway.

Human immunodeficiency virus

Acquired immune deficiency syndrome (AIDS) can affect the ear, nose and throat (ENT) system at any point during the disease. The initial seroconversion may present with the symptoms of glandular fever, which is followed by an asymptomatic period of variable length. In the pre-AIDS period, before the full-blown symptoms of the AIDS-related complex, many patients have minor upper respiratory tract symptoms that are often overlooked, such as otitis externa, rhinosinusitis and a non-specific pharyngitis. As the patient moves into the full-blown AIDS-related complex, a persistent, generalised lymphadenopathy is frequently found affecting the cervical nodes, which is usually due to follicular hyperplasia. However, patients may also develop tumours such as Kaposi's sarcoma, sometimes seen in the oral

cavity, and high-grade malignant B-cell lymphoma affecting the cervical lymph nodes and nasopharynx. In addition, multiple ulcers may be found in the oral cavity or pharynx associated with herpes infection. Severe candida may affect the oral cavity, pharynx, oesophagus or even larynx, and a hairy leucoplakia may affect the tongue (Fig. 45.26).

The globus syndrome

A wide variety of patients experience the feeling of a lump in the throat (from the Latin *globus* = lump). The symptom most commonly affects adults between 30 and 60 years of age. This feeling is not true dysphagia as there is no difficulty in swallowing. Most patients notice the symptom more if they swallow their own saliva, i.e. a forced, dry swallow, rather than when they eat or drink.

The aetiology of this common symptom is unknown, but some patients may have gastro-oesophageal reflux or spasm of their cricopharyngeus muscle.

The original name of 'globus hystericus' is unhelpful and although these patients may be anxious and at times introverted, they nonetheless require full examination to exclude local disease. Radiological and endoscopic investigation may be necessary to exclude an underlying cause.

Pharyngeal pouch

A pharyngeal pouch is a protrusion of mucosa though Killian's dehiscence, a weak area of the posterior pharyngeal wall between the oblique fibres of the thyropharyngeus and the transverse fibres of cricopharyngeus at the lower end of the inferior constrictor muscle (Fig. 45.27). These fibres, along with the circular fibres of the upper oesophagus, form the physiological upper oesophageal sphincter mechanism. Why the pouch forms is not yet clear, even with modern videofluoroscopic and manometric studies. Many patients with pharyngeal pouches have been demonstrated to have normal relaxation of the upper oesophageal sphincter mechanism in relation to swallowing, but others have been shown to have incomplete pharyngeal relaxation, early cricopharyngeal contraction and abnormalities of the pharyngeal contraction wave.

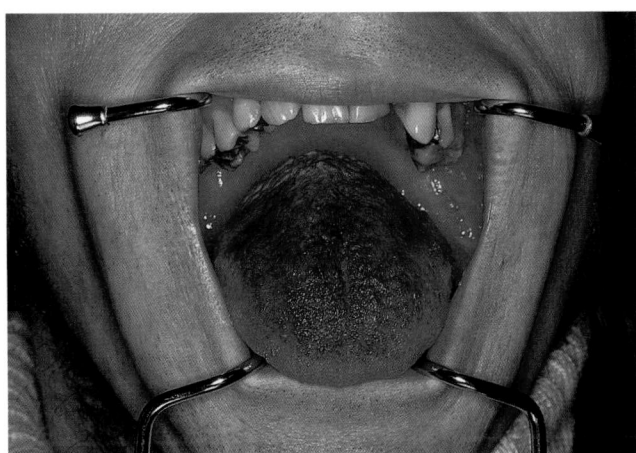

Figure 45.26 Intraoral view showing hairy tongue in a human immunodeficiency virus-positive patient.

CHAPTER 45 | PHARYNX, LARYNX AND NECK

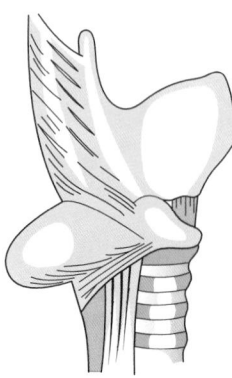

Figure 45.27 A pharyngeal pouch.

Clinical features

Patients suffering from this condition are commonly more than 60 years of age and it is twice as common in women as men. As the diverticulum enlarges, patients may experience regurgitation of undigested food, sometimes hours after a meal, particularly if they are bending down or turning over in bed at night. They sometimes wake at night with a feeling of tightness in the throat and a fit of coughing. Occasionally, they may present with recurrent, unexplained chest infections as a result of aspiration of the contents of the pouch. As the pouch increases in size, the patients may notice gurgling noises from the neck on swallowing and the pouch may become large enough to form a visible swelling in the neck.

Radiological examination

A thin emulsion of barium is given to the patient as a barium swallow (Fig. 45.28) or ideally as part of a videofluoroscopic swallowing study. Care should be exercised in patients who cough on swallowing, indicating they may have aspiration. A small volume of barium is sufficient to outline the pharynx, pouch and upper oesophagus. The videofluoroscopic study gives

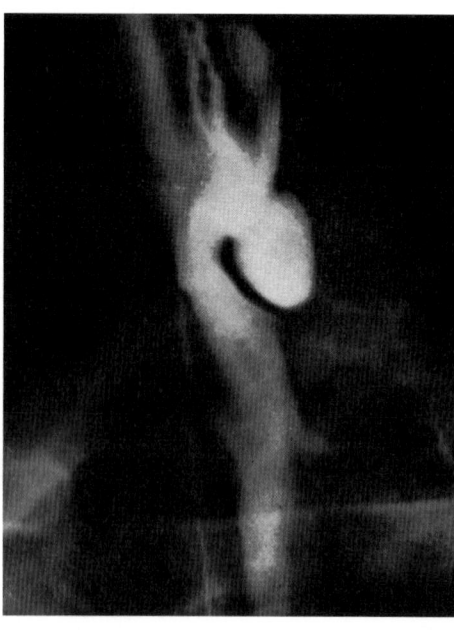

Figure 45.28 Barium swallow showing a pharyngeal pouch.

additional information about the pharyngeal contraction waves and the performance of the upper oesophageal sphincter.

Treatment

Surgery is indicated when the pouch is associated with progressive symptoms and particularly when a prominent cricopharyngeal bar of muscle associated with abnormality of the upper oesophageal sphincter mechanism causes considerable dysphagia. In elderly patients, a decision to operate may be influenced by their general condition. Preoperative chest physiotherapy and attention to the respiratory, cardiovascular and nutritional aspects of the patient are important. Perioperative antibiotics are recommended.

In the classic external operation, the opening to the pouch is first identified using a pharyngoscope and a nasogastric tube placed into the oesophageal lumen for postoperative nutrition. This initial endoscopy is often difficult because the normal oesophageal opening is small compared with the lumen of the pouch, but it may be better visualised using a Dohlmann's rigid endoscope. The pouch may be packed with ribbon gauze soaked in proflavin solution to further aid identification of its neck.

A lower neck incision along the anterior border of the left sternocleidomastoid muscle, or a transverse crease incision, is used and the muscle and carotid sheath are retracted laterally and the trachea and larynx medially. The pouch is found medially behind the lower pharynx and is carefully isolated and dissected back to its origin at Killian's dehiscence. It is then excised and the pharynx closed in two layers or, if it is small, the pouch may be invaginated into the pharyngeal lumen before closing the muscle layers. In all cases, a myotomy dividing the fibres of the cricopharyngeus muscle and the upper oesophageal circular muscle fibres must be performed. The wound is usually closed with drainage and the patient fed through a nasogastric tube for 3–7 days.

Complications

The classic operation has been associated with wound infection, mediastinitis, pharyngeal fistula formation and stenosis of the upper oesophagus. Variations have been tried which include simply hitching up the pouch into a superior position without excising it, thus allowing the fundus and body to empty continuously into the oesophagus. This is unsatisfactory with larger pouches, and upper oesophageal myotomy is still required.

Endoscopic operations

Endoscopic division of the bar of muscle forming the anterior wall of the pouch and the posterior aspect of the lumen of the oesophagus has been advocated for many years using Dohlmann's instruments or a carbon dioxide laser applied via a special pharyngoscope. An endoscopic stapling technique using a modified pharyngoscope to safely divide the anterior wall of the pouch and the posterior wall of the oesophagus is increasingly used. This completes a full myotomy and allows any food and fluid to drain from the pouch directly down the oesophagus. The endoscopic technique is associated with a high symptomatic success rate and a low morbidity which is particularly important in the elderly.

Sideropenic dysphagia

Prolonged iron deficiency anaemia may lead to dysphagia, particularly in middle-aged women. In addition, they may have koilonychia, cheilosis, angular stomatitis together with lassitude and poor exercise tolerance. The dysphagia is caused by a post-cricoid or upper oesophageal web and these patients have a higher incidence of post-cricoid malignancy. The syndrome is associated with the names of Plummer and Vinson, Paterson and Brown Kelly.

TUMOURS OF THE OROPHARYNX

Benign

Benign tumours of the oropharynx are rare, papillomas being the most common. These are usually incidental findings and are rarely of any importance.

Malignant

The most important epithelial tumour is squamous cell carcinoma, which constitutes approximately 90% of all epithelial tumours in the upper aerodigestive tract (Figs 45.29 and 45.30). In the oropharynx, the proportion is less (70%) because of the higher incidence of lymphoma (25%) and salivary gland tumours (5%).

Aetiology

Squamous carcinomas of the oropharynx are strongly associated with cigarette smoking and consumption of alcohol. In countries where the consumption of tobacco and alcohol are associated with poor oral hygiene, these malignancies assume major importance. Because of the rich lymphatic drainage of the oropharynx, cervical node metastases are common. They may be the only presenting feature with an apparent occult primary tumour often being unsuspected and missed in the tonsil or tongue base.

Treatment

Treatment varies with facilities around the world, but early tumours may be cured by radiotherapy, laser excision or more

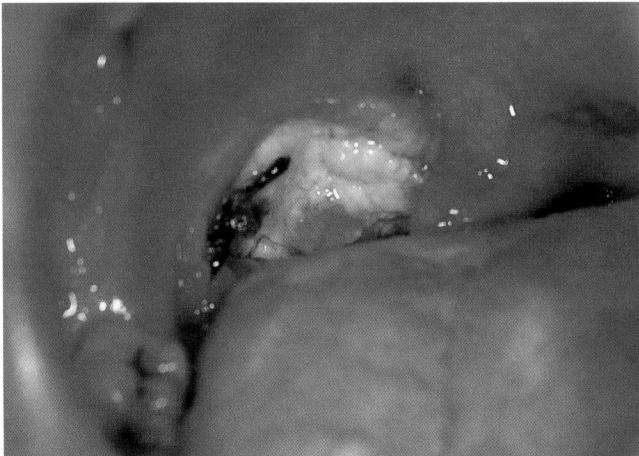

Figure 45.29 Squamous cell carcinoma of the right tonsil.

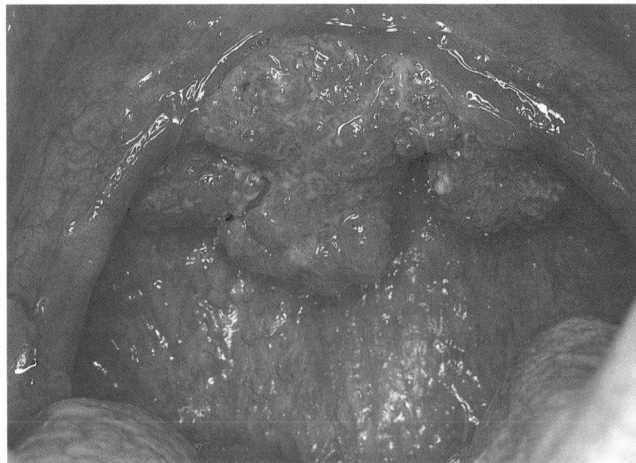

Figure 45.30 Squamous cell carcinoma of the soft palate.

conventional excision. Recurrent disease following radiotherapy is managed surgically and repair of the oropharynx may require regionally based myocutaneous flaps or free flaps with microvascular anastomosis. Neck dissection is required in a large proportion of cases of advanced disease. Postoperative dysphagia with aspiration as a result of interference in the complex neuromuscular control of the second phase of swallowing is a particular problem in these patients. This type of surgery is best carried out in a major centre undertaking this work on a regular basis.

Lymphoma of the head and neck

Lymphomas of the head and neck may arise in nodal or extra-nodal sites and both Hodgkin's disease and non-Hodgkin's lymphoma commonly present as lymph node enlargement in the neck. Hodgkin's disease is rare in the oropharynx, but non-Hodgkin's lymphoma accounts for 15–20% of tumours at this site in some countries. Most are of the B-cell type and have features in common with other tumours of MALT. Further evaluation with CT scanning of the thorax and abdomen, and bone marrow evaluation are essential.

Radiotherapy is the treatment of choice for localised non-Hodgkin's lymphoma and may give control rates as high as 75% at 5 years. For disseminated non-Hodgkin's lymphoma, systemic chemotherapy is preferred.

TUMOURS OF THE HYPOPHARYNX

Benign

Benign tumours of the hypopharynx are very rare, the most common being the fibroma and the leiomyoma. They show a smooth, constant mass lying in the lumen of the hypopharynx or oesophagus.

Malignant

Malignant tumours of the hypopharynx are almost exclusively squamous cell carcinomas with a predominance of moderate and poor differentiation. The tumours are usually classified according to their probable anatomical site of origin from the pyriform fossa,

CHAPTER 45 | PHARYNX, LARYNX AND NECK

post-cricoid region or posterior pharyngeal wall. Marked differences in the incidence of these tumours occur globally because of factors such as iron-deficiency anaemia (see Sideropenic dysphagia, p. 714). They may be associated with marked submucosal spread of 10 mm or more, which further complicates evaluation. Tumours arising from the pyriform fossa and posterior pharyngeal wall may spread to upper or lower cervical nodes. Tumours arising in the post-cricoid area typically metastasise to paratracheal and paraoesophageal nodes, which may not be palpable. As with oropharyngeal tumours, alcohol and tobacco are two principal carcinogens. Post-cricoid carcinoma, though rare, is more common in women than men.

The diagnosis of hypopharyngeal carcinoma should be considered in all patients presenting with dysphagia, hoarseness or referred otalgia, particularly if they have a history of iron-deficiency anaemia, smoking or significant alcohol consumption.

Laryngoscopy may show only subtle signs of disease such as oedema or pooling of saliva unilaterally in a pyriform fossa, or diminution of vocal fold mobility. All regions of the neck must be assessed in a systematic manner. Fine-needle aspirate is advocated for suspicious nodes. A suspected primary may require videofluoroscopy or barium swallow study, endoscopy and biopsy, and CT or MRI scanning if available. A chest radiograph should be taken to detect a second primary or metastasis.

Treatment

Squamous carcinoma of the hypopharynx commonly presents late and carries a poor prognosis. Early lesions may be treated with radiotherapy alone or transoral endoscopic carbon dioxide laser resection. Major open excisional surgery is generally used for recurrence after radiotherapy or as primary excision in advanced disease. Total pharyngolaryngectomy is commonly required (Fig. 45.31) and for lesions extending into the upper oesophagus, oesophagectomy and total thyroidectomy may additionally be needed. Myocutaneous flaps, transposed jejunum or stomach are used to reconstruct the pharynx. Swallowing and voice rehabilitation are necessary to support patients after this major surgery if they are to adjust and maintain some quality of life (Summary box 45.6).

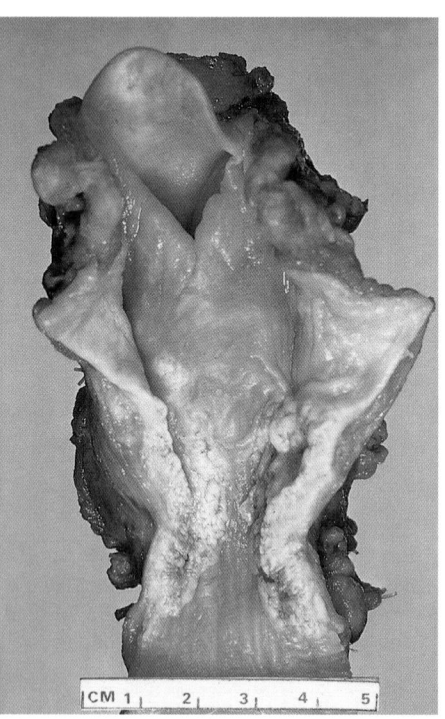

Figure 45.31 Total pharyngolaryngectomy specimen showing hypopharyngeal carcinoma (hypopharynx opened from posterior).

Summary box 45.6

Tumours of the hypopharynx

- Variable symptoms – discomfort, pain, dysphagia, hoarseness
- Awareness increased by history of smoking and alcohol
- Expert examination with nasendoscopy
- Referral to expert for detailed assessment and treatment – radiotherapy, laser or extensive surgery

---

DISEASES OF THE LARYNX

Emergencies

Stridor

Stridor means noisy breathing. It may be inspiratory or expiratory, or occurring in both phases of respiration. Inspiratory stridor is usually due to an obstruction at or above the vocal folds and is most commonly the result of an inhaled foreign body or acute infections such as epiglottitis. Expiratory stridor is usually from the lower respiratory tract and gives rise to a prolonged expiratory wheeze. It is most commonly associated with acute asthma or acute infective tracheobronchitis. Biphasic stridor is usually due to obstruction or disease of the tracheobronchial airway and distal lungs (Summary box 45.7).

Summary box 45.7

Stridor

Inspiratory
- Foreign body or epiglottitis

Expiratory
- Acute asthma or infective tracheobronchitis

Biphasic
- Obstruction, disease of tracheobronchial airway or distal lungs

---

Stridor in children

Infants and children presenting with stridor need careful assessment with a full history and examination as appropriate. If, on presentation, a child is cyanosed and severely unwell, the airway must be secured as soon as possible, but a brief history with important pointers can often be obtained from the parents.

History In infants in the first year of life, it is important to establish if the stridor is associated with particular activities such as swallowing, crying or movement. These may suggest congenital laryngomalacia or subglottic stenosis. If the stridor is exacerbated by feeding, particularly in the first 4 weeks of life, this suggests a vascular ring or tracheo-oesophageal fistula. If the cry is weak or abnormal, this suggests a vocal fold palsy. If the problem only occurs in association with an upper respiratory tract infection and, in particular, is biphasic, this would suggest congenital subglottic stenosis. In a young child, inspiratory stridor and drooling suggest acute epiglottitis, whereas biphasic stridor without drooling suggests laryngotracheobronchitis or croup (Summary box 45.8).

Summary box 45.8

Acute paediatric stridor

Congenital
    Laryngomalacia
    Laryngeal web
    Subglottic stenosis

Acquired
- Inflammatory
    Angioneurotic oedema
- Traumatic
    Impacted foreign body, laryngeal fracture
- Infective
    Epiglottis, laryngotracheobronchitis
- Neurological
    Vocal fold palsy
- Neoplasia
    Benign laryngeal papillomatosis

Examination It is important when possible to observe the child carefully at rest. Once a baby starts to cry, it may be impossible to study its resting respiratory pattern for some time. Ask the mother, not a nurse or a colleague, to move a baby or young child into different positions, such as face down and supine, and watch for changes in respiratory pattern and level of distress. Observe any drooling and, with neonates and infants, always try to watch the child being fed, listening to the trachea and chest with a stethoscope if possible. Always examine the whole child, looking for any evidence of congenital abnormalities before attempting any examination of the throat.

If a child is stridulous and drooling and sitting upright in its mother's arms or a chair, do not attempt to lay it down and do not attempt to look inside the mouth. These manoeuvres are potentially life-threatening as the child may aspirate a large quantity of thick saliva contained within the oral cavity. The child does not wish to attempt swallowing in the case of a retropharyngeal abscess, parapharyngeal abscess or acute epiglottitis as these conditions are so painful. It is particularly important in acute epiglottitis as the aspiration of thick saliva may be associated with further laryngeal spasm and a respiratory arrest. Restlessness, increasing tachycardia and cyanosis are important signs of hypoxia. If the child is not distressed and drooling, and not markedly stridulous, he/she may be cooperative enough that it is possible to look inside the mouth and check the palate, tongue and oropharynx. In stridulous children, particularly neonates and infants, a transcutaneous oximeter is invaluable. A resuscitation trolley with the necessary equipment for emergency intubation or tracheostomy should be close at hand if at all possible before commencing examination.

Investigation Plain lateral radiographs of the neck and a chest radiograph can be obtained but only if the child's condition permits. If a child is severely stridulous, they should *not* be sent to a radiography department without access to medical staff or resuscitation equipment.

Examination under anaesthesia is essential in all children whose diagnosis remains in doubt. This requires a high level of skill and appropriate rigid laryngoscopes, bronchoscopes, endoscopic Hopkins' rods and an operating microscope should be made available if possible. Equipment should be available at all times to undertake an urgent tracheostomy to establish or maintain an airway.

Acute epiglottitis

In children acute epiglottitis is of rapid onset. It tends to occur in children of 2 years of age and over. Stridor is usually associated with drooling of saliva. The condition is caused by *Haemophilus influenzae* infection, which initially causes a severe pharyngitis at the junction of the oro- and hypopharynx before producing inflammation and oedema of the laryngeal inlet. As it progresses, it involves the whole of the supraglottic larynx, with severe oedema of the aryepiglottic folds and epiglottis being the most notable component, hence the commonly used term 'acute epiglottitis'.

These children frequently require intensive management with emergency intubation or tracheostomy followed by oxygenation, humidification, continuous oximetry and antibiotics such as ampicillin or chloramphenicol. There may be associated septicaemia so blood cultures should be obtained. Attempted examination with a spatula into the mouth may precipitate a respiratory arrest and should be avoided.

Laryngotracheobronchitis (croup)

Croup is usually of slower onset than acute epiglottitis and occurs most commonly in children under 2 years of age. It is usually viral in origin and the cases often occur in clusters. The children have biphasic stridor, and are often hoarse with a typical barking cough. Airway intervention is required less often, but admission to hospital with oxygenation and humidification, coupled with antibiotics, may be necessary if there are signs of secondary infection.

Foreign bodies

Both children and adults may inhale foreign bodies. Young children will attempt to swallow a wide variety of objects, but coins, beads and parts of toys are particularly common. In adults, the aspiration is usually food, particularly inadequately chewed bones and meat. This is more common in elderly edentulous adults. Occasionally, portions of dentures may be inhaled, particularly in association with road traffic accidents.

Clinical features

The history is paramount and a history of foreign body ingestion or inhalation in a child, even though the pain, dysphagia, coughing, etc. may have settled, should always be taken seriously.

Adults usually have a clear recall, which facilitates diagnosis. Fish bones may lodge in the tonsils or base of tongue with minimal symptoms, but small fish bones may give rise to para- and retropharyngeal abscess formation.

Examination

Examination may be prevented by trismus, pain and anxiety, but the presence of a foreign body may be suspected by a salivary pool within the pyriform fossa or adjacent oedema and erythema of the pharyngolaryngeal mucosa.

Radiology

Radiology may be helpful but is not critical. Fish bones are often invisible on plain radiographs and a normal plain radiograph does not exclude a foreign body within the pharynx, larynx, oesophagus or lungs.

Specialised studies may help in cases of doubt, using a CT scan or a gastrografin swallow in the case of a suspected oesophageal foreign body.

Treatment

In the case of an inhaled foreign body causing severe stridor in a neonate or infant, it may be removed either by hooking it from the pharynx with a finger or by inverting the child carefully by the ankles and slapping his/her back. In a larger child, it may be more appropriate to bend them over your knee with their head hanging down and again strike them firmly between the shoulders. In the case of adults, an impacted laryngeal foreign body may be coughed out using a Heimlich manoeuvre. This involves standing behind the patient, clasping the arms around the lower thorax, such that the knuckles of the clasped hands come into contact with the patient's xiphisternum, and then a brief, firm compression of the lower thorax may aid instant expiration of the foreign body. If none of these immediate emergency measures removes the foreign body and the patient is cyanosed and severely stridulous, an immediate cricothyroidotomy or tracheostomy may be necessary. In less urgent cases, and when a foreign body is strongly suspected, endoscopy under general anaesthesia may be indicated.

Other causes of acute pharyngolaryngeal oedema

Angioneurotic oedema, radiotherapy, laryngeal trauma associated with road traffic accidents, corrosives, scalds and smoke ingestion may all cause significant pharyngolaryngeal oedema, in addition to the acute infective conditions mentioned elsewhere. Hoarseness is the predominant symptom along with dysphagia prior to the increase in dyspnoea. If laryngoscopic examination is possible, marked oedema of the supraglottis and pharynx can be seen. Humidified oxygen, adrenaline nebulisers, systemic antihistamines and steroids may be valuable. Morphine should not be given as it may cause respiratory depression and respiratory arrest. If the dyspnoea progresses, intubation or tracheostomy will be necessary.

TRACHEOSTOMY AND OTHER EMERGENCY AIRWAY MEASURES

This procedure relieves airway obstruction or protects the airway by fashioning a direct entrance into the trachea through the skin of the neck. Tracheostomy may be carried out as an emergency when the patient is *in extremis* and the larynx cannot be intubated, but it is not always an easy procedure, particularly in an obese patient. An easier alternative for the inexperienced is insertion of a large intravenous cannula or a small tube into the cricothyroid membrane, which lies in the midline immediately below the thyroid cartilage. Emergency intubation is a further option when the laryngotracheal airway is not obstructed and

tracheostomy may be performed thereafter. *The time to do a tracheostomy is when you first think it may be necessary.*

If time allows, the following should be undertaken:

- inspection and palpation of the neck to assess the laryngotracheal anatomy in the individual patient;
- indirect or direct laryngoscopy;
- assessment of pulmonary function.

Whenever possible, the procedure should be adequately explained to the patient beforehand, with particular emphasis on the inability to speak immediately following the operation. Ample reassurance is required that they will not have 'lost' their voice permanently. The indications for tracheostomy are shown in Summary box 45.9

Summary box 45.9

Indications for tracheostomy

Acute upper airway obstruction
- For example, an inhaled foreign body, a large pharyngolaryngeal tumour, or acute pharyngolaryngeal infections in children

Potential upper airway obstruction
- For example, after major surgery involving the oral cavity, pharynx, larynx or neck

Protection of the lower airway
- For example, protection against aspiration of saliva in unconscious patients as a consequence of head injuries, faciomaxillary injuries, comas, bulbar poliomyelitis or tetanus

Patients requiring prolonged artifical respiration

Emergency tracheostomy

If a skilled anaesthetist is unavailable, local anaesthesia is employed, but in desperate cases when the patient is unconscious, none is required. In patients who have suffered severe head and neck trauma and who may have an unstable cervical spine fracture, cricothyroidotomy may be more suitable. If it is possible, the patient should be laid supine with padding placed under the shoulders and the extended neck kept as steady as possible in the midline. This aids palpation of the thyroid and cricoid cartilage between the thumb and index finger of the free hand. The movements of the fingers of the free hand are important in this technique. The operation is more difficult in small children and thick-necked adults as the landmarks are difficult to palpate (Figs 45.32 and 45.33).

A vertical midline incision is made from the inferior aspect of the thyroid cartilage to the suprasternal notch and continued down between the infrahyoid muscles. There may be heavy bleeding from the wound at this point, particularly if the neck is congested as a result of the patient's efforts to breathe around an acute upper airway obstruction. No steps should be taken to control this haemorrhage, although an assistant and suction are valuable. The operator should feel carefully for the cricoid cartilage using the index finger of the free hand while retracting the skin edges by pressure applied by the thumb and middle finger. If the situation is one of extreme urgency, a further vertical incision straight into the trachea at the level of the second, third and

---

Henry Jay Heimlich, B. 1920, Thoracic Surgeon, Xavier University, Cincinnati, OH, USA.
in extremis is Latin for 'in the last things'.

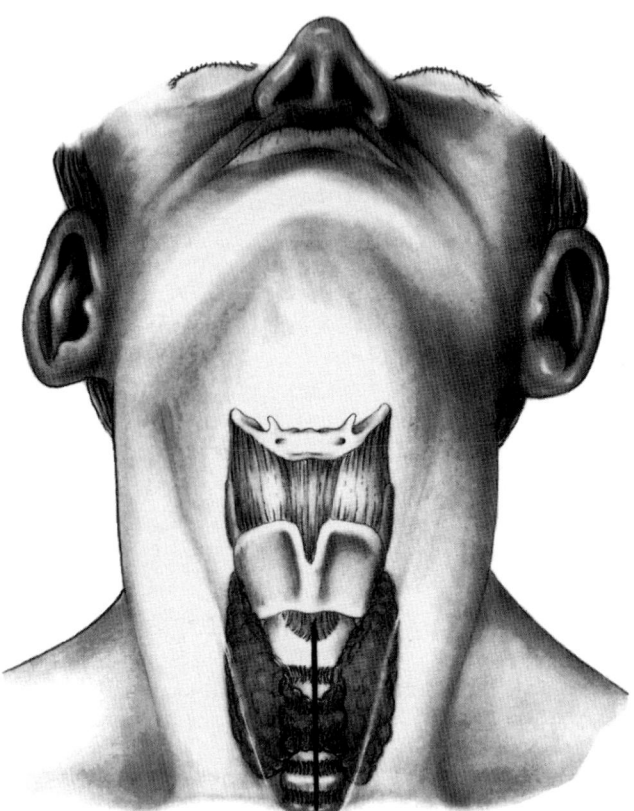

Figure 45.32 The position of skin incision in an emergency tracheostomy.

fourth ring should be made immediately without regard to the presence of the thyroid isthmus. The knife blade is rotated through 90°, thus opening the trachea. At this point the patient may cough violently as blood enters the airway. The operator should be aware of this possibility and avoid losing the position of the scalpel in the open trachea. Any form of available tube should be inserted into the trachea as soon as possible and blood and secretion sucked out. Once an airway has been established, haemostasis is then secured. With the emergency under control, the tracheostomy should be refashioned as soon as possible.

Should additional equipment and more time be available once the cricoid cartilage has been identified, blunt finger dissection inferiorly can be used to mobilise the thyroid isthmus, which should be divided between haemostats, clearing the trachea before making a vertical incision through the second to the fourth rings. A tracheal dilator is inserted through the tracheal incision and the edges of the tracheal wound are separated gently. In cases of suspected human immunodeficiency virus (HIV) infection or diphtheria, the surgeon places a swab over the wound so that the violent expiratory efforts which may follow do not contaminate the operator(s) with infected mucus and blood. When respiratory efforts have become less violent, a tracheostomy tube is inserted into the trachea and the dilator removed. It is important that the surgeon keeps a finger on the tube while the assistant ties the attached tapes around the patient's neck. Return the neck to a neutral position before tying the tapes firmly.

Elective tracheostomy

The advantage of an elective procedure is that there is complete airway control at all times, unhurried dissection and careful

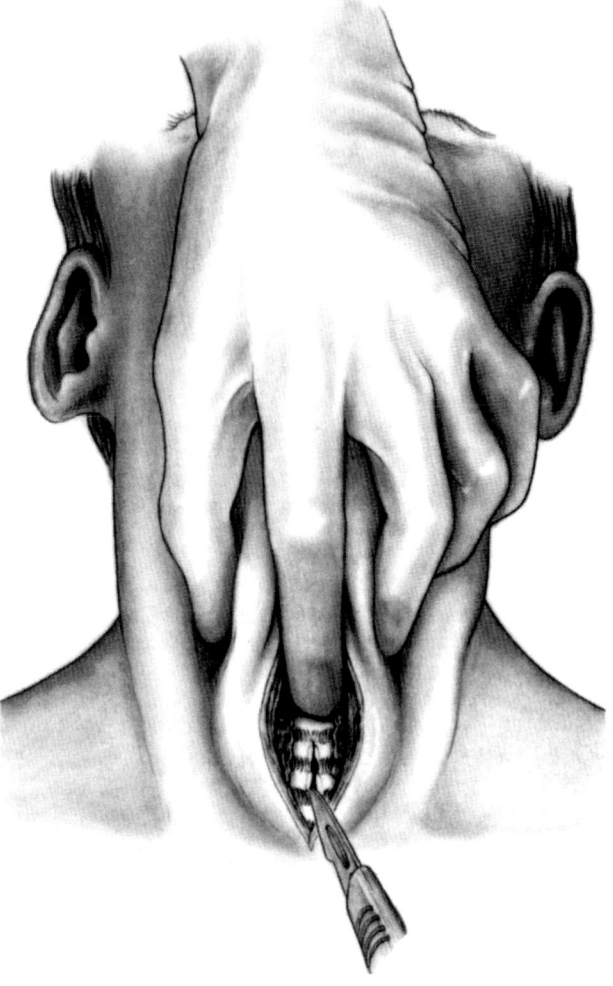

Figure 45.33 An incision in the trachea in an emergency tracheostomy.

placement of an appropriate tube. Close cooperation between the surgeon, anaesthetist and scrub nurse is essential, and attention to detail will markedly reduce possible complications and morbidity from the procedure.

Following induction of general anaesthesia and endotracheal intubation, the patient is positioned with a combination of head extension and placement of an appropriate sandbag under the shoulders (Fig. 45.34). There should be no rotation of the head. Children's heads should not be overextended as it is possible to enter the trachea in the fifth and sixth rings in these circumstances. Insertion of a bronchoscope in the trachea may help when performing tracheostomy in young children. A transverse incision may be used in the elective situation (Fig. 45.35). The tracheal isthmus is divided carefully and oversewn and tension sutures placed either side of the tracheal fenestration in children (Fig. 45.36). A Bjork flap may be used in adults (Figs 45.37 and 45.38).

The advantages of the Bjork method far outweigh the potential disadvantages and the method is particularly useful for those

Viking Olaf Bjork, **B. 1918, formerly Cardiac Surgeon, Karolinska Sjukset, Stockholm, Sweden.**

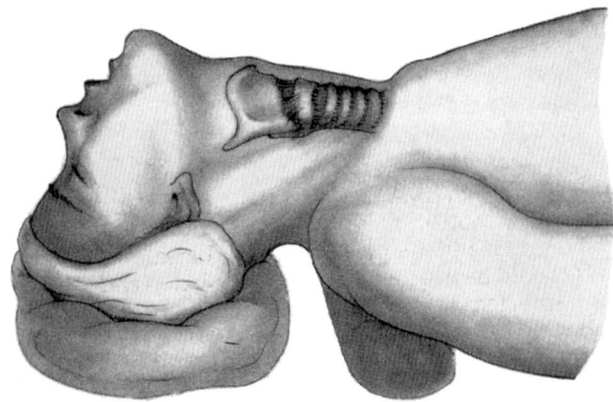

Figure 45.34 Position of the patient for elective tracheostomy.

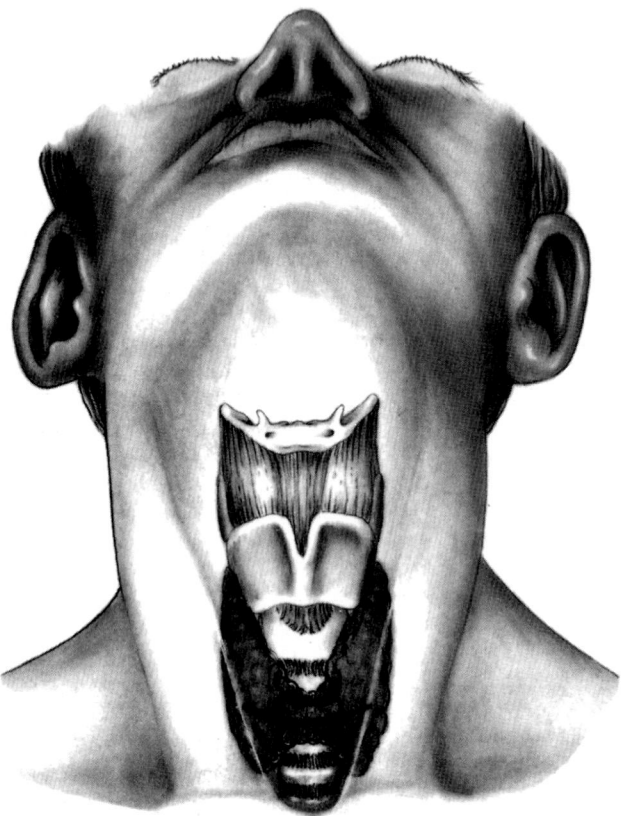

Figure 45.35 Position of a skin incision in an elective tracheostomy.

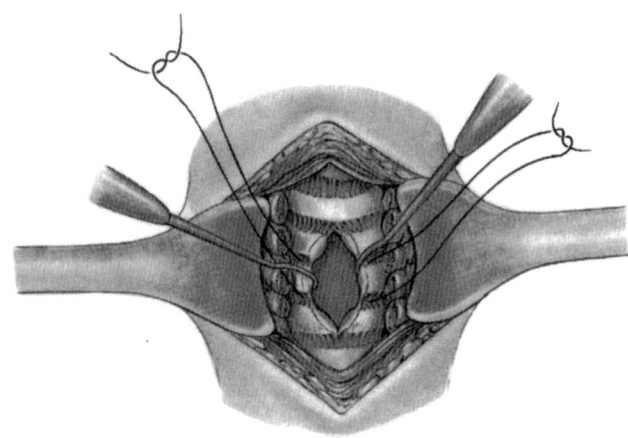

Figure 45.36 Tracheal fenestration in an elective tracheostomy.

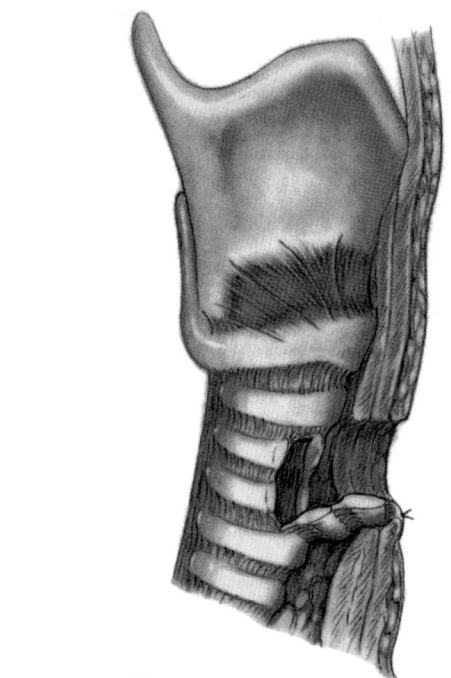

Figure 45.37 Bjork flap.

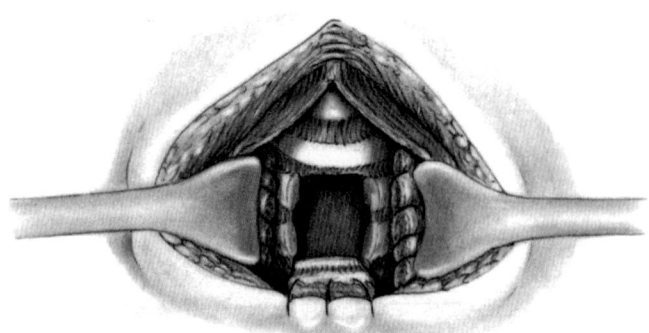

Figure 45.38 Fenestration in a Bjork flap.

surgeons who undertake occasional tracheostomy or when the level of skill and experience of the nursing staff is limited. Performed correctly, it is safe and allows reintroduction of a displaced tube with the minimum of difficulty.

The inferiorly based flap is begun at its apex with an incision on the superior aspects of the second ring and extends down either side through the second and third rings. The tip of the flap should be stitched to the inferior edge of the transverse skin incision using horizontal mattress sutures through the structure of the second ring. These sutures should be generous enough so that they will not cut out. The first tracheal ring should not be violated in any circumstances.

Tracheostomy tubes (Figs 45.39 and 45.40)

These are basically made of two materials: silver or plastic. Both materials have been used to make tubes of various sizes with varying curves, angles, cuffs, inner tubes and speaking valves. A cuffed tube is used initially, which may be changed after 3–4 days to a non-cuffed plastic or silver tube. The pressure within the tube cuff should be carefully monitored and should be low enough so as not to occlude circulation in the mucosal capillaries. When in position, the tube should be retained by double tapes passed around the patient's neck with a reef knot on either side. It is important that the patient's head is flexed when the tapes are tied, otherwise they may become slack when the patient is moved from the position of extension, thereby resulting in a possible displacement of the tube if the patient coughs.

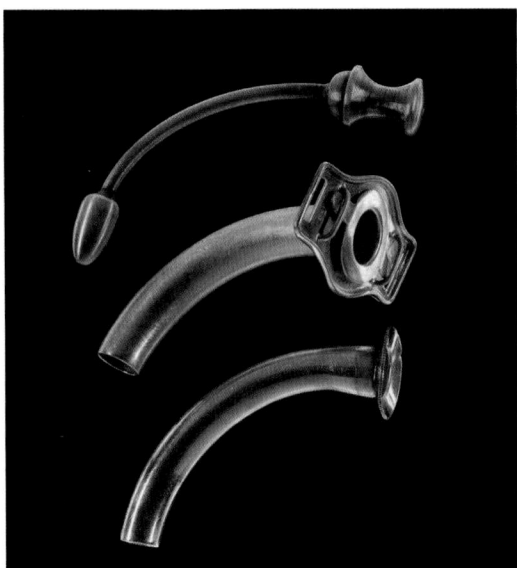

Figure 45.39 Silver tracheostomy tube. From above: introducer, outer tube and inner tube.

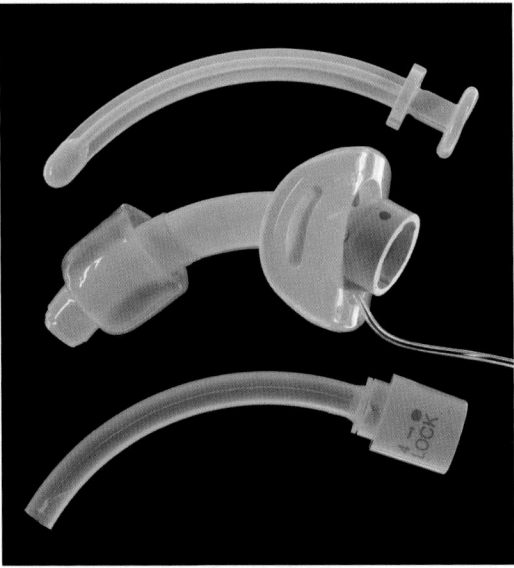

Figure 45.40 Modern plastic tracheostomy tube with introducer, low-pressure cuff and inner canula.

Alternatively, the flanges of the plastic tube may be stitched directly to the underlying neck skin.

All forms of tracheostomy and cricothyroidotomy bypass the upper airway and have the following advantages:

- the anatomical dead space is reduced by approximately 50%;
- the work of breathing is reduced;
- alveolar ventilation is increased;
- the level of sedation needed for patient comfort is decreased and, unlike endotracheal intubation, the patient may be able to talk and eat with a tube in place.

However, there are several disadvantages:

- loss of heat and moisture exchange performed in the upper respiratory tract;
- desiccation of tracheal epithelium, loss of ciliated cells and metaplasia;
- the presence of a foreign body in the trachea stimulates mucous production; where no cilia are present, this mucociliary stream is arrested;
- the increased mucus is more viscid and thick crusts may form and block the tube;
- although many patients with a tracheostomy can feed satisfactorily, there is some splinting of the larynx, which may prevent normal swallowing and lead to aspiration; this aspiration may not be apparent.

Postoperative treatment is designed to counteract these effects and frequent suction and humidification are most important. A trolley must be placed by the bed containing a tracheal dilator, duplicate tubes and introducers, retractors and dressings. Oxygen is at hand and, in the initial period, a nurse must be in constant attendance. Humidification will render the secretions less viscid and a sucker with a catheter attached should be on hand to keep the tracheobronchial tree free from secretions (Summary box 45.10).

Summary box 45.10

Tracheostomy: postoperative management

- Suction – efficient, sterile and as often as required
- Humidification (with or without oxygen)
- A warm, well-ventilated room
- Position of the tube and patient
- Spare tube, introducer, tapes, tracheal dilator
- Change of tube, inner tube, possible speaking valve
- Physiotherapy

Complications of tracheostomy

The intraoperative, early and late postoperative complications of tracheostomy are listed in Table 45.2.

OTHER EMERGENCY AIRWAY PROCEDURES

Fibreoptic endotracheal intubation

In most emergency situations, endotracheal intubation is the most direct and satisfactory method of securing the airway. Nasotracheal intubation in expert hands is also a well-established technique and is particularly useful if the patient has trismus, severe mandibular injuries, cervical spine rigidity or an obstructing mass within the oral cavity. Both forms of intubation can be

CHAPTER 45 | PHARYNX, LARYNX AND NECK

Table 45.2 Tracheostomy: complications

Intraoperative complications	Haemorrhage
	Injury to paratracheal structures, particularly the carotid artery, recurrent laryngeal nerve and oesophagus
	Damage to the trachea
Early postoperative complications	Apnoea caused by a fall in the P_{CO_2}
	Haemorrhage
	Subcutaneous emphysema, pneumomediastinum and pneumothorax
	Accidental extubation, anterior displacement of the tube, obstruction of the tube lumen and tip occlusion against the tracheal wall
	Infection
	Swallowing dysfunction
Late postoperative complications	Difficult decannulation
	Tracheocutaneous fistula
	Tracheo-oesophageal fistula, tracheoinnominate artery fistula with severe haemorrhage
	Tracheal stenosis

facilitated in case of difficulty by passing a fibreoptic endoscope through the centre of an endotracheal tube, hence guiding it into the larynx and trachea under direct vision.

Laryngeal mask airway

The laryngeal mask airway (LMA) is a wide-bore airway with an inflatable cuff at the distal end, which forms a seal in the pharynx around the laryngeal inlet. Provided the laryngotracheal airway is clear, the LMA provides a clear and secure airway. The technique can easily be learnt by non-anaesthetists and secures an airway in most cases. It comes in a range of sizes covering infants to large adults. It is particularly useful in cases of difficult intubation (Fig. 45.41).

Transtracheal ventilation

This technique is simple and effective and allows ventilation for periods in excess of 1 hour providing time to allow for more elective intubation. The cricothyroid membrane is located by palpation of the neck with the index finger, and a 14- or 16-gauge plastic sheathed intravascular needle and a 10-ml syringe containing a few millilitres of lignocaine are introduced in the midline and directed downwards and backwards into the tracheal lumen. The needle is advanced steadily and negative pressure is placed on the syringe until bubbles of air are clearly seen (Fig. 45.42). The tissues of the neck may be infiltrated with the anaesthetic if desired and the tracheal mucosa likewise partly anaesthetised by the introduction of 1–2 ml after gaining the lumen. The needle is removed and the plastic sheath cannula remains in the tracheal lumen and must be carefully held and fixed in place by the operator so that it does not come out of the lumen into the soft tissues of the neck. It is attached by means of a Luer connection to the high-pressure oxygen supply. Ventilation may be undertaken in a controlled manner with a jetting device with the chest being observed for appropriate movements.

If there is severe obstruction of the laryngopharynx by the foreign body or tumour, the exhaled outflow of gases can be aided

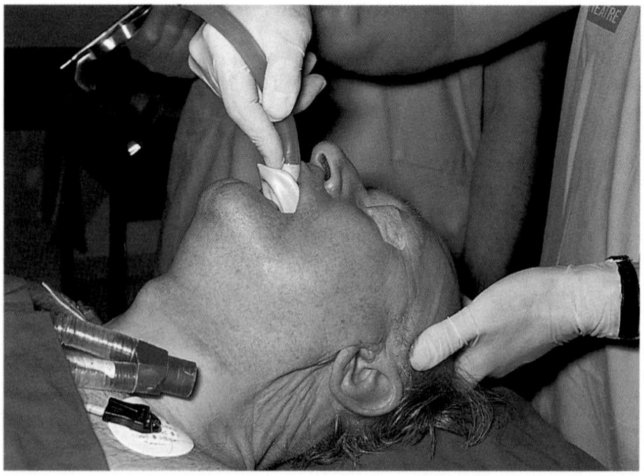

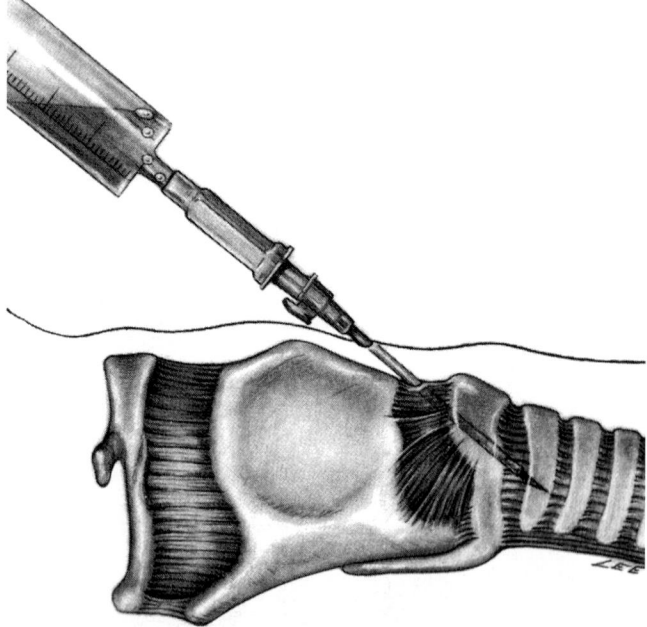

Figure 45.42 Transtracheal needle introduction.

Luer **was a German instrument maker who was working in Paris, France, at the end of the 19th century.**

Figure 45.41 Laryngeal mask airway being inserted.

by the placement of one or two further cannulae as exhalation ports. This procedure gains extremely rapid control of ventilation and requires a minimum of technical expertise. Its only notable complication is surgical emphysema of the neck tissues if the cannula dislodges from the tracheal lumen.

Cricothyroidotomy

Cricothyroidotomy has the advantages of speed and ease requiring little equipment and surgical expertise. However, its use for all but the briefest access to the airway remains controversial and there are conflicting reports with regard to the subsequent incidence of complications, particularly those of subglottic stenosis and long-term voice changes.

The patient's neck is extended and the area between the prominence of the thyroid cartilage and the cricoid cartilage below is palpated with the index finger of the free hand. In the emergency situation, a vertical skin incision is recommended with dissection rapidly carried down to the cricothyroid membrane. A 1-cm transverse incision is made through the membrane immediately above the cricoid cartilage and the scalpel twisted through a right angle to gain access to the airway. If available, artery forceps, dilator or tracheal hook will improve the aperture and insertion of an available tube (Figs 45.43 and 45.44).

Depending on the degree of emergency, it may be necessary for the surgeon to assess the results of the procedure by direct laryngoscopy and the authors recommend that careful consideration should be given to conversion of the cricothyroidotomy to a tracheostomy. Although there is debate about the frequency of subglottic stenosis following this procedure, there is general agreement that it is much increased if any long-term ventilation

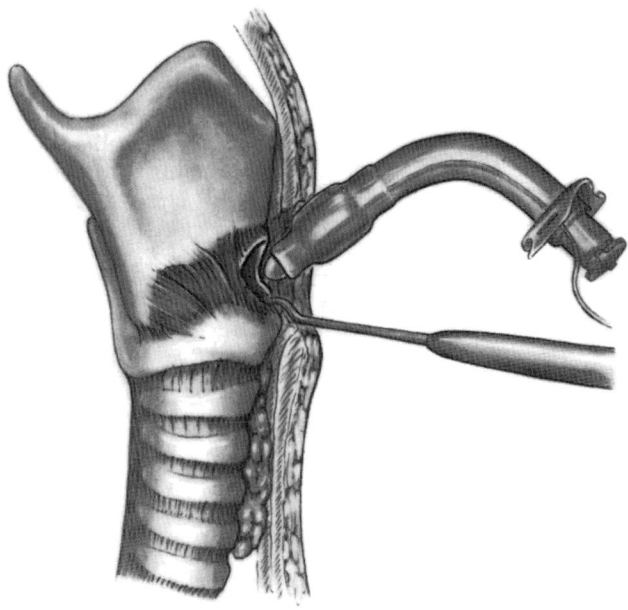

Figure 45.44 Insertion of a tube after cricothyroidotomy.

is undertaken via even a modestly size tracheostomy tube through the cricothyroid membrane.

LARYNGEAL DISEASE CAUSING VOICE DISORDERS

Vocal nodules

These are fibrous thickenings of the vocal folds at the junction of the middle and anterior third (Fig. 45.45), and are the result of vocal abuse; they are known as singers' nodules in adults and screamers' nodules in children. Speech therapy is therefore the preferred treatment and the lesions will resolve spontaneously in most cases. Occasionally, the nodules will need to be surgically removed using modern microlaryngoscopic dissection or laser techniques (Summary box 45.11).

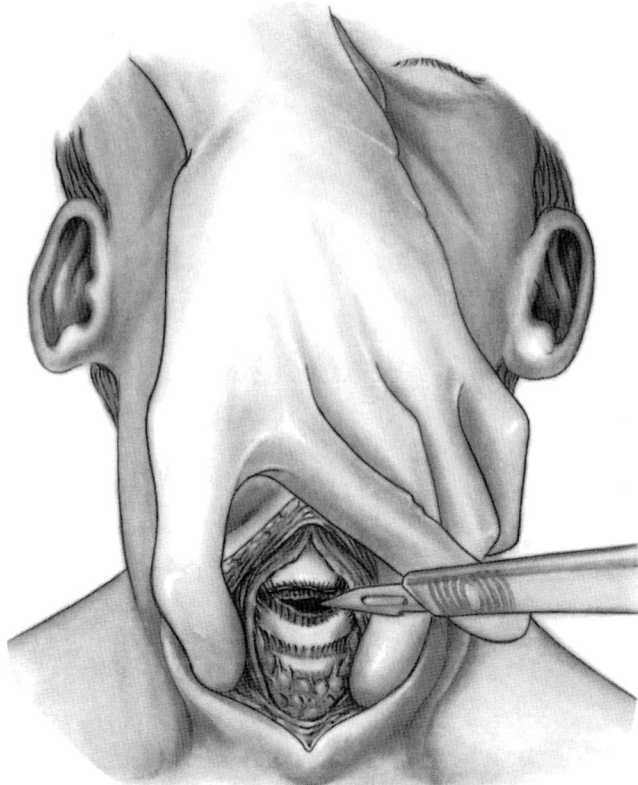

Figure 45.43 Incision in a cricothyroidotomy.

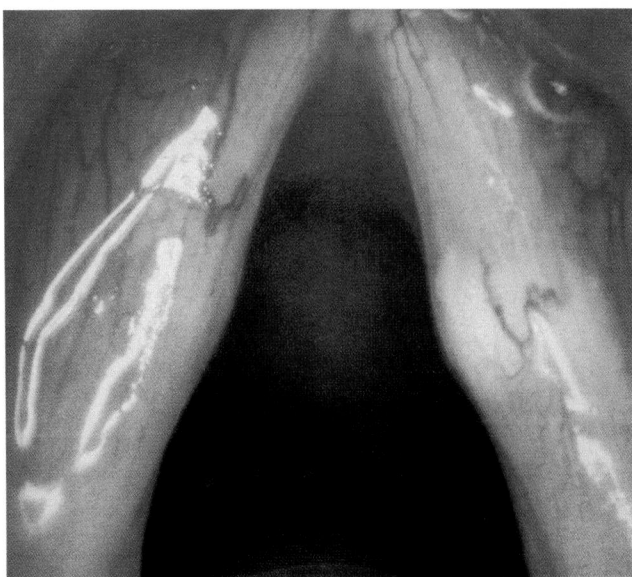

Figure 45.45 Vocal fold nodules.

Summary box 45.11

Causes of hoarseness

- Localised vocal fold pathology, e.g. vocal nodule, polyps or laryngeal papillomatosis, acute or chronic laryngitis
- Vocal fold palsy
- Laryngeal tumours
- Non-specific voice disorders, functional dysphonia

Vocal fold polyps

These are usually unilateral and may be associated with an acute infective episode, cigarette smoking and vocal abuse (Fig. 45.46). Speech therapy is again indicated, but they do usually require removal by microdissection or laser surgery.

Laryngeal papillomata

These occur mainly in children, but can also present in adults. They are most commonly found on the vocal folds, but may spread throughout the larynx and tracheobronchial airway (Fig. 45.47). They are caused by papillomaviruses and need removal by carbon dioxide laser or microsurgery to maintain a reasonable voice and airway. Anti-viral treatment is of doubtful value at present and new therapeutic vaccines are awaited.

Acute laryngitis

This often occurs in association with upper respiratory tract infections in association with a cough and pharyngitis. Usually viral, it may be localised to the larynx and it settles quickly if the voice is rested during the acute inflammation. Steam inhalations are soothing along with mild analgesia, but antibiotics are unnecessary (Summary box 45.12).

Summary box 45.12

Warning

- Hoarseness lasting for 3–4 weeks should always be referred for an ENT opinion, particularly in smokers

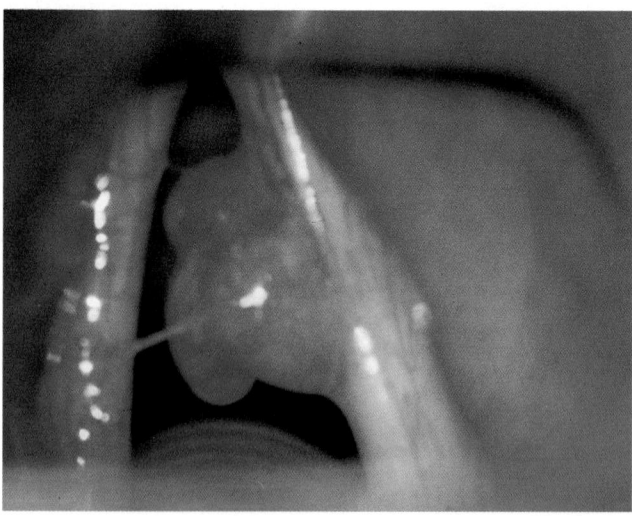

Figure 45.46 A vocal fold polyp.

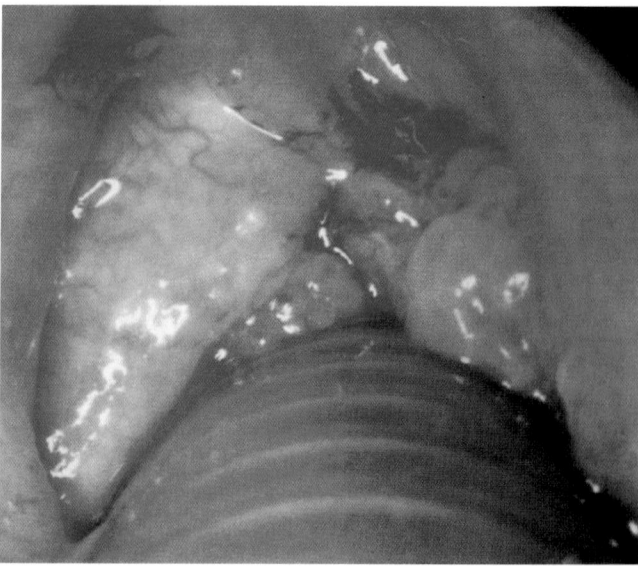

Figure 45.47 Laryngeal papillomata.

Chronic laryngitis

Chronic laryngitis may be specific and can be caused by mycobacteria, syphilis and fungi. Treatment is directed towards the causative organism. Non-specific laryngitis is common, the main predisposing factors being smoking, chronic upper and lower respiratory sepsis and voice abuse. Gastro-oesophageal reflux has been implicated as a factor in laryngitis, vocal fold nodules and polyps, but the evidence is controversial. There is, however, a vogue for treatment with anti-reflux medication and proton pump inhibitors. Diagnosis of chronic laryngitis should not be made unless the larynx has been fully evaluated by a laryngologist.

Vocal fold palsy

This may be unilateral or bilateral (Fig. 45.48), but a unilateral left vocal fold palsy is the most common because of the long intrathoracic course of the left recurrent laryngeal nerve, which arches around the aorta and may be commonly involved in inflammatory and neoplastic conditions involving the left hilum. Lung cancer is the most common cancer in many parts of the world, and should be considered the cause of a left vocal palsy until proved otherwise.

Other malignant lesions can cause a similar effect and may arise in the nasopharynx, thyroid gland or oesophagus. Bilateral vocal fold paralysis is uncommon and tends to occur after thyroid surgery or head injuries (Summary box 45.13).

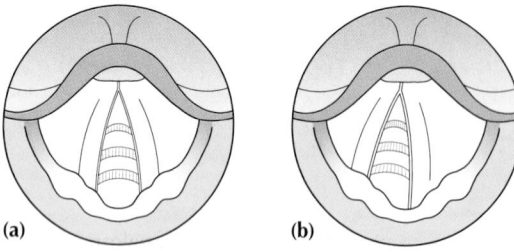

Figure 45.48 Vocal fold positions. (a) Normal; (b) unilateral vocal fold palsy.

Clinical features

Unilateral recurrent laryngeal nerve palsy of sudden onset produces hoarseness, difficulty in swallowing liquids and a weakened cough. These symptoms may be short-lived and the voice may return to normal within a few weeks as the muscles in the opposite vocal fold compensate and move it across the midline to meet the paralysed vocal fold, which usually lies in the paramedian position. Bilateral recurrent laryngeal nerve palsy is an occasional and serious complication of thyroidectomy. Acute dyspnoea occurs as a result of the paramedian position of both vocal folds, which reduce the airway to 2–3 mm and which tend to get sucked together on inspiration. In severe cases, tracheostomy or intubation is necessary immediately, otherwise death occurs from asphyxia.

Investigation of vocal fold paralysis is by a CT scan from skull base to diaphragm. Approximately 20–25% of vocal fold paralysis occurs without known pathology and spontaneous recovery may occur. When compensation does not occur, a unilateral paralysed fold may be medialised by a small external operation on the thyroid cartilage (thyroplasty).

In bilateral vocal fold palsy, surgery may be carried out to remove a small portion of the posterior aspect of one vocal fold or a portion of one arytenoid cartilage. These procedures are most easily performed endoscopically with a carbon dioxide laser. They increase the size of the posterior glottic airway, allowing the patient to be decannulated or even the avoidance of an initial tracheostomy.

TUMOURS OF THE LARYNX

Benign tumours of the larynx are extremely rare. Squamous carcinoma is the most common malignant tumour, being responsible for more than 90% of tumours within the larynx. It is the most common head and neck cancer and previously almost always occurred in elderly male smokers. However, over the past two decades, the incidence among women is rising as a consequence of increased smoking habits. The incidence of laryngeal cancer in the three compartments, supraglottis, glottis and subglottis, varies around the world. The glottis is generally the most common site for cancer in patients in the UK, followed by the supraglottis (Fig. 45.49).

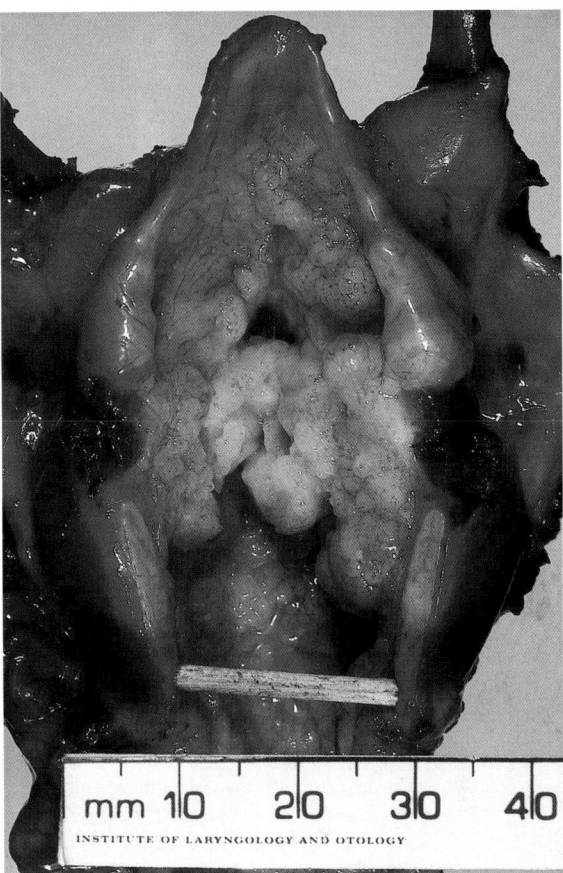

Figure 45.49 A total laryngectomy specimen with transglottic tumour.

Clinical features

Patients almost always present with hoarseness. If an early diagnosis can be made, i.e. confined to one vocal fold, treatment with radiotherapy or carbon dioxide laser excision is associated with a 5-year disease-free survival of approximately 90%. This rate drops dramatically once the lymphatically rich supraglottis or subglottis is involved because of spread to neck nodes. Tumour spread to just one neck gland halves the overall prognosis for the patient.

Investigations

Direct laryngoscopy, preferably a microlaryngoscopy, together with Hopkins' rod examination, allows precise determination of the extent of the tumour and biopsy confirms the histology. CT and MRI give further details of the extent of larger tumours, demonstrating spread outside the larynx and suspicious nodal involvement within the neck, which may not be obvious clinically. The tumour–node–metastasis (TNM) classification of laryngeal cancer is given in Table 45.3.

Treatment

Early supraglottic and glottic tumours, stages 1 and 2, are optimally treated with megavoltage radiotherapy. Five-year cure rates for stages 1 and 2 are approximately 90 and 70%, respectively, with excellent voice preservation. If radiotherapy is not feasible, tumours may be excised by means of endoscopic laser

Table 45.3 Tumour–node–metastasis (TNM) classification of laryngeal carcinoma

T – primary tumour

- TX   Primary tumour cannot be assessed
- T0   No evidence of primary tumour
- Tis   Carcinoma *in situ*
- Supraglottis
  - T1   Tumour limited to one subsite of supraglottis, with normal vocal fold mobility
  - T2   Tumour invades more than one subsite of supraglottis, with normal vocal fold mobility
  - T3   Tumour limited to larynx with vocal fold fixation and/or invades post-cricoid area, medial wall of piriform sinus or pre-epiglottic tissues
  - T4   Tumour invades through cartilage and/or extends to other tissues beyond the larynx, e.g. to oropharynx, soft tissues of neck
- Glottis
  - T1   Tumour limited to vocal fold(s) (may involve anterior or posterior commissures) with normal mobility
  - T1a   Tumour limited to one vocal fold
  - T1b   Tumour involves both vocal folds
  - T2   Tumour extends to supraglottis and/or subglottis, and/or with impaired vocal fold mobility
  - T3   Tumour limited to the larynx with vocal fold fixation
  - T4   Tumour invades through thyroid cartilage and/or extends to other tissues beyond the larynx, e.g. to oropharynx, soft tissues of the neck
- Subglottis
  - T1   Tumour limited to the subglottis
  - T2   Tumour extends to vocal fold(s) with normal or impaired mobility
  - T3   Tumour limited to the larynx with vocal fixation
  - T4   Tumour invades through thyroid cartilage and/or extends to other tissues beyond the larynx, e.g. to oropharynx, soft tissues of the neck

N – regional lymph nodes

- N0   No regional lymph node metastases
- N1   Metastasis in a single ipsilateral lymph node 3 cm or less in greatest diameter
- N2   Metastasis in a single ipsilateral lymph node more than 3 cm or in multiple ipsilateral nodes or in bilateral or contralateral nodes

M – distant metastasis

Stage grouping

Stage 0	Tis	N0	M0
Stage I	T1	N0	M0
Stage II	T2	N0	M0
Stage III	T1	N1	M0
	T2	N1	M0
	T3	N0, N1	M0
Stage IV	T4	N0, N1	M0
	Any T	N2, N3	M0
	Any T	Any N	M1

surgery or open partial laryngeal surgery. The latter may be in the form of a laryngofissure when the thyroid cartilage is opened anteriorly in the midline or, in the case of more extensive unilateral glottic and supraglottic growths, a vertical hemilaryngectomy (Fig. 45.50). This leaves a defect on one side of the larynx, which is usually reconstructed with adjacent strap muscles. With early bilateral supraglottic tumours, a horizontal laryngectomy may be undertaken, excising the supraglottic growth. The remaining glottis and supraglottis are then stitched to the tongue base.

Advanced laryngeal disease

Once the squamous carcinoma has caused fixation of the vocal fold or has infiltrated outside the larynx into adjacent structures such as the thyroid gland and strap muscles, some form of subtotal or total laryngectomy is required (Figs 45.51–45.53).

After the larynx has been removed, the remaining trachea is brought out onto the lower neck as a permanent tracheal stoma and the hypopharynx, which is opened at the time of the operation, is closed to restore continuity for swallowing. Thus the upper aero- and digestive tracts are permanently disconnected. Part or all of the thyroid gland and associated parathyroid glands may also be removed, depending on the extent of the disease.

Vocal rehabilitation

The loss of the larynx as a generator of sound does not prevent patients speaking as long as an alternative source of vibration can be created in the pharynx. This can be achieved in one of three ways:

1 An external device when applied to the soft tissues of the neck produces sound, which is turned into speech by the vocal tract comprising the tongue, pharynx, oral cavity, lips, teeth and nasal sinuses. These devices are usually battery powered.
2 Some patients may learn to swallow air into the pharynx and upper oesophagus. On regurgitating the air, a segment of the pharyngo-oesophageal mucosa vibrates to produce sound, which is modified by the vocal tract into speech (Fig. 45.54).
3 A small one-way valve may be inserted through the back wall of the tracheal stoma into the pharynx (Fig. 45.55). This allows air from the trachea to pass into the pharynx, but does not allow food and liquid to pass into the airway. These valves must not be confused with tracheostomy tubes. Like all foreign bodies, the speaking valves are associated with minor complications, such as the formation of granulations, bleeding or leakage of pharyngeal contents.

THE NECK

Lump in the neck

The correct diagnosis of a lump in the neck can often be made with a careful history and examination. The clinical signs of size, site, shape, consistency, fixation to skin or deep structures, pulsation, compressibility, transillumination or the presence of a bruit still remain as important as ever (Summary box 45.14).

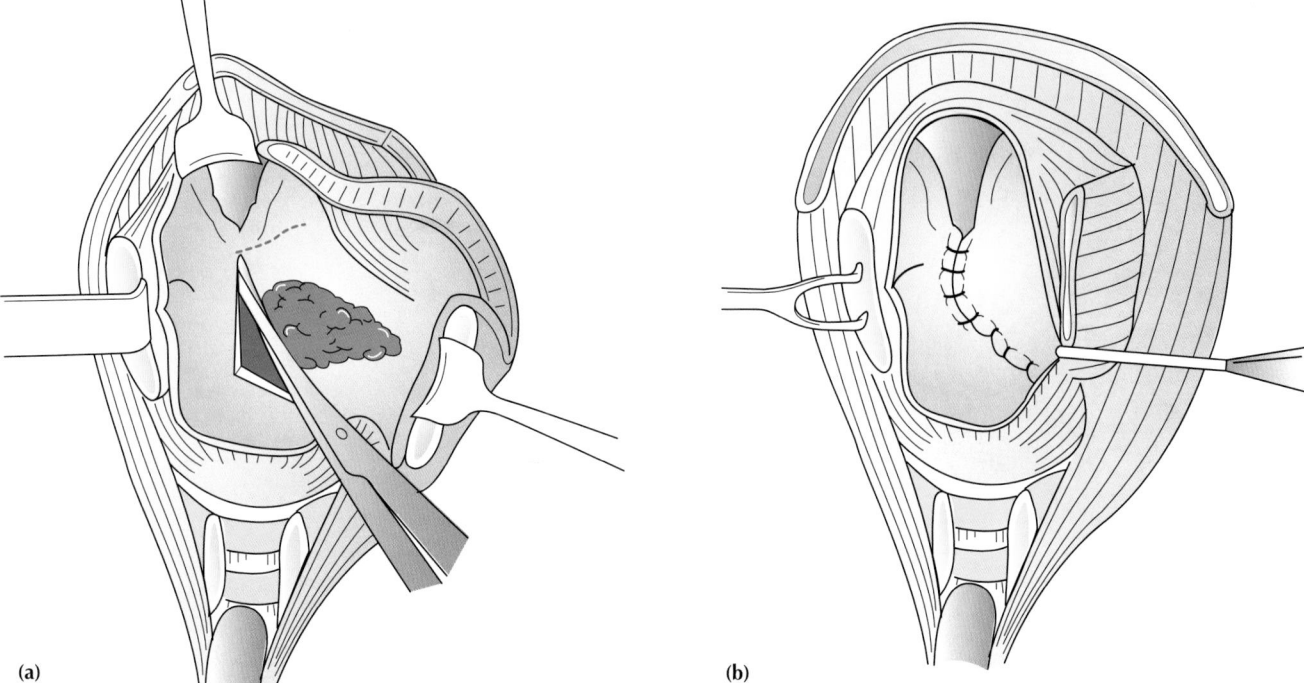

Figure 45.50 (a and b) Resection of tumour with left vertical partial hemilaryngectomy.

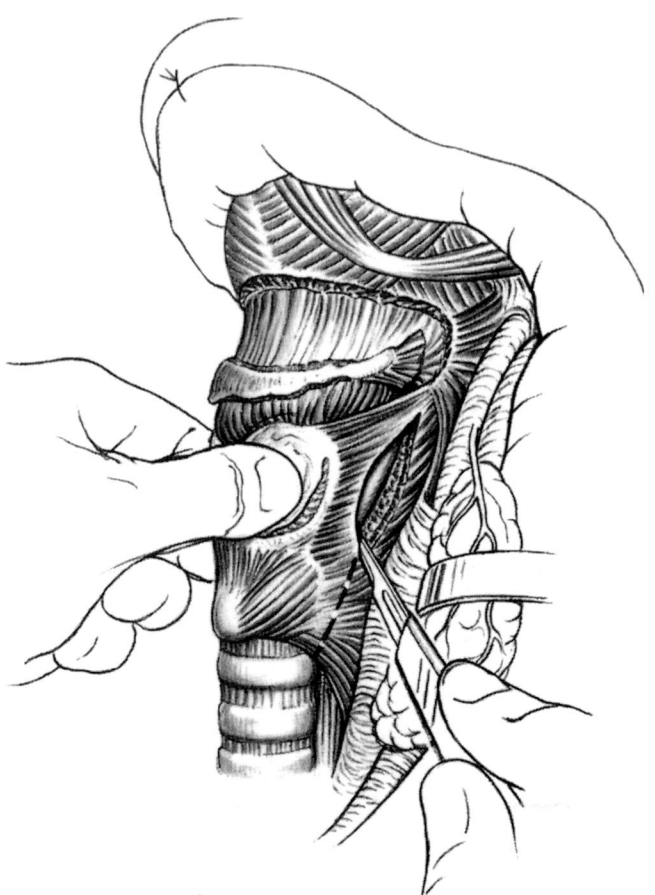

Figure 45.51 The stages of a total laryngectomy. Freeing of the specimen by division of the inferior constrictor muscle, after division of the strap muscles.

> **Summary box 45.14**
>
> **Diagnosis of a lump in the neck**
>
> *History*
>
> *Physical signs*
> - Size
> - Site
> - Shape
> - Surface
> - Consistency
> - Fixation: deep/superficial
> - Pulsatility
> - Compressibility
> - Transillumination
> - Bruit

Branchial cyst

A branchial cyst probably develops from the vestigial remnants of the second branchial cleft, is usually lined by squamous epithelium, and contains thick, turbid fluid full of cholesterol crystals. The cyst usually presents in the upper neck in early or middle adulthood and is found at the junction of the upper third and middle third of the sternomastoid muscle at its anterior border. It is a fluctuant swelling that may transilluminate and is often soft in its early stages so that it may be difficult to palpate.

If the cyst becomes infected it becomes erythematous and tender and, on occasions, it may be difficult to differentiate from a tuberculous abscess. Ultrasound and fine-needle aspiration both aid diagnosis and treatment is by complete excision, which is best undertaken when the lesion is quiescent. Although the anterior aspect of the cyst is easy to dissect, it may pass backwards and upwards through the bifurcation of the common carotid

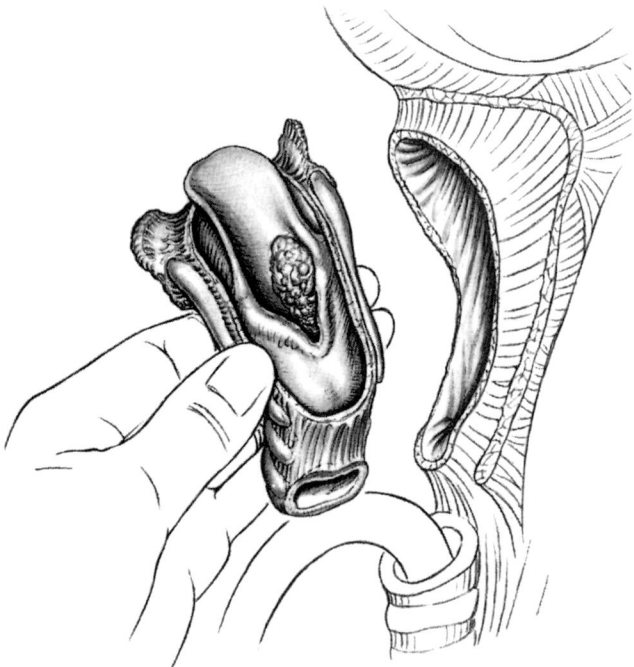

Figure 45.52 Removal of a laryngeal specimen.

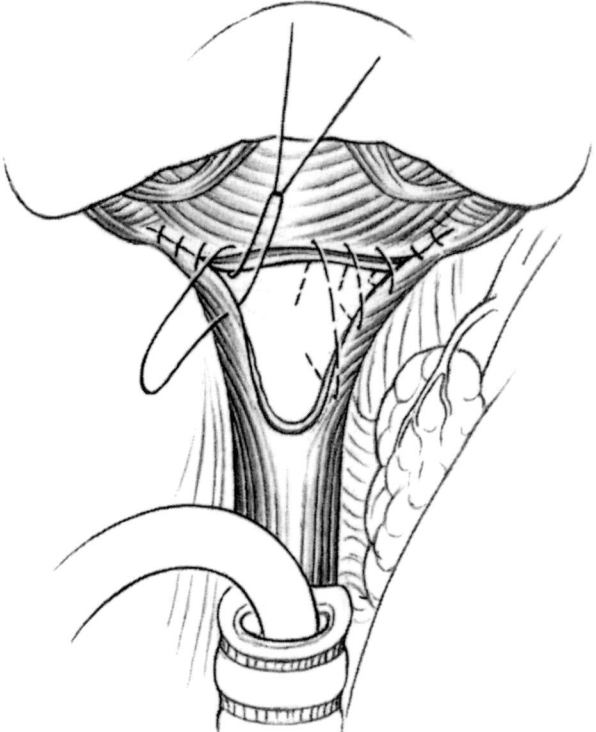

Figure 45.53 Transverse closure of the pharynx with an endo-tracheal tube in the end tracheostome.

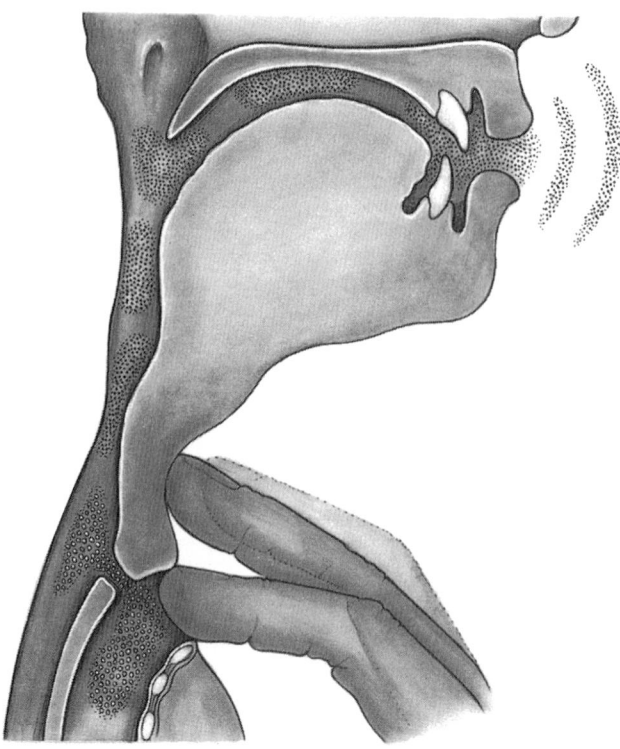

Figure 45.54 Production of oesophageal speech.

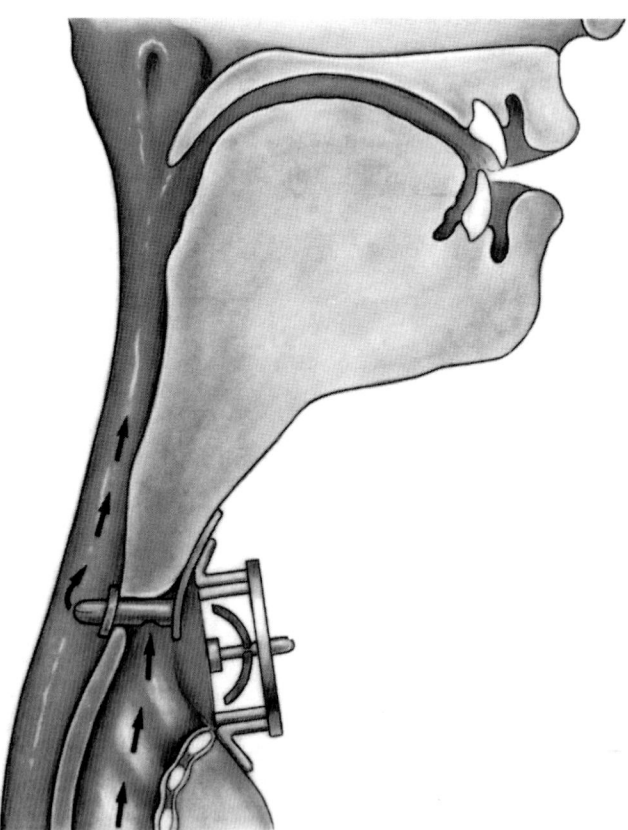

Figure 45.55 A Blom–Singer valve with a tracheo-oesophageal fistula and an outer stoma valve.

artery as far as the pharyngeal constrictors. It passes superficial to the hypoglossal and glossopharyngeal nerves, but deep to the posterior belly of the digastric. These structures and the spinal accessory nerve must be positively identified to avoid damage.

Branchial fistula (Fig. 45.56)

A branchial fistula may be unilateral or bilateral and is thought to represent a persistent second branchial cleft. The external orifice is nearly always situated in the lower third of the neck near the anterior border of the sternocleidomastoid, whilst the internal orifice is located on the anterior aspect of the posterior faucial pillar just behind the tonsil. However, the internal aspect of the tract may end blindly at or close to the lateral pharyngeal wall, constituting a sinus rather than a fistula. The tract is lined by ciliated columnar epithelium and, as such, there may be a small amount of recurrent mucous or mucopurulent discharge onto the neck. The tract follows the same path as a branchial cyst and requires complete excision, often by more than one transverse incision in the neck.

Cystic hygroma (Fig. 45.57)

Cystic hygroma usually present in the neonate or in early infancy, and occasionally may present at birth and be so large as to obstruct labour. The cysts are filled with clear lymph and lined by a single layer of epithelium with a mosaic appearance. Swelling usually occurs in the neck and may involve the parotid, submandibular, tongue and floor of mouth areas. The swelling may be bilateral and is soft and partially compressible, visibly increasing in size when the child coughs or cries. The characteristic that distinguishes it from all other neck swellings is that it is brilliantly translucent. The cheek, axilla, groin and mediastinum are other less frequent sites for a cystic hygroma.

The behaviour of cystic hygromas during infancy is unpredictable. Sometimes the cyst expands rapidly and occasionally respiratory difficulty ensues, requiring immediate aspiration and even occasionally a tracheostomy. The cyst may become infected.

Definitive treatment is complete excision of the cyst at an early stage. Injection of a sclerosing agent, for example picibanil (OK-432), may reduce the size of the cyst; however, they are commonly multicystic and if the injection is extracystic subsequent surgery may be more difficult.

Thyroglossal duct cysts

Embryology

The thyroid gland descends early in fetal life from the base of the tongue towards its position in the lower neck with the isthmus

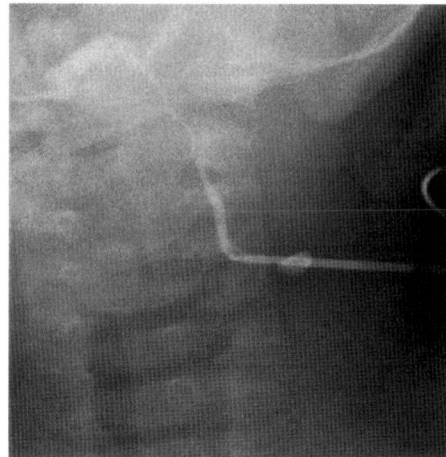

(a)

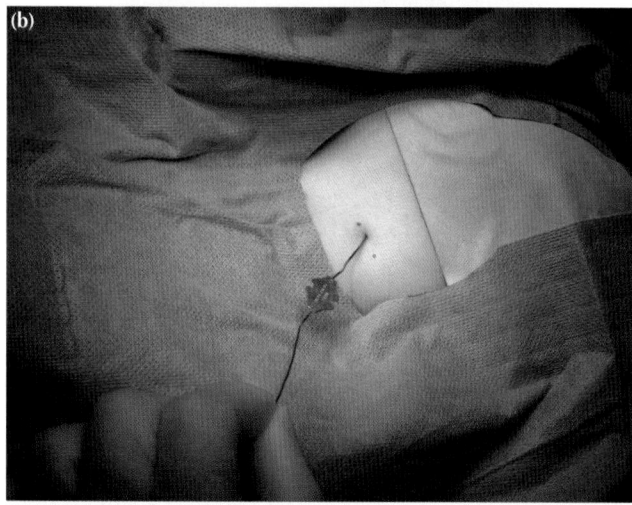

(b)

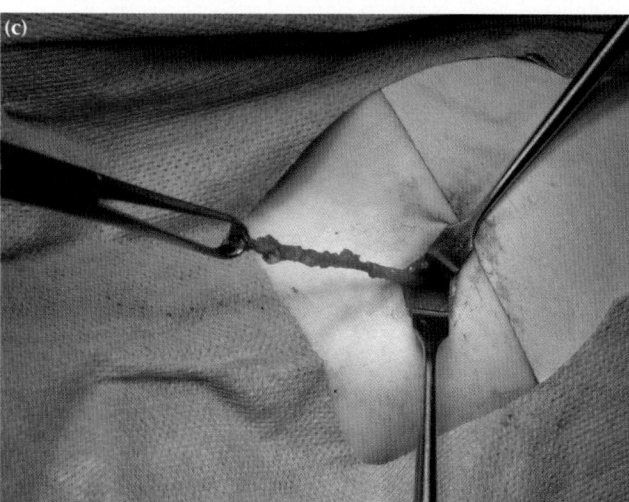

(c)

Figure 45.56 (a) Plain radiograph with radio-opaque dye in the fistula tract. (b) Probing of the fistula tract. (c) Excision of the fistula tract.

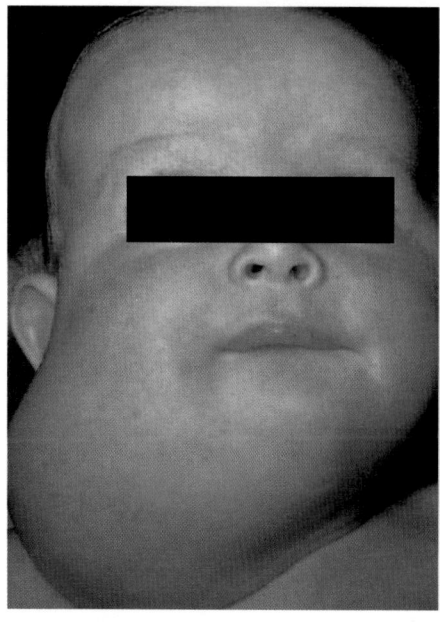

Figure 45.57 Cystic hygroma.

lying over the second and third tracheal rings. At the time of its descent, the hyoid bone has not been formed and the track of the descent of the thyroid gland is variable, passing in front, through or behind the eventual position of the hyoid body. Thyroglossal duct cysts represent a persistence of this track and may therefore be found anywhere in or adjacent to the midline from the tongue base to the thyroid isthmus. Rarely, a thyroglossal cyst may contain the only functioning thyroid tissue in the body.

Clinical features

The cysts almost always arise in the midline but, when they are adjacent to the thyroid cartilage, they may lie slightly to one side of the midline. Classically, the cyst moves upwards on swallowing and with tongue protrusion, but this can also occur with other midline cysts such as dermoid cysts, as it merely indicates attachment to the hyoid bone.

Thyroglossal cysts may become infected and rupture onto the skin of the neck presenting as a discharging sinus. Although they often occur in children, they may also present in adults, even as late as the sixth or seventh decade of life (Fig. 45.58).

Treatment

Treatment must include excision of the whole thyroglossal tract, which involves removal of the body of the hyoid bone and the suprahyoid tract through the tongue base to the vallecula at the site of the primitive foramen caecum, together with a core of

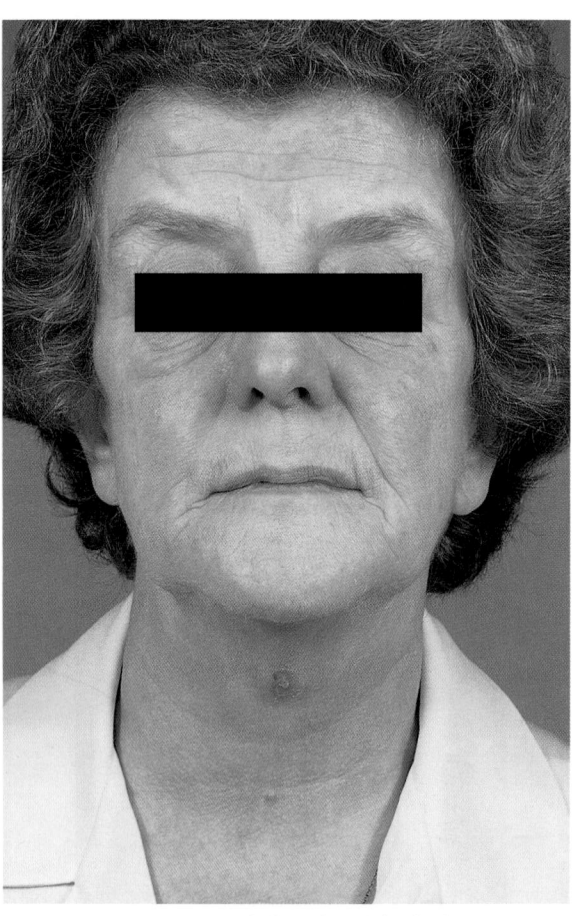

Figure 45.58 A patient with thyroglossal fistula from a cyst in the midline of the neck.

tissue on either side. This operation is known as Sistrunk's operation and prevents recurrence, most notably from small side branches of the thyroglossal tract.

TRAUMA TO THE NECK

Wounds above the hyoid bone

The cavity of the mouth or pharynx may have been entered and the epiglottis may be divided via the pre-epiglottic space. These wounds require repair with absorbable sutures on a formal basis under a general anaesthetic. If there is any degree of associated oedema or bleeding, particularly in relation to the tongue base or laryngeal inlet, it is advisable to perform a tracheostomy to avoid any subsequent respiratory distress.

Wounds of the thyroid and cricoid cartilage

Blunt crushing injuries or severe laceration injuries to the laryngeal skeleton can cause marked haematoma formation and rapid loss of the airway. There may be significant disruption of the laryngeal skeleton. These patients should not have an endotracheal intubation for any length of time, even if this is the initial emergency way of protecting the airway. The larynx is a delicate three-tiered sphincter and the presence of a foreign body in its lumen after severe disruption gives rise to major fibrosis and loss of laryngeal function. These injuries are frequently an absolute indication for a low tracheostomy, following which the larynx can be carefully explored, damaged cartilages repositioned and sutured, and the paraglottic space drained.

An indwelling stent of soft sponge shaped to fit the laryngeal lumen and held by a nylon retaining suture through the neck may be left in place for approximately 5 days. This stent can be removed endoscopically after cutting the retaining suture and, as the laryngeal damage heals, the patient may then be decannulated.

Division of the trachea

Wounds of the trachea are rare. They should all be formally explored and, in order to obtain adequate exposure, it is usually necessary to divide and ligate the thyroid isthmus. A small tracheostomy below the wound followed by repair of the trachea with a limited number of submucosal sutures is appropriate. In self-inflicted wounds, the recurrent laryngeal nerves, which lie protected in the tracheo-oesophageal grooves, are rarely injured. Primary repair is rarely possible but may be undertaken at the time of formal exploration of a major neck wound.

Neurovascular injury

Penetrating wounds of the neck may involve the common carotid or the external or internal carotid arteries. Major haemorrhagic shock may occur. Venous air embolism may occur as a result of damage to one of the major veins, most commonly the internal jugular. Compression, resuscitation and exploration under general anaesthetic, with control of vessels above and below the injury, and primary repair should be undertaken. All cervical nerves are vulnerable to injury, particularly the vagus and recurrent laryngeal nerves and cervical sympathetic chain.

Walter Ellis Sistrunk, Jr., **1880–1933**, Professor of Clinical Surgery, Baylor University College of Medicine, Dallas, TX, USA.

Thoracic duct injury

Wounds to the thoracic duct are rare and most often occur in association with dissection of lymph nodes in the left supraclavicular fossa. When damage to the duct is not recognised at the time of operation, chyle may subsequently leak from the wound in amounts up to $2\,l\,day^{-1}$ with profound effects on nutrition.

Treatment

Should the damage be recognised during an operation, the proximal end of the duct must be ligated. Ligation of the duct is not harmful because there are a number of anastomotic channels between the lymphatic and venous system in the lower neck. If undetected, chyle usually starts to discharge from the neck wound within 24 hours of the operation. On occasion, firm pressure by a pad to the lower neck may stop the leakage, but frequently this is unsuccessful and the wound should be re-explored and the damaged duct ligated.

Inflammatory conditions of the neck

Ludwig's angina

Ludwig described a clinical entity characterised by a brawny swelling of the submandibular region combined with inflammatory oedema of the mouth. It is these combined cervical and intraoral signs that constitute the characteristic feature of the lesion, as well as the accompanying putrid halitosis.

The infection is often caused by a virulent streptococcal infection associated with anaerobic organisms and sometimes with other lesions of the floor of the mouth such as carcinoma. The infection encompasses both sides of the mylohyoid muscle causing oedema and inflammation such that the tongue may be displaced upwards and backwards, giving rise to dysphagia and subsequently to painful obstruction of the airway. Unless treated, cellulitis may extend beneath the deep fascial layers of the neck to involve the larynx, causing glottic oedema and airway compromise.

Antibiotic therapy should be instituted as soon as possible using intravenous broad-spectrum antibiotics, such as amoxycillin or cefuroxime, combined with metronidazole to combat the anaerobes.

In advanced cases when the swelling does not subside rapidly with such treatment, a curved submental incision may be used to drain both submandibular triangles. The mylohyoid muscle may be incised to decompress the floor of the mouth and corrugated drains placed in the wound, which is then lightly sutured. This operation may be conducted under local anaesthetic. Rarely, a tracheostomy may be necessary.

Cervical lymphadenitis

Cervical lymphadenitis is common due to infection or inflammation in the oral and nasal cavities, pharynx, larynx, ear, scalp and face.

Acute lymphadenitis

The affected lymph nodes are enlarged and tender, and there may be varying degrees of general constitutional disturbance such as pyrexia, anorexia and general malaise. The treatment in the first instance is directed to the primary focus of infection, for example tonsillitis or a dental abscess.

Chronic lymphadenitis

Chronic, painless lymphadenopathy may be caused by tuberculosis in young children or adults, or be secondary to malignant disease, most commonly from a squamous carcinoma in older individuals. Lymphoma and/or HIV infection may also present in the cervical nodes (Summary box 45.15).

> **Summary box 45.15**
>
> **Causes of cervical lymphadenopathy**
>
> **Inflammatory**
> - Reactive hyperplasia
>
> **Infective**
> - Viral
>   For example, infectious mononucleosis, HIV
> - Bacterial
>   *Streptococcus, Staphylococcus*
>   Actinomycosis
>   Tuberculosis
>   Brucellosis
> - Protozoan
>   Toxoplasmosis
>
> **Neoplastic**
> - Malignant
>   Primary, e.g. lymphoma
>   Secondary, e.g. squamous cell carcinoma
>   Known primary
>   Occult primary

Tuberculous adenitis

The condition most commonly affects children or young adults, but can occur at any age. The deep upper cervical nodes are most commonly affected, but there may be a widespread cervical lymphadenitis with many matting together. In most cases, the tubercular bacilli gain entrance through the tonsil of the corresponding side as the lymphadenopathy. Both bovine and human tuberculosis may be responsible. In approximately 80% of patients, the tuberculous process is limited to the clinically affected group of lymph nodes, but a primary focus in the lungs must always be suspected.

As renal and pulmonary tuberculosis occasionally coexist, the urine should be examined carefully. Rarely, the patient may develop a natural resistance to the infection and the nodes may be detected at a later date as evidenced by calcification on radiography. This can also be seen after appropriate general treatment of tuberculosis adenitis. If treatment is not instituted, the caseated node may liquefy and break down with the formation of a cold abscess in the neck. The pus is initially confined by the deep cervical fascia, but after weeks or months, this may become eroded at one point and the pus flows through the small opening into the space beneath the superficial fascia. The process has now reached the well-known stage of a 'collar-stud' abscess. The superficial abscess enlarges steadily and, unless suitably treated, a discharging sinus results.

Treatment

The patient should be treated by appropriate chemotherapy, dependent on the sensitivities derived from the abscess contents.

Wilhelm Friedrich von Ludwig, 1790–1865, Professor of Surgery and Midwifery, Tubingen, Germany.

If an abscess fails to resolve despite appropriate chemotherapy and general measures, occasionally excision of the abscess and its surrounding fibrous capsule is necessary, together with the relevant lymph nodes. If there is active tuberculosis of another system, for example pulmonary tuberculosis, then removal of tuberculous lymph nodes in the neck is inappropriate. The nodes are commonly related to the internal jugular vein, common carotid and vagus nerve, and are usually associated with significant fibrosis making surgery difficult. A portion of the internal jugular vein may require excision, taking considerable care to avoid damage to the vagus or the cervical sympathetic trunk. To facilitate access, the sternocleidomastoid muscle should be divided, particularly if the disease is adjacent to the spinal accessory nerve or the hypoglossal nerve. The resected nodes should be sent for both histology and microbiology.

PRIMARY TUMOURS OF THE NECK

Neurogenic tumours

Chemodectoma (carotid body tumour)

This is a rare tumour that has a higher incidence in areas where people live at high altitudes because of chronic hypoxia leading to carotid body hyperplasia. The tumours most commonly present in the fifth decade and approximately 10% of patients have a family history. There is an association with phaeochromocytoma. The tumours arise from the chemoreceptor cells on the medial side of the carotid bulb and, at this point, the tumour is adherent to the carotid wall. The cells of the chemodectoma are not hormonally active and the tumours are usually benign with only a small number of cases producing proven metastases (Fig. 45.59).

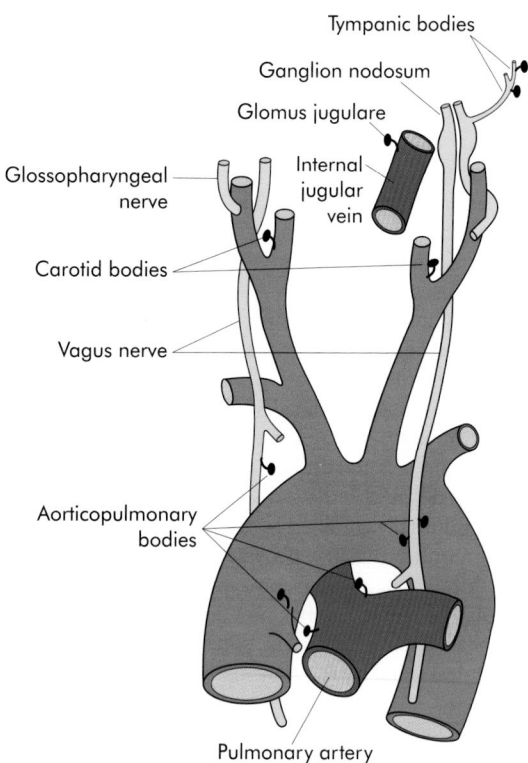

Tympanic bodies

Ganglion nodosum

Glomus jugulare

Glossopharyngeal nerve

Internal jugular vein

Carotid bodies

Vagus nerve

Aorticopulmonary bodies

Pulmonary artery

Figure 45.59 Sites for chemodectomas.

Clinical features

There is often a long history of a slowly enlarging, painless lump at the carotid bifurcation. About one-third of patients present with a pharyngeal mass that pushes the tonsil medially and anteriorly. The mass is firm, rubbery, pulsatile, mobile from side to side but not up and down, and can sometimes be emptied by firm pressure, after which it slowly refills in a pulsatile manner. A bruit may also be present. Swellings in the parapharyngeal space, which often displace the tonsil medially, should not be biopsied from within the mouth.

Investigations

When a chemodectoma is suspected, a carotid angiogram can be carried out to demonstrate the carotid bifurcation, which is usually splayed, and a blush, which outlines the tumour vessels. MRI scanning also provides excellent detail in most cases. This tumour must not be biopsied and fine-needle aspiration is also contraindicated.

Treatment

Because these tumours rarely metastasise and their overall rate of growth is slow, the need for surgical removal must be considered carefully as complications of surgery are potentially serious. The operation is best avoided in elderly patients. Radiotherapy has no effect. In some cases it may be possible to dissect the tumour away from the carotid bifurcation but, at times, when the tumour is large, it may not be separable from the vessels and resection will be necessary, such that all appropriate facilities should be available to establish a bypass while a vein autograph is inserted to restore arterial continuity in the carotid system.

Vagal body tumours

Vagal paragangliomas arise from nests of paraganglionic tissue of the vagus nerve just below the base of the skull near the jugular foramen. They may also be found at various sites along the nerve down to the level of the carotid artery bifurcation.

They also present as slowly growing and painless masses in the anterolateral aspect of the neck, and may also have a long history, commonly of 2–3 years, before diagnosis. They may spread into the cranial cavity. Diagnosis is confirmed by CT and MRI scanning and additional arteriography if necessary. Treatment is surgical excision.

Peripheral nerve tumours

Schwannomas are solitary and encapsulated tumours attached to or surrounded by nerve, although paralysis of the associated nerve is unusual. The vagus nerve is the most common site. Neurofibromas also arise from the Schwann cell and may be part of von Recklinghausen's syndrome of multiple neurofibromatosis. Multiple neurofibromatosis is an autosomal dominant, hereditary disease and the neurofibromata may be present at birth and often multiply.

Diagnosis requires CT or MRI scanning to differentiate them from other parapharyngeal tumours but, on occasions, the diagnosis must wait until excision.

Friedrich Theodor Schwann, 1810–1882, Professor of Anatomy and Physiology, successively at Louvain (1839–1848), and Liege (1848–1880), Belgium, described the neurilemma in 1839.
Friedrich Daniel von Recklinghausen, 1833–1910, Professor of Pathology, Strasbourg, France, described generalised neurofibromatosis in 1882.

Secondary carcinoma

Metastatic spread of squamous carcinoma to the cervical lymph nodes is a common occurrence from head and neck primary cancers. The nasopharynx, tonsil, tongue, pyriform fossa and supraglottic larynx must be carefully examined by panendoscopy for the primary growth before considering biopsy or any surgery on the neck. Investigation is further assisted by ultrasound and fine needle aspirate of the neck node.

Management

The management of malignant cervical lymph nodes depends on the overall treatment regime.

- If surgery is being used to treat the primary disease and the cervical nodes are palpable and > 3 cm, they may be excised with the primary lesion.
- If radiotherapy is used initially, as is always the case in carcinoma of the nasopharynx, then radiotherapy may also be given to the neck nodes, whatever their stage. In the case of the tongue, pharynx or larynx, however, if the node exceeds 3 cm in diameter, then surgery may be necessary for the neck nodes, even if the primary tumour is treated by chemoradiation.
- If radiotherapy is used initially with resolution of the primary tumour, but there is subsequent residual or recurrent nodal disease, then this situation will require cervical lymph node dissection.

Type of neck dissection

Classical radical neck dissection (Crile)

The classic operation involves resection of the cervical lymphatics and lymph nodes and those structures closely associated: the internal jugular vein, the accessory nerve, the submandibular gland and the sternocleidomastoid muscle. These structures are all removed *en bloc* and in continuity with the primary disease if possible. The main disability that follows the operation is weakness and drooping of the shoulder due to paralysis of the trapezius muscle as a consequence of excision of the accessory nerve.

Modified radical neck dissection

In selected cases, one or more of the three following structures are preserved: the accessory nerve, the sternocleidomastoid

> George Washington Crile, **1864–1943, Professor of Surgery, The Western Reserve University, and one of the Founders of the Cleveland Clinic, Cleveland, OH, USA.**

muscle or the internal jugular vein. Otherwise, all major lymph node groups and lymphatics are excised. Whichever structures are preserved should be clearly noted.

Selective neck dissection

In this type of dissection, one or more of the major lymph node groups is preserved along with the sternocleidomastoid muscle, accessory nerve and internal jugular vein. In these circumstances, the exact groups of nodes excised must be documented.

SUMMARY

The anatomical and physiological performance of the pharyngo-larynx is involved in the important mechanisms of breathing, coughing, voice production and swallowing. A variety of congenital, traumatic, infectious and neoplastic conditions disturb these functions, giving rise to the common symptoms of pain, swelling, hoarseness, dyspnoea and dysphagia.

Squamous carcinomas are the most common malignancies, accounting for approximately 80% of all head and neck tumours. Their incidence and anatomical site vary around the world, but they are mainly caused by the preventable aetiological agents of smoking and alcohol, although nasopharyngeal squamous carcinomas have additional genetic and environmental factors. These head and neck cancers have a high morbidity and mortality, and require expert treatment.

FURTHER READING

Bull, P. and Clarke, R. (2007) *Diseases of the Ear, Nose and Throat.* Blackwell, Oxford.

Hibbert, J. (ed.) (1997) *Scott Brown's Otolaryngology, Laryngology and Head and Neck Surgery*, 6th edn. Butterworth-Heinemann, Oxford.

Dhillon, R. and East, C. (2006) *Nose and Throat, Head and Neck Surgery.* Elsevier, Amsterdam.

Lund, V.J. and Howard, D.J. (1997) Ear, nose and throat emergencies, Part II. In: *Cambridge Textbook of Accident and Emergency Medicine.* Cambridge University Press, Cambridge.

Probst, R., Grevers, G. and Iro, H. (2006) *Basic Otorhinolaryngology.* Georg Thieme, Stuttgart.

Snow, J.B. (ed.) (2007) *Ballenger's Handbook of Otorhinolaryngology, Head and Neck Surgery*, 17th edn. B.C. Decker, Hamilton.

Wei, W. and Sham, J. (2000) *Cancer of the Larynx and Hypopharynx.* Isis Medical Media, Oxford.

CHAPTER 45 | PHARYNX, LARYNX AND NECK

Oropharyngeal cancer

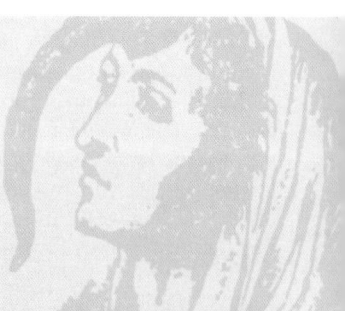

LEARNING OBJECTIVES

To understand:
- The relationship between oral cancers and the use of alcohol and tobacco
- The cardinal features of oropharyngeal cancer

- The investigation and treatment of patients with oropharyngeal cancer

INTRODUCTION AND EPIDEMIOLOGY

In the western world oral/oropharyngeal cancer is rare, accounting for 2–4% of all malignant tumours, although there is evidence that the incidence is on the increase, particularly among young people. In the Indian subcontinent, however, oropharyngeal cancer is the most common malignant tumour, accounting for 40% of all cancers.

Epidemiology

The principal aetiological agents are tobacco and alcohol. In Europe and North America this is mainly through cigarette smoking combined with alcohol abuse. Synergism between alcohol abuse and tobacco use in the development of squamous cell carcinoma (SCC) of the head and neck is well established. Risk factors associated with cancer of the head and neck are outlined in Summary box 46.1.

Summary box 46.1

Risk factors associated with cancer of the head and neck

- Tobacco
- Alcohol
- Areca nut/pan masala
- Human papillomavirus
- Epstein–Barr virus
- Plummer–Vinson syndrome
- Poor nutrition

Michael Anthony Epstein, **B.** 1921, formerly Professor of Pathology, The University of Bristol, Bristol, England.
Yvonne Barr, **B.** 1931, a Virologist who emigrated to Australia. Epstein and Barr discovered this virus in 1964.
Henry Stanley Plummer, **1874–1937**, Physician, The Mayo Clinic, Rochester, MN, USA, described this syndrome in 1912.
Porter Paisley Vinson, **1890–1959**, Physician, The Mayo Clinic, Rochester, MN, who later practised in Richmond, VA, USA.

In the Indian subcontinent, the use of 'pan' (a combination of betel nut, areca nut, lime and tobacco) as well as reverse smoking (smoking a cheroot with the burning end inside the mouth) are responsible for the high incidence of oropharyngeal cancer. Betel quid appears to be the major carcinogen, although there is also a relationship between slaked lime and the areca nut and cancer.

INCIDENCE

The incidence is greater in men than in women and it is predominantly a disease of the elderly (those over 60 years of age). The incidence in women is increasing, particularly in young patients, with oral tongue cancer being the cancer that is usually, but not exclusively, present. In Europe and North America the current trend of binge drinking and acute tobacco abuse has been observed to correlate with the rising incidence of tongue cancer in younger people.

ANATOMY

Lip and oral cavity

The oral cavity extends from the skin–vermilion border of the lips anteriorly to the junction of the soft palate superiorly and the line of the circumvallate papillae on the junction of the posterior one-third third and anterior two-thirds of the tongue posteriorly. The anatomical sites that are frequently involved in mouth cancer include the floor of the mouth, the lateral border of the anterior tongue and the retromolar trigone (Fig. 46.1). The retromolar trigone is defined as the attached mucosa overlying the ascending ramus of the mandible posterior to the last molar tooth and extending superiorly to the maxillary tuberosity.

Oropharynx

The oropharynx extends vertically from the oral surface of the soft palate to the superior surface of the hyoid bone (floor of vallecula). This includes the base of the tongue, the soft palate and the anterior and posterior tonsillar pillars, as well as the pharyngeal tonsils and the lateral and posterior pharyngeal walls.

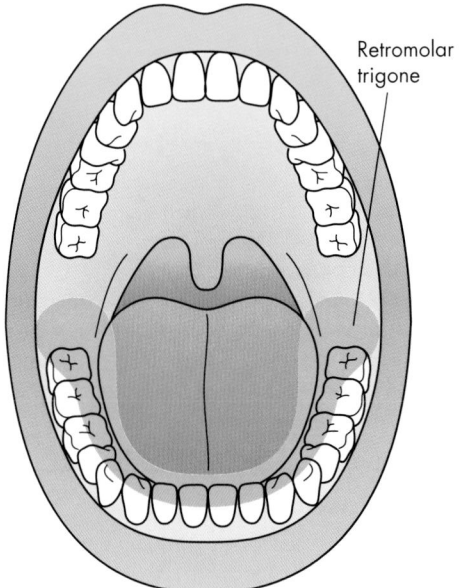

Figure 46.1 Common anatomical sites (blue) for oral squamous cell carcinoma.

Retromolar trigone

The lateral boundaries include the pharyngeal constrictor muscles and the medial aspect of the mandible.

PATHOLOGY

The anatomy of the oral cavity and the oropharynx is complex and the course of the nerves, blood vessels, lymphatic pathways and fascial planes influences the spread of disease. Fascial planes, including the periosteum, serve as barriers to the direct spread of tumours but contribute to the spread of tumours into the cervical lymph nodes. Perineural invasion acts as a conduit for the direct spread of tumours and profoundly impacts on prognosis and survival. Angio-invasion also carries a negative prognosis and correlates directly with distant metastases, particularly of oral tongue cancer.

Histology

SCC is the predominant histology for tumours arising in the oral cavity and oropharynx. Tumours mainly arise from the mucosal epithelium, although malignant salivary gland tumours from the minor salivary glands are a rare but important group of lesions. Lymphomas, particularly around the Waldeyer's ring (tonsils, tongue base, lingual tonsil regions, posterior one-third of the tongue), make up the last of the three principal pathological groups of oropharyngeal cancer.

Chronic exposure of the mucosal surface to carcinogenic substances, i.e. tobacco and alcohol, can produce multiple subclinical sites of carcinoma that can at any stage develop into malignant tumour. This pathological process supports the preventative measures of smoking cessation and alcohol rehabilitation in patients with head and neck cancer, thereby minimising the occurrence of synchronous and metachronous tumours (see below).

Heinrich Wilhelm Gottfried Waldeyer-Hartz, **1836–1921**, Professor of Pathological Anatomy, Berlin, Germany.

Pre-malignant lesions

The majority of oral carcinomas are not preceded by or associated with clinically obvious pre-malignant lesions. There are, however, a group of oral pathological conditions in which an association with malignant transformation exists (Summary box 46.2).

Summary box 46.2

Conditions associated with malignant transformation

High-risk lesions
- Erythroplakia
- Speckled erythroplakia
- Chronic hyperplastic candidiasis

Medium-risk lesions
- Oral submucous fibrosis
- Syphilitic glossitis
- Sideropenic dysphagia (Paterson–Kelly syndrome)

Low-risk/equivocal-risk lesions
- Oral lichen planus
- Discoid lupus erythematosus
- Discoid keratosis congenita

Clinical features

Pre-malignant lesions of the oral mucosa and oropharyngeal mucosa present as either:

- leucoplakia;
- speckled leucoplakia;
- erythroplakia/plasia.

Leucoplakia

Leucoplakia is defined as any white patch or plaque that cannot be characterised clinically or pathologically. It is purely a descriptive term with no histological correlation. Leucoplakia varies from a small, well-circumscribed, homogenous white plaque to an extensive lesion involving large surface areas of the oral mucosa. It may be smooth or wrinkled, fissured and vary in colour depending on the thickness of the lesion.

Speckled leucoplakia

This is a variation of leucoplakia arising on an erythematous base (Fig. 46.2). It has the highest rate of malignant transformation.

Erythroplakia

Erythroplakia is defined as any lesion of the oral mucosa that presents as a bright red plaque which cannot be characterised clinically or pathologically as any other recognisable condition. The lesions are irregular in outline and separated from adjacent normal mucosa (Fig. 46.3). The surfaces may be nodular. These lesions occasionally coexist with leucoplakia.

Donald Rose Paterson, **1863–1939**, Surgeon, The Ear, Nose and Throat Department, The Royal Infirmary, Cardiff, Wales.
Adam Brown Kelly, **1865–1941**, Surgeon, The Ear, Nose and Throat Department, The Royal Victoria Infirmary, Glasgow, Scotland.

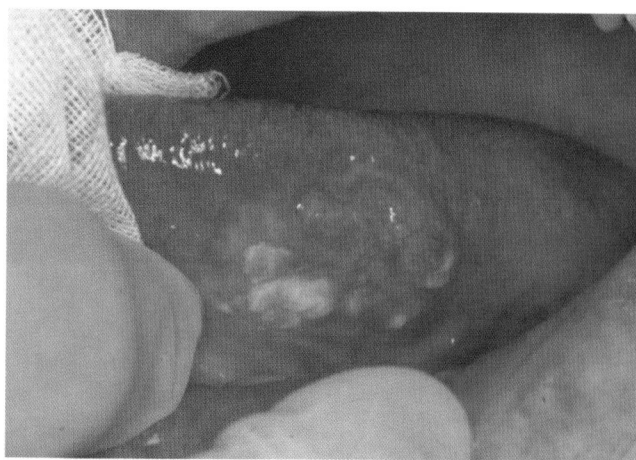

Figure 46.2 Speckled leucoplakia on the lateral border of the tongue. Histology confirms carcinoma *in situ*.

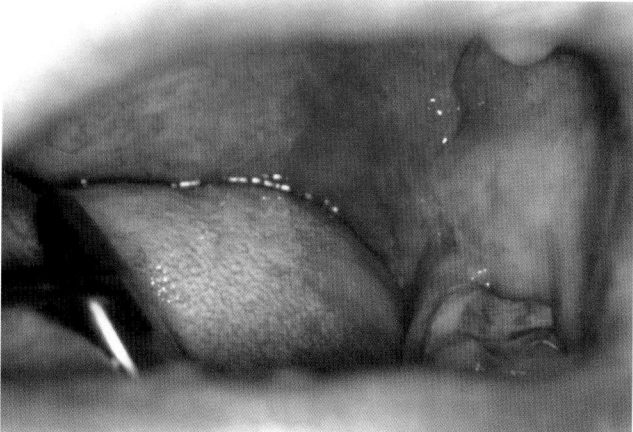

Figure 46.3 Erythroplakia of the left soft palate and lateral pharyngeal wall.

FIELD CHANGE AND SECOND PRIMARY TUMOURS

The diffuse and chronic exposure of the mucosa of the upper aerodigestive tract to carcinogenic substances, e.g. tobacco and alcohol, causes widespread adverse changes in the mucosal epithelium. The consequence of the diffuse exposure is the development of separate tumours at different anatomical sites. These may present simultaneously, within 6 months (synchronous) or may be delayed (metachronous). Slaughter, in 1950, first proposed the concept of field change or 'cancerisation'. Separate primary tumours may not represent distinct genetic mutational events but rather the same clonal origin of cells, which migrate to separate sites in the upper aerodigestive tract. Nevertheless, minimising exposure of the oropharyngeal tissues to potential insults is the cornerstone of long-term management for patients with head and neck cancer.

Patients who develop a first tumour in the oral cavity and the oropharynx are more likely to develop a second primary tumour in the upper oesophagus. The overall rate of second primary tumour development is 15%. In total, 80% of these are metachronous tumours, of which 50% develop within the first 2 years of initial presentation (Fig. 46.4). The prevalence of synchronous second primary tumours is 4%.

Potential for malignant change

The potential risk for malignant transformation:

- increases with increasing age of the patient;
- increases with increasing age of the lesion;
- is higher in smokers;
- increases with alcohol consumption;
- depends on the anatomical site of the pre-malignant lesion;
- is particularly high for leucoplakia on the floor of the mouth and ventral surface of the tongue, particularly in younger women, even in the absence of associated risk factors.

PRE-MALIGNANT CONDITIONS

Chronic hyperplastic candidiasis

Chronic hyperplastic candidiasis produces dense plaques of leucoplakia, particularly around the commissures of the mouth. The lesions occasionally extend on to the vermilion and even the facial skin (Fig. 46.5). These lesions have a high incidence of malignant transformation, thought to be the result of invasion of

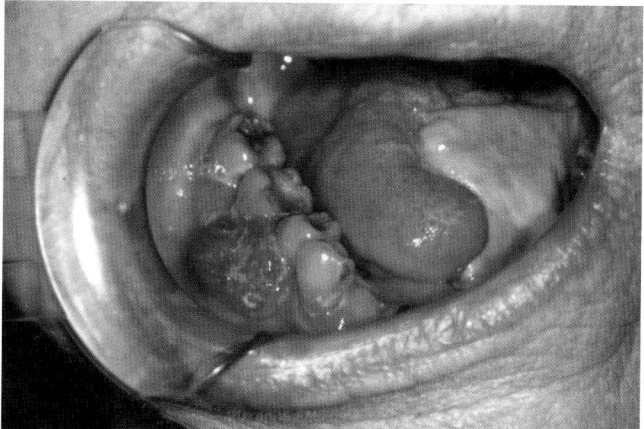

Figure 46.4 Metachronous tumour in the right mandibular alveolus after previous partial glossectomy and forearm flap reconstruction.

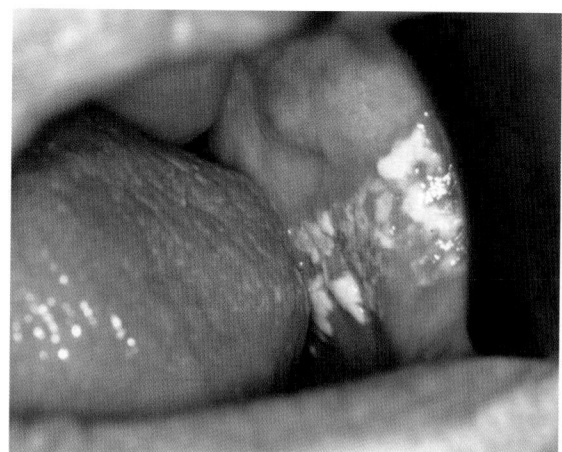

Figure 46.5 Chronic hyperplastic candidiasis of the left buccal mucosa.

the lesion by *Candida albicans*. A small percentage of patients have an associated immunological defect, which encourages the invasion of *C. albicans*, rendering the patient susceptible to malignant transformation. Specific management of chronic hyperplastic candidiasis includes prolonged (6 weeks) topical anti-fungal treatment or systemic anti-fungal treatment (2 weeks). If the lesions persist after medical therapy, surgical excision or laser vaporisation is strongly recommended.

Oral submucous fibrosis

Oral submucous fibrosis is a progressive disease in which fibrous bands form beneath the oral mucosa. Scarring produces contracture, resulting in limited mouth opening and restricted tongue movement. The condition is almost entirely confined to the Asian population and is characterised pathologically by epithelial fibrosis with associated atrophy and hyperplasia of the overlying epithelium (Fig. 46.6). The epithelium also shows changes of epithelial dysplasia. Restricted mouth opening can be treated with either intralesional steroids or surgical excision and skin grafts.

Research strongly indicates that oral submucous fibrosis is significantly associated with the use of pan masala areca nut, with or without concurrent alcohol use. Tobacco smoking alone is not associated with oral submucous fibrosis.

Sideropenic dysphagia (Plummer–Vincent and Paterson–Kelly syndromes)

There is a well-known relationship between sideropenia (iron deficiency in the absence of anaemia) and the development of oral cancer. Sideropenia is common in Scandinavian women and leads to epithelial atrophy, which renders the oral mucosa vulnerable to irritation from topical carcinogens. Correction of the sideropenia with iron supplements reduces the epithelial atrophy and risk of malignant transformation.

CLASSIFICATION AND STAGING

TNM staging

Staging of head and neck cancer is defined by the American Joint Committee on Cancer (AJCC) and follows the TNM system. The system also takes into account the pretreatment computerised tomography (CT) or magnetic resonance imaging (MRI) of the tumour. The T classification indicates the extent of the primary tumour and the N classification relates to the extent of regional neck metastases to the cervical lymph nodes; this is identical for all mucosal sites of the head and neck except for the nasopharynx. The M classification relates to distant metastasis. The risk of distant metastasis is dependent on nodal disease rather than the size of the primary tumour. Tumours close to the midline are at a greater risk of developing bilateral or contralateral cervical node metastasis.

The TNM staging system is outlined in Table 46.1.

Patterns of lymph node metastasis

The cervical lymph nodes are divided into five principal levels as outlined in Fig. 46.7.

The spread of tumour from the primary site has been well addressed. SCC in the oral cavity and lips tends to metastasise to lymph nodes at levels I, II and III. However, with SCC of the oral tongue there is a risk of skip metastasis directly to lymph node levels III or IV, without the involvement of higher-level lymph node groups. Tumours arising in the oropharynx commonly metastasise to lymph node levels II, III and IV, as well as retropharyngeal and contralateral nodal groups.

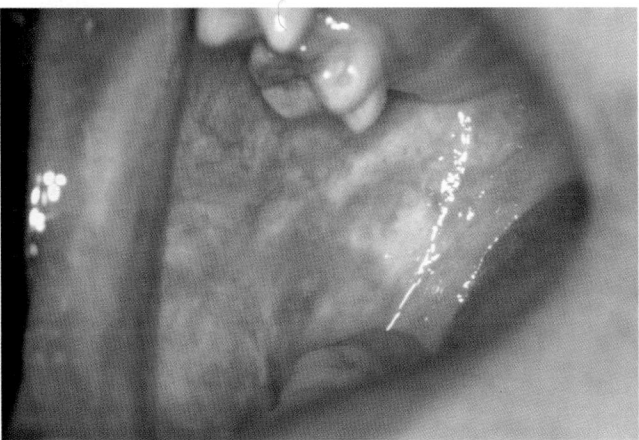

Figure 46.6 Oral submucous fibrosis of the right buccal mucosa and soft palate.

Table 46.1 The TNM staging system

Primary tumour (T)

TX	Primary tumour cannot be assessed
T0	No evidence of primary tumour
Tis	Carcinoma *in situ*
T1	Tumour < 2 cm in greatest dimension
T2	Tumour > 2 but < 4 cm
T3	Tumour > 4 cm but < 6 cm
T4	Tumour invades adjacent structures, e.g. mandible, skin

Regional lymph nodes (N)

NX	Regional lymph nodes cannot be assessed
N0	No regional lymph node metastasis
N1	Metastasis in a single ipsilateral lymph node < 3 cm in greatest dimension
N2a	Metastasis in a single ipsilateral lymph node > 3 cm but not more than 6 cm
N2b	Metastasis in multiple ipsilateral lymph nodes, none > 6 cm in greatest dimension
N2c	Metastasis in bilateral or contralateral lymph nodes, none greater than 6 cm in greatest dimension
N3	Metastasis in any lymph node > 6 cm

Distant metastasis

M0	No evidence of distant metastasis
M1	Evidence of distant metastasis

Stage

Stage	T	N	M
0	Tis	N0	M0
I	T1	N0	M0
II	T2	N0	M0
III	T3	N0	M0
	T1, T2, T3	N1	M0
IV	T4	N0	M0
	Any T	N2	M0
	Any T	N3	M0
	Any T	Any N	M1

CHAPTER 46 | OROPHARYNGEAL CANCER

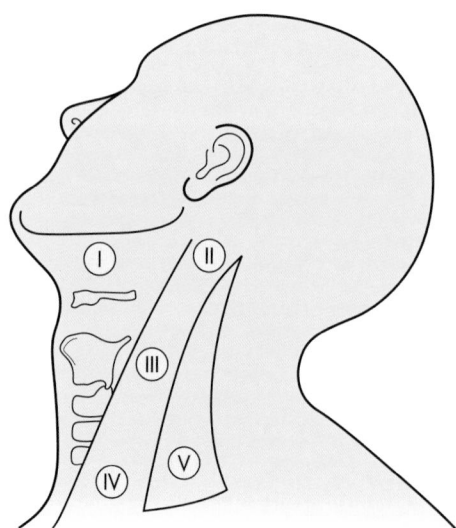

Figure 46.7 Cervical lymph nodes: (I) submandibular; (II) upper deep cervical; (III) mid-cervical; (IV) lower cervical; (V) posterior triangle.

Distant metastases are relatively uncommon but sites involved include lung, brain, liver, bone and skin.

CLINICAL FEATURES

Between 25% and 50% of patients with cancer of the oral cavity or oropharynx present late. Many of these patients are elderly and frail and delay visiting the doctor or the dentist partly because they wear dentures and are accustomed to the discomfort and associated ulceration. Occasionally, dental and medical practitioners fail to recognise that a lesion may be malignant and further delay referral. Moreover, early oral cancer is usually not painful until either the ulcer becomes infected or the tumour invades local sensory nerve fibres. Clinical presentation is markedly dependent on the anatomical site.

Lip cancer

Lip cancer presents early as it is readily visible to the patient. It usually arises as an ulcer on the vermilion border (Fig. 46.8). In total, 95% of carcinomas of the lip arise on the lower lip and 15%

arise in the central one-third and commissures. Tumours tend to spread laterally over the mucosal surface. Lymph node metastases, usually to the submental or submandibular nodes, occur late.

Oral cavity

Cancers of the oral cavity present in a variable way (Fig. 46.9) but are often associated with persisting swelling or ulceration within the oral cavity (Summary box 46.3).

> **Summary box 46.3**
>
> **Clinical features of oral cancer**
>
> ■ Persistent oral swelling for > 4 weeks
> ■ Mouth ulceration for > 4 weeks
> ■ Sore tongue
> ■ Difficulty swallowing
> ■ Jaw or facial swelling
> ■ Painless neck lump
> ■ Unexplained tooth mobility
> ■ Trismus

The duration of symptoms is highly variable, from several weeks to many months.

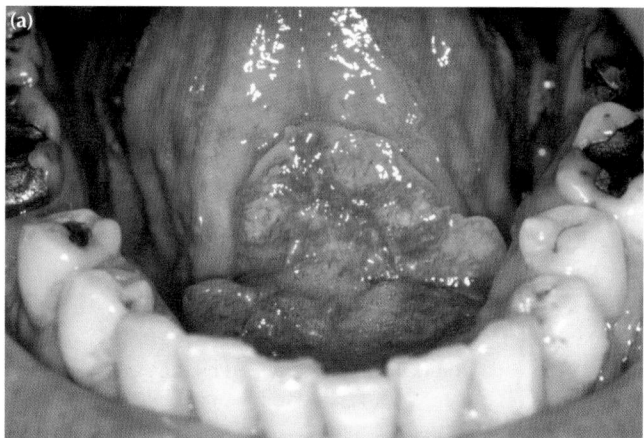

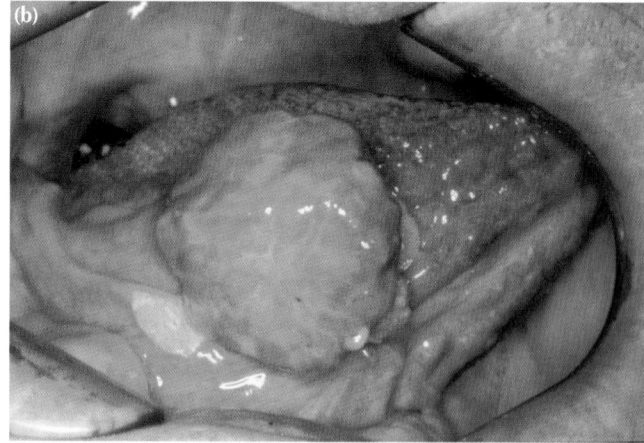

Figure 46.9 (a) Ulcerative squamous cell carcinoma of the anterior floor of the mouth. (b) Exophytic squamous cell carcinoma of the right lateral border of the tongue.

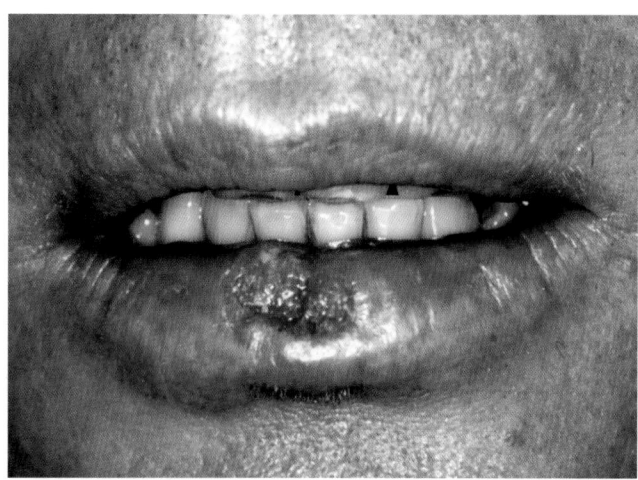

Figure 46.8 Squamous cell carcinoma of the lower lip.

Oropharynx

Cancer of the oropharynx frequently presents much later than cancer of the lip and oral cavity. An ipsilateral or contralateral lump in the neck may be the single presenting complaint from a patient with a carcinoma arising from the tongue base, tonsil or soft palate. Palpable asymmetry, particularly in the tonsil, often represents submucosal infiltration of tumour. Deeper infiltration of the tongue base, pterygoid muscles or adherence of the tumour to the jaw results in poor mobility of the tongue or palate. Common clinical features of oropharyngeal cancer are outlined in Summary box 46.4.

Summary box 46.4

Clinical features of oropharyngeal cancer

- Localised and persistent sore throat
- Difficulty and/or painful swallowing for > 4 weeks
- Painless neck lump
- Unilateral tonsillar enlargement or ulceration
- Otalgia

INVESTIGATIONS

When a clinical diagnosis of oropharyngeal cancer is suspected, a comprehensive protocol of investigations should be instituted. An incisional biopsy should be carried out in all cases. Formal examination under anaesthetic is preferred in the vast majority of cases, not only to carry out the biopsy, but also to palpate and examine the extent of the tumour, which can be exquisitely tender in the conscious patient. Under the same anaesthetic, extraction of teeth with a dubious prognosis can be performed. Where available, and when the diagnosis is clear-cut, insertion of a percutaneous endoscopic gastrostomy (PEG) should be performed to facilitate feeding in the treatment phase. The biopsy should be generous and include the most suspicious area of the lesion, as well as normal adjacent tissue. Areas of necrosis or gross infection should be avoided.

Radiography

Plain radiography of the jaw is of limited value but does provide an opportunity for dental assessment. Before examination under anaesthesia, an orthopantomogram of the jaws is helpful to assess bony invasion, particularly from tumours arising on the alveolus and maxillary antrum.

Magnetic resonance imaging

MRI is the investigation of choice for cancer of the oral cavity and oropharynx, as it is not distorted by metallic dental restorations and provides excellent visualisation of soft-tissue infiltration of the tumour (Fig. 46.10). Its specificity and sensitivity in diagnosing cervical node metastasis is similar to that of CT. Patients who suffer with claustrophobia may have difficulty in tolerating the investigation.

Computerised tomography

CT is much more widely available than MRI but has limited value in oral cavity and oropharyngeal cancer. It is useful when bony invasion is suspected. CT of the thorax and abdomen is also indicated for patients who have proven cervical lymph node

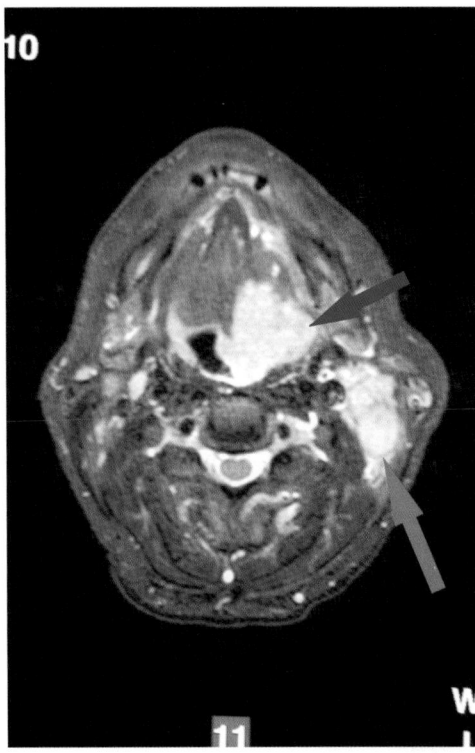

Figure 46.10 Magnetic resonance imaging of a primary tumour of the left tongue base (blue arrow) and neck node metastasis (red arrow).

metastasis or who have large-volume disease, in which the risk of distant metastasis is high.

Radionucleotide studies

A radioisotope bone scan of the facial skeleton adds little to the diagnosis and assessment of oropharyngeal cancer. The scan is not specific and tends to show increased uptake wherever there is increased metabolic activity in bone. A false-positive diagnosis is common and 'over-staging' of the disease frequent.

Fine-needle aspiration cytology

Fine-needle aspiration cytology (FNAC) is useful for the assessment and pathological diagnosis of enlarged cervical lymph nodes. It involves the use of a fine-needle puncture into the mass and immediate aspiration for cytological examination. It has few complications and does not spread tumour. It requires no specialist equipment other than a 21G or 23G needle and a 10 ml syringe. Aspiration should be carried out only when the needle enters the swelling. If the specimen can be assessed immediately by an expert cytologist, then it can be sent without fixation. If there is delay in microscopic examination, then the specimen, smeared on a microscope slide, should be fixed before transfer to the laboratory. The positive yield from FNAC is dependent not only on the quality of the aspirate, but also on the skill of the cytologist.

Ultrasound

Ultrasound has limited use in the management of oropharyngeal cancer. It is useful as an adjunct in FNAC to ensure accurate aspiration of a deeply seated neck node swelling. It also has a place in abdominal assessment, particularly when metastases of the liver are suspected.

TREATMENT

General principles

The two principal treatment modalities of oropharyngeal cancer are surgery and radiotherapy. Small tumours can be managed either by primary radiotherapy or surgery. Large-volume disease, i.e. advanced tumour, usually requires a combination of surgery and radiotherapy. There is an increasing move to manage extensive disease of the oropharynx with chemoradiotherapy, provided that patients are medically fit to tolerate the toxicity. Factors that need to be taken into consideration include:

- the site of disease;
- the stage;
- histology;
- concomitant medical disease;
- social factors.

The management of head and neck cancer involves a team approach, whereby patients are assessed objectively by several specialists who agree on an optimum treatment strategy.

Cancer of the oral cavity is frequently managed with primary surgery whereas cancer of the oropharynx can be treated with either primary radiotherapy or primary surgery, or a combination, i.e. surgery for neck nodes and radiotherapy for the primary site.

When the tumour invades bone, e.g. the mandible, primary surgery is deemed appropriate as radiotherapy is less effective in controlling disease. Surgery is also more appropriate for bulky advanced disease, usually followed by postoperative radiotherapy. Tumours of intermediate size, e.g. T2 and T3 tumours, are more problematic and treatment regimes more controversial, hence the need for planning by a multidisciplinary team.

Cervical node involvement

When cervical lymph node involvement occurs, treatment should be geared towards a single modality to deal simultaneously with the lymph node disease and the primary tumour.

Histology

The degree of differentiation of SCC does not normally influence the management of the tumour alone. Management of verrucous carcinoma, a variant of SCC, is identical to that of any other SCC.

Malignant tumours of the minor salivary glands require primary surgery whereas lymphoma is managed by radiotherapy or chemotherapy and radiotherapy, depending on the stage. Postoperative radiotherapy for minor salivary gland tumours is often indicated to reduce the risk of locoregional recurrence.

Age

Modern anaesthesia and postoperative critical care facilities have allowed major head and neck surgery to be carried out on patients with significant medical comorbidity. Advancing age is now not considered to be a contraindication to major head and neck cancer surgery. Conversely, young patients should not be denied radiotherapy for fear of inducing a second malignancy, e.g. sarcoma, in later life.

Previous radiotherapy

A second course of radiotherapy to a previously irradiated site is contraindicated as the tumour is likely to be radioresistant and re-irradiation will invariably result in extensive tissue necrosis.

Field change

Surgery is preferred when multiple tumours are present or there is extensive pre-malignant change of the oropharyngeal mucosa. Radiotherapy is unsatisfactory as the entire oral cavity requires treatment, causing severe morbidity. In addition, subsequent post-radiotherapy changes make the diagnosis of future pre-malignancy and malignancy more difficult.

Management of pre-malignant conditions

Elimination of associated aetiological factors is the basis of the management of pre-malignant oral mucosal lesions. Cessation of smoking, elimination of the areca nut/pan habit and reduction in alcohol consumption should be encouraged in all patients with pre-malignant lesions. A photographic record of the lesion is useful, particularly for long-term follow-up. All erythroplakia and speckled leucoplakia should undergo urgent incisional biopsy. Biopsy from more than one site provides a better representation of histological changes within a lesion.

Severe epithelial dysplasia and carcinoma in situ should be ablated by surgical excision or laser vaporisation. Small lesions, particularly on the lateral border of the tongue or buccal mucosa, may be managed with surgical excision and primary closure by undermining the adjacent mucosa. Larger defects can be managed with laser vaporisation and allowed to epithelialise spontaneously (Fig. 46.11). With mild to moderate epithelial dysplasia, treatment is facilitated by elimination of causative agents. Patients who continue to smoke should be managed as for severe dysplasia and carcinoma in situ. Patients who cease smoking and areca nut/pan habits may be followed up closely at 3-monthly intervals.

LIP CANCER

Surgery and external beam radiotherapy are highly effective methods of treatment for lip cancer. The cure rate approaches 90% for either modality.

Pre-malignant changes on the lower lip mucosa are frequently extensive and are best managed by a lower lip shave, in which the vermilion defect is closed by advancement of the lower labial mucosa.

Small tumours

Small tumours (< 2 cm) of the lip can be managed with either a V- or W-shaped excision under local or general anaesthesia. The defect, which should be no larger than one-third of the total lip size, is closed in three layers – mucosa, muscle and skin – with particular attention paid to the correct alignment of the vermilion border (Fig. 46.12).

Intermediate tumours

Larger tumours, which produce defects of between one-third and two-thirds the size of the lower lip, require local flaps for reconstruction. V or W excision will result in microstomia. Large central defects are best managed using the Johansen step technique (Fig. 46.13). This allows closure of the defect by symmetrical advancement of soft-tissue flaps, utilising the excess skin in the labio-mental grooves. Alternative techniques include the Bernard rotational flap.

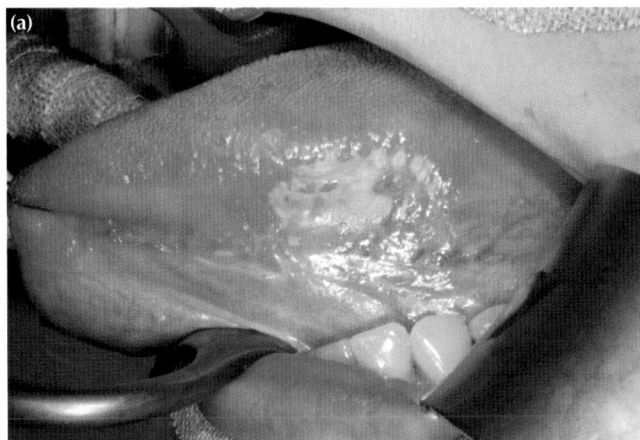

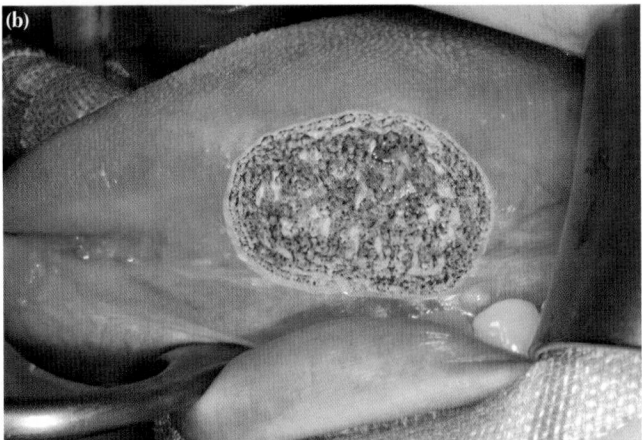

Figure 46.11 (a) Leucoplakia with severe dysplasia of the lateral border of the tongue. (b) Laser vaporisation.

Total lip reconstruction

Extensive tumours of the lower lip, which invade adjacent tissues (T4), have a high incidence of neck node metastasis. Patients with such advanced disease require surgery that may include unilateral or bilateral selective neck dissection and total excision of the lower lip and chin. The lower lip defect is best reconstructed with a forearm flap (Fig. 46.14).

TONGUE CANCER

Up to 30% of patients with a T1 (< 2 cm diameter) tumour (Fig. 46.15) have occult metastasis at presentation and should undergo simultaneous treatment of the neck by either selective neck dissection or radiotherapy. When performing surgical excision of the primary tumour, a 2-cm margin in all planes should be achieved to ensure a wide, complete excision. Resection resulting in partial or hemiglossectomy can be performed with either a cutting diathermy or laser if available. Advanced tumours (T3 and T4) often encroach upon the floor of the mouth and, occasionally, the mandible. In these circumstances a major resection of the tongue and floor of the mouth and mandible is required. T4 tumours of the oral tongue often cross the midline, for which total glossectomy is the only option to achieve adequate tumour clearance.

When a patient undergoes simultaneous neck dissection, the resection of the primary tumour should preferably be in continuity with the neck node specimen. This eliminates 'lingual' lymph nodes [lying between the primary tumour and submandibular (level I) nodes]; these nodes may contain micro-deposits of tumour, which may lead to local recurrence.

Access

Access for oropharyngeal cancer is important to allow accurate

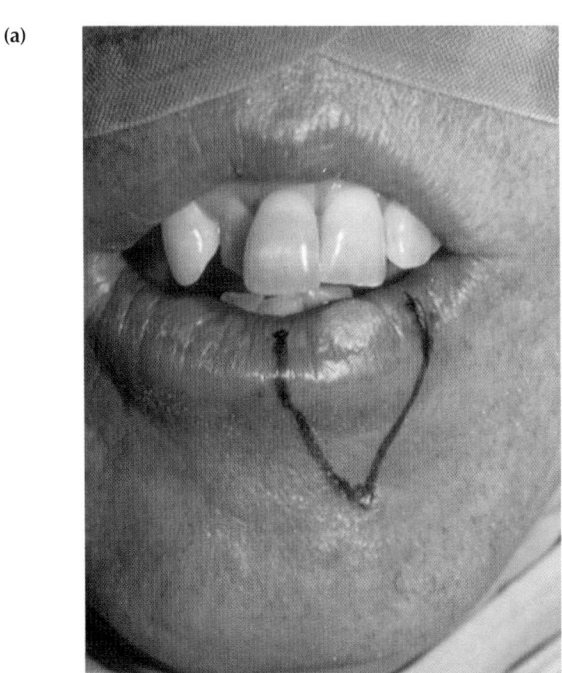

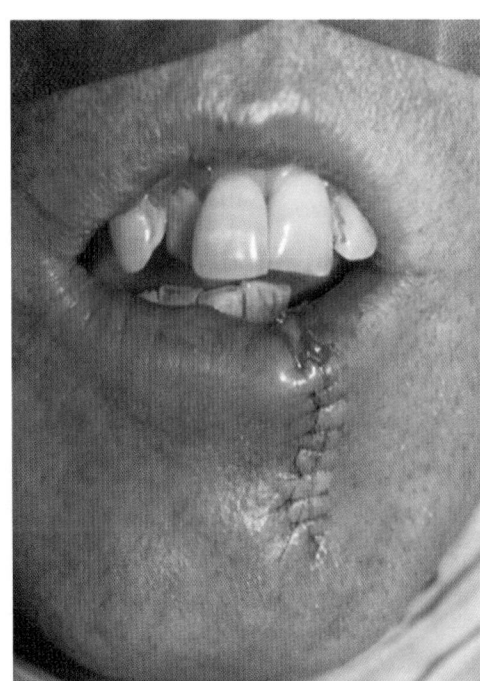

Figure 46.12 (a) Skin markings for wedge excision of the lower lip. (b) Primary closure.

CHAPTER 46 | OROPHARYNGEAL CANCER

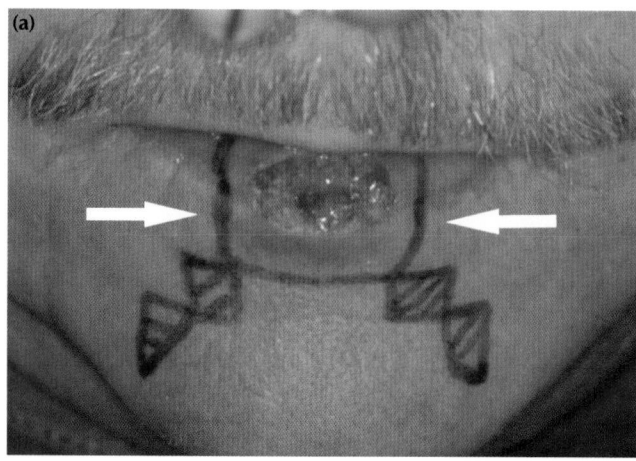

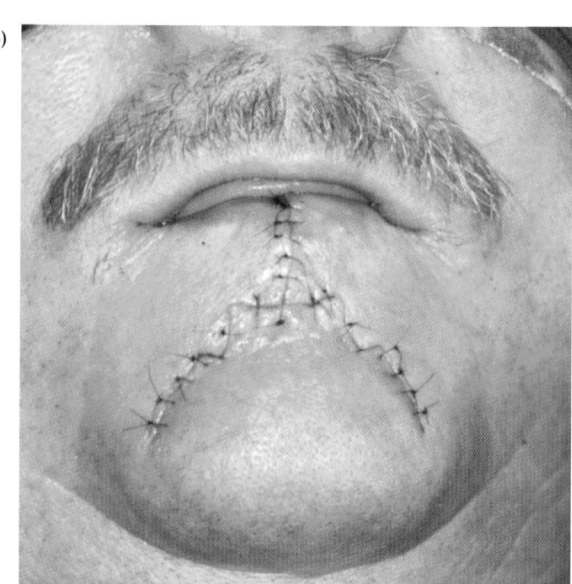

Figure 46.13 (a) Skin markings for Johansen step reconstruction. (b) Closure of lip and labio-mental steps.

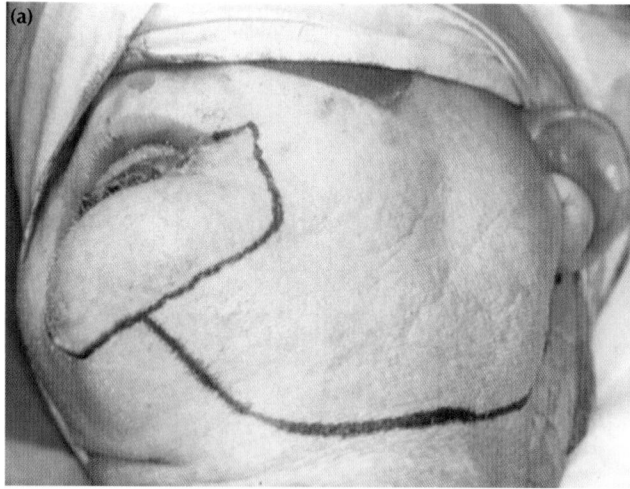

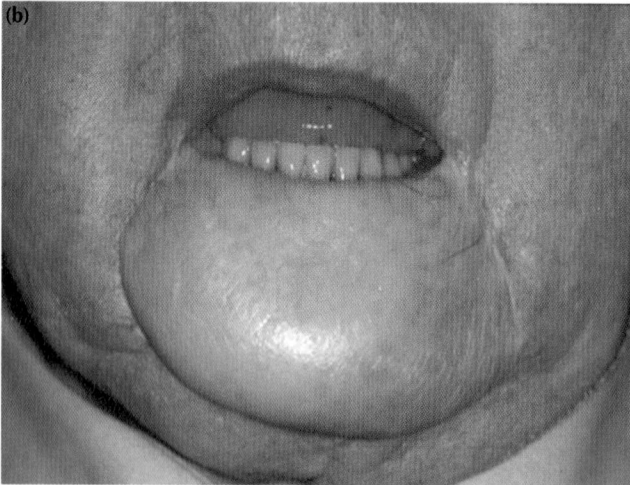

Figure 46.14 (a) Skin markings for total excision of the lower lip, chin and left selective neck dissection. (b) Postoperative view of the reconstructed lower lip using a radial artery forearm flap.

assessment and clear visualisation to enable tumour clearance to be achieved. Access techniques include:

- transoral – small anterior oral tumours only;
- lip-split technique and paramedian or median mandibulotomy (Fig. 46.16);
- visor incision (Fig. 46.17).

Reconstruction

Small defects of the lateral tongue can be managed by primary closure or allowed to heal by secondary intention. Larger defects, e.g. T2, T3 and T4 resections, require formal reconstruction to encourage good speech and swallowing. A radial forearm flap either with skin (Fig. 46.18) and/or fascia, utilising microvascular anastomosis, gives a good functional result. Large-volume defects including total glossectomy require more bulky flaps such as the rectus abdominus free flap. If feasible, the preservation of one or both hypoglossal nerves is useful to encourage floor of mouth function to help relearn swallowing.

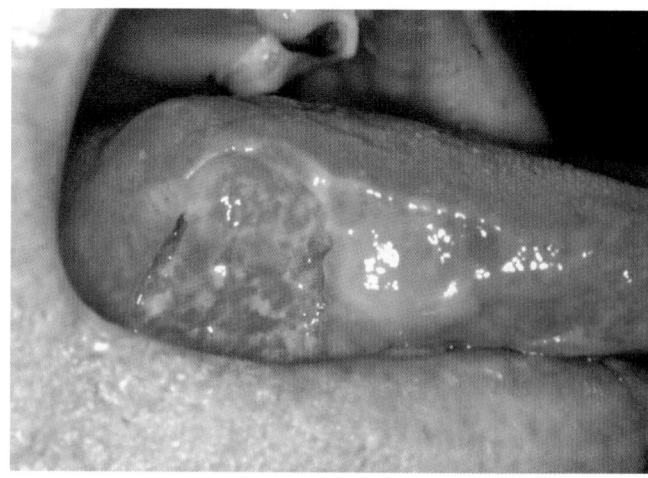

Figure 46.15 Ulcerative squamous cell carcinoma of the right lateral border of the tongue.

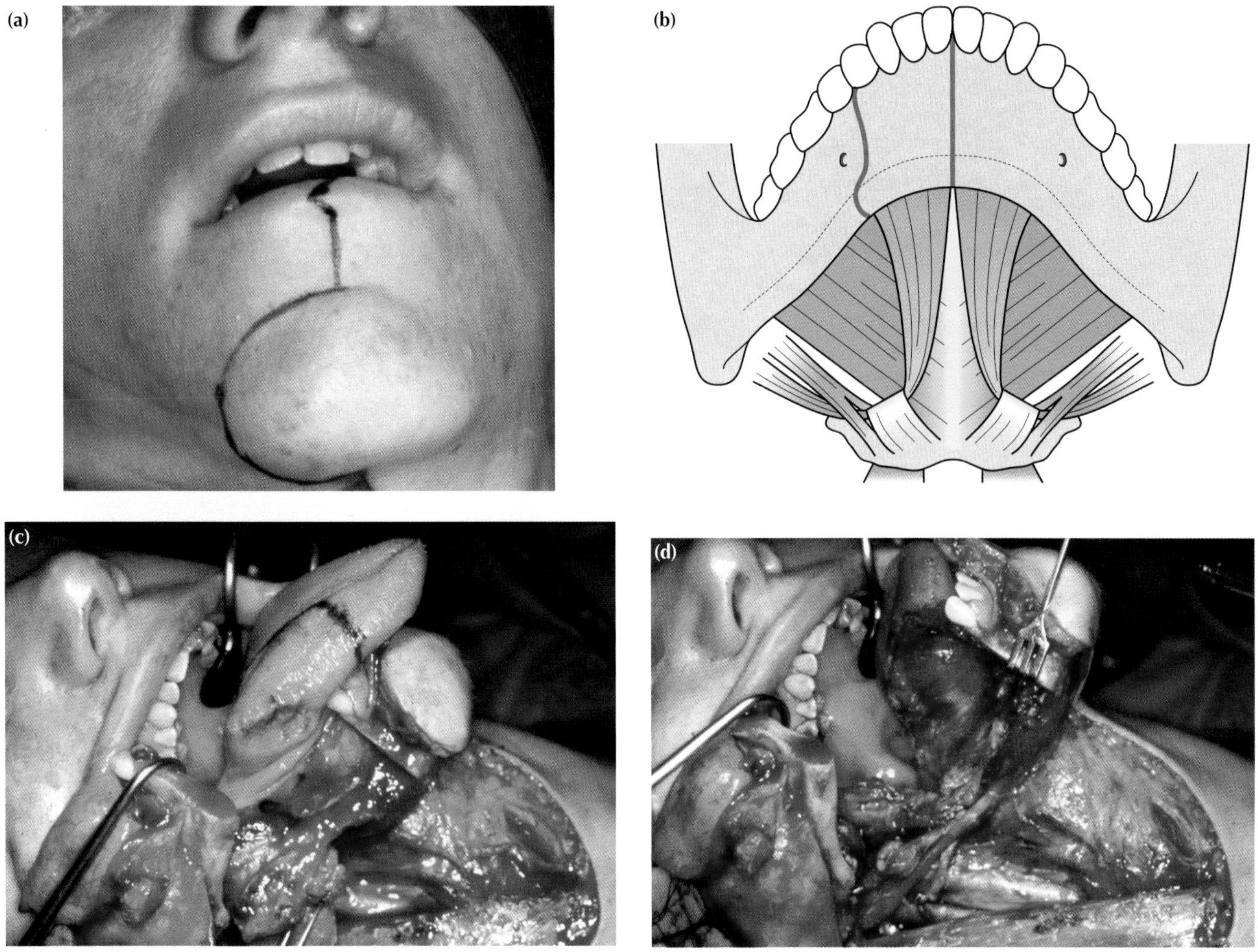

(a)

(b)

(c)

(d)

Figure 46.16 (a) Skin markings for lip split and mandibulotomy in continuity with neck dissection. (b) Paramedian and midline mandibulotomy. (c) Margins for primary tumour resection after mandibulotomy. (d) Tongue defect after right selective neck dissection, mandibulotomy and partial glossectomy.

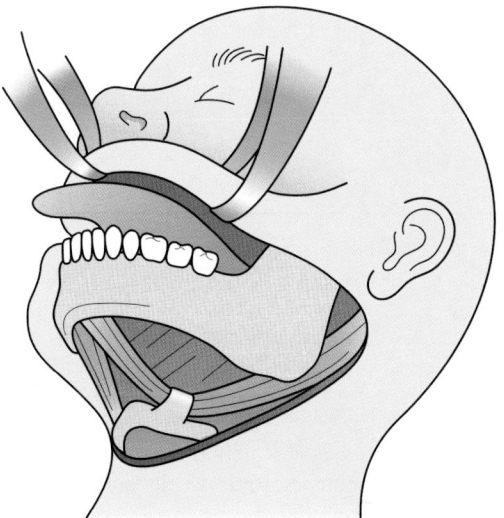

Figure 46.17 Visor approach to the anterior mandible/floor of the mouth and tongue.

FLOOR OF MOUTH

Carcinoma of the floor of the mouth can spread to the ventral surface of the anterior tongue or encroach upon the lower anterior alveolus (Fig. 46.19). Surgical excision may include a partial anterior glossectomy and anterior mandibular resection. Only very small tumours of the floor of mouth can be managed by simple excision. The visor procedure provides excellent access (see Fig. 46.17).

Reconstruction

Small tumours of the floor of the mouth frequently require formal reconstruction. It is unacceptable to advance the cut surface of the ventral tongue to the labial mucosa as severe difficulties with speech, swallowing and mastication ensue. Simple soft-tissue defects of the anterior floor of mouth are best reconstructed with a radial artery forearm flap. If a patient is unfit for microvascular free-flap surgery or the facilities are limited, bilateral nasolabial flaps tunnelled into the mouth and interdigitated provide an acceptable alternative (Fig. 46.20). Large defects that involve rim

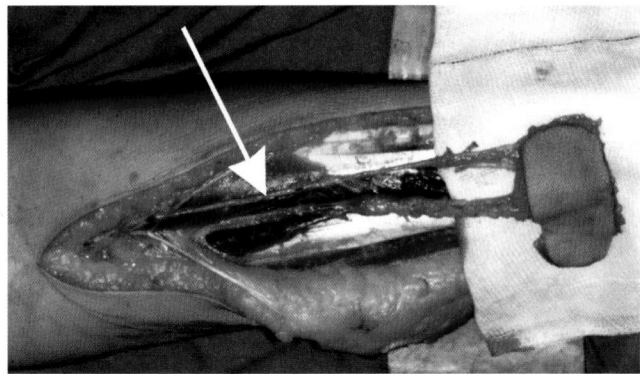

Figure 46.18 Radial artery forearm flap raised before division of vascular pedicle and cephalic vein (arrow).

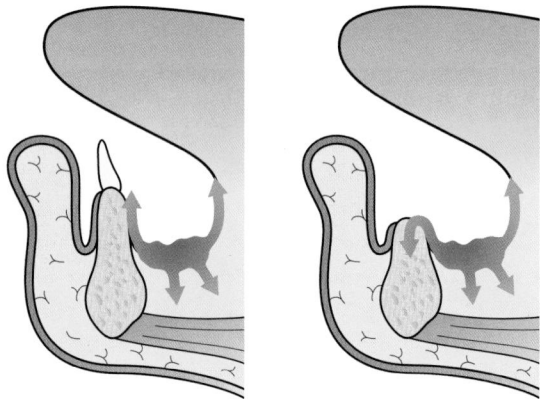

Figure 46.19 Spread of tumour from the anterior floor of the mouth showing the different patterns in a dentate (left) and edentulous (right) mandible.

resection of the anterior mandible may also be managed with soft-tissue reconstruction only. Full-thickness resection of the anterior mandible, however, requires immediate reconstruction to prevent severe functional defects or a cosmetic deformity. Vascularised bone with a soft-tissue component provides the most up-to-date method of reconstruction. A fibula flap or a vascularised iliac crest graft [deep circumflex iliac artery (DCIA)] are two options in the management of anterior mandible defects with simultaneous floor of mouth defects.

BUCCAL MUCOSA

SCC of the buccal mucosa (Fig. 46.21) should be excised widely, including the underlying buccinator muscle. Larger tumours occasionally extend onto the maxillary tuberosity, tonsillar fossa or mandibular alveolus. Facial skin involvement is rare but carries a poor prognosis. Although cervical node metastasis from buccal mucosa usually occurs less readily than in tongue and floor of mouth cancer, a simultaneous ipsilateral selective supraomohyoid neck dissection (levels I, II, III) is considered good practice.

Access for buccal carcinoma can be achieved either transorally for smaller lesions (T1, T2) or using the lip-splitting technique for larger lesions (T3, T4).

Reconstruction of the buccal mucosa prevents scarring and trismus. Options include the radial artery forearm flap or a temporalis muscle flap. Raw temporalis muscle inset into the

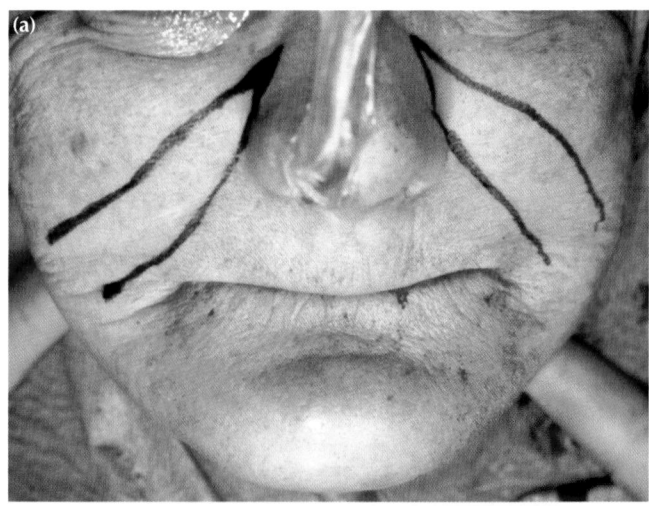

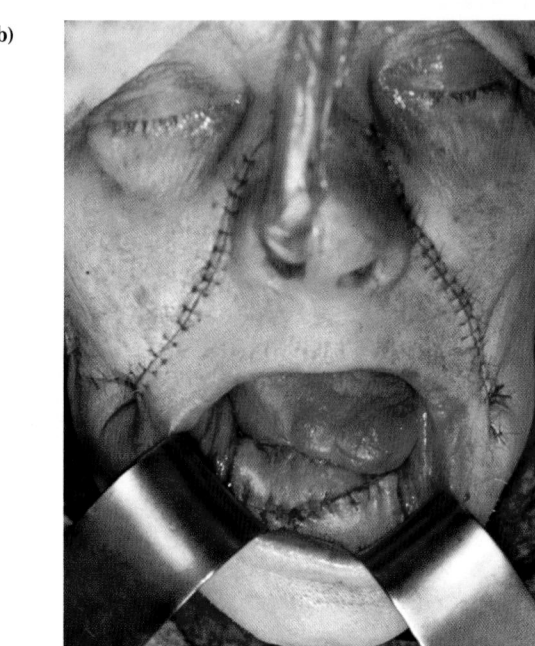

Figure 46.20 (a) Skin markings for bilateral nasolabial flaps. (b) Transposition of bilateral nasolabial flaps into the anterior floor of the mouth.

buccal mucosal defect will epithelialise spontaneously over several weeks.

LOWER ALVEOLUS

Surgery is the treatment of choice for tumours that involve the mandibular alveolus (Fig. 46.22a). Ipsilateral selective neck dissections should be performed for lateral tumours although the incidence of occult subclinical neck node metastasis is low. Bilateral selective neck dissection should be considered for anterior tumours. Bone invasion (Fig. 46.22b) demands segmental resection of the mandible in continuity with neck dissection. Primary or immediate reconstruction is preferred as the functional and cosmetic outcomes are usually superior to those of delayed reconstruction. Options for bony reconstruction are shown in Table 46.2. They include the fibula flap for the edentulous mandible (Fig. 46.22c, d) and the iliac crest (DCIA) for

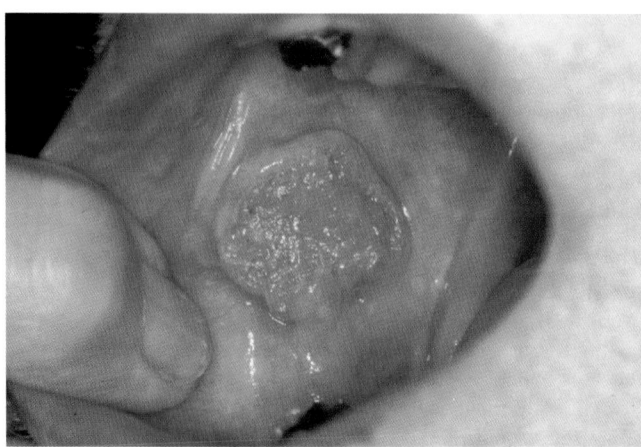

Figure 46.21 Exophytic squamous cell carcinoma of the right buccal mucosa.

Table 46.2 Mandibular reconstruction

Method	Technique
No reconstruction	Primary closure
Soft tissue only	Pectoralis major myocutaneous flap
Alloplastic material	2.4 mm reconstruction plate alone
Combination alloplastic/ soft tissue	2.4 mm reconstruction plate and pectoralis major flap
Non-vascularised bone grafts	Titanium tray and cancellous chips (iliac crest)
Vascularised bone grafts	Fibula (edentulous and dentate); iliac crest (dentate); scapula (concomitant large soft-tissue defect)

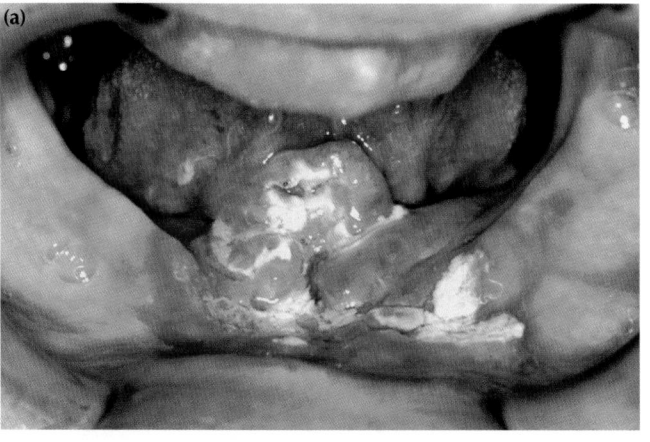

(a)

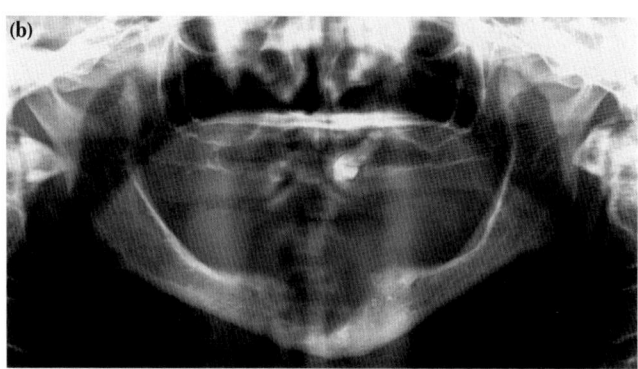

(b)

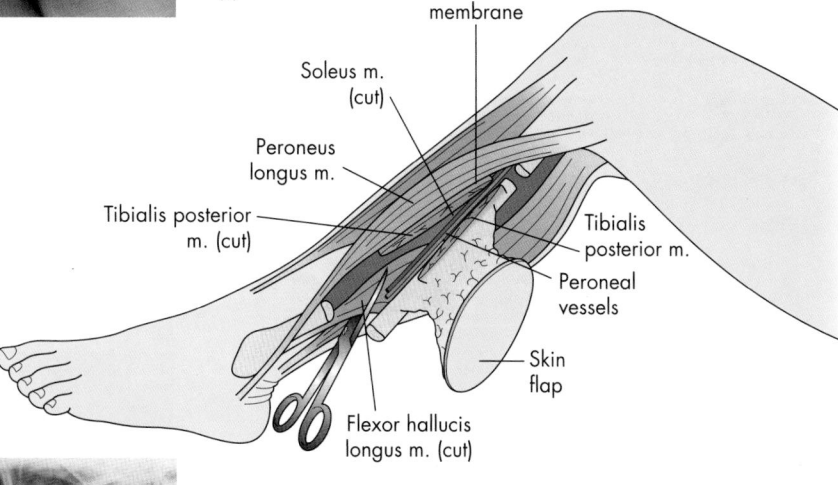

(c)

Interosseous membrane
Soleus m. (cut)
Peroneus longus m.
Tibialis posterior m. (cut)
Tibialis posterior m.
Peroneal vessels
Skin flap
Flexor hallucis longus m. (cut)

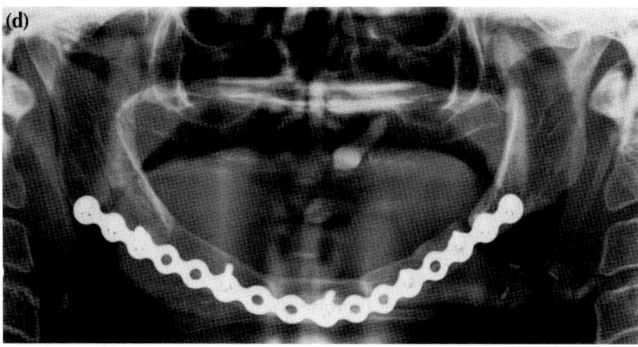

(d)

Figure 46.22 (a) Extensive squamous cell carcinoma of the anterior mandible involving the floor of the mouth. (b) Plain radiography (orthopantomogram) revealing bony destruction of the anterior mandible. (c) Osseocutaneous fibula flap. (d) Postoperative radiograph of the reconstructed mandible with fibula flap and reconstruction plate.

patients with a dentate mandible (Fig. 46.23). The vascularised iliac crest can be wrapped with internal oblique abdominal wall muscle, which epithelialises spontaneously. This intraoral epithelialisation provides an excellent surface for prosthetic replacement.

Although non-vascularised bone grafts have a place in mandibular reconstruction, the long-term success is frequently low as many patients receive postoperative radiotherapy, which results in the loss of the bone and dehiscence of the titanium tray or reconstruction plate.

RETROMOLAR PAD

Tumours at this site frequently, but not always, invade the ascending ramus of the mandible. They also spread medially into the soft palate or even the tonsillar fossa. Access for excision is carried out via a lip split and mandibulotomy (see Fig. 46.16 p. 743). Small defects are managed either with a temporalis muscle flap or a radial artery forearm flap. Segmental mandibular resections require vascularised bone to achieve adequate reconstruction.

HARD PALATE AND MAXILLARY ALVEOLUS

The maxillary alveolus and hard palate are relatively uncommon sites for SCC. A tumour arising in these areas may arise either from the oral mucosa per se or from the maxillary antrum penetrating the oral cavity. In the Indian subcontinent, carcinoma of the hard palate is particularly associated with reverse smoking. Occasionally, malignant tumours of minor salivary glands present as swellings of the hard palate. Small tumours of the maxillary alveolus can be managed by transoral partial maxillectomy. More

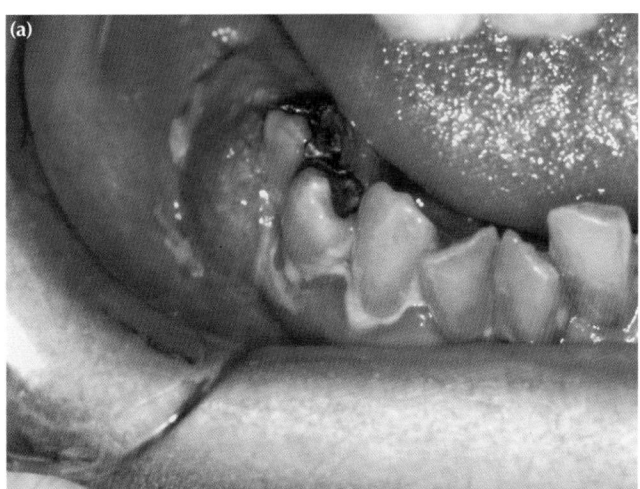

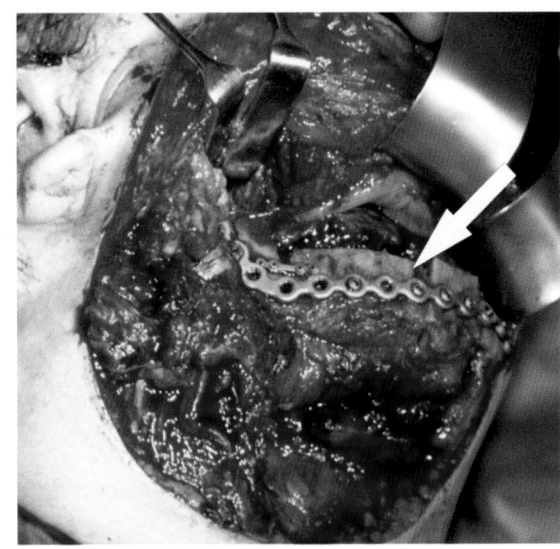

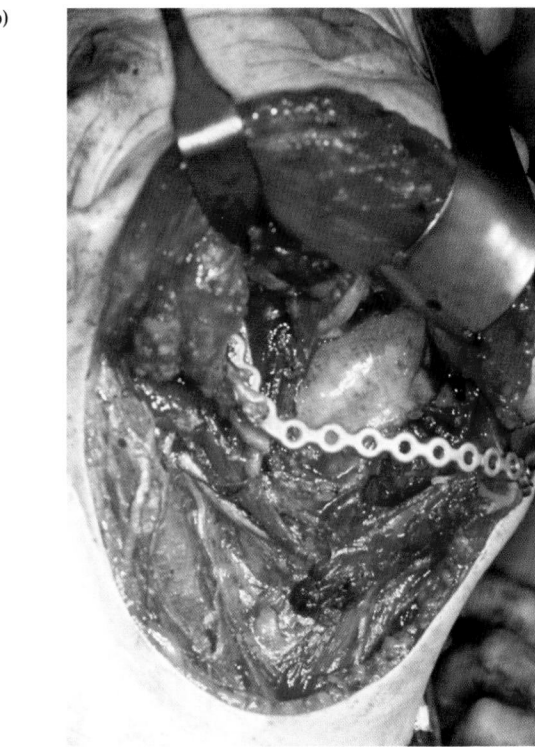

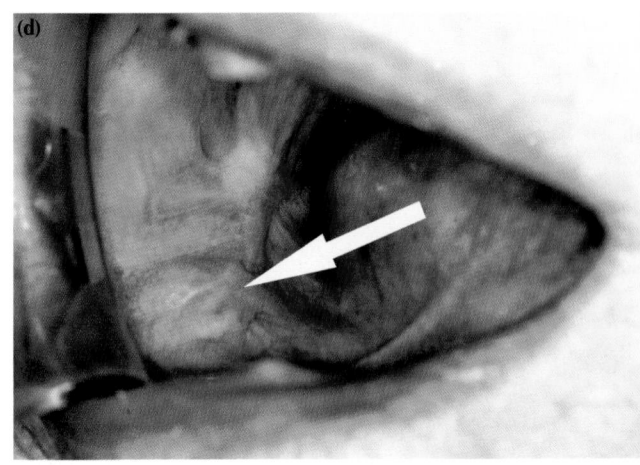

Figure 46.23 (a) Squamous cell carcinoma of the right mandibular alveolus. (b) Resection of the right mandible with reconstruction plate. (c) Vascularised (deep circumflex iliac artery) iliac crest (arrow) bone graft. (d) Right mandible with epithelialised abdominal muscle (arrow).

extensive tumours involving the floor of the maxillary sinus require wider access by a Weber–Ferguson incision (Fig. 46.24). If the preoperative investigations demonstrate extension of the disease into the pterygoid space or the infratemporal fossa, the prognosis is poor as surgical clearance is difficult if not impossible. Tumour extending into the orbit requires simultaneous orbital exenteration or even a combined neurosurgical resection. The vascularised iliac crest graft is the method of choice for immediate maxillary reconstruction although the fibula provides adequate bony replacement to maintain facial contour.

Microvascular free tissue transfer remains the method of choice for the management of defects in the oropharynx (Table 46.3). Free flaps are superior reconstructive options to pedicled or local flaps, which may be used for salvage procedures or recurrent disease. Each 'free' flap has a principal blood supply and a concomitant venous drainage. The flaps can be tailored to the defect to include skin, fascia, bone and muscle. The techniques of free tissue transfer demand specialist training and a microscope to connect blood vessels in the neck after neck dissection, e.g. facial artery to the prepared artery attached to the flap. The vascular anatomy of microvascular free flaps is highlighted in Table 46.4.

OROPHARYNX

Tumours of the oropharynx are frequently not amenable to surgery because of the morbid nature of the resection – small and intermediate (T1, T2) tongue base tumours may necessitate total glossectomy to achieve adequate clearance at the root of the tongue. Tumours of the soft palate and tonsil, however, can be managed with either primary surgery in continuity with neck dissection or primary radiotherapy. Subsequent defects of the

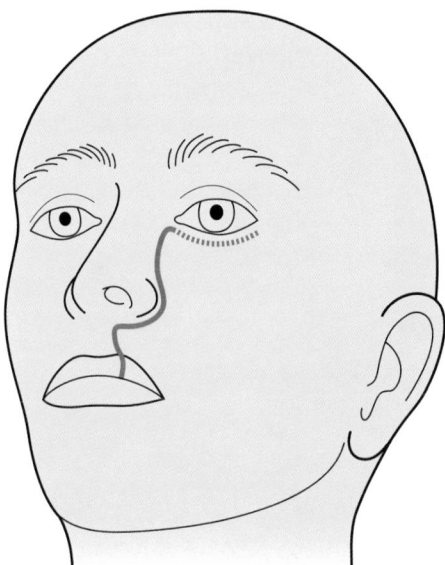

Figure 46.24 Weber–Ferguson incision for maxillectomy (lower eyelid extension is rarely required).

tonsillar area can be managed with a forearm flap. Defects of the soft palate, including total soft palate reconstruction, are best managed with a combined reconstruction consisting of a superiorly based pharyngeal flap to line the nasal surface and a forearm flap for the oral surface of the new soft palate. Chemoradiotherapy is now increasingly used to manage tumours of the oropharynx in which organ preservation, but not necessarily function, is the goal. In patients with large-volume neck

Table 46.3 Primary reconstructive options in oropharyngeal cancer

Anatomical site	Microvascular free flap	Alternative flaps
Floor of mouth	Forearm	Nasolabial flaps (bilateral)
Lateral tongue	Forearm	Platysma skin flap
Total tongue/glossectomy	Rectus abdominus	Pectoralis major
Buccal mucosa	Forearm	Temporalis muscle
Mandible		
Dentate	Iliac crest	Fibula
Edentulous	Fibula	Reconstruction plate and pectoralis major
Maxilla		
Low-level/hard palate	Temporalis muscle	Forearm
High	Iliac crest	Fibula
Soft palate/tonsil	Forearm	Temporalis muscle, galeal flap, pectoralis major
Tongue base	Forearm	Pectoralis major

Table 46.4 Microvascular 'free' flaps in oropharyngeal reconstruction

Flap	Blood supply	Common variants
Forearm	Radial artery	Skin only; fascia only
Composite forearm	Radial artery	Skin and bone (radius)
Anterolateral thigh	Perforator vessels of the profunda femoris artery	Skin only; skin and muscle
Rectus abdominus	Deep inferior epigastric artery	Skin and muscle; muscle only
Fibula	Peroneal artery	Bone and skin; bone only; bone and fascia/fat
Ilium	Deep circumflex iliac artery	Bone only; bone and muscle; bone, muscle and skin
Scapula	Subscapular artery	Bone and skin; bone and muscle

disease, e.g. N2 and N3, a combined modality of neck dissection followed by chemoradiotherapy to manage the tumour at the primary site and residual neck disease is the optimum strategy.

Chemotherapy

The role of chemotherapy has evolved over the last 20–30 years. It was initially reserved for treatment of recurrent and incurable disease, often using single-agent therapy. Combination chemotherapy, particularly platinum agents and 5-fluorouracil, is now more effective in controlling recurrent and incurable disease. However, combination chemotherapy is associated with more severe side-effects and a balance needs to be reached between efficacy, palliation and quality of life.

Chemotherapy also now has an important role in the treatment of locally advanced and previously untreated oropharyngeal carcinoma. There is compelling evidence that tumours of the tongue base may best be managed with primary chemoradiotherapy rather than radical surgery. The addition of chemotherapy with radiotherapy does, however, increase the morbidity and mortality rates. Patients who are frail or who have significant medical comorbidity may not tolerate the regime.

Chemoradiotherapy has been shown to improve survival in patients whose tumours are deemed unresectable, although organ preservation, i.e. swallowing and speech, is not always sustained.

There is good evidence for the superiority of chemoradiotherapy over radiotherapy alone; however, chemoradiotherapy is rarely effective in large-volume disease.

Management of the neck

The management of the cervical lymph nodes is highly dependent on the planned treatment of the primary tumour. When surgery is deemed appropriate for the primary tumour, simultaneous neck dissection should be considered. If radiotherapy is preferred, treatment to the neck should be contemplated, particularly when there is a high risk of occult metastases, e.g. tongue.

The clinically node-negative neck

The cervical lymph nodes contain occult metastases in up to 30% of patients. This is particularly significant with patients presenting with primary carcinomas of the tongue and, to a lesser extent, floor of mouth. Tumours arising in the buccal mucosa and mandibular alveolus are less likely to have occult metastasis. Nevertheless, increasing evidence exists that active treatment of cervical lymph nodes in the absence of obvious disease is considered good practice. Patients with carcinoma of the lateral tongue, floor of mouth and mandibular alveolus are best managed by supraomohyoid neck dissection (surgical removal of lymph node levels I, II and III in continuity with the primary tumour) (Fig. 46.25).

(a)

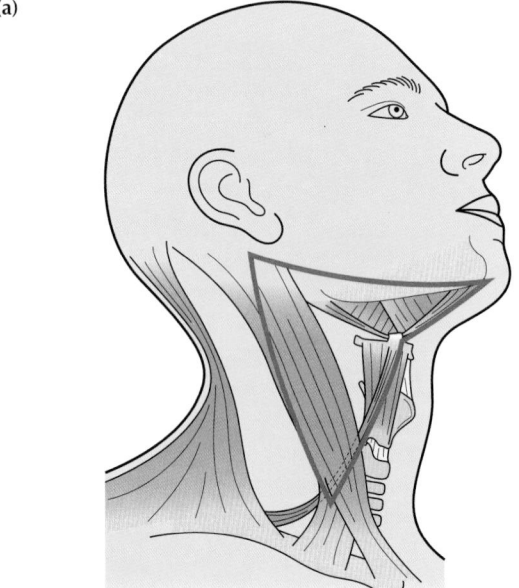

(c)

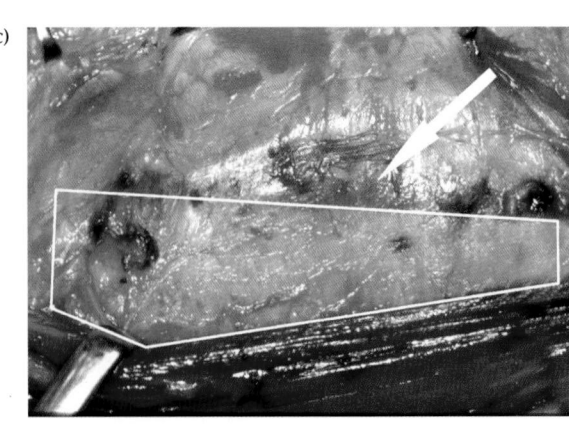

(b)

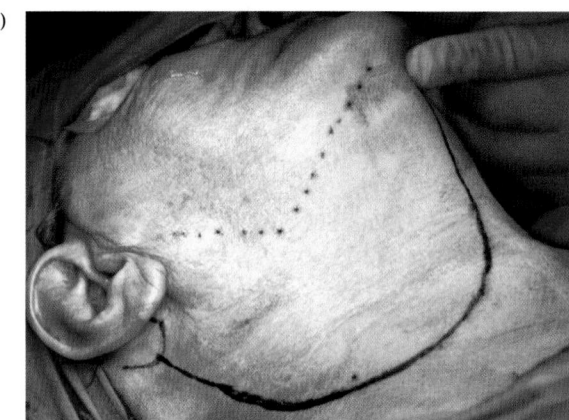

(d)

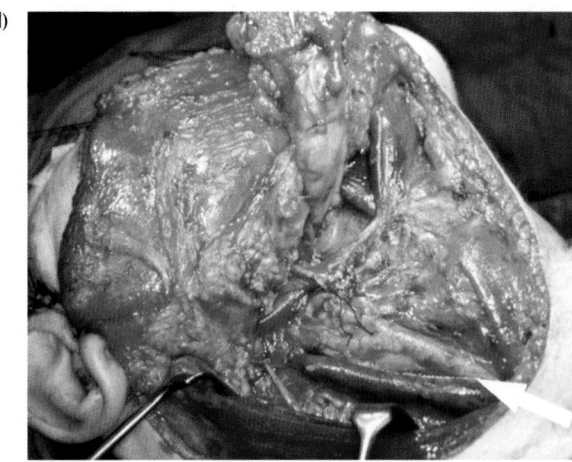

Figure 46.25 (a) Anatomical boundaries for supraomohyoid neck dissection (levels I, II, III). (b) Standard skin incision for neck dissection (solid line). (c) Deep cervical lymph nodes (box) posterolateral to the internal jugular vein (arrow). (d) Completed supraomohyoid neck dissection revealing great vessels of the neck (arrow).

(a)

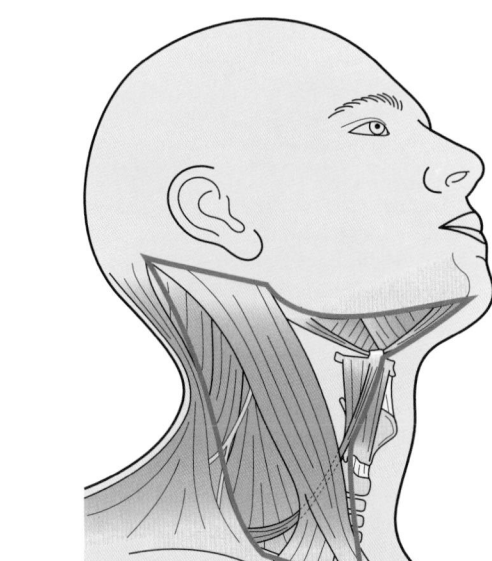

(b)

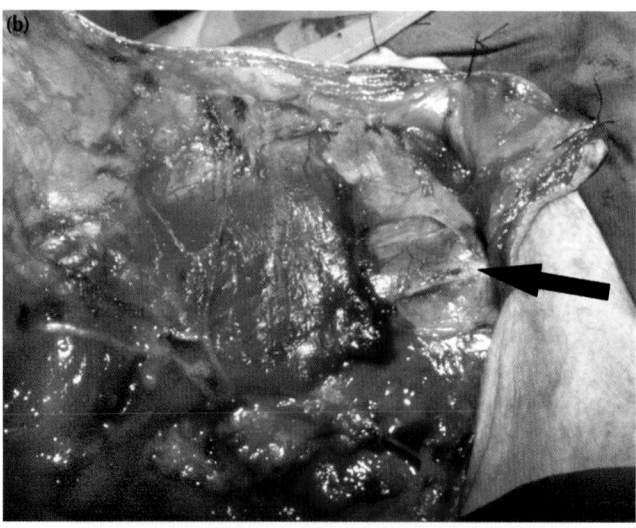

(c)

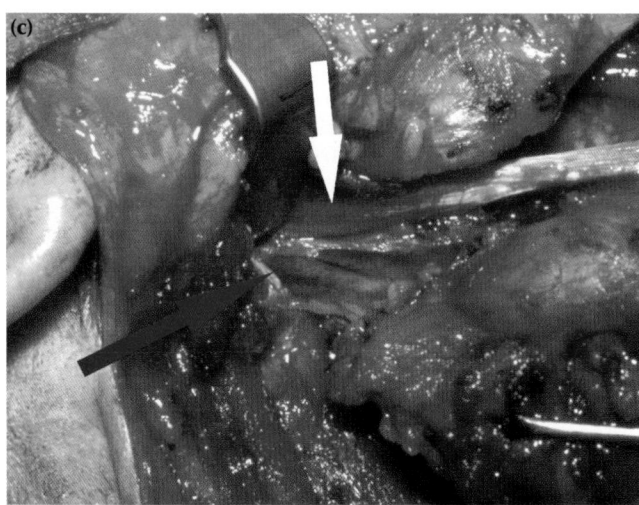

(d)

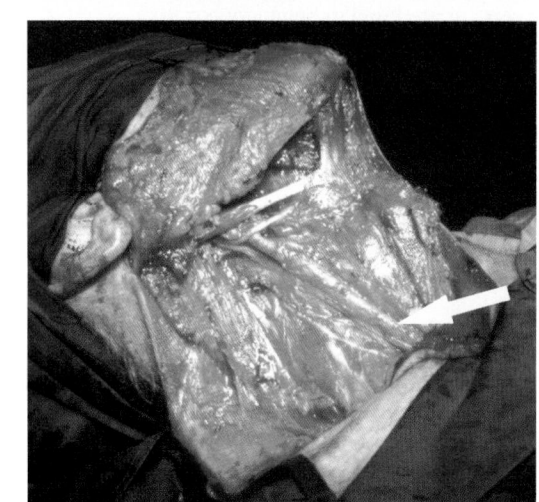

Figure 46.26 (a) Anatomical boundaries for radical neck dissection. (b) Lower end of the internal jugular vein exposed (arrow) by transection of the sternomastoid muscle. (c) Upper end of the internal jugular vein (blue arrow) isolated beneath digastric muscle (white arrow). (d) Appearance after radical neck dissection, revealing the common carotid artery system (arrow).

Good evidence exists that carcinoma of the tongue can produce occult cervical metastasis directly to lymph node level IV. Consequently, the extended supraomohyoid neck dissection removing lymph node levels I, II, III and IV is indicated for patients with carcinoma of the tongue with N0 neck disease. Selective neck dissection is regarded as a staging as much as a therapeutic procedure. Patients who have two or more positive nodes or evidence of extracapsular spread should be managed with postoperative radiotherapy to the neck and the primary site.

Elective external beam radiotherapy is an alternative when radiotherapy is planned for the primary site.

The clinically node-positive neck

The presence of an isolated ipsilateral cytologically positive lymph node of < 3 cm is now considered best managed by selective supraomohyoid neck dissection. There is good evidence that radical or modified radical neck dissection is not required for patients with N1 neck disease associated with oropharyngeal cancer.

N2a and N2b disease

Radical or modified radical neck dissection (Fig. 46.26), often followed by postoperative radiotherapy, is appropriate to control neck disease. Patients unfit for surgery can be offered external beam radiotherapy palliation.

N2c disease

Patients with mouth cancer presenting with bilateral nodes often have a large, inoperable, primary tumour. Bilateral neck dissection can be undertaken although morbidity is high. One internal jugular vein needs to be spared, usually on the side that is less involved with disease. Postoperative radiotherapy is indicated if there is multiple node involvement or extracapsular spread. Postoperative neck oedema and facial congestion occurs and may take months to resolve.

N3 disease

In N3 disease there is extensive involvement of the neck, often with fixation to the overlying skin. This is associated with advanced primary disease. Radical neck dissection may be feasible in such circumstances but strong consideration should be given to radiotherapy if there is evidence of tumour involving the internal carotid artery or the skull base.

The different types of neck dissection and their indications are summarised in Table 46.5.

COMPLICATIONS

Notwithstanding the general complications of major surgery, complications specifically associated with the treatment of oropharyngeal cancer are speech deficiencies, especially with resection of the anterior floor of the mouth and tongue; swallowing dysfunction and aspiration, especially after oropharyngeal resection; neurological injury, e.g. lingual nerve, hypoglossal nerve palsy; wound breakdown and cervical fistula formation; failure of internal fixation/reconstruction plates; failure of microvascular anastomosis; and flap failure. Other complications that may occur are listed in Summary box 46.5.

Summary box 46.5

Complications of treatment for oropharyngeal cancer

Surgical
- Accessory nerve palsy – shoulder dysfunction and pain
- Soft-tissue oedema, especially bilateral neck dissection
- Phrenic nerve injury
- Thoracic duct injury
- Cranial nerve injury
- Rupture of the carotid artery

Radiotherapy
- Osteoradionecrosis of the mandible
- Hypothyroidism
- Atherosclerosis of the carotid artery
- Neck and shoulder dysfunction
- Trismus
- Xerostomia
- Visual impairment
- Radiation neuritis

Chemotherapy
- Nausea and vomiting
- Diarrhoea
- Stomatitis
- Gastrointestinal upset
- Renal toxicity
- Leucopenia and thrombocytopenia

Patients undergoing treatment for oropharyngeal cancer frequently develop severe functional problems. The size and location of the tumour will dictate the extent of resection and the sacrifice of important structures.

Loss of tongue and floor of mouth musculature and the removal of bone and associated muscle attachments together with the sacrifice of sensory and motor cranial nerves all greatly affect not only appearance but also speech, swallowing and nutritional status. Psychological disturbance is universal in patients undergoing major head and neck cancer surgery and radiotherapy.

The techniques of immediate reconstruction, particularly with microvascular flaps, minimise the complications and side-effects but many patients are nevertheless radically changed for the remainder of their lives. Patients undergoing 'salvage' surgery following primary radiotherapy frequently undergo delayed wound healing, cervical fistula formation and, occasionally, carotid artery blowout/rupture. Skin anaesthesia associated with scar contracture creates additional problems, particular with neck mobility and trismus.

POST-TREATMENT MANAGEMENT

Patients with oropharyngeal cancer need to be followed up regularly not only to detect possible recurrence, but also to manage the morbidity associated with treatment. In total, 70% of recurrences occur in the first 12 months following treatment and 90% in the first 2 years. Patients who survive for 5 years are cured and discharged. Recurrence after extensive surgery and radiotherapy is frequently beyond any further treatment and palliative care is a logical pathway.

OUTCOME AND PROGNOSIS

Survival after oropharyngeal cancer is directly related to:

- the size of the primary tumour (T stage);
- the evidence of neck node metastasis (N stage);
- concomitant medical problems, e.g. cardiorespiratory disease.

Patients with large primary tumours are more likely to develop cervical node metastasis. Cervical node metastasis, particularly with extracapsular spread, is the most significant factor in determining prognosis for oropharyngeal cancer. The overall 5-year survival rates are shown in Table 46.6.

Supportive treatment is important for patients with oropharyngeal cancer, particularly in the form of speech and language support and dietetic and psychological input. Smoking

Table 46.5 Neck dissection in oropharyngeal cancer

Type of neck dissection	Lymph node levels removed	Indication
Selective		
Supraomohyoid	I–III	N0; N1; neck access for microsurgery
Extended supraomohyoid neck dissection	I–IV	Oral tongue cancer with N0 neck nodes; N1
Radical		
Full	I–V	N2; N3; neck recurrence after radiotherapy
Modified radical neck dissection	I–V, with preservation of internal jugular vein, accessory nerve and/or sternomastoid muscle	Involvement of neck skin; recurrence after selective neck dissection

cessation and a drastic reduction in alcohol intake reduces the risk of developing further metachronous carcinomas in the aerodigestive tract.

Table 46.6 Five-year survival rates for oropharyngeal cancer

Stage at presentation	Survival rate (%)
I	80–90
II	65–75
III	40–50
IV	30

FURTHER READING

Avery, B.S. (1998) Neck dissections. In: Langdon, J.D. and Patel, M.F. (eds). *Operative Maxillofacial Surgery.* Chapman & Hall, London, 295–302.

Brown, A.E. (1998) Reconstructive surgery: free flaps without bone. In: Langdon, J.D. and Patel, M.F. (eds). *Operative Maxillofacial Surgery.* Chapman & Hall, London, 125–39.

Langdon, J.D. and Henck, J.M. (1995) *Malignant Tumours of the Mouth, Jaws and Salivary Glands.* Arnold, London.

McGregor, A. and McGregor, F.M. (1986) *Cancer of the Face and Mouth.* Churchill Livingstone, Edinburgh.

Ord, R.A. (1998) Local resection and local reconstruction of oral carcinomas and jaw resection. In: Langdon, J.D. and Patel, M.F. (eds). *Operative Maxillofacial Surgery.* Chapman & Hall, London, 273–94.

Soutar, D.S. and Tiwari, R. (1994) *Excision and Reconstruction Head and Neck Cancer.* Churchill Livingstone, Edinburgh.

Urken, M.L., Cheney, M.L., Sullivan, M. and Biller, H.F. (1995) *Atlas of Regional and Free Flaps for Head and Neck Reconstruction.* Raven Press, New York.

Vaughan, E.D. (1998) Reconstructive surgery: free flaps with bone. In: Langdon, J.D. and Patel, M.F. (eds). *Operative Maxillofacial Surgery.* Chapman & Hall, London, 141–9.

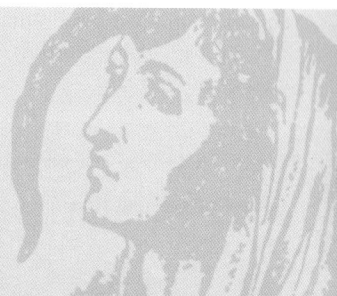

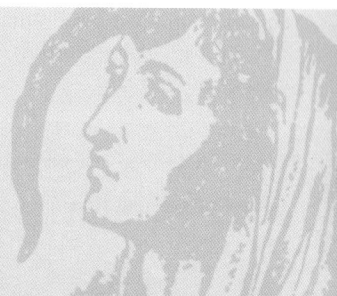

Disorders of the salivary glands

CHAPTER
47

LEARNING OBJECTIVES

To understand:
- The surgical anatomy of the salivary glands
- The presentation, pathology and investigation of salivary gland disease

- The medical and surgical treatment of stones, infections and tumours that affect salivary glands

---

There are four main salivary glands, two submandibular glands and two parotid glands. In addition, there are multiple minor salivary glands.

MINOR SALIVARY GLANDS

Anatomy

The mucosa of the oral cavity contains approximately 450 minor salivary glands. They are distributed in the mucosa of the lips, cheeks, palate, floor of the mouth and retromolar area. These minor salivary glands also appear in other areas of the upper aerodigestive tract including the oropharynx, larynx and trachea as well as the sinuses. They have a histological structure similar to that of mucous-secreting major salivary glands. Overall, they contribute to 10% of the total salivary volume (Summary box 47.1).

Summary box 47.1

Anatomy of salivary glands

- Two submandibular glands
- Two parotid glands
- Two sublingual glands
- Approximately 450 minor salivary glands

Common disorders of minor salivary glands

Cysts

Extravasation cysts are common and result from trauma to the overlying mucosa. They usually affect minor salivary glands within the lower lip, producing a variable swelling that is painless and usually, but not always, translucent (Fig. 47.1). Some resolve spontaneously, but most require formal surgical excision that includes the overlying mucosa and the underlying minor salivary gland. Recurrence is rare.

Tumours

Few tumours show more diversity in histological appearance and anatomical site than those that arise from mucous glands of the

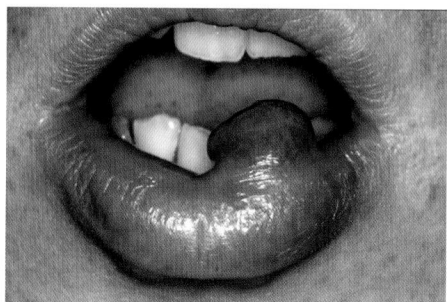

Figure 47.1 Mucous retention cyst. A translucent swelling on the lower lip is typical.

upper aerodigestive tract. Tumours of minor salivary glands are histologically similar to those of major glands; however, up to 90% of minor salivary gland tumours are malignant. Although tumours of minor salivary gland origin occur anywhere in the upper aerodigestive tract, common sites for tumour formation include the upper lip, palate and retromolar regions. Less common sites for minor salivary gland tumours include the nasal and pharyngeal cavities. Minor salivary gland tumours have also been reported in the paranasal sinuses and throughout the pharynx. These tumours arise in submucosal seromucous glands that are found throughout the upper aerodigestive tract. Very rarely, a muco-epidermoid carcinoma can present as an intraosseous tumour of the mandible.

Benign minor salivary gland tumours present as painless, firm, slow-growing swellings. Overlying ulceration is extremely rare. Minor salivary gland tumours of the upper lip are managed by excision to include the overlying mucosa, with primary closure (Fig. 47.2a–c).

Benign tumours of the palate, less than 1 cm in diameter, can be managed by excisional biopsy, and the defect is allowed to heal by secondary intention (Fig. 47.3a–d). Where tumours of the palate are greater than 1 cm in diameter, incisional biopsy is recommended to establish a diagnosis prior to formal excision.

Malignant minor salivary gland tumours are rare. They have a firm consistency, and the overlying mucosa may have a varied

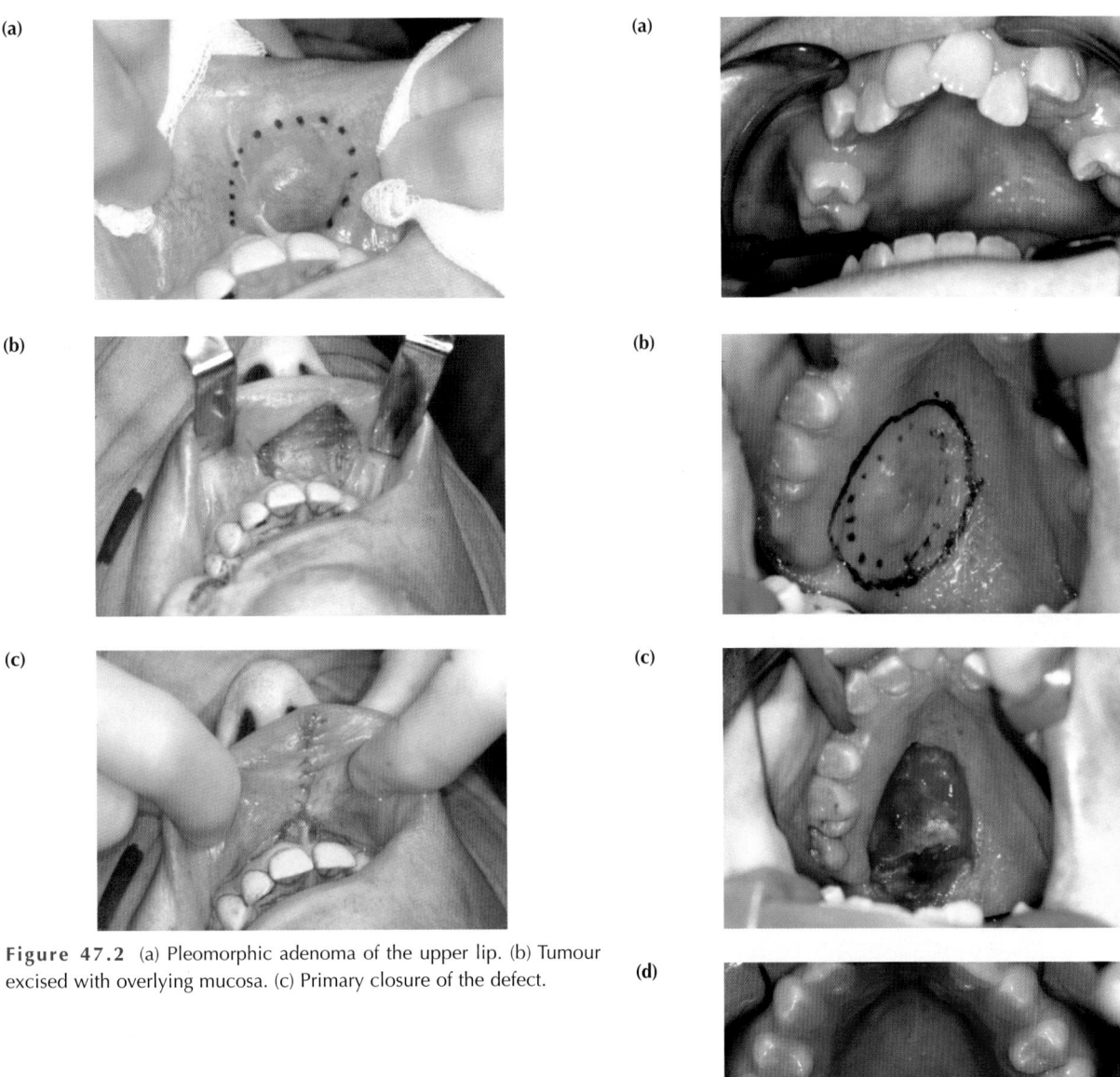

(a)

(b)

(c)

Figure 47.2 (a) Pleomorphic adenoma of the upper lip. (b) Tumour excised with overlying mucosa. (c) Primary closure of the defect.

(a)

(b)

(c)

(d)

Figure 47.3 (a) Pleomorphic adenoma in the right palate in a 12-year-old girl. (b) Tumour marked out with adequate margins including the overlying mucosa. (c) The subsequent defect. (d) Healing by secondary intention 3 years after surgery.

discolouration from pink to blue or black (Fig. 47.4). The tumour may become necrotic with ulceration as a late presentation.

Malignant minor salivary gland tumours of the palate are managed by wide excision which may involve partial or total maxillectomy. The subsequent defect can be managed by either prosthetic obturation or immediate reconstruction. Various microvascular flaps have been designed to reconstruct maxillectomy defects including radial forearm flap, fibular flap, rectus abdominus, latissimus dorsi and the vascularised iliac crest graft (Fig. 47.5a and b).

THE SUBLINGUAL GLANDS

Anatomy

The sublingual glands are a paired set of minor salivary glands lying in the anterior part of the floor of mouth between the mucous membrane, the mylohyoid muscle and the body of the mandible close to the mental symphysis. Each gland has numerous excretory ducts that open either directly into the oral cavity or indirectly via ducts that drain into the submandibular duct (Summary box 47.2).

Summary box 47.2

Sublingual glands

- Problems are rare
- Minor mucous retention cysts may need surgery
- Plunging ranula is a retention cyst that tunnels deep
- Nearly all tumours are malignant

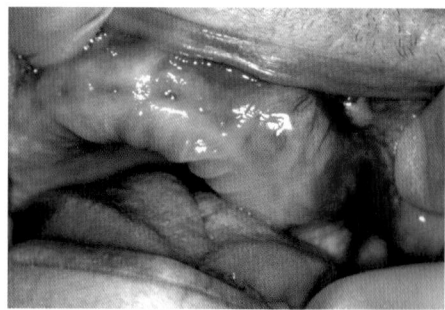

Figure 47.4 Adenoid cystic carcinoma of the left maxillary alveolus.

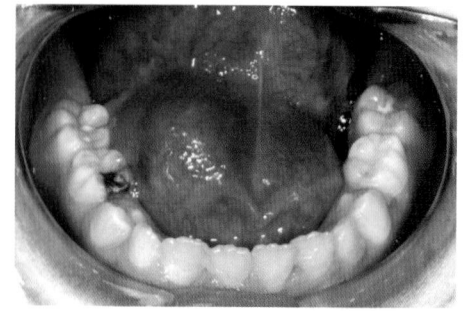

Figure 47.6 Large ranula affecting the floor of the mouth.

(a)

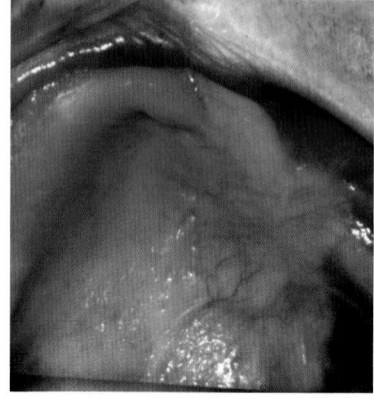

(b)

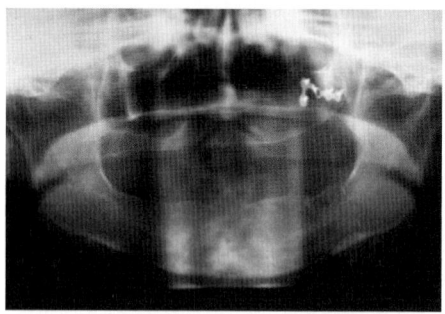

Figure 47.5 (a) Postoperative appearance following left maxillectomy and immediate reconstruction with a vascularised iliac crest graft and abdominal wall musculature (epithelialised). (b) Postoperative radiographic appearance of a reconstructed left maxilla with internal fixation.

Common disorders of the sublingual glands

Cysts

Minor mucous retention cysts develop in the floor of the mouth either from an obstructed minor salivary gland or from the sublingual salivary gland. The term 'ranula' should be applied only to a mucous extravasation cyst that arises from a sublingual gland. It produces a characteristic translucent swelling that takes on the appearance of a 'frog's belly' (ranula) (Fig. 47.6). A ranula can resolve spontaneously, but many also require formal surgical excision of the cyst and the affected sublingual gland. Incision and drainage, however tempting, usually results in recurrence.

Ranula **is derived from 'rana', the Latin for frog.**

Plunging ranula

Plunging ranula is a rare form of mucous retention cyst that can arise from both sublingual and submandibular salivary glands. Mucus collects within the cyst, which perforates through the mylohyoid muscle diaphragm to enter the neck. Patients present with a dumbbell-shaped swelling that is soft, fluctuant and painless in the submandibular or submental region of the neck (Fig. 47.7a and b). Diagnosis is made on ultrasound or magnetic resonance imaging (MRI) examination. Excision is usually performed via a cervical approach removing the cyst and both the submandibular and sublingual glands. Smaller plunging ranulas can be treated successfully by transoral sublingual gland excision with or without marsupialisation.

Tumours

Tumours involving the sublingual gland are extremely rare and are usually (85%) malignant. They present as a hard or firm painless swelling in the floor of the mouth Treatment requires wide excision involving the overlying mucosa and simultaneous neck dissection. Immediate reconstruction of the intraoral defect is recommended using, for example, a radial artery forearm flap.

(a)

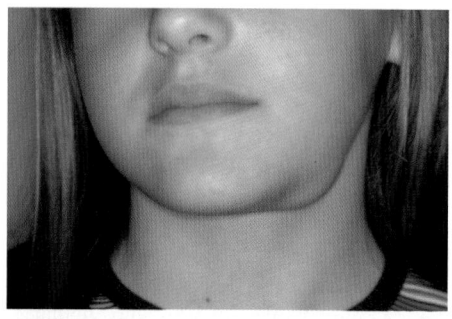

(b)

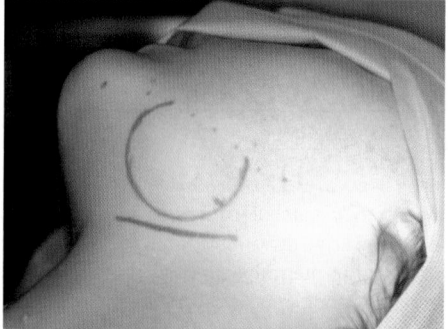

Figure 47.7 Plunging ranula in the left submandibular region.

THE SUBMANDIBULAR GLANDS

Anatomy

The submandibular glands are paired salivary glands that lie below the mandible on either side. They consist of a larger superficial and a smaller deep lobe that are continuous around the posterior border of the mylohyoid muscle. Important anatomical relations include the anterior facial vein running over the surface of the gland and the facial artery. The deep part of the gland lies on the hyoglossus muscle closely related to the lingual nerve and inferior to the hypoglossal nerve. The gland is surrounded by a well-defined capsule that is derived from the deep cervical fascia which splits to enclose it. The gland is drained by a single submandibular duct (Wharton's duct) that emerges from its deep surface and runs in the space between the hyoglossus and mylohyoid muscles. It drains into the anterior floor of the mouth at the sublingual papilla. There are several lymph nodes immediately adjacent and sometimes within the superficial part of the gland (Summary box 47.3).

> **Summary box 47.3**
>
> **Important anatomical relationships of the submandibular glands**
>
> - Lingual nerve
> - Hypoglossal nerve
> - Anterior facial vein
> - Facial artery
> - Marginal mandibular branch of the facial nerve

Ectopic/aberrant salivary gland tissue

The most common ectopic salivary tissue is the Stafne bone cyst. This presents as an asymptomatic, clearly demarcated radiolucency of the angle of the mandible, characteristically below the inferior dental neurovascular bundle (Fig. 47.8). It is formed by invagination into the bone on the lingual aspect of the mandible of an ectopic lobe of the juxtaposed submandibular gland. No treatment is required.

Inflammatory disorders of the submandibular gland

Inflammation of the submandibular gland is termed sialadenitis. Submandibular sialadenitis may be acute, chronic or acute on chronic.

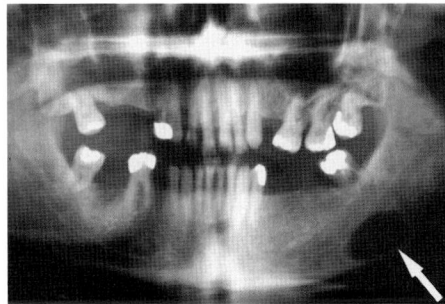

Figure 47.8 Plain radiographic appearance of a Stafne bone cyst.

Thomas Wharton, ?1616–1673, Physician, St. Thomas's Hospital, London, England, described the submandibular duct in 1656.
Edward C. Stafne, 1894–1981, Dental Surgeon, The Mayo Clinic, Rochester, MN, USA, described these cysts in 1942.

Common causes are:

1. Acute submandibular sialadenitis
   (a) *Viral.* The paramyxovirus (mumps) is a viral illness of the salivary glands that usually produces parotitis. The submandibular glands are occasionally involved, causing painful tender swollen glands. Other viral infections of the submandibular gland are extremely rare.
   (b) *Bacterial.* Bacterial sialadenitis is more common than viral sialadenitis and occurs secondary to obstruction. Following infection and despite control of acute symptoms with antibiotics, the gland frequently becomes chronically inflamed and requires formal excision.
2. Chronic submandibular sialadenitis.

Obstruction and trauma

The most common cause of obstruction within the submandibular gland is stone formation (sialothiasis) within the gland and its associated duct system. Eighty per cent of all salivary stones occur in the submandibular glands because their secretions are highly viscous. Eighty per cent of submandibular stones are radio-opaque and can be identified on plain radiography (Fig. 47.9).

Clinical symptoms

Patients usually present with acute painful swelling in the region of the submandibular gland, precipitated by eating (Fig. 47.10). The swelling occurs rapidly and often resolves spontaneously over 1–2 hours after the meal is completed. This classical picture occurs when the stone causes complete obstruction, usually at the opening of the submandibular duct. More frequently, the stone causes only partial obstruction when it lies within the hilum of the gland or within the duct in the floor of the mouth. In such circumstances, symptoms are more infrequent, producing minimal discomfort and swelling, not confined to mealtimes. Clinical examination reveals an enlarged firm submandibular gland, tender on bimanual examination. Pus may be visible, draining from

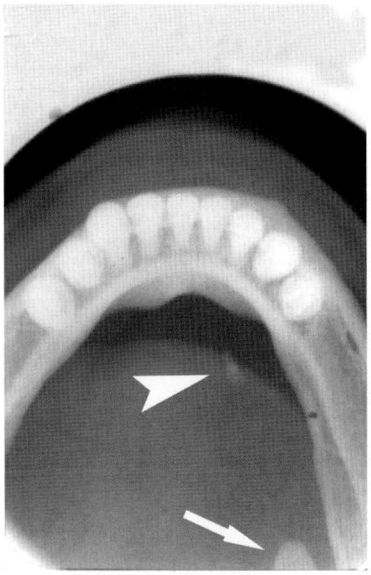

Figure 47.9 Lower occlusal X-ray highlighting a radio-opaque submandibular duct stone (arrowhead). Note the larger stone posteriorly located in the hilum of the gland (arrow).

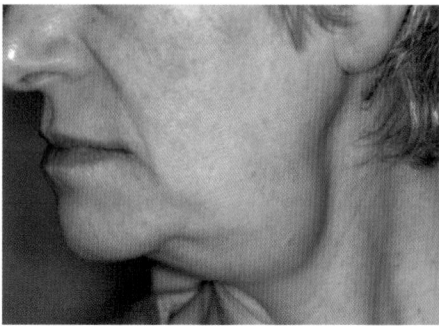

Figure 47.10 Acute left submandibular sialadenitis.

the sublingual papilla (Fig. 47.11), the consequence of chronic and non-specific bacterial infection.

Management

If the stone is lying within the submandibular duct in the floor of the mouth anterior to the point at which the duct crosses the lingual nerve (second molar region), the stone can be removed by incising longitudinally over the duct. Once the stone has been delivered, the wall of the duct should be left open to promote free drainage of saliva. Suturing the duct will lead to stricture formation and the recurrence of obstructive symptoms. Where the stone is proximal to the lingual nerve, i.e. at the hilum of the gland, stone retrieval via an intraoral approach should be avoided as there is a high risk of damage to the lingual nerve during exploration in the posterior lingual gutter. Treatment is by simultaneous submandibular gland excision and removal of the stone and ligation of the submandibular duct under direct vision.

Other causes of submandibular duct obstruction include external pressure, particularly trauma to the floor of the mouth. This may result from an overextended flange on a lower denture that impinges on the sublingual papilla and causes inflammation and subsequent stricture.

Submandibular gland excision

Submandibular gland excision is indicated for:

- sialadenitis;
- salivary tumours.

Excision of the submandibular gland involves four distinct phases:

Incision and exposure of gland

Surgery is usually performed under endotracheal general anaesthesia with moderate neck extension and the chin rotated to the

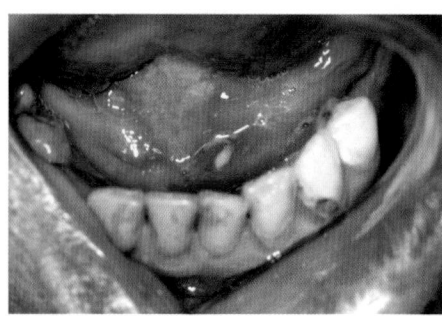

Figure 47.11 Acute suppurative submandibular sialadenitis. There is pus extruding from the left sublingual papilla.

opposite side. The incision should be marked at least 3–4 cm below the lower border of the mandible to avoid damage to the marginal mandibular branch of the facial nerve (Fig. 47.12a). The incision should be sited within the nearest skin crease and should be no more than 6 cm long. Infiltration with lidocaine with adrenaline is optional. Sharp dissection is performed down to the platysma muscle, which should be clearly identified to facilitate later closure (Fig. 47.12b). The muscle is incised and then retracted. The underlying investing layer of deep cervical fascia is then divided, and the marginal mandibular branch of the facial nerve that normally runs on the deep surface of the platysma muscle is preserved. Posteriorly, the incision approaches the angular tract where the deep cervical fascia splits to form the investing layer around the sternomastoid muscle. Superficial veins, including the anterior facial vein, require ligation.

Gland mobilisation

Deepening the incision divides the submandibular gland capsule. In inflammatory conditions, the submandibular gland is excised by intracapsular dissection, mobilising the gland by sharp dissection. For tumours of the submandibular gland, extracapsular dissection by suprahyoid neck dissection is performed.

The superficial lobe of the submandibular gland is first mobilised by retracting superiorly with Allis's forceps. As dissection proceeds, the posterior belly and anterior belly of the digastric muscle are identified. Dissection posteriorly identifies the facial artery (Fig. 47.13), which is divided to facilitate further mobilisation. The course of the facial artery is variable, sometimes penetrating the gland emerging on the upper border, and sometimes lying in a groove on the deeper aspect of the gland. The gland is further mobilised by blunt and sharp dissection. A

(a)

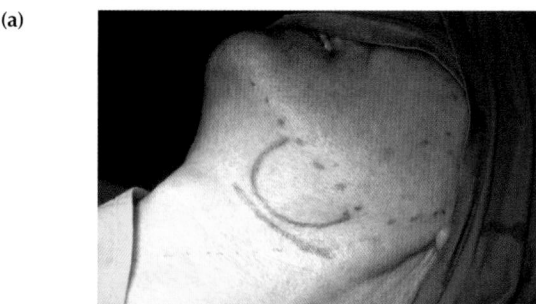

(b)

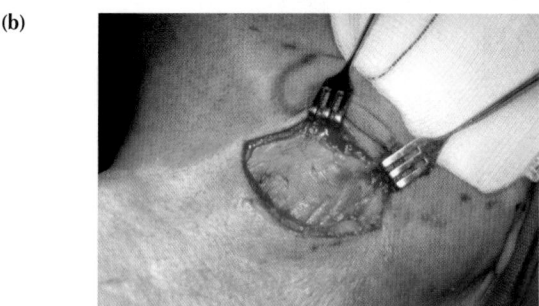

Figure 47.12 (a) Surface landmarks of submandibular gland excision. (b) Skin flaps elevated and platysma exposed.

Oscar Huntington Alis, **1836–1921, Surgeon, The Presbyterian Hospital, Philadelphia, PA, USA.**

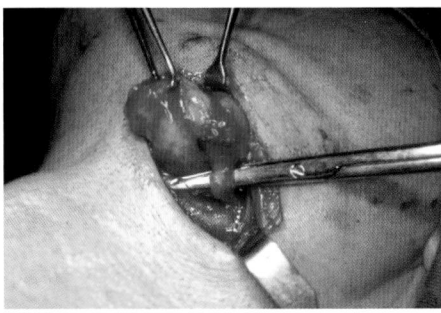

Figure 47.13 Submandibular gland mobilisation and exposure of the facial artery.

number of small arteries and veins are encountered, which require control with bipolar diathermy.

Dissection of the deep lobe and identification of the lingual nerve

An important landmark in submandibular gland dissection is the posterior border of the mylohyoid muscle. Once identified, it can be retracted forwards to reveal the deep lobe of the gland. Several veins are usually encountered, which need to be controlled with diathermy. The gland is then retracted inferiorly, invariably attached to the lingual nerve through parasympathetic secretor motor fibres. In the presence of chronic infection and subsequent fibrosis, identification of the lingual nerve on the deep aspect of the gland is sometimes difficult. It is imperative that the lingual nerve is formally identified prior to division of the parasympathetic fibres. The gland is then pedicled entirely on the submandibular duct, which, once identified, is ligated. The gland is delivered and sent for histological examination. The hypoglossal nerves lie deep to the submandibular capsule and should not be damaged during intracapsular dissection (Fig. 47.14).

Three cranial nerves are at risk during removal of the submandibular gland:

1 the marginal mandibular branch of the facial nerve;
2 the lingual nerve;
3 the hypoglossal nerve.

An adequate incision coupled with meticulous haemostasis allows the surgeon to identify these important structures during surgery.

Wound closure

Haemostasis is confirmed and a vacuum suction drain inserted. The wound is closed using a continuous resorbable suture to the

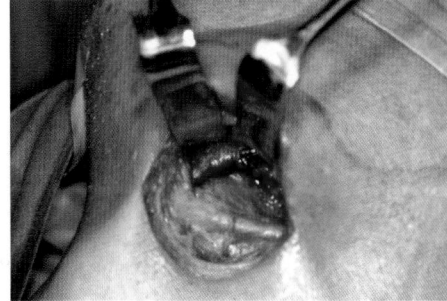

Figure 47.14 Bed of the submandibular triangle following submandibular gland removal, revealing the posterior edge of the mylohyoid muscle and the tendon of the digastric muscle.

platysma muscle, as the platysma muscle has a direct contribution to the depressor activity of the corner of the mouth. The skin may be closed with a subcuticular non-resorbable suture, removed 7 days after surgery. The drain remains for 24 hours.

Complications of submandibular gland excision

1 Haematoma;
2 wound infection;
3 marginal mandibular nerve injury;
4 lingual nerve injury;
5 hypoglossal nerve injury;
6 transection of the nerve to the mylohyoid muscle producing submental skin anaesthesia.

Tumours of the submandibular gland

Tumours of the submandibular gland are uncommon and usually present as a slow-growing, painless swelling within the submandibular triangle (Fig. 47.15). Only 50% of submandibular gland tumours are benign, in contrast to 80–90% of parotid gland tumours (Table 47.1). In many circumstances, the swelling cannot, on clinical examination, be differentiated from submandibular lymphadenopathy. Most salivary neoplasms, even malignant tumours, are often slow-growing, painless swellings. Unfortunately, pain is not a reliable indication of malignancy as benign tumours often present with pain in the affected gland, presumably due to capsular distension or outflow obstruction.

Clinical features of malignant salivary tumours

1 Facial nerve weakness;
2 rapid enlargement of the swelling;
3 induration and/or ulceration of the overlying skin;
4 cervical node enlargement.

Investigation

Computerised tomography (CT) and MRI scanning are the most helpful techniques for imaging tumours arising in the major salivary glands. The tumour is intrinsic to the gland, and its border can be imaged to highlight whether it is circumscribed and

Table 47.1 Salivary gland tumours – frequency and distribution

Type	Location	Frequency	Malignant
Major	Parotid	Common	10–20%
	Submandibular	Uncommon	50%
	Sublingual	Very rare	85%
Minor	Upper aerodigestive tract	Rare	90%

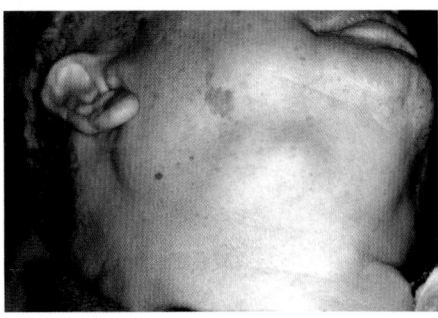

Figure 47.15 Benign tumour of the right submandibular gland.

probably benign or diffuse, invasive and probably malignant. The scan will highlight the relationship of the tumour to other anatomical structures, which is helpful in planning surgery.

Open surgical biopsy is contraindicated as this may seed the tumour into surrounding tissues, making it impossible to eradicate microscopic deposits of tumour cells.

Fine-needle aspiration biopsy is a safe alternative to open biopsy. There is evidence to suggest that, provided the needle gauge does not exceed 18G, there is no risk of seeding viable tumour cells. The role of fine-needle aspiration biopsy is, however, controversial as it rarely alters surgical management.

Management of submandibular gland tumours

As with all salivary gland tumours, surgical excision with a cuff of normal tissue is the goal. When the tumour is small and entirely encased within the submandibular gland parenchyma, straightforward intracapsular submandibular gland excision is appropriate. However, benign tumours that are large and project beyond the submandibular gland are best served by suprahyoid neck dissection, preserving the marginal mandibular branch of the facial nerve, lingual nerve and hypoglossal nerves. This entails a full clearance of the submandibular triangle, involving the development of a subplatysmal skin flap (Fig. 47.16a–e), dissection of periosteum along the lower border and inner aspect of the mandible, and delivery of the gland and tumour with a cuff of

normal tissue. In cases of overt malignancy, modified neck dissection or radical neck dissection is appropriate. This may necessitate sacrifice of the lingual and hypoglossal nerves if the tumour is adherent to the deep bed of the gland (Fig. 47.17a–d).

THE PAROTID GLAND

Anatomy

The parotid gland lies in a recess bounded by the ramus of the mandible, the base of the skull and the mastoid process. It lies on the carotid sheath and the XIth and XIIth cranial nerves and extends forward over the masseter muscle. The gland is enclosed in a sheath of dense deep cervical fascia. Its upper pole extends just below the zygoma and its lower pole into the neck.

Several important structures run through the parotid gland. These include:

1 branches of the facial nerve;
2 the terminal branch of the external carotid artery that divides into the maxillary artery and the superficial temporal artery;
3 the retromandibular vein;
4 intraparotid lymph nodes.

The gland is arbitrarily divided into deep and superficial lobes, separated by the facial nerve. Eighty per cent of the parotid gland

(a)

(b)

(c)

(d)

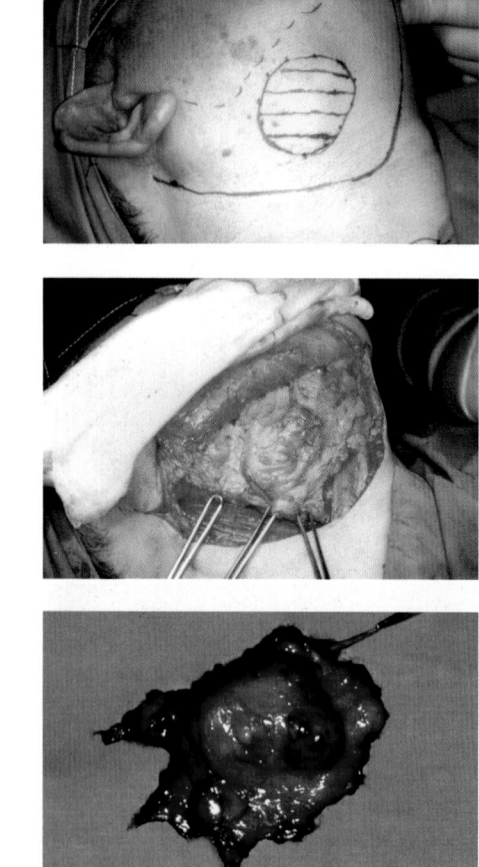

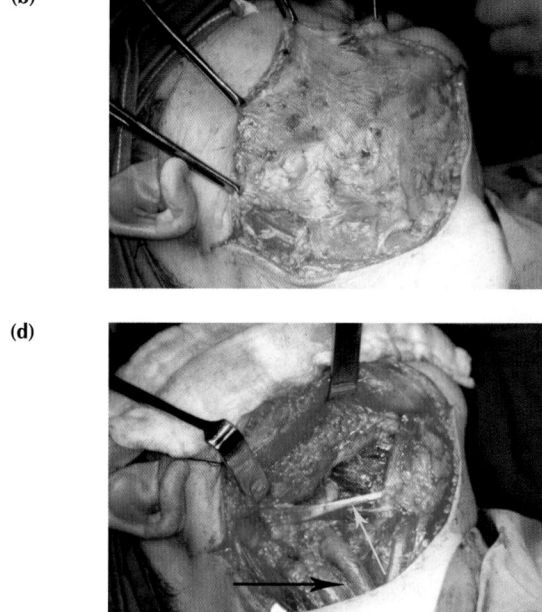

(e)

Figure 47.16 (a) Landmarks and incision for suprahyoid neck dissection to remove a large pleomorphic adenoma of the submandibular gland. (b) Skin flap raised at the subplatysmal level. (c) Mobilisation of the contents of the anterior triangle of the neck along the anterior border of the sternomastoid. (d) Suprahyoid neck dissection completed, revealing digastric tendon (yellow arrow) and great vessels (black arrow). (e) Specimen revealing tumour with a cuff of normal tissue with artery forceps attached to the submandibular duct.

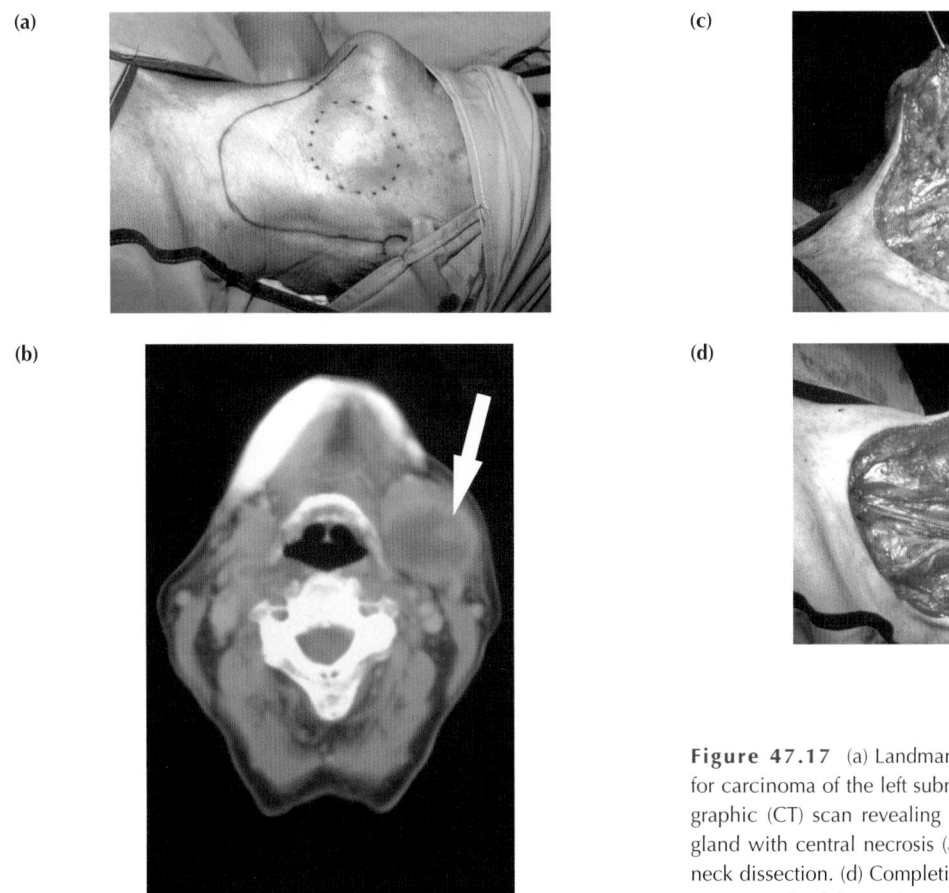

Figure 47.17 (a) Landmarks and incision for radical neck dissection for carcinoma of the left submandibular gland. (b) Computerised tomographic (CT) scan revealing a large tumour of the left submandibular gland with central necrosis (arrow). (c) Skin flap developed for radical neck dissection. (d) Completion of radical neck dissection revealing the great vessels of the neck (arrow).

lies superficial and 20% deep to the nerve entering. An accessory lobe is occasionally present.

Developmental disorders

Developmental disorders such as agenesis, duct atresia and congenital fistula are extremely rare.

Inflammatory disorders

Viral infections

Mumps is the most common cause of acute painful parotid swelling and predominantly affects children. It is spread via airborne droplets of infected saliva. The disease starts with a prodromal period of 1–2 days, during which the patient experiences fever, nausea and headache. This is followed by pain and swelling in one or both parotid glands. Parotid pain can be very severe and exacerbated by eating and drinking. Symptoms resolve within 5–10 days. The diagnosis is based on history and clinical examination: a recent contact with an infected patient with a painful parotid swelling is often sufficient to lead to a diagnosis. Atypical viral parotitis does occur and may present with predominantly unilateral swelling or even submandibular involvement. A single episode of infection confers lifelong immunity. Treatment of mumps is symptomatic with regular paracetamol and adequate oral fluid intake. Complications of orchitis, oophoritis, pancreatitis, sensorineural deafness and meningoencephalitis are rare, but are more likely to occur in adults.

Other viral agents that produce parotitis include Coxsackie A and B, parainfluenza 1 and 3, Echo and lymphocytic choriomeningitis.

Bacterial infections

Acute ascending bacterial sialadenitis is historically described in dehydrated elderly patients following major surgery. Reduced salivary flow secondary to dehydration results in ascending infection via the parotid duct into the parotid parenchyma. Acute bacterial parotitis is now more common with no obvious precipitating factors. The patient presents with a tender, painful parotid swelling that arises over several hours (Fig. 47.18). There is generalised malaise, pyrexia and occasional cervical lymphadenopathy.

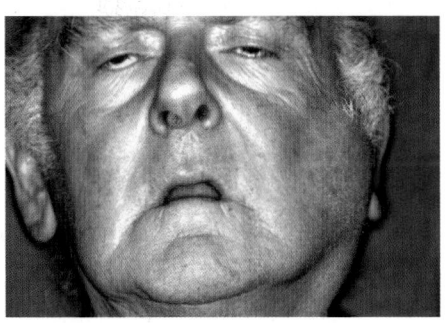

Figure 47.18 Acute left bacterial parotitis.

The pain is exacerbated by eating or drinking. The parotid swelling may be diffuse, but often localises to the lower pole of the gland. Intraoral examination may reveal pus exuding from the parotid gland papilla. The infecting organism is usually *Staphylococcus aureus* or *Streptococcus viridans*, and treatment is with appropriate intravenous antibiotics. If the gland becomes fluctuant, ultrasound may identify abscess formation within the gland that may require aspiration with a large-bore needle or formal drainage under general anaesthesia. In the latter procedure, the skin incision should be made low to avoid damage to the lower branch of the facial nerve. Blunt dissection using sinus forceps is preferred, and the cavity is opened to facilitate drainage. A drain is inserted and left *in situ* for 24–72 hours. Sialography is contraindicated during acute infection. Chronic bacterial sialadenitis is rare in the parotid gland.

Recurrent parotitis of childhood

Recurrent parotitis of childhood is a distinct clinical entity of unknown aetiology and variable prognosis. It is characterised by rapid swelling of one or both parotid glands, in which the symptoms are made worse by chewing and eating. Systemic upset with fever and malaise is variable. The symptoms usually last from 3 to 7 days, and are then followed by a quiescent period of weeks to several months. Children usually present between the ages of 3 and 6 years, although symptoms have been reported in infants as young as 4 months. The diagnosis is based on the characteristic history and can be confirmed by sialography. This shows a characteristic punctate sialectasis likened to a 'snowstorm' (Fig. 47.19). The condition usually responds to short courses of antibiotics although, if recurrence is frequent, prophylactic low-dose antibiotics may be required for several months or even years. Few children require formal parotidectomy. However, if the onset of symptoms is late, e.g. adolescence/early adulthood, fewer patients respond to conservative measures and may require total conservative parotidectomy.

Human immunodeficiency virus (HIV)-associated sialadenitis

Chronic parotitis in children is pathognomonic of HIV infection. The presentation of HIV-associated sialadenitis is very similar to

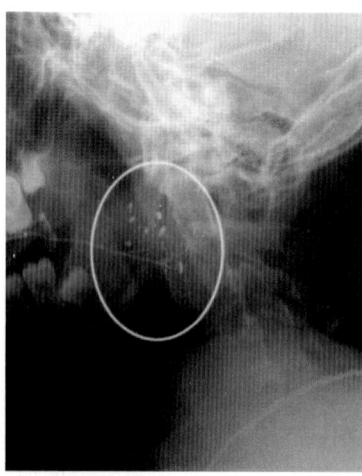

Figure 47.19 Characteristic 'snowstorm' appearance of recurrent parotitis of childhood (circled).

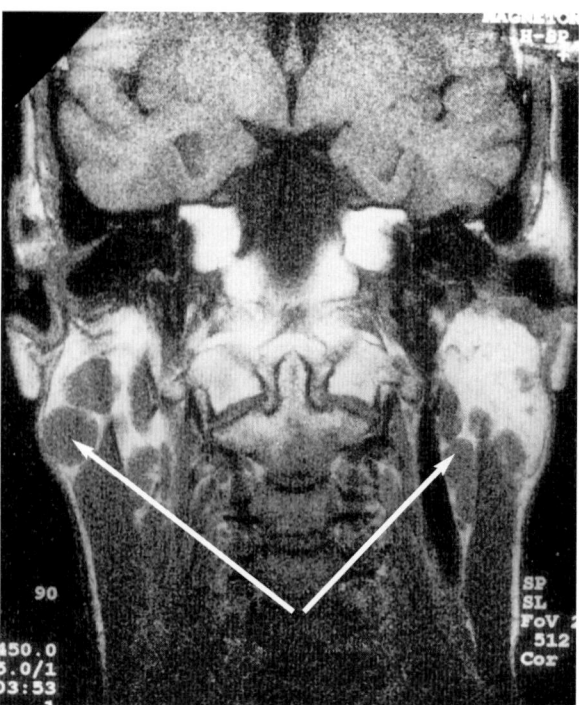

Figure 47.20 Magnetic resonance imaging (MRI) scan. Giant bilateral parotid cysts in human immunodeficiency virus (HIV) infection.

classical Sjögren's syndrome in adulthood. Although HIV-associated sialadenitis and Sjögren's syndrome are histologically similar, the former condition is usually associated with a negative autoantibody screen. Other presentations of salivary gland disease in HIV-positive patients include multiple parotid cysts, which cause gross parotid swelling and facial disfigurement. CT and MRI demonstrate the characteristic 'Swiss cheese' appearance of multiple large cystic lesions (Fig. 47.20). The glands are usually painless, although surgery may be indicated to improve the appearance.

Obstructive parotitis

There are several causes of obstructive parotitis, which produces intermittent painful swelling of the parotid gland, particularly at mealtimes.

Papillary obstruction

Obstructive parotitis is less common than obstructive submandibular sialadenitis but, nevertheless, can be caused by trauma to the parotid papilla through either an overextended upper denture flange or a fractured upper molar tooth. The subsequent inflammation and oedema obstructs salivary flow, particularly at mealtimes. The patient usually experiences rapid onset pain and swelling at mealtimes. If left untreated, progressive scarring and fibrosis in and around the parotid duct papilla will produce a permanent stenosis. Symptoms are unlikely to resolve unless a papillotomy is performed. This is a simple procedure performed under either local or general anaesthesia. The parotid duct is cannulated, and the distal parotid duct is laid open by

Henrik Samuel Conrad Sjögren, 1899–1986, Professor of Ophthalmology, Göthenburg, Sweden, described this condition in 1933.
A Swiss cheese is one with many holes in it.

incising longitudinally down onto the probe allowing free drainage of saliva.

Stone formation

Sialolithiasis is less common in the parotid gland (20%) than in the submandibular gland (80%). Parotid duct stones are usually radiolucent and rarely visible on plain radiography. They are frequently located at the confluence of the collecting ducts or located in the distal aspect of the parotid duct adjacent to the parotid papilla. Parotid gland sialography is usually required to identify the stone. A stone located in the collecting duct or within the gland requires surgical removal via a parotidectomy approach. The stone is identified by palpation and, once exposed, the surrounding parotid duct is incised longitudinally to release the stone.

Tumours of the parotid gland

The parotid gland is the most common site for salivary tumours. Most tumours arise in the superficial lobe and present as slow-growing, painless swellings below the ear (Fig. 47.21a), in front of the ear (Fig. 47.21b) or in the upper aspect of the neck. Less commonly, tumours may arise from the accessory lobe and present as persistent swellings within the cheek. Rarely, tumours may arise from the deep lobe of the gland and present as parapharyngeal masses (Fig. 47.21c and d). Symptoms include difficulty in swallowing and snoring. Clinical examination reveals a diffuse firm swelling in the soft palate and tonsil.

Some 80–90% of tumours of the parotid gland are benign, the most common being pleomorphic adenoma (Table 47.2).

Malignant salivary gland tumours are divided into two distinct sub-groups:

1 *Low-grade malignant tumours*, e.g. acinic cell carcinoma, are indistinguishable on clinical examination from benign neoplasms.
2 *High-grade malignant tumours* usually present as rapidly growing, often painless swellings in and around the parotid gland. The tumour presents as either a discrete mass with infiltration into the overlying skin (Fig. 47.22) or a diffuse but hard swelling of the gland with no discrete mass. Presentation with advanced disease is common, and cervical lymph node metastases may be present.

Investigations

CT and MRI scanning are the most useful imaging techniques (Fig. 47.23a and b). Fine-needle aspiration biopsy may aid in obtaining a preoperative diagnosis, but open surgical biopsy is contraindicated unless malignancy is suspected, and preoperative histological diagnosis is required as a prelude to radical parotidectomy.

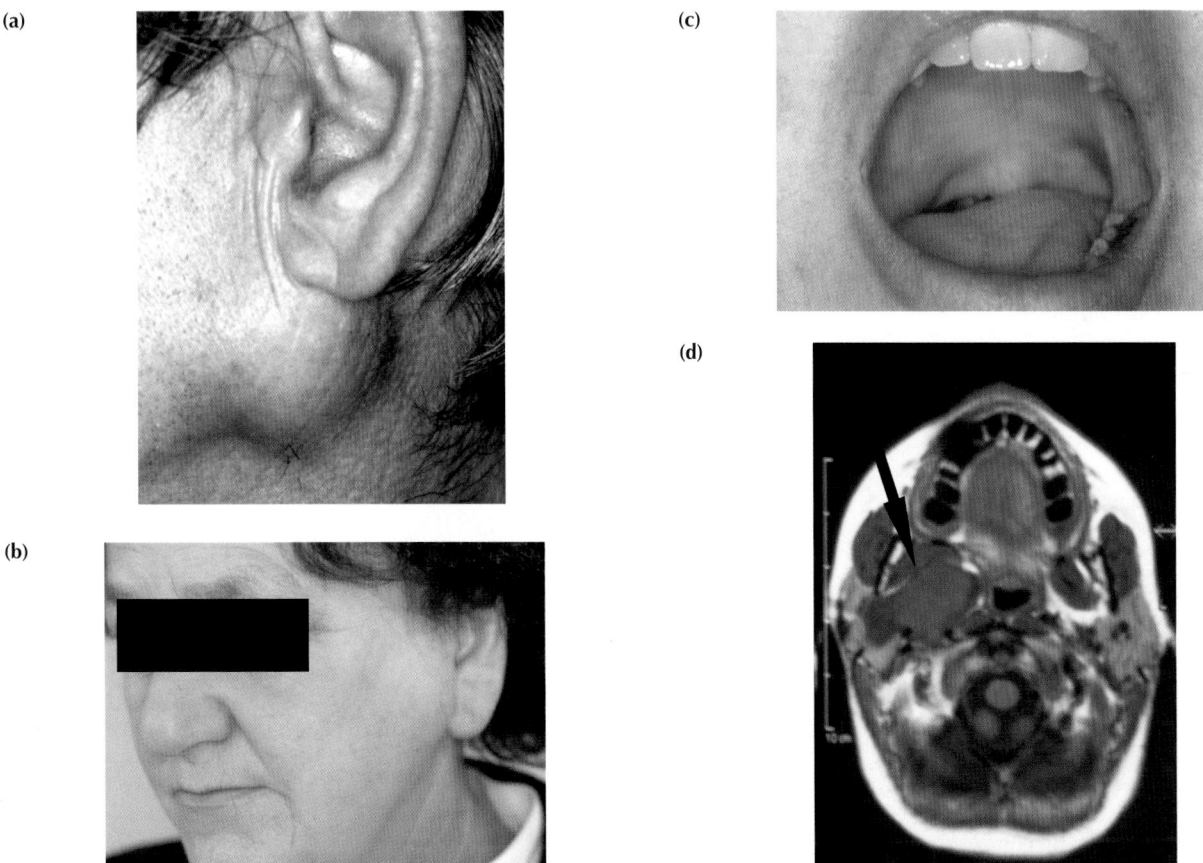

(a)

(b)

(c)

(d)

Figure 47.21 (a) Benign tumour of the left parotid gland producing characteristic deflection of the ear lobe. (b) Pleomorphic adenoma arising from the upper pole of the left parotid gland producing a pre-auricular swelling. (c) Deep lobe tumour of the right parotid presenting with a swelling of the right soft palate. (d) Magnetic resonance imaging (MRI) scan revealing a large deep lobe tumour (arrow) of the right parotid gland, occupying the parapharyngeal space.

Table 47.2 Classification of salivary gland tumours (simplified)

Type	Sub-group	Common examples
I Adenoma	Pleomorphic	Pleomorphic adenoma
	Monomorphic	Adenolymphoma (Warthin's tumour)
II Carcinoma	Low grade	Acinic cell carcinoma
		Adenoid cystic carcinoma
		Low-grade muco-epidermoid carcinoma
	High grade	Adenocarcinoma
		Squamous cell carcinoma
		High-grade muco-epidermoid carcinoma
III Non-epithelial tumours		Haemangioma, lymphangioma
IV Lymphomas	Primary lymphomas	Non-Hodgkin's lymphomas
	Secondary lymphomas	Lymphomas in Sjögren's syndrome
V Secondary tumours	Local	Tumours of the head and neck especially
	Distant	Skin and bronchus
VI Unclassified tumours		
VII Tumour-like lesions	Solid lesions	Benign lymphoepithelial lesion
		Adenomatoid hyperplasia
	Cystic lesions	Salivary gland cysts

All tumours of the superficial lobe of the parotid gland should be managed by superficial parotidectomy. There is no role for enucleation even if a benign lesion is suspected. The aim of superficial parotidectomy is to remove the tumour with a cuff of normal surrounding tissue. The term 'suprafacial parotidectomy' has been used as not all branches of the facial nerve need be formally dissected, particularly if a tumour lies in the lower pole of the parotid gland.

Parotidectomy

Superficial parotidectomy

Superficial parotidectomy is the commonest procedure for parotid gland pathology. Surgery is performed under endotracheal general anaesthesia, which may or may not be accompanied by hypotensive anaesthesia to facilitate dissection, improve the visual surgical field and reduce blood loss. The operation has several distinct phases.

Incision and development of a skin flap
The most commonly used incision is the 'lazy S' pre-auricular–mastoid–cervical (Fig. 47.24a). The incision is marked out and

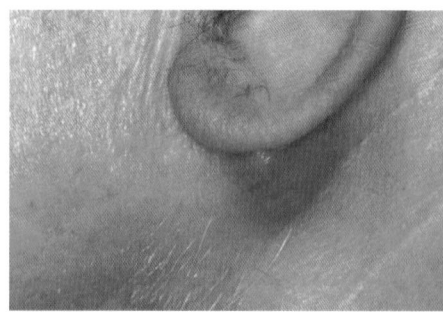

Figure 47.22 Malignant tumour of the left parotid gland with invasion of the overlying skin.

marked at three points along its length to facilitate closure. Infiltration with local anaesthetic and adrenaline is optional, but does aid in the development of the skin flap, improves visibility and reduces blood loss in the initial phase. The skin flap is developed in an anterior direction by either scalpel or scissors dissection. The plane of dissection is well below the hair follicles, just above the parotid fascia. The skin flap is developed forwards to the anterior border of the gland. Posterior undermining of the incision in the cervical region facilitates access to the anterior border of the sternomastoid muscle.

Mobilisation of the gland
This phase of the dissection aims to free the posterior margin of the gland, allowing identification of the facial nerve. Clips are applied along the fascia overlying the sternomastoid muscle, with the assistant applying traction anteriorly. By sharp dissection along the anterior border of the sternomastoid, an avascular plane is developed (Fig. 47.24b), which requires elective transection of the great auricular nerve. At the lower end of the dissection, the external jugular vein is often encountered and ligated. The gland is gradually mobilised by sharp dissection up to and on to the anterior aspect of the mastoid process, identifying the posterior belly of the digastric muscle.

A second avascular plane is developed along the anterior border of the cartilaginous and bony external auditory meatus immediately anterior to the tragus. The two avascular planes are then connected by blunt and sharp dissection. By developing two broad avascular planes, identification of the facial nerve trunk is facilitated (Fig. 47.24c). It is best achieved by scissors dissection

Aldred Scott Warthin, **1866–1931**, Professor of Pathology, University of Michigan, Ann Arbor, MI, USA.
Thomas Hodgkin, **1798–1866**, Curator of the Museum, and Demonstrator of Morbid Anatomy, Guy's Hospital, London, England, described lymphadenoma in 1832.

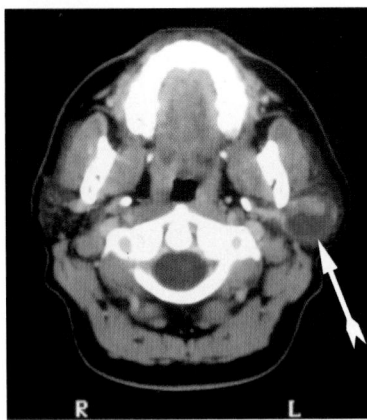

Figure 47.23 (a) Magnetic resonance imaging (MRI) scan revealing a space-occupying lesion (arrow) in the right parotid gland; histology revealed pleomorphic adenoma. (b) Computerised tomographic (CT) scan of the left parotid gland revealing a cystic lesion (arrow). Histology revealed acinic cell carcinoma.

in the line of the facial nerve trunk. A facial nerve stimulator is optional but helpful. Landmarks commonly used to aid identification of the trunk of the facial nerve are:

1 The inferior portion of the cartilaginous canal. This is termed Conley's pointer and indicates the position of the facial nerve, which lies 1 cm deep and inferior to its tip.
2 The upper border of the posterior belly of the digastric muscle. Identification of this muscle not only mobilises the parotid gland, but also exposes an area immediately superior, in which the facial nerve is usually located.

Location of the facial nerve trunk

Once the facial nerve trunk is identified, gentle traction anteriorly facilitates further mobilisation. Control of haemorrhage at this stage is vital as bleeding, no matter how minor, significantly impedes visibility for the surgeon. Haemostasis can be achieved with bipolar diathermy, although caution is necessary particularly when the facial nerve is approached. Damage to the stylomastoid artery, which lies immediately lateral to the nerve, can result in troublesome bleeding immediately prior to identification. Pledget swabs soaked in adrenaline are sometimes helpful in reducing the ooze associated with this phase of the dissection.

Dissection of the gland off the facial nerve

Once the facial nerve trunk is identified, further exposure of the branch of the facial nerve can be achieved by scissors dissection in the perineural plane immediately above the nerve. The tunnel thus created is then laid open, and divisions and branches of the facial nerve are followed to the periphery in a sequential manner, usually beginning with the upper division. The upper division divides into a temporal and a zygomatic branch, and the lower division into mandibular and cervical branches. In this way, the superficial lobe and its associated tumour are mobilised in a superior to inferior direction (Fig. 47.24d). The upper division of the nerve is frequently tortuous in its course and can be damaged unless great care is taken during perineural dissection. It is often not necessary to dissect all branches of the facial nerve completely, as adequate tumour clearance can be achieved with a more conservative resection of the superficial lobe. When a branch of the facial nerve is adherent to the tumour or running through the tumour, it may require elective division. With the exception of the buccal branch, the transected nerve should be repaired immediately with a cable graft, harvested from the great auricular nerve.

Closure

The patient is placed into a Trendelenburg position to identify any residual bleeding vessels. A suction drain is applied for a period of 24–48 hours, and the wound closed in layers (Fig. 47.24f).

Radical parotidectomy

Radical parotidectomy is performed for patients in whom there is clear histological evidence of a high-grade malignant tumour, e.g. squamous cell carcinoma. Low-grade malignant tumours can usually be managed by standard superficial parotidectomy. Radical parotidectomy involves removal of all parotid gland tissue and elective sectioning of the facial nerve, usually through the main trunk (Fig. 47.25a–f). The surgery inevitably removes the ipsilateral masseter muscle and may also require simultaneous neck dissection, particularly where there is clinical, radiological and cytological evidence of lymph node metastases in the ipsilateral neck.

Complications of parotid gland surgery

Complications of parotid gland surgery include:

1 haematoma formation;
2 infection;
3 temporary facial nerve weakness;
4 transection of the facial nerve and permanent facial weakness;
5 sialocele;
6 facial numbness;
7 permanent numbness of the ear lobe associated with great auricular nerve transection;
8 Frey's syndrome.

Frey's syndrome

Frey's syndrome (gustatory sweating) is now considered an inevitable consequence of parotidectomy, unless preventative measures are taken (see below). It results from damage to the autonomic innervation of the salivary gland with inappropriate regeneration

Friedrich Trendelenburg, **1844–1924, successively Professor of Surgery at Rostock (1875–1882), Bonn (1822–1895), and Leipzig, (1895–1911), Germany. The Trendelenburg Position was first described in 1885.**
Lucie Frey, **1896–1944, Physician, The Neurological Clinic, Warsaw, Poland.**

(a)

(b)

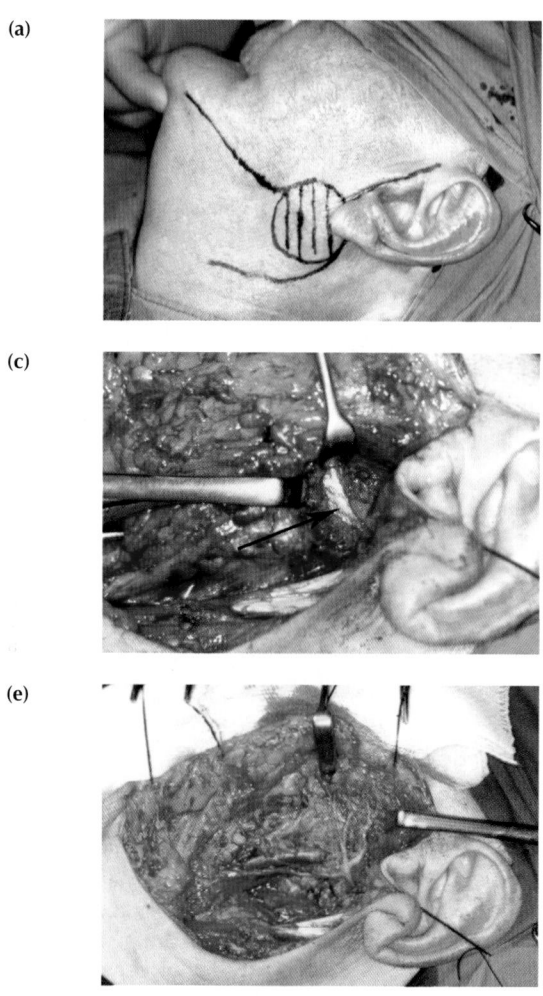

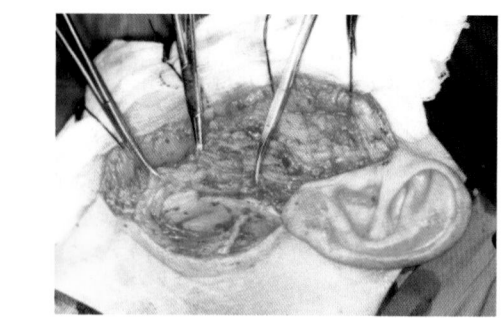

(c)

(d)

(e)

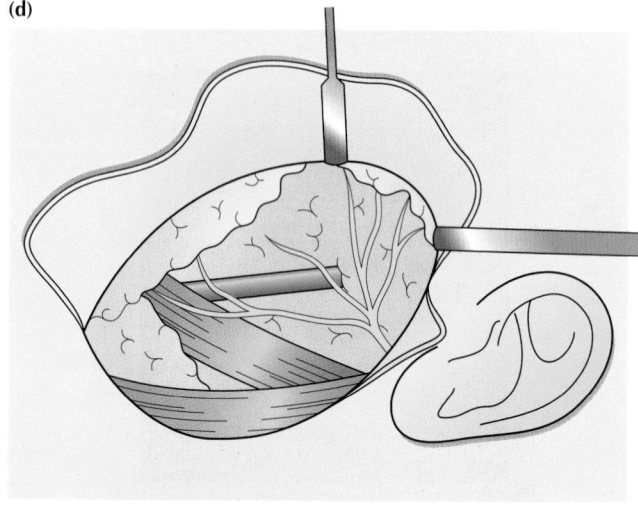

(f)

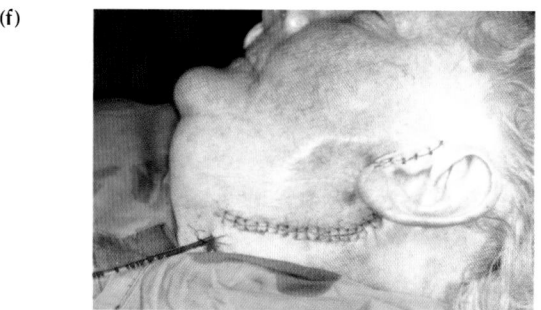

Figure 47.24 (a) Landmarks and cervical–mastoid pre-auricular incision for superficial parotidectomy. (b) Development of the avascular plane along the anterior border of the sternomastoid prior to sacrifice of the great auricular nerve. (c) Identification of the trunk of the facial nerve (arrow). (d) Diagram highlighting the anatomical landmarks of the parotid bed. (e) Branches of the facial nerve and retromandibular vein following delivery of the tumour. (f) Wound closure with a vacuum drain.

of parasympathetic nerve fibres that stimulate the sweat glands of the overlying skin. The clinical features include sweating and erythema over the region of surgical excision of the parotid gland as a consequence of autonomic stimulation of salivation by the smell or taste of food. The symptoms are entirely variable and are clinically demonstrated by a starch iodine test. This involves painting the affected area with iodine, which is allowed to dry before applying dry starch, which turns blue on exposure to iodine in the presence of sweat. Sweating is stimulated by salivary stimulation. The management of Frey's syndrome involves the prevention as well as the management of established symptoms.

Prevention

There are a number of techniques described to prevent Frey's syndrome following parotidectomy. These include:

- sternomastoid muscle flap;
- temporalis fascial flap;

- insertion of artificial membranes between the skin and the parotid bed.

All these methods place a barrier between the skin and the parotid bed to minimise inappropriate regeneration of autonomic nerve fibres.

Management of established Frey's syndrome

Methods of managing Frey's syndrome include:

- anti-perspirants, usually containing aluminium chloride;
- denervation by tympanic neurectomy;
- the injection of botulinum toxin into the affected skin.

The last is the most effective and can be performed as an out-patient.

Granulomatous sialadenitis

This is a group of rare conditions that affect the salivary glands producing a variety of signs and symptoms, particularly painless

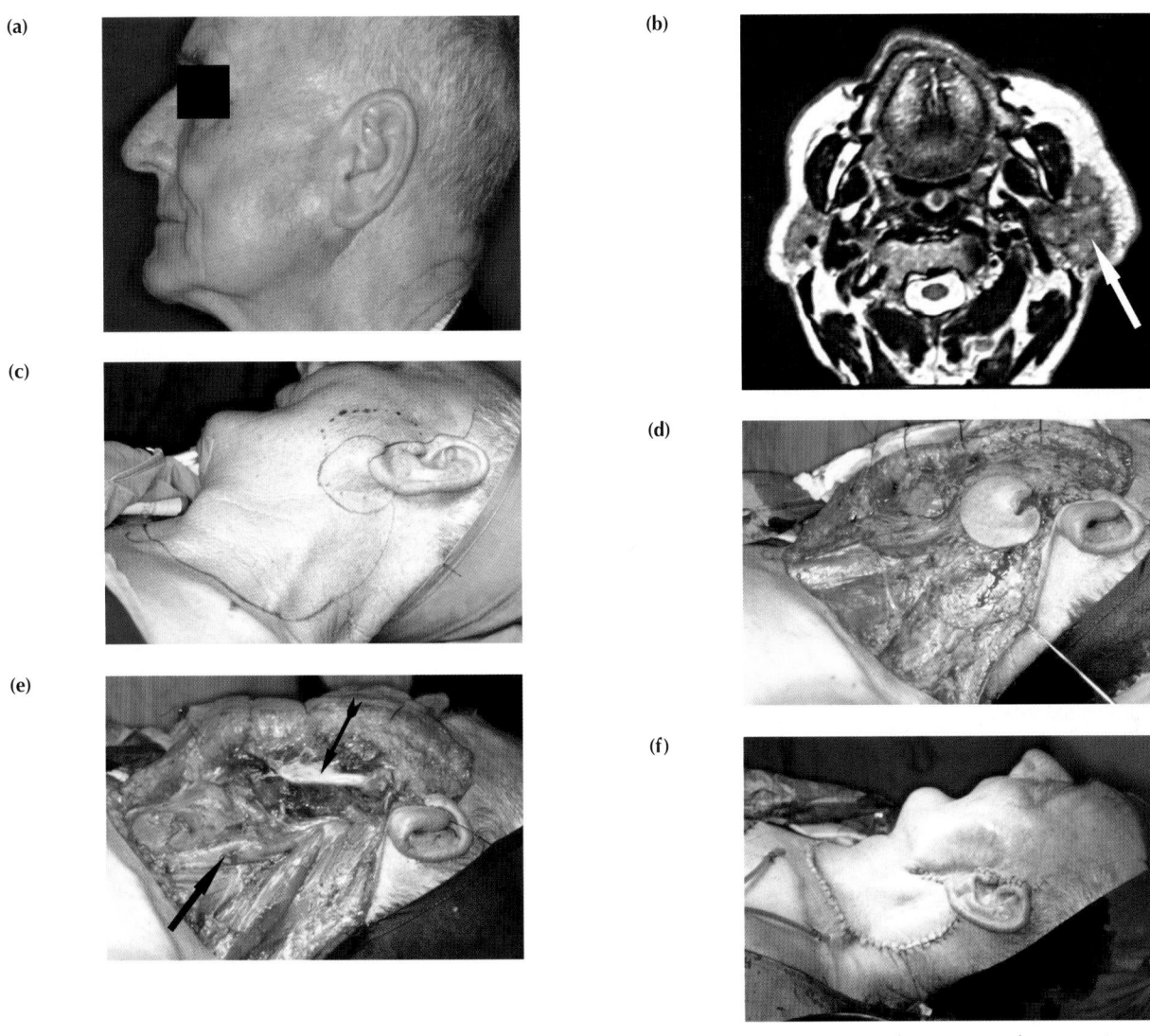

Figure 47.25 (a) High-grade malignant tumour in the left parotid gland. (b) Magnetic resonance imaging (MRI) scan demonstrating a diffuse infiltrative malignant tumour of the left parotid gland (arrow). (c) Skin incision outlined for radical neck dissection and left radical parotidectomy including the removal of overlying skin. (d) Skin flap developed. (e) Appearance after left radical neck dissection and left radical parotidectomy. Posterior mandible (upper arrow) and great vessels of the neck (lower arrow) are visible. (f) Wound closure after left radical neck dissection.

swellings of the parotid and/or submandibular glands. Systemic upset is variable. These include the following.

Mycobacterial infection

Tuberculosis and non-tuberculous sialadenitis typically present as a tumour-like swelling of the salivary gland. There is little pain and no fever. Preoperative investigations may be of some help, and the diagnosis is only confirmed when the swelling has been excised by either submandibular gland excision or formal parotidectomy.

Sarcoidosis

Sarcoidosis can affect the salivary tissue and presents with persistent salivary gland swelling that may be associated with xerostomia. Occasionally, the patient will present with a localised tumour-like swelling in one salivary gland, more commonly the parotid – the so called sarcoid pseudotumour. In such circumstances, the diagnosis is only likely to be made following surgical excision for a presumed neoplasm.

Heerfordt's syndrome is sarcoidosis that involves parotid swelling, anterior uveitis, facial palsy and fever.

Other

These include cat scratch disease, toxoplasmosis, syphilis, deep mycoses and Wegener's granulomatosis, allergic sialadenitis and sialadenitis associated with radiotherapy of the head and neck.

Tumour-like lesions

There is a group of pathological conditions that affect the salivary glands which do not fall into any particular classification or category and are often difficult to diagnose. These include such conditions as sialadenosis, adenomatoid hyperplasia and multifocal monomorphic adenomatosis.

> Christian Frederick Heerfordt, 1871–1953, a Danish Ophthalmologist, described this syndrome in 1909.
> Friedrich Wegener, 1907–1990, Professor of Pathology, Lübeck, Germany, described this form of granulomatosis in 1939.

Sialadenosis

Sialadenosis (sialosis) is used to describe non-inflammatory swelling particularly affecting the parotid gland. It is usually occurs in association with a variety of conditions including diabetes mellitus, alcoholism, other endocrine diseases, pregnancy, drugs, bulimia and other eating disorders, and idiopathic diseases.

Most patients present between 40 and 70 years of age, and the salivary swellings are soft and often symmetrical (Fig. 47.26). When the parotid glands are affected, patients may complain of a hamster-like appearance. Drug-induced sialosis is particularly common with sympathomimetic drugs. In many patients, no underlying disorder can be identified. Severe and prolonged malnutrition, as seen in eating disorders, produces sialadenosis by a process of glandular atrophy and fatty replacement. The pathological mechanism of sialadenosis can be associated with a process of neuropathy, which interferes with salivary gland function and subsequent acinar cell atrophy. This may be the case in diabetes mellitus, where autonomic neuropathy is a recognised complication as well as drug-induced sialosis.

The treatment of sialosis is unsatisfactory, but treatment is aimed at the correction of the underlying disorder. Drug-associated sialadenosis may regress when the drug responsible is withdrawn.

Degenerative conditions

Sjögren's syndrome

Sjögren's syndrome is an autoimmune condition causing progressive destruction of salivary and lacrimal glands. Primary Sjögren's syndrome differs from secondary Sjögren's syndrome in that xerostomia and keratoconjunctivitis sicca occur without the associated connective tissue disorder. However, the symptoms are often more severe, and the incidence of lymphomatous transformation (see below) in the primary group is higher than that in the secondary group (Table 47.3).

Table 47.3 Degenerative disorders

Primary Sjögren's syndrome	More severe xerostomia
	Widespread exocrine gland dysfunction
	No connective tissue disorder
Secondary Sjögren's syndrome	M:F: 1:10
	Middle age
	Underlying connective tissue disorder
Benign lymphoepithelial lesion	20% develop lymphoma
	Diffuse parotid swelling
	20% bilateral

Females are affected more than males in the ratio 10:1. Occasionally, there is enlargement of the salivary glands, more commonly the parotid rather than the submandibular glands. The glands are occasionally painful, and the patient sometimes develops a bacterial sialadenitis due to ascending infection from the associated xerostomia.

The characteristic pathological feature of Sjögren's syndrome is the progressive lymphocytic infiltration, acinar cell destruction and proliferation of duct epithelium in all salivary and lacrimal gland tissue. The diagnosis is based on the history as no single laboratory investigation is pathognomonic of either primary or secondary Sjögren's syndrome (Fig. 47.27).

Management

Management of Sjögren's syndrome remains symptomatic. No known treatment modifies or improves the xerostomia or keratoconjunctivitis sicca. An ophthalmological assessment is important, and artificial tears are essential to preserve corneal function. For dry mouth, various artificial salivary substitutes are available, but patients often consume large volumes of water, carrying a bottle of water with them at all times. In the dentate patient, the use of salivary substitutes with fluoride is important to counter the risk of accelerating dental caries. Other oral complications include oral candidosis and accelerated periodontal disease.

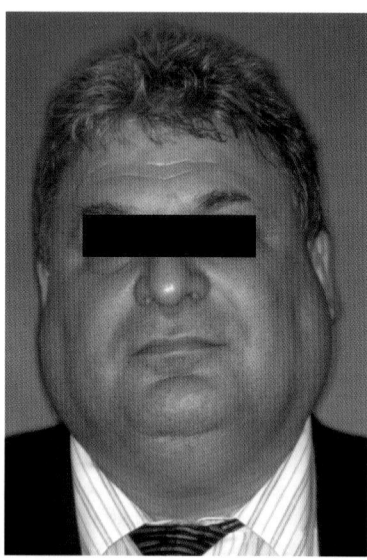

Figure 47.26 Sialosis of the parotid glands secondary to excess alcohol intake.

A hamster **is a small nocturnal Eurasian rodent.**

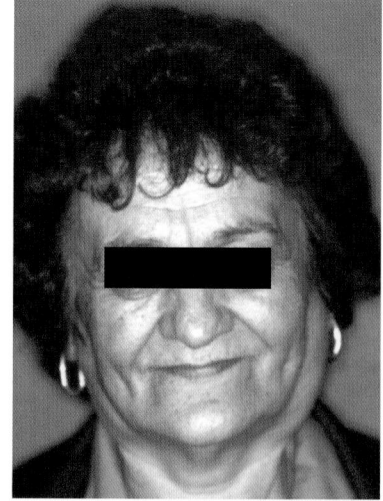

Figure 47.27 Clinical appearance of primary biliary cirrhosis associated with Sjögren's syndrome.

Complications of Sjögren's syndrome

There is an increased incidence of developing lymphoma (most commonly monocytoid B-cell lymphoma) in patients with Sjögren's syndrome. The risk is highest within the primary group, and the onset of lymphoma is heralded by immunological change within the blood.

Benign lymphoepithelial lesion

The use of the word 'benign' to describe this lesion is misleading because 20% of patients with benign lymphoepithelial lesion ultimately develop lymphoma. It is not possible to distinguish on histological grounds benign lymphoepithelial lesion from Sjögren's syndrome. Both are characterised by lymphocytic infiltration, acinar atrophy and ductal epithelial proliferation. Clinically, benign lymphoepithelial lesion presents as a diffuse swelling of the parotid gland. The swelling is firm, often painful and, in 20% of patients, the presentation is bilateral. Most patients are female and over 50 years of age. Parotidectomy is often undertaken to establish a diagnosis. Prolonged follow-up is essential.

Xerostomia

Xerostomia is a common symptom in many aspects of medical practice. Normal salivary flows decrease with age in both men and women, although many patients with xerostomia are post-menopausal women who also complain of a burning tongue or mouth. Common causes of xerostomia are:

1 chronic anxiety states and depression;
2 dehydration;
3 anti-cholinergic drugs, especially antidepressants;
4 salivary gland disorders – Sjögren's syndrome. Ascending parotitis is an occasional complication of xerostomia and is managed with antibiotics and increased fluid intake;
5 radiotherapy to the head and neck.

Sialorrhoea

Certain drugs and oral infection produce a transient increase in salivary flow rates. In healthy individuals, excess salivation is rarely a symptom as excess saliva is swallowed spontaneously. Uncontrolled drooling is usually seen in the presence of normal salivary production. It is seen in children with mental and physical handicap, notably cerebral palsy.

Management

Uncontrollable drooling is managed surgically, and many operations are available. Surgical options include:

- bilateral submandibular duct repositioning and simultaneous sublingual gland excision;
- bilateral submandibular gland excision;
- transposition of the parotid ducts and simultaneous submandibular gland excision.

Most resting salivary gland flow arises from the submandibular glands, and surgery should be focused on this gland to control uncontrolled sialorrhoea.

FURTHER READING

McGurk, M. and Renehan, A.E. (2001) *Controversies in the Management of Salivary Gland Disease*. Oxford University Press, Oxford.

CHAPTER 47 | DISORDERS OF THE SALIVARY GLANDS

PART 8 | Breast and endocrine

The thyroid and parathyroid glands

LEARNING OBJECTIVES

To understand:

- The development and anatomy of the thyroid and parathyroid glands
- The physiology and investigation of thyroid and parathyroid function
- The investigation of thyroid swelling
- The treatment of thyrotoxicosis and thyroid failure

- The indications for and technique of thyroid surgery
- The management of thyroid cancer
- The investigation and management of hyperparathyroidism
- The risks and complications of thyroid and parathyroid surgery

EMBRYOLOGY

The thyroglossal duct develops from the median bud of the pharynx. The foramen caecum at the base of the tongue is the vestigial remnant of the duct. This initially hollow structure migrates caudally and passes in close continuity with, and sometimes through, the developing hyoid cartilage. The parathyroid glands develop from the third and fourth pharyngeal pouches (Fig. 48.1). The thymus also develops from the third pouch. As it descends it takes the associated parathyroid gland with it, which explains why the inferior parathyroid arising from the third pouch normally lies inferior to the superior gland. However, the inferior parathyroid may be found anywhere along this line of descent. The developing thyroid lobes amalgamate with the structures arising in the fourth pharyngeal pouch, i.e. the superior parathyroid gland and the ultimobranchial body. Parafollicular cells (C cells) from the neural crest reach the thyroid via the ultimobranchial body.

SURGICAL ANATOMY (FIGS 48.2–48.4)

The normal thyroid gland weighs 20–25 g. The functioning unit is the lobule supplied by a single arteriole and consisting of 24–40 follicles lined with cuboidal epithelium. The follicle contains colloid in which thyroglobulin is stored (Fig. 48.2). The arterial supply is rich, and extensive anastomoses occur between the main thyroid arteries and branches of the tracheal and oesophageal arteries (Fig. 48.3). There is an extensive lymphatic network within the gland. Although some lymph channels pass directly to the deep cervical nodes, the subcapsular plexus drains principally to the central compartment juxtathyroid nodes – 'Delphian' (level 6) –

Delphi, a sacred site near the Gulf of Corinth in Greece, is the place where Pythia, the snake-woman oracle, resided. She sat on a tripod clutching the ribbons of the monolithic 'omphalos' of the world, and after inhaling sulphurous fumes, would utter meaningless jargon which was interpreted equivocally by the attendant priests for those who came to consult her. Formerly the purpose of these lymph nodes was uncertain, and they were therefore called 'Delphic'.

paratracheal nodes (level 7) and nodes on the superior and inferior thyroid veins, and from there to the deep cervical (levels 2, 3, 4 and 5) and mediastinal groups of nodes.

The normal parathyroid gland weighs up to 50 mg with a characteristic orange/brown colour and mobility within the surrounding fat and thymic tissue. Most adults have four parathyroid

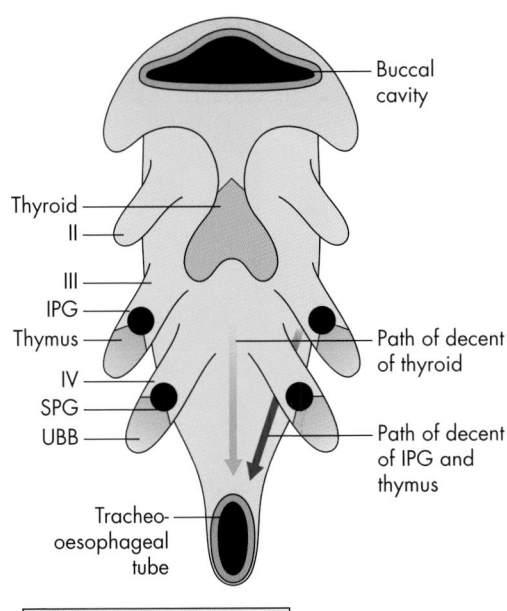

Figure 48.1 Embryology of the thyroid and parathyroid. Diagram of an anterior view of the pharynx in a four week embryo showing the relationship of the third and fourth pharyngeal pouches to final position of the thyroid and parathyroid glands.

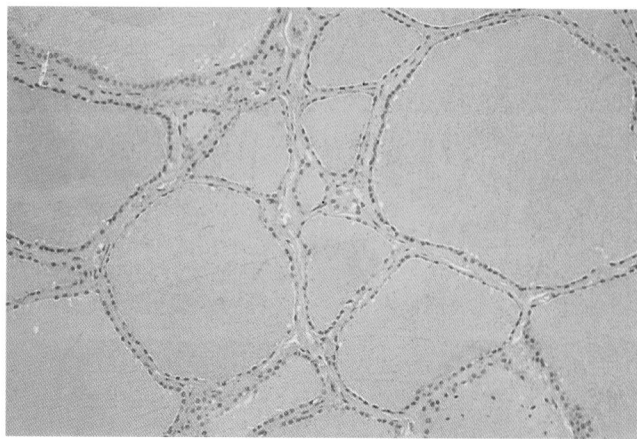

Figure 48.2 Histology of the normal thyroid.

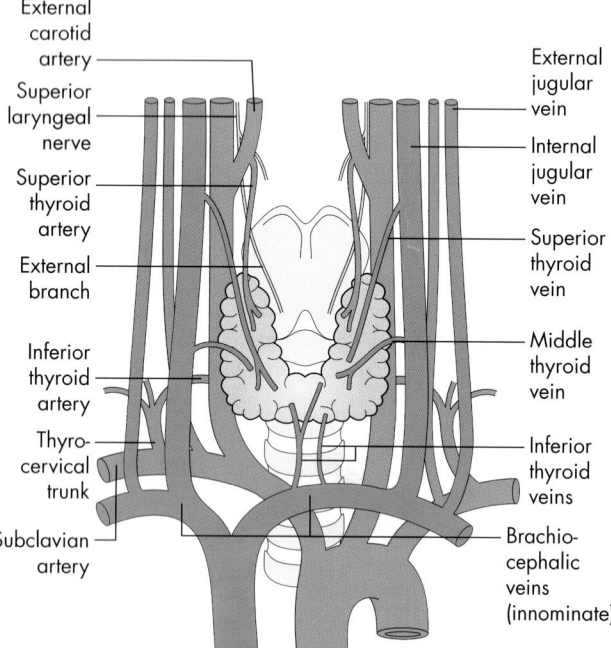

Figure 48.3 The thyroid gland from the front.

External carotid artery
Superior laryngeal nerve
Superior thyroid artery
External branch
Inferior thyroid artery
Thyro-cervical trunk
Subclavian artery

External jugular vein
Internal jugular vein
Superior thyroid vein
Middle thyroid vein
Inferior thyroid veins
Brachio-cephalic veins (innominate)

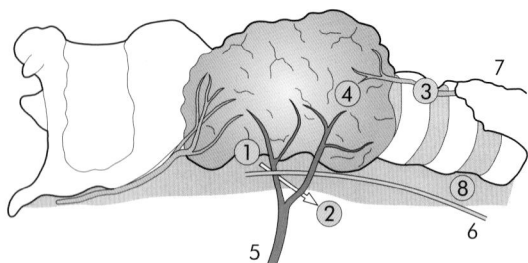

Figure 48.4 Surgical anatomy of the thyroid. The situation after mobilisation of the right lobe and the relationships of the recurrent laryngeal nerve, inferior thyroid artery and the parathyroid glands as they are usually found are shown. 1 and 2, common sites for the superior parathyroid gland – the arrow shows the tendency for an enlarged gland to migrate from position 1 to position 2, i.e. in an inferior direction, to lie posterior to the inferior thyroid artery (5) and oesophagus (8); 3 and 4, common sites for the inferior parathyroid gland (the upper horn of the thymus points like an index finger to the inferior parathyroid, which may lie under the 'fingernail'); 5, inferior thyroid artery; 6, recurrent laryngeal nerve; 7, thymus; 8, oesophagus (see Fig. 48.49a).

Summary box 48.1

Embryology and anatomy

- Know the embryology of the thyroid and parathyroid glands
- Know the surgical and radiological anatomy of the thyroid

PHYSIOLOGY

Thyroxine

The hormones tri-iodothyronine (T_3) and L-thyroxine (T_4) (extracted by E.C. Kendall in 1915) are bound to thyroglobulin within the colloid. Synthesis within the thyroglobulin complex is controlled by several enzymes, in distinct steps:

- trapping of inorganic iodide from the blood;
- oxidation of iodide to iodine;
- binding of iodine with tyrosine to form iodotyrosines;
- coupling of monoiodotyrosines and di-iodotyrosines to form T_3 and T_4.

When hormones are required, the complex is resorbed into the cell and thyroglobulin is broken down. T_3 and T_4 are liberated and enter the blood, where they are bound to serum proteins: albumin, thyroxine-binding globulin (TBG) and thyroxine-binding prealbumin (TBPA). The small amount of hormone that remains free in the serum is biologically active.

The metabolic effects of the thyroid hormones are due to unbound free T_4 and T_3 (0.03% and 0.3% of the total circulating hormones respectively). T_3 is the more important physiological hormone and is also produced in the periphery by conversion from T_4. T_3 is quick acting (within a few hours), whereas T_4 acts more slowly (4–14 days).

Edward Calvin Kendall, **1886–1972, Professor of Physiological Chemistry, The Graduate Medical School, The Mayo Foundation, Rochester, MN, USA. He shared the 1950 Nobel Prize for Physiology or Medicine with Hench and Reichstein 'for their discoveries concerning the suprarenal cortex hormones, their structure and biological effects'.**

---

glands but supernumerary glands occur and nests of parathyroid tissue are commonly found in the thymus. The superior parathyroid is more consistent in position than the inferior. The superior gland is commonly found in fat above the inferior thyroid artery and close to the cricothyroid articulation (Fig. 48.4). It should be noted that the anatomical and radiological site, usually described as above the artery and posterior to the recurrent laryngeal nerve (RLN), is different from the surgical anatomy when the thyroid lobe is mobilised and rotated anteriorly. When the superior gland enlarges it tends to pass behind the inferior thyroid artery and descend inferiorly behind the oesophagus. The inferior parathyroid gland is usually found under the capsule of the upper horn of the thymus or on the inferior pole of the thyroid lobe. A maldescended gland, however, can be found anywhere along the line of descent, virtually from the base of the skull to the aortopulmonary window (Summary box 48.1).

Parathyroid hormone

The parathyroid glands secrete the 84-amino-acid peptide parathyroid hormone (PTH), which controls the level of serum calcium and extracellular fluid. PTH is released in response to a low serum calcium or high serum magnesium level. PTH activates osteoclasts to resorb bone and increases calcium reabsorption from urine and renal activation of vitamin D, with subsequent increased gut absorption of calcium. Renal excretion of phosphate is also increased.

Calcitonin

The parafollicular C-cells of the thyroid are of neuroendocrine origin and arrive in the thyroid via the ultimobranchial body (see Fig. 48.1). They produce calcitonin, which is a serum marker for recurrence of medullary thyroid cancer.

The pituitary–thyroid axis

The synthesis and liberation of thyroid hormones from the thyroid is controlled by thyroid-stimulating hormone (TSH) from the anterior pituitary. Secretion of TSH depends upon the level of circulating thyroid hormones and is modified in a classic negative feedback manner. In hyperthyroidism, when hormone levels in the blood are high, TSH production is suppressed whereas in hypothyroidism it is stimulated. Regulation of TSH secretion also results from the action of thyrotrophin-releasing hormone (TRH) produced in the hypothalamus.

Thyroid-stimulating antibodies

A family of IgG immunoglobulins bind with TSH receptor sites (TSH-RAbs) and activate TSH receptors on the follicular cell membrane. They have a more protracted action than TSH (16–24 vs. 1.5–3 hours) and are responsible for virtually all cases of thyrotoxicosis not due to autonomous toxic nodules. Serum concentrations are very low but their measurement is not essential to make the diagnosis.

Therapeutic notes

T_4 is given once daily; an average replacement dose is $150\,\mu g$ and a suppressive dose is $200\,\mu g$. T_3 is given in divided doses, usually as a suppressive dose of 4–$60\,\mu g$. Recombinant human TSH is now available and is used to maximise (radioactive) iodine uptake as an alternative to thyroid hormone withdrawal.

TESTS OF THYROID FUNCTION

There is a large variety of available tests of thyroid function. In a surgical setting the investigations requested should be the minimum necessary to reach a diagnosis and formulate a management plan. Only a small number of parameters need to be measured as a routine, although this may require supplementation or the measurements may need to be repeated when inconclusive.

Serum thyroid hormones

Serum TSH

TSH levels can be measured accurately down to very low serum concentrations with an immunochemiluminometric assay. When the serum TSH level is in the normal range, measuring the T_3 and T_4 levels is redundant. Interpretation of deranged TSH levels, however, depends on knowledge of the T_3 and T_4 values (Table 48.1). In the euthyroid state, T_3, T_4 and TSH levels will all be within the normal range. Florid thyroid failure results in depressed T_3 and T_4 levels, with gross elevation of the TSH. Incipient or developing thyroid failure is characterised by low-normal values of T_3 and T_4 and elevation of TSH. In toxic states the TSH level is suppressed and undetectable.

Thyroxine (T_4) and tri-iodothyronine (T_3)

These are transported in plasma bound to specific proteins (TBG). Only a small fraction of the total (0.03% of T_4 and 0.3% of T_3) is free and physiologically active. Assays of total hormone for both are now obsolete because of the confounding effect of circulating protein concentrations, influenced by the level of circulating oestrogen and the nutritional state. Highly accurate radioimmunoassays of free T_3 and free T_4 are now routine. T_3 toxicity (with a normal T_4) is a distinct entity and may only be diagnosed by measuring the serum T_3, although a suppressed TSH level with a normal T_4 may suggest the diagnosis.

An appropriate combination to establish the functional thyroid status at initial assessment is measurement of serum TSH and assay of anti-thyroid antibodies, supplemented by free T_4 and T_3 evaluation when TSH is abnormal.

Thyroid autoantibodies

Serum levels of antibodies against thyroid peroxidase (TPO; previously referred to as thyroid microsomal antigen) and thyroglobulin are useful in determining the cause of thyroid dysfunction and swellings. Autoimmune thyroiditis may be associated with thyroid toxicity, failure or euthyroid goitre. Levels above 25 units ml^{-1} for TPO antibody and titres of greater than 1:100 for anti-thyroglobulin are considered significant, although a proportion of patients with histological evidence of lymphocytic (autoimmune) thyroiditis are seronegative. The presence of anti-thyroglobulin antibody interferes with assays of serum thyroglobulin with implications for the follow-up of thyroid cancers.

Thyroid imaging

Chest and thoracic inlet radiography (Fig. 48.5)

Simple radiographs of the chest and thoracic inlet will rapidly and economically confirm the presence of significant retrosternal goitre and clinically important degrees of tracheal deviation and compression. Chest radiographs tend to underestimate the extent of retrosternal extensions. Pulmonary metastases may also be detected.

Table 48.1 Results of thyroid function tests in normal and pathological states

Thyroid functional state	TSH (0.3–3.3 mU l^{-1})	Free T$_4$ (10–30 nmol l^{-1})	Free T$_3$ (3.5–7.5 µmol l^{-1})
Euthyroid	Normal	Normal	Normal
Thyrotoxic	Undetectable	High	High
Myxoedema	High	Low	Low
Suppressive T$_4$ therapy	Undetectable	High	High (may be normal)
T$_3$ toxicity	Low/undetectable	Normal	High

CHAPTER 48 | THE THYROID AND PARATHYROID GLANDS

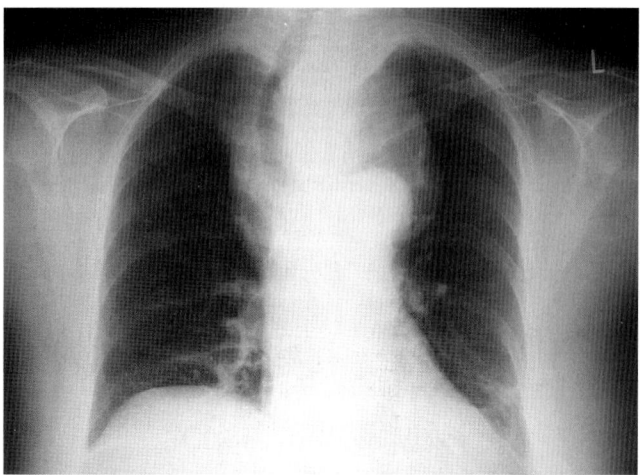

Figure 48.5 Chest radiograph showing a retrosternal goitre with tracheal displacement.

Ultrasound scanning (Fig. 48.6)

High-frequency ultrasound scanning gives good anatomical images of the thyroid and surrounding structures but, unfortunately, reveals more thyroid swellings than are clinically relevant. After a period of years in the relative doldrums ultrasound is enjoying a revival as a means of reducing the number of unsatisfactory aspiration cytology samples; it permits more targeted sampling, allowing the identification of parathyroid adenomas and nodes involved in thyroid cancer.

(a)

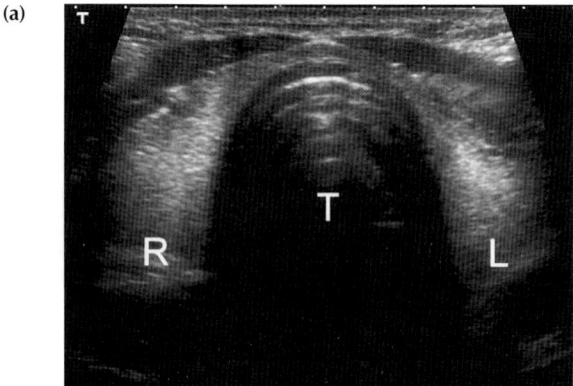

(b)

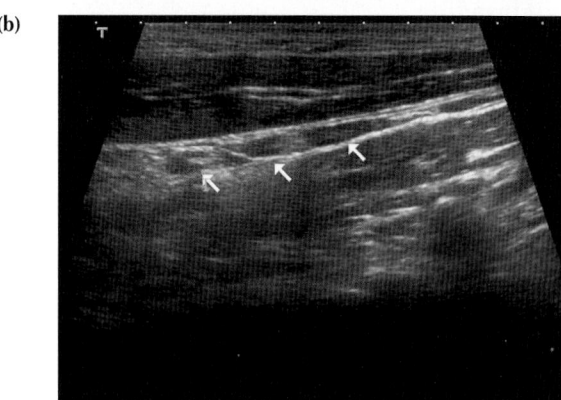

Figure 48.6 Ultrasound scanning. (a) Transverse scan of a normal thyroid. R, right lobe; L, left lobe; T, trachea. (b) Longitudinal scan of normal jugular lymph nodes (white arrows).

Computerised tomography, magnetic resonance imaging and positron emission tomography scanning (Fig. 48.7)

Like ultrasound scanning, routine computerised tomography (CT), magnetic resonance imaging (MRI) and positron emission tomography (PET) of unexceptional thyroid swellings are not indicated and are reserved for the assessment of known malignancy and to assess the extent of retrosternal and, occasionally, recurrent goitres. The appearance of a retrosternal goitre on CT can give a misleading impression of the operative difficulty in delivery through a neck incision.

Isotope scanning (Fig. 48.8)

The uptake by the thyroid of a low dose of either radiolabelled iodine (^{123}I) or the cheaper technetium (^{99m}Tc) will demonstrate the distribution of activity in the whole gland. Routine isotope scanning is unnecessary and inappropriate for distinguishing benign from malignant lesions because the majority (80%) of 'cold' swellings are benign and some (5%) functioning or 'warm' swellings will be malignant. Its principal value is in the toxic patient with a nodule or nodularity of the thyroid. Localisation of overactivity in the gland will differentiate between a toxic nodule with suppression of the remainder of the gland and toxic multinodular goitre

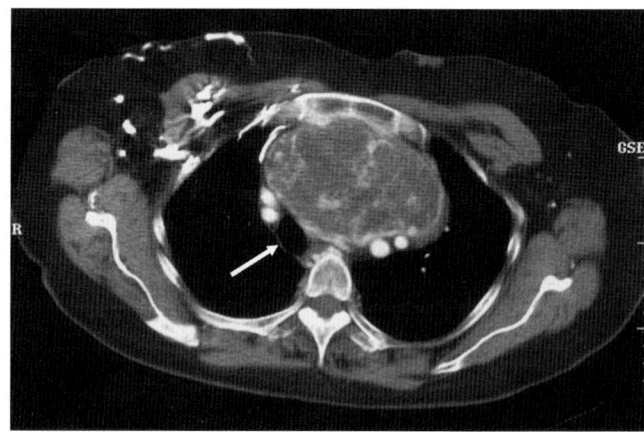

Figure 48.7 Computerised tomography scan of the chest showing a retrosternal goitre with tracheal displacement (arrowed).

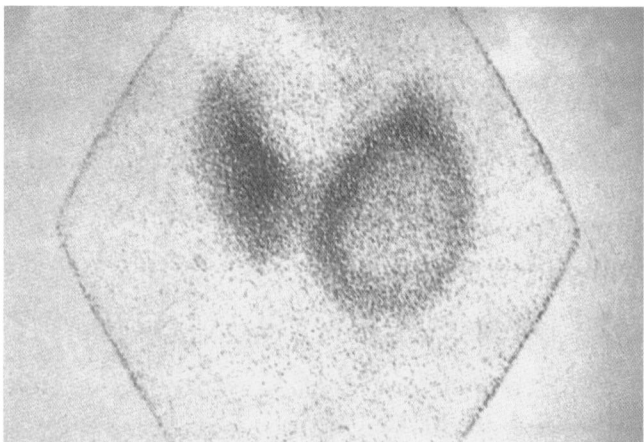

Figure 48.8 Technetium thyroid scan showing a 'cold' nodule that does not take up isotope expanding the left thyroid lobe.

with several areas of increased uptake, with important implications for therapy.

Whole-body scanning is used to demonstrate metastases but the patient must have all normally functioning thyroid tissue ablated, either by surgery or radioiodine, before the scan is performed, because thyroid cancer cannot compete with normal thyroid tissue in the uptake of iodine.

Fine-needle aspiration cytology

Fine-needle aspiration cytology (FNAC) is the investigation of choice for discrete thyroid swellings. FNAC has excellent patient compliance, is simple and quick to perform in the out-patient department and is readily repeated. This technique, developed in Scandinavia some 35 years ago, has become routine throughout the world in the last 25 years. FNAC results should be reported using standard terminology (Table 48.2). There is a trend to use ultrasound to guide the needle to achieve more accurate sampling and reduce the rate of unsatisfactory aspirates (Summary box 48.2).

Summary box 48.2

Thyroid investigations

Essential
- Serum: TSH (T_3 and T_4 if abnormal); thyroid autoantibodies
- FNAC of palpable discrete swellings; ultrasound guidance may reduce the 'Thy1' rate

Optional
- Corrected serum calcium
- Serum calcitonin (carcinoembryonic antigen may be used as an alternative screening test for medullary cancer)
- Imaging: chest radiograph and thoracic inlet if tracheal deviation/retrosternal goitre; ultrasound, CT and MRI scan for known cancer, some reoperations and some retrosternal goitres; isotope scan if discrete swelling and toxicity coexist

---

HYPOTHYROIDISM

A scheme for classifying hypothyroidism is given in Table 48.3.

Cretinism (fetal or infantile hypothyroidism)

Cretinism is the consequence of inadequate thyroid hormone production during fetal and neonatal development. 'Endemic cretinism' is due to dietary iodine deficiency, whereas sporadic cases are due to either an inborn error of thyroid metabolism or complete or partial agenesis of the gland. A hoarse cry, macroglossia and umbilical hernia in a neonate with features of thyroid failure suggests the diagnosis. Immediate diagnosis and treatment with thyroxine within a few days of birth are essential

Table 48.2 Classification of fine-needle aspiration cytology reports

Thy1	Non-diagnostic
Thy2	Non-neoplastic
Thy3	Follicular
Thy4	Suspicious of malignancy
Thy5	Malignant

Table 48.3 Classification of hypothyroidism

Autoimmune thyroiditis (chronic lymphocytic thyroiditis)
Non-goitrous: primary myxoedema
Goitrous: Hashimoto's disease

Iatrogenic
After thyroidectomy
After radioiodine therapy
Drug induced (anti-thyroid drugs, para-aminosalicylic acid and iodides in excess)

Dyshormonogenesis

Goitrogens

Secondary to pituitary or hypothalamic disease

Thyroid agenesis

Endemic cretinism
Often goitrous and due to iodine deficiency

---

to prevent damage *in utero* progressing and if physical and mental development are to be normal. In non-endemic areas and societies with iodised salt, sporadic hypothyroidism still occurs at a rate of 1:4000 live births, and biochemical screening of neonates for hypothyroidism using TSH and T_4 assays on a heel-prick blood sample is widespread. Women taking anti-thyroid drugs may give birth to a hypothyroid infant and radioactive iodine must never be given to pregnant women.

Adult hypothyroidism

The term myxoedema should be reserved for severe thyroid failure and not applied to the much commoner mild thyroid deficiency. The signs of thyroid deficiency are:

- bradycardia;
- cold extremities;
- dry skin and hair;
- periorbital puffiness;
- hoarse voice;
- bradykinesis, slow movements;
- delayed relaxation phase of ankle jerks.

The symptoms are:

- tiredness;
- mental lethargy;
- cold intolerance;
- weight gain;
- constipation;
- menstrual disturbance;
- carpal tunnel syndrome.

Hakaru Hashimoto, 1881–1934, Director of The Hashimoto Hospital, Mie, Japan described chronic lymphocytic thyroiditis in 1912. The link to an autoimmune basis was first defined by Roitt and his co-workers.
Ivan Maurice Roitt, (dates unknown), Professor of Immunology, The Middlesex Hospital, London, England.
in utero is Latin for 'in the uterus'.
Myxoedema was first described in 1873 by Sir William Withey Gull, 1816–1890, Physician, Guy's Hospital, London, England.

Comparison of the facial appearance with a previous photograph may be helpful. Delayed relaxation of the ankle jerk reflex is the most useful clinical sign in making the diagnosis.

Thyroid function tests

These show low T_4 and T_3 levels with a high TSH (except in the rare event of pituitary failure) (see Table 48.1). High serum levels of TPO antibodies are characteristic of autoimmune disease.

Treatment

Oral thyroxine (0.10–0.20 mg) as a single daily dose is curative. Caution is required in the elderly or those with cardiac disease; in such cases the replacement dose is commenced at 0.05 mg daily and increased cautiously. If a rapid response is required, tri-iodothyronine (20 μg t.d.s.) may be used.

Myxoedema (Fig. 48.9)

The signs and symptoms of hypothyroidism are accentuated. The facial appearance is typical; there is often supraclavicular puffi-ness, a malar flush and a yellow tinge to the skin. Myxoedema coma, characterised by altered mental state, hypothermia and a precipitating medical condition, for example cardiac failure or infection, carries a high mortality rate. Treatment comprises thyroid replacement, either a bolus of 500 mg of T_4 or 10 μg of T_3 either intravenously or orally every 4–6 hours. If the body tem-perature is less than 30°C the patient must be warmed slowly. Intravenous broad-spectrum antibiotics and hydrocortisone (in divided doses) are recommended.

Primary or atrophic myxoedema is considered to be an autoimmune disease similar to chronic lymphocytic (Hashi-moto's) thyroiditis (see below) but without goitre formation. Delay in diagnosis is common and the degree of hypothyroidism is usually more severe than in goitrous autoimmune thyroiditis.

Dyshormonogenesis

Genetic deficiencies in the enzymes controlling the synthesis of thyroid hormones account for a minority of cases of neonatal hypothyroidism and goitre. These are usually inherited in an autosomal recessive pattern and a family history is common. If

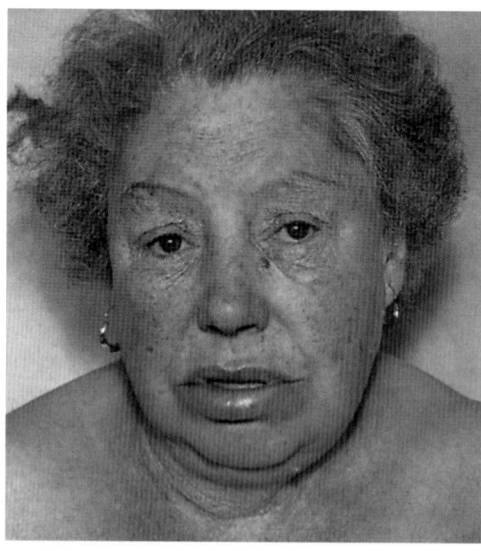

Figure 48.9 Myxoedema. Note the bloated look, the pouting lips and the dull expression (courtesy of Dr V.K. Summers, Liverpool, UK).

the biochemical effect is of moderate degree, thyroid enlargement may be the only manifestation; dyshormonogenesis should be considered in young patients presenting with euthyroid goitre. The most common abnormalities affect TPO activity and thyroglobulin synthesis. A classic example of dyshormonogenesis due to TPO deficiency is Pendred's syndrome, in which goitre is associated with severe sensorineural hearing impairment and abnormality of the bony labyrinth observed on CT examination of the temporal bones.

THYROID ENLARGEMENT

The normal thyroid gland is impalpable. The term goitre (from the Latin *guttur* = the throat) is used to describe *generalised* enlargement of the thyroid gland. A discrete swelling (nodule) in one lobe with no palpable abnormality elsewhere is termed an *isolated* (or *solitary*) swelling. Discrete swellings with evidence of abnormality elsewhere in the gland are termed *dominant* (Summary box 48.3).

> **Summary box 48.3**
>
> **Thyroid swellings**
>
> - Know how to describe thyroid swellings
> - Use appropriate investigations
> - Know the indications for surgery
> - Select the appropriate procedure
> - Describe and manage postoperative complications

A scheme for classifying thyroid enlargement is given in Table 48.4.

Simple goitre

Aetiology

Simple goitre may develop as a result of stimulation of the thyroid gland by TSH, either as a result of inappropriate secretion from a microadenoma in the anterior pituitary (which is rare) or in response to a chronically low level of circulating thyroid hor-mones. The most important factor in endemic goitre is dietary deficiency of iodine (see below), but defective hormone synthesis probably accounts for many sporadic goitres (see below).

TSH is not the only stimulus to thyroid follicular cell prolifera-tion; other growth factors, including immunoglobulins, exert an influence. The heterogeneous structural and functional response in the thyroid resulting in characteristic nodularity may be due to the presence of clones of cells that are particularly sensitive to growth stimulation.

Iodine deficiency

The daily requirement for iodine is about 0.1–0.15 mg. In nearly all districts where simple goitre is endemic there is a very low iodide content in the water and food. Endemic areas are found in the mountainous ranges, such as the Rocky Mountains, the Alps, the Andes and the Himalayas. In the UK endemic areas include Derbyshire and Yorkshire. Endemic goitre is also found in lowland

> Vaughan Pendred, **1869–1946, a General Practitioner of Durham, England,** described this syndrome in 1896. Exactly 100 years later the defect was mapped to chromosome 7q.

Table 48.4 Classification of thyroid swellings

Simple goitre (euthyroid)
Diffuse hyperplastic
　　Physiological
　　Pubertal
　　Pregnancy
Multinodular goitre

Toxic
Diffuse
　　Graves' disease
Multinodular
Toxic adenoma

Neoplastic
Benign
Malignant

Inflammatory
Autoimmune
　　Chronic lymphocytic thyroiditis
　　Hashimoto's disease
Granulomatous
　　De Quervain's thyroiditis
Fibrosing
　　Riedel's thyroiditis
Infective
　　Acute (bacterial thyroiditis, viral thyroiditis, 'subacute thyroiditis')
　　Chronic (tuberculous, syphilitic)
Other
　　Amyloid

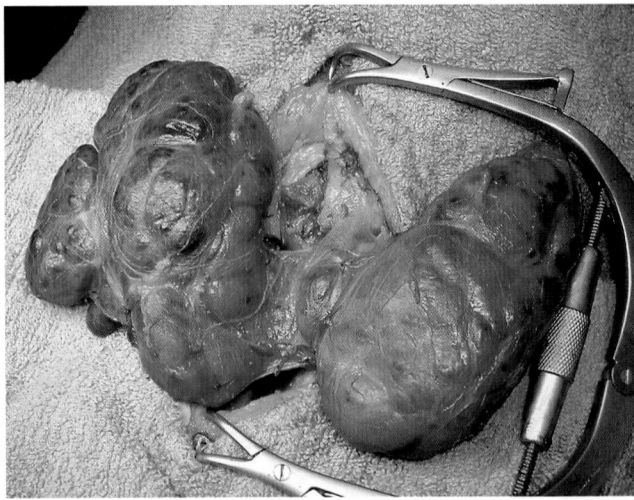

Figure 48.10 Total thyroidectomy for dyshormonogenetic goitre in a 14-year-old girl.

as para-aminosalicylic acid (PAS) and, of course, the anti-thyroid drugs. Thiocyanates and perchlorates interfere with iodide trapping whereas carbimazole and thiouracil compounds interfere with the oxidation of iodide and the binding of iodine to tyrosine.

Surprisingly enough, iodides in large quantities are goitrogenic because they inhibit the organic binding of iodine and produce an iodide goitre. Excessive iodine intake may be associated with an increased incidence of autoimmune thyroid disease.

The natural history of simple goitre

The stages in goitre formation are as follows:

- Persistent growth stimulation causes diffuse hyperplasia; all lobules are composed of active follicles and iodine uptake is uniform. This is a diffuse hyperplastic goitre, which may persist for a long time but is reversible if stimulation ceases.
- Later, as a result of fluctuating stimulation, a mixed pattern develops with areas of active lobules and areas of inactive lobules.
- Active lobules become more vascular and hyperplastic until haemorrhage occurs, causing central necrosis and leaving only a surrounding rind of active follicles.
- Necrotic lobules coalesce to form nodules filled with either iodine-free colloid or a mass of new but inactive follicles.
- Continual repetition of this process results in a nodular goitre. Most nodules are inactive, and active follicles are present only in the internodular tissue.

Diffuse hyperplastic goitre

Diffuse hyperplasia corresponds to the first stages of the natural history. The goitre appears in childhood in endemic areas but, in sporadic cases, it usually occurs at puberty when metabolic demands are high. If TSH stimulation ceases the goitre may regress; however, it tends to recur later at times of stress such as pregnancy. The goitre is soft, diffuse and may become large enough to cause discomfort. A colloid goitre is a late stage of diffuse hyperplasia when TSH stimulation has fallen off and when many follicles are inactive and full of colloid (Fig. 48.11).

Nodular goitre

Nodules are usually multiple, forming a multinodular goitre (Fig. 48.12). Occasionally, only one macroscopic nodule is found, but

areas where the soil lacks iodide or the water supply comes from far-away mountain ranges, e.g. the Great Lakes of North America, the plains of Lombardy, the Struma valley, the Nile valley and the Congo. Calcium is also goitrogenic and goitre is common in low-iodine areas on chalk or limestone, for example Derbyshire and southern Ireland. Although iodides in food and water may be adequate, failure of intestinal absorption may produce iodine deficiency.

Dyshormonogenesis

Enzyme deficiencies of varying severity may be responsible for many sporadic goitres, i.e. in non-endemic areas (Fig. 48.10). There is often a family history, suggesting a genetic defect. Environmental factors may compensate in areas of high iodine intake; for example, goitre is almost unknown in Iceland where the fish diet is rich in iodine. Similarly, a low intake of iodine encourages goitre formation in those with a metabolic predisposition.

Goitrogens

Well-known goitrogens are the vegetables of the brassica family (cabbage, kale and rape), which contain thiocyanate, drugs such

Bernhard Moritz Carl Ludwig Riedel, **1846–1916, Professor of Surgery, Jena, Germany, described this form of thyroiditis in 1896.**
Struma. **The River Struma arises in the mountains of Bulgaria and flows into the Aegean Sea. Along its banks, and those of its tributaries, dwell peoples of several nationalities amongst whom endemic goitre has long been prevalent. Struma is a European continental term for goitre.**

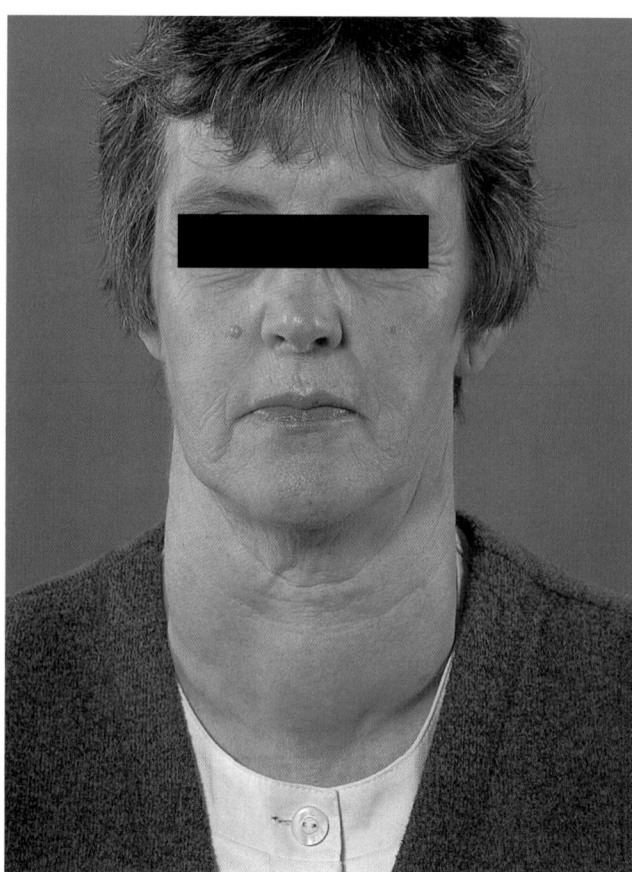

Figure 48.11 Colloid goitre.

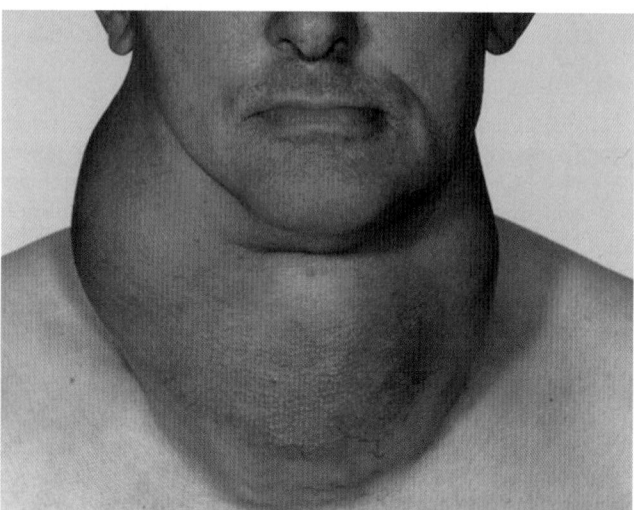

Figure 48.12 Large multinodular goitre.

microscopic changes will be present throughout the gland; this is one form of a clinically solitary nodule. Nodules may be colloid or cellular, and cystic degeneration and haemorrhage are common, as is subsequent calcification. Nodules appear early in endemic goitre and later (between 20 and 30 years) in sporadic goitre, although the patient may be unaware of the goitre until his or her late 40s or 50s. All types of simple goitre are more common in females than males because of the presence of oestrogen receptors in thyroid tissue.

Diagnosis

Diagnosis is usually straightforward. The patient is euthyroid, the nodules are palpable and often visible (smooth, usually firm and not hard) and the goitre is painless and moves freely on swallowing. Hardness and irregularity, due to calcification, may simulate carcinoma. A painful nodule or the sudden appearance or rapid enlargement of a nodule raises suspicion of carcinoma; however, such cases are usually due to haemorrhage into a simple nodule. Differential diagnosis from autoimmune thyroiditis may be difficult and the two conditions frequently coexist.

Investigations

Thyroid function should be assessed to exclude mild hyperthyroidism, and the presence of circulating thyroid antibodies tested to differentiate from autoimmune thyroiditis. Plain radiographs of the chest and thoracic inlet will rapidly demonstrate clinically significant tracheal deviation or compression. Ultrasound and CT give more detailed images but rarely influence clinical management. FNAC is only required for a dominant swelling in a generalised goitre.

Complications

Tracheal obstruction may occur because of gross lateral displacement or compression in a lateral or anteroposterior plane by retrosternal extension of the goitre (see Figs 48.5 and 48.7, p. 774). Acute respiratory obstruction may follow haemorrhage into a nodule impacted in the thoracic inlet.

Secondary thyrotoxicosis

Transient episodes of mild hyperthyroidism are common, occurring in up to 30% of patients.

Carcinoma

An increased incidence of cancer (usually follicular) has been reported from endemic areas. Dominant or rapidly growing nodules in longstanding goitres should always be subjected to aspiration cytology.

Prevention and treatment of simple goitre

In endemic areas, for example Switzerland, parts of the USA and Argentina, the incidence of goitre has been strikingly reduced by the introduction of iodised salt. In the early stages a hyperplastic goitre may regress if thyroxine is given at a dose of 0.15–0.2 mg daily for a few months.

Although the nodular stage of simple goitre is irreversible, more than half of benign nodules will regress in size over 10 years (Kuma). Most patients with multinodular goitre are asymptomatic and do not require operation. Operation may be indicated on cosmetic grounds, for pressure symptoms or in response to patient anxiety. Retrosternal extension with actual or incipient tracheal compression is also an indication for operation, as is the presence of a dominant area of enlargement that may be neoplastic.

There is a choice of surgical treatment in multinodular goitre. This includes *total thyroidectomy*, with immediate and lifelong replacement of thyroxine, or some form of partial resection, to conserve sufficient functioning thyroid tissue to subserve normal function while reducing the risk of hypoparathyroidism that accompanies total thyroidectomy. *Subtotal thyroidectomy* involves partial resection of each lobe, removing the bulk of the gland and leaving up to 8 g of relatively normal tissue in each remnant. The technique is essentially the same as described for toxic goitre, as are the postoperative complications. More often, however, the multinodular change is asymmetrically distributed, with one lobe more significantly involved than the other. In these circumstances, particularly in older patients, *total lobectomy* on the more affected side is the appropriate management, with either subtotal resection (Dunhill procedure) or no intervention on the less affected side.

In many cases the causative factors persist and recurrence is likely. Reoperation for recurrent nodular goitre is more difficult and hazardous and, for this reason, an increasing number of thyroid surgeons favour total thyroidectomy in younger patients. However, when the first operation comprised unilateral lobectomy alone for asymmetrical goitre, reoperation and completion of total thyroidectomy is straightforward if required for progression of nodularity in the remaining lobe.

After subtotal resection it has been customary to give thyroxine to suppress TSH secretion, with the aim of preventing recurrence. Whether this is either necessary or effective is uncertain, although the evidence of benefit in endemic areas is better than elsewhere. There is some evidence that radioactive iodine may reduce the size of recurrent nodular goitre after previous subtotal resection and, in some circumstances, this may be a safer alternative than reoperation, particularly if there has been more than one previous thyroid procedure.

Clinically discrete swellings

Discrete thyroid swellings (thyroid nodules) are common and are present in 3–4% of the adult population in the UK and USA. They are three to four times more frequent in women than men.

Diagnosis

A discrete swelling in an otherwise impalpable gland is termed *isolated* or *solitary*, whereas the preferred term is *dominant* for a similar swelling in a gland with clinical evidence of generalised abnormality in the form of a palpable contralateral lobe or generalised mild nodularity. About 70% of discrete thyroid swellings are clinically isolated and about 30% are dominant. The true incidence of isolated swellings is somewhat less than the clinical estimate. Clinical classification is inevitably subjective and overestimates the frequency of truly isolated swellings. When such a gland is exposed at operation or examined by ultrasonography, CT or MRI, clinically impalpable nodules are often detected. The true frequency of thyroid nodularity compared with the clinical detection rate by palpation is shown in Fig. 48.13. Establishing the presence of such minor abnormality is unnecessary because the management of discrete swellings, be they isolated or dominant, is similar.

The importance of discrete swellings lies in the increased risk of neoplasia compared with other thyroid swellings. Some 15% of isolated swellings prove to be malignant, and an additional 30–40% are follicular adenomas. The remainder are non-neoplastic, largely consisting of areas of colloid degeneration,

Sir Thomas Peel Dunhill, **1876–1957**, Surgeon, St. Bartholomew's Hospital, London, England.

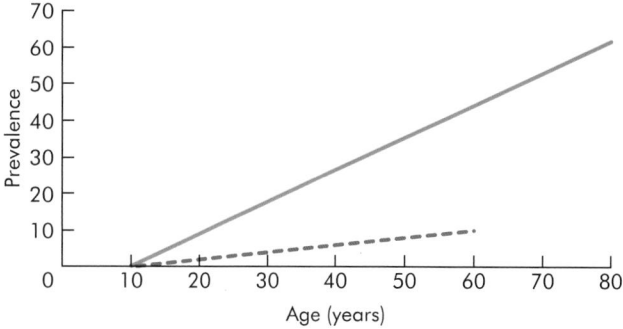

Figure 48.13 The prevalence of thyroid nodules detected on palpation (broken line) or by ultrasonography or post-mortem examination (solid line) (after Mazzaferri).

thyroiditis or cysts. Although the incidence of malignancy or follicular adenoma in clinically dominant swellings is approximately half of that of truly isolated swellings, it is substantial and cannot be ignored (Fig. 48.14).

Investigation

Thyroid function

Serum TSH and thyroid hormone levels should be measured. If hyperthyroidism associated with a discrete swelling is confirmed biochemically, it indicates either a 'toxic adenoma' or a manifestation of toxic multinodular goitre. The combination of toxicity and nodularity is important and is an indication for isotope scanning to localise the area(s) of hyperfunction.

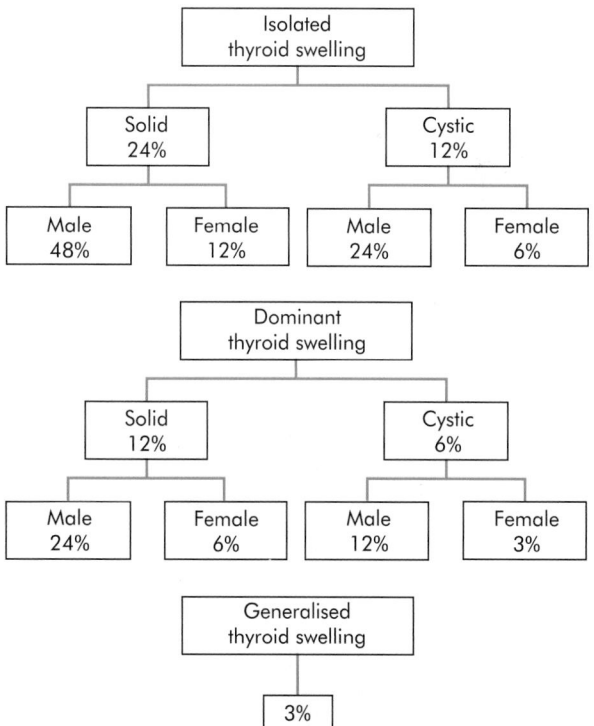

Figure 48.14 The risk of malignancy in thyroid swellings ('rule of 12'). The risk of cancer in a thyroid swelling can be expressed as a factor of 12. The risk is greater in isolated vs. dominant swellings, solid vs. cystic swellings and men vs. women.

Autoantibody titres

The autoantibody status may determine whether a swelling is a manifestation of chronic lymphocytic thyroiditis. The presence of circulating antibodies may increase the risk of thyroid failure after lobectomy.

Isotope scan

Isotope scanning used to be the mainstay of investigation of discrete thyroid swellings to determine the functional activity relative to the surrounding gland according to isotope uptake.

On scanning, swellings are categorised as 'hot' (overactive), 'warm' (active) or 'cold' (underactive). A hot nodule is one that takes up isotope while the surrounding thyroid tissue does not. Here, the surrounding thyroid tissue is inactive because the nodule is producing such high levels of thyroid hormones that TSH secretion is suppressed. A warm nodule takes up isotope, as does the normal thyroid tissue around it. A cold nodule does not take up isotope (see Fig. 48.8, p. 774).

About 80% of discrete swellings are cold, but only 15% prove to be malignant and the use of this criterion as an indication for operation lacks discrimination. Routine isotope scanning has been abandoned except when toxicity is associated with nodularity.

Ultrasonography

This was formerly widely used as a non-invasive supplement to clinical examination in determining the physical characteristics of thyroid swellings. Although ultrasonography can demonstrate subclinical nodularity and cyst formation, the former is clinically irrelevant and the latter apparent at aspiration, which should be routine in all discrete swellings. There was a decline in the use of ultrasound because it had a minimal impact on management; however, it is becoming more popular again as an adjunct to FNAC and in the assessment of malignant lymphadenopathy.

Fine-needle aspiration cytology

FNAC is the investigation of choice in discrete thyroid swellings. FNAC has excellent patient compliance, is simple and quick to perform in the out-patient department and is readily repeated.

Thyroid conditions that may be diagnosed by FNAC include colloid nodules (Fig. 48.15), thyroiditis, papillary carcinoma (Fig. 48.16), medullary carcinoma, anaplastic carcinoma and lymphoma. FNAC cannot distinguish between a benign follicular adenoma (Fig. 48.17) and follicular carcinoma, as this distinction is dependent not on cytology but on histological criteria, which include capsular and vascular invasion.

Although FNAC was reported as being highly accurate by Lowhagen and his colleagues (who were its pioneers) at the Karolinska Hospital, high accuracy has not always been reproducible, especially when results are analysed critically. There are very few false positives with respect to malignancy but there is a definite false-negative rate with respect to both benign and malignant neoplasia. In addition, there can be a high rate of unsatisfactory aspirates, particularly in cystic or partly cystic swellings. These often yield only cyst fluid with macrophages and degenerate cells with few thyroid follicular cells upon which to report. After aspiration, a further sample for cytology should be taken from the cyst wall. There has been a recent trend to use ultrasound to guide the needle to achieve more accurate sampling and reduce the rate of unsatisfactory aspirates.

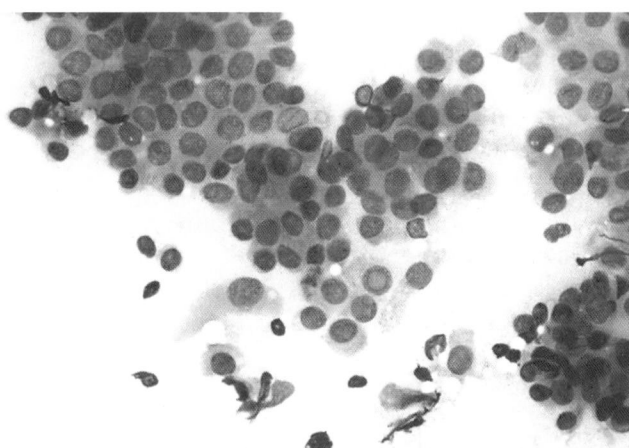

Figure 48.16 Thy5 aspiration cytology. Papillary carcinoma with typical cellular variability and nuclear inclusions.

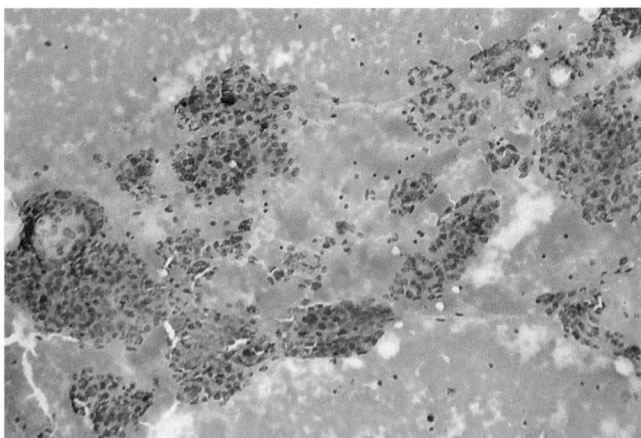

Figure 48.17 Thy3 aspiration cytology. Follicular neoplasm showing increased cellularity with a follicular pattern.

Torsten Lowhagen, **Cytologist, The Department of Tumour Pathology, The Karolinska Hospital, Stockholm, Sweden.**

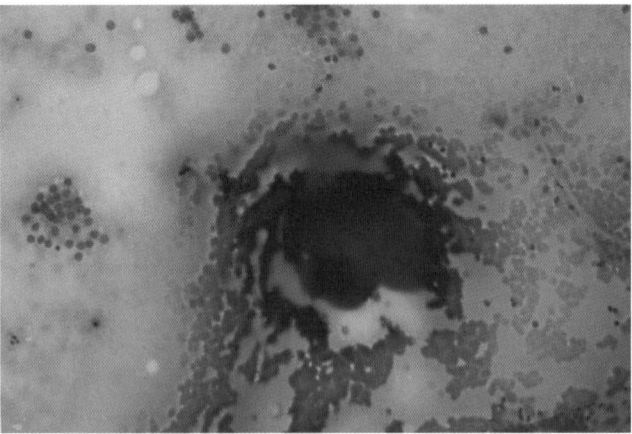

Figure 48.15 Thy2 aspiration cytology. Non-neoplastic appearances with scanty normal follicular cells together with colloid (= colloid nodule).

Relatively few cysts are permanently abolished by one or more aspirations and, because of the risk of malignancy, recurrent cysts should be removed.

Radiology

Chest and thoracic inlet radiographs may confirm tracheal deviation, compression or retrosternal extension and are required when either clinical suspicion or FNAC indicates malignancy.

Ultrasound scan

Although ultrasound gives additional information to supplement clinical examination it will also often reveal previously unsuspected nodularity, which raises the problem of managing such incidentally found lesions.

Other scans

CT and MRI scans give excellent anatomical detail of thyroid swellings but have no role in the first line of investigation. They are most useful in assessing retrosternal (see Fig. 48.7 p. 774) and recurrent swellings, particularly if initial surgery has been performed elsewhere. A PET scan (Fig. 48.18) may be useful, particularly in localising disease that does not take up radio-iodine.

Laryngoscopy

Flexible laryngosopy has rendered indirect laryngoscopy obsolete and is widely used preoperatively to determine the mobility of the vocal cords, although usually for medico-legal rather than clinical reasons. Nevertheless, the presence of a unilateral cord palsy coexisting with a swelling suggestive of malignancy is usually diagnostic.

Core biopsy

Core biopsy gives a strip of tissue for histological rather than cytological assessment. It has a high diagnostic accuracy but requires local anaesthesia and may be associated with complications such as pain, bleeding and tracheal and recurrent laryngeal nerve damage. It has little application in routine assessment except in locally advanced, surgically unresectable malignancy (either anaplastic carcinoma or lymphoma), when core biopsy may avoid operation. In some centres core biopsy is recommended in cases of Thy1 FNAC (inadequate cytology) specimens to avoid operating on patients in whom the risk of malignancy is very low. It is unlikely to be useful in differentiating Thy3 specimens (i.e. follicular lesions) because of sampling issues.

Treatment

The main indication for operation is the risk of neoplasia. The reason for advocating the removal of all follicular neoplasms is that it is seldom possible to distinguish between a follicular adenoma and a carcinoma except on the basis of histological evidence of capsular or vascular invasion. FNAC cannot make this distinction although, on occasion, cellular nuclear features may be so abnormal as to suggest malignant change. On this basis, some 50% of isolated swellings and 25% of dominant swellings should be removed on the grounds of neoplasia. Even when the cytology is negative, the age and sex of the patient and the size of the swelling may be relative indications for surgery, especially when a large swelling is symptomatic.

There are useful clinical criteria to assist in selection for operation according to the risk of neoplasia and malignancy. Hard texture alone is not reliable as tense cystic swellings may be suspiciously hard; however, a hard, irregular swelling with any apparent fixity, which is unusual, is highly suspicious. Evidence of recurrent laryngeal nerve paralysis, suggested by hoarseness and a non-occlusive cough and confirmed by laryngoscopy, is almost pathognomonic. Deep cervical lymphadenopathy along the internal jugular vein in association with a clinically suspicious swelling is almost diagnostic of papillary carcinoma. In most patients, however, such features are absent, but there are risk factors associated with sex and age. The incidence of thyroid carcinoma in women is about three times that in men; however, a discrete swelling in a man is much more likely to be malignant than a swelling in a woman and should be removed. The risk of carcinoma is increased at either end of the age range and a discrete swelling in a teenager of either sex must be provisionally diagnosed as carcinoma. The risk increases over the age of 50 years, more so in men.

Thyroid cysts

Routine FNAC (or ultrasonography) shows that over 30% of clinically isolated swellings contain fluid and are cystic or partly cystic. Tense cysts may be hard and mimic carcinoma. Bleeding into a cyst often presents with a history of sudden painful swelling, which resolves to a variable extent over a period of weeks if untreated. Aspiration yields altered blood but reaccumulation is frequent. About 50% of cystic swellings are the result of colloid degeneration or are of uncertain aetiology, because of an absence of epithelial cells in the lining. Although most of the remainder are the result of involution in follicular adenomas (Fig. 48.19), some 10–15% of cystic follicular swellings are histologically malignant

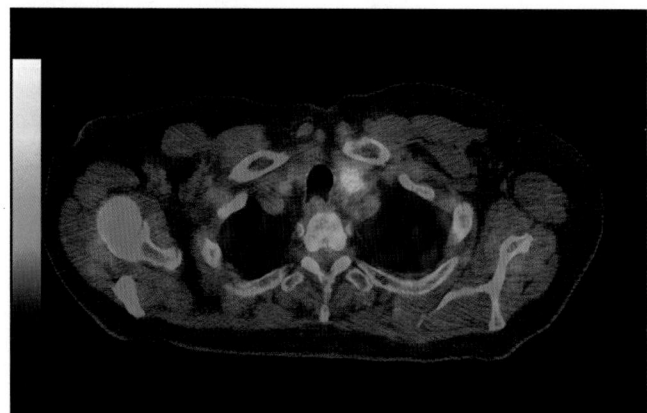

Figure 48.18 Fused computerised tomography and positron emission tomography scans showing a left-sided thyroid neoplasm (courtesy of Dr M. Brooks, Aberdeen, UK).

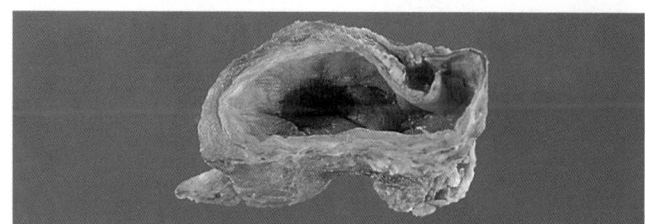

Figure 48.19 An apparently simple cystic thyroid swelling, the wall of which comprised follicular neoplastic tissue.

(30% in men and 10% in women). Papillary carcinoma is often associated with cyst formation (Fig. 48.20).

Most patients with discrete swellings, however, are women aged 20–40 years, in whom the risk of malignancy is low and the indications for operation are not clear. FNAC is the most appropriate investigation to aid selection.

The indications for operation in isolated or dominant thyroid swellings are listed in Table 48.5.

Selection of thyroid procedure

The choice of thyroid operation depends on:

- diagnosis (if known preoperatively);
- risk of thyroid failure;
- risk of RLN injury;
- risk of recurrence;
- Graves' disease;
- multinodular goitre;
- differentiated thyroid cancer (DTC);
- risk of hypoparathyroidism.

Total and near-total thyroidectomy do not conserve sufficient thyroid tissue for normal thyroid function and thyroid replacement therapy is necessary. In most patients with negative antithyroid antibodies, one thyroid lobe will maintain normal

Table 48.5 Indications for operation in thyroid swellings

Neoplasia
FNAC positive
Clinical suspicion, including:
Age
Male sex
Hard texture
Fixity
Recurrent laryngeal nerve palsy
Lymphadenopathy
Recurrent cyst
Toxic adenoma
Pressure symptoms
Cosmesis
Patient's wishes

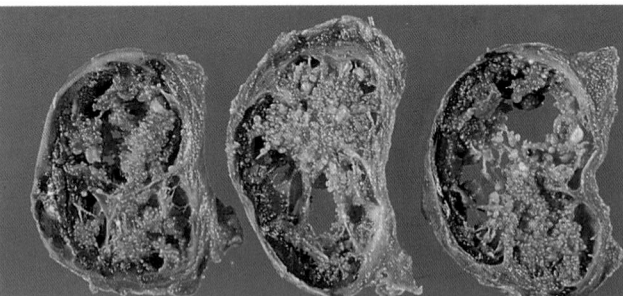

Figure 48.20 Cyst formation in a papillary carcinoma.

Robert James Graves, **Physician, The Meath Hospital, Dublin, Ireland, published an account of exophthalmic goitre in 1835.**

function. In subtotal thyroidectomy the volume of thyroid tissue preserved influences the risk of thyroid failure; larger remnants have a better chance of normal function but a higher risk of recurrence in Graves' disease.

Subtotal resections for colloid goitre run the risk of later growth of the remnant and, if a second operation is required years later, this greatly increases the risk to the RLN and parathyroid glands. In young patients, total thyroidectomy should be considered. It may be preferable to leave the least affected lobe untouched to permit a straightforward lobectomy in the future if required, rather than carry out subtotal resections.

In Graves' disease, preserving large remnants increases the risk of recurrence of the toxicity and, in these cases, it is better to err on the side of removing too much thyroid tissue than too little (Table 48.6). Thyroid failure need not be regarded as a failure of treatment but recurrent toxicity is.

The relative merits of routine total vs. selective total thyroidectomy in DTC are discussed below (Summary box 48.4).

Summary box 48.4

Thyroid operations

All thyroid operations can be assembled from three basic elements:

- Total lobectomy
- Isthmusectomy
- Subtotal lobectomy

Total thyroidectomy = 2 × total lobectomy + isthmusectomy

Subtotal thyroidectomy = 2 × subtotal lobectomy + isthmusectomy

Near-total thryroidectomy = total lobectomy + isthmusectomy + subtotal lobectomy

Lobectomy = total lobectomy + isthmusectomy

Retrosternal goitre

Very few retrosternal goitres arise from ectopic thyroid tissue; most arise from the lower pole of a nodular goitre. If the neck is short and the pretracheal muscles are strong, particularly in men, the negative intrathoracic pressure tends to draw these nodules into the superior mediastinum.

Clinical features

A retrosternal goitre is often symptomless and discovered on a routine chest radiograph (see Fig. 48.5, p. 774). There may, however, be severe symptoms:

- *Dyspnoea*, particularly at night, cough and stridor (harsh sound on inspiration). Many patients attend a chest clinic with a diagnosis of asthma before the true nature of the problem is discovered.
- *Dysphagia*.
- *Engorgement of facial, neck and superficial chest wall veins*; in severe cases there may be obstruction of the superior vena cava (Fig. 48.21).
- *Recurrent nerve paralysis* is rare; the goitre may also be malignant or toxic.

Table 48.6 Comparison of surgical options for Graves' disease

	Total thyroidectomy	Subtotal thyroidectomy
Control of toxicity	Immediate	Immediate
Return to euthyroid state	Immediate	Variable – up to 12 months
Risk of recurrence	None	Lifelong – up to 5%[a]
Risk of thyroid failure	100%	Lifelong – up to 25%[a]
Risk of permanent hypoparathyroidism	5%	1%
Need for follow-up	Minimal	Lifelong

[a] The risk of recurrence and late failure are a function of the size of the remnant as a proportion of the total gland weight. Large remnants in small glands have a higher risk of recurrence and a low risk of failure, and small remnants in large glands have a higher risk of thyroid failure but a low risk of recurrence.

Chest and thoracic inlet radiographs show a soft-tissue shadow in the superior mediastinum, sometimes with calcification and often causing deviation and compression of the trachea. A CT scan gives the most accurate and often dramatic anatomical visualisation (see Fig. 48.7 p. 774).

Significant tracheal compression and obstruction may be demonstrated objectively by a flow–volume loop pulmonary function test in which the rate of flow is plotted against the volume of air inspired and then expired. Deterioration in flow because of an increase in tracheal compression, either acutely or in the long term, may be used to monitor progression of the disease and indicate the need for surgery. The changes are reversed by operation (Fig. 48.22).

Treatment

If obstructive symptoms are present in association with thyrotoxicosis it is unwise to treat a retrosternal goitre with antithyroid drugs or radioiodine as these may enlarge the goitre. Resection can almost always be carried out from the neck, but median sternotomy is sometimes necessary (see Fig. 48.21b). The cervical part of the goitre should first be mobilised by ligation and division of the superior thyroid vessels and the middle thyroid vein. The retrosternal goitre can then be delivered by traction, which may be facilitated by inserting a series of sutures, a finger or, traditionally, a spoon. Haemorrhage is rarely a problem because the goitre takes its blood supply with it from the neck. The RLN should be identified before delivering the retrosternal goitre, as it may be considerably displaced and is particularly vulnerable to injury from traction or tearing. If a large retrosternal goitre cannot be delivered intact, piecemeal delivery is possible; however, this risks leaving a fragment of nodular goitre deep in the mediastinum, which may result in a very difficult reoperation many years later. Fragmentation must be avoided when malignancy is likely. These problems are avoided with a timely median sternotomy.

Thyroid incidentaloma

The increased use of imaging modalities for non-thyroid head and neck pathology has created the clinical conundrum of the '*thyroid incidentaloma*'. These are clinically unsuspected and impalpable thyroid swellings and, in some parts of the world, this has reached 'epidemic' proportions. Injudicious reporting generates needless anxiety if the possibility of malignancy is raised inappropriately. The vast majority of impalpable thyroid swellings can be safely managed expectantly by a single annual review, with no intervention unless certain criteria are met or the swelling becomes palpable (Fig. 48.23).

HYPERTHYROIDISM

Thyrotoxicosis

The term thyrotoxicosis is retained because hyperthyroidism, i.e. symptoms due to a raised level of circulating thyroid hormones, is not responsible for all manifestations of the disease. Clinical types are:

- diffuse toxic goitre (Graves' disease);
- toxic nodular goitre;
- toxic nodule;
- hyperthyroidism due to rarer causes.

Diffuse toxic goitre

Graves' disease, a diffuse vascular goitre appearing at the same time as the hyperthyroidism, usually occurs in younger women and is frequently associated with eye signs. The syndrome is that of primary thyrotoxicosis (Fig. 48.24); 50% of patients have a family history of autoimmune endocrine diseases. The whole of the functioning thyroid tissue is involved, and the hypertrophy and hyperplasia are due to abnormal thyroid-stimulating antibodies (TSH-RAbs) that bind to TSH receptor sites and produce a disproportionate and prolonged effect.

Toxic nodular goitre

A simple nodular goitre is present for a long time before the hyperthyroidism, usually in the middle-aged or elderly, and is very infrequently associated with eye signs. The syndrome is that of secondary thyrotoxicosis.

In many cases of toxic nodular goitre the nodules are inactive and it is the internodular thyroid tissue that is overactive. However, in some toxic nodular goitres, one or more nodules are overactive and here the hyperthyroidism is due to autonomous thyroid tissue as in a toxic adenoma.

Toxic nodule

A toxic nodule is a solitary overactive nodule, which may be part of a generalised nodularity or a true toxic adenoma. It is autonomous and its hypertrophy and hyperplasia are not due to TSH-RAb. TSH secretion is suppressed by the high level of circulating thyroid hormones and the normal thyroid tissue surrounding the nodule is itself suppressed and inactive.

Histology

The normal thyroid gland consists of acini lined with flattened cuboidal epithelium and filled with homogeneous colloid (see Fig. 48.2, p. 772). In hyperthyroidism (Fig. 48.25) there is hyperplasia

(a)

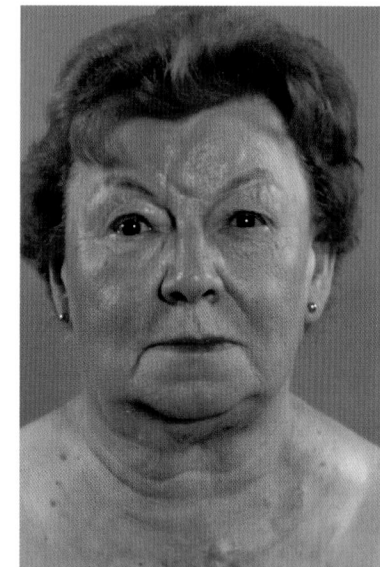

(b)

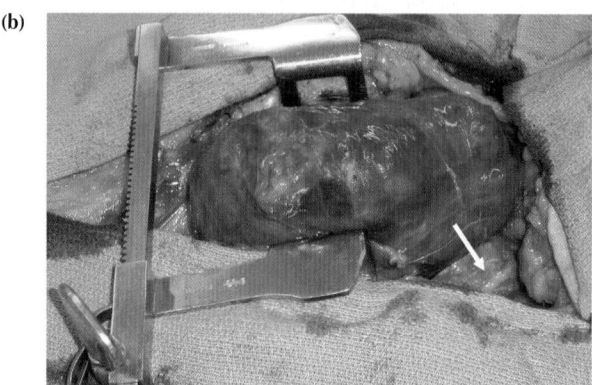

(c)

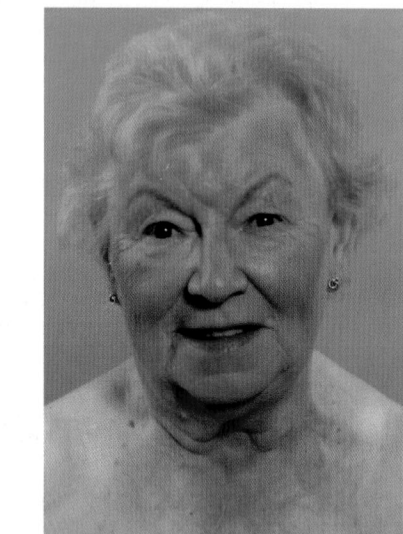

Figure 48.21 (a) Retrosternal goitre with superior vena cava obstruction. Preoperative appearance showing venous congestion. (b) Sternal split to deliver impacted left thyroid lobe. The recurrent laryngeal nerve is visible (arrow). (c) Postoperative appearance.

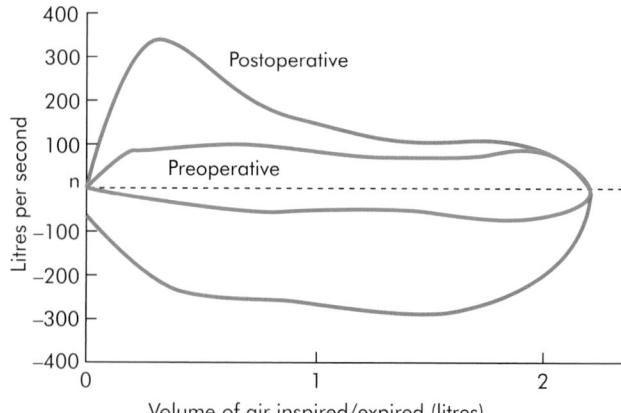

Figure 48.22 Flow–volume loops before and after operation on a goitre causing tracheal compression.

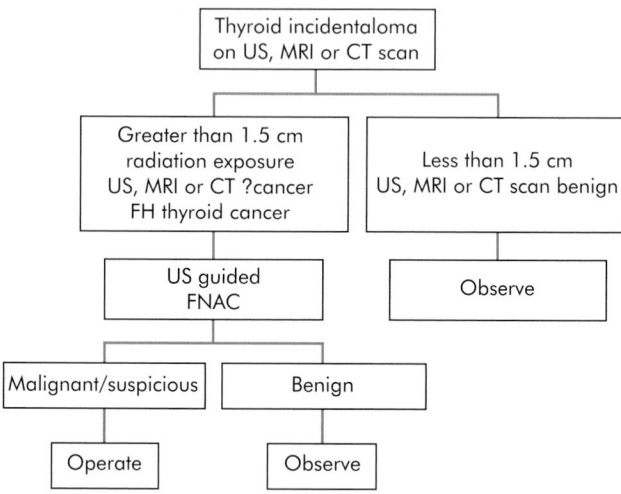

Figure 48.23 Management of thyroid incidentalomas. CT, computerised tomography; FH, family history; FNAC, fine-needle aspiration cytology; MRI, magnetic resonance imaging; US, ultrasound.

of acini, which are lined by high columnar epithelium. Many of them are empty and others contain vacuolated colloid with a characteristic 'scalloped' pattern adjacent to the thyrocytes.

Clinical features

The symptoms are:

- tiredness;
- emotional lability;
- heat intolerance;
- weight loss;
- excessive appetite;
- palpitations.

The signs of thyrotoxicosis are:

- tachycardia;
- hot, moist palms;
- exophthalmos;
- lid lag/retraction;
- agitation;
- thyroid goitre and bruit.

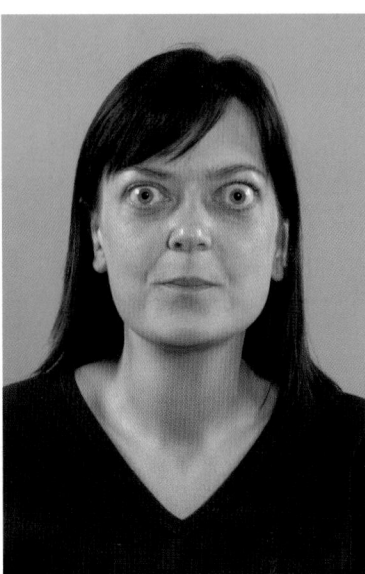

Figure 48.24 Graves' disease.

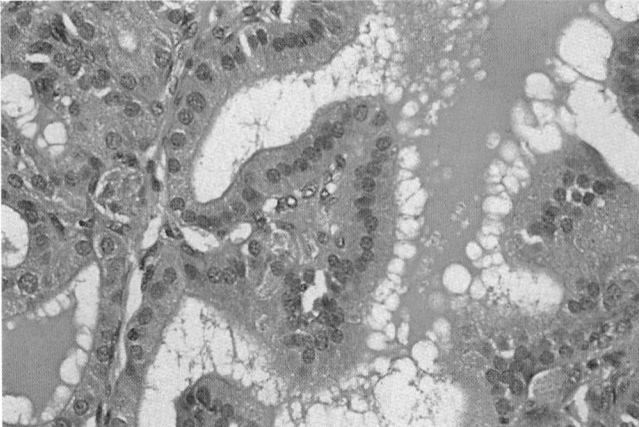

Figure 48.25 Histology of thyrotoxicosis.

Symptomatology

Thyrotoxicosis is eight times more common in women than in men. It may occur at any age. The most significant symptoms are loss of weight despite a good appetite, a recent preference for cold, and palpitations. The most significant signs are the excitability of the patient, the presence of a goitre, exophthalmos and tachycardia or cardiac arrhythmia.

The goitre in primary thyrotoxicosis is diffuse and vascular; it may be large or small, firm or soft, and a thrill and a bruit may be present. The onset is abrupt but remissions and exacerbations are not infrequent. Hyperthyroidism is usually more severe than in secondary thyrotoxicosis but cardiac failure is rare. Manifestations of thyrotoxicosis not due to hyperthyroidism *per se*, for example orbital proptosis, ophthalmoplegia and pretibial myxoedema, may occur in primary thyrotoxicosis.

In secondary thyrotoxicosis the goitre is nodular. The onset is insidious and may present with cardiac failure or atrial fibrillation. It is characteristic that the hyperthyroidism is not severe. Eye

per se **is Latin for 'through itself'.**

signs other than lid lag and lid spasm (due to hyperthyroidism) are very rare.

Cardiac rhythm

A fast heart rate, which persists during sleep, is characteristic. Cardiac arrhythmias are superimposed on the sinus tachycardia as the disease progresses, and they are more common in older patients with thyrotoxicosis because of the prevalence of coincidental heart disease. Stages of development of thyrotoxic arrhythmias are:

1 multiple extrasystoles;
2 paroxysmal atrial tachycardia;
3 paroxysmal atrial fibrillation;
4 persistent atrial fibrillation, not responsive to digoxin.

Myopathy

Weakness of the proximal limb muscles is commonly found if looked for. Severe muscular weakness (thyrotoxic myopathy), resembling myasthenia gravis, occasionally occurs. Recovery proceeds as hyperthyroidism is controlled.

Eye signs

Some degree of exophthalmos is common (see Fig. 48.24). It may be unilateral. True exophthalmos is a proptosis of the eye, caused by infiltration of the retrobulbar tissues with fluid and round cells, with a varying degree of retraction or spasm of the upper eyelid. (Lid spasm occurs because the levator palpebrae superioris muscle is partly innervated by sympathetic fibres.) This results in widening of the palpebral fissure so that the sclera may be seen clearly above the upper margin of the iris and cornea (above the 'limbus').

Spasm and retraction usually disappear when the hyperthyroidism is controlled. They may be improved by beta-adrenergic blocking drugs, for example guanethidine eye drops. Oedema of the eyelids, conjunctival injection and chemosis are aggravated by compression of the ophthalmic veins (Fig. 48.26). Weakness of the extraocular muscles, particularly the elevators (inferior oblique), results in diplopia. In severe cases papilloedema and corneal ulceration occur. When severe and progressive it is known as malignant exophthalmos (Fig. 48.27) and the eye may be destroyed. Graves' ophthalmopathy is an autoimmune disease in which there are antibody-mediated effects on the ocular muscles.

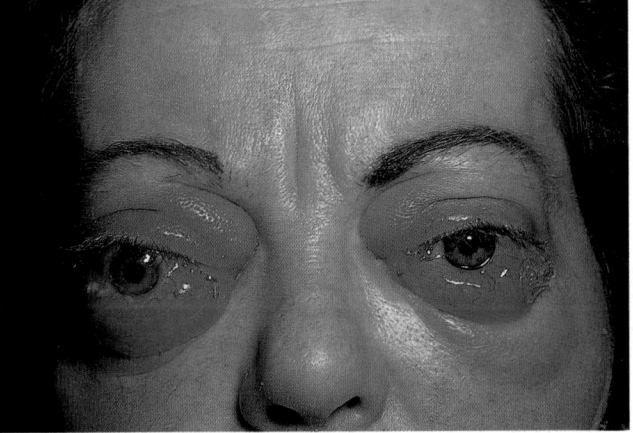

Figure 48.26 Severe Graves' ophthalmopathy (courtesy of Dr J.S. Bevan, Aberdeen, UK).

CHAPTER 48 | THE THYROID AND PARATHYROID GLANDS

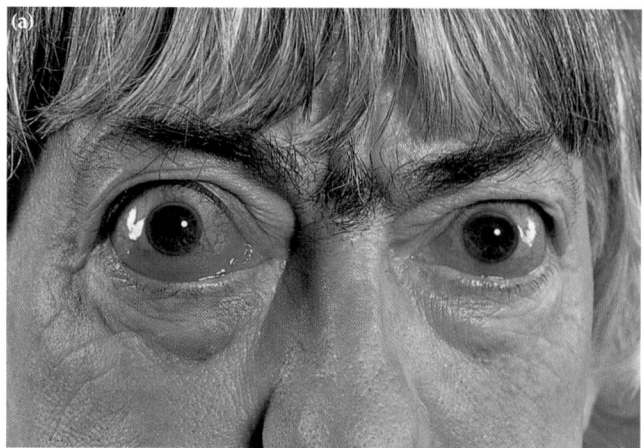

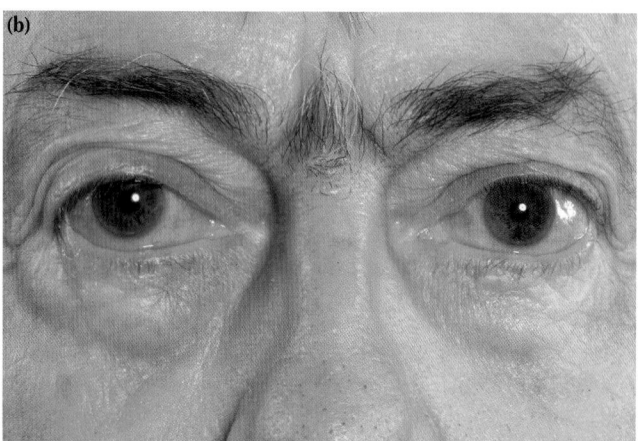

Figure 48.27 (a) Progressive (malignant) exophthalmos. (b) Following treatment with steroids, orbital radiotherapy and bilateral tarsorraphy (courtesy of Dr J.S. Bevan, Aberdeen, UK).

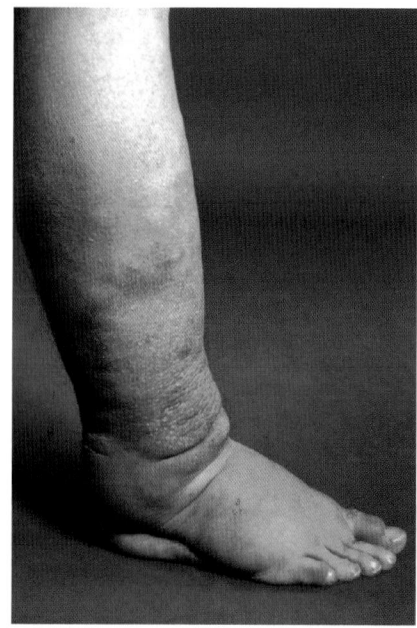

Figure 48.28 Thyroid dermopathy (pretibial myxoedema). It is usually symmetrical and minor degrees are not uncommon but are easily missed. The earliest stage is a shiny red plaque of thickened skin with coarse hair, which may be cyanotic when cold. In severe cases the skin of the whole leg below the knee is involved, together with that of the foot and the ankle, and there may be clubbing of the fingers and toes (thyroid acropachy).

Exophthalmos tends to improve with time. Sleeping propped up and lateral tarsorrhaphy will help to protect the eye but will not prevent progression. Hypothyroidism increases proptosis by a few millimetres and should be avoided.

Improvement has been reported with massive doses of prednisone. Intraorbital injection of steroids is dangerous because of the venous congestion, and total thyroid ablation has not proved effective. When the eye is in danger, orbital decompression may be required.

Thyroid dermopathy ('pretibial myxoedema') (Fig. 48.28) is a rare condition characterised by thickening of the skin, usually in areas of trauma, by deposition of hyaluronic acid in the dermis and subcutis. It usually occurs a few years after the onset of thyrotoxicosis and usually responds to treatment of the underlying thyroid disorder and topical steroids.

Diagnosis of thyrotoxicosis

Most cases are readily diagnosed clinically. Difficulty is most likely to arise in the differentiation of mild hyperthyroidism from an anxiety state when a goitre is present. In these cases the thyroid status is determined by the diagnostic tests described earlier. A TRH test is rarely indicated.

T_3 thyrotoxicosis is diagnosed by estimating the free T_3. It should be suspected if the clinical picture is suggestive but routine tests of thyroid function reveal a normal T_4 but suppressed TSH.

A thyroid scan is required to diagnose an autonomous toxic nodule and differentiate it from a dominant swelling in a toxic multinodular goitre.

Thyrotoxicosis should always be considered in:

- children with a growth spurt, behaviour problems or myopathy;
- tachycardia or arrhythmia in the elderly;
- unexplained diarrhoea;
- loss of weight.

Principles of treatment of thyrotoxicosis

Non-specific measures are rest and sedation; in established thyrotoxicosis these should be used only in conjunction with specific measures, i.e. the use of anti-thyroid drugs, surgery and radio-iodine.

Anti-thyroid drugs

Those in common use are carbimazole and propylthiouracil. β-Adrenergic blockers such as propranolol and nadolol are used to block the cardiovascular effects of the elevated T4. Iodides, which may reduce the vascularity of the thyroid, should be used only as immediate preoperative preparation in the 10 days before surgery. Anti-thyroid drugs are used to restore the patient to a euthyroid state and to maintain this for a prolonged period in the hope that a permanent remission will occur, i.e. that the production of TSH-RAbs will diminish or cease. Anti-thyroid drugs cannot cure a toxic nodule. The overactive thyroid tissue is autonomous and recurrence of the hyperthyroidism is certain when the drug is discontinued.

- *Advantages.* No surgery and no use of radioactive materials.
- *Disadvantages.* Treatment is prolonged and the failure rate is at

least 50%. The duration of treatment may be tailored to the severity of the toxicity, with milder cases being treated for only 6 months and severe cases for 2 years before stopping therapy.

It is impossible to predict which patient is likely to go into permanent remission although large gland size, severity of disease and TSH-RAb levels are indicators of poor prognosis.

Some goitres enlarge and become very vascular during treatment, even if thyroxine is given at the same time. This is probably due to TSH-RAb stimulation during the prolonged course of treatment and not a direct effect of the drug.

Very rarely there is a dangerous drug reaction, particularly agranulocytosis or aplastic anaemia. If a sore throat develops the patient should be instructed to discontinue treatment until the white cell count has been checked because of the risk of agranulocytosis.

Initially, 10 mg of carbimazole is given three or four times a day, with a latent interval of 7–14 days before clinical improvement is apparent. It is important to maintain a high concentration of the drug throughout a 24-hour period by spacing the doses at 8- or 6-hourly intervals. When the patient becomes biochemically euthyroid, a maintenance dose of 5 mg two or three times a day is given for 6–24 months. An alternative technique is to continue with the high dose of carbimazole and inhibit all T_3 and T_4 production by giving a maintenance dose of 0.1–0.15 mg of thyroxine daily. There is no risk of producing iatrogenic thyroid insufficiency and follow-up is less demanding ('block and replacement treatment').

The levels of TSH-RAbs usually fall during treatment and this accounts for the permanent cure that occurs in 50% of patients.

Surgery

In diffuse toxic goitre and toxic nodular goitre with overactive internodular tissue, surgery cures by reducing the mass of overactive tissue. Cure is probable if the thyroid tissue can be reduced below a critical mass but there is a risk of both permanent thyroid failure and recurrence of toxicity following subtotal resection. Operations may result in a reduction of TSH-RAbs or it may be that circulating TSH-RAbs, however high their levels, can only produce limited hypertrophy and hyperplasia when the mass of thyroid tissue is small. In the autonomous toxic nodule, and in toxic nodular goitre with overactive autonomous toxic nodules, surgery cures by removing all of the overactive thyroid tissue; this allows the suppressed normal tissue to function again.

- *Advantages.* The goitre is removed, the cure is rapid and the cure rate is high if surgery has been adequate.
- *Disadvantages.* Recurrence of thyrotoxicosis occurs in approximately 5% of cases if less than total thyroidectomy is carried out. There is a risk of permanent hypoparathyroidism and nerve injury. Young women tend to have a worse cosmetic result from the scar.

Every operation carries a risk, but with suitable preparation and an experienced surgeon the mortality is negligible and the morbidity low.

Postoperative thyroid insufficiency occurs in 20–45% of cases. Long-term follow-up is necessary as the few patients who develop recurrence may do so at any time in the future. In addition, although it is usually apparent within 1 or 2 years, thyroid failure may also be a late development.

Parathyroid insufficiency should be permanent in less than 5%.

Radioiodine

Radioiodine destroys thyroid cells and, as in thyroidectomy, reduces the mass of functioning thyroid tissue to below a critical level.

- *Advantages.* No surgery and no prolonged drug therapy.
- *Disadvantages.* Isotope facilities must be available.

The rate and timing of late thyroid failure are influenced by the dose selected (200–600 MBq). The higher dose is likely to result in thyroid failure in 6 months, whereas the lower dose may result in late thyroid insufficiency. This is due to sublethal damage to those cells not actually destroyed by the initial treatment and this eventually causes failure of cellular reproduction. Indefinite follow-up is essential.

There is no evidence that therapeutic radioiodine is carcinogenic or teratogenic. In some clinics, radioiodine is given to almost all patients over the age of 25 years, i.e. when development is complete. Follow-up requirements are reduced if a total ablative dose of radioiodine is administered followed by routine replacement treatment with thyroxine. In the UK, reluctance to prescribe radioiodine to those under the age of 45 years has faded. The response is slow but a substantial improvement is to be expected in 8–12 weeks. Accurate dosage is difficult and, should there be no clinical improvement after 12 weeks, a further dose is given. Two or more doses are necessary in 20–30% of patients.

Choice of therapy

Patients must be considered individually. Below are listed guiding principles on the most satisfactory treatment for a particular toxic goitre at a particular age; these must, however, be modified according to the facilities available and the personality, intelligence and wishes of the individual patient, business or family commitments and any other coexisting medical or surgical condition. Access to post-treatment care and availability of replacement thyroxine can be important considerations in the Third World.

In advising treatment, compliance, influenced by social and intellectual factors, is important; many patients cannot be trusted to take drugs regularly if they feel well, and indefinite follow-up, which is essential after radioiodine or subtotal thyroidectomy, is a burden for all.

Diffuse toxic goitre

In patients over 45 years, radioiodine is appropriate. In those under 45 years, surgery for the large goitre and anti-thyroid drugs or radioiodine for the small goitre is recommended. As mentioned above, radioiodine is being increasingly used in younger patients, particularly when their families are complete.

Toxic nodular goitre

Toxic nodular goitre is often large and uncomfortable and enlarges still further with anti-thyroid drugs. Large goitres should be treated surgically because they do not respond as well or as rapidly to radioiodine or anti-thyroid drugs as a diffuse toxic goitre.

Toxic nodule

Surgery or radioiodine treatment is appropriate. Resection is easy, certain and without morbidity. Radioiodine is a good alternative for those over the age of 45 years because the suppressed thyroid tissue does not take up iodine and there is thus no risk of delayed thyroid insufficiency.

Recurrent thyrotoxicosis after surgery

In general, radioiodine is the treatment of choice, but anti-thyroid drugs may be used in young women intending to have children. Further surgery has little place.

Failure of previous treatment with anti-thyroid drugs or radioiodine

In this case, surgery or thyroid ablation with ^{123}I is appropriate.

Special problems in treatment

Pregnancy

Radioiodine is absolutely contraindicated in pregnancy because of the risk to the fetus. The danger of surgery is miscarriage and the danger of anti-thyroid drugs is of inducing thyroid insufficiency in the mother and, because both TSH and anti-thyroid drugs cross the placenta, of the baby being born goitrous (Fig. 48.29) and hypothyroid. The risk of either surgery in the second trimester, in competent hands, or careful administration of anti-thyroid drugs is very small and the choice is exactly as in a non-pregnant woman.

Post-partum hyperthyroidism

Pregnancy may lead to an exacerbation of a variety of auto-immune diseases in the post-partum period. Post-partum hyperthyroidism may be a problem in a patient previously diagnosed with hyperthyroidism or may occur in a patient without any previous history of thyroid disease.

Children

Radioiodine is contraindicated because of the theoretical risk of inducing thyroid carcinoma. There is an increased risk of recurrence after thyroidectomy because thyroid cells are highly active in the young. Children and adolescents should be treated with anti-thyroid drugs until the late teens, failing which total or near-total thyroidectomy by an expert surgeon should be undertaken.

The thyrocardiac

This is a patient with severe cardiac damage due wholly or partly to hyperthyroidism. The patient is usually middle aged or elderly

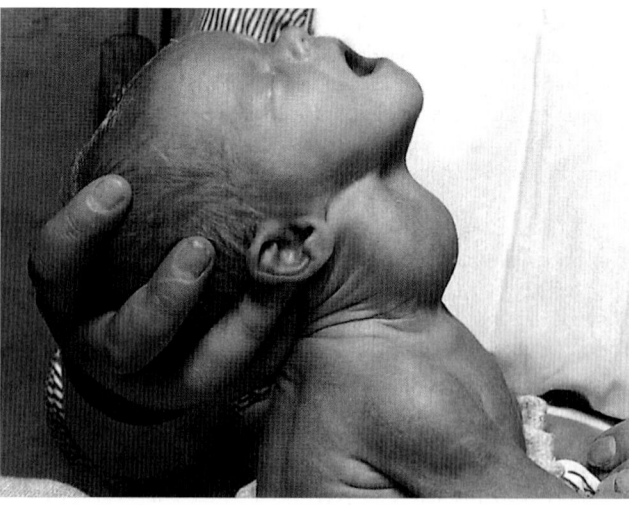

Figure 48.29 Transmitted thiouracil goitre. This does not occur if T$_3$ is given with anti-thyroid drugs as it too crosses the placenta.

with secondary thyrotoxicosis and the hyperthyroidism is not very severe; untreated Graves' disease sufficient to produce the level of emaciation and cardiomyopathy that was common before 1900 is rare in contemporary Western practice. The cardiac condition is far more significant than the hyperthyroidism, but this must be rapidly controlled to prevent further cardiac damage. β-Blockade (propranolol) can assist rapid control of cardiac effects.

Radioiodine is the treatment of choice together with anti-thyroid drugs started either before or after and continued until the radioiodine has had an effect (usually 6 weeks).

High titres of thyroid antibodies

The presence of high titres of thyroid antibodies indicates lymphatic infiltration of the goitre, i.e. a diffuse or focal thyroiditis, and a liability to spontaneous remission. These patients are best treated with anti-thyroid drugs but, if medical treatment fails, definitive treatment by operation or radioiodine is not contraindicated. Steroids may help to reduce pain and swelling.

Proptosis of recent onset

There is a view that treating thyrotoxicosis abruptly with radioiodine or surgery when proptosis is recent may induce malignant exophthalmos. It is reasonable to treat these patients with anti-thyroid drugs until the proptosis has been stable for 6 months.

Hyperthyroidism due to other causes

Thyrotoxicosis factitia

Hyperthyroidism may be induced by taking thyroxine, but only if the dosage exceeds the normal requirements of 0.15–0.25 mg day^{-1}. Doses below the normal requirements simply suppress normal hormone production by the thyroid.

Jod–Basedow thyrotoxicosis

In European countries diffuse toxic goitre is often called Basedow's disease or Jod–Basedow thyrotoxicosis (*Jod* = German for iodine + Basedow). Large doses of iodide given to a hyperplastic endemic goitre that is iodine avid may produce temporary hyperthyroidism and, very occasionally, persistent hyperthyroidism.

Subacute/acute forms of autoimmune thyroiditis or of de Quervain's thyroiditis

In subacute or acute forms of autoimmune thyroiditis or of de Quervain's thyroiditis (see later), mild hyperthyroidism may occur in the early stages because of the liberation of thyroid hormones from damaged tissue.

Secondary carcinoma

A large mass of secondary carcinoma will rarely produce sufficient hormone to induce mild hyperthyroidism.

Neonatal thyrotoxicosis

Neonatal thyrotoxicosis occurs in babies born to hyperthyroid mothers or to euthyroid mothers who have had thyrotoxicosis. High TSH-RAb titres are present in both mother and child because TSH-RAbs can cross the placental barrier. The

Karl Adolf Basedow, 1799–1854, a General Practitioner of Merseberg, Germany, published his account of exophthalmic goitre in 1840.
Friedrich Joseph de Quervain, 1868–1940, Professor of Surgery, Berne, Switzerland, described this form of thyroiditis in 1902.

hyperthyroidism gradually subsides after 3–4 weeks as the TSH-RAb titres in the baby's serum fall.

Surgery for thyrotoxicosis

Preoperative preparation

Traditional preparation aims to make the patient biochemically euthyroid at operation. The thyroid state is determined by clinical assessment, i.e. by improvement in previous symptoms and by objective signs such as weight gain and lowering of the pulse rate, and by serial estimations of the thyroid profile.

Preparation is as an out-patient and only rarely is admission to hospital necessary, because of severe symptoms at presentation, failure to control the hyperthyroidism or non-compliance with medication. Failure to control with anti-thyroid drugs is unusual but may be the result of uneven dosage, i.e. not taking the drug at 6- or 8-hourly intervals.

Carbimazole 30–40 mg day^{-1} is the drug of choice for preparation. When euthyroid (after 8–12 weeks), the dose may be reduced to 5 mg 8-hourly or a 'block and replace' regime used (see above). The last dose of carbimazole may be given on the evening before surgery. Iodides are not used alone because if the patient needs preoperative treatment a more effective drug should be given.

An alternative method of preparation is to abolish the clinical manifestations of the toxic state using β-blocking drugs. β-blockers act on the target organs and not on the gland itself. Propranolol inhibits the peripheral conversion of T$_4$ to T$_3$. This results in very rapid control and operation may be arranged within 1 week. The appropriate drugs are propranolol 40 mg t.d.s. or, preferably, a slow-release preparation once daily. Clinical response to β-blockade is rapid and the patient may be rendered clinically euthyroid and operation arranged in a few days rather than weeks. The dose of β-blocker is increased to achieve the required clinical response and quite often larger doses (propranolol 80 mg t.d.s. or nadolol 320 mg once daily) are necessary.

β-Blockers do not interfere with synthesis of thyroid hormones, and hormone levels remain high during treatment and for some days after thyroidectomy. It is therefore important to continue to give the drug for 7 days postoperatively.

Iodine may be given with carbimazole or β-blocker for the 10 days before operation. Iodide alone produces a transient remission and may reduce vascularity, thereby marginally improving safety. The use of iodine preparations is not universal because of more effective alternatives. Iodine gives an additional measure of safety in case the early morning dose of β-blocker is mistakenly omitted on the day of operation.

Propranolol or nadolol controls symptoms very rapidly and has additional value in combination with carbimazole in the immediate treatment of patients with very severe hyperthyroidism.

Surgery

Preoperative investigations to be carried out and recorded are:

- *Thyroid function tests.*
- *Laryngoscopy.* Whether this is routine is a matter for local protocols because every RLN must be routinely and obsessionally preserved.
- *Thyroid antibodies.*

> Carbimazole **also has an immunosuppressive action on TSH-RAb production.**

- *Serum calcium estimation.*
- An *isotope scan* before preoperative preparation in toxic nodular goitre if total thyroidectomy is not planned. The surgeon should know which nodules, if any, are autonomous and active in order to ensure their resection. A scan is of no value in diffuse toxic goitre when uptake, for practical purposes, is uniform. The diagnosis of a single toxic nodule can only be made by demonstrating that the nodule is active and the remaining thyroid tissue is suppressed.

The extent of the resection depends on the size of the gland, the age of the patient, the experience of the surgeon, the need to minimise the risk of recurrent toxicity and the wish to avoid postoperative thyroid replacement (see Table 48.6 p. 783). Thus, young patients with small glands are at greatest risk of recurrence even with very small remnant sizes. There is an increasing trend towards total thyroidectomy, which simplifies subsequent management and rapidly achieves a permanent euthyroid state on thyroxine replacement. In contrast, a patient with a large goitre who wishes to avoid postoperative medication is suitable for subtotal thyroidectomy.

Technique

General anaesthesia is administered through an endotracheal tube and good muscle relaxation obtained. The patient is supine on the operating table with the table tilted up 15° at the head end to reduce venous engorgement (reverse Trendelenburg). A gel pad or sandbag is placed transversely under the shoulders and the neck is extended (with care, particularly in the elderly) to make the thyroid gland more prominent and to apply tension to skin, platysma and strap muscles, which makes dissection easier.

A gently curved skin crease incision is made midway between the notch of the thyroid cartilage and the suprasternal notch; a lower incision is easier to hide but is more likely to result in a hypertrophic scar. Flaps of skin, subcutaneous tissue and platysma are raised upwards to the superior thyroid notch and downwards to the suprasternal notch. The deep cervical fascia is divided in the midline between the sternothyroid muscles down to the plane of the thyroid capsule. The strap muscles are not divided as a routine but may be if greater exposure is required. The sternothyroid muscle is mobilised off the thyroid lobes, taking care to stay close to the muscle and outside the capsule.

In 30% of patients, middle thyroid veins passing directly into the internal jugular vein require ligation and division. The plane between the medial aspect of the upper pole and the cricothyroid muscle is developed by keeping close to the thyroid to minimise the risk of trauma to the external branch of the superior laryngeal nerve. The branches of the superior thyroid artery splay out over the upper pole and our preference is to ligate these individually. This permits progressive downward delivery of even the highest upper pole. The lobe is then free to rotate medially out of its bed. The inferior thyroid arteries are not routinely ligated to preserve the parathyroid blood supply.

The RLN should be identified in its course in the operative field. It should first be sought below the level of the inferior thyroid artery as it passes obliquely upwards and forwards. This course (Fig. 48.30), oblique to the trachea and oesophagus, is accentuated by mobilisation of the thyroid lobe. If not immediately seen the nerve can usually be palpated as a taut strand crossing the tracheo-oesophageal groove. At a higher level, the nerve lies between the branches of the inferior thyroid artery. The

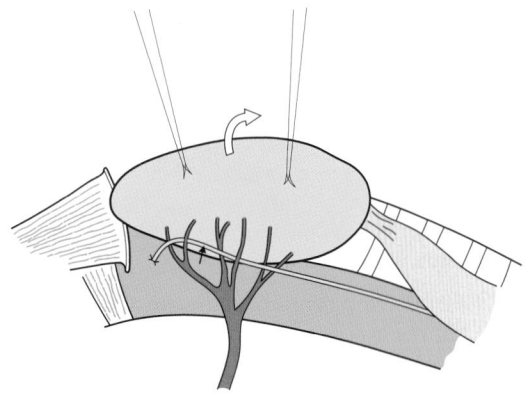

Figure 48.30 Identification of the recurrent laryngeal nerve (see text). Note how rotating the gland anteriorly (open arrow) kinks the nerve (closed arrow) that is normally intimately related to the terminal branches of the inferior thyroid artery.

nerve passes into the larynx under the inferior border of the inferior constrictor immediately behind the inferior cornu of the thyroid cartilage. If the right nerve cannot be found in its usual course, an anomalous (non-recurrent) nerve, present in 1% of cases, should be suspected; this arises from the vagus trunk, usually passes from behind the carotid sheath, curving medially, forwards and upwards, and may be mistaken for the inferior thyroid artery (Fig. 48.31).

The parathyroid glands are identified by careful inspection in the common sites (see Fig. 48.2, p. 772). The thymus is detached by serially dividing the inferior thyroid veins.

In subtotal thyroidectomy the isthmus is transected and the lobe resected obliquely from the medial and lateral aspects to produce a V-shaped surface. This facilitates subsequent suturing of the divided surface for haemostasis. Care is required to avoid devascularisation of the parathyroids and damage to the RLNs, particularly from the medial aspect. If a parathyroid gland is inadvertently or unavoidably excised or devascularised, it should be fragmented and autotransplanted immediately within the sternomastoid muscle.

Subtotal resection of each lobe is carried out, leaving a remnant of 4–5 g on each side. Absolute haemostasis is secured by ligation of individual vessels and by suture of the thyroid remnants to the tracheal fascia.

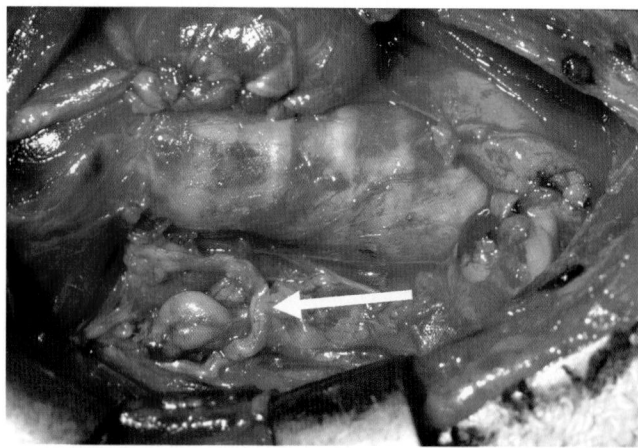

Figure 48.31 Operative photograph of non-recurrent laryngeal nerve (arrow). As is often the case, the inferior thyroid artery is absent.

Total thyroidectomy (see Fig. 48.10, p. 777) avoids transection of thyroid tissue by complete excision of the gland, including the pyramidal lobe, with preservation *in situ* or autotransplantation of as many parathyroids as can be identified.

The pretracheal muscles and cervical fascia are sutured and the wound closed. Randomised clinical trials have confirmed that routine drainage to the deep cervical space is not required.

New technology in thyroidectomy

The major immediate risk following thyroidectomy is haemorrhage. Conventionally, artery forceps, ligature and suture have been used to secure the meticulous haemostasis necessary to minimise the frequency of haemorrhage. Ultrasonic shears and enhanced bipolar diathermy are increasingly used in thyroid surgery and may be advantageous in complex procedures.

Postoperative complications

Haemorrhage A tension haematoma deep to the cervical fascia is usually due to reactionary haemorrhage from one of the thyroid arteries; occasionally, haemorrhage from a thyroid remnant or a thyroid vein may be responsible. This is a rare but desperate emergency requiring urgent decompression by opening the layers of the wound, not simply the skin closure, to relieve tension before urgent transfer to theatre to secure the bleeding vessel (Fig. 48.32).

A subcutaneous haematoma or collection of serum may form under the skin flaps and require evacuation in the following 48 hours. This should not be confused with the potentially life-threatening deep tension haematoma.

Respiratory obstruction This is very rarely due to collapse or kinking of the trachea (tracheomalacia). Most cases are caused by laryngeal oedema. The most important cause of laryngeal oedema is a tension haematoma. However, trauma to the larynx by anaesthetic intubation and surgical manipulation are important contributory factors, particularly if the goitre is very vascular, and may cause laryngeal oedema without a tension haematoma. Unilateral or bilateral recurrent nerve paralysis will not cause immediate postoperative respiratory obstruction unless laryngeal oedema is also present but it will aggravate the obstruction.

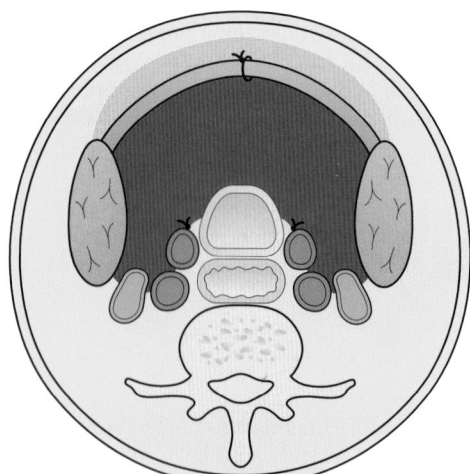

Figure 48.32 Postoperative haematoma. Subplatysmal haematoma (light grey) may need to be evacuated but tension haematoma (dark grey) deep to strap muscles requires urgent decompression and haemostasis.

If releasing the tension haematoma does not immediately relieve airway obstruction, the trachea should be intubated at once. An endotracheal tube can be left in place for several days; steroids are given to reduce oedema and a tracheostomy is rarely necessary. Intubation in the presence of laryngeal oedema may be very difficult and should be carried out by an experienced anaesthetist. Repeated unsuccessful attempts may aggravate the problem and, in a crisis, it is safer to perform a needle tracheostomy as a temporary measure; a large bore 12G intravenous cannula (diameter 2.3 mm) is satisfactory.

Recurrent laryngeal nerve paralysis and voice change RLN injury may be unilateral or bilateral, transient or permanent. Early routine postoperative laryngoscopy reveals a much higher incidence of transient cord paralysis than is detectable by simple assessment of the integrity of the voice and cough. Such temporary dysfunction is not clinically important, however, but voice and cord function should be assessed at the first follow-up 4 weeks postoperatively. An audit of the British Association of Endocrine Surgeons revealed an RLN palsy rate of 1.8% at 1 month declining to 0.5% at 3 months for first-time operations. Permanent paralysis is rare if the nerve has been identified at operation. Injury to the external branch of the superior laryngeal nerve is more common because of its proximity to the superior thyroid artery. This leads to loss of tension in the vocal cord with diminished power and range in the voice. Patients, particularly those who use their voices professionally, must be advised that any thyroid operation will result in change to the voice even in the absence of nerve trauma. Fortunately, for most patients the changes are subtle and only demonstrable on formal voice assessment.

Thyroid insufficiency Following subtotal thyroidectomy this usually occurs within 2 years; however, there is a small but progressive annual incidence over many years, which is often insidious and difficult to recognise. The incidence is considerably higher than was previously thought and rates of 20–45% at 10 years have been reported. This results from a change in the autoimmune response, from stimulation to destruction of the thyroid cells. There is a definite relationship between the estimated weight of the thyroid remnant and the development of thyroid failure after subtotal thyroidectomy for Graves' disease. Thyroid insufficiency is rare after surgery for a toxic adenoma because there is no autoimmune disease present.

Parathyroid insufficiency This is due to removal of the parathyroid glands or to infarction through damage to the parathyroid end artery; often, both factors occur together. Vascular injury is probably far more important than inadvertent removal. The incidence of permanent hypoparathyroidism should be less than 1% and most cases present dramatically 2–5 days after operation; however, very rarely the onset is delayed for 2–3 weeks or a patient with marked hypocalcaemia is asymptomatic.

Thyrotoxic crisis (storm) This is an acute exacerbation of hyperthyroidism. It occurs if a thyrotoxic patient has been inadequately prepared for thyroidectomy and is now extremely rare. Very rarely, a thyrotoxic patient presents in a crisis and this may follow an unrelated operation. Symptomatic and supportive treatment is for dehydration, hyperpyrexia and restlessness. This requires the administration of intravenous fluids, cooling the

patient with ice packs, the administration of oxygen, diuretics for cardiac failure, digoxin for uncontrolled atrial fibrillation, sedation and intravenous hydrocortisone. Specific treatment is with carbimazole 10–20 mg 6-hourly, Lugol's iodine 10 drops 8-hourly by mouth or sodium iodide 1 g intravenously. Propranolol intravenously (1–2 mg) or orally (40 mg 6-hourly) will block β-adrenergic effects.

Wound infection Cellulitis requiring prescription of antibiotics, often by the general practitioner, is more common than most surgeons appreciate. A significant subcutaneous or deep cervical abscess is exceptionally rare and should be drained.

Hypertrophic or keloid scar This is more likely to form if the incision overlies the sternum and in dark-skinned individuals. Intradermal injections of corticosteroid should be given at once and repeated monthly if necessary. Scar revision rarely results in significant long-term improvement.

Stitch granuloma This may occur with or without sinus formation and is seen after the use of non-absorbable, particularly silk, suture material. Absorbable ligatures and sutures must be used throughout thyroid surgery. Some surgeons use a subcuticular absorbable skin suture rather than the traditional skin clips or staples. Skin staples, if used, can be removed safely in less than 48 hours because the skin closure is supported by the platysma stitch.

Postoperative care

If the voice is normal and the cough occlusive it is not essential to carry out laryngoscopy before leaving hospital. Transient cord palsies are probably more common than generally appreciated. Even if routine cord visualisation is not part of the normal postoperative review, persisting voice change requires visualisation of the cords.

Hypocalcaemia depends not only on the identification but also on the preservation of the parathyroid glands with an intact blood supply. In addition, metabolic bone disease, 'hungry bones syndrome', results in the rapid influx of serum calcium into bones, particularly if preoperative preparation has been with β-blockade rather than normalisation of the serum T_4. Hypocalcaemia is more common after total than subtotal thyroidectomy and reflects the increased trauma to the parathyroids. About 25% of patients develop transient hypocalcaemia and oral calcium may be necessary (1 g three or four times daily). If associated symptoms are severe and the serum calcium less, 10 ml of 10% calcium gluconate (equivalent to 8.4 mg or 2.3 mmol calcium) should be given. To screen for parathyroid insufficiency the serum calcium should be measured at the first review attendance 4–6 weeks after operation.

After subtotal resection, stability in terms of thyroid function takes time. It is important that biochemical (subclinical) thyroid failure should not be an indication for treatment during the first year, as the majority of patients with early subclinical failure, which is common, ultimately regain normality. Even when there are clinical features of failure, thyroxine should be withheld if possible during the first 6 months. Most patients who develop thyroid failure do so within the first 2 years but there is a continuing incidence thereafter. Recurrent thyrotoxicosis may occur at

Jean Guillaume Lugol, **1786–1851**, Physician, Hôpital St. Louis, Paris, France.

any time after operation and follow-up should therefore be for life.

Once a stable situation has been achieved, follow-up after thyroid surgery should be carried out by an automated computerised system, which dramatically reduces the number of patient attendances at the thyroid clinic.

The incidences quoted for thyroid failure (20–45%) and recurrent thyrotoxicosis (5%) after subtotal thyroidectomy for Graves' disease refer to UK experience and may be different elsewhere in the world. In Iceland, for example, an area of high dietary iodine intake, the incidence of thyroid failure is much lower and that of recurrent toxicity much higher than in the UK (Summary box 48.5).

Summary box 48.5

Hyperthyroidism

- ■ **Describe the causes**
- ■ **Discuss the pros and cons of the three major treatment options**
- ■ **Know how to prepare a patient for operation**
- ■ **Describe appropriate surgical procedures**
- ■ **Know about early and late postoperative management**

NEOPLASMS OF THE THYROID

Thyroid neoplasms are classified in Table 48.7 and the relative incidence of malignancies is given in Table 48.8.

Table 48.7 Classification of thyroid neoplasms

Benign
Follicular adenoma

Malignant
Primary
Follicular epithelium – differentiated
  Follicular
  Papillary
Follicular epithelium – undifferentiated
  Anaplastic
Parafollicular cells
  Medullary
Lymphoid cells
  Lymphoma

Secondary
Metastatic
  Local infiltration

Table 48.8 Relative incidence of primary malignant tumour of the thyroid gland

Relative incidence	(%)	Relative incidence	(%)
Papillary carcinoma	60	Medullary carcinoma	5
Follicular carcinoma	20	Malignant lymphoma	5
Anaplastic carcinoma	10		

Benign tumours

Follicular adenomas present as clinically solitary nodules (Fig. 48.33) and the distinction between a follicular carcinoma and an adenoma can only be made by histological examination; in the adenoma there is no invasion of the capsule or of pericapsular blood vessels. Treatment is therefore by wide excision, i.e. lobectomy. The remaining thyroid tissue is normal so that prolonged follow-up is unnecessary. It is doubtful if there is such an entity as a papillary adenoma and all papillary tumours should be considered as malignant, even if encapsulated.

Malignant tumours

The vast majority of primary malignancies are carcinomas derived from follicular cells (Table 48.7). Dunhill classified them histologically as differentiated and undifferentiated; the differentiated carcinomas are further subdivided into follicular and papillary. Lymphoma makes up the remainder of primary malignancies. Metastases to the thyroid account for < 5% of malignancies. Secondary disease should be considered when there is a history of malignancy, particularly kidney and breast cancer, and when the cytology of a thyroid swelling is atypical. Direct invasion by upper aerodigestive squamous cancer is a rare but lethal event. Lymph node and blood-borne metastases to bone and lung occur and may be the mode of presentation (Figs 48.34 and 48.35).

Aetiology of malignant thyroid tumours

The single most important aetiological factor in differentiated thyroid carcinoma, particularly papillary carcinoma, is irradiation of the thyroid under 5 years of age. The incidence of childhood thyroid cancer in the Ukraine rose from 57 cases in the 5 years before the Chernobyl nuclear incident in 1986 to 577 cases in the subsequent 10 years. In the town of Gomel, the incidence rose from < 1 case per million population to 96 cases per million population.

Short-latency aggressive papillary cancer is associated with the *ret/PTC3* oncogene and later-developing, possibly less aggressive, cancers are associated with *ret/PTC1*. The incidence of follicular carcinoma is high in endemic goitrous areas, possibly as a result of TSH stimulation. Malignant lymphomas sometimes develop in autoimmune thyroiditis, and the lymphocytic infiltration in the autoimmune process may be an aetiological factor.

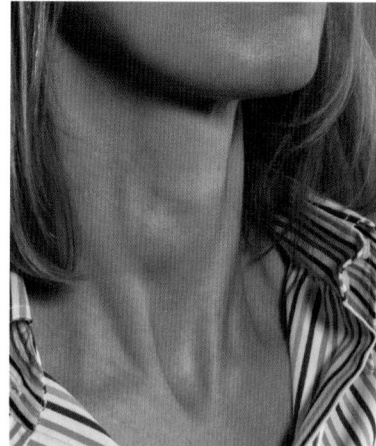

Figure 48.33 Isolated swelling in the upper pole of the right thyroid lobe.

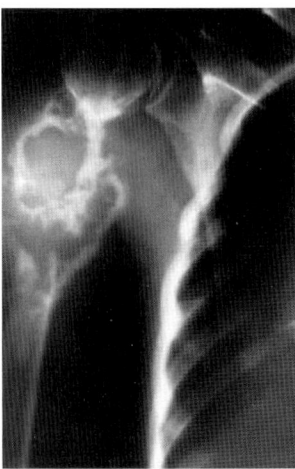

Figure 48.34 Metastasis in the humerus from a carcinoma of the thyroid (courtesy of D.S. Devadatta, Vellore, India).

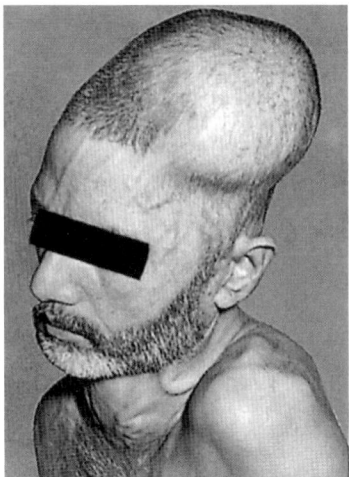

Figure 48.35 Metastasis in the left parietal bone from a carcinoma of the thyroid (courtesy of Professor A.K. Toufeeq, Lahore, Pakistan).

Clinical features of thyroid cancers

The annual incidence of thyroid cancers is about 3.7 cases per 100 000 population and the female–male sex ratio is 3:1. The overall mortality rate should be low because most patients are in a low-risk category; however, older patients have more aggressive disease with a worse prognosis. The most common presenting symptom is a thyroid swelling (Figs 48.33 and 48.36) and a 5-year history is not uncommon in differentiated growths. Enlarged cervical lymph nodes may be the presentation of papillary carcinoma. Recurrent laryngeal nerve paralysis is very suggestive of locally advanced disease.

Anaplastic growths are usually hard, irregular and infiltrating. A differentiated carcinoma may be suspiciously firm and irregular but is often indistinguishable from a benign swelling. Small papillary tumours may be impalpable, even when lymphatic metastases are present. Pain, often referred to the ear, is frequent in infiltrating growths.

Diagnosis of thyroid neoplasms

Diagnosis is obvious on clinical examination in most cases of anaplastic carcinoma, although Riedel's thyroiditis (see later) is

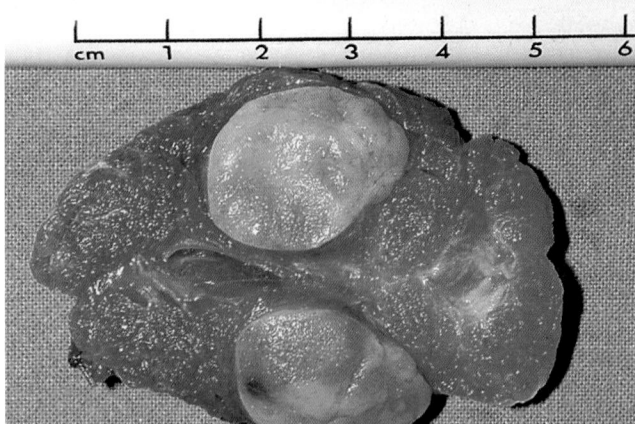

Figure 48.36 Follicular neoplasm of the thyroid presenting as an isolated swelling.

indistinguishable. The localised forms of granulomatous thyroiditis and lymphadenoid goitre may simulate carcinoma. It is not always easy to exclude a carcinoma in a multinodular goitre, and solitary nodules, particularly in a young male patient, are always suspect. Failure to take up radioiodine is characteristic of almost all thyroid carcinomas [only very rarely will differentiated carcinoma (primary or secondary) take up ^{123}I in the presence of normal thyroid tissue], but this also occurs in degenerating nodules and all forms of thyroiditis. TSH levels are often raised in carcinoma but this may be clouded by simultaneous elevation of anti-thyroid antibodies. The key role of FNAC in preoperative diagnosis has already been discussed. There is a false-negative rate with all investigations, and lobectomy is appropriate when there is a strong clinical suspicion. Incisional biopsy may cause seeding of cells and local recurrence and is not advised in a resectable carcinoma. In an anaplastic and obviously irremovable carcinoma, however, incisional or core needle biopsy is justified.

When a preoperative diagnosis is made, imaging with ultrasound, MRI or CT is required. As well as additional information on the extent of the primary tumour, imaging provides valuable information on nodal involvement (Figs 48.37 and 48.38), which permits preoperative planning for nodal dissection.

Frozen section histology has a limited role in thyroid surgery. It cannot reliably differentiate between encapsulated benign and malignant follicular neoplasms and is of more value in confirming whether nodes are involved with papillary cancer, thereby influencing the extent of nodal surgery.

Papillary carcinoma

Most papillary tumours contain a mixture of papillary and colloid-filled follicles and, in some, the follicular structure predominates. Nevertheless, if any papillary structure or characteristic cytology is present, the tumour will behave in a predictable fashion as a papillary carcinoma. Histologically the tumour shows papillary projections and characteristic pale empty nuclei (Orphan Annie-eyed nuclei) (Fig. 48.39). Papillary carcinomas are very seldom encapsulated.

Multiple foci may occur in the same lobe as the primary tumour or, less commonly, in both lobes. They may be due to lymphatic

Orphan Annie **is a character from a strip cartoon, who, along with others, such as Daddy Warbucks, are drawn with empty circles for eyes.**

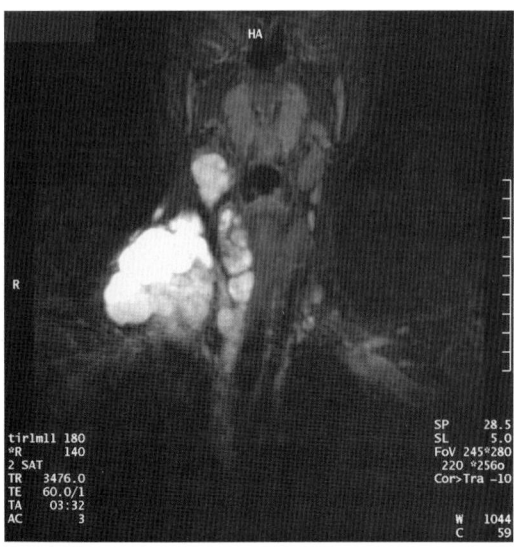

Figure 48.37 Magnetic resonance imaging scan of papillary cancer with multiple node metastases.

spread in the rich intrathyroidal lymph plexus or to multicentric growth. Spread to the lymph nodes is common but blood-borne metastases are unusual unless the tumour is extrathyroidal. The term extrathyroidal indicates that the primary tumour has infiltrated through the capsule of the thyroid gland, although minimal invasion of the sternothyroid muscle is much less significant than infiltration into the oesophagus or trachea.

Microcarcinoma (occult carcinoma)

The reported prevalence of tiny foci of papillary carcinoma is related to the care with which the thyroid is examined histologically. In an autopsy study from Finland in which the thyroid was examined serially in 2-mm slices, an incidence of up to 36% was reported. Clearly the majority of such tumours never progress to become a clinically significant entity. A small percentage of cancers present with enlarged lymph nodes in the jugular chain or pulmonary metastases with no palpable abnormality of the thyroid. The primary tumour may be no more than a few millimetres in size and is often termed occult. Foci of papillary carcinoma may also be discovered in thyroid tissue resected for other reasons, for example Graves' disease. The term 'occult' was formally applied to all papillary carcinomas of less than 1.5 cm in diameter but the preferred terminology now is microcarcinoma for cancers less

than 1 cm in diameter. These have a uniformly excellent prognosis although those presenting with nodal or distant metastases justify more aggressive therapy.

Follicular carcinoma

These appear to be macroscopically encapsulated but, microscopically, there is invasion of the capsule and of the vascular spaces in the capsular region (Fig. 48.40). Multiple foci are seldom seen and lymph node involvement is much less common than in papillary carcinoma. Blood-borne metastases (Fig. 48.41) are more common and the eventual mortality rate is twice that of papillary cancer.

Hürthle cell tumours are a variant of follicular neoplasm in which oxyphil (Hürthle, Askanazy) cells predominate histologically. Hürthle cell cancers are associated with a poorer prognosis and some hold that all Hürthle cell neoplasms are malignant.

Differences between papillary and follicular carcinoma

The major differences between papillary (including mixed papillary and follicular) and follicular carcinoma were set out by Cady on the basis of an analysis of 40 years' experience at the Lahey Clinic (Table 48.9).

Prognosis in differentiated thyroid carcinoma

Compared with most cancers the prognosis in differentiated thyroid carcinoma is excellent. Although influenced by histological type, prognosis is much more dependent on age at diagnosis, size of the tumour, metastatic disease and the presence of either extrathyroidal spread (in papillary cancer) or major capsular transgression (in follicular carcinoma). There is a multiplicity of

Table 48.9 Major differences between papillary and follicular carcinoma (after Cady)

	Papillary (%)	Follicular (%)
Male incidence	22	35
Lymph node metastases	35	13
Blood vessel invasion	40	60
Recurrence rate	19	29
Overall mortality rate	11	24
Location of recurrent carcinoma		
Distant metastases	45	75
Nodal metastases	34	12
Local recurrence	20	12

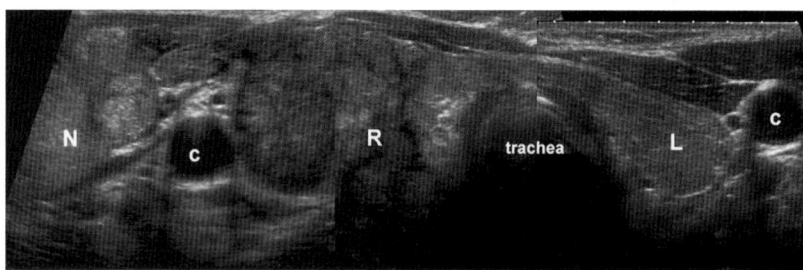

Figure 48.38 Composite ultrasound scan of papillary cancer of the right thyroid lobe with extensive nodal metastases. N, enlarged nodes; c, carotid artery, R, primary carcinoma in the right thyroid lobe; L, normal left thyroid lobe (courtesy Dr D. McAteer, Aberdeen, UK).

Karl Hürthle, 1866–1945, a German histopathologist who first drew attention to these cells.
Max Askanazy, 1865–1940, described these cells whilst working at the Pathological Anatomy Institute, Tubingen, Germany.

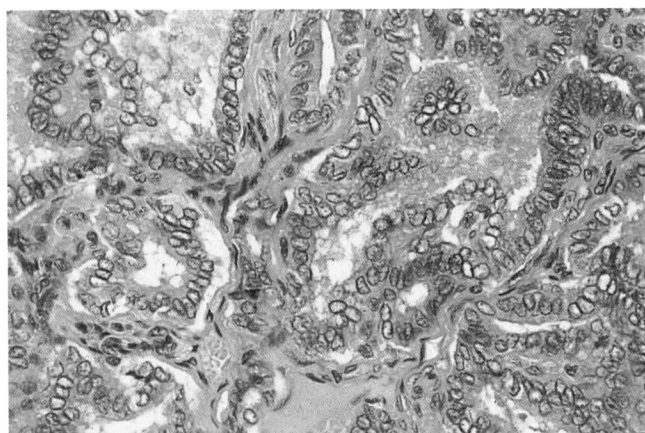

Figure 48.39 Histology of papillary thyroid carcinoma showing typical papillary projections and empty (Orphan Annie-eyed) nuclei (courtesy of Dr S.W.B. Ewen, Aberdeen, UK).

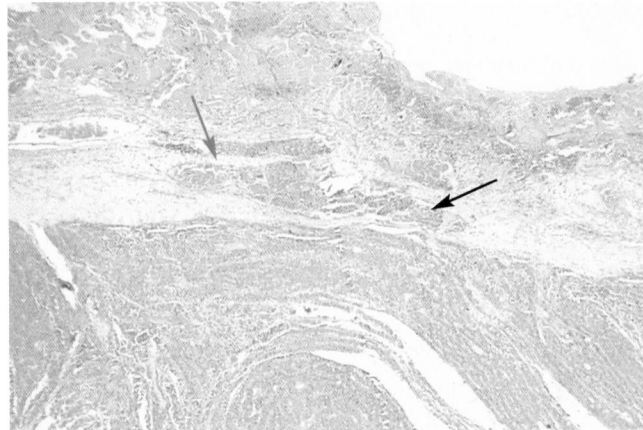

Figure 48.40 Histology of follicular thyroid carcinoma showing vascular (red arrow) and capsular (black arrow) invasion (courtesy of Dr S.W.B. Ewen, Aberdeen, UK).

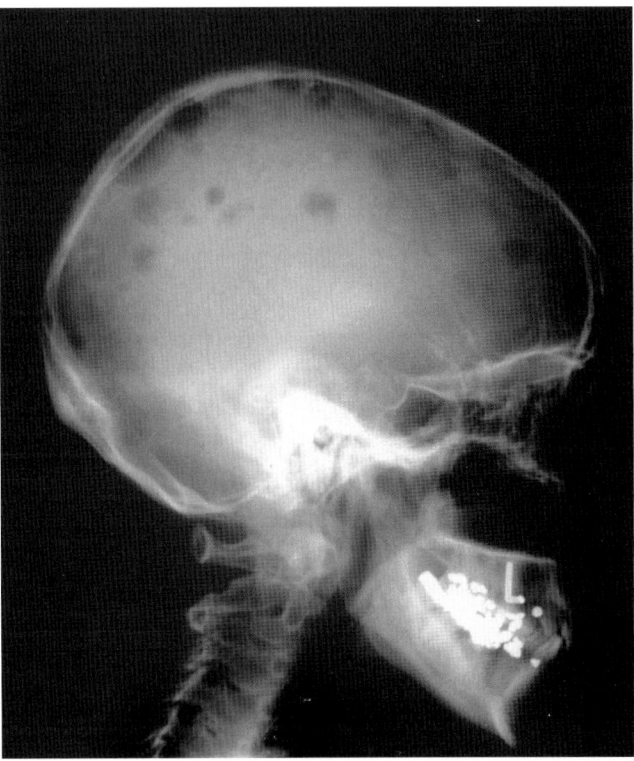

Figure 48.41 Follicular carcinoma of the thyroid with skull secondaries.

scoring systems available, all of which identify patients at high (40% at 20 years) or low (1% at 20 years) risk of death (Table 48.10). All patients should be tumour–node–metastasis (TNM) staged and this classification acknowledges the low risk of patients aged less than 45 years at presentation (Table 48.11). Approximately 80% of patients are at a low risk of dying of thyroid cancer but suboptimal treatment, i.e. failure to eradicate all

macroscopic disease at the first operation, may lead to increased recurrence and avoidable death many years after presentation. It is, however, important to avoid iatrogenic morbidity by overzealous treatment in those patients with a normal life expectancy.

Surgical treatment of differentiated thyroid carcinoma

There is agreement that patients with large, locally aggressive or metastatic DTC require total thyroidectomy, with excision of adjacent involved structures if necessary, and appropriate nodal surgery followed by radioiodine ablation with long-term TSH suppression. However, such 'high-risk' patients are in the minority and there is continuing disagreement on the most appropriate operation for 'low-risk' DTC, although contemporary guidelines increasingly recommend total thyroidectomy for virtually all cancers.

Table 48.10 Prognostic scoring in differentiated thyroid cancer

	Age	Sex	Size	Metastases	Nodes	Extrathyroid	Histological grade	Complete excision
AMES	+	+	+	+		+		
AGES	+		+	+		+	+	
MACIS	+		+	+		+		+
EORTC	+			+		+		
TNM	+	+	+	+	+	+		

AMES – age, metastases, extent, size.
AGES – age, grade, extent, size.
MACIS – metastases, age, completeness of excision, invasion, size.
EORTC – European Organisation for Research and Treatment of Cancer.
TNM – tumour, nodes, metastases – American Joint Committee on Cancer.

CHAPTER 48 | THE THYROID AND PARATHYROID GLANDS

Table 48.11 Tumour–node–metastasis staging (5th edition) of thyroid cancer

Tumour

TX	Primary cannot be assessed
T0	No evidence of primary
T1	Limited to thyroid, 1 cm or less
T2	Limited to thyroid, > 1 cm but < 4 cm
T3	Limited to thyroid, > 4 cm
T4	Extending beyond capsule, any size

Nodes

NX	Cannot be assessed
N0	No regional node metastases
N1	Regional node metastases

Metastases

MX	Cannot be assessed
M0	No metastases
M1	Metastases present

Stage	Under 45 years	Over 45 years
I	Any T, any N, M0	T1, N0, M0
II	Any T, any N, M1	T2, N0, M0 or T3, N0, M0
III		T4, N0, M0 or any T, N1, M0
IV		Any T, any N, M1

Note the effect of age on stage; only patients older than 45 years can have stage III or IV disease.

CHAPTER 48 | THE THYROID AND PARATHYROID GLANDS

The conservative approach reserves total thyroidectomy for specific indications (namely those in which there is a preoperative diagnosis of high-risk cancer, bilateral disease or when there is a clear indication for postoperative radioiodine therapy). 'Small' cancers confined to one lobe can be managed by lobectomy and TSH suppression. Unfortunately there is no consistent definition of a small cancer, with arbitrary limits of between 1 and 4 cm in use.

The radical approach advocates routine total thyroidectomy, often necessitating early reoperation and a second lobectomy following a diagnostic first lobectomy. Routine 'central compartment' node dissection is also advocated. Total thyroidectomy facilitates the use of radioiodine for postoperative scanning to detect and subsequently ablate metastases. It is unlikely that this policy will improve on the 99% survival rate regardless of primary surgical treatment in low-risk patients. It is argued that this policy will reduce local recurrence but this is based on an imperfect evidence base.

This argument cannot be resolved at present because of the long and changing natural history of DTC, the inherently good prognosis for the great majority of patients, the lack of randomised studies and the paucity of long-term prospective data.

The case for a policy of routine total thyroidectomy is based on large but retrospective studies of patients in whom the risk of local recurrence (particularly) and death was higher if therapy was less than total thyroidectomy with radioiodine ablation. It is argued that the prevalence of multifocality in papillary carcinoma and the risk from occult metastases justifies more radical treatment in all patients because it is not possible to identify low-risk patients reliably. If the low operative morbidity attributable to total thyroidectomy achieved in some expert centres, with negligible rates of hypoparathyroidism and recurrent nerve injury

(Delbridge), was universal, a small possible benefit in the long term would become more attractive. However, there are centres with large practices in thyroid surgery still reporting hypoparathyroidism rates of up to 30% after total thyroidectomy for cancer, particularly when combined with routine and more radical nodal surgery. Total thyroidectomy and permanent hypoparathyroidism requires long-term access to thyroxine, calcium and possibly vitamin D supplements. This may be a consideration in selecting treatment options in some countries. Similarly, there are cultural differences over the liberal use of radioactive iodine, which has become virtually routine in western countries.

Local recurrence in either the thyroid bed or the contralateral lobe should be exceptionally rare after total lobectomy, particularly in low-risk cases. The evidence that the long-term results of routine total thyroidectomy are better than a more conservative policy (selective total thyroidectomy) is based on the prolonged follow-up of cohorts of patients extending back over 50 years. There have been changes in the stage, and possibly the behaviour, of thyroid cancer over that time. In addition, the selection criteria for and the surgical technique of thyroidectomy are now more precise and better documented. A randomised trial would have to recruit several thousand patients and take 30 years to resolve this debate. For the foreseeable future, the risks of iatrogenic morbidity (recurrent nerve injury and hypoparathyroidism) associated with a policy of routine total thyroidectomy must be balanced against the knowledge that this will overtreat 95% of low-risk patients. Unfortunately, there is no reliable method of identifying those who will benefit.

The author's current practice when a *preoperative diagnosis* of DTC has been made, usually on FNAC, is to image the neck with MRI or CT. Total thyroidectomy is recommended for tumours greater than 2 cm and those with nodal involvement or metastases and lobectomy is recommended for the remainder. Functional selective node dissection (Watkinson) of involved node levels is performed as required. Lateral extension of the normal thyroidectomy incision generally gives adequate access to node levels 2–6. If access to level 2 is difficult, an additional higher skin crease incision or alternatively a J-shaped utility incision may be made.

Routine central compartment node clearance is not recommended for small tumours with negative imaging although a representative node biopsy may be assessed by frozen section histology. Preserving inferior parathyroid function is practically impossible with level 6/7 clearance. Very occasionally it may be necessary to sacrifice the RLN if it is completely encircled and, on even more rare occasions, extrathyroidal spread may require tracheal, oesophageal or laryngeal resection.

When the diagnosis of DTC is made *after diagnostic lobectomy*, TSH suppression and review can be recommended, with reoperation only for a clear indication. Indications for completion total

Leigh Walter Delbridge, **formerly Professor of Surgery, The University of Sydney, The Royal North Shore Hospital, Sydney, N.S.W. Australia.**
Radioactive iodine **was first used in the treatment of thyrotoxicosis in 1942 by Herz and Roberts.**
A. Roberts, **The Isotope Department, The Massachusetts Institute of Technology, Boston, MA, USA.**
John Carmel Watkinson, **Contemporary, Otolaryngologist, Queen Elizabeth Hospital, Birmingham, England.**

thyroidectomy are the development of a new swelling or rising thyroglobulin levels. This policy is based on the outcome of thyroid lobectomy in the author's unit in both low- and high-risk patients since 1977.

Additional measures

Thyroxine

On the basis that most tumours are TSH dependent it is standard practice to prescribe thyroxine (0.1–0.2 mg daily) for all patients after operation for differentiated thyroid carcinoma to suppress endogenous TSH production. Suppression of the TSH level should be confirmed by measurement. Failure of suppression to a level of $< 0.1 \, \text{mU} \, l^{-1}$ may indicate an inadequate dose of thyroxine or, more usually, that the patient is non-compliant. There is a trend to manage patients with undetectable thyroglobulin after radical treatment with a TSH level in the normal range because of some concern over the impact of long-term TSH suppression.

Thyroid hormone replacement is obviously necessary after total thyroidectomy and in the majority of patients after near-total thyroidectomy, and is usually given in the form of thyroxine. Patients with potential or actual distant metastases, who may require repeated radioiodine administration for scanning and therapy, should be given tri-iodothyronine (40–60 µg daily^{-1}) because it is much shorter acting and, on stopping it, increased TSH secretion and thyroid avidity for iodine recover quickly so that radioiodine may be given after several days. The patient is thereby spared weeks of developing thyroid insufficiency after stopping thyroxine before radioiodine may be given.

Radioiodine

If metastases take up radioiodine they may be detected by scanning and treated with large doses of radioiodine. For effective scanning all normal thyroid tissue must have been ablated, either by surgery or preliminary radioiodine, and the patient must be hypothyroid to improve uptake. Alternatively, synthetic recombinant TSH may be used to stimulate uptake. The indications for scanning after operation for differentiated carcinoma are also disputed, but radioactive iodine is indicated in patients with unresectable disease, local recurrence or metastatic disease, high-risk patients and in those with a rising serum thyroglobulin level. A whole body scan can be carried out 10 days after empirical treatment with high-dose radioactive iodine, to allow decay of activity (Fig. 48.42). Unfortunately, the more aggressive and de-differentiated the cancer, the less likely it is to take up radioactive iodine: those most in need of an effect are least likely to derive a benefit.

If metastases have been treated, the serum thyroglobulin level and local protocols will determine when the scan should be repeated and further therapeutic doses of radioiodine given if necessary. Solitary distant metastases may be treated by external radiotherapy.

Thyroglobulin

The measurement of serum thyroglobulin is of value in the follow-up and detection of metastatic disease in patients who have undergone surgery for DTC. It can be used after lobectomy, as after total thyroidectomy, provided that endogenous TSH production has been completely suppressed by T$_4$. This measurement reduces the need for serial radioactive iodine scanning but, when a rise occurs, imaging with neck ultrasound is appropriate.

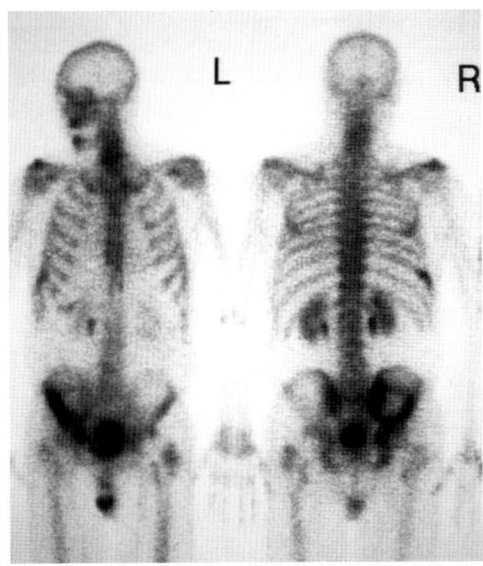

Figure 48.42 Whole-body scan after total thyroidectomy and high-dose radioiodine for follicular carcinoma showing metastases in the right shoulder, ribs and pelvis (courtesy of Dr M. Brooks, Aberdeen, UK).

Surgery or therapeutic radioiodine is then indicated, with a subsequent whole-body scan once activity has decayed. This will confirm and locate metastatic disease, which is iodine avid. The presence of circulating anti-thyroglobulin antibodies interferes with and invalidates thyroglobulin as a serum marker for recurrence and, occasionally, careful clinical palpation of the neck will be the first indication of local recurrence.

Undifferentiated (anaplastic) carcinoma

This occurs mainly in elderly women and is diagnosed much less often now than in the past, when many thyroid lymphomas were mistakenly classified histologically as anaplastic carcinomas. Local infiltration is an early feature of these tumours, with spread by lymphatics and by the bloodstream. They are extremely lethal tumours and survival is calculated in months. Complete resection is justified if the disease appears confined to the thyroid and possibly the strap muscles and is only possible in a minority of patients. Even then the survival rarely exceeds 6 months and the median is around 3 months for the whole group. Some of these aggressive lesions present in an advanced stage with tracheal obstruction and they require urgent tracheal decompression. The trachea may be decompressed and tissue obtained for histology by isthmusectomy. Tracheostomy is best avoided. Radiotherapy should be given in all cases and may provide a worthwhile period of palliation, but there is little evidence to support the use of chemotherapy.

Medullary carcinoma

These are tumours of the parafollicular cells (C cells) derived from the neural crest and not of cells of the thyroid follicle, as is the case for other primary thyroid carcinomas. The cells are not unlike those of a carcinoid tumour and there is a characteristic amyloid stroma (Fig. 48.43). High levels of serum calcitonin and carcinoembryonic antigen are produced by many medullary tumours. Levels fall after resection and rise again with recurrence making it a valuable tumour marker in the follow-up of patients with this disease. Diarrhoea is a feature in 30% of cases and this

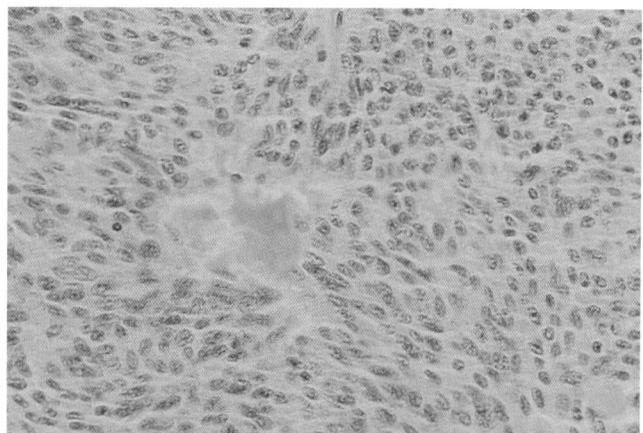

Figure 48.43 Histology of medullary carcinoma showing characteristic 'cell balls' and amyloid (courtesy of Dr S.W.B. Ewen, Aberdeen, UK).

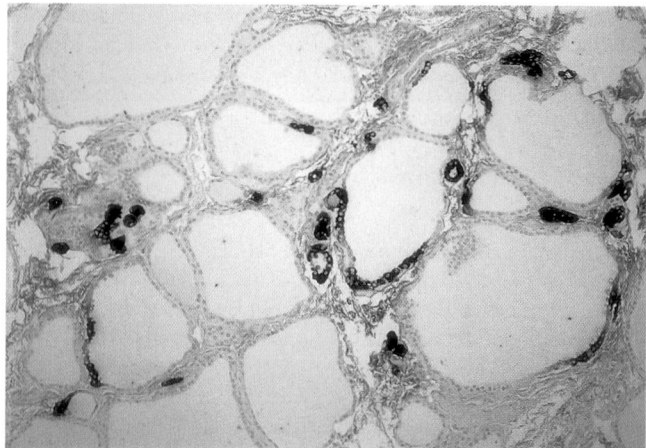

Figure 48.44 Hyperplasia of parafollicular C cells in a child from a family with medullary cancer (courtesy of Dr S.W.B Ewen, Aberdeen, UK).

may be due to 5-hydroxytryptamine or prostaglandins produced by the tumour cells.

Some tumours are familial, possibly accounting for 10–20% of all cases. Medullary carcinoma may occur in combination with adrenal phaeochromocytoma and hyperparathyroidism (HPT) (usually due to hyperplasia) in the syndrome known as multiple endocrine neoplasia type 2A (MEN-2A). The familial form of the disease frequently affects children and young adults, whereas sporadic cases occur at any age with no sex predominance. When the familial form is associated with prominent mucosal neuromas involving the lips, tongue and inner aspect of the eyelids, with a marfanoid habitus, the syndrome is referred to as MEN type 2B.

Involvement of lymph nodes occurs in 50–60% of cases of medullary carcinoma and blood-borne metastases are common. As would be expected, tumours are not TSH dependent and do not take up radioactive iodine. The prognosis is variable and depends on the stage at diagnosis. Any nodal involvement virtually eliminates the prospect of cure and, unfortunately, even small tumours confined to the thyroid gland may have spread by the time of diagnosis, particularly in familial cancers. In common with many endocrine tumours the progression of disease may be very slow with a characteristically indolent course and long survival, even in the absence of cure.

Treatment

Treatment is by total thyroidectomy and either prophylactic or therapeutic resection of the central and bilateral cervical lymph nodes.

Familial cases are now detected by genetic screening for *RET* gene mutations, which identifies individuals who will develop medullary cancer later in life (Fig. 48.44). The genetic tests are supplemented by estimating serum calcitonin levels in the basal state and after stimulation by either calcium or pentagastrin. A rise in calcitonin levels in these circumstances should lead to thyroidectomy, but even then the disease may be beyond the pre-invasive C-cell hyperplasia stage (Fig. 48.45). Prophylactic surgery is now recommended for infants with the genetic trait. A

Bernard Jean Antonin Marfan, **1858–1942, Physician, Hôpital des Enfants-Malades, Paris, France, described this syndrome in 1896.**

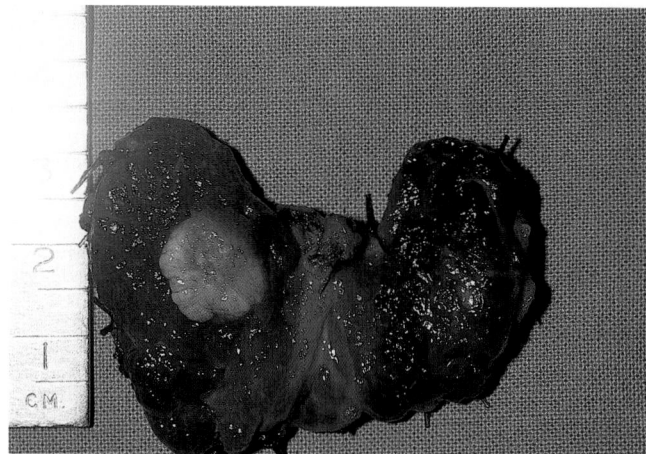

Figure 48.45 Total thyroidectomy specimen from a young girl undergoing surgery following genetic screening, showing a small medullary cancer in the right lobe.

recent refinement as a result of preoperative genetic differentiation between sporadic and familial cancers suggests that lobectomy might be adequate treatment for sporadic cases.

In all cases, before embarking upon thyroid surgery, phaeochromocytoma must be excluded by measurement of urinary catecholamine levels.

Malignant lymphoma

In the past, many malignant lymphomas were diagnosed as small round-cell anaplastic carcinomas. The response to irradiation is good (Fig. 48.46) and radical surgery is unnecessary once the diagnosis is established by biopsy. Although the diagnosis may be made or suspected on FNAC, sufficient material is seldom available for immunocytochemical classification and large-bore needle (Trucut) or open biopsy is usually necessary. In patients with tracheal compression, isthmusectomy is the most appropriate form of biopsy, although the response to therapy is so rapid that this should rarely be necessary unless there has been difficulty in making a histological diagnosis. The prognosis is good if there is no involvement of cervical lymph nodes. Rarely, the tumour is part of widespread malignant lymphoma disease, and the prognosis in

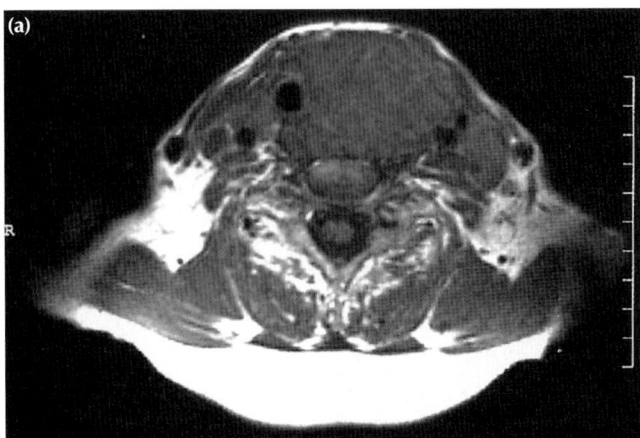

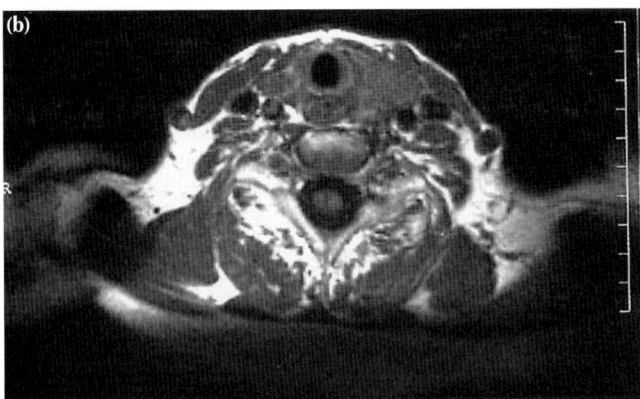

Figure 48.46 Magnetic resonance imaging scans of extensive malignant lymphoma (a) before and (b) after 7 days of external beam radiotherapy (courtesy of Dr F.W. Smith, Aberdeen, UK).

these cases is worse. Most lymphomas occur against a background of lymphocytic thyroiditis (Summary box 48.6).

Summary box 48.6

Thyroid cancer

- Know the different pathological types and their behaviour
- Use appropriate investigations
- Be aware of the controversies in treatment
- Know about risk stratification and the possible effect on treatment
- Describe total thyroidectomy and node dissection
- Know how to manage the complications
- Understand the role of postoperative radioiodine therapy

THYROIDITIS

Chronic lymphocytic (autoimmune) thyroiditis (Fig. 48.47)

This common condition is usually associated with raised titres of thyroid antibodies. Not infrequently there is a family history of other autoimmune disease. It commonly presents as a goitre, which may be diffuse or nodular with a characteristic 'bosselated' feel, or with established or subclinical thyroid failure. The diagnosis often follows investigation of a discrete swelling. Features of chronic lymphocytic (focal) thyroiditis are commonly present on

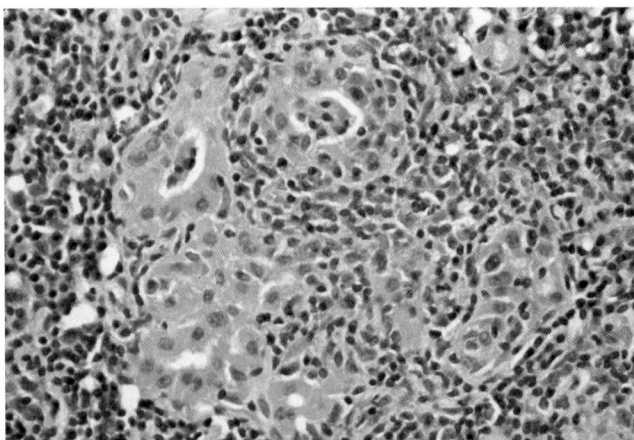

Figure 48.47 Autoimmune thyroiditis (Hashimoto's disease; struma lymphomatosa) showing intense lymphocytic plasma cell infiltration, acinar destruction and fibrosis. Compare with the normal histology shown in Figure 48.2, p. 772.

histological examination in association with other thyroid diseases, notably toxic goitre. Primary myxoedema without detectable thyroid enlargement represents the end-stage of the pathological process.

Clinical features

The onset, thyroid status and type of goitre vary profoundly from case to case. The onset may be insidious and asymptomatic or so sudden and painful that it resembles the acute form of granulomatous thyroiditis. Mild hyperthyroidism may be present initially, but hypothyroidism is inevitable and may develop rapidly or extremely slowly. The goitre is usually lobulated and may be diffuse or localised to one lobe. It may be large or small, and soft, rubbery or firm in consistency, depending on the cellularity and degree of fibrosis. The disease is most common in women at the menopause but may occur at any age. Papillary carcinoma and malignant lymphoma are occasionally associated with autoimmune thyroiditis.

Diagnosis

Biochemical tests of thyroid function vary with the thyroid status and are of diagnostic value only if hypothyroidism is present. Significantly, raised serum levels of one or more thyroid antibodies are present in over 85% of cases. Nevertheless, differential diagnosis from nodular goitre, carcinoma and malignant lymphoma of the thyroid is not always easy. FNAC is the most appropriate investigation although abundant lymphocytes may make the cytological distinction between autoimmune thyroiditis and lymphoma difficult. When there is doubt about neoplastic disease, which may coexist with thyroiditis, diagnostic lobectomy may be necessary.

Treatment

Full replacement dosage of thyroxine should be given for hypothyroidism and if the goitre is large or symptomatic because some (under TSH stimulation) may subside with hormone therapy. More minor manifestations of the condition, such as a small goitre with raised antibody titres, or histological evidence of thyroiditis in association with other thyroid disease, do not justify thyroxine replacement if thyroid function is biochemically normal; however, long-term surveillance is necessary because of the risk of late thyroid failure. Occasionally, the goitre increases in size despite hormone treatment and, in these circumstances, there may be a favourable response to steroid therapy. Thyroidectomy may be necessary if the goitre is large and causes discomfort. An increase in size of a longstanding lymphocytic goitre should be assessed urgently because of the possibility of the development of malignant lymphoma.

Granulomatous thyroiditis (subacute thyroiditis, de Quervain's thyroiditis)

Granulomatous thyroiditis is caused by a viral infection. In a typical subacute presentation there is pain in the neck, fever, malaise and a firm irregular enlargement of one or both thyroid lobes. There is a raised erythrocyte sedimentation rate and absent thyroid antibodies, the serum T_4 is high normal or slightly raised and the ^{123}I uptake of the gland is low. The condition is self-limiting and after a few months the goitre subsides and there may be a period of months of hypothyroidism before eventual recovery. In 10% of cases the onset is acute, the goitre is very painful and tender and there may be symptoms of hyperthyroidism. One-third of cases are asymptomatic but for the presence of the goitre. If diagnosis is in doubt it may be confirmed by FNAC, radioactive iodine uptake and a rapid symptomatic response to prednisone. The specific treatment for the acute case with severe pain is to give prednisone 10–20 mg daily for 7 days, with the dose gradually reduced over the next month. If thyroid failure is prominent, treatment with thyroxine may be required until function recovers.

Riedel's thyroiditis

Riedel's thyroiditis is very rare, accounting for 0.5% of goitres. Thyroid tissue is replaced by cellular fibrous tissue, which infiltrates through the capsule into muscles and adjacent structures, including the parathyroids, recurrent nerves and carotid sheath. It may occur in association with retroperitoneal and mediastinal fibrosis and is most probably a collagen disease. The goitre may be unilateral or bilateral and is very hard and fixed. The differential diagnosis from anaplastic carcinoma can be made with certainty only by biopsy, when a wedge of the isthmus should also be removed to free the trachea. If the condition is unilateral the other lobe is usually involved later and subsequent hypothyroidism is common. Treatment is with high-dose steroids and thyroxine replacement. A reduction in the size of the goitre and long-term improvement in symptoms are to be expected if treatment is commenced early (Summary box 48.7).

Summary box 48.7

Thyroiditis

- Be aware of the common and uncommon forms of thyroiditis
- Understand their effects on thyroid function

PARATHYROID HYPERPARATHYROIDISM

Primary hyperparathyroidism

Primary HPT is more commonly sporadic than familial. Hypercalcaemia in the presence of inappropriately raised serum PTH levels is due to enlargement of one or more glands and hypersecretion of PTH. The normal response to hypercalcaemia is PTH suppression.

Epidemiology

The prevalence of sporadic primary HPT increases with age and it affects women more than men. On biochemical screening approximately 1% of adults are hypercalcaemic.

Familial HPT occurs as part of the following genetically determined conditions:

- MEN-1 (multiple endocrine neoplasia type 1; Werner's syndrome)
- MEN-2A (Sipple's syndrome) and rarely MEN-2B.
- familial isolated HPT.

Pathology

The majority (85%) of patients with sporadic primary HPT have a single adenoma, approximately 13% have hyperplasia affecting all four glands and about 1% will have more than one adenoma or a carcinoma. In familial disease, multiple gland enlargement is the norm.

There is a weak correlation between the size of an adenoma and the level of PTH (Fig. 48.48). The histological differentiation between adenoma and hyperplasia can be difficult and the macroscopic findings are an important determinant in making the diagnosis. A single enlarged gland with three small normal glands is characteristic of a single adenoma, regardless of the histology, which may show considerable overlap between a hyperplastic and an adenomatous gland. Multiple adenomas occur more frequently in older patients. Parathyroid hyperplasia by definition affects all four glands (Fig. 48.49a and b).

Parathyroid carcinomas are large tumours and typically much more adherent or even frankly invasive than large adenomas. Histology demonstrates a florid desmoplastic reaction with dense fibrosis and capsular and vascular invasion.

Parathyroid cysts may be secondary to degeneration in nodules or adenomas, or developmental and, although some present as a

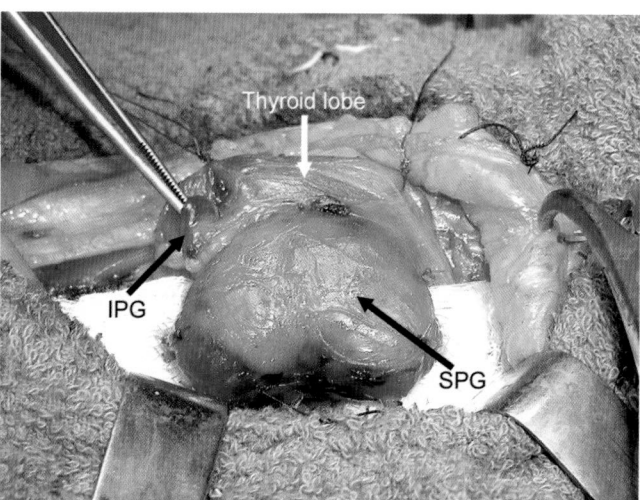

Figure 48.48 Parathyroid adenoma. Operative photograph showing the normal left inferior parathyroid (IPG) and large left superior parathyroid adenoma (SPG).

Otto Werner, **1879–1936**, a German Physician who had a practice in a small town near the German–Danish border.
John Sipple, **B. 1930**, Professor of Medicine, SUNY Medical Center, New York, NY, USA.

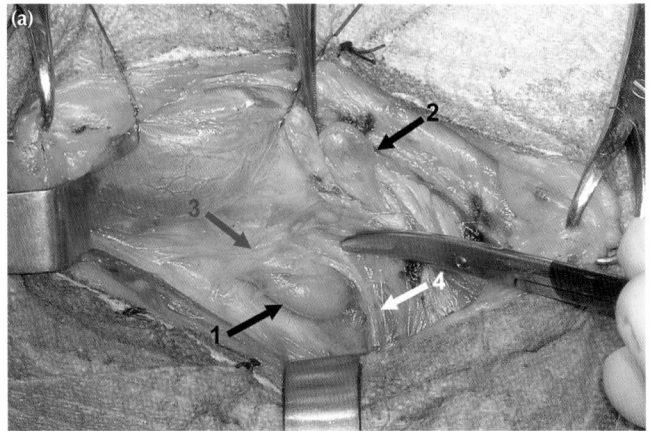

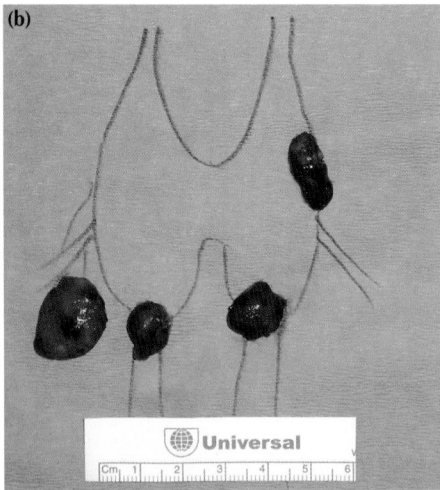

Figure 48.49 Parathyroid hyperplasia. (a) Mobilised right thyroid lobe showing enlarged superior (1) and inferior (2) parathyroid glands. Note how the superior gland has migrated posterior and inferior to the inferior thyroid artery (3). (4) Recurrent laryngeal nerve. (b) Total parathyroidectomy specimens.

palpable neck swelling, small cysts are most often noted as incidental findings during neck exploration. If aspirated preoperatively the diagnosis should be suspected from the watery clear fluid aspirated. The diagnosis is confirmed by a high PTH level in the aspirated fluid.

Clinical presentation

The classic quartet of 'stones, bones, abdominal groans and psychic moans' is rarely observed in developed countries where the diagnosis is usually made on serum calcium estimation well before the full picture of severe bone disease (von Recklinghausen's disease), renal calculi and calcinosis, pancreatitis and psychiatric disorder develops. Incidentally detected hypercalcaemia is rarely truly 'asymptomatic' and most patients experience an improved sense of well-being after surgery. Careful enquiry into family history is always appropriate and may reveal an index case for familial disease, including familial primary HPT, MEN syndromes and familial hypocalciuric hypercalcaemia.

Diagnosis

Although ionised calcium is the physiologically active circulating element, total serum calcium is a satisfactory measure. The effect of calcium binding to serum proteins must be corrected by upward or downward correction to a serum albumin level of $40\,\mathrm{g\,l^{-1}}$. Inappropriate (elevated or normal) PTH levels in the presence of high serum calcium are diagnostic of primary HPT. Hypophospataemia and elevated urine calcium excretion are confirmatory.

Other causes of hypercalcaemia must be considered and excluded (Table 48.12). Advanced malignancy is the most common cause of hypercalcaemia in hospital patients, resulting from parathyroid hormone-related peptide (PTHrP) or bone metastases. The PTH level is suppressed.

Familial hypocalciuric hypercalcaemia is an autosomal dominant disorder characterised by mild elevation of calcium and PTH levels secondary to a missense mutation in the cell membrane calcium receptor. The low urinary excretion of calcium will discriminate this from HPT. Parathyroidectomy is not required. However, neonatal HPT is rare but associated with severe hypercalcaemia in homozygous patients and urgent near-total parathyroidectomy is required.

Treatment of primary hyperparathyroidism

At present, surgery is the only curative option and should be offered to all patients with significant hypercalcaemia provided that they are otherwise fit for the procedure. There are a number of medical strategies and therapies, particularly in mild HPT, including simple expectant treatment until the calcium level or symptoms reach a level at which surgery becomes more attractive, a low-calcium diet, withdrawal of drugs (diuretics and lithium) that aggravate hypercalcaemia and, more recently, calcium-reducing agents such as bisphosphanates and the calcium receptor agonist cinacalcet.

Occasionally, patients present with a parathyroid crisis and severe hypercalcaemia (serum calcium greater than $3.5\,\mathrm{mmol\,l^{-1}}$). This results in confusion, nausea, abdominal pain, cardiac arrhythmias and hypotension with acute renal failure. Intravenous saline and bisphosphonate therapy (pamidronate) are required to correct the dehydration and hypercalcaemia. This is best done in a high-dependency unit or even an intensive therapy unit setting to monitor the major physiological fluxes that result.

Indications for operation

Conventional indications for operation are shown in Table 48.13; traditionally, endocrine surgeons have had a lower threshold for

Table 48.12 Causes of hypercalcaemia

Endocrine	Primary hyperparathyroidism
	Thyrotoxicosis
	Phaeochromocytoma
	Adrenal crisis
Renal failure	Tertiary hyperparathyroidism
Malignant disease	Skeletal secondaries
	Myeloma
Nutritional	Milk alkali syndrome
	Excess vitamin D intake
Granulomatous disease	Tuberculosis
	Sarcoidosis
Immobilisation	
Inherited disorders	Hypercalciuric hypercalcaemia

Table 48.13 Indications for parathyroidectomy in primary hyperparathyroidism

Urinary tract calculi
Reduced bone density
High serum calcium[a]
? All in younger age group < 50 years
Deteriorating renal function
Symptomatic hypercalcaemia

[a] Variously set between 2.85 and 3.00 mmol l[-1]

recommending operation than physicians. However, the widespread adoption of minimal access techniques for parathyroidectomy has changed many physicians' attitudes because of the perceived reduction in operative morbidity. There remains a cohort of patients with mild primary HPT and those with significant comorbidity in whom the decision for operation remains a matter of clinical judgement.

Preoperative localisation

There has been a paradigm shift in the use of preoperative imaging in primary HPT. Until a few years ago the maxim that the 'only localisation test necessary was to locate a good endocrine surgeon' (Doppman) was apposite when opinion favoured a conventional bilateral neck exploration. Skilled surgeons can achieve cure rates of about 98%, with lack of success the result of an ectopic adenoma not accessible through a cervical incision or occasionally the failure to recognise multiple gland disease. Although there should be minimal morbidity associated with a bilateral neck exploration, an image-guided targeted approach reduces this even further and has become routine in most major centres. Concerns remain that subtle abnormalities will be missed if all glands are not routinely visualised but, to date, these have not been translated into a significant clinical issue. There remains a cohort of patient in whom preoperative imaging does not localise an adenoma and the experience of the surgeon remains paramount in achieving a high cure rate.

High-frequency neck ultrasound is non-invasive and should

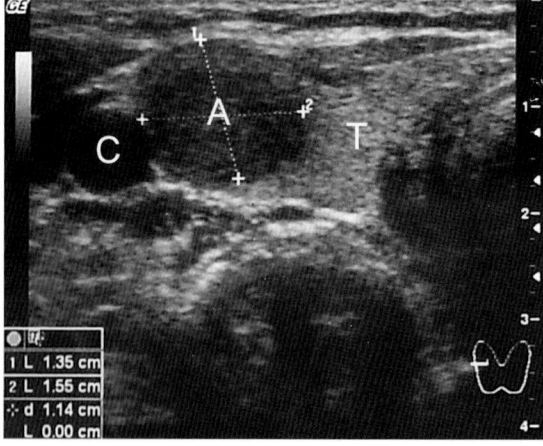

Figure 48.50 Ultrasound scan of a parathyroid adenoma at the upper pole of the right thyroid lobe. C, carotid artery; A, parathyroid adenoma; T, right thyroid lobe.

John L. Doppman, **Contemporary, Radiologist, Bethesda, USA.**

identify 75% of enlarged glands. It gives better resolution but reduced penetration and it cannot visualise the mediastinum (Fig. 48.50). Nodular thyroid disease is a confounding factor.

Technetium-99m (^{99m}Tc)-labelled sestamibi (MIBI) isotope scans (Fig. 48.51) also identify 75% of abnormal parathyroid glands. The area scanned must include the mediastinum to detect ectopic glands. Single-photon emission computerised tomography (SPECT) (Fig. 48.52) gives a three-dimensional image that may influence the surgical approach. Concordance between ultrasound and sestamibi scans permits a targeted approach with confidence. However, the size of the adenoma is important and imaging and concordance decline with glands weighing less than 500 mg.

CT, PET and MRI are not indicated prior to first-time neck exploration.

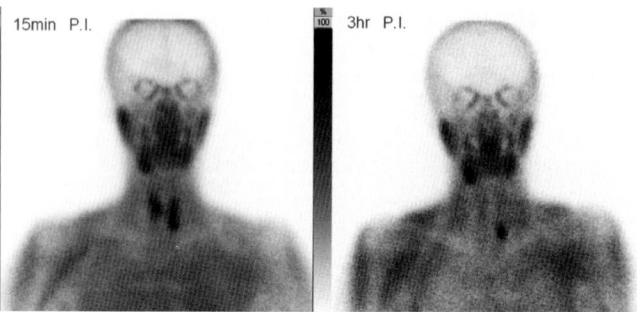

Figure 48.51 Technetium-99m-labelled sestamibi isotope scans 15 min and 3 hours after injection showing retention of isotope in a left inferior parathyroid adenoma.

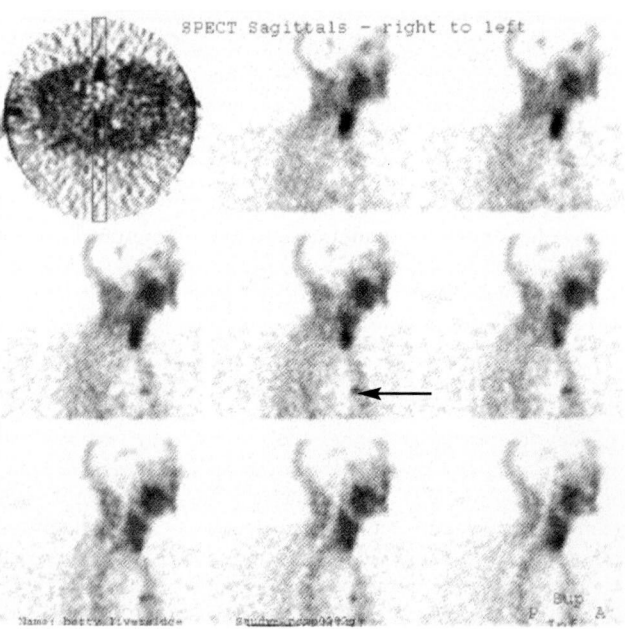

Figure 48.52 Technetium-99m-labelled sestamibi isotope scan with single photon emission computerised tomography showing a hot-spot in the anterior mediastinum (arrow) (courtesy of Mr B. Harrison, Sheffield, UK).

The noun isotope **is derived from the Greek Isos = equal and topos = place, meaning having an equal place on the periodic table.**

Operation for primary hyperparathyroidism

Preoperative discussion must include the possibility of:

- persistent HPT (5%);
- recurrent laryngeal nerve injury (1%);
- postoperative haemorrhage (1%);
- permanent hypoparathyroidism;
- recurrent HPT.

There are a number of surgical options available of which a targeted small incision approach and bilateral exploration using a conventional 'thyroidectomy' incision are the most frequently performed. Video-assisted (in which a video endoscope is used to reduce the size of incision and permit bilateral exploration) and totally endoscopic techniques with multiple punctures have not achieved much popularity. Preoperative intravenous infusion of methylene blue (5 mg kg^{-1} body weight in 500 ml of dextrose–saline) is used by some surgeons because it preferentially stains parathyroid tissue. The short serum half-life of PTH means that intraoperative measurements can be used to confirm that the source of excess PTH production has been excised, although this is of more value in reoperations than first-time operations. A gamma probe can be used to guide exploration following preoperative injection of MIBI.

Operative strategy and technique of parathyroidectomy

Targeted approach

General or local anaesthesia may be used. A head light and magnifying loupes are useful. Confident preoperative localisation permits a 2- to 3-cm incision located over the site of the adenoma (Fig. 48.53). This may be placed to permit extension to a formal bilateral exploration incision if the imaging is suboptimal. The subplatysmal plane is incised and a lateral approach to the strap muscles permits development of the plane between the thyroid capsule and carotid artery and jugular veins. The adenoma is easily identified in the anticipated site when imaging is concordant. It is carefully mobilised, staying close to but avoiding rupture of the capsule. Identification of the RLN is not routine and only bipolar diathermy should be used. Failure to immediately identify the gland may require an extended exploration, which can be accomplished through a unilateral limited incision. Conversion to a formal neck incision and bilateral exploration should rarely be required if preoperative assessment has been rigorous.

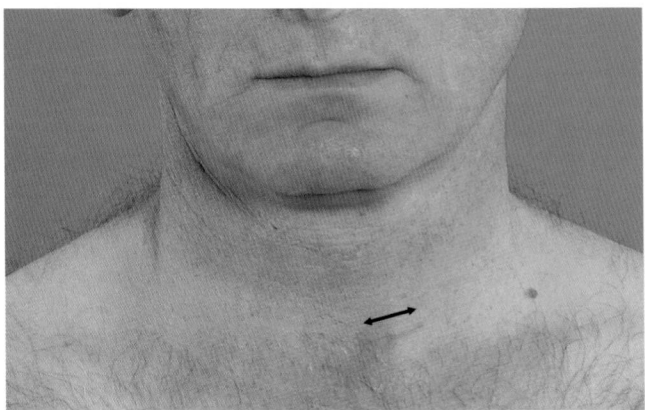

Figure 48.53 Targeted parathyroid surgery; a 2-cm incision over a left inferior parathyroid adenoma.

Conventional approach

The patient is positioned in reverse Trendelenburg with a silicone gel pad placed transversely under the shoulders to extend the neck and the head supported in a padded ring. A transverse collar incision is made, the subplatysmal plane is developed superiorly and inferiorly and the deep cervical fascia are incised in the midline between the strap muscles. The thyroid lobes are mobilised with division of the middle thyroid vein when present. It is not normally necessary to divide the superior thyroid vessels unless the exploration proves difficult. Medial rotation of the thyroid lobe exposes the inferior thyroid artery and RLN (see Fig. 48.49). The glands are identified in a systematic manner commencing with the common sites and working sequentially through to the rare locations. The superior gland is sought above the termination of the inferior thyroid artery, then inferiorly behind the inferior thyroid artery and oesophagus. The inferior gland is sought along the thyrothymic axis, on the surface of the inferior pole of the thyroid lobe, the upper horn of the thymus, the mediastinal thymus, then within the carotid sheath and finally within the thyroid lobe, which may require thyroid lobectomy. All abnormal glands are excised and, in the event of sporadic four-gland disease, subtotal parathyroidectomy is carried out, preserving approximately 50 mg of one gland. This must be marked with a non-absorbable suture to facilitate any possible future re-exploration.

In patients with four-gland disease, transcervical thymectomy is recommended to reduce the risk of persistent or recurrent HPT. In patients with MEN-1, total parathyroidectomy reduces the risk of recurrence.

Preoperative imaging will identify the 1% of patients with a mediastinal adenoma and permit a single curative operation (Fig. 48.54). This may be performed thoracoscopically rather than by a mediastinotomy.

Secondary hyperparathyroidism

Chronic renal failure results in *secondary HPT*. The kidney cannot convert vitamin D into the physiologically active 1,25-cholecalciferol. Reduced intestinal absorption of calcium resulting in a low serum calcium, and elevated phosphate due to renal failure to excrete phosphate, increases secretion of PTH. Prolonged stimulation results in parathyroid hyperplasia. Initially this is reversible following renal transplantation but when autonomous hyperfunction progresses after transplantation this is termed tertiary HPT.

Secondary HPT also occurs in vitamin D-deficient *rickets*, *malabsorption* and *pseudohypoparathyroidism*.

Clinical and biochemical features

These include bone pain, pruritus, muscle weakness, renal osteodystrophy and soft-tissue calcification (Fig. 48.55). Calciphylaxis (calcific uraemic arteriolopathy) is the end-stage of this condition with arteriolar occlusion resulting in cutaneous ulceration and gangrene. The systemic effects of these changes result in a high mortality rate and urgent parathyroidectomy may be required if the PTH is excessively high.

> Friedrich Trendelenburg, **1844–1924, Professor of Surgery, Rostock (1875–1882), Bonn (1882–1895), and Leipzig (1895–1911), Germany.** The Trendelenburg position was first described in 1885.

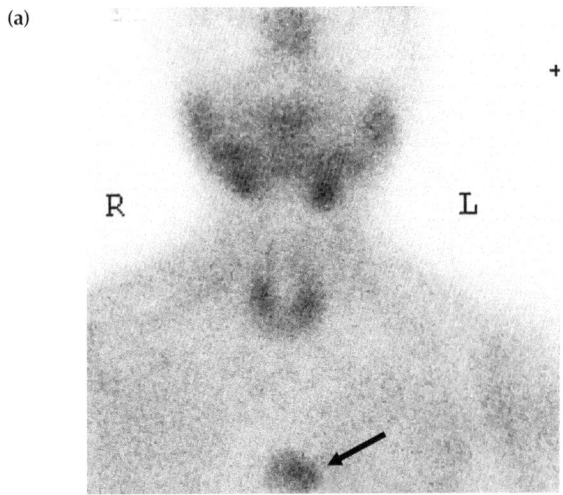

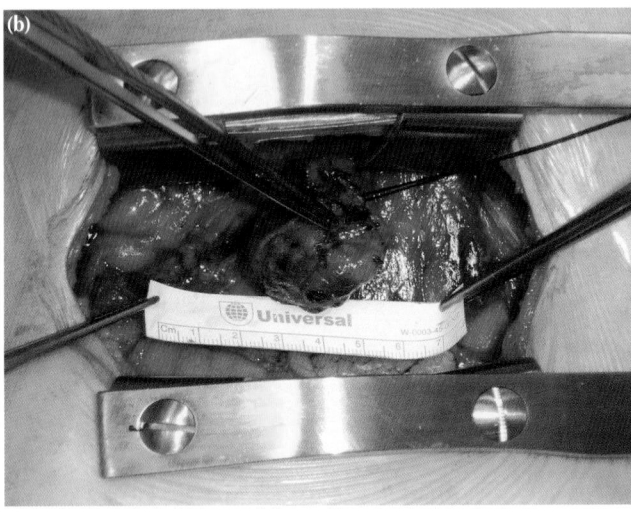

Figure 48.54 Mediastinal parathyroid adenoma (courtesy of Mr K. Buchan, Aberdeen, UK) (a) Preoperative technetium-99m-labelled sestamibi isotope scan with mediastinal adenoma (arrowed). (b) Operative photograph of a median sternotomy showing a 4-cm para-thyroid adenoma.

Treatment

Medical treatment of secondary HPT includes dietary phosphate restriction and calcium and vitamin D supplementation. Surgery is indicated when there is an excessive rise in the calcium/phosphate product and serum PTH. Patients are prepared with high-dose vitamin D (calcitriol) to reduce the severity of the profound hypocalcaemia that would otherwise follow parathyroidectomy. Preoperative dialysis is obligatory.

Operative strategy

Multiple-gland disease is usual although occasionally HPT secondary to single-gland disease is the cause rather than the consequence of renal failure. Options for management include total parathyroidectomy (see Fig. 48.49), total parathyroidectomy with autotransplantation of 50 mg of parathyroid tissue into the brachioradialis or subtotal parathyroidectomy. The last strategy is preferred if renal transplantation is likely. Transcervical thymectomy is indicated.

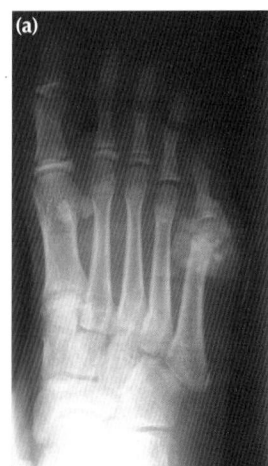

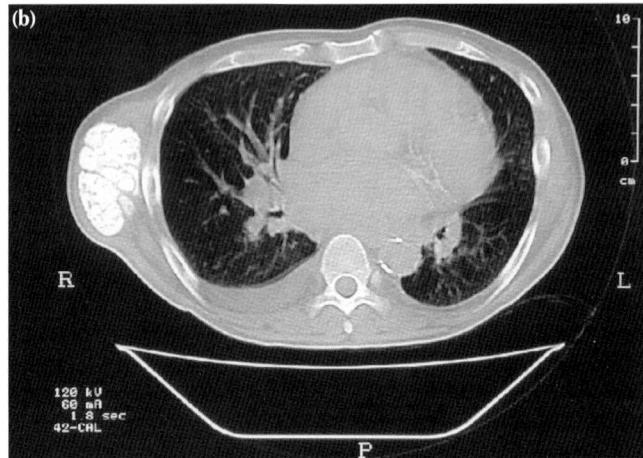

Figure 48.55 Secondary hyperparathyroidism. (a) Radiograph of ectopic calcification. (b) Computerised tomography scan showing ectopic calcification in the chest wall.

Postoperative hypocalcaemia is inevitable even after subtotal parathyroidectomy or autotransplantation. Preoperative preparation and oral vitamin D and calcium are essential. Intravenous calcium and magnesium are often required.

Parathyroid carcinoma

Cancer of the parathyroid is rare, accounting for 1% of cases of HPT. Typical features are very high calcium and PTH levels, often with a palpable neck swelling or occasionally lymphadenopathy. Scanning may support the diagnosis (Fig. 48.56). The diagnosis is rarely known at the time of exploration but, if suspected, operation should include excision of the tumour mass with *en bloc* thyroid lobectomy and node dissection when indicated. The diagnosis is difficult to make histologically and may only become apparent when recurrent disease presents with hypercalcaemia, increased serum PTH and evidence of local recurrence. Adjuvant or palliative radiotherapy may be indicated and overall survival, as in most endocrine cancers, is reasonable with a 5-year survival rate of 85%.

---

en bloc **is French for 'in a block'.**

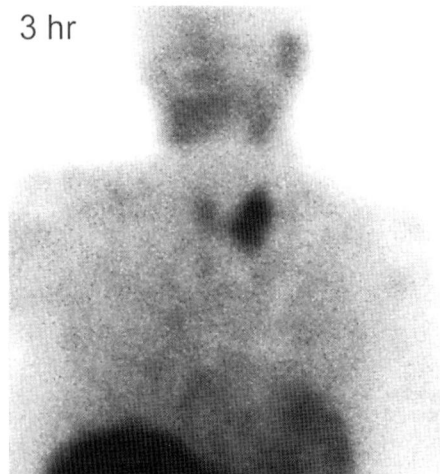

Figure 48.56 Technetium-99m-labelled sestamibi isotope scan at 3 hours showing a left superior parathyroid carcinoma.

Persistent hyperparathyroidism

The first operation is the best opportunity to cure HPT surgically and, when competently performed, should be successful in more than 95% of procedures. If hypercalcaemia persists after a first neck exploration the diagnosis, preoperative investigations, operative findings and pathology must be reviewed carefully. Referral to a specialist centre is prudent. If reoperation is appropriate, further investigation is required to localise the abnormal parathyroid tissue, usually a missed adenoma. This may be readily apparent but can require a combination of ultrasound, sestamibi, CT, MRI, PET, selective angiography (Fig. 48.57) and venous sampling for PTH. The results of this last technique may be difficult to interpret if normal venous drainage has been disrupted by previous operations.

When the site of an ectopic or missed adenoma is accurately identified, a second operation can be straightforward when performed through intact tissue planes. Re-exploration through previously explored tissues is more difficult and increases the risks to the RLNs and the risks of postoperative hypocalcaemia.

Recurrent hyperparathyroidism

Recurrent HPT is diagnosed when hypercalcaemia recurs more than 12 months after an initially curative operation. This may occur because of:

- missed pathology at the first operation;
- (rarely) development of a second adenoma;
- hyperplasia in autotransplanted tissue;
- parathyromatosis (disseminated nodules of parathyroid tissue within the soft tissues of the neck and superior mediastinum caused by rupture of abnormal parathyroid tissue at initial surgery).

Reoperative parathyroid surgery is associated with an increased risk of RLN injury and postoperative hypocalcaemia. Knowledge that surgical cure is achieved when a single gland has been removed obviates the need for further dissection. An intraoperative rapid PTH assay can be used to demonstrate the fall in PTH levels that occurs when all abnormal parathyroid tissue has been excised. If PTH levels fall to < 50% of baseline values at 15 min after specimen excision, the surgeon can terminate the intervention and

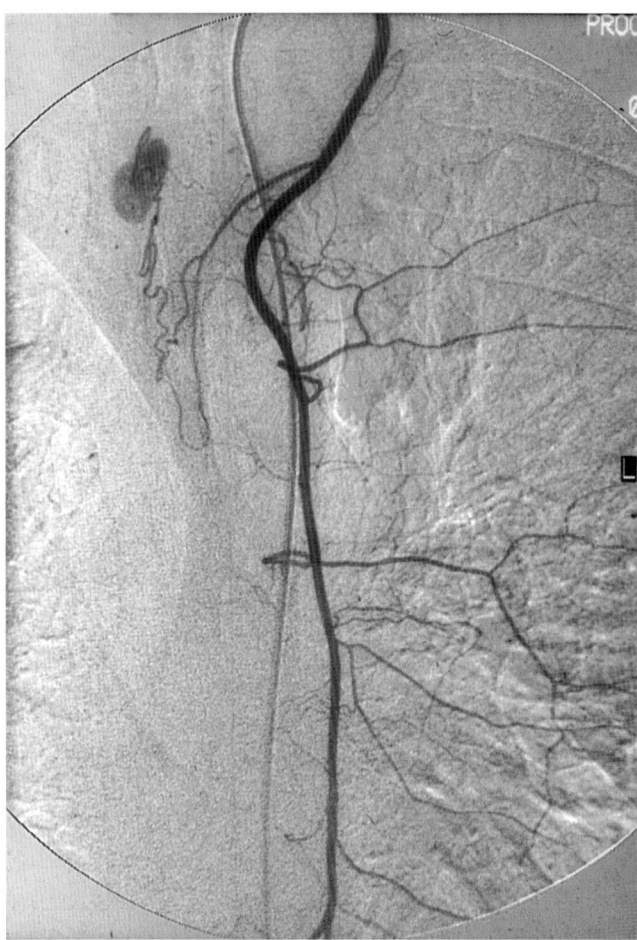

Figure 48.57 Selective arteriogram of the internal mammary artery showing parathyroid tumour blush in a patient who had undergone three previous neck explorations for hyperparathyroidism (courtesy of Mr B. Harrison, Sheffield, UK).

reduce the risk of surgical morbidity associated with further exploration of a scarred operative field.

HYPOPARATHYROIDISM

Although there are rare congenital (DiGeorge) and medical (autoimmune polyglandular and Wilson) syndromes causing hypoparathyroidism, for practical purposes, postoperative hypoparathyroidism is the dominant management issue in surgical practice. This results from trauma to or removal or devascularisation of the parathyroid glands, which may be deliberate but is more often inadvertent.

Symptoms and signs

The symptoms and signs of acute hypoparathyroidism are related to the level of serum calcium and range from mild circumoral and digital numbness and paraesthesia to tetanic symptoms with carpopedal or laryngeal spasms, cardiac arrhythmias and fits.

Angelo DiGeorge, **B. 1921, Professor of Paediatrics, Temple University, Philadelphia, PA, USA.**
Samuel Alexander Kinnier Wilson, **1878–1936, Professor of Neurology, King's College Hospital, London, England.**

CHAPTER 48 | THE THYROID AND PARATHYROID GLANDS

Chronic hypoparathyroidism can lead to abnormal bone deminerralisation, cataracts, calcification in basal ganglia and consequent extrapyramidal disorders.

Percussion of the facial nerve just below the zygoma causes contraction of the ipsilateral facial muscles (Chvostek's sign). Carpopedal spasm can be induced by occlusion of the arm with a blood pressure cuff for 3 min (Trousseau's sign). Electrocardiogram changes include prolonged QT intervals and QRS complex changes.

Treatment

Acute symptomatic hypocalcaemia is a medical emergency and requires urgent correction by intravenous injection of calcium. Magnesium supplements may also be required. Oral calcium (1 g three or four times daily) supplemented by 1–3 µg daily of 1-alpha-vitamin D if necessary should be given with a view to gradual withdrawal over the next 3–12 months (Summary box 48.8).

Summary box 48.8

Management of postoperative hypocalcaemia

- Check serum calcium within 24 hours of total thyroidectomy or earlier if symptomatic
- Medical emergency if the level is < 1.90 mmol l⁻¹: correct with 10 ml of 10% calcium gluconate intravenously; 10 ml of 10% magnesium sulphate intravenously may also be required
- Give 1 g of oral calcium three or four times daily
- Give 1–3 µg daily of oral 1-alpha-vitamin D if necessary

Frantisek Chvostek, **1835–1884, Physician, The Josefsacademie, Vienna, Austria.**
Armand Trousseau, **1801–1867, Physician, Hôtel Dieu, Paris, France.**

FURTHER READING

Kuma, K., Matsuzuka, F., Kobayashi, A. et al. (1992) Outcome of long-standing solitary thyroid nodules. *World J Surg* **16**: 583–7.

Mazzaferri, E.L. (1993) Management of a solitary thyroid nodule. *N Engl J Med* **328**: 55–9.

Mazzaferri, E.L., Harmer C., Mallick U.K. and Kendall-Taylor, P. (2006) *Practical Management of Thyroid Cancer*. Springer-Verlag, London.

McIver, B., Hay, I.D., Giuffrida, D.F. et al. (2001) Anaplastic thyroid cancer: a fifty year experience at a single institution. *Surgery* **130**: 1028–34.

Monfared A., Gorti G. and Kim D. (2002) Microsurgical anatomy of the laryngeal nerves as related to thyroid surgery. *Laryngoscope* **112**: 386–92.

Palazzo, F.F. and Delbridge, L.W. (2004) Minimal access/minimally invasive parathyroidectomy for primary hyperparathyroidism. *Surg Clin N Am* **84**: 717–34.

Ravetto, C., Colombo, L. and Dottorino, M.E. (2000) Usefulness of fine-needle aspiration in the diagnosis of thyroid carcinoma: a retrospective study of 37895 patients. *Cancer* **90**: 357–63.

Richards, M.L., Chisholm, R., Bruder, J. and Strodel, W.E. (2002) Is thyroid frozen section too much for too little? *Am J Surg* **184**: 510–14.

Tan, G.H. and Gahrib, H. (1997) Thyroid incidentalomas: management approaches to nonpalpable nodules discovered incidentally on thyroid imaging. *Ann Intern Med* **126**: 226–31.

Wanebo, H., Coburn, M., Teates, D. and Cole, B. (1998) Total thyroidectomy does not enhance disease control or survival even in high-risk patients with differentiated thyroid cancer. *Ann Surg* **227**: 912–21.

Adrenal glands and other endocrine disorders

LEARNING OBJECTIVES

To understand:
- The anatomy and function of the adrenal and other endocrine glands
- The diagnosis and management of endocrine disorders
- The role of surgery in the management of endocrine disorders

ADRENAL GLANDS

Anatomy

The weight of a normal adrenal gland is approximately 4 g. There are two distinct components of the gland: the inner adrenal medulla and the outer adrenal cortex (Fig. 49.1). The adrenal glands are situated at the upper poles of the kidneys in the retroperitoneum within Gerota's capsule. The right adrenal gland is located between the right liver lobe and the diaphragm, close to and partly behind the inferior vena cava. The left adrenal gland lies on the upper pole of the left kidney and reaches the renal pedicle. It is covered by the pancreatic tail and the spleen (Fig. 49.2).

The adrenal glands are well supplied by blood vessels. The arterial blood supply branches from the aorta and the diaphragmatic and renal arteries and varies considerably. A large adrenal

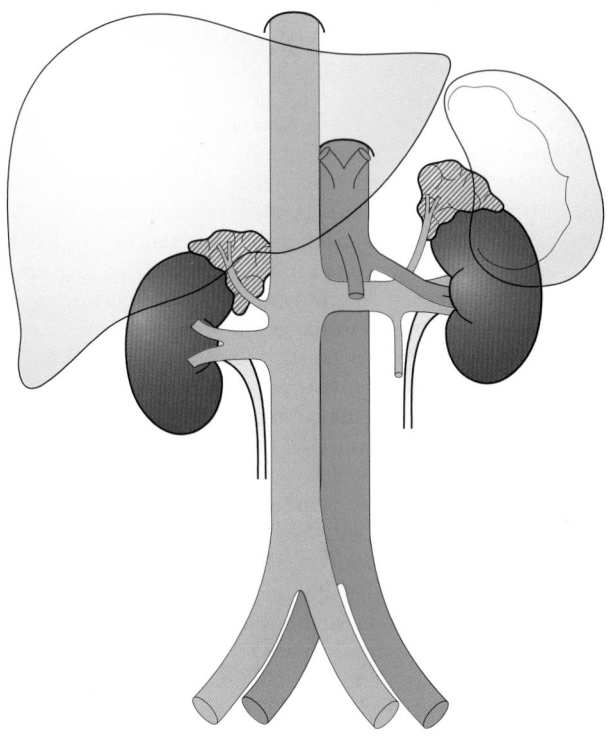

Figure 49.2 Position of the adrenal glands (hatched) in the retroperitoneum.

vein drains on the right side into the vena cava and on the left side into the renal vein.

Embryology

The two functional parts, the cortex and the medulla, arise from different blastodermic layers: mesodermal cells form the adrenal cortex and neuroectodermal cells migrate to the cortex during embryogenesis and form the adrenal medulla.

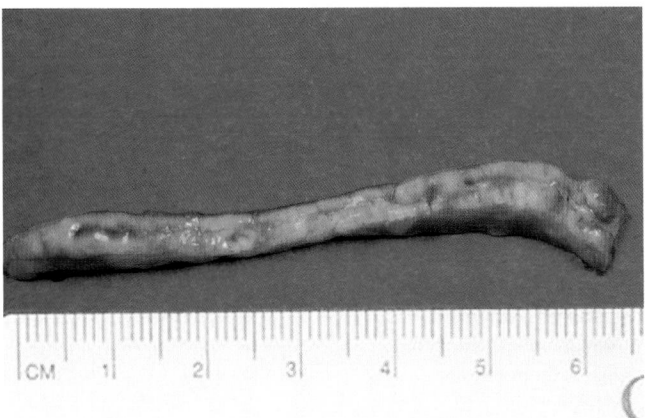

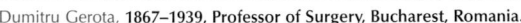

Figure 49.1 Cross-section of a normal adrenal gland. The inner, very thin layer between the two dark lines (zona reticularis) is the adrenal medulla.

Dumitru Gerota, **1867–1939, Professor of Surgery, Bucharest, Romania.**

Histology

The adrenal cortex is characterised by a zonal configuration. The outer zona glomerulosa contains small, compact cells. The zona fasciculata can be identified by the larger, lipoid cells, which are arranged in radial columns. Compact and pigmented cells characterise the inner zona reticularis. The adrenal medulla consists of a thin layer of large chromaffin cells, which store catecholamine granules.

Function of the adrenal glands

The adrenal glands play a pivotal role in the response to stress. Catecholamines are secreted by the adrenal medulla and corticosteroids, aldosterone and cortisol are synthesised in the adrenal cortex.

Cells of the adrenal medulla synthesise mainly adrenaline (epinephrine) but also noradrenaline (norepinephrine) and dopamine. These catecholamines act as hormones as they are secreted directly into the circulation. Their effects, which are mediated through α and β receptors on target organs, include activation of the cardiovascular system, resulting in an increase in blood pressure and heart rate; vasoconstriction of vessels in the splanchnic system and vasodilatation of vessels in the muscles; bronchodilatation; and increased glycogenolysis in liver and muscles.

Cells of the zona glomerulosa produce aldosterone, which regulates sodium–potassium homeostasis. The target organs of aldosterone are the kidneys, the sweat and salivary glands and the intestinal mucosa. Aldosterone promotes sodium retention and potassium excretion. The most important regulators of aldosterone secretion are the renin–angiotensin system and the serum potassium concentration. Renin produced by the juxtaglomerular cells in the kidneys acts on its substrate angiotensinogen to generate angiotensin I. Angiotensin I is converted by the angiotensin-converting enzyme (ACE) to the octapeptide angiotensin II, which is modified to angiotensin III. Both stimulate the secretion of aldosterone from the adrenal cortex. A decrease in renal blood flow (haemorrhage, dehydration, salt depletion, orthostasis, renal artery stenosis) or hyponatraemia increases renin secretion and leads to sodium retention, potassium excretion and an increase of plasma volume.

Cells of the zona fasciculata and zona reticularis synthesise cortisol and the adrenal androgens dehydroepiandrosterone (DHEA) and its sulphate DHEAS. DHEA and DHEAS are precursors of androgens and are converted by different peripheral tissues. Cortisol secretion is regulated by adrenocorticotrophic hormone (ACTH), which is produced by the anterior pituitary gland. The hypothalamus controls ACTH secretion by secreting corticotropin-releasing hormone (CRH). The cortisol level inhibits the release of CRH and ACTH via a closed-loop system.

Cortisol is the most important steroid and has numerous metabolic and immunological effects. It increases gluconeogenesis and lipolysis; decreases peripheral glucose utilisation, immunological response and muscular mass; affects fat distribution, wound healing and bone mineralisation; and alters mood (euphoria or, rarely, depression) and cortical awareness.

DISORDERS OF THE ADRENAL CORTEX

Incidentaloma

Definition

A clinically unapparent mass detected incidentally by imaging studies conducted for other reasons.

Incidence

The prevalence of adrenal masses in autopsy studies ranges from 1.4% to 8.7% and increases with age. Incidentalomas may be detected on imaging studies in 4% of patients. More than 75% are non-functioning adenomas but Cushing's adenomas, phaeochromocytomas and even adrenocortical carcinomas may be present (Table 49.1).

Diagnosis

When an incidentaloma is identified, a complete history and clinical examination are required. A biochemical work-up for hormone excess and sometimes additional imaging studies are also needed. The main goal is to exclude a functioning or malignant adrenal tumour.

Hormonal evaluation includes:

- morning and midnight plasma cortisol measurements;
- a 1-mg overnight dexamethasone suppression test;
- 24-hour urinary cortisol excretion (optional);
- 24-hour urinary excretion of catecholamines, metanephrines or plasma-free metanephrines;
- serum potassium, plasma aldosterone and plasma renin activity;
- serum DHEAS, testosterone or 17β-hydroxyestradiol (virilising or feminising tumour).

For evaluation of malignancy, computerised tomography (CT) or magnetic resonance imaging (MRI) should be performed in all patients with adrenal masses, followed by fine-needle aspiration cytology after a phaeochromocytoma has been excluded. The likelihood of an adrenal mass being an adrenocortical carcinoma increases with the size of the mass (25% > 4 cm). Adrenal metastases are likely in patients with a history of cancer elsewhere (Summary box 49.1).

Summary box 49.1

Adrenal gland biopsy

- Never biopsy an adrenal mass until phaeochromocytoma has been biochemically excluded
- The indication for adrenal gland biopsy is to confirm adrenal gland metastasis

---

Table 49.1 Prevalence of non-functioning and functioning tumours in patients with incidentalomas

Tumour	Prevalence (%)
Non-functioning adenoma	78
Cushing's adenoma	7
Adrenocortical carcinoma	4
Phaeochromocytoma	4
Myelolipoma	2
Cyst	2
Metastases	2
Conn's adenoma	1

Harvey Williams Cushing, **1869–1939, Professor of Surgery, Harvard University Medical School, Boston, MA, USA.**

Treatment

The treatment of functional adrenal tumours is described below. Any non-functioning adrenal tumour greater than 4 cm in diameter and smaller tumours that increase in size over time should undergo surgical resection. Non-functioning tumours smaller than 4 cm should be followed-up after 6, 12 and 24 months by imaging and hormonal evaluation.

Primary hyperaldosteronism

Incidence

Primary hyperaldosteronism (PHA) is defined by hypertension, hypokalaemia and hypersecretion of aldosterone. In PHA, plasma renin activity is suppressed. Among patients with hypertension the incidence of hypokalaemic PHA is approximately 2%. Recent studies have revealed that up to 12% of hypertensive patients have PHA with normal potassium levels.

Pathology

The most frequent cause of PHA with hypokalaemia is a unilateral adrenocortical adenoma (Conn's syndrome) (Fig. 49.3). In 20–40% of cases, bilateral micronodular hyperplasia is causative. Rare causes of PHA are bilateral macronodular hyperplasia, glucocorticoid-suppressible hyperaldosteronism or adrenocortical carcinoma. In the subset of patients with normokalaemic PHA, 70% have hyperplasia and 30% unilateral adenoma.

Clinical features

Most patients are between 30 and 50 years of age with a female predominance. Apart from hypertension and hypokalaemia, patients complain of non-specific symptoms: headache, muscle weakness, cramps, intermittent paralysis, polyuria, polydypsia and nocturia.

Diagnosis

The key feature of the biochemical diagnosis is the assessment of potassium level and the aldosterone to plasma renin activity ratio. Antihypertensive and diuretic therapy, which cause hypokalaemia and influence the renin–angiotensin–aldosterone system, have to be discontinued. Once the biochemical diagnosis is confirmed, MRI or CT should be performed to distinguish unilateral from bilateral disease. Conn's adenomas usually measure between 1 and 2 cm and are detected by CT with a sensitivity of 80–90% (Fig. 49.4). Micronodular changes and small adenomas are often underdiagnosed. An apparent unilateral mass could be a non-functioning tumour in a patient with bilateral micronodular hyperplasia. Therefore, selective adrenal vein catheterisation is warranted before a decision on non-surgical or surgical treatment is made. During selective adrenal vein catheterisation, samples are obtained from the vena cava and from both adrenal veins and the aldosterone to cortisol ratio (ACR) is determined in each sample. A significant difference in the ACR ratio on one side indicates unilateral disease.

Treatment

The first-line therapy for PHA with bilateral hyperplasia is medical treatment with spironolactone. In most cases supplemental antihypertensive medication is necessary.

Unilateral laparoscopic adrenalectomy is an effective therapy in patients with clear evidence of unilateral or asymmetrical bilateral disease. A subtotal resection is favoured in the case of a typical Conn's adenoma. In 10–30% of patients who undergo an adrenalectomy, hypertension persists despite adequate diagnostic work-up and treatment.

Cushing's syndrome

Definition

Hypersecretion of cortisol caused by endogenous production or excessive use of corticosteroids is known as Cushing's syndrome. It can be either ACTH-dependent or ACTH-independent in origin. The most common cause (85%) of ACTH-dependent Cushing's syndrome is Cushing's disease resulting from a pituitary adenoma that secretes an excessive amount of ACTH. Ectopic ACTH-producing tumours (small cell lung cancer, foregut carcinoid) and CRH-producing tumours (medullary thyroid

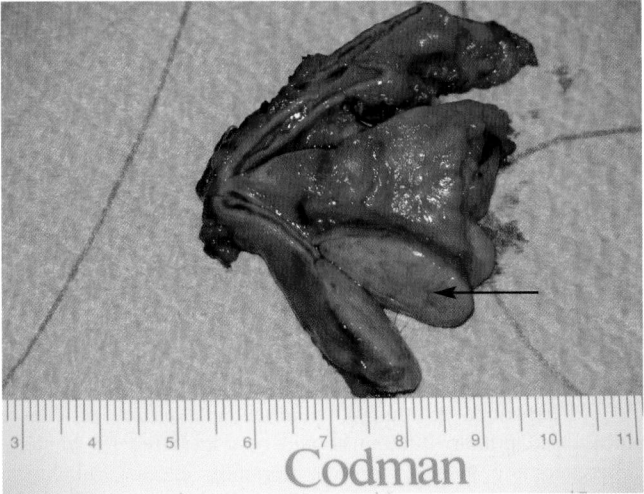

Figure 49.3 A Conn's adenoma (arrow) of the left adrenal gland; note the V-shaped normal adrenal tissue.

Jerome William Conn, **1907–1981**, Professor of Internal Medicine, The University of Michigan, Michigan, MI, USA.

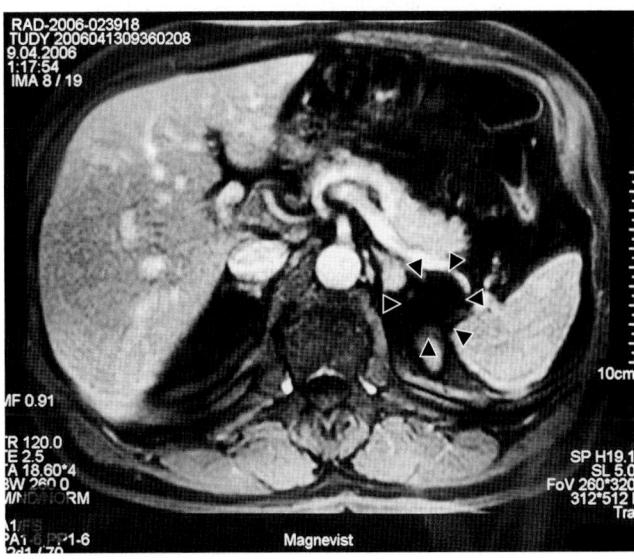

Figure 49.4 Computerised tomography scan of a Conn's adenoma of the left adrenal gland (arrowheads).

carcinoma, neuroendocrine pancreatic tumour) are more infrequent causes of ACTH-dependent Cushing's syndrome.

In about 15% of patients, an ACTH-independent Cushing's syndrome (low ACTH levels) is caused by a unilateral adrenocortical adenoma. Adrenocortical carcinoma and bilateral macronodular or micronodular hyperplasia represent rare causes of hypercortisolism.

Clinical symptoms

The clinical features of Cushing's syndrome are shown in Summary box 49.2. The typical patient is characterised by a facial plethora, a buffalo hump and a moon face in combination with hypertension, diabetes and central obesity (Figs 49.5 and 49.6). However, clinical signs can be minimal or absent in patients with subclinical Cushing's syndrome.

Summary box 49.2

Clinical features of Cushing's syndrome

- Weight gain/central obesity
- Diabetes
- Hirsutism
- Hypertension
- Skin changes (abdominal striae, facial plethora, ecchymosis, acne)
- Muscle weakness
- Menstrual irregularity/impotence
- Depression/mania
- Osteoporosis
- Hypokalaemia

Diagnosis

- Morning and midnight plasma cortisol levels are elevated, possibly with loss of diurnal rhythm.

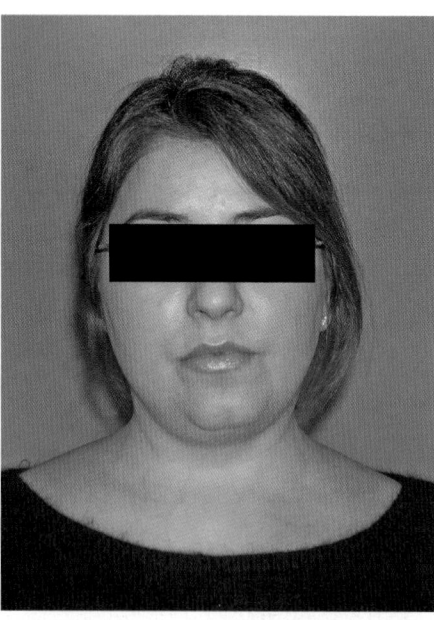

Figure 49.5 34-year-old patient with Cushing's syndrome whose symptoms included thickening of the face, weight gain and acne. Today patients with Cushing's syndrome rarely have the full-blown appearance as shown in older textbooks.

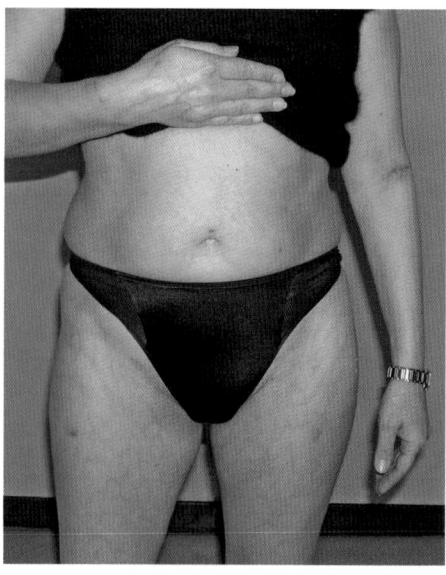

Figure 49.6 Discrete central obesity, ecchymosis and fragile skin in a patient with Cushing's syndrome.

- Dexamethasone fails to suppress 24-hour urinary cortisol excretion.
- Serum ACTH levels discriminate ACTH-dependent from ACTH-independent disease.

Elevated or normal ACTH levels provide evidence for an ACTH-producing pituitary tumour (85%) or ectopic ACTH production. Therefore, in patients with elevated ACTH, MRI of the pituitary gland must be performed. If MRI is negative and additional venous sampling from the inferior petrosal sinus has excluded a pituitary microadenoma, a CT scan of the chest and abdomen is warranted to detect an ectopic cortisol-producing tumour. In patients with suppressed ACTH levels, a CT or MRI scan is performed to assess the adrenal glands.

Subclinical Cushing's syndrome is diagnosed if clinical symptoms are absent and urinary cortisol excretion is in the normal range but a basal low ACTH level increases to normal after CRH stimulation.

Treatment

Medical therapy with metyrapone or ketoconazole reduces steroid synthesis and secretion and is used in patients with severe hypercortisolism or if surgery is not possible. ACTH-producing pituitary tumours are treated by trans-sphenoidal resection or radiotherapy. If an ectopic ACTH source is localised, resection will cure hypercortisolism.

A unilateral adenoma is treated by adrenalectomy. In cases of bilateral ACTH-independent disease (Fig. 49.7), bilateral adrenalectomy is the primary treatment. Patients with an ectopic ACTH-dependent Cushing's syndrome and an irresectable or unlocalised primary tumour should be considered for bilateral adrenalectomy as this controls hormone excess. Subclinical Cushing's syndrome caused by unilateral adenoma is treated by unilateral adrenalectomy.

Preoperative management

Patients with Cushing's syndrome are at an increased risk of hospital-acquired infection and thromboembolic and myocardial

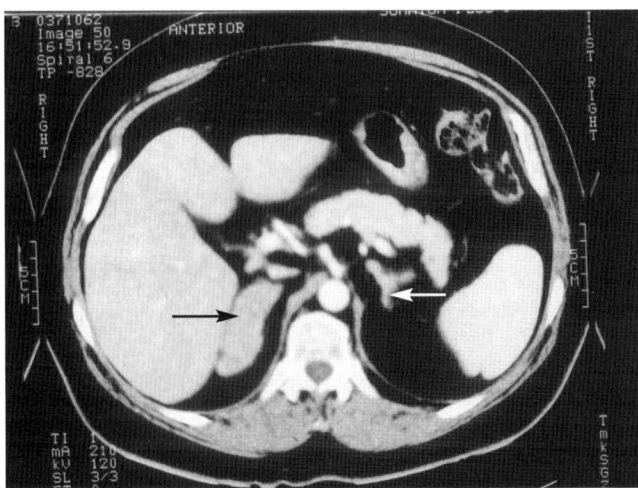

Figure 49.7 Bilateral asymmetrical hyperplasia of the adrenal glands (arrows) in a patient with Cushing's syndrome.

complications. Therefore, prophylactic anti-coagulation and the use of prophylactic antibiotics are essential. Cushing-associated diseases (diabetes, hypertension) must be controlled by medical therapy preoperatively.

Postoperative management

Supplemental cortisol should be given after surgery. In total, 15 mg h⁻¹ is required parenterally for the first 12 hours followed by a daily dose of 100 mg for 3 days, which is gradually reduced thereafter. After unilateral adrenalectomy, the contralateral suppressed gland needs up to 1 year to recover adequate function. In 10% of patients with Cushing's disease who undergo a bilateral adrenalectomy, the pituitary adenoma converts into an aggressive tumour (Nelson's syndrome).

Adrenal metastases

Adrenal metastases are discovered at autopsy in one-third of patients with malignant disease (less frequently during life). In declining frequency, the most common primary tumours are breast, lung, renal, gastric, pancreatic, ovarian and colorectal cancer. In selected cases an adrenalectomy can be performed.

Adrenocortical carcinoma

Incidence

Adrenocortical carcinoma is a rare malignancy with an incidence of 1–2 cases per 1 000 000 population per year and a variable but generally poor prognosis. A slight female predominance is observed (1.5:1). The age distribution is bimodal with a first peak in childhood and a second between the fourth and fifth decades.

Pathology

The differentiation between benign and malignant adrenal tumours is challenging, even in the hands of an experienced pathologist. Criteria for malignancy are tumour size, the presence of necrosis or haemorrhage and microscopic features such as capsular or vascular invasion. These should be assessed in terms of a

Don H. Nelson, **B. 1925, Professor of Medicine, The University of Utah, Salt Lake City, UT, USA.**

microscopic diagnostic score. Additional information is provided by immunohistochemistry. The macroscopic features are commonly multinodularity and heterogeneous structure (see Fig. 49.8).

Clinical presentation

Approximately 60% of patients present with evidence of steroid hormone excess (Cushing's syndrome). Patients with non-functioning tumours frequently complain of abdominal discomfort or back pain caused by large tumours. However, with increasing use of abdominal imaging, a growing number of adrenocortical carcinomas are detected incidentally.

Diagnosis

The diagnostic work-up should include measurements of DHEAS, cortisol and catecholamines to exclude a phaeochromocytoma and a dexamethasone suppression test. MRI and CT are equally effective in distinguishing adrenocortical adenoma from carcinoma (Fig. 49.9). MRI angiography is useful to exclude tumour thrombus in the vena cava, which must be excluded before adrenalectomy. As distant metastases are frequently

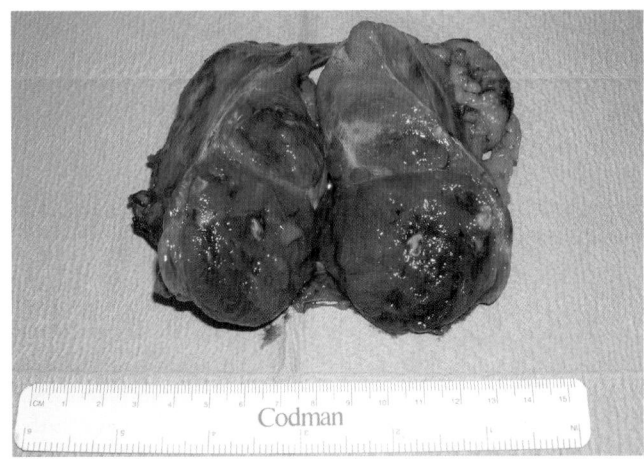

Figure 49.8 Adrenocortical carcinoma that caused Cushing's syndrome and virilisation in a female patient.

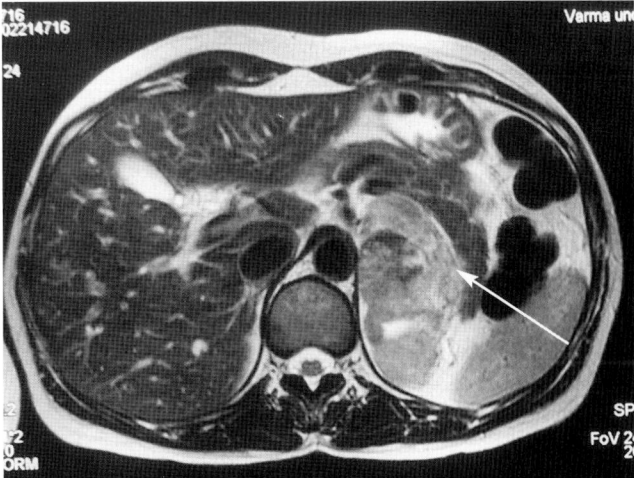

Figure 49.9 Magnetic resonance imaging of adrenocortical carcinoma (arrow) in a patient with cortisol and testosterone excess.

present, a CT scan of the lung is recommended. The World Health Organization classification of 2004 is based on the McFarlane classification and defines four stages: tumours < 5 cm (stage I) or > 5 cm (stage II), locally invasive tumours (III) or tumours with distant metastases (IV).

Treatment

Complete tumour resection (R0) is associated with favourable survival and should be attempted whenever possible. In order to prevent tumour spillage and implantation metastases, the capsule must not be damaged. *En bloc* resection with removal of locally involved organs is often required and in case of tumour thrombus in the vena cava the assistance of a cardiac surgeon is sometimes needed. Laparoscopic adrenalectomy is associated with a high incidence of local recurrence and cannot be recommended. Tumour debulking plays a role in functioning tumours to control hormone excess.

Patients should be treated postoperatively with mitotane alone or in combination with etoposide, doxorubicin and cis-platin in 30% and 50% of cases respectively. Adjuvant radiotherapy may reduce the rate of local recurrence. After surgery, restaging every 3 months is required as the risk of tumour relapse is high. Prognosis depends on the stage of disease and complete removal of the tumour. Patients with stage I or II disease have a 5-year survival rate of 25% whereas patients with stage III and stage IV disease have 5-year survival rates of 6% and 0% respectively.

Congenital adrenal hyperplasia (adrenogenital syndrome)

Virilisation and adrenal insufficiency in children are pathognomonic of congenital adrenal hyperplasia (CAH). This is an autosomal recessive disorder caused by a variety of enzymatic defects in the synthetic pathway of cortisol and other steroids from cholesterol. The most frequent defect (95%) is the 21-hydroxylase deficiency, which has an incidence of 1 in 5000 live births. Excessive ACTH secretion is caused by the loss of cortisol and this leads to an increase in androgenic cortisol precursors and to CAH. CAH may present in girls at birth with ambiguous genitalia or as late-onset disease at puberty. Hypertension and short stature, caused by the premature epiphyseal plate closure, are common symptoms. Affected patients are treated by replacement of cortisol and with fludrocortisone.

Adrenal insufficiency

Primary adrenal insufficiency is caused by the loss of function of the adrenal cortex (Summary box 49.3). It was first described by Thomas Addison in 1855. An early diagnosis is a clinical challenge, even today. Symptoms are only evident when about 90% of the adrenal cortex is destroyed. Secondary adrenal insufficiency is defined as a deficiency of pituitary ACTH secretion. Tertiary adrenal deficiency is provoked by a loss of hypothalamic CRH secretion and is caused by therapeutic glucocorticoid administration, a brain tumour or irradiation.

Summary box 49.3

Diseases associated with adrenal insufficiency

- Polyglandular autoimmune syndrome
- Tuberculosis
- After bilateral adrenalectomy
- Haemorrhage
- Metastases
- Systemic diseases (Boeck's disease, amyloidosis, Wilson's disease)
- Hereditary diseases (e.g. adrenoleukodystrophia, adrenogenital syndrome)
- HIV infection

Acute adrenal insufficiency

Acute adrenal insufficiency usually presents as shock in combination with fever, nausea, vomiting, abdominal pain, hypoglycaemia and electrolyte imbalance. The Waterhouse–Friderichsen syndrome is a bilateral adrenal infarction associated with meningococcal sepsis and is rapidly fatal unless immediately treated. Because of intestinal symptoms and fever, the so called Addisonian crisis is often misdiagnosed as an acute abdominal condition.

Chronic adrenal insufficiency

When symptoms develop over time, patients present with severe anorexia, weakness and nausea. As a result of negative feedback, ACTH and proopiomelanocortin (POMC) levels increase and cause hyperpigmentation of the skin and mucosa. Hypotension, hyponatraemia, hyperkalaemia and hypoglycaemia are commonly observed. The diagnosis of adrenal insufficiency is made using the ACTH stimulation test. Basal ACTH levels are found to be high with cortisol levels decreased.

Treatment

If a patient displays features of adrenal insufficiency, treatment must immediately be commenced, before the biochemical diagnosis. Initial blood samples can be used for later determinations of ACTH and cortisol levels. In addition to intravenous administration of hydrocortisone, 100 mg every 6 hours, 3 litres of saline is given in 6 hours under careful cardiovascular monitoring. Concomitant infections, which are frequently present, require aggressive treatment.

Chronic adrenal insufficiency is treated by replacement therapy with daily oral hydrocortisone (10 mg m^{-2} body surface area) and fludrocortisone (0.1 mg). Patients must be advised about the need to take lifelong glucocorticoid and mineralocorticoid replacement therapy. To prevent an Addisonian crisis, patients must be aware of the need to adjust the dose in case of illness or stress. If patients with adrenal insufficiency are scheduled for surgery, appropriate steroid cover must be administrated.

Caesar Peter Moller **Boeck**, 1845–1917, **Professor of Medicine, The University of Oslo, Norway.**
Samuel Alexander Kinnier **Wilson**, 1878–1936, **Professor of Neurology, King's College Hospital, London, England, described this condition in 1912.**
Rupert **Waterhouse**, 1873–1958, **Physician, The Royal United Hospital, Bath, England, described this syndrome in 1911.**
Carl **Friderichsen**, 1886–1979, **Medical Superintendent, Sundby Hospital, Copenhagen, Denmark, gave his account of the syndrome in 1918.**

---

en bloc is French for 'in a block'.
Thomas **Addison**, 1795–1860, **Physician, Guy's Hospital, London, England, described the effects of disease of the suprarenal capsules in 1849.**

DISORDERS OF THE ADRENAL MEDULLA

Phaeochromocytoma (adrenal paraganglioma)

Definition

This is a tumour of the adrenal medulla, which is derived from chromaffin cells and which produces catecholamines.

Aetiology

The prevalence of phaeochromocytoma in patients with hypertension is 0.1–0.6% with an overall prevalence of 0.05% in autopsy series. In total, 4% of incidentalomas are phaeochromocytomas. Sporadic phaeochromocytomas occur after the fourth decade whereas patients with hereditary forms are diagnosed earlier. Phaeochromocytoma is known as the '10% tumour' as 10% of tumours are inherited, 10% are extra-adrenal, 10% are malignant, 10% are bilateral and 10% occur in children. With the recent advent of detailed genetic tests, however, the incidence of hereditary phaeochromocytomas has been shown to be higher.

Hereditary phaeochromocytomas occur in several tumour syndromes:

- *Multiple endocrine neoplasia type 2 (MEN 2)*: an autosomal dominant inherited disorder that is caused by activating germline mutations of the *RET* proto-oncogene.
- *Familial paraganglioma (PG) syndrome*: glomus tumours of the carotid body and extra-adrenal paraganglioma are characteristic in this hereditary tumour syndrome, which is caused by germline mutations within the succinate dehydrogenase complex subunit B (*SDHB*) and *SDHD* genes.
- *von Hippel–Lindau (VHL) syndrome*: those affected can develop early-onset bilateral kidney tumours, phaeochromocytomas, cerebellar and spinal haemangioblastomas and pancreatic tumours. Patients have a germline mutation in the *VHL* gene.
- *Neurofibromatosis (NF) type 1*: phaeochromocytomas in combination with fibromas on the skin and mucosae ('café-au-lait' skin spots) are indicative of a germline mutation in the *NF1* gene.

Pathology

Phaeochromocytomas are greyish-pink on the cut surface and are usually highly vascularised. Areas of haemorrhage or necrosis are often observed (Fig. 49.10). Microscopically, tumour cells are polygonal but the configuration varies considerably. The differentiation between malignant and benign tumours is difficult, except if metastases are present. An increased PASS (phaeochromocytoma of the *adrenal gland scale score*) indicates malignancy as does a high number of Ki-67-positive cells, vascular invasion or a breached capsule.

Phaeochromocytomas may also produce calcitonin, ACTH, vasoactive intestinal polypeptide (VIP) and parathyroid hormone-related protein (PTHrP). In patients with MEN 2, the onset of phaeochromocytoma is preceded by adrenomedullary hyperplasia, usually bilateral. Phaeochromocytoma is rarely malignant in MEN 2.

Clinical features

Symptoms and signs are caused by catecholamine excess and can be continuous or intermittent (Table 49.2). In total, 90% of

Eugen von Hippel, **1867–1939, Professor of Ophthalmology, Göttingen, Germany.**
Arvid Lindau, **1892–1958, Professor of Pathology, Lund, Sweden.**

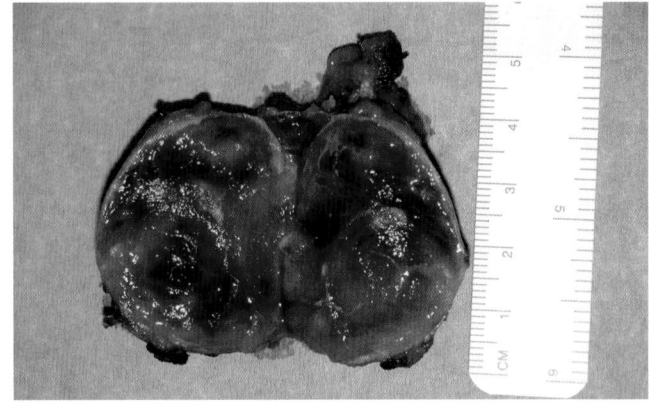

Figure 49.10 Gross appearance of a phaeochromocytoma.

Table 49.2 Clinical signs of phaeochromocytoma

Symptoms	Prevalence (%)
Hypertension:	80–90
Paroxysmal	50–60
Continuous	30
Headache	60–90
Sweating	50–70
Palpitation	50–70
Pallor	40–45
Weight loss	20–40
Hyperglycaemia	40
Nausea	20–40
Psychological effects	20–40

patients with the combination of headache, palpitations and sweating have a phaeochromocytoma. Paroxysms may be precipitated by physical training, induction of general anaesthesia and numerous drugs and agents (contrast media, tricyclic antidepressive drugs, metoclopramide and opiates). Hypertension may occur continuously, be intermittent or absent. A subset of patients is asymptomatic. More than 20% of apparently sporadic phaeochromocytomas are caused by germline mutations in the *RET, SDHB, SDHD* and *NF1* genes; genetic testing for these genes is therefore generally recommended.

Diagnosis

The first step in the diagnosis of a phaeochromocytoma is the determination of adrenaline, noradrenaline, metanephrine and normetanephrine levels in a 24-hour urine collection. Catecholamine levels that exceed the normal range by 2–40 times will be found in affected patients. Determination of plasma-free metanephrine and normetanephrine levels is a recently available test that has a high sensitivity. Biochemical tests should be performed at least twice. The biochemical diagnosis is followed by the localisation of the phaeochromocytoma and/or metastases. MRI is preferred because contrast media used for CT scans can provoke paroxysms. Classically, phaeochromocytomas show a 'Swiss cheese' configuration (Fig. 49.11). ^{123}I-MIBG (meta-iodobenzylguanidine) single-photon emission computerised tomography (SPECT) will identify about 90% of primary tumours and is essential for the detection of multiple extra-adrenal tumours and metastases (Fig. 49.12).

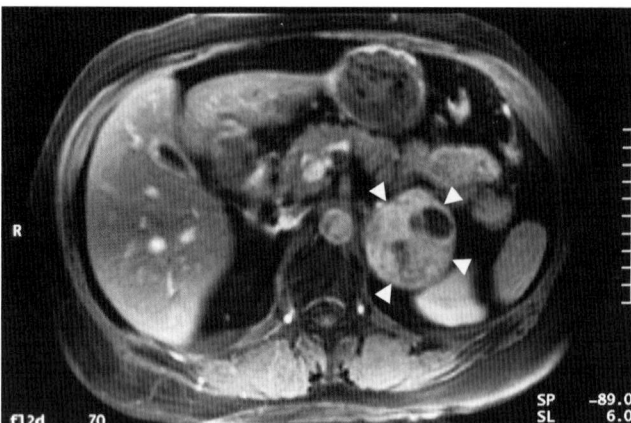

Figure 49.11 Magnetic resonance imaging of a sporadic phaeochromocytoma of the left adrenal gland (arrowheads).

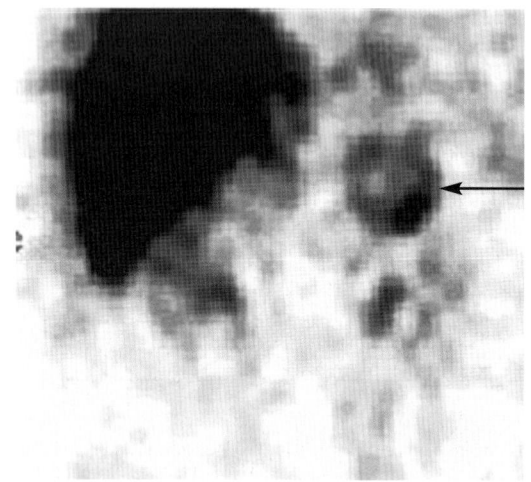

Figure 49.12 Meta-iodobenzylguanidine (MIBG) single-photon emission computerised tomography scan of a phaeochromocytoma of the left adrenal gland (arrow) in the same patient as in Figure 49.11.

Treatment

Laparoscopic resection is now routine in the treatment of phaeochromocytoma. If the tumour is larger than 8–10 cm or radiological signs of malignancy are detected an open approach should be considered.

Preoperative

Once a phaeochromocytoma has been diagnosed, an α-adrenoreceptor blocker (phenoxybenzamine) is used to block catecholamine excess and its consequences during surgery. With adequate medical pre-treatment, the perioperative mortality rate has decreased from 20–45% to less than 3%. A dose of 20 mg of phenoxybenzamine initially should be increased daily by 10 mg until a daily dose of 100–160 mg is achieved and the patient reports symptomatic postural hypotension. Additional β-blockade is required if tachycardia or arrhythmias develop; this should not be introduced until the patient is α-blocked.

Peroperative

With adequate α-blockade preoperatively, anaesthesia should not differ from that used in patients with a non-functioning adrenal tumour; however, in some patients, dramatic changes in heart rate and blood pressure may occur and require sudden administration of pressor or vasodilator agents. A central venous catheter and invasive arterial monitoring are essential. Special attention is required when the adrenal vein is ligated as a sudden drop in blood pressure may occur. Rarely, the infusion of large volumes of fluid or even administration of adrenaline can be necessary.

Postoperative

Patients should be observed for 24 hours in the intensive care unit (ICU) as hypovolaemia and hypoglycaemia may occur. Biochemical cure should be confirmed by an assessment of catecholamines 2–3 weeks postoperatively. Lifelong yearly biochemical tests should be performed to identify recurrent, metastatic or metachronous phaeochromocytoma (Summary box 49.4).

Summary box 49.4

Phaeochromocytoma

- Obtain a secure biochemical diagnosis
- Exclude family history
- Diagnosis confirmed, treat with α-blockers
- Plan surgical excision
- Yearly lifelong follow-up

Malignant phaeochromocytoma

Definition

Approximately 10% of phaeochromocytomas are malignant. This rate is higher in extra-adrenal tumours (paragangliomas). The diagnosis of malignancy implies metastases of chromaffin tissue, most commonly to lymph nodes, bone and liver. About 8% of patients with an apparently benign phaeochromocytoma subsequently develop metastases.

Treatment

Surgical excision is the only chance for cure. Even in patients with metastatic disease, tumour debulking can be considered to reduce the tumour burden and to control the catecholamine excess. Symptomatic treatment can be obtained with α-blockers. Mitotane should be started as adjuvant or palliative treatment. Treatment with ^{131}I-MIBG or combination chemotherapy has resulted in a partial response in 30% and an improvement of symptoms in 80% of patients. The natural history is highly variable with a 5-year survival rate of less than 50%.

Phaeochromocytoma in pregnancy

Phaeochromocytomas in pregnancy may imitate an amnion infection syndrome or pre-eclampsia. Without adequate α-blockade, mother and unborn child are threatened by hypertensive crisis during vaginal delivery. In the first and second trimesters the patient should be scheduled for laparoscopic adrenalectomy after adequate α-blockade; the risk of a miscarriage during surgery is high. In the third trimester, elective Caesarean with consecutive adrenalectomy should be performed. The maternal mortality rate is 50% when a phaeochromocytoma remains undiagnosed.

Neuroblastoma

Definition

A neuroblastoma is a malignant tumour that is derived from the sympathetic nervous system in the adrenal medulla (38%) or from any site along the sympathetic chain in the paravertebral sites of the abdomen (30%), chest (20%) and, rarely, the neck or pelvis.

Pathology

Neuroblastomas have a pale and grey surface, are encapsulated and show typical areas with calcification. With increased tumour size, necrosis and haemorrhage may be detected. They are characterised by the presence of immature cells derived from the neuroectoderm of the sympathetic nervous system. Mature cells are found only in ganglioneuroblastomas.

Clinical features

Predominantly newborn infants and young children (< 5 years of age) are affected. Symptoms are caused by tumour growth or by bone metastases. Patients present with a mass in the abdomen, neck or chest, proptosis, bone pain, painless bluish skin metastases, weakness or paralysis. Metastatic disease is present in 70% of patients. The catecholamine excess is asymptomatic and an excess of ACTH or VIP may occur.

Diagnosis

Biochemical evaluation should include urinary excretion (24-hour urine) of vanillylmandelic acid (VMA), homovanillic acid (HVA), dopamine and noradenaline, as increased levels are present in about 80% of patients. Accurate staging requires CT/MRI of the chest and abdomen, a bone scan, bone marrow aspiration and core biopsies as well as an MIBG scan. Staging is established according to the International Neuroblastoma Staging System (INSS).

Treatment

Prognosis can be predicted by the tumour stage and the age at diagnosis. Patients are classified as low, intermediate or high risk. Low-risk patients are treated by surgery alone (the addition of 6–12 weeks of chemotherapy is optional) whereas intermediate-risk patients are treated by surgery with adjuvant multi-agent chemotherapy (carboplatin, cyclophosphamide, etoposide, doxorubicin). High-risk patients receive high-dose multi-agent chemotherapy followed by surgical resection in responding tumours and myeloablative stem cell rescue. Patients assigned to the low-risk, intermediate-risk and high-risk groups have overall 3-year survival rates of 90%, 70–90% and 30% respectively.

Ganglioneuroma

Definition

A ganglioneuroma is a benign adrenal neoplasm that arises from neural crest tissue. Ganglioneuromas occur in the adrenal medulla and are characterised by mature sympathetic ganglion cells and Schwann cells in a fibrous stroma.

Clinical features

Ganglioneuroma is found in all age groups but is more common before the age of 60. Ganglioneuromas occur anywhere along the paravertebral sympathetic plexus and in the adrenal medulla (30%). Most often they are identified incidentally by CT or MRI performed for other indications.

Theodor Schwann, **1810–1882, Professor of Anatomy, Louvain (1839–1848), and later at Liège (1849–1880), described the neurilemma in 1839.**

Treatment

Treatment is by surgical excision, laparoscopic when adrenalectomy is indicated.

SURGERY OF THE ADRENAL GLANDS

Since its introduction in the 1990s, laparoscopic or retroperitoneoscopic adrenalectomy has become the 'gold standard' in the resection of adrenal tumours, except for tumours with signs of malignancy. The more popular approach is the laparoscopic transperitoneal approach, which offers a better view of the adrenal region and may be easier to learn. The advantage of the retroperitoneoscopic approach is the minimal dissection required by this extra-abdominal procedure. In the case of small, bilateral tumours or in patients with hereditary tumour syndromes a subtotal resection is warranted. The mortality rate ranges from 0 to 2% in specialised centres.

An open approach should be considered if radiological signs, distant metastases, large tumours (> 8–10 cm) or a distinct hormonal pattern suggest malignancy. The surgical access in such cases should be thoracoabdominal.

Laparoscopic adrenalectomy

Knowledge of the anatomy of the adrenal region is essential as anatomical landmarks guide the surgeon during operation. If these landmarks are respected, injury to the vena cava or renal vein, the pancreatic tail or the spleen can be avoided. Careful haemostasis is essential as small amounts of blood can impair the surgeon's view. To prevent tumour spillage, direct grasping of the adrenal tissue/tumour has to be avoided.

Right adrenalectomy

After mobilisation of the right liver lobe the adrenal vein is identified and divided. The dissection continues at the level of the periadrenal fat using careful coagulation and is finished by the complete or subtotal removal of the adrenal gland.

Left adrenalectomy

With the patient positioned on his or her right side, mobilisation of the spleen will displace the pancreatic tail medially. The incision of Gerota's fascia is followed by identification of the adrenal vein, which runs into the renal vein in the space between the medial aspect of the kidney and the posterior aspect of the pancreatic tail (Fig. 49.13). The resection is completed by the transection of the adrenal gland at the level of the periadrenal fat.

Retroperitoneoscopic adrenalectomy

The first port is placed at the distal end of the 12th rib with the patient in the prone position. After a digital dissection into the retroperitoneum, Gerota's fascia is displaced ventrally. The right adrenal vein is covered by the retrocaval posterior aspect of the adrenal gland. The left adrenal vein is usually located at the medial inferior pole of the adrenal gland.

Open adrenalectomy

An open adrenalectomy through a thoracoabdominal approach is almost exclusively performed when a malignant adrenal tumour is suspected. On the right side the hepatic flexure of the colon is mobilised and the right liver lobe is cranially retracted to achieve an optimal exposure of the inferior vena cava and the adrenal

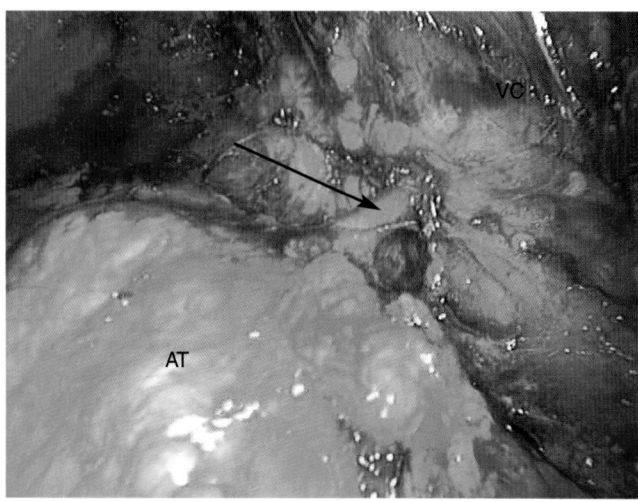

Figure 49.13 Laparoscopic view during a right adrenalectomy. Arrow indicates the adrenal vein. AT, adrenal tumour; VC, vena cava.

gland. On the left side the adrenal gland can be exposed after mobilisation of the splenic flexure of the colon, through the transverse mesocolon or through the gastrocolic ligament. The remaining dissection is the same as in laparoscopic adrenalectomy. A resection of regional lymph nodes is recommended in malignant adrenal tumours and should include resection of the tissue between the renal pedicle and the diaphragm.

PANCREATIC ENDOCRINE TUMOURS

Introduction

Pancreatic endocrine tumours (PETs) represent an important subset of pancreatic neoplasms. They account for 5% of all clinically detected pancreatic tumours. They consist of single or multiple, benign or malignant neoplasms and are associated in 10–20% of cases with multiple endocrine neoplasia type 1 (MEN 1). PETs present as either functional tumours, causing specific hormonal syndromes, or non-functional tumours, with symptoms similar to those in patients with pancreatic adenocarcinoma. This section focuses on insulinomas, gastrinomas and non-functioning tumours because they represent 90% of all PETs (Table 49.3).

Function of the endocrine pancreas

The endocrine cells of the pancreas are grouped in the islets of Langerhans, which constitute approximately 1–2% of the mass of the pancreas (Fig. 49.14). There are about one million islets in a healthy adult human pancreas and their combined weight is 1–1.5 g. There are four main types of cell in the islets of Langerhans, which can be classified according to their secretions:

- beta cells producing insulin (65–80% of the islet cells);
- alpha cells producing glucagon (15–20%);
- delta cells producing somatostatin (3–10%);
- pancreatic polypeptide (PP) cells containing polypeptide (1%).

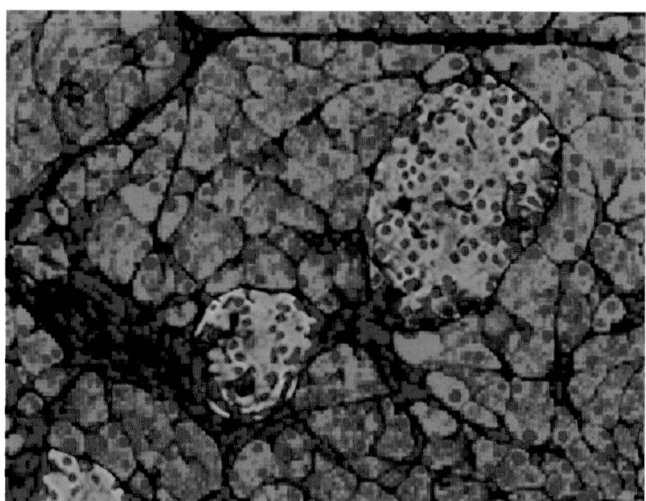

Figure 49.14 Immunofluorescent labelling of endocrine [insulin (green)] and exocrine [amylase (red)] pancreatic cells and the nuclear marker DAPI (blue) (courtesy of Dr Esni, Department of Surgery, University of Pittsburgh, USA).

Table 49.3 Neuroendocrine tumours of the pancreas

Tumour (syndrome)	Incidence (%)	Presentation	Malignancy (%)
Insulinoma	70–80	Weakness, sweating, tremor, tachycardia, anxiety, fatigue, dizziness, disorientation, seizures	< 10
Gastrinoma	20–25	Intractable or recurrent peptic ulcer disease (haemorrhage, perforation), complications of peptic ulcer, diarrhoea	60–80
Non-functional tumours	30–50	Obstructive jaundice, pancreatitis, epigastric pain, duodenal obstruction, weight loss, fatigue	60–90
VIPoma	4	Profuse watery diarrhoea, hypotension, abdominal pain	80
Glucagonoma	4	Migratory necrolytic skin rash, glossitis, stomatitis, angular cheilitis, diabetes, severe weight loss, diarrhoea	80
Somatostatinoma	< 5	Cholelithiasis, diarrhoea, neurofibromatosis	50
Carcinoid	< 1	Flushing, sweating, diarrhoea, oedema	90
ACTHoma	< 1	Cushing's syndrome	> 90
GRFoma	< 1	Acromegaly	30

ACTH, adrenocorticotrophic hormone; GRF, growth hormone-releasing factor; VIP, vasoactive intestinal polypeptide.

Paul Langerhans, **1847–1888**, Professor of Pathological Anatomy, Freiberg, Germany.

Insulinoma

Definition

This is an insulin-producing tumour of the pancreas causing Whipple's triad, i.e. symptoms of hypoglycaemia after fasting or exercise, plasma glucose levels $< 2.8\,\mathrm{mmol\,l^{-1}}$ and relief of symptoms on intravenous administration of glucose.

Incidence

Insulinomas are the most frequent of all the functioning PETs with a reported incidence of 2–4 cases per million population per year. Insulinomas have been diagnosed in all age groups with the highest incidence found in the fourth to the sixth decades. Women seem to be slightly more frequently affected.

Pathology

The aetiology and pathogenesis of insulinomas are unknown. No risk factors have been associated with these tumours. Virtually all insulinomas are located in the pancreas and tumours are equally distributed within the gland. Approximately 90% are solitary and about 10% are multiple and are always associated with MEN 1 syndrome.

Prognosis and predictive factors

No markers are available that reliably predict the biological behaviour of an insulinoma. Approximately 10% are malignant. Insulinomas of $< 2\,\mathrm{cm}$ in diameter without signs of vascular invasion or metastases are considered benign.

Clinical features

Insulinomas are characterised by fasting hypoglycaemia and neuroglycopenic symptoms. The episodic nature of the hypoglycaemic attacks is caused by intermittent insulin secretion by the tumour. This leads to central nervous system symptoms such as diplopia, blurred vision, confusion, abnormal behaviour and amnesia. Some patients develop loss of consciousness and coma. The release of catecholamines produces symptoms such as sweating, weakness, hunger, tremor, nausea, anxiety and palpitations.

Biochemical diagnosis

A fasting test that may last for up to 72 hours is regarded as the most sensitive test. Usually, insulin, proinsulin, C-peptide and blood glucose are measured in 1- to 2-hour intervals to demonstrate inappropriately high secretion of insulin in relation to blood glucose. About 80% of insulinomas are diagnosed by this test, most of them in the first 24 hours. Continuous C-peptide levels demonstrate the endogenous secretion of insulin and exclude factitious hypoglycaemia caused by insulin injection.

Differential diagnosis

The differential diagnosis of hypoglycaemia includes hormonal deficiencies, hepatic insufficiency, medication, drugs and enzyme defects. Occasionally, differentiating insulinoma from other causes of hypoglycaemia can be difficult. Nesidioblastosis is a rare disorder, mainly encountered in children, which is characterised by replacement of normal pancreatic islets by diffuse hyperplasia of islet cells.

Medical treatment of insulinoma

Medical management is reserved only for patients who are unable or unwilling to undergo surgical treatment or for unresectable metastatic disease. Diazoxide suppresses insulin secretion by direct action on the beta cells and offers reasonably good control of hypoglycaemia in approximately 50% of patients. When surgical options to treat malignant insulinomas cannot be applied, chemotherapeutic options include doxorubicin and streptozotocin.

Surgical treatment of insulinoma

Indications for operation

After a positive fasting test and exclusion of diffuse abdominal metastases by ultrasound or CT scan, all patients should undergo surgical excision of insulinoma.

Preoperative localisation studies

Intraoperative exploration of the pancreas is the best method to use for localisation of insulinoma. The author's experience of preoperative localisation in more than 40 patients has shown that insulinomas are detected in about 65% of cases by endoscopic ultrasound (EUS), 33% of cases by CT scan and abdominal ultrasound, 15% of cases by magnetic resonance tomography and not at all by somatostatin receptor scintigraphy (SRS). On the other hand, all tumours were identified and resected after surgical exploration and intraoperative ultrasound (IOUS) of the pancreas after extensive mobilisation of the gland. For preoperative localisation of an insulinoma, EUS has the highest sensitivity and should be used if laparoscopic resection is considered. If no lesion is identified and one can rely on the biochemical tests for diagnosis, laparotomy should follow.

Benign insulinoma

Surgical cure rates in patients with the biochemical diagnosis of insulinoma range from 90% to 100%. At surgical exploration the abdomen is initially explored for evidence of metastatic disease. Following this, an extended Kocher manoeuvre and mobilisation of the head and then the distal pancreas is performed to explore the whole gland. IOUS should then be used to confirm the presence of a tumour, to find non-palpable lesions and also to identify the relation of the tumour to the pancreatic duct (Fig. 49.15a). Tumour enucleation is the technique of choice (Fig. 49.15b). For superficial tumours, laparoscopic enucleation is undertaken (Fig. 49.16). Tumours located deep in the body or tail of the pancreas and those in close proximity to the pancreatic duct require distal pancreatectomy. Postoperatively, blood sugar levels begin to rise in most patients within the first few hours after removal of the tumour. To preserve pancreatic function and reduce the risk of iatrogenic diabetes mellitus, patients in whom tumour localisation is not successful at operation should not undergo blind resection.

Malignant insulinoma

Aggressive attempts at resection are recommended as these tumours are much less virulent than adenocarcinomas.

George Hoyt Whipple, **1878–1976, Professor of Pathology, The University of Rochester, Rochester, NY, USA, described this disease in 1907. He shared the 1934 Nobel Prize for Physiology or Medicine with George Richards Minot, and William Parry Murphy 'for their discoveries concerning liver therapy against anaemias'.**

Theodor Kocher, **1841–1917, Professor of Surgery, Berne, Switzerland, was awarded the Nobel Prize for Physiology or Medicine in 1909, 'for his work on the physiology, pathology, and surgery of the thyroid gland.'**

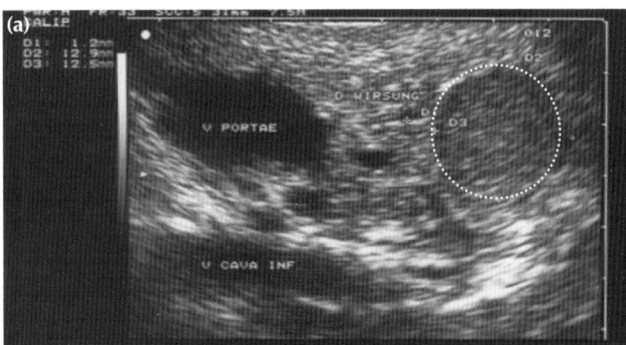

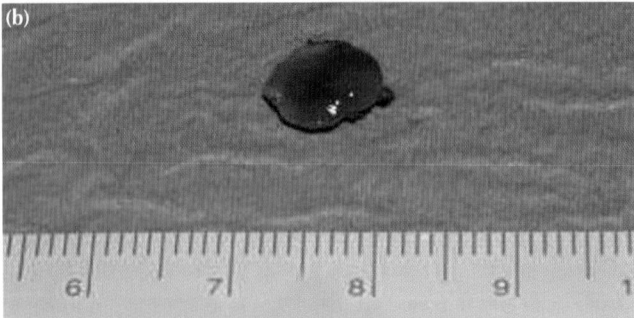

Figure 49.15 (a) Intraoperative ultrasound showing a typical insulinoma (dashed circle). v portae, portal vein; v cava inf, inferior vena cava; d wirsung, pancreatic duct. (b) Enucleated insulinoma.

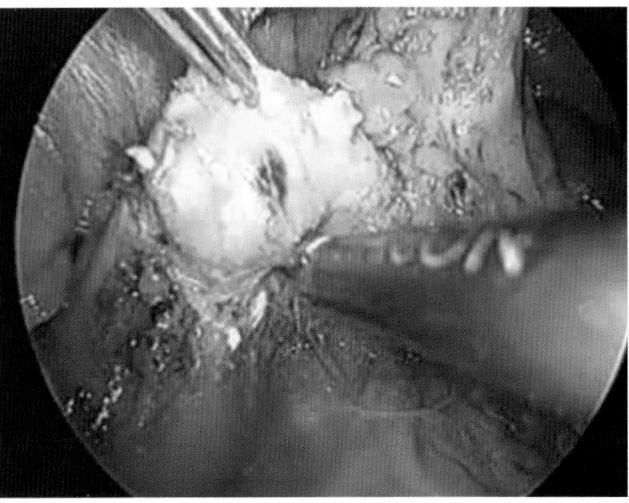

Figure 49.16 Laparoscopic enucleation of an insulinoma.

Gastrinoma (Zollinger–Ellison syndrome)

Definition

Zollinger–Ellison syndrome (ZES) is a condition that includes (1) fulminating ulcer diathesis in the stomach, duodenum or atypical sites; (2) recurrent ulceration despite adequate therapy; and (3) non-beta islet cell tumours of the pancreas (gastrinoma).

Robert Milton Zollinger, B. 1903, Professor of Surgery, The Ohio State University, Columbus, OH, USA.
Edwin Homer Ellison, 1918–1970, Professor of Surgery, Marquette University, WI, USA.
Zollinger and Ellison described this condition in a joint paper in 1955 when they were both working at The Ohio State University.

Incidence

Gastrinomas account for about 20% of PETs, second in frequency to insulinomas. Approximately 0.1% of patients with duodenal ulcers have evidence of ZES. The reported incidence is between 0.5 and 4 cases per million population per year. ZES is more common in males than in females. The mean age at the onset of symptoms is 38 years, and the range 7–83 years.

Pathology

The aetiology and pathogenesis of sporadic gastrinomas are unknown. At the time of diagnosis more than 60% of tumours are malignant. Pancreatic gastrinomas are mainly found in sporadic disease; most are found in the head of the pancreas. More than 70% of the gastrinomas in MEN 1 syndrome and most sporadic gastrinomas are located in the first and second part of the duodenum. Therefore, the anatomical area comprising the head of the pancreas, the superior and descending portion of the duodenum and the relevant lymph nodes has been called the 'gastrinoma triangle' because it harbours the vast majority of these tumours (Fig. 49.17).

Prognosis and predictive factors

In general, the progression of gastrinomas is relatively slow with a 5-year survival rate of 65% and a 10-year survival rate of 51%. Patients with complete tumour resection have excellent 5- and 10-year survival rates (90–100%). Patients with pancreatic tumours have a worse prognosis than those with primary tumours in the duodenum. There is no established marker to predict the biological behaviour of gastrinoma.

Clinical and biochemical features

Over 90% of patients with gastrinomas have peptic ulcer disease, often multiple or in unusual sites. Diarrhoea is another common symptom, caused by the large volume of gastric acid secretion. Abdominal pain from either peptic ulcer disease or gastro-oesophageal reflux disease (GORD) remains the most common symptom, occurring in more than 75% of patients.

Biochemical diagnosis

If the patient presents with a gastric pH below 2.5 and a serum gastrin concentration above 1000 pg ml⁻¹ (normal < 100 pg ml⁻¹)

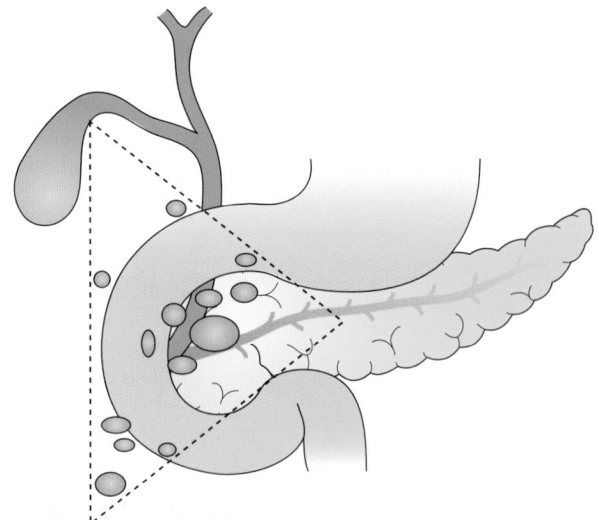

Figure 49.17 The gastrinoma triangle.

then the diagnosis of ZES is confirmed. Unfortunately, the majority of patients have serum gastrin concentrations between 100 and 500 pg ml^{-1} and in these patients a secretin test should be performed. The secretin test is considered positive if an increase in serum gastrin of > 200 pg ml^{-1} over the pre-treatment value is obtained; this also rules out other causes of hypergastrinaemia (e.g. atrophic gastritis).

Differential diagnosis

The most common misdiagnoses are idiopathic peptic ulcer disease, chronic idiopathic diarrhoea and GORD. Other reasons for hypergastrinaemia are chronic atrophic gastritis, gastric outlet stenosis and retained antrum after gastric resection.

Medical treatment of gastrinoma

In most patients with ZES, gastric hypersecretion can be treated effectively with proton pump inhibitors. Octreotide can also help to control acid hypersecretion. Systemic chemotherapy is utilised in patients with diffuse metastatic gastrinomas. Streptozotocin in combination with 5-fluorouracil or doxorubicin is the first-line treatment.

Surgical treatment of gastrinoma

Indications for operation

The only chance for cure is surgical resection and routine surgical exploration increases survival. Therefore, surgical exploration should be performed in all patients without diffuse metastases.

Preoperative localisation studies

Pancreatic gastrinomas are often larger than 1 cm in diameter whereas gastrinomas of the duodenum are usually smaller. Therefore, it is nearly impossible to identify duodenal gastrinomas by preoperative imaging. Pancreatic gastrinomas are detected by endoscopic ultrasound in about 80–90% of cases, and by CT in 39% of cases, and by MRI in 46% of cases. In approximately one-third of patients the results of conventional imaging studies are negative. On the basis of recent studies and the author's experience, either endoscopic ultrasound or CT and SRS should be performed preoperatively for staging.

Pancreatic gastrinomas

Most pancreatic gastrinomas are solitary, located in the head of the gland or uncinate process, and can be identified at operation. Enucleation with peripancreatic lymph node dissection is the procedure of choice. Rarely, tumours are situated in the body or tail and should be treated by enucleation or distal resection. Even if a tumour is found in the pancreas, duodenotomy is recommended to detect additional tumours.

Duodenal gastrinomas

The duodenum should be opened with a longitudinal incision and the posterior and anterior walls palpated separately (Fig. 49.18). Duodenal tumours smaller than 5 mm can be enucleated with the overlying mucosa; larger tumours are excised with full-thickness excision of the duodenal wall.

Non-functional endocrine pancreatic tumours

Definition

PETs are clinically classified as non-functioning (NF-PETs) when they do not cause a clinical syndrome.

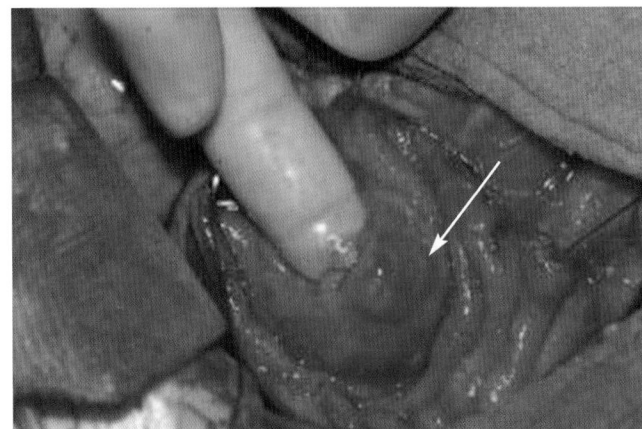

Figure 49.18 Palpation of a duodenal gastrinoma (arrow) after duodenotomy.

Incidence

NF-PETs account for 30–50% of all PETs. They are most often diagnosed in the fifth to sixth decades of life.

Pathology

NF-PETs cannot be differentiated from functional tumours by immunocytochemistry because they may also express hormones such as gastrin, insulin, etc. They usually stain positively for chromogranin A and synaptophysin. The tumours are usually large (> 5 cm) and unifocal except in MEN 1 syndrome. They are distributed throughout the pancreas with a head to body to tail ratio of 7:1:1.5.

Prognosis and predictive factors

About 70% of all NF-PETs are malignant. Overall 5- and 10-year survival rates of 65% and 49% respectively have been described. When comparing NF-PETs with functioning PETs, the NF-PETs have a worse prognosis.

Clinical features

Patients usually present late because of the lack of a clinical/hormonal marker of tumour activity. Therefore, in contrast to functioning PETs, patients with NF-PETs present with various non-specific symptoms, including jaundice, abdominal pain, weight loss and pancreatitis. In some cases liver metastases are the first presentation.

Biochemical diagnosis

Increased levels of chromogranin A have been reported in 50–80% of NF-PETs; the level of chromogranin A sometimes correlates with the tumour burden. The combination of elevated chromogranin A and PP measurements increases the sensitivity of diagnosis from 84% to 96% in NF-PETs.

Differential diagnosis

Differentiation from the more aggressive pancreatic adenocarcinoma is extremely important (Table 49.4). Recognition of NF-PETs is imperative because of their resectability and excellent long-term survival compared with their exocrine counterparts.

Table 49.4 Differences between pancreatic cancer and non-functioning endocrine pancreatic tumours (NF-PETs)

	Pancreatic cancer	**NF-PETs**
Tumour size	< 5 cm	> 5 cm
CT scan	Hypodensity	Hyperdensity
	No calcifications	Calcifications possible
Chromogranin A in blood	Negative	Positive
Somatostatin receptor scintigraphy	Negative	Positive

Medical treatment of non-functioning islet cell tumours

When surgical excision is not possible, chemotherapeutic options include streptozotocin, octreotide and interferon.

Surgical treatment of non-functioning islet cell tumours

Indications for operation

An aggressive surgical approach should be considered in malignant NF-PETs, even in the presence of distant metastases.

Preoperative localisation studies

Preoperative ultrasound or CT scan are the procedures of choice as these tumours are relatively large. Also, SRS should be performed to differentiate endocrine from non-endocrine pancreatic tumours.

Operative procedures

The major goal is a potentially curative resection. This may require partial pancreaticoduodenectomy as well as the synchronous or metachronous resection of liver metastases. Using an aggressive approach, curative resections are possible in up to 62% of cases and overall 5-year survival rates of around 65% can be achieved. Repeated resections for resectable recurrences or metastases are justified to improve survival.

NEUROENDOCRINE TUMOURS OF THE BRONCHI, STOMACH AND SMALL BOWEL

Definition and physiology

Neuroendocrine tumours (NET) of the gut and the pancreas arise from the diffuse neuroendocrine cell system, which can be found as single or clustered cells in the mucosa of the bronchi, stomach, gut, biliary tree, urogenital system and in the pancreas (see Chapters 67, 65 and 68 for NET of the appendix, colon and rectum respectively). This cell system was first recognised as the 'clear cell system' by Feyrter in the 1930s and is identical to the APUD (amine precursor uptake and decarboxylation) system described by Pearse in 1970. All cells of the system secrete different neuroendocrine markers, such as synaptophysin, chromogranin A and neurone-specific enolase (NSE), and produce peptide hormones that are stored in granules, e.g. serotonin, somatostatin, PP or gastrin. In clinical practice chromogranin A is utilised as a tumour marker. The main functional test for NET of the jejunum and ileum (the NET that are most often encoun-

Anthony Guy Everson Pearse, **1916–2003**, Professor of Histo-chemistry, The Royal Postgraduate Medical School, Hammersmith, London, England.

tered) is the measurement of the serotonin metabolite 5-hydroxyindoleacetic acid (5-HIAA) in urine.

Pathology

Neuroendocrine cells can form hyperplasias or tumours. Oberndorfer coined the term 'carcinoids' for tumours arising from these cells in 1907. Although the term carcinoid continues to be used in clinical practice, these tumours do not always grow in a well-differentiated pattern reflecting the rather benign 'carcinoma-like', i.e. 'carcinoid', tumour. They can show different growth patterns, from benign tumours to high-grade undifferentiated carcinomas having a poor prognosis (neuroendocrine carcinomas). Therefore, they should always be addressed as NET, including a description of their histological pattern (benign, low- or high-grade malignant) and their anatomical site (e.g. stomach, ileum) according to the World Health Organization (WHO) classification (2000). The relative distribution of NET in different organs is given in Table 49.5. Another classification based on embryological principles classifies NET as foregut (lung, stomach, pancreas), midgut (small bowel and appendix) and hindgut (colon and rectum) tumours.

Table 49.5 Relative distribution of neuroendocrine tumours in different organs

Site	Distribution (%)
Lung	10
Stomach	5
Duodenum	2
Small bowel	25
Appendix	40
Colon	6
Rectum	15

Neuroendocrine tumours of the bronchi

Aetiology and clinical features

About 1–2% of all lung tumours are NET. Their aetiology is unknown except in those diagnosed in patients with MEN 1 syndrome. In centrally located tumours, symptoms can be coughing, dyspnoea or fever if obstruction and pneumonia occur. NET situated in the peripheral parts of the lung do not cause symptoms for a long time. The WHO classification should be used for these tumours and should replace the former classification of typical or atypical 'carcinoid'.

Diagnosis and treatment

The diagnosis is made by radiography, CT scan, octreotide (SRS) scan and bronchoscopy and biopsy (Fig. 49.19). The treatment of choice is surgical resection. In benign or low-grade malignancy, a parenchyma-sparing resection without regional lymph node dissection should be performed. In highly undifferentiated NET, patients should be treated as in ordinary lung cancer. If there is metastatic disease, treatment with somatostatin analogues or chemotherapy (e.g. cisplatin and etoposide or streptozotocin and doxorubicin) is recommended.

Even in advanced disease and in the presence of liver metastases, patients do not suffer from 'carcinoid' syndrome ('flushing', etc.), as NET of the foregut do not secrete serotonin. This is also the reason why a 5-HIAA urine test cannot be used to help make a diagnosis.

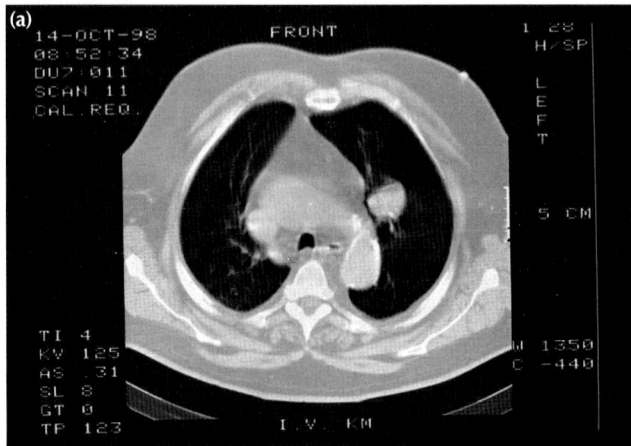

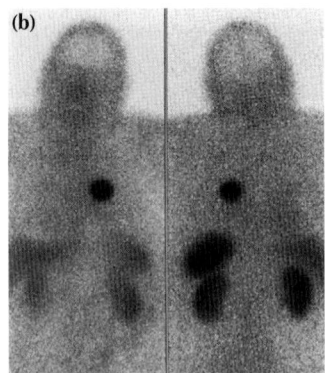

Figure 49.19 (a) Computerised tomography scan and (b) octreotide scan of a pulmonary (bronchial) neuroendocrine tumour.

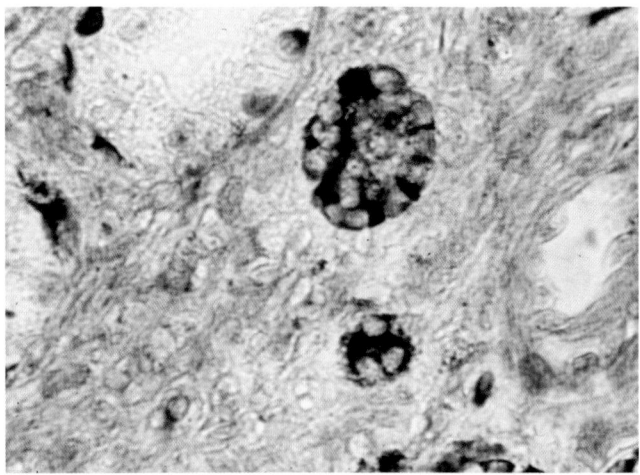

Figure 49.20 Immunostaining of chromogranin in micronodular hyperplasia of enterochromaffin-like (ECL) cells of the stomach associated with chronic atrophic gastritis.

Neuroendocrine tumours of the stomach

These tumours are rare. They comprise about 5% of all NET of the gastrointestinal tract and have an incidence of approximately 0.2 cases per 100 000 population per year. There are four different types of gastric NET (Table 49.6). Types 1 and 2 are small benign tumours that arise from the enterochromaffin-like (ECL) cells in the gastric mucosa and grow in either a linear or a nodular pattern (Fig. 49.20). Hypergastrinaemia may cause symptoms and the treatment of choice is endoscopic resection. Types 3 and 4 are almost always malignant and surgical resection should be undertaken if possible.

Pathogenesis, diagnosis and treatment

Type 1 tumours (ECLomas) are the most frequent NET of the stomach (approximately 80%); they occur mostly in elderly women. Chronic hypergastrinaemia is the result of chronic atrophic gastritis and achlorhydria, the alkaline pH being the stimulus for hypersecretion of gastrin. They do not cause symptoms and are usually detected during gastroscopy for other reasons. Endoscopic resection is the treatment of choice. Antrectomy and resection of ECLomas should be undertaken only if there is recurrent disease and multiple (more than six) tumours, with at least one measuring > 1 cm and infiltration of at least one into the submucosa.

The pathogenesis, diagnosis and treatment of type 2 tumours is similar to that of type 1. The only difference is the cause of the hypergastrinaemia, which in type 2 tumours is the result of MEN 1 syndrome, with multiple gastrinomas in the duodenum or, rarely, in the pancreas.

Type 3 tumours are rare, sporadic and solitary tumours of unknown origin. Serum gastrin is normal; upper gastrointestinal bleeding is the usual symptom that leads to endoscopy. Type 3 tumours are usually larger than 2cm (Fig. 49.21) and often have lymph node and liver metastases at the time of diagnosis. Gastrectomy and lymph node dissection and resection of liver metastases is the treatment of choice. Liver metastases can also be treated by chemoembolisation.

Type 4 tumours present as large ulcerating malignancies similar to adenocarcinomas and should be treated accordingly. The prognosis of types 3 and 4 is poor (Table 49.6).

Table 49.6 Classification of gastric neuroendocrine tumours

Type	Histological pattern	Size and location	Causative factor and prognosis
1	Benign, non-functional, well differentiated	Gastric corpus; < 1 cm; mucosa/submucosa	ECLomas in chronic atrophic gastritis, hypergastrinaemia
2	Benign or low-grade malignant, differentiated	1–2 cm; angio-invasion; mucosa/submucosa	ECLomas with hypergastrinaemia as a result of gastrinoma in MEN 1
3	Low-grade malignant, differentiated	2 cm; invasion beyond submucosa	Sporadic ECLomas not related to hypergastrinaemia
4	Intermediate or small cell type, high-grade malignant (neuroendocrine carcinoma)	Different sizes	Causative factor unknown; prognosis poor

ECL, enterochromaffin-like; MEN, multiple endocrine neoplasia.

CHAPTER 49 | ADRENAL GLANDS AND OTHER ENDOCRINE DISORDERS

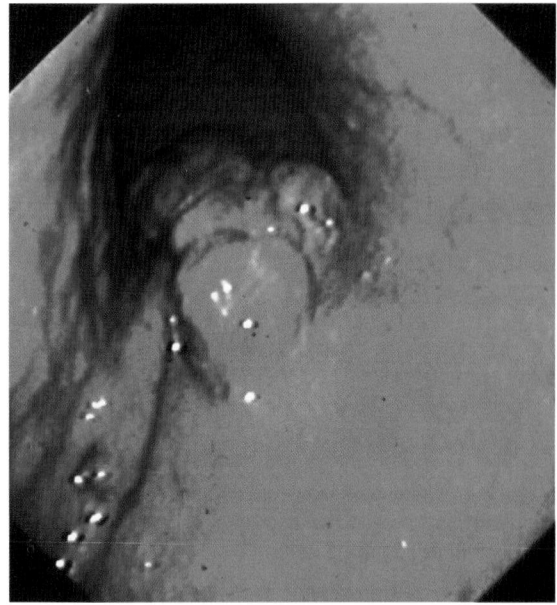

Figure 49.21 Type 3 gastric neuroendocrine tumour discovered after upper gastrointestinal bleeding.

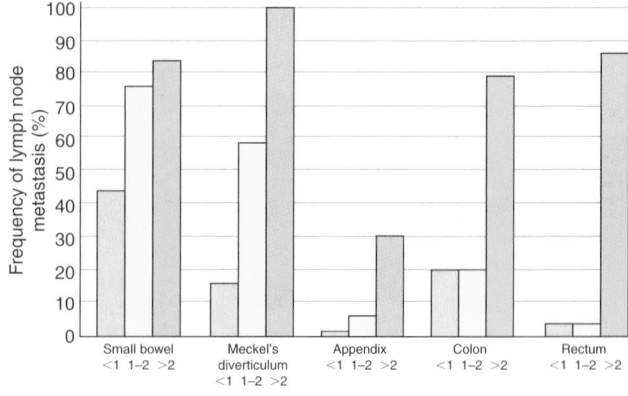

Figure 49.22 Relation of site and diameter of neuroendocrine tumours of the gut to frequency of lymph node metastasis.

Neuroendocrine tumours of the small bowel

Introduction

These are the tumours that are most commonly referred to as 'carcinoid' tumours, as most NET of the gastrointestinal tract are found in the small bowel. They are also called 'midgut' tumours (together with NET of the appendix and the right colon). These tumours produce serotonin and cause the 'carcinoid' syndrome, but only in patients who have a large volume of liver metastases or if there is advanced local tumour growth draining into the inferior vena cava and thereby bypassing the liver. NET of the duodenum (gastrinomas in MEN 1 syndrome, somatostatinomas and others) are very rare and are not discussed further.

Pathology

NET of the jejunum and ileum arise from a sub-group of cells of the diffuse neuroendocrine system, the enterochromaffin (EC) cells, which secrete serotonin and substance P. They are either solitary or more often multiple, are almost always malignant and metastasise early to the regional lymph nodes and the liver depending on the location of the primary tumour(s) (Fig. 49.22).

Clinical symptoms

Symptoms that lead to the diagnosis are caused by either the primary tumour or its lymph node metastases. Acute or chronic, recurrent or persistent abdominal pain, ileus or, rarely, lower gastrointestinal bleeding may occur. Symptoms may be due to liver metastases, such as sudden painful reddening of the face and chest ('flushing'), diarrhoea or bronchospasm. These symptoms constitute 'carcinoid' syndrome. About 60% of patients eventually develop cardiac symptoms because of stenosis and insufficiency of the pulmonary and, more rarely, the tricuspid valve, with enlargement and thickening of the wall of the right atrium. The aetiology is unknown but local effects of serotonin and kinins may contribute.

Abdominal symptoms are caused either by obstruction of the appendix by an appendiceal NET (leading to appendectomy) or by obstruction of the mesentery or the bowel lumen by growth of lymph node metastases in the mesentery near the bowel. Pain is caused by chronic ischaemia of the bowel (Fig. 49.23), resulting not only from mesenteric lymph node metastases but also from constriction of mesenteric arteries and fibrosis of the mesentery by a so-called desmoplastic reaction.

Primary tumours in the jejunum and ileum rarely cause symptoms such as bleeding or intussusception as they usually only measure from a few millimetres up to 1 cm or at the most 2 cm in diameter (Fig. 49.24). A polypoid NET of the terminal ileum may, however, cause ileocaecal intussusception.

Diagnosis

The diagnosis of NET of the small bowel is made by history, physical examination of the abdomen, imaging and an assessment of 5-HIAA in a 24-hour urine sample. It is positive in larger tumours only if metastases are present. Cross-sectional imaging, sonography, CT scan and MRI will not show the primary tumour but will show mesenteric lymph node and liver metastases.

The best method for staging of NET is an octreotide (SRS)

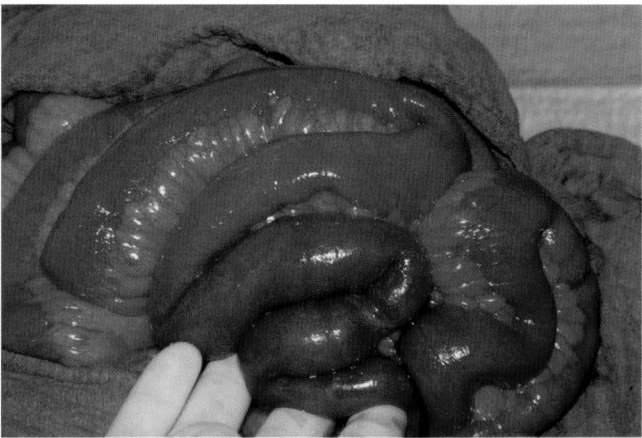

Figure 49.23 Chronic ischaemia of the small bowel caused by desmoplastic reaction and narrowing of vessels in the mesentery in a neuroendocrine tumour of the ileum.

Johann Friedrich Meckel (The Younger), **1781–1833, Professor of Anatomy and Surgery, Halle, Germany.**

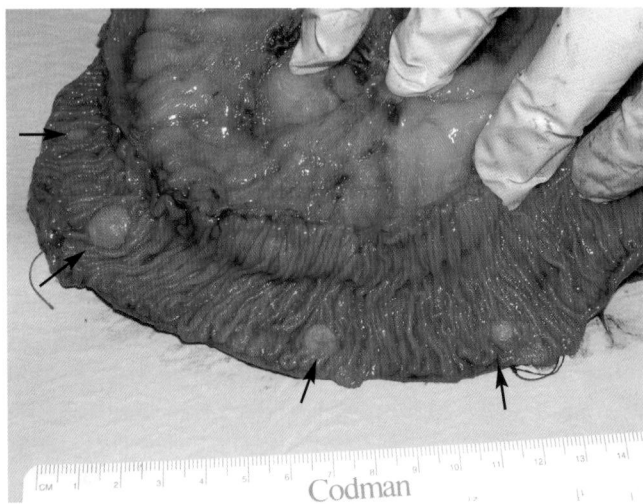

Figure 49.24 Multiple neuroendocrine tumours in the small bowel causing large lymph node metastases in the mesentery.

scan. This will show tumour deposits in all organs provided that they are large enough and have a high somatostatin receptor density (Fig. 49.25).

Surgical procedure

Surgery should be undertaken as soon as the diagnosis is made, even in the presence of liver metastases. The main goal is resection of the bowel primary tumour(s) and mesenteric lymph node metastases. This may entail resection of large amounts of bowel (100 cm or more), particularly if stage III or IV lymph node masses are found in the mesentery (Fig. 49.26). In the presence of liver metastases, extrahepatic disease should be resected

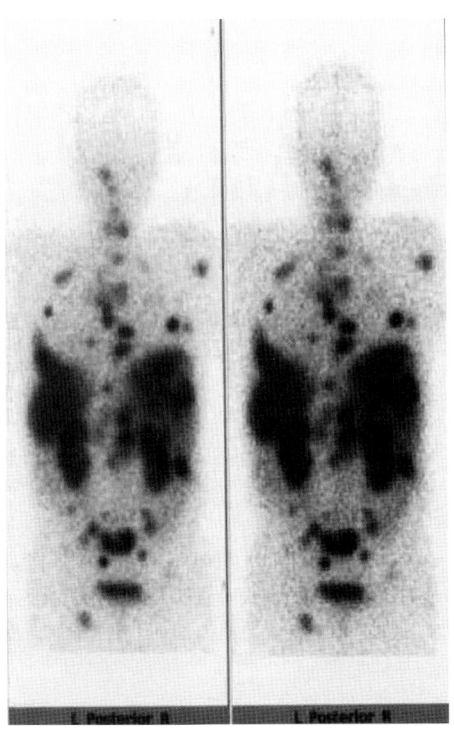

Figure 49.25 Octreotide scan of a patient with neuroendocrine tumour of the gut and diffuse metastases in different organs.

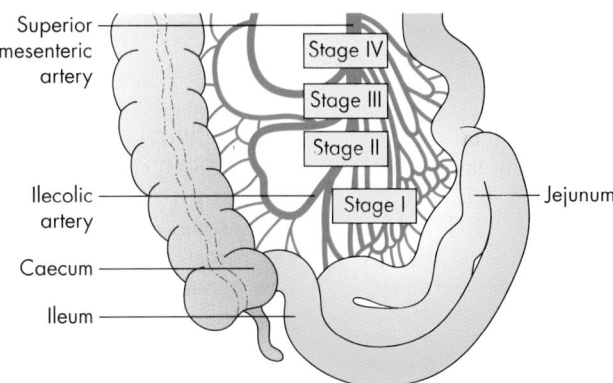

Figure 49.26 Bulky lymph node metastases can occur at different levels in the mesentery. To resect them completely, long segments of bowel must be resected, the closer to the mesenteric root the metastases are situated [adapted from Akerström, G., Hellman, P. and Öhrvall, U. (2001) Midgut and hindgut carcinoid tumours. In: Doherty, G.M. and Skogseid, B. (eds.). *Surgical Endocrinology*. Lippincott Williams & Wilkins, Philadelphia, PA, by kind permission].

whenever possible. Metastatic disease in the mesenteric root will lead to long-term pain in the abdomen or back and to a poor quality of life, whereas liver metastases can be treated by chemotherapy or embolisation.

Somatostatin and its analogues provide symptomatic treatment of the 'carcinoid' syndrome caused by a large volume of liver metastases. These drugs may also have an antiproliferative effect. Surgery to remove liver metastases is possible in approximately 10% of patients. In others, embolisation, chemoembolisation, SRS using radioactively labelled octreotide, chemotherapy, biotherapy and also liver transplantation can be performed.

MULTIPLE ENDOCRINE NEOPLASIAS

Introduction

Multiple endocrine neoplasias (MEN) are inherited syndromes characterised by a different pattern of benign and malignant tumours in different endocrine glands. There are two main types, type 1 (MEN 1) and type 2 (MEN 2). The mode of inheritance is autosomal dominant in both.

MEN 1 is characterised by the triad of tumours in the anterior pituitary gland, mostly presenting as prolactinomas or non-functioning tumours, hyperplasia of the parathyroids causing primary hyperparathyroidism (pHPT) and pancreaticoduodenal endocrine tumours (PETs). The syndrome was first described by Wermer in 1954 and is therefore also called Wermer's syndrome. It is caused by germline mutations in the *menin* gene, located on chromosome 11.

MEN 2 is divided into three subtypes: familial medullary thyroid carcinoma (FMTC), MEN 2a and MEN 2b. Medullary thyroid carcinoma (MTC) plays the key role in all subtypes. MEN 2 is caused by germline mutations in the *RET* proto-oncogene, located on chromosome 10. MEN 2a is characterised by the combination of MTC, pHPT and mostly bilateral phaeochromocytomas. MTC combined with phaeochromocytoma alone is called

Paul Wermer, **1898–1975, Physician, The Presbyterian Hospital, New York, NY, USA, described this condition in 1954.**

Sipple's syndrome. FMTC is characterised by distinct mutations in *RET* and MTC alone as the clinical manifestation. MEN 2b comprises MTC, phaeochromocytoma and characteristic facial and oral mucosal neurinomas and intestinal ganglioneuromatosis accompanied by a marfanoid habitus (Fig. 49.27).

The most important difference between MEN 1 and MEN 2, besides the different clinical pictures, is that MEN 2 is characterised by a well-understood genotype–phenotype correlation. This means that depending on the particular mutation in the *RET* proto-oncogene the phenotypic appearance and the onset of endocrine tumours will be different and can be predicted from the type of mutation. This is not the case in MEN 1 syndrome.

Multiple endocrine neoplasia type 1

Epidemiology

The prevalence of the syndrome is estimated to be around 0.04–0.2 cases per 1000 population per year. The penetrance is high with almost 100% of mutation carriers developing the syndrome. The disease is equally distributed between men and women.

Clinical presentation

The clinical presentation depends on the affected organs. Often tumours occur synchronously (Table 49.7). Most of the mutation carriers identified in screening programmes are asymptomatic.

Parathyroids

In total, 90–100% of patients suffering from MEN 1 develop pHPT and it is usually the first manifestation of the disease. MEN 1 pHPT is characterised by multiglandular disease so that all four parathyroids become hyperplastic in the course of the disease. The clinical presentation of MEN 1 pHPT is similar to that of the sporadic disease. Few patients have asymptomatic disease; most common in symptomatic disease is nephrolithiasis. Diagnosis is

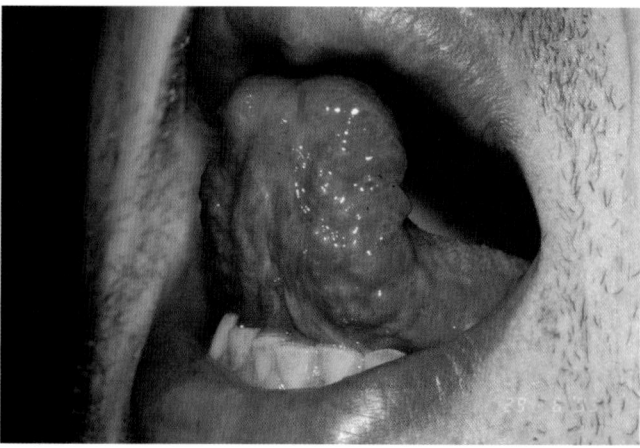

Figure 49.27 Neurinomas of the tongue in a patient with multiple endocrine neoplasia type 2b.

established by determination of parathyroid hormone (PTH) and calcium in serum.

Endocrine pancreas

PETs occur in around 50–60% of MEN 1 patients. In patients taking part in screening programmes, 70–90% are found to have non-functioning and functioning PETs. This high rate of detection of PETs is the result of the improvement in diagnostic procedures in the last decade, including EUS. MEN 1 PETs are the most common syndrome-associated cause of death. They are mostly multiple and often recur after surgery. Although most patients have multiple tumours, one hormone syndrome is usually dominant. The most common functional tumour is gastrinoma followed by insulinoma. VIPomas, glucagonomas and somatostatinomas are extremely rare. Non-functioning tumours can be asymptomatic for many years.

Table 49.7 Affected organs in multiple endocrine neoplasia type 1

Endocrine gland affected	Frequency (%)	Hormone	Clinical syndrome
Parathyroids	90	PTH	pHPT
Pancreas, duodenum (mostly multiple):	50–80		
Gastrinoma		Gastrin	Zollinger–Ellison syndrome
Insulinoma		Insulin	Hypoglycaemia syndrome
Non-functioning tumours		PP	–
VIPoma		VIP	Verner–Morrison syndrome
Glucagonoma		Glucagon	Glucagonoma syndrome
Anterior pituitary gland:	30–60		
Prolactinoma		Prolactin	Galactorrhea
Non-functioning adenoma		–	Non-specific
Other manifestations			
Adrenals	40–50	Cortisol?	Mostly non-functioning
NET in lung, thymus, stomach	3–10	–	–
Lipoma	5–10	–	–

NET, neuroendocrine tumours; pHPT, primary hyperparathyroidism; PP, pancreatic polypeptide; PTH, parathormone; VIP, vasoactive intestinal polypeptide.

John Sipple, **B. 1930, Physician, The State University of New York, New York, NY, USA.**
John V. Verner, **B. 1927, an American Physician.**
A.B. Morrison, **B. 1921, an American Physician.**

The diagnostic work-up is similar to that for sporadic PETs and includes laboratory tests, such as different hormone measurements, e.g. gastrin, insulin, PP, etc., and imaging.

Anterior pituitary gland

Tumours of the anterior pituitary gland are found in 30–60% of patients with MEN 1. These are mostly microadenomas that present as prolactinomas or non-functioning tumours. Most prolactinomas can be treated with anti-hormone medication.

Adrenal tumours and other organ manifestations

Adrenal involvement is common in MEN 1 patients and affects nearly 40–50% of patients. Mostly non-functioning bilateral adenomas are found. Very rarely adrenocortical carcinomas or phaeochromocytomas may develop.

Although very rare, manifestations of MEN 1 include NET of the lung, thymus, stomach, duodenum and small bowel. It is important to check for NETs of the thymus, as they are mostly malignant and are the main cause of death in MEN 1 patients.

Genetic screening

Identification of the MEN 1 (*menin*) gene in 1997 formed the basis for direct mutational analysis of the gene and for family screening. After genetic counselling of the index patient, family members can be screened. Mutation carriers can then be included in screening programmes that make early detection of endocrine tumours possible. Screening programmes should follow the consensus guidelines published by Brandi *et al.* in 2001. In cases of obviously sporadic endocrine tumours in patients younger than 40 years, genetic testing for MEN 1 seems to be useful.

Operative therapy

Parathyroids

The indications for surgery in MEN 1 pHPT follow the same criteria as in sporadic disease but the choice of procedure is different. As multiglandular disease is present in all cases, resection follows the same rules as in secondary HPT. Therefore, the most common procedures are total parathyroidectomy, including cervical thymectomy and autotransplantation of parathyroid tissue in the forearm, or 3½-gland resection, leaving approximately 50 mg of parathyroid tissue behind, and cervical thymectomy. Selective resection of enlarged glands is obsolete because of the high rates of recurrence.

Endocrine pancreas

Indications for surgery and its extent are controversial. Most experts agree that MEN 1 gastrinoma and insulinoma have to be operated on to prevent liver metastases and to control hormonal excess, provided that diffuse liver metastases are not present. MEN 1 gastrinomas are more often located in the duodenum as multiple small tumours than in the pancreas. For gastrinomas located in the duodenum or pancreatic head (gastrinoma triangle, Fig. 49.17), pylorus-preserving partial pancreaticoduodenectomy is recommended. In rare cases the gastrinoma is located in the body or tail of the pancreas. In such cases distal pancreatectomy with excision of tumours in the pancreatic head is the procedure of choice. In MEN 1 insulinoma the standard operative procedure is distal pancreatectomy with enucleation of tumours in the pancreatic head. Non-functioning PETs are operated on if they reach a size of 1 cm. Careful palpation and IOUS are essential in every pancreatic procedure for MEN 1 PETs.

Anterior pituitary gland

The indications for surgery in tumours of the anterior pituitary gland are the presence of symptomatic non-functional tumours or if medical therapy of prolactinoma fails. Most procedures can be performed through a trans-sphenoidal approach.

Adrenal tumours

Functional adrenal tumours in MEN 1 are rare and have to be operated on. Non-functioning tumours should be resected if they reach a size of 4 cm. Pre- and perioperative management follows the same rules as in sporadic adrenal tumours; therefore, phaeochromocytoma has to be ruled out in every patient. In most cases a laparoscopic or retroperitoneoscopic approach can be used. If there is evidence for a malignant tumour, open surgery is preferred.

Multiple endocrine neoplasia type 2

In most patients with MEN 2a, the disease is caused by mutations of the *RET* proto-oncogene in codon 634. MTC is almost always the first manifestation of the syndrome. If phaeochromocytoma and pHPT do not occur, one must suspect the presence of the FMTC subtype. Patients with MEN 2b do not develop pHPT and in 95% of cases mutations in codon 918 of the *RET* proto-oncogene are causative (Table 49.8).

Medullary thyroid carcinoma

MTC is characterised by multicentricity and is often accompanied by C-cell hyperplasia. These characteristics should lead to molecular diagnostic work-up (mutational analysis of the *RET* proto-oncogene) in patients with 'sporadic' MTC. In contrast to sporadic MTC, the diagnosis in families with known mutation of the *RET* gene is mostly made much earlier, possibly as the result of mutational screening and calcitonin measurements. MTC is most aggressive in MEN 2b. It occurs in early childhood, much earlier than in MEN 2a, with lymph node metastases present in the early stages.

Primary hyperparathyroidism

pHPT in MEN 2a is less common and has a milder clinical course than MEN 1 pHPT. It occurs in about 20–30% of patients with

Table 49.8 Frequency of diseases in multiple endocrine neoplasia type 2 related to mutation in different codons

Syndrome	Frequently affected codons in *RET*	MTC	pHPT	PCC
FMTC	533, 630, 768, 844	90–100%	–	–
MEN 2a	609, 634, 790, 804	90–100%	20–30%	10–50%
MEN 2b	883, 918	100%	–	10–50%

FMTC, familial medullary thyroid cancer; MEN 2a, multiple endocrine neoplasia type 2a; MEN 2b, multiple endocrine neoplasia type 2b; MTC, medullary thyroid cancer; PCC, phaeochromocytoma; pHPT, primary hyperparathyroidism; *RET*, *RET* proto-oncogene (RET = rearranged during transfection).

Table 49.9 Prophylactic thyroidectomy for medullary thyroid cancer depending on the site of mutation of the *RET* proto-oncogene in multiple endocrine neoplasia type 2 patients with normal calcitonin levels

| | | Risk group | |
	High	Medium	Low
Codon	883, 918, 922	609, 611, 618, 620, 634	768, 790, 791, 804, 891
Thyroidectomy at age (years)	< 1	6	< 20

MEN 2a. Most patients are asymptomatic but all parathyroid glands become hyperplastic, mostly metachronously. The disease develops after the third decade of life.

Phaeochromocytoma

The frequency of phaeochromocytoma in MEN 2 is around 10–50% and most tumours are bilateral. This can occur synchronously or metachronously. The tumours are almost always benign. Diagnostic work-up includes measurement of urinary catecholamines, abdominal CT or MRI, and ^{131}I-MIBG scintigraphy (see above).

Operative therapy

Medullary thyroid carcinoma

Operative therapy for MEN 2 MTC in patients detected by genetic screening is a good example of efficient prophylactic surgery, as the likelihood of developing MTC is 100% for most mutations. The mutation carriers can be operated on with no evidence of tumour in the thyroid, protecting them from MTC for the rest of their lives. Different *RET* mutations are associated with early or late onset of the disease. Risk groups have been defined to determine the appropriate age for thyroidectomy (Table 49.9).

Phaeochromocytoma

The operative approach is open surgery or laparoscopy or retroperitoneoscopy, depending on the manifestation of the disease in a given patient. Unilateral or bilateral subtotal resection may be feasible, which retains the healthy part of the gland and prevents postoperative dependence on cortisol and mineralocorticoid supplementation (see above) (Fig. 49.28).

Primary hyperparathyroidism

The clinical situation in MEN 2 pHPT is even more difficult than in MEN 1 pHPT because of the association with MTC in MEN 2. During neck surgery for MTC in a eucalcaemic patient, enlarged parathyroid glands should be removed. In cases in which neck surgery has already been performed for MTC, the surgical approach to MEN 2a pHPT should be more tailored to the individual patient. For example, in an older patient after thyroidectomy for MTC with mild asymptomatic hypercalcaemia, localisation procedures and a targeted approach with intraoperative parathormone measurement may be worthwhile, if possible.

FURTHER READING

Allolio, B. and Fassnacht, M. (2006) Clinical review: adrenocortical carcinoma: clinical update. *Journal of Clinical Endocrinology and Metabolism* 91: 2027–37.

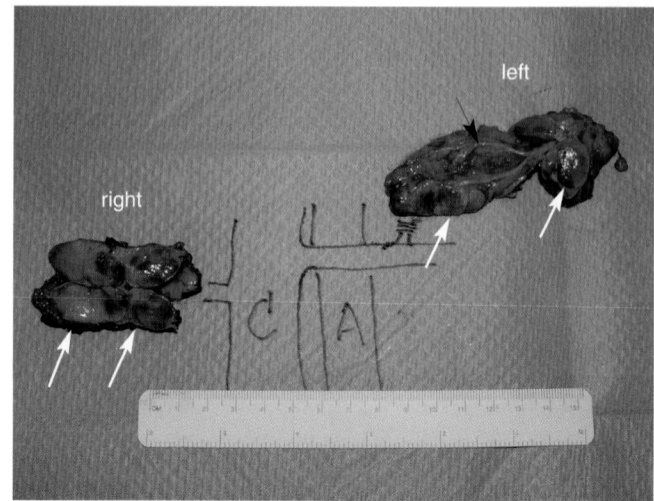

Figure 49.28 Bilateral multiple phaeochromocytomas in a patient with multiple endocrine neoplasia type 2a. A, aorta; C, vena cava; white arrows, tumours; black arrow, normal adrenal.

Bartsch, D.K., Fendrich, V., Langer, P., Celik, I., Kann, P.H. and Rothmund, M. (2005) Outcome of duodenopancreatic resections in patients with multiple endocrine neoplasia type 1. *Annals of Surgery* 242: 757–64.

Brandi, M.L., Gagel, R.F., Angeli, A. *et al.* (2001) Guidelines for diagnosis and therapy of MEN type 1 and type 2. *Journal of Clinical Endocrinology and Metabolism* 86: 5658–71.

Fendrich, V., Langer, P., Celik, I. *et al.* (2006) An aggressive surgical approach leads to long-term survival in patients with pancreatic endocrine tumors. *Annals of Surgery* 244: 845–51.

Ilias, I. and Pacak, K. (2005) Diagnosis and management of tumors of the adrenal medulla. *Hormone and Metabolic Research* 37: 717–21.

Kulke, M.H. and Mayer, R.J. (1999) Medical progress: carcinoid tumors. *New England Journal of Medicine* 340: 858–68.

Norton, J.A., Fraker, D.L., Alexander, H.R. *et al.* (2006) Surgery increases survival in patients with gastrinoma. *Annals of Surgery* 244: 410–19.

Rindi, G., Kloppel, G., Alhman, H. *et al*; and all other Frascati Consensus Conference participants; European Neuroendocrine Tumor Society (ENETS) (2006) TNM staging of foregut (neuro)endocrine tumors: a consensus proposal including a grading system. *Virchows Archiv* 449: 395–401.

Shen, W.T., Sturgeon, C. and Duh, Q.Y. (2005) From incidentaloma to adrenocortical carcinoma: the surgical management of adrenal tumors. *Journal of Surgical Oncology* 89: 186–92.

Young, W.F., Jr. (2007) Clinical practice: the incidentally discovered adrenal mass. *New England Journal of Medicine* 356: 601–10.

CHAPTER

50

LEARNING OBJECTIVES

To understand:
- Appropriate investigation of breast disease
- Breast anomalies and the complexity of benign breast disease
- The in-depth modern management of breast cancer

COMPARATIVE AND SURGICAL ANATOMY

The protuberant part of the human breast is generally described as overlying the second to the sixth ribs and extending from the lateral border of the sternum to the anterior axillary line. Actually, a thin layer of mammary tissue extends considerably further, from the clavicle above to the seventh or eighth ribs below and from the midline to the edge of the latissimus dorsi posteriorly. This fact is important when performing a mastectomy, the aim of which is to remove the whole breast. The anatomy of the breast is illustrated in Fig. 50.1.

The *axillary tail* of the breast is of surgical importance. In some normal subjects it is palpable and, in a few, it can be seen premenstrually or during lactation. A well-developed axillary tail is sometimes mistaken for a mass of enlarged lymph nodes or a lipoma.

The *lobule* is the basic structural unit of the mammary gland. The number and size of the lobules vary enormously: they are most numerous in young women. From 10 to over 100 lobules empty via ductules into a lactiferous duct, of which there are 15–20. Each lactiferous duct is lined with a spiral arrangement of contractile myoepithelial cells and is provided with a terminal ampulla, a reservoir for milk or abnormal discharges.

The *ligaments of Cooper* are hollow conical projections of fibrous tissue filled with breast tissue; the apices of the cones are attached firmly to the superficial fascia and thereby to the skin overlying the breast. These ligaments account for the dimpling of the skin overlying a carcinoma.

The *areola* contains involuntary muscle arranged in concentric rings as well as radially in the subcutaneous tissue. The areolar epithelium contains numerous sweat glands and sebaceous glands, the latter of which enlarge during pregnancy and serve to lubricate the nipple during lactation (Montgomery's tubercles).

The *nipple* is covered by thick skin with corrugations. Near its apex lie the orifices of the lactiferous ducts. The nipple contains smooth muscle fibres arranged concentrically and longitudinally; thus, it is an erectile structure, which points outwards.

The lymphatics of the breast drain predominantly into the axillary and internal mammary lymph nodes. The axillary nodes receive approximately 85% of the drainage and are arranged in the following groups:

- *lateral,* along the axillary vein;
- *anterior,* along the lateral thoracic vessels;
- *posterior,* along the subscapular vessels;
- *central,* embedded in fat in the centre of the axilla;
- *interpectoral,* a few nodes lying between the pectoralis major and minor muscles;
- *apical,* which lie above the level of the pectoralis minor tendon in continuity with the lateral nodes and which receive the efferents of all the other groups.

The apical nodes are also in continuity with the supraclavicular nodes and drain into the subclavian lymph trunk, which enters the great veins directly or via the thoracic duct or jugular trunk. The *sentinel node* is defined as the first lymph node draining the tumour-bearing area of the breast. The importance of the sentinel node is described later.

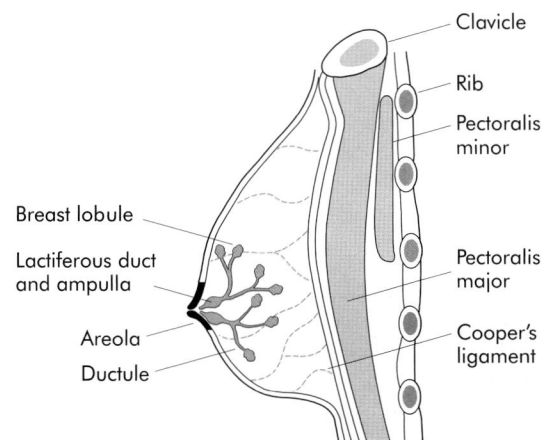

Figure 50.1 Cross-sectional anatomy of the breast.

Labels: Clavicle; Rib; Pectoralis minor; Pectoralis major; Cooper's ligament; Breast lobule; Lactiferous duct and ampulla; Areola; Ductule

Sir Astley Paston Cooper, **1768–1841, Surgeon, Guy's Hospital, London, England, described these ligaments in 1845.**
William Fetherston Montgomery, **1797–1859, Obstetrician, Dublin, Ireland, described these tubercles in 1837.**

The internal mammary nodes are fewer in number. They lie along the internal mammary vessels deep to the plane of the costal cartilages, drain the posterior third of the breast and are not routinely dissected although they were at one time biopsied for staging.

INVESTIGATION OF BREAST SYMPTOMS

Although an accurate history and clinical examination are important methods of detecting breast disease, there are a number of investigations that can assist in the diagnosis. Examination precedes palpation and requires careful observation of the patient both with the arms at rest and also elevated to lift the breast. Small lesions may betray their presence by dimpling or minor distortions when the patient moves.

Mammography

Soft tissue radiographs are taken by placing the breast in direct contact with ultrasensitive film and exposing it to low-voltage, high-amperage X-rays (Fig. 50.2). The dose of radiation is approximately 0.1 cGy and, therefore, mammography is a very safe investigation.

The sensitivity of this investigation increases with age as the breast becomes less dense. In total, 5% of breast cancers are missed by population-based mammographic screening programmes; even in retrospect, such carcinomas are not apparent. Thus, a normal mammogram does not exclude the presence of carcinoma. Digital mammography is being introduced, which allows manipulation of the images and computer-aided diagnosis. Tomo-mammography is also being assessed as a more sensitive diagnostic modality.

Ultrasound

Ultrasound is particularly useful in young women with dense breasts in whom mammograms are difficult to interpret, and in distinguishing cysts from solid lesions (Figs 50.3 and 50.4). It can also be used to localise impalpable areas of breast pathology. It is not useful as a screening tool and remains operator dependent. Increasingly, ultrasound of the axillary tissue is performed when a cancer is diagnosed and guided percutaneous biopsy of any suspicious glands may be performed.

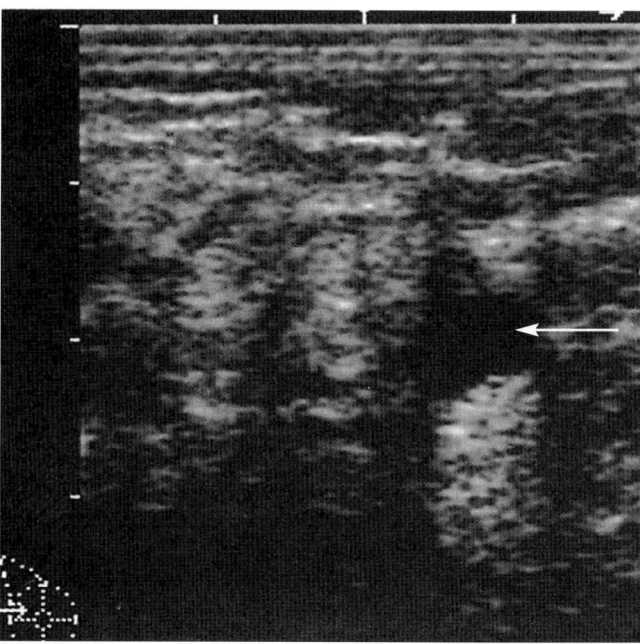

Figure 50.3 Ultrasound of the breast showing a cyst (arrow).

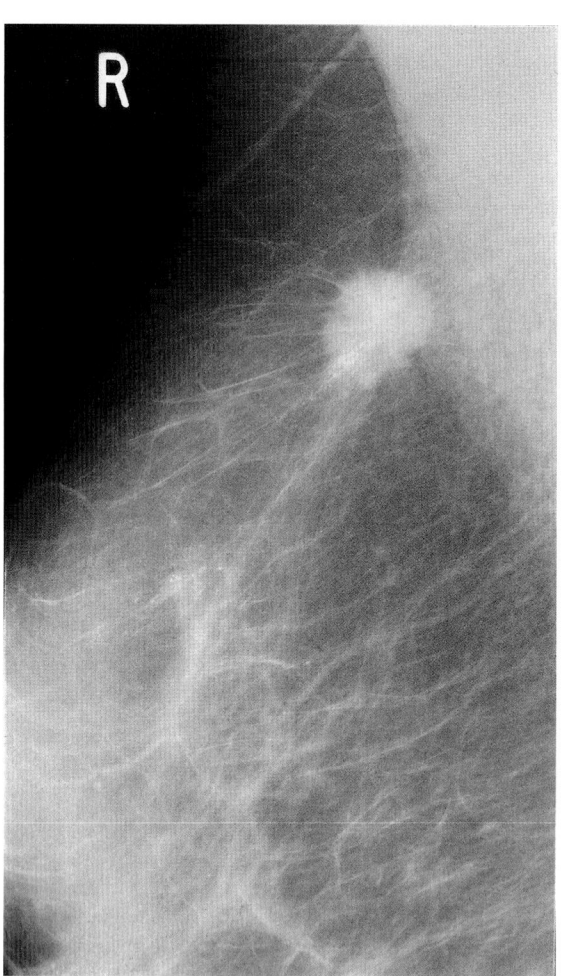

Figure 50.2 Mammogram showing a carcinoma.

Gy is short for Gray, the SI unit for the absorbed dose of ionizing radiation. Louis Harold Gray, 1905–1965, Director, The British Empire Cancer Campaign Research Unit in Radiobiology, Mount Vernon Hospital, Northwood, Middlesex, England.

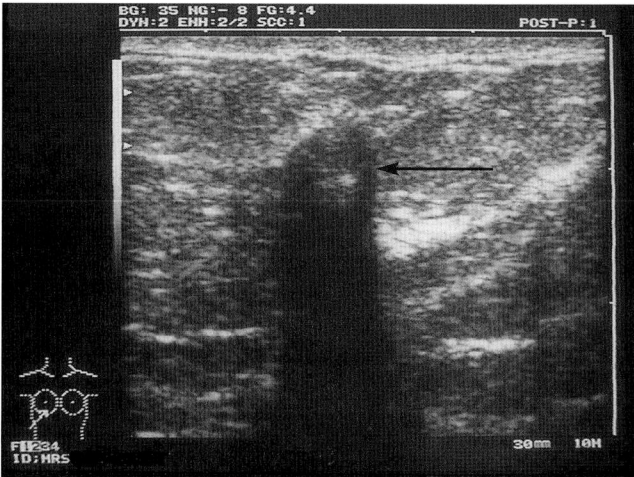

Figure 50.4 Ultrasound of the breast showing a carcinoma (arrow).

Magnetic resonance imaging

Magnetic resonance imaging (MRI) is of increasing interest to breast surgeons in a number of settings:

- It can be useful to distinguish scar from recurrence in women who have had previous breast conservation therapy for cancer (although it is not accurate within 9 months of radiotherapy because of abnormal enhancement).
- It is the best imaging modality for the breasts of women with implants.
- It has proven to be useful as a screening tool in high-risk women (because of family history).
- It is less useful than ultrasound in the management of the axilla in both primary breast cancer and recurrent disease (Fig. 50.5).

Although biopsies can be performed with MRI guidance this is complicated because of the configuration of the imaging system. With improved ultrasound equipment, an MRI-detected lesion can often be found on a second-look ultrasound and biopsied using this modality.

Needle biopsy/cytology

Histology can be obtained under local anaesthesia using a spring-loaded core needle biopsy device (Fig. 50.6). Cytology is obtained using a 21G or 23G needle and 10-ml syringe with multiple passes through the lump with negative pressure in the syringe. The aspirate is then smeared on to a slide, which is air dried or fixed (Fig. 50.7). Fine-needle aspiration cytology (FNAC) is the least invasive technique of obtaining a cell diagnosis and is rapid

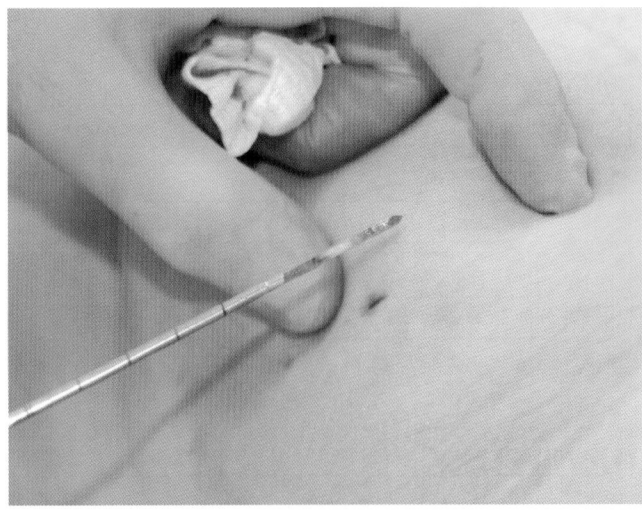

Figure 50.6 Corecut biopsy of breast.

and very accurate if both operator and cytologist are experienced. However, false negatives do occur, mainly through sampling error, and invasive cancer cannot be distinguished from *in situ* disease. A histological specimen taken by core biopsy allows a definitive preoperative diagnosis, differentiates between duct carcinoma *in situ* (DCIS) and invasive disease and also allows the tumour to be stained for receptor status. This is important before commencing neoadjuvant therapy.

Large-needle biopsy with vacuum systems

The sampling error decreases as the biopsy volume increases and using 8G or 11G needles allows more extensive biopsies to be taken. This is useful in the management of microcalcifications or in the complete excision of benign lesions such as fibroadenomas.

Triple assessment

In any patient who presents with a breast lump or other symptoms suspicious of carcinoma, the diagnosis should be made by a combination of clinical assessment, radiological imaging and a tissue sample taken for either cytological or histological analysis (Fig. 50.8), the so called triple assessment. The positive predictive value (PPV) of this combination should exceed 99.9%.

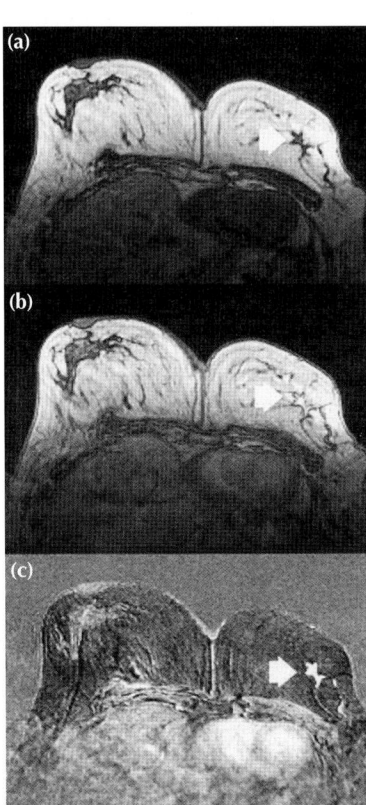

Figure 50.5 Magnetic resonance imaging scan of the breasts showing carcinoma of the left breast (arrows). (a) Pre-contrast; (b) post-gadolinium contrast; (c) subtraction image.

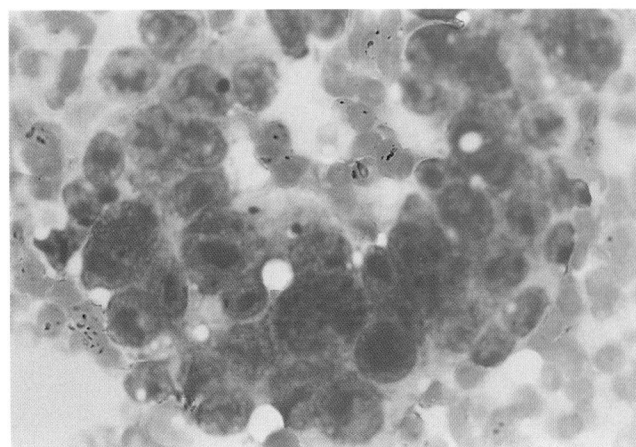

Figure 50.7 Fine-needle aspiration cytology (FNAC) showing grade III ductal carcinoma cells.

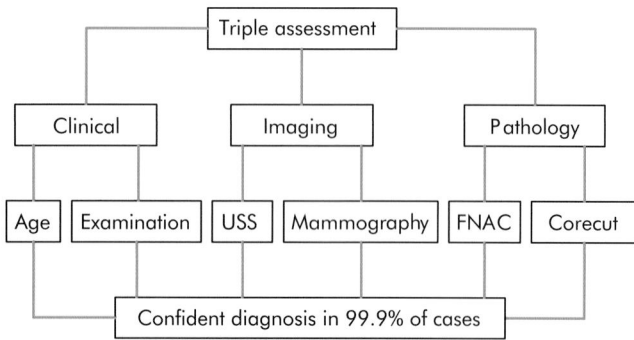

Figure 50.8 Triple assessment of breast symptoms. USS, ultrasound scan.

THE NIPPLE

Absence of the nipple is rare and is usually associated with amazia (congenital absence of the breast).

Supernumerary nipples not uncommonly occur along a line extending from the anterior fold of the axilla to the fold of the groin (Fig. 50.9). This constitutes the milk line of lower mammals.

Nipple retraction

This may occur at puberty or later in life. Retraction occurring at puberty, also known as *simple nipple inversion*, is of unknown aetiology (benign horizontal inversion). In about 25% of cases it is bilateral. It may cause problems with breast-feeding and infection can occur, especially during lactation, because of retention of secretions. Recent retraction of the nipple may be of considerable pathological significance. A slit-like retraction of the nipple may be caused by duct ectasia and chronic periductal mastitis (Fig. 50.10a), but circumferential retraction, with or without an underlying lump, may well indicate an underlying carcinoma (Fig. 50.10b).

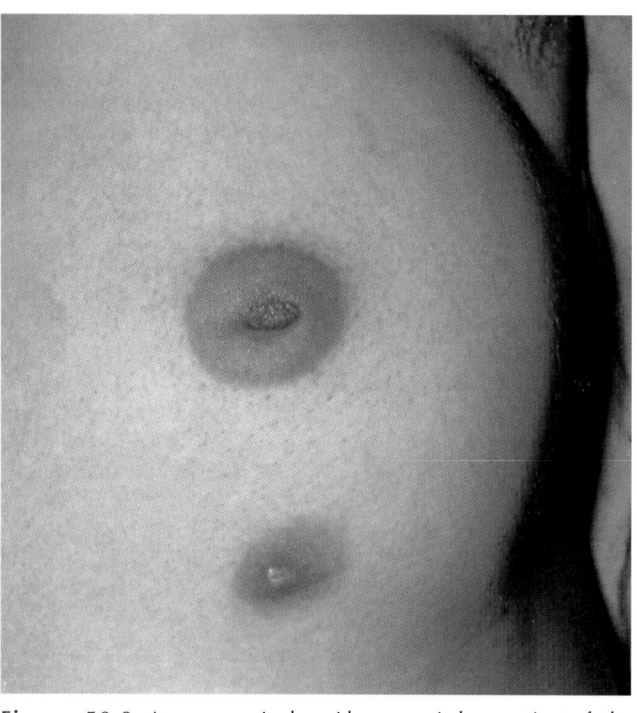

Figure 50.9 Accessory nipple with congenital retraction of the normal nipple.

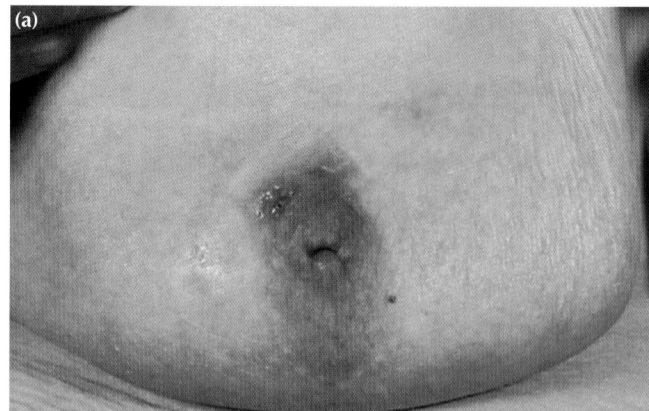

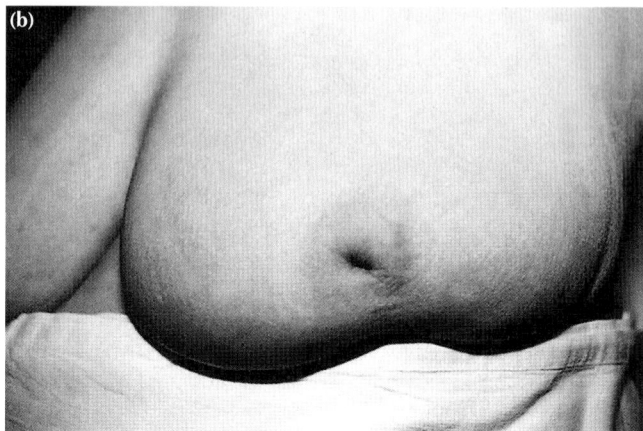

Figure 50.10 Recent nipple retraction. (a) Slit-like retraction of duct ectasia with mammary duct fistula. (b) Circumferential retraction with underlying carcinoma.

Treatment

Treatment is usually unnecessary and the condition may spontaneously resolve during pregnancy or lactation.

Simple cosmetic surgery can produce an adequate correction but has the drawback of dividing the underlying ducts. Mechanical suction devices have been used to evert the nipple, with some effect.

Cracked nipple

This may occur during lactation and be the forerunner of acute infective mastitis. If the nipple becomes cracked during lactation, it should be rested for 24–48 hours and the breast should be emptied with a breast pump. Feeding should be resumed as soon as possible.

Papilloma of the nipple

Papilloma of the nipple has the same features as any cutaneous papilloma and should be excised with a tiny disc of skin. Alternatively, the base may be tied with a ligature and the papilloma will spontaneously fall off.

Retention cyst of a gland of Montgomery

These glands, situated in the areola, secrete sebum and if they become blocked a sebaceous cyst forms.

Eczema

Eczema of the nipples is a rare condition and is often bilateral; it is usually associated with eczema elsewhere on the body. It is treated with 0.5% hydrocortisone (not a stronger steroid preparation).

Paget's disease

Paget's disease of the nipple must be distinguished from eczema. The former is caused by malignant cells in the subdermal layer. Eczema tends to occur in younger people who have signs of eczema elsewhere (look at the antecubital fossae).

Discharges from the nipple

Discharge can occur from one or more lactiferous ducts. Management depends on the presence of a lump (which should always be given priority in diagnosis and treatment) and the presence of blood in the discharge or discharge from a single duct. Mammography is rarely useful except to exclude an underlying impalpable mass. Cytology may reveal malignant cells but a negative result does not exclude a carcinoma.

- A *clear, serous discharge* may be 'physiological' in a parous woman or may be associated with a duct papilloma or mammary dysplasia. Multiduct, multicoloured discharge is physiological and the patient may be reassured.
- A *blood-stained discharge* may be caused by duct ectasia, a duct papilloma or carcinoma. A duct papilloma is usually single and situated in one of the larger lactiferous ducts; it is sometimes associated with a cystic swelling beneath the areola.
- A *black or green discharge* is usually the result of duct ectasia and its complications (Summary box 50.1).

Summary box 50.1

Discharges from the nipple (the principal causes are italicised)

Discharge from the surface
- Paget's disease
- Skin diseases (eczema, psoriasis)
- Rare causes (e.g. chancre)

Discharge from a single duct
Blood-stained:
- *Intraduct papilloma*
- *Intraduct carcinoma*
- *Duct ectasia*
Serous (any colour):
- *Fibrocystic disease*
- *Duct ectasia*
- Carcinoma

Discharge from more than one duct
Blood-stained:
- *Carcinoma*
- Ectasia
- Fibrocystic disease
Black or green:
- *Duct ectasia*
Purulent:
- *Infection*
Serous:
- *Fibrocystic disease*
- Duct ectasia
- Carcinoma
Milk:
- *Lactation*
- Rare causes (hypothyroidism, pituitary tumour)

Sir James Paget, 1814–1899, Surgeon, St. Bartholomew's Hospital, London, England, described this disease of the nipple in 1874.

Treatment

Treatment must firstly be to exclude a carcinoma by occult blood test and cytology. Simple reassurance may then be sufficient but, if the discharge is proving intolerable, an operation to remove the affected duct or ducts can be performed (microdochectomy).

Microdochectomy

It is important not to express the blood before the operation as it may then be difficult to identify the duct in theatre. A lacrimal probe or length of stiff nylon suture is inserted into the duct from which the discharge is emerging. A tennis racquet incision can be made to encompass the entire duct or a periareolar incision used and the nipple flap dissected to reach the duct. The duct is then excised. A papilloma is nearly always situated within 4–5 cm of the nipple orifice.

Ductoscopy (inspection of the internal structure of the duct system) using microendoscopes is technically feasible but generally disappointing. The affected duct may not be visualised and biopsy systems are currently rudimentary.

Cone excision of the major ducts (after Hadfield)

When the duct of origin of nipple bleeding is uncertain or when there is bleeding or discharge from multiple ducts, the entire major duct system can be excised for histological examination without sacrifice of the breast form. A periareolar incision is made and a cone of tissue is removed with its apex just deep to the surface of the nipple and its base on the pectoral fascia. The resulting defect may be obliterated by a series of purse-string sutures although a temporary suction drain will reduce the chance of long-term deformity. It is vital to warn the patient that she will be unable to breast-feed after this and may experience altered nipple sensation.

BENIGN BREAST DISEASE

This is the most common cause of breast problems; up to 30% of women will suffer from a benign breast disorder requiring treatment at some time in their lives. The most common symptoms are pain, lumpiness or a lump. The aim of treatment is to exclude cancer and, once this has been done, to treat any remaining symptoms.

Congenital abnormalities

Amazia

Congenital absence of the breast may occur on one (Fig. 50.11) or both sides. It is sometimes associated with absence of the sternal portion of the pectoralis major (Poland's syndrome). It is more common in males.

Polymazia

Accessory breasts (Fig. 50.12) have been recorded in the axilla (the most frequent site), groin, buttock and thigh. They have been known to function during lactation.

Mastitis of infants

Mastitis of infants is at least as common in boys as in girls. On the third or fourth day of life, if the breast of an infant is pressed

---

Geoffrey John Hadfield, Surgeon, Stoke Mandeville Hospital, Aylesbury, Buckinghamshire, England.
Alfred Poland, 1822–1872, Surgeon, Guy's Hospital, London, England described this condition in 1841.

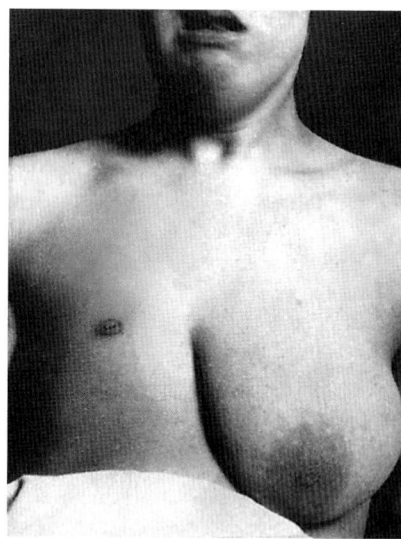

Figure 50.11 Congenital absence of the right breast.

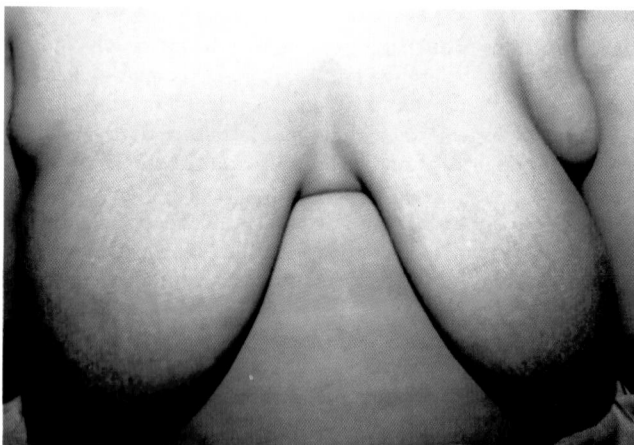

Figure 50.12 Bilateral accessory breasts.

lightly, a drop of colourless fluid can be expressed; a few days later, there is often a slight milky secretion, which disappears during the third week. This is popularly known as 'witch's milk' and is seen only in full-term infants. It is caused by stimulation of the fetal breast by prolactin in response to the drop in maternal oestrogens and is essentially physiological. True mastitis is uncommon and is predominately caused by *Staphylococcus aureus*.

Diffuse hypertrophy

Diffuse hypertrophy of the breasts occurs sporadically in otherwise healthy girls at puberty (benign virginal hypertrophy) and, much less often, during the first pregnancy. The breasts attain enormous dimensions and may reach the knees when the patient is sitting. The condition is rarely unilateral. This tremendous overgrowth is apparently caused by an alteration in the normal sensitivity of the breast to oestrogenic hormones and some success in treating it with anti-oestrogens has been reported. Treatment is otherwise by reduction mammoplasty.

Injuries of the breast

Haematoma

Haematoma, particularly a resolving haematoma, gives rise to a lump, which, in the absence of overlying bruising, is difficult to diagnose correctly unless it is biopsied.

Traumatic fat necrosis

Traumatic fat necrosis may be acute or chronic and usually occurs in stout, middle-aged women. Following a blow, or even indirect violence (e.g. contraction of the pectoralis major), a lump, often painless, appears. This may mimic a carcinoma, even displaying skin tethering and nipple retraction, and biopsy is required for diagnosis. A history of trauma is not diagnostic as this may merely have drawn the patient's attention to a pre-existing lump. A seatbelt may transect the breast with a sudden deceleration injury, as in a road traffic accident.

Acute and subacute inflammations of the breast

Bacterial mastitis

Bacterial mastitis is the most common variety of mastitis and is associated with lactation in the majority of cases.

Aetiology

Lactational mastitis is seen far less frequently than in former years. Most cases are caused by *Staphylococcus aureus* and, if hospital acquired, are likely to be penicillin resistant. The intermediary is usually the infant; after the second day of life, 50% of infants harbour staphylococci in the nasopharynx.

Although ascending infection from a sore and cracked nipple may initiate the mastitis, in many cases the lactiferous ducts will first become blocked by epithelial debris leading to stasis; this theory is supported by the relatively high incidence of mastitis in women with a retracted nipple. Once within the ampulla of the duct, staphylococci cause clotting of milk and, within this clot, organisms multiply.

Clinical features

The affected breast, or more usually a segment of it, presents the classical signs of acute inflammation. Early on this is a generalised cellulitis but later an abscess will form.

Treatment

During the cellulitic stage the patient should be treated with an appropriate antibiotic, for example flucloxacillin or co-amoxiclav. Feeding from the affected side may continue if the patient can manage. Support of the breast, local heat and analgesia will help to relieve pain.

If an antibiotic is used in the presence of undrained pus, an 'antibioma' may form. This is a large, sterile, brawny oedematous swelling that takes many weeks to resolve.

It used to be recommended that the breast should be incised and drained if the infection did not resolve within 48 hours or if after being emptied of milk there was an area of tense induration or other evidence of an underlying abscess. This advice has been replaced with the recommendation that repeated aspirations under antibiotic cover (if necessary using ultrasound) be performed. This often allows resolution without the need for an incision scar and will also allow the patient to carry on breast-feeding.

The presence of pus can be confirmed with needle aspiration and the pus sent for bacteriological culture. In contrast to the majority of localised infections, fluctuation is a late sign. Usually, the area of induration is sector shaped and, in early cases, about one-quarter of the breast is involved (Fig. 50.13); in many late cases the area is more extensive (Fig. 50.14). When in doubt an ultrasound scan may clearly define an area suitable for drainage.

Operative drainage of a breast abscess

This is less commonly needed as prompt commencement of antibiotics and repeated aspiration is usually successful. Incision of a lactational abscess is necessary if there is marked skin thinning and can usually be performed under local anaesthesia if an analgesic cream such as EMLA (lidocaine) is applied 30 min before surgery.

The usual incision is sited in a radial direction over the affected segment, although if a circumareolar incision will allow adequate access to the affected area this is preferred because it gives a better cosmetic result. The incision passes through the skin and the superficial fascia. A long artery forceps is then inserted into the abscess cavity. Every part of the abscess is palpated against the point of the artery forceps and its jaws are opened. All loculi that can be felt are entered.

Finally, the artery forceps having been withdrawn, a finger is introduced and any remaining septa are disrupted. The wound may then be lightly packed with ribbon gauze or a drain inserted to allow dependent drainage.

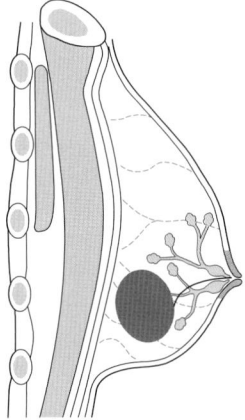

Figure 50.13 Intramammary breast abscess.

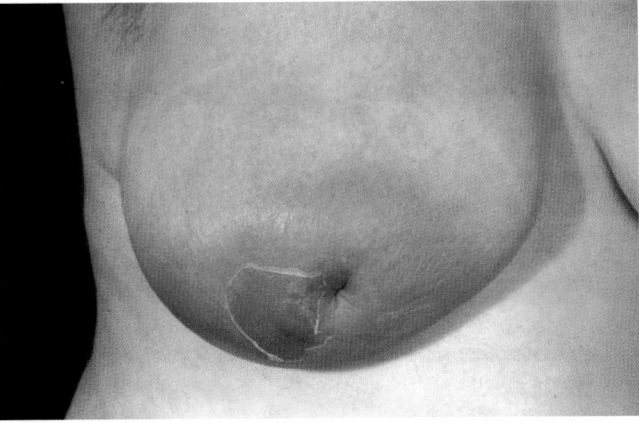

Figure 50.14 Large breast abscess.

Chronic intramammary abscess

A chronic intramammary abscess, which may follow inadequate drainage or injudicious antibiotic treatment, is often a very difficult condition to diagnose. When encapsulated within a thick wall of fibrous tissue the condition cannot be distinguished from a carcinoma without the histological evidence from a biopsy.

Tuberculosis of the breast

Tuberculosis of the breast, which is comparatively rare, is usually associated with active pulmonary tuberculosis or tuberculous cervical adenitis.

Tuberculosis of the breast (Fig. 50.15) occurs more often in parous women and usually presents with multiple chronic abscesses and sinuses and a typical bluish, attenuated appearance of the surrounding skin. The diagnosis rests on bacteriological and histological examination. Treatment is with anti-tuberculous chemotherapy. Healing is usual, although often delayed, and mastectomy should be restricted to patients with persistent residual infection.

Actinomycosis

Actinomycosis of the breast is rarer still. The lesions present the essential characteristics of faciocervical actinomycosis.

Mondor's disease

Mondor's disease is thrombophlebitis of the superficial veins of the breast and anterior chest wall (Fig. 50.16), although it has also been encountered in the arm.

In the absence of injury or infection, the cause of thrombophlebitis (like that of spontaneous thrombophlebitis in other sites) is obscure. The pathognomonic feature is a thrombosed subcutaneous cord, usually attached to the skin. When the skin over the breast is stretched by raising the arm, a narrow, shallow subcutaneous groove alongside the cord becomes apparent. The differential diagnosis is lymphatic permeation from an occult

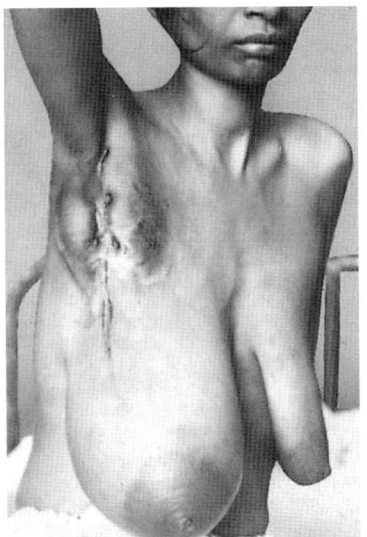

Figure 50.15 Tuberculosis of the breast with secondary suppurating axillary lymph nodes (courtesy of Professor A.K. Toufeeq, Lahore, Pakistan).

Henri Mondor, **1885–1962, Professor of Surgery, Paris, France.**

CHAPTER 50 | THE BREAST

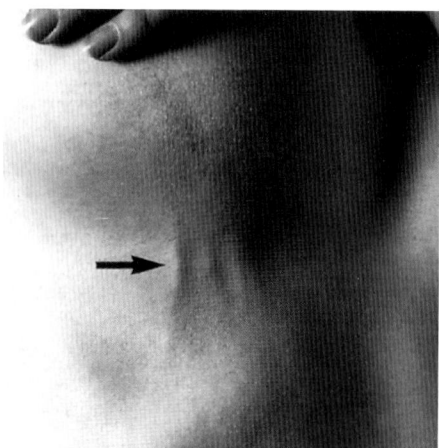

Figure 50.16 Mondor's disease under the right breast (arrow).

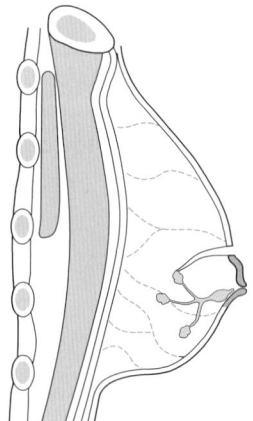

Figure 50.18 Mammary fistula originating in a chronic subareolar abscess.

carcinoma of the breast. The only treatment required is restricted arm movements and, in any case, the condition subsides within a few months without recurrence, complications or deformity. There are case reports of Mondor's disease being associated with subsequent development of malignancy although this has been unsubstantiated by others and is thought to be coincidental.

Duct ectasia/periductal mastitis

Pathology

This is a dilatation of the breast ducts, which is often associated with periductal inflammation. The pathogenesis is obscure and almost certainly not uniform in all cases, although the disease is much more common in smokers.

The classical description of the pathogenesis of duct ectasia asserts that the first stage in the disorder is a dilatation in one or more of the larger lactiferous ducts, which fill with a stagnant brown or green secretion. This may discharge. These fluids then set up an irritant reaction in surrounding tissue leading to periductal mastitis or even abscess and fistula formation (Figs 50.17 and 50.18). In some cases, a chronic indurated mass forms beneath the areola, which mimics a carcinoma. Fibrosis eventually develops, which may cause slit-like nipple retraction.

An alternative theory suggests that periductal inflammation is the primary condition and, indeed, anaerobic bacterial infection is found in some cases. A marked association between recurrent periductal inflammation and smoking has been demonstrated. This was thought by some to indicate that arteriopathy is a contributing factor in its aetiology although others believe that smoking increases the virulence of the commensal bacteria. It is certainly clear that cessation of smoking increases the chance of a long-term cure.

Clinical features

Nipple discharge (of any colour), a subareolar mass, abscess, mammary duct fistula and/or nipple retraction are the most common symptoms.

Treatment

In the case of a mass or nipple retraction, a carcinoma must be excluded by obtaining a mammogram and negative cytology or histology. If any suspicion remains the mass should be excised.

Antibiotic therapy may be tried, the most appropriate agents being co-amoxiclav or flucloxacillin and metronidazole. However, surgery is often the only option likely to bring about cure of this notoriously difficult condition; this consists of excision of all of the major ducts (Hadfield's operation). It is particularly important to shave the back of the nipple to ensure that all terminal ducts are removed. Failure to do so will lead to recurrence.

Aberrations of normal development and involution

Nomenclature

The nomenclature of benign breast disease is confusing. This is because over the last century a variety of clinicians and pathologists have chosen to describe a mixture of physiological changes and disease processes according to a variety of clinical, pathological and aetiological terminology. As well as leading to confusion, patients were often unduly alarmed or overtreated by ascribing a pathological name to a variant of physiological development. To sort out this confusion, a new system [Aberrations of Normal Development and Involution (ANDI)] has been developed and described by the Cardiff Breast Clinic. (Many alternative terms have been applied to this condition, including fibrocystic disease, fibroadenosis, chronic mastitis and mastopathy.)

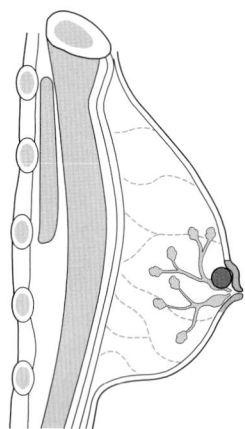

Figure 50.17 Subareolar abscess in duct ectasia.

Aetiology

The breast is a dynamic structure that undergoes changes throughout a woman's reproductive life and, superimposed upon this, cyclical changes throughout the menstrual cycle. This is illustrated in Fig. 50.19. The pathogenesis of ANDI involves disturbances in the breast physiology extending from a perturbation of normality to well-defined disease processes. There is often little correlation between the histological appearance of the breast tissue and the symptoms.

Pathology

The disease consists essentially of four features that may vary in extent and degree in any one breast.

- *Cyst formation.* Cysts are almost inevitable and very variable in size.
- *Fibrosis.* Fat and elastic tissues disappear and are replaced with dense white fibrous trabeculae. The interstitial tissue is infiltrated with chronic inflammatory cells.
- *Hyperplasia* of epithelium in the lining of the ducts and acini may occur, with or without atypia.
- *Papillomatosis.* The epithelial hyperplasia may be so extensive that it results in papillomatous overgrowth within the ducts.

Clinical features

The symptoms of ANDI are many as the term is used to encompass a wide range of benign conditions, but often include an area of lumpiness (seldom discrete) and/or breast pain (mastalgia).

- A benign discrete lump in the breast is commonly a cyst or fibroadenoma. True lipomas occur rarely.
- Lumpiness may be bilateral, commonly in the upper outer quadrant or, less commonly, confined to one quadrant of one breast. The changes may be cyclical, with an increase in both lumpiness and often tenderness before a menstrual period.
- Non-cyclical mastalgia is more common in peri-menopausal than post-menopausal women. It may be associated with ANDI or with periductal mastitis. It should be distinguished from referred pain, for example a musculoskeletal disorder. 'Breast' pain in post-menopausal women not taking hormone-replacement therapy (HRT) is usually derived from the chest wall.

About 5% of breast cancers exhibit pain at presentation.

Treatment of lumpy breasts

If the clinician is confident that he or she is not dealing with a discrete abnormality (and clinical confidence is supported by mammography and/or ultrasound scanning if appropriate), then initially the woman can be offered firm reassurance. It is perhaps

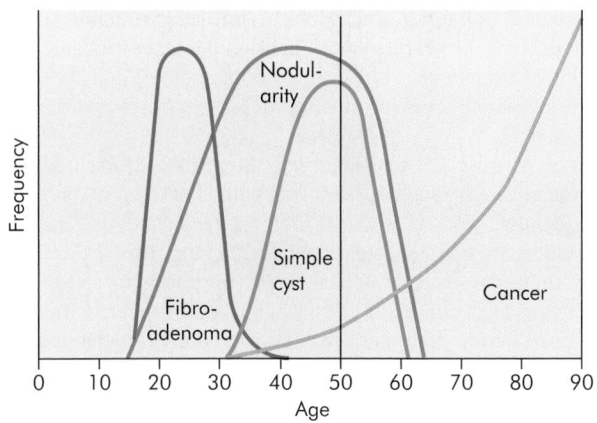

Figure 50.19 Normal breast changes throughout life. UK National Health Service Breast Screening Programme data.

worthwhile reviewing the patient at a different point in the menstrual cycle, for example 6 weeks after the initial visit, and often the clinical signs will have resolved by that time. There is a tendency for women with lumpy breasts to be rendered unnecessarily anxious and to be submitted to multiple random biopsies because the clinician lacks the courage of his or her convictions.

Treatment of mastalgia

Pronounced cyclical mastalgia may become a significant clinical problem if the pain and tenderness interfere with the woman's life, disturb her sleep and impair sexual activity. Initially, firm reassurance that the symptoms are not associated with cancer will help the majority of women. Acknowledgement that this is a real symptom, a non-dismissive attitude and an explanation of the aetiology are all helpful in managing this condition.

In the first instance, an appropriately fitting and supportive bra should be worn throughout the day and a soft bra (such as a sports bra) worn at night. Avoiding caffeine drinks is said to help, although the author remains unconvinced.

A patient symptom diary will help her to chart the pattern of pain throughout the month and thus determine whether this is cyclical mastalgia. This allows the majority of patients to adjust to the concept of a cyclical nature of their problem but, if reassurance is inadequate, then a planned escalation of treatment (Table 50.1) could be advised. Oil of evening primrose, in adequate doses given over 3 months, will help more than half of these women. It appears to achieve higher response rates in those over 40 years of age rather than younger women. For those with intractable symptoms, an anti-gonadotrophin, such as danazol, or a prolactin inhibitor, such as bromocriptine, may be tried. Very rarely it is necessary to prescribe an anti-oestrogen, for example

Table 50.1 Treatment of breast pain

Exclude cancer	
Reassure	Use pain chart if unsure if cyclical or non-cyclical. Also allows time for reassurance to become active!
Adequate support	Firm bra during the day and a softer bra at night
Exclude caffeine	Works for some although not very efficacious in author's practice
Consider medication	
Evening primrose oil (GLA)	Better effect in women over 40 years old than in younger women
Danazol, 100 mg t.d.s.	Start at 100 mg per day and increase (seldom used these days)
Tamoxifen	Not licensed for this indication but occasionally very helpful

tamoxifen, or a luteinising hormone-releasing hormone (LHRH) agonist to deprive the breast epithelium of oestrogenic drive. Ablative surgery should never be contemplated for breast pain and any patient seeking this treatment should be referred to a psychiatrist.

For non-cyclical mastalgia it is important to exclude extra-mammary causes such as chest wall pain. This is common in post-menopausal women who are not on HRT and the neck and shoulders are common sights of referred pain. It is seldom necessary these days to carry out a biopsy on a very localised tender area that might be harbouring a subclinical cancer as imaging is so much better. Treatment may be with non-steroidal analgesics or by injection with local anaesthetic on a 'trigger spot'.

Breast cysts

These occur most commonly in the last decade of reproductive life as a result of a non-integrated involution of stroma and epithelium. They are often multiple, may be bilateral and can mimic malignancy. Diagnosis can be confirmed by aspiration and/or ultrasound. They typically present suddenly and cause great alarm; prompt diagnosis and drainage provides immediate relief.

Treatment

A solitary cyst or small collection of cysts can be aspirated. If they resolve completely, and if the fluid is not blood-stained, no further treatment is required. However, 30% will recur and require reaspiration. Cytological examination of cyst fluid is no longer practised routinely. If there is a residual lump or if the fluid is blood-stained, a core biopsy or local excision for histological diagnosis is advisable, which is also the case if the cyst reforms repeatedly. This will exclude cystadenocarcinoma, which is more common in elderly women.

Galactocele

Galactocele, which is rare, usually presents as a solitary, sub-areolar cyst and always dates from lactation. It contains milk and in longstanding cases its walls tend to calcify.

Fibroadenoma

These usually arise in the fully developed breast between the ages of 15 and 25 years, although occasionally they occur in much older women. They arise from hyperplasia of a single lobule and usually grow up to 2–3 cm in size. They are surrounded by a well-marked capsule and can thus be enucleated through a cosmetically appropriate incision. A fibroadenoma does not require excision unless associated with suspicious cytology, it becomes very large or the patient expressly desires the lump to be removed.

Giant fibroadenomas occasionally occur during puberty. They are over 5 cm in diameter and are often rapidly growing but, in other respects, are similar to smaller fibroadenomas and can be enucleated through a submammary incision. They are more common in the Afro-Caribbean population.

Phyllodes tumour

These benign tumours, previously sometimes known as serocystic disease of Brodie or cystosarcoma phyllodes, usually occur in women over the age of 40 years but can appear in younger women. They present as a large, sometimes massive, tumour with an unevenly bosselated surface. Occasionally, ulceration of over-lying skin occurs because of pressure necrosis. Despite their size they remain mobile on the chest wall. Histologically, there is a wide variation in their appearance, with some of low malignant potential resembling a fibroadenoma and others having a higher mitotic index, which are histologically worrying. The latter may recur locally but, despite the name of cystosarcoma phyllodes, they are rarely cystic and only very rarely develop features of a sarcomatous tumour. These may metastasise via the bloodstream.

Treatment

Treatment for the benign type is enucleation in young women or wide local excision. Massive tumours, recurrent tumours and those of the malignant type will require mastectomy (Summary box 50.2).

Summary box 50.2

Benign breast disorder classification

Congenital disorders
- Inverted nipple
- Supernumerary breasts/nipples
- Non-breast disorders
- Tietze's disease (costochondritis)
- Sebaceous cysts and other skin conditions

Injury

Inflammation/infection

ANDI (aberations of normal differentiation and involution):
- Cyclical nodularity and mastalgia
- Cysts
- Fibroadenoma
Duct ectasia/periductal mastitis
Pregnancy-related:
- Galactocele
- Puerperal abscess

When the diagnosis of carcinoma is in doubt

There will always be cases when the clinician cannot be sure whether a particular lump in the breast is an area of mammary dysplasia, a benign tumour or an early carcinoma.

If there is doubt on clinical, cytological or radiological examination, it is essential to obtain a tissue diagnosis. This is often possible by needle biopsy. In the event of a negative result, open biopsy of the mass is necessary. Because of the possibility of reporting errors and because the histology is likely to be more difficult (if a diagnosis has not already been made), the author suggests that frozen-section reporting should be used rarely and certainly should not form the basis for a decision to undertake a mastectomy. Table 50.2 gives an algorithm for investigating any breast lump.

Risk of malignancy developing in association with benign breast pathology

The relative risks of malignancy developing according to different histological features found at biopsy are illustrated in Table 50.3.

Sir Benjamin Collins Brodie, **1783–1862, Surgeon, St. George's Hospital, London, England, described serocystic disease of the breast in 1840.**

Alexander Tietze, **1864–1927, Professor of Surgery, Breslau, Germany (now Wroclaw, Poland), described this condition in 1921.**

Table 50.2 Investigation of a breast lump (after imaging performed) using fine-needle aspiration with cytology

Cystic	Lump disappears; clear fluid (many colours)	Discharge patient
	Residual thickening; blood-stained fluid	Investigate – ?core biopsy
Solid	Benign	Offer excision or observe
	Atypical	Investigate – ?core biopsy
	Malignant	Treat for cancer

These were elucidated 30 years ago but remain pertinent and a recent single-centre review reinforces the conclusion that the histological classification of the benign lesion in combination with a family history of breast cancer are important predictors of risk.

CARCINOMA OF THE BREAST

Breast cancer is the most common cause of death in middle-aged women in western countries. In 2004 approximately one and a half million new cases were diagnosed worldwide. In England and Wales, 1 in 12 women will develop the disease during their lifetime.

Aetiological factors

Geographical
Carcinoma of the breast occurs commonly in the western world, accounting for 3–5% of all deaths in women. In developing countries it accounts for 1–3% of deaths.

Age
Carcinoma of the breast is extremely rare below the age of 20 years but, thereafter, the incidence steadily rises so that by the age of 90 years nearly 20% of women are affected.

Gender
Less than 0.5% of patients with breast cancer are male.

Genetic
It occurs more commonly in women with a family history of breast cancer than in the general population. Breast cancer related to a specific mutation accounts for about 5% of breast cancers yet has far-reaching repercussions in terms of counselling and tumour prevention in these women. This will be discussed more fully in a subsequent section.

Diet
Because breast cancer so commonly affects women in the 'developed' world, dietary factors may play a part in its causation. There is some evidence that there is a link with diets low in phytoestrogens. A high intake of alcohol is associated with an increased risk of developing breast cancer.

Endocrine
Breast cancer is more common in nulliparous women and breast-feeding in particular appears to be protective. Also protective is having a first child at an early age, especially if associated with late menarche and early menopause. It is known that in post-menopausal women, breast cancer is more common in the obese. This is thought to be because of an increased conversion of steroid hormones to oestradiol in the body fat. Recent studies have clarified the role of exogenous hormones, in particular the oral contraceptive pill and HRT, in the development of breast cancer. For most women the benefits of these treatments will far outweigh the small putative risk; however, long-term exposure to the combined preparation of HRT does significantly increase the risk of developing breast cancer.

Previous radiation
This was considered to be of historical interest, with the majority of women exposed to the atomic bombs at Hiroshima and

Table 50.3 Relative risk of invasive breast carcinoma based on pathological examination of benign breast tissue (American College of Pathologists Consensus Statement)[a]

No increased risk	Adenosis, sclerosing or florid
	Apocrine metaplasia
	Cysts, macro and/or micro
	Duct ectasia
	Fibroadenoma
	Fibrosis
	Hyperplasia
	Mastitis (inflammation)
	Periductal mastitis
	Squamous metaplasia
Slightly increased risk (1.5–2 times)	Hyperplasia, moderate or florid, solid or papillary
	Papilloma with a fibrovascular core
Moderately increased risk (5 times)	Atypical hyperplasia (ductal or lobular)
Insufficient data to assign a risk	Solitary papilloma of lactiferous sinus
	Radial scar lesion

After Page and Dupont (1978) by kind permission of the *Journal of the National Cancer Institute*, USA.
[a] A combination with positive family history significantly increases the risks shown above.

Nagasaki having died. It is, however, a real problem in women who have been treated with mantle radiotherapy as part of the management of Hodgkin's disease, in which significant doses of radiation to the breast are received. The risk appears about a decade after treatment and is higher if radiotherapy occurred during breast development. A surveillance programme has been organised in the UK with MRI and mammographic screening.

Pathology

Breast cancer may arise from the epithelium of the duct system anywhere from the nipple end of the major lactiferous ducts to the terminal duct unit, which is in the breast lobule. The disease may be entirely *in situ*, an increasingly common finding with the advent of breast cancer screening, or may be invasive cancer. The degree of differentiation of the tumour is usually described using three grades: well differentiated, moderately differentiated or poorly differentiated. Commonly, a numerical grading system based on the scoring of three individual factors (nuclear pleomorphism, tubule formation and mitotic rate) is used, with grade III cancers roughly equating to the poorly differentiated group.

Previously, descriptive terms were used to classify breast cancer ('scirrhous', meaning woody, or 'medullary', meaning brain-like). More recently, histological descriptions have been used. These have been shown to have clinical correlations in the way that the tumour behaves and are likely to be used for the near future. However, with the increasing application of molecular markers there will be a change in the way that breast cancers are classified and it is likely that much more information about an individual tumour will be routinely reported, such as its likelihood of metastasis and to which therapeutic agents it will be susceptible. Gene array analysis of breast cancers has identified five subtypes. Some of these correlate with known markers such as oestrogen receptor status. There are specific gene signatures that are said to correlate with response to chemotherapy or poor prognosis; trials based upon these differences are planned. A typical result of a multigene array is shown in Fig. 50. 20.

Current nomenclature

Ductal carcinoma is the most common variant with *lobular carcinoma* occurring in up to 15% of cases. There are subtypes of lobular cancer including the classical type, which carries a better prognosis than the pleomorphic type. Occasionally, the picture may be mixed with both ductal and lobular features. There are different patterns of spread depending on histological type. If there is doubt whether a tumour is predominantly lobular in type, immunohistochemical analysis using the e-cadherin antibody, which reacts positively in lobular cancer, will help in diagnosis.

Rarer histological variants, usually carrying a better prognosis, include *colloid carcinoma*, whose cells produce abundant mucin, *medullary carcinoma*, with solid sheets of large cells often associated with a marked lymphocytic reaction, and *tubular carcinoma*. Invasive lobular carcinoma is commonly multifocal and/or bilateral. Cases detected via the screening programme are often smaller and better differentiated than those presenting to the symptomatic service and are of a special type.

Inflammatory carcinoma is a fortunately rare, highly aggressive cancer that presents as a painful, swollen breast, which is warm with cutaneous oedema. This is the result of blockage of the subdermal lymphatics with carcinoma cells. Inflammatory cancer usually involves at least one-third of the breast and may mimic a breast abscess. A biopsy will confirm the diagnosis and show undifferentiated carcinoma cells. It used to be rapidly fatal but with aggressive chemotherapy and radiotherapy and with salvage surgery the prognosis has improved considerably.

In situ carcinoma is pre-invasive cancer that has not breached the epithelial basement membrane. This was previously a rare, usually asymptomatic, finding in breast biopsy specimens but is becoming increasingly common because of the advent of mammographic screening; it now accounts for over 20% of cancers detected by screening in the UK. *In situ* carcinoma may be ductal (DCIS) or lobular (LCIS), the latter often being multifocal and bilateral. Both are markers for the later development of invasive cancer, which will develop in at least 20% of patients. Although mastectomy is curative, this constitutes overtreatment in many cases. The best treatment for *in situ* carcinoma is the subject of a number of on-going clinical trials. DCIS may be classified using the Van Nuys system, which combines the patient's age, type of DCIS and presence of microcalcification, extent of resection margin and size of disease. Patients with a high score benefit from radiotherapy after excision, whereas those of low grade, whose tumour is completely excised, need no further treatment.

Staining for oestrogen and progesterone receptors is now considered routine, as their presence will indicate the use of adjuvant hormonal therapy with tamoxifen or the newer aromatase inhibitors (Fig 50.21). Tumours are also stained for c-erbB2 (a growth factor receptor) as patients who are positive can be treated with the monoclonal antibody trastuzumab (Herceptin), either in the adjuvant or relapse setting.

The pathologist is an important member of the breast cancer team and will increasingly help decide which adjuvant therapies will be appropriate.

Paget's disease of the nipple

Paget's disease of the nipple (Fig. 50.22a and b) is a superficial manifestation of an underlying breast carcinoma. It presents as an eczema-like condition of the nipple and areola, which persists despite local treatment. The nipple is eroded slowly and eventually disappears. If left, the underlying carcinoma will sooner or later become clinically evident. Nipple eczema should be biopsied if there is any doubt about its cause. Microscopically, Paget's disease is characterised by the presence of large, ovoid cells with

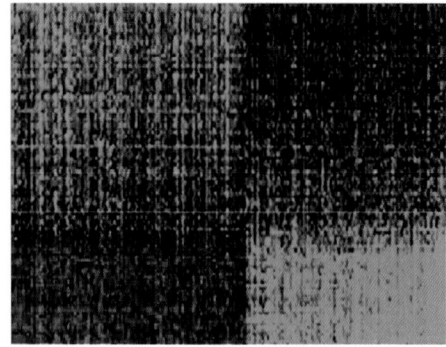

Figure 50.20 Gene array heat map of breast cancers.

Thomas Hodgkin, **1798–1866, Curator of the Museum, and Demonstrator of Morbid Anatomy, Guy's Hospital, London, England.**

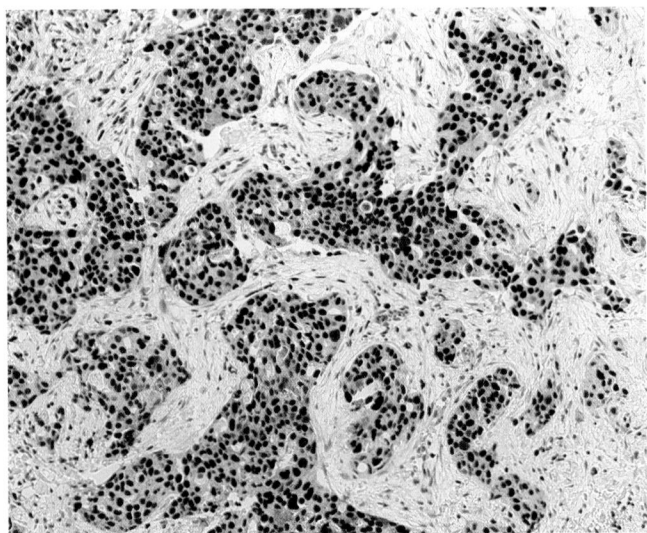

Figure 50.21 Immunohistochemical staining for oestrogen receptors.

abundant, clear, pale-staining cytoplasm in the Malpighian layer of the epidermis.

The spread of breast cancer

Local spread

The tumour increases in size and invades other portions of the breast. It tends to involve the skin and to penetrate the pectoral muscles and even the chest wall if diagnosed late.

Lymphatic metastasis

Lymphatic metastasis occurs primarily to the axillary and the internal mammary lymph nodes. Tumours in the posterior one-third of the breast are more likely to drain to the internal mammary nodes. The involvement of lymph nodes has both biological and chronological significance. It represents not only an evolutional event in the spread of the carcinoma but is also a marker for the metastatic potential of that tumour. Involvement of supraclavicular nodes and of any contralateral lymph nodes represents advanced disease.

Spread by the bloodstream

It is by this route that skeletal metastases occur, although the initial spread may be via the lymphatic system. In order of frequency the lumbar vertebrae, femur, thoracic vertebrae, rib and skull are affected and these deposits are generally osteolytic. Metastases may also commonly occur in the liver, lungs and brain and, occasionally, the adrenal glands and ovaries; they have, in fact, been described in most body sites.

Clinical presentation

Although any portion of the breast, including the axillary tail, may be involved, breast cancer is found most frequently in the upper outer quadrant (Figs 50.23 and 50.24). Most breast cancers will present as a hard lump, which may be associated with indrawing of the nipple. As the disease advances locally there may be skin involvement with peau d'orange (Fig. 50.25) or frank

Marcello Malpighi, 1628–1694, Professor of Physic successively at Bologna, Pisa and Messina, and in 1691 Physician to the Papal Court in Rome, Italy.
peau d'orange **is French for 'orange skin'.**

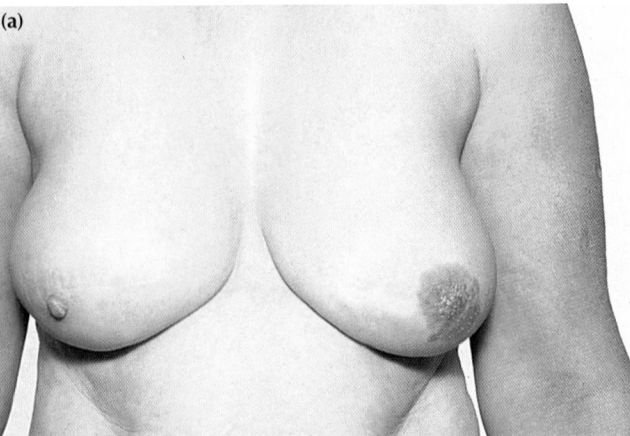

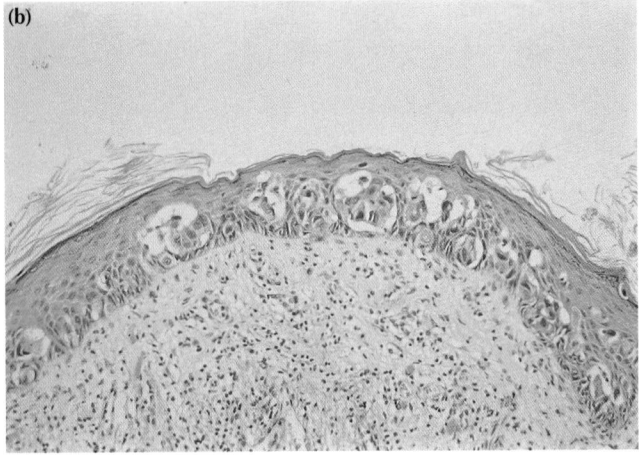

Figure 50.22 (a) Paget's disease of the nipple. (b) Histological appearance of Paget's disease.

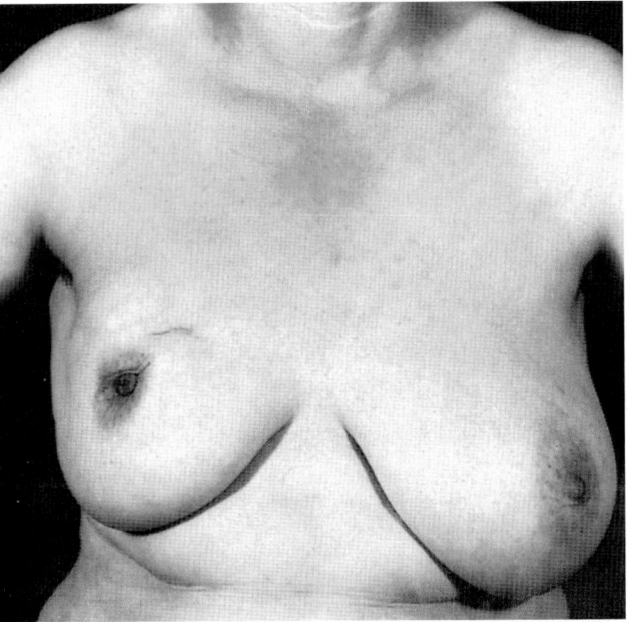

Figure 50.23 Invasive carcinoma of the right breast. Note the shrinking and elevation of the breast with nipple retraction.

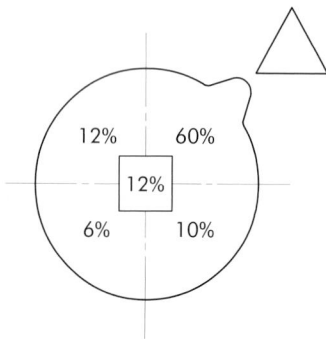

Figure 50.24 The relationship of carcinoma of the breast to the quadrants of the breast.

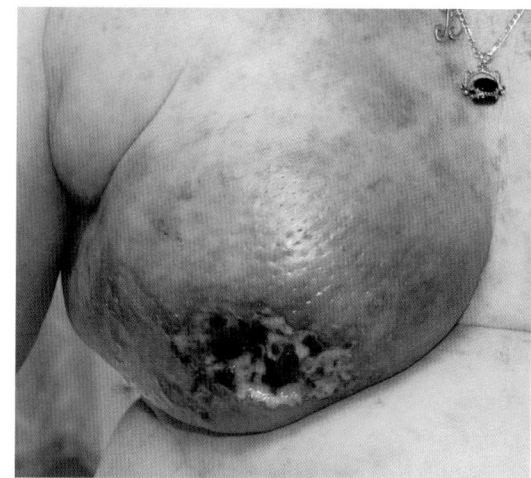

Figure 50.26 Ulcerated carcinoma of the right breast.

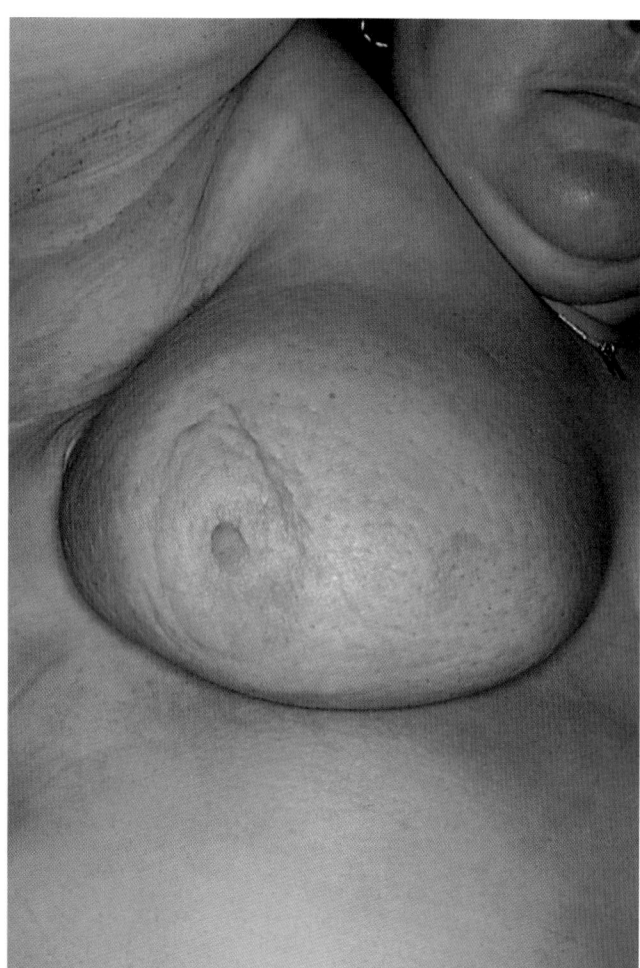

Figure 50.25 Peau d'orange of the breast.

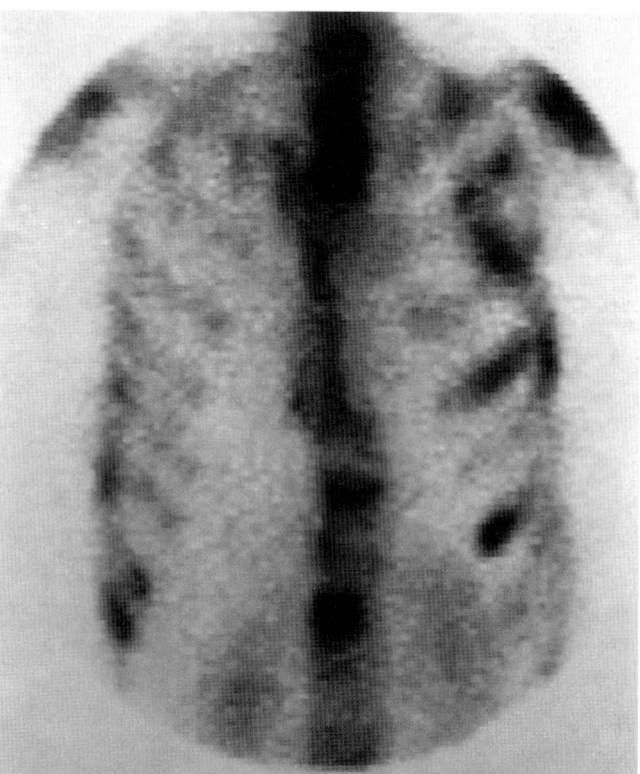

Figure 50.27 Skeletal isotope bone scan showing multiple 'hot-spots' due to metastases.

ulceration and fixation to the chest wall (Fig. 50.26). This is described as cancer-en-cuirasse when the disease progresses around the chest wall. About 5% of breast cancers in the UK will present with either locally advanced disease or symptoms of metastatic disease. This figure is much higher in the developing world. These patients must then undergo a staging evaluation so that the full extent of their disease can be ascertained. This will include a careful clinical examination, chest radiograph, computerised tomography (CT) of the chest and abdomen and an isotope bone scan (Fig. 50.27). This is important for both progno-

sis and treatment; a patient with widespread visceral metastases may obtain an increased length and quality of survival from systemic hormone therapy or chemotherapy but is unlikely to benefit from surgery as she will die from her metastases before local disease becomes a problem. In contrast, patients with relatively small tumours (< 5 cm in diameter) confined to the breast and ipsilateral lymph nodes rarely need staging beyond a good clinical examination as the pick-up rate for distant metastases is so low. Currently, a chest radiograph, full blood count and liver function tests are all that are recommended for screening of patients with early-stage breast cancer.

Staging of breast cancer

Classical staging of breast cancer by means of the TNM (tumour–node–metastasis) or UICC (Union Internationale Contre le Cancer) criteria is used less often as we gain more knowledge of the biological variables that affect prognosis. It is becoming increasingly clear that it is these factors (discussed in more detail below) rather than anatomical mapping that influence outcome and treatment. Perhaps a more pragmatic approach would be to classify patients according to the treatment that they require (Table 50.4). Treatment recommendations are summarised in consensus statements such as those from the American Society of Clinical Oncology (ASCO) and the St Gallen Conference.

Prognosis of breast cancer

The best indicators of likely prognosis in breast cancer remain tumour size and lymph node status; however, it is realised that some large tumours will remain confined to the breast for decades whereas some very small tumours are incurable at diagnosis. Hence, the prognosis of a cancer depends not on its chronological age but on its invasive and metastatic potential. In an attempt to define which tumours will behave aggressively, and thus require early systemic treatment, a host of prognostic factors have been described. These include the histological grade of the tumour, hormone receptor status, measures of tumour proliferation such as S-phase fraction, growth factor analysis and oncogene or oncogene product measurements. Many others are under investigation but have proved of little practical value in patient management. Prognostic indices (such as the Nottingham prognostic index) have combined these factors to allow subdivision of patients into discrete prognostic groups. More recently, a computer-aided program (adjuvant online; www.adjuvantonline.com) has been developed, which incorporates the putative benefits of treatment allowing oncologist and patient to visualise the benefits of therapy. There are commercial enterprises that are trying to combine a gene profile with classical prognostic indicators to give a recurrence score but these must be viewed as unproven at the moment. Other groups have developed 'gene signatures' said to be able to detect cancers of good or poor prognosis but there is little consistency between the various signatures developed by different groups and these approaches have not yet been translated into clinical practice.

Treatment of cancer of the breast

The two basic principles of treatment are to reduce the chance of local recurrence and the risk of metastatic spread. Treatment of early breast cancer will usually involve surgery with or without radiotherapy. Systemic therapy such as chemotherapy or hormone therapy is added if there are adverse prognostic factors such as lymph node involvement, indicating a high likelihood of metastatic relapse. At the other end of the spectrum, locally advanced or metastatic disease is usually treated by systemic therapy to palliate symptoms, with surgery playing a much smaller role. An algorithm for the management of breast cancer is shown in Summary box 50.3.

Summary box 50.3

Algorithm for management of operable breast cancer

Achieve local control

Appropriate surgery
- Wide local excision (clear margins) and radiotherapy, *or*
- Mastectomy ± radiotherapy (offer reconstruction – immediate or delayed)
- Combined with axillary procedure (see text)
- Await pathology and receptor measurements
- Use risk assessment tool; stage if appropriate

Treat risk of systemic disease
- Offer chemotherapy if prognostic factors poor; include Herceptin if Her-2 positive
- Radiotherapy as decided above
- Hormone therapy if oestrogen receptor or progesterone receptor positive

---

The multidisciplinary team approach

As in all branches of medicine, good doctor–patient communication plays a vital role in helping to alleviate patient anxiety. Participation of the patient in treatment decisions is of particular importance in breast cancer when there may be uncertainty as to the best therapeutic option and the desire to treat the patient within the protocol of a controlled clinical trial. As part of the preoperative and postoperative management of the patient it is often useful to employ the skills of a trained breast counsellor and also to have available advice on breast prostheses, psychological support and physiotherapy, when appropriate.

In many specialist centres the care of breast cancer patients is undertaken as a joint venture between the surgeon, medical oncologist, radiotherapist and allied health professionals such as the clinical nurse specialist. This has been shown to be good for the patient, to lead to higher trial entry and to improve the mental health of the professionals in the breast team. There are published guidelines for the optimal management of patients with breast cancer such as SIGN 84 (Scottish Intercollegiate Guidelines Network).

Table 50.4 A pragmatic classification of breast cancer

Group	Approximate 5-year survival rate	Example	Treatment
'Very low-risk' primary breast cancer	>90%	Screen-detected DCIS, tubular or special types	Local
'Low-risk' primary breast cancer	70–90%	Node negative with favourable histology	Locoregional with/without systemic
'High-risk' primary breast cancer	<70%	Node positive or unfavourable histology	Locoregional with systemic
Locally advanced	<30%	Large primary or inflammatory	Primary systemic
Metastatic	–	–	Primary systemic

DCIS, duct carcinoma *in situ*.

Local treatment of early breast cancer

Local control is achieved through surgery and/or radiotherapy (Summary box 50.4).

Summary box 50.4

Treatment of early breast cancer

The aims of treatment are:

- 'Cure': likely in some patients but late recurrence is possible
- Control of local disease in the breast and axilla
- Conservation of local form and function
- Prevention or delay of the occurrence of distant metastases

---

Surgery

Surgery still has a central role to play in the management of breast cancer but there has been a gradual shift towards more conservative techniques, backed up by clinical trials that have shown equal efficacy between mastectomy and local excision followed by radiotherapy.

It was initially hoped that avoiding mastectomy would help to alleviate the considerable psychological morbidity associated with breast cancer but recent studies have shown that over 30% of women develop significant anxiety and depression following both radical and conservative surgery. After mastectomy women tend to worry about the effect of the operation on their appearance and relationships, whereas after conservative surgery they may remain fearful of a recurrence.

Mastectomy is indicated for large tumours (in relation to the size of the breast), central tumours beneath or involving the nipple, multifocal disease, local recurrence or patient preference. The radical Halsted mastectomy, which included excision of the breast, axillary lymph nodes and pectoralis major and minor muscles, is no longer indicated as it causes excessive morbidity with no survival benefit. The modified radical (Patey) mastectomy is more commonly performed and is thus described below. Simple mastectomy involves removal of only the breast with no dissection of the axilla, except for the region of the axillary tail of the breast, which usually has attached to it a few nodes low in the anterior group.

Patey mastectomy The breast and associated structures are dissected *en bloc* (Fig. 50.28) and the excised mass is composed of:

- the whole breast;
- a large portion of skin, the centre of which overlies the tumour but which always includes the nipple;
- all of the fat, fascia and lymph nodes of the axilla.

The pectoralis minor muscle is either divided or retracted to gain access to the upper two-thirds of the axilla. The axillary vein and nerves to the serratus anterior and latissimus dorsi (the thoraco-dorsal trunk) should be preserved. The intercostal brachial nerves are usually divided in this operation and the

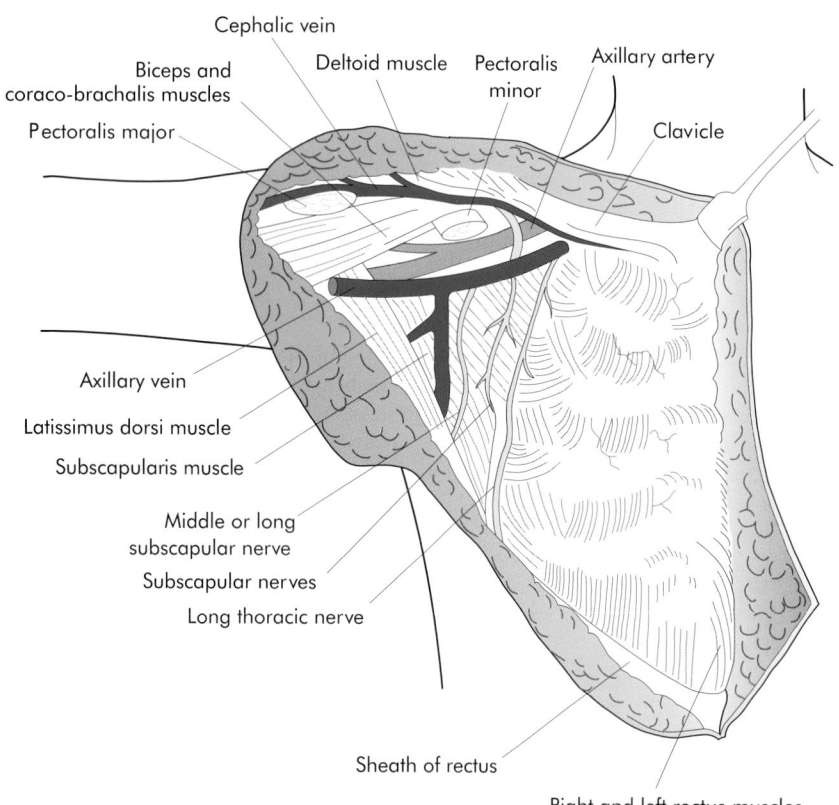

Figure 50.28 Radical mastectomy with pectoralis removed; the modified radical approach leaves the pectoralis major muscle intact.

William Stewart Halsted, 1852–1922, Professor of Surgery, Johns Hopkins Medical School, Baltimore, MD, USA.
David Howard Patey, 1899–1976, Surgeon, The Middlesex Hospital, London, England.

patient should be warned about sensation changes postoperatively.

The wound is drained using a wide-bore suction tube. Early mobilisation of the arm is encouraged and physiotherapy helps normal function to return very quickly; most patients are able to resume light work or housework within a few weeks.

Conservative breast cancer surgery This is aimed at removing the tumour plus a rim of at least 1 cm of normal breast tissue. This is commonly referred to as a wide local excision. The term lumpectomy should be reserved for an operation in which a benign tumour is excised and in which a large amount of normal breast tissue is not resected. A quadrantectomy involves removing the entire segment of the breast that contains the tumour. Both of these operations are usually combined with axillary surgery, usually via a separate incision in the axilla. There are various options that can be used to deal with the axilla, including sentinel node biopsy, sampling, removal of the nodes behind and lateral to the pectoralis minor (level II) or a full axillary dissection (level III).

There is a somewhat higher rate of local recurrence following conservative surgery, even if combined with radiotherapy, but the long-term outlook in terms of survival is unchanged. Local recurrence is more common in younger women and in those with high-grade tumours and involved resection margins. Patients whose margins are involved should have a further local excision (or a mastectomy) before going on to radiotherapy. Excision of a breast cancer without radiotherapy leads to an unacceptable local recurrence rate.

The role of axillary surgery is to stage the patient and to treat the axilla. The presence of metastatic disease within the axillary lymph nodes remains the best single marker for prognosis; however, treatment of the axilla does not affect long-term survival, suggesting that the axillary nodes act not as a 'reservoir' for disease but as a marker for metastatic potential. It used to be accepted that only pre-menopausal women should have their axilla staged by operation as there was a good case for giving chemotherapy to lymph node-positive patients; however, it is now clear that post-menopausal women also benefit from chemotherapy and so all patients require axillary surgery. In post-menopausal patients, tamoxifen was once given regardless of axillary lymph node status, but it is now known that all hormone receptor-positive patients, irrespective of age, benefit from this. If mastectomy is performed it is reasonable to clear the axilla as part of the operation, but if a wide local excision is planned the surgeon should dissect the axilla through a separate incision.

Axillary surgery should not be combined with radiotherapy to the axilla because of excess morbidity. Removal of the internal mammary lymph nodes is unnecessary.

Sentinel node biopsy This technique is currently becoming the standard of care in the management of the axilla in patients with clinically node-negative disease. The sentinel node is localised peroperatively by the injection of patent blue dye (Fig. 50.29) and radioisotope-labelled albumin in the breast. The recommended site of injection is in the subdermal plexus around the nipple although some still inject on the axillary side of the cancer. The marker passes to the primary node draining the area and is detected visually and with a hand-held gamma camera. The excised node can be sent for frozen-section histological analysis or touch imprint cytology (TIC) if preoperative diagnosis is sought. In some cases

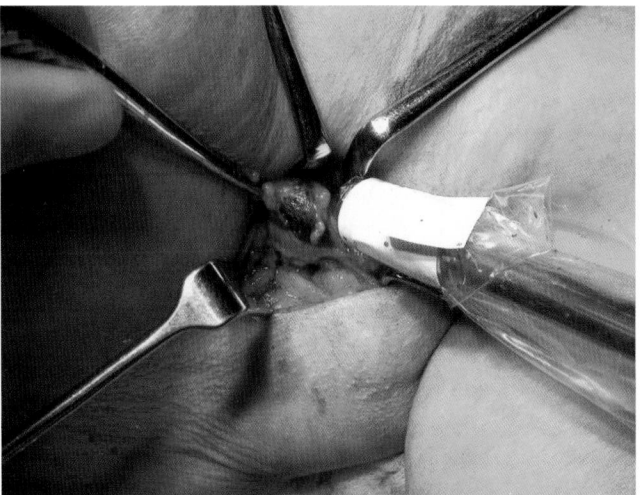

Figure 50.29 Sentinel node biopsy.

there are only subcapsular micrometastases that are missed at frozen section. In patients in whom there is no tumour involvement of the sentinel node, further axillary dissection can be avoided. A normogram outlining the chances of further axillary node positivity has been developed by the group at Memorial Sloan Kettering Hospital, New York, and is available on their website (www.mskcc.org/mskcc/html/15938.cfm).

Radiotherapy

Radiotherapy to the chest wall after mastectomy is indicated in selected patients in whom the risks of local recurrence are high. This includes patients with large tumours and those with large numbers of positive nodes or extensive lymphovascular invasion. There is some evidence that postoperative chest wall radiotherapy improves survival in women with node-positive breast cancer.

It is conventional to combine conservative surgery with radiotherapy to the remaining breast tissue. Recurrence rates are too high for treatment by local excision alone except in special cases (small node-negative tumours of a special type). Trials are under way to investigate whether radiotherapy can be given intraoperatively at one sitting or as an accelerated postoperative course. This would have considerable advantages in making conservative surgery available in areas where radiotherapy is not currently used. It would also relieve the burden of the current demand for radiotherapy, which accounts for up to 40% of activity in some departments.

Extrapolation from the Oxford overviews of systemic therapy (carried out every 5 years) suggests that for every four local recurrences one additional life will be spared at 15 years. This means that it is important to get the first treatments right and avoid local recurrence.

Adjuvant systemic therapy

Over the last 25 years there has been a revolution in our understanding of the biological nature of carcinoma of the breast. It is now widely accepted that the outcomes of treatment are predetermined by the extent of micrometastatic disease at the time of diagnosis. Variations in the radical extent of local therapy might influence local relapse but probably do not alter long-term mortality from the disease. However, systemic therapy targeted at these putative micrometastases might be expected to delay relapse and prolong survival. As a result of many international clinical trials and recent world overview analyses it can be stated with statistical confidence that the appropriate use of adjuvant chemotherapy or hormone therapy will improve relapse-free survival by approximately 30%, which ultimately translates into an absolute improvement in survival of the order of 10% at 15 years. Bearing in mind how common the disease is in northern Europe and the USA, these figures are of major public health importance.

Who to treat and with what are still questions for which absolute answers have yet to found, but the data from the overviews of recent trials show that lymph node-positive and many higher risk node-negative women should be recommended adjuvant combined chemotherapy. Women with hormone receptor-positive tumours will obtain a worthwhile benefit from about 5 years of endocrine therapy, either 20 mg daily of tamoxifen if pre-menopausal or the newer aromatase inhibitors (anastrozole, letrozole and exemestane) if post-menopausal. It is no longer appropriate to give hormone therapy to women who do not have oestrogen or progesterone receptor-positive disease.

Hormone therapy

Tamoxifen has been the most widely used 'hormonal' treatment in breast cancer. Its efficacy as an adjuvant therapy was first reported in 1983 and it has now been shown to reduce the annual rate of recurrence by 25%, with a 17% reduction in the annual rate of death. The beneficial effects of tamoxifen in reducing the risk of tumours in the contralateral breast have also been observed, as has its role as a preventative agent (IBIS-I and NSABP-P1 trials). Trials studying the optimal duration of treatment suggest that 5 years of treatment is preferable to 2 years.

Other hormonal agents that are also beneficial as adjuvant therapy have been developed. These include the LHRH agonists, which induce a reversible ovarian suppression and thus have the same beneficial effects as surgical or radiation-induced ovarian ablation in pre-menopausal receptor-positive women, and the oral aromatase inhibitors for post-menopausal women. The latter group of compounds are now licensed for treatment of recurrent disease, in which they have been shown to be superior to tamoxifen. A large trial comparing anastrazole to tamoxifen in the adjuvant setting has shown a beneficial effect for the aromatase inhibitor in terms of relapse-free survival, although the data are still immature for overall survival. There is an additional reduction in contralateral disease, which makes this drug suitable for a study of prevention, and the side-effect profile is different from that of tamoxifen. However, it is currently considerably more expensive.

Chemotherapy

Chemotherapy using a first-generation regimen such as a 6-monthly cycle of cyclophosphamide, methotrexate and 5-fluorouracil (CMF) will achieve a 25% reduction in the risk of relapse over a 10- to 15-year period. It is important to understand that this 25% reduction refers to the likelihood of an event happening. For example, a woman with a 96% chance of survival at, say, 5 years only has a 4% chance of death over this time and the absolute benefit from chemotherapy would be an increase in survival rate of 1%, to 97%. This would not be a sufficient gain to offset the side-effects of this potentially toxic therapy. However, for a woman with a 60% chance of dying (40% survival rate) a 25% reduction in risk would increase her likelihood of survival to 55% and thus treatment would be worthwhile. CMF is no longer

considered adequate adjuvant chemotherapy and modern regimens include an anthracycline (doxorubicin or epirubicin) and the newer agents such as the taxanes.

Chemotherapy was once confined to pre-menopausal women with a poor prognosis (in whom its effects are likely to be the result, in part, of a chemical castration effect) but is being increasingly offered to post-menopausal women with poor-prognosis disease as well. Chemotherapy may be considered in node-negative patients if other prognostic factors, such as tumour grade, imply a high risk of recurrence. The effect of combining hormone and chemotherapy is additive although hormone therapy is started after completion of chemotherapy to reduce side-effects.

High-dose chemotherapy with stem cell rescue for patients with heavy lymph node involvement has now been shown in controlled trials to offer no advantage and has been abandoned.

Primary chemotherapy (neoadjuvant) is being used in many centres for large but operable tumours that would traditionally require a mastectomy (and almost certainly postoperative adjuvant chemotherapy). The aim of this treatment is to shrink the tumour to enable breast-conserving surgery to be performed. This approach is successful in up to 80% of cases but is not associated with improvements in survival compared with conventionally timed chemotherapy. For older patients with breast cancers strongly positive for hormone receptors a similar effect can be seen with 3 months of endocrine treatment.

Newer 'biological' agents will be used more frequently as molecular targets are identified – the first of these, trastuzamab (Herceptin), is active against tumours containing the growth factor receptor c-erbB2. Other agents currently available include bevacizumab, a vascular growth factor receptor inhibitor, and lapitinab, a combined growth factor receptor inhibitor. It is unclear how and when these agents will be used, whether in combination or instead of standard chemotherapy agents.

Follow-up of breast cancer

Patients with breast cancer used to be followed for life to detect recurrence and dissemination. This led to large clinics with little value for either patient or doctor. It is current practice to arrange yearly or 2-yearly mammography of the treated and contralateral breast. There is a move to return the patient early to the care of the general practitioner with fast-track access back to the breast clinic if suspicious symptoms appear. There is currently no routine role for repeated measurements of tumour markers or imaging other than mammography.

Phenomena resulting from lymphatic obstruction in advanced breast cancer

Peau d'orange

Peau d'orange is caused by cutaneous lymphatic oedema. Where the infiltrated skin is tethered by the sweat ducts it cannot swell, leading to an appearance like orange skin. Occasionally, the same phenomenon is seen over a chronic abscess.

Late oedema of the arm is a troublesome complication of breast cancer treatment, fortunately seen less often now that radical axillary dissection and radiotherapy are rarely combined. However, it does still occur occasionally after either mode of treatment alone and appears at any time from months to years after treatment. There is usually no precipitating cause but recurrent tumour should be excluded because neoplastic infiltration of the axilla can cause arm swelling as a result of both lymphatic and venous blockage. This neoplastic infiltration is often painful because of brachial plexus nerve involvement.

An oedematous limb is susceptible to bacterial infections following quite minor trauma and these require vigorous antibiotic treatment. Antibiotics may need to be given for much longer than is normal and patients at risk of infection should have antibiotics readily available to enable treatment to be started promptly. Treatment of late oedema is difficult but limb elevation, elastic arm stockings and pneumatic compression devices can be useful.

Cancer-en-cuirasse

The skin of the chest is infiltrated with carcinoma and has been likened to a coat. It may be associated with a grossly swollen arm. This usually occurs in cases with local recurrence after mastectomy and is occasionally seen to follow the distribution of irradiation to the chest wall. The condition may respond to palliative systemic treatment but prognosis in terms of survival is poor.

Lymphangiosarcoma

Lymphangiosarcoma is a rare complication of lymphoedema with an onset many years after the original treatment. It takes the form of multiple subcutaneous nodules in the upper limb and must be distinguished from recurrent carcinoma of the breast. The prognosis is poor but some cases respond to cytotoxic therapy or irradiation. Interscapulothoracic (forequarter) amputation is rarely indicated.

Breast reconstruction

Despite an increasing trend towards conservative surgery, up to 50% of women still require, or want, a mastectomy. These women can now be offered immediate or delayed reconstruction of the breast. Few contraindications to breast reconstruction exist. Even those with a limited life expectancy may benefit from the improved quality of life; however, patients do require counselling before this procedure so that their expectations of cosmetic outcome are not unrealistic.

The easiest type of reconstruction is using a silicone gel implant under the pectoralis major muscle. This may be combined with prior tissue expansion using an expandable saline prosthesis first (or a combined device), which creates some ptosis of the new breast. If the skin at the mastectomy site is poor (e.g. following radiotherapy) or if a larger volume of tissue is required, a musculocutaneous flap can be constructed either from the latissimus dorsi muscle (an LD flap) (Fig. 50.30) or using the transversus abdominis muscle (a TRAM flap as shown in Fig. 50.31). The latter gives an excellent cosmetic result in experienced hands but is a lengthy procedure and requires careful patient selection. It is now usually performed as a free transfer using microvascular anastomosis, although the pedicled TRAM from the contralateral side is still used. Variations on the TRAM flap requiring less muscle harvesting, such as the DIEP flap (based on deep inferior epigastric vessels), are increasingly being used.

The timing of reconstruction is difficult. Impediments to immediate reconstruction include insufficient theatre time and a lack of experienced reconstructive surgeons. In addition, if a patient is likely to need postoperative radiotherapy then a delayed reconstruction using a flap often gives a better result.

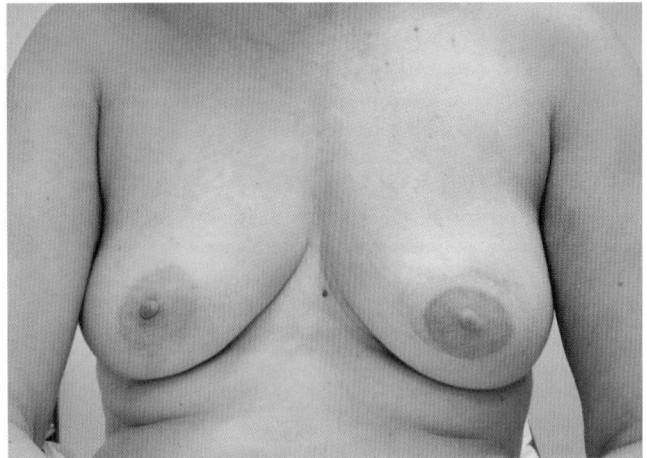

Figure 50.30 Reconstruction with latissimus dorsi flap.

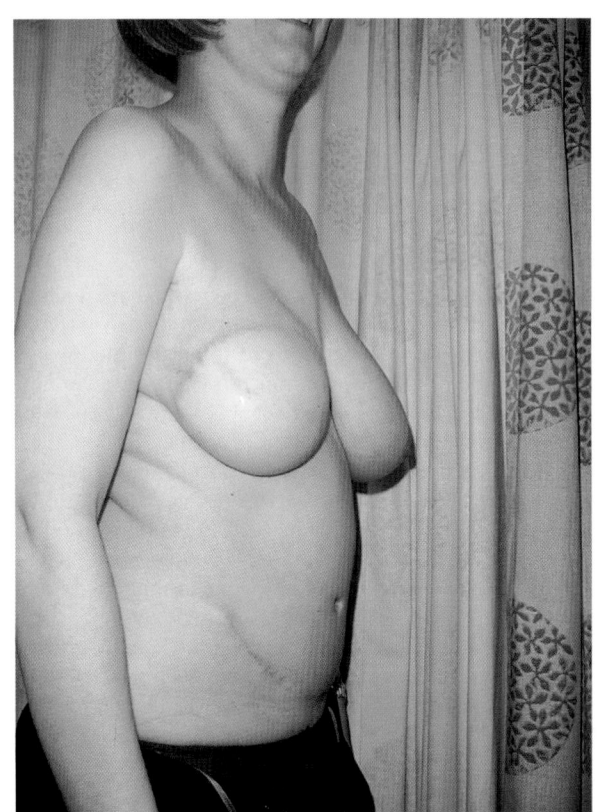

Figure 50.31 Transversus abdominus muscle flap.

Radiotherapy onto a prosthesis often leads to a high incidence of capsular contracture and unacceptable results.

Nipple reconstruction is a relatively simple procedure that can be performed under a local anaesthetic. Many different types of nipple reconstruction are described but the majority lose height with time. Tattooing of the reconstructed nipple is often required. Alternatively, the patient can be fitted with a prosthetic nipple. To achieve symmetry the opposite breast may require a cosmetic procedure such as reduction or augmentation mammoplasty, or mastopexy. A breast reconstructive service can be offered by a suitably trained breast surgeon, a plastic surgeon or, ideally, using a combined oncoplastic approach. The patient needs to be warned that breast reconstruction is seldom, if ever, one operation.

External breast prostheses that fit within the bra are the most common method of restoring volume fill and should be available for all women who do not have an immediate reconstruction.

Screening for breast cancer

Because the prognosis of breast cancer is closely related to stage at diagnosis it would seem reasonable to hope that a population screening programme that could detect tumours before they come to the patient's notice might reduce mortality from breast cancer. Indeed, a number of studies have shown that breast screening by mammography in women over the age of 50 years will reduce cause-specific mortality by up to 30%. Following the publication in 1987 of the Forrest report, the National Health Service in the UK launched a programme of 3-yearly mammographic screening for women between the ages of 50 and 64 years (now increased to 70 years). The introduction of this programme has undoubtedly improved the quality of breast cancer services but a number of questions remain unanswered, including the value of screening women under 50 years and the ideal interval between screenings. The psychological consequences of false alarms or false reassurances still need to be addressed and self-examination programmes that have failed to show any benefit for the population in terms of earlier detection of or decreased mortality from breast cancer remain controversial.

Familial breast cancer

Recent developments in molecular genetics and the identification of a number of breast cancer predisposition genes (*BRCA1*, *BRCA2* and *p53*) have done much to stimulate interest in this area. Yet women whose breast cancer is due to an inherited genetic change actually account for less than 5% of all cases of breast cancer, that is about 1250 cases per year in the UK and 9000 cases in the USA. A much larger number of women will have a risk that is elevated above normal because of an as yet unspecified familial inheritance. These women have a risk of developing breast cancer that is 2–10 times above baseline. The risks associated with family history are summarised in Table 50.5.

The *BRCA1* gene has been cloned and is located on the long arm of chromosome 17 (17q). The gene frequency in the population is approximately 0.0006. It does, however, occur with greater frequency in certain populations such as Ashkenazi Jews, in

whom there is often a common (founder) mutation. *BRCA2* is located on chromosome 13q and there is an association with male breast cancer. Women who are thought to be gene carriers may be offered breast screening (and ovarian screening in the case of *BRCA1*, which is known to impart a 50% lifetime risk of ovarian cancer), usually as part of a research programme, or genetic counselling and mutation analysis. Those who prove to be 'gene positive' have a 50–80% risk of developing breast cancer, predominantly while pre-menopausal. Many will opt for prophylactic mastectomy. Although this does not completely eliminate the risk, it does reduce it considerably. This work should be carried out in specialist centres.

For the great majority of women with a positive family history, who are unlikely to be carriers of a breast cancer gene, there are no currently proven breast cancer screening manoeuvres, although this is under investigation. Tamoxifen given for 5 years appears to reduce the risk of breast cancer by 30–50% and newer agents are currently under trial. Thus, these women are best served by being assessed and followed-up, preferably in a properly organised family history clinic.

Pregnancy

The effects of pregnancy on breast cancer are not well studied but it is thought that breast cancer presenting during pregnancy or lactation tends to be at a later stage, presumably because the symptoms are masked by the pregnancy; however, in other respects it behaves in a similar way to breast cancer in a non-pregnant young woman and should be treated accordingly. Thus, treatment is similar with some provisos: radiotherapy should be avoided during pregnancy, making mastectomy a more frequent option than breast conservation surgery; chemotherapy should be avoided during the first trimester but appears safe subsequently; most tumours are hormone receptor negative and so hormone treatment, which is potentially teratogenic, is not required. Becoming pregnant subsequent to a diagnosis of breast cancer appears not to alter the likely outcome, but women are usually advised to wait at least 2 years as it is within this time that recurrence most often occurs. The risk of developing breast cancer with oral contraceptive use is only slight, and disappears 10 years after stopping the oral contraceptive pill.

Hormone replacement therapy

HRT does increase the risk of developing breast cancer if taken for prolonged periods and in certain high-risk groups. HRT may also prolong symptoms of benign breast disorders such as cysts and mastalgia and make mammographic appearances more difficult to interpret.

Patients who develop breast cancer while on HRT appear to have a more favourable prognosis. The consequences in terms of recurrence in women using HRT following breast cancer are unknown.

Treatment of advanced breast cancer

Breast cancer may occasionally present as metastatic disease without evidence of a primary tumour (that is with an occult primary). The diagnosis is made partly by exclusion of another site for the primary tumour and may be confirmed by histology with special immunohistological stains of the metastatic lesions. Management should be aimed at palliation of the symptoms and treatment of the breast cancer, usually by endocrine manipulation with or without radiotherapy.

Table 50.5 Likelihood of genetic mutation with family history

No. of family cases < 50 years old	*BRCA1* (%)[a]	*BRCA2* (%)[b]
2	4	3
3	17	13
4	41	33
5	55	44

[a] BRCA1 is also associated with ovarian and, to a lesser extent, colorectal and prostate cancer.
[b] BRCA2 is associated with familial male breast cancer.

Sir Andrew Patrick McEwen Forrest, **Regius Professor of Clinical Surgery, The University of Edinburgh, Edinburgh, Scotland.**
Ashkenazi Jews **are Jews of Eastern or Central European descent.**

Locally advanced inoperable breast cancer

Locally advanced inoperable breast cancer, including inflammatory breast cancer, is usually treated with systemic therapy, either chemotherapy or hormone therapy.

Occasionally, 'toilet mastectomy' or radiotherapy is required to control a fungating tumour but often incision through microscopically permeated tissues results in a worse outcome.

Metastatic carcinoma of the breast

Metastatic carcinoma of the breast will also require palliative systemic therapy to alleviate symptoms. Hormone manipulation is often the first-line treatment because of its minimal side-effects. It is particularly useful for bony metastases. However, only about 30% of these tumours will be hormone responsive and, unfortunately, in time even these will become resistant to treatment. First-line hormone therapy for post-menopausal women is now anastrazole or one of the other third-generation aromatase inhibitors. Tamoxifen, ovarian suppression by surgery (for premenopausal women), radiotherapy and medical treatment are all in common use. When resistance to these has developed, other hormonal agents can prove useful, with about one-half of the response rate seen in the first-line therapy. The newer agents such as anti-progestins, pure anti-oestrogens and growth factor tyrosine kinase inhibitors are all candidates for this role.

Cytotoxic therapy is used particularly in younger women or those with visceral metastases and rapidly growing tumours. A variety of regimens is available and, although none prolongs survival, contrary to expectations, quality of life and symptom control is often better with more aggressive treatments, with responses being seen in up to 70% of patients.

Local treatment may also prove useful for some metastatic disease such as radiotherapy for painful bony deposits and internal fixation of pathological fractures.

THE MALE BREAST

Gynaecomastia

Idiopathic

Hypertrophy of the male breast may be unilateral or bilateral. The breasts enlarge at puberty and sometimes present the characteristics of female breasts (Fig. 50.32).

Hormonal

Enlargement of the breasts often accompanied stilbestrol therapy for prostate cancer, now rarely used. It may also occur as a result of a teratoma of the testis, in anorchism and after castration. Rarely, it may be a feature of ectopic hormonal production in bronchial carcinoma and in adrenal and pituitary disease. Body builders may use steroids to improve their physique, which may cause gynaecomastia. Some even go so far as to take tamoxifen to mask this symptom.

Associated with leprosy

Gynaecomastia is very common in men suffering from leprosy. This is possibly because of bilateral testicular atrophy, which is a frequent accompaniment of leprosy.

Associated with liver failure

Gynaecomastia sometimes occurs in patients with cirrhosis as a result of failure of the liver to metabolise oestrogens. It is

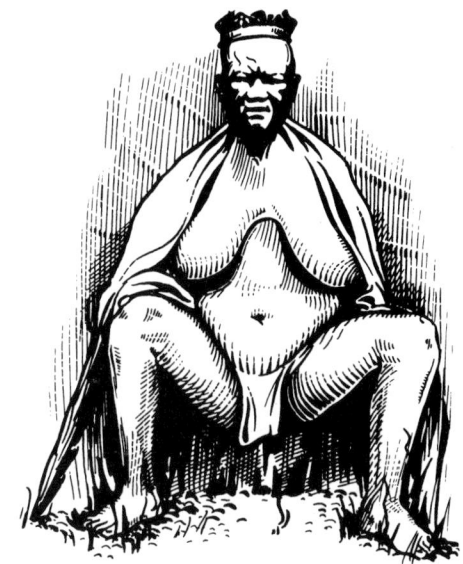

Figure 50.32 Chief Chengwayo, from a photograph by Schujelot.

associated with drugs that interfere with the hepatic metabolism of oestrogens. It is also seen with certain drugs such as cimetidine, digitalis and spironolactone.

Associated with Klinefelter syndrome

Gynaecomastia may occur in patients with Klinefelter's syndrome, a sex chromosome anomaly having 47XXY trisomy.

Treatment

Provided that the patient is healthy and comparatively young, reassurance may be sufficient. If not, mastectomy with

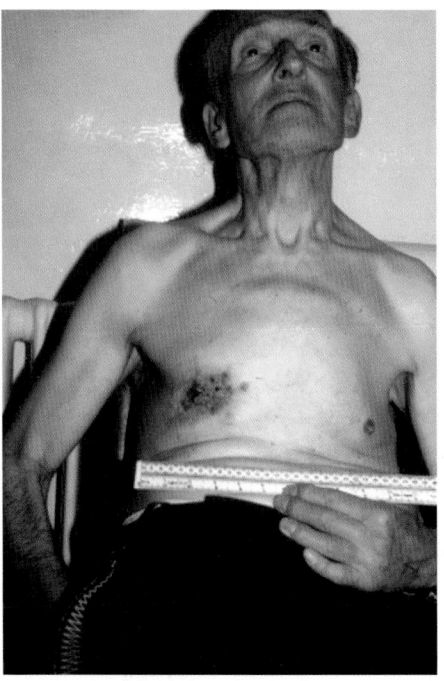

Figure 50.33 Carcinoma of the male breast.

Harry Fitch Klinefelter, Jr., **B. 1912, Physician of Baltimore, MD, USA, described this syndrome in 1942.**

preservation of the areola and nipple can be performed. The patient must be warned about the side-effects of this procedure, which are common and a cause of many medico-legal complaints in the UK.

Carcinoma of the male breast

Carcinoma of the male breast (Fig. 50.33) accounts for less than 0.5% of all cases of breast cancer. The known predisposing causes include gynaecomastia and excess endogenous or exogenous oestrogen. As in the female it tends to present as a lump and is most commonly an infiltrating ductal carcinoma.

Treatment

Stage for stage the treatment is the same as for carcinoma in the female breast and prognosis depends upon stage at presentation. Adequate local excision, because of the small size of the breast, should always be with a 'mastectomy'.

OTHER TUMOURS OF THE BREAST

Lipoma

A true lipoma is very rare.

Sarcoma of the breast

Sarcoma of the breast is usually of the spindle-cell variety and accounts for 0.5% of malignant tumours of the breast. Some of these growths arise in an intracanalicular fibroadenoma or may follow previous radiotherapy, e.g. for Hodgkin's lymphoma, many years previously. It may be impossible to distinguish clinically a sarcoma of the breast from a medullary carcinoma, but areas of cystic degeneration suggest a sarcoma and on incising the neoplasm it is pale and friable. Sarcoma tends to occur in younger women between the ages of 30 and 40 years. Treatment is by simple mastectomy followed by radiotherapy. The prognosis depends on the stage and histological type.

Metastases

On rare occasions cancer elsewhere may present with a metastasis in the breast. The breast is also occasionally infiltrated by Hodgkin's disease and other lymphomas.

FURTHER READING

Harris, J.R., Lippman, M., Morrow, M. and Hellman, S. (2006) *Diseases of the Breast*. Lippincott, Philadelphia, PA.

Hughes, L.E., Mansel, R.E. and Webster, D.J.T. (1989) *Benign Disorders and Diseases of the Breast*, 2nd edn. Baillière Tindall, London.

Sainsbury, R. (2006) Breast operations. In: Kirk, R. (ed.), *General Surgical Operations*. Churchill Livingstone.

SIGN 84 Management of breast cancer in women. A national clinical guideline. Available online at: www.sign.ac.uk

Cardiac surgery

INTRODUCTION

In 1925 Sir Henry Souttar reported the first mitral commissurotomy in the *British Medical Journal*. He wrote that the heart should be as amenable to surgery as any other organ and that many of the problems in heart disease were, to a large extent, mechanical. He saw the main problem as being maintenance of blood flow, particularly to the brain, while surgery was being performed. The first real advances occurred in the late 1940s and early 1950s, driven by surgeons who had gained confidence and experience under the pressures and opportunities provided by war. Further progress waited upon the development of cardiopulmonary bypass in the mid-1950s. Now the number, range and technical complexity of heart operations are remarkable; with the heart restored to good working order, the well-being and lifespan of patients with congenital, valvular and degenerative heart disease can be very much improved.

CARDIOPULMONARY BYPASS

Introduction

Cardiopulmonary bypass (CPB) was first used successfully in 1953 by Gibbon and has revolutionised cardiac surgical practice. It can be employed in any procedure in which the heart and lungs need to be stopped temporarily and their function replaced by artificial means (Box 51.1). Before Gibbon's work, valve surgery under direct vision would not have been possible nor would the precise reconstructions needed to treat extensive coronary artery disease. Much of the success of modern CPB is attributable to the development of new biomaterials and sophisticated oxygenating devices as well as a greater understanding of the pathophysiological consequences of CPB (Summary box 15.1).

Sir Henry Sessions Souttar, **1875–1964**, Surgeon, The London Hospital, London, England.
John Heysham Gibbon, **1903–1973**, worked at Jefferson University, Philadelphia, PA, USA.

Summary box 51.1

Alternative uses of CPB

- Rewarming from profound hypothermia
- Resuscitation in severe respiratory failure
- As an adjunct in pulmonary embolectomy
- In single- and double-lung transplantation
- In cardiopulmonary trauma
- In certain non-cardiac surgical procedures:
  Resection of highly vascular tumours
  Large complex arteriovenous malformations
  Tumours invading large blood vessels (e.g. renal or hepatic tumours extending into the inferior vena cava, right atrium or even pulmonary arteries)

Surgical approach to the heart

For most operations, the heart is approached by a median sternotomy. An incision is made from the jugular or suprasternal notch to the lower end of the xiphisternum. The sternum is divided and retracted to expose the thymus superiorly and the pericardium inferiorly. The thymus, although atrophic in adults, often remains relatively vascular. The thymus and pleurae are dissected from the pericardium, and the pericardium is opened. Before cannulation for CPB, the patient is fully heparinised.

Initiating cardiopulmonary bypass

Arterial cannulation

Conventionally, the great vessels are exposed and an aortic perfusion cannula is inserted into the ascending aorta, held in place by the purse-string suture. Air is excluded and the cannula connected to the bypass circuit. Alternatively, when it is inadvisable (aortic dissection), impractical (aortic root surgery) or impossible (severe adhesions) to cannulate the aorta, femorofemoral bypass can be employed. Arterial return is via the femoral artery.

Venous cannulation

A second purse-string suture is inserted into the right atrium by the appendage. A single 'two-stage' venous cannula placed in the right atrium establishes venous drainage. The venous pipe has end holes that sit in the inferior vena cava and side holes that sit in the right atrium (to take the drainage from the superior vena cava). Alternatively, the superior and inferior vena cavae may be cannulated separately to gain better control over the venous return and to facilitate surgery within the right atrium. Femorofemoral bypass with venous drainage from the femoral vein offers an alternative, particularly during thoracic aortic procedures.

Cardiopulmonary bypass circuit

Once the circuit is connected (Fig. 51.1) the CPB machine (the 'pump') takes over circulation and ventilation. Blood is pumped from a venous reservoir and oxygenated with a membrane oxygenator that allows gas exchange across a silicone membrane. To reduce the metabolic demands of the tissues the core systemic temperature may be lowered by passing the returning blood through a heat exchanger. The degree of cooling is according to the severity and complexity of the surgical procedure, as well as the surgeon's preference. The blood is also filtered to remove particulate emboli and infused back into the systemic arterial circulation via a roller pump. This returns blood to the patient at an even arterial perfusion pressure. The surgeon can now isolate the heart from the rest of the circulation with suction pumps to keep the area around the heart clear of blood. A vent suction pump may be used to decompress the heart.

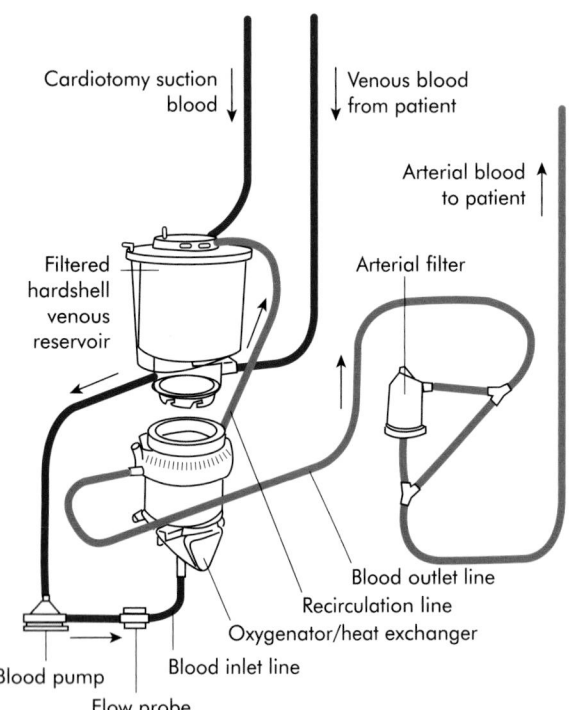

Figure 51.1 Components of the cardiopulmonary bypass (CPB) circuit. [Reproduced from Abraham, J.K. (2000) Cardiopulmonary bypass. *Surgery* **18**: 11, with permission from The Medical Publishing Company.]

Myocardial protection

To obtain a bloodless operative field, the ascending aorta is usually cross-clamped once CPB has been established and blood is diverted away from the heart. The heart ceases to eject and, as a result of inhibition of coronary blood flow, becomes anoxic. Permanent myocardial damage will develop within 30–45 min. Therefore, most cardiac operations require some form of myocardial protection. Techniques of myocardial protection and the operative management of the myocardium have had a significant impact on the complexity of cardiac surgery. The methods of myocardial protection include intracoronary infusion of a cardioplegic solution, intermittent cross-clamp fibrillation and total circulatory arrest.

Cardioplegic solutions vary in terms of temperature, pH, arresting agent, osmolality, presence of red cells and other factors. Most solutions contain potassium as the arresting agent. Potassium arrests the heart in diastole by depolarisation of the membrane. Cold (4–10°C) isotonic crystalloid or chilled blood solutions aid myocardial protection by reducing metabolic requirements through local hypothermia.

Intermittent cross-clamp fibrillation is a technique in which intermittent ventricular fibrillation is induced by a small electrical charge. The heart does not eject and is relatively still but not bloodless. The aorta is cross-clamped to render the heart ischaemic. The heart can tolerate short periods (10–20 min) of intermittent ischaemia, providing the heart is reperfused when the cross-clamp is released and allowed to beat following cardioversion for short periods during the operation.

Total circulatory arrest becomes a necessity when visibility and clarity of the operative area is crucial, as in paediatric surgery or in surgery of the ascending aorta and arch of the aorta. CPB is instituted and core systemic temperature reduced to 15–18°C (profound hypothermia). The metabolic rate of all organs of the body is reduced by 50% with every 7°C drop in temperature. So, with the pump switched off at 18°C, circulatory arrest can be tolerated for 20–30 min. Additional cerebral protection can be provided with ice packs placed around the head. Retrograde and antegrade cerebral perfusion techniques can also be used.

Discontinuing cardiopulmonary bypass

At the end of the procedure, air must be meticulously excluded from the cardiac chambers. Once perfusion is restored to the coronary arteries the heart may beat spontaneously or, if ventricular fibrillation is present, it may require a shock by a direct current (DC). Epicardial pacing wires may be placed to treat postoperative bradycardia or heart block. The patient is rewarmed, acidosis or hypokalaemia is corrected, and ventilation is restarted. The heart gradually takes over the circulation while the arterial flow from the CPB machine is reduced. When the blood pressure is acceptable and the surgeon is confident that the heart function is adequate, CPB is discontinued.

Complications of cardiopulmonary bypass

CPB is a complex technique and, as such, there are many potentially serious complications (Summary box 51.2). Increasingly, 'off-pump' coronary artery surgery is being used to avoid such complications.

CORONARY ARTERY BYPASS SURGERY

Introduction

Before the 1950s, surgical attempts to treat coronary artery disease (CAD) through augmentation of non-coronary flow to the myocardium via the creation of pericardial or omental adhesions met with limited success. By the 1960s, the importance of aortocoronary saphenous vein grafts and the value of the internal mammary or internal thoracic artery were increasingly recognised. From the start, the results of coronary artery bypass graft (CABG) surgery were carefully monitored. By the 1970s, three large, prospectively randomised, multicentre trials were being conducted. All of these studies showed that a subset of patients had improved survival after surgery. With the advent of percutaneous coronary intervention (PCI) in the 1980s, the patient population undergoing CABG has changed, becoming progressively sicker but often with the most to gain (Summary box 51.3).

Coronary artery anatomy

The coronary arteries are branches of the ascending aorta, arising from ostia in the aortic sinuses above the aortic valve, the right from the anterior sinus and the left from the left posterior sinus (Fig. 51.2).

Left coronary artery

The left main coronary artery, which arises from the aortic root, can be the site of significant stenosis ('left main stem disease') and carries the worst prognosis in terms of survival without surgery. The artery is inaccessible at its origin and therefore grafts are anastomosed to its branches, the left anterior descending artery (LAD) or anterior interventricular artery and obtuse/marginal (OM) branches of the circumflex artery. The LAD is the most frequently diseased coronary artery and most often bypassed during CABG surgery.

Right coronary artery

The right coronary artery (RCA) passes from its origin anteriorly between the right atrial appendage and the pulmonary trunk and courses in the atrioventricular groove around the margin of the right ventricle. It usually forms an anastomosis with the circumflex artery at the junction of the right and left atria and the

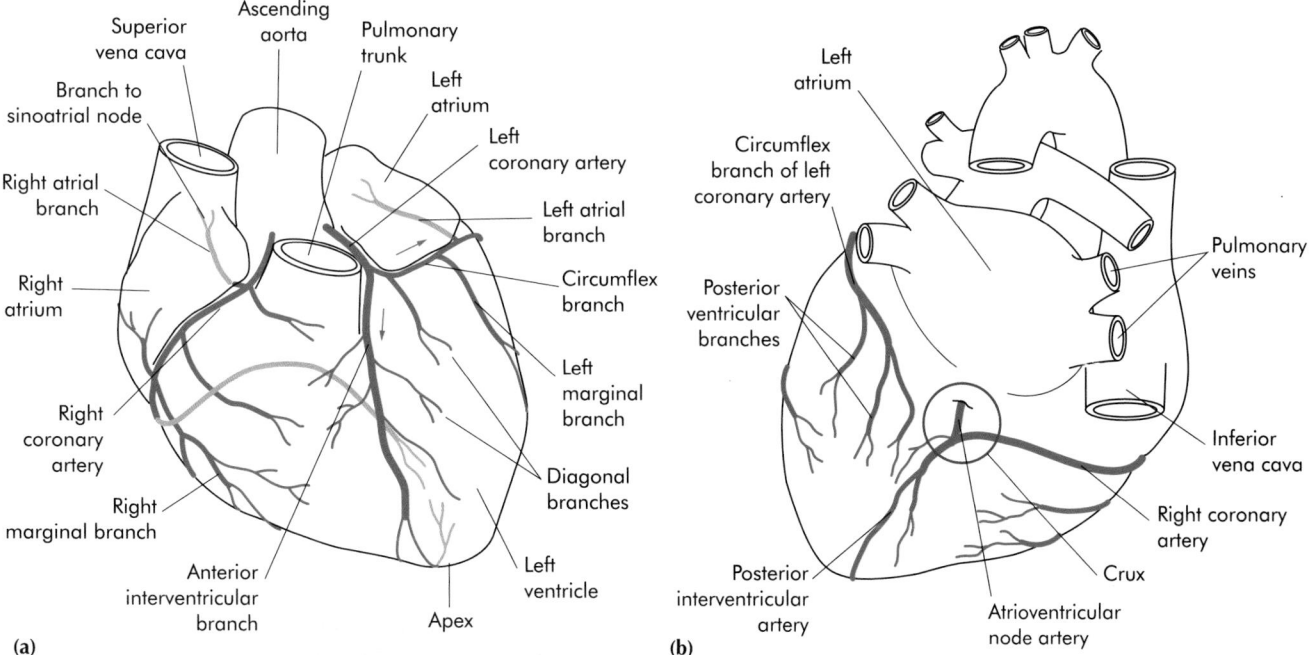

Figure 51.2 The heart, showing the distribution the of the left and right coronary arteries. (a) Anterior surface of the heart and (b) base and diaphragmatic surface of the heart.

CHAPTER 51 | CARDIAC SURGERY

interventricular septum (the crux). It continues as the posterior descending artery or interventricular artery. Common sites of stenosis of the RCA are in its proximal portion or at the bifurcation or crux. In the presence of disease at the bifurcation, a graft can be placed distally to the posterior descending artery.

The question of anatomical dominance is determined by the artery that supplies the posterior descending artery. In approximately 90% of cases the posterior descending artery arises from the RCA, a pattern referred to as right dominance. The posterior descending artery can also arise from the circumflex artery, a pattern referred to as left dominance, which occurs in approximately 10% of cases. A balanced pattern is one in which two posterior descending arteries, one arising from the right coronary artery and one from the circumflex artery, can exist (Fig. 51.2).

Ischaemic heart disease

Ischaemic heart disease (IHD) is a major cause of morbidity and mortality in developed countries. The underlying pathology is usually atherosclerosis of the coronary arteries.

Pathophysiology

Atherosclerosis is the process underlying the formation of focal obstructions or plaques in large- and medium-sized arteries. It is characterised by the presence of focal intimal thickening, these intimal elevations being made up of accumulations of cholesterol-rich 'gruel' (atherosis) and a proliferation of connective tissue (sclerosis). An essential component of atherogenesis is inflammation involving monocytes/macrophages, T lymphocytes and mast cells. Four stages are described in the pathogenesis of atherosclerosis:

- Initiation with deposition of foam cells to form fatty streaks.
- Progression into mature atherosclerotic or fibrolipid plaques.
- Destabilisation with rupture of the plaque, exposure of thrombogenic atheroma, and deposition of platelets and fibrin. This may lead to subsequent ischaemia, infarction or narrowing of the vessel through plaque repair.
- Plaque repair: many coronary thrombi eventually undergo a process of recanalisation with a degree of reperfusion.

Clinical manifestations

The principal symptoms of IHD are chest pain or angina, breathlessness, fatigue, swelling, palpitations and syncope. Severity of symptoms and the extent to which the symptoms interfere with everyday activities form a significant part of the clinical history. An assessment of risk factors should be included (Summary box 51.4). Clinical examination follows and, although often normal, any evidence of myocardial ischaemia or stigmata of associated disease such as diabetes or peripheral vascular disease should be noted.

Summary box 51.4

Risk factors for IHD

- Advancing age
- Male gender
- Hyperlipidaemia
- Diabetes mellitus
- Hypertension
- Smoking
- Family history of IHD
- Obesity
- Reduced physical activity

Investigations

Non-invasive methods of diagnosis

Resting electrocardiography

As a baseline test, a 12-lead resting electrocardiogram (ECG) often provides the first indication of ischaemic cardiac disease and is essential in the acute clinical setting. However, it is not necessarily abnormal even in the presence of severe multivessel coronary heart disease. Evidence of previous myocardial infarction is seen commonly, as Q waves and/or non-specific ST and T-wave changes.

Cardiac isoenzymes and troponins

These are useful in assessing patients with an acute coronary syndrome (ACS) when the diagnosis is in doubt. Standard enzyme measurement such as creatine kinase MB and lactate dehydrogenase usually take too long and may delay thrombolytic therapy. Troponin T and I, markers of myocardial damage, appear to be more specific and may aid rapid diagnosis as well as having prognostic implications.

Exercise tolerance testing

Exercise tolerance testing (ETT) is a valuable technique for assessing myocardial ischaemia, both for diagnostic purposes and as a prognostic tool. However, an abnormal exercise test must be interpreted in the light of the probability of coronary artery disease and the physiological response to exercise as measured by the percentage of the maximum predicted heart rate achieved. A positive test with evidence of ischaemia on the ECG (ST depression of ≤ 2 mm) does not always indicate IHD, and a negative test does not always exclude its presence.

Echocardiography

Performed either through a transthoracic or transoesophageal approach, it is valuable for the evaluation of ventricular function and regional wall motion abnormalities, as well as valvular lesions.

Stress echocardiography can detect regional wall motion abnormalities brought on by exercise or the use of dobutamine or dipyridamole. It is a reliable method of identifying viable myocardium. Impaired but recoverable myocardium possesses a functional reserve that allows it to be temporarily recruited into action, whereas scar tissue does not.

Radionuclide studies and cardiac magnetic resonance imaging

The two main types of radionuclide study available are perfusion and blood pool studies. They allow an assessment of the perfusion and cellular integrity of viable myocardium. Cardiac magnetic resonance imaging (MRI) can be performed to evaluate the structure and function of the heart and blood vessels and offers an alternative to angiography.

Positron emission tomography

Positron emission tomography (PET) provides information on myocardial perfusion, metabolism and cell membrane function. Positron-emitting isotopes are used to label physiological substances, after which the regional distribution of these substances can be measured. PET is valuable in the diagnosis of coronary artery disease, particularly when the more widely available imaging modalities are inconclusive. It can identify injured but viable myocardium that is potentially salvageable by revascularisation.

Computerised tomography

With the development of the latest computerised tomography (CT) scanners, which have the ability to correct for respiratory and cardiac movements, multislice high-resolution CT scanning may become an alternative to coronary angiography. It allows for the assessment of coronary disease, particularly proximal coronary artery disease, and gives some information about the degree of coronary artery calcification.

Invasive methods of diagnosis

Coronary angiography

Selective coronary angiography provides the means of accurately diagnosing the presence and extent of coronary artery disease and remains the 'gold standard' diagnostic technique (Fig. 51.3). In spite of the availability of newer imaging techniques such as cardiac MRI, selective coronary angiography provides high image quality, demonstrating the extent, severity and location of coronary artery stenoses and the quality and size of the distal coronary arteries. Any stenosis in an artery of > 70% of the diameter (90% reduction on cross-sectional area) is considered 'severe'. In addition, it allows assessment of ventricular function and provides the cardiac surgeon with information to determine operability, operative risk and probability of operative result. This test only outlines the coronary anatomy, does not demonstrate ischaemia and carries an overall complication rate of less than 1% (Summary box 51.5).

Summary box 51.5

Coronary angiography

- 'Gold standard' for imaging of anatomy
- Demonstrates extent, severity and location of stenoses
- Reduction in diameter of > 70% is considered severe (90% reduction in cross-sectional area)
- Demonstrates quality and size of distal arterial tree
- Aids diagnosis of ischaemia
- Evaluates suitability for surgery
- Aids in prognostic assessment

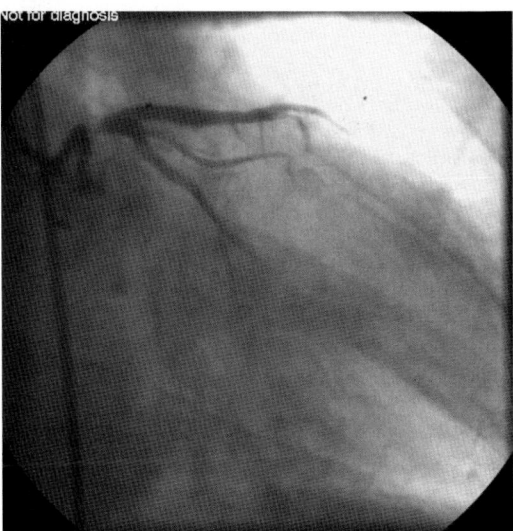

Figure 51.3 Coronary angiogram demonstrating severe stenosis in the left main stem prior to bifurcation of the left anterior descending and circumflex arteries.

Indications for surgery

Surgery for coronary artery disease may be indicated for *symptomatic* or *prognostic* reasons. The decision to advise CABG is based on the balance between the expected benefit and the risks that the patient faces. Studies have identified a subset of patients with certain angiographic features who have improved survival after surgery (Summary box 51.6).

Summary box 51.6

Survival is improved through surgery in patients with:

- > 50% stenosis of the left main stem ('critical left main stem disease')
- > 70% stenosis of the proximal left anterior interventricular artery
- All three main coronary arteries diseased ('triple-vessel disease')
- Poor ventricular function associated with coronary artery disease

---

Chronic stable angina

A common indication is for the relief of symptoms of angina despite adequate medical therapy. Percutaneous coronary angioplasty (PTCA) and coronary stents are increasingly used for treatment. In the presence of certain angiographic features, surgical revascularisation offers a better survival. Angina can be relieved by surgical revascularisation in most patients and symptomatic improvement can be expected for over 10 years.

Acute coronary syndromes

The majority of patients who are hospitalised with *unstable angina* become asymptomatic within 48 hours of the initiation of anti-anginal therapy, and ECG signs of transient ischaemia disappear. If, however, the patient develops recurrent angina and/or ECG changes despite medical therapy, surgical revascularisation has largely been superseded by thrombolysis and primary PTCA. If following an uncomplicated acute myocardial infarction (MI), the patient is a suitable candidate for surgical revascularisation, elective CABG should be carried out at least 6 weeks after the infarction to reduce the higher complication rate associated with recent acute MI.

Surgery for the complications of myocardial infarction

MI leads to myocyte necrosis, which may heal to form scar tissue or rupture if the ventricular wall gives way. Free rupture of the ventricle is usually fatal despite treatment. *Ventricular septal rupture* typically presents 3–7 days after infarction with pulmonary oedema, a pansystolic murmur and hypotension. The diagnosis is usually confirmed with echocardiography. Repair is with a pericardial or artificial Dacron patch.

Papillary muscle necrosis causes acute mitral regurgitation, a pansystolic murmur and pulmonary oedema. Diagnosis is made by echocardiography and right heart catheterisation (showing large V waves). Mitral valve replacement is usually necessary, but the mortality rate is higher than in valve replacement for rheumatic heart disease as a result of the associated coronary artery disease.

Ventricular aneurysm occurs following partial-thickness necrosis of the ventricular wall if the free wall is replaced with non-contractile fibrous tissue. Left ventricular function is affected because the fibrous wall balloons out during systole and reduces the actual stroke volume. Repair is undertaken using CPB, and CABG is undertaken at the same time if necessary.

Combined with valve replacement

Patients undergoing valve replacement usually have coronary bypass surgery to any significant coronary lesions. However, several variables need to be carefully evaluated when considering the choice of a combined procedure and the overall operative risk: these include age > 70 years, female sex and poor left ventricular function, as well as what the underlying valve pathology is and which valve is to be replaced.

Acute failure of percutaneous coronary angioplasty

Since the advent of intracoronary stents, the need for emergency CABG following complications of PTCA is low at < 1%. The mortality rate in this group is significantly higher than for elective CABG.

Contraindications to surgery

Few absolute contraindications exist, although the presence of significant cerebrovascular disease may require modification of surgical strategy. Other relative contraindications are recognised (Summary box 51.7).

Summary box 51.7

Contraindications for coronary artery bypass surgery

- Small, diffusely diseased arteries
- Diffuse disease and heart failure
- Acute myocardial infarction over 6 hours old
- Moribund patients after resuscitation

Preparation for surgery

Clinical assessment

Before CABG, the severity and stability of the patient's IHD, the presence of significant valvular disease and the status of left ventricular function should be properly evaluated.

Any comorbid risk factors for IHD should be documented and, in particular, the state of coexisting diseases assessed. Attention is paid to the presence of carotid artery disease, peripheral vascular disease, respiratory status, preoperative diabetic control and presence of associated diabetic complications, significant renal dysfunction or coagulopathy. All medications taken by the patient are noted. Ideally, some should be stopped before surgery, in particular any anti-platelet agents, including aspirin and anticoagulants, as well as oral hypoglycaemics. Others drugs, such as diuretics and angiotensin-converting enzyme (ACE) inhibitors, are stopped on the discretion of the surgeon. However, apart from the exceptions noted, as a general rule all cardiac and antihypertensive medications should be taken preoperatively.

Risk assessment

Risk assessment or stratification can be calculated using various scoring systems developed for cardiac surgery, including the EuroSCORE and PARSONNET. The common scoring systems

The Parsonnet score was developed by V. Parsonnet and others, at the Newark Beth Israel Medical Center, New Jersey, NJ, USA, and is based on the publication 'A Method of Uniform Stratification of Risk for Evaluating the Results of Surgery in Acquired Adult Heart Disease', (1989).

stratify risk factors that are recognised to be associated with poor outcome following surgery. An estimate of operative mortality can be calculated and allows informed consent by the patient.

Selection of conduit

Venous grafts

The long saphenous vein is the most common vein used as a conduit as it is straightforward to harvest, provides good length and is easy to handle.

The 10-year patency rate for long saphenous vein grafts is reported to be 50–60%, with 10–15% occluding in 1 year. Strategies to improve vein graft patency include smoking cessation following CABG, the use of lipid-lowering agents and the early use of anti-platelet agents such as low-dose aspirin. In assessing the patient preoperatively, the legs should be checked for varicose veins. Alternative vein conduits include the short saphenous vein or upper limb veins such as the cephalic vein.

Arterial grafts

The left internal mammary artery (LIMA), or internal thoracic artery, has become the conduit of choice for the LAD. Since the mid-1980s, 10-year patency rates of 90% have been reported, with improved long-term survival and fewer reoperations. As LIMA–LAD anastomosis avoids the late complication of vein graft atherosclerosis, particular interest has focused on the use of bilateral internal mammary artery (BIMA) grafts. It does have limitations, however, and may be particularly inappropriate in certain sub-groups of patients, such as the obese diabetic in whom sternal wound complications appear higher.

The use of the radial artery as a second or alternative arterial bypass graft has enjoyed a revival. This has been driven to some extent by the developing concept of total arterial revascularisation and the belief that this will help improve long-term results of coronary surgery. Patency rates appear at least as good if not better than for long saphenous vein grafts. In assessing a patient in whom a radial artery harvest is planned, an Allen's test is performed (Summary box 51.8).

Summary box 51.8

Allen's test

- The patient makes a tight fist while the surgeon compresses both distal and ulnar arteries digitally; this squeezes blood from the hand
- The hand is then relaxed and compression of the ulnar artery is released; the speed of returning colour to the hand is assessed
- If colour returns in 5–7 s, patency and collateral flow from the ulnar artery is confirmed

---

Alternative arterial bypass grafts include the gastroepiploic artery and the inferior epigastric artery.

The operation

Intraoperative monitoring includes monitoring of continuous central venous pressure and blood pressure (via a central line in

Edgar van Nuys Allen, 1900–1961, Professor of Medicine, The Mayo Clinic, Rochester, MN, USA.

the internal jugular or subclavian vein and radial artery line respectively), urine output via a urinary catheter, temperature using a probe positioned at the nasal septum, and the ECG.

The operation commences with harvesting of the long saphenous vein from the leg (Fig. 51.4) while the chest is opened via a median sternotomy and the LIMA is dissected from the chest wall (Fig. 51.5). The patient is typically placed on CPB after heparinising, the aorta is cross-clamped and the heart arrested with cardioplegia. The grafts are anastomosed to coronary arteries distal to the stenosis (Fig. 51.6).

The aortic cross-clamp is removed and the heart is reperfused with oxygenated blood. A side-biting clamp is applied to the ascending aorta and the proximal anastomoses are completed. The patient is warmed and weaned from CPB. The heparin is reversed and the patient is returned to the intensive care unit (ICU).

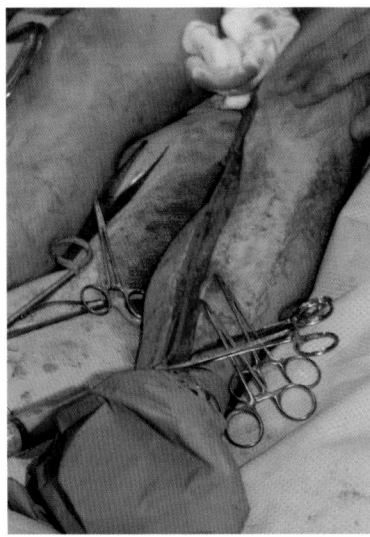

Figure 51.4 The long saphenous vein is exposed at the ankle, anterior to the medial malleolus, as far as the saphenofemoral junction (if required). The side branches are tied carefully and divided, and the vein is excised. Gentle distension of the vein through a cannula at its distal end allows inspection for leaks.

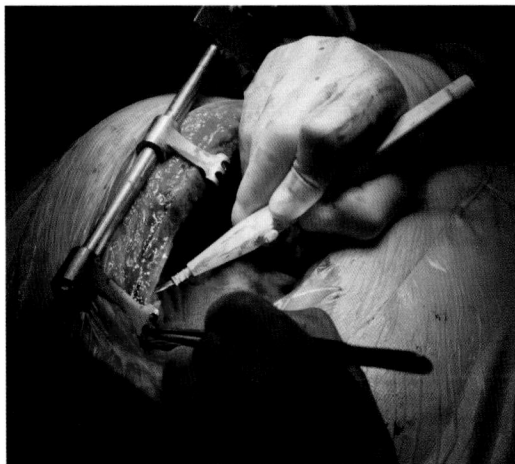

Figure 51.5 A pedicled left internal mammary artery is dissected off the chest wall and divided distally after systemic heparinisation. It is left attached to the subclavian artery proximally.

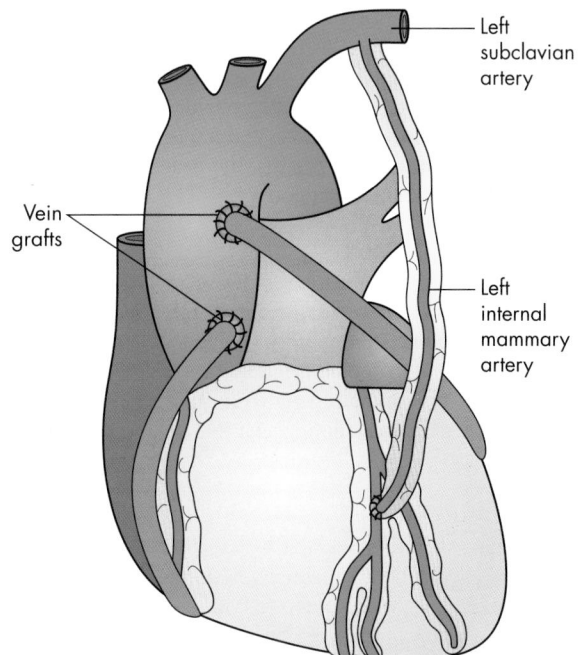

Figure 51.6 Completed coronary artery bypass grafts

Postoperative recovery

The majority of patients are extubated a few hours after returning from surgery and remain in the ICU for 24 hours or so. In some centres, 'fast tracking' appropriate patients allows for an earlier transfer to a recovery area or high-dependency unit (HDU). Discharge is routinely 5–8 days after surgery.

Postoperative complications

Bleeding

Significant bleeding occurs in approximately 3–5% of patients. Rarely, acute cardiac tamponade or profound hypotension may occur in the early postoperative period and requires emergency re-sternotomy.

Arrhythmias

The most common postoperative arrhythmia is sinus tachycardia, closely followed by atrial fibrillation (AF). It occurs in around 30% of patients undergoing CABG and often spontaneously reverts to sinus rhythm. Treatment includes correction of potassium ($> 4.5 \text{ mmol l}^{-1}$), the use of amiodarone or digoxin and, if necessary, cardioversion. Bradycardia is seldom seen, but temporary pacing via epicardial pacing wires inserted intraoperatively may be required in the postoperative period.

Poor cardiac output state

Myocardial function typically declines in the first few hours following cardiac surgery, presumably in response to an ischaemia/reperfusion-type injury. Often, inotropic agents are required at this time to support the heart and circulation. Occasionally, the patient develops a persistent low cardiac output state. The clinical manifestations of such a situation include poor peripheral perfusion, with poor urine output, a developing metabolic acidosis and low blood pressure.

There are several mechanisms that account for this complication in the early postoperative period, including depressed myocardial contractility, reduced preload, increased afterload and a disturbance in heart rate or rhythm.

Treatment is aimed at the underlying cause but generally includes oxygenation, optimising preload, reducing afterload, managing any rhythm disturbances and improving contractility. If the low cardiac output state persists, the heart may require pharmacological or mechanical support.

Pharmacological support

Inotropic drugs act in a variety of ways to alter the systemic vascular resistance, increase the heart rate and increase the force of myocardial contractility. Commonly used inotropes include isoprenaline, dopamine, dobutamine, adrenaline (epinephrine) and noradrenaline (norepine); they are often used in conjunction with vasodilating agents that decrease the afterload.

Mechanical support

If low cardiac output persists despite inotropic support, the heart may require mechanical support while it recovers its function. The intra-aortic balloon pump (IABP) is a device that is inserted, either percutaneously or under direct vision, into the common femoral artery. It is threaded into the aorta until its tip lies just distal to the arch vessels (Fig. 51.7). The balloon is triggered by the ECG, deflating during ventricular systole (thus reducing afterload) and inflating in diastole (displacing blood that perfuses the coronary arteries retrogradely). When the heart has recovered sufficiently, the balloon is removed.

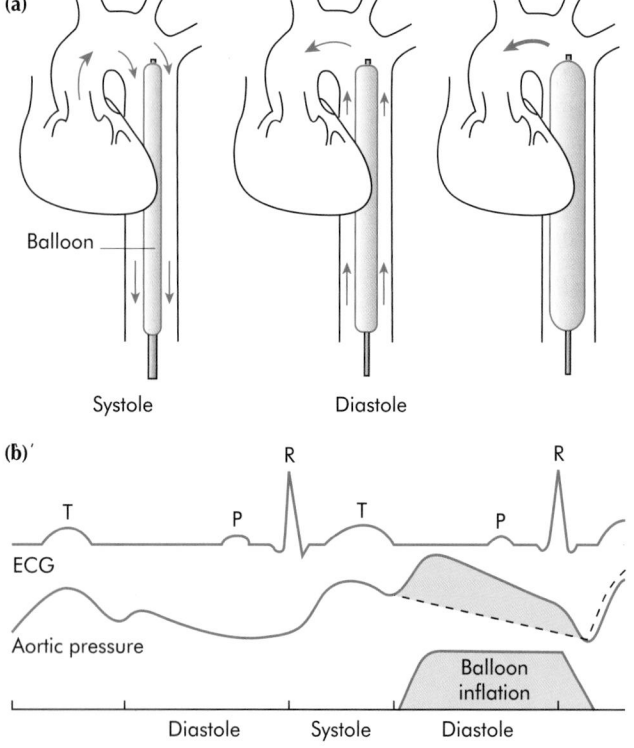

Figure 51.7 Intra-aortic balloon pump counterpulsation. (a) The balloon deflates during systole and thereby lowers systemic resistance. It inflates during diastole and increases coronary perfusion in addition to augmenting the systemic blood pressure. (b) The pressure changes and phases of the electrocardiogram (ECG) are shown.

Neurological dysfunction

Stroke leading to a focal neurological deficit occurs in approximately 2% of patients following CABG. Embolisation, probably originating from the aortic arch or heart chambers, is the most common mechanism for territorial infarcts, with hypoperfusion leading to watershed infarcts. Diffuse neurological injury may occur leading to more subtle cognitive abnormalities in memory, concentration and attention.

Wound infection

Significant deep wound infection resulting in sternal dehiscence and mediastinitis occurs in around 0.5–2% of patients. This can be associated with significant morbidity with a prolonged hospital stay and further surgical interventions for debridement and/or rewiring of the sternum. It still has a significant mortality rate of as high as 40%. Wound infections are more common in diabetics and the obese.

Mortality

In the UK, the overall mortality rate for patients undergoing CABG is 2–3%. Multiple factors have been demonstrated to affect mortality after CABG, including age, gender, left ventricular function, use of LIMA and complete revascularisation.

Surgical outcome

Relief of symptoms

If revascularisation is complete, CABG alleviates or improves anginal symptoms in more than 90% of patients at 1 year; this falls to 80% at 5 years and 60% at 10 years. This symptomatic deterioration usually reflects progression of atherosclerotic disease in vein grafts and native coronary arteries.

Survival

Early surgical versus medical studies have reported survival rates to be 95% at 1 year, 90% at 5 years, 75% at 10 years and 60% at 15 years. Through changes in surgical practice, such as an increased use of arterial conduits and the widespread use of aspirin and lipid-lowering statins, post-CABG survival may well improve in the future (Summary box 51.9).

Summary box 51.9

Coronary artery bypass surgery outcome

Mortality
- 2–3%

Peroperative infarct
- 2–3%

Angina
- Better in 90% at 1 year
- 80% at 5 years
- 60% at 10 years

Survival
- 95% at 1 year
- 90% at 5 years
- 75% at 10 years
- 60% at 15 years

Off-pump coronary artery surgery

CABG without the use of CPB is a well established and increasingly popular method that may be combined with a minimally invasive approach or carried out through a conventional sternotomy. It offers the advantages that it avoids the physiological stress associated with CPB and, to some extent, the aortic manipulation that can lead to neurological injury through atherosclerotic embolisation. Since the introduction of cardiac stabilising devices such as the Octopus (Fig. 51.8), off-pump coronary artery bypass (OPCAB) grafting has become widespread.

Minimal access surgery

Minimally invasive direct coronary artery bypass (MIDCAB) grafting is performed through a strategically placed minimal access incision and so avoids all invasive aspects of conventional CABG. Through an anterior submammary incision the LIMA can be dissected down with the aid of a thoracoscope and grafted to the LAD. More lateral MIDCAB incisions allow access to other coronary vessels including branches of the circumflex artery. Patient selection remains, at least at present, a restriction to the ever-increasing minimally invasive methods being developed. Although not yet critically evaluated, one particular approach is to combine MIDCAB (typically LIMA to LAD) with PCI to other less accessible coronary arteries ('hybrid' coronary revascularisation).

VALVULAR HEART DISEASE

Introduction

Early surgical management of valvular heart disease concentrated on valvular repair. The heroic early procedures for valve stenosis were closed and therefore 'blind' commissurotomies. They were replaced by open procedures with full visualisation allowing precise repair and replacement. The first prosthetic valve replacement was performed by Harken in 1960 replacing the aortic valve, followed by a mitral valve replacement by Starr

a year later. Continued improvements in perioperative care, myocardial protection and, in particular, the development of prosthetic heart valves have improved long-term haemodynamic effects, provided symptom relief and prolonged survival. The majority of valvular operations involve surgery on the aortic or mitral valve; tricuspid and pulmonary valve surgery is rarely undertaken.

Surgical anatomy

Heart valves function to maintain pressure gradients between cardiac chambers and so ensure unidirectional flow of blood without reflux through the heart. The aortic valve is tricuspid with semilunar leaflets attached to the aortic wall at the annulus with the aortic sinuses occurring above the base of each leaflet, two of which form the origin or ostium of the coronary arteries. The intrinsic shape of the aortic semilunar valve allows blood to leave the ventricle during systole and prevents its regurgitation during diastole. If disease leads to disruption of the leaflets or the annulus, valve function will be affected.

The mitral valve is bicuspid; the more anterior cusp is larger and lies between the orifices of the mitral and aortic valves. The leaflets, like those of the aortic valve, are attached to an annulus. The leaflets join at two commissures and are supported by a subvalvular apparatus consisting of chordae tendinae and papillary muscles. The papillary muscles contract in ventricular systole, pulling the cusps towards the atrioventricular orifice and holding blood within the ventricle. The proper functioning of the mitral valve depends on the integrity of the annulus, leaflets, chordae and papillary muscles. If surgical correction is required, emphasis is on the preservation of these structures when possible (Fig. 51.9).

Surgical options for heart valve disease

The decision of whether to repair or replace the diseased valve depends on the underlying pathology, the severity of disease, and quality and/or involvement of the surrounding supporting structures. Generally, repair is increasingly favoured when possible in mitral valve disease, particularly in mitral regurgitation in which it has been shown to have good long-term outcomes. Repair is the operation of choice in tricuspid valve disease, but aortic valve surgery generally involves replacing the diseased valve (Table 51.1).

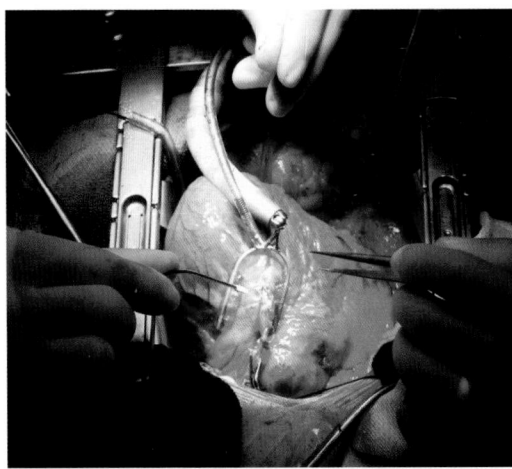

Figure 51.8 Off-pump coronary artery bypass using an Octopus stabiliser to perform the distal anastomosis.

Dwight Emary Harken, **B. 1910**, formerly Chief of Thoracic Surgery, The Peter Bent Brigham Hospital, Boston, MA, USA.
Albert Starr, **B. 1926**, formerly Professor of Surgery, The University of Oregon, Portland, OR, USA.

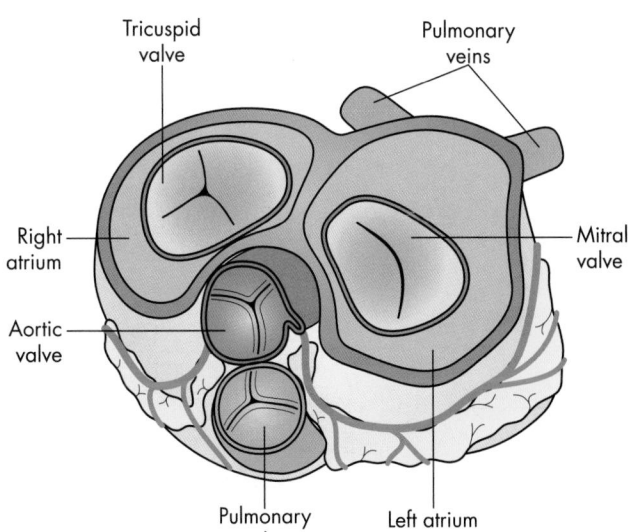

Figure 51.9 Four valves of the heart.

Table 51.1 Comparing options for heart valve surgery

	Advantages	Disadvantages
Valve repair	Preservation of integral structures	Technical difficulties
	Improved haemodynamics	Variable failure rate
	Avoids long-term anticoagulation	
Valve replacement		
Mechanical	Readily available	Needs lifelong anticoagulation
	Extensive experience of use	Susceptibility to infection
	Used in any age group	
	Durability, lifelong	
Biological		
Stented	Readily available	Limited lifespan
	Short period of anticoagulation	
Stentless	Readily available	Limited lifespan
	Probably better haemodynamics with less outflow tract obstruction	More difficult to insert
	Short period of anticoagulation	
Homograft	No anticoagulation	Not readily available
	Improved haemodynamics	Technical difficulties
	Long-term outcome uncertain	

Table adapted from Sharpe, D.A.C. and Das, S.R. (2000) Heart valve surgery. *Surgery* **18**: 265–9.

Important factors in selecting the type of procedure and prosthesis include the age of the patient and the need for anticoagulation. Because of uncertainties about its lifespan, there is debate about when a bioprosthetic valve should be used, with most accepting its use in those over 65 years. The need for anticoagulation may have an impact on choice of valve, particularly in women of childbearing age, in the elderly, in the presence of congenital or acquired bleeding diathesis and when there is the need for further major surgery.

Types of prosthetic valves

Mechanical valves

Mechanical valves can be used in any age group to replace any valve (Fig. 51.10). They are extremely durable but the components of the valve are thrombogenic and therefore the patient requires systemic anticoagulation, usually with warfarin. This subjects the patients to a lifetime of blood tests, medication and the constant threat of haemorrhagic complications (intracerebral, epistaxis, gastrointestinal bleed).

Biological valves

Biological valves include *homograft* (or *allograft*) valves, removed from cadavers; *autografts*, a patient's own valve; and, most commonly, *heterografts* (or *xenografts*) prepared from animal tissues. All share the basic design of three semilunar leaflets with central flow, so decreasing pressure gradients and minimising turbulence (Fig. 51.11). Heterograft 'tissue' valves are the most commonly used valves and can be stented with a limited durability of 10–15 years, whereas stentless (or frameless) valves are expected to have less late calcific degeneration but are more technically difficult to insert.

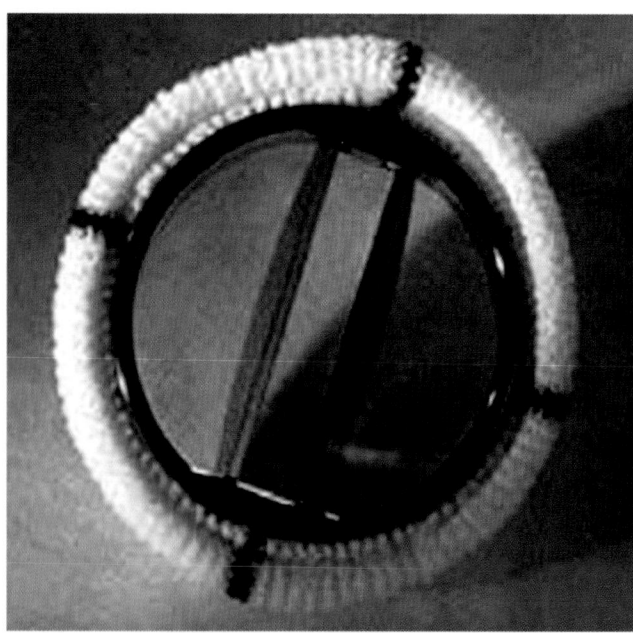

Figure 51.10 Bileaflet mechanical valve.

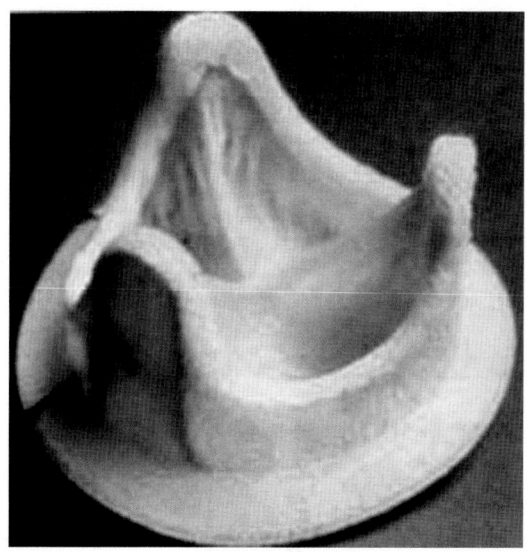

Figure 51.11 Porcine heterograft stented valve.

Prosthetic valve dysfunction and complications

Structural valve failure

Bioprosthetic valves are vulnerable to degenerative changes. Structural failure rates for biological valves, although rare in those over 70 years of age, can reach 60% after 15 years. Structural failure of a mechanical valve is generally uncommon.

Paravalvular leak

Early-onset paravalvular leaks usually result from technical difficulties at insertion. Late-onset leaks can occur and may be related to an episode of endocarditis or, in the presence of bioprostheses, leaflet degeneration. The leak can cause haemolytic anaemia or haemodynamic compromise and the valve may need replacement.

Thrombosis and thromboembolism

Thrombus formation on a prosthetic valve remains the most common complication of mechanical and biological valves (Fig. 51.12). The risk of thromboembolism is greater with a valve in the mitral position (mechanical or biological) than with one in the aortic position. Improved haemodynamic function lowers the probability of thromboembolism. The incidence of thromboembolism in current mechanical valves is 0.5–3% per patient-year.

Prosthetic valve endocarditis

The incidence of prosthetic valve endocarditis (PVE) is 2–4%. The risk is lifelong and at its greatest in the first 15 weeks after surgery. The incidence of PVE is higher with mechanical and bioprosthetic valves and lowest with homograft and autograft valves. The diagnosis is made by symptoms of septicaemia, appearance of a new murmur or a septic embolus. It is confirmed with echocardiography, which may show vegetations and even abscess formation. A high index of suspicion is required and early multiple blood cultures are needed to confirm the diagnosis, identify the infective organism and choose appropriate antibiotic therapy. The most common organisms that can lead to PVE are the *Staphylococcus* species, particularly *Staphylococcus epidermidis* in early PVE and *Staphylococcus aureus* (at least 50% of cases); the *Streptococcus* species, usually *Streptococcus viridans* but also *Streptococcus pneumoniae*; and, less commonly, Gram-negative bacilli, as well as fungal organisms.

The treatment of choice is early aggressive intravenous antibiotic therapy. Serial echocardiography to assess extent of infection into surrounding myocardial tissue as well as functional assessment of the infected valve may help in optimising decisions on timing of surgical intervention. The prognosis of PVE remains poor with an overall mortality rate of over 50%.

Postoperative management

Antibiotic prophylaxis

Valve surgery, like all cardiac procedures, requires perioperative and immediate postoperative antibiotic prophylaxis. If prosthetic infective endocarditis is to be avoided, further prophylaxis with appropriate antibiotics is required during dental and minor surgical procedures in all patients with prosthetic heart valves.

Anti-thrombotic therapy

All patients with mechanical valves require warfarin, usually started on the second postoperative day. The use of anticoagulation or anti-platelet therapy with biological valves is variable and depends on the patient's underlying rhythm postoperatively.

Mitral valve disease

Approximately one-third of all valve surgery performed in the UK is for mitral valve disease, with increasing emphasis on valve repair as the importance of preserving the mitral valve apparatus has become apparent.

Mitral regurgitation

Any pathological process affecting the mitral valve apparatus will lead to mitral regurgitation. As such, there are many causes of regurgitation and they can be broadly classified into five headings (Summary box 51.10).

Summary box 51.10

Causes of mitral regurgitation and likely pathology

Degenerative
- Mitral valve prolapse
- Floppy valve: degeneration of the leaflets with/without chordal rupture
- Senile calcification: calcified annulus
- Connective tissue disorders (e.g. Marfan's syndrome, Ehlers–Danlos' syndrome): disruption of mitral valve apparatus

Ischaemic
- Papillary muscle rupture: following myocardial infarction
- Dynamic mitral regurgitation: as a result of transient ischaemia
- Poor left ventricular function: most common 'functional' cause secondary to myocardial ischaemia

Rheumatic
- Previous acute rheumatic fever: stiffened leaflets unable to coapt

Infective
- Endocarditis: leaflet destruction

Functional
- Presence of reduced left ventricular function with increased ventricular size

Adapted from Hall, R. (1997) Mitral valve disease. *Medicine* **25**: 27.

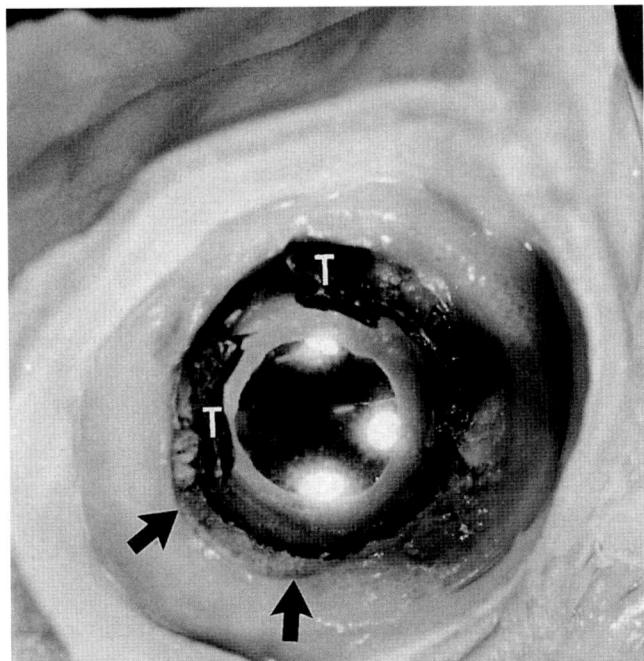

Figure 51.12 Thrombus (marked T and illustrated with the arrows) on the moving components of a ball-and-cage valve.

Pathophysiology

There is an important distinction between acute and chronic mitral regurgitation. The former is compared with chronic mitral regurgitation, usually as a result of ischaemic papillary muscle rupture or following infective endocarditis, whereas the latter is a result of myxomatous degeneration of the leaflets leading to a floppy valve.

In *acute mitral regurgitation*, the left ventricle ejects blood back into a small poorly compliant left atrium, imposing a sudden volume load on the left atrium during ventricular systole. This leads to an abrupt rise in left atrial pressure followed by a rise in pulmonary venous pressure and pulmonary oedema.

In *chronic mitral regurgitation*, the process is sufficiently slow to allow compensatory left ventricular dilatation and hypertrophy, and dilatation of the left atrium without any significant increase in pressure, so protecting the pulmonary circulation. As the disease advances and the left atrial dilatation can no longer cope, left atrial pressure begins to rise, leading to a rise in pulmonary venous pressure and progressive pulmonary congestion, and eventual congestive cardiac failure.

Clinical features

In acute mitral regurgitation, the patient is usually unwell, presenting with clinical and radiological evidence of acute pulmonary oedema and a loud apical pansystolic murmur. Patients with mild chronic mitral regurgitation are usually asymptomatic. With progressive pulmonary congestion and left ventricular failure, the patient develops fatigue, dyspnoea on exertion and orthopnoea. The development of atrial fibrillation with left atrial dilatation is common. The enlarged left ventricle leads to a heaving apical impulse and a pansystolic murmur.

Investigations

- *ECG* may show only left atrial hypertrophy (bifid P waves), left ventricular hypertrophy and atrial fibrillation.
- *Chest radiography.* There may be cardiomegaly with prominent pulmonary vasculature.
- *Echocardiography* is often combined with colour flow Doppler imaging, which shows the severity of the regurgitant jet of mitral regurgitation.

Indications for surgery

Indications for surgery include severe symptoms as assessed by the New York Heart Association (NYHA) functional classification system, a progressive increase in left ventricular volume leading to ventricular dysfunction, uncontrolled endocarditis and severe acute mitral regurgitation (Fig. 51.13). Timing of surgery is crucial, as surgery performed too late in the natural history of the condition does not benefit the patient because of the damage already done.

Mitral stenosis

The most common cause of mitral stenosis remains rheumatic fever, although the incidence of overt rheumatic fever in the developed world has decreased. During the healing phase of acute rheumatic fever, the valve leaflets become adherent to each other at their free border so that the commissures become

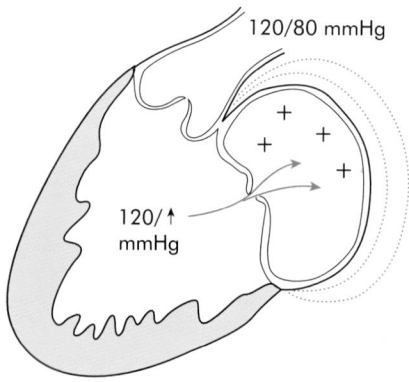

Figure 51.13 Features and pathophysiology of mitral regurgitation. There is a loud parasystolic murmur and the left atrium enlarges. The left ventricle enlarges as a consequence of volume overload.

obliterated and the valve orifice narrows. Symptoms from mitral stenosis usually develop more than 10 years after the acute attack.

Pathophysiology

Mitral stenosis slows ventricular filling during diastole and the pressure in the left atrium rises to maintain cardiac output. This leads to atrial hypertrophy and dilatation. Pulmonary congestion results from the rise in left atrial pressure but, with time, the lungs are protected against pulmonary oedema by constriction of the pulmonary vessels. However, this adaptive response, along with the passive 'back pressure' generated by the rise in left atrial pressure, leads to pulmonary hypertension. This leads to an increased demand on the right ventricle with eventual right heart failure and tricuspid regurgitation. The development of atrial fibrillation is common and can lead to a significant reduction in cardiac output. Atrial fibrillation predisposes to thrombi forming in the left atrium, which may embolise.

Clinical features

Patients may remain asymptomatic for years and then present with symptoms when the heart is stressed by an event such as pregnancy, fever or a chest infection, or with the onset of atrial fibrillation. The common symptoms are fatigue and dyspnoea on exertion, which result from the combination of reduced forward flow and increased back pressure. The resulting pulmonary congestion adds to the breathlessness and may produce a cough or haemoptysis. If mitral stenosis is advanced, there may also be a right ventricular heave due to right ventricular hypertrophy in response to pulmonary hypertension. Auscultation reveals an opening snap soon after the second heart sound, as the diseased valve is opened forcibly by the high pressure in the left atrium. The reverse happens when the valve closes and there is a loud 'tapping' first heart sound. In addition, a rumbling mid-diastolic murmur can be heard. The duration of the murmur is related to the severity of the mitral stenosis, increasing in length as the mitral stenosis becomes more severe.

Investigations

- *ECG* may show left atrial enlargement (P-mitrale) or AF. Right axis deviation and other ECG signs of right ventricular hypertrophy (tall QRS complexes in the right ventricular leads V_{1-3}) may also be present.

- *Chest radiography.* There is a small aortic outline and a prominent pulmonary artery. The left atrium is enlarged (sometimes to an enormous degree) along with upper lobe diversion as a result of the raised pulmonary venous pressure. The right ventricle also appears enlarged (Fig. 51.14).
- *Echocardiography*, in combination with colour flow Doppler imaging, allows assessment of the flow across the valve and, therefore, the degree of stenosis. Transoesophageal echocardiography (TOE) may be better at assessing valve morphology in detail and excluding the presence of an atrial clot.

Indications for surgery

Medical management includes the use of anticoagulation in patients with AF or left atrial enlargement. Prophylactic antibiotics for endocarditis should be administered before invasive procedures. Tachyarrhythmias, including fast AF, which may lead to decompensation and cardiac failure, should be avoided. Digoxin is the mainstay of treatment but other rate-controlling agents are increasingly used. Diuretics may provide some benefit.

Surgery is indicated for severe symptoms (NYHA class III or IV), moderate or severe mitral stenosis (mitral valve area ≤ 1.5 cm²) or systemic emboli. Prognosis is determined by the severity of the stenosis, the size of the atrium, the onset of AF, rising pulmonary artery pressure and the unpredictable risk of embolism from a large, fibrillating atrium (Fig. 51.15). Surgical options include commissurotomy or valvotomy, which may be closed or open, mitral valve repair or mitral valve replacement. Since the 1980s, percutaneous mitral balloon valvotomy (PMBV), a catheter-based approach, has become an accepted alternative to surgical approaches in selected patients (Summary box 51.11).

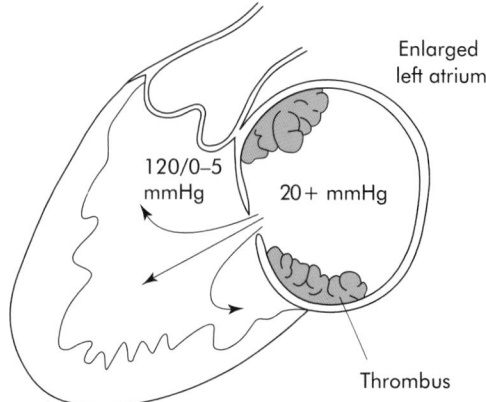

Figure 51.15 Features and pathophysiology of mitral stenosis. The aorta and left ventricle are relatively small because of chronically reduced cardiac output. The atrium is enlarged and may fibrillate, become stagnant and contain a thrombus. The ventricle fills with a turbulent jet that may be detected as a diastolic murmur or a thrill at the apex.

Summary box 51.11

Causes of mitral valve disease

Stenosis
- Rheumatic heart disease (common)
- Calcification of valve or chordae
- Congenital (rare)

Regurgitation
- Rheumatic heart disease
- Valve prolapse
- Left ventricular dilatation or hypertrophy
- Ischaemia
- Bacterial endocarditis

Mitral valve operations

Depending on the type of procedure and approach to the mitral valve, a median sternotomy or, occasionally, a left or right thoracotomy is completed. The mitral valve can be approached directly through the left atrium in the interatrial groove, through the right atrium and then the interatrial septum, or through the left atrial appendage.

Closed mitral valvotomy

Closed mitral valvotomy (or commissurotomy) was first carried out in the 1920s and by the 1950s was an accepted clinical procedure for the surgical treatment of mitral stenosis. The heart is approached through a left thoracotomy and purse-string sutures are placed at the apex of the left ventricle and in the left atrial appendage. A finger is introduced into the left atrial appendage and the mitral valve is assessed by direct palpation. A special dilator ('the Tubbs dilator') is inserted through the left ventricular apex and across the mitral valve. The dilator is opened and the fused commissures are split. Some regurgitation may occur and the process may have to be repeated after 10–15 years. In

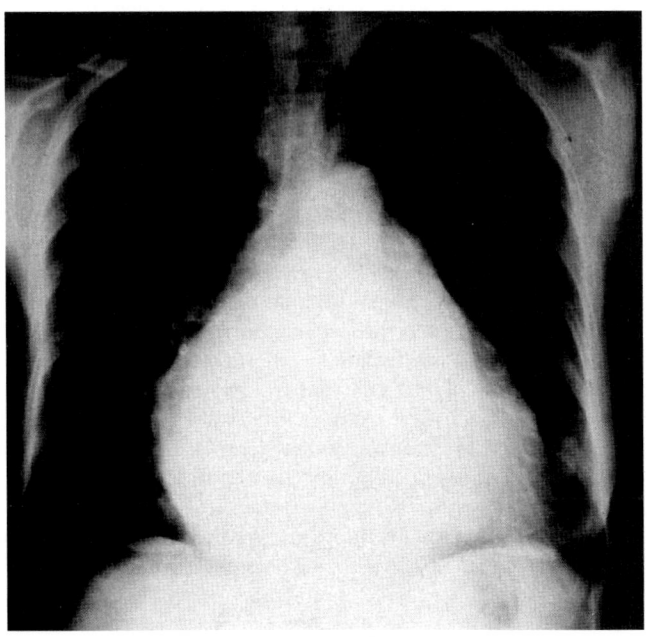

Figure 51.14 Chest radiograph of longstanding mitral stenosis, showing a massive left atrium.

Oswald Sydney Tubbs, **1908–1993, Cardiothoracic Surgeon, St. Bartholomew's Hospital, London, England.**

experienced hands, the mortality rate is < 1%. It is now uncommonly performed in developed countries as similar results can be achieved with PMBV.

Open mitral valvotomy

With the development of CPB in the 1960s, open mitral valvotomy (or commissurotomy) became accepted practice. It allows direct inspection of the mitral valve apparatus and, under direct vision, division of the commissures, splitting of fused chordae tendinae and papillary muscles, and debridement of calcium deposits. Amputation of the left atrial appendage may reduce the chance of subsequent thromboembolic events.

It has became clear that restoration of normal valve function is preferable to replacement and, as experience in open valvotomy has increased, there have been improvements in the complexity and variety of reconstructive mitral repair techniques available, particularly those to deal with mitral regurgitation.

Mitral valve repair

The functional classification system developed by Carpentier serves as a guideline in valve reconstruction. It allows classification of any mitral insufficiency into one of three groups according to the amplitude of the leaflet motion and provides a useful framework for the mechanisms of failure of the mitral valve. As a rule, several valvular lesions or abnormalities are involved in a functional abnormality, with specific techniques developed to correct each lesion.

At surgery, the anatomy of the valvular apparatus and subvalvular structures has to be carefully inspected. In particular, the extent of annular dilatation, leaflet prolapse and chordal dysfunction are assessed. The mitral valve reconstruction is completed using various techniques, including insertion of a prosthetic ring annuloplasty (Fig 51.16); quadrangular resection of the leaflet; use of a sliding plasty; chordal shortening; chordal transposition; and use of an Alfieri stitch.

The results of valve repair are better for regurgitant lesions than for stenotic lesions and repair is more likely with degenerative

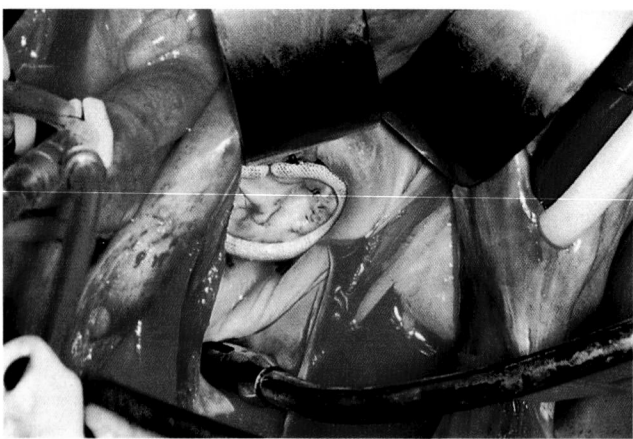

Figure 51.16 Operative view of the completed repair of a mitral valve using a Carpentier–Edwards annuloplasty ring (courtesy of A. Murday, FRCS).

Alain Carpentier, **Cardiothoracic Surgeon, Hôpital European Georges Pompidou, Paris, France.**
Ottavio R. Alfieri, **Cardiothoracic Surgeon, Ospedale San Raffaele, Milan, Italy.**

mitral lesions as opposed to rheumatic lesions or endocarditis. The operative mortality is 1–3%. Complication-free survival at 5 years ranges from 80 to 95%. Valve repair, although not conclusively demonstrated, offers better preservation of ventricular function and avoids the need for prolonged anticoagulation as well as avoiding valve-related complications such as PVE or structural dysfunction.

Mitral valve replacement

When valve repair is not possible mitral valve replacement is necessary. This usually involves a median sternotomy and access to the left atrium on CPB. The diseased valve is exposed, excised and a suitably sized mechanical or bioprosthetic valve is implanted. The atriotomy is closed following de-airing of the left heart. Intraoperative TOE can be used to assess adequate valve function.

The operative mortality rate for elective mitral valve replacement is approximately 5–6%. This depends largely on the state of the myocardium and the general condition (including age) of the patient. Common serious in-hospital complications include stroke (< 4%) and renal failure (3%), although any complication of heart surgery is possible. The longer-term prognosis for patients following mitral valve replacement is generally good in comparison with the natural history of mitral valve disease.

Aortic valve disease

Approximately two-thirds of all valve surgery performed in the UK is for aortic valve disease, which remains common despite a reduction in the incidence of rheumatic fever in the developed world.

Aortic stenosis

Aortic stenosis, as opposed to aortic sclerosis, is when a pressure gradient can be demonstrated across the valve. Therefore, the difference is not absolute, as sclerosis can progress to stenosis. The common cause of aortic stenosis in adults is an acquired, degenerative, calcific process that produces an immobilisation of the aortic valve cusps. Progressive fibrosis and calcification of a congenitally abnormal valve can mimic this degenerative process. The usual congenital abnormality is commissural fusion, leading to a bicuspid aortic valve, which occurs in approximately 1% of the population (Fig. 51.17).

Pathophysiology

A pressure gradient develops between the left ventricle and the aorta, with the left ventricle adapting to this systolic pressure overload by an increase in left ventricular wall thickness or hypertrophy. This adaptive response is an attempt to normalise left ventricular wall stress in the face of increased left ventricular systolic pressure, and may maintain a normal cardiac output, prevent left ventricular dilatation and avoid significant symptoms for a number of years. Eventually, myocardial function is affected and, together with insufficient left ventricular hypertrophy to normalise wall stress (load mismatch), ventricular contractility is reduced.

When aortic stenosis is severe and cardiac output is normal, a > 50 mmHg gradient between peak systolic left ventricular and aortic pressure exists. As aortic stenosis worsens, cardiac output cannot increase with exertion and eventually becomes insufficient at rest. The reduction in ventricular contractility leads to an irreversible decline in left ventricular function, with dilatation

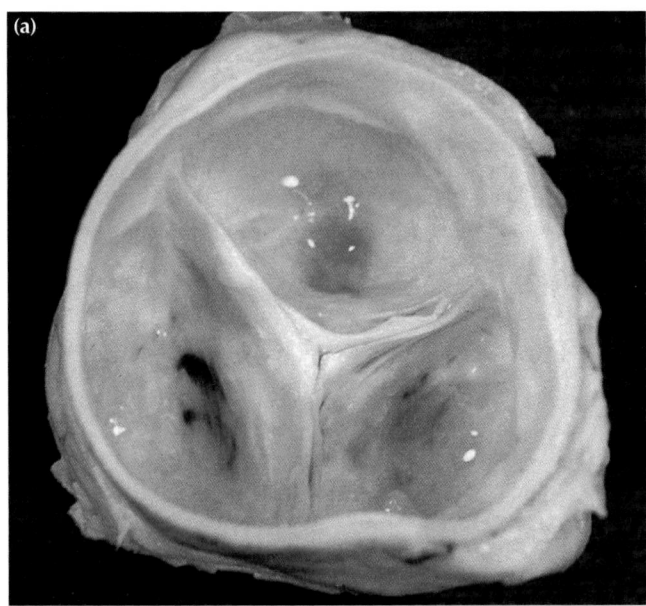

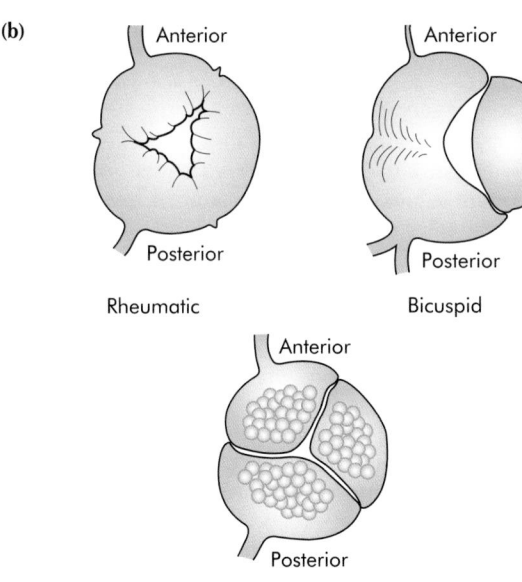

Figure 51.17 (a) Formaldehyde-treated aortic valve (normal tricuspid configuration). (b) Aortic stenosis, different pathologies.

and a rise in left ventricular end-diastolic pressure, to the point of overt left heart failure.

Clinical features

Patients are often asymptomatic until decompensation occurs, typically presenting with dyspnoea and angina, which is due to increased oxygen needs of the hypertrophied left ventricle, reduced coronary filling and inadequate cardiac output during exertion. Patients often describe a feeling of light-headedness or 'near' syncope on effort. Cardiac arrhythmias can also occur. Auscultation of the heart demonstrates a murmur that is typically harsh, ejection in nature and best heard over the aortic area with radiation to the carotids. With critical aortic stenosis and a fall in cardiac output, the murmur may become quieter. The apex beat may be displaced in late disease along with signs of cardiac congestion (Fig. 51.18).

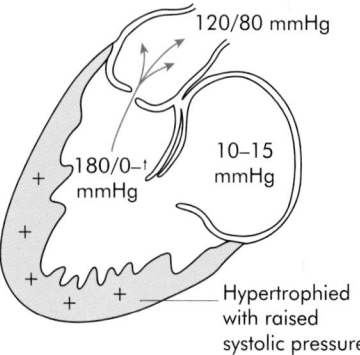

Figure 51.18 Features and pathophysiology of aortic stenosis. Haemodynamic changes in aortic stenosis. Aorta with post-stenotic dilatation.

Investigations

- *ECG.* There is left ventricular hypertrophy with tall R waves in the lateral leads and sometimes a 'strain pattern' (S–T depression with inverted T waves in the lateral leads).
- *Chest radiography.* May be normal. Cardiomegaly and pulmonary congestion can be seen in the presence of left ventricular failure. Post-stenotic dilatation of the aorta is occasionally seen (Fig. 51.19).
- *Echocardiography* confirms the diagnosis and, together with colour flow Doppler imaging, allows assessment of the aortic valve gradient, calculation of valve area, and evaluation of left ventricular dimensions and wall thickness.

Indications for surgery

Medical management focuses on the avoidance of systemic hypotension and arterial vasodilatation, which may reduce myocardial perfusion pressure and therefore provoke ischaemia.

The natural history of symptomatic patients with aortic stenosis is dismal, with a 10-year mortality rate of 80–90%. The patient is at risk of sudden death related to the severity of the stenosis.

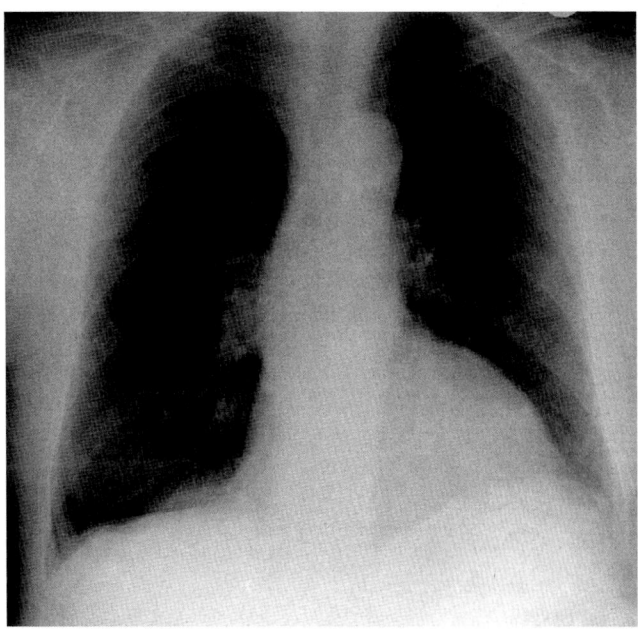

Figure 51.19 Chest radiograph in aortic stenosis.

An estimated or actual peak systolic gradient of > 6.7 kPa (50 mmHg) with left ventricular function is sufficient indication for aortic valve replacement.

Indications for surgery in asymptomatic patients with severe aortic stenosis are controversial. Most would consider surgery in patients with left ventricular dysfunction, concomitant coronary artery disease, in patients over 60–65 years, severe left ventricular hypertrophy, arrhythmias and silent ischaemia.

Aortic regurgitation

The causes of aortic regurgitation can be classified according to the speed of development of the regurgitant jet (acute or chronic) or according to the anatomical location of pathology (valve leaflet or aortic wall). The causes of acute aortic regurgitation include infective endocarditis, aortic dissection and trauma. The common causes of chronic aortic regurgitation include degeneration leading to aortic root and/or annular dilatation, congenital bicuspid valve and previous rheumatic fever or endocarditis (Summary box 51.12).

Summary box 51.12

Causes of aortic regurgitation according to predominant anatomical location of pathology

Valve leaflet disease
- Congenital, e.g. bicuspid valve leading to degenerative changes, with ventricular septal defect
- Rheumatic heart disease
- Infective endocarditis

Aortic wall pathology
- Inflammatory, e.g. connective tissue disorders such as ankylosing spondylitis, systemic lupus erythematosus, rheumatoid arthritis
- Systemic disease, e.g. tertiary syphilis
- Degenerative, e.g. Marfan's syndrome, aortic root dissection, senile aortopathy, leading to aortic root/annular dilatation

Adapted from Petch, M. (1997) Aortic valve disease. *Medicine* **25**: 31.

Pathophysiology

Acute aortic regurgitation imposes a volume load on the left ventricle because of backflow. It causes a sharp rise in left ventricular end-diastolic pressure, premature closure of the mitral valve and inadequate forward left ventricular filling. The result is sudden haemodynamic deterioration and acute respiratory compromise.

In chronic aortic regurgitation, volume load and left ventricular end-diastolic pressure increase gradually, leading to compensatory left ventricular dilatation and eccentric hypertrophy to maintain adequate cardiac output. Systolic and diastolic function is abnormal, and sudden deterioration can occur.

Clinical features

Longstanding aortic regurgitation is asymptomatic until the left ventricle begins to fail, when exertional dyspnoea may be the only symptom. Angina can also develop. A wide pulse pressure due to

a reduction in diastolic pressure and collapsing pulse (water-hammer pulse) are commonly seen. Other manifestations of the wide pulse pressure include visible capillary pulsation of the nail bed (Quincke's sign), pulsatile head bobbing (de Musset's sign), visible arterial pulsation in the neck (Corrigan's sign), a 'pistol-shot' sound on auscultating over the femoral artery (Traube's sign) and uvular pulsation (Müller's sign). The apex is displaced laterally, often visible and hyperdynamic or 'thrusting' in nature because of the left ventricular hypertrophy. Auscultation reveals a high-pitched early diastolic murmur best heard at the left sternal edge (Fig. 51.20).

Investigations

- *ECG*. There is left ventricular hypertrophy and sometimes a 'strain pattern'.
- *Chest radiography*. Cardiomegaly can be seen if the left ventricle is dilating; sometimes, the aortic shadow may also indicate dilatation.
- *Echocardiography*. This allows assessment of the underlying cause and severity of aortic regurgitation and enables the diameter of the aortic root as well as left ventricular dimensions to be determined. Colour flow Doppler imaging quantifies the size of the regurgitant jet.

Indications for surgery

Medical therapy with vasodilator drugs for the relief of dyspnoea or angina is designed to improve forward stroke volume and reduce regurgitant volume. However, symptomatic relief does not alter the need for valve surgery.

The indications for surgery are the onset of symptoms of NYHA class III or IV. Minor degrees of aortic regurgitation are well tolerated but if the left ventricle deteriorates and dilates it may be too late for surgery. An end-diastolic pressure of > 70 mmHg, an end-systolic pressure of > 50 mmHg, an end-systolic dimension of > 50 mm and an end-diastolic dimension of > 70 mm indicate severe pathology warranting surgical intervention, even in patients with mild symptoms (NYHA class II). Asymptomatic patients with left ventricular dysfunction during

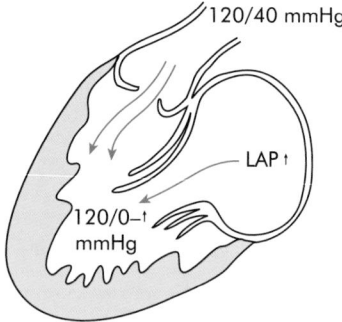

Figure 51.20 Haemodynamic consequences of aortic regurgitation. The left ventricle dilates and hypertrophies and there is a diastolic murmur. LAP, left atrial pressure.

Heinrich Irenaeus Quincke, **1842–1922, Professor of Medicine, Kiel, Germany.**
Louis Charles Alfred de Musset, **1810–1857, French poet and playwright in whom the sign, traditionally, was first noticed.**
Sir Dominic John Corrigan, **1802–1880, Physician, The Jervis Street Hospital, Dublin, Ireland.**
Ludwig Traube, **1818–1876, Physician, The Charité, Berlin, Germany.**
Friedrich von Müller, **1858–1941, a Physician of Munich, Germany.**

Bernard Jean Antonin Marfan, **1858–1942, Physician L'Hôpital des Enfants–Malades, Paris, France, described this syndrome in 1896.**

exercise should be followed up with regular echocardiography. Aortic valve replacement is recommended if there is progressive left ventricular dilatation or a fall in systolic function occurs (Summary box 51.13).

Summary box 51.13

Causes of aortic valve disease

Stenosis
- Congenital
- Rheumatic heart disease
- Acquired calcification and fibrosis of valve or chordae tendineae with age

Regurgitation
- Rheumatic heart disease
- Infective endocarditis
- Congenital
- Inflammatory:
    Systemic lupus erythematosus
    Rheumatic ankylosing spondylitis
- Dilatation of aortic root:
    Marfan's syndrome
    Dissection
- Systemic disease:
    Syphilis
    Ulcerative colitis

Aortic valve surgery

Unlike mitral valve surgery, there are few occasions when the aortic valve can be repaired and usually the valve requires replacement. However, in neonates and children, aortic valve repair or valvotomy is well established. Percutaneous aortic balloon valvotomy has a role in children, but appears to offer no benefits in adult aortic valve disease.

Aortic valve replacement

This is performed through a median sternotomy on CPB. The aorta is cross-clamped and opened proximally to reveal the diseased valve. Cardioplegic solution is infused into the coronary arteries to arrest the heart in diastole. The valve is then excised leaving the annulus *in situ* but removing as much calcific debris as possible. The annulus is sized and the mechanical or biological valve is then sutured into position at the level of the native annulus and the aortotomy is closed.

The operative mortality rate for elective aortic valve surgery is < 5%, but is higher in emergency surgery, in surgery for endocarditis and in older patients. The common serious in-hospital complications include stroke (2%), peroperative myocardial infarction (2%), renal failure requiring dialysis (0.7%) and heart block requiring a permanent pacemaker (< 1%). The major determinant of late survival after aortic valve surgery is preoperative left ventricular function. The 5-year survival rate is approximately 75–85%, with the majority of late deaths related to myocardial factors.

CONGENITAL HEART DISEASE

Introduction

Congenital heart diseases are abnormalities of cardiac structure that are present from birth. Such abnormalities in the development of the heart typically arise in the third to eighth week of gestation. The first operation for congenital heart disease was the ligation of a patent ductus arteriosus (PDA) by Gross in 1938. With the development of neonatal CPB, improved methods of myocardial protection and microsurgical techniques, an increasing number of corrective and palliative operations are possible.

Development of the heart and fetal circulation

By 12 weeks of fetal life the primitive vascular tube is fully developed. The fetal circulation differs from that of the adult in that the right and left ventricles pump blood in parallel rather than in series. Such an arrangement allows the heart and head to receive more highly oxygenated blood. In the fetus this is possible because of the presence of three structural shunts: the ductus venosus, the foramen ovale and the ductus arteriosus (Fig. 51.21).

Circulatory changes at birth

Soon after birth, pulmonary vascular resistance falls because of the action of breathing and the resulting pulmonary vasodilatation. In addition, within 30 min of delivery, the ductus arteriosus constricts in response to an increase in blood oxygen levels. The result is a reversal of the pulmonary–systemic pressure gradient and termination of blood flow from the pulmonary artery into the aorta.

After birth, the act of cutting and tying the umbilical cord stops venous blood flow from the placenta. This lowers the pressure in the inferior vena cava and, with the fall in pulmonary vascular resistance, right atrial pressure falls. The result is closure of the foramen ovale. The abolition of venous return from the placenta also causes the ductus venosus to close.

The closure of the fetal circulatory shunts in the few hours following birth is functional, with complete structural closure typically taking several months. In 20% of adults the structural closure of the foramen ovale remains incomplete, but is of no cardiovascular significance.

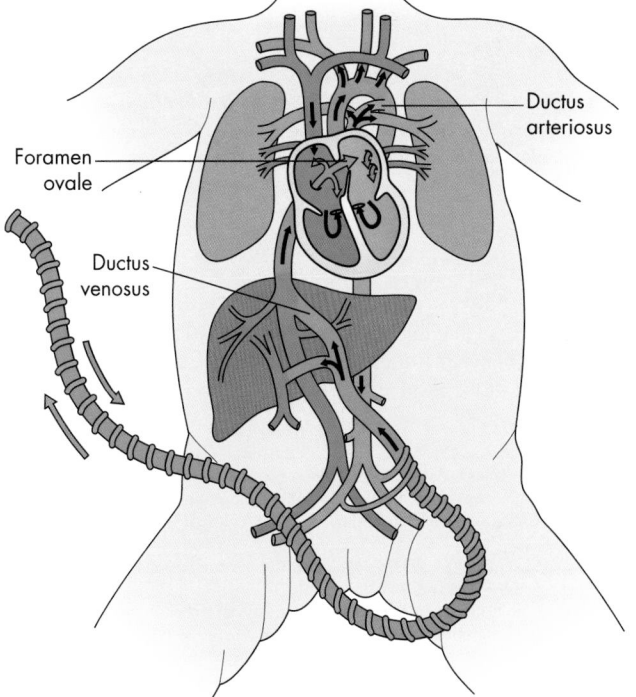

Figure 51.21 Fetal circulation.

Abnormalities of cardiac structure may arise from the persistence of normal fetal channels (PDA, patent foramen ovale), failure of septation (atrial septal defect, ventricular septal defect, tetralogy of Fallot), stenosis (intracardiac–supravalvular, valvular, infravalvular or extracardiac–coarctation of the aorta), atresia or abnormal connections (transposition of the great arteries, total anomalous venous drainage). Fetal echocardiography is now sufficiently sensitive to detect intracardiac lesions in the second trimester.

Incidence

Congenital heart disease is the most common congenital abnormality in the UK; the incidence of significant cardiac abnormalities is 8 cases per 1000 live births. Many spontaneous abortions or stillbirths have cardiac malformations or chromosomal abnormalities associated with structural heart defects. In neonates and children with congenital heart disease, 15% will have more than one cardiac abnormality and 15% will have another extracardiac abnormality.

Aetiology

There is often no obvious aetiology; most abnormalities appear to be multifactorial with both genetic and environmental influences. There are well-recognised associations (Summary box 51.14).

Summary box 51.14

Recognised associations with congenital heart disease

Maternal (environmental) factors
- Infection: rubella
- Disease: systemic lupus erythematosus, diabetes mellitus
- Drugs/medications: alcohol abuse, warfarin, phenytoin

Genetic factors
- Single gene defects: Marfan's, Noonan's and Holt–Oram's syndromes
- Chromosomal defects: trisomy 21 (Down's syndrome), trisomy 18 (Edwards' syndrome), trisomy 13 (Patau's syndrome), Turner's syndrome
- Deletions: DiGeorge's and Williams' syndromes

Diagnosis

Occasionally an antenatal diagnosis is possible, with severe congenital heart disease detected *in utero* at 16–18 weeks. If an infant is suspected of having a congenital heart disease, a diagnostic evaluation begins with an accurate history from the parents and specific questions about maternal health and drug intake during

Etienne Arthur Louis Fallot, 1850–1911, Professor of Medicine, Marseilles, France.
Jacqueline Anne Noonan, B. 1921, Pediatric Cardiologist, The University of Kentucky College of Medicine, Lexington, KY, USA, described this condition in 1963.
Mary Clayton Holt, 1924–1993, Cardiologist, The London Hospital for Women and Children, London, England.
Samuel Oram, 1913–1991, Cardiologist, King's College Hospital, London, England. Holt and Oram described this syndrome in a joint paper in 1960.
John Hilton Edwards, 1928–2007, Professor of Genetics, The University of Oxford, Oxford, England.
Angelo M. DiGeorge, B. 1921, Professor of Pediatrics, Temple University, Philadelphia, PA, USA.

pregnancy. A detailed family history is important because some defects are familial. Clinical examination may reveal a murmur, evidence of heart failure, failure to thrive and cyanosis. In addition, congenital heart disease can present with hypertension, an arrhythmia, evidence of polycythaemia or a thromboembolic event. Investigation is much the same as for the adult patient and, with fetal echocardiography available, cardiac catheterisation is now avoided whenever possible.

Classification

Congenital heart disease can be broadly classified according to the presence or absence of cyanosis, although the distinction is not always clear-cut. The presence of central cyanosis, blueness of the trunk and mucous membranes, results from levels of deoxygenated haemoglobin of $> 3–5\,\mathrm{g\,dl^{-1}}$ in the arterial circulation.

Cyanotic congenital heart diseases make up one-third of cases and are usually more complex, although they do include simple defects. Cyanotic congenital cardiac lesions can involve:

- A right-to-left shunt resulting in decreased pulmonary blood flow. Many of these lesions consist of a septal defect in conjunction with a right-sided obstructive lesion, producing an obligatory right-to-left shunt. The most common cause of this is tetralogy of Fallot.
- Parallel systemic and pulmonary blood flow rather than in series. If there is no mixing this is incompatible with life, so typically neonates have a patent foramen ovale that allows some mixing of the two circulations at this level. The most common example of this is transposition of the great vessels (TGV).
- Defects in the connections of the heart in which there is mixing of the systemic and pulmonary flows. An example of such a complex lesion is total anomalous pulmonary venous drainage.

Acyanotic congenital heart diseases represent the other two-thirds of cases and are usually less complex. Such defects result in an increase in the work imposed on the heart because of either:

- A left-to-right shunt with increased pulmonary blood flow, which causes an increase in volume work of the heart. Examples include PDA, atrial septal defect (ASD) and ventricular septal defect (VSD).
- Obstruction of the blood flow across a heart valve on the left side of the heart, such as aortic stenosis, or in the aorta itself, as occurs with coarctation of the aorta, leading to an increase in pressure and work of the heart.

Typically, acyanotic congenital heart disease presents as heart failure in infancy because of pulmonary congestion caused by increased pulmonary blood flow or increased pulmonary venous blood pressure resulting from an obstructive lesion. The common acyanotic cardiac defects can also present as a murmur in infancy or later.

Cyanotic congenital heart disease
Fallot's tetralogy

This is the most common cyanotic congenital heart disease found in children surviving to 1 year and accounts for about 4–6% of all congenital heart diseases. The four intracardiac lesions originally described (Fig. 51.22) were:

- VSD
- overriding aorta

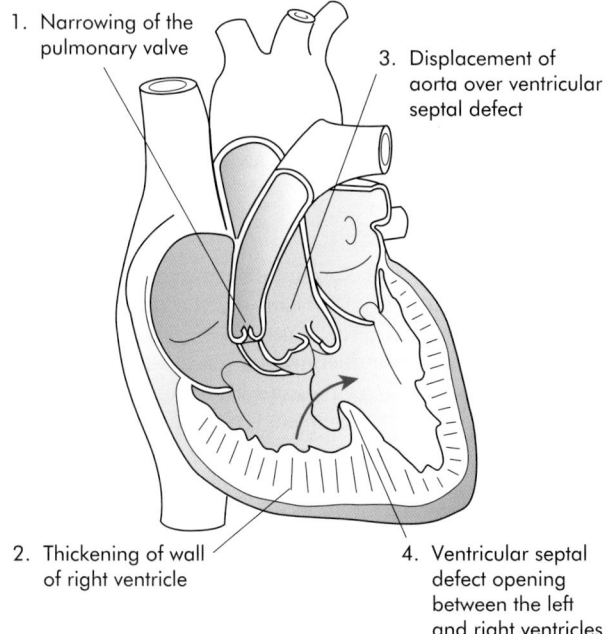

1. Narrowing of the pulmonary valve

3. Displacement of aorta over ventricular septal defect

2. Thickening of wall of right ventricle

4. Ventricular septal defect opening between the left and right ventricles

Figure 51.22 Fallot's tetralogy. Four abnormalities that result in insufficiently oxygentated blood being pumped to the body.

- pulmonary (typically infundibular or subpulmonary) stenosis
- right ventricular hypertrophy.

Clinically, there may be no signs initially but, as pulmonary stenosis progresses, cyanosis typically develops within the first year of life. Squatting is an adaptation by the child to hypoxic spells. This increases systemic vascular resistance and the venous return to the heart and consequently blood is diverted into the pulmonary circulation with increased oxygenation. Lethargy and tiredness are also common. Classically the chest radiograph demonstrates a 'boot-shaped' heart with poorly developed lung vasculature. The diagnosis is confirmed with echocardiography. Surgery to correct the tetralogy can be performed early as a single complete primary repair or later following an initial palliative shunt, which diverts systemic blood into the pulmonary circulation and may be used to improve oxygenation. The results of surgery are good, with a late survival rate at 5–10 years following correction of tetralogy of 95%, an operative mortality rate for a repair of between 5% and 10%, and an incidence of reoperation following tetralogy repair of 5–10%.

Transposition of the great vessels

The condition, first described by Morgagni, is the second most common cyanotic congenital heart disease and is the most common cause of cyanosis from a congenital cardiac defect discovered in the newborn period. TGV results from abnormal development and typically occurs when the aorta arises from the right ventricle and the pulmonary artery from the left ventricle (Fig. 51.23). The resulting transposition causes the pulmonary and systemic circulations to run in parallel rather than in series, so that oxygenated pulmonary venous blood returns back to the lungs and desaturated systemic venous blood is pumped around the body. The situation is incompatible with life and mixing of the blood must occur through associated shunts such as a patent foramen ovale or associated VSD. The most obvious presentation is severe central cyanosis ocurring in the first 48 hours of life.

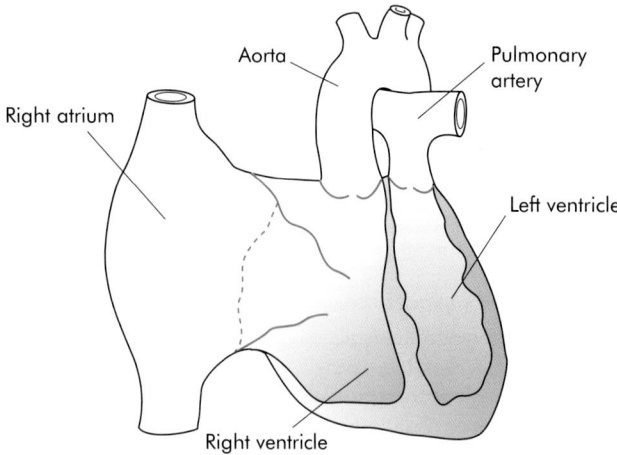

Aorta

Pulmonary artery

Right atrium

Left ventricle

Right ventricle

Figure 51.23 Transposition of the great vessels.

However, if there is a large ASD or VSD there may be minimal cyanosis initially. Typically, progress is poor and, as pulmonary vascular resistance declines in the neonatal period, high pulmonary flow develops, with cardiac enlargement and left ventricular failure.

The chest radiograph shows pulmonary plethora, with the heart having an 'egg on its side' appearance, with a small pedicle (aorta in front of pulmonary artery). Cardiac catheterisation and echocardiography confirm the diagnosis and delineate the anatomy. Initial palliation is by percutaneous (Rashkind) balloon atrial septostomy or, alternatively, intravenous prostaglandin to keep the ductus open. Definitive repair is usually by the arterial switch procedure, mostly carried out as a two-stage procedure, whereby the pulmonary artery is first banded to 'tone up' the left ventricle. However, the arterial switch procedure without prior pulmonary artery banding is increasingly being carried out in the newborn with TGV and an intact ventricular septum. The long-term results are impressive and it has replaced the atrial switch or baffle (Mustard or Senning) operations.

Total anomalous pulmonary venous drainage

Total anomalous pulmonary venous drainage (TAPVD) accounts for only 1–2% of congenital heart disease. In this condition the pulmonary venous drainage has become disconnected from the left atrium and drains into the systemic venous circulation at some other point (inferior vena cava, superior vena cava, coronary sinus or right atrium). Typically, TAPVD presents after the first week of life with cyanosis that is mild to moderate depending on pulmonary flow. Infants with high pulmonary flow develop cardiac failure, recurrent chest infections, failure to thrive and feeding difficulties. If high pulmonary flow is associated with a large ASD, cyanosis is often minimal and the lesion is tolerated well. If there is additional venous obstruction, cyanosis presents at birth with dyspnoea and pulmonary oedema. Echocardiography and cardiac (pulmonary) angiography are necessary to

William Jacobson Rashkind, **B. 1922, Surgeon, The Children's Hospital, Philadelphia, PA, USA.**
William T. Mustard, **formerly Associate Professor of Surgery, The Hospital for Sick Children, Toronto, Ontario, Canada.**
Ake Senning, **1915–2000, Professor of Surgery, The University Hospital, Zurich, Switzerland.**

confirm the diagnosis and establish the location of the anomalous drainage.

The surgical principle is to re-establish the pulmonary venous drainage into the left atrium. The exact operative technique depends on the anatomy and type of TAPVD. The long-term results for survivors of the operation are generally good. Late death following repair is uncommon but, when it occurs, it is often caused by intimal fibroplasia of the pulmonary veins away from the anastomosis.

Eisenmenger's syndrome

Eisenmenger's syndrome is becoming less common as corrective surgery is undertaken increasingly early and fewer patients develop a fixed increase in their pulmonary vascular resistance. It occurs following the reversal of a left-to-right shunt across a previous left-to-right shunt, such as with an ASD, VSD or posterior interventricular artery. These congenital anomalies cause an increase in flow and higher right-sided pressures, which lead to compensatory right ventricular hypertrophy and a subsequent rise in pulmonary artery pressure. Increasing pulmonary hypertension leads to equalisation of pressures either side of the shunt but, at some point, the right-sided pressures will exceed those on the left side, resulting in shunt reversal and desaturated blood entering the left side of the circulation. Cyanosis and dyspnoea are the most common clinical features. Closure of the shunt is contraindicated if pulmonary hypertension is irreversible because the right-to-left shunt now serves to decompress the pulmonary circulation.

Acyanotic congenital heart disease

Patent ductus arteriosus

The ductus arteriosus, a normal fetal communication, facilitates the transfer of oxygenated blood from the pulmonary artery to the aorta, shunting blood away from the lungs. Normally, functional closure of the ductus occurs within a few hours of birth; it is abnormal if it persists beyond the neonatal period. The ductus closes in response to an increase in peripheral oxygen saturation and a drop in the resistance of the pulmonary circulation as the lungs expand; this causes the ductal tissue to contract through a prostaglandin inhibition mechanism. Prostaglandins, such as indomethacin, may be used therapeutically to close the ductus in the first few weeks of life. In premature babies the ductus is more likely to remain patent for longer or permanently. In the isolated case of PDA, there is a left-to-right shunt of blood, resulting in a high pulmonary blood flow. Small shunts usually cause few symptoms and signs apart from the continuous machinery murmur in the left second intercostal space. Larger ducts cause cardiac failure and can uncommonly lead to shunt reversal with cyanosis and clubbing. The diagnosis is best confirmed by echocardiography with colour flow Doppler imaging. Cardiac catheterisation is performed only if additional lesions are suspected.

After 6 months of age, spontaneous closure of a PDA is rare. Most should be closed by preschool age, regardless of the absence of symptoms, if the risks of infective endocarditis, developing left ventricular failure or, rarely, Eisenmenger's syndrome are to be avoided. In the adult, surgical treatment is indicated if there is a persistent left-to-right shunt, even in the presence of pulmonary hypertension. In the premature infant, if medical treatment to close the ductus is unsuccessful, the lesion may be treated by interventional cardiology using an umbrella or coil duct occlusion device inserted percutaneously. If the lesion is very large or the patient very small, surgical closure via a left thoracotomy is preferred. This can be accomplished by either ligation or division of the PDA. The operative mortality rate is low and outcome generally very good.

Coarctation of the aorta

This accounts for 6–7% of congenital heart disease and is defined as a haemodynamically significant narrowing of the aorta, usually in the descending aorta just distal to the left subclavian artery, around the area of the ductus arteriosus (Fig. 51.24). The coarctation typically puts a pressure load on the left ventricle, which can ultimately fail. The upper body is well perfused but the lower body, including the kidneys, is poorly perfused, leading to fluid overload, excess renin secretion and acidosis. Coarctation usually affects boys and, if it occurs in girls, it is suggestive of Turner's syndrome.

In the neonatal period, coarctation, often referred to as 'infantile' or preductal coarctation, presents with symptoms of heart failure. The child may appear well in the first few days of life because the coarctation is bypassed by the ductus arteriosus and oxygenated blood reaches the entire systemic circulation. As the ductus closes, the child becomes progressively more unwell. In adult-type coarctation, which is often juxtaductal or slightly postductal, obstruction is gradual with complications developing in adolescence or early adulthood. Hypertension is a common presenting problem in older children, often upper body hypertension only with development of enormous collateral vessels that may cause rib-notching and flow murmurs over the scapula. Other

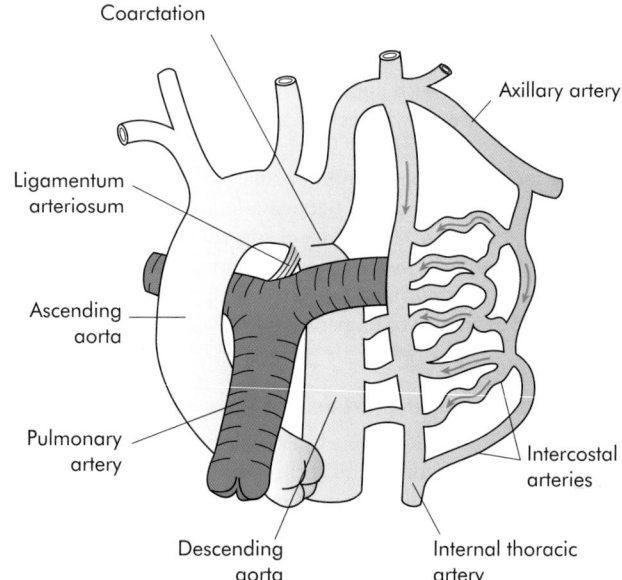

Figure 51.24 Coarctation of the aorta. Coarctation causes severe obstruction of blood flow in the descending thoracic aorta. The descending aorta and its branches are perfused by collateral channels from the axillary and internal thoracic arteries through the intercostal arteries (arrows).

Victor Eisenmenger, 1864–1932, German Physcian.

Henry Hubert Turner, 1892–1970, Professor of Medicine, The University of Oklahoma, Oklahoma City, OK, USA.

symptoms include prominent pulsation in the neck, tired legs or intermittent claudication on exercise. Clinical examination of the pulses may demonstrate a radiofemoral delay and a murmur that is continuous and heard best over the thoracic spine or below the left clavicle.

The chest radiograph classically demonstrates rib-notching from the age of 6–8 years because of dilated posterior intercostal vessels. The heart is usually of normal size in the older child and shows a classical 'three sign' replacing the typical aortic knuckle. The upper part of the three sign is the dilated left subclavian, the middle part is the narrowing at the coarctation site, and the lower part is the post-stenotic dilatation of the descending aorta. Echocardiography is diagnostic, with cardiac catheterisation performed if other anomalies are present. Infant coarctation typically presents with cardiac failure, often requiring vigorous medical treatment, including the administration of indomethacin to reopen the ductus and general resuscitation, before corrective surgery. Definitive treatment is usually surgical repair via a left thoracotomy. Coarctation presenting in the child or later typically requires surgical repair, as most patients die before the age of 40 years because of the associated complications. Percutaneous balloon dilatation is an alternative procedure in older children and adults and, in particular, for recoarctation. Without correction, the majority of deaths are caused by heart failure, infective endocarditis, rupture of the aorta or haemorrhagic stroke. The preoperative hypertension may not resolve despite surgical repair.

Atrial septal defects

An ASD is a defect in the septum between the left and right atria leading to a left-to-right shunt, the significance of which is determined by the size of the defect and the relative compliance of the ventricles. The development of the atrial septum is complex and abnormalities of development lead to three commonly recognised ASDs (Fig. 51.25).

The most common type is an *ostium secundum* ASD. The anomaly is caused by a defect in the floor of the fossa ovalis,

resulting in failure of the septum secundum to develop completely and cover the foramen ovale. Secundum defects are usually asymptomatic in childhood, with symptoms developing insidiously, typically presenting in middle age with congestive cardiac failure secondary to pulmonary hypertension or with atrial arrhythmias.

In *ostium primum* ASD the anomaly is a form of partial atrioventricular canal defect or endocardial cushion defect. The abnormalities are confined to the atrial septum and are caused by the endocardial cushions failing to develop and so close the ostium primum part of the interatrial septum. The defect is associated with abnormalities of the mitral valve, leading to mitral regurgitation. There is a relatively high incidence of this abnormality in trisomy 21 (Down's syndrome). Typically, the primum defect presents earlier than ostium secundum in childhood, with dyspnoea, recurrent chest infections and, if pulmonary hypertension develops, cyanosis.

A *sinus venosus* ASD is a rare defect and is the result of failure of partition of the pulmonary and systemic venous circulations. These defects are most commonly located high in the atrial septum at the junction of the superior vena cava and the right atrium. They are frequently associated with anomalous pulmonary venous drainage with right superior pulmonary veins draining into the superior vena cava or right atrium directly (Summary box 51.15).

> **Summary box 51.15**
>
> ### ASDs
>
> ***Common defects***
> - Ostium secundum: fossa ovalis defect (approximately 70% of ASDs)
> - Ostium primum: atrioventricular septal defect (approximately 20% of ASDs)
> - Sinus venosus defect: often associated with anomalous pulmonary venous drainage (approximately 10% of ASDs)
> - Patent foramen ovale: common in isolation, usually no left-to-right shunt (not strictly an ASD)
>
> ***Rarer defects***
> - Inferior vena cava defects: a low sinus venosus defect and may allow shunting of blood into the left atrium
> - Coronary sinus septal defect: also known as unroofed coronary sinus with the left superior vena cava draining to the left atrium as part of a more complex lesion

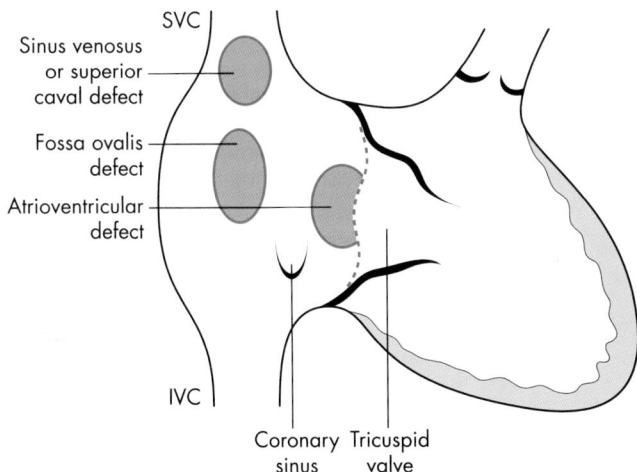

Figure 51.25 Atrial septum viewed from the right. The fossa ovalis is a useful reference point; the most common defect is in this area and is called a fossa ovalis (or ostium secundum) defect. A defect near the atrioventricular junction may be part of the spectrum of atrioventricular septal defects; if the defect is near the entry of the superior vena cava (SVC) it is commonly associated with anomalies of venous drainage into the atria. IVC, inferior vena cava.

Closure is performed during the first decade of life, even in the absence of symptoms, to avoid late-onset right ventricular failure, endocarditis and paradoxical emboli. In adults, closure is still appropriate for symptomatic improvement and avoidance of complications. The traditional method of closure involves open-heart surgery with CPB and closure of the defect either directly with sutures, as with most secundum defects, or, if the defect is large, using a pericardial or synthetic patch. Closure of small to moderate ASDs using percutaneous catheter-delivered devices in the cardiology catheter laboratory is increasingly common. Primum atrioventricular defect repairs may require additional mitral

John Langdon Haydon Down (sometimes given as Langdon-Down), **1828–1896**, Physician, The London Hospital, London, England.

valve repair. The operative mortality rate for isolated atrioventricular defect repairs is < 1%, with an excellent prognosis. Surgical correction of complete atrioventricular canal defects, with closure of the ASD and ventricular septal components and mitral valve repair, is possible with a higher surgical mortality rate.

Ventricular septal defects

A VSD is a defect in the interventricular septum that allows a left-to-right shunting of blood. VSDs account for 20–30% of congenital heart disease and affect approximately 2 in 1000 live births. They may occur in isolation or as part of a more complex set of cardiac abnormalities (e.g. tetralogy of Fallot, complete atrioventricular canal defect). Four major anatomical types of VSD are described, based on the anatomical subsections of the interventricular septum (Summary box 51.16 and Fig. 51.26).

Summary box 51.16

Types of VSD

Perimembranous defect
- Also called conoventricular VSD; the most common defect (70–80%), usually located within the membranous septum and may extend to the tricuspid valve annulus or base of the aortic valve

Muscular defect
- Also called trabecular VSD; occurs in 10% of cases and is located within the membranous septum and often multiple

Atrioventricular defect
- Also called atrioventricular canal-type defect; occurs in 5% of cases and is located in the atrioventricular canal beneath the tricuspid valve

Subarterial defect
- Also called infundibular or subarterial VSD; occurs in 5–10% of cases and lies within the conal septum immediately subaortic

---

The VSD permits a left-to-right shunt at the ventricular level, with subsequent right ventricular volume overload and increased pulmonary blood flow. This may lead to progressive pulmonary oedema and congestive cardiac failure. Persistently elevated pulmonary blood flow and pulmonary vascular resistance also lead to irreversible pulmonary hypertension. They may eventually result

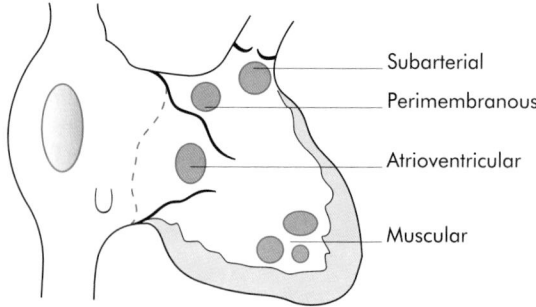

Figure 51.26 Ventricular septum viewed from the right, showing the characteristic sites of ventricular septal defects.

in reversal of flow across the defect and Eisenmenger's syndrome. The clinical presentation reflects the magnitude of the left-to-right shunt, which in turn depends on the size of the VSD and the pulmonary and systemic vascular resistances. Small defects may close or cause little systemic disturbance (maladie de Roger); infants are asymptomatic with normal development. In the first 5 years, up to 30–50% of VSDs close spontaneously. Clinically, a loud pansystolic murmur can be detected at the left sternal border because of high pressure flow between the ventricles. Large defects typically present with congestive cardiac failure in the first 2 months of life. Because of the size of the VSD, ventricular pressures are equalised and often only a soft systolic murmur is detected. If left untreated, pulmonary hypertensive changes start from about 1 year of age. Eisenmenger's syndrome, secondary to shunt reversal in such cases, may become evident in the second decade of life.

Echocardiography confirms the diagnosis and can estimate the degree of shunting across the defect. Cardiac catheterisation can quantify the various pressures within the cardiac chambers and so assess the degree of pulmonary hypertension, as well as demonstrating a step-up in oxygen saturation between left and right ventricles. Generally, surgical closure is indicated for large defects, when there is failure to respond to medical therapy, for left-to-right shunts of > 2:1, when there are signs of increasing pulmonary vascular resistance and in the presence of complications of VSD. These include (1) aortic regurgitation, which occurs in about 5% of defects; (2) infundibular stenosis, which tends to be progressive and leads to shunt reversal; and (3) infective endocarditis, often presenting with pneumonia or pleurisy as the infected 'emboli' in a VSD with a typical left-to-right shunt flows into the pulmonary circulation.

THE THORACIC AORTA

The most common pathology affecting the thoracic aorta is aneurysm formation or dissection.

Thoracic aortic aneurysms

A true aneurysm is a localised dilatation of a blood vessel involving all layers of the vessel, whereas a false aneurysm has compressed supporting tissue as its wall and is usually the result of a defect in the vessel intima (from trauma, dissection or previous surgery). Aneurysms are described as fusiform when the whole circumference is affected or saccular when only part of the circumference is involved.

Aortic aneurysms can develop anywhere along its length, but thoracic aortic aneurysms, including those that extend into the upper abdomen (thoracoabdominal aneurysms), account for 25%, typically occurring in men in the fifth to seventh decade or younger in those with connective tissue disorders.

Aetiology

The most common aetiology is atherosclerosis, but connective tissue disorders account for many aneurysms in the aortic root and ascending aorta now that tertiary syphilis is rare. Marfan's syndrome is associated with cystic medial degeneration involving the vessel wall and causes widening of the proximal aorta and aortic root, leading to aortic valve insufficiency. Other disorders

---

Henri Louis Roger, **1809–1891**, Physician, Hôpital Sainte-Eugene, Paris, France.

associated with aneurysm formation and dissection include Ehlers–Danlos's syndrome and osteogenesis imperfecta.

Trauma, typically following blunt chest injury, can lead to aneurysm formation, usually involving the descending aorta. However, these are usually false aneurysms containing haematoma from injury to the aortic vessel wall.

Clinical features

Many aneurysms are asymptomatic and are discovered incidentally on routine chest radiographs. Others present as a space-occupying lesion in the thorax with pain caused by pressure on adjacent structures (vertebra), hoarseness (left recurrent laryngeal nerve), dysphagia (oesophagus) and respiratory symptoms (left main bronchus). Aortic root aneurysms may lead to dilatation of the aortic root annulus and aortic regurgitation.

Rupture can lead to cardiac tamponade or haemorrhage into the left pleural space, leading to dyspnoea and, if the tracheobronchial airway or oesophagus is involved, haemoptysis or haematemesis respectively.

Investigations

The diagnosis is confirmed by CT or MRI. Arteriography is not necessary for diagnosis but is often required to demonstrate the relation of the arch vessels to the aneurysm.

Indications for surgery

Without treatment the aneurysm is likely to expand and ultimately rupture. Important factors to consider when planning treatment are age, comorbidity and coexisting coronary disease.

In ascending aneurysms, the presence of progressive aortic valve insufficiency is an important indication for surgery. Other indications in this group, including Marfan-related aneurysms, are a diameter of 5–6 cm and the presence of symptoms. In descending aneurysms, indications for surgery include symptoms, acute enlargement and a diameter of approximately 6 cm.

Surgical options

The approach adopted for surgical treatment depends on the location of the aneurysm, but typically involves a median sternotomy, CPB and cooling the patient to 18°C before cross-clamping the aorta above the aneurysm (Fig. 51.27). If the *aortic root* is involved, the aorta, together with its annulus and valve, is resected and a composite graft is sutured to the aortic root. The circulation is arrested and, after removal of the aortic cross-clamp, the distal anastomosis is completed. The coronary ostia require reimplantation into the graft (Bentall's operation). If the *ascending aorta* is involved, it is resected and replaced with a tube graft. For *aortic arch* aneurysms, surgery on this section of the aorta is a formidable undertaking because the cerebral and subclavian vessels have to be anastomosed to the graft, either separately or *en bloc*. Typically, it involves a period of circulatory arrest and some form of cerebral protection. Excision of a *descending aortic aneurysm* is with graft replacement under CPB with exposure via a left thoracotomy or

Edvard Ehlers, 1863–1937, Professor of Clinical Dermatology, Copenhagen, Denmark.
Henri Alexandre Danlos, 1844–1912, Dermatologist, Hôpital St. Louis, Paris, France, gave his account of this condition in 1908.
Hugh Henry Bentall, formerly Professor of Cardiac Surgery, The Royal Postgraduate Hospital, Hammersmith, London, England.

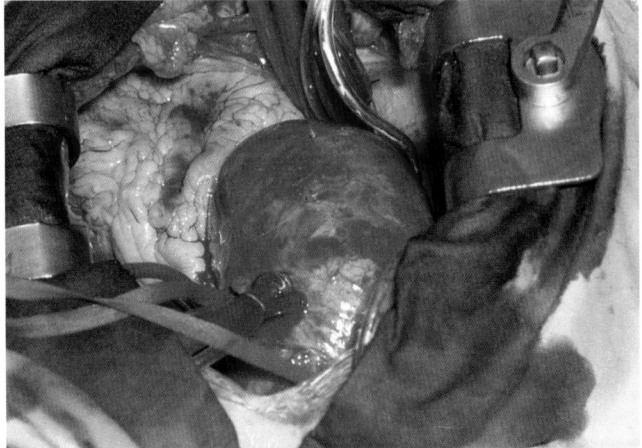

Figure 51.27 A large thoracic aortic aneurysm.

with a heparin-bonded shunt. Increasingly, thoracic aneurysms at the aortic arch or more distal are repaired using a percutaneous approach via the femoral artery with insertion of an endovascular stent under radiological guidance.

Surgical outcome

The operative mortality rate is variable depending on the location and type of repair required but electively is between 5% and 15%. An emergency repair has a considerably higher operative mortality rate. Long-term survival depends on underlying pathology but, for ascending aneurysm repairs, the 5-year survival rate is approximately 65%. The major complications of descending aneurysm repairs include paraplegia, renal failure and ventricular dysfunction.

Aortic dissection

This occurs when there is a defect or flap in the intima of the aorta, resulting in blood tracking into the aortic tissues splitting the medial layer and creating a false lumen. It most commonly occurs in the ascending aorta or less often just distal to the left subclavian artery. It is also more common in men, typically those aged 50–70 years, and in Afro-Caribbeans.

Aetiology

It usually occurs as a spontaneous or sporadic event, although very often a history of hypertension is noted. Other important associations include Marfan's syndrome and pregnancy (Summary box 51.17).

Summary box 51.17

Predisposing factors for aortic dissection

- Age
- Hypertension
- Marfan's syndrome
- Pregnancy
- Other connective tissue disorders, for example Ehlers–Danlos's syndrome, giant cell arteritis, systemic lupus erythematosus
- Coarctation of the aorta
- Turner's or Noonan's syndromes
- Aortotomy site

Clinical features

The presentation is often a tearing intrascapular pain not unlike the pain of myocardial ischaemia, and it may be difficult to distinguish between the two. The extent of arterial dissection may produce widespread symptoms and signs.

The dissection can extend distally down the aorta to involve:

- the renal arteries (renal pain and renal failure)
- the mesenteric arteries (abdominal pain and bowel ischaemia)
- the spinal arteries (paraplegia)
- the iliac arteries (leg pain, pallor, loss or reduced pulses and limb ischaemia).

The dissection may track proximally to involve:

- the head and neck vessels (symptoms and signs of a stroke or transient ischaemic attack)
- the coronary vessels (myocardial infarction)
- the aortic root (aortic regurgitation).

The aneurysm may rupture back into the lumen or externally into the pericardium (cardiac tamponade) or mediastinum (left haemothorax).

Classification

There are two classifications, both of which are limited in their application but widely used. The DeBakey classification is based on the pattern of dissection whereas the Stanford classification is based on whether the ascending aorta is involved (Fig. 51.28).

Investigations

The diagnosis is suspected when chest radiography demonstrates a widened mediastinum, often associated with fluid in the left costophrenic angle. Diagnosis is confirmed by whatever method is most readily at hand and includes echocardiography, ideally TOE, CT of the thorax or MRI (Fig. 51.29). Traditionally, aortography was the 'gold standard' technique and it still provides excellent information before surgery but, increasingly, advanced three-dimensional CT angiography and MRI are used when available.

Management

In the emergency situation, before further imaging, blood pressure (which is usually high at presentation) should be brought under control to prevent extension of the dissection.

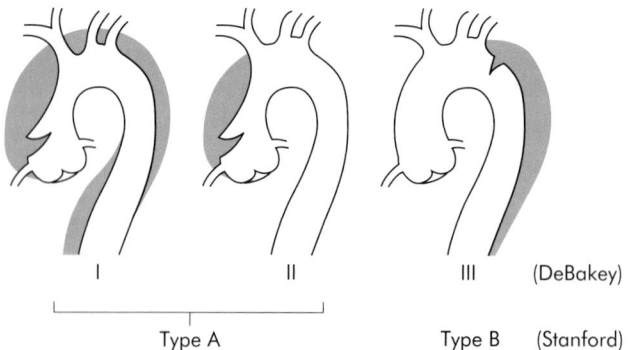

Figure 51.28 Stanford classification of aortic dissections according to whether the ascending aorta is involved (type A) or not (type B). This is simpler than the DeBakey classification (types I, II and III).

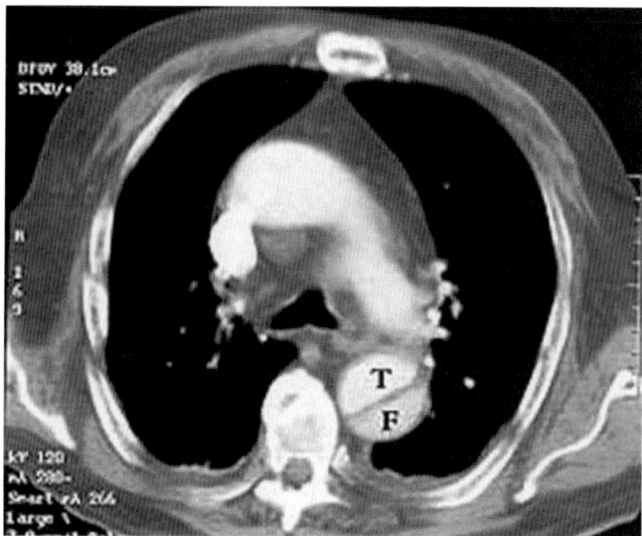

Figure 51.29 Computerised tomography scan showing acute dissection of the descending thoracic aorta. F, false lumen; T, true lumen.

Surgical options

Type A (or type I and II) dissections

Those involving the ascending aorta usually require surgical intervention. The chest is opened through a median sternotomy and CPB is started with core cooling down to 18°C. The aorta is cross-clamped as high as possible and opened. Cardioplegia solution is infused into the coronary ostia to arrest the heart in diastole. If the intimal tear is present and localised, the ascending aorta is excised with the tear and replaced with a synthetic graft. The distal anastomosis is performed with circulatory arrest.

Type B (or type III) dissections

Initially, these are best managed medically with antihypertensive drugs. Surgery is indicated if the pain increases (signalling impending rupture), the aneurysm is expanding on serial chest radiographs or complications, such as organ, limb or neurological symptoms, develop. The operation may be performed with a heparin-bonded shunt or under CPB. There is a real risk of paraplegia from this operation, which should be mentioned specifically to the patient before operation. Use of percutaneously placed endovascular stents is likely to increase in the future, although currently its role in the acute setting remains to be established.

Surgical outcome

If dissection is untreated, the mortality rate is 50% within 48 hours and 75% within 1–2 weeks. Almost all patients with type A dissections will die if not operated on, whereas patients with type B dissections have a better prognosis. The surgical mortality rate is variable but is around 15% for proximal aortic dissection. The overall survival rate for patients leaving hospital, regardless of the type of dissection, is around 80% at 5 years and 40% at 10 years.

PERICARDIAL DISEASE

There is a fibrous envelope covering the heart and separating it from the mediastinal structures. This fibrous structure includes a parietal layer and allows the heart to move with each beat. It is not essential for life because it can be left wide open after cardiac surgery without any ill-effects; however, there are a number of conditions affecting the pericardium that may present to the surgeon.

Pericardial effusion

There is a continuous production and resorption of pericardial fluid. If a disease process disturbs this balance a pericardial effusion may develop. If the pressure exceeds the pressure in the atria, compression will occur, venous return will fall and the circulation will be compromised. This state of affairs is called 'tamponade'. A gradual build-up of fluid (e.g. malignant infiltration) may be well tolerated for a long period before tamponade occurs, and the pericardial cavity may contain 2 litres of fluid. Acute tamponade (from penetrating trauma, during coronary angiography or postoperatively) may occur in minutes with small volumes of blood. The clinical features are low blood pressure with a raised jugular venous pressure and paradoxical pulse. Kussmaul's sign is a characteristic pattern that is seen when the jugular venous pressure rises with inspiration as a result of the impaired venous return to the heart.

Emergency treatment of pericardial tamponade is aspiration of the pericardial space. A wide-bore needle is inserted under local anaesthesia to the left of the xiphisternum, between the angle of the xiphisternum and the ribcage (Fig. 51.30). The needle is advanced towards the tip of the scapula into the pericardial space. An ECG electrode attached to the needle will indicate when the heart has been touched. This will relieve the situation temporarily until the cause of the tamponade is established. Penetrating wounds of the heart usually require exploration through a median sternotomy. Emergency room thoracotomy is rarely required. Chronic tamponade is usually a result of malignant infiltration of the pericardium (usually secondary carcinoma from breast or bronchus) or, very occasionally, uraemia or connective tissue disease. Treatment sometimes requires a pericardial window between the pericardial space and the pleural or peritoneal space.

Pericarditis

Infection and inflammation may also affect the pericardium. Acute pericarditis usually occurs following a viral illness. Treatment is with non-steroidal anti-inflammatory drugs and bed rest (in case there is an underlying myocarditis). Acute purulent pericarditis is uncommon but requires urgent drainage and intravenous antibiotics with attention to the underlying cause.

Chronic pericarditis is an uncommon condition in which the pericardium becomes thickened and non-compliant. The heart cannot move freely and the stroke volume is reduced by the constrictive process. The central venous pressure is raised and the liver becomes congested. Peripheral oedema and ascites are also a feature. Treatment is aimed at relieving the constriction.

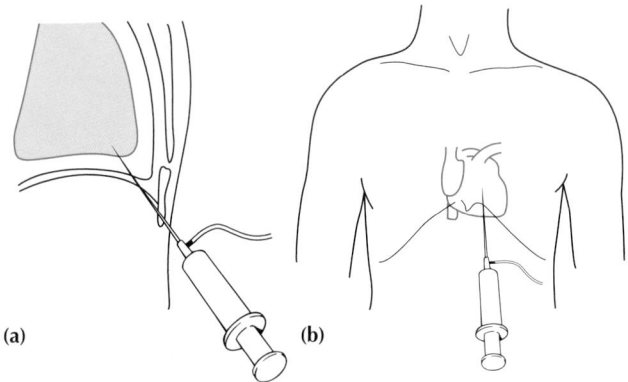

Figure 51.30 (a) Pericardial aspiration through the subxiphoid region. (b) Site of needle insertion for pericardial aspiration.

Adolf Kussmaul, 1822–1902, successively Professor of Medicine at Heidelberg, Erlangen, Freiburg and Strasbourg, Germany.

FURTHER READING

Treasure, T., Hunt, I., Keogh, B. and Pagano, D. (eds) (2004) *The Evidence for Cardiothoracic Surgery*. tfm, Shrewsbury, UK.

Bojar, R.M. (1999) *Manual of Perioperative Care in Cardiac Surgery*, 3rd edn. Blackwell Science, Oxford.

Henry Edmunds, L., Jr. (2003) *Cardiac Surgery in the Adult*, 2nd edn. Available online at: www.ctsnet.org/book/edmunds/

Kirklin, J. and Barratt-Boyce, B. (2003) *Cardiac Surgery*, 3rd edn. Churchill Livingstone, Edinburgh.

The thorax

LEARNING OBJECTIVES

To understand:
- The anatomy and physiology of the thorax

- Investigation of chest pathology
- Surgical oncology as applied to chest surgery

INTRODUCTION

Anatomical development of the lungs

The lungs are derived from an outpouching of the primitive foregut during the fourth week of intrauterine life. This bud becomes a two-lobed structure, the ends of which ultimately become the lungs. The lobar arrangement is defined early and is fairly constant but anomalies of fissures and segments are common.

The primitive lungs drain into the cardinal veins, which ultimately become the pulmonary veins draining into the left atrium. Variability in venous drainage is very common and is usually of little functional significance. At the most severe end of the spectrum is total anomalous drainage, which presents in early infant life because oxygenated blood is all directed back to the right heart.

Anatomy of the lungs

The left lung is divided by the oblique fissure, which lies nearer vertical than horizontal, so the upper and lower lobes could also be called anterior and posterior. On the right, the equivalent of the upper lobe is further divided to give the middle lobe. Each lobe is composed of segments, with anatomically defined and named bronchial, pulmonary arterial and venous connections (Fig. 52.1).

The right main bronchus is shorter, wider and nearly vertical compared with the left. As a consequence, inhaled foreign bodies are more likely to enter the right main bronchus than the left (Fig. 52.2). The trachea and bronchi have a systemic arterial blood supply delivered by the bronchial arteries, which arise directly from the nearby thoracic aorta.

Lymphatic drainage tends to follow the bronchi. Lymph nodes are both named and identified by numbered 'stations', which are of importance in staging of lung cancer (Fig. 52.3).

Mechanics of breathing

The intercostal muscles contract, causing the ribs to move upwards and outwards, thereby increasing the transverse and anteroposterior dimensions of the chest wall. The diaphragm contracts simultaneously and flattens, increasing the vertical dimension of the chest cavity. As the volume increases, the intrathoracic pressure falls and air flows in until the alveolar pressure is the same

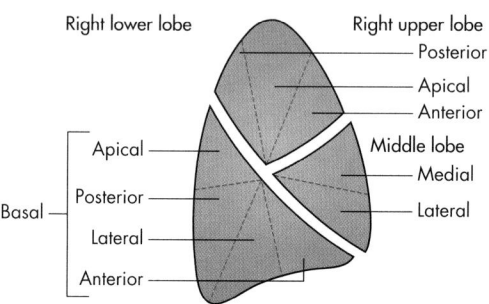

Figure 52.1 The lobar and segmental divisions of the lungs, right lung above and left lung below as if viewed from the side.

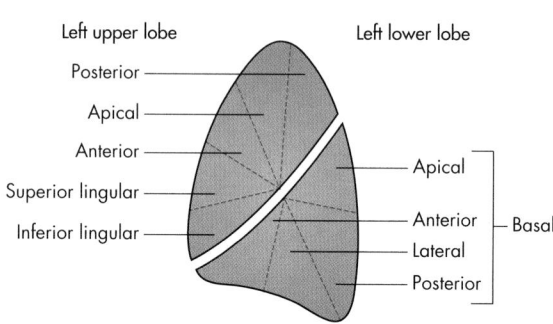

Figure 52.2 Surgical anatomy of the bronchial tree. To surgically remove the right lower lobe and conserve the middle lobe, the surgeon must be prepared to dissect and separately divide the apical bronchial segment (red line).

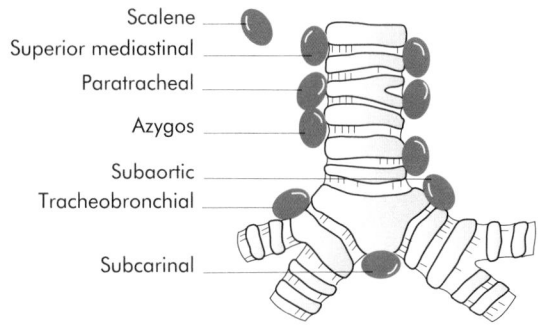

Scalene
Superior mediastinal
Paratracheal
Azygos
Subaortic
Tracheobronchial
Subcarinal

Figure 52.3 Lymph nodes related to the bronchial tree.

as the atmospheric pressure. The only force used in normal expiration is the elastic recoil of the lung.

Coughing to clear sputum is an essential part of recovery from surgery. In a vigorous cough, probably the only muscle in the body that is relaxπed is the diaphragm; as the abdomen and chest wall muscles contract, the limbs are braced and the sphincters are tightened. When the intrathoracic and abdominal pressure is built up, the glottis is opened and the diaphragm is forced up as a piston, or like the plunger of a syringe, to expel air at high velocity.

Investigation of the respiratory system

Any patient undergoing general anaesthesia requires some assessment of respiratory function. This may be a clinical appraisal of fitness but more detail is necessary for patients who are undergoing thoracotomy and lung resection.

Pulmonary function tests are useful in determining the functional capacity of the patient and the severity of pulmonary disease, and in predicting the response to various treatments. The tests range from simple clinic or bedside measurements to those only available in specialist centres. The simpler tests are listed below (Table 52.1).

Peak expiratory flow rate

Peak expiratory flow rate (PEFR) is measured by a Wright peak flow meter or a peak flow gauge. This is a reliable and reproducible test but has the disadvantage of being effort dependent, and it may therefore be affected by abdominal or thoracic wound pain.

Forced expiratory volume in 1 second

The forced expiratory volume in 1 s (FEV_1) is the amount of air forcibly expired in 1 s. It is low in obstructive lung disease and may be normal in patients with poor gas exchange.

Table 52.1 Respiratory values in lung disease

	Obstructive pattern	**Restrictive pattern**
PEFR	↓↓	Normal or ↓
FEV_1	↓↓	Normal or ↓
FVC	Normal or ↓	↓↓
FEV_1/FVC	< 70	> 80

FEV_1, forced expiratory volume in 1 s; FVC, forced vital capacity; PEFR, peak expiratory flow rate.

> Basil Martin Wright, **1912–2001, Member of the Scientific Staff of the Medical Research Council Research Centre, Northwick Park Hospital, Harrow, Middlesex, England.**

Forced vital capacity

The forced vital capacity (FVC) is the volume of air forcibly displaced following maximal inspiration to maximal expiration. The FEV_1 and the FVC can be measured using a Vitallograph and a ratio (FEV_1/FVC) can be calculated (Fig. 52.4). A low ratio indicates obstruction and the test should be repeated after bronchodilators. A normal ratio (FVC and FEV_1 reduced to the same extent) indicates a restrictive pathology.

Blood gases

Oxygen saturation can be measured non-invasively. The oxygen content of blood falls precipitously when saturation is less than 90% as an effect of the oxygen dissociation curve. Arterial blood gases provide a great deal of information (Table 52.2).

Fitness for lung resection

A patient with an $FEV_1 > 1.5$ litres is fit enough to undergo lobectomy; an $FEV_1 > 2.0$ litres is required for pneumonectomy. If the measurements are less than these they should be quoted as percentage predicted and further tests should be done.

The pleura

The key to many aspects of practical chest surgery is an understanding of the pleura and of the mechanics of breathing. Management of the essentially healthy pleural space is logical and simple and needs minimal technology. On the other hand, when pleural disease is advanced, for example when there is gross pleural sepsis surrounding a leaking and trapped lung, management is difficult and the patient may require prolonged care with repeated interventions.

The physiology of pleural fluid

The turnover of fluid in the human pleural space is about 1–2 litres in 24 hours, with only 5–10 ml of fluid present at any one time as a film, about 20 μm thick, between the visceral and parietal pleura. The quantities can only be measured indirectly because the very act of instrumenting the pleura to obtain a sample or measure the volume or pressure of fluid interferes with the physiological mechanisms that govern the flux of pleural fluid. For example, if there is a tube in the normal healthy pleural space it will drain 100–200 ml or more of fluid each day, which is simply part of the normal turnover; without the tube, the fluid would be absorbed.

Table 52.2 Blood gases

	Pao_2[a]	$Paco_2$[b]
Asthma		
Mild	↓	↓
Moderate	↓↓	Normal
Severe	↓↓↓	↑
Chronic bronchitis	↓↓	↑
Emphysema	Normal or ↓	↓
Fibrosing alveolitis (left ventricular failure or pulmonary embolus)	↓↓	↓ or normal
Type I respiratory failure	↓↓↓	Normal
Type II respiratory failure	↓↓↓	↓↓

[a] Arterial oxygen tension.
[b] Arterial carbon dioxide tension.

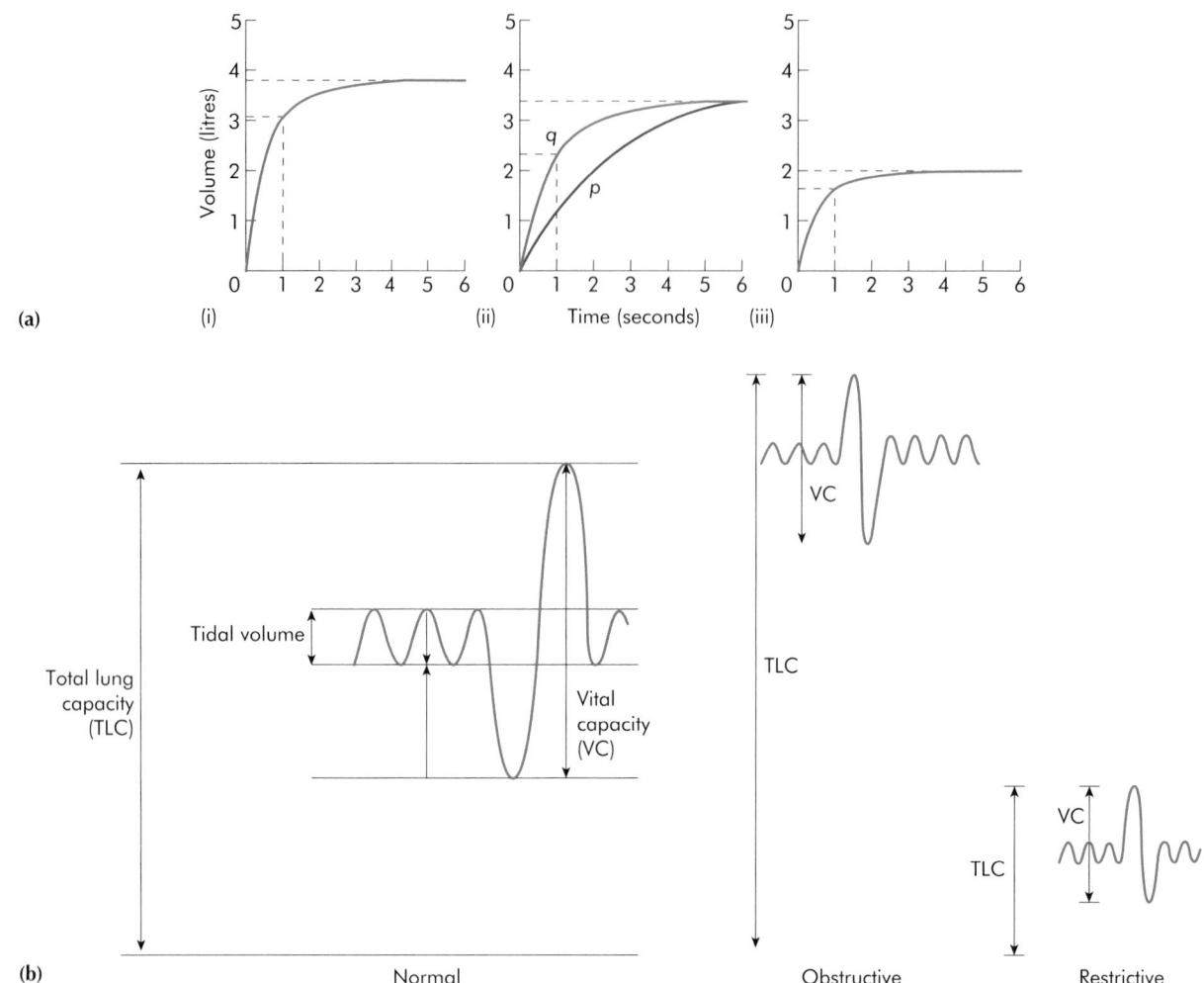

Figure 52.4 Spirometry. (a) Spirogram drawings obtained from a Vitallograph: (i) normal FEV$_1$ 31 litres, FVC 3.8 litres, FEV$_1$/FVC 82%; (ii) obstructive defect, reversible asthma, *p* before a bronchodilator, FEV$_1$ 1.4 litres, FVC 3.5 litres, FEV$_1$/FVC 40%; *q* after a bronchodilator, FEV$_1$ 2.5 litres, FVC 3.5 litres, FEV$_1$/FVC 71%; (iii) restrictive defect, fibrosing alveolitis, FEV$_1$ 1.8 litres, FVC 2.0 litres, FEV$_1$/FVC 90%. No change with bronchodilators. (b) Changes in lung volume in obstructive and restrictive lung disease. [Reproduced from H.H. Gray (1993) Pulmonary embolism. *Medicine International* **21**: 477, by kind permission of the Medicine Group (Journals) Ltd.]

The mechanisms and equations given are simplifications but serve to explain the clinical conditions encountered. The fluid is produced from the capillaries of the parietal pleura as a transudate, according to the Starling capillary loop pressures. However, there is a further negative force in the pleura. The elastic content of the lung causes it to recoil and collapse if not held open by the negative pressure in the pleura. This elastic recoil exerts about 4 mmHg negative pressure and favours accumulation of fluid. The secreting forces add up to about 11 mmHg in health. Pleural fluid is mainly reabsorbed (about 90%) by the visceral pleura, whose capillaries are part of the pulmonary circulation. The principal force in absorption of pleural fluid is oncotic pressure (approximately 25 mmHg) less the difference in mean capillary hydrostatic pressure of the pulmonary capillary (8 mmHg). Thus, the overall absorbing pressure is $25 - 8 = 17$ mmHg, producing a net drying effect $(17 - 11)$ of about 6 mmHg (Fig. 52.5).

Ernest Henry Starling, **1866–1927, Professor of Physiology, University College, London, England.**

Gas in the pleural space

There is normally no free gas in the pleural space because the same physiological mechanism that absorbs air from a pneumothorax prevents any gas accumulating.

The partial pressures (water as saturated vapour pressure) of the gases in venous/end-capillary blood are:

- P_{O_2} 40 mmHg   5.3 kPa
- P_{CO_2} 46 mmHg   6.1 kPa
- P_{N_2} 573 mmHg   76.4 kPa
- P_{H_2O} 47 mmHg   6.3 kPa

These partial pressures add up to less than atmospheric pressure (760 mmHg). Free gas is therefore absorbed into the blood and lost to the atmosphere through the lungs, with the gases moving in relation to their solubility (carbon dioxide quickest and nitrogen slowest) and relative concentrations in the pleural space and the blood. This does not favour nitrogen, which constitutes about 80% of atmospheric air. Breathing oxygen accelerates nitrogen removal by reducing the content of nitrogen in the blood and increasing the gradient for its absorption. Nitrous oxide anaesthesia is dangerous

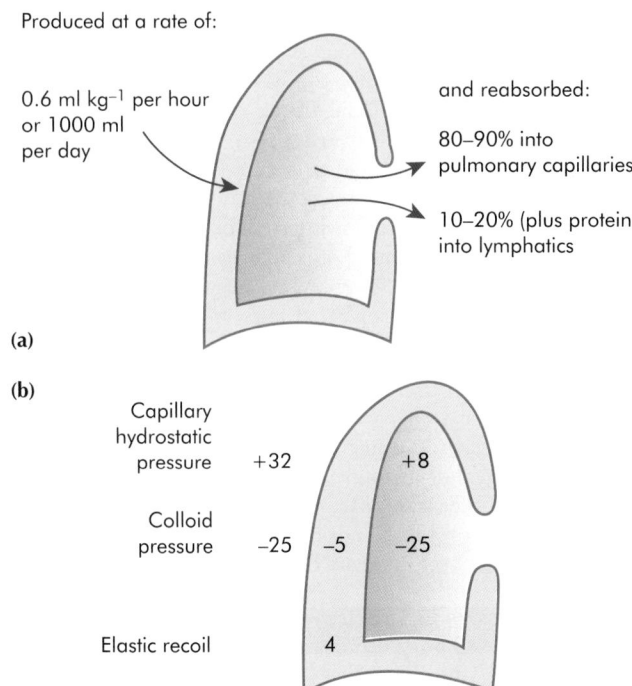

Produced at a rate of:

0.6 ml kg^{-1} per hour
or 1000 ml
per day

and reabsorbed:

80–90% into
pulmonary capillaries

10–20% (plus protein)
into lymphatics

(a)

(b)

Capillary
hydrostatic
pressure   +32   +8

Colloid
pressure   –25   –5   –25

Elastic recoil   4

Net drying effect 6 mmHg

Figure 52.5 (a) Production and absorption of pleural fluid. (b) Normal pleural physiology. (See the text for an explanation of this simplistic physiological model.)

in the presence of a pneumothorax; nitrous oxide is very soluble and, although not normally present in the pleural space, it will be rapidly transported into the space if the patient is given nitrous oxide to breathe.

PLEURAL DISEASE

Pneumothorax

Pneumothorax is the presence of air outside the lung, within the pleural space. It must be distinguished from bullae or air cysts within the lung. Bullae can be the cause of an air leak from the lung and can therefore coexist with pneumothorax.

Spontaneous pneumothorax occurs when the visceral pleura ruptures without an external traumatic or iatrogenic cause.

- Primary spontaneous pneumothorax is a disease in its own right.
- Secondary spontaneous pneumothorax occurs when the visceral pleura leaks as part of an underlying lung disease; any disease that involves the pleura may cause pneumothorax, including tuberculosis, any degenerative or cavitating lung disease and necrosing tumours.

Tension pneumothorax is when (independent of aetiology) there is a build-up of positive pressure within the hemithorax, to the extent that the lung is completely collapsed, the diaphragm is flattened and the mediastinum is distorted and, eventually, the venous return to the heart is compromised. Any pleural breach is inherently valve-like because air will find its way out through the alveoli but cannot be drawn back in because the lung tissue collapses around the hole in the pleura. Patients

being mechanically ventilated following trauma are at particular risk.

Surgical emphysema is the presence of air in the tissues. It requires a breach of an air-containing viscus in communication with soft tissues, and the generation of positive pressure to push the air along tissue planes. The most serious cause is a ruptured oesophagus. Mediastinal surgical emphysema can also occur with asthma or barotrauma from positive pressure ventilation. A poorly managed chest drain with intermittent build-up of pressure allows air to track into the chest wall through the point where the drain breaches the parietal pleura.

Primary spontaneous pneumothorax

This is a common disease characteristically seen in young people from their mid-teens to late-20s. About 75% of cases are in young men, who tend to be tall, and the condition runs in families. It is due to leaks from small blebs, vesicles or bullae, which may become pedunculated, typically at the apex of the upper lobe or on the upper border of the lower or middle lobes.

Usually, pneumothorax presents with sharp pleuritic pain and breathlessness. The pleura is exquisitely sensitive and the movement of the lung on and off the parietal pleura causes severe discomfort. As a result it is mild cases that are more painful, whereas complete collapse is usually painless but causes more breathlessness. Bleeding and tension pneumothorax can occur. They are usually self-limiting; careful observation is wiser than too-ready resort to a chest drain. If the patient is not in respiratory distress or hypoxic there is no urgency. Tension pneumothorax should be immediately relieved by inserting a cannula into the hemithorax in as safe a position as possible (Summary box 52.1).

Summary box 52.1

Pneumothorax

- **Patient comfortable:**
  - watch
  - Po_2 monitoring
- **Pneumothorax complete or patient breathless:**
  - aspirate
- **Aspiration fails or patient hypoxic:**
  - insert chest drain
- **Patient ill:**
  - immediate drainage

The best estimates of recurrence rates are:

- of patients who experience a first event, only about one-third experience recurrence;
- of those who have a second episode, about one-half go on to experience a third episode;
- those who have had three episodes will probably go on to have repeated recurrences.

Inserting and managing a chest drain

An intercostal tube connected to an underwater seal is central to the management of chest disease; however, the management of the pleura and of chest drains can be troublesome, even in experienced hands.

The safest site for insertion of a drain (Fig. 52.6) is in the triangle that lies:

- anterior to the mid-axillary line;
- above the level of the nipple;
- below and lateral to the pectoralis major muscle.

This will ideally find the fifth space. The technique includes the following:

- Meticulous attention to sterility throughout.
- Adequate local anaesthesia to include the pleura.
- Sharp dissection only to cut the skin.
- Blunt dissection with artery forceps down through the muscle layers; these should only be the serratus anterior and the intercostals.
- An oblique tract, so that the skin incision and the hole in the parietal pleura do not overlie each other and the drain is in a short tunnel, which reduces the chance of entraining air.

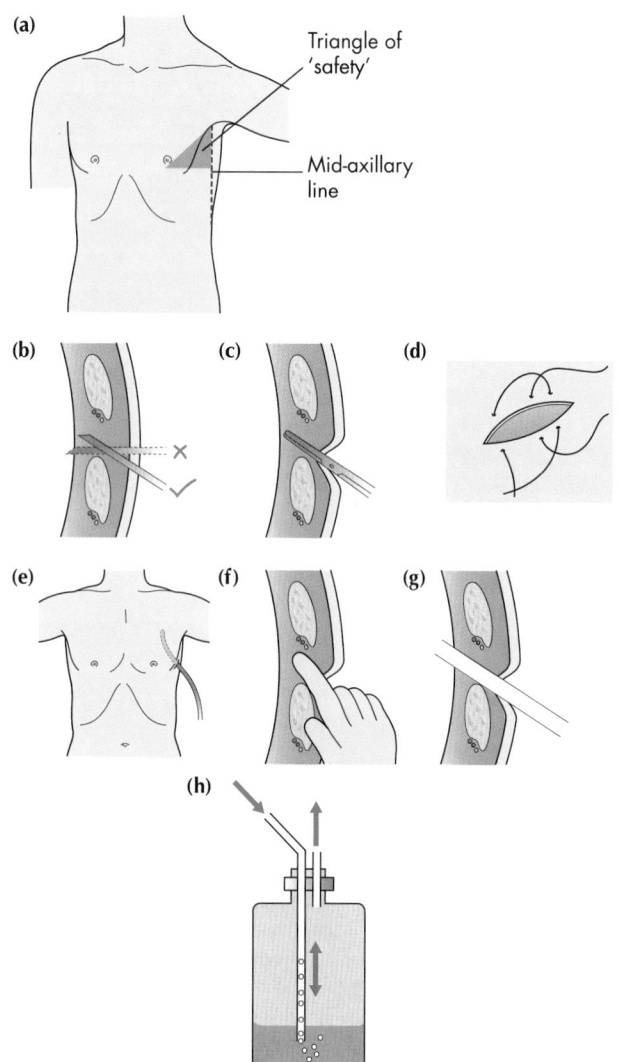

Figure 52.6 Insertion of chest drain: (a) triangle of safety; (b) penetration of the skin, muscle and pleura; (c) blunt dissection of the parietal pleura; (d) suture placement; (e) gauging the distance of insertion; (f) digital examination along the tract into the pleural space; (g) withdrawal of central trochar and positioning of drain; (h) underwater seal chest drain bottle.

- A drain for pneumothorax and haemothorax should aim towards the apex of the lung. A drain for pleural effusion or empyema should be nearer the base. The drain should pass over the upper edge of the rib to avoid the neurovascular bundle that lies beneath the rib.
- The retaining stitch should be secure but not obliterate the drain.
- A vertical mattress suture is inserted for later wound closure. This is vital for pneumothorax management but should be omitted if the drain is for empyema (provided there is adherence of the pleura) because that tract should lie open.
- After completion, check that the drain has achieved its objective by taking a chest radiograph.

It is preferable not to apply suction to the drain or to clamp it. The danger is that the clamp may be applied for transport and forgotten. Dangers of disconnection and siphoning are small or best averted in other ways apart from clamping. A bubbling drain should (almost) never be clamped. Remove the drain when it no longer has a function (Summary box 52.2).

> **Summary box 52.2**
>
> **Suction on a pleural tube**
>
> - Beware! Inserting the drain, and not the suction, is the life-saving manoeuvre
> - If the lung is reluctant to expand, the suction deviates the mediastinum
> - If the lung is fragile, it may worsen an air leak

Definitive management of pneumothorax

Pleurectomy and pleurodesis

Surgery for pneumothorax is best performed by video-assisted thoracoscopic surgery (VATS).

The object of the exercise is threefold:

1. to deal with any leaks from the lung;
2. to search for and obliterate any blebs and bullae;
3. to make the visceral pleura adherent to the parietal pleura so that any subsequent leaks are contained and the lung cannot completely collapse.

Pleural adhesion is achieved in one of three ways:

1. *Pleurectomy.* The conventional approach through thoracotomy is to systematically strip the parietal pleura from the chest wall. However, the intercostal veins are at risk, the subclavian vein can be torn at the apex and the sympathetic chain can be damaged, causing Horner's syndrome.
2. *Pleural abrasion.* A scourer is used to scrape off the slick surface of the parietal pleura. This has the same effect as pleurectomy, although it may not be as reliable.
3. *Chemical pleurodesis.* Talc insufflation is the preferred method. It carries much less risk and may well be as effective.

Pleural disease

Pleural effusion can be readily understood with reference to the physiological mechanisms governing the flux of pleural fluid given

Johann Friedrich Horner, 1831–1886, Professor of Ophthalmology, Zurich, Switzerland, described this syndrome in 1869.

above. Pleural effusions are divided into exudates and transudates, depending on protein content (more or less than 30 g l^{-1}), and characterised further according to glucose content, pH and lactate dehydrogenase content. The following are the most common ways in which the pleural fluid balance is disturbed:

- *Elevated pulmonary capillary pressure.* If left atrial pressure rises, the pulmonary capillary pressure must rise with it, whether as a result of impaired cardiac performance or an overloaded circulation.
- *Reduced intravascular oncotic pressure.* If the plasma proteins fall because of renal or hepatic disease or malnutrition, the absorption mechanism fails.
- *Accumulation of pleural protein* due to obstruction of the mediastinal lymphatics secondary to lymphoma or cancers that invade the lymphatic system.
- *Excessive permeability of the capillaries to fluid and protein* as in inflammatory diseases, particularly the collagen vascular diseases. Of particular importance to the surgeon is the fluid associated with pneumonia, which may result in empyema.

Malignant pleural effusion

Pleural effusion is a common complication of cancer. This may be due to:

- lung cancer;
- pleural involvement with primary or secondary malignancy;
- mediastinal lymphatic involvement.

Lung cancer

There may be direct involvement of the parietal and/or visceral pleura, collapse of the lung parenchyma and spread to the mediastinal lymphatics, or a combination of these, causing pleural fluid accumulation. It is usually regarded as a feature that puts lung cancer beyond surgical cure.

Pleural malignancy The only primary malignancy of the pleura seen with any regularity is malignant mesothelioma. This is a consequence of asbestos exposure with few exceptions. The peak of asbestos imports into the UK was from 1960 to 1975 and the incidence of mesothelioma is rising and is expected to peak in around 2010–20. Mesothelioma commonly presents with breathlessness because of pleural effusions, pain and systemic features of malignancy. Diffuse seeding of the parietal and visceral pleura is a common pattern of dissemination of cancers, particularly adenocarcinoma of any origin.

Mediastinal lymphatic involvement

In many instances, particularly in breast cancer, there is no evident disease in the pleura. The disease is in the mediastinal lymphatics, which are obstructed, and this upsets the balance of physiological forces that control pleural fluid.

Surgery for patients with malignant pleural effusion

The surgeon has two roles:

- to make the diagnosis;
- to achieve effective palliation by pleurodesis.

Diagnosis

Pleural biopsy can be obtained by a range of techniques. An unequivocally positive biopsy is useful but a negative biopsy may be a sampling error (Summary box 52.3).

Summary box 52.3

Biopsy of the pleura

- Cytological examination of the pleural fluid (low yield)
- Abrams' needle (low yield in malignancy)
- Computerised tomography (CT)-guided needle biopsy of a suspicious area
- VATS biopsy
- Open surgical biopsy

VATS is the preferred technique for mesothelioma but CT-guided biopsy is increasingly used and is effective.

Thoracoscopy or video-assisted thoracoscopic surgery

The direct-vision thoracoscope has been used for many years, but its use was limited mainly to performing biopsies. The instrument had a limited view and was uncomfortable to use for any length of time. All this has changed since the advent of video-assisted thoracoscopy (Fig. 52.7); the surgeon's hands are freed because the camera is attached to the thoracoscope, which can be operated by an assistant with the image displayed on a television screen. The surgeon is able to manipulate instruments with both hands to perform an impressive variety of procedures.

Pneumonectomy, lobectomy and empyema drainage are all possible, but thoracoscopic procedures for common, more minor problems is the area providing clear justification for this technique. Lung biopsy and the treatment of recurrent pneumothorax are the most frequent indications. The principal advantage is that a large incision is not required and therefore less postoperative pain and a more rapid recovery should result. Once mastered, the surgeon benefits from a better, well-lit and magnified view, and access to all parts of the chest cavity.

Empyema

Empyema is the end-stage of pleural infection from any cause; the pathological diagnosis requires the presence of thick pus with a thick cortex of fibrin and coagulum over the lung. It can occur as a complication of any thoracic operation. It is seen if a traumatic haemothorax becomes infected or in the course of management of pneumothorax or pleural effusions. It may be associated with pus under the diaphragm (Table 52.3).

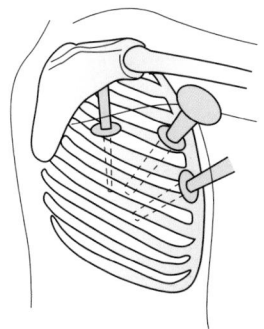

Figure 52.7 Video-assisted thoracoscopic surgery. In general, three ports are used: one camera and two operating.

Leon David Abrams, **formerly Cardiothoracic Surgeon, The United Birmingham Hospitals, Birmingham, England.**

Table 52.3 Conditions that predispose to empyema formation

Pulmonary infection	Unresolved pneumonia
	Bronchiectasis
	Tuberculosis
	Fungal infections
	Lung abscess
Aspiration of pleural effusion	Any aetiology
Trauma	Penetrating injury
	Surgery
	Oesophageal perforation
Extrapulmonary sources	Subphrenic abscess
Bone infections	Osteomyelitis of ribs or vertebrae

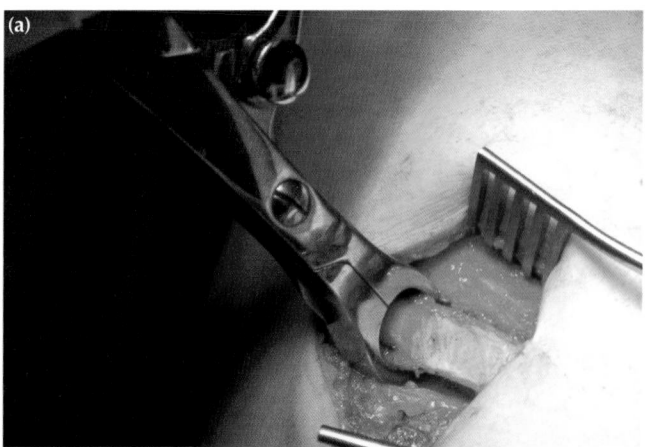

When empyema presents *de novo* it usually follows pneumonia and three phases are described:

1 In the exudative phase, there is protein-rich ($> 30 \, \text{g} \, \text{l}^{-1}$) effusion. If this becomes infected with the organisms from the lung (typically *Streptococcus milleri* and *Haemophilus influenzae* in children), the scene is set for empyema. At this stage antibiotics may be all that is required. Aspiration or drainage to dryness in addition is preferred.
2 Over the next days, the fluid thickens to what is known as the fibrinopurulent phase. Drainage at this stage is prudent.
3 The organising phase causes the lung to be trapped by a thick peel or 'cortex' for which surgical management may be required.

Rib resection and video-assisted thoracoscopic surgical biopsy

This method is used for open pleural biopsy and in the surgical treatment of empyema. To perform this procedure satisfactorily, a double-lumen tube (endotracheobronchial) is required. The patient is positioned with the diseased side uppermost. The presence of fluid at the site to be operated on is confirmed by needle aspiration.

- For malignant effusion, an approach via the fifth, sixth or seventh rib laterally is preferred.
- For empyema, a more posterior approach aiming for the lowest part of the empyema cavity as shown by ultrasound or computerised tomography (CT) is preferred.

A 3-cm incision over the selected rib is made and using diathermy it is deepened through the latissimus dorsi to the periosteum. The intercostal muscle is stripped off the upper surface of the rib. Care is required to free the periosteum from the groove in the lower border of the rib so that the nerve, artery and vein of the intercostal bundle come away uninjured with the intercostal muscle. The rib is divided with a ring-shaped rib cutter (costotome) that divides the rib easily without damage to other structures (Fig. 52.8).

- All fluid can be aspirated under direct vision or video-thoracoscopy.
- In the case of malignant effusion, a substantial full-thickness piece of parietal pleura is sent for histological examination (Fig. 52.9).

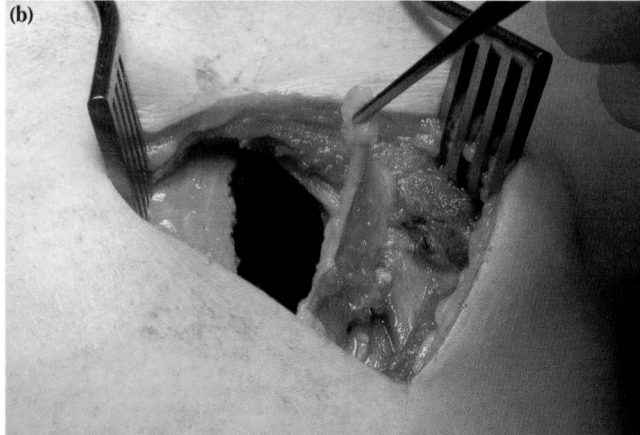

Figure 52.8 Resection of a short segment of rib to allow open pleural biopsy.

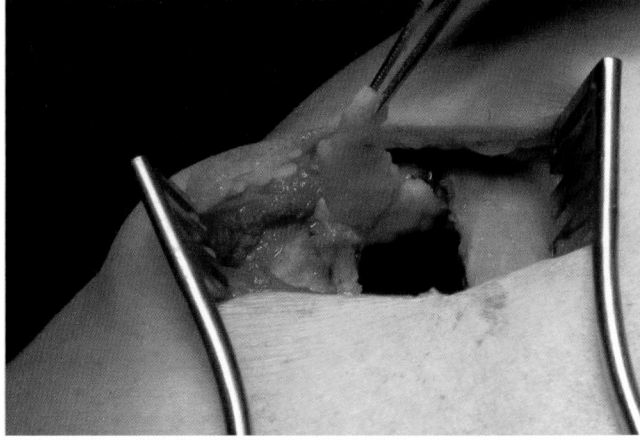

Figure 52.9 Full-thickness open pleural biopsy.

- In empyema, adequate specimens of pus, coagulum and pleura are sent for microbiological examination.
- In malignant effusion, talc is insufflated as a dry powder so that it coats the moist pleural surfaces.

Drainage

- A drain is inserted, which must lie in the bottom of the cavity.

- It should lie obliquely in its course through the skin and chest wall and into the pleura, or it will kink.
- The drain must exit the skin anterior to the mid-axillary line otherwise the patient will have to lie on it, causing pain and obstructing the tube.

Decortication

If the lung is trapped, there is space left and drainage is insufficient, the more radical operation of decortication is performed.

PRESENTATION OF LUNG DISEASE

Haemoptysis

Diseases causing repeated haemoptysis include carcinoma, bronchiectasis, carcinoid tumours and some infections. Severe mitral stenosis is now a rare cause. Patients with repeated haemoptysis should be investigated, at the very least by chest radiography and bronchoscopy. Haemoptysis following trauma may be from a lung contusion or injury to a major airway. Treatment depends on the underlying cause.

Common associated chest symptoms include cough with or without sputum, pain, breathlessness, hoarseness and more general symptoms of systemic upset, including fatigue and loss of weight. Occasionally, chest disease may cause palpitation due to atrial fibrillation. Any of these symptoms in association with haemoptysis requires urgent investigation.

Investigation

Bronchoscopy (Table 52.4)

Flexible bronchoscopy may be performed with the patient awake and the oropharynx anaesthetised with topical lignocaine (Fig. 52.10). The bronchoscope is passed into the nose and through the vocal folds under direct vision. As the scope is flexible, its tip can be directed into the segmental bronchi with ease. Tissue and sputum samples may be obtained for diagnostic purposes. There is a greater range of movement with this instrument, but the biopsies are relatively small and suction limited.

Rigid bronchoscopy requires general anaesthesia in most instances. It is ideal for therapeutic manoeuvres, such as removal of foreign bodies, aspiration of blood and thick secretions, and intraluminal surgery (laser resection or stent placement). The surgeon and the anaesthetist share control of the airway. Continuous electrocardiography (ECG) and pulse oximetry monitoring are now essential. The technique involves the operator standing

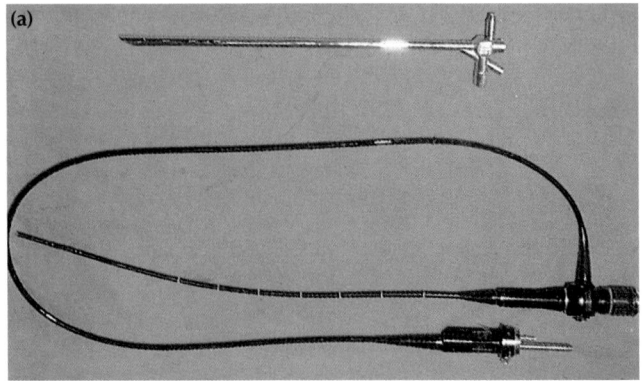

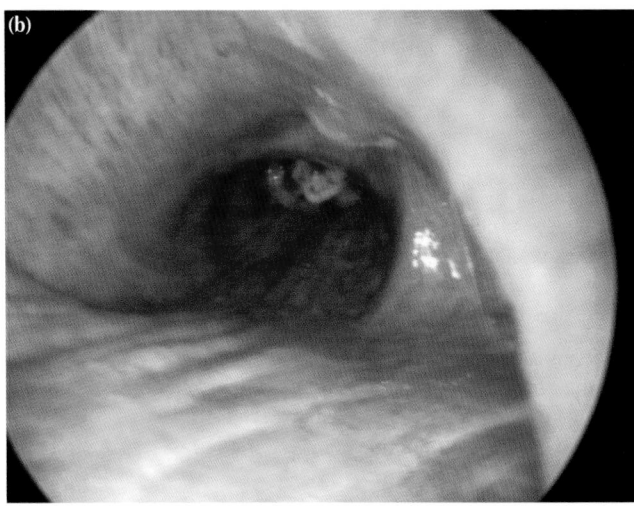

Figure 52.10 (a) Rigid and flexible bronchoscopes. (b) View past the carina into the left main bronchus with a tumour seen in the bronchial lumen.

behind the patient and lifting the maxilla by the upper teeth, using the middle finger and forefinger of the left hand. The bronchoscope rests on the left thumb as it is introduced over the tongue in the midline. Care must be taken not to trap the lips or tongue between the teeth and the bronchoscope, and the fulcrum should be the left thumb and not the teeth. The bronchoscope is passed under direct vision into the oropharynx, behind the epiglottis, until the vocal folds are seen. Turning the instrument through 90° will help to negotiate the vocal folds; only then should the neck be extended.

The tracheal rings and the carina should be easily seen. Advancing the bronchoscope into the right and left main bronchus reveals the orifices of the more peripheral bronchi. Operability is determined by the proximity of a lesion to the carina and whether or not the carina is widened (indicating inoperability from subcarinal lymph node involvement). Complications are rare but include bleeding, pneumothorax, laryngospasm and arrhythmia (Summary box 52.4).

Table 52.4 Uses of bronchoscopy

Diagnostic	Confirmation of disease: carcinoma of the bronchus; inflammatory process; infective process
Investigative	Tissue biopsy
Preoperative assessment	Before lung resection
	Before oesophageal resection
	Persistent haemoptysis
Therapeutic	Removal of secretions
	Removal of foreign bodies
	Stent placement, endobronchial resection, etc.

> **Summary box 52.4**
>
> **Biopsy hazards**
>
> - **Bleeding disorders**
> - **Systemic anticoagulation**
> - **Pulmonary hypertension**

CHAPTER 52 | THE THORAX

Other techniques of biopsy of intrathoracic lesions are often necessary to confirm diagnosis, stage disease and plan treatment. The options range from percutaneous needle biopsy under radiological control to open-lung biopsy. However, high-quality, contrast-enhanced, multislice helical CT scanning will reduce the requirement for invasive assessment.

Airway obstruction

Tracheal obstruction may present acutely as a life-threatening emergency or insidiously with little in the way of symptoms until critical narrowing and stridor occur. The more common causes of airway narrowing are outlined in Table 52.5.

Treatment depends on the underlying cause. Tracheostomy may be required to overcome the obstruction, but there are few indications to do this as an emergency. Tracheal replacement with artificial substitutes has so far been unsuccessful, but resection of up to 6 cm of trachea is now possible. Sleeve resections of the major bronchi are also possible.

Inhaled foreign bodies

This is a fairly common occurrence in small children and is often marked by a choking incident that then apparently passes. Surprisingly large objects can be inhaled and become lodged in the wider-calibre and more vertically placed right main bronchus. There are three possible presentations:

1 asymptomatic;
2 wheezing (from airway narrowing) with a persistent cough and signs of obstructive emphysema;
3 pyrexia with a productive cough from pulmonary suppuration.

A chest radiograph is vital; even if the object is not radio-opaque there may be other changes. An experienced anaesthetist is required. The procedure may be very difficult if there is a severe inflammatory reaction.

MALIGNANT TUMOURS

Primary lung cancer

Lung cancer is one of the most common cancers throughout the world. In the UK, there are 40 000 cases a year, making it the most common single cancer. From the time of diagnosis, 80% of patients are dead within 1 year and only 5% survive for 5 years.

Surgical resection has a limited role in curative treatment because at the time of presentation many cases are locally advanced or widely disseminated and are beyond surgical cure. The proportion of lung cancers in which resection is attempted varies from fewer than 10% in the UK to about 25% in the USA. However, the thoracic surgeon working in a cancer team has a role in diagnosis, staging and palliation apart from resection in

appropriate cases. The disease is so common that surgeons of all disciplines will encounter cases of lung cancer presenting with various manifestations.

Cigarette smoking is undoubtedly the major risk factor for developing bronchial carcinoma and accounts for 85–95% of all cases. To a lesser extent, atmospheric pollution and certain occupations (radioactive ore and chromium mining) contribute. The risk is related to the lifetime burden of cigarette smoking, which is commonly quoted as 'pack-years' (a 'pack' being 20 cigarettes): the number of packs smoked per day multiplied by the number of years of exposure. In the UK, the mortality rate from lung cancer for individuals smoking more than 40 cigarettes per day is over 210 deaths per 100 000 population per year. This compares with a mortality rate of less than 4 deaths per 100 000 population per year in non-smokers.

Pathological types

For practical purposes, lung cancers are divided into small cell and non-small cell lung cancer (NSCLC), which are seen in a ratio of about 1:4.

- The pattern of disease, the prognosis and the results of treatment for small cell (also known as oat cell) carcinoma differ from all other types sufficiently for these to be managed differently from the outset on the basis of the histological classification.
- Subdivisions of NSCLC according to histological characteristics are much less important, but pathological staging is critical to treatment and outcome.

Histological classification of lung cancer

Small cell lung cancers were known as oat cell cancers because of the packed nature of small dense cells. These represent about 20% of all lung cancer. They tend to metastasise early to lymph nodes and by blood-borne spread. The median survival is measured in months. The tumours are very responsive to chemotherapy such that median survival may be doubled (but is still short), but they are rarely, if ever, cured. Surgery has little place.

Adenocarcinoma is now the most common of the NSCLC types, having overtaken squamous cancer. The increasing incidence is partly due to an increasing incidence in women and may be the result, in part, of a move towards lower-tar cigarettes that are inhaled more deeply to get the same effect.

Squamous carcinoma typically appears as a cavitating tumour.

Large cell undifferentiated is a discrete histological type of NSCLC and is included within neuroendocrine tumours.

Bronchioalveolar carcinoma has a distinct pattern of growth following the pre-existing pulmonary architecture and is thus much less dense; it appears as a patchy diffuse shadow ('ground glass') on the radiograph rather than a solid mass and has a histological appearance to match. After resection, it can appear in another lobe or the other side.

Accurate diagnosis and staging of the tumour are vital if surgery is to be considered.

Clinical features

Clinical features of lung carcinoma depend on:

- the site of the lesion;
- the invasion of neighbouring structures;
- the extent of metastases.

Table 52.5 Causes of airway narrowing

Intraluminal	Inhaled foreign body
	Neoplasm
Intramural	Congenital stenosis
	Fibrous stricture (post-intubation or tuberculosis)
Extramural	Neoplasm (thyroid cancer, secondary deposits)
	Aortic arch aneurysm

Common symptoms include a persistent cough, weight loss, dyspnoea and non-specific chest pain.

- Haemoptysis occurs in fewer than 50% of patients presenting for the first time.
- Cough, or a changed cough, is a common presentation but non-specific in this population.
- Severe localised pain suggests chest wall invasion with the infiltration of an intercostal nerve. Invasion of the apical area may involve the brachial plexus, leading to Pancoast's syndrome.
- Dyspnoea may come from loss of functioning lung tissue, lymphatic invasion or the development of a large pleural effusion.
- Pleural fluid is an ominous feature and the presence of blood in a pleural effusion suggests that the pleura has been directly invaded.
- Clubbing (Fig. 52.11) and hypertrophic pulmonary osteoarthropathy accompany some lung cancers and may resolve with excision of the primary lesion.
- Invasion of the mediastinum may result in hoarseness (because of recurrent laryngeal nerve involvement), dysphagia (because of the involvement of, or extrinsic pressure on, the oesophagus) and superior vena caval obstruction.
- Small cell carcinoma is associated with the development of myopathies including the Eaton–Lambert syndrome, which is similar to myasthenia gravis (Summary box 52.5).

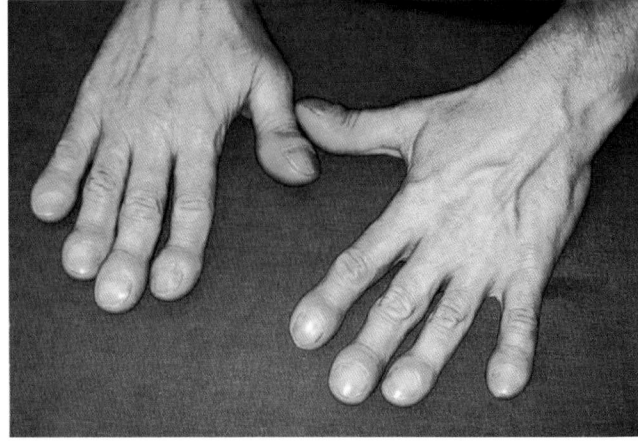

Figure 52.11 Example of finger clubbing in a patient with bronchogenic carcinoma.

Summary box 52.5

Symptoms of lung cancer

- Haemoptysis < 50% of patients
- Cough, new or changed pattern
- Pain
- Dyspnoea
- Clubbing
- Hoarseness
- Myopathies

Table 52.6 The international tumour–node–metastasis (TNM) staging system

Primary tumour (T)

TX Tumour proven by the presence of malignant cells and bronchial secretions, but not visualised by radiography or bronchoscopy

T0 No evidence of primary tumour

TIS Carcinoma *in situ*

T1 A tumour that is 3 cm or less in greatest dimension, surrounded by lung or visceral pleura and without evidence of invasion proximal to a lobar bronchus at bronchoscopy

T2 A tumour of more than 3 cm in greatest dimension or a tumour of any size that either invades the visceral pleura or has associated atelectasis or obstructive pneumonitis, which extends to the hilar region, but does not involve an entire lung; at bronchoscopy, the proximal extent of demonstrable tumour must be within a lobar bronchus or at least 2 cm distal to the carina

T3 A tumour of any size, with direct extension into the chest wall (including superior sulcus tumours), diaphragm, mediastinal pleura or pericardium, without involving the heart, great vessels, trachea, oesophagus or vertebral body, or a tumour in the main bronchus within 2 cm of the carina without involving the carina

T4 A tumour of any size, with invasion of the mediastinum or involving the heart, great vessels, trachea, oesophagus, vertebral body or carina, or the presence of malignant pleural effusion

Nodal involvement (N)

N0 No demonstrable metastasis or regional lymph node

N1 Metastasis to lymph nodes in the peribronchial or the ipsilateral hilar region, or both, including direct extension

N2 Metastasis to the ipsilateral, mediastinal and subcarinal lymph nodes

N3 Metastasis to the contralateral mediastinal lymph nodes, contralateral hilar lymph nodes, ipsilateral or contralateral scalene or supraclavicular lymph nodes

Distant metastasis (M)

M0 No known distant metastasis

M1 Distant metastasis present

CHAPTER 52 | THE THORAX

Henry Khunrath Pancoast, **1875–1939**, Professor of Radiology, The University of Pennsylvania, Philadelphia, PA, USA, described this condition in 1932.

Lee M. Eaton, **1905–1958**, a Neurologist who was a Professor at The Mayo Clinic, Rochester, MN, USA.

Edward H. Lambert, **B. 1915**, Professor of Physiology, The University of Minnesota, MN, USA. Eaton and Lambert described this condition in a joint paper in 1956.

Treatment of lung cancer

Careful investigation is required to determine which tumours are operable and will benefit from a major thoracic resection. The internationally agreed tumour–node–metastasis (TNM) staging system gives prognostic information on the natural history of the disease. Tumours graded up to T2, N1, M0 can be encompassed within an anatomical surgical resection and have a much improved prognosis when treated surgically so the tumour must be staged accurately before resection (Table 52.6). A number of non-tumour factors, including the general fitness of the patient and the results of lung function tests, help to determine the appropriate treatment. In patients with incurable disease, treatment is palliative to maximise quality of life and disease-free survival.

Survival

Carcinoma of the bronchus generally has a low survival rate after diagnosis (Table 52.7). Important factors in determining prognosis are the histological type of the tumour, the spread (stage) and the general condition of the patient. Early detection and surgical resection offer the best hope for cure.

Diagnosis and staging

There are three keys to diagnosis:

1 detecting the primary lesion;
2 tissue diagnosis;
3 staging (Table 52.8).

Table 52.7 Survival table following operation for carcinoma of the bronchus

5-year survival according to presurgical staging (%)	
Stage I	56–67
Stage II	39–55
Stage IIIa	23
Stage IIIb	< 10

5-year survival according to cell type (%)	
Squamous cell carcinoma	35–50
Adenocarcinoma	25–45
Adenosquamous carcinoma	20–35
Undifferentiated carcinoma	15–25
Small cell carcinoma	0–5

Table 52.8 Staging of carcinoma of the lung

Stage	Tumour	Nodal involvement	Distant metastasis	Operable/inoperable
Occult carcinoma	TX	N0	M0	Operable
Stage 0	TIS			
Stage I	T1	N0	M0	Operable
Stage II	T1	N1	M0	Operable
	T2	N1	M0	Operable
Stage IIIa	T3	N0	M0	Inoperable
	T3	N1	M0	Inoperable
	T1–3	N2	M0	Inoperable
Stage IIIb	Any T	N3	M0	Inoperable
	T4	Any N	M0	Inoperable
Stage IV	Any T	Any N	M1	Inoperable

Detection of the primary lesion

Chest radiography

A chest radiograph will detect most lung cancers but some, particularly early curable tumours, are hidden by other structures. Secondary effects such as pleural effusion, distal collapse and raised hemidiaphragm may be evident (Fig 52.12).

Computerised tomography

This is the first investigation in suspected lung cancer. The surgeon needs to know if the primary is resectable (T stage) and which if any lymph nodes are involved (N stage) (Fig. 52.13). Lymph nodes of more than 2 cm in diameter are likely to be

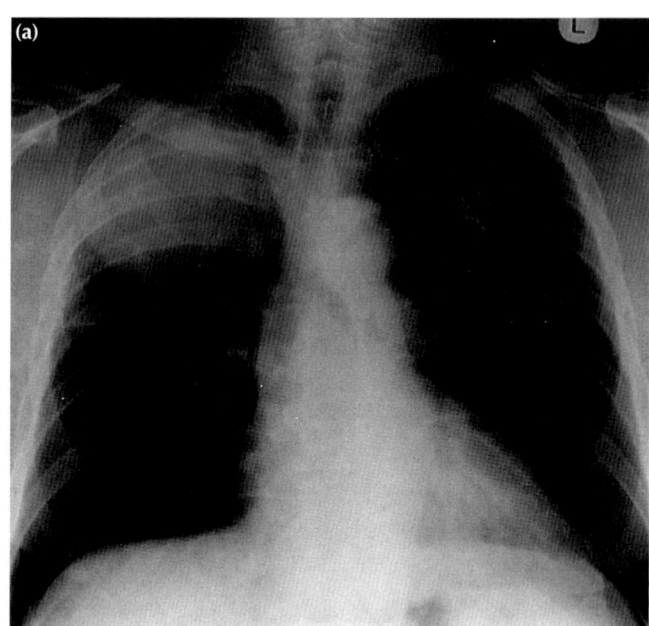

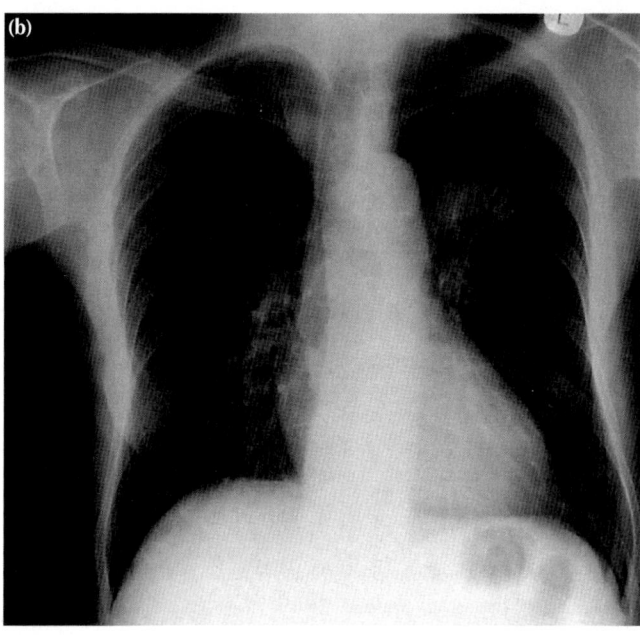

Figure 52.12 Chest radiographs of carcinoma of the lung. (a) This patient has a large mass in the right upper lobe, causing Horner's syndrome. (b) This patient has a left hilar mass and presented with haemoptysis.

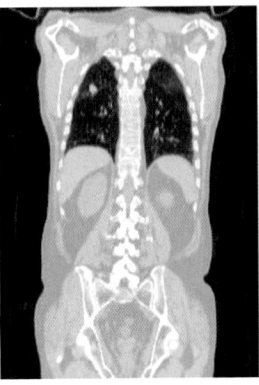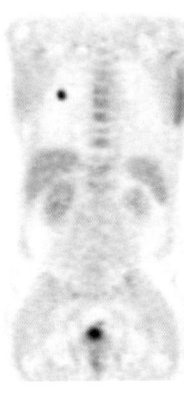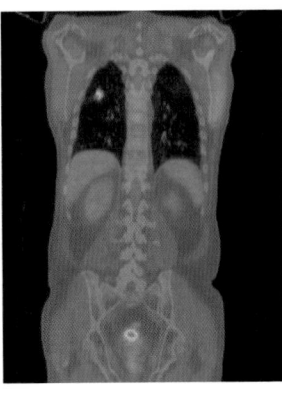

Figure 52.13 An FDG-avid bronchial carcinoma without metastases shown on a positron emission tomography/computerised tomography scan (courtesy of Dr Sally Barrington).

involved in the disease (70%) (Fig. 52.14) and those less than 1 cm in the shorter axis are very unlikely to be involved. If the presence of cancer in the nodes is critical to management, further evidence from positron emission tomography with fluorodeoxyglucose (FDG-PET) or biopsy (see below) is essential. Remote metastases to the liver, adrenals or elsewhere may be detected.

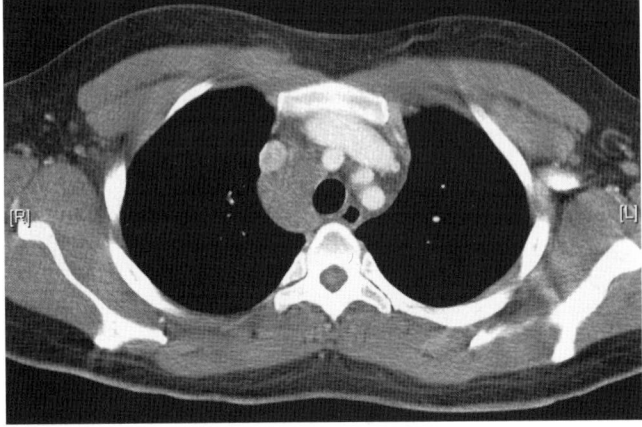

Figure 52.14 Paratracheal lymphadenopathy shown on a computerised tomography scan (courtesy of Dr Sheila Rankin).

Positron emission tomography

The patient is given radiolabelled FDG, which is taken up by all metabolising cells but more avidly by cancer cells. The FDG enters the Kreb's cycle but cannot complete it and accumulates in proportion to the glucose avidity of the cells. High accumulation is associated with lung cancers and secondaries. Infection or other inflammation, and lymphadenopathy secondary to it, are also FDG avid (Figs 52.13, 52.15 and 52.16).

Sputum cytology

Sputum cytology may reveal malignant cells but the false-negative rate is high.

Invasive procedures

Computerised tomography-guided biopsy

Percutaneous CT-guided fine-needle aspiration (FNA) may give a good yield of cells for cytological examination.

Alternatively, a core of tissue can be obtained for formal histology. These techniques are best for larger and more peripheral lesions. Pneumothorax is common (30%) but rarely requires intercostal tube drainage. The contraindications include poor respiratory reserve when even a small pneumothorax would be hazardous.

Thoracoscopy, mediastinoscopy, mediastinotomy and open-lung biopsy are aimed at establishing a tissue diagnosis and

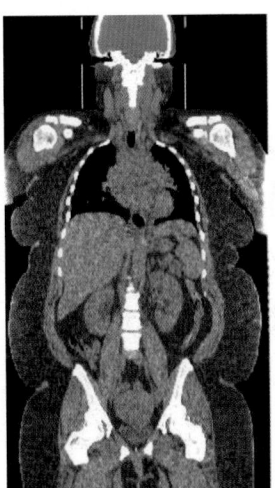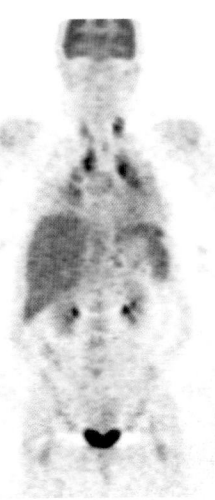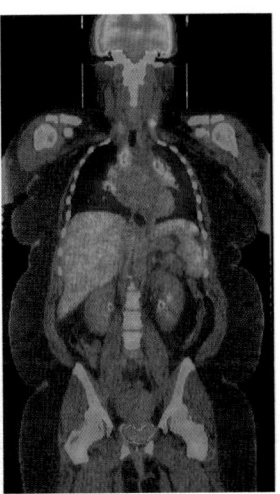

Figure 52.15 Multiple FDG-avid mediastinal lymph nodes shown on a positron emission tomography/computerised tomography scan (courtesy of Dr Sally Barrington).

CHAPTER 52 | THE THORAX

Sir Hans Adolf Krebs, **1900–1981**, Professor of Biochemistry, The University of Oxford, Oxford, England.

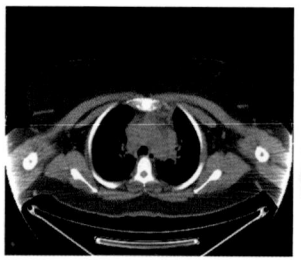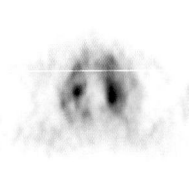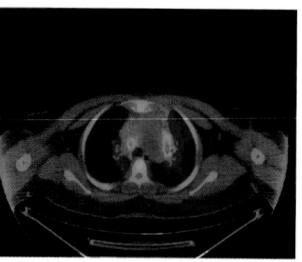

Figure 52.16 Bilateral mediastinal FDG-avid lymphodenopathy seen on a positron emission tomography/computerised tomography scan (courtesy of Dr Sally Barrington).

assessing the degree of spread (staging), which determines resectability. Histological proof of the status of mediastinal nodes may be important to avoid unavailing thoracotomy for incurable cancers and, conversely, to not deny surgery when the nodes are enlarged but not involved with cancer.

Mediastinoscopy

This procedure is performed under general anaesthesia with the patient supine and his or her neck extended (Fig. 52.17). A transverse incision is made 2 cm above the sternal notch and deepened until the strap muscles are reached. These are retracted laterally and the thyroid isthmus is retracted superiorly to reveal the pretracheal fascia. Careful blunt dissection in this plane allows access to the paratracheal and subcarinal nodes. A mediastinoscope is introduced for direct visualisation and biopsy. Great caution should be used in the presence of superior vena caval obstruction. Complications include pneumothorax and haemorrhage.

Mediastinotomy

An incision is made through the second intercostal space to gain access to some of the mediastinal lymph nodes on the affected side (Fig. 52.18; see also Fig. 52.3, page 877). Damage to the internal mammary artery and the phrenic nerve must be avoided. Mediastinal extension of tumour can also be assessed.

These techniques may also be used in the diagnosis of other mediastinal conditions, including:

- lymphoma;
- anterior mediastinal tumours;
- thymoma;
- sarcoid, tuberculosis or any other cause of lymphadenopathy.

Thoracotomy

Although the most frequent reason for thoracotomy is lung cancer, all surgeons dealing with trauma should be able to perform a thoracotomy if required. The standard route into the thoracic cavity is through a posterolateral thoracotomy. The incision is used for access to the:

- lung and major bronchi;
- thoracic aorta;
- oesophagus;
- posterior mediastinum.

A double-lumen endotracheal tube is used to allow ventilation of one lung while the other is collapsed, to facilitate surgery and to protect the non-operated lung and retain control of ventilation (Fig. 52.19).

The patient is turned to the lateral position with the affected

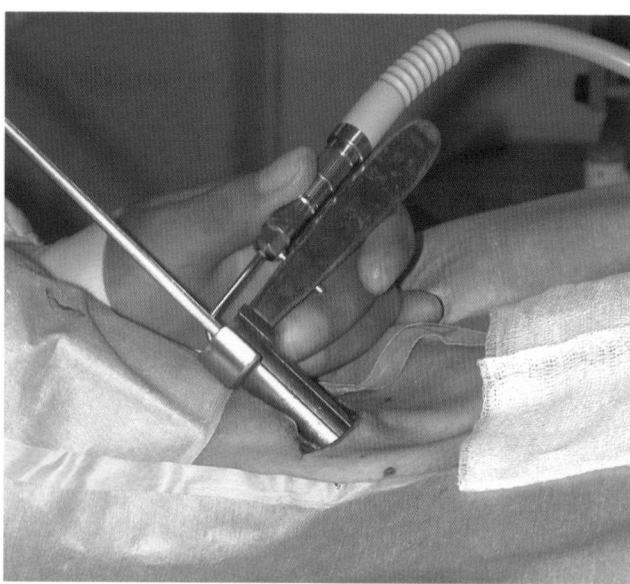

Figure 52.17 Mediastinoscopy. The mediastinoscope slides down immediately in front of the trachea, behind the aortic arch and behind and between the great vessels of the head and neck.

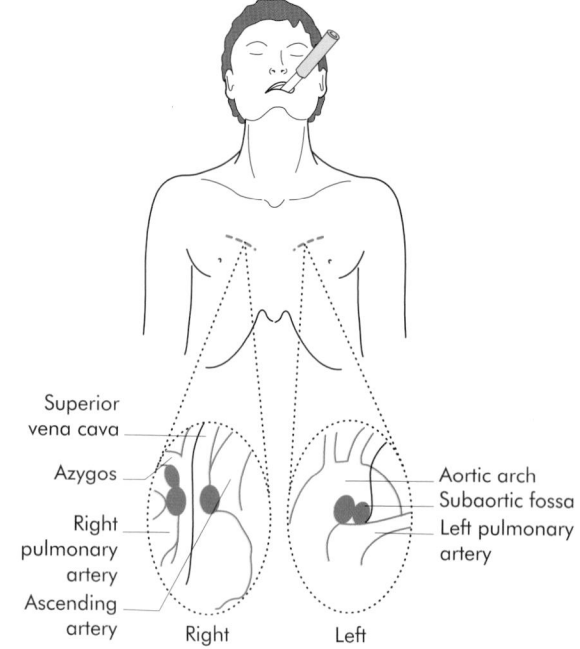

Figure 52.18 Mediastinotomy: structures accessible through anterior mediastinotomy.

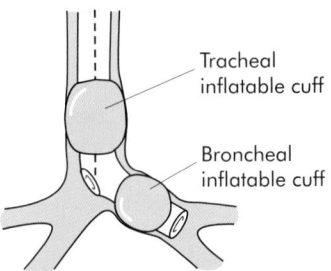

Figure 52.19 The double-lumen tube permits separate ventilation of the right and left lungs.

side up (Fig. 52.20). The lower leg is flexed at the hip and the knee, with a pillow between the legs. Table supports are used to maintain the position and additional strapping is used at the hips for stability. The upper arm may be supported by a bracket in a position of 90° flexion. The lower arm is flexed and positioned by the head. It is important for both the surgeon and the anaesthetist to be completely satisfied with the position of the patient and the tube and lines at this stage.

- The incision passes 1–2 cm below the tip of the scapula, and extends posteriorly and superiorly between the medial border of the scapula and the spine.
- The incision is deepened through the subcutaneous tissues to the latissimus dorsi. This muscle is divided with coagulating diathermy, taking care over haemostasis.
- A plane of dissection is developed by hand deep to the scapula and serratus anterior. The ribs can be counted down from the highest palpable rib (which is usually the second) and the sixth rib periosteum is scored with the diathermy near its upper border. A periosteal elevator is used to lift the periosteum off the superior border of the rib (Fig. 52.21).
- This reveals the pleura, which may be entered by blunt dissection. A rib spreader is inserted between the ribs and opened gently to prevent fracture.

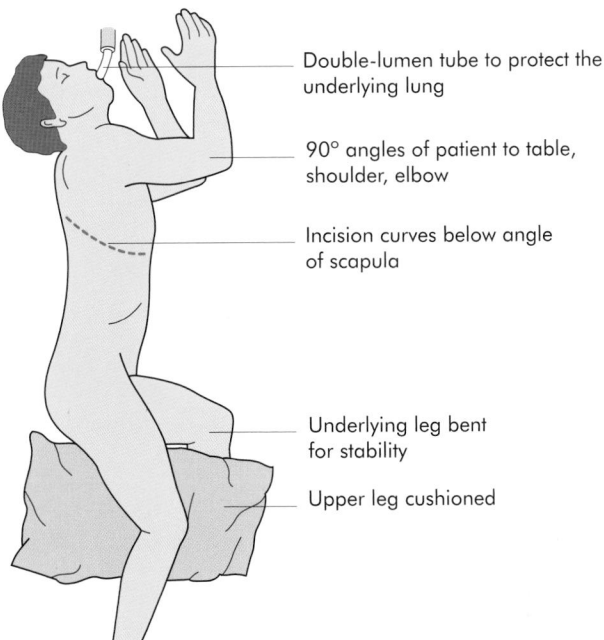

- Double-lumen tube to protect the underlying lung
- 90° angles of patient to table, shoulder, elbow
- Incision curves below angle of scapula
- Underlying leg bent for stability
- Upper leg cushioned

Figure 52.20 Correct positioning for thoracotomy.

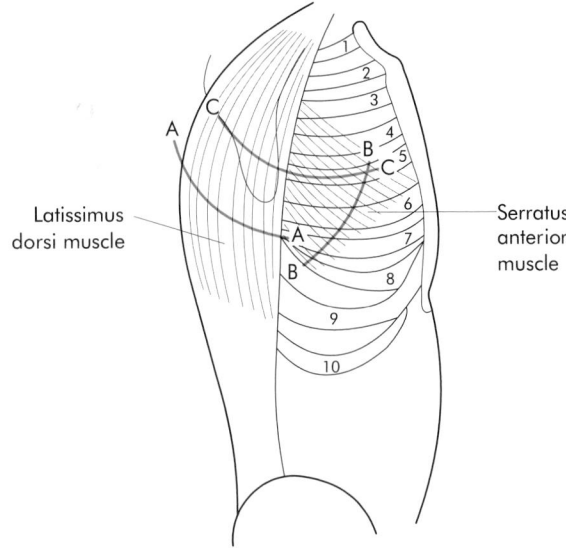

Latissimus dorsi muscle

Serratus anterior muscle

A–A The latissimus dorsi is divided in line with the skin incision
B–B If the serratus anterior is divided, it should be close to its attachment to ribs 6, 7 and 8. It can be left intact and mobilised along its inferior border.
C–C The intercostal muscles are stripped off the upper border of the rib

Figure 52.21 Incision and layers encountered during anterolateral thoracotomy.

- Exposure may be facilitated by dividing the rib at the costal angle or by dividing the costotransverse ligament. Resection of a rib is not usually required.
- The anaesthetist is now able to deflate the affected lung to allow a better view of the intrathoracic structures.
- In an emergency thoracotomy for penetrating wounds of the heart, a more anterior approach is used and no specialised supporting equipment is required (Fig. 52.22).

Chest drains

Large-calibre (24–28F) intercostal drains are usually inserted at the end of the procedure. It is best to make the exit site through the seventh or eighth intercostal space, anterior to the mid-axillary line, so that the patient does not lie on them. Even if the site to be drained is posterior, as in empyema, the drains are tunnelled to come out more anteriorly for easier management. The more anteriorly sited drain goes to the apex (the 'A' drain: anterior and apical for air) and the posteriorly placed drain goes to the lung base (the 'B' drain: basal and towards the back, for blood). A rib approximator is used to realign the ribs and the stripped periosteum and intercostal muscle are sutured to the intercostal muscle below the stripped rib with a continuous absorbable suture. The fascia and muscle layer are closed in layers using an absorbable suture. Skin closure is a matter of personal preference.

Analgesia is an important aspect of postoperative care and the process may be started intraoperatively by infiltrating the intercostal nerves in the region of the incision with a long-acting local anaesthetic. Various strategies have been developed to deliver analgesics postoperatively to facilitate a normal breathing pattern.

Surgical management

The principle of surgery is to remove all cancer (the primary and the regional lymph nodes) but to conserve as much lung as possible.

CHAPTER 52 | THE THORAX

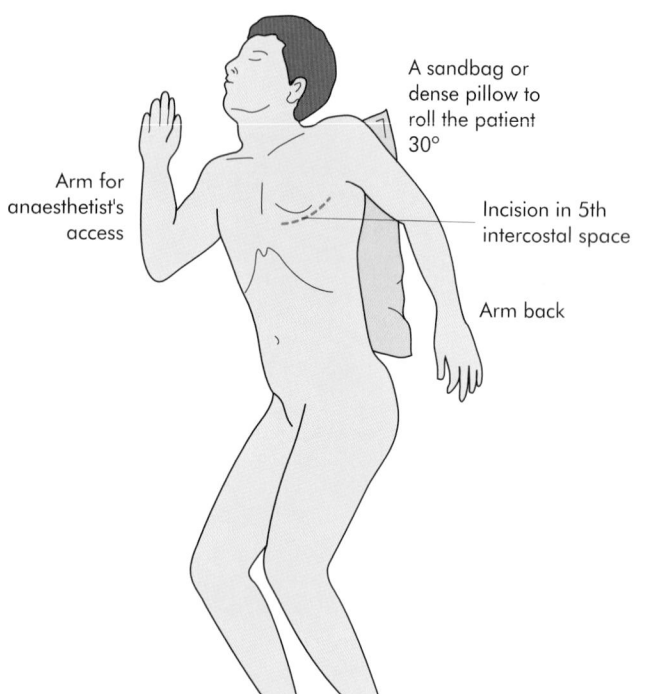

Figure 52.22 Emergency left anterior thoracotomy for access to the heart. Requires no special supports or devices.

Lobectomy

Following dissection of the fissure and hilar structures, the branches of the pulmonary artery and veins to the lobe are isolated and ligated. The bronchus is sewn or stapled according to preference.

At the completion of the operation, the remaining lung is reinflated. Some air leak is common (about 60% of cases) and usually settles within a few days. Intercostal drains are inserted to the base and apex of the space (see above). The patient does not need intensive care and postoperative ventilation is best avoided. The perioperative mortality rate is 2–3%.

Pneumonectomy

Pneumonectomy is removal of a whole lung and has a higher mortality rate (5–10%). The surgeon must be satisfied that the patient is fit to tolerate this procedure from the preoperative work-up. This procedure is reserved for either centrally placed tumours involving the main bronchus or those that straddle the fissure. At thoracotomy, an inspection of the lung and direct palpation of the mass will determine resectability and lymph node spread. Fixation of the tumour to the aorta, heart or oesophagus implies irresectability. Involvement of the mediastinal lymph chain is associated with a poor prognosis. With modern preoperative imaging, resection is abandoned in only about 3% of cases.

Pneumonectomy is anatomically more straightforward than lobectomy:

- The pulmonary artery is first dissected, divided and sutured.
- The pulmonary veins are then isolated, divided and sutured.
- The main bronchus is divided so that no blind stump remains (Fig. 52.23). The technique of stump closure is important if a bronchopleural fistula is to be avoided. The tissues are carefully handled and the stump is usually stapled.

Drainage of the space is a matter of debate. Most use a water-seal drain and either leave it unclamped or unclamp it for 1 min every hour until the drainage ceases; others prefer not to drain. The critical point is that no suction should be applied as there is now a sealed space with the mobile mediastinum on one side of it. The air in the pneumonectomy space is gradually absorbed and the fluid level within the space rises (Fig. 52.24).

Thoracoscopic lung resection

Minimally invasive surgery has become fashionable in recent years in all forms of surgery but, in reality, only a few per cent of all resections are performed this way.

Complications of lung resection

Bleeding Bleeding should be avoidable by the use of a careful surgical technique, but may be severe in the presence of dense adhesions.

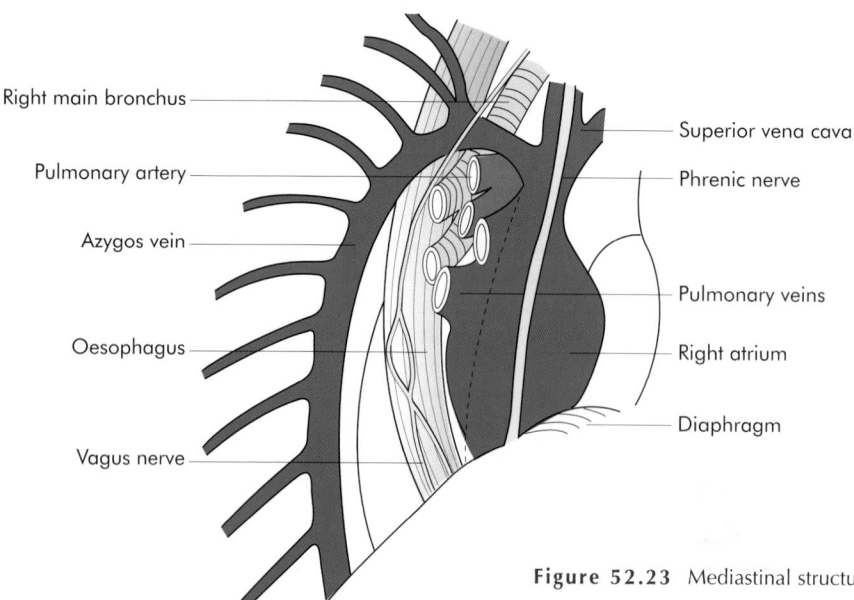

Figure 52.23 Mediastinal structures after removal of right lung.

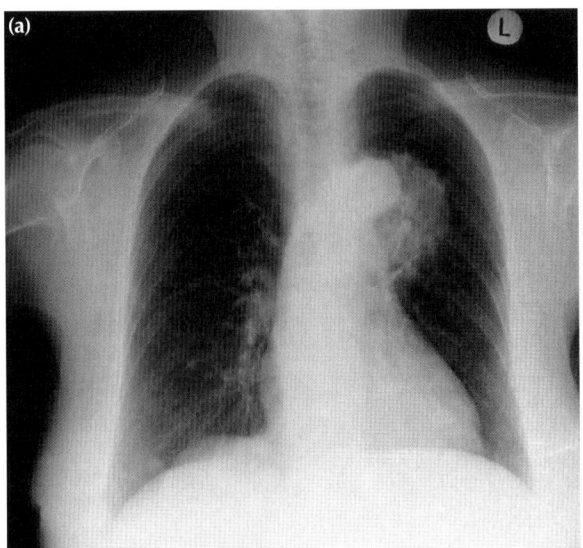

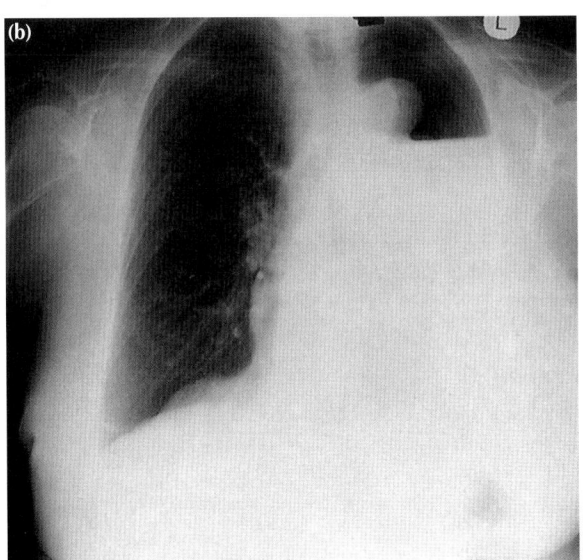

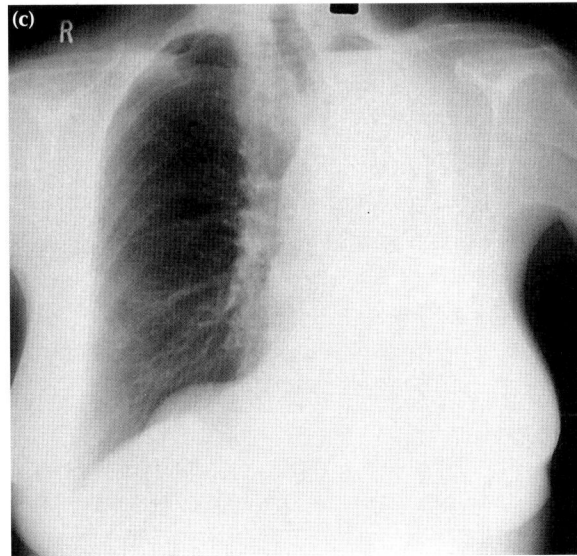

Figure 52.24 Chest radiographs (a) pre- and (b) post-pneumonectomy, with rising fluid level (c) in the left haemothorax.

Respiratory infection Many of these patients are ex-smokers and so basal collapse and hypoxaemia are common postoperatively.

Persistent air leak Chest drains are placed at the time of surgery to deal with the air leak. Rarely, the air leak persists and the remaining lung does not expand. Re-thoracotomy may then be necessary to seal the leak.

Bronchopleural fistula Bronchopleural fistula is a serious complication. Following pneumonectomy the space left behind is initially filled with air. This is slowly reabsorbed and the space fills with tissue fluid. The fluid level rises until the air is finally reabsorbed. Dehiscence of the bronchial stump leads to the development of a bronchopleural fistula and the fluid in the space (which is almost inevitably infected) is expectorated in large quantities. This complication has a high morbidity and mortality rate.

The patient is nursed sitting up and turned so that the affected space is dependent, to prevent infected fluid from entering the remaining lung while arrangements are made to site a pleural drain. This should be connected to an underwater seal but not suction. Bronchopleural fistulas are unlikely to resolve spontaneously and management is highly specialised.

Postoperative care

Patients have limited respiratory reserve following lung resection, so infection and fluid overload are to be avoided. Once air leaks have settled, the drains are removed. Mobilisation, breathing exercises and regular physiotherapy are begun as soon as the patient's condition permits.

Postoperative pain

It is important to deal with post-thoracotomy pain effectively so that a normal breathing pattern and gas exchange are achieved in the early postoperative period. Three strategies are routinely used in combination:

- patient-controlled analgesia (PCA) with intravenous boluses of opiates;
- paravertebral, extrapleural catheter-delivered local anaesthetic;
- background oral analgesia with paracetamol.

Long-term post-thoracotomy pain can be reduced by careful attention to detail during the operation. Sources of avoidable chronic pain include rib fracture and the entrapment of intercostal nerves during wound closure.

Benign tumours

Benign tumours of the lung are uncommon and account for fewer than 15% of solitary lesions seen on chest radiographs. A peripheral tumour usually causes no symptoms until it is large; a central tumour may present with haemoptysis and signs of bronchial obstruction while small. A tumour is likely to be benign if it has not increased in size on chest radiographs for more than 2 years or it has some degree of calcification; however, a tissue diagnosis is usually pursued.

Most benign nodules are *granulomas* (tuberculosis or histoplasmosis). The most common benign tumour is a *hamartoma*, a developmental abnormality containing mesothelial and endothelial elements. Diagnosis (and definitive treatment) is achieved by excision of the lesion. Any of the mesodermal elements of the lung may form a mesodermal tumour (chondroma, lipoma, leiomyoma). Deposits of amyloid may give similar radiographic appearances of a nodule (pseudotumour).

Bronchopulmonary carcinoid tumours

These carcinoid tumours are derived from the neuroendocrine cells of bronchial glands. Most (80%) are found in the major bronchi and are characteristically slow growing and highly vascular. They are currently classified within a spectrum of neuroendocrine tumours. Most behave in a benign way; however, approximately 15% metastasise. Surgical excision is preferred.

The mediastinum

Primary tumours of the mediastinum

Thymoma, neurogenic tumours, germ cell tumours and lymphoma are the usual primary tumours of the mediastinum (Fig. 52.25).

Thymoma This is the most common mediastinal tumour, accounting for 25% of the total (Fig. 52.26). Thymomas vary in behaviour from benign to aggressively invasive. The only reliable indicator of malignancy is capsular invasion. Diagnosis and treatment are best achieved by complete thymectomy.

Germ cell tumour Germ cell tumours account for 13% of all mediastinal masses and cysts and are usually found in the anterior mediastinum (Fig. 52.27). They contain elements from all three cell types (mesoderm, endoderm and ectoderm). They tend to present in young adults and 75% are benign and cystic, although they may cause compression of neighbouring structures; hence, dermoid cysts are best excised. Malignancy is suspected if elevated levels of serum alpha-fetoprotein, human chorionic gonadotrophin and carcinoembryonic antigen are detected.

Lymphoma Lymphoma is a common cause of a mediastinal mass lesion, particularly the anterior mediastinum, leading to obstruction of the superior vena cava.

Mesenchymal tumours Lipomas are common in the anterior mediastinum. Other mesenchymal tumours are very rare.

Thyroid Ectopic thyroid tissue (and parathyroid) may be found in the anterior mediastinum but usually the mass is an extension of a thyroid lesion.

Neural tumours These may derive from the sympathetic nervous system or the peripheral nerves and are more prevalent in the posterior mediastinum. They may be painful but are more often discovered accidentally on routine chest radiography (Fig. 52.28). They include neuroblastoma in childhood, and Schwannomas and neurofibromas in adults. Phaeochromocytoma arises from the sympathetic chain and produces the characteristic endocrine syndrome.

The mediastinal lymph nodes are commonly involved by metastatic tumour mimicking a primary mediastinal lesion. Symptoms are generally secondary to compression or invasion of a structure within the mediastinum.

MEDICAL CONDITIONS FOR WHICH SURGERY MAY BE REQUIRED

Bronchiectasis

This is chronic irreversible dilatation of the medium-sized bronchi, which may occur following a suppurative pneumonia or bronchial obstruction. It is the pathological end-stage of a range of conditions. If generalised it is almost never considered for surgical resection. Cases caused by whooping cough and measles are decreasing in frequency in developed countries.

Treatment

Removal of the bronchiectatic part of the lung for symptoms of bleeding, recurrent infection or copious symptoms can be very effective when the disease is localised.

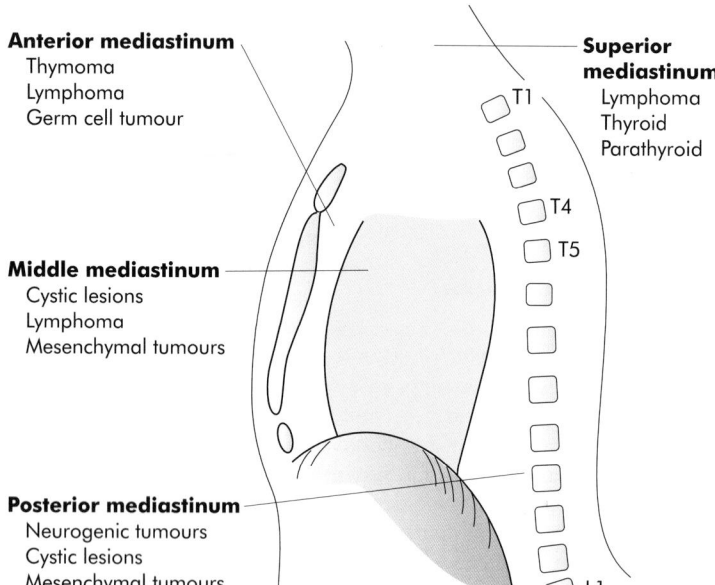

Anterior mediastinum
Thymoma
Lymphoma
Germ cell tumour

Middle mediastinum
Cystic lesions
Lymphoma
Mesenchymal tumours

Posterior mediastinum
Neurogenic tumours
Cystic lesions
Mesenchymal tumours

Superior mediastinum
Lymphoma
Thyroid
Parathyroid

T1
T4
T5
L1

Figure 52.25 Mediastinal pathology. Subdivisions of the mediastinum with the most common mediastinal masses.

Theodor Schwann, 1810–1882, Professor of Anatomy and Physiology successively at Louvain (1839–1848), and Liege, Belgium (1849–1888).

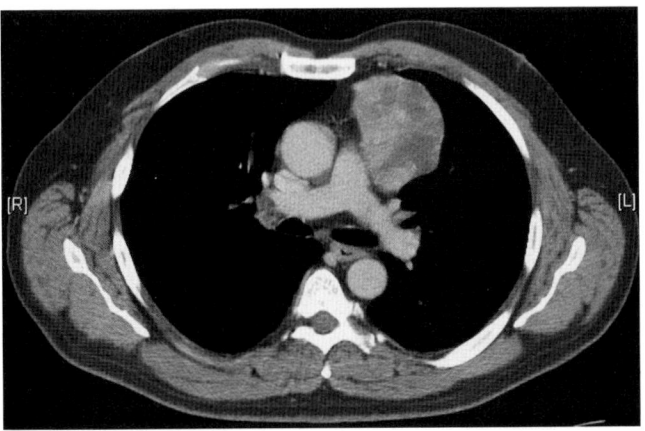

Figure 52.26 Computerised tomography scan showing a thymoma presenting as a mediastinal mass.

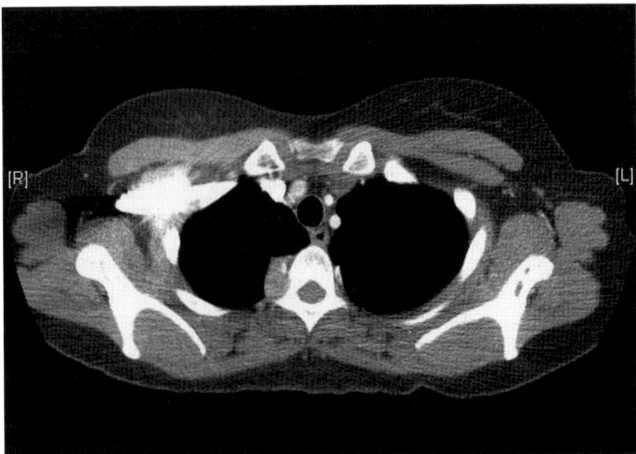

Figure 52.28 CT showing a right-sided paravertebral neural tumour.

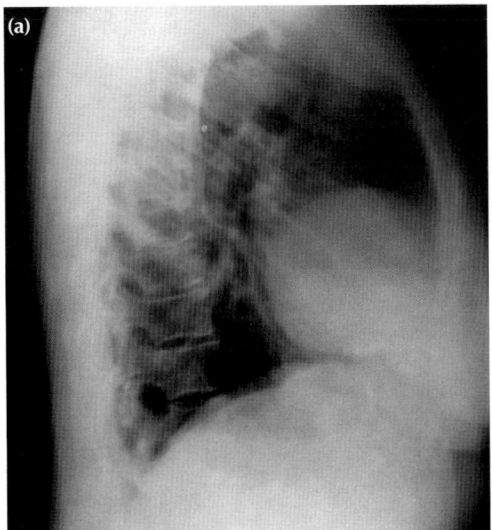

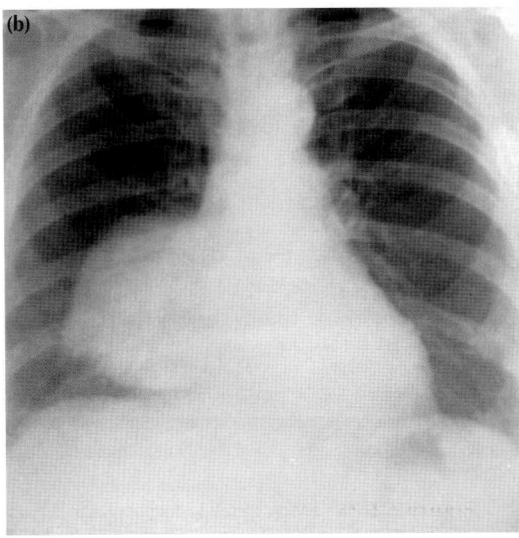

Figure 52.27 Lateral (a) and posteroanterior (b) radiographs of a patient with a mediastinal teratoma. The tumour lies anteriorly and extends into the right hemithorax.

Lung abscess

The causes of lung abscess are shown in Table 52.9. The chest radiograph shows a cavity with a fluid level or in myecetoma a fungal ball. Most acute abscesses resolve with appropriate antibiotic therapy and postural drainage. Surgery is avoided. Small radiologically sited drains are used sometimes in the intensive care unit.

Tuberculosis

Surgery is rarely indicated for tuberculosis in developed countries but, when it is, it must be combined with adequate anti-tubercular chemotherapy or the benefit of surgery will be lost (Summary box 52.6).

Table 52.9 Causes of lung abscess

Specific pneumonia	Streptococcal
	Staphylococcal
	Pneumococcal
	Klebsiella spp.
	Anaerobic
Bronchial obstruction	Carcinoma
	Carcinoid
	Foreign body
	Postoperative atelectasis
Chronic respiratory sepsis	Sinusitis
	Tonsillitis
	Dental infection
Septicaemia	
Penetrating lung injury	

Theodor Albrecht Edwin Klebs, **1834–1913, Professor of Bacteriology successively at Prague, The Czech Republic; Zurich, Switzerland; and The Rush Medical College, Chicago, IL, USA.**

Tuberculosis: indications for surgery

- Suspicious lesion on chest radiograph in which neoplasia cannot be excluded
- Chronic tuberculous abscess, resistant to chemotherapy
- Aspergilloma within a tuberculous cavity
- Life-threatening haemoptysis

Diagnosis

Surgical procedures may be necessary to establish the diagnosis if suspected clinically but sputum or pus cultures are persistently negative.

Complications such as an aspergilloma in a chronic cavity causing life-threatening haemoptysis may require lobectomy.

Pulmonary sequestration

This describes a section of lung separated from the normal bronchial connection with other abnormalities of development, which often include a direct systemic arterial supply from the aorta. The segment becomes cystic and infected. Interlobar sequestration occurs within the lung substance. It may present with recurrent chest infections and/or haemoptysis.

Lung cysts

Developmental lung cysts have a tendency to become infected. Acquired lung cysts may contain air or fluid and may be single or multiple. Pulmonary hydatid disease is a cause in endemic areas. Air cysts (bullae) may be spontaneous but may be secondary to emphysematous degeneration (Fig. 52.29).

LUNG TRANSPLANTATION

Lung transplantation is an established therapy for those with end-stage parenchymal or pulmonary vascular disease, which is limited by the number of donor lungs available.

CHEST TRAUMA

The approach to trauma must be methodical and exact, because the signs, particularly in the presence of other injury, may easily be missed. The general principles of resuscitation and ATLS (Advanced Trauma and Life Support) must be followed. Thoracic trauma is responsible for over 70% of all deaths following road traffic accidents. Blunt trauma to the chest in isolation is fatal in 10% of cases, rising to 30% if other injuries are present. Penetrating thoracic wounds vary according to the prevalence of civil violence, with a mortality rate of 3% for simple stabbing to 15% for gunshot wounds.

Early deaths after thoracic trauma are caused by hypoxaemia, hypovolaemia and tamponade. The first steps in treating such patients should be to diagnose and treat these problems as early as possible because they may be readily corrected. Young patients have a large physiological reserve, and serious injury may be overlooked until this reserve is used up, by which time the situation is critical and may be irretrievable. The best approach is to remain highly suspicious if life-threatening conditions are to be anticipated and treated. Early consultation with a regional thoracic centre is advised in cases of

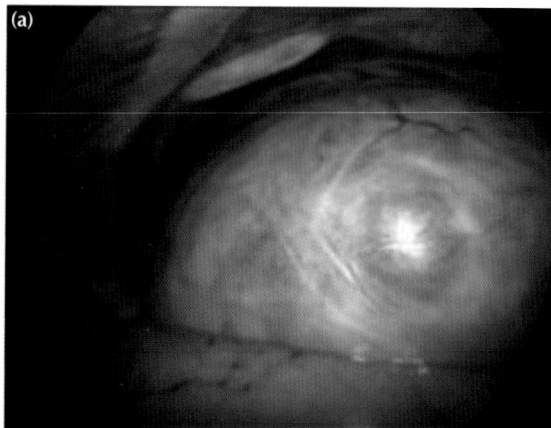

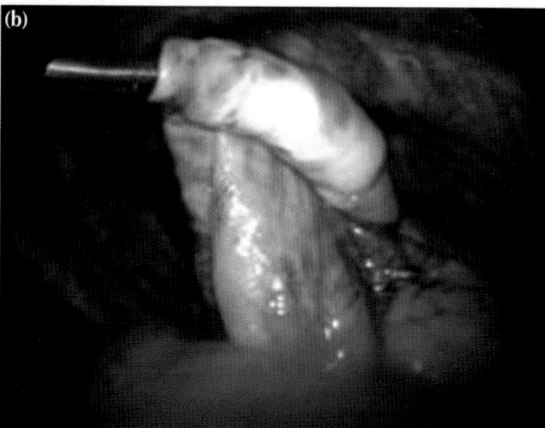

Figure 52.29 (a) A large solitary bulla seen on videothoracoscopy. (b) The bulla deflated and rolled in preparation for staple resection.

doubt. In an emergency it is essential that experienced help is summoned.

Management of chest trauma is covered in detail in Chapter 26.

THE DIAPHRAGM

The diaphragm is the fibromuscular structure separating the thorax from the abdomen (Fig. 52.30). There are two well-recognised congenital sites where abdominal viscera can herniate into the chest (Fig. 52.31):

- *the foramen of Morgagni*: a hernia in the anterior part of the diaphragm with a defect between the sternal and costal attachments. The most commonly involved viscus is the transverse colon.
- *the foramen of Bochdalek*: through the dome of the diaphragm posteriorly.

Traumatic rupture of the diaphragm may occur with blunt trauma. Unless there is severe bleeding or strangulation of the viscera it is best managed at an interval. In a severely injured

Giovanni Battista Morgagni, 1682–1771, Professor of Anatomy, Padua, Italy for 59 years. He is regarded as 'The Founder of Morbid Anatomy'.
Victor Alexander Bochdalek, 1801–1883, Professor of Anatomy, Prague, The Czech Republic.

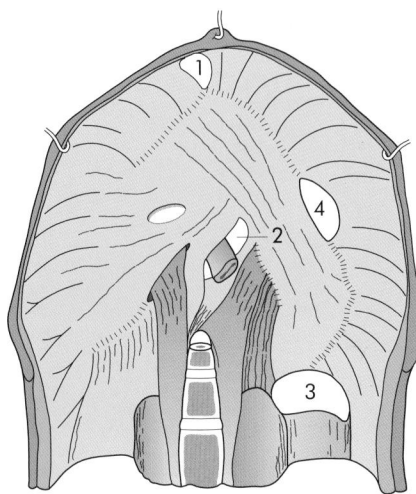

Figure 52.30 Diagram of sites of hernias. The usual sites of congenital diaphragmatic hernia: 1, foramen of Morgagni; 2, oesophageal hiatus; 3, foramen of Bochdalek (pleuroperitoneal hernia); and 4, dome.

patient being ventilated it can wait until other injuries are dealt with and weaning from the ventilator is being considered.

THE CHEST WALL

Tumours of the chest wall

These can be tumours of any component of the chest wall, i.e. bone, cartilage and soft tissue. They are treated similarly to those that occur in other sites and require specialist surgical input only if major resection and chest wall reconstruction are contemplated.

Other diseases of the chest wall

Congenital abnormalities are often incidental findings on chest radiography (bifid rib), but there are some important exceptions.

Cervical rib and thoracic outlet syndrome

This rib is usually represented by a fibrous band originating from the seventh cervical vertebra and inserting onto the first thoracic rib. It may be asymptomatic, but because the subclavian artery and brachial plexus course over it a variety of symptoms may occur. The lower trunk of the plexus (mainly T1) is compressed, leading to wasting of the interossei and altered sensation in the T1 distribution. Compression of the subclavian artery may result in a post-stenotic dilatation with thrombus and embolus formation. The diagnosis, assessment and surgery are fraught with uncertainties and are best left to those with a well-developed interest in this problem.

Pectus excavatum

The sternum is depressed, with a dish-shaped deformity of the anterior portions of the ribs on one or both sides. It is never a cause of respiratory problems.

Pectus carinatum (pigeon chest)

In this condition the sternum is elevated above the level of the ribs and treatment is offered for cosmetic reasons. The sternum is mobilised and allowed to fall back into place.

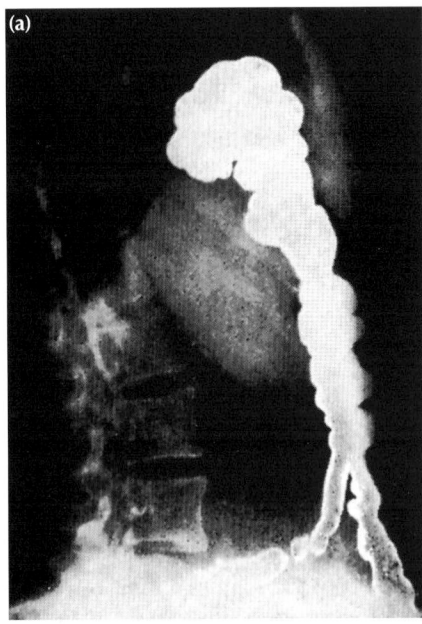

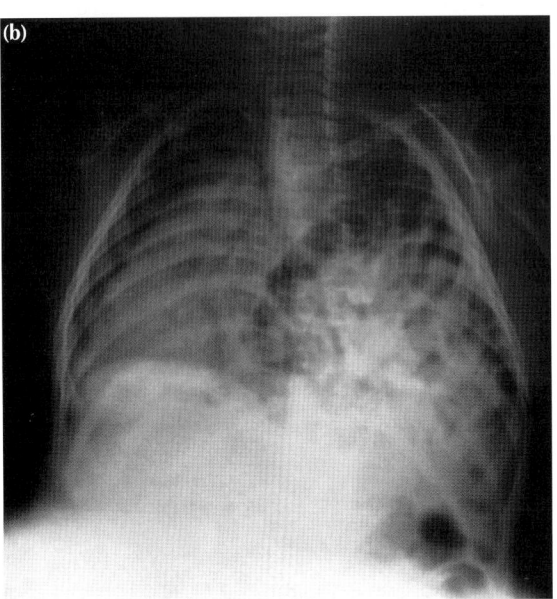

Figure 52.31 Chest radiograph of congenital diaphragmatic hernia. (a) Colon occupying a Morgagni hernia (courtesy of Dr Oliver Smith, Birmingham). (b) Foramen of Bochdalek hernia on the left side in an infant. The left pleural cavity is occupied by intestine, the mediastinum is displaced to the right and the right lung is aerated very little.

It often comes to light during the growth spurt at adolescence when, of course, the teenager is particularly sensitive about appearance. Most patients are asymptomatic and the only justification for treatment is on cosmetic grounds. Some surgeons make a very good case for this but the risk of morbidity and of a less than perfect result must be clearly spelt out to the patients and their parents. Surgery involves mobilising the sternum with the costal cartilages and holding this central panel anteriorly with a steel bar. Surgery is best left until the late teens, when further growth of the chest wall is unlikely.

FURTHER READING

British Thoracic Society (2001) *The Burden of Lung Disease*. A statistics report from the British Thoracic Society.

Miller, A.C. and Harvey, J.E. (1993) Guidelines for the management of spontaneous pneumothorax. Standards of Care Committee, British Thoracic Society. *Br Med J* **307**: 114–16.

PART
10 | Vascular

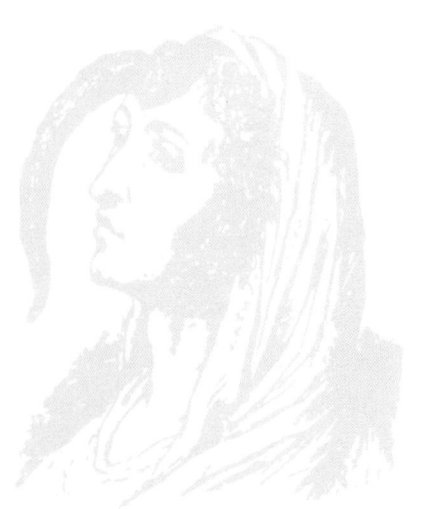

Arterial disorders

INTRODUCTION

Arterial disorders represent the most common cause of morbidity and death in western societies. Much of this is due to the effects of atheroma on the arteries supplying the heart muscle (coronary thrombosis and myocardial infarction) and brain (stroke), although atheroma is also common at other sites. This chapter addresses diseases that are typically the province of the vascular surgeon, namely those affecting the arteries of the body, excluding those of the heart and those within the cranium.

ARTERIAL STENOSIS AND OCCLUSION

Cause and effect

Arterial stenosis or occlusion is commonly caused by atheroma but can occur acutely as a result of emboli or trauma. Stenosis or occlusion produces symptoms and signs that are related to the organ supplied by the artery: e.g. lower limb – claudication, rest pain and gangrene; brain – transient ischaemic attacks and stroke; myocardium – angina and myocardial infarction; kidney – hypertension and renal failure (Fig. 53.1); intestine – abdominal pain and infarction. The severity of the symptoms is related to the size of the vessel occluded and the alternative routes (collaterals) available for blood flow (Fig. 53.2).

Features of arterial stenosis or occlusion in the leg

Intermittent claudication

Intermittent claudication is a cramp-like pain felt in the muscles that is:

- brought on by walking;
- not present on taking the first step (unlike osteoarthrosis);

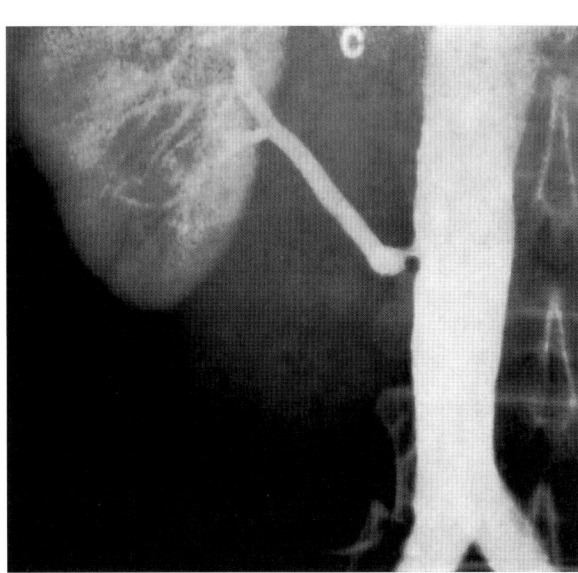

Figure 53.1 Renal artery stenosis. Angiogram by retrograde femoral catheterisation. Note the post-stenotic dilatation.

- relieved by standing still (unlike lumbar intervertebral disc nerve compression).

The distance that a patient is able to walk without stopping varies only slightly from day to day. It is altered by walking up hill, the speed of walking and changes in general health, such as anaemia or heart failure.

The pain of claudication is most commonly felt in the calf but it can affect the thigh or buttock. Buttock claudication plus sexual impotence resulting from arterial insufficiency is eponymously called Leriche's syndrome. Arm claudication is unusual

Claudication from the Latin *claudicare* – to limp. The Roman emperor Claudius, (10 BC to 54 AD) walked with a limp, which was possibly due to poliomyelitis.

Rene Leriche, 1879–1955, Professor of Surgery, Strasbourg, France, described this syndrome.

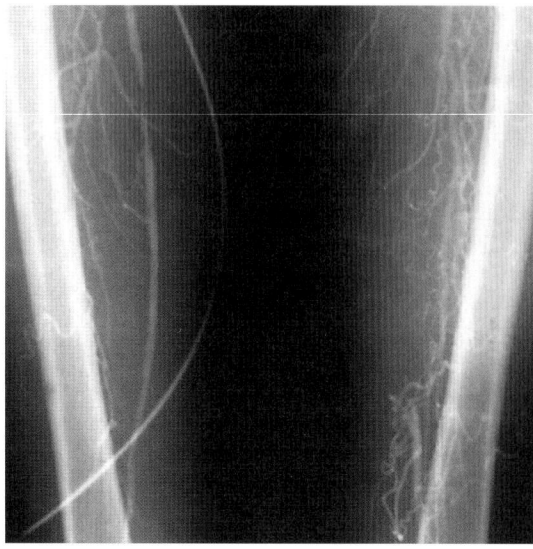

Figure 53.2 Right superficial femoral stenosis. Left superficial femoral occlusion with collateral vessels present, causing claudication.

but may be caused by subclavian, axillary or brachial artery obstruction.

Rest pain

Rest pain occurs with the limb (usually the leg) at rest; it is exacerbated by lying down or elevation of the foot. Characteristically, the pain is worse at night and it may be lessened by hanging the foot out of bed or by sleeping in a chair.

Coldness, numbness, paraesthesia and colour change

Coldness, numbness and paraesthesia are common in moderate and severe ischaemia but, in the absence of colour change (Fig. 53.3), a neurological cause should be excluded. Affected legs blanch on elevation and develop a purple discoloration on dependency.

Ulceration and gangrene

Ulceration occurs with severe arterial insufficiency and may present as a painful erosion between toes or as shallow, non-healing ulcers on the dorsum of the feet, on the shins and especially around the malleoli. The blackened mummified tissues of frank gangrene are unmistakable (Fig. 53.4).

Temperature sensation and movement

A severely ischaemic foot is usually cold, but an ischaemic limb tends to equilibrate with the temperature of its surroundings and may feel quite warm under the bedclothes. The acutely ischaemic limb is frequently paralysed and insensate; such a limb has a poor prognosis without treatment. Severe chronic ischaemia does not produce paralysis and is sensate. Ischaemic limbs must be handled gently.

Arterial pulsations

Pulsation distal to an arterial occlusion is usually absent or, in the presence of good collaterals, diminished. It is standard practice to feel for pulsation in the radial, carotid, common femoral, popliteal, posterior tibial and dorsalis pedis arteries and in the abdominal aorta. Diminution of a pulse can often be appreciated by comparing it with its opposite number. Expansile pulsation

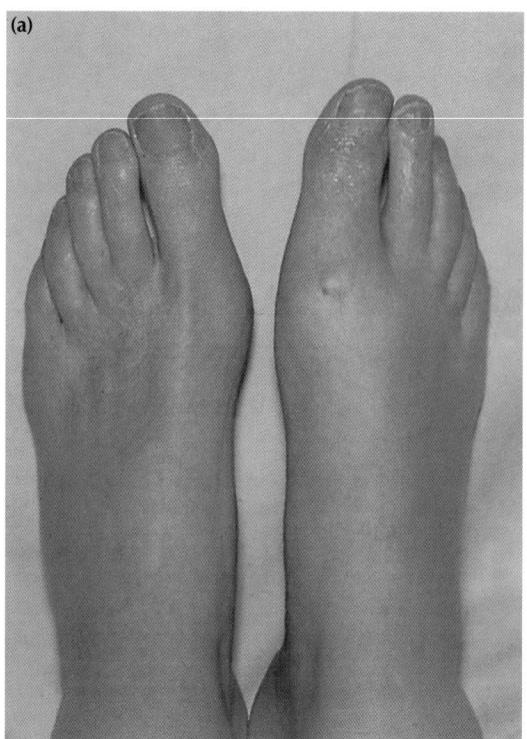

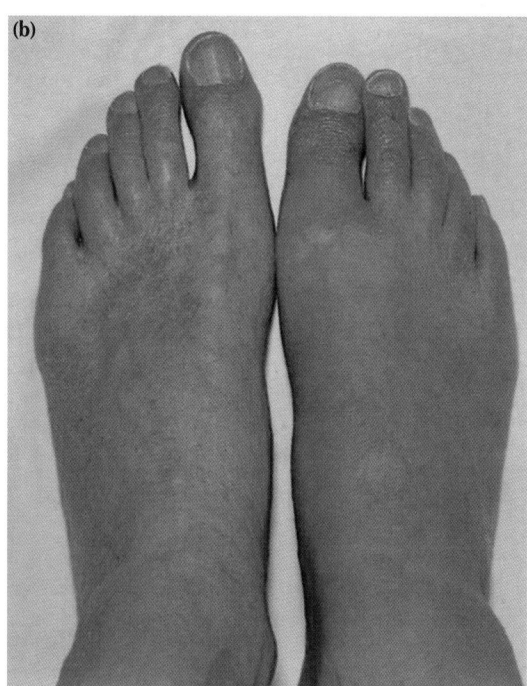

Figure 53.3 Colour changes with elevation (a) and dependency (b).

may indicate an aneurysm. Stenosis, or occlusion with a highly developed collateral circulation, may allow distal pulses to be normal to palpation. In this case, the sign of the 'disappearing pulse' may prove useful; after exercise to the point of claudication a previously palpable pulse disappears, reappearing after rest. The explanation is that exercise produces vasodilatation below the obstructing lesion and the arterial inflow cannot keep pace with the increasing vascular space; pressure falls and the pulse disappears.

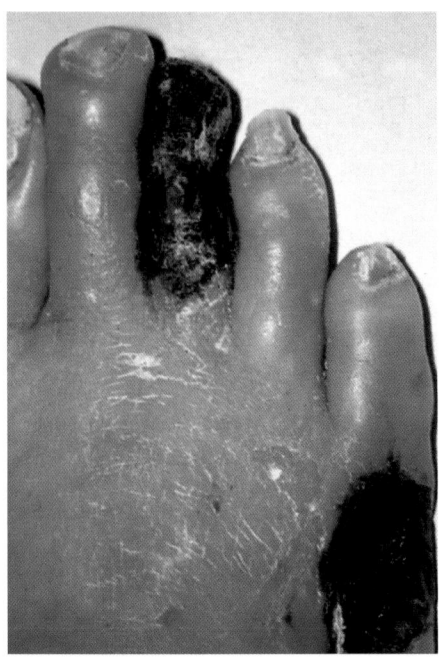

Figure 53.4 Severe chronic ischaemia with dry gangrene.

Table 53.1 Relationship of clinical findings to site of disease

Aortoiliac obstruction	Claudication in both buttocks, thighs and calves
	Femoral and distal pulses absent in both limbs
	Bruit over aortoiliac region
	Impotence common (Leriche)
Iliac obstruction	Unilateral claudication in the thigh and calf and sometimes the buttock
	Bruit over the iliac region
	Unilateral absence of femoral and distal pulses
Femoropopliteal obstruction	Unilateral claudication in the calf
	Femoral pulse palpable with absent unilateral distal pulses
Distal obstruction	Femoral and popliteal pulses palpable
	Ankle pulses absent
	Claudication in calf and foot

The best results from surgery are obtained by operation on the larger vessels, which allows a high volume of blood flow through bypass grafts. For instance, aorto-iliac bypass is longer lasting than femorotibial bypass.

Arterial bruits

Examination should include auscultation of the subclavian, carotid and femoral (at the groin and adductor canal) arteries and the abdominal aorta. A bruit indicates turbulence, suggesting stenosis, and is conducted distally. Bruits may occur at unusual sites; the patient with renal artery stenosis (see Fig. 53.1, page 899) had a bruit over the affected vessel. A continuous 'machinery' murmur over an artery usually indicates an arteriovenous fistula.

Venous refilling

The limb is elevated for 30 s and then laid flat. Normal venous refilling occurs within seconds and slow refilling indicates arterial insufficiency. Fast refilling and varicose veins suggest an arteriovenous fistula (Summary box 53.1).

Summary box 53.1

Features of lower limb arterial stenosis or occlusion

- Intermittent claudication
- Rest pain
- Cold, numb, paraesthesia, colour change
- Ulceration
- Gangrene
- Assumes ambient temperature
- Sensation decreased
- Movement diminished or lost
- Arterial pulsation diminished or absent
- Arterial bruit
- Slow venous refilling

Relationship of clinical findings to site of disease

Consideration of symptoms and signs should determine the site of any major arterial obstruction (Table 53.1). Furthermore, the presence of an additional obstruction can usually be inferred. For example, signs of iliac artery obstruction and ulceration of the foot suggest an additional obstruction, as collateral circulation around an isolated iliac artery obstruction is usually excellent. Such severe features indicate a second obstruction, typically in the femoral or popliteal artery.

Investigation of arterial occlusive disease

Most patients with symptoms of arterial disease do not need active treatment, such as angioplasty or surgical reconstruction, and the decision whether or not to intervene can often be made without recourse to special investigations.

General investigation

Patients with arterial disease tend to be elderly and atherosclerosis is a generalised disease; if active intervention is contemplated, full assessment is essential. Tests relevant to diabetes, abnormal lipid metabolism, anaemia and conditions causing high blood viscosity (e.g. polycythaemia and thrombocythaemia) include a full blood count (including platelets), plasma fibrinogen, blood and urine glucose, and a blood lipid profile (triglycerides, total cholesterol, and high- and low-density lipoprotein cholesterol). Cardiac failure, myocardial ischaemia, hypertension and age-related diseases such as chronic obstructive pulmonary disease and neoplasia should also be considered.

Although a normal electrocardiogram (ECG) does not exclude severe coronary artery disease, a grossly abnormal ECG may influence decision making. An exercise ECG gives a more accurate assessment but many patients are limited in their ability to exercise. In such circumstances radioisotope ventriculography or echocardiography may be attractive as a non-invasive method of assessing left ventricular function. Patients must also be assessed for lung disease by chest radiograph and, if necessary, pulmonary function tests. Tests for renal function (serum creatinine) are also required, especially if contrast agents are to be used at angiography, as they may adversely affect kidney function.

Doppler ultrasound blood flow detection

A hand-held Doppler ultrasound probe is most useful in the assessment of occlusive arterial disease; many consider it essential (Figs 53.5 and 53.6). A continuous-wave ultrasound signal is transmitted from the probe at an artery and the reflected beam is picked up by a receiver within the probe itself. The change in frequency in the reflected beam compared with that of the transmitted beam is due to the Doppler shift, resulting from the reflection of the beam by moving blood cells. The frequency change may be converted into an audio signal that is typically pulsatile. Doppler ultrasound equipment can be used as a very sensitive type of stethoscope in conjunction with a sphygmomanometer to assess systolic pressure in small vessels. This is possible even when the arterial pulse cannot be palpated. It is of the greatest importance to appreciate that, although a 'Doppler signal' indicates moving blood, it does not necessarily indicate that the blood flow detected is sufficient to prevent limb loss, i.e. a Doppler signal does not indicate viability.

The ankle–brachial pressure index (ABPI) is the ratio of systolic pressure at the ankle to that in the arm. The higher of the pressures in the dorsalis pedis and posterior tibial arteries serves as the numerator, with the higher systolic pressure between the brachials serving as the denominator. Resting ABPI is normally about 1.0; values below 0.9 indicate some degree of arterial obstruction and less than 0.3 suggests imminent necrosis. It must

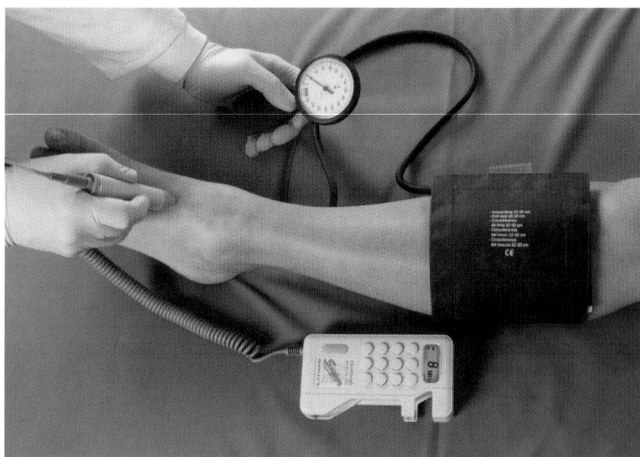

Figure 53.6 Hand-held Doppler probe and sphygmomanometer used to determine systolic pressure in the dorsalis pedis artery, as part of assessing the ankle–brachial pressure index.

be appreciated, however, that values approaching normality at rest may still be associated with intermittent claudication. Retesting after exercise is useful in this context as ABPI normally rises but occlusive disease may result in reduction. Artefacts are due especially to calcified arteries, which are often incompressible and lead to a falsely high pressure or ABPI result, especially in diabetics.

Duplex imaging

This is a major investigative technique in vascular disease. A duplex scanner uses B-mode ultrasound to provide an image of vessels (Figs 53.7 and 53.8). This image is created through the

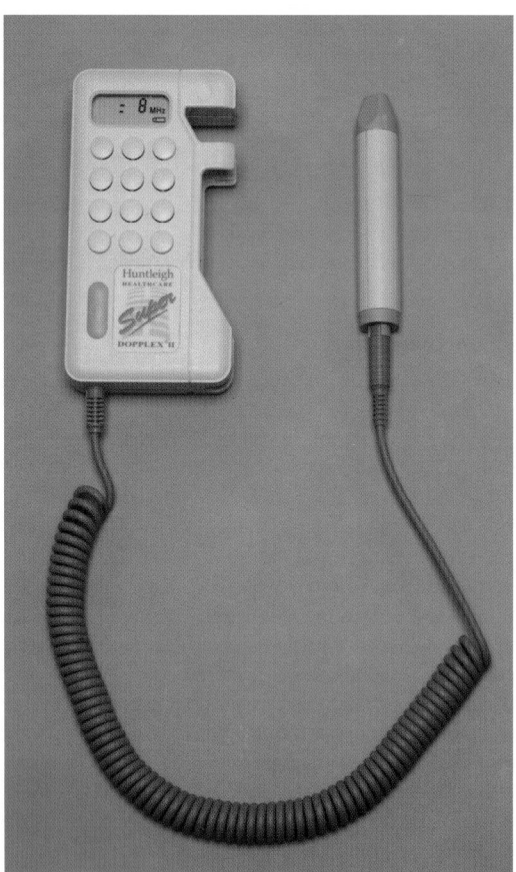

Figure 53.5 Simple hand-held Doppler ultrasound probe.

Christian Johann Doppler, **1803–1853, Professor of Experimental Physics, Vienna, Austria, enunciated the 'Doppler Principle' in 1842.**

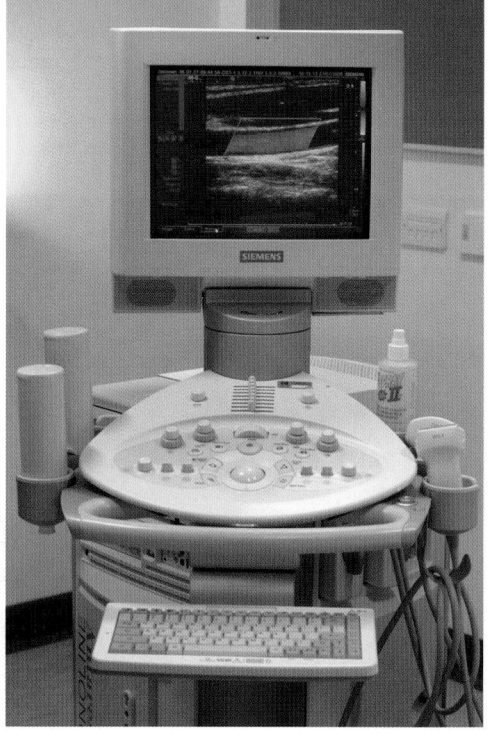

Figure 53.7 Colour duplex scanner.

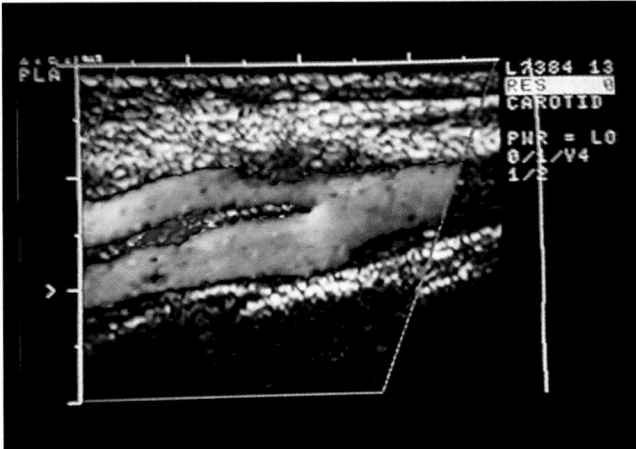

Figure 53.8 Colour duplex scan of carotid vessels in neck showing stenosis at common carotid bifurcation (courtesy of Dr Paul Allan, Royal Infirmary, Edinburgh, Scotland).

different abilities of different tissues to reflect the ultrasound beam. A second type of ultrasound, namely Doppler ultrasound, is then used to insonate the imaged vessels and the Doppler shift obtained is analysed by a computer in the duplex scanner. Such shifts can give detailed knowledge of vessel blood flow, turbulence, etc. Many scanners have the added sophistication of colour coding, which allows visualisation of blood flow on the image. The various colours indicate change in direction and velocity of flow; points of high flow generally indicate a stenosis (consider that rivers flow fast where they are narrow). Duplex scanning is at least as accurate as angiography in many circumstances. In terms of cost-effectiveness and safety, it is generally to be preferred to any type of angiography if the two tests are considered to be equally useful in any given clinical context.

Treadmill

Patients themselves are poor at assessing claudicating distance and it might be thought that a treadmill assessment would provide a useful objective measurement of distance to onset of pain. However, a simple measured walk along a hospital corridor is even more reliable. A good use for the treadmill (with a slight incline) is the detection of a fall in ABPI after exercise, indicating occult arterial stenosis (see above).

Angiography (synonym: arteriography)

In lower limb disease, symptoms and their severity determine whether intervention is needed. Angiography is only appropriate if intervention is being contemplated. Even then, it is often advisable to have a duplex scan first.

Classical angiography involves the injection of a radio-opaque solution into the arterial tree, generally by a retrograde percutaneous catheter method (Seldinger technique) usually involving the femoral artery (Figs. 53.9 and 53.10). Hazards include thrombosis, arterial dissection, haematoma, renal dysfunction and allergic reaction. Rather than taking simple films, nowadays a computer system digitises the images, allowing the image before injection of contrast agent to be subtracted from the contrast

Sven Ivar Seldinger, **1921–1998**, Radiologist, Karolinska Institute, Stockholm, Sweden, introduced percutaneous arterial catheterisation in 1953.

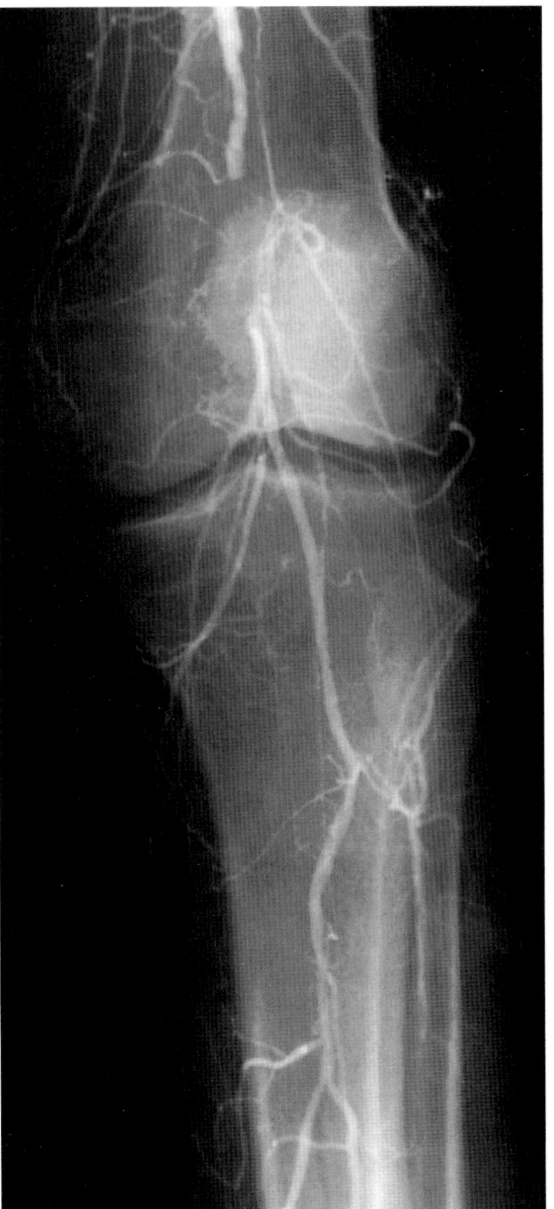

Figure 53.9 Arterial occlusion just above the knee causing claudication of the calf; good collateral circulation (arteriogram by the Seldinger technique).

image, thereby removing extraneous background and providing great clarity. Such digital subtraction angiography (DSA) may be carried out by arterial or venous injection of contrast agent. The former allows the use of fine catheters and relatively small amounts of contrast agent; although the latter avoids the need for arterial puncture completely, a high volume of contrast agent must be used.

The new millennium has seen the introduction of magnetic resonance angiography, which offers the prospect of multiplanar imaging without the need for ionising radiation or direct arterial puncture (Fig. 53.11). Although image quality is not as good as that of DSA, it is satisfactory for most purposes. Computerised tomography (CT) angiography is another recently introduced method that is gaining in popularity and, taken together, these two new techniques are gradually replacing DSA.

CHAPTER 53 | ARTERIAL DISORDERS

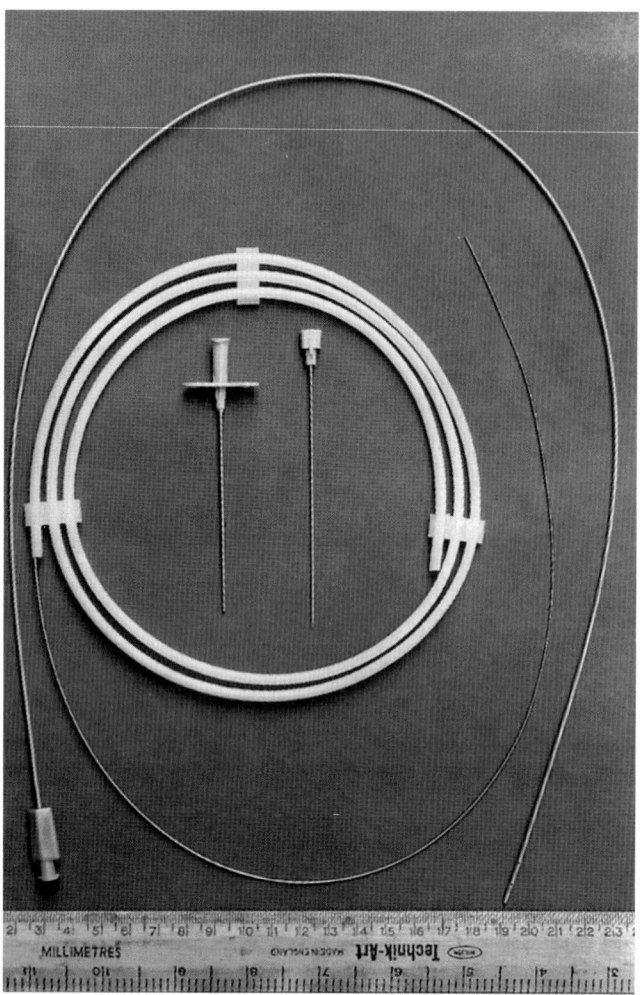

Figure 53.10 Seldinger needle and guidewire for introducing an arterial catheter.

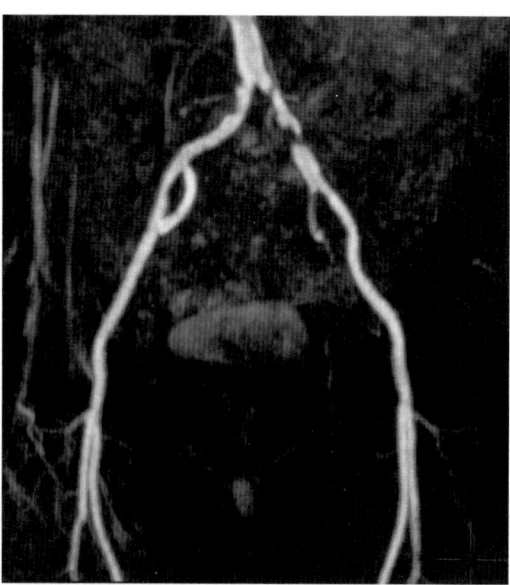

Figure 53.11 Magnetic resonance angiogram showing a tight stenosis at the midpoint of the left common iliac artery.

Non-surgical management of arterial stenosis or occlusion

General

When told that walking is not doing harm, many claudicants are content to live within the limitations imposed by their condition. Spontaneous improvement occurs in many patients over the first 6 months after an occlusive episode as collateral vessels develop. Lifestyle advice should be offered. Exercise is encouraged, particularly walking within the limits of the disability; supervised exercise programmes are ideal. Stopping smoking is essential. Dietary advice is required for those who are overweight and for those with high blood lipids. Care of the ischaemic foot is often required, especially in diabetics.

Drugs

Medication may be required for diseases associated with arterial disorders, such as hypertension and diabetes; some antihypertensives (particularly β-blockers) may exacerbate claudication. Raised blood lipids require active drug treatment but even when the lipid profile is normal a statin should be prescribed (e.g. 40 mg/day of pravastatin). An antiplatelet agent is also necessary, usually 75 mg day^{-1} of aspirin, with 75 mg day^{-1} of clopidogrel as an alternative for those who are aspirin intolerant. Other agents, such as vasodilators, are unlikely to prove beneficial.

Transluminal angioplasty and stenting

Arterial occlusive disease may be treated by inserting a balloon catheter into an artery and inflating it within a narrowed or blocked area (Figs 53.12 and 53.13). This is usually done percutaneously in the radiology department (Figs 53.14 and 53.15). Percutaneous transluminal angioplasty (PTA) has proved very successful in dilating the iliac arteries and, to a lesser extent, the arteries of the leg itself. The technique is also applicable at other sites (upper limb vessels, renal arteries, gastrointestinal arteries, carotid arteries) with variable outcomes. The basic method involves a (usually) femoral angiogram during which a guidewire is inserted through any stenosis or short occlusion to be treated. A balloon catheter is then inserted over the guidewire and the balloon positioned within the lesion, its position being confirmed by angiography. The balloon is then inflated for approximately 1 minute and deflated. This is repeated before withdrawal of the catheter.

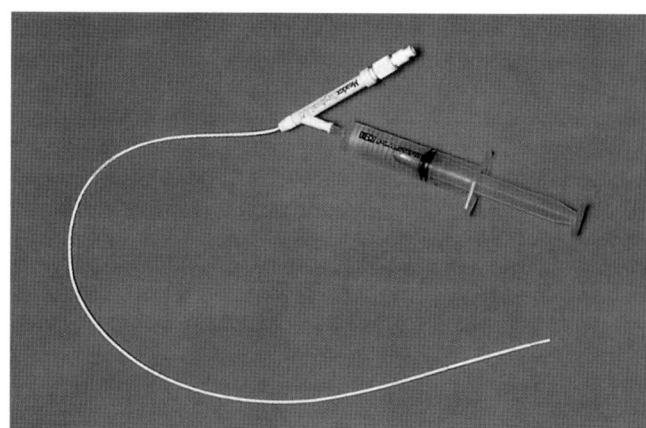

Figure 53.12 Balloon catheter for percutaneous transluminal angioplasty.

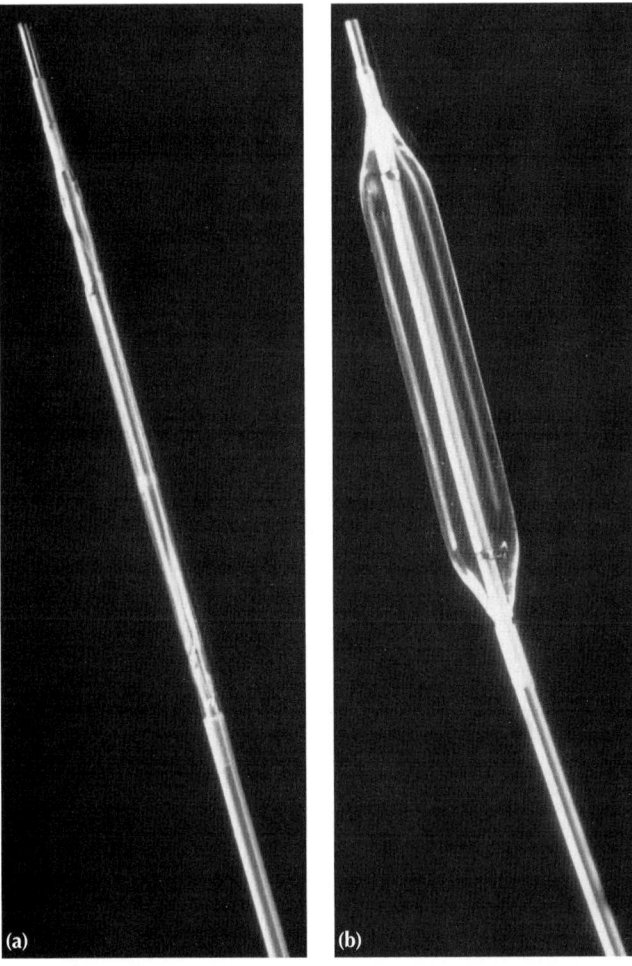

Figure 53.13 (a) Catheter balloon deflated; (b) balloon inflated.

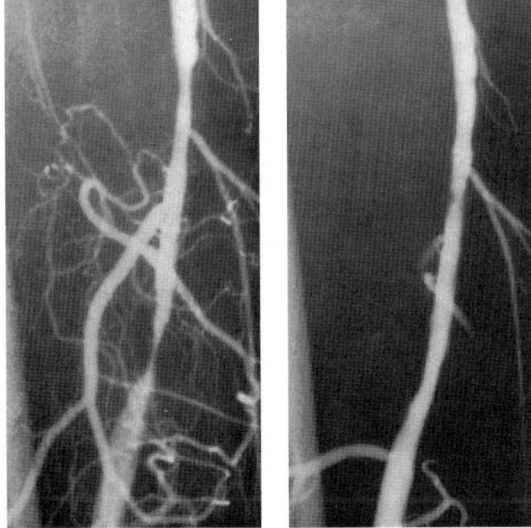

Figure 53.14 Narrowed superficial femoral artery before and after transluminal angioplasty (courtesy of J. McIvor, FRCR, London). The advantage of this technique is that it can be carried out under local anaesthesia using the Seldinger technique of percutaneous arterial puncture, and is therefore especially useful in the treatment of patients who are medically unfit for major surgery.

Should the vessel fail to stay adequately dilated, it may be possible to hold the lumen open using a metal stent (Figs 53.16 and 53.17). Such a device may be introduced on a balloon catheter, the balloon itself when inflated expanding the stent; the balloon is then deflated and the catheter removed. An alternative type of stent is held compressed by a sheath of plastic in a delivery system. The stent is positioned at the site of arterial dilatation and its sheath withdrawn to allow the device to self-expand and so hold the lumen open.

PTA of the carotid artery is currently topical. At this site the matter of microemboli at the time of dilatation as a cause of iatrogenic stroke cannot be ignored. Several techniques have been developed to try to reduce this problem, including umbrella-style catheters capable of trapping debris released at the point of balloon expansion. Whether or not carotid PTA will prove a sound alternative to carotid endarterectomy remains to be determined through randomised controlled trials.

Operations for arterial stenosis or occlusion

Site of disease and type of operation

Aortoiliac occlusion responds well to aortofemoral bypass (Fig. 53.18a, page 908), but this operation carries a mortality rate of about 5%. Today, PTA is usually a better alternative if technically possible. In a patient who is unable to withstand major surgery, who has pronounced ischaemia and who has no PTA option, a femorofemoral or iliofemoral crossover bypass may be considered (if only one iliac system is involved with disease) or an axillo-bifemoral bypass may be done (if both iliac segments are diseased).

Superficial femoral artery occlusive disease often produces unilateral symptoms. For claudication, conservative treatment is almost always the best plan but, if the block is short and favourably sited, PTA may be a resonable option. If the lesion is not favourable for PTA and the patient fully understands the risks and benefits of intervention, a femoropopliteal bypass may be considered (Fig. 53.18b, page 908); long-term graft patency is related to the quality of inflow and outflow, and graft length (common femoral to above-knee or below-knee popliteal). It is also related to the material used for the bypass. Autogenous saphenous vein gives the best results when used either as a reversed conduit or *in situ* after valve disruption. Some patients have a profunda femoris origin stenosis that can be overcome by a small vein or prosthetic patch angioplasty.

Occlusive disease below the popliteal artery may require bypass to a tibial vessel, even down to ankle level. Success is fair but the risk of early failure with limb loss is such that this femorotibial bypass is only appropriate for limb salvage or severe rest pain. The most successful conduit is the long saphenous vein used in the *in situ* fashion after disrupting the valves with a valvulotome. If the long saphenous vein is not available from either leg, short saphenous or arm veins may be used. A polytetrafluoroethylene (PTFE) graft may even be employed; many surgeons construct the lower anastomosis using a small collar of vein (Miller cuff) between the PTFE and the recipient artery, which may improve patency.

Prosthetic materials

Dacron is the favoured material for aortoiliac work (Fig. 53.19a); it gives excellent results. For bypass in the femoropopliteal region,

Justin H. Miller, **Vascular Surgeon, Royal Adelaide Hospital, Adelaide, SA, Australia.**

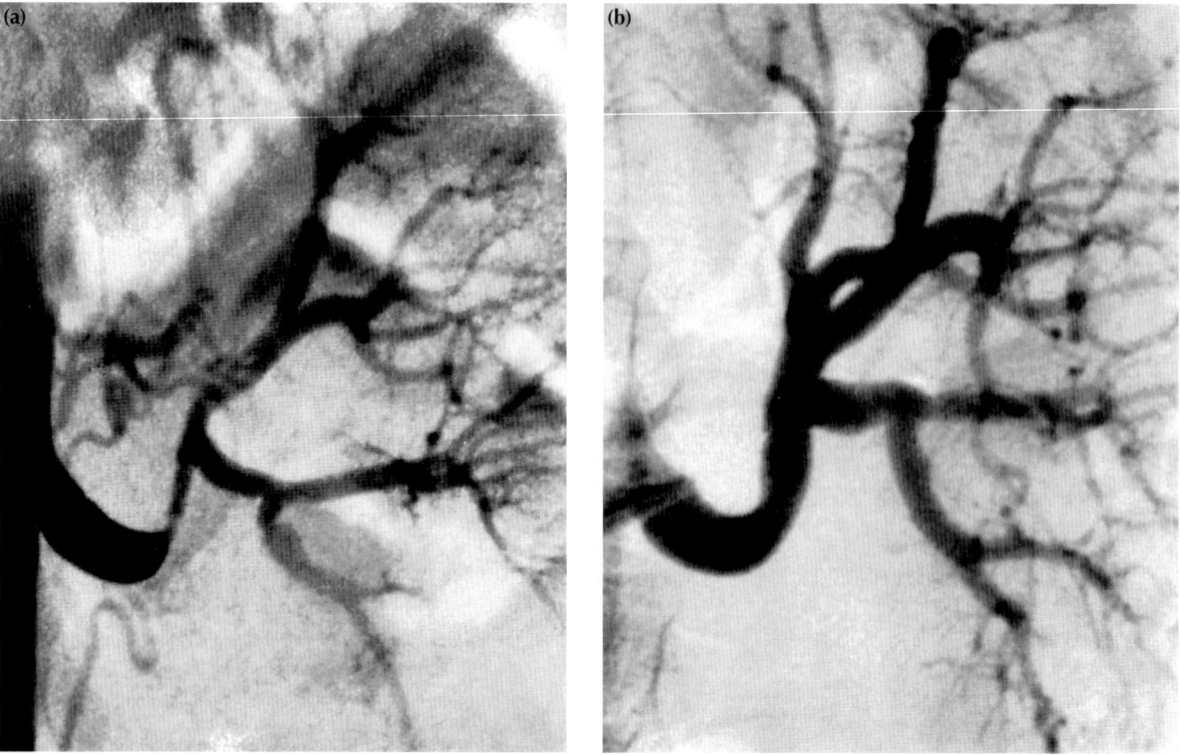

Figure 53.15 Before (a) and after (b) balloon dilatation of a severely stenosed left renal artery in a 20-year-old woman with uncontrollable hypertension. The blood pressure fell to normal after the procedure. The stenosis was probably due to fibromuscular hyperplasia, but no tissue was available for histological diagnosis.

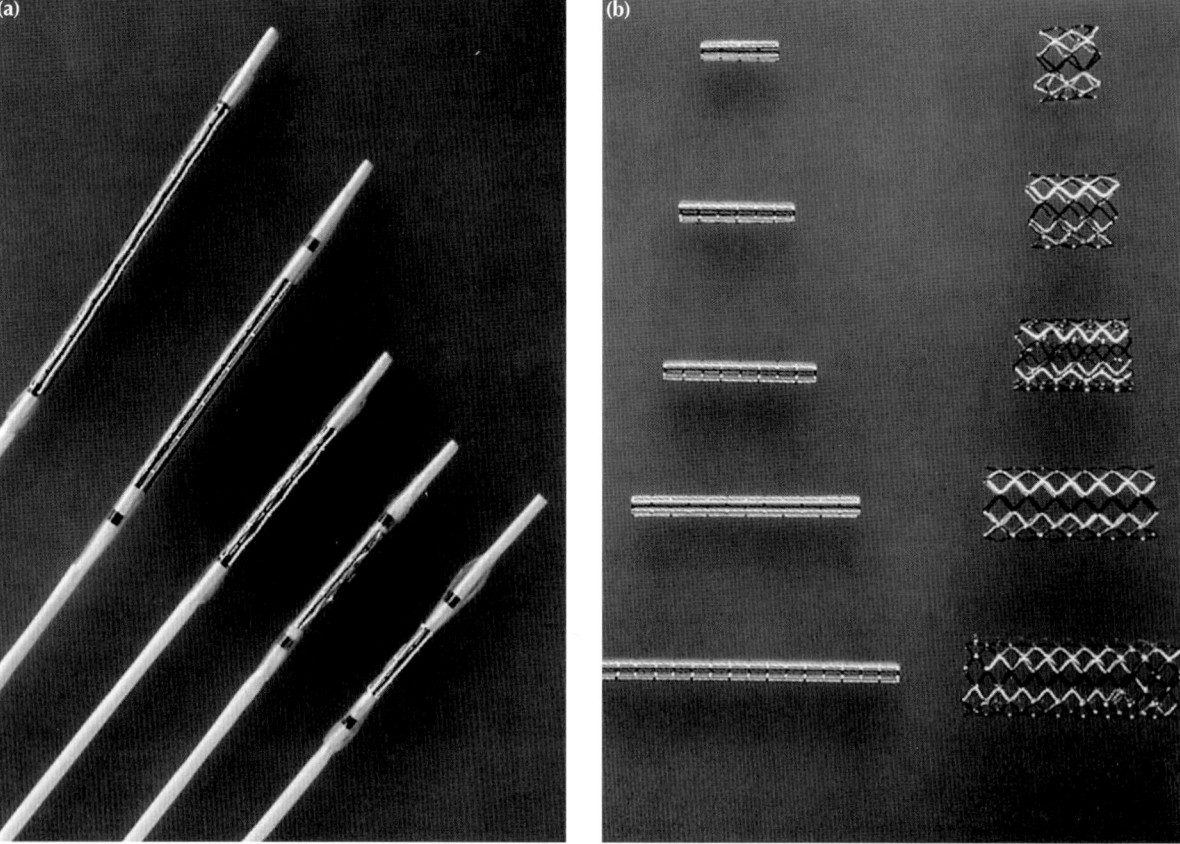

Figure 53.16 (a) Balloon catheters carrying stents; (b) non-expanded and expanded stents (courtesy of Johnson and Johnson Interventional Systems, Bracknell, Berks, England).

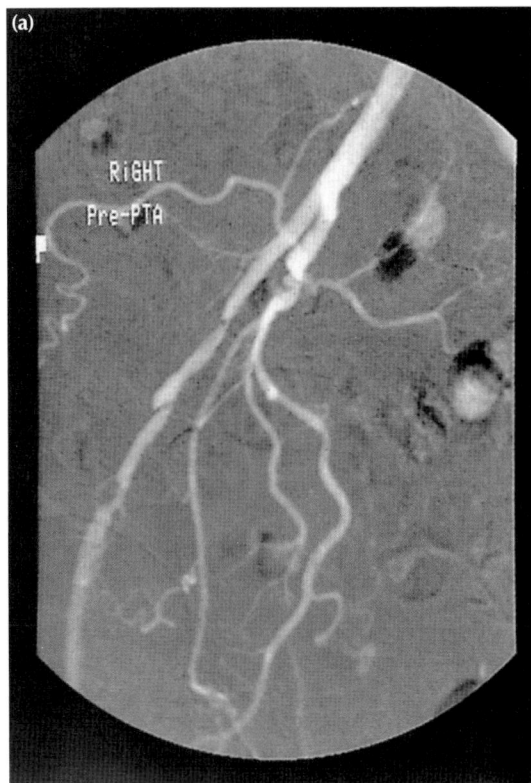

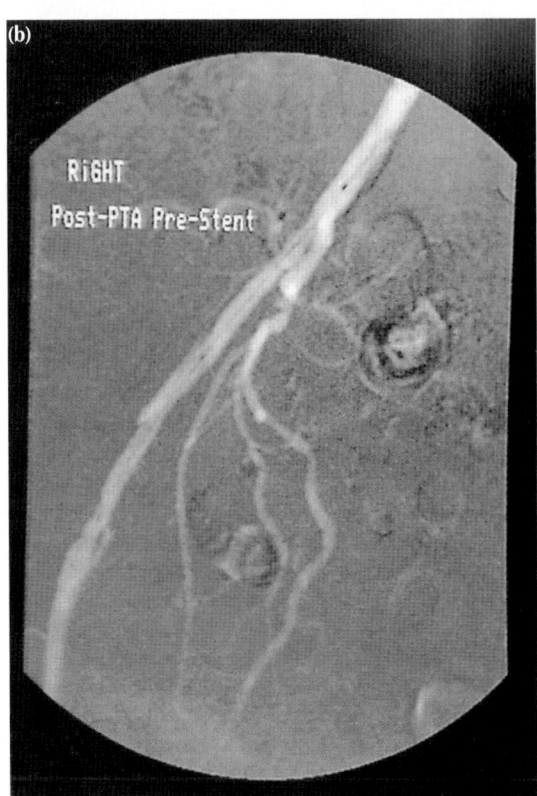

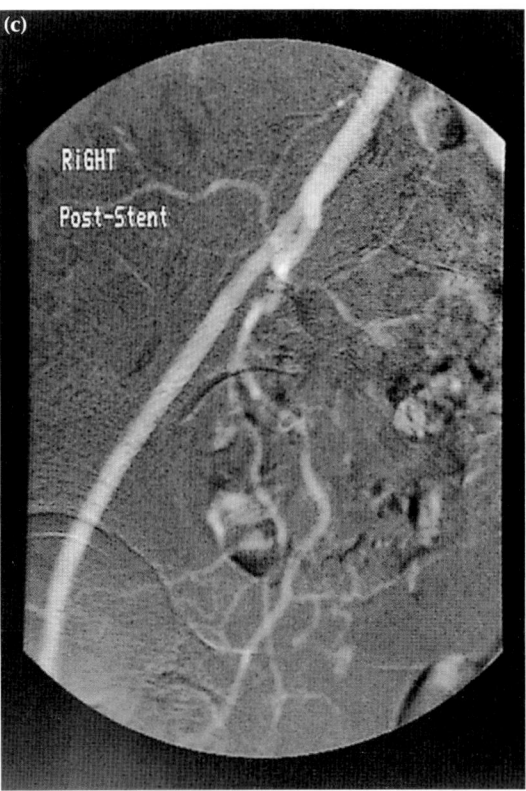

Figure 53.17 (a) External iliac artery stenosis before dilatation; (b) after dilatation by percutaneous transluminal angioplasty; and (c) dilated artery patency assured by stent (courtesy of Johnson and Johnson Interventional Systems, Bracknell, England, and Dr W. Shaw, Ninewells Hospital, Dundee, Scotland).

aorta it is usual to use 2/0 or 3/0 sutures and in the femoral artery at the groin 4/0 or 5/0 sutures. Finer sutures, up to 7/0, may be needed further down the limb.

Technical details

For aortofemoral bypass the aorta is approached through a midline or transverse abdominal incision. The common femoral arteries and their branches are exposed through vertical groin incisions. The small bowel is retracted to the right and the posterior peritoneum opened. Retroperitoneal tunnels are made from the aorta to the groins. Heparin (5000 U) is given intravenously and the vessels clamped. A vertical incision is made in the anterior aspect of the aorta to which an obliquely cut, bifurcated Dacron graft is sutured end-to-side. The graft limbs are then fed down to the groins where they are anastomosed end-to-side to the common femoral arteries or, if there is evidence of profunda stenosis, to an arteriotomy running from the common femoral vessel down into the profunda. The posterior peritoneum is closed over the Dacron to prevent adhesion of the graft to bowel. The abdomen and groin wounds are closed without drainage.

For femoropopliteal bypass the popliteal artery above or below the knee is exposed through a medial incision. The common femoral artery is exposed at groin level. The long saphenous vein may be treated in two different ways. First, it may be excised, and its tributaries tied, reversed and sutured into the limb as a bypass. Second, it may be left in place (*in situ*) and the valves disrupted with a valvulotome. The graft is then sutured to the femoral artery

if autogenous vein is not available, PTFE (Fig. 53.19b) or glutaraldehyde-tanned, Dacron-supported, human umbilical vein (Fig. 53.19c) may be employed. In general, any vein used requires a diameter of at least 3 mm. Monofilament sutures are used for vascular surgery; polypropylene is particularly popular. In the

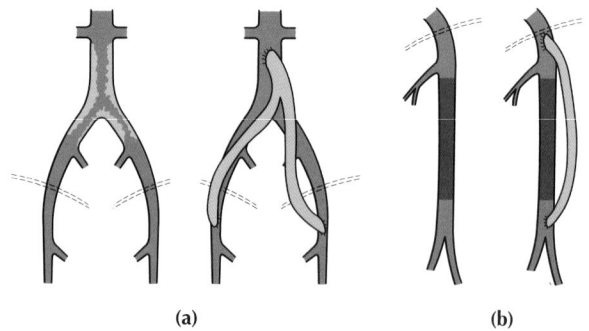

(a)   **(b)**

Figure 53.18 (a) Atherosclerotic narrowing of the aortic bifurcation. Aorto-bifemoral graft to bypass stenosis. (b) Superficial femoral artery occlusion with profunda femoris stenosis providing poor collateral circulation. Femoropopliteal graft used to bypass the occluded area into good 'run-off' below.

proximally and to the popliteal vessel distally. If no suitable vein is available, a prosthetic material (usually PTFE) may be used, with or without a small vein collar (Miller cuff) at its distal end (Fig. 53.20a). Suction drains are rarely necessary. Femorodistal bypass is usually carried out using the long saphenous vein in the *in situ* mode (Fig. 53.20b). For profundaplasty the common femoral artery and its branches are exposed and, after giving heparin and clamping the

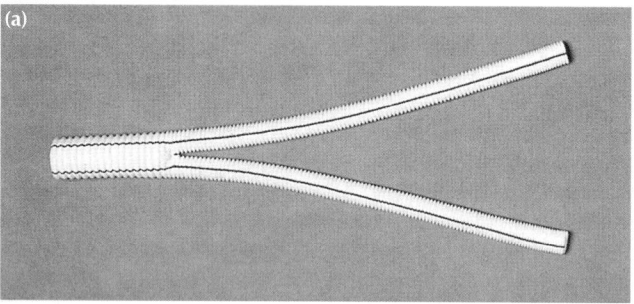

(a)

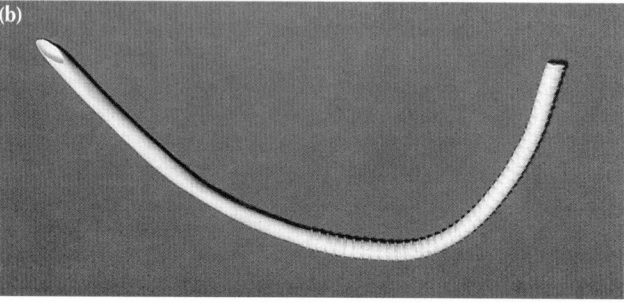

(b)

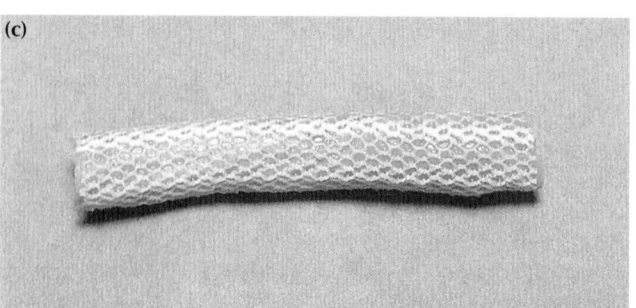

(c)

Figure 53.19 (a) Dacron bifurcation graft; (b) polytetrafluoroethylene graft; (c) human umbilical vein graft.

vessels in the usual way, an incision is made into the common femoral artery and carried down into the profunda, effectively dividing the stenotic profunda origin. The arteriotomy is then closed with a vein or prosthetic patch to widen the narrowed segment.

A femorofemoral crossover graft is useful for relieving an iliac artery occlusion when the other iliac artery is patent. A prosthetic graft is tunnelled subcutaneously above the pubis and anastomosed end-to-side to the common femoral arteries on each side. Blood from the patent iliac runs through the graft to the ischaemic limb. An axillofemoral graft is useful for salvaging a threatened limb in a poor-risk patient with bilateral iliac obstruction. A long prosthetic graft is tunnelled subcutaneously, from an end-to-side anastomosis with the axillary artery proximally, to reach the femoral artery of the involved limb in the groin where the distal anastomosis is made. The axillary artery will carry sufficient blood to maintain the circulation in both arm and leg. Short-term results are good; in these comorbid patients long-term patency is rarely important. An axillo-bifemoral bypass carries twice as much blood flow through its long limb as an axillo(uni)femoral bypass; the former is said to have a correspondingly improved patency rate. These axillary artery-based salvage operations should not be performed for intermittent claudication alone as limb loss may result if the operation fails.

Results of operation

Long-term results of aortoiliac reconstructive surgery are good, usually marred only by progressive infrainguinal disease. Femoropopliteal surgery is less successful. Immediate postoperative success for vein bypass exceeds 90% but many fail in the first 18 months after operation and, at the end of 5 years, the success rate is about 60%. PTFE bypass gives a poorer result than vein bypass, with 5-year success rates of less than 50%. Although the results of femorotibial bypass are even less satisfactory, such surgery can ensure limb salvage in patients who are generally debilitated and whose expected lifespan is limited; however, they are never appropriate for claudication.

Other sites of atheromatous occlusive disease

The principles of arterial surgery outlined above can be applied at other arterial sites. Carotid stenosis may cause transient ischaemic attacks (TIAs). These are recurrent and, by definition, short-lived mini-strokes. Resolution occurs within 24 hours (usually within minutes) but TIAs are a warning of impending major stroke. Patients should have a duplex scan and, if carotid occlusive disease of appropriate severity and at an appropriate site is confirmed (classically at the internal carotid artery origin) (Fig. 53.21), carotid endarterectomy should be offered. This involves clamping the vessels, an arteriotomy in the common carotid artery continued up into the internal carotid artery through the diseased segment, removal of the occlusive disease (endarterectomy) and closure of the arteriotomy, often with a patch. During clamping, some patients will have inadequate cerebral blood flow. Such a situation may be recognised by recording a low pressure in the distal internal carotid artery above the level of the clamp if general anaesthesia has been employed, or by a temporary neurological deficit if local anaesthesia has been used. It is necessary in such circumstances to insert a temporary silicone shunt over the arterial field being worked upon.

Subclavian artery stenosis may cause claudication in an arm or artery-to-artery embolisation, leading to digital ischaemia. It

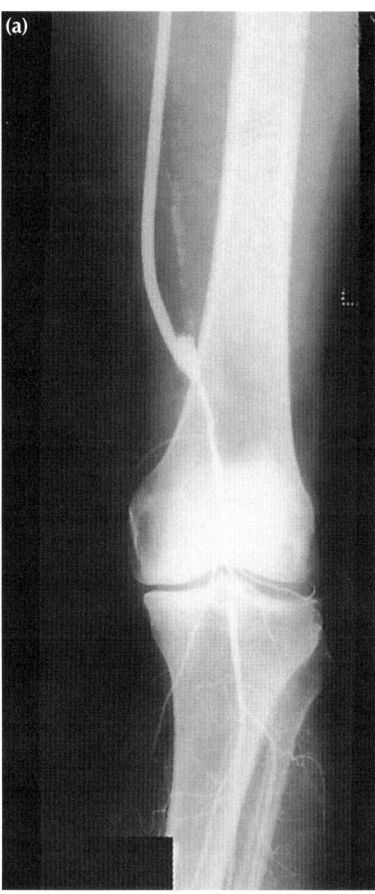 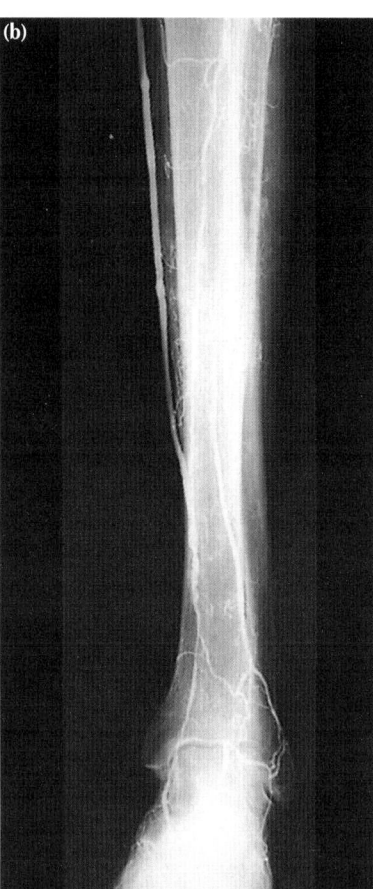

Figure 53.20 (a) Completion angiogram of femoro-popliteal bypass graft (with Miller cuff). (b) Completion angiogram of femorodistal bypass graft *in situ*.

may be treated by endarterectomy or bypass, but nowadays PTA is the treatment of choice. Sometimes subclavian artery lesions are associated with neck pathology, such as a cervical rib. Any underlying pathology must be corrected at the time of arterial repair. Subclavian steal syndrome may occur if it is the first part of the subclavian artery that is obstructed, with the vertebral artery providing a collateral circulation into the arm by reversing its direction of flow. This may cause periods of cerebral ischaemia. However, the classic syndrome of syncopal attack and visual disturbance associated with arm exercise and a diminished blood pressure in the affected limb is rare; asymptomatic reversal of flow in the vertebral artery is much more common. In symptomatic patients, PTA or operation is indicated.

Enteric artery occlusive disease may cause pain after eating that has no obvious diagnosis in a patient with known atheromatous disease and weight loss. In general, two of the three enteric vessels (coeliac axis, superior mesenteric artery, inferior mesenteric artery) must be occluded to produce 'intestinal claudication'. Great care must be taken to exclude all other diagnoses before contemplating PTA, endarterectomy or bypass.

Renal artery stenosis may cause hypertension and, eventually, loss of renal function. It is usually possible to control hypertension with drugs but, if renal failure seems likely, direct intervention is indicated. PTA is the method of choice, if feasible. Otherwise, a variety of operations are available (endarterectomy, aortorenal bypass, renal artery revascularisation using another vessel such as the splenic artery, renal autotransplantation).

ACUTE ARTERIAL OCCLUSION

Sudden occlusion of an artery is commonly caused by emboli. It may also happen when thrombosis occurs on a plaque of pre-existing atheroma, but in this case collaterals are likely to have built up in the face of chronic arterial stenosis, making the effect of the eventual occlusion less dramatic; such effects have been considered in the preceding section.

Embolic occlusion

An embolus is a body that is foreign to the bloodstream and which may become lodged in a vessel and cause obstruction. It is often a thrombus that has become detached from the heart or a more proximal vessel. Sources are the left atrium in cardiac arrhythmia (particularly atrial fibrillation) and a mural thrombus following myocardial infarction; less common sources are aneurysms and thrombi formed on atheromatous plaques (so called artery-to-artery embolism). Emboli may lodge in any organ and cause ischaemic symptoms.

- *Leg* – pain, pallor, paresis, pulselessness and paraesthesia (Fig. 53.22). Acute arterial occlusion due to an embolus differs from occlusion due to thrombosis on a pre-existing atheroma; in the latter case a collateral circulation has often built up over time (Figs 53.23 and 53.24). It is essential to differentiate between the two as they require different management.
- *Brain* – the middle cerebral artery (or its branches) is most commonly affected, resulting in major or minor (TIA) stroke.

CHAPTER 53 | ARTERIAL DISORDERS

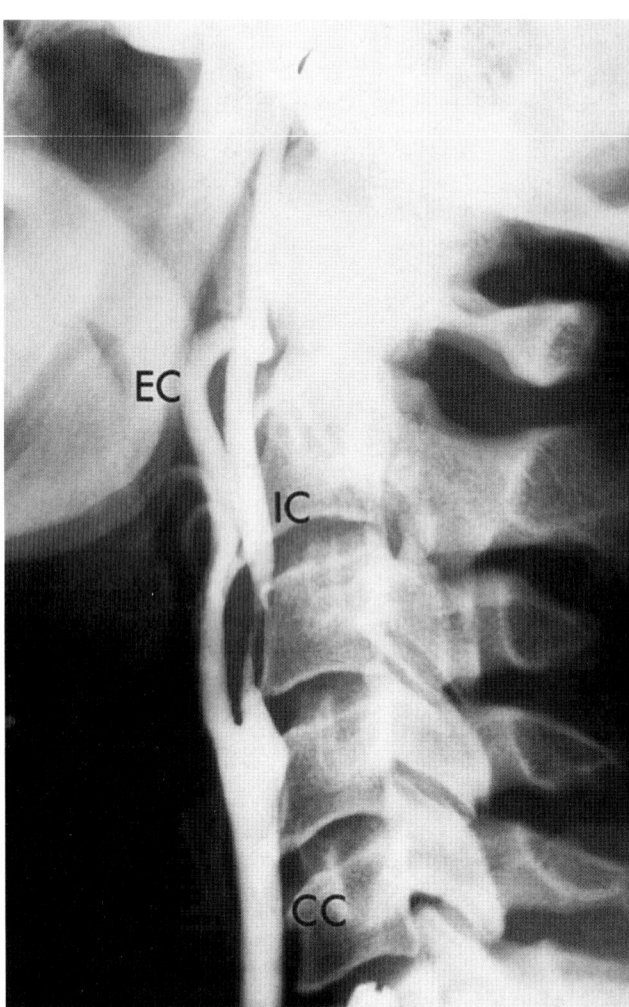

Figure 53.21 Carotid stenosis. A unilateral localised stenosis suitable for operation. CC, common carotid; EC, external carotid; IC, internal carotid.

- *Retina* – amaurosis fugax is fleeting blindness caused by a minute thrombus emanating from an atheromatous plaque in the carotid artery passing into the central retinal artery. Lasting obstruction causes permanent blindness.
- *Mesenteric vessels* – possible gangrene of the corresponding loop of intestine.
- *Spleen* – causing local pain.
- *Kidneys* – causing loin pain and haematuria.

Clinical features

Embolic arterial occlusion is an emergency that requires immediate treatment. The leg is often affected, with pain, pallor, paresis, loss of pulsation and paraesthesia (or anaesthesia) (see Fig. 53.22). The limb is cold and the toes cannot be moved, which contrasts with venous occlusion when muscle function is not affected. The diagnosis can be made clinically in a patient who has no history of claudication and has a source of emboli, who suddenly develops severe pain or numbness of the limb, which becomes cold and mottled. Movement becomes progressively more difficult and sensation is lost. Pulses are absent distally but the femoral pulse may be palpable, even thrusting, as distal occlusion results in forceful expansion of the artery with each pressure wave despite the lack of flow.

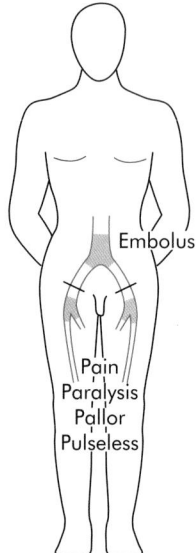

Figure 53.22 The symptoms and signs of embolism (four Ps). The fifth feature, anaesthesia, is often stated to be paraesthesia (the fifth P) but, in truth, complete loss of sensation in the toes and feet is characteristic.

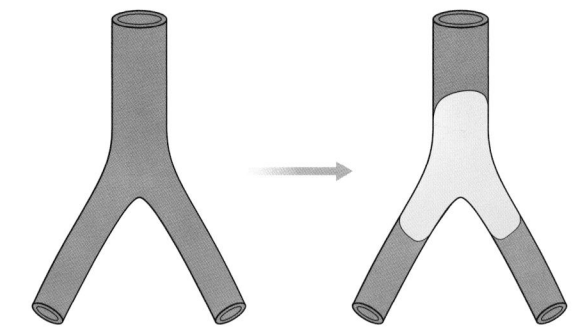

Figure 53.23 Aortic bifurcation embolus. Source of embolus is a recent myocardial infarct or atrial fibrillation. This causes severe, dramatic symptoms.

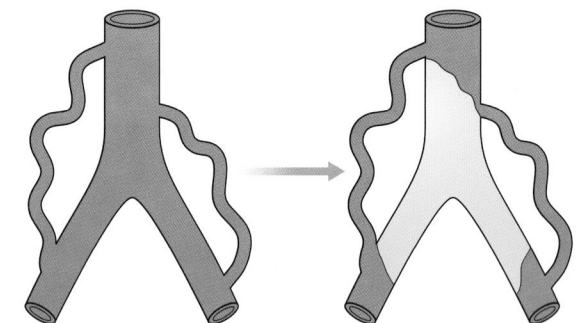

Figure 53.24 Aortic bifurcation thrombosis. No source of embolus but previous claudication. Claudication worse but no dramatic event.

Treatment

Because of the ensuing stasis, a thrombus can extend distally and proximally to the embolus. The immediate administration of 5000 U of heparin intravenously can reduce this extension and maintain patency of the surrounding (particularly the distal) vessels until the embolus can be treated. The relief of pain is essential because it is severe and constant. Embolectomy and thrombolysis are the treatments available for patients with limb emboli.

Embolectomy

Local or general anaesthesia may be used. The artery (usually the femoral), bulging with clot, is exposed and held in slings. Through a longitudinal or transverse incision the clot begins to extrude and is removed, together with the embolus (Fig. 53.25), with the help of a Fogarty balloon catheter. The catheter, with its balloon tip, is introduced both proximally and distally until it is deemed to have passed the limit of the clot. The balloon is inflated and the catheter withdrawn slowly, together with any obstructing material (Fig. 53.26). The procedure is repeated until bleeding occurs. Postoperatively, heparin therapy is continued until long-term anticoagulation with warfarin is established to reduce the chance of further embolism.

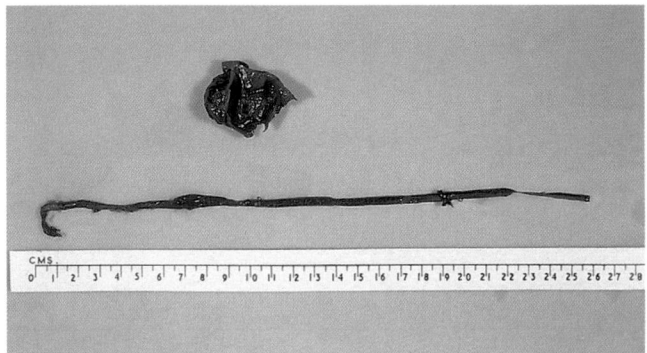

Figure 53.25 Embolic material removed from the common femoral artery, along with a long distal extension thrombus.

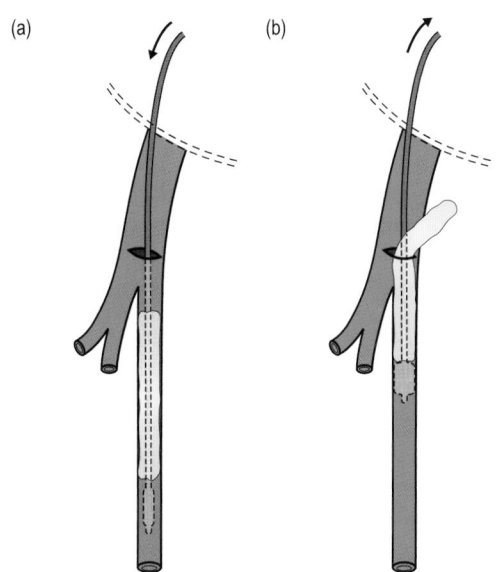

Figure 53.26 (a) A Fogarty catheter is inserted through an arteriotomy in the common femoral artery and fed distally down the superficial femoral artery and through the embolus. (b) The balloon is inflated and the catheter withdrawn, removing the embolus; the deep femoral and iliac arteries are similarly treated.

Thomas J. Fogarty, **Surgeon, University of Oregon Medical School, Portland, Oregon, USA.**

Compartment syndrome

In limbs that have been subject to sudden ischaemia followed by revascularisation, oedema is likely. Muscles swell within fixed fascial compartments and this can itself be a cause of ischaemia, with both local muscle necrosis and nerve damage due to pressure, and distal effects such as renal failure secondary to the liberation of myocyte breadown products. The treatment is urgent fasciotomy to release the compression. The usual site at which such surgery is necessary is the calf (especially the anterior tibial compartment), but compartment syndrome may occasionally affect the thigh and the arm.

Intra-arterial thrombolysis

If ischaemia is not so severe that immediate operation is essential, it may be possible to treat either embolus or thrombosis by intra-arterial thrombolysis (Fig. 53.27). At arteriography of the ischaemic limb (usually via the common femoral artery) a narrow catheter is passed into the occluded vessel and left embedded within the clot. Tissue plasminogen activator (TPA) is infused through the catheter and regular arteriograms are carried out to check on the extent of lysis, which, in successful cases, is achieved within 24 hours. The method should be abandoned if there is no progression of dissolution of clot with time. There are several contraindications to thrombolysis, the most important of which are recent stroke, bleeding diathesis and pregnancy, and results in those over 80 years old are poor.

Mesenteric artery occlusion

Acute mesenteric occlusion may be either thrombotic (following atheromatous narrowing) or embolic. Thrombotic occlusion follows progressive narrowing and so the symptoms also tend to be progressive with weight loss, abdominal pain (usually postprandial) and leucocytosis. Once the abdominal pain becomes severe, diarrhoea, systemic hypovolaemia and haemoconcentration occur. By this stage, the patient is ill out of proportion to the physical signs. Treatment is arteriography followed by percutaneous transluminal angioplasty or surgical bypass if the bowel has not already infarcted.

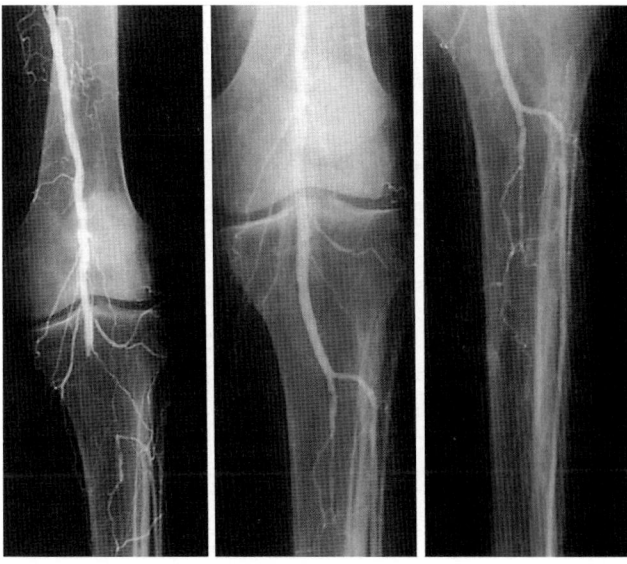

Figure 53.27 Angiogram of an occluded popliteal artery before thrombolysis (left), during successful lysis (middle) and after completion of lysis (right).

CHAPTER 53 | ARTERIAL DISORDERS

Embolic occlusion results in sudden, severe abdominal pain, with bowel emptying (vomiting and diarrhoea) and a source of emboli present (usually cardiac). Angiography and embolectomy, usually of the superior mesenteric artery, or bypass surgery can reduce the otherwise high mortality rate in these patients. A 'second look' laparotomy 24 hours later to check the viability of the bowel is often indicated.

Air embolism

Air may be accidentally injected into the venous circulation or sucked into an open vein. Venous air embolism is a rare complication of neck surgery if a large vein is inadvertently opened and it may be an accessory cause of death following a cut throat. Care should also be taken when infusing intravenous fluids, especially if a pressured system is used for rapid infusion, although a modern drip chamber with a plastic float should stop the injection when the fluid falls to a dangerously low level. If a large volume of air is allowed to reach the right side of the heart it may form an air lock within the pulmonary artery and cause right heart failure.

The treatment of air embolism is to put the patient in a head-down (Trendelenburg) position to encourage the air to enter the veins in the lower part of the body. The patient should also be placed on the left side to help the air to float to the ventricular apex, away from the ostium of the pulmonary artery. In extreme cases air may be aspirated from the heart through a needle introduced below the left costal margin. Oxygen should, of course, be administered.

Air may rarely enter the left side of the heart at open heart surgery or if a pulmonary vein is punctured when inducing a therapeutic pneumothorax. It may also enter via a patent foramen ovale (a common anomaly) as a paradoxical embolism. Air then may reach the coronary and/or the cerebral circulation. Treatment is along similar lines as for right heart air entry. Finally, air embolism may occur after fallopian tube insufflation or illegal abortion. Air may travel to the brain via the paravertebral veins.

Other forms of emboli

These include infective emboli of masses of bacteria or an infected clot, which may cause mycotic aneurysms, pyaemia or infected infarcts. Parasitic emboli, caused by the ova of *Taenia echinococcus* and *Filaria sanguinis hominis*, may occur in some countries; emboli of malignant cells (e.g. hypernephroma and cardiac myxoma) are rare but well recognised. Finally, fat embolism may follow major bony fractures. It is treated by the trauma or orthopaedic surgeon, rather than the vascular surgeon.

Therapeutic embolisation

This is used to arrest haemorrhage from the gastrointestinal, urinary (Fig. 53.28) and respiratory tracts, to treat arteriovenous malformations by blocking their arterial supply and to control the growth of unresectable tumours. Arterial embolisation requires accurate selective catheterisation using the Seldinger technique. A variety of materials may be used, including gelfoam sponge, plastic microspheres, balloons, ethyl alcohol, quick-setting plastics and metal coils.

Friedrich Trendelenburg, **1844–1924, Professor of Surgery successively at Rostock, Bonn and Leipzig, Germany.**
Gabrielle Falloppio (Fallopius), **1523–1563, Professor of Anatomy, Surgery and Botany, Padua, Italy,**

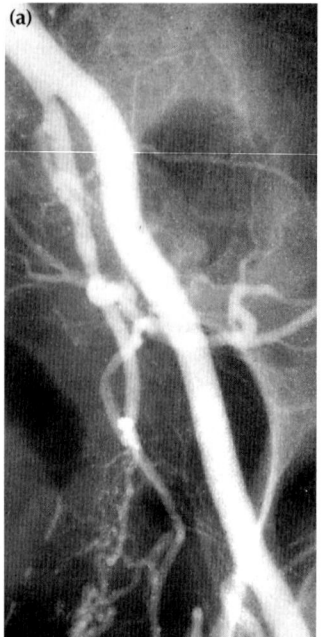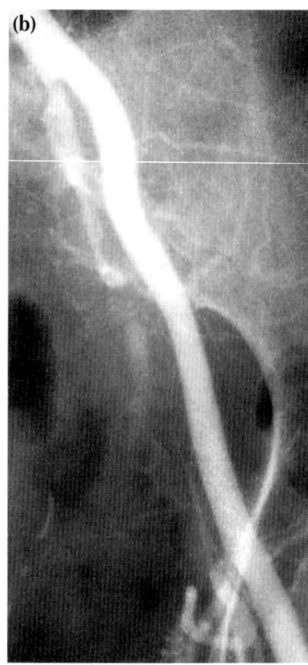

Figure 53.28 Before (a) and after (b) therapeutic embolisation of the internal iliac artery in a patient with gross haematuria from an ulcerating bladder carcinoma (courtesy of F. McIvor, FRCR, London, England).

GANGRENE

Gangrene implies death of macroscopic portions of tissue; the term necrosis may be used synonymously. It often affects the distal part of a limb because of arterial obstruction (from thrombosis, embolus or arteritis). This type of gangrene, which affects tissues that were initially sterile, must be distinguished from those forms of gangrene that derive mainly from infection (classically gas gangrene), although both may coexist.

Clinical features

A gangrenous part lacks arterial pulsation, venous return, capillary response to pressure, sensation, warmth and function. The colour of the part changes through a variety of shades according to circumstances (pallor, dusky grey, mottled, purple) until finally taking on the characteristic dark-brown, greenish-black or black appearance, which is caused by the disintegration of haemoglobin and the formation of iron sulphide.

Dry gangrene occurs when the tissues are desiccated by gradual slowing of the bloodstream; it is typically the result of atheromatous occlusion of arteries. The affected part becomes dry and wrinkled, discoloured from disintegration of haemoglobin, and greasy to the touch. Moist gangrene occurs when infection and putrefaction are present; the affected part becomes swollen and discoloured and the epidermis may be raised in blebs. Crepitus may be palpated as a result of infection by gas-forming organisms. This situation is quite common in the feet of diabetics.

Separation of gangrene

A zone of demarcation between the truly viable and the dead or dying tissue will eventually appear. Separation is achieved by the development of a layer of granulation tissue, which forms between the dead and the living parts. In dry gangrene, if the blood supply of the proximal tissues is adequate, the final line of demarcation appears in a matter of days and separation occurs neatly and with the minimum of infection (so called separation by aseptic ulceration). If bone is involved, complete separation takes longer than when soft tissues alone are affected, and the stump tends to be conical as the bone has a better blood supply than its coverings.

In moist gangrene there is significant infection and suppuration extends into the neighbouring living tissue, thereby causing the final line of demarcation to be more proximal than in dry gangrene (separation by septic ulceration). This is why dry gangrene must be kept as dry and aseptic as possible, and why every effort should be made to convert moist gangrene into the dry type.

Sometimes in gangrene from atheroma or embolism the line of final demarcation is very slow to form or does not develop. Unless the arterial supply to the living tissues can be improved, the gangrene will spread to adjacent tissues or will suddenly appear as 'skip' areas further up the limb. Skip lesions should always be carefully sought; black patches appear, perhaps on the other side of the foot, on the heel, on the dorsum of the foot or even in the calf. Infection may also cause gangrene to spread proximally into areas of extensive inflammation. To attempt local amputation in the phase of vague demarcation is to court failure, as gangrene reappears in the skin flaps.

Treatment of gangrene

The surgeon is generally concerned with how much of a limb or digit can be salvaged and this depends on the blood supply proximal to the gangrene. Sometimes this can be improved by radiological or surgical intervention. A good blood supply may allow a conservative excision or distal amputation, avoiding a major ablation, but a proximal life-saving amputation is required for rapidly spreading symptomatic gangrene and gas gangrene.

Sometimes, especially with digits, amputation can be avoided. Conservative treatment involves keeping the affected part absolutely dry. Exposure to the air and the use of a fan may assist in the desiccation process and may relieve pain. The limb must not be heated. Local pressure areas, e.g. the skin of the heel or the malleoli, must be protected if fresh patches of gangrene are not to occur in these places. Padded rings, foam blocks and air beds are useful preventative aids. Occasionally, the lifting of a crust or the removal of hard or desiccated skin helps demarcation or releases pus and relieves pain.

Specific varieties of gangrene

Diabetic gangrene

Diabetic gangrene is related to three factors: trophic changes from peripheral neuropathy, ischaemia as a result of atheroma, and low resistance to infection because of excess sugar in the tissues (Fig. 53.29). The neuropathy impairs sensation and thus favours the neglect of minor injuries and infections. Motor involvement is frequently accompanied by loss of reflexes and deformities (neuropathic joints). Thick callosities develop on the sole and amateur chiropody may allow the entry of infection. Whatever the portal, any infection can spread proximally with speed in subfascial planes in diabetic patients. Palpable dorsalis pedis and posterior tibial pulses, and the absence of rest pain and intermittent claudication, may signify that there is no associated major arterial disease. Bacteriological examination is made of any pus and a radiograph may reveal the extent of any osteitis.

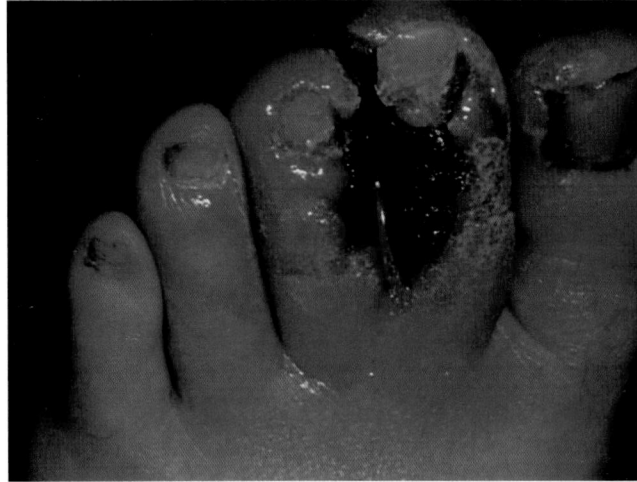

Figure 53.29 Diabetic gangrene.

Treatment consists of bringing the diabetes under control by diet and drugs. The gangrene is treated as described above, with a conservative approach if there is no major arterial obstruction. A rapid spread of infection requires drainage by incision and the removal of any obviously dead tissue. This may require quite extensive laying open of infected tissue planes. Good drainage and the control of infection should be followed by rapid healing if the blood supply is adequate.

Bedsores

A bedsore is gangrene caused by local pressure (Fig. 53.30). Bedsores are predisposed to by five factors: pressure, injury, anaemia, malnutrition and moisture. They can appear and extend rapidly in immobile patients and in those with debilitating illness. Prophylactic measures must be taken, including the avoidance of pressure over bony prominences by the use of foam blocks or similar, regular turning, and nursing on specially designed beds that reduce the pressure to the skin. A water bed or a ripple bed is sometimes desirable. Injury from wrinkled sheets and maceration of the skin by sweat, urine or pus must be prevented by skilled nursing and the use of an adhesive film dressing.

A bedsore can be expected if erythema appears that does not

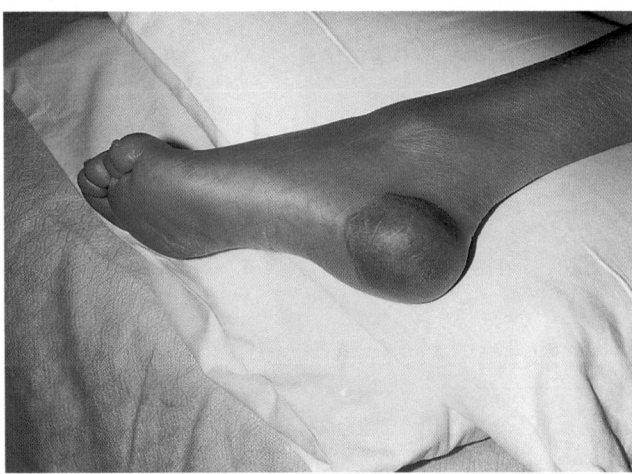

Figure 53.30 Bedsores typically appear over areas exposed to pressure, such as the sacrum and (as in this case) the heel.

change colour on pressure. The affected area must be kept dry and an aerosol silicone spray may be used. Once pressure sores develop, they are difficult to heal. They may be treated by lotions or by exposure to keep them as dry as possible. They should be kept clean and debrided if necessary. Advice from a plastic surgeon should be sought for major lesions; rotation flaps can be effective.

Drug abuse

Inadvertent arterial injection of drugs has become common in many countries with significant numbers of drug addicts. Usually, the femoral artery in the groin is involved and presentation is with pain and mottling distally in the leg. All pulses down to ankle level are generally retained but, if not, imaging and intra-arterial thrombolysis may be considered. If pulses are present, dextran and heparin may be given to help what is a microvascular pathology, but there is no firm evidence of their efficacy in this condition. Fortunately, most cases resolve and progression to gangrene is rare. It should be remembered that many of these patients carry the human immunodeficiency virus and/or various hepatitis viruses.

Frostbite

Frostbite is caused by exposure to cold. It is seen both in climbers at high altitudes and in the elderly or the vagrant during cold, windy spells (Fig. 53.31). Vessel walls are damaged, leading to transudation and oedema. The sufferer experiences a severe burning pain in the affected part, which later assumes a waxy appearance as the pain disappears. Blistering and then gangrene follow. Frostbitten parts must be warmed gradually; any temperature higher than that of the body is detrimental. The part should be wrapped in cotton wool and kept at rest. Friction, e.g. rubbing with snow, may damage already devitalised tissues. Warm drinks and clothing should be provided and powerful analgesics given to relieve the pain that heralds the return of circulation. Amputations should be conservative.

Ainhum

Ainhum (Fig. 53.32) is a disease of unknown aetiology that usually affects black men (and occasionally women) who have run barefoot in childhood. It is recorded in central Africa, central America and the Orient. A fissure appears at the level of the interphalangeal joint of a toe, usually of the little toe. The fissure is followed by a fibrous band that encircles the digit and causes necrosis. The treatment in the early stage is by Z-plasty and in the later stages by amputation.

Ergot

Ergot is a cause of gangrene in those who eat rye bread infected with *Claviceps purpurea*. Certain groups living on the Mediterranean coast or the Russian steppes are particularly at risk. It may also occur in migraine sufferers who take ergot preparations as prophylaxis over a long period (Fig. 53.33).

Venous gangrene

Although deep vein thrombosis is common, venous gangrene is surprisingly rare. It occurs when the circulation of a limb (usually the leg) is disrupted by overwhelming outflow obstruction and this requires massive deep vein thrombosis at a proximal site. Treatment in those at risk is by full anticoagulation with heparin and effective elevation of the swollen leg, preferably with the head and trunk level or even lowered. It is all too common to see futile

CHAPTER 53 | ARTERIAL DISORDERS

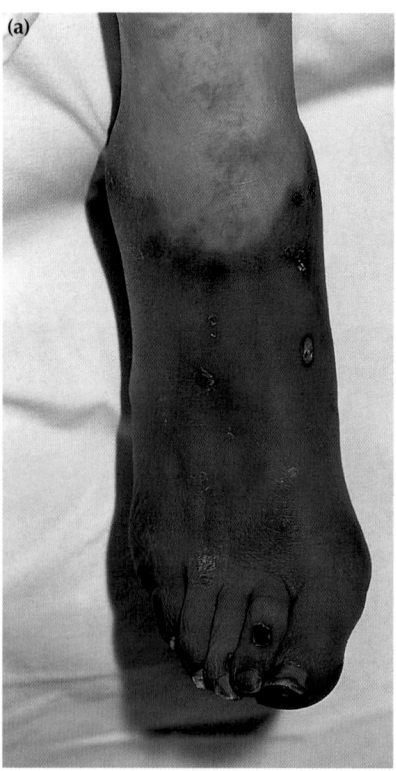

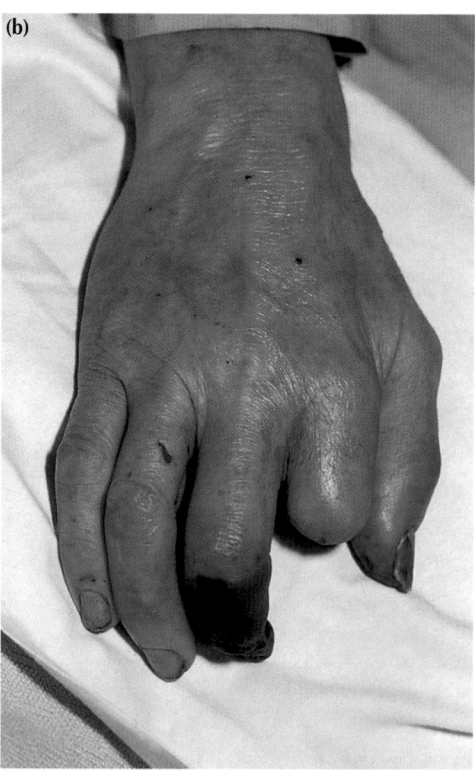

Figure 53.31 (a) Frostbite of the foot. Note the clear demarcation. (b) Frostbite of the middle finger in the same patient. The index finger was lost 2 years before, also from frostbite.

Airhum is the name given to the condition by the Yoruba people of Nigeria.

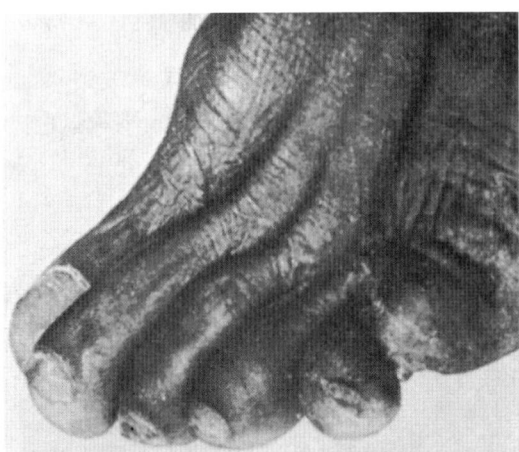

Figure 53.32 Ainhum (courtesy of Dennis Morrissey, FRCS, Birmingham).

attempts at treatment with the body in a 'jack-knife' position. This form of management prevents progression to gangrene in most cases. Systemic lytic therapy (e.g. with TPA) has not proved successful for the condition but some would advocate venous thrombectomy in extreme circumstances using a Fogarty catheter.

AMPUTATION

General

Amputation should be considered when part of a limb is dead, deadly or a dead loss. A limb is dead when arterial occlusive disease is severe enough to cause infarction of macroscopic portions of tissue, i.e. gangrene. The occlusion may be in major vessels (atherosclerotic or embolic occlusions) or in small peripheral vessels (diabetes, Buerger's disease, Raynaud's disease, inadvertent intra-arterial injection). If the obstruction cannot be reversed and the symptoms are severe, amputation is required.

A limb is deadly when the putrefaction and infection of moist gangrene spreads to surrounding viable tissues. Cellulitis and severe toxaemia are the result. Amputation is required as a life-

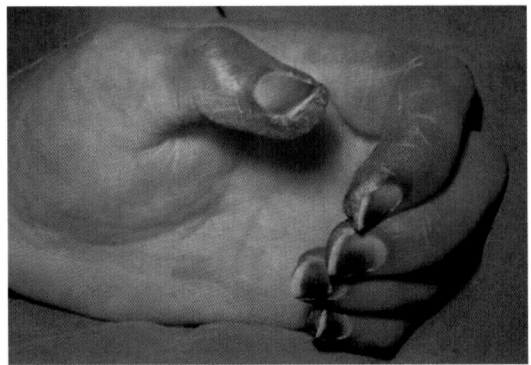

Figure 53.33 Gangrene due to ergot. The patient had taken repeated doses of ergotamine tartrate for 'migraine' while on a transatlantic flight.

Leo Buerger, 1879–1943, Professor of Urologic Surgery, New York Polyclinic Medical School, New York, USA, described thromboangitis obliterans in 1908.
Maurice Raynaud, 1834–1881, Physician, Hospital Lariboisiere, Paris, France, described this condition in 1862.

saving operation. Antibiotic cover should be broad and massive. Other life-threatening situations for which amputation may be required include gas gangrene (as opposed to simple infection), neoplasm (such as osteogenic sarcoma) and arteriovenous fistula.

A limb may be deemed a dead loss in the following circumstances: first, when there is relentless severe rest pain without gangrene – amputation will improve quality of life; second, when a contracture or paralysis makes the limb impossible to use and renders it a hindrance; and third, when there is major unrecoverable traumatic damage (Summary box 53.2).

Summary box 53.2

Indications for amputation

Dead limb
- Gangrene

Deadly limb
- Wet gangrene
- Spreading cellulitis
- Arteriovenous fistula
- Other (e.g. malignancy)

'Dead loss' limb
- Severe rest pain
- Paralysis
- Other (e.g. contracture, trauma)

Distal and transmetatarsal amputation

In patients with small-vessel disease, typically caused by diabetes, gangrene of the toes may occur with relatively good blood supply to the surrounding tissues. In such circumstances local amputation of the digits can result in healing. However, if the metatarsophalangeal joint region is involved, a ray excision is required, taking part of the metatarsal and cutting tendons back. The wound should not be sutured but loosely packed with gauze soaked in an antiseptic solution such as povidone iodine. Early mobility aids drainage provided that cellulitis is not present. For less extensive gangrene, if amputation is taken through a joint, healing is improved by removing the cartilage from the joint surface.

A transmetatarsal amputation can be used in circumstances similar to those meriting distal amputation, when several toes are affected and irreversible ischaemia has extended to the forefoot. A viable long plantar flap is essential for this operation to heal successfully (Fig. 53.34).

Major amputation

Preoperative preparation

The patient should, whenever possible, be given time to come to terms with the inevitability of amputation. Ideally, once the alternatives of a painful useless limb or a painless useful (artificial) one are explained, the patient will make the final decision. In gangrene of the foot, especially with 'skip' areas, this is the time for explanation of, and consent for, above-knee amputation should an attempt at below-knee section prove inadvisable on account of inadequate blood supply to the flaps. If there is time, the nutritional status of the patient should be optimised; certainly any anaemia should be corrected. Antibiotics should be given as required and especially immediately before operation to prevent clostridial infection.

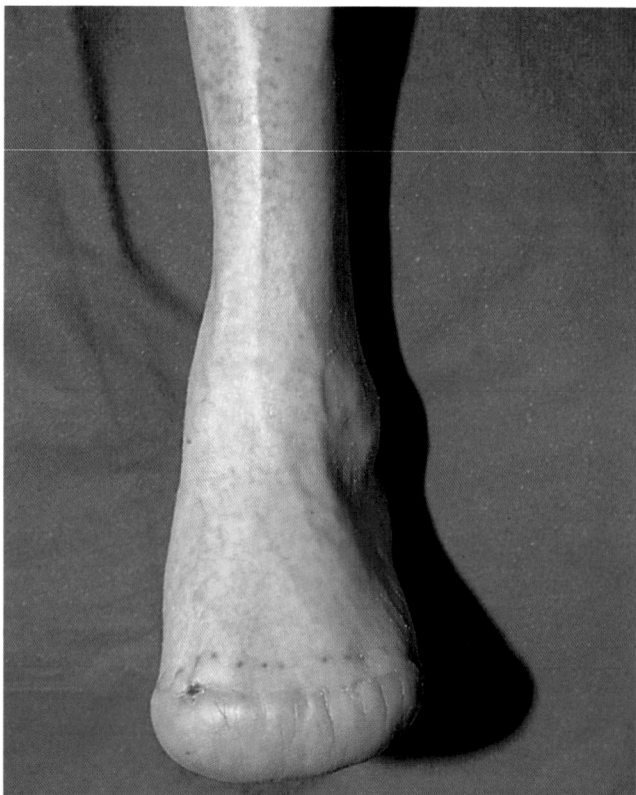

Figure 53.34 Transmetatarsal amputation for diabetic gangrene of the toes.

Choice of operation (Fig. 53.35)

Where good limb-fitting facilities exist, above- or below-knee amputations are preferable because the best cosmetic and functional results can be obtained with the resulting cone-bearing amputation stumps. If limb-fitting facilities are limited, however, an end-bearing amputation may be preferable (Syme's, through-knee, Gritti–Stokes) so that simple prostheses (peg leg or simple boot) can be used. Syme amputations are not suitable for severely ischaemic atheromatous limbs because of the poor healing of the heel flap.

For above- or below-knee amputations with a good stump shape, it is possible to hold a prosthesis in place simply by suction, without any cumbersome and unsightly straps. The stump should be of sufficient length to give the required leverage, i.e. not less than 8 cm below the knee (preferably 10–12 cm) and not less than 20 cm above the knee. There should be room for the artificial joint, i.e. the stump must not be too long; ideally 12 cm proximal to the knee joint above the knee and 8 cm proximal to the ankle joint below the knee are needed for the mechanism. A below-knee amputation is much better than an above-knee amputation in terms of eventual mobility. Every attempt should be made to preserve the knee joint if the extent of ischaemia allows.

James Syme, **1799–1871, Regius Professor of Clinical Surgery, University of Edinburgh, Scotland.**
Rocco Gritti, **1828–1920, Surgeon, Milan, Italy, described this operation in 1857.**
Sir William Stokes, **1839–1900, Surgeon, Dublin, Ireland, described his modification of Gritti's operation in 1870.**

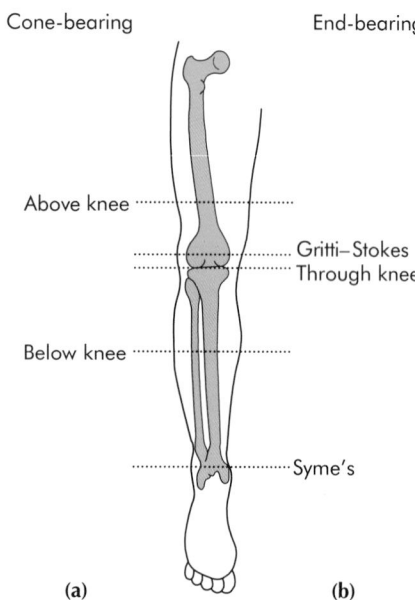

Figure 53.35 Choice of site: (a) cone-bearing and (b) end-bearing amputations.

Below-knee amputations

Two types of skin flap are commonly used: long posterior flap and skew flap. Skew flaps were described by K.P. Robinson. Whichever method is chosen, the total length of flap must be at least one and a half times the diameter of the leg at the point of bone section.

The long posterior flap amputation, although the older method, remains the more popular, probably because of its relative simplicity (Fig. 53.36). Anteriorly, the incision is deepened to bone and the lateral and posterior incisions are fashioned to leave the bulk of the gastrocnemius muscle attached to the flap, muscle and skin being transected together at the same level. If bleeding is inadequate, the amputation is refashioned at a higher level. Blood vessels are identified and ligated. Nerves are not clamped but pulled down gently and transected as high as possible. Vessels in nerves are ligated. The fibula is divided 2 cm proximal to the level of tibial division using bone cutters. The tibia is cleared and transected at the desired level, the anterior aspect of the bone being sawn obliquely before the cross-cut is made. This, with filing, gives a smooth anterior bevel, which prevents pressure necrosis of the flap. The long muscle/skin flap is tapered after removing the bulk of the soleus muscle (much of the gastrocnemius may be left unless it is very bulky). The area is washed with saline to remove bone fragments and the muscle and fascia are sutured with an absorbable material to bring the flap over the bone ends. A suction drain is placed deep to the muscle and brought out through a stab incision in the skin. The skin flap should lie in place with all tension taken by the deep sutures. Interrupted skin sutures are inserted. Gauze, wool and crepe bandages generally make up the stump dressing, although some surgeons prefer a rigid (plaster) dressing system.

The skew flap amputation makes use of anatomical knowledge of the skin blood supply. Equally long flaps are developed; they

Kingsley Peter Robinson, **formerly Surgeon, the Westminster Hospital, London, UK.**

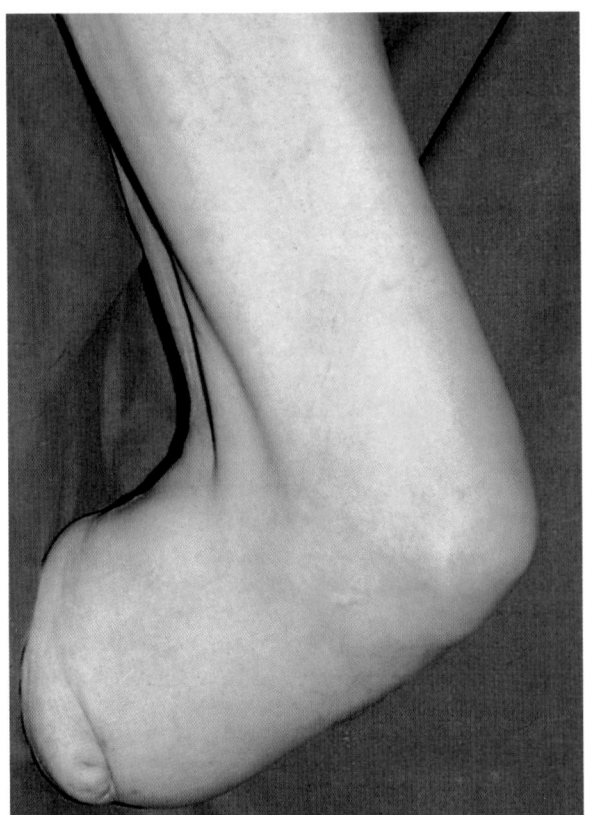

Figure 53.36 Classic long posterior flap type of below-knee amputation.

join anteriorly 2.5 cm from the tibial crest, overlying the anterior tibial compartment, and posteriorly at the exact opposite point on the circumference of the leg. After division of bone and muscle in a fashion similar to that described above, the gastrocnemius flap is sutured over the cut bone end to the anterior tibial periosteum with absorbable sutures. Finally, drainage and skin sutures are inserted and the limb dressed as for the long posterior flap operation.

Above-knee amputation

The site is chosen as indicated above but may need to be higher if bleeding is poor on incision of the skin. Equal curved anterior and posterior skin flaps are made of sufficient total length. Skin, deep fascia and muscle are transected in the same line. Vessels are ligated. The sciatic nerve is pulled down and transected cleanly as high as possible and the accompanying artery ligated. Muscle and skin are retracted and the bone cleared and sawn at the point chosen. Haemostasis is achieved. The muscle ends are united over the bone by absorbable sutures incorporating the fascia. A suction drain deep to the muscle is brought out through the skin clear of the wound. The fascia and subcutaneous tissues are further brought together so that the skin can be apposed by interrupted sutures. Gauze, wool and crepe bandages form the stump dressing.

Gritti–Stokes, through-knee and Syme's amputations

These are rarely carried out nowadays. For the femoral level Gritti–Stokes amputation, the section is transcondylar. Through-knee amputation is technically less complex. In Syme's amputation it is essential to preserve the blood supply to the heel flap by meticulous clean dissection of the calcaneus. The tibia and fibula are sectioned as low as possible to the top of the mortice joint. This type of procedure is rarely applicable in patients with occlusive vascular disease.

Postoperative care of an amputee

Opiate pain relief should be given regularly. Care of the good limb must not be forgotten as a pressure ulcer on the remaining foot will delay mobilisation, despite satisfactory healing of the stump. Exercise and mobilisation are of the greatest importance. After surgery, flexion deformity can be prevented by the use of a cloth placed over the stump with sand bags on each side to weight it down. Once the drain has been removed, exercises are started to build up muscle power and coordination. Daily stump bandaging in an attempt to mould the shape of the stump is now obsolete. Mobility is progressively increased with walking between bars and the use of an inflatable artificial limb, which allows weight-bearing to be started before a pylon or temporary artificial limb is ready (Fig. 53.37). This whole episode in the patient's life should be conducted in a positive manner through the various stages towards full independence. Early assessment of the home is part of the programme; it allows time for minor alterations, such as the addition of stair rails, movement of furniture to give support near doors and provision of clearance in confined passages.

Complications

Early complications include haemorrhage, which requires return to the operating room for haemostasis, haematoma, which requires evacuation, and infection, usually in association with a haematoma. Any abscess must be drained and appropriate antibiotics given. Gas gangrene can occur in a mid-thigh stump from faecal contamination. Wound dehiscence and gangrene of the flaps are caused by ischaemia; a higher amputation may well be

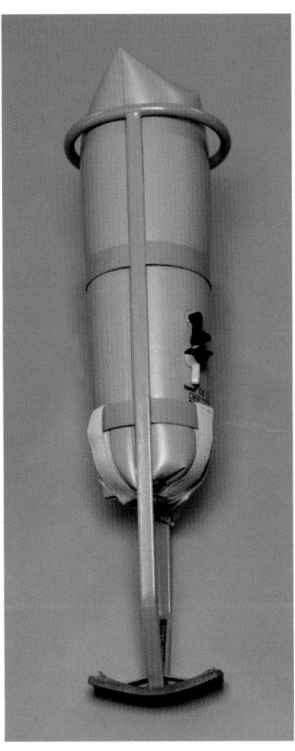

Figure 53.37 Inflatable artificial limb.

necessary. Amputees are at risk of deep vein thrombosis and pulmonary embolism in the early postoperative period and prophylaxis with subcutaneous heparin is essential for several weeks after operation.

Later complications include pain resulting from unresolved infection (sinus, osteitis, sequestrum), a bone spur, a scar adherent to bone and an amputation neuroma. Patients frequently remark that they can feel the amputated limb (phantom limb) and sometimes remark that it is painful (phantom pain). The surgeon's attitude should be one of firm reassurance that this sensation will almost certainly disappear with time; amitriptyline or gabapentin may help. Other late complications include ulceration of the stump because of pressure effects of the prosthesis or increased ischaemia.

ANEURYSM

General

Dilatations of localised segments of the arterial system are called aneurysms. They can either be true aneurysms, containing the three layers of the arterial wall (intima, media, adventitia) in the aneurysm sac, or false aneurysms, having a single layer of fibrous tissue as the wall of the sac, e.g. aneurysm following trauma. Aneurysms can also be grouped according to their shape (fusiform, saccular, dissecting) or their aetiology (atheromatous, traumatic, syphilitic, mycotic, etc.). The term mycotic is a misnomer because, although it indicates infection as a causal element in the formation of the aneurysm, this is due to bacteria, not fungi. Aneurysms occur all over the body in major vessels, including the aorta, and the iliac, femoral, popliteal, subclavian, axillary and carotid arteries. They may also occur in cerebral, mesenteric, splenic and renal arteries and their branches. The majority are true fusiform atherosclerotic aneurysms (Summary box 53.3).

Summary box 53.3

Classification of aneurysms

Wall
- True (three layers: intima, media, adventitia)
- False (single layer of fibrous tissue)

Morphology
- Fusiform
- Saccular
- Dissecting

Aetiology
- Atheromatous
- Mycotic (bacterial rather than fungal)
- Collagen disease
- Traumatic

Clinical features

All aneurysms can cause symptoms, as a result of expansion, thrombosis, rupture or the release of emboli. The symptoms relate to the vessel affected and the tissues it supplies. Most aneurysms of clinical significance can be palpated and, typically, an expansile pulsation is felt. Transmitted pulsation through a mass lesion, cyst or abscess lying adjacent to a large artery may be mistaken for aneurysmal pulsation. Before incising a swelling believed to be an abscess it is essential to make sure that it does not pulsate. Finally, a tortuous (and often ectatic) artery, usually the innominate or carotid, may seem like an aneurysm to the inexperienced clinician.

Abdominal aortic aneurysm

Abdominal aortic aneurysm is by far the commonest type of large vessel aneurysm and is found in 2% of the population at autopsy; 95% have associated atheromatous degeneration and 95% occur below the renal arteries. Symptomatic aneurysms may cause minor symptoms, such as back and abdominal discomfort, before sudden, severe back and/or abdominal pain develops from expansion and rupture. Asymptomatic aneurysms are found incidentally on physical examination, radiography or ultrasound investigation.

Ruptured abdominal aortic aneurysm

Abdominal aortic aneurysms can rupture anteriorly into the peritoneal cavity (20%) or posterolaterally into the retroperitoneal space (80%). Less than 50% of patients with rupture survive to reach hospital. Anterior rupture results in free bleeding into the peritoneal cavity; very few patients reach hospital alive. Posterior rupture on the other hand produces a retroperitoneal haematoma (Fig. 53.38). Often a brief period ensues when a combination of moderate hypotension and the resistance of the retroperitoneal tissues arrests further haemorrhage. The patient may remain conscious but in severe pain. If no operation is performed, death is virtually inevitable. Operation results in a better than 50% survival rate.

To achieve the best results, diagnosis and treatment must be rapid. A tender, pulsatile mass is usually palpable in the abdomen of a hypotensive patient. If there is doubt about the presence of an aneurysm an ultrasonogram may help, but this test is not of use to detect rupture. If there is doubt about rupture a CT scan is of more help, but it is still far from being foolproof. In practice, most diagnoses are reached on clinical grounds alone, without imaging.

Good venous access is needed for infusion of saline or volume-expanding fluids, but the systolic blood pressure should not be raised any more than is necessary to maintain consciousness and permit cardiac perfusion (< 100 mmHg). Elevation into the normotensive range may provoke further uncontrolled haemorrhage. A urinary catheter is passed. If the patient appears stable, surgery may be delayed until cross-matched blood is ready but the patient should still be transferred immediately to the operating room so that the procedure can commence immediately if haemodynamic instability develops. Always remember that the treatment of ruptured aneurysm is operation, not monitoring and resuscitation (Summary box 53.4).

Summary box 53.4

Management of ruptured abdominal aortic aneurysm

- Early diagnosis (abdominal/back pain, pulsatile mass, shock)
- Immediate resuscitation (oxygen, intravenous replacement therapy, central line)
- Maintain systolic pressure, but not > 100 mmHg
- Urinary catheter
- Cross-match six units of blood
- Rapid transfer to the operating room

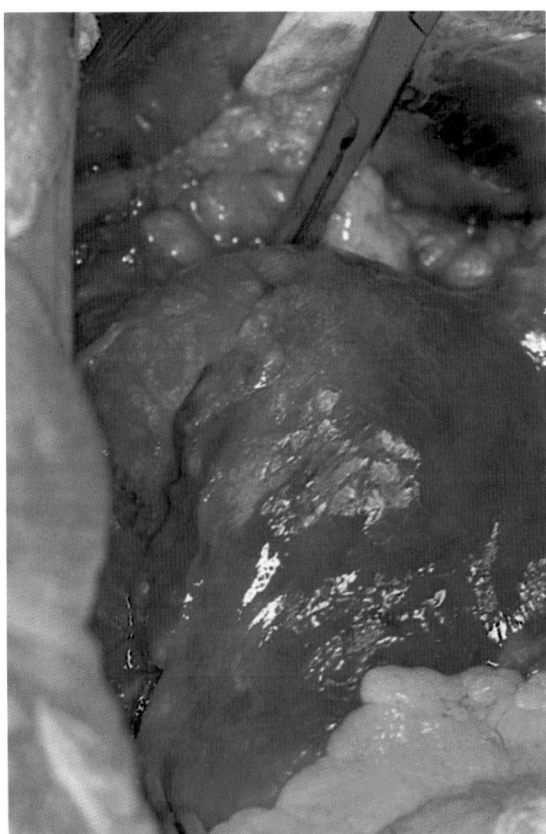

Figure 53.38 The retroperitoneal haematoma of a ruptured aortic aneurysm. The aortic pulsation is palpated through the haematoma at its upper limit and fingers are insinuated on each side of the aorta. With finger control, the upper clamp is positioned and closed on the aorta. The procedure is then as for a planned case. In this illustration, the clamp is at the proximal end of the aneurysm; the haematoma has spread from the left paracolic gutter to encircle the aneurysm and the aortic bifurcation.

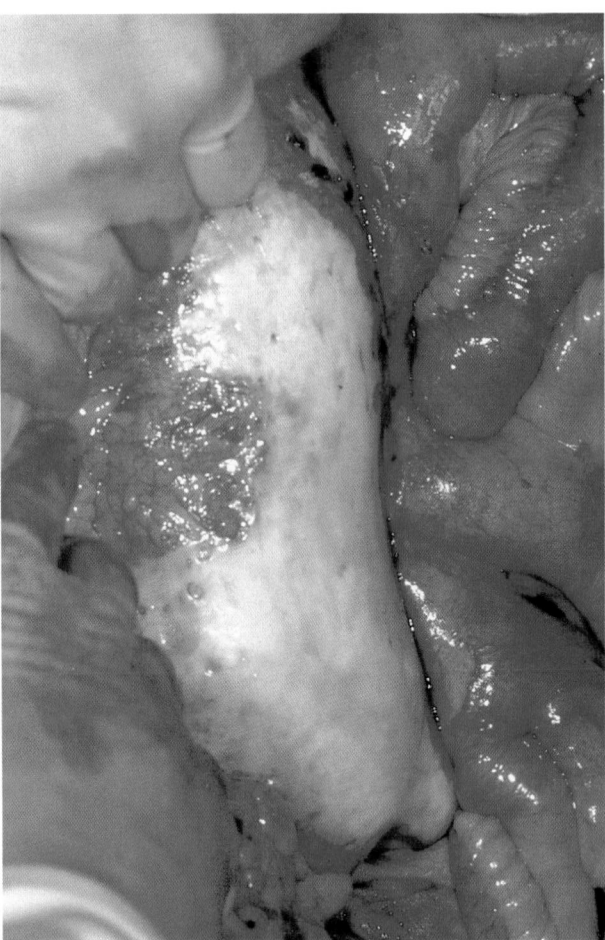

Figure 53.39 An inflammatory abdominal aortic aneurysm. Note the white 'icing' effect. Such lesions can be technically difficult to manage.

Symptomatic abdominal aortic aneurysm

Patients most commonly present with back and/or abdominal discomfort. Pain may also occur in the thigh and groin because of nerve compression. Gastrointestinal, urinary and venous symptoms can also be caused by pressure from an abdominal aneurysm. About 3% of all aneurysms cause pain as a result of inflammation of the aneurysm itself (Fig. 53.39). Finally, a few cause symptoms from distal embolisation of fragments of their intraluminal thrombus. It is said that without surgery, 80% of those with a symptomatic aneurysm will be dead in a year; with surgery, 80% will be alive. Therefore, an operation is indicated in patients who are otherwise reasonably fit. The risk of operation is particularly increased in the presence of hypertension, chronic airway disease, recent myocardial infarction and impaired renal function. Chronological age is not a bar to surgery but only a few patients are fit enough for this type of procedure once over the age of 80.

Asymptomatic abdominal aortic aneurysm

An aneurysm found incidentally on clinical examination, radiography or ultrasonography (Fig. 53.40) in an otherwise fit patient should be considered for repair if > 55 mm in diameter (measured by ultrasonography). The annual incidence of rupture rises from 1% or less in aneurysms that are < 55 mm in diameter to a significant level, perhaps as high as 20%, in those that are 70 mm in diameter. Assuming elective surgery carries a 5% mortality rate, the balance is in favour of elective operation once the diameter is > 55 mm, provided there is no major comorbidity. Regular ultrasonographic assessment is indicated for asymptomatic aneurysms < 55 mm in diameter (Summary box 53.5).

Summary box 53.5

Abdominal aortic aneurysm: indications for operation

Asymptomatic
- Aneurysm > 55 mm in anteroposterior diameter
- Patient fit for surgery (expected mortality rate < 5%)
- Indications for endoluminal operation are the same as for open operation

Symptomatic
- Aneurysm of any size that is painful or tender
- Aneurysm of any size that is causing distal embolisation
- Indications are wider than for an asymptomatic lesion (expected mortality rate 5–20%)

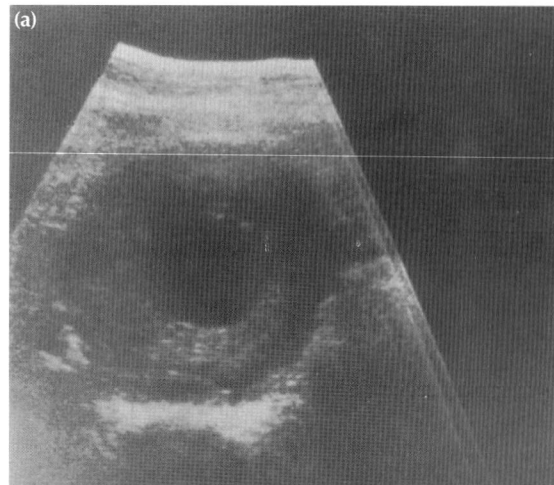

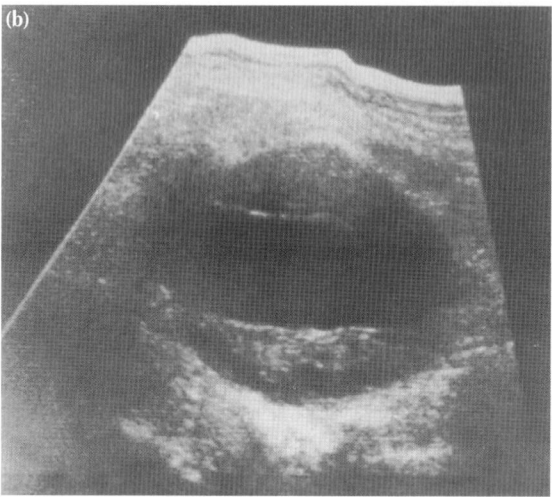

Figure 53.40 Ultrasonogram of an aortic aneurysm showing the large clot-filled sac with a small central lumen (transverse and longitudinal scans).

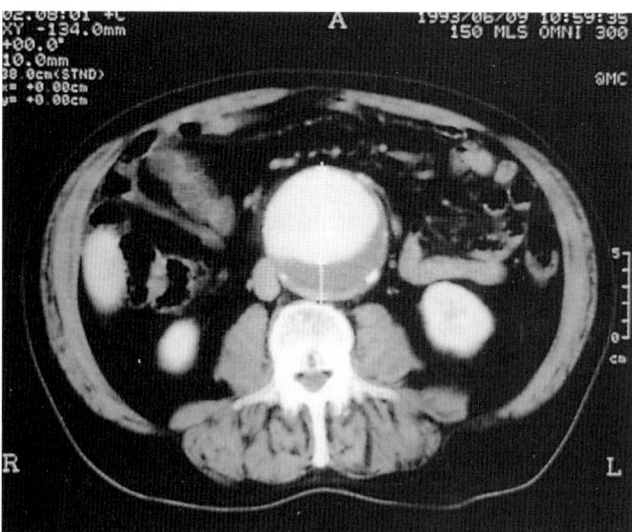

Figure 53.41 Computerised tomogram of the abdomen showing an aortic aneurysm. Blood flowing through the thrombus-containing sac is enhanced with contrast agent and appears white.

Investigations

Full blood count, electrolytes, liver function tests, coagulation tests and blood lipid estimation are carried out, with a cross-match if surgery is contemplated within a few days. Electrocardiography and cardiac assessment by echocardiography or isotope ventriculography are useful. Chest radiography and pulmonary function tests should also be carried out.

The morphology of the aneurysm is best assessed by CT scan (Figs 53.41 and 53.42) or magnetic resonance imaging. Although a digital subtraction or magnetic resonance angiogram may be useful in delineating any associated arterial occlusive

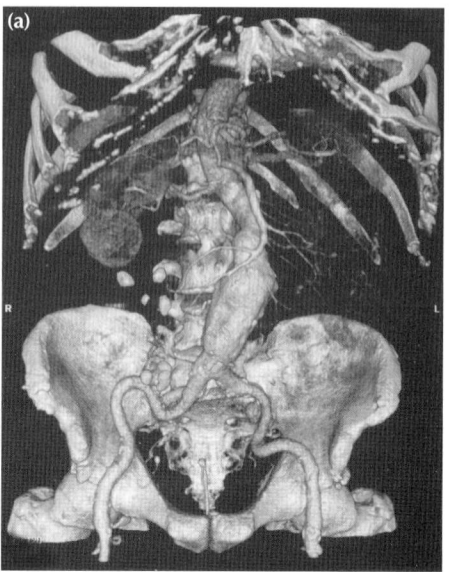

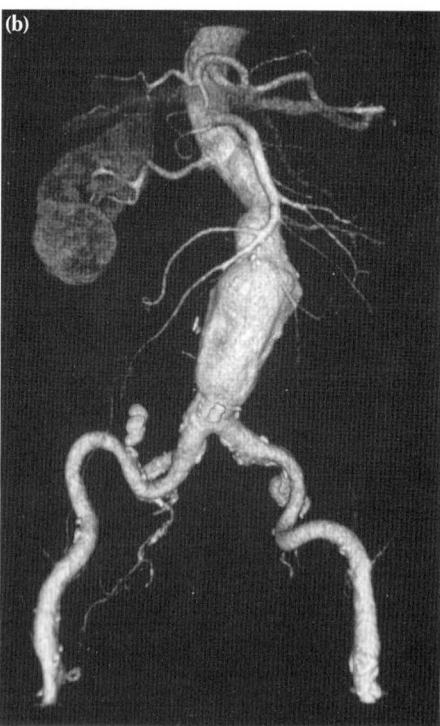

Figure 53.42 (a) Spiral computerised tomogram showing an infrarenal abdominal aortic aneurysm; (b) with the bony elements subtracted.

disease (Fig. 53.43), it should be appreciated that this does not permit an assessment of aneurysm diameter because the sac is usually filled with circumferential clot leading to a falsely narrow angiographic appearance (Fig. 53.44).

Open surgical procedure

Under general anaesthesia, with the patient lying supine, a full-length midline or supra-umbilical transverse incision is made. The small bowel is lifted to the patient's right and the aorta identified. The posterior peritoneum overlying the aorta is opened and the upper limit of the aneurysm identified. The aorta immediately above the dilatation is exposed; this is generally just inferior to the left renal vein and renal arteries (Fig. 53.45). The common iliac arteries are then exposed, heparin given and clamps applied above and below the lesion. The aneurysm is opened longitudinally and back-bleeding from lumbar and mesenteric vessels controlled by sutures placed from within the

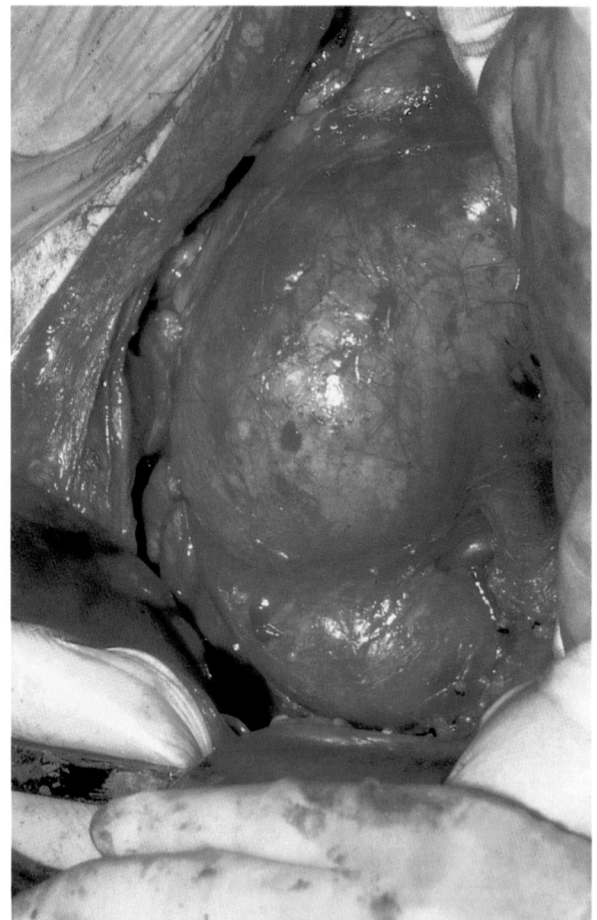

Figure 53.45 Operative appearance of a huge, non-ruptured infrarenal abdominal aortic aneurysm.

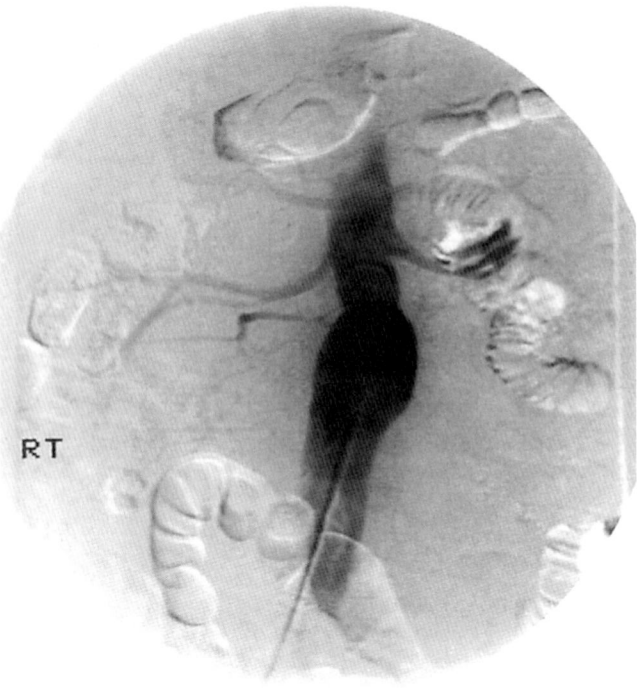

Figure 53.43 Angiogram of an abdominal aortic aneurysm. The neck of the aneurysm is inferior to the renal arteries.

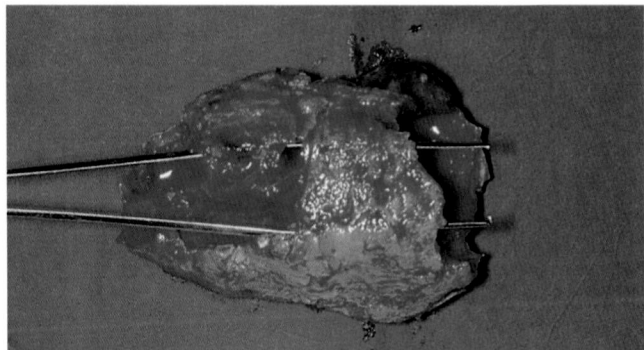

Figure 53.44 Thrombus removed from an abdominal aortic aneurysm; this thrombus is the reason an angiogram may give a false impression of aneurysm diameter.

sac. Upper and lower aortic necks are prepared to which an aortic prosthesis is then sutured end to end inside the sac with a monofilament non-absorbable suture (Fig. 53.46). Clamps are released slowly to prevent sudden hypotension. If haemostasis is satisfactory at this point, the aneurysm sac is closed round the prosthesis (Fig. 53.47) to exclude both it and the suture lines from the bowel to reduce the risk of adherence and potential fistula formation. The abdomen is then closed. Occasionally, when the iliac vessels are also involved with dilatation or severe atheroma, it is necessary to construct an aorto-bi-iliac or aorto-bifemoral bypass, rather than use a simple aorto-aortic tube.

Endoluminal procedure

This has gained in popularity over the last decade and most centres now routinely offer this minimally invasive treatment to elderly patients with suitable aortic morphology, generally on an elective or semi-elective basis. The aorta is accessed via the common femoral arteries, which are exposed surgically. Under radiological control, a delivery system is guided up into the aorta and an endovascular prosthesis (often termed a 'stent graft') placed within the aortic sac. The prosthesis is made from Dacron or PTFE with an integral metallic stent for support and to allow firm attachment to the vessels above and below the sac; most are modular, one part being an aortic body with one iliac attached and the other a separate single iliac stent graft. The larger component

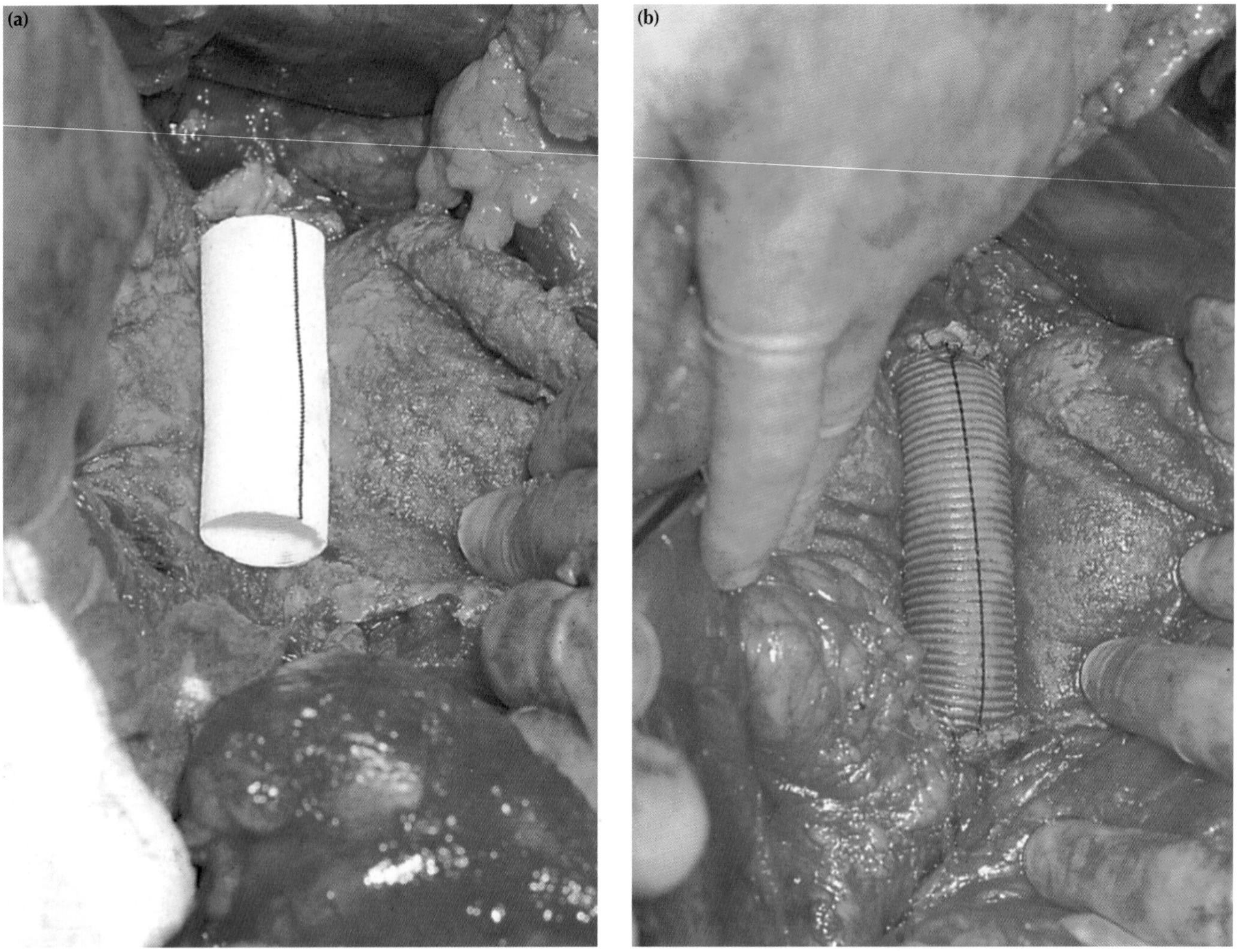

(a)

(b)

Figure 53.46 (a) Aneurysm sac opened. Note that the posterior wall of the aorta immediately above and below the sac is not divided. A Dacron tube graft is laid in place within the sac ready for suture. (b) Graft sutured in place and vascular clamps removed.

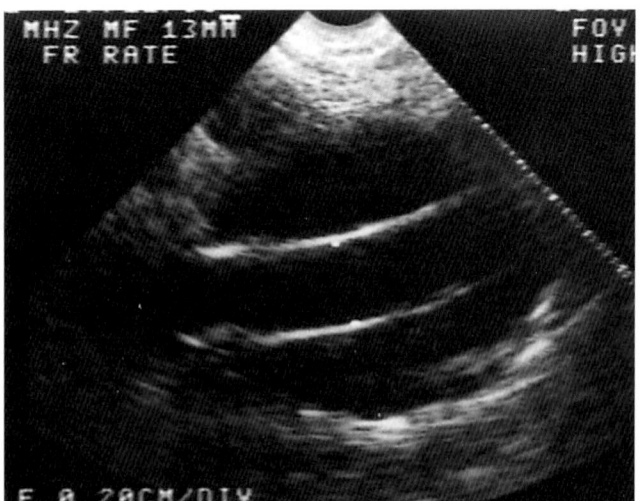

Figure 53.47 Aortic graft. Transverse scan showing the graft in the dilated aortic bed.

is inserted via one groin and the other via the opposite groin. Such modular stent-graft systems must be able to produce a blood-tight seal at the uppermost (infrarenal aortic) level of the graft, at both iliac levels distally and at the junction between the aorto-uni-iliac stent-graft module and its contralateral iliac partner. Although this technique has now been used in many thousands of patients worldwide, concerns remain about prosthetic fragmentation with the passage of time, displacement and leakage (endoleak) at the interface of vessel and stent graft or from patent lumbar arteries. These concerns mean that all patients require lifelong follow-up and regular imaging (Fig. 53.48), and there is a tendency to offer the endoluminal procedure to the older patient whose need for long-term prosthetic integrity is less.

Postoperative complications

The most common complications after open repair are respiratory (lower lobe consolidation, atelectasis and 'shock lung') and cardiac (ischaemia and infarction). A degree of colonic ischaemia because of lack of a collateral blood supply occurs in about 10% of patients but fortunately this usually resolves spontaneously.

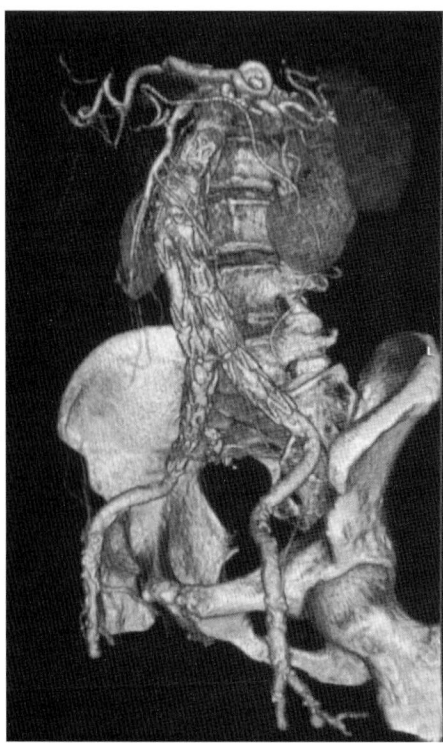

Figure 53.48 Spiral computerised tomogram showing an endoluminal aortoiliac 'stent graft'. The metallic stent structure is clearly observed.

Renal failure and infection of the graft are rare events after elective procedures but they may complicate procedures undertaken for rupture. Neurological complications include sexual dysfunction and spinal cord ischaemia. An aortoduodenal fistula is an uncommon but treatable complication of abdominal aortic replacement surgery. It should be suspected whenever haematemesis or melaena occurs in the months or years after operation. Prosthetic infection also occurs uncommonly and may require removal of the graft, limb revascularisation being achieved by simultaneous insertion of an axillo-bifemoral bypass.

Cardiac, respiratory, renal and neurological complications occur less often with the endovascular method but they are not obviated entirely by this minimally invasive technique. In the longer term, fistula and prosthetic infection remain rare but significant problems. Although the immediate mortality and morbidity rates of this method are less than those associated with open surgery, about 20% of patients need a secondary procedure to correct endoleaks or prosthetic migration, thrombosis or rupture.

Peripheral aneurysm

Popliteal aneurysm

Popliteal artery aneurysm accounts for 70% of all peripheral aneurysms; two-thirds are bilateral. Examination of the abdominal aorta is indicated if a popliteal aneurysm is found because one-third are accompanied by aortic dilatation. Popliteal aneurysms present as a swelling behind the knee or with symptoms caused by complications, such as severe ischaemia following thrombosis or distal ischaemic ulceration as a result of emboli. Urgent surgery, possibly with intra-arterial thrombolysis, is indicated in the acute situation. An asymptomatic aneurysm should be considered for elective repair to prevent future complications,

especially if it exceeds 25 mm in diameter. Ultrasonography and CT or magnetic resonance imaging can be helpful in confirming the diagnosis. Treatment is either a bypass with ligation of the aneurysm or an inlay graft.

Femoral aneurysm

True aneurysm of the femoral artery is uncommon. Complications occur in less than 3% so conservative treatment is generally indicated, but it is important to look for aneurysms elsewhere as over half are associated with abdominal or popliteal aneurysms. False aneurysm of the femoral artery occurs in 2% of patients after arterial surgery at this site. Some are infective in origin and rupture is possible; these require surgical correction. Local repair with reanastomosis at the groin under suitable antibiotic cover may be successful, but bypass, clear of the infected area, with subsequent excision of the infected graft is often the only way of preventing further problems.

Iliac aneurysm

This usually occurs in conjunction with aortic aneurysm and only rarely on its own. On its own, it is difficult to diagnose clinically so about half present already ruptured. Operation is indicated, with bypass and exclusion of the aneurysm by ligation above and below the dilatation.

Arteriovenous fistula

Communication between an artery and a vein (or veins) may be either a congenital malformation or the result of trauma. Arteriovenous fistulas for haemodialysis access are also created surgically. All arteriovenous communications have a structural and a physiological effect. The structural effect of arterial blood flow on the veins is characteristic; they become dilated, tortuous and thick walled (arterialised). The physiological effect, if the fistula is big enough, is an increase in cardiac output. In extreme circumstances this can cause left ventricular enlargement and even cardiac failure.

A pulsatile swelling may be present if the lesion is superficial. A thrill is detected on palpation and auscultation reveals a buzzing continuous bruit ('machinery murmur'). Dilated veins may be seen, in which there is a rapid blood flow. Pressure on the artery proximal to the fistula reduces the swelling and the thrill and bruit cease.

Duplex scan and/or angiography confirms the lesion, which is noteworthy for the speed with which venous filling occurs.

Management

Treatment is by embolisation. Excisional surgery can be advocated only rarely, perhaps for severe deformity or recurrent haemorrhage; the assistance of a plastic surgeon is wise. It is important to realise that ligation of a 'feeding' artery on its own is of no lasting value and is actually detrimental as it may preclude treatment by embolisation.

ARTERITIS AND VASOSPASTIC CONDITIONS

Thromboangiitis obliterans (Buerger's disease)

This is characterised by occlusive disease of the small- and medium-sized arteries (plantar, tibial, radial, etc.), thrombophlebitis of the superficial or deep veins, and Raynaud's syndrome; it occurs in male smokers, usually under the age of 30 years. Often, only one or two of the three manifestations are present. Histologically, there are inflammatory changes in the walls of arteries and veins, leading to thrombosis. Treatment is total abstinence from smoking, which arrests, but does not reverse, the disease. Established arterial occlusions are treated as for atheromatous disease, but amputations may eventually be required.

Other types of arteritis

Arteritis occurs in association with many connective tissue disorders, e.g. rheumatoid arthritis, systemic lupus erythematosus and polyarteritis nodosa. This is usually the province of the specialist physician but the surgeon may be called on to carry out minor amputations. Sympathectomy has previously been used but this is no longer advocated in this context.

Temporal arteritis is a disease in which localised infiltration with inflammatory and giant cells leads to arterial occlusion, ischaemic headache and tender, palpable, pulseless (thrombosed) arteries in the scalp. Irreversible blindness occurs if the ophthalmic artery becomes occluded. The surgeon may be required to perform a temporal artery biopsy, but this should not delay immediate steroid therapy to arrest and reverse the process before the ophthalmic artery is involved.

Takayasu's disease is an arteritis that obstructs major arteries, particularly the large vessels coming off the aorta. It usually pursues a relentless course.

Cystic myxomatous degeneration

This is typified by an accumulation of clear jelly (like a synovial ganglion) in the outer layers of a main artery, especially the popliteal artery. The lesion may narrow the vessel causing claudication. Duplex scan is the investigation of choice. Decompression, by removal of the myxomatous material, is often all that is required, but the 'ganglion' may recur, necessitating excision of part of the artery with interposition vein graft repair.

Raynaud's disease

This idiopathic condition usually occurs in young women and affects the hands more than the feet. There is abnormal sensitivity in the arteriolar response to cold. These vessels constrict and the digits (usually the fingers) turn white and become incapable of fine movements. The capillaries then dilate and fill with slowly flowing deoxygenated blood, resulting in the digits becoming swollen and dusky. As the attack passes off, the arterioles relax, oxygenated blood returns into the dilated capillaries and the digits become red. Thus, the condition is recognised by the characteristic sequence of blanching, dusky cyanosis and red engorgement, often accompanied by pain. Superficial necrosis is very uncommon. This condition must be distinguished from Raynaud's syndrome, which has similar features (see below). Treatment of Raynaud's disease consists of protection from cold and avoidance of pulp and nailbed infection. Calcium antagonists, such as nifedipine, may also have a role to play and electrically heated gloves can be useful in winter. Sympathectomy has been discredited in this condition.

Raynaud's syndrome

Although peripheral vasospasm may be noted in atherosclerosis, thoracic outlet syndrome, carpal tunnel syndrome, etc., the term

Raynaud's syndrome is most often used for a peripheral arterial manifestation of a collagen disease such as systemic lupus erythematosus or rheumatoid arthritis. The clinical features are as for Raynaud's disease but they may be much more aggressive. Raynaud's syndrome may also follow the use of vibrating tools. In this context it is a recognised industrial disease and is known as 'vibration white finger'.

Treatment is directed primarily at the underlying condition, although the conservative measures outlined above are often helpful. The syndrome when secondary to collagen disease leads frequently to necrosis of digits and multiple amputations. Sympathectomy yields disappointing results and should not be used. Nifedipine, steroids and vasospastic antagonists may all have a role in treatment. Patients with vibration white finger should avoid vibrating tools.

Acrocyanosis

Acrocyanosis may be confused with Raynaud's disease but it is painless and not episodic. It tends to affect young women and the mottled cyanosis of the fingers and/or toes may be accompanied by paraesthesia and chilblains.

Cervicodorsal sympathectomy

Open cervicodorsal sympathectomy was previously performed for vasospastic conditions affecting the hands and to treat palmar (sometimes axillary) hyperhidrosis. The operation is now obsolete, having been replaced by endoscopic transthoracic sympathectomy. Furthermore, it has been increasingly recognised that the vasospastic conditions do not respond to this form of treatment, rendering the endoscopic intervention a therapy that is suitable solely for hyperhidrosis.

An endoscope, often a rigid cystoscope, is used. The ipsilateral lung may be deflated by the anaesthetist and a cannula inserted into the chest wall to permit easy access for the scope. The sympathetic chain is visualised and a coagulating electrode used to ablate the ganglia below the stellate. The scope and cannula are then removed, the lung inflated and the small chest would closed.

Lumbar sympathectomy

Lumbar sympathectomy has been used to treat chronic lower limb ischaemia in the past. Lumbar sympathectomy by open operation has, however, been obsolete for several years and even chemical sympathectomy, its minimally invasive equivalent, can now be regarded as outdated. Chemical sympathectomy requires the injection of small quantities of dilute aqueous phenol into the lumbar sympathetic chain under radiographic control.

FURTHER READING

Ascher, E. and Haimovici, H. (eds) (2003) *Haimovici's Vascular Surgery*, 5th edn. Blackwell Publishing, Oxford.

Davies, A.H., Brophy, C.M. and Lumley, J. (eds) (2005) *Vascular Surgery*. Springer, Philadelphia, PA.

Moore, W.S. (ed.) (2005) *Vascular and Endovascular Surgery: A Comprehensive Review*, 7th edn. W.B. Saunders, Philadelphia, PA.

Ouriel, K. and Rutherford, W.B. (eds) (1998) *Atlas of Vascular Surgery: Operative Procedures*. W.B. Saunders, Philadelphia, PA.

Rutherford, R.B. (ed.) (2005) *Vascular Surgery*, 6th edn. W.B. Saunders, Philadelphia, PA.

Mikito Takayasu, **1860–1938, Japanese ophthalmologist, described this disease in 1908.**

Venous disorders

LEARNING OBJECTIVES

To understand:
- Venous anatomy and the physiology of venous return
- The pathophysiology of venous disease

- The clinical significance of varicose veins
- Deep venous thrombosis
- Venous insufficiency and venous ulceration

INTRODUCTION

The lower limb is the most common site of venous disorders. More than 5% of the population have varicose veins and 1% have, or have had, venous ulceration. At any one time, up to 200 000 people in the UK have active venous ulceration.

THE ANATOMY OF THE VENOUS SYSTEM OF THE LIMBS

Arterial blood flows through the main axial arteries of the upper and lower limbs before returning via the deep and superficial veins. All of the veins of the upper and lower limbs contain valves, which ensure that blood flows towards the heart.

The superficial venous trunks in the leg are the greater and lesser saphenous veins (Fig. 52.1a and b), which lie above the muscle fascia of the limb. The cephalic and basilic veins are the superficial venous trunks of the arm (Fig. 54.1c and d). The greater saphenous vein joins the femoral vein at a fixed point in the groin 2.5 cm below and lateral to the pubic tubercle, and the lesser saphenous vein terminates at a variable site in the popliteal fossa. Blood passing up the superficial veins enters the deep veins at the saphenopopliteal and saphenofemoral junctions.

In the calf and thigh there are a number of valved perforating (communicating) veins that join the superficial to the deep veins at inconstant sites and which allow blood to flow from the superficial to the deep venous system. The most important of these are the direct perforating veins of the medial and lateral calf and the communicating veins around the knee and in the mid-thigh.

The deep veins of the lower limb arise from three pairs of venae commitantes, which accompany the three crural arteries (anterior and posterior tibial and peroneal arteries). These six veins intercommunicate and join in the popliteal fossa to form the popliteal vein, which also receives the soleal and gastrocnemius veins.

The popliteal vein passes up through the adductor hiatus to enter the subsartorial canal as the femoral vein, which receives the deep (profunda) femoral vein (or veins) in the femoral triangle before passing behind the inguinal ligament to become the external iliac vein. The internal iliac vein joins with the external iliac vein in the pelvis to form the common iliac vein. The left common iliac vein passes behind the right common iliac artery to join the right common iliac vein on the right side of the abdominal aorta to form the inferior vena cava.

VENOUS PATHOPHYSIOLOGY

Blood enters the limb through the femoral arteries before passing through arterioles into the capillaries, which have a pressure of about 32 mmHg at their arterial ends. This pressure is reduced along the course of the capillaries and is approximately 12 mmHg at the venular end of the capillary.

The pressure continues to fall in the main veins and is as low as −5 mmHg at the upper end of the vena cava where it enters the right atrium.

The venous pressure in a foot vein on standing is equivalent to the height of a column of blood extending from the heart to the foot, e.g. approximately 100 mmHg (Fig. 54.2). To enable blood to be returned against gravity in the standing position an auxillary pump is required in the lower limb. This is the calf muscle pump, which is augmented to a lesser extent by the thigh and foot pumps. The deep veins of the calf are capacious and are joined by blind-ending sacks called the soleal sinusoids, which force blood into the popliteal and crural veins during calf muscle pump contraction, e.g. walking. The foot pump also ejects blood from the plantar veins during walking. As the calf muscles contract, the veins are compressed and the valves only allow blood to pass in the direction of the heart. The pressure within the calf compartment rises to 200–300 mmHg during muscle contraction. During muscle relaxation the pressure falls and blood from the superficial veins enters the deep veins through the saphenous junctions and the perforating veins. Each time this occurs the pressure falls in the superficial venous compartment until a threshold is reached, when the venous inflow keeps pace with ejection from the deep veins. This is normally around 30 mmHg, a fall of approximately two-thirds of the resting pressure. The reduction in the pressure of the superficial system is dependent on the presence of patent deep veins, perforating

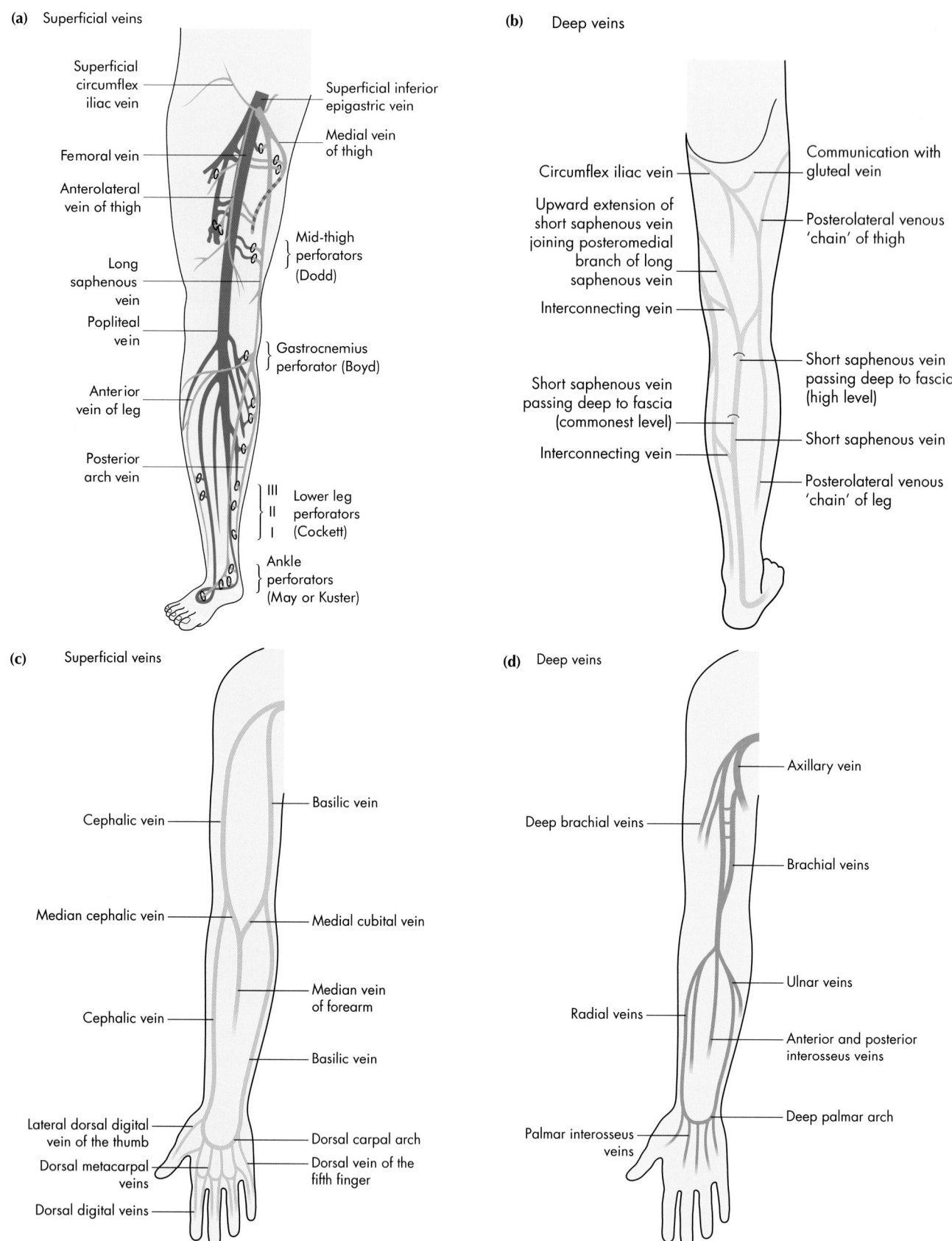

(a) Superficial veins

Superficial circumflex iliac vein

Superficial inferior epigastric vein

Medial vein of thigh

Femoral vein

Anterolateral vein of thigh

Long saphenous vein

Popliteal vein

Mid-thigh perforators (Dodd)

Anterior vein of leg

Gastrocnemius perforator (Boyd)

Posterior arch vein

III
II
I
Lower leg perforators (Cockett)

Ankle perforators (May or Kuster)

(b) Deep veins

Circumflex iliac vein

Communication with gluteal vein

Upward extension of short saphenous vein joining posteromedial branch of long saphenous vein

Posterolateral venous 'chain' of thigh

Interconnecting vein

Short saphenous vein passing deep to fascia (high level)

Short saphenous vein passing deep to fascia (commonest level)

Short saphenous vein

Interconnecting vein

Posterolateral venous 'chain' of leg

(c) Superficial veins

Cephalic vein

Basilic vein

Median cephalic vein

Medial cubital vein

Median vein of forearm

Cephalic vein

Basilic vein

Lateral dorsal digital vein of the thumb

Dorsal carpal arch

Dorsal metacarpal veins

Dorsal vein of the fifth finger

Dorsal digital veins

(d) Deep veins

Axillary vein

Deep brachial veins

Brachial veins

Radial veins

Ulnar veins

Anterior and posterior interosseus veins

Palmar interosseus veins

Deep palmar arch

Figure 54.1 (a and b) Anatomy of the superficial and deep veins of the lower limb. (c and d) Anatomy of the superficial and deep veins of the upper limb. (d) The principal deep veins of the lower limb. The innumerable branch veins and those lying within muscle are omitted. The tibial and peroneal veins are usually paired veins uniting in their upper parts.

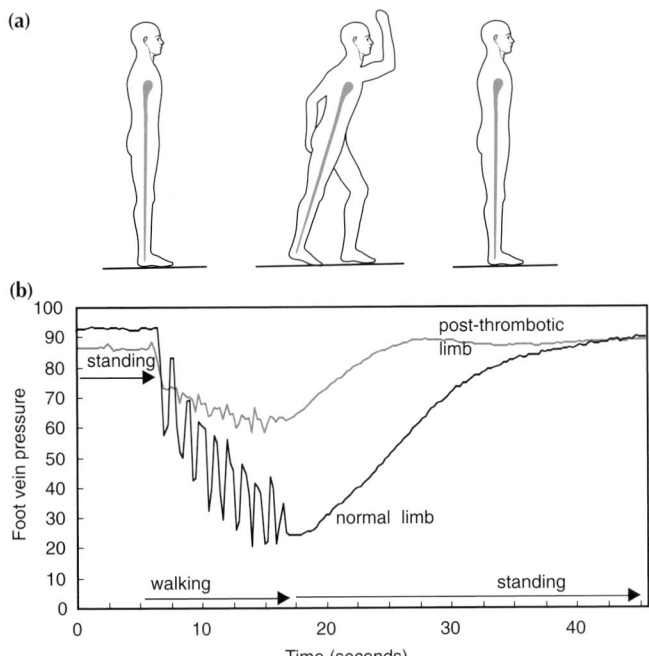

Figure 54.2 (a) Effect of exercise on the superficial venous pressure in health and disease; (b) Physiology of the calf muscle pump; pressure traces.

veins and superficial veins, which must contain competent valves. Ambulatory venous hypertension is a consequence of valve failure (reflux) or obstruction in the venous system and may eventually lead to lipodermatosclerosis and ulceration.

VARICOSE VEINS

These are defined as tortuous dilated veins. They affect 5% or more of the adult population of western countries. The gender prevalence was found to be nearly equal in the recent Edinburgh Vein Study. There is often a clear family history of the disorder, with some patients inheriting abnormalities in the *FOXC2* gene. The pathophysiology of varicose vein development is probably related to defective connective tissue and smooth muscle in the vein wall leading to a secondary incompetence of the valves rather than to a primary defect in the valves, which occurs in a small group of patients who have total venous avalvulosis. Varicose veins may develop secondarily in patients with post-thrombotic limbs and in patients with congenital abnormalities such as the Klippel–Trenaunay syndrome or multiple arterio-venous fistulae. Pregnancy and pelvic tumours are also well-recognised predisposing factors. Some of the other factors that may predispose to the development of varicose veins are:

- age;
- sex;
- race;
- weight;
- height;
- diet;
- side (left > right);
- bowel habit;
- occupation;
- heredity;
- clothes;
- erect stance.

Clinical features

Varicose veins rarely cause severe symptoms. Aching in the veins at the end of the day, after prolonged standing, is the most common complaint of patients referred to hospital, but many patients with severe varicose veins never consult a doctor. Other symptoms include ankle swelling, itching, bleeding, superficial thrombophlebitis, eczema, lipodermatosclerosis and ulceration. All of these symptoms are rare and it is not known why some patients with primary varicose veins develop the important complications of eczema, lipodermatosclerosis and ulceration.

Tortuous dilated veins in the subcutaneous tissue are indicative of varicose veins (Fig. 54.3). Most develop in the tributaries of the greater and lesser saphenous veins, which are usually dilated but rarely varicose themselves. Varicosities in the thigh are indicative of long saphenous incompetence, whereas varicosities on the back of the leg are suggestive of short saphenous incompetence. Some varicose veins join both systems and it is important to examine both the greater and lesser saphenous veins for the presence of valvular incompetence. Smaller varicosities are called reticular veins and are of dubious significance; the presence of these and thread veins within the skin is not necessarily associated with major varicose veins and is purely cosmetic. The Edinburgh Vein Study failed to show any evidence that the extent of valvular incompetence was related to the presence of symptoms.

Signs of varicose veins

A careful inspection and documentation of the site of the varicosities is extremely important. In addition, the termination of the long and short saphenous veins must be palpated, the latter with the knee slightly bent to relax the popliteal fascia. The

Maurice Klippel, **1858–1942, Neurologist, La Salpêtrière, Paris, France.**
Paul Trenaunay, **B. 1875, a French Neurologist.**
Klippel and Trenaunay described this condition in a joint paper in 1900.

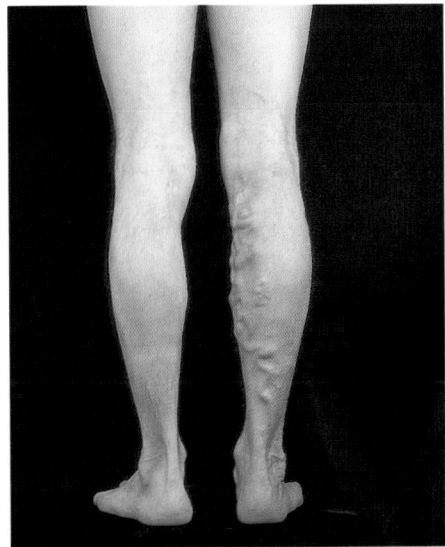

Figure 54.3 Varicose veins of the right leg.

presence of a dilated trunk can usually be detected if fingers are loosely placed over the trunk, which can be 'rolled back and forth'. Percussion over the varices may elicit an impulse tap by the fingers placed over the dilated trunk. A large varicosity in the groin (a saphena varix), often of the anterolateral thigh vein, may be visible (Fig. 54.4) and gentle palpation during coughing may elicit a cough thrill, which is a vibration experienced through the fingers caused by turbulent backflow within the varicosity.

Tourniquet tests have been abandoned by many clinicians. Complete control of all lower limb varicosities by a tourniquet placed around the upper thigh after elevation and emptying of the veins is, however, highly indicative of saphenofemoral incompetence. Release of the tourniquet leading to rapid refilling of varicosities is further confirmation of incompetence of the greater saphenous vein (Fig. 54.5). Greater saphenous incompetence is associated with 80% of all significant varicosities in the lower limbs. Abnormally distributed varices or a suspicion of lesser saphenous incompetence (e.g. varicosities on the back of the calf with a palpable dilated lesser saphenous trunk and control by a below-knee tourniquet) requires further assessment as the termination of the lesser saphenous vein is very variable.

Investigation

Many now believe that all patients with varicose veins should undergo an assessment by duplex scan. There is some evidence that this policy leads to a more accurate surgical approach and reduces the incidence of recurrence of the varicose veins. Duplex scanning is, however, not always available and clinical acumen combined with tourniquet tests and the use of a standard Doppler probe still suffices in many settings.

Standard Doppler examination

A standard Doppler probe emits a sound when blood flows past the transmitting and receiving crystals. A uniphasic signal indicates flow in one direction. A biphasic signal indicates forward and reverse flow and is indicative of blood refluxing down through incompetent valves. A Doppler probe is placed over the saphenofemoral junction. A calf squeeze is carried out and if a biphasic signal is obtained this confirms the presence of incompetence of the saphenofemoral junction. This diagnosis is further supported if all of the varices are controlled by a thigh tourniquet. The Doppler probe can be placed over distal varices when the tourniquet is released; retrograde flow is indicated by a rumbling noise as the blood refluxes down the long saphenous vein to fill the varices. This is not an accurate method of establishing incompetence of the lesser saphenous vein as its termination is variable and it is difficult to separate lesser saphenous incompetence from popliteal valvular incompetence. In all cases of short saphenous incompetence a further investigation is desirable; this is usually carried out by duplex scanning.

Duplex ultrasound imaging

The probe of a duplex scanner contains multiple emitting and receiving crystals. These allow a grey-scale image to be obtained in which the veins are seen as a black void in the subcutaneous and deep tissues. Directional flow can be shown as a colour image (red or blue) superimposed on the grey-scale image of the vessel (Fig. 54.6). Visible venous flow can only be seen when augmented by a calf squeeze. The B-mode grey-scale image allows the vein to be traced to its termination, while compression and relaxation, or a Valsalva manoeuvre, may demonstrate the presence of retrograde flow (reflux).

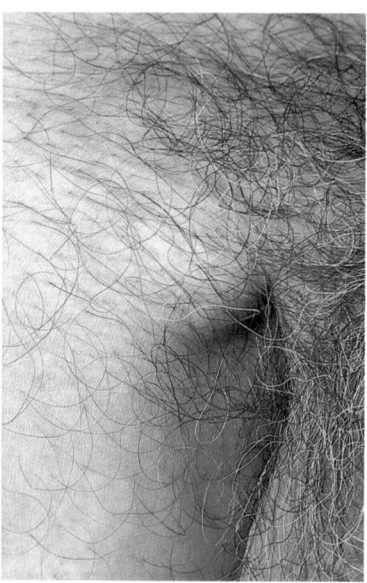

Figure 54.4 A saphena varix.

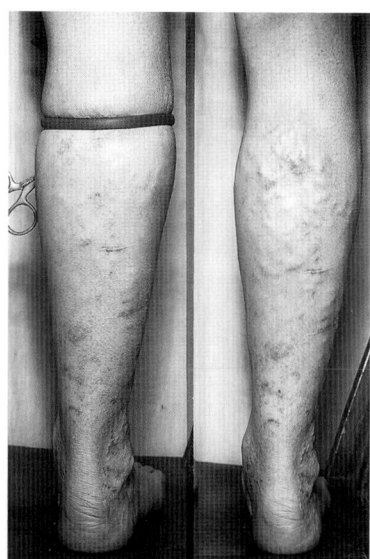

Figure 54.5 A tourniquet test.

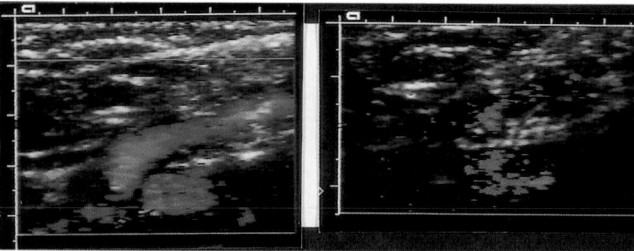

Figure 54.6 Duplex scan of the saphenofemoral junction showing antegrade and retrograde flow.

Christian Johann Doppler, **1803–1853, Professor of Experimental Physics, Vienna, Austria, enunciated the 'Doppler Principle' in 1842.**
Antonio Maria Valsalva, **1666–1723, Professor of Anatomy, Bologna, Italy.**

Varicography

In this investigation contrast is injected directly into surface varices. The contrast is non-thrombogenic, as it is non-ionic, and iso-osmolar with blood. This allows detailed mapping of the varices to their termination. This is an extremely useful investigation in patients with recurrent varicose veins or those with complex anatomy (Fig. 54.7).

Venography

In this investigation tourniquets are used to direct contrast injected into the superficial veins of the foot into the deep veins of the calf, thigh and pelvis. It is not used as a standard investigation in patients with varicose veins but is useful if the duplex scan indicates, but cannot confirm, the presence of post-thrombotic change (Fig. 54.8).

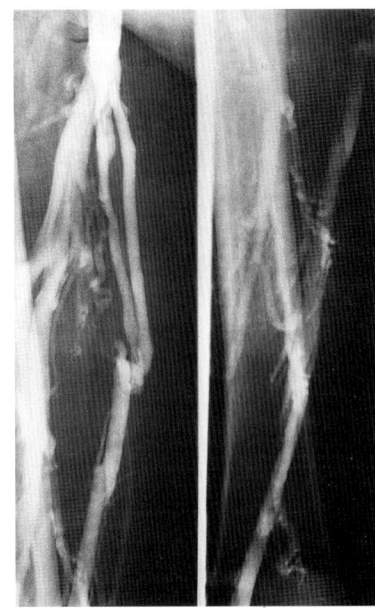

Figure 54.8 Venogram showing post-thrombotic venous occlusions with collateral pathways.

Management of patients with varicose veins

Many patients without symptoms or signs of lipodermatosclerosis or ulceration simply require reassurance. Others are concerned about the cosmetic appearance of their limbs and this may explain the female to male preponderance in patients presenting for treatment compared with the natural history studies (3:1 compared with 1:1).

Clear indications for intervention (see below) include recurrent episodes of haemorrhage and the development of skin changes (lipodermatosclerosis or ulceration) associated with an ankle flare indicative of venous hypertension (Fig. 54.9). In such patients a duplex scan and/or venography is essential.

Patients should be treated with elastic compression stockings if the varicose veins are found to be associated with post-thrombotic damage. Stockings can also be used to alleviate symptoms in elderly patients who do not wish to have surgery or other invasive forms of treatment. Most patients are prescribed class II stockings with an ankle pressure of around 30 mmHg decreasing to 10–15 mmHg at knee level. Above-knee stockings should never be prescribed as they are difficult to put on and tend to cut in and roll down. Class I stockings can be used to control simple varicose veins.

Injection sclerotherapy

In this technique a detergent is injected directly into the superficial veins. The most commonly used (and only sclerosant recognised for treatment in the UK) is sodium tetradecyl sulphate, although others are available on a named patient basis. The detergent destroys the lipid membranes of endothelial cells causing them to shed, leading to thrombosis, fibrosis and obliteration (sclerosis). Fegan stressed the importance of continued local compression following sclerosant injections to reduce the incidence and amount of superficial thrombosis and improve the

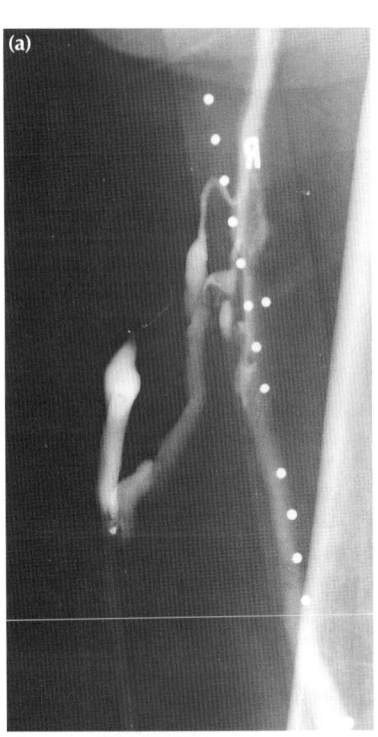

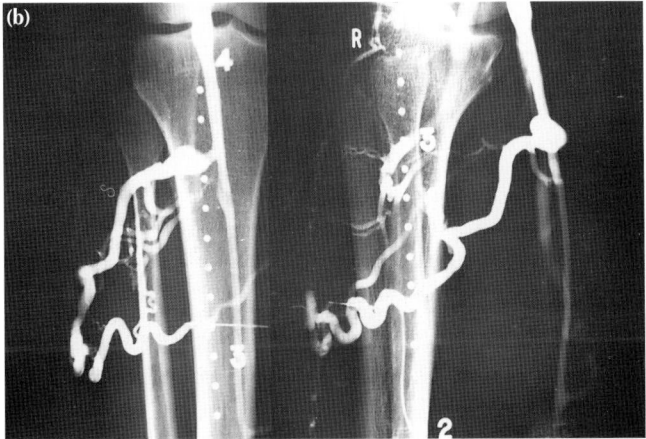

Figure 54.7 Varicograms. (a) A Hunterian perforator joining a divided long saphenous vein to the deep veins. (b) A varicose vein connecting the long and short saphenous veins.

William George Fegan, **a 20th Century Surgeon of Dublin, Ireland.**

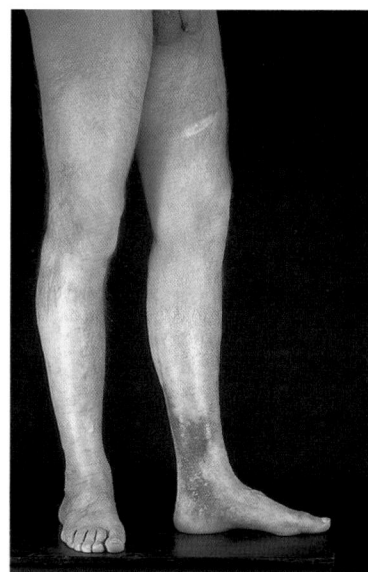

Figure 54.9 Lipodermatosclerosis of the calf skin associated with an ankle flare.

'sclerosis' of the vein. In trials carried out in the 1960s and 1970s injection sclerotherapy was not found to be effective at eradicating varicosities in the presence of major saphenous incompetence. It is, however, useful for dealing with minor varicosities and recurrences, especially in the calf and lower leg.

Ultrasound-guided foam sclerotherapy

This has recently become an alternative to the 'blind' sclerotherapy practised in the past and can be used to treat the main saphenous trunks. A needle is inserted into the vein that requires treatment under duplex ultrasound guidance and the sclerosant is made into foam. Foam sclerosants are available commercially or can be easily made by an air-mixing technique using a three-way tap. Ideally, polidocanol, another non-recognised detergent, is used rather than sodium tetradecyl sulphate. The foam is then injected under continued ultrasound monitoring, which can image the foam as it spreads up the vein. The top of the saphenous vein should be compressed by the ultrasound probe, preventing the majority of the foam from entering the deep veins until spasm in the main trunk develops. The leg can also be elevated to reduce spread of the foam into the axial deep veins. Using this technique both the greater and lesser saphenous veins can be obliterated. The distal varicosities can also be directly injected at the same time using the same technique, although many perform this at a separate session to limit the quantity of sclerosant that is administered.

Repeat duplex imaging confirms the presence of occlusion and over 90% of major trunks can be occluded by up to three treatments. As yet, there are no long-term results available for this technique and no controlled trials have been carried comparing this technique with other techniques for saphenous obliteration.

In any form of foam sclerotherapy, extravasation is associated with a risk of cutaneous ulceration and an escape of the sclerosant into the deep veins may cause deep vein thrombosis. More recently, severe headaches have been reported in some patients following foam sclerotherapy, which may be related to air entering the heart and passing through a right-to-left shunt before entering the brain. Some patients experience transient blindness and one stroke has been reported after a large quantity of foam had been administered. Recurrence rates are at present unknown.

Surgical treatment of varicose veins

Surgical treatment has always been used in the past to treat major long and short saphenous incompetence. The principles are to ligate the point of communication, the saphenofemoral and/or saphenopopliteal junctions, and to remove the major part of the incompetent trunk to prevent connections to the tributaries. The tributaries themselves are then individually removed by making minor cut-downs and teasing them out from under the skin (avulsions). The varicose veins must be carefully marked by tramlines of indelible marker pen to enable the sites of varicosity to be identified when the limbs are elevated. A careful consent is taken, explaining the risks of recurrence and minor nerve damage. The operation can be performed under general anaesthesia or local or regional (spinal/epidural) blockage.

Saphenofemoral junction ligation and greater saphenous stripping

An oblique incision is made in the groin centred 2.5 cm below and lateral to the pubic tubercle. The length of the incision depends on the build of the patient but must be adequate to expose the saphenofemoral junction safely. The greater saphenous vein is found in the superficial fat by blunt dissection and traced upwards to its T-shaped termination with the femoral vein. This must be clearly established before the vein is divided as disasters have befallen surgeons who have divided a femoral vein that has been mistaken for the greater saphenous vein in thin patients. As the vein is traced to its termination four tributaries are normally encountered. These are the superficial inferior epigastric vein, the superficial circumflex iliac vein and the deep and superficial external pudendal veins (see Fig. 54.1, p. 926). A number of anomalies can be present, the most common being a double saphenous vein, which normally receives large anterolateral thigh veins and posteromedial thigh veins. The long saphenous vein is not ligated until the T-junction has been confirmed and the femoral vein has been exposed for a centimetre in either direction. The saphenous trunk is then retrogradely stripped to the knee. Either a variation of Babcock's intraluminal stripper (Fig. 54.10) or a rigid metal 'pin' stripper is used which invaginates the vein and may cause less bruising. Stripping not only avulses the main vein trunk but also pulls out the termination of the tributaries. The posteromedial and anterolateral thigh veins should be separately divided and ligated if at all possible as this reduces bruising in the groin.

Avulsions

The tributaries are then avulsed and many surgeons attempt to do this after application of a tourniquet to reduce blood loss. Although not scientifically proven, the more accurate the avulsion of the tributaries, the better the long-term results. It is therefore very important to mark all of the tributary veins carefully. The avulsion incisions should be placed in Langer's lines and the

William Wayne Babcock, **1872–1963**, Professor of Surgery, Temple University Medical College, Philadelphia, PA, USA.
Karl Ritter von Edenberg Langer, **1819–1887**, Professor of Anatomy, Vienna, Austria described these lines in 1862.

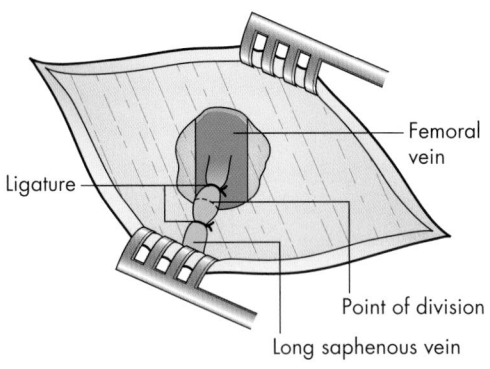

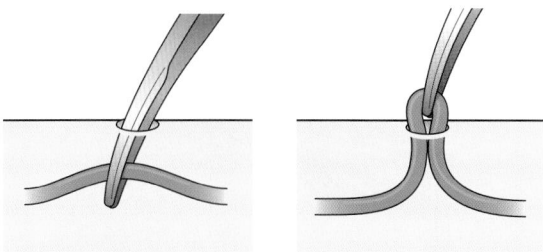

Figure 54.11 Avulsion of varicose tributaries.

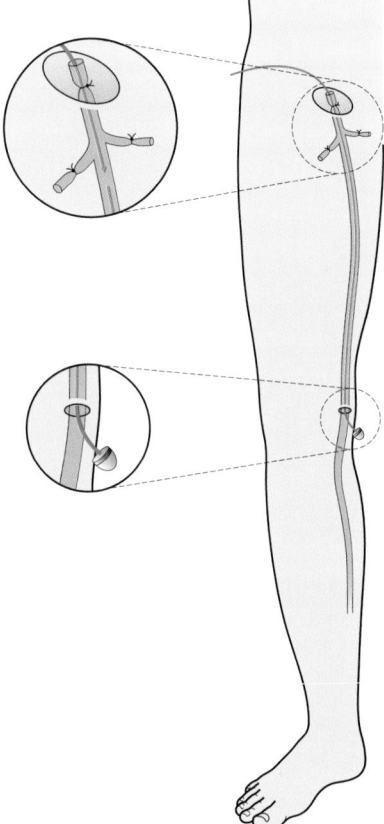

Figure 54.10 Long saphenous vein stripping.

through a vein of Giacomini, to join either the greater saphenous vein or the deep femoral vein in the upper thigh.

A transverse skin incision is made in the popliteal fossa just below the termination of the vein. The deep fascia is divided vertically. The vein is found and traced to the saphenopopliteal junction before it is divided (Fig. 54.12). It is disastrous to divide or damage the popliteal vein. Tributaries may enter the short saphenous vein near its termination. After the vein has been divided, a stripper is passed upwards from the ankle, carefully dissecting off the sural nerve to ensure that the whole of the lesser saphenous vein is removed. This obliterates the junction with the mid-calf perforating vein, which is responsible for many recurrences.

Postoperative care

Postoperatively the legs are elevated, analgesia is given and bandages are applied. Many patients have the surgery under local or spinal block and many can be treated as day cases.

Alternative techniques

A number of newer techniques have been developed to destroy the main saphenous trunks. The first was *radiofrequency ablation* in which a catheter is passed up the saphenous vein from the lower leg and withdrawn under ultrasound control while radiofrequency waves are used to destroy the endothelial lining through a series of metal prongs. Laser is also being used to cause endothelial damage (Fig. 54.13). This technique appears to be effective but is expensive. Long-term follow-up and controlled trials are not available.

Endovenous laser ablation is a more recent development. A laser probe is passed up inside a catheter inserted into the lower

vein must be teased out of the subcutaneous tissue using small hooks or mosquito forceps (Fig. 54.11). Long lengths of varicosity may be successfully teased out by careful surgeons who are not in a rush.

Saphenopopliteal junction ligation and lesser saphenous stripping

Preoperative ultrasound localisation of the junction should ideally be carried out. Approximately one-third of popliteal veins end in the lower part of the popliteal fossa, one-third end in the middle of the popliteal fossa and one-third extend up, often

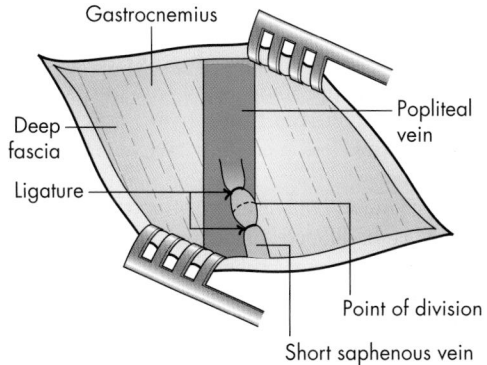

Figure 54.12 Short saphenous ligation.

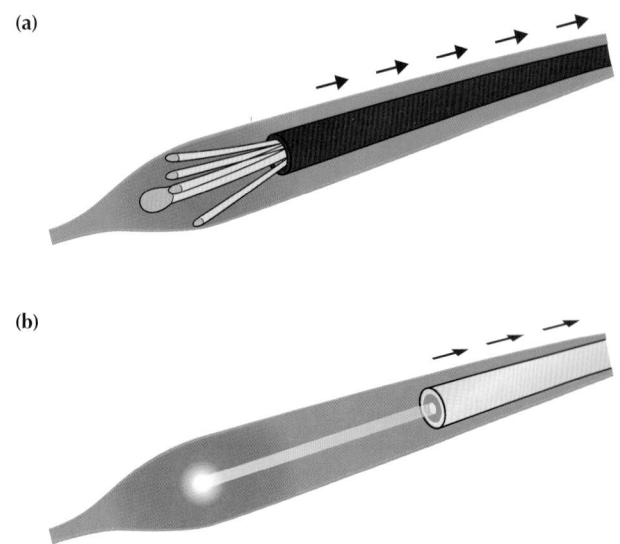

(a)

(b)

Figure 54.13 (a) VNUS closure; (b) laser.

part of the saphenous vein under ultrasound guidance (Fig. 54.14). It is very important that large amounts of crystalloid fluid containing local anaesthesia are placed around the vein to separate the skin from the laser probe and avoid cutaneous burns. A duplex ultrasound scan confirms that the laser probe is at the saphenofemoral junction and the laser is then withdrawn, administering a set number of joules to the endothelial lining of the saphenous veins. The laser probes are marginally less expensive than radiofrequency ablation.

Both laser and radiofrequency ablation do not provide 'flush' occlusion of the saphenous vein, often leaving tributaries that would always be divided at surgery. Long-term studies are required to ascertain the recurrence rate of both techniques.

Complications of varicose vein surgery

After surgery bruising and sensory nerve injury are common. The greater saphenous vein should only be stripped to just below the knee to avoid damage to the accompanying saphenous nerve, and the sural nerve must be carefully dissected off the lesser saphenous vein at the ankle. All patients should be warned that numbness and tingling are common but that they will invariably recover. Motor nerve injury should not occur if the anatomy is carefully displayed. Damage to the main veins and accompanying arteries is also avoidable if care is taken to display the anatomy. Deep vein thrombosis is rare unless there is iatrogenic damage to the deep veins. A previous deep vein thrombosis usually contraindicates varicose vein surgery but, if surgery is undertaken, subcutaneous low molecular weight heparin must be given.

The most common complication of varicose vein surgery is recurrence. This is difficult to define and should be divided into recurrence of a previously treated venous system and development of new varicosities arising in a hitherto untreated system. The latter of course cannot be prevented. Careful attention to detail and correct evaluation all reduce the risk of recurrence.

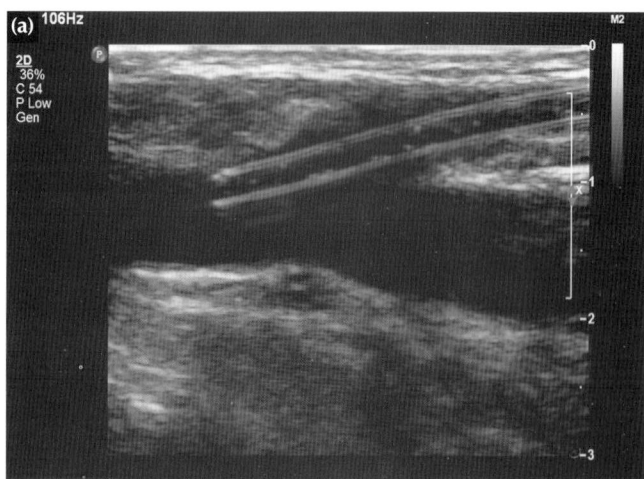

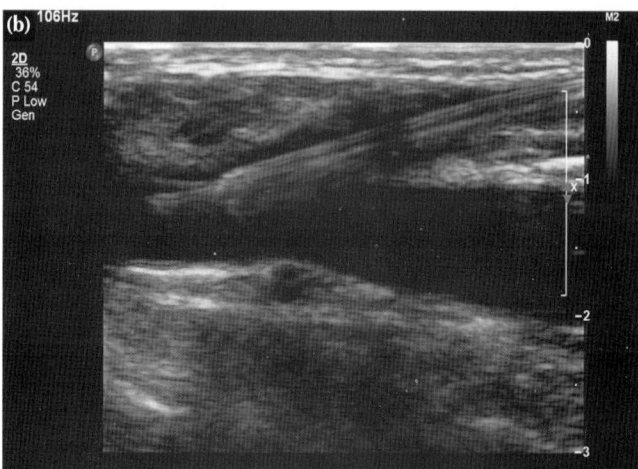

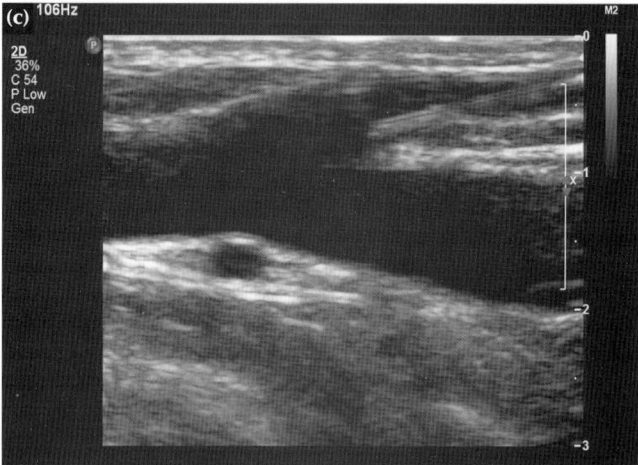

Figure 54.14 Laser probe inside long saphenous vein. (a) Sheath in femoral vein. (b) Sheath pulled back. (c) Laser probe causing heating (sclerosis) of vein.

DEEP VEIN INCOMPETENCE AND OBSTRUCTION

These problems usually follow a deep vein thrombosis, which almost never resolves completely without leaving obliterated segments of vein and damaged valves. Primary deep vein incompetence does occur but is rare. The exact incidence of primary deep vein incompetence is not known and many cases follow a subclinical thrombosis (see Post-thrombotic leg). Some venous obstruction may follow trauma, which includes iatrogenic injuries.

Post-thrombotic leg

A thrombus normally forms in the calf veins and extends upwards into the main axial veins. When it resolves, segments of vein remain obstructed, valves are destroyed or damaged and collateral veins dilate to bypass obstructed segments. Post-thrombotic damaged veins are often surrounded by fibrotic tissue and can no longer dilate in response to increased flow, which occurs during exercise. The lumen is often criss-crossed with thickened white tissue (synaechae), which is the scarred remains of a thrombosis.

Presentation

All patients who have had a deep vein thrombosis may develop signs of a post-thrombotic limb. These are variable and include leg swelling, discomfort on walking, oedema, varicose veins (which need not be present), the presence of an ankle flare, lipodermatosclerosis and eventually ulceration (Fig. 54.15). Patients should be questioned about previous fractures, childbirth, operations, etc. when a clear history of a deep vein thrombosis is lacking.

Investigations

These include duplex scanning to look for deep vein reflux and venography to demonstrate occluded/obstructed deep venous segments and the presence of collaterals.

Treatment

Treatment is usually by elastic compression hosiery, but bypass surgery and valve reconstruction should be considered in patients with severe symptoms who have clearly obstructed or refluxing veins.

Techniques of venous reconstruction

Venous bypasses may be carried out using the saphenous vein from the opposite limb as a crossover or free bypass (Fig. 54.16). Prosthetic grafts do poorly as venous flow is low and the patients are often highly thrombogenic. Venous valves may be tightened by external compression devices or internally reefed by sutures

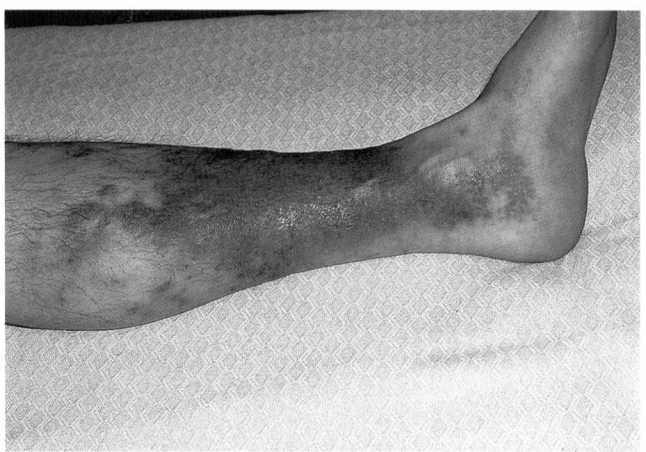

Figure 54.15 Post-thrombotic leg.

(Fig. 54.16). Valves may be transplanted from the upper limb and artificial valves may be inserted endovenously. None of these techniques is established apart perhaps from the 'Palma' cross-femoral bypass using the opposite long saphenous vein, which is tunnelled suprapubically and anastomosed to the femoral vein below the site of obstruction/occlusion (Fig. 54.16). Many patients continue to have symptoms of swelling and leg discomfort. They must continue to wear stockings to prevent ulceration and unfortunately there is a high incidence of recurrent thrombosis. Patients require lifelong anticoagulants if thromboses recur, especially if they have an associated thrombophilia such as antithrombin deficiency (see below).

The condition of patients with narrowed iliac veins (iliac vein compression) can be improved by inserting a metallic stent if the thrombus has been successfully lysed.

LEG ULCERATION

Venous disease is responsible for between 60% and 70% of all ulcers in the lower leg. There are many other causes of leg ulcers and these must be excluded in any patient presenting with ulceration:

- venous disease: superficial incompetence; deep venous damage (post-thrombotic);

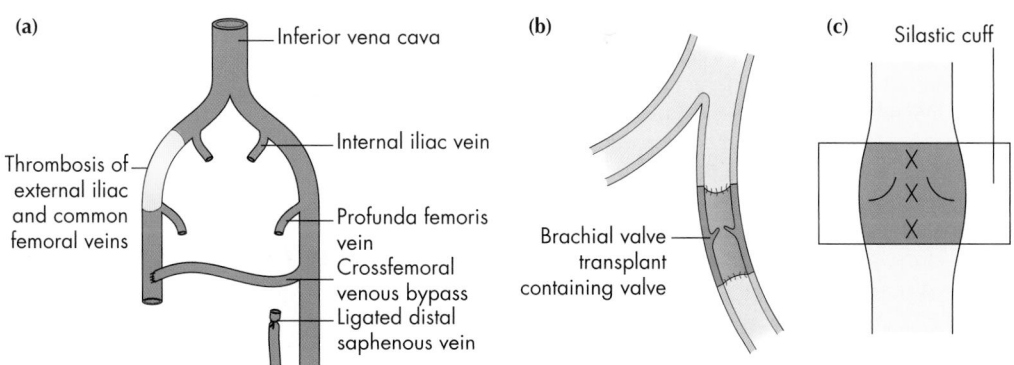

(a)
Inferior vena cava
Internal iliac vein
Thrombosis of external iliac and common femoral veins
Profunda femoris vein
Crossfemoral venous bypass
Ligated distal saphenous vein

(b)
Brachial valve transplant containing valve

(c) Silastic cuff

Figure 54.16 Various techniques for bypassing venous obstruction and improving valve competence. (a) Palma; (b) Taheri; (c) Lane.

- arterial ischaemic ulcers;
- rheumatoid ulcers;
- traumatic ulcers;
- neuropathic ulcers (diabetes);
- neoplastic ulcers (squamous cell carcinoma and basal cell carcinoma).

Up to 20% of patients have evidence of arterial disease, which may be the sole cause of ulceration or may be a mixed factor in the development of an ulcer in association with venous disease.

Aetiology of ulceration

The mechanism for ulcer development has not been established. Originally, it was thought that static blood within the superficial veins led to hypoxia, which caused tissue death (stasis ulcers). This was not confirmed by investigation of venous oxygen saturation, which was found to be higher in ulcerated limbs. This led to the concept of arteriovenous fistulae, which were thought to develop in response to the high venous pressure; however, this could not be confirmed. High venous pressure was found to be associated with a pericapillary infiltrate. This includes fibrin and other proteins, which are known to lead to fibrosis. It was hypothesised that these 'cuffs' could act as a diffusion block.

Leucocytes were found to decrease in the venous effluent coming out of dependent limbs. This decrease in leucocyte passage was shown to increase if short-term venous hypertension was induced by application of a tourniquet. This led to the concept of white cell 'trapping', which has not been confirmed by further investigation. Polymorphonuclear leucocytes were not found within the tissues but increased numbers of mast cells, monocytes and lymphocytes have been found in peri-ulcer tissues.

Reactive oxygen species are increased in the ulcer environment and these may generate free radicals, leading to tissue damage. Proteolytic enzymes are also increased in ulcers and the fibroblasts in the ulcer surrounds are also abnormal, being in a 'senescent' state. Growth factors may be inhibited, leading to poor repair, and their absence may also lead to ulceration. It is very difficult to prove whether any of these factors is the cause of or the result of an ulcer.

At present, ambulatory venous hypertension is the only accepted cause of ulceration. It is important to try and define the exact mechanism of ulcer development. The venous hypertension may be the result of primary valve incompetence of the saphenous veins, incompetence of the perforating veins or incompetence or obstruction of the deep veins.

Clinical features

The ulcer must be carefully examined. A venous ulcer has a gently sloping edge and the base contains granulation tissue covered by a variable amount of slough and exudate. Any elevation of the ulcer edge should indicate the need for a biopsy to exclude a carcinoma (squamous cell or basal cell carcinoma).

The venous ulcer of the leg characteristically develops in the skin of the gaiter region, the area between the muscles of the calf and the ankle. This is the region where many of the Cockett perforators join the posterior tibial vein to the surface vein,

---

A gaiter is a leather or cloth covering for the lower leg and ankle. The name is derived from the French 'guetre' for the same piece of clothing.
Frank Bernard Cockett, formerly Surgeon, St. Thomas's Hospital, London, England.

---

known as the posterior arch vein. The majority of ulcers develop on the medial side of the calf but ulcers associated with lesser saphenous incompetence often develop on the lateral side of the leg. Ulcers can develop on any part of the calf skin in patients with post-thrombotic legs; however, venous ulcers rarely extend on to the foot or into the upper calf and, if there is ulceration at these sites, other diagnoses should be seriously considered. Ulcers often develop in response to minor trauma; many patients notice some itching, perhaps associated with mast cell degranulation, before the ulcers develop. Almost all venous ulcers have surrounding lipodermatosclerosis (Fig. 54.17). This is thickening, pigmentation, inflammation and induration of the calf skin. The pigmentation comes from haemosiderin and melanin and the haemosiderin itself may be an important factor in the ulcer development. Another cause of ulceration should be considered if there is no evidence of lipodermatosclerosis or an ankle flare.

A full examination of the front and back of the limbs with the patient standing should be carried out to assess the presence of varicosities and truncal incompetence of the saphenous systems (note that venous ulcers are not always accompanied by varicose veins). The presence of an ankle flare suggests venous hypertension.

All patients should have their pulses palpated and, if there is any doubt, their Doppler pressures should be measured. Sensation and proprioception should be assessed to exclude neuropathy, especially in diabetic patients. A careful examination of the hand and other joints may confirm the presence of rheumatoid arthritis or osteoarthritis.

Investigation

Some clinicians will carry out a duplex scan when the patient with an ulcer is first seen to assess the state of the deep and superficial veins. The presence of reflux in these veins does not confirm a venous ulcer but supports the diagnosis in the absence of another cause.

All patients presenting for the first time with a new leg ulcer should have a full blood count, erythrocyte sedimentation rate (C-reactive protein) and sickle cell test if they have an appropriate

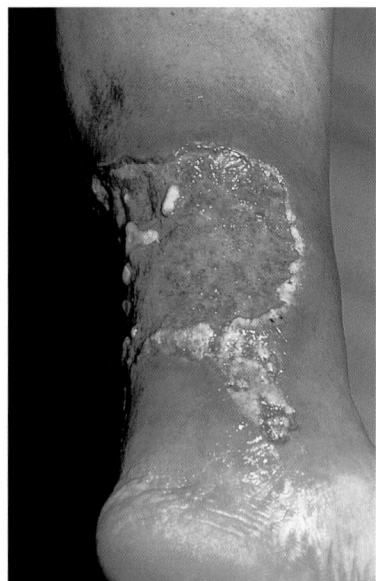

Figure 54.17 A venous ulcer.

racial background. Anaemia can both cause ulcers (e.g. sickle cell disease and pernicious anaemia) and result from ulceration (e.g. iron deficiency anaemia and the anaemia of chronic disease). Polycythaemia is a rare cause of ulceration. Any patient found to have evidence of an unexplained peripheral neuropathy or distal ischaemia should have their blood or urinary glucose measured to exclude diabetes. An antibody screen should be obtained if the ulcer appears 'atypical' or there is any suggestion of joint disease (e.g. rheumatoid arthritis). All patients presenting with a new ulcer should have their Doppler pressures measured to document the adequacy of the blood supply to the affected limbs, even when the foot pulses are easily palpable.

Once the ulcer has healed, there is no doubt that a duplex scan assessment (see Fig. 54.6, p. 928) of the veins of both lower limbs is essential to document the major sites of valvular incompetence. Bipedal ascending phlebography will often detect obstruction and post-thrombotic changes missed by the duplex scan (see Fig. 54.8, p. 929). These investigations are invaluable for arriving at a strategy to reduce the risk of re-ulceration.

Management

When the diagnosis of a 'probable venous ulcer' has been made, patients are initially treated by a compression bandaging regimen, which can be applied in a specialised clinic or by a district or practice nurse. Patients with new ulcers should ideally be assessed in a specialised ulcer clinic to confirm the diagnosis and agree the correct treatment regimen.

Many bandaging regimens have been described but three types usually suffice. A multilayered elastic compression bandaging system has been shown to be effective (Charing Cross four-layer bandage), as has a rigid multilayered system (Steripaste three-layer bandage). A low-compression regimen is desirable for mixed venous/arterial ulcers. The alternative to these bandaging regimens is to apply a bland absorbent leak-proof dressing beneath a graduated elastic compression stocking (class II).

These compression regimens are ideally applied by trained staff on a weekly basis until the ulcer is starting to heal and the amount of exudate is reduced. Longer periods between dressing changes can then be instituted. At each attendance ulcer size must be measured to monitor improvement. Measurement of the two maximal diameters is a satisfactory and cheap method of assessment, although other more sophisticated area measurements are often utilised. Antibiotics do not speed ulcer healing and all other specific ulcer-healing drugs are of dubious validity.

Failure to heal an ulcer may indicate that it has another cause (e.g. malignancy, rheumatoid arthritis or arterial ischaemia). Biopsies are indicated if malignancy is suspected and it is important to remember that a Marjolin's type of ulcer (a squamous cell or basal cell carcinoma) can develop in a chronic longstanding venous ulcer (Fig. 54.18).

Once these factors have been excluded, consideration must be given to healing the ulcer by excision and grafting. A number of biological dressings have been developed, including fetal keratinocytes and collagen meshes, which have been shown to improve healing; however, they are not cost-effective for the majority of ulcers and they have been shown to be of value only

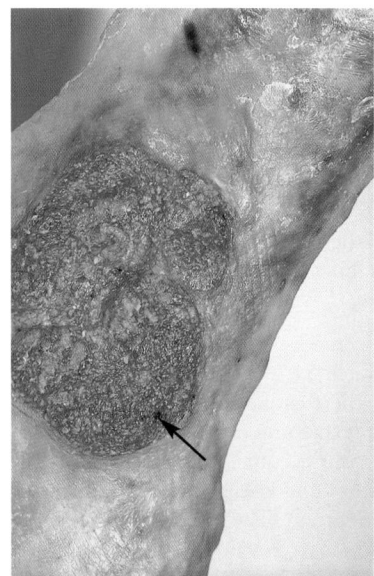

Figure 54.18 A Marjolin's ulcer (a squamous cell cancer arising in a chronic venous ulcer; arrow).

in the post hoc analysis of certain sub-groups. Pinch grafts and ulcer excision with mesh grafting have been shown to provide good early healing with moderate long-term results (50% healed at 5 years).

The recent Eschar trial has confirmed that surgery to sites of superficial venous incompetence does not speed ulcer healing and this practice should be abandoned unless new evidence is provided of its efficacy.

Prevention of recurrence

Once an ulcer has healed the patient must be re-evaluated in an attempt to prevent recurrence. Patients with normal deep veins should be offered treatment to obliterate any sites of saphenous or perforator reflux. The Eschar study has confirmed the results of other studies showing that this treatment is effective in reducing the incidence of ulcer recurrence in patients with *normal* deep veins. Some patients will decline treatment and others will be considered unsuitable for major interventions on their veins.

Elastic stockings should be prescribed for all patients with evidence of post-thrombotic deep vein damage and these remain an alternative treatment for patients with superficial venous disease who decline intervention. Further studies are required to determine whether laser ablation and foam sclerotherapy are as satisfactory as surgery in achieving prolonged ulcer-free periods.

Prognosis

All venous ulcers can be healed but, even in those who have successful surgery or wear their stockings religiously, there is a 20–30% incidence of re-ulceration by 5 years. The greatest risk of re-ulceration is in the post-thrombotic leg.

VENOUS THROMBOSIS

A venous thrombus is the formation of a semi-solid coagulum within flowing blood in the venous system. Venous thrombosis of the deep veins of the leg is complicated by the immediate risk of pulmonary embolus and sudden death. Subsequently, patients

---

Charing Cross. **This method of treating venous ulcers was introduced at Charing Cross Hospital, London, England.**
Jean-Nicholas Marjolin, 1780–1850, Surgeon, Paris, France, described the **development of carcinomatous ulcers in scars in 1828.**

are at risk of developing a post-thrombotic limb and venous ulceration.

Aetiology

The three factors described by Virchow over a century ago are still considered important in the development of venous thrombosis. These are:

- changes in the vessel wall (endothelial damage);
- stasis, which is diminished blood flow through the veins;
- coagulability of blood (thrombophilia).

There are many predisposing causes of venous thrombosis. These are listed in Table 54.1. The most important factor is a hospital admission for the treatment of a medical or surgical condition. Injury, especially fractures of the lower limb and pelvis, pregnancy and the oral contraceptive pill are other well-recognised predisposing factors. Endothelial damage is now recognised to be increasingly important. The interaction of the endothelium with inflammatory cells, or previous deep vein damage, may render the endothelial surface hypercoagulable and less fibrinolytic.

Stasis is a predisposing factor seen in many of the conditions described in Table 54.1, especially in the postoperative period, in patients with heart failure and in those with arterial ischaemia.

A number of conditions are associated with increased coagulability of the blood (thrombophilia) (Table 54.2). Deficiencies of anti-thrombin, activated protein C and protein S have all been

Table 54.1 Risk factors for venous thromboembolism

Patient factors	Age
	Obesity
	Varicose veins
	Immobility
	Pregnancy
	Puerperium
	High-dose oestrogen therapy
	Previous deep vein thrombosis or pulmonary embolism
	Thrombophilia (see Table 54.2)
Disease or surgical procedure	Trauma or surgery, especially of pelvis, hip and lower limb
	Malignancy, especially pelvic, and abdominal metastatic
	Heart failure
	Recent myocardial infarction
	Paralysis of lower limb(s)
	Infection
	Inflammatory bowel disease
	Nephrotic syndrome
	Polycythaemia
	Paraproteinaemia
	Paroxysmal nocturnal haemoglobinuria antibody or lupus anticoagulant
	Behçet's disease
	Homocystinaemia

Rudolf Ludwig Carl Virchow, **1821–1902, Professor of Pathology, Berlin, Germany.**

Table 54.2 Abnormalities of thrombosis and fibrinolysis that lead to an increased risk of venous thrombosis

Congenital	Deficiency of anti-thrombin III, protein C or protein S
	Antiphospholipid antibody or lupus anticoagulant
	Factor V Leiden gene defect or activated protein C resistance
	Dysfibrinogenaemias
Acquired	Antiphospholipid antibody or lupus anticoagulant

shown to predispose to venous thrombosis in young patients. Activated protein C deficiency is associated with inheritance of the factor V Leiden gene and may account for the higher incidence of venous thrombosis in Caucasian populations (being present in 6–7%). It results in a small increase in the risk of venous thrombosis, although it may act in concert with some of the other predisposing factors. A thrombophilic cause should be sought in any patient presenting with an episode of venous thrombosis who gives a family history of deep vein thrombosis.

Although the development of deep vein thrombosis is probably multifactorial, immobility remains one of the most important factors. Recently the term 'e-thrombosis' has been used to describe blood clots occurring in people sitting at their computers for long periods of time. Deep vein thrombosis has also been recognised as a complication of long-haul flights.

Pathology

A thrombus often develops in the soleal veins of the calf, initially as a platelet aggregate. Subsequently, fibrin and red cells form a mesh until the lumen of the vein wall occludes. The coralline thrombus then extends as a propagated loose red fibrin clot containing many red cells (Fig. 54.19). This is likely to extend up to

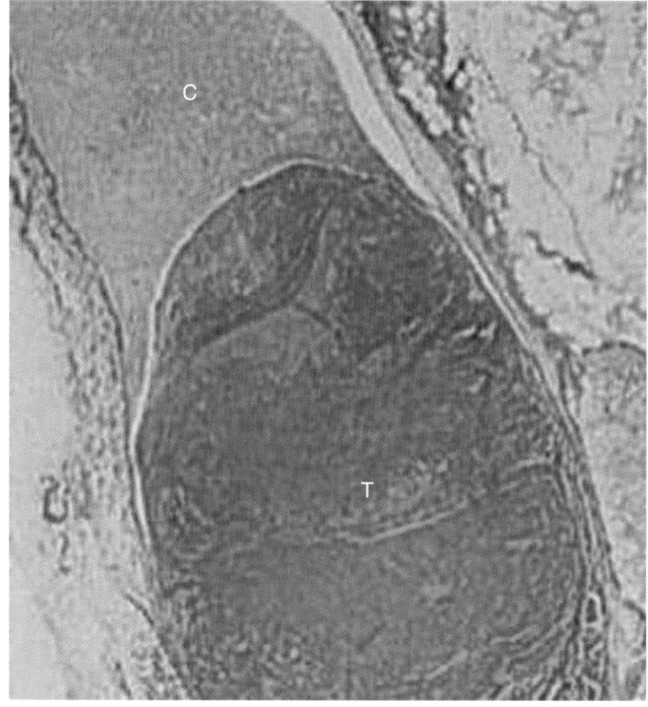

Figure 54.19 An organised thrombus. C, clot; T, thrombus.

the next large venous branch and is more likely to break off and embolise to the lung as a pulmonary embolism. In this situation the embolus arising from the lower leg veins becomes detached, passes through the large veins of the limb and vena cava, through the right heart and lodges in the pulmonary arteries. This may totally occlude perfusion to all or part of one or both lungs (pulmonary embolism). Acute right heart obstruction may lead to sudden collapse and death. Lung infarction is rare as the lung has a dual blood supply (bronchial and pulmonary arteries). Moderately sized emboli can cause pyramidal shaped infarcts.

Diagnosis

The most common presentation of a deep vein thrombosis is pain and swelling, especially in the calf of one lower limb. Bilateral deep vein thromboses are common, occurring in up to 30%. When the swelling is bilateral, deep vein thromboses must be differentiated from other causes of systemic oedema, such as hypoproteinaemia, renal failure and heart failure. Many patients have no symptoms of thrombosis and may first present with signs of a pulmonary embolism, e.g. pleuritic chest pain, haemoptysis and shortness of breath. Some patients also develop shortness of breath from chronic pulmonary hypertension. Sometimes the leg appears cellulitic and very occasionally it may be white or cyanosed: phlegmasia alba dolens and phlegmasia cerulia dolens. Patients presenting with venous gangrene (Fig. 54.20) often have an underlying neoplasm.

The physical signs may also be absent or ephemeral. Mild pitting oedema of the ankle, dilated surface veins, a stiff calf and tenderness over the course of the deep veins should be sought. Homans' sign – resistance (not pain) of the calf muscles to forcible dorsiflexion – is not discriminatory and should be abandoned. A low-grade pyrexia may be present, especially in a patient who is having repeated pulmonary emboli. Patients may have signs of cyanosis, dyspnoea, raised neck veins, a fixed split second heart sound and a pleural rub if they are having pulmonary emboli causing right heart strain, although these signs may be lacking.

Investigation

The diagnosis of deep vein thrombosis and pulmonary embolism should be established by special investigations as the symptoms and signs are non-specific and may be entirely lacking. In addition, treatment with anticoagulation is not without risk and the diagnosis must be made with certainty.

Patients who present to an accident and emergency department with an idiopathic thrombosis usually have a D-dimer measurement. If this is within the normal range there is no indication for further investigation but, if raised, a duplex ultrasound examination of the deep veins should be performed. The deep veins of the lower limb are located and compressed. Filling defects in flow and a lack of compressibility indicate the presence of a thrombosis (Fig. 54.21). Ascending venography, which shows a thrombus as a filling defect, is now rarely required unless other measures are being considered (Fig. 54.22).

Pulmonary embolism is diagnosed by ventilation–perfusion scanning, which shows mismatched defects (Fig. 54.23) by computerised tomographic (CT) scanning of the pulmonary arteries, which can show filling defects in the pulmonary arteries (Fig. 54.24). Pulmonary angiography is rarely required unless treatment is being instigated.

The differential diagnosis of a deep vein thrombosis includes a ruptured Baker's cyst, a calf muscle haematoma, a ruptured plantaris muscle, a thrombosed popliteal aneurysm and arterial

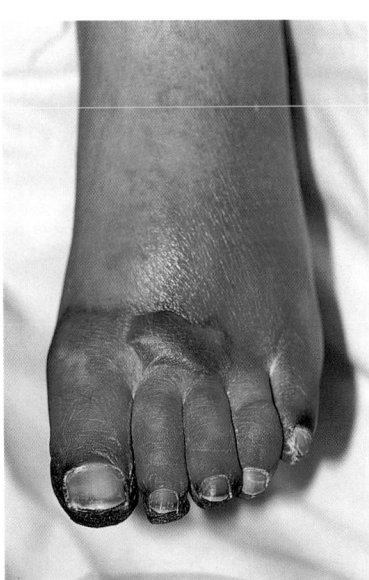

Figure 54.20 A foot with venous gangrene. The gangrene is symmetrical involving all of the toes. There is no clear-cut edge and there is marked oedema of the foot.

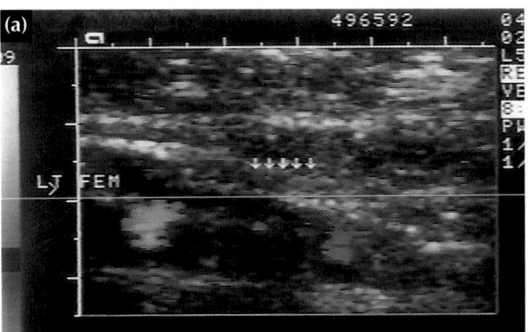

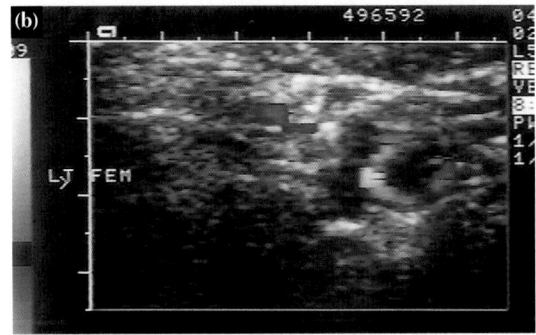

Figure 54.21 A longitudinal (a) and transverse (b) section of a duplex scan of a vein containing a thrombus.

John Homans, 1877–1954, Professor of Clinical Surgery, The Harvard University Medical School, Boston, MA, USA.

William Morrant Baker, 1839–1896, Surgeon, St. Bartholomew's Hospital, London, England, described these cysts in 1877.

CHAPTER 54 | VENOUS DISORDERS

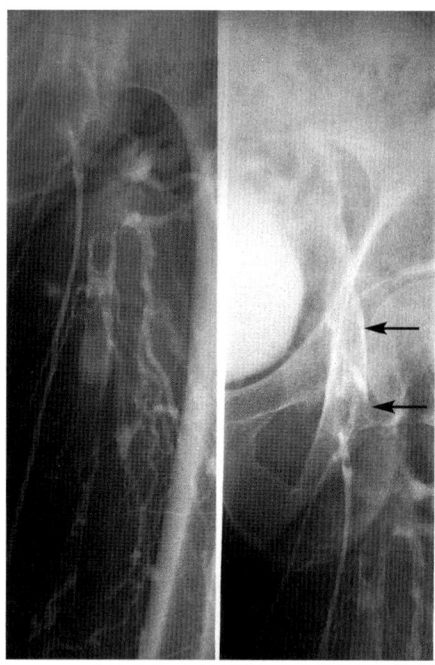

Figure 54.22 An ascending venogram of a deep vein thrombosis seen as filling defects (arrows) with contrast passing around the thrombus.

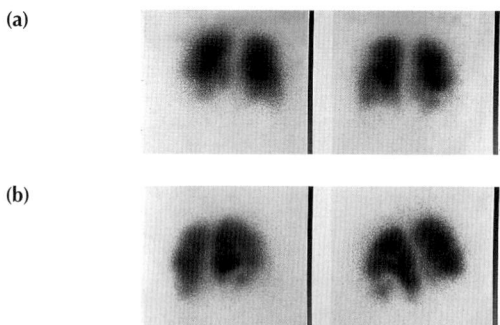

(a)

(b)

Figure 54.23 A ventilation–perfusion lung scan showing unmatched filling defects on the perfusion scan that are not present on the ventilation scan. (a) Ventilation, (b) perfusion.

ischaemia. Duplex scanning will detect many of these conditions but often patients present with non-specific pain in the calf that resolves with no firm diagnosis being made. The differential diagnosis of a pulmonary embolism includes myocardial infarction, pleurisy and pneumonia.

Prophylaxis

Patients who are being admitted for surgery can be graded as low, moderate or high risk. Low-risk patients are young, with minor illnesses, who are to undergo operations lasting 30 min or less. Those at moderate risk are patients over the age of 40 or those with a debilitating illness who are to undergo major surgery. High-risk patients are those over the age of 40 who have serious accompanying medical conditions, such as stroke or myocardial infarction, or who are undergoing major surgery with an additional risk factor such as a past history of venous thromboembolism or known malignant disease.

Prophylactic methods can be divided into mechanical and

pharmacological. A variety of mechanical methods have been tried but only the use of graduated elastic compression stockings and external pneumatic compression have stood the test of time. These mechanical measures reduce the incidence of thrombosis. Pharmacological methods are more effective than mechanical methods at reducing the risk of thrombosis, although they carry an increased risk of bleeding. In the past, low-dose unfractionated heparin was used both intravenously and subcutaneously. Most patients now start on low molecular weight heparin given subcutaneously, with the dose based on the patient's weight. This does not require monitoring and has a reduced risk of heparin-induced thrombocytopenia. It can be given once a day and probably has a lower risk of bleeding complications. Unfractionated heparin and warfarin are rarely used in the prophylaxis of deep vein thrombosis. A combination of mechanical and pharmacological treatment with heparin can be used in patients considered at high risk.

Treatment of a deep vein thrombosis

Patients who are confirmed to have a deep vein thrombosis on duplex imaging should be started on subcutaneous low molecular weight heparin and rapidly anticoagulated with warfarin unless there is a specific contraindication. Warfarin is usually started at a dose of 10 mg on day one, 10 mg on day two and 5 mg on day three. A prothrombin time taken on day three guides the maintenance dose of warfarin.

The great majority of patients are treated with heparin and warfarin in this way. Thrombolysis should be considered, however, in patients with an iliac vein thrombosis, especially if they are seen early and the limb is extremely swollen. Very few surgeons still carry out venous thrombectomy, although it may still be attempted in patients with pre-venous gangrene and phlegmasia cerulia dolens. A venous thrombectomy should be accompanied by an arteriovenous fistula to increase venous flow through the vein that has had the thrombus removed.

During thrombolysis the tissue plasminogen activator in most patients is administered directly into the thrombus, either via the popliteal vein or by direct puncture in the groin. New devices are being marketed that physically disrupt the thrombus at the same time as local lysis is carried out. Some thrombi can be compressed

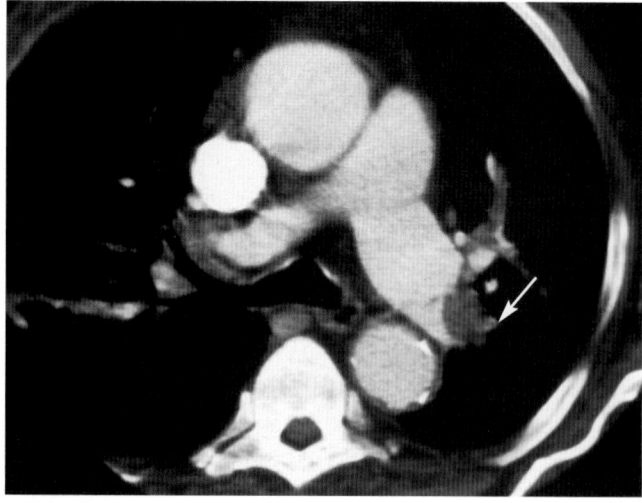

Figure 54.24 A computerised tomography scan showing pulmonary emboli as filling defects (arrow) in the pulmonary artery.

by stent grafting, allowing the venous lumen to be opened, especially in the iliac region. This technique is very good in patients with an anatomical obstruction from an 'iliac vein compression syndrome' (Fig. 54.25).

Treatment of pulmonary embolus

Most pulmonary emboli can be treated by anticoagulation and observation but severe right heart strain and shortness of breath indicates the need for fibrinolytic treatment. Rarely, patients who are on the point of cardiac arrest should undergo surgical pulmonary embolectomy.

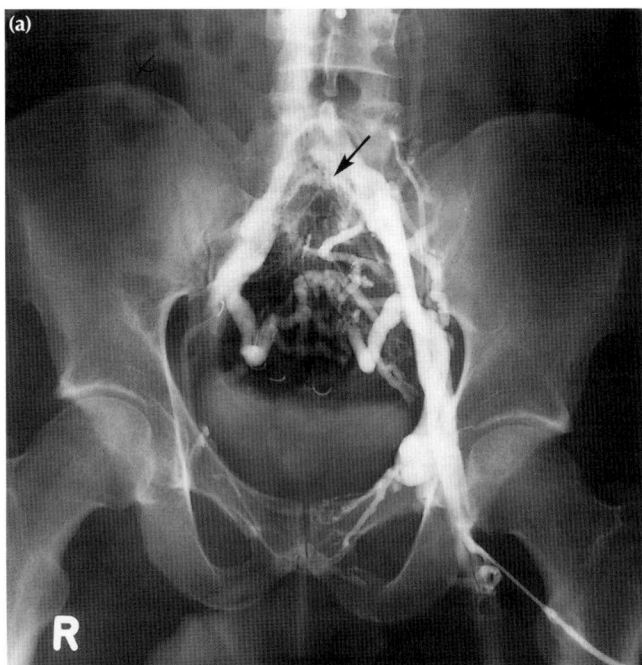

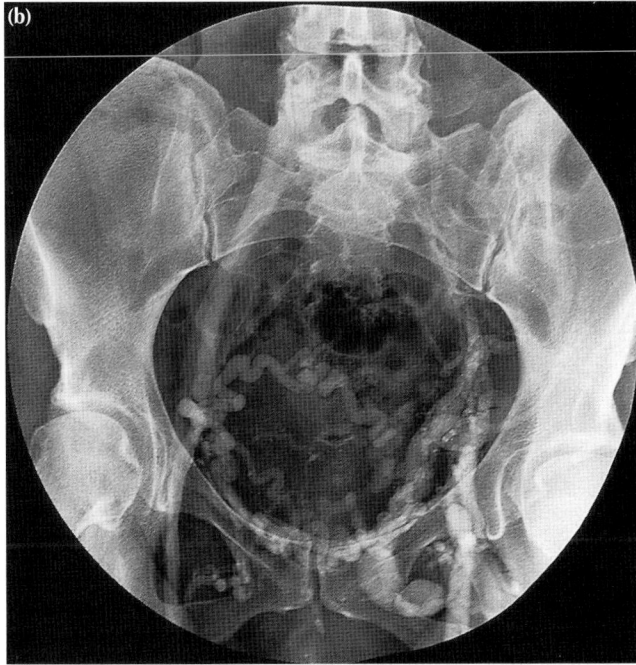

Figure 54.25 Venograms. (a) An iliac vein compression with collateral vessels. (b) An iliac vein thrombosis with cross-pubic collaterals.

Prophylaxis against pulmonary embolism

In patients who are considered at high risk of embolism or when anticoagulants are contraindicated, a vena cava filter may be inserted to prevent the onward passage of any emboli. Filters can also be placed in patients who continue to have pulmonary emboli despite adequate anticoagulation. A number of filters are now available, some of which are removable (temporary filters). There are no good randomised trials to determine which filter is best but the Greenfield filter has stood the test of time.

Superficial thrombophlebitis

This is a superficial venous thrombosis. The term 'thrombophlebitis' implies a major inflammatory component; however, this is rarely seen. Common causes include external trauma (especially to varicose veins), venepunctures and infusions of hyperosmolar solutions and drugs. The presence of an intravenous cannula for longer than 24–48 hours often leads to thrombosis. Some systemic diseases such as thromboangiitis obliterans (Buerger's disease) and malignancy, especially of the pancreas, can lead to a flitting thrombophlebitis (thrombophlebitis migrans), affecting different veins at different times. Finally, coagulation disorders such as polycythaemia, thrombocytosis and sickle cell disease are often associated, as is a concomitant thrombosis within the deep veins.

The surface vein feels solid and is tender on palpation. The overlying skin may be attached to the vein and in the early stages may be erythematous before gradually turning brown. A linear segment of vein of variable length can be easily palpated once the inflammation has died down.

A full blood count, coagulation screen and duplex scan of the deep veins should usually be obtained. Any suggestion of an associated malignancy should be investigated using appropriate endoscopy and imaging studies, such as an abdominal CT scan.

Most patients are treated with non-steroidal anti-inflammatory drugs and the condition resolves spontaneously. Rarely, infected thrombi require incision or excision. Ligation to prevent propagation into the deep veins is almost never required. Associated deep vein thrombosis or thrombophilias are treated by anticoagulation.

CONGENITAL VENOUS ANOMALIES

There are four main types of anomaly:

- aplasia;
- hypoplasia;
- duplication;
- persistence of vestigial vessels.

Aplasia is most commonly seen in the inferior vena cava and has a similar presentation to the post-thrombotic limb. Membranous occlusion of the left common iliac vein (May–Thurner–Cockett syndrome) often develops where the vein passes behind the right common iliac artery (iliac vein compression syndrome) (Fig. 54.25). This leads to an iliac vein thrombosis, which most

The Greenfield filter **was designed by L. Greenfield a 20th century American Surgeon.**
Leo Buerger, **1879–1943**, Professor of Urologic Surgery, The New York Polyclinic Medical School, New York, NY, USA, described thromboangiitis obliterans in 1908.

commonly affects the left common and external iliac veins. Membranes may also narrow the hepatic veins, which can become totally occluded, leading to Budd–Chiari syndrome.

Hypoplasia results in a narrow vein.

Duplications are quite common, with double vena cava, femoral and renal veins; they often present as an incidental finding.

Klippel–Trenaunay syndrome

This is a combined anomaly of a cutaneous naevus, persistent vestigial veins with varicose veins, and soft tissue and bone hypertrophy. The condition is a mesodermal abnormality that is not familial (Fig. 54.26).

Segments of the deep veins are often aplastic and there may be an associated obstruction of the lymphatics. The condition must be distinguished from the Parkes Weber syndrome, in which there are multiple arteriovenous fistulae causing venous hypertension, ulceration and high-output cardiac failure.

Most patients with Klippel–Trenaunay syndrome should be treated conservatively with elastic compression hosiery; however, some will benefit from laser ablation of the naevus, stapling of the bones to avoid leg length discrepancy and removal of large veins, provided the deep veins are normal. Low molecular weight heparin should be given to all patients having surgery as this syndrome is associated with an increased risk of deep vein thrombosis.

ENTRAPMENT OF VEINS

The axillary vein and the popliteal vein are the two veins that are most commonly compressed. The former is compressed at the thoracic outlet between the first rib and the clavicle, where it usually presents as an axillary vein thrombosis (see below) (Fig. 54.27a). The latter is compressed by an abnormal insertion of the gastrocnemius muscles. Entrapment may cause discomfort and swelling of the limb during exercise before thrombosis develops. Treatment is by surgical decompression, excising the first rib or dividing the abnormal musculature of the gastrocnemius insertion.

AXILLARY VEIN THROMBOSIS

Thrombosis of the axillary vein may occur following excessive exercise in a patient with an anatomically abnormal thoracic outlet. The vein may be compressed by a cervical rib if this is present (Fig. 54.27b). The arm is swollen and painful and, at an early stage, the thrombus can be removed by treatment with tissue plasminogen activator delivered through one of the arm veins. The vein must then be imaged to see if there is any compression on elevation of the arm. Thoracic outlet decompression can be carried out by resecting the cervical rib or first rib if this is confirmed.

George Budd, 1808–1882, Professor of Medicine, King's College Hospital, London, England, described this syndrome in 1845.
Hans Chiari, 1851–1916, Professor of Pathological Anatomy, Strasbourg, Germany, (Strasbourg was returned to France after the end of World War I, in 1918), gave his account of this condition in 1898.
Frederick Parkes Weber, 1863–1962, Physician, The German Hospital, Dalston, London, England.

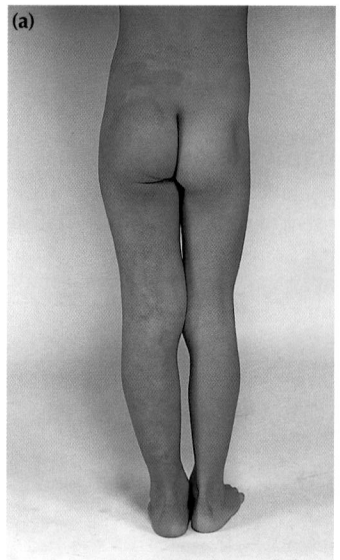

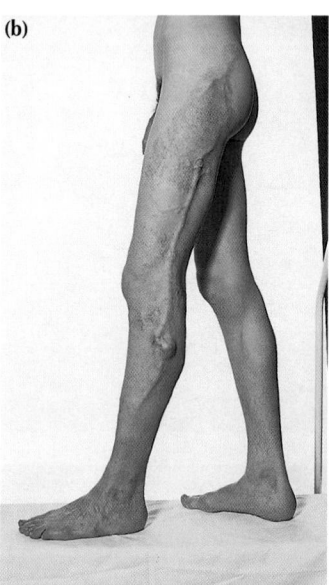

Figure 54.26 Two patients with Klippel–Trenaunay syndrome. (a) This patient has a longer leg and a capillary naevus. (b) This patient has a large lateral anomalous axial vein.

VENOUS INJURY

Blunt or penetrating trauma almost always damages some small- and medium-sized veins, which can be safely ignored or ligated without causing any problems. Larger axial venous channels have in the past been ligated when injured, but it is now recognised that these axial veins should be repaired whenever possible to reduce subsequent morbidity (pain and swelling in the tissues being drained) and limb loss when associated with a concomitant arterial injury. Many venous injuries remain undiagnosed at the time of injury, (e.g. crural vein damage associated with a fractured tibia) and only present many years later when post-thrombotic changes become apparent. Venous injuries occur from both civilian and military trauma but the incidence of venous military injuries has been particularly well documented. In total, 40–50%

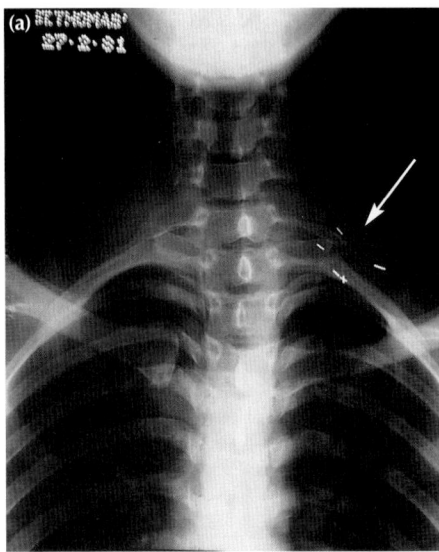

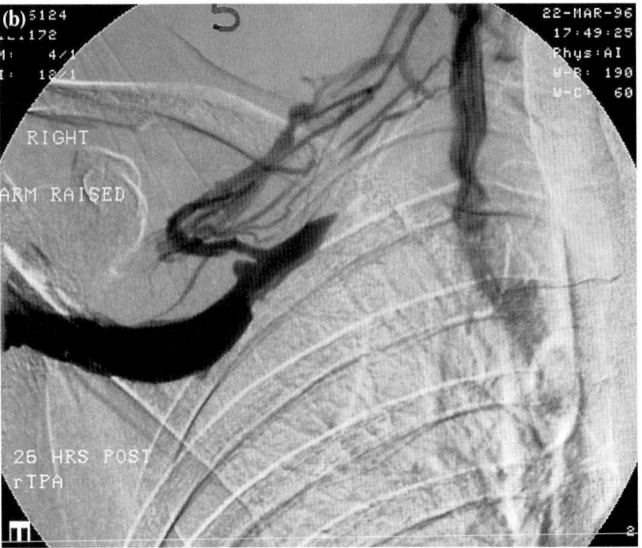

Figure 54.27 Thoracic outlet syndrome. (a) Cervical ribs; (b) elevation of the arm causing occlusion of the axillary vein with collateral fillings. The patient has had previous surgery on the left side.

of arterial injuries have concomitant venous injuries, especially in the popliteal fossa.

Classification

Venous injuries may be lacerated, contused or torn apart (stretched) (Fig. 54.28). Iatrogenic injuries result from damage at the time of surgery and from punctures caused by catheter insertion by radiologists and physicians.

Thrombosis, haemorrhage and embolisation are all common complications and arteriovenous fistulae may develop when a penetrating needle transfixes the vein and artery.

Associated injuries to soft tissue, arteries and bones often overshadow the venous injury. Massive haemorrhage from the pelvic bones or the inferior vena cava can rapidly lead to hypervolaemic shock and death if left untreated. Haematomas are common and engorgement, cyanosis and swelling are also indicative of a major venous injury.

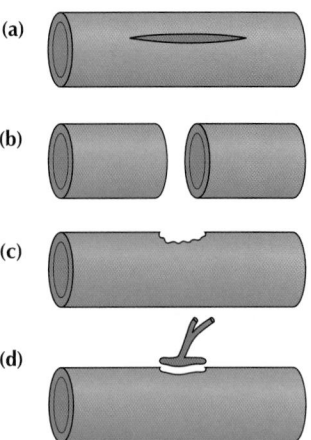

Figure 54.28 Types of venous damage. (a) Incision; (b) transection; (c) irregular laceration; (d) avulsion of a tributary.

Investigations are rarely helpful and rapid exploration is usually required. Embolisation and stent grafting can have a limited role, especially if the venous injury is relatively inaccessible or an arteriovenous fistula has developed.

The patient must be adequately resuscitated, have blood cross-matched and have good intravenous access obtained via a central venous pressure line if possible, provided that there are no injuries around the neck or thorax. Gentle wound exploration, under tourniquet control when possible, should assess the extent of the injuries before the vessels are dissected out and clamped. Different types of repair are shown in Fig. 54.29; the type of repair carried out depends on the extent of the venous injury, including how much venous wall has been lost or damaged. Lateral sutures and vein patches are ideal methods of repair and end-to-end anastomosis is satisfactory provided that it is not carried out under tension.

Vein replacement should be by autogenous tissue whenever possible, using vein harvested from another site, e.g. the internal jugular vein or the long saphenous vein from an undamaged limb. Artificial grafts with polytetrafluoroethylene (PTFE) are likely to get infected in contaminated wounds and have given poor results in recent conflicts. The use of anticoagulants and an arteriovenous fistula to reduce the risk of thrombosis in the vein graft are controversial and depend on the associated injuries that are present. In contaminated wounds, tetanus, toxoid and antibiotics should be given. A fasciotomy should always be considered if there is a concomitant arterial and venous injury.

Prognosis

It is now recognised that repair of a major axial vein can be carried out with a 70–80% success rate, reducing the morbidity of a combined arterial and venous injury considerably (especially limb loss). Complex repairs should not, however, be carried out if a patient's life is at risk, when ligation may have to suffice in the short term.

VENOUS TUMOURS

Cystic degeneration of the vein wall is an uncommon cause of venous occlusion. It may be detected by ultrasound. The cyst may be de-roofed or the venous segment excised.

CHAPTER 54 | VENOUS DISORDERS

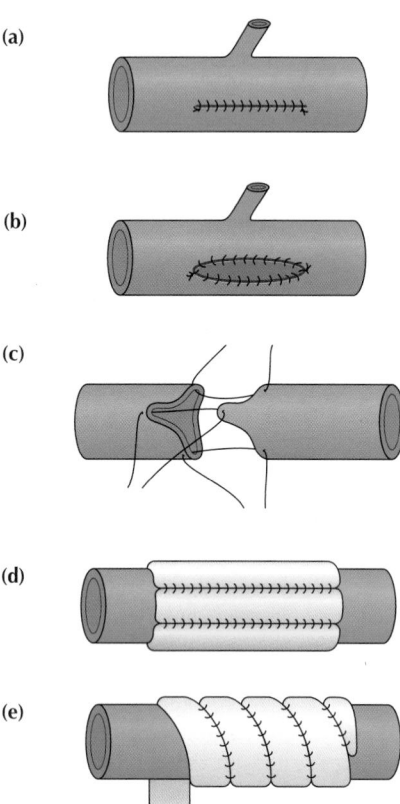

Figure 54.29 Types of venous repair. (a) Lateral suture; (b) patch graft; (c) Carrel triangulation technique of venous anastomosis; (d) panel graft; (e) spiral graft.

Venous malformation cavernous angioma/haemangioma

These malformations are common, often affecting the skin but also extending into the deep tissues, including bones and joints. They usually present with variable swelling and dilated veins beneath the skin. Occasionally, there is no visible mass and the complaint is one of pain. Haemorrhage and thrombophlebitis may exacerbate the pain. A soft compressible mass, which is venous in colour especially if it is under the skin, is usually present (Fig. 54.30a). A dark blue tinge is often apparent even if the malformation is deeply situated. Nodules within the mass usually represent previous episodes of thrombosis. The size and extent of the haemangioma are best visualised by nuclear magnetic resonance with a short tau inversion recovery (STIR) sequence (Fig. 54.30b) or CT scanning with contrast enhancement. Venography rarely shows an abnormality, but direct puncture with contrast injection shows the connections of the malformation.

Treatment options include surgical excision or sclerotherapy. Neither of these is entirely curative because it is difficult to remove all of the angiomatous tissue or sclerose the angioma completely. Sclerosis can be dangerous when the veins connect to the deep system.

Leiomyomas and leiomyosarcomas of the vein wall

These are extremely rare tumours that are usually slow growing. They present with pain and a mass with signs of venous obstruction,

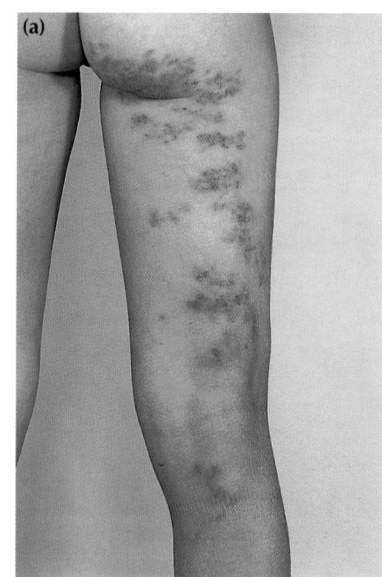

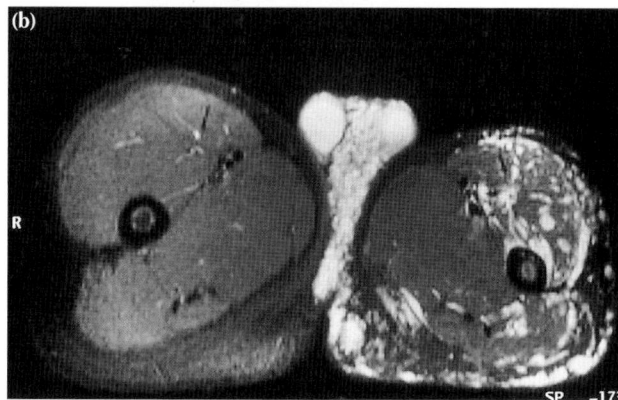

Figure 54.30 (a) Venous angioma of the leg. (b) Magnetic resonance with a short tau inversion recovery sequence showing angioma in white throughout the limb.

e.g. oedema and distended veins. Duplex scanning, CT (Fig. 54.31) and magnetic resonance imaging show a filling defect within the vein wall. Treatment is by resection with replacement by autogenous vein taken from another site. Rarely, a PTFE graft is required. When the tumour affects the vena cava it must be resected and replaced with a prosthetic graft.

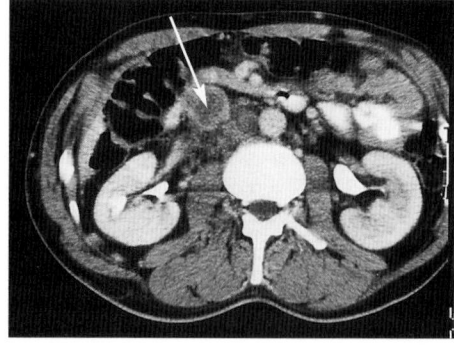

Figure 54.31 Inferior vena cava containing a filling defect from a leiomyosarcoma.

FURTHER READING

Bergan, J.J. and Kistner, R.L. (1992) *Atlas of Venous Surgery*. WB Saunders, Philadelphia, PA.

Bradbury, A., Evans, C., Allan, P., Lee, A., Ruckley, C.V. and Fowkes, F.G.R. (1999) What are the symptoms of varicose veins? Edinburgh Vein Study Cross-sectional Population Survey. *Br Med J* **318:** 353–6.

Browse, N.L. and Burnand, K.G. (1982) The cause of venous ulceration. *Lancet* **2:** 243–5.

Browse, N.L., Burnand, K.G., Irvine, A.T. and Wilson, N. (1999) *Diseases of the Veins*, 2nd edn. Arnold, London.

Callan, M.J., Ruckley, C.V., Harper, D.R. and Dale, J.J. (1985) Chronic venous ulceration of the leg: extent of the problem and provision of care. *Br Med J* **290:** 1855–6.

Cockett, F.B. (1956)The pathology and treatment of venous ulcers of the leg. *Br J Surg* **44:** 260–78.

Coleridge-Smith, P.D., Thomas, P., Scurr, J.H. and Dormandy, J.A. (1988) Causes of venous ulceration: a new hypothesis. *Br Med J* **296:** 1726–7.

Dodd, H. and Cockett, F.B. (1956) *The Pathology and Surgery of Veins of the Lower Limb*. EOS Livingstone, London.

Falanga, V. and Eaglestein, W.H. (1993) The 'trap' hypothesis of venous ulceration. *Lancet* **341:** 1006–8.

Gloviczki, P. and Bergan, J.J. (1998) *Atlas of Endoscopic Vein Surgery*. Springer, London.

Gloviczki, P. and Yao, J.S.T. (eds) (2001) *Handbook of Venous Disorders*, 2nd edn. Arnold: London.

Goldman, M.P., Bergan, J.J. and Guex, J.J. (2007) *Sclerotherapy*, 4th edn. Elsevier/Mosby, Philadelphia, PA.

Hill, R.D., Raskob, G.E. and Pineo, G.F. (1996) *Venous Thromboembolism. An Evidence-based Atlas*. Futura Armonk, London.

Hobson, R.W., Rich, N.M. and Wright, C.B. (1983) *Venous Trauma: Pathophysiology, Diagnosis and Surgical Management*. Futura Publishing, Mt Kisco, NY.

Venous Forum (1995) Classification and grading of chronic venous disease: a consensus statement. *J Vasc Surg* **21:** 635–45.

Lymphatic disorders

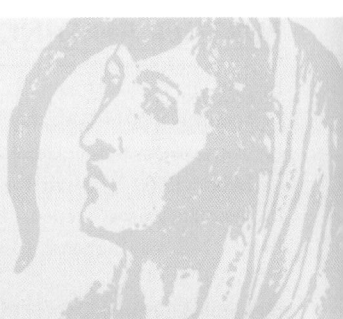

LEARNING OBJECTIVES

To understand:
- The main functions of the lymphatic system
- The development of the lymphatic system
- The various causes of limb swelling
- The aetiology, clinical features, investigations and treatment of lymphoedema

INTRODUCTION

The lymphatic system was first described by Erasistratus in Alexandria more than 2000 years ago. William Hunter, in the late eighteenth century, was the first to describe the function of the lymphatic system. Starling's pioneering work on the hydrostatic and haemodynamic forces controlling the movement of fluid across the capillary provided further insights into the function of the lymphatics. However, there is much about the lymphatic system that is not understood and debate continues over the precise aetiology of the most common abnormality of the system, namely lymphoedema.

ANATOMY AND PHYSIOLOGY OF THE LYMPHATIC SYSTEM

Functions

The principal function of the lymphatics is the return of protein-rich fluid to the circulation through the lymphaticovenous junctions in the jugular area. Thus, water, electrolytes, low-molecular-weight moieties (polypeptides, cytokines, growth factors) and macromolecules (fibrinogen, albumin, globulins, coagulation and fibrinolytic factors) from the interstitial fluid (ISF) return to the circulation via the lymphatics. Intestinal lymph (chyle) transports cholesterol, long-chain fatty acids, triglycerides and the fat-soluble vitamins (A, D, E and K) directly to the circulation, bypassing the liver. Lymphocytes and other immune cells also circulate within the lymphatic system.

Development and macroanatomy

In the human embryo lymph sacs develop at 6–7 weeks' gestation as four cystic spaces, one on either side of the neck and one in each groin. These cisterns enlarge and develop communications that permit lymph from the lower limbs and abdomen to drain via the cisterna chyli into the thoracic duct, which in turn drains into the left internal jugular vein at its confluence with the left subclavian vein. Lymph from the head and right arm drains via a separate lymphatic trunk, the right lymphatic duct, into the right internal jugular vein. Lymphatics accompany veins everywhere except in the cortical bony skeleton and central nervous system, although the brain and retina possess cerebrospinal fluid and aqueous humour respectively. The lymphatic system comprises lymphatic channels, lymphoid organs (lymph nodes, spleen, Peyer's patches, thymus, tonsils) and circulating elements (lymphocytes and other mononuclear immune cells). Lymphatic endothelial cells are derived from embryonic veins in the jugular and perimesonephric areas from where they migrate to form the primary lymph sacs and plexus. Both transcription (e.g. Prox1) and growth (e.g. VEGF-C) factors are essential for these developmental events.

Microanatomy and physiology

Lymphatic capillaries

Lymphatics originate within the ISF space from specialised endothelialised capillaries (initial lymphatics) or non-endothelialised channels such as the spaces of Disse in the liver. Initial lymphatics are unlike arteriovenous capillaries in that:

- they are blind-ended;
- they are much larger (50 mm);
- they allow the entry of molecules of up to 1000 kDa in size because the basement membrane is fenestrated, tenuous or even absent and the endothelium itself possesses intra- and intercellular pores;
- they are anchored to interstitial matrix by filaments. In the resting state, initial lymphatics are collapsed. When ISF volume and pressure increases, initial lymphatics and their pores are held open by these filaments to facilitate increased drainage.

Erasistratus of Chios c.300–250 B.C. of the Medical School at Alexandria in Egypt is regarded by many as the first Physiologist.
William Hunter, 1718–1783, Anatomist and Obstetrician who became the first Professor of Anatomy at the Royal Academy of Arts, London, England. He was the elder brother of John Hunter the Anatomist and Surgeon.
Ernest Henry Starling, 1866–1927, Professor of Physiology, University College, London, England.

Johann Conrad Peyer, 1653–1712, Professor of Logic, Rhetoric and Medicine, Schaffhausen, Switzerland, described the lymph follicles in the intestine (Peyer's Patches) in 1677.
Josef Disse, 1852–1912, a German Anatomist.

Terminal lymphatics

Initial lymphatics drain into terminal (collecting) lymphatics that possess bicuspid valves and endothelial cells rich in the contractile protein actin. Larger collecting lymphatics are surrounded by smooth muscle. Valves partition the lymphatics into segments (lymphangions) that contract sequentially to propel lymph into the lymph trunks.

Lymph trunks

Terminal lymphatics lead to lymph trunks, which have a structure similar to that of veins, namely a single layer of endothelial cells, lying on a basement membrane overlying a media comprising smooth muscle cells that are innervated with sympathetic, parasympathetic and sensory nerve endings. About 10% of lymph arising from a limb is transported in deep lymphatic trunks that accompany the main neurovascular bundles. The majority, however, is conducted against venous flow from deep to superficial in epifascial lymph trunks. Superficial trunks form lymph bundles of various sizes, which are located within strips of adipose tissue, and tend to follow the course of the major superficial veins.

Starling's forces

The distribution of fluid and protein between the vascular system and ISF depends on the balance of hydrostatic and oncotic pressures between the two compartments (Starling's forces), together with the relative impermeability of the blood capillary membrane to molecules over 70 kDa. In health there is net capillary filtration, which is removed by the lymphatic system.

Transport of particles

Particles enter the initial lymphatics through interendothelial openings and vesicular transport through intraendothelial pores. Large particles are actively phagocytosed by macrophages and transported through the lymphatic system intracellularly.

Mechanisms of lymph transport

Resting ISF is negative (-2 to $-6\,mmH_2O$), whereas lymphatic pressures are positive, indicating that lymph flows against a small pressure gradient. It is believed that prograde lymphatic flow depends upon three mechanisms:

1. transient increases in interstitial pressure secondary to muscular contraction and external compression;
2. the sequential contraction and relaxation of lymphangions;
3. the prevention of reflux because of valves.

Lymphangions are believed to respond to increased lymph flow in much the same way as the heart responds to increased venous return in that they increase their contractility and stroke volume. Contractility is also enhanced by noradrenaline, serotonin, certain prostaglandins and thromboxanes, and endothelin-1. Pressures of up to 30–50 mmHg have been recorded in normal lymph trunks and up to 200 mmHg in severe lymphoedema. Lymphatics may also modulate their own contractility through the production of nitric oxide and other local mediators. Transport in the thoracic and right lymph ducts also depends upon intrathoracic (respiration) and central venous (cardiac cycle) pressures. Therefore, cardiorespiratory disease may have an adverse effect on lymphatic function.

In summary, in the healthy limb, lymph flow is largely due to intrinsic lymphatic contractility, although this is augmented by exercise, limb movement and external compression. However, in lymphoedema, when the lymphatics are constantly distended with lymph, these external forces assume a much more important functional role.

ACUTE INFLAMMATION OF THE LYMPHATICS

Acute lymphangitis is an infection, often caused by *Streptococcus pyogenes* or *Staphylococcus aureus*, which spreads to the draining lymphatics and lymph nodes (lymphadenitis) where an abscess may form. Eventually this may progress to bacteraemia or septicaemia. The normal signs of infection (rubor, calor, dolor) are present and a red streak is seen in the skin along the line of the inflamed lymphatic (Fig. 55.1). The part should be rested to reduce lymphatic drainage and elevated to reduce swelling, and the patient should be treated with intravenous antibiotics based upon actual or suspected sensitivities. Failure to improve within 48 hours suggests inappropriate antibiotic therapy, the presence of undrained pus or the presence of an underlying systemic disorder (malignancy, immunodeficiency). The lymphatic damage caused by acute lymphangitis may lead to recurrent attacks of infection and lymphoedema; patients with lymphoedema are prone to so-called acute inflammatory episodes (see below).

LYMPHOEDEMA

Definition

Lymphoedema may be defined as abnormal limb swelling caused by the accumulation of increased amounts of high protein ISF secondary to defective lymphatic drainage in the presence of (near) normal net capillary filtration.

The scope of the clinical problem

At birth, 1 in 6000 persons will develop lymphoedema with an overall prevalence of 0.13–2%. The condition is not only associated with significant physical symptoms and complications but is also a frequent cause of emotional and psychological distress, which can lead to difficulties with relationships, education and work (Summary box 55.1).

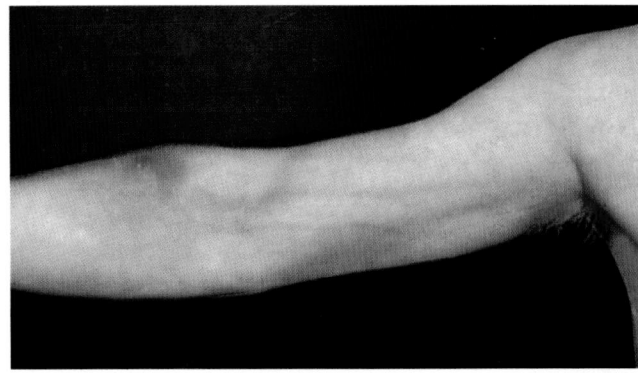

Figure 55.1 Acute lymphangitis of the arm. Erythematous streaks extend from the site of primary infection on the volar aspect of the forearm to epicondylar nodes at the elbow and from there to enlarged and tender axillary lymph nodes.

Summary box 55.1

Symptoms frequently experienced by patients with lymphoedema

- Constant dull ache, even severe pain
- Burning and bursting sensations
- General tiredness and debility
- Sensitivity to heat
- 'Pins and needles'
- Cramp
- Skin problems including flakiness, weeping, excoriation and breakdown
- Immobility, leading to obesity and muscle wasting
- Backache and joint problems
- Athlete's foot
- Acute infective episodes

Despite this significant impact on quality of life, many sufferers choose not to seek medical advice because of embarrassment and a belief that nothing can be done. Patients who do come forward for help, especially those with non-cancer-related lymphoedema, often find they have limited access to appropriate expertise and treatment. Lymphoedema is often misdiagnosed and mistreated by doctors, who frequently have a poor understanding of the importance of the condition, believing it to be primarily a cosmetic problem in the early stages. However, making an early diagnosis is important because relatively simple measures can be highly effective at this stage and can prevent the development of disabling late disease, which is often very difficult to treat. It is also an opportunity for patients to make contact with patient support groups (Summary box 55.2).

Summary box 55.2

What every patient with lymphoedema should receive

- An explanation of why the limb is swollen and the underlying cause
- Guidance on skin hygiene and care and the avoidance of acute infective episodes
- Anti-fungal prophylactic therapy to prevent athlete's foot
- Rapid access to antibiotic therapy if necessary, hospital admission for acute infective episodes
- Appropriate instructions regarding exercise therapy
- Manual lymphatic drainage (MLD)
- Multilayer lymphoedema bandaging (MLLB)
- Compression garments and, if appropriate, specialised footwear
- Advice on diet
- Access to support services and networks

The severity of unilateral limb lymphoedema can be classified as:

- mild: < 20% excess limb volume;
- moderate: 20–40% excess limb volume;
- severe: > 40% excess limb volume.

Pathophysiology

The ISF compartment (10–12 litres in a 70-kg man) constitutes 50% of the wet weight of the skin and subcutaneous tissues and, in order for oedema to be clinically detectable, its volume has to double. About 8 litres (protein concentration approximately $20–30\,g\,l^{-1}$, similar to ISF) of lymph is produced each day and travels in afferent lymphatics to lymph nodes. There, the volume is halved and the protein concentration doubled, resulting in 4 litres of lymph re-entering the venous circulation each day via efferent lymphatics. In one sense, all oedema is lymphoedema in that it results from an inability of the lymphatic system to clear the ISF compartment. However, in most types of oedema this is because the capillary filtration rate is pathologically high and overwhelms a normal lymphatic system, resulting in the accumulation of low-protein oedema fluid. In contrast, in true lymphoedema, when the primary problem is in the lymphatics, capillary filtration is normal and the oedema fluid is relatively high in protein. Of course, in a significant number of patients with oedema there is both abnormal capillary filtration and abnormal lymphatic drainage, as in chronic venous insufficiency (CVI) for example.

Lymphoedema results from lymphatic aplasia, hypoplasia, dysmotility (reduced contractility with or without valvular insufficiency), obliteration by inflammatory, infective or neoplastic processes, or surgical extirpation. Whatever the primary abnormality, the resultant physical and/or functional obstruction leads to lymphatic hypertension and distension, with further secondary impairment of contractility and valvular competence. Lymphostasis and lymphotension lead to the accumulation in the ISF of fluid, proteins, growth factors and other active peptide moieties, glycosaminoglycans and particulate matter, including bacteria. As a consequence, there is increased collagen production by fibroblasts, an accumulation of inflammatory cells (predominantly macrophages and lymphocytes) and activation of keratinocytes. The end result is protein-rich oedema fluid, increased deposition of ground substance, subdermal fibrosis and dermal thickening and proliferation. Lymphoedema, unlike all other types of oedema, is confined to the epifascial space. Although muscle compartments may be hypertrophied because of the increased work involved in limb movement, they are characteristically free of oedema.

Classification

Two main types of lymphoedema are recognised:

1 *primary lymphoedema*, in which the cause is unknown (or at least uncertain and unproven); it is thought to be caused by 'congenital lymphatic dysplasia';
2 *secondary or acquired lymphoedema*, in which there is a clear underlying cause.

Primary lymphoedema is usually further subdivided on the basis of the presence of family, age of onset and lymphangiographic findings (Tables 55.1 and 55.2) (see below).

Risk factors for lymphoedema

Although the true risk factor profile for lymphoedema is not currently known, a number of factors are thought to predispose an individual to its development and predict progression, severity and outcome of the condition (Table 55.3).

Symptoms and signs

In most cases, the diagnosis of primary or secondary lymphoedema can be made and the condition can be differentiated from other causes of a swollen limb on the basis of history and examination without recourse to complex investigation (Table 55.4). Unlike other types of oedema, lymphoedema characteristically

Table 55.1 Aetiological classification of lymphoedema

Primary lymphoedema	Congenital (onset < 2 years old): sporadic; familial (Nonne–Milroy's disease)
	Praecox (onset 2–35 years old): sporadic; familial (Letessier–Meige's disease)
	Tarda (onset after 35 years old)
Secondary lymphoedema	Parasitic infection (filariasis)
	Fungal infection (tinea pedis)
	Exposure to foreign body material (silica particles)
	Primary lymphatic malignancy
	Metastatic spread to lymph nodes
	Radiotherapy to lymph nodes
	Surgical excision of lymph nodes
	Trauma (particularly degloving injuries)
	Superficial thrombophlebitis
	Deep venous thrombosis

Table 55.2 Clinical classification of lymphoedema

Grade (Brunner)	Clinical features
Subclinical (latent)	There is excess interstitial fluid and histological abnormalities in lymphatics and lymph nodes, but no clinically apparent lymphoedema
I	Oedema pits on pressure and swelling largely or completely disappears on elevation and bed rest
II	Oedema does not pit and does not significantly reduce upon elevation
III	Oedema is associated with irreversible skin changes, i.e. fibrosis, papillae

involves the foot (Fig. 55.2). The contour of the ankle is lost through infilling of the submalleolar depressions, a 'buffalo hump' forms on the dorsum of the foot, the toes appear 'square' because of confinement of footwear and the skin on the dorsum of the toes cannot be pinched because of subcutaneous fibrosis (Stemmer's sign). Lymphoedema usually spreads proximally to knee level and less commonly affects the whole leg (Fig. 55.3). In the early stages, lymphoedema will 'pit' and the patient will report that the swelling is down in the morning. This represents a reversible component to the swelling, which can be controlled.

Failure to do so allows fibrosis, dermal thickening and hyperkeratosis to occur. In general, primary lymphoedema progresses more slowly than secondary lymphoedema. Chronic eczema, fungal infection of the skin (dermatophytosis) and nails (onychomycosis), fissuring, verrucae and papillae (warts) are frequently seen in advanced disease. Ulceration is unusual, except in the presence of chronic venous insufficiency.

Lymphangiomas are dilated dermal lymphatics that 'blister' onto the skin surface. The fluid is usually clear but may be blood-stained. In the long term, lymphangiomas thrombose and fibrose, forming hard nodules that may raise concerns about malignancy. If lymphangiomas are < 5 cm across, they are termed lymphangioma circumscriptum, and if they are more widespread, they are termed lymphangioma diffusum. If they form a reticulate pattern of ridges then it has been termed lymphoedema *ab igne*.

Table 55.3 Risk factors for lymphoedema

Upper limb/trunk lymphoedema	Lower limb lymphoedema
Surgery with axillary lymph node dissection, particularly if extensive breast or lymph node surgery	Surgery with inguinal lymph node dissection
Scar formation, fibrosis and radiodermatitis from postoperative axillary radiotherapy	Postoperative pelvic radiotherapy
Radiotherapy to the breast or to the axillary, internal mammary or subclavicular lymph nodes	Recurrent soft tissue infection at the same site
Drain/wound complications or infection	Obesity
Cording (axillary web syndrome)	Varicose vein stripping and vein harvesting
Seroma formation	Genetic predisposition/family history of chronic oedema
Advanced cancer	Advanced cancer
Obesity	Intrapelvic or intra-abdominal tumours that involve or directly compress lymphatic vessels
Congenital predisposition	Orthopaedic surgery
Trauma in an 'at-risk' arm (venepuncture, blood pressure measurement, injection)	Poor nutritional status
Chronic skin disorders and inflammation	Thrombophlebitis and chronic venous insufficiency, particularly post-thrombotic syndrome
Hypertension	Any unresolved asymmetrical oedema
Taxane chemotherapy	Chronic skin disorders and inflammation
Insertion of pacemaker	Concurrent illnesses such as phlebitis, hyperthyroidism, kidney or cardiac disease
Arteriovenous shunt for dialysis	Immobilisation and prolonged limb dependency
Air travel	Air travel
Living in or visiting an area for endemic lymphatic filariasis	Living in or visiting an area for endemic lymphatic filariasis

Reproduced with permission from: Lymphoedema Framework. *Best Practice Management of Lymphoedema*. International Consensus. London: MEP Ltd, 2006. © MEP Ltd 2006.

ab igne **is Latin for 'from fire'.**

Table 55.4 Differential diagnosis of the swollen limb

Non-vascular or lymphatic	General disease states	Cardiac failure from any cause
		Liver failure
		Hypoproteinaemia due to nephrotic syndrome, malabsorption, protein-losing enteropathy
		Hypothyroidism (myxoedema)
		Allergic disorders, including angioedema and idiopathic cyclic oedema
		Prolonged immobility and lower limb dependency
	Local disease processes	Ruptured Baker's cyst
		Myositis ossificans
		Bony or soft-tissue tumours
		Arthritis
		Haemarthrosis
		Calf muscle haematoma
		Achilles tendon rupture
	Retroperitoneal fibrosis	May lead to arterial, venous and lymphatic abnormalities
	Gigantism	Rare
		All tissues are uniformly enlarged
	Drugs	Corticosteroids, oestrogens, progestagens
		Monoamine oxidase inhibitors, phenylbutazone, methyldopa, hydralazine, nifedipine
	Trauma	Painful swelling due to reflex sympathetic dystrophy
	Obesity	Lipodystrophy
		Lipoidosis
Venous	Deep venous thrombosis	There may be an obvious predisposing factor, such as recent surgery
		The classical signs of pain and redness may be absent
	Post-thrombotic syndrome	Swelling, usually of the whole leg, due to iliofemoral venous obstruction
		Venous skin changes, secondary varicose veins on the leg and collateral veins on the lower abdominal wall
		Venous claudication may be present
	Varicose veins	Simple primary varicose veins are rarely the cause of significant leg swelling
	Klippel–Trenaunay's syndrome and other malformations	Rare
		Present at birth or develops in early childhood
		Comprises an abnormal lateral venous complex, capillary naevus, bony abnormalities, hypo(a)plasia of deep veins and limb lengthening
		Lymphatic abnormalities often coexist
	External venous compression	Pelvic or abdominal tumour including the gravid uterus
		Retroperitoneal fibrosis
	Ischaemia–reperfusion	Following lower limb revascularisation for chronic and particularly chronic ischaemia
Arterial	Arteriovenous malformation	May be associated with local or generalised swelling
	Aneurysm	Popliteal
		Femoral
		False aneurysm following (iatrogenic) trauma

Lymphangiomas frequently weep (lymphorrhoea, chylorrhoea), causing skin maceration, and they act as a portal for infection. Protein-losing diarrhoea, chylous ascites, chylothorax, chyluria and discharge from lymphangiomas suggest lymphangectasia (megalymphatics) and chylous reflux.

Ulceration, non-healing bruises and raised purple-red nodules should lead to suspicion of malignancy. Lymphangiosarcoma was originally described in post-mastectomy oedema (Stewart–Treves'

syndrome) and affects around 0.5% of patients at a mean onset of 10 years. However, lymphangiosarcoma can develop in any long-standing lymphoedema, but usually takes longer to manifest (20 years). It presents as single or multiple bluish/red skin and subcutaneous nodules that spread to form satellite lesions, which may then become confluent. The diagnosis is usually made late and confirmed by skin biopsy. Amputation offers the best chance of survival but, even then, most patients live for less than 3 years. It has been suggested that lymphoedema leads to an impairment of immune surveillance and so predisposes to other malignancies, although the causal association is not as definite as it is for lymphangiosarcoma (Summary box 55.3).

William Morrant Baker, 1839–1896, Surgeon, St. Bartholomew's Hospital, London, England, described these cysts in 1877.
Fred Waldorf Stewart, 1894–1991, an American Physician.
Norman Treves, 1894–1964, an American Surgeon.
Stewart and Treves reported this condition in a joint paper in 1948.

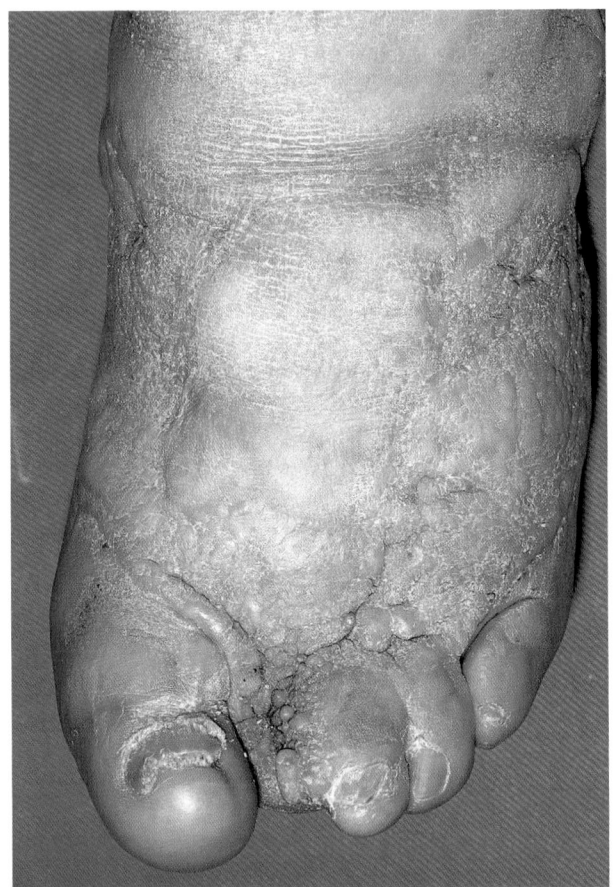

Figure 55.2 The foot of a patient with typical lymphoedema.

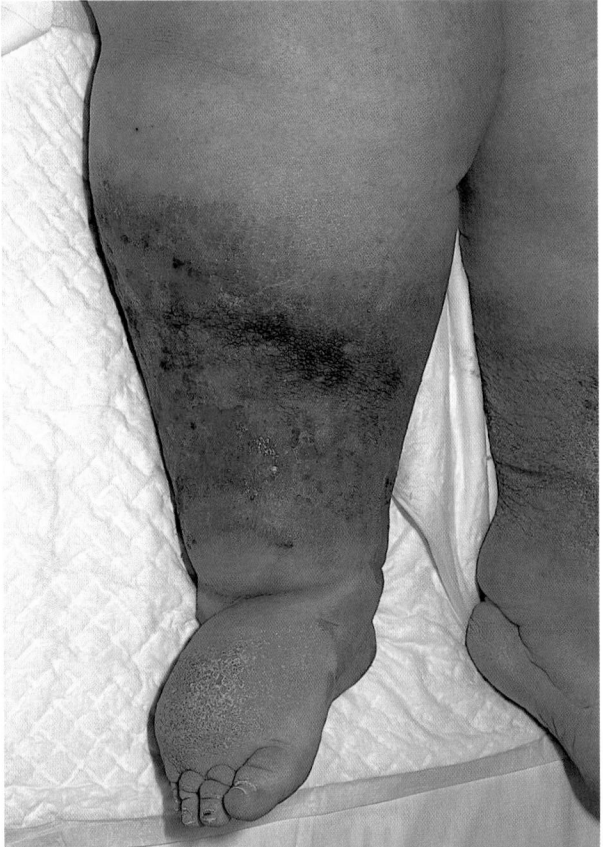

Figure 55.3 The lower leg of a patient with typical lymphoedema.

Summary box 55.3

Malignancies associated with lymphoedema

■ Lymphangiosarcoma (Stewart–Treves' syndrome)
■ Kaposi's sarcoma [human immunodeficiency virus (HIV)]
■ Squamous cell carcinoma
■ Liposarcoma
■ Malignant melanoma
■ Malignant fibrous histiocytoma
■ Basal cell carcinoma
■ Lymphoma

PRIMARY LYMPHOEDEMA

Aetiology

It has been proposed that all cases of primary lymphoedema are due to an inherited abnormality of the lymphatic system, sometimes termed 'congenital lymphatic dysplasia'. However, it is possible that many sporadic cases of primary lymphoedema occur in the presence of a (near-)normal lymphatic system and are actually examples of secondary lymphoedema for which the triggering events have gone unrecognised. These might include seemingly trivial (but repeated) bacterial and/or fungal infections, insect bites, barefoot walking (silica), deep venous thrombosis (DVT) or episodes of superficial thrombophlebitis. In animal models, simple excision of lymph nodes and/or trunks leads to acute lymphoedema, which resolves within a few weeks,

presumably because of the development of collaterals. The human condition can only be mimicked by inducing extensive lymphatic obliteration and fibrosis. Even then, there may be considerable delay between the injury and the onset of oedema. Primary lymphoedema is much more common in the legs than the arms. This may be because of gravity and a bipedal posture, the fact that the lymphatic system of the leg is less well developed, or the increased susceptibility of the leg to trauma and/or infection. Furthermore, loss of the venoarteriolar reflex (VAR), which protects lower limb capillaries from excessive hydrostatic forces in the erect posture, with age and disease (CVI, diabetes), may be important.

Classification

Primary lymphoedema is usually classified on the basis of apparent genetic susceptibility, age of onset or lymphangiographic findings. None of these is ideal and the various classification systems in existence can appear confusing and conflicting as various terms and eponyms are used loosely and interchangeably. This has hampered research and efforts to gain a better understanding of underlying mechanisms, the effectiveness of therapy and prognosis.

Genetic susceptibility

Primary lymphoedema is often subdivided into those cases in which there appears to be a genetic susceptibility or element to the disease, and those in which there is not. The former may be further divided into those cases that are familial (hereditary), when typically the only abnormality is lymphoedema and there is a family history, and those cases that are syndromic, when the lymphoedema is only one of several congenital abnormalities and is either inherited or sporadic. Syndromic lymphoedema may be sporadic and chromosomal [Turner's (XO karyotype), Klinefelter's (XXY), Down's (trisomy 21) syndrome] or clearly inherited and related to an identified or presumed single-gene defect [lymphoedema–distichiasis (autosomal dominant)], or of uncertain genetic aetiology (yellow-nail and Klippel–Trenaunay–Weber's syndromes). Familial (hereditary) lymphoedema can be difficult to distinguish from non-familial lymphoedema because a reliable family history may be unobtainable, the nature of the genetic predisposition is unknown and the genetic susceptibility may only translate into clinical disease in the presence of certain environmental factors. Although the distinction may not directly affect treatment, the patients are often concerned lest they be 'passing on' the disease to their children.

Two main forms of familial (hereditary) lymphoedema are recognised – Nonne–Milroy (type I) and Letessier–Meige (type II) – although it is likely that both eponymous diseases overlap and represent more than a single disease entity and genetic abnormality. Milroy's disease is estimated to be present in 1:6000 live births and is probably inherited in an autosomal dominant manner with incomplete (about 50%) penetrance. In some families, the condition may be related to abnormalities in the gene coding for a vascular endothelial growth factor (VEGF) on chromosome 5. The disease is characterised by brawny lymphoedema of both legs (and sometimes the genitalia, arms and face), which develops from birth or before puberty. The disease has been associated with a wide range of lymphatic abnormalities on lymphangiography. Meige's disease is similar to Milroy's disease, except that the lymphoedema generally develops between puberty and middle age (50 years). It usually affects one or both legs but may involve the arms. Some, but not all, cases appear to be inherited in an autosomal dominant manner. Lymphangiography generally shows aplasia or hypoplasia.

Age of onset

Lymphoedema congenita (onset at or within 2 years of birth) is more common in males and is more likely to be bilateral and involve the whole leg. Lymphoedema praecox (onset from 2 to 35 years) is three times more common in females, has a peak incidence shortly after menarche, is three times more likely to be unilateral than bilateral and usually only extends to the knee. Lymphoedema tarda develops, by definition, after the age of 35 years and is often associated with obesity, with lymph nodes being

replaced with fibrofatty tissue. The cause is unknown. Lymphoedema developing for the first time after 50 years should prompt a thorough search for underlying (pelvic, genitalia) malignancy. It is worth noting that, in such patients, lymphoedema often commences proximally in the thigh rather than distally (Fig. 55.4).

Lymphangiographic classification

Browse has classified primary lymphoedema on the basis of lymphangiographic findings (Table 55.5 and Figs 55.5 and 55.6). These findings may be related to the clinical presentations described above. Some patients with lymphatic hyperplasia possess megalymphatics in which lymph or chyle refluxes freely under the effects of gravity against the physiological direction of flow. The megalymphatics usually end in thin-walled vesicles on the skin, serous surfaces (chylous ascites, chylothorax), intestine (protein-losing enteropathy), kidney or bladder (chyluria) (Fig. 55.7).

SECONDARY LYMPHOEDEMA

This is the most common form of lymphoedema. There are several well-recognised causes including infection, inflammation, neoplasia and trauma (Table 55.6).

Filariasis

This is the most common cause of lymphoedema worldwide, affecting up to 100 million individuals. It is particularly prevalent in Africa, India and South America where 5–10% of the population may be affected. The viviparous nematode *Wucheria bancrofti*, whose only host is man, is responsible for 90% of cases and is spread by the mosquito. The disease is associated with poor sanitation. The parasite enters lymphatics from the blood and lodges in lymph nodes, where it causes fibrosis and obstruction, due

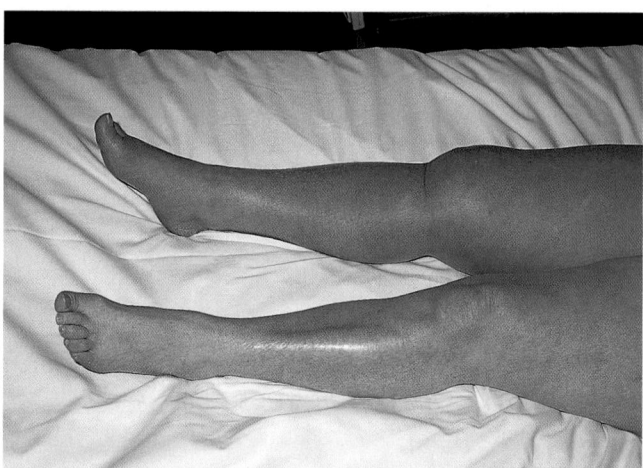

Figure 55.4 This patient, in her sixth decade, presented with rapid onset of lymphoedema of the right leg. On further investigation she was found to have locally advanced bladder carcinoma. Note that unlike most cases of lymphoedema the swelling is greater proximally than distally.

Henry Hubert Turner, 1892–1970, Professor of Medicine, The University of Oklahoma, OK, USA.
Harry Fitch Klinefelter, Jr. B. 1912, Associate Professor of Medicine, The Johns Hopkins University Medical School, Baltimore MD, USA, described this syndrome in 1942.
John Langdon Haydon Down, (sometimes given as Langdon-Down), 1828–1896, Physician, The London Hospital, London, England.
Maurice Klippel, 1858–1942, Neurologist, La Sêlpetrière, Paris, France.
Paul Trenaunay, B. 1875, a French Neurologist.
Klippel and Trenaunay described this condition in a joint paper in 1900.
Frederick Parkes Weber, 1863–1962, Physician, The German Hospital, Dalston, London, England.
Max Nonne, 1861–1959, a Neurologist of Hamburg, Germany, described this disease in 1891.
William Forsyth Milroy, 1855–1942, Professor of Clinical Medicine, Columbia University, New York, NY, USA, described the condition in 1892.
Henri Meige, 1866–1940, Physician, La Salpêtrière, Paris, France, gave his description of the disease in 1899.

Sir Norman Leslie Browse, Formerly Professor of Surgery, The United Medical and Dental Schools of Guy's and St. Thomas's Hospitals, London, England.
Otto Eduard Heinrich Wucherer, 1820–1873, a German Physician who practised in Brazil, South America.
Sir Joseph Bancroft, 1836–1894, an English Physician and Epidemiologist who worked in Brisbane, Queensland, Australia.

Table 55.5 Lymphangiographic classification of primary lymphoedema

	Congenital hyperplasia (10%)	Distal obliteration (80%)	Proximal obliteration (10%)
Age of onset	Congenital	Puberty (praecox)	Any age
Sex distribution	Male > female	Female > male	Male = female
Extent	Whole leg	Ankle, calf	Whole leg, thigh only
Laterality	Unilateral = bilateral	Often bilateral	Usually unilateral
Family history	Often positive	Often positive	No
Progression	Progressive	Slow	Rapid
Response to compression therapy	Variable	Good	Poor
Comments	Lymphatics are increased in number; although functionally defective, there is usually an increased number of lymph nodes. May have chylous ascites, chylothorax and protein-losing enteropathy	Absent or reduced distal superficial lymphatics. Also termed aplasia or hypoplasia	There is obstruction at the level of the aortoiliac or inguinal nodes. If associated with distal dilatation, the patient may benefit from lymphatic bypass operation. Other patients have distal obliteration as well

partly to direct physical damage and partly to the immune response of the host. Proximal lymphatics become grossly dilated with adult parasites. The degree of oedema is often massive, in which case it is termed elephantiasis (Fig. 55.8). Immature parasites (microfilariae) enter the blood at night and can be identified on a blood smear, in a centrifuged specimen of urine or in lymph itself. A complement fixation test is also available and is positive in present or past infection. Eosinophilia is usually present. Diethylcarbamazine destroys the parasites but does not reverse the lymphatic changes, although there may be some regression over time. Once the infection has been cleared, treatment is as for primary lymphoedema. Public health measures to reduce mosquito breeding, protective clothing and mosquito netting may be usefully employed to combat the condition (Summary box 55.4).

> **Summary box 55.4**
>
> **Features of filariasis**
>
> ***Acute***
> - Fever
> - Headache
> - Malaise
> - Inguinal and axillary lymphadenitis
> - Lymphangitis
> - Cellulitis, abscess formation and ulceration
> - Funiculo-epididymo-orchitis
>
> ***Chronic***
> - Lymphoedema of legs (arm, breast)
> - Hydrocele
> - Abdominal lymphatic varices
>   Chyluria
>   Lymphuria

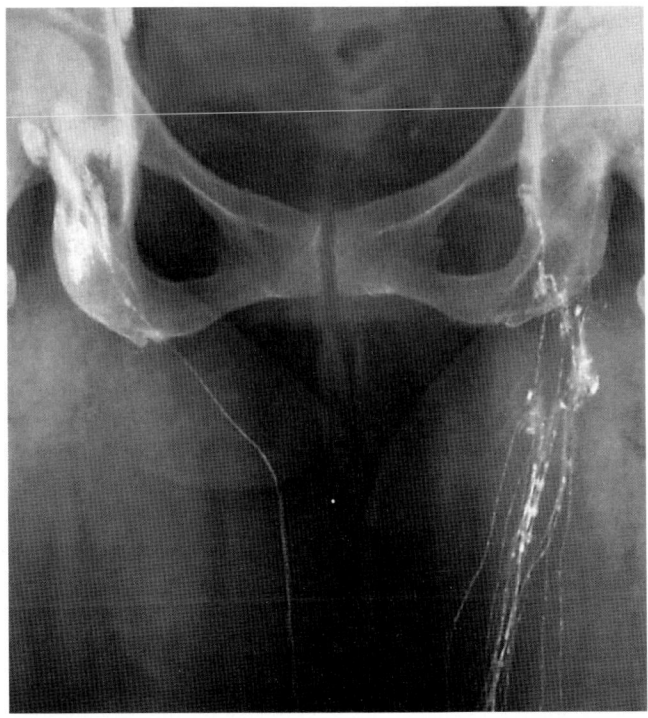

Figure 55.5 This patient presented with congenital lymphoedema of the right leg. The lymphangiogram shows lymphatic hypoplasia.

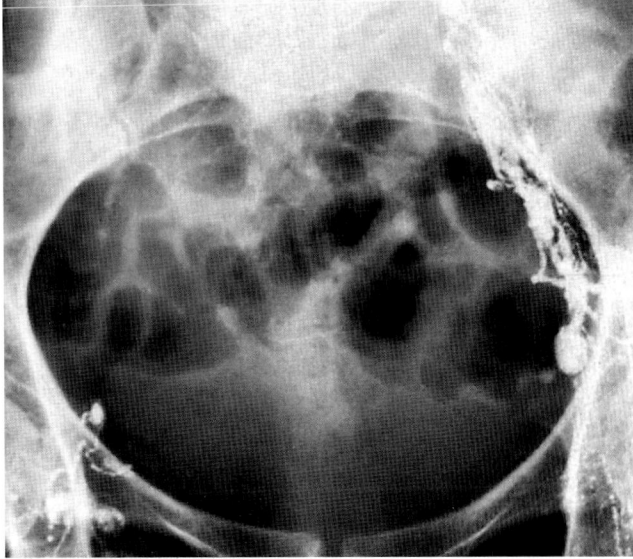

Figure 55.6 This patient presented with lymphoedema of the right leg. A bipedal lymphangiogram demonstrated normal lymphatics in the right leg up to the inguinal nodes, but no progression of contrast above the inguinal ligament – a case of proximal obstruction.

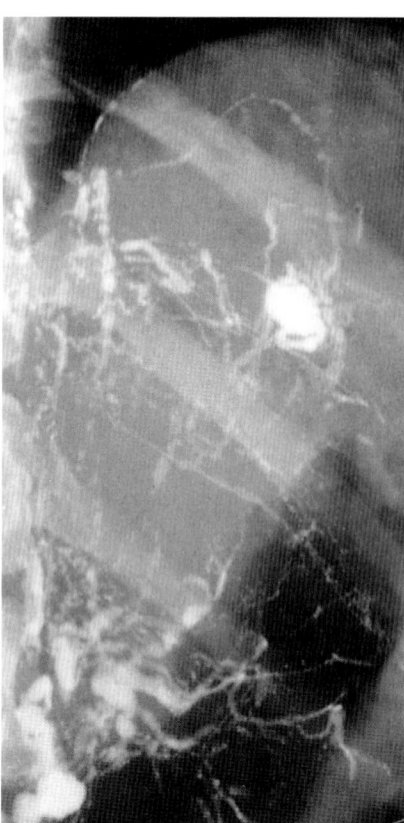

Figure 55.7 Lymphangiogram demonstrating reflux from dilated para-aortic vessels into the left kidney in a patient with filariasis who presented with chyluria.

Endemic elephantiasis (podoconiosis)

This is common in the tropics and affects more than 500 000 people in Africa. The barefoot cultivation of soil composed of alkaline volcanic rocks leads to destruction of the peripheral lymphatics by particles of silica, which can be seen in macrophages in draining lymph nodes. Plantar oedema develops in childhood and rapidly spreads proximally. The condition is prevented and its progression is slowed by the wearing of shoes.

Bacterial infection

Lymphangitis and lymphadenitis can cause lymphatic destruction that predisposes to lymphoedema complicated by further acute inflammatory episodes. Interestingly, in such patients, lymphangiography has revealed abnormalities in the contralateral, unaffected limb, suggesting an underlying, possibly inherited, susceptibility. Lymphatic and lymph node destruction by tuberculosis is also a well-recognised cause of lymphoedema, especially in developing countries.

Malignancy and its treatment

Treatment (surgery, radiotherapy) for breast carcinoma is the most common cause of lymphoedema in developed countries, but is decreasing in incidence as surgery becomes more conservative (see Chapter 50). Lymphoma may present with lymphoedema, as may malignancy of the pelvic organs and external genitalia. Kaposi's

> Moritz Kaposi, 1837–1902, Professor of Dermatology, Vienna, Austria, described pigmented sarcoma of the skin in 1872.

Table 55.6 Classification of causes of secondary lymphoedema

Classification	Example(s)
Trauma and tissue damage	Lymph node excision
	Radiotherapy
	Burns
	Variscose vein surgery/harvesting
	Large/circumferential wounds
	Scarring
Malignant disease	Lymph node metastases
	Infiltrative carcinoma
	Lymphoma
	Pressure from large tumours
Venous disease	Chronic venous insufficiency
	Venous ulceration
	Post-thrombotic syndrome
	Intravenous drug use
Infection	Cellulitis/erysipelas
	Lymphadenitis
	Tuberculosis
	Filariasis
Inflammation	Rheumatoid arthritis
	Dermatitis
	Psoriasis
	Sarcoidosis
	Dermatosis with epidermal involvement
Endocrine disease	Pretibial myxoedema
Immobility and dependency	Dependency oedema
	Paralysis
Factitious	Self harm

Reproduced with permission from: Lymphoedema Framework. *Best Practice Management of Lymphoedema*. International Consensus. London: MEP Ltd, 2006. © MEP Ltd 2006.

sarcoma developing in the course of HIV-related illness may cause lymphatic obstruction and is a growing cause of lymphoedema in certain parts of the world.

Trauma

It is not unusual for patients to develop chronic localised or generalised swelling following trauma. The aetiology is often multifactorial and includes disuse, venous thrombosis and lymphatic injury or destruction. Degloving injuries and burns are particularly likely to disrupt dermal lymphatics. Tenosynovitis can also be associated with localised subcutaneous lymphoedema, which can be a cause of troublesome persistent swelling following ankle and wrist 'sprains' and repetitive strain injury.

Lymphoedema and chronic venous insufficiency

It is important to appreciate the relationship between lymphoedema and CVI as both conditions are relatively common and so often coexist in the same patient, and it can be difficult to unravel which components of the patient's symptom complex are caused by each. There is no doubt that superficial venous thrombophlebitis (SVT) and DVT can both lead to lymphatic destruction and secondary lymphoedema, especially if recurrent. Lymphoedema is an important contributor to the swelling of the

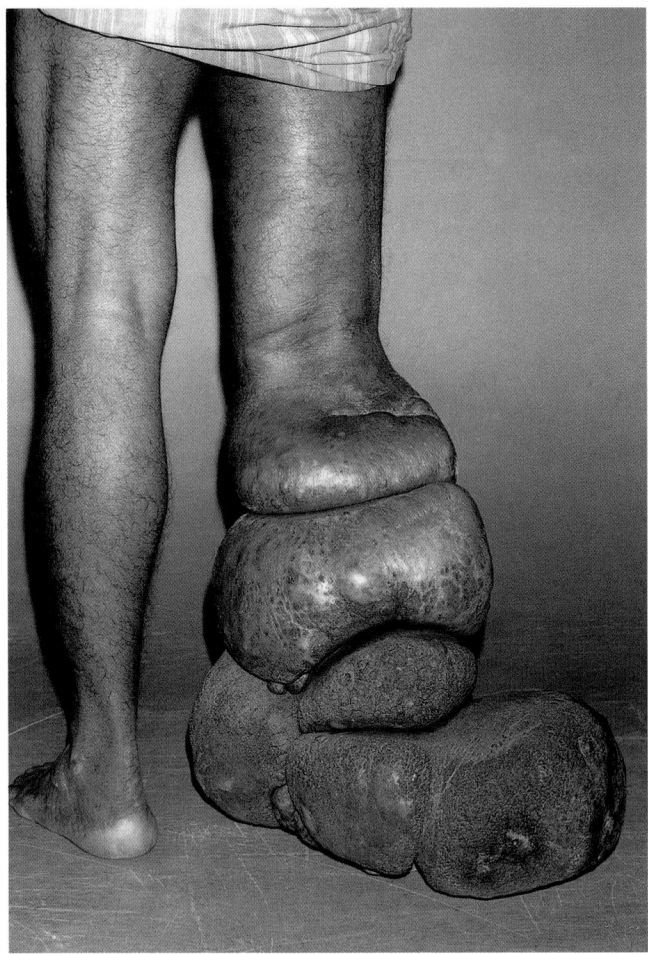

Figure 55.8 Elephantiasis due to filariasis.

post-phlebitic syndrome. It has also been suggested that lymphoedema can predispose to DVT, and possible SVT, through immobility and acute inflammatory episodes. Certainly, tests of venous function (duplex ultrasonography, plethysmography) are frequently abnormal in patients with lymphoedema.

It is not uncommon to see patients (usually women) with lymphoedema in whom a duplex ultrasound scan has revealed superficial reflux (such reflux is present subclinically in up to one-third of the adult population). Although isolated, superficial venous reflux rarely, if ever, leads to limb swelling; such patients are frequently misdiagnosed as having venous disease rather than lymphoedema, and are subjected mistakenly to varicose vein surgery. Not only will such surgery invariably fail to relieve the swelling, it will usually make it worse as saphenofemoral and saphenopopliteal ligation, together with saphenous stripping, will compromise still further drainage through the subcutaneous lymph bundles (which follow the major superficial veins) and draining inguinal and popliteal lymph nodes.

Miscellaneous conditions

Rheumatoid and psoriatic arthritis (chronic inflammation and lymph node fibrosis), contact dermatitis, snake and insect bites, and retroperitoneal fibrosis are all rare but well-documented causes of lymphoedema. Pretibial myxoedema is due to the obliteration of initial lymphatics by mucin.

Conditions mimicking lymphoedema

Factitious lymphoedema

This is caused by application of a tourniquet (a 'rut' and sharp cut-off is seen on examination) or 'hysterical' disuse in patients with psychological and psychiatric problems.

Immobility

Generalised or localised immobility of any cause leads to chronic limb swelling that can be misdiagnosed as lymphoedema, for example the elderly person who spends all day (and sometimes all night) sitting in a chair (armchair legs), the hemiplegic stroke patient and the young patient with multiple sclerosis.

Lipoedema

This presents almost exclusively in women and comprises bilateral, usually symmetrical, enlargement of the legs and, sometimes, the lower half of the body because of the abnormal deposition of fat. It may or may not be associated with generalised obesity. There are a number of features that help to differentiate the condition from lymphoedema but, of course, lipoedema may coexist with other causes of limb swelling. It has been proposed that lipoedema results from, or at least is associated with, fatty obliteration of lymphatics and lymph nodes (Summary box 55.5).

Summary box 55.5

Features of lipoedema that help differentiate it from lymphoedema

- Occurs almost exclusively in women
- Onset nearly always coincides with puberty
- Nearly always bilateral and symmetrical
- Involvement of trunk
- The feet are not involved, leading to an inverse shouldering effect at the malleoli
- No pitting
- No response to elevation or compression
- No skin changes of lymphoedema (negative Stemmer's sign)
- Magnetic resonance imaging shows subcutaneous fat but no fluid accumulation

---

INVESTIGATION OF LYMPHOEDEMA

Are investigations necessary?

It is usually possible to diagnose and manage lymphoedema purely on the basis of history and examination, especially when the swelling is mild and there are no apparent complicating features. In patients with severe, atypical and multifactorial swelling, investigations may help confirm the diagnosis, inform management and provide prognostic information.

'Routine' tests

These include a full blood count, urea and electrolytes, creatinine, liver function tests, thyroid function tests, plasma total protein and albumin, fasting glucose, urine dipstick including observation for chyluria, blood smear for microfilariae, chest radiograph and ultrasound.

Lymphangiography

Direct lymphangiography involves the injection of contrast medium into a peripheral lymphatic vessel and subsequent radiographic visualisation of the vessels and nodes. It remains the 'gold standard' for showing structural abnormalities of larger lymphatics and nodes (Fig. 55.9). However, it can be technically difficult, it is unpleasant for the patient, it may cause further lymphatic injury and, largely, it has become obsolete as a routine method of investigation. Few centres now perform this technique and those that do generally reserve it for preoperative evaluation of the rare patient with megalymphatics who is being considered for bypass or fistula ligation. Indirect lymphangiography involves the intradermal injection of water-soluble, non-ionic contrast into a web space, from where it is taken up by lymphatics and then followed radiographically. It will show distal lymphatics but not normally proximal lymphatics and nodes.

Isotope lymphoscintigraphy

This has largely replaced lymphangiography as the primary diagnostic technique in cases of clinical uncertainty. Radioactive technetium-labelled protein or colloid particles are injected into an interdigital web space and specifically taken up by lymphatics, and serial radiographs are taken with a gamma camera. The technique provides a qualitative measure of lymphatic function rather than quantitative function or anatomical detail. Quantitative lymphoscintigraphy is performed using a dynamic (exercise) component in addition to the static test and provides information on lymphatic transport.

Computerised tomography

A single, axial computerised tomography (CT) slice through the midcalf has been proposed as a useful diagnostic test for lymphoedema (coarse, non-enhancing, reticular 'honeycomb' pattern in an enlarged subcutaneous compartment), venous oedema (increased volume of the muscular compartment) and lipoedema (increased subcutaneous fat). CT can also be used to exclude pelvic or abdominal mass lesions.

Magnetic resonance imaging

Magnetic resonance imaging (MRI) can provide clear images of lymphatic channels and lymph nodes, and can be useful in the assessment of patients with lymphatic hyperplasia. MRI can also distinguish venous and lymphatic causes of a swollen limb, and detect tumours that may be causing lymphatic obstruction.

Ultrasound

Ultrasound can provide useful information about venous function including DVT and venous abnormalities.

Pathological examination

In cases in which malignancy is suspected, samples of lymph nodes may be obtained by fine-needle aspiration, needle core biopsy or surgical excision. Skin biopsy will confirm the diagnosis of lymphangiosarcoma.

MANAGEMENT OF LYMPHOEDEMA

Overview

The evaluation of the lymphoedema patient needs to be 'holistic' and their care delivered by a multiprofessional team comprising physical therapists, nurses, orthotists, physicians (dermatologists, oncologists, palliative care specialists), surgeons and social service professionals. Although surgery itself has a very small role, surgeons (especially those with breast and vascular interests) are frequently asked to oversee the management of these patients. Early diagnosis and institution of management are essential because at that stage relatively simple measures can be highly effective and will prevent the development of disabling late-stage disease, which is extremely difficult to treat. There is often a latent period of several years between the precipitating

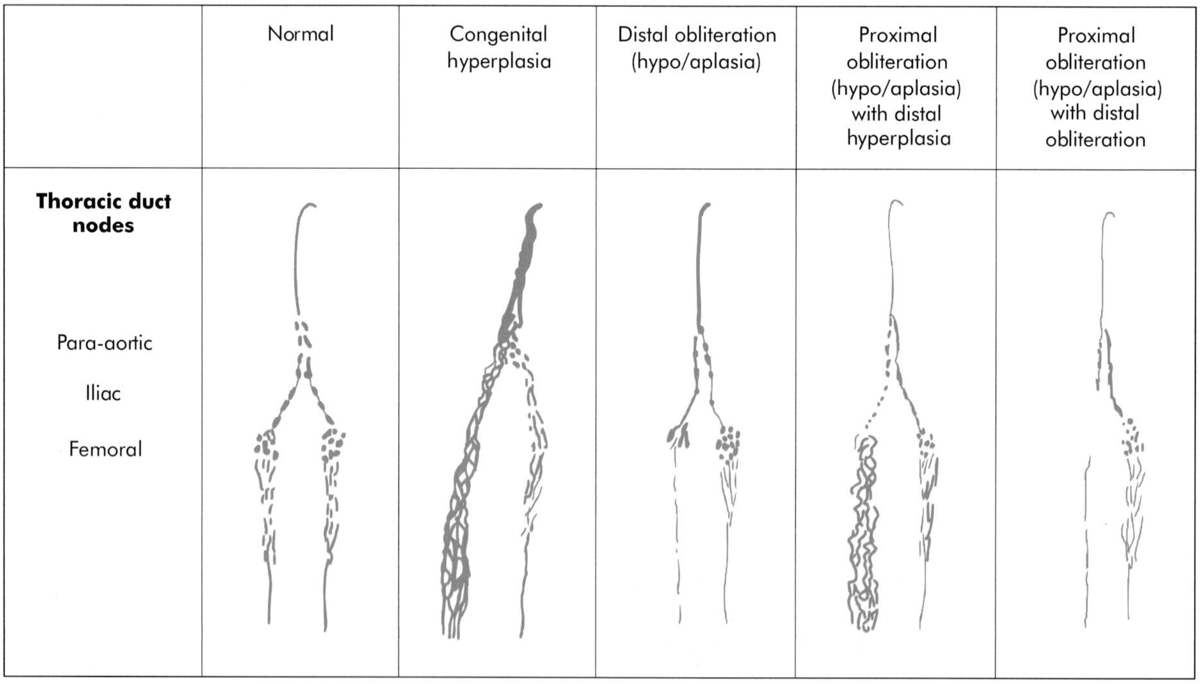

Figure 55.9 Lymphangiographic patterns of primary lymphoedema.

event and the onset of lymphoedema. The identification, education and treatment of such 'at-risk' patients can slow down, even prevent, the onset of disease. In patients with established lymphoedema, the three goals of treatment are to relieve pain, reduce swelling and prevent the development of complications (Summary box 55.6).

Summary box 55.6

Initial evaluation of the patient with lymphoedema

- History (age of onset, location, progression, exacerbating and relieving features)
- Past medical history including cancer history
- Family history
- Obesity (diet, height and weight, body mass index)
- Complications (venous, arterial, skin, joint, neurological, malignant)
- Assessment of physical, emotional and psychosocial symptoms
- Social circumstances (mobility, housing, education, work)
- Special needs (footwear, clothing, compression garments, pneumatic devices, mobility aids)
- Previous and current treatment
- Pain control
- Compliance with therapy and ability to self-care

Relief of pain

On initial presentation, 50% of patients with lymphoedema complain of significant pain. The pain is usually multifactorial and its severity and underlying cause(s) will vary depending on the aetiology of the lymphoedema. For example, following treatment for breast cancer, pain may arise from the swelling itself (radiation and surgery induced); nerve (brachial plexus and intercostobrachial nerve), bone (secondary deposits, radiation necrosis) and joint (arthritis, bursitis, capsulitis) disease; and recurrent disease. Treatment involves the considered use of non-opioid and opioid analgesics, corticosteroids, tricyclic antidepressants, muscle relaxants, anti-epileptics, nerve blocks, physiotherapy and adjuvant anti-cancer therapies (chemo-, radio- and hormonal therapy), as well as measures to reduce swelling if possible. In patients with non-cancer-related lymphoedema, the best way to reduce pain is to control swelling and prevent the development of complications. Whatever the cause, pain is a somatopsychic experience that is affected by mood and morale. These issues are important in patients with both cancer-related lymphoedema, who are concerned about recurrent disease, and non-cancer-related disease, who often have poor self-esteem and problems with body image and perception.

Control of swelling

Physical therapy for lymphoedema comprising bed rest, elevation, bandaging, compression garments, massage and exercises was first described at the end of the nineteenth century, and through the twentieth century various eponymous schools developed. Although there is little doubt that physical therapy can be highly effective in reducing swelling, its general acceptance and practice has been hampered by a lack of proper research and confusing terminology. The current preferred term is decongestive lymphoedema therapy (DLT), which comprises two phases. The first is a short intensive period of therapist-led care and the second is a

maintenance phase in which the patient uses a self-care regimen with occasional professional intervention. The intensive phase comprises skin care, MLD and MLLB, and exercises. The length of intensive treatment will depend upon the disease severity, the degree of patient compliance and the willingness and ability of the patient to take more responsibility for the maintenance phase. However, weeks rather than months should be the goal.

Skin care

The patient must be carefully educated in the principles and practice of skin care. The patient should inspect the affected skin daily, with special attention paid to skinfolds, where maceration may occur. The limb should be washed daily; the use of bath oil (e.g. Balneum) is recommended as a moisturiser and the limb must be carefully dried afterwards. A hair drier on low heat is more effective and hygienic, and less traumatic, than a towel. If the skin is in good condition daily application of a bland emollient (e.g. aqueous cream) is recommended to keep the skin hydrated. If the skin is dry and flaky then a bland ointment [e.g. 50:50 white soft paraffin/liquid paraffin (WSP/LP)] should be used twice daily and, if there is marked hyperkeratosis, a keratolytic agent, such as 5% salicylic acid, should be added. Many commercially available soaps, creams and lotions contain sensitisers (e.g. lanolin in E45 cream) and are best avoided as patients with lymphoedema are highly susceptible to contact dermatitis (eczema). Apart from causing intense discomfort, eczema acts as an entry point for infection. Management comprises avoidance of the allergen (patch testing may be required) and topical corticosteroids. Fungal infections are common, difficult to eradicate and predispose to acute inflammatory episodes. Chronic application of anti-fungal creams leads to maceration and it is better to use powders in shoes and socks. Ointment containing 3% benzoic acid helps prevent athlete's foot and can be used safely over long periods. Painting at-risk areas with an antiseptic agent such as eosin may be helpful. Lymphorrhoea is uncommon but extremely troublesome. Management comprises emollients, elevation, compression and sometimes cautery under anaesthetic (Summary box 55.7).

Summary box 55.7

Skin care

- Protect hands when washing up or gardening; wear a thimble when sewing
- Never walk barefoot and wear protective footwear outside
- Use an electric razor to depilate
- Never let the skin become macerated
- Treat cuts and grazes promptly (wash, dry, apply antiseptic and a plaster)
- Use insect repellent sprays and treat bites promptly with antiseptics and anti-histamines
- Seek medical attention as soon as the limb becomes hot, painful or more swollen
- Do not allow blood to be taken from, or injections to be given into, an affected arm (and avoid blood pressure measurement)
- Protect the affected skin from sun (shade, high-factor sun block)
- Consider taking antibiotics if going on holiday

Apart from lymphangiosarcoma, acute inflammatory episodes are probably the most serious complications of lymphoedema and frequently lead to emergency hospital admission. About 25% of primary and 5% of secondary lymphoedema patients are affected. Acute inflammatory episodes start rapidly, often without warning or a precipitating event, with tingling, pain and redness of the limb. Patients feel 'viral' and severe attacks can lead to the rapid onset of fever, rigors, headache, vomiting and delirium. Patients who have suffered previous attacks can usually predict the onset and many learn to carry antibiotics with them and self-medicate at the first hint of trouble. This may stave off a full-blown attack and prevent the further lymphatic injury that each acute inflammatory episode causes. It is rarely possible to isolate a responsible bacterium but the majority are presumed to be streptococcal and/or staphylococcal in origin. The diagnosis is usually obvious but dermatitis, thrombophlebitis and DVT are in the differential diagnosis. Benzyl (intravenous) or phenoxymethyl (oral) penicillin and flucloxacillin (or clindamycin in severe attacks) are the antibiotics of choice and should be given for 2 weeks. Rest will reduce lymphatic drainage and the spread of infection, elevation will reduce the oedema and heparin prophylaxis will reduce the risk of DVT. Co-amoxiclav can be taken by patients who self-medicate. The use of long-term prophylactic antibiotics is not evidence based, but is probably reasonable in patients who suffer frequent attacks. However, the benefits of scrupulous compliance with physical therapy and skin care cannot be underestimated.

Manual lymphatic drainage

Several different techniques of MLD have been described and the details are beyond the scope of this chapter. However, they all aim to evacuate fluid and protein from the ISF space, and stimulate lymphangion contraction. The therapist should perform MLD daily; they should also train the patient (and/or carer) to perform a simpler, modified form of massage termed simple lymphatic drainage (SLD). In the intensive phase, SLD supplements MLD and, once the maintenance phase is entered, SLD will carry on as daily massage.

Multilayer lymphoedema bandaging and compression garments

Elastic bandages provide compression, produce a sustained high resting pressure and 'follow in' as limb swelling reduces. However, the sub-bandage pressure does not alter greatly in response to changes in limb circumference consequent upon muscular activity and posture. By contrast, short-stretch bandages exert support through the production of a semi-rigid casing where the resting pressure is low but changes quite markedly in response to movement and posture.

It is generally believed that non-elastic MLLB is preferable (and arguably safer) in patients with severe swelling during the intensive phase of DLT, whereas compression (hosiery, sleeves) is preferable in milder cases and during the maintenance phase. Whether the aim is to provide support or compression, the pressure exerted must be graduated (100% ankle/foot, 70% knee, 50% mid-thigh, 40% groin) and, of course, the adequacy of the arterial circulation must be assessed. As it is rarely possible to feel pulses in the lymphoedematous limb, non-invasive assessment of the ankle–brachial pressure index (ABPI) using a hand-held Doppler ultrasound device is usually necessary. MLLB is highly skilled and to be effective and safe it needs to be applied by a specially trained therapist. It is also extremely labour intensive, needing to be changed daily.

Compression garments form the mainstay of management in most clinics. The control of lymphoedema requires higher pressures (30–40 mmHg arm, 40–60 mmHg leg) than are typically used to treat CVI. Confusingly, the British (classes I: 14–17 mmHg; II: 17–24 mmHg; III: 24–35 mmHg) and international (European) (classes I: 20–30 mmHg; II: 30–40 mmHg; III: 40–50 mmHg; IV: 50–60 mmHg) standards are different. The patient should put the stocking on first thing in the morning before rising. It can be difficult to persuade patients to comply. Putting lymphoedema-grade stockings on and off is difficult and many patients find them intolerably uncomfortable, especially in warm climates. Furthermore, although intellectually they understand the benefits, emotionally they may find wearing them presents a greater body image problem than the swelling itself.

Enthusiasm for pneumatic compression devices has waxed and waned. Unless the device being used allows the sequential inflation of multiple chambers up to > 50 mmHg, it will probably be ineffective for lymphoedema. The benefits to the patient are maximised and complications are minimised if these devices are used under the direction of a physical therapist as part of an overall package of care.

Exercise

Lymph formation is directly proportional to arterial inflow and 40% of lymph is formed within skeletal muscle. Vigorous exercise, especially if it is anaerobic and isometric, will tend to exacerbate lymphoedema and patients should be advised to avoid prolonged static activities, for example carrying heavy shopping bags or prolonged standing. In contrast, slow, rhythmic, isotonic movements (e.g. swimming) and massage will increase venous and lymphatic return through the production of movement between skin and underlying tissues (essential to the filling of initial lymphatics) and augmentation of the muscle pumps. Exercise also helps to maintain joint mobility. Patients who are unable to move their limbs benefit from passive exercises. When at rest, the lymphoedematous limb should be positioned with the foot/hand above the level of the heart. A pillow under the mattress or blocks under the bottom of the bed will encourage the swelling to go down overnight.

Drugs

There are considerable, and scientifically inexplicable, differences in the use of specific drugs for venous disease and lymphoedema between different countries. The benzpyrones are a group of several thousand naturally occurring substances, of which the flavonoids have received the most attention. Enthusiasts will argue that a number of clinical trials have shown benefit from these compounds, which are purported to reduce capillary permeability, improve microcirculatory perfusion, stimulate interstitial macrophage proteolysis, reduce erythrocyte and platelet aggregation, scavenge free radicals and exert an anti-inflammatory effect. Detractors will argue that the trials are small and poorly controlled with short follow-up and 'soft' endpoints, and that any benefits observed can be explained by a placebo effect. In the UK, oxerutins (Paroven) are the only such drugs licensed for venous disease and none has a license for lymphoedema. Diuretics are of no value in pure lymphoedema. Their chronic use is associated with side-effects, including electrolyte disturbance, and should be avoided.

Surgery

Only a small minority of patients with lymphoedema benefit from surgery. Operations fall into two categories: bypass procedures and reduction procedures.

Bypass procedures

The rare patient with proximal ilioinguinal lymphatic obstruction and normal distal lymphatic channels might benefit, at least in theory, from lymphatic bypass. A number of methods have been described including the omental pedicle, the skin bridge (Gillies), anastomosing lymph nodes to veins (Neibulowitz) and the ileal mucosal patch (Kinmonth). More recently, direct lymphaticovenular anastomosis has been carried out on vessels of 0.5–0.8 mm diameter using supermicrosurgical techniques, with promising results. The procedures are technically demanding and not without morbidity, and there is no controlled evidence to suggest that these procedures produce a superior outcome to best medical management alone.

Limb reduction procedures

These are indicated when a limb is so swollen that it interferes with mobility and livelihood. These operations are not 'cosmetic' in the sense that they do not create a normally shaped leg and are usually associated with significant scarring. Four operations have been described.

Sistrunk

A wedge of skin and subcutaneous tissue is excised and the wound closed primarily. This is most commonly carried out to reduce the girth of the thigh.

Homans

First, skin flaps are elevated, and then subcutaneous tissue is excised from beneath the flaps, which are then trimmed to size to accommodate the reduced girth of the limb and closed primarily. This is the most satisfactory operation for the calf (Fig. 55.10). The main complication is skin flap necrosis. There must be at least 6 months between operations on the medial and lateral sides of the limb and the flaps must not pass the midline. This procedure has also been used on the upper limb, but is contraindicated in the presence of venous obstruction or active malignancy.

Thompson

One denuded skin flap is sutured to the deep fascia and buried beneath the second skin flap (the so called 'buried dermal flap') (Fig. 55.11). This procedure has become less popular as pilonidal sinus formation is common. The cosmetic result is no better than that obtained with the Homans' procedure and there is no evidence that the buried flap establishes any new lymphatic connection with the deep tissues.

Sir Harold Delf Gillies, **1882–1960, Plastic Surgeon, St. Bartholomew's Hospital, London, England.**
John Bernard Kinmonth, **1916–1982, Surgeon, St. Thomas's Hospital, London, England.**
Walter Ellis Sistrunk, Jr., **1880–1933, Professor of Clinical Surgery, Baylor University College of Medicine, Houston, TX, USA.**
John Homans, **1877–1954, Professor of Clinical Surgery, The Harvard University Medical School, Boston, MA, USA.**
Frederick Thompson, **1910–1975, Plastic Surgeon, The Middlesex Hospital, London, England.**

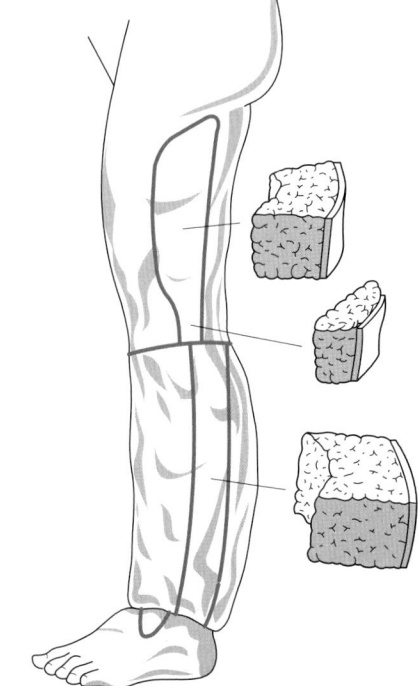

Figure 55.10 Homans' procedure involves raising skin flaps to allow the excision of a wedge of skin and a larger volume of subcutaneous tissue down to the deep fascia. Surgery to the medial and lateral aspects of the leg must be separated by at least 6 months to avoid skin flap necrosis.

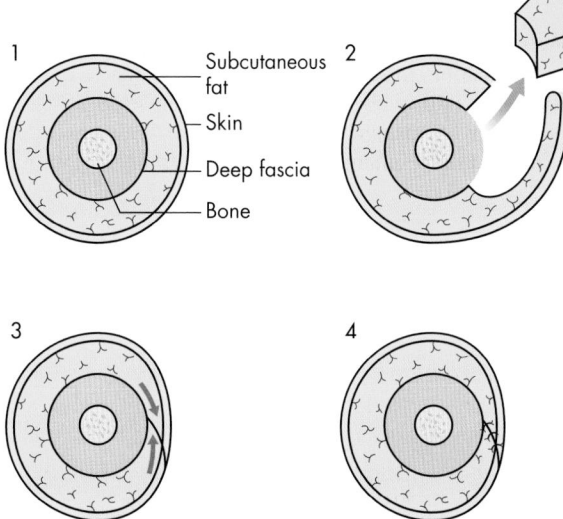

Figure 55.11 A cross-sectional representation of Thompson's reduction operation; the buried dermal flap.

Charles

This operation was initially designed for filariasis and involved excision of all of the skin and subcutaneous tissues down to the deep fascia, with coverage using split-skin grafts (Fig. 55.12). This leaves a very unsatisfactory cosmetic result and graft failure is not

Major-General Sir Richard Havelock Charles, **1887–1934, a Surgeon in The Indian Medical Service.**

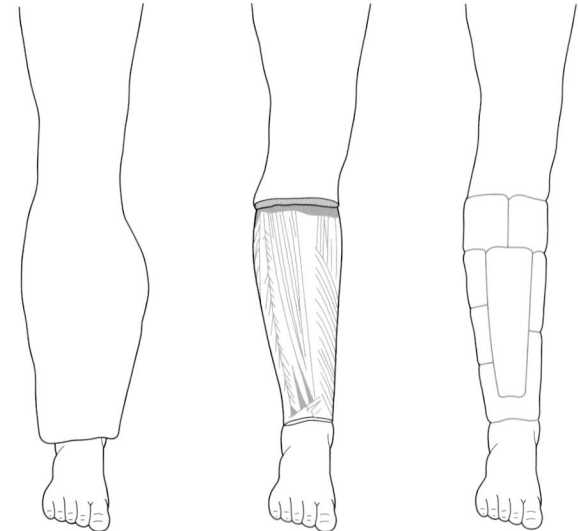

Figure 55.12 The Charles procedure involves circumferential excision of lymphoedematous tissue down to and including the deep fascia followed by split-skin grafting. This procedure gives a very poor cosmetic result but does allow the surgeon to remove very large amounts of tissue and is particularly useful in patients with severe skin changes.

uncommon. However, it does enable the surgeon to reduce greatly the girth of a massively swollen limb.

Chylous ascites and chylothorax

These are associated with megalymphatics. The diagnosis may be obvious if accompanied by lymphoedema and lymphangioma. However, some patients develop chylous ascites and/or chylothorax in isolation, in which case the diagnosis can be confirmed by aspiration and the identification of chylomicrons in the aspirate. Cytology for malignant cells should also be carried out. A CT scan may show enlarged lymph nodes and CT with guided biopsy, laparoscopy or even laparotomy and biopsy may be necessary to exclude lymphoma or other malignancy. Lymphangiography may indicate the site of a lymphatic fistula that can be surgically ligated. Even if no localised lesion is identified, it may be possible to control leakage at laparotomy or even remove a segment of affected bowel. If the problem is too diffuse to be corrected surgically, a peritoneal venous shunt may be inserted, although occlusion and infection are important complications. Medical treatment comprising the avoidance of fat in the diet and the prescription of medium-chain triglycerides (which are absorbed directly into the blood rather than via the lymphatics) may reduce swelling. Chylothorax is best treated by pleurodesis, but this may lead to death from lymph-logged lungs as the excess lymph has nowhere to drain.

Chyluria

Filariasis is the most common cause, with chyluria occurring in 1–2% of cases 10–20 years after initial infestation. It usually presents as painless passage of milky white urine, particularly after a fatty meal. The chyle may clot, leading to renal colic, and hypoproteinaemia may result. Chyluria may also be caused by ascariasis, malaria, tumour and tuberculosis. Intravenous urography and/or lymphangiography will often demonstrate the lymphourinary fistula. Treatment includes a low-fat and high-protein diet, increased oral fluids to prevent clot colic, and laparotomy and ligation of the dilated lymphatics. Attempts have also been made to sclerose the lymphatics either directly or via instrumentation of the bladder, ureter and renal pelvis.

FURTHER READING

Lymphoedema Framework (2006) *Best Practice for the Management of Lymphoedema. International Consensus*. MEP Ltd, London.

Szuba, A. and Rockson, S.G. (1997) Lymphedema: anatomy, physiology and pathogenesis. *Vasc Med* **2**: 321–6.

Twycross, R., Jenns, K. and Todd, J. (2000) *Lymphoedema*. Radcliffe Medical Press, Oxford.

PART 11 | Abdominal

History and examination of the abdomen

LEARNING OBJECTIVES

To understand:

- The importance of history-taking and abdominal examination in the overall assessment of the surgical patient
- The significance of a structured format for history-taking

- The mechanisms behind both the symptoms produced by abdominal conditions and the signs elicited from abdominal examination, in order to explain the underlying diagnosis

INTRODUCTION

An accurate history combined with a detailed and full examination is the mainstay of all good clinical assessment in surgery (as in all areas of medicine). In the case of the acute abdomen, this becomes even more important as time for reflection and review is limited and appropriate investigations may need to be organised quickly, along with any management decision for urgent surgery. Furthermore, although advanced imaging techniques, both static and dynamic, are now commonplace, providing very detailed information of diseased organs, a good understanding of the background clinical information is still required for accurate interpretation.

The importance of a good history and examination in the assessment of the acute abdomen was demonstrated in the 1970s by the late Tim de Dombal from Leeds and Tony Gunn from Scotland. Both authors developed and then examined the role of computer-aided diagnosis (CAD) systems in the assessment of acute abdominal pain. A detailed proforma of the patient's history and examination findings needed to be completed by the assessing clinician and entered into a computer, which then produced a list of the most probable diagnoses based on Bayesian reasoning. Repeated studies throughout the UK demonstrated an overall improvement in diagnostic accuracy of around 20% when CAD was used. Further studies subsequently showed that the diagnostic accuracy of medical students (assumed to be the most ignorant in the surgical assessment hierarchy!) using CAD was the same as that of hospital doctors when only the proforma was used (to collect the clinical details), which was not significantly different from clinicians using CAD. In other words,

Francis Timothy de Dombal, **1937–1995, Professor of Information Science, The University of Leeds, Leeds, England.**
Alexander Anton Gunn, **Surgeon, Bangour Village Hospital, Broxburn, West Lothian, Scotland.**
Thomas Bayes, **1702–1761, English Presbyterian Minister and Mathematician who published 'Essay towards solving a problem in the doctrine of chances' in 1763.**

the improvement in diagnostic accuracy, seen across the board, was related more to using the proforma, or structured data sheets, than to actually using the computer program, emphasising the importance of taking a good history and carrying out a thorough examination.

This chapter will therefore focus on the history-taking and examination requirements for the assessment of patients with both elective and emergency abdominal problems. It will not go into detailed pathological features of the various systems, as these are covered in their respective chapters, but will simply provide the reader with a template on which to base good clinical assessment (Summary box 56.1).

Summary box 56.1

The history

- ■ The single most important factor in obtaining a reliable diagnosis from the history is its comprehensiveness
- ■ History is also important in determining fitness for surgery
- ■ Previous surgery needs careful documentation as it affects the safety of laparoscopic procedures
- ■ If a comprehensive suite of investigations is not available, the history becomes even more important

HISTORY-TAKING

Basic structure

As in all areas of medical history-taking, the basic structure of *presenting complaint*, *history of presenting complaint* and *associated features* is an appropriate start to taking an abdominal surgical history. This is then followed by a review of the *past medical history* and the *systems*. For the former, details of previous operations are important, not just for reaching a diagnosis, but also in the influence these might have on any further operations required and whether a laparoscopic approach might be made more difficult or hazardous. When writing up a systems review, it is probably best to put into the *history of present complaint* and *associated features* section the information you have gathered in the system where the problem lies. For example, when taking the *history of the presenting complaint* in a patient complaining of dyspepsia, the questions associated with the *upper gastrointestinal system* should be asked at this point (dysphagia, early satiety, reflux, vomiting, etc). Thereafter, the standard history-taking format (Summary box 56.2) should take place covering all the usual areas of *drug allergies, family and social histories*. The importance of covering all areas of history-taking cannot be overemphasised for the surgeon. It is only by doing this that a complete picture of the patient's overall 'medical condition' can be appreciated and therefore contribute, not only to the differential diagnosis, but also to the assessment of their fitness for any possible surgery (Summary box 56.2).

Summary box 56.2

Format for surgical history-taking

- Presenting complaint
- History of presenting complaint
- Associated features (including systemic review of the relevant system, e.g. gastrointestinal, urological, etc.)
- Past medical and surgical history
- Systems review
- Drug/allergy history
- Family history
- Social history

History-taking in the presence of the acute abdomen, which is almost synonymous with 'acute abdominal pain', takes on an even greater importance. As already mentioned, time may be of the essence and, depending on where the patient is in the world, access to advanced investigative techniques may be limited at best, or completely unavailable at worst.

Abdominal pain

The complaint of abdominal pain is probably one of the more common surgical complaints of patients attending both an outpatient clinic and also as an emergency at hospital. The assessment of abdominal pain will be discussed as for 'acute abdominal pain', but the underlying history-taking and examination should be the same for both the 'elective' and the 'emergency' patient.

All the organs contained in the abdomen, pelvis and retroperitoneum can be the cause of abdominal pain. However, one must not forget that acute abdominal pain can also be caused by some acute medical problems (porphyria, diabetic ketoacidosis, etc.) in addition to both acute cardiac and pulmonary disorders (Summary box 56.3).

Summary box 56.3

Medical causes of abdominal pain

- Diabetic ketoacidosis
- Porphyria
- Pain arising from the heart or lungs

Understanding the mechanism behind the distribution of pain fibres within the abdomen and retroperitoneum helps to explain the clinical symptoms and signs of the acute abdomen. The parietal peritoneum lines the abdominal wall, and the visceral peritoneum invests the viscera. The parietal peritoneum is innervated by the relevant somatic nerves through spinal nerves in the distribution of the overlying dermatomes: the xiphisternum at the level of T4, the umbilicus at T8 and the inguinal ligament at T12. Pain is sharply localised to the point of inflammation of the parietal peritoneum. For example, an acutely inflamed sigmoid colon from diverticulitis causes irritation to the overlying parietal peritoneum, and pain is then localised to the left iliac fossa.

The viscera and visceral peritoneum is innervated by the autonomic nervous system with pain travelling back to the spinal cord along sympathetic fibres. However, the pain is localised or referred to the equivalent somatic distribution of that nerve root (from T1 to L2) (Fig. 56.1). This pain is therefore deep, poorly localised and usually associated with sympathetic symptoms such as sweating and nausea. The gastrointestinal tract is divided embryologically into the foregut, midgut and hindgut, each arising with its own blood and nerve supply. Pain from the foregut is localised to the epigastrium, from the midgut to the peri-umbilical region and from the hindgut to the lower abdomen (Table 56.1). As a result, early inflammation of a mobile part of the viscera, such as the appendix/small bowel, which does not result in parietal peritoneal inflammation, produces referred pain in the peri-umbilical pain region. As the inflammation reaches the parietal peritoneum, the pain localises to that dermatome, as supplied by the somatic nerve supply. In the case of the appendix, this will obviously be the right iliac fossa. Another example of referred pain occurs when the diaphragm is irritated. As the nerve supply comes from the phrenic nerve (C3, 4, 5), the pain is localised to those dermatomes supplied by the equivalent somatic nerves, and pain may be felt in the region of the shoulder (Summary box 56.4).

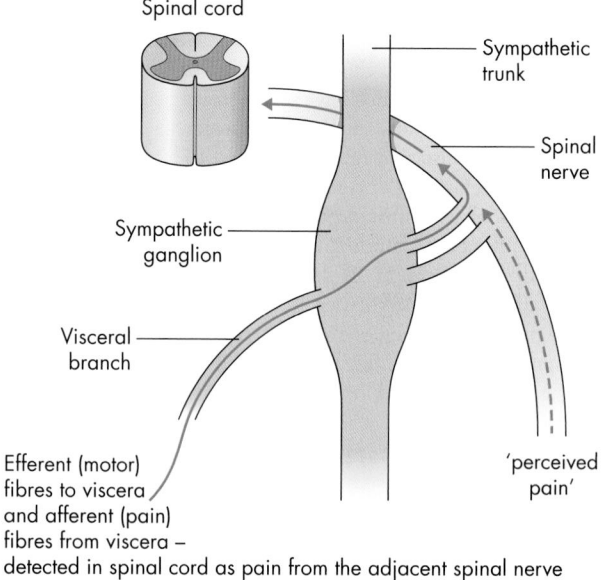

Figure 56.1 Pathways for parietal and visceral pain.

Table 56.1 Embryological division of the gastrointestinal tract

	Viscera
Foregut	Oesophagus
	Stomach
	Duodenum – first and second parts
	Pancreas
	Liver
	Gall bladder
Midgut	Duodenum – third and fourth parts
	Jejunum
	Ileum
	Right colon
	Transverse colon
	Appendix
Hindgut	Left colon
	Sigmoid colon
	Rectum

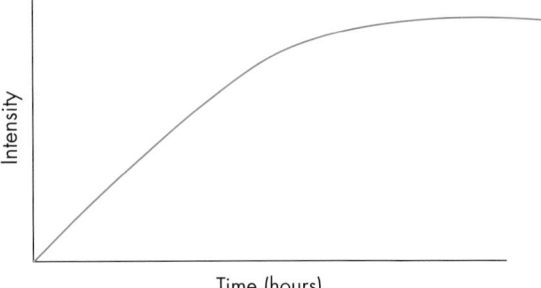

Figure 56.2 Time/intensity graph for the pain of inflammation.

pancreatitis, acute salpingitis (pelvic inflammatory disease) and mesenteric adenitis. The pain is initially often very non-specific, gradually increasing in intensity over a period of several hours or even days (Summary box 56.5; Fig. 56.2).

Summary box 56.4

Origins and presentation of abdominal pain

Source	Presentation
Parietal peritoneum	Well localised but can radiate forwards and backwards along the dermatome
Visceral peritoneum	Poorly localised; associated with sweating and nausea
Retroperitoneal structures	Pain in the back

The nature of the pain will change as the cause evolves

Summary box 56.5

Sources of pain that evolve over hours or days

- ■ Acute   Appendicitis
              Cholecystitis
              Salpingitis
              Mesenteric adenitis
- ■ Infarction
- ■ Free blood in the peritoneum

Pain due to parietal peritoneal inflammation may also radiate back or forwards along the line supplied by the somatic nerve, as is seen in acute cholecystitis, when pain spreads from the right subcostal region around to the back.

Inflammation of the retroperitoneal structures, such as the pancreas and kidney, causes irritation of the somatic spinal nerves, producing back pain. Similarly, an inflamed retrocaecal appendix will irritate the ilio-psoas muscle, producing pain in the right loin at times, especially when the psoas muscle is stretched.

Of course, most causes of abdominal pain will incorporate both visceral and parietal pain, producing a picture that changes as the inflammation increases and spreads. This evolving picture may be picked up within the history-taking process or subsequently by regular and repeated review of the patient. Pain from small bowel obstruction will usually be central and colicky in nature but, as the obstructed loop becomes ischaemic and starts to inflame the overlying peritoneum, the pain will become continuous, more widespread and be associated with signs of 'peritonitis' (see below).

The history of abdominal pain associated with specific disorders

Inflammation and infection

Common intra-abdominal inflammatory conditions include acute appendicitis, acute cholecystitis, acute diverticulitis, acute

Other conditions that cause abdominal pain through this mechanism include infarction (which may initially present as obstruction, see below) and haemorrhage, where the intraperitoneal blood irritates the parietal peritoneum.

Perforation

Perforation of an abdominal viscus usually results in the sudden onset of severe abdominal pain (Fig. 56.3). Identifying the viscus in question may be determined by a history of preceding abdominal symptoms or illness, such as constipation or peptic ulcer disease. In the early stages, the site of maximum tenderness may also indicate the organ that has perforated (upper or lower abdomen), but generalised peritonitis usually follows very quickly as the intra-abdominal structures have not had time to try and 'wall off' the diseased organ, as often occurs in 'inflammatory' conditions. The most common organs that perforate (excluding the appendix) are the stomach and duodenum (from peptic ulcer disease) and the colon (from diverticular disease or severe constipation).

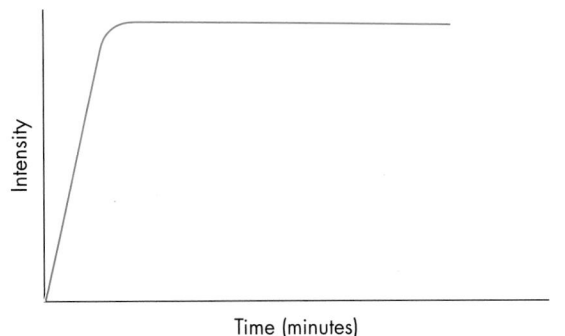

Figure 56.3 Time/intensity graph for the pain of perforation.

Of course, the endpoint of many of the conditions that produce visceral inflammation is perforation but, generally, these patients present with symptoms of the underlying disease first, rather than the short severe presentation associated with a sudden perforation (Summary box 56.6).

Summary box 56.6

Causes of sudden onset abdominal pain

- Perforation   Appendix
                    Stomach
                    Duodenum
                    Colon

Obstruction

Obstruction of any hollow viscus within the abdominal cavity usually causes acute abdominal pain. Obstruction of all viscera except the gall bladder tends to produce colicky pain (Fig. 56.4), while obstruction of the gall bladder (inaccurately termed 'biliary colic') usually presents with a more acute continuous type of pain, often punctuated by acute exacerbations, and is similar to that of inflammation, but may have a slightly quicker onset. Colicky pain classically resolves between short-lived episodes, and it is only when underlying inflammation or infection sets in that a more continuous background element to the pain is introduced. This can of course represent the development of a serious complication (such as ischaemia of the bowel) and, therefore, its recognition by the emergency surgeon is crucial to prompt treatment.

Specific characteristics of 'abdominal pain'

The site, onset, character and duration of the abdominal pain provide important pointers to the diagnosis. Radiation of the pain, progression or alteration of its site or character, factors that aggravate the pain or relieve it and any associated symptoms are also helpful in refining the diagnosis. The site of the abdominal pain is usually related to one of nine areas (Fig. 56.5). These regions are demarcated by the mid-clavicular lines in the vertical axis and by the transpyloric and transtubercular lines in the horizontal axis. Figure 56.5 also indicates some of the common organs and pathological processes that commonly cause pain experienced in these regions.

Obtaining information on aggravating or relieving factors can be particularly helpful to the assessing surgeon. Pain made worse by moving and coughing suggests peritoneal inflammation

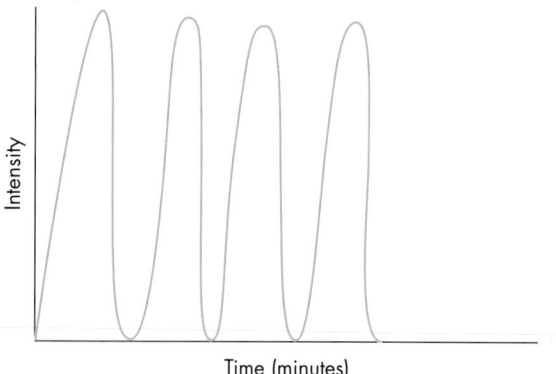

Figure 56.4 Time/intensity graph for the pain of obstruction.

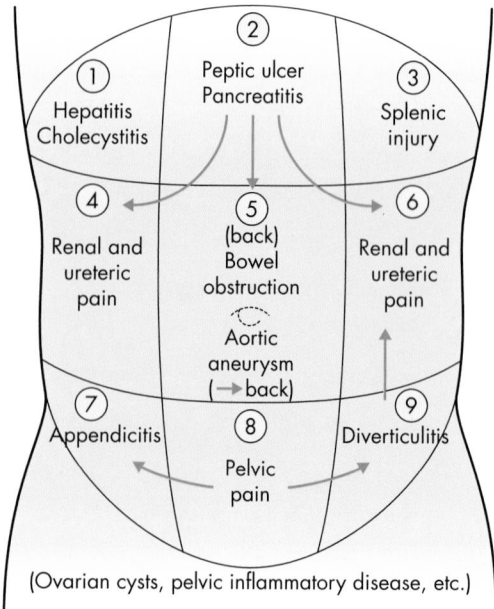

(Ovarian cysts, pelvic inflammatory disease, etc.)

1. Right subcostal
2. Epigastrium
3. Left subcostal
4. Right flank (loin is more posterior)
5. Peri-umbilical
6. Left flank loin
7. Right iliac fossa
8. Suprapubic/hypogastrium
9. Left iliac fossa

Figure 56.5 Nine sites of abdominal pain.

'peritonism', whereas pain which makes the patient roll around or double up is typical of 'colic' (Summary box 56.7).

Summary box 56.7

Aggravating features of pain

Aggravating feature	Interpretation
Moving or coughing	Peritoneal inflammation
Patient rolls around with pain	Colic (suggests obstruction of viscus)

Factors that aggravate or relieve pain are also important in making a diagnosis, and information on the influence of movement, injury, position, food, antacids, vomiting, bowel action and micturition on the pain must always be sought. A history of previous trauma, however minor, may also be important. At the same time, it is important to ask about associated symptoms such as vomiting, diarrhoea, dysuria or a missed period that preceded or followed the onset of the pain as these may again provide important diagnostic clues.

As mentioned earlier, true colic is a gripping pain of sudden onset, which rapidly reaches a crescendo before equally swiftly

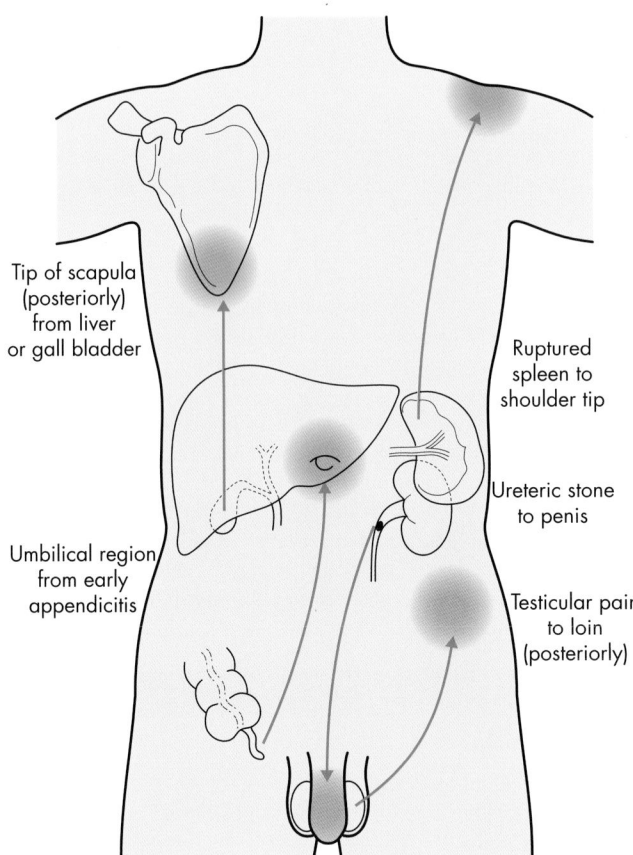

Tip of scapula
(posteriorly)
from liver
or gall bladder

Ruptured
spleen to
shoulder tip

Ureteric stone
to penis

Umbilical region
from early
appendicitis

Testicular pain
to loin
(posteriorly)

Figure 56.6 Common sites of radiation of abdominal pain.

dying away, usually completely. This description is true of intestinal and renal colic, but biliary colic is a misnomer (see above) as patients tend to complain of a continuous pain with exacerbations of severe pain. As already mentioned, strangulation should be suspected when intestinal colic alters to become a continuous pain.

Other common adjectives for abdominal pains include stabbing, wrenching, boring, burning and crushing, and these should all be taken into account with the other symptoms when trying to reach a diagnosis. Specific areas of radiation are characteristic of certain causes of abdominal pain and help to reach a diagnosis. Some of the classical sites of radiation are shown in Figure 56.6.

Identification of the 'best questions' to ask is obviously important and, in his studies on acute abdominal pain, de Dombal revealed not only how important enquiry into factors aggravating the pain was, but also that this simple question was omitted in half the patients being questioned in a single hospital.

Other surgical symptoms

Although each is important in its own right, the other symptoms that cause a patient to be referred for surgical assessment, in either the elective or the emergency setting, do not present the complex pictures associated with 'abdominal pain' and can therefore be pooled together for the purposes of this chapter. Clearly, the individual chapters in this textbook will focus on the individual symptoms that are important to diseases of that organ. Common symptoms are:

1 abdominal distension/bloating;
2 nausea/vomiting;

3 haematemesis/melaena;
4 abdominal lumps/masses (including groin and scrotal lumps);
5 jaundice;
6 weight loss/cachexia;
7 altered bowel habit and bleeding/mucous per rectum.

EXAMINATION

After taking a detailed history, the patient should be carefully examined. An abdominal examination must always be part of a 'general' examination, but must specifically include the general appearance of the patient, including cachexia, anaemia, pallor, cyanosis, jaundice, dehydration, fetor and pyrexia. In the acute setting, a rapid (and/or irregular) pulse and low blood pressure may be important.

The neck and chest should be examined next, looking especially for lymphadenopathy, breast tumours and signs of pulmonary disease, while examination of the cardiovascular system may reveal evidence of cardiac failure, valve disorders or peripheral vascular disease.

The abdominal examination is made easier by the preceding history, which should have alerted the clinician to the possible underlying differential diagnoses. However, the opportunity to identify additional findings, which might either confirm or refute these diagnoses, must not be missed by a less than thorough examination. In the assessment of the patient with acute abdominal pain, several good studies have demonstrated that examination, along with the patient's distress, is facilitated by early administration of adequate analgesia. The old adage that analgesia should be withheld until a patient with acute abdominal pain has been assessed by the surgeon should be banished from every surgical textbook (Summary box 56.8).

Summary box 56.8

Abdominal examination (inspection)

- Analgesia should not be withheld
- Observe the abdomen before palpation
- Make a careful check for scars

Inspection

The swellings caused by enlargements of the liver, spleen, kidneys and bladder or tumours of the bowel or ovary and other intra-abdominal or retroperitoneal structures may all be visible on careful inspection. The expansile pulsation of an abdominal aneurysm may also be seen. All abdominal scars must be noted (and subsequently tested for an incisional hernia). Distension, which is usually caused by ascites, intestinal obstruction or a large intra-abdominal tumour, might also be apparent. A careful inspection may also reveal skin eruptions (such as those caused by herpes zoster), distended veins from portal hypertension (or occlusion of the inferior vena cava) and visible peristalsis. The hernial orifices must be specifically inspected (and then examined) along with the male genitalia, looking especially for tenderness and masses within the scrotum.

Palpation

Palpation of the abdomen should not be carried out until full inspection has been completed. An initial *superficial* examination might reveal specific sites of a mass or maximum tenderness, which can then be further evaluated by deeper palpation, if appropriate (in the case of pain) (Summary box 56.9).

Summary box 56.9

Abdominal examination (palpation)

- Check for pain first with superficial palpation
- Masses can be localised by checking for mobility (while patient lifts legs)
- Rebound tenderness suggests peritoneal inflammation
- Board-like rigidity suggests generalised peritonitis

Abdominal masses

A mass arising within the anterior abdominal wall will usually be mobile with the patient relaxed. On contracting the abdominal wall muscles (such as by lifting the legs in the straight position), lumps superficial to the abdominal wall muscles will become more obvious, those attached to the deep fascia will become less mobile, whereas those arising within the muscle layer will become fixed and less obvious. Lumps arising deep to the abdominal wall (i.e. within the peritoneal cavity or retroperitoneum) will usually become impalpable on tensing the anterior abdominal wall muscles. Intraperitoneal lumps will usually have some degree of mobility, even if only movement on respiration (i.e. liver and spleen), depending on which organs are involved. Retroperitoneal masses are usually fixed, although an enlarged kidney may be 'ballotable'.

Guarding and rebound tenderness

In the presence of abdominal pain, the degree of abdominal wall rigidity and involuntary guarding should be assessed. *Guarding* represents contraction of the abdominal wall muscles over the area of pain. This might occur 'voluntarily' when the patient wishes to avoid the pain from examination, or 'involuntarily' when the muscles go into spasm as the inflamed viscus touches the parietal peritoneum, resulting in a reflex spasm contracting the overlying abdominal wall muscles. The presence of *rebound* tenderness indicates underlying peritoneal inflammation and is best examined using percussion, although pain on coughing is also indicative of rebound tenderness. When the underlying peritoneal inflammation becomes generalised, the abdomen becomes '*board-like*' to palpation, and selective tenderness can no longer be elicited. This sign represents widespread *involuntary guarding*. Specific pain due to *abdominal wall tenderness* is apparent as an increase in pain at the point of maximal abdominal tenderness when the abdominal muscles are contracted.

Ascites

The presence of fluid within the peritoneal cavity may be suspected from clinical examination, but will usually require confirmation by either ultrasonography or computerised tomography (CT). Percussion of the abdomen in a patient with significant ascites will reveal dull flanks and a resonant central area, where the bowels 'float' on the underlying fluid. If the patient is asked to turn onto their side, the area of dullness will move downwards over their abdominal wall, while the area of resonance will 'float' to the flank of the side facing upwards (Summary box 56.10).

Summary box 56.10

Ascites

- Produces distension and dullness to percussion in the flanks
- The dullness 'shifts' as the patient is rolled onto their side

---

Pelvic examination

In the assessment of a patient with any gastrointestinal symptoms, a rectal examination is required and, if there is suspicion of underlying anorectal disease, this should be followed by a proctoscopy and sigmoidoscopy. A stool sample for occult blood should also be obtained where possible. However, the role of the rectal examination in assessment of the acute abdomen has changed over the last decade following a large study from Edinburgh, which demonstrated that, in patients with right iliac fossa pain (i.e. suspected appendicitis), no further additional information was obtained if rebound tenderness had already been demonstrated. However, when a gynaecological diagnosis is suspected, or needs to be excluded, a gentle pelvic examination should be carried out (Summary box 56.11).

Summary box 56.11

Pelvic examination

- Palpation for tenderness
- Rectal examination for tenderness and blood
- Proctoscopy for haemorrhoids, fissure and anal tumour
- Sigmoidoscopy for rectal tumours, inflammation and ulceration

---

Auscultation

Listening to the noises emanating from within the abdominal cavity requires experience, and interpretation is highly subjective. However, additional useful information can be obtained in relation to the characteristic bowel sounds produced by intestinal obstruction (gurgling and high pitched) and the total absence of bowel sounds found in patients with a severe generalised peritonitis or a postoperative paralytic ileus. Abdominal bruits associated with underlying vascular disease may also be detected (Summary box 56.12).

Summary box 56.12

Source of change in bowel sounds

- Gurgling and high pitched = Obstruction
- Absent = Peritonitis or ileus
- Bruits = Vascular

Specific signs

There are a number of specific 'named' signs that are still used to describe specific abdominal conditions, and these are described in Table 56.2.

OBSERVATION AND REVIEW

In the case of acute abdominal pain, there is a group of patients in whom, after full clinical assessment, the admitting surgeon

Table 56.2 Specific signs in abdominal examination

Sign	Description	Pathology
Courvoisier	Palpable gall bladder and jaundice	Carcinoma of the head of the pancreas
Cullen	Peri-umbilical bruising	Haemorrhagic pancreatitis or ectopic pregnancy
Grey Turner	Bruising of flank	Haemorrhagic pancreatitis
Rovsing	Pain on extension of the hip joint (due to psoas irritation)	Retrocaecal appendicitis
Murphy	Right upper quadrant tenderness exacerbated by inspiration	Acute cholecystitis
Virchow	Palpable left supraclavicular fossa lymph node	Oesophagogastric carcinoma

considers that the need for an urgent operation is uncertain. This is probably the most difficult group to deal with compared with those in whom an urgent operation is either clearly required, or clearly not required, and undoubtedly the one in which the majority of errors occur. Further expeditious investigations are obviously essential in this group and are discussed in some detail elsewhere in this book. However, while these are taking place, a

Ludwig Courvoisier, **1843–1918, Professor of Surgery, Basle, Switzerland.**
Thomas Stephen Cullen, **1868–1953, Professor of Gynaecology, The Johns Hopkins University, Baltimore, MD, USA.**
George Grey Turner, **1877–1951, Professor of Surgery, The University of Durham (1927–1943), and at The Postgraduate Medical School, Hammersmith, London, England (1934–1945).**
Nils Thorkild Rosving, **1862–1927, Professor of Surgery, Copenhagen, Denmark.**
John Benjamin Murphy, **1857–1916, Professor of Surgery, The Northwestern University, Chicago, IL, USA.**
Rudolf Ludwig Karl Vichow, **1821–1902, Professor of Pathological Anatomy, Berlin, Germany.**

period of observation with regular review is essential, and the benefits have been clearly reported on several occasions by surgeons from Aberdeen. This has now become an integral part of the early management of patients with acute abdominal pain and has been further highlighted by a recent prospective trial of CT in the investigation of abdominal pain. In this study, the presumed diagnosis was recorded on admission and at 24 hours, with a further review at 6 months. Only 50% of diagnoses on admission were correct at 6-month follow-up, but 76% of the diagnoses at 24 hours were correct. This included patients in the CT arm and the standard treatment arm.

FURTHER READING

Paterson-Brown, S. (ed.) (2005) *A Companion to Specialist Surgical Practice – Core Topics in General and Emergency Surgery*, 3rd edn. Elsevier Science, London.

CHAPTER 56 | HISTORY AND EXAMINATION OF THE ABDOMEN

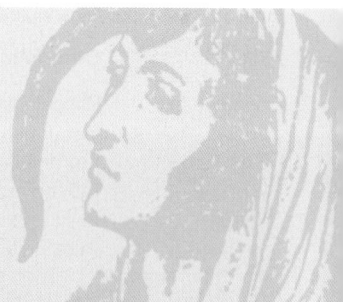

Hernias, umbilicus and abdominal wall

CHAPTER 57

HERNIA

No disease of the human body, belonging to the province of the surgeon, requires in its treatment a better combination of accurate anatomical knowledge with surgical skill than Hernia in all its varieties.

Sir Astley Paston Cooper (1804)

A hernia is a protrusion of a viscus or part of a viscus through an abnormal opening in the walls of its containing cavity. The external abdominal hernia is the most common form, the most frequent varieties being the inguinal, femoral and umbilical, accounting for 75% of cases (Fig. 57.1). The rarer forms constitute 1.5%, excluding incisional hernias.

General features common to all hernias

Aetiology

Any condition that raises intra-abdominal pressure, such as a powerful muscular effort, may produce a hernia. Whooping cough is a predisposing cause in childhood, whereas a chronic cough, straining on micturition or straining on defaecation may precipitate a hernia in an adult. Hernias are more common in smokers, which may be the result of an acquired collagen deficiency increasing an individual's susceptibility to the development of hernias. It should be remembered that the appearance of a hernia in an adult can be a sign of intra-abdominal malignancy. Stretching of the abdominal musculature because of an increase in contents, as in obesity, can be another factor. Fat acts to separate muscle bundles and layers, weakens aponeuroses and favours the appearance of paraumbilical, direct inguinal and hiatus hernias. A femoral hernia is rare in men and nulliparous women but more common in multiparous women due to stretching of the pelvic ligaments. An indirect hernia may occur in a congenital preformed sac – the remains of the processus vaginalis.

Peritoneal dialysis can cause the development of a hernia from a previously occult weakness or enlargement of a patent processus vaginalis (Summary box 57.1).

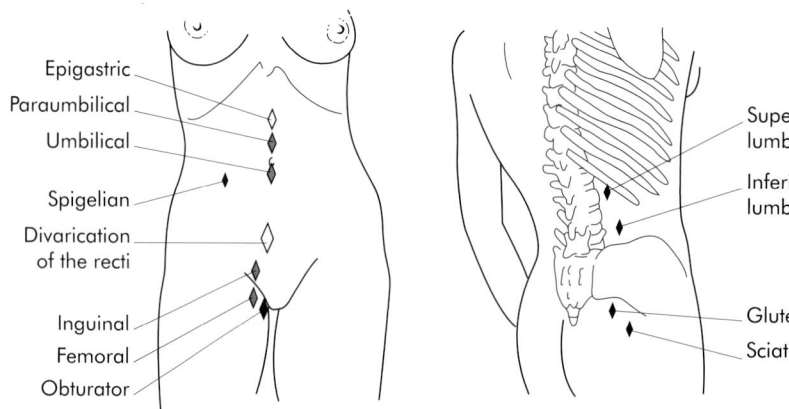

Figure 57.1 External hernias. Red = common; white = not unusual; black = rare.

Sir Astley Paston Cooper, **1768–1841, Surgeon, Guy's Hospital, London, England.**

CHAPTER 57 | HERNIAS, UMBILICUS AND ABDOMINAL WALL

Summary box 57.1

Causes of hernias

- Coughing
- Straining
- Obesity
- Intra-abdominal malignancy

Composition of a hernia

As a rule, a hernia consists of three parts – the sac, the coverings of the sac and the contents of the sac.

The sac

The sac is a diverticulum of peritoneum, consisting of mouth, neck, body and fundus. The neck is usually well defined but in some direct inguinal hernias and in many incisional hernias there is no actual neck. The diameter of the neck is important because strangulation of bowel is a likely complication when the neck is narrow, as in femoral and paraumbilical hernias.

The body of the sac varies greatly in size and is not necessarily occupied. In cases occurring in infancy and childhood, the sac is gossamer thin. In longstanding cases the wall of the sac may be comparatively thick.

The covering

Coverings are derived from the layers of the abdominal wall through which the sac passes. In longstanding cases they become atrophied from stretching and so amalgamated that they are indistinguishable from each other.

Contents

These can be:

- omentum = omentocele (synonym: epiplocele);
- intestine = enterocele; more commonly small bowel but may be large intestine or appendix;
- a portion of the circumference of the intestine = Richter's hernia;
- a portion of the bladder (or a diverticulum) may constitute part of or be the sole content of a direct inguinal, a sliding inguinal or a femoral hernia;
- ovary with or without the corresponding fallopian tube;
- a Meckel's diverticulum = a Littre's hernia;
- fluid, as part of ascites or as a residuum thereof.

Classification

Irrespective of site, a hernia can be classified into five different types (Summary box 57.2).

August Gottlieb Richter, **1742–1812**, Lecturer in Surgery, Göttingen, Germany described this form of hernia in 1777.
Gabriele Falloppio, (Fallopius), **1523–1563**, Professor of Anatomy, Surgery and Botany, Padua, Italy.
Johann Friedrich Meckel, (The Younger), **1781–1833**, Professor of Anatomy and Surgery, Halle, Germany, described the diverticulum in 1809.
Alexis Littre, **1658–1726**, Surgeon and Lecturer in Anatomy, Paris, France, described 'Meckel's Diverticulum' in a hernial sac in 1700, 81 years before Meckel was born.

Summary box 57.2

Types of hernia

- Reducible – contents can be returned to abdomen
- Irreducible – contents cannot be returned but there are no other complications
- Obstructed – bowel in the hernia has good blood supply but bowel is obstructed
- Strangulated – blood supply of bowel is obstructed
- Inflamed – contents of sac have become inflamed

Reducible hernias

The hernia either reduces itself when the patient lies down or can be reduced by the patient or the surgeon. The intestine usually gurgles on reduction and the first portion is more difficult to reduce than the last. Omentum, in contrast, is described as doughy and the last portion is more difficult to reduce than the first. A reducible hernia imparts an expansile impulse on coughing.

Irreducible hernia

In this case the contents cannot be returned to the abdomen but there is no evidence of other complications. It is usually due to adhesions between the sac and its contents or overcrowding within the sac. Irreducibility without other symptoms is almost diagnostic of an omentocele, especially in femoral and umbilical hernias. Note that any degree of irreducibility predisposes to strangulation.

Obstructed hernia

This is an irreducible hernia containing intestine that is obstructed from without or within, but there is no interference to the blood supply to the bowel. The symptoms (colicky abdominal pain and tenderness over the hernia site) are less severe and the onset more gradual than in strangulated hernias, but more often than not the obstruction culminates in strangulation. Usually there is no clear distinction clinically between obstruction and strangulation and the safe course is to assume that strangulation is imminent and treat accordingly.

Incarcerated hernia

The term 'incarceration' is often used loosely as an alternative to obstruction or strangulation but is correctly employed only when it is considered that the lumen of that portion of the colon occupying a hernial sac is blocked with faeces. In this case, the scybalous contents of the bowel should be capable of being indented with the finger, like putty.

Strangulated hernia

A hernia becomes strangulated when the blood supply of its contents is seriously impaired, rendering the contents ischaemic. Gangrene may occur as early as 5–6 hours after the onset of the first symptoms. Although inguinal hernia may be 10 times more common than femoral hernia, a femoral hernia is more likely to strangulate because of the narrowness of the neck and its rigid surrounds (Summary box 57.3).

Summary box 57.3

Natural history of hernias

- Irreducible hernias – there is a risk of strangulation at any time
- Obstructed hernias – usually go on to strangulation
- Strangulated hernias – gangrene can occur within 6 hours

Pathology

The intestine is obstructed and its blood supply impaired. Initially, only the venous return is impeded; the wall of the intestine becomes congested and bright red with the transudation of serous fluid into the sac. As congestion increases the wall of the intestine becomes purple in colour. The intestinal pressure increases, distending the intestinal loop and impairing venous return further. As venous stasis increases, the arterial supply becomes more and more impaired. Blood is extravasated under the serosa and is effused into the lumen. The fluid in the sac becomes blood-stained and the shining serosa dull because of a fibrinous, sticky exudate. At this stage the walls of the intestine have lost their tone and become friable. Bacterial transudation occurs secondary to the lowered intestinal viability and the sac fluid becomes infected. Gangrene appears at the rings of constriction (Fig. 57.2), which become deeply indented and grey in colour. The gangrene then develops in the anti-mesenteric border, the colour varying from black to green depending on the decomposition of blood in the subserosa. The mesentery involved by the strangulation also becomes gangrenous. If the strangulation is unrelieved, perforation of the wall of the intestine occurs, either at the convexity of the loop or at the seat of constriction. Peritonitis spreads from the sac to the peritoneal cavity.

Clinical features

Sudden pain, at first situated over the hernia, is followed by generalised abdominal pain, colicky in character and often located mainly at the umbilicus. Nausea and subsequently vomiting ensue. The patient may complain of an increase in hernia size. On examination the hernia is tense, extremely tender and irreducible, and there is no expansile cough impulse.

Unless the strangulation is relieved by operation, the spasms of pain continue until peristaltic contractions cease with the onset of ischaemia, when paralytic ileus (often the result of peritonitis) and septicaemia develop. Spontaneous cessation of pain must be viewed with caution, as this may be a sign of perforation (Summary box 57.4).

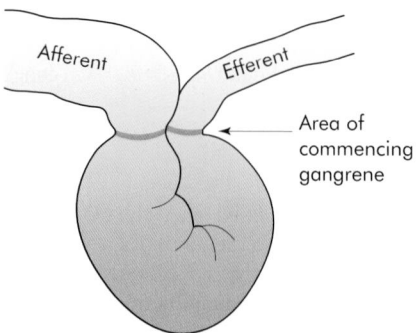

Figure 57.2 Gangrene commences at the areas of constriction and then at the anti-mesenteric border.

Summary box 57.4

Strangulated hernias

- Present with local then general abdominal pain and vomiting
- A normal hernia can strangulate at any time
- Most common in hernias with narrow necks such as femoral hernias
- Require urgent surgery

Richter's hernia

Richter's hernia is a hernia in which the sac contains only a portion of the circumference of the intestine (usually small intestine). It usually complicates femoral and, rarely, obturator hernias.

Strangulated Richter's hernia

Strangulated Richter's hernia (Fig. 57.3) is particularly noteworthy as operation is frequently delayed because the clinical features mimic gastroenteritis. The local signs of strangulation are often not obvious, the patient may not vomit and, although colicky pain is present, the bowels are often opened normally or there may be diarrhoea; absolute constipation is delayed until paralytic ileus supervenes. For these reasons, gangrene of the knuckle of bowel and perforation have often occurred before operation is undertaken.

Strangulated omentocele

The initial symptoms are in general similar to those of strangulated bowel. Vomiting and constipation may be absent as omentum, unlike intestine, can exist on a very meagre blood supply. The onset of gangrene is therefore delayed, occurring first in the centre of the fatty mass. Unrelieved, a bacterial invasion of the ischaemic contents of the sac will occur and an abscess eventually develops. In an inguinal hernia, infection usually terminates as a scrotal abscess, but extension from the sac to the general peritoneal cavity is always a possibility.

Inflamed hernia

Inflammation can occur from inflammation of the contents of the sac, e.g. acute appendicitis or salpingitis, or from external causes, e.g. the trophic ulcers that develop in the dependent areas of large umbilical or incisional hernias. The hernia is usually tender but not tense and the overlying skin red and oedematous. Treatment is based on treatment of the underlying cause.

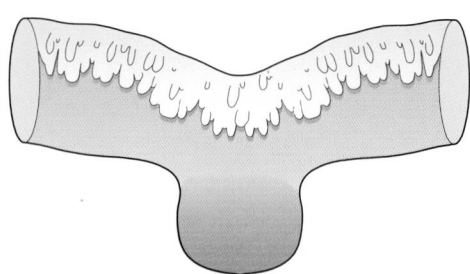

Figure 57.3 Diagrammatic representation of gangrenous Richter's hernia from a case of strangulated femoral hernia.

Inguinal hernia

Surgical anatomy

The superficial inguinal ring is a triangular aperture in the aponeurosis of the external oblique muscle and lies 1.25 cm above the pubic tubercle. The ring is bounded by a superomedial and an inferolateral crus joined by the criss-crossed intercrural fibres. Normally the ring will not admit the tip of the little finger.

The deep inguinal ring is a U-shaped condensation of the transversalis fascia and it lies 1.25 cm above the inguinal (Poupart's) ligament, midway between the symphysis pubis and the anterior superior iliac spine. The transversalis fascia is the fascial envelope of the abdomen and the competency of the deep inguinal ring depends on the integrity of this fascia.

The inguinal canal

In infants, the superficial and deep inguinal rings are almost superimposed and the obliquity of the canal is slight. In adults, the inguinal canal, which is about 3.75 cm long, is directed downwards and medially from the deep to the superficial inguinal ring. In the male, the inguinal canal transmits the spermatic cord, the ilioinguinal nerve and the genital branch of the genitofemoral nerve. In the female, the round ligament replaces the spermatic cord.

Figure 57.4 illustrates the canal, viewing the structures from superficial to deep as is seen at operation. The anterior boundary comprises mainly the external oblique aponeurosis with the conjoined muscle laterally. The posterior boundary is formed by the fascia transversalis and the conjoined tendon (internal oblique and transversus abdominus medially). The inferior epigastric vessels lie posteriorly and medially to the deep inguinal ring. The superior boundary is formed by the conjoined muscles (internal oblique and transversus) and the inferior boundary is the inguinal ligament.

An indirect hernia travels down the canal on the outer (lateral and anterior) side of the spermatic cord. A direct hernia comes out directly forwards through the posterior wall of the inguinal canal. Whereas the neck of the indirect hernia is lateral to the inferior epigastric vessels, the direct hernia usually emerges medial to this except in the saddle-bag or pantaloon type, which has both a lateral and a medial component. An inguinal hernia can be differentiated from a femoral hernia by ascertaining the relation of the neck of the sac to the medial end of the inguinal ligament and the pubic tubercle; i.e. in the case of an inguinal hernia the neck is above and medial, whereas that of a femoral hernia is below and lateral (Fig. 57.4). Digital control of the internal ring may help in distinguishing between an indirect and a direct inguinal hernia, although some reports have found that the preoperative diagnosis is incorrect as often as it is correct.

Indirect (synonym: oblique) inguinal hernia

This is the most common form of hernia (see Aetiology p. 968). Indirect hernias are most common in the young, whereas direct hernias are most common in the old. In the first decade of life, inguinal hernia is more common on the right side in the male. This is no doubt associated with the later descent of the right testis and a higher incidence of failure of closure of the processus vaginalis. In adult males, 65% of inguinal hernias are indirect and 55% are right-sided. The hernia is bilateral in 12% of cases. If both sides are explored in an infant presenting with one hernia,

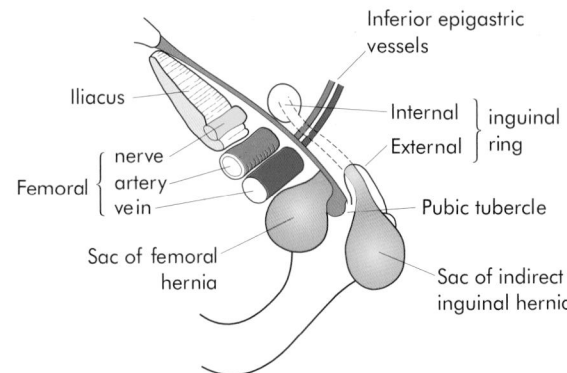

Figure 57.4 The relationships of an indirect inguinal and a femoral hernia to the pubic tubercle; the inguinal hernia emerges above and medial to the tubercle whereas the femoral hernia lies below and lateral to it.

the incidence of a patent processus vaginalis on the other side is 60% (Summary box 57.5).

Summary box 57.5

Natural history of inguinal hernias

- Inguinal hernias in babies are the result of a persistent processus vaginalis
- Indirect inguinal hernia is the most common hernia of all, especially in the young
- Direct inguinal hernia becomes more common in the elderly

Three types of indirect inguinal hernia occur (Fig. 57.5):

1 *Bubonocele.* The hernia is limited to the inguinal canal.
2 *Funicular.* The processus vaginalis is closed just above the epididymis. The contents of the sac can be felt separately from the testis, which lies below the hernia.
3 *Complete (synonym: scrotal).* A complete inguinal hernia is rarely present at birth but is commonly encountered in infancy. It also occurs in adolescence or in adulthood. The testis appears to lie within the lower part of the hernia.

Clinical features

Notes on examination The clinician examines the patient from the front with the patient standing with legs apart. The patient is instructed to look at the ceiling and cough. If the hernia will

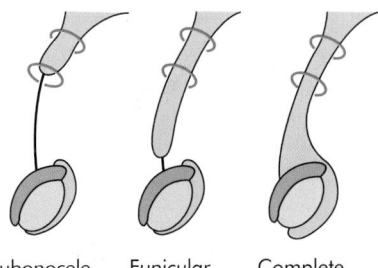

Figure 57.5 Types of oblique inguinal hernia. *Bubon* (Greek) = groin; *funiculus* (Latin) = a small cord.

come down, it usually does. The examiner looks and feels for the impulse and then addresses the following questions:

- Is the hernia right, left or bilateral?
- Is it an inguinal or femoral hernia?
- Is it a direct or an indirect hernia?
- Is it reducible or irreducible (the patient may have to lie down for this to be ascertained)?
- Is the inguinal hernia incomplete or complete?
- What are the contents?

Looking at all ages, males are 20 times more commonly affected than females. The patient complains of pain in the groin or pain referred to the testicle when performing heavy work or taking strenuous exercise. When asked to cough, a small transient bulging may be seen and felt together with an expansile impulse. When the sac is still limited to the inguinal canal, the bulge may be better seen by observing the inguinal region from the side or even looking down the abdominal wall while standing behind the relevant shoulder of the patient.

As an indirect inguinal hernia increases in size it becomes apparent when the patient coughs, and persists until reduced (Fig. 57.6). As time goes on, the hernia comes down as soon as the patient stands up. In large hernias there is a sensation of weight and dragging on the mesentery. This may produce epigastric pain. If the contents of the sac are reducible, the inguinal canal will be found to be commodious.

In infants the swelling appears when the child cries. It can be translucent in infancy and early childhood but never in an adult. In girls an ovary may prolapse into the sac.

Differential diagnosis in the male
In males the differential diagnosis includes the following:

- vaginal hydrocele (Fig. 57.7);
- encysted hydrocele of the cord;
- spermatocele;
- femoral hernia;
- incompletely descended testis in the inguinal canal – an inguinal hernia is often associated with this condition;
- lipoma of the cord – this is often a difficult but unimportant diagnosis and it is usually not settled until the parts are displayed by operation.

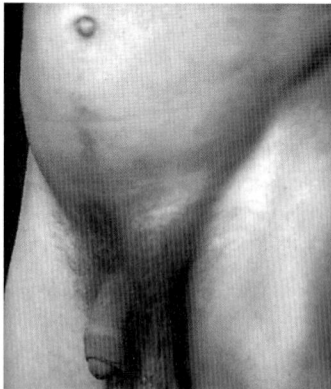

Figure 57.6 Oblique left inguinal hernia that became apparent when the patient coughed and persisted until it was reduced when he lay down.

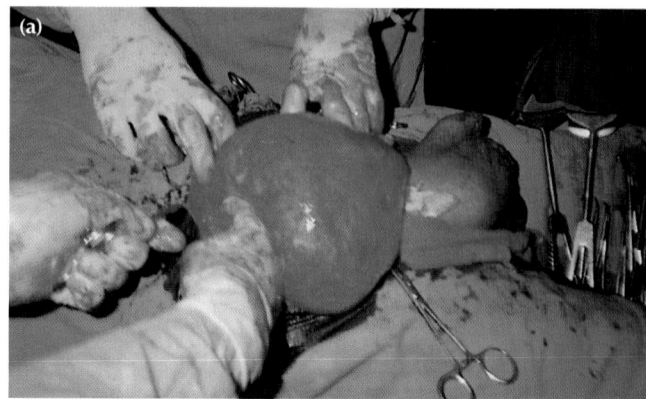

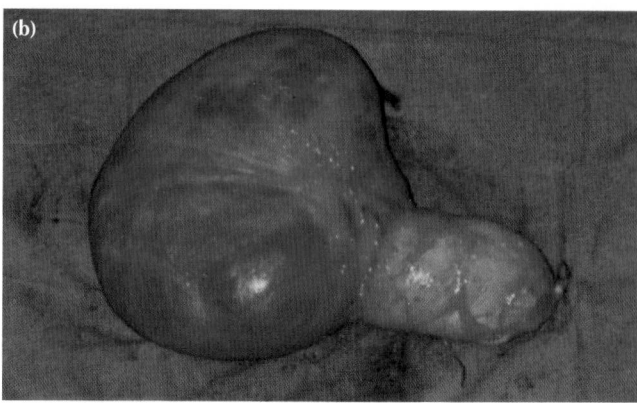

Figure 57.7 Large transilluminant cystic swelling present in the lower abdomen, extending down the inguinal canal in the scrotum. (a) Lesion being removed. (b) Excised specimen. It is not possible to distinguish between a complex scrotal hernia, a hydrocele of the cord and a vaginal hydrocele in such cases before exposing the anatomy; in this case the lesion was an abdominoscrotal hydrocele (courtesy of Drs D. Pratep and R. Sahai, Jhabsi, India).

Note that examination using finger and thumb across the neck of the scrotum will help to distinguish between a swelling of inguinal origin and one that is entirely intrascrotal.

Differential diagnosis in the female
In females the differential diagnosis includes the following:

- hydrocele of the canal of Nuck – this is the most common differential diagnostic problem;
- femoral hernia.

Treatment
Operation is the treatment of choice. It must be remembered that patients who have a bad cough from chronic bronchitis should not be denied an operation, for these are the very people who are in danger of developing a strangulated hernia. In adults, local, epidural or spinal, as well as general anaesthesia, can be used (Summary box 57.6).

Anton Nuck, 1650–1692, Professor of Anatomy and Medicine, Leiden, The Netherlands.

The basic operation is inguinal herniotomy, which entails dissecting out and opening the hernial sac, reducing any contents and then transfixing the neck of the sac and removing the remainder. It is employed either by itself or as the first step in a repair procedure (herniorrhaphy). By itself it is sufficient for the treatment of hernia in infants, adolescents and young adults. Any attempts at repair in such cases may, in fact, do more harm than good.

In infants it is not necessary to open the canal, as the internal and external rings are superimposed. Excellent results are obtained. The operation is usually now performed as a day case unless there are additional medical or social problems.

Herniotomy and repair (herniorrhaphy) consists of: (1) excision of the hernial sac; plus (2) repair of the stretched internal inguinal ring and the transversalis fascia; and (3) further reinforcement of the posterior wall of the inguinal canal. (2) and (3) must be achieved without tension resulting in the wound and various techniques exist to achieve this, e.g. Shouldice operation, fascial flaps or mesh implants.

Excision of the hernial sac (adult herniotomy) An incision[1] is made in the skin and subcutaneous tissue 1.25 cm above and parallel to the medial two-thirds of the inguinal ligament. In large, irreducible hernias the incision may be extended laterally or into the upper part of the scrotum. After dividing the superficial fascia and securing haemostasis, the external oblique aponeurosis and the superficial inguinal ring are identified. The external oblique aponeurosis is incised in the line of its fibres and the structures beneath carefully separated from its deep surface before completing the incision through the superficial inguinal ring. In this way, the ilioinguinal nerve is safeguarded. With the inguinal canal thus opened, the upper leaf of the external oblique muscle is separated from the internal oblique muscle by blunt dissection. In the same way, the lower leaf is separated from the contents of the inguinal canal until the inner aspect of the inguinal ligament is seen. The cremasteric muscle fibres may be divided longitudinally to display the spermatic cord, but this is by no means essential.

- *Excision of the sac.* The indirect sac may be distinguished as a pearly white structure lying on the outer side of the cord and, when the internal spermatic fascia has been incised longitudinally, it can usually be dissected out and then opened between artery forceps.
- *Variations in dissection.* If the sac is small it can be freed *in toto*. If it is of the long, funicular or scrotal type, or is extremely thickened and adherent, the fundus must not be sought because in doing so the blood supply to the testis may be compromised. The sac is freed within the inguinal canal and divided circumferentially such that the fundus remains in the

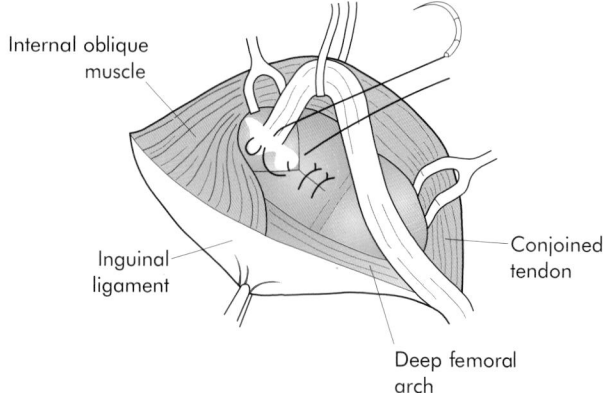

Figure 57.8 The Lytle method of repair of the stretched internal inguinal ring, which should be narrowed to admit the tip of the little finger. Lateral displacement of the cord is often advantageous (after F.S.A. Doran, FRCS, Bromsgrove, UK).

scrotum. Care must be taken to avoid damage to the vas and spermatic artery when freeing the sac posteriorly.

- An *adherent sac* can be separated from the cord by first injecting saline under the posterior wall from within (hydrodissection). A similar tactic is employed when dissecting the gossamer sac of infants and children.
- *Reduction of contents.* Intestine or omentum is returned to the peritoneal cavity. Omentum is often adherent to the neck or fundus of the sac: if adherent to the neck it is freed and if adherent to the fundus of a large sac it may be transfixed, ligated and cut across at a suitable point. The distal part of the omentum, like the distal part of a large scrotal sac, can be left *in situ* (the fundus should, however, not be ligated).
- *Isolation and ligation of the neck of the sac.* Whatever type of sac is encountered, it is necessary to free the neck by blunt dissection until the parietal peritoneum can be seen on all sides. The dissection is considered complete only when the extraperitoneal fat has been encountered and the inferior epigastric vessels have been seen on the medial side. It used to be considered essential to open the sac to ensure that no bowel or omentum was adherent to the neck. If the sac is obviously empty, it is sufficient to simply reduce it, close the internal ring and perform a herniorrhaphy if required. If the sac is opened, all contents should be reduced and the neck transfixed as high as possible before excising the sac.

Repair of the transversalis fascia and the internal ring When the internal ring is weak and stretched and the transversalis is bulging, the repair should include a technique of narrowing the deep ring, e.g. the Lytle method of narrowing the ring with lateral displacement of the cord (Fig. 57.8), or the Shouldice method, whereby the ring and fascia are incised and carefully separated from the deep inferior epigastric vessels and extraperitoneal fat before an overlapping repair ('double breasting') of the lower flap behind the upper flap is performed (Fig. 57.9). In the classic Shouldice operation, a third and fourth layer of tension-free suturing, using monofilament materials, polypropylene, polyamide or wire, are placed between the internal oblique aponeurosis arch and the inguinal ligament.

---

1   Prior to the skin incision in large inguinoscrotal hernias, the usual antiseptic preparation of the skin should not be extended to the perineal aspect of the scrotum because, by doing so, severe bacterial contamination of the operation is likely.

William James Lytle, 1896–1986, Surgeon, The Royal Infirmary, Sheffield, England.

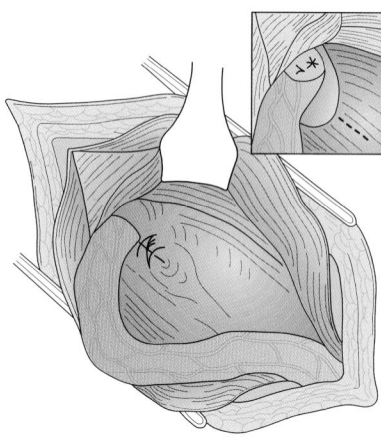

Figure 57.9 After the neck of the sac has been divided at the deep inguinal ring, the fascia transversalis of the deep opening is identified and assessed. If the ring is of normal size, the stump of the sac is reduced and no more need be done. If the ring is marginally dilated (stretched), it should be carefully dissected and possibly divided slightly (inset), and then sutured tightly around the medial side of the cord with polypropylene to reconstitute a competent deep inguinal ring.

Reinforcement of the posterior inguinal wall This is achieved by suturing without tension the tendinous aponeurotic arch of the internal oblique to the undersurface of the inguinal ligament and to the pubic tubercle (as described above in the Shouldice operation) or by reinforcing the posterior wall of the canal with a prosthetic mesh. Care is taken when suturing not to pick up the same tendinous bundle for each suture. Suturing of muscle bundles is of no value. The suturing method can include a rectus-relaxing incision (Halsted–Tanner). The Lichtenstein tension-free hernioplasty involves placement of an approximately 16 × 8 cm (tailored to the individual patient's requirements) mesh as an extra lamina, anterior to the posterior wall and overlapping it generously in all directions, including medially over the pubic tubercle (Fig. 57.10).

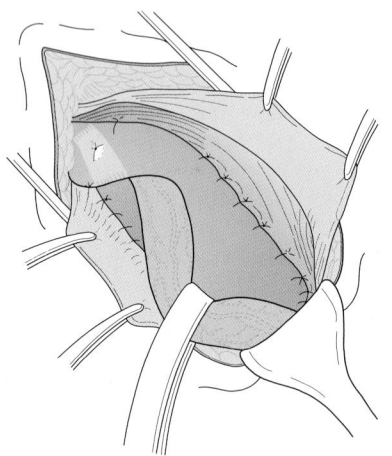

Figure 57.10 Lichtenstein repair. The 'tails' of the mesh are overlapped and crossed and a single suture is placed to create a new 'internal' ring.

William Stewart Halsted, **1852–1922, Professor of Surgery, Johns Hopkins Hospital Medical School, Baltimore, MD, USA.**
Norman Cecil Tanner, **1906–1982, Surgeon, Charing Cross Hospital, London, England.**

Other historical techniques, which should now be abandoned because of poor results, include overlapping the external oblique behind the cord (making it lie subcutaneously). Special care is needed to avoid excessive narrowing of the new external ring, which could jeopardise the vascular supply to and the venous return from the testis.

Completion of operation If desired, the cremasteric muscle can be reconstituted: the external oblique is directly sutured or overlapped, leaving a new external ring that should accommodate the tip of a finger.

A truss A truss may be used when operation is contraindicated or when operation is refused. Its use should be mainly historical, as there are very few contraindications to surgery with today's variety of anaesthetic techniques. If a truss is to be worn, the hernia must be reducible. A rat-tailed spring truss with a perineal band to prevent the truss slipping will, with due care and attention, control a small or moderately sized inguinal hernia. A truss must be worn continuously during waking hours, kept clean and in proper repair and renewed when it shows signs of wear. It must be applied before the patient gets up and while the hernia is reduced. A properly fitting truss must control the hernia when the patient stands with legs apart, stoops and coughs violently. If it does not it is a menace because it increases the risk of strangulation.

There is no place for trusses in the management of infant hernias. If an infant hernia becomes suddenly irreducible, urgent operative repair is indicated. Otherwise, the infant hernia can be left alone until the child is over 3 months old, when routine daycase repair can be performed.

Direct inguinal hernia

In adult males, 35% of inguinal hernias are direct. At presentation, 12% of patients will have a contralateral hernia in addition, and there is a fourfold increased risk of future development of a contralateral hernia if one is not present at the original presentation.

A direct inguinal hernia is always acquired. The sac passes through a weakness or defect of the transversalis fascia in the posterior wall of the inguinal canal. In some cases the defect is small and is represented by a discrete defect in the transversalis fascia, whereas in others there is a generalised bulge. Often the patient has poor lower abdominal musculature, as shown by the presence of elongated bulgings (Malgaigne's bulges). Women practically never develop a direct inguinal hernia (Brown). Predisposing factors are smoking and occupations that involve straining and heavy lifting. Damage to the ilioinguinal nerve (previous appendicectomy) is another cause, because of the resulting weakness of the conjoined tendon.

Direct hernias do not often attain a large size or descend into the scrotum (Fig 57.11). In contrast to an indirect inguinal hernia, a direct inguinal hernia lies behind the spermatic cord. The sac is often smaller than the hernial mass would indicate, the protruding mass mainly consisting of extraperitoneal fat. As the neck of the sac is wide, direct inguinal hernias do not often strangulate (Summary box 57.7).

Francis Robert Brown, **1889–1967, Surgeon, The Royal Infirmary, Dundee, Scotland.**
Joseph Francois Malgaigne, **1806–1865, Professor of Surgery, Paris, France.**

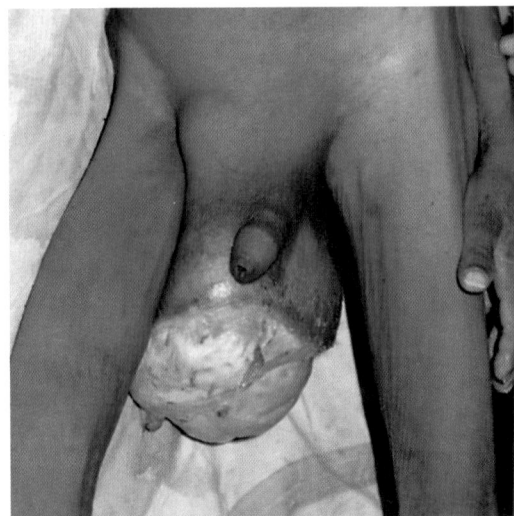

Figure 57.11 A huge inguinal hernia (direct) that has descended into the scrotum. The overlying skin has become gangrenous and sloughed away (courtesy of Dr Anupam Rai, Jabalpur, India).

Summary box 57.7

Direct inguinal hernias

- All are acquired
- They are most common in older men
- They rarely strangulate

Funicular direct inguinal hernia (synonym: prevesical hernia)

This is a narrow-necked hernia with prevesical fat and a portion of the bladder that occurs through a small oval defect in the medial part of the conjoined tendon just above the pubic tubercle. It occurs principally in elderly men and occasionally becomes strangulated. Unless there are definite contraindications, operation should always be advised.

Dual (synonym: saddle-bag, pantaloon) hernia

This type of hernia consists of two sacs that straddle the inferior epigastric artery, one sac being medial and the other lateral to this vessel. The condition is not rare and is a cause of recurrence, one of the sacs having been overlooked at the time of operation.

Operation for direct hernia

The principles of repair of direct hernias are the same as those of an indirect hernia, with the exception that the hernia sac can usually be simply inverted after it has been dissected free and the transversalis fascia reconstructed in front of it. This reconstruction of the posterior wall of the inguinal canal should be undertaken by the Shouldice repair or by using a mesh implant according to the Lichtenstein technique (see Figs 57.9 and 57.10). The 'Bassini' darn operation is no longer acceptable because of its high recurrence rate and slow rehabilitation.

Laparoscopic herniorrhaphy (see Chapter 19) Over the last 10 years, minimally invasive techniques have been developed for the treatment of inguinal hernias. Two techniques are described, a transabdominal approach (TAPP) and a preperitoneal approach (TEP). The TAPP approach establishes a pneumoperitoneum and places a synthetic mesh preperitoneally by dissecting the peritoneum off the hernial orifices and positioning the mesh beneath the peritoneum before closing the peritoneum over the mesh. The TEP approach is completely preperitoneal. The preperitoneal plane is opened by either balloon dissection or direct dissection via a paraumbilical incision. The hernial orifices can be identified bilaterally and any hernia sac reduced. Placing a large mesh over the hernial orifices in the preperitoneal plane completes the repair (Fig. 57.12). There is some discussion about the requirement for mesh fixation, and various techniques are available to fix the mesh in place. In the UK, there has been a general trend away from TAPP repairs as the incidence of complications is higher than with the TEP repair. However, the TEP repair is technically more difficult to perform and is associated with a longer learning curve. In experienced hands, the recurrence rate for TEP repairs is less than 1%.

Laparoscopic repairs can be applied to primary, bilateral and recurrent inguinal hernias as well as to femoral hernias. The National Institute for Clinical Excellence (NICE) in the UK has produced guidelines on the use of laparoscopic surgery for inguinal hernias and has recommended the consideration of the TEP laparoscopic technique for any inguinal hernia, unilateral, recurrent or bilateral, but only in laparoscopic centres where there are surgeons experienced in the technique.

Strangulated inguinal hernia

The pathological and clinical features of strangulated inguinal hernias have been described earlier in this chapter. Strangulation of an inguinal hernia occurs at any time during life and in both sexes. Indirect inguinal hernias strangulate more commonly, the direct variety not so often because of the wide neck of the sac. Sometimes a hernia strangulates on the first occasion that it descends; more often strangulation occurs in patients who have

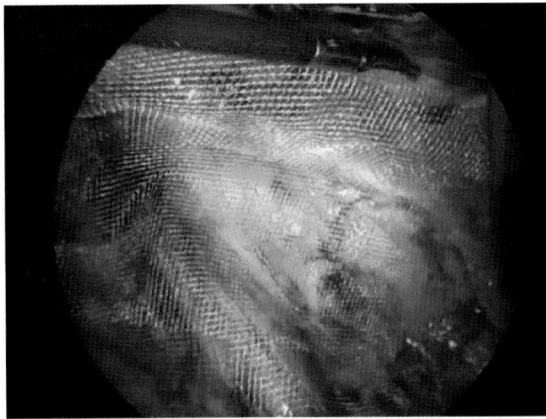

Figure 57.12 TEP repair. Laparoscopically placed preperitoneal mesh covering the myopectineal orifice. Extraperitoneal dissection has proceeded to reveal loose areolar tissue in the space of Retzius.

Edoardo Bassini, 1844–1924, Professor of Surgery, Padua, Italy, described this method of herniorrhaphy in 1889.

Robert Edward Gross, B. 1905, Ladd Professor of Children's Surgery, Harvard University Medical School, Boston, MA, USA.

worn a truss for a long time and in those with a partially reducible or an irreducible hernia.

In order of frequency, the constricting agent is: (1) the neck of the sac; (2) the external inguinal ring in children; and (3) adhesions within the sac (rarely).

Contents

Usually the small intestine is involved in the strangulation, with the next most frequent being the omentum; sometimes both are involved. It is rare for the large intestine to become strangulated in an inguinal hernia, even when the hernia is of the sliding variety.

Strangulation during infancy

The incidence of strangulation in infancy is 4% (Gross) and the ratio of girls to boys is 5:1. More frequently, the hernia is irreducible but not strangulated. In most cases of strangulated inguinal hernia occurring in female infants, the content of the sac is an ovary or an ovary plus its fallopian tube.

Treatment of strangulated inguinal hernia

The treatment of strangulated hernia is by emergency operation. Vigorous resuscitation with intravenous fluids, nasogastric aspiration and antibiotics is essential, although operation should not be unduly delayed in moribund patients. It is also advisable to empty the bladder, if necessary by catheterisation (Summary box 57.8).

Summary box 57.8

Preoperative treatment of strangulated inguinal hernias

- Resuscitate with adequate fluids
- Empty stomach with nasogastric tube
- Give antibiotics to contain infection
- Catheterise to monitor haemodynamic state

Inguinal herniotomy for strangulation An incision is made over the most prominent part of the swelling. The external oblique aponeurosis is exposed and the sac, with its coverings, is seen issuing from the superficial ring. In all but very large hernias it is possible to deliver the body and fundus of the sac together with its coverings and (in the male) the testis on to the surface (it is not necessary to deliver the testis if the fundus of the sac can be adequately exposed). Each layer covering the anterior surface of the body of the sac near the fundus is incised and, if possible, stripped off the sac. The sac is then incised and any fluid, which may be highly infective, drained effectively. The external oblique aponeurosis and the superficial inguinal ring are divided. A finger is then passed into the opening in the sac and, employing the finger as a guide, the sac is slit along its length. If the constriction lies at the superficial inguinal ring or within the canal, it is readily divided by this procedure. When the constriction is at the deep ring, by applying artery forceps to the cut edge of the neck of the sac and drawing them downwards, and at the same time retracting the internal oblique upwards, it may be possible to continue slitting the sac over the finger towards the point of constriction. When the constriction is too tight to admit a finger, a grooved dissector is inserted and the neck of the sac is divided with a knife in an upward and inward direction, i.e. parallel to the inferior epigastric vessels, under vision. Once the constriction has

been divided, the strangulated contents can be drawn down. Devitalised omentum is excised after being securely ligated. Viable intestine is returned to the peritoneal cavity. Doubtfully viable and gangrenous intestine is excised by localised resection. If the hernial sac is of moderate size and can be separated easily from its coverings, it is excised and closed by a purse-string suture. When the sac is large and adherent, much time is saved by cutting across the sac circumferentially, as described earlier. Having tied or sutured the neck of the sac, a repair can be made if the condition of the patient permits. If the incision has been soiled or gangrenous bowel resected, the use of prosthetic mesh may be questionable, although some authorities have successfully utilised polypropylene mesh with antibiotic cover. Biosynthetic meshes made from collagen or dermis are also available and, because they are totally absorbed, are more suited to use in a contaminated environment.

Conservative measures These are indicated only in infants. The child is given analgesics and placed in gallow's traction (the judgement of Solomon position). In 75% of cases reduction is effected and there appears to be no danger of gangrenous intestine being reduced (Irvine Smith).

Note that vigorous manipulation (taxis) has no place in modern surgery and is mentioned only to be condemned. Its dangers include:

- contusion or rupture of the intestinal wall;
- reduction-en-masse: 'The sac together with its contents is pushed forcibly back into the abdomen; as the bowel will still be strangulated by the neck of the sac, the symptoms are in no way relieved' (Treves);
- reduction into the a loculus of the sac;
- the sac may rupture at its neck and the contents are reduced, not into the peritoneal cavity but extraperitoneally (Summary box 57.9).

Summary box 57.9

Non-operative treatment of hernias

- Only indicated in children
- Forcible reduction must never be attempted

Maydl's hernia (synonym: hernia-in-W) Maydl's hernia is rare. The strangulated loop of the W lies within the abdomen, so local tenderness over the hernia is not marked. At operation, two comparatively normal-looking loops of intestine are present in the sac. After the obstruction has been relieved, the strangulated loop will become apparent if traction is exerted on the middle of the loops occupying the sac.

Results of operations for inguinal hernia

Recurrence

Reported recurrence rates vary between 0.2% and 15% depending on the technique employed. Only by using a meticulous

---

Irvine Battinson Smith, **Formerly Surgeon, Burton-on-Trent General Hospital, Burton-on-Trent, Staffordshire, England.**
en masse **is French for 'in a body'.**
Sir Frederick Treves, **1853–1923, Surgeon, The London Hospital, London, England.**
Karl Maydl, **1853–1903, Professor of Surgery, Prague, The Czech Republic.**

technique, principally concentrating on reinforcement of the posterior wall of the inguinal canal using the Shouldice technique or mesh hernioplasty, can a recurrence rate of less than 2% be achieved. Only 50% of recurrences will become apparent within 2 years. In a few cases 'false' recurrences occur, i.e. another type of hernia occurs – direct after indirect, femoral after inguinal. However, to the patient it is a recurrence! (Summary box 57.10.)

Summary box 57.10

Recurrence of hernias

- The recurrence rate after surgery should be less than 2%
- Some recurrences will be new hernias

The spermatic cord as a barrier to effective closure of the inguinal canal

Even in the elderly patient, removal of the testis and cord is very rarely required for effective repair, even in cases of recurrent inguinal hernia. In operations for multiple recurrences or when previous surgery has been associated with infections or excessive scarring, the operation should be approached through virgin territory, i.e. the preperitoneal route, by an experienced surgeon.

Sliding hernia (synonym: hernia-en-glissade) (Fig. 57.13)

As a result of slipping of the posterior parietal peritoneum on the underlying retroperitoneal structures, the posterior wall of the sac is not formed of peritoneum alone, but by the sigmoid colon and its mesentery on the left, the caecum on the right and, sometimes, on either side by a portion of the bladder. It should be clearly understood that the caecum, appendix or a portion of the colon wholly within a hernial sac does not constitute a sliding hernia. A small bowel sliding hernia occurs approximately once in 2000 cases, a sacless hernia once in 8000 cases.

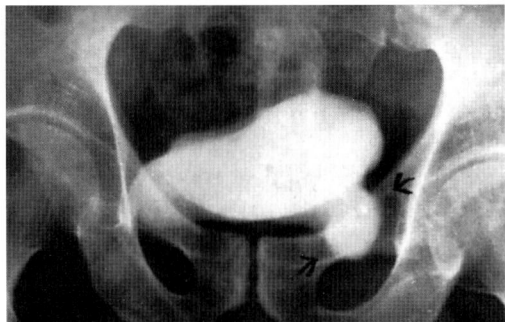

(a)

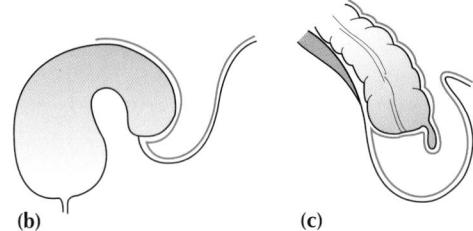

(b)   **(c)**

Figure 57.13 Sliding hernia. (a) Cystogram showing a left inguinal hernia involving a bladder. (b) Diagram of the same. (c) Caecum and appendix in a right sliding hernia.

Clinical features

A sliding hernia occurs almost exclusively in men. Five out of six sliding hernias are situated on the left side; bilateral sliding hernias are rare. The patient is nearly always over 40 years of age, the incidence rising with age. There are no clinical findings that are pathognomonic of a sliding hernia, but it should be suspected in a very large globular inguinal hernia descending well into the scrotum.

Occasionally, large intestine is strangulated in a sliding hernia; more often, non-strangulated large intestine is present behind the sac containing strangulated small intestine.

Treatment

A sliding hernia is impossible to control with a truss and, as a rule, the hernia is a cause of considerable discomfort. Consequently, operation is indicated and the results are very good.

Operation

It is unnecessary to remove any of the sliding hernial sac provided it is freed completely from the cord and the abdominal wall and that it is replaced deep to the repaired fascia transversalis. In some circumstances it is desirable to perform an orchidectomy to effect a secure repair. No attempt should be made to dissect the caecum or colon free from the peritoneum under the impression that these are adhesions. If this is attempted, peritonitis or a faecal fistula may result from necrosis of a devascularised portion of the bowel. This is especially liable to occur on the left side, as vessels in the mesocolon may be injured.

Femoral hernia

Femoral hernia is the third most common type of primary hernia. It accounts for about 20% of hernias in women and 5% in men. The over-riding importance of femoral hernia lies in the facts that it cannot be controlled by a truss and that of all hernias it is the most liable to become strangulated, mainly because of the narrowness of the neck of the sac and the rigidity of the femoral ring. Strangulation is the initial presentation of 40% of femoral hernias (Summary box 57.11).

Summary box 57.11

Femoral hernias

- More common in women
- Cannot be controlled with a truss
- Have a high incidence of strangulation
- Should be operated on as soon as possible

Surgical anatomy

The femoral canal occupies the most medial compartment of the femoral sheath and extends from the femoral ring above to the saphenous opening below. It is 1.25 cm long and 1.25 cm wide at its base, which is directed upwards. The femoral canal contains fat, lymphatic vessels and the lymph node of Cloquet. It is closed above by the septum crurale, a condensation of extraperitoneal tissue pierced by lymphatic vessels, and below by the cribriform fascia.

Jules Germain Cloquet, **1790–1883, Professor of Anatomy and Surgery, Paris, France.**

The femoral ring is bounded:

- anteriorly by the inguinal ligament;
- posteriorly by Astley Cooper's (iliopectineal) ligament, the pubic bone and the fascia over the pectineus muscle;
- medially by the concave knife-like edge of Gimbernat's (lacunar) ligament, which is also prolonged along the iliopectineal line, as Astley Cooper's ligament;
- laterally by a thin septum separating it from the femoral vein.

Sex incidence

The female to male ratio is about 2:1, but it is interesting that, whereas female patients are frequently elderly, male patients are usually between 30 and 45 years of age. The condition is more prevalent in women who have borne children than in nulliparae.

Pathology

A hernia passing down the femoral canal descends vertically as far as the saphenous opening. While it is confined to the inelastic walls of the femoral canal the hernia is necessarily narrow but, once it escapes through the saphenous opening into the loose areolar tissue of the groin, it expands, sometimes considerably. A fully distended femoral hernia assumes the shape of a retort and its bulbous extremity may be above the inguinal ligament. By the time the contents have pursued so tortuous a path, they are usually irreducible and apt to strangulate.

Clinical features

Femoral hernia is rare before puberty. Between 20 and 40 years of age the prevalence rises and this continues to old age. The right side (Fig. 57.14) is affected twice as often as the left and in 20% of cases the condition is bilateral. The symptoms to which a femoral hernia gives rise are less pronounced than those of an inguinal hernia; indeed, a small femoral hernia may be unnoticed by the patient or disregarded for years, perhaps until the day it strangulates. Adherence of the greater omentum sometimes causes a dragging pain. Rarely, a large sac is present.

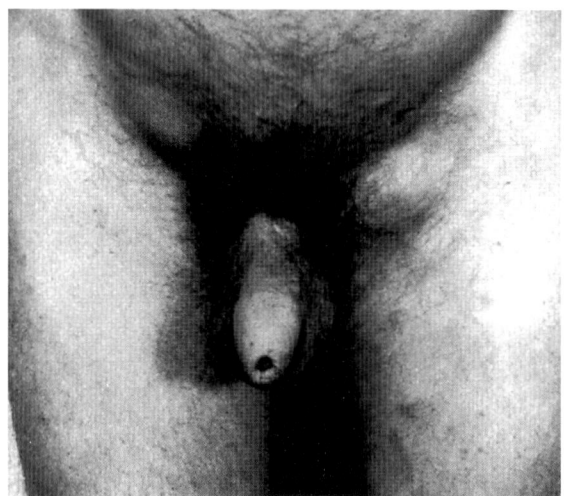

Figure 57.14 The patient has a left inguinal and a right femoral hernia (see Fig. 57.15).

Manoel Louise Antonio don Gimbernat, **1734–1816**, Professor of Anatomy, Barcelona, Spain, and later Director of the Royal College of Surgeons in Spain.

Differential diagnosis

A femoral hernia has to be distinguished from:

- *An inguinal hernia.* The neck of the sac lies above and medial to the medial end of the inguinal ligament at its attachment to the pubic tubercle. The neck of the sac of a femoral hernia lies below this (Fig. 57.15). The fundus of an inguinal or femoral hernia may follow the line of least resistance and occupy a variety of places; for instance, occasionally, the fundus of a femoral hernia sac overlies the inguinal ligament.
- *A saphena varix.* A saccular enlargement of the termination of the long saphenous vein, usually accompanied by other signs of varicose veins. The swelling disappears completely when the patient lies flat whereas a femoral hernia sac is usually still palpable. In both, there is an impulse on coughing. A saphena varix will, however, impart a fluid thrill to the examining fingers when the patient coughs or when the saphenous vein below the varix is tapped with the fingers of the other hand. Sometimes a venous hum can be heard when a stethoscope is applied over a saphena varix.
- *An enlarged femoral lymph node.* There may be other enlarged lymph nodes to aid the diagnosis. If Cloquet's lymph node alone is affected it may be impossible to distinguish from a femoral hernia sac unless there are other clues, such as an infected wound or abrasion on the corresponding limb or on the perineum.
- *Lipoma.*
- *A femoral aneurysm.* See Chapter 53.
- *A psoas abscess.* There is often a fluctuating swelling – an iliac abscess – which communicates with the swelling in question. If suspected, an examination of the spine and a radiograph will confirm the diagnosis.
- *A distended psoas bursa.* The swelling diminishes when the hip is flexed and osteoarthritis of the hip is present.
- *Rupture of the adductor longus with haematoma formation.* Suspected on clinical history.

Hydrocele of a femoral hernial sac

The neck of the sac becomes plugged with omentum or by adhesions and a hydrocele of the sac results.

Laugier's femoral hernia

This is a hernia through a gap in the lacunar (Gimbernat's) ligament. The diagnosis is based on the unusual medial position of a small femoral hernia sac. The hernia has nearly always strangulated.

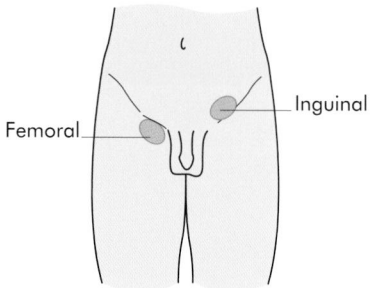

Figure 57.15 The essentials of the differential diagnosis between a femoral and an inguinal hernia (as in Fig. 57.14).

Stanislaus Laugier, **1799–1872**, Surgeon, Hôtel Dieu, Paris, France.

Narath's femoral hernia

This occurs only in patients with congenital dislocation of the hip and is the result of lateral displacement of the psoas muscle. The hernia lies hidden behind the femoral vessels.

Cloquet's hernia

Cloquet's hernia is one in which the sac lies under the fascia covering the pectineus muscle. Strangulation is likely. The sac may coexist with the usual type of femoral hernia sac.

Strangulated femoral hernia

A femoral hernia strangulates frequently and gangrene rapidly develops. This is explained by the narrow, unyielding femoral ring. In 40% of cases the obstructing agent is not the lacunar ligament but the neck of the femoral sac itself. A Richter's hernia is a frequent occurrence (see above).

Treatment of a femoral hernia

The constant risk of strangulation is sufficient reason to recommend operation, which should be carried out soon after the diagnosis has been made. A truss is contraindicated because of this risk.

Operative treatment

Several approaches to the femoral hernia have been advocated including the low operation (Lockwood), the high operation (McEvedy) and the inguinal operation (Lotheissen). In all cases the bladder must be emptied by catheterisation immediately before commencing surgery. To these well-described techniques may be added the laparoscopic approach – the TEP repair visualising the femoral canal and the iliac vessels from a preperitoneal approach, enabling safe reduction of the hernia sac while monitoring the iliac vessels under direct vision. It should be noted that throughout operations for the repair of a femoral hernia on the lateral side, the external iliac/femoral vein must be protected; on the medial side, great care must be taken not to injure the bladder, particularly as a portion of the bladder may form part of the wall of the sac (a sliding femoral hernia).

The low operation (Lockwood) The sac is dissected out below the inguinal ligament via a groin crease incision. It is essential to peel off the anatomical layers that cover the sac. These are often thick and fatty. After dealing with the contents (e.g. freeing adherent omentum), the neck of the sac is pulled down, ligated as high as possible and allowed to retract through the femoral canal. The canal may be closed by suturing the inguinal ligament to the iliopectineal line using three non-absorbable sutures. An alternative method of closure is to roll a sheet of polypropylene mesh into a cylinder and anchor the cylinder in the canal with non-absorbable sutures placed medially, superiorly and inferiorly.

The high (McEvedy) operation Classically, a vertical incision is made over the femoral canal and continued upwards above the inguinal ligament. An acceptable alternative that heals well and with less pain is to use a 'unilateral' Pfannenstiel incision, which can be extended to form a complete Pfannenstiel incision if formal laparotomy is required. This incision provides good access to the preperitoneal space. Through the lower part of the incision, the sac is dissected out. The upper part of the incision exposes the inguinal ligament and the rectus sheath. The superficial inguinal ring is identified and an incision 2.5 cm above the ring and parallel to the outer border of the rectus muscle is deepened until the extraperitoneal space is identified. By gauze dissection in this space, the hernial sac entering the femoral canal can easily be identified. If the sac is empty and small it may be drawn upwards; if it is large, the fundus is opened below and its contents, if any, dealt with appropriately before delivering the sac upwards from its canal. The sac is then freed from the extraperitoneal tissue and its neck ligated. An excellent view of the iliopectineal ligament is obtained and the conjoined tendon is sutured to it with non-absorbable sutures. An alternative repair, particularly suitable for recurrent femoral hernias, is to suture a sheet of polypropylene mesh over the femoral canal orifice, anchoring the mesh inferiorly to the iliopectineal ligament and medially to the rectus sheath.

An advantage of this approach is that, if resection of intestine is required, ample room can be obtained by opening the peritoneum. The disadvantage of this approach is that, if infection occurs, an incisional hernia may develop.

Lotheissen's operation The inguinal canal is opened as for inguinal herniorrhaphy. The transversalis fascia is incised to the medial side of the epigastric vessels and the opening is enlarged. The peritoneum is now in view; one must be certain that it is the peritoneum and not the bladder or a diverticulum thereof. The peritoneum is picked up with dissecting forceps and incised. It is now possible to ascertain if any intraperitoneal structure is entering the femoral sac. If the sac is empty, artery forceps are placed upon the edges of the opening into the peritoneum and, by gauze dissection, the sac is withdrawn from the femoral canal. An empty sac can be delivered easily. If strangulation is suspected, as soon as the external oblique has been exposed, the inferior margin of the wound is retracted, thereby displaying the swelling. The coverings of the sac are incised and peeled off, until the sac, dark from contained blood-stained fluid, is apparent. The sac is incised and the fluid that escapes is mopped up with care. The retractor is removed and the operation is continued above the inguinal ligament as described above. Once the peritoneum has been opened above the inguinal ligament, one can see exactly what is entering the sac. Should the obstruction lie in a narrow neck of the sac, the neck of the sac may be gently stretched by insertion of artery forceps.[2] The contents of the sac are delivered and dealt with appropriately. Sometimes, to facilitate reduction of the hernial contents, it is necessary to divide or digitally dilate part of the lacunar (Gimbernat's) ligament.

The Lotheissen repair is effected by suturing the conjoined tendon to the iliopectineal line to form a shutter. While protecting

---

2 An abnormal obturator artery is present on the medial or the lateral side of the neck of the sac in 28% of cases.

Albert Narath, **1864–1924, Professor of Surgery, Heidelberg, Germany.**
Charles Barrett Lockwood, **1856–1914, Surgeon, St. Bartholomew's Hospital, London, England.**
Peter George McEvedy, **1890–1951, Surgeon, Ancoats Hospital, Manchester, England.**

Hermann Johann Pfannenstiel, 1862–1909, Gynaecologist, Breslau, Germany, (now Wroclaw, Poland), described this incision in 1900.
George Lotheissen, 1868–1941, Surgeon, The Kaiser Franz Joseph Hospital, Vienna, Austria, described this operation in 1898.

the external iliac/femoral vein with the forefinger, non-absorbable sutures are passed through the periosteum and Cooper's ligament overlying the iliopectineal line. The retractor is removed and the long ends of the sutures are passed outwards from within, through the conjoined tendon and tied, thus approximating the conjoined tendon to the iliopectineal line. If there is any tension, a Tanner's slide will facilitate this step. The incised external oblique is sutured.

An alternative repair is to buttress the femoral canal with a sheet of polypropylene mesh. Once the sac has been dealt with, a sheet of mesh is inserted into the preperitoneal space and anchored inferiorly to the iliopectineal line, inferomedially to Cooper's ligament and superomedially to the rectus sheath. The transversalis fascia may then be approximated in front of the mesh and the incised external oblique repaired. It should be noted that the peritoneum must be closed before placement of the mesh.

Umbilical hernia

Exomphalos (synonym: omphalocele) occurs once in every 6000 births; it is due to failure of all or part of the midgut to return to the coelom during early fetal life. There is some debate as to whether gastroschisis represents a separate entity or is simply an exomphalos with ruptured membranes, but the debate has little practical importance because the principles of treatment are similar. When the sac remains unruptured it is semitranslucent (Fig. 57.16) and, although very thin, it consists of two layers – an outer layer of amniotic membrane and an inner layer of peritoneum. Omphaloceles may be divided into those with a fascial defect less than 4 cm and those with a defect greater than 4 cm. The former are termed herniation of the umbilical cord. In smaller defects a single loop of intestine may not be obvious and ligation of what was thought to be a normal umbilical cord will result in transection of the intestine, leaving the embarrassing problem of an umbilico-enteric fistula.

In large defects, the liver, spleen, stomach, pancreas, colon or bladder may be seen through the membrane. The intestine lies freely mobile within the intact sac without evidence of adhesions or inflammation. In contrast, the liver has dense adhesions to the sac, a fact that must be remembered during surgical repair.

Treatment

Small defects may be closed primarily soon after birth as there is usually no difficulty with disproportion between the size of the abdominal cavity and the volume of the sac contents.

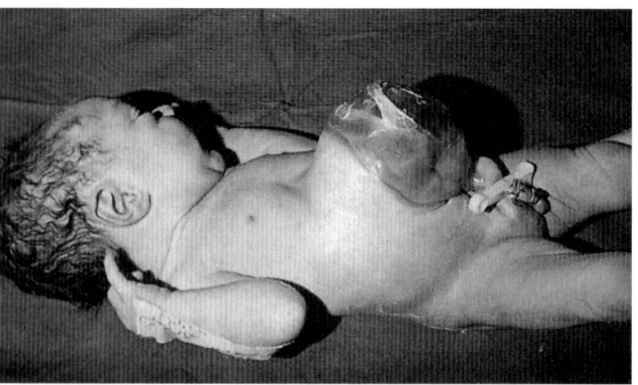

Figure 57.16 Exomphalos. The delicate sac ruptured soon afterwards.

Large defects present a more substantial problem and four techniques have been described: non-operative therapy, skin flap closure, staged closure and primary closure.

Non-operative therapy

This is appropriate for premature infants with a gigantic intact sac or those in whom associated anomalies make survival of a major operation unlikely. The intact sac is painted daily with a desiccating antiseptic solution and, if successful, an eschar forms over the sac. Eventually, granulation tissue grows in from the periphery and the subsequent ventral hernia can be repaired later.

Skin flap closure

The sac is gently trimmed away enabling inspection of the abdominal contents. The skin is freed from the fascial edges and undermined laterally. The umbilical vessels are ligated or one artery is cannulated for monitoring. The skin flaps are approximated in the midline with simple sutures and the ventral hernia is then closed at a later date (months to years later).

Staged closure

The sac is gently trimmed away from the skin edge and the skin further freed from the fascial attachments. The prosthetic material [polypropylene mesh or expanded polytetrafluoroethylene (PTFE)] is sutured with interrupted non-absorbable sutures circumferentially to the full thickness of the musculofascial abdominal wall to form a silo. The top of the silo is gathered and tied with umbilical tape. At daily intervals the silo is opened under strict aseptic conditions and the contents examined for infection or dehiscence. The viscera are pushed gently back in to the abdominal cavity and the infant observed for signs of raised intra-abdominal pressure. The silo is then tied at a reduced level and the cycle repeated until the sac is flush with the abdominal wall. At this stage the fascia may be closed with interrupted sutures and skin closed over the top.

Primary closure

The sac is gently dissected away from the skin edge and the underlying fascia. The intestine is then evacuated completely of meconium and fluid, distally and proximally, through a nasogastric tube. The abdominal wall is stretched gradually and repeatedly in quadrants, usually achieving a doubling of volume. The viscera are then replaced and the fascial layer closed primarily, usually under moderate tension. Intragastric pressure monitoring is helpful to prevent undue vena caval compression (Summary box 57.12).

Summary box 57.12
Exomphalmos
■ Small defects may result in the sac being tied off with cord
■ Large defects need a staged approach

Congenital umbilical hernia

Rarely, a fully developed umbilical hernia is present at birth, presumably due to intrauterine epithelialisation of a small exomphalos.

Umbilical hernia of infants and children

This is a hernia through a weak umbilicus, which may result partly from failure of the round ligament (obliterated umbilical

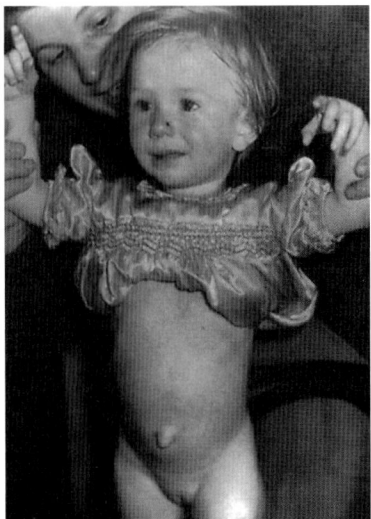

Figure 57.17 Infantile umbilical hernia.

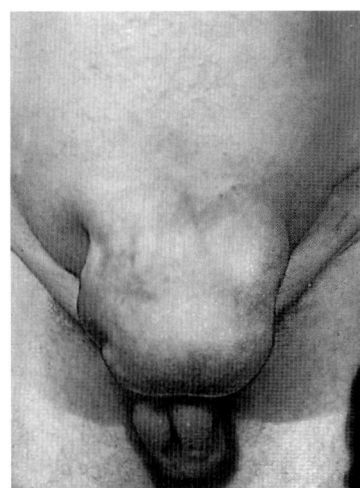

Figure 57.18 A large paraumbilical hernia.

vein) to cross the umbilical ring and partly from absence of the Richet fascia. Both sexes seem to be equally affected although there are significant racial differences; the incidence in black infants is reported to be up to eight times higher than that in white infants. The hernia is often symptomless but increases in size on crying and assumes a classical conical shape (Fig. 57.17). Obstruction or strangulation below the age of 3 years is extremely uncommon.

Treatment

Conservative treatment is indicated under the age of 2 years; when the hernia is symptomless, reassurance of the parents is all that is necessary, as 95% of hernias will disappear spontaneously. If the hernia persists at 2 years of age or older it is unlikely to resolve and herniorrhaphy is indicated.

Operation A small curved incision is made immediately below the umbilicus. The skin cicatrix is dissected upwards and the neck of the sac isolated. After ensuring that the sac is empty of contents, it is either inverted into the abdomen or ligated by transfixion and excised. The defect in the linea alba is closed with interrupted absorbable sutures (Summary box 57.13).

Summary box 57.13

Umbilical hernias in infants and children

- Rarely strangulate
- Most resolve spontaneously

Paraumbilical hernia (synonyms: supraumbilical hernia, infraumbilical hernia)

In adults the hernia does not occur through the umbilical scar but is a protrusion through the linea alba, just above or sometimes just below the umbilicus (Fig. 57.18). As it enlarges it becomes rounded or oval in shape, with a tendency to sag downwards.

Paraumbilical hernias can become very large. The neck of the sac is often remarkably narrow compared with the size of the sac and the volume of its contents, which usually consist of greater omentum often accompanied by small intestine and, alternatively or in addition, a portion of transverse colon. In long-standing cases the sac sometimes becomes loculated because of adherence of omentum to its fundus.

Clinical features

Women are affected five times more frequently than men. The patient is usually overweight and between the ages of 35 and 50. Increasing obesity, with flabbiness of the abdominal muscles, and repeated pregnancy are important aetiological factors. These hernias may become irreducible because of the formation of omental adhesions within the sac. Symptomatically, a large umbilical hernia causes a dragging pain because of its weight. Gastrointestinal symptoms are common and are probably due to traction on the stomach or transverse colon. Often there are transient attacks of intestinal colic because of partial intestinal obstruction. In long-standing cases, intertrigo of the adjacent surfaces of skin and trophic ulcers of the fundus are troublesome complications.

Treatment

If the hernia is untreated it increases in size and more and more of its contents become irreducible. Eventually, strangulation may occur. Thus, operation should be advised in nearly all cases. If the patient is obese and the hernia is symptomless, operation can be postponed until the patient has lost weight.

Umbilical herniorrhaphy If the defect is small, a primary herniorrhaphy can be performed. If the defect is large, the repair is best performed with prosthetic buttressing of the abdominal wall. The classic primary repair is that described by Mayo. A transverse elliptical incision is made around the umbilicus and the subcutaneous tissues are dissected off the rectus sheath to expose the neck of the sac. The neck is incised to expose the contents. Intestine is returned to the abdomen and any adherent omentum

Louis Alfred Richet, **1816–1891**, Professor of Clinical Surgery, The Faculty of Medicine, Paris, France.

William James Mayo, **1861–1939**, Surgeon, The Mayo Clinic, Rochester, MN, USA, described this operation in 1901.

CHAPTER 57 | HERNIAS, UMBILICUS AND ABDOMINAL WALL

freed. Excess adherent omentum can be removed with the sac if necessary. The sac is then removed and the peritoneum closed with an absorbable suture. The aponeurosis on both sides of the umbilical ring is mobilised from underlying tissue sufficiently to allow an overlap of 5 or 7.5 cm. Interrupted mattress sutures are then inserted into the aponeurosis as shown in Fig. 57.19. When this row of mattress sutures has been tied, the overlapping upper margin is stitched to the sheath of the rectus abdominis and the midline aponeurosis. A suction drain should be placed in the wound in fat patients, who ooze blood and liquid fat. The subcutaneous fat and skin are then approximated with deep sutures.

Paraumbilical hernioplasty In the case of very large primary umbilical hernias (fascial defects > 4 cm) or for recurrent paraumbilical hernias, the use of prosthetic material (polypropylene mesh) is recommended.

Additional lipectomy In patients with a paraumbilical hernia associated with a large, pendulous, fat-laden abdominal wall, the operation can, with great advantage, be combined with panniculectomy by fashioning the incisions to embrace a larger area of the fat-laden superficial layers of the abdominal wall.

Strangulation

Strangulation is a frequent complication of a large paraumbilical hernia in adults. Because of the narrow neck and the fibrous edge of the linea alba, gangrene is liable to supervene unless early operation is carried out. It should also be remembered that in large hernias the presence of loculi may result in a strangulated knuckle of the bowel in one part of an otherwise soft and non-tender hernia.

Operation In early cases the operation does not differ from that for non-strangulated cases. Gangrenous contents are dealt with as in other situations. If a portion of the transverse colon is gangrenous it should be exteriorised by the Paul–Mikulicz method and the gangrenous portion excised. If the ring is large enough to transmit the colon unhampered it is left alone; otherwise, it is enlarged. It is important that the small intestine is thoroughly scrutinised as a small loop may have been trapped and slipped back when the constriction was relieved. If non-viable gut is overlooked, peritonitis quickly supervenes and the symptoms are

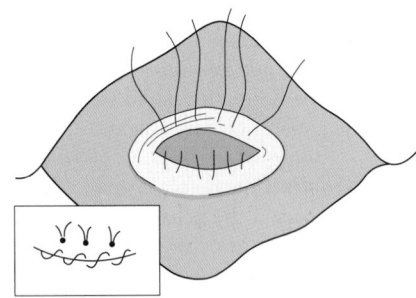

Figure 57.19 Mayo's operation for umbilical hernia. Interrupted sutures to provide an overlap are first inserted. Inset: the overlap has been made and completed with a continuous suture. It is important to denude the area of fat before stitching the flap into position.

Johann von Mikulicz-Radecki, **1850–1905, Professor of Surgery, Breslau, Germany, (now Wroclaw, Poland).**

ascribed to postoperative discomfort. The condition of the patient steadily deteriorates until he or she succumbs after a few days (Summary box 57.14).

Epigastric hernia (synonym: fatty hernia of the linea alba)

An epigastric hernia occurs through the linea alba anywhere between the xiphoid process and the umbilicus, usually midway between these structures. Such a hernia commences as a protrusion of extraperitoneal fat through the linea alba, and it was hypothesised that this protrusion occurred at the site where small blood vessels pierced the linea alba. However, only a minority of epigastric hernias are accompanied by blood vessels, and it is more likely that the defect occurs as a result of a weakened linea alba due to abnormal decussation of the fibres of the aponeurosis. More than one hernia may be present, and the most common cause of 'recurrence' is failure to identify a second defect at the time of original repair.

A swelling the size of a pea consists of a protrusion of extraperitoneal fat only (fatty hernia of the linea alba). If the protrusion enlarges, it drags a pouch of peritoneum after it and so becomes a true epigastric hernia. The mouth of the hernia is rarely large enough to permit a portion of hollow viscus to enter it; consequently, either the sac is empty or it contains a small portion of greater omentum.

It is likely that an epigastric hernia is the direct result of a sudden strain tearing the interlacing fibres of the linea alba. The patients are often manual workers between 30 and 45 years of age.

Clinical features

Symptomless

A small fatty hernia of the linea alba can be felt more easily than it can be seen and may be symptomless, discovered only in the course of routine abdominal palpation.

Painful

Sometimes such a hernia gives rise to attacks of local pain, worse on physical exertion, and tenderness to touch and light clothing. This may be because the fatty contents become nipped sufficiently to produce partial strangulation.

Referred pain

It is not uncommon to find that the patient, who may not have noticed the hernia, complains of pain suggestive of a peptic ulcer. However, as the majority of these hernias are asymptomatic, symptoms should not be ascribed to the hernia until any gastrointestinal pathology has been excluded.

Treatment

If the hernia is giving rise to symptoms, operation should be undertaken.

Operation An adequate vertical or transverse incision is made over the swelling, exposing the linea alba. The protruding extraperitoneal fat is cleared from the hernial orifice by gauze dissection. If the pedicle passing through the linea alba is slender, it is separated on all sides of the opening by blunt dissection. After ligating the pedicle, the small opening in the linea alba is closed with non-absorbable sutures in adults and with absorbable sutures in children. When a hernial sac is present, it is opened and any contents reduced, after which the sac neck is transfixed and the sac excised before repairing the linea alba. If smaller protrusions of fat are found above or below the hernia, these should also be dealt with. If the hernia is large (defect greater than 4 cm diameter), the repair should be reinforced with polypropylene mesh positioned in the retromuscular plane (Summary box 57.15).

Summary box 57.15

Epigastric hernias

- Too small to contain bowel
- Only need surgery if painful

Rare external hernias

Interparietal hernia (synonym: interstitial hernia)

An interparietal hernia has a hernial sac that passes between the layers of the anterior abdominal wall. The sac may be associated with, or communicate with, the sac of a concomitant inguinal or femoral hernia. Lack of knowledge of this condition is the cause of misdiagnosis and mismanagement.

Other varieties

1 *Preperitoneal* (20%). Usually the sac takes the form of a diverticulum from a femoral or inguinal hernia.
2 *Intermuscular* (60%). The sac passes between the muscular layers of the anterior abdominal wall, usually between the external oblique and internal oblique muscles. The sac is nearly always bilocular and is associated with an inguinal hernia.
3 *Inguino-superficial* (20%). The sac expands beneath the superficial fascia of the abdominal wall or the thigh. This type is commonly associated with an incompletely descended testis.

Clinical features
The patients (mostly male) present with intestinal obstruction caused by obstruction or strangulation of the hernia. In the preperitoneal variety swelling is unlikely to be apparent and delays in diagnosis occur; consequently the mortality rate is high.

Treatment
Operation is imperative because of intestinal obstruction.

Spigelian hernia

This is a variety of interparietal hernia occurring at the level of the arcuate line. It is very rare, with only 1000 cases reported in the literature. The fundus of the sac, clothed by extraperitoneal fat, may lie beneath the internal oblique muscle, where it is virtually impalpable. More often, it advances through that muscle and spreads out like a mushroom between the internal and external

oblique muscles and gives rise to a more evident swelling. The patient is often corpulent and usually over 50 years of age, men and women being equally affected. Typically, a soft, reducible mass will be encountered lateral to the rectus muscle and below the umbilicus. Diagnosis is confirmed by computerised tomography or ultrasound scanning. The latter has the advantage that it can be performed in the upright patient if no defect is visible in the reclining position. Because of the rigid fascia surrounding the neck, strangulation may occur.

Treatment
If a defect is palpable, a muscle-splitting approach is used. After isolating the sac, dealing with any contents, and ligating and excising it, the transversus and internal oblique and external oblique muscles are repaired by direct apposition. If no sac is palpable, a paramedian approach is used and the sac sought in the extraperitoneal space. The repair then proceeds as described above. A transabdominal laparoscopic approach may also be employed.

Lumbar hernia

Most primary lumbar hernia occur through the inferior lumbar triangle of Petit (Fig. 57.20), bounded below by the crest of the ilium, laterally by the external oblique muscle and medially by the latissimus dorsi. Less commonly, the sac comes through the superior lumbar triangle, which is bounded by the 12th rib above, medially by the sacrospinalis and laterally by the posterior border of the internal oblique muscle. Primary lumbar hernias are very rare, with only 300 cases reported. More commonly, lumbar hernias are secondary to renal operations, when extensive incisional sacs may be present.

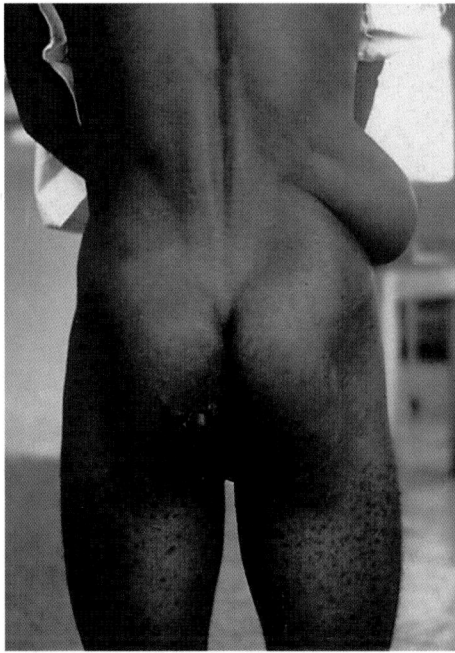

Figure 57.20 Inferior lumbar hernia, which contained caecum, appendix and small bowel. Note the filarial skin rash on the buttocks (courtesy of V.J. Hartfield, formerly of S.E. Nigeria).

Adrien Van der Spieghel, (Spigelius), **1578–1625, Professor of Anatomy, Padua, Italy.**

Jean Louis Petit, **1674–1750, Director of the Académie de Chirurgie, Paris, France.**

Differential diagnosis

A lumbar hernia must be distinguished from:

- a lipoma;
- a cold (tuberculous) abscess pointing to this position;
- phantom hernia due to local muscular paralysis – lumbar phantom hernia can result from any interference with the nerve supply of the affected muscles (e.g. poliomyelitis).

Treatment

Being small, a primary lumbar hernia is easily repaired. As the natural history is for these hernias to increase in size with time, any primary lumbar hernia should be repaired at presentation. Incisional lumbar hernias may be large and the defect is impossible to repair unless fascial flaps are used. The repair can be reinforced with a sheet of polypropylene mesh.

Perineal hernia

This type of hernia is very rare and includes:

- postoperative hernia through a perineal scar, which may occur after excision of the rectum;
- median sliding perineal hernia, which is a complete prolapse of the rectum (Chapter 68);
- anterolateral perineal hernia, which occurs in women and presents as a swelling of the labium majus;
- posterolateral perineal hernia, which passes through the levator ani to enter the ischiorectal fossa.

Treatment

A combined operation is generally the most satisfactory for the last two types of hernia. The hernia is exposed by an incision directly over it. The sac is opened and its contents are reduced. The sac is cleared from surrounding structures and the wound closed. With the patient in semi-Trendelenburg position, the abdomen is opened and the mouth of the sac is exposed. The sac is inverted, ligated and excised and the pelvic floor repaired by muscle apposition and, if indicated, buttressing of the repair with prosthetic mesh.

Obturator hernia

Obturator hernia, which passes through the obturator canal, occurs six times more frequently in women than in men. Most patients are over 60 years of age. The swelling is liable to be overlooked because it is covered by the pectineus. It seldom causes a definite swelling in Scarpa's triangle, but if the limb is flexed, abducted and rotated outwards, the hernia sometimes becomes more apparent. The leg is usually kept in a semi-flexed position and movement increases the pain. In more than 50% of cases of strangulated obturator hernia, pain is referred along the obturator nerve by its geniculate branch to the knee. On vaginal or rectal examination the hernia can sometimes be felt as a tender swelling in the region of the obturator foramen.

Cases of obturator hernia that present themselves have usually undergone strangulation, which is frequently of the Richter type.

Friedrich Trendelenburg, **1844–1924**, Professor of Surgery, Rostock (**1875–1882**), Bonn (**1882–1895**), and Leipzig (**1895–1911**), Germany.
Antonio Scarpa, **1747–1832**, Professor of Anatomy, Pavia, Italy.

Treatment

Operation is indicated. A lower laparotomy should be performed (on the side of the lesion, if known). The diagnosis is confirmed and a full Trendelenburg position adopted. The constricting agent is the obturator fascia. Taking every precaution to avoid spilling infected fluid from the hernial sac into the peritoneal cavity, this fascia can be stretched to allow reduction by inserting suitable forceps through the gap in the fascia and opening the blades with care. If incision of the fascia is required, it is made parallel to the obturator vessels and nerve. The contents of the sac are dealt with. The defect is repaired by stitching the broad ligament over the opening to prevent recurrence.

Gluteal and sciatic hernias

A gluteal hernia passes through the greater sciatic foramen, either above or below the piriformis. A sciatic hernia passes through the lesser sciatic foramen. Differential diagnosis must be made between these conditions and:

- a lipoma or fibrosarcoma beneath the gluteus maximus;
- a tuberculous abscess;
- a gluteal aneurysm.

All doubtful swellings in this situation should be explored by operation.

UMBILICUS

Inflammation of the umbilicus

Infection of the umbilical cord

In over 50% of babies born in maternity hospitals the stump of the umbilical cord is found to be carrying staphylococci by the third or fourth day post delivery. Less commonly the stump of the cord harbours streptococci, and epidemics of puerperal sepsis in maternity hospitals have been traced to the umbilical cord of one infant in the nursery thus infected. *Escherichia coli* and *Clostridium tetani* (causing neonatal tetanus) are other possible invaders. The chief prophylaxis is strict asepsis during severance of the cord and the use of 0.1% chlorhexidine locally for a few days (Summary box 57.16).

> **Summary box 57.16**
>
> **Infection of umbilical cord**
>
> - **Most become infected**
> - **Staff must wash hands between patients to prevent cross-infection**

Omphalitis

The incidence of an infected umbilicus is much higher in communities that do not practise aseptic severance of the umbilical cord. When the stump of the umbilical cord becomes inflamed, antibiotic therapy usually localises the inflammation. By employing warm, moist dressings, the crusts separate, giving exit to pus. Exuberant granulation tissue requires a touch of silver nitrate. In more serious cases infection is liable to spread along the defunct hypogastric arteries or umbilical vein when, in all probability, one or other of the following complications will supervene:

- *Abscess of the abdominal wall.* If gentle pressure is exerted above or below the navel and a bead of pus exudes at the navel, a deep abscess associated with one of the defunct umbilical vessels is present. This must be opened. A probe is passed into the sinus to determine its direction and this is followed by a grooved director on to which the skin and overlying tissues are incised in the midline.
- *Extensive ulceration of the abdominal wall.* Extensive ulceration of the abdominal wall due to synergistic infection is treated in the same way as postoperative subcutaneous gangrene (see below).
- *Septicaemia* can occur from organisms entering the bloodstream via the umbilical vein. Jaundice is often the first sign. An abscess in the abdominal wall above the umbilicus should be sought. In other respects, the treatment of this grave complication follows the usual lines.
- *Jaundice in the newborn.* Infection reaching the liver via the umbilical vein may cause a stenosing intrahepatic cholangiolitis, appearing some 3–6 weeks after birth.
- *Portal vein thrombosis and subsequent portal hypertension.*
- *Peritonitis* carries a bad prognosis.
- *Umbilical hernia.*

Umbilical granuloma

Chronic infection of the umbilical cicatrix that continues for weeks causes granulation tissue to pout at the umbilicus. There is no certain means of distinguishing this condition from an adenoma. Usually, an umbilical granuloma can be treated by one application of silver nitrate followed by dry dressings, but an adenoma soon recurs in spite of these measures.

Dermatitis of and around the umbilicus

This is common at all times of life. Fungus and parasitic infections are more difficult to eradicate from the umbilicus than from the skin of the abdomen. Sometimes the dermatitis is consequent upon a discharge from the umbilicus, as is the case when an umbilical fistula or a sinus is present. In overweight women, intertrigo occurs.

A deep, tender swelling in the midline below the umbilicus signifies that an abscess is present in the extraperitoneal fat; this is usually due to an infected urachal remnant. Exploration and proper drainage is necessary.

Pilonidal sinus

Pilonidal sinus (a sinus containing a sheath of hairs) is sometimes encountered. It should be excised.

Umbilical calculus (umbolith)

This is often black in colour and is composed of desquamated epithelium, which becomes inspissated and collects in the deep recess of the umbilicus. The treatment is to dilate the orifice and extract the calculus but, to prevent recurrence, it may be necessary to excise the umbilicus.

Umbilical fistulae

As the umbilicus is a central abdominal scar it is understandable that a slow leak from any viscus is liable to track to the surface at this point. Added to this, very occasionally, the vitellointestinal duct or the urachus remains patent; consequently, it has been aptly remarked that the umbilicus is a creek into which many fistulous streams may open.

For instance, an enlarged, inflamed gall bladder perforating at its fundus may discharge gallstones through the umbilicus. An unremitting flow of pus from a fistula at the umbilicus of a middle-aged woman led to the discovery of a length of gauze overlooked during a hysterectomy 5 years previously.

The vitellointestinal duct

The vitellointestinal duct occasionally persists and gives rise to one of the following conditions:

- It remains patent (Fig. 57.21a). The resulting umbilical fistula discharges mucus and, rarely, faeces. Often, a small portion only of the duct near the umbilicus remains unobliterated. This gives rise to a sinus that discharges mucus. The epithelial lining of the sinus often becomes everted to form an 'adenoma'.
- Sometimes both the umbilical and the intestinal ends of the duct close but the mucous membrane of the intervening portion remains and an intra-abdominal cyst develops (Fig. 57.21b).
- With its lumen obliterated or unobliterated the vitellointestinal duct provides an intraperitoneal band (Fig. 57.21c); this is a potential danger because intestinal obstruction is liable to occur. The obstruction results from a coil of small intestine passing under or over or becoming twisted around the band.
- Such a band may contract and pull a Meckel's diverticulum into a congenital umbilical hernia (Fig. 57.21d).
- A vitellointestinal cord connected to a Meckel's diverticulum, but not attached to the umbilicus, becomes adherent to or knotted around another loop of small intestine and so causes intestinal obstruction.
- Sometimes a band extending from the umbilicus is attached to the mesentery near its junction with a distal part of the ileum. In this case the band is probably an obliterated vitelline artery and is not necessarily associated with a Meckel's diverticulum.

Treatment

A patent vitellointestinal duct should be excised, together with a Meckel's diverticulum if present, preferably when the child is about 6 months old. When a vitellointestinal band gives rise to acute intestinal obstruction, after removing the obstruction by dividing the band it is expedient, when possible, to excise the band and bury the cut ends.

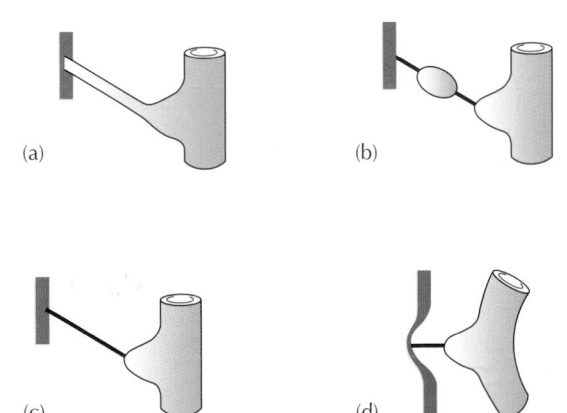

Figure 57.21 Anomalies connected with the vitellointestinal duct. (a) Umbilical fistula; (b) intra-abdominal cyst; (c) intraperitoneal band; (d) Meckel's diverticulum with a band adherent to the sac of a congenital umbilical hernia.

CHAPTER 57 | HERNIAS, UMBILICUS AND ABDOMINAL WALL

Patent urachus

A patent urachus seldom reveals itself until maturity or even old age. This is because the contractions of the bladder commence at the apex of the organ and pass towards the base. Because it opens into the apex of the bladder a patent urachus is closed temporarily during micturition and so the potential urinary stream from the bladder is cut off. Thus, the fistula remains unobtrusive until a time when the organ is overfull, usually due to some form of obstruction.

Treatment

Treatment is directed to removing the obstruction in the lower urinary tract. If, after this has been remedied, the leak continues or a cyst develops in connection with the urachus, umbilectomy and excision of the urachus down to its insertion into the apex of the bladder, with closure of the latter, is indicated.

Neoplasms of the umbilicus

Benign

Umbilical adenoma or raspberry tumour

This is commonly seen in infants (Fig. 57.22) but only occasionally later in life. It is due to a partially (occasionally a completely) unobliterated vitellointestinal duct. Mucosa prolapsing through the umbilicus gives rise to a raspberry-like tumour, which is moist and tends to bleed.

Treatment If the tumour is pedunculated, a ligature is tied around it and, in a few days, the polypus drops off. Should the tumour reappear after this procedure, umbilectomy is indicated. Sometimes a patent vitellointestinal duct, or more often a vitellointestinal band, will be found associated with a Meckel's diverticulum. The Meckel's diverticulum and the attached cord or duct should be excised at the same time as the umbilicus. Histologically, the tumour at the umbilicus consists of columnar epithelium rich in goblet cells.

Endometrioma

Endometrioma occurs in women between the ages of 20 and 45 years. On histological examination it is found to consist of endometrial glands occupying the same plane in the dermis as the sudoriferous glands and opening onto the surface in the same

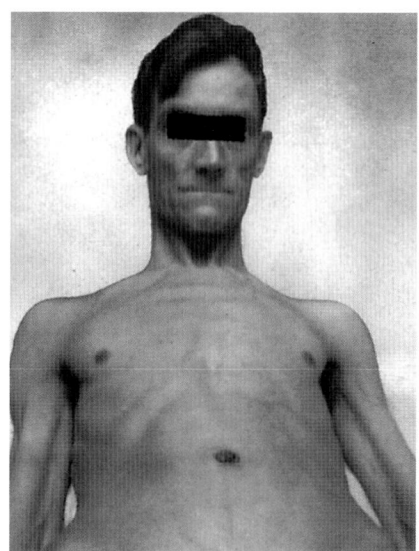

Figure 57.23 Secondary nodule at the umbilicus in a case of carcinoma of the stomach.

way. The umbilicus becomes painful and bleeds at each menstruation, when the small fleshy tumour between the folds of the umbilicus becomes more apparent. Occasionally, an umbilical endometrioma is accompanied by endometriomas in the uterus or ovary. When the tumour is solitary, as is usually the case, umbilectomy will cure the condition.

Malignant

Secondary carcinoma

Secondary carcinoma at the umbilicus (or Sister Joseph's nodule[3]) (Fig. 57.23) is quite common but is always a late manifestation of the disease. The primary neoplasm is often situated in the stomach, colon or ovary, but a metastasis from the breast, probably transmitted along the lymphatics of the round ligament of the liver, is sometimes located here.

THE ABDOMINAL WALL

Burst abdomen and incisional hernia

In 1–2% of cases, mostly between the sixth and eighth day after operation, an abdominal wound bursts open and viscera are extruded. The disruption of the wound tends to occur a few days beforehand when the sutures apposing the deep layers (peritoneum, posterior rectus sheath) tear through or even become untied. An incisional hernia usually starts as a symptomless partial disruption of the deeper layers during the immediate or early postoperative period, the event passing unnoticed if the skin wound remains intact after the skin sutures have been removed.

---

3   The neoplastic nodule sited at the umbilicus is known as Sister Joseph's nodule. Sister Joseph of the Mayo Clinic imparted this clinical observation to the late Dr William Mayo.

Sister Mary Joseph (nee Julia Dempsey), **Nursing Superintendent, St. Mary's Hospital, which became the Mayo Clinic, Rochester, MN, USA.**
The Mayo Clinic in Rochester, MN, USA, was founded in 1889 as the St. Mary's Hospital by William Worrall Mayo and his two sons, William James Mayo and Charles Horace Mayo, both of whom became surgeons to the hospital.

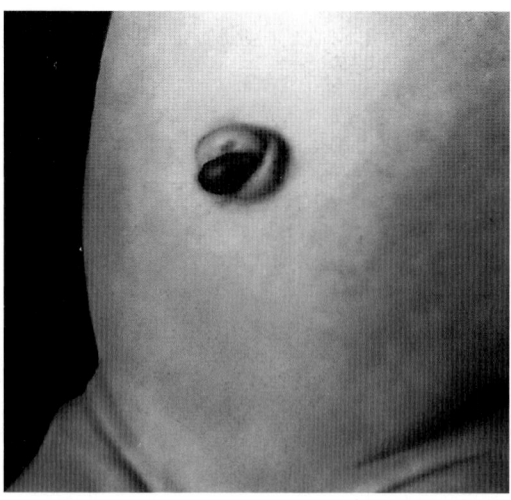

Figure 57.22 Adenoma (raspberry tumour) of the umbilicus.

Factors relating to the incidence of burst abdomen and incisional hernia

Technique of wound closure

Choice of suture material Catgut leads to a higher incidence of 'bursts' than the use of non-absorbable monofilament polypropylene, polyamide or wire, and should never be used.

Method of closure Interrupted suturing has a low incidence of bursts. Through and through suturing is good for the obstructed case. The incidence of burst hernia following one-layer closure is low but it is higher than that following a two-layered closure. Interrupted 'far and near' sutures are a recommended technique for single-layer mass closures. When continuous suturing of layers (one or two) is performed, a particular fault is the use of a short length of material pulled tightly; in an anaesthetised relaxed patient the incision is thus shortened and made taut so that when the patient is conscious and coughing the material will act as if it is a cheese-wire cutter. The golden rule is to insert a length of suture that is at least four times but less than five times the length of the incision. This ensures that the layers are gently apposed.

Drainage Drainage directly through a wound leads to a higher incidence of bursts than employing drainage through a separate (stab) incision.

Factors relating to incisions

Midline and vertical incisions have a greater tendency to burst than those that are transverse. Since the widespread use of non-absorbable suture materials, even midline vertical incisions are associated with a very low incidence of disruption.

Reasons for initial operation

Deep wound infection is notorious for causing burst abdomen and/or late incisional hernia. Operations on the pancreas, with leakage of enzymes, and on obstructed cases are other reasons for disruption.

Coughing, vomiting and distension

At the completion of an operation, any violent coughing set off by the removal of an endotracheal tube and suction of the laryngopharynx strains the sutures; likewise cough, vomiting and distension (e.g. due to ileus) in the early postoperative period. Overvigorous postoperative ventilation in sedated patients can lead to wound disruption.

General condition of the patient

Obesity, jaundice, malignant disease, hypoproteinaemia and anaemia are all factors conducive to disruption of a laparotomy wound. Abdominal wounds in pregnancy are notorious for a high risk of disruption; steroids delay healing (Summary box 57.17).

Summary box 57.17

Causes of burst abdomen

- Poor closure technique
- Deep wound infection
- Coughing or vomiting
- Poor metabolic state of patient

Burst abdomen (synonym: abdominal dehiscence)

Clinical features

A serosanguinous (pink) discharge from the wound is a forerunner of disruption in 50% of cases. It is the most pathognomonic sign of impending wound disruption and it signifies that intraperitoneal contents are lying extraperitoneally. Patients often volunteer the information that they 'felt something give way'. If skin sutures have been removed, omentum or coils of intestine may be forced through the wound and will be found lying on the skin. Pain and shock are often absent. It is important to note that there may be symptoms and signs of intestinal obstruction.

Treatment

An emergency operation is required to replace the bowel, relieve any obstruction and resuture the wound. While awaiting operation, reassure the patient and cover the wound with a sterile towel and, if necessary, administer appropriate analgesics. The stomach is emptied by a nasogastric tube and intravenous fluid therapy commenced.

Operation

Each protruding coil of intestine is washed gently with saline solution and returned to the abdominal cavity. The protruding greater omentum is treated similarly and spread over the intestine. Having cleansed the abdominal wall, all layers are approximated by through and through sutures of monofilament nylon, which may be passed through a soft rubber or plastic tube collar. The abdominal wall may be supported by strips of adhesive plaster encircling the anterior two-thirds of the circumference of the trunk. Antibiotic therapy is started.

Contrary to what might be thought, peritonitis rarely supervenes and, although the skin wound may become infected, healing is satisfactory. A second dehiscence rarely occurs. There is biochemical evidence that healing after disruption produces a stronger wound. This is because of the improvement in collagen metabolism in these circumstances. An incisional hernia is often a late sequel (see below).

Incisional hernia (synonym: postoperative hernia)

Aetiology

Incisional hernia occurs most often in obese individuals, and a persistent postoperative cough and postoperative abdominal distension are its precursors. There is a high incidence of incisional hernia following operations for peritonitis because, as a rule, the wound becomes infected. The placing of a drainage tube through a separate stab incision as opposed to bringing such a tube through the laparotomy wound reduces the frequency (see also General features common to all hernias, p. 968).

An incisional hernia usually starts as a symptomless partial disruption of the deeper layers of a laparotomy wound during the immediate or very early postoperative period. Often the event passes unnoticed if the skin wound remains intact after the stitches have been removed (or because subcuticular stitches have been used, which remain in place). A serosanguinous discharge is often the signal of dehiscence and resuture of the deeper layers of the incision obviates the more difficult repair of an established and much larger hernia later on.

Clinical features

There are great variations in the degree of herniation. The hernia may occur through a small portion of the scar, often the lower end. More frequently there is a diffuse bulging of the whole length of the incision. A postoperative hernia, especially one through a lower abdominal scar, usually increases steadily in size and more and more of its contents become irreducible. Sometimes the skin overlying it is so thin and atrophic that normal peristalsis can be seen in the underlying intestine. Attacks of partial intestinal obstruction are common and strangulation is liable to occur at the neck of a small sac or in a loculus of a large one. Nevertheless, most cases of incisional hernia are asymptomatic and broad-necked and do not need treatment (Summary box 57.18).

Summary box 57.18

Incisional hernias

- Rarely strangulate
- Large ones may be dangerous to reduce

Treatment

Palliative

An abdominal belt is sometimes satisfactory, especially in cases of a hernia through an upper abdominal incision.

Operation

Many procedures have been advocated, which is testimony to the fact that the repairs may be difficult to accomplish, but it is now clear that one technique is superior to all the others.

To obtain a lasting repair, very special preparation is required. If the patient is obese, weight reduction by dieting should precede the operation. To attempt to return the contents of a very large hernia to the main abdominal cavity if they have not been there for several years is to court danger, particularly if weight reduction has not been effected. In these circumstances there is not only a risk of failure of the hernioplasty but also a greatly increased risk of paralytic ileus from visceral compression and of pulmonary complications from elevation of the diaphragm. The repair of these large hernias is highly specialised surgery and should be performed only in centres with considerable experience in dealing with them. For example, one technique employed to enlarge the abdominal cavity is that of prolonged pneumoperitoneum, in which the intra-abdominal pressure is raised to 15–18 cmH$_2$O for up to several weeks preoperatively. The technique requires careful monitoring and patient counselling to be effective but, if employed correctly, can enable a primary repair to be successful.

Three techniques have been described: simple and complex apposition and plastic fibre mesh or net closures.

Simple apposition The hernial sac is dissected. It is then formally, if not already inadvertently, opened and the contents are reduced. Adherent omentum and bowel have to be freed by dissection before the mouth of the sac can be defined. The layers are repaired, usually with non-absorbable sutures: first the peritoneum and then the fascial (aponeurotic) layers. The lateral edges of the fascia are freed from the overlying muscles for some distance, and this fascial layer is approximated with interrupted sutures at the upper and lower ends of the wound. The muscles and the remaining fascial layer are approximated. Tension-relaxing incisions may be required and should be placed well laterally.

Complex apposition This consists of various types of layered closures (Mayo, 'Keel', da Silva) and should be considered obsolete and of historical interest only.

Plastic fibre mesh or net closures These techniques are now the method of choice for all but the smallest defects (< 4 cm). The sac is dealt with as above. The layers of the fascia are dissected out and, if above the umbilicus, the posterior rectus sheath edges apposed. A sheet of polypropylene mesh is then inserted between the posterior rectus sheath and the muscle fibres and anchored in place. If below the umbilicus, the mesh is placed in the preperitoneal space. The anterior rectus sheath is then apposed as above. If the defect is too large to close by simple apposition of the rectus sheath, advanced techniques involving muscle-relaxing incisions are employed, such as the Ramirez component separation technique, which enable either the anterior or posterior component of the rectus sheath to be closed and reinforced with an onlay prosthetic mesh.

Incisional and primary ventral hernias are also increasingly being repaired by the laparascopic placement of mesh. A laparoscopy and division of adhesions is initially performed and the hernia defect defined intraperitoneally. One of a variety of meshes specifically designed for intraperitoneal use is introduced through a port and fixed to the abdominal wall by tacks or transfascial sutures (Fig. 57.24). The critical steps of the laparoscopic approach are ensuring a sufficient circumferential overlap of the fascial defect (> 4 cm) and adequate fixation of the mesh to the anterior abdominal wall. Prospective trials are currently taking place to define the method and degree of optimum fixation.

Careful haemostasis and meticulous asepsis are essential during these operations. Postoperative collections of serum can be removed by drainage using plastic tubing that leads, via skin punctures lateral to the wound, into closed suction drainage bottles (e.g. RediVac).

Postoperative care

Gastric decompression and intravenous fluids are employed and nothing by mouth allowed until the bowels have functioned.

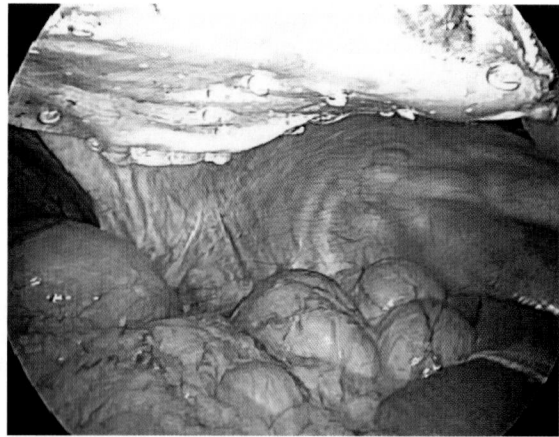

Figure 57.24 Laparoscopic repair of an incisional hernia. The position of the intraperitoneal mesh covering a fascial defect. After the contents of the sac have been reduced the hernial defect can be defined.

Early ambulation and gentle physical exercise is to be encouraged. The patient should not resume strenuous exercise for several weeks.

Results of treatment

Most series report recurrence of the hernia in 30–50% of patients, except where mesh inlay techniques have been employed in specialist centres, in which case recurrence rates may be as low as 10%.

Divarication of the rectus abdominis

Divarication of the rectus abdominis is seen principally in elderly multiparous patients. When the patient strains, a gap can be seen between the rectus abdominis, through which the abdominal contents bulge. When the abdomen is relaxed, the fingers can be introduced between the rectus.

Treatment

An abdominal belt is all that is required. There is no risk of strangulated intestinal contents. A similar condition is seen in babies, except that the divarication exists above the umbilicus. No treatment is necessary; as the child grows a spontaneous cure results.

Tearing of the inferior epigastric artery

Tearing of the inferior epigastric artery occurs in three dissimilar types of individual: elderly women, often thin and feeble; athletic, muscular men, usually below middle age; and pregnant women, mainly multiparae late in pregnancy. The site of the haematoma is usually at the level of the arcuate line, where the posterior sheath of the rectus abdominis is lacking.

Clinical features

The possibility of tearing of the epigastric vessels should always be considered when, following a bout of coughing or a sudden blow to the abdominal wall, an exquisitely tender lump appears in relation to the rectus abdominis. Occasionally a haematoma occurs within the muscles lateral to the rectus sheath. Unless there is bruising of the overlying skin, the diagnosis may be difficult.

Differential diagnosis

The conditions for which the haematoma is frequently mistaken are a twisted ovarian cyst in women and, when the lump is on the right side, an appendix abscess in both sexes. The sign most likely to be of value in differentiating a haematoma of the abdominal wall from these conditions, namely tensing of the abdominal musculature, is often unsatisfactory because of the pain it causes. The differential diagnosis between the haematoma and a strangulated Spigelian hernia may be difficult. The absence of vomiting suggests a haematoma and the presence of resonance over the swelling favours a Spigelian hernia; a plain radiograph of the abdomen sometimes gives positive evidence of the latter.

As a complication of pregnancy

Rupture of the inferior epigastric artery occurs occasionally during pregnancy. Surprisingly, haemorrhage into this closed space from this comparatively small artery has proved fatal.

Treatment

With rest, a comparatively small haematoma may resolve, but sometimes renewed haemorrhage causes the haematoma to

rupture into the peritoneal cavity. Thus, it is safer to operate early, evacuate the clot and ligate the artery (Summary box 57.19).

Summary box 57.19

Tear of epigastric artery

- Follows a bout of coughing
- May mimic intra-abdominal sepsis

Infections

Cellulitis can occur in any of the planes of the abdominal wall.

Superficial cellulitis is usually discovered when an abdominal wound is inspected following pyrexia. The earliest sign is when the stitches become embedded in the oedematous skin. Later there is a blush extending for a variable distance from the incision or the stitch holes. On palpation with the gloved hand, one area is usually found to be more indurated and tender than the remainder. A stitch should be removed from the immediate vicinity and if pus or seropus escapes it should be sent for bacteriological examination; treatment should then be commenced with a broad-spectrum antibiotic.

Deep cellulitis is characterised by brawny oedema towards one or both flanks, and not infrequently of the scrotum or vulva as well. Antibiotic therapy is the mainstay of treatment. When tenderness persists, an anatomical incision dividing the muscles carefully, layer by layer until pus or purulent fluid is encountered, is often advisable.

Progressive postoperative bacterial synergistic gangrene

Fortunately, this is a rare complication after laparotomy, usually for a perforated viscus (notably perforated appendicitis). It has also occurred after gall bladder operations, after colectomy for ulcerative colitis and even after drainage of an empyema thoracis. The condition is due to the synergistic action of microaerophilic non-haemolytic streptococci and, usually, a *Staphylococcus*. The skin in the immediate vicinity of the wound exhibits signs of cellulitis. Within a few hours, a central purplish zone with an outer brilliant red zone can be distinguished and the whole region is extremely tender. The condition advances with various degrees of rapidity (Fig. 57.25). The gangrenous skin liquefies, exposing underlying granulation tissue. If the condition persists, overwhelming septicaemia and associated multi-organ failure supervene.

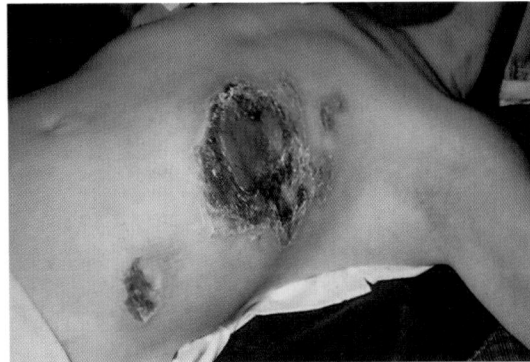

Figure 57.25 Bacterial synergistic gangrene of the chest and abdominal wall. The area has become gangrenous and looks like suede leather. Beware of amoebiasis cutis.

Treatment

Identification of the organisms and a report on their sensitivity to antibiotics is essential. Metronidazole should be given together with a powerful broad-spectrum antibiotic. Without vigorous and effective treatment, the gangrene spreads to the flanks and the patient may die of toxaemia. If the infection has become established, surgical debridement of all the necrotic and infected tissue should be performed. Hyperbaric oxygen, if available, can be life-saving. Cellulitis due to bacteroids may give no bacterial growth by conventional techniques and may be missed.

Amoebic cutis

The possibility of this potentially lethal complication of amoebic colitis, liver abscess or empyema should always be considered. Confirmation may be difficult and an immunofluorescence test necessary.

Subcutaneous gas-forming infection

This is described in Chapter 4 (under Gas gangrene).

Neoplasms of the abdominal wall

Desmoid tumour

A desmoid tumour is a tumour arising in the musculoaponeurotic structures of the abdominal wall, especially below the level of the umbilicus. It is a completely unencapsulated fibroma and is so hard that it creaks when it is cut. Some cases recur repeatedly in spite of apparently adequate excision.

Aetiology

About 80% of cases occur in women, many of whom have borne children, and the neoplasm occurs occasionally in scars of old hernial or other abdominal operation wounds. Consequently, trauma, for example the stretching of the muscle fibres during pregnancy or possibly a small haematoma of the abdominal wall, appears to be an aetiological factor. They can occur in cases of familial adenomatous polyposis (FAP).

Pathology

The tumour is composed of fibrous tissue containing multinucleated plasmodial masses resembling foreign body giant cells. Usually of very slow growth, it tends to infiltrate muscle in the immediate area. Eventually it undergoes a myxomatous change and it then increases in size more rapidly. Metastasis does not occur. Unlike fibroma elsewhere, no sarcomatous change occurs.

Treatment

Unless the tumour is excised widely, with a surrounding margin of at least 2.5 cm of healthy tissue, recurrence commonly takes place. After removal of a large tumour, repair of the defect in the abdominal wall by nylon mesh is required. These tumours are moderately radiosensitive. (Intraperitoneal desmoids are best left alone when possible.)

Fibrosarcoma of the abdominal wall

Fibrosarcoma of the abdominal wall is rare. It is resistant to radiotherapy and only in some cases can a wide excision with nylon mesh repair offer hope of a cure.

Adenocarcinoma

Adenocarcinoma of the colon or of other viscera may invade the abdominal wall. In such cases, the resection of this extension, along with the primary growth, may require special repair of the resulting defect.

Secondary implantation in the wound may follow any abdominal operation for carcinoma; bladder cancer is notorious for this propensity.

FURTHER READING

Kingsnorth, A.N. and LeBlanc, K.A. (2003) *Management of Abdominal Hernias*, 3rd edn. Hodder Arnold, London.

Nyhus, L.M. and Condon, R.E. (eds) (2001) *Hernia*, 5th edn. J.B. Lippincott, Philadelphia.

Schumpelick, V. and Kingsnorth, A.N. (eds) (1999) *Incisional Hernia*. Springer-Verlag, Berlin.

The peritoneum, omentum, mesentery and retroperitoneal space

CHAPTER

58

LEARNING OBJECTIVES

To recognise and understand:

- The clinical features of localised and generalised peritonitis
- The common causes and complications of peritonitis
- The principles of surgical management in patients with peritonitis

- The clinical presentations and treatment of abdominal/pelvic abscesses
- The clinical presentations of tuberculous peritonitis
- The causes and pathophysiology of ascites
- The spectrum of mesenteric and retroperitoneal conditions

THE PERITONEUM

The peritoneal membrane is conveniently divided into two parts – the visceral peritoneum surrounding the viscera and the parietal peritoneum lining the other surfaces of the cavity. The peritoneum has a number of functions (Summary box 58.1).

Summary box 58.1

Functions of the peritoneum

- Pain perception (parietal peritoneum)
- Visceral lubrication
- Fluid and particulate absorption
- Inflammatory and immune responses
- Fibrinolytic activity

The parietal portion is richly supplied with nerves and, when irritated, causes severe pain accurately localised to the affected area. The visceral peritoneum, in contrast, is poorly supplied with nerves and its irritation causes vague pain that is usually located to the midline.

The peritoneal cavity is the largest cavity in the body, the surface area of its lining membrane (2 m² in an adult) being nearly equal to that of the skin. The peritoneal membrane is composed of flattened polyhedral cells (mesothelium), one layer thick, resting upon a thin layer of fibroelastic tissue. Beneath the peritoneum, supported by a small amount of areolar tissue, lies a network of lymphatic vessels and rich plexuses of capillary blood vessels from which all absorption and exudation must occur. In health, only a few millilitres of peritoneal fluid is found in the peritoneal cavity. The fluid is pale yellow, somewhat viscid and contains lymphocytes and other leucocytes; it lubricates the viscera, allowing easy movement and peristalsis.

In the peritoneal space, mobile gas-filled structures float upwards, as does free air ('gas'). In the erect position, when free fluid is present in the peritoneal cavity, pressure is reduced in the upper abdomen compared with the lower abdomen. When air is introduced, it rises, allowing all of the abdominal contents to sink.

During expiration, intra-abdominal pressure is reduced and peritoneal fluid, aided by capillary attraction, travels in an upward direction towards the diaphragm. Experimental evidence shows that particulate matter and bacteria are absorbed within a few minutes into the lymphatic network through a number of 'pores' within the diaphragmatic peritoneum. This upward movement of peritoneal fluids is responsible for the occurrence of many subphrenic abscesses.

The peritoneum has the capacity to absorb large volumes of fluid: this ability is used during peritoneal dialysis in the treatment of renal failure. But the peritoneum can also produce an inflammatory exudate when injured (Summary box 58.2).

Summary box 58.2

Causes of a peritoneal inflammatory exudate

- Bacterial infection, e.g. appendicitis, tuberculosis
- Chemical injury, e.g. bile peritonitis
- Ischaemic injury, e.g. strangulated bowel, vascular occlusion
- Direct trauma, e.g. operation
- Allergic reaction, e.g. starch peritonitis

When a visceral perforation occurs, the free fluid that spills into the peritoneal cavity runs downwards, largely directed by the normal peritoneal attachments. For example, spillage from a perforated duodenal ulcer may run down the right paracolic gutter.

When parietal peritoneal defects are created, healing occurs not from the edges but by the development of new mesothelial cells throughout the surface of the defect. In this way, large defects heal as rapidly as small defects.

ACUTE PERITONITIS

Most cases of peritonitis are caused by an invasion of the peritoneal cavity by bacteria, so that when the term 'peritonitis' is used without qualification, bacterial peritonitis is implied. Bacterial peritonitis is usually polymicrobial, both aerobic and anaerobic organisms being present. The exception is primary peritonitis ('spontaneous' peritonitis), in which a pure infection with streptococcal, pneumococcal or *Haemophilus* bacteria occurs.

Bacteriology

Bacteria from the gastrointestinal tract

The number of bacteria within the lumen of the gastrointestinal tract is normally low until the distal small bowel is reached, whereas high concentrations are found in the colon. However, disease (e.g. obstruction, achlorhydria, diverticula) may increase proximal colonisation. The biliary and pancreatic tracts are normally free from bacteria, although they may be infected in disease, e.g. gallstones. Peritoneal infection is usually caused by two or more bacterial strains. Gram-negative bacteria contain endotoxins (lipopolysaccharides) in their cell walls that have multiple toxic effects on the host, primarily by causing the release of tumour necrosis factor (TNF) from host leucocytes. Systemic absorption of endotoxin may produce endotoxic shock with hypotension and impaired tissue perfusion. Other bacteria such as *Clostridium welchii* produce harmful exotoxins.

Bacteroides are commonly found in peritonitis. These Gram-negative, non-sporing organisms, although predominant in the lower intestine, often escape detection because they are strictly anaerobic and slow to grow on culture media unless there is an adequate carbon dioxide tension in the anaerobic apparatus (Gillespie). In many laboratories, the culture is discarded if there is no growth in 48 hours. These organisms are resistant to penicillin and streptomycin but sensitive to metronidazole, clindamycin, lincomycin and cephalosporin compounds. Since the widespread use of metronidazole (Flagyl), *Bacteroides* infections have greatly diminished.

Non-gastrointestinal causes of peritonitis

Pelvic infection via the fallopian tubes is responsible for a high proportion of 'non-gastrointestinal' infections.

Immunodeficient patients, for example those with human immunodeficiency virus (HIV) infection or those on immunosuppressive treatment, may present with opportunistic peritoneal infection, e.g. *Mycobacterium avium-intracellulare* (MAI) (Summary box 58.3).

Summary box 58.3

Bacteria in peritonitis

Gastrointestinal source
- *Escherichia coli*
- Streptococci (aerobic and anaerobic)
- *Bacteroides*
- *Clostridium*
- *Klebsiella pneumoniae*
- *Staphylococcus*

Other sources
- *Chlamydia*
- Gonococcus
- β-Haemolytic streptococci
- Pneumococcus
- *Mycobacterium tuberculosis*

Route of infection

Infecting organisms may reach the peritoneal cavity via a number of routes (Summary box 58.4).

Summary box 58.4

Paths to peritoneal infection

- Gastrointestinal perforation, e.g. perforated ulcer, diverticular perforation
- Exogenous contamination, e.g. drains, open surgery, trauma
- Transmural bacterial translocation (no perforation), e.g. inflammatory bowel disease, appendicitis, ischaemic bowel
- Female genital tract infection, e.g. pelvic inflammatory disease
- Haematogenous spread (rare), e.g. septicaemia

Even in patients with non-bacterial peritonitis (e.g. acute pancreatitis, intraperitoneal rupture of the bladder or haemoperitoneum), the peritoneum often becomes infected by transmural spread of organisms from the bowel, and it is not long (often a matter of hours) before a bacterial peritonitis develops. Most duodenal perforations are initially sterile for up to several hours, and many gastric perforations are also sterile at first; intestinal perforations are usually infected from the beginning. The proportion of anaerobic to aerobic organisms increases with the passage of time. Mortality reflects:

- the degree and duration of peritoneal contamination;
- the age of the patient;
- the general health of the patient;
- the nature of the underlying cause.

Localised peritonitis

Anatomical, pathological and surgical factors may favour the localisation of peritonitis.

Hans Christian Joachim Gram, 1853–1938, Professor of Pharmacology (1891–1900), and of Medicine (1900–1923), Copenhagen, Denmark, described this method of staining bacteria in 1884.
William Henry Welch, 1850–1934, Professor of Pathology, Johns Hopkins University, Baltimore, MD, USA, discovered the causative organism of gas gangrene in 1892.
William Alexander Gillespie, Formerly Professor of Clinical Bacteriology, The University of Bristol, Bristol, England.
Gabriele Falloppio, (Fallopius), 1523–1563, Professor of Anatomy, Surgery, and Botany, Padua, Italy.

Theodor Escherich, 1857–1911, Professor of Paediatrics, Vienna, Austria, discovered the Bacterium Coli Commune in 1886.
Theodor Albrecht Edwin Klebs, 1834–1913, Professor of Bacteriology successively at Prague, in the Czech Republic; Zurich, Switzerland, and The Rush Medical College, Chicago, IL, USA.

Anatomical

The greater sac of the peritoneum is divided into (1) the subphrenic spaces, (2) the pelvis and (3) the peritoneal cavity proper. The last is divided into a supracolic and an infracolic compartment by the transverse colon and transverse mesocolon, which deters the spread of infection from one to the other. When the supracolic compartment overflows, as is often the case when a peptic ulcer perforates, it does so over the colon into the infracolic compartment or by way of the right paracolic gutter to the right iliac fossa and hence to the pelvis.

Pathological

The clinical course is determined in part by the manner in which adhesions form around the affected organ. Inflamed peritoneum loses its glistening appearance and becomes reddened and velvety. Flakes of fibrin appear and cause loops of intestine to become adherent to one another and to the parietes. There is an outpouring of serous inflammatory exudate rich in leucocytes and plasma proteins that soon becomes turbid; if localisation occurs, the turbid fluid becomes frank pus. Peristalsis is retarded in affected bowel and this helps to prevent distribution of the infection. The greater omentum, by enveloping and becoming adherent to inflamed structures, often forms a substantial barrier to the spread of infection.

Surgical

Drains are frequently placed during operation to assist localisation (and exit) of intra-abdominal collections: their value is disputed. They may act as conduits for exogenous infection.

Diffuse peritonitis

A number of factors may favour the development of diffuse peritonitis:

- *Speed of peritoneal contamination* is a prime factor. If an inflamed appendix (Fig. 58.1) or other hollow viscus perforates before localisation has taken place, there is a gush of contents into the peritoneal cavity, which may spread over a large area almost instantaneously. Perforation proximal to an obstruction or from sudden anastomotic separation is associated with severe generalised peritonitis and a high mortality rate.

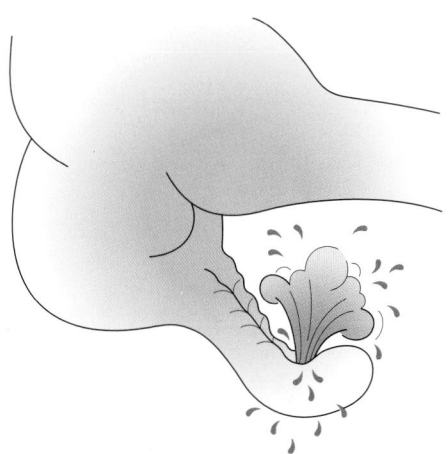

Figure 58.1 Sudden perforation, especially if engendered by purgation, often results in an immediate, widespread bacterial peritonitis.

- *Stimulation of peristalsis* by the ingestion of food or even water hinders localisation. Violent peristalsis occasioned by the administration of a purgative or an enema may cause the widespread distribution of an infection that would otherwise have remained localised.
- The *virulence of the infecting organism* may be so great as to render the localisation of infection difficult or impossible.
- *Young children* have a small omentum, which is less effective in localising infection.
- *Disruption of localised collections* may occur with injudicious handling, e.g. appendix mass or pericolic abscess.
- *Deficient natural resistance* ('immune deficiency') may result from use of drugs (e.g. steroids), disease [e.g. acquired immune deficiency syndrome (AIDS)] or old age.

Clinical features

Localised peritonitis

Localised peritonitis is bound up intimately with the causative condition, and the initial symptoms and signs are those of that condition. When the peritoneum becomes inflamed, the temperature, and especially the pulse rate, rise. Abdominal pain increases and usually there is associated vomiting. The most important sign is guarding and rigidity of the abdominal wall over the area of the abdomen that is involved, with a positive 'release' sign (rebound tenderness). If inflammation arises under the diaphragm, shoulder tip ('phrenic') pain may be felt. In cases of pelvic peritonitis arising from an inflamed appendix in the pelvic position or from salpingitis, the abdominal signs are often slight; there may be deep tenderness of one or both lower quadrants alone, but a rectal or vaginal examination reveals marked tenderness of the pelvic peritoneum. With appropriate treatment, localised peritonitis usually resolves; in about 20% of cases, an abscess follows. Infrequently, localised peritonitis becomes diffuse. Conversely, in favourable circumstances, diffuse peritonitis can become localised, most frequently in the pelvis or at multiple sites within the abdominal cavity.

Diffuse (generalised) peritonitis

Diffuse (generalised) peritonitis may present in differing ways dependent on the duration of infection.

Early

Abdominal pain is severe and made worse by moving or breathing. It is first experienced at the site of the original lesion and spreads outwards from this point. Vomiting may occur. The patient usually lies still. Tenderness and rigidity on palpation are found typically when the peritonitis affects the anterior abdominal wall. Abdominal tenderness and rigidity are diminished or absent if the anterior wall is unaffected, as in pelvic peritonitis or, rarely, peritonitis in the lesser sac. Patients with pelvic peritonitis may complain of urinary symptoms; they are tender on rectal or vaginal examination. Infrequent bowel sounds may still be heard for a few hours but they cease with the onset of paralytic ileus. The pulse rises progressively but, if the peritoneum is deluged with irritant fluid, there is a sudden rise. The temperature changes are variable and *can be subnormal*.

Late

If resolution or localisation of generalised peritonitis does not occur, the abdomen remains silent and increasingly distends.

Circulatory failure ensues, with cold, clammy extremities, sunken eyes, dry tongue, thready (irregular) pulse and drawn and anxious face (Hippocratic facies; Fig. 58.2). The patient finally lapses into unconsciousness. With early diagnosis and adequate treatment, this condition is rarely seen in modern surgical practice (Summary box 58.5).

Summary box 58.5

Clinical features in peritonitis

- Abdominal pain, worse on movement
- Guarding/rigidity of abdominal wall
- Pain/tenderness on rectal/vaginal examination (pelvic peritonitis)
- Pyrexia (may be absent)
- Raised pulse rate
- Absent or reduced bowel sounds
- 'Septic shock' [systemic inflammatory response syndrome (SIRS)] in later stages

---

Diagnostic aids

Investigations may elucidate a doubtful diagnosis, but the importance of a careful history and repeated examination must not be forgotten.

- A *radiograph of the abdomen* may confirm the presence of dilated gas-filled loops of bowel (consistent with a paralytic ileus) or show free gas, although the latter is best shown on an erect chest radiograph (Fig. 58.3). If the patient is too ill for an 'erect' film to demonstrate free air under the diaphragm, a lateral decubitus film is just as useful, showing gas beneath the abdominal wall.
- *Serum amylase estimation* may establish the diagnosis of acute pancreatitis provided that it is remembered that moderately raised values are frequently found following other

abdominal catastrophes and operations, e.g. perforated duodenal ulcer.
- *Ultrasound* and *computerised tomography (CT) scanning* are increasingly used to identify the cause of peritonitis (Fig. 58.4). Such knowledge may influence management decisions.
- *Peritoneal diagnostic aspiration* may be helpful but is usually unnecessary. Bile-stained fluid indicates a perforated peptic ulcer or gall bladder; the presence of pus indicates bacterial peritonitis. Blood is aspirated in a high proportion of patients with intraperitoneal bleeding (Summary box 58.6).

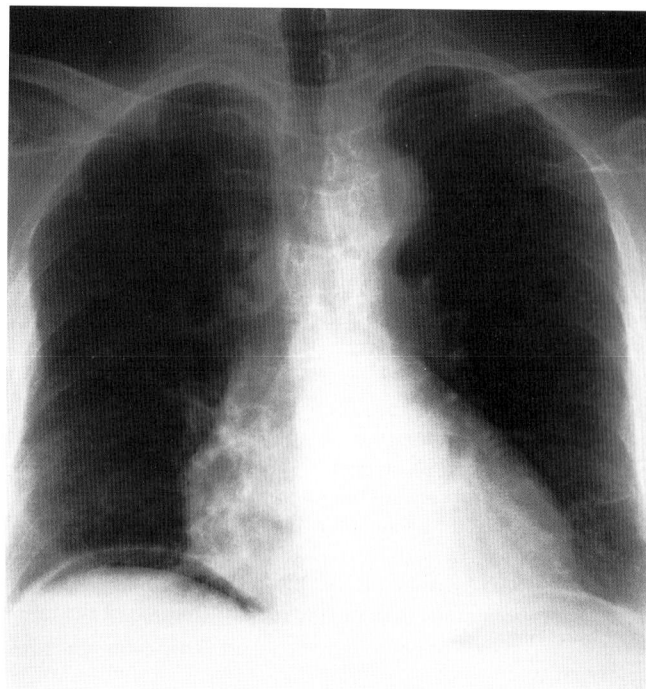

Figure 58.3 Gas under the diaphragm in a patient with free perforation and peritonitis (courtesy of Dr S. Padley, Chelsea and Westminster Hospital, London, UK).

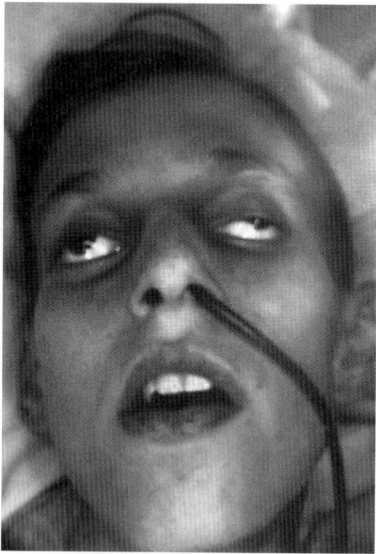

Figure 58.2 The Hippocratic facies in terminal diffuse peritonitis.

Hippocrates of Cos, a Greek Physician and Surgeon, and by common consent 'The Father of Medicine', was born on the island of Cos, off Turkey, about 460 BC and probably died in 375 BC.

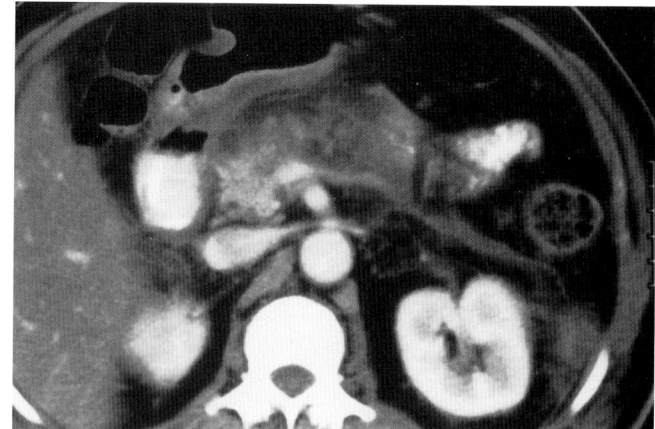

Figure 58.4 Acute pancreatitis seen on computerised tomography scanning with swelling of the gland and surrounding inflammatory changes (courtesy of Dr J. Healy, Chelsea and Westminster Hospital, London, UK).

Summary box 58.6

Investigations in peritonitis

- Raised white cell count and C-reactive protein are usual
- Serum amylase >4× normal indicates acute pancreatitis
- Abdominal radiographs are occasionally helpful
- Erect chest radiographs may show free peritoneal gas (perforated viscus)
- Ultrasound/CT scanning often diagnostic
- Peritoneal fluid aspiration (with or without ultrasound guidance) may be helpful

Treatment

In case of doubt, early surgical intervention is to be preferred to a 'wait and see' policy. This rule is particularly true for previously healthy patients and those with postoperative peritonitis. Caution is required in patients at high operative risk because of comorbidity or advanced age.

Treatment consists of:

- general care of the patient;
- specific treatment of the cause;
- peritoneal lavage when appropriate.

General care of the patient

The care of critically ill surgical patients is described in detail in Chapters 13, 16 and 20. Nutritional support is covered in Chapter 17 and anaesthesia and pain relief in Chapter 14.

Correction of circulating volume and electrolyte imbalance

Patients are frequently hypovolaemic with electrolyte disturbances. The plasma volume must be restored and electrolyte concentrations corrected. Central venous catheterisation and pressure monitoring may be helpful, particularly in patients with concurrent disease. Plasma protein depletion may also need correction as the inflamed peritoneum leaks large amounts of protein. If the patient's recovery is delayed for more than 7–10 days, intravenous nutrition is required.

Gastrointestinal decompression

A nasogastric tube is passed into the stomach and aspirated. Intermittent aspiration is maintained until the paralytic ileus has resolved. Measured volumes of water are allowed by mouth when only small amounts are being aspirated. If the abdomen is soft and not tender, and bowel sounds return, oral feeding may be progressively introduced. It is important not to prolong the ileus by missing this stage.

Antibiotic therapy

Administration of antibiotics prevents the multiplication of bacteria and the release of endotoxins. As the infection is usually a mixed one, initial treatment with parenteral broad-spectrum antibiotics active against aerobic and anaerobic bacteria should be given.

Correction of fluid loss

A fluid balance chart must be started so that daily output by gastric aspiration and urine is known. Additional losses from the lungs, skin and in faeces are estimated, so that the intake requirements can be calculated and seen to have been administered.

Throughout recovery, the haematocrit and serum electrolytes and urea must be checked regularly.

Analgesia

The patient should be nursed in the sitting-up position and must be relieved of pain before and after operation. If appropriate expertise is available, epidural infusion may provide excellent analgesia. Freedom from pain allows early mobilisation and adequate physiotherapy in the postoperative period, which help to prevent basal pulmonary collapse, deep vein thrombosis and pulmonary embolism.

Vital system support

Special measures may be needed for cardiac, pulmonary and renal support, especially if septic shock is present (see Chapter 2).

Specific treatment of the cause

If the cause of peritonitis is amenable to surgery, operation must be carried out as soon as the patient is fit for anaesthesia. This is usually within a few hours. In peritonitis caused by pancreatitis or salpingitis, or in cases of primary peritonitis of streptococcal or pneumococcal origin, non-operative treatment is preferred provided the diagnosis can be made with confidence.

Peritoneal lavage

In operations for general peritonitis it is essential that, after the cause has been dealt with, the whole peritoneal cavity is explored with the sucker and, if necessary, mopped dry until all seropurulent exudate is removed. The use of a large volume of saline (1–2 litres) containing dissolved antibiotic (e.g. tetracycline) has been shown to be effective (Matheson) (Summary box 58.7).

Summary box 58.7

Management of peritonitis

General care of patient:
- Correction of fluid and electrolyte imbalance
- Insertion of nasogastric drainage tube
- Broad-spectrum antibiotic therapy
- Analgesia
- Vital system support

Operative treatment of cause when appropriate with peritoneal debridement/lavage

Prognosis and complications

With modern treatment, diffuse peritonitis carries a mortality rate of about 10%. The systemic and local complications are shown in Summary boxes 58.8 and 58.9.

Summary box 58.8

Systemic complications of peritonitis

- Bacteraemic/endotoxic shock
- Bronchopneumonia/respiratory failure
- Renal failure
- Bone marrow suppression
- Multisystem failure

Summary box 58.9

Abdominal complications of peritonitis

- Adhesional small bowel obstruction
- Paralytic ileus
- Residual or recurrent abscess
- Portal pyaemia/liver abscess

Acute intestinal obstruction due to peritoneal adhesions

This usually gives central colicky abdominal pain with evidence of small bowel gas and fluid levels sometimes confined to the proximal intestine on radiography. Bowel sounds are increased. It is more common with localised peritonitis. It is essential to distinguish this from paralytic ileus.

Paralytic ileus

There is usually little pain, and gas-filled loops with fluid levels are seen distributed throughout the small and large intestines on abdominal imaging. In paralytic ileus, bowel sounds are reduced or absent.

Abdominal and pelvic abscesses

Abscess formation following local or diffuse peritonitis usually occupies one of the situations shown in Fig. 58.5. The symptoms and signs of a purulent collection may be vague and consist of nothing more than lassitude, anorexia and malaise; pyrexia (often low-grade), tachycardia, leucocytosis, raised C-reactive protein and localised tenderness are also common (Summary box 58.10).

Summary box 58.10

Clinical features of an abdominal/pelvic abscess

- Malaise
- Sweats with or without rigors
- Abdominal/pelvic (with or without shoulder tip) pain
- Anorexia and weight loss
- Symptoms from local irritation, e.g. hiccoughs (subphrenic), diarrhoea and mucus (pelvic)
- Swinging pyrexia
- Localised abdominal tenderness/mass

Later, a palpable mass may develop that should be monitored by marking out its limits on the abdominal wall and meticulous daily examination. More commonly, its course is monitored by repeat ultrasound or CT scanning. In most cases, with the aid of antibiotic treatment, the abscess or mass gradually reduces in size until, finally, it is undetectable. In others, the abscess fails to resolve or becomes larger, in which event it must be drained. In many situations, by waiting for a few days the abscess becomes adherent to the abdominal wall, so that it can be drained without opening the general peritoneal cavity. If facilities are available, ultrasound- or CT-guided drainage may avoid further operation. Open drainage of an intraperitoneal collection should be carried out by cautious blunt finger exploration to minimise the risk of an intestinal fistula.

Pelvic abscess

The pelvis is the commonest site of an intraperitoneal abscess because the vermiform appendix is often pelvic in position and the fallopian tubes are frequent sites of infection. A pelvic abscess can also occur as a sequel to any case of diffuse peritonitis and is common after anastomotic leakage following colorectal surgery. The most characteristic symptoms are diarrhoea and the passage of mucus in the stools. Rectal examination reveals a bulging of the anterior rectal wall, which, when the abscess is ripe, becomes softly cystic. Left to nature, a proportion of these abscesses burst into the rectum, after which the patient nearly always recovers rapidly. If this does not occur, the abscess should be drained deliberately. In women, vaginal drainage through the posterior fornix is often chosen. In other cases, when the abscess is definitely pointing into the rectum, rectal drainage (Fig. 58.6) is employed. If any uncertainty exists, the presence of pus should be confirmed by ultrasound or CT scanning with needle aspiration if indicated. Laparotomy is almost never necessary. Rectal drainage of a pelvic abscess is far preferable to suprapubic drainage, which risks exposing the general peritoneal cavity to infection. Drainage tubes can also be inserted percutaneously or via the vagina or rectum under ultrasound or CT guidance (Fig. 58.7).

Intraperitoneal abscess

Anatomy

The complicated arrangement of the peritoneum results in the formation of four intraperitoneal spaces in which pus may collect (Figs 58.8 and 58.9).

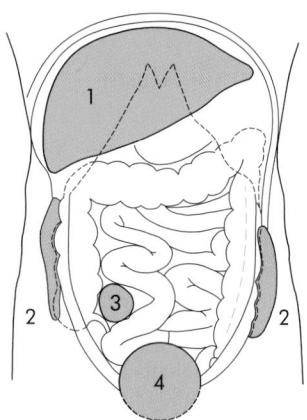

Figure 58.5 Common situations for residual abscesses: (1) subphrenic; (2) paracolic; (3) right iliac fossa; (4) pelvic.

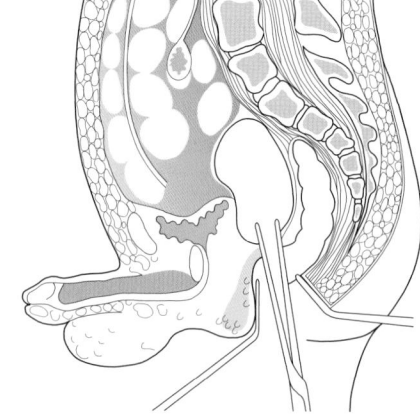

Figure 58.6 Opening a pelvic abscess into the rectum.

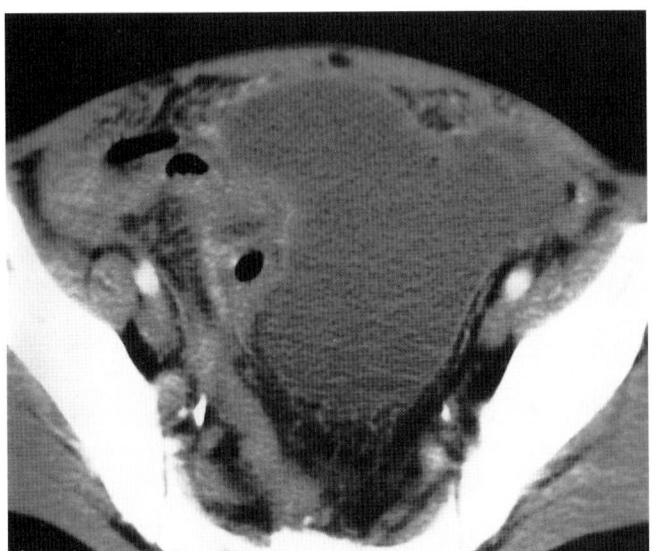

Figure 58.7 A pelvic abscess seen on computerised tomography scanning (courtesy of Dr J. Healy, Chelsea and Westminster Hospital, London, UK).

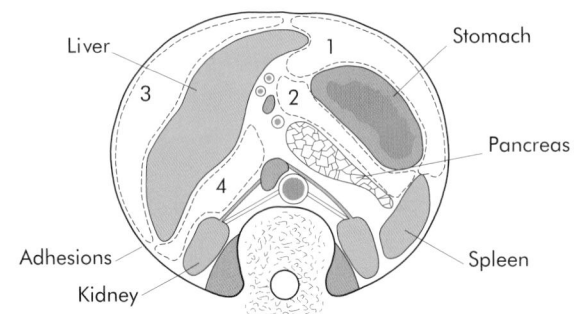

Figure 58.8 Intraperitoneal abscesses on transverse section. (1) The left subphrenic space; (2) left subhepatic space/lesser sac; (3) right subphrenic space; (4) right subhepatic space.

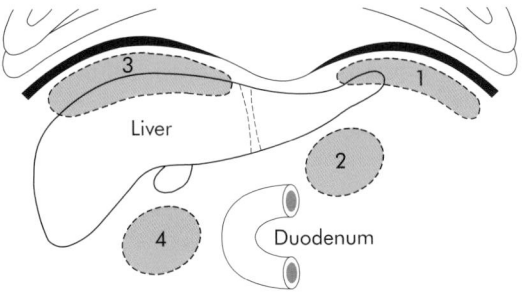

Figure 58.9 Intraperitoneal abscesses on sagittal section. (1) Left subphrenic; (2) left subhepatic/lesser sac; (3) right subphrenic; (4) right subhepatic.

Left subphrenic space

This is bounded above by the diaphragm and behind by the left triangular ligament and the left lobe of the liver, the gastrohepatic omentum and the anterior surface of the stomach. To the right is the falciform ligament and to the left the spleen, gastrosplenic omentum and diaphragm. The common cause of an abscess here is an operation on the stomach, the tail of the pancreas, the spleen or the splenic flexure of the colon.

Left subhepatic space/lesser sac

The commonest cause of infection here is complicated acute pancreatitis. In practice, a perforated gastric ulcer rarely causes a collection here because the potential space is obliterated by adhesions.

Right subphrenic space

This space lies between the right lobe of the liver and the diaphragm. It is limited posteriorly by the anterior layer of the coronary and the right triangular ligaments and to the left by the falciform ligament. Common causes of abscess here are perforating cholecystitis, a perforated duodenal ulcer, a duodenal cap 'blow-out' following gastrectomy and appendicitis.

Right subhepatic space

This lies transversely beneath the right lobe of the liver in Rutherford Morison's pouch. It is bounded on the right by the right lobe of the liver and the diaphragm. To the left is situated the foramen of Winslow and below this lies the duodenum. In front are the liver and the gall bladder and behind are the upper part of the right kidney and the diaphragm. The space is bounded above by the liver and below by the transverse colon and hepatic flexure. It is the deepest space of the four and the commonest site of a subphrenic abscess, which usually arises from appendicitis, cholecystitis, a perforated duodenal ulcer or following upper abdominal surgery.

Clinical features

The symptoms and signs of subphrenic infection are frequently non-specific and it is well to remember the aphorism, 'pus somewhere, pus nowhere else, pus under the diaphragm'.

Symptoms

A common history is that, when some infective focus in the abdominal cavity has been dealt with, the condition of the patient improves temporarily but, after an interval of a few days or weeks, symptoms of toxaemia reappear. The condition of the patient steadily, and often rapidly, deteriorates. Sweating, wasting and anorexia are present. There is sometimes epigastric fullness and pain, or pain in the shoulder on the affected side, because of irritation of sensory fibres in the phrenic nerve, referred along the descending branches of the cervical plexus. Persistent hiccoughs may be a presenting symptom.

Signs

A swinging pyrexia is usually present. If the abscess is anterior, abdominal examination will reveal some tenderness, rigidity or even a palpable swelling. Sometimes the liver is displaced downwards but more often it is fixed by adhesions. Examination of the chest is important and, in the majority of cases, collapse of the lung or evidence of basal effusion or even an empyema is found.

James Rutherford Morison, **1853–1939, Professor of Surgery, The University of Durham, Durham, England.**
Jacob Benignus Winslow, **1669–1760, Professor of Anatomy, Physic and Surgery, Paris, France.**

CHAPTER 58 | THE PERITONEUM, OMENTUM, MESENTERY AND RETROPERITONEAL SPACE

Investigations

A number of the following investigations may be helpful:

- *Blood tests* usually show a leucocytosis and raised C-reactive protein.
- A *plain radiograph* sometimes demonstrates the presence of gas or a pleural effusion. On screening, the diaphragm is often seen to be elevated (so called 'tented' diaphragm) and its movements impaired.
- *Ultrasound* or *CT scanning* is the investigation of choice and permits early detection of subphrenic collections (Fig. 58.10).
- *Radiolabelled white cell scanning* may occasionally prove helpful when other imaging techniques have failed.

Differential diagnosis

Pyelonephritis, amoebic abscess, pulmonary collapse and pleural empyema may give rise to diagnostic difficulty.

Treatment

The clinical course of suspected cases is monitored, and blood tests and imaging investigations are carried out at suitable intervals. If suppuration seems probable, intervention is indicated. If skilled help is available it is usually possible to insert a percutaneous drainage tube under ultrasound or CT control. The same tube can be used to instil antibiotic solutions or irrigate the abscess cavity. To pass an aspirating needle at the bedside through the pleura and diaphragm invites potentially catastrophic spread of the infection into the pleural cavity.

If an operative approach is necessary and a swelling can be detected in the subcostal region or in the loin, an incision is made over the site of maximum tenderness or over any area where oedema or redness is discovered. The parietes usually form part of the abscess wall so that contamination of the general peritoneal cavity is unlikely.

If no swelling is apparent, the subphrenic spaces should be explored by either an anterior subcostal approach or from behind after removal of the outer part of the 12th rib according to the position of the abscess on imaging. With the posterior approach, the pleura must not be opened and, after the fibres of the diaphragm have been separated, a finger is inserted beneath the diaphragm so as to explore the adjacent area. The aim with all techniques of drainage is to avoid dissemination of pus into the peritoneal or pleural cavities.

When the cavity is reached, all of the fibrinous loculi must be broken down with the finger and one or two drainage tubes must be fully inserted. These drains are withdrawn gradually during the next 10 days and the closure of the cavity is checked by sinograms or scanning. Appropriate antibiotics are also given.

SPECIAL FORMS OF PERITONITIS

Postoperative

The patient is ill with raised pulse and peripheral circulatory failure. Following an anastomotic dehiscence, the general condition of a patient is usually more serious than if the patient had suffered leakage from a perforated peptic ulcer with no preceding operation. Local symptoms and signs are less definite. Abdominal pain may not be prominent and is often difficult to assess because of normal wound pain and postoperative analgesia. The patient's deterioration may be attributed wrongly to cardiopulmonary collapse, which is usually concomitant.

Peritonitis follows abdominal operations more frequently than is realised. The principles of treatment do not differ from those of peritonitis of other origin. Antibiotic therapy alone is inadequate; no antibiotic can stay the onslaught of bacterial peritonitis caused by leakage from a suture line, which must be dealt with by operation.

In patients on treatment with steroids

Pain is frequently slight or absent. Physical signs are similarly vague and misleading.

In children

The diagnosis can be more difficult, particularly in the preschool child (see Chapter 6). Physical signs should be elicited by a gentle, patient and sympathetic approach.

In patients with dementia

Such patients can be fractious and unable to give a reliable history. Abdominal tenderness is usually well localised, but guarding and rigidity are less marked because the abdominal muscles are often thin and weak.

Bile peritonitis

Unless there is reason to suspect that the biliary tract was damaged during operation, it is improbable that bile as a cause of peritonitis will be thought of until the abdomen has been opened. The common causes of bile peritonitis are shown in Summary box 58.11.

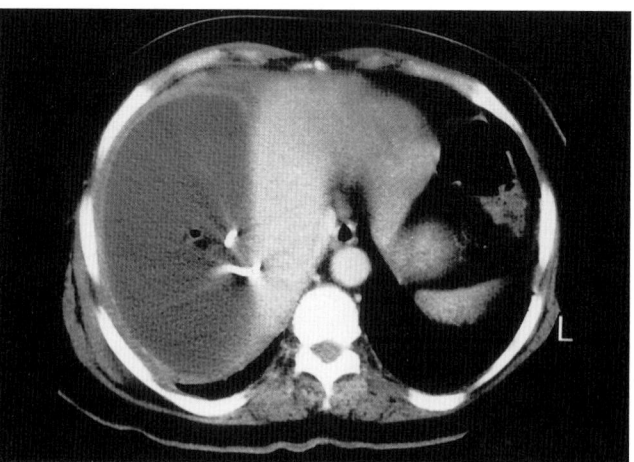

Figure 58.10 A subphrenic abscess drained under computerised tomography guidance (courtesy of Dr J. Healy, Chelsea and Westminster Hospital, London, UK).

> **Summary box 58.11**
>
> **Causes of bile peritonitis**
>
> - Perforated cholecystitis
> - Post cholecystectomy:
>   - Cystic duct stump leakage
>   - Leakage from an accessory duct in the gall bladder bed
>   - Bile duct injury
>   - T-tube drain dislodgement (or tract rupture on removal)
> - Following other operations/procedures:
>   - Leaking duodenal stump post gastrectomy
>   - Leaking biliary–enteric anastomosis
>   - Leakage around percutaneous placed biliary drains
> - Following liver trauma

Unless the bile has extravasated slowly and the collection becomes shut off from the general peritoneal cavity, there are signs of diffuse peritonitis. After a few hours a tinge of jaundice is not unusual. Laparotomy (or laparoscopy) should be undertaken with evacuation of the bile and peritoneal lavage. The source of bile leakage should be identified. A leaking gall bladder is excised or a cystic duct ligated. An injury to the bile duct may simply be drained or alternatively intubated; later, reconstructive operation is often required. Infected bile is more lethal than sterile bile. A 'blown' duodenal stump should be drained as it is too oedematous to repair, but sometimes it can be covered by a jejunal patch. The patient is often jaundiced from absorption of peritoneal bile, but the surgeon must ensure that the abdomen is not closed until any obstruction to a major bile duct has been either excluded or relieved. Bile leaks after cholecystectomy or liver trauma may be dealt with by percutaneous (ultrasound-guided) drainage and endoscopic biliary stenting to reduce bile duct pressure. The drain is removed when dry and the stent at 4–6 weeks.

Meconium peritonitis (see Chapter 6)

Pneumococcal peritonitis

Primary pneumococcal peritonitis may complicate nephrotic syndrome or cirrhosis in children. Otherwise healthy children, particularly girls between 3 and 9 years of age, may also be affected, and it is likely that the route of infection is sometimes via the vagina and fallopian tubes. At other times, and always in males, the infection is blood-borne and secondary to respiratory tract or middle ear disease. The prevalence of pneumococcal peritonitis has declined greatly and the condition is now rare.

Clinical features

The onset is sudden and the earliest symptom is pain localised to the lower half of the abdomen. The temperature is raised to 39°C or more and there is usually frequent vomiting. After 24–48 hours, profuse diarrhoea is characteristic. There is usually increased frequency of micturition. The last two symptoms are caused by severe pelvic peritonitis. On examination, abdominal rigidity is usually bilateral but is less than in most cases of acute appendicitis with peritonitis.

Differential diagnosis

A leucocytosis of $30\,000\,\mu l^{-1}$ ($30 \times 10^9\,l^{-1}$) or more with approximately 90% polymorphs suggests pneumococcal peritonitis rather than appendicitis. Even so, it is often impossible to exclude perforated appendicitis. The other condition that can be difficult to differentiate from primary pneumococcal peritonitis in its early stage is basal pneumonia. An unduly high respiratory rate and the absence of abdominal rigidity are the most important signs supporting the diagnosis of pneumonia, which is usually confirmed by a chest radiograph.

Treatment

After starting antibiotic therapy and correcting dehydration and electrolyte imbalance, early surgery is required unless spontaneous infection of pre-existing ascites is strongly suspected, in which case a diagnostic peritoneal tap is useful. Laparotomy or laparoscopy may be used. Should the exudate be odourless and sticky, the diagnosis of pneumococcal peritonitis is practically certain, but it is essential to perform a careful exploration to exclude other pathology. Assuming that no other cause for the peritonitis is discovered, some of the exudate is aspirated and sent to the laboratory for microscopy, culture and sensitivity tests. Thorough peritoneal lavage is carried out and the incision closed. Antibiotic and fluid replacement therapy are continued. Nasogastric suction drainage is essential. Recovery is usual.

Other organisms are now known to cause some cases of primary pneumococcal peritonitis in children, including *Haemophilus*, other streptococci and a few Gram-negative bacteria. Underlying pathology (including an intravaginal foreign body in girls) must always be excluded before primary peritonitis can be diagnosed with certainty.

Idiopathic streptococcal and staphylococcal peritonitis in adults

Idiopathic streptococcal and staphylococcal peritonitis in adults is fortunately rare. In streptococcal peritonitis, the peritoneal exudate is odourless and thin, contains some flecks of fibrin and may be blood-stained. In these circumstances pus is removed by suction, the abdomen closed with drainage and non-operative treatment of peritonitis performed. The use of intravaginal tampons has led to an increased incidence of *Staphylococcus aureus* infections: these can be associated with 'toxic shock syndrome' and disseminated intravascular coagulopathy.

Familial Mediterranean fever (periodic peritonitis)

Familial Mediterranean fever (periodic peritonitis) is characterised by abdominal pain and tenderness, mild pyrexia, polymorphonuclear leucocytosis and, occasionally, pain in the thorax and joints. The duration of an attack is 24–72 hours, when it is followed by complete remission, but exacerbations recur at regular intervals. Most of the patients have undergone appendicectomy in childhood. This disease, often familial, is limited principally to Arab, Armenian and Jewish populations; other races are occasionally affected. Mutations in the *MEFV* (Mediterranean fever) gene appear to cause the disease. This gene produces a protein called pyrin, which is expressed mostly in neutrophils but whose exact function is not known.

Usually, children are affected but it is not rare for the disease to make its first appearance in early adult life, with cases in women outnumbering those in men by two to one. Exceptionally, the disease becomes manifest in patients over 40 years of age. At operation, which may be necessary to exclude other causes but should be avoided if possible, the peritoneum – particularly in the vicinity of the spleen and the gall bladder – is inflamed. There is no evidence that the interior of these organs is abnormal. Colchicine therapy is used during attacks and to prevent recurrent attacks.

Starch peritonitis

Like talc, starch powder has found disfavour as a surgical glove lubricant. In a few starch-sensitive patients, it causes a painful ascites, fortunately of limited duration. Should laparotomy be performed, any small granulomas in, say, the omentum will be found to contain birefringent starch particles. Starch-free surgical gloves are now widely available.

TUBERCULOUS PERITONITIS

Acute tuberculous peritonitis

Tuberculous peritonitis sometimes has an onset that so closely resembles acute peritonitis that the abdomen is opened. Straw-coloured fluid escapes and tubercles are seen scattered over the peritoneum and greater omentum. Early tubercles are greyish and translucent. They soon undergo caseation and appear white or yellow and are then less difficult to distinguish from carcinoma. Occasionally, they appear like patchy fat necrosis. On opening the abdomen and finding tuberculous peritonitis, the fluid is evacuated, some being retained for bacteriological studies. A portion of the diseased omentum is removed for histological confirmation of the diagnosis and the wound closed without drainage.

Chronic tuberculous peritonitis

The condition presents with abdominal pain (90% of cases), fever (60%), loss of weight (60%), ascites (60%), night sweats (37%) and abdominal mass (26%) (Summary box 58.12).

Summary box 58.12

Tuberculous peritonitis

- Acute and chronic forms
- Abdominal pain, sweats, malaise and weight loss are frequent
- Caseating peritoneal nodules are common – distinguish from metastatic carcinoma and fat necrosis of pancreatitis
- Ascites common, may be loculated
- Intestinal obstruction may respond to anti-tuberculous treatment without surgery

---

Origin of the infection

Infection originates from:

- tuberculous mesenteric lymph nodes;
- tuberculosis of the ileocaecal region;
- a tuberculous pyosalpinx;
- blood-borne infection from pulmonary tuberculosis, usually the 'miliary' but occasionally the 'cavitating' form.

Varieties of tuberculous peritonitis

There are four varieties of tuberculous peritonitis: ascitic, encysted, fibrous and purulent.

Ascitic form

The peritoneum is studded with tubercles and the peritoneal cavity becomes filled with pale, straw-coloured fluid. The onset is insidious. There is loss of energy, facial pallor and some loss of weight. The patient is usually brought for advice because of distension of the abdomen. Pain is often absent; in other cases there is considerable abdominal discomfort, which may be associated with constipation or diarrhoea. On inspection, dilated veins may be seen coursing beneath the skin of the abdominal wall. Signs of ascites can be elicited readily (see below). In boys, congenital hydroceles sometimes appear, resulting from the patent processi vaginales becoming filled with ascitic fluid. Because of the increased intra-abdominal pressure, an umbilical hernia commonly occurs. On abdominal palpation, a transverse solid mass can often be detected. This is rolled-up greater omentum infiltrated with tubercles.

Diagnosis is seldom difficult except when it occurs in an acute form or when it first appears in an adult, in which case it has to be differentiated from other forms of ascites, especially malignancy. Laparoscopy is useful by allowing inspection of the peritoneal cavity, where the appearance is often diagnostic. The 'open' (Hasson) technique of trocar insertion should be used because of the risk of adhesions to the abdominal wall. Areas of caseation can be biopsied for histology and microbiological studies. The ascitic fluid is pale yellow, usually clear and rich in lymphocytes. The specific gravity is comparatively high, often 1.020 or more. Even after centrifugation, *Mycobacterium tuberculosis* can rarely be found, but its presence can be demonstrated by culture.

Once the diagnosis of tuberculous peritonitis has been made, it is always important to look for tuberculous disease elsewhere. The possibility of tuberculous salpingitis in females should be remembered. A chest radiograph should always be taken before laparoscopy or laparotomy is performed. If the general condition is good, the patient can return home and, if an adult, carry out light work before the course of anti-tuberculous therapy has been completed.

Encysted form

The encysted (loculated) form is similar to the ascitic form except that one part of the abdominal cavity alone is involved. Thus, a localised intra-abdominal swelling is produced, which may give rise to difficulty in diagnosis. In a woman above the age of puberty, when the swelling is in the pelvis, an ovarian cyst will probably be diagnosed. In the case of a child it is sometimes difficult to distinguish the swelling from a mesenteric cyst. For these reasons, operation is often performed and, if an encapsulated collection of fluid is found, it is evacuated and sent for microscopy and culture. Late intestinal obstruction is a possible complication.

Fibrous form

The fibrous (synonym: plastic) form is characterised by the production of widespread adhesions, which cause coils of intestine, especially the ileum, to become matted together and distended. These distended coils act as a 'blind loop' and give rise to steatorrhoea, wasting and attacks of abdominal pain. On examination, the adherent intestine with omentum attached, together with the thickened mesentery, may give rise to a palpable swelling or swellings. The first intimation of the disease may be subacute or acute intestinal obstruction. Sometimes the cause of the obstruction can be remedied easily by the division of bands. Small bowel bypass should be avoided to prevent development of a 'blind loop' syndrome. If the adhesions are accompanied by fibrous strictures of the ileum as well, it is best to excise the affected bowel, provided that not too much of the small intestine needs to be sacrificed. Anti-tuberculous therapy will often rapidly cure the condition without the need for surgery.

Purulent form

The purulent form is rare. When it occurs, usually it is secondary to tuberculous salpingitis. Amidst a mass of adherent intestine and omentum, tuberculous pus is present. Sizeable cold abscesses often form and point on the surface, commonly near

---

Harith Hasson, **Professor of Gynaecology, Chicago, USA.**

the umbilicus, or burst into the bowel. In addition to prolonged general treatment, operative treatment may be necessary for the evacuation of cold abscesses and possibly for intestinal obstruction. If a faecal fistula forms, it usually persists because of distal intestinal obstruction. Closure of the fistula must therefore be combined with some form of anastomosis between the segment of intestine above the fistula and an unobstructed area below. The prognosis of this variety of tuberculous peritonitis is relatively poor.

ASCITES

Ascites, an excess of serous fluid within the peritoneal cavity, can be recognised clinically only when the amount of fluid present exceeds 150 ml; in the obese a greater quantity than this is necessary before there is clear evidence. Ultrasound and CT scanning can detect much smaller volumes of ascitic fluid (Fig. 58.11).

Mechanism of ascites

The balanced effects of plasma and peritoneal colloid osmotic and hydrostatic pressures determine the exchange of fluid between the capillaries and the peritoneal fluid. Protein-rich fluid enters the peritoneal cavity when capillary permeability is increased, as in peritonitis and carcinomatosis peritonei. Capillary pressure may be increased because of generalised water retention, cardiac failure, constrictive pericarditis or vena cava obstruction. Capillary pressure is raised selectively in the portal venous system in the Budd–Chiari syndrome, cirrhosis of the liver or extrahepatic portal venous obstruction. Plasma colloid osmotic pressure may be lowered in patients with reduced nutritional intake, diminished intestinal absorption, abnormal protein losses or defective protein synthesis such as occurs in cirrhosis. Peritoneal lymphatic drainage may be impaired, resulting in the accumulation of protein-rich fluid.

Clinical features

The abdomen is distended evenly with fullness of the flanks, which are dull to percussion. Usually, shifting dullness is present but when there is a very large accumulation of fluid this sign is absent. In such cases, on flicking the abdominal wall, a characteristic fluid thrill is transmitted from one side to the other. In women, ascites must be differentiated from an enormous ovarian cyst.

Congestive heart failure, the commonest cause of ascites, results in increased venous pressure in the vena cava and consequent obstruction to the venous outflow from the liver. This increased pressure can be seen as engorgement of the veins of the neck – a striking sign in this condition. The ascitic fluid is light yellow and of low specific gravity, about 1.010, with a low protein concentration ($< 25\,g\,l^{-1}$). Patients with constrictive pericarditis (Pick's disease) have both peritoneal and pleural effusions because of engorgement of the venae cavae consequent upon the diminished capacity of the right side of the heart.

In cirrhosis, there is obstruction to the portal venous system, which is caused by obliterative fibrosis of the intrahepatic venous bed. Lymph flow may be increased. In the Budd–Chiari syndrome (see Chapter 61), thrombosis or obstruction of the hepatic veins is responsible for obstruction to venous outflow from the liver.

The ascites seen in patients with peritoneal metastases is caused by excessive exudation of fluid and lymphatic blockage. The fluid is dark yellow and frequently blood-stained. The specific gravity, 1.020 or over, and the protein content ($> 25\,g\,l^{-1}$) are high. Microscopic examination often reveals cancer cells, especially if large quantities of fluid are 'spun down' to produce a concentrated deposit for sampling.

Ascites occurs with low plasma albumin concentrations, for example in patients with albuminuria or starvation. The ascites in this instance is caused by alterations in the osmotic pressure of the capillary blood and has a low specific gravity.

Rarely, ascites and pleural effusion are associated with solid fibroma of the ovary (Meigs' syndrome). The effusions disappear when the tumour is excised (Summary box 58.13).

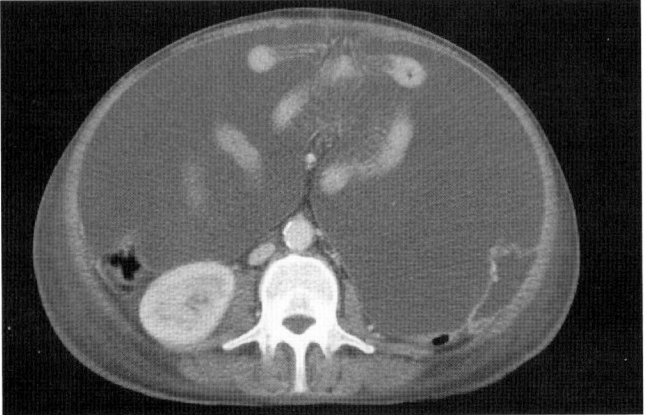

Figure 58.11 Computerised tomography scan showing gross ascites.

> **Summary box 58.13**
>
> ### Causes of ascites
>
> ***Transudates (protein < 25 g l⁻¹)***
> - Low plasma protein concentrations:
>   Malnutrition
>   Nephrotic syndrome
>   Protein-losing enteropathy
> - High central venous pressure:
>   Congestive cardiac failure
> - Portal hypertension:
>   Portal vein thrombosis
>   Cirrhosis
>
> ***Exudates (protein > 25 g l⁻¹)***
> - Tuberculous peritonitis
> - Peritoneal malignancy
> - Budd–Chiari syndrome (hepatic vein occlusion or thrombosis)
> - Pancreatic ascites
> - Chylous ascites
> - Meigs' syndrome

Treatment

Treatment of the specific cause is undertaken whenever possible; for example, if portal venous pressure is raised, it may be possible to lower it by treatment of the primary condition. Dietary sodium restriction to 200 mg day^{-1} may be helpful, but diuretics are usually required.

Paracentesis abdominis

The bladder having been emptied, puncture of the peritoneum is carried out under local anaesthetic using a moderately sized trocar and cannula at one of the points shown in Fig. 58.12. Alternatively, a peritoneal drain may be inserted under ultrasound guidance to minimise the risk of visceral injury. In cases where the effusion is caused by cardiac failure, the fluid must be evacuated slowly. Fluid is sent for microscopy, culture, including mycobacteria, and analysis of protein content and amylase. Unless other measures are taken the fluid soon reaccumulates, and repeated tappings remove valuable protein.

Permanent drainage of ascitic fluid

In rare cases in which ascites accumulates rapidly after paracentesis and the patient is otherwise fit, permanent drainage of the ascitic fluid via a peritoneovenous shunt (e.g. LeVeen, Denver) may render the patient more comfortable. Similar in concept to shunts for hydrocephalus (see Chapter 40), a catheter (e.g. of silicone) is constructed with a valve so as to allow one-way flow from the peritoneum to a central vein (e.g. internal jugular). A chamber placed subcutaneously over the chest wall may be included for manual compression. Insertion is relatively simple. The complications include overloading the venous system, cardiac failure and disseminated intravascular coagulopathy. The frequency of these complications may be reduced by evacuating ascitic fluid and partially replacing it with normal saline at the time of shunt insertion. The procedure may also be used for patients with terminal malignant ascites, giving improved quality of life despite the risk of further dissemination of malignant cells.

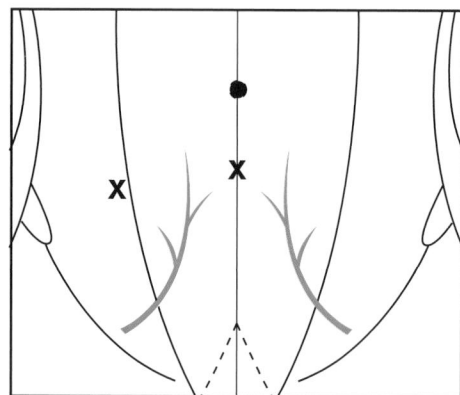

Figure 58.12 Usual points of puncture for tapping ascites. The bladder must be emptied by a catheter before the puncture is made. Note the relationship of the sites of the puncture to the inferior epigastric artery (red) (courtesy of Drs V.C. and V.V. Shah, Jamnagar, India).

Chylous ascites

In some patients the ascitic fluid appears milky because of an excess of chylomicrons (triglycerides). Most cases are associated with malignancy, usually lymphomas; other causes are cirrhosis, tuberculosis, filariasis, nephrotic syndrome, abdominal trauma (including surgery), constrictive pericarditis, sarcoidosis and congenital lymphatic abnormality. The prognosis is poor unless the underlying condition can be cured. In addition to other measures used to treat ascites, patients should be placed on a fat-free diet with medium-chain triglyceride supplements.

PERITONEAL LOOSE BODIES (PERITONEAL MICE)

Peritoneal loose bodies almost never cause symptoms. One or more may be found in a hernial sac or in the pouch of Douglas. The loose body may come from an appendix epiploica that has undergone axial rotation followed by necrosis of its pedicle and detachment but they are also found in those who suffer from subacute attacks of pancreatitis. These hyaline bodies attain the size of a pea or bean and contain saponified fat surrounded by fibrin.

NEOPLASMS OF THE PERITONEUM

Carcinoma peritonei

This is a common terminal event in many cases of carcinoma of the stomach, colon, ovary or other abdominal organs and also of the breast and bronchus. The peritoneum, both parietal and visceral, is studded with secondary growths and the peritoneal cavity becomes filled with clear, straw-coloured or blood-stained ascitic fluid.

The main forms of peritoneal metastases are:

- discrete *nodules* – by far the most common variety;
- *plaques* varying in size and colour;
- diffuse *adhesions* – this form occurs at a late stage of the disease and gives rise, sometimes, to a 'frozen pelvis'.

Gravity probably determines the distribution of free malignant cells within the peritoneal cavity. Cells not caught in peritoneal folds gravitate into the pelvic pouches or into a hernial sac, the enlargement of which is occasionally the first indication of the condition. Implantation occurs also on the greater omentum, the appendices epiploicae and the inferior surface of the diaphragm.

Differential diagnosis

Early discrete tubercles common in tuberculous peritonitis are greyish and translucent and closely resemble the discrete nodules of peritoneal carcinomatosis. Fat necrosis can usually be distinguished from a carcinomatous nodule by its opacity. Peritoneal hydatids can also simulate malignant disease after rupture of a hydatid cyst, with seeding of daughter cysts.

Treatment

Ascites caused by carcinomatosis of the peritoneum may respond to systemic or intraperitoneal chemotherapy or to endocrine therapy in the case of hormone receptor-positive tumours.

Harry LeVeen, **Professor of Surgery, The University of South Carolina, SC, USA.**

James Douglas, 1675–1742, Anatomist and Male Midwife, London, England.

Pseudomyxoma peritonei

This rare condition occurs more frequently in women. The abdomen is filled with a yellow jelly, large quantities of which are often encysted. The condition is associated with mucinous cystic tumours of the ovary and appendix. Recent studies suggest that most cases arise from a primary appendiceal tumour with secondary implantation on to one or both ovaries. It is often painless and there is frequently no impairment of general health. Pseudomyxoma peritonei does not give rise to extraperitoneal metastases. Although an abdomen distended with what seems to be fluid that cannot be made to shift should raise the possibility, the diagnosis is more often suggested by ultrasound and CT scanning or made at operation. At laparotomy, masses of jelly are scooped out. The appendix, if present, should be excised together with any ovarian tumour. Unfortunately, recurrence is inevitable, but patients may gain symptomatic benefit from repeated 'debulking' surgery. Occasionally, the condition responds to radioactive isotopes or intraperitoneal chemotherapy. The role of early radical peritoneal excision is uncertain.

Mesothelioma

As in the pleural cavity, this is a highly malignant tumour. Asbestos is a recognised cause. It has a predilection for the pelvic peritoneum. Chemocytotoxic agents are the mainstay of treatment.

Desmoid

This is considered under familial adenomatous polyposis (see Chapter 65).

LAPAROSCOPY (PERITONEOSCOPY)

Laparoscopic surgery has developed rapidly over recent years. The principles of the technique are discussed in Chapter 19 and numerous examples of its application for common procedures are given throughout the book.

THE OMENTUM

Rutherford Morison called the greater omentum 'the abdominal policeman'. The greater omentum attempts, often successfully, to limit intraperitoneal infective and other noxious processes (Fig. 58.13). For instance, an acutely inflamed appendix is often found wrapped in omentum, and this saves many patients from developing diffuse peritonitis. Some sufferers of herniae are also greatly indebted to this structure, for it often plugs the neck of a hernial sac and prevents a coil of intestine from entering and becoming strangulated.

The omentum is usually involved in tuberculous peritonitis and carcinomatosis of the peritoneum.

Torsion of the omentum

Torsion of the omentum is a rare emergency and consequently is seldom diagnosed correctly. It is usually mistaken for appendicitis with somewhat abnormal signs. It may be primary or secondary to an adhesion of the omentum, to an old focus of infection or to a hernia.

The patient is most frequently a middle-aged, obese man. A tender lump may be present in the abdomen. The blood supply having been jeopardised, the twisted mass sometimes becomes gangrenous, in which case bacterial peritonitis may follow.

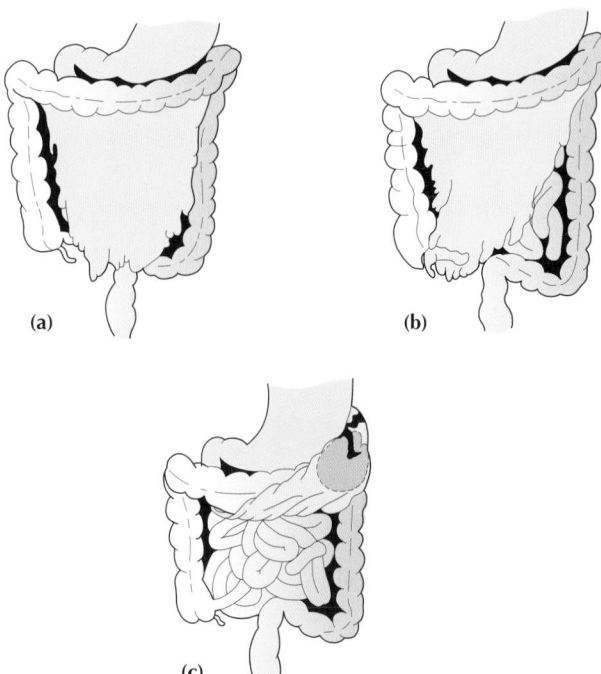

Figure 58.13 The greater omentum. (a) Normal; (b) in appendicitis; (c) in a (comparatively small) laceration of the spleen.

Treatment is surgical; the pedicle above the twist is ligated securely and the mass removed.

THE MESENTERY

Mesenteric injury

A wound of the mesentery can follow severe abdominal contusion and is a cause of haemoperitoneum.

Seatbelt syndrome

If a car accident occurs when a seatbelt is worn, sudden deceleration can result in a torn mesentery. This possibility should be borne in mind, particularly as multiple injuries may distract attention from this injury. If there is any bruising of the abdominal wall, or even marks of clothing impressed into the skin, laparotomy may be indicated.

Diagnostic peritoneal lavage

Diagnostic peritoneal lavage may be helpful in this situation. Under local anaesthesia, a subumbilical incision is made down to the peritoneum in a similar way to that used for 'open' laparoscopy. A purse-string suture is placed in the peritoneum, which is then incised. Free fluid, e.g. blood or intestinal contents, may be found but, if not, a peritoneal dialysis catheter is inserted and the purse-string suture tied. A litre of normal saline is run into the peritoneum and then drained off by placing the bag and tubing below the patient's abdomen. The presence of blood (>100 000 red blood cells per μl), bile or intestinal contents is an indication for laparotomy.

In about 60% of cases, the mesenteric laceration is associated with a rupture of the intestine. If the tear is a large one, and especially if it is transverse (Fig. 58.14a), the blood supply to the neighbouring intestine is cut off and a limited resection of gut is

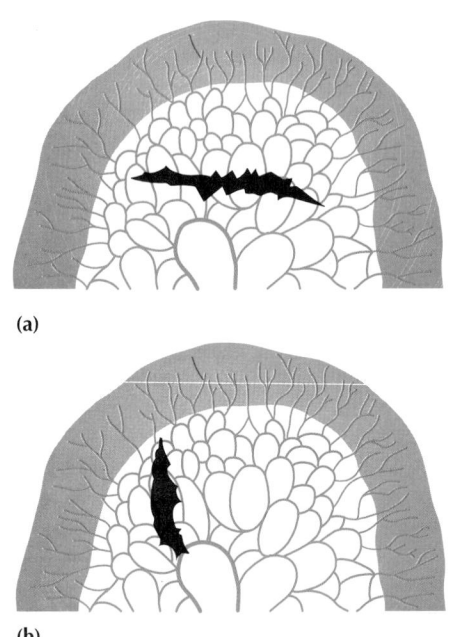

(a)

(b)

Figure 58.14 Laceration of the mesentery, a common injury in driving accidents. (a) A transverse tear often imperils the blood supply of a segment of intestine, making resection necessary; (b) a longitudinal tear can be closed by suture.

imperative. Small wounds and wounds in the long axis (Fig. 58.14b) should be sutured.

Torsion of the mesentery

See midgut volvulus and volvulus of the small intestine (see Chapter 66).

Embolism and thrombosis of mesenteric vessels

See Chapter 66.

Acute non-specific ileocaecal mesenteric adenitis

Aetiology

Non-specific mesenteric adenitis was so named to distinguish it from specific (tuberculous) mesenteric adenitis. It is now much more common than the tuberculous variety. The aetiology often remains unknown, although some cases are associated with *Yersinia* infection of the ileum. In other cases, an unidentified virus is blamed. In about 25% of cases, a respiratory infection precedes an attack of non-specific mesenteric adenitis. This self-limiting disease is never fatal but may be recurrent.

Pathology

There is a small increase in the amount of peritoneal fluid. The ileocaecal mesenteric lymph nodes are enlarged and can be seen and felt between the leaves of the mesentery. In very acute cases they are distinctly red, and many of them are the size of a walnut. The nodes nearest the attachment of the mesentery are the largest. They are not adherent to their peritoneal coats and, if a

small incision is made through the overlying peritoneum, a node is extruded easily.

Clinical features

During childhood, acute non-specific mesenteric adenitis is a common condition. The typical history is one of short attacks of central abdominal pain lasting from 10 to 30 min, and associated with circumoral pallor. Vomiting is common but there is no alteration of bowel habit. If vomiting is absent, it is more likely to be a case of mesenteric adenitis than appendicitis.

Examination
There are spasms of general abdominal colic, usually referred to the umbilicus, with intervals of complete freedom. The patient seldom looks ill. In more than half of the cases the temperature is elevated. Abdominal tenderness is poorly localised. When present, shifting tenderness is a valuable sign for differentiating the condition from appendicitis. The neck, axillae and groins should be palpated for enlarged lymph nodes.

Leucocyte count
There is often a leucocytosis of $10\,000-12\,000\,\mu l^{-1}$ ($10-12\times10^9\,l^{-1}$) or more on the first day of the attack, but this falls on the second day.

Treatment

When the diagnosis can be made with assurance, bed rest and simple analgesia is the only treatment necessary. If at a second examination a few hours later, acute appendicitis cannot be excluded, it is safer to perform either appendicectomy or diagnostic laparoscopy.

Tuberculosis of the mesenteric lymph nodes

Tuberculous mesenteric lymphadenitis is considerably less common than acute non-specific lymphadenitis. Tubercle bacilli, usually, but not necessarily, bovine, are ingested and enter the mesenteric lymph nodes by way of Peyer's patches. Sometimes only one lymph node is infected; usually there are several; occasionally massive involvement occurs.

Presentation

Demonstrated radiologically
The shadows cast by one or more calcified tuberculous lymph nodes are seen in a plain radiograph of the abdomen. They must be distinguished from other calcified lesions, e.g. renal or ureteric stones.

As a cause of general symptoms
The patient, usually a child under 10 years of age, loses their appetite, looks pale and there is some loss of weight; sometimes evening pyrexia occurs.

As a cause of abdominal pain
Sometimes abdominal pain is the cause of the patient being brought for advice; usually this pain is central, not severe but rather a discomfort, and is often constant. On examination the abdomen is somewhat protuberant and there is tenderness on

deep pressure to the right of the umbilicus. In these circumstances, the condition resembles acute non-specific mesenteric lymphadenitis. A normal leucocyte count favours tuberculosis and, in a child, a positive Mantoux test is confirmatory evidence of tuberculosis.

Symptoms indistinguishable from those of appendicitis

On occasions, the abdominal pain is acute and may be accompanied by vomiting. This, combined with tenderness and some rigidity in the right iliac fossa, makes the diagnosis from appendicitis almost impossible. When, as is sometimes the case, the tuberculous infection of the mesenteric lymph nodes becomes reactivated in adolescence or adulthood, the diagnostic difficulties are even greater. A radiograph may show calcified lymph nodes but, as such a condition can coexist with appendicitis, in some cases laparoscopy or laparotomy is necessary. If the mesentery is found to be in an inflamed state with caseation of some of the lymph nodes, the diagnosis of active tuberculosis is confirmed.

As a cause of intestinal obstruction

Remote, rather than recent, tuberculous mesenteric adenitis can be the cause of intestinal obstruction. For instance, a coil of small intestine becomes adherent to a caseating node and is thereby angulated or a free coil may become imprisoned in the tunnel beneath the site of adherence and the mesentery.

As a cause of pseudomesenteric cyst

When tuberculous mesenteric lymph nodes break down, the tuberculous pus may remain confined between the leaves of the mesentery and a cystic swelling having the characteristics of a mesenteric cyst is found. When such a condition is confirmed at operation, the tuberculous pus should be aspirated without soiling the peritoneal cavity, the wound closed, the sensitivity of the organism should be sought and medical treatment continued until the infection has been overcome.

As ileocaecal lymph nodes

At laparotomy, hard, enlarged lymph nodes may be found limited to the ileocaecal mesentery as a result of previous tuberculous infection.

Treatment

Therapy is similar to that of other tuberculous infections. Most cases subside but from time to time a local abscess forms, usually in the right iliac fossa, in which case the tuberculous pus should be evacuated and the abdomen closed without drainage.

Mesenteric cysts

Mesenteric cysts are classified as:

- chylolymphatic;
- simple (mesothelial);
- enterogenous;
- urogenital remnant;
- dermoid (teratomatous cyst).

Chylolymphatic cyst, the commonest variety, probably arises in congenitally misplaced lymphatic tissue that has no efferent

> Charles Mantoux, 1877–1947, Physician, Le Cannet, Alpes Maritimes, France, described the intra-dermal tuberculin test in 1908.

communication with the lymphatic system; it arises most frequently in the mesentery of the ileum. The thin wall of the cyst, which is composed of connective tissue lined by flat endothelium, is filled with clear lymph or, less frequently, with chyle varying in consistency from watered milk to cream. Occasionally, the cyst attains a great size. More often unilocular than multilocular, a chylolymphatic cyst is almost invariably solitary, although there is an extremely rare variety in which myriads of cysts are found in the various mesenteries of the abdomen. A chylolymphatic cyst has a blood supply that is independent from that of the adjacent intestine and, thus, enucleation is possible without the need for resection of gut.

Enterogenous cysts are believed to be derived either from a diverticulum of the mesenteric border of the intestine that has become sequestrated from the intestinal canal during embryonic life or from a duplication of the intestine (see Chapter 6). An enterogenous cyst has a thicker wall than a chylolymphatic cyst and it is lined by mucous membrane, sometimes ciliated. The content is mucinous and is either colourless or yellowish brown as a result of past haemorrhage. The muscle in the wall of an enteric duplication cyst and the bowel with which it is in contact have a common blood supply; consequently, removal of the cyst always entails resection of the related portion of intestine.

Clinical features of a mesenteric cyst

A mesenteric cyst is encountered most frequently in the second decade of life, less often between the ages of 1 and 10 years and, exceptionally, in infants under 1 year.

The patient presents on account of:

- A *painless abdominal swelling*. A cyst of the mesentery presents characteristic physical signs:
  - there is a fluctuant swelling near the umbilicus (Fig. 58.15a);
  - the swelling moves freely in a plane at right angles to the attachment of the mesentery (Fig. 58.15b);
  - there is a zone of resonance around the cyst.
- *Recurrent attacks of abdominal pain* with or without vomiting. The pain results from recurring temporary impaction of a food bolus in a segment of bowel narrowed by the cyst or possibly from torsion of the mesentery.
- An *acute abdominal catastrophe*, which arises as a result of:
  - torsion of that portion of the mesentery containing the cyst;
  - rupture of the cyst, often as a result of a comparatively trivial accident;
  - haemorrhage into the cyst;
  - infection.

Radiography

Ultrasound and CT scanning will demonstrate the lesion and may allow diagnosis of cyst type. A barium meal and follow-through may show displacement of the hollow viscera around the cyst and, not infrequently, some portion of the lumen of the small intestine will be narrowed.

Treatment

Many chylolymphatic cysts can be enucleated *in toto*.

When, after aspiration of about half the contents of the cyst, the major portion of the cyst has been dissected free, but one portion abutting on the intestine or a major blood vessel seems too dangerous to remove, this portion can be left attached and its lining destroyed by careful diathermy.

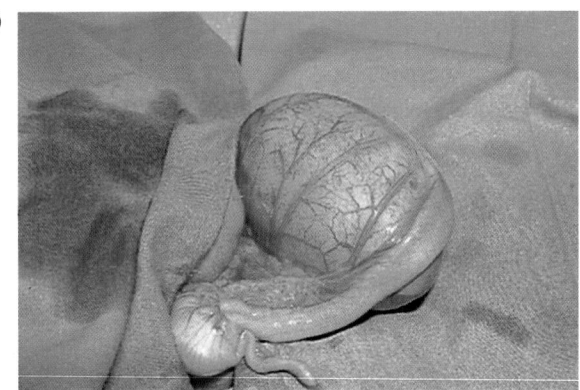

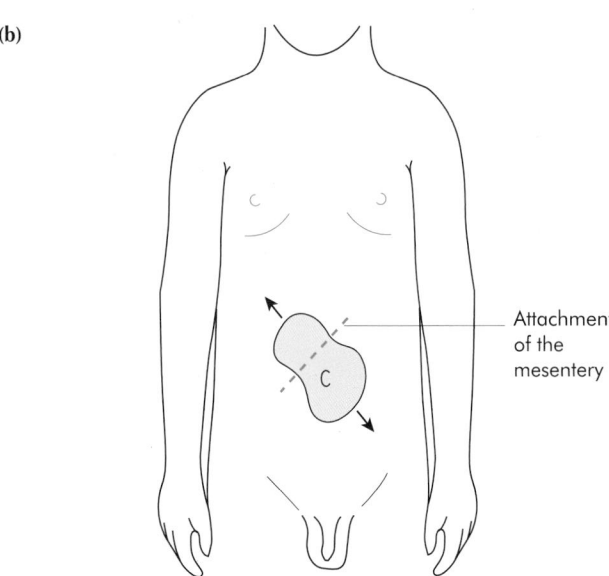

Figure 58.15 A mesenteric cyst (a) moves freely in the direction of the arrows, i.e. at right angles to the attachment of the mesentery (b).

In the case of an enterogenous cyst, enucleation must not be attempted. If a comparatively short segment of the intestine is involved, resection of the cyst with the adherent portion of the intestine, followed by intestinal anastomosis, is the correct course.

The older treatment of marsupialisation of a mesenteric cyst has little to recommend it; a fistula or recurrence results.

Omental cysts

Omental cysts occur nearly as frequently as mesenteric cysts. Preoperative differentiation is possible because a lateral radiograph, ultrasound or CT scan shows the cyst in front of the intestines. Treatment is omentectomy.

Cyst of the mesocolon

Cyst of the mesocolon is uncommon and is differentiated from a mesenteric cyst only at operation. The treatment is similar.

Cysts arising from a urogenital remnant

Cysts arising from a urogenital (wolffian or müllerian) remnant are essentially retroperitoneal but they are included in the

Kaspar Friedrich Wolff, 1733–1794, Professor of Anatomy and Physiology, St. Petersburg, Russia, described the mesonephric duct and body in 1759.
Johannes Peter Müller, 1801–1858, Professor of Anatomy and Physiology, Berlin, Germany, described the para-mesonephric duct in 1825.

classification because it is possible for such a cyst to project forward into the mesentery.

Other cysts

The following, although not being mesenteric cysts in the true meaning of the term, give rise to the same physical signs:

- *serosanguinous cyst*, probably traumatic in origin although a history of an accident is seldom obtained;
- *tuberculous abscess of the mesentery*;
- *hydatid cyst of the mesentery*.

Neoplasms of the mesentery

Mesenteric tumours are classified as:

- benign:
  - lipoma;
  - fibroma;
  - fibromyxoma;
- malignant:
  - lymphoma;
  - secondary carcinoma.

Tumours situated in the mesentery give rise to physical signs that are similar to those of a mesenteric cyst, the sole exception being that they sometimes feel solid.

If indicated, a benign tumour of the mesentery is excised in the same way as an enterogenous mesenteric cyst, i.e. with resection of the adjacent intestine. A malignant tumour of the mesentery usually requires biopsy confirmation and non-surgical treatment, e.g. chemotherapy for lymphoma (Summary box 58.14).

Summary box 58.14
Conditions of the mesentery
■ **Traumatic tears**
■ **Torsion**
■ **Embolism/thrombosis**
■ **Acute non-specific adenitis**
■ **Tuberculous adenitis**
■ **Cysts**
■ **Neoplasms – benign and malignant**

THE RETROPERITONEAL SPACE

Pus or blood in the retroperitoneal space tends to track to the corresponding iliac fossa. If a retroperitoneal abscess develops, it should be evacuated by the nearest route through the abdominal wall, avoiding opening the peritoneum. Should the retroperitoneal collection be found at laparotomy, it must be drained by a counterincision in the flank. Pus may develop from a renal or spinal source and is sometimes tuberculous ('cold abscess'); tracking can develop alongside the psoas muscle and appear in the groin, where it must be distinguished from other swellings (e.g. hernia; see Chapter 57). Retroperitoneal haematoma may be caused by a fractured spine or pelvis, a leaking abdominal aneurysm, acute pancreatitis or a ruptured kidney.

Retroperitoneal cyst

A cyst developing in the retroperitoneal space often attains very large dimensions and has first to be distinguished from a hydronephrosis. Even after the latter condition has been eliminated by scanning or urography, a retroperitoneal cyst can seldom be distinguished with certainty from a retroperitoneal tumour until displayed at operation. The cyst may be unilocular or multilocular. Many of these cysts are believed to be derived from a remnant of the wolffian duct, in which case they are filled with clear fluid. Others are either teratomatous and filled with sebaceous material or multicystic lymphangiomas.

Excision of these and other retroperitoneal swellings is best performed through a transperitoneal incision.

Idiopathic retroperitoneal fibrosis

This is one of a group of fibromatoses (others being Dupuytren's contracture and Peyronie's disease). Most cases are idiopathic but in other patients the cause is known (Summary box 58.15).

Summary box 58.15

Causes of retroperitoneal fibrosis

Benign
- Idiopathic (Ormond's disease)
- Chronic inflammation
- Extravasation of urine
- Retroperitoneal irritation by leakage of blood or intestinal content
- Aortic aneurysm ('inflammatory type')
- Trauma
- Drugs:
    Chemotherapeutic agents
    Methysergide
    β-Adrenoceptor antagonists

Malignant
- Lymphoma
- Carcinoid tumours
- Secondary deposits (especially from carcinoma of stomach, colon, breast and prostate)

Familial cases are known, involving mediastinal fibrosis, sclerosing cholangitis, Riedel's thyroiditis and orbital pseudotumour. Extensive collagen deposition surrounds the ureters, mostly at the level of the pelvic brim or below. Most patients present with ureteric obstruction, often with renal failure (see Chapter 71). Ureteric stenting and steroid therapy are often effective. Cases resulting from malignancy are treated appropriately according to the cause.

Primary retroperitoneal neoplasms arising from connective tissues

Retroperitoneal lipoma

The patient may seek advice on account of a swelling or because of indefinite abdominal pain. Women are more often

Baron Guillaume Dupuytren, 1777–1835, Surgeon in Chief, Hôtel Dieu, Paris, France, described this condition in 1831.
François de la Peyronie, 1678–1747, Surgeon to King Louis XIV of France, and Founder of the Royal Academy of Surgery, Paris, France.
J.K. Ormond, An American Urologist.
Bernard Moritz Carl Ludwig Riedel, 1864–1916, Professor of Surgery, Jena, Germany, described this form of Thyroiditis in 1896.

affected. These swellings sometimes reach an immense size. Diagnosis is usually by ultrasound and CT scanning. A retroperitoneal lipoma sometimes undergoes myxomatous degeneration, a complication that does not occur in a lipoma in any other part of the body. Moreover, a retroperitoneal lipoma is often malignant (liposarcoma) (Fig. 58.16) and may increase rapidly in size.

Retroperitoneal sarcoma

Retroperitoneal sarcoma presents signs that are similar to those of a retroperitoneal lipoma. Occasionally, the tumour, by pressure on the colon, causes symptoms of subacute intestinal obstruction. On examination, a smooth fixed mass, which is not tender, is palpated. The most likely original diagnosis is that of a neoplasm of the kidney. This is ruled out by scanning. The ureter, however, is liable to become displaced by the tumour. Exploratory laparotomy should be performed and, when possible, the tumour is removed. Often, it is found to be widely disseminated in the retroperitoneal space, rendering complete removal impossible, in which case a portion is excised for histology. Even when excised at a comparatively early stage, recurrence always takes place, and these tumours must be looked upon as being necessarily fatal. Radiotherapy sometimes keeps recurrence in abeyance for a time.

Removal of a retroperitoneal cyst or neoplasm

After the anterior abdominal wall has been opened and the diagnosis of a retroperitoneal tumour has been confirmed, the incision is extended as necessary. The small intestine is packed away in the upper abdomen or exteriorised and the caecum and the sigmoid colon are relegated to their respective fossae. The posterior peritoneum is then incised throughout its length over the area to be exposed, the incision being parallel to the left border of the aorta. The peritoneum is dissected from the tumour, which is removed as completely as possible.

Retroperitoneal tumours arising from specific organs

These may arise from:

- lymph nodes (Fig. 58.17) (see Chapter 55);
- adrenal gland (see Chapter 49);
- kidney and ureter (see Chapter 71);
- nervous tissue.

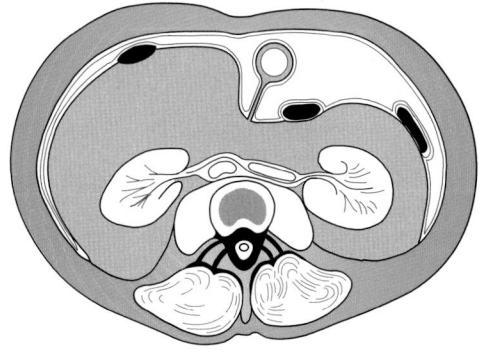

Figure 58.16 Rapidly growing retroperitoneal liposarcoma.

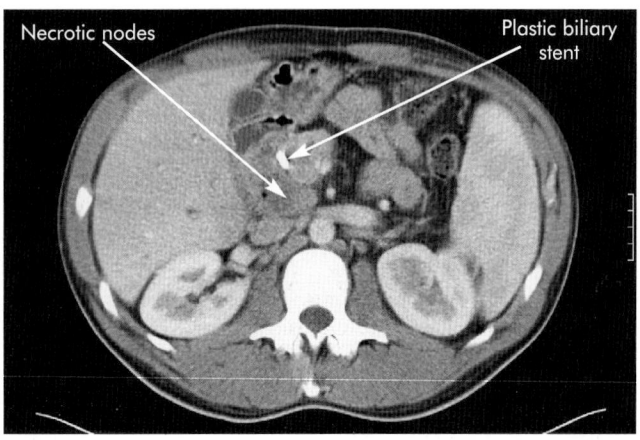

Figure 58.17 Computerised tomography scan showing enlarged necrotic retroperitoneal nodes in a patient with lymphoma. The nodes caused obstructive jaundice by compressing the bile duct; a plastic biliary stent has been inserted at endoscopic retrograde cholangiopancreatography to relieve jaundice.

FURTHER READING

Ellis, B.W. and Paterson-Brown, S. (eds) (2000) *Hamilton Bailey's Emergency Surgery*. Hodder Arnold, Oxford.

Jenkins, M.P, Alvaranga, J.C. and Thomas, J.M. (1996) The management of retroperitoneal soft tissue sarcomas. *Eur J Cancer* **32A**: 622–6.

Paterson-Brown, S. (ed.) (2006) *Core Topics in General and Emergency Surgery*, 3rd edn. Saunders, London.

Trentner, K.-H. and Schumpelick, V. (eds) (1997) *Peritoneal Adhesions*. Springer, Berlin.

The oesophagus

LEARNING OBJECTIVES

To understand:
- The anatomy and physiology of the oesophagus and their relationship to disease
- The clinical features, investigations and treatment of benign and malignant disease with particular reference to the common adult disorders

BACKGROUND

Surgical anatomy

The oesophagus is a muscular tube, approximately 25 cm long, mainly occupying the posterior mediastinum and extending from the upper oesophageal sphincter (the cricopharyngeus muscle) in the neck to the junction with the cardia of the stomach. The musculature of the upper oesophagus, including the upper sphincter, is striated. This is followed by a transitional zone of both striated and smooth muscle with the proportion of the latter progressively increasing so that, in the lower half of the oesophagus, there is only smooth muscle. It is lined throughout with squamous epithelium. The parasympathetic nerve supply is mediated by branches of the vagus nerve that has synaptic connections to the myenteric (Auerbach's) plexus. Meissner's submucosal plexus is sparse in the oesophagus.

The upper sphincter consists of powerful striated muscle. The lower sphincter is more subtle, and is created by the asymmetrical arrangement of muscle fibres in the distal oesophageal wall just above the oesophagogastric junction. It is helpful to remember the distances 15, 25 and 40 cm for anatomical location during endoscopy (Fig. 59.1).

Physiology

The main function of the oesophagus is to transfer food from the mouth to the stomach in a coordinated fashion. The initial movement from the mouth is voluntary. The pharyngeal phase of swallowing involves sequential contraction of the oropharyngeal musculature, closure of the nasal and respiratory passages, cessation of breathing and opening of the upper oesophageal sphincter. Beyond this level, swallowing is involuntary. The body of the oesophagus propels the bolus through a relaxed lower oesophageal sphincter (LOS) into the stomach, taking air with it (Fig. 59.2). This coordinated oesophageal wave that follows a conscious swallow is called primary peristalsis. It is under vagal control, although there are specific neurotransmitters that control the LOS.

The upper oesophageal sphincter is normally closed at rest and serves as a protective mechanism against regurgitation of oesophageal contents into the respiratory passages. It also serves to stop air entering the oesophagus other than the small amount that enters during swallowing.

The LOS is a zone of relatively high pressure that prevents gastric contents from refluxing into the lower oesophagus (Fig. 59.3). In addition to opening in response to a primary peristaltic wave, the sphincter also relaxes to allow air to escape from the stomach and at the time of vomiting. A variety of factors influence sphincter tone, notably food, gastric distension, gastrointestinal hormones, drugs and smoking. The arrangement of muscle fibres, their differential responses to specific neurotransmitters and the

Leopold Auerbach, 1828–1897, Professor of Neuropathology, Breslau, Germany, (now Wroclaw, Poland), described the myenteric plexus in 1862.
Georg Meissner, 1829–1905, Professor of Physiology, Göttingen, Germany, described the submucosal plexus in 1852.

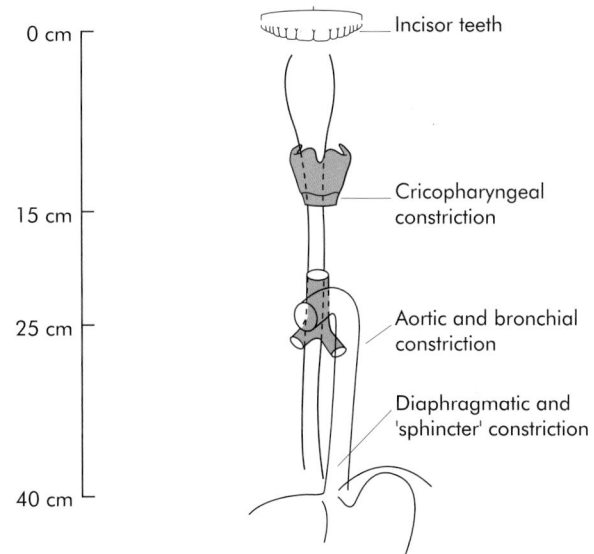

Figure 59.1 Endoscopic landmarks. Distances are given from the incisor teeth. They vary slightly with the build of the individual.

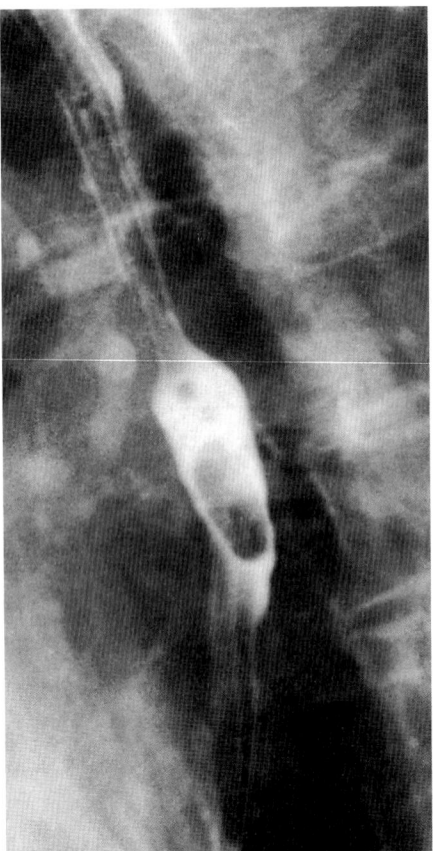

Figure 59.2 A bolus of barium or food usually takes air with it into the stomach.

relationship to diaphragmatic contraction all contribute to the action of the LOS. The presence of the physiological sphincter was first demonstrated by Code using manometry with small balloons. Nowadays, LOS pressure is measured by perfused tubes or micro-transducers. The normal LOS is 3–4 cm long and has a pressure of 10–25 mmHg. Accurate measurement of sphincter relaxation is achieved using a device (Dent sleeve) that straddles the high-pressure zone.

Manometry is also used to assess the speed and amplitude of oesophageal body contractions and ensure that peristalsis is propagated down the entire length of the oesophagus (Fig. 59.4). Secondary peristalsis is the normal reflex response to a stubborn food bolus or refluxed material designed to clear the oesophagus by a contraction that is not preceded by a conscious swallow. It is worth remembering that the majority of clearance swallows to neutralise refluxed gastric acid are, however, achieved by primary peristalsis, which carries saliva with its high bicarbonate content down to the lower oesophagus. Tertiary contractions are non-peristaltic waves that are infrequent (< 10%) during laboratory-based manometry, although readily detected if manometry is undertaken while the patient eats a meal (Fig. 59.5).

Symptoms (Summary box 59.1)

Summary box 59.1

Symptoms of oesophageal disease

- Difficulty in swallowing described as food or fluid sticking (oesophageal dysphagia)
    Must rule out malignancy
- Pain on swallowing (odynophagia)
    Suggests inflammation and ulceration
- Regurgitation or reflux (heartburn)
    Common in gastro-oesophageal reflux disease
- Chest pain
    Difficult to distinguish from cardiac pain

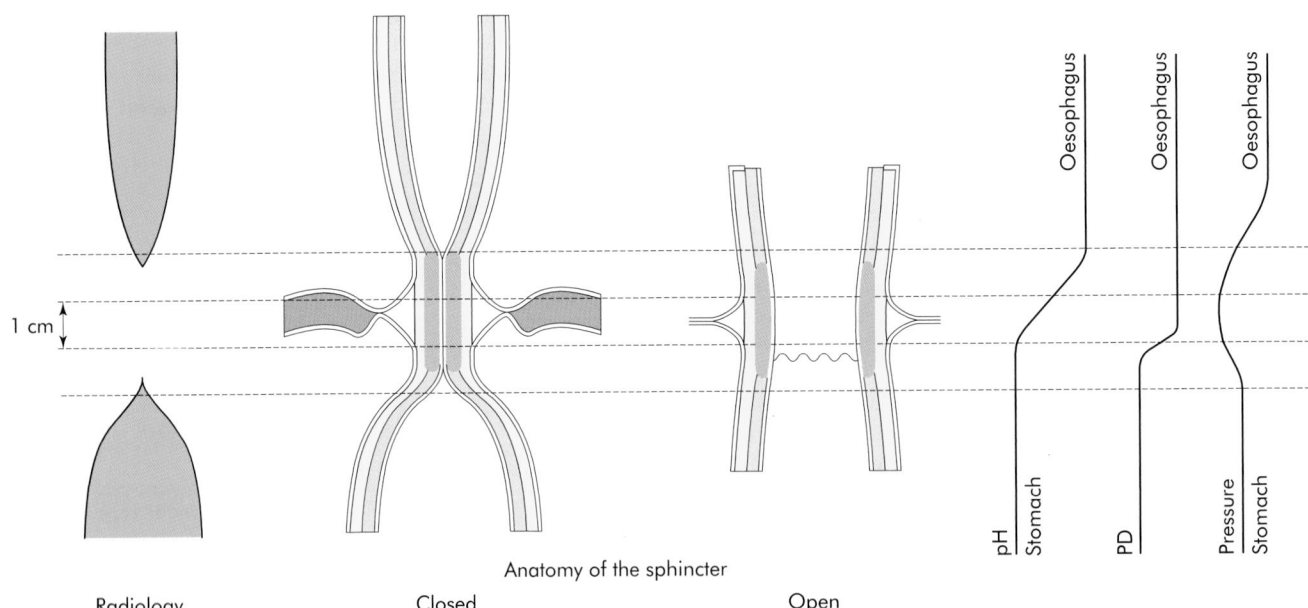

Radiology　　　Closed　　　Anatomy of the sphincter　　　Open

Figure 59.3 Correlation between the radiological appearances of a barium column and the lower oesophageal sphincter open and closed. The three curves on the right, set up vertically, show the pH gradient, the mucosal potential difference (PD) marking the junction of squamous and columnar epithelium and the high-pressure zone of the sphincter.

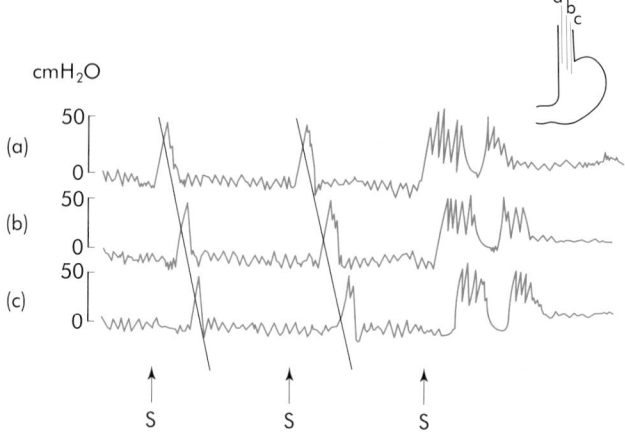

Figure 59.4 Triple water-perfused tube study of normal lower oesophagus and lower oesophageal sphincter. Note that the swallowing contractions (S) in the body of the oesophagus are sequential, i.e. peristaltic

Dysphagia

Dysphagia is used to describe difficulty with swallowing. When there is a problem with swallowing in the voluntary (oral or pharyngeal) phases, patients will usually say that they cannot swallow properly, but they do not characteristically describe 'food sticking'. Instead, when they try to initiate a conscious swallow, food fails to enter the oesophagus, stays in the mouth or enters the airway causing coughing or spluttering. Virtually all causes of this type of dysphagia are chronic neurological or muscular diseases. Oesophageal dysphagia occurs in the involuntary phase and is characterised by a sensation of food sticking. The nature of this type of dysphagia is often informative regarding a likely diagnosis. Dysphagia may occur acutely or in a chronic fashion, can affect solids and/or fluids and be intermittent or progressive. While many patients point to a site of impaction, this is unreliable.

Odynophagia

Odynophagia refers to pain on swallowing. Patients with reflux oesophagitis often feel retrosternal discomfort within a few seconds of swallowing hot beverages, citrus drinks or alcohol. Odynophagia is also a feature of infective oesophagitis and may be particularly severe in chemical injury.

Regurgitation and reflux

Regurgitation and reflux are often used synonymously. It is helpful to differentiate between them, although it is not always possible. Regurgitation should strictly refer to the return of oesophageal contents from above a functional or mechanical obstruction. Reflux is the passive return of gastroduodenal contents to the mouth as part of the symptomatology of gastro-oesophageal reflux disease (GORD). Loss of weight, anaemia, cachexia, change of voice due to refluxed material irritating the vocal cords and cough or dyspnoea due to tracheal aspiration may all accompany regurgitation and/or reflux.

Chest pain

Chest pain similar in character to angina pectoris may arise from an oesophageal cause, especially gastro-oesophageal reflux and motility disorders. Exercise-induced chest pain can be due to reflux.

Investigations

Radiography

Contrast radiography has been somewhat overshadowed by endoscopy but remains a useful investigation for demonstrating narrowing, space-occupying lesions, anatomical distortion or abnormal motility. An adequate barium swallow should be tailored to the problem under investigation. It may be helpful to give a solid bolus (bread or marshmallow) if a motility disorder is suspected. Video recording is useful to allow subsequent replay and detailed analysis. Barium radiology is, however, inaccurate in the diagnosis of gastro-oesophageal reflux, unless reflux is gross, and should not be used for this purpose. Plain radiographs will show some foreign bodies.

Cross-sectional imaging by computerised tomography (CT) scanning is now an essential investigation in the assessment of neoplasms of the oesophagus and can be used in place of a contrast swallow to demonstrate perforation. The role of CT and other cancer-specific tests is described later.

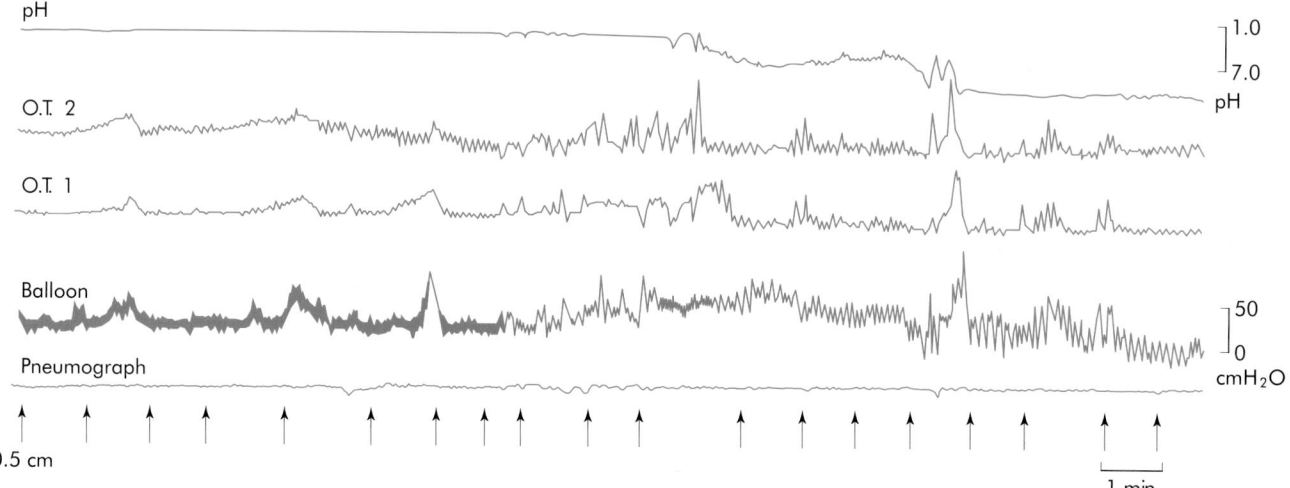

Figure 59.5 Manometric recording from the body of a normal oesophagus. Peristalsis is seen in the first and last panels, but other waves are simultaneous. Non-peristaltic simultaneous contractions are called 'tertiary contractions'.

Endoscopy

Endoscopy is necessary for the investigation of most oesophageal conditions. It is required to view the inside of the oesophagus and the oesophagogastric junction, to obtain a biopsy or cytology specimen, for the removal of foreign bodies and to dilate strictures. Traditionally, there are two types of instrument available, the rigid oesophagoscope and the flexible video endoscope, but the rigid instrument is now virtually obsolete.

For flexible video gastroduodenoscope, general anaesthesia is not required; most examinations can be done on an out-patient basis, and the quality of the magnified image is superb. The technology associated with video endoscopy continues to improve.

As a matter of routine, the stomach and duodenum are examined as well as the oesophagus. If a stricture is encountered, it may be helpful to dilate it to allow a complete inspection of the upper gastrointestinal tract, but this decision should be dictated by clinical circumstances and an appreciation of the perforation risk.

Endosonography

Endoscopic ultrasonography relies on a high-frequency (5–30 MHz) transducer located at the tip of the endoscope to provide highly detailed images of the layers of the oesophageal wall and mediastinal structures close to the oesophagus. Radial echoendoscopes have a rotating transducer that creates a circular image with the endoscope in the centre, and this type of scanner is widely used to create diagnostic transverse sectional images at right angles to the long axis of the oesophagus (Fig. 59.6). Linear echoendoscopes produce a sectoral image in the line of the endoscope and are used to biopsy submucosal oesophageal lesions or mediastinal masses such as lymph nodes (Fig. 59.7). Radial scanners without optical components are available for passage through narrow strictures over a guidewire, and there are even catheter probes that can be passed down the endoscope biopsy channel.

Oesophageal manometry

Manometry is now widely used to diagnose oesophageal motility disorders. Recordings are usually made by passing a multilumen catheter with three to eight recording orifices at different levels down the oesophagus and into the stomach. Electronic microtransducers that are not influenced by changes in patient position during the test have gradually supplanted perfusion systems. With either system, the catheter is withdrawn progressively up the oesophagus, and recordings are taken at intervals of 0.5–1.0 cm to measure the length and pressure of the LOS and assess motility in the body of the oesophagus during swallowing.

24-hour pH recording

Prolonged measurement of pH is now accepted as the most accurate method for the diagnosis of gastro-oesophageal reflux. It is particularly useful in patients with atypical reflux symptoms, those without endoscopic oesophagitis and when patients respond poorly to intensive medical therapy. A small pH probe is passed into the distal oesophagus and positioned 5 cm above the upper margin of the LOS, as defined by manometry. The probe is connected to a miniature digital recorder that is worn on a belt and allows most normal activities. Patients mark symptomatic events such as heartburn. A 24-hour recording period is usual, and the pH record is analysed by an automated computer program. An oesophageal pH < 4 at the level of the pH electrode is conventionally considered the cut-off value and, in most oesophageal laboratories, the total time when pH is < 4 in a 24-hour period does not exceed 4% in a healthy adult. Patterns of reflux and the correlation between symptoms and oesophageal pH < 4 can be calculated. Most laboratories use a scoring system (Johnson–DeMeester) to create a numerical value, above which reflux is considered pathological. Radiotelemetry pH probes are also available that can be fixed to the oesophageal wall endoscopically without the need for a transnasal catheter.

(a)

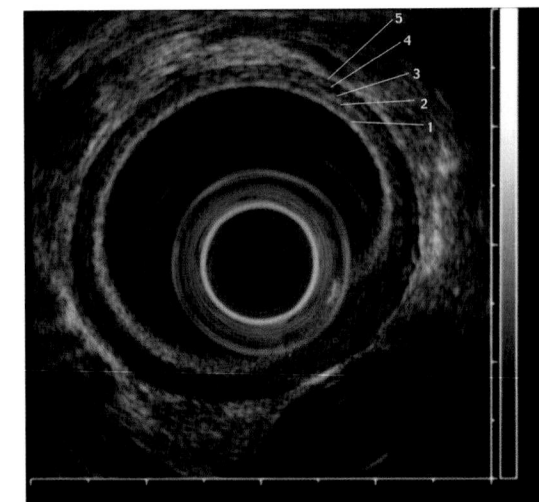

(b)

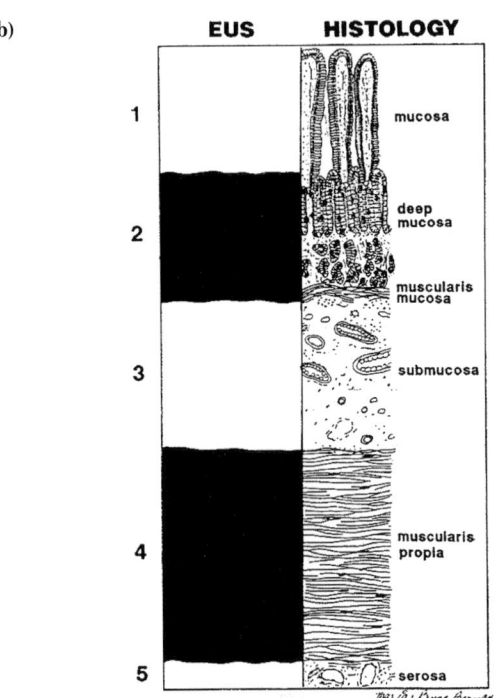

Figure 59.6 Radial endosonography indicating wall layers as alternating hyper- and hypoechoic bands.

Tom R. DeMeester, **Professor of Surgery, Los Angeles, CA, USA.**

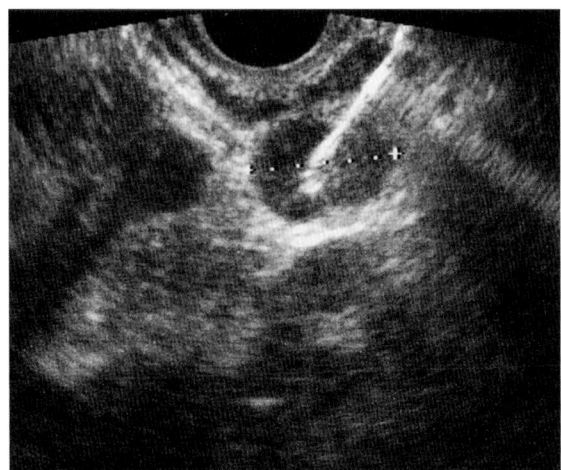

Figure 59.7 Linear endosonography with the needle traversing an ultrasound plane for guided biopsy.

Therapeutic procedures

Dilatation of strictures

Stricture dilatation is essentially undertaken for benign conditions and should be used with caution in the context of malignant disease. The risks associated with dilatation for malignant disease are discussed later. The advent of guidewire-directed dilatation of the oesophagus in the 1970s was a major advance over earlier blind dilatation systems. Their use is now considered standard practice. There are many different designs, but essentially they are solid dilators of increasing diameter. To restore normal swallowing, a stricture should be dilated to at least 16 mm in diameter. A guidewire is passed down the biopsy channel of an endoscope and through the stricture under vision. If the stricture is long or tortuous, this should be undertaken under radiological guidance to ensure that the guidewire passes easily into the stomach. The endoscope is withdrawn, leaving the guidewire in place, and graduated dilators are passed over the guidewire, sometimes with radiographic screening for safety purposes. The dilatation of reflux-induced strictures is usually straightforward. These strictures are nearly always short and at the oesophagogastric junction, so that the stomach is visible through the narrowed segment. Radiological control is rarely needed. Conversely, distal oesophageal adenocarcinomas extending into the stomach are often soft, friable and tortuous to negotiate.

Balloons with inflation diameters of 25–40 mm may also be used for dilatation. Pneumatic dilatation is widely used to disrupt the non-relaxing LOS in achalasia.

Thermal recanalisation

Various types of laser (mainly Nd-YAG), bipolar diathermy, injection of absolute alcohol or argon-beam plasma coagulation have all been used successfully to ablate tissue in order to recanalise the oesophagus.

CONGENITAL ABNORMALITIES

See Chapter 6.

FOREIGN BODIES IN THE OESOPHAGUS

All manner of foreign bodies have become arrested in the oesophagus (Fig. 59.8). Button batteries may be a troublesome problem in children. The most common impacted material is food, and this usually occurs above a significant pathological lesion (Fig. 59.9). Plain radiographs are often useful for foreign bodies, but modern denture materials are not always radiopaque. A contrast examination is not usually required and only makes endoscopy more difficult (Summary box 59.2).

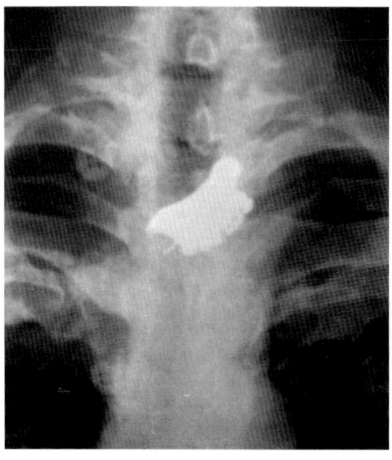

Figure 59.8 False teeth impacted in the oesophagus. (Note: modern dentures are usually radiolucent.)

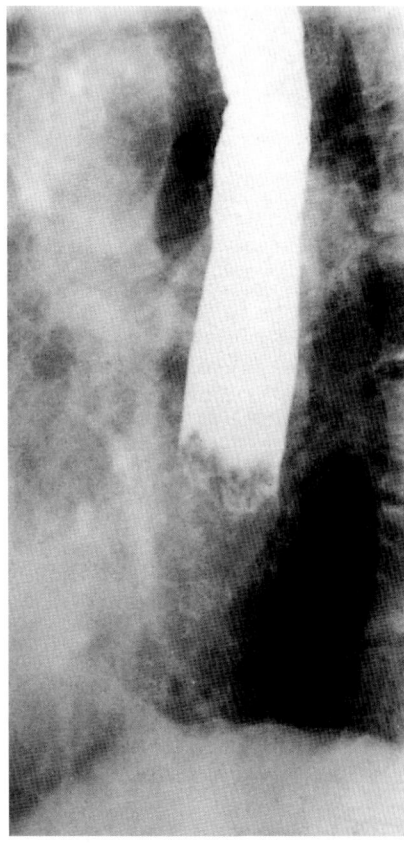

Figure 59.9 An impacted meat bolus at the lower end of the oesophagus. This may be the first presentation of a benign stricture or a malignant tumour.

Summary box 59.2

Foreign bodies

- The most common is a food bolus, which usually signifies underlying disease
- It is usually possible to remove foreign bodies by flexible endoscopy
- Beware of button batteries in the oesophagus

Foreign bodies that have become stuck in the oesophagus should be removed by flexible endoscopy using suitable grasping forceps, a snare or a basket. If the object may injure the oesophagus on withdrawal, an overtube can be used, and the endoscope and object can be withdrawn into the overtube before removal. Button batteries can be a particular worry as they are difficult to grasp, and it is tempting to push them on into the stomach. However, an exhausted battery may rapidly corrode in the gastrointestinal tract and is best extracted. A multiwire basket of the type used for gallstone retrieval nearly always works. An impacted food bolus will often break up and pass on if the patient is given fizzy drinks and confined to fluids for a short time. The cause of the impaction must then be investigated. If symptoms are severe or the bolus does not pass, it can be extracted or broken up at endoscopy.

PERFORATION

Perforation of the oesophagus is usually iatrogenic (at therapeutic endoscopy) or due to 'barotrauma' (spontaneous perforation). Many instrumental perforations can be managed conservatively, but spontaneous perforation is often a life-threatening condition that regularly requires surgical intervention (Summary box 59.3).

Summary box 59.3

Perforation of the oesophagus

- Potentially lethal complication due to mediastinitis and septic shock
- Numerous causes, but may be iatrogenic
- Surgical emphysema is virtually pathognomonic
- Treatment is urgent; it may be conservative or surgical, but requires specialised care

---

Barotrauma (spontaneous perforation, Boerhaave syndrome)

This occurs classically when a person vomits against a closed glottis. The pressure in the oesophagus increases rapidly, and the oesophagus bursts at its weakest point in the lower third, sending a stream of material into the mediastinum and often the pleural cavity as well. The condition was first reported by Boerhaave, who reported the case of a grand admiral of the Dutch fleet who was a glutton and practised autoemesis. Boerhaave syndrome is the most serious type of perforation

---

Hermann Boerhaave, 1668–1738, Professor of Medicine and Botany, The University of Leiden, The Netherlands. He was the creator of the modern method of clinical teaching.

---

because of the large volume of material that is released under pressure. This causes rapid chemical irritation in the mediastinum and pleura followed by infection if untreated. Barotrauma has also been described in relation to other pressure events when the patient strains against a closed glottis (e.g. defaecation, labour, weight-lifting).

Diagnosis of spontaneous perforation

The clinical history is usually of severe pain in the chest or upper abdomen following a meal or a bout of drinking. Associated shortness of breath is common. Many cases are misdiagnosed as myocardial infarction, perforated peptic ulcer or pancreatitis if the pain is confined to the upper abdomen. There may be a surprising amount of rigidity on examination of the upper abdomen, even in the absence of any peritoneal contamination.

The diagnosis can usually be suspected from the history and associated clinical features. A chest X-ray is often confirmatory with air in the mediastinum, pleura or peritoneum. Pleural effusion occurs rapidly either as a result of free communication with the pleural space or as a reaction to adjacent inflammation in the mediastinum. A contrast swallow or CT is nearly always required to guide management (Fig. 59.10).

Pathological perforation

Free perforation of ulcers or tumours of the oesophagus into the pleural space is rare. Erosion into an adjacent structure with fistula formation is more common. Aerodigestive fistula is most common and usually encountered in primary malignant disease of the oesophagus or bronchus. Coughing on eating and signs of aspiration pneumonitis may allow the problem to be recognised at a time when intervention may be appropriate and feasible. Covering the communication with a self-expanding metal stent is the usual solution. Erosion into a major vascular structure is invariably fatal.

Penetrating injury

Perforation by knives and bullets is uncommon, even in war, as the oesophagus is a relatively small target surrounded by other vital organs.

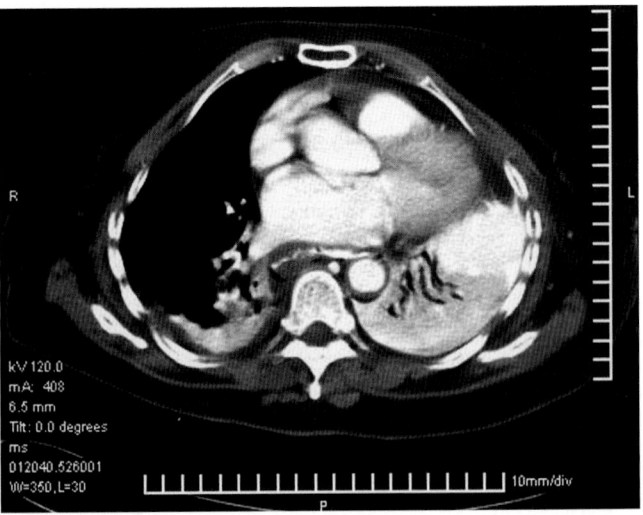

Figure 59.10 Computerised tomography scan showing the site of perforation in the lower oesophagus.

Foreign bodies

The oesophagus may be perforated during removal of a foreign body but, occasionally, an object that has been left in the oesophagus for several days will erode through the wall.

Instrumental perforation

Instrumentation is by far the most common cause of perforation. Modern instrumentation is remarkably safe, but perforation remains a risk that should never be forgotten (Summary box 59.4).

Summary box 59.4
Instrumental perforation
■ Prevention of perforation is better than cure

Perforation related to diagnostic upper gastrointestinal endoscopy is unusual with an estimated frequency of about 1:4000 examinations. Perforation can occur in the pharynx or oesophagus, usually at sites of pathology or when the endoscope is passed blindly. A number of patient-related factors are associated with increased risk, including large anterior cervical osteophytes, the presence of a pharyngeal pouch and mechanical causes of obstruction. Perforation may follow biopsy of a malignant tumour.

Patients undergoing therapeutic endoscopy have a perforation risk that is at least 10 times greater than those undergoing diagnostic endoscopy. The oesophagus may be perforated by guidewires, graduated dilators or balloons, or during the placement of self-expanding stents. The risk is considerably higher in patients with malignancy.

Diagnosis of instrumental perforation

In most cases, a combination of technical difficulties and an interventional procedure should lead to a high index of suspicion. History and physical signs may be useful pointers to the site of perforation.

Cervical perforation may result in pain localised to the neck, hoarseness, painful neck movements and subcutaneous emphysema. Intrathoracic and intra-abdominal perforations, which are more common, can give rise to immediate symptoms and signs either during or at the end of the procedure, including chest pain, haemodynamic instability, oxygen desaturation or visual evidence of perforation. Within the first 24 hours, patients may additionally complain of abdominal pain or respiratory difficulties. There may be evidence of subcutaneous emphysema, pneumothorax or hydropneumothorax. In some patients, the diagnosis may be missed and recognised only at a late stage beyond 24 hours, as unexplained pyrexia, systemic sepsis or the development of a clinical fistula.

Prompt and thorough investigation is the key to management. Careful endoscopic assessment at the end of any procedure combined with a chest X-ray will identify many cases of perforation immediately. If not recognised immediately, then early and late suspected perforations should be assessed by a water-soluble contrast swallow. If this is negative, a dilute barium swallow should be considered. A CT scan can be used to replace a contrast swallow or as an adjunct to accurately delineate specific fluid collections.

Treatment of oesophageal perforations

Perforation of the oesophagus usually leads to mediastinitis. The loose areolar tissues of the posterior mediastinum allow a rapid spread of gastrointestinal contents. The aim of treatment is to limit mediastinal contamination and prevent or deal with infection. Operative repair deals with the injury directly, but imposes risks of its own; non-operative treatment aims to limit the effects of mediastinitis and provide an environment in which healing can take place.

The decision between operative and non-operative management rests on four factors. These are:

1 the site of the perforation (cervical vs. thoracoabdominal oesophagus);
2 the event causing the perforation (spontaneous vs. instrumental);
3 underlying pathology (benign or malignant);
4 the status of the oesophagus before the perforation (fasted and empty vs. obstructed with a stagnant residue).

It follows that most perforations that can be managed non-operatively occur in the context of small instrumental perforations of a clean oesophagus without obstruction, where leakage is likely to be confined to the nearby mediastinum at worst (Table 59.1).

Instrumental perforations in the cervical oesophagus are usually small and can nearly always be managed conservatively. The development of a local abscess is an indication for cervical drainage preventing the extension of sepsis into the mediastinum.

The conservative management of an instrumental perforation in the thoracoabdominal parts of the oesophagus can be undertaken when the perforation is detected early and prior to oral alimentation. General guidelines for non-operative management include:

• pain that is readily controlled with opiates;
• absence of crepitus, diffuse mediastinal gas, hydropneumothorax or pneumoperitoneum;
• mediastinal containment of the perforation with no evidence of widespread extravasation of contrast material;
• no evidence of on-going luminal obstruction or a retained foreign body.

In addition, conservative management might be appropriate in patients who have remained clinically stable despite diagnostic delay. The principles of non-interventional management involve hyperalimentation, preferably by an enteral route, nasogastric suction and broad-spectrum intravenous antibiotics.

Surgical management is required whenever patients:

• are unstable with sepsis or shock;
• have evidence of a heavily contaminated mediastinum, pleural space or peritoneum;

Table 59.1 Management options in perforation of the oesophagus

Factors that favour non-operative management	Factors that favour operative repair
Small septic load	Large septic load
Minimal cardiovascular upset	Septic shock
Perforation confined to mediastinum	Pleura breached
Perforation by flexible endoscope	Boerhaave's syndrome
Perforation of cervical oesophagus	Perforation of abdominal oesophagus

- have widespread intrapleural or intraperitoneal extravasation of contrast material.

On-going luminal obstruction (often related to malignancy) in a frail patient considered unfit for major surgery can be dealt with by placement of a covered self-expanding stent. Expanding metal stents should be used with caution in patients with benign disease as they cause significant tissue reaction and some designs are impossible to remove at a later date. Biodegradable and removable stents are being developed and may be used alone or as a bridge to later definitive treatment where perforation accompanies obstruction.

For patients requiring surgery, the choice rests between direct repair, the deliberate creation of an external fistula or, rarely, oesophageal resection with a view to delayed reconstruction. Direct repair is preferred by many surgeons if the perforation is recognised early (within the first 4–6 hours) and the extent of mediastinal and pleural contamination is small. After 12 hours, the tissues become swollen and friable and less suitable for direct suture. The hole in the mucosa is always bigger than the hole in the muscle, and the muscle should be incised to see the mucosal edges clearly. It is essential that there should be no obstruction distal to the repair. A variety of local tissues (gastric fundus, pericardium, intercostal muscle) have been used to buttress such repairs.

Primary repair is inadvisable with late presentation and in the presence of widespread mediastinal and pleural contamination. These patients tend to be more ill as a result of the delay, and the aim of treatment should be to achieve wide drainage with the creation of a controlled fistula and distal enteral feeding. This can usually be achieved by placing a T-tube into the oesophagus along with appropriately located drains and a feeding jejunostomy. In unusual circumstances, for instance with extensive necrosis following corrosive ingestion, emergency oesophagectomy may be necessary. Oesophagostomy and gastrostomy should be performed with a view to delayed reconstruction.

MALLORY–WEISS SYNDROME

Forceful vomiting may produce a mucosal tear at the cardia rather than a full perforation. The mechanism of injury is different. In Boerhaave's syndrome, vomiting occurs against a closed glottis, and pressure builds up in the oesophagus. In Mallory–Weiss syndrome, vigorous vomiting produces a vertical split in the gastric mucosa, immediately below the squamocolumnar junction at the cardia in 90% of cases. In only 10% is the tear in the oesophagus (Fig. 59.11). The condition presents with haematemesis. Usually, the bleeding is not severe, but endoscopic injection therapy may be required for the occasional, severe case. Surgery is rarely required. There are two other injuries to the oesophagus that lie within the spectrum of the mucosal tear of Mallory–Weiss and the full-thickness tear of Boerhaave. Intramural rupture produces a dissection within the oesophageal wall that causes severe chest pain, often with odynophagia. It is best diagnosed by contrast radiology. Intramural haematoma is seen most often in elderly patients on

George Kenneth Mallory, B. 1926, Professor of Pathology, Boston University, Boston, MA, USA.
Soma Weiss, 1898–1942, Professor of Medicine, Harvard University Medical School, Boston, MA, USA.

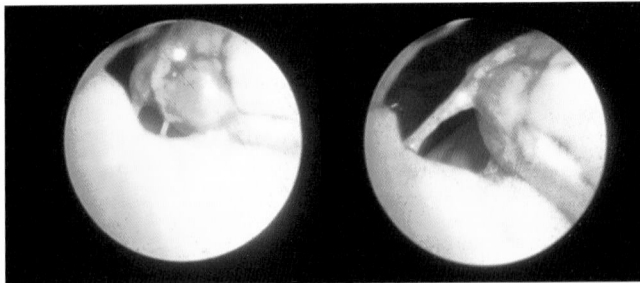

Figure 59.11 The endoscopic appearance of a mucosal tear at the cardia (Mallory–Weiss).

anticoagulants or patients with coagulation disorders, and usually follows an episode of vomiting. Large haematomas causing dysphagia can occur extending from the cardia up to the carina. The diagnosis is readily made on endoscopy. Both intramural rupture and intramural haematoma can be managed conservatively. Symptoms usually resolve in 7–14 days, and oral intake can be reinstituted as soon as symptoms allow.

CORROSIVE INJURY

Corrosives such as sodium hydroxide (lye, caustic soda) or sulphuric acid may be taken in attempted suicide. Accidental ingestion occurs in children and when corrosives are stored in bottles labelled as beverages. All can cause severe damage to the mouth, pharynx, larynx, oesophagus and stomach. The type of agent, its concentration and the volume ingested largely determine the extent of damage. In general, alkalis are relatively odourless and tasteless, making them more likely to be ingested in large volume. Alkalis cause liquefaction, saponification of fats, dehydration and thrombosis of blood vessels that usually leads to fibrous scarring. Acids cause coagulative necrosis with eschar formation, and this coagulant may limit penetration to deeper layers of the oesophageal wall. Acids also cause more gastric damage than alkalis because of the induction of intense pylorospasm with pooling in the antrum.

Symptoms and signs are notoriously unreliable in predicting the severity of injury. The key to management is early endoscopy by an experienced endoscopist to inspect the whole of the oesophagus and stomach (Fig. 59.12). Deep ulcers and the recognition of a grey or black eschar signify the most severe lesions with the greatest risk of perforation. Minor injuries with only oedema

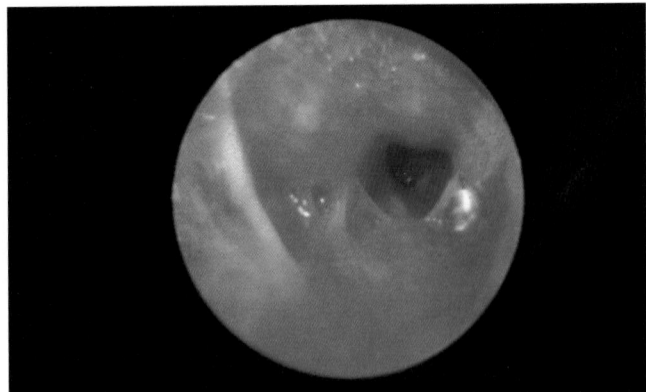

Figure 59.12 Acute caustic burn in the haemorrhagic phase.

of the mucosa resolve rapidly with no late sequelae. These patients can safely be fed. With more severe injuries, a feeding jejunostomy may be appropriate until the patient can swallow saliva satisfactorily. The widespread use of broad-spectrum antibiotics and steroids is not supported by evidence.

Regular endoscopic examinations are the best way to assess stricture development (Fig. 59.13). Significant stricture formation occurs in about 50% of patients with extensive mucosal damage (Fig. 59.14). The role and timing of repeat endoscopies with or without dilatation in such patients remains controversial. Other than the need for emergency surgery for bleeding or

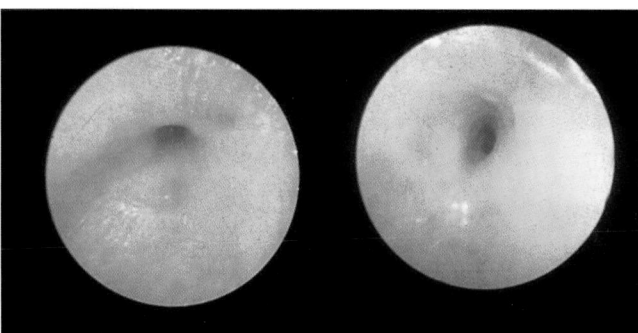

Figure 59.13 The late result of a caustic alkali burn with a high oesophageal stricture.

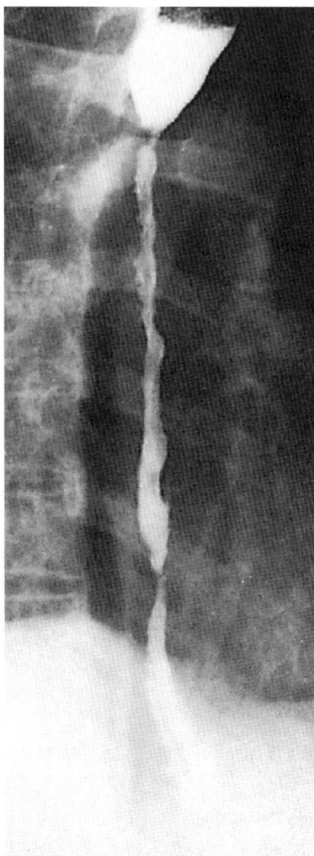

Figure 59.14 Caustic or lye stricture with marked stenosis high in the body of the oesophagus. The strictures are frequently multiple and difficult to dilate unless treated energetically at an early stage.

perforation, elective oesophageal resection should be deferred for at least 3 months until the fibrotic phase is established. Oesophageal replacement is usually required for very long or multiple strictures. Resection can be difficult because of peri-oesophageal inflammation in these patients. Because of associated gastric damage, colon may have to be used as the replacement conduit.

There is also controversy regarding the risk of developing carcinoma in the damaged oesophagus and stomach and how this might influence management. The lifetime risk is certainly less than 5%. Some surgeons advocate resection and replacement, while others believe that oesophageal bypass and endoscopic surveillance is preferable, as removal of the badly damaged oesophagus from a scarred mediastinum can be hazardous (Summary box 59.5).

> **Summary box 59.5**
>
> **Corrosive injury**
>
> ■ Skilled early endoscopy is mandatory

DRUG-INDUCED INJURY

Many medications, such as antibiotics and potassium preparations, are potentially damaging to the oesophagus, as tablets may remain for a long time, especially if taken without an adequate drink. Acute injury presents with dysphagia and odynophagia, which may be severe. The inflammation usually resolves within 2–3 weeks, and no specific treatment is required apart from appropriate nutritional support. A stricture may follow.

GASTRO-OESOPHAGEAL REFLUX DISEASE

Aetiology

Normal competence of the gastro-oesophageal junction is maintained by the LOS. This is influenced by both its physiological function and its anatomical location relative to the diaphragm and the oesophageal hiatus. In normal circumstances, the LOS transiently relaxes as a coordinated part of swallowing, as a means of allowing vomiting to occur and in response to stretching of the gastric fundus, particularly after a meal to allow swallowed air to be vented. Most episodes of physiological reflux occur during postprandial transient lower oesophageal sphincter relaxations (TLOSRs). In the early stages of GORD, most pathological reflux occurs as a result of an increased number of TLOSRs rather than a persistent fall in overall sphincter pressure. In more severe GORD, LOS pressure tends to be generally low, and this loss of sphincter function seems to be made worse if there is loss of an adequate length of intra-abdominal oesophagus.

The absence of an intra-abdominal length of oesophagus results in a sliding hiatus hernia. The normal condensation of peritoneal fascia over the lower oesophagus (the phreno-oesophageal ligament) is weak, and the crural opening widens allowing the upper stomach to slide up through the hiatus. The loss of the normal anatomical configuration exacerbates reflux, although sliding hiatus hernia alone should not be viewed as the cause of reflux. Sliding hiatus hernia is associated with GORD and may make it worse but, as long as the LOS remains competent, pathological GORD does not occur. Many GORD sufferers do not have a hernia, and many of those with a hernia do not have GORD. It should be noted that rolling or paraoesophageal hiatus hernia is a quite different and potentially dangerous condition (see below). A proportion of patients have a rolling hernia and symptomatic GORD or a mixed hernia with both sliding and rolling components. Reflux oesophagitis that is visible endoscopically is a complication of GORD and occurs in a minority of sufferers overall, but in around 40% of patients referred to hospital.

In western societies, GORD is the most common condition affecting the upper gastrointestinal tract. This is partly due to the declining incidence of peptic ulcer as the incidence of infection with *Helicobacter pylori* has reduced as a result of improved socioeconomic conditions along with a rising incidence of GORD in the last 20–30 years. The cause of the increase is unclear, but may be due in part to increasing obesity. The strong association between GORD, obesity and the parallel rise in the incidence of adenocarcinoma of the oesophagus represents a major health challenge for most western countries.

Clinical features

The classical triad of symptoms is retrosternal burning pain (heartburn), epigastric pain (sometimes radiating through to the back) and regurgitation. Most patients do not experience all three. Symptoms are often provoked by food, particularly those that delay gastric emptying (e.g. fats, spicy foods). As the condition becomes more severe, gastric juice may reflux to the mouth and produce an unpleasant taste often described as 'acid' or 'bitter'. Heartburn and regurgitation can be brought on by stooping or exercise. A proportion of patients have odynophagia with hot beverages, citrus drinks or alcohol. Patients with nocturnal reflux and those who reflux food to the mouth nearly always have severe GORD. Some patients present with less typical symptoms such as angina-like chest pain, pulmonary or laryngeal symptoms. Dysphagia is usually a sign that a stricture has occurred, but may be caused by an associated motility disorder.

Because GORD is such a common disorder, it should always be the first thought when a patient presents with oesophageal symptoms that are unusual or that defy diagnosis after a series of investigations.

Diagnosis

In most cases, the diagnosis is assumed rather than proven, and treatment is empirical. Investigation is only required when the diagnosis is in doubt, when the patient does not respond to a proton pump inhibitor (PPI) or if dysphagia is present. The most appropriate examination is endoscopy with biopsy. If the typical appearance of reflux oesophagitis, peptic stricture or Barrett's oesophagus is seen, the diagnosis is clinched, but visible oesophagitis is not always present, even in patients selected as above. This is compounded in clinical practice by the widespread use of PPIs, which cause rapid healing of early mucosal lesions. Many patients will have received such treatment before referral. The endoscopic appearances of the normal oesophagus, hiatus hernia, oesophagitis and stricture are shown in Figures 59.15–59.21. It is worth remembering that the correlation between symptoms and endoscopic appearances is poor. On the other hand, there is a strong correlation between worsening endoscopic appearances and the duration of oesophageal acidification on pH testing.

Norman Rupert Barrett, **1903–1979, Surgeon, St. Thomas's Hospital, London, England.**

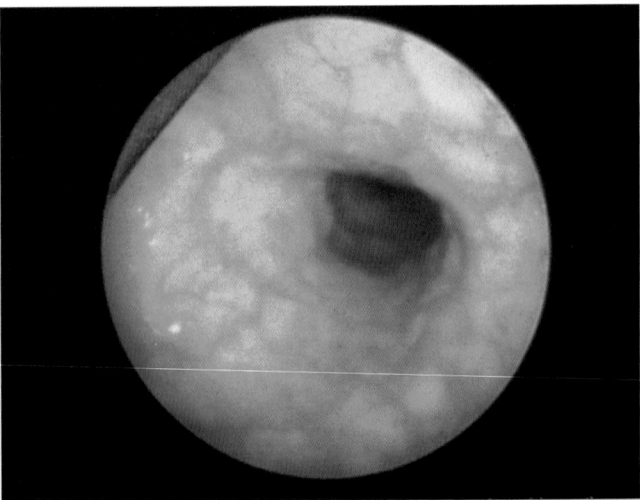

Figure 59.15 The endoscopic appearance of the normal squamous mucosa in the body of the oesophagus.

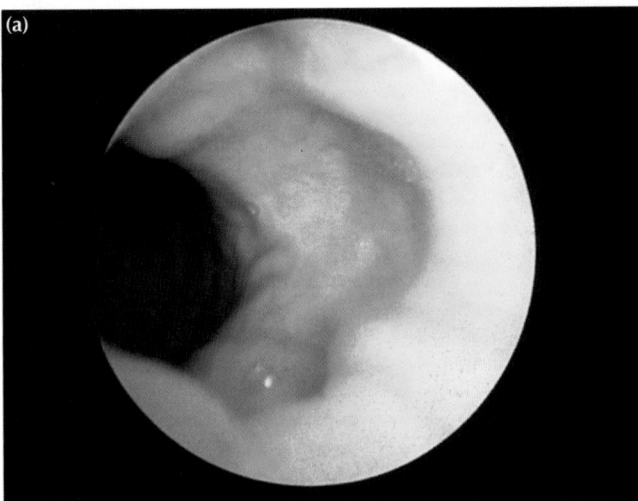

(a)

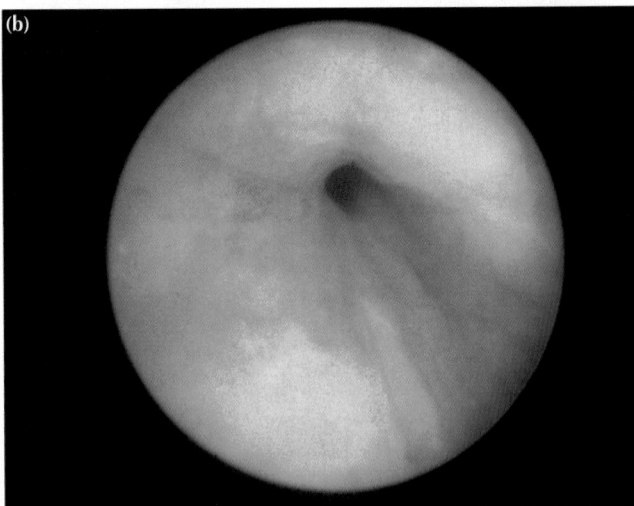

(b)

Figure 59.16 The normal lower oesophageal sphincter: (a) open; (b) closed.

In patients with atypical or persistent symptoms despite therapy, oesophageal manometry and 24-hour oesophageal pH recording may be justified to establish the diagnosis and guide management (Summary box 59.6).

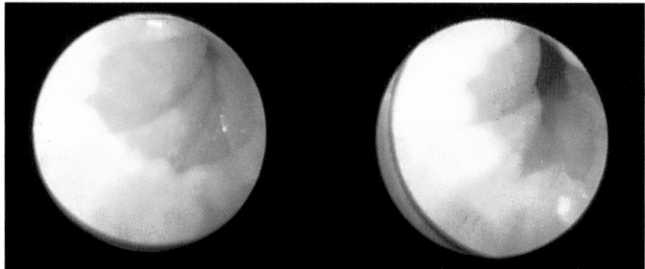

Figure 59.17 The squamocolumnar junction is clearly seen in the lower oesophagus with a normal sharp demarcation.

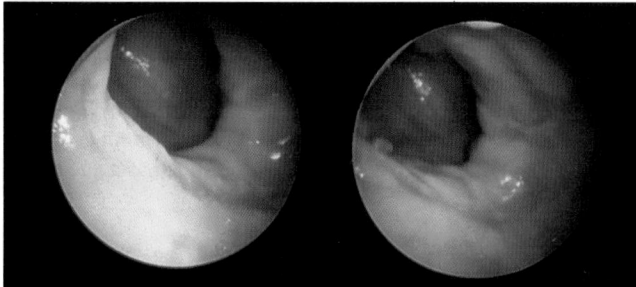

Figure 59.18 Sliding hiatus hernia. The diaphragm can be seen constricting the upper stomach.

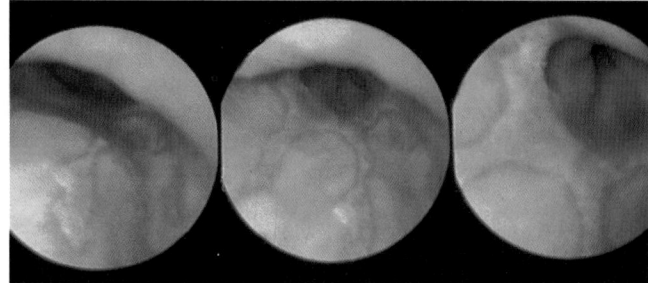

Figure 59.19 Reflux oesophagitis.

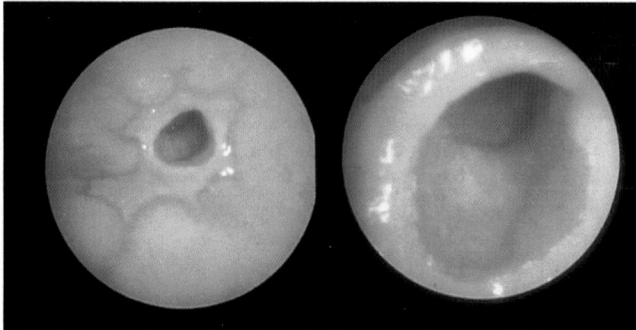

Figure 59.20 Benign stricture with active oesophagitis (left) and healed with columnar epithelium (right).

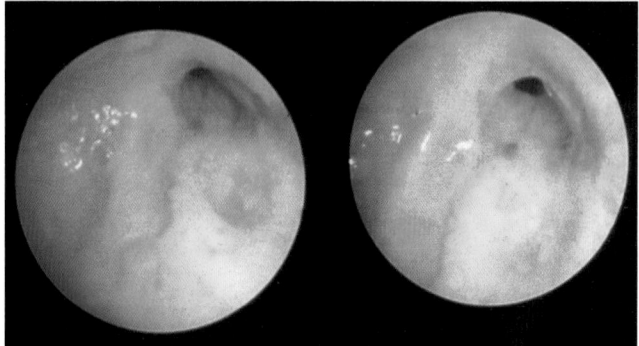

Figure 59.21 Ulceration associated with a benign peptic stricture.

Summary Box 59.6

Diagnostic measurement in GORD

- 24-hour pH recording is the 'gold standard' for diagnosis of GORD
- TLOSRs are the most important manometric findings in GORD
- The length and pressure of the LOS are also important

As a matter of routine, PPIs are stopped 1 week before oesophageal pH recording, but acid secretion is sometimes reduced for 2 weeks or more, and this can necessitate repeat examination after a prolonged interval without a PPI. Manometry and pH recording are also essential in patients being considered for anti-reflux surgery. While the main purpose of the test is objectively to quantify the extent of reflux disease, it is also used to rule out a diagnosis of achalasia. In the early stages of achalasia, chest pain can dominate the clinical picture and, when associated with intermittent swallowing problems and non-specific symptoms, it is easy to see how a clinical diagnosis of GORD might be made. Patients with achalasia can also have an abnormal pH study as a result of fermentation of food residue in a dilated oesophagus. Usually, the form of the pH trace is different from that of GORD, with slow undulations of pH rather than rapid bursts of reflux, but the complete absence of peristalsis on manometry is pathognomonic of achalasia.

Barium swallow and meal examination gives the best appreciation of gastro-oesophageal anatomy (Fig. 59.22). This may be important in the context of surgery for rolling or mixed hiatus hernias, but it is unimportant in most patients with GORD.

Management of uncomplicated GORD

Medical management

Most sufferers from GORD do not consult a doctor and do not need to do so. They self-medicate with over-the-counter medicines such as simple antacids, antacid–alginate preparations and H_2-receptor antagonists. Consultation is more likely when symptoms are severe, prolonged and unresponsive to the above treatments. Simple measures that are often neglected include advice about weight loss, smoking, excessive consumption of alcohol, tea or coffee, the avoidance of large meals late at night and a modest degree of head-up tilt of the bed. Tilting the bed has been shown to have an effect that is similar to taking an H_2-receptor antagonist. The common practice of using additional pillows has no significant effect.

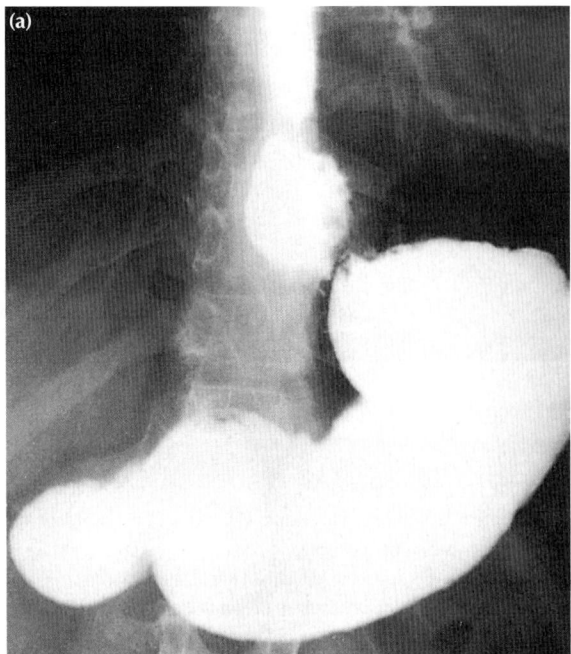

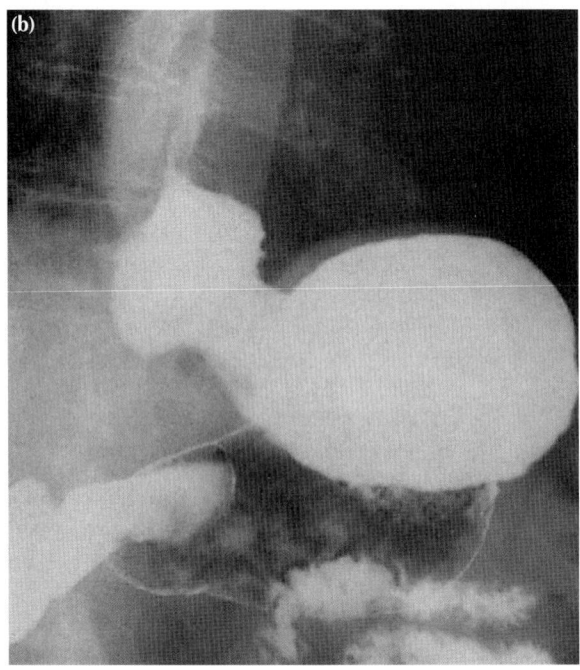

Figure 59.22 (a) Sliding hiatus hernia with a sphincter and diaphragmatic crural narrowing clearly shown. (b) Another sliding hernia in which the sphincter is lax, and the diaphragm is wide open. The patient is in the Trendelenburg position to demonstrate barium in the fundus. This unphysiological position may stimulate 'reflux' in those who do not have gastro-oesophageal reflux disease (GORD).

PPIs are the most effective drug treatment for GORD. Indeed, they are so effective that, once started, patients are very reluctant to stop taking them. Given an adequate dose for 8 weeks, most

Friedrich Trendelenburg, **1844–1924, successively Professor of Surgery at Rostock (1875–1882), Bonn (1882–1895), and Leipzig, Germany (1895–1911).**

patients have a rapid improvement in symptoms (within a few days), and more than 90% can expect full mucosal healing at the end of this time. For this reason, a policy of 'step-down' medical treatment is advocated based on the general advice outlined above and a standard dose of a PPI given for 8 weeks. At the end of that time, the dose of PPI is reduced to that which keeps the patient free of symptoms, and this might even mean the cessation of PPI treatment. Because most patients do not make major lifestyle changes and because PPIs are so effective, many remain on long-term treatment. For the minority who do not respond adequately to a standard dose, a trial at an increased dose or the addition of an H_2-receptor antagonist is recommended. If unsuccessful, these patients should be formally investigated.

PPI therapy is also important in patients with reflux-induced strictures, resulting in significant prolongation of the intervals between endoscopic dilatation. As yet, fears that chronic acid suppression might have serious long-term side-effects including the risk of gastric cancer seem unwarranted.

Surgery

Strictly speaking, the need for surgery should have been reduced as medication has improved so much. Paradoxically, the number of anti-reflux operations has remained relatively constant and may even be increasing. This is probably due partly to increased patient expectations and partly to the advent of minimal access surgery, which has improved the acceptability of procedures.

Endoscopic treatments

A number of endoscopic treatments have been tried in the last 10 years that attempt to augment a failing LOS. These involve endoscopic suturing devices that plicate gastric mucosa just below the cardia to accentuate the angle of His, radiofrequency ablation applied to the level of the sphincter and the injection of submucosal polymers into the lower oesophagus. The procedures have generally been applied to patients with only small hiatus hernias or none at all, so only a small proportion of patients who present to hospitals are suitable. While all methods produce some temporary improvement in symptoms and objective assessments of reflux, failure rates at 1 year are over 50%, and there are no large case series that have reported long-term outcomes.

Surgical treatments

The indication for surgery in uncomplicated GORD is essentially patient choice. The risks and possible benefits need to be discussed in detail. Risks include a small mortality rate (0.1–0.5%, depending on patient selection), failed operation (5–10%) and side-effects such as dysphagia, gas bloat or abdominal discomfort (10%). With current operative techniques, 85–90% of patients should be satisfied with the result of an anti-reflux operation. Patients who are asymptomatic on a PPI need a careful discussion of the risk side of the equation. Those who are symptomatic on a PPI need a careful clinical review to make sure that they will benefit from an operation. Reasons for failure on a PPI include 'volume' reflux (a good indication for surgery), a 'hermit' lifestyle in which the least deviation from lifestyle rules leads to symptoms (a good indication), psychological distress with intolerance of minor symptoms (a poor indication; these patients are likely to be dissatisfied with surgery), poor compliance (a good indication if the reason for poor compliance is the side-effects of treatment, otherwise a bad indication) and misdiagnosis of GORD.

Which operation?

There are many operations for GORD, but they are virtually all based on the creation of an intra-abdominal segment of oesophagus, crural repair and some form of wrap of the upper stomach (fundoplication) around the intra-abdominal oesophagus. The contribution of each component to operative success is widely debated, but it is clear that operations that fail to address all three components have inferior success rates. The major types of anti-reflux operation were all developed in the 1950s (Fig. 59.23). When performed correctly, these are all effective operations. Randomised clinical trials do not show a clear advantage for any one operation over the others.

Total fundoplication (Nissen) tends to be associated with slightly more short-term dysphagia but is the most durable repair in terms of long-term reflux control. Partial fundoplication, whether performed posteriorly (Toupet) or anteriorly (Dor, Watson), has fewer short-term side-effects at the expense of a slightly higher long-term failure rate. One disadvantage of total fundoplication is the creation of an overcompetent cardia, resulting in the 'gas bloat' syndrome in which belching is impossible. The stomach fills with air, the patient feels very full after small meals and passes excessive flatus. This does not seem to occur with partial fundoplication. The problem has been largely overcome by the 'floppy' Nissen technique in which the fundoplication is loose around the oesophagus and is kept short in length. While the other short-term side-effects of fundoplication usually resolve within 3 months of surgery, this is rarely the case for gas bloat. The problem is best remedied by conversion to a partial fundoplication.

As with primary surgery, a variety of revisional procedures

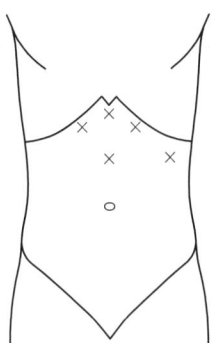

Figure 59.24 Laparoscope cannula sites for laparoscopic fundoplication.

have been described. For most patients, recurrent reflux relates to anatomical failure, so the solution is a revisional fundoplication. A very small proportion of patients may undergo more than two operations to correct recurrent reflux or unacceptable side-effects. Revisional surgery carries a lower chance of success and, in some patients, local revision is technically impossible. The final resort is partial gastrectomy with a Roux-en-Y reconstruction. This reduces gastric acid secretion and diverts bile and pancreatic secretions away from the stomach. Thus, the volume of potential refluxate in the stomach is reduced and, because of its changed composition, it is less damaging to the oesophagus.

For many years, the relative merits of thoracic and abdominal approaches were hotly debated. The introduction of minimal access surgery has made this debate practically obsolete, and most anti-reflux operations are now done with a laparoscopic approach.

Laparoscopic fundoplication

Five cannulae are inserted in the upper abdomen (Fig. 59.24). The cardia and lower oesophagus are separated from the diaphragmatic hiatus. An appropriate length of oesophagus is mobilised in the mediastinum. The fundus may be mobilised by dividing the short gastric vessels that tether the fundus to the spleen. The hiatus is narrowed by sutures placed behind the oesophagus. In total (Nissen) fundoplication, the fundus is drawn behind the oesophagus and then sutured to itself in front of the oesophagus (Fig. 59.25a). In partial fundoplication, the fundus is drawn either behind or in front of the oesophagus and sutured to it on each side, leaving a strip of exposed oesophagus either at the front (Fig. 59.25b) or at the back.

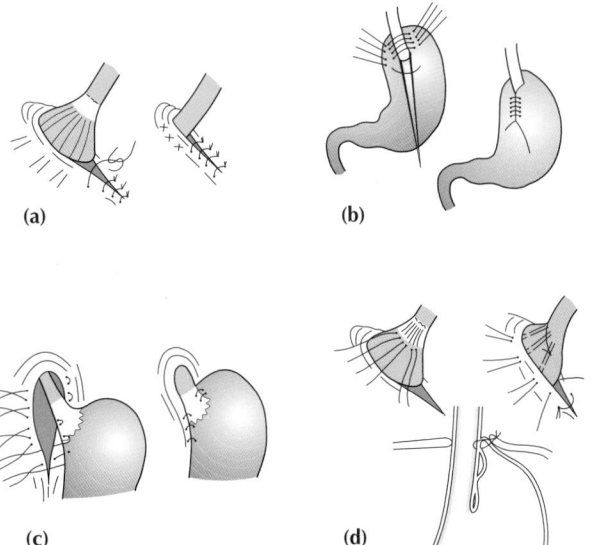

Figure 59.23 Various operations for the surgical correction of gastro-oesophageal reflux disease. (a) The original Allison repair of hiatus hernia (this is ineffective and is no longer done); (b) Nissen fundoplication; (c) Hill procedure; (d) Belsey mark IV operation.

Rudolph Nissen, **1896–1981, Professor of Surgery, Istanbul, Turkey, and later at Basle, Switzerland.**
A.M. Toupet, **a French Surgeon.**
Philip Rowland Allison, **1907–1974, Professor of Surgery, Oxford University, Oxford, England.**
Lucius Davis Hill, **Surgeon, The Mason Clinic, Seattle, MN, USA.**
Ronald Herbert Robert Belsey, **D. 2007, Thoracic Surgeon, The Frenchay Hospital, Bristol, England.**

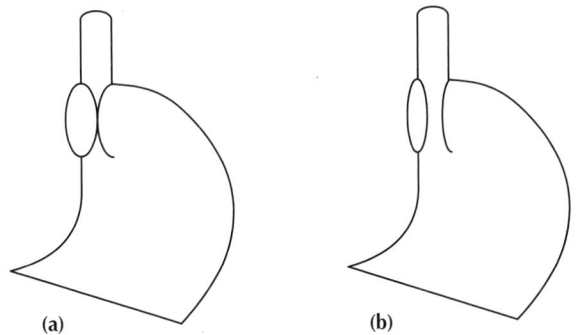

Figure 59.25 (a) Total (Nissen) fundoplication; (b) partial fundoplication (Toupet).

Cesar Roux, **1857–1934, Professor of Surgery and Gynaecology, Lausanne, Switzerland, described this method of forming a jejunal conduit in 1908.**

Complications of gastro-oesophageal reflux disease

Stricture

Reflux-induced strictures (see Fig. 59.21, p. 1019) occur mainly in the late middle-aged and the elderly, but they may present in children. It is important to distinguish a benign reflux-induced stricture from a carcinoma. This is not usually difficult on the basis of location (immediately above the oesophagogastric junction), length (only about 1–2 cm) and smooth mucosa, but sometimes a cancer spreads under the oesophageal mucosa at its upper margin, producing a benign-looking stricture.

Peptic strictures generally respond well to dilatation and long-term treatment with a PPI. As most patients are elderly, anti-reflux surgery is not usually considered. However, it is an alternative to long-term PPI treatment, just as in uncomplicated GORD in younger and fitter patients. Most patients do not require anything other than a standard operation (Summary box 59.8).

Summary box 59.8

Peptic stricture

- Day-case dilatation and PPI for peptic stricture

Oesophageal shortening

The issue of oesophageal shortening continues to provoke debate. There can be no doubt that, in the presence of a large sliding hiatus hernia, the oesophagus is short, but this does not necessarily mean that, with mobilisation from the mediastinum, it cannot easily be restored to its normal length. The extent to which severe inflammation in the wall of the oesophagus causes fibrosis and real shortening is less clear. If a good segment of intra-abdominal oesophagus cannot be restored without tension, a Collis gastroplasty should be performed (Fig. 59.26). This produces a neo-oesophagus around which a fundoplication can be done (Collis–Nissen operation) (Summary box 59.8).

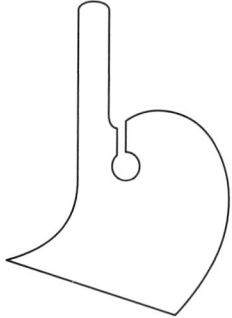

Figure 59.26 Collis gastroplasty to produce a neo-oesophagus around which a Nissen fundoplication is done. The operation may be performed by a laparoscopic as well as an open approach using circular and linear staplers.

John Leigh Collis, **1911–2003**, Professor of Thoracic Surgery, The University of Birmingham, Birmingham, England.

Summary box 59.8

GORD

- Is due to loss of competence of the LOS and is extremely common
- May be associated with a hiatus hernia, which may be sliding or, less commonly, rolling (paraoesophageal)
- The most common symptoms are heartburn, epigastric discomfort and regurgitation, often made worse by stooping and lying

Achalasia and GORD are diagnostically easily confused
- Dysphagia may occur, but a neoplasm must be excluded
- Diagnosis and treatment can be instituted on clinical grounds

Endoscopy may be required and 24-hour pH is the 'gold standard'
- Management is primarily medical (PPIs being the most effective), but surgery may be required; laparoscopic fundoplication is the most popular technique
- Stricture may develop in time

Barrett's oesophagus (columnar-lined lower oesophagus)

Barrett's oesophagus is a metaplastic change in the lining mucosa of the oesophagus in response to chronic gastro-oesophageal reflux (Fig. 59.27). Many of these patients do not have particularly severe symptoms, although they do have the most abnormal pH profiles. This adaptive response involves a mosaic of cell types, probably beginning as a simple columnar epithelium that becomes 'specialised' with time. The hallmark of 'specialised' Barrett's epithelium is the presence of mucus-secreting goblet cells (intestinal metaplasia). One of the great mysteries of GORD

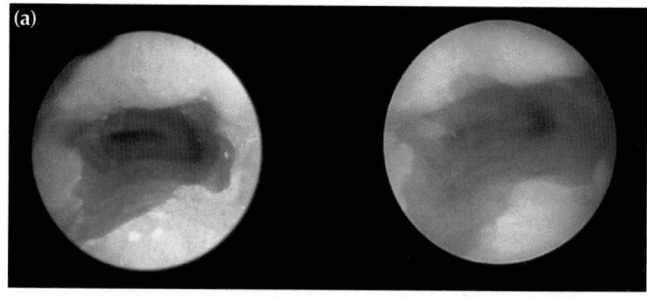

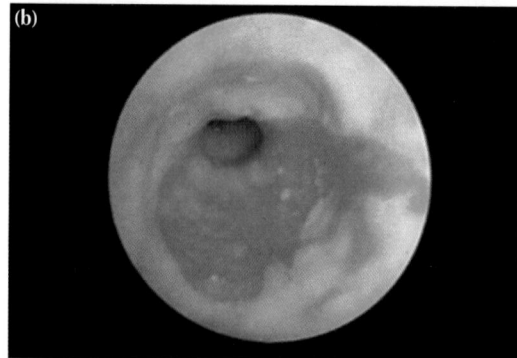

Figure 59.27 Barrett's oesophagus with proximal migration of the squamocolumnar junction (a) and with a view of the distal oesophagus (b).

is why some people develop oesophagitis and others develop Barrett's oesophagus, often without significant oesophagitis. In Barrett's oesophagus, the junction between squamous oesophageal mucosa and gastric mucosa moves proximally. It may be difficult to distinguish a Barrett's oesophagus from a tubular, sliding hiatus hernia during endoscopy, as the two often coexist (Fig. 59.28) or where the visible Barrett's segment is very short. The key is where the gastric mucosal folds end. The mucosa in the body of the stomach has longitudinal folds; the columnar lining of Barrett's oesophagus is smooth. Strictures can occur in Barrett's oesophagus and nearly always appear at the new squamocolumnar junction (Fig. 59.29). Rarely, a stricture may occur in the columnar segment after healing of a Barrett's ulcer (Fig. 59.30). When intestinal metaplasia occurs, there is an increased risk of adenocarcinoma of the oesophagus (Summary box 59.9), which is about 25 times that of the general population (Figs 59.30–32).

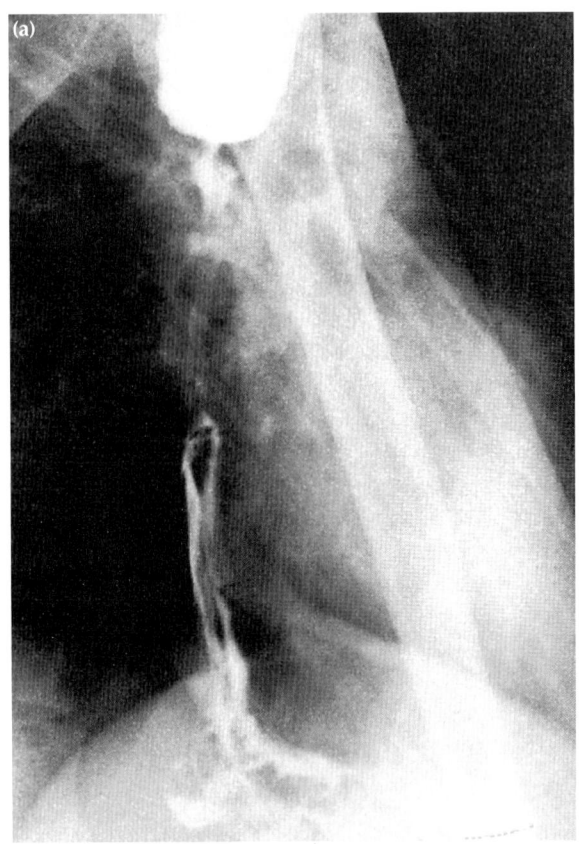

Summary box 59.9

Barrett's oesophagus

- Intestinal metaplasia is an important risk factor for the development of adenocarcinoma
- Do not confuse Barrett's ulcer with oesophagitis

Patients who are found to have Barrett's oesophagus may be submitted to regular surveillance endoscopy with multiple biopsies in the hope of finding dysplasia or *in situ* cancer rather than allowing invasive cancer to develop and cause symptoms. There is as yet no general agreement about the benefits of surveillance endoscopy, nor about its ideal frequency. Annual endoscopy has been widely practised, but 2-year intervals are probably adequate, provided no dysplasia has been detected. A significant problem is that the incidence of Barrett's oesophagus in the community is estimated to be at least 10 times the incidence discovered in dyspeptic patients referred for endoscopy. Thus, adenocarcinoma in Barrett's oesophagus often presents with invasive cancer without any preceding reflux symptoms.

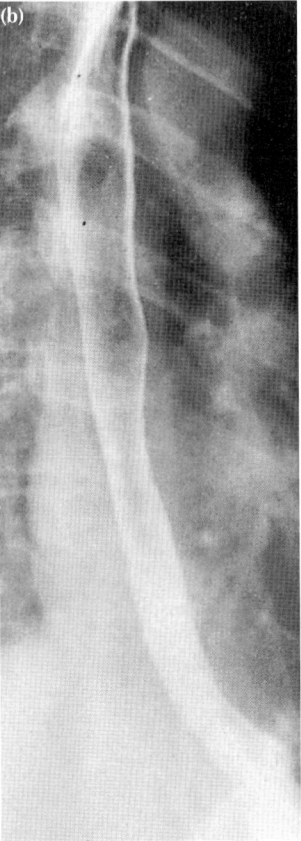

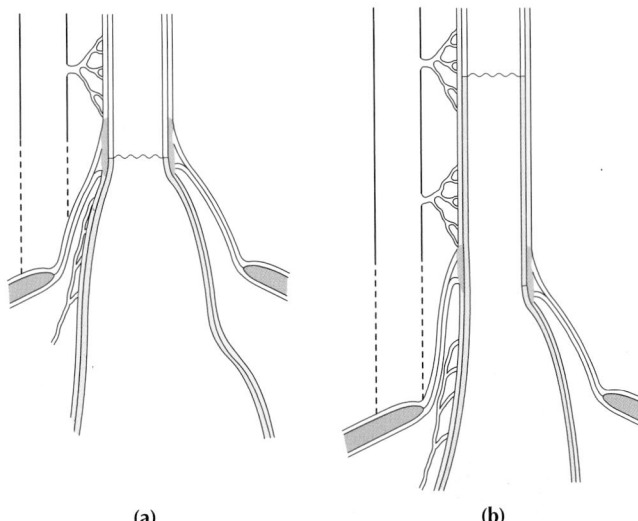

(a)   (b)

Figure 59.28 (a) The relationship between the lower oesophageal sphincter, the squamocolumnar junction and the diaphragm in sliding hiatus hernia. (b) Barrett's oesophagus and sliding hernia.

Figure 59.29 The radiological appearance of a mid-oesophageal stricture in a patient with Barrett's oesophagus (a) and in a patient with a normal lumen following dilatation (b).

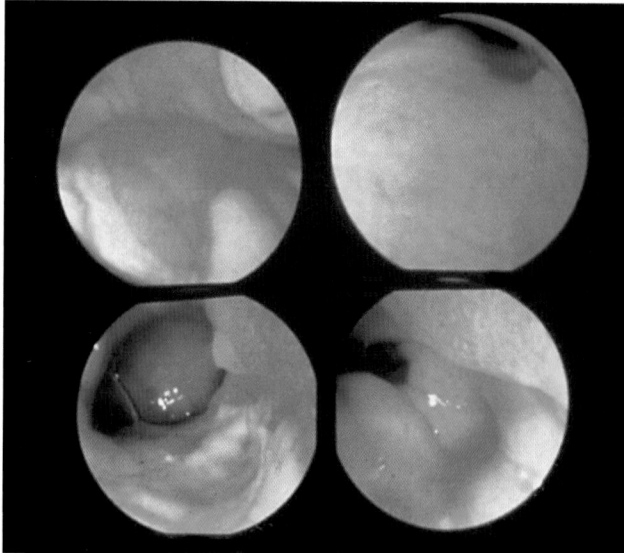

Figure 59.30 Barrett's ulcer in the columnar cell-lined oesophagus.

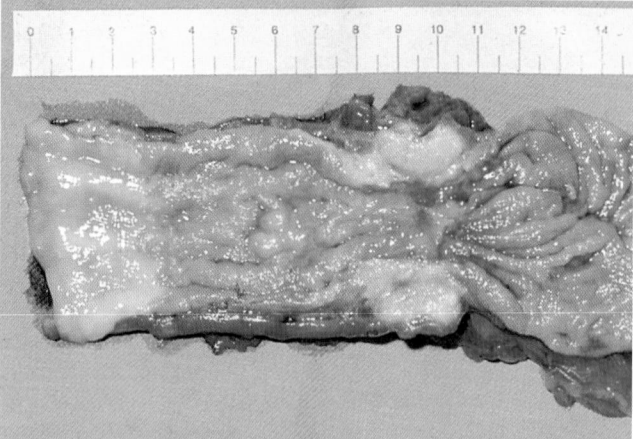

Figure 59.31 The macroscopic appearances of an adenocarcinoma in Barrett's oesophagus.

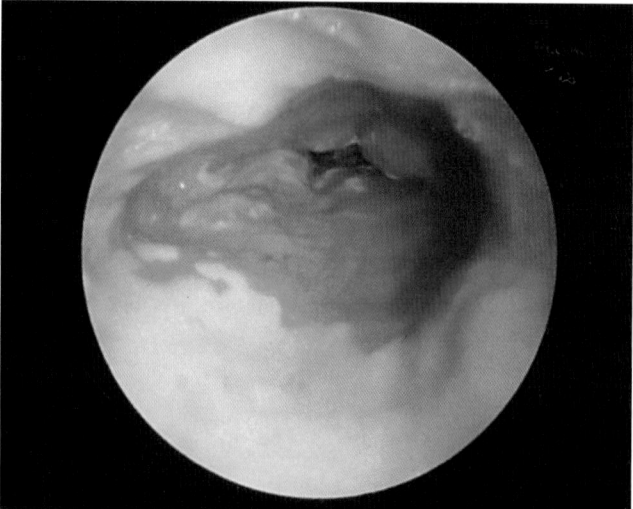

Figure 59.32 Endoscopic view of carcinoma in Barrett's oesophagus.

Until recently, Barrett's oesophagus was not diagnosed until there was at least 3 cm of columnar epithelium in the distal oesophagus. With the better appreciation of the importance of intestinal metaplasia, Barrett's oesophagus may be diagnosed if there is any intestinal metaplasia in the oesophagus. The relative risk of cancer probably increases with increasing length of abnormal mucosa. The following terms are widely used:

- *classic Barrett's* (3 cm or more columnar epithelium);
- *short-segment Barrett's* (less than 3 cm of columnar epithelium);
- *cardia metaplasia* (intestinal metaplasia at the oesophagogastric junction without any macroscopic change at endoscopy).

When Barrett's oesophagus is discovered, the treatment is that of the underlying GORD. There has been considerable interest in recent years in endoscopic methods of ablating Barrett's mucosa in the hope of eliminating the risk of cancer development. Laser, photodynamic therapy, argon-beam plasma coagulation and endoscopic mucosal resection (EMR) have all been used. In conjunction with high-dose PPI treatment or an anti-reflux operation, these endoscopic methods can result in a neosquamous lining. There is no evidence yet that any of these methods is reliable in eliminating cancer risk. Residual islands of Barrett's epithelium can persist, glands may be buried beneath the new lining, and damage to the oesophageal wall may cause stricturing.

PARAOESOPHAGEAL ('ROLLING') HIATUS HERNIA

True paraoesophageal hernias in which the cardia remains in its normal anatomical position are rare. The vast majority of rolling hernias are mixed hernias in which the cardia is displaced into the chest and the greater curve of the stomach rolls into the mediastinum (Fig. 59.33). Sometimes, the whole of the stomach lies in the chest (Fig. 59.34). Colon or small intestine may sometimes lie in the hernia sac. The hernia is most common in the elderly, but may occur in young fit people. As the stomach rolls up into the chest, there is always an element of rotation (volvulus) (Summary box 59.10).

Summary box 59.10
'Rolling' hiatus hernia
■ Potentially dangerous, because of volvulus

The symptoms of rolling hernia are mostly due to twisting and distortion of the oesophagus and stomach. Dysphagia is common. Chest pain may occur from distension of an obstructed stomach. Classically, the pain is relieved by a loud belch. Symptoms of GORD are variable. Strangulation, gastric perforation and gangrene can occur. Emergency presentation with any of these complications carries high mortality on account of a combination of late diagnosis, generally elderly patients with comorbid diseases and the complexity of surgery involved.

The hernia may be visible on a plain radiograph of the chest as a gas bubble, often with a fluid level behind the heart (Fig. 59.35). A barium meal is the best method of diagnosis. The endoscopic appearances may be confusing, especially in large hernias when it is easy to become disorientated.

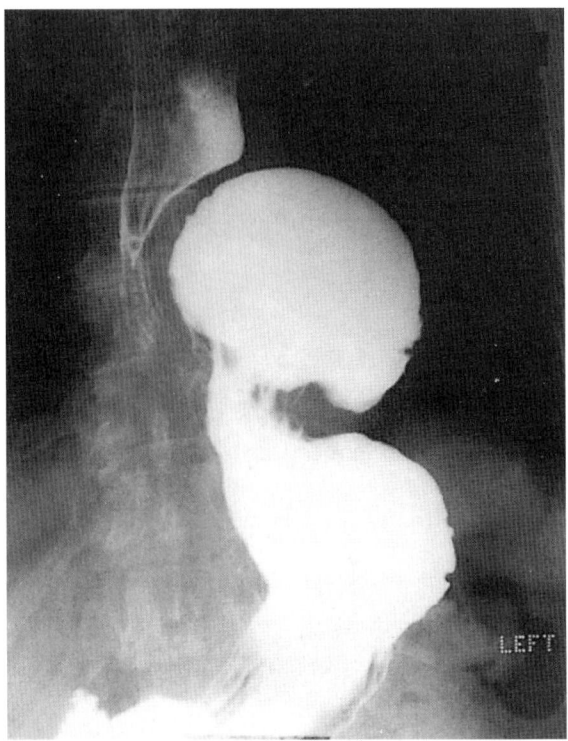

Figure 59.33 A paraoesophageal hernia showing the gastro-oesophageal junction just above the diaphragm and the fundus alongside the oesophagus, compressing the lumen.

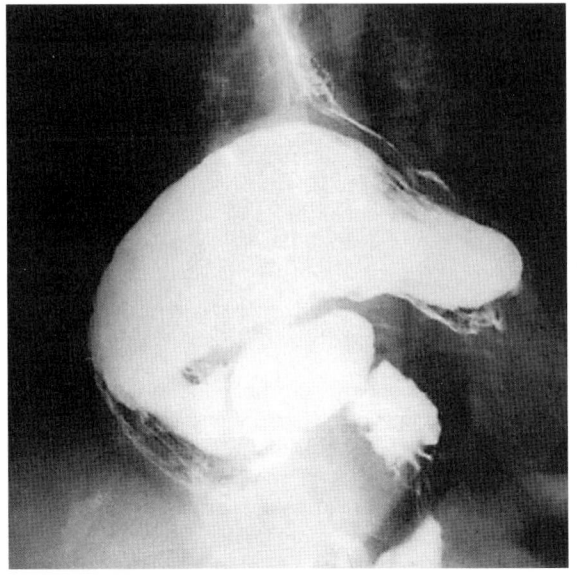

Figure 59.34 A huge paraoesophageal hernia with an upside-down stomach and the pylorus just below the hiatus.

Symptomatic rolling hernias nearly always require surgical repair as they are potentially dangerous. The risk of an asymptomatic patient developing a significant problem when a rolling hiatus hernia is discovered incidentally has probably been overestimated in the past. The annual risk is probably no more than 1%. Patients who present as an emergency with acute chest pain may be treated initially by nasogastric tube to relieve the distension that

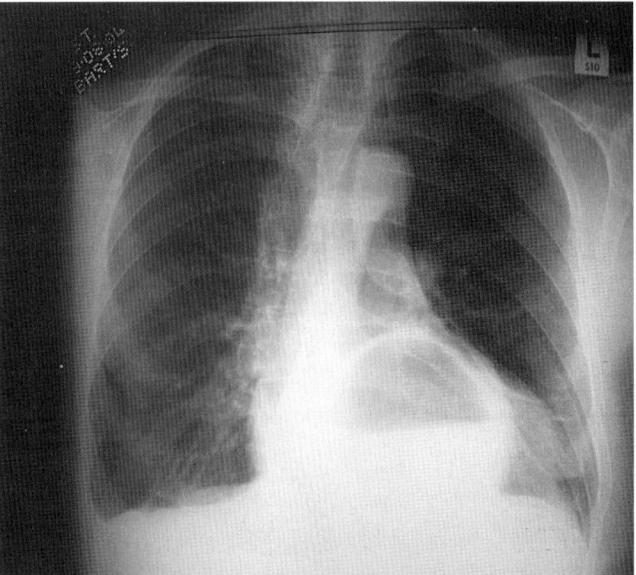

Figure 59.35 A gas bubble seen on a plain chest radiograph, showing the fundus of the stomach in the chest. Courtesy of Dr Stephen Ellis, Barts and the London NHS Trust.

causes the pain, followed by operative repair. If the pain is not relieved or perforation is suspected, immediate operation is mandatory.

Emergency surgery needs to be tailored to the problem encountered and the fitness of the patient. Elective surgery involves reduction of the hernia, excision of the sac, reducing the crural defect and some form of retention of the stomach in the abdomen. Some surgeons perform a fundoplication, arguing that this is a very effective means of maintaining reduction and that it deals with the associated GORD. Others argue that fundoplication should only be done if reflux can be conclusively demonstrated beforehand. Surprisingly, both philosophies achieve good results. Laparoscopic repair has recently become popular. Full anatomical repair of a large rolling hernia can be difficult by this approach and requires considerable expertise. Secure closure of the hiatal defect can be a problem, and some surgeons advocate mesh to reinforce the repair.

NEOPLASMS OF THE OESOPHAGUS

Benign tumours

Benign tumours of the oesophagus are relatively rare. True papillomas, adenomas and hyperplastic polyps do occur, but the majority of 'benign' tumours are not epithelial in origin and arise from other layers of the oesophageal wall [gastrointestinal stromal tumour (GIST), lipoma, granular cell tumour]. Most benign oesophageal tumours are small and asymptomatic, and even a large benign tumour may cause only mild symptoms (Fig. 59.36). The most important point in their management is usually to carry out an adequate number of biopsies to prove beyond reasonable doubt that the lesion is not malignant (Fig. 59.37).

Malignant tumours

Non-epithelial primary malignancies are also rare, as is malignant melanoma. Secondary malignancies rarely involve the oesophagus with the exception of bronchogenic carcinoma by direct invasion of either the primary and/or contiguous lymph nodes.

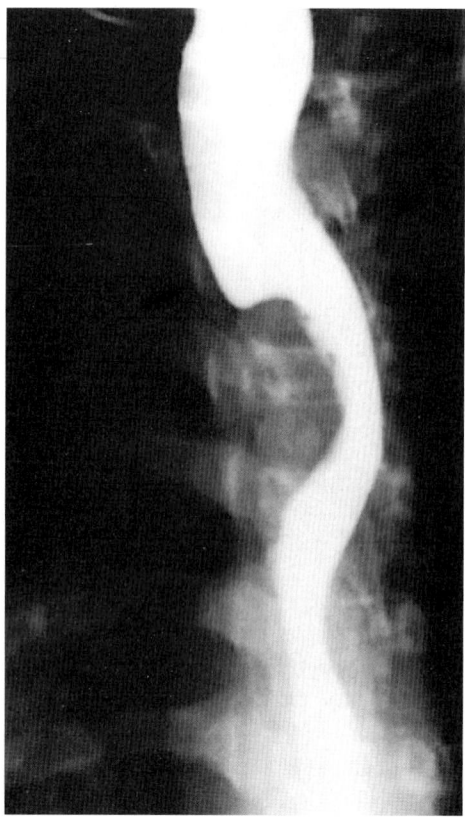

Figure 59.36 Classic appearance of a large oesophageal gastro-intestinal stromal tumour on barium swallow.

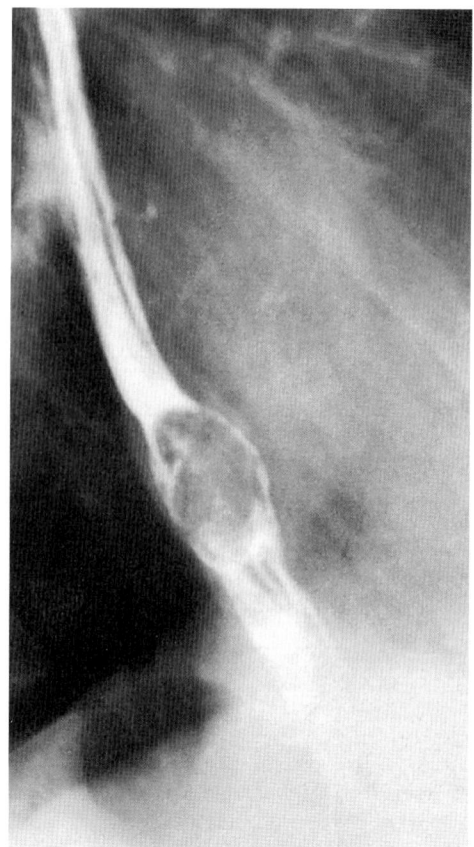

Figure 59.37 An intraluminal polyp that proved to be a leiomyosar-coma.

Carcinoma of the oesophagus

Cancer of the oesophagus is the sixth most common cancer in the world. In general, it is a disease of mid to late adulthood, with a poor survival rate. Only 5–10% of those diagnosed will survive for 5 years (Summary box 59.11).

Summary box 59.11

Carcinoma of the oesophagus

- Squamous cell usually affects the upper two-thirds; adenocarcinoma usually affects the lower third
- Common aetiological factors are tobacco and alcohol (squamous cell) and GORD (adenocarcinoma)
- The incidence of adenocarcinoma is increasing
- Lymph node involvement is a bad prognostic factor
- Dysphagia is the most common presenting symptom, but is a late feature
- Accurate pretreatment staging is essential in patients thought to be fit to undergo 'curative' treatment

---

Pathology and aetiology

Squamous cell cancer (Figs 59.38 and 59.39) and adenocarcinoma (Figs 59.40 and 59.41) are the most common types. Squamous cell carcinoma generally affects the upper two-thirds of the oesophagus and adenocarcinoma the lower one-third. Worldwide, squamous cell cancer is most common, but adeno-carcinoma predominates in the west and is increasing in incidence.

Geographical variation in oesophageal cancer

The incidence of oesophageal cancer varies more than that of any other cancer. Squamous cell cancer is endemic in the Transkei region of South Africa and in the Asian 'cancer belt' that extends across the middle of Asia from the shores of the Caspian Sea (in northern Iran) to China. The highest incidence in the world is in Linxian in Henan province in China, where it is the most common single cause of death, with more than 100 cases per 100 000 population per annum. The cause of the disease in the endemic areas is not known, but it is probably due to a combination of fungal contamination of food and nutritional deficiencies. In Linxian, supplementation of the diet with beta-carotene, vitamin E and selenium has been shown to reduce the incidence.

Away from the endemic areas, tobacco and alcohol are major factors in the occurrence of squamous cancer. Incidence rates vary from less than 5:100 000 in white people in the USA to 26.5:100 000 in some regions of France.

In many western countries, the incidence of squamous cell cancer has fallen or remained static, but the incidence of adeno-carcinoma of the oesophagus has increased dramatically since the mid-1970s at a rate of 5–10% per annum. The change is greater than that of any other neoplasm in this time. Adenocarcinoma now accounts for 60–75% of all oesophageal cancers in several countries. The reason for this change is not understood. A similar rate of increase in GORD over the same period, which mirrors an increase in obesity in the west, is likely to be an important factor, particularly through the link to Barrett's oesophagus.

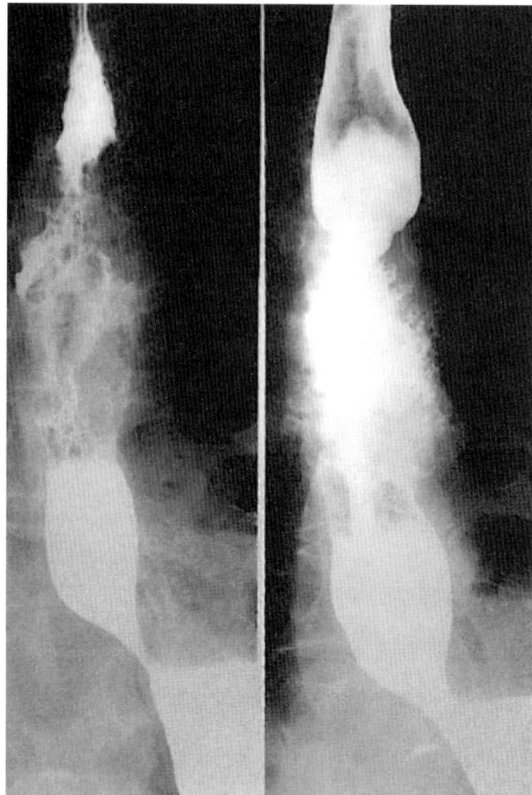

Figure 59.38 The classic appearances of a mid-oesophageal proliferative squamous cell carcinoma.

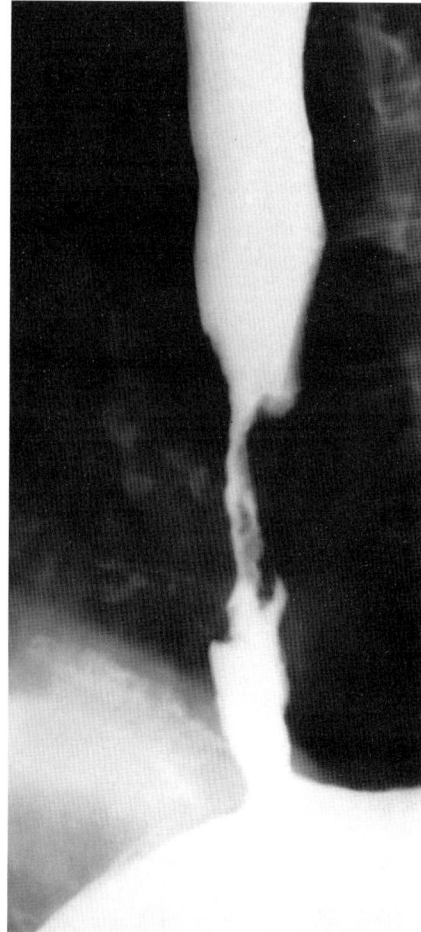

Figure 59.39 Squamous cell carcinoma of the oesophagus producing an irregular stricture with shouldered margins.

There has been a similar increase in the incidence of carcinoma of the cardia of the stomach, which suggests that cancer of the cardia and adenocarcinoma of the oesophagus may share common aetiological factors. With a falling incidence of cancer in the rest of the stomach, more than 60% of all upper gastrointestinal cancers in the west involve the cardia or distal oesophagus.

Both adenocarcinomas and squamous cell carcinomas tend to disseminate early. Sadly, the classical presenting symptoms of dysphagia, regurgitation and weight loss are often absent until the primary tumour has become advanced, and so the tumour is often well established before the diagnosis is made. Tumours can spread in three ways: invasion directly through the oesophageal wall, via lymphatics or in the bloodstream. Direct spread occurs both laterally, through the component layers of the oesophageal wall, and longitudinally within the oesophageal wall. Longitudinal spread is mainly via the submucosal lymphatic channels of the oesophagus. The pattern of lymphatic drainage is therefore not segmental, as in other parts of the gastrointestinal tract. Consequently, the length of oesophagus involved by tumour is frequently much longer than the macroscopic length of the malignancy at the epithelial surface. Lymph node spread occurs commonly. Although the direction of spread to regional lymphatics is predominantly caudal, the involvement of lymph nodes is potentially widespread and can also occur in a cranial direction. Any regional lymph node from the superior mediastinum to the coeliac axis and lesser curve of the stomach may be involved regardless of the location of the primary lesion within the oesophagus. Haematogenous spread may involve a variety of different organs including the liver, lungs, brain and bones. Tumours arising from the intra-abdominal portion of the oesophagus may also disseminate transperitoneally.

Clinical features

Most oesophageal neoplasms present with mechanical symptoms, principally dysphagia, but sometimes also regurgitation, vomiting, odynophagia and weight loss. Clinical findings suggestive of advanced malignancy include recurrent laryngeal nerve palsy, Horner's syndrome, chronic spinal pain and diaphragmatic paralysis. Other factors making surgical cure unlikely include weight loss of more than 20% and loss of appetite. Cutaneous tumour metastases or enlarged supraclavicular lymph nodes may be seen on clinical examination and indicate disseminated disease. Hoarseness due to recurrent laryngeal nerve palsy is a sign of advanced and incurable disease. Palpable lymphadenopathy in the neck is likewise a sign of advanced disease.

Patients with early disease may have non-specific dyspeptic symptoms or a vague feeling of 'something that is not quite right' during swallowing. Some are diagnosed during endoscopic surveillance of patients with Barrett's oesophagus and, while this does identify patients with the earliest stages of disease, such

Johann Friedrich Horner, 1831–1886, Professor of Ophthalmology, Zurich, Switzerland, described this syndrome in 1869.

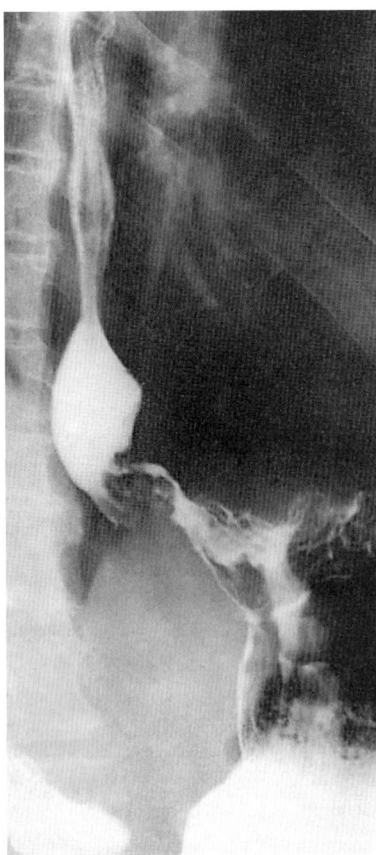

Figure 59.40 Adenocarcinoma of the lower oesophagus, spreading upwards from the cardia.

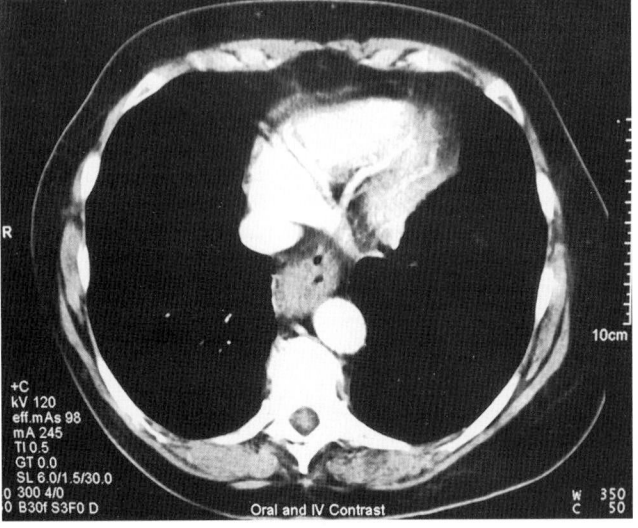

Figure 59.41 Computerised tomography scan showing a primary tumour of the lower oesophagus.

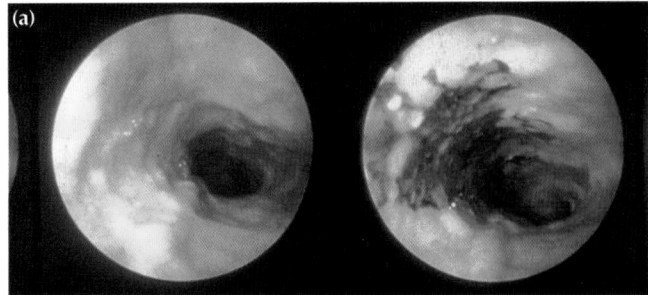

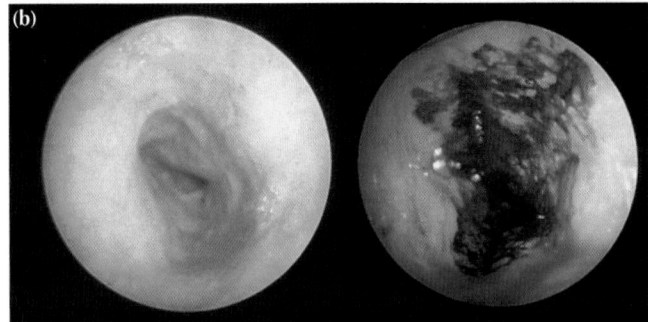

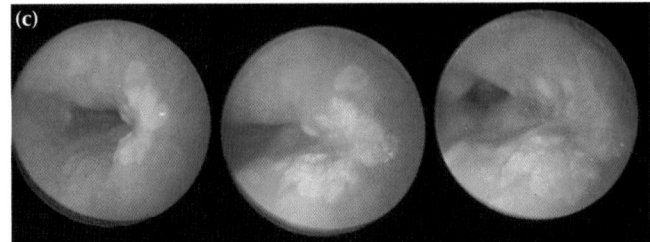

Figure 59.42 Carcinoma *in situ* showing the varied presentations: (a) occult form; (b) erythroplakia; (c) leucoplakia. The right-hand pictures in (a) and (b) demonstrate the use of vital staining with methylene blue.

programmes have little overall impact, as most patients with Barrett's oesophagus are unknown to the medical profession and make their first presentation with a symptomatic and therefore usually locally advanced oesophageal cancer. The widespread use of endoscopy as a diagnostic tool does nevertheless provide an opportunity for early diagnosis (Fig. 59.42). Biopsies should be taken of all lesions in the oesophagus (Figs 59.43 and 59.44), no matter how trivial they appear and irrespective of the indication for the examination.

Investigation

Endoscopy is the first-line investigation for most patients. It provides an unrivalled direct view of the oesophageal mucosa and any lesion allowing its site and size to be documented. Cytology and/or histology specimens taken via the endoscope are crucial for accurate diagnosis. The combination of histology and cytology increases the diagnostic accuracy to more than 95%. The chief limitation of conventional endoscopy is that only the mucosal surface can be studied and biopsied. Other investigations are therefore usually required to define the extent of local or distant spread. The improved image resolution of modern endoscopes and novel techniques involving magnification and the use of dyes to enhance surface detail may lead to more early lesions being recognised (see Fig 59.42).

General assessment and staging

Once the initial diagnosis of a malignant oesophageal neoplasm has been made, patients should be assessed first in terms of their general health and fitness for potential therapies. Their preferences should also be considered. Most potentially curative therapies

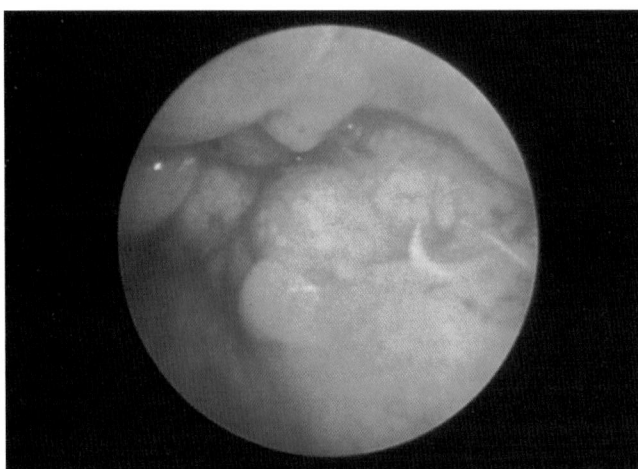

Figure 59.43 Endoscopic appearances of a mid-oesophageal squamous cell carcinoma.

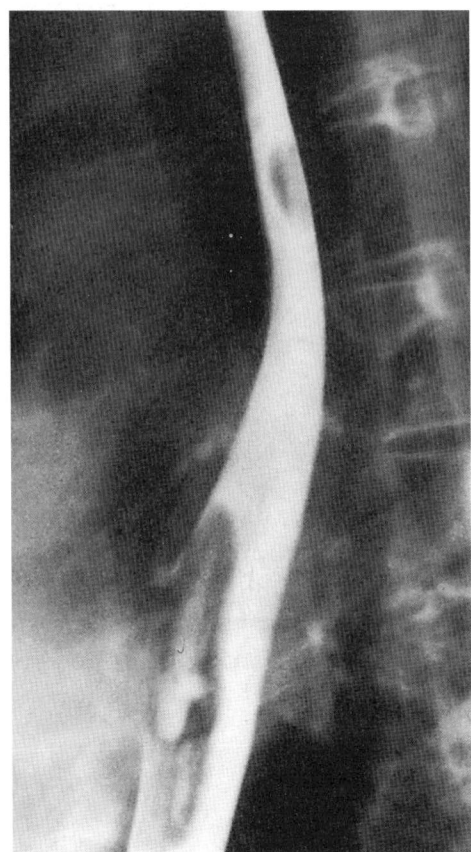

Figure 59.44 Beware the differential diagnosis of infection, for what appears to be a tumour. This mid-oesophageal mass was actually tuberculosis.

include radical surgery, although chemoradiotherapy is an alternative in squamous cell carcinoma. Patients who are unfit for, or who do not wish to contemplate, radical treatments should not be investigated further, but should be diverted to appropriate palliative therapies, depending on symptoms and current quality of life. Only those patients suitable for potentially curative therapies should proceed to staging investigations to rule out haematogenous spread

and then to assess locoregional stage [endoscopic ultrasound (EUS) ± laparoscopy]. This will distinguish between early (T1/T2, N0) and advanced lesions (T3/T4, N1) and indicate whether surgery alone or multimodal therapy is most appropriate. Where attempted cure is deemed possible, the aim should be to provide the best chance of cure while minimising perioperative risks. In general, surgery alone should be reserved for patients with early disease, and multimodal therapy should be used in patients with locally advanced disease, in whom the chance of cure by surgery alone is small (generally less than 20%).

The most widely used pathological staging system is the World Health Organization (tumour–nodes–metastasis TNM) classification.

Table 59.2 shows the TNM system for oesophageal cancer in its most updated form. Like all pathological systems, it is reliant on the nature and extent of the surgery performed. For example, performing more extensive radical surgical lymphadenectomy provides a more accurate assessment of the 'N' stage. There is evidence that many patients described as N0 in the past were probably N1, a phenomenon described as stage migration.

Staging information may be gathered before the commencement of therapy, during therapy (e.g. at open operation) or following treatment (histology or post-mortem). The techniques commonly used to provide preoperative staging data are described in Figure 59.45, along with a suggested algorithm.

Blood tests

These are of limited value. Blood tests reveal nothing about local invasion or regional lymph node spread and, to date, no reliable tumour marker for oesophageal cancer has been isolated from peripheral blood. The presence of abnormal liver function tests (LFTs) may suggest the presence of liver metastases, but this is generally too insensitive to be diagnostic. Many patients with known liver metastases have normal LFTs. At best, abnormal LFTs only reinforce the clinical suspicion of spread to the liver, and further imaging is usually required to confirm the diagnosis.

Transcutaneous ultrasound

It is difficult to visualise mediastinal structures with transcutaneous ultrasound. With the relatively low-frequency sound waves

Table 59.2 TNM staging scheme for oesophageal cancer

Tis	High-grade dysplasia
T1	Tumour invading lamina propria or submucosa
T2	Tumour invading muscularis propria
T3	Tumour invading beyond muscularis propria
T4	Tumour invading adjacent structures
Tx	Primary tumour cannot be assessed
N0	No regional lymph node metastases
N1	Regional lymph node metastases
Nx	Lymph nodes cannot be assessed
M0	No distant metastases
M1(a)	Coeliac node involved (for distal oesophageal tumours) Supraclavicular node involved (for proximal tumours)
M1(b)	Coeliac or supraclavicular node involved if not remote from tumour site (i.e. not 1a) All other distant metastases
Mx	Distant metastases cannot be assessed

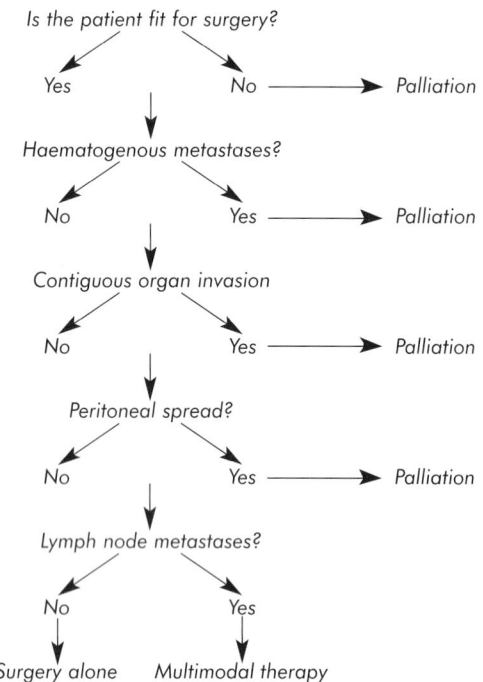

Is the patient fit for surgery?

Yes | No → Palliation

Haematogenous metastases?

No | Yes → Palliation

Contiguous organ invasion

No | Yes → Palliation

Peritoneal spread?

No | Yes → Palliation

Lymph node metastases?

No | Yes

Surgery alone | Multimodal therapy

Figure 59.45 Algorithm for the management of oesophageal cancer.

used, good depth of tissue penetration is achieved at the expense of poor image resolution. In addition, the mediastinal organs are surrounded by bone and air, which renders them largely inaccessible to external ultrasound. The technique is therefore used mainly to assess spread to the liver, the whole of which can be clearly visualised by standard transcutaneous ultrasound. Haematogenous spread can be more fully assessed by combining ultrasound with chest radiography, although this combination is less accurate than CT scanning.

Bronchoscopy

Many middle- and upper-third oesophageal carcinomas (and therefore usually squamous carcinomas) are sufficiently advanced at the time of diagnosis that the trachea or bronchi are already involved (Fig. 59.46). Bronchoscopy may reveal either impingement or invasion of the main airways in over 30% of new patients with cancers in the upper third of the oesophagus. In some cases, therefore, bronchoscopy alone can confirm that the tumour is locally unresectable.

Laparoscopy

This is a useful technique for the diagnosis of intra-abdominal and hepatic metastases. It has the advantage of enabling tissue samples or peritoneal cytology to be obtained and is the only modality reliably able to detect peritoneal tumour seedlings (Fig. 59.47). This is particularly important for tumours arising from the intra-abdominal portion of the oesophagus, cardia and where there is a potential communication between a full-thickness tumour and the peritoneal cavity, for instance where there is a hiatus hernia.

Computerised tomography

CT scanning is the modality most used to identify haematogenous metastases (Fig. 59.48). Distant organs are easily seen and metastases within them visualised with high accuracy (94–100%). The normal thoracic oesophagus is easily demonstrated by CT scanning. The mediastinal fat planes are usually clearly imaged in healthy individuals, and any blurring or distortion of these images is a fairly reliable indicator of abnormality. In cachectic patients with dysphagia and malnutrition, the mediastinal fat plane may be virtually absent, making local invasion difficult to assess. Spiral and thin-slice CT permit structures such as lymph nodes to be adequately imaged, down to a minimum diameter of about 5 mm. Smaller nodes cannot be reliably visualised, and it is not possible to distinguish between enlarged lymph nodes that have reactive changes only and metastatic nodes. Similarly, micrometastases within normal-sized nodes cannot be detected.

Magnetic resonance imaging scanning

Magnetic resonance imaging (MRI) does not expose the patient to ionising radiation and needs no intravascular contrast medium, although intraoesophageal air or contrast media may help to assess wall thickness. Distant metastases to organs such as the

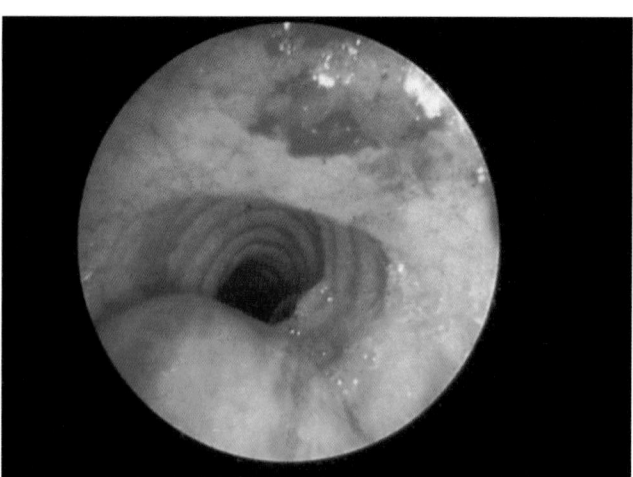

Figure 59.46 Invasion into the posterior wall of the trachea from an oesophageal carcinoma.

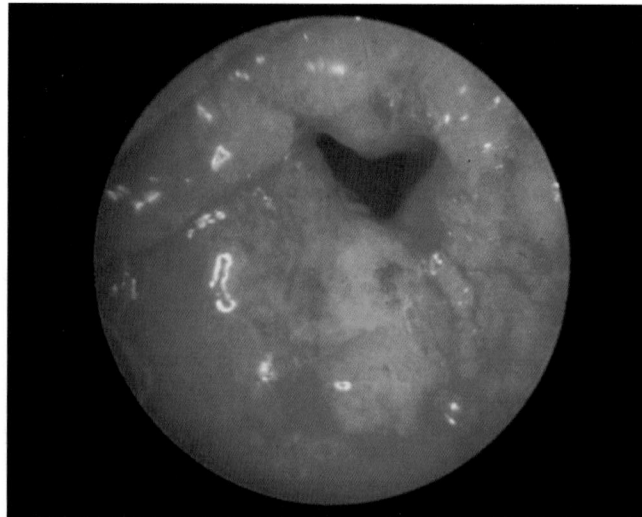

Figure 59.47 Adenocarcinoma of the cardia. Transcoelomic spread may occur with this type of lesion.

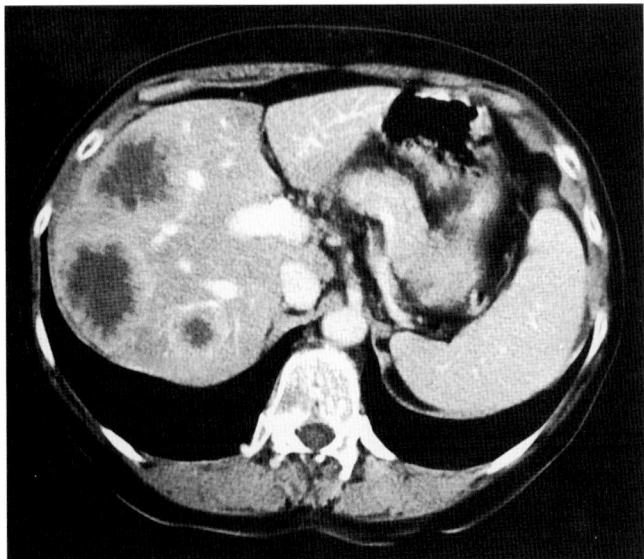

Figure 59.48 Computerised tomography scan demonstrating liver metastases.

liver are usually reliably identified by MRI but, at the moment, there do not seem to be additional benefits over CT.

Endoscopic ultrasound

After haematogenous spread, the two principal prognostic factors for oesophageal cancer are the depth of tumour penetration through the oesophageal wall and regional lymph node spread. Although CT will detect distant metastasis, its limited axial resolution precludes a reliable assessment of both the depth of wall penetration and lymph node involvement. EUS can determine the depth of spread of a malignant tumour through the oesophageal wall (T1–3), the invasion of adjacent organs (T4) and metastasis to lymph nodes (N0 or N1) (Figs 59.49–59.51). It can also detect contiguous spread downward into the cardia and more distant metastases to the left lobe of the liver.

EUS visualises the oesophageal wall as a multilayered structure. The layers represent ultrasound interfaces rather than true anatomical layers, but there is close enough correlation to allow

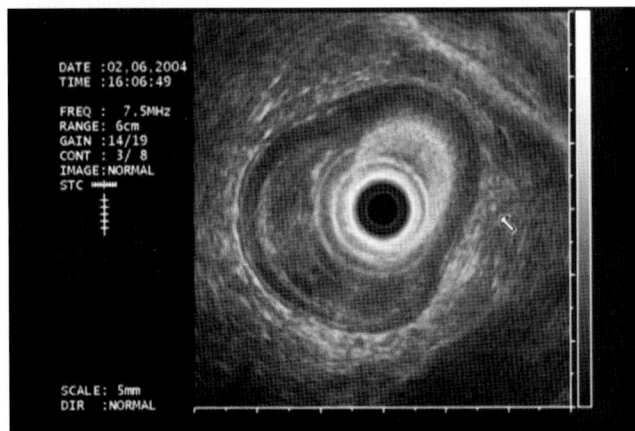

Figure 59.49 Endosonography demonstrating an 'early' tumour. Note the preservation of the outer dark wall layer that represents the muscle coat.

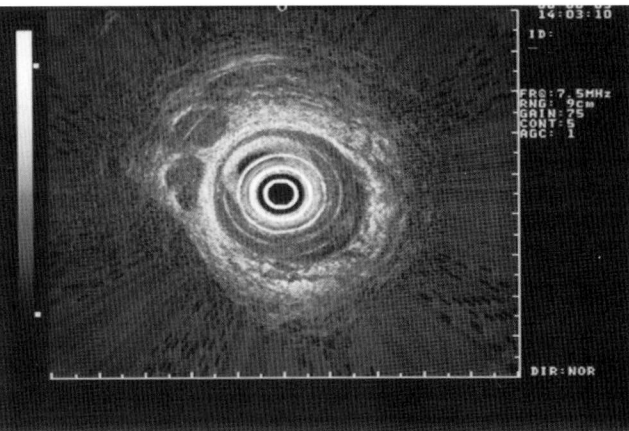

Figure 59.50 Endosonography demonstrating an 'advanced' local tumour. Note the breach of the outer white line that represents the interface between the oesophageal wall and the mediastinum.

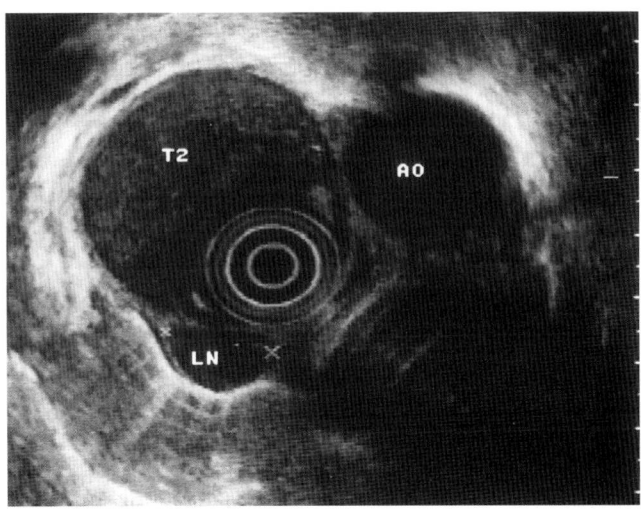

Figure 59.51 Endosonography demonstrating malignant nodes. These are usually large, hypoechoic and round compared with normal nodes.

accurate assessment of the depth of invasion through the oesophageal wall. Structures smaller than 5 mm can be clearly seen enabling very small nodes to be imaged. The EUS image morphology of such structures provides an additional means of distinguishing malignant from reactive or benign lymph nodes. For submucosal lesions, EUS can demonstrate the wall layer of origin of a lesion, suggesting the likely histological type.

Narrow EUS instruments are available for insertion over a guidewire to minimise the risk of technical failure, and linear array echoendoscopes can be used to biopsy lesions that might signify incurability outside the wall of the gastrointestinal tract (e.g. coeliac lymph nodes).

Positron emission tomography/computerised tomography scanning

Positron emission tomography (PET) in the context of cancer staging relies on the generally high metabolic activity (particularly in the glycolytic pathway) of tumours compared with normal tissues. The patient is given a small dose of the radiopharmaceutical agent ¹⁸F-fluorodeoxyglucose (FDG). This enters cells and is phosphorylated. FDG-6-phosphate cannot be metabolised further and, because it is a highly polar molecule, it cannot easily diffuse back out of the cell. After intravenous injection of FDG, it continuously accumulates in metabolically active cells. Primary oesophageal cancers are usually sufficiently active to be easily visible, and spatial resolution of positive PET areas occurs down to about 5–8 mm. When used in isolation, there are problems with the anatomical location of these areas. This has been significantly improved by combining PET with CT (Fig. 59.52). Although there are wide variations between centres, a change in stage is frequently reported in around 15% of patients. It has also been suggested that a reduction in PET activity following chemotherapy might be a way of predicting 'responders' to this approach.

Treatment of malignant tumours

Principles

At the time of diagnosis, around two-thirds of all patients with oesophageal cancer will already have incurable disease. The aim of palliative treatment is to overcome debilitating or distressing symptoms while maintaining the best quality of life possible for the patient. Some patients do not require specific therapeutic interventions, but do need supportive care and appropriate liaison with community nursing and hospice care services.

As dysphagia is the predominant symptom in advanced oesophageal cancer, the principal aim of palliation is to restore adequate swallowing. A variety of methods are available and, given the short life expectancy of most patients, it is important that the choice of treatment should be tailored to each individual. Tumour location and endoscopic appearance are important in this regard, as is the general condition of the patient.

Once oesophageal neoplasms reach the submucosal layer of the oesophagus, the tumour has access to the lymphatic system, meaning that, even at this early local stage, there is an incidence of nodal positivity for both squamous cell carcinoma and adenocarcinomas of between 10% and 50%. The principle of oesophagectomy is to deal adequately with the local tumour in order to minimise the risk of local recurrence and achieve an adequate lymphadenectomy to reduce the risk of staging error. Although studies in Japan would indicate that more extensive lymphadenectomy is associated with better survival, this may simply reflect more accurate staging. A number of studies support the view that the proximal extent of resection should ideally be 10 cm above the macroscopic tumour and 5 cm distal. When such a margin cannot be achieved proximally, particularly with

squamous cell carcinoma, there is evidence that postoperative radiotherapy can minimise local recurrence, although not improve survival.

Adenocarcinoma commonly involves the gastric cardia and may therefore extend into the fundus or down the lesser curve. Some degree of gastric excision is essential in order to achieve adequate local clearance and accomplish an appropriate lymphadenectomy. Excision of contiguous structures, such as crura, diaphragm and mediastinal pleura, needs to be considered as a method of creating negative resection margins.

The rarity of intramucosal cancer in symptomatic patients means that there are no randomised studies to compare different approaches to this type of very early disease. Even in Barrett's oesophagus, where high-grade dysplasia and early cancer coexist, most centres favour oesophagectomy in fit patients. Photodynamic therapy (PDT) is an alternative approach that has largely been used in patients who were either unfit or unwilling to undergo surgery. This endoscopic technique relies on the administration of a photosensitiser that is taken up preferentially by dysplastic and malignant cells followed by exposure of an appropriate segment of the oesophagus to laser light. The main drawback is skin photosensitisation, so patients must avoid sunlight exposure in the short term. PDT is also associated with a risk of stricture formation although, as the technique and photosensitising agents improve, these problems are reducing.

Surgery alone is best suited to patients with disease confined to the oesophagus (T1, T2) without nodal metastasis (N0). As a result of careful preoperative investigation, most of these patients are now identifiable and can be offered surgery alone, with a prospect of cure in between 50% and 80%. Patients with more advanced stages of disease require either multimodal approaches or entry into appropriate trials.

It is essential that oesophagectomy should be performed with a low hospital mortality and complication rate. Case selection, volume and experience of the surgical team are all important. Preoperative risk analysis has shown that this can play a major part in reducing hospital mortality. There are really no circumstances in the western world in which surgery should be undertaken if it is not part of an overall treatment plan aimed at cure (Summary box 59.12).

Summary box 59.12

Treatment of carcinoma of the oesophagus

- Radical oesophagectomy is the most important aspect of curative treatment
- Neoadjuvant treatments before surgery may improve survival in a proportion of patients
- Chemoradiotherapy alone may cure selected patients, particularly those with squamous cell cancers
- Useful palliation may be achieved by chemo/radiotherapy or endoscopic treatments

---

Treatments with curative intent

Surgery

Histological tumour type, location and the extent of the proposed lymphadenectomy all influence the operative approach. This is largely an issue of surgical preference, although it should be recognised that a left thoracoabdominal approach is limited proximally by the aortic arch and should be avoided when the primary

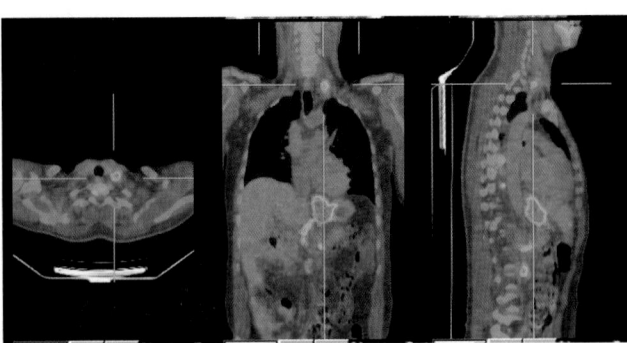

Figure 59.52 Positron emission tomography/computerised tomography demonstrating a primary tumour and a distant metastatic node.

tumour is at or above this level. Similarly, transhiatal oesophagectomy is unsuitable for most patients with squamous cell carcinoma because a complete mediastinal lymphadenectomy is not easily achieved by this approach. The most widely practised approach in the west is the two-phase Ivor Lewis (sometimes called Lewis–Tanner) operation (Fig. 59.53), with an initial laparotomy and construction of a gastric tube, followed by a right thoracotomy to excise the tumour and create an oesophagogastric anastomosis. The closer this is placed to the apex of the thoracic cavity, the fewer problems there are with reflux disease. Three-phase oesophagectomy (McKeown) may be more appropriate for more proximal tumours in order to achieve better longitudinal clearance, although the additional distance gained is less than many surgeons believe. A third cervical incision also permits lymphadenectomy in this region.

The extent of lymphadenectomy is highly controversial. For squamous cell carcinoma, because a higher proportion of patients will have middle- and upper-third tumours in the thoracic oesophagus, the rationale behind a three-phase operation with three-field lymphadenectomy is more understandable, even though this approach has not been widely adopted in the west. For adenocarcinoma, the incidence of metastases in the neck is relatively low in the context of patients who would otherwise be curable. For this reason, two-phase operations with two-field lymphadenectomy seem the most logical operations. While two-field lymphadenectomy does not substantially increase operative morbidity or mortality, the same cannot be said for more extended operations.

The introduction of minimal access techniques has been

pioneered in Australia by Gotley and Smithers and in North America by Luketich. In experienced hands, the open operation can be reproduced without significant compromise. As yet, benefits seem to be confined to reduced wound pain and the absence of specific complications associated with long incisions.

While many centres have reduced hospital mortality to single figures following oesophagectomy, the complication rate remains high. At least one-third of all patients will develop some significant complication after surgery. The most common of these is respiratory, followed by anastomotic leakage, chylothorax and injury to the recurrent laryngeal nerves. The most common late problem is benign anastomotic stricture, which seems to be higher with cervical rather than with intrathoracic anastomoses, although the problem is usually easily dealt with by endoscopic dilatation.

Lesions of the cardia that do not involve the oesophagus to any significant extent may be dealt with by extended total gastrectomy to include the distal oesophagus, or by proximal gastrectomy and distal oesophagectomy (Summary box 59.13).

> **Summary box 59.13**
>
> ### Oesophagogastric surgery
>
> - Beware of satellite nodules proximal to the primary lesion
> - Carefully preserve the blood supply of the stomach, both venous and arterial
> - Right thoracic approach gives easy access to the oesophagus

Two-phase oesophagectomy (abdomen and right chest, Ivor Lewis)

Mobilisation of the stomach must be done with care as it is essential to have a tension-free, well-vascularised stomach for transposition. The left gastric, short gastric and left gastroepiploic arteries are all divided. The viability of the transposed stomach mainly depends on the right gastroepiploic and, to a lesser extent, the right gastric vessels. It should be noted that venous drainage is as important as arterial supply, and it is essential to perform an accurate anatomical dissection that preserves the right gastroepiploic vein as well as the artery. The stomach is divided to remove the cardia and the upper part of the lesser curve, including the whole of the left gastric artery and its associated lymph nodes.

The approach to the oesophagus through the right chest is straightforward. A thoracotomy with entry above the fifth rib gives excellent access to the mediastinum and the thoracic inlet. The azygos vein is divided, and the whole of the intrathoracic oesophagus can be mobilised along with the thoracic duct (which is ligated by most surgeons) and the mediastinal lymph nodes. The oesophagus is divided just below the thoracic inlet. As most lesions are in the lower or middle thirds, this usually gives adequate proximal clearance of at least 5 cm. Carcinomas of the upper thoracic oesophagus are almost always incurable at the time of diagnosis, and invasion of the trachea is common. If one of these lesions is resectable, it is essential to use an incision in the neck (McKeown or three-phase operation) and to resect more of the oesophagus than is customary in the operation of subtotal oesophagectomy.

Oesophagogastric anastomosis may be performed equally well by hand or by stapler. Both methods require attention to detail. In experienced hands, clinical anastomotic leakage should be less than 5%. Most surgeons still prefer to keep the patient

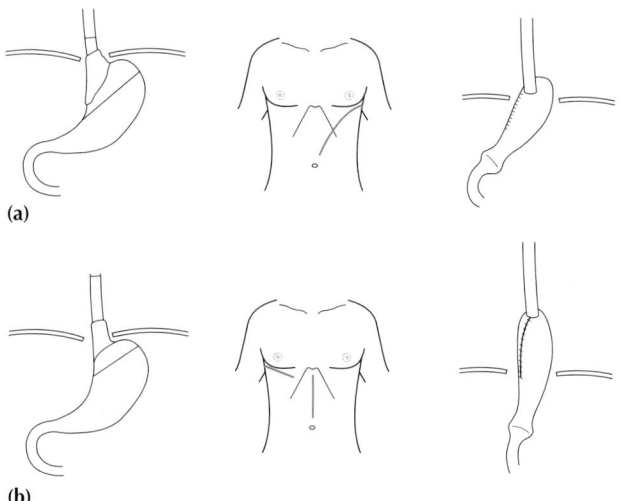

(a)

(b)

Figure 59.53 The two usual approaches for surgery of the oesophagus are the thoracoabdominal (a), which opens the abdominal and thoracic cavities together, and the two-stage Ivor Lewis approach (b), in which the abdomen is opened first, closed and then the thoracotomy is performed. In the McKeown operation, a third incision in the neck is made to complete the cervical anastomosis.

Ivor Lewis, 1895–1982, Surgeon, The North Middlesex Hospital, London, England, and later at Rhyl, North Wales.
Norman Cecil Tanner, 1906–1982, Surgeon, Charing Cross Hospital, London, England.
Kenneth Charles McKeown, 1912–1995, Surgeon, Darlington Memorial Hospital, Darlington, County Durham, England.

nil-by-mouth for 5–7 days. Most centres have abandoned the use of routine contrast swallows in patients who are clinically well. Conversely, aggressive investigation of a suspected leak is mandatory for any unexplained fever or clinical event. This may involve contrast radiology, CT scan or endoscopy to resolve the situation adequately.

Postoperative nutritional support remains controversial. There is general agreement that parenteral feeding is associated with more nosocomial infection, including pneumonia, than enteral feeding. It is also expensive. If nutritional support is given, a feeding jejunostomy is probably the best method.

Transhiatal oesophagectomy (without thoracotomy)

This approach was popularised for cancer by Orringer, adapting a technique developed in Brazil by Pinotti for the removal of Chagasic megaoesophagus (see the section on Achalasia, p. 1036). The stomach is mobilised through a midline abdominal incision, and the cervical oesophagus is mobilised through an incision in the neck. The diaphragm is then opened from the abdomen, and the posterior mediastinum is entered. The lower oesophagus and the tumour are mobilised under direct vision, and the upper oesophagus is mobilised by blunt dissection. This approach can provide an adequate removal of the tumour and lymph nodes in the lower mediastinum, but it is not possible to remove the nodes in the middle or upper mediastinum. It may be a useful procedure for lesions of the lower oesophagus, but is hazardous for a middle third lesion that may be adherent to the bronchus or to the azygos vein.

Neoadjuvant treatments with surgery

Apart from the earliest stages of disease, surgery alone produces relatively few cures in either squamous cell carcinoma or adenocarcinoma patients. This led to a number of trials throughout the 1980s and 1990s to investigate the value of chemotherapy and surgery or chemoradiotherapy and surgery compared with surgery alone. Some studies relate only to squamous cell cancer, and many are open to criticism on the grounds of trial design or patient numbers. Nevertheless, positive results in favour of neoadjuvant therapy for adenocarcinoma in two studies as well as a limited meta-analysis indicate that it is no longer appropriate to consider surgery alone as the 'gold standard' treatment for most patients who are surgical candidates with adenocarcinoma. The exact role of surgery in a multimodal approach to squamous cell carcinoma is an unresolved issue.

Gastro-oesophageal reflux following oesophagogastric resection

Gastro-oesophageal reflux may be a major problem following any operation that involves resecting the cardia. Reflux may present with the typical symptoms of GORD or with a peptic stricture at the site of the anastomosis. However, the presentation may be different with a miserable patient who fails to thrive following the operation and who is then suspected of having recurrent cancer. This atypical presentation is particularly common following total gastrectomy with an inadequate reconstruction that allows bile reflux (Summary box 59.14).

Mark Burton Orringer, **Surgeon**, Ann Arbor, MI, USA.
Walter Pinotti, **Professor of Surgery**, Sao Paulo, Brazil.
Carlos Justiniano Ribeiro Chagas, **1879–1934**, Director the Oswaldo Cruz Institute, and Professor of Tropical Medicine, The University of Rio de Janeiro, Brazil.

Summary box 59.14

Post oesophagectomy

- Reflux may be a problem following resection
- Symptoms may be atypical
- Reflux may be limited or avoided by subtotal oesophagectomy and gastric transposition high in the chest

Non-surgical treatments

Radiotherapy alone was widely used as a single-modality treatment for squamous cell carcinoma of the oesophagus until the late 1970s. The 5-year survival overall was 6%. As a result, multimodal approaches were adopted throughout the 1980s, initial trials indicating that similar long-term survival rates could be obtained with surgery. Subsequent randomised studies essentially confined to patients with squamous cell carcinoma have indicated significant survival advantages with chemoradiotherapy over radiotherapy alone. While it is clear that chemoradiotherapy does offer a prospect of cure for patients who may not be fit for surgery, particularly in squamous cell carcinoma, the high rate of locoregional failure has meant that surgery remains the mainstay of attempted curative treatments for both adenocarcinoma and squamous cell carcinoma in patients who have potentially resectable disease and are fit for oesophagectomy. In most western series, this represents about one-third of patients with adenocarcinoma and a slightly lower percentage of patients with squamous cell carcinoma. There has been no formal comparison of the results of radiotherapy and surgical resection, and it is therefore impossible to make dogmatic statements about the relative merits of each form of treatment (Summary box 59.15).

Summary box 59.15

Alternative therapeutic approaches

- Chemoradiotherapy may be a useful alternative to surgery, especially in unfit patients

Palliative treatment

Surgical resection and external beam radiotherapy may be used for palliation, but are not suitable when the expected survival is short, as most of the remainder of life will be spent recovering from the 'treatment'. Surgical bypass is likewise too major a procedure for use in a patient with limited life expectancy. A variety of relatively simple methods of palliation are now available that will produce worthwhile relief of dysphagia with minimal disturbance to the patient (Summary box 59.16).

Summary box 59.16

Palliation should be simple and effective

Intubation has been used for many years following the invention of the Souttar tube, which was made of coiled silver wire. A variety

Sir Henry Sessions Souttar, **1875–1964**, Surgeon, The London Hospital, London, England.

of rigid plastic or rubber tubes were developed for placement under endoscopic and/or radiological control. The technology of intubation has now moved on with the development of various types of expanding metal stent (Fig. 59.54). These are also inserted under radiographic or endoscopic control. The stent is collapsed during insertion and released when it is in the correct position. Expanding stents produce a wider lumen for swallowing than rigid tubes. More importantly, it is not necessary to dilate the oesophagus to beyond 8 mm to insert the unexpanded stent through the tumour, so there is a lower risk of injury to the oesophagus.

Endoscopic laser treatment may be used to core a channel through the tumour. It is based on thermal tumour destruction. It produces a worthwhile improvement in swallowing, but has the disadvantage that it has to be repeated every few weeks. Lasers may also be used to unblock a stent that has become occluded by tumour overgrowth. *Other endoscopic methods* include bipolar diathermy, argon-beam plasma coagulation and alcohol injection.

Brachytherapy is a method of delivering intraluminal radiation with a short penetration distance (hence the term brachy) to a tumour. An introduction system is inserted through the tumour, and the treatment is then delivered in a single session lasting approximately 20 min. The equipment is expensive to purchase, but running costs are low.

While the above methods are suitable for patients with very advanced disease, the elderly and those with significant comorbidities that would make more aggressive strategies inappropriate, an increasing proportion of patients (particularly with adenocarcinoma) are being treated by platinum-based chemotherapy. In general, this leads to only a modest prolongation of survival but a better quality of life than in those receiving an endoscopic treatment alone.

Malignant tracheo-oesophageal fistula

Malignant tracheo-oesophageal fistula is a sign of incurable disease. Some have advocated surgical bypass and oesophageal exclusion, but this is a major procedure. An expanding metal stent is probably the best treatment.

Post-cricoid carcinoma

Post-cricoid carcinoma is considered in Chapter 45 in neoplasms of the pharynx.

MOTILITY DISORDERS AND DIVERTICULA

Oesophageal motility disorders

A motility disorder can be readily understood when a patient has dysphagia in the absence of a stricture, and a barium-impregnated

food bolus is seen to stick in the oesophagus. If this can be correlated with a specific abnormality on oesophageal manometry, accepting that this is the cause of the patient's symptoms may be straightforward. Unfortunately, this is often not the case. Pain, with or without a swallowing problem, is frequently the dominant symptom, and patients often undergo extensive hospital investigation before the oesophagus is considered as a source of symptoms. Symptoms are often intermittent, and the correlation between symptoms and test 'abnormalities' is poor. Much harm may be done by inappropriate enthusiastic surgery for ill-defined conditions. It should also be remembered that oesophageal dysmotility may be only a feature of a general disturbance in gastrointestinal function (Summary box 59.17).

> **Summary box 59.17**
>
> ### Oesophageal motility disorders
>
> - May be part of a more diffuse gastrointestinal motility problem
> - May be associated with GORD

It is convenient to classify oesophageal motility disorders as in Table 59.3.

Functional pain and the oesophagus

Pain that is assumed to arise from dysfunction of the gastrointestinal tract may reflect abnormal motor activity, abnormal perception or a combination of the two. There is evidence that all three exist. Very high-pressure uncoordinated contractions ('spasm') have been shown to correlate with pain. Distension of a balloon in the oesophagus indicates that some patients have a low threshold for the sensation of pain (visceral hypersensitivity), and this itself may reflect local or central neuronal dysfunction. In practice, the difficulty is in understanding the relative

Table 59.3 Classification of oesophageal motility disorders

Disorders of the pharyngo-oesophageal junction
Neurological – stroke, motor neurone disease, multiple sclerosis, Parkinson's disease
Myogenic – myasthenia, muscular dystrophy
Pharyngo-oesophageal (Zenker's) diverticulum

Disorders of the body of the oesophagus
Diffuse oesophageal spasm
Nutcracker oesophagus

Autoimmune disorders – especially systemic sclerosis (CREST)
Reflux associated
Idiopathic

Allergic
Eosinophilic oesophagitis
Non-specific oesophageal dysmotility

Disorders of the lower oesophageal sphincter
Achalasia
Incompetent lower sphincter (i.e. GORD)

CREST, calcinosis, Raynaud's syndrome, (o)esophageal motility disorders, sclerodactyly and telangiectasia.
GORD, gastro-oesophageal reflux disease.

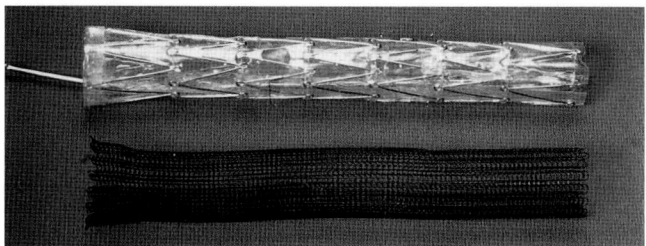

Figure 59.54 Expanding metal stents, covered and uncovered.

contributions of these elements, so that a logical treatment might follow.

Achalasia

Pathology and aetiology

Achalasia (Greek 'failure to relax') is uncommon, but merits prominence because it is reasonably understood and responds to treatment. It is due to loss of the ganglion cells in the myenteric (Auerbach's) plexus, the cause of which is unknown. In South America, chronic infection with the parasite *Trypanosoma cruzi* causes Chagas' disease, which has marked clinical similarities to achalasia. Achalasia differs from Hirschsprung's disease of the colon because the dilated oesophagus usually contains few ganglion cells, whereas the dilated colon contains normal ganglion cells proximal to a constricted, aganglionic segment. Histology of muscle specimens generally shows a reduction in the number of ganglion cells (and mainly inhibitory neurones) with a variable degree of chronic inflammation. In so called 'vigorous achalasia', which may be an early stage of the disease, there is inflammation and neural fibrosis, but normal numbers of ganglion cells (Summary box 59.18).

Summary box 59.18

Achalasia

- Is uncommon
- Is due to selective loss of inhibitory neurones in the lower oesophagus
- The causes dysphagia and carcinoma must be excluded
- Treatment is by either endoscopic dilatation or surgical myotomy

---

The physiological abnormalities are a non-relaxing LOS and absent peristalsis in the body of the oesophagus. In its earliest stages, the oesophagus is of normal calibre and still exhibits contractile (although non-peristaltic) activity. In some patients, these uncoordinated contractions result in pain as much as a sense of food sticking. With time, the oesophagus dilates and contractions disappear, so that the oesophagus empties mainly by the hydrostatic pressure of its contents. This is nearly always incomplete, leaving residual food and fluid. The gas bubble in the stomach is frequently absent, as no bolus with its accompanying normal gas passes through the sphincter. The 'megaoesophagus' becomes tortuous with a persistent retention oesophagitis due to fermentation of food residues (Fig. 59.55), and this may account for the increased incidence of carcinoma of the oesophagus (Summary box 59.19).

Summary box 59.19

Lower oesophageal stricture

- Beware pseudoachalasia; look for tumour

Pseudoachalasia is an achalasia-like disorder that is usually produced by adenocarcinoma of the cardia (Fig. 59.56), but has also

been described in relation to benign tumours at this level. It has been presumed that the inability of the sphincter to relax is linked to the loss of body peristalsis, but other cancers outside the oesophagus (bronchus, pancreas) have also been associated with pseudoachalasia.

Clinical features

The disease is most common in middle life, but can occur at any age. It typically presents with dysphagia, although pain (often mistaken for reflux) is common in the early stages. Patients often present late and, having had relatively mild symptoms, remain untreated for many years. Regurgitation is frequent, and there may be overspill into the trachea, especially at night.

Diagnosis

Achalasia may be suspected at endoscopy by finding a tight cardia and food residue in the oesophagus. Barium radiology may show hold-up in the distal oesophagus, abnormal contractions in the oesophageal body and a tapering stricture in the distal oesophagus, often described as a 'bird's beak' (see Fig. 59.55). The gastric gas bubble is usually absent. These typical features of well-developed achalasia are often absent, and endoscopy and radiology can be normal. A firm diagnosis is established by oesophageal manometry. Classically, the LOS does not relax completely on swallowing, there is no peristalsis and there is a raised resting pressure in the oesophagus (Fig. 59.57). The LOS pressure may be elevated, but is often normal.

Treatment

Alone among motility disorders, achalasia responds well to treatment. The two main methods are forceful dilatation of the cardia and Heller's myotomy.

Pneumatic dilatation

This involves stretching the cardia with a balloon to disrupt the muscle and render it less competent. The treatment was first described by Plummer. Many varieties of balloon have been used but, nowadays, plastic balloons with a precisely controlled external diameter are used. If the pressure in the balloon is too high, the balloon is designed to split along its length rather than expanding further. Balloons of 30–40 mm in diameter are available and are inserted over a guidewire (Fig. 59.58). Perforation is the major complication. With a 30-mm balloon, the incidence of perforation should be less than 0.5%. The risk of perforation increases with bigger balloons, and they should be used cautiously for progressive dilatation over a period of weeks. Forceful dilatation is curative in 75–85% of cases. The results are best in patients aged more than 45 years (Summary box 59.20).

Summary box 59.20

Achalasia

- Beware perforation due to dilatation of achalasia
- Beware postoperative reflux

Harald Hirschsprung, 1831–1916, Physician, The Queen Louise Hospital for Children, and Professor of Paediatrics, Copenhagen, Denmark, described congenital megacolon in 1888.

Ernst Heller, 1877–1964, Surgeon, St. George's Krankenhaus, Leipzig, Germany.
Henry Stanley Plummer, 1874–1937, Physician, The Mayo Clinic, Rochester, MN, USA.

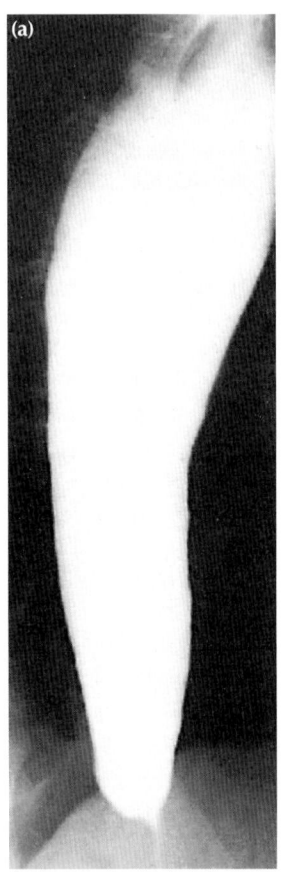

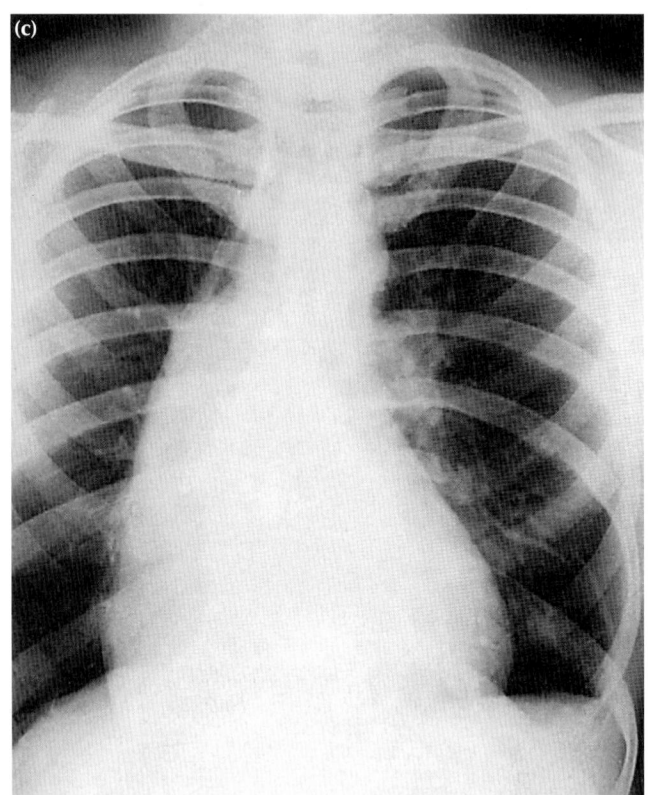

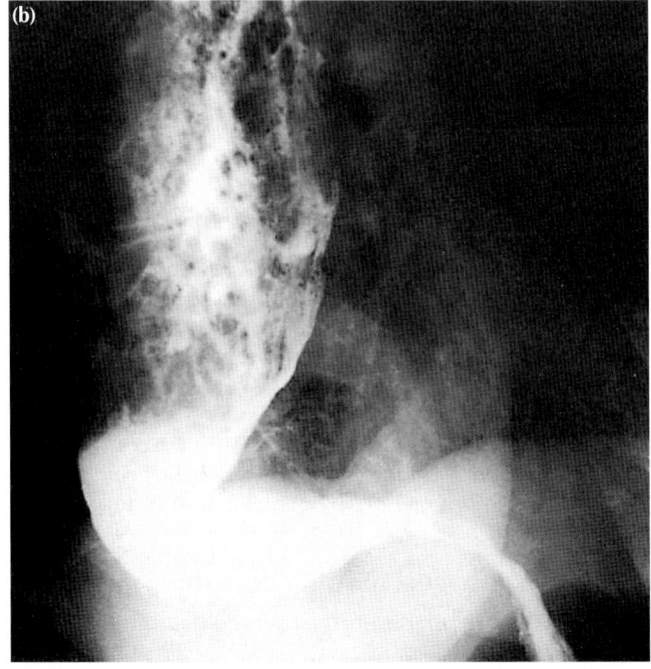

Figure 59.55 Achalasia of the oesophagus. (a) Barium swallow showing the smooth outline of the stricture, which narrows to a point at its lower end. (b) Tortuosity and sigmoid appearance of the lower oesophagus. (c) Mediastinal shadow due to a large, fluid-filled oesophagus.

Heller's myotomy

This involves cutting the muscle of the lower oesophagus and cardia (Fig. 59.59). The major complication is gastro-oesophageal reflux, and most surgeons therefore add a partial anterior fundoplication (Heller–Dor's operation). The procedure is ideally suited to a minimal access laparoscopic approach, and most surgeons use intraoperative endoscopy to judge the extent of the myotomy and to ensure that the narrow segment is abolished.

It is successful in more than 90% of cases and may be used after failed dilatation.

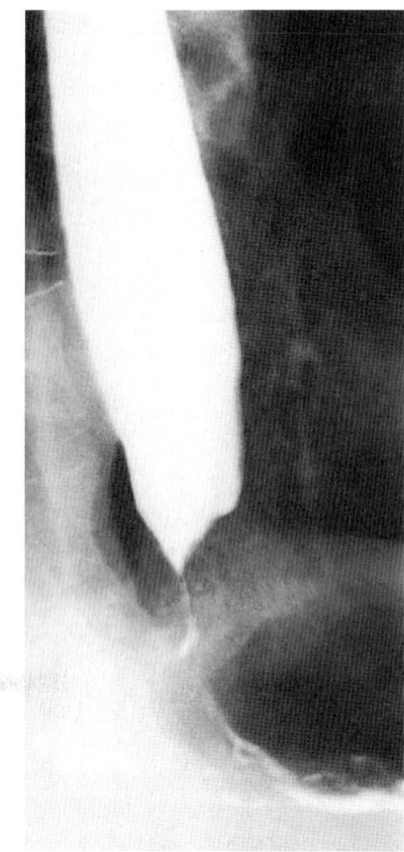

Figure 59.56 Almost achalasia, but note the irregularity of the taper, which indicates carcinoma of the cardia.

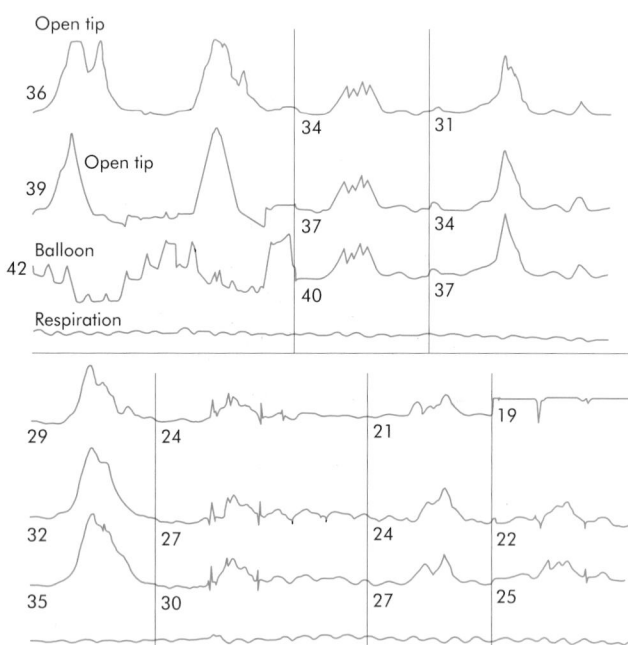

Figure 59.57 Manometry in achalasia, showing simultaneous contractions in the body of the oesophagus and incomplete relaxation of the lower oesophageal sphincter (LOS) in response to swallowing.

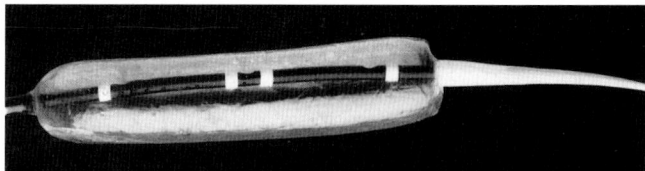

Figure 59.58 Balloon dilator for the treatment of achalasia by forceful dilatation.

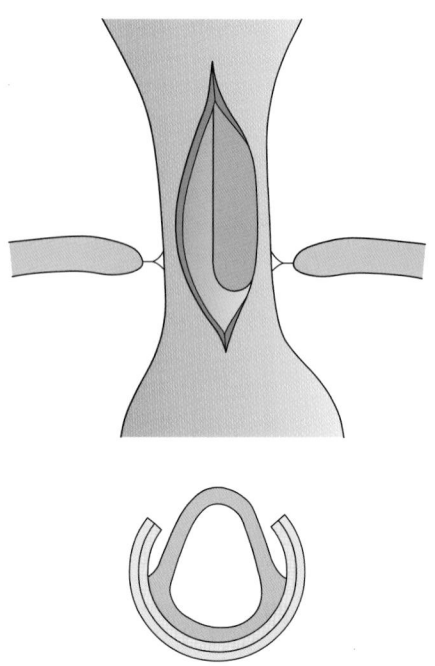

Figure 59.59 Heller's myotomy. The incision should not go too far on to the stomach. The lateral extent must enable the mucosa to pout out, to prevent the edges healing together.

Botulinum toxin

This is done by endoscopic injection into the LOS. It acts by interfering with cholinergic excitatory neural activity at the LOS. The effect is not permanent, and the injection usually has to be repeated after a few months. For this reason, its use is restricted to elderly patients with other comorbidities.

Drugs

Drugs such as calcium channel antagonists have been used but are ineffective for long-term use. However, sublingual nifedipine may be useful for transient relief of symptoms if definitive treatment is postponed.

Other oesophageal motility disorders

Disorders of the pharyngo-oesophageal junction

With the exception of Zenker's diverticulum (see below), most patients with oropharyngeal dysphagia have generalised neurological or muscular disorders with pharyngeal involvement. A small number of patients who have sustained a cerebrovascular accident benefit from myotomy of the cricopharyngeus to alleviate pooling of saliva and nocturnal aspiration, but they should

Friedrich Albert Zenker, **1825–1898, Professor of Pathology, Dresden, Germany.**

have good deglutition and phonation before this is performed. The operation is also effective in patients with oculopharyngeal muscular dystrophy.

Disorders of the body of the oesophagus

Diffuse oesophageal spasm and nutcracker oesophagus

Diffuse oesophageal spasm is a condition in which there are incoordinate contractions of the oesophagus, causing dysphagia and/or chest pain. The condition may be dramatic, with spastic pressures on manometry of 400–500 mmHg, marked hypertrophy of the circular muscle and a corkscrew oesophagus on barium swallow (Fig. 59.60). These abnormal contractions are more common in the distal two-thirds of the oesophageal body, and this may have some relevance to treatment. Making the diagnosis when chest pain is the only symptom may be difficult. Prolonged ambulatory oesophageal manometry that correlates episodes of chest pain with manometric abnormalities may establish the diagnosis.

There is no proven pharmacological or endoscopic treatment. Calcium channel antagonists, vasodilators and endoscopic dilatation have only transient effects. While the severity and frequency of symptoms may be tolerated by most patients, sometimes the combination of chest pain and dysphagia is sufficiently severe that malnutrition begins. In these patients, extended oesophageal myotomy up to the aortic arch may be required. Surgical treatment of diffuse spasm is more successful in improving dysphagia than chest pain, and caution should be exercised in patients in whom chest pain is the only symptom.

Nutcracker oesophagus is a condition in which peristaltic pressures of more than 180 mmHg develop. It is said to cause chest pain, but there is still some debate as to whether it is a real disorder.

Oesophageal involvement in autoimmune disease

Oesophageal involvement is mainly seen in systemic sclerosis, but may be a feature of polymyositis, dermatomyositis, systemic lupus erythematosus, polyarteritis nodosa or rheumatoid disease. While most involve weak peristalsis, swallowing difficulties may be compounded by pharyngeal problems in the disorders that primarily affect skeletal muscle (e.g. polymyositis) or extraoesophageal

problems such as involvement of the cricoarytenoid joint in rheumatoid disease or dry mouth in Sjögren's syndrome. In systemic sclerosis, smooth muscle atrophy causes hypoperistalsis (Fig. 59.61). The LOS is involved, leading to a loss of the anti-reflux barrier. A wide range of symptoms can follow from mild to severe dysphagia accompanied by regurgitation and aspiration. Reflux can be severe and is exacerbated by weak acid clearance so that strictures can occur. There are no drugs that specifically correct the motor disorder, and medical treatment is mainly directed at minimising reflux-induced damage with PPIs. A small number of patients may require anti-reflux surgery.

Eosinophilic oesophagitis is a disorder that occurs in children and adults either alone or as a manifestation of eosinophilic gastroenteritis. It is characterised by eosinophilic infiltration of the oesophageal wall, presumably of allergic or idiopathic origin. The commonest presenting symptom is dysphagia, and more than half have some history of atopy. The oesophagus often seems narrow and friable on endoscopy and may include mucosal rings. The most important feature is the development of deep ulcers leading to stricture development, especially in the proximal oesophagus. The diagnosis is established by endoscopic biopsy.

Elimination diets, topical and systemic steroids all seem to be helpful in the short term, but there is scant information on the long-term impact of any particular approach. Immunotherapy directed against interleukin (IL)-5, which has a major role in eosinophil recruitment, seems to be a promising innovative approach. Although endoscopic dilatation has been recommended, this can create deep ulcers and further scarring, so should be used with caution and only when the above therapies fail.

Pharyngeal and oesophageal diverticula

Most oesophageal diverticula are *pulsion* diverticula that develop at a site of weakness as a result of chronic pressure against an

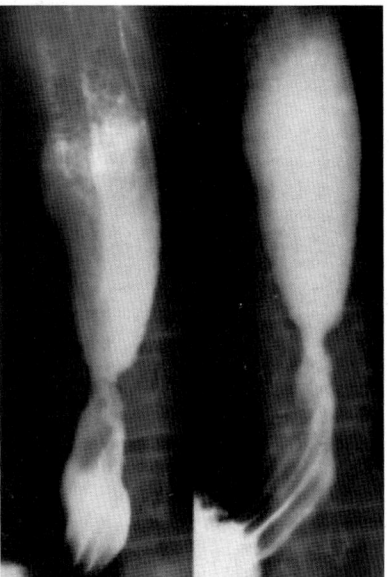

Figure 59.61 Advanced scleroderma of the oesophagus. The oesophagus dilates, and the lower oesophageal sphincter is widely incompetent.

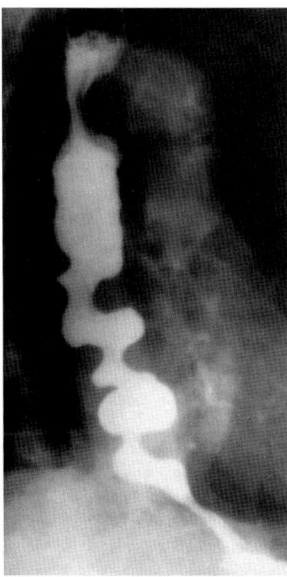

Figure 59.60 Corkscrew oesophagus in diffuse oesophageal spasm.

CHAPTER 59 | THE OESOPHAGUS

obstruction. Symptoms are mostly caused by the underlying disorder unless the diverticulum is particularly large. *Traction* diverticula (Fig. 59.62) are much less common. They are mostly a consequence of chronic granulomatous disease affecting the tracheobronchial lymph nodes due to tuberculosis, atypical mycobacteria or histoplasmosis. Fibrotic healing of the lymph nodes exerts traction on the oesophageal wall and produces a focal outpouching that is usually small and has a conical shape. There may be associated broncholithiasis, and additional complications may occur, such as aerodigestive fistulation (Fig. 59.63) and bleeding.

Zenker's diverticulum (pharyngeal pouch) is not really an oesophageal diverticulum as it protrudes posteriorly above the cricopharyngeal sphincter through the natural weak point (the dehiscence of Killian) between the oblique and horizontal (cricopharyngeus) fibres of the inferior pharyngeal constrictor (Figs 59.64 and 59.65). The exact mechanism that leads to its formation is unknown, but it involves loss of the coordination between pharyngeal contraction and opening of the upper sphincter. When the diverticulum is small, symptoms largely reflect this incoordination with predominantly pharyngeal dysphagia. As the pouch enlarges, it tends to fill with food on eating, and the fundus descends into the mediastinum. This leads to halitosis and oesophageal dysphagia. Treatment can be undertaken endoscopically with a linear cutting stapler to divide the

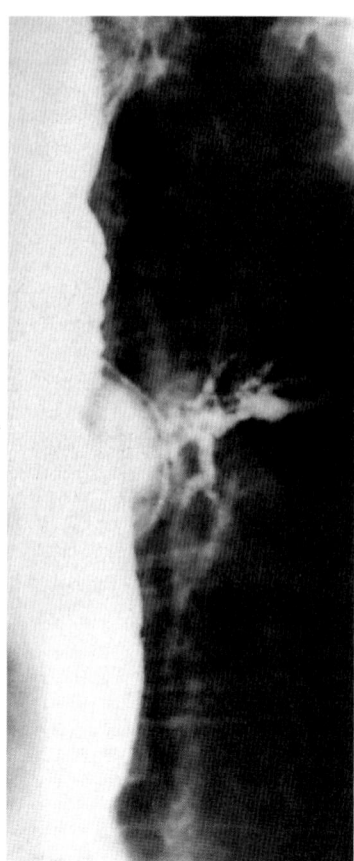

Figure 59.63 Mid-oesophageal diverticulum with a tracheo-oesophageal fistula.

septum between the diverticulum and the upper oesophagus, producing a diverticulo-oesophagostomy, or can be done by open surgery involving pouch excision, pouch suspension (diverticulopexy) and/or myotomy of the cricopharyngeus. All techniques have good results.

Mid-oesophageal diverticula are usually small pulsion diverticula of no particular consequence. The underlying motility disorder does not usually require treatment. Some pulsion diverticula may fistulate into the trachea (Fig. 59.63), but this is more common with traction diverticula in granulomatous disease.

Epiphrenic diverticula are pulsion diverticula situated in the lower oesophagus above the diaphragm (Fig. 59.66). They may be quite large, but cause surprisingly few symptoms. They again probably reflect some loss of coordination between an incoming pressure wave and appropriate relaxation of the LOS. This needs to be acknowledged in the surgical management of the patient. The diverticulum, in isolation, should not be assumed to account for a patient's illness just because it looks dramatic on a radiograph. Large diverticula may be excised, and this should be combined with a myotomy from the site of the diverticulum down to the cardia to relieve functional obstruction (Summary box 59.21).

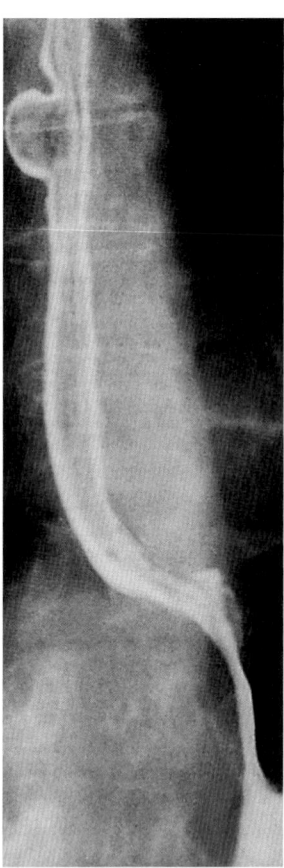

Figure 59.62 Mid-oesophageal traction diverticulum with the mouth facing downwards.

Gustav Killian, **1860–1921, Professor of Laryngology at Freiburg, and later at Berlin, Germany.**

Summary box 59.21

Oesophageal diverticula

■ **Diverticula are indicators of a motor disorder and not necessarily the cause of symptoms**

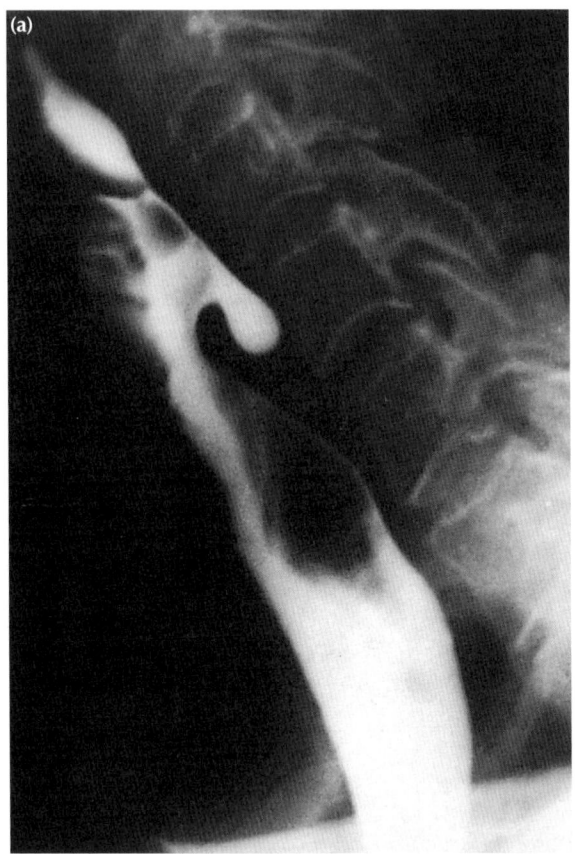

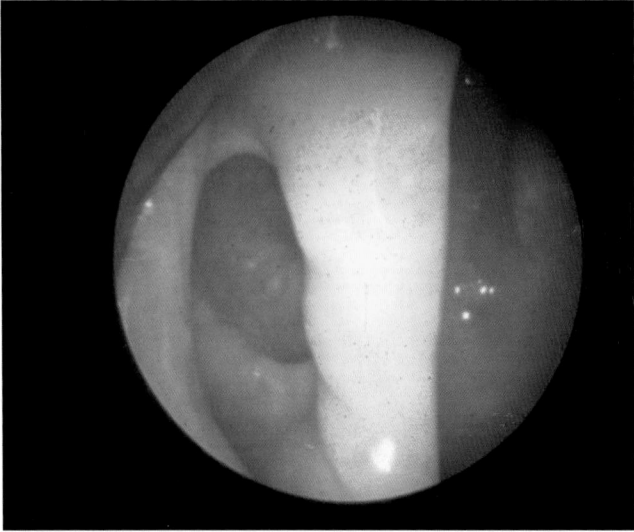

Figure 59.65 The endoscopic appearance of the mouth of a pharyngeal pouch posterior to the normal opening (left) of the oesophagus.

Diffuse intramural pseudodiverticulosis is a rare condition in which there are multiple tiny outpouchings from the lumen of the oesophagus. The pseudodiverticula are dilated excretory ducts of oesophageal sebaceous glands. It is questionable whether the condition produces any symptoms in its own right.

OTHER NON-NEOPLASTIC CONDITIONS

Schatzki's ring

Schatzki's ring is a circular ring in the distal oesophagus (Fig. 59.67), usually at the squamocolumnar junction. The cause is obscure, but there is a strong association with reflux disease. The core of the ring consists of variable amounts of fibrous tissue and cellular infiltrate. Most rings are incidental findings. Some are associated with dysphagia and respond to dilatation in conjunction with medical anti-reflux therapy.

Oesophageal infections

Bacterial infection of the oesophagus is rare, but fungal and viral infections do occur. They are particularly important in immunocompromised patients

Oesophagitis due to *Candida albicans* is relatively common in patients taking steroids (especially transplant patients) or those undergoing cancer chemotherapy. It may present with dysphagia or odynophagia. There may be visible thrush in the throat. Endoscopy shows numerous white plaques that cannot be moved, unlike food residues (Fig. 59.68). Biopsies are diagnostic. In severe cases, a barium swallow may show dramatic mucosal ulceration and irregularity that is surprisingly similar to the appearance of oesophageal varices (Figs 59.69 and 59.70). Treatment is with a topical antifungal agent.

Dysphagia and odynophagia can also be caused by herpes simplex virus and cytomegalovirus (CMV). With the former, there may be a history of a herpetic lesion on the lip some days earlier, and endoscopy may reveal vesicles or small ulcers with raised margins, usually in the upper half of the oesophagus. CMV

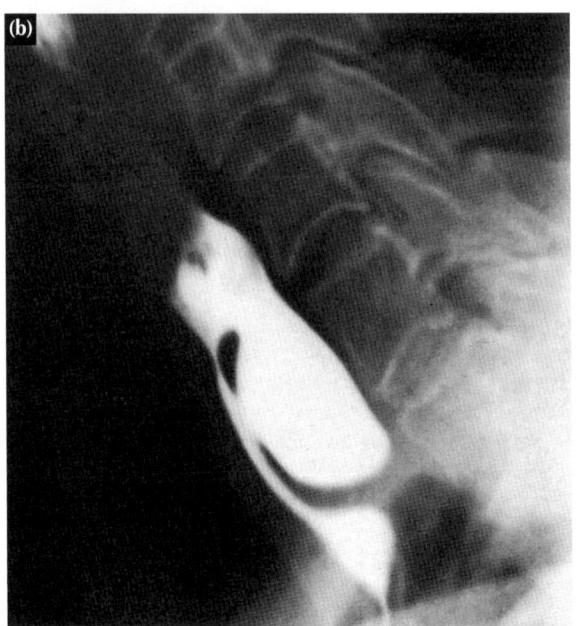

Figure 59.64 The typical appearances of: (a) a small pharyngeal pouch with a prominent cricopharyngeal impression and 'streaming' of barium, indicating partial obstruction; and (b) a large pouch extending behind the oesophagus towards the thoracic inlet.

Richard Schatski, **1901–1992, American Radiologist.**

CHAPTER 59 | THE OESOPHAGUS

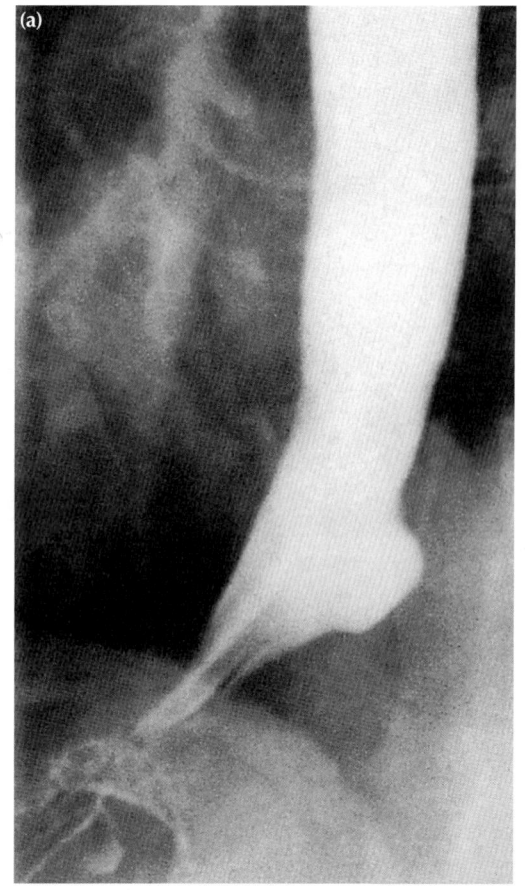

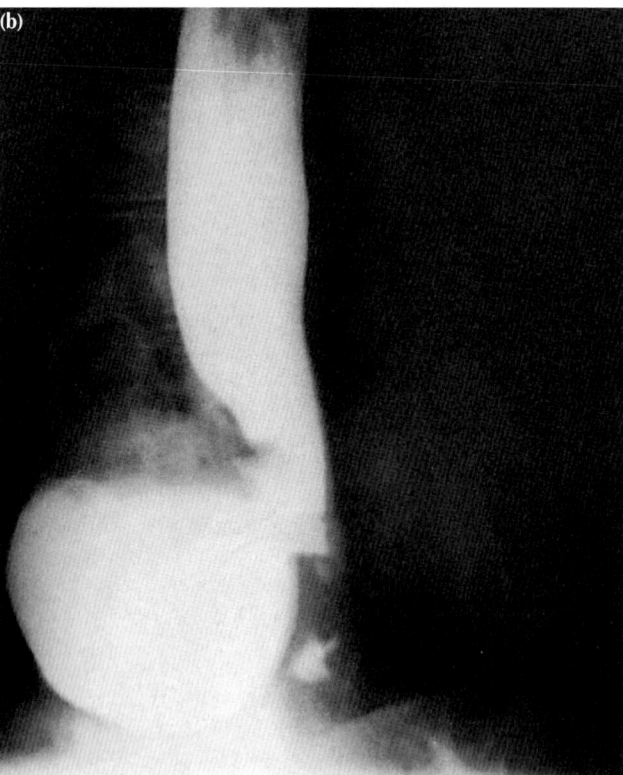

Figure 59.66 Epiphrenic diverticulum proximal to the gastro-oesophageal sphincter. (a) Small and asymptomatic; (b) large, symptomatic and appearing as a gas-filled bubble on the chest radiograph.

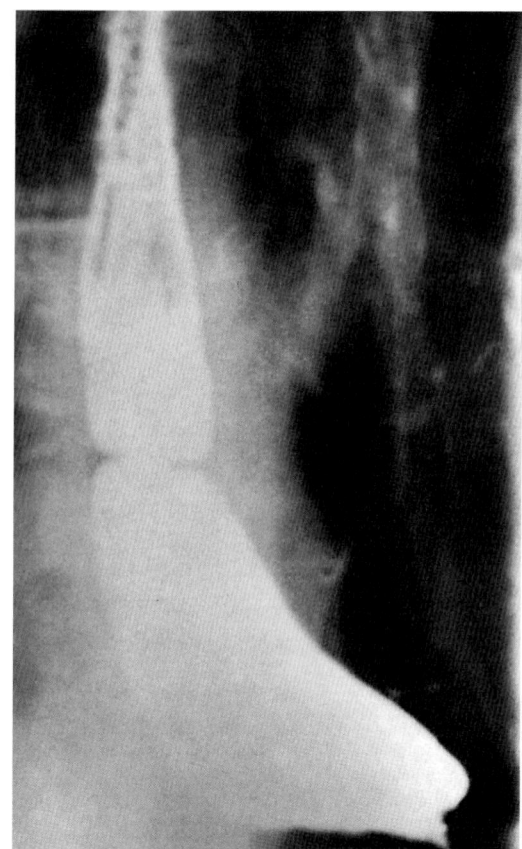

Figure 59.67 Schatzki's ring, a thin submucosal web completely encircling the whole of the lumen, usually situated at the squamocolumnar junction.

infection may be apparent in graft-versus-host disease following bone marrow transplantation. It has a characteristic endoscopic appearance with a geographical, serpiginous border. In both cases, endoscopic biopsy is diagnostic.

Chagas' disease

This condition is confined to South American countries, but is of interest because oesophageal symptoms occur that are similar to severe achalasia. It is caused by a protozoan, *Trypanosoma cruzi*, transmitted by an insect vector. Parasites reach the bloodstream and, after a long latent period, there is damage particularly to cardiac and smooth muscle. Destruction of both Auerbach's and Meissner's plexuses leads to acquired megaoesophagus.

Crohn's disease

The oesophagus is not commonly affected by symptomatic Crohn's disease. However, pathological studies indicate that it may be present in 20% of patients without symptoms. Symptoms are often severe, and a diagnosis of reflux oesophagitis is usually made on the basis of retrosternal pain and dysphagia. Endoscopy shows extensive oesophagitis that extends much further proximally than reflux oesophagitis. Biopsies may be diagnostic, but may show only non-specific inflammation. In severe cases, deep

Burrill Bernard Crohn, **1884–1983, Gastroenterologist, Mount Sinai Hospital, New York, NY, USA, described regional ileitis in 1932.**

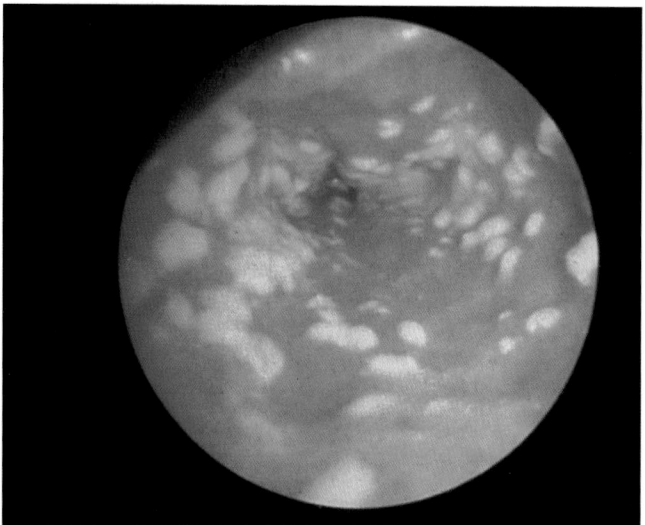

Figure 59.68 Endoscopic appearance of oesophageal candidiasis.

Plummer–Vinson syndrome

This is also called the Paterson–Kelly syndrome or *sideropenic dysphagia*. The original descriptions are vague and poorly supported by evidence of a coherent syndrome. Dysphagia is said to occur because of the presence of a post-cricoid web that is associated with iron deficiency anaemia, glossitis and koilonychia. The classical syndrome is rarely complete. Some patients may have oropharyngeal leucoplakia, and this may account for an alleged increased risk of developing hypopharyngeal cancer.

Webs certainly occur in the upper and middle oesophagus, usually without any kind of associated syndrome. They are nearly always thin diaphanous membranes identified coincidentally by contrast radiology. Even symptomatic webs that cause a degree of obstruction may be inadvertently ruptured at endoscopy. Few require formal endoscopic dilatation.

Vascular abnormalities affecting the oesophagus

Several congenital vascular anomalies may produce dysphagia by compression of the oesophagus. Classically, this results from an

sinuses occur, and fistulation has been described. Crohn's oesophagitis is said to respond poorly to medical treatment and, although balloon dilatation of strictures and surgical resection for multiple internal fistulae have both been described, these interventions should be used with great caution.

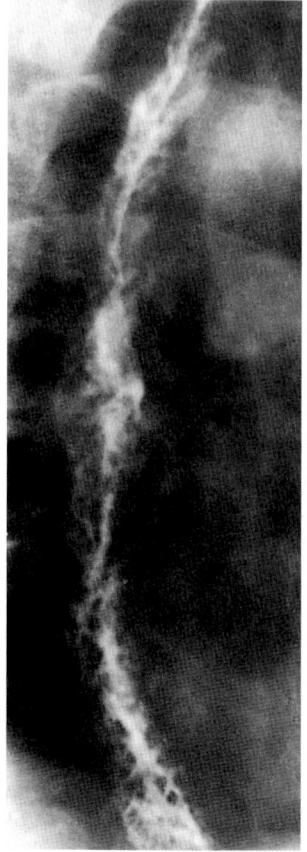

Figure 59.69 Oesophageal candidiasis with shaggy appearance of mucosal defects.

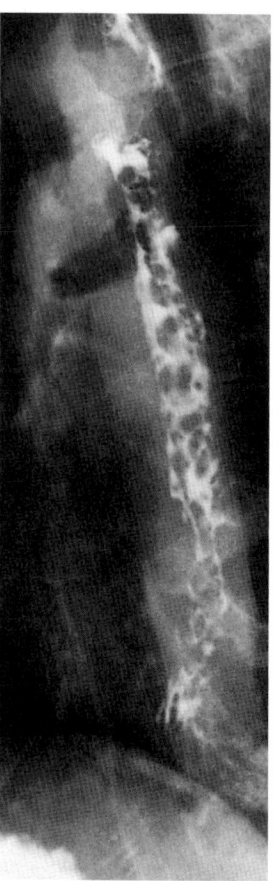

Figure 59.70 Oesophageal varices with smooth outline of the filling defects.

Porter Paisley Vinson, 1890–1959, Physician, The Mayo Clinic, Rochester, MN, who later practiced in Richmond, VA, USA.
Adam Brown Kelly, 1865–1941, Surgeon, The Ear, Nose and Throat Department, The Royal Victoria Infirmary, Glasgow, Scotland.
Donald Rose Paterson, 1863–1939, Surgeon, The Ear, Nose and Throat Department, The Royal Infirmary, Cardiff, Wales.
Vinson, Kelly and Paterson all described this syndrome independently in 1919.

CHAPTER 59 | THE OESOPHAGUS

aberrant right subclavian artery (arteria lusoria). However, the oesophagus is more commonly compressed by vascular rings, such as a double aortic arch. Dysphagia occurs in only a minority of cases and usually presents early in childhood, although it can occur in the late teens. Treatment is usually by division of the non-dominant component of the ring.

In adults, acquired causes include aneurysm of the aorta, diffuse cardiac enlargement and pressure from the left common carotid or vertebral arteries. It is rare that symptom severity justifies surgical intervention.

Mediastinal fibrosis

This rare condition can occur alone or in conjunction with retroperitoneal fibrosis. The cause is unknown and, while the major consequences are usually cardiovascular as a result of caval compression, dysphagia can occur. The existence of irreparable cardiovascular problems usually precludes surgical intervention on the oesophagus.

FURTHER READING

Castell, D.O. and Richter, J.E. (2003) *The Esophagus*, 4th edn. Lippincott, Williams & Wilkins.

Griffin, S.M. and Raimes, S.A. (2006) *Oesophago-gastric Surgery*, 3rd edn. Elsevier Saunders, London.

Jamieson, G.G. (1988) *Surgery of the Oesophagus*. Churchill Livingstone, Edinburgh.

Pearson, F.G. *et al.* (2002) *The Esophagus*, 2nd edn. Churchill Livingstone, Edinburgh.

Sharma, P. and Sampliner, R.E. (2006) *Barrett's oesophagus and esophageal adenocarcinomas*, 2nd edn. Blackwell, Oxford.

Stomach and duodenum

To recognise and understand:
- The anatomy and pathophysiology of the stomach in relation to disease
- The most appropriate investigations for gastroduodenal symptoms
- The importance of gastritis and *Helicobacter pylori*

- The investigations and treatment of peptic ulcer disease and its complications
- The presentation and treatment of gastric cancer
- The causes of duodenal obstruction and presentation of duodenal tumours

INTRODUCTION

The function of the stomach is to act as a reservoir for ingested food. It also serves to break down foodstuffs mechanically and commence the processes of digestion before these products are passed into the duodenum.

GROSS ANATOMY OF THE STOMACH AND DUODENUM

Blood supply

Arteries

The stomach has an arterial supply on both the lesser and greater curves (Fig. 60.1). On the lesser curve, the left gastric artery, a

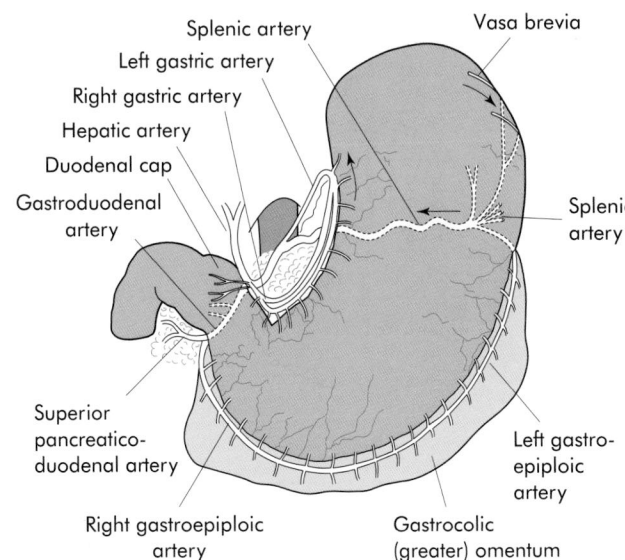

Splenic artery
Left gastric artery
Right gastric artery
Hepatic artery
Duodenal cap
Gastroduodenal artery
Vasa brevia
Splenic artery
Superior pancreatico-duodenal artery
Right gastroepiploic artery
Gastrocolic (greater) omentum
Left gastro-epiploic artery

Figure 60.1 The arterial blood supply of the stomach.

branch of the coeliac axis, forms an anastomotic arcade with the right gastric artery, which arises from the common hepatic artery. Branches of the left gastric artery pass up towards the cardia. The gastroduodenal artery, which is also a branch of the hepatic artery, passes behind the first part of the duodenum, highly relevant to the bleeding duodenal ulcer. Here it divides into the superior pancreaticoduodenal artery and the right gastroepiploic artery. The superior pancreaticoduodenal artery supplies the duodenum and pancreatic head, and forms an anastomosis with the inferior pancreaticoduodenal artery, a branch of the superior mesenteric artery. The right gastroepiploic artery runs along the greater curvature of the stomach, eventually forming an anastomosis with the left gastroepiploic artery, a branch of the splenic artery. This vascular arcade, however, is often variably incomplete. The fundus of the stomach is supplied by the vasa brevia (or short gastric arteries), which arise near the termination of the splenic artery.

Veins

In general, the veins are equivalent to the arteries, with those along the lesser curve ending in the portal vein and those on the greater curve joining via the splenic vein. On the lesser curve the coronary vein is particularly important. It runs up the lesser curve towards the oesophagus and then passes left to right to join the portal vein; it becomes markedly dilated in portal hypertension.

Lymphatics

The lymphatics of the stomach are of considerable importance in the surgery of gastric cancer and are described in detail in that section.

Nerves

As with all of the gastrointestinal tract, the stomach and duodenum possess both intrinsic and extrinsic nerve supplies. The intrinsic nerves exist principally in two plexuses, the myenteric plexus of Auerbach and the submucosal plexus of Meissner. Compared with the rest of the gut, the submucosal plexus of the stomach contains relatively few ganglionic cells, as does the myenteric plexus in the fundus. However, in the antrum, the ganglia of the myenteric plexus are well developed. The extrinsic supply is derived mainly from the vagus nerves, fibres of which originate in the brainstem. The vagal plexus around the oesophagus condenses into bundles that pass through the oesophageal hiatus (Fig. 60.2), the posterior bundle usually being identifiable as a large nerve trunk. Vagal fibres are both afferent (sensory) and efferent. The efferent fibres are involved in the receptive relaxation of the stomach and the stimulation of gastric motility, as well as having a secretory function. The sympathetic supply is derived mainly from the coeliac ganglia.

MICROSCOPIC ANATOMY OF THE STOMACH AND DUODENUM

The gastric epithelial cells are mucus producing and are turned over rapidly. In the pyloric part of the stomach, and also the duodenum, mucus-secreting glands are found. Most of the specialised cells of the stomach (parietal and chief cells) are found in the gastric crypts (Fig. 60.3). The stomach also has numerous endocrine cells.

Parietal cells

These are in the body (acid-secreting portion) of the stomach and line the gastric crypts, being more abundant distally. They are responsible for the production of hydrogen ions used to form hydrochloric acid. The hydrogen ions are actively pumped by the proton pump, a hydrogen–potassium-ATPase (Sachs), which exchanges intraluminal potassium for hydrogen ions. The potassium ions enter the lumen of the crypts passively, but the hydrogen ions are pumped against an immense concentration gradient (1 000 000:1).

Chief cells

These lie principally proximally in the gastric crypts and produce pepsinogen. Both forms of pepsinogen, pepsinogen I and II, are produced by chief cells, but pepsinogen I is produced only in the stomach. The ratio between pepsinogens I and II in the serum decreases with gastric atrophy. Pepsinogen is activated in the stomach to produce pepsin, the active enzyme.

Endocrine cells

The stomach has numerous endocrine cells, which are critical to its function. In the gastric antrum the mucosa contains G cells, which produce gastrin. Throughout the body of the stomach, enterochromaffin-like (ECL) cells are abundant and produce histamine, a key factor in driving gastric acid secretion. There are also large numbers of somatostatin-producing D cells throughout the stomach, and somatostatin has a negative regulatory role. The peptides and neuropeptides produced in the stomach are discussed later.

Duodenum

The duodenum is lined by a mucus-secreting columnar epithelium. In addition, Brunner's glands lie beneath the mucosa and are similar to the pyloric glands in the pyloric part of the stomach. Endocrine cells in the duodenum produce cholecystokinin and secretin.

PHYSIOLOGY OF THE STOMACH AND DUODENUM

The stomach mechanically breaks up ingested food and, together with the actions of acid and pepsin, forms chyme that passes into the duodenum. In contrast to the acidic environment of the stomach, that of the duodenum is alkaline, because of the secretion of bicarbonate ions from both the pancreas and the duodenum. This neutralises the acid chyme and adjusts the osmolarity

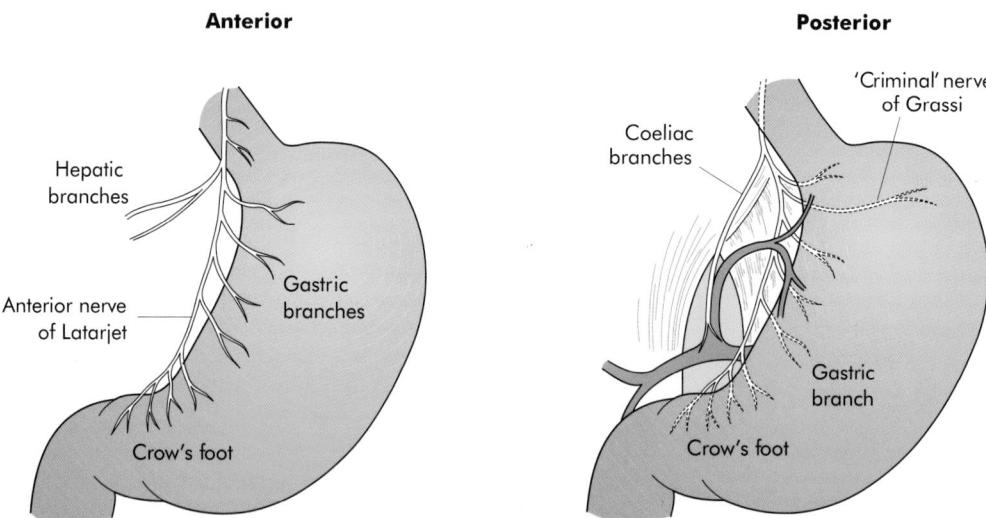

Figure 60.2 The anatomy of the anterior and posterior vagus nerves in relation to the stomach.

Leopold Auerbach, 1828–1897, Professor of Neuropathology, Breslau, Germany, (now Wroclaw, Poland), described the myenteric plexus in 1862.
Georg Meissner, 1829–1905, Professor of Physiology, Göttingen, Germany, described the submucosal plexus in 1852.
George Sachs, Professor of Medicine, CURE, Los Angeles, CA, USA.
Johann Conrad Brunner, 1653–1729, Professor of Anatomy, at Heidelberg, Germany and later at Strasbourg, France, described these glands in 1687.

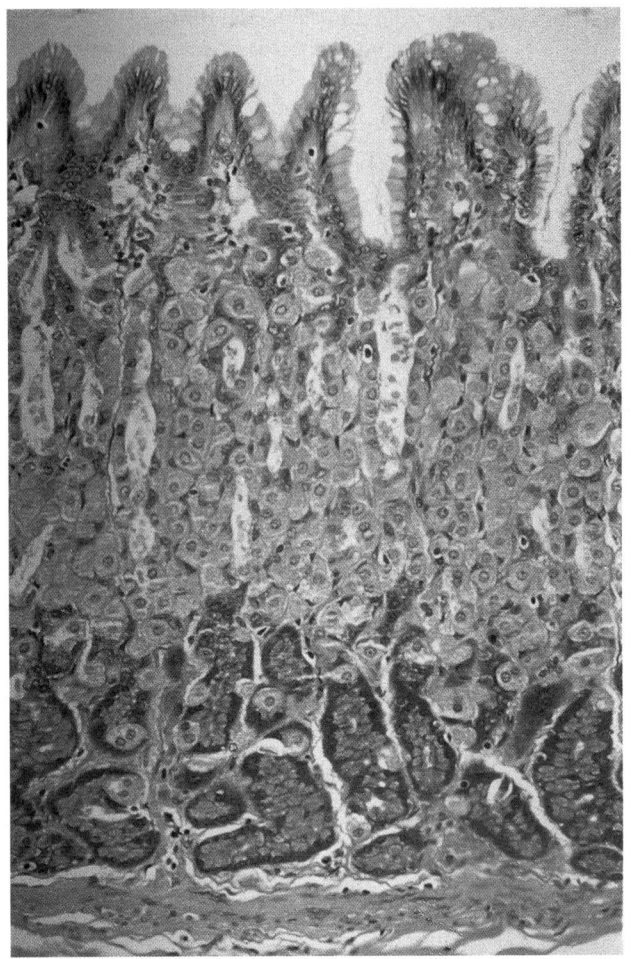

Figure 60.3 The histological appearance of a gastric gland. The mucus-secreting cells are seen at the mucosal surface, the eosinophilic parietal cells superficially in the glands, and the basophilic chief cells in the deepest layer.

to approximately that of plasma. Endocrine cells in the duodenum produce cholecystokinin, which stimulates the pancreas to produce trypsin and the gall bladder to contract. Secretin, produced by the endocrine cells of the duodenum, inhibits gastric acid secretion and promotes production of bicarbonate by the pancreas.

Gastric acid secretion

The secretion of gastric acid and pepsin tends to run in parallel, although the understanding of the mechanisms of gastric acid secretion is considerably greater than that of pepsin. Numerous factors are involved in gastric acid production. These include neurotransmitters, neuropeptides and peptide hormones, and several other factors. This complexity need not detract from the fact that there are basic principles which are easily understood (Fig. 60.4). Hydrogen ions are exported from parietal cells via the proton pump. Although numerous factors can act on parietal cells, the most important is histamine, which acts via the H_2-receptor. Histamine is produced, in turn, by the ECL cells of the stomach and acts in a paracrine (local) fashion on parietal cells. These relationships explain why proton pump inhibitors can abolish gastric acid secretion, as they act on the final common pathway of gastric secretion, and why H_2-receptor antagonists

have such profound effects on gastric acid secretion, even though this is not insurmountable (Fig. 60.4). The ECL cell produces histamine in response to a number of stimuli that include the vagus and gastrin. Gastrin is released by G cells in response to the presence of food in the stomach. The production of gastrin is inhibited by acid, hence creating a negative-feedback loop. Various other peptides, including secretin, inhibit gastric acid secretion.

Classically, three phases of gastric secretion are described. The *cephalic phase* is mediated by vagal activity, secondary to sensory arousal as first demonstrated by Pavlov. The *gastric phase* is a response to food within the stomach, which is mediated principally, but not exclusively, by gastrin. In the *intestinal phase*, the presence of chyme in the duodenum and small bowel inhibits gastric emptying and the acidification of the duodenum leads to the production of secretin, which also inhibits gastric acid secretion, along with numerous other peptides originating from the gut. The stomach also possesses somatostatin-containing D cells. Somatostatin is released in response to a number of factors including acidification. This peptide acts probably on the G cell, the ECL cell and the parietal cell itself to inhibit acid production.

Gastric mucus and the gastric mucosal barrier

The gastric mucus layer is essential to the integrity of the gastric mucosa. It is a viscid layer of mucopolysaccharides produced by the mucus-producing cells of the stomach and the pyloric glands. Gastric mucus is an important barrier that protects the gastric mucosa from mechanical damage and also from the effects of acid and pepsin. Its considerable buffering capacity is enhanced by the presence of bicarbonate ions within the mucus. Many factors can lead to the breakdown of this gastric mucous barrier. These include bile, non-steroidal anti-inflammatory drugs (NSAIDs), alcohol, trauma and shock. Tonometry studies have shown that, of all the gastrointestinal tract, the stomach is the most sensitive to ischaemia following a hypovolaemic insult and also the slowest

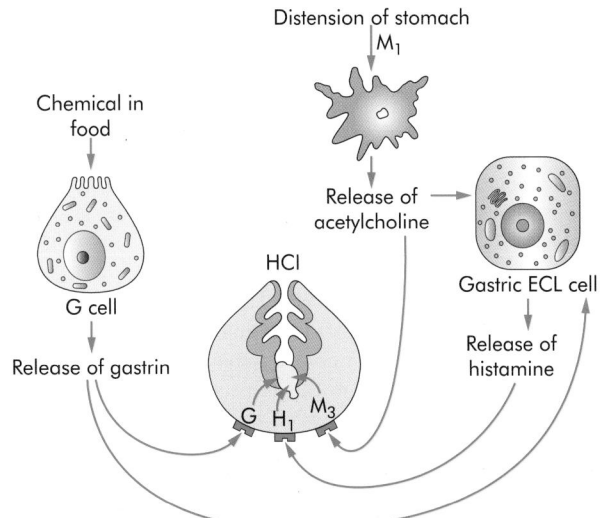

Figure 60.4 The parietal cell in relation to the mechanism of gastric acid secretion. ECL, enterochromaffin-like; G, gastrin receptor; H, histamine receptor; M, muscarinic receptor.

Ivan Petrovich Pavlov, **1849–1936, Professor of Physiology, The Medico-Chirurgical Academy, St. Petersburg, Russia.**

to recover. This may explain the high incidence of stress ulceration (Summary box 60.1).

Summary box 60.1

The anatomy and physiology of the stomach

- The stomach acts as a reservoir for food and commences the process of digestion
- Gastric acid is produced by a proton pump in the parietal cells, which in turn is controlled by histamine acting on the H$_2$-receptors
- Histamine is produced by the endocrine gastric ECL cells in response to a number of factors, particularly gastrin and the vagus
- Proton pump inhibitors abolish gastric acid production, whereas H$_2$-receptor antagonists only markedly reduce it
- The gastric mucous layer is essential to the integrity of the gastric mucosa

---

Peptides and neuropeptides in the stomach and duodenum

As with most of the gastrointestinal tract, the endocrine cells of the stomach produce peptide hormones and neurotransmitters. Previously, nerves and endocrine cells were considered distinct in terms of their products. However, it is increasingly realised that there is enormous overlap within these systems. Many peptides recognised as hormones may also be produced by neurones, hence the term neuropeptides. The term 'messenger' can be used to describe all such products. There are three conventional modes of action that overlap:

1. *Endocrine.* The messenger is secreted into the circulation where it affects tissues that may be remote from the site of origin (Bayliss and Starling).
2. *Paracrine.* Messengers are produced locally and have local effects on tissues. Neurones and endocrine cells both act in this way.
3. *Neurocrine* (classic neurotransmitter). Messengers are produced by the neurone via the synaptic knob and pass across the synaptic cleft to the target.

Many peptide hormones act on the intrinsic nerve plexus of the gut (see later) and influence motility. Similarly, neuropeptides may influence the structure and function of the mucosa. Some of these peptides, neuropeptides and neurotransmitters are shown in Table 60.1.

Gastroduodenal motor activity

The motility of the entire gastrointestinal tract is modulated to a large degree by its intrinsic nervous system. The migrating motor complex (MMC) is critical in this respect. In the small bowel in the fasted state, and after food has cleared, there is a period of quiescence lasting approximately 40 min (phase I). There follows a series of waves of electrical and motor activity, also lasting for about 40 min, propagated from the fundus of the stomach in a caudal direction at a rate of about three per minute (phase II). These pass as far as the pylorus but not beyond. Duodenal slow

Sir William Maddock Baylis, **1860–1924**, Professor of Physiology, University College, London, England.
Ernest Henry Starling, **1866–1927**, Professor of Physiology, University College, London, England.

waves are generated in the duodenum at a rate of about 10 per minute, which propagate down the small bowel. The amplitude of these contractions increases to a maximum in phase III, which lasts for about 10 min. This 90-min cycle of activity is then repeated. From the duodenum, the MMC moves distally at 5–10 cm min^{-1}, reaching the terminal ileum after 1.5 hours.

Following a meal, the stomach exhibits receptive relaxation, which lasts for a few seconds. Following this, adaptive relaxation occurs, which allows the proximal stomach to act as a reservoir. Most of the peristaltic activity is found in the distal stomach (the antral mill) and the proximal stomach demonstrates only tonic activity. The pylorus, which is most commonly open, contracts with the peristaltic wave and allows only a few millilitres of food through at a time. The antral contraction against the closed sphincter is important in the milling activity of the stomach. Although the duodenum is capable of generating 10 waves per minute, after a meal it only contracts after an antral wave reaches the pylorus. The coordination of the motility of the antrum, pylorus and duodenum means that only small quantities of food reach the small bowel at a time. Motility is influenced by numerous factors, including mechanical stimulation and neuronal and endocrine influences (Table 60.1).

Table 60.1 Function and source of peptides and neuropeptides in the stomach

Function	Source
Stimulate secretion	
Gastrin	G cells
Histamine	ECL cells
Acetylcholine	Neurones
Gastrin-releasing peptide	Neurones and mucosa
Cholecystokinin	Duodenal endocrine cells
Inhibit secretion	
Somatostatin	D cells and neurones
Secretin	Duodenal endocrine cells
Enteroglucagon	Small intestinal endocrine cells
Prostaglandins	Mucosa
Neurotensin	Neurones
GIP	Duodenal and jejunal endocrine cells
PYY	Small intestinal endocrine cells
Stimulate motility	
Acetylcholine	Neurones
5-HT	Neurones
Histamine	ECL cells
Substance P	Neurones
Substance K	Neurones
Motilin	Neurones
Gastrin	G cells
Angiotensin	
Inhibit motility	
Somatostatin	D cells and neurones
VIP	Neurones
Nitric oxide	Neurones and smooth muscle
Noradrenaline	Neurones
Encephalin	Neurones
Dopamine	Neurones

ECL, entrochromaffin-like; GIP, gastric inhibitory polypeptide; PYY, peptide YY; VIP, vasoactive intestinal peptide.

INVESTIGATION OF THE STOMACH AND DUODENUM

Flexible endoscopy

Among all of the methods used to investigate and image the stomach and duodenum, flexible endoscopy is now the 'gold standard'. The original flexible gastroscopes were fibreoptic (Hirschowitz), but now most use a solid-state camera mounted at the instrument's tip (Figs 60.5 and 60.6). Other members of the endoscopy team are able to see the image and this is useful when taking biopsies or performing interventional techniques, and also facilitates teaching and training.

Flexible endoscopy is more sensitive than conventional radiology in the assessment of the majority of gastroduodenal conditions. This is particularly the case with peptic ulceration, gastritis and duodenitis. In upper gastrointestinal bleeding, endoscopy is far superior to any other investigation and, in most circumstances, is the only imaging required.

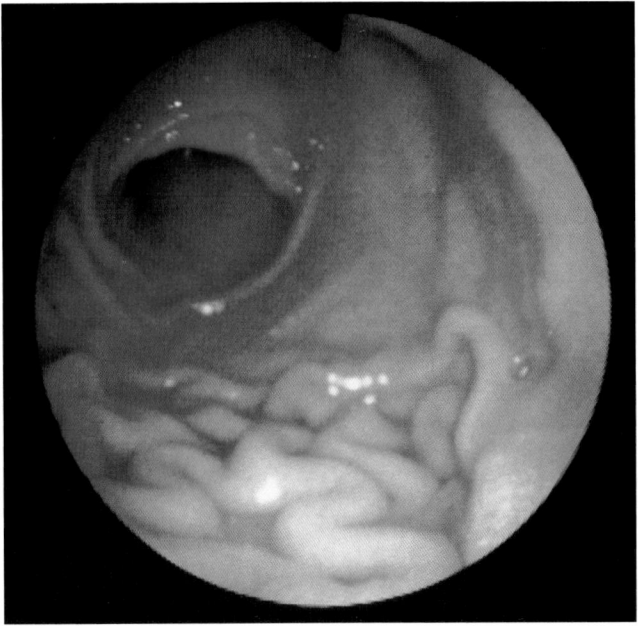

Figure 60.6 A view of the normal stomach during endoscopy (courtesy of G.N.J. Tytgat, Amsterdam, The Netherlands).

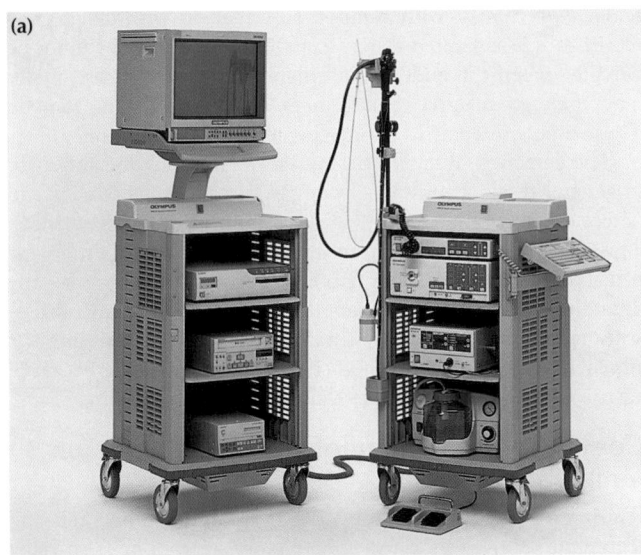

(a)

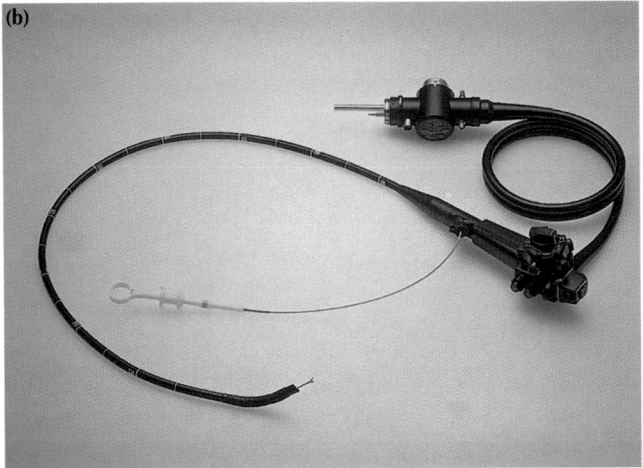

(b)

Figure 60.5 A video gastroscope [courtesy of KeyMed (Medical and Industrial Equipment) Ltd]. (a) The camera stack. (b) The gastroscope and biopsy forceps in the working channel.

Basil I. Hirschowitz, **Professor of Medicine, Birmingham, AL, USA.**

Fibreoptic endoscopy is generally a safe investigation but it is important that all personnel undertaking this procedure are adequately trained and that resuscitation facilities are always available. Although morbidity and mortality are extremely low, the technique is not without hazard. Careless and rough handling of the endoscope during intubation of a patient may result in perforations of the pharynx and oesophagus. An inadequately performed endoscopy is also dangerous as a serious condition may be overlooked. This is particularly the case in early and curable gastric cancer, the appearance of which may often be subtle and which therefore may be missed by inexperienced endoscopists. A more experienced endoscopist will have a higher index of suspicion for any mucosal abnormalities and will take more biopsies. Spraying the mucosa with dye endoscopically may allow better discrimination between normal and abnormal mucosa, allowing small cancers to be more easily seen. In the future, advances in technology may allow 'optical biopsy' to determine the nature of mucosal abnormalities in real time.

Upper gastrointestinal endoscopy is normally carried out under sedation, usually with incremental doses of a benzodiazepine until the patient is adequately sedated. Sedation is of particular concern in the case of gastrointestinal bleeding as it may have a more profound effect on cardiovascular stability. It has now become the standard to use pulse oximetry to monitor patients during upper gastrointestinal endoscopy, and nasal oxygen is also often administered. Buscopan is useful to abolish duodenal motility for examinations of the second and third parts of the duodenum. Examinations of this type are best carried out using a side-viewing endoscope.

Some patients are relatively resistant to sedation with benzodiazepines, particularly those who are accustomed to alcohol. Increasing the dose of benzodiazepines in these patients may not result in any useful sedation, but merely make the patient more restless and confused. Such patients are sometimes better endoscoped fully awake using a local anaesthetic throat spray and a narrow-gauge endoscope. Whatever the circumstances, it is important that resuscitation facilities are available, including agents that reverse the effects of benzodiazepines, such as flumazenil.

The technology associated with upper gastrointestinal endoscopy is continuing to advance. Instruments that allow both endoscopy and endoluminal ultrasound to be performed simultaneously (see later) are used routinely. Bleeding from the stomach and duodenum can be treated with a number of haemostatic measures. These include injection with various substances, diathermy, heater probes and lasers. These approaches appear to be useful in the treatment of bleeding ulcers, although there are few good controlled trials in this area. Currently, there is no good evidence that such interventional procedures work in patients who are bleeding from very large vessels, such as the gastroduodenal artery or splenic artery, although technology may overcome this problem in future.

Contrast radiology

Upper gastrointestinal radiology is now less frequently used as endoscopy is a more sensitive investigation for most gastric problems. Computerised tomography (CT) imaging with oral contrast has also replaced contrast radiology in areas where anatomical information is sought, e.g. large hiatus hernias of the rolling type and chronic gastric volvulus. In these conditions it may be difficult for the endoscopist to determine exactly the anatomy or, indeed, negotiate the deformity to see the distal stomach.

Ultrasonography

Standard ultrasound imaging can be used to investigate the stomach, but used conventionally it is less sensitive than other modalities. In contrast, endoluminal ultrasound and laparoscopic ultrasound are probably the most sensitive techniques available in the preoperative staging of gastric cancer. In endoluminal ultrasound, the transducer is usually attached to the distal tip of the instrument. However, devices have been developed that may be passed down the biopsy channel, albeit with poorer image quality. Five layers (Fig. 60.7) of the gastric wall may be identified on endoluminal ultrasound and the depth of invasion of a tumour can be assessed with exquisite accuracy [90% accuracy for the 'T' tumour component of the staging]. Enlarged lymph nodes can also be identified and the technique's accuracy in this situation is about 80%. Finally, it may be possible to identify liver metastases not seen on axial imaging. Laparoscopic ultrasound is also very

sensitive and is one of the most sensitive methods of detecting liver metastases from gastric cancer.

An additional use of ultrasound is in the assessment of gastric emptying. Swallowed contrast is utilised, which is designed to be easily seen using an ultrasound transducer. The emptying of this contrast is then followed directly. The accuracy of the technique is similar to that of radioisotope gastric emptying studies.

Computerised tomography scanning and magnetic resonance imaging

The resolution of CT scanners continues to improve and multi-slice CT is of increasing value in the investigation of the stomach, especially malignancies (Fig. 60.8). The presence of gastric wall thickening associated with a carcinoma of any reasonable size can be easily detected by CT, but the investigation lacks sensitivity in detecting smaller and curable lesions. It is much less accurate in 'T' staging than endoluminal ultrasound. Lymph node enlargement can be detected and, based on the size and shape of the lymph nodes, it is possible to be reasonably accurate in detecting nodal involvement with tumour. However, as with all imaging techniques, it is limited. Microscopic tumour deposits cannot be detected when the node is not enlarged and, in contrast, nodes may undergo reactive enlargement but not contain tumour. These problems apply to all imaging techniques.

The detection of small liver metastases is improving although, in general terms, metastases from gastric cancer are less easy to detect using CT than those, for instance, from colorectal cancer. This is because metastases from gastric cancer may be of the same density as liver and may not handle the intravenous contrast any differently. At present, magnetic resonance imaging (MRI) scanning does not offer any specific advantage in assessing the stomach, although it has a higher sensitivity for the detection of gastric cancer liver metastases than conventional CT imaging.

Computerised tomography/positron emission tomography

Positron emission tomography (PET) is a functional imaging technique that relies on the uptake of a tracer, in most cases by metabolically active tumour tissue. Fluorodeoxyglucose (FDG) is the most commonly used tracer. This tracer has a short half-life,

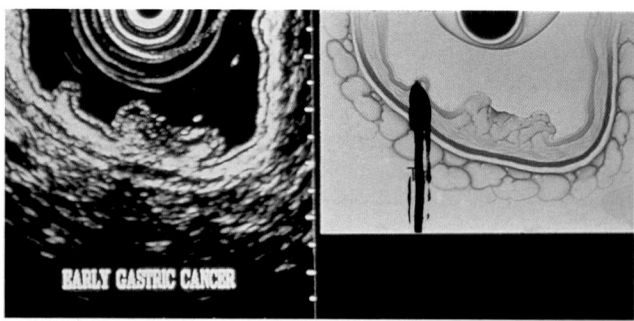

Figure 60.7 Endoscopic ultrasound of the stomach. Five layers can be identified in the normal stomach. A gastric cancer is shown invading the muscle of the gastric wall [courtesy of KeyMed (Medical and Industrial Equipment) Ltd].

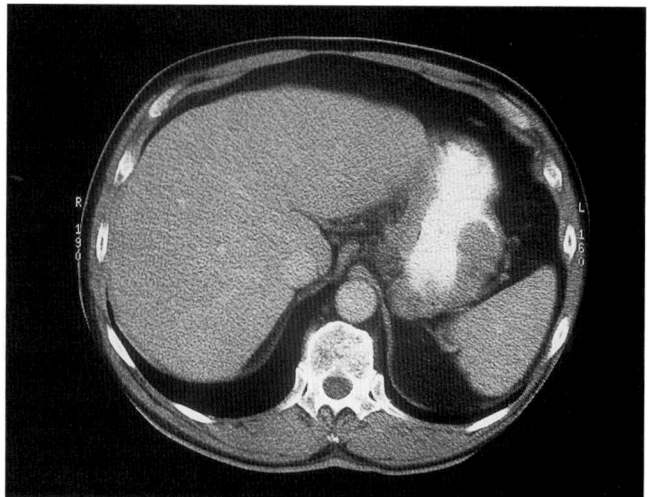

Figure 60.8 A computerised tomography scan of the abdomen showing a gastric cancer arising in the body of the stomach.

so manufacture and use have to be carefully coordinated. To be of value, anatomical and functional information need to be linked, hence CT/PET is now used universally. It is increasingly being used in the preoperative staging of gastro-oesophageal cancer, as it will often demonstrate occult spread, which renders the patient surgically incurable (Fig. 60.9).

Laparoscopy

This technique is now well used in the assessment of patients with gastric cancer. Its particular value is in the detection of peritoneal disease, which is difficult by any other technique unless the patient has ascites or bulky intraperitoneal disease. Its main limitation is in the evaluation of posterior extension but other techniques are available, especially CT and endoluminal ultrasound. Usually, laparoscopy is combined with peritoneal cytology unless laparotomy follows immediately.

Gastric emptying studies

These are useful for studying gastric dysmotility problems, particularly those that follow gastric surgery. The principle of the examination is that a radioisotope-labelled liquid and solid meal is ingested and the emptying of the stomach is followed on a gamma camera. This allows the proportion of activity in the remaining stomach to be assessed numerically, and it is possible to follow liquid and solid gastric emptying independently (Fig. 60.10).

Angiography

Angiography is used most commonly in the investigation of upper gastrointestinal bleeding that is not identified using endoscopy. Therapeutic embolisation may also be of value in the treatment of bleeding in patients in whom surgery is difficult or inadvisable (Summary box 60.2).

> **Summary box 60.2**
>
> ### The investigation of gastric disorders
>
> - Flexible endoscopy is the most sensitive and commonly used technique
> - Great care is necessary in performing endoscopy to avoid complications and missing important pathology
> - Axial imaging, particularly multislice CT, is useful in the staging of gastric cancer, although it may be less sensitive in the detection of liver metastases than other modalities
> - CT/PET is useful in staging gastric cancer
> - Endoscopic ultrasound is the most sensitive technique in the evaluation of the 'T' stage of gastric cancer and in the assessment of duodenal tumours
> - Laparoscopy is sensitive in detecting peritoneal metastases, and laparoscopic ultrasound provides an accurate evaluation of lymph node and liver metastases

PAEDIATRIC DISORDERS

Hypertrophic pyloric stenosis of infancy and duodenal atresia (see Chapter 6)

HELICOBACTER PYLORI

Over the last 20 years this organism has proved to be of overwhelming importance in the aetiology of a number of common gastroduodenal diseases, such as chronic gastritis, peptic ulceration and gastric cancer. The organism had unquestionably been observed by a number of workers since Bircher's first description in 1874, but it was not until 1980 that Warren and Marshall, with enthusiasm but perhaps a lack of caution, ingested the organism

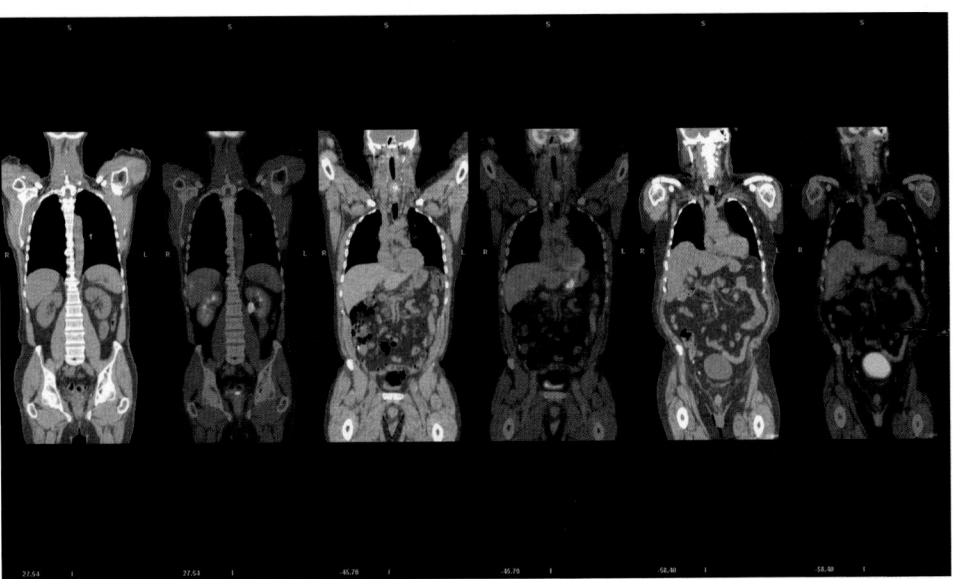

Figure 60.9 Computerised tomography/positron emission tomography of a patient with gastric cancer. The middle pair of images shows the primary tumour. The two images on the left show unsuspected liver metastases, whereas the two on the right show a left cervical node positive for metastases.

J. Robin Warren, **B. 1937**, Pathologist, The Royal Perth Hospital, Perth, WA, Australia.
Barry J. Marshall, **B. 1931**, Physician, The Royal Perth Hospital, WA, Australia.

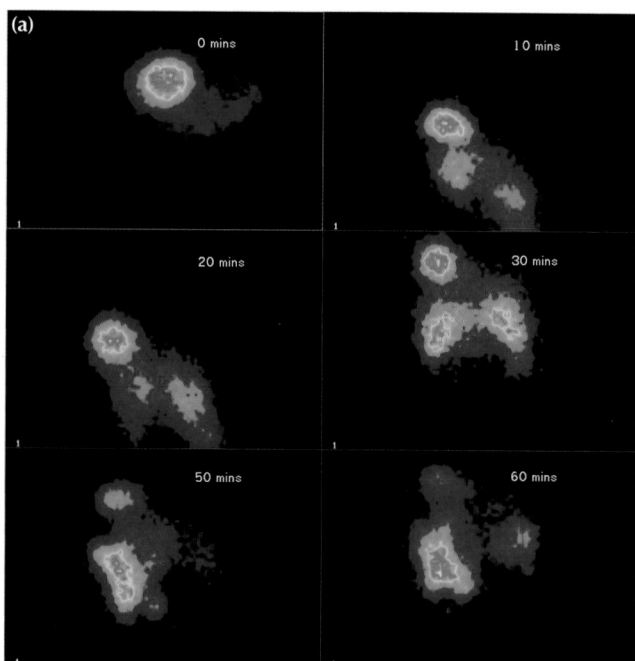

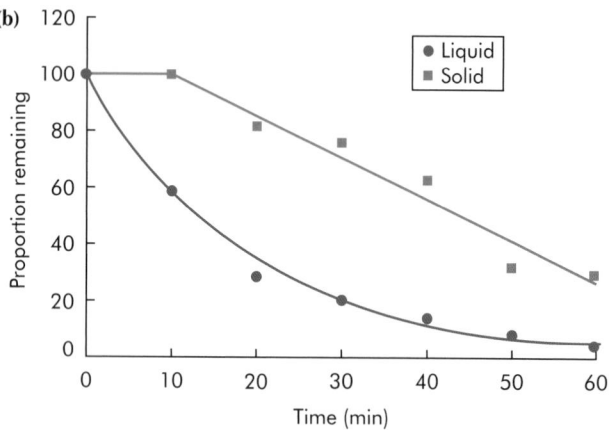

Figure 60.10 Dual-phase solid and liquid gastric emptying. The use of two isotopic labels allows the liquid and solid phases of the emptying to be followed separately. (a) Image acquisition. (b) Gastric emptying curves in a normal individual showing the typical lag period in the solid phase before linear emptying (courtesy of Dr V. Lewington, Southampton, England).

to confirm that Koch's postulates could be fulfilled with respect to the gastritis that they succeeded in causing in themselves. Eradication therapy was then employed with mixed success, but both received the Nobel Prize for Medicine and Physiology in 2005. The organism is spirally shaped and is fastidious in its requirements, being difficult to culture outside the mucus layer of the stomach.

One of the characteristics of the organism is its ability to hydrolyse urea, resulting in the production of ammonia, a strong alkali. The effect of ammonia on the antral G cells is to cause the release of gastrin via the previously described negative-feedback

loop. This is probably responsible for the modest, but inappropriate, hypergastrinaemia in patients with peptic ulcer disease, which, in turn, may result in gastric acid hypersecretion. The organism's obligate urease activity is utilised by various tests designed to detect the presence of the organism, including the ^{13}C and ^{14}C breath tests and the CLO test (a commercially available urease test kit), which is performed on gastric biopsies. The organism can also be detected histologically (Fig. 60.11), using the Giemsa or the Ethin–Starey silver stains, and cultured using appropriate media. Previous or current infection with the organism may also be detected serologically.

After infection with *H. pylori*, enzymes produced by the organism disrupt the gastric mucous barrier and the inflammation induced in the gastric epithelium is the basis of many of the associated disease processes. The association of the organism with chronic (type B) gastritis is not in doubt as Koch's postulates have been fulfilled. Some strains of *H. pylori* produce cytotoxins, notably the *cagA* and *vacA* gene products, and the production of cytotoxins seems to be associated with the ability of the organism to cause gastritis, peptic ulceration and cancer. The effect of the organism on the gastric epithelium is to incite a classic inflammatory response that involves the migration and degranulation of acute inflammatory cells, such as neutrophils, and also the accumulation of chronic inflammatory cells, such as macrophages and lymphocytes.

It is evident how *H. pylori* infection results in chronic gastritis and also how this may progress to gastric ulceration, but for a while it remained an enigma as to how the organism could be involved in duodenal ulceration, as the normal duodenum is not colonised. As mentioned above, the production of ammonia does increase the level of circulating gastrin and it has been subsequently shown that eradication of the organism in patients with duodenal ulcer disease will reduce the acid levels to normal. However, the overlap in gastric acid secretion between normal subjects and those with duodenal ulcers is considerable and the modestly increased acid levels in patients with *Helicobacter*-associated antral gastritis are insufficient to explain the aetiology of duodenal ulceration.

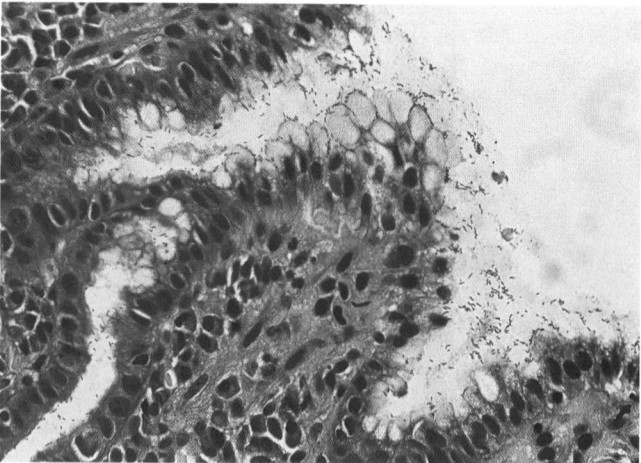

Figure 60.11 Antral mucosa showing colonisation with *Helicobacter pylori* (modified Giemsa stain).

The explanation can probably be found in the phenomenon of duodenal gastric metaplasia. Gastric metaplasia is the normal response of the duodenal mucosa to excess acidity. It can be thought of in the same way as any other metaplasia in the gastro-intestinal tract: an attempt by the mucosa to resist an injurious stimulus. Although normal duodenal mucosa cannot be infected with *H. pylori*, gastric metaplasia in the duodenum is commonly infected and this infection results in the same inflammatory process that is observed in the gastric mucosa. The result is duodenitis, which is almost certainly the precursor of duodenal ulceration.

Infection with *H. pylori* may be the most common human infection. The incidence of infection within a population increases with age and, in many populations, infection rates of 80–90% are not unusual. It appears that most infection is acquired in childhood and the probability of infection is inversely related to socio-economic group. The means of spread has not been identified but the organism can occur in the faeces and faeco-oral spread seems most likely. The organism is not normally found in saliva or dental plaque. There is evidence in different environments and in different population groups that the manifestations of the infection may be different. Predominantly antral gastritis, which is commonly seen in the west, results initially in increased levels of acid production and peptic ulcer disease, whereas gastritis affecting the body of the stomach, common in the developing world, may lead to hypochlorhydria and gastric neoplasia.

It has been known since 1984 that *Helicobacter* infection is amenable to treatment with antibiotics. The profound hypochlorhydria produced by proton pump inhibitors combined with antibiotics is also effective in eradicating the organism. Commonly used eradication regimes include a proton pump inhibitor and two antibiotics, such as metronidazole and amoxycillin. Very high eradication rates, in the region of 90%, can be achieved with combinations that include the antibiotic clarithromycin, although it may be that, in the future, antibiotic resistance will become a problem. Reinfection following successful eradication appears rare but incomplete eradication is a more important clinical problem.

At present, eradication therapy is recommended for patients with duodenal ulcer disease but not for patients with non-ulcer dyspepsia or in asymptomatic patients who are infected. However, recent data show that a proportion of patients with non-ulcer dyspepsia do respond to treatment. *Helicobacter pylori* is now classed by the World Health Organization as a class 1 carcinogen and it may be that further epidemiological studies on the risk of gastric cancer change the current advice on treatment.

GASTRITIS

The understanding of gastritis has increased markedly following elucidation of the role of *H. pylori* in chronic gastritis.

Type A gastritis

This is an autoimmune condition in which there are circulating antibodies to the parietal cell. This results in the atrophy of the parietal cell mass, resulting in hypochlorhydria and ultimately achlorhydria. As intrinsic factor is also produced by the parietal cell there is malabsorption of vitamin B12, which, if untreated, may result in pernicious anaemia. In type A gastritis, the antrum is not affected and the hypochlorhydria leads to the production of high levels of gastrin from the antral G cells. This results in chronic hypergastrinaemia. This, in turn, results in hypertrophy of the ECL cells in the body of the stomach, which are not affected by the autoimmune damage. Over time it is apparent that microadenomas develop in the ECL cells of the stomach, sometimes becoming identifiable tumour nodules. Very rarely, these tumours can become malignant. Patients with type A gastritis are predisposed to the development of gastric cancer, and screening such patients endoscopically may be appropriate.

Type B gastritis

There are abundant epidemiological data to support the association of this type of gastritis with *H. pylori* infection. Most commonly, type B gastritis affects the antrum, and it is these patients who are prone to peptic ulcer disease. *Helicobacter*-associated pangastritis is also a very common manifestation of infection, but gastritis affecting the corpus alone does not seem to be associated. However, there are some data to suggest that *Helicobacter* may be involved in the initiation of the process. Patients with pangastritis seem to be most prone to the development of gastric cancer.

Intestinal metaplasia is associated with chronic pangastritis with atrophy. Although intestinal metaplasia per se is common, intestinal metaplasia associated with dysplasia has significant malignant potential and, if this condition is identified, endoscopic screening may be appropriate.

Reflux gastritis

This is caused by enterogastric reflux and is particularly common after gastric surgery. Its histological features are distinct from those of other types of gastritis. Although commonly seen after gastric surgery, it is occasionally found in patients with no previous surgical intervention or who have had a cholecystectomy. Bile-chelating or prokinetic agents may be useful in treatment and as a temporising measure to avoid the consideration of revisional surgery. Operation for this condition should be reserved for the most severe cases.

Erosive gastritis

This is caused by agents that disturb the gastric mucosal barrier; NSAIDs and alcohol are common causes. The NSAID-induced gastric lesion is associated with inhibition of the cyclo-oxygenase type 1 (COX-1) enzyme, hence reducing the production of cytoprotective prostaglandins in the stomach. Many of the beneficial anti-inflammatory activities of NSAIDs are mediated by COX-2, and the use of specific COX-2 inhibitors reduces the incidence of these side-effects. However, taken in the long term, COX-2 inhibitors appear to be associated with cardiovascular complications, in common with many NSAIDs.

Stress gastritis

This is a common sequel of serious illness or injury and is characterised by a reduction in the blood supply to superficial mucosa of the stomach. Although common, it is not usually recognised unless stress ulceration and bleeding supervene, in which case treatment can be extremely difficult. The condition also sometimes follows cardiopulmonary bypass. Prevention of the stress bleeding from the stomach is much easier than treating it, hence the routine use of H_2-receptor antagonists, with or without barrier agents such as sucralfate, in patients who are in intensive care. These measures have been shown to reduce the incidence of bleeding from stress ulceration.

Ménétrier's disease

This is an unusual condition characterised by gross hypertrophy of the gastric mucosal folds, mucus production and hypochlorhydria. The condition is pre-malignant and may present with hypoproteinaemia and anaemia. There is no treatment other than a gastrectomy. The disease seems to be caused by overexpression of transforming growth factor alpha (TGFα). Like epidermal growth factor (EGF), this peptide also binds to the EGF receptor. The histological features of Ménétrier's disease may be reproduced in transgenic mice overexpressing TGFα.

Lymphocytic gastritis

This type of gastritis is seen rarely. It is characterised by the infiltration of the gastric mucosa by T cells and is probably associated with *H. pylori* infection. The pattern of inflammation resembles that seen in coeliac disease or lymphocytic colitis.

Other forms of gastritis

Eosinophilic gastritis appears to have an allergic basis and is treated with steroids and cromoglycate. Granulomatous gastritis is seen rarely in Crohn's disease and may also be associated with tuberculosis. Acquired immunodeficiency syndrome (AIDS) gastritis is secondary to infection with *Cryptosporidium*. Phlegmonous gastritis is a rare bacterial infection of the stomach found in patients with severe intercurrent illness. It is usually an agonal event (Summary box 60.3).

Summary box 60.3

Gastritis

- The spiral bacterium *H. pylori* is critical in the development of type B gastritis, peptic ulceration and gastric cancer
- Infection appears to be acquired mainly in childhood and the infection rate is inversely associated to socio-economic status
- Eradication, recommended specifically in patients with peptic ulcer disease, can be achieved in up to 90% of patients with a combination of a proton pump inhibitor and antibiotics, and reinfection is uncommon
- Erosive gastritis is usually related to the use of non-steroidal anti-inflammatory drugs (NSAIDs)
- Type A gastritis is an autoimmune process and is associated with the development of gastric cancer

---

PEPTIC ULCERS

Although the name 'peptic' ulcer suggests an association with pepsin, this is essentially unimportant as in the absence of acid, for instance in type A gastritis with atrophy, peptic ulcers do not occur. All peptic ulcers can be healed by using proton pump inhibitors, which can render a patient virtually achlorhydric.

Common sites for peptic ulcers are the first part of the duodenum and the lesser curve of the stomach, but they also occur on the stoma following gastric surgery, the oesophagus and even in a Meckel's diverticulum, which contains ectopic gastric epithelium. In general, the ulcer occurs at a junction between different types of epithelium, the ulcer occurring in the epithelium least resistant to acid damage.

In the past, much distinction has been made between acute and chronic peptic ulcers, but this difference can sometimes be difficult to determine clinically. It is probably best to consider that there is a spectrum of disease, from superficial gastric and duodenal ulcers, frequently seen at endoscopy, to deep chronic penetrating ulcers. This does not minimise the importance of acute stress ulceration; these ulcers can both perforate and bleed.

For many years, the cause of peptic ulceration remained an enigma. When comparing groups of patients having duodenal and pre-pyloric peptic ulcers with normal subjects, gastric acid levels are higher in the ulcer group, but the overlap is very considerable. Patients with gastric ulceration have relatively normal levels of gastric acid secretion. As peptic ulceration will occur in the presence of very high acid levels, such as those found in patients with a gastrinoma (Zollinger–Ellison syndrome), and as all ulcers can be healed in the absence of acid, it is clear that acid is important. In patients with a gastrinoma it may be the only aetiological factor, but this is not the case in the majority of patients. As with many diseases, genetic factors may be involved to a limited degree and social stress has also been implicated, although this has been shown to be false (Asher).

It is now widely accepted that infection with *H. pylori* is the most important factor in the development of peptic ulceration. The other factor of major importance at present is ingestion of NSAIDs. Cigarette smoking predisposes to peptic ulceration and increases the relapse rate after treatment with gastric antisecretory agents or, as carried out in the past, elective surgery. Multiple other factors may be involved in the transition between the superficial and the deep penetrating chronic ulcer, but they are of lesser importance.

Duodenal ulceration

Incidence

There have been marked changes in the last two decades in the demography of patients presenting with duodenal ulceration in the west. First, even before the introduction of H_2-receptor antagonists, the incidence of duodenal ulceration and the frequency of elective surgery for the condition were falling. This trend has continued and now, in the west, dyspeptic patients presenting with a duodenal ulcer at gastroscopy are uncommon. In part, this may relate to the widespread use of gastric antisecretory agents and eradication therapy for patients with dyspepsia. Second, the peak incidence is now in a much older age group than previously and, although it is still more common in men, the difference is less marked. These changes mirror the changes, at least in part, in the epidemiology of *H. pylori* infection. In Eastern

---

Pierre Eugene Menetrier, 1859–1935, a French Histopathologist who later became Professor of Medical History in the Faculty of Medicine, Paris, France.
Burrill Bernard Crohn, 1884–1983, Gastroenterologist, Mount Sinai Hospital, New York, NY, USA described regional ileitis in 1932.

Johann Friedrich Meckel, (The Younger), 1781–1833, Professor of Anatomy and Surgery, Halle, Germany, described the diverticulum in 1809.
Robert Milton Zollinger, B. 1903, Professor of Surgery, The Ohio State University, Columbus, OH, USA.
Edwin Horner Ellison, 1918–1970, Professor of Surgery, Marquette University, WI, USA.
Zollinger and Ellison described this condition in a joint paper in 1955 when they were both working at The Ohio State University.
Richard Asher, 1912–1969, Physician, The Central Middlesex Hospital, London, England.

Europe the disease remains common and, although previously uncommon, it is now observed more frequently in some developing nations. Again, the relationship with *H. pylori* appears convincing.

Pathology

Most duodenal ulcers occur in the first part of the duodenum (Figs 60.12 and 60.13). A chronic ulcer penetrates the mucosa and into the muscle coat, leading to fibrosis. The fibrosis causes deformities such as pyloric stenosis. When an ulcer heals, a scar can be observed in the mucosa. Sometimes there may be more than one duodenal ulcer. The situation in which there is both a posterior and an anterior duodenal ulcer is referred to as 'kissing ulcers'. Anteriorly placed ulcers tend to perforate and, in contrast, posterior duodenal ulcers tend to bleed, sometimes by eroding a large vessel such as the gastroduodenal artery. Occasionally, the ulceration may be so extensive that the entire duodenal cap is ulcerated and devoid of mucosa. With respect to the giant duodenal ulcer, malignancy in this region is so

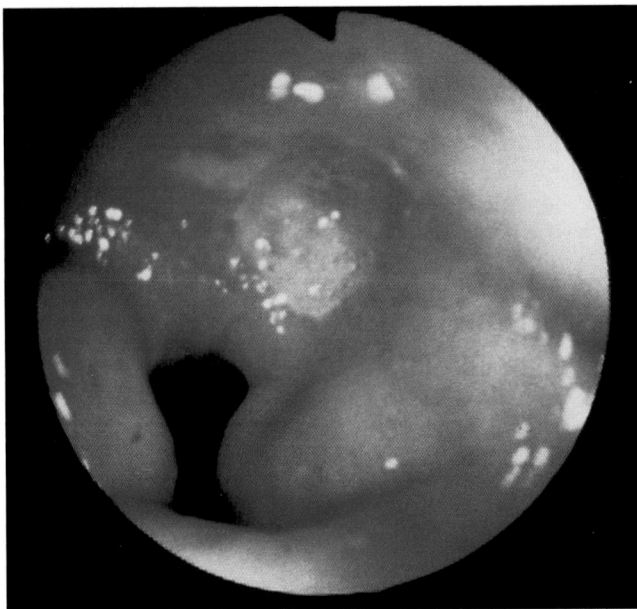

Figure 60.12 Duodenal ulcer at gastroduodenoscopy (courtesy of Dr G.N.J. Tytgat, Amsterdam, The Netherlands).

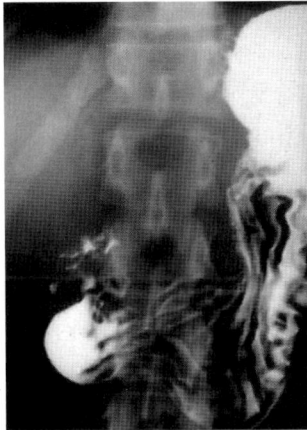

Figure 60.13 Duodenal ulcer shown by barium meal.

uncommon that, in normal circumstances, surgeons can be confident that they are dealing with benign disease, even though from external palpation it may not appear so. In the stomach the situation is different.

Histopathology

Microscopically, destruction of the muscular coat is observed and the base of the ulcer is covered with granulation tissue, with the arteries in this region showing the typical changes of endarteritis obliterans. Sometimes the terminations of nerves can be seen among the fibrosis. The pathological appearance of the healing ulcer must be carefully observed as some of the epithelial downgrowths can be misinterpreted as invasion. This is unlikely to be important in duodenal ulcers when malignancy rarely, if ever, occurs, but it is much more important in gastric ulcers.

Gastric ulceration

Incidence

As with duodenal ulceration, *H. pylori* and NSAIDs are the important aetiological factors in gastric ulceration. Gastric ulceration is also associated with smoking; other factors are of lesser importance.

There are marked differences between the populations affected by chronic gastric ulceration and those affected by duodenal ulceration. First, gastric ulceration is substantially less common than duodenal ulceration. The incidence of gastric ulcers is equal between the sexes and the population with gastric ulcers tends to be older. They are more prevalent in low socioeconomic groups and considerably more common in the developing world than in the west.

Pathology

The pathology of gastric ulcers is essentially similar to that of duodenal ulcers, except that gastric ulcers tend to be larger. Fibrosis, when it occurs, may result in the now rarely seen hourglass contraction of the stomach. Large chronic ulcers may erode posteriorly into the pancreas and, on other occasions, into major vessels such as the splenic artery. Less commonly, they may erode into other organs such as the transverse colon. Chronic gastric ulcers are much more common on the lesser curve (especially at the incisura angularis; Figs 60.14 and 60.15) than on the greater curve and, even when high on the lesser curve, they tend to be at the boundary between the acid-secreting and the non-acid-secreting epithelia. With atrophy of the parietal cell mass, non-acid-secreting epithelium migrates up the lesser curvature.

Malignancy in gastric ulcers

Chronic duodenal ulcers are not associated with malignancy but, in contrast, gastric ulcers are. Widely varying estimates are made of the incidence of gastric malignancy in gastric ulcers. The reason for this is that the authors reporting such diverse incidences are describing different clinical situations. Two clinical extremes must be distinguished to understand this problem. First, there is the situation in which a benign chronic gastric ulcer undergoes malignant transformation. This is known to happen, albeit rarely. The contrasting clinical extreme is the patient identified as having an ulcer in the stomach, either endoscopically or on contrast radiology, which is assessed as benign but biopsies reveal malignancy. In this situation the patient does not have, and probably never has had, chronic peptic ulceration in the stomach but has

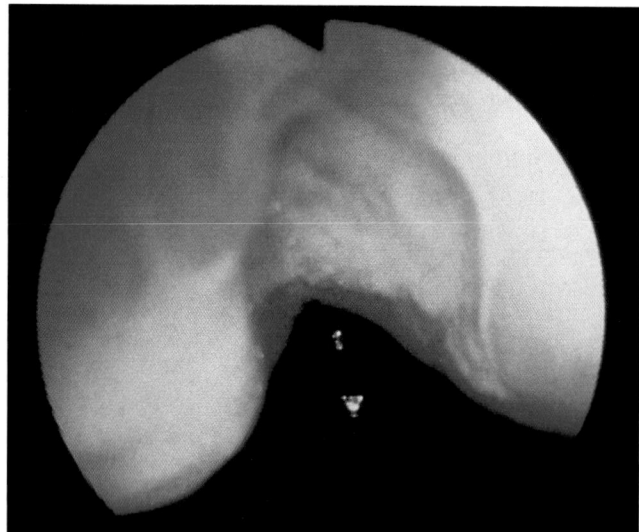

Figure 60.14 Benign incisural gastric ulcer shown at gastroscopy (courtesy of Dr G.N.J. Tytgat, Amsterdam, The Netherlands).

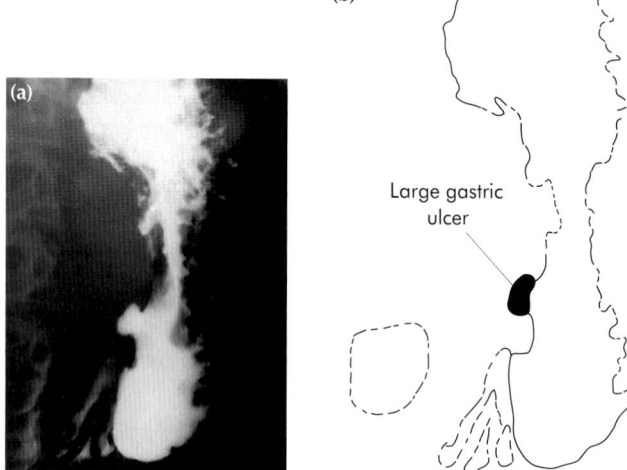

(b)

(a)

Large gastric ulcer

Figure 60.15 Benign gastric ulcer shown by barium meal. (a) Radiograph. (b) Diagrammatic outline.

presented with an ulcerated cancer. This situation is common, although whether a lesion found in the stomach is described as being benign or malignant on clinical grounds depends very much on the experience of the endoscopist or radiologist.

It is fundamental that any gastric ulcer should be regarded as being malignant, no matter how classically it resembles a benign gastric ulcer. Multiple biopsies should always be taken, perhaps as many as 10 well-targeted biopsies, before an ulcer can be tentatively accepted as being benign. Even then it is important that further biopsies are taken while the ulcer is healing and when healed. Modern anti-secretory agents can frequently heal the ulceration associated with gastric cancer but, clearly, are ineffective in treating the malignancy itself. At operation, even experienced surgeons may have difficulty distinguishing between the gastric cancer and a benign ulcer. Operative strategies differ so radically that it is essential, if at all possible, that a confident diagnosis is made before operation. The petechial haemorrhages found on the serosa of the patient with peptic ulceration are a

useful sign, but not entirely reliable. If at operation it is determined that the ulcer is probably benign, it should nonetheless be completely excised, if possible, and submitted for histological examination. It is not known whether a patient's survival is compromised by this approach if the ulcer turns out to be malignant on biopsy, as convincing data are not available.

Other peptic ulcers

The pre-pyloric gastric ulcer was difficult to treat in the past, a problem that has been overcome with the introduction of proton pump inhibitors. Pyloric channel ulcers are similar to duodenal ulcers. Both pre-pyloric and pyloric ulcers may be malignant, and biopsy is essential. Stomal ulcers occur after a gastroenterostomy or a gastrectomy of the Billroth II type. The ulcer is usually found on the jejunal side of the stoma.

Clinical features of peptic ulcers

Although many textbooks try to create differences in the clinical features of gastric and duodenal ulceration, detailed analysis has shown that they cannot be differentiated on the basis of symptoms. The demographic characteristics of groups of patients with gastric and duodenal ulceration do differ but this does not allow discrimination.

Pain

The pain is epigastric, often described as gnawing, and may radiate to the back. Eating may sometimes relieve the discomfort. The pain is normally intermittent rather than intractable.

Periodicity

One of the classic features of untreated peptic ulceration is periodicity. Symptoms may disappear for weeks or months to return again. This periodicity may be related to the spontaneous healing of the ulcer.

Vomiting

Although this occurs, it is not a notable feature unless stenosis has occurred.

Alteration in weight

Weight loss or, sometimes, weight gain may occur. Patients with gastric ulceration are often underweight but this may precede the occurrence of the ulcer.

Bleeding

All peptic ulcers may bleed. The bleeding may be chronic and presentation with anaemia is not uncommon. Acute presentation with haematemesis and melaena is discussed later.

Clinical examination

Examination of the patient may reveal epigastric tenderness but, except in extreme cases (for instance gastric outlet obstruction), there is unlikely to be much else to find.

Investigation of the patient with suspected peptic ulcer

Gastroduodenoscopy

This is the investigation of choice in the management of suspected peptic ulceration and, in the hands of a well-trained operator, is highly accurate.

In the stomach, any abnormal lesion should be multiply biopsied and, in the case of a suspected benign gastric ulcer, numerous biopsies must be taken to exclude, as far as possible, the presence of a malignancy. Commonly, biopsies of the antrum will be taken to see whether there is histological evidence of gastritis and a CLO test performed to determine the presence of *H. pylori*. A 'U' manoeuvre should be performed to exclude ulcers around the gastro-oesophageal junction. This is important as the increasing incidence of cancer at the gastro-oesophageal junction requires that all mucosal abnormalities in this region should undergo multiple biopsy. Similarly, if a stoma is present, for instance after gastroenterostomy or Billroth II gastrectomy, it is important to enter both afferent and efferent loops. Almost all stomal ulcers will be very close to the junction between the jejunal and gastric mucosa. Attention should be given to the pylorus to note whether there is any pre-pyloric or pyloric channel ulceration, and also whether it is deformed, which is often the case with chronic duodenal ulceration. In the duodenum, care must be taken to view all of the first part. It is not infrequent for an ulcer to be just beyond the pylorus and easily overlooked.

Treatment of peptic ulceration

The vast majority of uncomplicated peptic ulcers are treated medically. Surgical treatment of uncomplicated peptic ulceration has decreased markedly since the 1960s and is now seldom performed in the west. Surgical treatment was aimed principally at reducing gastric acid secretion and, in the case of gastric ulceration, removing the diseased mucosa. When originally devised, medical treatment also aimed to reduce gastric acid secretion, initially using highly successful H_2-receptor antagonists and, subsequently, proton pump inhibitors. This has now largely given way to eradication therapy.

Medical treatment

It is reasonable that a doctor managing a patient with an uncomplicated peptic ulcer should suggest modifications to the patient's lifestyle, particularly the cessation of cigarette smoking. This advice is rarely followed and pharmacological measures form the mainstay of treatment.

H_2-receptor antagonists and proton pump inhibitors

H_2-receptor antagonists (Black) revolutionised the management of peptic ulceration; most duodenal ulcers and gastric ulcers can be healed by a few weeks of treatment with these drugs provided that they are taken and absorbed. There remain, however, a group of patients who are relatively refractory to conventional doses of H_2-receptor antagonists. This is largely now irrelevant as proton pump inhibitors can effectively render a patient achlorhydric and all benign ulcers will heal using these drugs, the majority within 2 weeks. Symptom relief is impressively rapid, most patients being asymptomatic within a few days. Like H_2-receptor antagonists, proton pump inhibitors are safe and relatively devoid of serious side-effects. The problem with all gastric anti-secretory agents is that, following cessation of therapy, relapse is almost universal.

Eradication therapy

Eradication therapy is now routinely given to patients with peptic ulceration, and this is described earlier in this chapter (see *Helicobacter pylori*, p. 1051). Evidence suggests that if a patient has a peptic ulcer and *H. pylori* is the principal aetiological factor (essentially the patient not taking NSAIDs), complete eradication of the organism will cure the disease and reinfection as an adult is uncommon. Eradication therapy is therefore the mainstay of treatment for peptic ulceration. It is extremely economical by comparison with prolonged courses of anti-secretory agents or surgery. It is also considerably safer than surgical treatment.

There are some patients with peptic ulcers in whom eradication therapy may not be appropriate and this includes patients with NSAID-associated ulcers. Such patients should avoid these drugs if possible and, if not, they should be co-prescribed with a potent anti-secretory agent. Similarly, patients with stomal ulceration are not effectively treated with eradication therapy and require a prolonged course of anti-secretory agents. Patients with Zollinger–Ellison syndrome should be treated in the long term with proton pump inhibitors unless the tumour can be adequately managed by surgery.

Surgical treatment of uncomplicated peptic ulceration

From its peak in the 1960s, the incidence of surgery for uncomplicated peptic ulceration has fallen markedly, to the extent that peptic ulcer surgery is now of little more than historical interest. A description of operations used in the treatment of peptic ulcers is still necessary because surgery is commonly employed for the complicated ulcer and, in addition, many patients are left suffering from the consequences of the more destructive operations.

Operations for duodenal ulceration

Duodenal ulcer surgery (rationale)

Procedures devised for the treatment of duodenal ulcers have the common aim of excluding the damaging effects of acid from the duodenum. This has been achieved by diversion of the acid away from the duodenum, reducing the secretory potential of the stomach, or both. All of the operations devised achieved their aim to some extent, but with varying degrees of morbidity, mortality and postoperative side-effects. There is now no role for acid-reducing operations in the routine management of peptic ulcer disease but, occasionally, operations that involve gastrectomy have to be performed in the emergency situation. In addition, many patients have had such operations performed and suffer from the sequelae. Hence, it is important for the clinician to understand the anatomical and physiological consequences of surgery. The operations are described in historical sequence.

Billroth II gastrectomy

The first successful gastrectomy was performed by Billroth in January 1881, and Wolfler performed the first gastroenterostomy in the same year. The original Billroth operation consisted of a gastric resection with gastroduodenal anastomosis (Billroth I technique) (Fig. 60.16). The Billroth II operation was devised more by accident than design (Fig. 60.17). A gastroenterostomy (Fig. 60.18) was performed on a gravely ill patient with a pyloric

Sir James Whyte Black, **1924–2002, Professor of Analytical Pharmacology, King's College Hospital Medical School, London, England, introduced beta blockers and H receptor antagonists. For this work he shared the 1988 Nobel Prize for Physiology or Medicine with Gertrude Elion and George Hitchings.**

Christian Albert Theodor Billroth, **1829–1894, Professor of Surgery, Vienna, Austria.** Anton Wolfler, **1850–1917, Professor of Surgery, Prague, The Czech Republic.**

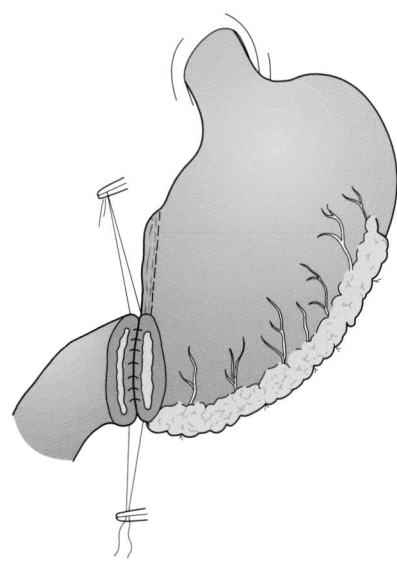

Figure 60.16 Billroth I gastrectomy. The lower half of the stomach is removed and the cut stomach anastomosed to the first part of the duodenum.

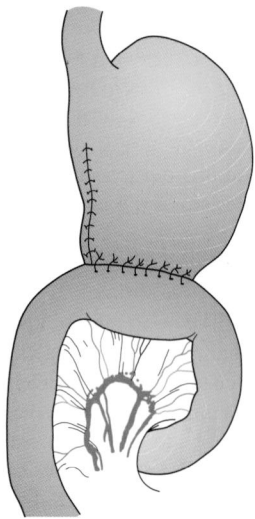

Figure 60.17 Billroth II. Two-thirds of the stomach are removed, the duodenal stump is closed and the stomach is anastomosed to the jejunum.

cancer, who was not expected to survive. Contrary to expectations, the patient improved and the stomach distal to the anastomosis was resected. It soon became evident that the use of gastrojejunal anastomosis after gastric resection could be safer and easier than the Billroth I procedure, and it became popular and effective in the surgical treatment of duodenal ulcer. Because of its disadvantages, such as higher operative mortality and morbidity, it has not been used for many years in the patient with an uncomplicated ulcer, but it is still used occasionally in the treatment of a complicated ulcer with a 'difficult' duodenum. In Billroth II gastrectomy, or its close relation Pólya gastrectomy, the

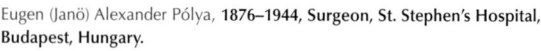

Eugen (Janö) Alexander Pólya, **1876–1944, Surgeon, St. Stephen's Hospital, Budapest, Hungary.**

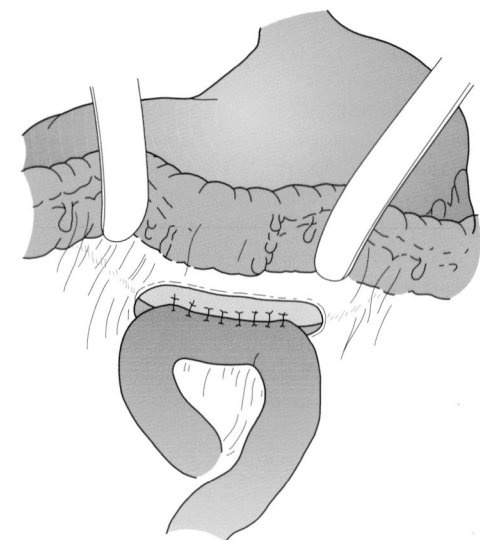

Figure 60.18 Gastroenterostomy. The jejunum is anastomosed to the posterior, dependent wall of the stomach.

antrum and distal body of the stomach are mobilised by opening the greater and lesser omentum and dividing the gastroepiploic arteries, right gastric artery and left gastric artery arcade at the limit of the resection. The duodenum is closed off either by suture or using staples, sometimes with difficulty in patients with a very deformed duodenum. Various techniques are available to close the difficult duodenum and, *in extremis*, a catheter may be placed in the duodenal stump, the duodenum closed around it and the catheter brought out through the abdominal wall. Following resection, the distal end of the stomach is narrowed by the closure of the lesser curve aspect of the remnant. The greater curve aspect is then anastomosed, usually in a retrocolic fashion, to the jejunum, leaving as short an afferent loop as feasible (see Fig. 60.17). Even when well performed, this procedure has an operative mortality rate of a few per cent and morbidity is not unusual. A common cause of morbidity is leakage from the duodenal stump, which is particularly associated with kinking of the afferent loop. Leakage from the gastrojejunal anastomosis is unusual unless it is under tension or the stomach has been devascularised during the mobilisation. The incidence of side-effects following gastrectomy is considerable, as shown in Table 60.2. Recurrence of the ulcer at the stoma is uncommon but can occur, especially as this procedure is traditionally not combined with vagotomy.

Gastrojejunostomy

Because of the potential for mortality after gastrectomy, the use of gastrojejunostomy alone in the treatment of duodenal ulceration was developed (Fig. 60.18). Reflux of alkali from the small bowel into the stomach reduced duodenal acid exposure and was often successful in healing the ulcer. However, because the jejunal loop was exposed directly to gastric acid, stomal ulceration was extremely common, hence the procedure in isolation was ineffective.

Truncal vagotomy and drainage

Truncal vagotomy was first introduced in 1943 by Dragstedt and, for many years, combined with drainage, was the mainstay of

Lester Reynold Dragstedt, **1893–1975, Professor of Surgery, Chicago, IL, USA.**

Table 60.2 Operative mortality, side effects and incidence of recurrence following duodenal ulcer operations

Operation	Operative mortality (%)	Significant side-effects (%)	Recurrent ulceration (%)
Gastrectomy	1–2	20–40	1–4
Gastroenterostomy alone	< 1	10–20	50
Truncal vagotomy and drainage	< 1	10–20	2–7
Selective vagotomy and drainage	< 1	10–20	5–10
Highly selective vagotomy	< 0.2	< 5	2–10
Truncal vagotomy and antrectomy	1	10–20	1

treatment of duodenal ulceration (Fig. 60.19). The principle of the operation is that section of the vagus nerves, which are critically involved in the secretion of gastric acid, reduces the maximal acid output by approximately 50%. Because the vagal nerves are conductors of motor impulses to the stomach, denervation of the antropyloroduodenal segment results in gastric stasis in a substantial proportion of patients on whom truncal vagotomy alone is performed. This was first noted by Dragstedt, who did not perform a drainage procedure when he first introduced the operation. The most popular drainage procedure was the Heineke–Mikulicz pyloroplasty (Fig. 60.20). It was simple to perform and involved the longitudinal section of the pyloric ring. The incision was closed transversely. Gastrojejunostomy (see Fig. 60.18) was the alternative drainage procedure to pyloroplasty. This was performed by opening the lesser sac and performing an anastomosis between the most dependent part of the antrum and the first jejunal loop. An isoperistaltic anastomosis was most commonly performed. The operation of truncal vagotomy and drainage was substantially safer than gastrectomy (Table 60.2). However, the side-effects of surgery were, in fact, little different from those that follow gastrectomy.

Highly selective vagotomy

In 1968 Johnston and Amdrup independently devised the operation of highly selective vagotomy in which only the parietal cell mass of the stomach was denervated (Fig. 60.21). This proved to be the most satisfactory operation for duodenal ulceration, with a low incidence of side-effects and acceptable recurrence rates when performed to a high technical standard. This operation became the 'gold standard' for the treatment of duodenal ulceration in the 1970s. The operative mortality rate was lower than

any other definitive operation for duodenal ulceration, in all probability because the gastrointestinal tract was not opened during this procedure. The unpleasant effects of surgery were largely avoided, although loss of receptive relaxation of the stomach did occur, leading to epigastric fullness and sometimes mild dumping. However, the severe symptoms that are seen after other more destructive gastric operations did not occur. It is often said that recurrent ulceration was the Achilles heel of this operation although, when performed well, recurrence was no more common than after truncal vagotomy. The operation disappeared from routine use with the advent of anti-secretory agents and eradication therapy.

Truncal vagotomy and antrectomy

For completeness this operation should be mentioned because at one stage it was popular in the USA. In addition to a truncal vagotomy, the antrum of the stomach was removed, thus eradicating the source of gastrin, and the gastric remnant was joined to the duodenum. The recurrence rates after this procedure were exceedingly low. However, the operative mortality rate was higher than after vagotomy and drainage (Table 60.2) and the incidence of unpleasant side-effects was similar.

Operations for gastric ulcer

In contrast to duodenal ulcer surgery, in which the principal objective was to reduce duodenal acid exposure, in gastric ulceration, the diseased tissue is usually removed as well. This has the advantage that malignancy can then be confidently excluded. As with duodenal ulceration, such surgery is not now performed except for complications of gastric ulcer.

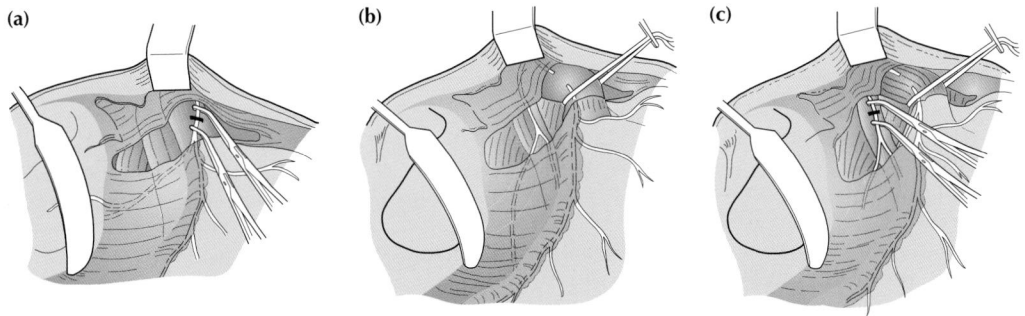

Figure 60.19 Truncal vagotomy. (a) Division of the anterior vagus. (b) Mobilisation of the oesophagus. (c) Division of the posterior vagus.

Walther Hermann Heineke, **1834–1901, Surgeon, of Erlangen, Germany.**
Johann von Mikulicz-Radecki, **1850–1905, Professor of Surgery, Breslau, Germany (now Wroclaw, Poland).**
David Johnston, **Professor of Surgery, The University of Leeds, Leeds, England.**
Eric Amdrup, **1923–1998, Professor of Surgery, Aarhus, Denmark.**

CHAPTER 60 | STOMACH AND DUODENUM

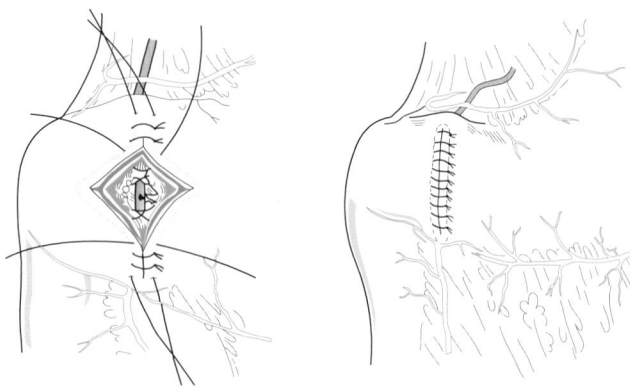

Figure 60.20 Pylroplasty.

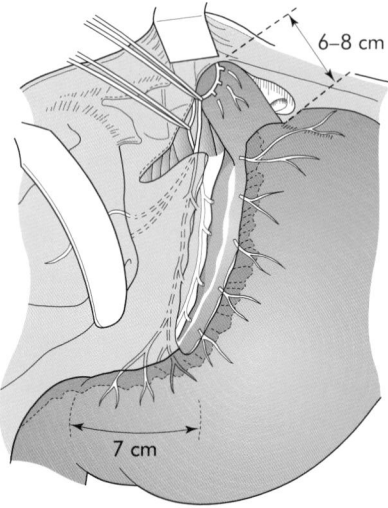

Figure 60.21 Highly selective vagotomy. The anterior and posterior vagus nerves are preserved but all branches to the fundus and body of the stomach are divided.

Billroth I gastrectomy

This was the standard operation (see Fig. 60.16) for gastric ulceration until medical treatments became prevalent. The distal stomach is mobilised and resected in the same way as in the Billroth II gastrectomy. This resection should include the ulcer, which is usually situated on the lesser curve. The cut edge of the remnant is then partially closed from the lesser curve aspect, leaving a stoma at the greater curve aspect, which should be similar in size to the duodenum. Reconstruction may be facilitated by mobilising the duodenum using Kocher's manoeuvre. The incidence of recurrent ulceration after this operation is low, but it carries with it the morbidity and mortality rates associated with any gastric resection.

Sequelae of peptic ulcer surgery

There are a number of sequelae of peptic ulcer surgery, which include recurrent ulceration, small stomach syndrome, bilious vomiting, early and late dumping, diarrhoea and malignant transformation. These sequelae principally follow the more destructive

operations, which are now seldom performed. However, a substantial number of patients suffer from side-effects from operations undertaken in the past. Approximately 30% of patients can expect to suffer a degree of dysfunction following peptic ulcer surgery (Table 60.2) and, in about 5% of such patients, the symptoms will be intractable.

Recurrent ulceration

Although mentioned first, this is by far the easiest problem to treat. Just as all peptic ulcers will heal with potent anti-secretory agents, so will ulcers that are recurrent after ulcer surgery.

As with other peptic ulcers, recurrent ulcers may present with complications, particularly bleeding and perforation. In this respect, the complication of gastrojejunal colic fistula requires a particular mention. In this rare condition, the anastomotic ulcer penetrates into the transverse colon. Patients suffer from diarrhoea that is severe and follows every meal. They have foul breath and may vomit formed faeces. Severe weight loss and dehydration are rapid in onset and, for this reason, the condition may be mistaken for malignancy. The major factor producing the nutritional disturbance is the severe contamination of the jejunum with colonic bacteria. A number of imaging techniques can be used to detect the fistula, most commonly CT with oral contrast or, indeed, a barium enema. Endoscopy may not convincingly demonstrate the fistula and, in about one-half of such cases, the barium meal will not reveal the problem. The treatment of gastro-colic fistula consists of first correcting the dehydration and malnutrition and then performing revisional surgery.

Small stomach syndrome

Early satiety follows most ulcer operations to some degree, including highly selective vagotomy, in which, although there is no anatomical disturbance of the stomach, there is a loss of receptive relaxation. Fortunately, this problem does tend to get better with time and revisional surgery is not necessary.

Bile vomiting

Bile vomiting can occur after any form of vagotomy with drainage or gastrectomy. Commonly, the patient presents with vomiting of a mixture of food and bile or sometimes bile alone after a meal. Often, eating will precipitate abdominal pain and reflux symptoms are common. Bile-chelating agents can be tried but are usually ineffective. In intractable cases, revisional surgery may be indicated. The nature of the revision depends very much on the original operation. Following gastrectomy, Roux-en-Y diversion is probably the best treatment. In patients with a gastroenterostomy, the drainage may be taken down and, in most circumstances, a small pyloroplasty can be performed. In patients with a pyloroplasty, reconstruction of the pylorus has been attempted but, in general terms, the results have been rather poor. Antrectomy and Roux-en-Y reconstruction may be the better option.

Early and late dumping

Although considered together because the symptoms are similar, early and late dumping have different aetiologies A common feature, however, is early rapid gastric emptying. Many patients have both early and late dumping.

Early dumping

Early dumping consists of abdominal and vasomotor symptoms, which are found in about 5–10% of patients following gastrectomy or vagotomy and drainage. It also affects a small percentage of patients following highly selective vagotomy because of the loss of receptive relaxation of the stomach. The small bowel is filled with foodstuffs from the stomach, which have a high osmotic load, and this leads to the sequestration of fluid from the circulation into the gastrointestinal tract. This can be observed by the rise in the packed cell volume while the symptoms are present. All of the symptoms shown in Table 60.3 can be related to this effect on the gut and the circulation.

Treatment The principal treatment is dietary manipulation. Small, dry meals are best, and avoiding fluids with a high carbohydrate content also helps. Fortunately, following operation, the syndrome tends to improve with time. For some reason, however, there is a group of patients who suffer intractable dumping regardless of any of these measures. The somatostatin analogue octreotide, given before meals, has been shown to be useful in some individuals and the long-acting preparation may also be useful. However, this treatment can lead to the development of gallstones and it does not help the diarrhoea from which many patients with dumping also suffer.

Revisional surgery may be occasionally required. In patients with a gastroenterostomy, the drainage may be taken down or, in the case of a pyloroplasty, repaired. Alternatively, antrectomy with Roux-en-Y reconstruction is often effective, although the procedure is of greater magnitude; following gastrectomy, it is the revisional procedure of choice.

Late dumping

This is reactive hypoglycaemia. The carbohydrate load in the small bowel causes a rise in the plasma glucose level, which, in turn, causes insulin levels to rise, causing a secondary hypoglycaemia. This can be easily demonstrated by serial measurements of blood glucose in a patient following a test meal. The treatment is essentially the same as for early dumping. Octreotide is very effective in dealing with this problem.

Post-vagotomy diarrhoea

This can be the most devastating symptom to afflict patients having peptic ulcer surgery. Most patients will suffer looseness of bowel action to some degree (with the exception of highly selective vagotomy) but, in about 5%, it may be intractable. Despite much investigation, the precise aetiology of the problem is uncertain. It is partly related to rapid gastric emptying. In all probability, the denervation of the upper gastrointestinal tract as a result of the vagotomy is also important. Exaggerated gastrointestinal peptide responses may also aggravate the condition.

The diarrhoea may take several forms. It may be severe and explosive, with the patient experiencing a considerable degree of urgency. The patient sometimes describes the diarrhoea as feeling like passing boiling water. At the other extreme, some patients only have minor episodes of diarrhoea, which are not as directly related to food.

Many authors regard diarrhoea and dumping as being essentially the same problem. However, many patients with severe diarrhoea do not have any of the other symptoms of dumping and, likewise, some patients with dumping do not experience any significant diarrhoea.

The condition is difficult to treat. The patient should be managed as for early dumping and anti-diarrhoeal preparations may be of some value. Octreotide is not effective in treating this condition and the results of revisional surgery are too unpredictable to make this an attractive option.

Malignant transformation

Many large studies now confirm that operations such as gastrectomy or vagotomy and drainage are independent risk factors for the development of gastric cancer. The increased risk appears to be approximately four times that of the control population.

It is not difficult to understand the increased incidence of gastric cancer, as bile reflux gastritis, intestinal metaplasia and gastric cancer are linked. The lag phase between operation and the development of malignancy is at least 10 years. Highly selective vagotomy does not seem to be associated with an increased incidence.

Nutritional consequences

Nutritional disorders are more common after gastrectomy than after vagotomy and drainage. Weight loss is common after gastrectomy and the patient may never return to their original weight. Eating small meals often may help.

Anaemia may result from either iron or vitamin B12 deficiency. Iron-deficiency anaemia occurs after both gastrectomy and vagotomy and drainage and is multifactorial in origin. Reduced iron absorption is probably the most important factor, although the loss of blood from the gastric mucosa may also be important. Vitamin B12 deficiency is prone to occur after total gastrectomy. However, because of the very large vitamin B12 stores, this may be very late in occurring. Vitamin B12 supplementation after total gastrectomy is essential. Rarely, vitamin B12 deficiency may occur after lesser forms of gastrectomy. The cause

Table 60.3 Features of early and late dumping

	Early	Late
Incidence	5–10%	5%
Relation to meals	Almost immediate	Second hour after meal
Duration of attack	30–40 min	30–40 min
Relieved by	Lying down	Food
Aggravated by	More food	Exercise
Precipitating factor	Food, especially carbohydrate-rich and wet	As for early dumping
Major symptoms	Epigastric fullness, sweating, light-headedness, tachycardia, colic, sometimes diarrhoea	Tremor, faintness, prostration

CHAPTER 60 | STOMACH AND DUODENUM

is a combination of reduced intrinsic factor production and, in some patients, bacterial colonisation, which results in the destruction of vitamin B12.

Bone disease is seen principally after gastrectomy and mainly in women. The condition is essentially indistinguishable from the osteoporosis commonly seen in post-menopausal women; it is only the frequency and magnitude of the disorder that distinguish it. Treatment is through dietary supplementation with calcium and vitamin D, and with exercise.

Gallstones

The development of gallstones is strongly associated with truncal vagotomy, in which the biliary tree as well as the stomach is denervated, leading to stasis and, hence, stone formation. Patients developing symptomatic gallstones will require cholecystectomy. However, this may induce or worsen other post-peptic ulcer surgery syndromes such as bilious vomiting and post-vagotomy diarrhoea.

The complications of peptic ulceration

The common complications of peptic ulcer are perforation, bleeding and stenosis. Bleeding and stenosis are considered below in the relevant sections.

Perforated peptic ulcer

Epidemiology

Despite the widespread use of gastric anti-secretory agents and eradication therapy, the incidence of perforated peptic ulcer has changed little. However, there has been a considerable change in the epidemiology of perforated peptic ulcer in the west over the last two decades. Previously, most patients were middle aged, with a ratio of 2:1 of men:women. With time, however, there has been a steady increase in the age of the patients suffering from this complication and an increase in the number of women affected, such that perforations now occur most commonly in elderly female patients. NSAIDs appear to be responsible for most of these perforations.

Clinical features

The classic presentation is instantly recognisable (Fig. 60.22). The patient, who may have a history of peptic ulceration, develops sudden-onset, severe, generalised abdominal pain as a result of the irritant effect of gastric acid on the peritoneum. Although the contents of an acid-producing stomach are relatively low in bacterial load, bacterial peritonitis supervenes over a few hours, usually accompanied by a deterioration in the patient's condition.

Initially, the patient may be shocked with a tachycardia but a pyrexia is not usually observed until some hours after the event. The abdomen exhibits a board-like rigidity and the patient is disinclined to move because of the pain. The abdomen does not move with respiration. Patients with this form of presentation need an operation, without which they will deteriorate with a septic peritonitis.

This classic presentation of the perforated peptic ulcer is observed less commonly than in the past. Very frequently, the elderly patient who is taking NSAIDs will have a less dramatic presentation, perhaps because of the use of potent anti-inflammatory drugs. The board-like rigidity seen in the abdomen of younger patients may also not be observed and a higher index of suspicion is necessary to make the correct diagnosis. In other patients, the leak from the ulcer may not be massive. They may present only with pain in the epigastrium and right iliac fossa as the fluid may track down the right paracolic gutter. Sometimes perforations will seal as a result of the inflammatory response and adhesion within the abdominal cavity, and so the perforation may be self-limiting. All of these factors may combine to make the diagnosis of perforated peptic ulcer difficult.

By far the most common site of perforation is the anterior aspect of the duodenum. However, the anterior or incisural gastric ulcer may perforate and, in addition, gastric ulcers may perforate into the lesser sac, which can be particularly difficult to diagnose. These patients may not have obvious peritonitis.

Investigations

An erect plain chest radiograph will reveal free gas under the diaphragm in more than 50% of cases (Fig. 60.23) but CT imaging is more accurate (see below). All patients should have serum amylase levels tested, as distinguishing between peptic ulcer perforation and pancreatitis can be difficult. Measuring the serum amylase, however, may not remove the diagnostic difficulty; it can be elevated following perforation of a peptic ulcer although, fortunately, the levels are not usually as high as the levels commonly seen in acute pancreatitis. Several other investigations are useful if doubt remains. A CT scan will normally be diagnostic in both conditions.

Treatment

The initial priorities are resuscitation and analgesia. Analgesia

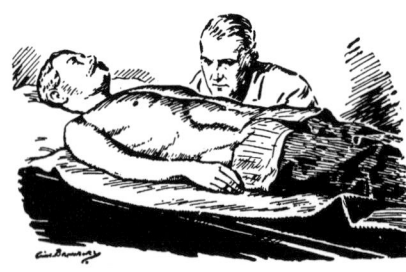

Figure 60.22 A sketch of Mr Hamilton Bailey watching for abdominal movement on respiration. In the case of a classically presenting perforated ulcer, the abdominal movement is restricted or absent.

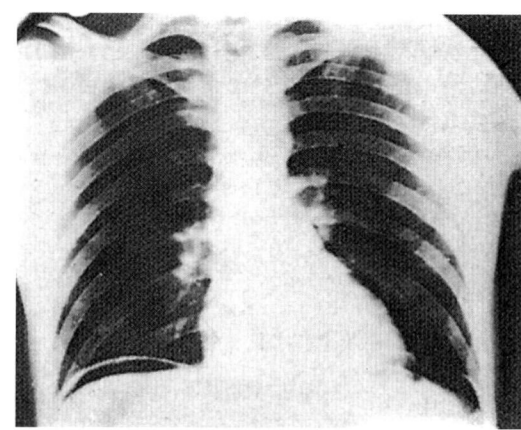

Figure 60.23 Plain abdominal radiograph of a perforated ulcer, showing air under the diaphragm.

should not be withheld for fear of removing the signs of an intra-abdominal catastrophe. In fact, adequate analgesia makes the clinical signs more obvious. It is important, however, to titrate the analgesic dose. Following resuscitation, the treatment is principally surgical. Laparotomy is performed, usually through an upper midline incision if the diagnosis of perforated peptic ulcer can be made with confidence. This is not always possible and, hence, it may be better to place a small incision around the umbilicus to localise the perforation with more certainty. Alternatively, laparoscopy may be used. The most important component of the operation is a thorough peritoneal toilet to remove all of the fluid and food debris. If the perforation is in the duodenum it can usually be closed by several well-placed sutures, closing the ulcer in a transverse direction as with a pyloroplasty. It is important that sufficient tissue is taken in the suture to allow the edges to be approximated, and the sutures should not be tied so tight that they tear out. It is common to place an omental patch over the perforation in the hope of enhancing the chances of the leak sealing. Gastric ulcers should, if possible, be excised and closed, so that malignancy can be excluded. Occasionally, a patient is seen who has a massive duodenal or gastric perforation such that simple closure is impossible; in these patients, a Billroth II gastrectomy is a useful operation.

All patients should be treated with systemic antibiotics in addition to a thorough peritoneal lavage. In the past, many surgeons performed definitive procedures such as either truncal vagotomy and pyloroplasty or, more recently and probably more successfully, highly selective vagotomy during the course of an operation for a perforation. Studies show that in well-selected patients and in expert hands this is a very safe strategy. However, nowadays, surgery is most commonly confined to first-aid measures and the peptic ulcer is treated medically, as described earlier in this chapter. Following operation, gastric anti-secretory agents should be started immediately.

Perforated peptic ulcers can often be managed by minimally invasive techniques if the expertise is available. The principles of operation are, however, the same; thorough peritoneal toilet is performed and the perforation is closed by intracorporeal suturing. Whichever technique is used, it is important that the stomach is kept empty postoperatively by nasogastric suction and that gastric anti-secretory agents are commenced to promote healing in the residual ulcer.

A great deal has been written about the conservative management of perforated ulcer. Some writers say that virtually all patients can be managed conservatively, whereas most surgeons have difficulty in understanding how a patient who is ill with widespread peritonitis and who has food debris widely distributed through the abdominal cavity will improve without an operation. There are undoubtedly patients who have small leaks from a perforated peptic ulcer and relatively mild peritoneal contamination who may be managed with intravenous fluids, nasogastric suction and antibiotics; however, these patients are in the minority.

Patients who have suffered one perforation may suffer another one. Therefore, they should be managed aggressively to ensure that this does not happen. In patients with *Helicobacter*-associated ulcers, eradication therapy is appropriate. Lifelong treatment with proton pump inhibitors is a reasonable option, especially in those who have to continue with NSAID treatment (Summary box 60.4).

Summary box 60.4

Peptic ulceration

- Most peptic ulcers are caused by *H. pylori* or NSAIDs and changes in epidemiology mirror changes in these principal aetiological factors
- Duodenal ulcers are more common than gastric ulcers, but the symptoms are indistinguishable
- Gastric ulcers may become malignant and an ulcerated gastric cancer may mimic a benign ulcer
- Gastric anti-secretory agents and *H. pylori* eradication therapy are the mainstay of treatment, and elective surgery is rarely performed now
- The long-term complications of peptic ulcer surgery may be difficult to treat
- The common complications of peptic ulcers are perforation, bleeding and stenosis
- The treatment of the perforated peptic ulcer is primarily surgical, although some patients may be managed conservatively

---

HAEMATEMESIS AND MELAENA

Upper gastrointestinal haemorrhage remains a major medical problem. Despite improvements in diagnosis and the proliferation in treatment modalities over the last few decades, an in-hospital mortality rate of 5% can be expected. In patients in whom the cause of bleeding can be found, the most common causes are bleeding peptic ulcer, erosions, Mallory–Weiss tear and bleeding oesophageal varices (Table 60.4).

Whatever the cause, the principles of management are identical. The patient should be first resuscitated and then investigated urgently to determine the cause of the bleeding. Only then should definitive treatment be instituted. For any significant gastrointestinal bleed, intravenous access should be established

Table 60.4 Causes of upper gastrointestinal bleeding

Condition	Incidence (%)
Ulcers	**60**
Oesophageal	6
Gastric	21
Duodenal	33
Erosions	**26**
Oesophageal	13
Gastric	9
Duodenal	4
Mallory–Weiss tear	*4*
Oesophageal varices	*4*
Tumour	*0.5*
Vascular lesions, e.g. Dieulafoy's disease	*0.5*
Others	*5*

George Kenneth Mallory, B. 1926, Professor of Pathology, Boston University, Boston, MA, USA.
Soma Weiss, 1898–1942, Professor of Medicine, Harvard University Medical School, Boston, MA, USA.

and, for those with severe bleeding, central venous pressure monitoring should be set up and bladder catheterisation performed. Blood should be cross-matched and the patient transfused as clinically indicated. As a general rule, most gastrointestinal bleeding will stop, albeit temporarily, but there are sometimes instances when this is not the case. In these circumstances, resuscitation, diagnosis and treatment should be carried out in quick succession. There are occasions when life-saving manoeuvres have to be undertaken without the benefit of an absolute diagnosis. For instance, in patients with known oesophageal varices and uncontrollable bleeding, a Sengstaken–Blakemore tube may be inserted before an endoscopy has been carried out. This practice is not to be encouraged, except *in extremis*. In some patients bleeding is secondary to a coagulopathy. The most important current causes of this are liver disease and inadequately controlled warfarin therapy. In these circumstances, the coagulopathy should be corrected, if possible, with fresh-frozen plasma.

Upper gastrointestinal endoscopy should be carried out by an experienced operator as soon as practicable after the patient has been stabilised. In patients in whom the bleeding is relatively mild, endoscopy may be carried out on the morning after admission. In all cases of severe bleeding it should be carried out immediately.

Bleeding peptic ulcers

The epidemiology of bleeding peptic ulcers exactly mirrors that of perforated ulcers. In recent years, the population affected has become much older and the bleeding is commonly associated with the ingestion of NSAIDs. Diagnosis can normally be made endoscopically although, occasionally, the nature of the blood loss precludes accurately identifying the lesion. However, the more experienced the endoscopist, the less likely this is to be a problem.

Medical and minimally interventional treatments

Medical treatment has limited efficacy. All patients are commonly started on a proton pump antagonist, but well-performed studies have failed to show that such treatments influence rebleeding, operation rate or mortality. However, meta-analyses of studies does suggest that tranexamic acid, an inhibitor of fibrinolysis, reduces the rebleeding rate.

Numerous endoscopic devices are now available that can be used to achieve haemostasis, ranging from expensive lasers and argon diathermy to inexpensive injection apparatus. There are few conclusive studies available but a review of the literature suggests that these treatments may have some value, although they will probably never be effective in patients who are bleeding from large vessels, with which the majority of the mortality is associated.

Surgical treatment

Criteria for surgery are well worked out. A patient who continues to bleed requires surgical treatment. The same applies to a significant rebleed. Patients with a visible vessel in the ulcer base, a spurting vessel or an ulcer with a clot in the base are statistically likely to require surgical treatment. Elderly and unfit patients are

more likely to die as a result of bleeding than younger patients; ironically, they should have early surgery. In general, a patient who has required more than 6 units of blood needs surgery. Various scoring systems have been devised, which predict the probability of rebleeding and mortality with some degree of accuracy.

The aim of the operation is to stop the bleeding. The advent of endoscopy has greatly helped in the management of upper gastrointestinal bleeding as a surgeon can usually be confident about the site of bleeding prior to operation. The most common site of bleeding from a peptic ulcer is the duodenum. In tackling this, it is essential that the duodenum is fully mobilised. This should be done before the duodenum is opened as it makes the ulcer much more accessible and also allows the surgeon's hand to be placed behind the gastroduodenal artery, which is commonly the source of major bleeding. Following mobilisation, the duodenum, and usually the pylorus, are opened longitudinally as in a pyloroplasty. This allows good access to the ulcer, which is usually found posteriorly or superiorly. Accurate haemostasis is important. It is the vessel within the ulcer that is bleeding and this should be controlled using well-placed sutures that under-run the vessel. The placing of more and more inaccurately positioned sutures is counter-productive. Following under-running, it is often possible to close the mucosa over the ulcer. The pyloroplasty is then closed with interrupted sutures in a transverse direction in the usual fashion.

The principles of management of bleeding gastric ulcers are essentially the same. The stomach is opened at an appropriate position anteriorly and the vessel in the ulcer under-run. If the ulcer is not excised then a biopsy of the edge needs to be taken to exclude malignant transformation. Sometimes the bleeding is from the splenic artery and if there is a lot of fibrosis then the operation may be challenging. However, most patients can be managed by conservative surgery. Gastrectomy for bleeding has been widely practised in the past but is associated with a high perioperative mortality, even if the incidence of recurrent bleeding is less.

Bearing in mind that most patients nowadays are elderly and unfit, the minimum surgery that stops the bleeding is optimal. Acid can be inhibited by pharmacological means and appropriate eradication therapy will prevent ulcer recurrence. Definitive acid lowering surgery is not now required. Patients on long-term NSAIDs can be managed as outlined earlier.

Stress ulceration

This commonly occurs in patients who have a major injury or illness, who have undergone major surgery or who have a major comorbidity. Many such patients are found in intensive care units. There seems little doubt that the incidence of this problem has reduced in recent years because of the widespread use of prophylaxis. Acid inhibition and the nasogastric or oral administration of sucralfate has been shown to reduce the incidence of stress ulceration. There is no doubt that it is far better to prevent this condition than to try to treat it once it occurs. Endoscopic treatment may be ineffective and operation may be required. The principles of management are the same as for the chronic ulcer.

Gastric erosions

Erosive gastritis has a variety of causes, especially the use of NSAIDs. Fortunately, most such bleeding settles spontaneously but when it does not it can be a major problem to treat. In

Robert William Sengstaken, B. 1923, Surgeon, Garden City, New York, NY, USA.
Arthur Hendley Blakemore, Associate Professor of Surgery, The Columbia College of Physicians and Surgeons, New York, NY, USA.

general terms, although there is a diffuse erosive gastritis, there is one (or more) specific lesion that has a significant-sized vessel within it. This should be dealt with appropriately, preferably endoscopically, although sometimes surgery is necessary.

Mallory–Weiss tear

This is a longitudinal tear below the gastro-oesophageal junction, which is induced by repetitive and strenuous vomiting. Doubtless, many such lesions occur and do not cause bleeding. When it is a cause of haematemesis, the lesion may often be missed; it can be difficult to see as it is just below the gastro-oesophageal junction, a position that can be difficult for the inexperienced endoscopist. Occasionally these lesions continue to bleed and require surgical treatment. Often, the situation arises in which the surgeon does not have guidance from the endoscopists regarding the site of bleeding, and a high index of suspicion in such circumstances is important. The stomach is opened by longitudinal gastrostomy and the upper section is carefully inspected. It is normally possible to palpate the longitudinal mucosal tear with a little induration at the edges, which gives a clue to the lesion's location. Under-running is all that is required.

Dieulafoy's disease

This is essentially a gastric arterial venous malformation that has a characteristic histological appearance. Bleeding as a result of this malformation is one of the most difficult types of upper gastrointestinal bleeding to treat. The lesion itself is covered by normal mucosa and, when not bleeding, it may be invisible. If it can be seen during the bleeding, all that may be visible is profuse bleeding coming from an area of apparently normal mucosa. If this occurs, the cause is instantly recognisable. If the lesion can be identified endoscopically there are various means of dealing with it, including the injection of sclerosant. If it is identified at operation then only a local excision is necessary. Occasionally, a lesion is only recognised after gastrectomy and sometimes not even then. The pathologist, as well as the endoscopist, may have difficulty in finding it.

Tumours

All of the gastric tumours described below may present with chronic or acute upper gastrointestinal bleeding. Bleeding is not normally torrential but can be unremitting. Gastric stromal tumours commonly present with bleeding and have a characteristic appearance, as the mucosa breaks down over the tumour in the gastric wall (Fig. 60.24). Whatever the nature, the tumours should be dealt with as appropriate.

Portal hypertension and portal gastropathy

The management of bleeding gastric varices is very challenging. Fortunately, most bleeding from varices is oesophageal and this is much more amenable to sclerotherapy, banding and balloon tamponade. Gastric varices may also be injected, although this is technically more difficult. Banding can also be used, again with difficulty. The gastric balloon of the Sengastaken–Blakemore tube can be used to arrest the haemorrhage if it is occurring from the fundus of the stomach. Octreotide reduces portal pressure in

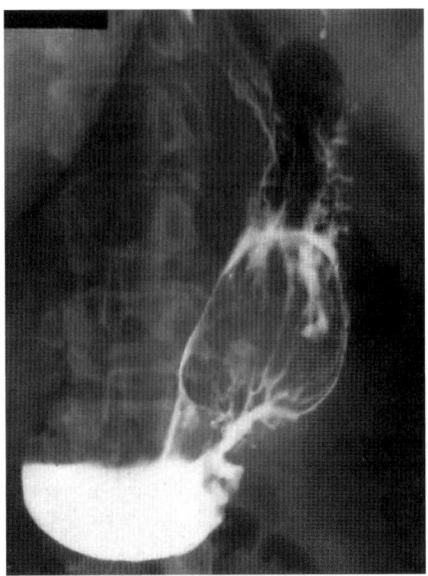

Figure 60.24 Gastric gastrointestinal stromal tumour with ulceration.

patients with varices, and trials suggest that it is of value in arresting haemorrhage in these patients, although its overall effect on mortality remains in doubt. Glypressin is also said to be of use.

Most surgeons prefer to avoid acute surgery on bleeding varices as, in contrast with elective operations for portal hypertension, acute shunts are attended by considerable operative mortality. For this reason, the acute TIPSS procedure (transjugular intrahepatic portosystemic shunt; see Chapter 61) can be an extremely useful, although technically demanding, procedure.

Portal gastropathy

Portal gastropathy is essentially the same disease process as described above. The mucosa is affected by the increased portal pressure and may exude blood, even in the absence of well-developed visible varices. The treatment is as above.

Aortic enteric fistula

This diagnosis should be considered in any patient with haematemesis and melaena that cannot be otherwise explained. Contrary to expectation, the bleeding from such patients is not always massive, although it can be. Very often there is nothing much to distinguish between the bleeding from the aortic enteric fistula and any other recurrent upper gastrointestinal bleeding. The vast majority of patients will have had an aortic graft and, in the absence of this, the diagnosis is unlikely. However, it is occasionally seen in patients with an untreated aortic aneurysm. A well-performed CT scan will commonly allow the diagnosis to be made with certainty. The condition should be managed by an expert vascular surgeon as, whether secondary or primary, the morbidity and mortality rates are high.

GASTRIC OUTLET OBSTRUCTION

The two common causes of gastric outlet obstruction are gastric cancer and pyloric stenosis secondary to peptic ulceration. Previously, the latter was more common. Now, with the decrease in the incidence of peptic ulceration and the advent of potent

CHAPTER 60 | STOMACH AND DUODENUM

medical treatments, gastric outlet obstruction should be considered malignant until proven otherwise, at least in the west.

The term 'pyloric stenosis' is normally a misnomer as the stenosis is seldom at the pylorus. Commonly, when the condition is due to underlying peptic ulcer disease the stenosis is found in the first part of the duodenum, the most common site for a peptic ulcer. True pyloric stenosis can occur as a result of fibrosis around a pyloric channel ulcer. However, in recent years, the most common cause of gastric outlet obstruction has been gastric cancer. In this circumstance, the metabolic consequences may be somewhat different from those of benign pyloric stenosis because of the relative hypochlorhydria found in patients with gastric cancer.

Clinical features

In benign gastric outlet obstruction there is usually a long history of peptic ulcer disease. Nowadays, as most patients with peptic ulcer symptoms are treated medically, it is easy to understand why the condition is becoming much less common. In some patients the pain may become unremitting and in other cases it may largely disappear. The vomitus is characteristically unpleasant in nature and is totally lacking in bile. Very often it is possible to recognise foodstuff taken several days previously. The patient commonly loses weight, and appears unwell and dehydrated. On examination it may be possible to see the distended stomach and a succussion splash may be audible on shaking the patient's abdomen.

Metabolic effects

These are most interesting as the metabolic consequences of benign pyloric stenosis are unique. The vomiting of hydrochloric acid results in hypochloraemic alkalosis but, initially, sodium and potassium levels may be relatively normal. However, as dehydration progresses, more profound metabolic abnormalities arise, partly related to renal dysfunction. Initially, the urine has a low chloride and high bicarbonate content, reflecting the primary metabolic abnormality. This bicarbonate is excreted along with sodium and so, with time, the patient becomes progressively hyponatraemic and more profoundly dehydrated. Because of the dehydration, a phase of sodium retention follows and potassium and hydrogen are excreted in preference. This results in the urine becoming paradoxically acidic and hypokalaemia ensues. Alkalosis leads to a lowering of the circulating ionised calcium, and tetany can occur.

Management

Treating the patient involves correcting the metabolic abnormality and dealing with the mechanical problem. The patient should be rehydrated with intravenous isotonic saline with potassium supplementation. Replacing the sodium chloride and water allows the kidney to correct the acid–base abnormality. Following rehydration it may become obvious that the patient is also anaemic, the haemoglobin being spuriously high on presentation.

It is notable that the metabolic abnormalities may be less if the obstruction is due to malignancy, as the acid–base disturbance is less pronounced.

The stomach should be emptied using a wide-bore gastric tube. A large nasogastric tube may not be sufficiently large to deal with the contents of the stomach and it may be necessary to pass an orogastric tube and lavage the stomach until it is completely emptied. This then allows investigation of the patient with endoscopy and contrast radiology. Biopsy of the area around the pylorus is essential to exclude malignancy. The patient should also have an anti-secretory agent, initially given intravenously to ensure absorption.

Early cases may settle with conservative treatment, presumably as the oedema around the ulcer diminishes as the ulcer is healed. Traditionally, severe cases are treated surgically, usually with a gastroenterostomy rather than a pyloroplasty. Endoscopic treatment with balloon dilatation has been practised and may be most useful in early cases. However, this treatment is not devoid of problems. Dilating the duodenal stenosis may result in perforation, and the dilatation may have to be performed several times and may not be successful in the long term (Summary box 60.5).

Summary box 60.5

Gastric outlet obstruction

- Gastric outlet obstruction is most commonly associated with longstanding peptic ulcer disease and gastric cancer
- The metabolic abnormality of hypochloraemic alkalosis is usually only seen with peptic ulcer disease and should be treated with isotonic saline with potassium supplementation
- Endoscopic biopsy is essential to determine whether the cause of the problem is malignancy
- Endoscopic dilatation of the gastric outlet may be effective in the less severe cases of benign stenosis
- Operation is normally required, with a drainage procedure being performed for benign disease and appropriate resectional surgery if malignant

---

Other causes of gastric outlet obstruction

Adult pyloric stenosis

This is a rare condition and its relationship to the childhood condition is unclear, although some patients have a long history of problems with gastric emptying. It is commonly treated by pyloroplasty rather than pyloromyotomy.

Pyloric mucosal diaphragm

The origin of this rare condition is unknown. It usually does not become apparent until middle life. When found, simple excision of the mucosal diaphragm is all that is required.

GASTRIC POLYPS

A number of conditions manifest as gastric polyps. Their main importance is that they may actually represent early gastric cancer. Biopsy is essential.

The most common type of gastric polyp is metaplastic. These are associated with H. pylori infection and regress following eradication therapy. Inflammatory polyps are also common. Fundic gland polyps deserve particular attention; they seem to be associated with the use of proton pump inhibitors and are also found in patients with familial polyposis.

None of the above polypoid lesions has proven malignant potential. True adenomas have malignant potential and should be removed, but they account for only 10% of polypoid lesions. Gastric carcinoids arising from ECL cells are seen in patients with pernicious anaemia and usually appear as small polyps.

GASTRIC CANCER

Carcinoma of the stomach is a major cause of cancer mortality worldwide. Its prognosis tends to be poor with cure rates little better than 5–10%, although better results are obtained in Japan where the disease is common. Gastric cancer is actually an eminently curable disease provided that it is detected at an appropriate stage and treated adequately. It rarely disseminates widely before it has involved the lymph nodes and, therefore, there is an opportunity to cure the disease prior to dissemination. Early diagnosis is therefore the key to success. Unfortunately, the late presentation of many cases is the cause of the poor overall survival figures. The only treatment modality able to cure the disease is resectional surgery.

Incidence

There are marked variations in the incidence of gastric cancer worldwide. In the UK the incidence is approximately 15 cases per 100 000 population per year, in the USA 10 cases per 100 000 population per year and in Eastern Europe 40 cases per 100 000 population per year. In Japan the disease is much more common, with an incidence of approximately 70 cases per 100 000 population per year, and there are small geographical areas in China where the incidence is double that in Japan. These underlying epidemiological data make it clear that this is an environmental disease. In general, men are more affected by the disease than women and, as with most solid organ malignancies, the incidence increases with age.

At present, marked changes are being observed in the west in terms of the incidence and sites of gastric cancer and the population affected, changes that to date have not been observed in Japan. First, the incidence of gastric cancer is continuing to fall, at a rate of about 1% per year, with the reduction exclusively affecting carcinomas arising in the body of the stomach and the distal stomach. In contrast, the incidence of carcinoma in the proximal stomach, particularly the oesophagogastric junction, appears to be increasing. Carcinoma of the distal stomach and body of the stomach is most common in low socio-economic groups, whereas the increase in proximal gastric cancer seems to affect principally higher socio-economic groups. Proximal gastric cancer does not seem to be associated with *H. pylori* infection, in contrast with carcinoma of the body of the stomach and the distal stomach.

Aetiology

Gastric cancer is a multifactorial disease (Correa). Epidemiological studies point to a role for *H. pylori*, although its importance is disputed. Studies reveal a correlation between the incidence of gastric cancer in various populations and the prevalence of *H. pylori* infection, but other factors are also important. There is insufficient evidence at the moment to support eradication programmes in asymptomatic patients who are infected with *H. pylori*, with a view to reducing the population incidence of gastric cancer. However, clinical trials may subsequently change this view. As mentioned above, *H. pylori* seems to be principally associated with carcinoma of the body of the stomach and the distal stomach rather than the proximal stomach. As *Helicobacter* is associated with gastritis, gastric atrophy and intestinal metaplasia, the association with malignancy is perhaps not surprising.

Several other risk factors have been identified as being important in the aetiology of gastric cancer. Patients with pernicious anaemia and gastric atrophy are at increased risk, as are those with gastric polyps. Patients who have had peptic ulcer surgery, particularly those who have had drainage procedures such as Billroth II or Pólya gastrectomy, gastroenterostomy or pyloroplasty, are at approximately four times the average risk. Presumably, duodenogastric reflux and reflux gastritis are related to the increased risk of malignancy in these patients. Intestinal metaplasia is a risk factor. Carcinoma is associated with cigarette smoking and dust ingestion from a variety of industrial processes. Diet appears to be important, as illustrated by the often quoted example of the change in the incidence of gastric cancer in Japanese families living in the USA. The high incidence of gastric cancer in some pockets in China is probably environmental and probably diet related. The ingestion of substances such as spirits may induce gastritis and, in the long term, cancer. Excessive salt intake, deficiency of antioxidants and exposure to *N*-nitroso compounds are also implicated. The aetiology of proximal gastric cancer remains an enigma. It is not associated with *Helicobacter* but is associated with obesity and higher socio-economic status. Genetic factors are also important but imperfectly elucidated (see below).

Clinical features

The features of advanced gastric cancer are usually obvious. However, curable gastric cancer has no specific features to distinguish it symptomatically from benign dyspepsia. The key to improving the outcome of gastric cancer is early diagnosis and, although in Japan there is a screening programme, most curable cases are picked up by the liberal use of gastroscopy in patients with dyspepsia. In the west, early diagnosis is much more difficult as the population incidence is much lower and, hence, the cost-effectiveness of performing gastroscopy for mild dyspeptic symptoms is low. However, a high index of suspicion is necessary, as endoscoping only patients with symptoms of advanced cancer is unlikely to be beneficial because such patients are not surgically curable. It is important to note that gastric anti-secretory agents will improve the symptoms of gastric cancer so the disease should be excluded preferably before therapy is started.

In advanced cancer, early satiety, bloating, distension and vomiting may occur. The tumour frequently bleeds, resulting in iron-deficiency anaemia. Obstruction leads to dysphagia, epigastric fullness or vomiting. With pyloric involvement the presentation may be of gastric outlet obstruction, although the alkalosis is usually less pronounced or absent compared with cases of duodenal ulceration leading to obstruction. Metastatic lymph nodes may be palpable, most notably in the left supraclavicular fossa (Virchow's node, Troisier's sign). In recent years, gastric outlet obstruction has been more commonly associated with malignancy than benign disease. Non-metastatic effects of malignancy are seen, particularly thrombophlebitis (Trousseau's sign) and deep venous thrombosis. These features result from the effects of the tumour on thrombotic and haemostatic mechanisms.

Rudolf Ludwig Carl Virchow, 1821–1902, Professor of Pathology, Berlin, Germany.
Charles Emil Troisier, 1844–1919, Professor of Pathology, Paris, France.
Armand Trousseau, 1801–1867, Physician, Hôtel Dieu, Paris. The sign led him to suspect that he had gastric cancer himself. He actually had pancreatic cancer which was diagnosed at post-mortem.

P. Correa, a Pathologist of New Orleans, LA, USA.

Site

The proximal stomach is now the most common site for gastric cancer in the west. Because so many malignancies occur at the oesophagogastric junction, and because the lower oesophagus is also a very common site of adenocarcinoma, it is artificial to separate the stomach from the oesophagus. Therefore, it is best to consider the whole of the upper gastrointestinal tract from the cricopharyngeus to the pylorus. The incidence of cancer at these various sites is shown in Fig. 60.25. It can be seen that just under 60% of all of the malignancies occurring in the oesophagus and stomach occur in proximity to the oesophagogastric junction. This high prevalence of proximal gastric cancer is not seen in Japan, where distal cancer still predominates, as it does in most of the rest of the world.

Pathology

The most useful classification of gastric cancer is the Lauren classification. In this system there are principally two forms of gastric cancer: intestinal gastric cancer and diffuse gastric cancer. In intestinal gastric cancer, the tumour resembles carcinomas found elsewhere in the tubular gastrointestinal tract and forms polypoid tumours or ulcers. It probably arises in areas of intestinal metaplasia. In contrast, diffuse gastric cancer infiltrates deeply into the stomach without forming obvious mass lesions but spreading widely in the gastric wall. Not surprisingly, this has a much worse prognosis. A small proportion of gastric cancers are of mixed morphology.

Gastric cancer can be divided into early gastric cancer and advanced gastric cancer. Early gastric cancer can be defined as cancer limited to the mucosa and submucosa with or without lymph node involvement (T1, any N); this classification is shown in Figs 60.26 and 60.27. In the Japanese classification, early gastric cancer can be protruding, superficial or excavated. Early gastric cancer is eminently curable, and even early gastric cancers associated with lymph node involvement have 5-year survival rates in the region of 90%. In Japan, approximately one-third of gastric cancers diagnosed are in this stage. However, in the UK it is uncommon to detect gastric cancers at this stage. A number of reasons probably still accounts for this. First, because gastric cancer is less common in the UK, dyspeptic patients are not always

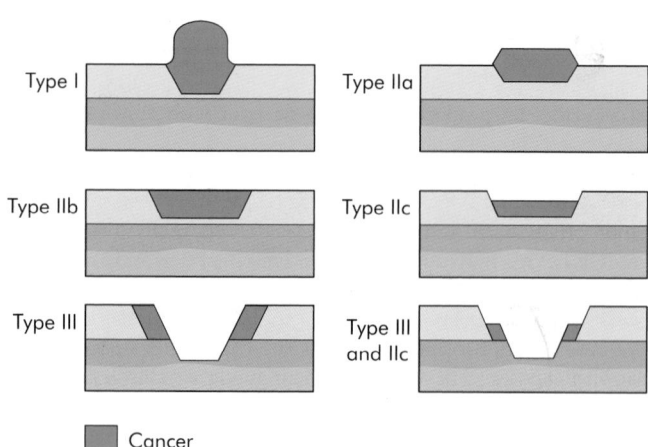

Figure 60.26 Japanese classification of early gastric cancer.

referred for endoscopy at an appropriate stage. Second, endoscopists are unfamiliar with the appearances of early gastric cancer and in all probability many such cases are missed.

Advanced gastric cancer involves the muscularis. Its macroscopic appearances have been classified by Bormann into four types (Figs 60.28 and 60.29). Types III and IV are commonly incurable.

The molecular pathology of gastric cancer

Although the molecular pathology of gastric cancer is less well worked out than that of colorectal cancer, several genetic events have been established, some of which have clinical relevance. Mutation or loss of heterozygosity in the APC gene or in the associated gene coding for β-catenin is found in approximately 50% and 30%, respectively, of cases of intestinal-type cancer. APC mutations are found less frequently in diffuse gastric cancer and not at all in patients with β-catenin mutations. In contrast, another related gene, E-cadherin, is mutated in 50% of cases of diffuse cancer. In some families, inherited diffuse gastric cancer has been shown to be related to a germline mutation in the E-cadherin gene. Inactivation of p53, a tumour-suppressor gene, is found in around 30% of both intestinal and diffuse gastric cancers. These findings serve to illustrate that there are important differences between the two types of cancer at a molecular level.

Errors in DNA replication manifesting as microsatellite instability (MSI) have been demonstrated in approximately 15% of cases of gastric cancer, with little distinction between the intestinal or diffuse types. This genetic phenotype is associated with the inherited cancer syndrome, hereditary non-polyposis colorectal cancer (HNPCC) or Lynch's syndrome. However, most cases of MSI are a result of an acquired mutation in the tumour itself.

Several growth factor receptors are overexpressed/amplified in gastric cancer; these include c-Met, k-Sam and c-ErbB2. Similarly, several growth factors may be overexpressed, including TGFα, EGF and vascular endothelial growth factor (VEGF).

Lastly, loss of heterozygosity in the BCL2 gene, an inhibitor of apoptosis, is associated with intestinal-type cancer.

Henry T. Lynch, **an Oncologist at the Creighton School of Medicine, Omaha, NE, USA.**

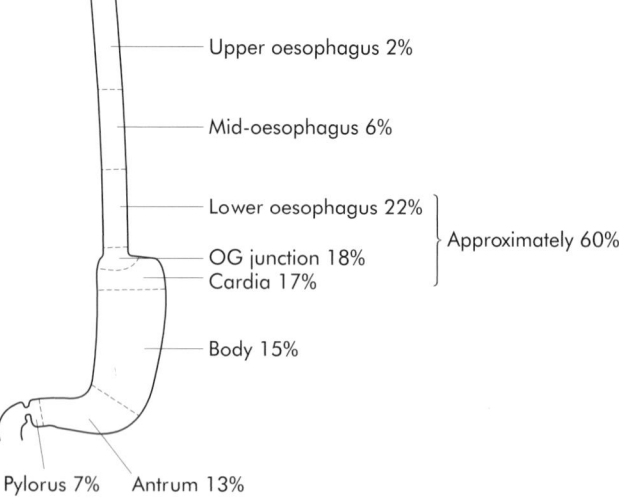

Figure 60.25 The incidence of cancer in the various parts of the upper gastrointestinal tract in the UK. OG, oesophagogastric.

Upper oesophagus 2%

Mid-oesophagus 6%

Lower oesophagus 22%

OG junction 18%

Cardia 17%

Approximately 60%

Body 15%

Pylorus 7%   Antrum 13%

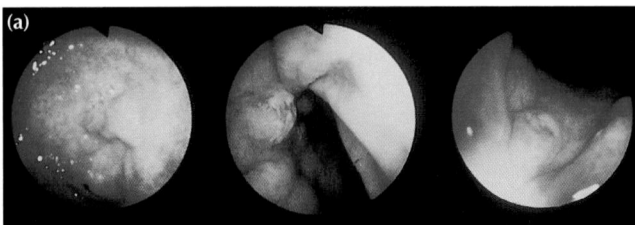

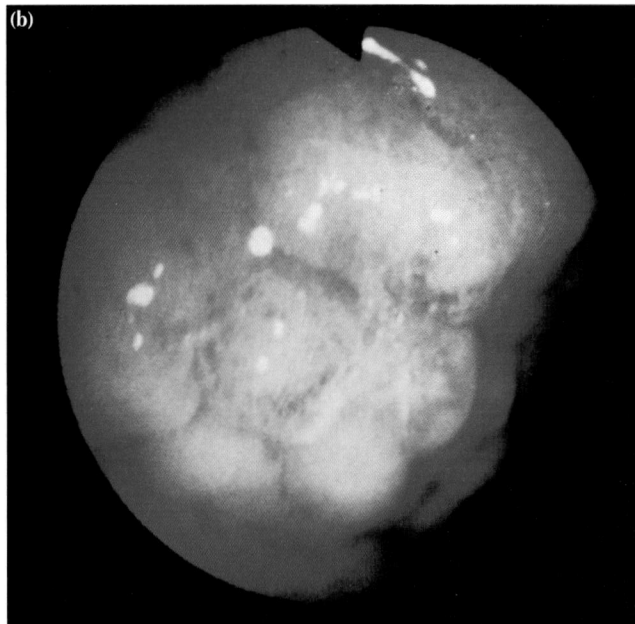

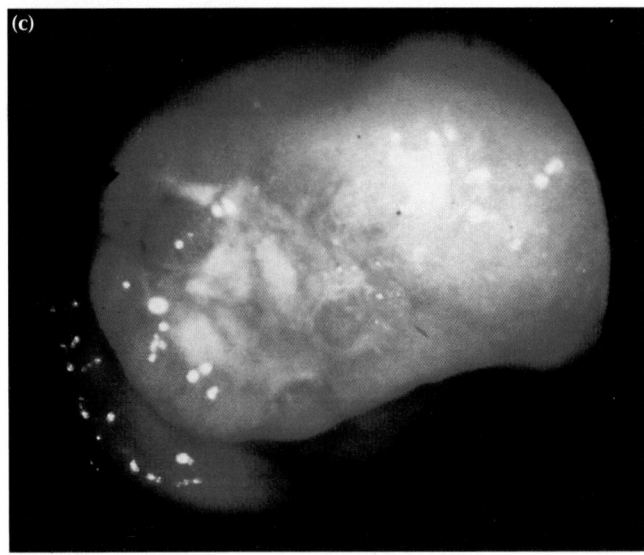

Figure 60.27 Early gastric cancer. (a) Type I; (b) type IIa; (c) type III (courtesy of Dr G.N.J. Tytgat, Amsterdam, The Netherlands).

These genetic changes may be involved in the familial predisposition to gastric cancer. Well-known syndromes such as HNPCC have gastric cancer as part of their spectrum.

Staging
The International Union Against Cancer (UICC) staging system is shown in Table 60.5.

Spread of carcinoma of the stomach
No better example of the various modes by which carcinoma spreads can be given than the case of stomach cancer. It is important to note that this distant spread is unusual before the disease spreads locally, and distant metastases are uncommon in the absence of lymph node metastases. The intestinal and diffuse types of gastric cancer spread differently. The diffuse type spreads via the submucosal and subserosal lymphatic plexus and it penetrates the gastric wall at an early stage.

Direct spread
The tumour penetrates the muscularis, serosa and ultimately adjacent organs such as the pancreas, colon and liver.

Lymphatic spread
This is by both permeation and emboli to the affected tiers (see below) of nodes. This may be extensive, with the tumour even appearing in the supraclavicular nodes (Troisier's sign). Unlike malignancies such as breast cancer, nodal involvement does not imply systemic dissemination.

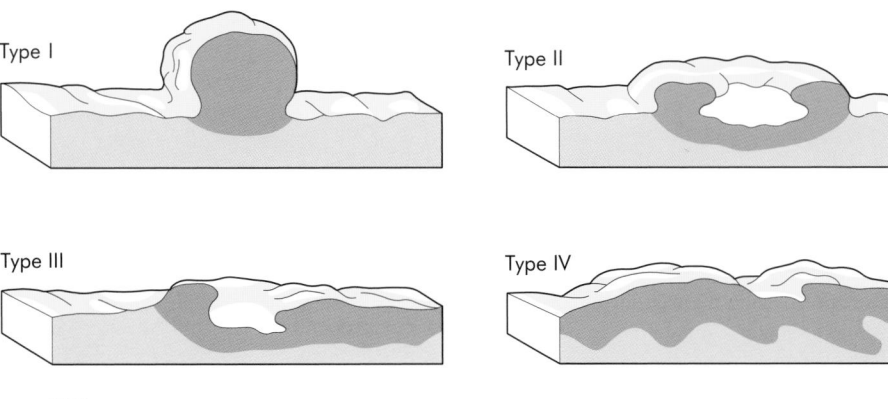

Figure 60.28 Borrmann classification of advanced gastric cancer.

CHAPTER 60 | STOMACH AND DUODENUM

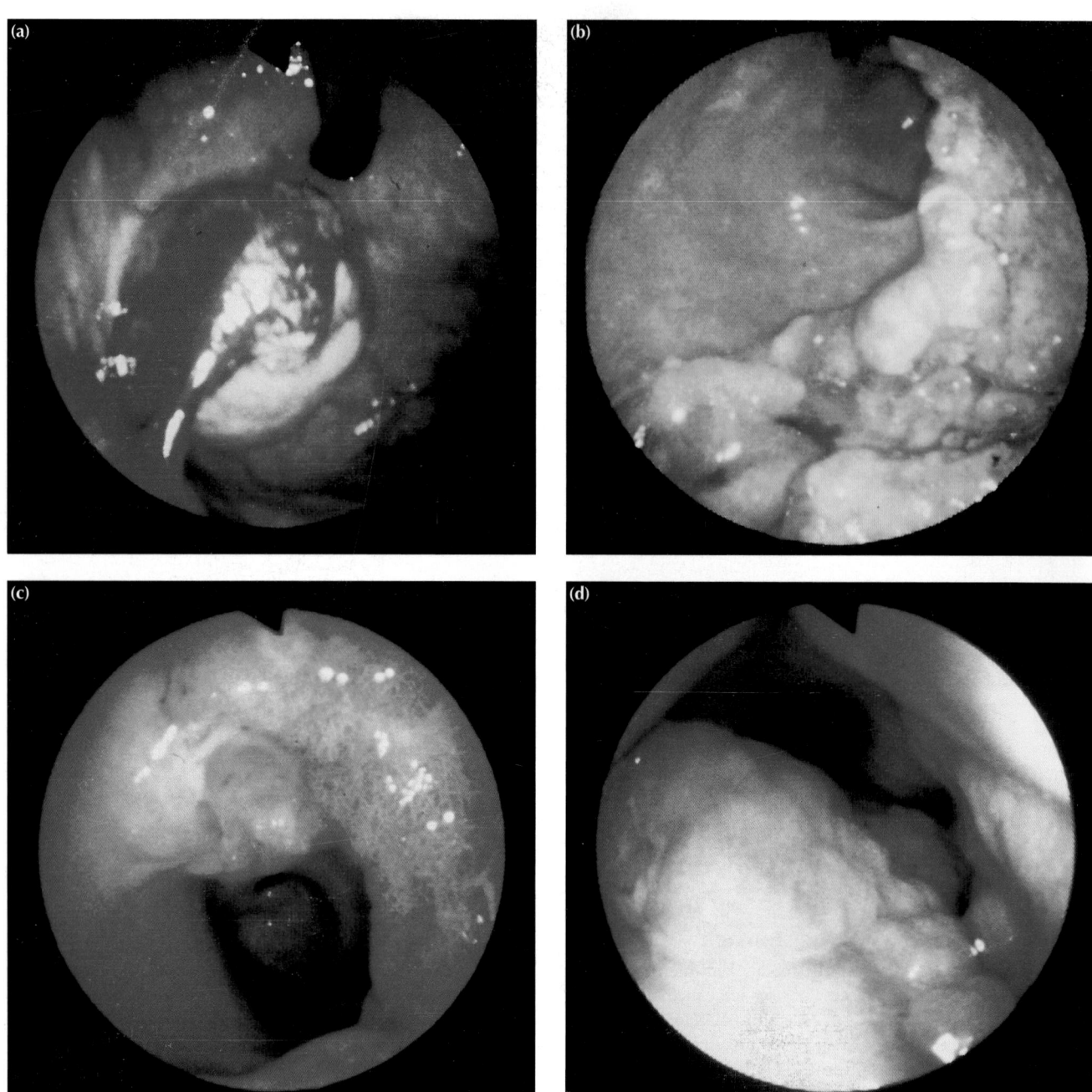

Figure 60.29 Advanced gastric cancer. (a) Type I; (b) type II; (c) type III; (d) type IV (linitus plastica) (courtesy of Dr G.N.J. Tytgat, Amsterdam, The Netherlands).

Blood-borne metastases

Blood-borne metastases occur first to the liver and subsequently to other organs, including lung and bone. They are uncommon in the absence of nodal disease.

Transperitoneal spread

This is a common mode of spread once the tumour has reached the serosa of the stomach and indicates incurability. Tumours can manifest anywhere in the peritoneal cavity and commonly give rise to ascites. Advanced peritoneal disease may be palpated either abdominally or rectally as a tumour 'shelf'. The ovaries may sometimes be the sole site of transcoelomic spread (Krukenberg's tumours). Tumour may spread via the abdominal cavity to the umbilicus (Sister Joseph's nodule). Transperitoneal spread of gastric cancer can be detected most effectively by laparoscopy and cytology.

Lymphatic drainage of the stomach

Understanding the lymphatic drainage of the stomach is the key to comprehending the radical surgery of gastric cancer. The

Friedrich Ernst Krukenberg, **1870–1946, Pathologist of Halle, Germany.**
Sister Mary Joseph, (née Julia Dempsey), **Nursing Superintendent, St. Mary's Hospital which became The Mayo Clinic, Rochester, MN, USA.**

Table 60.5 International Union Against Cancer (UICC) staging of gastric cancer

T1	Tumour involves lamina propria
T2	Tumour invades muscularis or subserosa
T3	Tumour involves serosa
T4	Tumour invades adjacent organs
N0	No lymph nodes
N1	Metastasis in 1–6 regional nodes
N2	Metastasis in 7–15 regional nodes
N3	Metastasis in more than 15 regional nodes
M0	No distant metastasis
M1	Distant metastasis (this includes peritoneum and distant lymph nodes)

Staging

IA	T1	N0	M0
IB	T1	N1	M0
	T2	N0	M0
II	T1	N2	M0
	T2	N1	M0
	T3	N0	M0
IIIA	T2	N2	M0
	T3	N1	M0
	T4	N0	M0
IIIB	T3	N2	M0
IV	T4	N1–3	M0
	T1–3	N3	M0
	Any T	Any N	M1

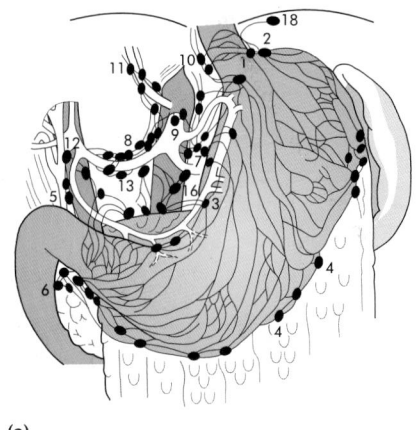

(a)

(b)

Figure 60.30 Lymphatic drainage of the stomach and nodal stations according to the Japanese classification. (a) The anterior view of the stomach. (b) The posterior view.

lymphatics of the antrum drain into the right gastric lymph node superiorly and the right gastroepiploic and subpyloric lymph nodes inferiorly. The lymphatics of the pylorus drain into the right gastric suprapyloric nodes superiorly and the subpyloric lymph nodes situated around the gastroduodenal artery inferiorly. The efferent lymphatics from the suprapyloric lymph nodes converge on the para-aortic nodes around the coeliac axis, whereas the efferent lymphatics from the subpyloric lymph nodes pass up to the main superior mesenteric lymph nodes situated around the origin of the superior mesenteric artery. The lymphatic vessels related to the cardiac orifice of the stomach communicate freely with those of the oesophagus.

The prognosis of operable cases of carcinoma of the stomach depends on whether or not there is histological evidence of regional lymph node involvement. Retrograde (downwards) spread may occur if the upper lymphatics are blocked. In Japan, lymph node dissection is highly advanced and the Japanese Research Society for Gastric Cancer has assigned a number to each lymph node station to aid the pathological staging (Fig. 60.30). Many centres in the west now perform surgery that involves a radical lymphadenectomy but, in other centres, both the staging and surgery are less developed.

Operability

It is important that patients with incurable disease are not subjected to radical surgery that cannot help them, hence the value of CT/PET (see Fig 60.9, p. 1051). Unequivocal evidence of incurability is haematogenous metastases, involvement of the distant peritoneum, N4 nodal disease and disease beyond the N4 nodes, and fixation to structures that cannot be removed. It is important to note that involvement of another organ per se does not imply incurability, provided that it can be removed. Controversies with respect to operability include N3 nodal involvement and involvement of the adjacent peritoneum; such surgery is performed in Japan but seldom elsewhere. Curative resection should be considered on the remaining patients.

Most operable patients should have neoadjuvant chemotherapy as described below, as this improves survival.

Total gastrectomy

This is best performed through a long upper midline incision. The stomach is removed *en bloc*, including the tissues of the entire greater omentum and lesser omentum (Fig. 60.31). In commencing the operation, the transverse colon is completely separated from the greater omentum. The dissection may then be commenced either proximally or, more usually, distally. The subpyloric nodes are dissected and the first part of the duodenum is divided, usually with a surgical stapler. The hepatic nodes are dissected down to clear the hepatic artery; this dissection also includes the suprapyloric nodes. The right gastric artery is taken on the hepatic artery. The lymph node dissection is continued to the origin of the left gastric artery, which is divided flush with its origin. The dissection is continued along the splenic artery,

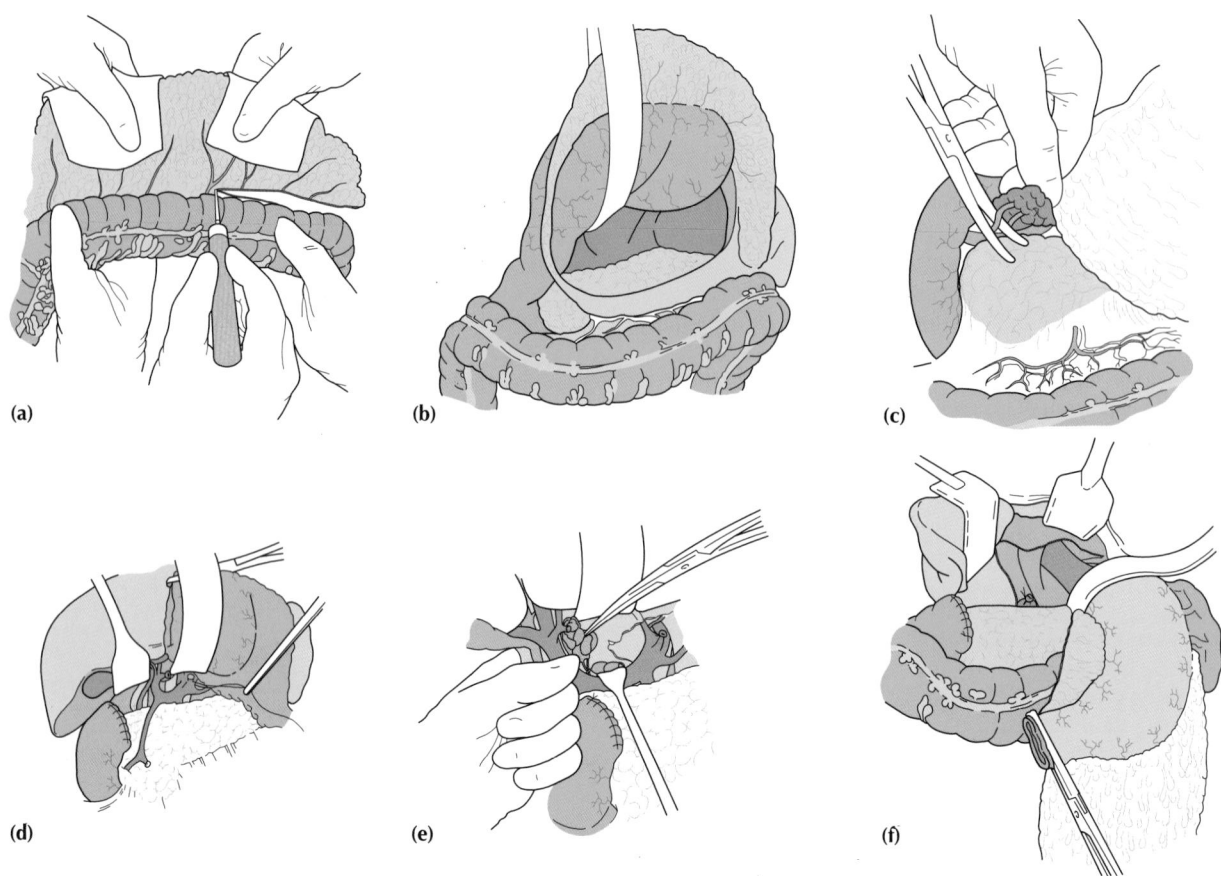

Figure 60.31 Radical total gastrectomy. (a) Dissection of omentum of the transverse colon; (b) exposure of the lesser sac; (c) splenectomy; (d) division and oversewing of the duodenum; (e) dissection of the left gastric artery nodes (group 17); (f) mobilisation of the oesophagus.

taking all of the nodes at the superior aspect of the pancreas and in the splenic hilum. Separation of the stomach from the spleen, if this organ is not going to be removed, is carried out and this then allows access to the nodal tissues around the upper stomach and oesophagogastric junction. The oesophagus can then be divided at an appropriate point using a combination of stay sutures and a soft non-crushing clamp, usually of the right-angled variety. It is important that the resection margins are well clear of the tumour. Involvement of either the proximal or distal resection margin carries an appalling prognosis and, if in doubt, frozen section should be performed. There is some controversy regarding the management of the spleen and distal pancreas in this procedure and this is discussed below.

Gastrointestinal continuity is reconstituted by means of a Roux loop. Other methods of reconstruction should be discouraged because of poor functional results. The Roux loop should be at least 50 cm long to avoid bile reflux oesophagitis. The simplest means of effecting the oesophagojejunostomy is to place a purse-string in the cut end of the oesophagus and, using a circular stapler introduced through the blind end of the Roux loop, staple the end of the oesophagus onto the side of the Roux loop. The blind open end of the Roux loop may then be closed either with sutures or, alternatively, with a linear stapler. The anastomosis can also be fashioned end-to-end. The Roux loop may be placed in either an anticolic or retrocolic position. The jejunojejunostomy is undertaken at a convenient point in the usual fashion (end-to-side, Fig. 60.32).

There remains some controversy about the extent of the lymphadenectomy required for the optimal treatment of curable gastric cancers. In Japan, at least a D2 gastrectomy (removal of the second tier of nodes) is performed on all operable gastric cancers and some centres are practising more radical surgery (D3 and even D4 resections). Certainly, the results of surgical treatment stage for stage in Japan are much better than those

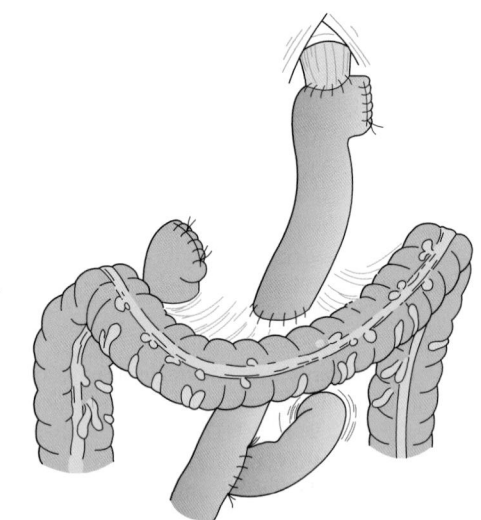

Figure 60.32 Oesophagojejunostomy Roux-en-Y.

commonly reported in the west, and the Japanese contention is that the difference is principally related to the staging and the quality of the surgery. It is observed that the physical proportions of the average Japanese patient, compared with the average patient in the west, favour the performance of more radical procedures. However, radical lymphadenectomies above D2 have not been subjected to any randomised controlled trials. In the UK and Europe, randomised trials have been set up to compare D1 and D2 gastrectomy but the results are difficult to interpret. One of the problems relates to standardisation of the operation. Overall, it seems that the oncological outcome may be better following a D2 gastrectomy, but this operation is associated with higher levels of morbidity and perioperative mortality. It is clear that most of this morbidity and mortality relates to the removal of the spleen with or without the distal pancreas. The traditional radical gastrectomy removes the spleen and distal pancreas *en bloc* with the stomach and, although this is indeed an adequate means of performing clearance of the lymph nodes around the splenic artery, there now seems little doubt that this substantially increases the complication rate. The Japanese D2 gastrectomy will commonly preserve the spleen and pancreas.

The differentiation between a D1 and a D2 operation depends upon the tiers of nodes removed. Different tiers need to be removed depending on the position of the primary tumour and this is outlined in Table 60.6. In general, a D1 resection involves the removal of the perigastric nodes and a D2 resection involves the clearance of the major arterial trunks.

Subtotal gastrectomy

For tumours distally placed in the stomach it appears unnecessary to remove the whole stomach. However, a subtotal gastrectomy is very similar to a total gastrectomy except that the proximal stomach is preserved, the blood supply being derived from the short gastric arteries. Following the resection, the simplest form of reconstruction is to close the stomach from the lesser curve, near the oesophagogastric junction, with either sutures or staples and then perform an anastomosis of the greater curve to the jejunum. Although the reconstruction can be performed as in a Billroth II-/Pólya-type gastrectomy, this may result in quite marked enterogastric reflux and bile reflux oesophagitis, and it is preferred to perform the reconstruction using a Roux loop.

Palliative surgery

In patients suffering from significant symptoms of either obstruction or bleeding, palliative resection is appropriate. A palliative gastrectomy need not be radical and it is sufficient to remove the tumour and reconstruct the gastrointestinal tract. Sometimes it is impossible to resect an obstructing tumour in the distal stomach and other palliative procedures need to be considered, although the prognosis in such patients, even in the short term, is poor. A high gastroenterostomy is a poor operation that very frequently does not allow the stomach to empty adequately and may produce the additional problem of bile reflux. A Roux loop with a wide anastomosis between the stomach and jejunum may be a better option, although even this may not allow the stomach to empty particularly well. Gastric exclusion and oesophagojejunostomy are practised by some surgeons. For inoperable tumours situated in the cardia, either palliative intubation, stenting or another form of recanalisation can be used (see Chapter 59). Recanalisation appears to offer better functional results.

Postoperative complications of gastrectomy

Radical gastrectomy is complex major surgery and predictably there are a large number of potential complications. Leakage of the oesophagojejunostomy should be uncommon in experienced hands. When it does occur it can often be managed conservatively as the Roux-en-Y reconstruction means that it is mainly saliva and ingested food that leaks. Some patients may establish a fistula from the wound or drain site and others may need radiological or surgically placed drains. It is unclear whether a nasoenteric tube should be used routinely; many surgeons do use such tubes routinely but this is not supported by any evidence base. It

Table 60.6 The lymph node (LN) stations (see Fig. 60.30) that need to be removed in a D1 (N1 nodes removed) or a D2 (N2 nodes removed) resection

LN number		Antrum	Middle	Site of cancer	
				Cardia	Cardia and oesophagus
1	Right cardia	N2	N1	N1	N1
2	Left cardia		N1	N1	N1
3	Lesser curve	N1	N1	N1	N1
4sa	Short gastric	N1	N1	N1	N1
4sb	Left gastroepiploic	N1	N1	N1	N1
4d	Right gastroepiploic	N1	N1	N2	N2
5	Suprapyloric	N1	N1	N2	N2
6	Infrapyloric	N1	N1	N2	N2
7	Left gastric artery	N2	N2	N2	N2
8a	Anterior hepatic artery	N2	N2	N2	N2
9	Coeliac artery	N2	N2	N2	N2
10	Splenic hilum		N2	N2	N2
11	Splenic artery		N2	N2	N2
19	Infradiaphragmatic				N2
20	Oesophageal hiatal			N2	N1
110	Lower oesophageal				N2
111	Supradiaphragmatic				N2

The nodes in stations 12–18 are not routinely removed in a D1 or D2 gastrectomy.

is common practice to perform a water-soluble contrast swallow 5–7 days after the operation to determine whether the anastomosis is intact, and it is not uncommon to find a small radiological leak. It is unusual to detect a major leak in the absence of clinical signs.

As with any gastrectomy, leakage from the duodenal stump can occur. This is usually due to a degree of distal obstruction and care must be taken when performing the Roux-en-Y anastomosis that there is no kinking. Paraduodenal collections can be drained radiologically, which will often convert the collection into an external fistula. Biliary peritonitis requires a laparotomy and peritoneal toilet, and in this circumstance it is best to leave a Foley catheter in the duodenum to establish a controlled duodenal fistula. If it is established that there is no distal obstruction, or if any such obstruction is managed, then with time the fistula will close.

The presence of septic collections along with a very radical vascular dissection may lead to catastrophic secondary haemorrhage from the exposed or divided blood vessels. This situation may be very difficult to manage, whether or not reoperation or interventional radiology is employed.

Long-term complications of surgery

Considering the radical nature of the total gastrectomy it is surprising that many patients, particularly younger ones, have good functional results. However, most patients will have a reduced capacity, particularly in the short term. They need to be given detailed nutritional advice, the substance of which is to eat small meals often while the jejunum or small gastric remnant adapts. In fact, there is very little functional difference between patients who have a total gastrectomy and those who have a subtotal gastrectomy. Various attempts have been made to try and improve the short-term functional results by forming a jejunal pouch and attaching this to the oesophagus; however, most surgeons do not perform this because, in the long term, there seems to be little functional advantage. It is surprising that these patients only infrequently suffer from the complications of gastric surgery, such as dumping and diarrhoea. Nutritional deficiencies may occur and the patient should be monitored with this in mind. The loss of the parietal mass leads to vitamin B12 deficiency and replacement should be given routinely.

Outlook after surgical treatment

The outlook after surgical treatment varies considerably between the west and Japan. In Japan, approximately 75% of patients will have a curative resection and, of these, the overall 5-year survival rate will be in the region of 50–70%. In contrast, in the west, most series show that only 25–50% of patients undergoing surgery will have a curative operation and the 5-year survival rate in such patients is only about 25–30%, although in some series it does approach Japanese levels. A combination of differences in staging and a higher standard of surgery in Japan probably accounts for these results. Staging is clearly crucial when survival figures are being compared. The more thorough the staging, the higher the stage is likely to be and, therefore, stage for stage, the outcome seems better in patients who are adequately staged pathologically. This phenomenon is termed 'stage migration'.

Frederic Eugene Basil Foley, **1891–1966**, Urologist, Anker Hospital, St. Paul, MN, USA.

Other treatment modalities

Because of the failure of radical surgery to cure advanced gastric cancer, there has been interest in the use of radiotherapy and chemotherapy.

Radiotherapy

The routine use of radiotherapy is controversial as the results of clinical trials are inconclusive. There are a number of radiosensitive tissues in the region of the gastric bed, which limits the dose that can be given. Radiotherapy has a role in the palliative treatment of painful bony metastases.

Chemotherapy

Gastric cancer may respond well to combination cytotoxic chemotherapy and neoadjuvant chemotherapy improves the outcome following surgery. Therefore, most patients should have chemotherapy before surgery. There are a number of well-investigated regimes but the best results are currently obtained using a combination of epirubicin, *cis*-platinum and infusional 5-fluorouracil (5-FU) or an oral analogue such as capecitabine. The same regimen is used as first line for patients with inoperable disease although oxaliplatin is being substituted for *cis*-platinum as it has fewer side-effects. Second-line treatment using combinations that include taxotere are increasingly being used. Chemotherapy for advanced disease is palliative.

Pattern of relapse following surgical treatment

As might be expected, the most common site of relapse following radical gastrectomy is the gastric bed, representing inadequate extirpation of the primary tumour. Widespread nodal intraperitoneal metastases, distant nodal metastases and liver metastases are all common. Dissemination to the lung and bones usually only occurs after liver metastases are already established (Summary box 60.6).

Summary box 60.6

Gastric cancer

- Gastric cancer is one of the most common causes of cancer death in the world
- The outlook is generally poor because of the advanced stage at presentation
- Better results are obtained in Japan, which has a high population incidence, screening programmes and high-quality surgical treatment
- The aetiology of gastric cancer is multifactorial; *H. pylori* is an important factor for distal but not proximal gastric cancer
- Early gastric cancer is associated with very high cure rates
- Gastric cancer can be classified into intestinal and diffuse types, the latter having a worse prognosis
- In the west, proximal gastric cancer is now more common than distal cancer and is usually of the diffuse type
- Spread may be by lymphatics, blood, transcoelomic or direct, but distant metastases are uncommon in the absence of lymph node involvement
- The treatment of curable cases is by radical surgery, and removal of the second tier of nodes (around the principal arterial trunks) may be advantageous
- Gastric cancer is chemosensitive and chemotherapy improves survival both in patients having curative surgery and with advanced disease

GASTROINTESTINAL STROMAL TUMOURS

Gastrointestinal stromal tumours (GISTs) commonly occur in the stomach and duodenum. Previously named leiomyoma and leiomyosarcoma, the term GIST is now used, recognising their particular distinct phenotype. The tumours are universally associated with a mutation in the tyrosine kinase *c-kit* oncogene. These tumours are sensitive to the tyrosine kinase antagonist imatinib, and an 80% objective response rate can be observed. Tumours with mutations in exon 11 of *c-kit* are particularly sensitive to this drug. The biological behaviour of these tumours is unpredictable but size and mitotic index are the best predictors of metastasis. Peritoneal and liver metastases are most common; spread to lymph nodes is extremely rare.

The incidence of the condition is unclear; small stromal tumours of the stomach are probably quite common but remain unnoticed. Clinically obvious tumours are considerably less common than gastric cancer.

The only way that many stromal tumours are recognised is either that the mucosa overlying the tumour ulcerates (see Fig. 60.24, p. 1065), leading to bleeding, or that they are noticed incidentally at endoscopy. Because the mucosa overlying the tumour is normal, endoscopic biopsy can be uninformative unless the tumour has ulcerated. Larger tumours present with non-specific gastric symptoms and, in many instances, it may initially be thought that they are gastric cancers (Fig. 60.33).

As the biological behaviour is difficult to predict, the best guide is to consider the size of the tumour. If easily resectable, surgery is the primary mode of treatment. Smaller tumours can be treated by wedge excision although the appropriate management of asymptomatic diminutive tumours found incidentally at endoscopy is unclear. Larger tumours may require a gastrectomy or duodenectomy (see Chapter 64) but lymphadenectomy is not required. Larger tumours that require multivisceral resection may be better treated for 3–6 months with imatinib before

operation as this will usually radically reduce their size and vascularity.

The prognosis of advanced metastatic GIST has been dramatically improved with imatinib chemotherapy but resection of metastases, especially from the liver, still has an important role.

GASTRIC LYMPHOMA

Gastric lymphoma is an interesting disease and some aspects of the management are controversial. It is first important to distinguish primary gastric lymphoma from involvement of the stomach in a generalised lymphomatous process. This latter situation is more common than the former. Unlike gastric carcinoma, the incidence of lymphoma seems to be increasing. Primary gastric lymphoma accounts for approximately 5% of all gastric neoplasms.

Gastric lymphoma is most prevalent in the sixth decade of life. The presentation is no different from gastric cancer, the common symptoms being pain, weight loss and bleeding. Acute presentations of gastric lymphoma such as haematemesis, perforation or obstruction are not common. Primary gastric lymphomas are B cell-derived, the tumour arising from the mucosa-associated lymphoid tissue (MALT). Primary gastric lymphoma remains in the stomach for a prolonged period before involving the lymph nodes. At an early stage, the disease takes the form of a diffuse mucosal thickening, which may ulcerate. Diagnosis is made as a result of the endoscopic biopsy and seldom on the basis of the endoscopic features alone, which are not specific.

Following diagnosis, adequate staging is necessary, primarily to establish whether the lesion is a primary gastric lymphoma or part of a more generalised process. CT scans of the chest and abdomen and bone marrow aspirate are required, as well as a full blood count.

Although the treatment of primary gastric lymphoma is somewhat controversial, it seems most appropriate to use surgery alone for the localised disease process. No benefit has been shown from adjuvant chemotherapy, although some oncologists contend that primary gastric lymphoma can be treated by chemotherapy alone. Chemotherapy alone is appropriate for patients with systemic disease.

Some of the more controversial aspects of gastric lymphoma concern the role of *H. pylori*. Lymphocytes are not found to any degree in normal gastric mucosa but are found in association with *Helicobacter* infection. It has also been shown that early gastric lymphomas may regress and disappear when the *Helicobacter* infection is treated (Isaacson).

Gastric involvement with the diffuse lymphoma

These patients are treated with chemotherapy, sometimes with dramatic and rapid responses. Surgeons are frequently asked to deal with the complications of gastric involvement. The two common complications are bleeding and perforation; both may occur at presentation, but more usually they may follow chemotherapy when there is rapid regression and necrosis of the tumour. These operations can be technically very challenging and normally require gastrectomy.

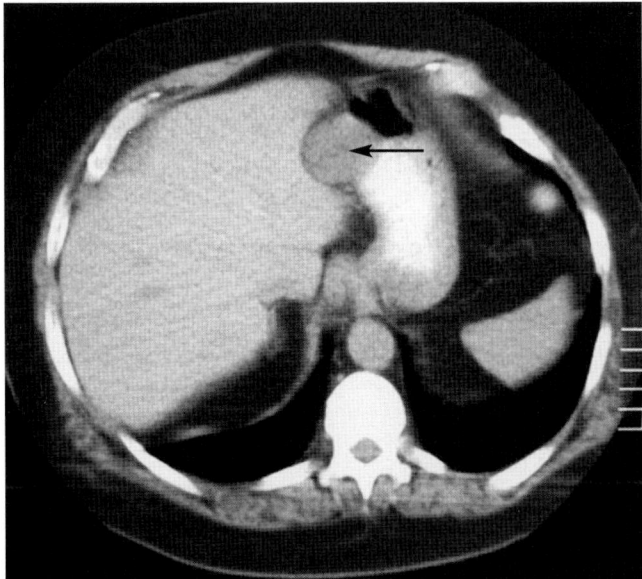

Figure 60.33 Computerised tomography (CT) of the upper abdomen showing a 3.5 cm gastrointestinal stromal tumour (GIST) arising from the gastric wall.

Peter Gersohn Isaacson, **Professor of Morbid Anatomy, University College, London, England.**

DUODENAL TUMOURS

Benign duodenal tumours

Duodenal villous adenomas occur principally in the periampullary region. Although generally uncommon, they are often found in patients with familial adenomatous polyposis. The appearances are similar to those of adenomas arising in the colon and, as they have malignant potential, they should be locally excised with histologically clear margins.

Duodenal adenocarcinoma

Although uncommon, this is the most common site for adenocarcinoma arising in the small bowel. Most tumours originate in the periampullary region and commonly arise in pre-existing villous adenomas. Patients present with anaemia because of ulceration of the tumour or obstruction as the polypoid neoplasm begins to obstruct the duodenum. Direct involvement in the ampulla leads to obstructive jaundice. Histologically, the lesion is a typical adenocarcinoma and the metastases are commonly to regional lymph nodes and the liver. At presentation, about 70% of the patients have resectable disease and, for those who survive operation, the 5-year survival rate is in the region of 20%, this approximately equating to cure. Poor prognostic features in the resected specimen include regional lymph node metastases, transmural involvement and perineural invasion. Curative surgical treatment will normally involve a pancreaticoduodenectomy (Whipple's procedure). Patients with familial polyposis, which is due to a mutation in the *APC* gene on chromosome 5, are predisposed to periampullary cancer, which is one of the most common causes of death in patients who have had their colon removed. Other duodenal malignancies include GISTs (see above) and neuroendocrine tumours.

Neuroendocrine tumours

A number of neuroendocrine neoplasms occurs in the duodenum. It is a common site for primary gastrinoma (Zollinger–Ellison syndrome). Non-functioning neuroendocrine tumours (usually called carcinoid tumours) also occur but uncommonly in comparison with the ileum.

Zollinger–Ellison syndrome

This syndrome is mentioned here because the gastrin-producing endocrine tumour is often found in the duodenal loop, although it also occurs in the pancreas, especially the head. It is a cause of persistent peptic ulceration. Before the development of potent gastric anti-secretory agents, the condition was recognised by the sometimes fulminant peptic ulceration that did not respond to gastric surgery short of total gastrectomy. It was also recognisable from gastric secretory studies in which the patient had a very high basal acid output but no marked response to pentagastrin, as the parietal cell mass was already nearly maximally stimulated by pathological levels of gastrin. The advent of proton pump inhibitors has rendered this extreme endocrine condition fully controllable, but also less easily recognised.

Gastrinomas may be either sporadic or associated with the autosomal dominantly inherited multiple endocrine neoplasia (MEN) type I (in which a parathyroid adenoma is almost invariably present). The tumours are most commonly found in the 'gastrinoma triangle' (Passaro) defined by the junction of the cystic duct and common bile duct superiorly, the junction of the second and third parts of the duodenum inferiorly, and the junction of the neck and body of the pancreas medially (essentially the superior mesenteric artery). Many are found in the duodenal loop, presumably arising in the G cells found in Brunner's glands. It is extremely important that the duodenal wall is very carefully inspected endoscopically and also at operation. Very often all that can be detected is a small nodule that projects into the medial wall of the duodenum.

Even malignant sporadic gastrinomas may have a very indolent course. The palliative resection of liver metastases may be beneficial and, as for other gut endocrine tumours, liver transplantation is practised in some centres with reasonable long-term results. However, the minority of tumours that are found to the left of the superior mesenteric artery (outside the 'triangle') seem to have a worse prognosis, with more having liver metastases at presentation. In MEN type I, the tumours may be multiple and the condition is incurable. Even in this situation, as with sporadic gastrinoma, surgical treatment should be employed to remove any obvious tumours and associated lymphatic metastases, as the palliation achieved may be good.

Duodenal obstruction

Duodenal obstruction in the adult is usually due to malignancy, and cancer of the pancreas is the most common cause. About one-fifth of patients with pancreatic cancer treated with endoscopic stenting will develop obstruction. Treatment is usually by gastroenterostomy but duodenal stenting is increasingly being used. In patients having a surgical biliary bypass for pancreatic cancer, gastric drainage may be necessary.

A variety of other malignancies can cause duodenal obstruction, including metastases from colorectal and gastric cancer. Primary duodenal cancer is much less common as a cause of obstruction than these other malignancies.

An annular pancreas may rarely cause duodenal obstruction. Obstruction usually follows an attack of pancreatitis and, on occasions, the obstruction may be mistaken for malignancy.

Arteriomesenteric compression is an ill-defined condition in which it is proposed that the fourth part of the duodenum is compressed between the superior mesenteric artery and the vertebral column; when it is convincingly demonstrated and causing weight loss, duodenojejunostomy may be performed (Summary box 60.7).

Summary box 60.7

Duodenal tumours

- Duodenal villous adenomas are commonly found around the ampulla of Vater and are pre-malignant
- Duodenal carcinoma is uncommon, but the commonest site for adenocarcinoma in the small intestine
- Both adenoma and carcinoma occur commonly in patients with familial polyposis and screening these patients is advised
- Pancreatic cancer is the most common cause of duodenal obstruction

---

Allen Oldfather Whipple, **1881–1963, Director of Surgical Services, The Presbyterian Hospital, and Professor of Surgery, The College of Physicians and Surgeons, Columbia University, New York, NY, USA.**

Edward Passaro, **Professor of Surgery, Los Angeles, CA, USA.**

GASTRIC OPERATIONS FOR MORBID OBESITY

Morbid obesity is defined as being 100% over the ideal weight for height or having a body mass index [(weight in kg)/(height in m)²] of greater than 45. It is an increasing and major health problem in the west, especially in the USA. A number of surgical treatments have been devised for morbid obesity, but none is free of problems. Selection of patients for operation should ideally be made by a team that includes a nutritionist/endocrinologist and a psychiatrist, as well as a surgeon, because it is important that major metabolic problems and severe psychiatric disorders are elucidated before operation. Morbidly obese patients as defined above have an excessive morbidity and mortality. The patient will often already have morbidity associated with severe obesity, such as hypertension, diabetes or osteoarthritis. Preoperative counselling should include discussion of the possibility of perioperative mortality. This is very much an elective procedure and the patient is at risk of postoperative respiratory problems and pulmonary thromboembolism. Thromboembolic prophylaxis is essential, as are antibiotics.

Increasingly, surgery is performed laparoscopically. The two most commonly performed procedures are the Lap Band procedure and gastric bypass. In the Lap Band procedure an inflatable cuff is placed laparoscopically just below the oesophagogastric junction (Fig. 60.34). The inflation of the band determines the level of restriction. However, very small differences in volume may result in complete dysphagia on the one hand and no significant weight loss on the other. Perioperative mortality is less than 1%. Band slippage may cause problems and the long-term results seem inferior to conventional surgery.

The operation that has the best long-term results is gastric bypass. This operation can be performed laparoscopically and, although technically difficult, it is becoming a standard procedure

(a)

(b)

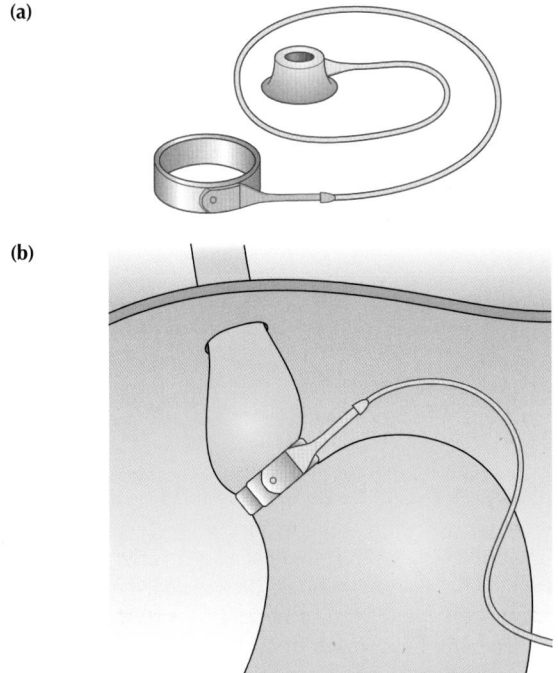

Figure 60.34 A gastric band (a) showing the cuff and injectable port and (b) in position around the upper part of the stomach.

for the severely obese (Fig. 60.35). Using a combination of circular and linear staplers, a gastric pouch is created as shown. The pouch has no connection to the rest of the stomach but is drained by a 70-cm Roux loop. The operative mortality is in the region of 2%.

After both procedures the patient must be managed in a high-dependency care unit until the possibility of apnoea and other complications are diminished. Epidural anaesthesia is useful as it decreases opiate requirements. The patient may be introduced to fluids and some food on the first postoperative day. Dietary advice is important; the patient must understand that liquidised food or high-calorie supplements are to be avoided. The patient should lose between one-third and one-half of their body weight over 2 years. Vomiting is common and vitamin supplementation is advised.

OTHER GASTRIC CONDITIONS

Acute gastric dilatation

This condition usually occurs in association with pyloroduodenal disorders or after surgery without nasogastric suction. The stomach, which may also be atonic, dilates enormously. Often the patient is also dehydrated and has electrolyte disturbances. Failure to treat this condition can result in a sudden massive vomit with aspiration into the lungs. The treatment is nasogastric suction with a large-bore tube, fluid replacement and treatment of the underlying condition.

Trichobezoar and phytobezoar

Trichobezoars (hair balls) (Fig. 60.36) are unusual and are almost exclusively found in female psychiatric patients, often young. They are caused by the pathological ingestion of hair, which remains undigested in the stomach. The hair ball can lead to ulceration and gastrointestinal bleeding, perforation or obstruction. The diagnosis is made easily at endoscopy or, indeed, from a plain radiograph. Treatment consists of removal of the trichobezoar, which may require open surgical treatment. Phytobezoars are made of vegetable matter and are found principally in patients who have gastric stasis. Often this follows gastric surgery.

Foreign bodies in the stomach

A variety of ingested foreign bodies reach the stomach and very often these can be seen on a plain radiograph. If possible they should be removed endoscopically but, if not, most can be left to pass. Even objects such as needles, about which there is understandable anxiety, will seldom cause harm. In general, an object that leaves the stomach will pass spontaneously. In contrast, attempted removal at laparotomy can be very difficult as the object may be much more difficult to find than might be expected. Most adults who swallow foreign bodies have ill-defined psychiatric problems and may appear to relish the attention associated with serial laparotomies. The treatment should therefore be expectant and intervention reserved for patients with symptoms in whom the foreign body is failing to progress.

Volvulus of the stomach

Rotation of the stomach usually occurs around the axis and between its two fixed points, i.e. the cardia and the pylorus. In theory, rotation can occur in the horizontal (organoaxial) or vertical (mesenteroaxial) direction but, commonly, it is the

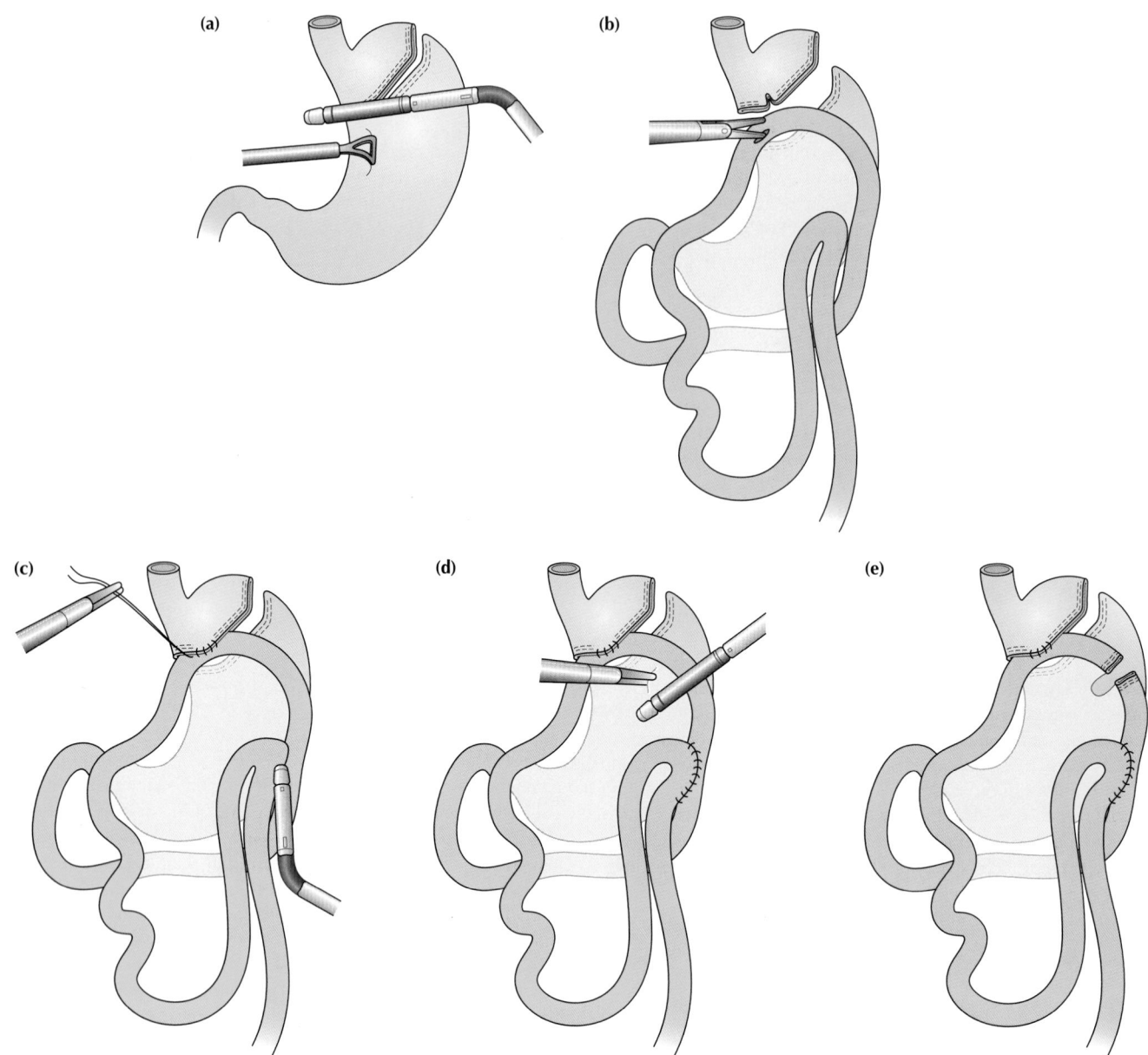

Figure 60.35 The technique of laparoscopic gastric bypass. (a) Formation of a gastric pouch; (b) anastomosis of the jejunum to the gastric pouch; (c) formation of the jejuno-jejunostomy; (d) completion of the jejuno-jejunostomy and division of the jejunum; (e) the completed procedure.

former that occurs. This condition is usually associated with a large diaphragmatic defect around the oesophagus (para-oesophageal herniation) (Fig. 60.37). What commonly happens is that the transverse colon moves upwards to lie under the left diaphragm, thus taking the stomach with it, and the stomach and colon may both enter the chest through the eventration of the diaphragm. The condition is commonly chronic, the patient presenting with difficulty in eating. An acute presentation with ischaemia may occur. It can be extremely difficult to sort out the anatomy endoscopically, and this is one situation in which contrast radiography is superior.

Treatment

If the problem is causing symptoms then surgical treatment is the only satisfactory approach. Traditionally, open surgery has been employed but this problem is suitable for laparoscopic treatment if appropriate skill is available. If there is a hernia, the sac and its contents (usually the stomach) should be reduced. The defect in the diaphragm should be closed, if necessary, with a mesh. It is advisable to separate the stomach from the transverse colon and then perform an anterior gastropexy to fix the stomach to the anterior abdominal wall. The results from this treatment are good.

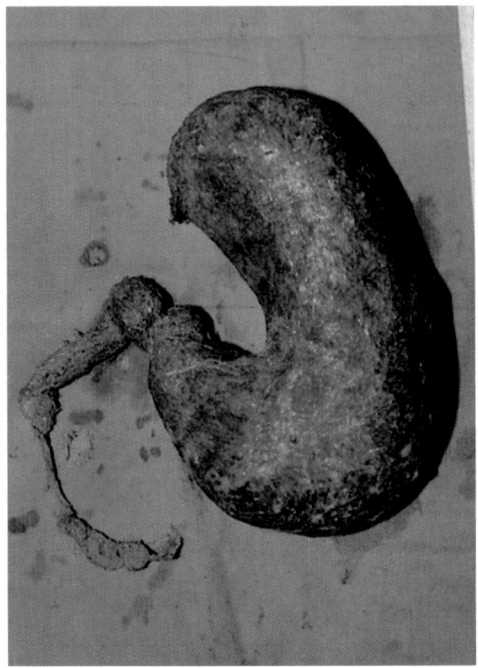

Figure 60.36 Trichobezoar of the stomach in a girl aged 15 years.

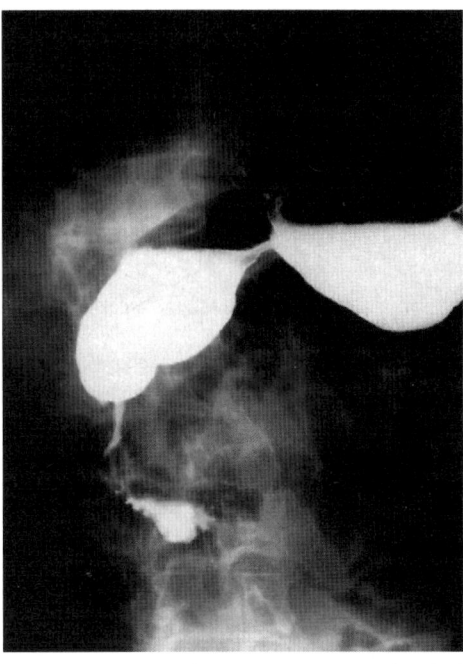

Figure 60.37 Barium meal showing organoaxial volvulus of the stomach associated with eventration of the diaphragm.

The liver

LEARNING OBJECTIVES

To understand:
- The anatomy of the liver
- The signs of acute and chronic liver disease

- The investigation of liver disease
- The management of liver trauma, infections, cirrhosis and tumours

INTRODUCTION

The liver is the largest organ in the body, weighing 1.5 kg in the average 70-kg man. The liver parenchyma is entirely covered by a thin capsule and by visceral peritoneum on all but the posterior surface of the liver, termed the 'bare area'. The liver is divided into a large right lobe, which constitutes three-quarters of the liver parenchyma, and a smaller left lobe. Surgical resection of these lobes would be termed a right or left lobectomy.

ANATOMY OF THE LIVER

Ligaments and peritoneal reflections

The liver is fixed in the right upper quadrant by peritoneal reflections that form ligaments. On the superior surface of the left lobe is the left triangular ligament. Dividing the anterior and posterior folds of this ligament allows the left lobe to be mobilised from the diaphragm and the left lateral wall of the inferior vena cava (IVC) to be exposed. The right triangular ligament fixes the entire right lobe of the liver to the undersurface of the right hemidiaphragm. Division of this ligament allows the liver to be mobilised from under the diaphragm and rotated to the left. Another major supporting structure is the falciform ligament (remnant of the umbilical vein), which runs from the umbilicus to the liver between the right and left lobes, passing into the interlobar fissure. From the fissure, it passes anteriorly on the surface of the liver, attaching it to the posterior aspect of the anterior abdominal wall. Division of the superior leaves of the falciform ligament allows exposure of the suprahepatic IVC, lying within a thin sheath of fibrous tissue. The final peritoneal reflection is between the stomach and the liver. This lesser omentum is often thin and fragile, but contains the hilar structures in its free edge.

Liver blood supply

The blood supply to the liver is unique, 80% being derived from the portal vein and 20% from the hepatic artery. The arterial blood supply in most individuals is derived from the coeliac trunk of the aorta, where the hepatic artery arises along with the splenic artery. After supplying the gastroduodenal artery, it branches at a very variable level to produce the right and left hepatic arteries.

The right artery supplies the majority of the liver parenchyma and is therefore the larger of the two arteries. There are many anatomical variations, knowledge of which is essential for safe surgery on the liver. The blood supply to the right lobe of the liver may be partly or completely supplied by a right hepatic artery arising from the superior mesenteric artery. This vessel passes posterior to the uncinate process and head of the pancreas, and runs to the liver on the posterior wall of the bile duct. Similarly, the arterial blood supply to the left lobe of the liver may be derived from the coeliac trunk via its left gastric branch. This vessel runs between the lesser curve of the stomach and the left lobe of the liver in the lesser omentum (Fig. 61.1).

Structures in the hilum of the liver

The hepatic artery, portal vein and bile duct are present within the free edge of the lesser omentum or the 'hepatoduodenal ligament'. To expose these structures requires division of the peritoneum overlying the hilar triad, followed by the division of small vessels and an extensive lymphatic plexus. The usual anatomical relationship of these structures is for the bile duct to be within the free edge, the hepatic artery to be above and medial, and the portal vein to lie posteriorly. Within this ligament, the common hepatic duct is joined by the cystic duct at a varying level to form the common bile duct. The common hepatic artery branches at a variable level within the ligament to form two, or often three, main arterial branches to the liver. The right hepatic artery often crosses the bile duct either anteriorly or posteriorly before giving rise to the cystic artery. Multiple small hepatic arterial branches provide blood to the bile duct, principally from the right hepatic artery. The portal vein arises from the confluence of the splenic vein and the superior mesenteric vein behind the neck of the pancreas. It has some important tributaries, including the left gastric vein which joins just above the pancreas.

Division of structures at the hilum

At the hilum, the major structures are divided into right and left branches. The right and left hepatic ducts arise from the hepatic parenchyma and join to form the common hepatic duct. The left duct has a longer extrahepatic course of approximately 2 cm. Once within the liver parenchyma, the duct accompanies the branches of

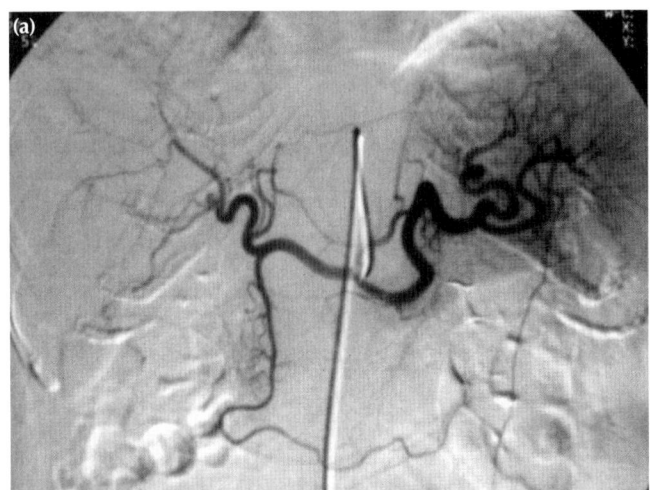

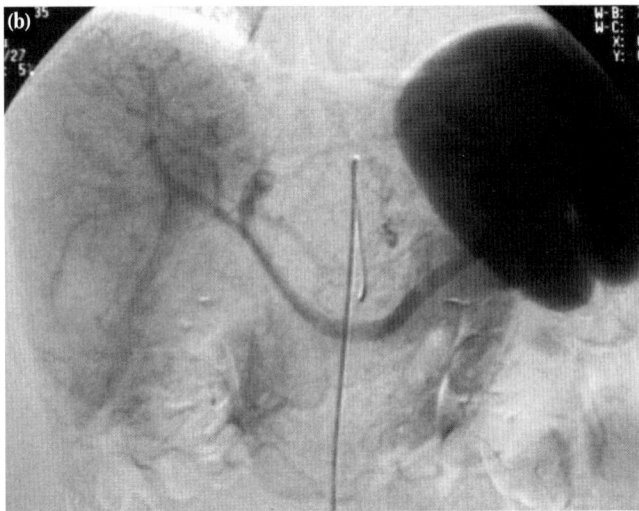

Figure 61.1 Hepatic angiography/conventional arterial anatomy. Arterial (a) and venous (b) phase of a selective hepatic angiogram. The hepatic artery usually arises from the coeliac trunk, along with the splenic artery, and gives rise to the gastroduodenal artery before dividing into the right and left hepatic arteries. The portal vein forms from the superior mesenteric and splenic veins, and divides into right and left branches in the hilum of the liver.

the hepatic artery and portal vein within a fibrous sheath. The portal vein often gives off two large branches to the right lobe, which are accessible outside the liver for a short length, before giving a left portal vein branch that runs behind the left hepatic duct.

Venous drainage of the liver

The venous drainage of the liver is via the hepatic veins into the IVC. The vena cava lies within a groove in the posterior wall of the liver. Above the liver, it immediately penetrates the diaphragm to join the right atrium, whereas below the liver parenchyma, there is a short length of vessel before the insertion of the renal veins. The inferior hepatic veins are short vessels that pass directly between the liver parenchyma and the anterior wall of the IVC. The major venous drainage is through three large veins that join the IVC immediately below the diaphragm. Outside the liver, these vessels are surrounded by a thin fibrous layer. The right hepatic vein can be exposed fully outside the

liver, but the middle and left veins usually join within the liver parenchyma. The right kidney and adrenal gland lie immediately adjacent to the retrohepatic IVC. The right adrenal vein drains into the IVC at this level, usually via one main branch. The IVC can be mobilised fully from the retroperitoneal tissues and, in the healthy state, there are no large vessels in this tissue plane.

THE INTERNAL ANATOMY OF THE LIVER

Understanding the internal anatomy of the liver has greatly facilitated safe liver surgery. Couinaud, a French anatomist, described the liver as being divided into eight segments (Fig. 61.2). Each of these segments can be considered as a functional unit, with a branch of the hepatic artery, portal vein and bile duct, and drained by a branch of the hepatic vein. The overall anatomy of the liver is divided into a functional right and left along the line between the gall bladder fossa and the middle hepatic vein (Cantlie's line). Liver segments (V–VIII), to the right of this line, are supplied by the right hepatic artery and the right branch of the portal vein, and drain bile via the right hepatic duct. To the

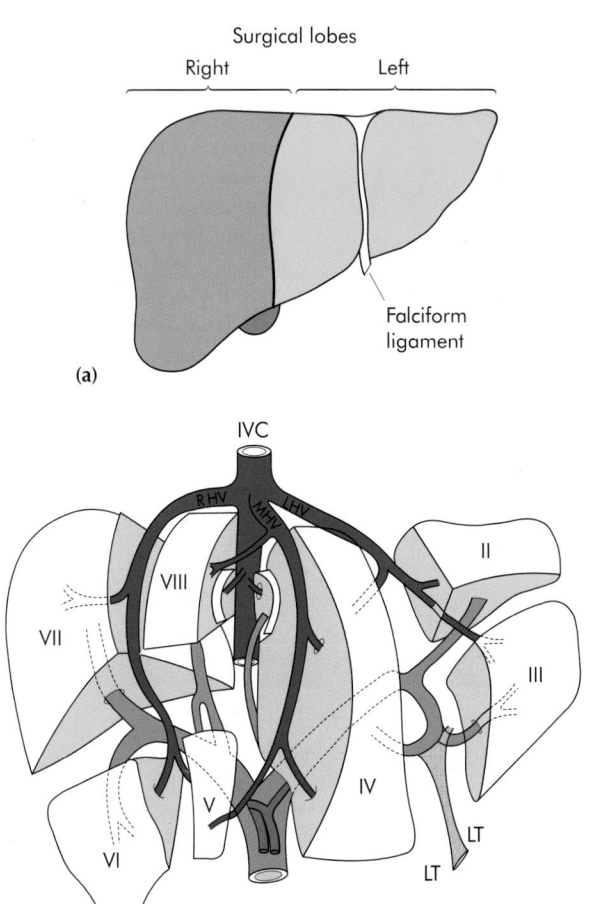

Figure 61.2 (a) The 'surgical' labels of the liver compared with the usual anatomical division into right and left lobes by the falciform ligament. (b) Segments of the liver (after Couinaud). IVC, inferior vena cava; RHV, right hepatic vein; LHV, left hepatic vein; LT, ligamentum teres; MHV, middle hepatic vein.

left of this line (segments I–IV), functionally, is the left liver, which is supplied by the left branch of the hepatic artery and the left portal vein branch, and drains bile via the left hepatic duct (Summary box 61.1).

Summary box 61.1

Liver anatomy

- The liver regenerates after partial resection
- There are two anatomical lobes with separate blood supply, bile duct and venous drainage
- Dual blood supply (20% hepatic artery and 80% portal vein)

The hepatic lobules

The functional units within the liver segments are the liver lobules. These comprise plates of liver cells separated by the hepatic sinusoids, large, thin-walled venous channels that carry blood to the central vein, a tributary of the hepatic vein, from the portal tracts, which contain branches of the hepatic artery and portal vein. During passage through the sinusoids, the many functions of the liver take place, including bile formation, which is channelled in an opposite direction to the blood flow to drain via the bile duct tributaries within the portal tracts.

Embryology

The liver is a foregut structure and forms as a small endodermal bud early in gestation. The cell population is bipotential, and cells may develop into hepatocytes or intrahepatic ductal cells. The liver endothelium is derived from the vitelline and umbilical veins, which merge with the endodermal bud to form the liver sinusoids. The supporting connective tissue, haemopoietic cells, important during intrauterine life, and Kupffer cells are derived from the mesoderm of the septum transversum.

ACUTE AND CHRONIC LIVER DISEASE

Liver function and tests

Adequate liver function is essential to survival; humans will survive for only 24–48 hours in the anhepatic state despite full supportive therapy. The liver is central to many key metabolic pathways (Summary box 61.2).

Summary box 61.2

Main functions of the liver

- Maintaining core body temperature
- pH balance and correction of lactic acidosis
- Synthesis of clotting factors
- Glucose metabolism, glycolysis and gluconeogenesis
- Urea formation from protein catabolism
- Bilirubin formation from haemoglobin degradation
- Drug and hormone metabolism
- Removal of gut endotoxins and foreign antigens

Karl Wilhelm von Kupffer, 1829–1902, Professor of Anatomy at Keil (1867), Königsberg (1875), and Münich, Germany (1880), described these 'stellate cells' in 1876.

An awareness of the currently available liver function tests and their significance is essential (Table 61.1).

Bilirubin is synthesised in the liver and excreted in the bile. Increased levels may be associated with increased haemoglobin breakdown, hepatocellular dysfunction resulting in impaired bilirubin transport and excretion, or biliary obstruction. In patients with known parenchymal liver disease, progressive elevation of bilirubin in the absence of a secondary complication suggests deterioration in liver function. The serum alkaline phosphatase is particularly elevated with cholestatic liver disease or biliary obstruction. The transaminase levels [aspartate transaminase (AST) and alanine transaminase (ALT)] reflect acute hepatocellular damage, as does the gamma-glutamyl transpeptidase (GGT) level, which may be used to detect the liver injury associated with acute alcohol ingestion. The synthetic functions of the liver are reflected in the ability to synthesise proteins (albumin level) and clotting factors (prothrombin time). The standard method of monitoring liver function in patients with chronic liver disease is serial measurement of bilirubin, albumin and prothrombin time.

Clinical signs of impaired liver function

These signs depend on the severity of dysfunction and whether it is acute or chronic.

Acute liver failure

Causes of acute liver failure

In the early stages there may be no objective signs, but with severe dysfunction the onset of clinical jaundice may be associated with neurological signs of liver failure, consisting of a liver flap, drowsiness, confusion and, eventually, coma (Summary box 61.3).

Summary box 61.3

Causes of acute liver failure

- Viral hepatitis (hepatitis A, B, C, D, E)
- Drug reactions [halothane, isoniazid–rifampicin, antidepressants, non-steroidal anti-inflammatory drugs, valproic acid]
- Paracetamol overdose
- Mushroom poisoning
- Shock and multiorgan failure
- Acute Budd–Chiari syndrome
- Wilson's disease
- Fatty liver of pregnancy

Treatment of acute liver failure

The overall mortality from acute liver failure is approximately 50%, even with the best supportive therapy (Summary box 61.4).

Table 61.1 Routinely available tests of liver function

Test	Normal range
Bilirubin	5–17 µmol l^{-1}
Alkaline phosphatase (ALP)	35–130 IU l^{-1}
Aspartate transaminase (AST)	5–40 IU l^{-1}
Alanine transaminase (ALT)	5–40 IU l^{-1}
Gamma-glutamyl transpeptidase (GGT)	10–48 IU l^{-1}
Albumin	35–50 g l^{-1}
Prothrombin time (PT)	12–16 s

Liver transplantation is appropriate for some patients with acute liver failure (Summary box 61.5), although the overall results are poor in comparison with liver transplantation for chronic liver disease.

Chronic liver disease

Lethargy and weakness are common features irrespective of the underlying cause. This often precedes clinical jaundice, which indicates the liver's inability to metabolise bilirubin. The serum bilirubin level reflects the severity of the underlying liver disease. Progressive deterioration in liver function is associated with a hyperdynamic circulation involving a high cardiac output, large pulse volume, low blood pressure and flushed warm extremities. Fever is a common feature, which may be related to underlying inflammation and cytokine release from the diseased liver or may be due to bacterial infection, to which patients with chronic liver disease are predisposed. Skin changes may be evident, including spider naevi, cutaneous vascular abnormalities that blanch on pressure, palmar erythema and white nails (leuconychia). Endocrine abnormalities are responsible for hypogonadism and gynaecomastia. The mental derangement associated with chronic liver disease is termed 'hepatic encephalopathy'. This is associated with memory impairment, confusion, personality changes, altered sleep patterns and slow, slurred speech. The most useful clinical sign is the flapping tremor demonstrated by asking the patient to extend his or her arms and hyperextend the wrist joint. Abdominal distension due to ascites is a common late feature. This may be suggested clinically by the demonstration of a fluid thrill or shifting dullness. Protein catabolism produces loss of muscle bulk and wasting, and a coagulation defect is suggested by the presence of skin bruising. A patient with the typical features of end-stage chronic liver disease is shown in Figure 61.3 (Summary box 61.6).

Classifying the severity of chronic liver disease

Classification is shown in Table 61.2.

Table 61.2 Child's classification of hepatocellular function in cirrhosis (using original units of measurement)

Group designation	A	B	C
Bilirubin (mg dl⁻¹)	< 2.0	2.0–3.0	> 3.0
Albumin (g dl⁻¹)	> 3.5	3.0–3.5	< 3.0
Ascites	None	Easily controlled	Poorly controlled
Neurological disorder	None	Minimal	Advanced
Nutrition	Excellent	Good	Wasting

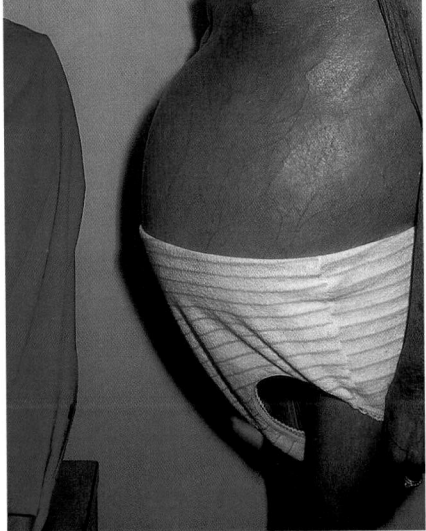

Figure 61.3 A patient with end-stage liver cirrhosis disease, demonstrating muscle wasting and gross abdominal distension due to ascites.

King's College Hospital London, England, **a pioneering centre for liver transplantation.**

IMAGING THE LIVER

The major advances that have taken place over recent years in surgical approaches to the liver and the enormous improvement in the safety of liver surgery are a result of the careful individualised planning of surgery achieved through improvements in preoperative imaging. The ideal choice of imaging modality is determined by the likely liver pathology and the locally available equipment and radiological expertise (Table 61.3).

Ultrasound

This is the first-line test owing to its safety and availability. It is entirely operator dependent. It is useful for determining bile duct dilatation, the presence of gallstones (Fig. 61.4) and the presence of liver tumours. Doppler ultrasound allows flow in the hepatic artery, portal vein and hepatic veins to be assessed. In some countries, it is used as a screening test for the development of primary liver cancers in a high-risk population. Ultrasound is useful in guiding the percutaneous biopsy of a liver lesion.

Computerised tomography

The current 'gold standard' for liver imaging is triple-phase, multislice, spiral computerised tomography (CT). This provides fine detail of liver lesions down to less than 1 cm in diameter and gives information on their nature (Fig. 61.5). Oral contrast enhancement allows visualisation of the stomach and duodenum in relation to the liver hilum. The early arterial phase of the intravenous contrast vascular enhancement is particularly useful for detecting small liver cancers, owing to their preferential arterial blood supply. The venous phase maps the branches of the portal vein within the liver and the drainage via the hepatic veins. Inflammatory liver lesions often exhibit rim enhancement with intravenous contrast, whereas the common haemangioma characteristically shows late venous enhancement. The density of any liver lesion can be measured, which can be useful in establishing the presence of a cystic lesion.

Table 61.3 Imaging the liver

Imaging modality	Principal indication
Ultrasound	Standard first-line investigation
Spiral CT	Anatomical planning for liver surgery
MRI	Alternative to spiral CT
MRCP	First-line, non-invasive cholangiography
ERCP	Imaging the biliary tract when endoscopic intervention is anticipated (e.g. ductal stones)
PTC	Biliary tract imaging when ERCP impossible or failed
Angiography	To detect vascular involvement by tumour
Nuclear medicine	To quantify biliary excretion and tumour spread
Laparoscopy/ laparoscopic ultrasound	To detect peritoneal tumour spread and superficial liver metastases

CT, computerised tomography; ERCP, endoscopic retrograde cholangiopancreatography; MRCP, magnetic resonance cholangiopancreatography; MRI, magnetic resonance imaging; PTC, percutaneous transhepatic cholangiography.

Christian Johann Doppler, 1803–1853, Professor of Experimental Physics, Vienna, Austria, enunciated the 'Doppler Principle' in 1842.

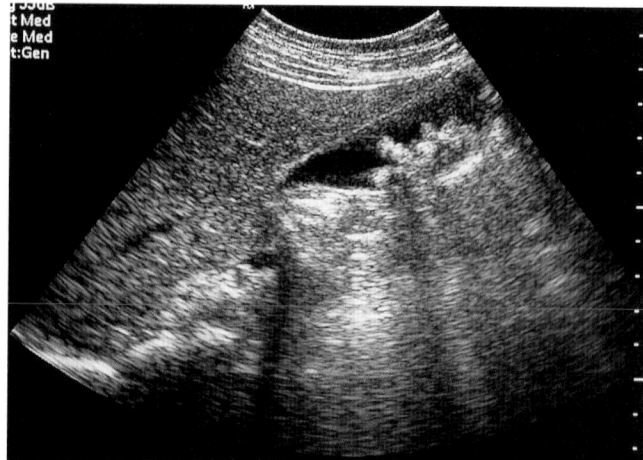

Figure 61.4 Ultrasound scan of the upper abdomen, showing the liver on the left and a gall bladder containing multiple gallstones centrally. The stones can be seen to cast an acoustic shadow.

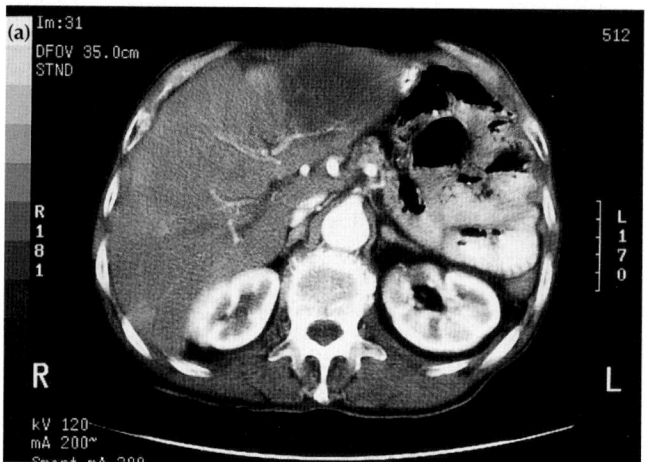

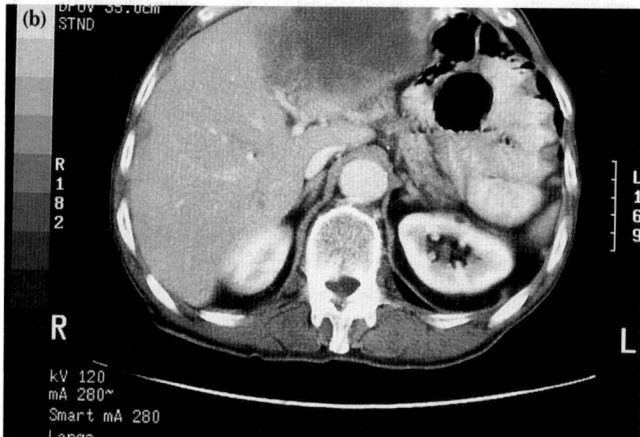

Figure 61.5 Computerised tomography (CT) scan of a patient with a liver tumour in the left lobe of the liver, using intravenous contrast enhancement. The vascularity of the lesion and, hence, its possible nature can be determined from the arterial (a) and venous (b) phases of the scan.

Magnetic resonance imaging

Magnetic resonance imaging (MRI) (Fig. 61.6) would appear to be as effective an imaging modality as CT in the majority of patients with liver disease. It does, however, offer several advantages. First, the use of iodine-containing intravenous contrast agents is precluded in many patients because of a history of allergy. These patients should be offered MRI rather than contrast CT. Second, magnetic resonance cholangiopancreatography (MRCP) provides excellent quality, non-invasive imaging of the biliary tract. The image quality is currently below that available from endoscopic retrograde cholangiopancreatography (ERCP) or percutaneous transhepatic cholangiography (PTC), but this is rapidly improving. It is useful for diagnostic questions when ERCP has failed or is impossible due to previous surgery. Magnetic resonance angiography (MRA) similarly provides high-quality images of the hepatic artery and portal vein, without the need for arterial cannulation. It is used as an alternative to selective hepatic angiography for diagnosis. It is particularly useful in patients with chronic liver disease and a coagulopathy in whom the patency of the portal vein and its branches is in question.

Endoscopic retrograde cholangiopancreatography

ERCP (Fig. 61.7a) is required in patients with obstructive jaundice who cannot undergo MRCP because of claustrophobia or where an endoscopic intervention is anticipated based on previous imaging [endoscopic removal of common bile duct (CBD) stones or insertion of a palliative biliary tract stent]. A

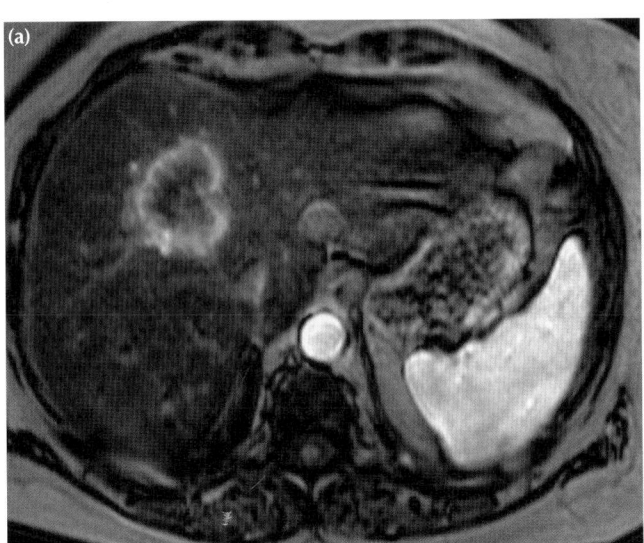

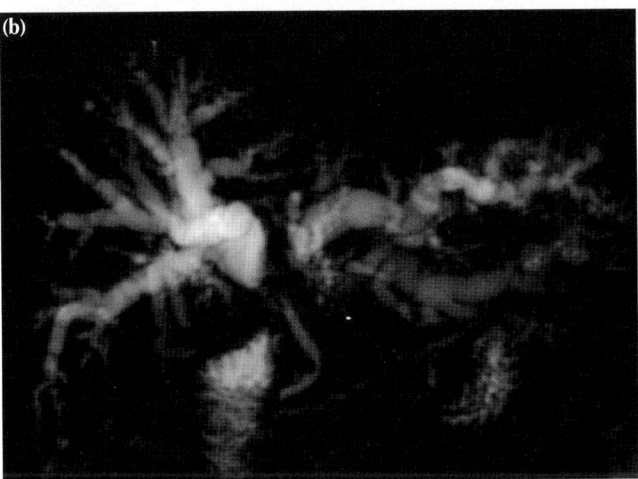

Figure 61.6 The role of magnetic resonance (MR) in liver disease. MR is increasingly used for imaging the liver. It may be used for cross-sectional imaging for staging liver cancers (MRI) (a), for non-invasive cholangiography to demonstrate a hilar stricture (magnetic resonance cholangiopancreatography, MRCP) (b) or for the non-invasive assessment of blood vessels (magnetic resonance angiography, MRA).

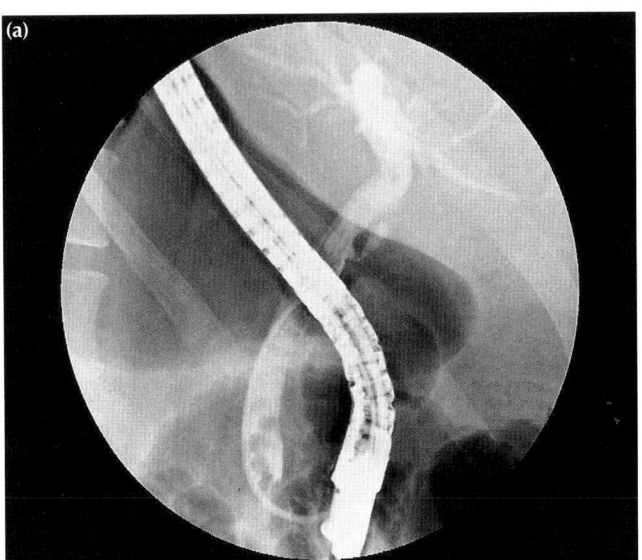

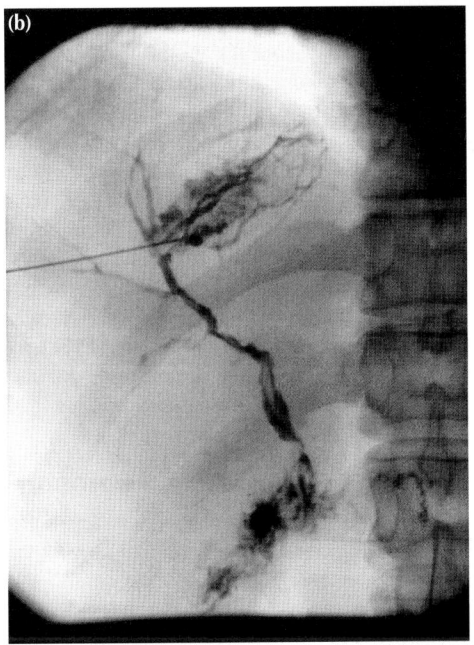

Figure 61.7 (a) Endoscopic retrograde cholangiopancreatography demonstrating the biliary tract with multiple stones in the distal common bile duct. (b) Percutaneous transhepatic cholangiography. Some contrast has extravasated at the site of hepatic puncture of the percutaneously placed needle, but the biliary tract is clearly demonstrated and shows the multiple strictures typical of primary sclerosing cholangitis.

CHAPTER 61 | THE LIVER

preoperative check of coagulation is essential, along with prophylactic antibiotics and an explanation of the main complications, which include pancreatitis, cholangitis and bleeding or perforation of the duodenum related to sphincterotomy.

Percutaneous transhepatic cholangiography

PTC is indicated where endoscopic cholangiography has failed or is impossible, e.g. in patients with previous pancreatoduodenectomy or Pólya gastrectomy. It is often required in patients with hilar bile duct tumours to guide external drainage of the bile ducts to relieve jaundice and to direct stent insertion (Fig. 61.7b).

Angiography

Selective visceral angiography (see Fig. 61.1, p. 1081) may be required for diagnostic purposes but, with improving cross-sectional imaging (CT and MR angiography), is usually employed for therapeutic intervention. Prior to liver resection, it may be used to visualise the anatomy of the hepatic artery to the right and left sides of the liver and to confirm patency or tumour involvement of the portal vein. It can also provide additional information on the nature of a liver nodule, as primary liver tumours have a well-developed arterial blood supply. Therapeutic interventions include the occlusion of arteriovenous malformations, the embolisation of bleeding sites in the liver and the treatment of liver tumours (transarterial embolisation, TAE).

Nuclear medicine scanning

Radioisotope scanning can provide diagnostic information that cannot be obtained by other imaging modalities. Iodoida is a technetium-99m (^{99m}Tc)-labelled radionuclide that is administered intravenously, removed from the circulation by the liver, processed by hepatocytes and excreted in the bile. Imaging under a gamma camera allows its uptake and excretion to be monitored in real time. These data are particularly useful when a bile leak or biliary obstruction is suspected and a non-invasive screening test is required. A sulphur colloid liver scan allows Kupffer cell activity in the liver to be determined. This may be particularly useful to confirm the nature of a liver lesion; adenomas and haemangiomas lack Kupffer cells and hence show no uptake of sulphur colloid.

18F-2-fluoro-2-deoxy-D-glucose positron emission tomography (FDG–PET) depends on the avid uptake of glucose by cancerous tissue in comparison with benign or inflammatory tissue. At present, it is mainly used to determine the nature of a mass lesion demonstrated on another form of imaging. Deoxyglucose is labelled with the positron emitter fluorine-18 (18FDG), and this is administered to the patient prior to imaging by PET. A three-dimensional image of the whole body is obtained, highlighting areas of increased glucose metabolism (Fig. 61.8).

Laparoscopy and laparoscopic ultrasound

Laparoscopy is useful for the staging of hepatopancreatobiliary cancers. Lesions overlooked by conventional imaging are mainly peritoneal metastases and superficial liver tumours. Approximately 10–30% of patients have additional lesions detected by laparoscopy, dependent on the quality of planar imaging by CT and MRI. Laparoscopic ultrasound may increase this figure and provides additional information for liver tumours on their proximity to the major vessels and bile duct branches.

Eugen (Janö) Alexander Pólya, **1876–1944, Surgeon, St. Stephen's Hospital, Budapest, Hungary.**

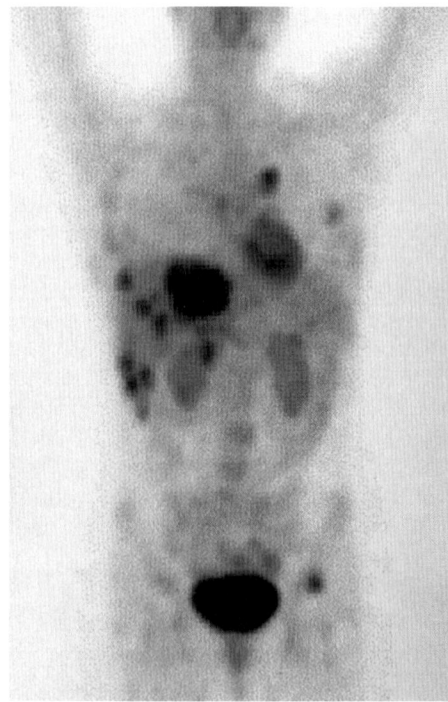

Figure 61.8 Whole-body positron emission tomography in a patient with colorectal metastases showing widespread areas of 18F-2-fluoro-2-deoxy-D-glucose uptake, indicating the sites of metastatic disease.

LIVER TRAUMA

General

Liver injuries are fortunately uncommon because of the position of the liver under the diaphragm where it is protected by the chest wall. However, when liver injury occurs, it is serious and can be associated with significant morbidity and mortality, even with prompt and appropriate management.

Liver trauma can be divided into blunt and penetrating injuries. Blunt injury produces contusion, laceration and avulsion injuries to the liver, often in association with splenic, mesenteric or renal injury. Penetrating injuries, such as stab and gunshot wounds, are often associated with chest or pericardial involvement (Summary box 61.7).

Summary box 61.7

Management of liver trauma

- Remember associated injuries
- At-risk groups
  Stabbing/gunshot in lower chest or upper abdomen
  Crush injury with multiple rib fractures
- Resuscitate
  Airway
  Breathing
  Circulation
- Assessment of injury
  Spiral CT with contrast
  Laparotomy if haemodynamically unstable
- Treatment
  Correct coagulopathy
  Suture lacerations
  Resect if major vascular injury
  Packing if diffuse parenchymal injury

Diagnosis of liver injury

The liver is an extremely well-vascularised organ, and blood loss is therefore the major early complication of liver injuries. Clinical suspicion of a possible liver injury is essential, as a laparotomy by an inexperienced surgeon with inadequate preparation preoperatively is doomed to failure. All lower chest and upper abdominal stab wounds should be suspect, especially if considerable blood volume replacement has been required. Similarly, severe crushing injuries to the lower chest or upper abdomen often combine rib fractures, haemothorax and damage to the spleen and/or liver. Patients with a penetrating wound will require a laparotomy and/or thoracotomy once active resuscitation is under way. Owing to the opportunity for massive on-going blood loss and the rapid development of a coagulopathy, the patient should be directly transferred to the operating theatre while blood products are obtained and volume replacement is taking place. Patients who are haemodynamically stable should have an oral and intravenous contrast-enhanced CT scan of the chest and abdomen. This will demonstrate evidence of parenchymal damage to the liver or spleen as well as associated traumatic injuries to their feeding vessels. Free fluid can also be clearly established and a diagnostic aspirate performed. The chest scan will help to exclude injuries to the great vessels and demonstrate damage to the lung parenchyma. Additional investigations that may be of value include peritoneal lavage, which can confirm the presence of haemoperitoneum, and laparoscopy, which can demonstrate an associated diaphragmatic rupture.

Initial management of liver injuries

Penetrating

The initial management of a patient with an upper abdominal penetrating injury is the basis of resuscitation. The initial survey assesses the patient's airway patency, breathing pattern and circulation. Peripheral venous access is gained with two large-bore cannulae and blood sent for cross-match of 10 units of blood, full blood count, urea and electrolytes, liver function tests, clotting screen, glucose and amylase. Initial volume replacement should be with colloid or O-negative blood if necessary. Arterial blood gases should be obtained and the patient intubated and ventilated if the gas exchange is inadequate. Intercostal chest drains should be inserted if associated pneumothorax or haemothorax is suspected. Once initial resuscitation has commenced, the patient should be transferred to the operating theatre, with further resuscitation performed on the operating table. The necessity for fresh frozen plasma and cryoprecipitate should be discussed with the blood transfusion service immediately the patient arrives, as these patients rapidly develop irreversible coagulopathies due to a lack of fibrinogen and clotting factors. Standard coagulation profiles are inadequate to evaluate this acute loss of clotting factors, and factors should be given empirically, aided by the results of thromboelastography (TEG), if available (Fig. 61.9).

Blunt trauma

With severe blunt injuries, the plan for resuscitation and management is as outlined above for penetrating injuries. For the patient who is haemodynamically stable, imaging by CT should be performed to further evaluate the nature of the injury. The basic surgical management differs between penetrating and blunt injuries thought to involve the liver; penetrating injuries should be explored, whereas blunt injuries can be treated conservatively.

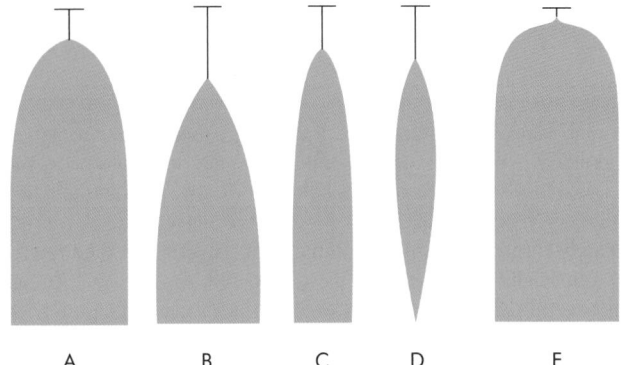

Figure 61.9 Thromboelastography (TEG). This dynamic form of assessing the coagulation status is being used increasingly for intraoperative monitoring. The shape of the TEG trace defines the nature of the underlying coagulation deficiency as shown. A, normal; B, delayed clot formation; C, reduced clot strength; D, clot lysis; E, hypercoagulable.

The indication for discontinuing conservative treatment for blunt trauma would be evidence of on-going blood loss despite correction of any underlying coagulopathy and the development of signs of generalised peritonitis.

The surgical approach to liver trauma

Good access is vital. A rooftop incision gives excellent visualisation of the liver and spleen and, if necessary, can be extended upwards for a median sternotomy. A stab incision in the liver can be sutured with a fine absorbable monofilament suture. If necessary, this may be facilitated by producing vascular inflow occlusion by placing an atraumatic clamp across the foramen of Winslow (the Pringle manoeuvre). Lacerations to the hepatic artery should be identified by placing an atraumatic bulldog clamp on the proximal vessel prior to repair with 5/0 or 6/0 Prolene suture. If unavoidable, the hepatic artery may be ligated, although parenchymal necrosis and abscess formation will result in some individuals. Portal vein injuries should be repaired with 5/0 Prolene, again with exposure of the vessel being facilitated by the placement of an atraumatic vascular clamp.

Deceleration injuries often produce lacerations of the liver parenchyma adjacent to the anchoring ligaments of the liver. These may be amenable to suture with an absorbable monofilament suture. Again, inflow occlusion may facilitate this suturing and, if necessary, the sutures can be buttressed to prevent them cutting through the liver parenchyma. With more severe deceleration injuries, a portion of the liver may be avulsed. These injuries are more complex as they are associated with a devitalised portion of the liver and, often, major injuries to the hepatic veins and IVC. Diffuse parenchymal injuries should be treated by packing the liver to produce haemostasis. This is effective for the majority of liver injuries if the liver is packed against the natural contour of the diaphragm by packing from below. Large abdominal packs should be used to ease their removal, and the abdomen closed to facilitate compression of the parenchyma. Care should be taken to avoid overzealous packing, as this may produce pressure necrosis of the liver parenchyma.

Jacob Benignus Winslow, **1669–1760, Professor of Anatomy, Physic, and Surgery, Paris, France.**
James Hogarth Pringle, **1863–1941, Surgeon, The Royal Infirmary, Glasgow, Scotland.**

Crush injuries to the liver often result in large parenchymal haematomas and diffuse capsular lacerations. Suturing is usually ineffective, and packing is the most useful method of providing haemostasis. Necrotic tissue should be removed, but poorly perfused, though viable, liver left *in situ*. If packing is necessary, the patient should have the packs removed after 48 hours, and usually no further surgical intervention is required. Antibiotic cover is advisable, and full reversal of any coagulopathy is essential. If a major liver vascular injury is suspected at the time of the initial laparotomy, then referral to a specialist centre should be considered. A common surgical approach in these circumstances would be to place the patient on veno-venous bypass using cannulae in the femoral vein via a long saphenous cut-down with the blood returned, using a roller pump, to the superior vena cava (SVC) via an internal jugular line. Veno-venous bypass allows the IVC to be safely clamped to facilitate caval or hepatic vein repair. A rapid infuser blood transfusion machine facilitates the delivery of large volumes of blood instantaneously. Once prepared, the patient is re-laparotomised via the rooftop incision with a midline extension to the xiphisternum. The liver is mobilised by division of the supporting ligaments, and complete vascular isolation of the liver is achieved by occluding the hilar inflow and the IVC above the renal veins and at the level of the diaphragm with atraumatic vascular clamps. Venous return is provided by the veno-venous bypass. Warm ischaemia of the liver is tolerated for up to 45 min, allowing sufficient time in a blood-free field for repair of injuries to the IVC or hepatic veins.

Other complications of liver trauma

A subcapsular or intrahepatic haematoma requires no specific intervention and should be allowed to resolve spontaneously. Abscesses may form as a result of secondary infection of an area of parenchymal ischaemia, especially after penetrating trauma. Treatment is with systemic antibiotics and aspiration under ultrasound guidance once the necrotic tissue has liquefied. Bile collections require aspiration under ultrasound guidance or percutaneous insertion of a pigtail drain. The site of origin of a biliary fistula should be determined by endoscopic or percutaneous cholangiography, and biliary decompression achieved by nasobiliary or percutaneous transhepatic drainage or endoprosthesis insertion. If this fails to control the fistula, the affected portion of the liver may require resection. Late vascular complications include hepatic artery aneurysm and arteriovenous or arteriobiliary fistulae (Fig. 61.10). These are best treated non-surgically by a specialist hepatobiliary interventional radiologist. The feeding vessel can be embolised transarterially.

Hepatic failure may occur following extensive liver trauma. This will usually reverse with conservative supportive treatment if the blood supply and biliary drainage of the liver are intact (Summary box 61.8).

Summary box 61.8
Other complications of liver trauma
■ Intrahepatic haematoma
■ Liver abscess
■ Bile collection
■ Biliary fistula
■ Hepatic artery aneurysm
■ Arteriovenous fistula
■ Arteriobiliary fistula
■ Liver failure

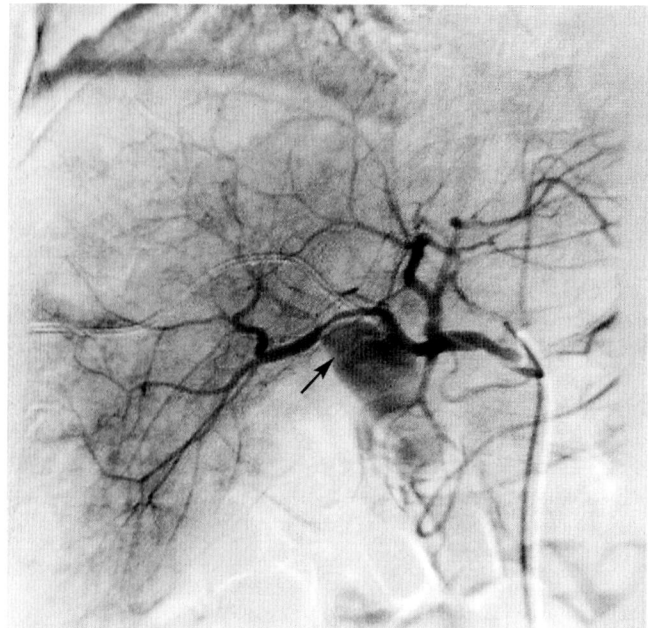

Figure 61.10 Hepatic aneurysm following liver trauma. An aneurysm arising from the right hepatic artery (arrow), which can be optimally treated by the interventional radiologist using transarterial embolisation.

Long-term outcome of liver trauma

The capacity of the liver to recover from extensive trauma is remarkable, and parenchymal regeneration occurs rapidly. Late complications are rare, but the development of biliary tract strictures many years after recovery from liver trauma has been reported. The treatment depends on the mode of presentation and the extent and site of stricturing. A segmental or lobar stricture, associated with atrophy of the corresponding area of liver parenchyma and compensatory hypertrophy of the other liver lobe, may be treated expectantly. A dominant extrahepatic bile duct stricture associated with obstructive jaundice may be treated initially with endobiliary balloon dilatation or stenting, but will usually require surgical correction using a Roux-en-Y hepatodochojejunostomy.

PORTAL HYPERTENSION

An elevation in portal pressure is most commonly found in the presence of liver cirrhosis, although it may be present in patients with extrahepatic portal vein occlusion, intrahepatic veno-occlusive disease or occlusion of the main hepatic veins [Budd–Chiari syndrome (BCS)]. As portal hypertension produces no symptoms, it is usually diagnosed following presentation with decompensated chronic liver disease and encephalopathy, ascites or variceal bleeding.

Management of bleeding varices
General resuscitation

Varices usually present with the acute onset of a large-volume haematemesis, the lower oesophagus being the most common site

Cesar Roux, 1857–1934, Professor of Surgery and Gynaecology, Lausanne, Switzerland, described this method of forming a jejunal conduit in 1908.

for variceal bleeding. The diagnosis may be suspected if the patient is known to have liver cirrhosis, but it needs to be confirmed following initial resuscitation of the patient. This involves obtaining peripheral and subsequently central venous access while adequate blood is obtained (initially 10 units). Liver function tests will reveal underlying liver disease, and a coagulation profile will reveal any underlying coagulopathy. Vitamin K is administered [10 mg intravenously (i.v.)], but correction of a coagulopathy will require the administration of fresh frozen plasma (FFP). An associated thrombocytopenia is usually secondary to hypersplenism due to cirrhosis and is treated if the platelet count falls below $50 \times 10^9 \, l^{-1}$. Variceal bleeding is often associated with hepatic encephalopathy and, in these circumstances, endoscopic evaluation may require sedation and mechanical ventilation. Bronchial aspiration is a frequent complication of variceal bleeding (Summary box 61.9).

Summary box 61.9

Management of bleeding oesophageal varices

- Blood transfusion
- Correct coagulopathy
- Oesophageal balloon tamponade (Sengstaken–Blakemore tube)
- Drug therapy (vasopressin/octreotide)
- Endoscopic sclerotherapy or banding
- Assess portal vein patency (Doppler ultrasound or CT)
- Transjugular intrahepatic portosystemic stent shunts (TIPSS)
- Surgery
    - Portosystemic shunts
    - Oesophageal transection
    - Splenectomy and gastric devascularisation

If the rate of blood loss prohibits endoscopic evaluation, a Sengstaken–Blakemore tube may be inserted to provide temporary haemostasis. This is shown diagrammatically in Figure 61.11. Once inserted, the gastric balloon is inflated with 300 ml of air and retracted to the gastric fundus, where the varices at the oesophagogastric junction are tamponaded by the subsequent inflation of the oesophageal balloon to a pressure of 40 mmHg. The two remaining channels allow gastric and oesophageal aspiration. A radiograph is used to confirm the position of the tube. The balloons should be temporarily deflated after 12 hours to prevent pressure necrosis of the oesophagus.

Drug treatment for variceal bleeding

This may be as effective as sclerotherapy in the initial control of variceal haemorrhage. Vasopressin has been the most extensively used drug for the initial control of variceal haemorrhage (20 U in 10 ml of 5% dextrose i.v. over 10 min). Octreotide, the long-acting somatostatin analogue, may be equally effective.

Endoscopic treatment of varices

Initial treatment of oesophageal varices in most centres is endoscopic sclerotherapy, using ethanolamine oleate or butyl

Robert William Sengstaken, B. 1923, Surgeon, Garden City, New York, NY, USA.
Arthur Hendley Blakemore, Associate Professor of Surgery, The Columbia College of Physicians and Surgeons, New York, NY, USA.

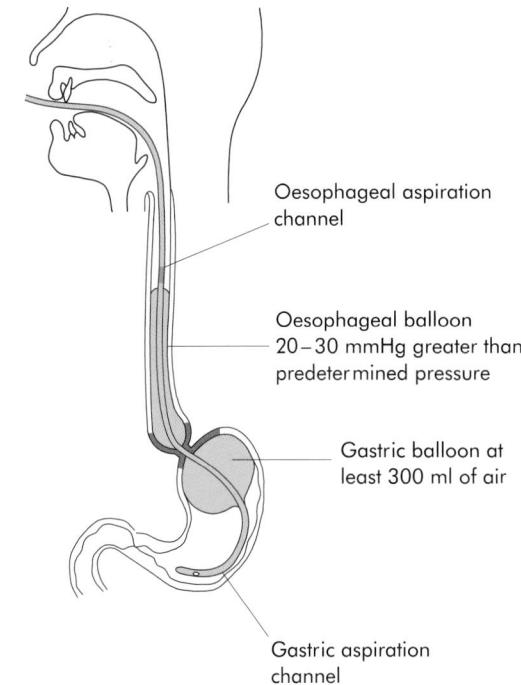

Oesophageal aspiration channel

Oesophageal balloon 20–30 mmHg greater than predetermined pressure

Gastric balloon at least 300 ml of air

Gastric aspiration channel

Figure 61.11 Oesophageal balloon tamponade.

cyanoacrylate. Banding may be equally effective and is associated with a lower incidence of oesophageal ulceration. The majority of variceal bleeds will respond to a single course. An early rebleed is less likely to be controlled by further sclerotherapy and a third bleed only rarely.

Transjugular intrahepatic portosystemic stent shunts

The emergency management of variceal haemorrhage has been revolutionised by the introduction of transjugular intrahepatic portosystemic stent shunts (TIPSS) in 1988. Over a short period, it has become the main treatment of variceal haemorrhage that has not responded to drug treatment and endoscopic therapy. The shunts are inserted under local anaesthetic, analgesia and sedation using fluoroscopic guidance and ultrasonography. Via the internal jugular vein and SVC, a guidewire is inserted into a hepatic vein and through the hepatic parenchyma into a branch of the portal vein. The track through the parenchyma is then dilated with a balloon catheter to allow insertion of a metallic stent, which is expanded once a satisfactory position is achieved (Fig. 61.12). A satisfactory drop in portal venous pressure is usually associated with good control of the variceal haemorrhage. The main early complication of this technique is perforation of the liver capsule, which can be associated with fatal intraperitoneal haemorrhage. TIPSS occlusion may result in further variceal haemorrhage and occurs more commonly in patients with well-compensated liver disease and good synthetic function. Post-shunt encephalopathy is the confusional state caused by the portal blood bypassing the detoxification of the liver. It occurs in about 40% of patients, a similar incidence to that found after surgical shunts. If severe, the lumen of the TIPSS can be reduced by insertion of a smaller stent. The main contraindication to TIPSS is portal vein occlusion. The main long-term complication of TIPSS is stenosis of the shunt, which is common (approximately 50% at 1 year) and may present as further variceal haemorrhage.

CHAPTER 61 | THE LIVER

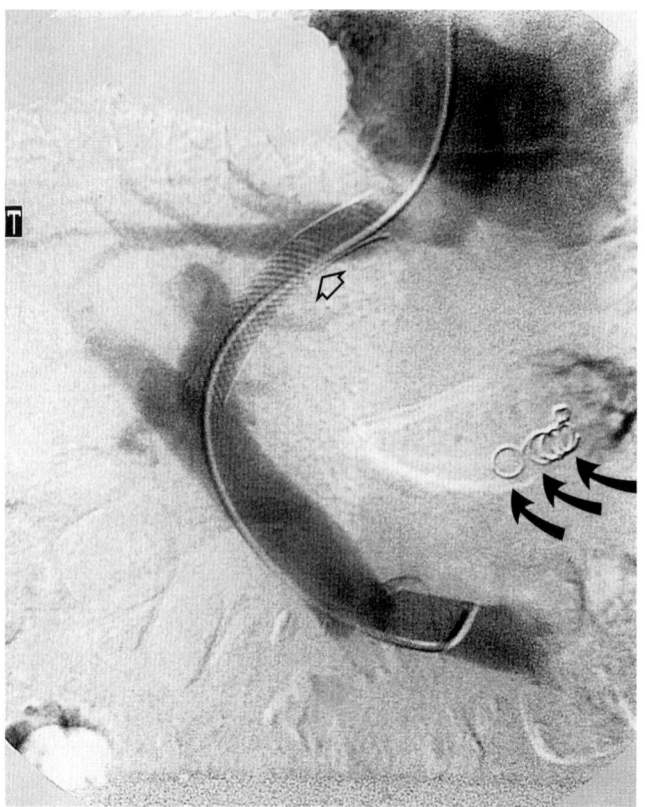

Figure 61.12 A check angiogram following insertion of a transjugular intrahepatic portosystemic stent shunt (open arrow). Injection of contrast into the portal vein flows through the metallic stent and outlines the right hepatic vein. Pressure measurements are taken from within the portal vein before and after insertion. Solid arrows indicate coils placed at the site of previous embolisation.

Surgical shunts for variceal haemorrhage

The increasing availability of liver transplantation and TIPSS has greatly reduced the indications for surgical shunts. It is rarely considered for the acute management of variceal haemorrhage, as the morbidity and mortality in these circumstances are high. The main current indication for a surgical shunt is a patient with Child's grade A cirrhosis, in whom the initial bleed has been controlled by sclerotherapy. Long-term β-blocker therapy and chronic sclerotherapy or banding are the main alternatives.

Surgical shunts are an effective method of preventing rebleeding from oesophageal or gastric varices, as they reduce the pressure in the portal circulation by diverting the blood into the low-pressure systemic circulation. Shunts may be divided into selective (e.g. splenorenal) and non-selective (e.g. portocaval), the former attempting to preserve blood flow to the liver while decompressing the left side of the portal circulation responsible for giving rise to the oesophageal and gastric varices. Selective shunts may be associated with a lower incidence of portal systemic encephalopathy (PSE), a confusional state commonly found in patients with chronic liver disease who have undergone radiological or surgical portosystemic shunts. The different types of surgical shunt are shown in Figure 61.13. There is no evidence that prophylactic shunting is beneficial in patients with varices that have not bled.

Oesophageal stapled transection

This technique for the management of bleeding oesophageal varices uses the circular stapling device, initially used for anastomosis of the rectum, for stapling and resecting a doughnut ring of the lower oesophagus. As with surgical shunts in the acute situation, it was associated with a high peroperative mortality and has been largely abandoned in centres where TIPSS is available.

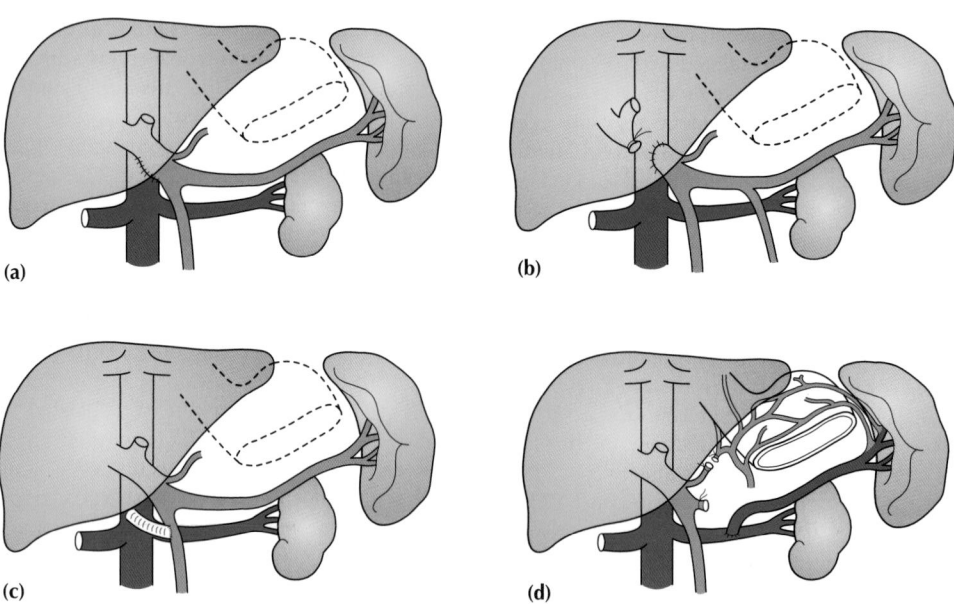

Figure 61.13 (a–d) Surgical shunts. Surgical shunts for portal hypertension involve shunting portal blood into the systemic veins. This commonly involves a side-to-side portocaval anastomosis (a) or end-to-side portocaval (b), mesocaval (c) or splenorenal (d) anastomoses.

C. G. Child, **Surgeon, Michigan, USA.**

Management of recurrent variceal bleeds secondary to splenic or portal vein thrombosis

Treatment is by splenectomy and gastro-oesophageal devascularisation, in which the blood supply to the greater and lesser curve of the stomach and lower oesophagus is divided. Splenic vein thrombosis may be seen secondary to chronic pancreatitis, and portal vein thrombosis is a common late complication of liver cirrhosis.

Variceal bleeding and orthotopic liver transplantation

The management of variceal bleeding should always take into account the possibility of liver transplantation when this is available. Age > 65 years or a history of ischaemic heart disease, heart failure or chronic respiratory disease would contraindicate transplantation. TIPSS would be the preferred management for bleeds resistant to sclerotherapy, as long as placement is optimal. Previous surgical shunts greatly increase the morbidity associated with orthotopic liver transplantation and probably the mortality.

Ascites

The accumulation of free peritoneal fluid is a common feature of advanced liver disease independent of the aetiology. The fluid accumulation is usually associated with abdominal discomfort and a dragging sensation. Development is usually insidious. The aetiology of the ascites must be established (Summary box 61.10).

Summary box 61.10

Determining the cause of ascites

Imaging (ultrasound or CT)
- Irregular cirrhotic liver
- Portal vein patency
- Splenomegaly of cirrhosis

Aspiration
- Culture and microscopy
- Protein content
- Cytology
- Amylase level

Imaging by CT will confirm the ascites and demonstrate the irregular and shrunken nature of a cirrhotic liver and associated splenomegaly. Intravenous contrast enhancement will allow abdominal varices to be demonstrated and patency of the portal vein, as portal vein thrombosis is a common predisposing factor to the development of ascites in chronic liver disease. In patients without evidence of liver disease, malignancy is a common cause, and the primary site may also be established on CT. Aspiration of the peritoneal fluid allows the measurement of protein content to determine whether the fluid is an exudate or transudate, and an amylase estimation to exclude pancreatic ascites. Cytology will determine the presence of cancerous cells, and both microscopy and culture will exclude primary bacterial peritonitis and tuberculous peritonitis. Urinary sodium excretion is used as a guide to diuretic therapy in cirrhosis.

Treatment of ascites in chronic liver disease

The initial treatment is to restrict additional salt intake and commence diuretics using either spironolactone or urosemide. This should be combined with advice on avoiding any precipitating factors for impaired liver function, such as alcohol intake in patients with alcoholic cirrhosis. Patients on diuretics should be monitored for the development of hyponatraemia and hypokalaemia (Summary box 61.11).

Summary box 61.11

Treatment of ascites in chronic liver disease
- Salt restriction
- Diuretics
- Abdominal paracentesis
- Peritoneovenous shunting
- TIPSS
- Liver transplantation

Abdominal paracentesis

Patients who fail to respond to diuretic treatment may require repeated percutaneous aspiration of the ascites (abdominal paracentesis), combined with volume replacement using salt-poor or standard human albumin solution, dependent on the serum sodium level. Paracentesis provides only short-term symptomatic relief.

Peritoneovenous shunting

The Le Veen shunt is designed for the relief of ascites due to chronic liver disease. One end of the silastic tube is inserted into the ascites within the peritoneal cavity and the other end is tunnelled subcutaneously to the neck, where it is inserted under direct vision into the internal jugular vein and fed into the SVC. Owing to a one-way valve within the tubing, peritoneal fluid is drawn from the abdomen and drained to the circulation due to the lower pressure in the SVC in comparison with the abdomen during the respiratory cycle. Complications include occlusion, displacement and infection. In an attempt to prevent the high occlusion rate, a further development was the insertion of a chamber placed over the costal margin to allow digital pressure and evacuation of any debris within the peritoneovenous shunt (Denver shunt).

TIPSS for ascites

The procedure and its limitations are as outlined above for the emergency treatment of bleeding varices secondary to portal hypertension. The use of TIPSS for ascites is for symptomatic relief, and the procedure is associated with considerable risks, including death from haemorrhage, renal failure or heart failure. Post-stent encephalopathy is common (about 40%), and the majority of stents will stenose on follow-up (approximately 50% by 1 year). Although a useful treatment modality, it has not become widely used because ascites is of itself not life-threatening. More encouraging results have been obtained in those with persistent chylothorax.

Liver transplantation for ascites

Diuretic-resistant ascites is an indication for liver transplantation if associated with deterioration in liver function (rising bilirubin, dropping albumin, prolonged prothrombin time). The patient's

Harry LeVeen, **Professor of Surgery, The University of South Carolina, SC, USA.**

age, underlying aetiology of liver disease and associated medical problems will be the major factors determining suitability for liver transplantation. In those considered inappropriate for liver transplantation, management is aimed at symptomatic control of ascites.

CHRONIC LIVER CONDITIONS

There are several chronic liver conditions, which, although rare, are important to recognise because they require a specific plan for investigation and treatment, and may present mimicking a more common clinical condition (Table 61.4).

Budd–Chiari syndrome

This is a condition principally affecting young females, in which the venous drainage of the liver is occluded by hepatic venous thrombosis or obstruction from a venous web. As a result of venous outflow obstruction, the liver becomes acutely congested, with the development of impaired liver function and, subsequently, portal hypertension, ascites and oesophageal varices. In an acute thrombosis, the patient may rapidly progress to fulminant liver failure but, in the majority of cases, abdominal discomfort and ascites are the main presenting features. If chronic, the liver progresses to established cirrhosis. The cause of the venous thrombosis needs to be established, and an underlying myeloproliferative disorder or pro-coagulant state is commonly found, such as anti-thrombin 3, protein C or protein S deficiency. The diagnosis is commonly suspected in a patient presenting with ascites, in whom a CT scan shows a large congested liver (early stage, Fig. 61.14) or a small cirrhotic liver in which there is gross enlargement of segment I (the caudate lobe). This feature results from preservation and hypertrophy of the segment with direct venous drainage to the IVC in the face of atrophy of the rest of the liver due to venous obstruction (Fig. 61.15). IVC compression or occlusion from the segment I hypertrophy is also a common feature, as is thrombosis of the portal vein. Confirmation of the suspected diagnosis is by hepatic venography via a transjugular approach, which demonstrates occlusion of the hepatic veins and may allow a transjugular biopsy.

Treatment of BCS must be tailored to the individual patient and, in particular, to the stage of disease at presentation. Patients presenting in fulminant liver failure should be considered for liver transplantation, as should those with established cirrhosis and

Table 61.4 Important chronic liver conditions

Condition	Common presentations
Budd–Chiari syndrome	Ascites
Primary sclerosing cholangitis (PSC)	Abnormal LFTs or jaundice
Primary biliary cirrhosis (PBC)	Malaise, lethargy, itching, abnormal LFTs
Caroli's disease	Abdominal pain, sepsis
Simple liver cysts	Coincidental finding, pain
Polycystic liver disease	Hepatomegaly, pain

LFTs, liver function tests.

George Budd, 1808–1882, Professor of Medicine, King's College Hospital London, England, described this syndrome in 1845.
Hans Chiari, 1851–1916, Professor of Pathological Anatomy, Strasbourg, Germany, (Strasbourg was returned to France in 1918 at the end of the First World War), gave his account of this condition in 1898.

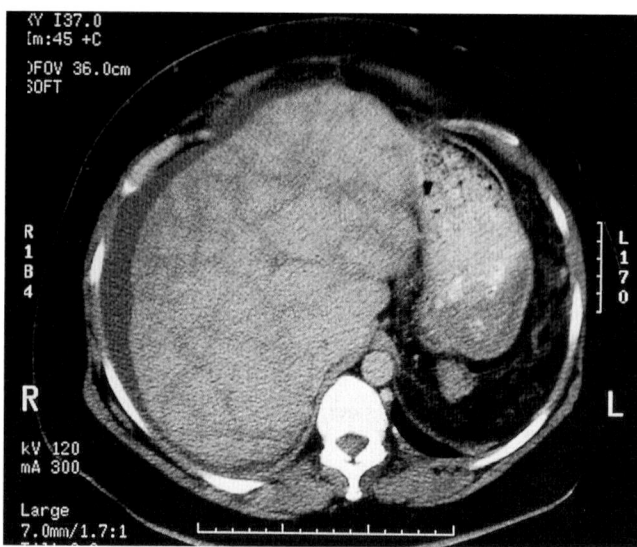

Figure 61.14 Computerised tomography scan in early Budd–Chiari syndrome.

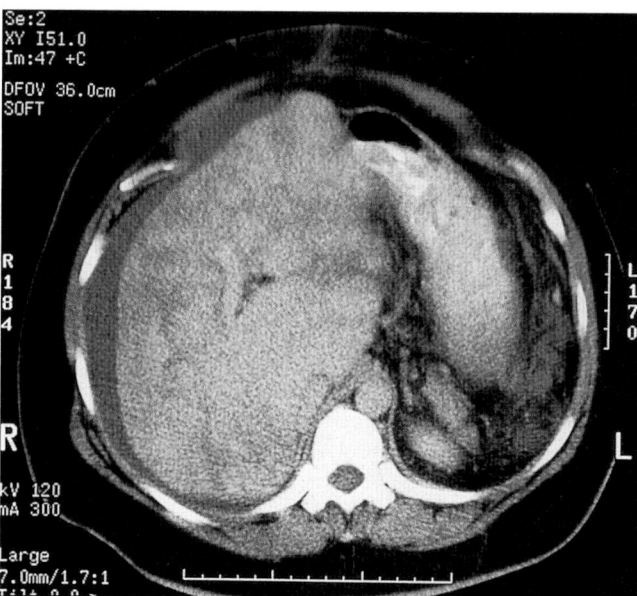

Figure 61.15 Segment I hypertrophy with Budd–Chiari syndrome.

the complications of portal hypertension. Those in whom cirrhosis is not established may be considered for portosystemic shunting by TIPSS, portocaval shunt or mesoatrial shunting. IVC compression may be relieved by the insertion of a retrohepatic expandable metallic stent. If the BCS is treated satisfactorily, the prognosis of this patient group is largely dependent on the underlying aetiology and whether this is amenable to treatment. Patients are usually left on lifelong anticoagulation with warfarin.

Primary sclerosing cholangitis

This condition often presents in young adults with mild non-specific symptoms, and biliary disease is suggested by the finding of abnormal liver function tests. Rarely, the first presentation is with jaundice due to biliary obstruction. The disease process results in progressive fibrous stricturing and obliteration of both the intrahepatic and the extrahepatic bile ducts. Although the aetiology is unknown, a genetic predisposition is likely owing to its association with chronic ulcerative colitis (UC). In patients with primary sclerosing cholangitis (PSC) and UC, the condition usually progresses even if the diseased colon is removed. The diagnosis is principally based on the findings at cholangiography, in which irregular, narrowed bile ducts are demonstrated in both the intrahepatic and the extrahepatic biliary tree (Fig. 61.16). If the radiological appearances are equivocal, a liver biopsy is required to demonstrate the fibrous obliteration of the biliary tracts. There is no specific treatment that can reverse the ductal changes, and the patients usually slowly progress to progressive cholestasis and death from liver failure. There is a strong predisposition to cholangiocarcinoma, and this should be considered in any patient with PSC in whom a new or dominant stricture is demonstrated on cholangiography.

Diagnosis of cancers in PSC is greatly facilitated by biliary brush cytology, as imaging rarely shows evidence of a mass lesion even in patients with advanced cancers. Patients with good liver function, no dominant strictures and negative biliary cytology may simply be monitored for disease progression. The only useful treatment modality is liver transplantation, which is associated with excellent results if carried out before bile duct cancer has developed. Temporary relief of obstructive jaundice due to a dominant bile duct stricture can be achieved by biliary stenting, although there is considerable risk of cholangitis from the introduction of bacteria to the biliary tract.

Primary biliary cirrhosis

As with PSC, the presentation of patients with primary biliary cirrhosis (PBC) is often hidden, with general malaise, lethargy

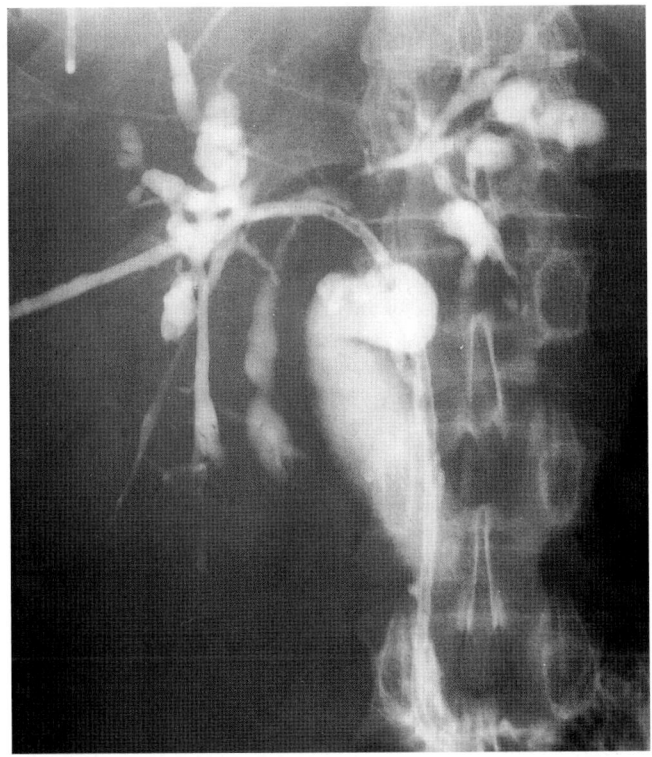

Figure 61.16 Primary sclerosing cholangitis (PSC). Percutaneous cholangiography showing the characteristic extensive bile duct strictures and dilatations associated with PSC.

and pruritus prior to the development of clinical jaundice or the finding of abnormal liver function tests. The condition is largely confined to females. Diagnosis is suggested by the finding of circulating anti-smooth muscle antibodies and, if necessary, is confirmed by liver biopsy. The condition is slowly progressive, with deterioration in liver function resulting in lethargy and malaise. It may be complicated by the development of portal hypertension and the secondary complications of ascites and variceal bleeding. The mainstay of treatment is liver transplantation, which should be considered when the patient's general condition starts to deteriorate with inability to lead a normal lifestyle.

Caroli's disease

This is congenital dilatation of the intrahepatic biliary tree, which is often complicated by the presence of intrahepatic stone formation. Presentation may be with abdominal pain or sepsis. Imaging is usually diagnostic, with the finding on ultrasound or CT of intrahepatic biliary lakes containing stones. Biliary stasis and stone formation combine to predispose to biliary sepsis, which may be life-threatening. Another well-recognised complication is the development of carcinoma. No specific treatment is available. Acute infective episodes are treated with antibiotics. Obstructed and septic bile ducts may be drained either radiologically or surgically. Malignant change within the ductal system results in cholangiocarcinoma, which may be amenable to resection. Segmental involvement of the liver by Caroli's disease may be treated by resection of the affected part, although the ductal dilatation is usually diffuse. Transplantation is a radical but definitive treatment for a patient whose liver function is generally well preserved.

Simple cystic disease

Liver cysts are a common coincidental finding in patients undergoing abdominal ultrasound. Radiological findings to suggest that a cyst is simple are that it is regular, thin walled and unilocular, with no surrounding tissue response and no variation in density within the cyst cavity. If these criteria are confirmed and the cyst is asymptomatic, no further tests or treatment are required. Large cysts may be associated with symptoms of abdominal discomfort, possibly related to stretching of the overlying liver capsule. Aspiration of the cyst contents under radiological guidance provides a sample for culture, microscopy and cytology, and allows the symptomatic response to cyst drainage to be assessed. Aspiration alone is usually associated with cyst and symptom recurrence, in which case more definitive treatment is required. Laparoscopic de-roofing is the treatment of choice for large symptomatic cysts and is associated with good long-term symptomatic relief.

Polycystic liver disease

This is a congenital abnormality associated with cyst formation within the liver and often other abdominal organs, principally the pancreas and kidney. Those associated with renal cysts may have autosomal dominant inheritance. The cysts are often asymptomatic and incidental findings on ultrasound. They usually have no effect on organ function and require no specific treatment. Occasionally, multiple liver cysts give rise to liver discomfort. This often responds to treatment with simple analgesics. Severe

Jacques Caroli, **B. 1901**, Professor of Medicine, Paris, France.

pain often indicates haemorrhage into a cyst, which may be confirmed by ultrasound or CT scan. Cyst discomfort that is not adequately controlled by oral analgesics may be treated by open or laparoscopic fenestration of the liver cysts, although the results are less favourable than with simple cysts.

LIVER INFECTIONS

Viral hepatitis

Viral hepatitis is a major world health problem. In addition to the well-recognised acute and chronic liver diseases produced by hepatitis A, B and C, other hepatitis viruses have been isolated, including hepatitis D, which is usually detected only in patients with hepatitis B virus (HBV) infection, and hepatitis E, which produces a self-limiting hepatitis due to faeco-oral spread similar to hepatitis A (Table 61.5).

Hepatitis A presents with anorexia, weakness and general malaise for several weeks prior to the development of clinical jaundice, often accompanied by tenderness on palpation of an enlarged liver. The condition is spread by the faeco-oral route and often spreads rapidly in closed communities. Liver function tests will be compatible with an acute hepatitis, with elevation of bilirubin and transaminases. Diagnosis is confirmed by the antibody titre to hepatitis A. The condition is virtually always self-resolving, although rarely the viral hepatitis can lead to fulminant liver failure. Once the clinical condition resolves, the liver tends to recover fully, with no functional deficit and no long-term sequelae.

Hepatitis B is a more serious condition in most respects than hepatitis A. Although it can also produce an acute self-resolving hepatitis, the virus is often not cleared and produces long-term liver damage, with the development of liver cirrhosis and primary liver cancers. Therefore, patients may present acutely with malaise, anorexia, abdominal pain and clinical jaundice due to active hepatitis, or at a late stage owing to the complications of cirrhosis, most commonly ascites or variceal bleeding. Treatment for acute hepatitis is supportive. In patients with cirrhosis, treatment is initially dictated by the specific complication at presentation (see sections on the treatment of ascites and variceal bleeding above). In established cirrhosis, liver transplantation may be considered if viral eradication or suppression can be achieved with anti-viral agents (e.g. lamivudine). Without viral suppression, death from reinfection of the transplanted liver is common. The hepatitis virus greatly increases the risk of primary liver cancers, which usually appear at the stage when the liver parenchyma has become cirrhotic. The assessment and management of HBV cirrhosis with hepatocellular carcinoma (HCC) is discussed in the section on 'Liver tumours' below.

Hepatitis C has become one of the most common causes of chronic liver disease worldwide and, in many countries, a large percentage of the population has been exposed; 1% of blood donors worldwide are hepatitis C virus (HCV) positive. Transmission is often related back to blood transfusion, and routine screening of blood for HCV has only recently been introduced in many countries. As with hepatitis B, it may present as an acute hepatitis or remain hidden until the development of cirrhosis and the complications of portal hypertension. Acute hepatitis C proceeds to cirrhosis in about 20% of cases. Deterioration in liver function, encephalopathy, ascites or bleeding in a patient with known HCV cirrhosis necessitates an urgent assessment for liver transplantation, if available. Although reinfection of the graft is common, it generally results in a mild hepatitis from which the graft and patient fully recover and is associated with a good long-term outcome.

Ascending cholangitis

Ascending bacterial infection of the biliary tract is usually associated with obstruction and presents with clinical jaundice, rigors and a tender hepatomegaly. The diagnosis is confirmed by the finding of dilated bile ducts on ultrasound, an obstructive picture of liver function tests and the isolation of an organism from the blood on culture. The condition is a medical emergency, and delay in appropriate treatment results in organ failure secondary to septicaemia. Once the diagnosis has been confirmed, the patient should be commenced on a first-line antibiotic (e.g. third-generation cephalosporin) and rehydrated, and arrangements should be made for endoscopic or percutaneous transhepatic drainage of the biliary tree. Biliary stone disease is a common predisposing factor, and the causative ductal stones may be removed at the time of endoscopic cholangiography by endoscopic sphincterotomy.

Pyogenic liver abscess

The aetiology of a pyogenic liver abscess is unexplained in the majority of patients. It has an increased incidence in the elderly, diabetics and the immunosuppressed, who usually present with anorexia, fevers and malaise, accompanied by right upper quadrant discomfort. The diagnosis is suggested by the finding of a multiloculated cystic mass on ultrasound or CT scan (Fig. 61.17) and is confirmed by aspiration for culture and sensitivity. The

Table 61.5 Liver infections and their treatment

Condition	Causative agent	Treatment
Viral hepatitis	Hepatitis A, B, C	Supportive, anti-viral agents (lamivudine, interferon, ribavirin)
		Liver transplant for cirrhosis
Ascending cholangitis	Enteric bacteria	Antibiotics (cephalosporin)
		Relieve obstruction
Pyogenic liver abscess	*Streptococcus milleri*	Antibiotics
	Escherichia coli	Aspiration
	Streptococcus faecalis	Drainage
Amoebic liver abscess	Entamoeba	Metronidazole
Hydatid liver disease	Echinococcus	Mebendazole
		Resection/omentoplasty

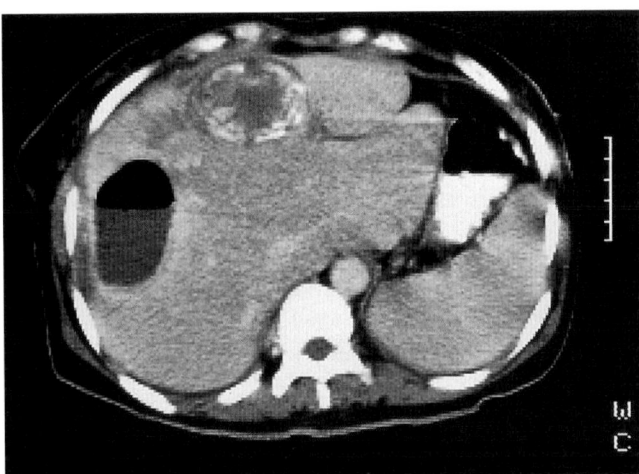

Figure 61.17 Liver abscess. Computerised tomography scan showing an air–fluid level and rim enhancement with intravenous contrast typical of a liver abscess. In the adjacent liver is a calcified hydatid cyst.

most common organisms are *Streptococcus milleri* and *Escherichia coli*, but other enteric organisms such as *Streptococcus faecalis*, *Klebsiella* and *Proteus vulgaris* also occur, and mixed growths are common. Opportunistic pathogens include staphylococci. Treatment is with antibiotics and ultrasound-guided aspiration. First-line antibiotics to be used are a penicillin, aminoglycoside and metronidazole or a cephalosporin and metronidazole. Percutaneous drainage without ultrasound guidance should be avoided as an empyema may follow drainage through the pleural space. A source for the liver abscess should be sought, particularly from the colon. Atypical clinical or radiological findings should raise the possibility of a necrotic neoplasm.

Amoebic liver abscess

Entamoeba histolytica is endemic in many parts of the world. It exists in vegetative form outside the body and is spread by the faeco-oral route. The most common presentation is with dysentery, but it may also present with an amoebic abscess, the common sites being paracaecal and in the liver. The amoebic cyst is ingested and develops into the trophozoite form in the colon, and then passes through the bowel wall and to the liver via the portal blood. Diagnosis is by isolation of the parasite from the liver lesion or the stool and confirming its nature by microscopy. Often patients with clinical signs of an amoebic abscess will be treated empirically with metronidazole (750 mg t.d.s. for 5–10 days) and investigated further only if they do not respond.

Hydatid liver disease

This is a very common condition in countries around the Mediterranean. The causative tapeworm, *Echinococcus granulosus*, is present in the dog intestine, and ova are ingested by humans and pass in the portal blood to the liver. Liver abscesses are often large by the time of presentation with upper abdominal discomfort or may present after minor abdominal trauma as an acute abdomen

due to rupture of the cyst into the peritoneal cavity. Diagnosis is suggested by the finding of a multiloculated cyst on ultrasound and is further supported by the finding of a floating membrane within the cysts on CT scan (Fig. 61.18). Active cysts contain a large number of smaller daughter cysts (Fig. 61.19), and rupture can result in these implanting and growing within the peritoneal cavity. Liver cysts can also rupture through the diaphragm, producing an empyema, into the biliary tract, producing obstructive jaundice, or into the stomach. Clinical and radiological diagnosis can be supported by serology for antibodies to hydatid antigen in the form of an enzyme-linked immunosorbent assay (ELISA). Treatment is indicated to prevent progressive enlargement and rupture of the cysts. In the first instance, a course of albendazole or mebendazole may be tried. Failure to respond to medical treatment usually requires surgical intervention, although percutaneous treatments with hypertonic saline and alcohol have been attempted. The surgical options range from liver resection or local excision of the cysts to de-roofing with evacuation of the contents.

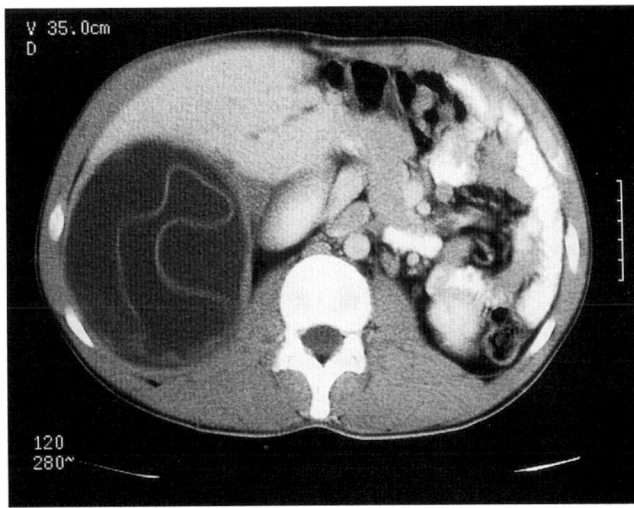

Figure 61.18 Hydatid liver cyst. Active hydatid disease usually produces a non-calcified liver cyst and, within the cyst, floating layers of the germinal membrane can be seen.

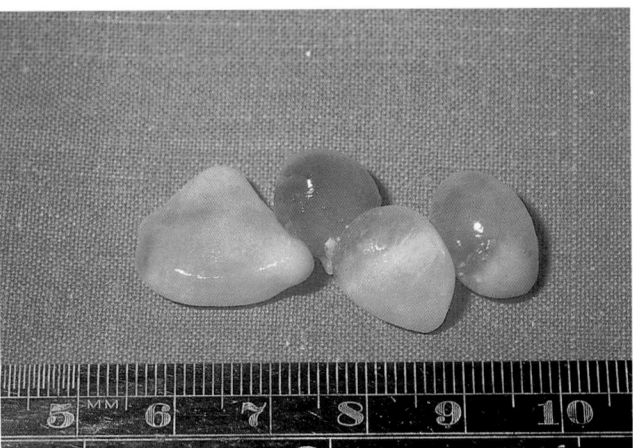

Figure 61.19 Hydatid 'daughter' cysts. These were removed from the bile duct of a patient presenting with obstructive jaundice due to a hydatid liver cyst communicating with the bile duct. Endoscopic removal should also be considered.

Contamination of the peritoneal cavity at the time of surgery with active hydatid daughters should be avoided by continuing drug therapy with albendazole and adding peroperative praziquantel. This should be combined with packing of the peritoneal cavity with hypertonic (2 mol l⁻¹) saline-soaked packs and instilling 2 mol l⁻¹ saline into the cyst before it is opened. A biliary communication should be actively sought and sutured. The residual cavity may become infected, and this may be reduced, as may bile leakage, by packing the space with pedicled greater omentum (an omentoplasty). Calcified cysts may well be dead. If doubt exists as to whether a suspected cyst is active, it can be followed on ultrasound, as active cysts gradually become larger and more superficial in the liver. Rupture of daughter hydatids into the biliary tract may result in obstructive jaundice or acute cholangitis. This may be treated by endoscopic clearance of the daughter cysts prior to cyst removal from the liver.

LIVER TUMOURS

Surgical approaches to resection of liver tumours

Adequate exposure of the liver is an absolute prerequisite to safe liver surgery. A rooftop or transverse abdominal incision provides excellent access to the liver if adequate retraction of the costal margin is employed using a costal margin retractor. Thoracoabdominal incisions are no longer required. The procedure for complete mobilisation of the liver is described, although this will not be necessary in all cases. There are many variations in surgical technique.

Mobilisation of the liver

The falciform ligament is first divided and followed along the anterior surface of the liver towards the suprahepatic IVC. The left triangular ligament is divided, facilitated by placing an abdominal pack in front of the oesophagogastric junction. The right triangular ligament is then divided by retraction of the diaphragm away from the right lobe parenchyma. On exposure of the bare area of the liver, the IVC can be seen as it passes behind the liver, and this can be slung above the renal veins below the liver and at the level of the main hepatic veins. Mobilisation of the liver is completed by division of the lesser omentum. Removing the liver from the IVC is achieved by lifting the liver anteriorly to expose the multiple small veins passing between the liver parenchyma and the IVC. These should be suture ligated to ensure haemostasis. This proceeds from above the renal veins until the main hepatic veins are reached below the diaphragm.

Dissection of the hilum

The peritoneum overlying the hilar triad is divided. The CBD is then exposed on the free edge of the lesser omentum, mobilisation being facilitated by ligation and division of the cystic duct and artery followed by removal of the gall bladder. Slinging the CBD with an elastic sling allows exposure of the common hepatic artery and dissection of the main right and left branches. These again may be slung to allow the remaining lymphatic tissue surrounding the portal vein to be ligated and divided. The possibility of an aberrant right hepatic artery should be sought lying posterior to the bile duct, and an accessory left hepatic artery from the left gastric artery in the lesser omentum. Dissection of the hilar bile ducts requires careful retraction on segment IV of the liver, and division of the small vessels and bile duct branches passing between segment IV and the confluence of the right and left hepatic ducts.

Division of the parenchyma

Once the liver has been adequately mobilised and the hilar vessels have been exposed, the main inflow vessels and bile duct can be divided to the liver lobe to be resected. The arterial branch may be ligated, but the bile duct should be transfixed with 4/0 PDS and the portal vein branch with a 4/0 Prolene suture. Division of the inflow vessels produces a line of demarcation between the right and left liver, passing to the right of and parallel with the falciform ligament. The parenchyma is divided along this plane of demarcation commencing by diathermy of the liver capsule. The ultrasound (Cusa) dissector is the most common method used for division of the parenchyma. This allows the parenchyma to be divided, leaving the vessels and bile duct branches to be diathermied or ligated depending on their size. Dissection continues on an even plane until the hepatic vein branches are approached from within the liver parenchyma, when they are ligated and divided (Fig. 61.20).

Segmental and local resections

These are considered in patients whose liver tumours can be excised with an adequate margin (generally considered to be 1 cm) without a formal right or left lobe liver resection. The segments that can be removed individually are those shown in Figure 61.2 (p. 1081). Each carries its own blood supply, venous drainage and bile drainage. The extent of mobilisation of the liver required (described above) depends on the segment to be resected. Hilar dissection may not be necessary. Segmental resections are used particularly in patients with HCC and underlying liver disease (e.g. HBV or HCV) to minimise the risk of postoperative liver failure (Fig. 61.21). Local resections are principally used for patients with liver metastases when removal of the tumour mass with a minimum margin of 1 cm of normal liver parenchyma is required.

Blood loss and transfusion

The reduction of blood loss during liver surgery has been one of the major achievements in the last decade, and resection without

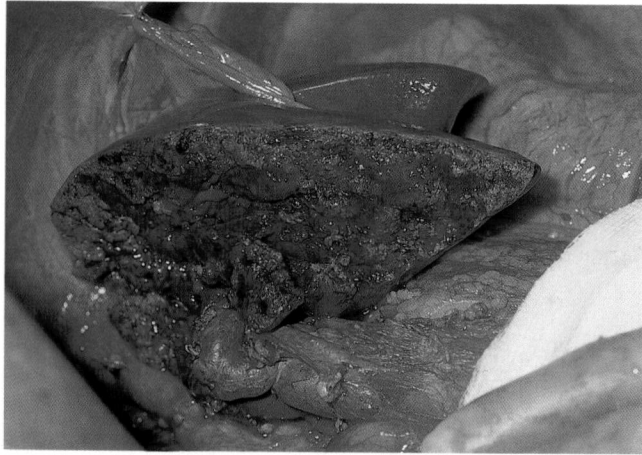

Figure 61.20 Hepatectomy post resection. Cut surface of the residual liver following a right hepatectomy in which segments V–VIII have been removed. On the lower edge, the portal vein and bile duct can be visualised.

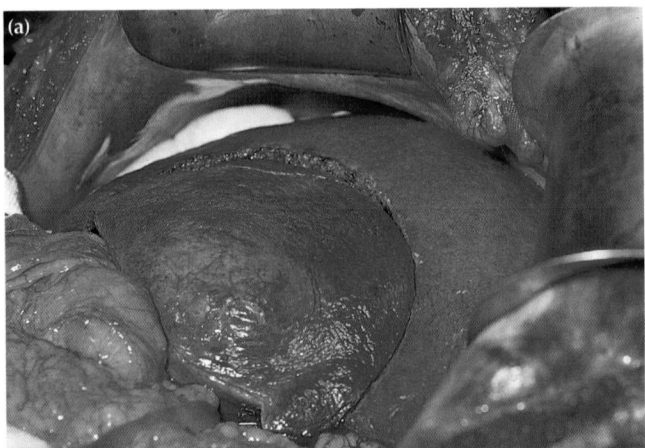

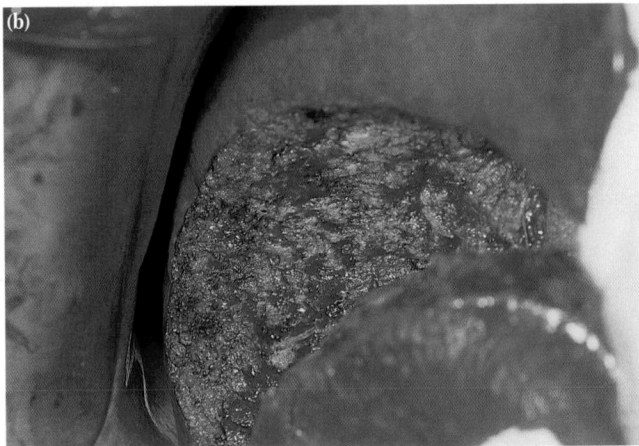

Figure 61.21 Segmental resection. Removal of a primary liver tumour by resection of liver segment VI (a and b) in a patient with well-compensated liver cirrhosis.

blood transfusion is often possible. The ultrasound dissector has been one of the main advances. Preoperative venesection, intraoperative haemodilution, reducing central venous pressure and the intraoperative cell saver have all helped to reduce the necessity for autologous blood transfusion. Better control of the coagulation cascade has been achieved using TEG (see Fig. 61.9 p. 1087), and the anti-fibrinolytic drug aprotinin has significantly reduced bleeding in patients with liver disease and an underlying coagulopathy. Oozing from the resected surface can be reduced by the topical application of fibrin glue or fibrin-impregnated collagen fleece. The main alternative is use of the argon-beam coagulator.

Benign liver tumours

Haemangiomas

These are the most common liver lesions, and their reporting has increased with the widespread availability of diagnostic ultrasound. They consist of an abnormal plexus of vessels, and their nature is usually apparent on ultrasound. If diagnostic uncertainty exists, CT scanning with delayed contrast enhancement shows the characteristic appearance of slow contrast enhancement due to small-vessel uptake in the haemangioma. Often, haemangiomas are multiple. Lesions found incidentally require confirmation of their nature and no further treatment. The management of 'giant' haemangiomas is more controversial. Occasional reports of rupture of

haemangiomas have led some to consider resection for the large lesions, especially if they appear to be symptomatic. They have little if any malignant potential, and this is no indication for surgery. Percutaneous biopsy of these lesions should be avoided as they are vascular lesions and may bleed profusely into the peritoneal cavity.

Hepatic adenoma (Fig. 61.22)

These are rare benign liver tumours. Imaging by CT demonstrates a well-circumscribed and vascular solid tumour. They usually develop in an otherwise normal liver. Unfortunately, there are no characteristic radiological features to differentiate these lesions from malignant tumours. Angiography will demonstrate a well-developed peripheral arterialisation of the tumour. Confirmation of the nature of these lesions is required by either percutaneous biopsy or resection with histological confirmation. These tumours are thought to have malignant potential, and resection is therefore the treatment of choice. Owing to their vascularity, bleeding following percutaneous biopsy is well recognised. An association with sex hormones (including the oral contraceptive pill) is well recognised, and regression of symptomatic adenomas on withdrawal of hormone stimulation is well documented.

Focal nodular hyperplasia

This is an unusual benign condition of unknown aetiology in which there is a focal overgrowth of functioning liver tissue supported by fibrous stroma. Patients are usually middle-aged females, and there

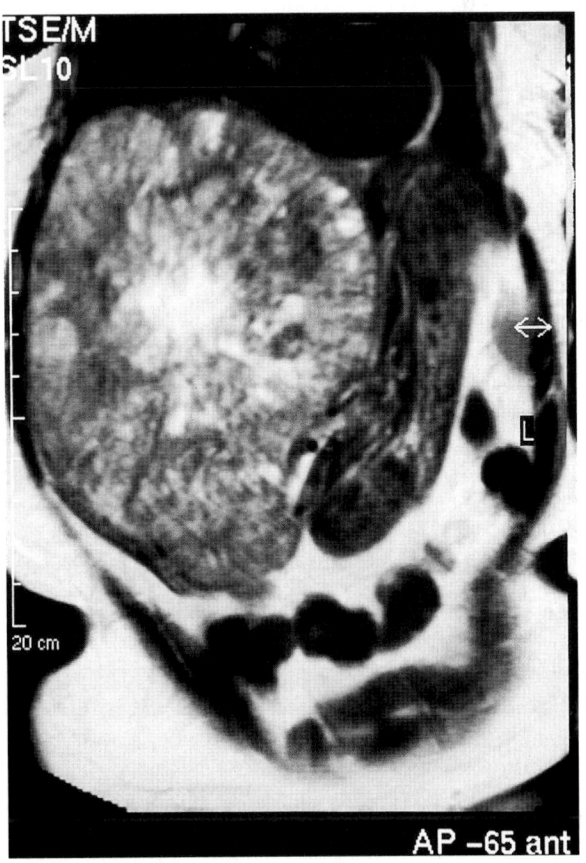

Figure 61.22 Hepatic adenoma. Magnetic resonance imaging scan of a giant hepatic adenoma. These lesions are thought to be pre-malignant, they may haemorrhage and, in some cases, their growth is sex hormone sensitive. Withdrawal of hormone preparations may allow spontaneous regression.

is no association with underlying liver disease. Ultrasound shows a solid tumour mass but does not help in discrimination. Contrast CT may show central scarring and evidence of a well-vascularised lesion. Again, these appearances are not specific for focal nodular hyperplasia (FNH). A sulphur colloid liver scan may be useful. FNH contain both hepatocytes and Kupffer cells. The latter take up the colloid allowing differentiation of FNH from either a benign adenoma or a primary or metastatic cancer, neither of which contains a significant number of Kupffer cells.

Surgery for liver metastases

Outcome

The role of surgery in the treatment of colorectal liver metastases is now well established, based on prospective data on resected patients compared with unresected patients with a similar stage of disease. The role of resection of liver metastases from other primary sites has not been defined. The expected patient survival rate for resection of solitary colorectal metastases is approximately 35% at 5 years, with few cancer-related deaths beyond this period. Multiple unilobar and bilobar liver metastases may also be considered for resection, although cure rates are significantly lower (Summary box 61.12).

Summary box 61.12

Prognostic factors in patients undergoing resection of colorectal liver metastases

- Stage of primary
- Time from primary resection
- Carcinoembryonic antigen (CEA) level
- Size of largest lesion
- Number of lesions

Staging

This involves defining the extent of the liver involvement with metastases and excluding extrahepatic disease. A standard work-up would involve oral and intravenous contrast CT scans of the liver and abdomen, chest CT scan and colonoscopy to look for locally recurrent or synchronous colonic cancers. MRI and PET scanning are useful in the clarification of equivocal lesions. This information should be taken in parallel with a general medical evaluation before deciding on the suitability for surgery of an individual patient. The typical appearance of colorectal liver metastases on contrast CT is shown in Figure 61.23. These patients usually have normal liver parenchyma and therefore tolerate a 60–70% resection of liver parenchyma without showing evidence of liver failure (Summary box 61.13).

Summary box 61.13

Staging and assessment with colorectal liver metastases

- General medical assessment
- CT, PET-CT or MRI of the abdomen/pelvis with contrast (? resectability)
- Chest CT
- Review histology of primary (? risk of local recurrence)
- Colonoscopy
- Liver function tests and tumour markers

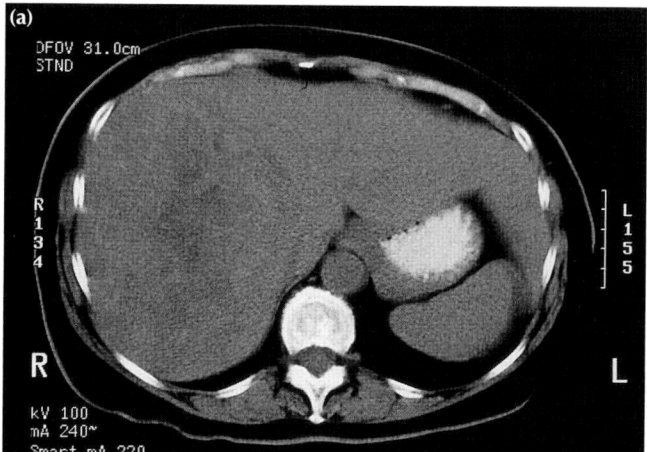

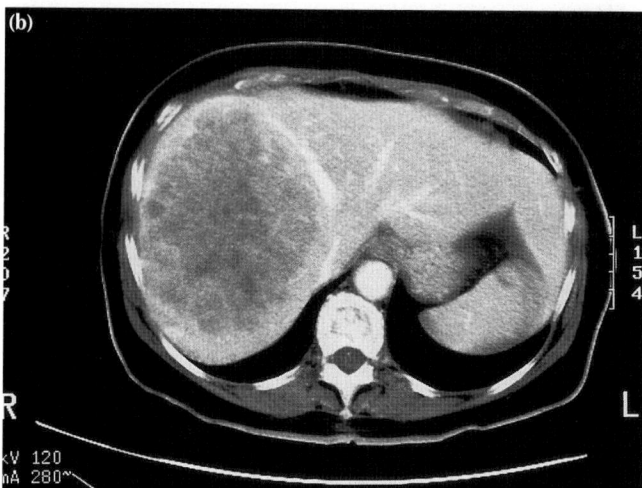

Figure 61.23 Colorectal liver metastases on computerised tomography (CT) scan: (a) after oral contrast CT; (b) after intravenous contrast. The colorectal liver metastasis occupying the entire right lobe of the liver is difficult to visualise on oral contrast CT. The addition of intravenous contrast shows its lack of enhancement and its relationship to the hepatic veins.

Surgical approach

The basic surgical approach to liver resection is outlined above. A search for local recurrent disease, peritoneal deposits and regional lymph node involvement should be made at the start of the laparotomy. Planar imaging often overlooks peritoneal or superficial liver metastatic deposits. Coeliac node involvement in patients with liver metastases considerably reduces the overall survival whether or not the liver and nodal disease is resected.

The treatment of unresectable disease

There have been major advances in the management of patients with colorectal liver metastases who, until recently, would have been considered 'unresectable' due to the size or distribution of their metastases. Chemotherapy with 5-fluorouracil (5FU) and folinic acid produces a response rate of approximately 30% but, when combined with oxaloplatinum, the response rate increases to 50–60%, often with a dramatic size reduction of the lesions. The combination of chemotherapy with monoclonal antibodies (mAbs) that recognise vascular endothelial growth factor (VEGF) receptor or the epidermal growth factor receptor (EGFR) may provide additional benefit. Long-term follow-up of patients downstaged with chemotherapy, who have proceeded to resection of their cancers, have shown 5-year survival rates of 30–40%.

Patients with bilobar metastases with a lesion centrally within the right lobe and a second lesion peripherally in the left lobe may have resection of their metastases in two stages to allow for regeneration of the liver parenchyma between the procedures. Good long-term survival has been reported for this group of patients.

Portal vein embolisation is a third development to affect patients previously deemed unresectable. Patients who require a right or extended right hepatectomy and in whom the left lobe volumes are congenitally small (< 30% of functioning parenchyma) have an increased risk of post-resection liver failure. This can be reduced by preoperative (3–6 weeks) percutaneous embolisation of the right portal vein branch, which produces atrophy of the affected lobe and hypertrophy of the contralateral lobe.

In patients who cannot be rendered resectable, systemic chemotherapy has been shown to produce survival and quality of life benefit. Many techniques are now available that produce local ablation of the tumours, including interstitial laser hyperthermia, radiofrequency ablation (RFA), microwave therapy, focused ultrasound and electrolytic therapy. These techniques may produce survival benefit along with chemotherapy in the palliative setting, but there is little objective evidence of long-term survival, and they should therefore be restricted to patients who cannot be offered surgical resection (Summary box 61.14).

Summary box 61.14

Strategies for 'unresectable' colorectal liver metastases

- Neoadjuvant oxaloplatinum/5-fluorouracil systemic chemotherapy
- Anti-VEGF or EGFR monoclonal antibody therapy
- Two-stage liver resection
- Portal vein embolisation

Hepatocellular carcinoma

Primary liver cancer (HCC) is one of the world's most common cancers, and its incidence is expected to rise rapidly over the next decade due to the association with chronic liver disease, particularly HBV and HCV. Many patients known to have chronic liver disease are now being screened for the development of HCC by serial ultrasound scans of the liver or serum measurements of alphafetoprotein (AFP). Patients often present in middle age, either because of the symptoms of chronic liver disease (malaise, weakness, jaundice, ascites, variceal bleed, encephalopathy) or with the anorexia and weight loss of an advanced cancer. The surgical treatment options include resection of the tumour and liver transplantation. Which option is most appropriate for an individual patient depends on the stage of the underlying liver disease, the size and site of the tumour, the availability of organ transplantation and the management of the immunosuppressed patient.

Staging and clinical assessment of HCC

In addition to a general assessment of the patient's fitness for surgery, crucial information is the severity of the underlying liver disease, based on Child's classification (see Table 61.2 p. 1083) and the size and site of the tumour. As chronic liver disease predisposes to these tumours, they are often multifocal by the time of diagnosis. Extensive liver resections in patients with advanced cirrhosis are associated with a high mortality due to liver failure and sepsis. In contrast, extensive resections for HCC in a non-cirrhotic liver are associated with a low risk of liver failure, and resection rather than transplantation would be the treatment option of choice. Tumours often metastasise to the lung and bone and, therefore, a chest CT scan and a bone scan are useful staging investigations. Evidence of intraperitoneal disease is difficult to determine by CT scan, and laparoscopy may be useful for this purpose. The intrahepatic distribution of HCC is equally difficult to determine within the cirrhotic liver. Ultrasound, early arterial phase enhanced spiral CT scan and contrast MRI are the most useful investigations that are currently available.

Surgical approach to HCC

The surgical approach should remove the known cancer with a 1- to 2-cm margin of unaffected liver tissue. In patients with associated chronic liver disease, the volume of liver resected should be minimised to reduce the incidence of postoperative liver failure. Local or segmental resections are preferred to major resections (see Fig. 61.21 p. 1097).

Non-surgical therapy for hepatocellular carcinoma

The majority of patients diagnosed with HCC will not be amenable to surgical resection because of the advanced stage of the cancer or the severity of the underlying liver disease. These patients can be offered local ablative treatments such as transarterial embolisation (TAE), transarterial chemoembolisation (TACE), percutaneous ethanol ablation (PEA) or RFA (Fig. 61.24).

Follow-up and adjuvant treatment

There is little evidence that adjuvant chemotherapy will improve the prognosis of patients following resection of HCC, and it may damage the function of the liver in those with underlying chronic liver disease. AFP is a clinically useful tumour marker for

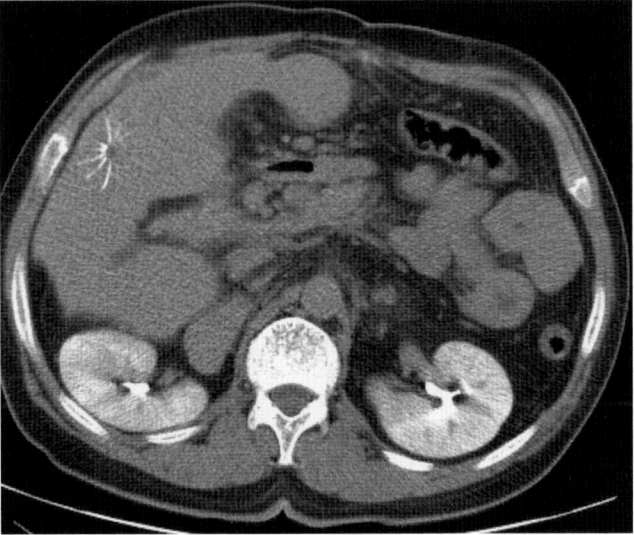

Figure 61.24 Computerised tomography scan after radiofrequency ablation for hepatocellular carcinoma.

follow-up, although its low sensitivity would suggest that imaging should also be used.

Cholangiocarcinoma

Presentation, pathology and natural history

Bile duct cancers typically present with painless obstructive jaundice. Elderly patients are frequently affected, but patients with PSC may develop these tumours at a much earlier age. These tumours are typically slow growing and often arise at the confluence of the right and left hepatic ducts (Klatskin tumours), eventually invading the liver parenchyma. Cancers at this site are usually fibrous and produce tight duct strictures. Distal bile duct cholangiocarcinomas are more frequently polypoidal and obstruct the lumen of the duct. Investigation, staging and management of bile duct and gall bladder malignancies are discussed in Chapter 63.

FURTHER READING

Bircher, J., Benhamou, J.-P., McIntyre, N., Rizzetto, M. and Rodes, J. (eds) (1999) *Oxford Textbook of Clinical Hepatology*, 2nd edn. Oxford University Press, Oxford.

Blumgart, L.H. (2006) *Surgery of the Liver, Biliary Tract and Pancreas*, 4th edn. W.B. Saunders, Philadelphia.

Sherlock, S. and Dooley, J.S.D. (eds) (2002) *Diseases of the Liver and Biliary Tract*, 11th edn. Blackwell Publishing, Oxford.

Townsend, C,M, (2004) *Sabiston Textbook of Surgery*, 17th edn. W.B. Saunders, Philadelphia.

The spleen

To understand:
- The function of the spleen
- The common pathologies involving the spleen
- The principles and potential complications of splenectomy

- The potential advantages of laparoscopic splenectomy
- The importance of prophylaxis against infection following splenectomy

EMBRYOLOGY, ANATOMY AND PHYSIOLOGY

Embryology

Fetal splenic tissue develops from condensations of mesoderm in the dorsal mesogastrium. This peritoneal fold attaches the dorsal body wall to the fusiform swelling in the foregut that develops into the stomach. This condensation divides the mesogastrium into two parts, one between the fetal splenic tissue and the stomach to form the gastrosplenic ligament and the other between it and the left kidney to form the lienorenal ligament.

Anatomy

The weight of the normal adult spleen is 75–250 g. It lies in the left hypochondrium between the gastric fundus and the left hemidiaphragm, with its long axis lying along the 10th rib. The hilum sits in the angle between the stomach and the kidney and is in contact with the tail of the pancreas. The concave visceral surface lies in contact with these structures, and the lower pole extends no further than the mid-axillary line. There is a notch on its inferolateral border, and this may be palpated when the spleen is enlarged.

The tortuous splenic artery arises from the coeliac axis and runs along the upper border of the body and tail of the pancreas, to which it gives small branches. The short gastric and left gastroepiploic branches pass between the layers of the gastrosplenic ligament. The main splenic artery generally divides into superior and inferior branches, which, in turn, subdivide into several segmental branches.

The splenic vein is formed from several tributaries that drain the hilum. The vein runs behind the pancreas, receiving several small tributaries from the pancreas before joining the superior mesenteric vein at the neck of the pancreas to form the portal vein.

The lymphatic drainage comprises efferent vessels in the white pulp that run with the arterioles and emerge from nodes at the hilum. These nodes and lymphatics drain via retropancreatic nodes to the coeliac nodes.

Sympathetic nerve fibres run from the coeliac plexus and innervate splenic arterial branches.

Physiology

The splenic parenchyma consists of white and red pulp that is surrounded by serosa and a collagenous capsule with smooth muscle fibres. These penetrate the parenchyma as trabeculae of dense connective tissue fibres rich in collagen and elastic tissue. These, with the reticular framework, support the cells of the spleen and surround the vessels in the splenic pulp. The white pulp comprises a central trabecular artery surrounded by nodules with germinal centres and periarterial lymphatic sheaths that provide a framework filled with lymphocytes and macrophages. Arteries from the central artery and the peripheral 'penicillar' arteries pass into the marginal zone that lies at the edge of the white pulp. Plasma-rich blood that has passed through the central lymphatic nodules is filtered as it passes through the sinuses within the marginal zone, and particles are phagocytosed. Immunoglobulins produced in the lymphatic nodules enter the circulation through the sinuses in the marginal zone, beyond which lies the red pulp, which consists of cords and sinuses. Cell-concentrated blood passes in the trabecular artery through the centre of the white pulp to the red pulp cords. Red cells must elongate and become thinner to pass from the cords to the sinuses, a process that removes abnormally shaped cells from the circulation (Fig. 62.1). As 90% of the blood passing through the spleen moves through an open circulation in which blood flows from arteries to cords, and thence sinuses, splenic pulp pressure reflects the pressure throughout the portal system. The remaining 10% of the blood flow through the spleen bypasses the cords and sinuses by direct arteriovenous communications, and the overall flow rate is about 300 ml min^{-1}.

FUNCTIONS OF THE SPLEEN

Although the spleen was previously thought to be dispensable, increasing knowledge of its function has led to a conservative approach in the management of conditions involving the spleen.

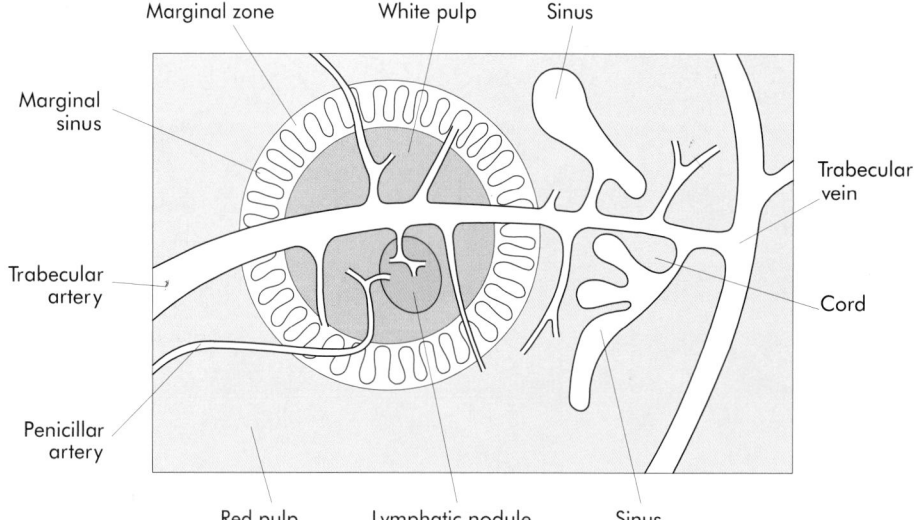

Marginal zone   White pulp   Sinus

Marginal
sinus

Trabecular
vein

Trabecular
artery

Cord

Penicillar
artery

Red pulp   Lymphatic nodule   Sinus

Figure 62.1 A central trabecular artery passing through the white pulp into the surrounding red pulp. A blood flow skimming effect results in most of the plasma passing down the branches of the artery while the cells pass in the central trabecular artery directly into the red pulp (courtesy of Professor T.G. Allen-Mersh, Westminster and Charing Cross Hospitals, London, UK).

It is now recognised that an incidental splenectomy during the course of another operative procedure increases the risk of complication and death. The surgeon should normally endeavour to preserve the spleen to maintain the following functions:

- *Immune function.* The spleen processes foreign antigens and is the major site of specific immunoglobulin M (IgM) production. The non-specific opsonins, properdin and tuftsin, are synthesised. These antibodies are of B- and T-cell origin and bind to the specific receptors on the surface of macrophages and leucocytes, stimulating their phagocytic, bactericidal and tumoricidal activity.
- *Filter function.* Macrophages in the reticulum capture cellular and non-cellular material from the blood and plasma. This will include the removal of effete platelets and red blood cells. This process takes place in the sinuses and the splenic cords by the action of the endothelial macrophages. Iron is removed from the degraded haemoglobin during red cell breakdown and is returned to the plasma. Removed non-cellular material may include bacteria and, in particular, pneumococci.
- *Pitting.* Particulate inclusions from red cells are removed, and the repaired red cells are returned to the circulation. These include Howell–Jolly and Heinz bodies, which represent nuclear remnants and precipitated haemoglobin or globin subunits respectively.
- *Reservoir function.* This function is less marked than in other species, but the spleen does contain approximately 8% of the red cell mass. An enlarged spleen may contain a much larger proportion of the blood volume.

William Henry Howell, **1860–1945, Professor of Physiology, Johns Hopkins University, Baltimore, MD, USA.**
Justin Marie Jules Jolly, **1870–1953, Professor of Histopathology, College de France, Paris, France.**
Robert Heinz, **1865–1924, Professor of Pharmacology and Toxicology, Erlangen, Germany.**

- *Cytopoiesis.* From the fourth month of intrauterine life, some degree of haemopoiesis occurs in the fetal spleen. Stimulation of the white pulp may occur following antigenic challenge, resulting in the proliferation of T and B cells and macrophages. This may also occur in myeloproliferative disorders, thalassaemias and chronic haemolytic anaemias (Summary box 62.1).

> **Summary box 62.1**
>
> **Functions of the spleen**
>
> ■ **Immune**
> ■ **Filter function**
> ■ **Pitting**
> ■ **Reservoir**
> ■ **Cytopoiesis**
> ■ **Splenectomy harms the patient**

INVESTIGATION OF THE SPLEEN

Conditions that result in splenomegaly can be diagnosed on the basis of the history and examination findings and from laboratory examination. In haemolytic anaemia, a full blood count, reticulocyte count and tests for haemolysis will determine the cause of the anaemia. Splenomegaly associated with portal hypertension caused by cirrhosis is diagnosed on the history, physical signs of liver dysfunction, abnormal tests of liver function and endoscopic evidence of oesophageal varices. Sinistral or segmental portal hypertension may result from isolated occlusion of the splenic vein by pancreatic inflammation or tumour. As many conditions that cause splenomegaly are associated with lymphadenopathy, investigation should be directed at those disease processes known to be associated with both physical signs. Lymph node biopsy may be required.

Radiological imaging

Plain radiology is rarely used in investigation, but the incidental finding of calcification of the splenic artery or spleen may raise the possible diagnosis of a splenic artery aneurysm, an old infarct, a benign cyst or hydatid disease. Multiple areas of calcification may suggest splenic tuberculosis. Ultrasonography can determine the size and consistency of the spleen, and whether a cyst is present. However, a computerised tomography (CT) scan with contrast enhancement is more commonly undertaken to better characterise the nature of the suspected splenic pathology and to exclude other intra-abdominal pathology. Magnetic resonance image (MRI) scanning may be similarly useful. Radioisotope scanning is used occasionally to provide information about the spleen. The use of technetium-99m (^{99m}Tc)-labelled colloid is normally restricted to determining whether the spleen is a significant site of destruction of red blood cells.

CONGENITAL ABNORMALITIES OF THE SPLEEN

Splenic agenesis is rare but is present in 10% of children with congenital heart disease. Polysplenia is a rare condition resulting from failure of splenic fusion.

Splenunculi are single or multiple accessory spleens that are found in approximately 10–30% of the population. They are located near the hilum of the spleen in 50% of cases and are related to the splenic vessels or behind the tail of the pancreas in 30%. The remainder are located in the mesocolon or the splenic ligaments. Their significance lies in the fact that failure to identify and remove these at the time of splenectomy may give rise to persistent disease.

Hamartomas are rarely found in life and vary in size from 1 cm in diameter to masses large enough to produce an abdominal swelling. One form is mainly lymphoid and resembles the white pulp, whereas the other resembles the red pulp.

Non-parasitic *splenic cysts* are rare. True cysts form from embryonal rests and include dermoid and mesenchymal inclusion cysts (Fig. 62.2). These are lined by flattened epithelium and should be differentiated from false cysts that may result from trauma and contain serous or haemorrhagic fluid. The walls of such degenerative cysts may be calcified and therefore resemble the radiological appearances of a hydatid cyst. The spleen is also a common site for pseudocyst development following a severe attack of pancreatitis (Fig. 62.3). Pseudocysts can easily be diagnosed on scanning, and intervention is normally required for symptomatic lesions that persist following a period of observation.

SPLENIC ARTERY ANEURYSM, INFARCT AND RUPTURE

Splenic artery aneurysm

Aneurysms involving the splenic artery are estimated to occur at 0.04–1% of post-mortem examinations. They are twice as common in the female and are usually situated in the main arterial trunk. Although these are generally single, more than one aneurysm is found in a quarter of cases. These may be a consequence of intra-abdominal sepsis and pancreatic necrosis in particular. They are more likely to be associated with arteriosclerosis in elderly patients.

The aneurysm is symptomless unless it ruptures and is more likely to be detected on a plain abdominal radiograph or scan. It is unlikely to be palpable, although a bruit may be present. Rupture is unsuspected in the majority of cases and, as it will generally rupture into the peritoneal cavity, the symptoms mimic those of splenic rupture. Almost half the cases of rupture occur in patients younger than 45 years of age, and a quarter are in pregnant women, usually in the third trimester of pregnancy or at labour.

The treatment of choice previously consisted of splenectomy and removal of the diseased artery. Some surgeons advocate ligation of the proximal and distal ends of the sac to allow thrombosis of the aneurysm and partial or complete splenectomy if necessary. The procedure has been performed laparoscopically. Embolisation or endovascular stenting following selective splenic artery angiography can be considered. In the younger patient with an asymptomatic splenic artery aneurysm, surgery or interventional radiology is indicated depending on local expertise after CT scan, MRI or selective coeliac angiography has confirmed the diagnosis (Fig. 62.4). In the elderly patient with a calcified

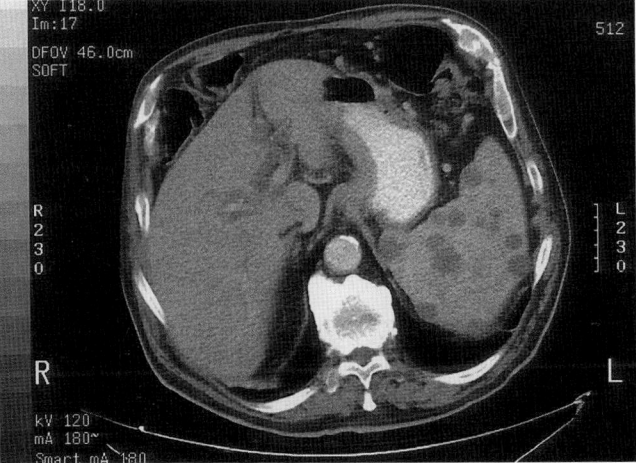

Figure 62.2 Computerised tomographic scan showing multiple low-density areas in the spleen consistent with multiple benign splenic cysts.

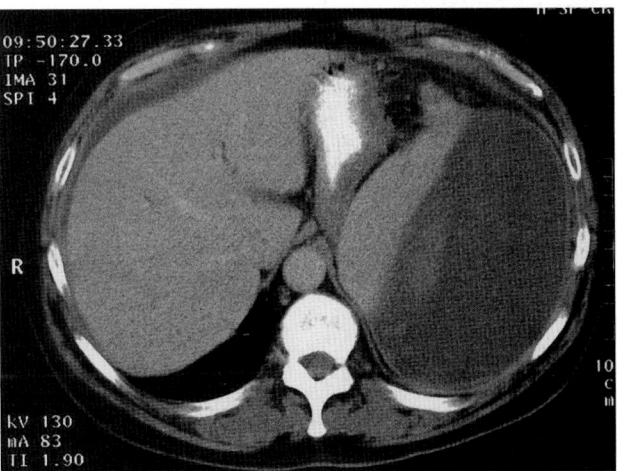

Figure 62.3 Computerised tomographic scan showing a large pseudocyst involving the spleen. There is displacement of the stomach medially, and a trace of ascitic fluid is present above the liver.

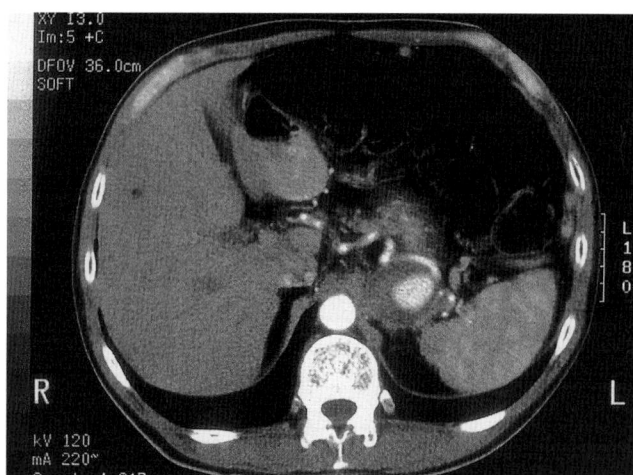

Figure 62.4 Computerised tomographic scan showing a pool of contrast in a pseudoaneurysm situated in the tail of the pancreas adjacent to the spleen.

aneurysm, there is less risk of rupture, and observation may be preferred. In patients with pancreatic necrosis, the treatment will include drainage of the septic focus.

Splenic infarction

This condition commonly occurs in patients with a massively enlarged spleen from myeloproliferative syndrome, portal hypertension or vascular occlusion produced by pancreatic disease, splenic vein thrombosis or sickle cell disease. The infarct may be asymptomatic or give rise to left upper quadrant and left shoulder tip pain. A contrast-enhanced CT scan will show the characteristic perfusion defect in the enlarged spleen (Fig. 62.5). Treatment is conservative, and splenectomy should be considered only when a septic infarct causes an abscess.

Splenic rupture

Splenic rupture (see Chapter 26) should be considered in any case of blunt abdominal trauma, particularly when the injury

occurs to the left upper quadrant of the abdomen. Iatrogenic injury to the spleen remains a frequent complication of any surgical procedure, particularly those in the left upper quadrant when adhesions are present.

Rupture of a malarial spleen

In tropical countries, this is not uncommon, and the delayed type of presentation following 'trivial' injury is not infrequent. In such patients, splenectomy should be considered before a perisplenic haematoma ruptures, a complication that is associated with a worse prognosis.

Surgery in such patients is challenging, and early ligation of the splenic vessels along the superior border of the pancreatic body should be considered before disturbing the haematoma.

SPLENOMEGALY AND HYPERSPLENISM

Splenomegaly is a common feature of many disease processes (Table 62.1). It should be borne in mind, however, that many conditions affecting the spleen, such as idiopathic thrombocytopenic purpura, may be associated with enlargement, but the gland is seldom palpable. Few of the conditions causing splenomegaly will require splenectomy as part of their treatment.

Hypersplenism is an indefinite clinical syndrome that is characterised by splenic enlargement, any combination of anaemia, leucopenia or thrombocytopenia, compensatory bone marrow hyperplasia and improvement after splenectomy. Careful clinical judgement is required to balance the long- and short-term risks of splenectomy against continued conservative management.

Splenic abscess

Splenic abscess may arise from an infected splenic embolus or in association with typhoid and paratyphoid fever, osteomyelitis, otitis media and puerperal sepsis. In general surgical practice, it may be associated with pancreatic necrosis or other intra-abdominal infection (Fig. 62.6). An abscess may rupture and form a left subphrenic abscess or result in peritonitis. The treatment involves that of the underlying cause and drainage of the splenic abscess by percutaneous means under radiological guidance.

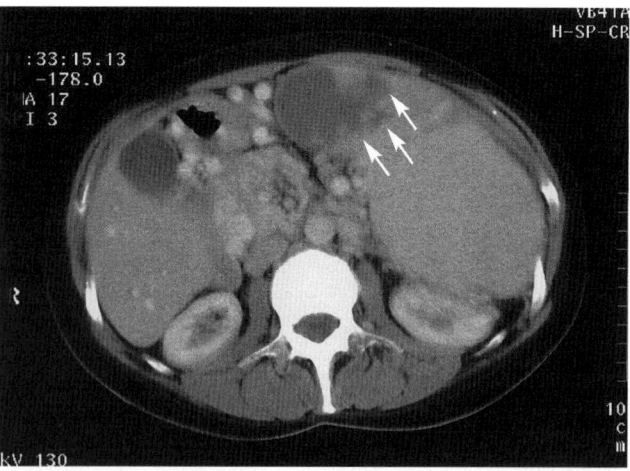

Figure 62.5 Computerised tomographic scan showing a splenic infarct (arrows) in a patient with splenomegaly and hypersplenism secondary to portal hypertension and portal vein thrombosis. The varices are evident at the hilus and at the greater curvature of the stomach.

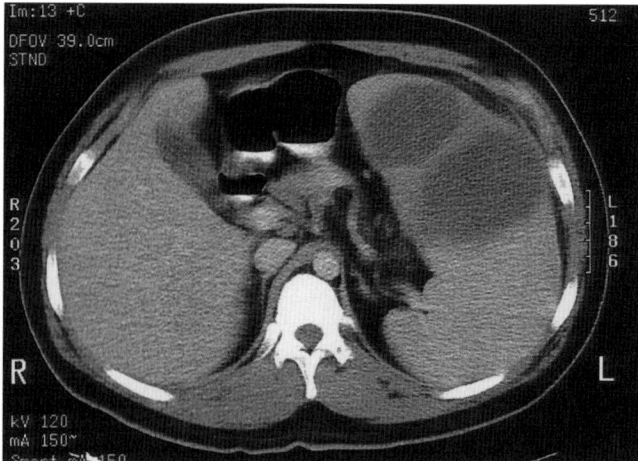

Figure 62.6 Computerised tomographic scan showing a multiloculated abscess in the enlarged spleen. This was managed successfully by percutaneous drainage under ultrasound guidance.

Table 62.1 Causes of splenic enlargement

Infective	Bacterial	Typhoid and paratyphoid
		Typhus
		Tuberculosis[a]
		Septicaemia
		Splenic abscess[b]
	Spirochaetal	Weil's disease
		Syphilis
	Viral	Infectious mononucleosis
		HIV-related thrombocytopenia[b]
		Psittacosis
	Protozoal and parasitic	Malaria
		Schistosomiasis[a]
		Trypanosomiasis
		Kala-azar
		Hydatid cyst[c]
		Tropical splenomegaly[a]
Blood disease	Acute leukaemia	Idiopathic thrombocytopenic purpura[c]
	Chronic leukaemia	Hereditary spherocytosis[a]
	Pernicious anaemia	Autoimmune haemolytic anaemia[a]
	Polycythaemia vera	Thalassaemia[a]
	Erythroblastosis fetalis	Sickle cell disease[a]
Metabolic	Rickets	
	Amyloid	
	Porphyria	
	Gaucher's disease[b]	
Circulatory	Infarct	
	Portal hypertension	
	Segmental portal hypertension[b]	(Pancreatic carcinoma, splenic vein thrombosis)
Collagen disease	Still's disease	
	Felty's syndrome[a]	
Non-parasitic cysts	Congenital	
	Acquired	
Neoplastic	Angioma	
	Primary fibrosarcoma	
	Hodgkin's lymphoma[b]	
	Other lymphomas	
	Myelofibrosis[b]	

HIV, human immunodeficiency virus.
[a] Often benefited by splenectomy.
[b] Splenectomy may be indicated.
[c] Benefited by splenectomy.

Tuberculosis

The diagnosis of tuberculosis should be considered in young adults with splenomegaly presenting with asthenia, loss of weight and fever. Tuberculosis of the spleen may produce portal hypertension or, rarely, cold abscess. Treatment with anti-tuberculous drugs will normally produce improvement. Splenectomy is not normally required and is made difficult by the inflammatory adhesions.

Tropical splenomegaly

Massive splenic enlargement frequently occurs in the tropics from malaria, kala-azar and schistosomiasis. Occasionally, splenomegaly cannot be fully attributed to these diseases. It may result from occult infection or be related to malnutrition. The massive splenomegaly observed in this condition may require removal for those patients disabled by anaemia or local symptoms. Lifelong antimalarial therapy is indicated in malaria-endemic areas.

Adolph Weil, **1848–1916**, Physician, Dorpat (now Tartu), Estonia, described leptospirosis icterohaemorrhagica in 1886.
Sir George Frederic Still, **1868–1941**, Professor of Diseases of Children, King's College Hospital, London, UK, described chronic articular rheumatism in children in 1896.

Schistosomiasis

This condition is prevalent in Africa, Asia and South America. It is caused by infection with *Schistosoma mansoni* in 75% of cases and by *Schistosoma haematobium* in the remainder. The splenic enlargement may result from portal hypertension associated with hepatic fibrosis, but can result from hyperplasia induced by the phagocytosis of disintegrated worms, ova and toxin. The splenomegaly can occur at any age. The diagnosis is based on examination of the urine and faeces for ova, abnormal liver function tests and the presence of hypochromic anaemia.

Successful medical treatment of established cases does not result in regression of splenomegaly, and removal of the painful and bulky spleen is indicated where there is no evidence of hepatic or renal insufficiency.

Leukaemia

This condition should be considered in the differential diagnosis of splenomegaly and is made by examining a blood or marrow film. Splenectomy is reserved for hypersplenism that occurs during the chronic phase of chronic granulocytic leukaemia.

Idiopathic thrombocytopenic purpura

In most cases of idiopathic thrombocytopenic purpura (ITP), the low platelet count results from the development of antibodies to specific platelet membrane glycoproteins that damage the patient's own platelets. It is also known as immune and auto-immune thrombocytopenic purpura. It is defined as isolated thrombocytopenia with normal bone marrow and the absence of other causes of thrombocytopenia. Two distinct clinical types are evident: the acute condition in the child and a chronic condition in the adult. Acute ITP often follows an acute infection and has a spontaneous resolution within 2 months. Chronic ITP persists longer than 6 months without a specific cause being identified. Approximately 50–75 cases per million arise each year in adults compared with 50 cases per million each year in children.

Clinical features

The adult form normally affects females between the ages of 15 and 50 years, although it can be associated with other conditions, including systemic lupus erythematosus, chronic lymphatic leukaemia and Hodgkin's disease. The childhood form is distributed equally between males and females and commonly presents before the age of 5 years. Purpuric patches (ecchymoses) occur on the skin and mucous membranes. Following trauma or pressure, examination often reveals numbers of petechial haemorrhages in the skin. There is a tendency to spontaneous bleeding from mucous membranes (e.g. epistaxis); in women, menorrhagia and the prolonged bleeding of minor wounds are common. Haemorrhage from the urinary and gastrointestinal tracts and haemarthrosis are rare. Although intracranial haemorrhage is also uncommon, it is the most frequent cause of death. The diagnosis is made based upon the presence of cutaneous ecchymoses and a positive tourniquet test. The spleen is palpable in fewer than 10% of patients, and the presence of gross splenic enlargement should raise the suspicion of an alternative diagnosis.

Sir Patrick Manson, 1844–1922, practised in Formosa (now Taiwan) and Hong Kong before becoming Physician to the Dreadnought Hospital, Greenwich, London, UK. He is regarded as 'The Father of Tropical Medicine'.
Thomas Hodgkin, 1798–1866, Lecturer in Morbid Anatomy and Curator of the Museum, Guy's Hospital, London, UK, described lymphadenoma in 1832.

Investigations

Coagulation studies are normal, and a bleeding time is not helpful in diagnosis. Platelet count in the peripheral blood film is reduced (usually $< 60 \times 10^9 \, l^{-1}$). Bone marrow aspiration reveals a plentiful supply of platelet-producing megakaryocytes.

Treatment

The course of the disease differs in children and adults. The disease regresses spontaneously in 75% of paediatric cases following the initial attack. Short courses of corticosteroids in both adult and child are usually followed by recovery. Prolonged steroid therapy should not be continued if this does not produce remission. Splenectomy is usually recommended if a patient has two relapses on steroid therapy or if the platelet count remains low. Generally, this is indicated where the ITP has persisted for more than 6–9 months.

Up to two-thirds of patients will be cured by surgical intervention, and 15% will be improved, but no benefit will be derived in the remainder. The response to steroids predicts a good response to splenectomy. In the acute setting, if severe bleeding has not been controlled by steroid therapy, fresh blood transfusion or transfusion with platelet concentrates before operation is necessary, although these are generally withheld until the splenic vessels have been controlled at operation.

Haemolytic anaemias

There are four causes of haemolytic anaemia that are generally amenable to splenectomy.

Hereditary spherocytosis

This autosomal dominant hereditary disorder is characterised by the presence of spherocytic red cells. Four abnormalities in red cell membrane proteins have been identified, but spectrin deficiency is the most common. Spherocytosis arises essentially from an increase in permeability of the red cell membranes to sodium. As this ion leaks into the cell, the osmotic pressure rises, resulting in swelling and increased fragility of the spherocyte. As the sodium pump has to work harder to rid the cells of sodium, there is greater loss of membrane phospholipid, resulting in an increased fragility of the membrane, and the energy and oxygen requirements increase. A large number of red cells are destroyed in the spleen, where there is a relative deficiency of both glucose and oxygen.

The clinical presentation is generally in childhood but may be delayed until later life. Mild intermittent jaundice is associated with mild anaemia, splenomegaly and gallstones. The circulating bilirubin is not conjugated with glucuronic acid, and is not therefore excreted in the urine as it is bound to albumin. Excretion of the resulting bilirubin complex by the liver favours the formation of pigment gallstones. Once the disease manifests itself, spontaneous remissions are uncommon; the patient is often pale and jaundiced at presentation and, in established cases, lassitude and undue fatigue are present.

In some families, the disease is characterised by a severe crisis of red blood cell destruction, during which the erythrocyte count may fall from 4.5×10^6 to $1.5 \times 10^6 \, ml^{-1}$ within a week. Such crises are characterised by the onset of pyrexia, abdominal pain, nausea, vomiting and extreme pallor followed by increased jaundice. These episodes may be precipitated by acute infection. Any child with gallstone disease should be investigated for hereditary spherocytosis and a family history sought.

Examination reveals splenomegaly, and the liver may also be palpable. Chronic leg ulcers may arise in adults with the disease.

Haematological investigations include the fragility test. Erythrocytes begin to haemolyse in 0.47% saline solution but, in this condition, haemolysis may occur in 0.6% or even stronger solutions. Immature red blood cells (reticulocytes), which differ from adult cells by possessing a reticulum, are discharged into the circulation by the bone marrow to compensate for the loss of erythrocytes by haemolysis.

Faecal urobilinogen is increased as this route excretes most of the urinobilinogen.

Radioactive chromium (^{51}Cr) labelling of the patient's own red cells will demonstrate the severity of red cell destruction. Daily scanning over the spleen will show the degree of red cell sequestration by the spleen. The presence of high levels of splenic radioactivity generally predicts a good response to splenectomy, but this test is used less commonly.

All patients with hereditary spherocytosis should be treated by splenectomy but, in juvenile cases, this is generally delayed until 6 years of age to minimise the risk of post-splenectomy infection, but before gallstones have had time to form. Ultrasonography should be performed preoperatively to determine the presence or absence of gallstones.

Acquired autoimmune haemolytic anaemia

This condition may arise following exposure to agents such as chemicals, infection or drugs, e.g. alpha-methyldopa, or be associated with another disease (e.g. systemic lupus erythematosus). In most instances, the cause is unknown, and red cell survival is reduced because of an immune reaction triggered by immunoglobulin or complement on the red cell surface. This condition is more common in women after the age of 50 years. In half the patients, the spleen is enlarged and, in 20% of cases, pigment gallstones are present.

Anaemia is invariably present and may be associated with spherocytosis because of red cell membrane damage. Antibody, which coats the red cells, can be detected by agglutination when anti-human globulin is added to a suspension of the patient's erythrocytes (Coombs test positive). The disease runs an acute self-limiting course, and no treatment is necessary. Splenectomy should, however, be considered if corticosteroids are ineffective, when the patient is developing complications from long-term steroid treatment or if corticosteroids are contraindicated. Eighty per cent of patients respond to splenectomy.

Thalassaemia (synonyms: Cooley's anaemia, Mediterranean anaemia)

This condition results from a defect in haemoglobin peptide chain synthesis and is transmitted as a dominant trait. The disease is really a group of related diseases, alpha, beta and gamma, depending upon which haemoglobin peptide chain's rate of synthesis is reduced. Most patients suffer from beta-thalassaemia, in which a reduction in the rate of beta-chain synthesis results in a decrease in haemoglobin A. Intracellular precipitates (Heinz bodies) contribute to premature red cell destruction.

Graduations of the disease range from heterozygous thalassaemia minor to homozygous thalassaemia major, which is associated with chronic anaemia, jaundice and splenomegaly. Patients with homozygous thalassaemia major frequently develop clinical signs in the first year of life, and these include retarded growth, enlarged head with slanting eyes and depressed nose, leg ulcers, jaundice and abdominal distension secondary to splenomegaly.

Red cells are small, thin and misshapen and have a characteristic resistance to osmotic lysis. In the more severe forms, nucleated red cells and other immature blood cells are seen. The final diagnosis is by haemoglobin electrophoresis.

Blood transfusion may be required to correct profound anaemia, but the patient may become transfusion dependent because of the development of hypersplenism. Splenectomy is therefore of benefit in patients who require frequent blood transfusion and if haemolytic antibodies have developed as a result.

Sickle cell disease

Sickle cell disease is a hereditary haemolytic anaemia occurring mainly among those of African origin in whom the normal haemoglobin A is replaced by haemoglobin S (HbS). The HbS molecule crystallises when the blood oxygen tension is reduced, thus distorting and elongating the red cell. The resulting increased blood viscosity may obstruct the flow of blood in the spleen. Splenic microinfarcts are therefore common.

The sickle cell trait can be detected in 9% of those of African origin, but most are asymptomatic; sickle cell disease occurs in about 1% of Africans. Depending upon the vessels affected by vascular occlusion, patients may complain of bone or joint pain, priapism, neurological abnormalities, skin ulcers or abdominal pain due to visceral blood stasis. The diagnosis is made by the finding of characteristic sickle-shaped cells on blood film, although this investigation has largely been replaced by haemoglobin electrophoresis.

Hypoxia that provokes a sickling crisis should be avoided and is particularly relevant in patients undergoing general anaesthesia. Adequate hydration and partial exchange transfusion may help in a crisis. Splenectomy is of benefit in a few patients in whom excessive splenic sequestration of red cells aggravates the anaemia. Chronic hypersplenism usually occurs in late childhood or adolescence, although *Streptococcus pneumoniae* infection may precipitate an acute form in the first 5 years of life.

Porphyria

Porphyria is a hereditary error of haemoglobin catabolism in which porphyrinuria occurs. Abdominal crises characterised by severe intestinal colic and constipation can be precipitated by the administration of barbiturates. The patient is anaemic and may suffer from photosensitivity; in advanced forms of the disease, neurological and mental symptoms are present. The splenomegaly associated with this condition may be overlooked. The urine may be orange and develops a port-wine colour after a few hours of exposure to the air. Splenectomy has little role to play in the management of this condition.

Gaucher's disease

This lipid storage disease is characterised by storage of glucocerebroside in the reticuloendothelial system and in the spleen.

Robin Royston Amos Coombs, **1921–2006, Quick Professor of Immunology, University of Cambridge, Cambridge, UK, described this test in 1945.**
Thomas Benton Cooley, **1871–1945, Professor of Pediatrics, Wayne University, Detroit, MI, USA, described this type of anaemia in 1927.**

Philippe Charles Ernest Gaucher, **1854–1918, Physician, Hôpital St Louis, Paris, France, described familial splenic anaemia in 1882.**

Enormous splenic enlargement may be associated with yellowish-brown discolouration of the skin on the hands and face, anaemia and conjunctival thickening (pinguecula). Slavonic and Jewish races are more prone to the disease, and the detection of Gaucher cells in the bone marrow confirms the diagnosis. Splenectomy is indicated only for severe symptoms related to the splenomegaly.

Hypersplenism due to portal hypertension

Splenomegaly is an invariable feature of portal hypertension (Fig. 62.7) and results in the thrombocytopenia and granulocytopenia observed in these patients. These may be improved if the portal hypertension is relieved by shunt surgery or liver transplantation. Splenectomy would normally be required only in those patients whose segmental portal hypertension has resulted in symptomatic oesophagogastric varices.

Felty's syndrome

Patients with rheumatoid arthritis may develop leucopenia. This is referred to as Felty's syndrome if it is extreme and associated with splenomegaly. There is no definite relationship between the severity of the arthritic changes and the leucopenia and splenomegaly. Splenectomy produces only a transient improvement in the blood picture, but rheumatoid arthritis may respond to steroid therapy to which it had previously become resistant.

NEOPLASMS

Haemangioma is the most common benign tumour of the spleen and may rarely develop into a haemangiosarcoma that is managed by splenectomy. The spleen is rarely the site of metastatic disease. Lymphoma is the most common cause of neoplastic enlargement, and splenectomy may play a part in its management. Splenectomy may be required to achieve a diagnosis in the absence of palpable lymph nodes or to relieve the symptoms of gross splenomegaly. However, the need for staging laparoscopy

has largely receded with the advent of CT scanning. Its use has been restricted to those patients in whom a definite histological diagnosis of intra-abdominal disease will affect management. Thus, selected patients with stage IA or IIA Hodgkin's disease may be candidates for staging laparotomy or laparoscopy. In the absence of obvious liver or intra-abdominal nodal disease, splenectomy is an integral part of the staging procedure to exclude splenic involvement, which would alter the method of treatment.

Myelofibrosis results from an abnormal proliferation of mesenchymal elements in the bone marrow, spleen, liver and lymph nodes. Most patients present over the age of 50 years, and the spleen may produce pain owing to its gross enlargement (Fig. 62.8) or from splenic infarcts. Splenectomy reduces the need for transfusion and may relieve the discomfort resulting from the splenomegaly.

SPLENECTOMY

The common indications for splenectomy are:

- trauma resulting from an accident or during a surgical procedure, as for example during mobilisation of the oesophagus, stomach, distal pancreas or splenic flexure of the colon;
- removal *en bloc* with the stomach as part of a radical gastrectomy or with the pancreas as part of a distal or total pancreatectomy;
- to reduce anaemia or thrombocytopenia in spherocytosis, idiopathic thrombocytopenic purpura or hypersplenism;
- in association with shunt or variceal surgery for portal hypertension (Summary box 62.2).

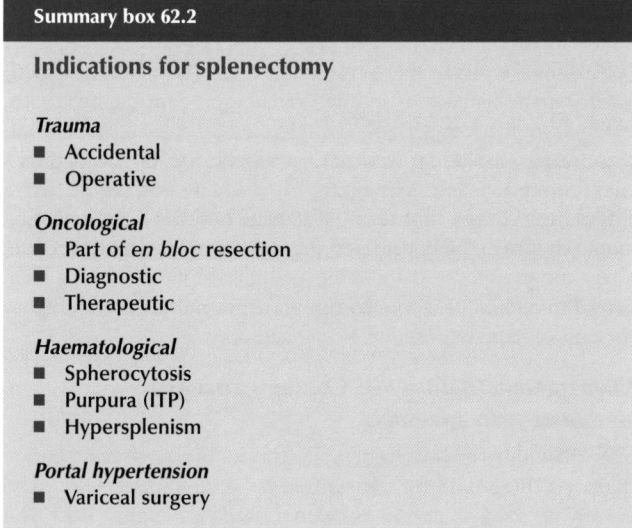

Summary box 62.2

Indications for splenectomy

Trauma
- Accidental
- Operative

Oncological
- Part of *en bloc* resection
- Diagnostic
- Therapeutic

Haematological
- Spherocytosis
- Purpura (ITP)
- Hypersplenism

Portal hypertension
- Variceal surgery

Preoperative preparation

In the presence of a bleeding tendency, transfusion of blood, fresh-frozen plasma, cryoprecipitate or platelets may be required. Coagulation profiles should be as near normal as possible at operation, and platelets should be available for patients with thrombocytopenia at operation and in the early postoperative period.

Antibiotic prophylaxis appropriate to the operative procedure should be given, and consideration should be given to the risk of post-splenectomy sepsis (see below).

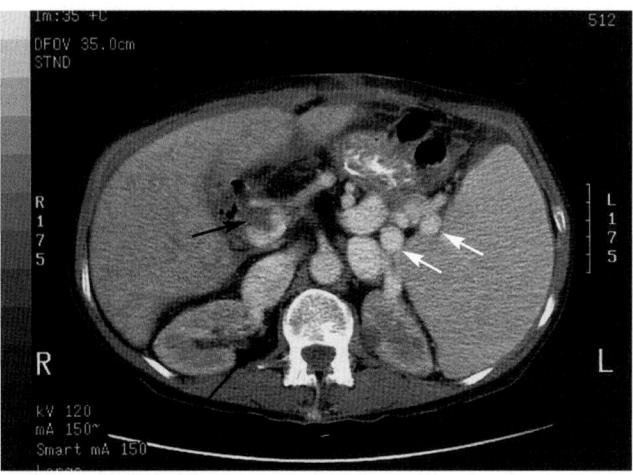

Figure 62.7 Computerised tomographic scan showing an enlarged spleen in a patient with portal hypertension secondary to portal vein thrombosis. Clot is evident within the lumen of the portal vein (black arrow), and large varices (white arrows) are present at the splenic hilus.

Augustus Roi Felty, **1895–1964**, Physician, Hartford Hospital, Hartford, CT, USA, described this disease in 1924.

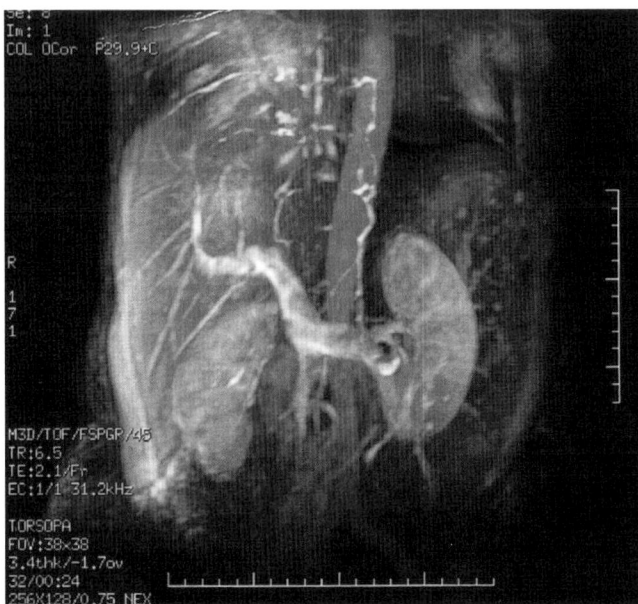

Figure 62.8 Magnetic resonance imaging (MRI) scan showing massive hepatosplenomegaly secondary to myelofibrosis. Note the prominent portal system and the left kidney, which is superimposed over the grossly enlarged spleen.

Technique of open splenectomy

Most surgeons use a midline or transverse left subcostal incision for open splenectomy. Rarely, a thoracoabdominal incision may be necessary for a massive spleen that is adherent to the diaphragm. Passage of a nasogastric tube following induction of the anaesthetic enables the stomach to be emptied.

In elective splenectomy, the gastrosplenic ligament is opened up, and the short gastric vessels are divided. The splenic vessels at the superior border of the pancreas are suture-ligated. The posterior surface of the spleen is exposed, the posterior leaf of the lienorenal ligament divided with long curved scissors, and the spleen rotated medially along with the tail and body of the pancreas (Fig. 62.9). The pancreas is separated from the hilar vessels, which are ligated and divided. Accessory splenic tissue in the splenic hilum or omentum should be excluded by a careful search at operation. There is no need to drain the wound if haemostasis is secured adequately.

Technique of laparoscopic splenectomy

The patient is placed on the right side with the space between the left ilium and costal margin exposed. Placement of access ports is often determined by the size of the patient and the spleen. Insufflation of the abdomen can be performed once access is obtained through an incision 1 cm from the costal margin at the left mid-clavicular line. A further trocar is inserted close to the costal margin below the xiphoid. A 12-mm trocar is inserted at a similar distance from the costal margin at the posterior axillary line. The splenocolic ligament is divided to give access to the lower splenic pole. The spleen is separated from the kidney and diaphragm before the gap between the splenic hilum and the tail of the pancreas is enlarged. The spleen is elevated to expose the splenic hilum, which is secured and divided with an endoscopic vascular stapler (Fig. 62.10). Two or three applications of the instrument may be required to secure the hilum and the short

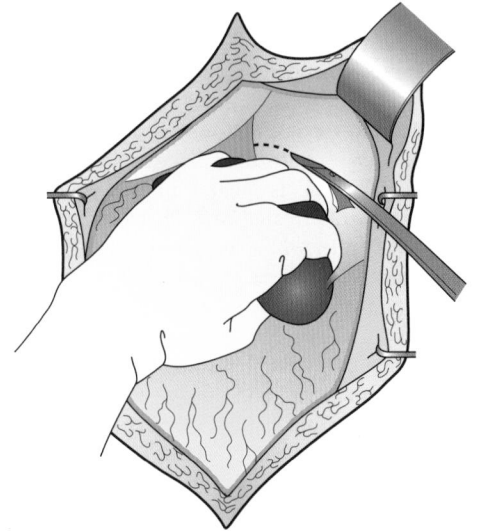

Figure 62.9 Diagrammatic view of the approach required to divide the short gastric vessels anteriorly and the lienorenal ligament posteriorly.

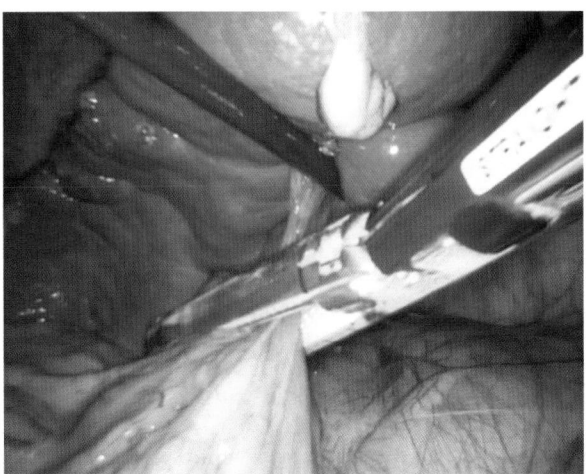

Figure 62.10 Photograph showing a stapling gun across the hilus of spleen for division of the splenic vessels during laparoscopic splenectomy.

gastric vessels. Any remaining attachments to the diaphragm are divided before a self-retaining opening bag is introduced through the incision of the open laparoscopy after removal of the 12-mm port. The spleen is placed in the bag, the mouth of which is pulled out of the abdominal opening before the spleen is crushed and retrieved with an instrument. The operation may be undertaken as a hand-assisted procedure.

Postoperative complications

Immediate complications specific to splenectomy include haemorrhage resulting from a slipped ligature. Haematemesis from gastric mucosal damage and gastric dilatation is uncommon. Left basal atelectasis is common, and a pleural effusion may be present. Adjacent structures at risk during the procedure include the stomach and pancreas. A fistula may result from damage to the greater curvature of the stomach during ligation of the short gastric vessels. Damage to the tail of the pancreas may result in

CHAPTER 62 | THE SPLEEN

pancreatitis, a localised abscess or a pancreatic fistula. The blood platelet count may rise and, if this exceeds $1 \times 10^6\,\mathrm{ml}^{-1}$, prophylactic aspirin is recommended to prevent axillary or other venous thrombosis.

Post-splenectomy septicaemia may result from *Streptococcus pneumoniae*, *Neisseria meningitides*, *Haemophilus influenzae* and *Escherichia coli*. The risk is greater in the young patient, in splenectomised patients treated with chemoradiotherapy and in patients who have undergone splenectomy for thalassaemia, sickle cell disease and autoimmune anaemia or thrombocytopenia.

Opportunist post-splenectomy infection (OPSI) is a major concern. Published guidelines emphasise that most infections after splenectomy could be avoided through measures that include offering patients appropriate and timely immunisation, antibiotic prophylaxis, education and prompt treatment of infection. The benefit of prophylactic antibiotics in this setting remains controversial. It is thought that children who have undergone splenectomy before the age of 5 years should be treated with a daily dose of penicillin until the age of 10 years. Prophylaxis in older children should be continued at least until the age of 16 years, but its use is less well defined in adults. Furthermore, compliance is problematic in the long term but, as the risk of overwhelming sepsis is greatest within the first 2–3 years after splenectomy, it seems reasonable to give prophylaxis during this time. However, all patients with compromised immune function should receive prophylaxis. Satisfactory oral prophylaxis can be obtained with penicillin, erythromycin or amoxicillin, or co-amoxiclav. Suspected infection can be treated intravenously with these same antibiotics and cefotaxime, ceftriaxone or chloramphenicol in patients allergic to penicillin and cephalosporins.

If elective splenectomy is planned, consideration should be given to vaccinating against pneumococcus, meningococcus (both repeated every 5 years) and *H. influenzae* (repeated every 10 years). Yearly influenza vaccination has been recommended as there is some evidence that it may reduce the risk of secondary bacterial infection. Such vaccinations should be administered at least 2 weeks before elective surgery and as soon as possible after recovery from surgery but before discharge from hospital in all other cases. Pneumococcal vaccination is recommended in those patients aged over 2 years. *Haemophilus influenzae* type b vaccination is recommended irrespective of age. Meningococcal vaccination is not recommended routinely unless the individual is considering travel to areas where there is a risk of group A infection, in local outbreaks and for contacts with infected cases.

Albert Ludwig Siegmund Neisser, **1855–1916, Director of the Dermatological Institute, Breslau, Germany (now Wroclaw, Poland).**
Theodor Escherich, **1857–1911, Professor of Paediatrics, Vienna, Austria.**

Meningococcal vaccination only offers protection of short duration, and group B and C infection is commoner. The improved immunogenic properties of the newer group C conjugate vaccine may confer greater protection to the patient. It is also recommended that influenza vaccine be given to asplenic patients as influenza has been implicated as a risk factor for secondary bacterial infection in both general and meningococcal disease.

In the trauma victim, vaccination can be given in the postoperative period, and the resulting antibody levels will be protective in the majority of cases. Antibody levels are, however, less than 50% of those achieved if vaccination is given in the presence of an intact spleen. Protection following vaccination is not always guaranteed (Summary box 62.3).

Summary box 62.3

Splenectomy

- Remember preoperative immunisation
- Prophylactic antibiotics in the long term
- OPSI is a real clinical danger

Patients who have undergone splenectomy and are travelling to countries where malaria is present are strongly advised to use all physical anti-mosquito barriers as well as antimalarial therapy.

FURTHER READING

Bisharat, N., Omari, H., Lavi, I. and Raz, R. (2001) Risk of infection and death among post-splenectomy patients. *J Infect* **43**: 182–6.

Davies, J.M., Barnes, R. and Milligan, D. (2002) Update of guidelines for the prevention and treatment of infection in patients with an absent or dysfunctional spleen. *Clin Med* **2**: 440–3.

Glasgow, R.E. and Mulvihill, S.J. (1999) Laparoscopic splenectomy. *World J Surg* **23**: 384–8.

Society for Surgery of the Alimentary Tract. Prophylaxis against post-splenectomy sepsis guidelines. Available online at: http://www.ssat.com/guidelines/spleen7.htm.

Guidelines for the prevention and treatment of infection in patients with an absent or dysfunctional spleen. Available online at: http://www.ssat.com/guidelines/spleen7.htm

http://www.scotland.gov.uk/health/cmobulletin/hb591-09.asp

Weatherall, D.J. (1997) The hereditary anaemias. *Br Med J* **314**: 492–6.

Working Party of the British Committee for Standards in Haematology – Clinical Haematology Task Force (1996) Guidelines for the prevention and treatment of infection in patients with an absent or dysfunctional spleen. *Br Med J* **312**: 430–4.

The gall bladder and bile ducts

LEARNING OBJECTIVES

To understand:
- The techniques used for imaging the biliary tree
- The management of gallstones
- Unusual disorders of the biliary tree
- Malignant disease of the biliary tree

SURGICAL ANATOMY AND PHYSIOLOGY

The gall bladder lies on the underside of the liver in the main liver scissura at the junction of the right and left lobes of the liver. The relationship of the gall bladder to the liver varies between being embedded within the liver substance to suspended by a mesentery. It is a pear-shaped structure, 7.5–12 cm long, with a normal capacity of about 35–50 ml. The anatomical divisions are a fundus, a body and a neck that terminates in a narrow infundibulum. The muscle fibres in the wall of the gall bladder are arranged in a crisscross manner, being particularly well developed in its neck. The mucous membrane contains indentations of the mucosa that sink into the muscle coat; these are the crypts of Luschka.

The *cystic duct* is about 3 cm in length but variable. Its lumen is usually 1–3 mm in diameter. The mucosa of the cystic duct is arranged in spiral folds known as the valves of Heister. Its wall is surrounded by a sphincteric structure called the sphincter of Lütkens. While the cystic duct joins the common hepatic duct in its supraduodenal segment in 80% of cases, it may extend down into the retroduodenal or even retropancreatic part of the bile duct before joining. Occasionally, the cystic duct may join the right hepatic duct or even a right hepatic sectorial duct.

The *common hepatic duct* is usually less than 2.5 cm long and is formed by the union of the right and left hepatic ducts. The *common bile duct* is about 7.5 cm long and is formed by the junction of the cystic and common hepatic ducts. It is divided into four parts:

- the *supraduodenal portion*, about 2.5 cm long, running in the free edge of the lesser omentum;
- the *retroduodenal portion*;
- the *infraduodenal portion*, which lies in a groove, but at times in a tunnel, on the posterior surface of the pancreas;
- the *intraduodenal portion*, which passes obliquely through the wall of the second part of the duodenum, where it is surrounded by the sphincter of Oddi, and terminates by opening on the summit of the ampulla of Vater.

Hubert von Luschka, **1820–1875, Professor of Anatomy, Tübingen, Germany.**
Ruggero Oddi, **1845–1906, Physiologist, Perugia, who later worked in Rome, Italy, described this sphincter in 1887.**
Abraham Vater, **1684–1751, Professor of Anatomy and Botany, (1719) and later of Pathology and Therapeutics, Wittenburg, Germany.**

The cystic artery, a branch of the right hepatic artery, is usually given off behind the common hepatic duct (Fig. 63.1). Occasionally, an accessory cystic artery arises from the gastroduodenal

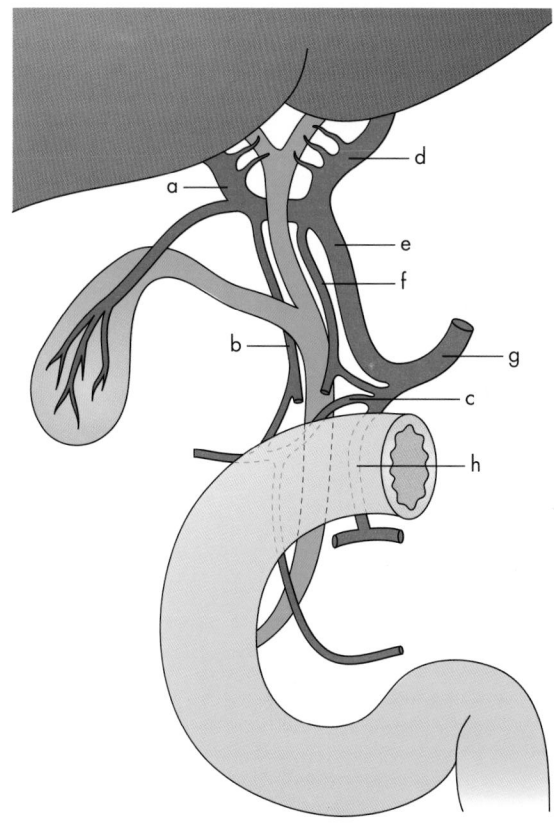

Figure 63.1 The anatomy of the gall bladder and bile ducts. Note the arrangement of the arterial tree: (a) right hepatic artery; (b) right choledochal artery; (c) retroduodenal artery; (d) left branch of hepatic artery; (e) hepatic artery; (f) left choledochal artery; (g) common hepatic artery; (h) gastroduodenal artery.

Berkeley George Andrew Moynihan, (Lord Moynihan of Leeds), **1865–1936, Professor of Clinical Surgery, the University of Leeds, Leeds, England.**

artery. In 15% of cases, the right hepatic artery and/or the cystic artery cross in front of the common hepatic duct and the cystic duct. The most dangerous anomalies are where the hepatic artery takes a tortuous course on the front of the origin of the cystic duct, or the right hepatic artery is tortuous and the cystic artery short. The tortuosity is known as the 'caterpillar turn' or 'Moynihan's hump' (Fig. 63.2). This variation is the cause of many problems during a difficult cholecystectomy with inflammation in the region of the cystic duct. Inadvertent damage to the right hepatic artery is most difficult to control laparoscopically.

Lymphatics

The lymphatic vessels of the gall bladder (subserosal and submucosal) drain into the cystic lymph node of Lund (the sentinel lymph node). This lies in the fork created by the junction of the cystic and common hepatic ducts. Efferent vessels from this lymph node go to the hilum of the liver and to the coeliac lymph nodes. The subserosal lymphatic vessels of the gall bladder also connect with the subcapsular lymph channels of the liver, and this accounts for the frequent spread of carcinoma of the gall bladder to the liver.

Surgical physiology

Bile, as it leaves the liver, is composed of 97% water, 1–2% bile salts and 1% pigments, cholesterol and fatty acids. The liver excretes bile at a rate estimated to be approximately 40 ml h^{-1}. The rate of bile secretion is controlled by cholecystokinin (CCK),

which is released from the duodenal mucosa. With feeding, there is increased production of bile.

FUNCTIONS OF THE GALL BLADDER

The gall bladder is a reservoir for bile. During fasting, resistance to flow through the sphincter is high, and bile excreted by the liver is diverted to the gall bladder. After feeding, the resistance to flow through the sphincter of Oddi is reduced, the gall bladder contracts, and the bile enters the duodenum. These motor responses of the biliary tract are in part effected by the hormone CCK.

The second main function of the gall bladder is concentration of bile by active absorption of water, sodium chloride and bicarbonate by the mucous membrane of the gall bladder. The hepatic bile that enters the gall bladder becomes concentrated 5–10 times, with a corresponding increase in the proportion of bile salts, bile pigments, cholesterol and calcium.

The third function of the gall bladder is the secretion of mucus – approximately 20 ml is produced per day. With total obstruction of the cystic duct in a healthy gall bladder, a mucocele develops on account of this function of the mucosa of the gall bladder.

RADIOLOGICAL INVESTIGATION OF THE BILIARY TRACT

Plain radiograph

A plain radiograph of the gall bladder will show radio-opaque gallstones in 10% of patients with gallstones (Fig. 63.3). Rarely, the centre of a stone may contain radiolucent gas in a triradiate or biradiate fissure, and this gives rise to characteristic dark shapes on a radiograph – the 'Mercedes-Benz' or 'seagull' sign.

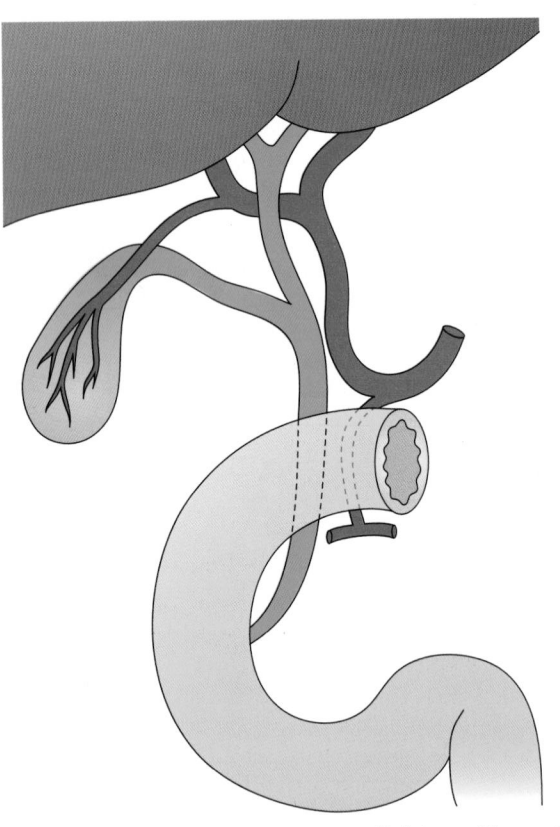

Figure 63.2 Tortuous hepatic artery (so called 'caterpillar turn' or 'Moynihan's hump'), a frequent cause of inadvertent arterial damage or bleeding during cholecystectomy.

Fred Bates Lund, **1865–1950, Surgeon, the Boston City Hospital, Boston, MA, USA.**

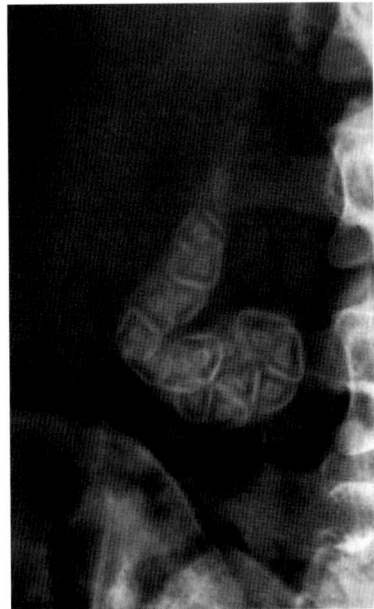

Figure 63.3 Plain radiograph showing radio-opaque stones in the gall bladder. Radio-opaque stones are uncommon (10%).

The Mercedes-Benz sign **takes its name from the insignia displayed on the bonnet of a Mercedes-Benz car.**
A Seagull **is a medium sized bird related to the Terns and Skuas, which is found world-wide and scavenges for its food.**

A plain X-ray may also show the rare cases of calcification of the gall bladder, a so called 'porcelain' gall bladder (Fig. 63.4). The importance of this appearance is an association with carcinoma in up to 25% of patients. It is therefore an indication for cholecystectomy. Gas may be seen in the wall of the gall bladder (emphysematous cholecystitis). Gas in the biliary tree may be seen after endoscopic sphincterotomy or surgical anastomosis (Summary box 63.1).

Summary box 63.1

Investigation of the biliary tree

- Ultrasound: stones and biliary dilatation
- Plain radiograph: calcification
- Magnetic resonance cholangiopancreatography: anatomy and stones
- Multidetector row computerised tomography scan: anatomy, liver, gall bladder and pancreas cancer
- Radioisotope scanning: function
- Endoscopic retrograde cholangiopancreatography: anatomy, stones and biliary strictures
- Percutaneous transhepatic cholangiography: anatomy and biliary strictures
- Endoscopic ultrasound: anatomy and stones

Oral cholecystography and intravenous cholangiography

Oral and intravenous cholecystography are of historical interest only as they are relatively inaccurate and have been discarded and replaced by more accurate imaging modalities.

Ultrasonography

Transabdominal ultrasonography (Figs 63.5–63.8) is the initial imaging modality of choice as it is accurate, readily available, inexpensive and quick to perform. However, it is operator dependent and may be suboptimal due to excessive body fat and intraluminal bowel gas. It can demonstrate biliary calculi, the size of the gall bladder, the thickness of the gall bladder wall, the presence of inflammation around the gall bladder, the size of the

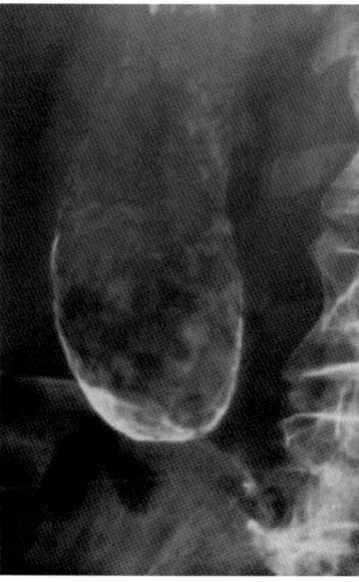

Figure 63.4 Porcelain gall bladder.

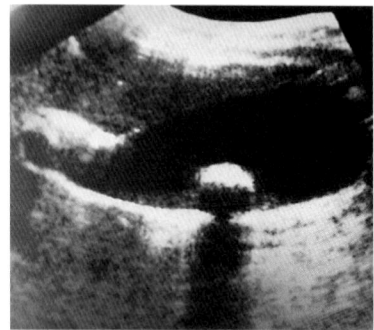

Figure 63.5 Ultrasound examination. Single large gallstone casting an 'acoustic shadow' (courtesy of James McIvor, FDS, FRCR, London, UK).

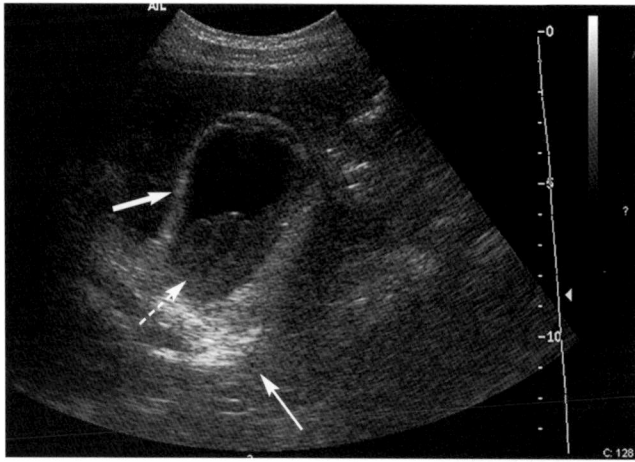

Figure 63.6 Cholecystitis. Ultrasound demonstrates pericholecystic fluid (thin arrow), gall bladder wall (thick arrow) and biliary sludge (broken arrow).

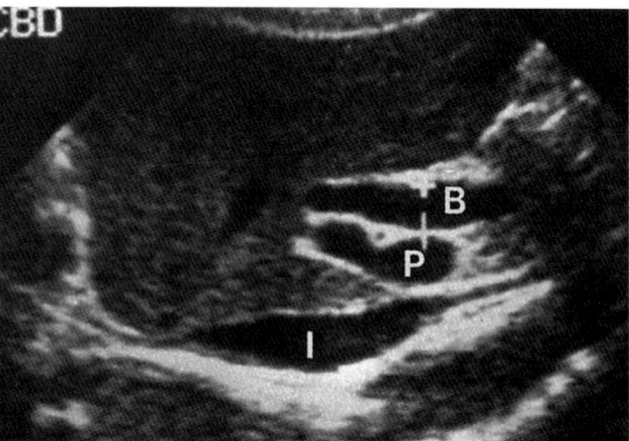

Figure 63.7 Ultrasound examination. Longitudinal scan through the hilum of the liver showing the dilated common bile duct (B). P, portal vein; I, inferior vena cava (courtesy of Dr J.E. Boultbee, Charing Cross Hospital, London, UK).

common bile duct and, occasionally, the presence of stones within the biliary tree. It may even show a carcinoma of the pancreas occluding the common bile duct.

In the patient who presents with obstructive jaundice, ultrasonography is particularly helpful as it can identify intra- and

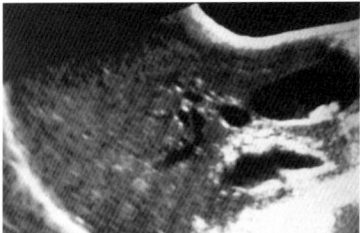

Figure 63.8 Ultrasound examination. Dilatation of the intrahepatic and common bile ducts due to a calculus impacted at the sphincter of Oddi. There are calculi visible in the gall bladder (courtesy of James McIvor, FDS, FRCR, London, UK).

extrahepatic biliary dilatation and the level of obstruction. In addition, the cause of the obstruction may also be identified, such as gallstones in the gall bladder, common hepatic or common bile duct stones or lesions in the wall of the duct suggestive of a cholangiocarcinoma or enlargement of the pancreatic head indicative of a pancreatic carcinoma.

Endoscopic ultrasonography (Figs 63.9 and 63.10) uses a specially designed endoscope with an ultrasound transducer at its tip, which allows visualisation of the liver and biliary tree from within the stomach and duodenum. It provides accurate imaging of the common bile duct and is particularly useful in detecting stones within the bile ducts, choledocholithiasis. In addition, it has been shown to be highly accurate in diagnosing and staging both pancreatic and periampullary cancers.

Radioisotope scanning

Technetium-99m (^{99m}Tc)-labelled derivatives of iminodiacetic acid (HIDA, IODIDA) are, when injected intravenously, selectively taken up by the retroendothelial cells of the liver and excreted into bile. This allows visualisation of the biliary tree and gall bladder. The gall bladder is visualised within 30 min of isotope injection in 90% of normal individuals and within 1 hour in the remainder (Fig. 63.11). The bowel is usually seen within 1 hour in the majority of patients. Non-visualisation of the gall bladder is suggestive of acute cholecystitis. If the patient has a

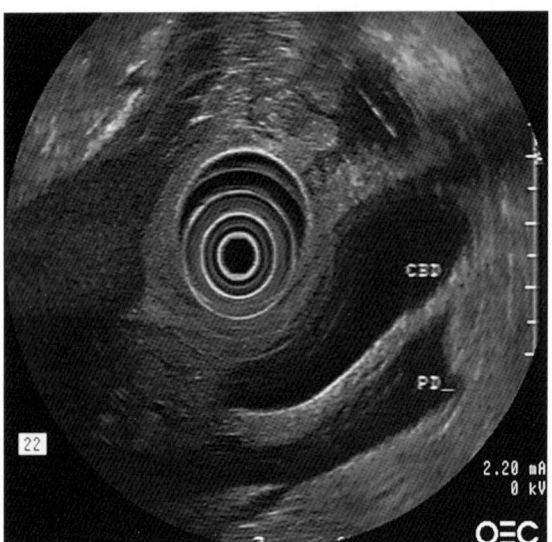

Figure 63.9 Endoscopic ultrasonography demonstrating the common bile duct and pancreatic duct.

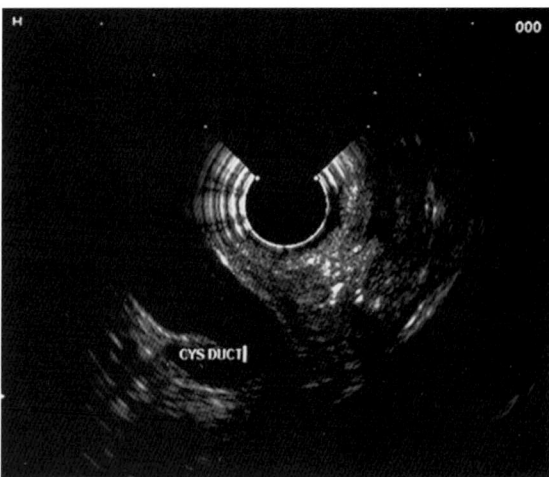

Figure 63.10 Endoscopic ultrasound showing the junction of the cystic duct with the common bile duct.

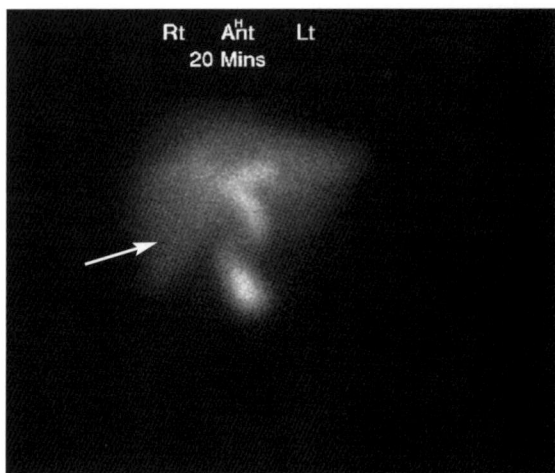

Figure 63.11 Dimethyl iminodiacetic acid (HIDA) scan demonstrating at 20 min non-visualisation of the gall bladder (arrow), suggestive of acute cholecystitis.

contracted gall bladder, as often occurs in chronic cholecystitis, gall bladder visualisation may be reduced or delayed.

Biliary scintigraphy may also be helpful in diagnosing bile leaks and iatrogenic biliary obstruction. When there is a suspicion of a bile leak following a cholecystectomy, radioisotope imaging should be performed. Scintigraphy can confirm the presence and quantify the leak, thus helping the surgeon to determine whether or not an operative or conservative approach is warranted.

Computerised tomography

This imaging modality allows visualisation of the liver, bile ducts, gall bladder and pancreas. It is particularly useful in detecting hepatic and pancreatic lesions and is the modality of choice in the staging of cancers of the liver, gall bladder, bile ducts and pancreas. It can identify the extent of the primary tumour and defines its relationship to other organs and blood vessels (Fig. 63.12). In addition, the presence of enlarged lymph nodes or metastatic disease can be seen.

For benign biliary diseases, standard computerised tomography (CT) is not that useful an investigation. Gallstones are

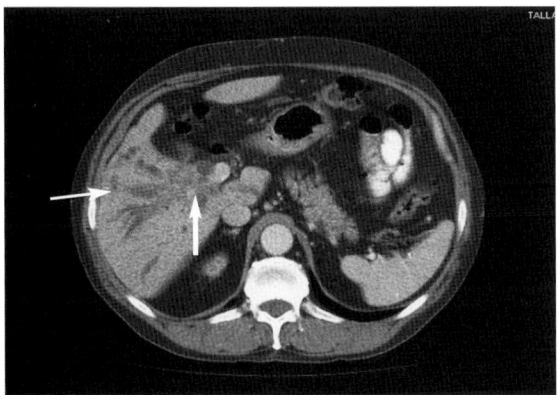

Figure 63.12 Computerised tomography scan demonstrating a hilar mass (thick arrow) and biliary dilation (thin arrow).

often not visualised, and cholecystitis is underdiagnosed. However, improvements in CT technology such as multidetector helical scanners that allow for three-dimensional reconstruction of the biliary tree have led to greater diagnostic accuracy and may increase the use of this modality in the future.

Magnetic resonance cholangiopancreatography

Magnetic resonance cholangiopancreatography (MRCP) is an imaging technique based on the principles of nuclear magnetic resonance used to image the gall bladder and biliary system. It is non-invasive and can provide either cross-sectional (Fig. 63.13) or projection (Fig. 63.14) images. Contrast is not required and, using appropriate techniques, excellent images can be obtained of the biliary tree that demonstrate ductal obstruction, strictures or other intraductal abnormalities. The images obtained are comparable to those from endoscopic retrograde cholangiopancreatography (ERCP) or percutaneous transhepatic cholangiography (PTC) without the potential complications of either technique.

Endoscopic retrograde cholangiopancreatography

This technique remains widely used. Using a side-viewing endoscope, the ampulla of Vater can be identified and cannulated. Injection of water-soluble contrast directly into the bile duct provides excellent images of the ductal anatomy (Fig. 63.15) and can identify causes of obstruction such as stones (Fig. 63.16) or

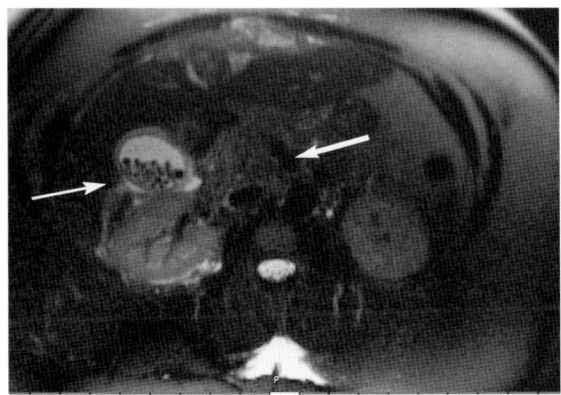

Figure 63.13 Cross-sectional magnetic resonance image demonstrating a hilar mass (thick arrow) (same as Fig. 63.12) and associated gallstones (thin arrow).

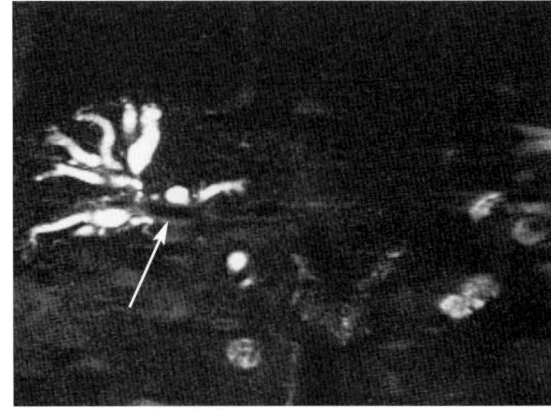

Figure 63.14 Magnetic resonance cholangiopancreatography demonstrating hilar obstruction as seen in Figures 63.12 and 63.13.

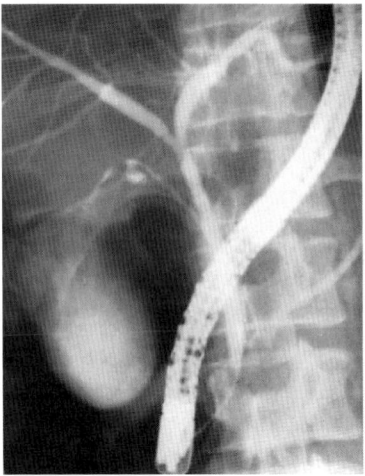

Figure 63.15 Endoscopic retrograde cholangiopancreatography: normal cholangiogram.

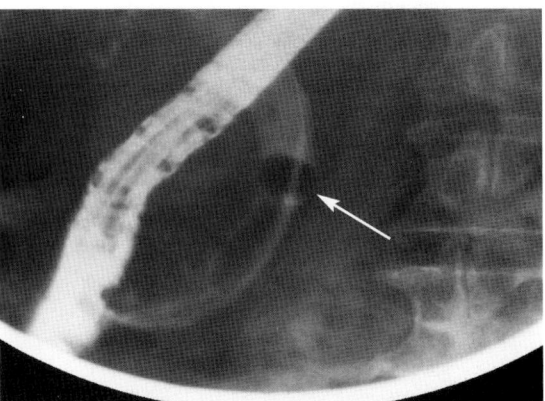

Figure 63.16 Endoscopic retrograde cholangiopancreatography demonstrating stone obstructing the common bile duct (arrow).

malignant strictures (Fig. 63.17). While the widespread availability of ultrasound and MRCP has limited the diagnostic use of ERCP, the technique has a role in the assessment of the jaundiced patient. In this group, it is especially useful in determining the cause and level of obstruction. Bile can be sent for cytological and

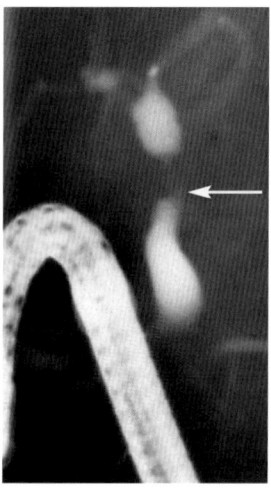

Figure 63.17 Endoscopic retrograde cholangiopancreatography: partial occlusion of the bile duct by a malignant stricture (arrow).

microbiological examination, and brushings can be taken from strictures for cytological studies. Therapeutic interventions such as stone removal or stent placement to relieve the obstruction can be performed. Thus, ERCP has evolved into a mainly therapeutic rather than a diagnostic technique.

Percutaneous transhepatic cholangiography

This is an invasive technique in which the bile ducts are cannulated directly. It is only undertaken once a bleeding tendency has been excluded and the patient's prothrombin time is normal. Antibiotics should be given prior to the procedure. Usually, under fluoroscopic control, a needle (the Chiba or Okuda needle) is introduced percutaneously into the liver substance. Under

radiological control (either ultrasound or CT), a bile duct is cannulated. Successful entry is confirmed by contrast injection or aspiration of bile. Water-soluble contrast medium is injected to demonstrate the biliary system. Multiple images can be taken demonstrating areas of strictures or obstruction (Fig. 63.18). Bile can be sent for cytology. In addition, PTC enables the placement of a catheter into the bile ducts to provide external biliary drainage or the insertion of indwelling stents. The scope of this procedure can be further extended by leaving the drainage catheter *in situ* for a number of days and then dilating the track sufficiently for a fine flexible choledochoscope to be passed into the intrahepatic biliary tree in order to diagnose strictures, take biopsies or remove stones.

In general, in the jaundiced patient, if a malignant stricture at the level of the confluence of the right and left hepatic ducts or higher is suspected, a PTC is preferred to an ERCP as successful drainage is more likely.

Peroperative cholangiography

During open or laparoscopic cholecystectomy, a catheter can be placed in the cystic duct and contrast injected directly into the biliary tree. The technique defines the anatomy and is mainly used to exclude the presence of stones within the bile ducts (Figs 63.19–63.21). A single X-ray plate or image intensifier can be used to obtain and review the images intraoperatively.

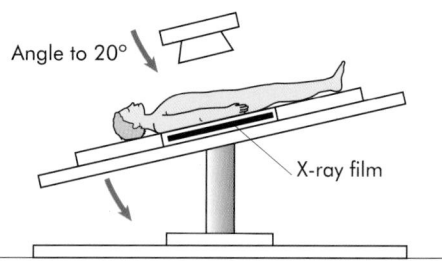

Figure 63.19 Peroperative cholangiography using a radiolucent table-top

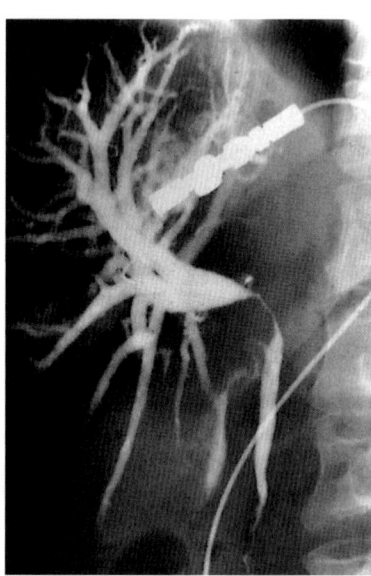

Figure 63.18 Transhepatic cholangiogram showing a stricture of the common hepatic duct (courtesy of Miss Phyllis George, FRCS, London, UK).

Kunio Okuda, **Professor of Medicine, The University of Chiba, East Honshu, Japan.**

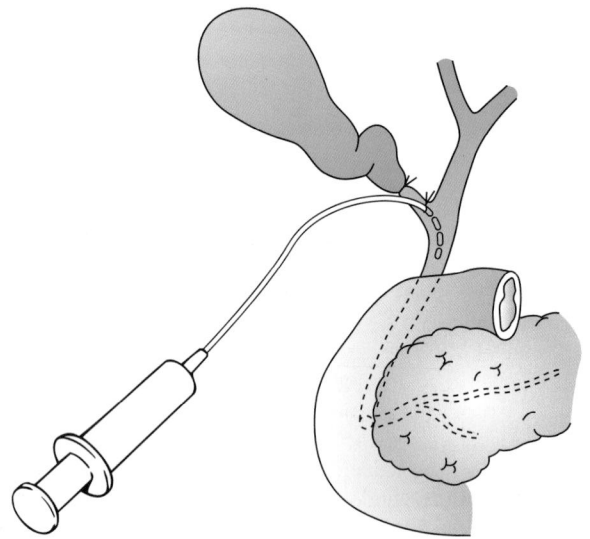

Figure 63.20 Peroperative cholangiography. Technique of introducing contrast.

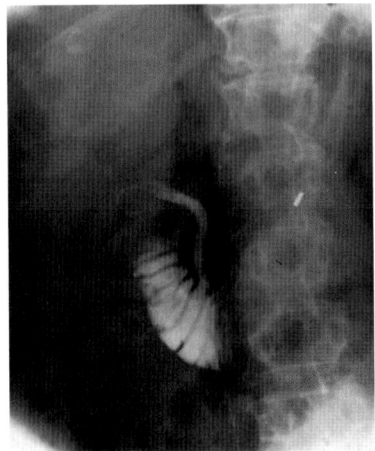

(a)

(b)

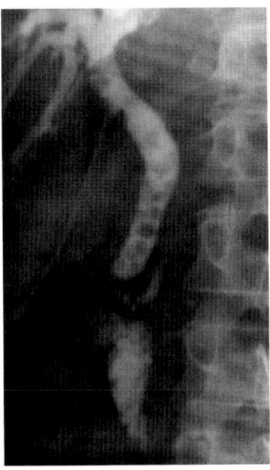

Figure 63.21 Peroperative cholangiography. (a) A normal duct: contrast passes without hindrance into the duodenum. (b) Dilated biliary system with multiple stones in the common bile duct and reflux of contrast into the pancreatic duct. Sphincterotomy was performed.

Irrespective of the technique used, the operating table should be tilted head down approximately 20° to facilitate filling of the intrahepatic ducts. In addition, care should be taken when injecting contrast not to introduce air bubbles into the system, as these may give the appearance of stones and lead to a false-positive result.

Operative biliary endoscopy (choledochoscopy)

At operation, a flexible fibreoptic endoscope can be passed down the cystic duct into the common bile duct enabling stone identification and removal under direct vision. The technique can be combined with an X-ray image intensifier to ensure complete clearance of the biliary tree. After exploration of the bile duct, a tube can be left in the cystic duct remnant or in the common bile duct (a T-tube) and drainage of the biliary tree established. After 7–10 days, a track will be established. This track can be used for the passage of a choledochoscope to remove residual stones in the awake patient in an endoscopy suite. This technique is invaluable in the management of difficult stone disease and prevents the excessive prolongation of an operative exploration of the common bile duct.

CONGENITAL ABNORMALITIES OF THE GALL BLADDER AND BILE DUCTS

Embryology

The hepatic diverticulum arises from the ventral wall of the foregut and elongates into a stalk to form the choledochus. A lateral bud is given off, which is destined to become the gall bladder and cystic duct. The embryonic hepatic duct sends out many branches, which join up the canaliculi between the liver cells. As is usual with embryonic tubular structures, hyperplasia obliterates the lumina of this ductal system; normally, recanalisation subsequently occurs and bile begins to flow. During early fetal life, the gall bladder is entirely intrahepatic.

Absence of the gall bladder

Occasionally, the gall bladder is absent. Failure to visualise the gall bladder is not necessarily a pathological problem.

The Phrygian cap

The Phrygian cap (Fig. 63.22) is present in 2–6% of cholecystograms and may be mistaken for a pathological deformity of the organ. 'Phrygian cap' refers to hats worn by the people of Phrygia, an ancient country of Asia Minor; it was rather like a liberté cap of the French Revolution.

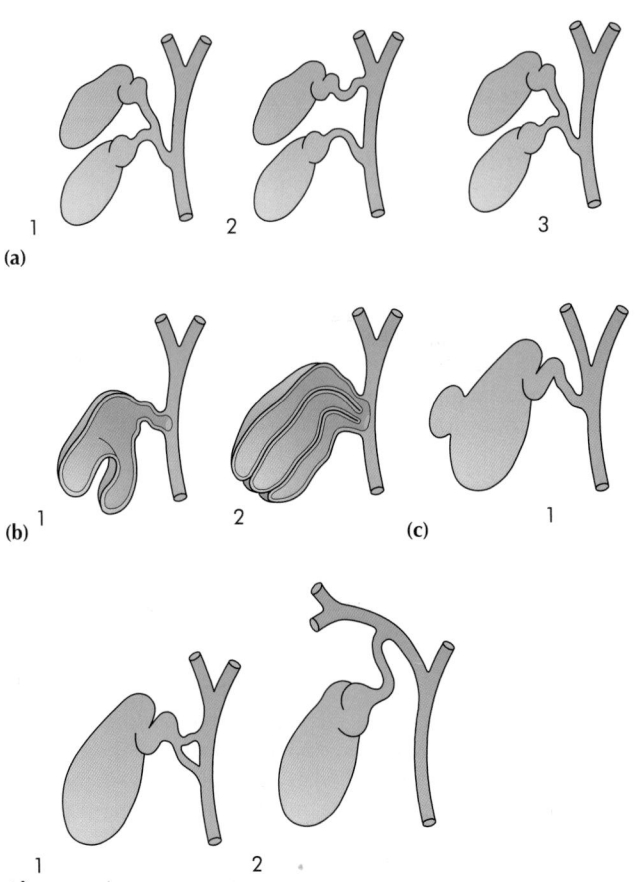

(a)

(b) 1   2   (c) 1

(d) 1   2

Figure 63.22 The main variations in gall bladder and cystic duct anatomy. (a) Double gall bladder. (b) Septum of the gall bladder; 1 is the most common, the so called 'Phrygian cap'. (c) Diverticulum of the gall bladder. (d) Variations in cystic duct insertion.

Floating gall bladder

The organ may hang on a mesentery, which makes it liable to undergo torsion.

Double gall bladder

Rarely, the gall bladder is duplicated. One may be intrahepatic.

Absence of the cystic duct

This is usually a pathological, as opposed to an anatomical, anomaly and indicates the recent passage of a stone or the presence of a stone at the lower end of the cystic duct, which is ulcerating into the common bile duct. The main danger at surgery is damage to the bile duct, and particular care to identify the correct anatomy is essential before division of any duct.

Low insertion of the cystic duct

The cystic duct opens into the common bile duct near the ampulla. All variations of this anomaly can occur (Fig. 63.23). At operation, they are not important. Dissection of a cystic duct that is inserted low in the bile duct should be avoided, as removal will damage the blood supply to the common bile duct and can lead to stricture formation.

An accessory cholecystohepatic duct

Ducts passing directly into the gall bladder from the liver do occur and are probably not uncommon. Nevertheless, larger ducts should be closed but, before doing so, the precise anatomy should be carefully ascertained (Fig. 63.23).

EXTRAHEPATIC BILIARY ATRESIA

Aetiology and pathology

Atresia is present in approximately 1:12 000 live births and affects males and females equally. The extrahepatic bile ducts are progressively destroyed by an inflammatory process, which starts around the time of birth. The aetiology is unclear. Intrahepatic changes also occur and eventually result in biliary cirrhosis and portal hypertension. Untreated, death from the consequences of liver failure occurs before the age of 3 years.

The inflammatory destruction of the bile ducts has been classified into three main types (Fig. 63.24):

- type I: atresia restricted to the common bile duct;
- type II: atresia of the common hepatic duct;
- type III: atresia of the right and left hepatic ducts.

Associated anomalies include, in about 20% of cases, cardiac lesions, polysplenia, situs inversus, absent vena cava and a preduodenal portal vein.

Clinical features

About one-third of patients are jaundiced at birth. In all, however, jaundice is present by the end of the first week and deepens progressively. The meconium may be a little bile-stained, but later the stools are pale and the urine is dark. Prolonged steatorrhoea gives rise to osteomalacia (biliary rickets). Pruritus is severe. Clubbing and skin xanthomas, probably related to a raised serum cholesterol, may be present.

Differential diagnosis

This includes any form of jaundice in a neonate giving a cholestatic picture. Examples are alpha-1-antitrypsin deficiency, cholestasis

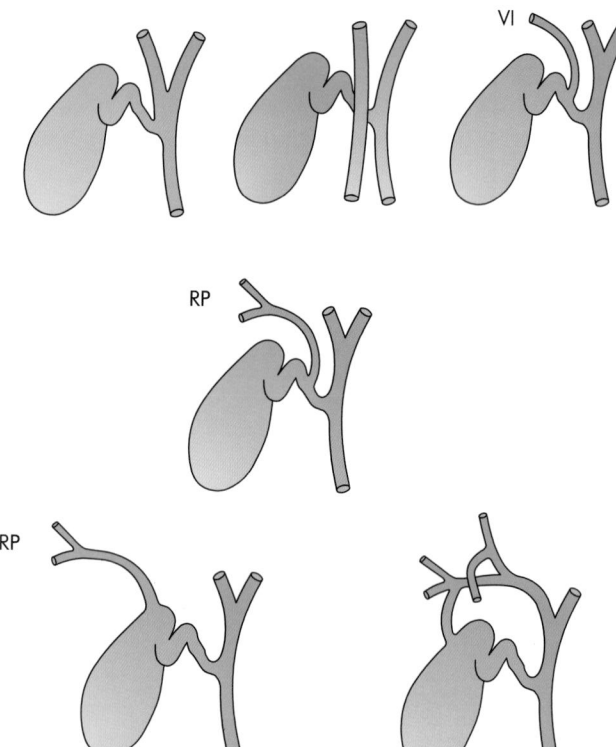

Figure 63.23 Patterns of cystic duct anatomy – note segment VI drainage into the cystic duct and the drainage of the right posterior sectorial duct (RP) into the neck of the gall bladder, or an accessory duct, the so called duct of Luschka.

associated with intravenous feeding, choledochal cyst and inspissated bile syndrome. Neonatal hepatitis is the most difficult to differentiate. Both extrahepatic biliary atresia and neonatal hepatitis are associated with giant cell transformation of the hepatocytes. Liver biopsy and radionuclide excretion scans are essential.

Treatment

Patent segments of proximal bile duct are found in 10% of type I lesions. A direct Roux-en-Y hepaticojejunostomy will achieve bile flow in 75%, but progressive fibrosis results in disappointing long-

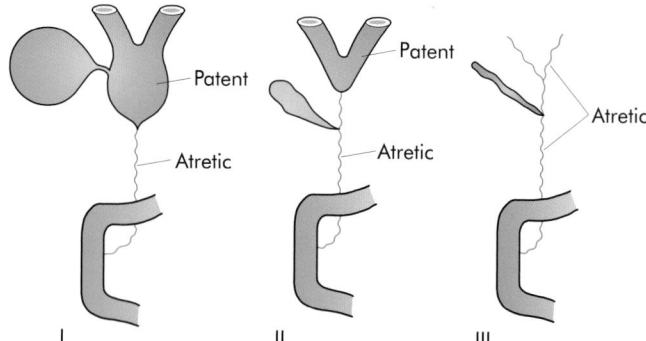

Figure 63.24 Classification of biliary atresia. Gall bladder filling provides a clue to the type of atresia.

Cesar Roux, 1857–1934, Professor of Surgery and Gynaecology, Lausanne, Switzerland, described this method of forming a jejunal conduit in 1908.

term results. A simple biliary–enteric anastomosis is not possible in the majority of cases in which the proximal hepatic ducts are either very small (type II) or atretic (type III). These are treated by the Kasai procedure, in which radical excision of all bile duct tissue up to the liver capsule is performed. A Roux-en-Y loop of jejunum is anastomosed to the exposed area of liver capsule above the bifurcation of the portal vein creating a portoenterostomy. The chances of achieving effective bile drainage after portoenterostomy are maximal when the operation is performed before the age of 8 weeks. Approximately 90% of children whose bilirubin falls to within the normal range can be expected to survive 10 years or more. Early referral for surgery is critical.

Postoperative complications include bacterial cholangitis, which occurs in 40% of patients. Repeated attacks lead to hepatic fibrosis, and 50% of long-term survivors develop portal hypertension, with one-third having variceal bleeding.

Liver transplantation should be considered in children in whom a portoenterostomy is unsuccessful. Results are improving with 70–80% alive 2–5 years following transplantation.

CONGENITAL DILATATION OF THE INTRAHEPATIC DUCTS (CAROLI'S DISEASE)

This rare condition is characterised by multiple irregular saccular dilatations of the intrahepatic ducts separated by segments of normal or stenotic ducts with a normal extrahepatic biliary system. The aetiology is unknown, but it is considered to be hereditary. It can be divided into a simple and a periportal fibrotic type. The periportal fibrotic type presents in childhood and is associated with biliary stasis, stone formation and cholangitis. In contrast, the simple type presents later with episodes of abdominal pain and biliary sepsis. Associated conditions include congenital hepatic fibrosis, polycystic liver and, rarely, cholangiocarcinoma. The mainstays of treatment are antibiotics for the cholangitis and the removal of calculi. As the condition can be limited to one lobe of the liver, lobectomy may be indicated.

Choledochal cyst

Cystic disease of the biliary system is rare. Choledochal cysts are congenital dilatations of the intra- and/or extrahepatic biliary system. The pathogenesis is unclear. Anomalous junctions of the biliary pancreatic junction are frequently observed, but whether or not these play a role in the pathogenesis of the condition is unclear. Todani and colleagues proposed a classification of cystic disease of the biliary tract (Fig. 63.25). Type I cysts are the most common and account for approximately 75% of patients.

Patients may present at any age with jaundice, fever, abdominal pain and a right upper quadrant mass on examination. However, 60% of cases are diagnosed before the age of 10 years. Pancreatitis is a not infrequent presentation in adults. Patients with choledochal cysts have an increased risk of developing cholangiocarcinoma with the risk varying directly with the age at diagnosis.

Ultrasonography will confirm the presence of an abnormal cyst and magnetic resonance imaging (MRI/MRCP) will reveal the anatomy, in particular the relationship between the lower end of the bile duct and the pancreatic duct. CT is also useful for delineating the extent of the intra- or extrahepatic dilatation.

Radical excision of the cyst is the treatment of choice with

Morio Kasai, **formerly Professor of Surgery, The University of Tokyo, Tokyo, Japan.**

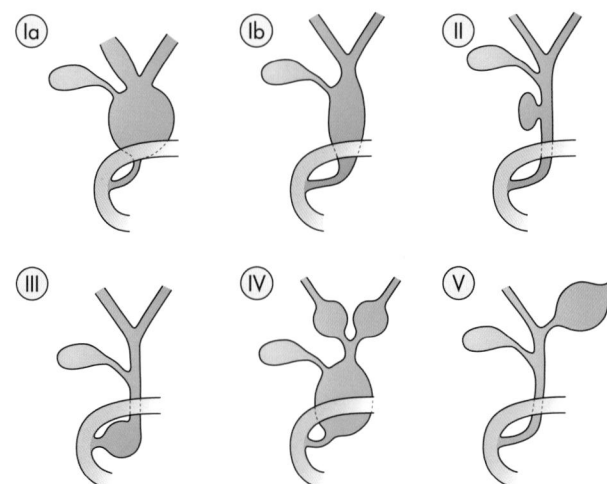

Figure 63.25 Classification of types of choledochal cyst. Type Ia and b: diffuse cystic. Note extension into the pancreas of type Ib. Type II: diverticulum of the common bile duct. Type III: diverticulum within the pancreas. Type IV: extension into the liver. Type V: cystic dilatation only of the intrahepatic ducts.

reconstruction of the biliary tract using a Roux-en-Y loop of jejunum. Complete resection of the cyst is important because of the association with the development of cholangiocarcinoma. Resection and Roux-en-Y reconstruction is also associated with a reduced incidence of stricture formation and recurrent cholangitis.

TRAUMA

Injuries to the gall bladder and extrahepatic biliary tree are rare. They occur as a result of blunt or penetrating abdominal trauma. Operative trauma is perhaps more frequent than external trauma. The physical signs are those of an acute abdomen. Management depends on the location and extent of the biliary and associated injury. In the stable patient, a transected bile duct is best repaired by a Roux-en-Y choledochojejunostomy. Injuries to the gall bladder can be dealt with by cholecystectomy.

TORSION OF THE GALL BLADDER

This is very rare and requires a long mesentery. It occurs most often in an older patient with a large mucocele of the gall bladder. The patient presents with extreme pain and an acute abdomen. Immediate exploration and cholecystectomy are indicated.

GALLSTONES (CHOLELITHIASIS)

Gallstones are the most common biliary pathology. It is estimated that gallstones are present in 10–15% of the adult population in the USA. They are asymptomatic in the majority (> 80%). In the UK, the prevalence of gallstones at the time of death is estimated to be 17% and may be increasing. Approximately 1–2% of asymptomatic patients will develop symptoms requiring cholecystectomy per year, making cholecystectomy one of the most common operations performed by general surgeons.

Aetiology of gallstones

Gallstones can be divided into three main types: cholesterol, pigment (brown/black) or mixed stones. In the USA and Europe,

80% are cholesterol or mixed stones, whereas in Asia, 80% are pigment stones. Cholesterol or mixed stones contain 51–99% pure cholesterol plus an admixture of calcium salts, bile acids, bile pigments and phospholipids.

Cholesterol, which is insoluble in water, is secreted from the canalicular membrane in phospholipid vesicles. Whether cholesterol remains in solution depends on the concentration of phospholipids and bile acids in bile and the type of phospholipid and bile acid. Micelles formed by the phospholipid hold cholesterol in a stable thermodynamic state. When bile is supersaturated with cholesterol or bile acid concentrations are low, unstable unilamellar phospholipid vesicles form, from which cholesterol crystals may nucleate, and stones may form. The process of gallstone formation is complex (Fig. 63.26). Obesity, high-calorie diets and certain medications can increase the secretion of cholesterol and supersaturate the bile, increasing the lithogenicity of bile. Nucleation of cholesterol monohydrate crystals from multilamellar vesicles is a crucial step in gallstone formation. Abnormal emptying of the gall bladder may promote the aggregation of nucleated cholesterol crystals; hence, removing gallstones without removing the gall bladder inevitably leads to gallstone recurrence.

Pigment stone is the name used for stones containing less than 30% cholesterol. There are two types – black and brown. Black stones are largely composed of an insoluble bilirubin pigment polymer mixed with calcium phosphate and calcium bicarbonate. Overall, 20–30% of stones are black. The incidence rises with age. Black stones accompany haemolysis, usually hereditary spherocytosis or sickle cell disease. For unclear reasons, patients with cirrhosis have a higher instance of pigmented stones.

Brown pigment stones contain calcium bilirubinate, calcium palmitate and calcium stearate, as well as cholesterol. Brown stones are rare in the gall bladder. They form in the bile duct and are related to bile stasis and infected bile. Stone formation is related to the deconjugation of bilirubin deglucuronide by bacterial β-glucuronidase. Insoluble unconjugated bilirubinate precipitates. Brown pigment stones are also associated with the presence of foreign bodies within the bile ducts such as endopros-

thesis (stents) or parasites such as *Clonorchis sinensis* and *Ascaris lumbricoides*.

Clinical presentation

Patients typically complain of right upper quadrant or epigastric pain, which may radiate to the back. This may be described as colicky, but more often is dull and constant. Other symptoms include dyspepsia, flatulence, food intolerance, particularly to fats, and some alteration in bowel frequency. Biliary colic is typically present in 10–25% of patients. This is described as a severe right upper quadrant pain that ebbs and flows associated with nausea and vomiting. Pain may radiate to the chest. The pain is usually severe and may last for minutes or even several hours. Frequently, the pain starts during the night, waking the patient. Minor episodes of the same discomfort may occur intermittently during the day. Dyspeptic symptoms may coexist and be worse after such an attack. As the pain resolves, the patient is able to eat and drink again, often only to suffer further episodes. It is of interest that the patient may have several episodes of this nature over a period of a few weeks and then no more trouble for some months (Summary box 63.2).

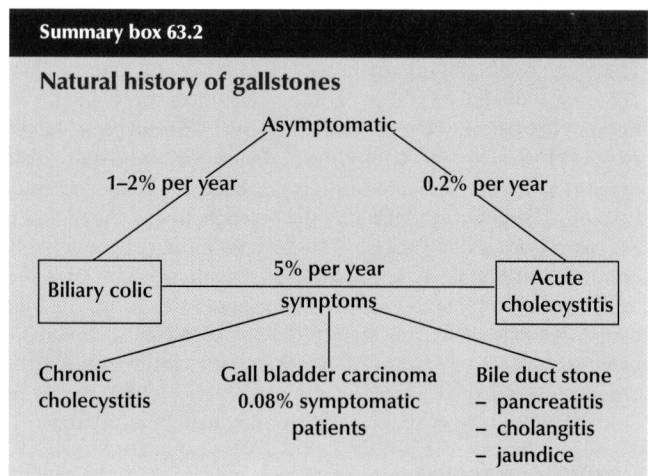

Summary box 63.2

Natural history of gallstones

Asymptomatic

1–2% per year   0.2% per year

Biliary colic — 5% per year symptoms — Acute cholecystitis

Chronic cholecystitis   Gall bladder carcinoma 0.08% symptomatic patients   Bile duct stone
– pancreatitis
– cholangitis
– jaundice

The natural history of gallstones is shown in Summary box 63.3. Jaundice may result if a stone migrates from the gall bladder and obstructs the common bile duct. Rarely, a gallstone can lead to bowel obstruction (gallstone ileus).

Summary box 63.3

Effects and complications of gallstones

In the gallbladder
■ Biliary colic
■ Acute cholecystitis
■ Chronic cholecystitis
■ Empyema of the gall bladder
■ Mucocele
■ Perforation

In the bile ducts
■ Biliary obstruction
■ Acute cholangitis
■ Acute pancreatitis

In the intestine
■ Intestinal obstruction (gallstone ileus)

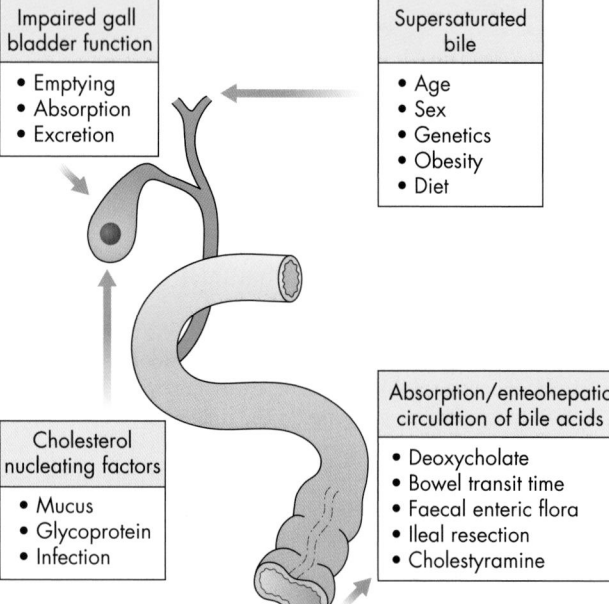

Impaired gall bladder function
• Emptying
• Absorption
• Excretion

Supersaturated bile
• Age
• Sex
• Genetics
• Obesity
• Diet

Cholesterol nucleating factors
• Mucus
• Glycoprotein
• Infection

Absorption/enteohepatic circulation of bile acids
• Deoxycholate
• Bowel transit time
• Faecal enteric flora
• Ileal resection
• Cholestyramine

Figure 63.26 Factors associated with gallstone formation.

When symptoms do not resolve, but progress to continued pain with fever and leucocytosis, the diagnosis of acute cholecystitis should be considered. The differential diagnosis is given in Summary box 63.4.

Summary box 63.4

Differential diagnosis of cholecystitis

Common
- Appendicitis
- Perforated peptic ulcer
- Acute pancreatitis

Uncommon
- Acute pyelonephritis
- Myocardial infarction
- Pneumonia – right lower lobe

Ultrasound scan aids diagnosis

Uncertain diagnosis – do CT scan

Diagnosis

A diagnosis of gallstone disease is based on the history and physical examination with confirmatory radiological studies such as transabdominal ultrasonography and radionuclide scans (see above). In the acute phase, the patient may have right upper quadrant tenderness that is exacerbated during inspiration by the examiner's right subcostal palpation (Murphy's sign). A positive Murphy's sign suggests acute inflammation and may be associated with a leucocytosis and moderately elevated liver function tests. A mass may be palpable as the omentum walls off an inflamed gall bladder. Fortunately, in the majority of cases, this process is limited by the stone slipping back into the body of the gall bladder and the contents of the gall bladder escaping by way of the cystic duct. This achieves adequate drainage of the gall bladder and enables the inflammation to resolve.

If resolution does not occur, an empyema of the gall bladder may result. The wall may become necrotic and perforate, with the development of localised peritonitis. The abscess may then perforate into the peritoneal cavity with a septic peritonitis – however, this is uncommon, because the gall bladder is usually localised by omentum around the perforation.

A palpable, non-tender gall bladder (Courvoisier's sign) portends a more sinister diagnosis. This usually results from a distal common duct obstruction secondary to a peripancreatic malignancy. Rarely, a non-tender, palpable gall bladder results from complete obstruction of the cystic duct with reabsorption of the intraluminal bile salts and secretion of uninfected mucus secreted by the gall bladder epithelium, leading to a mucocele of the gall bladder.

Treatment

Most authors would suggest that it is safe to observe patients with asymptomatic gallstones, with cholecystectomy only being performed for those patients who develop symptoms or complications of their gallstones. However, prophylactic cholecystectomy

---

John Benjamin Murphy, **1857–1916, Professor of Surgery, The Northwestern University, Chicago, IL, USA.**
Ludwig Courvoisier, **1843–1918, Professor of Surgery, Basle, Switzerland.**

---

should be considered in diabetic patients, those with congenital haemolytic anaemia and those due to undergo bariatric surgery for morbid obesity, as these groups are at increased risk of complications from gallstones.

For patients with biliary colic or cholecystitis, cholecystectomy is the treatment of choice in the absence of medical contra-indications. The timing of surgery in acute cholecystitis remains controversial. Many units favour early intervention, whereas others suggest that a delayed approach is preferable.

Conservative treatment followed by cholecystectomy

Experience shows that, in more than 90% of cases, the symptoms of acute cholecystitis subside with conservative measures. Non-operative treatment is based on four principles:

1 Nil per mouth (NPO) and intravenous fluid administration.
2 Administration of analgesics.
3 Administration of antibiotics. As the cystic duct is blocked in most instances, the concentration of antibiotic in the serum is more important than its concentration in bile. A broad-spectrum antibiotic effective against Gram-negative aerobes is most appropriate (e.g. cefazolin, cefuroxime or gentamicin).
4 Subsequent management. When the temperature, pulse and other physical signs show that the inflammation is subsiding, oral fluids are reinstated followed by regular diet. Ultrasonography is performed to ensure that no local complications have developed, that the bile duct is of a normal size and that no stones are contained in the bile duct. Cholecystectomy may be performed on the next available list, or the patient may be allowed home to return later when the inflammation has completely resolved.

Conservative treatment must be abandoned if the pain and tenderness increase; depending on the status of the patient, operative intervention and cholecystectomy should be performed (Fig. 63.27). If the patient has serious comorbid conditions, a percutaneous cholecystostomy can be performed under ultrasound control, which will rapidly relieve symptoms. A subsequent cholecystectomy is usually required.

Routine early operation

As noted above, some surgeons advocate urgent operation as a routine measure in cases of acute cholecystitis. Provided that the

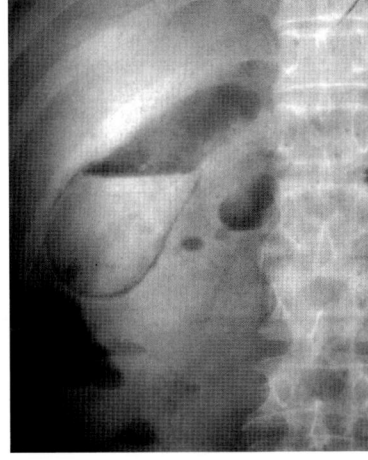

Figure 63.27 Gas in the gall bladder and gall bladder wall (*Clostridium perfringens*). Emergency surgery is indicated.

operation is undertaken within 5–7 days of the onset of the attack, the surgeon is experienced and excellent operating facilities are available, good results are achieved. Nevertheless, the conversion rate in laparoscopic cholecystectomy is five times higher in acute than in elective surgery. If an early operation is not indicated, one should wait approximately 6 weeks for the inflammation to subside before proceeding to operate.

EMPYEMA OF THE GALL BLADDER

The gall bladder appears to be filled with pus. It may be a sequel of acute cholecystitis or the result of a mucocele becoming infected. The treatment is drainage and, later, cholecystectomy.

Acalculous cholecystitis

Acute and chronic inflammation of the gall bladder can occur in the absence of stones and give rise to a clinical picture similar to calculous cholecystitis. Some patients have non-specific inflammation of the gall bladder, whereas others have one of the cholecystoses. Acute acalculous cholecystitis is seen particularly in patients recovering from major surgery (e.g. coronary artery bypass), trauma and burns. In these patients, the diagnosis is often missed, and the mortality rate is high.

THE CHOLECYSTOSES (CHOLESTEROSIS, POLYPOSIS, ADENOMYOMATOSIS AND CHOLECYSTITIS GLANDULARIS PROLIFERANS)

This is a not uncommon group of conditions affecting the gall bladder, in which there are chronic inflammatory changes with hyperplasia of all tissue elements.

Cholesterosis ('strawberry gall bladder')

In the fresh state, the interior of the gall bladder looks something like a strawberry; the yellow specks (submucous aggregations of cholesterol crystals and cholesterol esters) correspond to the seeds (Fig. 63.28). It may be associated with cholesterol stones.

Cholesterol polyposis of the gall bladder

Cholecystography shows negative shadows in a functioning gall bladder, or there is a well-defined polyp present on ultrasound.

These are either cholesterol polyposis or adenomatous change. With improving ultrasonography, they are seen more frequently, and surgery is advised only if they change in size or are longer than 1 cm.

Cholecystitis glandularis proliferans (polyp, adenomyomatosis and intramural diverticulosis)

Figure 63.29 summarises the varieties of this condition. A polyp of the mucous membrane is fleshy and granulomatous. All layers of the gall bladder wall may be thickened, but sometimes an incomplete septum forms that separates the hyperplastic from the normal. Intraparietal 'mixed' calculi may be present. These can be complicated by an intramural, and later extramural, abscess. If symptomatic, the patient is treated by cholecystectomy.

Diverticulosis of the gall bladder

Diverticulosis of the gall bladder is usually manifest as black pigment stones impacted in the outpouchings of the lacunae of Luschka. Diverticulosis of the gall bladder may be demonstrated by cholecystography, especially when the gall bladder contracts after a fatty meal. There are small dots of contrast medium just within and outside the gall bladder (Fig. 63.30). A septum may

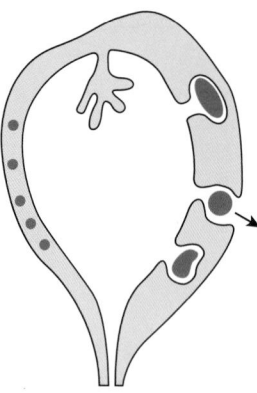

Figure 63.29 Types of cholecystitis glandularis proliferans (polypus, intramural or diverticular stones and fistula).

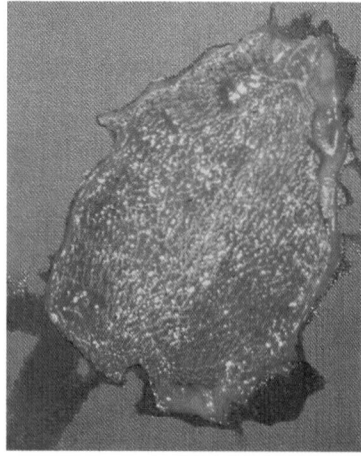

Figure 63.28 The interior of a strawberry gall bladder (cholesterosis) (courtesy of Dr Sanjay P. Thakur, Patna, India).

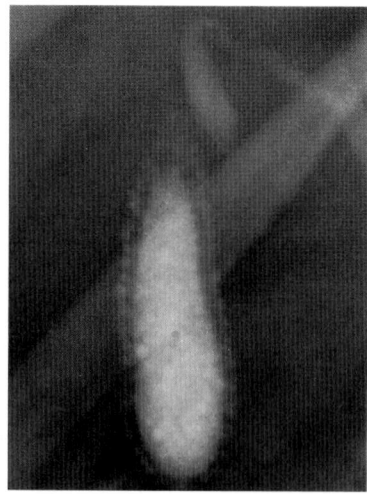

Figure 63.30 Cholecystogram showing diverticulosis with dots of contrast medium in the gall bladder wall.

also be present [to be distinguished from the Phrygian cap (see Fig. 63.22, p. 1117)]. The treatment is cholecystectomy.

Typhoid gall bladder

Salmonella typhi ('Typhoid Mary', a cook-general who passed *Salmonella typhi* in her faeces and urine, was responsible for nearly a score of epidemics of typhoid in and around New York City) or, occasionally, *Salmonella typhimurium* can infect the gall bladder. Acute cholecystitis can occur. More frequently, chronic cholecystitis occurs, and the patient, being a typhoid carrier, excretes the bacteria in the bile. Gallstones may be present (surgeons should not give patients their stones after their operation if there is any suspicion of typhoid!). It is debatable whether the stones are secondary to the *Salmonella* cholecystitis or whether pre-existing stones predispose the gall bladder to chronic infection. Salmonellae can, however, frequently be cultured from these stones. Ampicillin and cholecystectomy are indicated.

CHOLECYSTECTOMY

Preparation for operation

An appropriate history is taken, and the patient's fitness for the procedure is assessed. This includes investigation of the cardiovascular and respiratory systems, and a full blood count and biochemical profile are performed to exclude anaemia or abnormal liver function. Blood coagulation is checked if there is a history of jaundice. The patient is given prophylactic antibiotics either with pre-medication or at the time of anaesthetic induction. A second-generation cephalosporin is appropriate. Subcutaneous heparin or anti-embolic stockings are prescribed. The patient must sign a consent form to indicate that he or she is fully aware of the procedure being undertaken, the risks involved and the complications that may occur (Summary box 63.5).

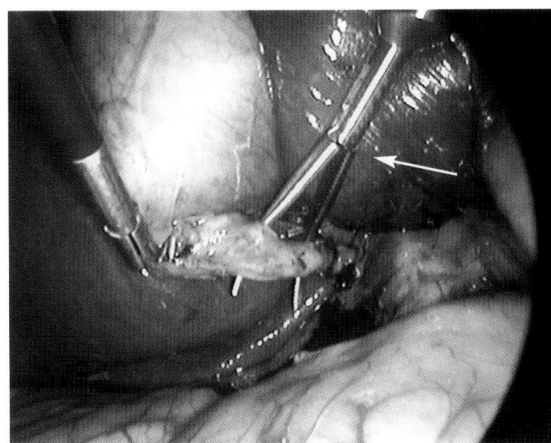

Figure 63.31 Operative image of a laparoscopic cholecystectomy. Forceps (arrowed) are dissecting the cystic duct.

The Phrygian Cap **refers to the hats worn by the people of Phrygia, an ancient country of Asia Minor. The cap was like the Liberté Cap of the French Revolutionaries.**
Typhoid Mary **was the name given to a cook-general who passed Salmonella typhi in her faeces and urine, and was responsible for nearly twenty epidemics of typhoid in, and around, New York City, in the United States.**

Summary box 63.5
Preparation for operation
■ **Full blood count**
■ **Renal profile and liver function tests**
■ **Prothrombin time**
■ **Chest X-ray and electrocardiogram (if over 45 years or medically indicated)**
■ **Antibiotic prophylaxis**
■ **Deep vein thrombosis prophylaxis**
■ **Informed consent**

Laparoscopic cholecystectomy

The preparation and indications for cholecystectomy are the same whether it is performed by laparoscopy or by open techniques. Laparoscopic cholecystectomy is the procedure of choice for the majority of patients with gall bladder disease (Fig. 63.31). The key, as in open surgery, is identification and safe dissection of Calot's triangle.

The patient is placed supine on the operating table. Following induction and maintenance of a general anaesthetic, the abdomen is prepared in a standard fashion. Pneumoperitoneum is established. A number of techniques are described. The author's preference is to use an open subumbilical cut-down with direct visualisation of the peritoneum to place the initial port. This port will function as the camera port. Many surgeons use a 'closed' technique using a Verres needle to establish pneumoperitoneum prior to placing the initial trocar.

Additional operating ports are inserted in the subxiphoid area and in the right subcostal area. The patient is placed in a reverse Trendelenburg position, slightly rotated to the left. This exposes the fundus of the gall bladder, which is retracted towards the diaphragm. The neck of the gall bladder is then retracted towards the right iliac fossa exposing Calot's triangle. This area is laid wide open by dividing the peritoneum on the posterior and anterior aspects. The cystic duct is carefully defined, as is the cystic artery. The gall bladder is separated from the liver bed for about 2 cm to allow for confirmation of the anatomy. Unless there are specific indications (see below), a routine cholangiogram is not performed. However, if doubt exists regarding the anatomy, a cholangiogram is warranted. Once the anatomy is clearly defined and the triangle of Calot has been laid wide open, the cystic duct and artery are clipped and divided. The gall bladder is then removed from the gall bladder bed by sharp dissection and, once free, removed via the umbilicus. An endobag may be used for extraction of the gall bladder to prevent contamination of the umbilical wound. Recovery after laparoscopic cholecystectomy is rapid – 80% of patients are discharged within 24 hours and the remainder by day 2. Any untoward symptoms require immediate investigation (Summary box 63.6).

Jean Francois Calot, **1861–1944, Surgeon, The Rothschild Hospital, Berck-sur-Mer, Pas-de-Calais, France.**
Janos Verres, **1903–1979, Chest Physician, and Chief of the Department of Internal Medicine, The Regional Hospital, Kapuvar, Hungary.**
Friedrich Trendelenburg, **1844–1924, Professor of Surgery, Rostock (1875–1882), Bonn, (1882–1895), and Leipzig, (1895–1911), Germany. The Trendelenburg position was first described in 1885.**

> **Summary box 63.6**
>
> **Post-cholecystectomy discomfort**
> - If there is a delay in recovery after cholecystectomy, exclude bile duct or bowel injury
> - Incidence of bile duct injury is 0.05%

Serious complications of laparoscopic cholecystectomy fall into two major areas: access complications or bile duct injuries. In the main, access complications occur during the insertion of the Verres needle to establish pneumoperitoneum or the insertion of trocars. If insertion is performed blindly or is found to be difficult, visceral injury should be excluded. If either a visceral or a bile duct injury is suspected, conversion to an open technique is recommended by most surgeons.

Open cholecystectomy

For patients in whom a laparoscopic approach is not indicated or in whom conversion from a laparoscopic approach is required, an open cholecystectomy is performed.

A short right upper transverse incision is made centred over the lateral border of the rectus muscle. The gall bladder is appropriately exposed, and packs are placed on the hepatic flexure of the colon, the duodenum and the lesser omentum to ensure a clear view of the anatomy of the porta hepatis. These packs may be retracted using the hand of the assistant ('It is the left hand of the assistant that does all the work' – Moynihan), or a stabilised ring retractor is used to keep the packs in position. A Duval forceps is placed on the infundibulum of the gall bladder, and the peritoneum overlying Calot's triangle is placed on a stretch. The peritoneum is then divided close to the wall of the gall bladder, and the fat in Calot's triangle is carefully dissected away to expose the cystic artery and the cystic duct. The cystic duct is dissected to the common bile duct, whose position is clearly ascertained. The cystic artery is tied and divided. The whole of the triangle of Calot is displayed to ensure that the anatomy of the ducts is clear, and the cystic duct is then divided between ligatures (Fig. 63.32). The gall bladder is then dissected away from the gall bladder bed.

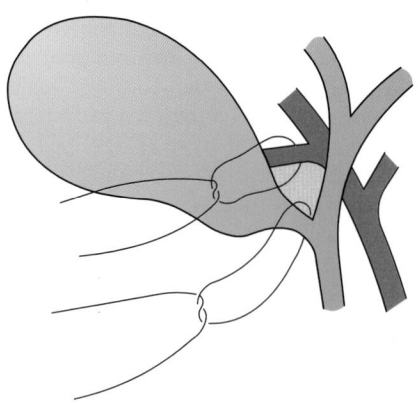

Figure 63.32 Ligatures passed and tied around the cystic artery and cystic duct. The grey shaded area represents Calot's triangle.

Pierre Duval, **B. 1874, a Surgeon, of Paris, France.**

Some golden rules in case of difficulty:

- When the anatomy of the triangle of Calot is unclear, blind dissection should stop.
- Bleeding adjacent to the triangle of Calot should be controlled by pressure and not by blind clipping or clamping.
- When there is doubt about the anatomy, a 'fundus-first' or 'retrograde' cholecystectomy dissecting on the gall bladder wall down to the cystic duct can be helpful.
- If the cystic duct is densely adherent to the common bile duct and there is the possibility of a Mirizzi syndrome (a gallstone ulcerating through into the common duct), the infundibulum of the gall bladder should be opened, the stone removed and the infundibulum oversewn.
- A cholecystostomy is rarely indicated but, if necessary, as many stones as possible should be extracted, and a large Foley catheter (14F) placed in the fundus of the gall bladder with a direct track externally. By so doing, should stones be left behind in the gall bladder, these can be extracted with a choledochoscope.

Indications for choledochotomy

In a situation in which sophisticated preoperative imaging or per-operative cholangiography is not available, it is well to remember the traditional indications for choledochotomy, which are:

1 palpable stones in the common bile duct;
2 jaundice, a history of jaundice or cholangitis;
3 a dilated common bile duct;
4 abnormal liver function tests, in particular a raised alkaline phosphatase.

Unless the expertise is available, it is probably inadvisable to perform a choledochotomy laparoscopically; rather, one should rely on postoperative endoscopic techniques or convert to an open operation. The incidence of symptomatic stones in the bile duct varies from 5% to 8%. These can, in the main, be dealt with endoscopically without resort to opening the duct. However, current trials suggest that, in experienced hands, the morbidity of the two techniques is similar.

Late symptoms after cholecystectomy

In 15% of patients, cholecystectomy fails to relieve the symptoms for which the operation was performed. Such patients may be considered to have a 'post-cholecystectomy' syndrome. However, such problems are usually related to the preoperative symptoms and are merely a continuation of those symptoms. Full investigation should be undertaken to confirm the diagnosis and exclude the presence of a stone in the common bile duct, a stone in the cystic duct stump or operative damage to the biliary tree. This is best performed by MRCP or ERCP. The latter has the added advantage that, if a stone is found in the common bile duct, it can be removed.

Management of bile duct obstruction following cholecystectomy

Patients with symptoms developing either immediately or delayed after a cholecystectomy, particularly if jaundice is present, need urgent investigation. This is especially true if the jaundice is associated with infection, a condition called cholangitis.

P. L. Mirizzi, **an Argentinian Physician, described this syndrome in 1948.**
Frederic Eugene Basil Foley, 1891–1966, Urologist, Anker Hospital, St. Paul, MN, **USA.**

The first step in management is to undertake an immediate ultrasound scan. This will demonstrate whether there is intra- or extrahepatic ductal dilatation. The anatomy needs to be defined by either an ERCP or an MRCP. The latter investigation will also allow for therapeutic manoeuvres such as removal of an obstructing stone or insertion of a stent across a biliary leak. If a fluid collection is present in the subhepatic space, drainage catheters may be required. These can be inserted under radiological control or, if this expertise is not available, at open operation. Small biliary leaks will usually resolve spontaneously, especially if there is no distal obstruction. Should the common bile duct be damaged, the patient should be referred to an appropriate expert for reconstruction of the duct.

About 15% of injuries to the bile ducts are recognised at the time of operation. In 85% of cases, the injury declares itself postoperatively by: (1) a profuse and persistent leakage of bile if drainage has been provided, or bile peritonitis if such drainage has not been provided; and (2) deepening obstructive jaundice. When the obstruction is incomplete, jaundice is delayed until subsequent fibrosis renders the lumen of the duct inadequate.

Any change in bilirubin or suggestion of duct damage requires investigation and the nature of the bile duct injury clarified. The surgical repair and subsequent outcome is related to the level of injury, which is determined using the Bismuth classification (Table 63.1).

Treatment

In the debilitated patient, temporary external biliary drainage may be achieved by passing a catheter percutaneously into an intrahepatic duct. Also, stents may be passed through strictures at the time of ERCP and left to drain into the duodenum. When the general condition of the patient has improved, definitive surgery can be undertaken. The principles of surgical repair are maintenance of duct length and restoration of biliary drainage. For benign stricture or duct transection, the preferred treatment is immediate Roux-en-Y choledochojejunostomy by an experienced surgeon. For a stricture of recent onset through which a guidewire can be passed, balloon dilatation with insertion of a stent is an acceptable alternative provided that the services of an experienced endoscopist are available. The outcome of such surgery is good, with 90% of patients having no further cholangitis or stricture formation.

Stones in the bile duct

Duct stones may occur many years after a cholecystectomy (Fig. 63.33) or be related to the development of new pathology, such as infection of the biliary tree or infestation by *Ascaris lumbricoides* or *Clonorchis sinensis*. Any obstruction to the flow of bile can give rise to stasis with the formation of stones within the duct. The consequence of duct stones is either obstruction to bile flow or infection. Stones in the bile ducts are more often associated with infected bile (80%) than are stones in the gall bladder.

Table 63.1 Bismuth classification

Type I	Low common bile duct; stump > 2 cm
Type II	Middle common hepatic duct; stump < 2 cm
Type III	Hilar – confluence of right and left ducts intact
Type IV	Right and left ducts separated
Type V	Involvement of the intrahepatic ducts

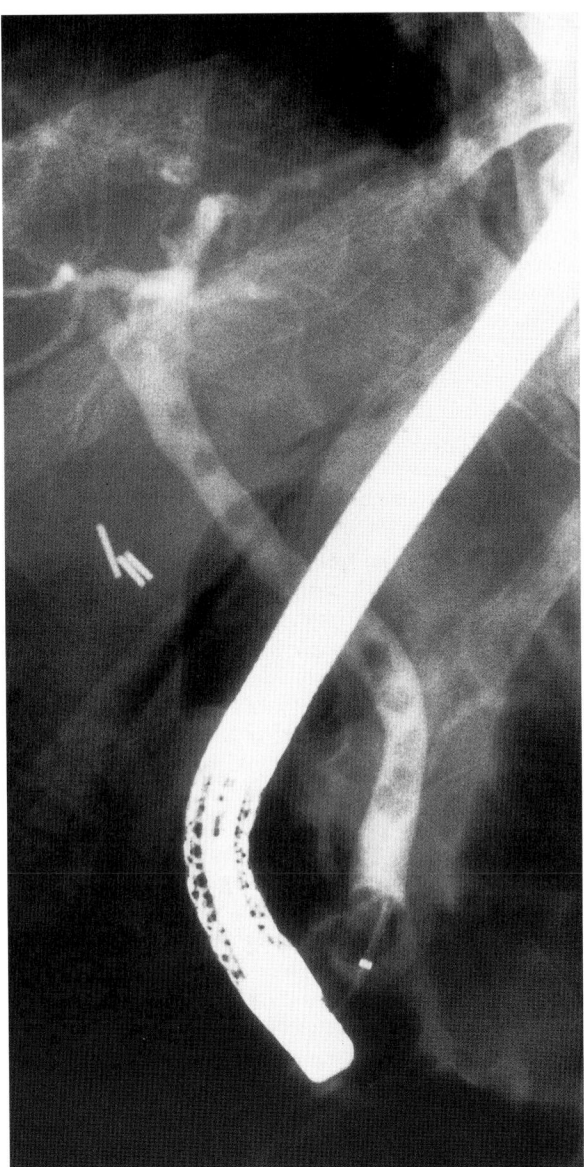

Figure 63.33 Endoscopic retrograde cholangiopancreatography: the patient presented with jaundice 4 days after laparoscopic cholecystectomy. The bile duct contained multiple stones.

Symptoms

The patient may be asymptomatic but usually has bouts of pain, jaundice and fever. The patient is often ill and feels unwell. The term 'cholangitis' is given to the triad of pain, jaundice and fevers, sometimes known as 'Charcot's triad'.

Signs

Tenderness may be elicited in the epigastrium and the right hypochondrium. In the jaundiced patient, it is useful to remember Courvoisier's law – in obstruction of the common bile duct due to a stone, distension of the gall bladder seldom occurs; the organ is usually already shrivelled. In obstruction from other causes, distension of the gall bladder is common by comparison.

Jean Martin Charcot, **1825–1893, Physician, La Salpêtrière, Paris, France.**

Management

It is essential to determine whether the jaundice is due to liver disease, disease within the duct, such as sclerosing cholangitis, or obstruction of the biliary tree. Ultrasound scanning, liver function tests, liver biopsy (if the ducts are not dilated) and MRI or ERCP will delineate the nature of the obstruction.

The patient may be ill. Pus may be present within the biliary tree, and liver abscesses may develop. Full supportive measures are required with rehydration, correction of clotting abnormalities and treatment with appropriate broad-spectrum antibiotics. Once the patient has been resuscitated, relief of the obstruction is essential. Endoscopic papillotomy is the preferred first technique with a sphincterotomy, removal of the stones using a Dormia basket or the placement of a stent if stone removal is not possible. If this technique fails, percutaneous transhepatic cholangiography can be performed to provide drainage and subsequent percutaneous choledochoscopy. Surgery, in the form of choledochotomy, is now rarely used for this situation, as most patients can be managed by minimally invasive techniques (Figs 63.34 and 63.35).

Choledochotomy

When faced with a sick patient whose investigations show that the cause of the cholangitis is stones in the duct, and minimally invasive techniques for stone extraction are not available, the surgeon has no alternative but to undertake a laparotomy. The aim of this surgery is to drain the common bile duct and remove the stones by a longitudinal incision in the duct. When the duct is clear of stones, a T-tube is inserted and the duct closed around it; the long limb of the T-tube is brought out on the right side, and the bile is allowed to drain externally. When the bile has become clear and the patient has recovered, a cholangiogram is performed, usually 7–10 days following operation. If residual stones are found, the T-tube is left in place for 6 weeks so that the track is 'mature'. The retained stones can be removed percutaneously by an interventional radiologist (Burhenne technique) (Fig. 63.35).

Stricture of the bile duct

The causes of benign biliary stricture are given in Summary box 63.7.

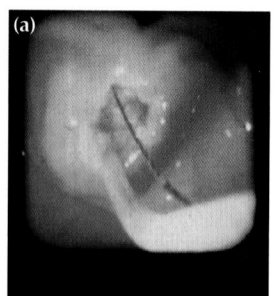 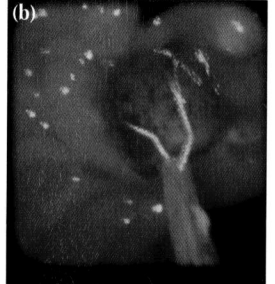

Figure 63.34 (a) Endoscopic sphincterotomy; (b) extraction of a stone from the bile duct through the ampulla.

Joachim Burhenne, **a Radiologist of Vancouver, Canada.**

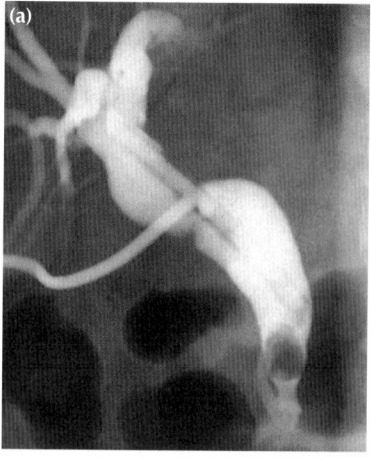

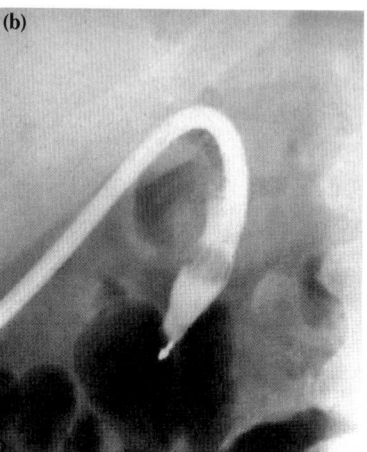

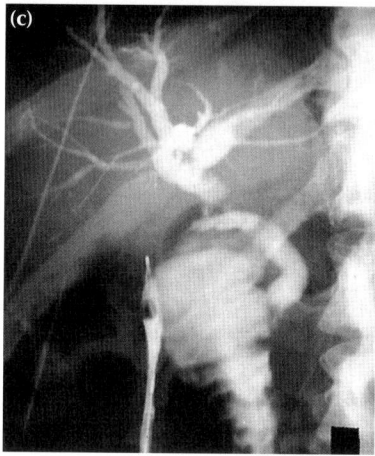

Figure 63.35 Extraction of a stone from the common bile duct by the Burhenne technique. (a) A T-tube *in situ* with a stone in the duct. (b) A steerable catheter has been manipulated into the duct and a basket placed around the stone. (c) The stone being extracted from the bile duct along the T-tube track.

THE GALL BLADDER AND BILE DUCTS

CHAPTER 63 |

Summary box 63.7

Causes of benign biliary stricture

Congenital
- Biliary atresia

Bile duct injury at surgery
- Cholecystectomy
- Choledochotomy
- Gastrectomy
- Hepatic resection
- Transplantation

Inflammatory
- Stones
- Cholangitis
- Parasitic
- Pancreatitis
- Sclerosing cholangitis
- Radiotherapy

Trauma

Idiopathic

Bile duct strictures may be investigated radiologically (Summary box 63.8).

Summary box 63.8

Radiological investigation of biliary strictures

- Ultrasonography
- Cholangiography via T-tube, if present
- ERCP
- MRCP
- PTC (see Figs 63.20 and 63.21, pp. 1116 and 1117)
- Multidetector row CT

PRIMARY SCLEROSING CHOLANGITIS

Primary sclerosing cholangitis is an idiopathic fibrosing inflammatory condition of the biliary tree that affects both intrahepatic and extrahepatic ducts. It is of unknown origin, but association with hypergammaglobulinaemia and elevated markers such as smooth muscle antibodies and anti-nuclear factor suggests an immunological basis. The majority of patients are between 30 and 60 years of age. There appears to be a male predominance and a strong association with inflammatory bowel disease, especially ulcerative colitis.

Common symptoms include right upper quadrant discomfort, jaundice, pruritus, fever, fatigue and weight loss. Investigation reveals a cholestatic pattern in liver function tests with elevation of serum alkaline phosphatase and gamma-glutamyl transferase and smaller rises in the aminotransferases. Bilirubin values can be variable and may fluctuate. Imaging studies such as MRCP or ERCP may demonstrate stricturing and beading of the bile ducts (Fig. 63.36). A liver biopsy is helpful in confirming the diagnosis and may help to guide therapy by excluding cirrhosis. The important differential diagnoses are secondary sclerosing cholangitis and cholangiocarcinoma. The latter condition may be very difficult to

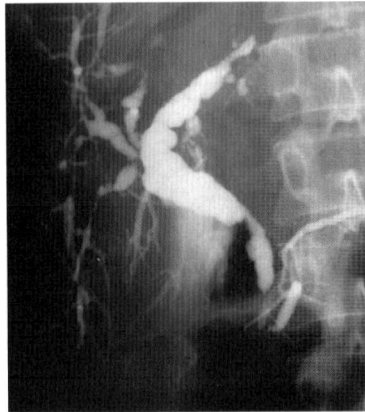

Figure 63.36 Sclerosing cholangitis in a patient with ulcerative colitis visualised by endoscopic retrograde cholangiopancreatography.

diagnose, and a high index of suspicion is required especially in the setting of an unexplained deterioration.

Medical management with antibiotics, vitamin K, cholestyramine, steroids and immunosuppressants such as azathioprine is generally unsuccessful. Endoscopic stenting of dominant strictures and, in selected patients with predominantly extrahepatic disease, operative resection may be worthwhile. For patients with cirrhosis, liver transplantation is the best option. Five-year survival following transplantation is in excess of 80%.

PARASITIC INFESTATION OF THE BILIARY TRACT

Biliary ascariasis

The round worm, *Ascaris lumbricoides,* commonly infests the intestine of inhabitants of Asia, Africa and Central America. It may enter the biliary tree through the ampulla of Vater and cause biliary pain. Complications include strictures, suppurative cholangitis, liver abscesses and empyema of the gall bladder. In the uncomplicated case, anti-spasmodics can be given to relax the sphincter of Oddi, and the worm will return to the small intestine to be dealt with by antihelminthic drugs. Operation may be necessary to remove the worm or deal with complications. Worms can be extracted via the ampulla of Vater by ERCP.

Clonorchiasis (Asiatic cholangiohepatis)

The disease is endemic in the Far East. The fluke, up to 25 mm long and 5 mm wide, inhabits the bile ducts, including the intrahepatic ducts. Fibrous thickening of the duct walls occurs. Many cases are asymptomatic. Complications include biliary pain, stones, cholangitis, cirrhosis and bile duct carcinoma. Choledochotomy and T-tube drainage and, in some cases, choledochoduodenostomy are required. Because a process of recurrent stone formation is set up, a choledochojejunostomy with Roux loop affixed to the abdominal parietes is performed in some centres to allow easy subsequent access to the duct system.

Hydatid disease

A large hydatid cyst may obstruct the hepatic ducts. Sometimes, a cyst will rupture into the biliary tree and its contents cause obstructive jaundice or cholangitis, requiring appropriate surgery (see Chapters 5 and 61).

TUMOURS OF THE BILE DUCT

Benign tumours of the bile duct

These are uncommon and need to be distinguished from other benign conditions such as choledocholithiasis, sclerosing cholangitis, Caroli's disease and choledochal cysts. They account for less than 0.1% of biliary tract operations.

The duration of symptoms may vary from a few days to months, and their clinical presentation may in fact mimic the more common conditions such as cholecystitis, choledocholithiasis, cancer of the bile duct and pancreatic cancer.

Benign neoplasms causing biliary obstruction may be classified as follows:

- papilloma and adenoma;
- multiple biliary papillomatosis;
- granular cell myoblastoma;
- neural tumours;
- leiomyoma;
- endocrine tumours.

Papilloma and adenoma

The most common benign neoplasm arises from the glandular epithelium lining the bile ducts. It can occur throughout the biliary system but is more common in the periampullary area, where a papilloma or adenoma may protrude through the ampulla of Vater and be visible at endoscopy. Jaundice is the commonest symptom occurring in more than 90% of cases. Coexisting gallstones are uncommon.

Treatment depends on the age, general status of the patient and site of the disease but, in general, it should consist of total resection. In some cases, a wide local resection can be performed, particularly for periampullary lesions.

Papillomatosis

This rare condition is characterised by the presence of multiple mucus-secreting tumours of the biliary epithelium. Patients present with obstructive jaundice, which may be intermittent and often complicated by cholangitis. These tumours have a malignant potential and should be resected if possible. This may involve liver resection if the disease is confined to a hepatic lobe. If both lobes are affected, then liver transplantation may be required.

Granular cell myoblastoma, neural tumours, leiomyomata and endocrine tumours are extremely uncommon. In general, if biliary obstruction occurs, it should be relieved by resection, bypass or endoscopic stenting.

Malignant tumours of the bile duct

Carcinoma may arise at any point in the biliary tree, from the common bile duct to the small intrahepatic ducts (Summary box 63.9).

Summary box 63.9
Bile duct cancer
■ Rare, but incidence increasing
■ Presents with jaundice and weight loss
■ Diagnosis by ultrasound and CT scanning
■ Jaundice relieved by stenting
■ Surgical excision possible in 5%
■ Prognosis poor – 90% mortality in 1 year

Jacques Caroli, **Professor of Medicine, Paris, France.**

Incidence

This is a rare malignancy accounting for 1–2% of new cancers in a western practice. The overall annual incidence is 1–1.5:100 000 with two-thirds of patients being older than 65 years.

Histologically, the tumour is usually an adenocarcinoma (cholangiocarcinoma), predominantly in the extrahepatic biliary system.

Associations

Patients with a history of ulcerative colitis, hepatolithiasis, choledochal cyst or sclerosing cholangitis are at increased risk of developing the disease. It is estimated that a longstanding history of sclerosing cholangitis increases the risk of developing biliary tract cancer by 20-fold compared with the normal population. In addition, liver fluke infestations in the Far East are also associated with cholangiocarcinoma. *Opisthorchis viverrini* infestation is important in Thailand, Laos and western Malaysia. These parasites induce DNA changes and mutations through production of carcinogens and free radicals, which stimulate cellular proliferation in the intrahepatic bile ducts and can ultimately lead to invasive cancer.

Clinical features

Biliary tract cancers tend to be slow-growing tumours that invade locally and metastasise to local lymph nodes. Distant metastases to the peritoneal cavity, liver and lung do occur. Jaundice is the most common presenting feature. Abdominal pain, early satiety and weight loss are also commonly seen. On examination, jaundice is evident, cachexia often noticeable and a palpable gall bladder is present if the obstruction is in the distal common bile duct (Courvoisier's sign).

Investigations

Biochemical investigations will confirm the presence of obstructive jaundice (elevated bilirubin, alkaline phosphatase and gamma-glutamyl transferase). The tumour marker CA19-9 may also be elevated. Non-invasive studies such as ultrasound and CT scanning define the level of biliary obstruction, the locoregional extent of disease and the presence of metastases (Fig. 63.37). For proximal tumours, percutaneous transhepatic cholangiography is the most useful modality. This outlines the anatomy of the tumour and the intrahepatic biliary system. In addition, it allows percutaneous biliary drainage, and samples can be obtained for cytology to confirm the diagnosis. For distal tumours, an ERCP is preferred as an endobiliary stent can be placed across the obstructing lesion. Again, cytology or biopsies can be taken for diagnosis.

Treatment

The treatment depends on the site and extent of disease. Most patients are inoperable, but 10–15% are suitable for surgical resection, which offers the only hope for long-term survival. Depending on the site of disease, resection may involve partial hepatectomy and reconstruction of the biliary tree. The perioperative mortality rate is now less than 5%. Distal common duct tumours may require a pancreaticoduodenectomy. Overall, the median survival is 18 months, with 20% of patients surviving 5 years post resection. Survival appears to be better for distal tumours compared with those involving the upper third of the biliary tree. Adjuvant chemotherapy or radiotherapy has a limited role and is not considered standard therapy.

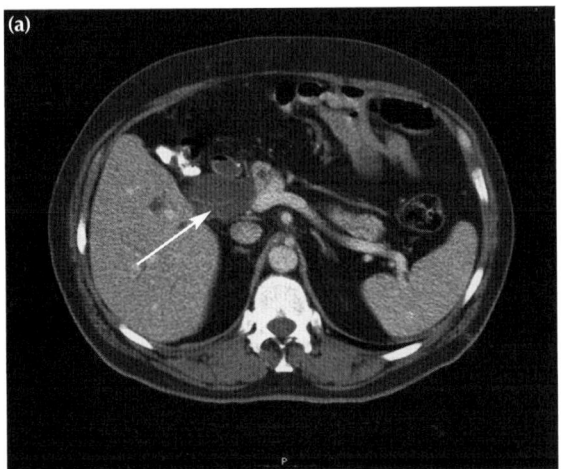

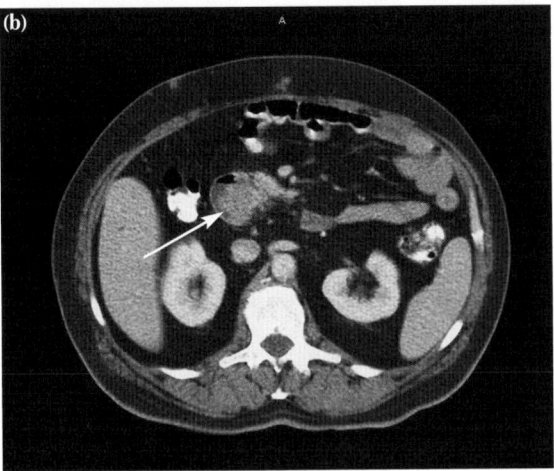

Figure 63.37 Computerised tomography scan demonstrating a distal common bile duct tumour with biliary obstruction (a; arrow) and duodenal infiltration (b; arrow).

Carcinoma of the gall bladder

Incidence

This is a rare disease, but extremely variable by geographical region and racial/ethnic groups. The highest incidence is in Chileans, American Indians and in parts of northern India, where it accounts for as much as 9.1% of all biliary tract disease. In western practice, gall bladder cancer accounts for less than 1% of new cancer diagnoses. The patients are usually older, in their sixties or seventies. The aetiology is unclear, but there may be an association with preexisting gallstone disease. Calcification of the gall bladder is associated with cancer (see Fig. 63.4, p. 1113) in 10–25% cases. Infection may promote the development of cancer as the risk of carcinoma in typhoid carriers is significantly increased (Summary box 63.10).

Summary box 63.10

Gall bladder cancer

- Rare
- Presents as for benign biliary disease (gallstones)
- Diagnosis by ultrasound and CT scanning
- Excision in less than 10% – remainder palliative treatment
- Prognosis poor – 95% mortality in 1 year

Pathology

The majority of cases are adenocarcinoma (90%). Grossly, carcinomas are difficult to differentiate from chronic cholecystitis; the tumour is most commonly nodular and infiltrative, with thickening of the gall bladder wall, often extending to the whole gall bladder. The tumour spreads by direct extension into the liver, seeding of the peritoneal cavity and involvement of the perihilar lymphatics and neural plexuses. At the time of presentation, the majority of tumours are advanced.

Clinical features

Patients may be asymptomatic at the time of diagnosis. If symptoms are present, they are usually indistinguishable from benign gall bladder disease such as biliary colic or cholecystitis, particularly in the older patient. Jaundice and anorexia are late features. A palpable mass is a late sign.

Investigation

Laboratory findings may be consistent with biliary obstruction or non-specific findings such as anaemia, leucocytosis, mild elevation in transaminases and increased erythrocyte sedimentation rate (ESR) or C-reactive protein (CRP). The level of serum CA19-9 is elevated in 80% of patients. The diagnosis is made on ultrasonography and defined by a multidetector row CT scan, with a percutaneous biopsy confirming the histological diagnosis. In selected patients, laparoscopy is useful in staging the disease, as it can detect peritoneal or liver metastases that would preclude further surgical resection.

Treatment and prognosis

Occasionally, the diagnosis is made by histological examination of a gall bladder removed for 'benign' gallstone disease. For early-stage disease confined to the mucosa or muscle of the gall bladder, no further treatment is indicated. However, for transmural disease, a radical *en bloc* resection of the gall bladder fossa and surrounding liver along with the regional lymph nodes should be performed. The disease has a very poor prognosis with the median survival less than 6 months and a 5-year survival of 5%. The value of adjuvant therapy is unproven.

FURTHER READING

Blumgart, L.H. and Fong, Y. (eds) (2000) *Surgery of the Liver and Biliary Tract*, 3rd edn. W.B. Saunders, London.

Carter, D.C., Russell, R.C.G., Pitt, H.A. and Bismuth, H. (eds) (1996) *Rob and Smith's Operative Surgery: Hepatobiliary and Pancreatic Surgery*. Chapman & Hall, London.

Poston, G.J. and Blumgart, L.H. (eds) (2002) *Surgical Management of Hepatobiliary and Pancreatic Diseases*. Informa Healthcare, London.

Sherlock, S. and Dooley, J. (eds) (2001) *Diseases of the Liver and Biliary System*, 11th edn. Blackwell Publishing, Oxford.

CHAPTER 63 | THE GALL BLADDER AND BILE DUCTS

CHAPTER
64

The pancreas

ANATOMY AND PHYSIOLOGY

Anatomy

The name 'pancreas' is derived from the Greek 'pan' (all) and 'kreas' (flesh). For a long time, its glandular function was not understood, and it was thought to act as a cushion for the stomach. The pancreas is situated in the retroperitoneum. It is divided into a head, which occupies 30% of the gland by mass, and a body and tail, which together constitute 70%. The head lies within the curve of the duodenum, overlying the body of the second lumbar vertebra and the vena cava. The aorta and the superior mesenteric vessels lie behind the neck of the gland. Coming off the side of the pancreatic head and passing to the left and behind the superior mesenteric vein is the uncinate process of the pancreas. Behind the neck of the pancreas, near its upper border, the superior mesenteric vein joins the splenic vein to form the portal vein (Figs 64.1 and 64.2). The tip of the pancreatic tail extends up to the splenic hilum.

The pancreas weighs approximately 80 g. Of this, 80–90% is composed of exocrine acinar tissue, which is organised into lobules. The main pancreatic duct branches into interlobular and intralobular ducts, ductules and, finally, acini. The main duct is lined by columnar epithelium, which becomes cuboidal in the ductules. Acinar cells are clumped around a central lumen, which communicates with the duct system. Clusters of endocrine cells, known as islets of Langerhans, are distributed throughout the pancreas. Islet cells consist of differing cell types: 75% are B cells (producing insulin); 20% are A cells (producing glucagon); and the remainder are D cells (producing somatostatin) and a small number of pancreatic polypeptide cells. Within an islet, the B cells form an inner core surrounded by the other cells. Capillaries draining the islet cells drain into the portal vein, forming a pancreatic portal system.

There are nine key processes that occur during pancreatic embryogenesis (Table 64.1). Malrotation of the ventral bud in the fifth week results in an annular pancreas, while the mode of

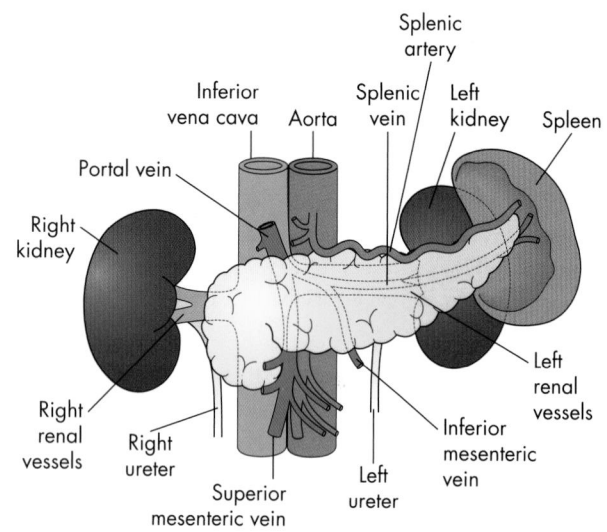

Figure 64.1 The posterior relations of the pancreas.

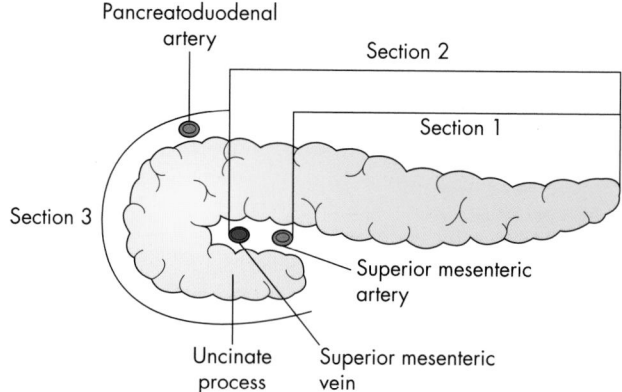

Figure 64.2 Transverse section of the pancreas. Section 1, body and tail of pancreas; section 2, neck of pancreas; section 3, head of pancreas. Note the position of the uncinate process behind the vessels.

Paul Langerhans, 1847–1888, Professor of Pathological Anatomy, Freiberg, Germany, described the islets in 1869.

Table 64.1 Steps in the development of the pancreas

1	Day 26	Dorsal pancreatic duct arises from the dorsal side of the duodenum
2	Day 32	Ventral bud arises from the base of the hepatic diverticulum
3	Day 37	Contact occurs between the two buds. Fusion by the end of week 6
4	Week 6	Ventral bud the produces the head and uncinate process
5	Week 6	Ducts fuse
6	Week 6	Ventral duct and distal portion of the dorsal duct form the main duct (duct of Wirsung)
7	Week 6	Proximal dorsal duct forms the duct of Santorini
8	Month 3	Acini appear
9	Months 3–4	Islets of Langerhans appear and become biologically active

ductule fusion in the seventh week produces the various possible ductular patterns. Between the 12th and 40th weeks of fetal life, the pancreas differentiates into exocrine and endocrine elements. The primitive ducts and their ductules are responsible for the lobular arrangement of the pancreas. Congenital anomalies of the pancreas are varied and arise during the early phase of development (Summary box 64.1). The anatomy of the pancreatic duct is variable as a result of the primordial bud development. The dorsal duct is expressed in a variable manner in the adult, as outlined in Figure 64.3. Approximately 10% of patients will have a significant flow from the main duct through the accessory papilla. The anatomy of the main duodenal papilla, also known as the ampulla of Vater, is also variable (Fig. 64.4). The outlet of each duct is protected by a complex sphincter mechanism (sphincter of Oddi) (Fig. 64.5).

Summary box 64.1

Anomalies of the pancreas

- Aplasia
- Hypoplasia
- Hyperplasia
- Hypertrophy
- Dysplasia
- Variations and anomalies of the ducts[a]
    Pancreas divisum
    Rotational anomalies
- Annular pancreas[a]
- Pancreatic gall bladder
- Polycystic disease[a]
- Congenital pancreatic cysts, cystic fibrosis[a] von Hippel–Lindau syndrome
- Ectopic pancreatic tissue, accessory pancreas[a]
- Vascular anomalies
- Choledochal cysts[a]
- Horseshoe pancreas

[a] The more frequent anomalies encountered in surgical practice.

Johann Georg Wirsung, ?–1643, Professor of Anatomy, Padua, Italy, described the pancreatic duct in 1642.

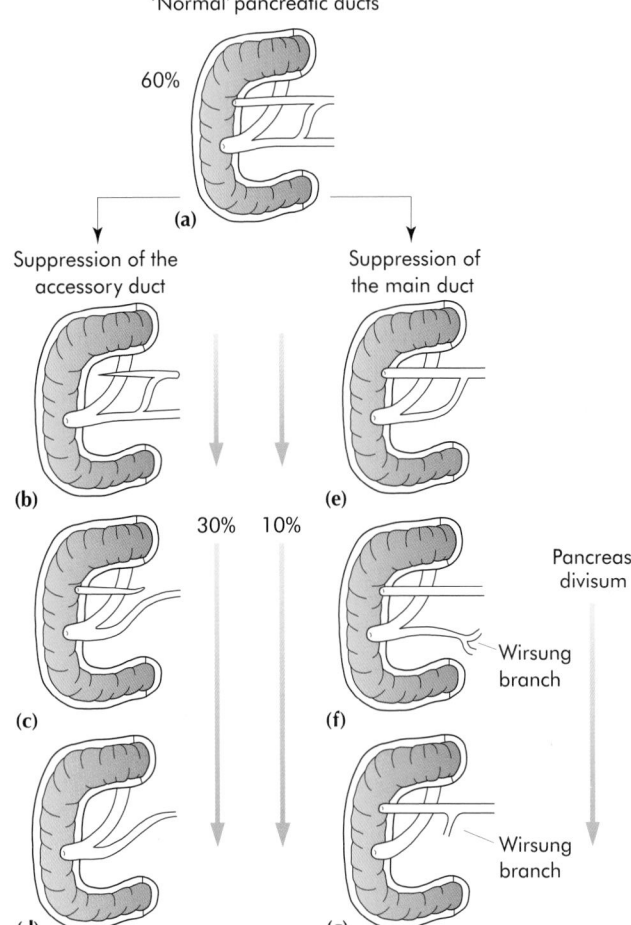

'Normal' pancreatic ducts

60%

(a)

Suppression of the accessory duct

Suppression of the main duct

(b)

(e)

30% 10%

(c)

Pancreas divisum

Wirsung branch

(f)

(d)

Wirsung branch

(g)

Figure 64.3 Variations in the pancreatic ducts. (a) The usual configuration. (b–d) Progressive suppression of the accessory duct (30%). (e–g) Progressive suppression of the main duct (10%). (f) Pancreas divisum – the ventral duct drains only the uncinate process.

Physiology

In response to a meal, the pancreas secretes digestive enzymes in an alkaline (pH 8.4) bicarbonate-rich fluid. Spontaneous secretion is minimal; the hormone secretin, which is released from the duodenal mucosa, evokes a bicarbonate-rich fluid. Cholecystokinin (CCK) (synonym: pancreozymin) is released from the duodenal mucosa in response to food. CCK is responsible for enzyme release. Vagal stimulation increases the volume of secretion. Protein is synthesised at a greater rate (per gram of tissue) in the pancreas than in any other tissue, with the possible exception of the lactating mammary gland. About 90% of this protein is exported from the acinar cells as a variety of digestive enzymes. Approximately 6–20 g of digestive enzymes enters the duodenum each day. Nascent proteins are synthesised as preproteins and undergo modification in a sequence of steps. The proteins move from the rough endothelial endoplasmic reticulum to the Golgi complex, where lysosomes and mature zymogen storage granules containing proteases are stored, and then to the ductal surface of the cell, from which they

Camillo Golgi, 1844–1926, Professor of Anatomy and Histology at Pavia, and later at Sienna, Italy.

CHAPTER 64 | THE PANCREAS

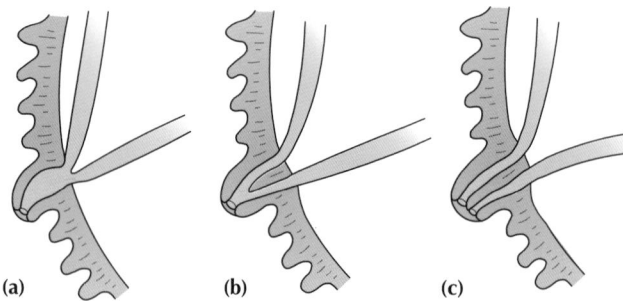

Figure 64.4 Variations in the relation of the common bile duct and main pancreatic duct at the main duodenal papilla. In (a), there is a common channel with no sphincter mechanism protecting flow between the ducts. In (b), there is a partial common channel, while in (c), there is separation of the two channels. Gallstone pancreatitis is more likely with (a) and (b).

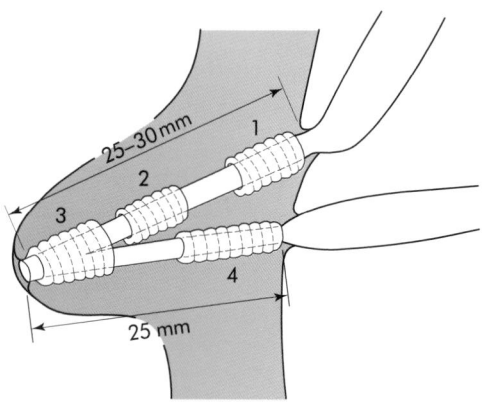

Figure 64.5 The complexity of the sphincter of Oddi. (1) Superior choledochal sphincter; (2) inferior choledochal sphincter; (3) ampullary sphincter; (4) pancreatic sphincter.

are extruded by exocytosis. During this phase, the proteolytic enzymes are in an inactive form, the maintenance of which is important in preventing pancreatitis.

INVESTIGATIONS (TABLE 64.2)

Estimation of pancreatic enzymes in body fluids

When the pancreas is damaged, enzymes such as amylase, lipase, trypsin, elastase and chymotrypsin are released into the serum. Measurement of serum amylase is the most widely used test of

Table 64.2 Investigation of the pancreas

Serum enzyme levels
Pancreatic function tests
Morphology
 Ultrasound scan
 Computerised tomography
 Magnetic resonance imaging
 Endoscopic retrograde cholangiopancreatography
 Endoscopic ultrasound
 Plain radiography
  Chest
  Upper abdomen

pancreatic damage. The serum amylase rises within a few hours of pancreatic damage and declines over the next 4–8 days. A markedly elevated serum level is highly suspicious but not diagnostic of acute pancreatitis. Urinary amylase and amylase–creatinine clearance ratios add little to diagnostic accuracy. If confirmation of the diagnosis is required, computerised tomography (CT) of the pancreas is of greater value (Summary box 64.2).

> **Summary box 64.2**
>
> **Causes of raised serum amylase level other than acute pancreatitis**
>
> - Upper gastrointestinal tract perforation
> - Mesenteric infarction
> - Torsion of an intra-abdominal viscus
> - Retroperitoneal haematoma
> - Ectopic pregnancy
> - Macroamylasaemia
> - Renal failure
> - Salivary gland inflammation

Pancreatic function tests

Pancreatic exocrine function can be assessed by directly measuring pancreatic secretion in response to a standardised stimulus. The stimulus to secretion can be physiological, e.g. ingestion of a test meal, as in the Lundh test, or pharmacological, e.g. intravenous injection of a hormone such as secretin or CCK. Duodenal intubation has to be performed with a triple-lumen tube so that the gastric and duodenal juices can be aspirated, and a non-absorbable marker such as polyethylene glycol is used to assess the completeness of the aspiration. The nitroblue tetrazolium–*para*-aminobenzoic acid (NBT–PABA) test provides an indirect measure of pancreatic function. The substance is administered orally and degraded in the gut by a pancreatic enzyme, and the breakdown product (PABA) is absorbed by the intestine and excreted in the urine; its urinary level is measured. The Pancreolauryl test works on a similar principle. These tests are cheap and easy to perform, but are non-specific, especially following gastrectomy and in conditions that may alter gastrointestinal transit and intestinal absorptive capacity. Measurement of the enzyme elastase in stool is simple and specific. Absence indicates exocrine insufficiency.

Imaging investigations

Ultrasonography

Ultrasonography is the initial investigation of choice in patients with jaundice to determine whether or not the bile duct is dilated, the coexistence of gallstones or gross disease within the liver such as metastases. It may also define the presence or absence of a mass in the pancreas (Fig. 64.6). However, obesity and overlying bowel gas often make interpretation of the pancreas itself unsatisfactory.

Computerised tomography

Most significant pathologies within the pancreas can be diagnosed on high-quality CT scans, with three-dimensional reconstruction if necessary. A specific pancreatic protocol should be followed. An initial unenhanced CT scan is essential to determine the presence of calcification within the pancreas and gall bladder (Fig. 64.7). Then, following rapid injection of intravenous contrast, scanning

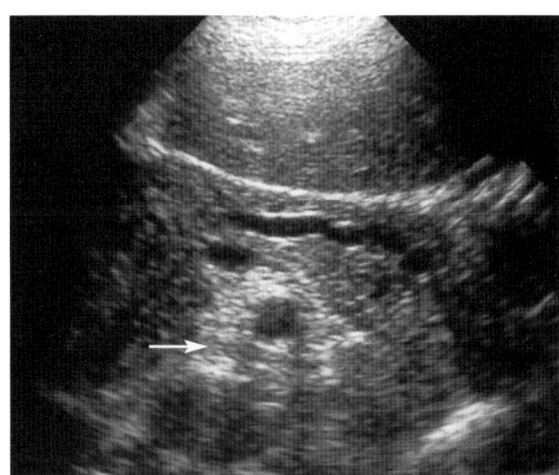

Figure 64.6 Ultrasound scan showing a mass in the head of the pancreas (marked by an arrow) and a dilated pancreatic duct in the body of the gland (courtesy of Dr Alison McLean).

(a)

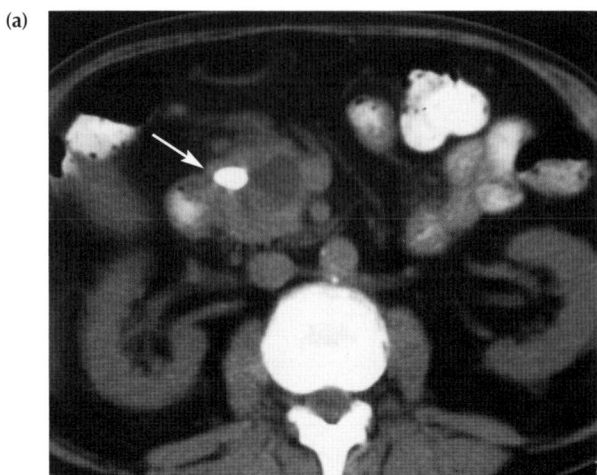

(b)

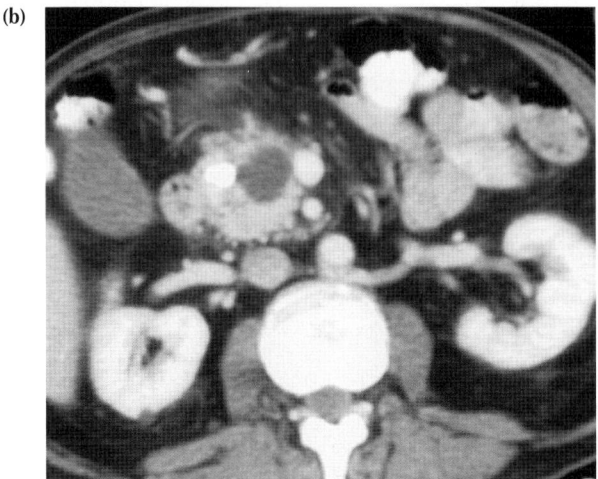

Figure 64.7 (a) Unenhanced computerised tomography scan of a man with chronic pancreatitis, showing a focus of calcification (marked by an arrow) in the head of the pancreas and a cyst adjacent to that. Oral contrast has been administered. (b) The same area after injection of intravenous contrast.

is performed in the arterial and venous phases. The stomach and duodenum should be outlined with water and distended to define the duodenal loop. Pancreatic carcinomas of 1–2 cm in size can usually be demonstrated whether in the head, body or tail of the pancreas (Fig. 64.8). Endocrine tumours are also well imaged on CT (Fig. 64.9). In patients with pancreatitis, necrotic areas within the gland can be identified by the absence of contrast enhancement on CT. Inflammatory collections and pseudocysts can be seen (Fig. 64.10). CT-guided drainage is helpful in the treatment of pancreatic collections, cysts and pseudocysts, and facilitates percutaneous fine-needle or Trucut biopsy.

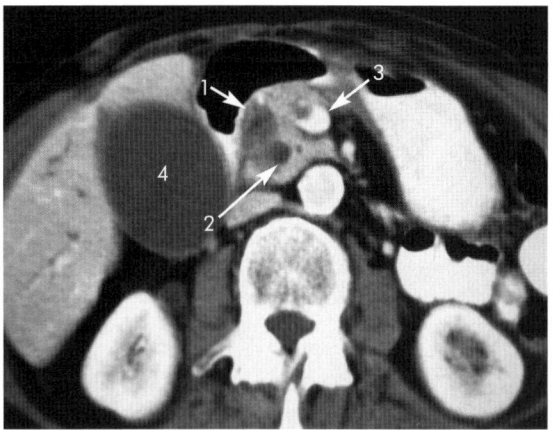

Figure 64.8 Contrast-enhanced computerised tomography scan of a patient with a carcinoma of the pancreatic head. The main bulk of the tumour lies inferior to the section shown here. The dilated bile duct (1) and main pancreatic duct (2) can be seen, with tumour infiltration around them. There is a thrombus in the superior mesenteric vein (3). The gall bladder is distended (4).

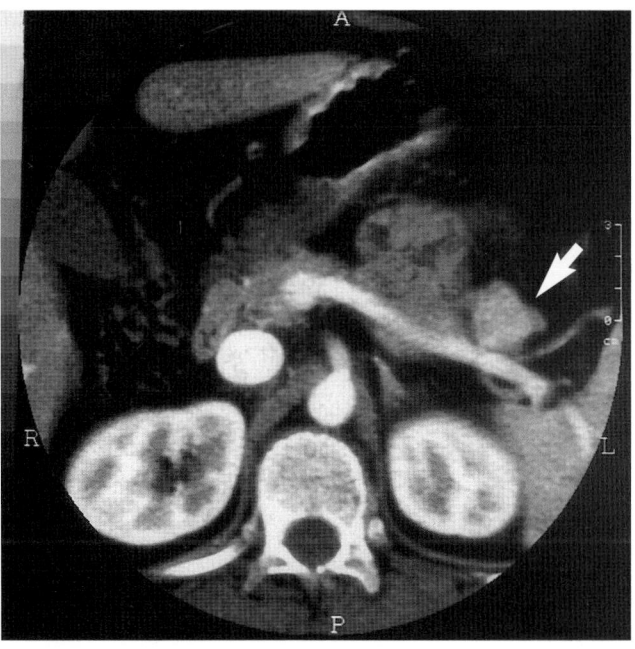

Figure 64.9 Computerised tomography scan showing a hypervascular insulinoma adjacent to the splenic vein. Local excision of the tumour resulted in normoglycaemia.

CHAPTER 64 | THE PANCREAS

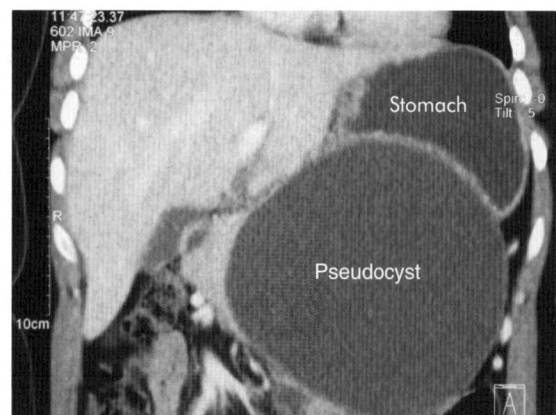

Figure 64.10 Computerised tomography scan of a large pseudocyst in relation to the body and tail of the pancreas.

Magnetic resonance imaging

With magnetic resonance imaging (MRI), the pancreas can be clearly identified, and clear images of the bile duct and the pancreatic duct, together with fluid collections, can be defined. Magnetic resonance cholangiography and pancreatography (MRCP) may well replace *diagnostic* endoscopic cholangiography and pancreatography (ERCP) as it is non-invasive and less expensive (Fig. 64.11). Using the technique in conjunction with intravenous injection of secretin, emptying of the pancreatic duct can be demonstrated to show the absence or presence of obstruction.

Endoscopic retrograde cholangiopancreatography

ERCP is performed using a side-viewing fibreoptic duodeno-scope. The ampulla of Vater is intubated, and contrast is injected into the biliary and pancreatic ducts to display the anatomy radiologically (Fig. 64.12). In pancreatic carcinoma, the main

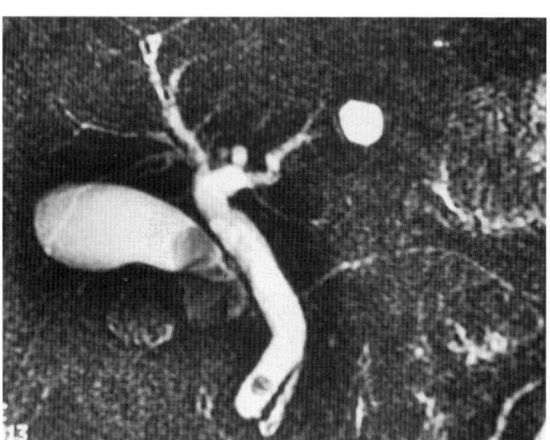

Figure 64.11 Magnetic resonance cholangiopancreatography in a patient with obstructive jaundice. A dilated common bile duct was seen on ultrasound, but no pancreatic mass lesion was visible on computerised tomography. The bile duct and the main pancreatic duct are seen very well, with a stone visible in the lower part of the bile duct and another in the neck of the gall bladder.

Abraham Vater, 1684–1751, Professor of Anatomy and Botany, and later of Pathology and Therapeutics, Wittenberg, Germany.

pancreatic duct may be narrowed or completely obstructed at the site of the tumour (Fig. 64.13), or the distal bile duct may be narrowed. Concurrent narrowing of both ducts results in the so called double duct sign (Fig. 64.14). Changes seen in chronic pancreatitis include the presence of pancreatic duct strictures, dilatation of the main pancreatic duct with stones,

(a)

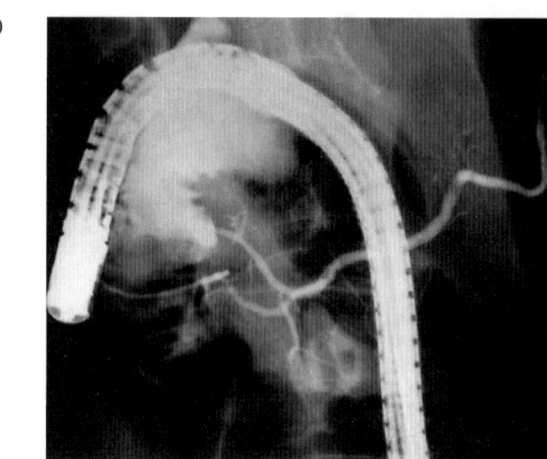

(b)

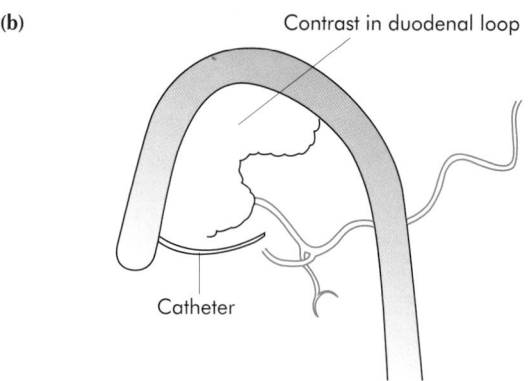

Figure 64.12 (a) Endoscopic retrograde cholangiopancreatography: normal pancreatic duct with filling of the duct of Santorini from the duct of Wirsung. (b) Diagrammatic outline of (a).

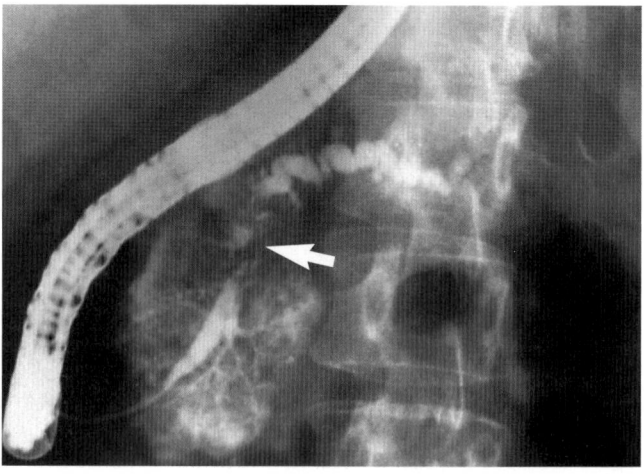

Figure 64.13 Endoscopic retrograde cholangiopancreatography: pancreatic carcinoma. Irregular stricture of the main pancreatic duct (marked by an arrow) with dilatation distal to the obstruction.

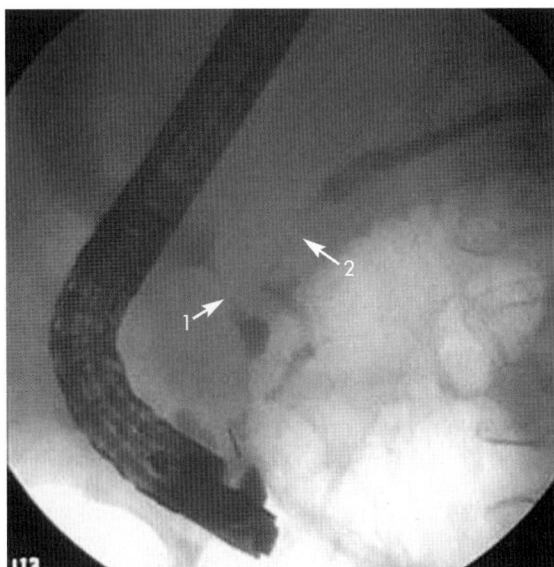

Figure 64.14 Endoscopic retrograde cholangiopancreatography depicting a malignant stricture in the lower part of the common bile duct and in the main pancreatic duct, an appearance referred to as the double duct sign (courtesy of Dr George Webster).

abnormalities of pancreatic duct side branches, communication of the pancreatic duct with cysts, and bile duct strictures (Figs 64.15–64.17). A plain radiograph before contrast studies is essential to delineate calcification (Fig. 64.18). In addition to imaging, bile or pancreatic fluid and brushings from duct strictures can yield cells that confirm the suspected diagnosis of carcinoma (Fig. 64.19). ERCP also allows the placement of biliary and pancreatic stents.

Endoscopic ultrasound

Endoscopic ultrasound (EUS) is performed using a special endoscope that has a high-frequency ultrasonic transducer at its tip. When the endoscope is in the lumen of the stomach or duodenum, the pancreas and its surrounding vasculature and lymph nodes can be assessed (Fig. 64.20). This is particularly useful in identifying small tumours that may not show up well on CT or MRI, and in demonstrating the relationship of a pancreatic tumour to major vessels nearby. EUS can clarify the relationship of a neuroendocrine tumour to the main pancreatic duct (important if

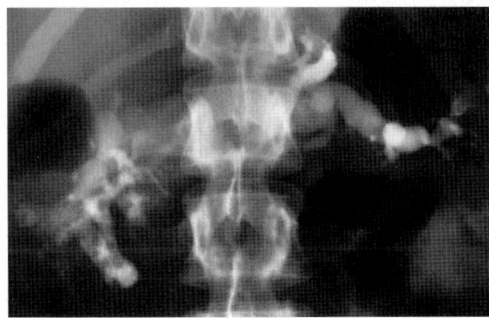

Figure 64.15 Endoscopic retrograde cholangiopancreatography: chronic pancreatitis. Most of the opacities lie within the duct system and are stones. Gross dilatation of ducts in the body and tail are due to obstructions by stones in the head of the pancreas.

(a)

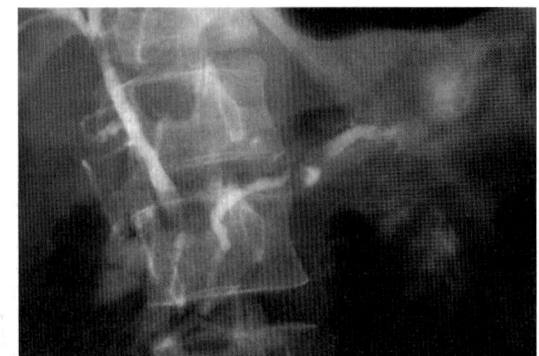

(b)

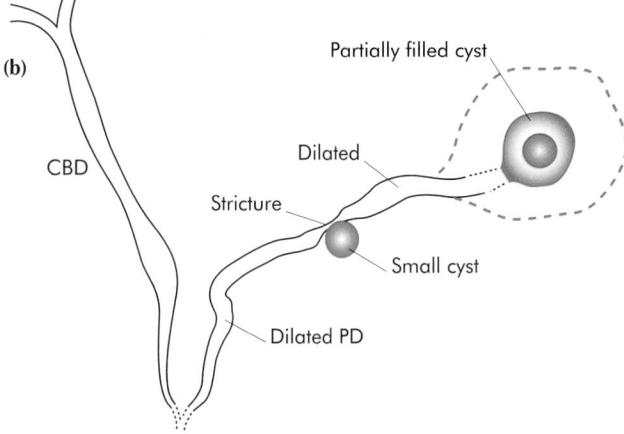

Figure 64.16 (a) Endoscopic retrograde cholangiopancreatography: relapsing acute pancreatitis. Normal biliary tree. Pancreatogram shows stricture of the main duct in the body with distal dilatation and cyst formation. (b) Diagrammatic outline of (a). CBD, common bile duct; PD, pancreatic duct.

enucleation is being considered). It helps to distinguish cystic tumours from pseudocysts. Transduodenal or transgastric fine-needle aspiration (FNA) or Trucut biopsy performed under EUS guidance avoids spillage of tumour cells into the peritoneal cavity.

CONGENITAL ABNORMALITIES

Cystic fibrosis

This is inherited as an autosomal recessive condition. It occurs most frequently among Caucasians, in whom it is the most common inherited disorder (incidence of 1:2000 live births in the UK). Cystic fibrosis (CF) develops when there is a mutation in the *CFTR* (cystic fibrosis transmembrane conductance regulator) gene on chromosome 7. This gene creates a cell membrane protein that helps to control the movement of chloride across the cell membrane.

CF is a multisystem disorder of exocrine glands that affects the lungs, intestines, pancreas and liver, and is characterised by elevated sodium and chloride ion concentrations in sweat. The mother may notice that the child is salty when kissed.

Most of the organ damage is due to blockage of the narrow passages by thickened secretions. Chronic pulmonary disease arises from plugging of bronchi and bronchioles. CF is the most common cause of chronic lung disease among children in

CHAPTER 64 | THE PANCREAS

(a)

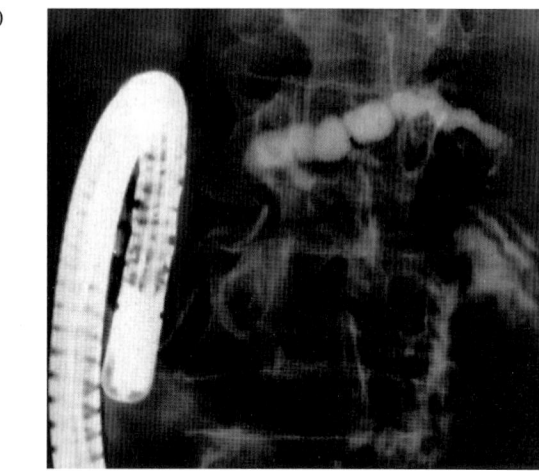

(b)

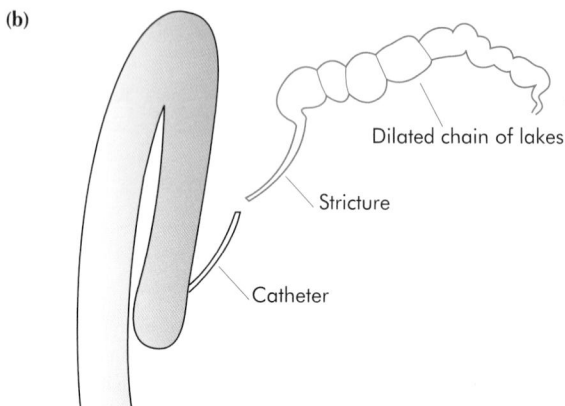

Dilated chain of lakes

Stricture

Catheter

Figure 64.17 (a) Endoscopic retrograde cholangiopancreatography: chronic pancreatitis. Long stricture of the pancreatic duct in the head; distal pancreatic duct shows sacculation with intervening short strictures, 'chain of lakes'. (b) Diagrammatic outline of (a).

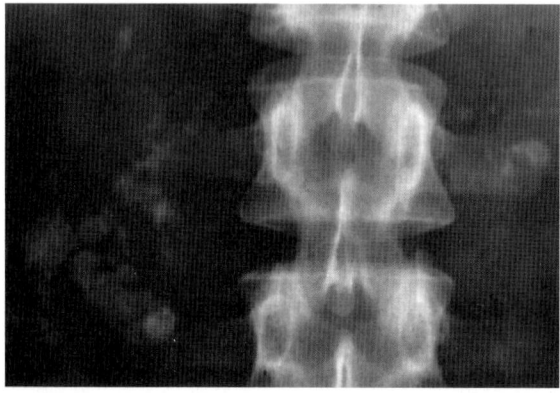

Figure 64.18 Plain abdominal radiograph: chronic pancreatitis. Multiple opacities can be seen in the region of the head and tail of the pancreas.

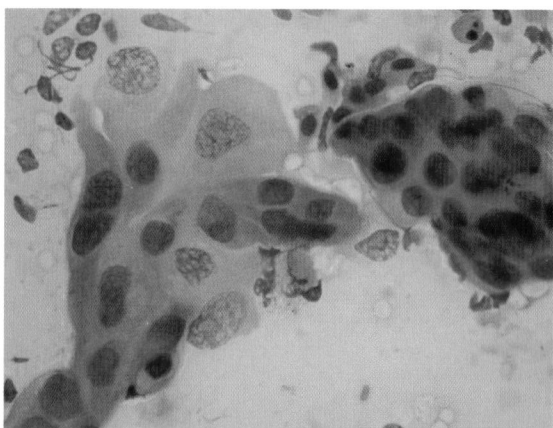

Figure 64.19 A group of adenocarcinoma cells identified in pancreatic juice collected at the time of endoscopic retrograde cholangiopancreatography (courtesy of Professor Roger Feakins).

(a)

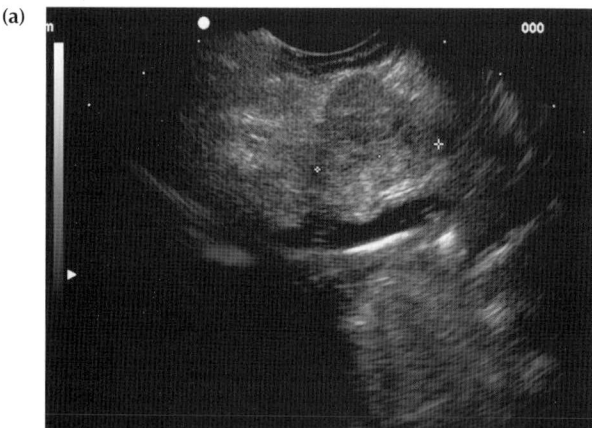

(b)

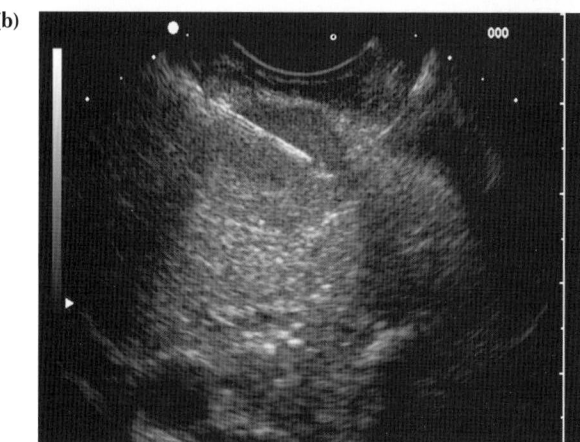

Figure 64.20 (a) Carcinoma of the pancreatic head as seen on endoscopic ultrasound (EUS). (b) Aspiration biopsy carried out under EUS guidance: needle seen entering the tumour (courtesy of Dr Peter Fairclough).

developed countries. Cor pulmonale may develop later. At birth, the meconium may set in a sticky mass and produce intestinal obstruction (meconium ileus) (see Chapter 6). Secretions precipitate in the lumen of the pancreatic duct causing blockage, which results in duct ectasia and fatty replacement of exocrine acinar tissue. Pancreatic exocrine insufficiency leads to fat malabsorp-

tion. Steatorrhoea is usually present from birth, resulting in stools that are bulky, oily and offensive. The islets of Langerhans usually appear normal, but diabetes mellitus can occur in older patients. The liver may become cirrhotic as a result of bile duct plugging, and signs of portal hypertension may appear. Infertility is common, due to the absence of the vas deferens in men and thick cervical mucus in women.

Outside the newborn period, the earliest clinical signs of CF are poor growth, poor appetite, rancid greasy stools, abdominal distension, chronic respiratory disease and finger clubbing. The appearance of secondary sexual characteristics may be delayed. The diagnosis can be made by genetic testing (which may be part of prenatal or newborn screening) and by the sweat test. Levels of sodium and chloride ions in the sweat above 90 mmol l^{-1} confirm the diagnosis.

Treatment is aimed at control of the secondary consequences of the disease. Pulmonary function is preserved with aggressive physiotherapy and antibiotics. Malabsorption is treated by administration of oral pancreatic enzyme preparations. The diet should be low in fat but contain added salt to replace the high losses in the sweat. With early diagnosis and optimal treatment, patients in the western world can now expect to survive to their mid-thirties. Those with end-stage lung disease may be considered for lung transplantation. Heterozygous carriers of the various gene mutations are asymptomatic but can be identified by DNA analysis. There is a suggestion that such patients may develop pancreatitis later in life.

Annular pancreas

This is the result of failure of complete rotation of the ventral pancreatic bud during development, so that a ring of pancreatic tissue surrounds the second or third part of the duodenum. It is most often seen in association with congenital duodenal stenosis or atresia and is therefore more prevalent in children with Down's syndrome. Duodenal obstruction typically causes vomiting in the neonate (see Chapter 6). The usual treatment is bypass (duodenoduodenostomy). The disease may occur in later life as one of the causes of pancreatitis, in which case resection of the head of the pancreas is preferable to lesser procedures.

Ectopic pancreas

Islands of ectopic pancreatic tissue can be found in the submucosa in parts of the stomach, duodenum or small intestine (including Meckel's diverticulum), the gall bladder, adjoining the pancreas, in the hilum of the spleen and within the liver. Ectopic pancreas may also be found in the wall of an alimentary tract duplication cyst (see Chapter 6).

Congenital cystic disease of the pancreas

This sometimes accompanies congenital disease of the kidneys and liver, and occurs as part of the von Hippel–Lindau syndrome.

INJURIES TO THE PANCREAS

External injury

Presentation and management

The pancreas, thanks to its somewhat protected location in the retroperitoneum, is not frequently damaged in blunt abdominal

trauma. If there is damage to the pancreas, it is often concomitant with injuries to other viscera, especially the liver, the spleen and the duodenum. Occasionally, a forceful blow to the epigastrium may crush the body of the pancreas against the vertebral column. Penetrating trauma to the upper abdomen or the back carries a higher chance of pancreatic injury. Pancreatic injuries may range from a contusion or laceration of the parenchyma *without* duct disruption to major parenchymal destruction *with* duct disruption (sometimes complete transection) and, rarely, massive destruction of the pancreatic head. The most important factor that determines treatment is whether the pancreatic duct has been disrupted.

Blunt pancreatic trauma usually presents with epigastric pain, which may be minor at first, with the progressive development of more severe pain due to the sequelae of leakage of pancreatic fluid into the surrounding tissues. The clinical presentation can be quite deceptive; careful serial assessments and a high index of suspicion are required. A rise in serum amylase occurs in most cases. A CT scan of the pancreas will delineate the damage that has occurred to the pancreas (Fig. 64.21). If there is doubt about duct disruption, an urgent ERCP should be sought. MRCP may also provide the answer, but the images can be difficult to interpret. Support with intravenous fluids and a nil by mouth regimen should be instituted while these investigations are performed. There is no need to rush to a laparotomy if the patient is haemodynamically stable, without peritonitis. It is preferable to manage conservatively at first, investigate and, once the extent of the damage has been ascertained, undertake appropriate action. Operation is indicated only if there is disruption of the main pancreatic duct; in almost all other cases, the patient will recover with conservative management.

In penetrating injuries, especially if other organs are injured and the patient's condition is unstable, there is a greater need to perform an urgent surgical exploration. Assessment of pancreatic damage and duct disruption at the time of surgery can be difficult, because the bruising associated with the retroperitoneal damage

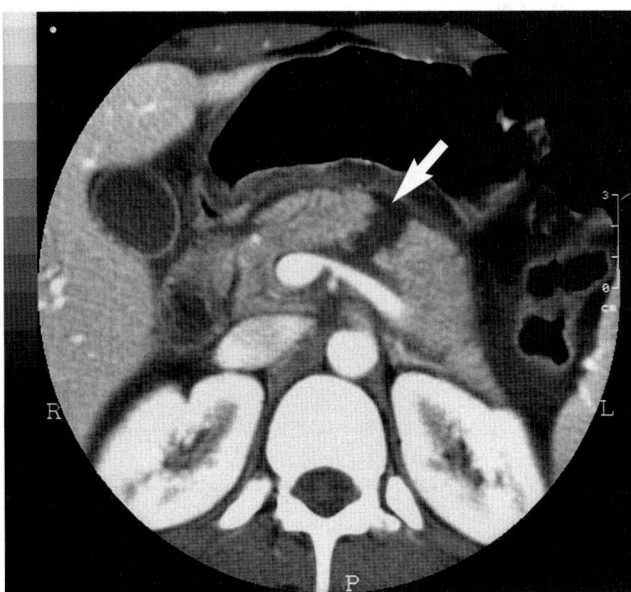

Figure 64.21 Computerised tomography scan showing a pancreatic transection due to a bicycle handlebar injury. A distal pancreatectomy was performed.

prevents clear visualisation of the pancreas. A patient and thorough examination of the gland should be carried out. Haemostasis and closed drainage is adequate for minor parenchymal injuries. If the gland is transected in the body or tail, a distal pancreatectomy should be performed, with or without splenectomy. If damage is purely confined to the head of the pancreas, haemostasis and external drainage is normally effective. In the emergency setting, in an unstable patient with concomitant injuries, a surgeon unaccustomed to pancreatic surgery should refrain from trying to ascertain whether the duct in the pancreatic head is intact or embarking on a major resection. However, if there is severe injury to the pancreatic head and duodenum, then a pancreatoduodenectomy may be necessary (Summary box 64.3).

Summary box 64.3

External injury to the pancreas

- Other organs are likely to be injured
- It is important to ascertain whether the pancreatic duct has been disrupted
- CT and ERCP are the most useful tests
- Surgery is indicated if the main pancreatic duct is disrupted

---

Prognosis

The most common cause of death in the immediate period is bleeding, usually from associated injuries. Once the acute phase has passed, the mortality and morbidity related to the pancreatic injury itself are treatable, with a complete return to normal activity the usual outcome.

Persistent drain output occurs in up to a third of patients (see the section on pancreatic fistulae below). Sometimes, in the aftermath of trauma that has been treated conservatively, duct stricturing develops, leading to recurrent episodes of pancreatitis. The appropriate treatment in such cases is resection of the tail of the pancreas up to the site of duct disruption.

Also, a pancreatic pseudocyst may develop. If the main duct is intact, the cyst can be aspirated percutaneously in the first instance; it may not be necessary to undertake a cystgastrostomy. If the cyst develops in the presence of complete disruption of the pancreas, there is no alternative but to undertake a distal resection or, occasionally, a pancreatojejunostomy with a Roux-en-Y loop. In a patient who presents with a peripancreatic cyst and a history of previous blunt abdominal trauma, do not assume that it is a post-traumatic pseudocyst. The possibility of a cystic neoplasm should be considered and excluded.

Iatrogenic injury

This can occur in several ways:

- Injury to the tail of the pancreas during splenectomy, resulting in a pancreatic fistula.
- Injury to the accessory pancreatic duct (Santorini), which is the main duct in 7% of patients, during Billroth II gastrectomy.

Cesar Roux, 1857–1934, Professor of Surgery and Gynaecology, Lausanne, Switzerland, described this method of forming a jejunal conduit in 1908.
Giandomenico (Giovanni Domenico) Santorini, 1681–1737, Professor of Anatomy and Medicine, Venice, Italy.
Christian Albert Theodor Billroth, 1829–1894, Professor of Surgery, Vienna, Austria.

A pancreatogram performed by cannulating the duct at the time of discovery of such an injury will demonstrate whether it is safe to ligate and divide the duct. If no alternative drainage duct can be demonstrated, then the duct should be reanastomosed to the duodenum.

- Enucleation of islet cell tumours of the pancreas can result in fistulae.
- Duodenal or ampullary bleeding following sphincterotomy. This injury may require duodenotomy to control the bleeding.

Pancreatic fistula

Pancreatic fistula usually follows operative trauma to the gland or may occur as a complication of acute or chronic pancreatitis. It is important to define the site of the fistula and the epithelial structure with which it communicates (e.g. externally to skin, or internally to bowel). If there is uncertainty about whether the fluid issuing from a drain site or a wound is pancreatic, measurement of the amylase content will be diagnostic.

Management includes correction of metabolic and electrolyte disturbances and adequate drainage of the fistula into a stoma bag with protection of the skin. Investigation of the cause of the fistula is required as the underlying cause must be treated before the fistula will close. Frequently, the cause is related to obstruction within the pancreatic duct, which can be overcome by the insertion of a stent or catheter endoscopically into the pancreatic duct. While waiting for closure of the fistula, the patient should be given parenteral or nasojejunal nutritional support (as opposed to nasogastric or oral feeding; the rationale is that parenteral or nasojejunal feeding reduces the volume of pancreatic secretion). The use of octreotide will also suppress pancreatic secretion (Summary box 64.4).

Summary box 64.4

Management of pancreatic fistulae

Tests
- Measure amylase level in fluid
- Determine the anatomy of the fistula
- Check whether the main pancreatic duct is blocked or disrupted

Measures
- Correct fluid and electrolyte imbalances
- Protect the skin
- Drain adequately
- Parenteral or nasojejunal feeding
- Octreotide to suppress secretion
- Relieve pancreatic duct obstruction if possible (ERCP and stent)
- Treat underlying cause

PANCREATITIS

Pancreatitis is inflammation of the gland parenchyma of the pancreas. For clinical purposes, it is useful to divide pancreatitis into acute, which presents as an emergency, and chronic, which is a prolonged and frequently lifelong disorder resulting from the development of fibrosis within the pancreas. It is probable that acute pancreatitis is but a phase of chronic pancreatitis.

Acute pancreatitis is defined as an acute condition presenting with abdominal pain and is usually associated with raised pancreatic enzyme levels in the blood or urine as a result of pancreatic inflammation. Acute pancreatitis may recur.

The underlying mechanism of injury in pancreatitis is thought to be premature activation of pancreatic enzymes within the pancreas, leading to a process of autodigestion. Anything that injures the acinar cell and impairs the secretion of zymogen granules, or damages the duct epithelium and thus delays enzymatic secretion, can trigger acute pancreatitis. Once cellular injury has been initiated, the inflammatory process can lead to pancreatic oedema, haemorrhage and, eventually, necrosis. As inflammatory mediators are released into the circulation, systemic complications can arise, such as haemodynamic instability, bacteraemia (due to translocation of gut flora), acute respiratory distress syndrome and pleural effusions, gastrointestinal haemorrhage, renal failure and disseminated intravascular coagulation (DIC).

Acute pancreatitis may be categorised as mild or severe. *Mild acute pancreatitis* is characterised by interstitial oedema of the gland and minimal organ dysfunction. Eighty per cent of patients will have a mild attack of pancreatitis, the mortality from which is around 1%. *Severe acute pancreatitis* is characterised by pancreatic necrosis, a severe systemic inflammatory response and often multi-organ failure. In those who have a severe attack of pancreatitis, the mortality varies from 20% to 50%. About one-third of deaths occur in the early phase of the attack, from multiple organ failure, while deaths occurring after the first week of onset are due to septic complications.

Chronic pancreatitis is defined as a continuing inflammatory disease of the pancreas characterised by irreversible morphological change typically causing pain and/or permanent loss of function. Many patients with chronic pancreatitis have exacerbations, but the condition may be completely painless.

Acute pancreatitis

Incidence

Acute pancreatitis accounts for 3% of all cases of abdominal pain among patients admitted to hospital in the UK. The hospital admission rate for acute pancreatitis is 9.8 per year per 100 000 population in the UK, although worldwide, the annual incidence may range from 5 to 50 per 100 000. The disease may occur at any age, with a peak in young men and older women.

Aetiology

The two major causes of acute pancreatitis are biliary calculi, which occur in 50–70% of patients, and alcohol abuse, which accounts for 25% of cases. Gallstone pancreatitis is thought to be triggered by the passage of gallstones down the common bile duct. If the biliary and pancreatic ducts join to share a common channel before ending at the ampulla, then obstruction of this passage may lead to reflux of bile or activated pancreatic enzymes into the pancreatic duct. Patients who have small gallstones and a wide cystic duct may be at a higher risk of passing stones. The proposed mechanisms for alcoholic pancreatitis include the effects of diet, malnutrition, direct toxicity of alcohol, concomitant tobacco smoking, hypersecretion, duct obstruction or reflux, and hyperlipidaemia. The remaining cases may be due to rare causes or be idiopathic (Summary box 64.5).

Summary box 64.5

Possible causes of acute pancreatitis

- Gallstones
- Alcoholism
- Post ERCP
- Abdominal trauma
- Following biliary, upper gastrointestinal or cardiothoracic surgery
- Ampullary tumour
- Drugs (corticosteroids, azathioprine, asparaginase, valproic acid, thiazides, oestrogens)
- Hyperparathyroidism
- Hypercalcaemia
- Pancreas divisum
- Autoimmune pancreatitis
- Hereditary pancreatitis
- Viral infections (mumps, coxsackie B)
- Malnutrition
- Scorpion bite
- Idiopathic

Among patients who undergo ERCP, 1–3% develop pancreatitis, probably as a consequence of duct disruption and enzyme extravasation. Patients with sphincter of Oddi dysfunction or a history of recurrent pancreatitis, and those who undergo sphincterotomy or balloon dilatation of the sphincter, carry a higher risk of developing post-ERCP pancreatitis. Patients who have undergone upper abdominal or cardiothoracic surgery may develop acute pancreatitis in the postoperative phase, as may those who have suffered blunt abdominal trauma.

Hereditary pancreatitis is a rare familial condition associated with mutations of the cationic trypsinogen gene. Patients have a tendency to suffer acute pancreatitis while in their teens, progress to chronic pancreatitis in the next two decades and have a high risk (possibly up to 40%) of developing pancreatic cancer by the age of 70 years.

Occasionally, tumours at the ampulla of Vater may cause acute pancreatitis. It is important to check the serum calcium level, a fasting lipid profile, autoimmune markers and viral titres in patients with so called idiopathic acute pancreatitis. It is equally important to take a detailed drug history and remember the association of corticosteroids, azathioprine, asparaginase and valproic acid with acute pancreatitis. A careful search for the aetiology must be made in all cases, and no more than 20% of cases should fall into the idiopathic category (Summary box 64.6).

Summary box 64.6

Aetiology of acute pancreatitis

- It is essential to establish the aetiology
- Investigate thoroughly before labelling it as 'idiopathic'
- After the acute episode resolves, remember further management of the underlying aetiology
- If the aetiology is gallstones, cholecystectomy is desirable during the same admission

---

Ruggero Oddi, **1845–1906**, Physiologist, Perugia, Italy.

Clinical presentation

Pain is the cardinal symptom. It characteristically develops quickly, reaching maximum intensity within minutes rather than hours and persists for hours or even days. The pain is frequently severe, constant and refractory to the usual doses of analgesics. Pain is usually experienced first in the epigastrium but may be localised to either upper quadrant or felt diffusely throughout the abdomen. There is radiation to the back in about 50% of patients, and some patients may gain relief by sitting or leaning forwards. The suddenness of onset may simulate a perforated peptic ulcer, while biliary colic or acute cholecystitis can be mimicked if the pain is maximal in the right upper quadrant. Radiation to the chest can simulate myocardial infarction, pneumonia or pleuritic pain. In fact, acute pancreatitis can mimic most causes of the acute abdomen and should seldom be discounted in differential diagnosis.

Nausea, repeated vomiting and retching are usually marked accompaniments. The retching may persist despite the stomach being kept empty by nasogastric aspiration. Hiccoughs can be troublesome and may be due to gastric distension or irritation of the diaphragm.

On examination, the appearance may be that of a patient who is well or, at the other extreme, one who is gravely ill with profound shock, toxicity and confusion. Tachypnoea is common, tachycardia is usual, and hypotension may be present. The body temperature is often normal or even subnormal, but frequently rises as inflammation develops. Mild icterus can be caused by biliary obstruction in gallstone pancreatitis, and an acute swinging pyrexia suggests cholangitis. Bleeding into the fascial planes can produce bluish discolouration of the flanks (Grey Turner's sign) or umbilicus (Cullen's sign). Neither sign is pathognomonic of acute pancreatitis; Cullen's sign was first described in association with rupture of an ectopic pregnancy. Subcutaneous fat necrosis may produce small, red, tender nodules on the skin of the legs.

Abdominal examination may reveal distension due to ileus or, more rarely, ascites with shifting dullness. A mass can develop in the epigastrium due to inflammation. There is usually muscle guarding in the upper abdomen, although marked rigidity is unusual. A pleural effusion is present in 10–20% of patients. Pulmonary oedema and pneumonitis are also described and may give rise to the differential diagnosis of pneumonia or myocardial infarction. The patient may be confused and exhibit the signs of metabolic derangement together with hypoxaemia.

Investigations

Typically, the diagnosis is made on the basis of the clinical presentation and an elevated serum amylase level. A serum amylase level three to four times above normal is indicative of the disease. A normal serum amylase level does not exclude acute pancreatitis, particularly if the patient has presented a few days later. If the serum lipase level can be checked, it provides a slightly more sensitive and specific test than amylase. If there is doubt, and other causes of acute abdomen have to be excluded, contrast-enhanced CT is probably the best single imaging investigation (see below) (Summary box 64.7).

Summary box 64.7

Investigations in acute pancreatitis should be aimed at answering three questions:

- Is a diagnosis of acute pancreatitis correct?
- How severe is the attack?
- What is the aetiology?

Assessment of severity

On account of the difference in outcome between patients with mild and severe disease, it is important to define that group of patients who will develop severe pancreatitis. Various scoring systems have been introduced, such as the Ranson and Glasgow scoring systems (Table 64.3). The APACHE II scoring system, used in intensive care units, can also be applied. A severe attack

---

Table 64.3 Scoring systems to predict the severity of acute pancreatitis: in both systems, disease is classified as severe when three or more factors are present

Ranson score	Glasgow scale
On admission	**On admission**
Age > 55 years	Age > 55 years
White blood cell count > $16 \times 10^9 \, l^{-1}$	White blood cell count > $15 \times 10^9 \, l^{-1}$
Blood glucose > 10 mmol l^{-1}	Blood glucose > 10 mmol l^{-1} (no history of diabetes)
LDH > 700 units l^{-1}	Serum urea > 16 mmol l^{-1} (no response to intravenous fluids)
AST > 250 Sigma Frankel units per cent	Arterial oxygen saturation (PaO_2) < 8 kPa (60 mmHg)
Within 48 hours	**Within 48 hours**
Blood urea nitrogen rise > 5 mg%	Serum calcium < 2.0 mmol l^{-1}
Arterial oxygen saturation (PaO_2) < 8 kPa (60 mmHg)	Serum albumin < 32 g l^{-1}
Serum calcium < 2.0 mmol l^{-1}	LDH > 600 units l^{-1}
Base deficit > 4 mmol l^{-1}	AST/ALT > 600 units l^{-1}
Fluid sequestration > 6 litres	

AST, aspartate aminotransferase; ALT, alanine aminotransferase; LDH, lactate dehydrogenase; PaO_2, arterial oxygen tension.

George Grey Turner, **1877–1951, Professor of Surgery, The University of Durham, Durham (1927–1934), and at the Postgraduate Medical School, Hammersmith, London, England (1934–1945).**
Thomas Stephen Cullen, **1868–1953, Professor of Gynecology, The Johns Hopkins University, Baltimore, MD, USA.**
John H.C. Ranson, **Professor of Surgery, The New York University School of Medicine, New York, NY, USA.**

may be heralded by an initial clinical impression of a very ill patient and an APACHE II score above 8. At 48 hours after the onset of symptoms, a Glasgow score of 3 or more, a C-reactive protein level greater than 150 mg l^{-1} and a worsening clinical state with sepsis or persisting organ failure indicate a severe attack. Severity stratification should be performed in all patients within 48 hours of diagnosis. Patients with a body mass index over 30 are at higher risk of developing complications.

Imaging

Plain erect chest and abdominal radiographs are not diagnostic of acute pancreatitis, but are useful in the differential diagnosis. Non-specific findings in pancreatitis include a generalised or local ileus (sentinel loop), a colon cut-off sign and a renal halo sign. Occasionally, calcified gallstones or pancreatic calcification may be seen. A chest radiograph may show a pleural effusion and, in severe cases, a diffuse alveolar interstitial shadowing may suggest acute respiratory distress syndrome.

Ultrasound does not establish a diagnosis of acute pancreatitis. The swollen pancreas may be seen, but ultrasonography should be performed within 24 hours in *all* patients to detect gallstones as a potential cause, rule out acute cholecystitis as a differential diagnosis and determine whether the common bile duct is dilated.

CT is not necessary for all patients, particularly those deemed to have a mild attack on prognostic criteria. But a contrast-enhanced CT is indicated in the following situations:

- if there is diagnostic uncertainty;
- in patients with severe acute pancreatitis, to distinguish interstitial from necrotising pancreatitis (Fig. 64.22). In the first 72 hours, CT may underestimate the extent of necrosis. The severity of pancreatitis detected on CT may be staged according to the Balthazar criteria;

- in patients with organ failure, signs of sepsis or progressive clinical deterioration;
- when a localised complication is suspected, such as fluid collection, pseudocyst or a pseudoaneurysm.

Cross-sectional MRI can yield similar information to that obtained by CT. EUS and MRCP can help in detecting stones in the common bile duct and directly assessing the pancreatic parenchyma, but are not widely available. ERCP allows the identification and removal of stones in the common bile duct in gallstone pancreatitis. In patients with severe acute gallstone pancreatitis and signs of ongoing biliary obstruction and cholangitis, an urgent ERCP should be sought (see below).

The presentation is so variable that sometimes even an experienced clinician can be mistaken. While this is not desirable, occasionally the diagnosis is only made at laparotomy. The appearances at laparotomy are characteristic (Fig. 64.23).

Management

If after initial assessment a patient is considered to have a mild attack of pancreatitis, a conservative approach is indicated with intravenous fluid administration and frequent, but non-invasive, observation. A brief period of fasting may be sensible in a patient who is nauseated and in pain, but there is little physiological justification for keeping patients on a prolonged 'nil by mouth' regimen. Antibiotics are not indicated. Apart from analgesics and anti-emetics, no drugs or interventions are warranted, and CT scanning is unnecessary unless there is evidence of deterioration. However, if a stable patient meets the prognostic criteria for a severe attack of pancreatitis, then a more aggressive approach is

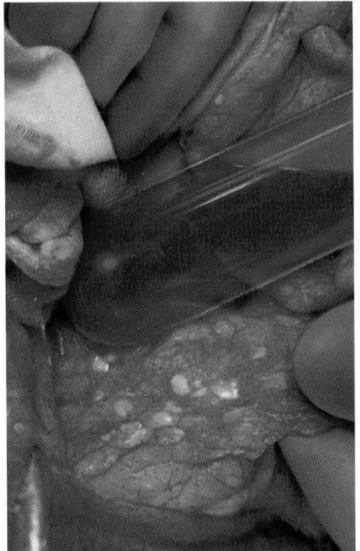

Figure 64.23 Widespread fat necrosis of the omentum. A test tube has been filled with blood-stained peritoneal fluid. This specimen was rich in amylase. Fat necroses are dull, opaque, yellow-white areas suggestive of drops of wax. They are most abundant in the vicinity of the pancreas, but are widespread in the greater omentum and the mesentery. At necropsy, they can sometimes be demonstrated beneath the pleura and pericardium, and even in the subsynovial fat of the knee joint. Fat necroses consist of small islands of saponification caused by the liberation of lipase, which splits into glycerol and fatty acids. Free fatty acids combine with calcium to form soaps (fatty necrosis) (courtesy of Dr G.D. Adhia, Mumbai, India).

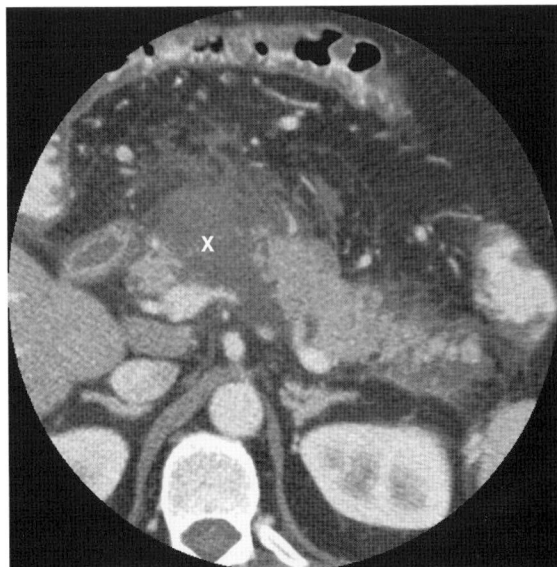

Figure 64.22 Contrast-enhanced computerised tomography scan showing acute necrotising pancreatitis. Note the area of reduced enhancement in the pancreas (marked **X**), the peripancreatic oedema and stranding of the fatty tissues (courtesy of Dr Niall Power).

Emil J. Balthazar, **Contemporary, Professor Emeritus, The Department of Radiology, The New York University, New York, NY, USA.**

CHAPTER 64 | THE PANCREAS

required, with the patient being admitted to a high-dependency or an intensive care unit and monitored invasively.

Patients with a severe attack should be admitted to an intensive care or high-dependency unit (Table 64.4). Adequate analgesia should be administered. Aggressive fluid resuscitation is important, guided by frequent measurement of vital signs, urine output and central venous pressure. Supplemental oxygen should be administered and serial arterial blood gas analysis performed. The haematocrit, clotting profile, blood glucose and serum levels of calcium and magnesium should be closely monitored.

A nasogastric tube is not essential but may be of value in patients with vomiting. Specific treatments such as aprotinin, somatostatin analogues, platelet-activating factor inhibitors and selective gut decontamination have failed to improve outcome in numerous clinical trials and should not be given. There are no data to support a practice of 'resting' the pancreas and feeding only by the parenteral or nasojejunal routes. If nutritional support is felt to be necessary, enteral nutrition (e.g. feeding via a nasogastric tube) is should be used.

There is some evidence to support the use of prophylactic antibiotics (intravenous cefuroxime, or imipenem, or ciprofloxacin plus metronidazole) in patients with severe acute pancreatitis for the prevention of local and other septic complications. The duration of antibiotic prophylaxis should not exceed 14 days. Additional antibiotic use should be guided by microbiological cultures.

If gallstones are the cause of an attack of predicted or proven severe pancreatitis, or if the patient has jaundice, cholangitis or a dilated common bile duct, urgent ERCP should be carried out within 72 hours of the onset of symptoms. There is evidence that sphincterotomy and clearance of the bile duct can reduce the incidence of infective complications in these patients. In patients with cholangitis, sphincterotomy should be carried out or a biliary stent placed to drain the duct. ERCP is an invasive procedure and carries a small risk of worsening the pancreatitis.

Systemic complications

Pancreatitis may involve all organ systems (Table 64.5) and place demands on the surgeon beyond his or her skills. Patients with systemic complications should be managed by a multidisciplinary team that includes intensive care specialists. When there is organ failure, appropriate supportive therapies may include inotropic support for haemodynamic instability, haemofiltration in the event of renal failure, ventilatory support for respiratory failure and correction of coagulopathies (including DIC). There is no role for surgery during the initial period of resuscitation and stabilisation; surgical intervention is contemplated only in the patient who deteriorates as a result of local complications following successful stabilisation.

Local complications and their management

Once the acute phase has been survived, usually by the end of the first week, and major organ failure is under control, then local complications become pre-eminent in the management of these patients. The course of the patient should be followed carefully and, if clinical resolution does not take place or signs of sepsis develop, a CT scan should be performed. It is important to be clear about the definitions. Certain terms are confusing, such as *phlegmon*, which may refer to an abscess or to an inflammatory mass in the pancreas. Local complications in pancreatic disease are serious and carry a significant mortality. The management approach is conservative on the whole, with surgery restricted to situations in which conservative management has failed.

Acute fluid collection

This occurs early in the course of acute pancreatitis and is located in or near the pancreas. The wall encompassing the collection is ill defined. The fluid is sterile, and most such collections resolve. No intervention is necessary unless a large collection causes symptoms or pressure effects, in which case it can be percutaneously aspirated under ultrasound or CT guidance. Transgastric drainage under EUS guidance is another option. An acute fluid collection that does not resolve can evolve into a pseudocyst or an abscess if it becomes infected.

Sterile and infected pancreatic necrosis

The term pancreatic necrosis refers to a diffuse or focal area of non-viable parenchyma that is typically associated with peripancreatic fat necrosis. Necrotic areas can be identified by an absence of contrast enhancement on CT. These are sterile to begin with, but can become subsequently infected, probably due to translocation of gut bacteria. Infected necrosis is associated with a mortality rate of up to 50%. Sterile necrotic material should not be drained or interfered with. But if the patient shows signs of sepsis, then one should determine whether the

---

Table 64.4 Early management of severe acute pancreatitis

Admission to HDU/ICU

Analgesia

Aggressive fluid rehydration

Oxygenation

Invasive monitoring of vital signs, central venous pressure, urine output, blood gases

Frequent monitoring of haematological and biochemical parameters (including liver and renal function, clotting, serum calcium, blood glucose)

Nasogastric drainage

Antibiotic prophylaxis can be considered (imipenem, cefuroxime)

CT scan essential if organ failure, clinical deterioration or signs of sepsis develop

ERCP within 72 hours for severe gallstone pancreatitis or signs of cholangitis

Supportive therapy for organ failure if it develops (inotropes, ventilatory support, haemofiltration, etc.)

If nutritional support is required, consider enteral (nasogastric) feeding

CT, computerised tomography; ERCP, endoscopic retrograde cholangiopancreatography; HDU, high-dependency unit; ICU, intensive care unit.

Table 64.5 Complications of acute pancreatitis

Systemic	Local
(*More common in the first week*)	(*Usually develop after the first week*)
Cardiovascular	Acute fluid collection
Shock	Sterile pancreatic necrosis
Arrhythmias	Infected pancreatic necrosis
Pulmonary	Pancreatic abscess
ARDS	Pseudocyst
Renal failure	Pancreatic ascites
Haematological	Pleural effusion
DIC	Portal/splenic vein thrombosis
Metabolic	Pseudoaneurysm
Hypocalcaemia	
Hyperglycaemia	
Hyperlipidaemia	
Gastrointestinal	
Ileus	
Neurological	
Visual disturbances	
Confusion, irritability	
Encephalopathy	
Miscellaneous	
Subcutaneous fat necrosis	
Arthralgia	

ARDS, acute respiratory distress syndrome; DIC, disseminated intravascular coagulation.

necrotic pancreas or the peripancreatic fluid is infected (Fig. 64.24). A CT scan should be performed and a needle passed into the area under CT guidance, choosing a path that does not traverse hollow viscera. This may be done under ultrasonographic guidance as well. If the aspirate is purulent, percutaneous drainage of the infected fluid should be carried out. The tube drain inserted should have the widest bore possible. The aspirate should be sent for microbiological assessment, and appropriate antibiotic therapy should be commenced as per the sensitivity report. The fluid can be quite viscous with particulate matter, and the drain may need regular flushing with full aseptic precautions. Often, repeated imaging and repeated insertion of drains is necessary.

If the sepsis worsens despite this, then a pancreatic necrosectomy should be considered. This is a challenging operation that carries a high morbidity and mortality, and is best carried out in a specialist unit. The overwhelming majority of patients with peripancreatic sepsis can be successfully treated by conservative means, and necrosectomy should be necessary in a very small proportion of patients. The surgical approach may be through a midline laparotomy, especially if the area involved is around the head of the gland. The duodenocolic and gastrocolic ligaments should be divided and the lesser sac opened. Thorough debridement of the dead tissue around the pancreas should be carried out. If the body and tail of the gland are primarily involved (Fig. 64.25), a retroperitoneal approach though a left flank incision may be more appropriate. The tissues are inevitably friable, and one should be careful not to precipitate excessive bleeding or inadvertently breach the bowel wall. Blunt dissection is preferable to sharp dissection. A feeding jejunostomy may be a useful adjunct to the procedure. If gallstones are the precipitating factor of the pancreatitis, a cholecystectomy should be included. Some prefer a minimally invasive approach to a formal laparotomy. A rigid laparoscope is inserted into the peripancreatic area through a retroperitoneal approach, and vigorous irrigation and suction is combined with a gradual nibbling away of the necrotic debris.

Once a necrosectomy has been completed, further necrotic tissue may form. There are several possible ways of dealing with this (listed below), none of which has been proved to be more effective than the others. The last two approaches make greater logistic demands as one is committed to a re-exploration every 48–72 hours.

- *Closed continuous lavage*: Tube drains are left in and the raw area flushed (Beger) (Fig. 64.26).
- *Closed drainage*: The incision is closed, but the cavity is packed with gauze-filled Penrose drains and closed suction drains. The Penrose drains are brought out through the flank and slowly pulled out and removed after 7 days.

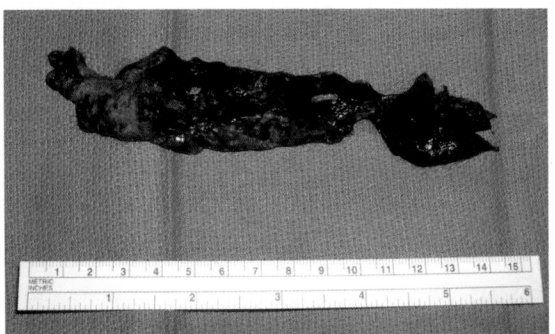

Figure 64.25 Necrotic body and tail of the pancreas removed as an intact specimen rather than piecemeal. The patient had suffered severe necrotising gallstone pancreatitis complicated by persistent pancreatic sepsis. Necrosectomy was carried out through a left flank retroperitoneal approach.

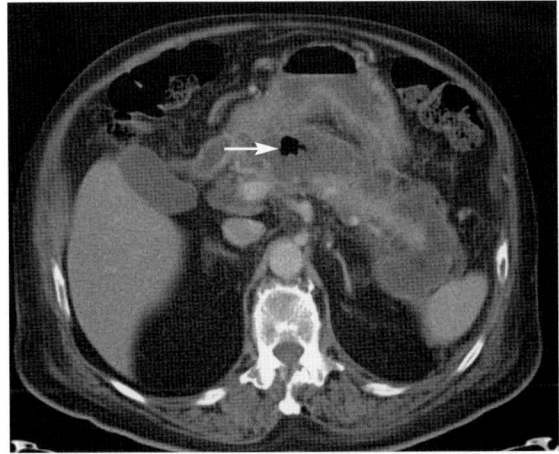

Figure 64.24 Infected pancreatic necrosis in an elderly patient. Note the areas of reduced enhancement in the pancreas and the peripancreatic fluid collection with pockets of gas within it (arrow). This resolved after percutaneous drainage and antibiotic therapy.

Hans Beger, **Contemporary, Emeritus Professor of Surgery, Ulm, Germany.**
Charles Bingham Penrose, **1862–1925, Professor of Gynecology, The University of Pennsylvania, Philadelphia, PA, USA.**

CHAPTER 64 | THE PANCREAS

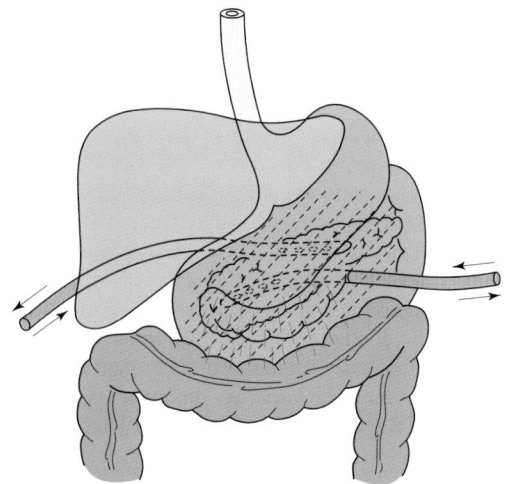

Figure 64.26 Continuous postoperative closed lavage of the lesser sac as advised by Beger. Lavage is carried out through several double-lumen and single-lumen catheters. Each time, 1 litre of saline is infused through and then drained over a period of hours, and the process is repeated.

- *Open packing*: The incision is left open, and the cavity is packed with the intention of returning to the operating room at regular intervals and repacking until there is a clean granulating cavity.
- *Closure and relaparotomy*: The incision is closed with drains with the intention of performing a series of planned relaparotomies every 48–72 hours until the raw area granulates (Bradley).

There is a sub-group of patients who respond initially to percutaneous treatment but then develop recurrent sepsis that requires repeated insertion of drains, and fail to thrive. Necrosectomy should be considered in these patients, but it can be a difficult judgement call.

Patients with peripancreatic sepsis are ill for long periods of time, and may require management in an intensive care unit. Nutritional support is essential. The parenteral and nasojejunal approaches are more popular (on the assumption that they rest the pancreas), although there is little evidence to show that nasogastric feeding, if tolerated, is harmful in any way.

Pancreatic abscess

This is a circumscribed intra-abdominal collection of pus, usually in proximity to the pancreas. It may be an acute fluid collection or a pseudocyst that has become infected. The principles of diagnosis and management are as outlined above for infected pancreatic necrosis. Percutaneous drainage with the widest possible drains placed under imaging guidance is the treatment, along with appropriate antibiotics and supportive care. Repeated scans may be required depending on the progress of the patient, and drains may need to be flushed, repositioned or reinserted. Very occasionally, open drainage of the abscess may be necessary.

Edward Bradley III, **Contemporary, Professor, The Department of Clinical Sciences, Florida State University College of Medicine, FL, USA.**

Pancreatic ascites

This is a chronic, generalised, peritoneal, enzyme-rich effusion usually associated with pancreatic duct disruption. Paracentesis will reveal turbid fluid with a high amylase level. Adequate drainage with wide-bore drains placed under imaging guidance is essential. Measures that can be taken to suppress pancreatic secretion include parenteral or nasojejunal feeding and administration of octreotide. An ERCP may allow demonstration of the duct disruption and placement of a pancreatic stent.

Pancreatic effusion

This is an encapsulated collection of fluid in the pleural cavity, arising as a consequence of acute pancreatitis. Concomitant pancreatic ascites may be present, or there may be a communication with an intra-abdominal collection. Percutaneous drainage under imaging guidance is necessary.

Haemorrhage

Bleeding may occur into the gut, into the retroperitoneum or into the peritoneal cavity. Possible causes include bleeding into a pseudocyst cavity, diffuse bleeding from a large raw surface, or a pseudoaneurysm. The last is a false aneurysm of a major peripancreatic vessel confined as a clot by the surrounding tissues and often associated with infection. Recurrent bleeding is common, often culminating in fatal haemorrhage. CT, angiography or MR angiography helps to make the diagnosis. Treatment involves embolisation or surgery.

Portal or splenic vein thrombosis

This may often develop silently and is identified on a CT scan. A marked rise in the platelet count should raise suspicions. In the context of acute pancreatitis, treatment is usually conservative. The patient should be screened for pro-coagulant tendencies. If varices or other manifestations of portal hypertension develop, they will require treatment, such as endoscopic injection or banding, β-blockade, etc. Thrombocytosis may mandate the use of aspirin or other anti-platelet drugs for a period. Systemic anticoagulation, if instituted early in the process, may achieve recanalisation of the vein, but it is not routinely used as it carries considerable risks in a patient with on-going pancreatitis.

Pseudocyst

A pseudocyst is a collection of amylase-rich fluid enclosed in a wall of fibrous or granulation tissue. Pseudocysts typically arise following an attack of acute pancreatitis, but can develop in chronic pancreatitis or after pancreatic trauma. Formation of a pseudocyst requires 4 weeks or more from the onset of acute pancreatitis (Fig. 64.27; see also Fig. 64.10, p. 1134). They are often single but, occasionally, patients will develop multiple pseudocysts. If carefully investigated, more than half will be found to have a communication with the main pancreatic duct.

A pseudocyst is usually identified on ultrasound or a CT scan. It is important to differentiate a pseudocyst from an acute fluid collection or an abscess; the clinical scenario and the radiological appearances should allow that distinction to be made. Occasionally, a cystic neoplasm may be confused with a chronic pseudocyst. EUS and aspiration of the cyst fluid is very useful in such a situation. The fluid should be sent for

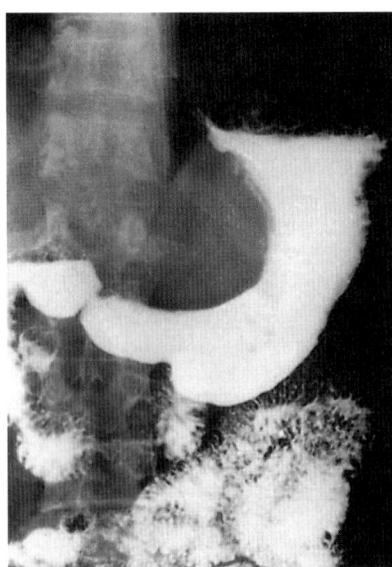

Figure 64.27 Barium meal. Pseudocyst displacing the stomach (courtesy of Professor V.K. Kapoor, Lucknow, India).

measurement of carcinoembryonic antigen (CEA) levels, amylase levels and cytology. Fluid from a pseudocyst typically has a low CEA level, and levels above 400 ng ml⁻¹ are suggestive of a mucinous neoplasm. Pseudocyst fluid usually has a high amylase level, but that is not diagnostic, as a tumour that communicates with the duct system may yield similar findings. Cytology typically reveals inflammatory cells in pseudocyst fluid. If there is no access to EUS, then percutaneous FNA is acceptable (just aspiration, *not* percutaneous insertion of a drain). ERCP and MRCP may demonstrate communication of the cyst with the pancreatic duct system, demonstrate ductal anomalies or diagnose chronic pancreatitis and thus help in planning treatment.

Pseudocysts will resolve spontaneously in most instances, but complications can develop (Table 64.6). Pseudocysts that are thick-walled or large (over 6 cm in diameter), have lasted for a long time (over 12 weeks) or have arisen in the context of chronic pancreatitis are less likely to resolve spontaneously, but these

Table 64.6 Possible complications of a pancreatic pseudocyst

Process	Outcomes
Infection	Abscess
	Systemic sepsis
Rupture	
Into the gut	Gastrointestinal bleeding
	Internal fistula
Into the peritoneum	Peritonitis
Enlargement	
Pressure effects	Obstructive jaundice from biliary compression
	Bowel obstruction
Pain	
Erosion into a vessel	Haemorrhage into the cyst
	Haemoperitoneum

factors are not specific indications for intervention. Therapeutic interventions are advised only if the pseudocyst causes symptoms, if complications develop or a distinction has to be made between a pseudocyst and a tumour.

There are three possible approaches to draining a pseudocyst: percutaneous, endoscopic and surgical. Percutaneous drainage to the exterior under radiological guidance should be avoided. It carries a very high likelihood of recurrence. Moreover, it is not advisable unless one is absolutely certain that the cyst is not neoplastic and that it has no communication with the pancreatic duct (or else a pancreatico-cutaneous fistula will develop). A percutaneous transgastric cystgastrostomy can be done under imaging guidance, and a double-pigtail drain placed with one end in the cyst cavity and the other end in the gastric lumen. This requires specialist expertise but, in experienced hands, the recurrence rates are no more than 15%. Endoscopic drainage usually involves puncture of the cyst through the stomach or duodenal wall under EUS guidance, and placement of a tube drain with one end in the cyst cavity and the other end in the gastric lumen. The success rates depend on operator expertise. Occasionally, ERCP and placement of a pancreatic stent across the ampulla may help to drain a pseudocyst that is in communication with the duct. Surgical drainage involves internally draining the cyst into the gastric or jejunal lumen (Fig. 64.28). Recurrence rates should be no more than 5%, and this still remains the standard against which the evolving radiological and endoscopic approaches are measured. Pseudocysts that have developed complications are best managed surgically (Summary box 64.8).

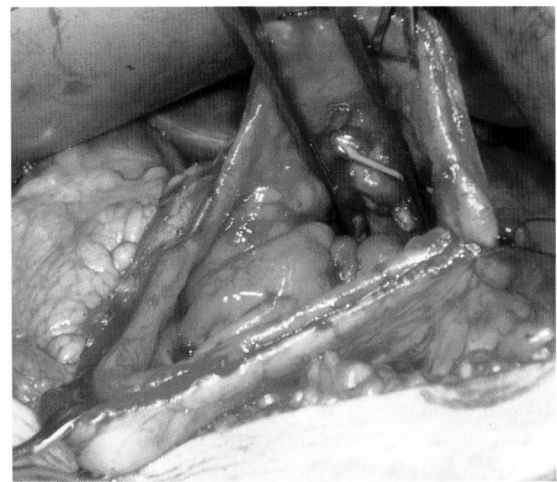

Figure 64.28 Cystgastrostomy for the pancreatic pseudocyst shown in Figure 64.10 (p. 1134). The anterior wall of the stomach has been opened and the edges drawn back, held by Babcock's forceps. An opening has been made through the posterior wall of the stomach into the pseudocyst, and the tips of the dissecting forceps are in the cavity of the pseudocyst, which is lined by slough and granulation tissue. The tip of a nasogastric tube is visible. A running stitch will next be placed along the edges of this opening, suturing the full thickness of the posterior gastric wall to the capsule of the pseudocyst.

William Wayne Babcock, **1872–1963, Surgeon, Philadelphia, PA, USA.**

> **Summary box 64.8**
>
> **Distinguishing a pseudocyst from a cystic neoplasm**
>
> - History
> - Appearance on CT and ultrasound
> - FNA of fluid, preferably under EUS guidance
>   CEA (high level in mucinous tumours)
>   Amylase (level usually high in pseudocysts, but
>   occasionally in tumours)
>   Cytology

Outcomes and follow-up of acute pancreatitis

The overall mortality from acute pancreatitis has remained at 10–15% over the past 20 years. There is a clear responsibility before the patient is discharged to determine the aetiology of the attack of pancreatitis, and the causes listed in Summary box 64.5 (p. 1139) must be looked for and excluded. Failure to remove a predisposing factor could lead to a second attack of pancreatitis, which could be fatal. A proportion of patients in the idiopathic group who suffer repeated attacks may prove to have biliary microlithiasis, which can be identified only by bile sampling at ERCP or by endoscopic ultrasound. In a patient who has gallstone pancreatitis, the gallstones should be removed as soon as the patient is fit to undergo surgery and, preferably, before discharge from hospital.

Chronic pancreatitis

Chronic pancreatitis is a chronic inflammatory disease in which there is irreversible progressive destruction of pancreatic tissue. Its clinical course is characterised by severe pain and, in the later stages, exocrine and endocrine pancreatic insufficiency. In the early stages of its evolution, it is frequently complicated by attacks of acute pancreatitis, which are responsible for the recurrent pain that may be the only clinical symptom. The incidence of chronic pancreatitis in several European, North American and Japanese studies ranges from 2 to 10 new cases per 100 000 population per year, with a prevalence of around 13 cases per 100 000, although there are suspicions that the prevalence is actually higher. The disease occurs more frequently in men (male to female ratio of 4:1), and the mean age of onset is about 40 years.

Aetiology and pathology

High alcohol consumption is the most frequent cause of chronic pancreatitis, accounting for 60–70% of cases, but only 5–10% of people with alcoholism develop chronic pancreatitis. The exact mechanism of how alcohol causes chronic inflammation in these patients is unclear; genetic and metabolic factors may be at play.

Other causes include pancreatic duct obstruction resulting from stricture formation after trauma, after acute pancreatitis or even occlusion of the duct by pancreatic cancer. Congenital abnormalities, such as pancreas divisum and annular pancreas, if associated with papillary stenosis, are rare causes of chronic pancreatitis.

Hereditary pancreatitis, CF, infantile malnutrition and a large unexplained idiopathic group make up the remainder. Hereditary pancreatitis is an autosomal dominant disorder with an 80% penetrance, associated with mutations in the cationic trypsinogen gene on chromosome 7. Idiopathic chronic pancreatitis accounts for approximately 30% of cases and has been subdivided into early-onset and late-onset forms. Among the idiopathic group are those who live in warm climates such as Kerala in southern India and appear to have a high incidence of pancreatitis. In this case, the pancreatitis begins at a young age and is associated with a high incidence of diabetes mellitus and stone formation. The importance of hereditary pancreatitis and pancreatitis occurring at a young age is that there is a markedly increased risk of developing pancreatic cancer, particularly if the patient smokes tobacco. Hyperlipidaemia and hypercalcaemia can lead to chronic pancreatitis.

Autoimmune pancreatitis has been described relatively recently. Features include diffuse enlargement of the pancreas, diffuse and irregular narrowing of the main pancreatic duct and a possible association with other autoimmune diseases. The changes may be confused with neoplasia. Autoantibodies may be present, and the immunoglobulin (Ig)G4 concentrations are elevated.

At the onset of the disease when symptoms have developed, the pancreas may appear normal. Later, the pancreas enlarges and becomes hard as a result of fibrosis. The ducts become distorted and dilated with areas of both stricture formation and ectasia. Calcified stones weighing from a few milligrams to 200 mg may form within the ducts. The ducts may become occluded with a gelatinous proteinaceous fluid and debris, and inflammatory cysts may form. Histologically, the lesions affect the lobules, producing ductular metaplasia and atrophy of acini, hyperplasia of duct epithelium and interlobular fibrosis.

Clinical features

Pain is the outstanding symptom in the majority of patients. The site of pain depends to some extent on the main focus of the disease. If the disease is mainly in the head of the pancreas, then epigastric and right subcostal pain is common, whereas if it is limited to the left side of the pancreas, left subcostal and back pain are the presenting symptoms. In some patients, the pain is more diffuse. Radiation to the shoulder, usually the left shoulder, occurs. Nausea is common during attacks, and vomiting may occur. The pain is often dull and gnawing. Severe flare-ups of pain may occur superimposed on background discomfort. All the complications of acute pancreatitis can occur with chronic pancreatitis. Weight loss is common, because the patient does not feel like eating. The pain prevents sleep and time off work is frequent. The number of hospital admissions for acute exacerbations is a pointer towards the severity of the disease. Analgesic use and abuse is frequent. This, too, gives an indication of the severity of the disability. The patient's lifestyle is gradually destroyed by pain, analgesic dependence, weight loss and inability to work. Loss of exocrine function leads to steatorrhoea in more than 30% of patients with chronic pancreatitis. Loss of endocrine function and the development of diabetes are not uncommon, and the incidence increases as the disease progresses. Complications frequently bring the patient to the attention of the surgeon. Infection is not infrequent, possibly related to the diabetes mellitus.

Investigations

Only in the early stages of the disease will there be a rise in serum amylase. Tests of pancreatic function merely confirm the presence of pancreatic insufficiency or that more than 70% of the gland has been destroyed.

Pancreatic calcifications may be seen on abdominal X-ray (see Fig. 64.18, p. 1136). CT or MRI scan will show the outline of the gland, the main area of damage and the possibilities for surgical correction (Fig. 64.29; see also Fig. 64.7, p. 1133). Calcification is

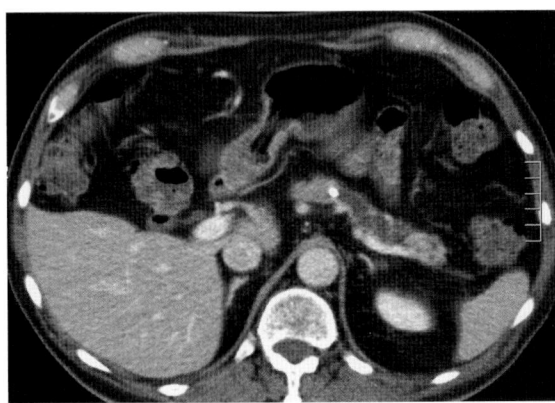

Figure 64.29 Computerised tomography scan in a patient with chronic pancreatitis. Stone obstructing the main pancreatic duct in the body of the gland; duct markedly dilated upstream.

seen very well on CT but not on MRI. An MRCP will identify the presence of biliary obstruction and the state of the pancreatic duct (Fig. 64.30). The use of intravenous secretin during the study may demonstrate a pancreatic duct stricture that is not apparent on a standard MRCP, but a normal-looking pancreas on CT or MRI does not rule out chronic pancreatitis. ERCP is the most accurate way of elucidating the anatomy of the duct and, in conjunction with the whole organ morphology, can help to determine the type of operation required, if operative intervention is indicated (Figs 64.15 and 64.17, p. 1136). Histologically proven chronic pancreatitis can, however, occur in the setting of normal findings on pancreatography. EUS can also be very useful. Sonographic findings characteristic of chronic pancreatitis include the presence of stones, visible side branches, cysts, lobularity, an irregular main pancreatic duct, hyperechoic foci and strands, dilation of the main pancreatic duct and hyperechoic margins of the main pancreatic duct. The presence of four or more of these features is highly suggestive of chronic pancreatitis.

Treatment

Most patients can be managed with medical measures. There is no single therapeutic agent that has been shown to relieve symptoms (Summary box 64.9).

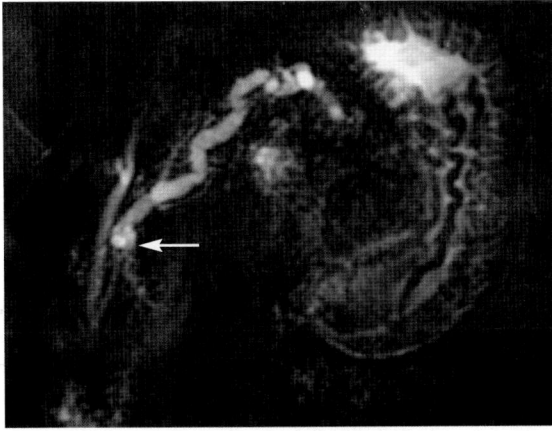

Figure 64.30 Magnetic resonance cholangiopancreatography in a patient with chronic pancreatitis. Stricture of the pancreatic duct in the body of the gland (arrow), with dilatation upstream.

Endoscopic, radiological or surgical interventions are indicated mainly to relieve obstruction of the pancreatic duct, bile duct or the duodenum, or in dealing with complications (e.g. pseudocyst, abscess, fistula, ascites or variceal haemorrhage). Decompressing an obstructed pancreatic duct can provide pain relief in some patients (the assumption is that ductal hypertension causes the pain).

Summary box 64.9

Medical treatment of chronic pancreatitis

Treat the addiction
- Help the patient to stop alcohol consumption and tobacco smoking
- Involve a dependency counsellor or a psychologist

Alleviate abdominal pain
- Eliminate obstructive factors (duodenum, bile duct, pancreatic duct)
- Escalate analgesia in a stepwise fashion
- Refer to a pain management specialist
- For intractable pain, consider CT/EUS-guided coeliac axis block

Nutritional and digestive measures
- Diet: low in fat and high in protein and carbohydrates
- Pancreatic enzyme supplementation with meals
- Correct malabsorption of the fat-soluble vitamins (A, D, E, K) and vitamin B12
- Medium-chain triglycerides in patients with severe fat malabsorption (they are directly absorbed by the small intestine without the need for digestion)
- Reducing gastric secretions may help

Treat diabetes mellitus

Endoscopic pancreatic sphincterotomy might be beneficial in patients with papillary stenosis and a high sphincter pressure and pancreatic ductal pressure. Patients with a dominant pancreatic duct stricture and upstream dilatation may benefit by placement of a stent across the stricture. The stent should be left in for no more than 4–6 weeks as it will block. The complication rate is high, and less than two-thirds of patients experience pain relief, but those who do get relief may benefit from a surgical bypass. Pancreatic duct stones may be extracted at ERCP, and this may sometimes be combined with extracorporeal shock wave lithotripsy. Pseudocysts may be drained internally under EUS guidance. Percutaneous or transgastric drainage of pseudocysts under ultrasound or CT guidance may be performed.

The role of surgery is to overcome obstruction and remove mass lesions. Some patients have a mass in the head of the pancreas, for which either a pancreatoduodenectomy or a Beger procedure (duodenum-preserving resection of the pancreatic head) is appropriate. If the duct is markedly dilated, then a longitudinal pancreatojejunostomy or Frey procedure can be of value (Fig. 64.31). The natural evolution of the disease may not be altered significantly, but around half the patients get long-term pain relief. The rare patient with disease limited to the tail will be cured by a distal pancreatectomy. Patients with intractable pain and diffuse

Charles Frederick Frey, **B. 1929, Professor of Surgery, The University of California, Davids, CA, USA.**

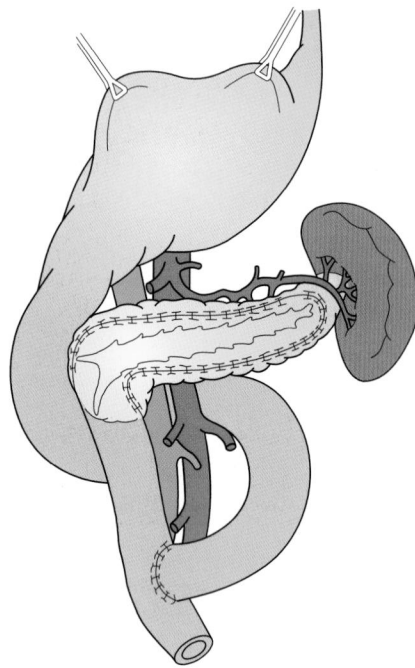

Figure 64.31 Pancreatojejunostomy. The pancreatic duct is opened longitudinally, and a loop of jejunum is sutured to the duct. In the Frey procedure, the superficial part of the head of the pancreas is removed to achieve drainage.

disease may plead for a total pancreatectomy in the expectation that removing the offending organ will relieve their pain. However, one should keep in mind that pancreatic function and quality of life are significantly impaired after this procedure, and the operative mortality rate is around 10%. Moreover, there is no guarantee of pain relief (approximately a third of patients get resolution, a third show some benefit, and a third see no benefit at all). Total pancreatectomy and islet autotransplantation has been reported in selected patients.

Prognosis

Chronic pancreatitis is a difficult condition to manage. Patients often suffer a gradual decline in their professional, social and personal lives. The pain may abate after a surgical or percutaneous intervention, but tends to return over a period of time. In a proportion of patients, the inflammation may gradually burn out over a period of years, with disappearance of the pain, leaving only the exocrine and endocrine insufficiencies. Development of pancreatic cancer is a risk in those who have had the disease for more than 20 years. New symptoms or a change in the pattern of symptoms should be investigated and malignancy excluded.

Sphincter of Oddi dysfunction

Separate mention is warranted of this condition, which should be considered in the differential diagnosis of chronic biliary or pancreatic pain. The sphincter of Oddi is 6–10 mm long and lies within the duodenal wall. A part of it encircles the common channel, and then there are separate biliary and pancreatic components (see Fig. 64.5, p. 1132). Scarring or stenosis of the sphincter can result from passage of stones, pancreatitis or prior endoscopic sphincterotomies. Sphincter of Oddi dyskinesia or dysfunction (SOD) is a clinical syndrome in which pain,

biochemical abnormalities and dilatation of the bile duct and/or pancreatic duct are attributed to abnormal function of the sphincter of Oddi. The true incidence of SOD is unknown. Females are more commonly affected than males.

There are two types of SOD. Biliary-type SOD is characterised by biliary pain, which may be accompanied by abnormally raised liver enzymes and/or dilation of the bile duct. It may be a cause of persistent post-cholecystectomy symptoms. A predominance of pancreatic problems, especially recurrent episodes of acute pancreatitis, is known as pancreatic-type SOD. The biliary and pancreatic sphincters can be evaluated at the time of ERCP with manometry, and high sphincter pressures may be demonstrated. Sphincterotomy and/or stenting of the involved duct system may be performed if deemed appropriate. SOD is however associated with a particularly high risk of post-ERCP pancreatitis, and such treatments are best carried out in tertiary units by expert gastroenterologists.

In a small sub-group of patients who have experienced significant but short-lived relief with sphincterotomy or stenting, surgical transduodenal sphincteroplasty may be considered. Although SOD can cause severe symptoms (and the patient may therefore be keen to have something done), it is not fatal. But post-ERCP pancreatitis and surgery both carry a small but definite risk of mortality.

CARCINOMA OF THE PANCREAS

Pancreatic cancer is the sixth leading cause of cancer death in the UK, and the incidence is 10 cases per 100 000 population per year. Worldwide, it constitutes 2–3% of all cancers and, in the USA, is the fourth highest cause of cancer death. The incidence has declined slightly over the last 25 years. There is no simple screening test; however, patients with an increased inherited risk of pancreatic cancer (Table 64.7) should be referred to specialist units for screening and counselling.

Pathology

More than 85% of pancreatic cancers are ductal adenocarcinomas. The remaining tumours constitute a variety of pathologies with individual characteristics. Endocrine tumours of the pancreas are rare. They are covered in Chapter 49.

Ductal adenocarcinomas arise most commonly in the head of the gland. They are solid, scirrhous tumours, characterised by neoplastic tubular glands within a markedly desmoplastic fibrous stroma. Fibrosis is also a characteristic of chronic pancreatitis, and histological differentiation between tumour and pancreatitis can cause diagnostic difficulties. Ductal adenocarcinomas infiltrate locally, typically along nerve sheaths, along lymphatics and into blood vessels. Liver and peritoneal metastases are common. Proliferative lesions in the pancreatic ducts can precede invasive ductal adenocarcinoma. These are termed pancreatic intraepithelial neoplasia or PanIN, and can demonstrate a range of structural complexity and cellular atypia.

Cystic tumours of the pancreas may be serous or mucinous. Serous cystadenomas are typically found in older women, and are large aggregations of multiple small cysts, almost like bubble-wrap. They are benign. Mucinous tumours, on the other hand, have the potential for malignant transformation. They include mucinous cystic neoplasms (MCNs) and intraductal papillary mucinous neoplasms (IPMNs). MCNs are seen in perimenopausal women, show up as multilocular thick-walled cysts in

Table 64.7 Risk factors for the development of pancreatic cancer

Demographic factors
Age (peak incidence 65–75 years)
Male gender
Black ethnicity

Environment/lifestyle
Cigarette smoking

Genetic factors and medical conditions
Family history
    Two first-degree relatives with pancreas cancer: relative risk
        increases 18- to 57-fold
    Germline *BRCA2* mutations in some rare high-risk families
Hereditary pancreatitis (50- to 70-fold increased risk)
Chronic pancreatitis (5- to 15-fold increased risk)
HNPCC
Ataxia telangiectasia
Peutz–Jeghers syndrome
Familial breast–ovarian cancer syndrome
Familial atypical multiple mole melanoma
Familial adenomatous polyposis – risk of ampullary/duodenal
    carcinoma
Diabetes mellitus

HNPCC, hereditary non-polyposis colorectal cancer.

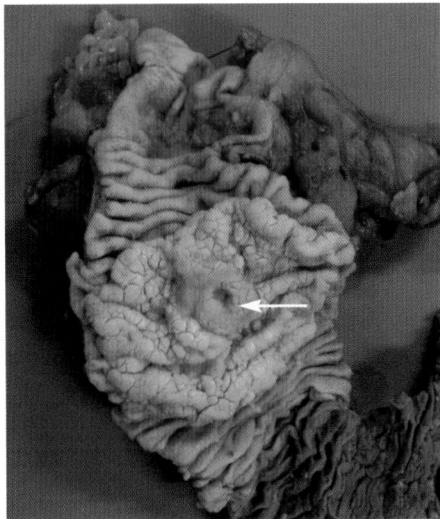

Figure 64.32 A large ampullary adenoma that turned into an adeno-carcinoma; the arrow indicates the ampulla. Photograph taken after resection in the form of a pancreatoduodenectomy (courtesy of Dr Joanne Chin-Aleong).

the pancreatic body or tail and, histologically, contain an ovarian-type stroma. IPMNs are more common in the pancreatic head and in older men, but an IPMN arising from a branch duct can be difficult to distinguish from an MCN. IPMNs arising within the main duct are often multifocal and have a greater tendency to prove malignant. Thick mucus seen extruding from the ampulla at ERCP is diagnostic of a main duct IPMN. Mucinous tumours can be confused with pseudocysts (see Summary box 64.8, p. 1146). Occasionally, lymphoepithelial cysts, lymphangiomas, dermoid cysts and intestinal duplication cysts can show up in the pancreas. Solid pseudopapillary tumour is a rare, slowly progressive but malignant tumour, seen in women of childbearing age, and manifests as a large, part-solid, part-cystic tumour.

Tumours arising from the ampulla or from the distal common bile duct can present as a mass in the head of the pancreas, and constitute around a third of all tumours in that area. Adenomas of the ampulla of Vater are diagnosed at endoscopy as polypoid submucosal masses covered by a smooth epithelium. They can harbour foci of invasive carcinoma; the larger the adenoma, the greater the risk. Biopsies taken at endoscopy may not always include the malignant focus. Endoscopic surveillance, endoscopic resection or even surgical transduodenal ampullary excision should be considered (Fig. 64.32). Patients with familial adenomatous polyposis (FAP) can present with multiple duodenal polyps. Malignant transformation in a duodenal polyp is a significant cause of mortality in these patients, mandating endoscopic follow-up and pancreatoduodenectomy in selected patients with high-grade dysplasia within the polyp.

Ampullary adenocarcinomas often present early with biliary

obstruction. Their natural history is distinctly more favourable compared with pancreatic ductal adenocarcinoma. Ampullary carcinomas are relatively small when diagnosed, which may account for their better prognosis. Occasionally, other malignant neoplasms can arise at the ampulla, such as carcinoid tumours and high-grade neuroendocrine carcinomas.

Clinical features

Jaundice secondary to obstruction of the distal bile duct is the most common symptom that draws attention to ampullary and pancreatic head tumours. It is characteristically painless jaundice but may be associated with nausea and epigastric discomfort. Pruritus, dark urine and pale stools with steatorrhoea are common accompaniments of jaundice. In the absence of jaundice, symptoms are often non-specific, namely vague discomfort, anorexia and weight loss, and are frequently dismissed by both patient and doctor. Upper abdominal symptoms in a recently diagnosed diabetic, especially in one above 50 years of age, with no family history or obesity, should raise suspicion. Occasionally, a patient will present with an unexplained attack of pancreatitis; all such patients should have follow-up imaging of the pancreas. Tumours of the body and tail of the gland often grow silently, and present at an advanced unresectable stage. Back pain is a worrying symptom, raising the possibility of retroperitoneal infiltration.

On examination, there may be evidence of jaundice, weight loss, a palpable liver and a palpable gall bladder. Courvoisier first drew attention to the association of an enlarged gall bladder and a pancreatic tumour in 1890, when he noted that, when the common duct is obstructed by a stone, distension of the gall bladder (which is likely to be chronically inflamed) is rare; when the duct is obstructed in some other way, such as a neoplasm, distension of the normal gall bladder is common. Other signs of intra-abdominal malignancy should be looked for with care, such as a palpable mass, ascites, supraclavicular nodes and tumour deposits in the pelvis; when present, they indicate a grim prognosis.

John Law Augustine Peutz, **1886–1968, Chief Specialist for Internal Medicine, St. John's Hospital, The Hague, The Netherlands.**
Harold Joseph Jeghers, **1904–1990, Professor of Internal Medicine, The New Jersey College of Medicine and Dentistry, Jersey City, NJ, USA.**

Ludwig Courvoisier, **1843–1918, Professor of Surgery, Basle, Switzerland.**

Investigation

In a jaundiced patient, the usual blood tests and ultrasound scan should be performed. Ultrasound will determine whether or not the bile duct is dilated. If it is, and there is a genuine suspicion of a tumour in the head of the pancreas, the preferred test is a contrast-enhanced CT scan (see Fig. 64.8, p. 1133). In the majority of instances, this should establish if there is a tumour in the pancreas and if it is resectable. The presence of hepatic or peritoneal metastases, lymph node metastases distant from the pancreatic head, encasement of the superior mesenteric, hepatic or coeliac artery by tumour are clear contraindications to surgical resection. Tumour size, continuous invasion of the duodenum, stomach or colon, and lymph node metastases within the operative field are not contraindications. If the tumour abuts or minimally invades the portal or superior mesenteric vein, this is not a contraindication to surgery (as part of the vein can be resected if necessary), but complete encasement and occlusion of the vein is. MRI and MR angiography can provide information comparable to CT.

ERCP and biliary stenting should be carried out if there is any suggestion of cholangitis, if there is diagnostic doubt (small ampullary lesions may not be seen on CT, and ERCP is the best way to identify them) or if there is likely to be a delay between diagnosis and surgery and the patient is deeply jaundiced with distressing pruritus. It relieves the jaundice and can also provide a brush cytology or biopsy specimen to confirm the diagnosis (see Figs 64.13, 64.14 and 64.19, pp. 1134, 1135 and 1136). Otherwise, however, preoperative ERCP and biliary stenting is not mandatory in patients with resectable disease; there is evidence to suggest that it is associated with a slightly higher incidence of infective complications after surgery. The prothrombin time should be checked, and clotting abnormalities should be corrected with vitamin K or fresh frozen plasma prior to ERCP. If a stent is placed in a patient who may undergo resection, it should be a plastic stent rather than a metal self-expanding one.

EUS is useful if CT fails to demonstrate a tumour, if tissue diagnosis is required prior to surgery (e.g. a mass has developed on a background of chronic pancreatitis and a distinction needs to be made between inflammation and neoplasia), if vascular invasion needs to be confirmed and in separating cystic tumours from pseudocysts (Fig. 64.33; see also Fig. 64.20, p. 1136). Transduodenal or transgastric FNA or Trucut biopsy performed under EUS guidance avoids spillage of tumour cells into the peritoneal cavity. Percutaneous transperitoneal biopsy of potentially resectable pancreatic tumours should be avoided as far as possible. Histological confirmation of malignancy is desirable but not essential, particularly if the imaging clearly demonstrates a resectable tumour. The lack of a tissue diagnosis should not delay appropriate surgical therapy. In patients judged to have unresectable disease, tissue diagnosis should be obtained prior to starting palliative therapy.

Diagnostic laparoscopy prior to an attempt at resection can spare a proportion of patients an unnecessary laparotomy by identifying small peritoneal and liver metastases. It can be combined with laparoscopic ultrasonography. The tumour marker CA19-9 is not highly specific or sensitive, but a baseline level should be established; if it is initially raised, it can be useful later in identifying recurrence.

Management

At the time of presentation, more than 85% of patients with ductal adenocarcinoma are unsuitable for resection because the

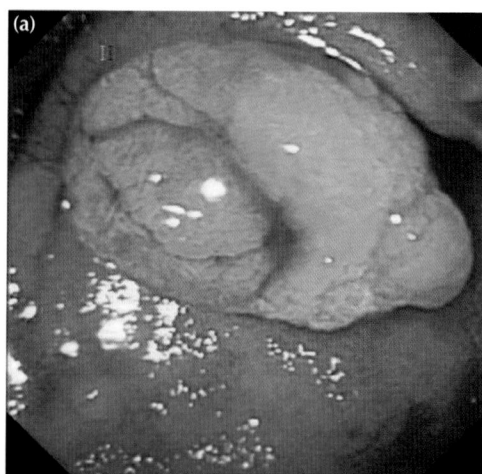

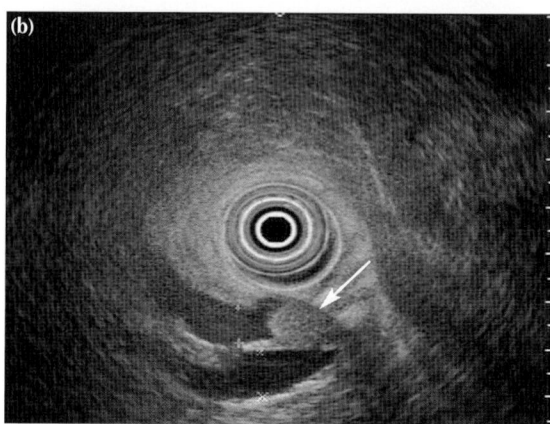

Figure 64.33 (a) Carcinoma of the ampulla as seen at endoscopy. (b) Appearance of the same tumour (arrow) on endoscopic ultrasound (courtesy of Dr Peter Fairclough).

disease is too advanced. If imaging shows that the tumour is potentially resectable, the patient should be considered for surgical resection, as that offers the only (albeit small) chance of a cure. Comorbidities should be carefully taken into account. Biological rather than chronological age should be the consideration. If a cystic tumour is encountered, no matter how large, surgical resection should be considered, as it carries a reasonable chance of cure. Tumours of the ampulla have a good prognosis and should, if at all possible, be resected. Some of the rare tumours and the neuroendocrine lesions should also be resected if at all possible. For those patients who have inoperable disease, palliative treatment should be offered.

Surgical resection

The standard resection for a tumour of the pancreatic head or the ampulla is a pylorus-preserving pancreatoduodenectomy (PPPD). This involves removal of the duodenum and the pancreatic head, including the distal part of the bile duct. The original pancreatoduodenectomy as proposed by Whipple included resection of the gastric antrum. Preserving the antrum and the pylorus is thought to yield a more physiological outcome with no difference in

Allen Oldfather Whipple, **1881–1963**, Director of Surgical Services, The Presbyterian Hospital, and Professor of Surgery, The College of Physicians and Surgeons, Columbia University, New York, NY, USA.

survival or recurrence rates. The Whipple procedure is now reserved for situations in which the entire duodenum has to be removed (e.g. in FAP) or where the tumour encroaches on the first part of the duodenum or the distal stomach and a PPPD would not achieve a clear resection margin. Total pancreatectomy is warranted only in situations where one is dealing with a multifocal tumour (e.g. a main duct IPMN), or the body and tail of the gland are too inflamed or too friable to achieve a safe anastomosis with the bowel. The PPPD procedure includes a local lymphadenectomy. Extended lymphadenectomy has not been shown to be beneficial in improving survival and is associated with increased morbidity. If the tumour is adherent to the portal or superior mesenteric vein, but can still be removed by including a patch or a short segment of vein in the resection, with an appropriate reconstruction of the vessel, then that should be done. This is not associated with an increase in the morbidity or mortality of the procedure, and the outcomes are similar.

For tumours of the body and tail, distal pancreatectomy with splenectomy is the standard. Infiltration of the splenic artery or vein by the tumour is not a contraindication to resection. When resecting the pancreatic tail for a benign lesion, one may attempt to preserve the spleen if possible. When removing the spleen, prior vaccinations against pneumococci, meningococci and *Haemophilus influenzae* B should be administered, and subsequent antibiotic prophylaxis given (see Chapter 62).

Attempts to downstage unresectable disease with chemotherapy or chemoradiation and render it resectable are rarely successful. Neoadjuvant chemotherapy or chemoradiation for resectable disease should only be considered within a clinical trial; it carries the risk that the disease may progress despite the neoadjuvant therapy and become unresectable.

Pancreatoduodenectomy

The clotting should be checked preoperatively and adequate hydration ensured. The patient should be aware of the diagnosis, the gravity of the operation and the risks involved. The operation has three distinct phases:

- exploration and assessment;
- resection;
- reconstruction.

A cholecystectomy is performed. The bile duct and hepatic artery are exposed, removing the lymphatic tissue in this area. Exposure of the hepatic artery enables division of the gastroduodenal artery and visualisation of the portal vein. The distal part of the gastric antrum is mobilised. The duodenum and right colon are mobilised from the retroperitoneal tissues. The superior mesenteric vein is exposed inferior to the pancreatic neck. Careful dissection into the plane between the vein and the pancreatic substance (see Fig. 64.2, p. 1130) will reveal whether the tumour is adherent to the vein. The fourth part of the duodenum is dissected and freed from the ligament of Treitz so that the upper jejunum can be brought into the supracolic compartment. At this juncture, a decision has to be made whether to proceed to the next phase of resection or not. If resection is to be performed, the jejunum is divided 20–30 cm downstream from the duodenojejunal flexure, and the mesentery of the proximal jejunum is

> Wenzel Treitz, **1819–1872**, Professor of Anatomy and Pathology, at Krakow, Poland, and later at Prague, The Czech Republic.

detached. The first part of the duodenum is divided. The neck of the pancreas is divided, and then the uncinate process is separated from the superior mesenteric artery and vein working up towards the upper bile duct, which is divided, releasing the specimen (Fig. 64.34). Retroperitoneal lymph nodes within the operative field are completely removed with the specimen. Reconstruction is carried out as in Figure 64.35. The pancreatic stump, the divided bile duct and the duodenal stump are anastomosed on to jejunum, in that order. Some surgeons prefer to anastomose the pancreas to the posterior wall of the stomach instead; others prefer to create a separate Roux loop of the jejunum and anastomose the pancreas to that. The operation should take between 3 and 6 hours. Blood loss should be low, and transfusion is often not necessary. The patients are usually nursed in a high-dependency area for the first 24–48 hours after surgery. Prolonged nasogastric drainage is unnecessary, and early feeding can be commenced.

Resection for pancreatic cancer should be carried out in specialist units. There is a clear correlation between higher caseload volume and lower hospital mortality and morbidity. PPPD should

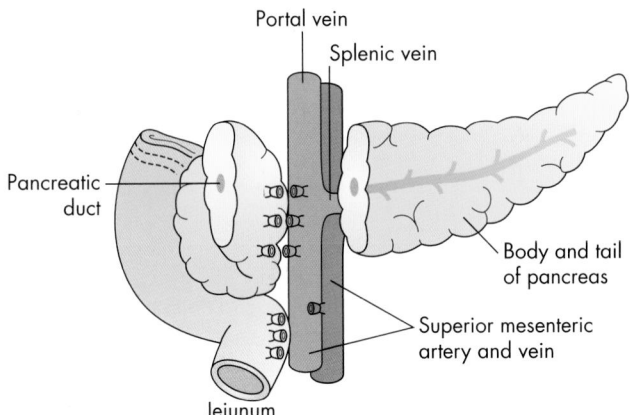

Figure 64.34 Resection of the head of the pancreas in a pylorus-preserving pancreatoduodenectomy.

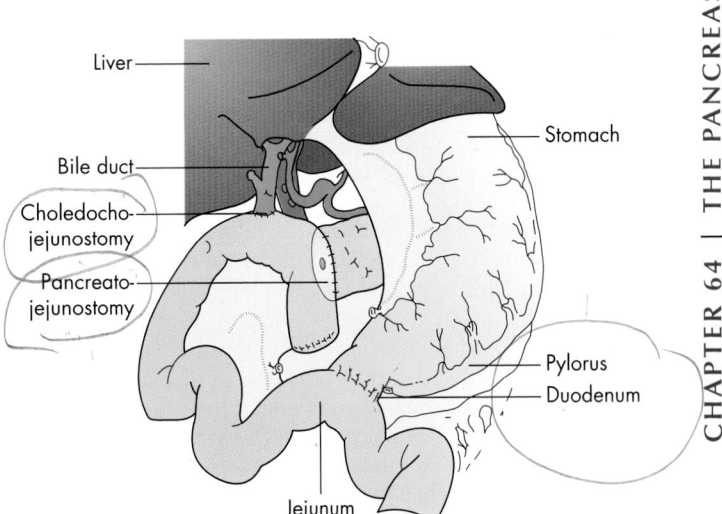

Figure 64.35 Reconstruction after a pylorus-preserving pancreatoduodenectomy.

carry a mortality of no more than 3–5%. The morbidity remains high, with some 30–40% of patients developing a complication in the postoperative period. These complications are usually infective, but a leak from the anastomosis between the pancreas and the bowel is known to occur in at least 10% of patients, and this may give rise to major complications. Octreotide may be administered in the perioperative period to suppress secretion and reduce the likelihood of a leak, but the evidence for its efficacy is still debatable. Following surgical resection, the pathological tumour–node–metastasis stage should be documented.

Adjuvant therapy

The reported 5-year survival following resection of a pancreatic adenocarcinoma ranges from 7% to 25%. The median survival is 11–20 months. Considering that, at best, 15% of patients have resectable disease to begin with, this means only two or three out of 100 patients with this disease can expect to survive to 5 years. Moreover, recurrences can and do show up even beyond the 5-year cut-off. It should be emphasised, however, that these depressing statistics apply to ductal adenocarcinomas. Patients with resected ampullary tumours have a 5-year survival of 40%, and cystic tumours and neuroendocrine tumours can often be cured by surgical resection.

The high recurrence rate following resection has inevitably led to the consideration of adjuvant treatments to improve outcome. In a large multicentre European study (ESPAC-1), adjuvant radiotherapy or chemoradiotherapy was shown to confer no advantage, but chemotherapy with 5-fluorouracil (5-FU) provided an overall benefit (median survival with chemotherapy was 20 months compared with 16 months without). Further trials are in progress, using gemcitabine and 5-FU in combination, and other agents. Most patients with resected ductal adenocarcinoma are now offered adjuvant chemotherapy. Some centres continue to offer chemoradiotherapy, particularly in patients with involved (R1) resection margins, and further trials of adjuvant chemoradiation are also in progress.

Palliation

The median survival of patients with unresectable, locally advanced, non-metastatic pancreatic cancer is 6–10 months and, in patients with metastatic disease, it is 2–6 months.

If unresectable disease is found in the course of a laparotomy that was commenced with the intent to resect, a choledochoenterostomy and a gastroenterostomy should be carried out to relieve (or pre-empt) jaundice and duodenal obstruction. The bile duct may be anastomosed to the duodenum, or to a loop of jejunum. It is preferable to use the bile duct rather than the gall bladder. Cholecystojejunostomy is easier to perform, but the bile must then drain through the cystic duct, which is narrow and, if the cystic duct is inserted low into the bile duct, it is vulnerable to occlusion by tumour growth. A coeliac plexus block can also be administered. A transduodenal Trucut biopsy of the tumour should be obtained.

In patients found to have unresectable disease on imaging, jaundice is relieved by stenting at ERCP (Fig. 64.36b). Stents may be made of plastic or self-expanding metal mesh. Plastic stents are cheaper but tend to occlude faster and, if the patient is likely to have a longer life expectancy, a metal stent can be used. If the patient is not a suitable candidate for endoscopic biliary stenting, a percutaneous transhepatic stent can be placed (Fig. 64.36a). Obstruction of the duodenum occurs in approximately 15% of cases. If this occurs early in the course of the disease, surgical bypass by gastrojejunostomy is appropriate but, if it is late in the

course of the disease, then the use of expanding metal stents inserted endoscopically is preferable, as many of these patients have prolonged delayed gastric emptying following surgery (Fig. 64.36c). If both biliary and duodenal metal stents are to be placed endoscopically, the biliary one should be placed first.

If no operative procedure is undertaken, an EUS-guided or percutaneous biopsy of the tumour should be performed before consideration of chemotherapy or chemoradiation. The role of chemotherapy in the management of pancreatic cancer remains ill defined. If the tumour is a lymphoma, then benefit is without doubt. Lymphomas of the pancreas are rare and constitute less than 3% of all pancreatic cancers. For patients with ductal adenocarcinoma, 5-FU or gemcitabine will produce a remission in 15–25%, while the remainder will receive no benefit from the therapy. No long-term cures have been described with chemotherapy or radiotherapy.

Steatorrhoea is treated with enzyme supplementation. Diabetes mellitus, if it develops, is treated with oral hypoglycaemics or insulin as appropriate, and pain with either analgesics or an appropriate nerve block (Summary box 64.10).

Summary box 64.10

Palliation of pancreatic cancer

Relieve jaundice and treat biliary sepsis
- Surgical biliary bypass
- Stent placed at ERCP or percutaneous transhepatic cholangiography

Improve gastric emptying
- Surgical gastroenterostomy
- Duodenal stent

Pain relief
- Stepwise escalation of analgesia
- Coeliac plexus block
- Transthoracic splanchnicectomy

Symptom relief and quality of life
- Encourage normal activities
- Enzyme replacement for steatorrhoea
- Treat diabetes

Consider chemotherapy

FURTHER READING

Ayub, K., Imada, R. and Slavin, J. (2004) Endoscopic retrograde cholangiopancreatography in gallstone-associated acute pancreatitis. *Cochrane Reviews* (2): CD003630.

Blumgart, L.H. (2006) *Surgery of the Liver, Biliary Tract and Pancreas*, 4th edn. Saunders.

Pancreatic Section, British Society of Gastroenterology; Pancreatic Society of Great Britain and Ireland; Association of Upper Gastrointestinal Surgeons of Great Britain and Ireland; Royal College of Pathologists; Special Interest Group for Gastro-Intestinal Radiology (2005) Guidelines for the management of patients with pancreatic cancer, periampullary and ampullary carcinomas. *Gut* 54 (Suppl V):1–16.

Moss, A.C., Morris, E. and MacMathuna, P. (2006) Palliative biliary stents for obstructing pancreatic carcinoma. *Cochrane Reviews* (2): CD004200.

(a)

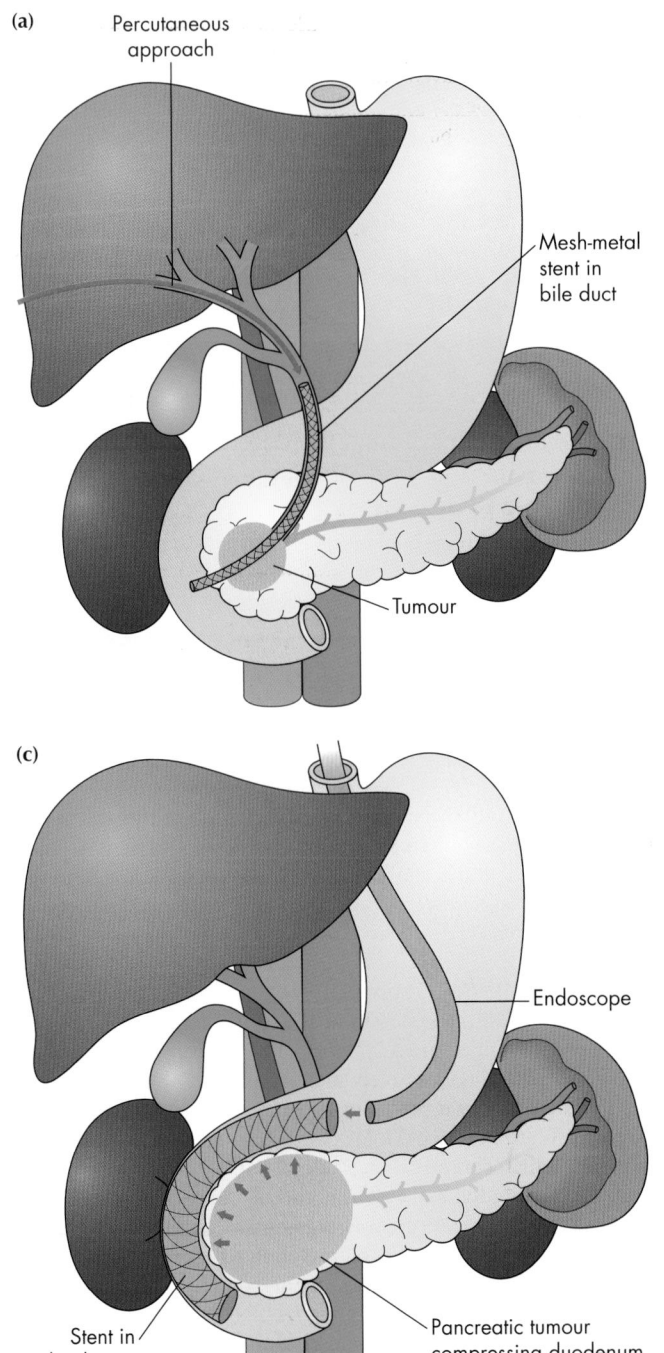

(b)

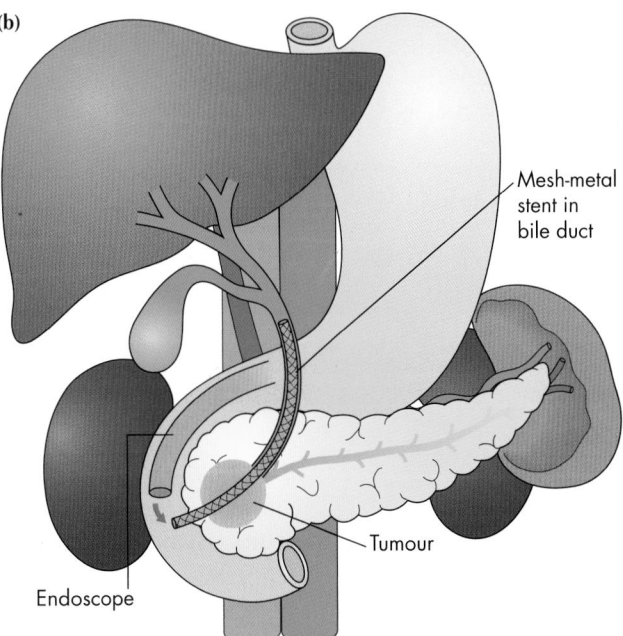

(c)

Figure 64.36 Approaches to biliary and duodenal stenting. (a) PTC: Percutaneous transhepatic cholangiography followed by cannulation of the biliary system and percutaneous placement of a biliary stent (mesh metal in this instance); (b) ERCP: Endoscopic retrograde cholangiography and placement of a biliary stent; (c) Endoscopic placement of a duodenal stent (mesh metal).

Sewnath, M.E., Karsten, T.M., Prins, M.H., Rauws, E.J.A., Obertop, H. and Gouma, D.J. (2002) A meta-analysis on the efficacy of preoperative biliary drainage for tumors causing obstructive jaundice. *Ann Surg* **236**:17–27.

Working Party of the British Society of Gastroenterology; Association of Surgeons of Great Britain and Ireland, Pancreatic Society of Great Britain and Ireland; Association of Upper GI Surgeons of Great Britain and Ireland. (2005) UK guidelines for the management of acute pancreatitis. *Gut* **54** (Suppl III):1–9.

Yip, D., Karapetis, C., Strickland, A., Steer, C.B. and Goldstein, D. (2006) Chemotherapy and radiotherapy for inoperable advanced pancreatic cancer. *Cochrane Reviews* (3): CD002093.

The small and large intestines

CHAPTER

65

LEARNING OBJECTIVES

To appreciate:
- The anatomy of the small and large intestines
- The investigation and treatment of the range of conditions that may affect the small and large intestines

To understand:
- That diseases of the intestines may involve functional or anatomical problems

- The principles behind the different types of surgery for the small and large intestines

To be able to deal with:
- Acute surgical problems of the small and large intestines

To know that:
- The surgical management of small and large intestinal disease is best conducted within a multidisciplinary team

ANATOMY OF THE SMALL AND LARGE INTESTINES

Small intestine

The small intestine starts at the pylorus and extends to the ileo-caecal valve. It is approximately 7 m in length and is divided into the duodenum, jejunum and ileum. Its main function is in the breakdown and absorption of food products. The small bowel is present in the central and lower portion of the abdominal cavity. Its relations consist of the greater omentum and abdominal wall anteriorly. Posteriorly, it is fixed to the vertebral column by way of its mesentery.

The duodenum is present proximally and is about 25 cm in length. It has no mesentery and, therefore, is the most fixed part of the small bowel. It merges into the jejunum at the duodeno-jejunal flexure. The remainder of the small bowel is made up of the jejunum and ileum. The jejunum makes up the proximal two-fifths and is wider, thicker and more vascular than the ileum. It also consists of circular folds of mucous membrane (valvulae conniventes) that can be used to distinguish it from the ileum. The ileum contains larger lymph node aggregates (Peyer's patches), and these can sometimes be lead points in cases of intussusception in the young.

The arterial supply of the duodenum consists of the right gastric, the superior pancreaticoduodenal branch of the hepatic artery and the inferior pancreaticoduodenal branch of the superior mesenteric artery. The veins drain into the leinal and superior mesenteric. The nerves are supplied from the coeliac plexus. The jejunum and ileum

are vascularised by the superior mesenteric artery through a rich plexus of vessels. The veins run a similar course. The nerve supply to the small intestines arises from sympathetic nerves around the superior mesenteric artery. Pathology such as obstruction causes visceral pain, which is felt in the peri-umbilical region.

Large intestine

The large intestine extends from the ileum to the anus. Rectal anatomy is described in Chapter 68. The colon is approximately 1.5 m in length. It is relatively more fixed than the small bowel. It also differs in that it possesses appendices epiploicae on its surface, which are peritoneal folds containing fat, and the presence of taenia, which consist of longitudinal bands of the outer muscle coat. It can be divided into the caecal, ascending, transverse, descending and sigmoid colonic segments.

The blood supply of the colon is derived from ileocolic, right colic and middle colic branches of the superior mesenteric vessels. The descending colon receives its blood supply from the left colic branch from the inferior mesenteric but also communicates with the superior mesenteric system via the marginal artery of Drummond. The veins run in a similar distribution. The nerve supply is derived from the sympathetic plexus surrounding the superior and inferior mesenteric arteries. Visceral pain is felt in the peri-umbilical region in the proximal colon and in the hypogastric region in the distal colon.

FUNCTIONAL ABNORMALITIES

Megacolon and non-megacolon constipation

There is no single definition of constipation; however, a bowel frequency of less than one every 3 days would be considered

---

Valvulae conniventes, **describes a fold of mucous membrane that passes transversely across two-thirds of the bowel circumference.**
Johann Conrad Peyer, **1653–1712, Professor of Logic, Rhetoric and Medicine, Schaffhausen, Switzerland, described the lymph follicles in the intestine in 1677.**

Drummond, **1852–1932, English Physician.**

abnormal by some. This group of conditions can be divided into:

1 megacolon:
   a Hirschsprung's disease;
   b non-Hirschsprung's megarectum and megacolon;
2 non-megacolon:
   a slow transit;
   b normal transit.

Hirschsprung's disease

See Chapter 6 for this and other congenital disorders.

Idiopathic megarectum and megacolon

This is a rare condition and the cause is not known, although in some it may result from poor toilet training during infancy and in others from a congenital abnormality of the intestinal myenteric plexus.

Clinical features

It presents usually in the first 20 years with severe constipation. Patients with idiopathic megarectum often present with faecal incontinence due to rectal faecal loading that requires manual evacuation. Patients with megacolon are more likely to present with abdominal distension and pain. On clinical examination, there may be a hard faecal mass arising out of the pelvis and, on rectal examination, there is a large faecaloma in the lumen. The anus is usually patulous, perianal soiling is common, and sigmoidoscopy is usually impossible but may show melanosis coli if the patient has been taking laxatives over many years.

Investigation

Imaging

As there is an enlarged rectum, often with distension of the colon over a variable length, a radiograph should be taken without prior bowel preparation, using a small quantity of water-soluble contrast to prevent barium impaction. There is usually gross faecal loading of the enlarged rectum and colon and, when a contrast examination is carried out, the width of the colon measured at the pelvic brim is usually more than 6.5 cm (Fig. 65.1).

Anorectal physiology tests

Anorectal physiology tests demonstrate delayed first sensation and raised maximum tolerated volume. Full-thickness rectal biopsy shows normal ganglion cells, a finding that definitively distinguishes this condition from Hirschsprung's disease.

Medical treatment

This is directed at emptying the rectum and keeping it empty with enemas, washouts and sometimes manual evacuation under anaesthesia. Thereafter, the patient is encouraged to develop a regular daily bowel habit, with the use of osmotic laxatives to help the passage of semiformed stool. Rectal evacuation with suppositories and biofeedback therapy may be useful in resistant cases.

Surgical treatment

Surgical treatment is sometimes necessary if medical therapy fails. Options that are available include:

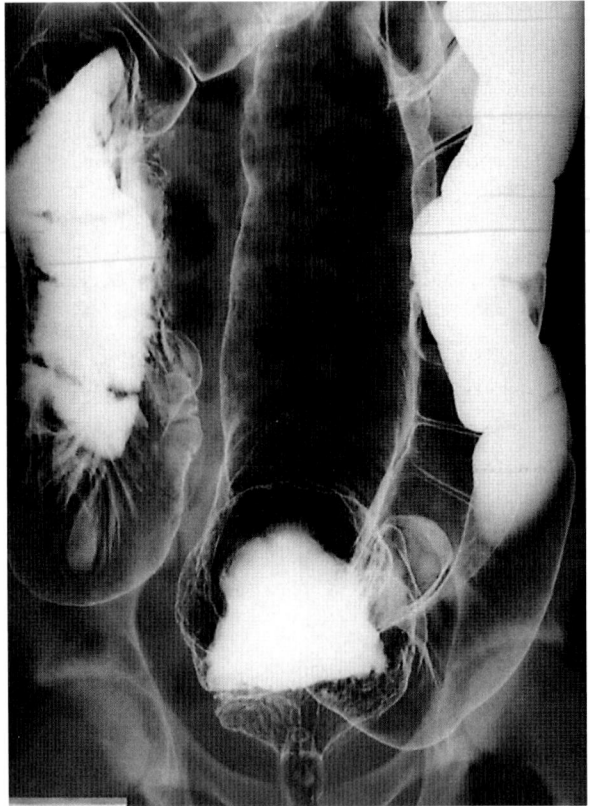

Figure 65.1 Double-contrast barium enema showing megarectum and a huge megasigmoid with normal left colon alongside for comparison (courtesy of Dr D. Nolan, John Radcliffe Hospital, Oxford, UK).

1 resection of the dilated rectum and colon (Fig. 65.2) back to normal-diameter colon with normal ganglion cells confirmed by frozen section at the time of surgery, which is followed by reconstruction with a coloanal anastomosis;
2 colectomy with the formation of an ileorectal anastomosis;
3 restorative proctocolectomy;
4 vertical reduction rectoplasty, which is a new procedure designed to reduce the volume of the rectum by at least 50% (Williams);

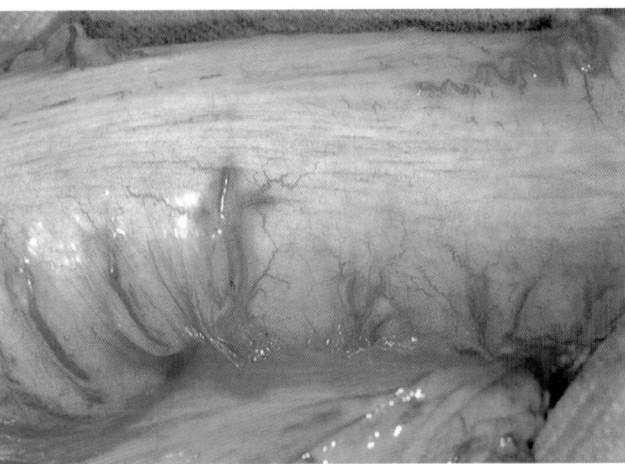

Figure 65.2 Megacolon.

5 stoma formation, which may be used either as a salvage operation for failure of previous surgery or as a primary intervention.

Non-megacolon constipation

Although constipation is often regarded as a trivial symptom, some patients are greatly disabled by abdominal pain, distension, reliance on laxatives and difficulty with defaecation. However, it is extremely prevalent complaint in western society. Some reports have put the annual prescription sales for laxatives in the UK at just under £50 million. These are usually otherwise healthy individuals who seek help for constipation but eat a normal diet and have a normal colon on endoscopy and barium enema.

Its cause is thought to involve slow whole-gut transit or a rectal evacuation problem. Factors influencing bowel transit time include:

- drugs: opiates, anti-cholinergics and ferrous sulphate;
- diseases: neurological conditions (Parkinson's disease, multiple sclerosis and diabetic nephropathy):
  - hypothyroidism;
  - hypercalcaemia.

Investigation

Whole-gut transit time can be measured by asking the patient to stop all laxatives and take a capsule containing radio-opaque markers (Fig. 65.3). Retention of more than 80% of the shapes, 120 hours after ingestion, is abnormal.

Defaecating proctography may be helpful if the main complaint is difficulty in evacuating stools.

Treatment

This can be done in several ways:

1 *Dietary fibre.* This is the first-line treatment for people with mild constipation. Constipation only resolves after several weeks of therapy and usually needs to be continued in the long term.
2 *Laxatives.* It is important that patients do not fall into a cycle of laxative abuse. A number of types are available which include bulk, osmotic and stimulant agents.
3 *Biofeedback.* This involves conditioning and coordination of the abdominal and pelvic compartments. It has been shown to be effective in those with a rectal evacuation problem and has also been used in slow transit with some response.

Idiopathic slow-transit constipation

This disorder is usually seen in women and results from infrequent bowel actions, which may have been present since childhood or may suddenly follow abdominal or pelvic surgery. Marker studies will reveal delayed transit, and the patient may or may not be able to empty the rectum normally (Fig. 65.3).

This is a difficult condition to treat medically; dietary measures are usually unsuccessful, and surgical treatment is justified only after careful studies and when medical treatment has been exhausted. Total colectomy and ileorectal anastomosis is the preferred procedure, but the results are unpredictable. Studies show complications of intermittent small bowel obstruction (60%),

James Parkinson, 1755–1824, a General Practitioner of Shoreditch, London, UK, published 'An Essay on the Shaking Palsey' in 1817.

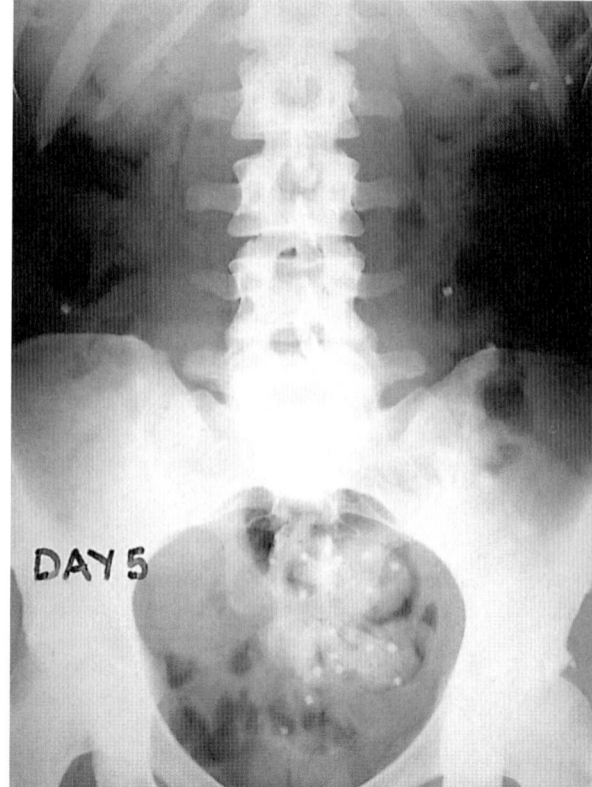

Figure 65.3 Whole-gut transit studied using radio-opaque markers. More than 80% should have passed by day 5, demonstrating delayed transit here (courtesy of Dr D. Nolan, John Radcliffe Hospital, Oxford, UK).

further surgery (30%), constipation (25%), diarrhoea (25%) and incontinence (10%). This may be explained in part by the argument that colectomy does not address the functional problem of the remaining bowel. Patients need to be carefully selected for surgery. Other types of surgery performed include stoma creation and segmental resection, but results are variable.

VASCULAR ANOMALIES (ANGIODYSPLASIA)

Capillary or cavernous haemangiomas are a cause of haemorrhage from the colon at any age. In the middle-aged or elderly patient, haemangioma needs to be distinguished from other causes of sudden massive haemorrhage, such as diverticulitis, ulcerative colitis (UC) or ischaemic colitis. Angiodysplasia is a vascular malformation associated with ageing. Its true incidence is probably not known because of the spectrum of disease severity, with ranges in the literature from 5 to 25% over the age of 60 years. With the advent of more sophisticated investigative tools, this may rise. Angiodysplasias occur particularly in the ascending colon and caecum of elderly patients. The malformations consist of dilated tortuous submucosal veins and, in severe cases, the mucosa is replaced by massive dilated deformed vessels.

Clinical features

In the majority, the symptoms are subtle and patients can present with anaemia. About 10–15% can have brisk bleeds, which may present as melaena or significant per rectum bleeding that is often intermittent.

In many patients in whom rectal bleeding has previously been attributed to diverticular disease, bleeding was probably, in fact, from angiodysplasia in the caecum. There is an association with aortic stenosis. Heyde's syndrome describes the association of aortic valve stenosis with gastrointestinal bleeding from colonic angiodysplasia. A mild form of von Willebrand's disease has been thought to be involved. This is caused by increased breakdown of von Willebrand factor by a natural enzyme called ADAMTS13 around sites of high shear stress such as a stenosed valve. The coagulation abnormality resolves after aortic valve replacement.

Investigation

Barium enema is usually unhelpful and should be avoided, not least because it may mask the lesion at subsequent endoscopy. Provided that the bleeding is not too brisk, colonoscopy may show the characteristic lesion in the right colon. The lesions are only a few millimetres in size and appear as reddish, raised areas at endoscopy. 'Pill' endoscopy is a relatively new technology that may detect small bowel lesions. Selective superior and inferior mesenteric angiography shows the site and extent of the lesion by a blush. If this fails, a radioactive test using technetium-99m (^{99m}Tc)-labelled red cells may confirm and localise the source of haemorrhage.

Treatment

The first principle is to stabilise an unstable circulation. Following this, the bleeding needs to be localised by colonoscopy. This allows simple therapeutic procedures such as cauterisation to be carried out. In severe uncontrolled bleeding, surgery becomes necessary. On-table colonoscopy is carried out to confirm the site of bleeding. Angiodysplastic lesions are sometimes demonstrated by transillumination through the caecum (Fig. 65.4). If it is still not clear exactly which segment of the colon is involved, then a total abdominal colectomy with ileorectal anastomosis may be necessary.

BLIND LOOP SYNDROME

It has been shown in dogs that, if a blind loop of the small intestine is made (Fig. 65.5), defects of absorption will appear. If this occurs in the upper intestine, the defect is chiefly of fat absorption; if in the lower intestine, there is vitamin B12 deficiency. This has been found to occur in humans and is referred to as the blind loop syndrome.

Essentially, the stasis produces an abnormal bacterial flora, which prevents proper breakdown of the food (especially fat) and mops up the vitamins that are present. Sometimes, the only manifestation is anaemia, resulting from vitamin B12 deficiency but, if steatorrhoea occurs, other serious malabsorption features follow. In general, high loops produce steatorrhoea, whereas low loops tend to produce anaemia.

Temporary improvement will follow the use of antibiotics to

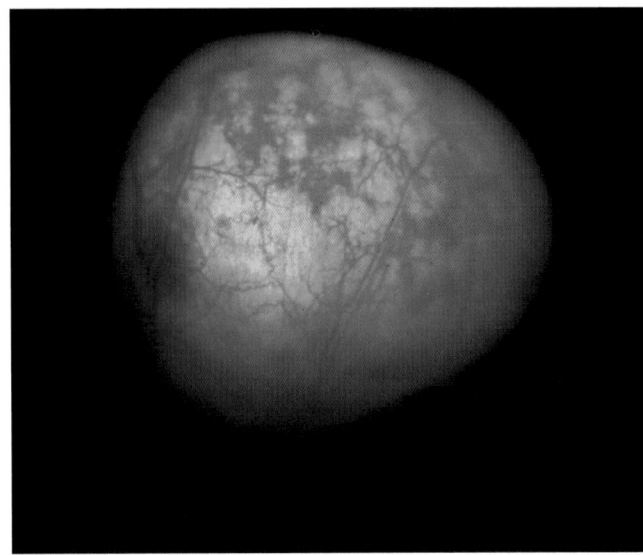

Figure 65.4 Angiodysplasia of the caecum demonstrated by transillumination with a colonoscope intraoperatively.

destroy the bacteria causing the trouble, but the main treatment is surgical extirpation of the cause of the stasis where applicable.

DIVERTICULAR DISEASE

Types

Diverticula can occur in a wide number of positions in the gut, from the oesophagus to the rectosigmoid. There are two varieties:

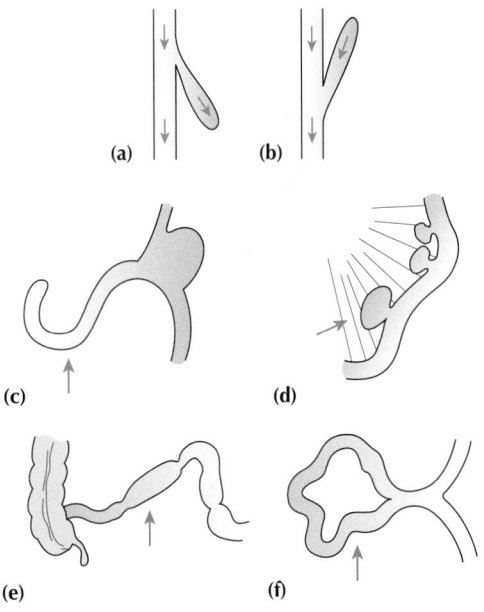

Figure 65.5 Common types of blind loop. (a) Self-filling: deficiency occurs. (b) Self-emptying: no deficiency occurs. (c) Long afferent loop stasis in Pólya gastrectomy. (d) Jejunal diverticula. (e) Intestinal stricture causing stasis. (f) 'Stenosis–anastomosis loop' syndrome.

CHAPTER 65 | THE SMALL AND LARGE INTESTINES

1 *Congenital.* All three coats of the bowel are present in the wall of the diverticulum, e.g. Meckel's diverticulum.
2 *Acquired.* The wall of the diverticulum lacks a proper muscular coat. Most alimentary diverticula are thought to be acquired.

Small intestine

Most of these diverticula arise from the mesenteric side of the bowel, probably as the result of mucosal herniation through the point of entry of blood vessels.

Duodenal diverticula

There are two types:

1 *Primary.* Mostly occurring in older patients on the inner wall of the second and third parts (Fig. 65.6), these diverticula are found incidentally on barium meal and are usually asymptomatic. They can cause problems locating the ampulla during endoscopic retrograde cholangiopancreatography (ERCP).
2 *Secondary.* Diverticula of the duodenal cap result from long-standing duodenal ulceration (Fig. 65.7).

Jejunal diverticula

These are usually of variable size and multiple (Fig. 65.8). Clinically, they may (1) be symptomless, (2) give rise to abdominal pain, (3) produce a malabsorption syndrome or (4) present as an acute abdomen with acute inflammation and occasionally perforation. They are more common in patients with connective tissue disorders. In patients with major malabsorption problems giving rise to anaemia, steatorrhoea, hypoproteinaemia or vitamin B12 deficiency, resection of the affected segment with end-to-end anastomosis can be effective.

Meckel's diverticulum

Meckel's diverticulum is present in 2% of the population; it is situated on the anti-mesenteric border of the small intestine, commonly 60 cm from the ileocaecal valve, and is usually 3–5 cm long. Many variations occur (2% – 2 feet – 2 inches is a useful aide-mémoire) (Figs 65.9 and 65.10). It represents the patent intestinal end of the vitellointestinal duct (Summary box 65.1).

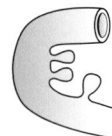

Figure 65.6 Primary diverticula of the second and third parts of the duodenum.

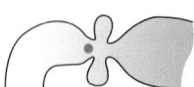

Figure 65.7 Secondary diverticula of the duodenal cap.

Johann Friedrich Meckel (the Younger), **1781–1833, Professor of Anatomy and Surgery, Halle, Germany.**

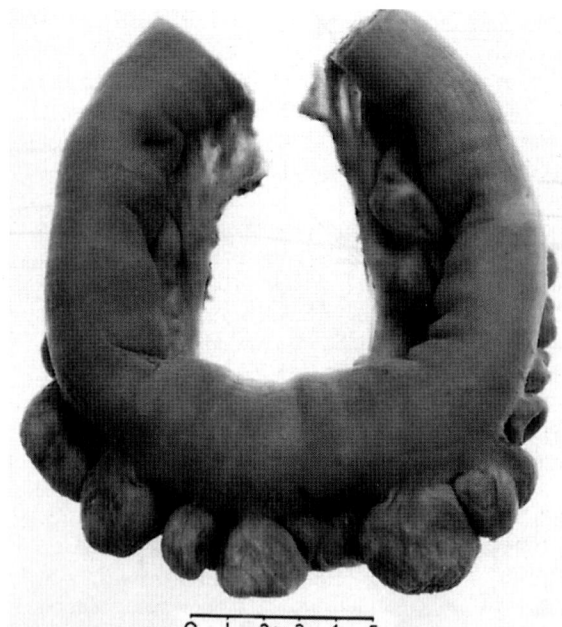

Figure 65.8 Jejunal diverticula.

Summary box 65.1

Meckel's diverticulum

■ Occurs in 2% of patients, are usually 2 inches (5 cm) in length and are situated 2 feet (60 cm) from the ileocaecal valve
■ It should be sought when a normal appendix is found at surgery for suspected appendicitis
■ If a silent Meckel's is found incidentally during the course of an operation, it can be left alone provided it is wide mouthed and not thickened
■ If ectopic gastric epithelium is present within the diverticulum, it may be the source of gastrointestinal bleeding

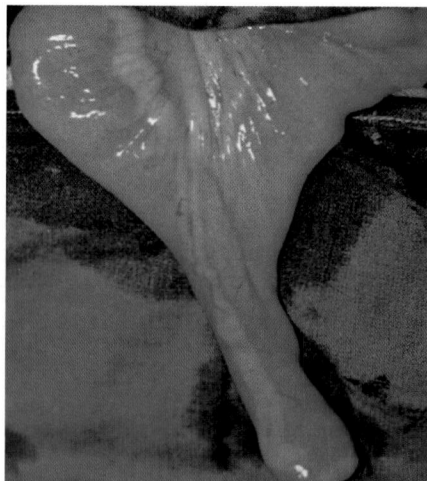

Figure 65.9 Meckel's diverticulum.

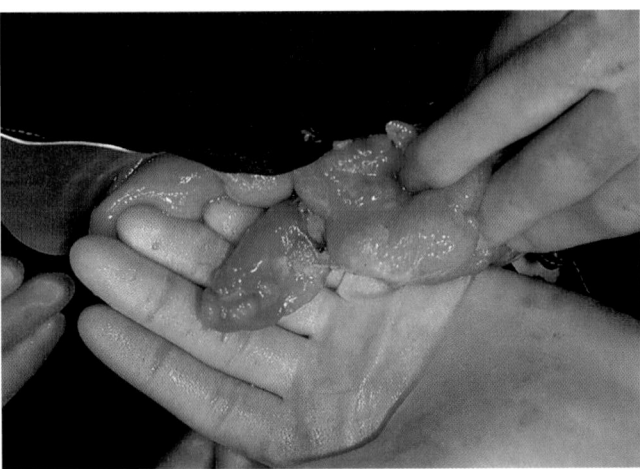

Figure 65.10 Gangrenous Meckel's diverticulitis.

A Meckel's diverticulum possesses all three coats of the intestinal wall and has its own blood supply. It is therefore vulnerable to infection and obstruction in the same way as the appendix. Indeed, when a normal appendix is found at surgery for suspected appendicitis, a Meckel's diverticulum should be sought by inspection of an appropriate length of terminal ileum. In 20% of cases, the mucosa contains heterotopic epithelium, namely gastric, colonic or sometimes pancreatic tissue. In order of frequency, these symptoms are as follows:

1 *Severe haemorrhage*, caused by peptic ulceration. Painless bleeding occurs per rectum and is maroon in colour. An operation is sometimes required for serious progressive gastrointestinal bleeding. When no lesion in the stomach or duodenum can be found, the terminal 150 cm of ileum should be carefully inspected.
2 *Intussusception*. In most cases, the apex of the intussusception is the swollen, inflamed, heterotopic epithelium at the mouth of the diverticulum.
3 *Meckel's diverticulitis* may be difficult to distinguish from the symptoms of acute appendicitis. When a diverticulum perforates, the symptoms may simulate those of a perforated duodenal ulcer. At operation, an inflamed diverticulum should be sought as soon as it has been demonstrated that the appendix and fallopian tubes are not at fault.
4 *Chronic peptic ulceration*. As the diverticulum is part of the mid-gut, the pain, although related to meals, is felt around the umbilicus.
5 *Intestinal obstruction*. The presence of a band between the apex of the diverticulum and the umbilicus may cause obstruction either by the band itself or by a volvulus around it.

Imaging

Meckel's diverticulum can be very difficult to demonstrate by contrast radiology; small bowel enema would be the most accurate investigation. Technetium-99m scanning may be useful in identifying Meckel's diverticulum as a source of gastrointestinal bleeding.

'Silent' Meckel's diverticulum

An aphorism attributed to Dr Charles Mayo is: 'a Meckel's diverticulum is frequently suspected, often sought and seldom found'. A Meckel's diverticulum usually remains symptomless throughout life and is found only at necropsy. When a silent Meckel's diverticulum is encountered in the course of an abdominal operation, it can be left provided it is wide mouthed and the wall of the diverticulum does not feel thickened. Where there is doubt and it can be removed without appreciable additional risk, it should be resected.

Exceptionally, a Meckel's diverticulum is found in an inguinal or a femoral hernia sac – Littre's hernia.

Meckel's diverticulectomy

A Meckel's diverticulum that is broad based should not be amputated at its base and invaginated in the same way as a vermiform appendix, because of the risk of stricture. Furthermore, this does not remove heterotopic epithelium when it is present. The steps of diverticulectomy are shown in Figure 65.11. Alternatively, a linear stapler device may be used. Where there is induration of the base of the diverticulum extending into the adjacent ileum, it is advisable to resect a short segment of ileum containing the diverticulum, restoring continuity with an end-to-end anastomosis.

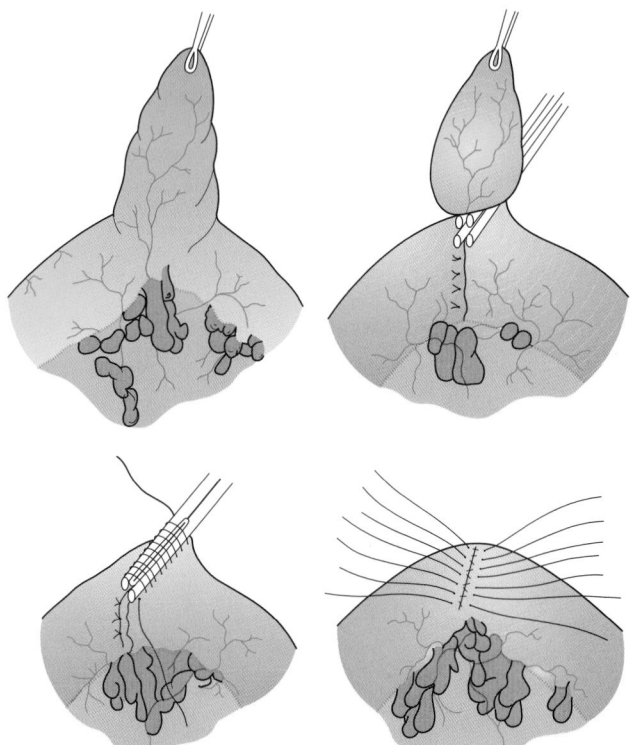

Figure 65.11 Steps in the performance of Meckelian diverticulectomy.

Colon

Introduction

The prevalence of diverticular disease in the western world is 60% over the age of 60 years. The condition is found in the sigmoid colon in 90% of cases, but the caecum can also be involved and, on occasion, the entire large bowel can be affected. Interestingly in South-east Asia, right-sided diverticular disease is twice as common as the left. The main morbidity of the disease is due to sepsis.

Aetiology

Diverticula of the colon are acquired herniations of colonic mucosa, protruding through the circular muscle at the points where the blood vessels penetrate the colonic wall. They tend to occur in rows between the strips of longitudinal muscle, sometimes partly covered by appendices epiploicae. The rectum with its complete muscle layers is not affected. It is thought to be related to reduced fibre in the western diet. This results in low stool bulk with resulting segmentation and hypertrophy of the colonic wall musculature, thus causing increased intraluminal pressure. Diverticular disease is rare in Africans and Asians, who eat a diet that is rich in natural fibre.

Diverticulosis

It is important to distinguish between diverticulosis, which may be asymptomatic, and clinical diverticular disease in which the diverticula are causing symptoms. On histological investigation, the diverticulum consists of a protrusion of mucous membranes covered with peritoneum. There is thickening of the circular muscle fibres of the intestine, which develops a concertina or saw-tooth appearance on barium enema (Fig. 65.12).

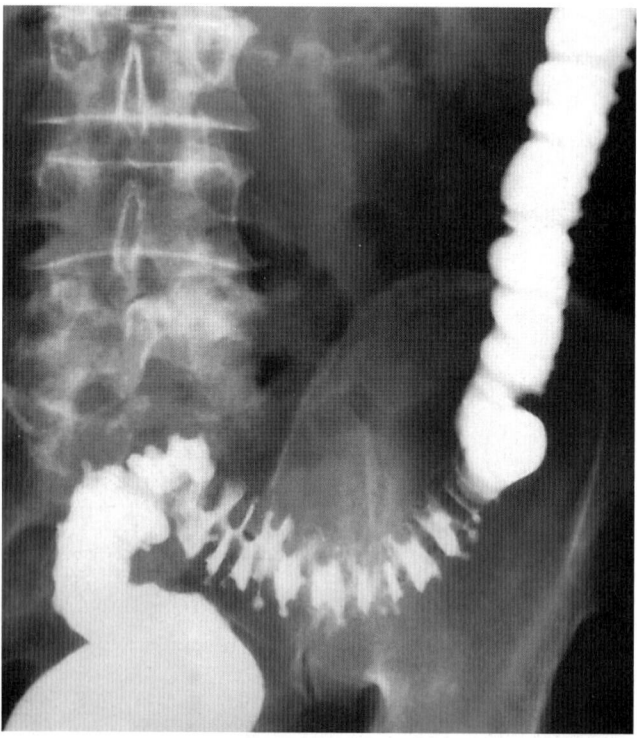

Figure 65.12 Barium enema showing sigmoid diverticular disease 'saw-teeth' and diverticula (courtesy of Dr D. Nolan, John Radcliffe Hospital, Oxford, UK).

Diverticulitis

Diverticulitis is the result of inflammation of one or more diverticula, usually with some pericolitis. It is not a precancerous condition, but cancer may coexist (Summary box 65.2).

Summary box 65.2

Complications of diverticular disease

- Diverticulitis
- Pericolic abscess
- Peritonitis
- Intestinal obstruction
- Haemorrhage
- Fistula formation

The complications are the following:

1 Recurrent periodic inflammation and pain – in some patients, these episodes may be clinically silent.
2 Perforation leading to general peritonitis or local (pericolic) abscess formation.
3 Intestinal obstruction:
  a in the sigmoid as a result of progressive fibrosis causing stenosis;
  b in the small intestine caused by adherent loops of small intestine on the pericolitis.
4 Haemorrhage: diverticulitis may present with profuse colonic haemorrhage in 17% of cases, often requiring blood transfusions.
5 Fistula formation (vesicocolic, vaginocolic, enterocolic, colocutaneous) occurs in 5% of cases, with vesicocolic being the most common.

Clinical features

Elective

In mild cases, symptoms such as distension, flatulence and a sensation of heaviness in the lower abdomen may be indistinguishable from those of irritable bowel syndrome.

Emergency

Persistent lower abdominal pain, usually in the left iliac fossa, with or without peritonitis, could be caused by diverticulitis. Fever, malaise and leucocytosis can differentiate diverticulitis from painful diverticulosis. The patient may pass loose stools or may be constipated; the lower abdomen is tender, especially on the left, but occasionally also in the right iliac fossa if the sigmoid loop lies across the midline. The sigmoid colon is often palpable, tender and thickened. Rectal examination may, but does not usually, reveal a tender mass. Any urinary symptoms may herald the formation of a vesicocolic fistula, which leads to pneumaturia (flatus in the urine) and even faeces in the urine.

Classification of contamination

Studies have shown that the degree of sepsis has a major impact on outcome. Those with inflammatory masses have a lower mortality than those with perforation (3% vs. 33%). Classification systems have been developed for acute diverticulitis, of which Hinchey is the most commonly used (Table 65.1).

E.F. Hinchey, P.G.H. Schaol and G.K. Richards. **Treatment of perforated diverticular disease of the colon.** *Adv Surg* 1978; 12: 85–109.

Table 65.1 Classification of diverticulitis

Stage	Severity	Pain	Systemic	Investigation	Management
1	Pericolic abscess or phlegmon	LIF	Possibly no change	Delayed barium enema, endoscopy	Bowel rest, IV antibiotic, DVT prophylaxis and fluids
2	Pelvic or intra-abdominal abscess	Severe, fullness in LIF	Mild toxic	CT	Percutaneous drainage
3	Non-faeculent peritonitis	Peritonitis	Toxic	CT	Resuscitation + operation
4	Faeculent peritonitis	Peritonitis	Severe toxicity, shock	Proceed to operation	Resuscitation + immediate operation

DVT, deep venous thrombosis; IV, intravenous; CT, computerised tomography; LIF, left iliac fossa.

Diagnosis

Radiology

Although the diagnosis of acute diverticulitis is made on clinical grounds, it can be confirmed during the acute phase by computerised tomography (CT). It is particularly good at identifying bowel wall thickening, abscess formation and extraluminal disease. The specificity is high and it is able to demonstrate other pathology. It has revolutionised the assessment of complicated diverticular disease. On identification of abscesses in stable patients, drainage may be carried out percutaneously. Such an option may delay or postpone further operative procedures.

Barium enemas (Fig. 65.13) and sigmoidoscopy are usually reserved for patients who have recovered from an attack of acute diverticulitis, for fear of causing perforation or peritonitis. Water-soluble contrast enemas may, however, be helpful in sorting out patients with large bowel obstruction. In the acute situation, it is good at detecting intraluminal changes and leakage. The sensitivity for this is of the order of 90%. Barium radiology is carried out to exclude a carcinoma and to assess the extent of the disease.

Where the sigmoid colon is thickened and narrowed, a 'saw-tooth' appearance may be seen. Some strictures can be very difficult to distinguish by radiology alone and, in those circumstances, colonoscopy will be necessary to rule out a carcinoma. Vesicocolic fistulae should be evaluated with cystoscopy and biopsy in addition to colonoscopy. Contrast examinations may show the fistula itself. The differential diagnosis for vesicocolic fistulae (and other fistulae) includes cancer, radiation damage, Crohn's disease (CD), tuberculosis and actinomycosis.

Colonoscopy

Colonoscopy may reveal the necks of diverticula within the bowel lumen (Fig. 65.14). A narrowed area of diverticulitis can be entered but, on occasion, not passed because of the severity of disease. The differential diagnosis from a carcinoma can be impossible if a tight stenosis prevents colonoscopy. In equivocal cases, biopsies may be taken.

Management

Non-complicated

Diverticulosis should be treated with a high-residue diet containing roughage in the form of wholemeal bread, flour, fruit and vegetables. The evidence for this is not of a high quality. Bulk formers such as bran, Celevac, Isogel and Fybogel may be given

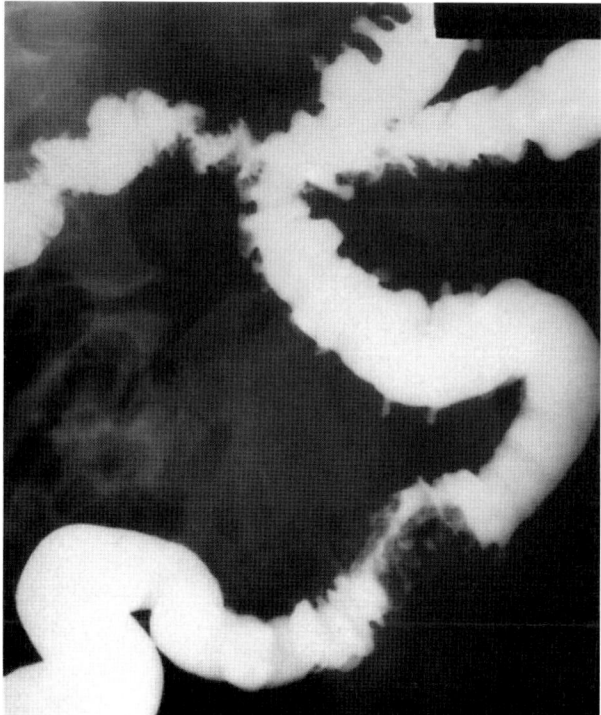

Figure 65.13 Barium enema showing a large filling defect in the sigmoid colon caused by a pericolic abscess (courtesy of Dr D. Nolan, John Radcliffe Hospital, Oxford, UK).

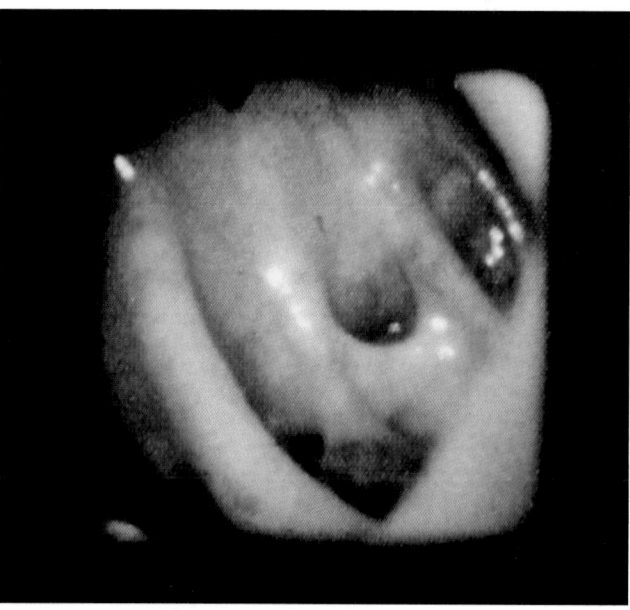

Figure 65.14 Colonoscopic view of sigmoid diverticula. Note the mouths of diverticula between the hypertrophied colonic walls.

CHAPTER 65 | THE SMALL AND LARGE INTESTINES

until the stools are soft. Painful diverticular disease may require antispasmodics.

Acute diverticulitis is treated by bed rest and intravenous antibiotics (usually cefuroxime and metronidazole). After the acute attack has subsided, and if the diagnosis has not already been confirmed by CT, a barium enema should be administered (Summary box 65.3).

Operative procedures for diverticular disease

The aim of surgery is to control sepsis in the peritoneum and circulation. Indications for operation include general peritonitis and failure to resolve on conservative treatment. Surgery, especially in the acute setting, has considerable risk. Postoperative mortality and reoperation rate for elective resection are 5% and 12%, respectively, which compares with 17% and 16% for emergency surgery. There is controversy as to whether a more radical approach should be adopted. Historically, data have shown that mortality was lower in patients in whom the inflamed colon was resected. However, two randomised comparative trials have shown that mortality is lower in the group in which a proximal defunctioning stoma is performed. The decision needs to be made by the individual surgeon based on the general state of the patient.

The risk of recurrence in patients with moderate diverticulitis is only 14%. This compares with 39% for severe diverticulitis. Therefore, a policy of monitoring can be used in elderly patients following an acute attack that settles. Younger patients unfortunately have a higher risk of recurrence (below the age of 50 years, the risk of recurrence is 25%). Surgery may be indicated for young patients with more than two attacks of inflammation. Some 10% of patients require an operation either for recurrent attacks, which make life a misery, or for the complications of diverticulitis.

1 The ideal operation carried out as an interval procedure after careful preparation of the gut is a one-stage resection. This involves removal of the affected segment and restoration of continuity by end-to-end anastomosis. Careful dissection will allow eventual mobilisation of the rectosigmoid out of the pelvis exposing the normal rectum, and greater mobility will allow an easier anastomosis.

2 If there is obstruction, inflammatory oedema and adhesions or the bowel is loaded with faeces, a Hartmann's operation is the procedure of choice (Fig. 65.15). This removes the risk of anastomotic leak. However, complications may ensue if the stoma is under tension, or the rectal stump breaks down. The involved area is resected. The rectum is closed at the peritoneal reflection, and the left colon brought out as a left iliac fossa colostomy. The once popular staged procedures using a preliminary transverse colostomy are now rarely used except by inexperienced surgeons because of the high mortality associated with them. In selected obstructed cases, the bowel can be cleaned by on-table lavage, making anastomosis much safer.

3 In acute perforation, peritonitis soon becomes general and may be purulent, with a mortality rate of about 15%. Gross faecal peritonitis carries a mortality rate of more than 50% and pneumoperitoneum is usually present; the diagnosis may not be confirmed until emergency laparotomy. There is a choice of procedures:

a primary resection and Hartmann's procedure (see above);
b primary resection and anastomosis after on-table lavage in selected cases;
c exteriorisation of the affected bowel, which is then opened as a colostomy, a procedure now rarely used.

4 Fistulae can be cured only by resection of the diseased bowel and closure of the fistula. In the case of a colovesical fistula, it

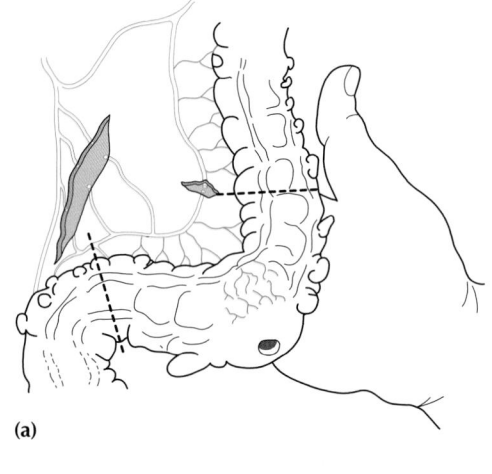

(a)

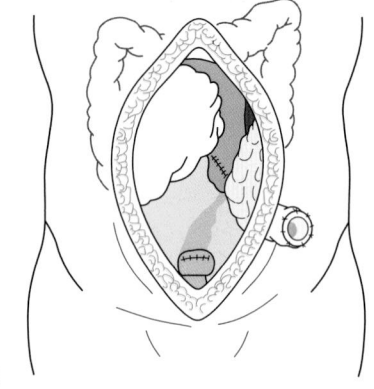

(b)

Figure 65.15 (a) Perforated sigmoid diverticular disease. (b) The Hartmann procedure – oversewn rectal stump and left iliac fossa colostomy.

is usually possible to 'pinch off' the affected bowel from the bladder, close it and then resect the sigmoid. In very difficult cases, a staged procedure with a preliminary defunctioning stoma may be necessary.

5   Haemorrhage from diverticulitis must be distinguished from angiodysplasia. It usually responds to conservative management and occasionally requires resection. On-table lavage and colonoscopy may be necessary to localise the bleeding site. If the source cannot be located, then subtotal colectomy and ileostomy is the safest option.

Diverticular disease and carcinoma coexist in 12% of cases. Exploration may be necessary but, even then, differentiation may be difficult until histological investigations are available (Table 65.2). Weight loss, falling haemoglobin and persistently positive occult blood are sinister features.

Solitary diverticulum of the caecum and ascending colon is rare and congenital, and may present with symptoms and signs identical to those of acute appendicitis.

Laparoscopic surgery

In selected cases, laparoscopic surgery has been used for sigmoid resection. This has the benefit of decreased hospital stay and costs. However, there is little high-quality research in the field to advocate its true merits.

ULCERATIVE COLITIS

Aetiology

The cause of UC is unknown. There is probably a genetic contribution with no clear Mendelian pattern of inheritance. It has been shown that 15% of patients with UC have a first-degree relative with inflammatory bowel disease. UC is more common in Caucasians than in blacks or Asians. In spite of intensive bacteriological studies, no organisms or group of organisms can be incriminated. Relapse of colitis has, however, been reported in association with bacterial dysenteries. Smoking seems to have a protective effect. Patients often comment that relapses are associated with periods of stress at home or at work, but personality and psychiatric profiles are the same as those of the normal population.

Studies show that mucosal permeability increases with the presence of inflammation. This may be due to a combination of genetic susceptibility or damage by toxins. The resulting passage of antigens that trigger inflammation may cause an influx of neutrophils and lymphocytes. This inflammation is usually dampened down in normal tissue, but this is lost in UC. There may be loss of tolerance to self-antigens. UC is thought to be an immune disorder in individuals with yet unknown susceptibility genes or a hypersensitivity reaction to an external antigen.

Epidemiology

There are 10–15 new cases per 100 000 population a year in the UK. This is higher in people of Jewish origin. The prevalence is 160 per 100 000 population. There are approximately 96 000 people with UC in the UK. The incidence has not changed over the last 20 years. The disease has been rare in eastern populations but is now being reported more commonly, suggesting an environmental cause that has developed as a result of an increasing 'westernisation' of diet and/or social habits and better diagnostic facilities. The sex ratio is equal in the first four decades of life. From the age of 40 years, the incidence in females falls whereas it remains the same in males. It is uncommon before the age of 10 years, and most patients are between the ages of 20 and 40 years at diagnosis.

Pathology

In 95% of cases, the disease starts in the rectum and spreads proximally. The rectum is involved in all circumstances except in those using topical rectal preparations (rectal sparing). It is a diffuse inflammatory disease, primarily affecting the mucosa and superficial submucosa, and only in severe disease are the deeper layers of the intestinal wall affected. There are multiple minute ulcers, and microscopic evidence proves that the ulceration is almost always more severe and extensive than the gross appearance indicates. When the disease is chronic, inflammatory polyps (pseudopolyps) occur in up to 20% of cases and may be numerous. In severe fulminant colitis, a section of the colon, usually the transverse colon, may become acutely dilated, with the risk of perforation ('toxic megacolon'). On microscopic investigation, there is an increase in inflammatory cells in the lamina propria, the walls of crypts are infiltrated by inflammatory cells and there are crypt abscesses. There is depletion of goblet cell mucin. With time, these changes become severe, and precancerous changes can develop (= severe dysplasia or carcinoma *in situ*).

Symptoms

The first symptom is watery or bloody diarrhoea; there may be a rectal discharge of mucus that is either blood-stained or purulent. Pain as an early symptom is unusual. In most cases, the disease is

Table 65.2 Differentiation of diverticulitis from carcinoma of the colon

	Diverticulitis	**Carcinoma**
History	Long	Short
Pain	More common	25% painless
Mass	25% have tenderness	
Bleeding	17% often profuse, periodic	65% – usually small amounts persistently
Radiograph	Diffuse change	Localised: no relaxation with propantheline bromide
Sigmoidoscopy	Inflammatory change over an area	No inflammation until ulcer reached
Colonoscopy	No carcinoma seen	Carcinoma seen and biopsied

Gregor Johann Mendel, **1822–1884, an Austrian monk and naturalist who became Abbott of the Augustinian Monastery at Brunn, Czechoslovakia, and discovered the laws of inheritance by studying the edible pea.**

CHAPTER 65 | THE SMALL AND LARGE INTESTINES

chronic and characterised by relapses and remissions. In general, a poor prognosis is indicated by (1) a severe initial attack, (2) disease involving the whole colon and (3) increasing age, especially after 60 years. If the disease remains confined to the left colon, the outlook is better.

Proctitis

About 50% have rectal inflammation. As most of the colon is healthy, the stool is formed or semiformed, and the patient is often severely troubled by tenesmus and urgency. There is usually no systemic upset, no effect on growth in children, and extra-alimentary manifestations are rare. In 5–10%, there is spread to involve the rest of the colon.

Colitis (Fig. 65.16)

Diarrhoea usually implies that there is active disease proximal to the rectum. There is an increased tendency to systemic upset. Protein loss is associated with bleeding, which results in weight loss. There is a greater risk of extra-alimentary manifestations and cancer. Approximately 30% of patients have inflammation extending to the sigmoid colon, and spread proximal to the splenic flexure occurs in 20%. The clinical pattern is one of recurrent severe attacks of bloody diarrhoea up to 20 times a day, dehydration and fluid electrolyte losses. Anaemia and hypoproteinaemia are common.

Disease severity

Disease severity can be graded as:

1 mild – rectal bleeding or diarrhoea with four or fewer motions per day and the absence of systemic signs of disease;
2 moderate – more than four motions per day but no systemic signs of illness;
3 severe – more than four motions a day together with one or more signs of systemic illness: fever over 37.5°C, tachycardia more than 90 min⁻¹, hypoalbuminaemia less than $30\,\text{g}\,\text{l}^{-1}$, weight loss more than 3 kg.

Complications of severe disease

Fulminating colitis and toxic dilatation (megacolon) (Fig. 65.17)

Patients with severe disease should be admitted to hospital for intensive treatment. This occurs in 5–10% of patients. The

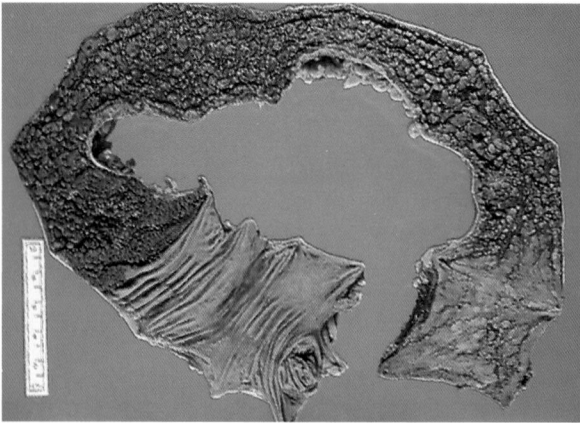

Figure 65.16 Extensive, active ulcerative colitis (the rectum is spared, which is unusual in the absence of treatment) (courtesy of Dr I. Talbot, St Mark's Hospital, London, UK).

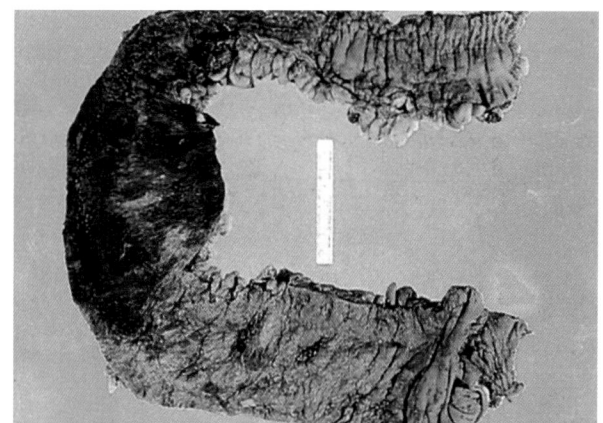

Figure 65.17 Fulminating ulcerative colitis with toxic dilatation of the transverse colon.

patient will have severe rectal symptoms with systemic upset such as weight loss and dehydration. A third will come to urgent surgery. Dilatation should be suspected in patients with active colitis who develop severe abdominal pain. It is an indication that inflammation has gone through all the muscle layers of the colon. In patients on intensive treatment such as steroids, there may be few symptoms. The diagnosis is confirmed by the presence on a plain abdominal radiograph of the colon with a diameter of more than 6 cm. The condition must be differentiated from dysentery, typhoid and amoebic colitis. Plain abdominal radiographs should be obtained daily in patients with severe colitis, and a progressive increase in diameter in spite of medical therapy is an indication for surgery (Summary box 65.4; Fig. 65.18).

Summary box 65.4
Complications of UC
Acute
■ Toxic dilatation
■ Perforation
■ Haemorrhage
Chronic
■ Cancer
■ Extra-alimentary manifestations: skin lesions, eye problems, liver disease

Perforation

Colonic perforation in UC is a grave complication with a mortality rate of 50% or more. Steroids may mask the physical signs. Perforation can sometimes occur without toxic dilatation. Generally, patients with severe attacks should be managed so that they do not develop these complications.

Severe haemorrhage

Severe rectal bleeding is uncommon and may occasionally require transfusion and, rarely, surgery.

Investigations

A plain abdominal film can often show the severity of disease. Faeces are present only in parts of the colon that are normal or only mildly inflamed. Mucosal islands can sometimes be seen.

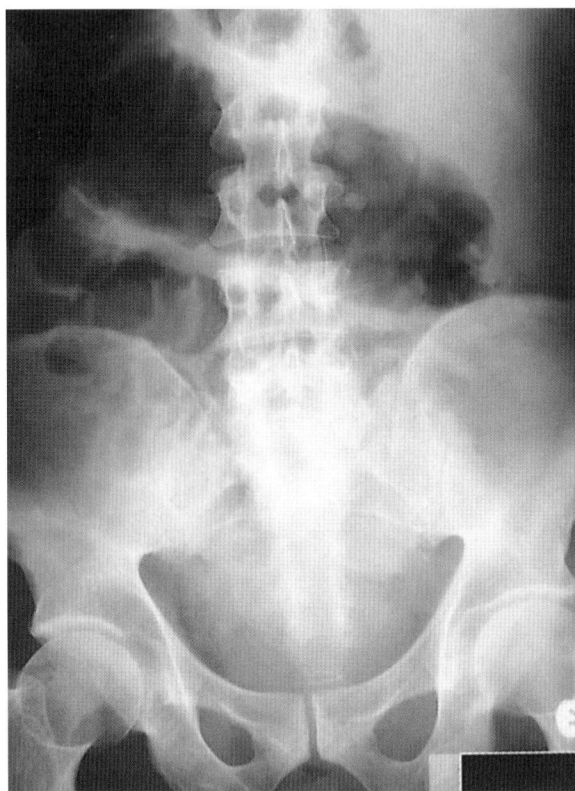

Figure 65.18 Supine abdominal radiograph in toxic megacolon. The transverse colon is dilated (7 cm), there is no formed residue in the colon, and large mucosal islands are present in the ascending colon and hepatic flexure. No haustration is present in the transverse colon, which distinguishes this from ileus of obstruction. Mucosal islands are due to oedematous remnants or mucosa where there has been extensive ulceration (courtesy of Dr C. Bartram, St Mark's Hospital, London, UK).

Small bowel loops in the right lower quadrant may be a sign of severe disease.

Barium enema

The principal signs are (Fig. 65.19):

- loss of haustration, especially in the distal colon;
- mucosal changes caused by granularity;
- pseudopolyps;
- in chronic cases, a narrow contracted colon.

In some centres, an instant enema is used with a water-soluble medium for contrast instead of barium and no bowel preparation to avoid aggravating any underlying colitis (Fig. 65.20).

Sigmoidoscopy

Sigmoidoscopy is essential for diagnosis of early cases and mild disease not showing up on a barium enema. The initial findings are those of proctitis: the mucosa is hyperaemic and bleeds on touch, and there may be a pus-like exudate. Where there has been remission and relapse, there may be the presence of regeneration nodules or pseudopolyps. Later, tiny ulcers may be seen that appear to coalesce. This is different from the picture of amoebic dysentery, in which there are large, deep ulcers with intervening normal mucosa.

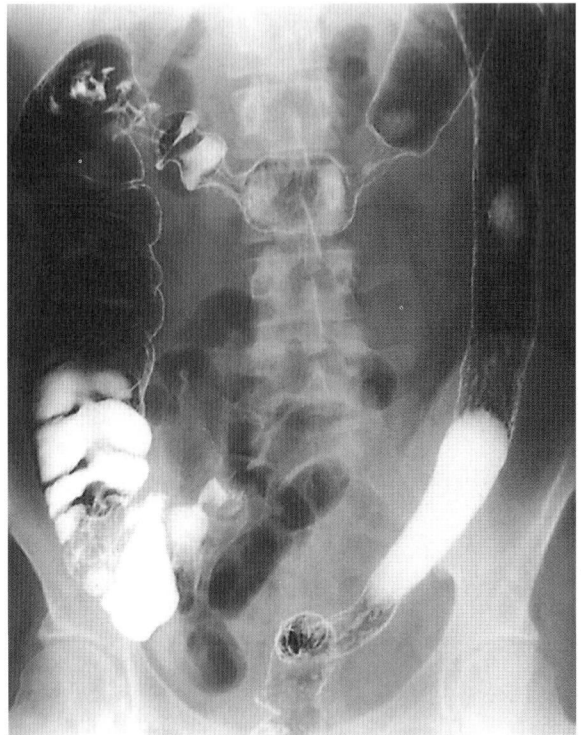

Figure 65.19 Double-contrast barium enema showing left-sided ulcerative colitis with a tubular left colon compared with a normal right colon (courtesy of Dr D. Nolan, John Radcliffe Hospital, Oxford, UK).

Colonoscopy and biopsy

This has an important place in management:

1 to establish the extent of inflammation;
2 to distinguish between UC and Crohn's colitis;
3 to monitor response to treatment;
4 to assess longstanding cases for malignant change.

Although it may occasionally be helpful, colonoscopy is not usually used in acute cases for fear of aggravating the disease or perforation.

Bacteriology

Campylobacter is the commonest cause of infective colitis in the UK. Pathologically, it is difficult to distinguish from UC. A stool specimen needs to be sent for microbiology analysis when UC is suspected. Other infective causes include *Shigella* and amoebiasis. Pseudomembranous colitis occurs in hospital patients on antibiotic treatment and non-steroidal anti-inflammatory drugs (NSAIDs). The causative organism is *Clostridium difficile*. Immunocompromised patients are at risk of infective proctocolitis from cytomegalovirus and cryptosporidia.

The cancer risk in colitis

Although this is an important complication, the overall risk is only about 3.5%. It is much less in early cases but increases with duration of disease. At 10 years, the risk of cancer in all patients

Burrill Bernard Crohn, 1884–1956, Gastroenterologist, Mount Sinai Hospital, New York, NY, USA, described regional ileitis in 1932.
Kiyoshi Shiga, 1870–1957, a Japanese Bacteriologist, reported his discovery of the dysentery bacillus in 1898.

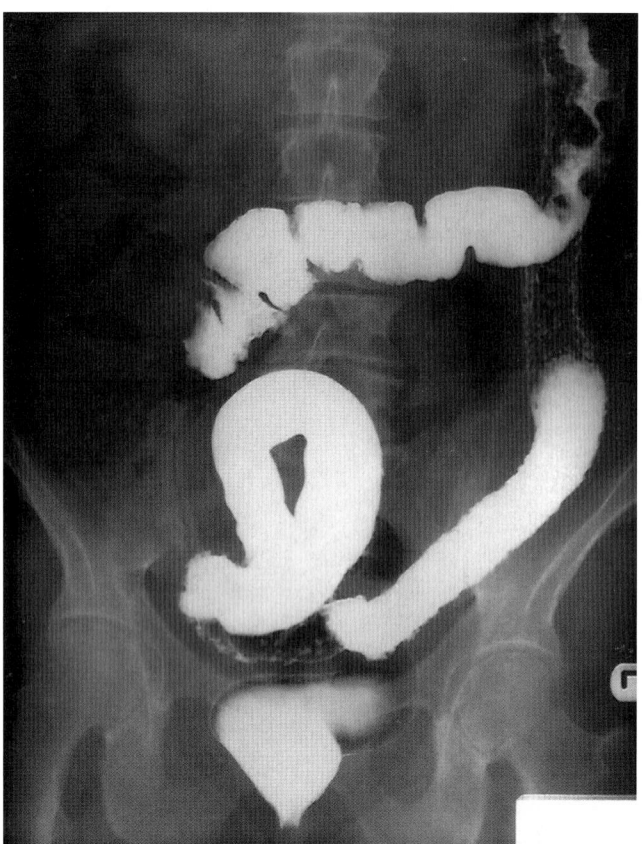

Figure 65.20 Instant enema in acute ulcerative colitis. The rectum shows a granular mucosa with ulceration extending from the proximal sigmoid into the splenic flexure region. The ulcers are seen tangentially as collar-stud projections from the mucosal line. Formed residue is present in the ascending colon and hepatic flexure. The colitis extends into the mid-transverse colon but is most active in the descending colon (courtesy of Dr C. Bartram, St Mark's Hospital, London, UK).

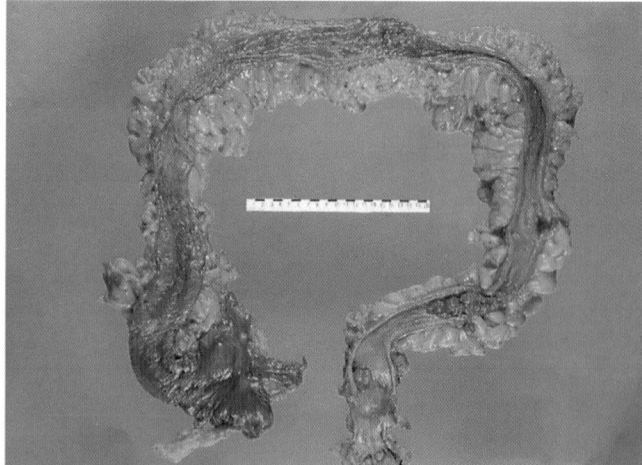

Figure 65.21 Resection specimen from a patient with longstanding ulcerative colitis showing a narrow tubular colon with areas of cancerous change in the rectum and sigmoid (courtesy of Dr B. Warren, John Radcliffe Hospital, Oxford, UK).

with UC, irrespective of disease extent, is 2%. This increases to 8% at 20 years and 18% at 30 years. Carcinoma is more likely to occur if the whole colon is involved and if the disease started in early life (Fig. 65.21). Carcinomatous change, often atypical and high grade, may occur at many sites at once. The colon is involved rather than the rectum, and the maximal incidence is during the fourth decade.

The golden rule is that, when the disease has been present for 10 years or more, regular colonoscopic checks must be carried out to check for dysplasia, even if the disease is clinically quiescent. If on biopsy, there is severe epithelial dysplasia, which is a marker for impending or frank carcinomatous change, surgery is indicated. Annual colonoscopy and biopsy is then part of cancer surveillance. In the rare patients with a fibrous stricture, the stricture should be examined especially carefully for the presence of an underlying carcinoma.

Extraintestinal manifestations

Arthritis occurs in around 15% of patients and is of the large joint polyarthropathy type, affecting knees, ankles, elbows and wrists. Sacroiliitis and ankylosing spondylitis are 20 times more common in patients with UC.

Bile duct cancer is a rare complication, and colectomy does not appear to reduce the risk of subsequent bile duct cancer or sclerosing cholangitis. Other manifestations include:

- *skin lesions*: erythema nodosum, pyoderma gangrenosum or aphthous ulceration;
- *eye problems*: iritis;
- *liver disease*: sclerosing cholangitis has been reported in up to 70% of cases. Diagnosis is by ERCP, which demonstrates the characteristic alternating stricturing and bleeding of the intrahepatic and extrahepatic ducts.

Treatment

It is important to appreciate the multidisciplinary approach to the management of UC. This involves the gastroenterologist, nurses, nutritionist, stomatherapist and social worker as well as the surgeon.

Medical treatment of an acute attack

Corticosteroids are the most useful drugs and can be given either locally for inflammation of the rectum or systemically when the disease is more extensive. One of the 5-aminosalicylic acid (5-ASA) derivatives can be given both topically and systemically. Their main function is in maintaining remission rather than treating an acute attack. Non-specific anti-diarrhoeal agents have no place in the routine management of UC (Summary box 65.5).

Summary box 65.5

Principles of management of UC

- Many patients can be adequately maintained for years on medical therapy
- Toxic dilatation must be suspected in any colitic patient who develops severe abdominal pain; missed colonic perforation is associated with a high mortality
- Colitic patients are at increased risk of developing cancer; those with pancolitis of long duration are most at risk

Mild attacks

Patients with a mild attack and limited disease will usually respond to rectally administered steroids. In those with more extensive disease, oral prednisolone 20–40 mg day^{-1} is given over a 3- to 4-week period. One of the 5-ASA compounds should be given concurrently.

Moderate attacks

These patients should be treated with oral prednisolone 40 mg day^{-1}, twice-daily steroid enemas and 5-ASA. Failure to achieve remission as an out-patient is an indication for admission.

Severe attacks

These patients must be regarded as medical emergencies and require immediate admission to hospital. Their appearance is often misleading, and they must be examined at least twice a day. It is important to monitor vital signs (pulse, temperature and blood pressure). Weight needs to be recorded at admission and twice a week while in hospital. A stool chart should be kept. Increasing abdominal girth is a potential sign of megacolon developing. A plain abdominal radiograph is taken daily and inspected for dilatation of the transverse colon of more than 5.5 cm. The presence of mucosal islands or intramural gas on plain radiographs (see Fig. 65.18), increasing colonic diameter or a sudden increase in pulse and temperature may indicate a colonic perforation. Fluid and electrolyte balance is maintained, anaemia is corrected and adequate nutrition is provided, sometimes intravenously in severe cases. If the patient is not having immediate surgery, then oral nutrition is important. High calories are required. If severe malnourishment is present, then parenteral nutrition may be indicated. The patient is treated with intravenous hydrocortisone 100–200 mg four times daily. This can be supplemented with a rectal infusion of prednisolone. There is no evidence that antibiotics modify the course of a severe attack. Some patients are treated with azathioprine or ciclosporin A to induce remission. If there is failure to gain an improvement within 3–5 days, then surgery must be seriously considered. Prolonged high-dose intravenous steroid therapy is fraught with danger. Patients who have had weeks of treatment, during which the colonic wall has become friable and disintegrates at laparotomy, are now fortunately rare.

Indications for surgery

The risk of colectomy is 20% overall, ranging from 5% in those patients with proctitis to 50% in those patients with a very severe attack. The need for surgery is highest in the first year after the disease onset, for:

- severe or fulminating disease failing to respond to medical therapy;
- chronic disease with anaemia, frequent stools, urgency and tenesmus;
- steroid-dependent disease – here, the disease is not severe but remission cannot be maintained without substantial doses of steroids;
- the risk of neoplastic change: patients who have severe dysplasia on review colonoscopy;
- extraintestinal manifestations;
- rarely, severe haemorrhage or stenosis causing obstruction.

Operations

The patient is placed in a position to allow access to the rectum. In the emergency situation, the 'first aid procedure' is a total abdominal colectomy and ileostomy. The rectal stump is left long but runs the risk of on-going haemorrhage. The rectum can either be brought out at the lower end of the wound as a mucous fistula or closed just beneath the skin. This has the advantage that the patient recovers quickly, the histology of the resected colon can be checked, and restorative surgery can be contemplated at a later date when the patient is no longer on steroids and in optimal nutritional condition. The alternative, division of the rectum below the sacral promontory, can result in breakdown and pelvic abscess, and makes subsequent identification of the stump more difficult. This is more likely to occur in patients in a poor condition or those on long-term steroids.

Proctocolectomy and ileostomy

This is the procedure associated with the lowest complication rate. It is indicated in patients who are not candidates for restoration. The patient is left with a permanent ileostomy. There is, however, a 20% long-term risk of adhesional obstruction (the reoperation rate is, however, very low) and 5–10% of the perineal wounds are slow to heal. The late result will be a chronic perineal sinus that may require repeated currettage or excision. The obvious disadvantage is an ileostomy and, although many patients cope remarkably well with satisfactory objective measures of quality of life, there is a psychological and social 'cost'. Problems that may arise with a stoma include stricture formation, prolapse, retraction and herniation.

Rectal and anal dissection

Refinements of the procedure have included a close rectal dissection to minimise damage to the nervi erigenti and hence erectile dysfunction, which may occur in 0.5–2%, and intersphincteric excision of the anus, which results in a smaller perineal wound and fewer healing problems.

Restorative proctocolectomy with an ileoanal pouch (Parks)

In this operation, a pouch is made out of ileum (Fig. 65.22) as a substitute for the rectum and sewn or stapled to the anal canal. This avoids a permanent stoma. It is reserved for patients with adequate anal sphincters and should be avoided when CD is a possibility. It should not initially be considered for poorly patients. Various pouch designs have been described, but the 'J' is the most popular and the most easily made using staplers (Fig. 65.23). The 'S' (three loop) has been associated with evacuation difficulties due to the short efferent spout. The 'W' (four loop) pouch has a larger reservoir, which results in less bowel frequency. There is some controversy over the correct technique for ileoanal anastomosis. In the earliest operations, the mucosa from the dentate line up to midrectum was stripped off the underlying muscle, but it is now known that a long muscle cuff is not needed. A mucosectomy of the upper anal canal with an anastomosis at the dentate line is claimed to remove all of the at-risk mucosa and any problem of subsequent cancer. It may also result in imperfect continence with nocturnal seepage. The alternative is an anastomosis double-stapled to the top of the anal canal, preserving the upper anal canal mucosa. Continence appears to be better, but the theoretical risk of leaving inflamed mucosa remains. The procedure can be carried out in stages. In most cases, a covering loop

---

Sir Alan Guyatt Parks, **1920–1982, Surgeon, St Mark's Hospital and the London Hospital, London, UK.**

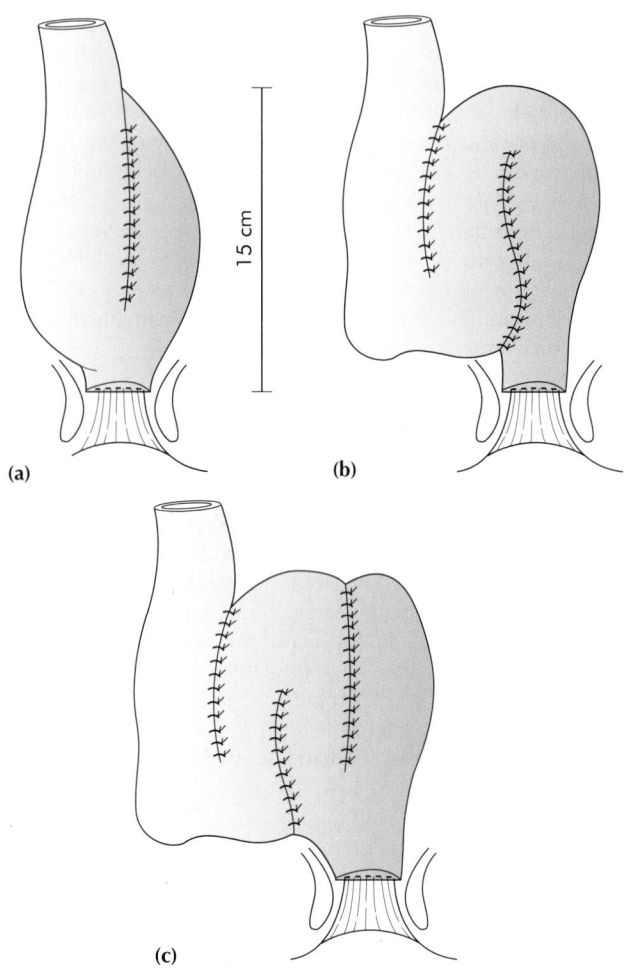

15 cm

(a) (b)

(c)

Figure 65.22 Ileoanal anastomosis with pouch. A substitute rectum is made from joined folds of ileum to form an expanded pouch of small intestine. The pouch is then joined directly to the anus at the level of the dentate line, all other rectal mucosa having been removed. Three ways of forming a pouch are illustrated: (a) a simple reversed 'J'; (b) an 'S' pouch; (c) a 'W' pouch.

ileostomy is used. Complications include pelvic sepsis – usually resulting from a leak at the ileoanal anastomosis – small bowel obstruction and pouch vaginal fistula. Frequency of evacuation is determined by pouch volume, completeness of emptying, reservoir inflammation and intrinsic small bowel motility, but can be between three and six evacuations daily. Increased frequency, urgency and faecal incontinence can be seen (20%, 5% and 5% respectively), but these reduce with time. Although associated with a higher complication rate, it is rapidly becoming the operation of choice in younger patients, avoiding a permanent ileostomy. The failure rate in the first year is 5–15%, the main reasons being pelvic sepsis (50%), poor function (30%) and pouchitis or inflammation of the pouch (10%). It is also important for women to realise that they may suffer from reduced fertility. So women yet to have children may elect for a colectomy with ileostomy or colectomy and ileorectal anastomosis if the rectum is spared in the first instance. There are much higher failure rates in CD when compared with UC (50% vs. 10%), and the operation is not to be recommended in this disease.

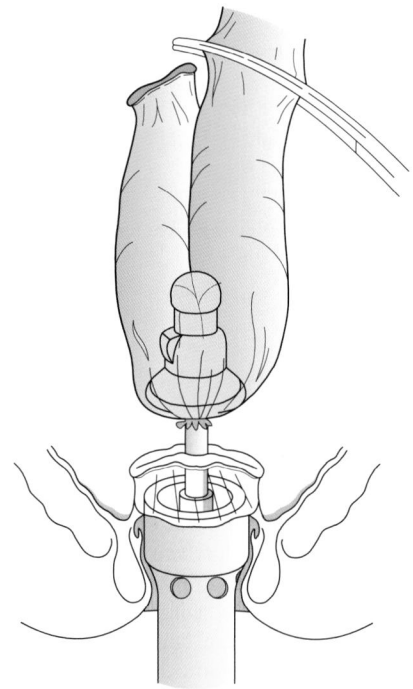

Figure 65.23 Stapled 'J' pouch with stapler creating a pouch–anus anastomosis.

Colectomy and ileorectal anastomosis

If there is minimal rectal inflammation, this can occasionally be used, although the surgeon should not be falsely reassured that the rectum has been relatively 'spared' in a patient using steroid enemas. If the rectum is preserved, then annual rectal inspection is advocated. Although it has the advantage of stoma avoidance and minimal risk to sexual function associated with rectal dissection, it has largely been superseded by restorative proctocolectomy. A number of series have shown low mortality and morbidity, but it has fallen out of favour due to the on-going risk of persisting inflammation and malignancy.

Ileostomy with a continent intra-abdominal pouch (Kock's procedure)

A reservoir is made from 30 cm of ileum and, just beyond this, a spout is made by inverting the efferent ileum into itself to give a continent valve just below skin level. The pouch is emptied by the patient inserting a catheter through the valve; this procedure is now rarely used. Complications include early leak with formation of fistulae, which can occur in 10–20%, and late subluxation of the valve, which can occur in 20%. Pouch survival at 10 years was 87% in one study.

Ileostomy

End-ileostomy (Brooke)

In those patients with a permanent ileostomy, there must be scrupulous attention to detail during the operation to ensure a good functional result. The position of the ileostomy should be

Nils Kock, **Swedish Surgeon, pioneered the creation of artificial reservoirs within the abdomen from loops of small intestine in the 1970s.**
Bryan Nicholas Brooke, **1915–1998, Professor of Surgery, St George's Hospital, London, UK.**

carefully chosen by the patient with the help of a stoma care nurse specialist. There is an argument for making the trephine incision before entering the abdomen to prevent any problems of distortion of the abdominal wall after opening. The ileum is normally brought through the rectus abdominis muscle. Careful attention to the terminal ileal mesentery should be taken to ensure that it is supplied by the marginal artery in order to reduce mesenteric bulk. The use of a spout (Fig. 65.24) was originally described by Bryan Brooke; this should project some 4 cm from the skin surface. A disposable appliance is placed over the ileostomy so that it is a snug fit at skin level.

Loop ileostomy

This is often used to defunction a pouch ileoanal procedure. A knuckle of ileum is pulled out through a skin trephine in the right iliac fossa. An incision is made in the distal part of the knuckle, and this is then pulled over the top of the more proximal part to create a spout on the proximal side of the loop with a flush distal side still in continuity. This allows near-perfect defunction, but also the possibility of restoration of continuity by taking down the spout and reanastomosing the partially divided ileum.

Ileostomy care

During the first few postoperative days, fluid and electrolyte balance must be adjusted with great care. There may be an 'ileostomy flux' while the ileum adapts to the loss of the colon, and the fluid losses can amount to 4 or 5 litres day^{-1}. The stools thicken in a few weeks and are semisolid in a few months. The help, skill and advice of the stoma care nurse specialist are essential. Modern appliances have transformed stoma care, and skin problems are unusual (Fig. 65.25).

Complications of an ileostomy include prolapse, retraction, stenosis, bleeding, fistula and paraileostomy hernia.

CROHN'S DISEASE (REGIONAL ENTERITIS)

CD became widely recognised following the report in 1932 by Crohn, Ginzburg and Oppenheimer describing young adults with a chronic inflammatory disease of the ileum. It can affect any part of the gastrointestinal tract from the lips to the anal margin, but ileocolonic disease is the most common presentation.

Epidemiology

It is most common in North America and northern Europe with an incidence of 5 per 100 000. This has increased over the last 30 years but is now thought to be levelling off. Prevalence rates as high as 56 per 100 000 have been reported in the UK. Over the last four decades, there seems to have been a rise in the incidence,

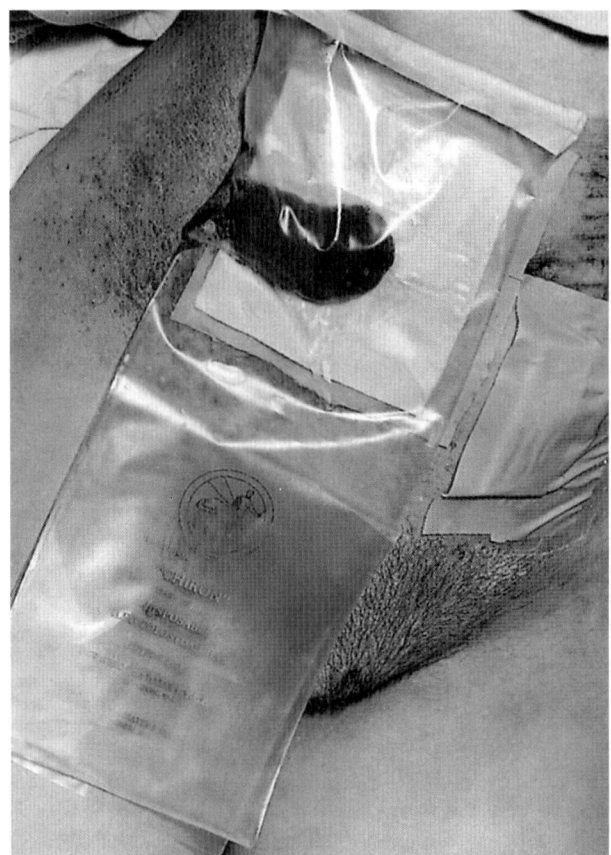

Figure 65.25 Disposable ileostomy bag (courtesy of B.N. Brooke, FRCS, London, UK).

which cannot be accounted for by increased diagnosis. It is slightly more common in women than in men, but is most commonly diagnosed in young patients between the ages of 25 and 40 years. There does, however, seem to be a second peak of incidence around the age of 70 years. Migration seems to increase the risk of developing CD as seen from the increased risk in migrant communities compared with their native countries.

Aetiology

Although CD has some features suggesting chronic infection, no causative organism has ever been found; similarities between CD and tuberculosis have focused attention on mycobacteria. Studies have found DNA of *Mycobacterium paratuberculosis* in the intestines of 60% of patients with CD as opposed to 10% of control subjects. However, no immunology reaction has been detected against this organism, and anti-tuberculosis treatment has no effect. Focal ischaemia has also been postulated as a causative factor, possibly originating from a vasculitis arising through an immunological process. A wide variety of foods has now been implicated, but none conclusively. Smoking increases the risk threefold, which is contrary to the protective effect seen in UC.

Genetic factors are thought to play a part. About 10% of patients have a first-degree relative with the disease, and concordance has been shown to approach 50% in monozygotic twins. Inheritance is thought to involve multiple genes with low

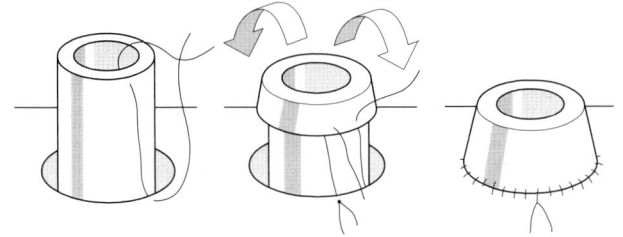

Figure 65.24 Ileostomy formation. Suturing the free extremity of the proximal ileum to the skin edges after eversion to form a spout (after Brooke).

A first-degree relative, **defined as the individual's parents, siblings or children.**

penetrance. The *NOD2/CARD15* gene has excited some interest recently. Certain variants of this gene have been shown to have strong associations with CD.

There is an association with ankylosing spondylitis. As with UC, it is now believed that CD can predispose to cancer, although the incidence of malignant change is not nearly as high as in UC and is most manifest in the ileum.

Pathogenesis

As in UC, there is thought to be an increased permeability of the mucous membrane. This leads to increased passage of antigens, which are thought to induce a cell-mediated inflammatory response. This results in the release of cytokines, such as interleukin-2 and tumour necrosis factor, which coordinate local and systemic responses. In CD, there is thought to be a defect in suppressor T cells, which usually act to prevent escalation of the inflammatory process.

Pathology

Ileal disease is the most common, accounting for 60% of cases; 30% of cases are limited to the large intestine, and the remainder are in patients with ileal disease alone or more proximal small bowel involvement. Anal lesions are common. CD of the mouth, oesophagus, stomach and duodenum is uncommon. Resection specimens show a fibrotic thickening of the intestinal wall with a narrow lumen (Fig. 65.26). There is usually dilated gut just proximal to the stricture and, in the strictured area, there are deep mucosal ulcerations with linear or snake-like patterns. Oedema in the mucosa between the ulcers gives rise to a cobblestone appearance. The transmural inflammation leads to adhesions, inflammatory masses with mesenteric abscesses and fistulae into adjacent organs. The serosa is usually opaque, there is thickening in the mesentery, and mesenteric lymph nodes are enlarged. The condition is discontinuous, with inflamed areas separated from normal intestine, so called skip lesions. Under the microscope, there are focal areas of chronic inflammation involving all layers of the intestinal wall. There are non-caseating giant cell granulomas, but these are only found in 60% of patients. They are most common in anorectal disease. The earliest mucosal lesions are discrete aphthous ulcers. Recent studies have also shown multifocal arterial occlusions in the muscularis propria.

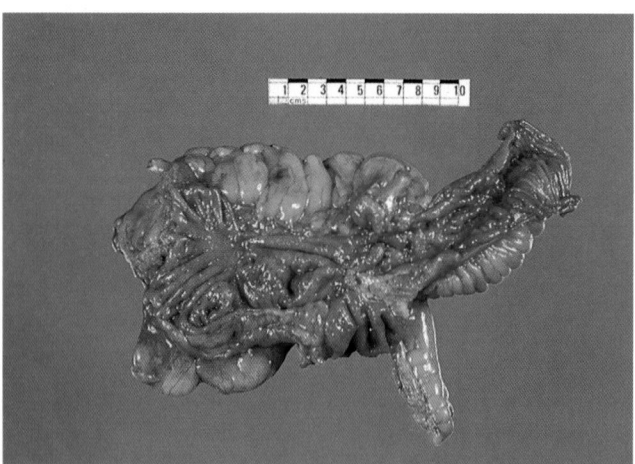

Figure 65.26 Crohn's disease of the ileocaecal region showing typical thickening of the wall of the terminal ileum with narrowing of the lumen (courtesy of Dr B. Warren, John Radcliffe Hospital, Oxford, UK).

Clinical features

Presentation depends upon the area of involvement.

Acute Crohn's disease

Acute CD occurs in only 5% of cases. Symptoms and signs resemble those of acute appendicitis, but there is usually diarrhoea preceding the attack. Rarely, there could be a free perforation of the small intestine, resulting in a local or diffuse peritonitis. Acute colitis with or without toxic megacolon can occur in CD but is less common than in UC.

Chronic Crohn's disease

There is often a history of mild diarrhoea extending over many months, occurring in bouts accompanied by intestinal colic. Patients may complain of pain, particularly in the right iliac fossa, and a tender mass may be palpable. Intermittent fevers, secondary anaemia and weight loss are common. A perianal abscess or fissure may be the first presenting feature of CD; the cause is often an infected anal crypt associated with concomitant diarrhoea but, as the disease becomes chronic, specific fistulae resulting from the CD itself can develop.

After months of repeated attacks with acute inflammation, the affected area of intestine begins to narrow with fibrosis, causing obstructive symptoms. Children developing the illness before puberty may have retarded growth and sexual development.

With progression of the disease, adhesions and transmural fissuring, intra-abdominal abscesses and fistula tracts can develop.

1 *Enteroenteric fistulae* can occur into adjacent small bowel loops or the pelvic colon, and *enterovesical fistulae* may cause repeated urinary tract infections and pneumaturia.
2 *Enterocutaneous fistulae* rarely occur spontaneously and usually follow previous surgery.

Anal disease

In the presence of active disease, the perianal skin appears bluish. Superficial ulcers with undermined edges are relatively painless and can heal with bridging of epithelium. Deep cavitating ulcers are usually found in the upper anal canal; they can be painful and cause perianal abscesses and fistulae, discharging around the anus and sometimes forwards into the genitalia. The most distressing feature of anal disease is sepsis from secondary abscesses and perianal fistulae. Remarkably, the rectal mucosa is often spared and may feel normal on rectal examination. If it is involved, however, it will feel thickened, nodular and irregular.

Investigation

Laboratory

A full blood count needs to be performed to exclude anaemia. There is usually a fall in albumin, magnesium, zinc and selenium, especially in active disease. Protein levels that correspond to disease activity include C-reactive protein and orosomucoid.

Endoscopy

Sigmoidoscopic examination may be normal or show minimal involvement. However, ulceration in the anal canal will be readily seen.

As a result of the discontinuous nature of CD, there will be areas of normal colon or rectum. In between these, there are areas of inflamed mucosa that are irregular and ulcerated, with a mucopurulent exudate. The earliest appearances are aphthoid-like ulcers surrounded by a rim of erythematous mucosa. These become larger and deeper with increasing severity of disease. In colonic CD, there may be stricturing, and it is important to exclude malignancy in these sites (Fig. 65.27). At the ileocolic anastomosis of a patient having had previous ileocaecal resection, recurrent disease is usually seen on the ileal side of the anastomosis.

Upper gastrointestinal symptoms may have to be investigated by way of upper gastrointestinal endoscopy, which may reveal deep longitudinal ulcers and cobblestone mucosa. Capsule endoscopy may also have a useful role in those with chronic gastrointestinal bleeding.

Imaging

Barium enema will show similar features to those of colonoscopy in the colon. The best investigation of the small intestine is small bowel enema (Fig. 65.28). This will show up areas of delay and dilatation. The involved areas tend to be narrowed, irregular and, sometimes, when a length of terminal ileum is involved, there may be the string sign of Kantor. Sinograms are useful in patients with enterocutaneous fistulae. CT scans are used in patients with fistulae and those with intra-abdominal abscesses and complex involvement (Fig. 65.29).

Magnetic resonance imaging (MRI) has been shown to be useful in assessing perianal disease.

Phenotyping

The Vienna classification was introduced by the World Congress of Gastroenterology in 1998. This was born out of the observation that, following presentation, the location and behaviour of the CD varied. This has relevance in studies carrying out genetic analysis of CD as there are different sub-categories with varied disease progression. Points that are recorded at presentation include age of onset, disease site in the gut, behaviour and data such as sex, ethnic origin, family history of inflammatory bowel disease and extraintestinal manifestations.

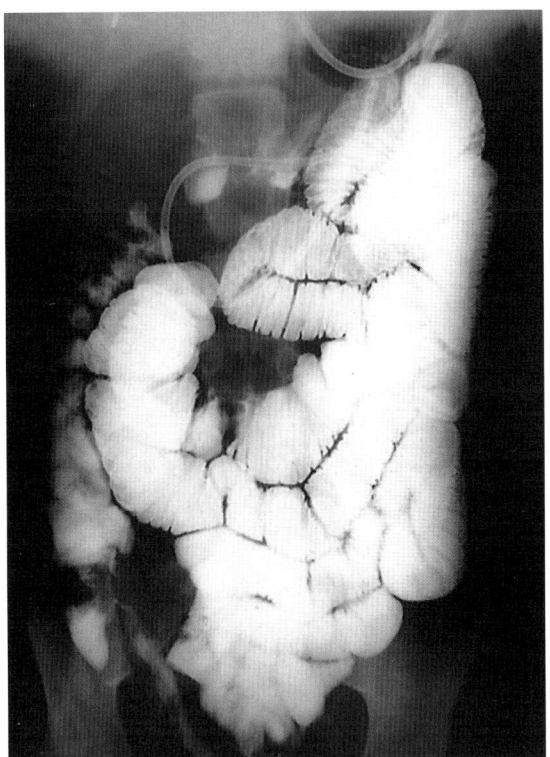

Figure 65.28 Small bowel enema examination showing a narrowed terminal ileum involved with Crohn's disease – the 'string' sign of Kantor.

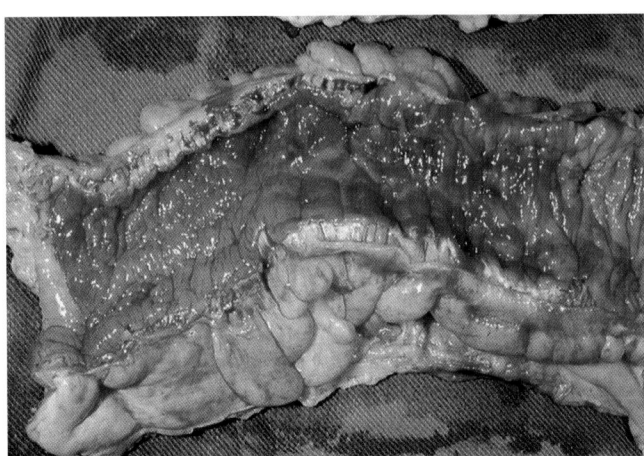

Figure 65.27 Colonic Crohn's disease. Note the normal mucosa on either side of the inflammatory stricture (courtesy of Dr B. Warren, John Radcliffe Hospital, Oxford, UK).

John Leonard Kantor, **1890–1947, Gastroenterologist, the Presbyterian Hospital, New York, NY, USA.**

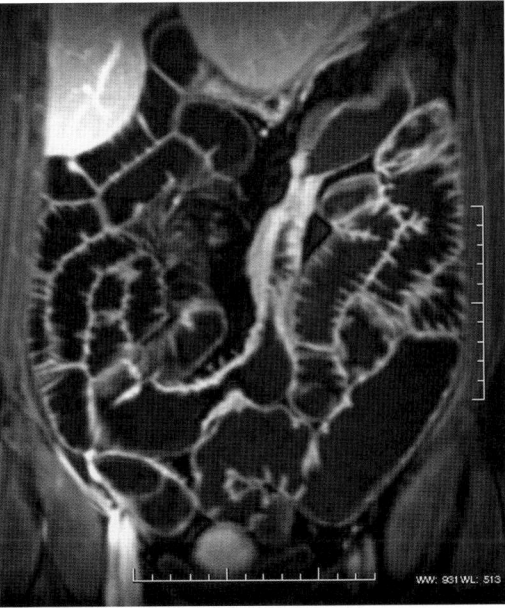

Figure 65.29 Computerised tomography enteroclysis showing small bowel dilatation secondary to strictured terminal ileum involved with Crohn's disease (courtesy of Dr H. Bungay, John Radcliffe Hospital, Oxford, UK).

CHAPTER 65 | THE SMALL AND LARGE INTESTINES

Treatment

Medical therapy

Steroids

Steroids are the mainstay of treatment. These are effective in inducing remission in moderate to severe disease in 70–80% of cases. Steroids can also be used as topical agents in the rectum with reduced systemic bioavailability, but long-term use causes adrenal suppression. They are better at inducing remission than mesalamine but has no role in maintenance. Patients suffering a relapse are treated with up to 40 mg of prednisolone orally daily, supplemented by 5-ASA compounds in those patients with colonic involvement, although there is some evidence that this may help small bowel disease as well. Meta-analysis has shown that aminosalicylates can be used after remission to reduce the absolute risk of recurrence.

Antibiotics

Those who have symptoms and signs of a mass or an abscess are also treated with antibiotics. Metronidazole is used, especially in perianal disease. Its mechanism is unknown and is thought to play a role in suppressing cell-mediated immunity. In a randomised controlled trial, it reduced disease activity in ileocolonic and colonic disease, but not small bowel disease.

Immunomodulatory agents

Azathioprine is used for its additive and steroid-sparing effect and is now standard maintenance therapy. It is a purine analogue, which is metabolised to 6-mercaptopurine and works by inhibiting cell-mediated events. It may take up to 12 weeks to have an effect. Ciclosporin acts by inhibiting cell-mediated immunity. Short-course intravenous treatment is associated with 80% remission; however, there is relapse after completion of treatment.

Monoclonal antibody

Infliximab, the murine chimeric monoclonal antibody directed towards tumour necrosis factor alpha, targets patients with severe, active disease who are refractory to 'conventional' treatments and who are at high risk of surgical interventions. A placebo-controlled trial reported the effects of single-dose infliximab on induction of remission in CD. Response after 1 month was 65% in the CD group. This compared with 17% in the placebo group. After 3 months the effects were 41% and 12% respectively. With maintenance regimes, this benefit was still apparent after a year. Infliximab is also effective in the treatment of fistulae (treatment group had a 60% reduction in fistulae compared with 26% in the placebo group). This benefit is reduced after a year. Long-term safety issues have yet to be resolved. There is a potential risk of malignancy.

Nutritional support

Nutritional support is essential. Severely malnourished people may require intravenous feeding or nasoenteric feeding regimens. Anaemia, hypoproteinaemia and electrolyte, vitamin and metabolic bone problems must all be addressed. It has been shown that parenteral nutrition can induce remission in up to 80% of patients, which is comparable to steroids, but there is no synergism or additive effect. However, relapse is high after a short duration (Summary box 65.6).

Indications for surgery

Surgical resection will not cure CD. Surgery is therefore focused on the complications of the disease. As many of these indications for surgery may be relative, joint management by an aggressive physician and a conservative surgeon is thought to be ideal. These complications include:

- recurrent intestinal obstruction;
- bleeding;
- perforation;
- failure of medical therapy;
- intestinal fistula;
- fulminant colitis;
- malignant change;
- perianal disease.

Surgery

In patients with active CD, prompt surgery is important when medical treatment fails. The main surgical principle is to preserve functional gut length and maintain gut function. Resection is kept to a minimum so as to deal with the local problem. The whole of the gastrointestinal tract has to be examined carefully at the time of laparotomy. If, on occasion, CD is diagnosed during the course of an operation for suspected appendicitis, the appendix should be removed. If the ileum is thick, rigid and pipe-like, senior help should be sought so that an ileocaecal resection can be carried out.

The course of the disease after surgery is unpredictable, but recurrence is common. It does not seem to be related to the presence of disease at the resection line. Recurrence rates vary from site to site, but the cumulative probability of recurrence requiring surgery for ileal disease is of the order of 20%, 40%, 60% and 80% at 5, 10, 15 and 20 years, respectively, after previous resection. Restorative operations have a higher incidence of recurrence than, for example, proctocolectomy and ileostomy. Preoperative factors that are imperative include adequate bowel preparation, deep venous thrombosis prophylaxis, steroid cover, nutritional support and consideration of stoma in those who are malnourished.

1   *Ileocaecal resection* is the usual procedure for ileocaecal disease with a primary anastomosis between the ileum and the ascending or transverse colon depending on the extent of the disease.
2   *Segmental resection.* Short segments of small or large bowel involvement can be treated by segmental resection. The usual indication is stricture.

3 *Colectomy and ileorectal anastomosis.* In patients with widespread colonic disease with rectal sparing and a normal anus, this can be a useful option.

4 *Emergency colectomy.* This accounts for 8% of operations for acute colonic disease. The indications are similar to those for UC. If medical treatment induces remission, then delayed surgery is sensible because of the high risk of recurrent active disease.

5 *Laparoscopic surgery.* Resections and diversion are safe in uncomplicated CD. This is coupled with extracorporeal anastomosis and results in small peri-umbilical incisions. The advantages include better cosmesis and early discharge.

6 *Temporary loop ileostomy.* This can be used either in patients with acute distal CD, allowing remission and later restoration of continuity, or in patients with severe perianal or rectal disease.

7 *Proctocolectomy.* Patients with colonic and anal disease failing to respond to medical treatment or defunction will eventually require a permanent ileostomy.

8 *Strictureplasty.* Multiple strictured areas of CD (Fig. 65.30) can be treated by a local widening procedure, strictureplasty, to avoid excessive small bowel resection (Fig. 65.31) (Lee).

9 *Anal disease* is usually treated conservatively by simple drainage of abscesses, placing setons around any fistulae and, occasionally in patients with inactive disease, primary repair of a rectovaginal or high fistula-*in-ano* could be attempted.

The differences between UC and CD are given in Summary box 65.7.

Summary box 65.7

Differences between UC and CD

- UC affects the colon; CD can affect any part of the gastrointestinal tract, but particularly the small and large bowel
- UC is a mucosal disease whereas CD affects the full thickness of the bowel wall
- UC produces confluent disease in the colon and rectum whereas CD is characterised by skip lesions
- CD more commonly causes stricturing and fistulation
- Granulomas may be found on histology in CD but not in UC
- CD is often associated with perianal disease whereas this is unusual in UC
- CD affecting the terminal ileum may produce symptoms mimicking appendicitis, but this does not occur in UC
- Resection of the colon and rectum cures the patient with UC, whereas recurrence is common after resection in CD

INFECTIONS

Intestinal amoebiasis

Amoebiasis is an infestation with *Entamoeba histolytica*. This parasite has a worldwide distribution and is transmitted mainly in contaminated drinking water.

Emanuel Cecil Gruebel Lee, 1933–1986, Surgeon, the Radcliffe Infirmary, Oxford, UK.

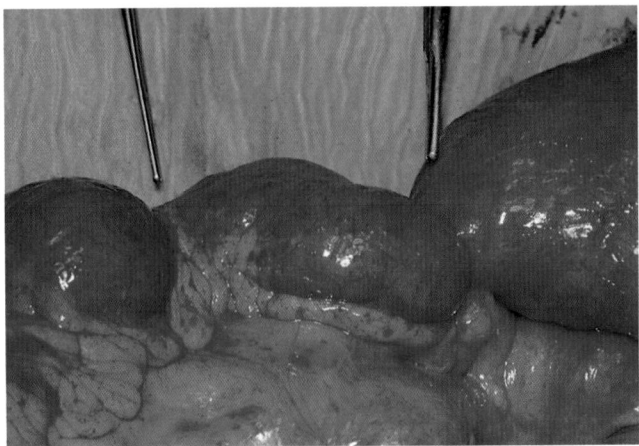

Figure 65.30 Small bowel strictures in Crohn's disease with dilatation between strictures.

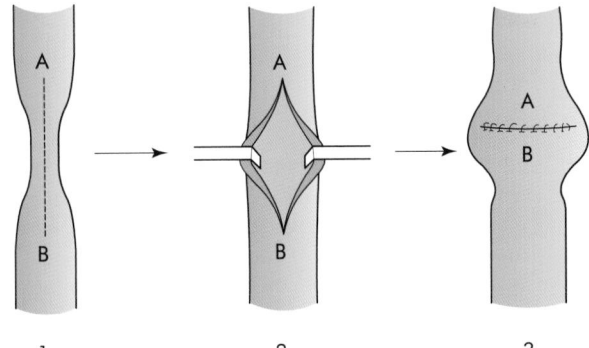

Figure 65.31 Strictureplasty. (1) A strictured length of intestine is incised along its length. (2) The bowel is opened and the walls are retracted as shown. (3) The bowel is resutured transversely to widen the narrowed segment.

Pathology

The ulcers, which have been described as 'bottlenecked' because of their considerably undermined edges, have a yellow necrotic floor, from which blood and pus exude. In 75%, they are confined to the lower sigmoid and upper rectum.

Biopsy

Endoscopic biopsies or fresh hot stools are examined carefully to look for the presence of amoebae. It is important to emphasise, however, that the presence of the parasite does not indicate that it is pathogenic (Fig. 65.32).

Clinical features

Dysentery is the principal manifestation of the disease, but it may come in various other guises.

Appendicitis or amoebic caecal mass

In tropical countries where amoebiasis is endemic, this is a constantly recurring problem. To operate on a patient with amoebic dysentery without precautions may prove fatal. The bowel is friable, and satisfactory closure of the appendix stump becomes difficult or impossible, especially in cases where a palpable mass is present. When there is an amoebic mass, there

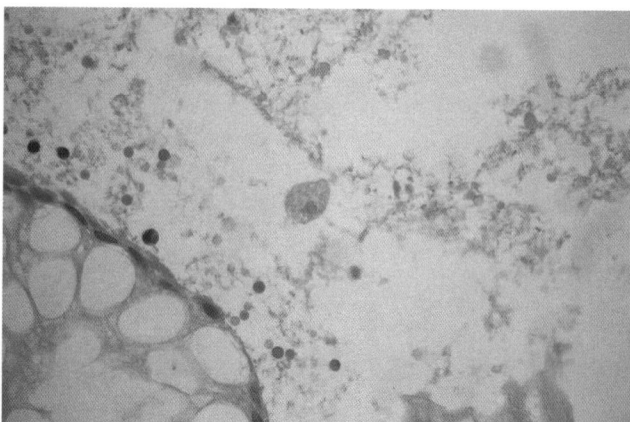

Figure 65.32 An amoeba in a rectal biopsy.

tends to be tenderness on deep palpation over the caecum and the sigmoid.

Perforation

The most common sites are the caecum and rectosigmoid; usually, perforation occurs into a confined space where adhesions have formed previously, and a pericolic abscess results, which eventually needs draining. When there is sudden faecal flooding into the general peritoneal cavity, drainage of the region of the perforation, gastrointestinal aspiration, intravenous fluid, antibiotics and a full course of emetine are sometimes successful.

Severe rectal haemorrhage as a result of separation of the slough is liable to occur.

Granuloma

Progressive amoebic invasion of the wall of the rectum or colon, with secondary inflammation, can produce a granulomatous mass indistinguishable from a carcinoma.

Ulcerative colitis

A search for amoebae should always be made in the stools of patients believed to have UC.

Other

Other presentations include the following:

- Fibrous stricture may follow the healing of extensive amoebic ulcers.
- Intestinal obstruction is a common complication of amoebiasis, and the obstruction is the result of adhesions associated with pericolitis and large granuloma.
- Paracolic abscess, ischiorectal abscess and fistula occur from perforation by amoebae of the intestinal wall followed by secondary infection.

Treatment

High-dose intravenous steroids in this situation can be catastrophic. Metronidazole (Flagyl) is the first-line drug, 800 mg three times daily for 7–10 days. Diloxanide furoate is best for chronic infections associated with the passage of cysts in stools. Intestinal antibiotics improve the results of the chronic stages, probably by coping with superadded infection.

Typhoid and paratyphoid

Typhoid

Paralytic ileus is the most common complication of typhoid. Intestinal haemorrhage may be the leading symptom. Other surgical complications of typhoid and parathyroid include:

- haemorrhage;
- perforation;
- cholecystitis;
- phlebitis;
- genitourinary inflammation;
- arthritis;
- osteomyelitis.

Typhoid ulcer

Perforation of a typhoid ulcer usually occurs during the third week and is occasionally the first sign of the disease. The ulcer is parallel to the long axis of the gut and is usually situated in the lower ileum.

Paratyphoid B

Perforation of the large intestine sometimes occurs in paratyphoid B infection; vigorous intravenous antibiotic therapy is given. Occasionally, surgery may be required to defunction the colon. In cases where severely diseased bowel is present, a colectomy may be necessary, as for UC.

Tuberculosis of the intestine

Tuberculosis can affect any part of the gastrointestinal tract from the mouth to the anus. The sites affected most often are the ileum, proximal colon and peritoneum. There are two principal types.

Ulcerative tuberculosis

Ulcerative tuberculosis is secondary to pulmonary tuberculosis and arises as a result of swallowing tubercle bacilli. There are multiple ulcers in the terminal ileum, lying transversely, and the overlying serosa is thickened, reddened and covered in tubercles.

Clinical features

Diarrhoea and weight loss are the predominant symptoms, and the patient will usually be receiving treatment for pulmonary tuberculosis.

Radiology

A barium meal and follow-through or small bowel enema will show the absence of filling of the lower ileum, caecum and most of the ascending colon as a result of narrowing and hypermotility of the ulcerated segment (Fig. 65.33).

Treatment

A course of chemotherapy is given. Healing often occurs provided the pulmonary tuberculosis is adequately treated. An operation is only required in the rare event of a perforation or intestinal obstruction.

Hyperplastic tuberculosis

This usually occurs in the ileocaecal region, although solitary and multiple lesions in the lower ileum are sometimes seen. This is caused by the ingestion of *Mycobacterium tuberculosis* by patients

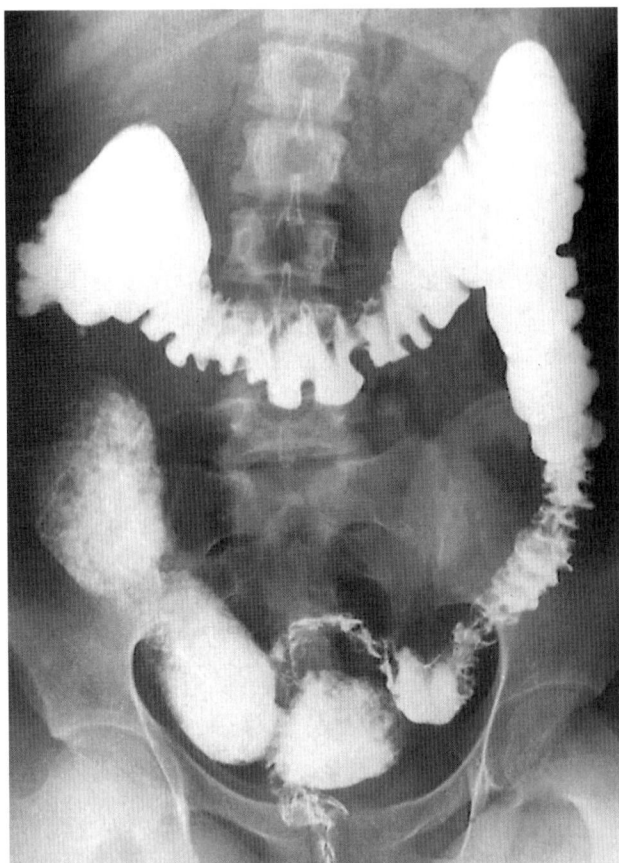

Figure 65.33 Ileocaecal tuberculosis; absent ascending colon and caecum with dilatation of terminal ileum (courtesy of Dr V.K. Kapoor, Delhi, India).

with a high resistance to the organism. The infection establishes itself in lymphoid follicles, and the resulting chronic inflammation causes thickening of the intestinal wall and narrowing of the lumen. There is early involvement of the regional lymph nodes, which may caseate. Unlike CD, with which it shares many similarities, abscess and fistula formation is rare.

Clinical features

Attacks of abdominal pain with intermittent diarrhoea are the usual symptoms. The ileum above the partial obstruction is distended, and the stasis and consequent infection lead to steatorrhoea, anaemia and loss of weight. Sometimes, the presenting picture is of a mass in the right iliac fossa in a patent with vague ill health. The differential diagnosis is that of an appendix mass, carcinoma of the caecum, CD, tuberculosis or actinomycosis of the caecum.

Radiology

A barium follow-through or small bowel enema will show a long narrow filling defect in the terminal ileum.

Treatment

When the diagnosis is certain and the patient has not yet developed obstructive symptoms, treatment with chemotherapy is advised and may cure the condition. Where obstruction is present, operative treatment is required and ileocaecal resection is best.

Actinomycosis of the ileocaecal region

Abdominal actinomycosis is rare. Unlike intestinal tuberculosis, narrowing of the lumen of the intestine does not occur and mesenteric nodes do not become involved. However, a local abscess spreads to the retroperitoneal tissues and the adjacent abdominal wall, becoming the seat of multiple indurated discharging sinuses. The liver may become involved via the portal vein.

Clinical features

The usual history is that appendicectomy has been carried out for an appendicitis. Some 3 weeks after surgery, a mass is palpable in the right iliac fossa and, soon afterwards, the wound begins to discharge. At first, the discharge is thin and watery, but later it becomes thicker and malodorous. Other sinuses may form and a secondary faecal fistula may develop. Pus should be sent for bacteriological examination, which will reveal the characteristic sulphur granules.

Treatment

Penicillin or cotrimoxazole treatment should be prolonged and in high dosage.

TUMOURS OF THE SMALL INTESTINE

Compared with the large intestine, the small intestine is rarely the seat of a neoplasm, and these become progressively less common from the duodenum to the terminal ileum.

Benign

Adenomas, submucous lipomas and gastrointestinal stromal tumours (GISTs) occur from time to time, and sometimes reveal themselves by causing an intussusception. The second most common complication is intestinal bleeding from an adenoma, in which event the diagnosis is frequently long delayed because the tumour is overlooked at barium radiology, endoscopy and even surgery.

Peutz–Jeghers syndrome

This is an autosomal dominant disease. The gene *STK11* on chromosome 19 has been found in a proportion of patients with this condition. This consists of:

- intestinal hamartomatosis is a polyposis affecting the whole of the small bowel and colon, where it is a cause of haemorrhage and often intussusception;
- melanosis of the oral mucous membrane and the lips.

The melanosis takes the form of melanin spots sometimes present on the digits and the perianal skin, but pigmentation of the lips is the *sine qua non* (Fig. 65.34).

Long-term follow-up of patients with Peutz–Jeghers syndrome has shown reduced survival secondary to complications of recurrent bowel cancer and the development of a wide range of cancers. These include colorectal, gastric, breast, cervical, ovarian,

John Law Augustine Peutz, **1886–1968, Chief Specialist for Internal Medicine, St John's Hospital, The Hague, The Netherlands.**
Sine qua non, **an indispensible condition, Latin for 'without which not'.**

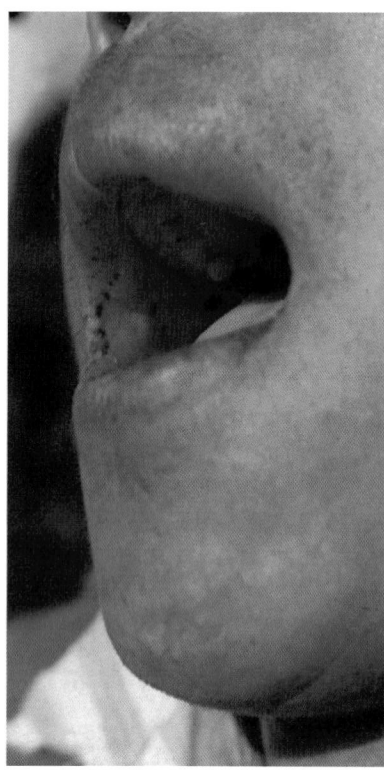

Figure 65.34 Melanin spots on the lips of a patient afflicted with Peutz–Jeghers syndrome (courtesy of Major P.C.M. Manta, Indian Medical Service).

pancreatic and testicular cancer. It is therefore important to keep these patients under surveillance. This can be done by endoscopy or contrast examinations every 3 years to detect early gastro-intestinal cancers. It is also important to make sure that female patients attend cervical and breast screening programmes.

Histology

The polyps can be likened to trees. The trunk and branches are smooth muscle fibres and the foliage is virtually normal mucosa.

Treatment

As malignant change rarely occurs, resection is only necessary for serious bleeding or intussusception. Large single polyps can be removed by enterotomy, or short lengths of heavily involved intestine can be resected. The incidence of further lesions developing problems in the future can be reduced by thorough intra-operative examination at the time of the first laparotomy. Using on-table enteroscopy, polyps suitable for removal can be identified. Those lesions within reach can be snared by colonoscopy.

Malignant

Lymphoma

There are three main types, as follows:

1 *Western-type lymphoma.* These are annular ulcerating lesions, which are sometimes multiple. They are now thought to be non-Hodgkin's B-cell lymphoma in origin. They may present

Thomas Hodgkin, 1798–1866, Lecturer in Morbid Anatomy and Curator of the Mueseum, Guy's Hospital, London, described lymphadenoma in 1832.

with obstruction and bleeding, perforation, anorexia and weight loss.

2 *Primary lymphoma associated with coeliac disease.* There is an increased incidence of lymphoma in patients with coeliac disease; this is now regarded as a T-cell lymphoma. Worsening of the patient's diarrhoea, with pyrexia of unknown origin together with local obstructive symptoms, are the usual features.

3 *Mediterranean lymphoma.* This is found mostly in North Africa and the Middle East and is associated with α-chain disease.

Unless there are particular surgical complications these conditions are usually treated with chemotherapy.

Carcinoma

Like small bowel tumours, these can present with obstruction, bleeding or diarrhoea. Complete resection offers the only hope of cure (Fig. 65.35).

Carcinoid tumour

These tumours occur throughout the gastrointestinal tract, most commonly in the appendix, ileum and rectum in decreasing order of frequency. They arise from neuroendocrine cells at the base of intestinal crypts. The primary is usually small but, when they metastasise, the liver is usually involved, with numerous secondaries, which are larger and more yellow than the primary; when this has occurred, the carcinoid syndrome will become evident. The tumours can produce a number of vasoactive peptides, most commonly 5-hydroxytryptamine (serotonin), which may be present as 5-hydroxyindoleacetic acid (5-HIAA) in the urine during attacks.

The clinical syndrome itself consists of reddish-blue cyanosis, flushing attacks, diarrhoea, borborygmi, asthmatic attacks and, eventually, sometimes pulmonary and tricuspid stenosis. Classically, the flushing attacks are induced by alcohol.

Treatment

Most patients with gastrointestinal carcinoids do not have carcinoid syndrome. Surgical resection is usually sufficient. In the cases found incidentally at appendicectomy, nothing further is required. In patients with metastatic disease, multiple enucleations of hepatic metastases or even partial hepatectomy can be carried out. The treatment has been transformed by the use of octreotide (a somatostatin analogue), which reduces both

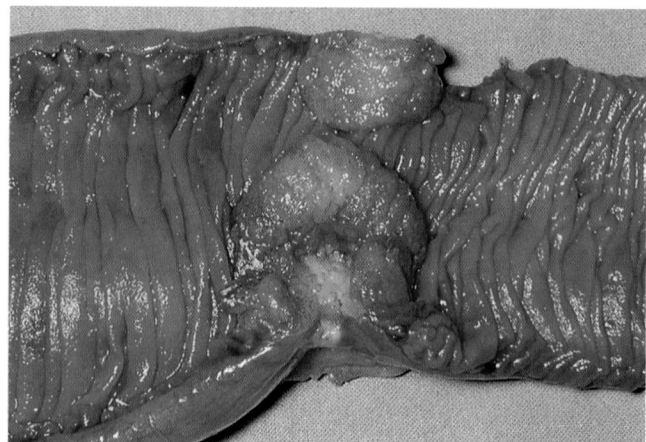

Figure 65.35 Small bowel adenocarcinoma.

flushing and diarrhoea, and octreotide cover is usually used in patients with a carcinoid syndrome who have surgery to prevent a carcinoid crisis. Carcinoid tumours generally grow more slowly than most metastatic malignancies; the patients may live with the syndrome of metastatic disease for many years.

Gastrointestinal stromal tumours

These tumours can be either benign or malignant. Increased size is associated with malignant potential. GIST is a type of sarcoma that develops from connective tissue cells. It is found most commonly in the stomach but can be found in other sites of the gut. It occurs most commonly in the 50- to 70-year age group. Although its cause is unknown, patients with neurofibromatosis have an increased risk of developing these types of tumour.

Symptoms

Patients may be asymptomatic. Other symptoms include lethargy, pain, nausea, haematemesis or melaena.

Treatment

Surgery is the most effective way of removing GISTs as they are radioresistant. Glivec (imatinib) is a tyrosine kinase inhibitor that has been shown to be effective in advanced cases.

TUMOURS OF THE LARGE INTESTINE

Benign

The term 'polyp' is a clinical description of any elevated tumour. It covers a variety of histologically different tumours shown in Table 65.3.

Polyps can occur singly, synchronously in small numbers or as part of a polyposis syndrome. In familial adenomatous polyposis (FAP), more than 100 adenomas are present. It is important to be sure of the histological diagnosis because adenomas have significant malignant potential.

Adenomatous polyps

Adenomatous polyps vary from a tubular adenoma (Fig. 65.36), rather like a raspberry on a stalk, to the villous adenoma, a flat spreading lesion. Solitary adenomas are usually found during the investigation of colonic bleeding or sometimes fortuitously. Villous tumours more usually give symptoms of diarrhoea, mucus discharge and occasionally hypokalaemia. The risk of malignancy developing in an adenoma increases with increasing size of

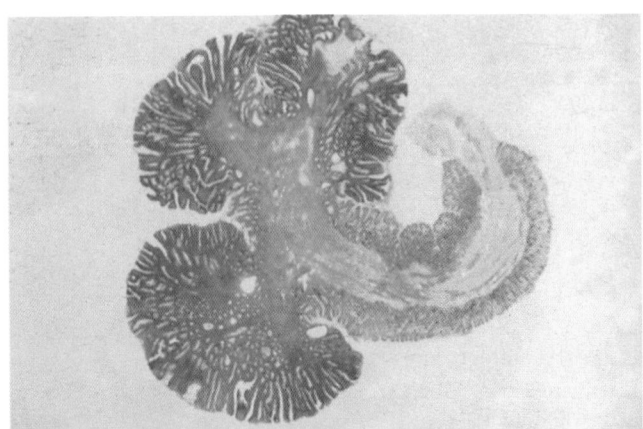

Figure 65.36 Pedunculated adenomatous polyp of the large intestine, longitudinal section (courtesy of Dr P. Millard, John Radcliffe Hospital, Oxford, UK).

tumour; for example, in 1-cm-diameter tubular adenomas there is a 10% risk of cancer, whereas with villous adenomas over 2 cm in diameter, there may be a 15% chance of carcinoma. Adenomas larger than 5 mm in diameter are usually treated because of their malignant potential. Colonoscopic snare polypectomy or diathermy obliteration with hot biopsy forceps can be used. Huge villous adenomas of the rectum can be difficult to remove even with techniques per anus, and occasionally proctectomy is required; the anal sphincter can usually be preserved.

Familial adenomatous polyposis

FAP is clinically defined by the presence of more than 100 colorectal adenomas. Over 80% of cases come from patients with a positive family history. However, 20% arise as a result of new mutations in the adenomatous polyposis coli gene (APC). This has been identified on the short arm of chromosome 5 (Bodmer). It is less common than hereditary non-polyposis colorectal cancer (HNPCC) and accounts for less than 1% of colorectal cancer. Although the large bowel is mainly affected, polyps can occur in the stomach, duodenum and small intestine. The main risk is large bowel cancer, but duodenal and ampullary tumours have been reported. It is inherited as a Mendelian dominant condition. The risk of colorectal cancer is 100% in patients with FAP. Males and females are equally affected. It can also occur sporadically without any previous sign or history, presumably by new mutations. There is often, in these cases, a history of large bowel cancer occurring in young adulthood or middle age, suggesting pre-existing adenomatosis.

FAP can be associated with benign mesodermal tumours such as desmoid tumours and osteomas. Epidermoid cysts can also occur (Gardner's syndrome); desmoid tumours in the abdomen invade locally to involve the intestinal mesentery and, although non-metastasising, they can become unresectable (Summary box 65.8).

Table 65.3 Classification of polyps of the large intestine

Class	Varieties
Inflammatory	Inflammatory polyps
Metaplastic	Metaplastic or hyperplastic polyps
Harmartomatous	Peutz–Jeghers polyp
	Juvenile polyp
Neoplastic	Adenoma
	– Tubular
	– Tubulovillous
	– Villous
	Adenocarcinoma
	Carcinoid tumour

Sir Walter Fred Bodmer, **Geneticist, University of Oxford, Director of Research, Imperial Cancer Research Fund, London, UK.**
Eldon John Gardner, **1909–1989, Geneticist, the University of Utah, Salt Lake City, UT, USA, described this syndrome in 1950.**

CHAPTER 65 | THE SMALL AND LARGE INTESTINES

> **Summary box 65.8**
>
> **FAP**
>
> ■ Autosomal dominant inherited disease due to mutation of the *APC* gene
> ■ More than 100 colonic adenomas are diagnostic
> ■ Surgery is the only means of preventing colonic cancer
> ■ Polyps and malignant tumours can develop in the duodenum and small bowel

Clinical features

Polyps are usually visible on sigmoidoscopy by the age of 15 years and will almost always be visible by the age of 30 years. Carcinoma of the large bowel occurs 10–20 years after the onset of the polyposis. One or more cancers will already be present in two-thirds of those patients presenting with symptoms.

Symptomatic patients

These are either patients in whom a new mutation has occurred or those from an affected family who have not been screened. They may have loose stools, lower abdominal pain, weight loss, diarrhoea and the passage of blood and mucus. Polyps are seen on sigmoidoscopy, and the number and distribution of polyps, and usually cancers if they are symptomatic, are shown on a double-contrast barium enema. If in doubt, colonoscopy is performed with biopsies to establish the number and histological type of polyps. If over 100 adenomas (Fig. 65.37) are present, the diagnosis can be made confidently, but it is important not to confuse this with non-neoplastic forms of polyposis.

Asymptomatic patients

Direct genetic testing will reveal mutations in 80% of cases. In the presence of an identified mutation in a family with FAP, any resulting negative tests for this can be interpreted to mean that these individuals do not carry the mutation. They can therefore be withdrawn from surveillance programmes and warned that they are at normal population 'risk' of developing colorectal cancer. In those families where a mutation cannot be identified, then surveillance is recommended annually.

The site of the mutation within the gene has important effects on the phenotype. Truncations of the carboxy end of the APC

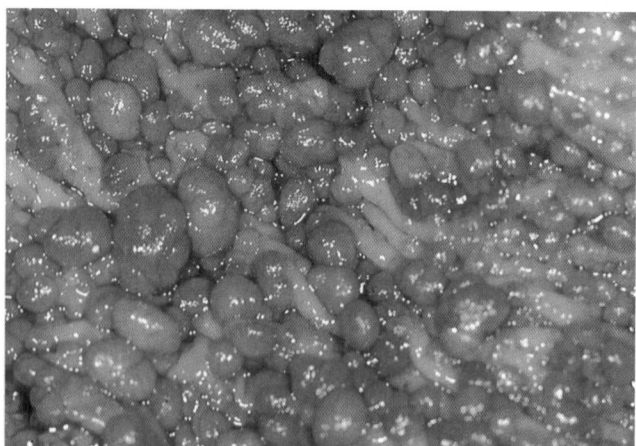

Figure 65.37 Familial adenomatous polyposis.

protein have a smaller effect on tumour suppressor function. This results in the attenuated FAP variant.

If there are no adenomas by the age of 30 years, FAP is unlikely. If the diagnosis is made during adolescence, operation is usually deferred to the age of 17 or 18 years or when symptoms or multiple polyps develop.

Screening policy

1 At-risk family members are offered genetic testing in their early teens.
2 At-risk members of the family should be examined at the age of 10–12 years, repeated every year.
3 Most of those who are going to get polyps will have them at 20 years, and these require operation.
4 If there are no polyps at 20 years, continue with 5-yearly examination until age 50 years; if there are still no polyps, there is probably no inherited gene. Carcinomatous change may exceptionally occur before the age of 20 years. Examination of blood relatives, including cousins, nephews and nieces, is essential, and a family tree should be constructed and a register of affected families maintained.

Treatment

Colectomy with ileorectal anastomosis has in the past been the usual operation because it avoids an ileostomy in a young patient and the risks of pelvic dissection to nerve function. The rectum is subsequently cleared of polyps by snaring or fulguration. The patients are examined by flexible sigmoidoscopy at 6-monthly intervals thereafter. In spite of this, a proportion of patients develop carcinoma in the rectal stump. The risk of carcinoma in the St Mark's series was 10% over a period of 30 years.

The alternative is a restorative proctocolectomy with an ileoanal anastomosis. This has a higher complication rate than ileorectal anastomosis. It is indicated in patients with serious rectal involvement with polyps, those who are likely to be poor at attending for follow-up and those with an established cancer of the rectum or sigmoid. However, it is now used more frequently for less severe cases. There have been reports of cancers developing after stapled anastomosis when a small remnant of rectal mucosa is left behind.

Postoperative surveillance

Because of the risk of further tumour formation, follow-up is important and takes the form of rectal/pouch surveillance. Gastroscopies are carried out to detect upper gastrointestinal tumours.

Hereditary non-polyposis colorectal cancer (Lynch's syndrome)

This syndrome is characterised by increased risk of colorectal cancer and also cancers of the endometrium, ovary, stomach and small intestines. It is an autosomal dominant condition that is caused by a mutation in one of the DNA mismatch repair genes – *MLH1*, *MSH2*, *MSH6*, *PMS* and *PMS2*. Most people with this syndrome have mutations in the *MLH1* and *MSH2* genes.

The lifetime risk of developing colorectal cancer is 80%, and the mean age of diagnosis is 44 years. Most cancers develop in the

> St. Mark's Hospital, **Harrow, UK**, was founded in 1835 and is recognised as a **national and international referral centre for intestinal and colorectal disorders.**

proximal colon. Females with HNPCC have a 30–50% lifetime risk of developing endometrial cancer. The average age of diagnosis is 46 years in this group.

Diagnosis

HNPCC can be diagnosed by genetic testing or Amsterdam criteria II:

- three or more family members with a HNPCC-related cancer, one of whom is a first-degree relative of the other two;
- two successive affected generations;
- one or more of the HNPCC-related cancers diagnosed before the age of 50 years;
- exclusion of FAP.

Malignant

Epidemiology

Colonic cancer can be diagnosed at operation as involving the large bowel proximal to where the two anti-mesenteric taenia converge (this represents the beginning of the rectum). In the UK, colorectal cancer accounted for 16 000 deaths in 2003 according to Cancer Research UK statistics. It represents a large part of the general surgeon's elective and emergency workload. About 22 000 patients are diagnosed with colonic cancer every year. Over the last four decades, the 5-year survival rate has improved from 30% to about 45%.

Genetics

There has been an explosion of information on the molecular genetics of sporadic colorectal cancer. *APC* mutations occur in two-thirds of colonic adenomas and carcinomas and are thought to present early in the carcinogenesis pathway. *K-RAS* mutations result in activation of cell signalling pathways. They are more common in larger lesions, thus implying that they are later events in the mutagenesis pathway. Other genes involved include *p53*.

However, it must be noted that the pathway is not one of a simple stepwise progression of mutations but a complicated array of multiple gene changes, which result in an outcome of cancer. No single mutation is a common theme for all colorectal cancer cases. However, knowledge of certain mutations can be used to assess prognosis and direct adjuvant therapy.

Aetiology

Other factors that have been implicated in the development of cancer have included dietary fibre. The hypothesis is that increased roughage is associated with reduced transit times, and this in turn reduces the exposure of the mucosa to carcinogens. This has been supported by population questionnaire studies. There have also been studies linking increased dietary animal fat, smoking and alcohol to colorectal cancer. There is some evidence that links cholecystectomy, and therefore increased bile acid secretion, to an increased risk of colorectal cancer.

The role of irritable bowel disease (IBD) in colorectal cancer is discussed elsewhere in this chapter.

Adenocarcinoma of the colon

Pathology

Microscopically, the neoplasm is a columnar cell carcinoma originating in the colonic epithelium. Macroscopically, the tumour may take one of four forms (Fig. 65.38). Type 4 is the least malignant form. It is likely that all carcinomas start as a benign

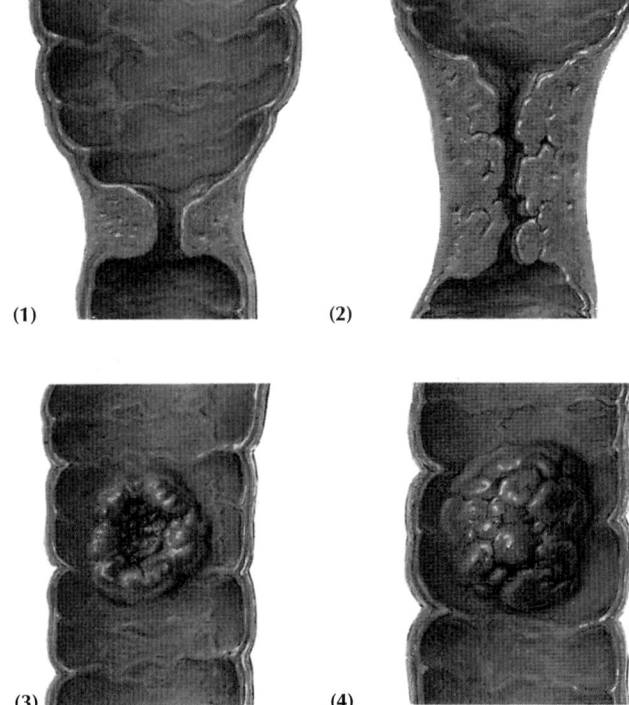

Figure 65.38 The four common macroscopic varieties of carcinoma of the colon. (1) Annular; (2) tubular; (3) ulcer; (4) cauliflower.

adenoma, the so called 'adenoma–carcinoma sequence'. This is supported by the observation that the prevalence of adenomas correlates with carcinoma. The distribution of adenoma in the colon also mirrors that of carcinoma. The annular variety tends to give rise to obstructive symptoms, whereas the others will present more commonly with bleeding. The sites and distribution of cases of cancer are shown in Figure 65.39. Tumours are more common in the left colon and rectum.

The spread of carcinoma of the colon

Generally this is a comparatively slow-growing neoplasm.

Local spread

The tumour can spread in a longitudinal, transverse or radial direction; it spreads round the intestinal wall and usually causes intestinal obstruction before it invades adjacent structures. The

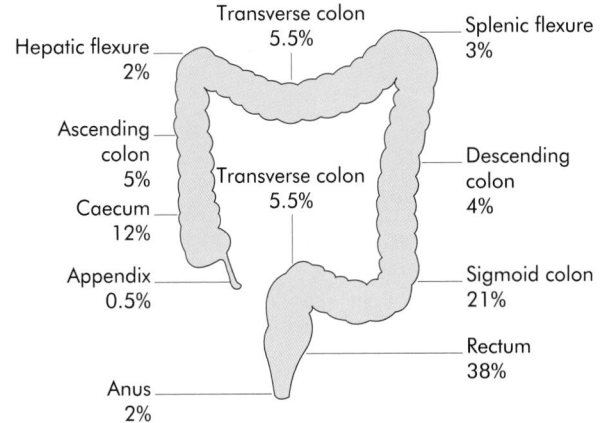

Figure 65.39 Distribution of colorectal cancer by site.

ulcerative type more commonly invades locally, and an internal fistula may result, for example into the bladder. There may also be a local perforation with an abscess or even an external faecal fistula. This type of radial spread to adjacent organs has the largest impact on prognosis. The progression of invasion occurs across the submucosa into the muscularis propria and thence out into the serosa and fat, lymphatics and veins in the mesentery alongside the bowel wall.

Lymphatic spread

Lymph nodes draining the colon are grouped as follows:

N1: nodes in the immediate vicinity of the bowel wall;
N2: nodes arranged along the ileocolic, right colic, midcolic, left colic and sigmoid arteries;
N3: the apical nodes around the superior and inferior mesenteric vessels where they arise from the abdominal aorta. Involvement of the lymph nodes by the tumour progresses in a gradual manner from those closest to the growth along the course of the lymphatic vessels to those placed centrally.

Bloodstream spread

This accounts for a large proportion (30–40%) of late deaths. Metastases are carried to the liver via the portal system, sometimes at an early stage before clinical or operative evidence is detected (occult hepatic metastases).

Transcoelomic spread

Rarely, colorectal cancer can spread by way of cells dislodging from the serosa of the bowel or via the subperitoneal lymphatics to other structures within the peritoneal cavity.

Staging colon cancer

There are several staging systems that are used such as Dukes, tumour–node–metastasis (TNM) and Jass. All of them can be used in order to predict prognosis and standardise treatment. Dukes' classification was originally described for rectal tumours (see Chapter 68) but has been adopted for histopathological reporting of colon cancer as well. There have been numerous modifications of the original system, leading to some confusion but, in its most basic form, Dukes' classification for colon cancer is as follows:

A: confined to the bowel wall;
B: through the bowel wall but not involving the free peritoneal serosal surface;
C: lymph nodes involved.

Dukes himself never described a D stage, but this is often used to describe either advanced local disease or metastases to the liver.

TNM classification

The TNM classification is more detailed and accurate but more demanding:

- T   Tumour stage;
- T1 Into submucosa;
- T2 Into muscularis propria;
- T3 Into pericolic fat but not breaching serosa;
- T4 Breaches serosa or directly involving another organ;
- N   Nodal stage;

Cuthbert Esquire Dukes, 1890–1977, Pathologist, St Mark's Hospital, London, UK.

- N0 No nodes involved;
- N1 One or two nodes involved;
- N2 Three or more nodes involved;
- M   Metastases;
- M0 No metastases;
- M1 Metastases;
- Ly Lymphatic invasion;
- L0 No lymphatic vessels involved;
- L1 Lymphatics involved;
- V   Venous invasion;
- V0 No vessel invasion;
- V1 Vessels invaded;
- R   Residual tumour;
- R0 No residual tumour;
- R1 Margins involved, residual tumour present.

Clinical features

Carcinoma of the colon usually occurs in patients over 50 years of age, but it is not rare earlier in adult life. Twenty per cent of cases present as an emergency with intestinal obstruction or peritonitis. In any case of colonic bleeding in patients over the age of 40 years, a complete investigation of the colon is required. A careful family history should be taken. Those with first-degree relatives who have developed colorectal cancer at the age of 45 years or below are at high risk and may be part of one of the colorectal cancer family syndromes.

Carcinoma of the left side of the colon

Most tumours occur in this location. They are usually of the stenosing variety.

Symptoms

The main symptoms are those of increasing intestinal obstruction. This includes lower abdominal pain, which may be colicky in nature, and abdominal distension. The patient may have a change in bowel habit with alternating diarrhoea and constipation (Summary box 65.9).

Summary box 65.9

Symptoms and signs of colorectal cancer

- **Right-sided tumours: iron deficiency anaemia, abdominal mass**
- **Left-sided tumours: rectal bleeding, alteration in bowel habit, tenesmus, obstruction**
- **Metastatic disease: jaundice, ascites, hepatomegaly; other symptoms and signs from rarer sites of metastasis**
- **There may be considerable overlap between these symptoms**

Carcinoma of the sigmoid

In addition to symptoms of intestinal obstruction, a low tumour may give rise to a feeling of the need for evacuation, which may result in tenesmus accompanied by the passage of mucus and blood. *Bladder symptoms* are not unusual and, in some instances, may herald a colovesical fistula.

Carcinoma of the transverse colon

This may be mistaken for a carcinoma of the stomach because of the position of the tumour together with anaemia and lassitude.

Carcinoma of the caecum and ascending colon

This may present with the following:

- anaemia, severe and unyielding to treatment;
- the presence of a mass in the right iliac fossa; colonoscopy may be needed to confirm the diagnosis;
- a carcinoma of the caecum can be the apex of an intussusception presenting with the symptoms of intermittent obstruction.

Metastatic disease

Patients may present for the first time with liver metastases and an enlarged liver, ascites from carcinomatosis peritonei and, more rarely, metastases to the lung, skin, bone and brain.

Methods of investigation of colon cancer

Flexible sigmoidoscopy

The 60-cm, fibreoptic, flexible sigmoidoscope is increasingly being used in the out-patient clinic or in special rectal bleeding clinics. The patient is prepared with a disposable enema and sedation is not usually necessary. This is particularly useful in supplementing barium investigations where diagnosis is difficult due to diverticular disease.

Colonoscopy

This is now the investigation of choice if colorectal cancer is suspected provided the patient is fit enough to undergo the bowel preparation. It has the advantage of not only picking up a primary cancer but also having the ability to detect synchronous polyps or even multiple carcinomas, which occur in 5% of cases. Ideally, every case should be proven histologically before surgery. Full bowel preparation and sedation are necessary. However, one must be aware of a small risk of perforation and also the failure to get to the caecum in 10% of cases, even by experienced endoscopists.

Radiology

Double-contrast barium enema is used when colonoscopy is contraindicated. It shows a cancer of the colon as a constant irregular filling defect (Fig. 65.40). False positives occur in 1–2% of cases and false negatives in 7–9% of cases.

Ultrasonography is often used as a screening investigation for liver metastases over the size of 1.5 cm, and CT is used in patients with large palpable abdominal masses, to determine local invasion, and is particularly used in the pelvis in the assessment of rectal cancer.

Spiral CT is particularly useful in elderly patients when contrast enemas or colonoscopy are not diagnostic or are contraindicated. In some centres, it is standard investigation above the age of 80 years. With the advent of technology in this field, there has been the introduction of virtual colonoscopy, which is effective in picking up polyps down to size of 6 mm (Fig. 65.41). This may even replace colonoscopy as the standard investigation in the future.

Urograms have a role in left-sided tumours where there is evidence of hydronephrosis on CT or ultrasound.

Treatment

Preoperative preparation

Recent literature has suggested that no bowel preparation is safe for right-sided colonic surgery. The most commonly used method

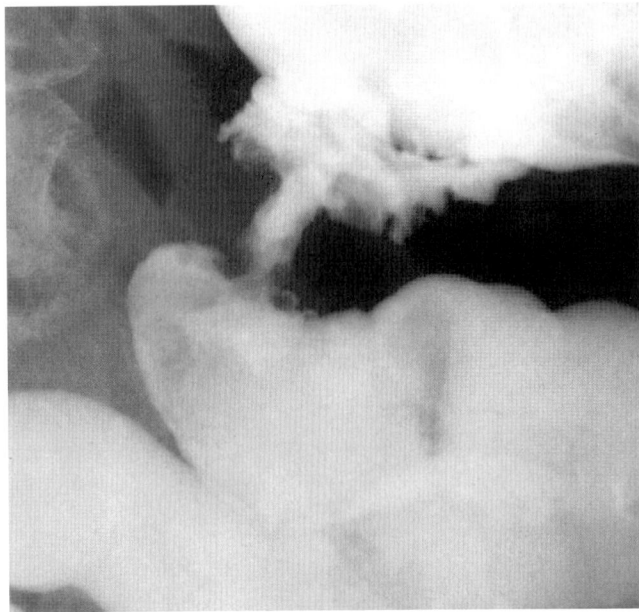

Figure 65.40 Barium enema showing a carcinoma of the sigmoid colon. It may have an 'apple core' appearance, i.e. a short, irregular stenosis with sharp shoulders at each end.

is dietary restriction to fluids only for 48 hours before surgery; on the day before the operation, two sachets of Picolax (sodium picosulphate) are taken to purge the colon. In addition, a rectal washout may be necessary. A stoma site is carefully discussed with the stoma care nursing specialist and anti-embolus stockings are fitted; the patient is started on prophylactic subcutaneous heparin, and intravenous prophylactic antibiotics are given at the start of surgery.

When intestinal obstruction is present, preparation in this way may precipitate abdominal pain, and it may be safer to use an on-table lavage technique at the time of the operation (Summary box 65.10).

Summary box 65.10

Principles of management of colorectal cancer

- Assessment of local and distant tumour spread should be performed both preoperatively and intraoperatively to allow planning of surgery
- Synchronous tumours occur in about 5% of patients and should be excluded preoperatively
- Operations are planned to remove the primary tumour and its draining locoregional lymph nodes
- Histological examination of resected tumours contributes to decision making regarding the need for adjuvant therapy

---

The test of operability

The abdomen is opened and the tumour assessed for resectability.

1. The liver is palpated for secondary deposits, the presence of which is not necessarily a contraindication to resection because the best palliative treatment for carcinoma of the colon is removal of the tumour.
2. The peritoneum, particularly the pelvic peritoneum, is

(a)

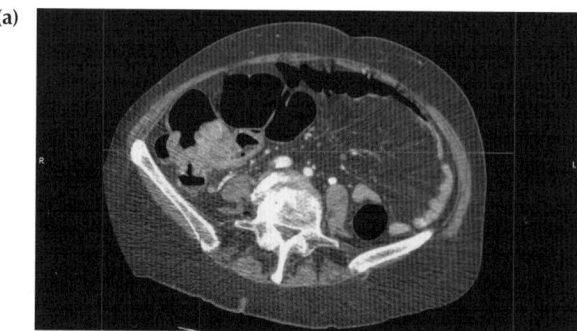

(b)

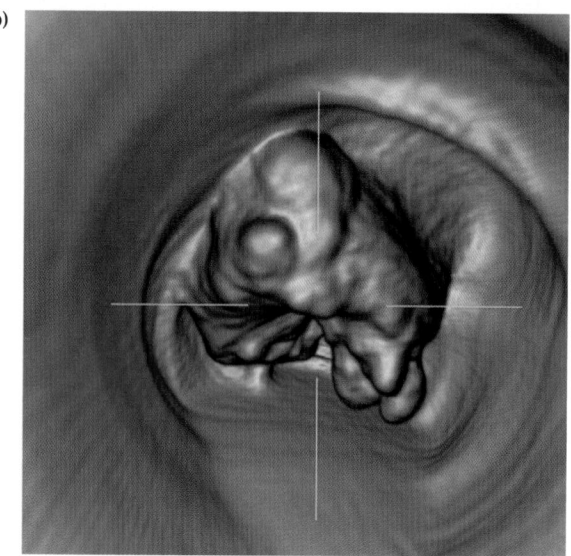

Figure 65.41 Virtual colonoscopy of the right colon. (a) Computerised tomography scan of the abdomen showing a caecal tumour. (b) Formatted 'virtual' image of the same lesion as in (a) (courtesy of Dr A. Slater, John Radcliffe Hospital, Oxford, UK).

inspected for signs of small, white, seed-like, neoplastic implantations. Similar changes can occur in the omentum.

3 The various groups of lymph nodes that drain the involved segment are palpated. Their enlargement does not necessarily mean that they are invaded by metastases, because the enlargement may be inflammatory.

4 The neoplasm is examined with a view to mobility and operability. Local fixation, however, does not always imply local invasion because some tumours excite a brisk inflammatory response.

Operations

The operations to be described are designed to remove the primary tumour and its draining locoregional lymph nodes, which may be involved by metastases. Lesser resections are indicated, however, should hepatic metastases render the condition incurable surgically. There is some evidence that early division of major blood vessels supplying the involved colon (no-touch technique – Turnbull) can slightly improve the number of curative

R. Turnbull, **Irish** surgeon, Cleveland Clinic, Ohio, reported the presence of cancer cells in the portal vein of patients undergoing resection for colon cancer. He then described in his Moynihan lecture a 'no-touch' isolation technique to reduce the manipulation of colonic tumours at surgery.

operations. The use of stapling and hand-suturing techniques for colonic anastomosis has been compared, and there is little difference in leak rate between the two.

Carcinoma of the caecum

Carcinoma of the caecum or ascending colon (Fig. 65.42) is treated when resectable by right hemicolectomy (Fig. 65.43).

The abdomen is opened, the peritoneum lateral to the ascending colon is incised, and the incision is carried around the hepatic flexure. The right colon is elevated, with the leaf of peritoneum containing its vessels and lymph nodes, from the posterior abdominal wall, taking care not to injure the ureter, spermatic vessels in the male or the duodenum. The peritoneum is separated medially near the origin of the ileocolic artery, which is divided together with the right colic artery when this has a separate origin from the superior mesenteric. The mesentery of the last 30 cm of ileum and the leaf of raised peritoneum attached to the caecum, ascending colon and hepatic flexure, after ligation of the mesenteric blood vessels, is divided as far as the proximal

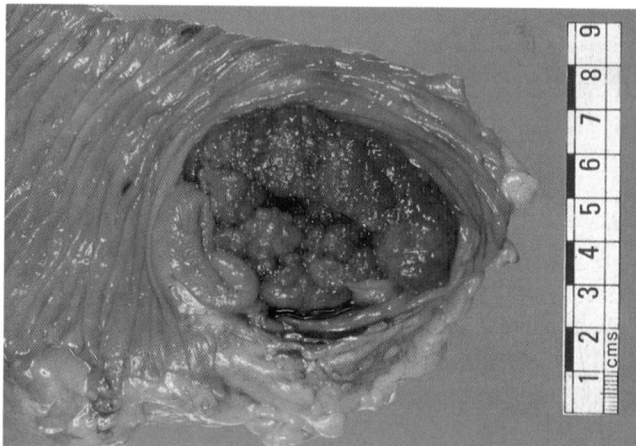

Figure 65.42 Large villous tumour of the caecum with malignant change.

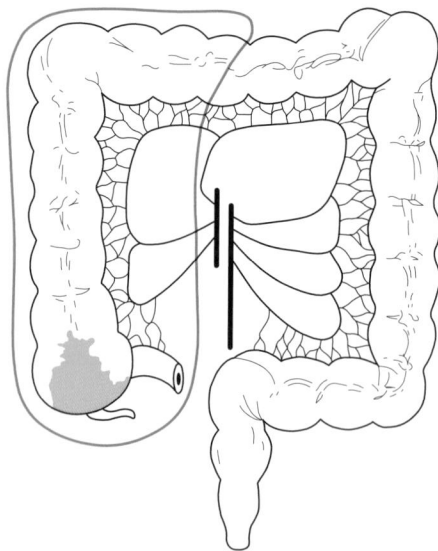

Figure 65.43 Area to be resected when the growth is situated in the caecum.

third of the transverse colon. When it is clear that there is an adequate blood supply at the resection margins, the right colon is resected, and an end-to-end anastomosis is fashioned between the ileum and the transverse colon.

Carcinoma of the hepatic flexure
When the hepatic flexure is involved, the resection must be extended correspondingly (Fig. 65.44).

Carcinoma of the transverse colon
When there is no obstruction, excision of the transverse colon and the two flexures together with the transverse mesocolon and the greater omentum, followed by end-to-end anastomosis, can be used. An alternative is an extended right hemicolectomy (Fig. 65.44).

Carcinoma of the splenic flexure or descending colon
The extent of the resection is from right colon to descending colon. Sometimes, removal of the colon up to the ileum, with an ileorectal anastomosis, is preferable.

Carcinoma of the pelvic colon
The left half of the colon is mobilised completely (Fig. 65.45). So that the operation is radical, the inferior mesenteric artery below its left colic branch, together with the related paracolic lymph nodes, must be included in the resection. This entails carrying the dissection as far as the upper third of the rectum. Many surgeons advocate flush ligation of the inferior mesenteric artery on the aorta (high ligation). Provided that there is no obstruction, primary anastomosis is the rule. Occasionally, a protecting upstream stoma may be necessary. The methods of dealing with large bowel obstruction as a result of colon cancer are described in Chapter 66.

Laparoscopic surgery
This has been heralded as the next major advance in colorectal surgery. However, its role needs to be accepted with an element of caution. It is technically demanding with a long learning curve.

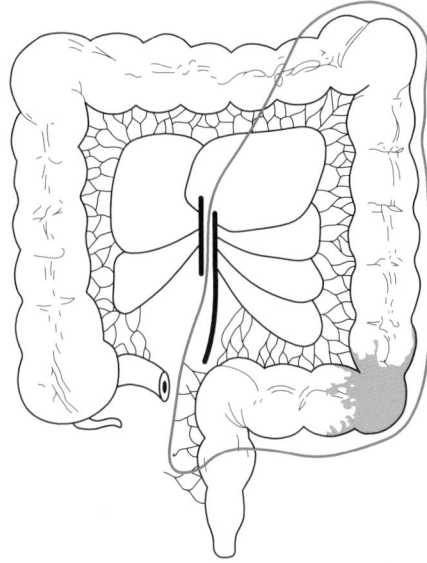

Figure 65.45 Area to be resected in the case of a carcinoma of the pelvic colon.

Patients undergoing such surgery need to be entered into clinical trials. Important technical issues are traction and adequate vision, which are vital, as for open conventional procedures. Hand-assisted methods can be used in particularly difficult cases, but this takes away some of the benefits of the minimal approach. Specimen retrieval is via small incisions. Techniques and technology are rapidly evolving.

When a growth is found to be inoperable
In the upper part of the left colon, an ileostomy is performed. In the pelvic colon, a left iliac fossa colostomy is preferable. With an inoperable growth in the ascending colon, a bypass using an ileocolic anastomosis is the best procedure. A total colectomy needs to be considered for multiple tumours. Over 95% of colonic carcinomas can, however, be resected.

Adjuvant therapy
See Chapter 68.

Screening
There is now good evidence from controlled trials that regular bowel screening using faecal occult blood testing of people aged 60–69 years can reduce the mortality risk of colorectal cancer by about 15%. Those who test positive for faecal occult blood tests are then offered colonoscopy. These data have prompted the setting up of the National Health Service Bowel Cancer Screening Programme in the UK. Flexible sigmoidoscopy can also be used as the initial screening tool, and early results from a clinical trial look promising.

Hepatic metastases
It is important not to biopsy hepatic metastases as this may cause tumour dissemination (Fig. 65.46). Hepatic resection is usually performed as a staged procedure after recovery from colonic resection. Most wait 12 weeks before restaging. By doing this, those with aggressive disease are excluded from further drastic surgery. Reports have shown 30% 5-year survival following hepatectomy for colorectal cancer metastases. Radiological imaging

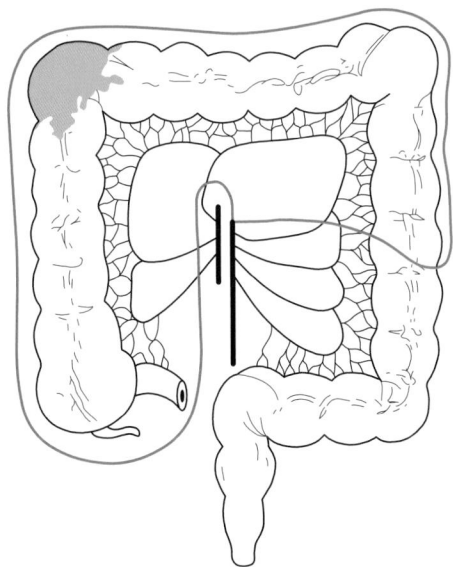

Figure 65.44 Area to be resected when the growth is situated at the hepatic flexure.

CHAPTER 65 | THE SMALL AND LARGE INTESTINES

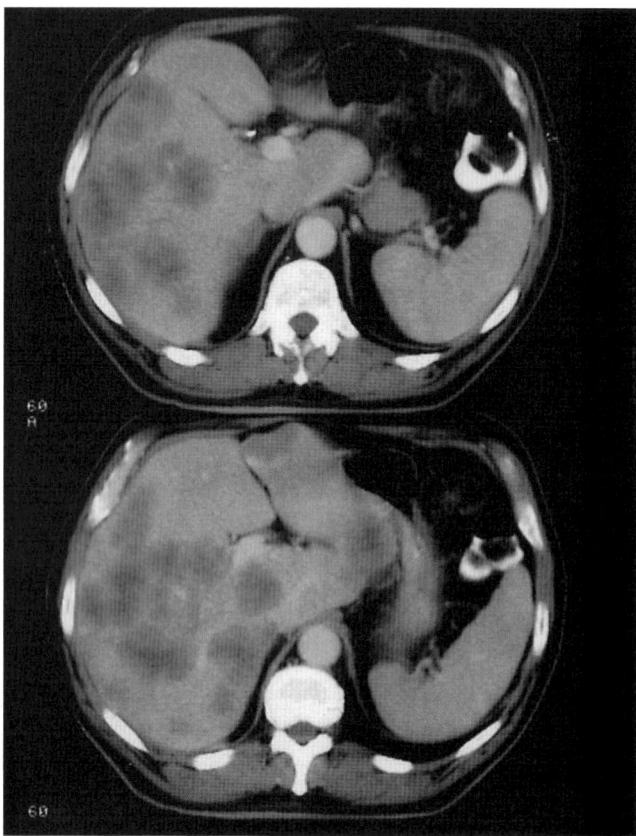

Figure 65.46 Computerised tomography scan of the liver showing multiple metastases from carcinoma of the colon.

will usually correctly identify colorectal metastases and assess patients suitable for liver resection. At present, the criterion for resection is fewer than three lesions in one lobe of liver. Irresectable symptomatic hepatic metastases may be suitable for other treatments including cytotoxic drugs or ablative treatments.

OTHER DISORDERS

Traumatic rupture

The intestine can be ruptured with or without an external wound – so called blunt trauma (Fig. 65.47). The most common cause of this is a blow to the abdomen that crushes the bowel against the vertebral column or sacrum; also, a rupture is more likely to occur where part of the gut has been fixed, for example in a hernia, or where a fixed part of the gut joins a mobile part such as the duodenojejunal flexure. Here, the damage may be retroperitoneal and easily overlooked.

In small perforations, the mucosa may prolapse through the hole and partly seal it, making the early signs misleading. In addition, there may be a laceration in the mesentery. The patient will then have a combination of intra-abdominal bleeding and release of intestinal contents into the abdominal cavity, giving rise to peritonitis.

Traumatic rupture of the large intestine is much less common. In blast injuries of the abdomen following the detonation of a bomb, the pelvic colon is particularly at risk of rupture. Compressed air rupture can follow the dangerous practical joke of turning on an airline carrying compressed air near the victim's anus.

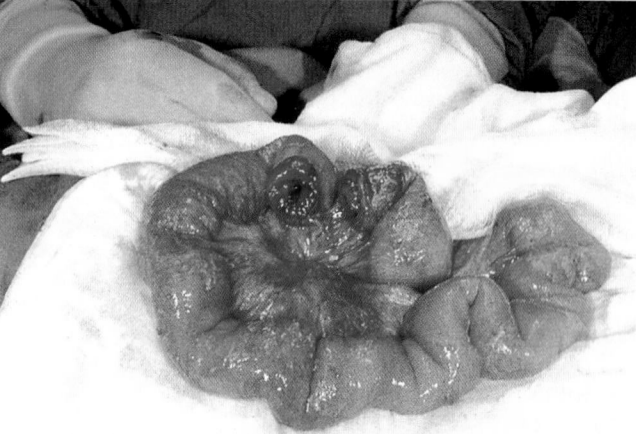

Figure 65.47 Traumatic rupture of the small intestine as a result of blunt abdominal trauma.

Rupture of the upper rectum can occur during sigmoidoscopy and occasionally during the placement of rectal catheters for barium radiology. Traumatic rupture of the colon can occur during colonoscopy. The most common site is the sigmoid colon, where the formation of a sigmoid loop pushes against the antimesenteric border of the sigmoid colon, stretching it out and eventually perforating it.

Gunshot wounds and impalement injuries to the bowel have more serious consequences because of the introduction of debris from the patient's clothing or the missile itself mixing with the bacteria in the patient's gut. High-velocity missiles may cause extensive damage to the bowel over a much wider area than just the entry and exit wounds.

Treatment

Where rupture is suspected, a plain radiograph in the erect or lateral decubitus position will demonstrate the presence of free air in the peritoneal cavity or indeed in the retroperitoneal tissues. In almost all cases, an abdominal exploration must be performed and, in many instances, simple closure of the perforation is all that is required. In others, for example where the mesentery is lacerated and the bowel is not viable, resection may be necessary. In the case of the large intestine, small, clean tears can be closed primarily; if there is a large tear with damage to the surrounding structures and the adjacent mesentery, resection and exteriorisation may be used. Much depends on the amount of intra-abdominal soiling.

In the case of retroperitoneal portions of the intestine, for example the duodenum, perforations can involve the front and back walls, and the duodenum in particular has to be carefully mobilised to check that a concealed tear is not overlooked. In all cases, the abdomen is washed out with saline and broad-spectrum intravenous antibiotics are given.

Enterocutaneous or faecal fistula

An external fistula communicating with the caecum sometimes follows an operation for gangrenous appendicitis or the draining of an appendix abscess. A faecal fistula can occur from necrosis of a gangrenous patch of intestine after the relief of a strangulated hernia, or from a leak from an intestinal anastomosis. The opening of an abscess connected with chronic diverticulitis or carcinoma of the colon frequently results in a faecal fistula. Radiation damage is also another cause of fistula formation. The most common cause of enterocutaneous fistula is, however, previous surgery. This happens most often in patients with adhesions following previous operations. Damage to the small intestine occurs inadvertently during dissection of the adhesions and, because of an associated subacute obstruction or abscess, the fistula 'blows' postoperatively. Enterocutaneous fistulae can be divided into:

- those with a high output, more than 1 litre day^{-1};
- those with a low output, less than 1 litre day^{-1}.

They can also be described anatomically as simple, with a direct communication between the gut and the skin, or complex, i.e. those with one or more tracts that are tortuous and sometimes associated with an intervening abscess cavity half way along the tract.

The discharge from a fistula connected with the duodenum or jejunum is bile-stained and causes severe excoriation of the skin. When the ileum or caecum is involved, the discharge is fluid faecal matter; when the distal colon is the affected site, it is solid or semisolid faecal matter. The site of leakage and the length of the fistula can be determined by small bowel enema and barium enema, by fistulography and, most importantly, by CT of the abdomen will show up any associated abscesses (Fig. 65.48).

Treatment

This can be very challenging in patients with a high-output fistula. Low-output fistulae can be expected to heal spontaneously, provided there is no distal obstruction. Reasons for failure of spontaneous healing also include:

- epithelial continuity between the gut and the skin;
- the presence of active disease where, for example, there is CD or carcinoma at the site of the anastomosis or in the tract;
- an associated complex abscess.

The abdominal wall must be protected from erosion by the use of appliances. The patient must remain nil by mouth; intravenous nutrition is started and signs of a decrease in fistula output are sought. The higher the fistula in the intestinal tract, the more skin excoriation must be expected, and this is worst in the case of a duodenal fistula. High-output fistulae cause rapid dehydration and hypoproteinaemia. Vigorous fluid replacement and nutritional

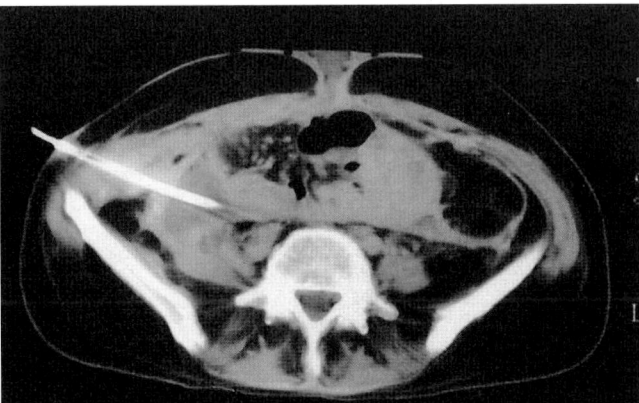

Figure 65.48 Computerised tomography scan in a patient with a complex enterocutaneous fistula and an intra-abdominal abscess being drained with a CT-guided catheter.

support are essential. The drainage of an intra-abdominal abscess can be life-saving. This can be achieved by either CT-guided drainage or, occasionally, laparotomy. In patients with a complex fistula, it may be necessary to bring out a defunctioning stoma upstream of the fistula site, even if this results in a high-output stoma.

Operative treatment

Operative repair should be attempted only after a trial of conservative management. The surgery can on occasion be extremely technically demanding, and an anastomosis should not be fashioned in the presence of continuing intra-abdominal sepsis or when the patient is hypoproteinaemic.

STOMAS

Colostomy

A colostomy is an artificial opening made in the large bowel to divert faeces and flatus to the exterior, where it can be collected in an external appliance. Depending on the purpose for which the diversion has been necessary, a colostomy may be temporary or permanent (Summary box 65.11).

Summary box 65.11

Stomas

- May be colostomy or ileostomy
- May be temporary or permanent
- Temporary or defunctioning stomas are usually fashioned as loop stomas
- An ileostomy is spouted; a colostomy is flush
- Ileostomy effluent is usually liquid whereas colostomy effluent is usually solid
- Ileostomy patients are more likely to develop fluid and electrolyte problems
- An ileostomy is usually sited in the right iliac fossa
- A temporary colostomy may be transverse and sited in the right upper quadrant
- End-colostomy is usually sited in the left iliac fossa
- All patients should be counselled by a stoma care nurse before operation
- Complications include skin irritation, prolapse, retraction, necrosis, stenosis, parastomal hernia, bleeding and fistulation

---

Temporary colostomy

A transverse loop colostomy has in the past been most commonly used to defunction an anastomosis after an anterior resection. It is now less commonly employed as it is fraught with complications and is difficult to manage; a loop ileostomy is preferred.

A loop left iliac fossa colostomy is still sometimes used to prevent faecal peritonitis developing following traumatic injury to the rectum, to facilitate the operative treatment of a high fistula-in-ano and incontinence.

A temporary loop colostomy is made, bringing a loop of colon to the surface, where it is held in place by a plastic bridge passed through the mesentery. Once the abdomen has been closed, the colostomy is opened, and the edges of the colonic incision are sutured to the adjacent skin margin (Fig. 65.49). When firm adhesion of the colostomy to the abdominal wall has taken place, the bridge can be removed after 7 days.

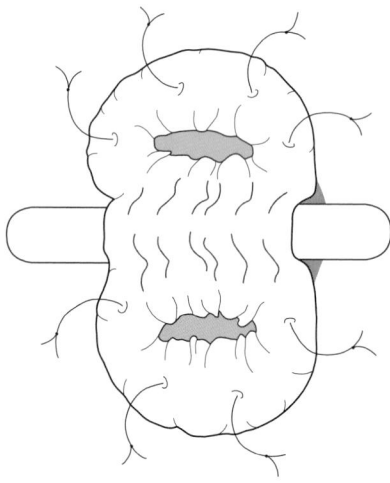

Figure 65.49 Usual temporary (loop) colostomy opened over a rod, and immediate suture of the colon wall to surrounding skin (many new rods are designed to lie beneath the skin's surface; alternatively, a skin bridge is used).

Following the surgical cure or healing of the distal lesion for which the temporary stoma was constructed, the colostomy can be closed. It is usual to perform a contrast examination (distal loopogram) to check that there is no distal obstruction or continuing problem at the site of previous surgery. Colostomy closure is most easily and safely accomplished if the stoma is mature, i.e. after the colostomy has been established for 2 months. Closure is usually performed by an intraperitoneal technique, which is associated with fewer closure breakdowns with faecal fistulae.

Double-barrelled colostomy

This colostomy was designed so that it could be closed by crushing the intervening 'spur' using an enterotome or a stapling device. It is rarely used now, but occasionally the colon is divided so that both ends can be brought to the surface separately, ensuring that the distal segment is completely defunctioned.

Permanent colostomy

This is usually formed after excision of the rectum for a carcinoma by the abdominoperineal technique.

It is formed by bringing the distal end (end-colostomy) of the divided colon to the surface in the left iliac fossa, where it is sutured in place, joining the colonic margin to the surrounding skin.

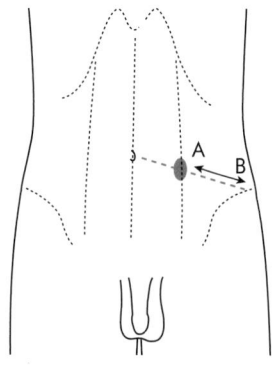

Figure 65.50 Usual site of a permanent (end) colostomy in the left iliac fossa. Note the distance A–B: 2.5 cm at least.

The point at which the colon is brought to the surface must be carefully selected to allow a colostomy bag to be applied without impinging on the bony prominence of the anterosuperior iliac spine. The best site is usually through the lateral edge of the rectus sheath, 6 cm above and medial to the bony prominence (Fig. 65.50).

Closure of the lateral space between the intraperitoneal segment of the sigmoid colon and the peritoneum of the pelvic wall, to prevent internal herniation or strangulation of loops of small bowel through the deficiency, has been practised, but there is no good evidence that it is effective.

Colostomy bags and appliances (Fig. 65.51)

Faeces from a permanent colostomy are collected in disposable adhesive bags. A wide range of such bags is currently available.

(a)

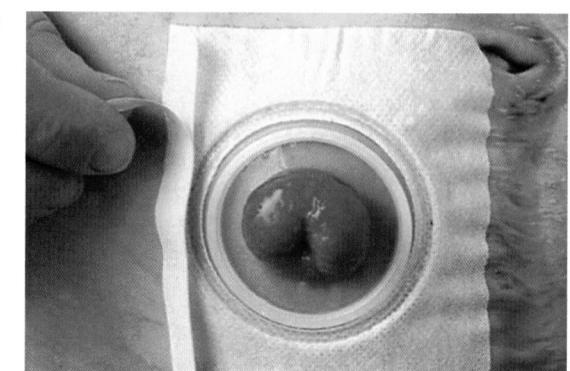

(b)

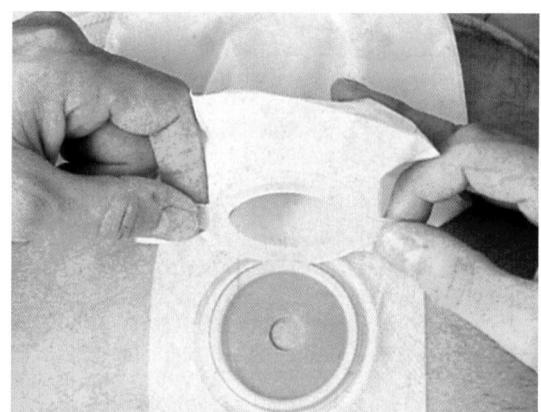

(c)

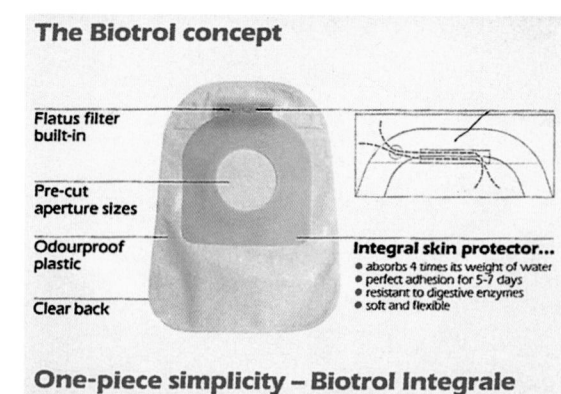

Figure 65.51 (a) The usual long-term backing ('stomahesive') and flange, onto which the bag is placed (b). (c) The desirable features incorporated in modern systems, e.g. the Biotrol concept as shown.

Many now incorporate a stomahesive backing, which can be left in place for several days. In most hospitals, a stoma care service is available to offer advice to patients, to acquaint them with the latest appliances and to provide the appropriate psychological and practical help.

Complications of colostomies
The following complications can occur to any colostomy but are more common after poor technique or siting of the stoma:

- prolapse;
- retraction;
- necrosis of the distal end;
- fistula formation;
- stenosis of the orifice;
- colostomy hernia;
- bleeding (usually from granulomas around the margin of the colostomy);
- colostomy 'diarrhoea': this is usually an infective enteritis and will respond to oral metronidazole 200 mg three times daily.

Many of these complications require revision of the colostomy. Sometimes, this can be achieved with an incision immediately around the stoma but, on occasion, reopening the abdomen and freeing up the colostomy may be necessary. Occasionally, transfer to the opposite side of the abdomen may be necessary.

Loop ileostomy

An ileostomy is now often used as an alternative to colostomy, particularly for defunctioning a low rectal anastomosis. The creation of a loop ileostomy from a knuckle of terminal ileum has already been described. The advantages of a loop ileostomy over a loop colostomy are the ease with which the bowel can be brought to the surface and the absence of odour. Care is needed, when the ileostomy is closed, that suture line obstruction does not occur.

Caecostomy

This is rarely used now. In desperately ill patients with advanced obstruction, a caecostomy may be useful. In late cases of obstruction, the caecum may become so distended and ischaemic that rupture of the caecal wall may be anticipated. This can occur spontaneously, giving rise to faecal peritonitis, or at operation, when an incision in the abdominal wall reduces its supportive role and allows the caecum to expand. In such a situation, it should be decompressed by suction as soon as the abdomen is opened. In thin patients, it may then be possible to carry out direct suture of the incised or perforated caecal wall to the abdominal skin of the right iliac fossa, although a resection of this area is really the best treatment. Following on-table lavage, via the appendix stump, the irrigating catheter can be left in place as a tube caecostomy. Caecostomy is only a short-term measure to allow a few days for the condition of the patient to improve. Reoperation should normally follow soon thereafter and a definitive procedure should be carried out.

FURTHER READING

Allan, R.N., Keighley, M.R.B., Alexander, J. and Hawkins, E. (1990) *Inflammatory Bowel Diseases*. Churchill Livingstone, Edinburgh.

Keighley, M.R.B. and Williams, N.S. (1999) *Surgery of the Anus, Rectum and Colon*, 2nd edn. W.B. Saunders, London.

Phillips, R.K.S. (2006) *A Companion to Specialist Surgical Practice*, 3rd edn. Elsevier Saunders, Philadelphia.

CHAPTER 65 | THE SMALL AND LARGE INTESTINES

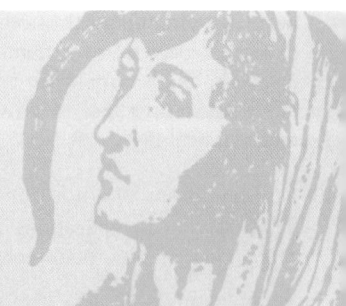

Intestinal obstruction

LEARNING OBJECTIVES

To understand:

- The pathophysiology of dynamic and adynamic intestinal obstruction
- The cardinal features on history and examination

- The causes of small and large bowel obstruction
- The indications and contraindications for conservative management in bowel obstruction

CLASSIFICATION

Intestinal obstruction may be classified into two types:

- *Dynamic*, in which peristalsis is working against a mechanical obstruction. It may occur in an acute or a chronic form (Fig. 66.1; Summary boxes 66.1 and 66.2).
- *Adynamic*, in which peristalsis may be absent (e.g. paralytic ileus) or it may be present in a non-propulsive form (e.g. mesenteric vascular occlusion or pseudo-obstruction). In both types a mechanical element is absent (Summary box 66.1).

Summary box 66.1

Causes of intestinal obstruction

Dynamic
- ■ Intraluminal
     Impaction
     Foreign bodies
     Bezoars
     Gallstones
- ■ Intramural
     Stricture
     Malignancy
- ■ Extramural
     Bands/adhesions
     Hernia
     Volvulus
     Intussusception

Adynamic
- ■ Paralytic ileus
- ■ Mesenteric vascular occlusion
- ■ Pseudo-obstruct

Summary box 66.2

Mechanisms of obstruction

- ■ Volvulus
- ■ Incarceration
- ■ Obstruction
- ■ Intussusception

PATHOPHYSIOLOGY

Irrespective of aetiology or acuteness of onset, in dynamic (mechanical) obstruction the proximal bowel dilates and develops an altered motility. Below the obstruction the bowel exhibits normal peristalsis and absorption until it becomes empty, at which point it contracts and becomes immobile. Initially, proximal peristalsis is increased to overcome the obstruction, in direct proportion to the distance of the obstruction. If the obstruction is not relieved, the bowel begins to dilate, causing a reduction in

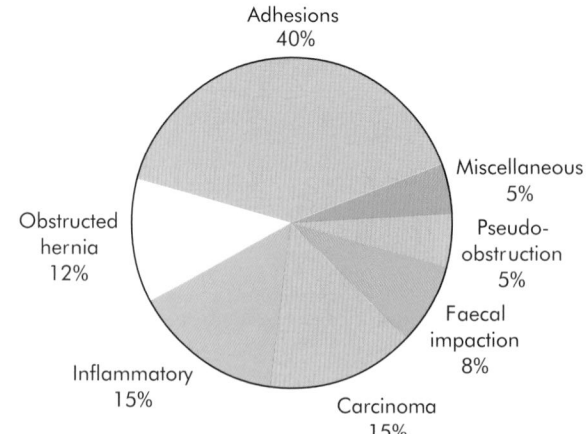

Figure 66.1 Pie chart showing the common causes of dynamic intestinal obstruction and their relative frequencies.

peristaltic strength, ultimately resulting in flaccidity and paralysis. This is a protective phenomenon to prevent vascular damage secondary to increased intraluminal pressure.

The distension proximal to an obstruction is produced by two factors:

- *Gas:* there is a significant overgrowth of both aerobic and anaerobic organisms, resulting in considerable gas production. Following the reabsorption of oxygen and carbon dioxide, the majority is made up of nitrogen (90%) and hydrogen sulphide.
- *Fluid:* this is made up of the various digestive juices. Following obstruction, fluid accumulates within the bowel wall and any excess is secreted into the lumen, whilst absorption from the gut is retarded. Dehydration and electrolyte loss are therefore due to:
  - reduced oral intake;
  - defective intestinal absorption;
  - losses as a result of vomiting;
  - sequestration in the bowel lumen.

STRANGULATION

When strangulation occurs, the viability of the bowel is threatened secondary to a compromised blood supply (Summary box 66.3).

Summary box 66.3
Causes of strangulation
External
■ Hernial orifices
■ Adhesions/bands
Interrupted blood flow
■ Volvulus
■ Intussusception
Increased intraluminal pressure
■ Closed-loop obstruction
Primary
■ Mesenteric infarction

The venous return is compromised before the arterial supply. The resultant increase in capillary pressure leads to local mural distension with loss of intravascular fluid and red blood cells intramurally and extraluminally. Once the arterial supply is impaired, haemorrhagic infarction occurs. As the viability of the bowel is compromised there is marked translocation and systemic exposure to anaerobic organisms with their associated toxins. The morbidity of intraperitoneal strangulation is far greater than with an external hernia, which has a smaller absorptive surface.

The morbidity and mortality associated with strangulation are dependent on age and extent. In strangulated external hernias the segment involved is short and the resultant blood and fluid loss is small. When bowel involvement is extensive the loss of blood and circulatory volume will cause peripheral circulatory failure.

Closed-loop obstruction

This occurs when the bowel is obstructed at both the proximal and distal points (Fig. 66.2). It is present in many cases of intestinal

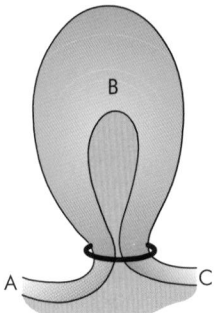

Figure 66.2 Distension. Closed-loop obstruction with no proximal (A) or distal (C) distension and impending strangulation (B).

strangulation. Unlike cases of non-strangulating obstruction, there is no early distension of the proximal intestine. When gangrene of the strangulated segment is imminent, retrograde thrombosis of the mesenteric veins results in distension on both sides of the strangulated segment.

A classic form of closed-loop obstruction is seen in the presence of a malignant stricture of the right colon with a competent ileocaecal valve (present in up to one-third of individuals). The inability of the distended colon to decompress itself into the small bowel results in an increase in luminal pressure, which is greatest at the caecum, with subsequent impairment of blood supply. Unrelieved, this results in necrosis and perforation (Fig. 66.3)

SPECIAL TYPES OF MECHANICAL INTESTINAL OBSTRUCTION

Internal hernia

Internal herniation occurs when a portion of the small intestine becomes entrapped in one of the retroperitoneal fossae or in a congenital mesenteric defect.

The following are potential sites of internal herniation:

- the foramen of Winslow;
- a hole in the mesentery;

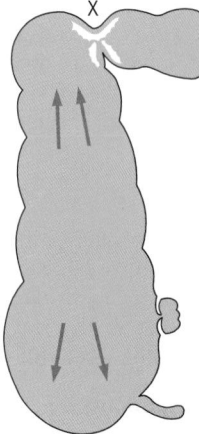

Figure 66.3 Carcinomatous stricture (X) of the hepatic flexure: closed-loop obstruction.

Jacob Benignus Winslow, **1669–1760, Professor of Anatomy, Physic and Surgery, Paris, France.**

- a hole in the transverse mesocolon;
- defects in the broad ligament;
- congenital or acquired diaphragmatic hernia;
- duodenal retroperitoneal fossae – left paraduodenal and right duodenojejunal;
- caecal/appendiceal retroperitoneal fossae – superior, inferior and retrocaecal;
- intersigmoid fossa.

Internal herniation in the absence of adhesions is uncommon and a preoperative diagnosis is unusual. The standard treatment for a hernia is to release the constricting agent by division. This should not be undertaken in cases of herniation involving the foramen of Winslow, mesenteric defects and the paraduodenal/duodenojejunal fossae as major blood vessels run in the edge of the constriction ring. The distended loop in such circumstances must first be decompressed with minimal contamination and then reduced.

Obstruction from enteric strictures

Small bowel strictures usually occur secondary to tuberculosis or Crohn's disease. Malignant strictures associated with lymphoma are common, whereas carcinoma and sarcoma are rare. Presentation is usually subacute or chronic. Standard surgical management consists of resection and anastomosis. In Crohn's disease, strictureplasty may be considered in the presence of short multiple strictures without active sepsis.

Bolus obstruction

Bolus obstruction in the small bowel may be caused by food, gallstones, trichobezoar, phytobezoar, stercoliths and worms.

Gallstones

This type of obstruction tends to occur in the elderly secondary to erosion of a large gallstone through the gall bladder into the duodenum. Classically, there is impaction about 60 cm proximal to the ileocaecal valve. The patient may have recurrent attacks as the obstruction is frequently incomplete or relapsing as a result of a ball-valve effect. A radiograph will show evidence of small bowel obstruction with a diagnostic air–fluid level in the biliary tree. The stone may not be visible. At laparotomy it may be possible to crush the stone within the bowel lumen, after milking it proximally. If not, the intestine is opened and the gallstone removed. If the gallstone is faceted, a careful check for other enteric stones should be made. The region of the gall bladder should not be explored.

Food

Bolus obstruction may occur after partial or total gastrectomy when unchewed articles can pass directly into the small bowel. Fruit and vegetables are particularly liable to cause obstruction. The management is similar to that for gallstone, with intraluminal crushing usually being successful.

Trychobezoars and phytobezoars

These are firm masses of undigested hair balls and fruit/vegetable fibre respectively. The former is due to persistent hair chewing or

sucking, and may be associated with an underlying psychiatric abnormality. Predisposition to phytobezoars results from a high fibre intake, inadequate chewing, previous gastric surgery, hypochlorhydria and loss of the gastric pump mechanism. When possible, the lesion may be kneaded into the caecum, otherwise open removal is required.

Stercoliths

These are usually found in the small bowel in association with a jejunal diverticulum or ileal stricture. Presentation and management are identical to that of gallstones.

Worms

Ascaris lumbricoides may cause low small bowel obstruction, particularly in children, the institutionalised and those near the tropics (Fig. 66.4). An attack frequently follows the initiation of anti-helminthic therapy. Debility is frequently out of proportion to that produced by the obstruction. If worms are not seen in the stool or vomitus the diagnosis may be indicated by eosinophilia or the sight of worms within gas-filled small bowel loops on a plain radiograph (Naik). At laparotomy it may be possible to knead the tangled mass into the caecum; if not it should be removed. Occasionally, worms may cause a perforation and peritonitis, especially if the enteric wall is weakened by such conditions as ameobiasis.

Obstruction by adhesions and bands

Adhesions

In western countries where abdominal operations are common, adhesions and bands are the most common cause of intestinal obstruction. Furthermore, in the early postoperative period, the onset of such a mechanical obstruction may be difficult to differentiate from paralytic ileus.

The causes of intraperitoneal adhesions are shown in Table 66.1. Any source of peritoneal irritation results in local fibrin production, which produces adhesions between apposed surfaces. Early fibrinous adhesions may disappear when the cause is removed or they may become vascularised and be replaced by mature fibrous tissue.

There are several factors that may limit adhesion formation (Summary box 66.4).

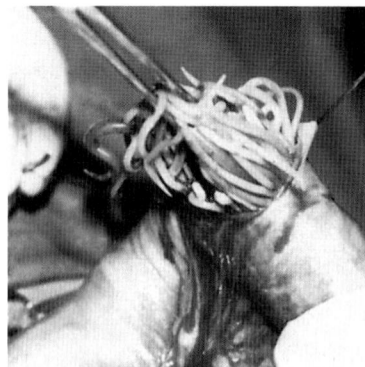

Figure 66.4 Obstruction of the small intestine due to *Ascaris lumbricoides* (courtesy of Asal Y. Izzidien, Nenavah, Iraq).

Table 66.1 The common causes of intra-abdominal adhesions

Ischaemic areas	Sites of anastomoses, reperitonealisation of raw areas, trauma, vascular occlusion
Foreign material	Talc, starch, gauze, silk
Infection	Peritonitis, tuberculosis
Inflammatory conditions	Crohn's disease
Radiation enteritis	

Summary box 66.4

Prevention of adhesions

Factors that may limit adhesion formation include:

- Good surgical technique
- Washing of the peritoneal cavity with saline to remove clots, etc.
- Minimising contact with gauze
- Covering anastomosis and raw peritoneal surfaces

Numerous substances have been instilled in the peritoneal cavity to prevent adhesion formation, including hyaluronidase, hydrocortisone, silicone, dextran, polyvinylpropylene (PVP), chondroitin and streptomycin, anticoagulants, anti-histamines, non-steroidal anti-inflammatory drugs and streptokinase. Currently, no single agent has been shown to be particularly effective.

Adhesions may be classified into various types by virtue of whether they are early (fibrinous) or late (fibrous) or by underlying aetiology. From a practical perspective there are only two types – 'easy' flimsy ones and 'difficult' dense ones.

Postoperative adhesions giving rise to intestinal obstruction usually involve the lower small bowel. Operations for appendicitis and gynaecological procedures are the most common precursors and are an indication for early intervention.

Bands

Usually only one band is culpable. This may be:

- congenital, e.g. obliterated vitellointestinal duct;
- a string band following previous bacterial peritonitis;
- a portion of greater omentum, usually adherent to the parietes.

Acute intussusception

This occurs when one portion of the gut becomes invaginated within an immediately adjacent segment; almost invariably, it is the proximal into the distal.

The condition is encountered most commonly in children, with a peak incidence between 5 and 10 months of age. About 90% of cases are idiopathic but an associated upper respiratory tract infection or gastroenteritis may precede the condition. It is believed that hyperplasia of Peyer's patches in the terminal ileum may be the initiating event. Weaning, loss of passively acquired

---

Johann Conrad Peyer, 1653–1712, Professor of Logic, Rhetoric and Medicine, Schaffhausen, Switzerland, described the lymph follicles in the intestine in 1677.

---

maternal immunity and common viral pathogens have all been implicated in the pathogenesis of intussusception in infancy.

Children with intussusception associated with a pathological lead point such as Meckel's diverticulum, polyp, duplication, Henoch–Schönlein purpura or appendix are usually older than those with idiopathic disease. After the age of 2 years, a pathological lead point is found in at least one-third of affected children. Adult cases are invariably associated with a lead point, which is usually a polyp (e.g. Peutz–Jeghers syndrome), a submucosal lipoma or other tumour.

Pathology

An intussusception is composed of three parts (Fig. 66.5):

- the entering or inner tube;
- the returning or middle tube;
- the sheath or outer tube (intussuscipiens).

The part that advances is the apex, the mass is the intussusception and the neck is the junction of the entering layer with the mass.

An intussusception is an example of a strangulating obstruction as the blood supply of the inner layer is usually impaired. The degree of ischaemia is dependent on the tightness of the invagination, which is usually greatest as it passes through the ileocaecal valve.

Intussusception may be anatomically defined according to the site and extent of invagination (Table 66.2). In most children, the intussusception is ileocolic (see Chapter 6, Fig. 6.13). In adults, colocolic intussusception is common (Summary box 66.5).

Summary box 66.5

Intussusception

- Most common in children
- Primary or secondary to intestinal pathology, e.g. polyp, Meckel's diverticulum
- Ileocolic is the commonest variety
- Can lead to an ischaemic segment
- Radiological reduction is indicated in most cases
- The remainder require surgery

Volvulus

A volvulus is a twisting or axial rotation of a portion of bowel about its mesentery. When complete it forms a closed loop of obstruction with resultant ischaemia secondary to vascular occlusion.

Volvuli may be primary or secondary. The primary form occurs secondary to congenital malrotation of the gut, abnormal mesenteric attachments or congenital bands. Examples include volvulus neonatorum, caecal volvulus and sigmoid volvulus. A secondary volvulus, which is the more common variety, is due to

---

Johann Friedrich Meckel, (The Younger), 1781–1833, Professor of Anatomy and Surgery, Halle, Germany, described the diverticulum in 1809.
Eduard Heinrich Henoch, 1820–1910, Professor of Diseases of Children, Berlin, Germany, described this form of purpura in 1868.
Johann Lucas Schönlein, 1793–1864, Professor of Medicine, Berlin, Germany, gave his account of this disease in 1837.
John Law Augustine Peutz, 1886–1968, Chief Specialist for Internal Medicine, St. John's Hospital, The Hague, The Netherlands.
Harold Joseph Jeghers, 1904–1990, Professor of Internal Medicine, New Jersey College of Medicine and Dentistry, Jersey City, NJ, USA.

rotation of a piece of bowel around an acquired adhesion or stoma. (Summary box 66.6).

Summary box 66.6

Volvulus

- May involve the small intestine, caecum or sigmoid colon; neonatal midgut volvulus secondary to midgut malrotation is life-threatening
- The commonest spontaneous type in adults is sigmoid
- Sigmoid volvulus can be relieved by decompression per anum
- Surgery is required to prevent or relieve ischaemia

Volvulus neonatorum

This occurs secondary to intestinal malrotation (see Chapter 6) and is potentially catastrophic.

Sigmoid volvulus

This is rare in Europe and the USA but more common in Eastern Europe and Africa. Indeed, it is the most common cause of large bowel obstruction in the indigenous black African population. Rotation nearly always occurs in the anticlockwise direction. The predisposing medical causes are summarised in Fig. 66.6. Other predisposing factors include a high residue diet and constipation.

Compound volvulus

This is a rare condition also known as ileosigmoid knotting. The long pelvic mesocolon allows the ileum to twist around the sigmoid colon, resulting in gangrene of either or both segments of bowel. The patient presents with acute intestinal obstruction,

Table 66.2 Types of intussusception in children (after R.E. Gross) (*n* = 702)

	Percentage of series
Ileoileal	5
Ileocolic	77
Ileoileocolic	12
Colocolic	2
Multiple	1
Retrograde	0.2
Others	2.8

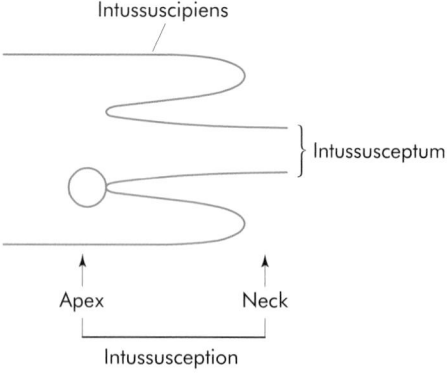

Figure 66.5 Mechanism and nomenclature of intussusception.

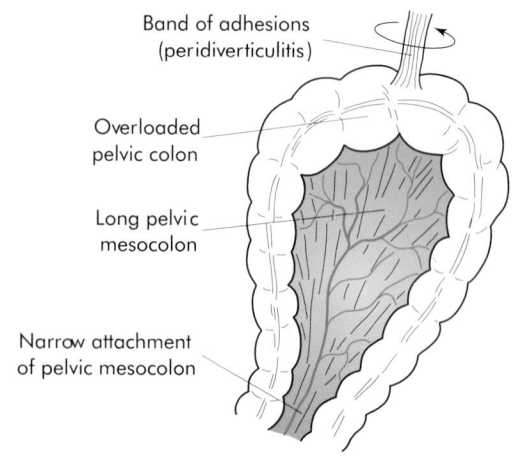

Figure 66.6 Causes predisposing to volvulus of the sigmoid colon. Idiopathic megacolon usually precedes the volvulus in African people.

but distension is comparatively mild. Plain radiography reveals distended ileal loops in a distended sigmoid colon. At operation, decompression, resection and anastomosis are required.

CLINICAL FEATURES OF INTESTINAL OBSTRUCTION

Dynamic obstruction

The diagnosis of dynamic intestinal obstruction is based on the classic quartet of pain, distension, vomiting and absolute constipation. Obstruction may be classified clinically into two types:

- small bowel obstruction – high or low;
- large bowel obstruction (Summary box 66.7).

Summary box 66.7

Features of obstruction

- In *high small bowel obstruction*, vomiting occurs early and is profuse with rapid dehydration. Distension is minimal with little evidence of fluid levels on abdominal radiography
- In *low small bowel obstruction*, pain is predominant with central distension. Vomiting is delayed. Multiple central fluid levels are seen on radiography
- In *large bowel obstruction*, distension is early and pronounced. Pain is mild and vomiting and dehydration are late. The proximal colon and caecum are distended on abdominal radiography

---

The nature of the presentation will also be influenced by whether the obstruction is:

- acute;
- chronic;
- acute on chronic;
- subacute.

Acute obstruction usually occurs in small bowel obstruction, with sudden onset of severe colicky central abdominal pain, distension and early vomiting and constipation (Summary box 66.8).

Summary box 66.8

Cardinal clinical features of acute obstruction

- Abdominal pain
- Distension
- Vomiting
- Absolute constipation

Chronic obstruction is usually seen in large bowel obstruction, with lower abdominal colic and absolute constipation followed by distension. In *acute on chronic obstruction* there is a short history of distension and vomiting against a background of pain and constipation. *Subacute obstruction* implies an incomplete obstruction.

Presentation will be further influenced by whether the obstruction is:

- simple – in which the blood supply is intact;
- strangulating/strangulated – in which there is direct interference to blood flow, usually by hernial rings or intraperitoneal adhesions/bands.

The common causes of intestinal obstruction in western countries and their relative frequencies are shown in Fig. 66.1 (see page 1188). The underlying mechanisms are shown in Summary box 66.2 (see page 1188).

The clinical features vary according to:

- the location of the obstruction;
- the age of the obstruction;
- the underlying pathology;
- the presence or absence of intestinal ischaemia.

Late manifestations of intestinal obstruction that may be encountered include dehydration, oliguria, hypovolaemic shock, pyrexia, septicaemia, respiratory embarrassment and peritonism. In all cases of suspected intestinal obstruction, all hernial orifices must be examined.

Pain

Pain is the first symptom encountered; it occurs suddenly and is usually severe. It is colicky in nature and is usually centred on the umbilicus (small bowel) or lower abdomen (large bowel). The pain coincides with increased peristaltic activity. With increasing distension, the colicky pain is replaced by a mild constant diffuse pain.

The development of severe pain is indicative of the presence of strangulation. Pain may not be a significant feature in postoperative simple mechanical obstruction and does not usually occur in paralytic ileus.

Vomiting

The more distal the obstruction, the longer the interval between the onset of symptoms and the appearance of nausea and vomiting. As obstruction progresses the character of the vomitus alters from digested food to faeculent material, as a result of the presence of enteric bacterial overgrowth.

Distension

In the small bowel the degree of distension is dependent on the site of the obstruction and is greater the more distal the lesion. Visible peristalsis may be present (Fig. 66.7). Distension is delayed

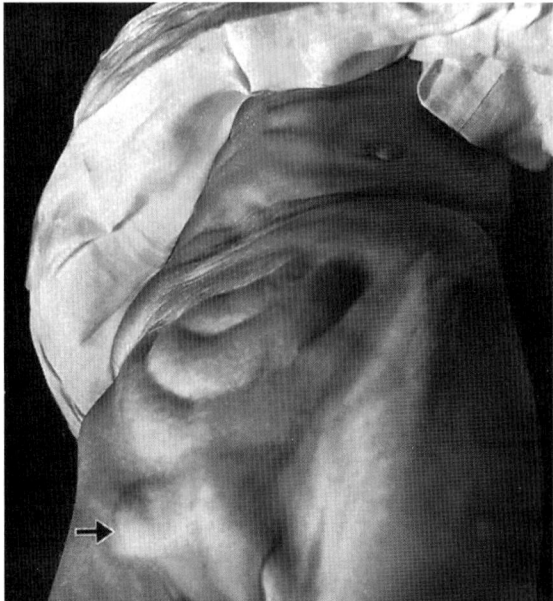

Figure 66.7 Visible peristalsis. Intestinal obstruction due to a strangulated right femoral hernia, to which the arrow points.

in colonic obstruction and may be minimal or absent in the presence of mesenteric vascular occlusion.

Constipation

This may be classified as absolute (i.e. neither faeces nor flatus is passed) or relative (where only flatus is passed). Absolute constipation is a cardinal feature of complete intestinal obstruction. Some patients may pass flatus or faeces after the onset of obstruction as a result of the evacuation of the distal bowel contents. The rule that constipation is present in intestinal obstruction does not apply in:

- Richter's hernia;
- gallstone obturation;
- mesenteric vascular occlusion;
- obstruction associated with pelvic abscess;
- partial obstruction (faecal impaction/colonic neoplasm) in which diarrhoea may often occur.

Other manifestations

Dehydration

Dehydration is seen most commonly in small bowel obstruction because of repeated vomiting and fluid sequestration. It results in dry skin and tongue, poor venous filling and sunken eyes with oliguria. The blood urea level and haematocrit rise, giving a secondary polycythaemia.

Hypokalaemia

Hypokalaemia is not a common feature in simple mechanical obstruction. An increase in serum potassium, amylase or lactate dehydrogenase may be associated with the presence of strangulation, as may leucocytosis or leucopenia.

August Gottlieb Richter, 1742–1812, Lecturer in Surgery, Göttingen, Germany, described this form of hernia in 1777.

Pyrexia

Pyrexia in the presence of obstruction may indicate:

- the onset of ischaemia;
- intestinal perforation;
- inflammation associated with the obstructing disease.

Hypothermia indicates septicaemic shock.

Abdominal tenderness

Localised tenderness indicates pending or established ischaemia. The development of peritonism or peritonitis indicates overt infarction and/or perforation.

Clinical features of strangulation

It is vital to distinguish strangulating from non-strangulating intestinal obstruction because the former is a surgical emergency. The diagnosis is entirely clinical; the clinical features are shown in Summary box 66.9.

Summary box 66.9

Clinical features of strangulation

- **Constant pain**
- **Tenderness with rigidity**
- **Shock**

In addition to the features above, it should be noted that:

- the presence of shock indicates underlying ischaemia;
- in impending strangulation, pain is never completely absent;
- symptoms usually commence suddenly and recur regularly;
- the presence and character of any local tenderness are of great significance and, however mild, tenderness requires frequent reassessment.

In non-strangulated obstruction there may be an area of localised tenderness at the site of the obstruction; in strangulation there is always localised tenderness associated with rigidity/rebound tenderness:

- Generalised tenderness and the presence of rigidity are indicative of the need for early laparotomy.
- In cases of intestinal obstruction in which pain persists despite conservative management, even in the absence of the above signs, strangulation should be diagnosed.
- When strangulation occurs in an external hernia, the lump is tense, tender and irreducible, there is no expansile cough impulse and it has recently increased in size.

Clinical features of intussusception

The classical presentation of intussusception is with episodes of screaming and drawing up of the legs in a previously well male infant. The attacks last for a few minutes and recur repeatedly. During attacks the child appears pale, whereas between episodes he may be listless. Vomiting may or may not occur at the outset but becomes conspicuous and bile-stained with time. Initially, the passage of stool may be normal, whereas, later, blood and mucus are evacuated – the 'redcurrant jelly' stool.

Whenever possible, examination should be undertaken between episodes of colic, without disturbing the child. Classically, the abdomen is not initially distended; a lump that hardens on palpation may be discerned but this is present in only 60% of cases (Fig. 66.8). There may be an associated feeling of emptiness in the right iliac fossa (the sign of Dance). On rectal examination, blood-stained mucus may be found on the finger. Occasionally, in extensive ileocolic or colocolic intussusception, the apex may be palpable or even protrude from the anus.

Unrelieved, progressive dehydration and abdominal distension from small bowel obstruction will occur, followed by peritonitis secondary to gangrene. Rarely, natural cure may occur as a result of sloughing of the intussusception.

Differential diagnosis

Acute gastroenteritis

Although abdominal pain and vomiting are common in acute gastroenteritis, with occasional blood and mucus in the stool, diarrhoea is a leading symptom and faecal matter or bile is always present in the stool.

Henoch–Schöenlein purpura

Henoch–Schöenlein purpura is associated with a characteristic rash and abdominal pain but intussusception may also occur.

Rectal prolapse

This may be easily differentiated by the fact that the projecting mucosa can be felt in continuity with the perianal skin whereas in intussusception the finger may pass indefinitely into the depths of a sulcus.

Clinical features of volvulus

Volvulus of the small intestine

This may be primary or secondary and usually occurs in the lower ileum. It may occur spontaneously in African people, particularly following the consumption of a large volume of vegetable matter, whereas in the west it is usually secondary to adhesions passing to the parietes or female pelvic organs.

Caecal volvulus

This may occur as part of volvulus neonatorum or *de novo* and is usually a clockwise twist. It is more common in females and usually presents acutely with the classic features of obstruction. At first the obstruction may be partial, with the passage of flatus and faeces. In 25% of cases, examination may reveal a palpable tympanic swelling in the midline or left side of the abdomen.

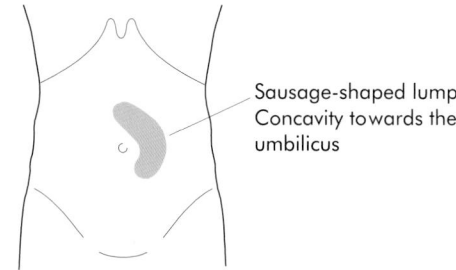

Sausage-shaped lump. Concavity towards the umbilicus

Figure 66.8 The physical signs as recorded by Hamilton Bailey in a typical case of intussusception in an infant.

Jean Baptiste Hippolyte Dance, **1797–1832, Physician, Hôpital Cochin, Paris, France.**
Henry Hamilton Bailey, **1894–1961, Surgeon, The Royal Northern Hospital, London, England.**

Sigmoid volvulus

The symptoms are of large bowel obstruction, which may initially be intermittent followed by the passage of large quantities of flatus and faeces. Presentation varies in severity and acuteness, with younger patients appearing to develop the more acute form. Abdominal distension is an early and progressive sign, which may be associated with hiccough and retching; vomiting occurs late. Constipation is absolute. In the elderly, a more chronic form may be seen.

IMAGING

Erect abdominal films are no longer routinely obtained and the radiological diagnosis is based on a supine abdominal film (Fig. 66.9). An erect film may subsequently be requested when further doubt exists.

When distended with gas, the jejunum, ileum, caecum and remaining colon have a characteristic appearance in adults and older children that allows them to be distinguished radiologically. The diameter of the distended viscus is not diagnostic (Summary box 66.10).

Summary box 66.10

Radiological features of obstruction

- The obstructed small bowel is characterised by straight segments that are generally central and lie transversely. No gas is seen in the colon
- The jejunum is characterised by its valvulae conniventes, which completely pass across the width of the bowel and are regularly spaced, giving a 'concertina' or ladder effect
- Ileum – the distal ileum has been piquantly described by Wangensteen as featureless
- Caecum – a distended caecum is shown by a rounded gas shadow in the right iliac fossa
- Large bowel, except for the caecum, shows haustral folds, which, unlike valvulae conniventes, are spaced irregularly, do not cross the whole diameter of the bowel and do not have indentations placed opposite one another

---

In intestinal obstruction, fluid levels appear later than gas shadows as it takes time for gas and fluid to separate (Fig. 66.10). These are most prominent on an erect film. In adults, two inconstant fluid levels – one at the duodenal cap and the other in the terminal ileum – may be regarded as normal. In infants (less than 1 year old), a few fluid levels in the small bowel may be physiological. In this age group it is difficult to distinguish large from small bowel in the presence of obstruction, because the characteristic features seen in adults are not present or are unreliable.

During the obstructive process, fluid levels become more conspicuous and more numerous when paralysis has occurred. When fluid levels are pronounced, the obstruction is advanced. In the small bowel, the number of fluid levels is directly proportional to the degree of obstruction and to its site, the number increasing the more distal the lesion.

In contrast, low colonic obstruction does not commonly give rise to small bowel fluid levels unless advanced, whereas high

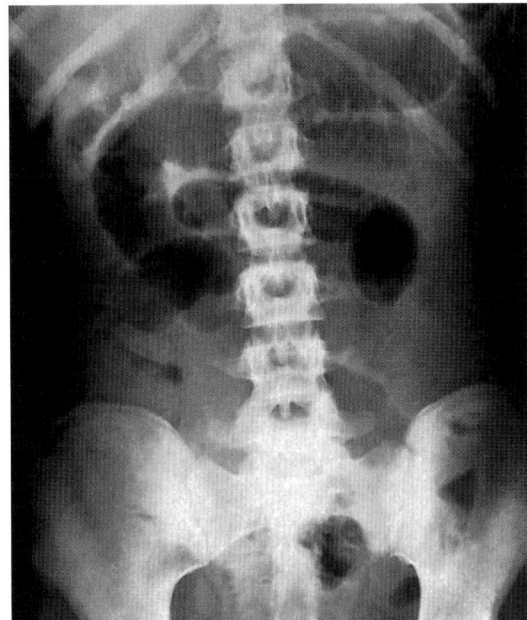

Figure 66.9 Gas-filled small bowel loop; patient supine.

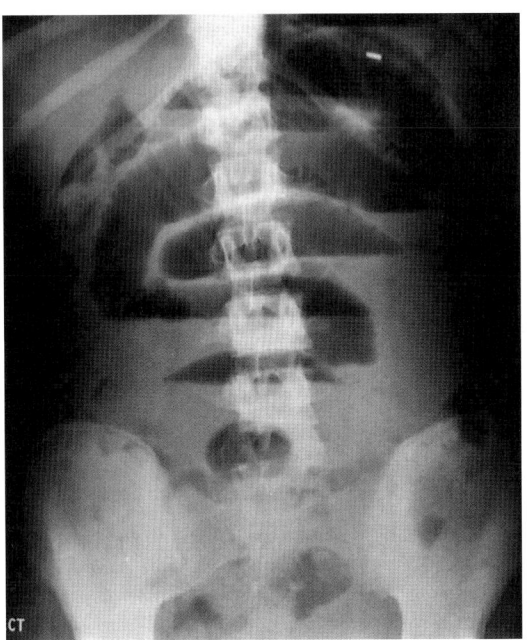

Figure 66.10 Fluid levels with gas above; 'stepladder pattern'. Ileal obstruction by adhesions; patient erect.

colonic obstruction may do so in the presence of an incompetent ileocaecal valve. Colonic obstruction is usually associated with a large amount of gas in the caecum. A limited water-soluble enema should be undertaken to differentiate large bowel obstruction from pseudo-obstruction. A barium follow-through is contraindicated in the presence of acute obstruction and may be life-threatening.

Impacted foreign bodies may be seen on abdominal radiographs. In gallstone ileus, gas may be seen in the biliary tree, with the stone visible, usually in the right iliac fossa, in 25% of cases.

It is noteworthy that gas-filled loops and fluid levels in the small and large bowel can also be seen in established paralytic ileus and pseudo-obstruction. The former can, however, normally be distinguished on clinical grounds whereas the latter can be confirmed radiologically. Fluid levels may also be seen in non-obstructing conditions such as inflammatory bowel disease, acute pancreatitis and intra-abdominal sepsis.

Imaging in intussusception

A plain abdominal field usually reveals evidence of small or large bowel obstruction with an absent caecal gas shadow in ileocolic cases. A soft tissue opacity is often visible in children. A barium enema may be used to diagnose the presence of an ileocolic intussusception (the claw sign) (Fig. 66.11) but does not demonstrate small bowel intussusception. An abdominal ultrasound scan has a high diagnostic sensitivity in children, demonstrating the typical doughnut appearance of concentric rings in transverse section. A computerised tomography (CT) scan is also useful in equivocal cases.

Imaging in volvulus

In caecal volvulus, radiography may reveal a gas-filled ileum and occasionally a distended caecum. A barium enema may be used to confirm the diagnosis, with an absence of barium in the caecum and a bird beak deformity.

In sigmoid volvulus, a plain radiograph shows massive colonic distension. The classic appearance is of a dilated loop of bowel running diagonally across the abdomen from right to left, with two fluid levels seen, one within each loop of bowel.

In volvulus neonatorium, the abdominal radiograph shows a variable appearance. Initially, it may appear normal or show evidence of duodenal obstruction but, as the intestinal strangulation progresses, the abdomen becomes relatively gasless.

TREATMENT OF ACUTE INTESTINAL OBSTRUCTION

There are three main measures used to treat acute intestinal obstruction (Summary box 66.11).

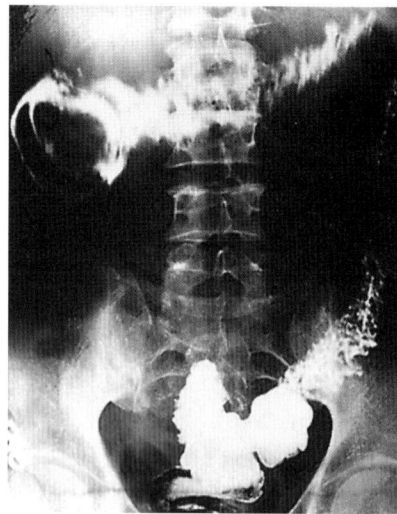

Figure 66.11 'Claw' sign of iliac intussusception. The barium in the intussusception is seen as a claw around a negative shadow of the intussusception (courtesy of R.S. Naik, Durg, India).

Summary box 66.11

Treatment of acute intestinal obstruction

- Gastrointestinal drainage
- Fluid and electrolyte replacement
- Relief of obstruction
- Surgical treatment is necessary for most cases of intestinal obstruction but should be delayed until resuscitation is complete, provided there is no sign of strangulation or evidence of closed-loop obstruction

---

The first two steps are always necessary before attempting the surgical relief of obstruction and are the mainstay of postoperative management. In a proportion of cases, particularly adhesive obstruction, they may be used exclusively.

The three principles of surgical intervention are shown in Summary box 66.12.

Summary box 66.12

Principles of surgical intervention for obstruction

Management of:
- The segment at the site of obstruction
- The distended proximal bowel
- The underlying cause of obstruction

Supportive management

Nasogastric decompression is achieved by the passage of a non-vented (Ryle) or vented (Salem) tube. The tubes are normally placed on free drainage with 4-hourly aspiration but may be placed on continuous or intermittent suction. As well as facilitating decompression proximal to the obstruction, they also reduce the risk of subsequent aspiration during induction of anaesthesia and post-extubation.

The basic biochemical abnormality in intestinal obstruction is sodium and water loss, and therefore the appropriate replacement is Hartmann's solution or normal saline. The volume required varies and should be determined by clinical haematological and biochemical criteria.

Antibiotics are not mandatory but many clinicians initiate broad-spectrum antibiotics early in therapy because of bacterial overgrowth. Antibiotic therapy is mandatory for all patients undergoing small or large bowel resection.

Surgical treatment

The timing of surgical intervention is dependent on the clinical picture. There are several indications for early surgical intervention (Summary box 66.13).

John Alfred Ryle, **1889–1950**, Regius Professor of Physic, The University of Cambridge, and later Professor of Social Medicine, The University of Oxford, England, introduced the Ryle's tube in 1921.
Henri Albert Charles Antoine Hartmann, **1860–1952**, Professor of Clinical Surgery, The Faculty of Medicine, The University of Paris, France.

Indications for early surgical intervention

- Obstructed or strangulated external hernia
- Internal intestinal strangulation
- Acute obstruction

The classic clinical advice that 'the sun should not both rise and set' on a case of unrelieved acute intestinal obstruction is sound and should be followed unless there are positive reasons for delay. Such cases may include obstruction secondary to adhesions when there is no pain or tenderness, despite continued radiological evidence of obstruction. In these circumstances, conservative management may be continued for up to 72 hours in the hope of spontaneous resolution.

If the site of obstruction is unknown, adequate exposure is best achieved by a midline incision. Assessment is directed to:

- the site of obstruction;
- the nature of the obstruction;
- the viability of the gut.

Identification and assessment of the caecum is the best initial manoeuvre. If it is collapsed, the lesion is in the small bowel and may be identified by careful retrograde assessment. A dilated caecum indicates large bowel obstruction. To display the cause of obstruction, distended loops of small bowel should be displaced with care and covered with warm moist abdominal packs.

Operative decompression may be required if dilatation of bowel loops prevents exposure, the viability of the bowel wall is compromised or subsequent closure will be compromised. Its benefits should be balanced against the potential risk of septic complications from spillage. Decompression may be performed using Savage's decompressor within a seromuscular purse-string suture. Alternatively, with a large-bore nasogastric tube in place, the small bowel contents may be gently milked in a retrograde manner to the stomach for aspiration. All volumes of fluid removed should be accurately measured and appropriately replaced.

The type of surgical procedure required will depend upon the cause of obstruction – division of adhesions (enterolysis), excision, bypass or proximal decompression.

Following relief of obstruction, the viability of the involved bowel should be carefully assessed (Table 66.3). Although frankly infarcted bowel is obvious, the viability status in many cases may be difficult to discern. If in doubt, the bowel should be wrapped in hot packs for 10 min with increased oxygenation and then reassessed. The state of the mesenteric vessels and pulsation in adjacent arcades should be sought. Nevertheless, non-occlusive vascular insufficiency may occur despite adequate pulsation. In doubtful cases, following resection, both ends of the bowel should be raised as stomas. This is not only safe but also allows regular assessment of the bowel. When no resection has been undertaken or there are multiple ischaemic areas (mesenteric vascular occlusion), a second-look laparotomy at 24–48 hours may be required.

Special attention should always be paid to the sites of constriction at each end of an obstructed segment. If of doubtful viability they should be infolded by the use of a seromuscular suture and covered with omentum.

The surgical management of massive infarction in the form of superior mesenteric artery occlusion is dependent on the patient's overall prognostic criteria. In the elderly, infarction of the small bowel from the duodenojejunal flexure and the right colon may be considered incurable, whereas in the young, with the potential for long-term intravenous alimentation and small bowel transplantation, a less conservative policy may be justified.

Whenever the small bowel is resected, the exact site of resection, the length of the resected segment and that of the residual bowel should be recorded.

Treatment of adhesions

Initial management is based on intravenous rehydration and nasogastric decompression; occasionally, this treatment is curative. Although an initial conservative regimen is considered appropriate, regular assessment is mandatory to ensure that strangulation does not occur. Conservative treatment should not be prolonged beyond 72 hours.

When, as is usual, laparotomy is required, although multiple adhesions may be found, only one may be causative. This should be divided and the remaining adhesions left *in situ* unless severe angulation is present. Division of these adhesions will only cause further adhesion formation.

When obstruction is caused by an area of multiple adhesions, the adhesions should be freed by sharp dissection. To prevent recurrence, the bare area should be covered with omental grafts.

Following the release of band obstruction, the constriction sites that have suffered direct compression should be carefully assessed and, if they show residual colour changes, invaginated.

Laparoscopic adhesiolysis may be considered in highly selected cases of chronic subacute obstruction (Summary box 66.14).

Table 66.3 Differentiation between viable and non-viable intestine

	Viable	Non-viable
Circulation	Dark colour becomes lighter	Dark colour remains
	Mesentery bleeds if pricked	No bleeding if mesentery is pricked
Peritoneum	Shiny	Dull and lustreless
Intestinal musculature	Firm	Flabby, thin and friable
	Pressure rings may or may not disappear	Pressure rings persist
	Peristalsis may be observed	No peristalsis

Paul Thwaites Savage, **formerly Surgeon, The Whittington Hospital, London, England.**

Summary box 66.14

Treatment of adhesive obstruction

- Initially treat conservatively provided there are no signs of strangulation; should rarely continue conservative treatment for longer than 72 hours
- At operation, divide only the causative adhesion(s) and limit dissection
- Cover serosal tears; invaginate (or resect) areas of doubtful viability
- Laparoscopic adhesiolysis may have a role in chronic cases

Treatment of recurrent intestinal obstruction caused by adhesions

Several procedures may be considered in the presence of recurrent obstruction including:

- repeat adhesiolysis (enterolysis) alone;
- Noble's plication operation (Fig. 66.12);
- Charles–Phillips transmesenteric plication (Fig. 66.13);
- intestinal intubation (Fig. 66.14).

Postoperative intestinal obstruction

Differentiation between persistent paralytic ileus and early mechanical obstruction may be difficult in the early postoperative period. In practice, the latter is probably more common. Early evidence of obstruction (days 1–5) is usually due to non-strangulating causes such as fibrinous adhesions and oedema. Obstruction is usually incomplete and the majority settle with continued conservative management. Late postoperative obstruction (> 7 days) is usually more significant in nature, and timely surgical intervention is usually required.

Treatment of intussusception

In the infant with ileocolic intussusception, after resuscitation with intravenous fluids, broad-spectrum antibiotics and nasogastric drainage, non-operative reduction can be attempted using an air or barium enema (see Chapter 6, Fig. 6.14). Successful reduction can only be accepted if there is free reflux of air or barium into the small bowel, together with resolution of symptoms and signs in the patient. Non-operative reduction is contraindicated if there are signs of peritonitis or perforation, there is a known pathological lead point or in the presence of profound shock. In experienced units, more than 70% of intussusceptions can be reduced non-operatively. Strangulated bowel and pathological lead points are unlikely to reduce. Perforation of the colon during pneumatic or hydrostatic reduction is a recognised hazard but is rare. Recurrent intussusception occurs in up to 10% of patients after non-operative reduction.

Surgery is required when radiological reduction has failed or is contraindicated. After resuscitation, a transverse right-sided abdominal incision provides good access. Reduction is achieved by gently compressing the most distal part of the intussusception toward its origin (Fig. 66.15), making sure not to pull. The last part of the reduction is the most difficult (Fig. 66.16). After reduction, the terminal part of the small bowel and the appendix will be seen to be bruised and oedematous. The viability of the whole bowel should be checked carefully. An irreducible intussusception or one complicated by infarction or a pathological lead point requires resection and primary anastomosis.

Acute intestinal obstruction of the newborn

Neonatal intestinal obstruction has many potential causes. Congenital atresia and stenosis are the most common. Intestinal

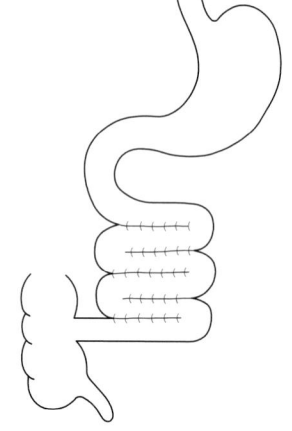

Figure 66.12 Noble's plication.

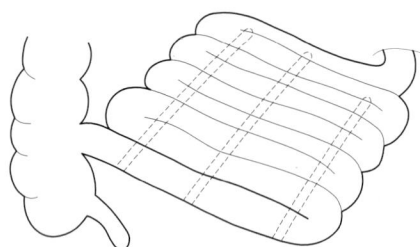

Figure 66.13 The Charles–Phillips procedure.

Thomas Benjamin Noble, **1895–1965, Surgeon, The Community Hospital, Indianapolis, IN, USA.**
Richard V. Phillips, **Surgeon, Albuquerque, NM, USA.**

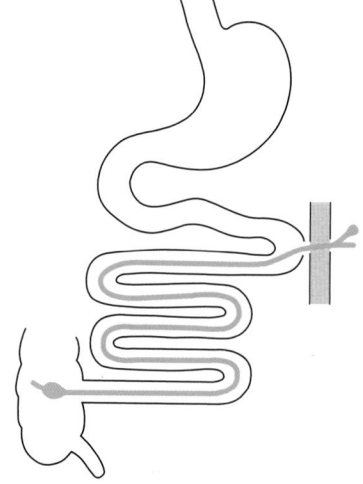

Figure 66.14 A Baker's tube inserted via a Witzel jejunostomy. A gastrostomy may also be used.

Friedrich Oskar Witzel, **1856–1925, a Surgeon at Bonn, Germany.**

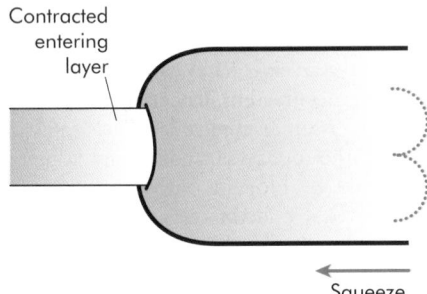

Figure 66.15 Diagram showing the method used to reduce an intussusception.

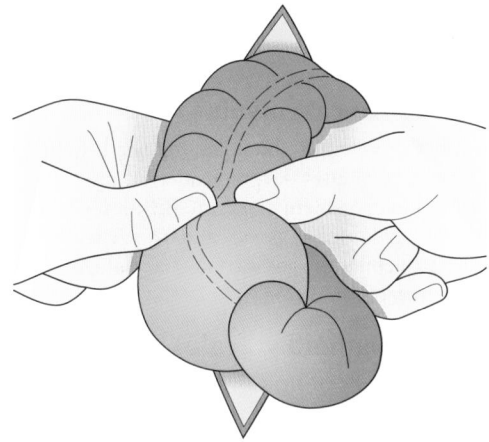

Figure 66.16 Reducing the terminal part of the intussusception (after R.E. Gross).

malrotation with midgut volvulus, meconium ileus, Hirschprung's disease, imperforate anus, necrotising enterocolitis and an incarcerated inguinal hernia may also be responsible. Many of these conditions are discussed in Chapter 6.

Intestinal atresia

Duodenal atresia and stenosis are the commonest forms of intestinal obstruction in the newborn (see Chapter 6). Jejunal or ileal atresias are next in frequency whereas colonic atresia is rare. The possibility of multiple atresias makes intraoperative assessment of the whole small and large bowel mandatory. As with all congenital anomalies, associated malformations are common and should be excluded.

There are four main types of jejunal/ileal atresia, ranging from an obstructing membrane with continuity of the bowel wall, through blind-ended segments of bowel separated by a fibrous cord or V-shaped mesenteric defect (including the so called apple-peel atresia) (Fig. 66.17), to multiple atresias ('string of sausages'). The obstructed proximal bowel is at risk of perforation, which may happen prenatally causing meconium peritonitis in the fetus.

Small bowel atresias present with intestinal obstruction soon after birth. Bilious vomiting is the dominant feature in jejunal atresia whereas abdominal distension is more prominent with ileal atresia. A small amount of pale meconium may be passed despite the atresia.

Plain abdominal radiographs show a variable number of dilated loops of bowel and fluid levels according to the level of obstruction.

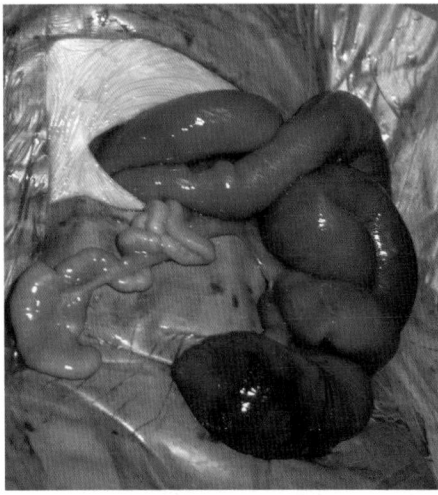

Figure 66.17 Apple-peel jejunal bowel atresia with obstructed proximal jejunum and collapsed distal ileum coiled round a remnant ileocolic artery (courtesy of M.D. Stringer, Leeds, UK).

In a stable infant, a contrast enema may be required to clarify the cause of a distal bowel obstruction.

Surgery

Duodenal atresia is corrected by a duodenoduodenostomy. In most cases of jejunal/ileal atresia, the distal end of the dilated proximal small bowel is resected and a primary end-to-end anastomosis is possible. If the proximal bowel is extremely dilated it may need to be tapered to the distal bowel before anastomosis. Occasionally, a temporary stoma is required before definitive repair.

Meconium ileus

Cystic fibrosis is almost always the underlying cause of this condition. Meconium is normally kept fluid by the action of pancreatic enzymes. In meconium ileus the terminal ileum becomes filled with thick viscid meconium, resulting in progressive intestinal obstruction. A sterile meconium peritonitis may have occurred *in utero*.

Visibly dilated loops of bowel are often palpable in the newborn with meconium ileus. An abdominal radiograph may show a dilated small intestine with mottling. Fluid levels are generally not seen. Unlike ileal atresia there is no abrupt termination of the gas-filled intestine. A contrast enema shows an unused microcolon. As the condition is caused by an autosomal recessive genetic defect, a family history may be present. Further assessment includes gene mutation analysis and, beyond the neonatal period, a sweat test, which shows elevated sodium and chloride levels ($> 70\,mmol\,l^{-1}$).

Uncomplicated meconium ileus may respond to treatment with a hyperosmolar gastrografin enema; this draws fluid into the gut lumen and also has detergent properties, which help to liquefy the meconium. Infants treated in this way need extra intravenous fluids to compensate for fluid shifts. Meconium ileus complicated by intestinal perforation, volvulus or atresia, or unresponsive to enemas, demands surgery. Various surgical procedures are used including intestinal resection and temporary stoma formation, resection and primary anastomosis, and, in uncomplicated cases, enterotomy and irrigation of the bowel. The

Bishop–Koop operation (Fig. 66.18) with its irrigating stoma is now only rarely used.

TREATMENT OF ACUTE LARGE BOWEL OBSTRUCTION

Large bowel obstruction is usually caused by an underlying carcinoma or occasionally diverticular disease, and presents in an acute or chronic form. The condition of pseudo-obstruction should always be considered and excluded by a limited contrast study or a CT air scan to confirm organic obstruction.

After full resuscitation, the abdomen should be opened through a midline incision. Distension of the caecum will confirm large bowel involvement. Identification of a collapsed distal segment of the large bowel and its sequential proximal assessment will readily lead to identification of the cause. When a removable lesion is found in the caecum, ascending colon, hepatic flexure or proximal transverse colon, an emergency right hemicolectomy should be performed. If the lesion is irremovable, a proximal stoma (colostomy or ileosotomy if the ileocaecal valve is incompetent) or ileotransverse bypass should be considered. Obstructing lesions at the splenic flexure should be treated by an extended right hemicolectomy with ileodescending colonic anastomosis.

For obstructing lesions of the left colon or rectosigmoid junction, immediate resection should be considered unless there are clear contraindications (Summary box 66.15).

Summary box 66.15

Management of left-sided large bowel obstruction

Contraindications to immediate resection include:

- Inexperienced surgeon
- Moribund patient
- Advanced disease

In rare instances, or when caecal perforation is imminent, additional time to improve the patient's clinical condition can be bought by performing an emergency caecostomy (or ileosotomy in the presence of an incompetent ileocaecal valve).

In the absence of senior clinical staff it is safest to bring the proximal colon to the surface as a colostomy. When possible the distal bowel should be brought out at the same time (Paul–Mikulicz procedure) to facilitate subsequent extraperitoneal closure. In the majority of cases, the distal bowel will not reach and is closed and returned to the abdomen (Hartmann's procedure). A second-stage colorectal anastomosis can be planned when the patient is fit.

If an anastomosis is to be considered using the proximal colon, in the presence of obstruction, it must be decompressed and cleaned by an on-table colonic lavage. Nevertheless, the subsequent anastomosis should still be protected with a covering stoma.

Treatment of caecal volvulus

At operation the volvulus should be reduced. Sometimes, this can only be achieved after decompression of the caecum using a needle. Further management consists of fixation of the caecum to the right iliac fossa (caecopexy) and/or a caecostomy. If the caecum is ischaemic or gangrenous, a right hemicolectomy should be performed.

Treatment of sigmoid volvulus

Flexible sigmoidoscopy or rigid sigmoidoscopy and insertion of a flatus tube should be carried out to allow deflation of the gut. Success, as long as ischaemic bowel is excluded, will provide temporary respite, allowing resuscitation and an elective procedure. Failure results in an early laparotomy, with untwisting of the loop and per anum decompression (Fig. 66.19). When the bowel is viable, fixation of the sigmoid colon to the posterior abdominal wall may be a safer manoeuvre in inexperienced hands. Resection is preferable if it can be achieved safely. A Paul–Mikulicz procedure is useful, particularly if there is suspicion of impending gangrene (Fig. 66.20); an alternative procedure is a sigmoid colectomy and, when anastomosis is considered unwise, a Hartmann's procedure with subsequent reanastomosis can be carried out.

CHRONIC LARGE BOWEL OBSTRUCTION

The symptoms of chronic intestinal obstruction may arise from two sources – the cause and the subsequent obstruction.

The causes of obstruction may be organic:

- intramural – faecal impaction;
- mural – colorectal cancer, diverticulitis, strictures (Crohn's disease, ischaemia), anastomotic stenosis;
- extramural – metastatic deposits, endometriosis;

or functional:

- Hirschsprung's disease, idiopathic megacolon, pseudo-obstruction.

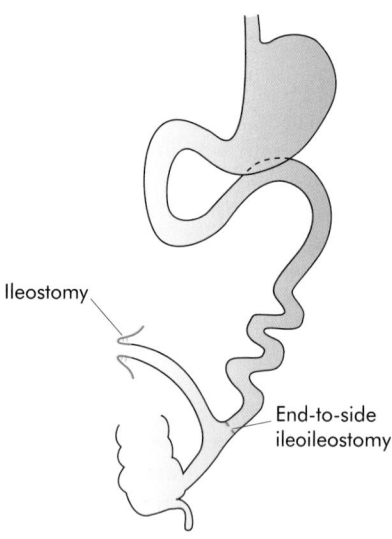

Figure 66.18 Bishop–Koop operation. This shows the completed procedure after grossly distended ileum has been resected. Because intestinal continuity is preserved, early closure of the ileostomy is not essential.

Ileostomy

End-to-side ileoileostomy

Frank Thomas Paul, 1851–1941, Surgeon, The Royal Infirmary, Liverpool, England.
Johann von Mikulicz-Radecki, 1850–1905, Professor of Surgery, Breslau, Germany, (now Wroclaw, Poland).
Harald Hirschsprung, 1830–1916, Physician, The Queen Louise Hospital for Children, Copenhagen, Denmark, described congenital megacolon in 1887.

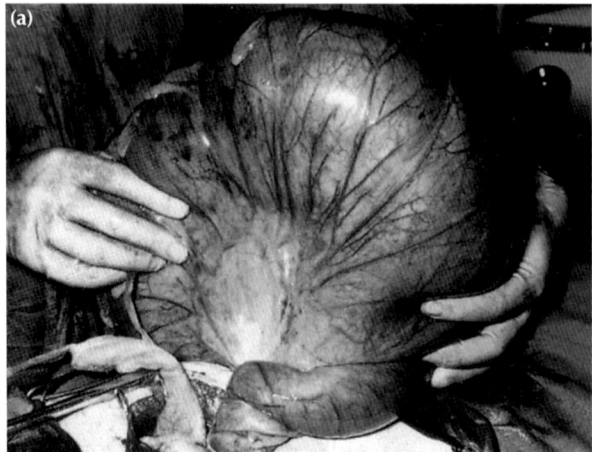

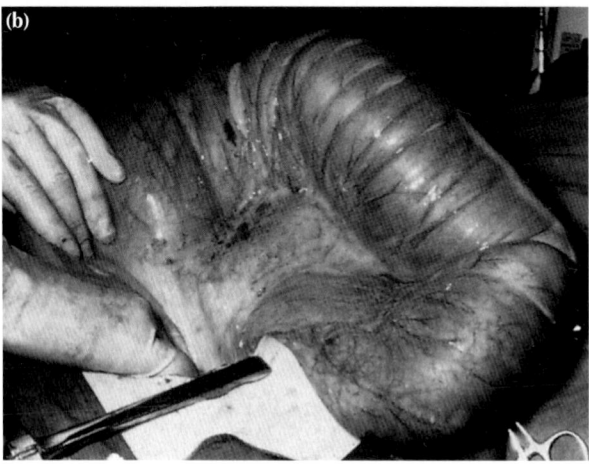

Figure 66.19 Volvulus of the sigmoid colon (a) before and (b) after untwisting (courtesy of S.U. Rahman, Manchester, England).

The symptoms of chronic obstruction differ in their predominance, timing and degree from acute obstruction. Constipation appears first. It is initially relative and then absolute, associated with distension. In the presence of large bowel disease, the point of greatest distension is in the caecum, and this is heralded by the onset of pain. Vomiting is a late feature and therefore dehydration is exceptional. Examination is unremarkable, save for confirmation of distension and the onset of peritonism in late cases. Rectal examination may confirm the presence of faecal impaction or a tumour.

Investigation

Plain abdominal radiography may confirm the presence of large bowel obstruction. All such cases should be confirmed by a subsequent single-contrast water-soluble enema study to rule out functional disease (Summary box 66.16).

Summary box 66.16

Principles of investigation of possible large bowel obstruction

- In the presence of large bowel obstruction, a single-contrast water-soluble enema or CT should be undertaken to exclude a functional cause

---

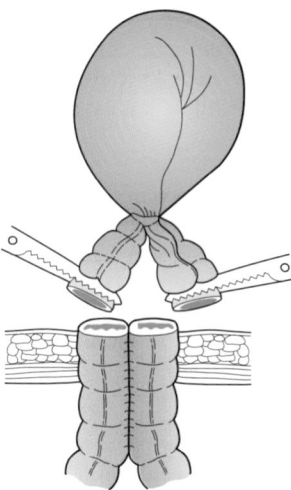

Figure 66.20 The Paul–Mikulicz operation applied to volvulus of the pelvic colon.

Organic disease requires a laparotomy, whereas functional disease requires colonoscopic decompression and conservative management. In the presence of organic obstruction, surgical management after resuscitation depends on the underlying cause and the relevant chapters in this book should be consulted.

ADYNAMIC OBSTRUCTION

Paralytic ileus

This may be defined as a state in which there is failure of transmission of peristaltic waves secondary to neuromuscular failure [i.e. in the myenteric (Auerbach's) and submucous (Meissner's) plexuses]. The resultant stasis leads to accumulation of fluid and gas within the bowel, with associated distension, vomiting, absence of bowel sounds and absolute constipation.

Varieties

The following varieties are recognised.

- *Postoperative*: a degree of ileus usually occurs after any abdominal procedure and is self-limiting, with a variable duration of 24–72 hours. Postoperative ileus may be prolonged in the presence of hypoproteinaemia or metabolic abnormality (see below).
- *Infection*: intra-abdominal sepsis may give rise to localised or generalised ileus. Resultant adhesions may contribute a mechanical element to the initial neurogenic aetiology.
- *Reflex ileus*: this may occur following fractures of the spine or ribs, retroperitoneal haemorrhage or even the application of a plaster jacket.
- *Metabolic*: uraemia and hypokalaemia are the most common contributory factors.

Clinical features

Paralytic ileus takes on a clinical significance if, 72 hours after laparotomy:

- there has been no return of bowel sounds on auscultation;
- there has been no passage of flatus.

Leopold Auerbach, **1828–1897**, Professor of Neuropathology, Breslau, Germany, (now Wroclaw, Poland), described the myenteric plexus in 1862.
Georg Meissner, **1829–1905**, Professor of Physiology, Gottingen, Germany, described the submucous plexus of the alimentary tract in 1852.

Abdominal distension becomes more marked and tympanitic. Pain is not a feature. In the absence of gastric aspiration, effortless vomiting may occur. Radiologically, the abdomen shows gas-filled loops of intestine with multiple fluid levels.

Management

The essence of treatment is prevention, with the use of nasogastric suction and restriction of oral intake until bowel sounds and the passage of flatus return. Electrolyte balance must be maintained. The use of an enhanced recovery programme with early introduction of fluids and solids is, however, becoming increasingly popular.

Specific treatment is directed towards the cause, but the following general principles apply:

- The primary cause must be removed.
- Gastrointestinal distension must be relieved by decompression.
- Close attention to fluid and electrolyte balance is essential.
- There is no place for the routine use of peristaltic stimulants. Rarely, in resistant cases, medical therapy with an adrenergic blocking agent in association with cholinergic stimulation, e.g. neostigmine (the Catchpole regimen), may be used, provided that an intraperitoneal cause has been excluded.
- If paralytic ileus is prolonged and threatens life, a laparotomy should be considered to exclude a hidden cause and facilitate bowel decompression.

Pseudo-obstruction

This condition describes an obstruction, usually of the colon, that occurs in the absence of a mechanical cause or acute intra-abdominal disease. It is associated with a variety of syndromes in which there is an underlying neuropathy and/or myopathy and a range of other factors (Summary box 66.17).

Summary box 66.17

Factors associated with pseudo-obstruction

Idiopathic
- Metabolic
  Diabetes: intermittent porphyria
  Acute hypokalaemia
  Uraemia
  Myxodoema
- Severe trauma (especially to the lumbar spine and pelvis)
- Shock
  Burns
  Myocardial infarction
  Stroke

Septicaemia
- Retroperitoneal irritation
  Blood
  Urine
  Enzymes (pancreatitis)
  Tumour
- Drugs
  Tricyclic antidepressants
  Phenothiazines
  Laxatives
- Secondary gastrointestinal involvement
  Scleroderma
  Chagas' disease

Carlos Justiniano Ribeiro Chagas, 1879–1934, Director of The Oswald Cruz Institute, and Professor of Tropical Medicine, The University of Rio de Janeiro, Brazil.

Small intestinal pseudo-obstruction

This condition may be primary (i.e. idiopathic or associated with familial visceral myopathy) or secondary. The clinical picture consists of recurrent subacute obstruction. The diagnosis is made by the exclusion of a mechanical cause. Treatment consists of initial correction of any underlying disorder. Metoclopramide and erythromycin may be of use.

Colonic pseudo-obstruction

This may occur in an acute or a chronic form. The former, also known as Ogilvie's syndrome, presents as acute large bowel obstruction. Abdominal radiographs show evidence of colonic obstruction, with marked caecal distension being a common feature. Indeed, caecal perforation is a well-recognised complication. The absence of a mechanical cause requires urgent confirmation by colonoscopy or a single-contrast water-soluble barium enema or CT. Once confirmed, pseudo-obstruction should be treated by colonoscopic decompression. It may recur in 25% of cases, necessitating further colonoscopy with simultaneous placement of a flatus tube. When colonoscopy fails or is unavailable, a tube caecostomy may be required. Continued symptoms may benefit from surgical intervention with subtotal colectomy and ileorectal anastomosis.

Acute mesenteric ischaemia

Mesenteric vascular disease may be classified as acute intestinal ischaemia – with or without occlusion – venous, chronic arterial, central or peripheral. The superior mesenteric vessels are the visceral vessels most likely to be affected by embolisation or thrombosis, with the former being most common. Occlusion at the origin of the superior mesenteric artery (SMA) is almost invariably the result of thrombosis, whereas emboli lodge at the origin of the middle colic artery. Inferior mesenteric involvement is usually clinically silent because of a better collateral circulation.

Possible sources for the embolisation of the SMA include a left atrium associated with fibrillation, a mural myocardial infarction, an atheromatous plaque from an aortic aneurysm and a mitral valve vegetation associated with endocarditis.

Primary thrombosis is associated with atherosclerosis and thromboangitis obliterans. Primary thrombosis of the superior mesenteric veins may occur in association with factor V Leiden, portal hypertension, portal pyaemia and sickle cell disease and in women taking the contraceptive pill.

Irrespective of whether the occlusion is arterial or venous, haemorrhagic infarction occurs. The mucosa is the only layer of the intestinal wall to have little resistance to ischaemic injury. The intestine and its mesentery become swollen and oedematous. Blood-stained fluid exudes into the peritoneal cavity and bowel lumen. If the main trunk of the SMA is involved, the infarction covers an area from just distal to the duodenojejunal flexure to the splenic flexure. Usually, a branch of the main trunk is implicated and the area of infarction is less.

Clinical features

The most important clue to an early diagnosis of acute mesenteric ischaemia is the sudden onset of severe abdominal pain in a patient with atrial fibrillation or atherosclerosis. The pain is typically central and out of all proportion to physical findings.

Sir William Heneage Ogilvie, 1887–1971, Surgeon, Guy's Hospital, London, England.

Persistent vomiting and defaecation occur early, with the subsequent passage of altered blood. Hypovolaemic shock rapidly ensues. Abdominal tenderness may be mild initially with rigidity being a late feature.

Investigation will usually reveal a profound neutrophil leucocytosis with an absence of gas in the thickened small intestine on abdominal radiographs. The presence of gas bubbles in the mesenteric veins is rare but pathognomonic.

Treatment needs to be tailored to the individual. In conjunction with full resuscitation, embolectomy via the ileocolic artery or revascularisation of the SMA may be considered in early embolic cases. The majority of cases, however, are diagnosed late. In the young, all affected bowel should be resected, whereas in the elderly or infirm the situation may be deemed incurable. Anti-coagulation should be implemented early in the postoperative period.

After extensive enterectomy it is usual for patients to require intravenous alimentation. The young, however, may sometimes develop sufficient intestinal digestive and absorptive function to lead relatively normal lives. In selected cases consideration may be given to small bowel transplantation.

Infarction of the large intestine alone is relatively rare. Involvement of the middle colic artery territory should be treated by transverse colectomy and exteriorisation of both ends, with an extended right hemicolectomy in selected cases.

Ischaemic colitis describes the structural changes that occur in the colon as a result of the deprivation of blood. They are most common in the splenic flexure, whose blood supply is particularly tenuous. They have been classified by Marston into gangrenous, transient and stricturing forms; only stricturing forms cause obstruction and only a few such patients require resection.

FURTHER READING

Becker, J.M. and Stucchi, A.F. (2004) Intra-abdominal adhesion prevention: are we getting any closer? *Ann Surg* **240**: 202–4.

Bickell, N.A., Federman, A.D. and Aufses, A.H. (2005) Influence of time on risk of bowel resection in complete small bowel obstruction. *J Am Coll Surg* **201**: 847–54.

Fazio, V.W., Cohen, Z., Fleshman, J.W., van Goor, H., Bauer, J.J., Wolff, B.G. *et al.* (2006) Reduction in adhesive small-bowel obstruction by Seprafilm (R) stop adhesion barrier after intestinal resection. *Dis Colon Rectum* **49**: 1–11.

Fevang, B.T., Fevang, J., Lie, S.A., Soreide, O., Svanes, K. and Viste, A. (2004) Long-term prognosis after operation for adhesive small bowel obstruction. *Ann Surg* **240**: 193–201.

Sajja, S.B. and Schein, M. (2004) Early postoperative small bowel obstruction. *Br J Surg* **91**: 683–91.

Williams, S.B., Greenspon, J., Young, H.A. and Orkin, B.A. (2005) Small bowel obstruction: conservative vs. surgical management. *Dis Colon Rectum* **48**: 1140–6.

Jeffery Adrian Priestley Marston, **formerly Surgeon, The Middlesex Hospital, London, England.**

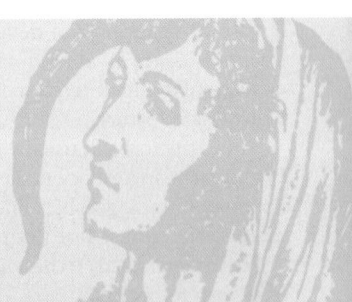

The vermiform appendix

LEARNING OBJECTIVES

To understand:
- The aetiology and surgical anatomy of acute appendicitis
- The clinical signs and differential diagnoses of appendicitis
- The management of postoperative problems
- Basic surgical techniques, both open and laparoscopic
- Less common conditions occasionally encountered

The vermiform appendix is considered by most to be a vestigial organ; its importance in surgery results only from its propensity for inflammation, which results in the clinical syndrome known as acute appendicitis. Acute appendicitis is the most common cause of an 'acute abdomen' in young adults and, as such, the associated symptoms and signs have become a paradigm for clinical teaching. Appendicitis is sufficiently common that appendicectomy (termed appendectomy in North America) is the most frequently performed urgent abdominal operation and is often the first major procedure performed by a surgeon in training. Notwithstanding advances in modern radiographic imaging and diagnostic laboratory investigations, the diagnosis of appendicitis remains essentially clinical, requiring a mixture of observation, clinical acumen and surgical science. In an age accustomed to early and accurate preoperative diagnosis, acute appendicitis remains an enigmatic challenge and a reminder of the art of surgical diagnosis.

ANATOMY

The vermiform appendix is present only in humans, certain anthropoid apes and the wombat. It is a blind muscular tube with mucosal, submucosal, muscular and serosal layers. Morphologically, it is the undeveloped distal end of the large caecum found in many lower animals. At birth, the appendix is short and broad at its junction with the caecum, but differential growth of the caecum produces the typical tubular structure by about the age of 2 years (Condon). During childhood, continued growth of the caecum commonly rotates the appendix into a retrocaecal but intraperitoneal position (Fig. 67.1). In approximately one-quarter of cases, rotation of the appendix does not occur, resulting in a pelvic, subcaecal or paracaecal position. Occasionally, the tip of the appendix becomes extraperitoneal, lying behind the caecum or ascending colon. Rarely, the caecum does not migrate

A wombat is a nocturnal, burrowing Australian marsupial.
Robert E. Condon, **Contemporary, Emeritus Professor of Surgery, The Medical College of Wisconsin, WI, USA.**

Retrocaecal 74%
Preileal 1%
Postileal 0.5%
Paracaecal 2%
Subcaecal 1.5%
Pelvic 21%

Figure 67.1 The various positions of the appendix (after Sir C. Wakeley, London, formerly PRCS).

during development to its normal position in the right lower quadrant of the abdomen. In these circumstances, the appendix can be found near the gall bladder or, in the case of intestinal malrotation, in the left iliac fossa, causing diagnostic difficulty if appendicitis develops (Fig. 67.2).

The position of the base of the appendix is constant, being found at the confluence of the three taeniae coli of the caecum, which fuse to form the outer longitudinal muscle coat of the appendix. At operation, use can be made of this to find an elusive appendix, as gentle traction on the taeniae coli, particularly the anterior taenia, will lead the operator to the base of the appendix.

The mesentery of the appendix or mesoappendix arises from the lower surface of the mesentery or the terminal ileum and is itself subject to great variation. Sometimes, as much as the distal one-third of the appendix is bereft of mesoappendix. Especially in childhood, the mesoappendix is so transparent that the contained blood vessels can be seen (Fig. 67.3). In many adults, it becomes laden with fat, which obscures these vessels. The appendicular artery, a branch of the lower division of the ileocolic artery, passes behind the terminal ileum to enter the mesoappendix a short distance from the base of the appendix. It then comes

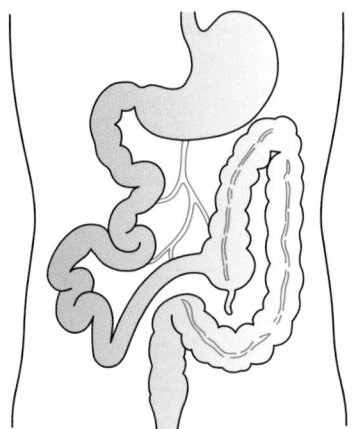

Figure 67.2 Left-sided caecum and appendix due to intestinal mal-rotation (after Findley and Humphreys).

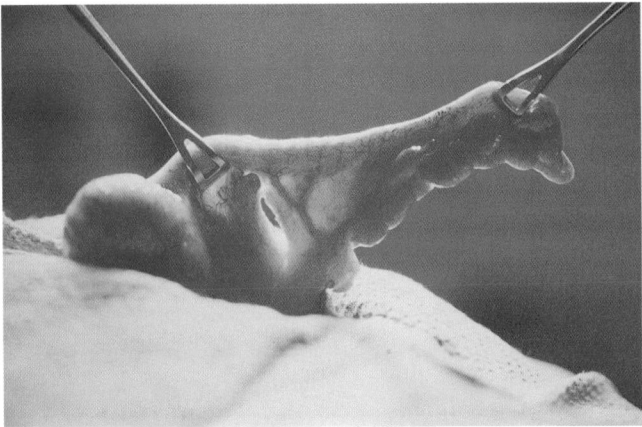

Figure 67.3 Mesoappendix displayed demonstrating the appendicular artery.

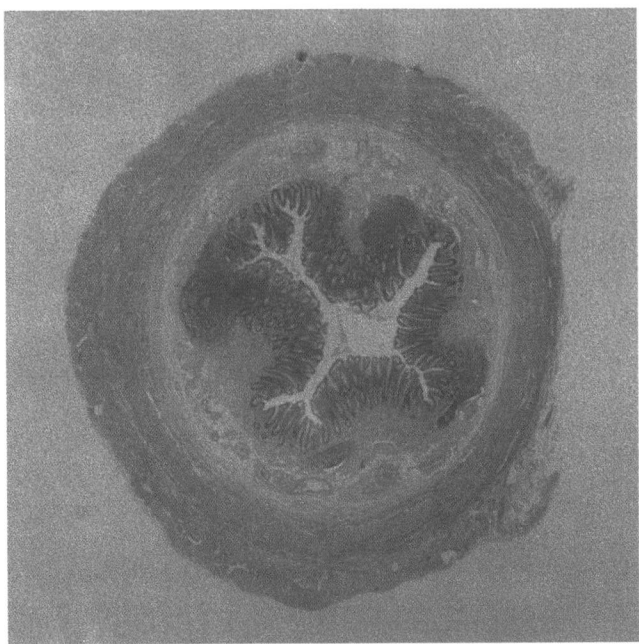

Figure 67.4 Normal vermiform appendix. The narrow lumen is bounded by mucosa which may be arranged in folds. There is usually abundant lymphoid tissue in the mucosa, especially in younger individuals. This may encroach on and further narrow the lumen. The mucosa is bounded by a relatively thin muscularis mucosa (courtesy of Dr P. Kelly, FRCPath, Dublin, Ireland).

to lie in the free border of the mesoappendix. An accessory appendicular artery may be present but, in most people, the appendicular artery is an 'end-artery', thrombosis of which results in necrosis of the appendix (synonym: gangrenous appendicitis). Four, six or more lymphatic channels traverse the mesoappendix to empty into the ileocaecal lymph nodes.

Microscopic anatomy

The appendix varies considerably in length and circumference. The average length is between 7.5 and 10 cm. The lumen is irregular, being encroached upon by multiple longitudinal folds of mucous membrane lined by columnar cell intestinal mucosa of colonic type (Fig. 67.4). Crypts are present but are not numerous. In the base of the crypts lie argentaffin cells (Kulchitsky cells), which may give rise to carcinoid tumours (see below). The appendix is the most frequent site for carcinoid tumours, which may present with appendicitis due to occlusion of the appendiceal lumen. The submucosa contains numerous lymphatic aggregations or follicles. While no discernible change in immune

function results from appendicectomy, the prominence of lymphatic tissue in the appendix of young adults seems to be important in the aetiology of appendicitis (see below).

ACUTE APPENDICITIS

While there are isolated reports of perityphlitis (fatal inflammation of the caecal region) from the late 1500s, recognition of acute appendicitis as a clinical entity is attributed to Reginald Fitz, who presented a paper to the first meeting of the Association of American Physicians in 1886 entitled 'Perforating inflammation of the vermiform appendix'. Soon afterwards, Charles McBurney described the clinical manifestations of acute appendicitis including the point of maximum tenderness in the right iliac fossa that now bears his name.

The incidence of appendicitis seems to have risen greatly in the first half of this century, particularly in Europe, America and Australasia, with up to 16% of the population undergoing appendicectomy. In the past 30 years, the incidence has fallen dramatically in these countries, such that the individual lifetime risk of appendicectomy is 8.6% and 6.7% among males and females respectively.

Nikolai Kulchitsky, 1856–1925, Professor of Histology, Kharkov, Ukraine, who left Russia after the Revolution of 1917, and later worked at University College, London. He described these cells in 1897.

Reginald Heber Fitz, 1843–1913, Professor of Medicine, Harvard University, Boston, MA, USA.
Charles McBurney, 1854–1913, Professor of Surgery, Columbia College of Physicians and Surgeons, New York, NY, USA. In 1889 McBurney published a paper on appendicitis in which he stated 'I believe that in every case the seat of greatest pain "determined by the pressure of one finger" has been very exactly between an inch and a half and two inches from the anterior spirious process of the ilium on a straight line drawn from that process to the umbilicus.'

Acute appendicitis is relatively rare in infants, and becomes increasingly common in childhood and early adult life, reaching a peak incidence in the teens and early 20s. After middle age, the risk of developing appendicitis is quite small. The incidence of appendicitis is equal among males and females before puberty. In teenagers and young adults, the male–female ratio increases to 3:2 at age 25; thereafter, the greater incidence in males declines.

Aetiology

There is no unifying hypothesis regarding the aetiology of acute appendicitis. Decreased dietary fibre and increased consumption of refined carbohydrates may be important. As with colonic diverticulitis, the incidence of appendicitis is lowest in societies with a high dietary fibre intake. In developing countries that are adopting a more refined western-type diet, the incidence continues to rise. This is in contrast to the dramatic decrease in the incidence of appendicitis in western countries observed in the past 30 years. No reason has been established for these paradoxical changes; however, improved hygiene and a change in the pattern of childhood gastrointestinal infection related to the increased use of antibiotics may be responsible.

While appendicitis is clearly associated with bacterial proliferation within the appendix, no single organism is responsible. A mixed growth of aerobic and anaerobic organisms is usual. The initiating event causing bacterial proliferation is controversial. Obstruction of the appendix lumen has been widely held to be important, and some form of luminal obstruction, either by a faecolith or a stricture, is found in the majority of cases.

A faecolith is composed of inspissated faecal material, calcium phosphates, bacteria and epithelial debris (Fig. 67.5). Rarely, a foreign body is incorporated into the mass. The incidental finding of a faecolith is a relative indication for prophylactic appendicectomy (Fig. 67.6). A fibrotic stricture of the appendix usually indicates

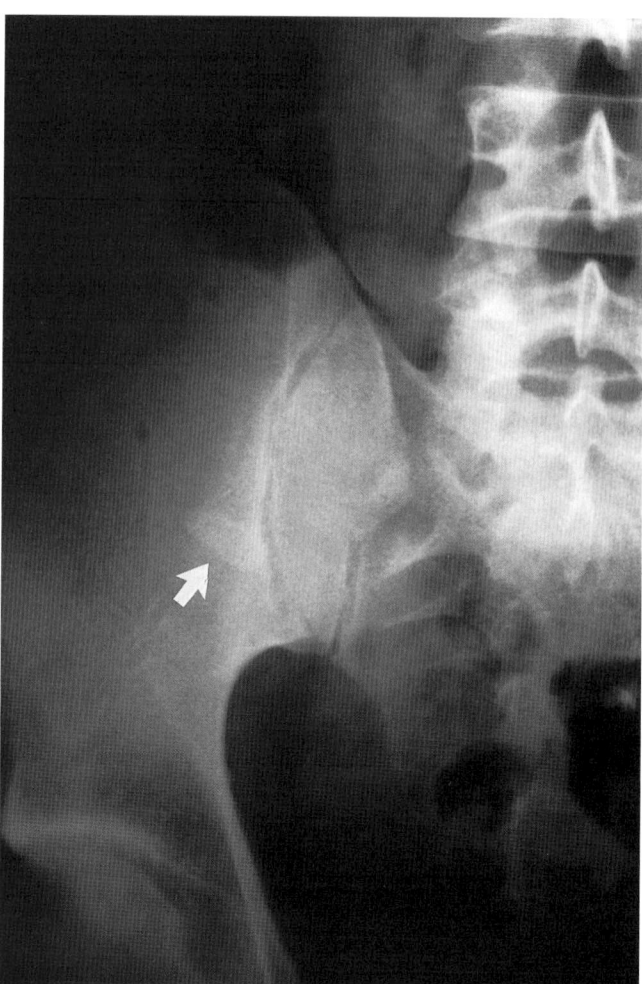

Figure 67.6 Supine abdominal radiograph showing the presence of a large faecolith in the right iliac fossa (arrow).

previous appendicitis that resolved without surgical intervention (Fig. 67.7). Obstruction of the appendiceal orifice by tumour, particularly carcinoma of the caecum, is an occasional cause of acute appendicitis in middle-aged and elderly patients. Intestinal parasites, particularly *Oxyuris vermicularis* (pinworm), can proliferate in the appendix and occlude the lumen.

Pathology

Obstruction of the appendiceal lumen seems to be essential for the development of appendiceal gangrene and perforation. Yet, in many cases of early appendicitis, the appendix lumen is patent despite the presence of mucosal inflammation and lymphoid hyperplasia. Occasional clustering of cases among children and young adults suggests an infective agent, possibly viral, which initiates an inflammatory response. Seasonal variation in the incidence is also observed, with more cases occurring between May and August in northern Europe than at other times of the year.

Lymphoid hyperplasia narrows the lumen of the appendix, leading to luminal obstruction. Once obstruction occurs, continued mucus secretion and inflammatory exudation increase intraluminal pressure, obstructing lymphatic drainage. Oedema and mucosal ulceration develop with bacterial translocation to the submucosa. Resolution may occur at this point either spontaneously or in response to antibiotic therapy. If the condition

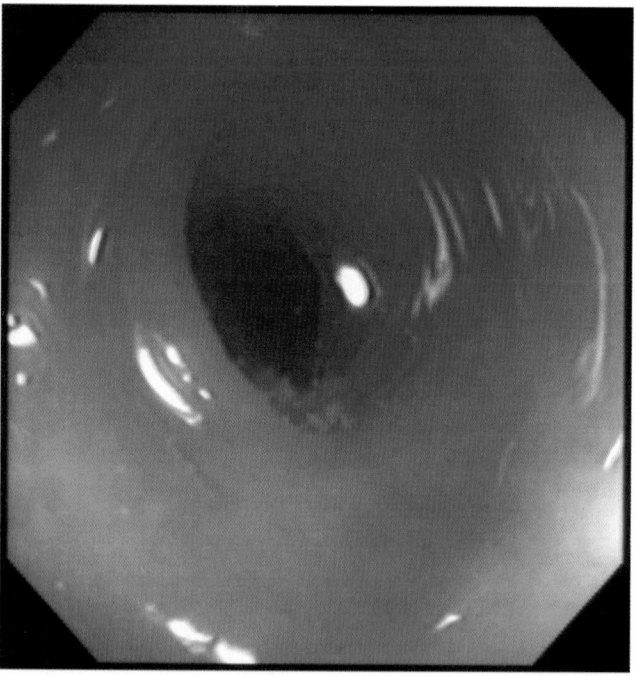

Figure 67.5 Colonoscopic view of the lumen of the appendix showing intraluminal debris (courtesy of Mr D. Winter, FRCSI, Dublin, Ireland).

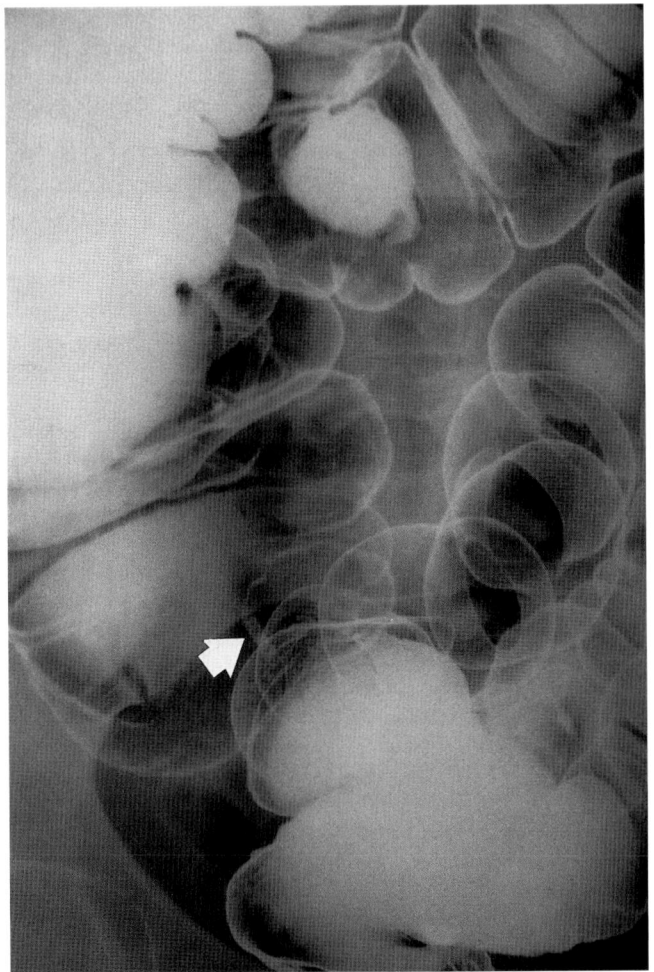

Figure 67.7 Barium enema radiograph demonstrating faecoliths of the appendix (arrow) with distal stricture of the appendix.

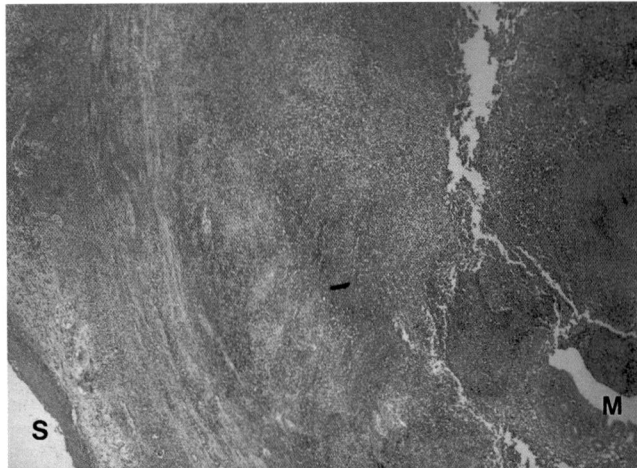

Figure 67.8 Acute appendicitis. A heavy acute inflammatory infiltrate extends through the full thickness of the wall of the appendix, destroying the mucosa, of which only a small island (M) remains, and the smooth muscle. The inflammation extends to involve the serosa (S) (courtesy of Dr P. Kelly, FRCPath, Dublin, Ireland).

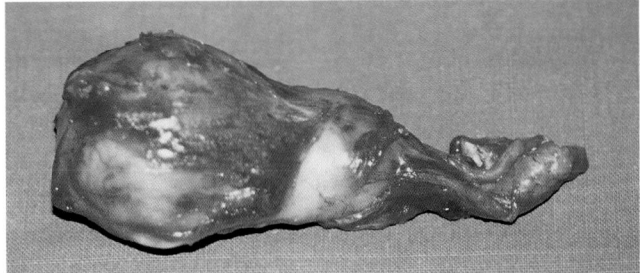

Figure 67.9 Mucocele of the appendix, following excision.

progresses, further distension of the appendix may cause venous obstruction and ischaemia of the appendix wall. With ischaemia, bacterial invasion occurs through the muscularis propria and submucosa, producing acute appendicitis (Fig. 67.8). Finally, ischaemic necrosis of the appendix wall produces gangrenous appendicitis, with free bacterial contamination of the peritoneal cavity. Alternatively, the greater omentum and loops of small bowel become adherent to the inflamed appendix, walling off the spread of peritoneal contamination, and resulting in a phlegmonous mass or paracaecal abscess. Rarely, appendiceal inflammation resolves, leaving a distended mucus-filled organ termed a mucocele of the appendix (Fig. 67.9).

It is the potential for peritonitis that is the great threat of acute appendicitis. Peritonitis occurs as a result of free migration of bacteria through an ischaemic appendicular wall, the frank perforation of a gangrenous appendix or the delayed perforation of an appendix abscess. Factors that promote this process include extremes of age, immunosuppression, diabetes mellitus and faecolith obstruction of the appendix lumen, a free-lying pelvic appendix and previous abdominal surgery that limits the ability of the greater omentum to wall off the spread of peritoneal contamination. In these situations, a rapidly deteriorating clinical course is accompanied by signs of diffuse peritonitis and systemic sepsis syndrome (Summary box 67.1).

Summary box 67.1

Risk factors for perforation of the appendix

- Extremes of age
- Immunosuppression
- Diabetes mellitus
- Faecolith obstruction
- Pelvic appendix
- Previous abdominal surgery

Clinical diagnosis

History

The classical features of acute appendicitis begin with poorly localised colicky abdominal pain. This is due to mid-gut visceral discomfort in response to appendiceal inflammation and obstruction. The pain is frequently first noticed in the peri-umbilical region and is similar to, but less intense than, the colic of small bowel obstruction. Central abdominal pain is associated with anorexia, nausea and usually one or two episodes of vomiting that follow the onset of pain (Murphy). Anorexia is a useful and

John Benjamin Murphy, 1857–1916, Professor of Surgery, Northwestern University, Chicago, IL, USA.

constant clinical feature, particularly in children. The patient often gives a history of similar discomfort that settled spontaneously. A family history is also useful as up to one-third of children with appendicitis have a first-degree relative with a similar history (Summary box 67.2).

Summary box 67.2

Symptoms of appendicitis

- Peri-umbilical colic
- Pain shifts to the right iliac fossa
- Anorexia
- Nausea

With progressive inflammation of the appendix, the parietal peritoneum in the right iliac fossa becomes irritated, producing more intense, constant and localised somatic pain that begins to predominate. Patients often report this as an abdominal pain that has shifted and changed in character. Typically, coughing or sudden movement exacerbates the right iliac fossa pain.

The classic visceral–somatic sequence of pain is present in only about half of those patients subsequently proven to have acute appendicitis. Atypical presentations include pain that is predominantly somatic or visceral and poorly localised. Atypical pain is more common in the elderly, in whom localisation to the right iliac fossa is unusual. An inflamed appendix in the pelvis may never produce somatic pain involving the anterior abdominal wall, but may instead cause suprapubic discomfort and tenesmus. In this circumstance, tenderness may be elicited only on rectal examination and is the basis for the recommendation that a rectal examination should be performed on every patient who presents with acute lower abdominal pain.

During the first 6 hours, there is rarely any alteration in temperature or pulse rate. After that time, slight pyrexia (37.2–37.7°C) with a corresponding increase in the pulse rate to 80 or 90 is usual. However, in 20% of patients, there is no pyrexia or tachycardia in the early stages. In children, a temperature greater than 38.5°C suggests other causes, e.g. mesenteric adenitis (see below).

Typically, two clinical syndromes of acute appendicitis can be discerned, *acute catarrhal (non-obstructive)* appendicitis and *acute obstructive* appendicitis. The latter is characterised by a much more acute course. The onset of symptoms is abrupt, and there may be generalised abdominal pain from the start. The temperature may be normal and vomiting is common, so that the clinical picture may mimic acute intestinal obstruction. Once recognised, urgent surgical intervention is required because of the more rapid progression to perforation.

Signs

The diagnosis of appendicitis rests more on thorough clinical examination of the abdomen than on any aspect of the history or laboratory investigation. The cardinal features are those of an unwell patient with low-grade pyrexia, localised abdominal tenderness, muscle guarding and rebound tenderness. Inspection of the abdomen may show limitation of respiratory movement in the lower abdomen. The patient is then asked to point to where the pain began and where it moved (the pointing sign). Gentle superficial palpation of the abdomen, beginning in the left iliac fossa moving anticlockwise to the right iliac fossa will detect muscle

guarding over the point of maximum tenderness, classically McBurney's point. Asking the patient to cough or gentle percussion over the site of maximum tenderness will elicit rebound tenderness (Summary box 67.3).

Summary box 67.3

Clinical signs in appendicitis

- Pyrexia
- Localised tenderness in the right iliac fossa
- Muscle guarding
- Rebound tenderness

Deep palpation of the left iliac fossa may cause pain in the right iliac fossa, Rovsing's sign, which is helpful in supporting a clinical diagnosis of appendicitis. Occasionally, an inflamed appendix lies on the psoas muscle, and the patient, often a young adult, will lie with the right hip flexed for pain relief (the psoas sign). Spasm of the obturator internus is sometimes demonstrable when the hip is flexed and internally rotated. If an inflamed appendix is in contact with the obturator internus, this manoeuvre will cause pain in the hypogastrium (the obturator test; Zachary Cope). Cutaneous hyperaesthesia may be demonstrable in the right iliac fossa, but is rarely of diagnostic value (Summary box 67.4).

Summary box 67.4

Signs to elicit in appendicitis

- Pointing sign
- Rovsing's sign
- Psoas sign
- Obturator sign

Special features, according to position of the appendix

Retrocaecal

Rigidity is often absent, and even application of deep pressure may fail to elicit tenderness (silent appendix), the reason being that the caecum, distended with gas, prevents the pressure exerted by the hand from reaching the inflamed structure. However, deep tenderness is often present in the loin, and rigidity of the quadratus lumborum may be in evidence. Psoas spasm, due to the inflamed appendix being in contact with that muscle, may be sufficient to cause flexion of the hip joint. Hyperextension of the hip joint may induce abdominal pain when the degree of psoas spasm is insufficient to cause flexion of the hip.

Pelvic

Occasionally, early diarrhoea results from an inflamed appendix being in contact with the rectum. When the appendix lies entirely within the pelvis, there is usually complete absence of abdominal rigidity, and often tenderness over McBurney's point is also lacking. In some instances, deep tenderness can be made out just above and to the right of the symphysis pubis. In either event,

---

Thorkild Rovsing, **1862–1937, Professor of Surgery, Copenhagen, Denmark.**
Sir Vincent Zachary Cope, **1881–1975, Surgeon, St. Mary's Hospital, London, England.**

a rectal examination reveals tenderness in the rectovesical pouch or the pouch of Douglas, especially on the right side. Spasm of the psoas and obturator internus muscles may be present when the appendix is in this position. An inflamed appendix in contact with the bladder may cause frequency of micturition. This is more common in children.

Postileal

In this case, the inflamed appendix lies behind the terminal ileum. It presents the greatest difficulty in diagnosis because the pain may not shift, diarrhoea is a feature and marked retching may occur. Tenderness, if any, is ill defined, although it may be present immediately to the right of the umbilicus.

Special features, according to age

Infants

Appendicitis is relatively rare in infants under 36 months of age and, for obvious reasons, the patient is unable to give a history. Because of this, diagnosis is often delayed, and thus the incidence of perforation and postoperative morbidity is considerably higher than in older children. Diffuse peritonitis can develop rapidly because of the underdeveloped greater omentum, which is unable to give much assistance in localising the infection.

Children

It is rare to find a child with appendicitis who has not vomited. Children with appendicitis usually have complete aversion to food.

The elderly

Gangrene and perforation occur much more frequently in elderly patients. Elderly patients with lax abdominal walls or obesity may harbour a gangrenous appendix with little evidence of it, and the clinical picture may simulate subacute intestinal obstruction. These features, coupled with coincident medical conditions, produce a much higher mortality for acute appendicitis in the elderly.

The obese

Obesity can obscure and diminish all the local signs of acute appendicitis. Delay in diagnosis, coupled with the technical difficulty of operating in the obese, makes it wiser to consider operating through a midline abdominal incision. Laparoscopy is particularly useful in the obese as it may obviate the need for a large abdominal incision.

Pregnancy

Appendicitis is the most common extrauterine acute abdominal condition in pregnancy, with a frequency of 1:1500–2000 pregnancies. Diagnosis is complicated by delay in presentation as early non-specific symptoms are often attributed to the pregnancy. Obstetric teaching has been that the caecum and appendix are progressively pushed to the right upper quadrant of the abdomen as pregnancy develops during the second and third trimesters. However, pain in the right lower quadrant of the abdomen remains the cardinal feature of appendicitis in pregnancy. Fetal loss occurs in 3–5% of cases, increasing to 20% if perforation is found at operation.

Differential diagnosis

Although acute appendicitis is the most common abdominal surgical emergency, the diagnosis can be extremely difficult at times. There are a number of common conditions that it is wise to consider carefully and, if possible, exclude. The differential diagnosis differs in patients of different ages; in women, additional differential diagnoses are diseases of the female genital tract (Table 67.1).

Children

The diseases most commonly mistaken for acute appendicitis are *acute gastroenteritis* and *mesenteric lymphadenitis*. In mesenteric lymphadenitis, the pain is colicky in nature and cervical lymph nodes may be enlarged. It may be impossible to clinically distinguish *Meckel's diverticulitis* from acute appendicitis. The pain is similar; however, signs may be central or left sided. Occasionally, there is a history of antecedent abdominal pain or intermittent lower gastrointestinal bleeding.

It is important to distinguish between acute appendicitis and *intussusception*. Appendicitis is uncommon before the age of 2 years, whereas the median age for intussusception is 18 months. A mass may be palpable in the right lower quadrant, and the preferred treatment of intussusception is reduction by careful barium enema.

Henoch–Schönlein purpura is often preceded by a sore throat or respiratory infection. Abdominal pain can be severe and can be confused with intussusception or appendicitis. There is nearly always an ecchymotic rash, typically affecting the extensor surfaces of the limbs and on the buttocks. The face is usually spared. The platelet count and bleeding time are within normal limits. Microscopic haematuria is common.

Lobar pneumonia and pleurisy, especially at the right base,

Table 67.1 Differential diagnosis of acute appendicitis

Children	Adult	Adult female	Elderly
Gastroenteritis	Regional enteritis	Mittelschmerz	Diverticulitis
Mesenteric adenitis	Ureteric colic	Pelvic inflammatory disease	Intestinal obstruction
Meckel's diverticulitis	Perforated peptic ulcer	Pyelonephritis	Colonic carcinoma
Intussusception	Torsion of testis	Ectopic pregnancy	Torsion appendix epiploicae
Henoch–Schönlein purpura	Pancreatitis	Torsion/rupture of ovarian cyst	Mesenteric infarction
Lobar pneumonia	Rectus sheath haematoma	Endometriosis	Leaking aortic aneurysm

James Douglas, 1675–1742, Anatomist and Man-midwife who practised in London, England, described this pouch in 1730.
Johann Friedrich Meckel, 1781–1883, Professor of Anatomy and Surgery, Halle, Germany.
Eduard Heinrich Henoch, 1820–1910, Professor of Diseases of Children, Berlin, Germany, described this form of purpura in 1868.
Johann Lucas Schönlein, 1793–1864, Professor of Medicine, Berlin, Germany, described this form of purpura in 1837.

CHAPTER 67 | THE VERMIFORM APPENDIX

may give rise to right-sided abdominal pain and mimic appendicitis. Abdominal tenderness is minimal, pyrexia is marked, and chest examination may reveal a pleural friction rub or altered breath sounds on auscultation. A chest radiograph is diagnostic.

Adults

Terminal ileitis in its acute form may be indistinguishable from acute appendicitis unless a doughy mass of inflamed ileum can be felt. An antecedent history of abdominal cramping, weight loss and diarrhoea suggests regional ileitis rather than appendicitis. The ileitis may be non-specific, due to Crohn's disease or *Yersinia* infection. *Yersinia enterocolitica* causes inflammation of the terminal ileum, appendix and caecum with mesenteric adenopathy. If suspected, serum antibody titres are diagnostic, and treatment with intravenous tetracycline is appropriate. If *Yersinia* infection is suspected at operation, a mesenteric lymph node should be excised and divided, with half submitted for microbiological culture (including tuberculosis) and half for histological examination.

Ureteric colic does not commonly cause diagnostic difficulty, as the character and radiation of pain differs from that of appendicitis. Urinalysis should always be performed, and the presence of red cells should prompt a supine abdominal radiograph. Renal ultrasound or intravenous urogram is diagnostic.

Right-sided acute pyelonephritis is accompanied and often preceded by increased frequency of micturition. It may cause difficulty in diagnosis, especially in women. The leading features are tenderness confined to the loin, fever (temperature 39°C) and possibly rigors and pyuria.

In perforated peptic ulcer, the duodenal contents pass along the paracolic gutter to the right iliac fossa. As a rule, there is a history of dyspepsia and a very sudden onset of pain that starts in the epigastrium and passes down the right paracolic gutter. In appendicitis, the pain starts classically in the umbilical region. Rigidity and tenderness in the right iliac fossa are present in both conditions but, in perforated duodenal ulcer, the rigidity is usually greater in the right hypochondrium. An erect chest radiograph will show gas under the diaphragm in 70% of patients. An abdominal computerised tomography (CT) examination is valuable when there is diagnostic difficulty.

Testicular torsion in a teenage or young adult male is easily missed. Pain can be referred to the right iliac fossa, and shyness on the part of the patient may lead the unwary to suspect appendicitis unless the scrotum is examined in all cases.

Acute pancreatitis should be considered in the differential diagnosis of all adults suspected of having acute appendicitis and, when appropriate, should be excluded by serum or urinary amylase measurement.

Rectus sheath haematoma is a relatively rare but easily missed differential diagnosis. It usually presents with acute pain and localised tenderness in the right iliac fossa, often after an episode of strenuous physical exercise. Localised pain without gastrointestinal upset is the rule. Occasionally, in an elderly patient, particularly one taking anticoagulant therapy, a rectus sheath haematoma may present as a mass and tenderness in the right iliac fossa after minor trauma.

Burrill Bernard Crohn, 1884–1983, Gastroenterologist, Mount Sinai Hospital, New York, NY, USA, described regional ileitis in 1932.
Alexandre Emile Yersin, 1863–1943, Bacteriologist, Paris, France.

Adult female (see also Chapter 76)

It is in women of childbearing age that pelvic disease most often mimics acute appendicitis. A careful gynaecological history should be taken in all women with suspected appendicitis, concentrating on menstrual cycle, vaginal discharge and possible pregnancy. The most common diagnostic mimics are pelvic inflammatory disease (PID), Mittelschmerz, torsion or haemorrhage of an ovarian cyst and ectopic pregnancy.

Pelvic inflammatory disease

PID comprises a spectrum of diseases that include salpingitis, endometritis and tubo-ovarian sepsis. The incidence of these conditions is increasing, and the diagnosis should be considered in every young adult female. Typically, the pain is lower than in appendicitis and is bilateral. A history of vaginal discharge, dysmenorrhoea and burning pain on micturition is a helpful differential diagnostic point. The physical findings include adnexal and cervical tenderness on vaginal examination. When suspected, a high vaginal swab should be taken for *Chlamydia trachomatis* and *Neisseria gonorrhoeae* culture, and the opinion of a gynaecologist should be obtained. Treatment is usually a combination of ofloxacin and metronidazole. Transvaginal ultrasound can be particularly helpful in establishing the diagnosis. When serious diagnostic uncertainty persists, diagnostic laparoscopy should be undertaken.

Mittelschmerz

Midcycle rupture of a follicular cyst with bleeding produces lower abdominal and pelvic pain, typically midcycle. Systemic upset is rare, a pregnancy test is negative, and symptoms usually subside within hours. Occasionally, diagnostic laparoscopy is required. Retrograde menstruation may cause similar symptoms.

Torsion/haemorrhage of an ovarian cyst

This can prove a difficult differential diagnosis. When suspected, pelvic ultrasound and a gynaecological opinion should be sought. If encountered at operation, untwisting of the involved adnexa and ovarian cystectomy should be performed, if necessary, in women of childbearing years. Documented visualisation of the contralateral ovary is an essential medico-legal precaution prior to oophorectomy for any reason.

Ectopic pregnancy

It is unlikely that a *ruptured* ectopic pregnancy, with its well-defined signs of haemoperitoneum, will be mistaken for acute appendicitis, but the same cannot be said for a right-sided tubal abortion, or still more for a right-sided unruptured tubal pregnancy. In the latter, the signs are very similar to those of acute appendicitis, except that the pain *commences* on the right side and stays there. The pain is severe and continues unabated until operation. Usually, there is a history of a missed menstrual period, and a urinary pregnancy test may be positive. Severe pain is felt when the cervix is moved on vaginal examination. Signs of intraperitoneal bleeding usually become apparent, and the patient should be questioned specifically regarding referred pain in the shoulder. Pelvic ultrasonography should be carried out in all cases in which an ectopic pregnancy is a possible diagnosis.

Elderly

Sigmoid diverticulitis

In some patients with a long sigmoid loop, the colon lies to the right of the midline, and it may be impossible to differentiate between diverticulitis and appendicitis. Abdominal CT scanning is particularly useful in this setting and should be considered in the management of all patients over the age of 60 years. A trial of conservative management with intravenous fluids and antibiotics is often appropriate, with a low threshold for exploratory laparotomy in the face of deterioration or lack of clinical response.

Intestinal obstruction

The diagnosis of intestinal obstruction is usually clear; the subtlety lies in recognising acute appendicitis as the occasional cause in the elderly. As with diverticulitis, intravenous fluids, antibiotics and nasogastric decompression should be instigated, with early resort to laparotomy.

Carcinoma of the caecum

When obstructed or locally perforated, carcinoma of the caecum may mimic or cause obstructive appendicitis in adults. A history of antecedent discomfort, altered bowel habit or unexplained anaemia should raise suspicion. A mass may be palpable (see below) and barium enema diagnostic.

Rare differential diagnoses

Preherpetic pain of the right 10th and 11th dorsal nerves is localised over the same area as that of appendicitis. It does not shift and is associated with marked hyperaesthesia. There is no intestinal upset or rigidity. The herpetic eruption may be delayed for 3–8 hours.

Tabetic crises are now rare. Severe abdominal pain and vomiting usher in the crisis. Other signs of tabes confirm the diagnosis.

Spinal conditions are sometimes associated with acute abdominal pain especially in children and the elderly. These may include tuberculosis of the spine, metastatic carcinoma, osteoporotic vertebral collapse and multiple myeloma. The pain is due to compression of nerve roots and may be aggravated by movement. There is rigidity of the lumbar spine and intestinal symptoms are absent.

The abdominal crises of *porphyria* and *diabetes mellitus* need to be remembered. A urinalysis should be undertaken in every abdominal emergency. In cyclical vomiting of infants or young children, there is a history of previous similar attacks and abdominal rigidity is absent. Acetone is found in the urine but is not diagnostic as it may accompany starvation.

Typhlitis or leukaemic ileocaecal syndrome is a rare but potentially fatal enterocolitis occurring in immunosuppressed patients. Gram-negative or *clostridial* (especially *Clostridium septicum*) septicaemia can be rapidly progressive. Treatment is with appropriate antibiotics and haematopoietic factors. Surgical intervention is rarely indicated.

Investigation

The diagnosis of acute appendicitis is essentially clinical; however, a decision to operate based on clinical suspicion alone can lead to the removal of a normal appendix in 15–30% of cases. The premise that it is better to remove a normal appendix than to delay diagnosis does not stand up to close scrutiny, particularly in the elderly. A number of clinical and laboratory-based scoring systems have been devised to assist diagnosis. The most widely used is the Alvarado score (Table 67.2). A score of 7 or more is strongly predictive of acute appendicitis.

Alfredo Alvarado, **Contemporary, Surgeon, Plantation, FL, USA.**

Table 67.2 The Alvarado (MANTRELS) score

Symptoms	Score
Migratory RIF pain	1
Anorexia	1
Nausea and vomiting	1
Signs	
Tenderness (RIF)	2
Rebound tenderness	1
Elevated temperature	1
Laboratory	
Leucocytosis	2
Shift to left	1
Total	10

RIF, right iliac fossa; MANTRELS, Migration of pain, Anorexia, Nausea or vomiting, Tenderness, Rebound pain, Elevation of temperature, Leucocytosis, Shift to left (segmented neutrophils).

In patients with an equivocal score (5–6), abdominal ultrasound or contrast-enhanced CT examination further reduces the rate of negative appendicectomy. Abdominal ultrasound examination is more useful in children and thin adults, particularly if gynaecological pathology is suspected, with a diagnostic accuracy in excess of 90% (Fig. 67.10). Contrast-enhanced CT scan (Fig. 67.11) is most useful in patients in whom there is diagnostic uncertainty, particularly older patients, in whom acute diverticulitis, intestinal obstruction and neoplasm are likely differential diagnoses. Selective use of CT scanning may be cost-effective by reducing both the negative appendicectomy rate and the length of hospital stay (Summary box 67.5).

> **Summary box 67.5**
>
> **Preoperative investigations in appendicitis**
>
> **Routine**
> - **Full blood count**
> - **Urinalysis**
>
> **Selective**
> - **Pregnancy test**
> - **Urea and electrolytes**
> - **Supine abdominal radiograph**
> - **Ultrasound of the abdomen/pelvis**
> - **Contrast-enhanced CT scan of the abdomen**

Treatment

The treatment for acute appendicitis is appendicectomy. There is a perception that urgent operation is essential to prevent the increased morbidity and mortality of peritonitis. While there should be no unnecessary delay, all patients, particularly those most at risk of serious morbidity, benefit by a short period of intensive preoperative preparation. Intravenous fluids, sufficient to establish adequate urine output (catheterisation is needed only in the very ill), and appropriate antibiotics should be given. There is ample evidence that a single peroperative dose of antibiotics reduces the incidence of postoperative wound infection. When peritonitis is suspected, therapeutic intravenous antibiotics to cover Gram-negative bacilli as well as anaerobic cocci should be given. Hyperpyrexia in children should be treated with salicylates

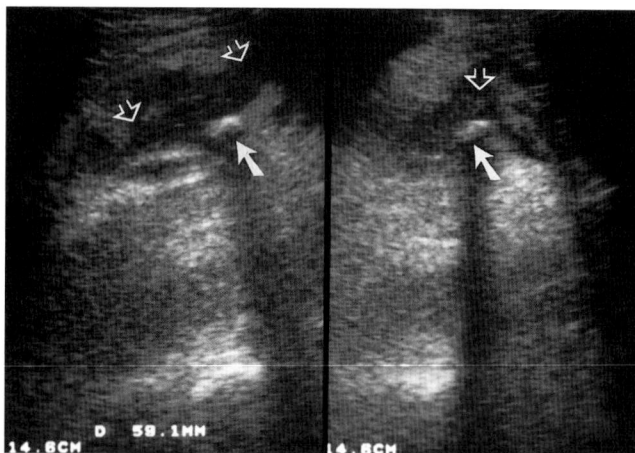

Figure 67.10 Abdominal ultrasound examination showing features of acute appendicitis, distended oedematous appendix (open arrows), longitudinal scan (left) and transverse scan (right). A faecolith is seen (closed arrow) (courtesy of Dr M. Behan, FRCR, Dublin, Ireland).

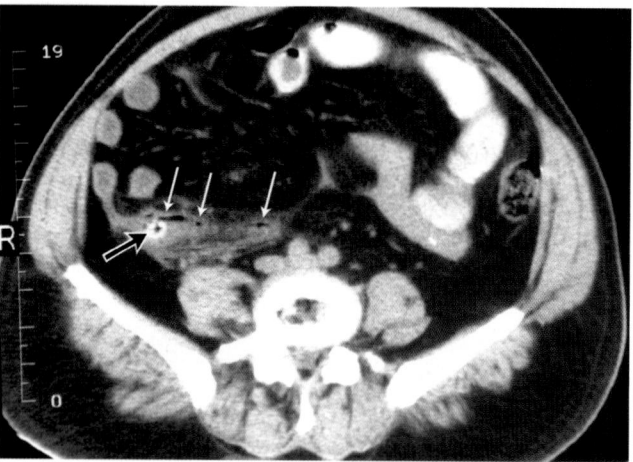

Figure 67.11 Abdominal contrast-enhanced computerised tomography scan showing a faecolith (open arrow) at the base of a distended (> 0.6 cm) appendix with intramural gas (white arrows) (courtesy of Dr H. Fenlon, FRCR, Dublin, Ireland).

in addition to antibiotics and intravenous fluids. With appropriate use of intravenous fluids and parenteral antibiotics, a policy of deferring appendicectomy after midnight to the first case on the following morning does not increase morbidity. However, when acute obstructive appendicitis is recognised, operation should not be deferred longer than it takes to optimise the patient's condition.

Appendicectomy

Claudius Amyand successfully removed an acutely inflamed appendix from the hernial sac of a boy in 1736. The first surgeon to perform deliberate appendicectomy for acute appendicitis was Lawson Tait in May 1880. The patient recovered; however, the

case was not reported until 1890. Meanwhile, Thomas Morton was the first to diagnose appendicitis, drain the abscess and remove the appendix with recovery, publishing his findings in 1887.

Appendicectomy should be performed under general anaesthetic with the patient supine on the operating table. When a laparoscopic technique is to be used, the bladder must be empty (ensure that the patient has voided before leaving the ward). Prior to preparing the entire abdomen with an appropriate antiseptic solution, the right iliac fossa should be palpated for a mass. If a mass is felt, it may, on occasion, be preferable to adopt a conservative approach (see below). Draping of the abdomen is in accordance with the planned operative technique, taking account of any requirement to extend the incision or convert a laparoscopic technique to an open operation.

Conventional appendicectomy

When the preoperative diagnosis is considered reasonably certain, the incision that is widely used for appendicectomy is the so called gridiron incision (gridiron: a frame of cross-beams to support a ship during repairs). The gridiron incision (described first by McArthur) is made at right angles to a line joining the anterior superior iliac spine to the umbilicus, its centre being along the line at McBurney's point (Fig. 67.12). If better access is required, it is possible to convert the gridiron to a Rutherford Morison incision (see below) by cutting the internal oblique and transversus muscles in the line of the incision.

In recent years, a transverse skin crease (Lanz) incision has become more popular, as the exposure is better and extension, when needed, is easier. The incision, appropriate in length to the size and obesity of the patient, is made approximately 2 cm below the umbilicus centred on the mid-clavicular–midinguinal line (Fig. 67.13). When necessary, the incision may be extended medially, with retraction or suitable division of the rectus abdominis muscle.

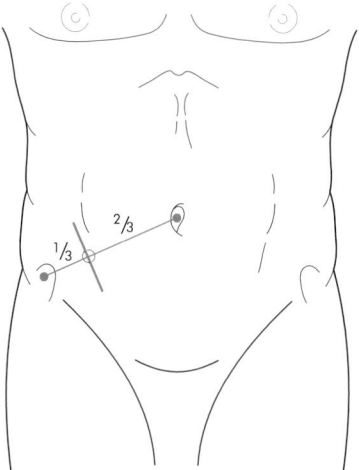

Figure 67.12 Gridiron incision for appendicitis, at right angles to a line joining the anterior superior iliac spine and umbilicus, centred on McBurney's point (courtesy of Mr M. Earley, FRSCI, Dublin, Ireland).

Claudius Amyand, **1685–1740**, Surgeon, St. George's Hospital, London, England.
Robert Lawson Tait, **1845–1899**, Surgeon, The Hospital for Diseases of Women, Birmingham, England.

Thomas George Morton, **1835–1903**, Surgeon, Philadelphia, PA, USA.
Lewis Linn McArthur, **1858–1934**, Surgeon, St. Luke's Hospital, Chicago, IL, USA.
James Rutherford Morison, **1853–1939**, Professor of Surgery, The University of Durham, Durham, England.
Otto Lanz, **1865–1935**, Surgeon, Amsterdam, The Netherlands.

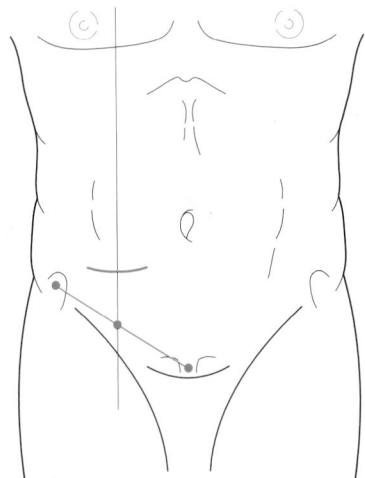

Figure 67.13 Transverse or skin crease (Lanz) incision for appendicitis, 2 cm below the umbilicus, centred on the mid-clavicular–midinguinal line (courtesy of Mr M. Earley, FRSCI, Dublin, Ireland).

When the diagnosis is in doubt, particularly in the presence of intestinal obstruction, a lower midline abdominal incision is to be preferred over a right lower paramedian incision. The latter, although widely practised in the past, is difficult to extend, more difficult to close and provides poorer access to the pelvis and peritoneal cavity.

Rutherford Morison's incision is useful if the appendix is para- or retrocaecal and fixed. It is essentially an oblique muscle-cutting incision with its lower end over McBurney's point and extending obliquely upwards and laterally as necessary. All layers are divided in the line of the incision.

Removal of the appendix

The caecum is identified by the presence of taeniae coli and, using a finger or a swab, the caecum is withdrawn. A turgid appendix may be felt at the base of the caecum. Inflammatory adhesions must be gently broken with a finger, which is then hooked around the appendix to deliver it into the wound. The appendix is conveniently controlled using a Babcock or Lane's forceps applied in such a way as to encircle the appendix and yet not damage it. The base of the mesoappendix is clamped in artery forceps, divided and ligated (Fig. 67.14a). When the mesoappendix is broad, the procedure must be repeated with a second or, rarely, a third artery forceps. The appendix, now completely freed, is crushed near its junction with the caecum in artery forceps, which is removed and reapplied just distal to the crushed portion. An absorbable 2/0 ligature is tied around the crushed portion close to the caecum. The appendix is amputated between the artery forceps and the ligature (Fig. 67.14b). An absorbable 2/0 or 3/0 purse-string or 'Z' suture may then be inserted into the caecum about 1.25 cm from the base (Fig. 67.14c). The stitch should pass through the muscle coat, picking up the taeniae coli. The stump of the appendix is invaginated (Fig. 67.14d) while the purse-string or 'Z' suture is tied, thus burying the appendix stump. Many surgeons believe invagination of the appendiceal stump is unnecessary.

William Wayne Babcock, **1872–1963**, Surgeon, Philadelphia, PA, USA.
Sir William Arbuthnot Lane, **1856–1943**, Surgeon, Guy's Hospital, London, England.

Methods to be adopted in special circumstances

When the caecal wall is oedematous, the purse-string suture is in danger of cutting out. If the oedema is of limited extent, this can be overcome by inserting the purse-string suture into more healthy caecal wall at a greater distance from the base of the appendix. Occasions may arise when, because of the extensive oedema of the caecal wall, it is better not to attempt invagination.

When the base of the appendix is inflamed, it should not be crushed, but ligated close to the caecal wall just tightly enough to occlude the lumen, after which the appendix is amputated and the stump invaginated. Should the base of the appendix be gangrenous, neither crushing nor ligation should be attempted. Two stitches are placed through the caecal wall close to the base of the gangrenous appendix, which is amputated flush with the caecal wall, after which these stitches are tied. Further closure is effected by means of a second layer of interrupted seromuscular sutures.

Retrograde appendicectomy

When the appendix is retrocaecal and adherent, it is an advantage to divide the base between artery forceps. The appendiceal vessels are then ligated, the stump ligated and invaginated, and gentle traction on the caecum will enable the surgeon to deliver the body of the appendix, which is then removed from base to tip. Occasionally, this manoeuvre requires division of the lateral peritoneal attachments of the caecum.

Drainage of the peritoneal cavity

This is usually unnecessary provided adequate peritoneal toilet has been done. If, however, there is considerable purulent fluid in the retrocaecal space or the pelvis, a soft silastic drain may be inserted through a separate stab incision. The wound should be closed using absorbable sutures to oppose muscles and aponeurosis.

Laparoscopic appendicectomy

The most valuable aspect of laparoscopy in the management of suspected appendicitis is as a diagnostic tool, particularly in women of child-bearing age. The placement of operating ports may vary according to operator preference and previous abdominal scars. The operator stands to the patient's left and faces a video monitor placed at the patient's right foot (Fig. 67.15). A moderate Trendelenburg tilt of the operating table assists delivery of loops of small bowel from the pelvis. The appendix is found in the conventional manner by identification of the caecal taeniae and is controlled using a laparoscopic tissue-holding forceps. By elevating the appendix, the mesoappendix is displayed (Fig. 67.16a). A dissecting forceps is used to create a window in the mesoappendix to allow the appendicular vessels to be coagulated or ligated using a clip applicator. The appendix, free of its mesentery, can be ligated at its base with an absorbable loop ligature (Fig. 67.16b), divided (Fig. 67.16c) and removed through one of the operating ports. It is not usual to invert the stump of the appendix (Fig. 67.16d). A single absorbable suture is used to close the linea alba at the umbilicus, and the small skin incisions may be closed with subcuticular sutures.

Patients who undergo laparoscopic appendicectomy are likely to have less postoperative pain and to be discharged from hospital and return to activities of daily living sooner than those who have undergone open appendicectomy. While the incidence of

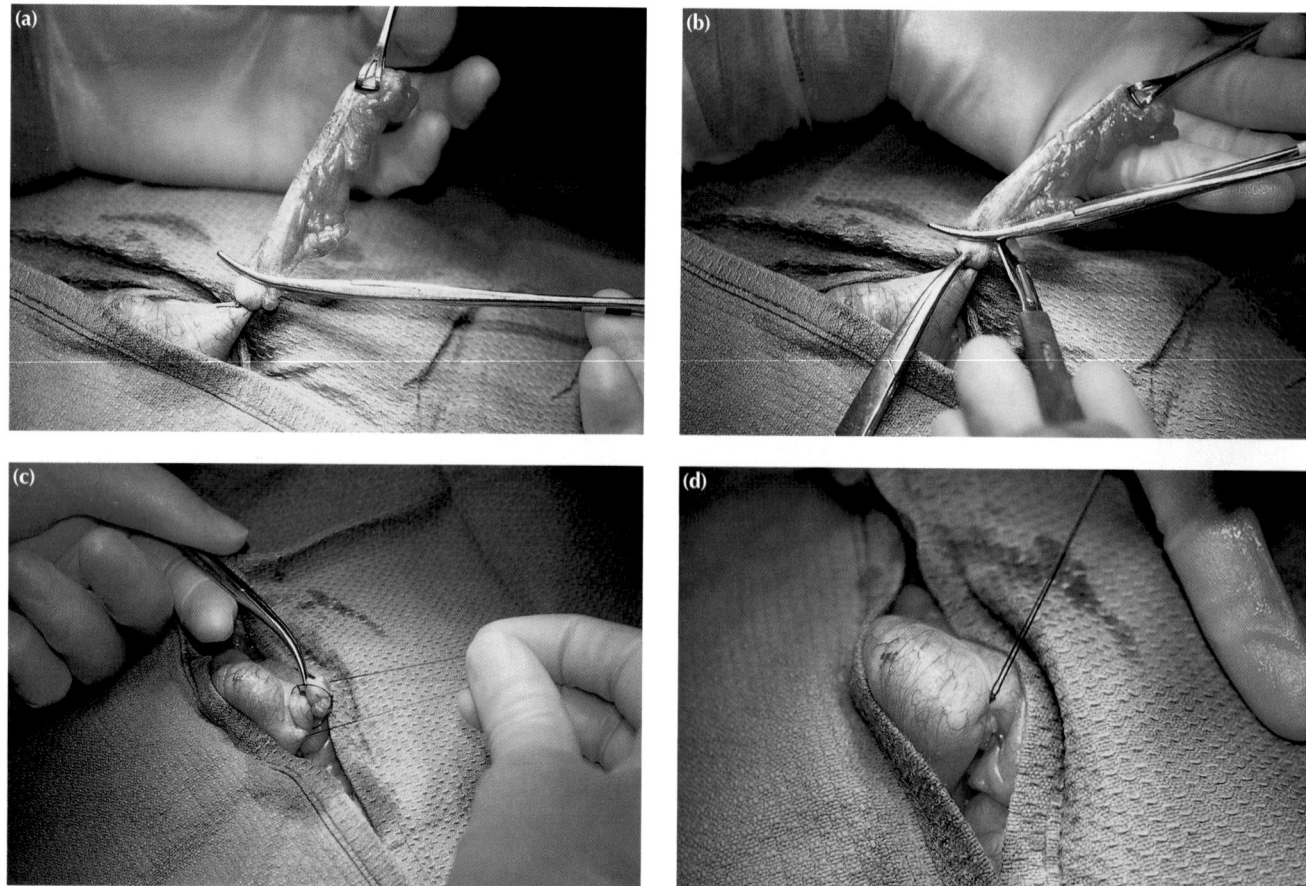

Figure 67.14 (a) Mesoappendix divided between artery forceps and ligated. (b) Appendix crushed and ligated at its base and about to be divided. (c) 'Z' suture inserted prior to inversion of the appendiceal stump. (d) Appendiceal stump inverted, the 'Z' suture having been tied.

postoperative wound infection is lower after the laparoscopic technique, the incidence of postoperative intra-abdominal sepsis may be higher in patients operated on for gangrenous or perforated appendicitis. There may be an advantage for laparoscopic over open appendicectomy in obese patients.

Instrument trolley

TV

Scrub nurse

X = 10 mm port
x = 5 mm port

Surgeon   **Camera operator**

Figure 67.15 Position of surgeon, assistants and equipment for laparoscopic appendicectomy.

Problems encountered during appendicectomy

A normal appendix is found

This demands careful exclusion of other possible diagnoses, particularly terminal ileitis, Meckel's diverticulitis and tubal or ovarian causes in women. It is usual to remove the appendix to avoid future diagnostic difficulties, even though the appendix is macroscopically normal, particularly if a skin crease or gridiron incision has been made. A case can be made for preserving the macroscopically normal appendix seen at diagnostic laparoscopy, although approximately one-quarter of seemingly normal appendices show microscopic evidence of inflammation.

The appendix cannot be found

The caecum should be mobilised, and the taeniae coli should be traced to their confluence on the caecum before the diagnosis of 'absent appendix' is made.

An appendicular tumour is found

Small tumours (under 2.0 cm in diameter) can be removed by appendicectomy; larger tumours should be treated by a right hemicolectomy.

An appendix abscess is found and the appendix cannot be removed easily

This should be treated by local peritoneal toilet, drainage of any abscess and intravenous antibiotics. Very rarely, a caecectomy or

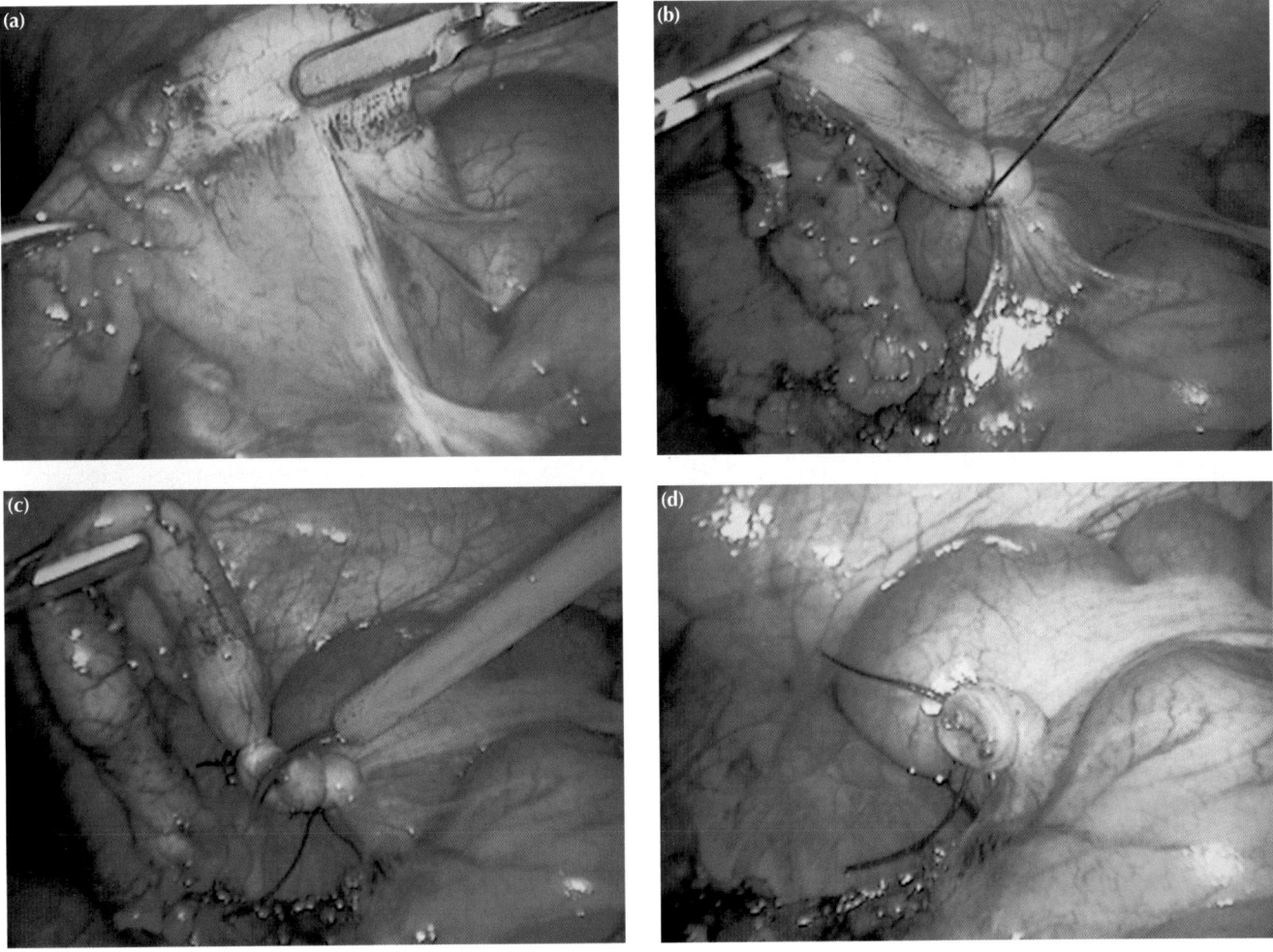

Figure 67.16 Laparoscopic appendicectomy. (a) Mesoappendix displayed. (b) Ligation at the base of the appendix. (c) Division of base. (d) Appendicectomy complete (courtesy of Mr O. McAnena, FRCSI, Galway, Ireland).

partial right hemicolectomy is required. (The first recorded operation for an appendix abscess was by Henry Hancock of Charing Cross Hospital, London, in 1848.)

Appendicitis complicating Crohn's disease

Occasionally, a patient undergoing surgery for acute appendicitis is found to have concomitant Crohn's disease of the ileocaecal region. Providing that the caecal wall is healthy at the base of the appendix, appendicectomy can be performed without increasing the risk of an enterocutaneous fistula. Rarely, the appendix is involved with the Crohn's disease. In this situation, a conservative approach may be warranted, and a trial of intravenous corticosteroids and systemic antibiotics can be used to resolve the acute inflammatory process.

Appendix abscess

Failure of resolution of an appendix mass or continued spiking pyrexia usually indicates that there is pus within the phlegmonous appendix mass. Ultrasound or abdominal CT scan may identify an area suitable for the insertion of a percutaneous drain. Should this prove unsuccessful, laparotomy though a midline incision is indicated.

Pelvic abscess

Pelvic abscess formation is an occasional complication of appendicitis and can occur irrespective of the position of the appendix within the peritoneal cavity. The most common presentation is a spiking pyrexia several days after appendicitis; indeed, the patient may already have been discharged from hospital. Pelvic pressure or discomfort associated with loose stool or tenesmus is common. Rectal examination reveals a boggy mass in the pelvis, anterior to the rectum, at the level of the peritoneal reflection (Fig. 67.17). Pelvic ultrasound or CT scan will confirm. Treatment is transrectal drainage under general anaesthetic.

Management of an appendix mass

If an appendix mass is present and the condition of the patient is satisfactory, the standard treatment is the conservative Ochsner–Sherren regimen. This strategy is based on the premise that the inflammatory process is already localised and that

> Albert John Ochsner, 1858–1925, Professor of Clinical Surgery, The University of Illinois College of Medicine, Chicago, IL, USA.
> James Sherren, 1872–1945, Surgeon, The London Hospital, London, England.

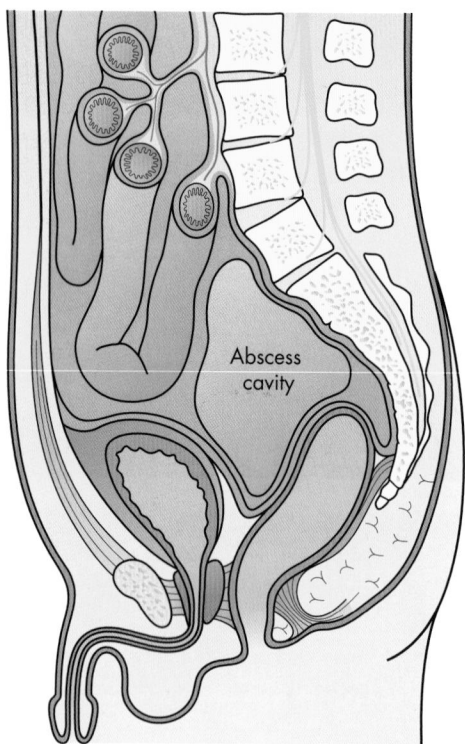

Figure 67.17 Appendix abscess involving the pelvis. Note the relationship to the rectum.

inadvertent surgery is difficult and may be dangerous. It may be impossible to find the appendix and, occasionally, a faecal fistula may form. For these reasons, it is wise to observe a non-operative programme but to be prepared to operate should clinical deterioration occur (Summary box 67.6).

Summary box 67.6

Criteria for stopping conservative treatment of an appendix mass

- A rising pulse rate
- Increasing or spreading abdominal pain
- Increasing size of the mass

Careful recording of the patient's condition and the extent of the mass should be made and the abdomen regularly re-examined. It is helpful to mark the limits of the mass on the abdominal wall using a skin pencil. A contrast-enhanced CT examination of the abdomen should be performed and antibiotic therapy instigated. An abscess, if present, should be drained radiologically. Temperature and pulse rate should be recorded 4-hourly and a fluid balance record maintained. Clinical deterioration or evidence of peritonitis is an indication for early laparotomy. Clinical improvement is usually evident within 24–48 hours. Failure of the mass to resolve should raise suspicion of a carcinoma or Crohn's disease. Using this regimen, approximately 90% of cases resolve without incident. The great majority of patients will not develop recurrence, and it is no longer considered advisable to remove the appendix after an interval of 6–8 weeks.

Postoperative complications

Postoperative complications following appendicectomy are relatively uncommon and reflect the degree of peritonitis that was present at the time of operation and intercurrent diseases that may predispose to complications (Summary box 67.7).

Summary box 67.7

Check-list for unwell patient following appendicectomy

- Examine the wound and abdomen for an abscess
- Consider a pelvic abscess and perform a rectal examination
- Examine the lungs – pneumonitis or collapse
- Examine the legs – consider venous thrombosis
- Examine the conjunctivae for an icteric tinge and the liver for enlargement, and enquire whether the patient has had rigors (pylephlebitis)
- Examine the urine for organisms (pyelonephritis)
- Suspect subphrenic abscess

Wound infection

Wound infection is the most common postoperative complication, occurring in 5–10% of all patients. This usually presents with pain and erythema of the wound on the fourth or fifth postoperative day, often soon after hospital discharge. Treatment is by wound drainage and antibiotics when required. The organisms responsible are usually a mixture of Gram-negative bacilli and anaerobic bacteria, predominantly *Bacteroides* species and anaerobic streptococci.

Intra-abdominal abscess

Intra-abdominal abscess has become a relatively rare complication after appendicectomy with the use of peroperative antibiotics. Postoperative spiking fever, malaise and anorexia developing 5–7 days after operation suggest an intraperitoneal collection. Interloop, paracolic, pelvic and subphrenic sites should be considered. Abdominal ultrasonography and CT scanning greatly facilitate diagnosis and allow percutaneous drainage. Laparotomy should be considered in patients suspected of having intra-abdominal sepsis but in whom imaging fails to show a collection, particularly those with continuing ileus.

Ileus

A period of adynamic ileus is to be expected after appendicectomy, and this may last a number of days following removal of a gangrenous appendix. Ileus persisting for more than 4 or 5 days, particularly in the presence of a fever, is indicative of continuing intra-abdominal sepsis and should prompt further investigation (see above). Rarely, early during postoperative recovery, a Richter's type of hernia may occur at the site of a laparoscopic port insertion and may be confused with a postoperative ileus. A CT scan is usually definitive.

Respiratory

In the absence of concurrent pulmonary disease, respiratory complications are rare following appendicectomy. Adequate

---

August Gottlieb Richter, **1742–1812, Lecturer in Surgery, Göttingen, Germany.**

postoperative analgesia and physiotherapy, when appropriate, reduce the incidence.

Venous thrombosis and embolism

These conditions are rare after appendicectomy, except in the elderly and in women taking the oral contraceptive pill. Appropriate prophylactic measures should be taken in such cases.

Portal pyaemia (pylephlebitis)

This is a rare but very serious complication of gangrenous appendicitis associated with high fever, rigors and jaundice. It is caused by septicaemia in the portal venous system and leads to the development of intrahepatic abscesses (often multiple). Treatment is with systemic antibiotics and percutaneous drainage of hepatic abscesses as appropriate.

Faecal fistula

Leakage from the appendicular stump occurs rarely, but may follow if the encircling stitch has been put in too deeply or if the caecal wall was involved by oedema or inflammation. Occasionally, a fistula may result following appendicectomy in Crohn's disease. Conservative management with low-residue enteral nutrition will usually result in closure.

Adhesive intestinal obstruction

This is the most common late complication of appendicectomy. At operation, a single band adhesion is often found to be responsible. Occasionally, chronic pain in the right iliac fossa is attributed to adhesion formation after appendicectomy. In such cases, laparoscopy is of value in confirming the presence of adhesions and allowing division.

Recurrent acute appendicitis

Appendicitis is notoriously recurrent. It is not uncommon for patients to attribute such attacks to 'biliousness' or dyspepsia. The attacks vary in intensity and may occur every few months, and the majority of cases ultimately culminate in severe acute appendicitis. If a careful history is taken from patients with acute appendicitis, many remember having had milder but similar attacks of pain. The appendix in these cases shows fibrosis indicative of previous inflammation (Fig. 67.18). Chronic appendicitis, per se, does not exist; however, there is evidence of altered neuroimmune function in the myenteric nerves of patients with so called recurrent appendicitis (Büchler).

Neoplasms of the appendix

Carcinoid tumour (synonym: argentaffinoma)

Carcinoid tumours arise in argentaffin tissue (Kulchitsky cells of the crypts of Lieberkühn) and are most common in the vermiform appendix. Carcinoid tumour is found once in every 300–400 appendices subjected to histological examination and is 10 times more common than any other neoplasm of the appendix. In many instances, the appendix had been removed because of symptoms of subacute or recurrent appendicitis. The tumour can occur in any part of the appendix, but it is frequently found in the distal third. The neoplasm feels moderately hard and, on sectioning the

Marcus Büchler, **Contemporary, Professor of Surgery, Heidelberg, Germany.**
Johann Nathaniel Lieberkühn, **1711–1756, Physician and Anatomist, Berlin, Germany, described these glands in 1745.**

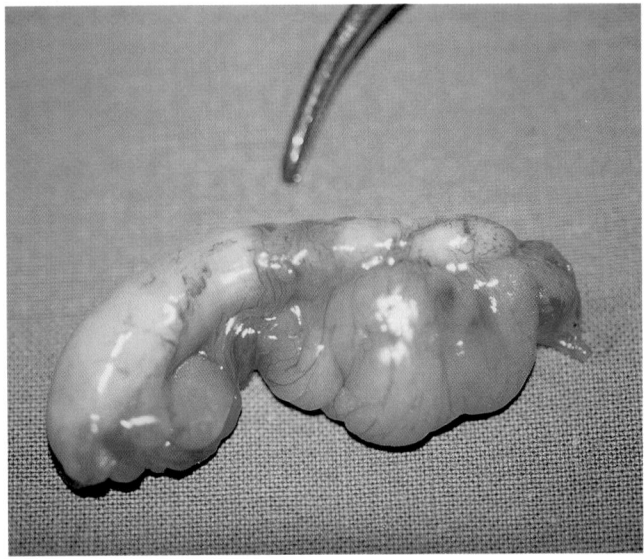

Figure 67.18 Excised appendix showing the point of luminal obstruction with distal fibrosis.

appendix, it can be seen as a yellow tumour between the intact mucosa and the peritoneum. Microscopically, the tumour cells are small, arranged in small nests within the muscle and have a characteristic pattern using immunohistochemical stain for chromogranin B (Fig. 67.19). Unlike carcinoid tumours arising in other parts of the intestinal tract, carcinoid tumour of the appendix rarely gives rise to metastases. Appendicectomy has been shown to be sufficient treatment, unless the caecal wall is involved, the tumour is 2 cm or more in size or involved lymph nodes are found, when right hemicolectomy is indicated.

Primary adenocarcinoma

Primary adenocarcinoma of the appendix is extremely rare. It is usually of the colonic type and should be treated by right

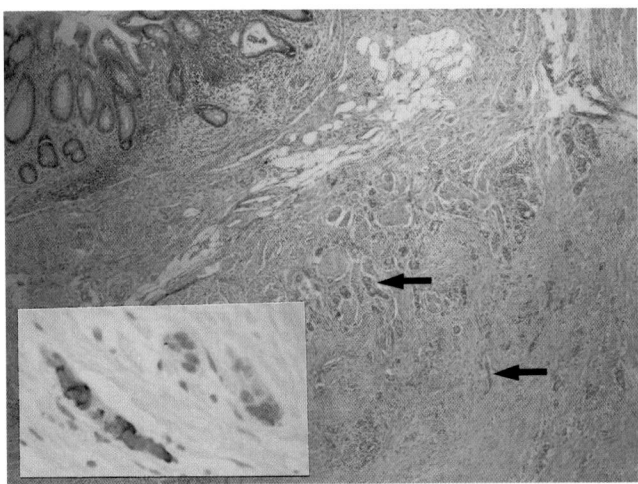

Figure 67.19 Carcinoid tumour. A small incidental carcinoid tumour of the appendix. The tumour cells infiltrate the muscle arranged in small nests and trabeculae (arrows). Tumour cells are small and have inconspicuous nuclei. Inset: higher magnification of an immunohistochemical stain for chromogranin B shows a strong positive reaction (brown) of tumour cells (courtesy of Dr P. Kelly, FRCPath, Dublin, Ireland).

CHAPTER 67 | THE VERMIFORM APPENDIX

hemicolectomy (as a second-stage procedure if the condition is not recognised at the first operation). A mucus-secreting adenocarcinoma of the appendix may rupture into the peritoneal cavity, seeding it with mucus-secreting malignant cells. Presentation is often delayed until the patient has gross abdominal distension as a result of pseudomyxoma peritoneii, which may mimic ascites. Treatment consists of radical resection of all involved parietal peritoneal surfaces and aggressive intraperitoneal chemotherapy (Sugarbaker).

FURTHER READING

Andersen, B.R., Kallehave, F.L. and Andersen, H.K. (2005) Antibiotics versus placebo for prevention of postoperative infection after appendicectomy. *Cochrane Database of Systematic Reviews* Issue 3, Art. No. CD001439. DOI: 10.1002/14651858.CD001439.pub2. (http://www.cochrane.org).

Berry, J. and Malt, R.A. (1984) Appendicitis near its centenary. *Am J Surg* **200**: 567–75.

Kaminski, A., Liu, I.L., Applebaum, H. et al. (2005) Routine interval appendectomy is not justified after initial non-operative treatment of acute appendicitis. *Arch Surg* **140**: 897–901.

Murphy, E.M.A., Farquharson, S.M. and Moran, B.J. (2006) Management of an unexpected appendiceal neoplasm. *Br J Surg* **93**: 783–92.

Rao, P.M., Rhea, J.T., Rattner, D.W. *et al.* (1999) Introduction of appendiceal CT: impact on negative appendectomy and appendiceal perforation rates. *Ann Surg* **229**: 334–49.

Rothrock, S.G. and Pagane, J.P. (2000) Acute appendicitis in children: emergency department diagnosis and management. *Ann Emerg Med* **36**: 39–51.

Sauerland, S., Lefering, R. and Neugebauer, E.A.M. (2004) Laparoscopic versus open surgery for suspected appendicitis. *Cochrane Database of Systematic Reviews* Issue 4, Art. No. CD001546. DOI: 10.1002/14651858.CD001546.pub2. (http://www.cochrane.org).

The rectum

LEARNING OBJECTIVES

To understand:
- The anatomy of the rectum and its relationship to surgical disease and its treatment
- The pathology, clinical presentation, investigation, differential diagnosis and treatment of diseases that affect the rectum

To appreciate that:
- Carcinoma of the rectum is common and its symptoms are similar to those of benign disease and, hence, patients with such symptoms must be carefully evaluated

ANATOMY

Surgical anatomy

The rectum begins where the taenia coli of the sigmoid colon join to form a continuous outer longitudinal muscle layer at the level of the sacral promontory. The rectum follows the curve of the sacrum, to end at the anorectal junction. The puborectalis muscle encircles the posterior and lateral aspects of the junction, creating the anorectal angle (normally 120°). The rectum has three lateral curvatures: the upper and lower are convex to the right, and the middle is convex to the left. On the luminal aspect, these three curves are marked by semicircular folds (Houston's valves) (Fig. 68.1). That part of the rectum that lies below the middle valve has a much wider diameter than the upper third and is known as the ampulla of the rectum.

The adult rectum is approximately 12–18 cm in length and is conveniently divided into three equal parts: the upper third, which is mobile and has a peritoneal coat; the middle third where the peritoneum covers only the anterior and part of the lateral surfaces; and the lowest third, which lies deep in the pelvis surrounded by fatty mesorectum and has important relations to fascial layers.

The lower third of the rectum is separated by a fascial condensation – Denonvilliers' fascia – from the prostate/vagina in front, and behind by another fascial layer – Waldeyer's fascia – from the coccyx and lower two sacral vertebrae (Table 68.1). These fascial layers are surgically important as they are a barrier to malignant invasion (Summary box 68.1).

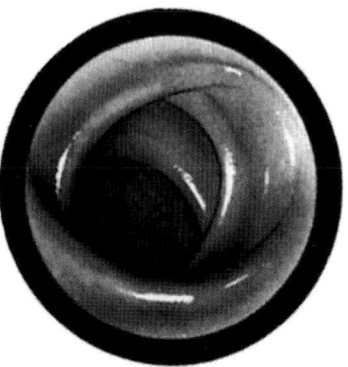

Figure 68.1 Houston's valves as seen through a sigmoidoscope.

Table 68.1 Relations of the rectum

	Male	Female
Anterior	Bladder	Pouch of Douglas
	Seminal vesicles	Uterus
	Ureters	Cervix
	Prostate	Posterior vaginal wall
	Urethra	
Lateral	Lateral ligaments	Lateral ligaments
	Middle rectal artery	Middle rectal artery
	Obturator internus muscle	Obturator internus muscle
	Side wall of pelvis	Side wall of pelvis
	Pelvic autonomic plexus	Pelvic autonomic plexus
	Levator ani muscle	Levator ani muscle
Posterior	Sacrum and coccyx	Sacrum and coccyx
	Loose areolar tissue	Loose areolar tissue
	Fascial condensation	Fascial condensation
	Superior rectal artery	Superior rectal artery
	Hypogastric nerves	Hypogastric nerves
	Lymphatics	Lymphatics

John Houston, **1802–1845, Physician, City of Dublin Hospital and Lecturer in Surgery, Dublin, Ireland.**
Charles Pierre Denonvilliers, **1808–1872, Professor of Anatomy and later of Surgery, Paris, France.**
Heinrich Wilhelm Gottfried Waldeyer-Hartz, **1836–1921, Professor of Pathological Anatomy, Berlin, Germany.**

James Douglas, **1675–1742, Anatomist and Male Midwife, London, UK.**

> **Summary box 68.1**
>
> **Anatomy of the rectum**
>
> - The rectum measures approximately 15 cm in length
> - It is divided into lower, middle and upper thirds
> - The blood supply consists of inferior, middle and superior rectal vessels
> - Although the lymphatic drainage follows the blood supply, the principal route is upwards along the superior rectal vessels to the para-aortic nodes

Blood supply

The superior rectal artery is the direct continuation of the inferior mesenteric artery and is the main arterial supply of the rectum. The arteries and their accompanying lymphatics lie within the loose fatty tissue of the mesorectum, surrounded by a sheath of connective tissue (the mesorectal fascia).

The *middle rectal artery* arises on each side from the internal iliac artery (Fig. 68.2) and passes to the rectum in the lateral ligaments. It is usually small and breaks up into several terminal branches.

The *inferior rectal artery* arises on each side from the internal pudendal artery as it enters Alcock's canal. It hugs the inferior surface of the levator ani muscle as it crosses the roof of the ischiorectal fossa to enter the anal muscles (Fig. 68.2).

Venous drainage

The superior haemorrhoidal veins draining the upper half of the anal canal above the dentate line pass upwards to become the rectal veins: these unite to form the *superior rectal vein,* which later becomes the *inferior mesenteric vein.* This forms part of the portal venous system and ultimately drains into the splenic vein. Middle rectal veins exist but are small, unimportant channels unless the normal paths are blocked.

Lymphatic drainage

The lymphatics of the mucosal lining of the rectum communicate freely with those of the muscular layers. The usual drainage flow is *upwards,* and only to a limited extent laterally and downwards. For this reason, surgical ablation of malignant disease concentrates mainly on achieving wide clearance of proximal lymph nodes. However, if the usual upwards routes are blocked (e.g. by

carcinoma), flow can reverse, and it is then possible to find metastatic lymph nodes on the side walls of the pelvis (along the middle rectal vessels) or even in the inguinal region (along the inferior rectal artery).

CLINICAL FEATURES OF RECTAL DISEASE

Symptoms

Rectal diseases are common and serious and can occur at any age. The symptoms of many of them overlap. In general, the inflammations affect younger age groups, while the tumours occur in the middle-aged and elderly. But no age is exempt from any of the diseases, however young: ulcerative colitis has been reported in the newborn and rectal cancer can occur in young people. The common symptoms of rectal disease are shown in Summary box 68.2.

> **Summary box 68.2**
>
> **Main symptoms of rectal disease**
>
> - Bleeding per rectum
> - Altered bowel habit
> - Mucus discharge
> - Tenesmus
> - Prolapse

Bleeding

This is often bright red in colour but may be darker, and should be carefully investigated at any age.

Altered bowel habit

Early-morning stool frequency ('spurious diarrhoea') is a symptom of rectal carcinoma, while blood-stained frequent loose stools characterise the inflammatory diseases.

Discharge

Mucus and pus are associated with rectal pathology.

Tenesmus

Often described by the patient as 'I feel I want to go but nothing happens', this is normally an ominous symptom of rectal cancer but can occur with any rectal pathology.

Prolapse

This usually indicates either mucosal or full-thickness rectal wall descent.

Loss of weight

This usually indicates serious or advanced disease, e.g. hepatic metastases.

Signs

Because the rectum is accessible via the anus, these can be elicited by systematic examination. The patient is either positioned in the left lateral (Sims') position or examined in the knee–elbow position (Fig. 68.3).

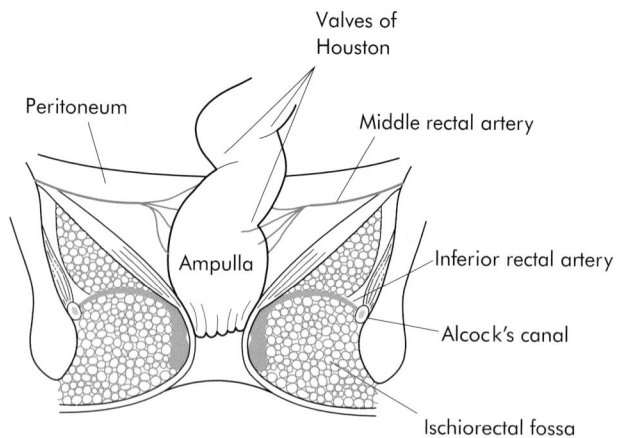

Figure 68.2 The rectum lying in the pelvis (coronal view). Note the curvatures corresponding to Houston's valves.

> James Marion Sims, 1813–1883, Gynaecological Surgeon, the State Hospital for Women, New York, NY, USA, introduced this position to give access to the anterior vaginal wall during operations for the closure of vagino-vesical fistulae.

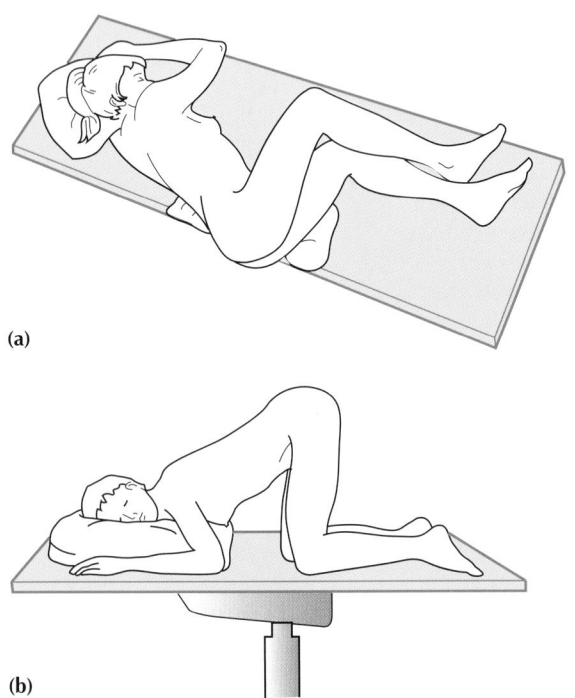

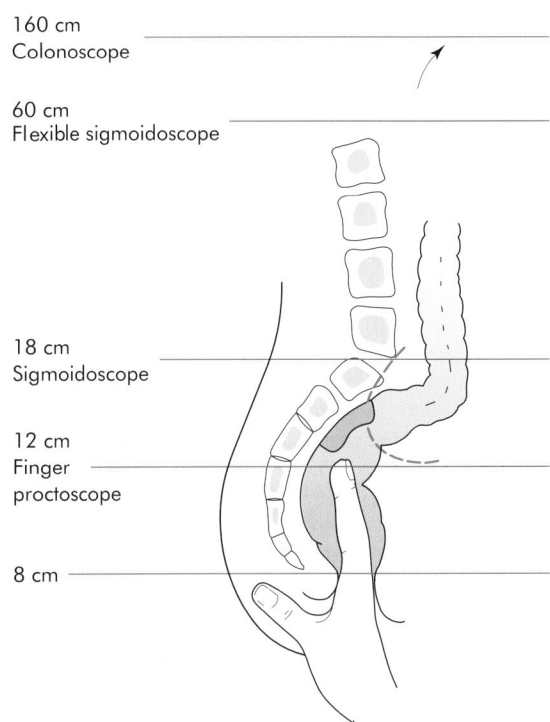

Figure 68.3 Positions for digital rectal examination. (a) Left lateral (Sims). (b) Knee–elbow. [Redrawn with permission from Corman, M.L. (1992) *Colon and Rectal Surgery*, 3rd edn. J.B. Lippincott Co., London].

Figure 68.4 Illustration showing how the various methods of examining the rectum reach different levels. Note that even cancers in the upper part of the rectum can be felt with the index finger, especially if the patient is asked to 'strain down' (courtesy of C.V. Mann).

Inspection

Visual examination of the anus precedes rectal examination to exclude the presence of anal disease, e.g. fissure or fistula.

Digital examination

The index finger used with gentleness and precision remains a valuable test for rectal disease (Fig. 68.4). Tumours in the lower and middle thirds of the rectum can be felt and assessed; by asking the patient to strain, even some tumours in the upper third can be 'tipped' with the finger. After it is removed, the finger should be examined for tell-tale traces of mucus, pus or blood. It

is always useful to note the normal as well as the abnormal findings on digital examination, e.g. the prostate in the male. Digital findings can be recorded as intraluminal (e.g. blood, pus), intramural (e.g. tumours, granular areas, strictures) or extramural (e.g. enlarged prostate, uterine fibroids).

Proctoscopy

This procedure can be used to inspect the anus, anorectal junction and lower rectum (up to 10 cm) (Fig. 68.5). Biopsy can be performed of any suspicious areas.

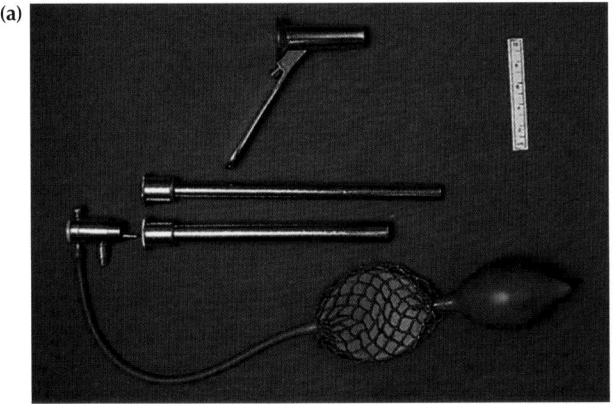

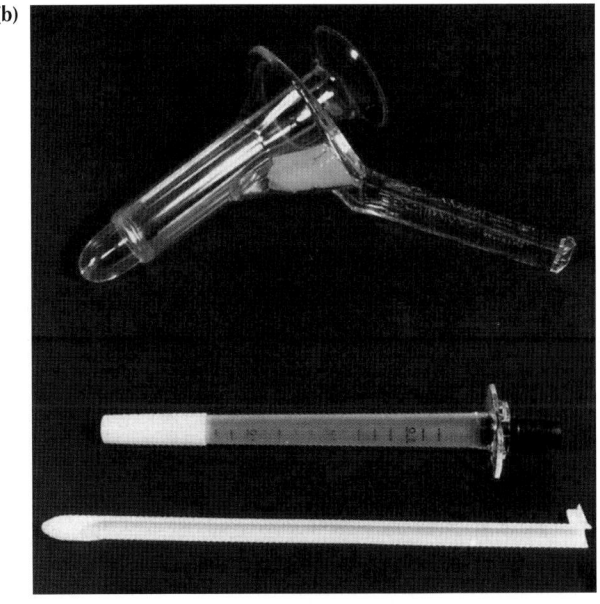

Figure 68.5 (a) A metal proctoscope and two different-sized metal Lloyd-Davies rigid sigmoidoscopes – small (diameter 20 mm). Since the advent of greater awareness of transmitted infection, disposable proctoscopes and sigmoidoscopes (b) have replaced the re-usable metal types.

CHAPTER 68 | THE RECTUM

Sigmoidoscopy

The sigmoidoscope was in the past a rigid stainless steel instrument of variable diameter and normally 25 cm in length (Fig. 68.5). This has in the main been replaced by a disposable plastic instrument. The rectum must be empty for proper inspection with a sigmoidoscope. Gentleness and skill are required for its use, and perforations can occur if care is not exercised.

Flexible sigmoidoscope

The 'flexiscope' can be used to supplement or replace rigid sigmoidoscopy (Fig. 68.6). It requires special skill and experience, and the lower bowel should be cleaned out with preliminary enemas. In addition to the rectum, the whole sigmoid colon is within visual reach of this instrument. The instrument is expensive and requires careful maintenance (Summary box 68.3).

Summary box 68.3

Examination of the rectum

- Visual inspection of the perineum
- Digital examination
- Proctoscopy
- Sigmoidoscopy – rigid or flexible

INJURIES

The rectum or anal canal may be injured in a number of ways, all uncommon:

- by falling in a sitting posture onto pointed object: the upturned leg of a chair, handle of a broom, floor-mop, pitchfork or a broken shooting stick have all resulted in rectal impalement;
- by penetrating injury (including gunshots) to the buttocks;
- by sexual assault or sexual activity involving anal penetration;
- by the fetal head during childbirth, especially forceps-assisted.

Diagnosis

The anus should be inspected and the abdomen palpated. If rigidity or tenderness is present, early laparotomy is imperative. A water-soluble contrast enema or computerised tomography (CT) scan with rectal contrast is useful to identify perforation. Prior to the operation, a urethral catheter is passed, but if there is any possibility of urethral injury (suggested by difficulty passing urine or haematuria), a urethrogram should be performed (see Chapters 72 and 74).

Treatment

If perforation is suspected, the rectum is examined under general anaesthetic with a finger and a speculum, particular attention being directed to the anterior wall. If penetrating injury is confirmed, lower laparotomy is then performed. If an intraperitoneal rupture of the rectum is found, the perforation is closed with sutures. After closing the laparotomy wound, a defunctioning colostomy is usually required, constructed in the left iliac fossa. If the rectal injury is below the peritoneal reflection, wide drainage from below is indicated, with rectal washout and a defunctioning colostomy. If the defect in the rectum is very large, resection may have to be contemplated, usually in the form of a Hartmann's procedure. Care must be taken to preserve sphincter function during debridement of the perineal wounds. Antibiotic cover must be provided against both aerobic and anaerobic organisms.

FOREIGN BODIES IN THE RECTUM

The variety of foreign bodies that have found their way into the rectum is hardly less remarkable than the ingenuity displayed in their removal (Fig. 68.7). A turnip has been delivered per anum by the use of obstetric forceps. A large soft rubber sex toy has been withdrawn by inserting a myomectomy screw into its lower end. A tumbler, mouth looking downwards, has been extracted by filling the interior with a wet plaster of Paris bandage, leaving the end of the bandage protruding and allowing the plaster to set.

If insurmountable difficulty is experienced in grasping any foreign body in the rectum, a laparotomy is usually necessary, which allows that object to be pushed from above into the assistant's fingers in the rectum. If there is considerable laceration of the mucosa, a temporary colostomy is advisable (Summary box 68.4).

Summary box 68.4

Injuries to the rectum are serious and invariably require surgery

- A temporary colostomy is often necessary
- There is a serious risk of associated necrotising fasciitis, and broad-spectrum antibiotics are mandatory
- There may be associated bladder or urethral damage

PROLAPSE

Mucosal prolapse

The mucous membrane and submucosa of the rectum protrude outside the anus for approximately 1–4 cm. When the prolapsed mucosa is palpated between the finger and thumb, it is evident that it is composed of no more than a double layer of mucous membrane (cf. full-thickness prolapse) (Summary box 68.5).

Henri Albert Charles Antoine Hartmann, **1860–1952. Professor of Clinical Surgery, Paris, France.**

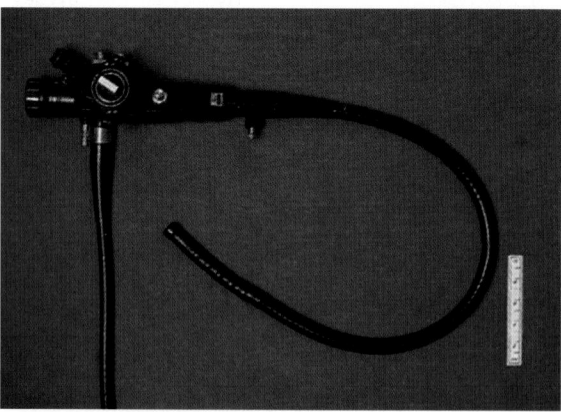

Figure 68.6 The flexible (60 cm) endoscope ('flexiscope').

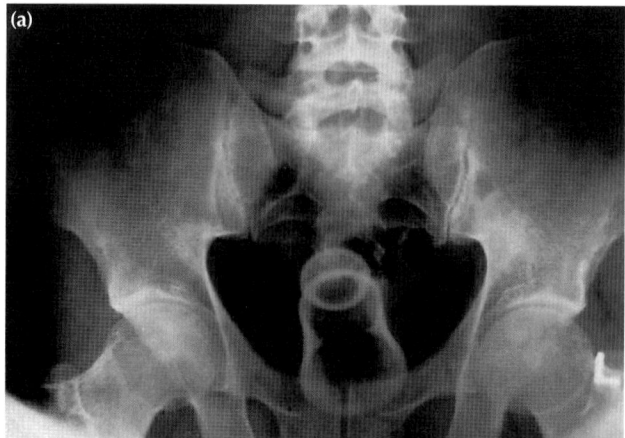

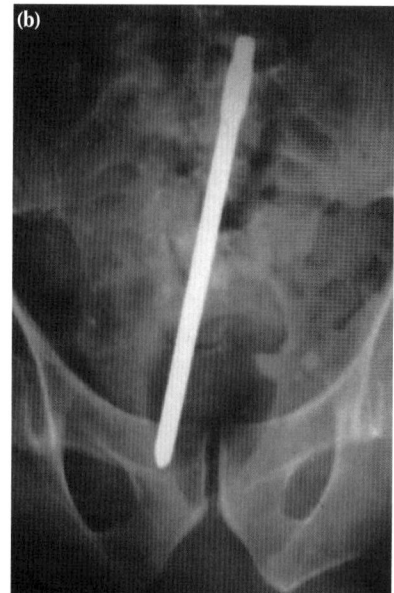

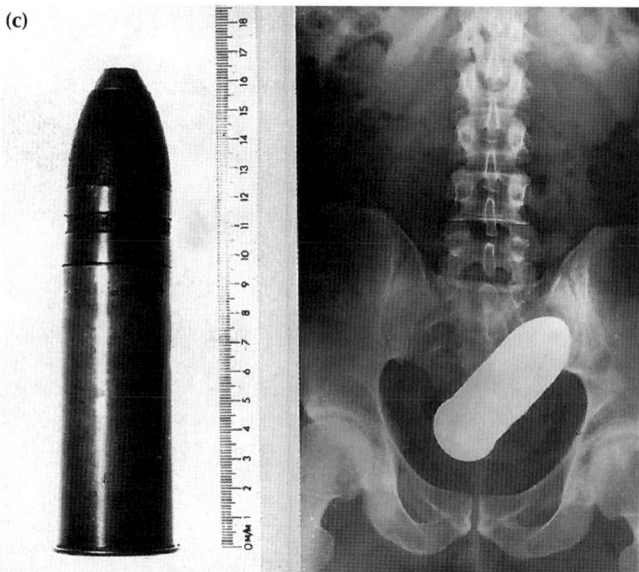

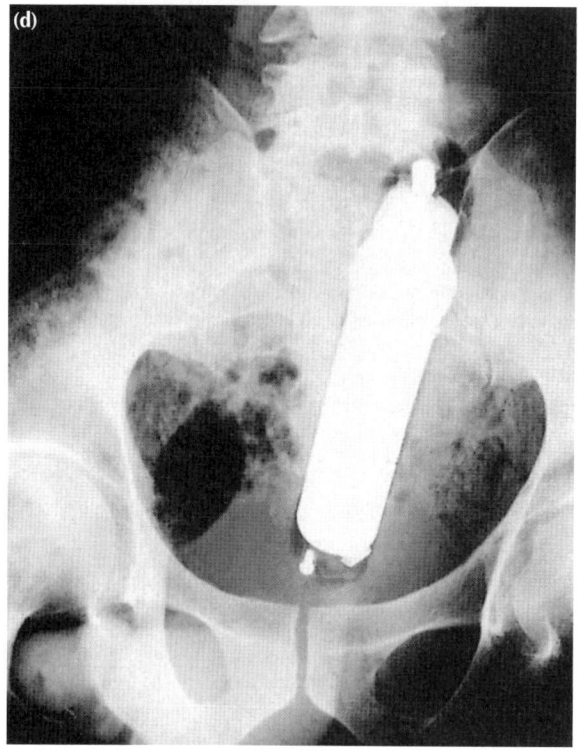

Figure 68.7 (a) Pepper pot in the rectum. On removal, it was found to be inscribed 'A present from Margate' (courtesy of Dr L.S. Carstairs, Royal Northern Hospital, London). (b) A screwdriver with a plastic handle (courtesy of Dr A.K. Sharma, Agra, India). (c) A live shell, which needed careful handling. (d) A large vibrator, which had pierced the lateral intraperitoneal rectal wall and caused peritonitis.

Summary box 68.5

Rectal prolapse

- It may be mucosal or full thickness
- If full thickness, the whole wall of the rectum is included
- It commences as a rectal intussusception
- In children, the prolapse is usually mucosal and should be treated conservatively
- In the adult, the prolapse is often full thickness and is frequently associated with incontinence
- Surgery is necessary for full-thickness rectal prolapse
- The operation is performed either via the perineum or via the abdomen

In infants

The direct downward course of the rectum, due to the as yet undeveloped sacral curve (Fig. 68.8), predisposes to this condition, as does the reduced resting anal tone, which offers diminished support to the mucosal lining of the anal canal (Mann).

In children

Mucosal prolapse often commences after an attack of diarrhoea, or from loss of weight and consequent loss of fat in the ischiorectal

Charles Victor Mann, Formerly Surgeon, St Mark's Hospital and the Royal London Hospital, London, UK.

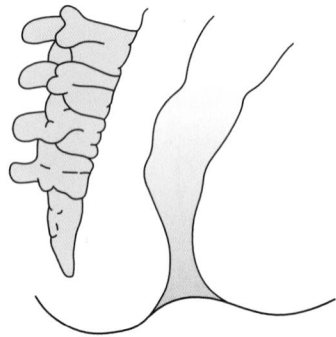

Figure 68.8 The absence of the normal sacral curve predisposes to rectal prolapse in an infant.

fossae. It may also be associated with fibrocystic disease, neurological causes and maldevelopment of the pelvis.

In adults

The condition in adults is often associated with third-degree haemorrhoids. In the female a torn perineum, and in the male straining from urethral obstruction, predisposes to mucosal prolapse. In old age, both mucosal and full-thickness prolapse are associated with atony of the sphincter mechanism, but whether this is the cause of the problem or secondary to it is unknown.

Partial prolapse may follow an operation for fistula *in ano* where a large portion of muscle has been divided. Here, the prolapse is usually localised to the damaged quadrant and is seldom progressive.

Prolapsed mucous membrane is pink; prolapsed internal haemorrhoids are plum coloured and more pedunculated.

Treatment

In infants and young children

Digital repositioning

The parents are taught to replace the protrusion, and any underlying causes are addressed.

Submucosal injections

If digital repositioning fails after 6 weeks' trial, injections of 5% phenol in almond oil are carried out under general anaesthestic. As a result of the aseptic inflammation following these injections, the mucous membrane becomes tethered to the muscle coat.

Surgery

Occasionally, surgery is required and, in such cases, the child is placed in the prone jack-knife position, the retrorectal space is entered, and the rectum is sutured to the sacrum.

In adults

Local treatments

Submucosal injections of phenol in almond oil or the application of rubber bands are sometimes successful in cases of mucosal prolapse.

Excision of the prolapsed mucosa

When the prolapse is unilateral, the redundant mucosa can be excised or, if circumferential, an endoluminal stapling technique can be used.

Full-thickness prolapse

Full-thickness prolapse (synonym: procidentia) is less common than the mucosal variety. The protrusion consists of all layers of the rectal wall and is usually associated with a weak pelvic floor. The prolapse is thought to commence as an intussusception of the rectum, which descends to protrude outside the anus. The process starts with the anterior wall of the rectum, where the supporting tissues are weakest, especially in women. It is more than 4 cm and commonly as much as 10–15 cm in length (Fig. 68.9). On palpation between the finger and thumb, the prolapse feels much thicker than a mucosal prolapse, and obviously consists of a double thickness of the entire wall of the rectum. Any prolapse over 5 cm in length contains anteriorly between its layers a pouch of peritoneum (Fig. 68.10). When large, the peritoneal pouch contains small intestine, which returns to the general peritoneal cavity with a characteristic gurgle when the prolapse is reduced. The anal sphincter is characteristically patulous and gapes widely on straining to allow the rectum to prolapse. Complete prolapse is uncommon in children. In adults, it can occur at any age, but it is more common in the elderly. Women are affected six times more often than men, and it is commonly associated with prolapse of the uterus. In the Middle East and Asia, complete rectal prolapse is not uncommon in young males. In approximately 50% of adults, faecal incontinence is also a feature.

Differential diagnosis

In the case of a child with abdominal pain, prolapse of the rectum must be distinguished from *ileocaecal intussusception* protruding from the anus. Figures 68.11 and 68.12 make the differential

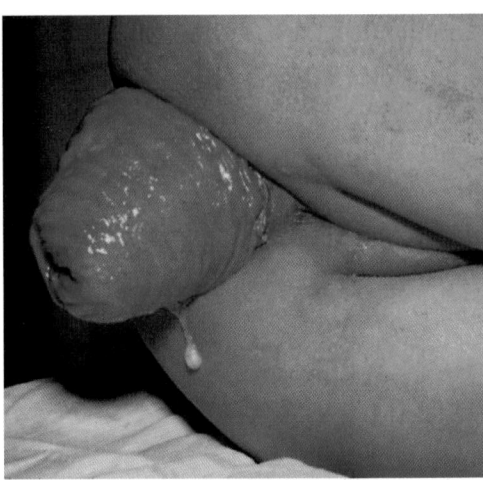

Figure 68.9 Full-thickness rectal prolapse (courtesy of G.D. Adhia, Bombay, India).

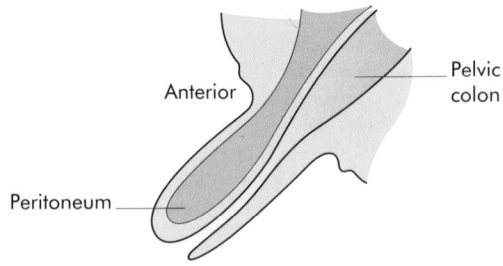

Figure 68.10 Rectal prolapse containing a pouch of peritoneum.

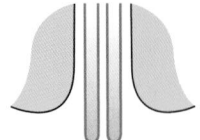

Figure 68.11 Intussusception protruding from the anus.

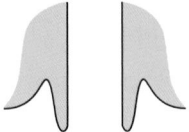

Figure 68.12 Partial prolapse of the rectum.

diagnosis clear. In *rectosigmoid intussusception* in the adult, there is a deep groove (5 cm or more) between the emerging protruding mass and the margin of the anus, into which the finger can be placed.

Treatment

Surgery is required, and the operation can be performed via the perineal or the abdominal approaches. An abdominal rectopexy has a lower rate of recurrence but, when the patient is elderly and very frail, a perineal operation is indicated. As an abdominal procedure risks damage to the pelvic autonomic nerves, resulting in possible sexual dysfunction, a perineal approach is also usually preferred in young men.

Perineal approach
These procedures have been used most commonly.

Thiersch operation
This procedure, which aimed to place a steel wire or, more commonly, a silastic or nylon suture around the anal canal, has become obsolete. The reasons for its lack of popularity were that the suture would often break or cause chronic perineal sepsis, or both, or the anal stenosis so created would produce severe functional problems. Delorme's operation is now the preferred perineal operation.

Delorme's operation (Fig. 68.13)
In this procedure, the rectal mucosa is removed circumferentially from the prolapsed rectum over its length. The underlying muscle is then plicated with a series of sutures, such that, when these are tied, the rectal muscle is concertinaed towards the anal canal. The anal canal mucosa is then sutured circumferentially to the rectal mucosa remaining at the tip of the prolapse. The prolapse is reduced, and a ring of muscle is created above the anal canal, which prevents recurrence.

Altemeier's procedure
This consists of excision of the prolapsed rectum and associated sigmoid colon from below, and construction of a coloanal anastomosis.

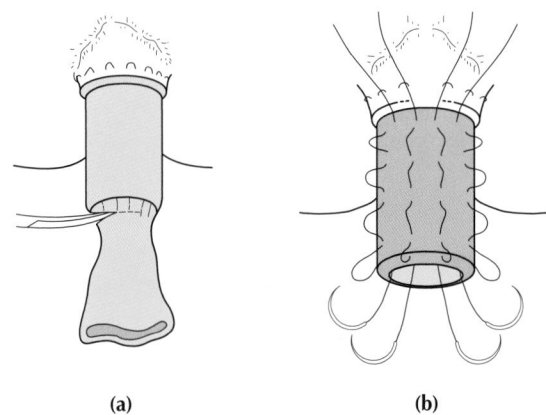

(a)   (b)

Figure 68.13 Delorme's operation for rectal prolapse. (a) The mucosa has been removed from the prolapse. (b) Interrupted sutures have been placed in the underlying muscle so that, when tied, the muscle is plicated. [Redrawn with permission from Keighley, M.R.B. and Williams, N.S. (1999) *Surgery of the Anus, Rectum and Colon*. W.B. Saunders, London].

Abdominal approach
The principle of all abdominal operations for rectal prolapse is to replace and hold the rectum in its proper position. They are recommended in patients with complete prolapse who are otherwise in good health. Many variations have been described: in *Wells' operation*, the rectum is fixed firmly to the sacrum by inserting a sheet of polypropylene mesh between them; *Ripstein's operation* involves hitching up the rectosigmoid junction by a Teflon sling to the front of the sacrum (Fig. 68.14); many surgeons simply suture the mobilised rectum to the sacrum using four to six interrupted non-absorbable sutures – so called sutured rectopexy. Recently, the technique has been performed laparoscopically, thus reducing the operative trauma and limiting the time in hospital.

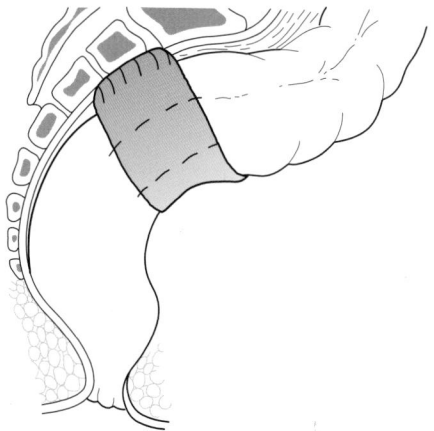

Figure 68.14 Abdominal rectopexy for rectal prolapse. The rectum is mobilised and fixed to the sacrum with a sheet of polypropylene mesh. [Redrawn with permission from Corman, M.L. (1992) *Colon and Rectal Surgery*, 3rd edn. J.B. Lippincott Co., London].

As an abdominal rectopexy may lead to severe constipation, some surgeons recommend combining this procedure with resection of the sigmoid colon (Goldberg), so called resection rectopexy. Approximately 50% of adult patients with a complete rectal prolapse are incontinent, and rectopexy cures only about one-third.

PROCTITIS

Inflammation is sometimes limited to the rectal mucosa; in other cases, it is associated with a similar condition in the colon (proctocolitis). The inflammation can be acute or chronic. The symptoms are tenesmus and the passage of blood and mucus and, in severe cases, of pus also. Although the patient has a frequent intense desire to defaecate, the amount of faeces passed at a time is small. Acute proctitis is usually accompanied by malaise and pyrexia. On rectal examination, the mucosa feels swollen and is often tender. Proctoscopy is seldom sufficient, and sigmoidoscopy is the more valuable method of examination. If the diagnosis is confirmed, colonoscopy with multiple biopsies is mandatory, to determine the extent of the inflammatory process. Skilled pathological assessment is required to establish or exclude the diagnosis of specific infection by bacteriological examination and culture of the stools, examination of scrapings or swabs from ulcers and serological tests.

Non-specific proctitis is an inflammatory condition affecting the mucosa and, to a lesser extent, the submucosa, confined to the distal rectum. In 10% of cases, the condition extends to involve the whole colon (total ulcerative colitis) (Summary box 68.6).

Summary box 68.6

Proctitis

- May be non-specific or related to a specific infective agent
- Non-specific proctitis usually remains confined to the distal bowel, but can spread to the proximal colon
- Causes bleeding, diarrhoea and tenesmus
- Treatment is usually conservative

Aetiology

This is unknown. The concept that the condition is a mild and limited form of ulcerative colitis (although actual ulceration is often not present) is the most acceptable hypothesis.

Clinical features

The patient is usually middle-aged and complains of slight loss of blood in the motions. Often, the complaint is one of diarrhoea but, on closer questioning, it transpires that usually one relatively normal action of the bowels occurs each day, although it is accompanied by some blood. During the day, the patient attempts to defaecate, with the passage of flatus and a little blood-stained faecal matter, which is interpreted as diarrhoea. On rectal examination, the mucosa feels warm and smooth. Often, there is some blood on the examining finger. Proctoscopic and sigmoidoscopic examination shows inflamed mucosa of the rectum, but usually no ulceration. The inflammation usually extends for only 5–15 cm from the anus, with the mucosa above this level being normal.

Treatment

The condition is usually self-limiting, but treatment with topical 5-aminosalicylic acid compounds (5-ASA) (Asacol, Penasa) in the form of suppositories or foam enemas is effective. Topical steroids are a less effective alternative. In very severe resistant cases, oral steroids may have to be used to obtain remission. Rarely, surgical treatment is required as a last resort when the patient is desperate for relief of symptoms.

Ulcerative proctocolitis

Proctitis is present in a high percentage of cases of ulcerative colitis, and the degree of severity of the rectal involvement may influence the type of operative procedure (see Chapter 65).

Proctitis due to Crohn's disease

Crohn's disease can occasionally affect the rectum, although classically it is spared. Sigmoidoscopic characteristics differ from those in non-specific proctitis. The inflammatory process tends to be patchy rather than confluent, and there may be fissuring, ulceration and even a cobblestone appearance. Rectal Crohn's disease is often associated with severe perineal disease characterised by fistulation. Skip lesions are also often present in the rest of the colon or small bowel, or both.

Proctitis due to specific infections
Clostridium difficile

An acute form of proctocolitis caused by infection with *Clostridium difficile* can follow broad-spectrum antibiotic administration. A 'membrane' can sometimes be seen on proctoscopy ('pseudomembranous' colitis).

Bacillary dysentery

The appearance is that of an acute purulent proctitis with multiple small, shallow ulcers. The examination of a swab taken from the ulcerated mucous membrane is more certainly diagnostic than stool microscopy.

Amoebic dysentery

The infection is more liable to be chronic, and exacerbations after a long period of freedom from symptoms often occur. Proctoscopy and sigmoidoscopy are not painful. The appearance of an amoebic ulcer is described in Chapter 65. Scrapings from the ulcer should be immersed in warm isotonic saline solution and sent to the laboratory for immediate microscopic examination.

Amoebic granuloma

This presents as a soft mass, usually in the rectosigmoid region. This lesion is frequently mistaken for a carcinoma. Sigmoidoscopy shows an ulcerated surface, but the mass is less friable than a carcinoma. A scraping should be taken, preferably with a small, sharp spoon on a long handle, and the material sent for immediate microscopic examination, as detailed above. A biopsy can also help. Treatment is as described in Chapter 65. Amoebic granuloma of the rectum is encountered from time to time in a patient who has never visited a country in which the disease is endemic.

Burrill Bernard Crohn, 1884–1956, Gastroenterologist, Mount Sinai Hospital, New York, NY, USA, described regional ileitis in 1932.

Tuberculous proctitis

This is nearly always associated with active pulmonary tuberculosis or tuberculous ulceration of the anus. Submucous rectal abscesses burst and leave ulcers with an undermined edge. A hypertrophic type of tuberculous proctitis occurs in association with tuberculous peritonitis, or tuberculous proctitis occurs in association with tuberculous peritonitis or tuberculous salpingitis. This type of tuberculous proctitis requires biopsy for confirmation of the diagnosis.

Gonococcal proctitis

Gonococcal proctitis occurs in both sexes as the result of rectal coitus and, in the female, from direct spread from the vulva. In the acute stage, the mucous membrane is hyperaemic, and thick pus can be expressed as the proctoscope is withdrawn. In the early stages, the diagnosis can be readily established by bacteriological examination but, later, when the infection is mixed, it is more difficult to recognise. Systemic treatment is so effective that local treatment is unnecessary.

Lymphogranuloma venereum

The modes of infection are similar to those of gonococcal proctitis but, in the female, chlamydial infection spreading from the cervix uteri via lymphatics to the pararectal lymph nodes is common. The proctological findings are similar to those of gonococcal proctitis. The diagnosis of lymphogranuloma venereum should be suspected when the inguinal lymph nodes are greatly enlarged, although the enlargement may be subsiding by the time proctitis commences.

Acquired immunodeficiency syndrome

Acquired immunodeficiency syndrome (AIDS) may present with a particularly florid type of proctitis. In such patients, unusual organisms such as cytomegalovirus (CMV), herpes simplex virus and organisms such as *Cryptosporidium* are often found.

'Strawberry' lesion of the rectosigmoid

This results from an infection by *Spirochaeta vincenti* and *Bacillus fusiformis*. The leading symptom is diarrhoea, often scantily blood-stained. Occasionally, the diagnosis can be made by the demonstration of the specific organisms in the stools. More often, sigmoidoscopy is required. The characteristic lesion is thickened, somewhat raised mucosa with superficial ulceration in the region of the rectosigmoid. The inflamed mucous membrane oozes blood at numerous pinpoints, giving the appearance of an over-ripe strawberry. A swab should be taken from the lesion and examined for Vincent's and fusiform organisms. Swabs from the gums and the throat are also advisable.

Rectal bilharziasis

Rectal bilharziasis is caused by *Schistosoma mansoni*, which is endemic in many tropical and subtropical countries, and particularly in the delta of the Nile.

In stage 1, a cutaneous lesion develops at the site of entrance of the cercariae (parasites of freshwater snails). Stage 2 is characterised by pyrexia, urticaria and a high eosinophilia. Both these

stages are frequently overlooked. Stage 3 results from deposition of the ova in the rectum (much more rarely in the bladder; Chapter 72) and is manifested by bilharzial dysentery. On examination in the later stages, papillomas are frequently present. The papillomas, which are sessile or pedunculated, contain the ova of the trematode, the life cycle of which resembles that of *Schistosoma haematobium*.

Untreated, the rectum becomes festooned, and prolapse of the diseased mucous membrane is usual. Multiple fistulae *in ano* are prone to develop.

Treatment

The primary treatment is systemic and should be undertaken by a specialist in tropical medicine. When the papillomas persist in spite of general treatment, they should be treated by local destruction.

Proctitis due to herbal enemas

This is a well-known clinical entity to those practising in tropical Africa. Following an enema consisting of a concoction of ginger, pepper and bark, administered by a witch doctor, a virulent proctitis sets in. Pelvic peritonitis frequently supervenes. Not infrequently, a complete gelatinous cast of the mucous membrane of the rectum is extruded. Very large doses of morphine, together with streptomycin, often prevent a fatal outcome if commenced early (Bowesman). Temporary colostomy is often advisable.

Treatment

General treatments should include bed rest in extreme cases. The stools should be kept soft. Suppositories of 5-ASA are often beneficial. Infective causes require specific treatment.

SOLITARY RECTAL ULCER

This is becoming a more commonly diagnosed problem. Classically, it takes the form of an ulcer on the anterior wall of the rectum. In this form, it must be differentiated from a rectal carcinoma or inflammatory bowel disease, particularly Crohn's disease. In recent years, it has been appreciated that the ulceration may heal, leaving a polypoid appearance. A variety of explanations as to its cause has been suggested, including persistent trauma by anal digitation. However, recent proctographic studies indicate that it may be due to a combination of internal intussusception or anterior rectal wall prolapse and an increase in intrarectal pressure. This combination of factors is usually caused by chronic straining as a result of constipation. The histological appearances confirm the diagnosis (Morson) and are similar to the appearances of biopsies from a full-thickness overt rectal prolapse. The condition, although benign, is difficult to treat. Symptomatic relief from bleeding and discharge may sometimes be achieved by preventing the internal prolapse by biofeedback, an intrarectal stapling procedure or an abdominal rectopexy. In rare cases, rectal excision may be required.

Jean Hyacinthe Vincent, 1862–1950, Professor of Epidemiology, Val-de-Grace Military Hospital, Paris, France.

Theodor Maximillan Bilharz, 1825–1862, Professor of Zoology, Cairo, Egypt.
Charles Bowesman, ?1907–1993, Surgical Specialist, Colonial Medical Service, Kumasi, Ghana.

BENIGN TUMOURS

The rectum, along with the sigmoid colon, is the most frequent site of polyps (and cancers) in the gastrointestinal tract. Adenomatous polyps of the colon and rectum have the potential to become malignant. The chance of developing invasive cancer is enhanced if the polyp is more than 1 cm in diameter. Removal of all polyps is recommended to give complete histological examination and exclude (or confirm) carcinoma, and also to prevent local recurrence. This is best done using endoscopic hot biopsy or snare polypectomy techniques. If one or more rectal polyps are discovered on sigmoidoscopic examination, a colonoscopy must be performed, as further polyps are frequently found in the colon and treatment may be influenced. *No rectal polyp should be removed until the possibility of a proximal carcinoma has been ruled out, otherwise local implantation of cancer cells may occur in the distally situated rectal wound.*

The rectum shares substantially the same spectrum of polyps as the colon. Polyps are described chiefly in terms of their tissue organisation. Certain polyps that have features relevant to the rectum are now described.

Polyps relevant to the rectum

Juvenile polyp

This is a bright-red glistening pedunculated sphere ('cherry tumour'), which is found in infants and children. Occasionally, it persists into adult life. It can cause bleeding, or pain if it prolapses during defaecation. It often separates itself, but can be removed easily with forceps or a snare. A solitary juvenile polyp has virtually no tendency to malignant change, but should be treated if it is causing symptoms. It has a unique histological structure of large mucus-filled spaces covered by a smooth surface of thin rectal cuboidal epithelium (Fig. 68.15). The rare autosomal dominantly inherited syndrome juvenile polyposis does confer an increased risk of gastrointestinal cancers. It is characterised by multiple juvenile polyps and a positive family history (Summary box 68.7).

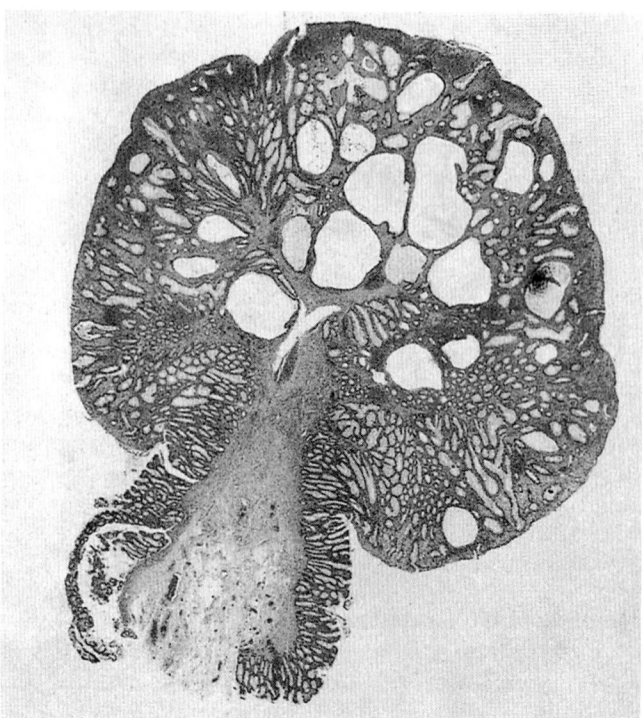

Figure 68.15 Microscopic appearance of a juvenile polyp.

Summary box 68.7
Polyps in the rectum
■ Are either single or multiple
■ Adenomas are the most frequent histological type
■ Villous adenomas may be extensive and undergo malignant change more commonly than tubular adenomas
■ All adenomas must be removed to avoid carcinomatous change
■ All patients must undergo colonoscopy to determine whether further polyps are present
■ Most polyps can be removed by endoscopic techniques, but sometimes major surgery is required

Hyperplastic polyps

These are small, pinkish, sessile polyps, 2–4 mm in diameter and frequently multiple. They are harmless.

Inflammatory pseudopolyps

These are oedematous islands of mucosa. They are usually associated with colitis in the UK, but most inflammatory diseases (including tropical diseases) can cause them. They are more likely to cause radiological difficulty as the sigmoidoscopic appearances are usually associated with obvious signs of the inflammatory cause.

Villous adenomas

These have a characteristic frond-like appearance. They may be very large, and occasionally fill the entire rectum. These tumours have an enhanced tendency to become malignant – a change that can sometimes be detected by palpation with the finger; any hard area should be assumed to be malignant and should be biopsied.

Rarely, the profuse mucous discharge from these tumours, which is rich in potassium, causes dangerous electrolyte and fluid losses (Fig. 68.16).

Provided cancerous change has been excluded, these tumours can be removed by submucosal resection endoscopically, surgically per anum or by sleeve resection from above. Only very occasionally is rectal excision required. A recent technique known as transanal endoscopic microsurgery (TEM) has been developed (Buess), which has improved the endoanal approach for the local removal of villous adenomas. The method requires the insertion of a large operating sigmoidoscope. The rectum is distended by carbon dioxide insufflation, the operative field is magnified by a camera inserted via the sigmoidoscope, and the image is displayed on a monitor (Fig. 68.17). The lesion is excised using specially designed instruments. The technique is highly specialised and takes a considerable amount of time to master.

Familial adenomatous polyposis

This autosomal dominantly inherited condition is characterised by the development of multiple rectal and colonic polyps around

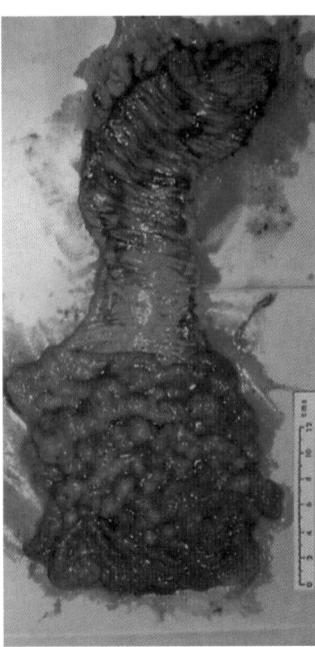

Figure 68.16 Huge villous adenoma which occupied the lower half of the rectum and caused hypokalaemia.

puberty. A colonoscopy and biopsy will confirm the diagnosis. Recently, the adenomatous polyposis coli (APC) gene responsible for the disease has been isolated on chromosome 5 (Bodmer), and its sequence has been determined. This discovery makes the screening of affected families far more straightforward. As this condition is pre-malignant, a total colectomy must be performed; often, the rectum can be preserved, but regular flexible endoscopy and removal of polyps before they develop carcinoma are required. The operation of restorative proctocolectomy with pouch–anus anastomosis is an alternative if proctectomy is required: the rectum is replaced by a 'pouch' of folded ileum (Chapter 65). A pan-proctocolectomy with permanent ileostomy is necessary in some instances, especially when patient follow-up may be impractical.

Treatment

Colonoscopic polypectomy is satisfactory in the case of most adenomas. For large lesions, especially the sessile variety, transanal excision or even excision of the rectum may be the only curative treatment. Follow-up is required, the frequency depending on the number, size and histological type of adenomas.

Benign lymphoma

This occurs as a circumscribed movable nodule, firm but not hard, greyish-white to pink in colour and essentially submucosal. This rare neoplasm, which occurs at all ages and in both sexes, has no definite capsule. Complete local excision is curative.

Endometrioma

Endometrioma is rare and may be misdiagnosed as a carcinoma. The focus of ectopic endometrial tissue produces either a constricting lesion of the rectosigmoid or a tumour invading the

Sir Walter Fred Bodmer, **Geneticist, Director of Research, Imperial Cancer Research Fund, London, UK.**

(a)

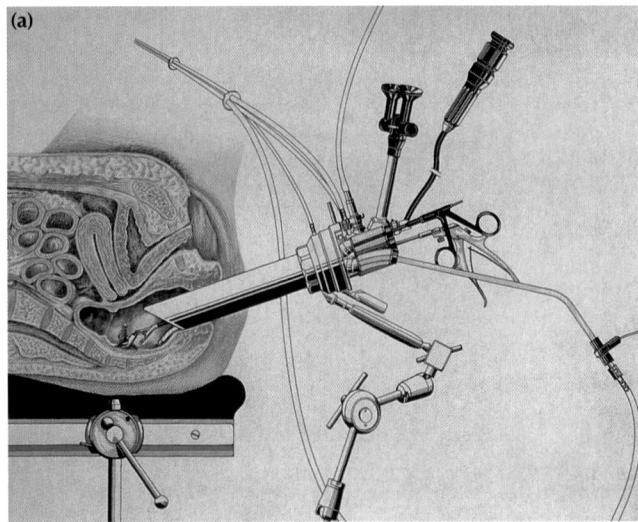

(b)

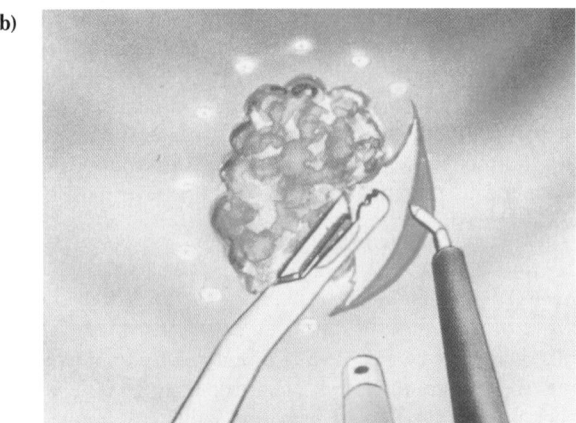

(c)

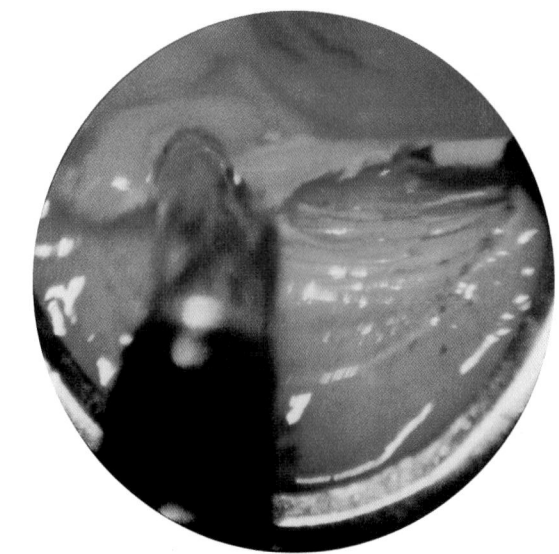

Figure 68.17 (a–c) Transanal endoscopic microsurgery technique (see text).

rectum from the rectovaginal septum. The latter variety gives rise to a very tender submucous elevation of the rectal wall. Endometrioma occurs usually between 20 and 40 years of age, less often at the menopause. Dysmenorrhoea and rectal bleeding

CHAPTER 68 | THE RECTUM

(particularly coinciding with the menses) are the main symptoms. On sigmoidoscopy, endometriosis involving the rectosigmoid junction usually presents as a stricture, with the mucous membrane intact. Hormonal manipulation is the first line of therapy, but sometimes total abdominal hysterectomy and bilateral salpingoophorectomy is required.

Haemangioma

Haemangioma of the rectum is an uncommon cause of serious haemorrhage. When localised in the lower part of the rectum or anal canal, a haemangioma can be excised. When the lesion is diffuse, or lying in the upper part of the rectum, the symptoms simulate ulcerative colitis, and the diagnosis is often missed for a long period, or it is mistakenly thought to be a carcinoma. Selective angiography and embolisation may be helpful, but excision of the rectum is sometimes required.

Gastrointestinal stromal tumour

Smooth muscle tumours of the rectum are rare. If the mitotic rate is high, and if there is variation in nuclear number, size and shape, hyperchromasia and frequent bizarre cells, these tumours are likely to metastasise. In these circumstances, they should be classified as malignant gastrointestinal stromal tumours (formerly leiomyosarcomas). The uncertainty in their behaviour means that treatment should, whenever possible, be by radical excision.

CARCINOMAS

Overall, colorectal cancer is the second most common malignancy in western countries, with approximately 18 000 patients dying per annum in the UK. The rectum is the most frequent site involved.

Origin

It is now accepted that colorectal cancer arises from adenomas in a stepwise progression in which increasing dysplasia in the adenoma is due to an accumulation of genetic abnormalities (the adenoma–carcinoma sequence; Vogelstein). In approximately 5% of cases, there is more than one carcinoma present. Usually, these carcinomas present as an ulcer, but polypoid and infiltrating types are also common.

Types of carcinoma spread

Local spread

Local spread occurs circumferentially rather than in a longitudinal direction. It is thought that a period of 6 months is required for involvement of a quarter of the circumference, and 18 months to 2 years for complete encirclement. After the muscular coat has been penetrated, the growth spreads into the surrounding mesorectum, but is initially limited by the mesorectal fascia. If penetration occurs anteriorly, the prostate, seminal vesicles or bladder become involved in the male; in the female, the vagina or the uterus is invaded. In either sex, if the penetration is lateral, a ureter may become involved, while posterior penetration may reach the sacrum and the sacral plexus. Downward spread for more than a few centimetres is rare.

Lymphatic spread

Lymphatic spread from a carcinoma of the rectum above the peritoneal reflection occurs almost exclusively in an upward direction; below that level, the lymphatic spread is still upwards, but when the neoplasm lies within the field of the middle rectal artery, primary lateral spread along the lymphatics that accompany it is not infrequent.

Downward spread is exceptional, with drainage along the subcutaneous lymphatics to the groins being confined, for practical purposes, to the lymph nodes draining the perianal rosette and the epithelium lining the distal 1–2 cm of the anal canal.

Metastasis at a higher level than the main trunk of the superior rectal artery occurs only late in the disease. A radical operation should ensure that the high-lying lymph nodes are removed by ligating the inferior mesenteric artery at a high level.

Atypical and widespread lymphatic permeation can occur in highly undifferentiated neoplasms.

Venous spread

The principal sites for blood-borne metastases are liver (34%), lungs (22%) and adrenals (11%). The remaining 33% are divided among the many other locations where secondary carcinomatous deposits tend to lodge, including the brain.

Peritoneal dissemination

This may follow penetration of the peritoneal coat by a high-lying rectal carcinoma.

Stages of progression

Dukes classified carcinoma of the rectum into three stages (Fig. 68.18).

Dukes' staging

A The growth is limited to the rectal wall (15%): prognosis excellent.

B The growth is extended to the extrarectal tissues, but no metastasis to the regional lymph nodes (35%): prognosis reasonable.

C There are secondary deposits in the regional lymph nodes (50%). These are subdivided into C1, in which the local pararectal lymph nodes alone are involved, and C2, in which the nodes accompanying the supplying blood vessels are implicated up to the point of division. This does not take into account cases that have metastasised beyond the regional lymph nodes or by way of the venous system: prognosis is poor.

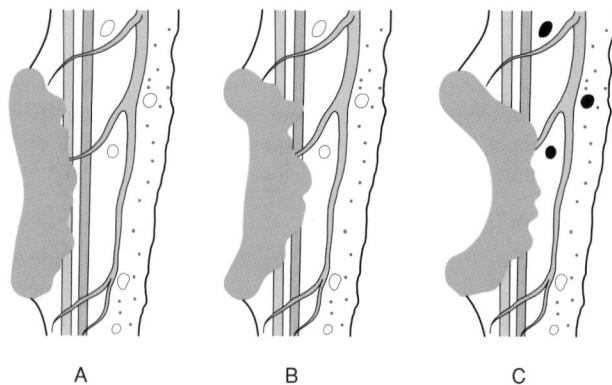

Figure 68.18 The three cardinal stages of progression of the neoplasm (after C. Dukes, FRCS).

A stage D is often included, which was not described by Dukes. This stage signifies the presence of widespread metastases, usually hepatic.

Other staging systems have been developed (e.g. Astler–Coller, TNM) to improve prognostic accuracy, but the tumour–node–metastasis (TNM) classification is now recognised internationally as the optimum classification for staging.

TNM staging

T represents the extent of local spread and there are four grades:

- T1 tumour invasion through the muscularis mucosae, but not into the muscularis propria;
- T2 tumour invasion into but not through the muscularis propria;
- T3 tumour invasion through the muscularis propria, but not through the serosa (on surfaces covered by peritoneum) or mesorectal fascia;
- T4 tumour invasion through the serosa or mesorectal fascia.

N describes nodal involvement:

- N0 no lymph node involvement;
- N1 1–3 involved lymph nodes;
- N2 4 or more involved lymph nodes.

M indicates the presence of distant metastases:

- M0 no distant metastases;
- M1 distant metastases.

The prefix 'p' indicates that the staging is based on histopathological analysis, and 'y' that it is the stage after neoadjuvant treatment, which may have resulted in downstaging.

Histological grading

In the great majority of cases, carcinoma of the rectum is a columnar-celled adenocarcinoma. The more nearly the tumour cells approach normal shape and arrangement, the less malignant the tumour is. Conversely, the greater the percentage of cells of an undifferentiated type, the more malignant the tumour is:

- Low grade = well-differentiated   11%   prognosis good;
- Average grade   64%   prognosis fair;
- High grade = anaplastic tumours   25%   prognosis poor.

Vascular and perineural invasion are poor prognostic features, as is the presence of an infiltrating (rather than pushing) margin. In a small number of cases, the tumour is a primary mucoid carcinoma. The mucus lies within the cells, displacing the nucleus to the periphery, like the seal of a signet ring. Primary mucoid carcinoma gives rise to a rapidly growing bulky growth that metastasises very early and the prognosis of which is very poor (Summary box 68.8).

> **Summary box 68.8**
>
> **Pathology and staging of rectal cancer**
>
> - Tumours are adenocarcinomas and are well, moderately or poorly differentiated
> - They spread by local, lymphatic, venous and transperitoneal routes
> - Circumferential local spread is the most important as this profoundly affects surgical treatment
> - Although lymphatic spread follows the blood supply of the rectum, most occurs in an upwards direction via the superior rectal vessels to the para-aortic nodes
> - The TNM classification is the internationally recognised staging system

Clinical features

Carcinoma of the rectum can occur early in life, but the age of presentation is usually above 55 years, when the incidence rises rapidly. Often, the early symptoms are so insignificant that the patient does not seek advice for 6 months or more (Summary box 68.9), and the diagnosis is often delayed in younger patients as these symptoms are attributed to benign causes. Initial rectal examination and a low threshold for investigating persistent symptoms are essential to prevent this.

> **Summary box 68.9**
>
> **Early symptoms of rectal cancer**
>
> - Bleeding per rectum
> - Tenesmus
> - Early morning diarrhoea

Bleeding

Bleeding is the earliest and most common symptom. There is nothing characteristic about the time at which it occurs, nor is the colour or the amount of blood distinctive; often, the bleeding is slight in amount and occurs at the end of defaecation, or is noticed because it has stained underclothing. Indeed, more often than not, the bleeding in every respect simulates that of internal haemorrhoids (haemorrhoids and carcinoma sometimes coexist).

Sense of incomplete defaecation

The patient's bowels open, but there is the sensation that there are more faeces to be passed (*tenesmus*, a distressing straining to empty the bowels without resultant evacuation). This is a very important early symptom and is almost invariably present in tumours of the lower half of the rectum. The patient may endeavour to empty the rectum several times a day (spurious diarrhoea), often with the passage of flatus and a little blood-stained mucus ('bloody slime').

Alteration in bowel habit

This is the next most frequent symptom. The patient may find it necessary to start taking an aperient or to supplement the usual dose. A patient who has to get up early in order to defaecate, or one who passes blood and mucus in addition to faeces ('early-morning bloody diarrhoea'), is usually found to be suffering from carcinoma of the rectum. Often, it is the patient with an annular carcinoma at the rectosigmoid junction who suffers with increasing constipation, and the one with a growth in the ampulla of the rectum who has early-morning diarrhoea (Bruce).

Pain

Pain is a late symptom, but pain of a colicky character may accompany advanced tumours of the rectosigmoid, and is caused by some degree of intestinal obstruction. When a deep carcinomatous ulcer of the rectum erodes the prostate or bladder, there may be severe pain. Pain in the back, or sciatica, occurs when the cancer invades the sacral plexus.

Weight loss is suggestive of hepatic metastases.

Investigation

Abdominal examination

Abdominal examination is normal in early cases. Occasionally, when an advanced annular tumour is situated at the rectosigmoid junction, signs of obstruction of the large intestine are present. By the time the patient seeks advice, metastases in the liver may be palpable. When the peritoneum has become studded with secondary deposits, ascites results.

Rectal examination

In many cases, the neoplasm can be felt digitally: in early cases as a nodule with an indurated base. When the centre ulcerates, a shallow depression will be found, the edges of which are raised and everted. On bimanual examination, it may be possible to feel the lower extremity of a carcinoma situated in the rectosigmoid junction. After the finger has been withdrawn, if it has been in direct contact with a carcinoma, it is smeared with blood or mucopurulent material tinged with blood. When a carcinomatous ulcer is situated in the lower third of the rectum, involved lymph nodes can sometimes be felt as one or more hard, oval swellings in the mesorectum posteriorly or posterolaterally above the tumour. In females, a vaginal examination should be performed and, when the neoplasm is situated on the anterior wall of the rectum, with one finger in the vagina and another in the rectum, very accurate palpation can be carried out.

Proctosigmoidoscopy

Proctosigmoidoscopy will always show a carcinoma, if present, provided that the rectum is emptied of faeces beforehand.

Biopsy

Using biopsy forceps (Fig. 68.19) via a sigmoidoscope, a portion of the edge of the tumour can be removed. If possible, another

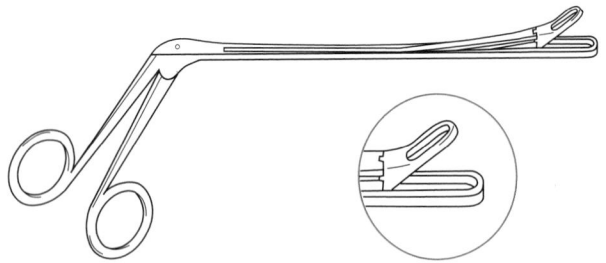

Figure 68.19 Yeoman's biopsy forceps.

Sir John Bruce, **1905–1975, Professor of Surgery, Edinburgh, UK.**

specimen from the more central part of the growth should also be obtained.

Colonoscopy

A colonoscopy is required if possible in all patients to exclude a synchronous tumour, be it an adenoma or a carcinoma. If a proximal adenoma is found, it can be conveniently snared and removed via the colonoscope. If a synchronous carcinoma is present, the operative strategy will need changing. If a full colonoscopy is not possible, a CT colonography or barium enema can be performed.

When a stenosing carcinoma is present, it may not be possible using these investigations, especially colonoscopy, to visualise the proximal colon. However, in view of the high incidence of synchronous tumours, it is imperative that a colonoscopy is always performed either before or within a few months of surgical resection.

Differential diagnosis

When an adenoma shows evidence of induration or unusual friability, it is almost certain that malignancy has occurred, even in spite of biopsy findings to the contrary. On the other hand, biopsy is invaluable in distinguishing carcinoma from an inflammatory stricture or an amoebic granuloma. The possibility of a neoplasm being an endometrioma should always be considered in patients with dysmenorrhoea. The possibility of a carcinoid tumour in atypical cases must be remembered. In the last four instances, biopsy should establish the correct diagnosis. The solitary ulcer syndrome has already been alluded to above (Summary box 68.10).

Summary box 68.10

Diagnosis and assessment of rectal cancer

All patients with suspected rectal cancer should undergo:
- Digital rectal examination
- Sigmoidoscopy and biopsy
- Colonoscopy if possible (or CT colonography or barium enema)

All patients with proven rectal cancer require staging by:
- Imaging of the liver and chest, preferably by CT
- Local pelvic imaging by magnetic resonance imaging and/or endoluminal ultrasound

---

Treatment

Some form of excision of the rectum is essential, if at all possible, because of the extreme suffering entailed if the neoplasm remains. However, before surgery is embarked upon, it is necessary to assess:

- the fitness of the patient for operation;
- the extent of spread of the tumour.

The findings will affect the surgical approach.

Assessment of spread should include CT of the chest and abdomen to exclude distant metastases (Fig. 68.20). Ultrasonography of the liver and a chest radiograph are decreasingly used alternatives. Positron emission tomography (PET) scanning can be helpful in identifying metastases if imaging is otherwise equivocal.

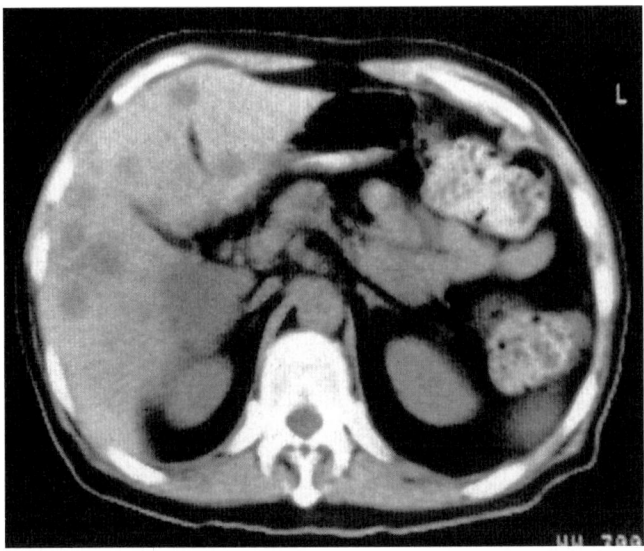

Figure 68.20 Computerised tomography scan of the liver in a patient with a rectal cancer showing multiple liver metastases.

Endoluminal ultrasound, whereby a probe is placed in the rectal lumen, can be used to assess the local spread of the tumour (Fig. 68.21), and is particularly accurate in staging the degree of penetration through the rectal wall in early tumours. CT is not particularly accurate in local staging, which is usually performed using magnetic resonance imaging (MRI), which allows assessment of the proposed circumferential resection margin and adjacent structures (Fig. 68.22).

Principles of surgical treatment

Radical excision of the rectum, together with the mesorectum and associated lymph nodes, should be the aim. Even in the presence of widespread metastases, a rectal excision should be considered, as this is often the best means of palliation. The presence of liver metastases does not necessarily rule out the feasibility of a radical excision. The results of surgery for liver metastases have

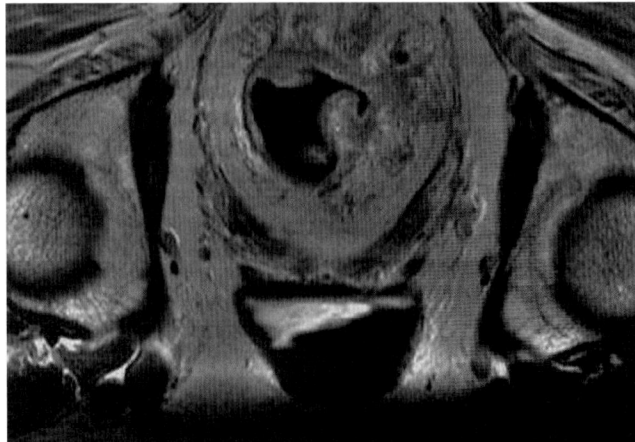

Figure 68.22 Magnetic resonance imaging scan of pelvis showing extensive T3 rectal carcinoma invading the left side of the mesorectum.

greatly improved, with long-term survival being achieved in over a third of patients.

When a tumour appears to be locally advanced (i.e. invading a neighbouring structure or threatening to breach the circumferential resection margin), the administration of a course of preoperative chemoradiotherapy may reduce its size and make curative surgery possible. Recent evidence suggests that the administration of preoperative 'short-course' neoadjuvant radiotherapy in resectable rectal cancer cases significantly reduces the incidence of local recurrence (Pahlman).

For patients who are unfit for radical surgery or who have widespread metastases, a local procedure such as transanal excision, laser destruction or interstitial radiation should be considered.

When a rectal excision is possible, whenever feasible, the aim should be to restore gastrointestinal continuity and continence by preserving the anal sphincter. A sphincter-saving operation (anterior resection) is usually possible for tumours whose lower margin is two or more centimetres above the anal canal. Although removal of the rectum with a permanent colostomy (abdominoperineal excision) was often required for tumours of the lower third of the rectum in the past, the introduction of the stapling gun has enabled many more of these patients to be treated by a sphincter-saving procedure. Provided a minimum distal margin of clearance of 2 cm can be secured, it is safe to restore gastrointestinal continuity (Williams).

The principles of the operation involve radical excision of the neoplasm, removal of the mesorectum and high proximal ligation of the inferior mesenteric lymphovascular pedicle. Once the rectum has been adequately mobilised, it is removed, and the rectal stump is washed out. Restoration of continuity by direct end-to-end anastomosis (manually or by stapling) must be carried out by a meticulous technique to reduce the risks of suture line breakdown.

Rectosigmoid tumours and those in the upper third of the rectum are removed by 'high anterior resection', in which the rectum and mesorectum are taken to a margin 5 cm distal to

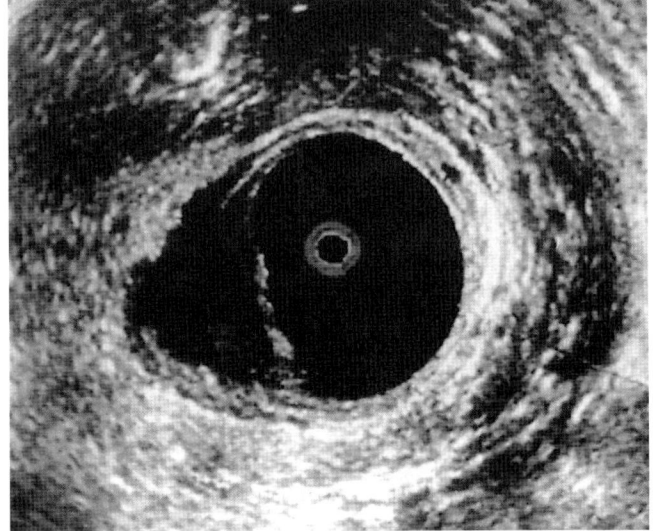

Figure 68.21 Endoluminal ultrasound. The probe is in the rectal lumen and shows a rectal tumour invading through the rectal wall.

Norman Stanley Williams, **Contemporary, Professor of Surgery, Barts and The London School of Medicine and Dentistry,** London, UK.

CHAPTER 68 | THE RECTUM

the tumour, and a colorectal anastomosis is performed. This does not usually require defunctioning. The retention of at least a part of the rectum results in good postoperative function.

For tumours in the middle and lower thirds of the rectum, complete removal of the rectum and mesorectum is required, i.e. total mesorectal excision (TME) (Heald). A temporary protecting stoma is usually formed after TME (see later).

Preoperative preparation

The bowel is prepared by mechanical cleansing using a combination of diet, purgatives and enemas (e.g. senna, Picolax). Prophylactic systemic antibiotics are given peroperatively. The antibiotic regimen must be active against both aerobic and anaerobic organisms. At present, a suitable prescription would be cefuroxime 750 mg plus metronidazole 500 mg given on induction of anaesthesia. If a patient comes to surgery with a loaded colon, on-table intraoperative irrigation can be performed.

All patients should see a stoma care nurse preoperatively and be sited for a temporary or permanent ileostomy or colostomy. They must also be counselled as to the complications of the procedure, and particularly about the risks of pelvic autonomic nerve damage causing bladder and sexual disturbance, especially impotence.

Blood and electrolyte deficiencies are corrected. Before commencing the operation, an indwelling catheter is inserted into the bladder (Summary box 68.11).

Summary box 68.11

Preoperative preparation

- Mechanical bowel preparation
- Counselling and siting of stomas
- Correction of anaemia and electrolyte disturbance
- Cross-matching of blood
- Prophylactic antibiotics
- Deep vein thrombosis prophylaxis
- Insertion of urethral catheter

Combined (abdominal and perineal) excision of the rectum

This operation is still required for some tumours of the lower third of the rectum, which are unsuitable for a sphincter-saving procedure. It has the advantage for difficult tumours of the lower rectum of two surgeons operating from the abdominal and perineal approaches simultaneously. A large catheter is passed to allow easy identification of the urethra and, with the patient in the Trendelenburg lithotomy position, the legs being supported in special supports (Lloyd-Davies–Allen), access is afforded to the abdomen and the perineum at the same time.

The abdominal surgeon makes a midline incision. The liver and the peritoneum are examined for metastases. The small intestine is packed away from the pelvis. A self-retaining retractor is placed in the wound, and the sigmoid colon is freed by dividing the peritoneal reflection on the left side. The sigmoid colon is mobilised to the midline on its mesentery, and the left

ureter and testicular or ovarian vessels are identified. The mesocolon is now divided at the site of the proposed division of the colon and the trunk of the inferior mesenteric artery (Fig. 68.23), ligated and divided distal to the first branch. (Some surgeons emphasise 'flush ligation' of the artery at its origin from the aorta.) Most surgeons prefer to divide the sigmoid colon at this point, and this is usually done with a linear stapling cutting instrument. The rectosigmoid mesentery is further divided and separated from the sacrum by sharp dissection with scissors or, more usually, diathermy. Great care is exercised to ensure that the hypogastric nerves are identified and preserved. It is essential that, as the distal dissection proceeds, the surgeon remains outside the posterior margin of the mesorectum and stays within the bloodless plane between the mesorectum and the sacrum, i.e. 'the holy plane' (Heald). In this way, the sacrum is cleared almost down to the coccyx.

The peritoneal incision is carried anteriorly around the rectum and deepened, and the seminal vesicles or the vaginal wall are identified so that Denonvilliers' fascia behind them is cleared by a dissection leading down to the prostate or perineal body. The condensations of fascia that attach the rectum to the pelvic side walls and are known as the lateral ligaments are dissected by diathermy. This tissue contains the middle rectal vessels, which sometimes require separate ligation and division.

When the abdominal surgeon has made certain that the condition is operable, the perineal surgeon closes the anus with purse-string sutures of stout silk or nylon. An elliptical incision between the tip of the coccyx and the central perineal point is

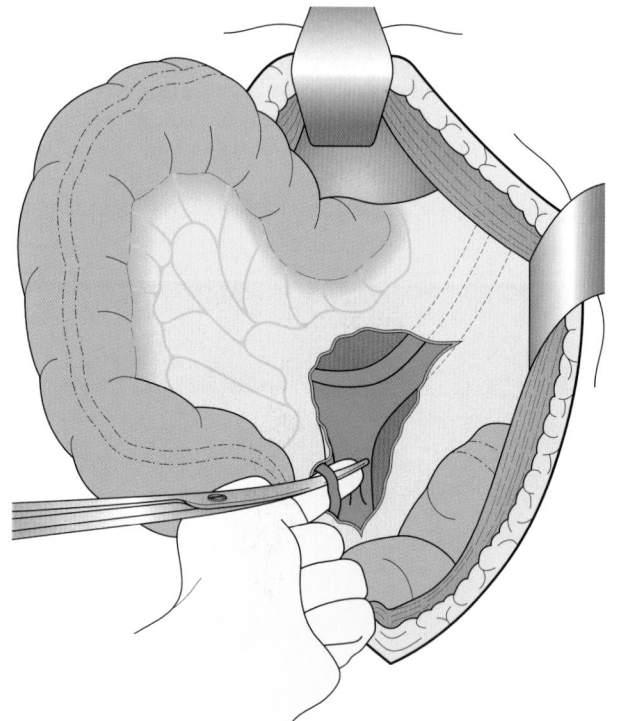

Figure 68.23 Exposure and division of the inferior mesenteric vessels flush with the aorta (high tie) in the course of an abdominoperineal excision of the rectum. [Redrawn with permission from Keighley, M.R.B. and Williams, N.S. (1999) *Surgery of the Anus, Rectum and Colon*. W.B. Saunders, London.]

made around the anus and deepened. The left forefinger is insinuated into the levator ani, which is divided lateral to the finger, first on one side and then on the other (Fig. 68.24). The dissection is deepened posteriorly by incising Waldeyer's fascia, which is a thick condensation of pelvic fascia lying between the rectum and the sacrum. Contact is made with the abdominal surgeon. The apex of skin anterior to the anus is grasped in artery forceps, which serves as a retractor, and by scissors or diathermy and gauze dissection, the wound is deepened, when the catheter within the membranous urethra will be felt. A plane of cleavage will be found between the rectum and the prostate in the male or between the rectum and the vagina in the female. This plane having been carefully determined, Denonvilliers' fascia is divided, after which the rectum can be stripped from the prostate or the vagina. The posterior wall of the vagina is frequently excised with the rectum. When the abdominal surgeon has cleared the rectum laterally, the whole of the anus and rectum can be drawn downwards and removed through the perineal wound.

Haemostasis must be secured and the perineal wound closed in layers. It is usual to use laterally situated suction drains brought out through each ischiorectal fossa to keep the large perineal cavity from filling up with blood and serous exudate. These drains can be removed after several days.

The site for the colostomy in the left iliac fossa should have been marked preoperatively by the stoma care nurse in consultation with the patient. If this has not been possible, it should be sited equidistant from the umbilicus and the left anterior superior iliac spine at the linea semilunaris, about 2.5 cm above the spinoumbilical line. A circular piece of skin and fascia, about 3 cm in diameter, is excised and this trephine deepened. The rectus sheath and muscle layers are split, and the peritoneum divided. The stapled end of the colon is now passed through this incision

and the colostomy formed (usually after closure of the abdominal wound) by suturing the colon directly to the skin. The paracolic gutter may be closed with sutures – this will close the 'lateral space'. An adherent plastic colostomy bag is then fitted in position, and the dressings are placed on the abdominal wound.

Care of the colostomy

This is much the same as care of an ileostomy (Chapter 65). Within a very short time, the colostomy acts once or twice a day. The patient soon learns which foods cause diarrhoea and therefore avoids them. Many patients are now taught to empty their lower colon by irrigation through the colostomy: this has many advantages for the patient who requires an inactive colostomy while at work. Occlusive caps are also available, which fit in the end of the stoma and allow some degree of continence.

Stenosis of the colostomy is usually avoided by the removal of a circle of skin and subcutaneous tissues at the colostomy site. Dilators may be necessary if there is any tendency for stenosis to occur.

Laparoscopic abdominoperineal excision

Recently, it has been demonstrated that the operation can be carried out laparoscopically. The rectum is mobilised completely from above, using the laparoscope. The perineal part of the procedure is unchanged. After transecting the midsigmoid colon with an endoscopic stapler–cutter instrument, the specimen containing the carcinoma is delivered through the perineal wound. A trephine incision is made in the left iliac fossa, and the sigmoid colon is brought out as an end-colostomy. Although the operative technique has been shown to be quite feasible and reduces postoperative pain and time in hospital, there is concern that it may not be as curative as the standard 'open' technique. The concern

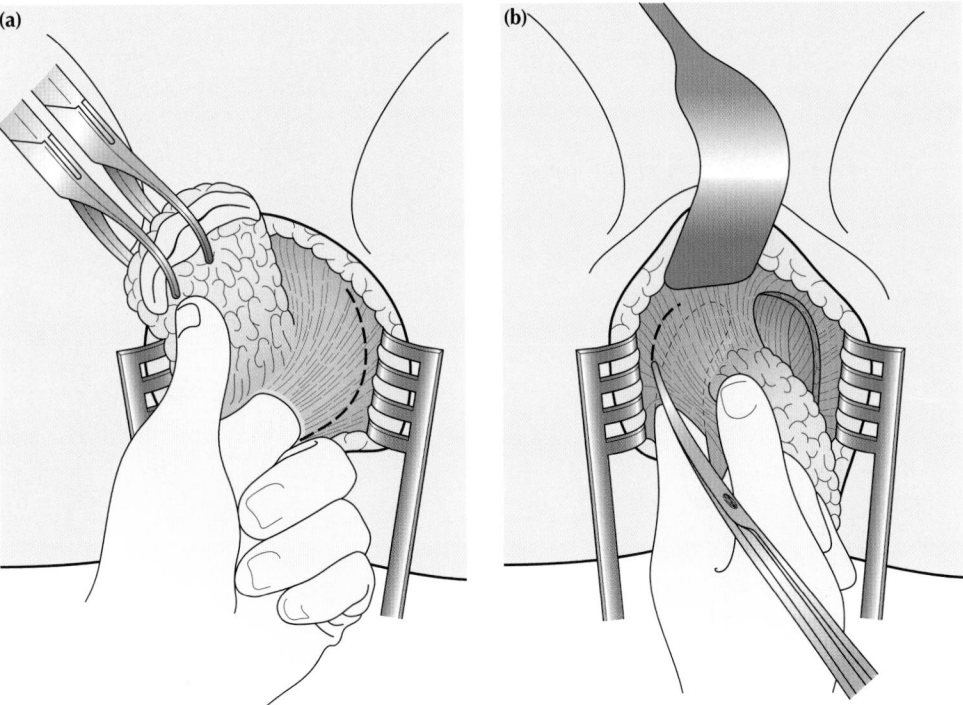

Figure 68.24 (a and b) Separation and division of the pubococcygeus and puborectalis muscles in the course of the perineal phase of an abdominoperineal excision of the rectum. [Redrawn with permission from Keighley, M.R.B. and Williams, N.S. (1999) *Surgery of the Anus, Rectum and Colon*. W.B. Saunders, London.]

surrounds the degree of clearance that can be achieved via the laparoscope, and the risk of free cancer cells being disseminated around the peritoneal cavity and implanting, particularly at the 'port' sites. Controlled trials will be needed to determine whether the laparoscopic approach is safe and as effective as the open technique, and these are in progress.

Anterior resection

As discussed previously, in the last two decades, there has been a move to extend sphincter-saving operations to treat most tumours of the middle third of the rectum, and indeed many in the lower third. The introduction of the circular stapling instruments, with their detachable heads, has made such procedures far more feasible.

The operation of low anterior resection proceeds in the same manner as the abdominal part of abdominoperineal excision. The rectum is mobilised to the pelvic floor, and a right-angled clamp is placed at least 2 cm below the tumour. The rectal stump can then be stapled transversely, using an appropriate instrument. After the rectum and sigmoid colon have been excised, continuity is re-established by the method depicted in Figure 68.25. Although a single loop of colon is often used for the anastomosis, a short J-shaped colonic pouch may be constructed with the aim of increasing neorectal capacity and thus reducing postoperative bowel frequency and urgency (Parc). Some surgeons are concerned that the anastomotic leakage rate will be increased if the technique of cross-stapling of the rectal stump is used. They prefer to place a purse-string suture in the rectal stump lumen, as well as in the proximal colon. After the stapling gun is fired and removed, it is essential that the head of the instrument is

detached and the 'doughnuts' are examined. A break in the circumference of one or both 'doughnuts' signifies a defect in the anastomosis, and the latter should be sought and repaired with interrupted sutures. In these circumstances, a covering stoma will also be required to allow safe healing of the anastomosis. Some surgeons believe that such a stoma is required for all colorectal and coloanal anastomoses that are constructed below the peritoneal reflection.

Occasionally, although the rectum, together with its tumour, can be removed adequately, continuity cannot be restored by a stapling technique. In such cases, it may still be possible to restore continuity by bringing the colon down to the anal canal and constructing a coloanal anastomosis via the transanal route (Fig. 68.26) (the so called abdominotransanal–coloanal operation first described by Parks).

In each of the procedures, it is essential to ensure that any free tumour cells released by mobilisation of the rectum are destroyed by irrigation of the rectal lumen with a cancercidal solution such as 1% cetrimide. By so doing, the implantation of such cells and subsequent local recurrence is prevented. However, it should be realised that, although a small percentage of local recurrences are due to implantation of shed cells, the majority result from inadequate removal of the tumour at the time of the initial operation. Although it is usual for the surgeon to remove all macroscopic tumour, he or she is often unable to remove all microscopic tumour. Particular interest has recently focused on local microscopic spread. It is now known that micrometastases are present in the mesorectum, and these are the most likely cause of local recurrence after rectal excision (Quirke). Heald has emphasised

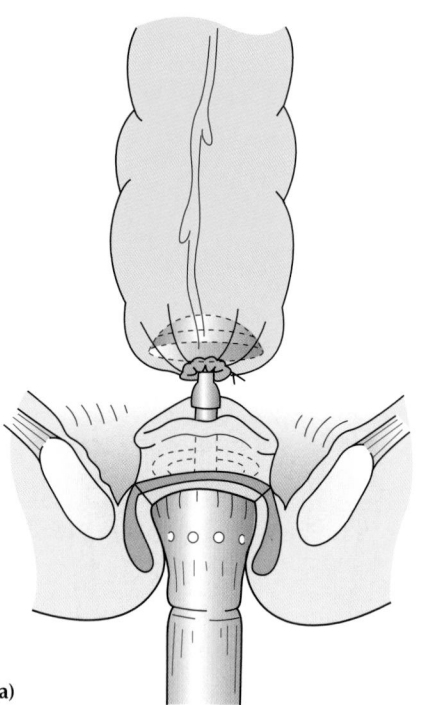
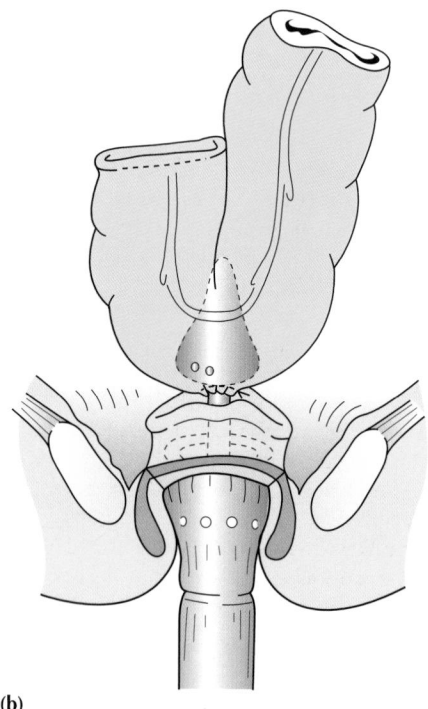

(a)   (b)

Figure 68.25 Low anterior resection by the double stapling method. The rectum has been excised, and the distal anorectal stump has been transected with a transverse stapling device. A circular stapling gun is used to construct (a) a straight low coloanal anastomosis or (b) a colonic pouch–anus anastomosis.

Sir Alan Guyatt Parks **Surgeon, St Mark's Hospital and the London Hospital, London, UK.**

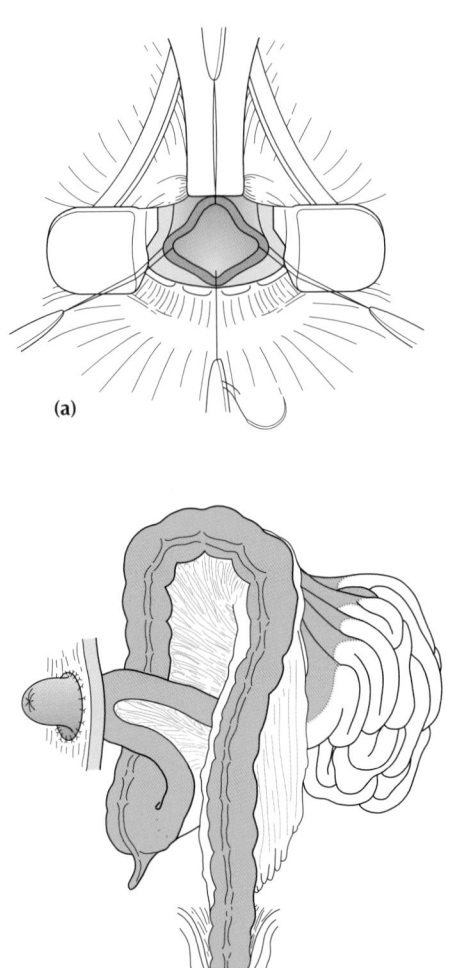

(a)

(b)

Figure 68.26 Abdominotransanal–coloanal anastomosis. (a) The rectum has been excised, and the mucosa from the distal anorectal stump has been removed, leaving the rectal muscle intact. The proximal colon has been brought down through the rectal muscular cuff to be anastomosed to the anal mucosa via the transanal route. (b) The completed coloanal anastomosis. A covering ileostomy has been performed, to allow the anastomosis to heal.

how important it is to remove all the mesorectum during anterior resection or abdominoperineal excision, the procedure known as TME. TME is now being practised worldwide and appears to reduce the risks of local recurrence substantially (Fig. 68.27). However, it is unlikely that surgery alone will deal adequately with all the micrometastases in the pelvis. Consequently, neoadjuvant radiotherapy may have added benefit (see below).

Laparoscopic anterior resection

It is now possible to perform anterior resection using the laparoscope, the anastomosis being performed using a circular stapling gun. Considerable skill and experience is required but, with improvements in technology, such procedures may become more commonplace. Nevertheless, like laparoscopic abdominoperineal excision, there is concern that these operations may be less curative than the standard operations.

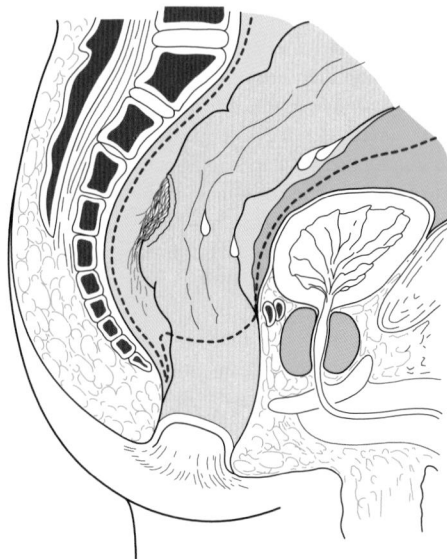

Figure 68.27 Plane of dissection for total mesorectal excision.

Hartmann's operation

This is an excellent procedure in an old and frail patient who would not stand a lengthy anterior resection, or in whom there is concern about anal sphincter function or the viability of an anastomosis. Through an abdominal incision, the rectum is excised, the anorectal stump is transected, usually with a stapler, a colostomy is performed and the peritoneum is oversewn to cover the pelvic defect in the usual way.

Palliative colostomy

This is indicated only in cases giving rise to intestinal obstruction, or where there is gross infection of the neoplasm. It is sometimes possible to resect the growth later (e.g. after chemoradiotherapy) and, in some cases, cure, rather than palliation, is achieved.

Other palliative procedures

Occasionally, a neodymium:yttrium–aluminium–garnet (Nd: YAG) laser can be used to deal with an obstructing or bleeding lesion. Intraluminal stents can also be inserted endoscopically in high, stenosing rectal cancers to palliate a tumour that is causing obstruction.

Local operations

For small, low-grade mobile lesions, which are often Dukes' A (T1) tumours, local removal should be curative. For these tumours, especially in the unfit or in patients who will not accept a colostomy, local removal has been used. Such operations are only suitable for lesions within 10 cm of the anal verge. Turnbull advocated local diathermy removal, while York-Mason developed a trans-sphincteric approach, but a peranal approach is usually possible, with full-thickness excision of the lesion. More recently, the TEM technique has been used for these tumours. This involves inserting a large-calibre operating sigmoidoscope transanally, through which carbon dioxide is infused to produce rectal distension. Using specially designed instruments and an

Rupert B. Turnbull, Jr, **1913–1981, Surgeon, the Cleveland Clinic, Cleveland, OH, USA.**
Aubrey York-Mason, **1910–1993, Surgeon, St Helier Hospital, Carshalton, Surrey, UK.**

CHAPTER 68 | THE RECTUM

endoluminal camera inserted through the sigmoidoscope, the rectal carcinoma can be excised and the defect closed under direct vision by magnification of the image on a video monitor.

There is considerable doubt, however, as to whether such local techniques should be used for potentially curable lesions as they do not allow full histopathological staging or deal with the mesorectal or lymphatic spread of the tumour. Combined local excision with c°hemotherapy and radiotherapy has been suggested as a curative treatment for T1 and T2 tumours, but is not widely accepted.

More extensive operations

When the carcinoma of the rectum has spread to contiguous organs, the radical operation can often be extended to remove these structures. Thus, in the male, in whom spread is usually to the bladder, a cystectomy and resection of the rectum can be effected. In the female, the uterus acts as a barrier, preventing spread from the rectum to the bladder. Accordingly, a hysterectomy should be undertaken in addition to excision of the rectum. Should the bladder base be involved, then pelvic exenteration must include that structure. Pelvic evisceration for carcinoma of the rectum is justifiable only when the surgeon is reasonably confident that the growth can be *completely* removed.

Pelvic exenteration (Brunschwig's operation)

The aim is to remove all the pelvic organs, together with the internal iliac and the obturator groups of lymph nodes (Fig. 68.28). The Trendelenburg lithotomy position facilitates the procedure, and ligation of both internal iliac arteries diminishes the blood loss. A rectus abdominis flap can be used to fill the empty pelvis. Special care must therefore be taken to suture the perineal skin accurately, and to avoid pressure necrosis of the perineal incision by nursing the patient on alternate sides. Some form of urinary diversion is necessary, usually an ileal conduit.

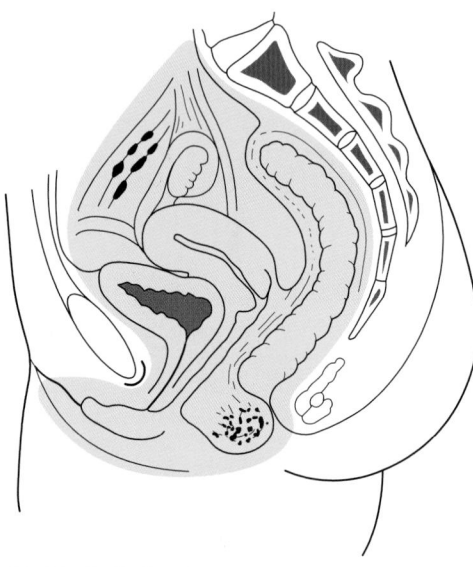

Figure 68.28 Radical pelvic exenteration, indicating the extent of the dissection and the viscera removed. [Redrawn with permission from Keighley, M.R.B. and Williams, N.S. (1999) *Surgery of the Anus, Rectum and Colon*. W.B. Saunders, London].

Alexander Brunschwig, **1901–1969**, Gynaecologist, the Memorial Hospital for the Treatment of Cancer, New York, NY, USA.

Liver resection

Single or several well-localised liver metastases can now be resected with relatively low mortality and morbidity. Provided the patients are carefully selected, a reasonable long-term survival rate can be achieved (approximately 40% in some series). Such surgery is usually carried out in a specialised liver unit, and it is generally advised that it takes place after the primary lesion has been dealt with (Summary box 68.12).

> **Summary box 68.12**
>
> **Surgery for rectal cancer**
>
> - Surgery is the mainstay of curative therapy
> - The primary resection consists of rectal excision with TME
> - Most cases can be treated by anterior resection with the colorectal anastomosis being achieved with a circular stapling gun
> - A smaller group of low, extensive tumours require an abdominoperineal excision with a permanent colostomy
> - Preoperative radiotherapy can reduce local recurrence
> - Adjuvant chemotherapy can improve survival in node-positive disease
> - Liver resection in carefully selected patients offers the best chance of cure for single or well-localised liver metastases

Radiotherapy

With modern techniques, some adenocarcinomas now respond to radiotherapy. Various controlled trials have been performed to investigate the effect of adjuvant radiotherapy given either pre- or postoperatively. The overall results of these trials suggest that, provided an adequate dose is given, neoadjuvant radiotherapy can reduce the incidence of local recurrence; however, long-term survival is not affected. Recent studies have combined radiotherapy with chemotherapy in an attempt to shrink an extensive tumour prior to surgical excision. In some cases using this combined therapy, the results can be spectacular, and it has become the standard initial treatment for locally advanced tumours, allowing potentially curative resection in cases that would otherwise be inoperable.

Palliative irradiation can be given for inoperable primary tumours or local recurrence, especially when painful. Papillon refined a technique of intracavity radiation that applies the treatment direct to the tumour from the rectal lumen. In a selected series of early cases, the results were good (5-year survival rates of more than 70%). Intraoperative irradiation is also being evaluated as an adjuvant therapy.

Chemotherapy

A variety of drugs has been tried both as an adjuvant therapy and for the treatment of disseminated disease. The most frequently used drug is 5-fluorouracil (5-FU). Up until recently, the results of various trials using 5-FU, either alone or in combination, were disappointing. However, there is now good evidence that the combination of systemic 5-FU and folinic acid (leucovorin) has a small, yet significant effect on survival when combined with surgery in node-positive disease. Similarly, studies in which 5-FU has been infused into the portal vein during and immediately after the primary operation (Taylor) have shown a small benefit. Such intraportal adjuvant therapy is thought to kill malignant cells, which are released into the circulation during operative manipulation of tumour, and thus prevent the formation of metastases.

Some exciting new drugs have become available recently, the most notable being irinotecan and oxaliplatin. Both agents have been shown to have a moderate but beneficial effect in disseminated disease, but it remains to be seen whether they will be effective in an adjuvant setting.

Results of surgery for rectal cancer

In specialised centres, the resectability rate may be as high as 95%, with an operative mortality of less than 5%. Overall, 5-year survival rate is about 50%, but it may be a little higher in these centres. The most likely reason for this difference is the higher proportion of advanced and emergency cases treated in non-specialised hospitals. However, another contributing reason is that, in specialised centres, there is a concentration of expertise that is not readily available in district hospitals. Survival rates are influenced by Dukes' stage, with stage C patients doing worse than those with A and B lesions (Fig. 68.29). The degree of mobility also influences survival, with fixed lesions having a worse prognosis than mobile lesions. The lower the tumour is in the rectum, the worse the outlook. Histological grade also influences outcome, with anaplastic lesions having the worse prognosis. Interestingly, despite the more frequent use of sphincter-saving resection compared with abdominoperineal excision, survival has not been affected.

Local recurrence

Local recurrence after rectal excision is a major problem. The patient often presents with persistent pelvic pain, which radiates down the legs if the sacral roots are involved. Bladder problems may occur. If recurrence develops after abdominoperineal excision, a swelling or induration may be present in the perineum,

or an abscess or discharging sinus may develop. Occasionally, the presence of a large recurrence in the pelvis may lead to bilateral leg oedema caused by pressure or invasion of lymphatics or veins. After sphincter-saving resection, local recurrence may produce a change in bowel habit or the passage of blood per rectum. Sigmoidoscopic examination after sphincter-saving resection may reveal friable tissue at the anastomosis which, when biopsied, confirms the diagnosis. However, the recurrence is usually situated extrarectally, and is detected either as induration on digital examination or by endoluminal ultrasonography, CT or MRI. These investigations can also detect recurrence before it causes symptoms. Local recurrence rates vary between 2% and 25% and are higher after abdominoperineal excision than after sphincter-saving resection. The most common cause is inadequate removal of all the tumour at the initial operation. This is due to the presence of microscopic tumour deposits in the tissues surrounding the rectum. Heald has shown that, if the mesorectum is removed in its entirety, the local recurrence rate can be reduced to less than 5%.

Other possible causes of local recurrence include implantation of viable cells on the suture line and the development of a new primary tumour. Although both mechanisms may occur, inadequate removal of the tumour is far and away the most important reason for recurrence. Eighty per cent of all local recurrences develop within 2 years following surgery, and they are very difficult to treat. The best prospect of salvage is by surgical resection. However, it is possible to achieve apparently complete removal in only a minority of cases. It was hoped that serial measurements of carcinoembryonic antigen might identify those patients who might benefit from early radical surgery, but this has been found not to be the case (Northover). The mainstay of therapy for local recurrence is radiotherapy, which is invariably palliative. Surgery is occasionally indicated and will usually involve hysterectomy, bladder resection and even partial sacrectomy.

Carcinoid tumour

Like benign lymphoma, carcinoid tumour originates in the submucosa, with the mucous membrane over it being intact. Consequently, it seldom produces evidence of its presence in the early stages, when it presents as a small plaque-like elevation. The incidence of clinical malignancy, i.e. the occurrence of metastases, is 10%. This is much less than that for carcinoid tumour of the small intestine, but it is greater than that for carcinoid tumour of the appendix. Multiple primary carcinoid tumours of the rectum are not infrequent. The neoplasm is of slow progression, and usually metastasises late. Large carcinoids (over 2 cm) are almost always malignant.

Treatment

Local excision is sufficient treatment for small carcinoids. Resection of the rectum is advisable if the growth is more than 2.5 cm in diameter, if recurrence follows local excision or if the growth is fixed to the perirectal tissues. Even when metastases are present, resection may prolong life.

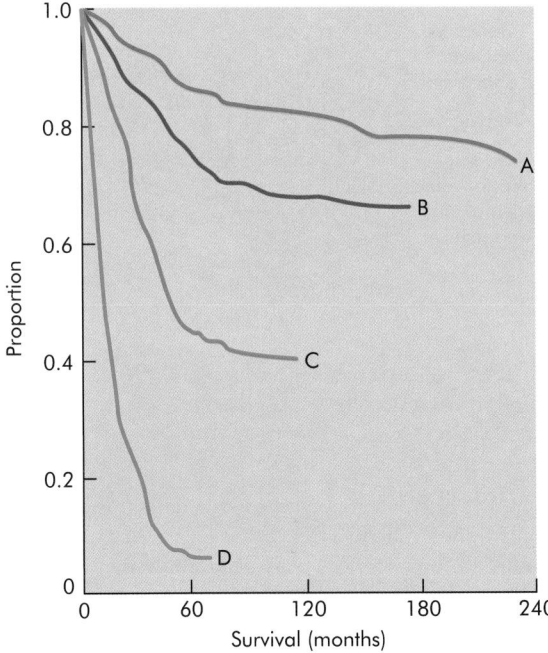

Figure 68.29 Cancer-specific survival rates following surgery for rectal cancer according to Dukes' stages. [Redrawn with permission from Keighley, M.R.B. and Williams, N.S. (1999) *Surgery of the Anus, Rectum and Colon*. W.B. Saunders, London].

FURTHER READING

Keighley, M.R.B. and Williams, N.S. (eds) (1999) *Surgery of the Anus, Rectum and Colon*, 2nd edn. W.B. Saunders, London.

Phillips, R.K.S. (ed.) (2005) *A Companion to Specialist Surgical Practice: Colorectal Surgery*, 3rd edn. Elsevier Saunders, London.

The anus and anal canal

LEARNING OBJECTIVES

To understand

- The anatomy of the anus and anal canal and their relationship to surgical disease and its treatment
- The pathology, clinical presentation, investigation, differential diagnosis and treatment of diseases that affect the anus and anal canal

- That anal disease is common and its treatment tends to be conservative, although surgery may be required
- That too aggressive or inappropriate surgery may render the patient permanently disabled

ANATOMY AND PHYSIOLOGY

Surgical anatomy

The anal canal commences at the level where the rectum passes through the pelvic diaphragm and ends at the anal verge. The muscular junction between the rectum and anal canal can be felt with the finger as a thickened ridge – the anorectal 'bundle' or 'ring'.

Anal canal anatomy (Fig. 69.1)

The anorectal ring

The anorectal ring marks the junction between the rectum and the anal canal. It is formed by the joining of the puborectalis muscle (Fig. 69.2), the deep external sphincter, conjoined longitudinal muscle and the highest part of the internal sphincter. The anorectal ring can be clearly felt digitally, especially on its posterior and lateral aspects.

The puborectalis muscle

Puborectalis, part of the funnel-shaped muscular pelvic diaphragm, maintains the angle between the anal canal and rectum and hence is an important component in the continence mechanism (Fig. 69.2). The muscle derives its nerve supply from the sacral somatic nerves, and is functionally indistinct from the external anal sphincter. The position and length of the anal canal, as well as the angle of the anorectal junction, depend to a major extent on the integrity and strength of the puborectalis muscle sling. It gives off fibres that contribute to the longitudinal muscle layer.

The external sphincter

The external sphincter forms the bulk of the anal sphincter complex and, although traditionally it has been subdivided into deep, superficial and subcutaneous portions, it is a single muscle

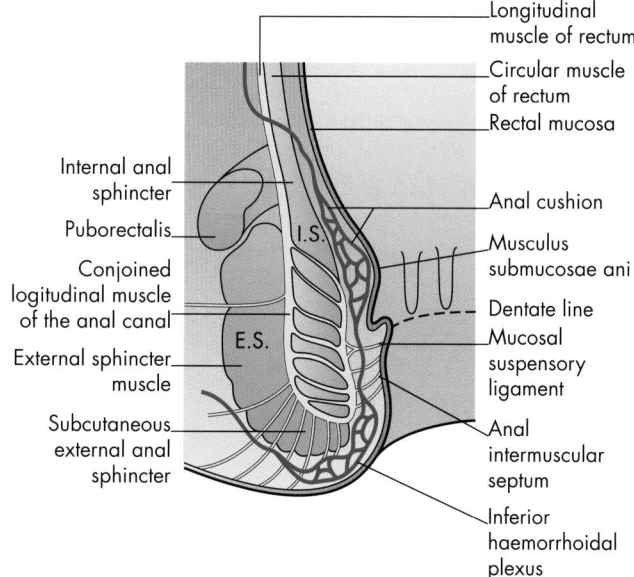

Figure 69.1 Relevant anatomy of the anus. [Redrawn with permission from Mann, C.V. (2002) *Surgical Treatment of Haemorrhoids*. Springer, London.]

(Goligher), which is variably divided by lateral extensions from the longitudinal muscle layer. Some of its fibres are attached posteriorly to the coccyx, whereas anteriorly they fuse with the perineal muscles. Being a somatic voluntary muscle, the external sphincter is red in colour and is innervated by the pudendal nerve.

John Cedric Goligher, **1912–1998, Professor of Surgery, University of Leeds, Leeds, UK.**

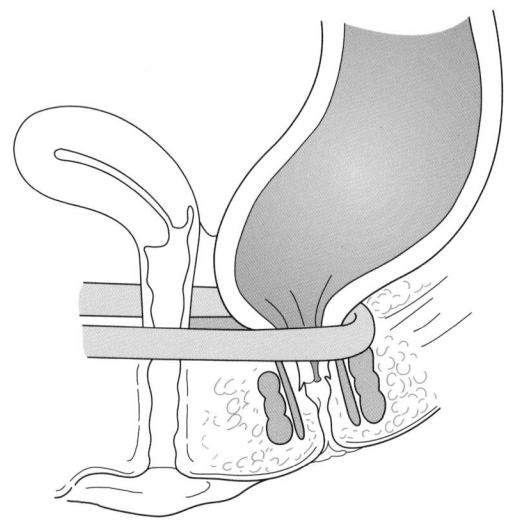

Figure 69.2 The disposition of the puborectalis muscle. Note how it maintains the rectoanal angle.

The intersphincteric plane

Between the external sphincter muscle laterally and the longitudinal muscle medially exists a potential space, the intersphincteric plane. This plane is important as it contains intersphincteric anal glands (see below) and is also a route for the spread of pus, which occurs along the extensions from the longitudinal muscle layer. The plane can be opened up surgically to provide access for operations on the sphincter muscles.

The longitudinal muscle

The longitudinal muscle is a direct continuation of the smooth muscle of the outer muscle coat of the rectum, augmented in its upper part by striated muscle fibres originating from the medial components of the pelvic floor. Most of the muscle continues caudally before splitting into multiple terminal septa that surround the muscle bundles of the subcutaneous portion of the external sphincter to insert into the skin of the lowermost part of the anal canal and adjacent perianal skin. Milligan and Morgan named the most medial of these septa, passing around the inferior border of the internal sphincter, the 'anal intermuscular septum'. As it descends, however, it gives off fibres that pass medially across the internal sphincter to reach the submucosal space, and laterally across the external sphincter and ischiorectal space to reach the fascia of the pelvic side walls. As well as providing a supportive mesh for the anal canal and other muscular components, its ramifications provide potential pathways for the spread of infection. During defaecation, its contraction widens the anal lumen, flattens the anal cushions, shortens the anal canal and everts the anal margin; subsequent relaxation allows the anal cushions to distend and thus contribute to an airtight seal.

The internal sphincter

The internal sphincter is the thickened (2–5 mm) distal continuation of the circular muscle coat of the rectum, which has

Edward Thomas Campbell Milligan, **1886–1972, Surgeon, St Mark's Hospital, London, UK.**
Sir Clifford Naughton Morgan, **1901–1986, Surgeon, St Mark's Hospital and St Bartholomew's Hospital, London, UK.**

developed special properties and which is in a tonic state of contraction. This involuntary muscle commences where the rectum passes through the pelvic diaphragm and ends above the anal orifice, its lower border palpable at the intersphincteric groove, below which lie the most medial fibres of the subcutaneous external sphincter, and separated from it by the anal intermuscular septum. When exposed during life, it is pearly-white in colour and its circumferentially placed fibres can be seen clearly. Although innervated by the autonomic nervous system, it receives intrinsic non-adrenergic and non-cholinergic (NANC) fibres, stimulation of which causes release of the neurotransmitter nitric oxide, which induces internal sphincter relaxation.

The epithelium and sub-epithelial structures

The pink columnar epithelium lining the rectum extends through the anorectal ring into the surgical anal canal. Passing downwards the mucous membrane becomes cuboidal and redder in colour (Fig. 69.3) whereas above the anal valves it is plum coloured. Just below the level of the anal valves there is an abrupt, albeit wavy, transition to stratified squamous epithelium, which is parchment coloured. This wavy junction constitutes the dentate line. The dentate line is a most important landmark both morphologically and surgically, representing the site of fusion of the proctodaeum and post-allantoic gut, and being the site of the crypts of Morgagni (synonym: anal crypts, sinuses). The latter are small pockets between the inferior extremities of the columns of Morgagni through which anal ducts that communicate with deeper placed anal glands open into the anal lumen. The squamous epithelium lining the lower anal canal is thin and shiny and is known as the anoderm; it differs from the true skin in that it has no epidermal appendages, i.e. hair and sweat glands. At the dentate line, the anoderm is attached more firmly to deeper structures. The mucosa and submucosa above the dentate line is uneven and thrown into folds, the so called anal cushions. There are variations in the numbers and positions of these cushions but there are usually three, corresponding to those seen in later life. These are described classically as occupying the left lateral, right posterior and right anterior positions, and they continue proximally as the primary rectal foldings. Secondary foldings (the rectal columns of Morgagni) lie both over and between the primary folds. This area is the caudal limit of the so called epithelial

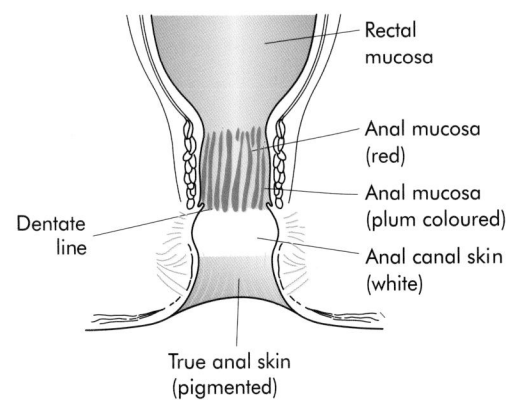

Figure 69.3 The lining membrane of the anal canal (after Sir Clifford Naunton Morgan, London).

Giovani Battista Morgagni, **Professor of Anatomy, Padua, Italy, for 59 years. He is regarded as the founder of morbid anatomy.**

transitional zone, below which the stratified squamous epithelium is richly innervated by sensory nerve endings serving several modalities including touch, pain and temperature. The bulk of the anal cushions themselves, situated in the upper part of the anal canal, receive only visceral afferent innervation and, although there is perception of stretching, sensitivity to noxious stimuli is much more blunted than distally.

Between the epithelial layer and the internal sphincter lies the submucosa, consisting of vascular, muscular and connective tissue supportive elements. From the longitudinal muscle, medial extensions cross the internal anal sphincter and form part of the supporting meshwork of the submucosa, blending with the true submucosal smooth muscle layer and thereby supporting the mucosa itself. Parks described the increased density of fibres that insert into the mucosa of the anal crypts at the level of the dentate line, termed the 'mucosal suspensory ligament'. One feature of this structure is that it separates the superior (portal) and inferior (systemic) haemorrhoidal plexuses, another is that the mucosa is more firmly tethered to underlying tissues at this level than above. It is important to appreciate that the meshwork of supporting tissues (muscle fibres and connective tissue) within the subepithelial space is intimately linked to deeper structures within the anal sphincter complex, including the internal sphincter, longitudinal muscle layer and external anal sphincter, and indeed structures beyond the sphincter complex. With age, the smooth muscle component of this mesh is reduced and muscle fibres are gradually replaced with fibroelastic connective tissue, which in turn becomes fragmented.

Blood supply

In addition to the meshwork support of the lining of the anal canal, the subepithelial space contains venous dilatations supported by the same fibroelastic connective tissue and smooth muscle scaffolding. Debate has centred on the nature of the vascular component of haemorrhoids, but the seminal anatomical studies of Thomson have clarified this issue. Venous dilatations are seen in the submucosa both above and below the level of the dentate line; they are much more numerous above although tend to be larger below. The historical description of the blood supply to the upper anal canal as constant, with bifurcation of the main trunk of the superior rectal artery into right and left branches and with subsequent division of the former into anterior and posterior divisions thereby determining the sites of haemorrhoids around the anal circumference, was questioned by Thomson. He demonstrated that the divisions of the superior rectal artery were not constant and that, furthermore, the anal submucosa in a proportion of his specimens received a blood supply from the middle and inferior rectal arteries. He was also able to show the presence of free communications between tributaries of the superior, middle and inferior rectal veins, as well as tiny direct arteriovenous communications with the submucosal venous dilatations. These communications have been shown both histologically and radiologically, and the oxygen tension of the blood contained within the venous dilatations (as well as the colour) is more arterial than venous.

Sir Alan Guyatt Parks, 1920–1962, Surgeon, St Mark's Hospital and the London Hospital, London, UK.
William Hamish Fearon Thomson, Surgeon, The Gloucestershire Royal Infirmary, Gloucester, England.

Venous drainage

The anal veins are distributed in a similar fashion to the arterial supply. The upper half of the anal canal is drained by the superior rectal veins, tributaries of the inferior mesenteric vein and thus the portomesenteric venous system, and the middle rectal veins, which drain into the internal iliac veins. The inferior rectal veins drain the lower half of the anal canal and the subcutaneous perianal plexus of veins: they eventually join the internal iliac vein on each side.

Lymphatic drainage

Lymph from the upper half of the anal canal flows upwards to drain into the postrectal lymph nodes and from there goes to the para-aortic nodes via the inferior mesenteric chain. Lymph from the lower half of the anal canal drains on each side first into the superficial and then into the deep inguinal group of lymph glands. However, if the normal flow is blocked, e.g. by tumour, the lymph can be diverted into the alternative route (Summary box 69.1).

Summary box 69.1

Anal canal anatomy

- The internal sphincter is composed of circular, non-striated involuntary muscle supplied by autonomic nerves
- The external sphincter is composed of striated voluntary muscle supplied by the pudendal nerve
- Extensions from the longitudinal muscle layer support the sphincter complex
- The space between sphincters is known as the intersphincteric plane
- The superior part of the external sphincter fuses with the puborectalis muscle, which is essential for maintaining the anorectal angle, necessary for continence
- The lower part of the anal canal is lined by sensitive squamous epithelium
- Blood supply to the anal canal is via superior, middle and inferior rectal vessels
- Lymphatic drainage of the lower half of the anal canal goes to inguinal lymph nodes

---

The anal glands

Anal glands (which are not vestigial remnants of sexual scent glands) may be found in the submucosa and intersphincteric space (Fig. 69.4), and normally number between 0 and 10 in an individual. They drain via ducts into the anal sinuses at the level of the dentate line. Not all sinuses have a duct draining into them and, occasionally, more than one gland can discharge into the same sinus. Their function is unknown although they secrete mucin (distinct from that secreted by the rectal epithelium), which perhaps lubricates the anal canal to ease defaecation. The importance of intersphincteric anal glands is that they are widely considered to be the potential source of anal sepsis, either acute, presenting as perianal, ischiorectal or even pelvic sepsis, or chronic, presenting as a cryptoglandular (non-specific) anal fistula.

EXAMINATION OF THE ANUS

Careful clinical examination will be diagnostic in the vast majority of patients complaining of anal symptoms but it requires a

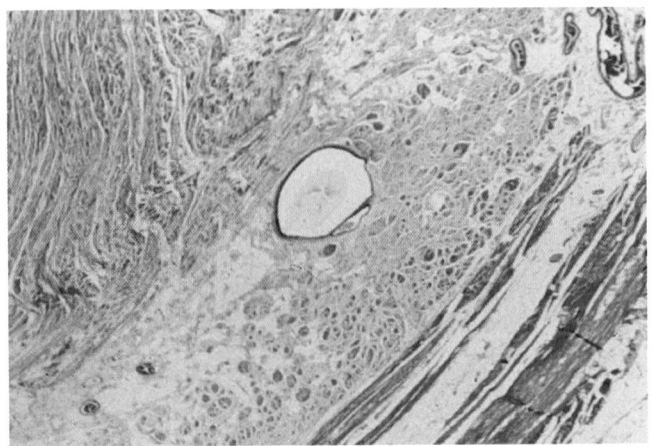

Figure 69.4 Intersphincteric anal gland lying between the voluntary muscle of the external sphincter and the longitudinal muscle. The internal sphincter is also seen. [Reproduced with permission from Nicholls, R.J. and Dozois, R.R. (1997) *Surgery of the Colon and Rectum*. Churchill Livingstone, Edinburgh.]

relaxed patient who is informed of what the examination will entail, a private environment, a chaperone (for the security of both parties) and good light. Most commonly, the patient is examined in the left lateral (Sims) position with the buttocks overlying the edge of the examination couch and with the axis of the torso crossing, rather than parallel with, the edge of the couch. Alternatively, in younger patients, the prone jack-knife or knee–elbow positions may be used (Fig. 69.5). The examining couch should be of sufficient height to allow easy inspection and access for any necessary manoeuvres. A protective glove should be worn.

Inspection

The buttocks are gently parted to allow inspection of the anus and perineum: the presence of any skin lesions and whether they are confined to the perineum or evident elsewhere on general examination, e.g. psoriasis, lichen planus, or on genital examination, e.g. warts, candidiasis, lichen sclerosus et atrophicus, the vesicles of herpes simplex virus (HSV); evidence of anal leakage; whether the anus is closed or patulous; and the position of the anus and perineum at rest and on bearing down (the latter may reveal prolapse of haemorrhoids or even the rectum). Pain on parting the buttocks, perhaps together with the presence of a sentinel tag, may indicate the presence of an underlying fissure, but may also prompt the need for examination under anaesthesia to exclude more suspicious pathology, for example squamous cell carcinoma of the anal canal.

Digital examination with the index finger

With an adequately lubricated index finger, the soft tissues around the anus are palpated for induration, tenderness and subcutaneous lesions. The index finger is then introduced gently into the anal canal along its posterior aspect. At the apex of the canal, the sling of puborectalis is felt posteriorly; supralevator induration feels bony hard and is more easily appreciated if unilateral. The posterior surface of the prostate gland with its median sulcus can be palpated anteriorly in male patients; in female patients, the uterine cervix can be palpated. The presence of any distal intrarectal, intra-anal or extraluminal mass is recorded. Sphincter length, resting tone and voluntary squeeze are assessed. On withdrawal the examining finger is inspected for the presence of mucus, blood or pus and to identify stool colour.

Proctoscopy (Fig. 69.6)

Proctoscopy, performed with the patient in the same position, allows a detailed inspection of the distal rectum and anal canal. Minor procedures can also be carried out through this instrument, e.g. treatment of haemorrhoids by injection or banding (see below) and biopsy. Asking the patient to bear down on slow withdrawal of the proctoscope may reveal a descending intussusception.

(a)

(b)

James Marion Sims, 1813–1883, Gynaecological Surgeon, the State Hospital for Women, New York, USA. Introduced this position to give access to the anterior vaginal wall during operations for the closure of vesico-vaginal fistulae.

(c)

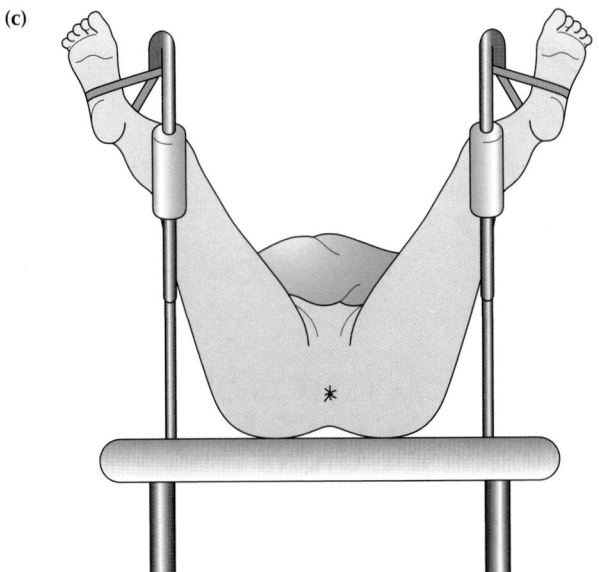

Figure 69.5 The left lateral, knee–elbow and lithotomy positions for examination. [Redrawn with permission from Mann, C.V. (2002) *Surgical Treatment of Haemorrhoids*. Springer, London.]

CHAPTER 69 | THE ANUS AND ANAL CANAL

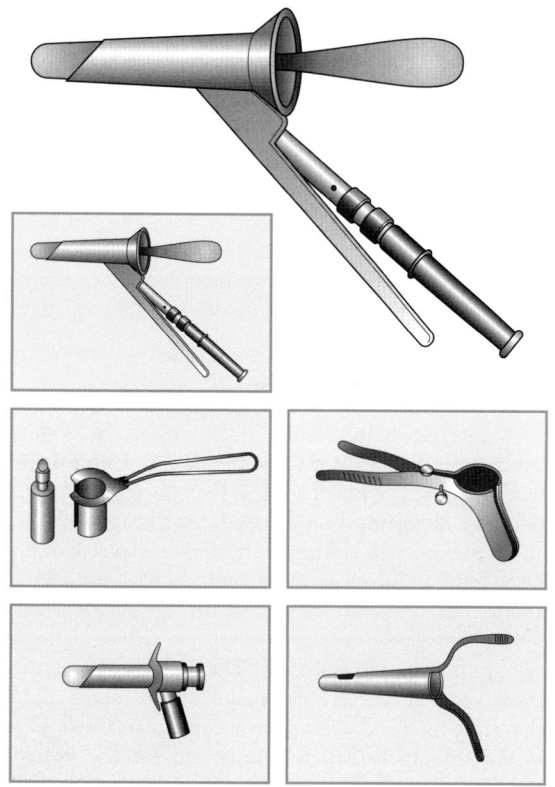

Figure 69.6 Various types of proctoscope. [Redrawn with permission from Mann, C.V. (2002) *Surgical Treatment of Haemorrhoids*. Springer, London.]

Sigmoidoscopy (see Chapter 68)

Although this is strictly an examination of the rectum, it should always be carried out even when an anal lesion has been confirmed. Rectal pathology, e.g. colitis or carcinoma, is frequently associated with an anal lesion, e.g. fissure or haemorrhoids. Not infrequently, rectal pathology is found that is independent of the anal lesion and which requires treatment (Summary box 69.2).

Summary box 69.2

Examination of anal canal

- A rectal examination is essential for any patient with anorectal and/or bowel symptoms – 'If you don't put your finger in, you might put your foot in it'
- A proctosigmoidoscopy is essential in any patient with bowel symptoms, and particularly if there is rectal bleeding

---

PHYSIOLOGICAL ASPECTS OF THE ANAL SPHINCTERS AND PELVIC FLOOR, AND SPECIAL INVESTIGATIONS

Anal continence and defaecation are highly complex processes that necessitate the structural and functional integrity of the cerebral, autonomic and enteric nervous systems, the gastrointestinal tract (especially the rectum) and the pelvic floor and anal sphincter complex, any of which may be compromised and lead to disturbances of function of varying severity. The sphincter

mechanism provides the ultimate barrier to leakage and its integrity can be assessed fairly simply and objectively in the physiology laboratory (Swash and Henry). Perineal position and degree of descent on straining (markers of pelvic floor and pudendal nerve function) can be quantified, and functional anal canal length, resting tone (reflective predominantly of internal sphincter activity) and squeeze increment (reflective of external sphincter function) can be measured by a variety of simple manometric techniques (Fig. 69.7). The structural integrity of the sphincters can be visualised with endoluminal ultrasound (Fig. 69.8), and neuromuscular function can be measured by assessment of conduction velocity along the pudendal nerve on each side, or, more painfully, by needle electromyogram (EMG) studies (Figs 69.9 and 69.10). In the elderly especially, but also in younger patients, disorders relating to rectal sensorimotor dysfunction can lead to 'overflow' of rectal contents through what may be an otherwise normal sphincter. The dynamics of defaecation can also be assessed radiologically by evacuation proctography, in which radio-opaque pseudo-stool is inserted into the rectum and the patient asked to rest, squeeze and then bear down to evacuate the rectal contents under real-time imaging. Proctography can be combined with synchronous EMG and pressure studies (Williams) (Fig. 69.11) to yield more information about possible reasons [mechanical (rectocoele, intussusception) or functional (anismus, lack of effort)] for disordered defaecation in an individual. Results of all physiological tests have to be compared with a normal range and within the context of the patient's symptoms, and are used to guide rational rather than empirical treatment strategies.

CONGENITAL ABNORMALITIES

Early in embryonic life there is a common chamber – the cloaca – into which the hind gut and the allantois open. This endoderm-lined chamber is separated from the surface ectoderm of the embryo by the cloacal membrane. The cloaca becomes divided into two parts, dorsal (rectum) and ventral (urogenital sinus), by the downgrowth of a septum. The dorsal part of the cloacal

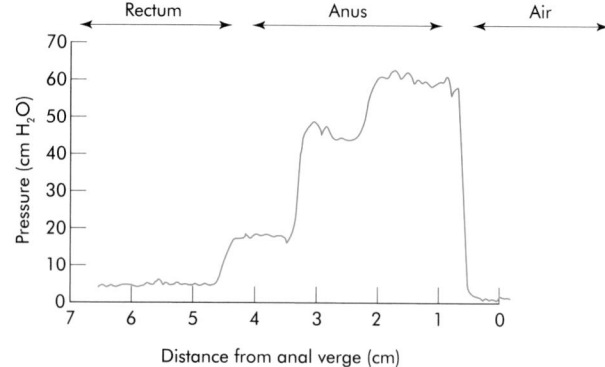

Figure 69.7 A typical, normal 'pull-through' manometric study of the anal canal (3.5 cm long; maximal pressure approximately 60 cmH$_2$O).

Michael Swash, **Formerly Professor of Neurology, St Bartholomew's and The Royal London Hospital, London, England.**
Michael Meldrum Henry, **Surgeon, The Chelsea and Westminster Hospital, London, England.**
Norman Stanley Williams, **Contemporary, Professor of Surgery, St Bartholomew's and the Royal London Hospital, London, UK.**

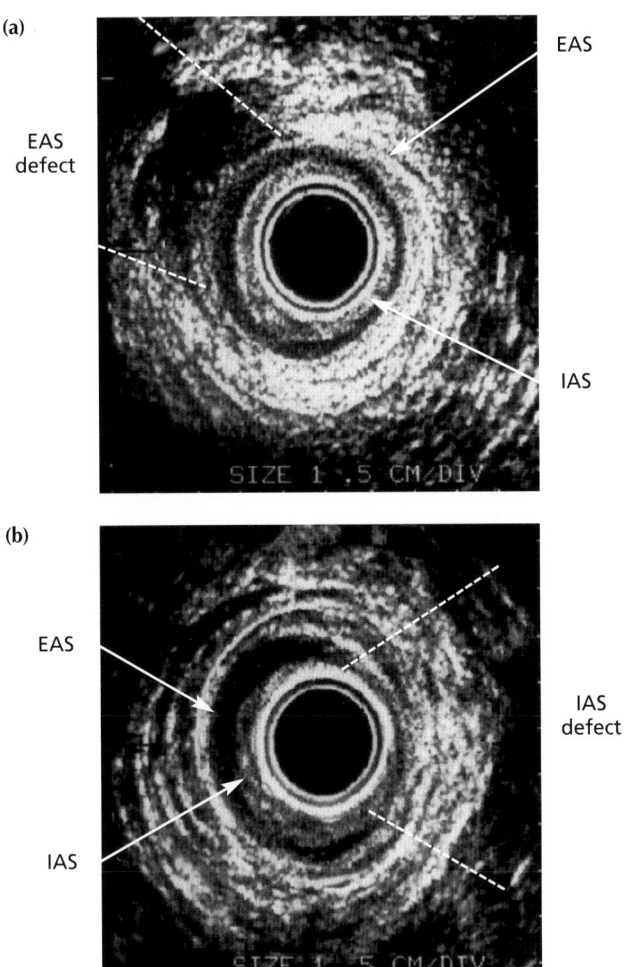

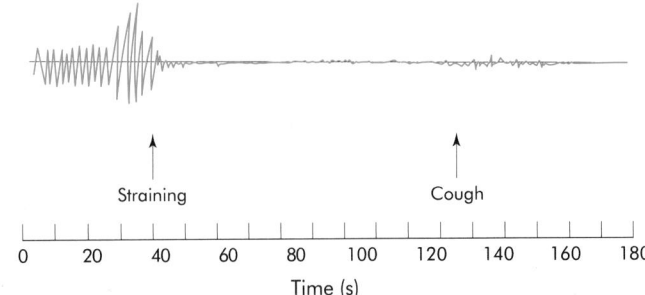

Figure 69.10 An electromyographic study of the external sphincter showing prolonged inhibition on straining and absent cough reflex. This is typical of a denervated patulous sphincter.

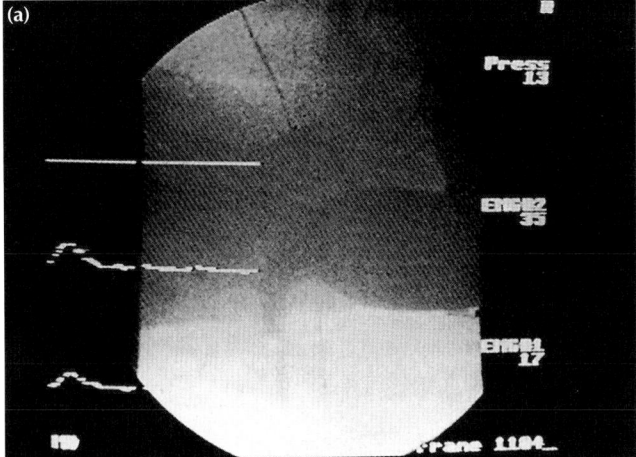

Figure 69.8 Endoanal ultrasonography. (a) External anal sphincter (EAS) defect caused by obstetric injury. (b) Internal anal sphincter (IAS) defect post-sphincterotomy.

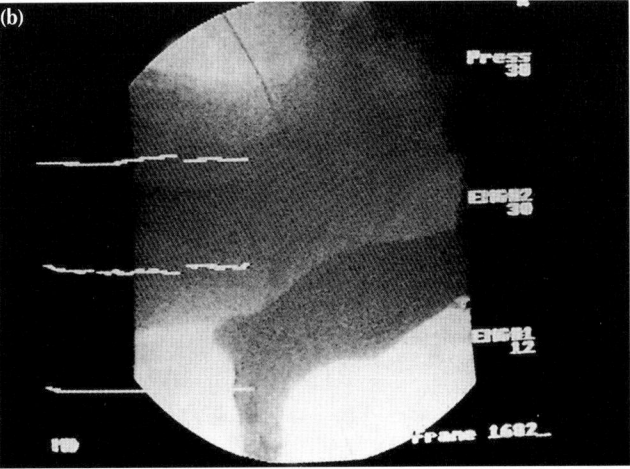

Figure 69.11 Integrated dynamic proctography. (a) At rest; (b) during evacuation. Visualisation of the rectum is achieved using barium-impregnated 'synthetic stool'. The effects of straining and evacuation on the electromyographic activity of the sphincter muscles and intrarectal pressure can be simultaneously recorded (Williams).

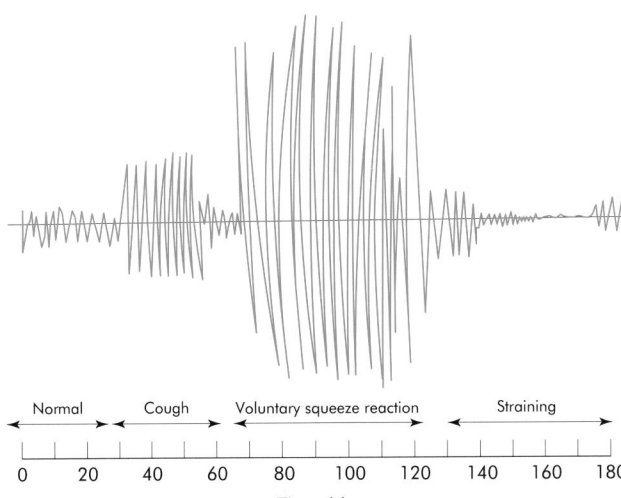

Figure 69.9 A typical, normal electromyographic study of the external sphincter during various activities.

membrane, known as the anal membrane, is thus composed of an outer layer of ectoderm and an inner layer of endoderm. Resorption of this anal membrane by the eighth week of embryonic life creates the anal canal.

CHAPTER 69 | THE ANUS AND ANAL CANAL

Imperforate anus (see Chapter 6)

Imperforate anus (strictly, it should be anal 'agenesis' or 'atresia') has historically been divided into two main groups – high and low – depending on the level of termination of the rectum in relation to the pelvic floor. Treatment and prognosis are influenced by any associated abnormalities of the sacrum and genitourinary systems. In both sexes, low defects embrace rectoperineal fistula (Fig. 69.12), covered anus and anal membrane. The most frequent defect in boys with imperforate anus is one in which the distal rectum is sited within the puborectalis sling but terminates as a fistula into the bulbar urethra (Fig. 69.13) (see also Chapter 6, Fig. 6.22) or prostatic urethra above the main anal sphincter complex. Boys with a fistula into the bladder neck (a high defect) have the poorest prognosis because of the underdevelopment of the sacrum and pelvic and anal musculature. The most common defect in girls is a rectovestibular fistula, in which the fistula opens into the posterior vestibule (not the vagina) (Fig. 69.12). The finding of a single perineal orifice indicates a persistent cloaca in which the rectum, vagina and urinary tract form a confluence (Fig. 69.13); the longer the common channel, the greater the likelihood of more complex defects, including vaginal and uterine septation, duplication or atresia. An anterior anus, although not imperforate, is not fully located within the sphincter mechanism and is regarded as part of the spectrum of anorectal malformations (Fig. 69.12).

Clinical management

Careful perineal examination will usually provide the most important clues about the neonate's type of malformation. The presence of meconium on the perineum indicates a low defect and meconium in the urine is evidence of a urinary tract fistula. During the first 24 hours the baby should receive intravenous fluids and antibiotics, and should be evaluated for associated congenital anomalies. By 24 hours, the distal limit of air within the rectum, seen on a lateral prone radiograph, indicates the distance between the rectal stump and perineum (Fig. 69.14).

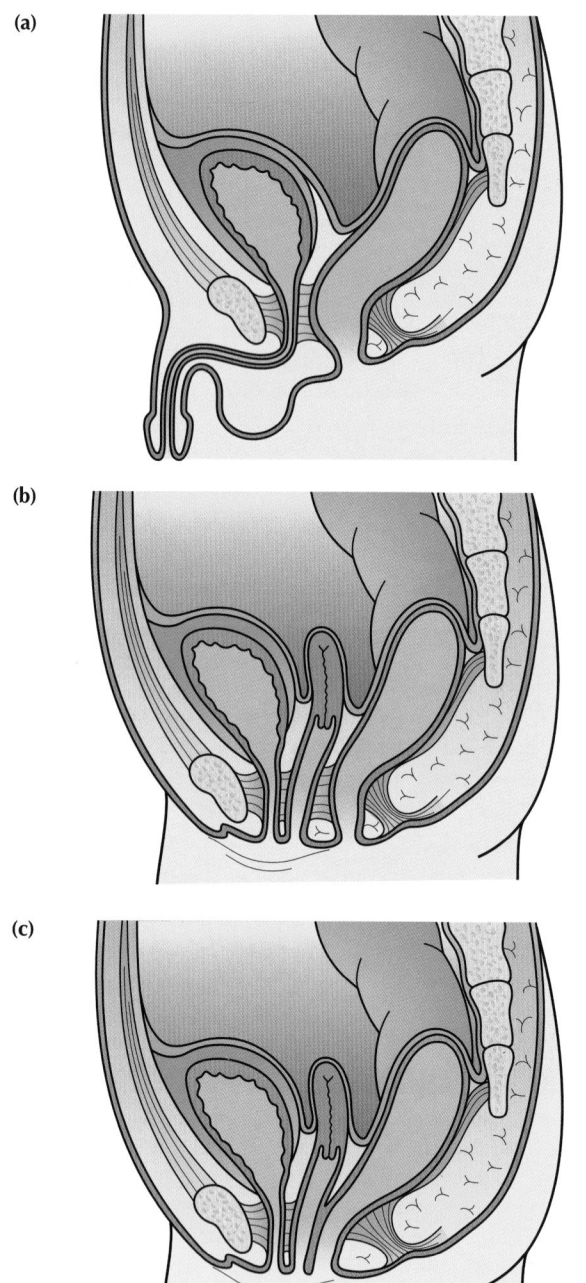

Figure 69.12 Low anorectal malformations. (a) Rectoperineal fistula in a boy; (b) rectoperineal fistula in a girl (anterior anus); (c) rectovestibular fistula (courtesy of Alberto Pena and Springer-Verlag. From 'Atlas of Surgical Management of Anorectal Malformations' by Alberto Pena, 1990. Copyright Springer-Verlag.

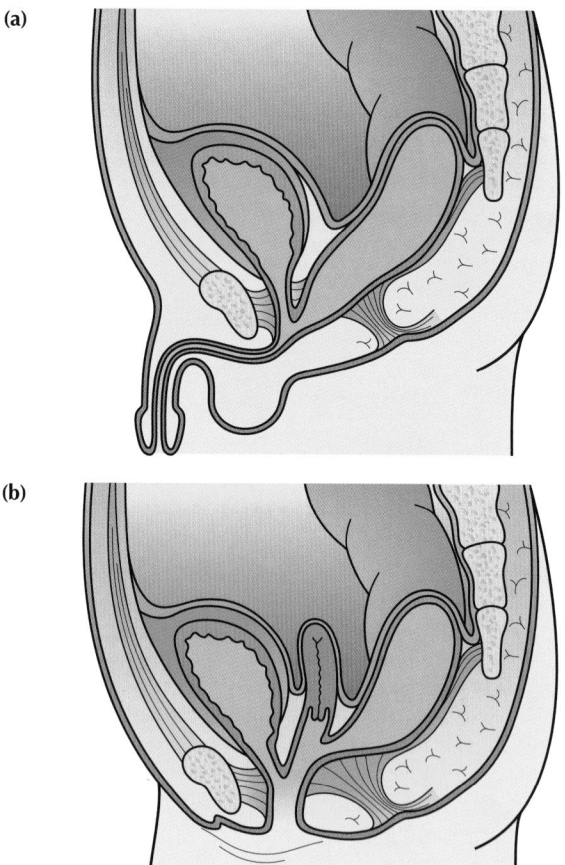

Figure 69.13 More complex anorectal malformations. (a) Rectobulbar fistula; (b) cloacal malformation (courtesy of Alberto Pena and Springer-Verlag. From 'Atlas of Surgical Management of Anorectal Malformations' by Alberto Pena, 1990. Copyright Springer-Verlag.

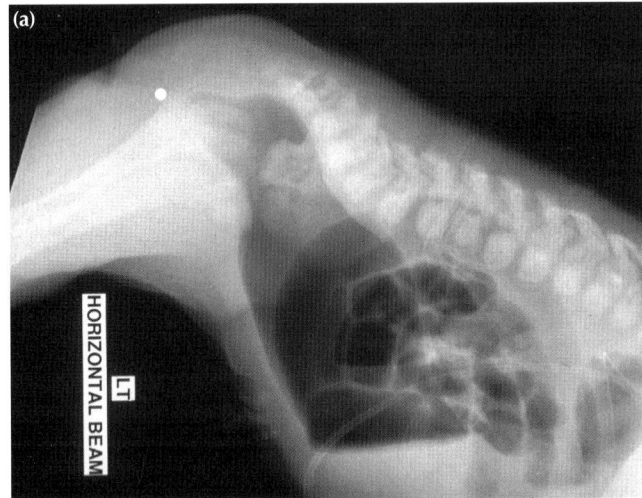

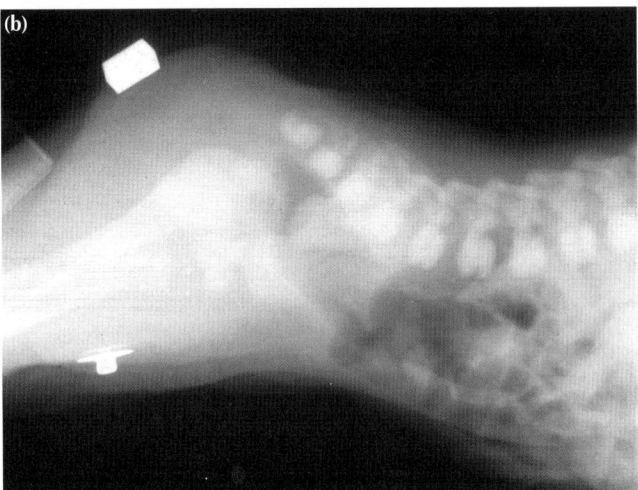

Figure 69.14 Lateral prone shoot-through radiograph of a neonate with (a) low and (b) high anorectal malformation. A radio-opaque marker has been placed on the anal dimple (courtesy of Mark D. Stringer, Leeds, UK).

Treatment

Low anomalies with a perineal fistula can be treated by an anoplasty. More complex malformations require early colostomy, with definitive repair performed several months later. This may involve posterior sagittal anorectoplasty (PSARP, Pena, with or without transabdominal mobilisation of the left colon and division of any communication with the urinary tract. In girls with a cloaca and long common channel, urinary and vaginal reconstruction is also required. Postoperatively, a programme of anal dilatation is instituted, and any residual colostomy is closed at a later date. Ultimate bowel function (voluntary bowel movements, continence, constipation) is related to the type of anorectal abnormality and the presence of associated defects, especially sacral (Summary box 69.3).

Alberto Pena, **Contemporary, Professor of Pediatric Surgery, Schneider Children's Hospital, New York, NY, USA.**

Summary box 69.3

Imperforate anus

- A rare congenital disorder
- Classified as being high or low depending on the site of the rectal termination in relation to the pelvic floor
- Low defects: relatively easy to correct but prone to constipation
- High defects: more difficult to correct and prone to faecal incontinence

Post-anal dermoid

The space in front of the lower part of the sacrum and coccyx may be occupied by a soft, cystic swelling – a post-anal dermoid cyst. Hidden in the hollow of the sacrum it is unlikely to be discovered unless a sinus communicating with the exterior is present or it develops as a result of inflammation. Such a cyst usually remains asymptomatic until adult life, when it is prone to becoming infected. Exceptionally, because of its size, it gives rise to difficulty in defaecation. The cyst is easily palpable on rectal examination.

Differential diagnosis

Especially in a child, an anterior sacral meningocele must be excluded. This enlarges when the child cries and is frequently associated with paralysis of the lower limbs and incontinence. When a discharging sinus is present, a post-anal dermoid will probably be mistaken for a pilonidal sinus or even an anal fistula. Pressure over the sacrococcygeal region with a finger in the rectum may cause a flow of sebaceous material, and injection of contrast media followed by radiography reveals a bottle-necked cyst in front of the coccyx.

Treatment

Treatment involves complete excision of the cyst and, if present, the sinus. In the case of large cysts it is necessary to remove the coccyx to gain access. The coccyx should also be removed *en bloc* in any child with a presacral dermoid because of the risk of sacrococcygeal teratoma.

Post-anal dimple (synonym: fovea coccygea)

A dimple in the skin beneath the tip of the coccyx, sometimes amounting to a short blind pit, is noticed from time to time in the course of a clinical examination and is of no consequence.

Pilonidal sinus

The term pilonidal sinus describes a condition found in the natal cleft overlying the coccyx, consisting of one or more, usually non-infected, midline openings, which communicate with a fibrous track lined by granulation tissue and containing hair lying loosely within the lumen. A common affliction amongst the military, it has been referred to as 'jeep disease'.

Aetiology and pathology

Although acquired theories of development are better accepted than the more historical congenital theories, exact mechanisms

A jeep is a small military, general purpose, vehicle with hard springing, which gives its occupants a very bouncy ride when driven over rough terrain.

of development are speculative. Evidence that supports the acquired theory of origin of pilonidal sinuses can be summarised as follows:

- Interdigital pilonidal sinus is an occupational disease of hairdressers, the hair within the interdigital cleft or clefts being the customers'. Pilonidal sinuses of the axilla and umbilicus have also been reported.
- The age incidence of the appearance of pilonidal sinus (82% occur between the ages of 20 and 29 years) is at variance with the age of onset of congenital lesions.
- Hair follicles have almost never been demonstrated in the walls of the sinus.
- The hairs projecting from the sinus are dead hairs, with their pointed ends directed towards the blind end of the sinus.
- The disease mostly affects men, in particular hairy men.
- Recurrence is common, even though adequate excision of the track is carried out.

It is thought that the combination of buttock friction and shearing forces in that area allows shed hair or broken hairs which have collected there to drill through the midline skin, or that infection in relation to a hair follicle allows hair to enter the skin by the suction created by movement of the buttocks, so creating a subcutaneous, chronically infected, midline track. From this primary sinus, secondary tracks may spread laterally, which may emerge at the skin as granulation tissue-lined, discharging openings. Usually, but not invariably (when diagnosis may be confused with anal fistula or hidradenitis suppurativa), the sinus runs cephalad. Carcinoma arising in chronic pilonidal disease has been described but is exceedingly rare.

Clinical features

The condition is seen much more frequently in men than women, usually after puberty and before the fourth decade of life, and is characteristically seen in dark-haired individuals rather than those with softer blond hair (Oldham). Patients complain of intermittent pain, swelling and discharge at the base of the spine but little in the way of constitutional symptoms. There is often a history of repeated abscesses that have burst spontaneously or which have been incised, usually away from the midline. The primary sinus may have one or many openings, all of which are strictly in the midline between the level of the sacrococcygeal joint and the tip of the coccyx.

Conservative treatment

As the natural history of the condition is usually one of regression, in those whose symptoms are relatively minor, simple cleaning out of the tracks and removal of all hair, with regular shaving of the area and strict hygiene, may be recommended.

Treatment of an acute exacerbation (abscess)

If rest, baths, local antiseptic dressings and the administration of a broad-spectrum antibiotic fail to bring about resolution, the abscess should be drained through a small longitudinal incision made over the abscess and off the midline, with thorough curettage of granulation tissue and hair. This procedure may or may not be associated with complete resolution.

Surgical treatment of chronic pilonidal disease

The multitude of surgical procedures advocated to eradicate pilonidal disease, combined with the lack of prospective trials, attests to the lack of overall superiority of one method over the others. Time spent off work and perceived recurrence rates, but more usually surgeon preference, influence the choice of method, which includes the laying open of all tracks with or without marsupialisation, the excision of all tracks with or without primary closure, and the excision of all tracks and then closure by some other means designed to avoid a midline wound [Z-plasty, Karydakis procedure (Fig 69.15)]. Bascom's procedure involves an incision lateral to the midline to gain access to the sinus cavity, which is rid of hair and granulation tissue (Fig. 69.16), and excision and closure of the midline pits (Fig. 69.17). The lateral wound is left open (Fig. 69.18). Irrespective of procedure, postoperative wound care is important and centres around elimination of hair (ingrown, local or other) from the wound.

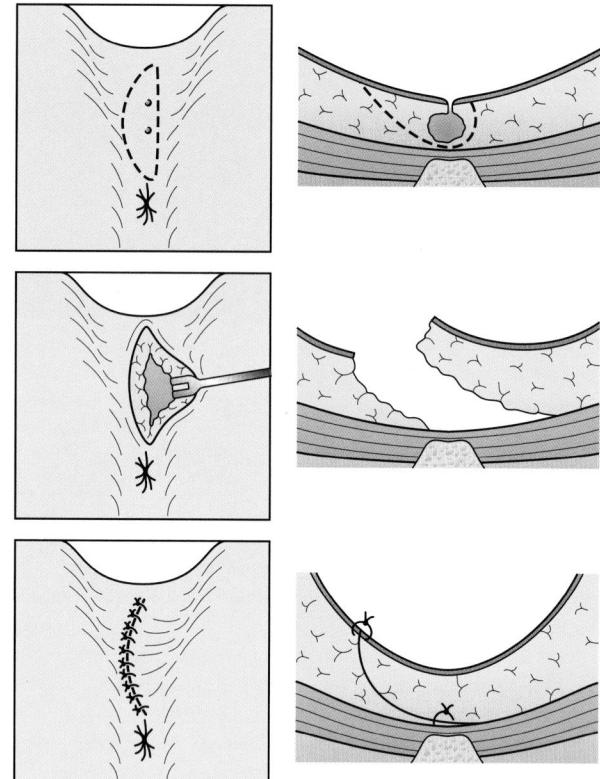

Figure 69.15 Karydakis's operation for pilonidal sinus. A semilateral incision is made around the sinus complex, the diseased component excised and the flap mobilised to allow tension-free closure of the wound off the midline. [Reproduced with permission from Nicholls, R.J. and Dozois, R.R. (1997) *Surgery of the Colon and Rectum*. Churchill Livingstone, Edinburgh.]

James Bagot Oldham, **1899–1977, Surgeon, the United Liverpool Hospitals, Liverpool, UK.**

Col Dr Karydakis, **Surgeon, Athens, Greece.**
J. Bascom, **American Surgeon.**

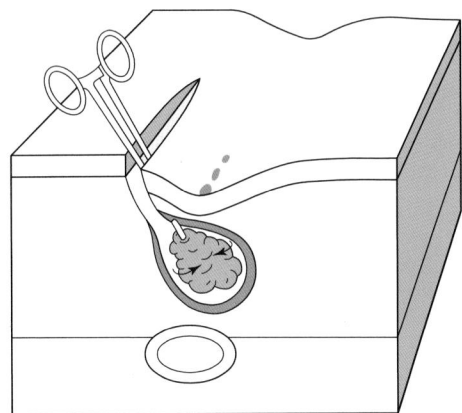

Figure 69.16 Bascom's technique for pilonidal sinus: 1.

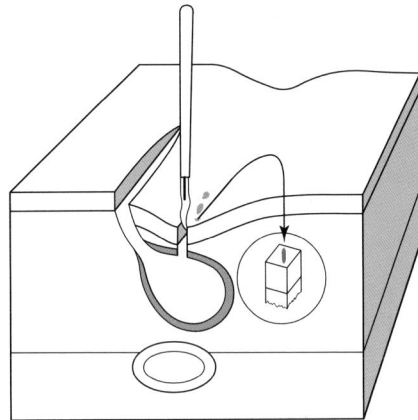

Figure 69.17 Bascom's technique for pilonidal sinus: 2.

Recurrent pilonidal sinus

Three possibilities account for this disappointment:

- part of the sinus complex has been overlooked at the primary operation;
- new hairs enter the skin or the scar;
- there is persistence of a midline wound caused by shearing forces and scarring; in this situation, revisional surgery may include re-excision followed by wound closure and obliteration of the natal cleft either by myocutaneous rotational buttock flap or cleft closure (Bascom).

ANAL INCONTINENCE

Aetiology

As continence is dependent upon the structural and functional integrity of both the neurological pathways and the gastrointestinal tract, the risk factors for anal incontinence are many (Summary box 69.4). Patients complaining of the involuntary loss of rectal contents require a comprehensive assessment of the nature and severity of symptoms; past history, especially of gastrointestinal disease, neurological conditions, obstetric events and anal surgery; and careful clinical examination (in the elderly, incontinence is often one of overflow secondary to rectal impaction, and proctitis may lead to such an irritable rectum that even the strongest sphincter is occasionally overwhelmed). A combination of history and examination will usually be diagnostic, but special investigations are then usually required to clarify the exact cause, including exclusion of an underlying malignancy, and to direct management.

Summary box 69.4

Causes of anal incontinence

Congenital/childhood
- Anorectal anomalies
- Spina bifida
- Hirschsprung's disease
- Behavioural

Acquired/adulthood
- Diabetes mellitus
- Cerebrovascular accident
- Parkinson's disease
- Multiple sclerosis
- Spinal cord injury
- Other neurological conditions:
  - Myotonic dystrophy
  - Shy–Drager syndrome
  - Amyloid neuropathy
- Gastrointestinal infection
- Irritable bowel syndrome
- Metabolic bowel disease
- Inflammatory bowel disease
- Megacolon/megarectum
- Anal trauma
- Abdominal surgery:
  - Small bowel resection
  - Colonic resection
- Pelvic surgery:
  - Hysterectomy
  - Rectal excision
- Pelvic malignancy
- Pelvic radiotherapy
- Rectal prolapse
- Rectal evacuatory disorder:
  - Mechanical, e.g. rectocoele, intussusception
  - Functional, i.e. pelvic floor dyssynergia
- Anal surgery:
  - Haemorrhoidectomy
  - Surgery for fistula
  - Surgery for fissure
  - Rectal disimpaction
- Obstetric events

General
- Ageing
- Dependence of nursing care
- Obesity
- Psycho-behavioural factors
- Intellectual incapacity
- Drugs:
  - Primary constipating and laxative agents
  - Secondary effects

Sphincteric causes of incontinence may be classified as structural, in which there is disruption (or atrophy) of part of the sphincter muscles, neuropathic (previously termed idiopathic), in which the nerve supply to the sphincters is damaged, usually by chronic straining or complicated vaginal delivery (prolonged second stage), or a combination of the two. The commonest causes of

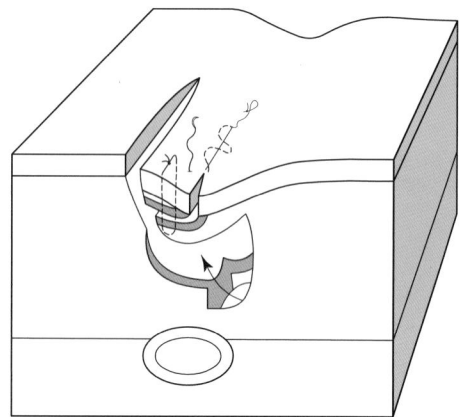

Figure 69.18 Bascom's technique for pilonidal sinus: 3.

sphincteric disruption are obstetric damage, anal surgery (following haemorrhoidectomy, dilatation or sphincterotomy for anal fissure, and fistulotomy for anal fistula) and trauma (including anal intercourse, forced or otherwise).

In general, conservative measures to reduce symptoms are employed initially. These may be in the form of stool bulking or constipating agents, nurse-led bowel retraining including specific biofeedback programmes, or anal plugs, which expand within and thus seal the anal canal. Failure of such measures and severity of symptoms may result in selection for surgery.

Operations to reunite divided sphincter muscles

In situations in which there is a discrete disruption of the sphincters, the ends of the divided muscle are found and reunited by a double overlap repair (Fig. 69.19).

Operations to reef the external sphincter and puborectalis muscle

If the sphincter muscles are stretched and patulous (as they often are in old age and in cases of rectal prolapse) they may be tightened by a post-anal repair, which, through the use of darns of absorbable material to narrow down and plicate the external sphincter and the puborectalis sling (Fig. 69.20), aims to recreate the anorectal angle and to restore length to the anal canal and strength to the anal sphincter. The approach is usually through the intersphincteric plane. The operation is now much less popular because long-term outcomes have been reported as poor.

Operations to augment the anal sphincters

If the degree of sphincter disruption or weakness is such that restoration of function cannot be achieved by direct means, the sphincter can be augmented by using muscle transposed from nearby (gluteus maximus or gracilis) or by using an artificial sphincter. Transposition of the gracilis muscle around the anal canal is followed by electrical stimulation, with conversion from a fast-twitch to a less fatiguable slow-twitch muscle by an implanted pacemaker (Williams) (Fig. 69.21). Because of its magnitude this technique is performed only in highly selected and motivated patients, most of whom have had more conventional treatment that has failed to cure their incontinence; it is effective in approximately 60% of patients in the long term. A simpler means of augmenting the sphincter, developed initially for urinary incontinence, is the placement of an inflatable silastic cuff around

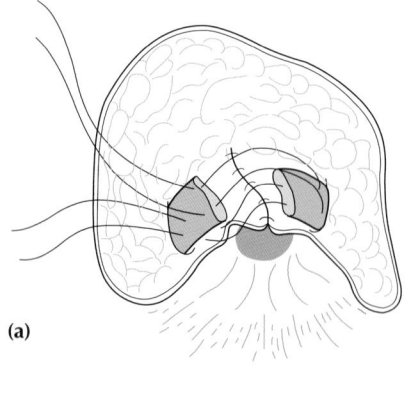

(a)

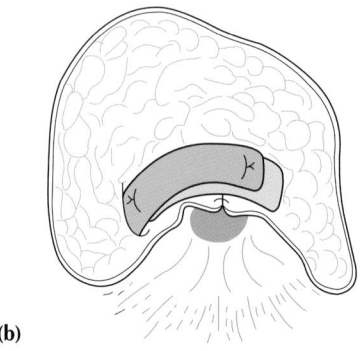

(b)

Figure 69.19 Direct sphincter repair in which (a) the sphincter defect is excised and (b) the remaining muscle is overlapped. [Redrawn with permission from Mann, C.V. and Glass, R.E. (1991) *Surgical Treatment of Anal Incontinence*. Springer, New York.]

the anal canal. When evacuation is required the cuff is deflated by squeezing a small balloon positioned in the scrotum or labia, the balloon being attached to a subcutaneous reservoir (Fig. 69.22). However, because this device is a foreign body that exerts pressure on the bowel wall, erosion and infection have been found to be common problems. To reduce the risk of septic complications the operation should be covered by antibiotics active against both aerobic and anaerobic organisms. Paradoxically, all of these methods used to treat incontinence may be associated with difficulties in rectal evacuation.

More recently, again as a result of its use in urinary incontinence, sacral nerve stimulation has been used to treat faecal incontinence, with encouraging short-term results. Rather than any direct action on sphincter strength, this technique appears to work by sensorimotor neurophysiological modulation of the hindgut through electrical stimulation of the sacral nerve roots via a needle positioned through one of the posterior sacral foramina (Fig. 69.23). A potential advantage of this technique is its relatively non-invasive nature, as well as the fact that its effects can be tested by temporary stimulation using an external stimulator before the expensive permanent pacemaker is implanted.

For some patients, and in those in whom quality of life remains poor despite attempts at restoring continence, a colostomy can provide relief from a condition which is both disabling and socially isolating.

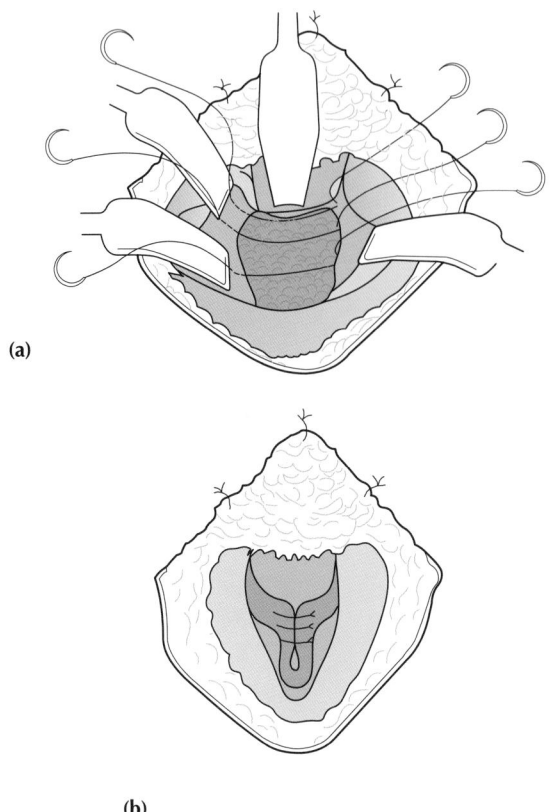

(a)

(b)

Figure 69.20 Post-anal repair in which (a) the sphincter muscle is plicated posterior to the anal canal, thus restoring the anorectal angle. (b) The completed repair. [Redrawn with permission from Mann, C.V. and Glass, R.E. (1991) *Surgical Treatment of Anal Incontinence.* Springer, New York.]

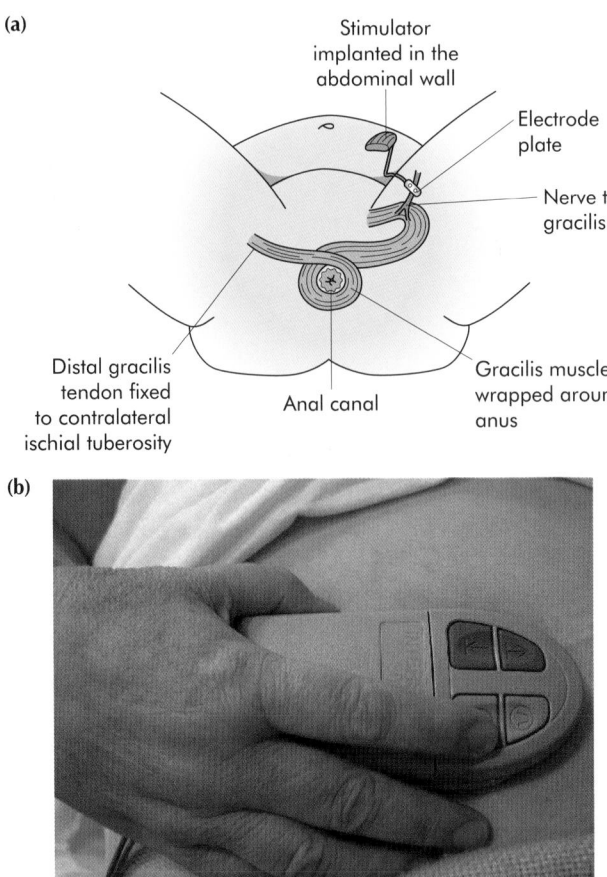

(a)

Stimulator implanted in the abdominal wall

Electrode plate

Nerve to gracilis

Gracilis muscle wrapped around anus

Anal canal

Distal gracilis tendon fixed to contralateral ischial tuberosity

(b)

Figure 69.21 (a) The electrically stimulated gracilis neosphincter or dynamic graciloplasty. (b) Hand-held radiotelemetry controller, which allows the patient to turn the stimulator on and off.

ANAL FISSURE

Definition

An anal fissure (synonym: fissure-*in-ano*) is a longitudinal split in the anoderm of the distal anal canal (Fig. 69.24), which extends from the anal verge proximally towards, but not beyond, the dentate line.

Aetiology

The cause of an anal fissure, and particularly the reason why the posterior midline is so frequently affected, is not completely understood. Classically, acute anal fissures arise from the trauma caused by the strained evacuation of a hard stool or, less commonly, from the repeated passage of diarrhoea. The location in the posterior midline perhaps relates to the exaggerated shearing forces acting at that site at defaecation, combined with a less elastic anoderm endowed with an increased density of longitudinal muscle extensions in that region of the anal circumference. Anterior anal fissure is much more common in women and may arise following vaginal delivery. Perpetuation and chronicity may result from repeated trauma, anal hypertonicity and vascular insufficiency, either secondary to increased sphincter tone or because the posterior commisure is less well perfused than the remainder of the anal circumference.

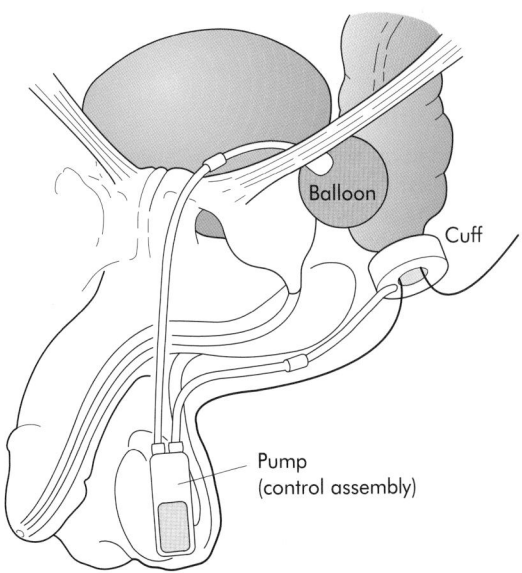

Balloon

Cuff

Pump (control assembly)

Figure 69.22 Artificial bowel sphincter. A cuff is placed around the anal canal. An inflatable pump control assembly is placed in the scrotum and the balloon reservoir is placed under the symphysis pubis.

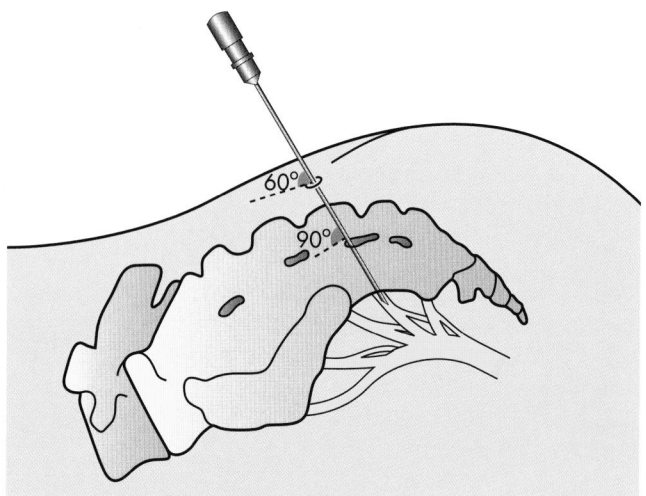

Figure 69.23 Diagram showing the placement of the electrode through a sacral foramen in sacral nerve stimulation.

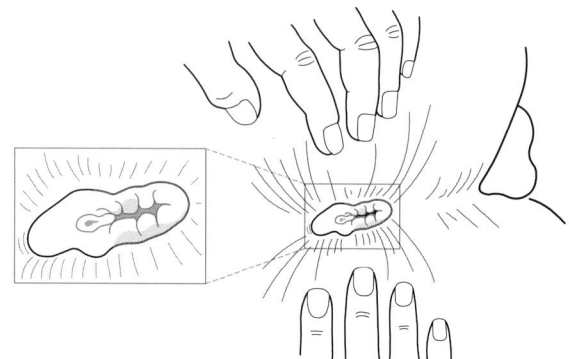

Figure 69.24 The appearance of an anal fissure. If the buttocks are gently parted, the presence of an anal fissure can usually be detected as an ulcer of variable depth with the skin tag and an anal papilla. [Redrawn with permission from Keighley, M.R.B. and Williams, N.S. (1999) *Surgery of the Anus, Colon and Rectum*, 2nd edn. W.B. Saunders, Philadelphia, PA.]

Clinical features

Although simple epithelial splits, acute anal fissures are, because of their location involving the exquisitely sensitive anoderm, characterised by severe anal pain associated with defaecation, which usually resolves spontaneously after a variable time only to recur at the next evacuation, as well as the passage of fresh blood, normally noticed on the tissue after wiping. Chronic fissures are characterised by a hypertrophied anal papilla internally and a sentinel tag externally (both consequent upon attempts at healing and breakdown), between which lies the slightly indurated anal ulcer overlying the fibres of the internal sphincter. When chronic, patients may also complain of itching secondary to irritation from the sentinel tag, discharge from the ulcer or discharge from an associated intersphincteric fistula, which has arisen through infection penetrating via the fissure base. Although most sufferers are young adults, the condition can affect any age, from infants to the elderly. Men and women are affected equally. Anterior fissures account for about 10% of those encountered in women but only 1% in men. A fissure sited

elsewhere around the anal circumference or with atypical features should raise the suspicion of a specific aetiology, and failure of adequate examination in the clinic should prompt early examination under anaesthesia, with biopsy and culture to exclude Crohn's disease, tuberculosis, sexually transmitted or human immunodeficiency virus (HIV)-related ulcers (syphilis, *Chlamydia*, chancroid, lymphogranuloma venereum, HSV, cytomegalovirus, Kaposi's sarcoma, B-cell lymphoma) and squamous cell carcinoma (Summary box 69.5).

Summary box 69.5
Anal fissure
■ Acute or chronic
■ Ischaemic ulcer in the midline of the anal canal
■ Ectopic site suggests a more sinister cause
Symptoms:
■ Pain on defaecation
■ Bright-red bleeding
■ Mucous discharge
■ Constipation

Treatment

After confirmation of the diagnosis in the clinic or under anaesthesia, with exclusion of secondary causes of anal ulceration, conservative management should result in the healing of almost all acute and the majority of chronic fissures. Emphasis must be placed on normalisation of bowel habits such that the passage of stool is less traumatic. The addition of fibre to the diet to bulk up the stool, stool softeners and adequate water intake are simple and helpful measures. Warm baths and topical local anaesthetic agents relieve pain; however, providing patients with anal dilators is usually associated with low compliance and consequently little effect. The mainstay of current conservative management is the topical application of pharmacological agents that relax the internal sphincter, most commonly nitric oxide donors (Scholefield); by reducing spasm, pain is relieved, and increased vascular perfusion promotes healing. Such agents include glyceryl trinitrate (GTN) 0.2% applied four times per day to the anal margin (although this may cause headaches) and diltiazem 2% applied twice daily.

Operative measures

Historically, under regional or general anaesthesia, forceful manual (four- or eight-digit) sphincter dilatation was used to reduce sphincter tone; however, this was achieved in an uncontrolled fashion with potential disruption at multiple sites of the internal (and even external) sphincter. The risk of incontinence following this procedure has now made it unpopular, although more conservative controlled stretching is still practised in young men with very high sphincter tone.

Fissure healing can also be achieved by a posterior division of the exposed fibres of the internal sphincter in the fissure base, but this is associated with prolonged healing, as well as passive anal

Burrill Bernard Crohn, **1884–1983**, Gastroenterologist, Mount Sinai Hospital, New York, NY, USA.
Moritz Kaposi, **1837–1902**, Professor of Dermatology, Vienna, Austria, described pigmented sarcoma of the skin in 1872.
John Howard Scholefield, **Contemporary**, Professor of Surgery, The University of Nottingham, Nottingham, England.

leakage thought mainly to be due to the resulting keyhole gutter deformity; however, it may be indicated if there is an associated intersphincteric fistula.

Lateral anal sphincterotomy (Notaras)

In this operation, the internal sphincter is divided away from the fissure itself – usually either in the right or the left lateral positions. The procedure can be carried out using an open or a closed method, under local, regional or general anaesthesia, and with the patient in the lithotomy or prone jack-knife position. The distal internal sphincter is palpated with a bivalved speculum at the intersphincteric groove. In the closed method a small longitudinal incision is made over this, and the submucosal and intersphincteric planes are carefully developed to allow precise division of the internal sphincter with a knife or scissors to the level of the apex of the fissure; the wound is then closed with absorbable sutures. Alternatively, either plane can be entered using a scalpel (no. 11 blade), with the blade advanced parallel to the sphincter and then rotated such that the sharp edge faces the internal sphincter, which can then be divided along its distal third. Pressure should be applied to the wound for a few minutes to prevent haematoma formation. In the open technique, the anoderm overlying the distal internal sphincter is divided longitudinally to expose the sphincter, which is divided, and the wound is closed with absorbable sutures. Although the fissure needs no specific attention, problematic papillae and external tags can be excised concomitantly.

Early complications of sphincterotomy include haemorrhage, haematoma, bruising, perianal abscess and fistula. Despite low recurrence rates the most important complication is incontinence of a variable nature and severity, which may affect up to 30% of patients, particularly women, who have weaker, shorter sphincter complexes and in whom there may already have been covert sphincter compromise incurred by childbirth.

Anal advancement flap

The recognition of the risk to continence following internal sphincterotomy has led some to advocate a different approach, especially in women and those with normal or low resting anal pressures, developed from the treatment of anal stenosis. After excision of the edges of the fissure and, if necessary, its base overlying the internal sphincter, an inverted house-shaped flap of perianal skin is carefully mobilised on its blood supply and advanced without tension to cover the fissure, and then sutured with interrupted absorbable sutures. The patient is maintained on stool softeners and bulking agents postoperatively, and usually also on topical sphincter relaxants; minor breakdown of one anastomotic edge does not herald ultimate failure (Summary box 69.6).

Summary box 69.6
Treatment of an anal fissure
■ Conservative initially, consisting of stool-bulking agents and softeners, and chemical agents in the form of ointments designed to relax the anal sphincter and improve blood flow
■ Surgery if above fails, consisting of lateral internal sphincterotomy or anal advancement flap

Mitchell James Notaras, **Surgeon, Barnet General Hospital, Barnet, England.**

Hypertrophied anal papilla

Anal papillae occur at the dentate line and are remnants of the ectodermal membrane that separated the hindgut from the proctodaeum. As these papillae are present in 60% of patients examined proctologically they should be regarded as normal structures. Anal papillae can become elongated, as they frequently do in the presence of an anal fissure. Occasionally, an elongated anal papilla may be the cause of pruritus. An elongated anal papilla associated with pain and/or bleeding at defaecation is sometimes encountered in infancy. Haemorrhage into a hypertrophied anal papilla can cause sudden rectal pain. A prolapsed papilla may become nipped by contraction of the sphincter mechanism after defaecation. Occasionally, a red oedematous papilla is encountered, with local pain and a purulent discharge from the associated crypt. This condition of 'cryptitis' may be cured by laying open the mouth of the infected anal gland and excising the papilla. Troublesome papillae may be simply excised.

Proctalgia fugax

This problem is characterised by attacks of severe pain arising in the rectum, recurring at irregular intervals and apparently unrelated to organic disease. The pain is described as cramp-like, often occurs when the patient is in bed at night, usually lasts only for a few minutes and disappears spontaneously. It may follow straining at stool, sudden explosive bowel action or ejaculation. It seems to occur more commonly in patients suffering from anxiety or undue stress, and it is also said to afflict young doctors. The pain may be unbearable – it is possibly caused by segmental cramp in the pubococcygeus muscle. It is unpleasant and incurable but is fortunately harmless and gradually subsides. A more chronic form of the disease has been termed the 'levator syndrome' and can be associated with severe constipation. Biofeedback techniques have been used to help such patients; in the past some surgeons tried severing the puborectalis muscle, but this can cause incontinence and should never be carried out.

HAEMORRHOIDS

The prevalence of haemorrhoids when patients are assessed proctoscopically far outweighs the prevalence of symptoms, and the term should only be used when patients have symptoms referable to them. Occasionally, patients with portal hypertension develop rectal varices, but these should not be confused with haemorrhoids as the consquences may be disastrous. Internal haemorrhoids (Greek: *haima* = blood, *rhoos* = flowing; synonym: piles, Latin: *pila* = a ball) are symptomatic anal cushions and characteristically lie in the 3, 7 and 11 o'clock positions (with the patient in the lithotomy position). In addition, haemorrhoids may be observed between the main pile masses, in which case they are internal haemorrhoids at the secondary position. External haemorrhoids relate to venous channels of the inferior haemorrhoidal plexus deep in the skin surrounding the anal verge and are not true haemorrhoids; they are usually only recognised as a result of a complication, which is most typically a painful solitary acute thrombosis. External haemorrhoids associated with internal haemorrhoids ('intero-external piles') result from progression of the latter to involve both haemorrhoidal plexuses and are best thought of as being external extensions of internal haemorrhoids. Secondary internal haemorrhoids arise as a result of a specific condition, although the mechanisms involved may be the same as those involved in the formation of primary internal haemorrhoids. The most important cause, albeit relatively uncommon, is carcinoma of the anorectum (Fig. 69.25) but there are may other causes, which may be categorised as follows:

- local, e.g. anorectal deformity, hypotonic anal sphincter;
- abdominal, e.g. ascites;
- pelvic, e.g. gravid uterus, uterine neoplasm (fibroid, carcinoma of the uterus or cervix), ovarian neoplasm, bladder carcinoma;
- neurological, e.g. paraplegia, multiple sclerosis.

Primary internal haemorrhoids

Theories of development

Portal hypertension and varicose veins

Misconceptions concerning the vascular anatomy of the anal canal (specifically the lack of appreciation of communications between portal and systemic systems and the 'normality' of venous dilatations) led to theories of development of primary internal haemorrhoids that lasted for several centuries. Man's upright posture (we know little about haemorrhoidal problems in animals), lack of valves in the portal venous system and raised abdominal pressure were thought to contribute to the development of anal varicosities. If raised portal venous pressure were indeed the cause, one would expect a high incidence in subjects suffering from portal hypertension; however, although such patients have a higher incidence of anorectal varices, these are a separate anatomical and clinical entity from haemorrhoids, which are seen no more frequently than in those without cirrhosis, portal hypertension and oesophageal varices.

Other vascular causes

Historically, some considered haemorrhoids to be haemangiomatous or to result from changes in the erectile tissue that forms part

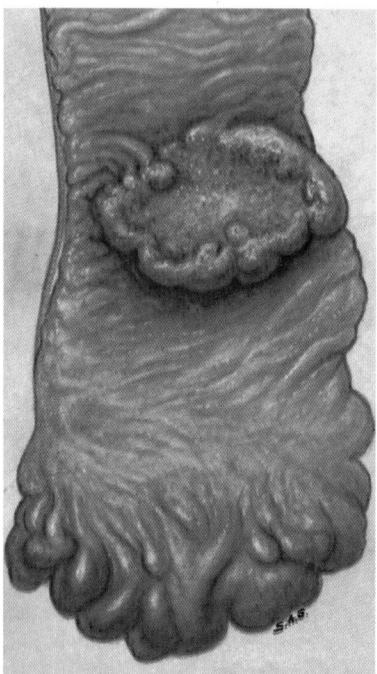

Figure 69.25 Carcinoma of the rectum associated with haemorrhoids, a not infrequent diagnostic pitfall.

of the continence mechanism, such as hyperplasia of the 'corpus cavernosum recti'.

Infection

Repeated infection of the anal lining, secondary to trauma at defaecation, has been postulated as a cause of weakening and erosion of the walls of the veins of the submucosa. This hypothesis is difficult to accept, as one of the truly incredible properties of the anal canal is its resistance to infection, as well as the ability of its mucosa to heal after surgical intervention despite the torrent of micro-organisms passing over it.

Diet and stool consistency

Much emphasis has been placed on the role of constipation in the development of haemorrhoids and, indeed, much of the management of sufferers involves attempts to 'normalise' bowel habits. A fibre-deficient diet results in a prolonged gut transit time, which is associated with the passage of smaller, harder stools that require more straining to expel. The presence of a hard faecal mass in the rectum could obstruct venous return, resulting in engorgement of the anal veins with the act of straining at stool or sitting for prolonged periods on the lavatory with a relaxed perineum, causing a disturbance of vascular flow. However, the epidemiological pattern of constipation is different from that of haemorrhoidal disease and, indeed, an association has been demonstrated between haemorrhoids and diarrhoeal disorders.

Anal hypertonia

The association between raised anal canal resting pressure and haemorrhoids is well known, but whether anal hypertonia causes symptoms attributable to haemorrhoids or whether anal cushion hypertrophy causes anal hypertonia is a subject of debate. The fact that surgical haemorrhoidectomy restores resting pressures to the normal range is not absolute evidence that the pile masses themselves are the cause of the hypertonia. It should be remembered, however, that there are a significant proportion of patients who suffer haemorrhoidal symptoms in whom the anal canal is relatively patulous, and there is mucosal prolapse, which is associated with perineal descent and pudendal neuropathy.

Ageing

In contrast to the anal cushion of early life, with age, the supporting structures show a higher proportion of collagen than muscle fibres and are fragmented and disorganised. Presumably, these changes arise over time with continued use of the anal canal for defaecation; however, similar changes are noted histologically in surgically excised haemorrhoids in younger patients.

Current view

Shearing forces acting on the anus (for a variety of reasons) lead to caudal displacement of the anal cushions and mucosal trauma. With time, fragmentation of the supporting structures (a normal consequence of ageing but perhaps accelerated in those with haemorrhoids) leads to loss of elasticity of the cushions such that they no longer retract following defaecation.

Clinical features

Bleeding, as the name haemorrhoid implies, is the principal and earliest symptom. The nature of the bleeding is characteristically separate from the motion and is seen either on the paper on wiping or as a fresh splash in the pan. Very rarely, the bleeding may be sufficient to cause anaemia. Pain is not commonly associated with the bleeding and its presence should make the clinician alert to the possibility of another diagnosis; however, pain may result from congestion of pile masses below a hypertonic sphincter. Piles associated with bleeding alone are called first-degree haemorrhoids (Summary box 69.7).

Summary box 69.7

Haemorrhoids: clinical features

- Haemorrhoids or piles are symptomatic anal cushions
- They are more common when intra-abdominal pressure is raised, e.g. in obesity, constipation and pregnancy
- Classically, they occur in the 3, 7 and 11 o'clock positions with the patient in the lithotomy position
- Symptoms of haemorrhoids:
  - bright-red, painless bleeding
  - mucus discharge
  - prolapse
  - pain only on prolapse

Patients may complain of true 'piles', lumps that appear at the anal orifice during defaecation and which return spontaneously afterwards (second-degree haemorrhoids), piles that have to be replaced manually (third-degree haemorrhoids) (Fig. 69.26) or piles that lie permanently outside (fourth-degree haemorrhoids). By this stage there is often a significant cutaneous component to the pile masses, which arise through repeated congestion and oedema. In addition to the main symptoms of pain and prolapse, patients may complain of anal irritation, which may occur as a result of mucus secretion from the caudally displaced rectal mucosa, minor leakage through a now imperfect anal seal or difficulties in cleaning after defaecation because of the irregularity of the anal verge (Summary box 69.8).

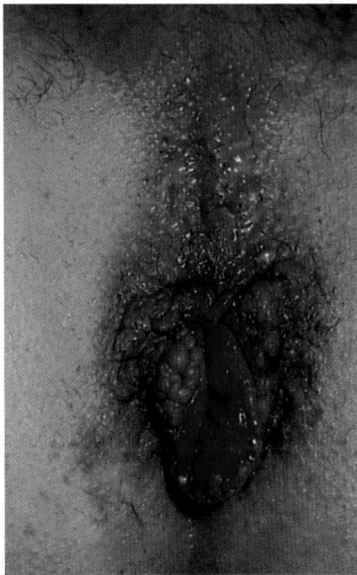

Figure 69.26 Third-degree haemorrhoids (courtesy of C.V. Mann, The Royal London Hospital, London).

Summary box 69.8

Four degrees of haemorrhoids

- First degree – bleed only, no prolapse
- Second degree – prolapse but reduce spontaneously
- Third degree – prolapse and have to be manually reduced
- Fourth degree – permanently prolapsed

Complications

Profuse haemorrhage is not rare. The bleeding mainly occurs externally but it may continue internally after the bleeding haemorrhoid has retracted or has been returned. In these circumstances the rectum is found to contain blood (Summary box 69.9).

Summary box 69.9

Complications of haemorrhoids

- Strangulation and thrombosis (Fig. 69.27)
- Ulceration
- Gangrene
- Portal pyaemia
- Fibrosis

Treatment of complications

Strangulation, thrombosis and gangrene In these cases it was formerly believed that surgery would promote portal pyaemia. However, if adequate antibiotic cover is given from the start, this is not found to be so, and immediate surgery can be justified in many patients. The other risk if surgery is performed at this stage, that of postoperative stenosis, results in some surgeons reviewing the situation much later and carrying out haemorrhoidectomy only if necessary. Besides adequate pain relief, bed rest with frequent hot baths and warm or cold saline compresses with firm pressure usually cause the pile mass to shrink considerably in 3–4 days. An anal dilatation technique has in the past been used as an alternative treatment to surgery for painful 'strangulated' haemorrhoids. However, because of the risk of incontinence this is no longer advised.

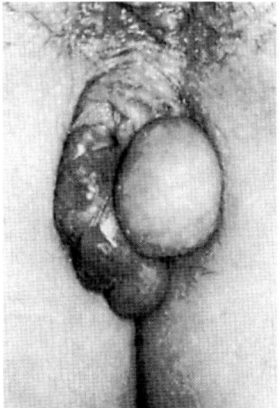

Figure 69.27 An attack of piles. Prolapsed strangulated piles, as commonly seen, on the left. A less common mass on the right with fibro-fatty covering.

Severe haemorrhage The cause usually lies in a bleeding diathesis or the use of anticoagulants. If such causes are excluded, a local compress containing adrenaline solution, with an injection of morphine and blood transfusion if necessary, will usually suffice. However, after adequate blood replacement, ligation and excision of the piles may be required.

Management

Exclusion of other causes of rectal bleeding, especially colorectal malignancy, is the first priority. In the absence of a specific predisposing cause, important measures include attempts at normalising bowel and defaecatory habits: only evacuating when the natural desire to do so arises, adopting a defaecatory position to minimise straining, and the addition of stool softeners and bulking agents to ease the defaecatory act. Various proprietary creams can be inserted into the rectum from a collapsible tube fitted with a nozzle, at night and before defaecation. Suppositories are also useful.

In those with first- or second-degree piles whose symptoms are not improved by conservative measures, injection sclerotherapy (Mitchell), the submucosal injection of 5% phenol in arachis oil or almond oil, may be advised. Any invasive treatment, however, must be with full agreement of the patient, who should be informed of the potential risks of such interventions. The aim is to create fibrosis, cause obliteration of the vascular channels and hitch up the anorectal mucosa. With the awake patient in the left lateral position and under direct vision with a proctoscope, about 5 ml of sclerosant is injected into the apex of the pile pedicle (Fig. 69.28) using a (now) disposable needle and syringe (Fig. 69.29). The procedure is repeated for each pile and the patient reassessed after 8 weeks; if necessary, the injections are repeated. Pain upon injection means that the needle is in the wrong place and should be withdrawn. Injections that are too superficial are heralded by the rapid bulging of the musosa, which turns white; this leads to superficial ulceration but rarely serious septic sequelae. However, injections placed too deeply can have disastrous consequences, including pelvic sepsis, prostatitis, impotence and rectovaginal fistula.

For more bulky piles, banding has been shown to be efficacious, but it is associated with more discomfort. The Barron's bander is a commonly available device used to slip tight elastic bands

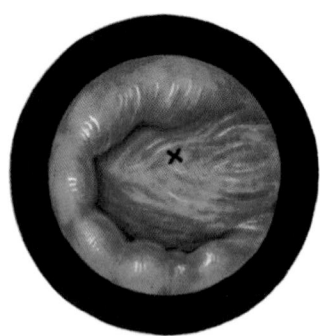

Figure 69.28 Correct site (cross) for injecting a haemorrhoid (after W.B. Gabriel, London).

Clinton Mitchell **of Illinois, IL, USA** was the first to use carbolic acid for injecting haemorrhoids. Itinerant irregular practitioners exploited the method. John Baron, **Surgeon, Chicago, IL., USA.**

(a)

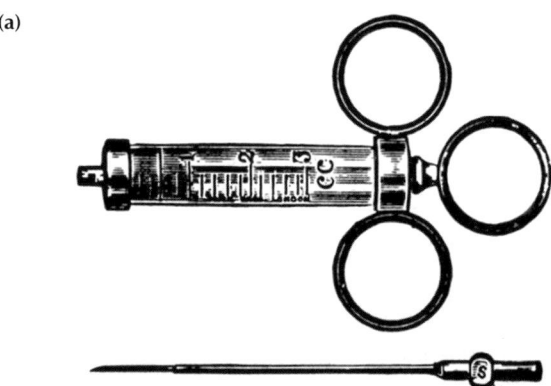

(b)

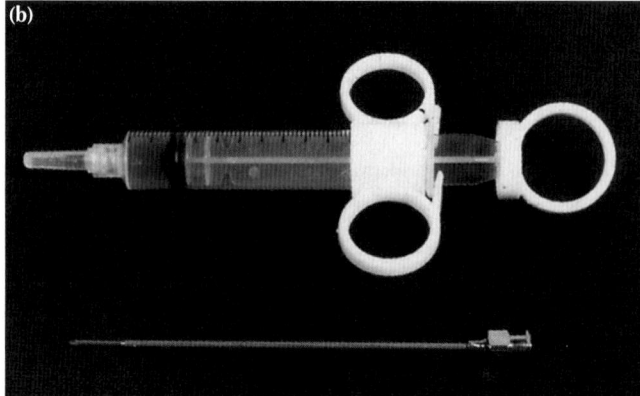

Figure 69.29 Gabriel's syringe (a) has now been replaced by disposable syringes (b).

onto the base of the pedicle of each haemorrhoid (Fig. 69.30). The bands cause ischaemic necrosis of the piles, which slough off within 10 days; this may be associated with bleeding, about which the patient must be warned. As with sclerotherapy, three piles may be treated at one session, and the process may be repeated after several weeks if necessary. The techniques of cryotherapy (Lloyd Williams) and infrared photocoagulation (Leicester) are not often used nowadays.

Operation

Indications

The indications for haemorrhoidectomy include:

- third- and fourth-degree haemorrhoids;
- second-degree haemorrhoids that have not been cured by non-operative treatments;
- fibrosed haemorrhoids;
- intero-external haemorrhoids when the external haemorrhoid is well defined.

If there is any doubt about the diagnosis of haemorrhoids, examination under anaesthesia and, if indicated, biopsy are necessary.

William Bashall Gabriel, 1893–1975, Surgeon, St Mark's Hospital and the Royal Northern Hospital, London, UK.
Kenneth Lloyd Williams, Dcd, Surgeon, The Royal United Hospitals, Bath, England.
Roger James Leicester, Formerly Surgeon, St George's Hospital, London, England.

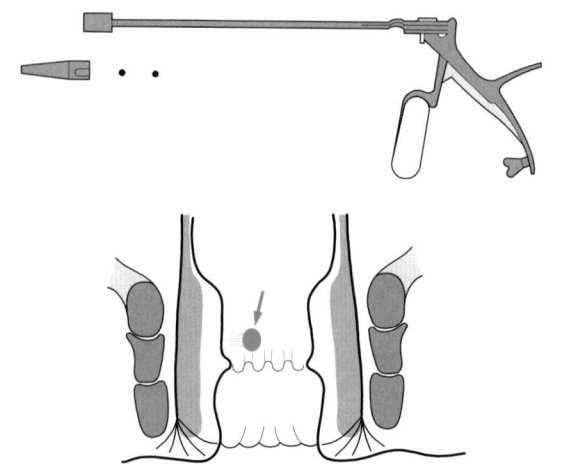

Figure 69.30 Barron's banding apparatus, with the appearance of a typical 'banded' haemorrhoid.

The other strong indication for surgery is haemorrhoidal bleeding sufficient to cause anaemia. Beyond these, the indications summarised above are more relative than absolute, because in these situations surgery aims simply to improve symptoms and, of course, is not without risk. For instance, elderly multiparous women with hypotonic sphincters who are just continent before haemorrhoidectomy may find that the procedure results in frank incontinence, a far worse condition than that for which they originally sought help.

Technique

It is usual for the patient to have been taking stool softeners in the days before surgery and a preoperative enema to empty the rectum is administered. The procedure is usually performed under general or regional anaesthesia with the patient in the lithotomy or prone jack-knife position. The perianal skin is shaved and a formal examination performed. Haemorrhoidectomy can be performed using an open or a closed technique. The open technique is most commonly used in the UK and is known as the Milligan–Morgan operation – named after the surgeons who described it. The closed technique is the popular technique in the USA. Both involve ligation and excision of the haemorrhoid but in the open technique the anal mucosa and skin are left open to heal by secondary intention, and in the closed technique the wound is sutured.

Open technique The anoderm and subcutaneous tissues between the pile masses may be injected with dilute adrenaline (epinephrine; 1:300 000 dilution) to reduce bleeding and aid preservation of the skin bridges left following excision. Artery forceps are applied to the skin-covered external components of the piles and traction exerted to reveal the internal components, which are also grasped by artery forceps. When held out by the assistant these pairs of artery forceps form a triangle (Fig. 69.31a). The operator takes the left lateral pair of artery forceps in the palm of the hand and places the extended forefinger in the anal canal to support the internal haemorrhoid. In this way traction is applied to the skin of the anal margin. With scissors or cutting diathermy, a V-shaped cut is made through the skin and those fibres inserting into it around the skin-holding artery forceps. Traction by both operator and assistant, combined with careful dissection,

will expose the lower border of the internal sphincter. The dissection proceeds up the anal canal, with the sides of the mucosal dissection converging towards the pile apex and with the internal sphincter visible and separate from the dissected pile (Fig. 69.31b). A transfixion ligature of strong Vicryl is applied to the pedicle at this level (Fig. 69.31c), the pile is excised well distal to the ligature and, after ensuring haemostasis, the ligature is cut long. Each haemorrhoid is dealt with in this manner, taking care to leave mucocutaneous bridges. If there are significant secondary haemorrhoids under these bridges they can be filleted out by scissor dissection. Haemostasis must be absolute at the end of the procedure, when a soft absorbable anal dressing is inserted. The margins of the skin wounds are trimmed so as not to leave overhanging edges (Fig. 69.32). Bleeding subcutaneous arteries having been secured, the areas denuded of skin are dressed with three pieces of petroleum jelly gauze. A pad of gauze and wool and a firmly applied T-bandage complete the operation.

Closed technique The haemorrhoid is excised, together with the overlying mucosa, as illustrated in Fig. 69.33a. The haemorrhoid is dissected carefully from the underlying sphincter and artery forceps is achieved. The pedicle is transfixed and ligated with 3/0 Vicryl or Dexon. Any residual small haemorrhoids should be removed by filleting them out after undermining the edges of the cut mucosa. The mucosal defect is then closed completely with a continuous suture using the same stitch that was employed to ligate the haemorrhoid pedicle. The remaining haemorrhoids are excised and ligated in a similar fashion, ensuring that there are adequate mucosal and skin bridges between each area of excision to avoid a subsequent stenosis.

With the aim of symptom relief but preservation of the anal cushions, the technique of stapled haemorrhoidopexy (Longo), which utilises a purpose-designed stapling gun (PPH, Ethicon Inc.), has recently been described. This procedure excises a strip of mucosa and submucosa (together with the vessels travelling within them) circumferentially, well above the dentate line. Activation of the gun also simultaneously repairs the cut mucosa and submucosa by stapling the edges together (Fig. 69.34). This procedure is quick to perform, and controlled trials suggest that it is less painful and less traumatic than conventional haemorrhoidectomy and, at least in the short term, it seems to be equally efficacious. However, its efficacy in the long term is unknown (Summary box 69.10).

Summary box 69.10

Treatment of haemorrhoids

- Symptomatic – advice about defaecatory habits, stool softeners and bulking agents
- Injection of sclerosant
- Banding
- Haemorrhoidectomy

Postoperative care

In these days of economic stringencies, the patient is discharged from hospital within a day or two of the operation. In the USA,

A. Longo, **Surgeon, Sicily, Italy.**

(a)

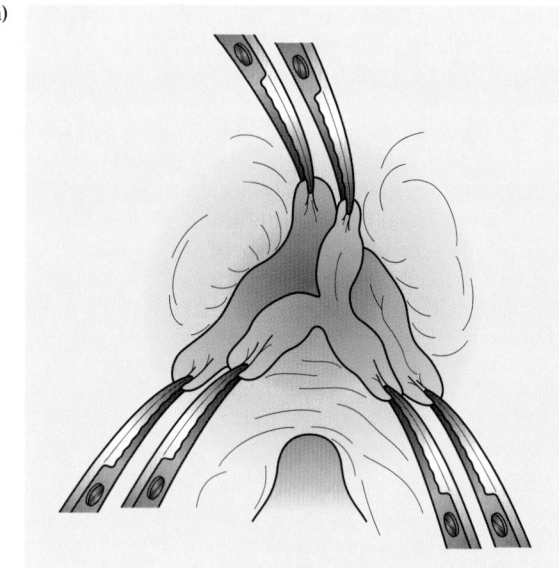

(b)

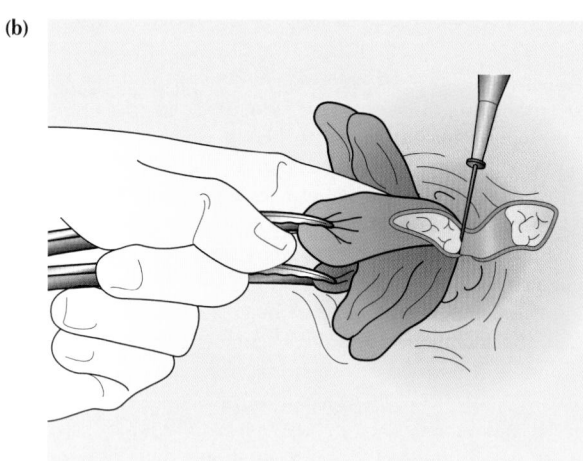

(c)

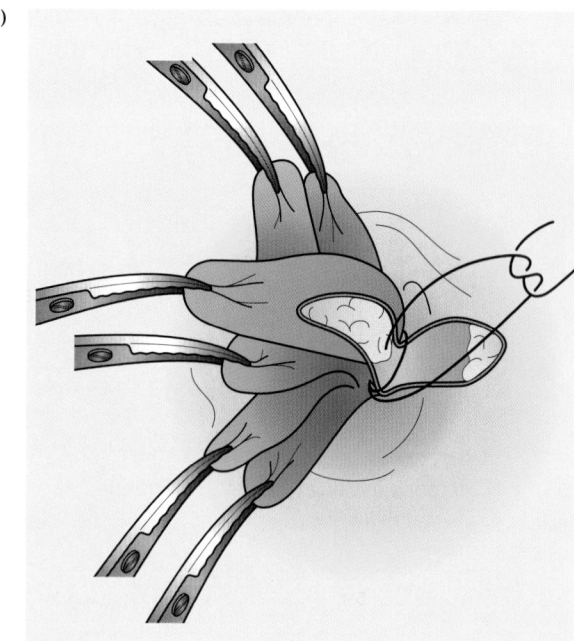

Figure 69.31 Ligation and excision of haemorrhoids. Open technique: (a) the artery forceps have been applied; (b) dissection of the left lateral pedicle; (c) transfixion of the pedicle. [Reproduced with permission from Nicholls, R.J. and Dozois, R.R. (1997) *Surgery of the Colon and Rectum*. Churchill Livingstone, Edinburgh.]

the procedure is often performed on a day-care basis. The patient is instructed to take two warm baths each day and is given a bulk laxative to take twice daily together with appropriate analgesia. Dry dressings are applied as necessary, a sterile sanitary towel usually being ideal. The patient is seen again 3–4 weeks after discharge and a rectal examination is performed. If there is evidence of stenosis, the patient is encouraged to use a dilator.

Postoperative complications

Postoperative complications may be early or late. Early complications include pain, which may require opiate analgesia; retention of urine, especially in men, which rarely may need relief by catheterisation; and reactionary haemorrhage, which is much more common than secondary haemorrhage. The haemorrhage may be mainly or entirely concealed but will become evident on examining the rectum. If persistent following adequate analgesia, the patient must be taken to the operating theatre and the bleeding point secured by careful diathermy or under-running with a

ligature on a needle, care being taken to avoid damage to the internal sphincter. Should a definite bleeding point not be found, the anal canal and rectum are packed.

Late postoperative complications include:

- *Secondary haemorrhage*. This is uncommon, occurring about the seventh or eighth day after operation. It is usually controlled by morphine but, if the haemorrhage is severe, an anaesthetic should be given and the bleeding controlled.
- *Anal stricture*, which must be prevented at all costs. A rectal examination at the postoperative review will indicate whether stricturing is to be expected. It may then be necessary to give a general anaesthetic and dilate the anus. After that, daily use of the dilator should give a satisfactory result.
- *Anal fissures and submucous abscesses*.
- *Incontinence*, especially if there has been inadvertent damage to the underlying internal sphincter. Although uncommon, this is obviously a very serious problem that is difficult to treat (Summary box 69.11).

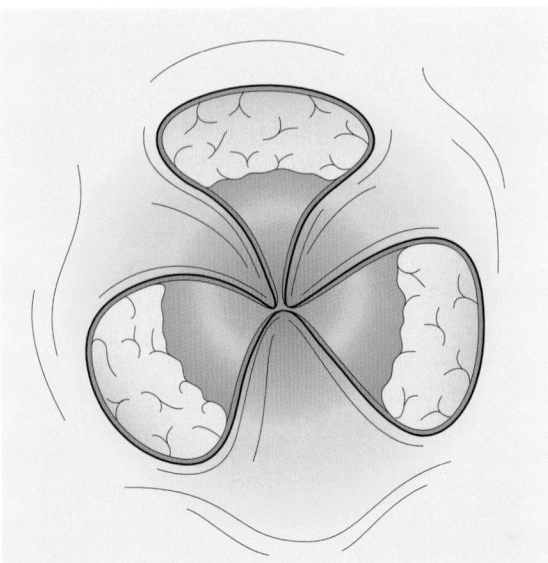

Figure 69.32 The appearance of the anus at the conclusion of the operation. (Note that to avoid stricture formation it is necessary to ensure that a bridge of skin and mucous membrane remains between each wound.) 'If it looks like a clover the trouble is over, if it looks like a dahlia, it is surely a failure.' [Reproduced with permission from Nicholls, R.J. and Dozois, R.R. (1997) *Surgery of the Colon and Rectum*. Churchill Livingstone, Edinburgh.]

Summary box 69.11

Complications of haemorrhoidectomy

Early
- Pain
- Acute retention of urine
- Reactionary haemorrhage

Late
- Secondary haemorrhage
- Anal stricture
- Anal fissure
- Incontinence

External haemorrhoids

A thrombosed external haemorrhoid relates anatomically to the veins of the superficial or external haemorrhoidal plexus and is commonly termed a perianal haematoma. It presents as a sudden-onset, olive-shaped, painful blue subcutaneous swelling at the anal margin and is usually consequent upon straining at stool, coughing or lifting a heavy weight (Fig. 69.35). The thrombosis is usually situated in a lateral region of the anal margin. If the patient presents within the first 48 hours the clot may be evacuated under local anaesthesia. Untreated it may resolve, suppurate, fibrose and give rise to a cutaneous tag, burst and the clot extrude, or continue bleeding. In the majority of cases, resolution or fibrosis occurs. Indeed, this condition has been called 'a 5-day, painful, self-curing lesion' (Milligan).

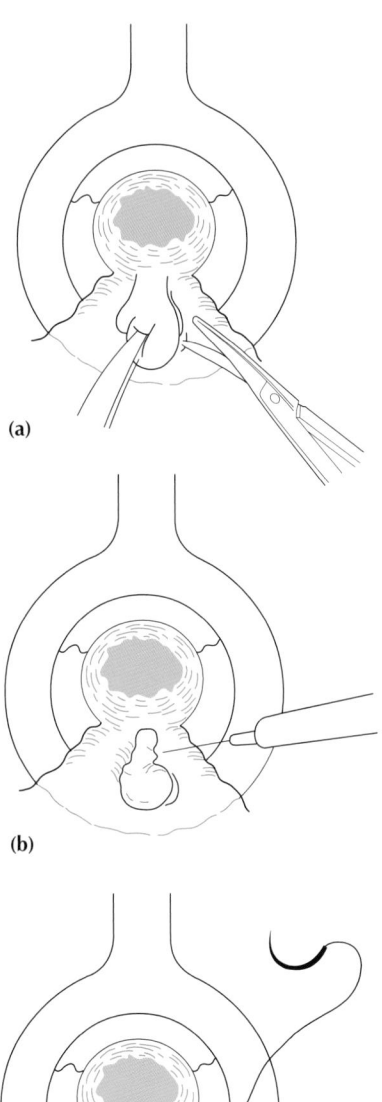

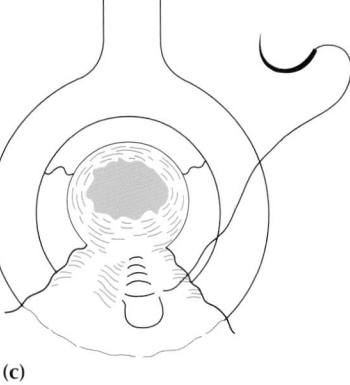

Figure 69.33 Closed technique of haemorrhoidectomy. (a) The haemorrhoidal tissue is excised. (b) Bleeding is controlled by diathermy. (c) The defect is closed with a continuous suture after first undermining the anoderm on each side. [Redrawn with permission from Keighley, M.R.B. and Williams, N.S. (1999) *Surgery of the Anus, Colon and Rectum*, 2nd edn. W.B. Saunders, Philadelphia, PA.]

PRURITUS ANI

This is intractable itching around the anus, a common and embarrassing condition. Usually, the skin is reddened and hyperkeratotic and it may become cracked and moist.

CHAPTER 69 | THE ANUS AND ANAL CANAL

(a)

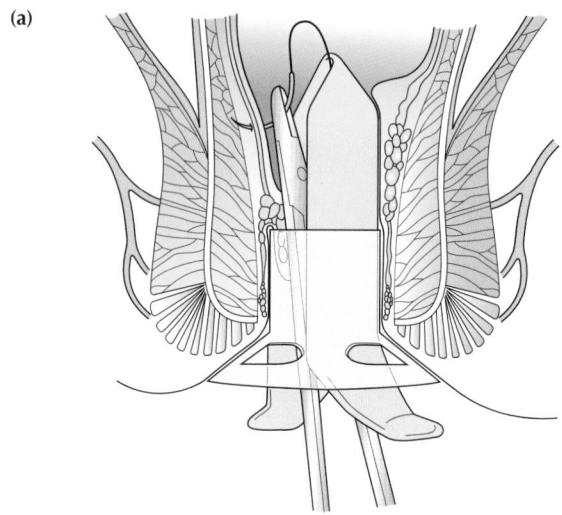

(b)

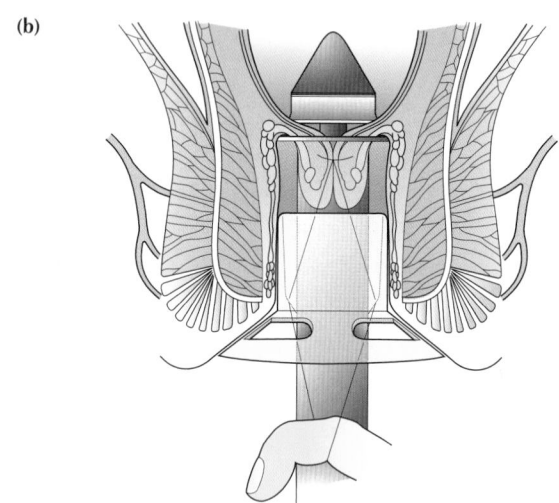

(c)

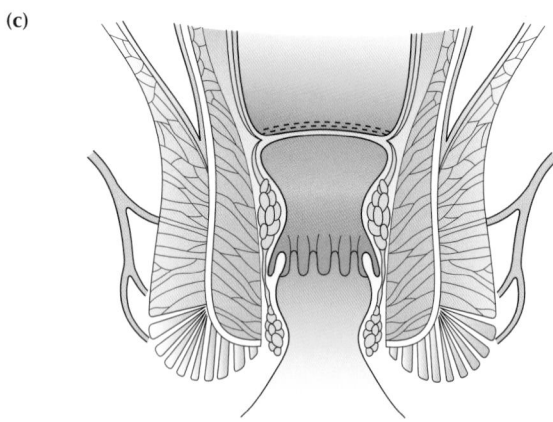

Figure 69.34 Stapled haemorrhoidectomy. (a) The purse-string suture is placed several centimetres above the dentate line. (b) The anvil of the fully opened stapling gun is inserted endoanally so that it is above the purse-string suture, which is then tied around the shaft of the gun. The gun is closed and fired. (c) After firing, a 3–4 cm strip of mucosa and submucosa containing the haemorrhoids is excised and the mucosal edges are simultaneously stapled together.

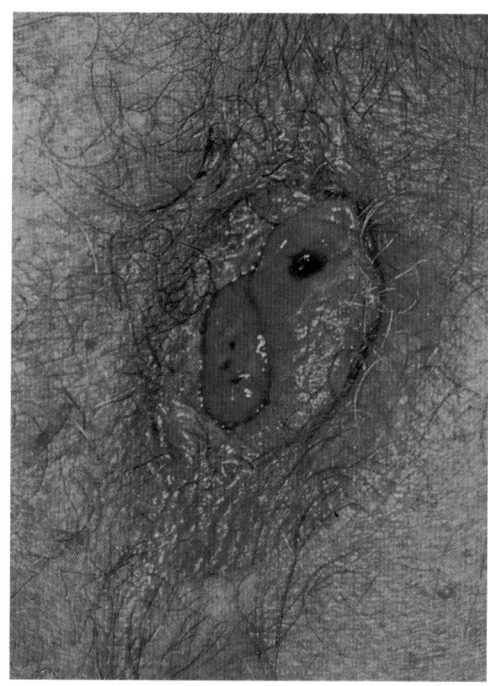

Figure 69.35 A thrombosed external haemorrhoid that has burst. There is also a mucosal prolapse, which is separate from the cutaneous lesion.

Causes

The causes are numerous. A useful mnemonic is 'pus, polypus, parasites, piles, psyche':

- *Lack of cleanliness*, excessive sweating and wearing rough or woollen underclothing.
- An *anal or perianal discharge* that renders the anus moist. The causative lesions include an anal fissure, fistula-*in-ano*, prolapsed internal or external haemorrhoids, genital warts and excessive ingestion of liquid paraffin. A mucous discharge is an intense pruritic agent and a polyp can be the cause.
- A *vaginal discharge*, especially caused by *Trichomonas vaginalis* infection.
- *Parasitic causes*. Threadworms should be excluded, especially in young subjects. Children suffering from threadworms should wear gloves at night, lest they scratch the perianal region and are reinfested with ova by nail biting – 'parasites lost, parasites regained'. Scabies and pediculosis pubis may infest the anal region.
- *Epidermophytosis* is a common cause, especially if the skin between the toes is also infected; microscopic and cultural examinations are essential. Half-strength Whitfield's ointment quickly gives relief and is the sheet anchor of treatment.
- *Allergy* is sometimes the cause, in which case there is likely to be a history of other allergic manifestations, such as urticaria, asthma or hay fever. Antibiotic therapy may be the precipitating factor.
- *Skin diseases* localised to the perianal skin: psoriasis, lichen planus and contact dermatitis.

Arthur Whitfield, **1867–1967, Professor of Dermatology, Kings College Hospital, London, UK. Whitfield's ointment is 'compound ointment of benzoic acid'.**

- *Bacterial infection*, such as intertrigo resulting from a mixed bacterial infection. Erythrasma caused by *Corynebacterium minutissimum* is responsible for some cases and its presence is detected by ultraviolet light, which induces a pink fluorescence.
- A *psychoneurosis*. It is alleged that in a few instances neurotic individuals become so immersed in their complaint that a pain–pleasure complex develops, the pleasure being the scratching. Possibly this is true, but such a syndrome should not be assumed without firm grounds for coming to this conclusion.
- *Diabetes* can sometimes present with pruritus ani, and the urine should be tested in all patients.

Treatment

The cause is treated. Symptomatic treatment includes the following:

- *Hygiene measures.* Cotton wool should be substituted for toilet paper. Soap is avoided and replaced by water alone, and the area pat-dried rather than rubbed. These measures alone, combined with wearing cotton underwear and the application of calamine lotion or zinc and castor oil, are all that is necessary to cure some cases. If there is much anal hair trapping the moisture and discharge, shaving can be very helpful.
- *Hydrocortisone.* In patients with dermatitis, and only in patients with dermatitis, the topical application of 0.5% or 1% prednisolone cream is often beneficial; sometimes after discontinuation of the therapy, the pruritus is liable to return, in which case 5% lidocaine hydrochloride (Xylocaine) ointment can be substituted for a time.
- *Strapping the buttocks* keeps moist opposing surfaces apart but is not well tolerated. If the moistness originates from anal discharge, a cotton wool anal plug will seal the anal orifice.

Operative treatment

This may be necessary for a concomitant lesion of the anorectum that is thought to initiate or contribute to the pruritus. Otherwise, surgery is not indicated (Summary box 69.12).

Summary box 69.12

Pruritus ani

- Common
- Numerous causes including skin diseases, parasites (threadworm), anal discharge, allergies, diabetes
- Treat the cause if possible
- Symptomatic treatment is the mainstay

ANORECTAL ABSCESSES

Acute sepsis in the region of the anus is common. A fundamental distinction that has to be made is whether the sepsis is in that area by chance (simple boil, skin appendage infection) or whether it has arisen as a consequence of the presence of the anorectum, specifically the anal glands. Overall, anorectal sepsis is more common in men than women, although infections with skin-type organisms (and thus unrelated to fistula) are evenly distributed. The cryptoglandular theory of intersphincteric anal gland infection (Parks) holds that, upon infection of a gland, pus, which

travels along the path of least resistance, may spread caudally to present as a perianal abscess, laterally across the external sphincter to form an ischiorectal abscess or, rarely, superiorly above the anorectal junction to form a supralevator intermuscular or pararectal abscess (depending on its relation to the longitudinal muscle), as well as circumferentially in any of the three planes: intersphincteric/intermuscular, ischiorectal or pararectal supralevator (Fig. 69.36). Sepsis unrelated to anal gland infection may occur at the same or at other sites (Fig. 69.37), including

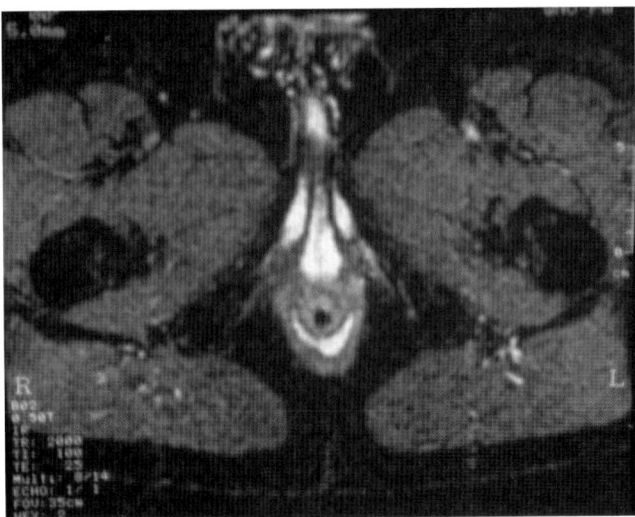

Figure 69.36 Axial magnetic resonance imaging (MRI) scan (STIR sequence) showing posterior horseshoe spread of sepsis within the intersphincteric space.

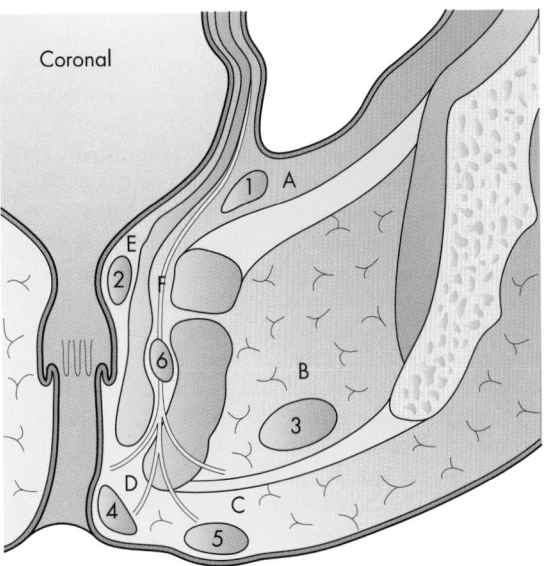

Figure 69.37 Diagram showing the spaces in relation to the anus and types of anorectal abscess in coronal section: A, pelvirectal supralevator space; B, ischiorectal space; C, perianal or superficial ischiorectal space; D, marginal or mucocutaneous space; E, submucous space; F, anorectal intermuscular (intersphincteric) space; 1, pelvirectal supralevator abscess; 2, submucous abscess; 3, ischiorectal abscess; 4, marginal abscess; 5, perianal abscess; 6, intersphincteric abscess. [Reproduced with permission from Nicholls, R.J. and Dozois, R.R. (1997) *Surgery of the Colon and Rectum.* Churchill Livingstone, Edinburgh.]

submucosal abscess (following haemorrhoidal sclerotherapy, which usually resolve spontaneously), mucocutaneous or marginal abscess (infected haematoma), ischiorectal abscess (foreign body, trauma, deep skin-related infection) and pelvirectal supralevator sepsis originating in pelvic disease. Underlying rectal disease, such as neoplasm and particularly Crohn's disease, may be the cause. Similarly, patients with generalised disorders, such as diabetes and acquired immunodeficiency syndrome (AIDS), may present with an anorectal abscess; in these patients, abscesses may run an aggressive course.

Presentation

A perianal abscess, confined by the terminal extensions of the longitudinal muscle, is usually associated with a short (2–3 day) history of increasingly severe, well-localised pain and a palpable tender lump at the anal margin. Examination reveals an indurated hot tender perianal swelling. Patients with infection in the larger fatty-filled ischiorectal space, in which tissue tension is much lower, usually present later, with less well localised symptoms but more constitutional upset and fever. On examination, the affected buttock is diffusely swollen with widespread induration and deep tenderness. If sepsis is higher, deep rectal pain, fever and sometimes disturbed micturition may be the only features, with nothing evident on external examination but tender supralevator induration palpable on digital examination above the anorectal junction.

Differential diagnosis

The only conditions with which an anorectal abscess is likely to be confused are abscesses connected with a pilonidal sinus, Bartholin's gland or Cowper's gland.

Management

Management of acute anorectal sepsis is primarily surgical, including careful examination under anaesthesia, sigmoidoscopy and proctoscopy, and adequate drainage of the pus. For perianal and ischiorectal sepsis (with an incidence of 60% and 30% respectively), drainage is through the perineal skin, usually through a cruciate incision over the most fluctuant point, with excision of the skin edges to de-roof the abscess (Fig. 69.38). Pus is sent for microbiological culture (Grace) and tissue from the wall is sent for histological appraisal to exclude specific causes. With a finger in the anorectum to avoid creation of a false opening, the cavity is carefully curetted. A gentle search may be made for an underlying fistula if the surgeon is experienced and, if obvious, a loose draining seton may be passed; injudicious probing in the acute stage is, however, potentially dangerous and may lead to a much more difficult situation. Unless by highly experienced hands, immediate fistulotomy should not be performed. After irrigation of the cavity, the wound is lightly tucked; antibiotics are prescribed if there is surrounding cellulitis and especially in those less resistant to infection, such as diabetics. If the pus subsequently cultures skin-type organisms there will be no underlying fistula and the patient can be reassured. If gut flora are cultured, it is likely, but not inevitable, that there is an underlying fistula.

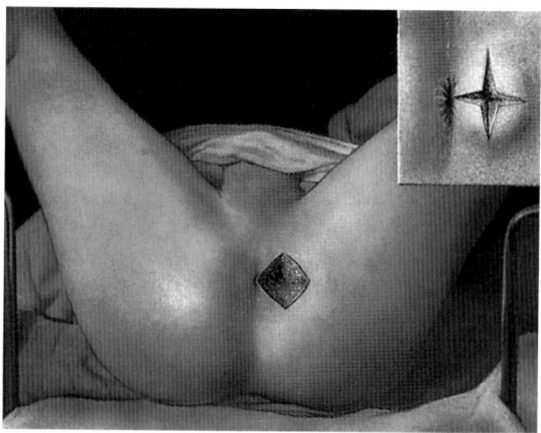

Figure 69.38 Incision of an ischiorectal abscess. The cavity is explored and, if septa exist, they should be broken down gently with a finger and the necrotic tissue lining the walls of the abscess removed by the finger wrapped in gauze. It is wise to biopsy the wall and send the pus for culture. Nothing further is done at this stage.

The management of supralevator sepsis is dependent upon its exact anatomy (within or outside the rectal wall) and its origin. Sepsis originating in pelvic disease necessitates appropriate management of the underlying cause (appendiceal, gynaecological, diverticular, Crohn's disease, malignancy), although intrarectal drainage may be apt to avoid creation of an extrasphincteric fistula. Cephalad extension of an intersphincteric fistula can be safely drained into the rectum, whereas supralevator extension of a trans-sphincteric fistula should be drained via the skin of the buttock. Rarely, a colostomy may be necessary to control severe sepsis, especially in the immunocompromised individual (Summary box 69.13).

Summary box 69.13

Anorectal abscess

- Usually produces a painful, throbbing swelling in the anal region. The patient often has swinging pyrexia
- Subdivided according to anatomical site into perianal, ischiorectal, submucous and pelvirectal
- Underlying conditions include fistula-*in-ano* (most common), Crohn's disesase, diabetes, immunosuppression
- Treatment is drainage of pus in first instance, together with appropriate antibiotics
- Always look for a potential underlying problem

FISTULA-*IN-ANO*

A fistula-*in-ano*, or anal fistula, is a chronic abnormal communication, usually lined to some degree by granulation tissue, which runs outwards from the anorectal lumen (the internal opening) to an external opening on the skin of the perineum or buttock (or rarely, in women, to the vagina). Anal fistulae may be found in association with specific conditions, such as Crohn's disease, tuberculosis, lymphogranuloma venereum, actinomycosis, rectal duplication, foreign body and malignancy (which may also very rarely arise within a longstanding fistula), and suspicion of these should be aroused if clinical findings are unusual. However, the majority are termed non-specific, idiopathic or cryptoglandular,

Caspar Bartholin, Secundus, 1655–1709, Professor of Medicine, Anatomy and Physics, Copenhagen, Denmark, described these glands in 1677.
William Cowper, 1666–1709, London surgeon, described these glands in 1697.
Roger Hew Grace, Formerly Professor of Colorectal Surgery, The Royal Wolverhampton Hospital, Wolverhampton, England.

and intersphincteric anal gland infection is deemed central to them.

Presentation

For reasons that are unknown, non-specific anal fistulae are more common in men than women. The overall incidence is about 9 cases per 100 000 population per year in western Europe, and those in their third, fourth and fifth decades of life are most commonly affected. Patients usually complain of intermittent purulent discharge (which may be bloody) and pain (which increases until temporary relief occurs when the pus discharges). There is often, but not invariably, a previous episode of acute anorectal sepsis that settled (incompletely) spontaneously or with antibiotics, or which was surgically drained. The passage of flatus or faeces through the external opening is suggestive of a rectal rather than an anal internal opening.

Classification

The most widespread and useful classification of anal fistulae is that proposed by Parks, based on the centrality of intersphincteric anal gland sepsis (the internal opening is usually at the dentate line), which results in a primary track whose relation to the external sphincter defines the type of fistula and which influences management (Fig. 69.39). Classifications based simply on level are less practical because they mean different things to different people, although the description of a fistula as high, indicating a high risk of incontinence if laid open, or low, with a lower but still some risk to function, is often used. Similarly, 'simple' and 'complex' are commonly used adjectives – complexity may be endowed by the level at which the primary track crosses the sphincters, the presence of secondary extensions or the difficulties faced in treatment. The vast majority of fistulae are intersphincteric or trans-sphincteric.

Intersphincteric fistulae (45%) do not cross the external sphincter (bar, for the purist, the most medial subcutaneous fibres running below the distal border of the internal sphincter); most commonly they run directly from the internal to the external openings across the distal internal sphincter, but may extend proximally in the intersphincteric plane to end blindly with or without an abscess, or enter the rectum at a second internal opening.

Trans-sphincteric fistulae (40%) have a primary track that crosses both internal and external sphincters (the latter at a variable level) and which then passes through the ischiorectal fossa

to reach the skin of the buttock. The primary track may have secondary tracks arising from it, which often reach the roof of the ischiorectal fossa, which may rarely pass through the levators to reach the pelvis and which may spread circumferentially (horseshoe). Circumferential spread of sepsis may occur in the intersphincteric and pararectal planes, as well as in the ischiorectal plane.

Suprasphincteric fistulae are very rare, are thought by some to be iatrogenic and are difficult to distinguish from high-level transsphincteric tracks (for which, fortunately, management strategies are similar). Extrasphincteric fistulae run without specific relation to the sphincters and usually result from pelvic disease or trauma.

Clinical assessment

A full medical (including obstetric, gastrointestinal, anal surgical and continence) history and proctosigmoidoscopy are necessary to gain information about sphincter strength and to exclude associated conditions. The key points to determine are the site of the internal opening; the site of the external opening(s); the course of the primary track; the presence of secondary extensions; and the presence of other conditions complicating the fistula. Palpable induration between external opening and anal margin suggests a relatively superficial track, whereas supralevator induration suggests a primary track above the levators or high in the roof of the ischiorectal fossa, or a high secondary extension. Intersphincteric fistulae usually have an external opening close to the anal verge. Goodsall's rule (Fig. 69.40), used to indicate the likely position of the internal opening according to the position of the external opening(s), is helpful but not infallible. The site of the internal opening may be felt as a point of induration or seen as an enlarged papilla. Probing in an awake patient is painful, unhelpful and can be dangerous. Full examination under anaesthesia should be repeated before surgical intervention. Dilute hydrogen peroxide, instilled via the external opening, is a very useful way of demonstrating the site of the internal opening; gentle use of probes (Fig. 69.41) and a finger in the anorectum usually delineates primary and secondary tracks and their relations to the sphincters. Any concerns about fistula topography at clinical examination or examination under anaesthesia (more common after previous unsuccessful surgery) should prompt further investigations before surgical intervention.

Special investigations

A successful outcome after fistula surgery requires an accurate assessment of the fistula itself, the sphincter through which it passes and patient expectations (especially in terms of risk to continence). Clinical examination will give some indication of functional anal sphincter length, resting tone and voluntary squeeze;

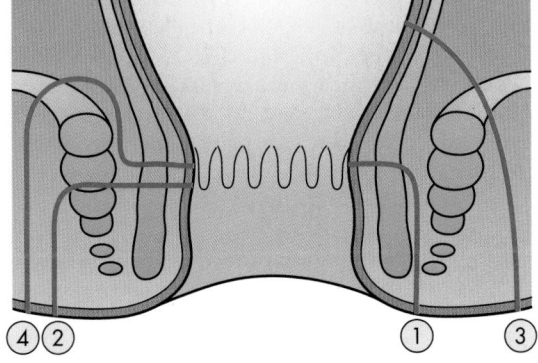

Figure 69.39 Types of anal fistula (Parks' classification): 1, intersphincteric; 2, trans-sphincteric; 3, suprasphincteric; and 4, extrasphincteric primary tracks.

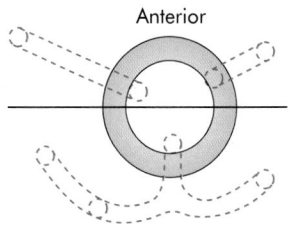

Anterior

Figure 69.40 Goodsall's rule.

David Henry Goodsall, 1843–1906, Surgeon, St Mark's Hospital, London, UK.

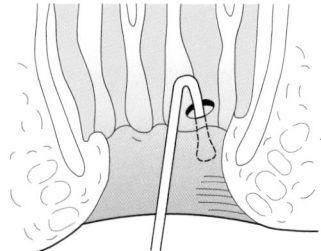

Figure 69.41 Retrograde probing of an anal canal sometimes reveals the internal orifice of the fistula.

these may be more objectively assessed by manometry whereas endoanal ultrasound gives useful information about sphincter integrity – the knowledge so gained may well influence surgical strategy. Endoanal ultrasound, especially with hydrogen peroxide, can also be used to delineate fistulae, although definition of sepsis outside or above the sphincters is limited by the probe's focal range and scarring makes interpretation difficult. Nonetheless, ultrasound, which is more accurate than clinical examination, is useful to determine whether a fistula is relatively straightforward or not. Magnetic resonance imaging (MRI) is acknowledged to be the 'gold standard' for fistula imaging but it is limited by availability and cost and is usually reserved for difficult recurrent cases. The great advantage of MRI is its ability to demonstrate secondary extensions, which may be missed at surgery and which are the cause of persistence (Fig. 69.42). Fistulography and computerised tomography (CT) both have limitations but are useful techniques if an extrasphincteric fistula is suspected.

Surgical management

Patients with minimal symptoms, especially if they have compromised sphincters, may be managed expectantly. Eradication of sepsis requires surgery, the aim of which must be balanced with

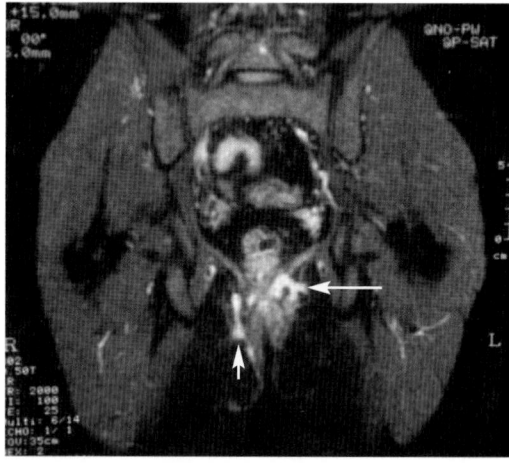

Figure 69.42 Coronal magnetic resonance imaging (MRI) scan (STIR sequence) demonstrating a primary track running up the right ischiorectal space (short white arrow), which then crosses the sphincters to open into the anal canal just below the puborectalis. However, there is a blind secondary extension (long white arrow) passing to the contralateral side in the roof of the left ischiorectal fossa (and involving the levators), which was missed at surgery and which was the cause of fistula persistence.

the preservation of continence. Most fistulae are relatively straightforward to deal with; however, a minority are extremely problematic and are not the realm of the 'occasional proctologist'. The multitude of strategies advocated attests to these difficult situations; comparisons between techniques are difficult to make because of the heterogeneity of patient groups, the variability in classification, the inapplicability of certain techniques in some situations, inadequate reporting of functional outcomes, inadequate follow-up and surgeon preference over-riding entry into prospective randomised trials.

Fistulotomy

That the fistulous track must be laid open from its termination to its source was a rule promulgated by John of Arderne more than 600 years ago. Fistulotomy, or laying open, is the surest way of getting rid of a fistula, but, by definition, it involves division of all those structures lying between the external and internal openings. It is therefore applied mainly to intersphincteric fistulae and trans-sphincteric fistulae involving less than 30% of the voluntary musculature (but not anteriorly placed fistulae in women); however, even then, it is not immune to postoperative defects in continence. After full examination under anaesthesia in the lithotomy or prone jackknife position, during which the internal opening should have been identified, a grooved fistula probe is passed from the external to the internal opening (Fig. 69.43), the amount of sphincter below and above the probe is noted and, if indicated, the track is laid open over the probe. Granulation tissue is curetted and sent for histological appraisal and the wound edges are trimmed. Secondary tracks, often identified as granulation tissue that persists despite curettage, should be laid open or drained. Marsupialisation reduces wound size and speeds up healing. Primary tracks crossing the external sphincter more deeply have been managed with good outcomes by fistulotomy and immediate reconstitution of the divided muscle – failure to eradicate all sepsis and subsequent breakdown of the repair, however, are very problematic. Alternatively, a staged fistulotomy may be carried out in which secondary tracks are laid open and only part of the sphincter enclosed by the primary track is divided, with the remainder encircled by a loose seton. After sufficient time for healing of the wound and fibrosis, the seton-enclosed track is divided at a second stage.

Fistulectomy

This technique involves coring out of the fistula, usually by diathermy cautery; it allows better definition of fistula anatomy than fistulotomy, especially the level at which the track crosses the sphincters and the presence of secondary extensions. If the sphincteric component of the fistula is deemed low enough to allow safe fistulotomy, then this may proceed (at the expense of longer healing times than conventional fistulotomy). If laying open is not advisable, then the sphincteric component can be managed by another method.

Setons

Setons (Latin: *seta* = bristle) have been used in a variety of ways in fistula surgery and it is important for surgeons to be clear about

---

John of Arderne, **1307–1390**, was the first English surgeon of note. He practised at Newark-upon-Trent, Nottinghamshire and, from 1370, in London, UK. He described his operation for the treatment of fistula in about 1376.

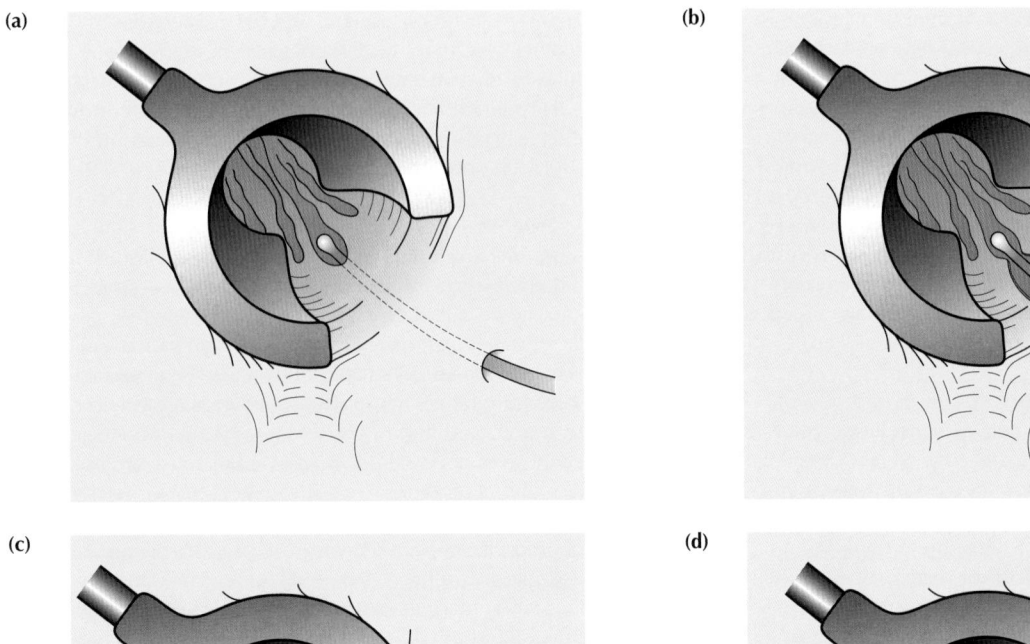

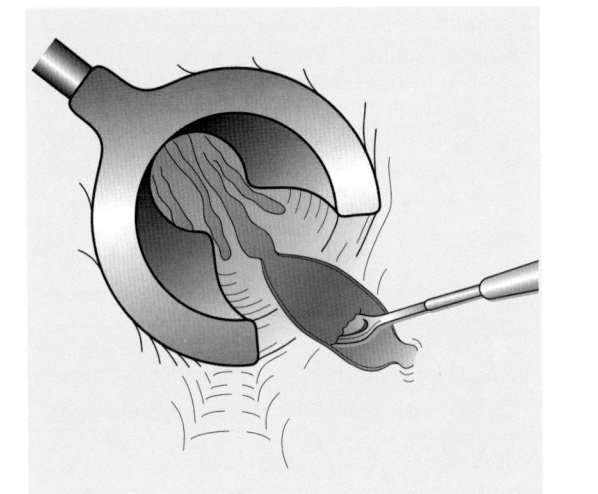
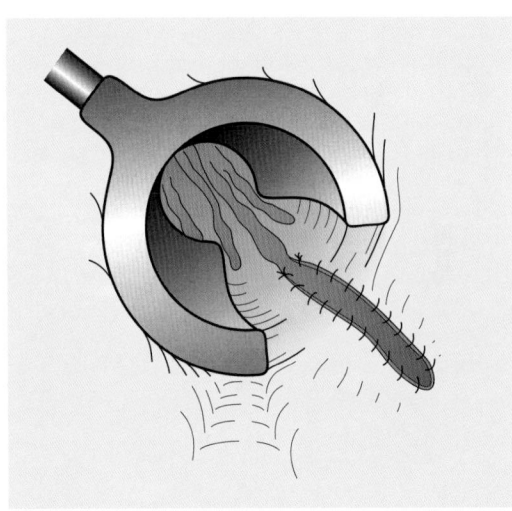

Figure 69.43 Fistulotomy. A grooved probe is passed from the external to internal openings and the track laid open over the probe. The track is curetted to remove granulation tissue, the edges of the wound are trimmed and the wound may then be marsupialised. [Reproduced with permission from Nicholls, R.J. and Dozois, R.R. (1997) *Surgery of the Colon and Rectum.* Churchill Livingstone, Edinburgh.]

what they are trying to achieve in a particular situation. *Loose* setons are tied such that there is no tension upon the encircled tissue; there is no intent to cut the tissue. A variety of materials have been used but the seton should be non-absorbable, non-degenerative and comfortable. *Tight* or *cutting* setons are placed with the intention of cutting through the enclosed muscle.

Uses of loose setons
1. For *long-term palliation* to avoid septic and painful exacerbations by establishing effective drainage; most often in Crohn's disease and in those with problematic fistulae not wishing to countenance the possibility of incontinence.
2. Used *before 'advanced' techniques* (fistulectomy, advancement flap, cutting seton); acute sepsis and secondary extensions are eradicated and a loose seton is passed across the sphincteric component of the primary track to simplify the fistula and allow fibrosis.
3. As part of a *staged fistulotomy.*
4. As part of a therapeutic strategy to *preserve the external sphincter* in trans-sphincteric fistulae. Secondary tracks in the ischiorectal fossa are laid open. Access to the site where the

primary track crosses the external sphincter may sometimes necessitate division of the anococcygeal ligaments to reach the deep post-anal space. The internal sphincter is laid open to the level of the internal opening (or higher if there is a cephalad intersphincteric extension) to eradicate the presumed source and the sepsis in the intersphincteric space. A seton is then passed along the residual track around the denuded external sphincter and tied loosely, and the wounds are dressed. Initial postoperative management includes daily wound irrigation and light wound redressing. The seton is left in place for 3 months and, if there is evidence of good healing, simply removed. Such a strategy certainly protects against the consequences of external sphincter division, with an incidence of healing in the short term of 50–60%.

Uses of cutting setons
Cutting setons aim to achieve the high fistula eradication rates associated with fistulotomy but without the degree of functional impairment endowed by division of the sphincters at a single stage. The enclosed muscle is gradually severed ('cheese wiring through ice') such that the divided muscles do not spring apart,

and the site of the fistula track is replaced by a thin line of fibrosis as it is brought down. Some recommend prior internal sphincter division, others incorporation of the internal sphincter within the cutting seton. A variety of seton material has been used, either elastic and 'self-cutting' or non-elastic and tightened at intervals, with the sphincter being divided at varying speeds. In eastern parts of the world the same aim has been achieved by chemical cautery using an Ayurvedic method, known in India as Kshara sutra, in which a specially prepared seton thread burns through the enclosed tissue. This out-patient method has been shown to be equivalent to one-stage fistulotomy in patients with intersphincteric and distal trans-sphincteric fistulae.

Advancement flaps

When the sphincter complex is not too indurated and adequate intra-anal access can be obtained, the advancement flap technique can be employed, which aims to preserve both anatomy and function. The principles are prior elimination of acute sepsis and secondary tracks, with ideally a direct track from internal to external openings; coring out of the entire track; and closure of the communication with the anal lumen with an adequately vascularised flap consisting of mucosa and internal sphincter, sutured without tension to the anoderm, well distant from the site of the (excised) internal opening. Modifications include flap orientation (proximally or distally based) and thickness (mucosal, partial or full-thickness internal sphincter), and treatment of the external wound.

Glues

The functional consequences of fistulotomy and the poorer eradication rates of sphincter-preserving techniques has led to a search for agents that, once the fistula has been adequately rid of lining granulation tissue and epithelium, essentially plug and seal the track and allow ingrowth of healthy tissue to replace it. Results with fibrin glue have shown short-term promise but there is currently insufficient evidence concerning indications for use, technique and long-term outcomes. Nevertheless, research into biological agents must continue if outcomes for the patient with an anal fistula are to be improved (Summary box 69.14).

Summary box 69.14

Anorectal fistulae

- Are common and may be simple or complex
- Are classified according to their relationship to the anal sphincters
- May be associated with underlying disease such as tuberculosis or Crohn's disease
- Laying open is the surest method of eradication, but sphincter division may result in incontinence

---

HIDRADENITIS SUPPURATIVA

This is a chronic suppurative condition of apocrine gland-bearing skin, which is found in the axillae, submammary regions, nape of the neck, groin, mons pubis, inner thighs and sides of the scrotum, as well as the perineum and buttocks, and is a source of considerable physical and psychological morbidity. There is no confirmatory test or specific characteristic for diagnosis, which makes definition difficult. Acne, pilonidal sinus and chronic scalp folliculitis may co-exist with hidradenitis suppurativa in the condition 'follicular occlusion tetrad'.

Pathology

Occlusion of gland ducts leads to bacterial proliferation, gland rupture and spread of infection and epithelial components into the surrounding soft tissue and to adjacent glands. Secondary infection (with *Staphylococcus aureus*, *Streptococcus milleri* and anaerobes) causes further local extension, skin damage and deformity, with multiple communicating subcutaneous fistulae. There is some evidence that the disease may be related to a relative androgen excess.

Presentation

The condition is not seen before puberty and rarely presents after the fourth decade of life. Overall, it is three times more common in women than men, although anogenital disease is more common in men, and obesity is a common association. When affecting the perineum, lesions begin as multiple raised boils, with recurrent lesions within the same vicinity leading to sinus tract formation, bridged scarring and multiple points of discharge. Rarely, it may involve the anal canal anoderm but it does not extend above the dentate line or involve the sphincter muscles themselves.

Differential diagnosis

In the early stages distinction from furunculosis can be difficult. Crohn's disease, cryptoglandular fistula, pilonidal sinus, tuberculosis, actinomycosis, lymphogranuloma venereum and granuloma inguinale must be considered when later stages present.

Treatment

In the early stages, general measures, including weight reduction and antiseptic soaps, may be helpful. Antibiotics may induce remission but often the disease relapses and progresses, at which point surgery is indicated. Inadequate treatment may lead to prolonged morbidity but any surgery should be less debilitating than the condition. Surgical intervention ranges from simple incision and drainage of acute sepsis to radical excision of all apocrine gland-bearing skin. Careful laying open of all tracts, possibly as a staged procedure according to anatomical location, is an option that appeals to many patients. Radical excision requires closure by skin graft or rotation flap and, occasionally, a defunctioning colostomy to allow healing.

CONDYLOMATA ACCUMINATA (ANAL WARTS)

There is increasing evidence that sexually transmitted infection with human papillomavirus (HPV) forms the aetiological basis of anal and perianal warts, anal intraepithelial neoplasia (AIN) and squamous cell carcinoma of the anus. In those area of the world where sexual promiscuity (especially anal intercourse) is more common, and in immunocompromised individuals (HIV-infected individuals and transplant recipients), there have been dramatic increases in the incidence of these conditions over the last 30

The Ayurvedic method **is derived from the Ayurveda, the most ancient system of Hindu medicine whose origin is ascribed to Brahma and dates from circa 1400 to 1200 BC.**

years, most importantly of AIN and anal cancers. Similar virally induced changes have been noted in the genital tracts of women [vulval intraepithelial neoplasia (VIN), cervical intraepithelial neoplasia (CIN) and cancers]. There are over 80 subtypes of HPV but certain subtypes (16, 18, 31, 33) are associated with a greater risk of progression to dysplasia and malignancy.

Condylomata accuminata is the most common sexually transmitted disease encountered by colorectal surgeons and is most frequently observed in homosexual men. Associated warts on the penis and along the female genital tract are common.

Presentation

Many are asymptomatic but pruritus, discharge, bleeding and pain are usual presenting complaints. In the early stages, examination reveals separate pinkish-white warts close to the anal margin and also often on the anoderm within the distal anal canal. Later, the warts enlarge, coalesce and carpet the skin. Rarely, relentless growth results in giant condylomata (Buschke–Löwenstein tumour), which may obliterate the anal orifice. The diagnosis is aided by aceto-whitening upon application of acetic acid but confirmed by biopsy, which will also indicate the presence or absence of dysplasia.

Treatment

Because of the field effect endowed by viral skin infection, long-term resolution can be problematic. Careful serial application of 25% podophyllin to discrete warts on the perianal skin is often used; however, it cannot be used intra-anally. Surgical excision under local, regional or general anaesthesia involves raising and separating the lesions with local infiltration of dilute adrenaline, which allows more accurate scissor or electrocautery excision to maximise the preservation of normal skin.

ANAL INTRAEPITHELIAL NEOPLASIA

AIN (Fig. 69.44) is virally induced dysplasia of the perianal or intra-anal epidermis. The incidence is unknown but it is being detected with increasing frequency in those areas where anoreceptive intercourse and HIV are prevalent. Patients are often asymptomatic and the diagnosis is often a histological surprise, although increasing numbers in high-risk groups are picked up on anal cytology. It is classified according to the degree of dysplasia on biopsy into AIN I, AIN II and AIN III, according to the lack of keratocyte maturation and extension of the proliferative zone from the lower third (AIN I) to the full thickness of the epithelium (AIN III), in the same manner as cervical or vulval dysplasia. The natural history is uncertain but progression from AIN II to AIN III to invasive carcinoma has been observed, notably in the immunocompromised. The term Bowen's disease should probably be avoided.

Presentation

AIN is often subclinical but is found in up to 30% of patients with anal warts. Suspicious areas are raised, scaly, white, erythematous, pigmented or fissured.

Abraham Buschke, 1868–1943, a German Dermatologist.
L. W. Löwenstein described this condition in 1939.
John Templeton Bowen, 1857–1941, Professor of Dermatology, Harvard University Medical School. Boston, MA, USA, described this intradermal precancerous skin lesion in 1912.

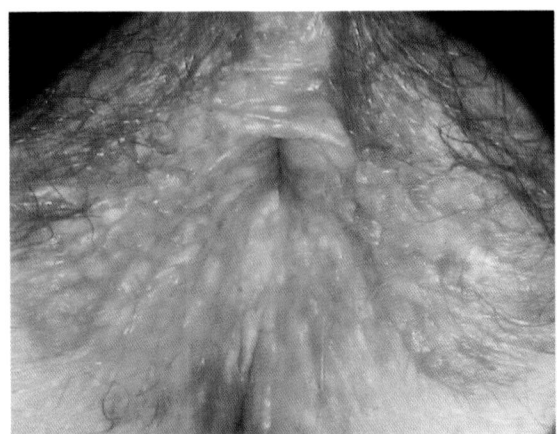

Figure 69.44 Extensive anal intraepithelial neoplasia (AIN), which extends intra-anally.

Diagnosis and management

A high index of suspicion and targeted biopsy yields the diagnosis, whereas multiple (mapping) biopsies give an indication of the extent and overall severity of the disease. AIN II and III should be regularly monitored clinically and, if necessary, by repeat biopsy to exclude invasive disease. Focal disease may be excised. More widespread disease can be dealt with surgically by wide local excision and closure of the resultant defect by flap or skin graft, with or without covering colostomy (especially if there is intra-anal disease). Topical imiquimod or oral retinoids have some effect on the progression of dysplasia.

NON-MALIGNANT STRICTURES

Spasmodic

An anal fissure causes spasm of the internal sphincter. Rarely, a spasmodic stricture accompanies secondary megacolon, possibly as a result of the chronic use of laxatives.

Organic

Postoperative stricture

This sometimes follows a haemorrhoidectomy performed incorrectly. Low coloanal anastomoses, especially if a stapling gun is used, can narrow down postoperatively.

Irradiation stricture

This is an aftermath of irradiation.

Senile anal stenosis

A condition of chronic internal sphincter contraction is sometimes seen in the elderly. Increasing constipation is present, with pronounced straining at stool. Faecal impaction is liable to occur. The muscle is rigid and feels like a tight rubber ring. There is no evidence of a fissure-in-ano. The treatment is dilatation at frequent intervals.

Lymphogranuloma inguinale (see Chapter 68)

This is by far the most frequent cause of a tubular inflammatory stricture of the rectum and 80% of the sufferers are women. Frei's

Wilhelm Sigmund Frei, 1885–1943, Professor of Dermatology, the State Hospital, Spandau, Berlin, who later settled in New York, NY, USA, described his test for lymphogranuloma inguinale in 1925.

reaction is usually positive. This variety of rectal stricture is particularly common in black populations and may be accompanied by elephantiasis of the labia majora. In the early stages, antibiotic treatment may lead to cure. In advanced cases, excision of the rectum is required.

Inflammatory bowel disease

Stricture of the anorectum may complicate Crohn's disease and, in this instance, the stricture is annular and often more than one is present. Occasionally, an anal stricture may occur in ulcerative colitis. Until a biopsy is obtained, a carcinoma should be suspected if a stricture is found.

Endometriosis

Endometriosis of the rectovaginal septum may present as a stricture. There is usually a history of frequent menstrual periods with severe pain during the first 2 days of the menstrual flow.

Neoplastic

When free bleeding occurs after dilatation of a supposed inflammatory stricture, carcinoma should be suspected (Grey Turner) and a portion of the stricture should be removed for biopsy. Sometimes in these cases, repeated biopsies show inflammatory tissue only. If, however, the symptoms show a marked progression, malignancy should be strongly suspected.

Clinical features

Increasing difficulty in defaecation is the leading symptom. The patient finds that increasingly large doses of aperients are required and, if the stools are formed, they are 'pipe-stem' in shape. In cases of inflammatory stricture, tenesmus, bleeding and the passage of mucopus are superadded. Sometimes the patient comes under observation only when subacute or acute intestinal obstruction has supervened.

Rectal examination

The finger encounters a sharply defined shelf-like interruption of the lumen. If the calibre is large enough to admit the finger, it should be noted whether the stricture is annular or tubular. Sometimes this point can be determined only after dilatation. A biopsy of the stricture must be taken.

Treatment

Prophylactic

The passage of an anal dilator during convalescence after haemorrhoidectomy greatly reduces the incidence of postoperative

stricture. Efficient treatment of lymphogranuloma inguinale in its early stages should lessen the frequency of stricture from that cause.

Dilatation by bougies

For anal and many rectal strictures, dilatation by bougies at regular intervals is all that is required.

Anoplasty

The stricture is incised and a rotation or advancement flap of skin and subcutaneous tissue replaces the defect and enlarges the anal orifice (Fig. 69.45). This technique is particularly useful for postoperative strictures.

Colostomy

Colostomy must be undertaken when a stricture is causing intestinal obstruction and in advanced cases of stricture complicated by fistulae-in-ano. In selected cases, this can be followed by restorative resection of the stricture-bearing area. If this step is anticipated, a loop ileostomy is constructed.

Rectal excision and coloanal anastomosis

When the strictures are at or just above the anorectal junction and are associated with a normal anal canal, but irreversible changes necessitate removal of the area, excision can be followed by a coloanal anastomosis with good functional results (Summary box 69.15).

Summary box 69.15

Benign anal stricture

- May be spasmodic or organic
- May be iatrogenic, e.g. after haemorrhoidectomy or repair of imperforate anus
- Biopsy must be taken to rule out malignancy
- Can usually be managed by regular dilatation

MALIGNANT TUMOURS

Malignant lesions of the anus and anal canal

Anal malignancy is rare and accounts for less than 2% of all large bowel cancers. Those arising below the dentate line are usually squamous, whereas those above are variously termed basaloid,

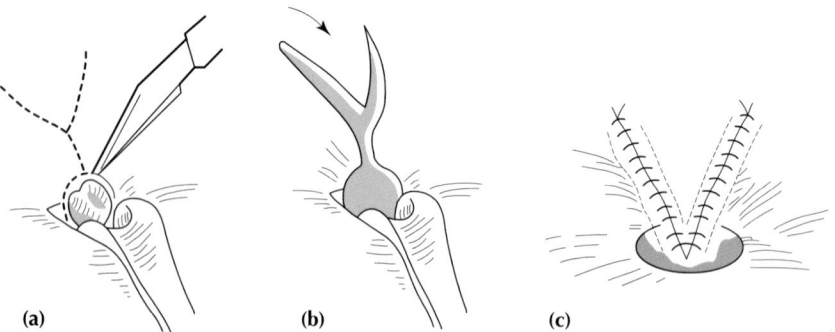

(a) (b) (c)

Figure 69.45 (a–c) Y–V advancement flap for anal stenosis.

George Grey Turner, **1877–1951, Professor of Surgery, University of Durham, Durham (1927–1934) and then at the Postgraduate Medical School, London (1934–1945).**

cloacogenic or transitional. Collectively they are known as epidermoid carcinomas, to distinguish them from those of non-squamous cell origin (adenocarcinoma, melanoma, lymphoma, sarcoma).

Squamous cell carcinoma

Although rare, the incidence of anal squamous cell carcinoma (SCC) is rising, with a direct association with HPV infection, AIN and immunosuppression. Thus, high-risk groups are those infected with HPV (especially subtypes 16, 18, 31 or 33) (Fig. 69.46), those with HIV infection, recipients of organ transplants (renal transplant patients have a 100-fold increased risk) and those with a past history of cancers at 'sexually accessible' sites (usually genital). Pain and bleeding are the most common symptoms and the disease is thus often initially misdiagnosed as a benign condition, highlighting the need for a level of suspicion and adequate examination. A mass, pruritus or discharge is less common. Advanced tumours may cause faecal incontinence by invasion of the sphincters and, in women, anterior extension may result in anovaginal fistulation. On examination, anal margin tumours look like malignant ulcers. There may be associated HPV lesions. Anal canal tumours are palpable as irregular indurated tender ulceration. Sphincter involvement may be evident.

Management

Historically, early anal margin tumours were treated by local excision and anal canal tumours by abdominoperineal excision of the rectum. Nowadays, primary treatment is by chemoradiotherapy [combined modality therapy (CMT); Nigro], the chemotherapy sually including a combination of 5-fluorouracil (5-FU) with mitomycin C or cisplatin. The surgeon, however, has an important role in management: initial diagnosis is surgical; small marginal tumours are still best treated by local excision; radical surgery is indicated in those with persistent or recurrent disease following CMT; and a defunctioning stoma may be indicated for those in whom treatment and disease regression is associated with radionecrosis, incontinence or fistula.

Other anal malignancies

Adenocarcinomata within the anal canal are usually extensions of distal rectal cancers. Rarely, adenocarcinoma may arise from anal glandular epithelium or develop within a longstanding (usually complex) anal fistula; treatment is as for low rectal cancers [i.e. abdominoperineal excision of the rectum (APER) with or without previous radiotherapy or chemoradiotherapy] but prognosis is less good.

Melanocytes can be found in the transitional zone of the anal canal. Malignant melanoma of the anus is very rare and usually presents as a bluish-black soft mass that may mimic a thrombosed external pile, although it may be amelanotic (Fig. 69.47). The prognosis, irrespective of treatment, is extremely poor. Perianal Paget's disease is exceedingly rare (Summary box 69.16).

Summary box 69.16

Anal cancer

- Uncommon tumour, which is usually a squamous cell carcinoma
- Associated with HPV
- More prevalent in patients with HIV infection
- May affect the anal verge or anal canal
- Lymphatic spread is to the inguinal lymph nodes
- Treatment is by chemoradiotherapy in the first instance
- Major ablative surgery is required if the above fails

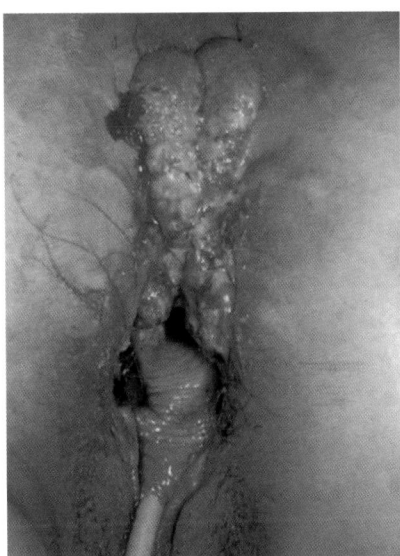

Figure 69.46 Neglected papillomas of the anus that have become malignant.

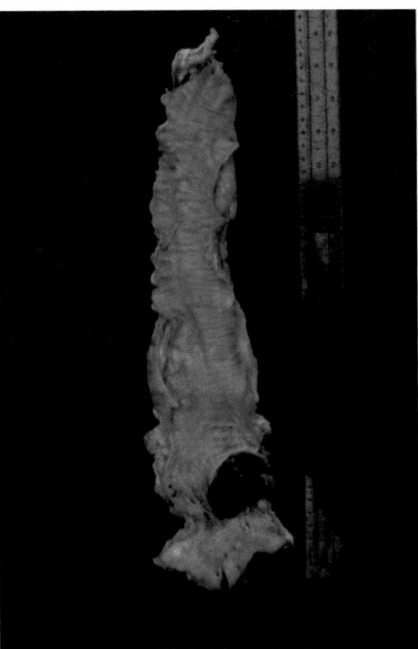

Figure 69.47 Malignant melanoma of the anal canal (courtesy of Mr B. Thomas, Kalushi, Zambia).

N. Nigro, **Surgeon, Wayne State University, Detroit, MI, USA.**

Sir James Paget, 1814–1899, Surgeon, St Bartholomew's Hospital, London, UK, described this disease in 1874.

FURTHER READING

Fielding, L.P. and Goldberg, S. (eds) (1999) *Robb and Smith's Operative Surgery. Surgery of the Colon, Rectum and Anus*, 2nd edn. Chapman & Hall, London.

Keighley, M.R.B. and Williams, N.S. (1999) *Surgery of the Anus, Rectum and Colon*, 2nd edn. W.B. Saunders, London.

PART
12 | Genitourinary

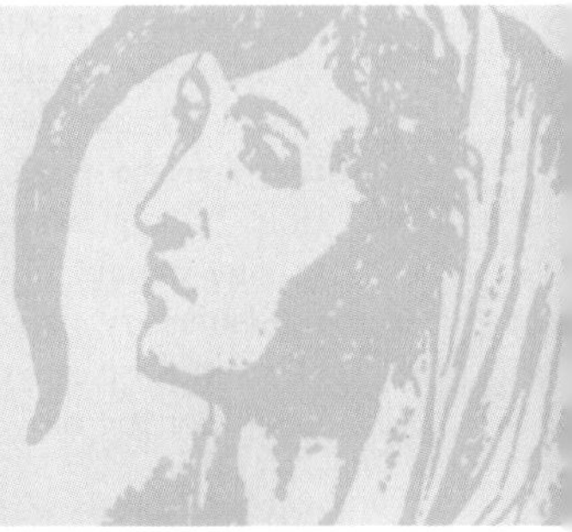

Urinary symptoms and investigations

To recognise and understand:
- The major symptoms of urological disease

- The most commonly used investigations for urological conditions

URINARY SYMPTOMS

Haematuria

The presence of blood in the urine (haematuria) may be the only indication of pathology in the urinary tract (Fig. 70.1). Tiny amounts of blood that are insufficient to stain the urine (microscopic haematuria) may be detected by dipstick testing as part of a routine health check. A substantial haemorrhage into the urinary tract will give the urine a red or brownish tinge (macroscopic haematuria) and the patient may pass blood clots. False-positive stick tests and the discoloured urine caused by beetroot and some drugs [e.g. Dindevan (phenindione), Pyridium (phenazopyridine) and Furadantin (nitrofurantoin)] can be distinguished from haematuria by the absence of red blood cells on urinary microscopy.

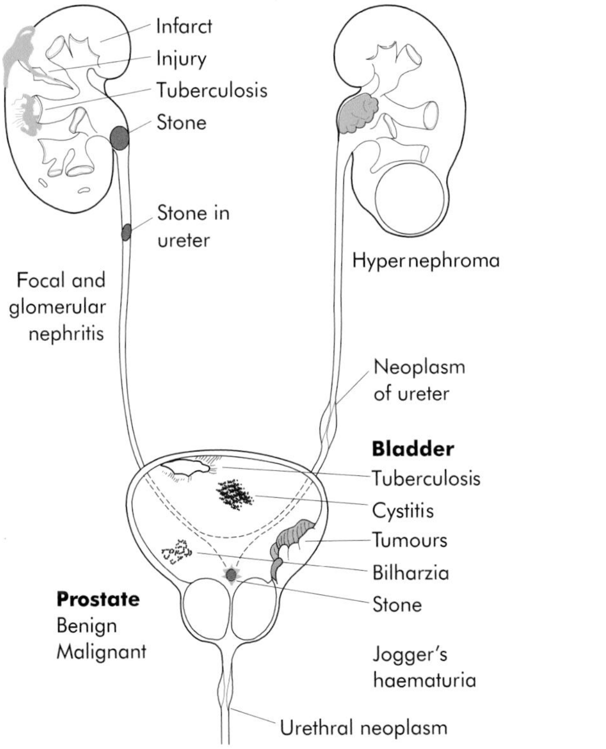

Haematuria may be intermittent or persistent. Blood appearing at the beginning of the urinary stream indicates a lower urinary tract cause, whereas uniform staining throughout the stream points to a cause higher up. Terminal haematuria is typical of severe bladder irritation caused stone or infection. If the patient experiences pain with haematuria, the characteristics of the pain may help to identify the source of the bleeding. If there is a malignant cause for the haematuria there is usually no pain.

None of these variations in the presentation of haematuria is sufficient in itself to diagnose the cause of bleeding, and all patients with haematuria should be investigated even if they are taking anticoagulant drugs. In a significant proportion, all tests will be negative: the chance of finding a urological cause in patients under 40 years of age with microscopic haematuria is particularly small. However, bleeding into the urinary tract may be caused by an occult nephropathy so it is important to check for significant proteinuria and hypertension in these patients (Summary box 70.1).

Blood dyscrasias
Purpura
Sickle cell trait
Anti-coagulants

Renal tumours
Transitional cell carcinoma
Wilm's tumour

Infarct
Injury
Tuberculosis
Stone

Stone in ureter

Focal and glomerular nephritis

Hypernephroma

Neoplasm of ureter

Bladder
Tuberculosis
Cystitis
Tumours
Bilharzia
Stone

Prostate
Benign
Malignant

Jogger's haematuria

Urethral neoplasm

Figure 70.1 The more common causes of haematuria.

Summary box 70.1

Haematuria

- Is always abnormal whether microscopic or macroscopic
- May be caused by a lesion anywhere in the urinary tract
- Is investigated by:
  - examination of midstream specimen for infection
  - cytological examination of a urine specimen
  - intravenous urogram and/or urinary tract ultrasound scan
  - flexible or rigid cystoscopy
- Is commonly caused by urinary infection, especially in young women

Pain (Summary boxes 70.2 and 70.3)

Renal pain

Inflammation and acute obstruction to the flow of urine from the renal pelvis are liable to cause pain that is typically felt as a deep-seated, sickening ache in the loin. It is probably the result of stretching of the capsule of the kidney. However, calculi in the kidney can also be painful in the absence of infection, although they may be too small or peripherally placed to cause obstruction. Slow-growing masses such as tumours or cysts are not usually painful unless they are very large. When the cause is inflammatory, there may be local deep tenderness and occasionally reflex spasm of the psoas muscle, leading to involuntary flexion of the hip joint.

Ureteric colic

This is an acute pain felt in the loin and radiating to the ipsilateral iliac fossa and genitalia. The patient often rolls around in agony as waves of excruciating sharp pain are imposed upon a continuing background of discomfort. Contrast this with the patient suffering from peritoneal pain, who lies still to avoid exacerbating the pain by movement.

Ureteric colic is usually caused by the passage of a stone, but blood clot or sloughed renal papilla may give identical pain. The site of the pain is a partial guide to the progress of a stone: the more the pain radiates into the groin, the more distal the stone. Local tenderness is much less than would be expected from the severity of the pain.

Summary box 70.2

Pain from the upper urinary tract

- When caused by acute obstruction of the renal pelvis, is typically fixed deep in the loin and 'bursting' in character
- When caused by acute ureteric obstruction (usually by a stone), is colicky with sharp exacerbations against a constant background
- Is liable to be referred to the groin, scrotum or labium as calculus obstruction moves distally in the ureter

---

Bladder pain

Bladder pain is felt as a suprapubic discomfort made worse by bladder filling. In men, a sharp pain misleadingly referred to the tip of the penis may be the result of irritation of the trigone of the bladder. Severe inflammation of the bladder can cause an extreme wrenching discomfort at the end of micturition. This symptom of bladder stone was recognised by the old lithotomists, who called it strangury.

Perineal pain

This is experienced as a penetrating ache in the perineum and rectum, sometimes with associated inguinal discomfort. The patient is characteristically exasperated and depressed by pain that has a peculiarly relentless nature. Pelvic pain is often blamed on 'chronic prostatitis', 'prostadynia' or 'chronic prostate pain syndrome', but it occurs in both men and women. It is notoriously difficult to treat successfully, a characteristic shared with various chronic scrotal pain syndromes.

Urethral pain

Urethral pain is a scalding or burning felt in the vulva or penis, especially during voiding.

Summary box 70.3

Pain from the lower urinary tract

- Is commonly felt as subrapubic discomfort, worsening as the bladder fills
- When caused by cystitis, typically has a burning or scalding character felt in the urethra on micturition
- May be referred to the tip of the penis in men, even when lesion is in the bladder

---

Altered bladder function

The normal bladder has two distinct phases of function. During the *filling phase* the bladder acts as a reservoir to collect urine until it is emptied in the *voiding phase*. Inappropriate contraction of the bladder detrusor muscle during filling (instability) is perceived as a sensation of urgency to pass urine. The patient may have frequency of micturition and a tendency to urge incontinence. Sleep may be disturbed by nocturia. Instability may be idiopathic in both sexes or part of the bladder response to outflow obstruction, notably in men with enlargement of the prostate. When detrusor instability has a demonstrable neurological cause, it is known as hyperreflexia.

Symptoms of impaired emptying are most commonly the result of bladder outflow obstruction, but detrusor failure presents a similar picture. The patient has difficulty initiating voiding (hesitancy) and the stream is variable or slow. Abdominal straining improves the weak flow. When the act of micturition is completed, there may be a feeling that urine remains in the bladder so the patient tries again (pis-en-deux). With time, the bladder becomes chronically overfilled. Urine spills out, typically at night when sleep halts constant trips to the lavatory (chronic retention with overflow) (Summary box 70.4).

Summary box 70.4

Altered bladder function

- Failure of the storage function of the bladder leads to urgency and frequency of micturition, often by day and by night
- Failure of the emptying function of the bladder is most commonly caused by obstruction to the bladder outflow (e.g. by prostatic enlargement) but can also be caused by weakness of the detrusor muscle
- Chronic retention of urine may present as nocturnal bedwetting

---

INVESTIGATION OF THE URINARY TRACT

With the exception of renal and scrotal masses or tenderness, a palpable bladder or an abnormal prostate on digital rectal examination, urological conditions are most likely to be diagnosed from the history or by investigations.

Urine

Dipsticks impregnated with chemicals that change colour in the presence of blood, protein or nitrites (Multistix, Labstix) are a

---

pis-en-deux **is French for to urinate twice.**

convenient way to screen urine for the presence of abnormalities. They can be read mechanically so that the clinician is provided with a paper readout of the results. When the urine is macroscopically clear and negative on dipstick testing, the chances of finding an abnormality on microscopy and culture of a midstream clean-catch specimen are small. Indeed, some bacteriological laboratories decline further examination of the urine in these circumstances on the grounds that it is not cost-effective. The presence of protein and nitrites (which are a product of the activity of organisms in the urine) indicates the likelihood of infection. The significance of microscopic haematuria is discussed above. Some dipsticks also give an indication of the pH and specific gravity of the urine.

Microscopy is essential to confirm the presence of white and red blood cells in the urine, and bacteria may also be visible under light microscopy. The presence of protein casts suggests disease affecting the renal parenchyma, as does red cell dysmorphia seen on phase contrast microscopy. Schistosoma ova have a typical appearance (Fig. 70.2), and vegetable or meat fibres may be present if there is a fistula connecting the bowel with the urinary tract.

Cytological examination of the urinary sediment is sensitive and specific for poorly differentiated transitional cell tumours anywhere in the urinary tract. However, false negatives are common in the 50% of these cancers that are well differentiated. A new chemical test (BTA-Bard) detects a bladder tumour antigen in the urine, and its findings can complement cytological examination of the urine.

Bacteriological culture of a clean-catch midstream specimen of the urine is the standard means of identifying urinary pathogens. The presence of organisms at a level of $> 10^5\,\mathrm{ml}^{-1}$ is deemed to indicate the presence of infection rather than contamination of the urine by bacteria. If there are pus cells in the urine but there is no growth on the routine culture media (sterile pyuria), it is worth testing for more fastidious organisms. The centrifuged sediment of multiple early-morning urine specimens must be cultured on Löwenstein–Jensen medium to detect urinary tract tuberculosis. *Chlamydia* is another common urinary pathogen that will not be detected on routine culture.

Biochemical examination for electrolytes, glucose, bilirubin, haemoglobin and myoglobin is essential to detect abnormal amounts of these substances in the urine. Analysis of a 24-hour specimen of urine will quantify the rate of loss, and is especially useful in the investigation of calculus disease caused by abnormal excretion of calcium, oxalate, uric acid and other products of metabolism (Summary box 70.5).

> **Summary box 70.5**
>
> **Microscopic, cytological, bacteriological and biochemical examination of urine**
>
> - Abnormalities found on Multistik testing of the urine should be confirmed by microscopy and culture
> - The presence of greater than 10^5 organisms per ml of urine is deemed to indicate the presence of a significant urinary infection
> - Cytological examination of the urine is likely to be abnormal when there is a poorly differentiated transitional cell tumour in the bladder

Tests of renal function

More than 70% of kidney function must be lost before renal failure becomes evident: there is a large functional reserve. It follows that renal damage must be extensive before changes occur in blood constituents whose level is controlled by renal excretion. Such damage is of three main types: reduction of renal plasma flow, destruction of glomeruli and impairment of tubular function. In severe hypertension or renal artery stenosis, the plasma flow is impaired. In glomerulonephritis or acute cortical necrosis, there is a loss of glomeruli, whereas in pyelonephritis, tubular function is most severely affected. In obstructive nephropathy, back pressure on the renal parenchyma causes all three types of damage.

Levels of blood urea and serum creatinine can be affected by various factors but, in practice, when taken together they serve as a useful clinical guide to overall renal function. A creatinine clearance test will give an approximate value for glomerular filtration rate but is prone to error. A more accurate assessment of glomerular function can be obtained from an estimate of the clearance of chromium-51-labelled ethylenediaminetetraacetic acid. Surgeons will usually call on their nephrological colleagues for more detailed investigations of tubular function and renal blood flow.

The specific gravity of the urine is fixed at a low level when the kidney loses the power to concentrate because of renal tubular dysfunction. Estimation of the urinary loss of sodium, β_2-microglobulin or the tubular enzyme N-acetylglucosamine (NAG) will further define the nature of any functional impairment (Summary box 70.6).

> **Summary box 70.6**
>
> **Tests of renal function**
>
> - Elevated blood urea and serum creatinine levels usually indicate a significant impairment of renal function
> - More sophisticated renal assessment is required to quantify the functional deficit

Imaging

A plain abdominal radiograph showing the kidneys, ureters and bladder (the KUB) can disclose a wealth of useful information.

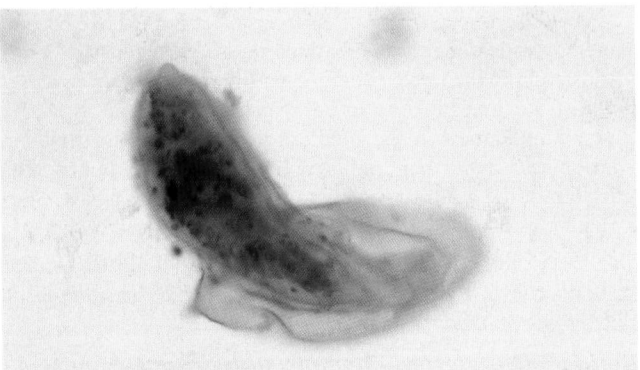

Figure 70.2 Schistosoma ovum (courtesy of Dr Nawal Derius).

Ernst Lowenstein, **b. 1878**, Pathologist, Vienna, Austria.
Carl Oluf Jensen, **1864–1934**, Veterinary Surgeon and Pathologist, Copenhagen, Denmark.

With the film properly orientated (with the liver on the right and gastric air bubble on the left unless there is situs invertus!) a glance at the spine and bony structures may reveal the presence of scoliosis, spina bifida, degenerative disease of the spine, metastases, fractures and arthritis. All of these may have relevance to the urological diagnosis. The soft-tissue shadows of the kidneys, outlined to a greater or lesser extent by their more radiolucent fatty coverings, overlie the upper attachments of the psoas muscles. A full bladder often presents a hazy outline arising from the pelvis.

Most urinary calculi absorb X-rays and should be sought in the region of the renal shadows and along the course of each ureter. These normally follow the tips of the transverse processes of the vertebrae, cross the sacroiliac joints and head for the ischial spine before hooking medially towards the bladder base. Stones with a low calcium content and those overlying bony structures may be difficult to see on the plain film. Pelvic phleboliths are very common and can look like lower ureteric calculi. Uric acid stones are the most common radiolucent calculi (Summary box 70.7).

Summary box 70.7

Straight abdominal radiograph

- Most urinary calculi are radiodense
- Uric acid calculi are typically radiolucent

Intravenous urography (urography) (Fig. 70.3)

Excretion renography has been a mainstay of urological investigation since the introduction of intravenous contrast media in the 1930s. These are organic chemicals to which iodine atoms are attached to absorb X-rays. When such a chemical is injected, usually into a vein in the antecubital fossa, it is filtered from the blood by the glomeruli and does not undergo tubular absorption. As a result, it rapidly passes through the renal parenchyma into the urine, which it renders radio-opaque.

Although intravenous urography (IVU) gives excellent images of the urinary tract, its use should be restricted because in a few patients the iodine in the contrast medium may provoke a potentially life-threatening anaphylactic reaction. Patients with a history of allergy, atopy and eczema are particularly vulnerable, but severe reactions may occur without warning. Less invasive and dangerous imaging techniques are clearly to be preferred if they are able to give comparable diagnostic information (Summary box 70.8).

Summary box 70.8

Intravenous urography

- IVU can cause a dangerous hypersensitivity reaction in a small number of patients

---

Preparation

It is usual to give a laxative to clear faeces that might otherwise obscure details of urinary tract anatomy. Modest fluid restriction is permissible, but dehydration is dangerous because it may precipitate acute renal failure.

Technique

The patient is observed carefully while the first few drops of contrast medium (Urografin or Niopam 370) are injected. The earliest films, taken within minutes of the injection, show the renal parenchyma opacified by contrast medium – the nephrogram phase. A delayed nephrogram on one side indicates unilateral functional impairment. Distortion of the renal outline or failure of part of the kidney to function suggests a space-occupying lesion.

After a few minutes, the contrast is excreted into the collecting system, opacifying the calyces and the renal pelvis. Later films show the ureters and, at the end of the study, the patient is asked to pass urine and a final film is taken to show detail of the bladder area. It is important to bear in mind that the static images of IVU provide only snapshots of dynamic events in the urinary tract. The appearance of a normal ureter changes as peristaltic waves of contraction pass along it.

IVU is particularly valuable to demonstrate tumours and calculi within the urinary tract, which are sometimes difficult to see on ultrasonography. It may also be useful to show details of abnormal anatomy that are difficult to interpret on an ultrasonogram.

As ultrasonography and other forms of scanning have become more sophisticated, the indications for the urogram are fewer. Obstruction to the upper urinary tract interferes with transport of contrast medium into the urine, which will show up as a non-functioning kidney on the standard urogram films. In these circumstances, a further radiograph taken many hours after injection of the contrast medium may show hazy opacification of a dilated system. Distortion of the calyces or the renal outline can equally be caused by a tumour or by harmless simple cysts. In each of these cases, more information can be obtained from ultrasonography or computerised tomography (CT).

Retrograde ureteropyelography (synonym: retrograde ureterogram)

A fine ureteric catheter can be passed into the ureteric orifice through a cystoscope (Fig. 70.4). Contrast medium injected through the catheter will demonstrate the anatomy of the upper urinary tract. The procedure is particularly useful if there is doubt

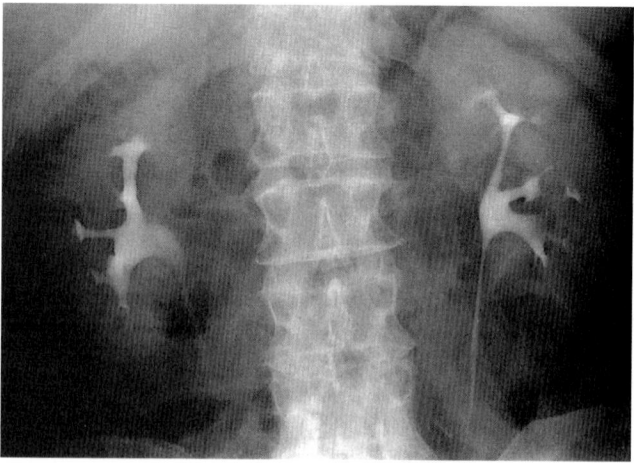

Figure 70.3 Normal intravenous urogram showing the outline of both kidneys with the collecting system and upper ureters highlighted by the contrast medium.

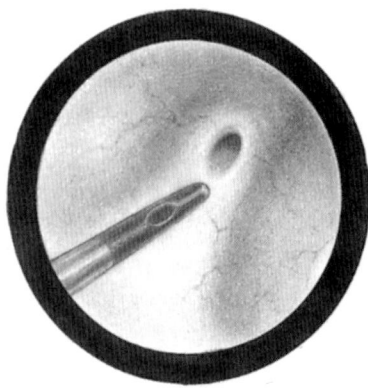

Figure 70.4 A ureteric catheter about to enter the left ureteric orifice. Cystoscopic view.

about an intraluminal lesion (Fig. 70.5) or if renal function is deficient (before surgery for pelviureteric junction obstruction, for instance). When a transitional tumour is found, it can be sampled by aspiration of urine from the upper tract or by brush biopsy. Retrograde ureteropyelography is possible under topical urethral anaesthesia using a flexible cystoscope. Introducing infection into a poorly draining part of the system carries a serious risk of septicaemia. If there is to be any delay in correcting the blockage surgically, facilities must be available to decompress the kidney by retrograde stenting or percutaneous nephrostomy.

Antegrade pyelography

Percutaneous puncture of a dilated renal collecting system is a reasonably simple procedure for the experienced interventional radiologist. The most common indication is the placement of a nephrostomy tube to drain an obstructed infected kidney or to provide access for percutaneous nephrolithotomy. Antegrade pyelography – in which contrast medium is introduced through the nephrostomy – can be helpful when retrograde studies are prevented by obstruction at the extreme lower end of the ureter.

Digital subtraction arteriography

Refinements in radiological imaging have now almost eliminated the need for translumbar aortography. Satisfactory imaging of the renal vessels can even be achieved by digital subtraction angiography after intravenous injection of contrast medium. More precise information can be obtained by intra-arterial injection through a fine catheter inserted into the femoral artery using the Seldinger technique. Arteriography is now rarely used to demonstrate tumour vasculature in a hypernephroma (Fig. 70.6), but a flush venogram is useful when CT suggests tumour invasion of the renal vein and vena cava.

Cystography

Cystography is now most commonly a component of video-urodynamic assessment (see Chapter 72). Its role in assessing ureteric reflux in children has been largely superseded by radioisotope scanning and dynamic ultrasonography.

Urethrography

Ascending urethrography is valuable to demonstrate the extent of a urethral stricture (Fig. 70.7) and the presence of false

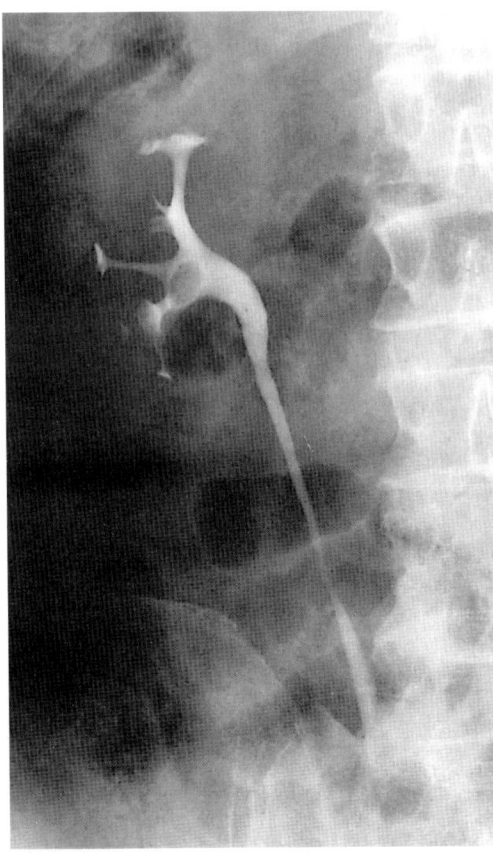

Figure 70.5 Retrograde ureterogram demonstrating the collecting system. The radiolucent filling defect in the renal pelvis is caused by a uric acid calculus.

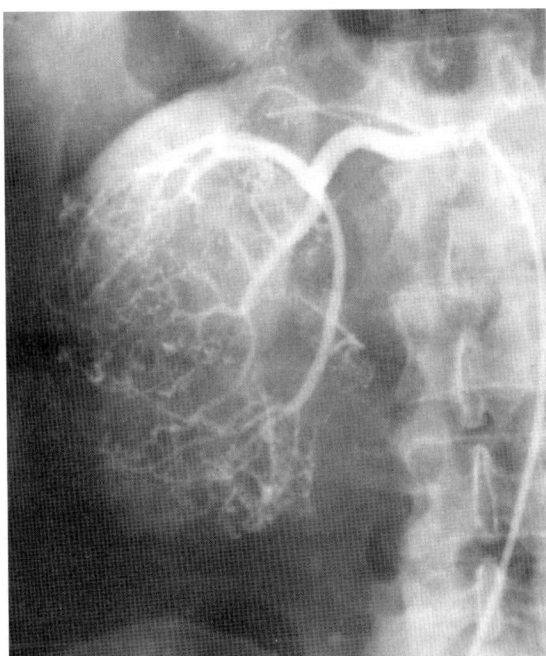

Figure 70.6 A selective renal arteriogram showing abnormal vessels in a renal cell carcinoma.

Sven Ivar Seldinger, b. 1921, Radiologist, Karolinska Sjukhuset, Stockholm, Sweden.

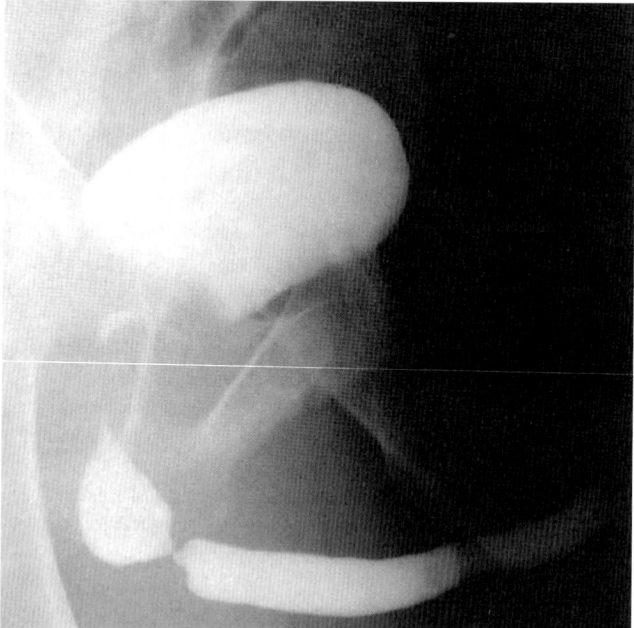

Figure 70.7 Ascending urethrogram demonstrating a tight stricture in the bulbar urethra. Above the stricture the contrast outlines the prostatic urethra and bladder.

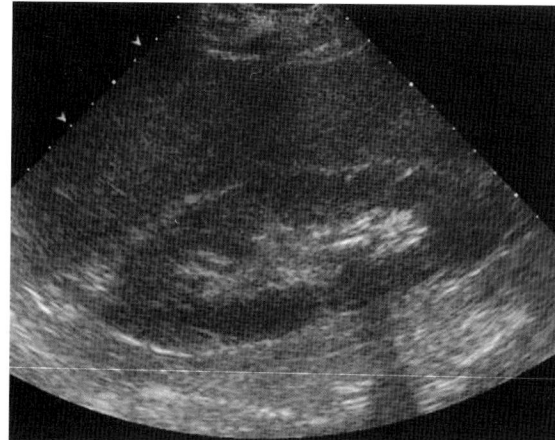

Figure 70.8 A calculus in the kidney casts an acoustic shadow (courtesy of Dr Matthew Matson).

passages and diverticula associated with it. A urethrogram can be used to assess the extent of urethral trauma, but there is a serious danger that contrast medium may pass into the circulation. Lipiodol carries the danger of fat embolus and should never be used, and death has followed the use of barium emulsion. Umbradil viscous V is a radio-opaque water-soluble gel that contains the local anaesthetic lignocaine. It can be injected gently and safely using Knutsson's apparatus even if the urothelium is breached.

Venography

Because extension of a renal carcinoma from the renal vein into the vena cava can usually be demonstrated by ultrasound, venography is now infrequently used for this purpose.

Ultrasonography

High-resolution ultrasonography is perhaps the imaging technique most widely used in urology. The size of the kidney, the thickness of its cortex and the presence and degree of hydronephrosis can be measured with great accuracy. Intrarenal masses can be diagnosed as smooth walled and fluid filled (simple cysts) or solid and complex (possible tumours). Stones produce a bright ultrasonic reflection and cast an acoustic shadow (Fig. 70.8). The volume of urine in the bladder before and after micturition can be calculated, and even tiny filling defects within it detected. Scrotal contents can be displayed in great detail. Only the lower ureter resists effective investigation by transabdominal ultrasonography because of its small calibre and its proximity to the large bones of the pelvis and spine (Summary box 70.9).

Folke Knutsson, **Director, The Roentgen Department, The University Hospital,** Uppsala, Sweden.

<table>
<tr><td>Summary box 70.9</td></tr>
</table>

Ultrasonography

■ Ultrasound scanning provides broadly similar anatomical information to an intravenous urogram but without the risks

---

Transrectal ultrasonography

This has become a routine component of the investigation of suspected carcinoma of the prostate. Most commonly, suspicion has arisen because the level of prostate-specific antigen is raised or there is an abnormality of the texture or outline of the prostate on digital rectal examination. The features of carcinoma or benign enlargement of the prostate, although not absolutely specific, are sufficiently well recognised to allow an experienced ultrasonographer to identify promising sites for transrectal fine-needle biopsy.

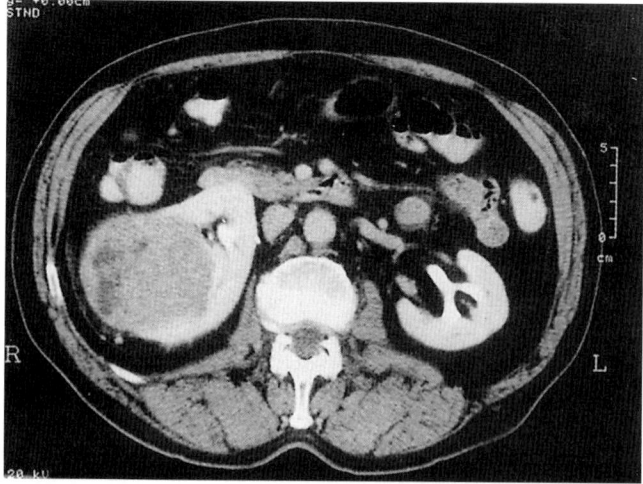

Figure 70.9 Computerised tomography showing renal cell carcinoma of the right kidney.

Computerised tomography

CT is particularly useful to assess structures in the retroperitoneum (Fig. 70.9). In renal carcinoma it will show:

- the size and site of the tumour and the degree of invasion of adjacent tissue;
- the presence of enlarged lymph nodes at the renal hilum;
- invasion of the renal vein and vena cava.

CT is of crucial importance in the initial staging and follow-up of men with testicular cancer, in whom the presence of retroperitoneal lymph node masses is a feature of advanced disease. It has also been used to stage bladder and prostate cancer, but its value is less clear-cut in these diseases. Non-contrast CT is also used routinely in the diagnosis of urinary calculi (Figs 70.10 and 70.11).

Magnetic resonance imaging and positron emission tomography

These technologies give information about the function of organs as well as detailed structural images. It is likely that as they become more widely available, they will replace many of the routine imaging techniques.

Radioisotope scanning

Radioisotope scanning is used in particular to obtain information about function in individual renal units. Diethyltriaminepentaacetic acid (DTPA) behaves in the kidney like inulin: it is filtered by the glomeruli and not absorbed by the tubules. Using a gamma camera, DTPA labelled with technetium-99m can be followed during its transit through individual kidneys to give a dynamic representation of renal function. A ^{99m}Tc-DTPA scan is particularly useful to prove that collecting system dilatation is caused by obstruction. In obstruction, radioactivity will remain in the kidney even if urine flow is stimulated by administration of a diuretic like frusemide (furosemide). Other substances [dimercaptosuccinic acid (DMSA), mercaptoacetylglycine (MAG-3) and sodium orthoiodohippurate (Hippuran)] labelled with suitable radioactive isotopes have similarly been used to investigate renal function (Fig. 70.12).

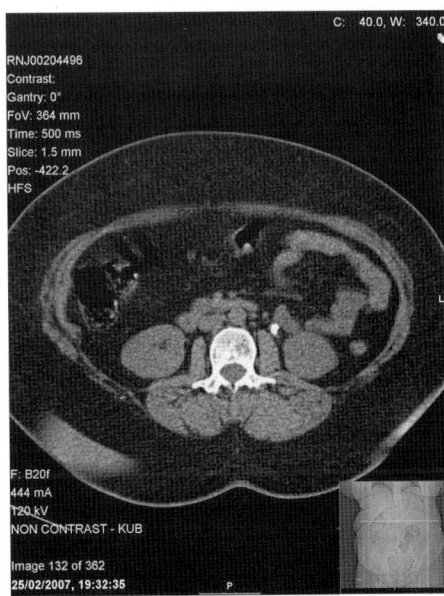

Figure 70.10 A non-contrast CT clearly shows a calculus in the left upper ureter (courtesy of Dr Matthew Matson).

Isotope bone scanning is fundamental to the staging of kidney and prostate cancers, which typically metastasise to the skeleton.

Endoscopy

Effective visual inspection of the lower urinary tract has been possible since 1877, when Nitze invented his cystoscope. A second leap forward in urological endoscopy came with the introduction by Hopkins of the rod lens telescope and fibreoptic illumination. This permitted the development of a family of endoscopes, which allow the urologist to visualise the upper and lower urinary tracts for diagnosis and therapy. Finally, in the early 1980s, the small-calibre flexible fibrescopic cystoscope was introduced. This allows simple diagnostic cystourethroscopy, bladder biopsy and retrograde ureterography to be performed under topical urethral anaesthesia with minimal discomfort to the patient (Summary box 70.10).

> **Summary box 70.10**
>
> ### Diagnostic examination
>
> - Diagnostic examination of the bladder is performed painlessly under local anaesthesia using a flexible cystoscope

ANURIA

Anuria is defined as the complete absence of urine production. Oliguria is present when less than 300 ml of urine is excreted in a day (Summary box 70.11).

> **Summary box 70.11**
>
> ### Diagnosing anuria
>
> - Check that the bladder is empty before diagnosing anuria
> - Ultrasound the bladder

The maintenance of renal function and urine production depends upon perfusion of the kidneys with oxygenated blood. Reduced renal blood flow or hypoxia impairs renal function. When both are present, the danger of acute renal failure is even greater.

Renal failure is traditionally divided into:

- prerenal;
- renal;
- postrenal (obstructive).

Prerenal

Prerenal causes of acute renal failure include:

- hypovolaemia;
- blood loss;
- sepsis;
- cardiogenic shock;
- anaesthesia;
- hypoxia.

> Max Nitze, 1848–1906, Urological Surgeon, Vienna, Austria.
> Harold Horace Hopkins, 1918–1994, Professor of Applied Optics, The University of Reading, Reading, England.

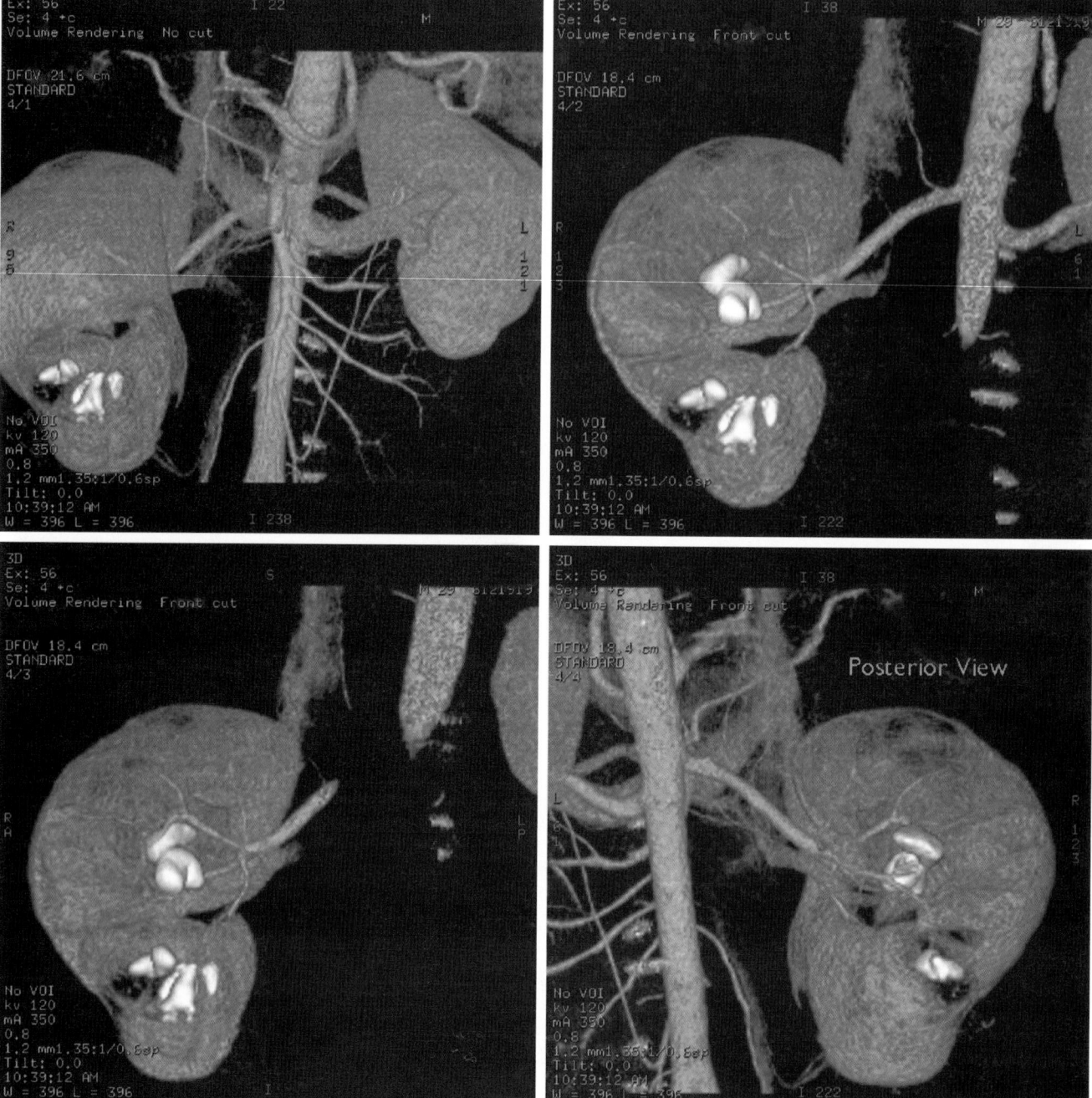

Figure 70.11 Reconstructed spiral computerised tomography scan showing calculi in the right kidney (courtesy of Professor R. Resnek).

Hypovolaemia

This may result from inadequate fluid intake or from excessive loss of body water. Dehydration, prolonged vomiting, diarrhoea and other abnormal gastrointestinal fluid losses, burns and excessive sweating are all common causes of hypovolaemia.

Blood loss

This is usually caused by trauma or surgery, but acute blood loss from the gastrointestinal tract or haemorrhage associated with childbirth may be sufficient to cause hypovolaemic renal impairment.

Sepsis

Gram-negative septicaemia from a urinary tract source is a particularly potent cause of bacteraemic shock. Sepsis from the biliary tract and overwhelming infection from other sites, especially in the immunocompromised individual, are also associated with acute renal failure.

Cardiogenic shock

Acute dysrhythmia secondary to myocardial infarction, cardiac tamponade and pulmonary embolus may all result in reduced cardiac output of often poorly oxygenated blood.

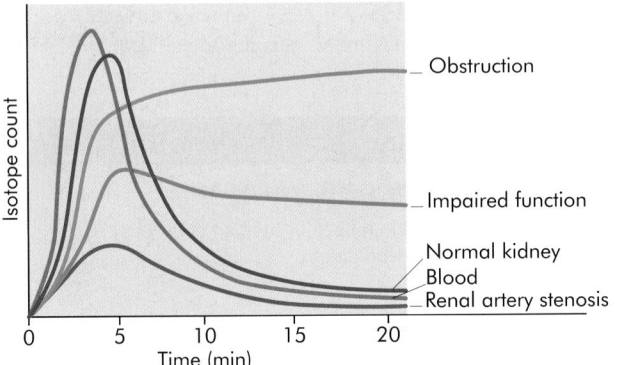

Figure 70.12 Radioisotope renogram.

Anaesthesia

Hypotension is a hazard of epidural and spinal anaesthesia.

Hypoxia

Prolonged hypoxia from any cause may occasionally be responsible.

Renal

Renal causes of acute renal failure include:

- drugs;
- poisons;
- contrast media;
- eclampsia;
- myoglobinuria;
- incompatible blood transfusion;
- disseminated intravascular coagulation.

It is uncommon for patients with established glomerulonephritis to develop acute oliguria; however, such patients are more prone to rapid deterioration of remaining renal function should any renal insult occur.

Drugs

Aminoglycosides, cephalosporins and diuretics can be nephrotoxic, particularly if used in combination. They are quite commonly used in patients whose renal function is already compromised by sepsis or circulatory abnormalities. Prolonged use of non-steroidal anti-inflammatory drugs (NSAIDs) can cause a chronic interstitial nephritis and papillary necrosis; they also reduce renal plasma flow and therefore have nephrotoxic properties. Angiotensin-converting enzyme inhibitors used for the control of hypertension can cause a rapid reduction in the glomerular filtration rate; this is particularly liable to occur in patients who have a reduced renal blood flow.

Poisons

Some of these are nephrotoxic.

Contrast media

Even modern contrast media may cause renal failure when injected into a dehydrated patient with compromised renal function.

Eclampsia

The early recognition of pre-eclampsia is vital to avoid the nephrotoxic consequences of toxaemia and uncontrolled hypertension.

Myoglobinuria

The presence of myoglobin in the urine is associated with the 'crush' syndrome after major trauma. Less severe injuries can also cause the syndrome, especially if a compartment syndrome is unrecognised or pressure areas break down.

Incompatible blood transfusion

This may lead to renal failure with myoglobinuria.

Disseminated intravascular coagulation

Disseminated intravascular coagulation usually follows major sepsis or massive blood transfusion and may occur post-partum.

Obstructive

Obstructive causes of acute renal failure include:

- calculi;
- pelvic malignancy;
- surgery;
- retroperitoneal fibrosis;
- bilharzia;
- crystalluria.

Calculi

Renal calculus disease is probably the most common cause of acute obstruction leading to anuria. The patient is likely to have unilateral renal colic against a background of non-function of the contralateral kidney, often due to previous surgery or pre-existing obstruction by calculus.

Pelvic malignancy

Carcinomas arising from the bladder, prostate, cervix, ovary or rectum can all lead to obstruction of one or both ureters. A history of haematuria and vaginal or rectal bleeding signpost the diagnosis. A large pelvic mass is commonly palpable on bimanual examination.

Surgery

The ureters are vulnerable to damage during pelvic and retroperitoneal surgery, but injury should be avoided if proper care is taken. It is unusual, but not impossible, to damage both ureters.

Retroperitoneal fibrosis

For details of retroperitoneal fibrosis see Chapter 71.

Bilharzia (see Chapter 5)

Schistosomiasis may lead to ureteric fibrosis and stenosis, and may be responsible for the development of squamous cell carcinoma of the bladder.

Crystalluria

Crystalluria causing urinary tract obstruction used to be associated with sulphonamide medications but this is now rare. However, uric acid crystalluria can develop in patients receiving chemotherapy for leukaemia or lymphoma unless they are given prophylactic treatment with allopurinol.

Theodor Maximilian Bilharz, **1825–1862, Professor of Zoology, Cairo, Egypt.**

Clinical aspects

Answers to the following questions should indicate the probable cause of reduced urine output.

- *Is urine being produced?* Catheterisation of the bladder is essential if a voided sample cannot be obtained. If urine is available, check the specific gravity, look for the presence of casts (implying a renal cause), test for myoglobinuria and send a sample for culture and microscopy.
- *Is there an obvious prerenal cause?* This can usually be answered by clinical examination, assessment of the patient's vital signs, examination of the fluid balance chart and measurement of the arterial oxygen concentration.
- *Is there ureteric obstruction?* Hydronephrosis may not be marked in acute obstruction, but ultrasonography will usually show some degree of ureteric dilatation. A plain abdominal radiograph should be checked for calculi.
- *What drugs have been given recently?* If a drug is thought to be responsible for renal impairment, it should obviously be withdrawn unless its use is vital.
- *Is this a progression to chronic renal failure?* The presence of shrunken kidneys on ultrasound, normochromic anaemia and hypertension suggest progression to a chronic state even if a previous history of renal failure is not available.

Management and treatment

Renal failure caused by acute tubular necrosis may progress through three recognisable phases:

- oliguria;
- the diuretic phase;
- recovery.

The initial management is aimed at prompt restoration of the circulating volume deficit and correction of tissue hypoxia. Most patients will require a level of care that is available only in a specialised unit. As a minimum, monitoring with a pulse oximeter and central venous pressure measurements will supplement basic observations. For patients with hypovolaemia or sepsis, inotropic support with dopamine may improve cardiac efficiency and increase renal blood flow. If urine production is not promptly restored, frusemide (furosemide) can be given but this is not always successful and the drug itself may be nephrotoxic. Mannitol may be used as a plasma expander and osmotic diuretic, but care must be taken not to overload the circulation. The aim is to achieve the best possible blood pressure, with a central venous pressure of $7–9\,cmH_2O$. It may be that 100% oxygen is needed to maintain the oxygen tension (PO_2).

If these measures fail, acute tubular necrosis has supervened. Excess fluid loads must be avoided and fluid input restricted to match the reduced output plus insensible losses (500–800 ml per 24 hours depending on ambient conditions). Abnormal losses due to vomiting, nasogastric aspiration, diarrhoea or fistulae will be monitored and replaced.

A hyperkalaemic acidosis is the characteristic metabolic abnormality of the oliguric phase of renal failure. Correction of the metabolic acidosis with intravenous bicarbonate is tempting but not always advisable. Rising serum potassium is life-threatening and requires effective intervention. A calcium resonium enema is the simplest remedy. The ion-exchange resin can also be administered orally but is unpalatable. Cautious use of intravenous dextrose and insulin should be considered if ion exchange fails. The help of a renal physician is highly desirable because urgent dialysis may become necessary to save life (Summary box 70.12).

Summary box 70.12

Shared management with nephrologist

- Enlist the help of a nephrologist at an early stage in the management of renal failure

---

The diuretic phase traditionally occurs between the eighth and 10th day but may be delayed as long as 6 weeks. Glomerular filtration recommences but tubular function takes longer to recover. A heavy loss of sodium and potassium can be expected, and fluid and electrolyte requirements must be carefully judged. In most patients the diuretic phase is followed by the recovery phase, but some never recover and will need renal replacement therapy if they are to survive.

Factors that influence the outcome of acute renal failure include the need for artificial ventilation, the need for inotropic support and the presence of jaundice. There is a significant mortality rate.

Nutritional support

Many patients are unable to eat. If enteral feeding is impossible, parenteral nutrition must be administered, with extreme care to avoid circulatory overload.

Infection

These patients are at increased risk of generalised infection. Swabs taken from the nose and throat, sputum specimens and urine, if available, should be sent for culture. If antibiotics are required, they should be non-nephrotoxic.

General nursing care

Meticulous recording of fluid balance is obviously central to the successful management of these patients. Patients who are seriously ill or comatose need regular turning and care of pressure areas if they are to avoid pressure sores. Physiotherapy to the chest and extremities will aid recovery.

Renal support

Renal replacement is needed for those patients in whom the oliguric or anuric phase is associated with significant uraemic symptoms (vomiting, muscular twitching, itching and altered states of consciousness) or uncontrollable hyperkalaemia (Summary box 70.13).

Summary box 70.13

Life-threatening hyperkalaemia

- In acute renal failure, significant hyperkalaemia is life-threatening and should be corrected at an early stage

---

Peritoneal dialysis

Provided that the patient has not had recent abdominal surgery, peritoneal dialysis can be performed by insertion of a fenestrated catheter under local anaesthesic. This is placed just inferior to the umbilicus in the midline. Sterile dialysis fluid is then run into the peritoneal cavity, where it equilibrates with the extracellular fluid using the peritoneum as a dialysis membrane. After a variable time, the fluid is drained into a closed drainage system. The process is repeated in cycles. Occasionally, when anuria is prolonged, a cuffed catheter needs to be inserted, as used in chronic ambulatory peritoneal dialysis. The disadvantages of acute peritoneal dialysis are the potential for introducing infection into the peritoneum and the rather slow rate of correcting metabolic imbalance, particularly hyperkalaemia.

Haemodialysis

A few sessions of haemodialysis may be life saving. A double-lumen catheter is placed over a guidewire into one of the great veins (jugular, subclavian or femoral). Between sessions of dialysis the lines are kept patent by filling them with heparin solution. Haemodialysis can result in a rapid correction of metabolic abnormalities but also tends to result in considerable fluctuations of the overall fluid balance. The other disadvantage is that heparinisation is necessary, and this may be undesirable after a recent surgical procedure.

Haemofiltration

This, like haemodialysis, requires the use of an extracorporeal machine but causes much less haemodynamic upset. This may be of critical importance for the acutely ill patient.

Obstructive renal failure

When the patient is too ill for surgery to remove the cause of obstruction to the upper urinary tract, the treatment of obstructive renal impairment is drainage, either externally using a nephrostomy or internally using an indwelling stent (Summary box 70.14).

Summary box 70.14

Catheterisation and stents

- Urethral or suprapubic catheterisation will relieve obstruction distal to the bladder
- Indwelling stents to relieve ureteric obstruction can be inserted cystoscopically or percutaneously

---

Percutaneous nephrostomy

Under ultrasonographic guidance and local anaesthetic, a fine-bore hollow needle is introduced via the flank through the parenchyma and into the expanded collecting system of the obstructed kidney. Once it penetrates the system, contrast medium can be injected through the needle to define its exact position. A wire passed through the lumen of the needle is used to guide the insertion of a series of dilators, which enlarge the track until it will accept a suitably sized nephrostomy tube (Fig. 70.13). This will drain urine and pus, provided that the latter is not too viscous. The tube is anchored firmly in place to allow continued drainage as renal function recovers.

Insertion of a J-stent

The ureter can be drained into the bladder by the insertion of a pigtail- or J-stent (see Fig. 70.13). The procedure begins with a retrograde ureterogram under fluoroscopic control to provide an image of the ureter. This will often give an indication of the cause

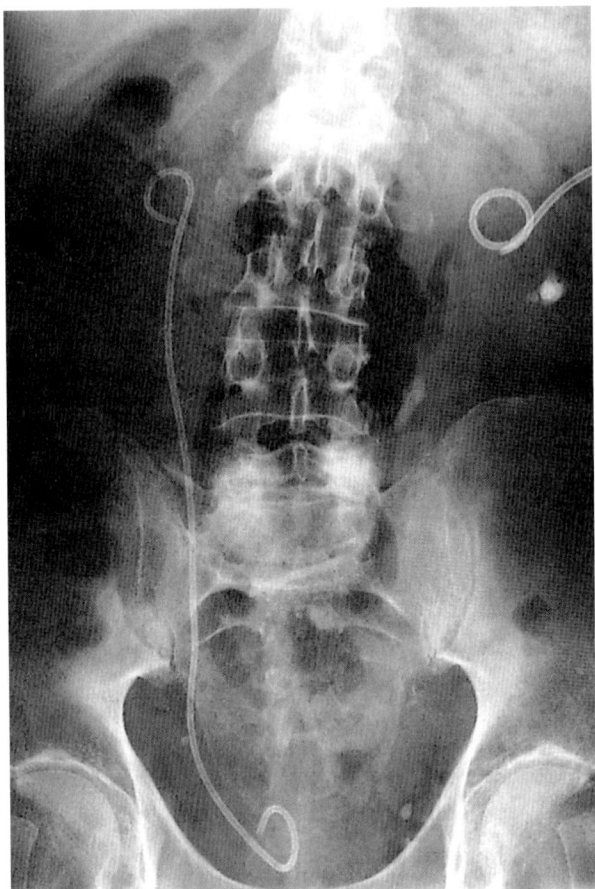

Figure 70.13 Radiograph showing a left-sided, pigtail nephrostomy tube draining a kidney obstruction by a ureteric calculus, seen at the level of L3–4. A J-stent is in the right ureter, which has been cleared of stones.

of the obstruction. A guidewire is introduced through the ureteric orifice and guided up the ureter into the renal pelvis. The stent is rail-roaded over the guidewire until its distal end also lies within the renal pelvis above the obstruction. When the guidewire is removed, the ends of the stent curl to form a J-shape or a pigtail to secure the device against migration. Stents can be placed under topical urethral anaesthesia using the flexible cystoscope and may be safely left in position for several months. They are a foreign body in the urinary tract and are prone to infection and encrustation if neglected. It is vital to keep careful records to account for all stents inserted.

If the J-stent cannot be inserted cystoscopically, it may be placed from above through a nephrostomy.

Open surgery

This is a rarity when the minimally invasive methods described above are available. Retrograde insertion of a nephrostomy through an incision in the renal pelvis is the preferred method because it can be surprisingly difficult to locate even dilated calyces by blind puncture of the renal parenchyma.

FURTHER READING

Blandy, J.P. and Kaisary, A.V. (2007) *Lecture Notes: Urology*, 6th edn. Blackwell, Oxford.

Tanagho, E.A. and McAnich, J.W. (eds) (2000) *Smith's General Urology*, 15th edn. McGraw-Hill/Appleton & Lange, New York.

Wein, A.J., Kavoussi, L.R., Novick, A.C., Partin, A.W. and Peters, C.A. (2007) *Campbell–Walsh Urology*, 9th edn. W.B. Saunders, Philadelphia, PA.

Weiss, G., Weiss, R.M. and O'Reilly, P.H. (eds) (2001) *Comprehensive Urology*. Elsevier Science, Amsterdam.

The kidneys and ureters

EMBRYOLOGY

A bud from the lower end of the mesonephric (wolffian) duct grows backwards behind the peritoneum to the sacral region. The stalk of the bud forms the ureter and its dilated upper extremity, the renal pelvis. From 6 weeks to 8 months of gestation, the primitive pelvis bifurcates repeatedly to form first the calyces and, after several subsequent divisions, the collecting ducts.

The renal parenchyma is derived from the metanephros, which is the most caudal of a series of embryonic renal masses: the primitive pronephros regresses as its function is supplanted by the mesonephros, which in turn is succeeded by the metanephros. The continuity of the glomerular apparatus and nephric tubules formed within the metanephros is established through connection with the collecting ducts. Between weeks 5 and 8 of embryonic development, each kidney ascends the posterior abdominal wall to reach its normal position in the loin. At the same time it rotates so that its hilum faces medially instead of forwards as it previously did.

In humans, the lobulation of the fetal kidney is usually lost as the lobules become bonded together by the growth of new cortex and the renal capsule. In some mammals, e.g. oxen and bears, fetal lobulation is retained.

SURGICAL ANATOMY

The parenchyma of each kidney usually drains into seven calyces, three upper, two middle and two lower calyces (Fig. 71.1). Each

Kaspar Friedrich Wolff, **1733–1794, Professor of Anatomy and Physiology, St Petersburg, Russia, described the mesonephric duct and body in 1759.**

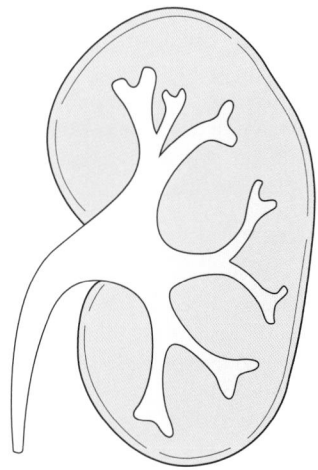

Figure 71.1 The arrangement of renal calyces.

of the three segments represents an anatomical and physiologically distinct unit with its own blood supply.

CONGENITAL ABNORMALITIES OF THE KIDNEY (TABLE 71.1)

Absence of one kidney

The prevalence of unilateral renal agenesis is about 1:1400 and it is usually discovered incidentally. If the mesonephric duct has failed to bud, the ureter will be absent. Alternatively, the ureter and renal pelvis are present but the kidney is absent. In either

Table 71.1 Congenital abnormalities of the kidney and ureter

Renal agenesis	
Renal ectopia	Pelvic kidney
	Horseshoe kidney
	Crossed dystopia
	Infantile polycystic disease
	Unilateral multicystic dysplastic kidney
Aberrant renal vessels	Multiple renal arteries and veins
Duplication	Duplex kidney
	Duplex renal pelvis
	Duplex kidney and ureter
Others	Congenital hydronephrosis
	Retrocaval ureter
	Congenital megaureter

case, the solitary contralateral kidney is likely to be hypertrophied (Summary box 71.1).

Summary box 71.1

Absence of one kidney

- About 1:1400 people has an absent kidney
- It is usually symptomless and often discovered by accident
- When planning a nephrectomy the surgeon should consider the possibility that the other kidney is congenitally absent

---

Renal ectopia

In approximately 1:1000 people the kidney does not ascend. Ectopic kidneys are usually found near the pelvic brim and are usually left sided. The contralateral kidney is generally in its normal position. Disease in an ectopic kidney may present diagnostic problems and an unwary surgeon may be tempted to remove it as an unexplained pelvic mass.

Horseshoe kidney

When the medial subdivisions of the mesonephric bud meet and fuse, the normal ascent of the kidneys is impeded by midline structures. The result is a pair of ectopic kidneys, usually fused at their lower poles, lying in front of the fourth lumbar vertebra and great vessels. Horseshoe kidney is found in 1:1000 necropsies and is commoner in men. Upper pole fusion is rare.

Clinical features

Horseshoe kidneys are liable to disease, possibly because the ureters angulate as they pass over the fused isthmus (Fig. 71.2).

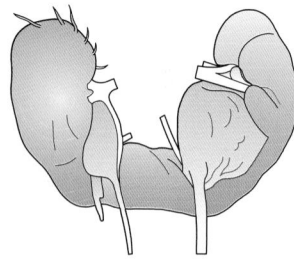

Figure 71.2 Horseshoe kidney. Note the ureters passing in front of the fused lower poles.

This may lead to urinary stasis with consequent infection and nephrolithiasis. Sometimes there is a true pelviureteric junction obstruction (see below), which has the same consequences. Horseshoe kidney is usually a radiological diagnosis. The most frequent appearance on the urogram shows the lower pole calyces on both sides being directed towards the midline. More rarely, all or most of the calyces are reversed (Fig. 71.3). Horseshoe kidney is not a contraindication to pregnancy but urinary complications are more frequent.

Division of the isthmus between the kidneys is usually only indicated in the course of surgery for abdominal aortic aneurysm. Although the tissue is often less vascular than normal renal parenchyma, the vascular supply of the horseshoe is typically eccentric, springing unpredictably from adjacent major vessels (Summary box 71.2).

Summary box 71.2

Horseshoe kidneys

- Horseshoe kidneys are liable to pelviureteric obstruction, infection and stone formation
- If not recognised, a pelvic kidney may cause diagnostic confusion during surgery

---

Unilateral fusion

Unilateral fusion (synonyms: crossed dystopia, cross fused renal ectopia) is rare but the urogram appearance is striking. Both kidneys are in one loin and are usually fused. The ureter of the lower kidney crosses the midline to enter the bladder on the contralateral side. Both renal pelves can lie one above each other medial to the renal parenchyma (unilateral long kidney) or the pelvis of the crossed kidney faces laterally (unilateral S-shaped kidney; Fig. 71.4).

Congenital cystic kidneys

Congenital cystic kidneys (synonym: polycystic kidneys) are hereditary and potentially lethal, and can be transmitted by either parent as an autosomal dominant trait. Thus, the risk of an offspring inheriting the condition can be as high as one in two depending upon the penetrance of the gene. The disease is not usually detectable on standard imaging until the second and third

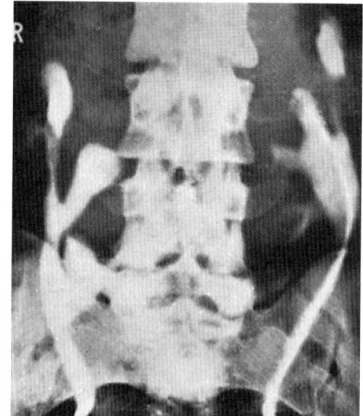

Figure 71.3 Urogram of a horseshoe kidney. Only rarely are all the calyces directed towards the spinal column.

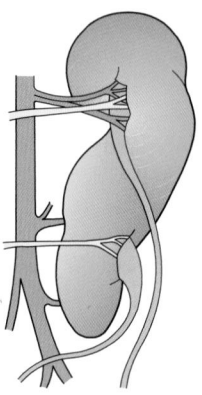

Figure 71.4 Unilateral S-fusion of the kidneys.

decades of life and does not usually manifest itself clinically before the age of 30 years.

Pathology

The kidneys are huge: the cysts distort the renal capsule. The renal parenchyma is riddled with cysts of varying size containing clear fluid, thick brown material or coagulated blood. There may be a congenital cystic disease of the liver. The aetiology of all renal cysts is uncertain although theories abound.

Clinical features in the adult

The condition is slightly more common in women than men. There are six clinical features:

- an irregular upper quadrant abdominal mass;
- loin pain;
- haematuria;
- infection;
- hypertension;
- uraemia.

Renal enlargement

The bilateral knobbly enlargement is unmistakable. Less florid examples may be revealed unexpectedly at laparotomy or on abdominal imaging. Unilateral renal swelling, in which one kidney contains larger cysts than the other, may be confused clinically with a cystic renal tumour.

Pain

Pain, felt as dull loin ache, is thought to be caused by the weight of the organ dragging upon its pedicle or by stretching of the renal capsule by the cysts. Haemorrhage into a cyst may cause more severe pain, as may the passage of a calculus from the diseased kidney.

Haematuria

Rupture of a cyst into the renal pelvis may cause recurrent haematuria. Profuse haematuria is uncommon.

Infection

Pyelonephritis is common in patients with congenital cystic kidney, presumably because of urinary stasis.

Hypertension

Hypertension is present in up to 75% of patients with polycystic kidneys over the age of 20 years.

Uraemia

Patients with congenital cystic kidneys pass large volumes of urine of low specific gravity containing a trace of albumin but no casts or cells. The non-specific symptoms of chronic renal failure develop as functioning renal tissue is replaced progressively by cysts. Severe anaemia is common. Signs of end-stage renal failure often begin suddenly during middle life and the patient is unlikely to survive without renal replacement therapy.

Imaging

Renal imaging shows multiple cysts in both kidneys and sometimes cysts in the liver and other organs. Blood and debris in the cysts may mimic the heterogeneity of a cystic adenocarcinoma. Simple cysts are usually solitary and have smooth thin walls and homogeneous contents (Fig. 71.5). Doubt about the diagnosis can be resolved by cytological examination of cyst fluid obtained by fine-needle aspiration.

Polycystic kidneys have a typical appearance on urography: the renal shadows are enlarged in all directions; the renal pelvis is compressed and elongated; and the calyces are stretched over the cysts ('big, bizarre and bilateral') (Fig. 71.6).

Treatment

As kidney failure develops, a low-protein diet will help to postpone the inevitability of renal replacement therapy. Infection, anaemia, hypertension and disturbances of calcium metabolism also need appropriate treatment by a nephrologist.

Surgery to uncap the cysts (Rovsing's operation) is rarely indicated because few now accept that this can preserve renal function by relieving pressure on the parenchyma (Summary box 71.3).

> **Summary box 71.3**
>
> **Polycystic kidney disease**
>
> - Inherited as an autosomal dominant trait
> - An important cause of end-stage renal failure in adults
> - Pain, haematuria, infection and hypertension are common
> - Liable to be fatal in early middle age

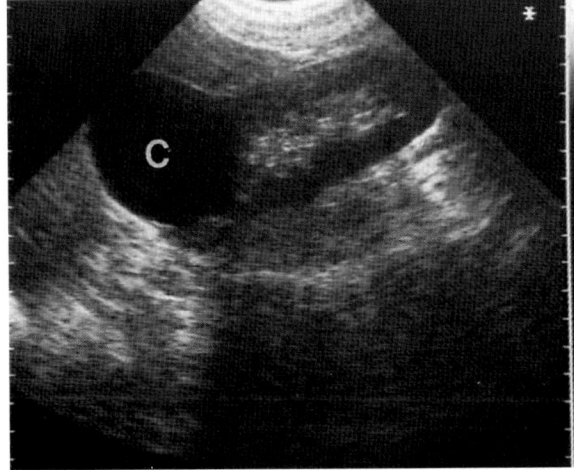

Figure 71.5 Simple cyst (C) of the lower pole shown on a longitudinal ultrasound scan of the kidney.

Nils Thorkild Rovsing, **1862–1927, Professor of Surgery, Copenhagen, Denmark.**

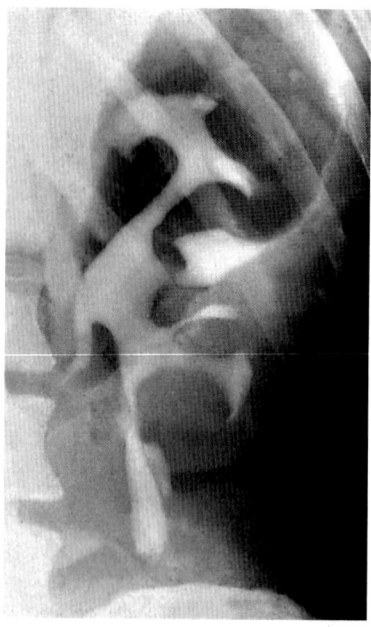

Figure 71.6 Polycystic kidney: urographic appearance. Note the length of the kidney and the bell-like calyces stretched over the cysts.

Infantile polycystic disease

Infantile polycystic disease is a rare autosomal recessive condition. The kidneys are large and may obstruct birth. Many patients are stillborn or die from renal failure early in life. In some children, associated congenital hepatic fibrosis is a major problem.

Unilateral multicystic disease

Multicystic dysplastic kidney is much more common. It presents as a mass in the flank. Excision is the treatment of choice. Wilms' tumour (see below), neuroblastoma and congenital hydronephrosis are all rarer causes of flank masses in childhood.

Simple cyst of the kidney (Fig. 71.5)

Simple cysts in one or both kidneys are often discovered incidentally on imaging of the upper abdomen: they rarely give symptoms and are often multiple. A palpable mass, pain from haemorrhage into the cyst and infection are uncommon presentations. Occasionally, a cyst in the hilum of the kidney (a parapelvic cyst) presses on the pelviureteric junction and causes obstruction.

The true nature of a cyst will be apparent by its characteristic appearance on ultrasound or computerised tomography (CT). Percutaneous cyst puncture for cytology is rarely necessary with modern imaging (Summary box 71.4).

Summary box 71.4

Simple renal cysts

- Common
- Often multiple
- Diagnosed on ultrasound
- Rarely require treatment
- Treat only if causing obstruction

Max Wilms, 1867–1918, Professor of Surgery, Heidelburg, Germany, described the embryoma of the kidney in 1899.

Differential diagnosis

In sheep-rearing districts, hydatid cysts of the kidney are common. On the right side they are liable to be mistaken for a hydatid cyst of the liver. Occasionally, the patient complains of passing 'grape skins' (ruptured daughter cysts) in the urine. Removal of the cyst must follow the principles used in excision of hydatid cyst of the liver, i.e. the scolices must be killed by injection of a scolicide (e.g. formalin solution) before the cyst is handled. If the cyst is large, nephrectomy may be the safest course.

Aberrant renal vessels

Two or more renal arteries are most common on the left. The main importance of the abnormality is as a source of potential error during operations in the retroperitoneum, especially those on the kidney. The renal arteries are functional end-arteries, so division of an aberrant lower pole artery leads to infarction of the section of parenchyma that it supplies. Renal veins, by contrast, have extensive collaterals and an aberrant vein can be divided with impunity. Aberrant vessels probably do not cause hydronephrosis, although a hydronephrotic renal pelvis may bulge between renal vessels, making them particularly noticeable (Fig. 71.7).

CONGENITAL ABNORMALITIES OF THE RENAL PELVIS AND URETER

Duplication of a renal pelvis

Duplication of a renal pelvis (Fig. 71.8) is found in about 4% of patients. It is usually unilateral and left sided. The small upper renal pelvis drains the upper group of calyces; the larger lower renal pelvis drains the middle and lower groups of calyces.

Duplication of a ureter

Duplication of a ureter is found in about 3% of urograms. The ureters often join in the lower third of their course (Fig. 71.9) and have a common ureteric orifice. When the ureters open independently into the bladder the ureter from the upper pelvis opens distal and medial to its fellow (Fig. 71.10).

Clinical features

Duplication of the renal pelvis or ureter is often a chance finding on renal imaging, but infection, calculus formation and pelviureteric

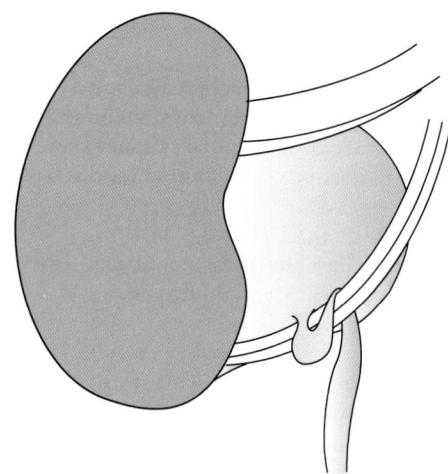

Figure 71.7 Aberrant accessory renal artery with hydronephrosis. The dilated renal pelvis bulges over the vessel.

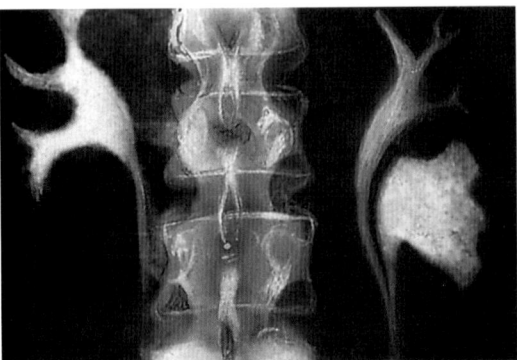

Figure 71.8 Urogram showing a left kidney with double pelvis.

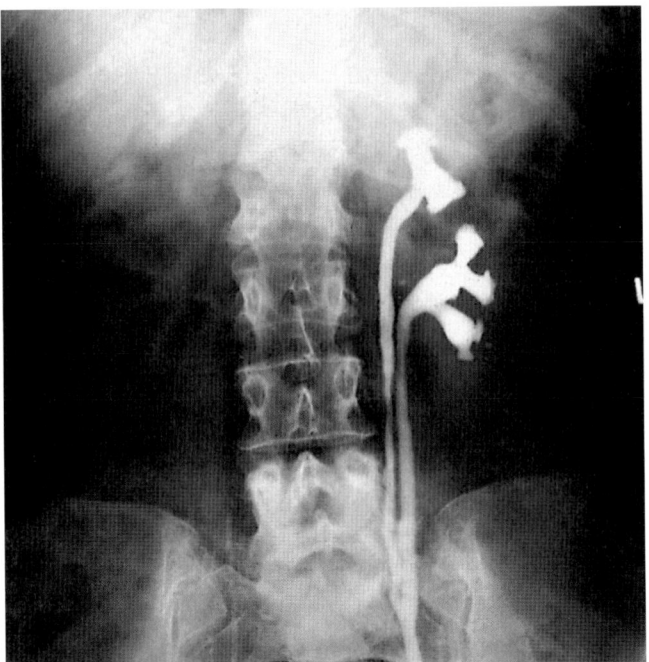

Figure 71.9 Retrograde ureterogram showing a double ureter on the left.

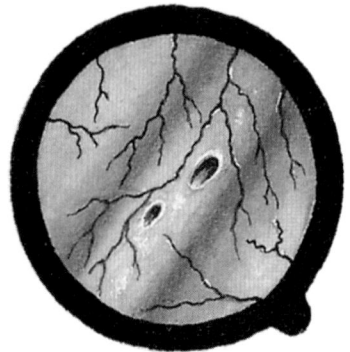

Figure 71.10 Complete ureteric duplication. Two ureteric orifices are seen on cystoscopy: the lower and more medial drains the upper renal pelvis.

a seminal vesicle or in an ejaculatory duct is likely to be functionally abnormal, and infection is common.

Treatment

Asymptomatic duplication of the kidney is harmless and does not require treatment. If one moiety is severely diseased or atrophic, partial nephrectomy is usually simple and effective. A refluxing ureter may need reimplanting. An ectopic ureter in the female frequently drains hydronephrotic and chronically infected renal tissue, which is best excised. Rarely, the incontinence can be cured and renal function preserved by implanting the ectopic ureter into the bladder or contralateral ureter (Summary box 71.5).

Summary box 71.5

Duplication of the kidneys and ureters

- Is relatively common and often asymptomatic and harmless
- One or both moieties of the duplex may be dysplastic
- Abnormalities of the insertion of the ureter into the bladder may cause urinary reflux, incontinence or obstruction

---

junction obstruction are more common than in normal kidneys. One of the moieties may be dysplastic and non-functioning. When the two ureters open separately, both may be abnormal in function, position or both. In children, this may result in a refluxing lower pole ureter and an upper pole ureter terminating in a ureterocele. In such cases, the duplex kidney is at risk of infection and/or obstruction.

An ectopic second ureteric opening is a rarity but it may cause puzzling symptoms. In the female, an ectopic ureter opens either into the urethra below the sphincter (Fig. 71.11) or into the vagina. The diagnosis can often be made from the history alone and is confirmed by urography. A girl or woman who voids normally but who has dribbled urine for as long as she can remember probably has an ectopic ureteric orifice. The orifice is difficult to see because it is guarded by a valve: it may help to give an intravenous injection of a dye such as indigocarmine to colour the urine leaking from it.

In the male patient, the aberrant opening is above the external urethral sphincter so the patient is continent. The ureteric orifice at the apex of the trigone, the posterior urethra, in

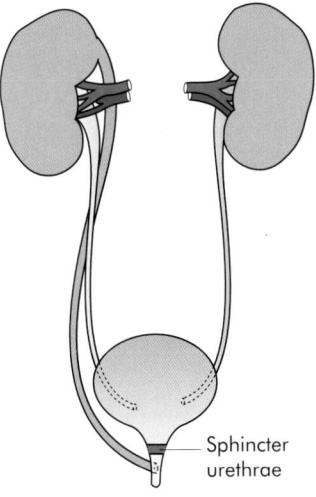

Figure 71.11 In women, one ureteric orifice may open below the sphincter, causing intractable incontinence of urine.

Congenital megaureter

Congenital megaureter is a rare oddity that may be bilateral and associated with other congenital anomalies. Functional obstruction at the lower end of the ureter may lead to progressive dilatation and infection. The ureteric orifice appears normal and a ureteric catheter passes easily. Reflux is not a feature of the untreated condition but is almost inevitable if the ureteric orifice is opened endoscopically. Spontaneous improvement can occur but infection or deteriorating function will require refashioning and reimplantion of the affected ureter.

Post-caval ureter

The right ureter passes behind the vena cava instead of lying to the right of it. If this causes obstructive symptoms, the ureter can be divided and rejoined in front of the cava using a long oblique anastomosis without tension. Unusually, the retrocaval portion of the ureter is fibrotic and must be excised.

Ureterocele

Ureterocele is a cystic enlargement of the intramural ureter, which is thought to result from congenital atresia of the ureteric orifice. Although present from childhood, the condition is often unrecognised until adult life. The 'adder head' on excretory urography (Fig. 71.12) is typical. Usually the cyst wall is composed of urothelium only and the diagnosis is confirmed by the cystoscopic appearance of a translucent cyst enlarging and collapsing as urine flows in from above (Fig. 71.13). Treatment should be

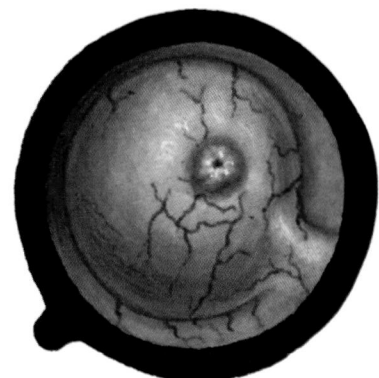

Figure 71.13 Ureterocele on cystoscopy.

avoided unless there are symptoms arising from infection and/or stone formation. Ureterocele is most common in women; occasionally, the cyst may cause obstruction to the bladder outflow by prolapsing into the internal urethral opening.

Endoscopic diathermy incision is usually all that is required for treatment of a symptomatic ureterocele, although a micturating cystogram is advisable to detect postoperative urinary reflux. In advanced unilateral cases with hydronephrosis or pyonephrosis, nephrectomy may be appropriate.

INJURIES TO THE KIDNEY

In civilian life, injuries to the kidney result most often from either blows or falls on the loin or crushing injury to the abdomen, typically in a road traffic accident. Haematuria after trivial injury to the kidney should suggest the possibility of a pre-existing disease, e.g. calculus, hydronephrosis or tuberculosis.

The degree of injury varies considerably from a small subcapsular haematoma to a complete tear through the kidney (Fig. 71.14). The kidney may be partially or wholly avulsed from its vascular pedicle; one pole may be completely detached.

Closed renal injury is usually extraperitoneal. In young children who have very little extraperitoneal fat, the peritoneum, which is closely applied to the kidney, can tear with the renal capsule, leaking blood and urine into the peritoneum (Summary box 71.6).

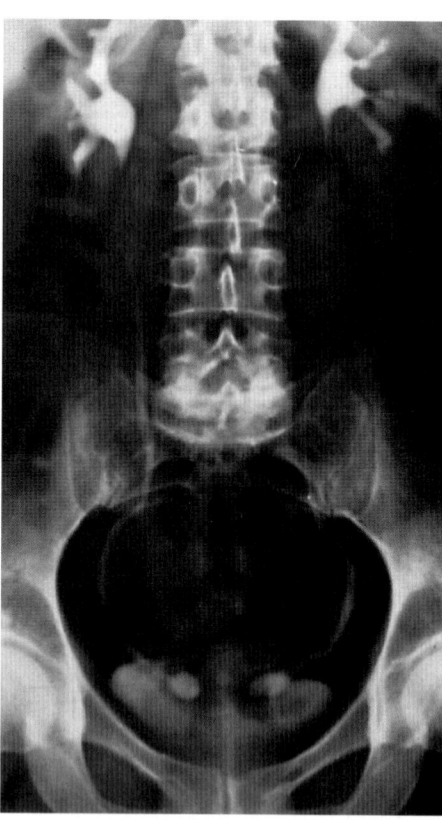

Figure 71.12 Adder-head appearance of a ureterocele.

> Adder head. **An adder is a venomous snake of the family Viperidae which is found in the UK and other parts of the world. It has a triangular shaped head.**

Summary box 71.6
Haemorrhage
■ Life-threatening haemorrhage is a serious risk in closed or open trauma to the kidney

Clinical features of closed renal trauma

Superficial soft-tissue bruising can be absent but there is local pain and tenderness.

Haematuria

Haematuria is the sign of a damaged kidney but it may not appear until some time after the injury. Profuse bleeding may cause clot colic.

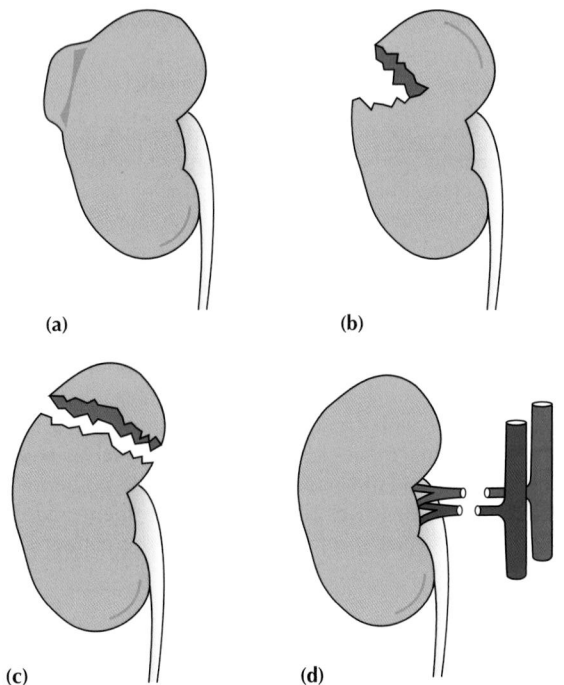

(a)　　　　　　　**(b)**

(c)　　　　　　　**(d)**

Figure 71.14 Types of closed renal trauma: (a) subscapular haematoma; (b) laceration; (c) avulsion of one pole; (d) avulsion of the renal pedicle.

Severe delayed haematuria

Sudden profuse haematuria between the third day and the third week after the accident in a patient who appears to be progressing well is caused by a clot becoming dislodged.

Meteorism

Abdominal distension 24–48 hours after renal injury is probably a result of retroperitoneal haematoma implicating splanchnic nerves (Summary box 71.7).

Summary box 71.7

Clinical features of closed renal trauma

- There may be no external bruising
- Haematuria indicates that the kidney has been damaged and should prompt careful monitoring of vital signs and urgent investigation
- Delayed haemorrhage may occur days after injury

Management and treatment

Conservative watchful treatment of closed renal trauma is usually successful. The possibility of injury to other organs must be considered at an early stage.

- Blood should be cross-matched for transfusion if there is evidence of hypovolaemic shock or continuing haemorrhage. Intravenous access should be established.
- The patient should stay in bed while there is macroscopic haematuria and activity must be curtailed for a week after the urine clears.
- Morphine analgesia may be appropriate.
- Hourly pulse and blood pressure charts must be kept.

- Antibiotics should be given to prevent infection of the haematoma.
- Each sample of urine passed should be checked for haematuria and the result charted.
- Intravenous urography (IVU) or contrast-enhanced CT should be performed urgently to assess the damage to the kidney and to show that the other kidney is normal.
- Blood should be sent for grouping and serum saved for cross-matching.

Surgical exploration

Surgical exploration is necessary in less that 10% of closed injuries; it is indicated if there are signs of progressive blood loss or there is an expanding mass in the loin. The aim is to stop bleeding while conserving as much renal tissue as possible; a renal arteriogram performed preoperatively can be helpful in framing a strategy for doing this. A radiologist may be able to stop the haemorrhage by embolisation if a bleeding vessel can be identified.

The possibility of damage to other abdominal organs is checked during a transperitoneal approach. Release of the tamponading effect of the perirenal haematoma can result in massive haemorrhage and the surgeon must be fully prepared for this. When the kidney is irretrievably ruptured or avulsed from its pedicle, nephrectomy is the only course. Small tears can be sutured over a haemostatic sponge or a piece of detached muscle. Large single rents in the kidney are best dealt with by passing a tube nephrostomy through the defect and suturing the renal tissue around it. If the laceration is confined to one pole of the kidney, partial nephrectomy may be practicable.

When a solitary kidney is sufficiently damaged to need exploration, it must be repaired. Failing this, the wound is packed firmly with gauze to stop the bleeding in the hope that some renal function may be retained when the ruptured kidney heals (Summary box 71.8).

Summary box 71.8

Surgical treatment in closed renal trauma

- Exploration of the kidney may be associated with massive blood loss as the haematoma is opened
- Nephrectomy is a possibility so it is important to establish that the contralateral kidney is functioning

---

Complications

Heavy haematuria may lead to clot retention requiring bladder washout through a catheter or a cystoscope.

Pararenal pseudohydronephrosis may occur over the course of a few weeks after injury as a result of a combination of complete cortical tear and ureteric obstruction caused by scarring.

Hypertension resulting from renal fibrosis may occur long after injury. It is often refractory to medical treatment and nephrectomy may be necessary.

Post-traumatic aneurysm of the renal artery (Fig. 71.15) is rare. There is pain in the loin and a non-tender swelling may be felt if the aneurysm is large. Congestion of the parenchyma leads to intermittent haematuria. Aortography is diagnostic. Excision or nephrectomy is urgently indicated to prevent fatal rupture of the aneurysm.

CHAPTER 71 | THE KIDNEYS AND URETERS

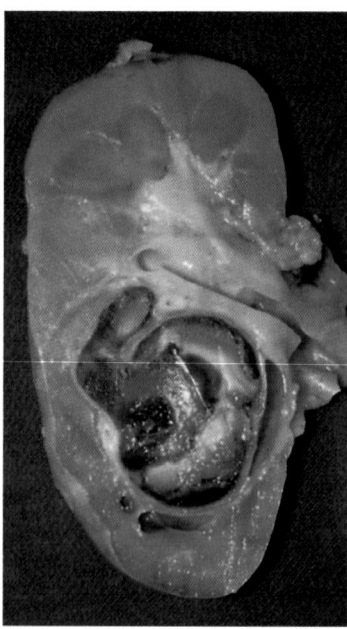

Figure 71.15 Aneurysm of the renal artery containing lamellated thrombus.

INJURIES TO THE URETER

Rupture of the ureter

This is an uncommon result of a hyperextension injury of the spine. The diagnosis is rarely made until there is swelling in the loin or iliac fossa associated with a reduction of urine output. An excretion urogram or contrast-enhanced CT shows extravasation of contrast from the injured ureter.

Injury to one or both ureters during pelvic surgery

This occurs most often during vaginal or abdominal hysterectomy when the ureter is divided, ligated, crushed or excised, usually inadvertently. Pre-emptive ureteric catheterisation prevents such accidents as the catheters make it easier to identify the ureters.

Injury recognised at the time of operation

Ureterovesical continuity should be restored by one of the methods described below unless the patient's condition is poor. Deliberate ligation of the proximal ureter and temporary percutaneous nephrostomy is then the best course until the patient is well enough for a repair (Summary box 71.9).

Summary box 71.9

Ureteric injury during operation

- The most common cause of injury to the ureters is surgical trauma during hysterectomy or other pelvic surgery
- Preoperative catheterisation of the ureters makes them easier to protect during surgery
- Injuries discovered at the time of surgery should be repaired immediately

---

Injury not recognised at the time of operation

Unilateral injuries

There are three possibilities:

- *No symptoms.* Secure ligation of a ureter may simply lead to silent atrophy of the kidney. The injury may be unsuspected until the patient undergoes urological imaging some time later.
- *Loin pain and fever*, possibly with pyonephrosis, occur with infection of the obstructed system. Urography shows no function, which will be permanent unless steps are taken quickly to relieve the obstruction by inserting a percutaneous nephrostomy.
- A *urinary fistula* develops through the abdominal or vaginal wound. The urogram or contrast-enhanced CT shows extravasation with or without obstruction of one or both ureters. Nephrostomies may be inserted and repair postponed until oedema and inflammation have subsided. The traditional delayed repair leaves the patient incontinent and demoralised. Early repair is safe provided that the patient is fit for surgery.

Bilateral injury

Ligation of both ureters leads to anuria. Ureteric catheters will not pass and urgent relief of obstruction by nephrostomy or immediate surgery is essential.

Repair of the injured ureter (Table 71.2)

If the cut ends of the ureter can be apposed without tension, they should be joined by a spatulated anastomosis over a double-pigtail catheter. If it is possible to insert a stent endoscopically past a partial ureteric obstruction, an open repair may be avoidable.

If the division is very low down, the bladder may be hitched up so that the ureter can be reimplanted into it. Extra length may be obtained by mobilising the kidney.

In the Boari operation (Fig. 71.16), a flap of bladder wall is fashioned into a tube to replace the lower ureter. The disadvantage of implanting the ureter end to side into the contralateral ureter (a transureteroureterostomy) is that it risks converting a unilateral injury into a bilateral one.

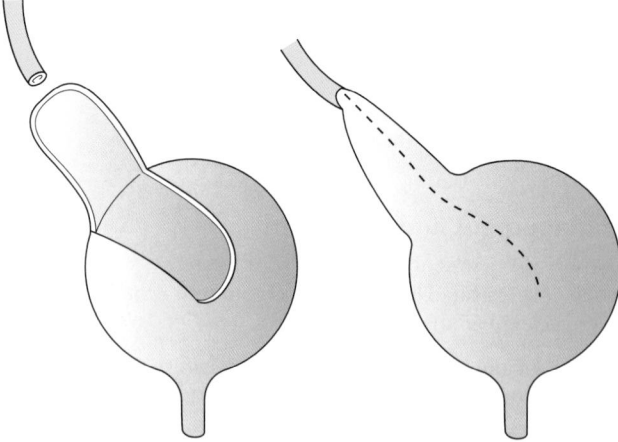

Figure 71.16 Boari operation: a strip of bladder wall is fashioned into a tube to bridge the gap between the cut ureter and the bladder.

Achille Boari, nineteenth century Italian Surgeon.

Table 71.2 Methods for repairing a damaged ureter

If there is no loss of length	Spatulation and end-to-end anastomosis without tension
If there is little loss of length	Mobilise kidney Psoas hitch of bladder Boari operation
If there is marked loss of length	Transureteroureterostomy Interposition of isolated bowel loop or mobilised appendix Nephrectomy

Nephrectomy may be the best course when the patient's outlook is poor and the other kidney is normal. When conservation of all renal tissue is vital, replacement of the damaged ureter by a segment of ileum is necessary (Summary box 71.10).

Summary box 71.10

Repair of the injured ureter

When surgical damage to a ureter is discovered postoperatively:

■ Repair need not be delayed if the patient is fit
■ A variety of techniques may be needed to ensure successful repair, and surgery should be performed by a urologist

HYDRONEPHROSIS

Hydronephrosis is an aseptic dilatation of the kidney caused by obstruction to the outflow of urine.

Unilateral hydronephrosis

See Summary box 71.11.

Summary box 71.11

Causes of unilateral ureteric obstruction

Extramural obstruction
■ Tumour from adjacent structures, e.g. carcinoma of the cervix, prostate, rectum, colon or caecum
■ Idiopathic retroperitoneal fibrosis
■ Retrocaval ureter

Intramural obstruction
■ Congenital stenosis, physiological narrowing of the pelviureteric junction leading to pelviureteric junction obstruction
■ Ureterocele and congenital small ureteric orifice
■ Inflammatory stricture following removal of ureteric calculus, repair of a damaged ureter or tuberculous infection
■ Neoplasm of the ureter or bladder cancer involving the ureteric orifice

Intraluminal obstruction
■ Calculus in the pelvis or ureter
■ Sloughed papilla in papillary necrosis (especially in diabetics, analgesic abusers and those with sickle cell disease) may obstruct the ureter

Bilateral hydronephrosis

Bilateral hydronephrosis is usually the result of urethral obstruction, but the lesions described above may occur on both sides.

When due to lower urinary obstruction, the cause may be:

- congenital:
  - posterior urethral valves;
  - urethral atresia;
- acquired:
  - benign prostatic enlargement or carcinoma of the prostate;
  - postoperative bladder neck scarring;
  - urethral stricture;
  - phimosis.

Urethral obstruction tends to lead to detrusor hypertrophy, which can lead to obstruction of the ureters in their intramural course.

Pathology

There is calyceal dilatation and the renal parenchyma is destroyed by pressure atrophy. A kidney destroyed by long-standing hydronephrosis is a thin-walled, lobulated, fluid-filled sac.

Clinical features

Unilateral hydronephrosis

Unilateral hydronephrosis (commonly caused by idiopathic pelviureteric junction obstruction or calculus) is more common in women and on the right.

Presenting features include the following:

- *Mild pain or dull aching* in the loin, often with a sensation of dragging heaviness made worse by excessive fluid intake. The kidney may be palpable.
- Attacks of *acute renal colic* may occur with no palpable swelling.
- *Intermittent hydronephrosis* (Dietl's crisis). A swelling in the loin is associated with acute renal pain. Some hours later the pain is relieved and the swelling disappears when a large volume of urine is passed.
- *Antenatal detection* in the fetus by ultrasound scan. Many of these cases are benign but postnatal investigation is required to detect those with significant pelviureteric junction obstruction (Summary box 71.12).

Summary box 71.12

Idiopathic pelviureteric obstruction

■ May be asymptomatic
■ May be present as intermittent loin pain exacerbated by a fluid load

Bilateral hydronephrosis

From lower urinary obstruction
Symptoms of bladder outflow obstruction predominate. The kidneys are unlikely to be palpable because renal failure intervenes before the kidneys become sufficiently large.

Joseph Dietl, 1804–1878, Professor of Pathology and Therapeutics, Krakau, Poland.

From bilateral upper urinary tract obstruction

This is rare compared with unilateral lesions although idiopathic retroperitoneal fibrosis affects both ureters and idiopathic pelviureteric junction obstruction can be bilateral. Although both systems are obstructed, symptoms may be referred to one side.

From pregnancy

Dilatation of the ureters and renal pelves occurs early in pregnancy and becomes more marked until the 20th week. It results from the effects on the ureteric smooth muscle of high levels of circulating progesterone and it may be considered as part of normal pregnancy. The ureters return to their normal size within 12 weeks of delivery. This physiological condition is associated with an increased liability to infection and there is a possibility that abdominal pain during pregnancy may be erroneously ascribed to ureteric obstruction (Summary box 71.13).

Summary box 71.13

Ureteric dilatation in pregnancy

- Physiological dilatation of the ureter is common in pregnancy

---

Imaging

Ultrasound scanning (Fig. 71.17) is the least invasive means of detecting hydronephrosis and is regularly used to diagnose pelviureteric junction obstruction *in utero*.

Excretion urography is only helpful if there is significant function in the obstructed kidney. The extrarenal pelvis is dilated and the minor calyces lose their normal cupping and become 'clubbed'. If the level of obstruction is in doubt, it can help to take follow-up films up to 36 hours after the contrast has been injected. The radio-opaque medium slowly diffuses to fill the obstructed system down to the blockage.

Isotope renography is the best test to establish that dilatation

of the renal collecting system is caused by obstruction. A substance [usually diethylenetriaminepenta-acetic acid (DTPA) or MAG-3] that is filtered by the glomeruli and not absorbed is injected intravenously. The DTPA is labelled with technetium-99m, a gamma-ray emitter, so that the passage of ^{99m}Tc-labelled DTPA through the kidneys can be tracked using a gamma camera. ^{99m}Tc-DTPA is quickly cleared from a normal kidney but is trapped in the renal pelvis on the obstructed side and will not be washed out even if the flow of urine is increased by administering furosemide (frusemide) (Fig. 71.18).

Very occasionally, a Whitaker test is indicated. A percutaneous puncture of the kidney is made through the loin and fluid is infused at a constant rate with monitoring of intrapelvic pressure. An abnormal rise in pressure confirms obstruction. Retrograde pyelography (Fig. 71.19) is rarely indicated but will confirm the site of obstruction immediately before corrective surgery (Summary box 71.14).

Summary box 71.14

Imaging

- Obstruction of the ureter is diagnosed by a combination of ultrasound scanning and isotope renography
- An obstructed kidney is worth preserving if the isotope renogram shows that it is contributing more than 20% of total renal function

---

Treatment

The indications for operation are bouts of renal pain, increasing hydronephrosis, evidence of parenchymal damage and infection. Conservation of renal tissue is the aim; nephrectomy should be considered only when the renal parenchyma has been largely destroyed. Mild cases should be followed by serial ultrasound scans and operated upon if dilatation is increasing.

Pyeloplasty

The Anderson–Hynes operation (Fig. 71.20) is appropriate when a reasonable thickness of functioning parenchyma

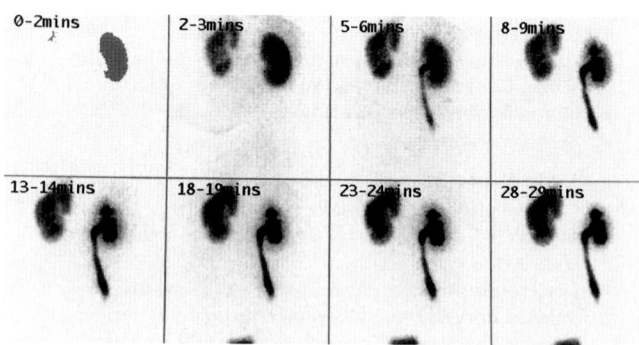

Figure 71.18 Isotope renogram series shows a late accumulation and persistence of radioactivity in the left kidney (the image is a posterior view).

Robert Whitaker, Urologist, Addenbrooke's Hospital, Cambridge, England.
James Christie Anderson, 1899–1984, Urologist, the Royal Hallamshire Hospital, Sheffield, England.
Wilfred Hynes, 1903–1991, Plastic Surgeon, the Plastic and Jaw Department, the Royal Sheffield Hospital, Sheffield, England.

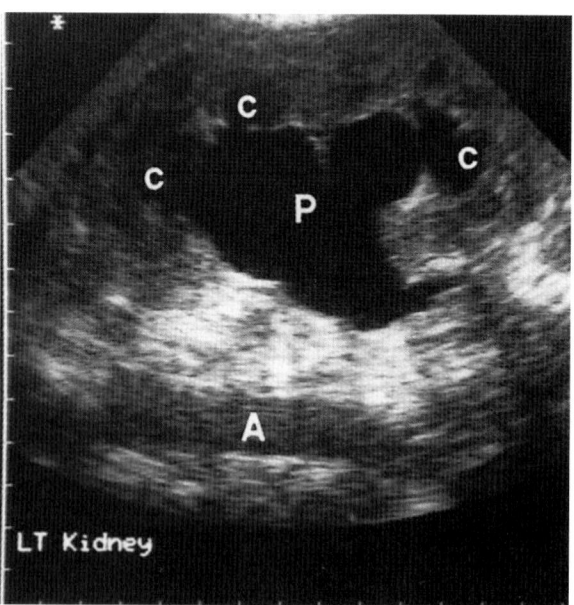

Figure 71.17 Ultrasound of a hydronephrotic kidney. A, artery; C, calyces; P, pelvis.

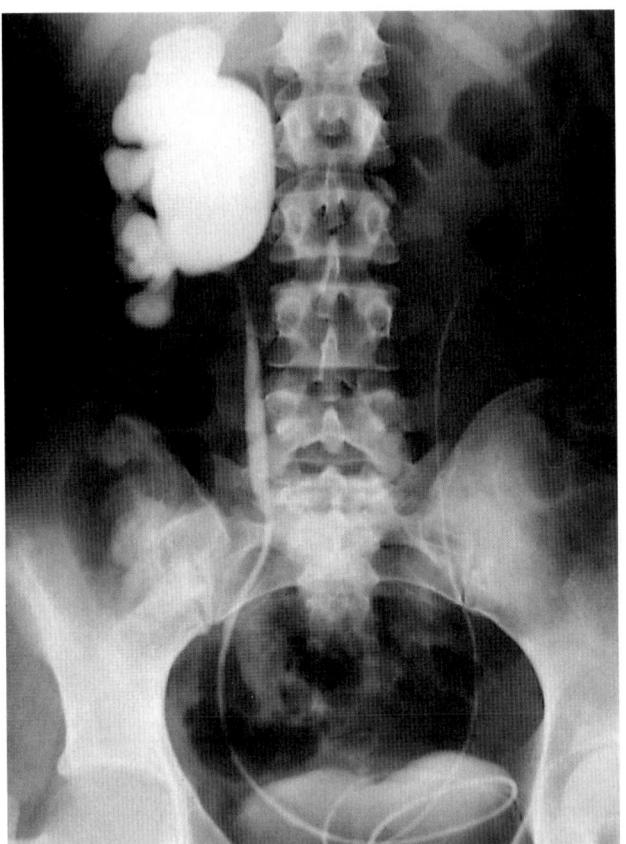

Figure 71.19 Retrograde ureteropyelogram showing hydronephrosis with greatly enlarged pelvis and dilated 'clubbed' calyces.

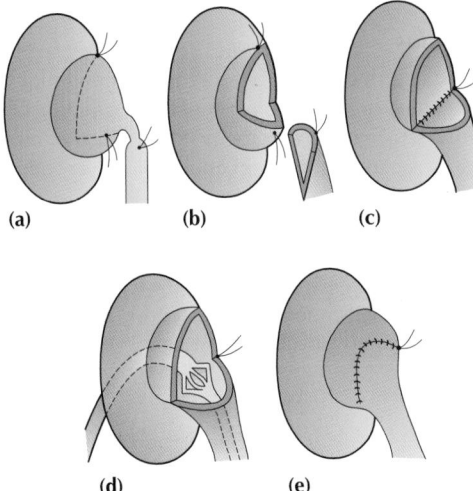

(a)   (b)   (c)

(d)   (e)

Figure 71.20 (a–e) Anderson–Hynes disjunction pyeloplasty.

remains. The upper third of the ureter and the renal pelvis are carefully mobilised. A renal vein overlying the distended pelvis can be divided, but an artery in this situation should be preserved to avoid infarction of the territory that it supplies. The anastomosis is made in front of such an artery using absorbable stitches to avoid calculus formation on the suture line. It is usual to protect the anastomosis with a nephrostomy tube or a ureteric stent.

Endoscopic pyelolysis

Disruption of the pelviureteric junction by a balloon passed up the ureter and distended under radiographic control has been used to treat idiopathic pelviureteric junction obstruction. The long-term efficacy of this and various forms of endoscopic pyelotomy has still to be proved.

RENAL CALCULI

Aetiology

This subject is complex and the following represents a brief summary of current opinion.

Dietetic

Deficiency of vitamin A causes desquamation of epithelium. The cells form a nidus on which a stone is deposited. It is uncertain whether this mechanism is of importance other than in the formation of bladder calculi.

Altered urinary solutes and colloids

Dehydration increases the concentration of urinary solutes until they are liable to precipitate. Reduction of urinary colloids, which adsorb solutes, or mucoproteins, which chelate calcium, might also result in a tendency for crystal and stone formation.

Decreased urinary citrate

The presence of citrate in urine, 300–900 mg 24 h^{-1} (1.6–4.7 mmol 24 h^{-1}) as citric acid, tends to keep otherwise relatively insoluble calcium phosphate and citrate in solution. The urinary excretion of citrate is under hormonal control and decreases during menstruation.

Renal infection

Infection favours the formation of urinary calculi. Clinical and experimental stone formation are common when urine is infected with urea-splitting streptococci, staphylococci and especially *Proteus* spp. The predominant bacteria found in the nuclei of urinary stones are staphylococci and *Escherichia coli*.

Inadequate urinary drainage and urinary stasis

Stones are liable to form when urine does not pass freely.

Prolonged immobilisation

Immobilisation from any cause, e.g. paraplegia, is liable to result in skeletal decalcification and an increase in urinary calcium favouring the formation of calcium phosphate calculi.

Hyperparathyroidism

Hyperparathyroidism leading to hypercalcaemia and hypercalciuria is found in 5% or less of those who present with radio-opaque calculi. In cases of recurrent or multiple stones, this cause should be eliminated by appropriate investigations (see Chapter 48). Hyperparathyroidism results in a great increase in the elimination of calcium in the urine. These patients 'pass their skeletons in their urine'. A parathyroid adenoma should be removed before definitive treatment for the urinary calculi.

Theodor Escherich, **1857–1911**, Professor of Paediatrics, Vienna, Austria, discovered the bacterium coli commune in 1886.

Types of renal calculus

Oxalate calculus (calcium oxalate) (Fig. 71.21)

Oxalate stones are irregular in shape and covered with sharp projections, which tend to cause bleeding. The surface of the calculus is discoloured by altered blood. A calcium oxalate monohydrate stone is hard and radiodense.

Phosphate calculus

A phosphate calculus [calcium phosphate often with ammonium magnesium phosphate (struvite)] is smooth and dirty white. It tends to grow in alkaline urine, especially when urea-splitting *Proteus* organisms are present. As a result, the calculus may enlarge to fill most of the collecting system, forming a staghorn calculus (Fig. 71.22). Even a very large staghorn calculus may be clinically silent for years until it signals its presence by haematuria, urinary infection or renal failure. Because they are large, phosphate calculi are usually easy to see on radiographic films.

Uric acid and urate calculi

These are hard, smooth and often multiple. They vary from yellow to reddish brown and sometimes have an attractive, multifaceted appearance. Pure uric acid stones are radiolucent and appear on an excretion urogram as a filling defect, which can be mistaken for a transitional tumour of the upper urinary tract. The presence of uric acid stones is confirmed by CT. Most uric acid stones contain some calcium, so they cast a faint radiological shadow. In children, mixed stones of ammonium and sodium urate are sometimes found. They are yellow, soft and friable. They are radiolucent unless they are contaminated with calcium salts.

Cystine calculus

These uncommon stones appear in the urinary tract of patients with a congenital error of metabolism that leads to cystinuria. Hexagonal, translucent, white crystals of cystine appear only in acid urine. They are often multiple and may grow to form a cast of the collecting system. Pink or yellow when first removed, they change to a greenish colour when exposed to air. Cystine stones are radio-opaque because they contain sulphur, and they are very hard.

Xanthine calculus

These are extremely rare. They are smooth and round, brick-red in colour, and show lamellation on cross-section.

Clinical features

Renal calculi are common. Approximately 50% of patients present between the ages of 30 and 50 years. The male–female ratio is 4:3.

Symptoms are variable and the diagnosis sometimes remains obscure until the stone is discovered on a radiograph (Summary box 71.15).

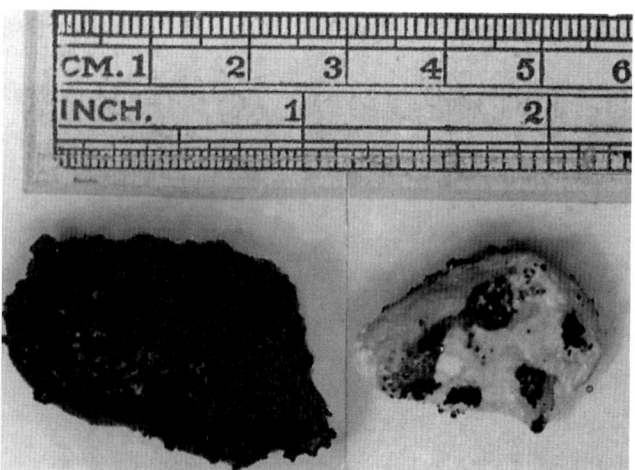

Figure 71.21 Oxalate calculi. The larger one removed from the right kidney is blackened by the deposition of altered blood.

Summary box 71.15

Renal stones

- Are common
- May be clinically silent even when large
- Are usually visible on a plain abdominal radiograph
- May be radiolucent when composed of uric acid

Silent calculus

Even large staghorn calculi may cause no symptoms for long periods, during which time there is progressive destruction of the renal parenchyma. Uraemia may be the first indication of bilateral calculi, although secondary infection usually produces symptoms first.

Pain

Pain is the leading symptom in 75% of people with urinary stones. Fixed renal pain is located posteriorly in the renal angle (Fig. 71.23), anteriorly in the hypochondrium, or in both. It may be worse on movement, particularly on climbing stairs.

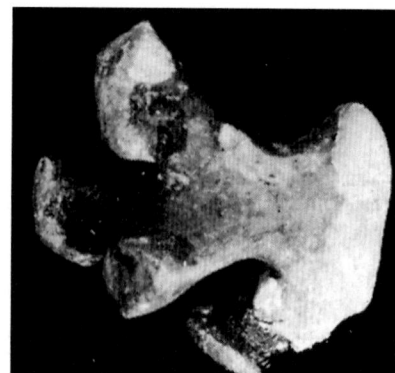

Figure 71.22 Staghorn calculus.

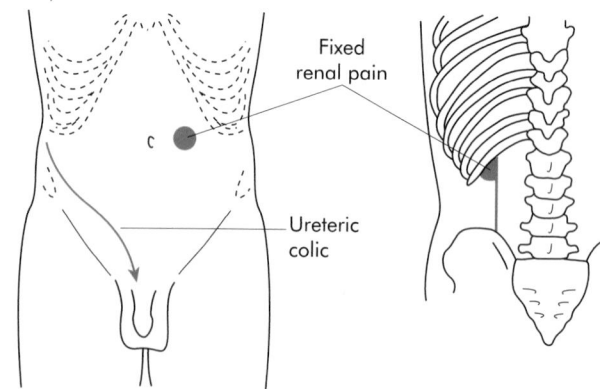

Figure 71.23 The usual distribution of renal pain.

Ureteric colic is an agonising pain passing from the loin to the groin. Typically, it starts suddenly causing the patient to writhe to find comfort. Pain resulting from renal stones rarely lasts more than 8 hours in the absence of infection. There is no pyrexia, although the pulse rate rises because of the severe pain. Ureteric colic is often caused by a stone entering the ureter but it may also occur when a stone becomes lodged in the pelviureteric junction. The severity of the colic is not related to the size of the stone (Summary box 71.16).

Summary box 71.16

Ureteric colic

- There is a pattern of severe exacerbation on a background of continuing pain
- Radiates to the groin, penis, scrotum or labium as the stone progresses down the ureter
- The severity of pain is not related to the size of the stone
- The pain is almost invariably associated with haematuria
- There may be few physical signs

Abdominal examination

During an attack of ureteric colic there is rigidity of the lateral abdominal muscles but not, as a rule, of the rectus abdominis. Percussion over the kidney produces a stab of pain and there may be tenderness on gentle deep palpation. Hydronephrosis or pyonephrosis leading to a palpable swelling in the loin is rare.

Haematuria

Haematuria is sometimes a leading symptom of stone disease and occasionally the only one. As a rule, the amount of bleeding is small.

Pyuria

Infection is likely in the presence of stones and is particularly dangerous when the kidney is obstructed. As pressure builds in the dilated collecting system, organisms are injected into the circulation and a life-threatening septicaemia can quickly develop.

The mechanical effect of stones irritating the urothelium may cause pyuria even in the absence of infection.

Investigation of suspected urinary stone disease

Radiography

The 'KUB' film shows the kidney, ureters and bladder. When a renal calculus is branched, there is no doubt about the diagnosis (Fig. 71.24). An opacity that maintains its position

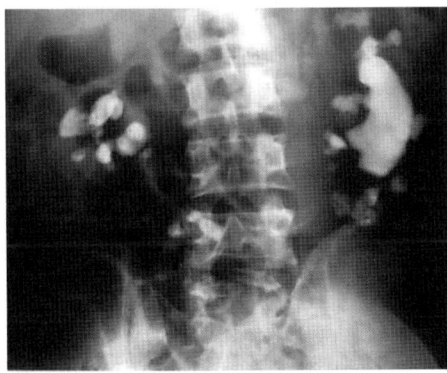

Figure 71.24 Plain abdominal radiograph showing complete staghorn calculi.

relative to the urinary tract during respiration is likely to be a calculus.

Calcified mesenteric nodes and opacities within the alimentary tract can sometimes be shown to be anterior to the vertebral bodies on a lateral radiograph and hence outside the urinary tract (Summary box 71.17).

Summary box 71.17

Opacities on a plain abdominal radiograph that may be confused with renal calculus

- Calcified mesenteric lymph node
- Gallstones or concretion in the appendix
- Tablets or foreign bodies in the alimentary canal [e.g. cyclopenthiazide (Navidrex-K)]
- Phleboliths – calcification in the walls of veins, especially in the pelvis
- Ossified tip of the 12th rib
- Calcified tuberculous lesion in the kidney
- Calcified adrenal gland

Contrast-enhanced computerised tomography

CT, preferably spiral, has become the mainstay of investigation for acute ureteric colic.

Excretion urography

Urography will establish the presence and anatomical site of a calculus. It also gives some important information about the function of the other kidney.

Ultrasound scanning

Ultrasound scanning is of most value in locating stones for treatment by extracorporeal shock wave lithotripsy (ESWL) (see below).

Surgical treatment of urinary calculi

Conservative management

Calculi smaller than 0.5 cm pass spontaneously unless they are impacted. Any surgical intervention carries the risk of complications and needless intervention should be avoided. Small renal calculi may cause symptoms by obstructing a calyx or acting as a focus for secondary infection. However, most can be safely observed until they pass (Summary box 71.18).

Summary box 71.18

Management of small stones

- Most small urinary calculi will pass spontaneously and can be treated conservatively
- The presence of infection in an upper urinary tract obstructed by stone is dangerous and is an indication for urgent surgical intervention

---

Preoperative treatment

If urinary infection is present, appropriate antibiotic treatment is started and continued during and after surgery as necessary.

Operation for stone

In developed countries, most stones are treated by urologists using minimal access and minimally invasive techniques. Open operations are still needed when appropriate expertise is not available or newer techniques have failed to clear the calculus (Summary box 71.19).

Modern methods of stone removal

Kidney stones

Percutaneous nephrolithotomy (Fig. 71.25) This involves the placement of a hollow needle into the renal collecting system through the soft tissue of the loin and the renal parenchyma. A wire inserted through the needle is used to guide the passage of a series of dilators, which expand the track into the kidney until it is large enough to take the nephroscope used to visualise the stone. Small stones may be grasped under vision and extracted whole. Larger stones must be fragmented by an ultrasound, laser or electrohydraulic probe and removed in pieces.

The aim is to remove all fragments if possible, and this may take some time if the calculus is large. When the operation is over, a nephrostomy drain is left in the system. This decompresses the kidney and allows repeated access if stone particles remain. Percutaneous nephrolithotomy is sometimes combined with ESWL in the treatment of complex (stag-horn) calculi. The surgeon removes the central part of the stone percutaneously and the more peripheral fragments are treated by ESWL.

Complications of percutaneous nephrolithotomy include (1) haemorrhage from the punctured renal parenchyma – this may be profuse and difficult to control; (2) perforation of the collecting system with extravasation of saline irrigant; (3) perforation of the colon or pleural cavity during placement of the percutaneous track.

Extracorporeal shock wave lithotripsy A urinary calculus has a crystalline structure. Bombarded with shock waves of sufficient energy it disintegrates into fragments. The principle is seen at its simplest in the original Dornier machine, in which shock waves were generated by an electrical discharge placed at one focus of an ellipsoid mirror. The patient was positioned under radiographic control so that the calculus was subjected to the full force of the shock waves concentrated at the second focus of the mirror. As shock waves are poorly transmitted through air, both the patient and the shock-wave generators were immersed in a bath of water.

Modern ESWL machines do not have a water bath; the fluid is confined to the path that the shock waves must follow to reach the kidney. The shocks may be generated by the discharge of an array of piezoelectric cells, and they may be aimed by ultrasound

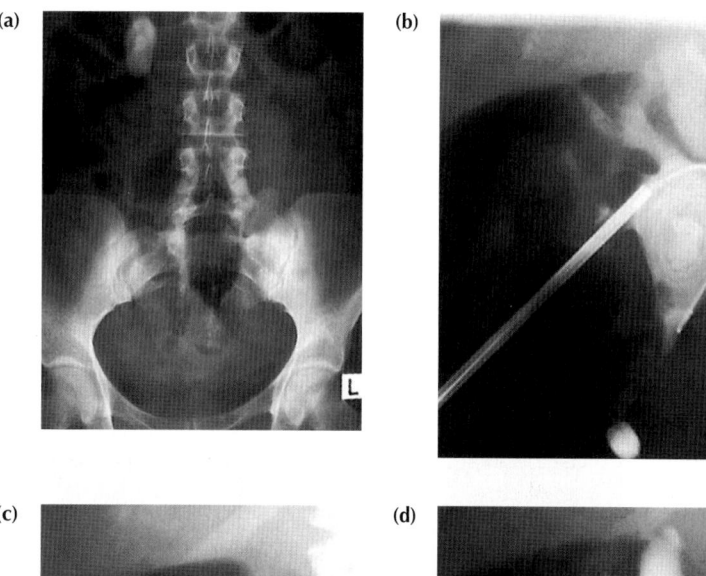

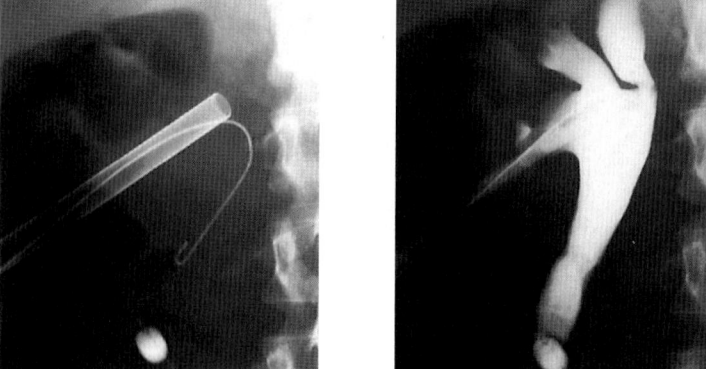

Figure 71.25 Percutaneous renal stone removal. (a) The stone is in the right renal pelvis. (b) Placement of a cannula under radiological control into the renal pelvis and through it a balloon catheter to stop fragments migrating into the upper ureter. (c) The stone is disrupted by contact lithotripsy and the fragments have been successfully removed by irrigation. (d) A nephrostogram confirms that the renal pelvis is intact.

rather than radiographic imaging (Fig. 71.26). The devices also differ in the strength of the disruptive force that they can develop. Less powerful machines are less effective in breaking stones, and several treatments may be necessary to clear a stone. Weaker shocks hurt less and treatment can be given without general anaesthesia.

When ESWL is successful, the stone fragments must pass down the ureter. Ureteric colic is common after ESWL, and the patient needs analgesia, usually in the form of a non-steroidal anti-inflammatory drug such as diclofenac. The bulky fragments of a large stone may impact in the ureter, causing obstruction. To avoid this, a stent should be placed in the ureter so that the kidney can drain while the pieces of stone pass. Occasionally, impacted fragments have to be removed ureteroscopically (see below).

The principal complication of ESWL is infection. Many calculi contain bacteria, which are released from the broken stone. It is wise to give prophylactic antibiotics before ESWL, and an obstructed system should be decompressed by the insertion of a ureteric stent or percutaneous nephrostomy before treatment.

The clearance of stone from the kidney will depend upon the consistency of the stone and its site. Most oxalate and phosphate stones fragment well and, if lying in the renal pelvis, will clear within days. The results with harder stones, especially cystine stones, are less satisfactory. When treating calyceal stones, the patients should be warned that the clearance of fragments may take months.

There is currently great interest in the long-term outcome of patients treated by ESWL. Certainly, some stones recur, especially if small fragments remain after treatment.

Open surgery for renal calculi (Fig. 71.27)

Operations for kidney stone are usually performed via a loin or lumbar approach. All of the procedures are difficult unless the kidney is fully mobilised and its vascular pedicle controlled. A sling should be placed around the upper ureter to stop stones migrating downwards.

Pyelolithotomy Pyelolithotomy is indicated for stones in the renal pelvis. When the wall of the renal pelvis has been dissected free from its surrounding fat, an incision is made in its long axis directly on to the stone. The stone is removed with gallstone forceps, taking care not to break it because fragments may be difficult to retrieve. Stone fragments in peripheral calyces may be detected by direct palpation or by intraoperative radiography or nephroscopy. If there is no infection, the pelvic incision is closed with interrupted absorbable sutures. If there is gross sepsis, a nephrostomy is essential to drain the system.

Extended pyelolithotomy The plane between the renal sinus and the wall of the collecting system is developed on the posterior surface of the kidney. This avoids major vessels and allows incisions to be made into the calyces so that even large staghorn stones can be removed intact.

Nephrolithotomy If there is a complex calculus branching into the most peripheral calyces, it may be necessary to make incisions into the renal parenchyma to clear the kidney. Nephrolithotomy may also be necessary when the adhesions resulting from previous surgery make access to the renal pelvis difficult. The renal pedicle must be temporarily cross-clamped to reduce bleeding from the highly vascular renal tissue. Incisions are made just posterior and parallel to the most prominent part of the convex renal border, where the territories of the anterior and posterior branches of the renal artery meet (Brödel's line). Cooling the kidney with ice packs or cooling coils extends the time that the kidney can remain ischaemic without permanent damage. All the incisions must be carefully closed with haemostatic sutures

CHAPTER 71 | THE KIDNEYS AND URETERS

(a)

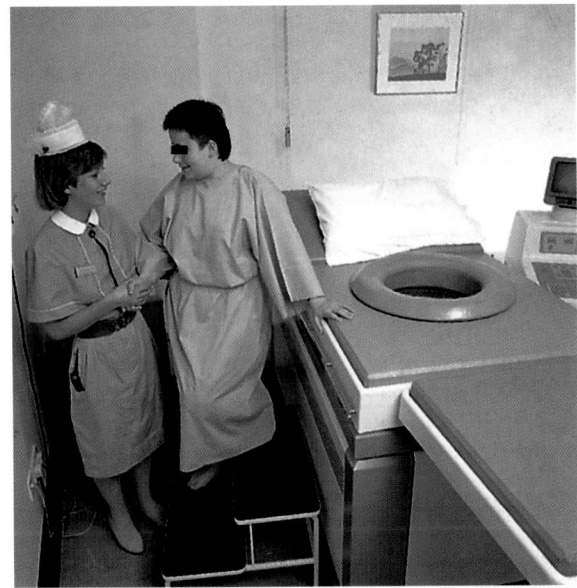

(b)

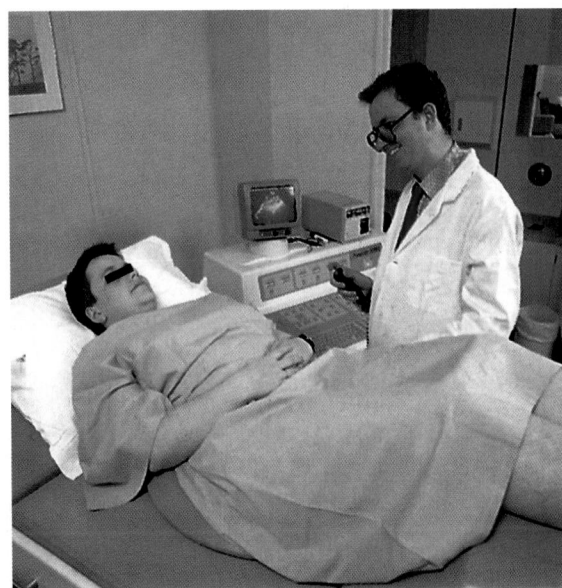

Figure 71.26 Extracorporeal shock wave lithotripsy. (a) The patient being placed on the ultrasound lithotripter. (b) Positioning of the patient being checked by ultrasound.

Max Brödel, 1870–1941, Medical artist who founded 'The Department of Art as Applied to Medicine' at the Johns Hopkins Hospital, Baltimore, MD, USA.

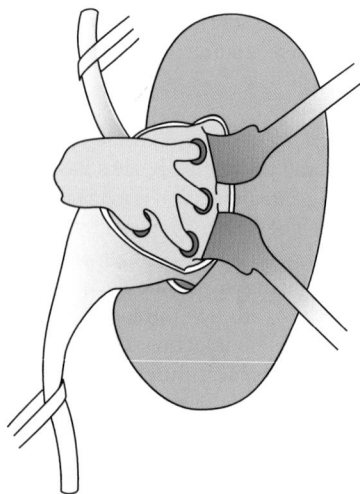

Figure 71.27 Open operations for renal calculus.

and the patient observed after the operation for signs of reactionary haemorrhage.

Partial nephrectomy is sometimes preferable when the stone is present in the lowermost calyx and there is associated infective damage to the adjacent parenchyma.

A kidney destroyed by obstruction and infection associated with stone disease should be removed, particularly when there is xanthogranulomatous pyelonephritis. This stone-related inflammatory mass must be removed with particular care because it is liable to be attached to adjacent structures such as the colon.

Treatment of bilateral renal stones Usually the kidney with better function is treated first unless the other kidney is more painful or there is pyonephrosis, which needs urgent decompression.

Silent bilateral staghorn calculi in the elderly and infirm may be treated conservatively. The patient should be encouraged to maintain a high fluid intake.

Prevention of recurrence

Ideally, all stone formers should be investigated to exclude metabolic factors, although the diagnostic yield is low in patients with a single small stone. The urine of all patients with stones should be screened for infection. The following investigations are appropriate in bilateral and recurrent stone formers:

- serum calcium, measured fasting on three occasions to exclude hyperparathyroidism;
- serum uric acid;
- urinary urate, calcium and phosphate in a 24-hour collection; the urine should also be screened for cystine;
- analysis of any stone passed.

Dietary advice is not usually helpful in avoiding stone recurrence in people who have a balanced diet. The enthusiast for excessive amounts of milk products (calcium stones), rhubarb, strawberries, plums, spinach and asparagus (calcium oxalate stones) should be advised to be more moderate.

Patients with hyperuricaemia should avoid red meats, offal and fish, which are rich in purines, and should be treated with allopurinol. Eggs, meat and fish are high in sulphur-containing proteins and should be restricted in cystinuria.

Stone sufferers should take the advice of Hippocrates and drink plenty to keep their urine dilute. Fluid intake should be increased appropriately to take account of increased losses.

Drug treatment is largely ineffective except in those few patients who are shown to have idiopathic hypercalciuria. Bendroflumethiazide (5 mg) and a calcium-restricted diet reduce urinary calcium (Summary box 71.20).

Summary box 71.20

Recurrent stone formation

- Calculus formation is more common in those who have had a previous urinary stone
- Unless calculi are caused by a specific biochemical abnormality, high fluid intake is the best way to discourage recurrent stone formation

---

URETERIC CALCULUS

A stone in the ureter usually comes from the kidney. Most are single small stones that are passed spontaneously.

Clinical features

The presence of a stone passing down the ureter often causes intermittent attacks of ureteric colic.

Ureteric colic

As the stone progresses to the lower ureter, the waves of agonising loin pain are typically referred more to the groin, external genitalia and the anterior surface of the thigh. The testis may be retracted by cremasteric spasm. When the stone is in the intramural ureter, the pain can be referred to the tip of the penis. Strangury, the painful passage of a few drops of urine, typically occurs with the stone in the intramural part of the ureter.

Impaction

Most stones pass spontaneously from the ureter but there are five sites of narrowing where the stone may be arrested (Fig. 71.28). When the stone becomes impacted, the attacks of colic give way to a more consistent dull pain, often felt in the iliac fossa. The pain may be increased by exercise and lessened by rest. Distension of the renal pelvis because of obstruction may cause pain and discomfort in the loin. The stone may become embedded as the adjacent ureteric wall becomes eroded and oedematous as a result of pressure ischaemia. Perforation of the ureter and extravasation of urine is a rare complication.

Severe renal pain subsiding after a day or so suggests complete ureteric obstruction. If obstruction persists after 1–2 weeks, the calculus should be removed because prolonged distension of the kidney will eventually lead to atrophy of the renal parenchyma.

Haematuria

Almost every attack of ureteric colic is associated with microscopic haematuria, which lasts for a day or so. More profuse

---

Hippocrates, c460–375 BC. A Greek Physician and Surgeon, who is regarded as 'The Father of Medicine'. He was born on the Greek island of Cos off the Turkish coast about 460 BC, and probably died in 375 BC.

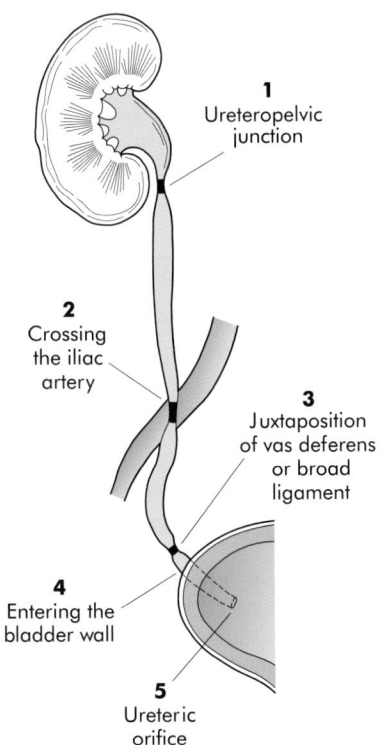

Figure 71.28 Normal anatomical narrowings (1–5) of the ureter.

1 Ureteropelvic junction
2 Crossing the iliac artery
3 Juxtaposition of vas deferens or broad ligament
4 Entering the bladder wall
5 Ureteric orifice

bleeding is uncommon and should raise the suspicion that the colic is due to passage of a clot.

Abdominal examination

There is tenderness and some rigidity over some part of the course of the ureter. The principal difficulty on the right side is to distinguish symptoms and signs of ureteric colic from those of acute appendicitis or acute cholecystitis. The presence of haematuria does not rule out appendicitis, because an inflamed appendix can give rise to a local ureteritis leaking some red cells into the urine. The patient with acute ureteric colic is usually in greater pain and less systemically ill.

Imaging

Most urinary calculi are visible on a plain abdominal radiograph. The stone may not be seen along the line of the ureter if it is small or if it is obscured by bowel contents or the shadows cast by nearby bones. Intravenous urography performed while the patient has pain can confirm the diagnosis, although spiral CT is increasingly used for this purpose. In ureteric colic there will probably be little or no excretion on the affected side. Occasionally, there is an extravasation of contrast from the dilated system. Late radiographs, taken up to 36 hours after the injection of contrast, may show dilatation of the ureter down to an obstructing calculus. A radiolucent uric acid stone may be demonstrated as a filling defect in the contrast-filled system.

Analgesic abusers occasionally fake symptoms to obtain drugs, and emergency imaging is useful in excluding renal colic. If the CT or urogram is normal during an attack, the patient does not have renal colic. The absence of blood in the urine makes colic less likely but its presence can be simulated by those desperate for drugs.

Cystoscopy is not indicated routinely but may reveal oedema and petechiae of the urothelium around the ureteric orifice when the stone is nearby. The stone may be visible in the orifice as it passes into the bladder.

Retrograde ureterography is performed as an immediate preliminary to an endoscopic operation to remove a calculus.

Treatment

Pain

Non-steroidal anti-inflammatory drugs such as diclofenac and indomethacin have replaced opiates as the first line of treatment for renal colic. The value of smooth muscle relaxants such as propantheline (Pro-Banthine) is debatable.

Removal of the stone (Summary box 71.21)

Expectant treatment is appropriate for small stones that are likely to pass naturally. This may take many months and, as long as the patient is not disabled by recurrent attacks of colic, progress can be followed by radiographs every 6–8 weeks.

Summary box 71.21

Indications for surgical removal of a ureteric calculus

- Repeated attacks of pain and the stone is not moving
- Stone is enlarging
- Complete obstruction of the kidney
- Urine is infected
- Stone is too large to pass
- Stone is obstructing solitary kidney or there is bilateral obstruction

---

Endoscopic stone removal

Dormia basket The use of wire baskets under image intensifier control has been replaced by ureteroscopic techniques but they may be useful when the necessary instruments and expertise are not available (Fig. 71.29). There is a significant danger of ureteric injury near the ureteric orifice, even with small stones.

Ureteric meatotomy Stones often lodge in the intramural part of the ureter. Endoscopic incision using a diathermy knife can

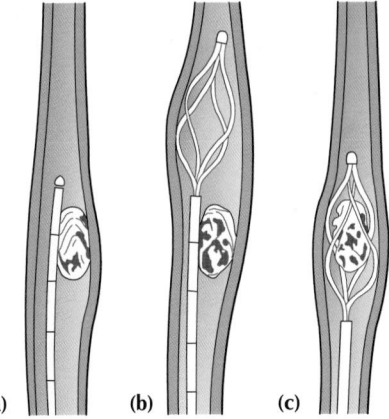

(a)   (b)   (c)

Figure 71.29 Dormia stone-catching basket in use: (a) basket introduced past stone; (b) opened; and (c) enclosing stone, ready for withdrawal.

Dormia, **formerly Assistant Professor of Urology, The University of Milan, Milan, Italy.**

---

enlarge the opening and free the stone. The procedure may lead to urinary reflux but this rarely causes problems.

Ureteroscopic stone removal

A ureteroscope is a long thin endoscope passed transurethrally across the bladder into the ureter (Fig. 71.30). The ureteroscope is used to remove stones that are impacted in the ureter. Stones that cannot be caught in baskets or endoscopic forceps under direct vision are fragmented using an electrohydraulic, percussive or laser lithotripter.

Push bang A stone in the middle or upper part of the ureter can often be flushed back into the kidney using a ureteric catheter. A J-stent secures the repositioned calculus in the kidney for subsequent treatment with ESWL.

A flexible fibreoptic ureteroscope can be used for laser destruction of calculi in the renal collecting system or ureter and to retrieve small stones from the kidney.

Lithotripsy *in situ*

A stone in a part of the ureter that can be identified by the imaging system of the lithotripter can be fragmented *in situ*. This form of treatment is not appropriate if there is complete obstruction or if the stone has been impacted for a long time.

Open surgery

Ureterolithotomy

A radiograph confirms the position of the stone immediately before surgery.

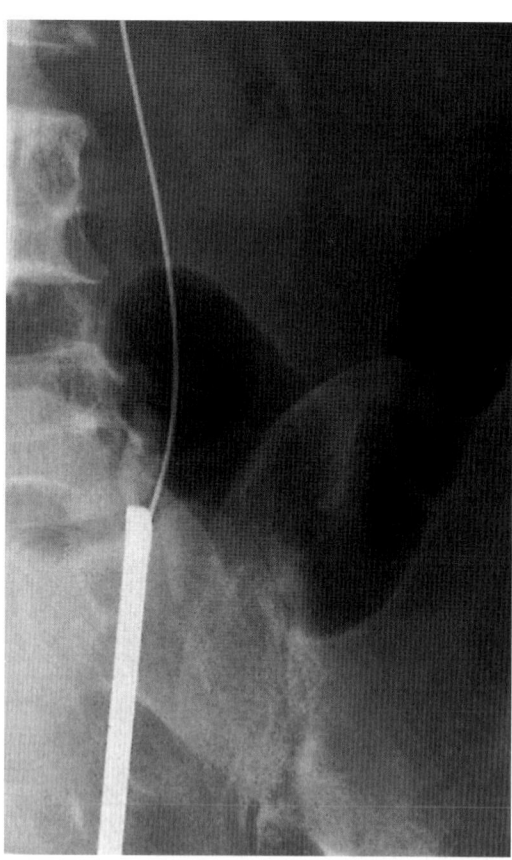

Figure 71.30 Ureteroscopy. Radiograph showing a ureteroscope and guidewire in the lower ureter.

The incision must be appropriate for the position of the stone. Calculi in the upper third of the ureter are approached through a loin or upper quadrant transverse incision as used for a stone in the renal pelvis. Access to midureteric stones is through a muscle-cutting iliac fossa incision; lower ureteric stones are best reached through a Pfannenstiel incision. For stones close to the bladder, exposure is improved by ligating and dividing the superior vesical vascular pedicle. The ureter is exposed in the retroperitoneum and slings are applied above and below the calculus to stop it from escaping. The ureter is incised longitudinally, directly on to the stone, which is freed from adhesions by blunt dissection and removed with stone forceps. Soft catheters are passed upwards and downwards to ensure that the ureter is clear. The ureterotomy is closed with interrupted absorbable sutures and a drain left in place for a day or so to drain urine leakage.

IDIOPATHIC RETROPERITONEAL FIBROSIS

In this rare condition one or both ureters are bound up in a progressive fibrosis of the retroperitoneal tissues. Most cases are idiopathic but some may be drug related. A similar clinical picture occurs in patients with leaking aortic aneurysm and infiltrating retroperitoneal malignancy.

The patient complains of backache, which is unremitting for several months. The onset of anuria and renal failure prompts investigation of the renal tract, which reveals hydronephrosis, usually on both sides. The excretion urogram typically shows medial displacement of the obstructed ureters and the appearances on CT are diagnostic. The sedimentation rate is markedly raised.

Treatment

It may be possible to insert ureteric stents as a temporary measure while renal function recovers. If not, percutaneous nephrostomies will allow the obstructed kidneys to drain. Some patients need renal replacement by dialysis. Some advocate conservative treatment with high-dose steroids. Surgical treatment involves dissection of the ureters from their fibrous jacket (ureterolysis). Wrapping omentum around the freed ureters discourages recurrent obstruction.

KIDNEY INFECTIONS (SUMMARY BOX 71.22)

Aetiology

Renal infections arise in the following ways:

- *Haematogenous infection* from a primary site in the tonsils or carious teeth or from cutaneous infections, particularly boils or a carbuncle. Renal tuberculosis occurs by bloodborne spread from lymph nodes in the neck, chest or abdomen.
- *Ascending infection* in the urinary tract is the most common route, and it is most likely to occur when there is vesicoureteric reflux. Urinary stasis and the presence of calculi are common contributory factors.

Herman Johann Pfannenstiel, **1862–1909, Gynaecologist, Breslau, Germany, (now Wroclaw, Poland) described this incision in 1900.**

Summary box 71.22

Kidney infection

- Acute pyelonephritis:
    In childhood
    In pregnancy
    With urinary obstruction
- Chronic pyelonephritis:
    Reflux nephropathy
- Pyonephrosis
- Renal abscess
- Perinephric abscess

Bacteriology

Escherichia coli and other Gram-negative organisms are commonly responsible. When *Streptococcus faecalis* is present it is usually accompanied by other organisms. In *E. coli* and streptococcal infections the urine is acidic. *Proteus* spp. and staphylococci split urea to form ammonia, which makes the urine alkaline and promotes the formation of calculi.

Acute pyelonephritis

Acute pyelonephritis is more common in females, especially during childhood, at puberty, after intercourse (as a complication of 'honeymoon cystitis'), during pregnancy and during menopause. It occurs more on the right and is frequently bilateral.

Clinical features

There may be prodromal symptoms of headache, lassitude and nausea, but the onset of pain is usually sudden, often with a rigor and vomiting. There is acute pain in the flank and hypochondrium. In a few cases the pain resembles renal colic. The remitting temperature rises to 39.0°C or more. The symptoms of cystitis commonly set in, with urgency, frequency and scalding dysuria. There is tenderness in the hypochondrium and in the loin. Rarely, in cases of severe bilateral pyelonephritis, especially when there is an associated obstruction, renal dysfunction may be sufficient to cause uraemia. The risk of life-threatening septicaemia is ever present (Summary box 71.23).

Summary box 71.23

Clinical features of kidney infections

- More common in women
- Often associated with septicaemia leading to pyrexia and rigors
- Associated with pyuria and occasionally haematuria
- Should be initially treated with broad-spectrum parenteral antibiotics
- Extremely dangerous if the kidney is obstructed

Bacteriological examination of the urine

A midstream urine specimen should be collected into a sterile container; the urine is centrifuged and the sediment examined microscopically. In early acute pyelonephritis, there are usually

Hans Christian Joachim Gram, **1853–1938**, Professor of Pharmacology (1891–1900), and of Medicine (1900–1923), Copenhagen, Denmark, described this method of staining bacteria in 1884.

pus cells and many bacteria. The urine may be misleadingly clear to the eye until the infection becomes established, when the urine is cloudy and full of pus. Culture and sensitivity testing of the causative organisms allows a rational choice of antibiotic, but parenteral treatment with a broad-spectrum antibiotic should be started before the results are available.

Severe cases

There are repeated rigors and a temperature of 40°C or more, often without a corresponding rise in pulse rate. There is vomiting, sweating and thirst; the patient feels awful. The blood culture is usually positive, especially if the specimen has been taken during a rigor.

Differential diagnosis

When the symptoms and signs are typical the diagnosis is straightforward. In other circumstances it may be difficult to be sure that the patient does not have pneumonia, acute appendicitis or acute cholecystitis. The urgent need is to distinguish acute pyelonephritis from appendicitis, and the site of pain and the presence of marked peritonism are usually helpful in identifying the latter. A plain abdominal radiograph may show the outline of a swollen kidney and, if the infection is severe, a skilled ultrasonographer may be able to detect the typical appearances of pyelonephritis.

Special cases

Pyelonephritis of pregnancy

Pyelonephritis of pregnancy usually occurs between the fourth and sixth months of gestation in women who have a past history of recurrent urinary infection. In about 10% of cases the disease runs a severe and protracted course and occasionally leads to abortion or premature birth.

Urinary infection in childhood

Urinary infection in childhood is important to recognise because it may damage the growing kidney. In young children, symptoms are often non-specific but the child may pass cloudy or offensive urine. The possibility of urinary sepsis should always be considered if a child fails to thrive or suffers unexplained pyrexia. Pain or screaming on micturition may occur. The older child may complain of loin pain and may develop urinary frequency and secondary enuresis.

Up to 50% of children with urinary infection have an underlying anatomical abnormality (e.g. reflux or obstruction). The diagnosis of infection is confirmed by examination of a clean-catch specimen or a specimen obtained by suprapubic needle puncture. On culture, a pure growth of more than 10^5 organisms/ml with a significant pyuria is evidence of infection. Such children should be investigated by ultrasound scan and other modalities to identify underlying urinary tract abnormalities and to assess renal function and scarring.

Vesicoureteric reflux of urine is detectable in about 35% of children with recurrent urinary infection. In some patients the reflux is caused by high pressure in a neuropathic bladder. It may be intermittent and is often more marked when there is active infection. Renal damage results from the combination of reflux and urinary infection early in life, and reflux nephropathy is the most common cause of end-stage renal failure in the UK. Long-term prophylactic antibiotic treatment has become the favoured treatment for recurrent urinary infections resulting from reflux. Surgical reimplantation of the ureters is reserved for those in whom conservative measures fail. However, reimplantation in these patients may fail to cure reflux (Summary box 71.24).

Acute pyelonephritis associated with urinary retention

Acute pyelonephritis is a relatively uncommon complication of chronic urinary retention. Often the organisms are introduced during instrumentation. Patients who have a significant post-micturition urinary residue should be given prophylactic antibiotics to cover transurethral procedures.

Treatment

The treatment of acute pyelonephritis should be prompt, appropriate and prolonged. A full investigation to exclude underlying abnormalities in the urinary tract should be undertaken when the acute illness subsides.

The patient will usually feel like lying in bed. While awaiting the bacteriological report and the results of sensitivity tests, an antimicrobial with a wide range of activity, such as amoxicillin or gentamicin, should be administered, parenterally if necessary. If the urine is acidic, as it is in the common coliform infections, alkalinisation of the urine by potassium citrate may help by inhibiting the growth of these organisms and relieving dysuria. When pain is severe, a morphine-like analgesic drug may be necessary if non-steroidal anti-inflammatory agents are ineffective. The patient should drink copiously; if this is not possible because of nausea and vomiting, an intravenous infusion should be set up.

Most urinary infections acquired outside hospital are sensitive to relatively cheap agents such as trimethoprim and amoxicillin. Hospital-acquired infections are much more likely to be resistant and more expensive second-line antibiotics may be needed. Gentamicin and carbenicillin are suitable for combating infections with more resistant strains of *Pseudomonas pyocyanea*, *Proteus* spp. and *Klebsiella* spp. Ciprofloxacin is particularly useful against *Pseudomonas* spp. in patients who do not have septicaemia. Despite the efficacy of modern antibacterial drugs, recurrent infection is likely if there is an untreated underlying abnormality of the urinary tract such as a stone, vesicoureteric reflux, fistula to the gastrointestinal tract or retention of urine.

Chronic pyelonephritis

Chronic pyelonephritis is so often associated with vesicoureteric reflux that some feel that it is better named 'reflux nephropathy'. It is an important cause of renal damage and death from end-stage renal failure.

Pathology

There is interstitial inflammation and scarring of the renal parenchyma with a patchy distribution. The renal tubules are atrophic and dilated. The glomeruli retain their normal structure until the final stages of the disease.

Clinical features

The condition is almost three times as common in women as it is in men. Two-thirds of female patients are under 40 years of age, whereas 60% of male patients are over 40.

It is possible, but unusual, for chronic pyelonephritis to remain clinically silent until the symptoms of advanced renal insufficiency appear.

Lumbar pain, dull and non-specific in character, is present in 60% of cases. Increased urinary frequency and dysuria are common. Hypertension, present in 40% of cases, may be of the accelerated ('malignant') type. Constitutional symptoms of lassitude, malaise, anorexia, nausea and headache constitute the main complaint in 30% of cases. The true cause of these non-specific symptoms may elude diagnosis for years.

Attacks of low-grade fever often prompt the urinary tract investigations that bring the condition to light.

Normochromic anaemia due to unsuspected renal impairment is an occasional presenting feature (Summary box 71.25).

Investigations

As the glomeruli are relatively preserved, proteinuria is less marked than in glomerulonephritis (< 3 g daily). Casts are not usually present but white cells are plentiful.

Escherichia coli, *Streptococcus faecalis*, *Proteus* spp. or *Pseudomonas* spp are found in the urine.

Treatment

Treatment is aimed at eradicating predisposing contributory factors such as obstruction or stones and treating the infection, often with repeated courses of antibiotic. Unfortunately, once the parenchyma has been scarred it becomes vulnerable to blood-borne organisms and reinfection is likely, sometimes with a different and resistant organism. Consequently, antibiotics confer only temporary benefit and progressive renal damage is common.

Surgical treatment is indicated only when the disease is confined to one kidney. This is unusual but in such cases nephrectomy or partial nephrectomy may stop the symptoms of infection and make hypertension easier to control. Patients with end-stage renal failure require renal replacement therapy.

Pyonephrosis

The kidney becomes a multilocular sac containing pus or purulent urine. Pyonephrosis results from infection of a hydronephrosis, follows acute pyelonephritis or, most commonly, arises as a complication of renal calculus disease. Pyonephrosis is usually unilateral.

Clinical features

The classical triad of symptoms is anaemia, fever and a swelling in the loin. When the condition arises as an infected hydronephrosis, the swelling may be very large and the pyrexia very high and associated with rigors. Symptoms of cystitis may be prominent.

Investigations

Imaging may show a calculus and will demonstrate dilatation of the pus-filled collecting system.

Treatment

Pyonephrosis is a surgical emergency because the patient is threatened with permanent renal damage and lethal septicaemia. Parenteral antibiotics should be given immediately and the kidney drained. If the pus is too thick to be aspirated through a large percutaneous nephrostomy, consider open nephrostomy. In cases in which there is a stone, the stone should be removed. Nephrectomy may be appropriate when the kidney is destroyed and function on the other side is good.

Renal carbuncle

An abscess may form in the renal parenchyma as the result of blood-borne spread of organisms, especially coliforms or *Staphylococcus aureus*. Occasionally, the condition results from infection of a haematoma following a blow to the kidney. Renal carbuncle is most commonly seen in diabetics, intravenous drug abusers, those debilitated by chronic disease and patients with acquired immunodeficiency.

Pathology

The renal parenchyma contains an encapsulated necrotic mass.

Clinical features

There is an ill-defined tender swelling in the loin, persistent pyrexia and leucocytosis, signs that closely simulate those of perinephric abscess. In early cases there is no pus or bacteria in the urine, but these appear later. The space-occupying lesion in the kidney may be confused with a renal adenocarcinoma (Fig. 71.31).

Treatment

Resolution by antibiotic treatment alone is unusual. Formal open incision of the abscess may be necessary if the pus is too thick to be drained by percutaneous aspiration.

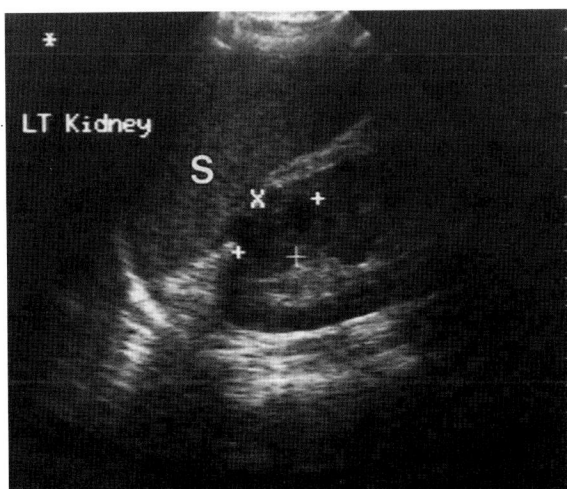

Figure 71.31 Longitudinal ultrasound scan through the upper pole of the left kidney demonstrates a renal carbuncle, outlined by crosses. S, spleen.

Perinephric abscess

The common causes of perinephric abscess are shown in Fig. 71.32. Other causes are infection of a perirenal haematoma and perinephric discharge of an untreated pyonephrosis or renal carbuncle. A mycobacterial perinephric abscess may arise by extension from a nearby tuberculous vertebra.

Clinical features

In perinephric abscess there is a high swinging pyrexia, abdominal tenderness and fullness in the loin (Fig. 71.33). Local signs present early if the infection starts in the lower part of the perinephric fat. Infection at the upper pole is masked by the lower ribs and signs in the loin are less. The white cell count is always markedly raised but there are characteristically no pus cells or organisms in the urine.

Imaging

The psoas shadow is obscured on the plain abdominal radiograph. There may be a reactionary scoliosis – with the concavity toward the abscess – and elevation and immobility of the diaphragm on the affected side. A calculus may be present. Ultrasonography and CT are diagnostic.

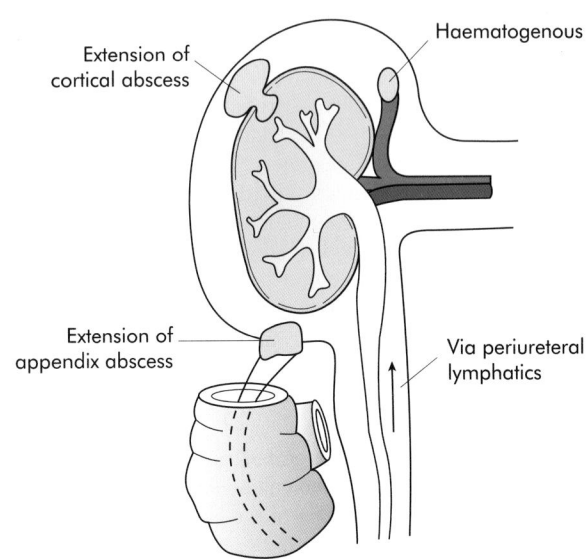

Figure 71.32 Sources of perinephric abscess.

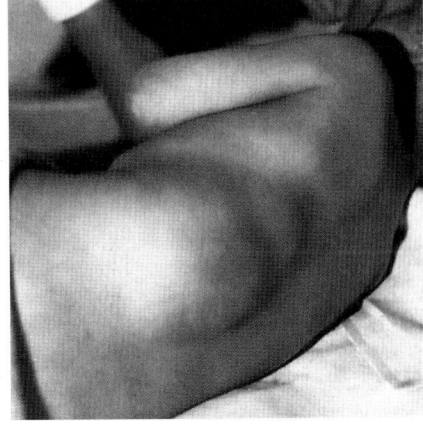

Figure 71.33 A large perinephric abscess.

Treatment

Open drainage may be necessary if the abscess cannot be aspirated through a large percutaneous needle. A lumbar incision is made under antibiotic cover. This should be large enough to allow the surgeon to open pockets of pus and to explore for an unruptured cortical abscess, which may also be present. A specimen of pus is sent for culture and the wound is closed over a tube drain (Summary box 71.26).

Summary box 71.26

Management of perinephric abscess

- Collections of pus in or around the kidney should be drained surgically if they cannot be aspirated by percutaneous needling

---

Renal tuberculosis

Aetiology and pathology

Tuberculosis of the urinary tract arises from haematogenous infection from a distant focus that is often impossible to identify. The lesions are usually confined to one kidney. Tuberculous granulomas in a renal pyramid coalesce to form an ulcer. Mycobacteria and pus cells discharge into the urine. Untreated lesions enlarge and a tuberculous abscess may form in the parenchyma. The necks of the calyces and the renal pelvis stenosed by fibrosis confine the infection so that there is tuberculous pyonephrosis, sometimes localised to one pole of the kidney. Extension of pyonephrosis or tuberculous renal abscess leads to perinephric abscess and the kidney is progressively replaced by caseous material (putty kidney), which may be calcified (cement kidney). At any stage, the plain radiograph may show areas of calcification (pseudocalculi). Less commonly, the kidneys may be bilaterally affected as part of the generalised process of miliary tuberculosis (Fig. 71.34).

Renal tuberculosis is often associated with tuberculosis of the bladder and typical tuberculous granulomas may be visible in the bladder wall. In the male, tuberculous epididymo-orchitis may occur without apparent infection of the bladder.

Clinical features

Renal tuberculosis usually occurs between 20 and 40 years of age, and is twice as common in men as in women; the right kidney is affected slightly more often than the left.

Urinary frequency is often the earliest symptom and may be the only one. The patient complains of a progressive increase in both daytime and night-time frequency.

'Sterile' pyuria

In early cases the urine is pale and slightly opalescent. Routine urine culture is negative.

Pain

Painful micturition is a feature as soon as tuberculous cystitis sets in. First, there is a suprapubic pain if voiding is delayed; later, a burning pain accompanies micturition. When there is secondary infection, a superadded agonising pain referred to the tip of the penis or to the vulva is often associated with haematuria and strangury.

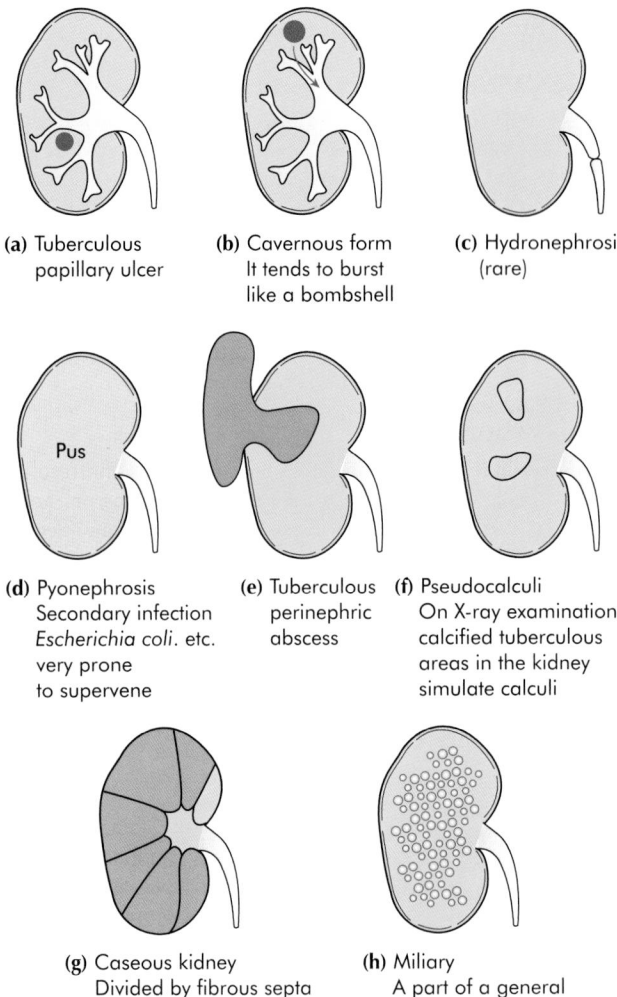

(a) Tuberculous papillary ulcer

(b) Cavernous form
It tends to burst like a bombshell

(c) Hydronephrosis (rare)

(d) Pyonephrosis
Secondary infection *Escherichia coli*. etc. very prone to supervene

(e) Tuberculous perinephric abscess

(f) Pseudocalculi
On X-ray examination, calcified tuberculous areas in the kidney simulate calculi

(g) Caseous kidney
Divided by fibrous septa

(h) Miliary
A part of a general tuberculous process

Figure 71.34 Types of lesion in renal tuberculosis.

Renal pain is often minimal but there may be a dull ache in the loin.

Haematuria

In 5% of cases, the first symptom is haematuria occurring from an ulcer on a renal papilla. The tuberculous lesion may be difficult to detect radiologically and mycobacteria may not be cultured from the urine until the onset of more suggestive symptoms months later.

A tuberculous kidney is oedematous and friable and is more liable to damage than a normal kidney.

Malaise and weight loss are usual and a low-level evening pyrexia is typical. A high temperature suggests secondary infection or dissemination, i.e. miliary tuberculosis.

On examination

It is unusual for a tuberculous kidney to be palpable. The prostate, seminal vesicles, vasa and scrotal contents should be examined for nodules or thickening (Summary box 71.27).

Investigation

Bacteriological

Bacteriological examination of at least three complete specimens of early-morning urine should be sent for microscopy and culture before specific chemotherapy is started. Staining of the urine sediment with the Ziehl–Neelsen stain occasionally shows the presence of acid-fast bacilli, but proof that these are pathological mycobacteria must await prolonged culture on Löwenstein–Jensen medium. When the clinical picture is convincing it is permissible to start anti-tuberculous therapy in anticipation of the culture results some 6 weeks later.

Radiography

An abdominal radiograph may show calcified lesions.

Intravenous urography

Early in the disease, the normally clear-cut outline of a renal papilla may be rendered indistinct by the presence of ulceration. Later, there may be calyceal stenosis (Fig. 71.35) and/or hydronephrosis caused by stricture of the renal pelvis or the ureter draining the affected kidney; this may be more easily demonstrable by retrograde ureterography (Fig. 71.36). A tuberculous abscess appears as a space-occupying lesion, which causes adjacent calyces to splay out. The bladder may appear shrunken, with its wall irregular or thickened. In late stages there may be dilatation of the contralateral ureter from obstruction where the ureter passes through a thickened and oedematous bladder wall.

Cystoscopy

Cystoscopy is not routine in the investigation of urinary tuberculosis but is often performed because there has been haematuria or unexplained bladder symptoms. There may be little to see in the first stages of the disease, but later the urothelium is studded with granulomas that cluster particularly around the ureteric orifices. The tubercles may coalesce to produce a tuberculous ulcer. As the bladder wall fibroses, the bladder capacity decreases. Contraction of the fibrosed ureter tugs at the ureteric orifice, which is displaced upwards, its mouth wide open (the so called 'golf-hole' orifice).

Chest radiography

A chest radiograph is indicated to exclude an active lung lesion.

Treatment

Anti-tuberculous chemotherapy is best managed by a physician with experience of the most modern drug regimens and their potential adverse effects. The surgeon must ensure that the state of the urinary tract is reviewed during the first few weeks of therapy because the renal pelvis and ureter may stricture *after* treatment has started.

Prognosis in renal tuberculosis is good if the patient completes the course of chemotherapy.

Operative treatment

Operative treatment should be conservative, aiming to remove large foci of infection, which are difficult to treat with drugs, and correct the obstruction caused by fibrosis. The optimum time for surgery is between 6 and 12 weeks after the start of anti-tuberculous chemotherapy.

The surgeon needs a repertoire of procedures to deal with

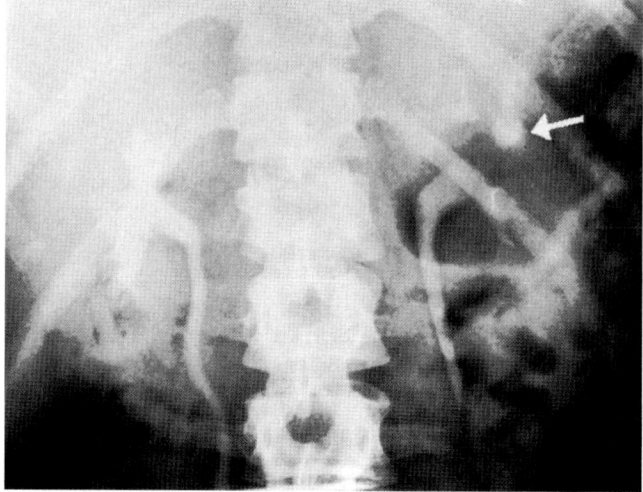

Figure 71.35 Intravenous urogram showing a small localised tuberculous lesion with hydrocalyx (arrow). Healing took place with conservative treatment.

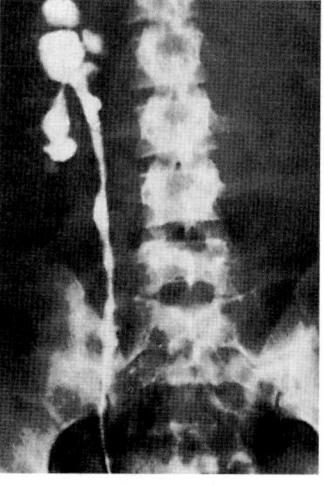

Figure 71.36 Retrograde ureterogram showing advanced tuberculosis of the right kidney. Right retrograde study shows multiple ureteric strictures and gross distortion of the internal architecture of the affected kidney.

various potential effects of urinary tuberculosis. An obstructed lower pole calyx may be drained into the upper ureter. A strictured renal pelvis needs a pyeloplasty. Ureteric stenosis and shortening may require a Boari operation or a bowel interposition, depending on the level and extent of the fibrosis. If the kidney has no function it is best to perform a nephroureterectomy (Fig. 71.37). A bladder too contracted to function as a reservoir for urine may be replaced with a neobladder fashioned from a loop of bowel in a substitution cystoplasty.

NEOPLASMS OF THE KIDNEY (SUMMARY BOX 71.28)

Summary box 71.28

Renal neoplasms

Benign neoplasms
- Adenoma
- Angioma
- Angiomyolipoma

Malignant neoplasms
- Wilms' tumour (nephroblastoma in children)
- Grawitz's tumour (adenocarcinoma, hypernephroma)
- Transitional cell carcinoma of the renal pelvis and collecting system
- Squamous carcinoma of the renal pelvis

Benign neoplasms

Adenoma

Pea-like cortical adenomas are occasionally discovered at post-mortem examination or incidentally during radiological imaging. They are asymptomatic and defined as benign.

Angioma

Angioma may cause profuse haematuria, often in young adults. The source of the bleeding may be difficult to diagnose without renal angiography.

Angiomyolipoma

Angiomyolipoma is an unusual tumour of the kidney that is often but not always associated with tuberous sclerosis. Its high fat content gives it a typical appearance on CT. Malignant elements are present in about one-quarter of them and may lead to metastasis.

Malignant neoplasms

Renal neoplasm in children

Wilms' tumour (synonym: nephroblastoma) (Fig. 71.38)

This is a mixed tumour containing blastemal, stromal and epithelial elements arising from embryonic nephrogenic tissue. The tumours are usually discovered during the first 5 years of life, usually in one pole of one kidney. Bilateral tumours pose a difficult clinical problem.

Pathology The cut surface of the tumour is tan coloured. A rapidly growing tumour is likely to be soft and friable in consistency.

Clinical features An abdominal tumour grows rapidly while the general well-being of the child deteriorates. The mass may be enormous compared with the tiny patient. Some patients are hypertensive.

Haematuria denotes extension of the tumour into the renal pelvis and the prognosis is less good.

Imaging by ultrasonography, CT or magnetic resonance imaging (MRI) confirms a solid space-occupying lesion in the kidney, with or without venous invasion, contralateral disease and distant spread.

(a)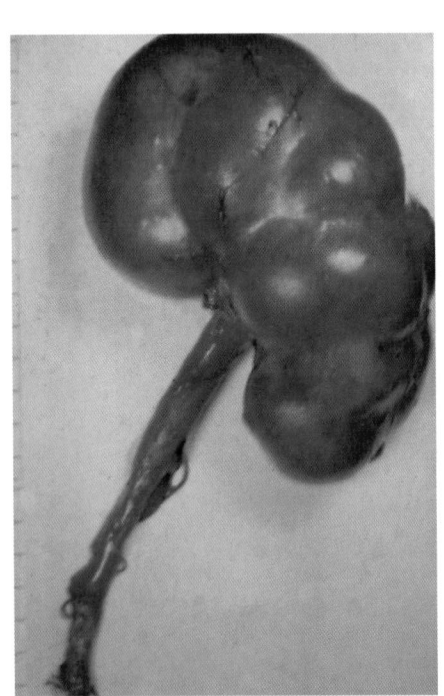

(b)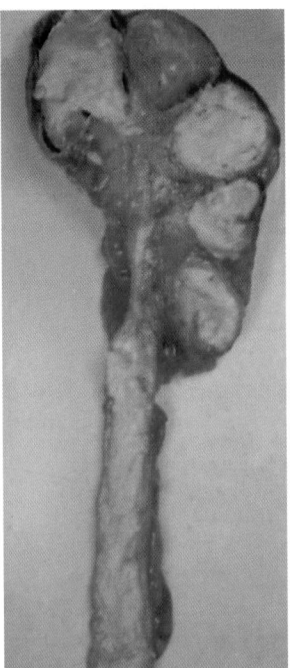

Figure 71.37 (a and b) Nephroureterectomy specimen from a patient with a kidney destroyed by tuberculous pyonephrosis.

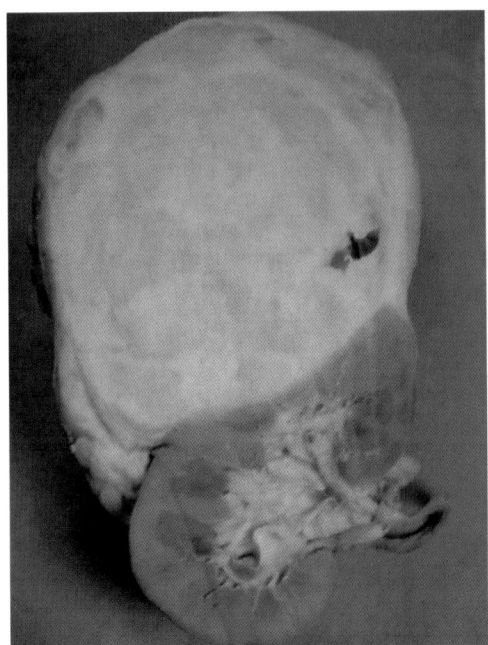

Figure 71.38 Wilms' tumour.

Metastasis to the lungs occurs early. Liver, bone and brain metastases are rare. Lymphatic spread is uncommon.

Treatment These children are best treated in specialist paediatric oncology units. Most unilateral tumours are treated by chemotherapy followed by nephrectomy. Partial nephrectomy may be possible in patients with bilateral disease.

Prognosis With modern chemotherapy and surgery, long-term survival can be expected in more than 80% of patients. The prognosis is worse in those with metastases and in older children (Summary box 71.29).

Summary box 71.29

Nephroblastoma (Wilms' tumour)

- Usually presents in the first 5 years of life
- Typically presents with an abdominal mass
- May cause haematuria, abdominal pain or fever
- Metastasises to the lung
- Is best treated in a specialist paediatric oncology unit

Renal neoplasm in adults

Hypernephroma (synonym: Grawitz's tumour)

This adenocarcinoma, the most common neoplasm of the kidney (75% incidence), arises from renal tubular cells. Whether carcinoma arises in pre-existing adenomas is uncertain.

Pathology Moderate-sized tumours are spherical and often occupy the poles of a single kidney, most commonly the upper pole. Hilar tumours are less common. The cut surface is usually yellowish or dull white, semi-transparent, with areas of haemorrhage (Fig.

Paul Albert Grawitz, **1850–1932, Professor of Pathology, Greifswald, Germany, described adeno-carcinoma of the kidney in 1884.**

71.39). The tumour is often divided into lobules, some of which are cystic. Larger tumours are irregular in shape with central haemorrhage and necrosis.

Microscopic structure The most common pattern is of solid areas of polyhedral or cubical clear cells with deeply stained, small, rounded nuclei and abundant cytoplasm containing lipids, cholesterol and glycogen. The cells are occasionally arranged as papillary cysts or tubules. Less commonly, the cells are granular (dark), and both clear and dark cells may be represented in the same tumour. The scanty stroma is richly vascular.

Spread The tumour is prone to grow into the renal vein. Cells are swept into the circulation and end up in the lungs, where they grow to form cannonball secondary deposits (Fig. 71.40).

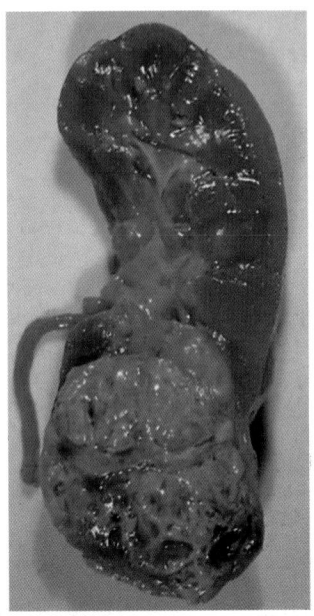

Figure 71.39 Adenocarcinoma of the kidney (Grawitz's tumour).

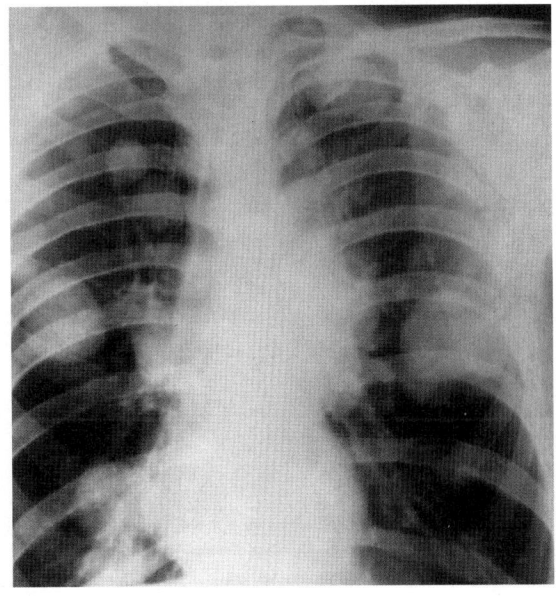

Figure 71.40 Cannonball secondaries from a hypernephroma.

Metastasis to bone also occurs and a secondary deposit in a long bone may be the only sign of distant spread for a year or more. Highly vascular metastases may pulsate. Tumour extending beyond the renal capsule is liable to metastasise via the lymph nodes in the hilum of the kidney to the para-aortic nodes and beyond.

Clinical features Adenocarcinoma of the kidney is twice as common in men as in women. Haematuria is usually the presenting symptom, sometimes with clot colic. There may be a dragging discomfort in the loin or the patient may detect a mass. In men, a rapidly developing varicocele is a rare but impressive sign, occurring most often on the left side because the left gonadal vein is obstructed where it joins the left renal vein.

Atypical presentations In 25% of cases there are no local symptoms. The patient presents with symptomatic secondary deposits in bone (Fig. 71.41) or the lung (persistent cough or haemoptysis).

Occasionally, persistent pyrexia (37.8–38.9°C) with no evidence of infection is the only symptom. Pyrexia after nephrectomy suggests metastases.

A few patients present with constitutional symptoms and anaemia.

Polycythaemia occurs in 4% of cases as a result of the production of erythropoietin by tumour cells. The erythrocyte sedimentation rate is always raised above the 1–2 mm found in idiopathic polycythaemia vera. The blood count returns to normal after nephrectomy unless there are metastases. Other hormones, such as renin and calcitonin, may be produced by the tumour. Hypercalcaemia is common.

Nephrotic syndrome has been reported as a rare presentation of hypernephroma.

Investigation Intravenous urography is still an important component of the investigation of haematuria. The plain radiograph may show abnormal calcification in the tumour and distortion of the renal outline, which will be confirmed on the nephrographic film. The calyces may be stretched and distorted. It is important to know whether the contralateral kidney is working (Fig. 71.42).

Once a mass has been demonstrated in the kidney, a scan is needed to decide whether it is solid or cystic. Ultrasound will give this information. CT with enhancement will demonstrate the extent of the lesion more clearly and will show whether the hilar lymph nodes or renal vein are involved (Fig. 71.43).

Enthusiasm for renal angiography and preoperative embolisation has waned. Occasionally, a flush inferior cavagram is helpful

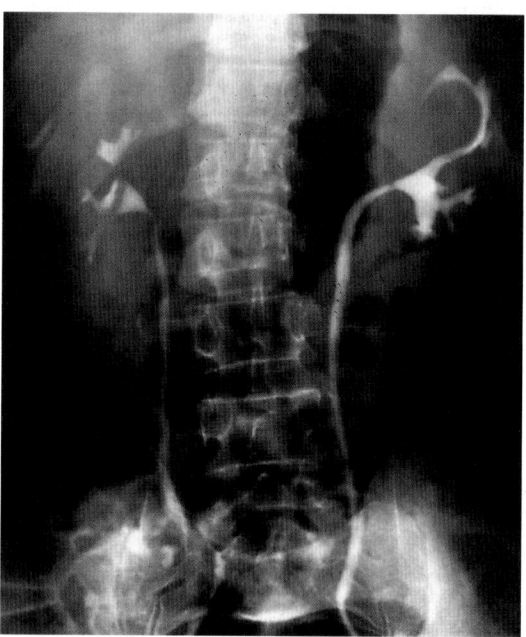

Figure 71.42 Intravenous urogram in a case of hypernephroma of the left kidney. The only symptom was one attack of painless haematuria. Note the displacement of the upper pole calyces by the mass.

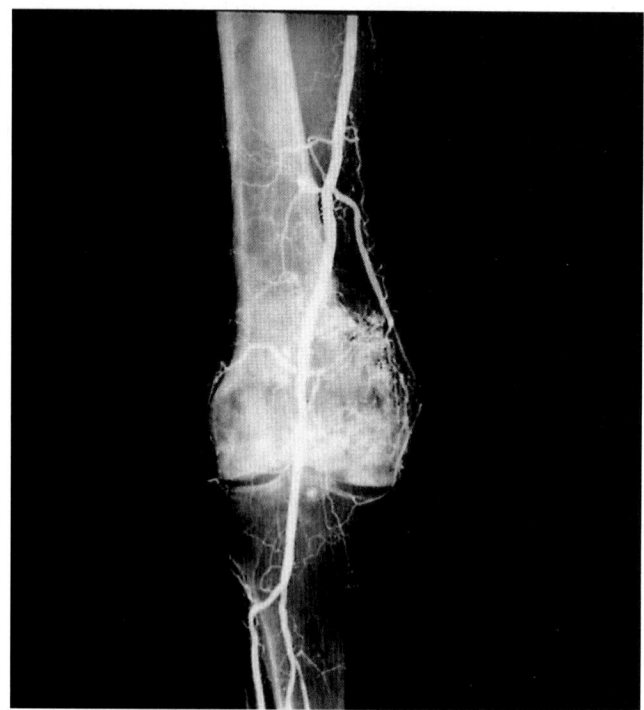

Figure 71.41 Arteriogram showing a vascular 'blush' due to metastasis in the femur from a Grawitz's tumour.

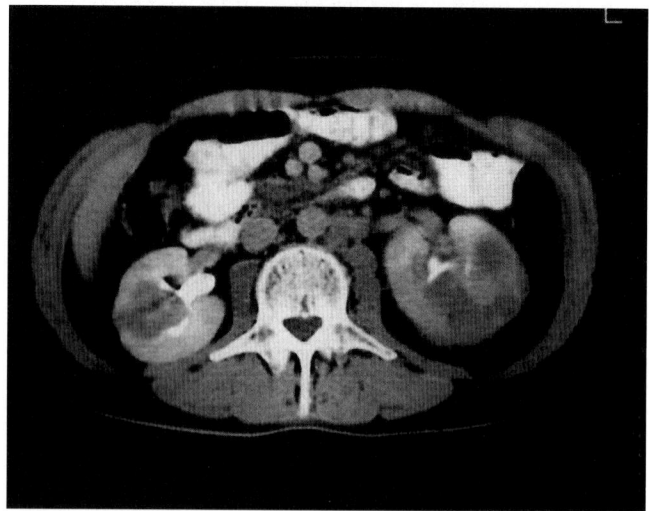

Figure 71.43 Computerised tomography scan showing large bilateral renal adenocarcinomas.

to show the extent of caval involvement by tumour growing in from the renal vein.

A chest radiograph is essential to detect lung secondaries. An isotope bone scan will reveal deposits in bone.

Treatment If the tumour is confined to the kidney, treatment is nephrectomy with removal of the perinephric fat. Nephrectomy can be performed through a loin or a transverse or oblique upper abdominal incision. The transabdominal approach has the advantage that the renal pedicle and the inferior vena cava can be widely exposed.

The vascular pedicle should be ligated before the kidney is mobilised because handling the tumour may cause malignant cells to be released into the circulation. The first step in the procedure is to clean the renal artery and ligate it in continuity. This may be more difficult from an anterior approach because the artery lies behind the vein. However, once the artery is occluded, the tumour loses most of its profuse blood supply and massive bleeding during mobilisation becomes less likely. Gentle palpation of the renal vein ensures that there is no tumour in its lumen. An empty vein can be divided between ligatures. The renal artery is then divided and the kidney mobilised within its coverings. Aberrant vessels feeding the tumour must be carefully ligated or coagulated to avoid troublesome bleeding. The ureter is then traced downwards as far as is safe and divided between ligatures.

If the renal vein or the inferior vena cava is invaded, the surgeon must obtain control of the cava above and below the tumour extension as a first priority. If there is extension into the thorax, the cardiac team may be needed to put the patient on cardiac bypass so that tumour can, if necessary, be removed from the right side of the heart.

Adenocarcinoma of the kidney responds poorly to radiotherapy or conventional chemotherapy. There have been early promising results from clinical trials of the cytokine interleukin-2 in this condition.

Prognosis Removal of even the largest neoplasm may cure the patient. In operable cases, 70% of patients are well after 3 years and 60% after 5 years. Macroscopic involvement of the renal vein or its tributaries, invasion beyond the capsule and lymphatic involvement all worsen the prognosis (Summary box 71.30).

Summary box 71.30

Adenocarcinoma of the kidney

- Often presents with haematuria
- May be associated with pyrexia of unknown origin, polycythaemia, hypercalcaemia, anaemia and other paraneoplastic symptoms
- Metastasises via the bloodstream to bone, liver and lung (cannonball secondaries)
- Renal vein extension may embolise to the pulmonary circulation during nephrectomy

---

Papillary transitional cell tumours of the renal pelvis (Fig. 71.44)

These resemble those of the bladder but are much less common. They may invade the renal parenchyma and have a tendency to be multifocal and to distant spread. Multiple ureteric tumours are thought to arise from a field change that renders the whole

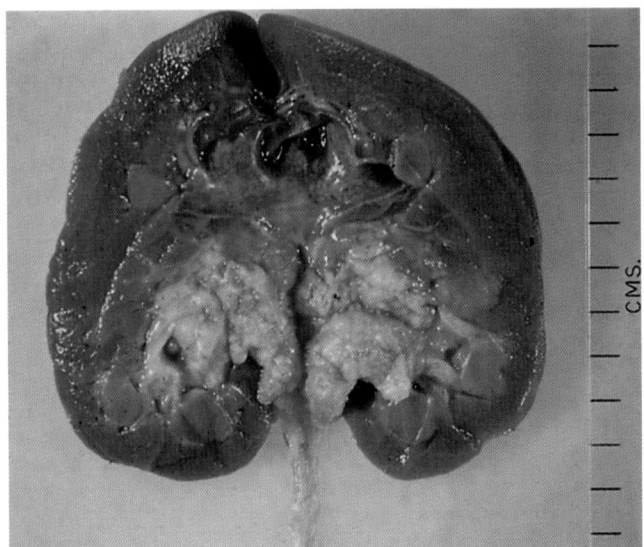

Figure 71.44 Papillary transitional cell tumour of the renal pelvis.

urothelium liable to metaplasia rather than seeding down the ureter. Whether the carcinogen is chemical or viral is uncertain.

Clinical features Haematuria is the most common symptom and usually causes the patient to seek help before the tumour mass becomes palpable.

The presence of malignant cells in the urine may indicate whether the tumour is well or poorly differentiated. There is some evidence that those with poorly differentiated tumours do better if they have a short course of radiotherapy before surgery. It is therefore useful to obtain cells from the tumour by sampling using a brush or catheter passed up the ureter under radiological control.

Intravenous urography usually demonstrates the tumour (Fig. 71.45). Retrograde pyelography may be helpful if the urogram is indistinct.

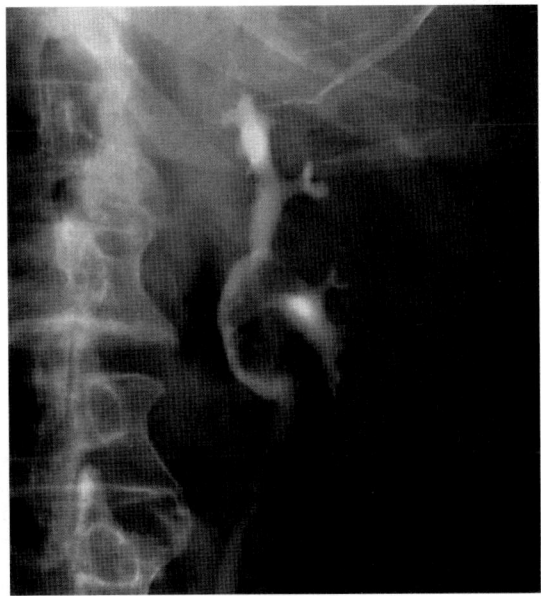

Figure 71.45 Intravenous urogram showing a filling defect in the left renal pelvis due to transitional cell carcinoma.

Treatment Conventional surgical treatment is by nephroureterectomy. The ureter must be disconnected with a cuff of bladder wall. If this is done by open surgery a second incision is needed to remove the kidney. Alternatively, the ureteric orifice can be widely resected with a resectoscope and the ureter delivered by a somewhat perilous blunt dissection from the upper abdominal wound used to remove the kidney. Some urologists argue that well-differentiated upper urinary tract transitional tumours should be treated conservatively by resection with appropriate steps taken to avoid the growth of tumour seeded in the percutaneous track.

Squamous cell carcinoma of the renal pelvis

This is rare and often associated with chronic inflammation and leucoplakia resulting from stone. The tumours are radiosensitive but metastasise early and the prognosis is poor.

Transitional cell tumours of the ureter

These are rare. They behave like tumours of the renal pelvis. Treatment is by nephroureterectomy.

About half of patients with tumours of the upper urinary tract will have tumours in the bladder at some stage. Follow-up by cystoscopy with regular urography is therefore necessary to detect recurrent tumours.

Balkan nephropathy Transitional cell tumours of the upper urinary tract have a very high incidence in certain areas of the Balkans. The same population has a high incidence of a form of primary nephropathy. The causative agent has not been identified with certainty but there seems to be an association with the consumption of grain products stored in a damp environment. Tumours that develop against a background of Balkan nephropathy should

> The Balkans are the countries which occupy an area in the south-east of Europe. They lie south of the Danube and Sava rivers, and form a peninsula bounded on the east by the Aegean and Black Seas, on the west by the Adriatic and Ionian Seas, and on the south by the Mediterranean.

be treated by nephron-sparing surgery in view of the impaired overall renal function.

Nephrectomy for benign disease

Nephrectomy is now rarely performed for benign disease but may be necessary if the kidney is atrophic or dysplastic or the cause of accelerated hypertension. Non-functioning kidneys resulting from longstanding obstruction or stone disease are a potential site for infection and even malignancy. In a simple nephrectomy, the kidney is dissected free through the convenient plane between the capsule and its fatty coverings. If this plane is obscured by the scarring of previous surgery, a subcapsular nephrectomy may be safer. Laparoscopic nephrectomy is sometimes possible for small kidneys destroyed by benign disease but the technique requires special skills and the costs and benefits are under evaluation.

Hypertension and a unilateral renal lesion

Ischaemia of the renal parenchyma leads to the release of pressor agents that cause arterial hypertension. When a renal lesion is discovered during the investigation of hypertension, nephrectomy may make the hypertension more amenable to drug treatment.

FURTHER READING

Blandy, J.P. and Kaisary, A.V. (2007) *Lecture Notes: Urology*, 6th edn. Blackwell, Oxford.

Tanagho, E.A. and McAnich, J.W. (eds) (2000) *Smith's General Urology*, 15th edn. McGraw-Hill/Appleton & Lange, New York.

Wein, A.J., Kavoussi, L.R., Novick, A.C., Partin, A.W. and Peters, C.A. (2007) *Campbell–Walsh Urology*, 9th edn. W.B. Saunders, Philadelphia, PA.

Weiss, G., Weiss, R.M. and O'Reilly, P.H. (eds) (2001) *Comprehensive Urology*. Elsevier Science, Amsterdam.

Wessells, H. and McAninch, J. (2004) *Urological Emergencies*. Humana Press, Totowa, NJ.

The urinary bladder

LEARNING OBJECTIVES

To understand:
- The anatomy, vascular supply and innervation of the bladder in relation to function and disease
- The principles of management of bladder trauma, incontinence and fistulae

- The common causes of acute and chronic urinary retention and management
- The different types of bladder cancer and the principles of management

SURGICAL ANATOMY OF THE BLADDER

- It is lined by transitional epithelium covering the connective tissue lamina propria, which contains a rich plexus of vessels and lymphatics.
- When the detrusor muscle hypertrophies, the inner layer, covered by urothelium, stands out, resulting in the appearance of trabeculation.
- Over the trigone is a thin layer of smooth muscle to which the epithelium is closely adherent and which extends as a sheath around the lower ureters and into the proximal urethra.
- Around the male bladder neck is the smooth muscle internal sphincter innervated by adrenergic fibres, which prevents retrograde ejaculation.
- The distal urethral sphincter is a horseshoe-shaped mass of striated muscle that lies anterior and distal to the prostate, or in the proximal two-thirds of the female urethra. It is distinct from the pelvic floor and is supplied by S2–S4 fibres via the pudendal nerve and by somatic fibres passing through the inferior hypogastric plexus.

Fascial and ligamentous supports of the bladder

At the posterolateral bladder neck, condensations of fascia pass forward medially and laterally to the ureter to join with the prostatic fascia; this fascia needs to be divided during cystectomy. The puboprostatic ligaments are well-defined condensations of the anterior endopelvic fascia; they stretch from the front of the prostate to the periosteum of the pubis and lie lateral to the dorsal vein complex. The urachus and obliterated hypogastric arteries, together with the folds of peritoneum overlying them, are called the median and lateral umbilical ligaments. Condensations of fascia also occur around the superior and inferior vascular pedicles.

Arteries

The superior and inferior vesical arteries are derived from the anterior trunk of the internal iliac artery. Branches from the obturator and inferior gluteal arteries (and from the uterine and vaginal arteries in females) also help to supply the bladder.

Veins

The veins form a plexus on the lateral and inferior surfaces of the bladder. In the male the prostatic plexus is continuous with the vesical plexus, which drains into the internal iliac vein. In the female similar large veins are continuous with the vaginal plexus.

Lymphatics

These accompany the veins and drain to nodes along the internal iliac vessels and then to the obturator and external iliac chains. Some lymphatics pass to nodes that are situated posteriorly to the internal iliac artery (hypogastric nodes).

INNERVATION (FIG. 72.1)

The parasympathetic input

This is derived from the anterior primary divisions of the second, third and fourth sacral segments (mainly S2 and S3). Fibres pass through the pelvic splanchnic nerves to the inferior hypogastric plexus, from where they are distributed to the bladder. The pelvic plexus can be damaged during deep pelvic operations.

The sympathetic input

This arises in the 11th thoracic to the second lumbar segments; fibres pass via the presacral hypogastric nerve (rather than via the sympathetic chains) to the inferior hypogastric plexus.

Somatic innervation

A somatic innervation passes to the distal sphincter mechanism via the pudendal nerves and also via fibres that pass through the inferior hypogastric plexus.

Functional aspects

Sympathetic nerves convey afferents from the fundus. Afferents

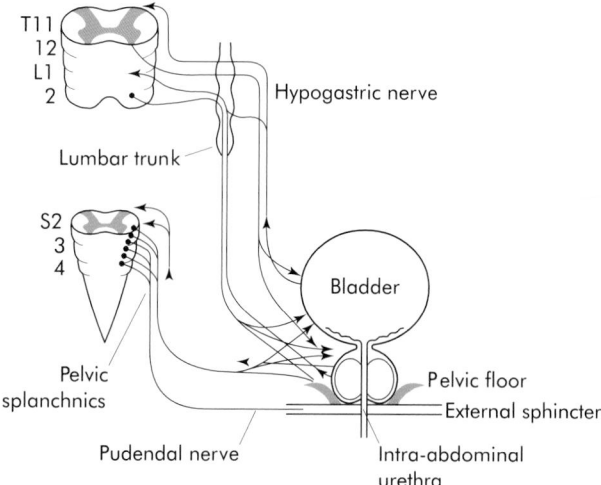

Figure 72.1 The nervous control of the bladder. Micturition is partly a reflex and partly a voluntary act.

arise from the mucosa, where they respond to touch, temperature and pain, and from the detrusor and lamina propria, where they convey stretch information. Afferents pass via the inferior hypogastric plexus to the posterior roots of S2–S4. Some aspects of micturition are centred in the pons, where detrusor contraction is coordinated with inhibition of the distal sphincter. Interruption of this pathway below the pons with preservation of the sacral cord is likely to result in a contractile detrusor and tonically active distal sphincter that will not relax during voiding (detrusor–sphincter dyssynergia).

CONGENITAL DEFECTS OF THE BLADDER

Bladder exstrophy (Fig. 72.2)

Clinical features

Bladder exstrophy occurs in 1:50 000 births (male–female ratio 4:1). In the male, the penis is broad and short, and bilateral

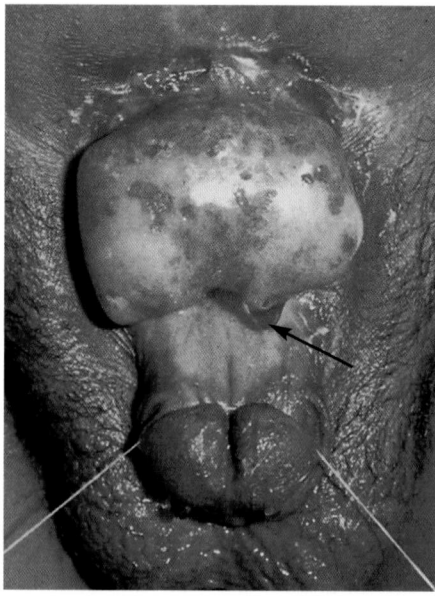

Figure 72.2 Ectopia vesicae in a male. A drop of urine (arrow) is seen at the left ureteric orifice, the corona glandis being retracted by threads (courtesy of G.D. Adhia, Bombay, India).

inguinal herniae may be present. There is separation of the pubic bones (Fig. 72.3). In epispadias alone, the pubes are united and external genitalia are almost normal, although in the female the clitoris is bifid (Fig. 72.4).

Treatment

The bladder is closed in the first year of life, usually following osteotomy of both iliac bones just lateral to the sacroiliac joints. Later, reconstruction of the bladder neck and sphincters is required. In some patients the reconstructed bladder remains small and requires augmentation. One-stage reconstruction is being practised in some major centres.

Less satisfactorily, urinary diversion can be carried out by means of ureterosigmoid anastomosis, an ileal or colonic conduit, or continent urinary diversion. Long-term complications include: (1) stricture at the site of anastomosis with bilateral hydronephrosis and infection; (2) hyperchloraemic acidosis; and (3) an increased (20-fold) risk of tumour formation (adenoma and adenocarcinoma) at the site of a ureterocolic anastomosis.

BLADDER TRAUMA

Bladder rupture

This can be intraperitoneal (20%) or extraperitoneal (80%) (Figs 72.5 and 72.6). Intraperitoneal rupture is usually secondary to a blow or fall on a distended bladder, more rarely to surgical damage. Extraperitoneal rupture is caused by blunt

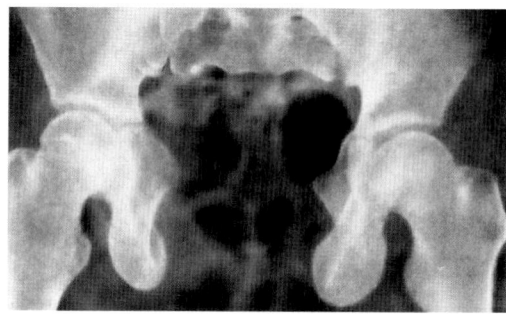

Figure 72.3 Separation of the pubes in a case of ectopia vesicae (courtesy of the late Professor Grey Turner, London, England).

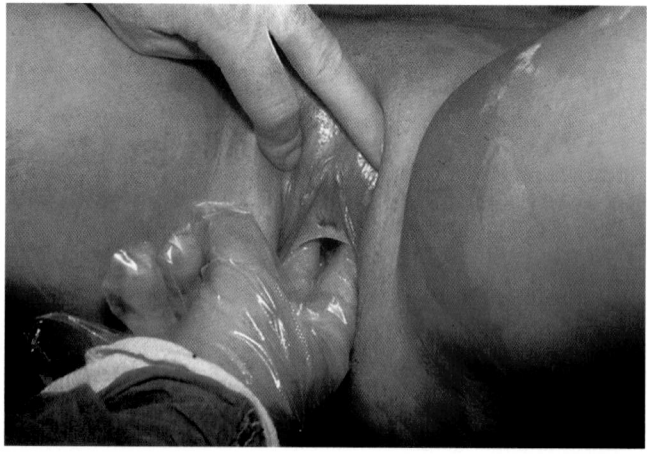

Figure 72.4 Female epispadias showing deficient sphincter and bifid clitoris.

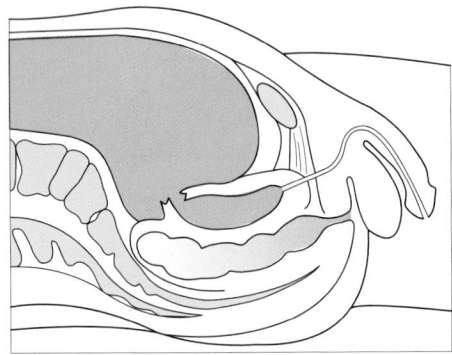

Figure 72.5 Intraperitoneal extravasation of urine.

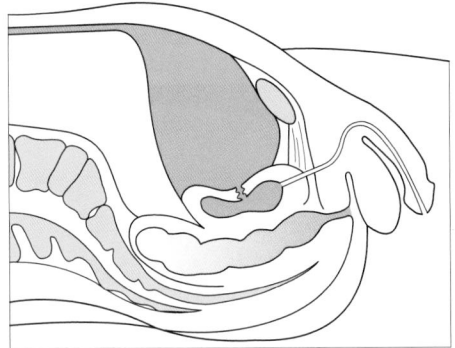

Figure 72.6 Extraperitoneal extravasation of urine.

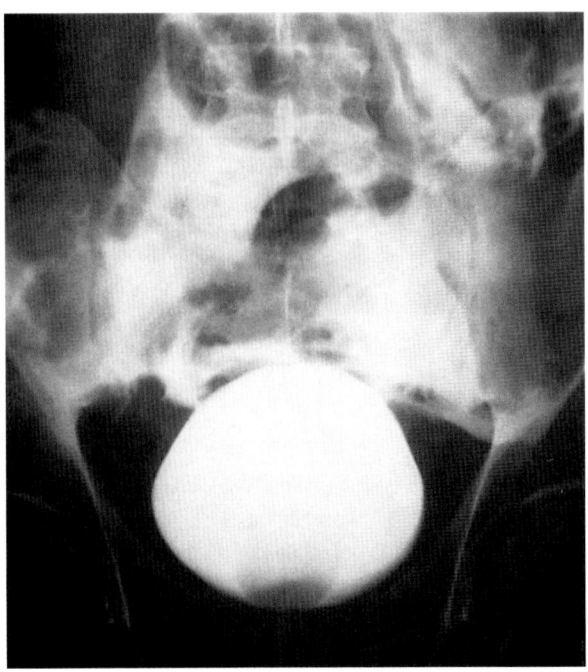

Figure 72.7 Cystogram of a patient who has fallen over and developed severe abdominal pain. Leakage of contrast into the peritoneal cavity is seen.

trauma or surgical damage. Gross haematuria can be absent. It may be difficult to distinguish extraperitoneal rupture from rupture of the membranous urethra (see Chapter 74). Intraperitoneal rupture is associated with sudden severe pain in the hypogastrium, often accompanied by syncope. The shock subsides and the abdomen distends and there is no desire to micturate. Peritonitis does not follow immediately if the urine is sterile; varying degrees of rigidity are present on examination.

Investigation

Computerised tomography (CT) is ideal. Plain erect radiographs may show a ground-glass appearance (fluid). Intravenous urography (IVU) may confirm a leak. Retrograde cystography will confirm the diagnosis (Fig. 72.7). It is important to image the patient after drainage of contrast as the full bladder may mask extravasation (Summary box 72.1).

Summary box 72.1

Bladder trauma

- Intraperitoneal or extraperitoneal
- Suspected if there is trauma and damage to the pelvis
- May be diagnosed by retrograde cystography

Treatment of intraperitoneal rupture

A lower midline laparotomy should be performed; the edges of the rent are trimmed and sutured with a single-layer 2/0 absorbable suture. A suprapubic and a urethral catheter are placed. Very rarely, the rupture will be through an unsuspected tumour; a biopsy can be taken before suturing the defect. Laparoscopic approaches are also now being used.

Injury to the bladder during operation

The bladder may be injured in: (1) inguinal or femoral herniotomy; (2) hysterectomy; and (3) excision of the rectum. If the injury is recognised, the bladder must be repaired and catheter drainage maintained for 7 days. If it is not recognised, the treatment is similar to that of rupture of the bladder.

When accidental extraperitoneal perforation of the bladder occurs during endoscopic resection, drainage of the bladder with a urethral catheter and the administration of antibiotics usually suffice. If a mass of extravasated fluid is present it is best to place a small drain through a stab incision. A laparotomy will usually be required if an intraperitoneal perforation is caused by transurethral resection (Summary box 72.2).

Summary box 72.2

Management of bladder trauma

- Extravesical injury – catheter drainage for 10 days
- Intraperitoneal injury – laparotomy, repair and bladder drainage

---

RETENTION OF URINE (SEE ALSO CHAPTER 73)

Acute retention

There are many possible causes of acute retention of urine (Summary box 72.3).

CHAPTER 72 | THE URINARY BLADDER

Summary box 72.3

The most frequent causes of acute retention

Male
- Bladder outlet obstruction (the commonest cause)
- Urethral stricture
- Acute urethritis or prostatitis
- Phimosis

Female
- Retroverted gravid uterus
- Bladder neck obstruction (rare)

Both
- Blood clot
- Urethral calculus
- Rupture of the urethra
- Neurogenic (injury or disease of the spinal cord)
- Smooth muscle cell dysfunction associated with ageing
- Faecal impaction
- Anal pain (haemorrhoidectomy)
- Intensive postoperative analgesic treatment
- Some drugs
- Spinal anaesthesia

Clinical features

- No urine is passed for several hours.
- Pain is present.
- The bladder is visible, palpable, tender (Fig. 72.8) and dull to percussion.
- Potential neurological causes should be excluded by checking reflexes in the lower limbs and perianal sensation.

Treatment

Treatment is to pass a fine urethral catheter (14F – French gauge is defined as the circumference in millimetres) and arrange urological management. Occasionally, in postoperative retention a warm bath can help (Figs 72.9–72.12).

Urethral catheterisation

Following a thorough hand wash, sterile gloves are donned. The genitalia are cleaned using soapy antiseptic. Lignocaine gel is inserted into the urethra, warning the patient that this may create stinging. The jelly should be massaged posteriorly in an

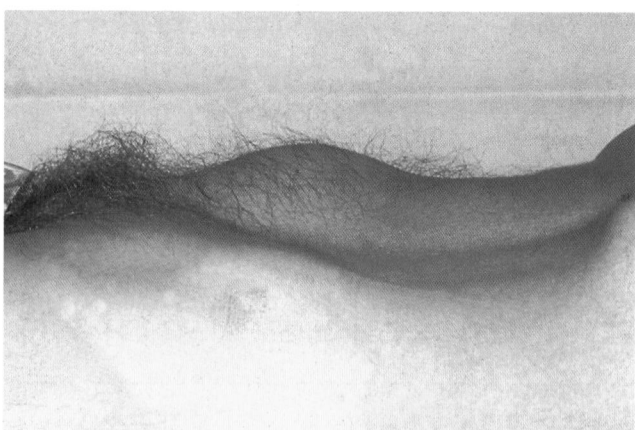

Figure 72.8 Distended bladder in a man who presented with retention of urine.

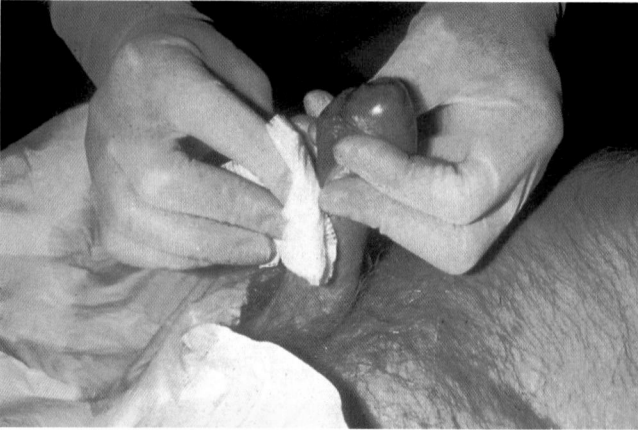

Figure 72.9 Cleaning of the penis before catheterisation.

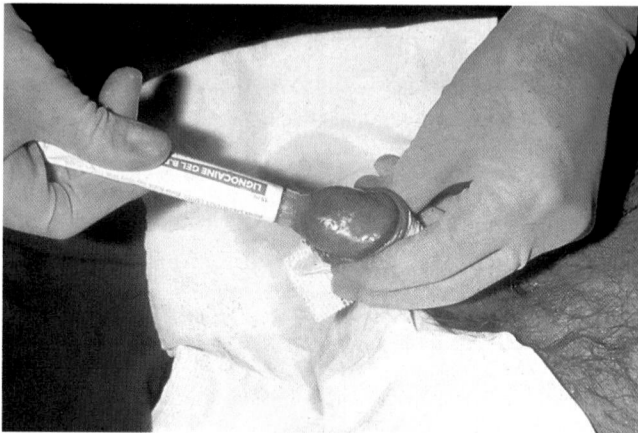

Figure 72.10 Insertion of local anaesthetic before insertion of a catheter.

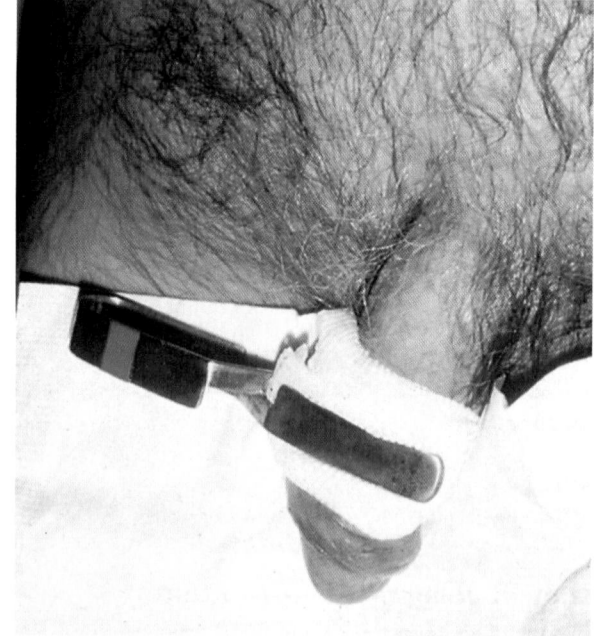

Figure 72.11 The use of a penile clamp to ensure that sufficient time is given to allow the anaesthetic to work before the catheter is inserted.

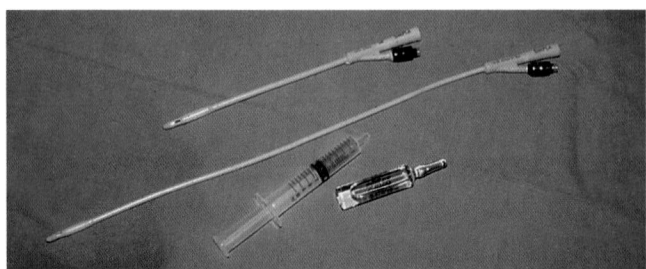

Figure 72.12 A selection of silicone catheters.

attempt to anaesthetise the sphincter region, and it is of advantage to place a penile clamp for several minutes. A small Foley catheter should be passed while the penis is held taut. In a female patient, the labia should be parted using the middle and index fingers of the left hand, which should not be moved once cleaning has been performed. Providing a stricture is not the cause, the catheter should pass freely. Once urine begins to drain it is wise to pass a few more centimetres of catheter into the bladder before the balloon is inflated to avoid inflation in the prostate. Force must not be used (Summary box 72.4).

Summary box 72.4

Catheterisation for acute retention of urine

Following catheterisation:

- Record the volume of urine drained
- Examine the abdomen to exclude other pathology (rupture of an aortic aneurysm, ureteric colic or diverticulitis can cause confusion)

If the catheter will not pass, it is usually due to poor technique, lack of anaesthesia, traumatisation of the urethra or a urethral stricture. Occasionally, a large prostatic middle lobe may prevent the catheter entering the bladder; sometimes a coudé catheter will pass. If a catheter cannot be passed the following plan should be pursued.

Suprapubic puncture

Suprapubic puncture with commercially available catheters such as Cystofix or Lawrence Add-a-Cath catheters is straightforward provided that the bladder is palpable. The skin, fascia and retropubicspace are anaesthetised with 0.5% lignocaine. Correct placement is confirmed by aspiration. A large-bore needle is then placed into the bladder, down which a fine catheter is passed (Cystofix) and then secured in position. The other option is to place a plastic suprapubic trocar and cannula, which has a removable plastic strip on the side. A standard 12F Foley catheter can be passed down the cannula, the balloon is inflated, the cannula is extracted and the strip is pulled away from the catheter (Add-a-Cath). If urine cannot be aspirated through the fine-bore needle, passing a suprapubic trocar should not be attempted.

If these devices are not available, a catheter can be placed in the bladder under direct vision through a small incision under local anaesthetic.

Frederic Eugene Basil Foley, **1891–1966, Urologist, Anker Hospital, St Paul, MN, USA.**

Urethral instrumentation

In a patient with a known stricture, an experienced urologist may elect to dilate the stricture or to take the patient to theatre to carry out an optical urethrotomy (see Chapter 74).

Chronic retention

In chronic retention there is no pain. These patients are at risk of upper tract dilatation because of high intravesical tension – they require urgent urological referral. Men with impaired renal function may develop postobstructive diuresis following catheterisation. Such men need careful monitoring, with replacement of inappropriate urinary losses by intravenous saline; they are also at risk of haematuria as the distended urinary tract empties. Often it is several days before full renal recovery occurs.

Retention with overflow

The patient is incontinent with small amounts of urine passing involuntarily from the distended bladder. It usually follows a neglected retention.

Indwelling catheters and closed systems of catheter drainage

The risk of ascending infection is decreased by connecting the catheter to sterile tubing connected to a collecting bag. Irrigations should be avoided unless clot retention occurs. When a catheter has been *in situ* for a few days, some degree of urethritis and bacteriuria is likely; changing a catheter then entails risks of severe infection if prophylactic antibiotics are not used (Fig. 72.13).

Acute retention due to drugs

A number of drugs can induce retention, including antihistamines, anti-hypertensives, anti-cholinergics and tricyclic antidepressants.

The acute neuropathic bladder

1 Immediately after spinal cord injury, 'spinal shock' occurs (see Chapter 33), which may last for days or months. The detrusor is not able to contract, the bladder distends and overflow incontinence occurs. Neglected bladder distension will lead to

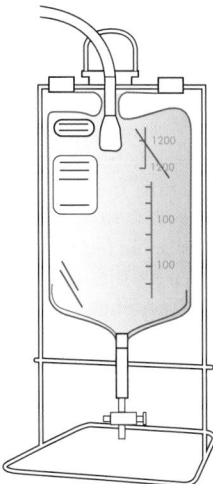

Figure 72.13 Modern Simpla bag used for continuous bladder drainage. (The nurse who is emptying the bag should be wearing disposable gloves to avoid contaminating the hands with organisms.)

damage to the detrusor, infection and ultimately renal failure. Management is as follows:

2 The bladder must be emptied by aseptic intermittent catheterisation performed two or three times daily or the use of an indwelling urethral catheter on continuous drainage, making sure that the patient has a high urinary output (3 litres per day) to combat infection. Currently, intermittent catheterisation is preferred as soon as the patient's spinal injury is stable.

3 Neurological examination must be performed to assess the level of sensory and motor loss. Ischaemic necrosis of the cord may extend below the upper level of cord injury. When sensory loss below the upper level is total, recovery is unlikely. Incomplete lesions may recover somatic and bladder function.

4 Demonstration of intact bulbocavernosus and anal reflexes indicates that the sacral cord and nerves are intact and that reflex bladder contractions are likely to develop, though they may be insufficient to empty the bladder. If there is persistent total loss of reflexes and perineal sensation then either the sacral cord or cauda equina is damaged. In such circumstances an acontractile bladder is likely. In cauda equina lesions there may be sensory, motor or mixed loss.

5 Full urodynamic assessment of bladder function should be undertaken when the injury is stable. This allows an accurate assessment of bladder and sphincter activity and will enable decisions to be made about further management; the prime aim is to prevent upper tract damage by promoting good bladder emptying (Summary box 72.5).

Summary box 72.5

Clinical management of spinal injury

- The bladder should be emptied during spinal shock by catheterisation
- Encourage high fluid intake
- Commence intermittent catheterisation
- When the patient is stable undertake full urodynamic evaluation

---

The following situations represent the typical patterns of bladder function seen after spinal cord injury.

Lesions above T10

Usually leads to an 'upper motor neurone' bladder with reflexes intact but isolated from higher control mechanisms. Such patients are at risk of autonomic dysreflexia.

Because of detrusor–sphincter dyssynergia, bladder contractions are high pressure and ineffective in producing bladder emptying; the bladder neck is normally open. If left untreated, upper tract dilatation and renal failure may result. Bladder capacity is usually decreased with the development of trabeculation and a typical 'fir-tree' appearance. Patients are incontinent during high-pressure phasic contractions because the sphincter resistance suddenly diminishes.

Some patients with low-pressure bladders that empty may be managed by means of condom drainage. Others will require clean intermittent self-catheterisation (CISC), popularised by Lapides. Patients with poor emptying, low bladder capacity and upper tract dilatation require treatment with endoscopic sphincterotomy and condom drainage. Some carefully selected patients may require bladder reconstruction.

Lesions involving the sympathetic outflow (T11, T12, L1, L2)

These patients are usually similar to the group with lesions above T10.

Damage to the sacral centre S2, S3, S4 and cauda equina lesions

Usually leads to a 'lower motor neurone' bladder, also found in spina bifida (myelodysplasia); the detrusor is acontractile. Abdominal straining can produce reasonable emptying but the mainstay is CISC. Some patients may have sensation of filling through the hypogastric nerves if T11 and T12 are intact. The bladder capacity may be good, but some patients have high resting pressures and high increases during bladder filling, which means that there is a risk to the upper urinary tract. The bladder neck is usually open and the distal sphincter mechanisms may be paralysed but of fixed resistance. Vesicoureteric reflux is common and upper tract damage is frequent in neglected cases. Patients who can achieve satisfactory bladder emptying by means of CISC usually have reasonable continence.

Bladder dysfunction after excision of the rectum or radical hysterectomy

Between 10% and 15% of patients undergoing radical rectal excision for cancer sustain damage to the inferior hypogastric plexus, leading to impotence in the male and neurogenic bladder dysfunction. This type of bladder dysfunction is similar to the cauda equina lesion. Postoperative retention in other patients may also be caused by simple bladder outlet obstruction. The best plan is to catheterise the patient to allow postoperative recovery and then carry out urodynamic investigation to determine the appropriate treatment.

INCONTINENCE OF URINE

Overall, urinary incontinence occurs in 5% of men and 20% of women. Up to 40% of women over the age of 60 years and 50% of institutionalised elderly patients experience regular episodes of urinary incontinence. Health problems include skin breakdown and depression, and loss of esteem and sexual activity. Continence is dependent on normal mobility and brain function allowing a perception of when it is socially acceptable to void, normal bladder sensation, normal voluntary detrusor contraction producing good bladder emptying, a normally competent sphincter mechanism, which relaxes appropriately during a voluntary detrusor contraction allowing good bladder emptying, and good bladder capacity with normally low pressures during filling. This is clearly a fine balance and several factors can cause incontinence. Several investigations are required for diagnosis of urinary incontinence (Summary box 72.6).

Summary box 72.6

Diagnosis of urinary incontinence

The following investigations are required:

- A careful history and physical examination and completion of frequency voiding charts
- Urodynamic testing in most patients and in all patients in whom surgical intervention is proposed
- Urine culture to exclude infection and measurement of serum creatinine

In selected cases IVU is carried out if a ureteric fistula is suspected, although ultrasound examination will often provide adequate details

---

Urodynamic testing

The key to the practical management of lower urinary tract dysfunction, and particularly incontinence, lies with urodynamic investigation. The principle is to artificially simulate bladder filling and emptying while obtaining pressure measurements (Fig. 72.14).

The patient attends with a full bladder and is allowed to void in private to measure the maximum urinary flow rate. After voiding, the residual urine is measured by ultrasound. A pair of catheters or a twin-lumen catheter is passed into the bladder, which allows the bladder to be filled at a rate of 50 ml min^{-1} while a continuous recording of intravesical pressure is made. To obtain 'true' detrusor pressure, a second channel is required to assess intra-abdominal pressure, measured by means of a small intra-rectal or intravaginal balloon. The bladder is filled until the patient states that the bladder is full. Radiographic screening may be carried out to assess bladder neck closure and urinary leakage during movement or coughing (stress incontinence) or during bouts of phasic detrusor pressure (detrusor instability). The patient is then asked to void at the end of bladder filling after the filling catheter has been removed (Fig. 72.15).

The normal bladder will accept approximately 400–550 ml when filled at room temperature at a rate of < 50 ml min^{-1}. The pressure increase in the bladder should be less than 15 cmH$_2$O. In addition, phasic pressure increases should not be seen. The normal voiding pressure should not exceed 60 cmH$_2$O in men and about 40 cmH$_2$O in women, with a flow rate of between 20 and 25 ml s^{-1}.

Common abnormalities identified during urodynamic testing in incontinence

Detrusor instability

Phasic increases in pressure give rise to urgency and urge incontinence (detrusor instability; Fig. 72.16). This abnormality is found in patients with neurogenic bladder dysfunction, such as in multiple sclerosis (MS) or Parkinson's disease or following a

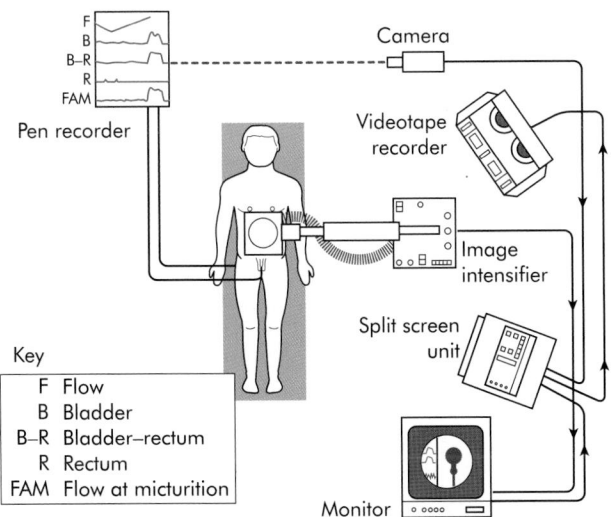

Figure 72.14 Urodynamic study.

Key
F	Flow
B	Bladder
B–R	Bladder–rectum
R	Rectum
FAM	Flow at micturition

James Parkinson, **1755–1824, a General Practitioner of Shoreditch, London, England, published 'An Essay on the Shaking Palsy' in 1817.**

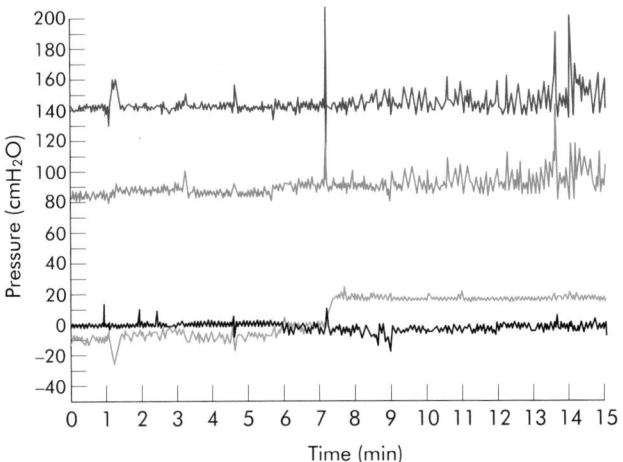

Figure 72.15 A section of an ambulatory, natural-fill urodynamic trace. The rectal pressure is in red, the bladder pressure in blue and the subtracted detrusor trace in black. The orange trace is the output of an electronic nappy, which records urinary leakage. A cough is shown, which results in genuine stress incontinence.

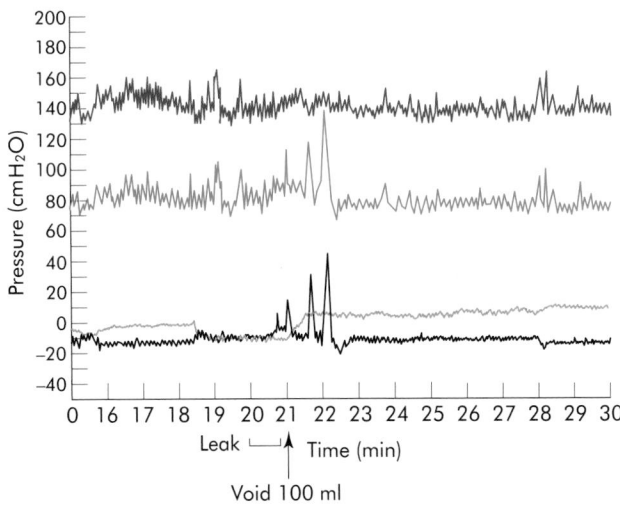

Figure 72.16 A section of an ambulatory, natural-fill urodynamic trace. The rectal pressure is in red, the bladder pressure in blue and the subtracted detrusor trace in black. The orange trace is the output of an electronic nappy which records urinary leakage. Phasic activity is shown, which is detrusor instability resulting in urge incontinence.

stroke or spinal injury, when it is known as detrusor hyperreflexia. About 50% of men with bladder outflow obstruction have detrusor instability, and in about half of them the instability resolves after prostatectomy. Idiopathic detrusor instability is common and must be distinguished from genuine stress incontinence (GSI) in women before performing bladder neck suspension procedures.

Genuine stress incontinence

This is defined as urinary leakage occurring during increased bladder pressure when this is solely due to increased abdominal pressure and not to increased true detrusor pressure (see Fig. 72.15). It is caused by sphincter weakness.

Chronic urinary retention

Chronic urinary retention with overflow incontinence is recognised by a large residual volume of urine (Fig. 72.17) and is usually associated with high pressures during bladder filling.

Bladder outflow obstruction

Bladder outflow obstruction is associated with increased voiding pressures, often in excess of 90 cmH$_2$O (Fig. 72.18), coupled with low urinary flow rates.

Neurogenic dysfunction

Neurogenic bladder dysfunction may also be identified (Summary box 72.7).

Summary box 72.7

Uses of urodynamic testing

- To distinguish GSI (due to sphincter weakness) from detrusor instability in women (see Fig. 72.15)
- For the classification of neurogenic bladder dysfunction
- To distinguish bladder outflow obstruction from idiopathic detrusor instability in men
- To investigate incontinence or other lower urinary tract symptoms

---

Causes of incontinence

There are various ways of classifying the causes of incontinence.

- *Problems of social control.* Patients with dementia often have incontinence because of uninhibited detrusor hyperreflexia and impaired social perception.
- *Storage problems.* Patients with a small bladder capacity owing to fibrosis (tuberculosis, radiotherapy or interstitial cystitis) can develop incontinence. Patients with a small functional capacity owing to severe detrusor instability, neurogenic dysfunction or infection can develop incontinence.
- *Impairment of emptying.* Patients with chronic retention or neurogenic bladder dysfunction have small functional bladder capacities with detrusor overactivity causing incontinence, despite having large residual volumes of urine.
- *Weak sphincter.* This leads to GSI.

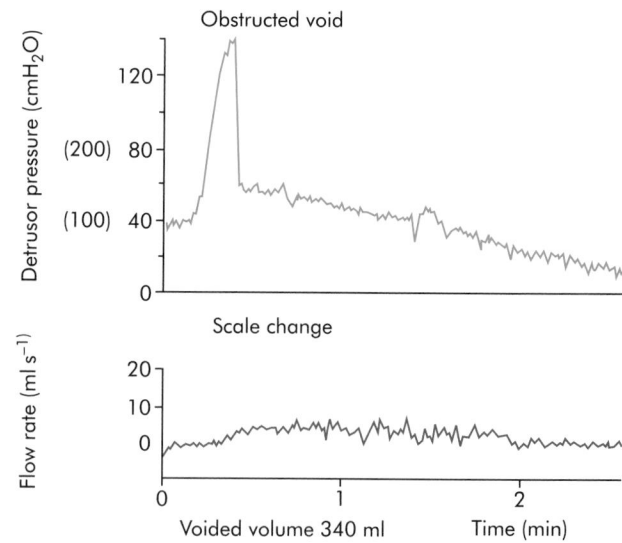

Figure 72.18 A conventional urodynamic trace showing detrusor pressure during voiding. There has been a change of scale because the pressure was so high; voiding pressures are increased with a low flow rate, which is diagnostic of bladder outflow obstruction.

- *Fistulae.* Leakage from fistulae or upper tract duplication with an ectopic ureter.

The common causes may be classified into male, female or mixed-sex groups.

Male incontinence

Chronic urinary retention with overflow

This may be due to benign prostatic hypertrophy, carcinoma of the prostate, urethral stricture and, in younger men, hypertrophy of the bladder neck. Examination may reveal that the bladder is distended, and it can be confirmed by ultrasound scanning. The treatment is discussed in Chapter 73.

Post-prostatectomy

Post-prostatectomy incontinence may result from injury to the external sphincter mechanism. Treatment may necessitate insertion of an artificial urethral sphincter (Fig. 72.19).

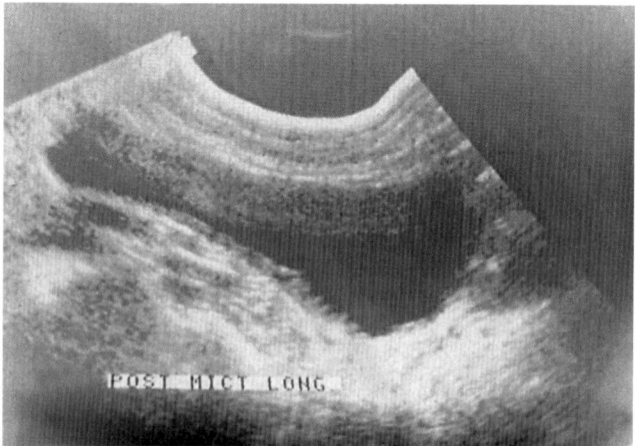

Figure 72.17 An ultrasound scan showing a large post-void residual urine.

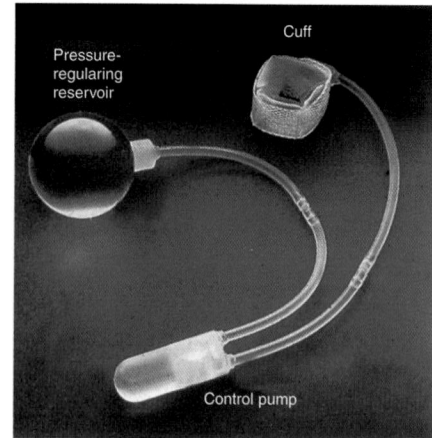

Figure 72.19 The artificial urinary sphincter made by American Medical Systems.

Female incontinence

Stress incontinence

The most common cause is GSI although, in some parts of the world, vesicourethral fistulae as a result of neglected labour are common. It is usually found in multiparous women with a history of difficult labour. It can be found in normal young women who indulge in competitive trampolining and in patients with epispadias. The classical symptom is urine loss during coughing, laughing, sneezing or a sudden change of posture. The symptoms may change with the menstrual cycle. The volume of urine loss can be measured during an exercise test, which is performed by putting the patient through a standard set of tests with 300 ml of fluid in the bladder; in GSI the fluid losses usually range from 10 to 50 ml. Urinary frequency and urgency are often found in such patients as they try to avoid incontinence by frequent voiding.

Idiopathic detrusor instability can mimic GSI and coexist with it. It is important to make a correct preoperative diagnosis by urodynamic measurements, as the outcome of surgery is suboptimal in women with idiopathic detrusor instability.

Minor to moderate stress urinary incontinence can be controlled by pelvic floor exercises. However, if this fails, surgery is indicated. Standard operations include open colposuspension or the use of a minimally invasive approach involving the insertion of a transvaginal tape (TVT procedure).

Open colposuspension

This operation is carried out through a Pfannenstiel incision with the patient in the Lloyd-Davies position. The vaginal fascia is identified by sweeping the bladder off the vagina and three sutures are placed on each side between the vaginal fascia and the iliopubic ligament. A suprapubic catheter is placed. Voiding difficulties are frequent but usually temporary. It is best to warn women with large bladder capacities and low voiding pressures that this complication may occur and that they may be required to carry out CISC for a period. The operation is very successful for the treatment of GSI, with good results at 1 year in 90% of patients, which are maintained in about 80% of patients at 5 years.

Modifications of bladder neck suspension can also be achieved by minimally invasive approaches such as the transvaginal sling. This technique does reduce both hospital stay and postoperative morbidity.

Incontinence common to both sexes

Idiopathic detrusor overactivity

Phasic increases in bladder pressure may occur during filling in otherwise normal patients (idiopathic) or it may be found in neurogenic bladder dysfunction (when it is known as detrusor hyperreflexia) and bladder outflow obstruction. Idiopathic detrusor overactivity may be symptomless but usually results in symptoms of frequency, urgency, urge incontinence, nocturia or nocturnal incontinence (enuresis) depending on the severity of the instability. It must be distinguished from GSI and from bladder outflow obstruction before surgical treatment. Infection, tuberculosis or carcinoma *in situ* (CIS) should be excluded. The mainstay of treatment is the use of various anti-cholinergic

medications (oxybutynin and tolterodine). Severe symptoms resistant to conventional conservative treatment resulting in major impairment of quality of life may need more aggressive treatment such as enterocystoplasty or the injection of small doses of botulinum toxin (the toxin from *Clostridium botulinum*), known as BoTox, which blocks cholinergic neuromuscular transmission, at least for a time.

Ageing

Ageing can result in smooth muscle cell dysfunction, which can cause combinations of small functional capacity, detrusor overactivity, impaired bladder emptying and symptoms of lower urinary tract dysfunction.

Congenital

Congenital causes include ectopic vesicae and severe epispadias. The abnormal entry of an ectopic ureter distal to the sphincter complex or into the vagina in a female patient should theoretically result in total urinary incontinence. This is discussed in Chapters 6 and 71.

Trauma

Trauma, whether from pelvic surgery or associated with pelvic fracture, may result in disruption of the nerve supply to the bladder or urethra, or in fistula formation.

Infection

Lower urinary tract infection (UTI) may be sufficient to induce urinary incontinence. A history of frequency, burning and a fever should prompt the diagnosis. Symptoms will usually settle with a course of antibiotics, but in the case of recurrent infection further investigation of the urinary tract will clearly be indicated.

Neoplasia

Locally advanced cancers in the pelvis, particularly carcinoma of the cervix in a woman and carcinoma of the prostate in a man, may result in direct invasion of the sphincter mechanism causing incontinence; occasionally, fistula formation may occur in women.

Other causes

Constant dribbling of urine coupled with normal micturition

This occurs when there is a ureteric fistula or an ectopic ureter associated with a duplex system opening into the urethra beyond the urethral sphincter in females or into the vagina. The history is diagnostic, and intravenous pyelography or ultrasound scanning may reveal the upper pole segment, which is often poorly functioning. Treatment is by excision of the aberrant ureter and portion of kidney. A ureteric fistula can be difficult to diagnose and its demonstration may require retrograde ureterography and a high degree of suspicion.

Nocturnal enuresis

This is a condition of young children and young adults. Of course, the time at which children become dry at night varies and, in some, nocturnal enuresis is merely a delayed onset of continence. In others, it persists until late adolescence and is classified into primary and secondary nocturnal enuresis.

Hermann Johann Pfannenstiel, **1862–1909**, Gynaecologist, Breslau, Germany, (now Wroclaw, Poland), described this incision in 1900.
Oswald Lloyd-Davies, **1905–1987**, Surgeon, St Mark's Hospital and The Middlesex Hospital, London, England.

Primary nocturnal enuresis occurs in patients with nocturnal enuresis alone and with no daytime symptoms. Often, they have been dry for a period, and the vast majority of patients will eventually become dry. In the meantime, a sympathetic approach to these children is essential. They often respond to a system of rewards using a 'star' chart. In addition, the use of DDAVP (a vasopressin analogue) can produce increased urinary concentration at night with a decrease in nocturnal incontinence. Other treatments include the use of amitriptyline and an alarm that wakes the child (or at least the child's parents) when incontinence occurs.

Treatments for incontinence

Treatments are listed below. Management is dependent on making a correct diagnosis.

Management and treatment

Problems of social functioning

Patients with dementia may respond to regular toileting. Anticholinergic agents can cause increased confusion in these patients and often, in severe cases, an indwelling catheter is needed.

Storage problems

Patients with a small bladder capacity because of fibrosis may require augmentation cystoplasty. Detrusor overactivity will require treatment with anti-cholinergic medication but, in severe cases, particularly in neuropathic patients at high risk of upper tract dilatation, bladder substitution (near-total supratrigonal cystectomy followed by the need for detubularised ileocaecal segment bladder substitution) or augmentation (enterocystoplasty) may be needed. These procedures should be carried out only after careful assessment in units used to dealing with such problems. Patients with very impaired mobility and MS may require ileal conduit diversion. The use of intravesical injections of BoTox has provided good improvements, and it may avoid or delay the need for major surgery.

Impaired bladder emptying

Patients with overflow incontinence because of bladder outflow obstruction will usually respond well to prostatectomy. Patients with impaired bladder emptying because of neurogenic bladder dysfunction should be treated in the first place by means of CISC.

Weak sphincter

Patients with GSI should be treated by means of pelvic floor exercises initially. Duloxetine can be used now as medical treatment for GSI. Bulking agents, such as macroplastique, can be used and can provide good temporary solutions. Surgical treatment by means of colposuspension or TVT may be needed. Those with post-prostatectomy incontinence or neurogenic bladder dysfunction may need to be fitted with an artificial urinary sphincter (Fig. 72.19), if they are well motivated and mobile, but careful assessment is required.

Use of appliances

An indwelling catheter drained constantly into a leg urinal may be a satisfactory solution although, in some instances, diversion via an ileal conduit is necessary. In men, a condom urinary appliance may be satisfactory and can avoid an indwelling catheter.

More major surgical treatments

Various types of urinary diversion

Urinary diversion may be required for the treatment of end-stage incontinence that is not otherwise treatable (see later in this chapter).

Bladder substitution procedures

The principle behind these operations is the creation of a low-pressure, large-capacity reservoir, which can be made using any segment of bowel isolated on its vascular pedicle (Figs 72.20–72.22). This is then detubularised by dividing its anti-mesenteric border and suturing this into a plate, which is then reconfigured into a spherical structure. This reservoir can then be anastomosed to the bladder remnant after excision of the fundus above the trigone. If necessary, the ureters can be reimplanted into the bowel segment. This new bladder will need to be emptied by means of CISC in up to 30% of cases.

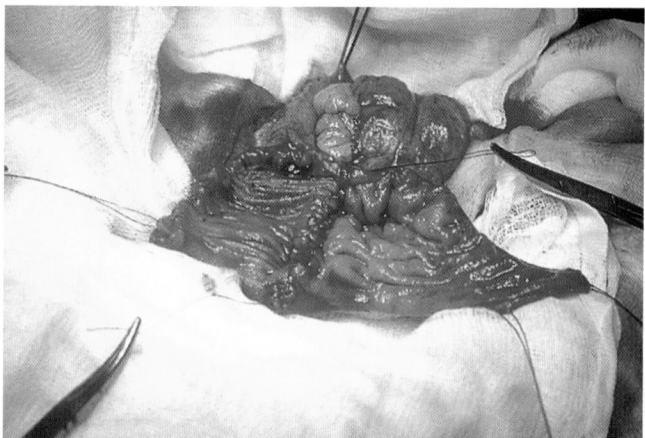

Figure 72.20 A vascularised ileocaecal segment being detubularised.

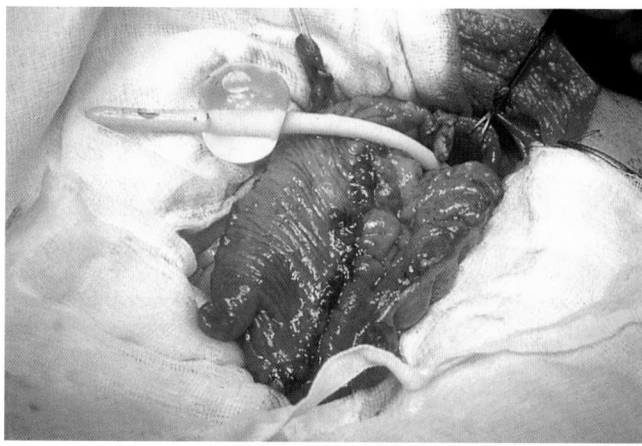

Figure 72.21 An ileocaecal segment being anastomosed to the trigone after near-total cystectomy; the left ureter is about to be implanted by means of a Camay–Le Duc anastomosis.

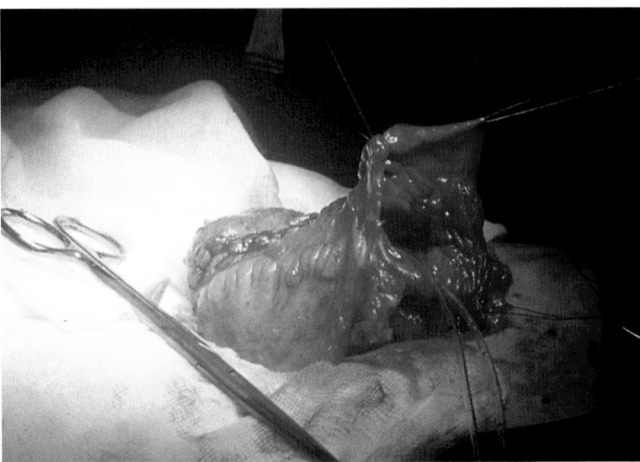

Figure 72.22 A capacious ileocaecal reservoir to be used in a patient requiring bladder substitution. These segments may be used for total bladder replacement, bladder substitution and the construction of continent diversion with a Mitrofanoff-type anti-incontinence mechanism (see later in the chapter).

'Clam' enterocystoplasty

This procedure was originally described by Bramble for the treatment of nocturnal enuresis. It has been used in the treatment of idiopathic detrusor instability. (Fig. 72.23). This procedure can also be used as an augmentation procedure in patients with neurogenic bladder dysfunction and a reasonable bladder capacity (approximately 300 ml).

Fitment of artificial urinary sphincter

See Fig. 72.19.

Summary

Treatments for incontinence can be summarised as follows:

1 *Devices for collection*: external penile condom, or an indwelling urethral or suprapubic catheter.

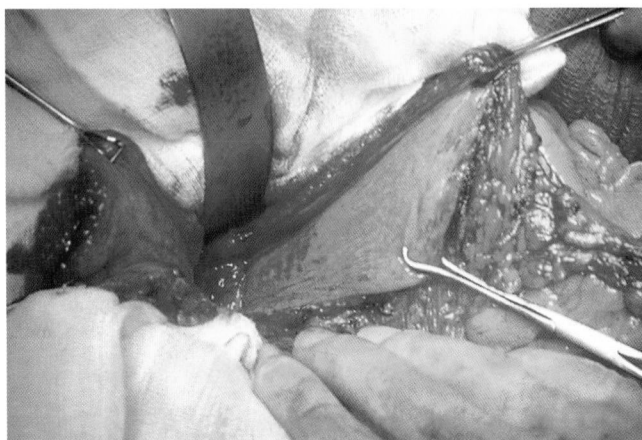

Figure 72.23 A 'clam' cystoplasty being performed. The ureteric orifices can be seen with the interureteric bar; the defect will be filled by a segment of detubularised ileum, performing a bladder augmentation.

Frank James Bramble, **formerly Urologist, The Royal Victoria Hospital, Bournemouth, England.**

2 *Drugs*: to decrease the strength of the bladder neck (e.g. α-adrenergic blockers); with mixed action on the bladder neck and central nervous system (e.g. tricyclic drugs); to inhibit bladder activity (e.g. anti-cholinergic drugs). Botulinum toxin is used in carefully selected patients. Duloxetine can now be used as medical treatment for GSI – it is a serotonin–noradrenaline (norepinephrine) reuptake inhibitor.

3 *Intermittent self-catheterisation*: to improve emptying.

4 *Increasing outlet*: pelvic floor physiotherapy; resistance colposuspension or TVT tapes or slings; periurethral injections of 'bulking agents' such as cross-linked collagen or other particles; use of the artificial urinary sphincter.

5 *Denervation of bladder*: S3 sacral nerve blockade, neurectomy or surgical transection of the bladder to inhibit bladder activity and improve functional capacity. These are rarely used nowadays because of the use of botulinum toxin and the clam cystoplasty or S3 nerve stimulation (see point 6).

6 *Sacral nerve stimulation devices* can improve incontinence. They involve percutaneous insertion of electrodes through the sacral foramina under radiological control and implantation of an electronic stimulator.

7 *Augmentation of bladder*: 'clam' enterocystoplasty, bladder capacity substitution with detubularised bowel segment.

8 *Urinary diversion*: ileal conduit, continent urinary diversion.

BLADDER STONES

Definition

A primary bladder stone is one that develops in sterile urine; it often originates in the kidney. A secondary stone occurs in the presence of infection, outflow obstruction, impaired bladder emptying or a foreign body.

Incidence

Until the twentieth century, bladder stone was a prevalent disorder among poor children and adolescents. Because of improved diet, especially an increased protein–carbohydrate ratio, primary vesical calculus is rare.

Composition and cystoscopic appearance

Most vesical calculi are mixed. An oxalate calculus is a primary calculus that grows slowly; usually, it is of moderate size and solitary, and its surface is uneven (Fig. 72.24). Although calcium oxalate is white, the stone is usually dark brown or black because of the incorporation of blood pigment. Uric acid calculi are round or oval, smooth and vary in colour from yellow to brown (Fig. 72.25). They occur in patients with gout but are also found in patients with ileostomies or with bladder outflow obstruction. A cystine calculus occurs only in the presence of cystinuria and is radio-opaque because of its high sulphur content. A triple phosphate calculus is composed of ammonium, magnesium and calcium phosphates and occurs in urine infected with urea-splitting organisms. It tends to grow rapidly. In some instances it occurs on a nucleus of one of the other types of calculus; more rarely it occurs on a foreign body (Figs 72.26 and 72.27). It is dirty white in colour and of chalky consistency.

A bladder stone is usually free to move in the bladder and it gravitates to the lowest part of the bladder. Less commonly, the stone is wholly or partially in a diverticulum, where it may be hidden from view.

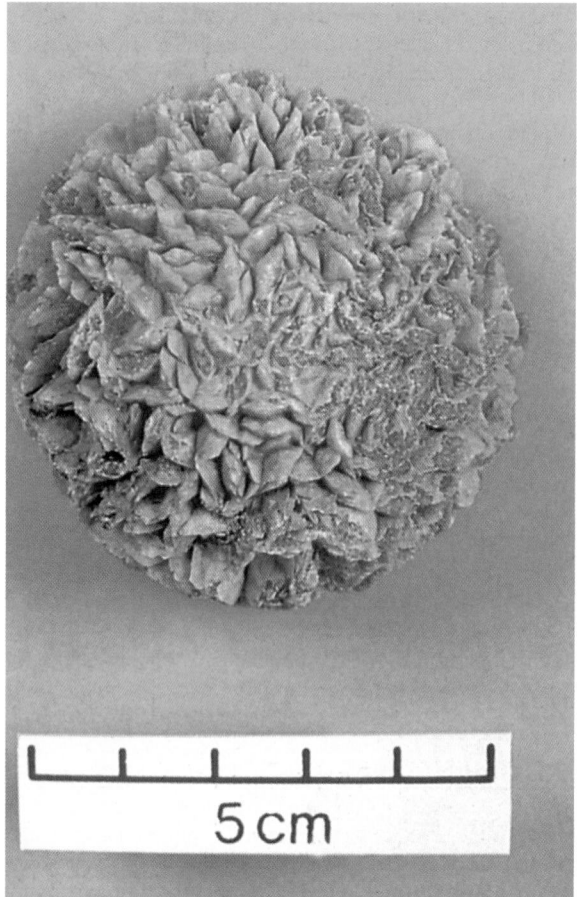

Figure 72.24   A rough bladder stone.

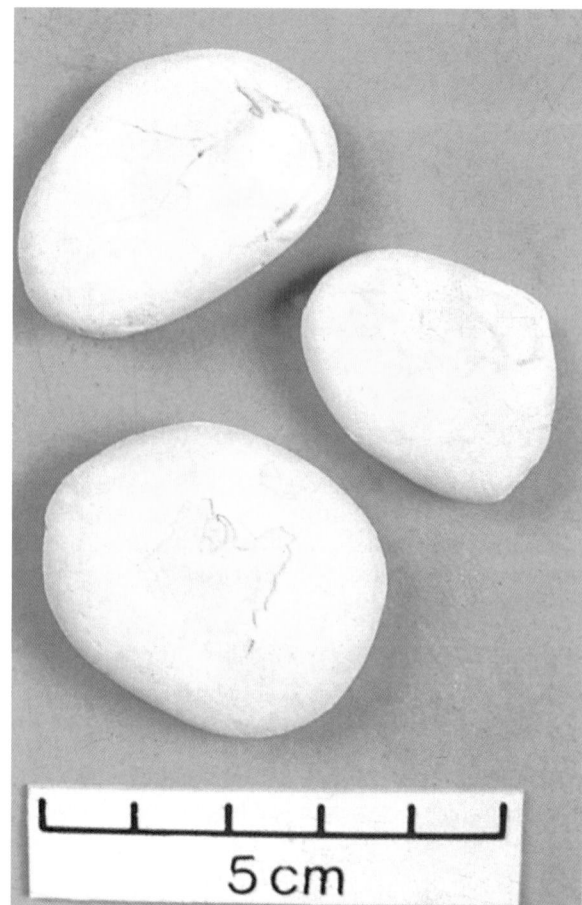

Figure 72.25   Smooth uric acid-type stones.

Clinical features

Men are affected eight times more frequently than women. Stones may be asymptomatic and found incidentally.

Symptoms

Frequency is the earliest symptom and there may be a sensation of incomplete bladder emptying. Pain (strangury) is most often found in patients with a spiculated oxalate calculus. It occurs at the end of micturition and is referred to the tip of the penis or to the labia majora; more rarely it is referred to the perineum or suprapubic region. The pain is worsened by movement. In young boys, screaming and pulling at the penis with the hand at the end of micturition are indicative of bladder stone. Haematuria is characterised by the passage of a few drops of bright-red blood at the end of micturition, and is due to the stone abrading the vascular trigone. Interruption of the urinary stream is due to the stone blocking the internal meatus. Urinary infection is a common presenting symptom.

Examination

Rectal or vaginal examination is normal; occasionally, a large calculus is palpable in the female. Examination of the urine reveals microscopic haematuria, pus or crystals that are typical of the calculus, for example envelope-like in the case of an oxalate stone or hexagonal plates in the case of cystine calculi. In most patients the stone is visible on ultrasound or on a plain radiogram (Fig. 72.28). Imaging of the whole of the urinary tract should be undertaken to exclude an upper tract stone. Nearly all stones can be

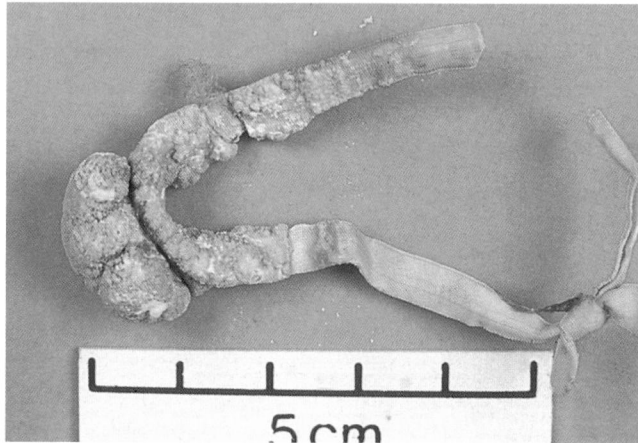

Figure 72.26   Stone on a vaginal sling that had eroded into the bladder.

dealt with endoscopically. In men with bladder outflow obstruction, endoscopic resection of the prostate should be performed at the same time as the stone is dealt with.

Treatment

The cause of the stone should be sought and treated; this may include bladder outflow obstruction or incomplete bladder emptying in patients with neurogenic bladder dysfunction.

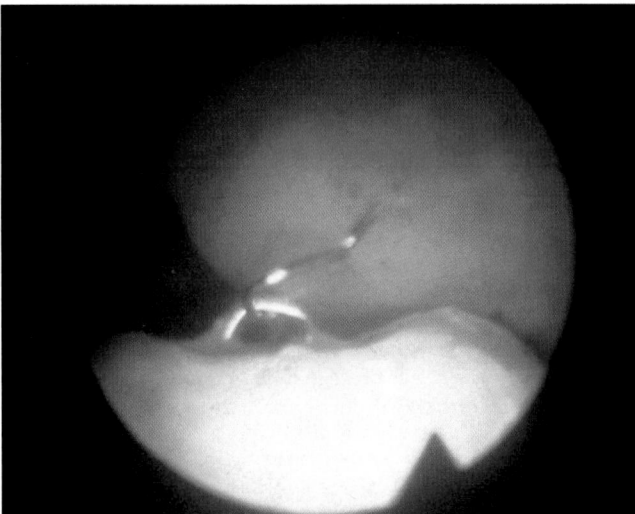

Figure 72.27 Uric acid stones that had formed on metal staples used to construct a colonic bladder augmentation.

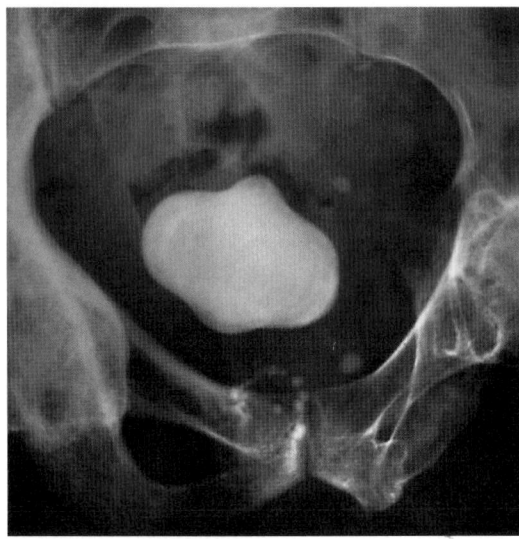

Figure 72.28 Radiograph showing a vesical calculus (no contrast has been used).

Litholapaxy

The blind lithotrite (Fig. 72.29) was an early type of minimally invasive technique. Standard management now includes the optical lithotrite, electrohydraulic lithotrite, Holmium laser or ultrasound probe (Fig. 72.30). Other devices include the stone punch, which is useful to crush small fragments further so that they can be evacuated with an Ellik evacuator. Contraindications to perurethral litholapaxy are extremely rare:

- *urethral*: a urethral stricture that cannot be dilated sufficiently; when a patient is aged below 10 years;
- *bladder*: a contracted bladder;
- *stone characteristics*: a very large stone.

Ultrasound lithotripsy is extremely safe but appropriate only for small stones. Laser lithotripsy with the holmium laser can deal

Milo Ellik, **B. 1905, American Urologist.**

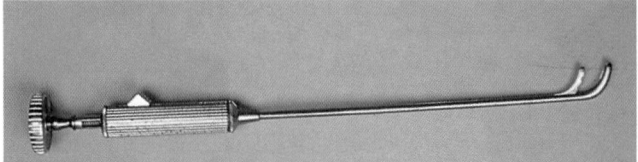

Figure 72.29 'Blind' lithotrite used to crush bladder stones.

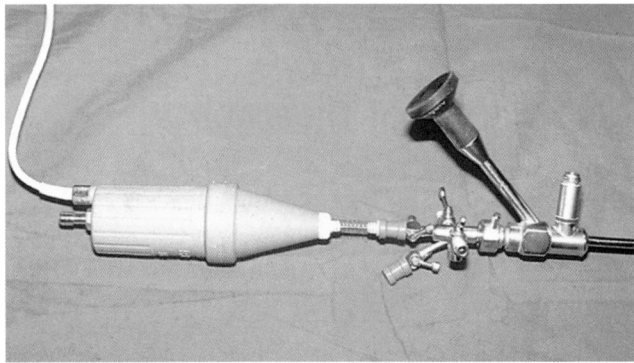

Figure 72.30 An endoscopic ultrasound probe, which is used to fragment bladder or kidney stones.

with most large stones. Once small fragments are produced, the optical lithotrite can be used to finish the job. For evacuation of the fragments, fluid (200 ml) is introduced into the bladder. The evacuator, filled with solution, is fitted on to the sheath. The bulb is compressed slowly and then permitted to expand; the returning solution carries with it fragments of stone.

Percutaneous suprapubic litholapaxy

It is possible to insert a needle into the bladder and then pass a guidewire. As in percutaneous nephrolithotomy, Alken metal dilators can be passed over the guidewire to dilate the track and an Amplatz sheath inserted followed by a large-bore nephroscope. This is the best method to use if it is not possible to carry out litholapaxy per urethram because of a narrow urethra.

Removal of a retained Foley catheter

A retained Foley catheter is usually caused by the channel that connects the balloon to the side arm becoming blocked, usually at the end near the balloon. The best way of dealing with this problem is to further inflate the balloon with 20 ml of water and then burst the balloon percutaneously using a needle under ultrasound screening. If the balloon bursts, it is important to subsequently cystoscope the patient to ensure that any fragments are removed before they can form a foreign body calculus. Cutting off the side arm and attempting to clear the channel with a wire is only occasionally successful.

FOREIGN BODIES IN THE BLADDER

The most common foreign body in the bladder is a fragment of catheter balloon (see above). Occasionally, a foreign body enters through the wall of the bladder, for example non-absorbable

P. Alken, **Urologist, The University of Heidelberg, Germany.**

sutures used in an extravesical pelvic operation. Complications include:

- lower UTI;
- perforation of the bladder wall;
- bladder stone.

Treatment

A small foreign body can usually be removed per urethram by means of an operating cystoscope. Occasionally, a suprapubic approach using the percutaneous insertion of a cystoscope is needed.

DIVERTICULAE OF THE BLADDER

Definition

The normal intravesical pressure during voiding is about 35–50 cmH$_2$O; however, pressures as great as 150 cmH$_2$O may be reached by a hypertrophied bladder endeavouring to force urine past an obstruction. This pressure causes the lining between the inner layer of hypertrophied muscle to protrude, forming multiple saccules. If one or more, but usually one, saccule is forced through the bladder wall, it becomes a diverticulum (Fig. 72.31). Congenital diverticula are the result of a developmental defect.

Aetiology of diverticulae

Congenital diverticulae

These are situated in the midline anterosuperiorly and represent the unobliterated vesical end of the urachus.

Pulsion diverticula

The usual cause is bladder outflow obstruction.

Pathology

The mouth of the diverticulum is situated above and to the outer side of one ureteric orifice. Exceptionally, it is near the midline behind the interureteric ridge. The size varies from 2 to 5 cm, but they may be larger. Diverticula are lined by bladder mucosa and the wall is composed of fibrous tissue only (compare with a traction diverticulum). A large diverticulum enlarges in a downward direction and sometimes may obstruct a ureter – probably because of peridiverticular inflammation.

Complications

Recurrent urinary infection

As the pouch cannot empty itself efficiently, there remains a stagnant pool of urine within it. Peridiverticulitis can cause dense adhesions between the diverticulum and surrounding structures. Squamous cell metaplasia and leucoplakia are infrequent complications.

Bladder stone

This develops as a result of stagnation and infection. The stone often protrudes into the bladder.

Hydronephrosis and hydroureter

This is extremely rare and is a consequence of peridiverticular inflammation and fibrosis.

Neoplasm

Neoplasm arising in a diverticulum is an uncommon complication (< 5%). The prognosis is dependent on the stage of the tumour (see below).

Clinical features

An uninfected diverticulum of the bladder usually causes no symptoms. The patient is nearly always male (95%) and over 50 years of age. Symptoms are those of associated urinary tract obstruction, recurrent infection and pyelonephritis. Haematuria (due to infection, stone or tumour) is a symptom in about 30%. In a few patients micturition occurs twice in rapid succession (the second act may follow a change of posture).

Diagnosis

Diverticula are usually discovered incidentally on cystoscopy or ultrasound (Figs 72.32–72.34).

Indications for operation

Operation is necessary only for the treatment of complications. Provided the diverticulum is small and associated outflow obstruction has been dealt with by prostate resection, there is no reason to resect the diverticulum. Even a large diverticulum may not require treatment in the absence of infection or other complications.

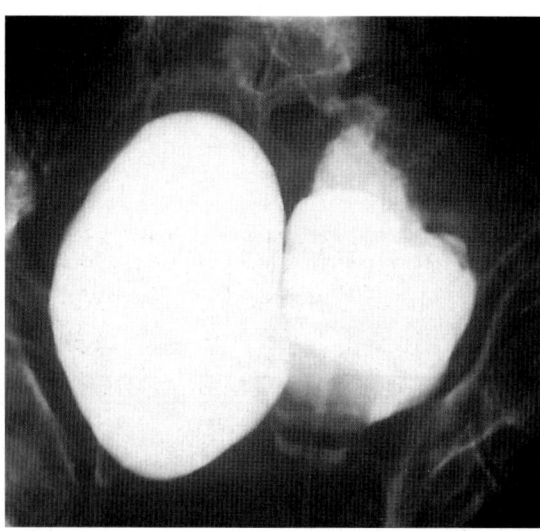

Figure 72.31 Cystogram showing a large diverticulum of the bladder.

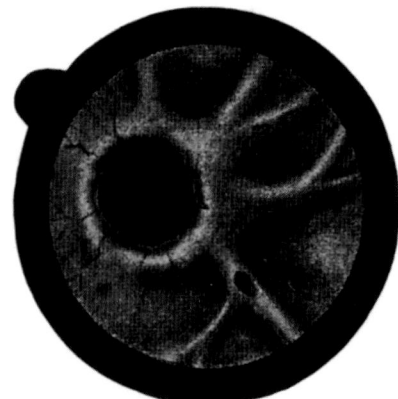

Figure 72.32 Cystoscopic appearance of the orifice of a diverticulum and trabeculation of the bladder.

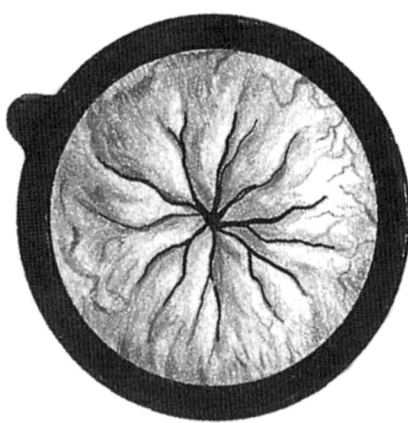

Figure 72.33 Occasional appearance of a diverticulum with inadequate distension of the bladder.

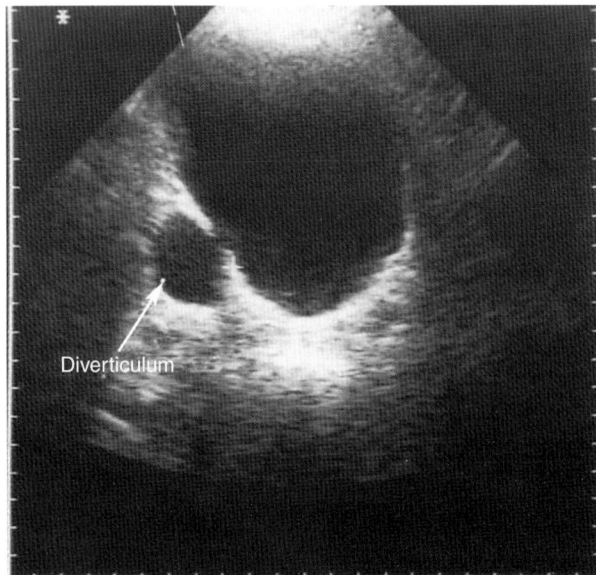

Figure 72.34 Bladder diverticulum demonstrated by ultrasound.

Combined intravesical and extravesical diverticulectomy

A ureteric stent is passed up the ureter on the affected side and the anterior bladder wall is exposed through a suprapubic incision. The bladder is incised in the midline and the diverticulum is packed with a strip of gauze. The neck of the diverticulum is separated from the ureter and when the pouch is free it is severed from the bladder. The resulting defect is closed in a single layer with 2/0 absorbable sutures. A suprapubic catheter is left in place and an extravesical drain is inserted. An alternative method, if the sac is densely adherent, is to carry the incision in the bladder down to the rim of the diverticular orifice, then to detach the diverticulum together with its fibrous rim. The incision in the bladder is closed and the diverticulum left in position with a corrugated drain placed into it for 2–3 days. The track fibroses rapidly after removal of the drain. If bladder outlet obstruction is present, prostatectomy should be carried out at the same time as the diverticulectomy, using any appropriate method [transurethral resection of the prostate (TURP), laser or open] (Summary box 72.8).

Traction diverticulum (synonym: hernia of the bladder)

A portion of the bladder protruding through the inguinal or femoral hernial orifice occurs in 1.5% of such herniae treated by operation (Fig. 72.35).

URINARY FISTULAE

Congenital urinary fistulae

The causes of congenital urinary fistulae include:

- Ectopia vesicae.
- A patent urachus – the presence of a urinary leak from the umbilicus, present at birth or commencing soon after, suggests this diagnosis. In adult life, infection in a urachal cyst may produce a fistula and adenocarcinoma may occur (Figs 72.36 and 72.37). Treatment is by means of excision of the urachal tract and closure of the bladder once distal obstruction has been excluded.
- In association with imperforate anus (see Chapters 6 and 69).

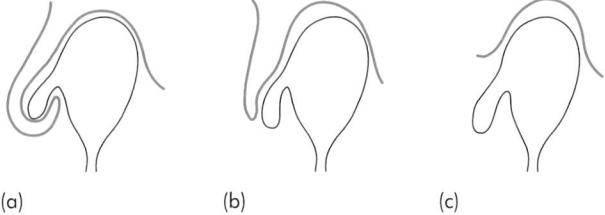

(a)   (b)   (c)

Figure 72.35   (a) Intraperitoneal, (b) paraperitoneal and (c) extraperitoneal hernia of the bladder, in relation to a hernial sac.

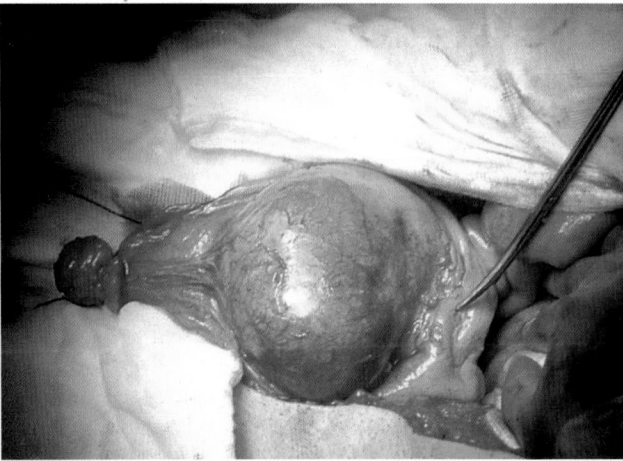

Figure 72.36 An operative photograph showing a large urachal cyst in which adenocarcinoma formation has occurred. A partial cystectomy with total removal of the urachal remnant is about to be carried out.

CHAPTER 72 | THE URINARY BLADDER

(a)

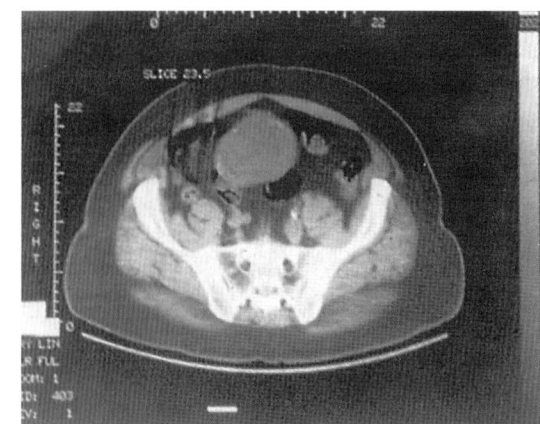

(b)

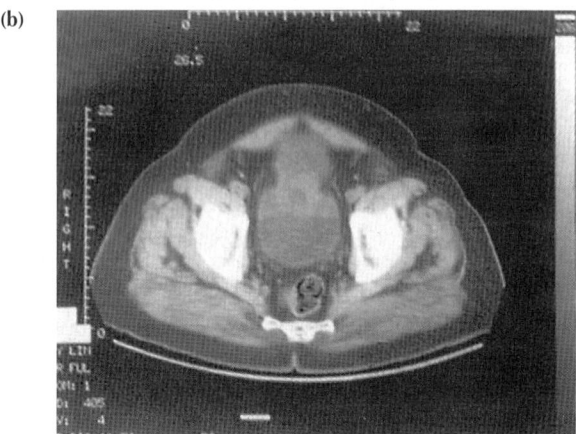

Figure 72.37 A computerised tomography scan of the same patient as in Figure 72.36, showing a large urachal cyst closely approximated to the dome of the bladder.

Traumatic urinary fistulae

Perforating wounds, damage not recognised during surgery or poor healing and avascular necrosis following radiotherapy and surgery may lead to fistula formation. Also, clot retention occurring after an open bladder operation may lead to dehiscence of the wound and a fistula, which will heal quickly provided the bladder is kept empty with an indwelling catheter.

Vesicovaginal fistulae

Aetiology

- *Obstetric.* The usual cause is protracted or neglected labour.
- *Gynaecological.* The operations chiefly causing this complication are total hysterectomy and anterior colporrhaphy.
- *Radiotherapy.*
- *Direct neoplastic infiltration.* Exceptionally, carcinoma of the cervix ulcerates through the anterior fornix to implicate the bladder.

When an injury to the bladder is recognised and repaired, leakage is uncommon, but escape of urine will quickly follow if such damage passes unnoticed. However, most vesicovaginal fistulae are the result of ischaemic necrosis of the bladder because of prolonged pressure of the fetal head in obstetric cases. In gynaecological cases, the ischaemia is brought about by grasping the bladder wall in an artery forceps, including the bladder wall in a suture or perhaps even by local oedema or haematoma. Leakage

because of necrosis of tissue seldom manifests itself before 7 days after the operation. An intractable fistula following radiotherapy for carcinoma of the cervix uteri may arise from avascular necrosis years after the apparent cure of the original lesion.

Clinical features

There is leakage of urine from the vagina and excoriation of the vulva. Vaginal examination may reveal a localised thickening on its anterior wall or in the vault. On inserting a vaginal speculum, urine will be seen escaping from an opening in the anterior vaginal wall.

The 'three-swab test'

The differential diagnosis between a ureterovaginal and vesicovaginal fistula can be made by placing a swab in the vagina and injecting a solution of methylene blue through the urethra; the vaginal swab becomes coloured blue if a vesicovaginal fistula is present. Cystoscopy and bilateral retrograde ureterography provide a more reliable demonstration. An IVU should be performed to exclude a coincidental ureterovaginal fistula (ureterovaginal fistula occurs with vesicovaginal fistula in about 10% of cases). Usually, the IVU shows some upper tract dilatation resulting from partial obstruction.

Treatment

Just occasionally, conservative management of a vesicovaginal fistula following hysterectomy, by urethral bladder drainage, is successful; however, the majority of fistulae will require definitive surgical repair. A low fistula (subtrigonal) is best repaired per vaginam. The fistula is exposed, the bladder is closed using absorbable sutures and the vagina subsequently closed with a separate layer. A urethral catheter should be left *in situ* for at least 10 days. For higher (supratrigonal) fistulae a transvaginal approach can be difficult. These patients should always be cystoscoped before the repair procedure and bilateral ureterograms performed. For high fistulae a suprapubic approach is the best method in most hands; however, some experts will aim to carry out vaginal closure in most cases that have not involved complex surgery or radiotherapy.

To repair a ureterovaginal fistula, an extraperitoneal approach to the ureter via the previous Pfannenstiel incision is made. Considerable adhesions will be encountered, but the ureter can usually be found above the level of the injury and followed down. Reimplantation into the bladder is often required. Depending on the amount of ureter lost, it may be possible to achieve reimplantation with a psoas hitch procedure. If the gap is too large a Boari flap of anterior bladder wall should be cut and brought over to meet the ureter and a reimplant performed. The most important principle of ureteric reimplantation is that there should be no tension on the repair.

Fistulae from renal pelvis to skin or gut

Tuberculosis of a kidney may result in a fistula to the duodenum, colon or skin. Similarly, a pyonephrosis may discharge into the gut or onto the skin. Duodenal ulcer involving the pelvis of the right kidney, Crohn's disease involving the renal pelvis or ureter,

Achille Boari, **nineteenth century Italian Surgeon.**
Burrill Bernard Crohn, **1884–1983,** Gastroenterologist, Mount Sinai Hospital, New York, NY, USA, **described regional ileitis in 1932.**

or cases of xanthogranulomatous pyelonephritis may cause fistulae. A longstanding urinoma will occasionally fistulate into the gut.

Fistulae arising from infection

The most common cause is diverticulitis of the colon. Fistulae may also follow Crohn's disease, appendix abscess or pelvis sepsis after acute salpingitis, or pelvic surgery.

The onset of a fistula from diverticular disease may well be treated as a simple urinary infection. The diagnosis can be difficult to make, but on cystoscopy a patch of oedema on the left side of the vault is suggestive and bubbles of gas may be seen (Fig. 72.38). A cystogram may reveal the fistula. The passage of gas per urethram in a patient is most suggestive (provided that diabetes resulting in urinary infection with a gas-forming organism is excluded).

Treatment of fistulae caused by diverticular disease

In most patients a single-stage operation is indicated provided that the surgeon is experienced in colonic surgery. At laparotomy, the communication is separated, the hole in the bladder being closed and patched with omentum, and the segment of diseased bowel resected; it is most important to ensure that the left colon and, if necessary, the splenic flexure are fully mobilised to facilitate a tension-free, well-vascularised anastomosis. The bladder is drained by a urethral catheter.

Fistulae caused by carcinoma

By the time that a fistula between the bowel and the bladder has developed, the tumour is usually locally advanced but may be operable.

Urethral fistulae in the male

These occur as the result of infection above a stricture producing a paraurethral abscess that ruptures into the urethra, allowing extravasation to occur suddenly into the scrotum and perineum. Urine and infection extend into the upper 2.5 cm of the thigh and lower abdominal wall. Widespread cellulitis and tissue necrosis (which may lead to Fournier's gangrene) may occur unless drainage of urine is achieved by suprapubic cystotomy and the tissue planes are freely drained by inguinal and scrotal incisions.

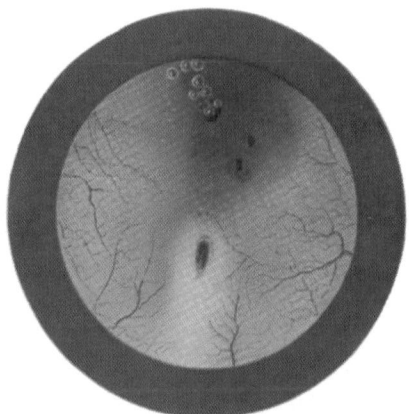

Figure 72.38 Cystoscopic view of a vesicointestinal fistula. Bubbles of gas can be seen issuing from the orifice of the fistula.

Jean Alfred Fournier, **1832–1915**, French Syphilologist, and Founder of the Venereal and Dermatological Clinic, Hôpital St Louis, Paris, France.

Neoplastic fistulae

Primary bladder tumours very rarely produce fistulae. Involvement of the bladder by tumours of the cervix, uterus, colon and rectum can produce fistulae, as may sarcoma of the small gut. Carcinoma of the prostate rarely produces a rectal fistula. Treatment is difficult and in most cases only palliative relief can be given. It is rarely in the patient's interest to carry out urinary diversion, although minimally invasive techniques such as placement of ureteric stents can be helpful in palliating symptoms (Summary box 72.9).

Summary box 72.9

Fistulae

- A fistula is a communication between two epithelium-lined surfaces
- Most urinary fistulae are vesicovaginal and result from obstetric trauma; an associated ureterovaginal fistulae occurs in about 10% of cases
- A 'three-swab test' is used to aid the diagnosis. An examination under anaesthesia, vaginoscopy, and cystoscopy and IVU should be performed and, if necessary, retrograde ureterography
- Conservative management is rarely successful
- The principles of repair include good exposure, excision of diseased tissue and tension-free vascularised repair in anatomic layers
- Fistulae caused by radiation, cancer and sepsis can be complex with multiple tracts
- The persistence of a fistula on the skin implies the presence of distal obstruction, chronic infection, such as tuberculosis, or a foreign body, such as a stone or non-absorbable ligature

---

LOWER URINARY TRACT INFECTION AND CYSTITIS

Infection of the bladder gives rise to symptoms of frequency, urgency, suprapubic discomfort, dysuria and cloudy offensive urine. These symptoms are often known as 'cystitis'. Lower UTIs are much more common in women than in men, particularly in the under 50s. It should be remembered that a lower UTI is often associated with upper tract colonisation and the presence of associated loin pain, pyrexia, rigors and malaise (these symptoms represent complicated infection and should be taken seriously as serious sepsis can ensue).

Isolated infection

A single episode of lower tract infection occurs frequently in females and is rarely complicated.

Recurrent infection

Recurrent infection may be associated with an underlying predisposing cause or may be a result of bacterial resistance. In healthy women, infection after intercourse can occur without any demonstrable abnormality of the urinary tract. Repeated attacks of UTI in women, or a single attack in a man or a child of either sex, should always be followed by investigation to discover and treat the cause; sometimes, however, no cause can be found. Asymptomatic bacteriuria is common and investigation may fail to demonstrate any underlying cause.

Infection in males

Although more common in female adults, the incidence of infection is higher in male infants as underlying urinary tract abnormalities are more frequent. Complicated or recurrent infection in adult males warrants prompt antibiotic therapy and investigation to exclude an underlying cause.

Infection in pregnancy

The incidence of asymptomatic bacteriuria in pregnant women is twice as high as in non-pregnant women. Simple uncomplicated infection can be treated following urine culture with an appropriate antibiotic that is not contraindicated in pregnancy, such as cephalosporin or ampicillin. Non-responsive infection may require intravenous therapy and an ultrasound scan.

Predisposing causes of urinary tract infection

- Incomplete emptying of the bladder, secondary to bladder outflow obstruction, a bladder diverticulum, neurogenic bladder dysfunction or decompensation of the detrusor muscle.
- A calculus, foreign body or neoplasm.
- Incomplete emptying of the upper tract, dilatation of the ureters associated with pregnancy, or vesicoureteric reflux. In childhood, the mainstay of treatment of vesicoureteric reflux is antibiotic therapy; operation is reserved for those with recurrent infection despite antibiotics or with severe upper tract dilatation.
- Oestrogen deficiency, which may give rise to lowered local resistance.
- Colonisation of the perineal skin by strains of *Escherichia coli* expressing molecules that facilitate adherence to mucosa.
- Diabetes.
- Immunosuppression.

Avenues of infection

Ascending infection from the urethra is the most common route (see Chapter 70). The organisms originate in the bowel, contaminate the vulva and reach the bladder. The passage of urethral instruments may cause infection in either sex, especially when the bladder contains residual urine (Fig. 72.39). Other routes are less common and include descending infection from the kidney (tuberculosis), haematogenous spread, lymphogenous spread and spread from adjoining structures (fallopian tube, vagina or gut).

Bacteriology

Bacterial virulence factors affect the ability of a pathogen to infect the host. The possession of pili (rod-shaped structures) that project from the outer membrane increases adhesiveness. The type of pilus can be used to classify the pathogen involved. *Escherichia coli* is the most common organism followed by *Proteus mirabilis*, *Staphylococcus epidermidis* and *Streptococcus faecalis*. Infection with other organisms or infection with mixed organisms is found in patients with neurogenic bladder dysfunction or those with a longstanding indwelling urethral catheter. These organisms include *Pseudomonas*, *Klebsiella*, *Staphylococcus aureus* and

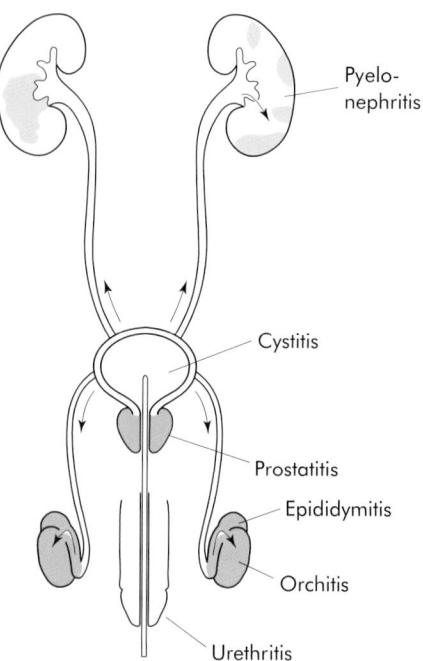

Figure 72.39 Complications liable to follow the changing of a urethral catheter in the presence of urethritis (courtesy of C.G. Scorer, FRCS, London, England).

various streptococci. Tuberculous infection is considered below. The presence of pus cells without organisms calls for examination for *Mycobacterium tuberculosis* and *Neisseria gonorrhoeae*. Having eliminated these possibilities, the underlying condition may be abacterial cystitis, CIS, renal papillary necrosis, stones or incomplete treatment of a urinary infection.

Clinical features

These include frequency, pain, haematuria and pyuria. Pyrexia and rigors are not associated with a simple UTI but are a sign of upper tract infection or septicaemia.

Examination

On examination there is tenderness over the bladder. Initial and midstream urine specimens should be collected in a male as acute prostatitis may be present (see below), which will lead to threads in the initial specimen. The midstream specimen must be subjected to microscopy and culture, and the sensitivity of any organisms assessed.

Treatment

Treatment should be commenced immediately and modified if necessary when the bacteriological report is to hand. The patient is urged to drink. Appropriate first-line antibiotics depend on local likely sensitivities but would include trimethoprim or one of the quinolones. Failure to respond indicates the need for further investigation to exclude predisposing factors. It is important to check for associated allergies or other drugs or conditions that might preclude the use of some antibiotics [e.g. concomitant administration of methotrexate and trimethoprim (both inhibit tetrahydrofolate reductase)].

Investigation

Investigation may be needed in the male or when recurrent infection occurs. This includes measurement of urinary flow rates and post-void residual urine. IVU, ultrasound scan or CT scanning will usually be carried out together with cystoscopy. Difficult cases may require urodynamic investigation (Summary box 72.10).

Summary box 72.10

UTI in adults

- Isolated UTI in adults is not infrequent and is more common in women
- Recurrent or complicated infection (haematuria, rigors) warrants appropriate antimicrobial therapy and investigation
- Investigation to exclude a predisposing cause includes urinalysis, microscopy and culture, upper tract imaging and cystoscopy
- *Mycobacterium tuberculosis, Neisseria gonorrhoeae* or *Mycoplasma genitalium* should be suspected if pus cells are present but urine culture is negative
- Cancer, especially CIS, masquerading as infection may be diagnosed as abacterial cystitis

---

SPECIAL FORMS OF LOWER URINARY TRACT INFECTION

Acute abacterial cystitis (acute haemorrhagic cystitis)

The patient presents with severe UTI. Pus is present in the urine but no organism can be cultured. It is commonly sexually acquired but tuberculous infection and CIS must be ruled out. The underlying causative organism may be *Mycoplasma* or herpes simplex virus. Cyclophosphamide can also cause this problem.

Frequency–dysuria syndrome (urethral syndrome)

This consists of symptoms of lower tract infection but with negative urine cultures. CIS, tuberculosis and interstitial cystitis should be excluded. Most urologists advise patients to adopt general measures such as wearing cotton underwear, using simple soaps, adopting general perineal hygiene measures and voiding after intercourse. Other treatments include cystoscopy and urethral dilatation, although the benefits remain doubtful.

Tuberculous urinary infection

Tuberculous urinary infection is secondary to renal tuberculosis. Early tuberculosis of the bladder commences around the ureteric orifice or trigone, the earliest evidence being pallor of the mucosa due to submucous oedema. Subsequently, tubercles may be seen and, in longstanding cases, there is marked fibrosis and the capacity of the bladder is greatly reduced (Fig. 72.40).

Treatment

Tuberculous infection usually responds rapidly to anti-tuberculous drugs but occasionally the involved kidney and ureter have to be removed. If the bladder remains of low capacity, patients will have severe symptoms and the upper tracts are at risk because of high filling pressures and vesicoureteric reflux. Such patients, after

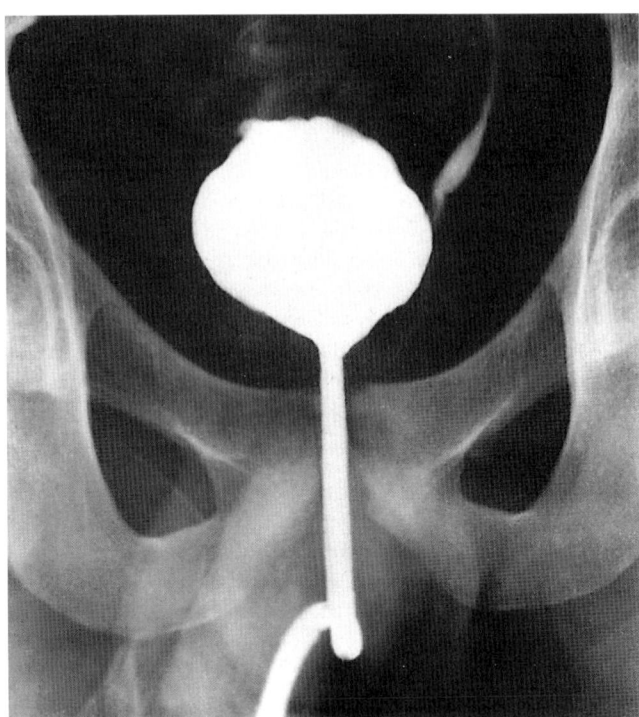

Figure 72.40 Retrograde cystograph showing an exceedingly contracted ('thimble') bladder in a case of tuberculous cystitis.

appropriate chemotherapy, respond well to bladder augmentation. The ureters may need reimplantation.

Bladder augmentation by ileocystoplasty or caecocystoplasty

The fibrosed supratrigonal bladder is removed and the bladder augmented with a segment of bowel. This may consist of intact caecum, a detubularised segment of ileum or a detubularised ileocaecal segment (see Figs 72.20–72.22, p. 1322–3).

Interstitial cystitis (Hunner's ulcer)

For practical purposes, this is confined to women. The first symptom is increased frequency; pain, relieved by micturition and aggravated by jarring and overdistension of the bladder, is another characteristic symptom. In most patients pyuria and urinary infection are absent. Haematuria also occurs. The aetiology remains as obscure as it was when Guy Hunner described the condition in 1914. It consists of a chronic pancystitis, often with marked infiltration with lymphocytes and macrophages. Fibrosis of the vesical musculature and areas of avascular atrophy of the epithelium occur. Ulceration of the mucosa occurs in the fundus of the bladder. In severe cases the bladder capacity is reduced to 30–60 ml. The characteristic linear bleeding ulcer is caused by splitting of the mucosa when the bladder is distended under anaesthesia. Inflammation of all coats of the bladder is present with granulation tissue in the submucosa underlying the ulcer. The muscularis is hypertrophied and the peritoneum in proximity to the area of maximum disease is thickened. The inflammation may involve the trigone, the urethra and, in severe cases, the

---

Guy Leroy Hunner, 1868–1951, Gynaecologist, The Johns Hopkins Hospital, Baltimore, MD, USA.

peritoneum. Pronounced mast cell infiltration is seen but is not specific. It is important to check urinary cytology and to biopsy the mucosa to exclude underlying neoplastic disease.

On cystoscopy the characteristic ulcer is found in the fundus, but it may be absent. This area bleeds readily as the bladder is decompressed. Treatment is difficult and unsatisfactory. Hydrostatic dilatation under anaesthesia may give relief for some months. Instillation of dimethylsulphoxide results in improvement in some patients. Other drugs that have been tried include intravesical heparin, oral ranitidine and steroid therapy. Patients with severe symptoms may well require cystectomy and orthotopic bladder substitution. In patients with severe inflammation involving the trigone and urethra, this operation may not result in complete relief and some type of urinary diversion may be needed.

Alkaline encrusting cystitis

Alkaline encrusting cystitis is rare and is due to urea-splitting organisms causing phosphatic encrustations on the bladder mucosa of elderly women. There are symptoms of chronic UTI and a plain radiograph shows the bladder outline. The encrustations may be removed by bladder irrigation and the infection treated with appropriate antibiotics.

Cystitis cystica

Under the influence of chronic inflammation the surface epithelium sends down buds, resulting in minute cysts filled with clear fluid, most abundant on the trigone. This is frequently found in patients with recurrent frequency and dysuria.

SCHISTOSOMIASIS OF THE BLADDER (SEE CHAPTER 5)

Geographical distribution

The disease is endemic in Egypt, parts of Africa, Israel, Syria, Saudi Arabia, Iran, Iraq and the shores of China's great lakes. Dwellers of the Nile valley have suffered for centuries. Marshes or slow-running fresh water provide the habitat for the freshwater snail (*Bulinus truncatus*) that is the intermediate host.

Mode of infestation

The disease is acquired through exposure of the skin to infected water, which usually occurs while bathing. The free-swimming, bifid-tailed embryos (cercariae) of the trematode *Schistosoma haematobium* penetrate the skin. Shedding their tails, they enter blood vessels and are swept to all parts of the body but they flourish in the liver where they live on erythrocytes and develop into male and female worms. Sexual maturity having been attained, the nematodes leave the liver and enter the portal vein. The male worm bends into the shape of a gutter (the gynaecophoric canal) into which a female worm nestles, and the pair makes its way towards the inferior mesenteric vein. *Schistosoma haematobium* has an affinity for the vesical venous plexus, which it reaches through the portosystemic anastomotic channels.

Having reached the bladder the female worm eventually enters a submucous venule which is so small that she completely blocks it. She now proceeds to lay about 20 ova in a chain; each ovum is provided with a terminal spine that penetrates the vessel wall. A heavily infected subject passes hundreds of ova a day. If the ova reach fresh water, the low osmotic pressure causes rupture and the ciliated miracidium emerges. To survive, it must reach and penetrate the intermediate snail host within 36 hours. Within the snail's liver, the miracidium enlarges and gives rise to myriads of daughter cysts, which are set free on the death of the snail. A single miracidium begets thousands of cercariae to complete the life cycle.

Clinical features

After penetration of the skin, urticaria lasting about 5 days can occur (swimmer's itch). Following an incubation period of 4–12 weeks, a high evening temperature, sweating and asthma, together with leucocytosis and eosinophilia, occur. Usually, an asymptomatic period of several months supervenes before the ova are released, causing the typical early sign and symptom of intermittent, painless, terminal haematuria. Men are affected three times more frequently than women.

Examination of the urine

The last few millilitres of an early-morning urine specimen are collected and centrifuged. Examination on several consecutive days may be required, but a negative result does not exclude bilharziasis, especially in patients no longer resident in bilharzial districts. Antibody detection by enzyme-linked immunoabsorbent assay (ELISA) using *Schistosoma mansoni* adult microsomal antigen (MAMA) can be performed. The test is positive 1 month after infection and is specific for *Schistosoma mansoni* and *Schistosoma haematobium*.

Cystoscopy

Depending on the length of time for which the disease has remained untreated, cystoscopy will reveal one or more of the following:

1 *Bilharzial pseudotubercles* are the earliest specific appearance of the disease. (Fig. 72.41).
2 *Bilharzial nodules* (Fig. 72.42) are caused by the fusion of tubercles.
3 '*Sandy patches*' are the result of calcified dead ova with degeneration of the overlying epithelium (Fig. 72.43).
4 *Ulceration* is the result of sloughing of the mucous membrane containing dead ova (Fig. 72.44).
5 *Fibrosis* is mainly the result of secondary infection.
6 *Granulomas*. Bilharzial masses are caused by the aggregation of nodules.
7 *Papillomas* are more pedunculated (Fig. 72.45).
8 *Carcinoma* is a common end result in grossly infected bilharziasis of the bladder that has been neglected for years.

Treatment

Safe and effective drugs are available for the treatment of schistosomiasis, including praziquantel taken in three doses of 20 mg kg^{-1} (total 60 mg kg^{-1}) 4 hours apart. It takes many months for dead ova to be expelled and, even after repeated courses and healing of the bladder lesion, living bilharzial worms have been found at necropsy in the portal system.

Theodor Maximilian Bilharz, 1825–1862, Professor of Zoology, Cairo, Egypt.
Sir Patrick Manson, 1844–1922, practised in Formosa (now Taiwan), and Hong Kong before becoming Physician to the Dreadnought Hospital, Greenwich, London, England. He is regarded as The Founder of Tropical Medicine.

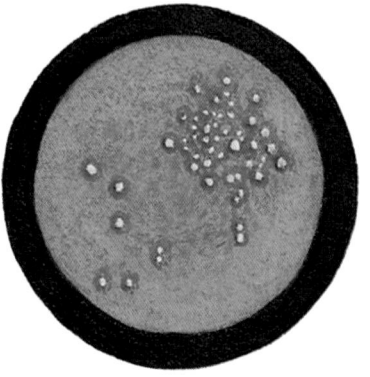

Figure 72.41 Bilharzial tubercles (courtesy of N. Makar).

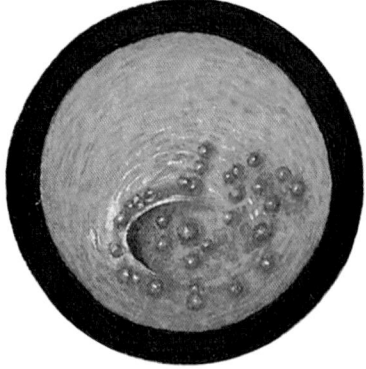

Figure 72.42 Bilharzial nodules (courtesy of N. Makar).

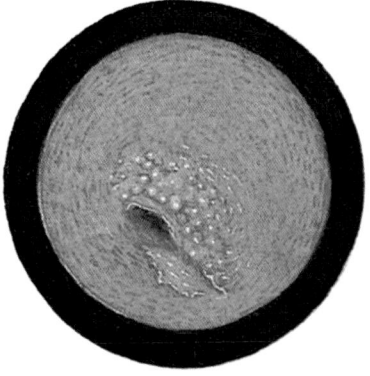

Figure 72.43 'Sandy patches' (courtesy of N. Makar).

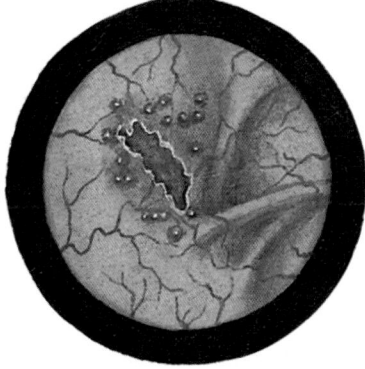

Figure 72.44 Bilharzial ulcer (courtesy of N. Makar).

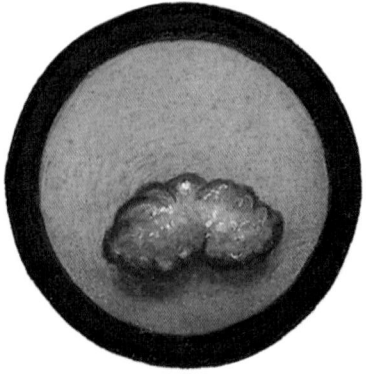

Figure 72.45 Bilharzial papilloma (courtesy of N. Makar).

Other complications, requiring specific treatment, include the following:

- urinary calculi;
- stricture of the ureters;
- prostatoseminal vesiculitis;
- fibrosis of the bladder and bladder neck (Fig. 72.46);
- bilharzial urethral strictures;
- squamous bladder cancer.

NEOPLASMS OF THE BLADDER

In total, 95% of primary bladder tumours originate in transitional epithelium; the remainder arise from connective tissue (angioma, myoma, fibroma and sarcoma) or are extra-adrenal phaeochromocytomas.

Secondary tumours of the bladder are common and most frequently arise from the sigmoid and rectum, the prostate, the uterus or the ovaries, although bronchial neoplasms may also spread to the bladder.

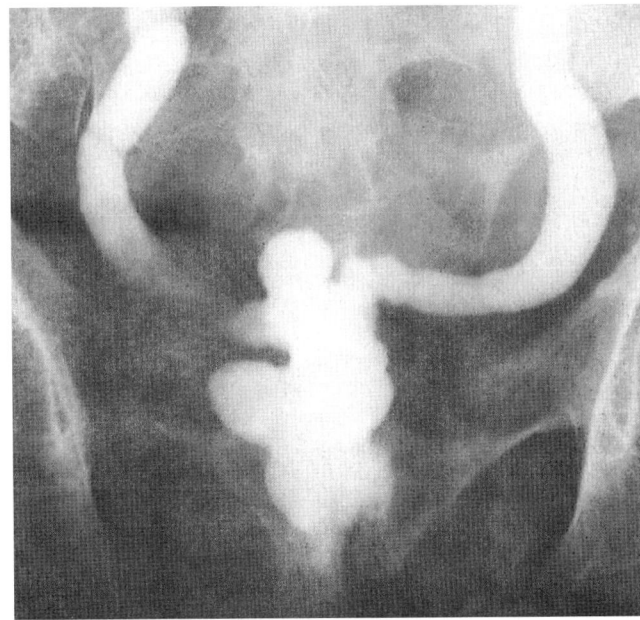

Figure 72.46 Bilharzial contracture of the bladder, with ureteric reflux (courtesy of H. Talib, Baghdad, Iraq).

Pathology

Benign papillary tumours

The papilloma consists of a single frond with a central vascular core with villi; it looks like a red sea anemone (Figs 72.47 and 72.48). Inverted papilloma is a condition in which the proliferative cells penetrate under normal mucosa so that the lesion is covered with smooth urothelium. It is benign.

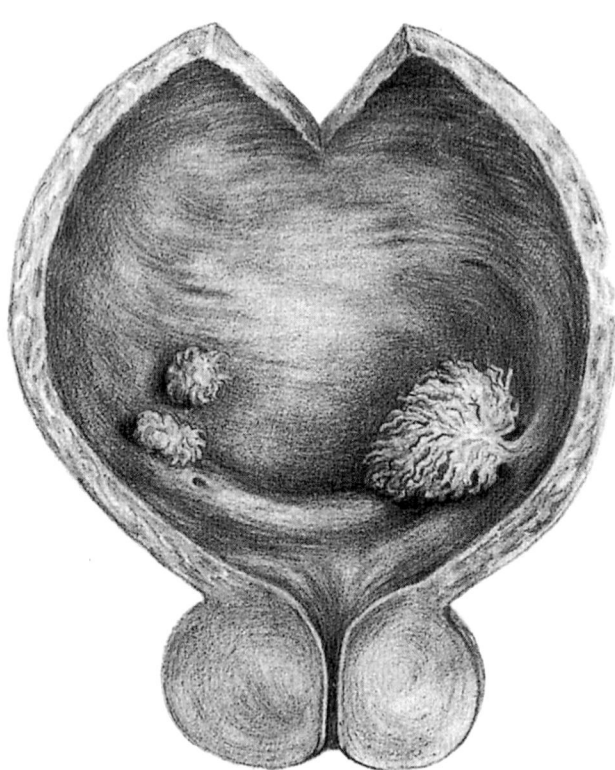

Figure 72.47 Papillary tumour with daughter implantation ('kiss' cancer).

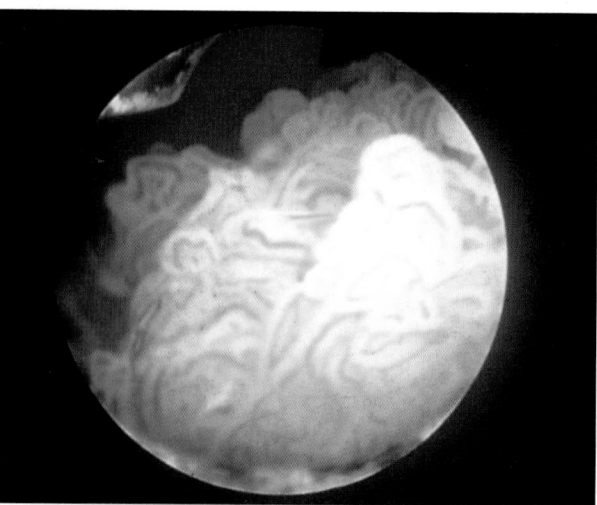

Figure 72.48 Endoscopic photograph of a pTa bladder tumour about to be resected.

CARCINOMA OF THE BLADDER

Histological types of bladder cancer include urothelial, squamous and adenocarcinoma [or mixed, as a result of metaplasia in a transitional cell carcinoma (TCC)]. Over 90% are urothelial in origin. Pure squamous carcinoma is uncommon (approximately 5%), except in areas where bilharzia is endemic. Primary adenocarcinoma, which arises either from the urachal remnant or from areas of glandular metaplasia, accounts for 1–2% of cases.

Urothelial cell carcinoma

Aetiology

Cigarette smoking is the main aetiological factor (40% of cancers). Occupational exposure to urothelial carcinogens remains common. The first suspicion of a chemical cause for bladder cancer was raised by Rehn in 1895 when he recorded a series of tumours in workers in aniline dye factories. Hueper showed that 2-naphthylamine was carcinogenic in dogs. Subsequent investigation demonstrated that the following compounds may be carcinogenic:

- 2-naphthylamine;
- 4-aminobiphenyl;
- benzidine;
- chlornaphazine;
- 4-chloro-*o*-toluidine;
- *o*-toluidine;
- 4,4'-methylene bis(2-choloroaniline);
- methylene dianiline;
- benzidine-derived azo dyes.

Occupations associated with an increased risk of bladder cancer are:

- textile workers;
- dye workers;
- tyre rubber and cable workers;
- petrol workers;
- leather workers;
- shoe manufacturers and cleaners;
- painters;
- hairdressers;
- lorry drivers;
- drill press operators;
- chemical workers;
- rodent exterminators and sewage workers.

Bladder cancer became a prescribed industrial disease (No. 39) in 1953, and previously exposed workers may be entitled to compensation. Balkan nephropathy is associated with an increased incidence of upper tract urothelial tumours (see Chapter 71).

A series of genetic events has been clearly implicated in cancer formation but is outside the remit of this chapter. Activation of dominantly acting oncogenes such as *ras* and *c-erbB*-1 and -2, and transcription factors such as E2F3, have been reported in bladder cancer, as has the inactivation of tumour-suppressor genes such as *p53*, *p21*, *p16* and the retinoblastoma gene. Activation of many other genes occurs including those coding for

Ludwig Rehn, **1849–1930**, Surgeon, Frankfurt am Main, Germany.
The Balkans are the countries which occupy an area in the south-east of Europe. They are south of the Danube and the Sava rivers, and form a peninsula bounded on the east by the Aegean and Black seas, on the west by the Adriatic and Ionian seas, and on the south by the Mediterranean.

enzymes that dissolve the basement membrane, such as the metalloproteinases (stromelysin, collagenases and elastase), lysosomal enzymes such as the cathepsins and others including urinary plasminogen activators; angiogenic factors [e.g. vascular endothelial growth factor (VEGF)] and other peptide growth factors such as the epidermal growth factor and its receptor also have a role to play. These changes are common to several tumour types, including prostate cancer (Summary box 72.11).

Summary box 72.11

Urothelial cell carcinoma of the bladder

- The fourth most common non-dermatological malignancy in men (male–female ratio 3:1)
- Strongly associated with smoking and chemical exposure in western societies
- Strongly associated with *Schistosoma haematobium* infection (bilharzial bladder cancer) in regions where the parasite is endemic
- Reducing in incidence in countries where smoking is decreasing

---

Tumour staging and grading

Study of the biological behaviour of transitional cell cancer of the bladder shows that cancers fall into the three following groups. Depth of invasion (T) from the tumour–node–metastasis (TNM) classification and grade (World Health Organization I, II or III) are important factors in planning treatment and determining prognosis in bladder cancer.

- Non-muscle-invasive pTa (Fig. 72.48) and pT1 tumours account for 70% of all new cases; these are known as 'superficial' bladder cancer. It is crucial to distinguish pTa tumours from superficially invasive pT1 disease. Histological examination may reveal invasion of the lamina propria (pT1) but not of the muscle or no invasion of lamina propria (pTa). These tumours may be single or multiple – single papillary pTa tumours account for a significant proportion of bladder cancers and carry an excellent prognosis.
- Muscle-invasive disease accounts for 25% of new cases. Such tumours carry a much worse prognosis as they are subject to local invasion and distant metastasis.
- Flat, non-invasive CIS (primary CIS) accounts for 5% of new cases. Unless diagnosed and treated promptly it carries a poor prognosis (Summary box 72.12).

Summary box 72.12

Bladder cancer staging

- Cystoscopy and resection of tumour with separate resection of the tumour base is essential for accurate analysis of invasion into detrusor muscle
- Bimanual examination should be performed after resection of the tumour
- Upper tract imaging by IVU is essential. CT to stage invasive disease for lymph node metastasis is preferred

---

Superficial bladder cancer (pTa and pT1)

These are usually papillary tumours that grow in an exophytic fashion into the bladder lumen (Figs 72.47 and 72.48). They may be single or multiple and may appear pedunculated, arising on a stalk with a narrow base, but if the tumours are less well differentiated they are more solid with a wider base. The mucosa around the tumour is often rather oedematous, with angry-looking, dilated blood vessels. These areas may contain *in situ* changes (concomitant CIS).

The urothelium elsewhere in the bladder may appear rather oedematous and velvety; this suggests a generalised 'field change' with the presence of widespread CIS. The most common sites for superficial tumours are the trigone and lateral walls of the bladder.

After initial complete treatment by endoscopic transurethral resection (TURT), patients with pTa or pT1 disease may develop two problems:

- About 50–70% develop recurrent tumours that may be single or multiple, and the recurrences may occur on one or on many occasions. The recurrent tumours are usually of the same stage or grade as the primary tumour. High-grade, multiple tumours with concomitant CIS are most likely to develop recurrent disease.
- About 15% will develop a recurrent tumour that invades the bladder muscle. The risk of such progression increases with high-grade disease, pT1 disease, multiple primary disease and concomitant CIS. Many urologists now regard the presence of pT1 grade 3 tumours as an indication for offering the patient immediate cystectomy because of the excellent outcome.

This behaviour provides the rationale for performing check cystoscopies. The factors that result in an increased recurrence and progression rate are:

- high grade;
- pT1 disease;
- concomitant CIS;
- multiple primary tumours;
- recurrent disease at the first check cystoscopy 3 months after diagnosis.

Patients presenting with a solitary grade 1 or grade 2 pTa tumour without concomitant CIS, which does not recur within the first 6 months, have an excellent outcome.

Patients with high-grade pTa or pT1 disease are at high risk and should be counselled very carefully. The options include a course of bacille Calmette–Guérin (BCG) followed by careful assessment or immediate cystectomy. The presence of persistent disease after a single course of BCG is reason to offer cystectomy (Summary box 72.13).

Summary box 72.13

Superficial bladder cancer

- Does not invade the detrusor muscle but can extend to the lamina propria
- Extension to the lamina propria (pT1) is a significant risk factor for progression to invasive disease, especially if associated with high-grade disease and CIS
- The incidence of recurrence of this disease can be reduced by intravesical chemotherapy and immunotherapy
- High-risk superficial disease (any grade 3 disease) is best managed by BCG immunotherapy followed by radical treatment if disease persists

---

Albert Leon Charles Calmette, **1863–1933, and** Jean-Marie Camille Guérin, **1872–1961, Microbiologists at the Institute Pasteur, at Lille in France, introduced the Bacille Calmette-Guérin in 1908.**

Muscle-invasive transitional cell carcinoma

Muscle-invasive tumours are nearly always solid (Fig. 72.49) although there may be a low tufted surface. These tumours are often large and broad based, having an irregular, ulcerated, appearance within the bladder. The incidence of metastases, whether from lymphatic invasion in the pelvis or blood-borne to the lung, liver or bones, is much more common and will cause the death of 30–50% of patients (Summary box 72.14).

Summary box 72.14

Invasive bladder cancer

- Invasive bladder cancer should be staged by an accurate bimanual examination performed under anaesthesia before and after resection of the tumour
- CT or magnetic resonance imaging should be performed to identify lymph node involvement and distant spread
- Radical therapy in the form of radical cystectomy and thorough lymph node dissection is the primary treatment
- Neoadjuvant cisplatin-based chemotherapy improves survival rates
- External beam radiotherapy is an option for patients who are unfit for, or who decline, cystectomy
- Locally advanced disease may be downstaged by radiotherapy or chemotherapy to enable salvage cystectomy

---

In situ carcinoma

The histological appearance of irregularly arranged cells with large nuclei and a high mitotic index replacing the normally well-ordered urothelium is known as CIS. It may occur alone (primary CIS) or in association with a new tumour (concomitant CIS) or it may occur later in a patient who has previously had a tumour (secondary CIS). It can only be diagnosed when a biopsy is examined under the microscope. It may cause severe symptoms of dysuria, suprapubic pain and frequency (hence its old name of malignant cystitis). It carries a risk for the patient of developing a malignant muscle-invasive cancer. Without treatment, 50% will die of bladder cancer.

Pure squamous cell carcinoma of the bladder

Squamous cell tumours tend to be solid and are nearly always associated with muscle invasion. This is the most prevalent form

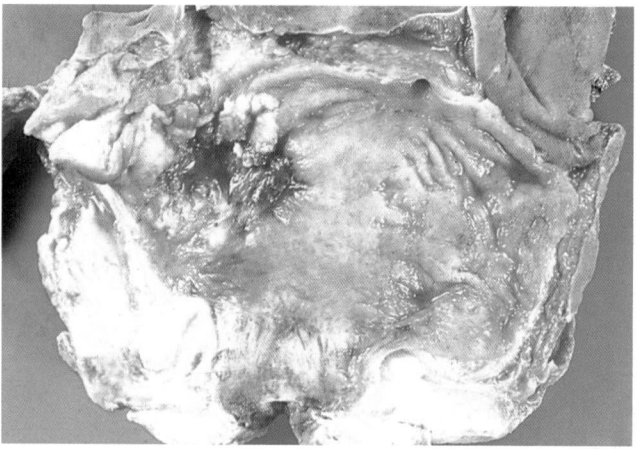

Figure 72.49 Radical cystectomy specimen showing a large solid bladder cancer with total removal of the bladder and prostate.

of bladder cancer in areas where bilharzia is endemic. Squamous cell tumours may be associated with chronic irritation caused by stone disease in the bladder as a result of metaplasia.

Pure adenocarcinoma

Adenocarcinoma accounts for approximately 1–2% of all bladder cancers. It usually arises in the fundus of the bladder at the site of the urachal remnant. Occasionally, primary adenocarcinomas arise at other sites and probably originate from areas of glandular metaplasia. Such tumours need to be distinguished from secondary cancer.

CLINICAL FEATURES OF BLADDER CARCINOMA

Painless gross haematuria is the most common symptom and is indicative of a bladder carcinoma until proven otherwise. Often, however, the patient fails to declare the symptom to their GP. The bleeding may give rise to clot formation and clot retention.

Constant pain in the pelvis usually heralds extravesical spread. There is often frequency and discomfort associated with urination. Pain in the loin or pyelonephritis may indicate ureteric obstruction and hydronephrosis. A late manifestation is nerve involvement causing pain that is referred to the suprapubic region, groins, perineum, anus and into the thighs.

It is also important to assess the patient as a whole. Many are elderly men who have been lifelong smokers and who suffer from chronic obstructive airway disease or cardiovascular disease. Their suitability for major surgery must be borne in mind.

INVESTIGATION OF BLADDER CARCINOMA

Urine

Urine should be cultured and examined cytologically for malignant cells. This is not a good screening test but a positive result is highly specific. New tests are being developed based on the presence of antigens such as nuclear matrix proteins (NMP22) or mini-chromosome maintenance (MCM) proteins, which may be able to detect new or recurrent tumours.

Blood

Estimation of haemoglobin and the level of serum electrolytes and urea should be carried out.

IVU or ultrasound scanning

This should be performed on all patients with painless haematuria. Occasionally, the preliminary film shows a faint shadow of an encrusted neoplasm of the bladder. The most common radiological sign is a filling defect (Fig. 72.50). Occasionally, irregularity of the bladder wall may herald the presence of an invasive tumour. Hydronephrosis may occur if a superficial tumour grows up the intramural ureter or if direct invasion of the ureteric wall occurs. Ultrasound scanning should be carried out if the kidney is non-functioning.

Cross-sectional imaging

Non-contrast CT is being used in some centres instead of IVU or ultrasound scanning for the immediate management of patients

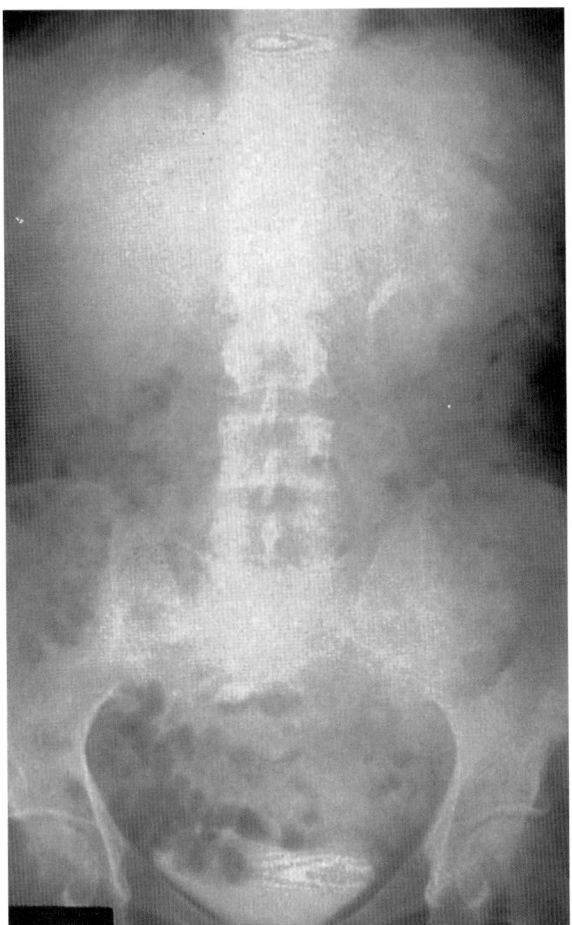

Figure 72.50 Intravenous urography showing a filling defect in the region of the right ureteric orifice.

(a)

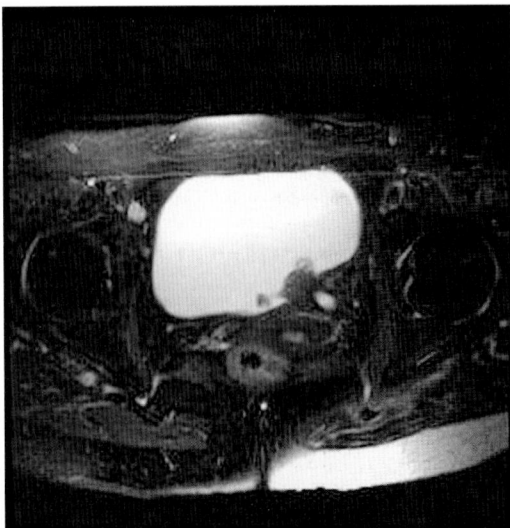

(b)

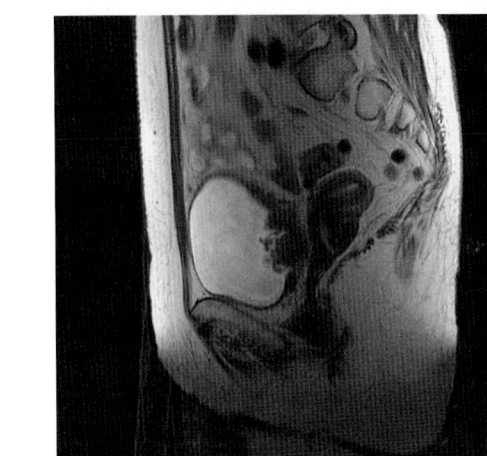

Figure 72.51 (a) Cross-sectional magnetic resonance imaging showing a 'cystogram' and a bladder cancer. (b) Cross-sectional magnetic resonance imaging showing invasive bladder cancer.

with gross painless haematuria. For staging when a muscle-invasive bladder cancer is suspected, contrast-enhanced CT is used, ideally before TURT. False-positive pT3 disease can be diagnosed if a CT scan is carried out soon after TURT. Magnetic resonance imaging is being used more frequently (Fig. 72.51) and can demonstrate lymph node metastasis or muscle invasion.

Cystourethroscopy

Cystourethroscopy is the mainstay of diagnosis and should always be performed on patients with haematuria. It can be carried out with a rigid instrument under general anaesthesia or with a flexible instrument under local anaesthesia. The urethra is inspected at the initial insertion of the instrument (urethroscopy) and the bladder is then examined in a systematic fashion (cystoscopy).

Bimanual examination

A bimanual examination with the patient fully relaxed under general anaesthesia should be performed both before and after endoscopic surgical treatment of these tumours. The bladder should be empty. Once there is muscle invasion the differentiation between pT2 and pT3 disease depends on whether a mass is palpable bimanually at the end of the procedure (pT3). When invasion has spread into the prostate in a man or the vagina in a woman it is classified as pT4a. If the tumour is fixed to the lateral pelvic side wall it is staged as pT4b.

TREATMENT FOR CARCINOMA OF THE BLADDER

Superficial tumours

Endoscopic surgery

The tumour should be carefully resected in layers using a resectoscope. The base of the tumour is sent separately for histological examination. Small pinch biopsies are taken near to and distant from the primary lesion when CIS is suspected (inflamed or velvety appearance). After removal of the tumour, two or three further loops of tissue from the base should be sent separately so that the pathologist can accurately determine whether there is lamina propria or muscle invasion. The base of the tumour is then coagulated, so achieving haemostasis. The appearance of pale-yellow glistening fat will indicate a perforation of the bladder. Should this occur before the resection is complete, it may be prudent to stop the resection and place a catheter in the bladder for a few days. In this instance the procedure could be completed some 2 weeks later. The bimanual examination is repeated at the end of the endoscopic procedure. Following these procedures, an irrigating catheter is left *in situ* for 48 hours to prevent clot retention of urine. There is good evidence that a single dose of mitomycin (Mitomycin C; 40 mg in 60 ml of fluid) instilled into the bladder before catheter removal decreases the risks of recurrence in patients with pTa and pT1 grade 1 and 2 disease.

Patients with larger solid tumours should have adequate material resected for histological staging and grading. If possible and straightforward, the mass of the tumour should be resected as completely as possible – even when pT2 or pT3 disease is suspected.

Follow-up

Most urologists agree that patients with a single low- or medium-grade pTa tumour can safely be treated by resection alone plus a single instillation of mitomycin, followed up with regular cystoscopies.

The treatment of patients with multiple low- or medium-grade pTa tumours can be by either resection alone or resection followed by a 6-week course of intravesical chemotherapy with mitomycin, doxorubicin or epirubicin.

The treatment of pT1 disease is difficult. Approximately 30% of tumours are understaged at first resection. For this reason, a repeat cystoscopy and resection of the tumour base is advocated within 6 weeks. Many urologists would offer immediate cystectomy to a patient with a high-grade pT1 tumour, particularly if it were multiple or accompanied by CIS, because of the 30–50% risk of progression to muscle invasion. Others will treat such patients by endoscopy followed by immunotherapy with intravesical BCG. The most effective treatment of solitary medium-grade pT1 disease remains uncertain, but a reasonable approach would be endoscopic resection followed by reresection of the area after 6 weeks, followed by intravesical BCG.

Follow-up cystoscopies are essential; they may be carried out under local anaesthesia with a flexible cystoscope or under general anaesthesia if the urologist feels that the patient is at high risk of recurrence. They should be performed at 3-monthly intervals over the first year; following this the time interval between cystoscopies can be determined according to the presence or absence of further disease. In total, 30% of patients will never develop another tumour so that, if the bladder has remained clear after 2 years, annual inspection may be adequate. For patients who go on to develop multiple recurrences within the bladder at each examination, the cystoscopies need to be maintained at frequent intervals so that the growths can be resected. These patients are at a greater risk of their disease progressing; although intravesical chemotherapy can decrease the recurrence rate, no reduction in progression rates has been found.

Open surgical excision

This should be totally avoided. If by some error a bladder containing a tumour is entered, then the tumour may be removed with a diathermy needle and the base coagulated and the bladder closed. Postoperative radiotherapy to the wound will diminish the chance of tumour implantation.

Invasive tumours

The treatment of cancer with proven muscle invasion remains a subject for debate. Whatever the modality of treatment employed, few centres have 5-year survival figures of more than 50%. There is a move towards primary surgical treatment in most centres. The use of systemic chemotherapy with a combination of agents – cisplatin, methotrexate, doxorubicin and vinblastine (M-VAC) or cisplatin plus gemcitabine given before (neoadjuvant) radical cystectomy – has been shown to be of benefit. The current evidence is that neoadjuvant chemotherapy improves survival by about 5–7%.

Radiotherapy

External beam radiotherapy

External beam radiotherapy is usually given at 60 Gy over a 4- to 6-week period. There is a complete response rate of 40–50%. Unfortunately, some patients do not respond and others exhibit only a partial response, with pTa or pT1 tumour remaining in the bladder giving rise to a risk of recurrence. Patients with residual disease after radiotherapy should be offered 'salvage cystectomy' if they are fit. Proponents of radiotherapy claim that it avoids the need to remove the bladder in some patients and allows men to retain potency. Radiotherapy is not without complications, and during the course of treatment will cause urinary frequency and also diarrhoea. Late complications can leave the bladder contracted and fibrosed, in which case it may need to be removed for palliative reasons. Late complications affecting the rectum should be uncommon, especially if lateral fields of irradiation are employed.

Surgery

Partial cystectomy

This should be limited to the treatment of small adenocarcinomas of the bladder.

Radical cystectomy and pelvic lymphadenectomy

This is now standard treatment for localised pT2–pT3 disease without evidence of secondary spread or of CIS that has not responded to BCG. Before contemplating radical surgery to remove the bladder, it is important to have evidence that surgical cure is attainable. A CT scan of the pelvis may locally overstage the bladder if a recent resection has been carried out, although the finding of grossly enlarged pelvic, iliac or para-aortic nodes or liver metastases will alter the decision for cystectomy. A bone scan [using technetium-99m (^{99m}Tc)] will help to show whether there is spread to bone.

Operation

Alternative drainage for urine is necessary following removal of the bladder. The standard procedure is to perform an ileal conduit. Male patients should be counselled about the onset of erectile impotence and absent ejaculation following the operation; they should also be told about alternative forms of urinary diversion, which include continent urinary diversions and orthotopic bladder replacement.

Patients should be seen by a stoma care therapist, who will help to advise the patient and will try different ileostomy bags to ensure that the correct site is chosen, avoiding skin creases so that one does not end up with the disaster of a leaking urinary ileostomy. A decision is made about whether the male urethra is to be removed (depending on the estimated risk of recurrence within the urethra); a urethrectomy is usually indicated in patients with primary CIS or those with tumour invading the prostate stroma. Many surgeons are now offering total replacement of the bladder after cystectomy.

The patient should receive prophylactic antibiotics including metronidazole, cefuroxime and amoxicillin, and low-dose heparin.

The abdomen is opened through a long midline incision extending down to the symphysis pubis. The liver and the retroperitoneum are checked for evidence of metastases, and the operability of the bladder is assessed. A bilateral pelvic lymphadenectomy is performed, removing external iliac nodes, internal iliac nodes and the nodes in the obturator fossae. The vessels passing to the bladder from the side wall are ligated in continuity; these include the obliterated hypogastric vessels, the superior vesical artery, the middle vesical veins, and the inferior vesical arteries and veins. The ureters are then divided. The posterior ligaments extending from the pararectal area to the back of the bladder are ligated and divided, and the layer posterior to Denonvilliers's fascia is opened up. The endopelvic fascia is then divided on each side and the puboprostatic ligaments are divided. A ligature is passed between the dorsal vein complex and the urethra, and the former is ligated and divided. The urethra is then mobilised and divided. The ligaments lateral to the prostate are divided and the bladder is removed. In women, the uterus and anterior vaginal wall need to be included. Women must be counselled about the loss of ovarian and uterine function.

An isolated loop of ileum is then prepared on its own mesentery, and continuity of the small bowel restored. The ureters are then implanted into the bowel and the ileostomy is created. Meticulous care must be taken to close all mesenteric windows, thus avoiding internal hernias. If the bladder is to be replaced orthotopically, a reservoir made from detubularised bowel (usually an ileocaecal segment or ileum) is created and anastomosed to the urethra after implantation of the ureters.

The operative mortality rate associated with cystectomy used to be considerable but is now < 2%. Late complications include urethral recurrence (about 5–8%), which is increased in the presence of multifocal tumours, CIS and, particularly, invasion of prostatic stroma (Fig. 72.52).

Leucoplakia

This condition is simply squamous metaplasia of the bladder. Profuse production of keratin may result in the passing of white particles in the urine. It cannot be treated easily. Localised areas may be resected endoscopically. Diffuse leucoplakia of the bladder is pre-malignant and results in squamous cancer of the bladder. Careful cystoscopic assessment is required and the condition may require cystectomy.

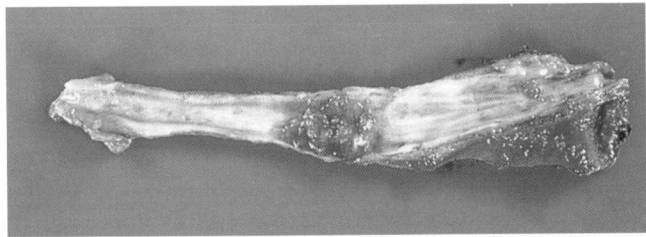

Figure 72.52 Urethrectomy specimen from a patient who has previously undergone a radical cystectomy showing new transitional cell tumour formation in the urethra.

Charles Pierre Denonvilliers, **1808–1872, Professor of Anatomy, and later of Surgery, Paris, France.**

Endometriosis

Endometriosis within the bladder wall is rare but can have the appearance of a vascular bladder tumour or a tumour that contains chocolate-coloured or bluish cysts. The swelling enlarges and bleeds during menstruation. If medical management fails, by means of danazol or luteinising hormone-releasing hormone (LHRH) agonists, further treatment is usually by means of partial cystectomy or full-thickness endoscopic resection, depending on its site. The condition may be part of more widespread disease. Endometriosis is also a cause of ureteric stricture.

INTERNAL AND EXTERNAL URINARY DIVERSION

Indications

Diversion of the urine may be either a temporary expedient to relieve distal obstruction or a permanent procedure when the bladder has been removed or has lost normal neurological control and in cases of incurable fistula or irremovable obstruction.

Methods of urinary diversion

Temporary methods use prosthetic materials, the most common being a urinary catheter. In elderly patients unfit for prostatectomy, and in some patients with terminal carcinoma of the prostate, an indwelling silicone urethral Foley catheter changed every 3 months is a satisfactory method of drainage. A suprapubic placement is an alternative to urethral placement. The major drawback of long-term catheterisation is infection secondary to the associated bacteriuria that invariably develops. Ureteric obstruction can be relieved by placement of internal 'double-J' pigtail ureteric stents, which can remain for 4–5 months but are usually changed every 3 months. As an alternative, a nephrostomy tube, inserted percutaneously by ultrasound and fluoroscopic imaging, is effective when internal stent placement is not feasible.

Permanent urinary diversion

External diversion

Ileal conduit

Permanent urinary tract diversion is most commonly performed by conduit diversion. The ureters are implanted into a short, isolated segment of ileum (Fig. 72.53a) or, less commonly, colon. The conduit diverts the urine onwards to a cutaneous stoma for collection in an ileostomy bag. This form of diversion is well established and associated with a low complication rate of less than 10%. The main complication is ureteroileal stricture, which can be limited by spatulation of the distal ureters and an end-to-end anastomosis as described by Wallace (Fig. 72.53a). Stenosis at the ileocutaneous site is less frequent, and a short isoperistaltic conduit limits the formation of a residual urine volume, reducing infection and avoiding the problems of reabsorption of urine. In some cases, when the pelvic area has been subjected to radiation, the lower ureters may be unhealthy; a high division with insertion of the ureters into an ileal loop above the root of the mesentery may then be wiser (Fig. 72.54).

The site for the stoma must be chosen before operation, in

David Mitchell Wallace, **1913–1992, Urologist, St Peter's Hospital, London, England.**

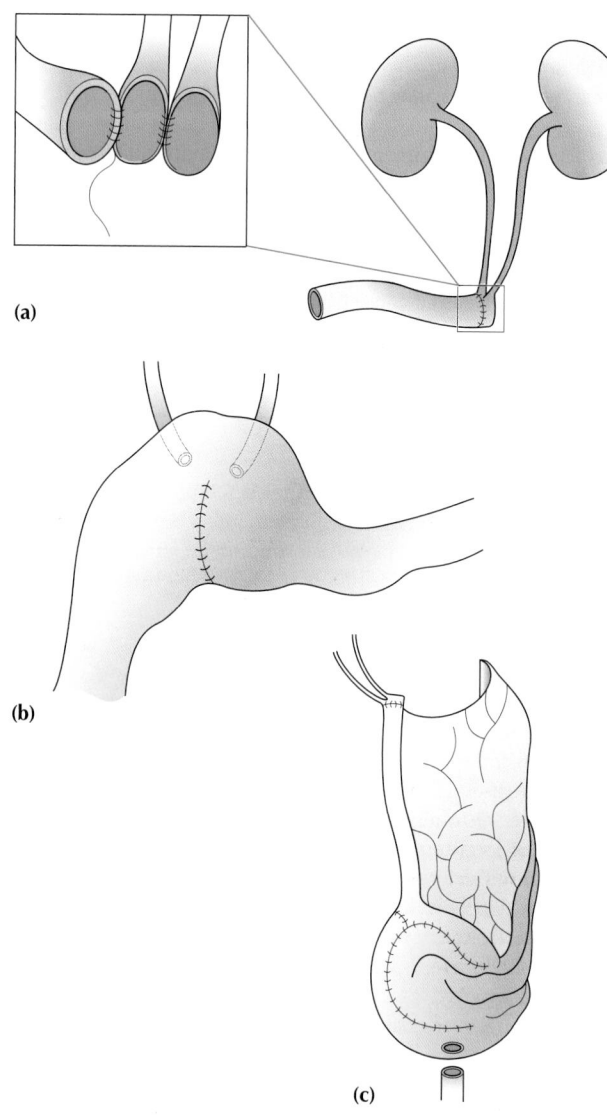

Figure 72.53 Diversion of urine. Favoured methods: (a) ileal conduit; the ureters are spatulated and anastomosed to ileum end-to-side (insert); (b) ureterosigmoidostomy; (c) ileal neobladder with anti-reflux long afferent limb.

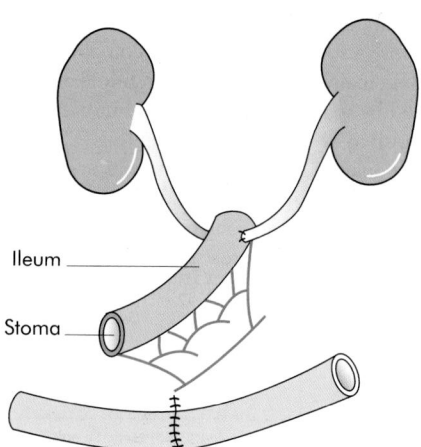

Figure 72.54 Ureteroileostomy (after D.M. Wallace, FRCS).

consultation with a stoma care therapist; the site is marked indelibly on the skin.

Operative details A coil of ileum, approximately 15–20 cm long and 30 cm from the ileocaecal valve, with its blood supply intact, is isolated. The left ureter is brought behind the mesorectum. The ureters may be joined to the ileum either end-to-side or end-to-end after anastomosing of the distal spatulated ureters to form a plate (Wallace). The distal end of the coil is brought out through an incision made at the site identified before operation; a disc of skin and fat is removed, a cruciate incision is made in the fascia and the muscle is split. The stoma is made about 2–3 cm long. It is evaginated initially by means of four sutures passing through the skin, the ileal loop as it passes through the opening and the cut edge of the ileum.

Internal urinary diversion

Colon and rectum

The advantage of diverting urine into the colon is that no collecting apparatus is necessary. Clearly, however, the anal sphincter must be competent. Before ureterosigmoidostomy is undertaken, the patient must prove that he or she can control at least 200 ml of fluid in the rectum. The disadvantage of the operation is that the renal tract is exposed continuously to infection from the faeces; this can be minimised by constructing an anti-reflux procedure. Various diversions are described; the Mainz II ureterosigmoidostomy creates a cul-de-sac type low-pressure reservoir in the sigmoid into which the ureters are placed (see Fig. 72.53b). This reduces reflux, and bowel content, although in contact with urine, takes a direct route to the rectum. In the long term, cancer can develop at long-standing ureterocolic junctions (Fig. 72.55).

Bladder reconstruction

Over the past decade, several techniques have been developed to allow a near-spherical urinary reservoir to be formed out of various lengths of bowel that are detubularised. These may consist of ileum, ileum and caecum or sigmoid colon (see Fig. 72.53c). The ureters can then be reimplanted in these reservoirs in an anti-reflux manner and the reservoir anastomosed to the membranous urethra in the male (see Figs 72.20–72.22,

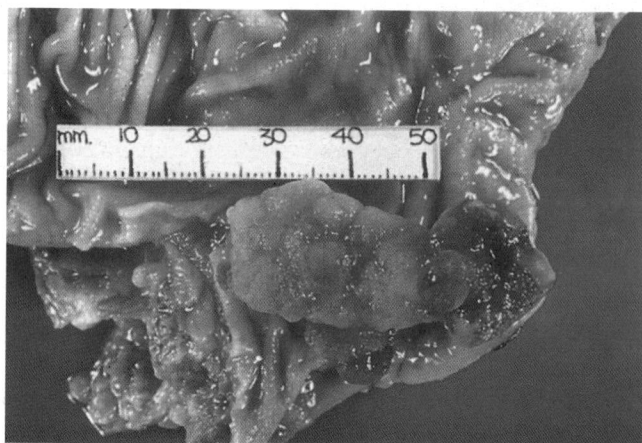

Figure 72.55 An anterior resection of the rectum specimen in a patient aged 18 years who has previously undergone ureterosigmoidostomy for the treatment of bladder exstrophy.

p. 1322–3). About 15–30% of patients cannot empty the neo-bladder completely and will need to perform intermittent self-catheterisation. The results are good in selected younger patients after radical cystectomy.

Continent urinary diversion

A similar concept is used in the construction of continent diversions. A urinary reservoir is made as described above and the ureters are attached to the reservoir. A continence mechanism is then made to connect the reservoir to the skin. This is the complication-prone part of the operation. The continence mechanism may be made of an invaginated loop of ileum supported by three rows of staples (Kock pouch) or from the appendix, buried in an anti-reflux manner in a submucosal tube (Mitrofanoff; Fig. 72.56). Alternatively, a length of ileum can be made into a tube (of a similar size to the appendix) after excision of the anti-mesenteric ileum and buried in a submucosal tunnel in an anti-reflux way. Clearly, these operations are complex, with the potential for increased postoperative complications.

Bladder substitution and augmentation

In patients with contraction of the bladder because of tuberculosis or with neuropathic dysfunction and a small bladder capacity, the bladder may need to be augmented. Similar techniques to those used to perform a bladder replacement can be utilised to make a near-spherical pouch from detubularised bowel, which can then be attached to the trigone or bladder neck after a near-total cystectomy (see Figs 72.20–72.22, p. 1322–3). The ureters are then reimplanted. The facility to provide a continence mechanism must be available if needed in the neuropathic patient. This may comprise an artificial urinary sphincter or a colposuspension in the female.

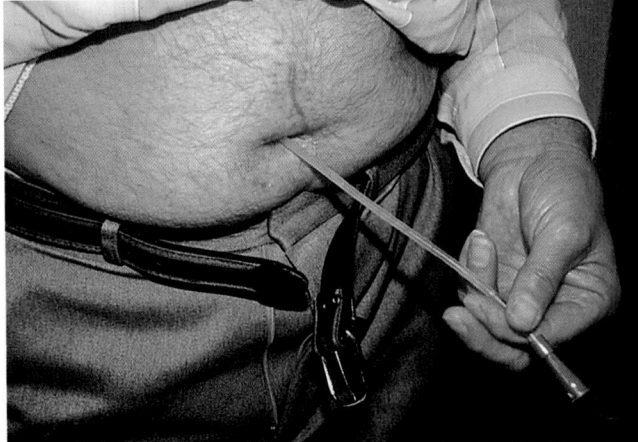

Figure 72.56 A patient with a pT3a bladder cancer who has previously undergone cystoprostatectomy and urethrectomy. A detubularised ileocaecal reservoir has been made with the ureters implanted in submucosal tunnels. The appendix has been implanted within the reservoir in a submucosal tunnel to provide the continence mechanism. The appendix has been brought to the umbilicus and is catheterised 4- to 6-hourly to empty the reservoir.

Nils G. Kock, **B. 1924, Professor of Surgery, The University of Goteborg, Sweden.**
Paul Mitrofanoff, **B. 1934, Professor of Paediatric Surgery, Rouen, France.**

Complications of internal diversion

Stricture

Ureterosigmoidostomy was first used by Chaput in 1894. Subsequent modifications included those made by Coffey and Grey Turner. In these methods the ureters were cut obliquely and pulled into the gut by a stitch – the ends were not stitched to the gut wall – and stenosis was common. Nesbit, Cordonnier and Leadbetter all recognised that these strictures could be prevented by anastomosing mucosa to mucosa.

Reflux of urine

High-pressure activity within a segment of gut can cause reflux of potentially infected urine at high pressure to the kidneys. In the long term, this can cause renal impairment. The principle of a low-pressure reservoir for both neobladder and ureterosigmoidostomy (Mainz II) reduces this. In addition, an anti-reflux mechanism, used in neobladder construction, is created by anastomosing the ureters to a non-detubularised 20-cm segment of small bowel, which is in continuity with the neobladder (see Fig. 72.53c).

Metabolic consequences of internal diversion

Resorption of solutes

This depends upon the following factors: (1) the area of bowel that is exposed to urine; and (2) the length of time that the urine is in contact with the bowel epithelium.

The biochemical changes associated with urinary diversion are due to a combination of reabsorption of chloride and urea and progressively diminishing tubular function as a result of pyelonephritis. Diarrhoea with loss of potassium-containing mucus may exacerbate the loss of potassium. The typical changes of a hyperchloraemic acidosis with potassium depletion occur more frequently with ureterosigmoid diversion than with a colonic and ileal neobladder. When severe, the patient develops loss of appetite, weakness, thirst and diarrhoea. Coma may ensue. Mild acidosis, unrecognised over a long period, produces osteomalacia. Bone pain and even pathological fracture can occur. Renal impairment from pyelonephritis and reabsorption from the mucosa are seen less frequently after ileal or colonic conduit formation, continent urinary diversion or orthotopic bladder substitution. In fact, they are seen very infrequently except in patients with pre-existing renal impairment and unsatisfactory emptying of the urinary reservoir. Malabsorption can occur with the loss of terminal ileum and small bowel. The loss of terminal ileum can result in vitamin B12 deficiency and so monitoring of vitamin B12 and folate is recommended after the first year.

Treatment

Patients should be instructed to empty the rectum or continent reservoir or neobladder 3-hourly by day. In patients who have undergone ureterosigmoidostomy and in whom acidosis is present, a rectal tube should be inserted at night to drain the urine continuously. The patient should take a mixture of potassium citrate and sodium bicarbonate three times a day (2 g of each, either as crystals

Henri Chaput, **B. 1857, Surgeon, La Salpêtrière, Paris, France.**
Robert Calvin Coffey, **1869–1933, Surgeon, Nashville, TN, USA.**
George Grey Turner, **1877–1951, Professor of Surgery, The University of Durham (1927–1934), and at The Postgraduate Medical School, Hammersmith, London, England (1934–1945).**

or as tablets). Regular serum biochemical analyses, including calcium, are required.

Established hyperchloraemic acidosis is usually associated with marked dehydration and the mainstay of treatment is administration of intravenous saline. The patient may be given small doses of sodium bicarbonate to half-correct the pH deficit if it is severe and additional intravenous potassium. This should be coupled with appropriate systemic antibiotic treatment.

Risk of malignancy

There is a risk of cancer developing in bowel used to reconstruct the urinary tract. When the urine is not mixed with faeces, the incidence is small, becoming significant after 15–18 years. The major risk of malignancy was discovered when ureterosigmoidostomy construction enabled free mixing of urine and faeces. The development of sigmoid reservoirs into which the ureters are inserted has reduced this risk.

FURTHER READING

Cardozo, L., Staskin, D.R. (2006) *Textbook of Female Urology and Urogynecology*, 2nd edn. Informa Healthcare, Abingdon.

George, N.J., Fitzpatrick, J., Mundy, A.R. and Neal, D.E. (1999) *Basic Science in Urology*. Isis Publications, Oxford.

Vogelzan, N.J., Scardino, P.T., Shipley, W.U., Debruyne, F.M.J., Marston Linehan, W. (2006) *Comprehensive Textbook of Genitourinary Oncology*, 3rd edn. Lippincott Williams & Wilkins, Philadelphia, PA.

Walsh, P.C., Retik, A.B., Vaughan, E.D., Wein, A.J., Kavoussi, L.R., Novick, A.C., Partin, A.W. and Peters, C.A. (2002) *Campbell's Urology*. Saunders, Philadelphia, PA.

The prostate and seminal vesicles

EMBRYOLOGY

From the primitive urethra, a series of solid epithelial buds develop and become canalised in a matter of weeks. The surrounding mesenchyme forms the muscular and connective tissue of the gland and has a major role in differentiation (stromal epithelium interactions). Skene's tubules, which open on either side of the female urethra, are the homologue of the prostate.

SURGICAL ANATOMY

The contemporary classification of the prostate into different zones was based on the work of McNeal (Fig. 73.1). He showed that it is divided into the peripheral zone (PZ), which lies mainly posteriorly and from which most carcinomas arise, and a central zone (CZ), which lies posterior to the urethral lumen and above the ejaculatory ducts as they pass through the prostate; the two zones are rather like an egg in an eggcup. There is also a peri-urethral transitional zone (TZ), from which most benign prostatic hyperplasia (BPH) arises. Smooth muscle cells are found throughout the prostate but, in the upper part of the prostate and bladder neck, there is a separate sphincter muscle that subserves a sexual function, closing during ejaculation. Resection of this tissue during prostatectomy is responsible for retrograde ejaculation. The distal striated urethral sphincter muscle is found at the junction of the prostate and the membranous urethra; it is horseshoe shaped with the bulk lying anteriorly and is quite distinct from the muscle of the pelvic floor (Fig. 73.1).

The glands of the peripheral zone (Fig. 73.2), lined by columnar epithelium, lie in the fibromuscular stroma, and their ducts, which are long and branched, open into posterolateral grooves on

Alexander Johnston Chalmers Skene, **1828–1900, Professor of Gynecology, Long Island Hospital, Brooklyn, New York, NY, USA.**

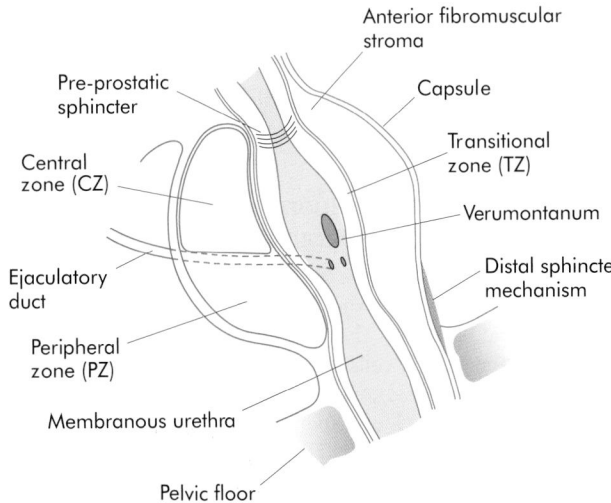

Figure 73.1 Sagittal diagram of the prostate just lateral to the urethra showing the division into the different zones described by McNeal. The transitional zone is the area from which most benign prostatic hyperplasia (BPH) arises.

either side of the verumontanum. The glands of the CZ and TZ are shorter and unbranched. All these ducts, the common ejaculatory ducts and the prostatic utricle open into the prostatic urethra.

BPH starts in the periurethral transitional zone and, as it increases in size, it compresses the outer PZ of the prostate, which becomes the false capsule. There is also the outer true fibrous anatomical capsule, and external to this lie condensations of endopelvic fascia known as the periprostatic sheath of endopelvic fascia. Between the anatomical capsule and the prostatic sheath lies the abundant prostatic venous plexus. The prostatic sheath is

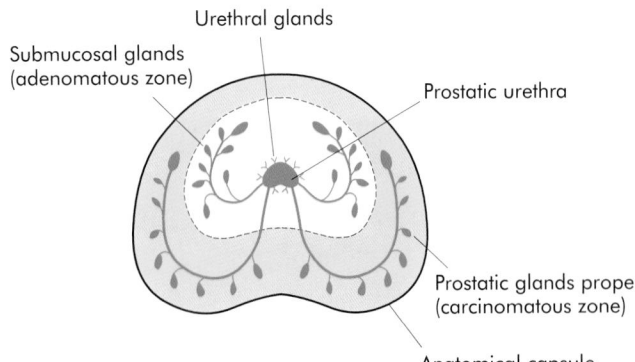

Figure 73.2 A transverse section of the prostate. The peripheral zone is the area from which most prostate cancers arise. The 'adenomatous' zone comprises the central and transitional zones.

contiguous with the fascia of Denonvilliers, which separates the prostate and its coverings from the rectum. The neurovascular bundles supplying autonomic innervation to the corpora of the penis are in very close relationship to the posterolateral aspect of the prostatic capsule and are at risk of damage during radical cystoprostatectomy or radical prostatectomy; inadvertent diathermy in the region of these nerves may be the cause of uncommon erectile impotence after transurethral prostatectomy.

PHYSIOLOGY

The prostate has a sexual function, but it is unclear how important its secretions are to human fertility. That the normal adult prostate undergoes atrophy after castration was known to John Hunter.

Systemic hormonal influences (endocrine) and local growth factors (paracrine and autocrine)

The growth of the prostate is governed by many local and systemic hormones whose exact functions are not yet known. The main hormone acting on the prostate is testosterone, which is secreted by the Leydig cells of the testes under the control of luteinising hormone (LH), itself secreted from the anterior pituitary under the control of hypothalamic luteinising hormone-releasing hormone (LHRH). LHRH has a short half-life and is released in a pulsatile manner. This pulsatile release is important, as receptors for LHRH will become desensitised if permanently occupied. The administration of LHRH analogues in a continuous, non-pulsatile manner exploits the concept of receptor desensitisation and forms the basis for androgen deprivation therapy in prostate cancer. Testosterone is converted to 1,5-dihydrotestosterone (DHT) by the enzyme 5α-reductase, which is found in high concentration in the prostate and the perigenital skin (type II). Other androgens are secreted by the adrenal cortex, but their effects are minimal in the normal male. Oestrogenic steroids are also secreted by the adrenal cortex and, in the ageing male, may play a part in disrupting the delicate balance between DHT and local peptide growth factors, and

Charles Pierre Denonvilliers, 1808–1872, Professor of Anatomy, and later of Surgery, Paris, France.
John Hunter, 1728–1793, Surgeon, St George's Hospital, London, England. He is regarded as 'The Father of Scientific Surgery'.
Franz von Leydig, 1821–1908, Professor of Histology successively at Wurzburg, Tubingen and Bonn, Germany.

hence increase the risk of BPH. Increased levels of serum oestrogens, by acting on the hypothalamus, decrease the secretion of LHRH (and hence LH) and thereby decrease serum testosterone levels. Thus, pharmacological levels of oestrogens cause atrophy of the testes and prostate by means of reductions in testosterone.

Other locally acting peptides are secreted by the prostatic epithelium and mesenchymal stromal cells in response to steroid hormones. These include epidermal growth factor, insulin-like growth factors, basic fibroblast growth factor and transforming growth factors alpha and beta. These undoubtedly play a part in normal and abnormal prostatic growth, but as yet their functions are unclear (Summary box 73.1).

> **Summary box 73.1**
>
> **Androgenic hormones**
>
> - Androgenic hormones, which drive prostate growth, are derived from several sources
> - The majority of testosterone (90%) is secreted by the Leydig cells of the testes under the control of LH, secreted from the anterior pituitary
> - Metabolised adrenal androgen accounts for the remaining 5–10% of testosterone
> - Testosterone is converted to DHT by the enzyme 5α-reductase type II, which is found in high concentration in the prostate and the perigenital skin
> - DHT has five times the potency of testosterone

Elaboration and secretion of prostate-specific antigen and acid phosphatases

Prostate-specific antigen (PSA) is a glycoprotein that is a serine protease. Its function may be to facilitate liquefaction of semen, but it is a marker for prostatic disease. It is measured by an immunoassay, and the normal range can differ a little from laboratory to laboratory. There is no real normal upper limit. The levels increase with age, with prostate cancer and with BPH. There are age-related values but, in general, in men aged 50–69 years, a level of about 3–4 ng ml^{-1} would prompt a discussion about the need for prostate biopsy. Its level in men with metastatic prostate cancer is usually increased to > 30 ng ml^{-1} and falls to low levels after successful androgen ablation. Men with locally confined prostate cancer usually have serum PSA levels < 10–15 ng ml^{-1}. Although PSA is a reliable marker for the progression of advanced disease, it is neither specific nor sensitive in the differential diagnosis of early prostate cancer and BPH, as both diseases are compatible with PSA in the range of 3–15 ng ml^{-1}. PSA measurement has superseded measurement of serum acid phosphatase. In summary, about 25% of men with a PSA of 4–10 ng ml^{-1} have prostate cancer (i.e. it is not very specific), and about 15–20% of men with a PSA of 1–4 ng ml^{-1} have prostate cancer. In general, one would advise men aged 50–69 years to undergo prostate biopsy if the PSA was more than ~ 3 ng ml^{-1}. The threshold would be lower in younger men with a strong family history.

BENIGN PROSTATIC HYPERPLASIA

Aetiology of benign prostatic hyperplasia
Hormones

Serum testosterone levels slowly but significantly decrease with advancing age; however, levels of oestrogenic steroids are not decreased equally. According to this theory, the prostate enlarges because of increased oestrogenic effects. It is likely that the secretion of intermediate peptide growth factors plays a part in the development of BPH (Summary box 73.2).

Summary box 73.2

Benign prostatic hyperplasia (BPH)

■ Occurs in men over 50 years of age; by the age of 60 years, 50% of men have histological evidence of BPH
■ Is a common cause of significant lower urinary tract symptoms in men and is the most common cause of bladder outflow obstruction in men > 70 years of age

---

Pathology

BPH affects both glandular epithelium and connective tissue stroma to variable degrees. These changes are similar to those occurring in breast dysplasia (see Chapter 50), in which adenosis, epitheliosis and stromal proliferation are seen in differing proportions. BPH typically affects the submucous group of glands in the transitional zone, forming a nodular enlargement. Eventually, this overgrowth compresses the PZ glands into a false capsule and causes the appearance of the typical 'lateral' lobes.

When BPH affects the subcervical CZ glands, a 'middle' lobe develops that projects up into the bladder within the internal sphincter (Fig. 73.3). Sometimes, both lateral lobes also project into the bladder, so that, when viewed from within, the sides and back of the internal urinary meatus are surrounded by an intravesical prostatic collar.

Effects of benign prostatic hyperplasia

It is important to realise that the relationship between anatomical prostatic enlargement, lower urinary tract symptoms (LUTS) and urodynamic evidence of bladder outflow obstruction (BOO) is complex (Fig. 73.4). Pathophysiologically, BOO may be caused in part by increased smooth muscle tone, which is under the control of α-adrenergic agonists (Summary box 73.3).

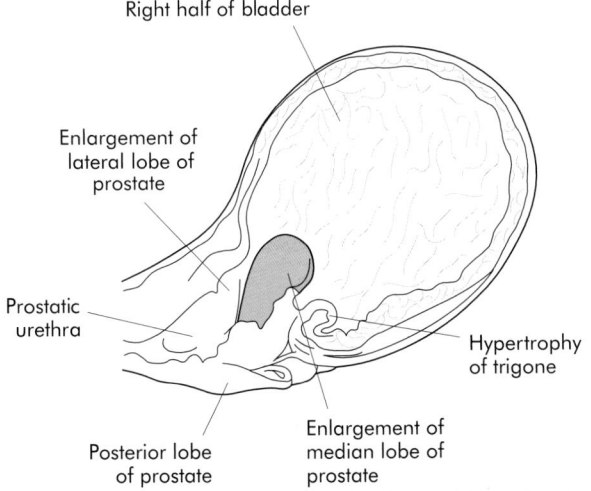

Figure 73.3 Diagram of late-stage bladder outflow obstruction (BOO) showing enlargement of the prostate from benign prostatic hyperplasia (BPH), trabeculation of the bladder with smooth muscle hypertrophy and fibrosis.

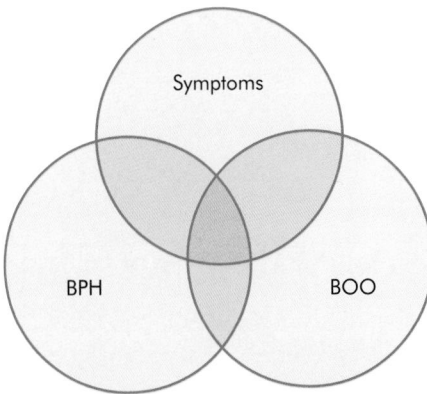

Figure 73.4 Diagrammatic representation of the relation between symptoms of prostatism, benign prostate hyperplasia (BPH) and urodynamically proven bladder outflow obstruction (BOO).

Summary box 73.3

Consequences of BPH

■ No symptoms, no BOO
■ No symptoms, but urodynamic evidence of BOO
■ Lower urinary tract symptoms, no evidence of BOO
■ Lower urinary tract symptoms and BOO
■ Others (acute/chronic retention, haematuria, urinary infection and stone formation)

Anatomically, the effects are as follows:

• *Urethra.* The prostatic urethra is lengthened, sometimes to twice its normal length, but it is not narrowed anatomically. The normal posterior curve may be so exaggerated that it requires a curved catheter to negotiate it. When only one lateral lobe is enlarged, distortion of the prostatic urethra occurs.
• *Bladder.* If BPH causes BOO, the musculature of the bladder hypertrophies to overcome the obstruction and appears trabeculated (Fig. 73.5). Significant BPH is associated with increased blood flow, and the resultant veins at the base of the bladder are apt to cause haematuria.

Lower urinary tract symptoms (LUTS)

In both sexes, non-specific symptoms of bladder dysfunction become more common with age, probably owing to impairment of smooth muscle function and neurovesical coordination. Not all symptoms of disturbed voiding in ageing men should therefore be attributed to BPH causing BOO. Urologists prefer the term LUTS and discourage the use of the descriptive term 'prostatism'.

The following conditions can coexist with BOO, leading to difficulty in diagnosis and in predicting the outcome of treatment:

• idiopathic detrusor overactivity (see Chapter 72);
• neuropathic bladder dysfunction as a result of diabetes, strokes, Alzheimer's disease or Parkinson's disease (see Chapter 72);

Alois Alzheimer, 1864–1915, a Neurologist who worked at Heidelberg and Munich, before being appointed Professor of Psychiatry at Breslau, Germany, (now Wrocław, Poland).
James Parkinson, 1755–1824, a General Practitioner of Shoreditch, London, England who published 'An Essay on the Shaking Palsy' in 1817.

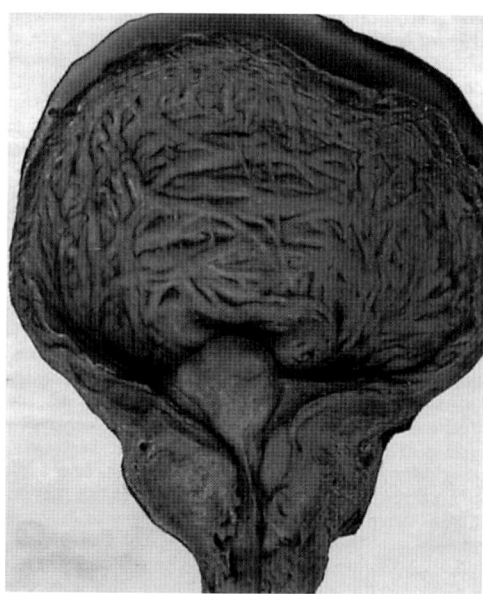

Figure 73.5 Trabeculation of the bladder from prostatic obstruction. When viewed from within, bands of muscle fibres can be seen – trabeculation. Between these hypertrophied bundles, there are shallow depressions, i.e. sacculations. Sometimes, one of the saccules (rarely two or more) continues to enlarge and forms a diverticulum (courtesy of the late Professor K.A.L. Aschoff, Freiburg, Germany).

- degeneration of bladder smooth muscle giving rise to impaired voiding and detrusor instability;
- BOO due to BPH.

Lower urinary tract symptoms can be described as:

- voiding
  - hesitancy (worsened if the bladder is very full);
  - poor flow (unimproved by straining);
  - intermittent stream – stops and starts;
  - dribbling (including after micturition);
  - sensation of poor bladder emptying;
  - episodes of near retention.
- storage
  - frequency;
  - nocturia;
  - urgency;
  - urge incontinence;
  - nocturnal incontinence (enuresis).

LUTS are usually assessed by means of scoring systems, which give a semi-objective measure of severity. However, some symptoms do not give an accurate picture of the underlying pathophysiological problem. For instance, a man with severe detrusor instability may void only small volumes and hence he will have a sensation of poor flow because low voided volumes (< 100 ml) are associated with low flow rates.

Severe irritative symptoms are usually associated with detrusor instability. Post-micturition dribbling is now known not to be a consequence of BOO and is not usually improved by prostatectomy.

Bladder outflow obstruction

This is a urodynamic concept based on the combination of low flow rates in the presence of high voiding pressures. It can be diagnosed definitively only by pressure–flow studies. This is because symptoms are relatively non-specific and can result from detrusor instability, neurological dysfunction and weak bladder contraction. Even low measured peak flow rates (< 10–12 ml s^{-1}) are not absolutely diagnostic because, in addition to BOO, weak detrusor contractions or low voided volumes (owing to instability) can be the cause. Nonetheless, flow rates provide a useful guide for everyday clinical management.

Urodynamically proven BOO may result from:

- BPH;
- bladder neck stenosis;
- bladder neck hypertrophy;
- prostate cancer;
- urethral strictures;
- functional obstruction due to neuropathic conditions.

The primary effects of BOO on the bladder are as follows:

- *Urinary flow rates decrease* (for a voided volume > 200 ml, a peak flow rate of > 15 ml s^{-1} is normal (Fig. 73.6), one of 10–15 ml s^{-1} is equivocal and one < 10 ml s^{-1} is low (Fig. 73.7).
- *Voiding pressures increase* (pressures > 80 cmH$_2$O are high (Fig. 73.8), pressures between 60 and 80 cmH$_2$O are equivocal and pressures < 60 cmH$_2$O are normal).

The long-term effects of bladder outflow obstruction are as follows:

1 The bladder may decompensate so that detrusor contraction becomes progressively less efficient and a residual urine develops.
2 The bladder may become more irritable during filling with a decrease in functional capacity partly caused by detrusor overactivity (see Chapter 76), which may also be caused by neurological dysfunction or ageing, or may be idiopathic.

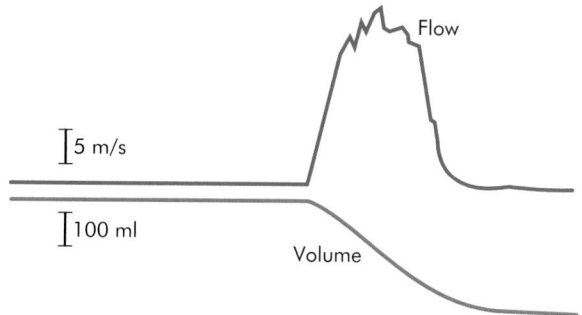

Figure 73.6 Normal flow rate. The voided volume is well in excess of 350 ml, and the maximum flow rate is in excess of 25 ml s^{-1}.

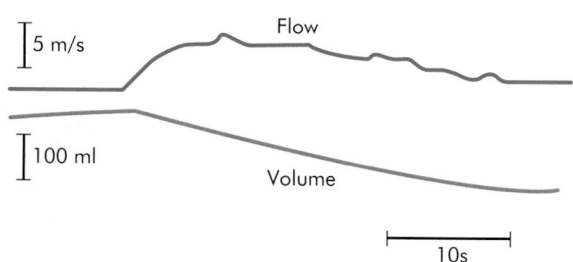

Figure 73.7 Diagram of a low flow rate showing a rather low voided volume of about 200 ml, but with markedly decreased flow rate. Such a flow rate could be caused by a urethral stricture, bladder outflow obstruction or a weak detrusor.

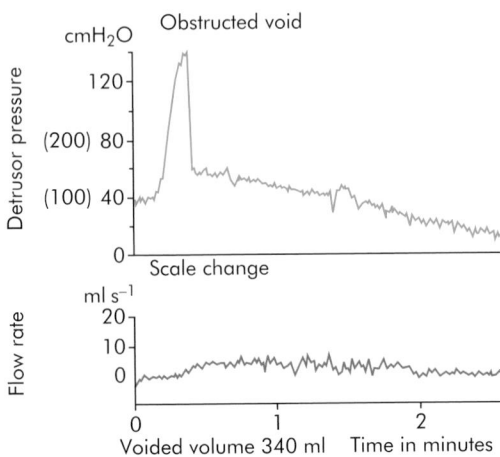

Figure 73.8 Conventional urodynamic trace showing detrusor pressure during voiding. There has been a change in scale because the pressure was so high; voiding pressures are increased with a low flow rate. This is diagnostic of bladder outflow obstruction.

Aside from symptoms, the complications of BOO are as follows:

1 *Acute retention* of urine is sometimes the first symptom of BOO. Postponement of micturition is a common precipitating cause; overindulgence in beer and confinement to bed on account of intercurrent illness or operation are other causes.

2 *Chronic retention.* In patients in whom the residual volume is > 250 ml or so (Fig. 73.9), the tension in the bladder wall increases owing to the combination of a large volume of residual urine and increased resting and filling bladder pressures (a condition known as high-pressure chronic retention). The increased intramural tension results in functional obstruction of the upper urinary tract with the development of bilateral hydronephrosis (Figs 73.10 and 73.11). As a result, upper tract infection and renal impairment may develop. Such men may present with overflow incontinence, enuresis and renal insufficiency. These symptoms should alert the doctor to the presence of this condition.

3 *Impaired bladder emptying.* If the bladder decompensates with the development of a large volume of residual urine, urinary infection and calculi are prone to develop.

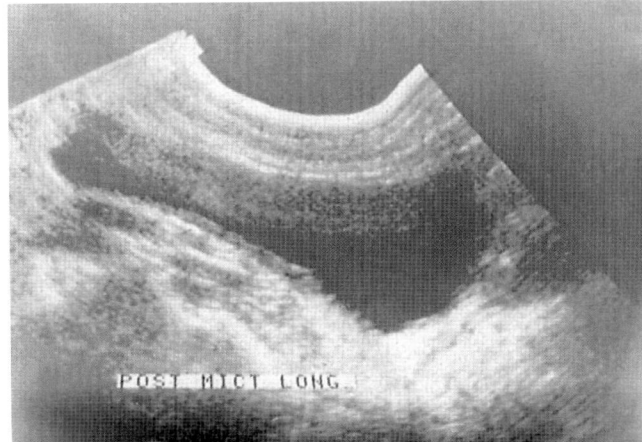

Figure 73.9 An ultrasonogram showing a large post-void residual urine.

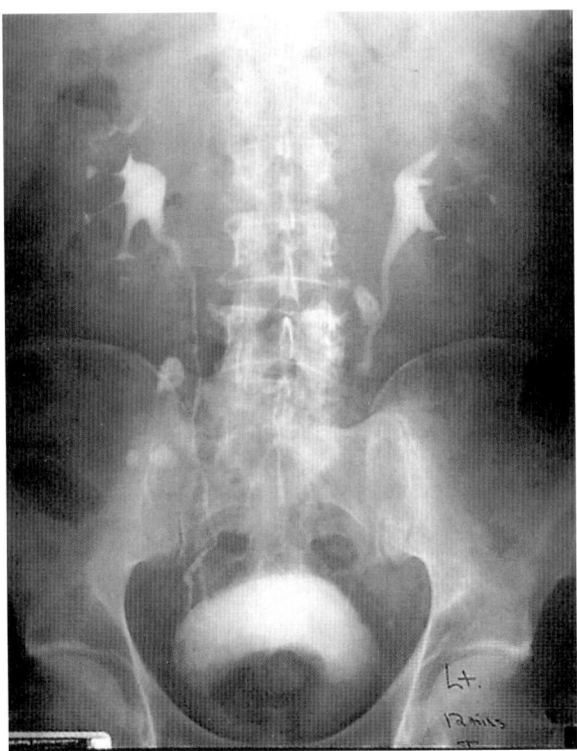

Figure 73.10 Intravenous urogram from a patient with symptoms of outflow obstruction and a moderate post-micturition residual urine. The patient did not undergo treatment.

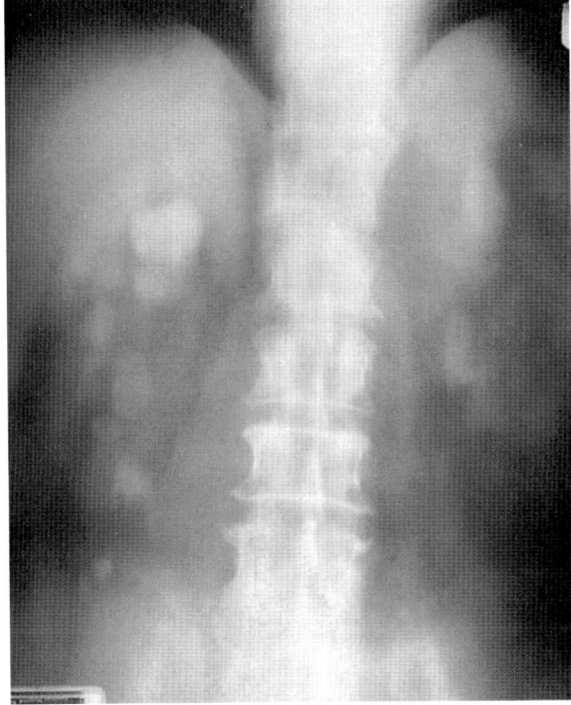

Figure 73.11 Intravenous urogram from the same patient as in Figure 73.10 but carried out some years later. The patient had developed chronic urinary retention and renal impairment owing to upper urinary dilatation.

CHAPTER 73 | THE PROSTATE AND SEMINAL VESICLES

4 *Haematuria*. This may be a complication of BPH. Other causes must be excluded by carrying out an intravenous urography (IVU), cystoscopy, urine culture and urine cytological examination.

5 Other than pain from retention, pain is not a symptom of BOO, and its presence should prompt the exclusion of acute retention, urinary infection, stones, carcinoma of the prostate and carcinoma *in situ* of the bladder.

ASSESSMENT OF THE PATIENT WITH LOWER URINARY TRACT SYMPTOMS

History

Symptom score sheets such as the International Prostate Symptom Score (IPSS) assign a score which gives information regarding the severity of symptoms at the outset and changes over time and following intervention. The IPSS assessment should include an assessment of quality of life, which is a reflection of the degree of 'bother' caused by a patient's symptoms. In addition to the IPSS, a frequency–volume diary completed by the patient before attending the clinic is invaluable in revealing fluid intake habits, diurnal variation in outputs and low-volume, frequent voiding. These assessments are routinely performed at lower urinary tract clinics but can be elicited by a thorough clinical history (Summary box 73.4).

Summary box 73.4

Investigations of men with LUTS

Essential investigations
■ Urine analysis by dipstick for blood, glucose and protein
■ Urine culture for infection
■ Serum creatinine
■ Urinary flow rate and residual volume measurement

Additional investigations
■ PSA if indicated
■ Pressure–flow studies

Abdominal examination

Abdominal extension is usually normal. In patients with chronic retention, a distended bladder will be found on palpation, on percussion and sometimes on inspection with loss of the transverse suprapubic skin crease. General physical examination may demonstrate signs of chronic renal impairment with anaemia and dehydration. The external urinary meatus should be examined to exclude stenosis, and the epididymides are palpated for signs of inflammation.

Rectal examination

In benign enlargement, the posterior surface of the prostate is smooth, convex and typically elastic, but the fibrous element may give the prostate a firm consistency. The rectal mucosa can be made to move over the prostate. Residual urine may be felt as a fluctuating swelling above the prostate. It should be noted that, if there is a considerable amount of residual urine present, it pushes the prostate downwards, making it appear larger than it is.

The nervous system

The nervous system is examined to eliminate a neurological lesion. Diabetes mellitus, tabes dorsalis, disseminated sclerosis,

cervical spondylosis, Parkinson's disease and other neurological states may mimic prostatic obstruction. If these are suspected then a pressure–flow urodynamic study should be carried out to diagnose BOO. Examination of perianal sensation and anal tone is useful in detection of an S2 to S4 cauda equina lesion.

Serum prostate-specific antigen

The difficulty here is the uncertain benefit of early detection and radical treatment of prostate cancer – this is dealt with in the section on prostate cancer. Certainly, men should be informed about the test, the risks of the prostate biopsy that might be required and the risks of the detection of a cancer that we are not certain how best to treat, as well as the positive aspects of the early discovery of a small prostate cancer. After suitable counselling, measurement of serum PSA may be helpful. Men in whom a diagnosis of early prostate cancer might influence treatment option (such as those under 70 years or those with a positive family history who might be offered radical treatment) should be offered a PSA measurement. If this is in excess of 2.5–4 nmol l^{-1}, then transrectal ultrasound scanning (TRUS) plus multiple transrectal biopsies (10 biopsies) should be considered.

If rectal examination is quite normal with no suspicion of cancer, and if no change in treatment policy would in any case result from the diagnosis of early prostate cancer, then there is little point in the routine measurement of PSA in men with uncomplicated BOO. However, because of the fear of future litigation, many find it easier to offer a PSA test.

Flow rate measurement

For this to be meaningful, two or three voids should be recorded, and the voided volume should be in excess of 150–200 ml. This usually means the patient attending a special flow rate clinic. A typical history and a flow rate < 10 ml s^{-1} (for a voided volume of > 200 ml; Fig. 73.7) will be sufficient for most urologists to recommend treatment. Usually, a flow rate measurement will be coupled with ultrasound measurement of post-void residual urine.

There are pitfalls in the measurement of flow rates. The machine must be accurately calibrated. The patient must void volumes in excess of 150 ml, and two or three recordings are needed to obtain a representative measurement. Decreased flow rates and symptoms of prostatism may be seen in:

• BOO;
• low voided volumes (characteristically in men with detrusor instability);
• men with weak bladder contractions (low pressure–flow voiding).

Pressure–flow urodynamic studies (Fig. 73.8)

Details of these studies are outlined in Chapter 72. They should be performed on the following patients:

• men with suspected neuropathy (Parkinson's disease, dementia, longstanding diabetes, previous strokes, multiple sclerosis);
• men with a dominant history of irritative symptoms and men with lifelong urgency and frequency;
• men with a doubtful history and those with flow rates in the near normal range (~ or > 15 ml s^{-1});
• men with invalid flow rate measurements (because of low voided volumes).

Blood tests

Serum creatinine, electrolytes and haemoglobin should be measured.

Examination of urine

The urine is examined for glucose and blood; a midstream specimen should be sent for bacteriological examination, and cytological examination may be carried out if carcinoma *in situ* is thought possible.

Upper tract imaging

Most urologists no longer carry out imaging of the upper tract in men with straightforward symptoms. Obviously, if infection or haematuria is present, then the upper tract should be imaged by means of intravenous urogram or ultrasound scan.

Cystourethroscopy

Inspection of the urethra, the prostate and the urothelium of the bladder should always be done immediately prior to prostatectomy, whether it is being done transurethrally or by the open route to exclude a urethral stricture, a bladder carcinoma and the occasional non-opaque vesical calculus. The decision of whether to perform prostatectomy must be made before cystoscopy. This should be based on the patient's symptoms, signs and investigations. Direct inspection of the prostate is a poor indicator of BOO and the need for surgery.

Transrectal ultrasound scanning

There is no need to carry this out routinely. Accurate estimation of prostatic size is also possible by means of transrectal or transabdominal ultrasound scanning.

MANAGEMENT OF MEN WITH BENIGN PROSTATIC HYPERPLASIA OR BLADDER OUTFLOW OBSTRUCTION

Strong indications for treatment (usually prostatectomy) include:

1 *Acute retention* (see Chapter 72) in fit men with no other cause for retention (drugs, constipation, recent operation, etc.) (accounts for 25% of prostatectomies).
2 *Chronic retention and renal impairment*: a residual urine of 200 ml or more, a raised blood urea, hydroureter or hydronephrosis demonstrated on urography and uraemic manifestations (accounts for 15% of prostatectomies).
3 *Complications of bladder outflow obstruction*: stone, infection and diverticulum formation.
4 *Haemorrhage*: occasionally, venous bleeding from a ruptured vein overlying the prostate will require prostatectomy to be performed.
5 *Elective prostatectomy for severe symptoms*: this accounts for about 60% of prostatectomies. Increasing difficulty in micturition, with considerable frequency day and night, delay in starting and a poor stream are the usual symptoms for which prostatectomy is advised. Frequency alone is not a strong indication for prostatectomy. The natural progression of outflow obstruction is variable and rarely gets worse after 10 years.

Severe symptoms, a low maximum flow rate ($< 10\ \mathrm{ml\ s^{-1}}$) and an increased residual volume of urine (100–250 ml) are relatively strong indications for operative treatment. The exact cut-off for operative or non-operative treatment will depend on careful discussion between the patient and the urologist (Summary box 73.5).

Summary box 73.5

Options for treatment of LUTS secondary to BPH

- ■ Conservative measures include watchful waiting in conjunction with fluid restriction and reduction in caffeine intake
- ■ Drug therapy is with α-blockers or, in men with a large prostate, a 5α-reductase inhibitor, or both
- ■ Interventional measures include transurethral resection of the prostate (TURP), which remains the 'gold standard'; consider open prostatectomy for large glands

---

Acute retention

The management of retention is discussed in detail in Chapter 72. Once the bladder has been drained by means of a catheter, the patient's fitness for treatment is determined. If retention was not caused by drugs or constipation, then prostatectomy would usually be the correct management. Unfit men or those with dementia may be treated by means of indwelling prostatic stents or a catheter. Similar comments apply to men with chronic retention once renal function has been stabilised by catheterisation. The role of α-adrenergic drugs followed by a trial of catheter has been tested and found to be successful in certain groups with a short history and a low residual volume of urine, but the recurrence rate becomes cumulatively high.

Special problems in the management of chronic retention (see Chapter 72 for general management of retention)

Men with chronic retention who have relatively low volumes of residual urine and who do not have symptoms suggestive of coexistent infection and with good renal function do not necessarily require catheterisation before proceeding to prostatectomy on the next available list. For those who are uraemic, urgent catheterisation is mandatory to allow renal function to recover and stabilise. Haematuria often occurs following catheterisation owing to collapse of the distended bladder and upper tract, but settles within a couple of days.

Uraemic patients with chronic retention are often dehydrated at the time of admission. Owing to the chronic back pressure on the distal tubules within the kidney, there is loss of the ability to reabsorb salts and water. The result, following release of this pressure, may be an enormous outflow of salts and water, which is known as post-obstructive diuresis. It is for this reason that a careful fluid chart, daily measurements of the patient's weight and serial estimations of creatinine and electrolytes are essential. Intravenous fluid replacement is required if the patient is unable to keep up with this fluid loss. These patients are often anaemic and may require a blood transfusion once fluid balance is stabilised (if haemoglobin is $< 9\ \mathrm{g\ l^{-1}}$).

Indications for elective treatment in men with LUTS secondary to BPH

Following careful assessment (see section on the assessment of men with LUTS), the following questions should be answered:

1 Have they failed a preliminary trial of medical therapy? Commonly, men will have been treated with α-blockers or 5α-reductase inhibitors and will have failed treatment. They are then referred by their general practitioner to the urologist.

2 Is BOO present? In many cases, the findings of significant symptoms (assessed by symptom scoring), a benign prostate supplemented by the finding of a low maximum flow rate [< 10–12 ml s^{-1} for a good voided volume (> 200 ml)] will suffice to make a reasonable working diagnosis of BOO. In some men, particularly those with irritative symptoms, suspected neurological disease or those with technically imperfect flow rate measurements, pressure–flow studies will need to be performed.

3 How severe are the symptoms and what are the risks of doing nothing? Severe symptoms and a large residual volume of urine will usually require treatment. Men with mild symptoms, good flow rates (> 15 ml s^{-1}) and good bladder emptying (residual urine < 100 ml) may be safely managed by reassurance and review: such patients rarely develop severe complications such as retention in the long term.

4 Is the man fit for operative treatment?

5 What treatments are available, what are the outcomes and do the side-effects justify treatment?

Treatment

Men with symptoms attending for elective treatment (excluding acute and chronic retention)

Conservative treatment

It is in men with relatively mild symptoms, reasonable flow rates (> 10 ml^{-1}) and good bladder emptying (residual urine < 100 ml) that careful discussion over the merits and side-effects of operative treatment is warranted. Waiting for a period of 6 months after careful discussion of the diagnosis is indicated. After this, a repeat assessment of symptoms, flow rates and ultrasound scan is helpful; many men with stable symptoms will elect to leave matters be. Advice over limiting fluid intake in the evening and careful use of propantheline to help with irritative symptoms is also useful.

Drugs

In men who are very concerned about the development of sexual dysfunction after transurethral resection of the prostate (TURP), the use of drugs may be helpful. Two classes of drug have been used in the treatment of men with BOO. α-Adrenergic blocking agents inhibit the contraction of smooth muscle that is found in the prostate. The other class of drug is the 5α-reductase inhibitors, which inhibit the conversion of testosterone to DHT, the most active form of androgen. These drugs, when taken for a year, result in a 25% shrinkage of the prostate gland. Both groups of drugs are effective; however, α-blockers work more quickly and, although the 5α-reductase inhibitors have fewer side-effects, they need to be taken for at least 6 months, and their effect is greatest in patients with large (> 50 g) glands. Drug therapy results in improvements in maximum flow rates by about 2 ml s^{-1} more than placebo and results in mild (20%) improvement in symptom scores. TURP, however, results in improvements in maximum flow rates from 9 to 18 ml s^{-1} and a 75% improvement in symptom scores. These drugs are expensive in comparison with their effectiveness, and a significant proportion of men who try these drugs will subsequently undergo TURP. They may be best targeted at men who have failed an initial trial of watchful waiting and who wish to avoid surgery for a period.

Operative treatment

Apart from the strong indications for operative treatment mentioned above, the most common reason for TURP is a combination of severe symptoms and a low flow rate < 12 ml s^{-1}. The key is to assess symptoms carefully and to counsel men about side-effects and likely outcome before advising operative treatment.

Counselling men undergoing prostatectomy

Men undergoing prostatectomy need to be advised about the following:

1 *Retrograde ejaculation*. This occurs in about 65% of men after prostatectomy.

2 *Erectile impotence*. This occurs in about 5% of men, usually those whose potency is waning.

3 *The success rate*. On the whole, men with acute and chronic retention do well from the symptomatic point of view. Ninety per cent of men undergoing elective operation for severe symptoms and urodynamically proven BOO do well in terms of symptoms and flow rates. Only about 65% of those with mild symptoms or those with weak bladder contraction as the cause of their symptoms do well. Men with unobstructed detrusor instability do not respond well to TURP. This is the reason for carefully documenting the severity of symptoms and flow rates (supplemented when necessary by pressure–flow studies) before deciding on treatment.

4 *The risk of reoperation*. After TURP, this is about 15% after 8–10 years.

5 *The morbidity rate*. Death after TURP is infrequent (< 0.5%), severe sepsis is found in about 6% and severe haematuria requiring transfusion of more than 2 units of blood occurs in about 3%. After discharge, about 15–20% of men subsequently require antibiotic treatment for symptoms of urinary infection. Risk factors for complications include admission with retention, prostate cancer, renal impairment and advanced age.

Methods of performing prostatectomy

The prostate can be approached (1) transurethrally (TURP), (2) retropubically (RPP), (3) through the bladder (transvesical; TVP) or (4) from the perineum (Fig. 73.12).

Transurethral resection of the prostate

TURP has largely replaced other methods unless diverticulectomy or the removal of large stones necessitates open operation; over 95% of men being treated by urologists can be dealt with by TURP. Perhaps the greatest advance in the history of transurethral surgery was marked by the development of the rigid lens system of Professor Harold Hopkins. His lenses, illuminated by a fibreoptic light source, permit unparalleled visualisation of

Harold Horace Hopkins, **1918–1994, Professor of Applied Optics, The University of Reading, Reading, England.**

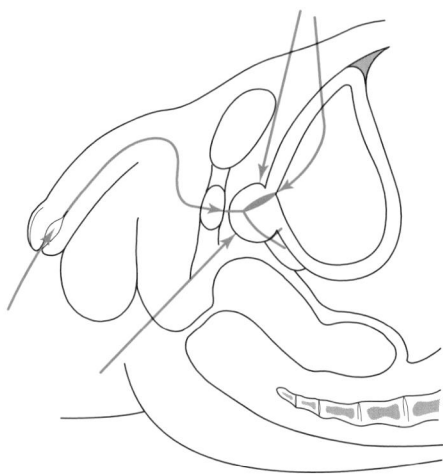

Figure 73.12 The surgical approaches to the prostate.

the working field. Men with indwelling catheters, those with recent urinary infection, those with chronic retention or those with prosthetic material or heart valves should receive broad-spectrum prophylactic antibiotics with amoxicillin plus cefuroxime or gentamicin intravenously at induction of anaesthesia.

Strips of tissue are cut from the bladder neck down to the level of the verumontanum (Fig. 73.13). Cutting is performed by a high-frequency diathermy current, which is applied across a loop mounted on the hand-held trigger of the resectoscope. Coagulation of bleeding points can be accurately achieved, and damage to the external sphincter is avoided provided one uses the verumontanum as a guide to the most distal point of the resection. The 'chips' of prostate are then removed from the bladder using an Ellik evacuator. The risks of hyponatraemia are reduced by using 1.5% isotonic glycine for irrigation, and the recent introduction of continuous-flow resectoscopes makes the procedure swift and safe in experienced hands. At the end of the procedure, careful haemostasis is performed, and a three-way,

self-retaining catheter irrigated with isotonic saline is introduced into the bladder to prevent any further bleeding from forming blood clots. Irrigation is continued until the outflow is pale pink, and the catheter is usually removed on the second or third postoperative day. In men with small prostates or bladder neck dyssynergia or stenosis, it is better to divide the bladder neck and prostatic urethra with a diathermy 'bee-sting' electrode.

Retropubic prostatectomy (Millin)

Using a low, curved transverse suprapubic Pfannenstiel incision, which includes the rectus sheath, the recti are split in the midline and retracted to expose the bladder. With the patient in the Trendelenburg position, the surgeon separates the bladder and the prostate from the posterior aspect of the pubis. In the space thus obtained, the anterior capsule of the prostate is incised with diathermy below the bladder neck, care being taken to obtain complete control of bleeding from divided prostatic veins by suture ligation. The prostatic adenoma is exposed and enucleated with a finger. A wedge is taken out of the posterior lip of the bladder neck to prevent secondary stricture in this region. The exposure of the inside of the prostatic cavity is good, and control of haemorrhage is achieved with diathermy and suture ligation of bleeding points before closure of the capsule over a Foley catheter (inserted per urethram) draining the bladder.

Transvesical prostatectomy

The bladder is opened, and the prostate enucleated by putting a finger into the urethra, pushing forwards towards the pubes to separate the lateral lobes, and then working the finger between the adenoma and the false capsule. In Freyer's operation (1901), the bladder was left open widely and drained by a suprapubic tube with a 16-mm lumen in order to allow free drainage of blood and urine. Harris (1934) advocated control of the prostatic arteries by lateral stitches inserted with his boomerang needle, the bladder wall was closed and the wound drained.

Perineal prostatectomy (Young)

This has now been abandoned for the treatment of BPH.

After treatment

Most urologists irrigate the bladder with sterile saline by means of a three-way Foley catheter for 24 hours or so.

Complications

Local

Haemorrhage is a major risk following prostatectomy whatever the surgical approach. Care should be taken in diathermising

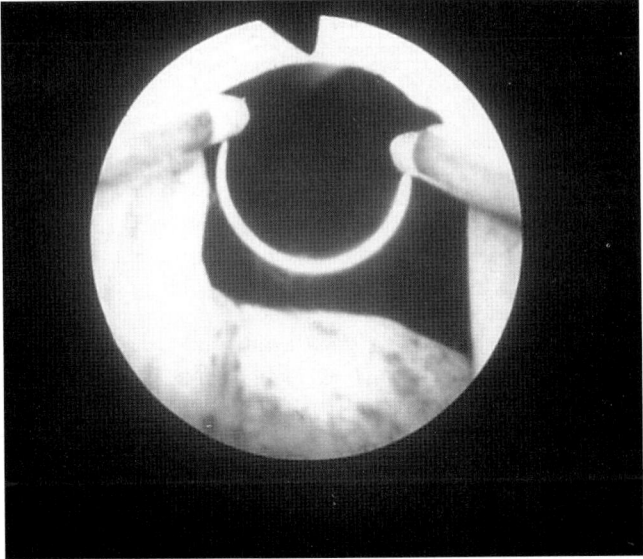

Figure 73.13 Endoscopic photograph of transurethral prostatectomy.

Milo Ellik, **a twentieth century American Urologist.**

Terence John Millin, **1903–1980, Surgeon, The Westminster Hospital, London, England, described the operation of retropubic prostatectomy in 1945.**
Hermann Johann Pfannenstiel, **1862–1909, Gynaecologist, Breslau, Germany, (now Wroclaw, Poland), described this incision in 1900.**
Friedrich Trendelenburg, **1844–1924, Professor of Surgery, Rostock (1875–1882), Bonn (1882–1895), and Leipzig (1895–1911), Germany. The Trendelenburg Position was first described in 1885.**
Frederic Eugene Basil Foley, **1891–1966, Urologist, Ankher Hospital, St Paul, MN, USA.**
Sir Peter Johnston Freyer, **1852–1921, Surgeon, St Peter's Hospital for Stone, London, England.**
Samuel Harry Harris, **1881–1937, Urologist, Lewisham Hospital, Sydney, NSW, Australia.**
Hugh Hampton Young, **1870–1945, Director, The James Buchanan Brady Urological Institute, Baltimore, MD, USA.**

arterial bleeding points after TURP; they are often better seen when the rate of inflow of fluid is decreased. In the recovery room, one should check that the bladder is draining adequately; if it is not, this may indicate that a clot is blocking the eye of the catheter. The bladder should be promptly washed out using strict aseptic technique. The catheter should be changed by the surgeon. Only rarely is it necessary to return the patient to the operating room.

Secondary haemorrhage tends to occur after the patient has been discharged. All men should be warned about this possibility and given appropriate advice to rest and to have a high fluid intake. It is usually minor in degree but if clot retention occurs, the patient will need to be readmitted, a catheter will have to be passed and the bladder washed out.

Perforation of the bladder or the prostatic capsule can occur at the time of transurethral surgery. This usually occurs from a combination of inexperience in association with a large prostate or heavy blood loss. If the field of vision becomes obscured by heavy blood loss, it is often prudent to achieve adequate haemostasis and abandon the operation, swallowing one's pride on the understanding that a second attempt may be necessary. A large perforation with marked extravasation may require the insertion of a small suprapubic drain. Rectal perforation should be extremely rare.

Sepsis

Bacteraemia is common even in men with sterile urine and occurs in over 50% of men with infected urine, prolonged catheterisation or chronic retention. Septicaemia can occur in these patients shortly after operation or when the catheter is removed. In men at high risk, the use of prophylactic antibiotics is recommended. Wound infection following open prostatectomy is common if a urethral catheter has been *in situ* for a number of days before the operation. The most worrying aspect of infection is the early rigor following surgery. If left undetected and untreated, this may progress to frank septicaemia with profound hypotension. A blood culture should be taken and antibiotics given parenterally, e.g. amoxicillin plus cefuroxime, or gentamicin.

Incontinence

Incontinence is inevitable if the external sphincter mechanism is damaged. The bladder neck is rendered incompetent by any prostatectomy and, therefore, an intact distal sphincter mechanism is essential for continence. Damage to the sphincter may occur at open prostatectomy and following transurethral surgery if the resection extends beyond the verumontanum. If pelvic floor physiotherapy is ineffective, then the only satisfactory treatment is the fitting of an artificial urinary sphincter. In some patients, detrusor instability contributes to the incontinence. The use of anti-cholinergic agents or imipramine or duloxetine may help.

Retrograde ejaculation and impotence

Impotence in men with good sexual function before surgery is uncommon, but retrograde ejaculation occurs commonly (> 50%) because of disruption to the bladder neck mechanism.

Urethral stricture

This may be secondary to prolonged catheterisation, the use of an unnecessarily large catheter, clumsy instrumentation or the presence of the resectoscope in the urethra for too long a period. These strictures arise either just inside the meatus or in the bulbar urethra. An early stricture can usually be managed by simple

bouginage but, later on, it may be necessary to cut the densely fibrotic stricture with the optical urethrotome. The routine use of an Otis urethrotomy prior to TURP reduces the incidence of postoperative stricture.

Bladder neck contracture

Occasionally, a dense fibrotic stenosis of the bladder neck occurs following overaggressive resection of a small prostate. It may be due to the overuse of coagulating diathermy. Transurethral incision of the scar tissue is necessary.

Reoperation

It is now well known that, after 8 years, 15–18% of men with BPH will undergo repeat TURP (the rate after open prostatectomy is about 5%). The reasons include a technically imperfect primary procedure and a speculative repeat operation in men with symptoms who are cystoscoped after operation.

General complications

Death occurs in about 0.2–0.3% of men undergoing elective prostatectomy. In very elderly men, in men with prostate cancer admitted as an emergency with acute or chronic retention or in those with very large prostates, the 30-day death rate may be in the order of 1%.

Cardiovascular

Pulmonary atelectasis, pneumonia, myocardial infarction, congestive cardiac failure and deep venous thrombosis are all potentially life-threatening conditions that can affect this elderly and often frail group of men.

Water intoxication

The absorption of water into the circulation at the time of transurethral resection can give rise to congestive cardiac failure, hyponatraemia and haemolysis. Accompanying this, there is frequently confusion and other cerebral events often mimicking a stroke. The incidence of this condition has been reduced since the introduction of isotonic glycine for performing the resections and the use of isotonic saline for postoperative irrigation. The treatment consists of fluid restriction.

Osteitis pubis

This is rare.

Newer treatments

In general, newer, minimally invasive treatments occupy a position intermediate between TURP and drug treatment. In the last decade, technological innovations led to the introduction of novel minimally invasive treatments for prostatectomy. Tissue ablative techniques using hyperthermia and laser energy were associated with minimal morbidity and could often be performed as out-patient procedures. Many of the initial studies reporting treatment success were poorly designed and over a short duration. Longer-term follow-up and randomised controlled trials have failed to confirm significant benefit from these techniques. More recently, the holmium laser, a pulsed solid-state laser, has been used to enucleate the prostate adenoma. This approach involves excision of parts of the prostate using a cutting laser and

---

Fessenden Nott Otis, 1825–1900, a nineteenth century American Urologist.

then morcellating the excised prostate fragments, which fall back into the bladder so that they can be removed. Morbidity with this procedure is low and short-term results favourable; long-term follow-up will be necessary to determine whether this treatment will have a role to play in the management of BOO. The green light laser is now being used to vaporise the prostate tissue, but has not yet been shown to be as durable as holmium laser treatment or TURP, because the amount of tissue removed is usually less.

Intraurethral stents (Fig. 73.14)

These devices are possibly helpful in the management of men with retention who are grossly unfit (classified by the American Society of Anesthesiologists as ASA grade IV). These men are rare cases.

BLADDER OUTFLOW OBSTRUCTION CAUSED BY THE BLADDER NECK

Aetiology

This condition usually occurs in men, but can rarely affect children of both sexes and women. It may be due to muscular hypertrophy or fibrosis of the tissues at the bladder neck following TURP.

Clinical syndromes

Owing to muscle hypertrophy or dyssynergia

Marion described a series of cases in which muscular hypertrophy of the internal sphincter in a young person had resulted in the development of a vesical diverticulum or hydronephrosis (Marion's disease or 'prostatism sans prostate'). It is thought that dyssynergic contraction of the smooth muscle of the bladder neck (bladder neck dyssynergia) may account for some cases of BOO.

Owing to fibrosis

The symptoms are similar to those of prostatic enlargement but are a consequence of scarring after TURP.

Treatment

The management of these patients depends on achieving an accurate diagnosis. For this, urodynamic investigation is often necessary, which should demonstrate raised voiding pressures and diminished flow rate.

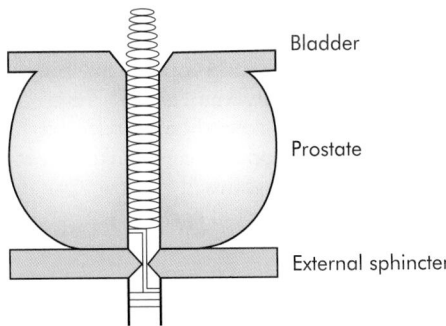

Figure 73.14 Diagram showing one type of prostatic stent *in situ*.

Bladder

Prostate

External sphincter

Jean Baptiste Camile Marion, **1869–1932, Professor of Urology, The Faculty of Medicine, Paris, France.**

Drugs

The presence of α-adrenergic receptors in the region of the bladder neck and prostatic urethra allows pharmacological manipulation of the outflow to the bladder.

α-Blocking drugs

Alfuzosin, 2.5 mg b.d. to t.d.s. (to a total maximum of 10 mg day⁻¹), doxazosin, 1 mg nocte (up to a maximum of 8 mg day⁻¹), indoramin, 20 mg b.d. (increased to a total maximum of 100 mg day⁻¹ in divided doses), prazosin 500 mg b.d. (maintenance up to 2 mg day⁻¹) and terazosin, 1 mg nocte (to a total maximum of 10 mg day⁻¹), can be very useful, causing relaxation of the bladder neck. These drugs are not target specific, and patients must be warned of the possibility of postural hypotension.

Transurethral incision

Transurethral incision of the bladder neck is the operation of choice. Sometimes symptoms recur, but this is usually due to inadequate division of the fibres of the bladder neck.

Congenital valves of the prostatic urethra

See Chapter 74.

PROSTATIC CALCULI

Prostatic calculi are of two varieties: endogenous, which are common, and exogenous, which are comparatively rare.

An exogenous prostatic calculus is a urinary (commonly ureteric) calculus that becomes arrested in the prostatic urethra. This is considered in Chapter 71.

Endogenous prostatic calculi are usually composed of calcium phosphate combined with about 20% organic material.

Clinical features

Prostatic calculi are usually symptomless, being discovered on TRUS, on radiography of the pelvis, during prostatectomy or associated with carcinoma of the prostate or chronic prostatitis. In cases associated with severe chronic prostatic infection, the associated fibrosis and nodularity are difficult to differentiate from carcinoma. On radiographs or ultrasound scans, these stones are often seen to form a horseshoe (Fig. 73.15) or a circle.

Treatment of prostatic calculi

They usually require no treatment.

Conservative measures

Associated chronic prostatic infection may be treated by means of ciprofloxacin or trimethoprim.

Transurethral resection

Transurethral resection will often release small calculi as the strips of prostatic tissue are excised. Others are passed per urethram at a later date.

Corpora amylaceae

Corpora amylaceae are tiny calcified lamellated bodies found in the glandular alveoli of the prostates of elderly men and apes, but not in the prostates of animals lower in the phylogenetic scale than anthropoids. Corpora amylaceae are probably the forerunners of endogenous prostatic calculi.

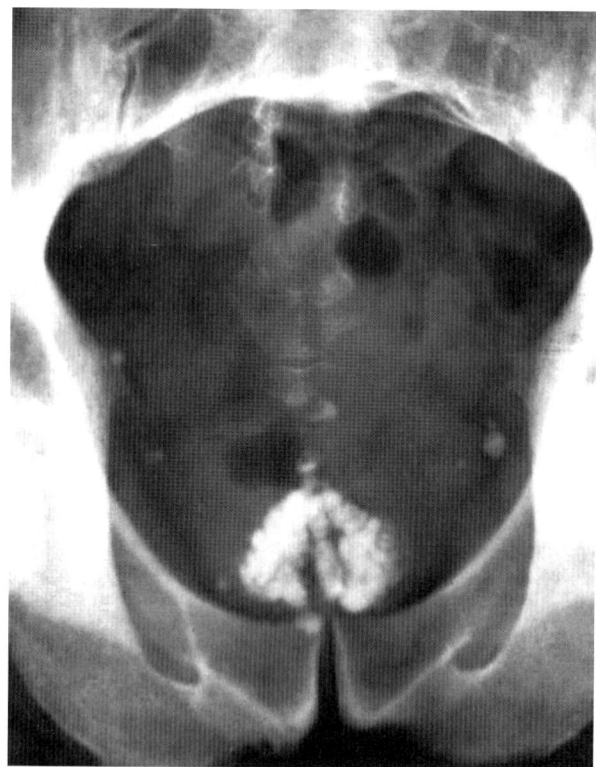

Figure 73.15 Endogenous prostatic calculi.

CARCINOMA OF THE PROSTATE

Carcinoma of the prostate is the most common malignant tumour in men over the age of 65 years. In England and Wales in 2004, 30 000 men were registered and 10 000 died from it; the corresponding figures in the USA were 260 000 and 35 000 respectively. If histological section of prostates at autopsy is performed, increasingly frequent foci of microscopic prostate cancers are found with increasing age. These foci of prostate cancer have variable potential for progressing clinically to metastatic disease. About 10–15% of younger men who develop prostate cancer have a positive family history of the disease, but the aetiology is unclear. Throughout the world, rates of microscopic foci of prostate cancer are constant, but rates of clinically evident disease are low in men in Japan and China. Carcinoma of the prostate usually originates in the PZ of the prostate (Fig. 73.2), so 'prostatectomy' for benign enlargement of the gland confers no protection from subsequent carcinoma.

Pathology

Serial sections of prostates obtained at routine necropsy demonstrate prostate carcinoma in 25% of men between 50 and 65 years of age. The incidence in men over 80 years is in the region of 70% (Franks). Most of these neoplasms are tiny and (if life had continued) might have remained latent for years.

The following types of prostate cancer occur:

- microscopic latent cancer found on autopsy or at cystoprostatectomy;
- tumours found incidentally during TURP (T1a and T1b) or following screening by PSA measurement (T1c);

- early, localised prostate cancer (T2);
- advanced local prostate cancer (T3 and T4);
- metastatic disease, which may arise from a clinically evident tumour (T2, T3 or T4) or from an apparently benign gland (T0, T1), i.e. occult prostate cancer.

It should be noted that only the last two groups cause symptoms, and such tumours are not curable. Only screening or the treatment of incidentally found tumours can result in cure of the disease. The problem is that many such tumours would never progress during the patient's lifetime; herein lies the problem with prostate cancer (Summary box 73.6).

Summary box 73.6

Prostate cancer detection

- The incidence has increased, and opportunistic PSA testing has enabled the detection of early-stage disease
- It is not yet clear whether national screening programmes for prostate cancer should be instigated
- Patients should be counselled about the investigations and treatment options available before a PSA test is performed

---

Screening for prostate cancer

The cancer detection rate using measurement of PSA is between 2% and 4%, and approximately 30% of men with an elevated PSA will have prostate cancer confirmed by biopsy. Unfortunately, 20% of men with clinically significant prostate cancer will have PSA values within the normal range. There is therefore controversy over the usefulness of PSA alone as a screening procedure. Currently, a number of prospective trials aimed at determining whether or not PSA testing reduces the disease-specific mortality of prostate cancer are under way. At present, in Europe, population-based screening is performed only within the confines of clinical trials.

Histological appearances

The prostate is a glandular structure consisting of ducts and acini; thus, the histological pattern is one of an adenocarcinoma. The prostatic glands are surrounded by a layer of myoepithelial cells. The first change associated with carcinoma is the loss of the basement membrane, with glands appearing to be in confluence. As the cell type becomes less differentiated, more solid sheets of carcinoma cells are seen. A classification of the histological pattern based on the degree of glandular de-differentiation and its relation to stroma has been devised by Gleason. Prostate cancers exhibit heterogeneity within tissue, and so two histological areas of prostate are each scored between 1 and 5. The scores are added to give an overall Gleason score of between 2 and 10; this (and the volume of the cancer) appears to correlate well with the likelihood of spread and the prognosis.

Local spread

Locally advanced tumours tend to grow upwards to involve the seminal vesicles, the bladder neck and trigone and, later, the

---

Donald F. Gleason, **b. 1920, Pathologist, University of Minnesota, Minneapolis, MN, USA.**

tumours tend to spread distally to involve the distal sphincter mechanism. Further upward extension obstructs the lower end of one or both ureters, obstruction of both resulting in anuria. The rectum may become stenosed by tumour infiltrating around it, but direct involvement is rare.

Spread by the bloodstream

Spread by the bloodstream occurs particularly to bone; indeed, the prostate is the most common site of origin for skeletal metastases, followed in turn by the breast, the kidney, the bronchus and the thyroid gland. The bones involved most frequently by carcinoma of the prostate are the pelvic bones and the lower lumbar vertebrae. The femoral head, rib cage and skull are other common sites.

Lymphatic spread

Lymphatic spread may occur (1) via lymphatic vessels passing to the obturator fossa or along the sides of the rectum to the lymph nodes beside the internal iliac vein and in the hollow of the sacrum and (2) via lymphatics that pass over the seminal vesicles and follow the vas deferens for a short distance to drain into the external iliac lymph nodes. From retroperitoneal lymph nodes, the mediastinal nodes and occasionally the supraclavicular nodes may become implicated.

Staging using the tumour, node, metastasis (TNM) system (Fig. 73.16)

1   *T1a, T1b and T1c.* These are incidentally found tumours in a clinically benign gland after histological examination of a prostatectomy specimen. T1a is a tumour involving less than 5% of the resected specimen; these tumours are usually well or moderately well differentiated. T1b is a tumour involving > 5% of the resected specimen. T1c tumours are impalpable tumours found following investigation of a raised PSA.
2   *T2a* disease presents as a suspicious nodule (Fig. 73.17) on rectal examination confined within the prostate capsule and involving one lobe. T2b disease involves both lobes.
3   *T3* tumour extends through the capsule (T3a, uni- or bilateral extension. T3b, seminal vesical extension).

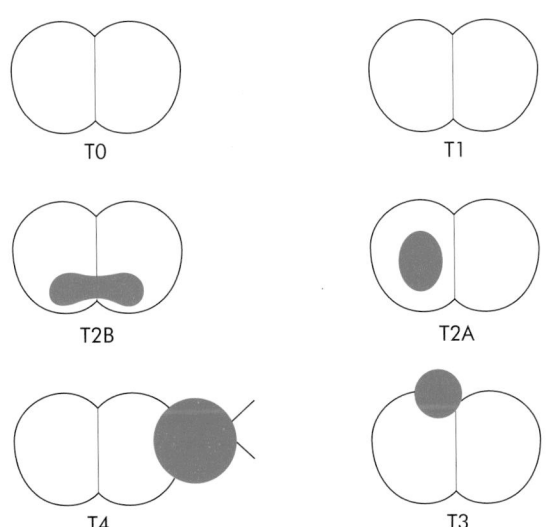

Figure 73.16 Tumour, node, metastasis (TNM) staging system for prostate cancer.

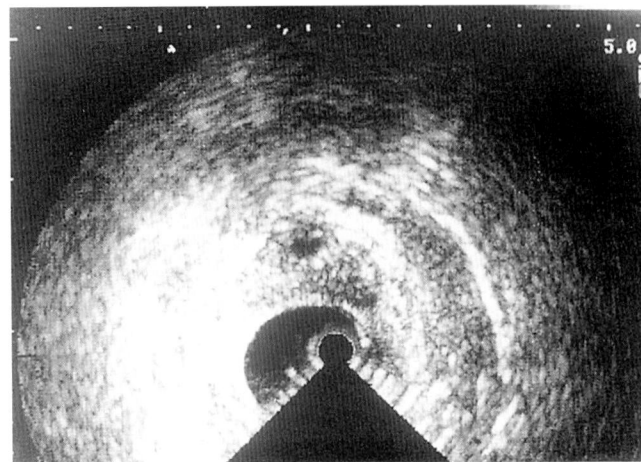

Figure 73.17 Transrectal ultrasound scan of a T2 nodule in the prostate.

4   *T4* is a tumour that is fixed or invading adjacent structures other than seminal vesicles – rectum or pelvic side wall (Summary box 73.7).

> **Summary box 73.7**
>
> **The natural history of prostate cancer**
>
> This depends on the stage and grade of disease:
>
> *T1 and T2*
> - The progression rate of well-differentiated T1a prostate cancer is very low: 10–14% after 8 years. For moderately differentiated tumours, the rate is about 20%
> - For T1b and T2 tumours, the rate is in excess of 35%
>
> *T3 and T4 (M0)*
> - About 50% progress to bony metastases after 3–5 years
>
> *M1*
> - The median survival of men with metastatic disease is about 3 years

Clinical features

Only advanced disease gives rise to symptoms, but even advanced disease may be asymptomatic. Symptoms of advanced disease include:

- BOO;
- pelvic pain and haematuria;
- bone pain, malaise, 'arthritis', anaemia or pancytopenia;
- renal failure;
- locally advanced disease or even asymptomatic metastases, which may be found incidentally on investigation of other symptoms.

Early prostate cancer is asymptomatic and may be found:

- incidentally following TURP for clinically benign disease (T1);
- as a nodule (T2) on rectal examination (Summary box 73.8).

> **Summary box 73.8**
>
> **The presentation of men with prostate cancer**
>
> - Often men are asymptomatic, and detection is by opportunistic PSA testing
> - Cancer is detected in men describing LUTS or may present with symptoms from metastatic disease

CHAPTER 73 | THE PROSTATE AND SEMINAL VESICLES

Rectal examination

Rectal examination can detect nodules within the prostate and advanced disease. TRUS may be used to access the local stage and can be combined with a needle core biopsy (Fig. 73.18). Irregular induration, characteristically stony hard in part or in the whole of the gland (with obliteration of the median sulcus), suggests carcinoma. Extension beyond the capsule up into the bladder base and vesicles (Fig. 73.19 demonstrates normal vesicles) is diagnostic, as is local extension through the capsule (Fig. 73.20).

Prostatic biopsy

If there is suspicion of prostate cancer, because of local findings, a raised PSA or metastatic disease, then a transrectal biopsy

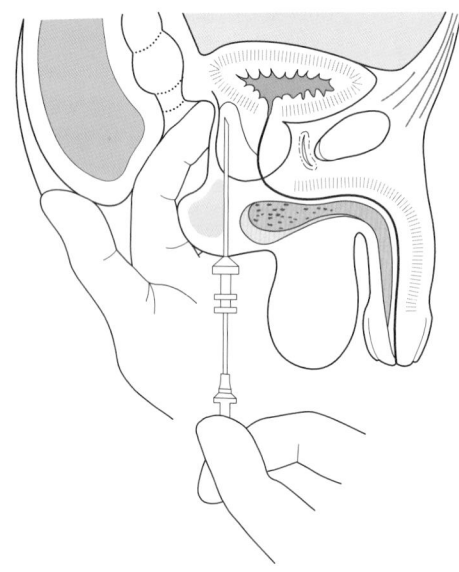

Figure 73.18 Obtaining a specimen of prostatic tissue by means of a TruCut biopsy needle.

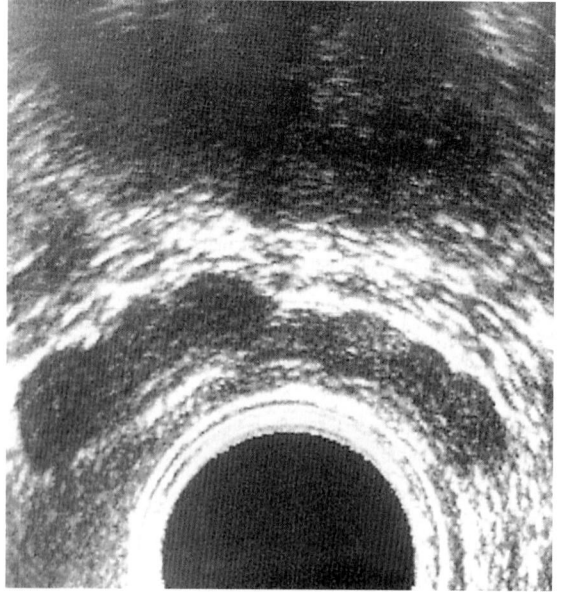

Figure 73.19 Transrectal ultrasound scan showing normal seminal vesicles.

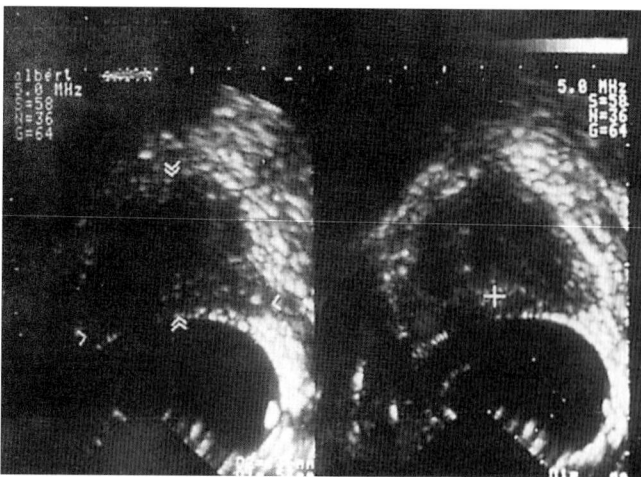

Figure 73.20 Transrectal ultrasound scan showing local extension of a T3 prostate cancer.

using an automated gun is recommended. Routine local anaesthetic is used to decrease pain. About 10 systematic biopsy cores are obtained as well as biopsy of any suspicious areas. Broadspectrum antibiotic cover is given to all patients to reduce the incidence of sepsis. If there are associated symptoms of BOO, then either:

- a TURP can be performed, which will provide diagnostic material and symptomatic relief;
- a transrectal biopsy can be carried out. If the diagnosis is positive and there is locally advanced disease, then hormone ablation can provide good symptomatic relief without the need for operation.

General blood tests

These are normal in early disease but, in metastatic disease, there may be leuco-erythroblastic anaemia secondary to extensive marrow invasion, or anaemia may be secondary to renal failure. There may be thrombocytopenia and evidence of disseminated intravascular coagulopathy with increased fibrinogen degradation products (FDPs).

Liver function tests

These will be abnormal if there is extensive metastatic invasion of the liver. The alkaline phosphatase may be raised from either hepatic involvement or secondaries in the bone. These can be distinguished by measurement of isoenzymes or gammaglutamyltransferase.

Prostate-specific antigen

This is discussed earlier in this chapter. It is good at following the course of advanced disease. It is lacking in sensitivity and specificity in the diagnosis of early localised prostate cancer. Nevertheless, the finding of a PSA > 10 nmol ml^{-1} is suggestive of cancer and > 35 ng ml^{-1} is almost diagnostic of advanced prostate cancer. A decrease in PSA to the normal range following hormonal ablation is a good prognostic sign.

Acid phosphatase

Acid phosphatase has been superseded by measurement of PSA.

Radiological examination

Radiographs of the chest may reveal metastases in either the lung fields or the ribs. An abdominal radiograph may show the characteristic sclerotic metastases in lumbar vertebrae and pelvic bones (Fig. 73.21). The bone appears dense and coarse, and it is sometimes difficult to distinguish the change from that in Paget's disease of bone. Nevertheless, osteolytic metastases are very common in prostate cancer and may coexist with sclerotic ones. Information about the upper urinary tracts can be obtained by excretion urography or ultrasound.

Cross-sectional imaging with magnetic resonance imaging and TRUS

Magnetic resonance imaging (MRI) with a high tesla magnet (1.5–3 T) is the most accurate method of staging local disease.

Transrectal ultrasound scanning can also be used. Locally extensive disease (T2) can be diagnosed with increased sensitivity by TRUS (Fig. 73.17) compared with rectal examination, but many tumours will still be missed. This problem remains a real one in screening for early prostate cancer; in comparison with breast cancer, with mammography detecting 70–80% of tumours, TRUS plus rectal examination and measurement of PSA will detect only 30–50% of cancers that are known to be present on autopsy studies (although it may detect the larger, more significant cancers).

Bone scan

Once the diagnosis has been established, it would be normal to perform a bone scan as part of the staging procedure if the PSA were > 10 nmol ml^{-1} or if the biopsy showed high-grade cancer. If the PSA is < 10 nmol ml^{-1}, then a bone scan would be performed only on clinical indications. The bone scan is performed by the injection of technetium-99m, which is then monitored using a gamma camera. It is more sensitive in the diagnosis of metastases (Fig. 73.22) than a skeletal survey, but false positives occur in areas of arthritis, osteomyelitis or a healing fracture.

Lymphangiography

This is no longer carried out. If accurate information is required, then pelvic lymphadenectomy can be performed by means of laparoscopic surgery.

Bone marrow aspiration

Sometimes, examination of the bone marrow will reveal the presence of metastatic carcinoma cells.

Treatment of carcinoma of the prostate

Early disease

Curative treatment can only be offered to patients with early disease (T1a, T1b, T1c and T2). T1a disease found incidentally at TURP is by definition low volume and usually well differentiated. This stage can often be managed by active surveillance, with 3- to 6-monthly digital rectal examination (DRE) and PSA measurement, considering treatment if there is evidence of disease progression. The options available for T1b, T1c and T2 disease need to take into account patient age, performance status and lifestyle preferences. The treatment of patients with advanced disease (T3, T4 or any M0) is only palliative (Summary box 73.9).

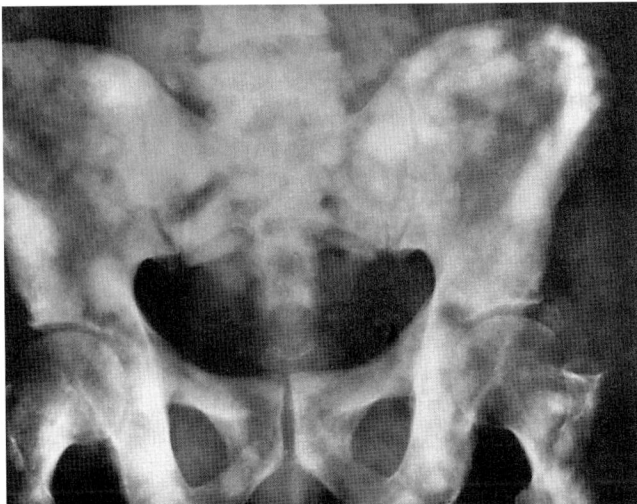

Figure 73.21 Osseous metastases of the pelvic bones in carcinoma of the prostate (courtesy of L.N. Pyrah, Leeds, UK).

Sir James Paget, 1814–1899, Surgeon, St Bartholomew's Hospital, London, England, described osteitis deformans in 1877.

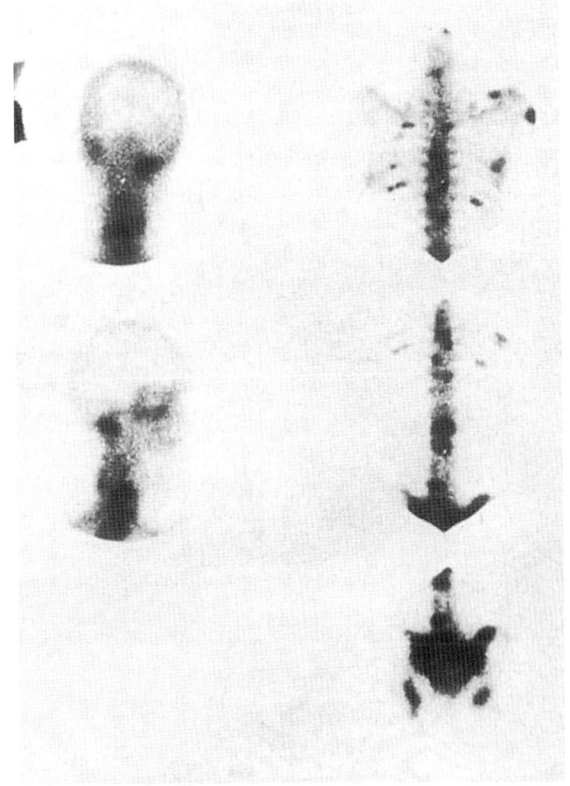

Figure 73.22 Bone scan showing multiple hot-spots suggestive of metastatic disease in a man with prostate cancer.

Radical prostatectomy

Radical prostatectomy is only suitable for localised disease (T1 and T2) and should be carried out only in men with a life expectancy of > 10 years. Exclusion of metastases would require a negative bone scan, chest radiograph and a serum PSA < 20 nmol ml^{-1}. It is a procedure that should be performed only by experienced surgeons when there is a high chance of cure. It results in a high incidence of impotence, but a low incidence of severe stress incontinence (< 2%), which may require the fitting of an artificial urinary sphincter. It involves removal of the prostate down to the distal sphincter mechanism in addition to the seminal vesicles (Fig. 73.23). The bladder neck is reconstituted and anastomosed to the urethra. Recent modifications to this operation by Professor Patrick Walsh of the Johns Hopkins Hospital in Baltimore have led to the realisation that careful dissection in early-stage disease can lead to preservation of the neurovascular bundles that lie behind the prostate. This modification has led to the preservation of erectile function in about 60–70% of cases. Recently, laparoscopic approaches to radical prostatectomy, sometimes supported by robotic techniques, have been introduced.

Radical radiotherapy for early prostate cancer

External beam radiotherapy (EBRT) can be administered in fields that conform to the contours of the prostate, thereby limiting exposure of adjacent tissues. Survival rates following the treatment of T1 and low-volume T2 disease are not greatly different from those following radical prostatectomy, although histological evidence of persistent tumour is found within the prostate in about 30% of treated patients. Patients with locally advanced disease (T3) may be treated by radiotherapy, but most urologists treat such patients by means of androgen ablation. The treatment requires the patient to attend hospital on a daily basis for between 4 and 6 weeks. Some local complications are inevitable, namely irritation of the bladder with urinary frequency, urgency and sometimes urge incontinence and similar problems affecting the rectum with diarrhoea and, occasionally, late radiation proctitis. Development of erectile dysfunction occurs less frequently than following radical prostatectomy, but is present in up to 30% of cases.

Brachytherapy

Under transrectal ultrasound guidance, radioactive seeds are permanently implanted into the prostate. A computer program converts accurate ultrasound measurements of the prostate gland to construct a plan of the gland. Under anaesthesia, the patient is placed in the lithotomy position and, according to the template plan, seeds are placed through transperineal needles. The radioisotopes commonly used are iodine-125 and palladium-103. These isotopes deliver an intense, confined radiation dose, which falls off rapidly to spare the surrounding structures. Brachytherapy is gaining widespread acceptance for the treatment of lower grade low-volume T1 disease. A major factor is the reduced peroperative complications and generally low morbidity. Long-term cancer survival results from institutions specialising in the procedure are encouraging.

Advanced disease

There is still debate about the timing of androgen ablation treatment in patients with locally advanced or metastatic disease without symptoms. The options are androgen deprivation at diagnosis or careful review, reserving active treatment for the later development of symptoms. Patients with poorly differentiated disease are at risk of a catastrophic event such as spinal cord compression; in these patients, early androgen ablation can prolong the time to complications. Also, patients with local or general symptoms should be offered androgen deprivation.

Orchidectomy

Orchidectomy is performed to carry out androgen ablation in the treatment of locally advanced (T3 or T4) disease or of metastatic disease. In 1941, prostate cancer was shown to be responsive to such treatment by Charles Huggins, the only urologist to win a Nobel Prize. Bilateral orchidectomy, whether total or subcapsular, will eliminate the major source of testosterone production.

Medical castration

Medical forms of androgen ablation have been available since the discovery of stilbestrol. The other commonly available treatment to reduce testosterone levels to the castrate range is LHRH agonists. These agents initially stimulate hypothalamic LHRH receptors but, because of their constant presence (rather than the

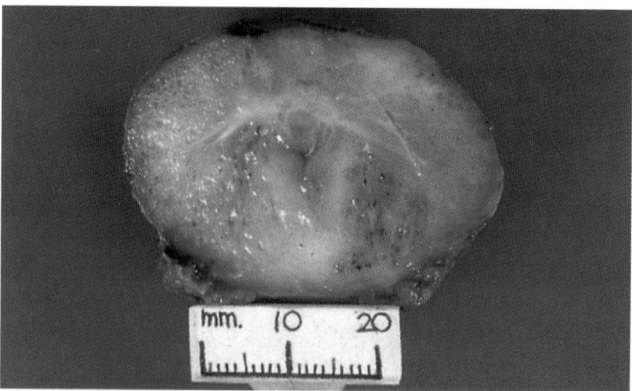

Figure 73.23 Radical prostatectomy specimen for a T2a prostate cancer. Preoperative PSA was 6 ng l^{-1}; postoperative levels remained undetectable at 8 years. The patient is fully continent.

Patrick C. Walsh, **Professor of Urology, Johns Hopkins Hospital, Baltimore, MD, USA.**

Charles Brenton Huggins, **1901–1997, Professor of Surgery, The University of Chicago, IL, USA, shared the 1966 Nobel Prize for Physiology or Medicine for his work on cancer of the prostate.**

normal diurnal rhythm), they then downregulate them, resulting in cessation of pituitary LH production and, hence, a decrease in testosterone production. In the first 10 days or so, serum testosterone levels may increase, and it is wise to give flutamide, bicalutamide or cyproterone acetate for this period. LHRH agonists may be given by monthly or 3-monthly depot injection.

Other treatments that block the androgen receptor have become available recently. Cyproterone acetate also has some progestogenic effect, while flutamide and bicalutamide are pure anti-androgen. In general, oral anti-androgen monotherapy has not been shown to be as good as LHRH agonists or orchidectomy.

Complete androgen blockade

Complete androgen blockade has been advocated as being likely to result in increased life expectancy and an increased time to progression in a fitter sub-group of men with advanced prostate cancer. The concept is that of abolishing the testicular secretion of testosterone by means of orchidectomy or the use of LHRH therapy and then inhibiting the effects of adrenal androgenic steroids by means of androgen receptor blockade with flutamide, bicalutamide or the use of cyproterone acetate. Recent overviews of randomised trials do not confirm earlier reports of effectiveness.

General radiotherapy

Radiotherapy for symptomatic metastases is an excellent form of palliative treatment, often producing dramatic pain relief in men with hormone-relapsed prostate cancer that can last up to 6 months. When multiple sites are involved, intravenous radiopharmaceuticals such as strontium-89 can be employed. Strontium is a bone-seeking isotope that delivers effective radiotherapy to metastatic areas. It appears to be as effective as hemibody irradiation in the treatment of men with metastatic hormone-relapsed disease; however, the duration of response has been disappointing.

Chemotherapy

Cytotoxic agents in the treatment of these men have proved disappointing, but whether this is because the tumour is inherently insensitive or because these elderly men will not tolerate effective doses is uncertain. Recent trials of docetaxel have shown improvements in survival, but only by a few months.

Summary of treatment

1 *Incidentally diagnosed T1a and T1b disease.* For men in their 70s, conservative treatment would usually be the correct approach. Radical surgical treatment might be considered in the younger (< 70 years) man with this form of the disease, although even in this group, some men will elect to pursue a conservative course when counselled about risks vs. benefits.
2 *Localised T1c and T2 disease.* In younger, fitter men (< 70 years), this may be treated by radical prostatectomy or radical radiotherapy. Active monitoring remains an option, particularly for more elderly patients with low-grade disease. In the elderly patient with outflow obstruction, transurethral resection with or without hormone therapy is indicated. The benefit of radical treatment over a conservative approach is likely to be about 25%, given that progression to metastatic disease is of this order of magnitude after 10 years.
3 *Locally advanced T3 and T4 disease.* These patients are at significant risk of disease progression. Early androgen ablation is favoured if close follow-up is not possible. For the sexually active, a careful conservative approach with the adoption of androgen ablation when symptoms arise is reasonable. Androgen ablation coupled with radiotherapy is standard treatment for younger men with T3 disease.
4 *Metastatic disease.* Once metastases have developed, the outlook is poor. For patients with symptoms, there is no dilemma; androgen ablation will provide symptomatic relief in over two-thirds of patients. For patients with asymptomatic metastases, the timing of treatment is less clear. Systemic chemotherapy with docetaxel should be considered in younger, fitter men.

PROSTATITIS

In both acute and chronic prostatitis, the seminal vesicles and posterior urethra are usually also involved.

Acute prostatitis

Aetiology

Acute prostatitis is common, but underdiagnosed. The usual organism responsible is *Escherichia coli*, but *Staphylococcus aureus*, *Staphylococcus albus*, *Streptococcus faecalis*, *Neisseria gonorrhoeae* or *Chlamydia* may be responsible. The infection may be haematogenous from a distant focus, or it may be secondary to acute urinary infection.

Clinical features

General manifestations overshadow the local: the patient feels ill, shivers, may have a rigor, has 'aches' all over, especially in the back, and may easily be diagnosed as having influenza. The temperature may be up to 39°C. Pain on micturition is usual, but not invariable. The urine contains threads in the initial voided sample, which should be cultured. Perineal heaviness, rectal irritation and pain on defaecation can occur; a urethral discharge is rare. Frequency occurs when the infection involves the bladder. Rectal examination reveals a tender prostate; one lobe may be swollen more than the other, and the seminal vesicles may be involved. A frankly fluctuant abscess is uncommon.

Treatment

Treatment must be rigorous and prolonged or the infection will not be eradicated and recurrent attacks may ensue. Spread of infection to the epididymides and testes may occur. Prolonged treatment with an antibiotic that penetrates the prostate well is indicated (trimethoprim or ciprofloxacin).

Prostatic abscess

In addition to the foregoing symptoms and signs, the advent of a prostatic abscess is heralded by the temperature rising steeply with rigors. Antibiotics disguise these features. Severe, unremitting perineal and rectal pain with occasional tenesmus often cause the condition to be confused with an anorectal abscess. Nevertheless, if a rectal examination is performed, the prostate will be felt to be enlarged, hot, extremely tender and perhaps fluctuant. Retention of urine is likely to occur and, in such men, suprapubic catheterisation is best.

Albert Ludwig Siegmund Neisser, 1855–1916, Director of the Dermatological Institute, Breslau, Germany (now Wrocław, Poland).

Treatment

The abscess should be drained without delay:

1 The abscess can be drained by perurethral resection – unroofing the whole cavity.
2 The perineal route is rarely indicated unless there is marked periprostatic spread.

Chronic prostatitis

Many urologists find the diagnosis of chronic prostatitis and 'prostatodynia' very difficult, for many men present with perigenital pain, testicular pain, prostatic pain exacerbated by sexual intercourse or pain that apparently renders sexual intercourse out of the question. Psychosexual dysfunction in such patients may be the underlying problem. The diagnosis of chronic prostatitis has to be based on:

- persistent threads in voided urine;
- prostatic massage showing pus cells with or without bacteria in the absence of urinary infection.

Aetiology

This is thought to be the sequel of inadequately treated acute prostatitis. While pus is present in the prostatic secretion, the responsible organism is often difficult to find. Other organisms such as *Chlamydia* species may be responsible for chronic abacterial prostatitis.

Clinical features

The clinical features are extremely varied. Only men with symptoms of posterior urethritis, prostatic pain and perigenital pain accompanied by intermittent fever and pus cells or bacteria in the post-prostatic massage specimen should be diagnosed as having chronic prostatitis.

Diagnosis

The three-glass urine test is valuable. If the first glass with the initial voided sample shows urine containing prostatic threads, prostatitis is present.

Rectal examination of the prostate may be normal or may show a soft, boggy and tender prostate.

Examination of the prostatic fluid obtained by prostatic massage should show pus cells and bacteria.

Urethroscopy may reveal inflammation of the prostatic urethra, and pus may be seen exuding from the prostatic ducts. The verumontanum is likely to be enlarged and oedematous. In many men with the symptoms described above, all investigations are normal.

Treatment

Antibiotic therapy should be administered only in accordance with bacteriological sensitivity tests. Trimethoprim penetrates well into the prostate. If *Trichomonas* or anaerobes are the responsible agent, a rapid response is obtained from administration of flagyl (metronidazole, 200 mg t.d.s. for 7 days to both partners). If *Chlamydia* is suspected, doxycycline is the antibiotic treatment of choice. It is uncertain whether prostatic massage helps in eradicating the infection.

Prostatodynia

This diagnosis is made by the presence of perigenital pain in the absence of any objective evidence of prostatic inflammation.

Whether the syndrome has any relationship with the prostate is unclear.

TUBERCULOSIS OF THE PROSTATE AND SEMINAL VESICLES

Tuberculosis of the prostate and seminal vesicles is rare and associated with renal tuberculosis. In 30% of cases, there is a history of pulmonary tuberculosis within 5 years of the onset of genital tuberculosis.

Tuberculosis of one or both seminal vesicles may be found when examining a patient with chronic tuberculous epididymitis, no symptoms being referable to the internal genitalia. On rectal examination, the affected vesicle is found to be nodular.

When the prostate is involved, rectal examination reveals nodules in one or both lateral lobes. Patients with tuberculous prostatitis usually present with the following:

- urethral discharge;
- painful, sometimes blood-stained, ejaculation;
- mild ache in the perineum;
- infertility;
- dysuria;
- abscess formation.

Special forms of investigation

Radiography sometimes displays areas of calcification in the prostate and/or the seminal vesicles.

Bacteriological examination of the seminal fluid yields positive cultures for tubercle bacilli.

Treatment

The general treatment is that for tuberculosis. If a prostatic abscess forms, it should be drained transurethrally.

SEMINAL VESICLES

Acute seminal vesiculitis

Acute seminal vesiculitis occurs in association with prostatitis. Prior to the antibiotic treatment of gonorrhoea, gonococcal vesiculitis was common.

Chronic seminal vesiculitis

Chronic seminal vesiculitis usually presents with haematospermia and pain on intercourse. TRUS demonstrates the features of distension and thickening and the presence of turbid fluid. The treatment is the same as for chronic prostatitis.

Tuberculous seminal vesiculitis

The clinical features and treatment have been discussed above.

Diverticulum of the seminal vesicle

Diverticulum of the seminal vesicle occurs occasionally. In such cases, the kidney of that side is absent, and the diverticulum represents an abortive ureteric bud. It is a cause of persistent infection.

Cyst of the seminal vesicle

A cyst of the seminal vesicle is uncommon and rarely requires treatment. It may be removed by dissection through an incision similar to that for perineal prostatectomy, if it is large or giving rise to symptoms.

FURTHER READING

George, N.J., Fitzpatrick, J., Mundy, A.R. and Neal, D.E. (1999) *Basic Science in Urology*. Isis Publications, Oxford.

Vogelzan, N.J., Scardino, P.T., Shipley, W.U., Debruyne, F.M.J. and Marston Linehan, W. (2006) *Comprehensive Textbook of Genitourinary Oncology*, 3rd edn. Lippincott Williams & Wilkins, Philadelphia, PA.

Wein, A.J., Kavoussi, L.R., Novick, A.C., Partin, A.W. and Peters, C.A. (2007) *Campbell's Urology*, 9th edn. Saunders, Philadelphia, PA.

Urethra and penis

LEARNING OBJECTIVES

To recognise and understand:
- The common congenital abnormalities of the urethra
- The management of urethral trauma and urethral stricture

- The common diseases of the penis and the principles of their surgical management

THE MALE URETHRA

Anatomy

The male urethra is a tubular structure extending from the bladder neck to the external urinary meatus at the tip of the glans penis. During its course through the prostate it is compressed from each side by the lateral lobes of the prostate, giving it a slit-like configuration. The verumontanum is a small hillock of tissue indented at its crown by a pit called the utriculus masculinus. The verumontanum marks the proximal extent of the external urethral sphincter and is an important landmark for urologists performing transurethral resection of the prostate. The distal urethra is invested by erectile tissue of the corpus spongiosus. It is normally flattened anteroposteriorly but distends when filled with fluid. The most proximal section distends most and is known as the urethral bulb.

The external urethral sphincter is composed of striated muscle within the urethral wall. In the female it extends for almost the whole length of the short urethra.

Congenital abnormalities

Urethral stricture

This rare condition may be associated with duplication of the urethra. Usually, symptoms are delayed until adolescence, when it may be indistinguishable from a stricture due to unrecognised urethral injury in childhood. A single treatment by optical urethrotomy or dilatation is usually effective.

Posterior urethral valves

These folds of urothelium cause obstruction to the urethra of boys. They are usually just distal to the verumontanum but they may be within the prostatic urethra. They are flap valves and so, although urine does not flow normally, a urethral catheter can be passed without difficulty. Dilatation of the urinary tract now commonly leads to diagnosis by ultrasound scanning before birth. Other cases present with urinary infection in the neonatal period. Sometimes the valves are incomplete and the patient is symptom free until adolescence or adulthood. Posterior urethral valves need to be detected and treated as early as possible to avoid the development of renal failure.

The valves can be difficult to see on urethroscopy because the flow of irrigant sweeps them into the open position. If the bladder is filled with contrast medium, the dilatation of the urethra above the valves can be demonstrated on a voiding cystogram. The bladder is hypertrophied and often shows diverticula. Typically, there is vesicoureteric reflux into dilated upper tracts (Summary box 74.1).

> **Summary box 74.1**
>
> **Congenital urethral valves**
>
> - Posterior urethral valves cause obstruction to the urinary tract in young boys
> - Antenatal ultrasound scanning typically shows urinary tract dilatation in affected boys

Treatment

A suprapubic catheter is inserted to relieve the back pressure and allow the effects of renal failure to subside before definitive treatment by transurethral resection of the valves.

Hypospadias (see also Chapter 6)

Hypospadias occurs in one in 200–300 boys and is the most common congenital malformation of the urethra. The external meatus opens on the underside of the penis or the perineum, and the ventral aspect of the prepuce is poorly developed ('hooded prepuce').

Hypospadias is classified according to the position of the meatus:

- *Glanular hypospadias.* This is common and does not usually require treatment. The normal site of the external meatus is marked by a blind pit, although it occasionally connects by a channel to the ectopic opening on the underside of the glans.

- *Coronal hypospadias.* The meatus is placed at the junction of the underside of the glans and the body of the penis.
- *Penile and penoscrotal hypospadias.* The opening is on the underside of the penile shaft (Fig. 74.1).
- *Perineal hypospadias.* This is the most severe abnormality. The scrotum is bifid and the urethra opens between its two halves. There may be testicular maldescent, which may make it difficult to determine the sex of the child.

The more severe varieties of hypospadias represent an absence of the urethra and corpus spongiosum distal to the ectopic opening. The absent structures are represented by a fibrous cord, which deforms the penis in a downward direction (chordee).

Treatment

Glanular hypospadias does not need treatment unless the meatus is stenosed, in which case a meatotomy is performed. Surgery is indicated for other forms of hypospadias to improve sexual function, to correct problems with the urinary stream and for cosmetic reasons. A variety of plastic surgical procedures is described to correct the chordee and to re-site the urethral opening. Most procedures use preputial skin and so circumcision should be avoided until the hypospadias has been repaired. Operations for hypospadias are best performed by a paediatric urologist (Summary box 74.2).

Summary box 74.2

Hypospadias

- Avoid circumcision as prepuce may be used in procedures to correct the abnormality

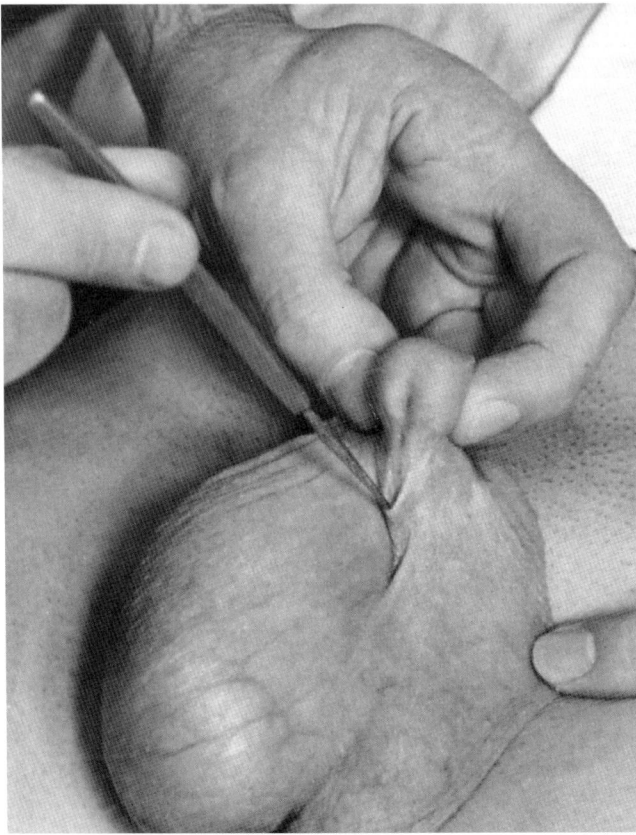

Figure 74.1 Penile hypospadias. The patient passes urine through the orifice demonstrated by the probe.

Epispadias

Epispadias is very rare. In penile epispadias, the opening on the dorsum is associated with upward curvature of the penis (Fig. 74.2). Epispadias usually coexists with bladder exstrophy and other severe developmental defects.

Injuries to the male urethra

Rupture of the bulbar urethra

There is a history of a blow to the perineum, usually due to a fall astride a projecting object. In the days of sailing ships, the common cause was falling astride a spar; the modern equivalent is seen among workers losing their footing on scaffolding. Cycling accidents, loose manhole covers (Fig. 74.3) and gymnasium accidents astride the beam account for a number of cases.

Clinical features

The signs of a ruptured bulbar urethra are retention of urine, perineal haematoma and bleeding from the external urinary meatus (Summary box 74.3).

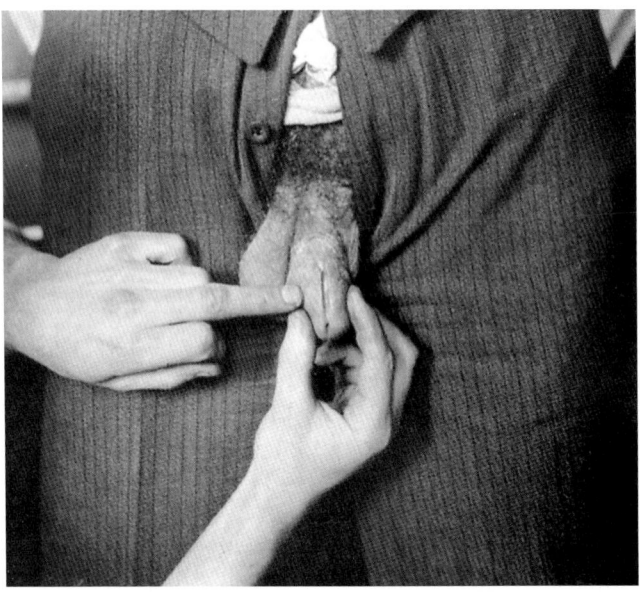

Figure 74.2 Glandular epispadias.

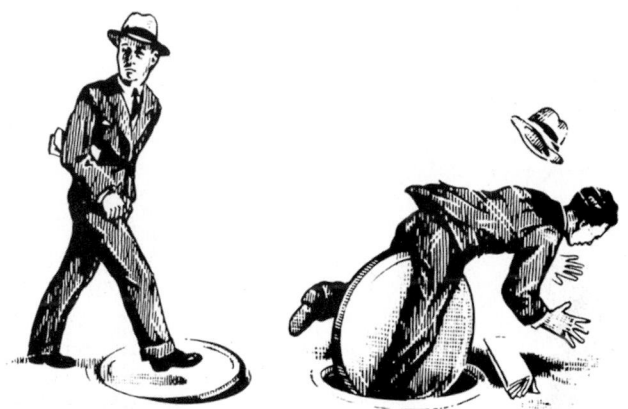

Figure 74.3 The type of accident that results in a ruptured bulbar urethra (after V.J. O'Connor).

> **Summary box 74.3**
>
> **Urethral injury**
>
> Suspect urethral injury after blunt perineal trauma when:
>
> - The man goes into retention
> - There is massive perineal swelling
> - There is blood at the urethral meatus

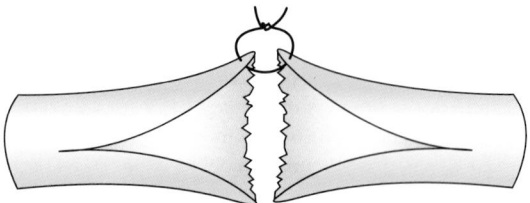

Figure 74.5 Open repair of a ruptured bulbar urethra.

Preliminary assessment and treatment

The patient should be treated with appropriate analgesic drugs. He should be discouraged from passing urine if rupture of the urethra is suspected. A full bladder should be drained with a catheter placed by percutaneous suprapubic puncture (Fig. 74.4). This reduces urinary extravasation and allows investigations to establish the extent of the urethral injury. If the patient has passed urine when first seen and there is no extravasation, the rupture, if any, is partial and a catheter is not needed. In any case, it is probably wise to administer a course of prophylactic antibiotics.

Treatment

The main worry is that injudicious urethral catheterisation will convert a partial tear into a complete transection of the urethra. The initial treatment described above is to be recommended for those who go into urinary retention after the accident, especially if there is bleeding from the urethra. More information may be obtained by an ascending urethrogram or even a flexible cystoscopy to assess the injury. Very occasionally, if the facilities for passing a percutaneous suprapubic catheter are not available, it may be permissible to try to pass a soft, small-calibre urethral catheter without force. This may allow a few patients to avoid the open placement of a suprapubic tube into the bladder.

If the urethral tear is complete, the suprapubic catheter should remain until arrangements can be made to repair it. Some surgeons advocate early open repair of the urethra with excision of the traumatised section and spatulated end-to-end reanastomosis of the urethra (Fig. 74.5). Others wait longer before embarking upon a repair operation but may attempt to find a way across the gap in the urethra using a urethroscope. This allows a urethral catheter to be placed so that the ends of the urethra are aligned while healing occurs (Summary box 74.4).

> **Summary box 74.4**
>
> **Urethral trauma**
>
> - It is safest to insert a suprapubic catheter before referral to a urologist

Complications

Subcutaneous extravasation of urine occurs in complete rupture if the patient attempts to pass urine.

Stricture is a common sequel to urethral trauma, whether there is a partial or complete tear or simply periurethral bruising. Infection may also play a part.

Rupture of the membranous urethra

Intrapelvic rupture of the membranous urethra occurs near the apex of the prostate (Fig. 74.6). Like extraperitoneal rupture of the bladder, it may be caused by penetrating wounds, but it is most usually a result of pelvic fracture.

Fracture of the pubic and ischial rami is most likely to result when sudden force is applied to one lower limb in a car accident or in landing on one leg after falling from a height. There is an associated disruption of the sacroiliac joint so that one half of the pelvis and ischiopubic ramus is pushed up above the other. This applies a traction force on the prostate, which is firmly bound by ligaments to the back of the symphysis pubis. The torn ends of the urethra may be widely displaced by this type of injury.

In another type of pelvic fracture the patient suffers a front-to-back compression of the pelvis in a blow directly from the front. A 'butterfly fracture' of the pubic rami on each side occurs. When the compressive force is relieved, the pubic fragment springs back so that the ends of the torn urethra are close. About 10–15% of cases of fractured pelvis have associated urethral injury.

Clinical features

The most common causes of pelvic fracture are road traffic accidents, severe crush injuries and falls. Often, the management of

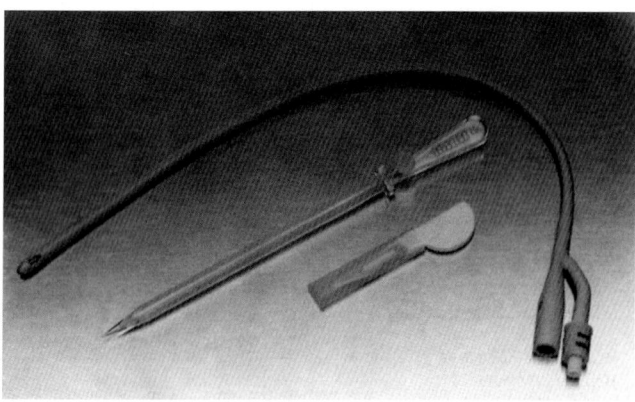

Figure 74.4 Kit for percutaneous suprapubic drainage of the bladder.

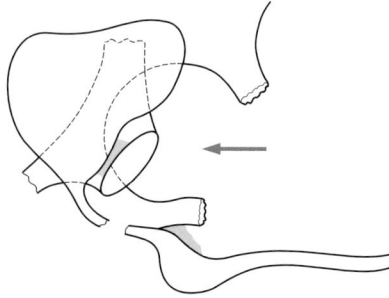

Figure 74.6 Intrapelvic rupture of the urethra. Note the displacement of the bladder.

injuries to the head, thorax and abdomen and long bones must take precedence and the overriding priority is to keep the patient alive by appropriate resuscitation.

A suprapubic catheter should be inserted as soon as practicable. The type of urethral injury can often be deduced from the plain radiograph – a major urethral disruption is almost certain if there is significant displacement of the pubic bones. If the prostate is displaced, it may be out of reach or 'high' on rectal examination. An ascending urethrogram with water-based contrast may be justified if there is doubt.

There may be associated injury to the bladder with either an intraperitoneal or extraperitoneal rupture. The former is associated with the onset of peritonitis and, if suspected, demands exploration and repair of the bladder even if laparotomy is not indicated by other injuries. Extraperitoneal rupture of the bladder causes symptoms that are difficult to distinguish from those of rupture of the membranous urethra. There is pain, bruising and dullness to percussion above the umbilicus. If there is a significant bladder rupture it must be repaired, a suprapubic catheter inserted and the retroperitoneal space drained (Summary box 74.5).

Summary box 74.5

Lower urinary tract injury in pelvic trauma

When the lower urinary tract is injured in a patient who has suffered multiple trauma:

- ■ Definitive treatment can usually be deferred if a suprapubic catheter is in place
- ■ Exploration is needed if there is evidence of rupture of the bladder, especially if it is intraperitoneal

---

Complications

Stricture The main complication of urethral trauma is urethral stricture. When the injury is severe and the disrupted ends of the urethra are far apart, the stricture is likely to be very difficult to treat. Because of this worry, some surgeons urge that an attempt should be made to realign the urethra as soon as the emergency is over. Often this will coincide with an attempt to reposition the pelvic fragments with the possibility of external fixation. If a way through the stricture can be found with a flexible or rigid urethroscope, a urethral catheter may be inserted. Alternatively, an open repair of the urethra can be attempted. Some experts prefer to allow a longer period of recovery before attempting to correct the urethral injury.

Many of these patients need a full-scale urethroplasty, especially if the ends of the urethra are poorly aligned. Often the ends of the urethra are widely displaced and there is extensive fibrosis and even ectopic calcification the gap. Occasionally, the ends are so far apart that they can be apposed only by cutting away the pubic bone. The management of a severe urethral stricture should be in the hands of a specialist.

Urinary incontinence If the external urethral sphincter is destroyed, continence of urine will depend upon the bladder neck mechanism. Subsequent surgical manoeuvres such as prostatectomy, which destroys the bladder neck, may cause incontinence.

Impotence Erectile impotence is common after pelvic fracture with urethral injury and is presumed to be the result of damage to the nerve supply of the penis. Some patients can achieve erection with prostaglandin injections, a vacuum device or an orally active agent such as sildenafil.

Orthopaedic For management of the fractured pelvis see Chapter 27.

Extravasation of urine Superficial extravasation is likely with complete rupture of the bulbar urethra and in ruptured urethral abscess. The extravasated urine is confined in front of the mid-perineal point by the attachment of Colles' fascia to the triangular ligament and by the attachment of Scarpa's fascia just below the inguinal ligament. The external spermatic fascia stops it getting into the inguinal canals. Extravasated urine collects in the scrotum and penis and beneath the deep layer of superficial fascia in the abdominal wall. Treatment is by urgent operation to drain the bladder by suprapubic cystostomy. Deep extravasation occurs with extraperitoneal rupture of the bladder or intrapelvic rupture of the urethra. It can also occur if the ureter is damaged or if there is perforation of the prostatic capsule or bladder during transurethral resection. Urine extravasates in the layers of the pelvic fascia and the retroperitoneal tissues. Treatment is by suprapubic cystostomy and drainage of the retropubic space.

Inflammation of the urethra

Inflammatory conditions of the urethra include:

- meatal ulcer;
- urethritis:
  - gonococcal urethritis;
  - non-specific urethritis;
  - Reiter's disease.

Ulceration of the urethral meatus

Meatal ulcer is quite common in circumcised boys and may be delayed for up to 2 years from circumcision. Lack of protection by the prepuce seems to be the excitatory cause, with friction from clothing and ammoniacal dermatitis contributory factors. Devascularisation caused by ligation of the frenular artery may possibly play a part. The ulcer forms a scab that blocks the meatus and the child can pass urine only by bursting the scab. This hurts, so the boy screams; a tiny amount of blood may be passed as well. The process causes fibrosis, which can result in an acquired pinhole meatus. Meatal stenosis may also follow hypospadias repair or be a complication of phimosis caused by balanitis xerotica obliterans. With a pinhole meatus, spraying or dribbling is common and there is a risk of chronic retention of urine with renal impairment.

Treatment

Local measures to soften the scab and alkalinise the urine are often curative. A few need meatotomy. The meatus is opened by cutting on to a fine probe placed in the anterior urethra. The cut edges of urothelium and skin are sewn together with an

---

Abraham Colles, 1773–1843, Professor of Surgery, The Royal College of Surgeons in Ireland, and Surgeon, Dr. Steevens' Hospital, Dublin, Ireland.
Antonio Scarpa, 1747–1832, Professor of Anatomy, Pavia, Italy.
Hans Conrad Julius Reiter, 1881–1969, President of the Health Service and Honorary Professor of Hygiene, Berlin, Germany, described this condition in 1916.

absorbable suture. If the stenosis recurs a skin flap can be laid in as a meatoplasty to widen the meatus (Fig 74.7).

Gonorrhoeal urethritis

Gonorrhoea is a sexually transmitted disease caused by *Neisseria gonorrhoeae* (gonococcus), a Gram-negative kidney-shaped diplococcus that infects the anterior urethra in men, the urethra and cervix in women and the oropharynx, rectum and anal canal in both sexes, but especially men.

Gonorrhoea in men usually declares itself by urethral discomfort and urethral discharge up to 10 days after exposure. There is often scalding dysuria. In some there may be no symptoms other than slight discharge.

Investigations

Pus and gonococci are present in the Gram-stained urethral smear. The passage of pus in the first part of the urinary stream can be demonstrated as haziness in the first glass of a two-glass test. Treatment should not wait upon the results of urethral culture when the clinical picture and urethral smear are typical.

Complications

Complications are uncommon in the UK and are all prevented by effective treatment. Local complications include posterior urethritis, prostatitis (acute or chronic), acute epididymoorchitis, periurethral abscess and urethral stricture. Gonococcal arthritis, iridocyclitis, septicaemia and endocarditis are even more unusual.

Treatment

Treatment is with antibiotics, usually ciprofloxacin or penicillin, and will usually be in the hands of a genitourinary physician.

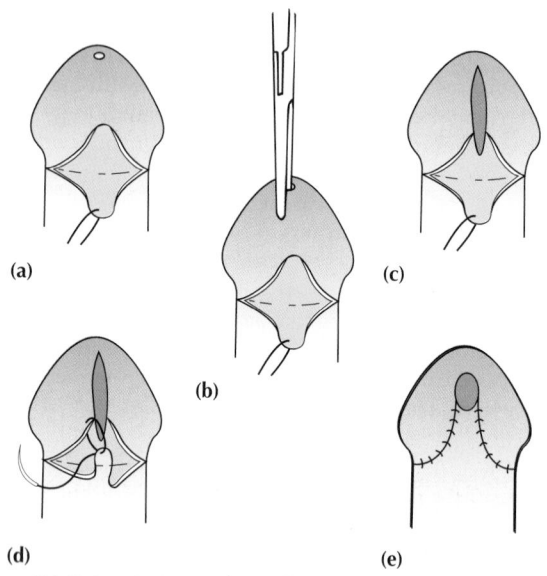

(a)

(b)

(c)

(d)

(e)

Figure 74.7 (a–e) Meatoplasty. The strictured meatus is incised and a flap of penile skin is laid in to form a funnel-shaped meatal opening.

Albert Ludwig Siegmund Neisser, **1855–1916**, Director of the Dermatological Institue, Breslau, Germany (now Wroclaw, Poland).
Hans Christian Joachim Gram, **1853–1938**, Professor of Pharmacology (1891–1900), and of Medicine (1900–1923), Copenhagen, Denmark, described this method of staining bacteria in 1884.

Contact tracing is important in controlling the spread of the disease.

Gonorrhoea in women affects primarily the urethra and cervix and is often symptomless. It can never be diagnosed on clinical grounds alone. Almost three-quarters of all female patients attend initially as a result of contact tracing. Symptoms, which are present in 50% or less, consist of a mild dysuria or slight urethral discharge, which can go unnoticed by the patient. If Skene's tubules are emptied by milking the urethra against the posterior pubic ramus, a bead of pus may appear at the urethral meatus. There may be some reddening or erosion of the cervix with a mucopurulent cervical plug, but copious vaginal discharge is more likely to be due to concomitant trichomonal vaginitis.

Complications

Gonococcal proctitis occurs in at least 60–70% of cases and is usually symptomless. About 10% suffer from salpingitis, which, if bilateral, may lead to infertility.

Gonorrhoea in the newborn

This is now rare but it used to be an important cause of blindness.

Non-specific urethritis (synonym: non-gonococcal urethritis)

This is a form of urethritis that is diagnosed by exclusion of gonorrhoea and other known infections. Some 40% of cases are due to *Chlamydia trachomatis* and some are shown to be caused by *Ureaplasma urealytica*. The causative agent in up to 50% of cases is unknown.

Clinical features

Dysuria and a mucopurulent urethral discharge appear up to 6 weeks after sexual intercourse. The urine is usually grossly clear but may contain 'threads' or pus cells. Epididymitis is not uncommon and urethral stricture rarely results. In women, the condition presents as a form of urethrotrigonitis and may be very resistant to diagnosis.

Treatment

Treatment with oxytetracycline or doxycycline is usually effective although relapse is common, especially in men, in whom the prostate may act as a reservoir of infection. It is important to treat both partners as reinfection is probable if this is not done. Urethroscopy is not indicated.

Reiter's disease

Reiter's disease (synonym: sexually acquired reactive arthritis) is usually sexually transmitted in the UK but elsewhere is more commonly dysenteric in origin. Subacute urethritis 4–6 weeks after contact is associated with a clear, viscid discharge that is free from organisms. A few days later, conjunctivitis, unilateral then bilateral, occurs in 50% of cases. In more severe cases there is anterior uveitis. Usually, in 10 days to 2 weeks, arthritis supervenes, but it is not an invariable feature of the condition. Another concurrent manifestation is keratoderma blennorrhagicum, consisting of nodules, vesicles and pustules, frequently found on the sole of the foot (Fig. 74.8).

Alexander Johnston Chalmers Skene, **1828–1900**, Professor of Gynecology, Long Island Hospital, Brooklyn, New York, NY, USA.

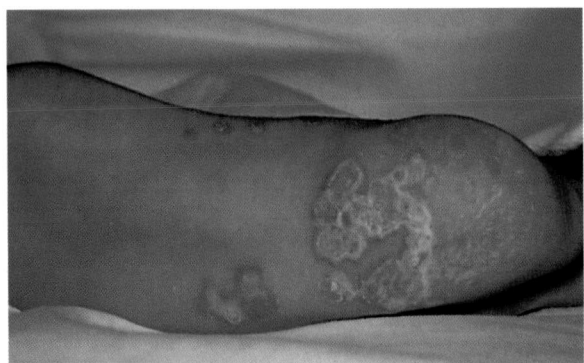

Figure 74.8 Reiter's disease – keratoderma blennorrhagicum of the heel.

Differential diagnosis

This is principally from gonorrhoea, which must be excluded by blood culture. In Reiter's disease, the urethritis and arthritis are milder and the incubation period is longer than that of gonorrhoea.

Prognosis

The urethritis and conjunctivitis frequently subside after a few weeks but the arthritis may persist for months. Severe anterior uveitis and frequently recurrent attacks suggest a poor outlook.

Treatment

The ophthalmic complications are treated with eye baths and shades. Mydriatics and topical steroids are indicated for iritis. Other symptoms may prove difficult to control, and patients with severe disease should be under the care of a specialist in genitourinary medicine.

Urethral stricture

Causes of urethral stricture

The causes of urethral stricture are:

- inflammatory:
  – post-gonorrhoeal;
- congenital;
- traumatic;
- instrumental:
  – indwelling catheter;
  – urethral endoscopy;
- postoperative:
  – open prostatectomy;
  – amputation of penis.

Post-gonorrhoeal stricture

This is less common since the introduction of effective antibiotic treatment for gonorrhoea. The stricture is most commonly in the bulbar urethra but post-meatal strictures are also seen.

Pathology Infection in the periurethral glands persists after inadequately treated gonorrhoea. The infection spreads to cause a periurethritis, which heals by fibrosis. Most strictures appear within 1 year of infection but may not cause difficulty in micturition for 10–15 years.

Clinical features The first symptoms are usually those of bladder outflow obstruction with straining to void and poor urinary stream. The relative youthfulness of the patient often rules out prostatic enlargement, which characteristically occurs after the age of 50. As the stream becomes narrower micturition is prolonged and is followed by dribbling as a result of urine trickling from the dilated urethra proximal to the stricture. Urinary frequency by day and night is also common and is due to incomplete bladder emptying, infection or both.

A well-established stricture may be palpable as scarring along the line of the urethra. If the stricture is tight enough, the patient will go into acute retention. If this happens there is a danger that ham-fisted attempts to pass a urethral catheter will result in a false passage. If a patient has gone into retention because of a urethral stricture, its lumen will be too narrow to pass even a tiny catheter.

Urethroscopy allows the stricture to be viewed as a circumferential scar (Fig. 74.9). Openings of false passages commemorate misguided attempts to pass a urethral catheter.

Urethrography using a water-miscible gel containing contrast medium will show the extent and severity of the stricture or failure of the medium to pass beyond the tightness, indicating complete stenosis (Figs 74.10 and 74.11).

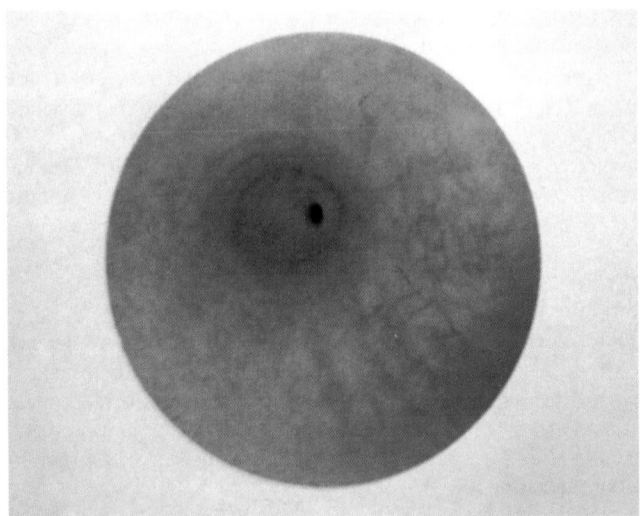

Figure 74.9 Urethroscopic appearance of a urethral stricture.

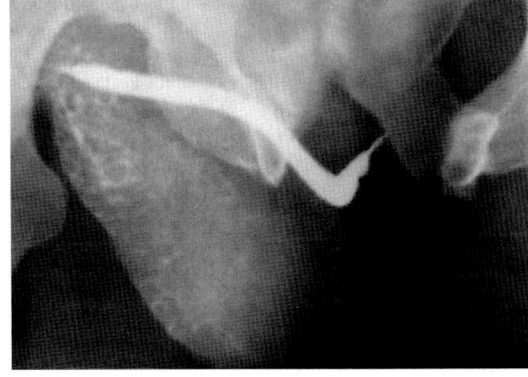

Figure 74.10 Ascending urethrogram showing urethral stricture of the membranous urethra following fracture of the pelvis.

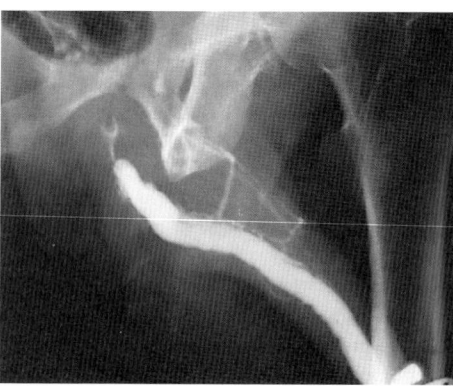

Figure 74.11 Gonorrhoeal stricture of the bulbar urethra. Note that some of the contrast has entered the penile veins.

Congenital stricture

This has been considered previously.

Traumatic stricture

The stricture that follows neglected or untreated rupture of the membranous urethra is sometimes a complete loss of continuity. In patients with a traumatic stricture, a transpubic urethroplasty is often needed to bridge the gap.

Post-instrumental stricture

This follows endoscopy or catheterisation and may affect any part of the urethra. Some surgeons recommend prophylactic dilatation or urethrotomy before transurethral surgery to try to avoid this complication. Some cases of stricture seem to be due to sensitivity to chemicals from a catheter, but most are the result of a combination of trauma, infection and pressure necrosis.

Stricture after prostatectomy

Postoperative stricture follows 4% of prostatectomies, irrespective of the method employed. The stricture is usually in the proximal part of the prostatic urethra and is also known as bladder neck stenosis. If it cannot be managed by dilatation, bladder neck stenosis should be treated by transurethral incision and resection of the stricture.

Postoperative stricture is also a complication of amputation of the penis (see below).

Complications of urethral stricture

Complications include:

- retention of urine;
- urethral diverticulum;
- periurethral abscess;
- urethral fistula;
- hernia, haemorrhoids and rectal prolapse caused by abdominal straining to void urine.

Treatment of urethral stricture

Treatment of urethral stricture is by:

- dilatation:
  - gum-elastic bougie;
  - filiform and follower;
  - metal sounds;
  - self-dilatation with Nélaton catheter;
- urethrotomy:
  - internal visual urethrotomy;
- urethroplasty:
  - excision and end-to-end anastomosis;
  - patch urethroplasty.

Dilatation is the old treatment for stricture. Under aseptic conditions, the urethra is stretched using graduated dilators. With care and gentleness the procedure can be performed under local urethral anaesthesia with lignocaine gel. The drawback of dilatation is that it is performed 'blind', so there is always a danger of making the stricture worse by causing a false passage. This is most likely with an inexperienced operator unfamiliar with the complexities of an individual patient's urethra. With any urinary tract instrumentation, infection is a danger, and fatal septicaemia can follow a supposedly straightforward dilatation. Urethral dilatation still has a place in elderly men with short strictures that recur infrequently. In these patients, occasional bouginage may be preferable to more complex procedures. Some patients can dilate their own urethras by intermittently passing a soft Nélaton catheter (Summary box 74.6).

Summary box 74.6

Urethral dilatation

■ Urethral dilatation for stricture is liable to cause additional urethral damage if performed inexpertly

---

Instruments

Strictures have been treated by surgeons for centuries and there are many different dilating instruments. A simple stricture may be dilated using metal sounds (Fig. 74.12), so called because they were originally used to 'sound' for stones in the bladder, or gum-elastic bougies (Fig. 74.13). These must be wielded with great care as it is easy to make a false passage. Filiforms are gum-elastic filaments that can be passed through the lumen of a urethral stricture (Fig. 74.14). This is usually best done under direct vision using a urethroscope. Once the lumen has been located with its tip, the other end of the filiform is screwed on to a 'follower', a gum-elastic bougie with a

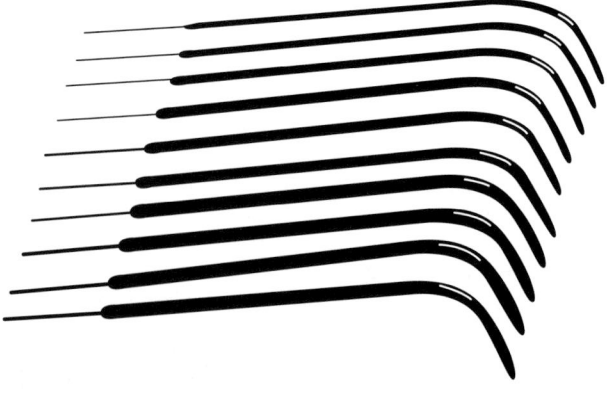

Figure 74.12 Metal dilators ('sounds').

Auguste Nélaton, 1807–1873, Professor of Surgery, Paris, France.

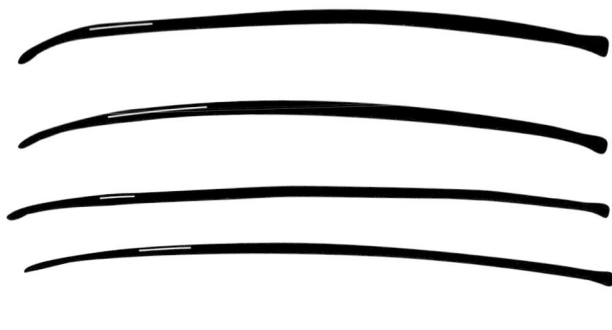

Figure 74.13 Gum-elastic bougies.

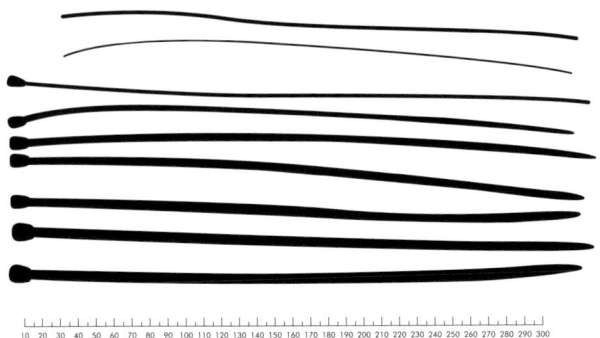

Figure 74.14 Filiform bougies with followers.

screw thread at its tip for the purpose. As the follower is advanced, the filiform guides it safely through the stricture. Once the stricture has been partially dilated by followers of increasing size, it is often safe to change to metal dilators. Patients who have had an optical urethrotomy are sometimes taught to keep the stricture open by regular self-dilatation with a urethral catheter of a suitable size.

Operative treatment

Internal urethrotomy is performed using the optical urethrotome. The stricture is cut under visual control using a knife passed through the sheath of a rigid urethroscope. The stricture is usually cut at the 12 o'clock position, taking care not to cut too deeply into the vascular spaces of the corpus spongiosum that surrounds the urethra. Other cuts can be made until there is a wide passage through the strictured segment of urethra. Many surgeons leave a catheter for 1–2 days afterwards but there is no evidence that this makes a significant difference to the effectiveness of the procedure. A single urethrotomy seems to give a permanent cure of uncomplicated stricture in about 50% of patients. The main complications are infection and bleeding. It is possible to get lost when trying to cut a way through a very tight stricture. This is especially true when there are false passages because of previous dilatation attempts. It helps to pass a guidewire to establish the true lumen of the urethra (Summary box 74.7).

Summary box 74.7

Endoscopic urethrotomy

- Cures about 50% of simple strictures
- May be supplemented by intermittent self-dilatation postoperatively with improved success rate

---

Urethroplasty

The simplest urethroplasty involves excision of the stenosed length of urethra and reanastomosis of the spatulated cut end (see Fig. 74.5, p. 1364). This operation is possible only if the stricture is relatively short because there must be no tension at the suture line. If end-to-end anastomosis is not feasible, a large number of different plastic surgical procedures are available to replace the fibrosed urethra using free full-thickness or pedicled skin grafts. The Orandi–Blandy operation makes use of a myocutaneous patch of perineal skin and dartos muscle (Fig. 74.15) whereas Turner-Warwick favoured penile skin. Buccal mucosa, readily harvested as a free graft, has the advantage of flourishing in both wet and dry conditions.

Urethroplasty should be considered when simpler means fail. The procedure can be very demanding, especially when the stricture is the result of pelvic trauma and the urethra is encased in hard fibrosis. A prolonged hospital stay is usual while the graft heals.

Diverticulum of the male urethra (synonym: urethral pouch)

This is usually congenital and represents a partial duplication of the urethra. Acquired cases are uncommon. They are sometimes seen as a result of increased intraurethral pressure behind a stricture. Others are caused by the longstanding presence of a foreign body such as a stone or calculus in the urethra.

Treatment is by excision of the diverticulum and removal of the cause if possible.

Periurethral abscess

Periurethral abscesses can be penile, bulbar or chronic.

Penile periurethral abscess

A penile periurethral abscess arises as an acute gonococcal infection of one of the glands of Littre. The tender induration felt on

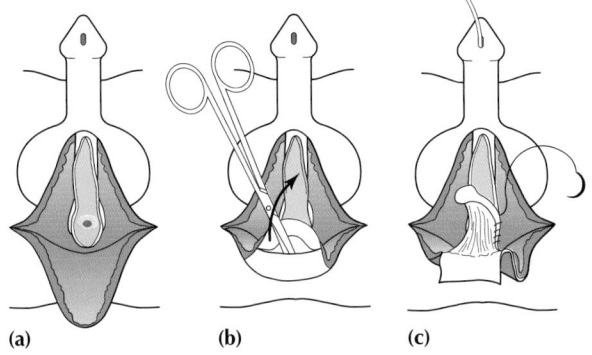

Figure 74.15 The pedicled patch urethroplasty of Orandi and Blandy. (a) A U-shaped incision in the perineum is developed to form a flap. The strictured urethra is incised. (b) A patch of skin attached to the underlying dartos muscle is separated from the tip of the U-shaped flap. (c) The patch is sutured in place to widen the strictured urethra. The blood supply to the patch comes from the underlying dartos muscle.

Ahmad Orandi, Urological surgeon, Fergus Falls, MN, USA.
John Peter Blandy, Contemporary, Formerly Professor of Urology, The London Hospital Medical College, London, England.
Richard Trevor Turner-Warwick, Contemporary, Formerly Urologist, The Middlesex Hospital, London, England.
Alexis Littre, 1658–1726, Surgeon, and Lecturer in Anatomy, Paris, France.

the underside of the penis points and discharges externally, often leaving a fistula.

Treatment

An anterior urethrotomy will encourage the abscess to burst into the urethra. When the abscess lies behind a stricture, it should be opened externally.

Bulbar periurethral abscess

A bulbar periurethral abscess is a spreading cellulitis caused by infection with streptococci and anaerobic organisms, possibly associated with a stricture. Extravasation of urine is not unusual.

Clinical features

There is perineal pain with pyrexia, rigors and tachycardia. Tenderness and swelling rapidly spread from the perineum to the penis and the anterior abdominal wall.

Treatment

Antibiotics are essential. Collections of pus should be drained and the urethra should be defunctioned by a suprapubic urinary catheter.

Chronic periurethral abscess

A chronic periurethral abscess sometimes results from a long-standing urethral stricture (Fig. 74.16). The multiple loculi of pus should be drained and the stricture treated. Urethral fistula occurs either spontaneously or as a result of incision of the abscess.

Urethral fistula

The most frequent cause of urethral fistula is bursting or incision of a periurethral abscess. If the fistulae arise behind a tight stricture there may be multiple openings (watering-can perineum). A fistula can also follow urethroplasty if there is necrosis of part of the graft.

Treatment

If the stricture is cured, some fistulae heal themselves. Occasionally, urethroplasty is indicated.

Urethral calculi

Urethral calculi can arise primarily behind a stricture or in an infected urethral diverticulum. More commonly, the stone is a renal calculus that has migrated to the urethra via the bladder.

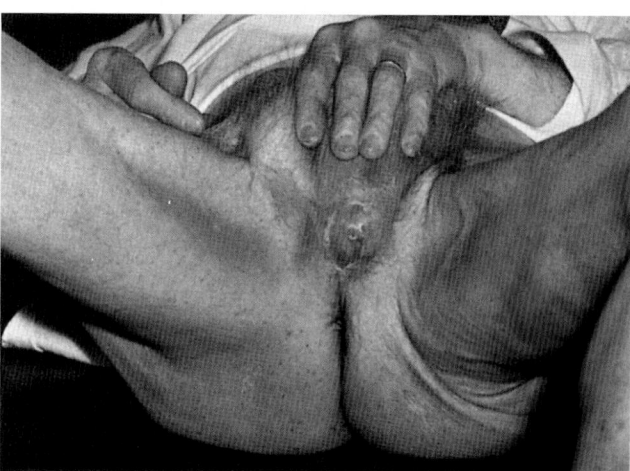

Figure 74.16 Chronic periurethral abscess.

Clinical features

Migratory calculi cause sudden pain in the urethra soon after an attack of ureteric colic. There is blockage to the flow of urine and, if the stone is small, the force of the jet will expel it from the external urethral meatus. Larger stones get stuck and must be removed endoscopically. It is sometimes possible to feel the calculus as a hard lump in the urethra, but if there is doubt the diagnosis is confirmed by urethroscopy.

A stone formed within the urethra is less likely to cause recognisable symptoms and is usually detected during urethroscopy or bouginage.

Treatment

A stone in the prostatic urethra is displaced back into the bladder and treated by lithopaxy or suprapubic cystotomy as if it were a bladder stone. Calculi in more distal parts of the urethra are removed by basketing under vision or fragmented in situ using the electrohydraulic or ultrasonic lithotripter. It may be necessary to perform a meatotomy to deliver the stone. Open removal by external urethrotomy is rarely necessary.

Neoplasms

Polyps are a relatively common finding in the prostatic urethra, where they may result from chronic infection.

Genital warts acquired by sexually transmitted infection are sometimes found in the anterior urethra as an extension of warts on the skin of the glans penis.

Angioma of the urethra is a very rare cause of urethral bleeding.

Carcinoma of the urethra is relatively rare. Multifocal transitional cell cancers of the bladder are sometimes associated with tumours in the prostatic urethra and occasionally more distally. Though superficial and susceptible to local ablation by diathermy or laser, they are associated with a tendency to distant spread. Squamous carcinoma can develop in an area of squamous metaplasia sometimes seen with a urethral stricture. It carries a poor prognosis even if the patient is treated by radical surgery. Bloody urethral discharge without infection should raise the suspicion that the patient has a urethral tumour.

THE FEMALE URETHRA

Abnormalities of the female urethra include:

- prolapse;
- stricture;
- diverticulum;
- caruncle;
- papillomata acuminata;
- carcinoma.

Prolapse

Prolapse occurs in later life and is usually symptomless. Prolapse of the urethral lining also occurs as a congenital abnormality, when it causes discomfort proportional to the degree of prolapse.

Stricture

This is uncommon in women but follows urethritis or, more commonly, the trauma of a difficult labour. Urinary retention, usually chronic, is an occasional result. True urethral strictures in women respond well to dilatation and should not be confused with a spasm of the urethral muscle of obscure cause, which sometimes causes retention in women, particularly after they have had unrelated surgery. The condition, which was described by Fowler and Kirby, is associated with an abnormal myotonic discharge in the urethral sphincter, which can be detected on an electromyogram. The patients remain in retention after urethral dilatation and many of them require intermittent self-catheterisation for life.

Diverticulum (synonym: urethrocele)

Diverticulum is more common in women than men. Some seem to be congenital. Others are acquired by rupture of a distended urethral gland or injury of the urethra during childbirth. Urine within the diverticulum becomes infected, causing local pain and repeated bouts of cystitis. Purulent urine is discharged if the urethra is compressed with a finger placed in the vagina. Excision of the diverticulum through the anterior vaginal wall is effective, but care must be taken not to damage the urethral sphincter.

Caruncle

This is common in elderly women. It presents as a soft, raspberry-like, pedunculated granulomatous mass about the size of a pea, attached to the posterior urethral wall near the external meatus. It is composed of highly vascular connective tissue stroma infiltrated with pus cells.

Clinical features

There may be frequency of micturition and pain afterwards. Occasionally, there is bleeding. A urethral prolapse is less tender and is not pedunculated.

Treatment

Treatment is by excision and diathermy coagulation of the base of the stalk. The patient should be given antibiotics to treat the underlying chronic urethritis.

Papillomata acuminata

Papillomata acuminata are the same as the sexually transmitted warts that occur on the penis. They are treated in the same way. In African women, papillomata acuminata are common and may grow to such a large size during pregnancy that they obstruct labour and necessitate a Caesarean section (Bowesman).

Carcinoma of the urethra

This occurs twice as often in women as in men. Whether a caruncle can become malignant is disputed, but caruncles and tumours often occur close together. Malignant swellings of the urethra feel harder than benign ones.

Treatment by radiotherapy or radical surgery is often ineffective. The overall prognosis is poor.

THE PENIS

Phimosis (see also Chapter 6)

Phimosis is overdiagnosed. The physiological adhesions between the foreskin and the glans penis may persist until 6 years of age or

Clare Juliet Fowler, **Contemporary**, Professor of Uro-neurology, The National Hospital for Nervous Diseases, Queen Square, London, England.
Roger Sinclair Kirby, **Contemporary**, Professor of Urology, St George's Hospital, London, England.
Charles Bowesman, **1907–1993**, Professor of Surgery, Kumasi, Ghana.

more, giving the false impression that the prepuce will not retract. Rolling back the prepuce causes its inner lining to pout and the meatus comes into view. This condition should not be confused with true phimosis in boys, with scarring of the prepuce, which will not retract without fissuring. In these cases the aperture in the prepuce may be so tight as to cause urinary obstruction. Urinary difficulty with residual urine and back pressure effects on the ureters and kidney is far more commonly caused by meatal stenosis, which may be masked by the prepuce. Phimosis occurs as a result of balanitis xerotica obliterans (BXO), a curious condition in which the normally pliant foreskin becomes thickened and will not retract. It is difficult to keep the penis clean and there is both a problem with hygiene and, in later life, an increased susceptibility to carcinoma.

Treatment is by circumcision.

Circumcision

Apparently, circumcision did not originate among the Jewish people: they took the practice either from the Babylonians or from African tribes, probably the latter. It had been practised in West Africa for over 5000 years.

Indications

In infants and young boys, circumcision is most usually performed at the request of the parents for social or religious reasons. Medical indications for circumcision in boys include true phimosis caused by BXO (rare under the age of 5 years); recurrent attacks of balanoposthitis; and recurrent urinary tract infections with an abnormal upper urinary tract. Phimosis may result from misguided attempts by parents to expose the glans forcibly.

In adults, circumcision is indicated because of an inability to retract for intercourse, for splitting of an abnormally tight frenulum, for balanitis and sometimes before radiotherapy for carcinoma of the penis (Summary box 74.8).

> **Summary box 74.8**
>
> **Circumcision**
>
> - Is most commonly performed for cultural reasons
> - Is not indicated for failure of retraction caused by congenital adhesions between the glans penis and the prepuce
> - Is indicated when there is true phimosis with balanoposthitis or obstruction to urinary flow

Technique in an infant

Applying a clamp or bone forceps across the prepuce distal to the glans with blind division of the foreskin is to be condemned. To see one boy with partial or total amputation of the glans is enough to realise the folly of this technique. It is far better to perform a proper circumcision under direct vision as in an adult.

The Plastibel (Hollister) is used as shown in Fig. 74.17: the ring separates between 5 and 8 days postoperatively.

Technique in adolescents and adults

In adolescents and adults the following method is preferable. The prepuce is held in artery forceps and put on a gentle stretch. A circumferential incision in the penile skin is made at the level of the corona using a knife. The prepuce is then slit up the midline dorsally to within 1 cm of the corona. This converts the foreskin

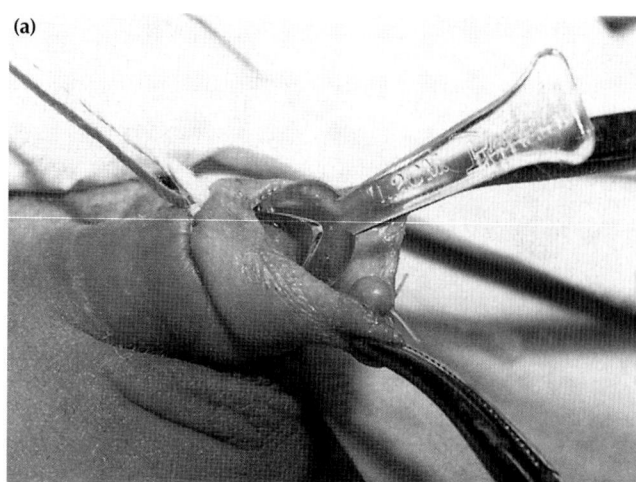

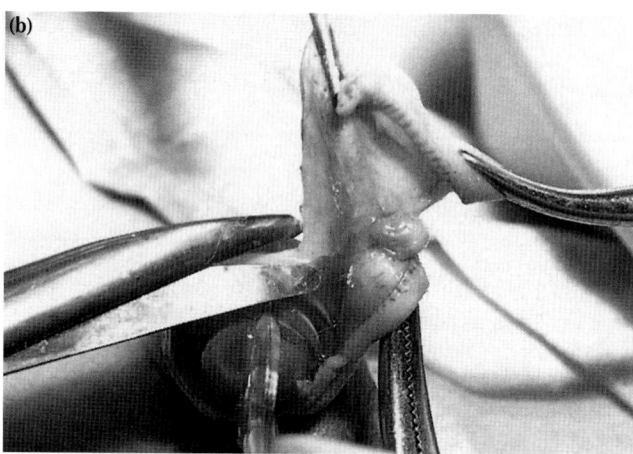

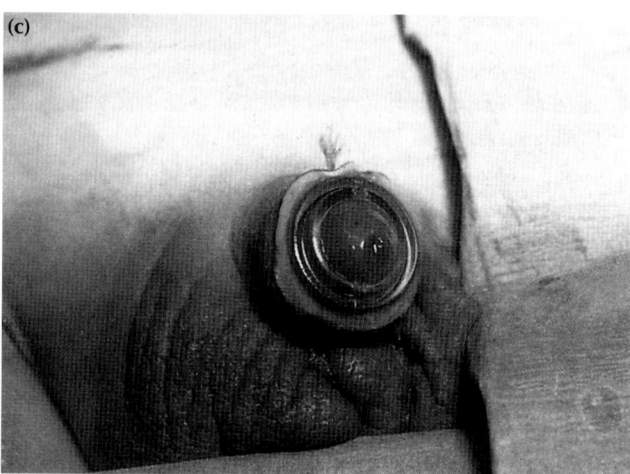

Figure 74.17 The Plastibel (Hollister) device for circumcision in infants. (a) The foreskin is freed and retracted. (b) After the Plastibel device has been slipped into place over the glans penis, the foreskin is ligated over the groove of the bell and redundant foreskin is cut away. (c) This shows the completed operation (courtesy of Professor Asal Y. Izzidien Al-Samarrai, King Saud University, Riyadh, Saudi Arabia).

into two flaps connected at the midline anteriorly. When the undersurface of the prepuce has been separated from the glans, the inner layer of each flap is incised with a second circumferential incision, leaving about 0.5 cm of the inner layer of the

prepuce distal to the corona. Cutting the remaining connective tissue completes the excision (Fig. 74.18). Monopolar diathermy must be avoided in operations on the penis in small boys because there is a danger that the small current path will cause coagulation at the base of the penis. Haemostasis is important in circumcision, however, and vessels should be secured by bipolar diathermy or ligated with non-absorbable material. The cut edges of the skin are approximated using interrupted sutures and the layers in the immediate region of the frenulum are brought neatly together using a mattress suture (Fig. 74.19) (Summary box 74.9).

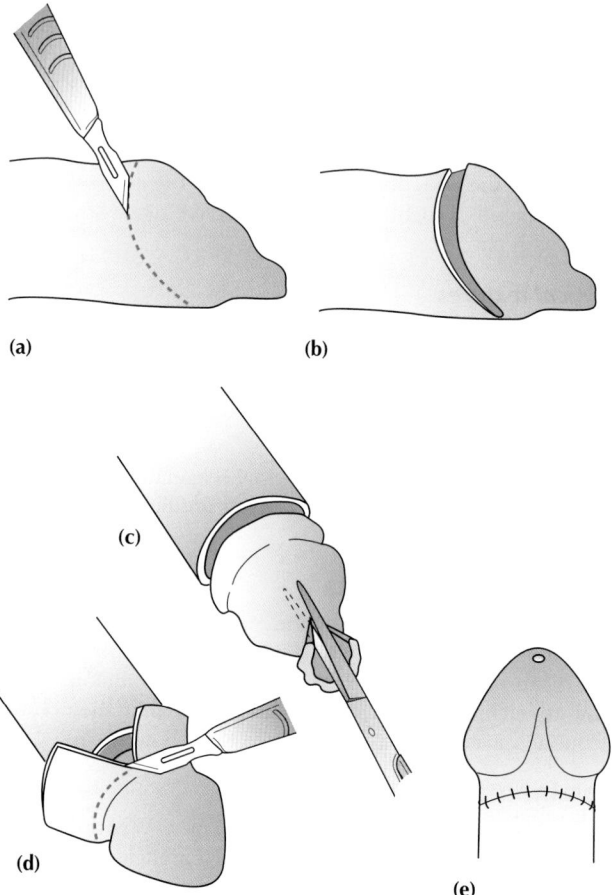

Figure 74.18 (a–e) Stages in circumcision.

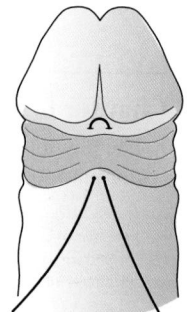

Figure 74.19 The 'four in one' frenular stitch.

Preputial calculi

Late in life, chronic posthitis may lead to adhesions between the prepuce and the glans and closure of the orifice of the preputial sac. Preputial calculi result from the accumulation beneath a non-retractable foreskin of inspissated smegma, urinary salts or both.

Injuries

Avulsion of the skin of the penis

Entanglement of clothing in rotating machinery is the usual cause. Repair is effected by burying the shaft of the penis in the scrotum (Fig. 74.20) with subsequent release at the time of a definitive plastic surgical repair.

Fracture of the penis

Fracture of the penis is an uncommon accident, usually occurring when the erect penis is bent violently downwards during intercourse. The extravasation of blood causes great pain and swelling. In early cases, incision and drainage of the clot with suture of the defect in the tunica of the ruptured corpus cavernosum gives acceptable results.

Strangulation of the penis

Strangulation of the penis by rings placed on the penis, usually for sexual reasons, can cause venous engorgement which prevents their removal. It may help to aspirate the corpora cavernosa but often the ring must be cut off with a ring cutter or hacksaw.

Paraphimosis

A tight foreskin once retracted may be difficult to return and a paraphimosis results. In this condition, the venous and lymphatic return from the glans and distal foreskin is obstructed and these structures swell, causing even more pressure within the obstructing ring of prepuce. Icebags, gentle manual compression and injection of a solution of hyaluronidase in normal saline may help to reduce the swelling. Such patients can be treated by circumcision if careful manipulation fails. A dorsal slit of the prepuce under local anaesthetic may be enough in an emergency.

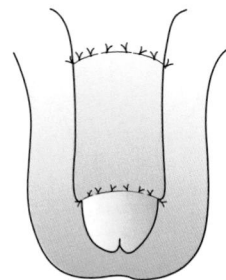

Figure 74.20 Covering the denuded shaft of the penis by burying it in a scrotal tunnel.

Inflammations

Balanoposthitis

Inflammation of the prepuce is known as posthitis; inflammation of the glans is balanitis. The opposing surfaces of the two structures are often involved, hence the term balanoposthitis. Skin conditions such as lichen planus and psoriasis affect the penis and, indeed, may be localised there. Drug hypersensitivity reactions can affect the skin of the penis.

In mild cases, the only symptoms are itching and some discharge. In more severe inflammation, the glans and foreskin are red-raw and pus exudes. Balanoposthitis is associated with penile cancer, diabetes and phimosis. Monilial infections are quite common under the prepuce.

Treatment is by broad-spectrum antibiotics and local hygiene measures.

Other abnormalities

Chordee

Chordee (French = corded) is a fixed bowing of the penis caused by hypospadias or, more rarely, chronic urethritis. Erection is deformed and sexual intercourse may be impossible. Treatment is usually surgical.

Peyronie's disease

Peyronie's disease is a relatively common cause of deformity of the erect penis. On examination, hard plaques of fibrosis can usually be palpated in the tunica of one or both corpora cavernosa. The plaques may be calcified (Fig. 74.21). The presence of the unyielding plaque tissue within the normally elastic wall of the corpus cavernosum causes the erect penis to bend, often dramatically, towards the side of the plaque. The aetiology is uncertain but it may be a result of past trauma – there is an association with Dupuytren's contracture.

Treatment is difficult. Some cases continue to progress. Others seem to remit after 3–5 years. Various drug treatments have been suggested but their beneficial effect is hard to prove in such a chronic condition. When the deformity of the penis is causing distress, it may be possible to straighten it by placing non-absorbable sutures in the corpus cavernosum opposite the plaque. This reduces the elasticity in this region to balance that caused by the plaque (Nesbitt's operation) (Summary box 74.10).

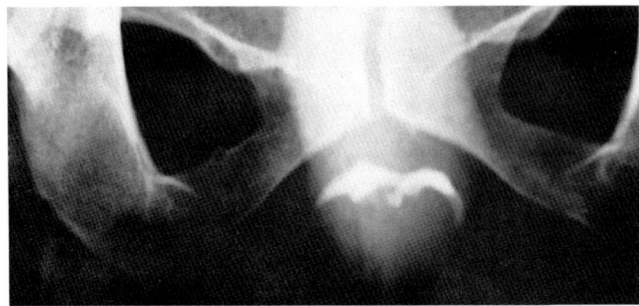

Figure 74.21 Penile calcification in Peyronie's disease (courtesy of Dr S.S. Rawat, Riyadh, Saudi Arabia).

Francois de la Peyronie, 1678–1747, Surgeon to King Louis XIV of France, and Founder of the Royal Academy of Surgery, Paris, France.
Baron Guillaume Dupuytren, 1777–1835, Surgeon, Hôtel Dieu, Paris, France, described this condition in 1831.
Thomas Nesbitt, Urological Surgeon, Nashville, TN, USA.

> **Summary box 74.10**
>
> **Peyronie's disease**
>
> - ■ Medical treatments are often ineffective
> - ■ The disease is typically self-limiting
> - ■ Surgery may be indicated to correct deformity that interferes with sexual function

Persistent priapism

The penis remains erect and becomes painful. This is a pathological erection and the glans penis and corpus spongiosum are not involved. The condition is usually seen as a complication of a blood disorder such as sickle cell disease or leukaemia. However, it can sometimes follow therapeutic injection of papaverine or even an abnormally prolonged bout of otherwise normal sexual activity. A tiny proportion is caused by malignant disease in the corpora cavernosa or the pelvis. Priapism is rarely seen as a consequence of spinal cord disease.

Treatment

An underlying cause should be excluded. The patient should be referred for specialist urological care. If aspiration of the sludged blood in the corpora cavernosa fails to cause detumescence, and repeated injection of metaraminol or 1:100 000 adrenaline (epinephrine) solution is ineffective, it may be necessary to decompress the penis by an anastomosis between the corpus spongiosum and one of the corpora cavernosa. The outlook for normal erectile function is poor (Summary box 74.11).

> **Summary box 74.11**
>
> **Prolonged priapism**
>
> - ■ Prolonged priapism is associated with erectile dysfunction, especially if surgical decompression by shunt formation is performed

Carcinoma

Aetiology

Circumcision soon after birth confers immunity against carcinoma of the penis. Later circumcision does not seem to have the same effect. Chronic balanoposthitis is known to be a contributory factor, and there are definite precarcinomatous states:

- leucoplakia of the glans, similar to the condition seen on the tongue;
- longstanding genital warts, which may rarely be the site of malignant change;
- Paget's disease of the penis.

Paget's disease of the penis (synonym: erythroplasia of Queyrat)

Paget's disease of the penis is 'a persistent rawness of the glans like a longstanding balanitis followed by cancer of the substance of the penis' (Sir James Paget). Treatment is by circumcision, observation and excision if the lesion does not resolve.

Pathology

Carcinoma of the penis may be flat and infiltrating or papillary (Fig. 74.22). The former often starts as leucoplakia and the latter results from an existing papilloma. Local growth continues for months or years. The earliest lymphatic spread is to the inguinal and then to the iliac nodes. Once the growth breaches the partial barrier formed by the fascial sheath of the corpora cavernosa it spreads rapidly and iliac lymph node involvement is common (Fig. 74.23). Distant metastatic deposits are infrequent.

Clinical features

About 40% of patients are under 40 years of age. Mild discomfort and light discharge are often neglected and the disease progresses slowly. By the time the patient presents, the growth is often large and secondary infection causes a foul bloody discharge. There is little or no pain.

In total, 60% present with inguinal lymph node enlargement but in half of these this is caused by sepsis. In most, the prepuce

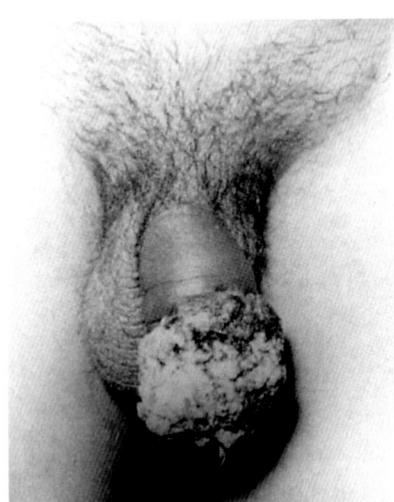

Figure 74.22 Carcinoma of the penis (courtesy of Dr V.K. Kapoor, All India Institute of Medical Sciences, Delhi, India).

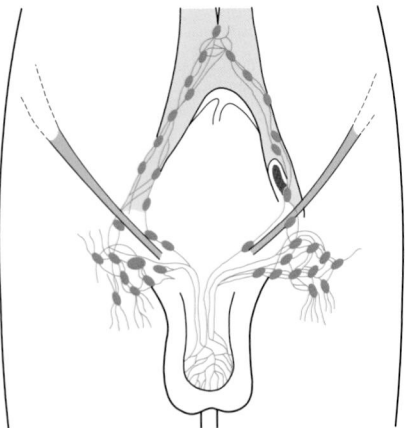

Figure 74.23 The lymphatic drainage of the penis. Superficial lymphatics drain to the inguinal and deep lymphatics to the iliac lymph nodes (after Archie L. Dean).

> Sir James Paget, 1814–1899, Surgeon, St Bartholomew's Hospital, London, England.
> Auguste Queyrat, B. 1872, Dermatologist, Paris, France, described this condition in 1911.

is non-retractile and must be split to view the lesion. A biopsy should be performed to make the diagnosis.

Untreated, the whole glans may be replaced by a fungating offensive mass. Later, the inguinal nodes erode the skin of the groin and the death of the patient may result from erosion of the femoral or external iliac artery.

Treatment

Radiotherapy is effective (60–70% survival rate at 5 years) for small cancers. Circumcision precedes treatment, which may be delivered by implanted radioactive tantalum wires, by external beam radiation or by means of a radioactive mould applicator applied externally to the penis.

Surgery is for large anaplastic growths, if there is infiltration of the shaft and when radiotherapy fails. Partial amputation is used for distal growths when adequate clearance of the tumour is possible. When an advanced, infiltrating or anaplastic lesion is present, total amputation is necessary.

Treatment of associated enlarged inguinal lymph nodes should usually be delayed until at least 3 weeks after local treatment of the primary lesion. Enlargement caused by infection will usually show signs of subsiding with antibiotic treatment if necessary. Block dissection is indicated if there is persistent enlargement that needle aspiration biopsy shows to be caused by tumour. The 5-year survival rate falls to 35% in these cases. If surgery to the nodes is impossible, radiotherapy may cause a worthwhile temporary regression (Summary box 74.12).

> **Summary box 74.12**
>
> **Carcinoma of the penis**
> - Relatively uncommon
> - Enlargement of superficial inguinal lymph nodes may be caused by infection or metastatic spread
> - May be treated by a combination of surgery and radiotherapy

Buschke–Löwenstein tumour

Buschke–Löwenstein tumour is uncommon. It has the histological pattern of a verrucous carcinoma. It is locally destructive and invasive but appears not to spread to lymph nodes or to metastasise. Treatment is by surgical excision.

Secondary cancer of the penis

Secondary cancer of the penis as a result of spread from a primary tumour of the bladder, rectum or prostate is uncommon.

SEXUALLY TRANSMITTED GENITAL INFECTIONS

Genital herpes

Genital herpes is caused by sexual transmission of the herpesvirus hominis (type 2, occasionally type 1). Recurrent attacks occur in 50% or more of cases. Pain along the distribution of the sensory nerve, usually genitofemoral, precedes the eruption by 2 days and

may be particularly severe around the anus. A group of tiny vesicles rapidly erodes to form shallow yellow- or red-based ulcers. In female patients, the ulcers often spread on to the thighs during the attack. Involvement of the urethra may cause retention of urine, which may persist for up to 14 days if there is radiculitis of the S2 and S3 nerve roots. Aciclovir has been shown to be effective in treating genital herpes but it does not prevent recurrences.

A child born to a mother with active infection is susceptible to a fatal generalised herpes infection in the neonatal period. Caesarean section should be considered in these circumstances. There is an increased risk of carcinoma of the cervix and annual cytology for life is recommended.

Lymphogranuloma venereum

Lymphogranuloma venereum is a sexually transmitted tropical disease caused by *Chlamydia trachomatis* (*Chlamydia A*) types L1–L3. The primary lesion is a fleeting, painless, genital papule or ulcer often unnoticed by the patient.

The inguinal glands become enlarged and painful in both sexes between 2 weeks and 4 months after infection. The masses of nodes mat together above and below the inguinal ligament to give the 'sign of the groove'. The overlying skin reddens and there may be fluctuation. In women, there may be a proctitis, which can go on to produce a rectal stricture if untreated. Lymphatic obstruction leads to lymphoedema in the perineum and occasionally the lower limbs. Urethritis and urethral stricture occur in men.

Confirmation is by isolating *Chlamydia A* from the lesion and by immunological tests to detect antibodies against the organism.

Treatment is by a combination of antibiotics, which may include sulphonamide, oxytetracycline and erythromycin. The multilocular bubo should not be incised; aspiration is permissible to reduce discomfort.

Granuloma inguinale

This is a chronic and slowly progressive ulcerative tropical disease affecting the genitals and surrounding tissue but occasionally occurring elsewhere in the body. It is usually sexually transmitted and is most common among socially deprived people. The incubation period varies greatly but is frequently 7–30 days.

Clinical course

A painless vesicle or indurated papule, usually on the external genitals but occasionally elsewhere on the skin, gradually erodes into a slowly extending ulcer with a beefy-red, granulomatous base. More chronic lesions may become greyish, especially at the edges, where, after months or years, malignant change may develop. The ulcerated area may bleed if touched but is surprisingly painless. Without treatment healing is only partial and keloid is common.

Diagnosis is by microscopy of material from the edges of the ulcer, which shows the presence of short Gram-negative rods within the cytoplasm of the large mononuclear cells.

Treatment is by oxytetracycline, streptomycin or co-trimoxazole.

A Caesarean section **is the operation of delivering the foetus by an incision into the uterus, usually through the abdominal wall.**

CHAPTER 74 | URETHRA AND PENIS

Condylomata acuminata (synonym: genital warts)

Genital warts are caused by infection with human papillomavirus and are sexually transmitted. Ordinary skin warts can occur on the genitals by direct contact with a finger lesion, but they are less moist and soft and less often pedunculated than the genital variety. The lesions most commonly occur under the prepuce in the coronal sulcus but may be found elsewhere, including inside the urinary meatus (Fig. 74.24). In women, genital warts are most commonly found on the vulva but they may line the vagina and occur on the cervix. Perianal warts are common.

Other associated sexually transmitted diseases should be excluded: in women mainly candidiasis and *Trichomonas* infection and in men syphilis or gonorrhoea. Genital warts may complicate human immunodeficiency virus (HIV) infection.

Treatment is by chemical or physical means. Podophyllin 25% in spirit is often effective as a topical application. It is applied to the wart taking great care to avoid the surrounding skin and washed off after 6 hours or so.

If chemical methods fail, the warts can be excised or they can be ablated with cryosurgery, electrosurgery or laser. Circumcision is sometimes advised if there are florid lesions under the foreskin.

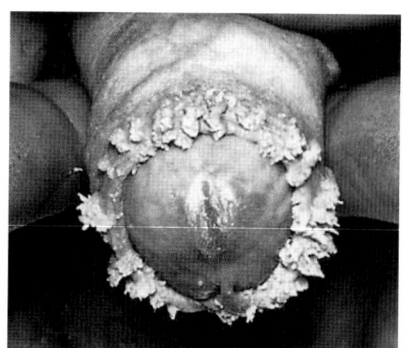

Figure 74.24 Penile warts.

FURTHER READING

Blandy, J.P. and Kaisary, A.V. (2007) *Lecture Notes: Urology*, 6th edn. Blackwell, Oxford.

Wein, A.J., Kavoussi, L.R., Novick, A.C., Partin, A.W. and Peters, C.A. (2007) *Campbell–Walsh Urology*, 9th edn. W.B. Saunders, Philadelphia, PA.

Testis and scrotum

LEARNING OBJECTIVES

To recognise and understand:
- Imperfect testicular descent and appreciate the main indications for intervention
- Testicular torsion as a urological emergency

- The principles of the management of varicocele, hydrocele and epididymal cysts
- The classification and management of testicular tumours
- The treatment options for infertile men

DEFINITIONS

Incomplete descent of the testis

The testis is arrested in some part of its path to the scrotum.

Ectopic testis

The testis is abnormally placed outside this path.

ANATOMY OF THE TESTIS

The testes develop in the retroperitoneum below the kidneys in early fetal life. About the same time as the wolffian duct becomes the epididymis and vas deferens, the precursor of the gubernaculum develops as a fold of peritoneum. The processus vaginalis starts as a dimple of peritoneum in about the 10th week of gestation and precedes the testis in its journey through the abdominal wall down to the scrotum. The fully developed gubernaculum contains muscle fibres but it is still not clear what part it plays in testicular descent. Maternal chorionic gonadotrophin stimulates growth of the testis and may stimulate its migration. Imperfectly developed testes tend to descend incompletely.

The anatomy of the adult testis reflects its embryonic development. The testicular arteries originate high up in the retroperitoneum, from the abdominal aorta on the left and from the renal artery on the right. The venous drainage finds its way to the left renal vein and the inferior vena cava. For much of their course the testicular artery and vein run parallel to the ipsilateral ureter, for which they may be mistaken during retroperitoneal surgery.

The epididymis extends as a fleshy strip on the posterior aspect of the testis and is palpable as a separate structure. The vas deferens takes its origin from the epididymis. It can be felt above

the testis as a firm tubular structure entering the external inguinal ring. In the inguinal canal, the vas deferens is invested by the cremasteric muscle along with the other components of the spermatic cord.

INCOMPLETELY DESCENDED TESTIS (SEE ALSO CHAPTER 6)

Incidence

About 4% of boys are born with one or both testes incompletely descended. About half of these reach the scrotum during the first month of life, but full descent after that is uncommon. The condition is sometimes missed at birth and discovered later in life. In a few cases, the presence of a hernia, testicular pain or acute torsion directs attention to the abnormality. In 10% of unilateral cases there is a family history.

Pathology

Incompletely descended testes are often macroscopically normal in early childhood but by puberty the testis is poorly developed compared with its intrascrotal counterpart. The epithelial elements are immature histologically and by late puberty irreversible destructive changes halt spermatogenesis and limit the production of androgens.

An incompletely descended testis brought down in early childhood often functions satisfactorily (Summary box 75.1).

Summary box 75.1

Undescended testis

- **Testes absent from the scrotum after 3 months of age are unlikely to descend fully**
- **An incompletely descended testis tends to atrophy as puberty approaches**
- **Early repositioning of an incompletely descended testis can preserve function**

Kaspar Friedrich Wolff, 1733–1794, Professor of Anatomy and Physiology, St Petersburg, Russia.

Clinical features

The condition is more common on the right and is bilateral in 20% of cases. Secondary sexual characteristics are typically normal.

The testis may be:

- intra-abdominal, lying extraperitoneally above the internal inguinal ring;
- inguinal, in which case it may or may not be palpable (Fig. 75.1);
- in the superficial inguinal pouch, in which case it must be distinguished from retractile testis.

During childhood the testes are mobile and the cremasteric reflex is active. In some boys, any stimulation of the skin of the scrotum or thigh causes the testis to disappear into the inguinal canal. Simply exposing the parts can also do this so that the testis is never seen in an intrascrotal position. The scrotum is normal as opposed to underdeveloped, which is usually seen with true incomplete descent. When the cremaster relaxes, the tell-tale bulge of the testis reappears only to vanish when the scrotal skin is touched again. A retractile testis can be gently milked from its position in the inguinal region to the bottom of the scrotum. A diagnosis of true incomplete descent should be made only if this is not possible. In infancy, most inapparent testes are retractile. They are normal and require no treatment (Summary box 75.2).

> **Summary box 75.2**
>
> **Retractile testis**
>
> - Retractile testes are more common than incompletely descended testes and require no treatment

Hazards of incomplete descent are:

- sterility in bilateral cases (especially intra-abdominal testes);
- pain as a result of trauma;
- an associated indirect inguinal hernia is often present and may cause symptoms;
- torsion;
- epididymo-orchitis in an incompletely descended right testis can mimic appendicitis;

- atrophy of an inguinal testis before puberty may possibly be caused by recurrent minor trauma;
- increased liability to malignant disease; cancer is more common in an incompletely descended testes – orchidopexy may or may not diminish the risk but it does improve the prospect of early diagnosis (Summary box 75.3).

> **Summary box 75.3**
>
> **Orchidopexy**
>
> - An increased liability to malignant disease is not necessarily corrected by orchidopexy but early diagnosis of a tumour is easier

Surgical treatment

Orchidopexy is usually performed after the age of 1 year to avoid the risks of operating on a tiny patient. Testes should be brought down into the scrotum before the boy starts school. In bilateral cases it is usual to operate on one side at a time.

Orchidopexy

In orchidopexy (synonym: orchiopexy), the testis and spermatic cord are mobilised and the testis is repositioned in the scrotum. The operation is performed through a short incision over the deep inguinal ring. The inguinal canal is exposed by division of the external oblique aponeurosis in the direction of its fibres.

Mobilisation begins with isolation of the indirect inguinal hernial sac, which lies anterior to the cord. The sac is fragile but with care it can be swept laterally to reveal filmy strands that join the neck of the sac to the cord. The fibrous strands are divided and the spermatic vessels are dissected free of the peritoneum until there is a sufficient length of liberated cord to place the testis in the scrotum without tension. Division of the cremaster and the coverings of the cord may give more length, but the tiny vas and testicular vessels are vulnerable to injury. The empty hemiscrotum is stretched with a finger passed into it through the inguinal incision to give enough room for the testis.

The testis is placed in a pouch constructed between the dartos muscle and the skin (Fig. 75.2). An alternative to the

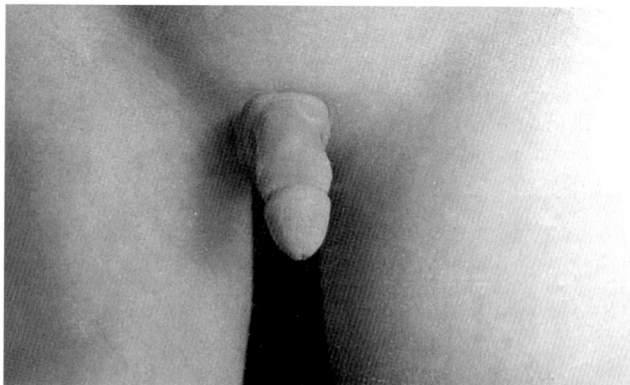

Figure 75.1 A cryptorchid in a boy aged 12 years. Note the retracted underdeveloped scrotum. In cases of retractile testis, the scrotum is relatively well developed.

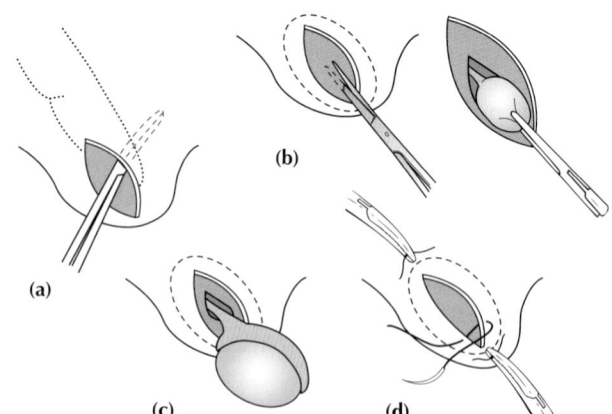

Figure 75.2 The testis is mobilised and retained in a pouch constructed between the dartos muscle and skin.

dartos pouch is to take the testis through the scrotal septum (Ombrédanne's operation).

Failure to bring the testis down

Sometimes a two-stage procedure is successful: the testis is mobilised as far as possible and anchored with a suture and the mobilisation is completed 6 months later. Orchidectomy should be considered if the incompletely descended testis is atrophic, particularly if the patient is past puberty and the other testis is normal.

Hormone treatment with human chorionic gonadotrophin is appropriate only when there is established hypogonadism.

ECTOPIC TESTIS

The sites of ectopic testis are:

- at the superficial inguinal ring;
- in the perineum;
- at the root of the penis;
- in the femoral triangle.

An ectopic testis is usually fully developed. The main hazard is liability to injury.

INJURIES TO THE TESTIS

Rupture by a blow is uncommon because of the testis's mobility within the scrotum. Contusion and rupture are associated with a collection of blood around the testis and cannot usually be distinguished with certainty without exploration. The haematocele (Fig. 75.3) should be drained and the tunica albuginea repaired after evacuation of haematoma. A severely damaged testis may have to be removed.

Traumatic displacement occasionally follows a blow. The displaced testis usually lies in one of the sites of ectopic testis and can be returned to its normal position by manipulation before it becomes anchored by fibrosis (Summary box 75.4).

Summary box 75.4

Scrotal trauma

- Scrotal exploration should be considered when there is massive swelling and pain after scrotal trauma

---

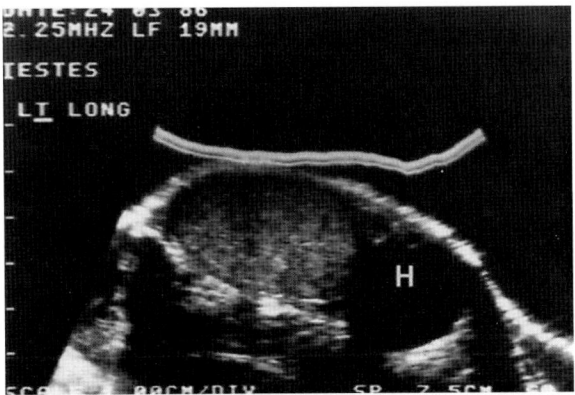

Figure 75.3 Longitudinal scan of testicle with haematocele (H) at lower pole.

Louis Ombrédanne, 1871–1956, Surgeon, Hôpital des Enfants Malades, Paris, France.

ABSENT TESTIS

'Vanishing' testis describes a condition in which a testis develops but disappears before birth. The most likely cause for this is prenatal torsion. True agenesis of the testis is rarer. Laparoscopy is useful in distinguishing these causes of clinically absent testis from intra-abdominal maldescent.

TORSION OF THE TESTIS

Predisposing causes

Torsion of the testis is uncommon because the normal testis is anchored and cannot rotate. For torsion to occur one of several abnormalities must be present:

- Inversion of the testis is the most common predisposing cause. The testis is rotated so that it lies transversely or upside down.
- High investment of the tunica vaginalis causes the testis to hang within the tunica like a clapper in a bell (Fig. 75.4).
- Separation of the epididymis from the body of the testis permits torsion of the testis on the pedicle that connects the testis with the epididymis (Fig. 75.5).

Normally, when there is a contraction of the abdominal muscles, the cremaster contracts as well. In the presence of one of the abnormalities described above, the spiral attachment of the cremaster favours rotation of the testis around the vertical axis. Straining at stool, lifting a heavy weight and coitus are all possible precipitating factors. Alternatively, torsion may develop spontaneously during sleep.

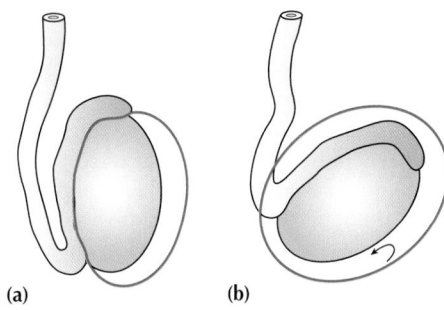

(a)   (b)

Figure 75.4 Testicular torsion. (a) Normal attachment. (b) An abnormally high attachment of the tunica vaginalis predisposes to torsion – the 'bell-clapper'.

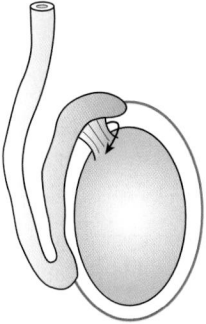

Figure 75.5 Testicular torsion. Separation of the testis from the epididymis – torsion about the pedicle between them.

Clinical features

Testicular torsion is most common between 10 and 25 years of age although a few cases occur in infancy. Symptoms vary with the degree of torsion. Most commonly there is sudden agonising pain in the groin and the lower abdomen. The patient feels nauseated and may vomit.

Torsion of a fully descended testis is usually easily recognised. The testis seems high and the tender twisted cord can be palpated above it. In mumps orchitis the cord is not particularly thickened. The onset of redness of the skin and a mild pyrexia may result in the condition being confused with epididymo-orchitis in the older patient; however, in epididymo-orchitis there will usually be dysuria associated with the accompanying urinary infection. Elevation of the testis reduces the pain in epididymo-orchitis and makes it worse in torsion. Very occasionally, torsion can be convincingly mimicked by a small tense strangulated inguinal hernia compressing the cord and causing compression of the pampiniform plexus.

Doppler ultrasound scan will confirm the absence of the blood supply to the affected testis, but performing this test may squander vital minutes. If there is any doubt about the diagnosis, the scrotum should be explored without delay.

An empty oedematous hemiscrotum suggests that a tender lump at the external inguinal ring is a torted testis rather than a strangulated hernia.

Treatment

In the first hour or so it may be possible to untwist the testis by gentle manipulation. If manipulation is successful, pain subsides and the testis is out of danger. Arrangements should be made for early operative fixation to avoid recurrent torsion.

Exploration for torsion can be performed through a scrotal incision. If the testis is viable when the cord is untwisted it should be prevented from twisting again by fixation with non-absorbable sutures between the tunica vaginalis and the tunica albuginea. The other testis should also be fixed because the anatomical predisposition is likely to be bilateral. An infarcted testis should be removed – the patient can be counselled later about a prosthetic replacement. It is not possible to recover the testis that has been torted for several days and little is gained by immediate exploration. The affected testis will become woody-hard and atrophy to a fibrous nodule. The other testis should be fixed (Summary box 75.5).

Summary box 75.5

Testicular torsion

- **Prompt exploration, untwisting and fixation is the only way to save the torted testis**
- **The patient should be counselled and consented for orchidectomy before exploration**
- **The anatomical abnormality is bilateral and the contralateral testis should also be fixed**

Torsion of a testicular appendage is sometimes mistaken for acute epididymo-orchitis and cannot be distinguished with certainty

from testicular torsion. The most common structure to twist is the appendix of the testis (the pedunculated hydatid of Morgagni). Immediate operation with ligation and amputation of the twisted appendage cures the condition.

Idiopathic scrotal oedema is an oddity that occurs between the age of 4 and 12 years and must be differentiated from torsion. The scrotum is very swollen but there is little pain or tenderness. The swelling may extend into the perineum, groin and penis. It is thought to be an allergic phenomenon; occasionally there is eosinophilia. The swelling subsides after a day or so but may recur (Fig. 75.6).

VARICOCELE

A varicocele is a varicose dilatation of the veins draining the testis.

Surgical anatomy

The veins draining the testis and the epididymis form the pampiniform plexus. The veins become fewer as they traverse the inguinal canal and at or near the inguinal ring they join to form one or two testicular veins, which pass upwards behind the peritoneum. The left testicular vein empties into the left renal vein, the right into the inferior vena cava below the right renal vein. The testicular veins may have valves near their terminations, but these are often absent. There is an alternative (collateral) venous return from the testes through the cremasteric veins, which drain mainly into the inferior epigastrics.

Aetiology

Most varicoceles present in adolescence or early adulthood, usually on the left. In many cases the dilated vessels are cremasteric veins and not part of the pampiniform plexus.

Obstruction of the left testicular vein by a renal tumour or after nephrectomy is a cause of varicocele in later life; characteristically, the varicocele does not decompress in the supine position.

Clinical features

Varicocele is usually symptomless but there may be an annoying dragging discomfort that is worse if the testis is unsupported. The scrotum on the affected side hangs lower than normal (Fig. 75.7), and on palpation, with the patient standing, the varicose plexus

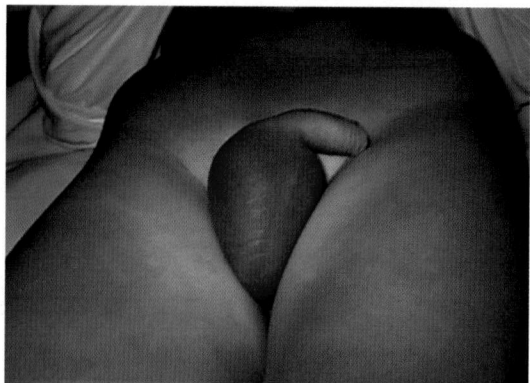

Figure 75.6 Oedema of the scrotum.

Christian Johann Doppler, **1803–1853**, Professor of Experimental Physics, Vienna, Austria, enunciated the 'Doppler Principle' in 1842.

Giovanni Battista Morgagni, **1682–1771**, Professor of Anatomy, Padua, Italy for 59 years. He is regarded as the Founder of Morbid Anatomy.

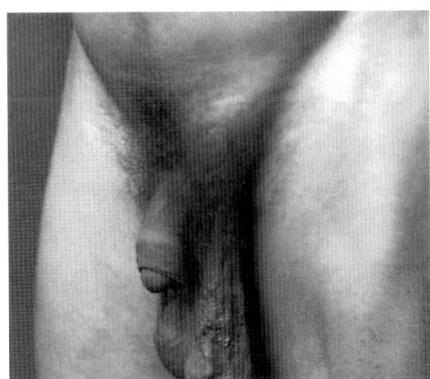

Figure 75.7 Large varicocele in a pendulous scrotum. Note the left inguinal hernia.

feels like a bag of worms. There may be a cough impulse. If the patient lies down the veins empty by gravity and this provides an opportunity to ensure that the underlying testis is normal to palpation. In longstanding cases the affected testis is smaller and softer than its fellow owing to a minor degree of atrophy. It is widely believed that varicocele causes infertility but the evidence is inconclusive.

Varicocele and spermatogenesis

Of all the possible causes of primary infertility, oligospermia is one of the most difficult to treat. Because varicocele is relatively common, some of those with oligospermia have a varicocele, and it is tempting to blame this for the infertility. Perhaps the presence of the unilateral varicocele somehow interferes with the normal temperature control of the scrotum, which keeps the testes at some 2.5°C below rectal temperature. Unfortunately, there is little evidence that varicocelectomy improves semen quality or the rate of conception (Summary box 75.6).

Summary box 75.6
Varicocele
■ Varicocele is a common condition and tends to recur after surgical treatment. Its association with subfertility is difficult to prove

Treatment

Operation is not indicated for asymptomatic varicocele. The simplest procedure is laparoscopic ligation of the testicular vein above the inguinal ligament where the pampiniform plexus has coalesced into one or two vessels. However, when facilities are available, embolisation of the testicular vein under radiographic control is probably the treatment of choice. Because of the presence of plentiful collateral veins, recurrence is common after all types of varicocele surgery.

HYDROCELE

A hydrocele is an abnormal collection of serous fluid in a part of the processus vaginalis, usually the tunica. Acquired hydroceles are primary or idiopathic, or secondary to testicular disease.

Aetiology

A hydrocele can be produced in four different ways (Fig. 75.8):

- by excessive production of fluid within the sac, e.g. secondary hydrocele;
- by defective absorption of fluid; this appears to be the explanation for most primary hydroceles although the reason why the fluid is not absorbed is obscure;
- by interference with lymphatic drainage of scrotal structures;
- by connection with the peritoneal cavity via a patent processus vaginalis (congenital).

Hydrocele fluid contains albumin and fibrinogen. If the contents of a hydrocele are allowed to drain into a collecting vessel, the liquid does not clot; however, the fluid coagulates if mixed with even a trace of blood that has been in contact with damaged tissue.

Clinical features

Hydroceles are typically translucent and it is possible to 'get above the swelling' on examination of the scrotum.

Primary vaginal hydrocele is most common in middle and later life but can also occur in older children. The condition is particularly common in hot countries. Because the swelling is usually painless it may reach a prodigious size before the patient presents for treatment. The testis may be palpable within a lax hydrocele, but an ultrasound scan is necessary to visualise the testis if the hydrocele sac is tense. Be wary of an acute hydrocele in a young man; there may be a testicular tumour (Summary box 75.7).

Summary box 75.7
Testicular malignancy and hydrocele
■ Testicular malignancy is an uncommon cause of hydrocele that can be excluded by ultrasound examination of the scrotum

About 5% of inguinal hernias are associated with a vaginal hydrocele on the same side.

In congenital hydrocele, the processus vaginalis is patent and connects with the peritoneal cavity. The communication is usually too small to allow herniation of intra-abdominal contents. Pressure on the hydrocele does not always empty it but the hydrocele fluid may drain into the peritoneal cavity when the child is lying down; thus, the hydrocele is often intermittent. Ascites should be considered if the swellings are bilateral.

Encysted hydrocele of the cord is a smooth oval swelling near the spermatic cord, which is liable to be mistaken for an inguinal

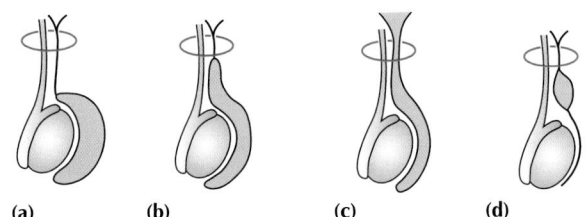

(a)　　　**(b)**　　　**(c)**　　　**(d)**

Figure 75.8 (a) Vaginal hydrocele (very common). (b) 'Infantile' hydrocele. (c) Congenital hydrocele. (d) Hydrocele of the cord.

hernia. The swelling moves downwards and becomes less mobile if the testis is pulled gently downwards.

Hydrocele of the canal of Nuck is a similar condition in females. The cyst lies in relation to the round ligament and is always at least partially within the inguinal canal.

Complications of hydrocele

- Rupture is rare.
- Transformation into a haematocele occurs after trauma or if there is spontaneous bleeding into the sac.
- The sac may calcify.

Treatment

Congenital hydroceles are treated by herniotomy if they do not resolve spontaneously (see Chapter 6).

Established acquired hydroceles often have thick walls. Unless great care is taken to stop bleeding after excision of the wall, haemorrhage from the cut edge is liable to cause a large scrotal haematoma. Lord's operation is suitable when the sac is reasonably thin-walled (Fig. 75.9). There is minimal dissection and the risk of haematoma is reduced. Eversion of the sac with placement of the testis in a pouch prepared by dissection in the fascial planes of the scrotum is an alternative (Jaboulay's procedure) (Fig. 75.10).

Cannula drainage of the hydrocele fluid is simple, but it always

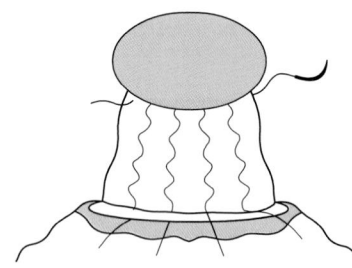

Figure 75.9 Lord's operation. A series of interrupted absorbable sutures is used to plicate the redundant tunica vaginalis. When these are tied, the tunica bunches at its attachment to the testis.

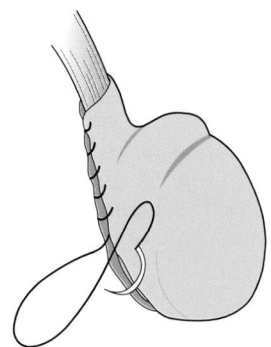

Figure 75.10 Jaboulay's procedure. The hydrocele sac is everted and anchored with sutures.

Anton Nuck, 1650–1692, Professor of Anatomy and Medicine, Leiden, The Netherlands.
Peter Herent Lord, Contemporary, Formerly Surgeon, Wycombe General Hospital, High Wycombe, Buckinghamshire, England.
Mathieu Jaboulay, 1860–1913, Professor of Surgery, Lyons, France.

reaccumulates within a week or so (see Gibbon below). It may be suitable for men unfit for scrotal surgery even under regional anaesthesia. Injection of sclerosants such as tetracycline is effective but painful.

Secondary hydrocele is most frequently associated with acute or chronic epididymo-orchitis. It is also seen with torsion of the testis and with some testicular tumours. A secondary hydrocele is usually lax and of moderate size: the underlying testis is palpable. If a tumour is suspected, the hydrocele should not be punctured for fear of needle-track implantation of malignant cells. A secondary hydrocele subsides when the primary lesion resolves.

Post-herniorrhaphy hydrocele

Post-herniorrhaphy hydrocele is a relatively uncommon complication of inguinal hernia repair.

Hydrocele of a hernial sac

Hydrocele of a hernial sac occurs when the neck of the sac is occluded by adhesions or an omental plug.

Filarial hydroceles and chyloceles

Filarial hydroceles and chyloceles account for up to 80% of hydroceles in tropical countries where the parasite *Wucheria bancrofti* is endemic. Filarial hydroceles follow repeated attacks of filarial epididymo-orchitis. They vary in size and may develop slowly or very rapidly. Occasionally, the fluid contains liquid fat, which is rich in cholesterol. This is caused by rupture of a lymphatic varix with discharge of chyle into the hydrocele. In longstanding chyloceles there are dense adhesions between the scrotum and its contents. Filarial elephantiasis supervenes in a small number of cases.

Treatment is by rest and aspiration. The more usual chronic cases are treated by excision of the sac.

Haematocele

Haematocele usually results from vessel damage during needle drainage of a hydrocele. Prompt refilling of the sac, pain, tenderness and reduced transillumination confirm the diagnosis. Acute haemorrhage into the tunica vaginalis sometimes results from testicular trauma with or without testicular rupture. If the haematocele is not drained, a clotted haematocele usually results.

Clotted haematocele

Clotted hydrocele may result from a slow spontaneous ooze of blood into the tunica vaginalis. It is usually painless and may be mistaken for a testicular tumour. Indeed, a tumour may present as a haematocele.

Treatment is by orchidectomy unless the testis is indubitably benign. As a rule, it is impossible to be certain until the mass has been bisected. The testis is often compressed and relatively useless (Fig. 75.11).

Edward Gibbon, 1737–1794, the author of 'The Decline and Fall of the Roman Empire', was greatly embarrassed by a large hydrocele. The second time that it was tapped it became infected, and Gibbon died a few days later. The hydrocele was associated with a large scrotal hernia which had probably been punctured.
Otto Eduard Heinrich Wucherer, 1820–1873, a German Physician who practised in Brazil, South America.
Joseph Bancroft, 1836–1894, an English Physician working in Australia.

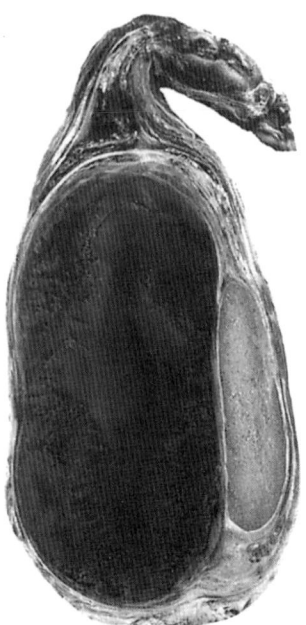

Figure 75.11 A longstanding haematocele. The testis has been flattened by prolonged pressure.

CYSTS ASSOCIATED WITH THE EPIDIDYMIS

There are several types of cyst associated with the epididymis (Summary box 75.8).

Summary box 75.8

Cysts associated with the epididymis

- Are separate from the testis on palpation
- Unless large or uncomfortable may be treated conservatively when diagnosed with certainty using ultrasound

---

Epididymal cysts

These are filled with a crystal-clear fluid. They are very common, usually multiple and vary in size at presentation. They represent cystic degeneration of the epididymis.

Clinical features

Cysts of the epididymis are usually found in middle age and are often bilateral. The clusters of tense cysts feel like a tiny bunches of grapes. They should be brilliantly transilluminable. The presence of a scrotal mass always raises the possibility of a testicular neoplasm, but epididymal cysts are almost always quite separate from the testis proper and this is a reassuring sign.

Treatment

Aspiration is useless because the cysts are multilocular. If they are causing discomfort they should be excised. Excision may interfere with the export of sperm from the testis on that side.

Cysts of a testicular appendage

Cysts of a testicular appendage are usually unilateral and are felt as small globular upper pole swellings. Such cysts are liable to torsion and should be removed if they cause symptoms.

Spermatocele

This is a unilocular retention cyst derived from some portion of the sperm-conducting mechanism of the epididymis.

Clinical features

A spermatocele typically lies in the epididymal head above and behind the upper pole of the testis. It is usually softer and laxer than other cystic lesions in the scrotum but, like them, it transilluminates. The fluid contains spermatozoa and resembles barley water in appearance. Spermatoceles are usually small and unobtrusive.

Treatment

Small spermatoceles can be ignored. Larger ones should be aspirated or excised through a scrotal incision.

EPIDIDYMO-ORCHITIS

Inflammation confined to the epididymis is epididymitis; infection spreading to the testis is epididymo-orchitis.

Acute disease

Mode of infection

Infection reaches the epididymis via the vas from a primary infection of the urethra, prostate or seminal vesicles. In men with outflow obstruction, epididymitis may result from a secondary urinary infection – a high pressure in the prostatic urethra causes reflux of infected urine up the vasa. In young men, the most common sexually transmitted infection causing epididymitis is now *Chlamydia*, but gonococcal epididymitis is still prevalent; both cause urethritis. Blood-borne infections of the epididymis are less common but may be suspected when there is *Escherichia coli*, streptococcal, staphylococcal or *Proteus* infection without evidence of urinary infection.

Clinical features

The initial symptoms are those of urinary infection. Later, an ache in the groin and a fever herald the onset of epididymitis. The epididymis and testis swell and become painful. The scrotal wall, at first red, oedematous and shiny, may become adherent to the epididymis. Resolution may take 6–8 weeks to complete. Occasionally, an abscess may form and discharge of pus may occur through the scrotal skin.

Acute epididymo-orchitis can follow any form of urethral instrumentation. It is particularly common when an indwelling catheter is associated with infection of the prostate. The incidence of acute postoperative epididymitis after prostatectomy has been greatly reduced by closed drainage, catheter care and the early use of antibiotics.

Acute tuberculous epididymitis should be considered when the vas is thickened and there is little response to the usual antibiotics.

Acute epididymo-orchitis develops in about 18% of males suffering from mumps, usually as the parotid swelling is waning. The main complication is testicular atrophy, which may cause infertility if the condition is bilateral (which is not usual). Partial

---

Theodor Escherich, **1857–1911, Professor of Paediatrics, Vienna, Austria,** discovered the bacterium coli commune in 1886.

atrophy is associated with persistent testicular pain. Mumps epididymitis sometimes occurs in the absence of parotitis, especially in infants. The epididymis and testis may be involved by infection with other enteroviruses and in brucellosis and lymphogranuloma venereum.

Treatment

Doxycycline (100 mg daily) is the treatment of choice for young men with chlamydial infection. If an organism is isolated from the urine, this simplifies the choice of antibiotic. Otherwise, treatment is with an agent that is active against a broad spectrum of urinary tract pathogens. The patient should drink plenty of fluid. Local measures can help to reduce pain. The scrotum is supported on a sling made of broad adhesive tape attached between the thighs. The inflamed organ rests on a pad of cotton wool placed on the sling.

Antibiotic treatment should continue for 2 weeks or until the inflammation has subsided. If suppuration occurs, drainage is necessary. The patient should be warned that the testis may atrophy (Summary box 75.9).

Summary box 75.9

Acute epididymo-orchitis

- May be secondary to urinary infection or urethritis
- Is a complication of catheterisation or instrumentation of the urinary tract
- May need aggressive treatment with parenteral antibiotics

Chronic disease

Chronic tuberculous epididymo-orchitis usually begins insidiously.

Aetiology

The frequency with which the lower pole is attacked first indicates that the infection is retrograde from a tuberculous focus in the seminal vesicles.

Clinical features

Typically, there is a firm discrete swelling of the lower pole of the epididymis, which aches a little. The disease progresses until the whole epididymis is firm and craggy behind a normal-feeling testis. There is a lax secondary hydrocele in 30% of cases, and a characteristic beading of the vas may be apparent as a result of subepithelial tubercles. The seminal vesicle feels indurated and swollen. In neglected cases, a tuberculous 'cold' abscess forms, which may discharge. The body of the testis may be uninvolved for years but the contralateral epididymis often becomes diseased.

In two-thirds of cases there is evidence of renal tuberculosis or previous disease. Otherwise, patients typically appear healthy.

The urine and semen should be examined repeatedly for tubercle bacilli in all patients with chronic epididymo-orchitis. An intravenous urogram and a chest radiograph should be performed.

Treatment

Secondary tuberculous epididymitis may resolve when the primary focus is treated.

Treatment with anti-tuberculous drugs is less effective in genital tuberculosis than in urinary tuberculosis. If resolution does not occur within 2 months, epididymectomy or orchidectomy is advisable. A course of anti-tuberculous chemotherapy should be completed even if there is no evidence of disease elsewhere.

Chronic non-tuberculous epididymitis usually follows the failure of an acute attack to resolve. The condition is difficult to distinguish from tuberculosis but the swelling may be larger and smoother. It is essential to exclude urethral stricture causing reflux of urine down the vas. If alternative granulomatous conditions such as sarcoidosis have been eliminated, chronic epididymitis should be treated with antibiotics. Epididymectomy or orchidectomy should be considered if there is no resolution after 4–6 weeks of conservative treatment.

ORCHITIS

Syphilitic orchitis is now uncommon. There are three types:

- bilateral orchitis, which is a feature of congenital syphilis;
- interstitial fibrosis, which causes painless destruction of the testis;
- gumma of the testis, which presents as a unilateral painless swelling of the testis that grows slowly; it is very difficult to distinguish from a neoplasm without surgical exploration.

Leprous orchitis causes testicular atrophy in over 25% of male lepers.

TUMOURS OF THE TESTES

The lymphatic drainage of the testes is to the para-aortic lymph nodes near the origin of the gonadal vessel. Lymphatics from the medial side of the testis may run with the artery to the vas and drain into a node at the bifurcation of the common iliac artery. The contralateral para-aortic lymph nodes are sometimes involved by tumour spread, but the inguinal lymph nodes are affected only if the scrotal skin is involved.

Most testicular neoplasms are malignant; testicular neoplasm is one of the most common forms of cancer in young men. Maldescent undoubtedly predisposes to malignancy. Even when the testis is located in the scrotum, tumours often escape detection until they have metastasised. Campaigns for regular testicular self-examination help raise awareness of the condition and may lead to earlier diagnosis (Summary box 75.10).

Summary box 75.10

Testis tumours

- A scrotal lump that cannot be felt separately from the testis may be a malignant tumour
- Lymphatic spread is to the retroperitoneal and intrathoracic lymph nodes
- Pulmonary metastases suggest that the tumour is a teratoma

Tumours of the testis are classified according to their predominant cellular type:

- seminoma (40%);
- teratoma (32%);

- combined seminoma and teratoma (14%);
- interstitial tumours (1.5%);
- lymphoma (7%);
- other tumours (5.5%).

Teratomas tend to occur in younger men, with the peak incidence being between 20 and 35 years, whereas the peak incidence of seminoma is between 35 and 45 years. Seminoma is rare before puberty.

Seminoma

A seminoma compresses neighbouring testicular tissue (Fig. 75.12). The enlarged testis is smooth and firm. The cut surface is homogeneous and pinkish cream in colour. Occasionally, fibrous septa form lobules. In rapidly growing tumours there may be areas of necrosis.

A seminoma consists of oval cells with clear cytoplasm and large, rounded nuclei with prominent acidophilic nucleoli. Sheets of cells resembling spermatocytes are separated by a fine fibrous stroma. Active lymphocytic infiltration of the tumour suggests a good host response and a better prognosis.

Seminomas metastasise via the lymphatics (Fig. 75.13) and haematogenous spread is uncommon.

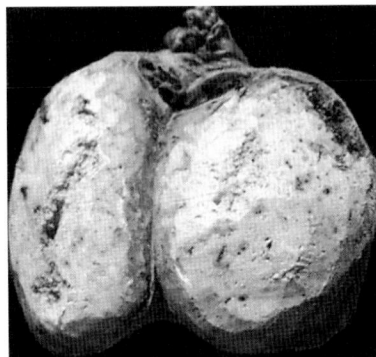

Figure 75.12 Seminoma of the testis.

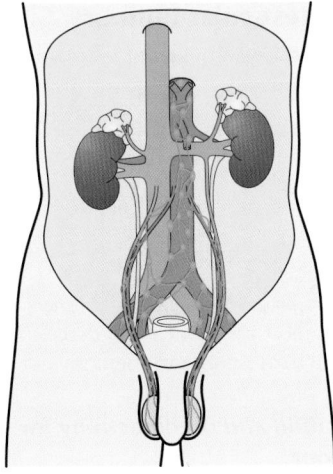

Figure 75.13 Lymphatic drainage of the testes to para-aortic lymph nodes.

Teratoma

A teratoma arises from totipotent cells in the rete testis and often contains a variety of cell types, of which one or more predominate. The tumour may be tiny but can reach the size of a coconut. Even a large tumour is moulded by the tunica albuginea so that the overall outline of the testis is maintained although the surface may be distorted.

The usual type of teratoma is yellowish in colour with cystic spaces containing gelatinous fluid (Fig. 75.14). Nodules of cartilage are often present.

Histology

- *Teratoma differentiated* (TD) (uncommon): has no histologically recognisable malignant components but it can metastasise. The best known is a dermoid cyst, which may contain cartilage and muscle as well as glandular elements.
- *Malignant teratoma intermediate, teratocarcinoma* (MTI; types A and B) (most common): contains definitely malignant and incompletely differentiated components. There is mature tissue in type A but not in type B.
- *Malignant teratoma anaplastic* (MTA), *embryonal carcinoma*: contains anaplastic cells of embryonal origin. Cells presumed to be from the yolk sac are often responsible for elevated alpha-fetoprotein levels. MTA is not always radiosensitive.
- *Malignant teratoma trophoblastic* (MTT) (uncommon): contains within other cell types a syncytial cell mass with malignant villous or papillary cytotrophoblasts (choriocarcinoma). It often produces human chorionic gonadotrophin (HCG). Spread by the bloodstream and lymphatics is early. It is one of the most malignant tumours known.

Interstitial cell tumours

Interstitial cell tumours arise from Leydig or Sertoli cells. A Leydig cell tumour masculinises; a Sertoli cell tumour feminises.

Prepubertal interstitial cell tumours excrete androgens, which

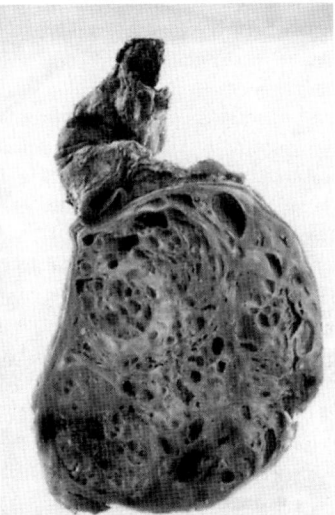

Figure 75.14 Teratoma of the testis – note the solid and cystic areas (courtesy of Dr Keith Simpson, London).

Franz von Leydig, 1821–1908, Professor of Histology successively at Würzburg, Tübingen, and Bonn, Germany.
Enrico Sertoli, 1842–1910, Professor of Experimental Physiology, Milan, Italy.

cause sexual precocity and extreme muscular development. Regression of the symptoms after orchidectomy may be incomplete because of hypertrophy of the contralateral testis.

Postpubertal interstitial cell tumours usually arise from Sertoli cells with output of feminising hormones leading to gynaecomastia, loss of libido and aspermia. As a rule, the tumour is benign and orchidectomy cures.

Clinical features

The patient may not seek advice for several months after first noticing that he has a testicular lump. A sensation of heaviness occurs when the testis is two or three times its normal size, but a minority of patients experience pain. Recent trauma to the affected side calls attention to the testicular enlargement but does not initiate the neoplasm.

The testis is enlarged, smooth, firm and heavy. Later, one or more softer protruberances may be palpable. Testicular sensation is often lost, but the sign should be elicited with care to avoid disseminating the disease. If present, a lax secondary hydrocele does not usually obscure the underlying tumour. The epididymis becomes more difficult to feel when it is flattened or incorporated in the growth. The vas is never thickened and rectal examination is normal. The diagnosis is confirmed by ultrasound scanning of the testis (Fig. 75.15).

Secondary retroperitoneal deposits may be palpable, especially just above the umbilicus on the ipsilateral tumour. There may be hepatic enlargement. Sometimes, an enlarged supraclavicular node is the presenting sign of a testicular tumour (Fig. 75.16). A chest radiograph may show pulmonary metastases especially when the primary tumour is a teratoma (Fig. 75.17).

Occasionally, the predominant symptoms are those of metastatic disease. Intra-abdominal disease may cause abdominal or lumbar pain and the mass may be discovered in the epigastrium. Lung metastases are usually silent but they can cause chest pain, dyspnoea and haemoptysis in the later stages of the disease. The primary tumour may not have been noticed by the patient, and indeed may be so tiny that it can be detected only by ultrasonography or operative exploration.

Atypical cases may simulate epididymo-orchitis; there may even be a urinary infection. All testicular swellings should be

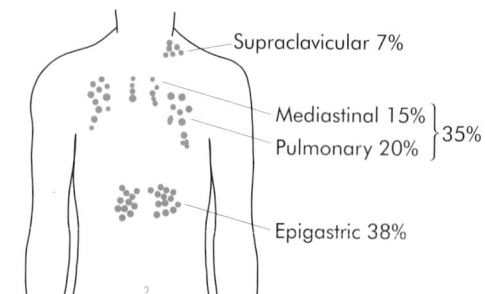

Figure 75.16 Distribution of metastases in teratoma of the testis.

Supraclavicular 7%
Mediastinal 15%
Pulmonary 20% } 35%
Epigastric 38%

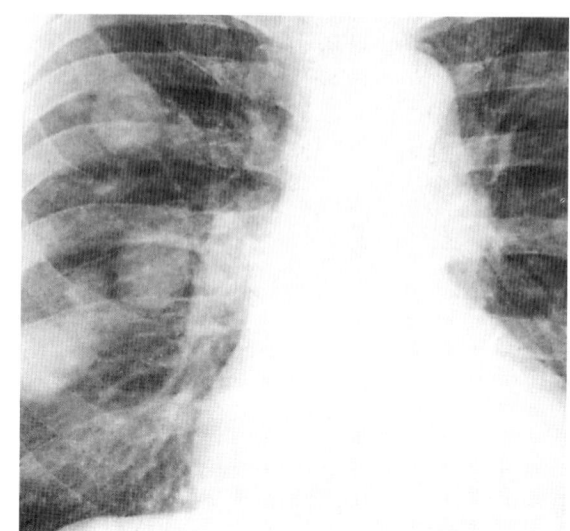

Figure 75.17 Cannonball metastases from carcinoma of the testis.

treated with suspicion, and failure to respond to antibiotics raises the possibility of a cancer. Rarely, patients present with severe pain and acute enlargement of the testis because of haemorrhage into a neoplasm. Between 1% and 5% of cases have gynaecomastia (mainly the teratomas).

The hurricane tumour is a malignancy that kills in a matter of weeks. A few teratomas grow slowly with increasing enlargement of the testis over 2 or 3 years.

Treatment of testicular tumours

Staging is an essential step in planning treatment:

- *Blood* is collected to enable the levels of tumour markers (HCG, alpha-fetoprotein and lactate dehydrogenase) to be measured. Tumour marker levels can be used to monitor the response to treatment.
- A *chest radiograph* shows whether there are pulmonary deposits.
- *Orchidectomy* is essential to remove the primary tumour and to obtain histology.
- *Computerised tomography* (CT) and *magnetic resonance imaging* (MRI) are the most useful means of detecting secondaries and for monitoring the response to therapy.

Scrotal exploration and orchidectomy for suspected testicular tumour

The spermatic cord is displayed by dividing the external oblique aponeurosis through a groin incision. A soft clamp placed across

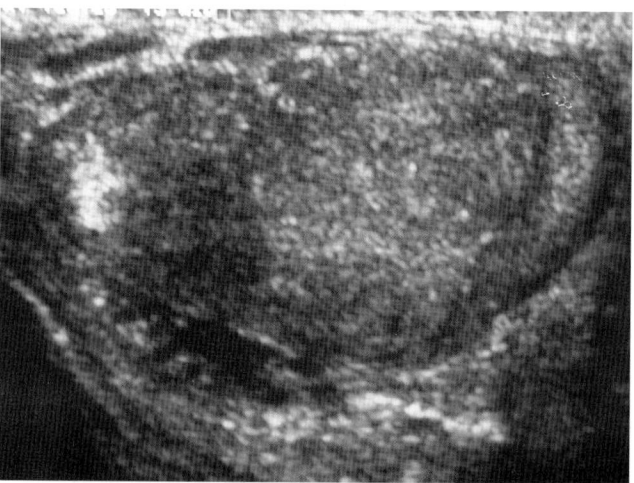

Figure 75.15 Testicular ultrasound: the homogeneous tissue of the testicular teratoma on the left of the image produces multiple ultrasound reflections.

the cord stops dissemination of malignant cells as the testis is mobilised into the wound. If necessary, the testis should be bisected along its anterior convexity to examine its internal structure. If there is a tumour or doubts still remain even after frozen section, the cord should be double ligated and divided at the level of the inguinal ring and the testis removed.

Staging of testicular tumours

The stages are:

- stage 1: testis lesion only – no spread;
- stage 2: nodes below the diaphragm only;
- stage 3: nodes above the diaphragm;
- stage 4: pulmonary or hepatic metastases.

Management by staging and histological diagnosis (after orchidectomy)

Seminomas are radiosensitive and excellent results have been obtained by irradiating stage 1 and stage 2 tumours. More recently, the tumour has been shown to be highly sensitive to cisplatin, which is already being used for patients with metastatic disease. Experts are divided as to whether patients with stage 1 disease should be treated with adjuvant chemotherapy.

Teratomas are less sensitive to radiation. Stage 1 tumours can be managed by monitoring the levels of serum markers and by repeated CT. Teratomas at stages 2–4 are managed by chemotherapy. Cisplatin, methotrexate, bleomycin and vincristine have been used in combination with great success. There are also those who advocate adjuvant chemotherapy for stage 1 teratomas, arguing that effective prophylaxis is less troublesome to the patient than prolonged surveillance.

Retroperitoneal lymph node dissection is sometimes needed when retroperitoneal masses remain after chemotherapy (Fig. 75.18). The tissue removed may contain only necrotic tissue, but some patients have foci of mature teratoma or active malignancy. The operation can be formidable if the tumour is large, and retrograde ejaculation is likely unless steps are taken to preserve the sympathetic outflow to the bladder neck.

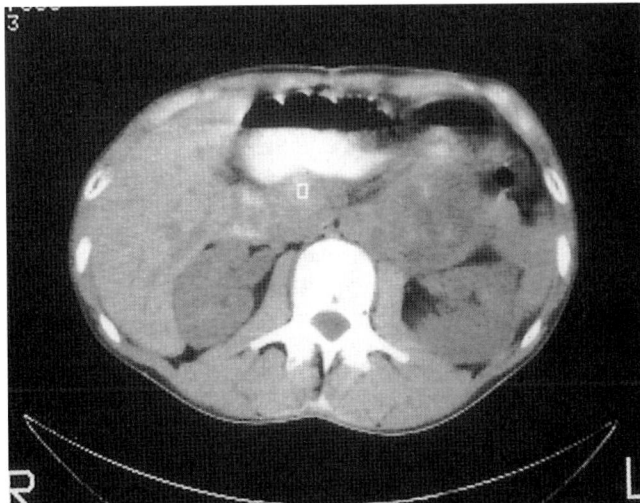

Figure 75.18 Computerised tomography scan showing a large residual retroperitoneal mass after chemotherapy.

Prognosis

Prognosis of testicular tumours depends on the histological type and the stage of the growth.

Seminoma

If there are no metastases, 95% of patients will be alive 5 years after orchidectomy and radiotherapy or chemotherapy. If there are metastases, the survival rate drops to 75%.

Teratoma

A 5-year survival rate of more than 85% is achievable in patients with stage 1 or 2 teratoma. Among patients with stage 3 and 4 disease, the 5-year survival rate is about 60% and getting better with improvements in chemotherapy (Summary box 75.11).

Summary box 75.11

Testis tumour markers and prognosis

- ■ Tumour markers help to make the diagnosis and to follow the effectiveness of treatment
- ■ Prognosis is excellent when the patient is treated with combination chemotherapy in a cancer centre

---

Testicular tumours in children

These are usually anaplastic teratomas. They occur before the age of 3 years and are often rapidly fatal.

TUMOURS OF THE EPIDIDYMIS

These may be benign mesothelioma or malignant sarcoma or secondary carcinoma. They are extremely rare but should not be forgotten when the patient presents with a non-cystic lump in the epididymis.

THE SCROTUM

Idiopathic scrotal oedema

This is described above (see under Torsion of the testis p. 1379).

Idiopathic scrotal gangrene

Idiopathic scrotal gangrene (synonym: Fournier's gangrene) is an uncommon and nasty condition (Fig. 75.19). It is a vascular disaster of infective origin that is characterised by:

- sudden scrotal inflammation;
- rapid onset of gangrene leading to exposure of the scrotal contents;
- the absence of any obvious cause in over half the cases.

The condition can follow minor injuries or procedures in the perineal area, such as a bruise, scratch, urethral dilatation, injection of haemorrhoids or opening of a periurethral abscess.

Haemolytic streptococci (sometimes microaerophilic) are associated with other organisms (*Staphylococcus*, *E. coli*, *Clostridium welchii*) in a fulminating inflammation of the subcutaneous

Jean Alfred Fournier, 1832–1915, Syphilologist, Founder of the Venereal and Dermatological Clinic, Hôpital St Louis, Paris, France.
William Henry Welch, 1850–1934, Professor of Pathology, Johns Hopkins University, Baltimore, MD, USA.

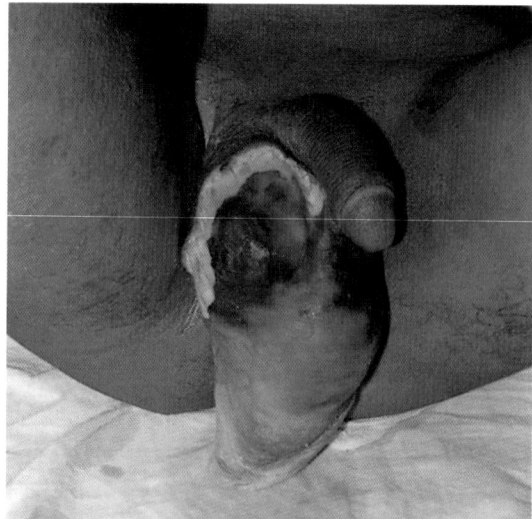

Figure 75.19 Fournier's gangrene.

tissues, which results in an obliterative arteritis of the arterioles to the scrotal skin (cf. gangrene of the abdominal wall).

Clinical features

There is sudden pain in the scrotum, prostration, pallor and pyrexia. Cellulitis spreads until the entire scrotal coverings slough, leaving the testes exposed but healthy.

Treatment

Expert microbiological advice should be obtained. The organisms are usually sensitive to gentamicin and a cephalosporin, which are given until the bacteriological report is available. Wide excision of the necrotic scrotal skin provides the best possible drainage and stops the spread of the gangrene. Many patients die despite active treatment (Summary box 75.12).

Summary box 75.12

Fournier's gangrene

■ Idiopathic scrotal gangrene (Fournier's gangrene) requires early and aggressive treatment if the patient is to survive

---

Filarial elephantiasis of the scrotum

Filarial elephantiasis of the scrotum is caused by obstruction of the pelvic lymphatics by *W. bancrofti* with superadded infection and lymphangitis. In longstanding cases, the enormously swollen scrotum may bury the penis (Fig. 75.20). There is no medical treatment available for this condition. The principle of surgical treatment is the construction of new lymphatic pathways using plastic surgery. In very advanced cases, excision of the affected skin with implantation of the testes into the thighs and a skin graft to the penis may be the only curative treatment.

Non-filarial elephantiasis

Non-filarial elephantiasis can result from fibrosis of the lymphatics caused by lymphogranuloma venereum.

Sebaceous cysts

Sebaceous cysts are common in the scrotal skin. They are usually small and multiple (Fig. 75.21).

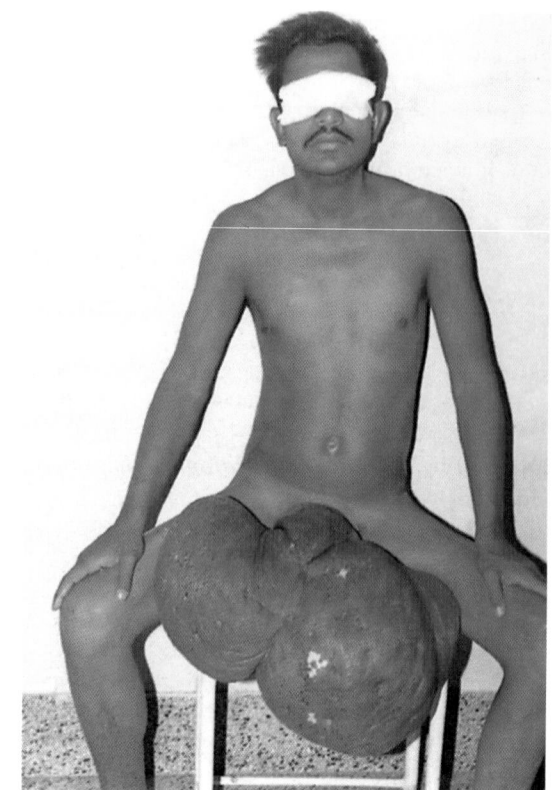

Figure 75.20 Elephantiasis of the scrotum burying the penis (courtesy of Mr S. Bhattacharjee, Lucknow, India).

Carcinoma of the scrotum

Known in the nineteenth century as an occupational hazard for chimney sweeps (described by Pott) and mule spinners, the majority of modern cases of squamous carcinoma of the scrotum arise with no obvious aetiological factor. Unlike carcinoma of the penis, carcinoma of the scrotum is almost unknown in India and Asiatic countries.

Clinical features

The growth starts as a wart or ulcer (Fig. 75.22) and as it grows it may involve the testis.

Treatment

The growth is excised with a margin of healthy skin. If associated enlargement of the inguinal nodes does not subside with antibiotics, a bilateral block dissection should be carried out up to the external nodes.

MALE INFERTILITY

Testicular failure

The semen may contain no sperm (azoospermia), few sperm (oligospermia) or predominantly abnormal sperm. The cause is

---

Percival Pott, 1714–1788, Surgeon, St Bartholomew's Hospital, London, England, described chimney sweeps' cancer of the scrotum in 1775. In those days the chimney sweep's apprentice climbed up inside the chimney.

levels of luteinising hormone and follicle-stimulating hormone will be high. In some patients with azoospermia, the testicular biopsy shows a failure of sperm development. Many treatments have been attempted but the results have been disappointing.

Obstruction

Azoospermia may also be caused by obstruction of the pathway of spermatozoa from the testis to the ejaculatory ducts via the epididymis. Testicular biopsy will show active spermatogenesis. If the site of the obstruction can be identified by vasography it may be possible to perform a bypass operation. Unfortunately, even in the best hands, the results of epididymovasostomy are poor.

In some couples there appears to be an immunological basis for the infertility, with clumping of sperm exposed to serum or cervical mucus.

Intracytoplasmic sperm injection (ICSI) has revolutionised the management of male factor infertility. Spermatozoa harvested from the ejaculate, by aspiration of the epididymis or even from testicular biopsy can be injected *in vitro* into ova obtained from the mother. Embryos are then transferred into the mother's uterus at the four- to six-cell stage (Summary box 75.13).

> **Summary box 75.13**
>
> **Male infertility**
>
> - Atrophy of the testis is associated with raised levels of gonadotrophin in the blood
> - Testicular biopsy will show whether azoospermia is a result of obstruction or failure of sperm maturation
> - If spermatozoa can be harvested they can be used in ICSI with a fertility rate of around 30%

Vasectomy for sterilisation

Vasectomy for sterilisation is a common and effective contraceptive procedure. It should be undertaken only after the couple has been carefully counselled. Both partners need to know that the operation is performed to make the man permanently sterile. They should be warned that normal contraceptive precautions should continue until the success of the operation is confirmed by semen analysis performed 12–16 weeks after surgery. They should also be warned of the possibility of spontaneous recanalisation, which may restore fertility unexpectedly (Summary box 75.14).

> **Summary box 75.14**
>
> **Vasectomy**
>
> - Counselling before vasectomy should include mention of the irreversibility of the procedure, the possibility of spontaneous recanalisation and the risk of chronic scrotal pain postoperatively

Vasectomy is easily and painlessly performed under local anaesthetic. The vasa are delivered through tiny bilateral scrotal incisions or through a single midline scrotal incision. For medico-legal reasons it is wise to remove a segment of each vas to prove that it has been successfully divided. Burying the cut ends or turning them back on themselves probably helps to prevent them rejoining.

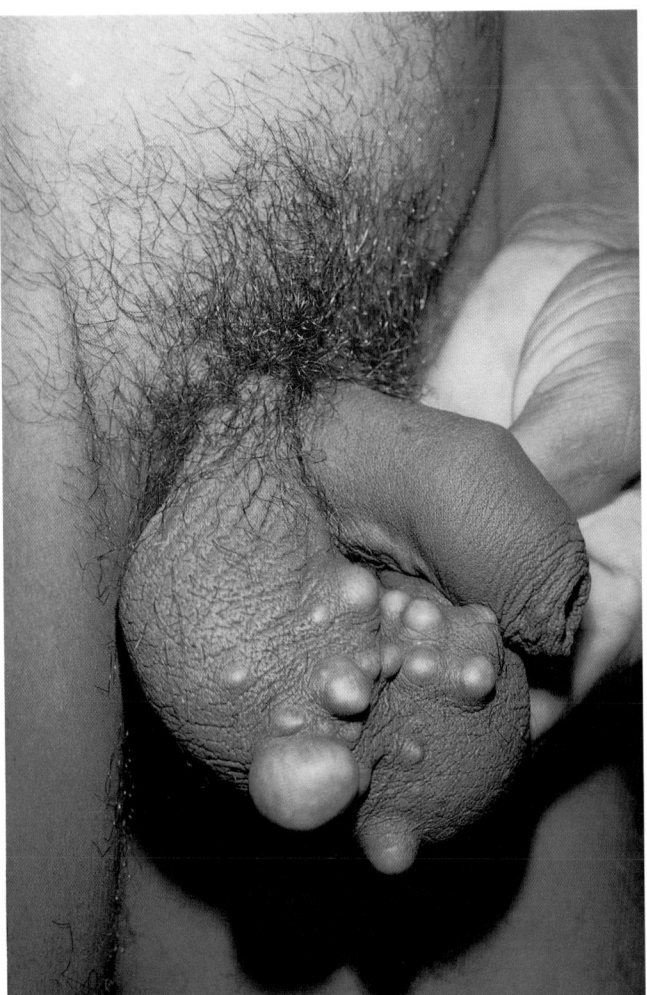

Figure 75.21 Sebaceous cysts of the scrotum (courtesy of Dr R. Kaje MS, Jimper, India).

presumably some form of testicular dysfunction, which may follow mumps infection, exposure to radiation or testicular trauma but is more often of unknown aetiology. The normal feedback mechanism to control the production of gonadotrophic hormones is disturbed if there is testicular atrophy and the serum

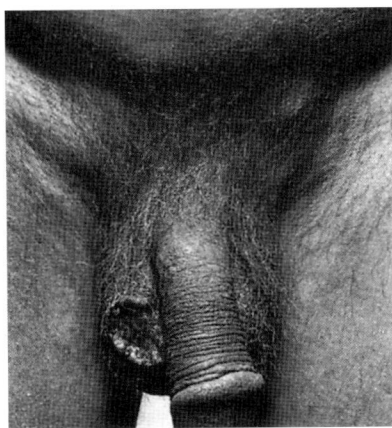

Figure 75.22 Carcinoma of the scrotum with bilateral enlargement of the inguinal lymph nodes (courtesy of Department of Medical Photography, Cardiff Royal Infirmary, Cardiff, UK).

Reversal of vasectomy may not restore fertility even if technically successful because of the presence of autoantibodies developed against the sequestered sperm. A success rate of 60–80% may be possible if the operation is performed within 3–4 years of vasectomy.

FURTHER READING

Blandy, J.P. and Kaisary, A.V. (2007) *Lecture Notes: Urology*, 6th edn. Blackwell, Oxford.

Tanagho, E.A. and McAnish, J.W. (eds) (2000) *Smith's General Urology*, 15th edn. McGraw-Hill/Appleton & Lange, New York.

Wein, A.J., Kavoussi, L.R., Novick, A.C., Partin, A.W. and Peters, C.A. (2007) *Campbell–Walsh Urology*, 9th edn. W.B. Saunders, Philadelphia, PA.

Weiss, G., Weiss, R.M. and O'Reilly, P.H. (eds) (2001) *Comprehensive Urology*. Elsevier Science, Amsterdam.

Gynaecology

76

To understand:
- Pelvic anatomy and reproductive physiology
- The common causes of vaginal bleeding and acute pain in early pregnancy
- The surgical management of acute pelvic inflammatory disease, endometriosis, uterine fibroids and ovarian tumours

ANATOMY

The female external genitalia are described as the vulva, which is bordered by the mons veneris anteriorly and the labio-crural folds posterolaterally. The introitus tends to be open in parous women but otherwise appears closed by the apposing labia majora. The labia minora are folds of skin that fuse anteriorly to form the clitoris, which contains erectile tissue similar to the penis. The fourchette is the posterior part of the introitus, which must stretch considerably to allow the delivery of a baby.

The vagina is an elastic, distensible tube, approximately 10 cm long, passing upwards and backwards from the introitus. The cervix protrudes into the vault of the vagina, dividing it into anterior, posterior and lateral fornices. Pelvic structures can be felt in the posterior and lateral fornices on bimanual examination, as the vaginal vault sits just below the pouch of Douglas (the area at the bottom of the pelvic cavity bordered by the uterus anteriorly and rectum posteriorly). The urethra and bladder neck sit above the anterior wall of the vagina; the perineal body and rectum behind the posterior wall (Fig. 76.1).

The uterus, consisting of a body and a cervix, is a pear-shaped structure that is flattened anteroposteriorly giving its cavity a flat, triangular shape. The uterus is supported partly by ligaments attached to the cervix (transverse cervical, pubocervical and uterosacral) consisting of condensed connective tissue. The cervix is a canal, approximately 2 cm long, connecting the external os, which can be seen on speculum examination, to the internal os, where the cervix enters the uterine cavity. The length of the uterine cavity, including the cervical canal, is approximately 6 cm in nulliparous women and approximately 8 cm in parous women. The walls of the uterus are 1–2 cm thick and composed of muscular tissue (myometrium). The uterine cavity is lined with endometrium, a tissue that undergoes cyclical changes in response to ovarian hormones (see the next section).

At the uterine fundus, on either side, are the cornua by which the uterus is connected to each fallopian tube. These are thin, muscular tubes, approximately 10 cm long, which connect the peritoneal and uterine cavities. They are divided into four parts: intramural, isthmus, ampulla and fimbriated opening, which picks up the oocyte following its release at the time of ovulation. The tubes are very narrow in the isthmic and intramural parts but they widen in the ampullary region. Each tube is contained within the upper part of the broad ligament, a fold of peritoneum on either side of the uterus, which also contains blood vessels and the round and ovarian ligaments. The fimbriated opening and part of the ampulla, however, are free and closely associated with the ovary on either side. The ovaries are flattened, ovoid structures, approximately 3–4 cm long, suspended from the back of the broad ligament on either side of the pelvis. The ovarian blood vessels are contained within the infundibulopelvic ligaments, which are continuations of the broad ligaments to the pelvic brim on either side.

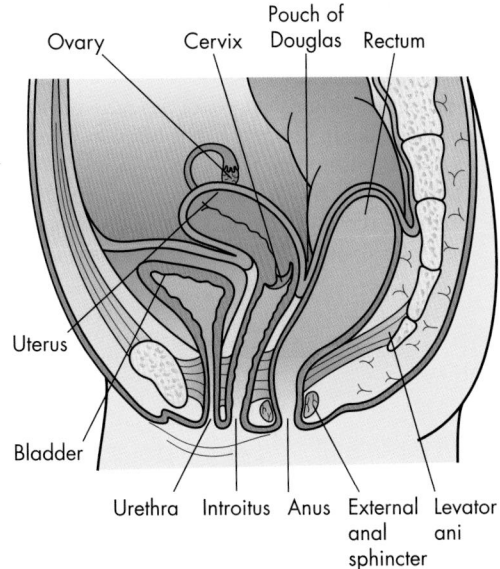

Figure 76.1 Female anatomy.

James Douglas, 1675–1742, Anatomist and Male Midwife, London, England.

Gabriele Falloppio, (Falloppius), 1523–1563, Professor of Anatomy, Surgery and Botany, Padua, Italy.

CHAPTER 76 | GYNAECOLOGY

The cervix is located in the centre of the bony cavity of the pelvis and the uterus can be pivoted around this point. It is usually angled forwards (anteverted) at approximately 90° relative to the vagina. It is usually freely mobile but filling of the bladder or changes in position may rotate it backwards. In some women the uterus is retroverted, either because of weak ligaments or because the uterus becomes adherent as the result of a disease process such as endometriosis. The uterus may also be angled forward (anteflexed) relative to the cervix when anteverted or backwards (retroflexed) when retroverted, in which case it can usually be felt in the pouch of Douglas on vaginal examination. The commonest cause of an enlarged uterus, aside from pregnancy, is the presence of fibroids (benign tumours of the myometrium) growing inside or outside the uterus. When fibroids are present, the overall size of the uterus is described in terms of weeks of pregnancy as it expands forwards and upwards into the abdominal cavity with increasing gestational age (Fig. 76.1).

REPRODUCTIVE PHYSIOLOGY

The menstrual cycle is under the control of circulating hormones produced within the hypothalamic–pituitary–ovarian axis. Thus, gonadotrophin-releasing hormone (GnRH) produced in the hypothalamus stimulates the pituitary to produce follicle-stimulating hormone (FSH) and luteinising hormone (LH), which in turn control how the ovary produces an oocyte on a monthly basis and also the hormones oestrogen and progesterone. These hormones have an effect on many structures in the body but principally on the endometrium, which prepares itself to receive a fertilised egg during the course of the menstrual cycle. In the first half (proliferative or follicular phase) of the cycle, following menstruation, the endometrium starts to regrow or proliferate in response to oestrogen produced by the growing ovarian follicle. The endometrium becomes thick and spongy during this phase of the cycle, associated with considerable angiogenesis.

Ovulation occurs at midcycle, on approximately day 14 (day 1 of the cycle is defined as the first day of menstruation), following which the follicle is transformed into the corpus luteum. In the second half (secretory or luteal phase) of the cycle the endometrium thickens even more in response to the hormone progesterone, produced by the corpus luteum (Fig. 76.2).

If fertilisation occurs the fertilised egg is transported along a fallopian tube into the uterine cavity and then implants in the endometrium. If fertilisation does not occur or if the fertilised egg fails to implant, the endometrium is shed and menstruation occurs. Bleeding (a 'period') tends to last for 4 days but can range from 2–6 days. Typically, about 40 ml of blood is lost during each period; if the bleeding is heavy (i.e. greater than 80 ml), blood clots may form. The whole process then starts again in the next menstrual cycle.

If fertilisation does occur, the duration of the pregnancy (gestational age) is traditionally calculated from the first day of the last menstrual period (LMP); however, ovulation may occur earlier or considerably later than day 14 or the woman's recollection of the date of the LMP may be incorrect, which means that calculating gestational age on the basis of the LMP alone may be inaccurate. This explains the alternative practice of calculating gestational age using ultrasound measurements of fetal size.

VAGINAL BLEEDING IN EARLY PREGNANCY

A miscarriage is defined as the spontaneous loss of an intrauterine pregnancy at less than 24 weeks' gestation. A miscarriage usually starts with painless vaginal bleeding, at which point it is defined as a *threatened miscarriage*. The bleeding may then become heavier with associated uterine cramps, at which point it becomes an *inevitable miscarriage*. Blood clots and products of conception (i.e. fetal and placental tissue) are then passed through the cervical os until the uterus is emptied (defined as a *complete miscarriage*). Sometimes, not all of the products of conception are passed spontaneously (defined as an *incomplete miscarriage*) and the woman may require an evacuation of retained products of conception (ERPC) to remove what is left of the pregnancy. The operation involves passing a plastic suction curette through the cervix into the uterine cavity. The current Royal College of Obstetricians and Gynaecologists (RCOG) recommendations are for ERPC to be considered if there is persistent excessive bleeding, haemodynamic instability, evidence of infected retained tissue or suspected gestational trophoblastic disease. Serious operative complications, which are fortunately rare, include uterine perforation with, possibly, intra-abdominal trauma (e.g. bowel damage), cervical tears and haemorrhage.

In the case of a miscarriage, on vaginal examination there is typically no cervical excitation (pain on moving the cervix) or tenderness in the vaginal fornices, which are signs associated with an ectopic pregnancy. The uterus feels the right size or smaller for the gestational age. The internal cervical os, by definition, is closed if the miscarriage is threatened or complete and open if the miscarriage is inevitable or incomplete. If the fetus has not developed (defined as a *missed abortion*) the uterus will feel small for the gestational age and there may have been no bleeding, in which case the os will be closed. In such circumstances the os will need to be dilated before performing the ERPC.

An ultrasound scan is usually performed to determine whether there is a viable intrauterine pregnancy present. It may not be possible to determine the precise location of the pregnancy because the woman has had a complete miscarriage, the pregnancy is not sufficiently advanced or she has an ectopic

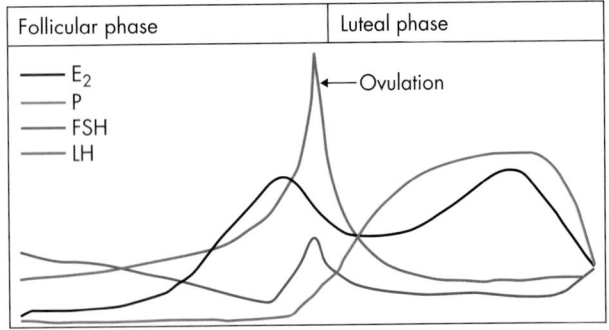

Figure 76.2 Endocrine cycle. E$_2$, oestrogen; FSH, follicle-stimulating hormone; LH, luteinising hormone; P, progesterone.

RCOG, The Royal College of Obstetricians and Gynaecologists, London, England.

pregnancy that is not visible on ultrasound. For these reasons it is important to establish the gestational age as accurately as possible, on the basis of the LMP and the length of the menstrual cycle as well as with any other relevant information, e.g. fertility treatment. It is still not uncommon, especially in early pregnancy, to make the diagnosis of a miscarriage on clinical grounds alone, for example in the case of:

- heavy vaginal bleeding with clots and associated uterine cramps;
- no history of abdominal pain;
- no cervical excitation or tenderness in the vaginal fornices;
- no risk factors for an ectopic pregnancy, e.g. a past history of pelvic inflammatory disease (PID) or previous tubal surgery.

Vaginal bleeding in early pregnancy may also result from a local cause such as a cervical lesion (which may first manifest as bleeding after intercourse) or, rarely, trauma.

VAGINAL BLEEDING IN THE NON-PREGNANT STATE

Bleeding in the non-pregnant state may occur at the time of an expected menstrual period, between periods (intermenstrual bleeding) or after intercourse (post-coital bleeding). It may also occur after surgical instrumentation of the uterus and/or cervix, including insertion of an intrauterine contraceptive device (IUCD). The principal causes of these types of bleeding are shown in Table 76.1.

The mainstay of management is to identify and treat pathology (except in women < 40 years old with heavy, menstrual periods in whom pathology is very rarely found; these women tend to be treated symptomatically). This usually involves ultrasound examination and an endometrial biopsy, either under direct vision at hysteroscopy or blindly with a Pipelle. The indications for endometrial biopsy are shown in Summary box 76.1.

Summary box 76.1

Indications for endometrial biopsy

Endometrial biopsy should be considered in the following women:

- All women > 40 years old with abnormal bleeding
- Younger women with major risk factors for endometrial hyperplasia/cancer:
    Polycystic ovarian syndrome
    Obesity
    Tamoxifen treatment
- Unopposed oestrogen therapy
- Family history of endometrial/colon cancer, especially hereditary non-polyposis colorectal cancer
- Younger women who fail to respond to conventional treatment

---

Women taking tamoxifen – the selective oestrogen receptor modulator used in breast cancer treatment – represent a special group because the drug can induce endometrial polyps, hyperplasia, cancer and, rarely, uterine sarcomas, which are much more aggressive. Tamoxifen treatment results in a doubling of the risk of endometrial cancer after 1–2 years of treatment and a

Table 76.1 Causes of vaginal bleeding in the non-pregnant state

Menstrual	Endometrial polyp/malignancy[a]
	Fibroids
Intermenstrual	Vaginal trauma/malignancy
	Cervical polyp/malignancy
	Endometrial polyp/malignancy
Post-coital	Vaginal malignancy[a]
	Cervical ectropion/polyp/malignancy

[a] These cancers occur principally in post-menopausal women.

quadrupling after 5 years. The relationship is time dependent and dose independent and the risk does not decrease after stopping treatment. There is no clear consensus regarding the need for screening and which method to use; the alternative, more common, approach is to investigate only those women who develop post-menopausal bleeding with tamoxifen use. Aromatase inhibitors such as anastrozole, letrozole and exemestane, which are also used in the treatment of breast cancer but whose effects are not mediated via the oestrogen receptor, are associated with less endometrial pathology than tamoxifen and it has even been suggested that aromatase inhibitors may reverse abnormalities induced by tamoxifen.

Women with hereditary non-polyposis colorectal cancer (HNPCC) and those who are at high risk of developing HNPCC are another special group as the lifetime risk of developing endometrial cancer is as high as 60%. Unlike sporadic cases of endometrial cancer, which are usually diagnosed during the sixth and seventh decades, the mean age at diagnosis in HNPCC patients is the fifth decade. However, it appears that 5-year survival rates in HNPCC patients with endometrial cancer are similar to those in women with sporadic disease. International guidelines suggest that these women should be screened annually from the age of 35 with transvaginal ultrasound, to measure endometrial thickness and look for polyps, and with endometrial biopsy.

Menstrual bleeding may be excessively heavy, irregular or frequent in the absence of pathology; this is known as dysfunctional uterine bleeding. Medical treatments used to reduce the amount of menstrual loss include tranexamic acid, mefenamic acid and the combined oral contraceptive (COC). It may be necessary to stop the bleeding completely using high-dose progestagens, the COC taken continuously or a GnRH agonist, which induces a menopause-like state. Increasingly, an intrauterine system (IUS) similar to a conventional coil, which releases levonorgestrel, is offered to patients as an alternative; it has the added advantage of being a reliable contraceptive.

The surgical treatments for excessive bleeding and their principal operative complications are described in Table 76.2; they are divided into those procedures that retain the uterus and those that do not. The ovaries may or may not be removed at the same time depending upon the woman's age and any co-existing pathology. The aim of all of the ablation methods is to reduce menstrual bleeding by ablating the endometrial layer and some of the underlying myometrium using electrical, thermal or laser energy. Amenorrhoea is not guaranteed but the procedures are less invasive and costly than hysterectomy. Clearly, none of these surgical treatments is suitable for women who wish to conceive.

CHAPTER 76 | GYNAECOLOGY

Table 76.2 Surgical treatments for excessive vaginal bleeding

Treatment	Route	Major operative risks
Removal of uterus: hysterectomy		
Subtotal (cervix retained)	Abdominal; laparoscopic	Damage to ureter, bladder or bowel; may result in fistula; risks of laparoscopy
Total (cervix removed)	Abdominal; vaginal; laparoscopic; laparoscopic-vaginal	
Retention of uterus: endometrial ablation		
Thermal balloon	Device inserted into uterine cavity	Uterine perforation
Cryotherapy	Device inserted into uterine cavity	Uterine perforation
Microwave	Device inserted into uterine cavity	Uterine perforation; thermal damage to pelvic organs (especially bowel)
Transcervical resection of endometrium	Hysteroscopic	Bleeding; fluid overload; uterine perforation; thermal damage to pelvic organs (especially bowel)

Abnormal bleeding can also be caused by invasive carcinoma of the cervix, the incidence of which has been reduced by screening programmes that aim to detect the precancerous state – cervical intraepithelial neoplasia (CIN) – using cervical cytology. In the UK, this is carried out every 3–5 years in women aged between 20 and 65 years. Infection with certain human papillomavirus (HPV) serotypes (16, 18, 31 and 33) is associated with an increased risk of invasive disease. Abnormalities in cervical cytology are followed up by microscopic examination of the cervix (colposcopy). CIN may be treated with local ablation (cryocautery, cold coagulation, electrodiathermy or laser) or excision [large loop excision of the transformation zone (LLETZ)].

ACUTE PELVIC PAIN IN EARLY PREGNANCY

Ectopic pregnancy

An ectopic pregnancy is one that grows outside the uterine cavity, almost always in a fallopian tube (rare sites include the ovary, cervix and broad ligament). As the ectopic grows the placenta infiltrates blood vessels within the fallopian tube, which can cause bleeding within the tube and bleeding into the peritoneal cavity. Further growth of the ectopic pregnancy can rupture the fallopian tube causing substantial intraperitoneal blood loss. It is the commonest cause of maternal death in the first trimester and accounts for 9% of maternal deaths in the UK. The major risk factors for ectopic pregnancy are shown in Summary box 76.2.

> **Summary box 76.2**
>
> ### Risk factors for ectopic pregnancy
>
> - **Previous pelvic inflammatory disease**
> - **Smoking**
> - **Older age**
> - **Previous spontaneous miscarriage**
> - **Previous medical termination**
> - **History of infertility**
> - **Previous use of an intrauterine contraceptive device**

An ectopic pregnancy may be suspected on clinical grounds but making the diagnosis can be difficult because the presentation is so variable and can mimic that of a miscarriage (Summary box 76.3).

> **Summary box 76.3**
>
> ### Differential diagnoses for acute pain in early pregnancy
>
> - **Ectopic pregnancy**
> - **Miscarriage**
> - **Urinary tract infection**
> - **Ovarian accident**
> - **Pain unrelated to pregnancy e.g. acute appendicitis**

There may be a history of lower abdominal pain with a small amount of vaginal bleeding at 4–6 weeks' gestation. On vaginal examination there may be cervical excitation and tenderness in the vaginal fornices; the cervical os is closed. Alternatively, the woman may not have any symptoms or physical findings. The urinary pregnancy test is usually positive. Modern monoclonal antibody-based urine tests can detect the beta subunit of human chorionic gonadotropin (β-hCG) at levels of 25 IU l^{-1}, which are reached 9 days post-conception, i.e. on day 23 of the menstrual cycle assuming ovulation occurred on day 14.

A transvaginal ultrasound scan should be performed if the diagnosis is suspected. The complete absence of an intrauterine gestational sac with a positive pregnancy test increases the probability of an ectopic pregnancy unless the pregnancy is not sufficiently advanced for the sac to be seen on ultrasound in the uterus. An ectopic pregnancy is more likely if fluid is seen in the pelvis or an adnexal mass is seen on ultrasound.

In equivocal cases, measuring serum levels of β-hCG can help to establish the diagnosis. β-hCG levels double every 48 hours if the pregnancy is viable and intrauterine. Levels tend to be static or the rise is less than double over a 48-hour period if the pregnancy is ectopic. A single level above approximately 1500 IU l^{-1} in association with an empty uterus on ultrasound is highly suggestive of an ectopic pregnancy. The best diagnostic test is laparoscopy (Fig. 76.3); occasionally, however, if the pregnancy is not sufficiently advanced, the ectopic pregnancy is too small to be seen in the fallopian tube. There is also a view that a laparoscopy should only be performed once a miscarriage has been excluded because of the surgical and anaesthetic risks associated with the procedure.

Once an ectopic pregnancy has been diagnosed at laparoscopy, a salpingectomy is usually performed. A salpingostomy

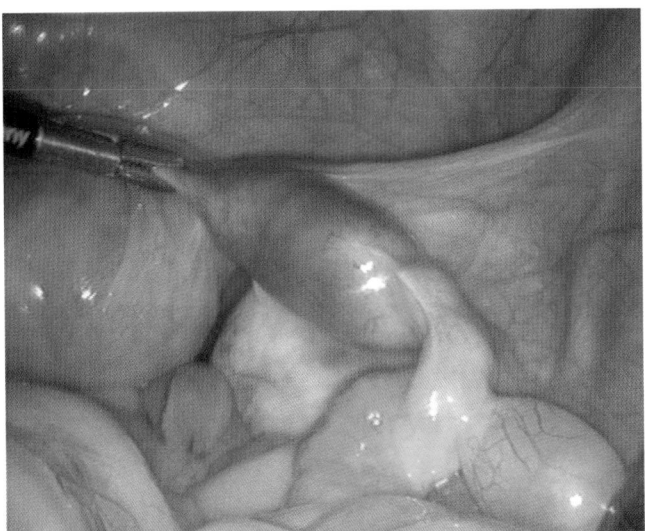

Figure 76.3 Laparoscopy showing an ectopic pregnancy.

may be performed instead as some gynaecologists maintain that subsequent intrauterine pregnancy rates are higher and recurrent ectopic rates lower following conservative surgery. Laparoscopy is the preferred approach because it is associated with shorter operation times, less intraoperative blood loss, shorter hospital stays and similar subsequent intrauterine pregnancy rates.

In practice, the type of operation chosen depends on factors such as the following:

- *The amount of bleeding*: an immediate laparotomy may be required if the woman has lost a great deal of blood.
- *The state of the tube*, i.e. the size of the ectopic pregnancy and whether or not it has ruptured (in general, if the ectopic pregnancy is too large the chances of conservative surgery being successful are small; if it has ruptured there is little point in trying to be conservative).
- *The state of the other tube*: one usually tries to be as conservative as possible if the other tube has been affected by PID (i.e. it is closed or densely adherent to other pelvic organs).
- *Previous ectopic pregnancy or tubal surgery*: one usually performs a salpingectomy if a woman has ad a previous ectopic pregnancy or tubal surgery in the same tube.
- *The woman's fertility intentions*: one usually performs a salpingectomy if a woman does not want more children.

Sometimes, the ectopic pregnancy is located at the very end of the tube, in which case it may be possible simply to 'milk' it out, thereby conserving the tube. The principal disadvantage of this method is that some residual trophoblastic tissue can be left inside the tube. The tissue often survives and continues to grow, which can cause intra-abdominal bleeding. The best method for determining whether all of the tissue has been removed at surgery is to measure serial serum β-hCG levels, which should fall to zero over time if all of the tissue has been removed; β-hCG levels remain constant or rise if there is residual trophoblastic tissue, which may necessitate another laparoscopy to remove the tube.

In the USA, many women avoid surgery altogether by being treated with intramuscular injections of methotrexate, which is toxic to trophoblastic tissue. The drug has some side-effects and the treatment carries the risks associated with residual trophoblastic tissue, namely internal bleeding and the eventual need for a laparoscopy. In the UK, methotrexate seems to be used only in those patients who are at increased surgical risk (e.g. the morbidly obese or those with extensive pelvic adhesions).

After treatment, the patient who still has one or both tubes should be warned that she is at increased risk of another ectopic pregnancy. She should therefore be encouraged to present as early as possible in a subsequent pregnancy to rule out this diagnosis.

INFECTION

The overwhelming majority of cases of acute PID are caused by ascending infection, which is often sexually transmitted. Rarer causes include spread from other pelvic organs, e.g. the appendix. *Chlamydia trachomatis* is the most common organism responsible for PID; the prevalence of *Neisseria gonorrhoeae* varies depending upon the locality. Infection involves the upper genital tract, particularly the endometrium and fallopian tubes. Risk factors include young age at first sexual activity, a high number of sexual partners and current use of an IUCD; infection may also follow a surgical procedure, e.g. termination of pregnancy.

There are no definitive criteria for the diagnosis of acute PID. Most clinicians rely instead upon the presence of one or more of the following features, which are suggestive of the diagnosis:

- lower abdominal pain and tenderness;
- deep dyspareunia (pain on intercourse);
- abnormal vaginal or cervical discharge;
- cervical excitation and adnexal tenderness;
- fever > 38°C.

The differential diagnoses include endometriosis, urinary tract infection, appendicitis and gastrointestinal dysfunction. A raised neutrophil count and an elevated erythrocyte sedimentation rate (ESR) or C-reactive protein (CRP) level support the diagnosis. Ultrasound may be useful if there appear to be hydrosalpinges present and/or tubo-ovarian abscesses. All women with suspected PID should be screened for *N. gonorrhoeae* and *C. trachomatis* by taking endocervical with or without urethral swabs. *Chlamydia trachomatis* is an intracellular organism; therefore, samples obtained for diagnostic purposes should contain cellular material. It is important to wipe off any discharge before inserting the swab inside the cervical os and firmly rotating it against the endocervix.

The RCOG guidelines recommend a low threshold for empirical treatment because the consequences of failing to treat acute PID effectively are so significant. Treatment should commence as soon as samples have been obtained for culture even though the results are unavailable; it should include a broad-spectrum antibiotic against coliforms and anaerobic species, which are responsible for secondary infection. Contact tracing and treatment, if possible, are essential (Summary box 76.4).

Albert Ludwig Siegmund Neisser, **1855–1916, Director of the Dermatological Institute Breslau, Germany, (now Wroclaw, Poland).**

CHAPTER 76 | GYNAECOLOGY

Summary box 76.4

Treatment of pelvic inflammatory disease

- Because of the lack of definitive clinical diagnostic criteria, a low threshold for the empirical treatment of PID is recommended.
- Women with suspected PID should be screened for gonorrhoea and *Chlamydia*. Testing for gonorrhoea should be with an endocervical specimen, tested via culture (direct inoculation on to a culture plate or transport of the swab to the laboratory within 24 hours) or using a nucleic acid amplification test (NAAT). Screening for *Chlamydia* should also be from the endocervix, preferably using a NAAT. Taking an additional sample from the urethra increases the diagnostic yield for gonorrhoea and *Chlamydia*. A first-catch urine sample provides an alternative sample.
- Out-patient antibiotic treatment should be commenced as soon as the diagnosis is suspected. Treatment should be based on one of the following regimens:
  - 400 mg oral ofloxacin twice a day plus 400 mg oral metronidazole twice a day for 14 days; or
  - 250 mg intramuscular ceftriaxone immediately or 2 g intramuscular cefoxitin immediately with 1 g oral probenecid, followed by 100 mg oral doxycycline twice a day plus 400 mg metronidazole twice a day for 14 days
- Admission to hospital is appropriate in the following circumstances:
  - surgical emergency cannot be excluded
  - clinically severe disease
  - tubo-ovarian abscess
  - PID in pregnancy
  - lack of response to oral therapy
  - intolerance to oral therapy
- In more severe cases, in-patient antibiotic treatment should be based on intravenous therapy, which should be continued until 24 hours after clinical improvement and followed by oral therapy. Recommended regimens are:
  - 2 g intravenous cefoxitin three times a day plus 100 mg intravenous doxycycline twice a day (oral doxycycline may be used if tolerated), followed by 100 mg oral doxycycline twice a day plus 400 mg oral metronidazole twice a day for a total of 14 days; or
  - 900 mg intravenous clindamycin three times a day plus intravenous gentamicin: 2 mg kg^{-1} loading dose followed by 1.5 mg kg^{-1} three times a day (a single daily dose of 7 mg kg^{-1} may be substituted), followed by 450 mg oral clindamycin four times a day to complete 14 days or 100 mg oral doxycycline twice a day plus 400 mg oral metronidazole twice a day to complete 14 days or 400 mg intravenous ofloxacin twice a day plus 500 mg intravenous metronidazole three times a day for 14 days

Inadequate or inappropriate treatment is associated with a significant risk of developing infertility, ectopic pregnancy, Fitz-Hugh–Curtis syndrome (an extrapelvic manifestation of PID associated with right upper quadrant pain, which probably results from inflammation of the liver capsule and diaphragm) and

Thomas Fitz-Hugh, Jr, 1894–1963, Physician, Chief of the Hematological Section, The University Hospital, The University of Pennsylvania, Philadelphia, PA, USA.
Arthur H. Curtis, 1881–1955, Professor of Obstetrics and Gynecology, The Northwestern Medical School, Chicago, IL, USA.

chronic pelvic pain in the future. The risk of infertility is obviously of great concern. Approximately 20% of women treated for PID will become infertile because of tubal damage; > 50% of tubal infertility cases are due to *Chlamydia* although, interestingly, many of these women do not report a history of PID (Summary box 76.5). In total, 6% of women will have an ectopic pregnancy in the first pregnancy following an episode of acute PID, a figure that is approximately 10 times greater than the rate in the general population.

Summary box 76.5

Chlamydia and gonorrhoea testing

There is a need to test women (especially those sexually active under the age of 25) who present with:

- Purulent vaginal discharge
- Post-coital/intermenstrual bleeding
- Mucopurulent cervicitis
- Inflamed/friable cervix (which may bleed on contact)
- Urethritis
- Suspected pelvic inflammatory disease
- Reactive arthritis

The majority of suspected cases are treated in the community but hospital admission is advisable if there is doubt about the diagnosis or symptoms/signs are severe. In hospital, antibiotics should be given intravenously until 24 hours after clinical improvement. If there is an intrauterine contraceptive device *in situ*, it should be removed with adequate counselling regarding pregnancy risk and future contraception.

Severe PID manifests as a tubo-ovarian abscess, so named because the fallopian tube and ovary become blended into a single, pus-filled, inflammatory mass, which is usually adherent to the uterus and surrounding bowel. The infection may have progressed from a milder form of PID or, increasingly, it may result from the introduction of infection or bowel damage at transvaginal oocyte aspiration in a patient undergoing *in vitro* fertilisation (IVF). Modern medical practice is to manage tubo-ovarian abscesses (Fig. 76.4) conservatively unless the patient fails to

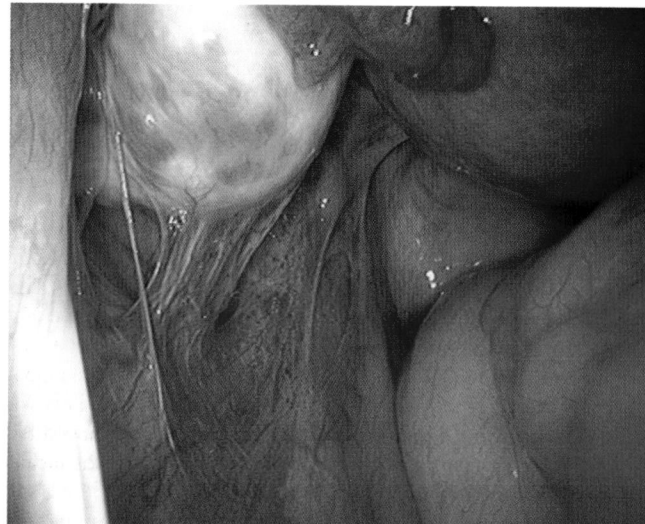

Figure 76.4 Pelvic inflammatory disease.

respond to intravenous antibiotics and systemic support. The response is judged to be inadequate if the woman remains systemically unwell, her symptoms do not improve, fever is not reduced, the white blood cell count does not fall and there is no evidence on ultrasound of the abscess becoming smaller. In such circumstances, surgical treatment is necessary, i.e. adhesiolysis and drainage of the abscess, at laparotomy or laparoscopy. As most women with a tubo-ovarian abscess are in the reproductive years, the intention is always to be as conservative as possible at surgery. Rarely, however, if the abscess has ruptured (Fig. 76.5) and the patient is extremely ill, then hysterectomy and bilateral salpingo-oophorectomy may be necessary.

Abscess drainage under radiological guidance, e.g. a transgluteal approach via the greater sciatic foramen under computerised tomography (CT) guidance, is sometimes performed. Transvaginal ultrasound-guided aspiration has also been advocated. It is clearly less invasive and there are claims that the method is as effective as surgery; however, it carries additional risks such as bowel damage.

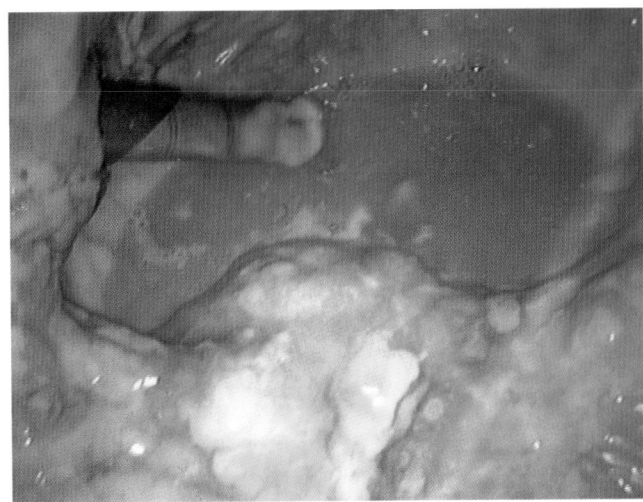

Figure 76.5 Pelvic inflammatory disease with rupture of a pelvic abscess.

UTEROVAGINAL PROLAPSE

Congenital weakness of the pelvic floor ligaments and fascia may be found in conditions such as spina bifida and bladder exstrophy. Far more common, however, are the acquired forms of pelvic floor damage caused by prolonged or difficult labour and multiparity. A gradual increase in denervation of the striated muscle of the pelvic floor with age and oestrogen deficiency at the menopause can also occur in nulliparous women (Fig. 76.6).

A minor degree of prolapse may be asymptomatic but with more significant degrees the patient complains of 'something coming down'. A cystocele (bladder prolapse) and a cystourethrocele lead to the sensation of a lump in the vagina and may also be associated with incontinence and recurrent urinary infections. Uterine descent can lead to backache; with complete prolapse of the uterus (procidentia) there may be vaginal discharge, ulceration of the vaginal skin and bleeding. A rectocele (prolapse of the rectum into the vagina) may cause difficulties with defaecation or a sensation of incomplete defaecation, which is relieved by digital reduction of the prolapse.

Non-surgical management of uterovaginal prolapse is with physiotherapy, hormone replacement therapy and the use of vaginal rings and pessaries. The vinyl ring is inserted between the posterior fornix and the pubic bone. The main complication is vaginal ulceration and infection leading to discharge and bleeding; it is advisable, therefore, to replace the rings frequently. The aims of surgical management are usually to correct the prolapse, treat any associated incontinence and preserve coital function if appropriate. The surgical procedures are intended to restore the uterovaginal anatomy and position. They may be carried out using a vaginal or abdominal approach or increasingly by a laparoscopic or minimal access approach with the use of vaginal slings and tapes (Table 76.3).

Table 76.3 Surgical treatments for uterovaginal prolapse

Condition	Treatment
Urethrocele/cystocele (Fig. 76.6a)	Traditionally, an anterior vaginal wall repair (anterior colporrhaphy) was performed vaginally; now replaced by vaginally inserted tape [transvaginal tape (TVT) or transobturator tape (TOT)] or mesh slings
Uterine prolapse (Fig. 76.6b)	If family complete, a vaginal hysterectomy with an anterior vaginal wall repair if necessary. If the uterus is to be preserved use either amputation of the cervix with suturing of the transverse cervical ligaments vaginally (Manchester repair) or laparoscopic plication of the uterosacral ligaments (McCall suture)
Enterocele (Fig. 76.6c)	Similar technique to repair of a hernia. The vaginal skin is opened and the hernial sac repaired
Vault prolapse (Fig. 76.6d)	Sacrospinous fixation or sacrocolpopexy; the vault is attached to the sacrum using a non-absorbable suture
Rectocele (Fig. 76.6e)	Posterior colporrhaphy: the posterior vaginal wall is opened, the rectum returned to its normal position and redundant vaginal skin is excised. A laparoscopic approach to repairing the defect in the pelvic floor with or without the use of a mesh is now more popular and as there is no resulting scarring in the vaginal skin the incidence of post-surgery dyspareunia is less

The Manchester repair **was introduced at St Mary's Hospital for Women and Children, Manchester, England.**

CHAPTER 76 | GYNAECOLOGY

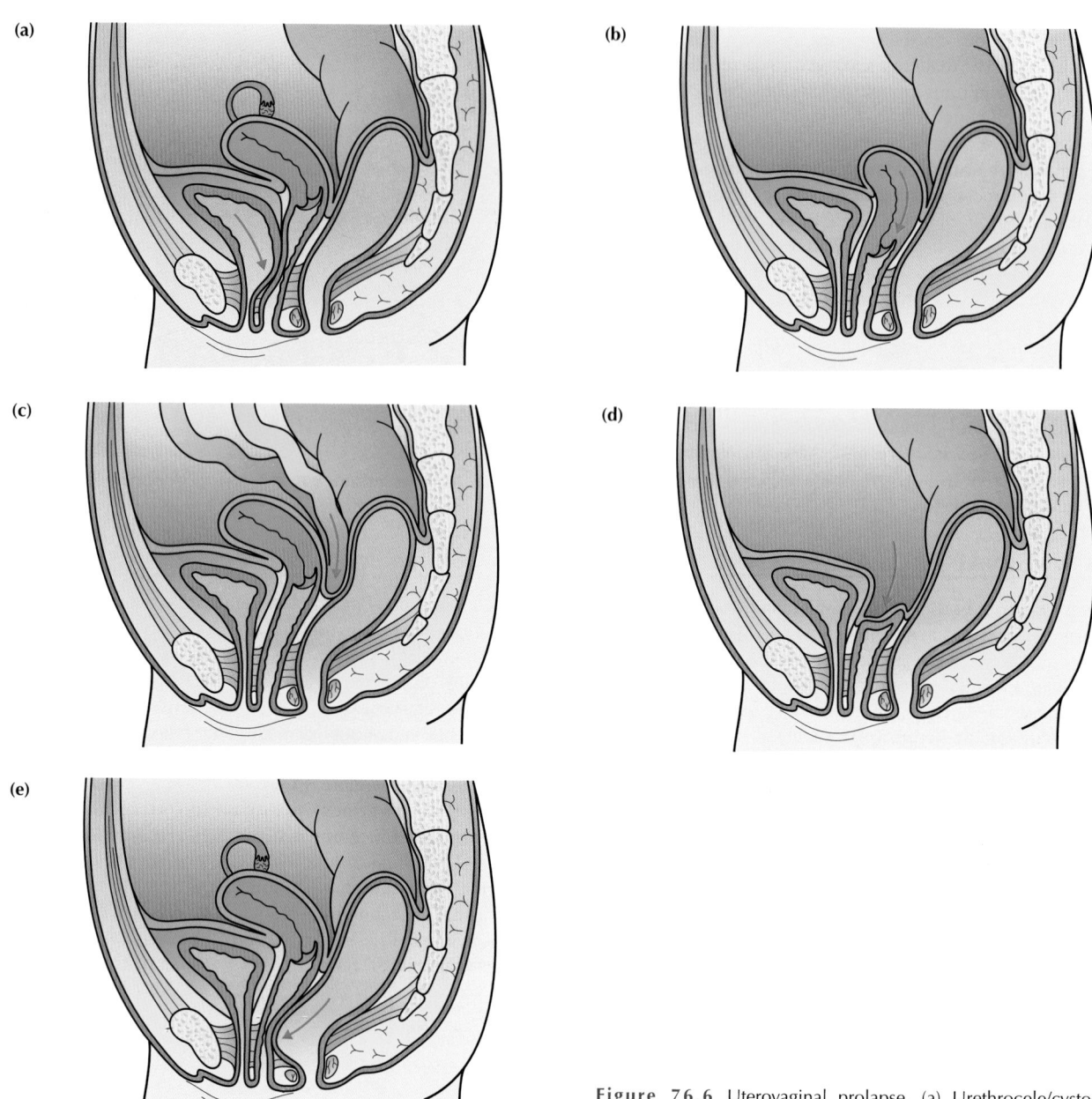

Figure 76.6 Uterovaginal prolapse. (a) Urethrocele/cystocele; (b) uterine prolapse; (c) enterocele; (d) vaginal vault prolapse; (e) rectocele.

TUMOURS

Uterine fibroids (leiomyomas)

Fibroids are benign, well-circumscribed, smooth muscle tumours of the uterus. Most women will have more than one fibroid, varying in diameter from 1–10 cm, which are typically found in the following locations (Fig. 76.7):

- *Subserosal* – may cause pressure symptoms (see below); if pedunculated, they can be difficult to distinguish from an ovarian tumour.
- *Intramural* – may similarly cause pressure symptoms; associated with infertility and heavy periods.
- *Submucosal* – associated with infertility, recurrent pregnancy loss and heavy periods; if pedunculated, may occasionally extrude through the cervical os.
- *Rare sites* include the broad ligament and cervix.

Women with uterine fibroids will present with heavy and/or irregular menstrual bleeding, pressure symptoms or problems conceiving, especially if there is a fibroid in the uterine cavity. The pressure symptoms include pelvic discomfort, urinary incontinence, frequency and retention, constipation and backache. When large fibroids are present, back pressure may cause or exacerbate varicosities. Although these symptoms are common, it is important to note that some women with fibroids are asymptomatic. Rarely, women may present acutely with pain arising from torsion of a pedunculated fibroid or red degeneration, especially in pregnancy.

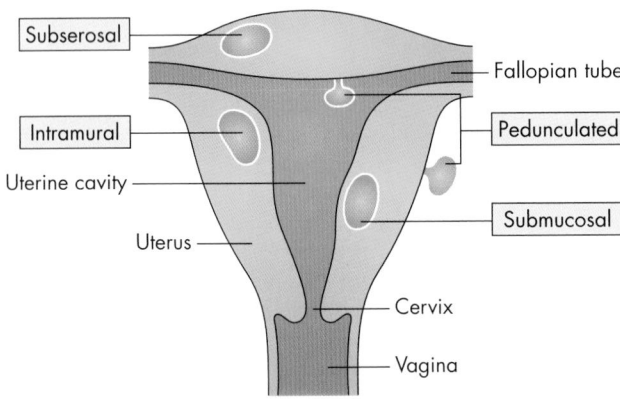

Figure 76.7 Uterine fibroids.

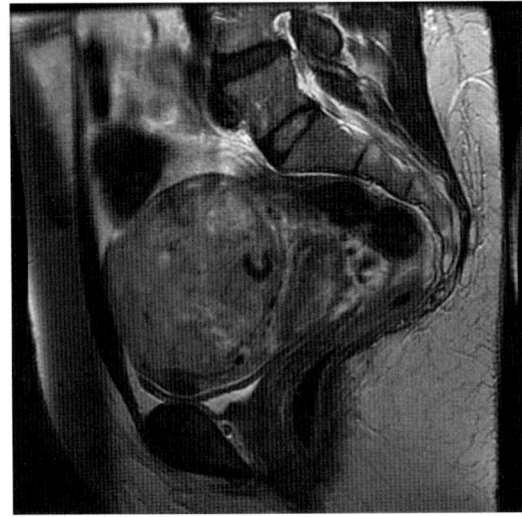

Figure 76.8 Magnetic resonance imaging of uterine fibroids.

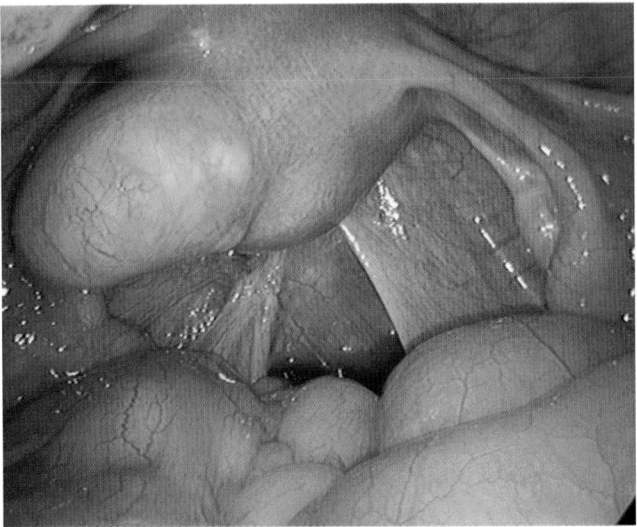

Figure 76.9 Laparoscopic view of a fibroid of the uterine fundus.

The diagnosis is usually apparent on bimanual and/or abdominal examination, on the basis of finding an enlarged uterus with attached swellings. The principal differential diagnosis is an ovarian tumour; as a general rule, the uterus is felt separately on vaginal examination if an ovarian tumour is present although not if the structures are adherent to each other. Ultrasound can usually distinguish fibroids from ovarian tumours; if not, magnetic resonance imaging (MRI) is clinically useful (Fig. 76.8) but, sometimes, it may be necessary to perform a laparoscopy to distinguish between the two pathologies (Fig. 76.9)

Emergency surgical treatment is only required if there is substantial menstrual bleeding or uncontrollable pain; these are rare events. Otherwise, the woman has time to consider her treatment options, which include shrinkage of the fibroids by inducing a hypo-oestrogenic state with a GnRH agonist, uterine artery embolisation (UAE), myomectomy (removal of the individual fibroids) and hysterectomy. The choice depends upon the woman's age and fertility intentions, the size and number of fibroids and their location (it is particularly important to know if there are fibroids in the cavity, especially if the woman is trying to conceive).

A GnRH agonist will usually shrink fibroids but this class of

drug has the disadvantage that treatment cannot be continued indefinitely because of the associated effect on bone mineral density; in addition, the fibroids tend to regrow to their original size when treatment is discontinued. UAE is becoming increasingly popular as an alternative to surgery. It involves blocking the blood supply to the fibroids using an angiographic technique, in which particles are embolised into each uterine artery via an angiographic catheter in a similar manner to the well-established technique for treating massive post-partum haemorrhage. Following embolisation the fibroids usually shrink, bringing symptomatic relief, i.e. decreased menstrual bleeding and fewer pressure symptoms. Complications include arterial injury at the site of catheter insertion, severe pain as a result of uterine ischaemia, infection, and ovarian damage and thromboembolism (a small number of deaths have been reported from uterine infection and pulmonary embolism). There is no consensus regarding the suitability of the technique for women who wish to conceive. Numerous pregnancies have been reported in women who have had UAE but concern still exists regarding the possible adverse effects on myometrial strength and ovarian function, which might affect a woman's chances of conceiving, carrying the pregnancy and delivering normally.

Myomectomy (performed at laparotomy or increasingly at laparoscopy) involves the removal of pedunculated, subserosal and/or intramural fibroids and closure of any defects left in the uterine wall. Surgical complications are unusual; in exceptional circumstances, however, a hysterectomy may be necessary because of uncontrollable blood loss. Fibroids in the uterine cavity should be removed hysteroscopically; the risks of the procedure are similar to those for transcervical resection of the endometrium (TCRE) (see above).

Endometriosis

Endometriosis – defined as the presence of endometrial-like tissue in extrauterine sites – is a complex genetic trait that affects up to 10% of women in the reproductive years. The symptoms associated with the disease include severe dysmenorrhoea, chronic pelvic pain, ovulation pain, deep dyspareunia, cyclical symptoms related to the involvement of other organs (e.g. bowel or bladder) with or without abnormal bleeding, infertility and chronic fatigue. However, the predictive value of any one symptom or set of symptoms remains uncertain as each can have other causes (e.g. irritable bowel syndrome) and a significant proportion of affected women are asymptomatic.

The most commonly affected sites are the pelvic organs and peritoneum, although distant sites such as the lungs are occasionally affected (resulting in symptoms such as recurrent haemoptysis at the time of menstruation). The extent of the disease varies from a few, small lesions on otherwise normal pelvic organs to large, ovarian, endometriotic cysts (endometriomas). There can be extensive fibrosis in structures such as the uterosacral ligaments (Fig. 76.10) and adhesion formation causing marked distortion of pelvic anatomy (Fig. 76.11). Disease severity can be assessed simply by describing the operative findings or, quantitatively, using various classification systems, but there is little correlation between such systems and the type or severity of pain symptoms.

Endometriosis typically appears as superficial 'powder-burn' or 'gunshot' lesions on the ovaries, serosal surfaces and peritoneum – black, dark-brown or bluish puckered lesions, nodules or small cysts containing old haemorrhage surrounded by a variable extent of fibrosis (Fig. 76.12). Atypical or 'subtle' lesions are also common, including red implants (petechial, vesicular, polypoid, haemorrhagic, red flame-like) and serous or clear vesicles. Other appearances include white plaques or scarring and yellow-brown peritoneal discolouration of the peritoneum. Ovarian endometriomas usually contain thick fluid like tar. They are distinguishable from simple haemorrhagic ovarian cysts because, typically, they are densely adherent to the peritoneum of the ovarian fossa. The surrounding fibrosis may involve the bowel. Deeply infiltrating endometriotic nodules represent another disease type. They extend more than 5 mm beneath the peritoneum and may grow into the uterosacral ligaments, vagina, bowel, bladder or ureters; when such lesions grow into the vagina they may be visible on speculum examination as 'blue-domed' cystic lesions in the posterior fornix.

The diagnosis of endometriosis is usually made on visual inspection of the pelvis at laparoscopy; non-invasive diagnostic tools, such as ultrasound scanning, can reliably detect only severe forms of the disease, i.e. endometriomas. The treatment options are limited because the cause is uncertain; treatments include hormonal drugs to suppress ovarian function and surgical ablation of endometriotic lesions with, if necessary, total abdominal hysterectomy and bilateral salpingo-oophorectomy. Women may require multiple admissions for surgery and/or prolonged treatment with costly drugs that have problematic side-effects. Lastly, patients with endometriosis may be at increased risk of ovarian cancer (especially endometrioid and clear-cell types) and non-Hodgkin's lymphoma, which adds to the burden of the disease.

Finding pelvic tenderness, a fixed retroverted uterus, tender

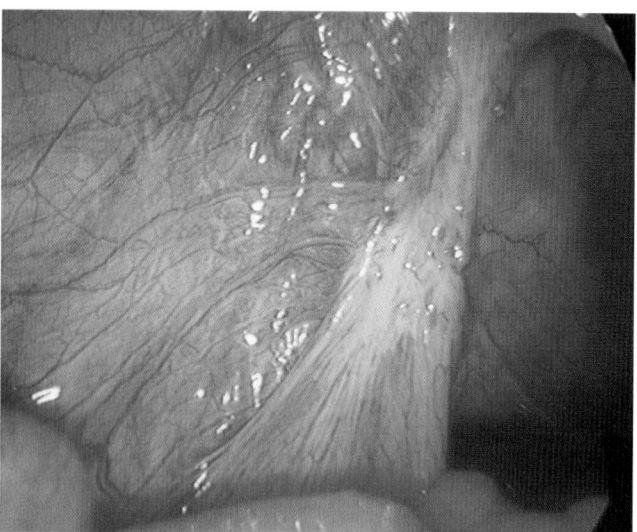

Figure 76.10 Endometriosis seen on the uterosacral ligament.

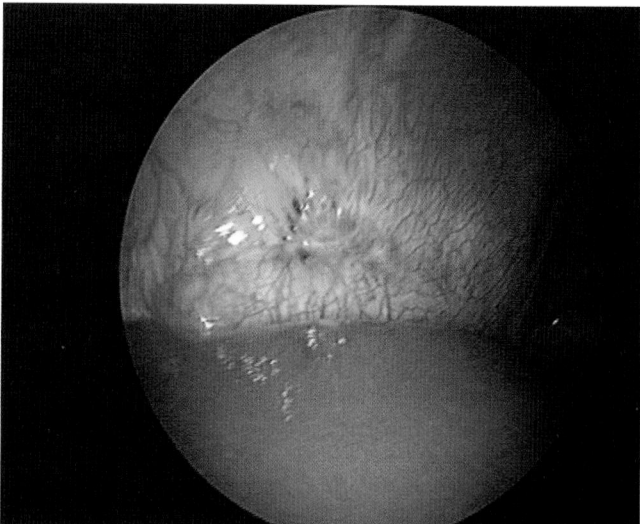

Figure 76.12 Endometriosis seen on the peritoneal surface of the diaphragm.

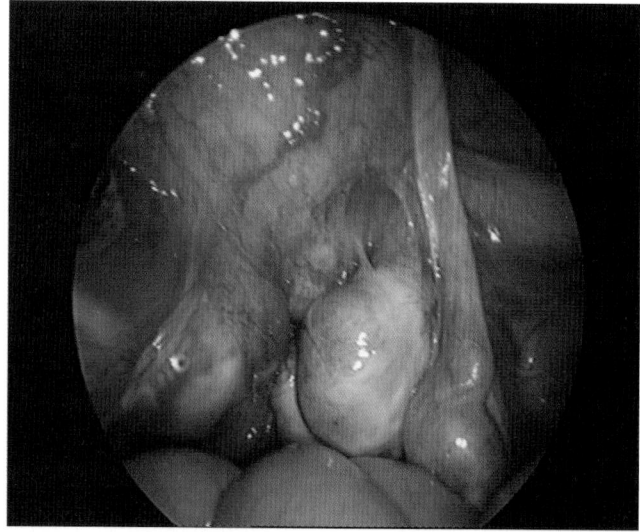

Figure 76.11 Bilateral ovarian endometriosis with pelvic adhesions.

Thomas Hodgkin, 1798–1866, Curator of the Museum, and Demonstrator of Morbid Anatomy, Guy's Hospital, London, England.

uterosacral ligaments or enlarged ovaries on examination is suggestive of endometriosis. The diagnosis is more certain if deeply infiltrating nodules are found on the uterosacral ligaments or in the pouch of Douglas and/or visible lesions are seen in the vagina or on the cervix. The findings may, however, be normal.

For a woman who has completed her family, hysterectomy plus bilateral salpingo-oophorectomy and removal of all the endometriosis present offers a good chance of cure. However, surgical treatment in a woman who wishes to conceive in the future aims to be as conservative as possible, ensuring in particular that ovarian function is preserved. The aim is to remove all of the endometriotic tissue and restore anatomy to normal by lysing adhesions. The standard (preferably laparoscopic) methods used are ovarian cystectomy and tissue excision or ablation with electrodiathermy, thermal coagulation or laser. The surgical risks include those for any laparoscopic procedure, as well as damage to the ureters and bowel; the risks are increased if deeply infiltrating disease is present, particularly if there is bowel wall involvement.

Benign ovarian tumour and cysts

Overall, 90% of ovarian tumours are benign although there is an increased risk of malignancy in older women. Ovarian tumours are subdivided into five main categories according to the World Health Organization's classification system (Table 76.4).

The most common solid tumours in young women are cystic teratomas (known more commonly as dermoid cysts), which typically contain a variety of tissues including hair, teeth and bone. Benign ovarian tumours are often asymptomatic and may present coincidentally, for example when an abdominal radiograph reveals the appearance of a tooth in the abdomen or pelvis. Conversely, they may present with pain, abdominal swelling and pressure effects. The pain may be the result of torsion or bleeding inside the cysts. Management will depend to some extent on the age of the woman and the characteristics of the cyst. In older women a conservative approach is reasonable only if the risks of malignancy are low (see Ovarian cancer). In younger women (< 35 years) the cyst can be followed by serial ultrasound scanning as many will regress – haemorrhagic corpus luteal cysts, for example, will often shrink after 3–4 months treatment with a COC. If there is uncontrollable pain, haemodynamic collapse or a suspicion of torsion, or the cyst does not regress, then laparoscopic ovarian cystectomy with conservation of ovarian tissue is the treatment of choice. As the vast majority of oocytes lie within 5 mm of the surface of the ovary, a carefully carried out cystectomy can leave a normally functioning ovary (Fig. 76.13) (Summary box 76.6).

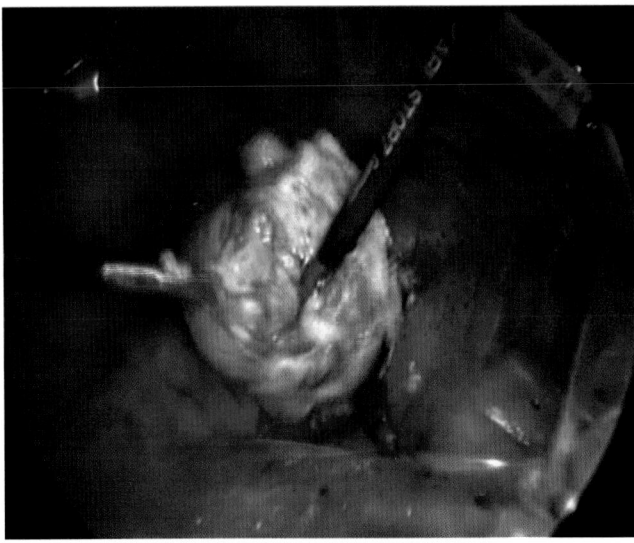

Figure 76.13 Ovarian cystectomy.

Summary box 76.6

Management of benign ovarian cysts

- Masses are usually detected incidentally but may be suggested by symptoms and signs
- A pregnancy test is done to exclude ectopic pregnancy
- Transvaginal ultrasonography can usually confirm the diagnosis. If results are indeterminate, MRI or CT may help. Masses with radiographic characteristics of cancer (e.g. cystic and solid components, surface excrescences, multilocular appearance, irregular shape) require excision
- Tumour markers may help in the diagnosis of specific tumours
- In women of reproductive age, simple, thin-walled cystic adnexal masses of 5–8 cm (usually follicular) without characteristics of cancer do not require further investigation unless they persist for more than three menstrual cycles
- Most ovarian cysts < 8 cm resolve without treatment; serial ultrasonography is carried out to document resolution. Cyst removal (ovarian cystectomy) via laparoscopy or laparotomy may be necessary for cysts ≥ 8 cm, cysts that persist for more than three menstrual cycles and haemorrhagic corpus luteum cysts with peritonitis
- Cystic teratomas require removal via cystectomy if possible. Oophorectomy is carried out for fibromas, cystadenomas, cystic teratomas > 10 cm and cysts that cannot be surgically removed from the ovary

---

Table 76.4 Classification of ovarian tumours

Epithelial tumours	Represent about 75% of all ovarian tumours and 90–95% of ovarian malignancies
Sex cord–stromal tumours	Represent about 5–10% of all ovarian neoplasms
Germ cell tumours	Represent about 15–20% of all ovarian neoplasms
Metastatic tumours	Represent about 5% of ovarian malignancies; usually arise from breast, colon, endometrium, stomach and cervical cancers
Other	A small number of other types of neoplasms, which develop from ovarian soft tissue or non-neoplastic processes

CHAPTER 76 | GYNAECOLOGY

Ovarian cancer

Ovarian cancer is the sixth most common malignancy amongst women worldwide and the leading gynaecological cause of death in the developing world. In the UK, over 6000 women die annually from ovarian cancer. Over 90% of cancers arise from the surface epithelium of the ovary (which has the same embryological origins as the peritoneum); the majority are sporadic rather than inherited. The peak incidence is in the age range of 60–70 years. The overall 5-year survival rate is less than 50% because approximately two-thirds of women present with advanced disease. The usual presenting symptoms are:

- abdominal distension and/or pain;
- weight gain and increased girth (ascites);
- urinary obstruction.

However, over half of all women present initially to a speciality other than gynaecology, with often vague symptoms caused by metastatic disease, e.g. shortness of breath, gastrointestinal disturbance or a change in bowel habit. Consequently, it is important to include ovarian cancer in the differential diagnosis of any woman presenting with recent onset of persistent, non-specific, abdominal symptoms (including those whose abdomen and pelvis appears normal on clinical examination).

Ultrasound is the first-line investigation if an ovarian mass is suspected on clinical grounds. The features suggestive of malignancy on ultrasound include the presence of:

- cyst complexity (number of locules, wall structure, thickness of septae, fluid echogenicity);
- solid papillary projections into the cyst;
- bilateral lesions;
- ascites;
- intra-abdominal metastases.

The level of cancer antigen 125 (CA-125; a glycoprotein expressed on tissue derived from coelomic and müllerian epithelia) in serum is measured; the normal cut-off value is 35 U ml^{-1}. Elevated levels are found in 50% of patients with stage I disease and > 90% of those with advanced disease. However, CA-125 levels are also elevated in other cancers, e.g. pancreas, breast, lung and colon. Levels may even be raised during menstruation; in benign conditions such as endometriosis, PID and liver disease; if ascites or other effusions are present; and after a recent laparotomy. The value of combining the ultrasound and CA-125

measurements is such that a post-menopausal woman with a simple, unilateral, unilocular cyst of < 5 cm in diameter and a normal serum CA-125 level should be managed conservatively (Summary box 76.7).

Summary box 76.7

Basic tests on suspicion of ovarian malignancy

- Ultrasonography: findings that suggest cancer include a solid component, surface excrescences, size > 6 cm, irregular shape and low vascular resistance on transvaginal Doppler flow studies
- A pelvic mass plus ascites usually indicates ovarian cancer but sometimes indicates Meigs' syndrome (a benign fibroma with ascites and right hydrothorax)
- CT or MRI is usually carried out before surgery to determine the extent of the cancer
- Tumour markers, including the ℝ subunit of human chorionic gonadotropin (ℝ-hCG), lactate dehydrogenase, ℝ-fetoprotein, inhibin and CA-125, are also measured
- CA-125 is elevated in 80% of advanced epithelial ovarian cancers but may be mildly elevated in endometriosis, pelvic inflammatory disease, pregnancy, fibroids, peritoneal inflammation and non-ovarian peritoneal cancer

---

Unfortunately, there are still no effective screening methods for ovarian cancer for the general population. Hence, the results of the UK Collaborative Trial of Ovarian Cancer Screening are eagerly awaited. The study aims to randomise 200 000 post-menopausal women to a control arm or one of two screening strategies: primary screening using measurement of serum CA-125 levels followed by transvaginal ultrasound as a second-line test or transvaginal ultrasound alone.

There is also no consensus regarding how women who are at high risk because of a family history should be screened, i.e. those with a first-degree relative affected by cancer within a family that meets one of the following criteria:

- two or more individuals with ovarian cancer, who are first-degree relatives of each other;
- one individual with ovarian cancer at any age and one with breast cancer diagnosed at < 50 years, who are first-degree relatives of each other (or second-degree relatives if the transmission is paternal);

Table 76.5 Staging of ovarian cancer

Stage I	Growth limited to the ovaries
Stage II	Growth involving one or both ovaries with pelvic extension
Stage III	Tumour involving one or both ovaries with histologically confirmed peritoneal implants outside the pelvis and/or positive retroperitoneal or inguinal nodes. Superficial liver metastasis equals stage III. Tumour is limited to the true pelvis but with histologically proven extension to the small bowel or omentum
Stage IV	Growth involving one or both ovaries with distant metastases. If pleural effusion is present there must be positive cytology to classify a case as stage IV. Parenchymal liver metastasis equals stage IV

Johannes Peter Müller, 1801–1858, Professor of Anatomy and Physiology, Berlin, Germany, described the paramesonephric duct in 1825.
Christian Johann Doppler, 1803–1853, Professor of Experimental Physics, Vienna, Austria, enunciated the 'Doppler Principle' in 1842.
Joe Vincent Meigs, 1892–1964, Gynaecolgical Surgeon, Massachusetts General Hospital, Boston, MA, USA.
A first degree relationship is that between parent and child.
A second degree relationship is that between siblings (ie via the parent), and between a grand-parent and a grand-child.

- one relative with ovarian cancer at any age and two with breast cancer diagnosed at < 60 years, who are connected by first-degree relationships (or second-degree relationships if the transmission is paternal);
- known carrier of relevant cancer gene mutations (e.g. *BRCA1* or *BRCA2*);
- untested first-degree relative of a predisposing gene carrier;
- three or more family members with colon cancer or two with colon cancer and one with stomach, ovarian, endometrial, urinary tract or small bowel cancer in two generations. One of these cancers must be diagnosed at < 50 years;
- an individual with both breast and ovarian cancer.

Some genetic mutations are known to predispose women to ovarian cancer: *BRCA1* and *BRCA2* and the mismatch repair genes associated with HNPCC families. *BRCA1* mutations confer a 30% lifetime risk of ovarian cancer up to the age of 60; the figure for *BRCA2* mutations is 27% up to the age of 70. The mismatch repair genes confer an increased lifetime risk of ovarian cancer of 9–12%, in addition to the increased risk of endometrial cancer (see Vaginal bleeding in the non-pregnant state, p. 1393). Referral to a specialist cancer genetics service is advisable. Women at high risk of ovarian cancer may be offered prophylactic oophorectomy, especially as they may also be at increased risk of breast cancer and there is some evidence to suggest that oophorectomy reduces breast cancer risk in these women. Unfortunately, there is no proven role for screening in women at high risk.

Staging (Table 76.5) is performed at laparotomy via a midline incision if disease is suspected preoperatively by:

- careful evaluation of all peritoneal surfaces;
- four washings of the peritoneal cavity: diaphragm, right and left abdomen, pelvis;
- infracolic omentectomy;
- selected lymphadenectomy of the pelvic and para-aortic lymph nodes;
- biopsy and/or resection of any suspicious lesions, masses and any adhesions;
- random blind biopsies of normal peritoneal surfaces, including that from the undersurface of the right hemidiaphragm, bladder reflection, cul-de-sac, right and left paracolic recesses and both pelvic side walls;
- total abdominal hysterectomy and bilateral salpingo-oophorectomy;
- appendicectomy for mucinous tumours; if a routine appendicectomy results in an intraoperative suspicion of a mucinous tumour, the surgeon should take washings and a biopsy from any suspicious area.

Surgery is the mainstay of treatment for ovarian cancer. The staging laparotomy and histological findings provide accurate information about prognosis and postoperative therapy. The general principle is cytoreductive surgery followed by combination chemotherapy; only a minority of patients with ovarian cancer need bowel resected during the primary procedure or surgery for recurrent disease. The only exception to this rule is a young woman with stage I disease or a borderline tumour who requests unilateral oophorectomy to conserve her fertility.

Stage IA or IB/grade 1 epithelial adenocarcinoma requires no postoperative therapy. Stage IA or IB/grade 2 or 3 cancers and stage II cancers require six courses of chemotherapy (typically, paclitaxel and carboplatin). Stage III or IV cancer requires six courses of similar chemotherapy. Intraperitoneal chemotherapy or high-dose chemotherapy with bone marrow transplantation is under study. Radiation therapy is used infrequently. Even if chemotherapy results in a complete clinical response (i.e. normal physical examination, normal serum CA-125 and negative CT scan of the abdomen and pelvis), about 50% of such patients with stage III or IV cancer will have residual tumour. Of patients with persistent elevation of CA-125, 90–95% have residual tumour.

Ovarian stimulation with ooctye or embryo freezing has been reported in patients with low-grade tumours (grade 1A/B) who wish to preserve fertility but the effect of this on the underlying disease is as yet unknown and it must therefore be carried out with caution.

FURTHER READING

Epithelial ovarian cancer. Available online at: http://www.sign.ac.uk/guidelines/fulltext/75/index.html.

FIGO Committee on Gynecologic Oncology (2000) Staging classifications and clinical practice guidelines for gynaecological cancers. Available online at: http://www.figo.org/Staging%20Booklet.pdf.

NLH Women's Health Specialist Library. Available online at: http://www.library.nhs.uk/womenshealth/.

RCOG Green-top guidelines on acute pelvic inflammatory disease, early pregnancy loss, endometriosis, ovarian cysts in postmenopausal women, pregnancy and breast cancer, and tubal pregnancy. Available online at: http://www.rcog.org.uk/index.asp?PageID=1042.

Scottish Intercollegiate Guidelines Network (2003) Epithelial ovarian cancer: a national clinical guideline. No.75. SIGN, Edinburgh. Available online at:http://www.sign.ac.uk/guidelines/fulltext/75/index.html.

PART 13 | Transplantation

Transplantation

HISTORICAL PERSPECTIVE

Since early times the idea of tissue and organ transplantation has captured the imagination of successive generations and, over the centuries, numerous fanciful descriptions of successful transplants have been recorded. One of the most widely cited early examples is that of the Christian Arab Saints Cosmas and Damian who, around 300 AD, were reputed to have successfully replaced the diseased leg of a patient with that from another man who had recently died (Fig. 77.1).

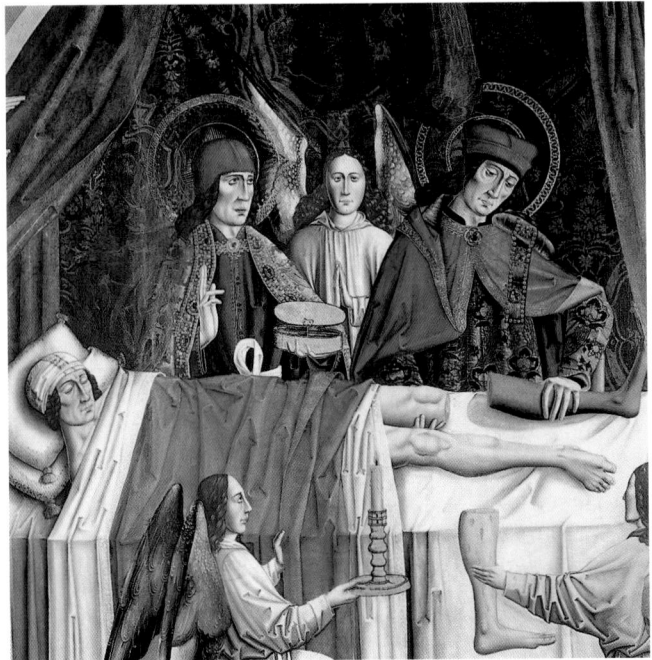

Figure 77.1 Depiction of Saints Cosmas and Damian performing a miraculous transplantation of the leg. Oil painting attributed to the Master of Los Balbases (courtesy of Wellcome Institute Library, London).

The modern era of transplantation began in the 1950s (Table 77.1) and relied on surgical techniques for anastomosing blood vessels that had been developed at the beginning of the twentieth century by Jaboulay and Carrel. The first successful kidney transplant was a living donor transplant performed in 1954 between identical twins by Murray and colleagues at the Brigham Hospital in Boston. This, and other kidney transplants between identical twins, demonstrated the technical feasibility of kidney transplantation, but attempts to perform renal transplantation when the donor and recipient were not genetically identical failed because no effective immunosuppression was available (Fig. 77.2). Then, in 1959, Schwartz and Dameshek discovered that 6-mercaptopurine had immunosuppressive properties, and Calne showed that azathioprine, a derivative of 6-mercaptopurine, prevented the rejection of canine kidney transplants. From the early 1960s, a combination of azathioprine and corticosteroids was used with moderate success to prevent graft rejection after kidney transplantation. These agents were sometimes supplemented with a polyclonal anti-lymphocyte antibody given at the time of transplantation to initiate immunosuppression or used to treat an episode of graft rejection.

The ciclosporin era began in the late 1970s following the discovery of this new agent by Borel and the demonstration by Calne of its potent immunosuppressive properties in clinical studies. The

Mathieu Jaboulay, **1860–1913, Professor of Surgery, Lyons, France.**
Alexis Carrel, **1873–1944, was a Surgeon from Lyons in France who worked at the Rockefeller Institute for Medical Research in New York, NY, USA. He received the Nobel Prize for Physiology or Medicine in 1912 'In recognition of his works on vascular suture and the transplantation of blood vessels and organs'.**
Joseph E. Murray, **Professor Emeritus of Plastic Surgery, The Harvard University Medical School, Boston, MA, USA. He shared the 1990 Nobel Prize for Physiology or Medicine with E. Donnall Thomas for his work on kidney transplantation.**
Robert S. Schwartz, **Professor of Medicine, The Tufts University School of Medicine, Boston, MA, USA.**
William Dameshek, **1900–1969, an American Physician and Haematologist.**
Jean-François Borel, **a Research Scientist working in Switzerland.**
Sir Roy Yorke Calne, **Emeritus Professor of Surgery, The University of Cambridge, Cambridge, England.**

CHAPTER 77 | TRANSPLANTATION

Table 77.1 Milestones in organ transplantation

1954	Murray performed successful kidney transplants between identical twins (Boston, MA, USA)
1962	Calne demonstrated the efficacy of azathioprine in preventing rejection of kidney allografts (Boston, MA, USA)
1963	Starzl performed the first human liver transplant (Denver, CO, USA)
1966	Starzl and colleagues used anti-lymphocyte globulin immunosuppression (Denver, CO, USA)
1966	Lillehei and Kelly performed the first human whole-organ pancreas transplant (along with a kidney transplant) (Minneapolis, MN, USA)
1967	Barnard performed the first human heart transplant (Cape Town, South Africa)
1968	Derom performed the first human lung transplant (Ghent, Belgium)
1969	Collins developed Collins' solution, a new kidney preservation solution
1974	Sutherland and Najarin performed the first human pancreatic islet transplant (Minneapolis, MN, USA)
1978	Calne introduced ciclosporin into clinical practice (Cambridge, UK)
1981	Reitz and Shumway performed the first successful human heart–lung transplant (Stanford, CA, USA)
1981	Cosimi and colleagues reported the first use of a therapeutic monoclonal antibody (OKT3) in transplantation
1987	Belzer and colleagues developed University of Wisconsin (UW) solution, a new liver and pancreas preservation solution (Wisconsin, USA)
1989	Starzl demonstrated the clinical efficacy of FK506 (tacrolimus) (Pittsburgh, PA, USA)
1995	Ratner and colleagues first described laparoscopic living donor nephrectomy (Johns Hopkins University, Baltimore, MD, USA)

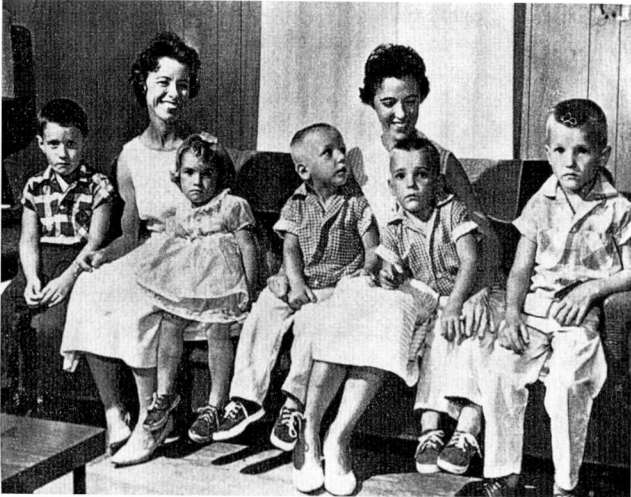

Figure 77.2 One of the early Boston recipients of a kidney transplant from an identical twin, shown here with her twin sister and their children.

introduction of ciclosporin was a major advance and ciclosporin (usually given together with azathioprine and steroids) not only improved the results of renal transplantation but also allowed transplantation of the heart and liver to be undertaken with acceptable results. Organ transplantation is now well established as an effective treatment for selected patients with end-stage organ failure. Kidney, liver, pancreas, heart and lung transplantation are all routine procedures having a good outcome, and transplantation of the small intestine is becoming more widely practised. Transplant activity is limited only by the shortage of cadaveric organs.

Definitions of common terms used in the area of organ transplantation are given in Summary box 77.1.

Summary box 77.1

Definitions

- *Allograft*: an organ or tissue transplanted from one individual to another
- *Xenograft*: a graft performed between different species
- *Orthotopic graft*: a graft placed in its normal anatomical site
- *Heterotopic graft*: a graft placed in a site different from that where the organ is normally located
- *Alloantigen*: transplant antigen
- *Alloantibody*: transplant antibody
- *HLA*: human leucocyte antigen, the main trigger of graft rejection

---

GRAFT REJECTION

Allografts provoke a powerful immune response that results in rapid graft rejection unless immunosuppressive therapy is given. The pioneering studies of Medawar in the 1940s and 1950s firmly established that allograft rejection was due to an immune response and not a non-specific inflammatory response and subsequent studies demonstrated that T lymphocytes play an essential role in mediating rejection.

Allografts trigger a graft rejection response because of allelic differences at polymorphic genes that give rise to histocompatibility antigens (transplant antigens), of which ABO blood group antigens and human leucocyte antigens (HLA) are the most important.

ABO blood group antigens

The ABO blood group antigens are expressed not only by red blood cells but also by most other cell types. For all types of organ allograft it is vitally important to ensure that recipients receive a graft that is ABO blood group compatible otherwise naturally occurring anti-A or anti-B antibodies will likely cause hyperacute graft rejection.

Permissible transplants are:

- group O donor to group O, A, B or AB recipient;
- group A donor to group A or AB recipient;
- group B donor to group B or AB recipient;
- group AB donor to group AB recipient.

There is no need to take account of Rhesus antigen compatibility.

Sir Peter Brian Medawar, 1915–1987, a Zoologist and Immunologist and who was Director of The National Institute for Medical Research, London, England. He shared the 1960 Nobel Prize for Physiology or Medicine with Sir (Frank) Macfarlane Burnett for his research into immunological tolerance.

HLA antigens

Allograft rejection (in blood group-compatible grafts) is directed predominantly against HLA – a group of highly polymorphic cell surface molecules. HLA are strong transplant antigens by virtue of their special physiological role as antigen recognition units, which act to display antigens from foreign pathogens for recognition by T lymphocytes. It was through their role in stimulating graft rejection responses that the existence of these molecules was first demonstrated by Dausset in 1958, hence their description as major histocompatibility antigens (Summary box 77.2).

Summary box 77.2

HLA antigens

- Are the most common cause of graft rejection
- Their physiological function is to act as antigen recognition units
- Are highly polymorphic (amino acid sequence differs widely between individuals)
- HLA-A, -B (class I) and -DR (class II) are the most important in organ transplantation
- Anti-HLA antibodies may cause hyperacute rejection

There are two types of HLA molecule: HLA class I and HLA class II (Table 77.2). They are broadly similar in structure (Fig. 77.3) but have different cell expression profiles. HLA class I antigens are present on all nucleated cells, whereas HLA class II antigens have a more restricted distribution and are expressed most strongly on antigen-presenting cells, such as dendritic cells, macrophages and B lymphocytes. T cells recognise HLA molecules via their T-cell receptors but full T-cell activation also requires an additional or second signal delivered by the interaction of co-stimulatory molecules on the surfaces of the antigen-presenting cell and T cell (Fig. 77.4).

Table 77.2 Human leucocyte antigen (HLA) class I and class II molecules

	Class I	Class II
HLA loci	HLA-A, -B and -C	HLA-DR, -DP and -DQ
Structure	Heavy chain and β_2-microglobulin	α- and β-chain
Distribution	All nucleated cells	B cells, dendritic cells, macrophages

Effector mechanisms of rejection

HLA antigens expressed by graft cells activate T cells and stimulate them to proliferate in response to interleukin-2 (IL-2) and other T-cell growth factors. Activated CD4 T cells, through the release of cytokines, play a central role in orchestrating the various effector mechanisms that are responsible for graft rejection (Fig. 77.5). The cellular effectors of graft rejection include cytotoxic CD8 T cells, which recognise donor HLA class I antigens expressed by the graft and cause target cell death by releasing lytic molecules such as perforin and granzyme. Graft-infiltrating CD4 T cells, which recognise donor HLA class II antigens, mediate direct target cell damage and are also able, by releasing cytokines such as interferon-γ, to recruit and activate macrophages that act as non-specific effector cells. Finally, CD4 T cells provide essential T-cell help for B lymphocytes that differentiate into plasma cells and produce alloantibodies which bind to graft antigen and induce target cell injury directly or through antibody-dependent, cell-mediated cytotoxicity.

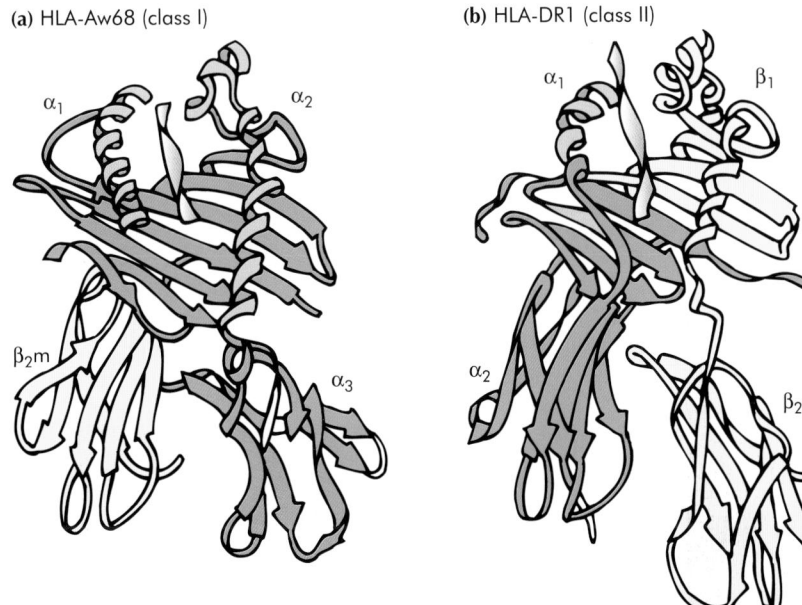

(a) HLA-Aw68 (class I)   **(b)** HLA-DR1 (class II)

Figure 77.3 The three-dimensional structure of the extracellular domains of human leucocyte antigen (HLA) class I and class II. The α_1 and α_2 domains of class I and the α_1 and β_1 domains of class II form a cleft that is floored by a β-pleated sheet and walled by two α-helices. The cleft binds an antigenic peptide and displays it on the cell surface for recognition by a T lymphocyte. (Redrawn with permission from Stern, L.J. and Wiley, D.C. (1994) Antigenic peptide binding by class I and class II histocompatibility proteins. *Structure* **2**: 245–51. Copyright Elsevier.)

Jean Dausset, B. 1916, a French Immunologist who was Professor of Experimental Medicine at The College of France, Paris, France. He shared the 1980 Nobel Prize for Physiology or Medicine with George Snell and Baruj Benacerraf for his discovery of the HLA antigens.

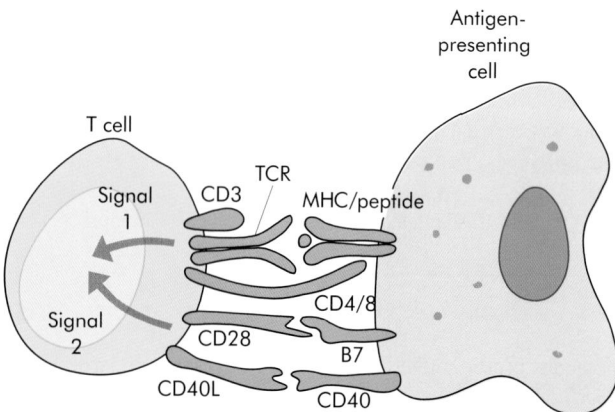

Figure 77.4 Molecular events involved in T-cell activation by an antigen-presenting cell. T-cell activation requires the delivery of two distinct signals to the T cell. The first signal is delivered by ligation of the T-cell receptor (TCR/CD3) complex with the major histocompatibility complex (MHC/peptide) complex. The second signal is delivered following the interaction between pairs of co-stimulatory molecules such as CD28/B7 and CD40L/CD40.

Types of allograft rejection

Allograft rejection can be divided into three types:

- hyperacute (occurs immediately);
- acute (usually occurs in the first 6 months);
- chronic (occurs months and years after transplantation).

Allograft rejection manifests as functional failure of the transplant and is confirmed histologically. Biopsy material is obtained from renal and pancreatic grafts by needle biopsy and from hepatic grafts by percutaneous or transjugular liver biopsy. Cardiac grafts are biopsied by transjugular endomyocardial biopsy and lung grafts by transbronchial biopsy. After small intestinal transplantation, mucosal biopsies are obtained from the graft stoma or more proximally by endoscopy. A standardised histological grading system, the Banff classification (named after the Canadian town where the initial scientific workshop was held), defines the

presence and severity of allograft rejection after solid organ transplantation (Summary box 77.3).

Summary box 77.3

Types of graft rejection

Hyperacute
- Immediate graft destruction due to ABO or pre-formed anti-HLA antibodies.
- Characterised by intravascular thrombosis

Acute
- Occurs during the first 6 months
- T-cell dependent, characterised by mononuclear cell infiltration
- Usually reversible

Chronic
- Occurs after the first 6 months
- Most common cause of graft failure
- Non-immune factors may contribute to pathogenesis
- Characterised by myo-intimal proliferation in graft arteries leading to ischaemia and fibrosis

---

Hyperacute rejection

This is due to the presence in the recipient of pre-formed antibodies against HLA class I antigens expressed by the donor. These arise from a previous blood transfusion, a failed transplant or pregnancy. This type of rejection also occurs if an ABO blood group-incompatible organ graft is performed. After revascularisation of the graft, antibodies bind immediately to the vasculature, activate the complement system and cause extensive intravascular thrombosis and graft destruction within minutes and hours. Kidney transplants are particularly vulnerable to hyperacute graft rejection, whereas heart and liver transplants are relatively resistant. Hyperacute rejection can be avoided by ensuring ABO blood group compatibility and by performing a cross-match test on recipient serum to ensure that there are no antibodies directed against HLA antigens expressed by a prospective kidney donor. If recipient serum contains antibodies to donor HLA class I antigens,

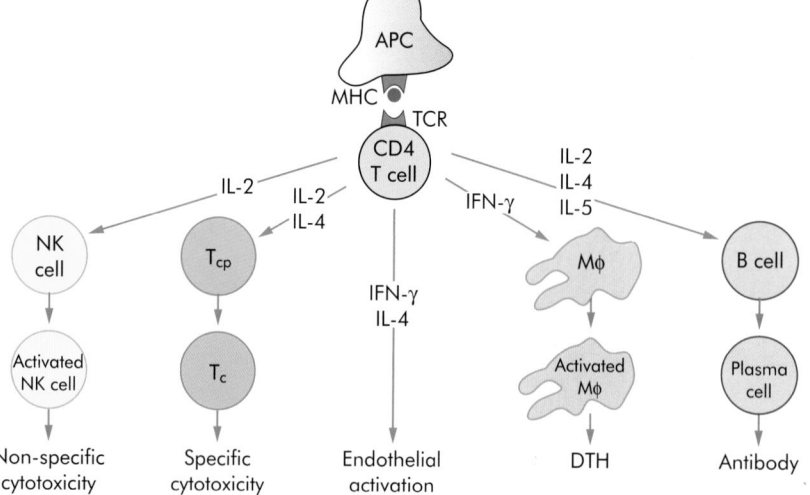

Figure 77.5 The central role of the CD4 T cell in orchestrating the various effector mechanisms responsible for allograft rejection. APC, antigen-presenting cell; DTH, delayed-type hypersensitivity; IFN-γ, interferon-gamma; IL, interleukin; MΦ, macrophage; MHC, major histocompatability complex; NK, natural killer; T_c, T cytotoxic cell; T_{cp}, T cytotoxic precursor cell; TCR, T-cell receptor.

Banff **is in Alberta, Canada.**

the cross-match test is positive and transplantation should not proceed. Antibodies directed against HLA class II antigens do not usually cause hyperacute rejection but are associated with an increased likelihood of acute rejection and a poor clinical outcome. Patients waiting for a kidney transplant should be screened for the development of HLA antibodies on a regular basis and especially after potential priming to HLA antigens by blood transfusion.

Patients awaiting heart transplantation are also screened for the presence of HLA antibodies and those with pre-formed antibodies are subjected to a prospective cross-match test. Although heart allografts rarely undergo hyperacute rejection, cardiac transplantation in the presence of a positive cross-match is associated with a high incidence of graft loss from accelerated acute rejection.

Even in the presence of a strongly positive cross-match test, liver transplants rarely undergo hyperacute rejection, although their long-term survival is inferior. It is not clear why the liver is resistant to hyperacute rejection. One factor may be that it is less susceptible to ischaemia than the kidney by virtue of its dual blood supply: 60% of the hepatic blood supply is derived from the portal vein and 40% from the hepatic artery.

Acute rejection

This usually occurs during the first 6 months of transplantation but may occur later. It is mediated predominantly by T lymphocytes but alloantibodies may also play an important role. Acute rejection is characterised by mononuclear cell infiltration of the graft (Fig. 77.6). The mononuclear cell infiltrate is heterogeneous and includes cytotoxic T cells, B cells, natural killer (NK) cells and activated macrophages. Antibody-mediated damage may also be present as evidenced by the deposition of the complement component C4d within the graft microvasculature. All types of organ allograft are susceptible to acute rejection and, although relatively common (occurring in around 20–30% of grafts), most episodes of acute rejection can be reversed by additional immunosuppressive therapy.

Chronic rejection

This usually occurs after the first 6 months. All types of transplant are susceptible and it is the major cause of allograft failure. Interestingly, however, the liver appears to be more resistant than other solid organs to the destructive effects of chronic rejection.

The pathophysiology of chronic rejection is not completely understood. The underlying mechanisms are immunological, and both alloantibodies and cellular effector mechanisms appear to be involved. However, alloantigen-independent factors also play an important role in the pathogenesis. A number of risk factors have been identified for chronic rejection of a kidney transplant. These are:

- previous episodes of acute rejection;
- poor HLA match;
- long cold ischaemia time;
- cytomegalovirus (CMV) infection;
- raised blood lipids;
- inadequate immunosuppression (including poor compliance).

The two most important risk factors for chronic rejection after kidney transplantation are acute rejection with vascular inflammation and recurrent episodes of acute rejection. Because non-immune factors often contribute significantly to the long-term failure of a kidney transplant, the term 'chronic allograft nephropathy' is usually used in preference to 'chronic rejection'.

The histological picture of chronic rejection after organ transplantation is dominated by vascular changes, with the development of myo-intimal proliferation in arteries, which results in ischaemia and fibrosis (Fig. 77.7). In addition to vasculopathy there are organ-specific features of chronic graft rejection. These are:

- *kidney*: glomerular sclerosis and tubular atrophy;
- *pancreas*: acinar loss and islet destruction;
- *heart*: accelerated coronary artery disease (cardiac allograft vasculopathy);
- *liver*: vanishing bile duct syndrome;
- *lungs*: obliterative bronchiolitis.

Chronic rejection causes functional deterioration in the graft, resulting after months or years in graft failure. Unfortunately, currently available immunosuppressive therapy has little effect in preventing chronic rejection.

Graft-versus-host disease

Although the main immunological problem after transplantation is graft rejection, the reciprocal problem of graft-versus-host

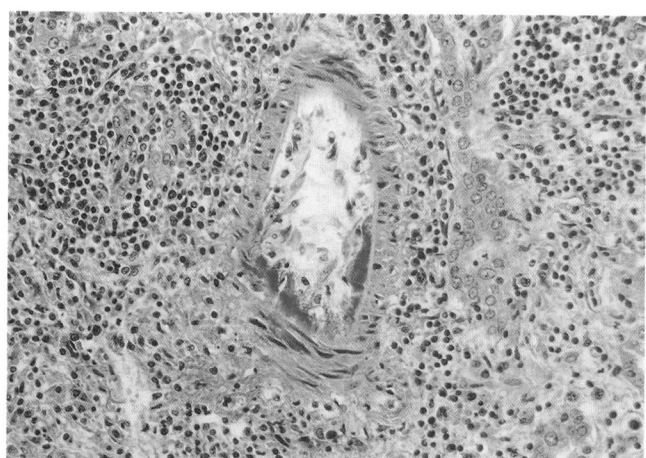

Figure 77.6 Severe acute renal allograft rejection with a heavy mononuclear cell infiltrate and intimal arteritis.

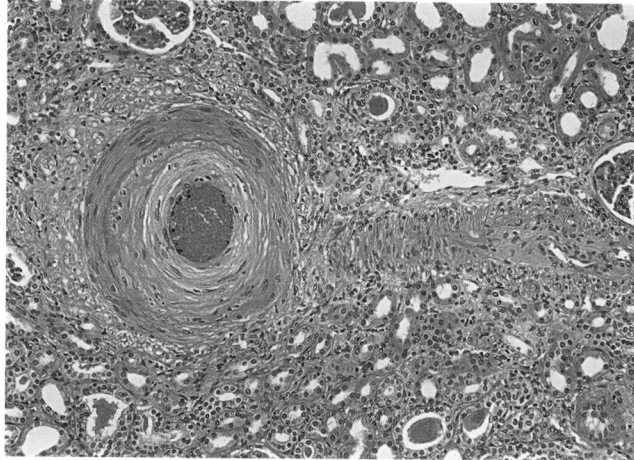

Figure 77.7 Chronic renal allograft rejection. The arteriole shows severe myo-intimal proliferation and luminal narrowing, resulting in ischaemic fibrosis.

reaction is occasionally seen following certain types of organ transplantation. The donor liver and small bowel both contain large numbers of immunocompetent lymphocytes and these may react against HLA antigens expressed by recipient tissues leading to graft-versus-host disease (GVHD). When GVHD develops it frequently involves the skin, causing a characteristic rash on the palms and soles. It may also involve the liver (after small bowel transplantation) and the gastrointestinal tract (after liver transplantation). GVHD is a serious and sometimes fatal complication.

HLA MATCHING

HLA molecules are encoded by the major histocompatibility complex (MHC), a cluster of genes situated on the short arm of chromosome 6 (Fig. 77.8). The HLA class I antigens comprise HLA-A, -B and -C, and the HLA class II antigens comprise HLA-DR, -DP and -DQ. The expression of MHC genes is co-dominant, i.e. the genes on both the maternally derived and the paternally derived chromosomes are expressed. Consequently, an individual may express between 6 and 12 different HLA antigens, depending on the degree of homozygosity (shared genes) at individual loci.

The HLA haplotype inherited from each parent is usually inherited as a complete haplotype according to simple mendelian genetics (Fig. 77.9). The HLA or 'tissue type' of an individual is determined by DNA typing techniques.

In deceased donor renal transplantation (but not other types of solid organ transplantation) attempts are usually made to match the donor and recipient for as many of the relevant HLA antigens as possible. In addition to reducing the risk of graft loss from rejection, a well-matched kidney allograft that subsequently fails is less likely to cause sensitisation to the HLA antigens that it expresses. It is particularly important in children and young adults to avoid, whenever possible, grafts that are mismatched for common HLA antigens because if re-transplantation is required subsequently it may be difficult to find an organ donor

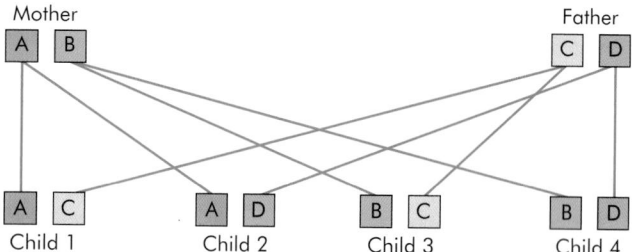

Figure 77.9 Human leucocyte antigen (HLA) inheritance. Children acquire one HLA haplotype (depicted as A–D) from each parent. As shown, child 1 shares one HLA haplotype (haploidentical) with child 2 and child 3, but does not share either haplotype with child 4. The chances that two siblings will share the same parental haplotypes, or that they will share neither HLA haplotype, is one in four. The chance that they will share one HLA haplotype is one in two.

who does not express the antigens to which the recipient has become sensitised. In terms of organ transplantation, HLA-A, -B and -DR are the most important antigens to take into account when matching donor and recipient in an attempt to reduce the risk of graft rejection (Fig. 77.10).

HLA matching has a relatively small but definite beneficial effect on renal allograft survival (HLA-DR > HLA-B > HLA-A). Recipients who receive well-matched renal allografts may require less intensive immunosuppression and also are troubled less by rejection episodes. It is common practice to express the degree of HLA matching between the donor and recipient in terms of whether or not there are mismatches at each locus for HLA-A, -B and -DR. A '000 mismatch' is a 'full house' or complete match, whereas a '012 mismatch' is matched at the HLA-A loci, has one mismatched HLA-B antigen and is mismatched for both HLA-DR antigens. Cadaveric kidneys are allocated in some countries, including the UK, by a points system that optimises HLA matching but also takes into account other factors, such as time on the waiting list, sensitisation to HLA antigens and the age relationship between the donor and recipient. Allocation of organs for transplantation must also take into account the relative size of donor and recipient. This is not an issue in renal transplantation in which adult kidneys can be readily used for paediatric recipients (and vice versa). However, in the case of heart, lung, liver and small bowel transplantation, it is important to consider size compatibility. In the case of liver transplants, HLA matching does not confer an advantage and, although it is beneficial in cardiac transplantation, it is not practicable because of the relatively small size of the recipient pool and the short permissible cold ischaemic time.

IMMUNOSUPPRESSIVE THERAPY

When considering immunosuppressive therapy for organ transplantation the surgeon is faced with an increasing range of agents from which to choose (Table 77.3). The agents used to prevent rejection act predominantly on T cells and the different classes of agent act at different sites during T-cell activation (Fig. 77.11). Most immunosuppressive protocols use a combination of agents. Individual agents can be classified according to their principal mode of action in preventing the T cell-dependent rejection response.

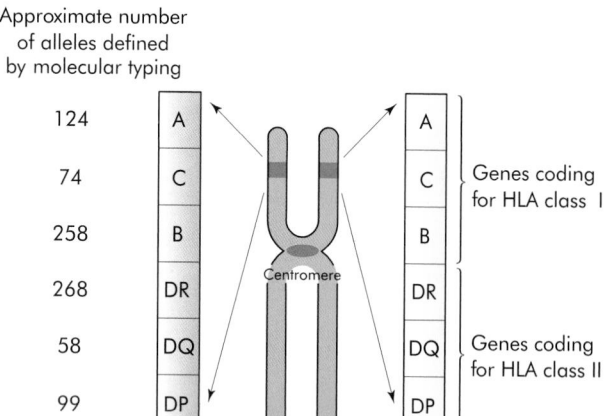

Approximate number of alleles defined by molecular typing

124	A
74	C
258	B
268	DR
58	DQ
99	DP

Genes coding for HLA class I

Genes coding for HLA class II

Centromere

Figure 77.8 The human leucocyte antigen (HLA) system on the short arm of chromosome 6.

Gregor Johann Mendel, **1822–1884, an Austrian monk and naturalist who became Abbot of the Augustinian Monastery at Brunn, The Czech Republic, and discovered the laws of inheritance by studying the edible pea.**

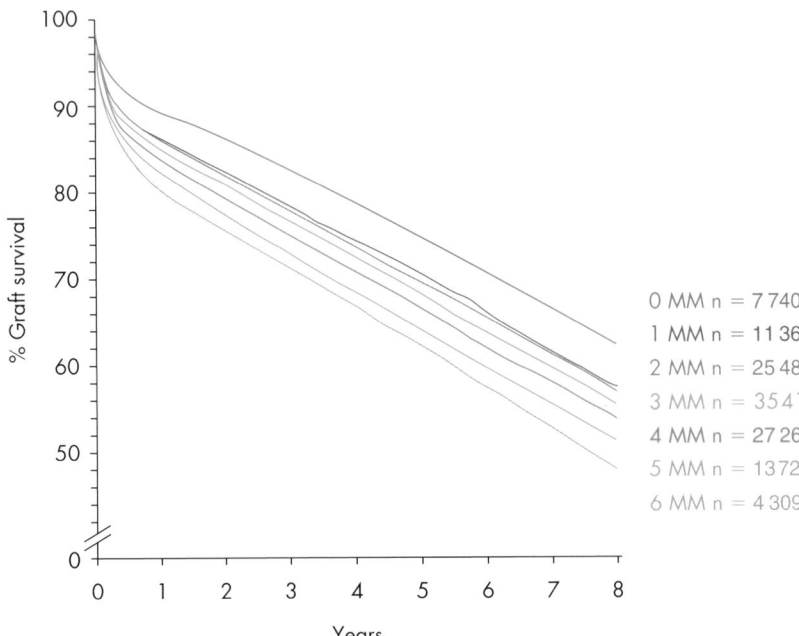

0 MM n = 7 740
1 MM n = 11 361
2 MM n = 25 481
3 MM n = 35 416
4 MM n = 27 264
5 MM n = 13 720
6 MM n = 4 309

Figure 77.10 Beneficial effect of human leuco-cyte antigen (HLA) matching (HLA-A, -B and –DR) on first deceased donor renal allograft survival (courtesy of Gerhard Opelz, Collaborative Transplant Study, CTC-K21101, Feb 2007). MM, antigen mis-match.

Table 77.3 Immunosuppressive agents

Agent	Principal mode of action
Corticosteroids	Widespread anti-inflammatory effects
Azathioprine	Prevents lymphocyte proliferation
Mycophenolate mofetil	Prevents lymphocyte proliferation
Ciclosporin	Blocks IL-2 gene transcription
Tacrolimus	Blocks IL-2 gene transcription
Sirolimus/everolimus	Blocks IL-2 receptor signal transduction
OKT3 monoclonal antibody	Depletion and blockade of T cells
ALG/ALS	Depletion and blockade of lymphocytes
Anti-CD25 monoclonal antibody	Targets activated T cells

ALG, anti-lymphocyte globulin; ALS, anti-lymphocyte serum; IL-2, interleukin-2.

Calcineurin blockers (ciclosporin and tacrolimus)

Ciclosporin and tacrolimus are the mainstay of most modern immunosuppressive protocols. Although structurally distinct, they exert their principal immunosuppressive effect through the same intracellular pathway. Each of the two agents binds within the T cell to a particular cytoplasmic protein or immunophilin (ciclosporin binds to cyclophilin and tacrolimus to FK-binding protein). The resulting immunophilin–drug complex then blocks the activity of calcineurin (a phosphatase) within the cytoplasm of the T cell. Calcineurin plays a critical role in facilitating the transcription of IL-2, the main T-cell growth factor, and other cytokines after T-cell activation. By blocking cytokine synthesis, ciclosporin and tacrolimus exert a potent immunosuppressive effect. The agents share a number of side-effects, the most notable of which is nephrotoxicity (Table 77.4). Cosmetic side-effects may be particularly distressing for the patient (Fig. 77.12). The calcineurin blockers have a relatively small therapeutic window. Their immunosuppressive action, as well as their side-effects, are dependent on their blood concentration, and monitoring of whole-blood drug levels is an important guide to optimal therapy. If, after renal transplantation, the graft fails to function immediately because of acute tubular necrosis,

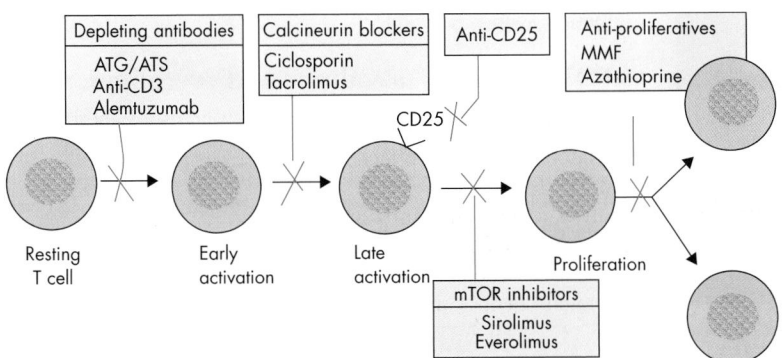

Figure 77.11 Site of action of immunosuppressive agents on the T cell. ATG, anti-thymocyte globulin; ATS, anti-lymphocyte serum; MMF, myophenolate mofetil; mTOR, mammalian target of rapamycin.

Table 77.4 Side effects of immunosuppressive agents used in organ transplantation

Agent	Side-effect
Corticosteroids	Hypertension, dyslipidaemia, diabetes, osteoporosis, avascular necrosis, cushingoid appearance
Azathioprine	Leucopenia, thrombocytopenia, hepatotoxicity, gastrointestinal symptoms
Mycophenolate mofetil	Leucopenia, thrombocytopenia, gastrointestinal symptoms
Ciclosporin	Nephrotoxicity, hypertension, dyslipidaemia, hirsutism, gingival hyperplasia
Tacrolimus	Nephrotoxicity, hypertension, dyslipidaemia, neurotoxicity, diabetes
Sirolimus/everolimus	Thrombocytopenia, dyslipidaemia, pneumonitis, impaired wound healing
ALG/ALS	Leucopenia, thrombocytopenia
OKT3 monoclonal antibody	Cytokine release syndrome, pulmonary oedema, leucopenia
Anti-CD25 monoclonal antibody	None described

ALG, anti-lymphocyte globulin; ALS, anti-lymphocyte serum.

calcineurin blockers may be reduced temporarily to avoid drug-induced nephrotoxicity. The relative efficacy of ciclosporin and tacrolimus in preventing rejection is broadly similar, and the choice between the two is dependent on the preference of the unit and on individual patient tolerance to the different side-effects.

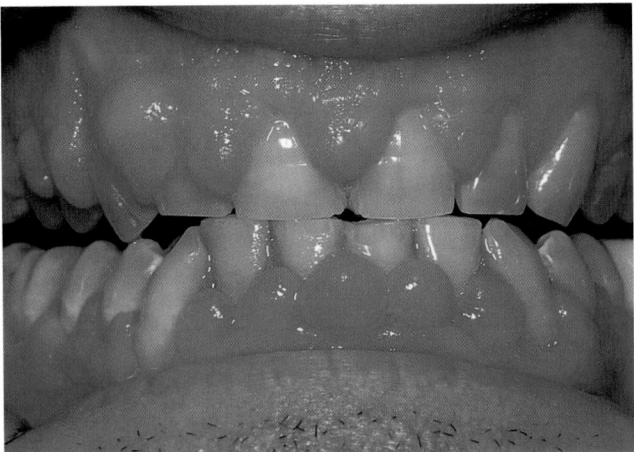

Figure 77.12 Gingival hyperplasia as a result of ciclosporin treatment.

Anti-proliferative agents (azathioprine and mycophenolate)

Lymphocytes are among the most rapidly proliferating cells in the body, and lymphocyte proliferation and clonal expansion are an integral part of the immune response to an allograft. The antiproliferative agents available for immunoprophylaxis are azathioprine and mycophenolate mofetil (MMF). Azathioprine is converted in the liver to its active metabolite, 6-mercaptopurine, which blocks purine metabolism and thereby inhibits cellular proliferation. Mycophenolate is a newer anti-proliferative agent and has now replaced azathioprine as the agent of choice in many transplant centres. After ingestion, MMF is converted to its active metabolite, mycophenolic acid. It inhibits the enzyme inosine monophosphate dehydrogenase, which is the rate-limiting enzyme in the *de novo* pathway of purine nucleotide synthesis. Because lymphocytes do not have a salvage pathway for purine synthesis, their ability to proliferate is selectively impaired. The main side effects of azathioprine and MMF are bone marrow suppression and gastrointestinal symptoms.

Steroids

Steroids have always been an important component of immunosuppressive regimens. Glucocorticoids are potent anti-inflammatory agents and have wide-ranging effects on the immune response. Because of their numerous and well-known side-effects, some centres attempt to gradually withdraw steroids from patients who have stable graft function after transplantation, but this sometimes precipitates a rejection episode and necessitates continuation of treatment.

Antibody therapies

Monoclonal antibodies directed against the IL-2 receptor on T lymphocytes (CD25) are commonly given at the time of transplantation to temporarily augment the effects of calcineurin blockade during the early post-transplant period. Their effect lasts for a few weeks only and they lack any significant agent-specific side-effects. Polyclonal antibody preparations [anti-lymphocyte globulin (ALG) or anti-lymphocyte serum (ALS)] are also widely used as a more potent and alternative induction agent. They cause a temporary depletion of circulating lymphocytes, which reduces rejection but may lead to an increase in infection and malignancy. In addition to their use as induction agents, polyclonal antibody preparations may be used to treat acute rejection episodes that fail to respond to steroid therapy. Depleting monoclonal antibodies directed against CD3 on T cells are little used now but a newer depleting antibody (alemtuzumab) directed against CD52 (expressed on T cells and dendritic cells) is used by a small but increasing number of units as an induction agent.

mTOR inhibitors (sirolimus and everolimus)

Sirolimus and its structural analogue everolimus are members of a relatively new class of potent immunosuppressive agent. Like tacrolimus, they are macrolides that bind within T lymphocytes to FK-binding protein. However, their mode of action is completely different from that of both ciclosporin and tacrolimus. They act by inhibiting an intracellular kinase called mammalian

de novo **is Latin for 'again from the beginning'.**

target of rapamycin (mTOR) and thereby interfere with intracellular signalling from the IL-2 receptor and arrest T-cell division in the G1 phase. In contrast to calcineurin blockers they are not nephrotoxic. However, their side-effect profile includes lymphocele formation, impaired wound healing, an adverse effect on the blood lipid profile, thrombocytopenia and very occasionally a potentially serious pneumonitis. mTOR inhibitors may have anti-tumour activity and the potential value of this effect in transplant patients is under investigation.

Immunosuppressive regimens

When selecting an immunosuppressive regimen, the challenge is to provide levels of immunosuppression that are sufficient to protect the graft from rejection without exposing the recipient to excessive risk from infection and malignancy as a result of non-specific immunosuppression (Summary box 77.4).

Summary box 77.4

Principles of immunosuppression

- Principles are the same for all types of organ transplantation
- The aim is to maximise graft protection and minimise side-effects
- Most regimens are based on calcineurin blockade and include steroids and an anti-proliferative agent
- The need for immunosuppression is highest in the first 3 months but indefinite treatment is needed
- Immunosuppression increases the risk of infection and malignancy

---

Immunosuppressive therapy is started at the time of transplantation and is continued indefinitely (as maintenance), although the requirement for immunosuppression is highest in the first few weeks after transplantation when the risk of acute rejection is greatest. Immunosuppressive protocols for different types of organ transplant vary somewhat between centres and within centres, but almost all use a combination of immunosuppressive agents acting at different points in the pathway of lymphocyte activation. Nearly all include a calcineurin blocker (ciclosporin or tacrolimus) as the main agent and often this is supplemented with anti-CD25 monoclonal antibody induction therapy. Calcineurin blockers are usually combined with an anti-proliferative agent (most often MMF) and steroids, so called 'triple therapy'. Less often, a calcineurin blocker is used with an anti-proliferative agent alone or with steroids alone (dual therapy). When there is particular concern about acute rejection, polyclonal antibody preparations are administered followed by a calcineurin blocker, an anti-proliferative agent and steroids (quadruple therapy).

The principles of immunoprophylaxis are similar for all types of organ transplantation. However, there is a tendency to use more intensive immunosuppression after thoracic organ transplantation than after kidney transplantation, in part because loss of a heart or lung graft from rejection almost inevitably culminates in death. Interestingly, liver grafts seem to be less susceptible to graft rejection for reasons that are still unclear. The mTOR inhibitors have been shown to be effective immunosuppressive agents for preventing acute rejection following kidney transplantation and they provide a non-nephrotoxic alternative to calcineurin inhibitors for maintenance therapy. They have a similar safety profile to calcineurin blockers in terms of post-transplant infection but some of their agent-specific side-effects are of potential concern and their clinical niche is still to be determined.

Acute rejection during the first 6 months of transplantation occurs in up to 30% of transplant recipients. Fortunately, the majority of episodes respond to a short course of high-dose steroid therapy. If the response to treatment is inadequate or if acute rejection recurs, rejection can often be treated successfully by anti-lymphocyte antibody therapy.

COMPLICATIONS OF IMMUNOSUPPRESSION

As well as the agent-specific side-effects already mentioned, the immunosuppressive agents used in organ transplantation cause non-specific immunosuppression and increase the risk of both infection and malignancy (Summary box 77.5).

Summary box 77.5

Side effects of non-specific immunosuppression

Infection
- Transplant recipients are at high risk of opportunistic infection, especially by viruses
- Viral infection may result from reactivation of latent virus or from primary infection
- CMV is a major problem
- Bacterial and fungal infections are also common
- Risk of infection is highest during first 6 months after transplantation
- Chemoprophylaxis is important in high-risk patients
- Pre-transplant vaccination against community-acquired infection should be considered

Malignancy
- Recipients are at risk of post-transplant lymphoproliferative disorder
- There is a high risk of squamous cancer of the skin and recipients should be reviewed regularly

---

Infection

Transplant recipients receiving immunosuppressive therapy are at high risk from opportunistic infection, especially by viruses. This is a potential problem in all recipients but those receiving aggressive immunosuppressive therapy after liver, heart, lung and small bowel transplantation are most at risk. Chemoprophylaxis is important in high-risk recipients, and early recognition followed by prompt and aggressive treatment of infection is essential. Pre-transplant vaccination against community-acquired infections should be considered.

Bacterial infection

The risk of bacterial infection is highest during the first month after transplantation. Recipients are at risk of bacterial infections in the wound, respiratory tract and urinary tract. It is standard practice to give a broad-spectrum antibiotic to cover the perioperative period as prophylaxis against wound infection and possible bacterial contamination of the donor organ. The risk of bacterial infection is greatest in transplant recipients who are critically ill before or after surgery and who are in the intensive care unit with indwelling catheters and lines. After recovery from surgery the risk of bacterial infection is much reduced. Tuberculosis is a concern in patients who have previously had mycobacterial infection and in patients from the Indian subcontinent. It is usual to give immunoprophylaxis to these individuals for a period of 6–12 months after transplantation.

Viral infection

The risk of viral infection is highest during the first 6 months after transplantation and the most common problem is CMV infection. CMV disease may arise because of reactivation of latent infection or because of primary infection that can be transmitted by an organ from a CMV-positive donor. The recipients at most risk from CMV infection are those who are CMV seronegative (i.e. those who have not been infected previously with CMV) who receive an organ from a CMV-seropositive donor. Matching seronegative donors with seronegative recipients is an effective strategy for reducing the risk of CMV infection but is not practicable. CMV disease typically presents with a high swinging fever, lethargy and leucopenia. The severity of the disease is variable and the clinical picture depends on the organ system most affected. It may present as:

- pneumonia;
- gastrointestinal disease;
- hepatitis;
- retinitis;
- encephalitis.

Severe CMV disease is potentially fatal. Prophylaxis for CMV consists of passive immunisation using hyperimmune immunoglobulin or, more commonly now, the administration of anti-viral agents in the form of aciclovir, valaciclovir, ganciclovir or valganciclovir. A diagnosis of active CMV infection can be confirmed by serology, detection of CMV antigenaemia, CMV culture, detection of viral DNA using the polymerase chain reaction (PCR), and histological examination of biopsy material. Treatment is with anti-viral agents and is more effective when given pre-emptively on the basis of increased viral load as judged, for example, by quantitative PCR analysis of CMV.

Herpes simplex virus (HSV) infection is common after transplantation and is usually due to reactivation of latent infection. It causes mucocutaneous lesions around the mouth and sometimes the genitalia. These usually respond to topical treatment with aciclovir but, in severe cases, systemic anti-viral therapy is needed. Disseminated HSV infection is rare.

Herpes zoster infection, as a result of reactivation of latent varicella zoster virus, occurs more frequently in transplant patients and should be treated with systemic anti-viral therapy. Primary varicella zoster virus infection (chickenpox) is potentially very serious in immunosuppressed patients but is relatively uncommon as most adults have acquired immunity.

Protozoal infection

Pneumocystis carinii is the most important protozoal infection seen after transplantation. It occurs during the first few months post-transplant and presents with respiratory symptoms. The diagnosis is made by examination of bronchoalveolar lavage fluid or lung biopsy material for evidence of parasite infection. Prophylaxis with co-trimoxazole is effective and is continued for up to 6 months after transplantation.

Fungal infection

Invasive fungal infections are uncommon in renal transplant recipients but infection with Candida or Aspergillus is more common after other types of solid organ transplantation. Fungal infection usually occurs in the first 3 months after transplantation, and early diagnosis and aggressive treatment are essential to avoid fatal infection.

Malignancy

After transplantation there is an increased risk of developing most types of malignancy but the risk is particularly high for those types of tumour in which viral infection plays an aetiological role. The risk is particularly high for skin cancer and a condition called post-transplant lymphoproliferative disorder (PTLD). Most of the skin cancers seen are squamous cell carcinomas, but basal cell carcinoma and malignant melanoma are also more common than in the general population. The risk of skin cancer after transplantation rises with age and with exposure to sunlight, and it has been predicted that 50% of transplant patients will develop a skin malignancy within 20 years of transplantation. Patients must be warned of this risk before they undergo transplantation and advised to take precautions to protect their skin from excessive sunlight. They should undergo a regular review of their skin to detect early malignancy, and when malignant lesions occur they must be treated promptly and aggressively.

PTLD is an abnormal proliferation of B lymphocytes, usually in response to Epstein–Barr virus infection. The condition presents in a variety of ways including as an infectious mononucleosis-type illness, as lymphadenopathy or with involvement of extranodal sites such as the tonsils, gastrointestinal tract, lung, liver or the transplanted organ (Fig. 77.13). PTLD occurs in around 1–3% of kidney and liver transplant recipients and the incidence is considerably higher in children. Patients at most risk are those who have received aggressive immunosuppression. PTLD is a serious condition with a mortality rate of up to 50%. If it is identified at an early stage, reduction or cessation of immunosuppressive therapy may cause disease regression and result in a cure. Chemotherapy is often given and anti-viral therapy, surgery and radiotherapy may also have a role in treating established disease. Disseminated PTLD and central nervous system (CNS) involvement have a poor prognosis.

Transplant patients also have a 300-fold increased risk of developing Kaposi's sarcoma, although this malignancy is still very uncommon after transplantation.

ORGAN DONATION

Most of the organs used for transplantation are obtained from brainstem-dead, heart-beating deceased donors and in the majority of cases multiple organs are procured. However, the number of organs required to satisfy the needs of transplantation far exceeds the number of deceased donor organs available. This has prompted a relaxation in the organ-specific donor selection criteria and in the use of organs from so called 'marginal donors'.

Michael Anthony Epstein, B. 1921, formerly Professor of Pathology, The University of Bristol, Bristol, England.
Yvonne Barr, B. 1931, a Virologist who emigrated to Australia.
Epstein and Barr discovered this virus in 1964.
Moritz Kaposi, 1837–1902, Professor of Dermatology, Vienna, Austria, described pigmented sarcoma of the skin in 1872.

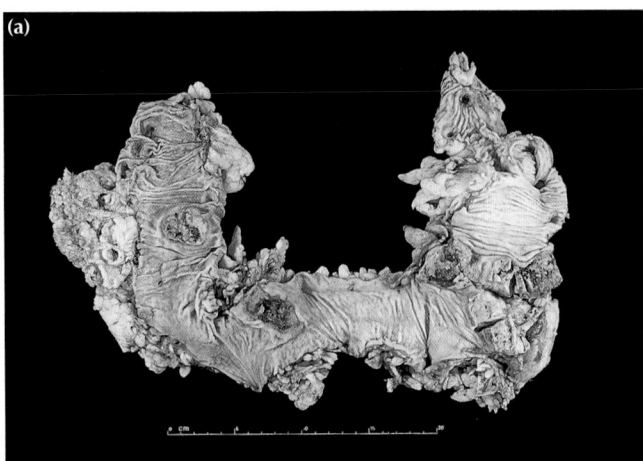

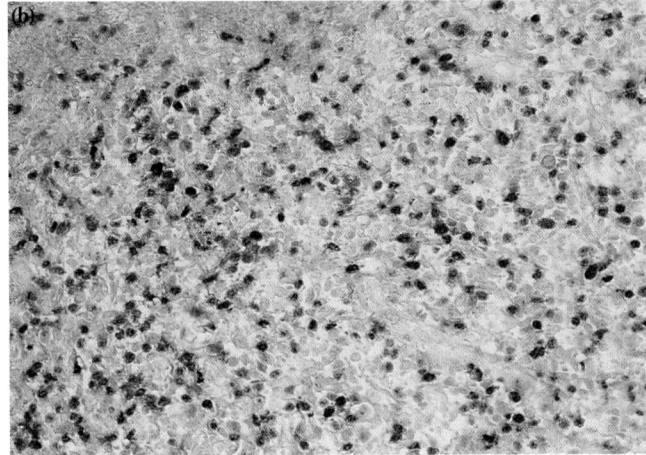

Figure 77.13 (a) Intestinal post-transplant lymphoproliferative disease. Note multiple lesions in the terminal ileum and colon. (b) Atypical B lymphocytes stained positive with a probe for Epstein–Barr virus DNA (courtesy of C. Watson, R. Chavez-Cartaya and D. Wight).

In the case of kidney transplantation there is a trend towards increased living donor transplantation and the use of kidneys from non-heart-beating deceased donors (Summary box 77.6).

Summary box 77.6

Overcoming the shortage of organs for transplantation

- Maximising heart-beating deceased donation
- Use of marginal heart-beating deceased donors
- Use of non-heart-beating donors
- Use of split-liver transplantation
- Increased living donor kidney (and liver) transplantation

Determination of brainstem death

Brain death occurs when severe brain injury causes irreversible loss of the capacity for consciousness combined with the irreversible loss of the capacity for breathing. In most countries it is accepted that the condition of brain death equates in medical, legal and religious terms with death of the patient. The concept of brain death arose through necessity in the management of

patients with irreversible brain damage on life support when there was no prospect of recovery. It was not in the interests of such patients, their relatives or the hospital in which they were being treated to delay their inevitable demise by continuing with futile life support. Acceptance of the concept of brain death had major implications for organ transplantation as it allowed the possibility of removal of viable organs from brain-dead patients before their circulation failed.

In many countries brain death is defined in terms of permanent functional death of the brainstem as neither consciousness nor spontaneous respiration is possible in the absence of a functional brainstem. A diagnosis of brainstem death should be considered only when certain preconditions have been met. The patient must have suffered major brain damage of known aetiology, be deeply unconscious and require artificial ventilation. Traumatic head injury and sudden intracranial haemorrhage are the most common causes of brainstem death. Particular care must be taken to ensure that muscle relaxant agents and drugs with known CNS depressant effects are not contributing to the clinical picture. Hypothermia, profound hypotension and metabolic or hormonal conditions that may contribute to CNS depression and confound the diagnosis of brainstem death must also be excluded. When the necessary preconditions have been satisfied, formal clinical assessment of the brainstem reflexes can be undertaken (Summary box 77.1). The UK guidelines state that the tests should be performed on two separate occasions by two clinicians experienced in this area. At least one of the two clinicians should be a consultant and neither should be connected with the transplant team. The time that must elapse between the two sets of brainstem tests is not specified in the guidelines and is determined on the basis of clinical judgement. In the UK there is no requirement to perform electrophysiological or brain perfusion studies to aid the diagnosis of brainstem death. Particular care is required in the diagnosis of brainstem death in neonates and infants (Summary box 77.7).

Summary box 77.7

Clinical testing for brainstem death

Absence of cranial nerve reflexes
- Pupillary reflex
- Corneal reflex
- Pharyngeal (gag) and tracheal (cough) reflex
- Oculovestibular (caloric) reflex

Absence of motor response
- The absence of a motor response to painful stimuli applied to the head/face and the absence of a motor response within the cranial nerve distribution to adequate stimulation of any somatic area is an indicator of brainstem death
- The presence of spinal reflexes does not preclude brainstem death

Absence of spontaneous respiration
- After pre-ventilation with 100% oxygen for at least 5 min, the patient is disconnected from the ventilator for 10 min to confirm absence of respiratory effort, during which time the arterial P_{CO_2} level should be > 8 kPa (60 mmHg) to ensure adequate respiratory stimulation.
- To prevent hypoxia during the apnoeic period, oxygen (6 l min⁻¹) is delivered via an endotracheal catheter

Evaluation of the deceased donor

After a brainstem-dead donor has been referred to the transplant team with a view to organ donation, the general suitability of the potential organ donor must be carefully assessed. Particular care must be taken to assess the donor from the point of view of transmissible infectious agents and malignancy. The medical history should be scrutinised and evidence sought of risk factors for human immunodeficiency virus (HIV), such as intravenous drug abuse. The presence of HIV infection and Creutzfeldt–Jakob disease (CJD) are absolute contraindications to organ donation. Hepatitis B (in most countries) and active systemic sepsis are also contraindications to donation. The presence of malignancy within the past 5 years is usually an absolute contraindication with the exception of primary tumours of the CNS, non-melanotic skin tumours and carcinoma *in situ* of the uterine cervix. If there are no general contradictions to organ donation, consideration is then given to organ-specific selection criteria.

Because of the high demand for donors there has been a progressive relaxation of the organ-specific selection criteria. The chronological age of the donor is less important than the physiological function of the organs under consideration for transplantation. As a rough guide, acceptable donor age ranges for each of the commonly transplanted organs are:

- kidney: 2 years to no upper age limit;
- liver: no age limit;
- heart: 1–65 years;
- lung: 5–65 years;
- pancreas: 10–60 years.

The donated organs should be free from primary disease. Potential kidney donors should have a reasonable urine output and relatively normal serum urea and creatinine levels, although acute terminal elevations are acceptable. Liver donors should not have hepatic disease, although impaired liver function tests are common in deceased donors and do not necessarily preclude donation. Heart donors should have a normal electrocardiogram and, in doubtful cases, echocardiography may be necessary. For lung donors the chest radiograph and gas exchange should be satisfactory, and bronchial aspirates should be free from fungal and bacterial infection. Elevations of blood glucose and serum amylase are not uncommon in deceased donors and do not preclude pancreas donation.

Organ procurement

When brainstem death has been confirmed, management of the donor is aimed at preserving the functional integrity of the organs to be procured. Brainstem death produces profound metabolic and neuroendocrine disturbances leading to cardiovascular instability. Careful monitoring and management of fluid balance is essential. Inotropic support is given and there may be a role for the use of tri-iodothyronine (T_3) and argipressin.

Procurement of multiple organs from a cadaveric donor requires cooperation between the thoracic and abdominal surgical teams. A midline abdominal incision and median sternotomy are used to obtain access. After dissection of the organs to be procured they are perfused *in situ*. The heart is perfused with cold cardioplegia solution via a cannula in the ascending aorta and the lungs are perfused via a cannula in the pulmonary artery. The abdominal organs are perfused with chilled organ preservation solution via an aortic and portal cannula. Blood and perfusate are vented from the left atrial appendage and the inferior vena cava. This produces rapid cooling of the organs, reduces their metabolic activity and preserves their viability. Additional surface cooling of the abdominal organs may be achieved by application of saline ice slush. The heart and lungs are excised followed by the liver and pancreas and then the kidneys, either *en bloc* or separately. The extent to which the abdominal organs are dissected prior to cold flush depends on the preference of the surgical team. Some surgeons perform minimal dissection prior to cold perfusion and complete the dissection of the abdominal organs *in situ* or on the back table after the organs have been removed *en bloc*. During procurement of the liver, care is taken to ensure that if there is an aberrant hepatic artery arising from the superior mesenteric artery it is included in the aortic patch. Similarly, care is taken to ensure that any polar renal arteries are included on an aortic patch with the renal artery (Fig. 77.14). A length of the donor iliac artery is excised for use in reconstructing the arterial supply of the pancreas prior to implantation.

After removal from the donor, the organs may undergo a further flush with chilled preservation solution and are then placed in two sterile bags and stored at 0–4°C by immersion in ice during transportation to the recipient centre. Once the donor organs have been excised, samples of donor spleen and mesenteric lymph nodes are obtained for determination of tissue type and use in the cross-match test.

Various organ preservation solutions are available for flushing organs before simple cold storage. They all contain impermeants to limit cell swelling, buffers to counter acidosis and electrolytes, the composition of which reflects that of intracellular rather than extracellular fluid. Commonly used preservation solutions include University of Wisconsin (UW) solution and Euro-Collins solution, but there are many others. The use of UW solution (Table 77.5) (developed by Belzer and colleagues) is particularly effective for liver grafts and after perfusion with UW solution the liver can be stored safely for up to 24 hours. The amount of time

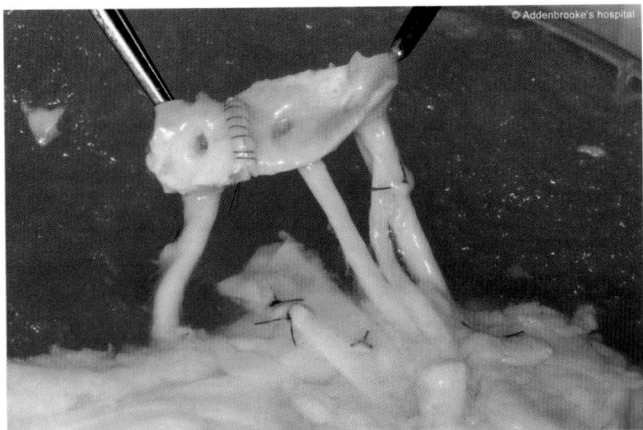

Figure 77.14 Deceased donor kidney with multiple renal arteries on an aortic patch. The aortic patch has been shortened to limit the length of the anastomosis needed when joining the donor patch to the side of the recipient external iliac artery (courtesy of Medical Photography, Addenbrooke's Hospital).

in situ **is Latin for 'in the place'.**
en bloc **is French for 'in a block'.**
The University of Wisconsin **is at Madison, WI, USA.**
Fokert O. Belzer, **1931–1995, a Surgeon of Madison, WI, USA.**

Table 77.5 Composition of University of Wisconsin solution

Potassium lactobionate (mmol l⁻¹)	100
Sodium phosphate (mmol)	25
Magnesium sulphate (mmol)	5
Adenosine (mmol l⁻¹)	5
Allopurinol (mmol l⁻¹)	1
Glutathione (mmol l⁻¹)	3
Raffinose (mmol l⁻¹)	30
Hydroxyethyl starch (g l⁻¹)	50
Insulin (U l⁻¹)	100
Dexamethasone (mg l⁻¹)	8
Potassium (mmol l⁻¹)	135
Sodium (mmol l⁻¹)	35
Osmolality (mosmol l⁻¹)	320
pH	7.4

for which an organ can be stored before transplantation varies depending on its type (Table 77.6). After arriving at the recipient transplant centre any necessary bench surgery is undertaken prior to implantation.

Non-heart-beating (asystolic) donors

There is an increasing use of kidneys and more recently livers from non-heart-beating (asystolic) donors (NHBD) in an attempt to address the shortage of organs for transplantation. Kidneys may be procured from patients who are dead on arrival at the hospital or who have died after withdrawal of support or following unsuccessful resuscitation.

NHBD can be grouped according to the Maastricht classification as follows:

- category 1: dead on arrival at hospital;
- category 2: unsuccessful resuscitation in hospital;
- category 3: 'awaiting cardiac arrest' after withdrawal of support;
- category 4: cardiac arrest while brain dead.

Maastricht category 1 and 2 donors are sometimes referred to as uncontrolled NHBD. The warm ischaemic time of kidneys from these two categories of donor is usually longer and less predictable than in the case of category 3 (controlled) donors. The majority of NHBD organs used for transplantation are from category 3 donors. To minimise the warm ischaemic time in NHBD, a

Table 77.6 Maximum and optimal cold storage times (approximate)ᵃ

Organ	Optimal storage time (hours)	Safe maximum storage time (hours)
Kidney	< 24	48
Liver	< 12	24
Pancreas	< 10	24
Small intestine	< 4	8
Heart	< 3	6
Lung	< 3	8

ᵃ Assuming zero warm ischaemic time and organs obtained from a non-marginal donor.

Maastricht **is a city in the Province of Limburg, in The Netherlands.**

double-balloon catheter may be introduced into the aorta via a femoral cut-down and chilled perfusate used to cool the kidneys *in situ*, preferably within 30 min of circulatory arrest (Fig. 77.15). However, it is more common (except in the case of category 1 and 2 donors) to allow a period of 10–15 min to elapse after cessation of heart beat and formal diagnosis of death before the patient is rapidly transferred to the operating room and the abdomen opened to allow cannulation of the aorta and cold perfusion of the kidneys. Kidneys obtained from NHBD invariably suffer a degree of ischaemic damage, and delayed graft function is more common (typically 50% for category 3 NHBD) than for kidneys obtained from heart-beating cadaveric donors. Irreversible ischaemic necrosis occasionally occurs and the graft never functions adequately (primary non-function). However, overall graft survival results for NHBD kidneys appear similar to those of kidneys obtained from heart-beating deceased donors. NHBD are not generally suitable for organs other than the kidney and liver. To minimise additional ischaemic damage it is essential that organs from NHBD are transplanted with the minimum possible cold storage time.

Living kidney donors

Currently, living donor renal transplants account for around 25–30% of the total renal transplant activity in the UK, but in some countries (notably the Scandinavian countries and the USA) this figure is much higher (> 50%). The justification for living donor renal transplantation is based on the shortage of deceased donor transplants and the superior results obtained. Traditionally, most living donor transplants were between genetically related individuals. However, living donor kidney transplants performed between genetically unrelated individuals also fare better than even well-matched deceased donor grafts, and this observation gave rise to a steady increase in living unrelated kidney transplantation activity, usually between partners. In all

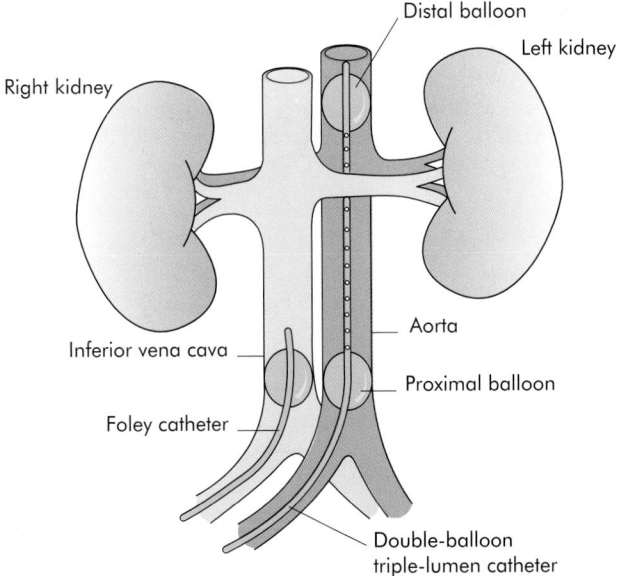

Figure 77.15 *In situ* perfusion of kidneys in a non-heart-beating donor (donation after cardiac death DCD). A double-balloon aortic catheter is introduced through a groin incision and 10–15 litres of chilled preservation solution are administered. The perfusate is vented through a Foley catheter introduced into the femoral vein.

cases of living donation it is essential to ensure that the prospective donor is fully informed and is free from coercion to donate and that the risk is small. In the UK, all living donor transplants require prior approval by the Human Tissue Authority (HTA). An independent practitioner approved by the HTA must provide confirmation to the HTA that the donor and recipient understand the implications of the operation and that there is no evidence of coercion or financial inducement.

Live donation should proceed only after the prospective donor has undergone rigorous assessment to ensure that they are suitable. Before the donation it is essential to perform imaging (usually magnetic resonance angiography or computerised tomography-guided angiography) to delineate the anatomy of the arterial supply to the kidneys. If the left kidney has a single renal artery (10% of kidneys have two or more renal arteries) it is usually chosen for transplantation because it has a longer renal vein, which simplifies the transplant operation. The presence of multiple arteries does not necessarily preclude donation although implantation of living donor kidneys with multiple arteries may increase the chances of vascular complications developing after implantation.

Donor nephrectomy was traditionally undertaken either through a loin incision and retroperitoneal approach or through a midline abdominal incision and transperitoneal approach. In many units laparoscopic donor nephrectomy is now undertaken routinely (Fig. 77.16). After removal from the donor the kidney is flushed immediately with chilled organ preservation solution (Fig. 77.17). The mortality rate for live donation is less than 0.05%; around one-half of reported deaths are due to pulmonary emboli so it is essential to ensure prophylaxis. The major complication rate is around 2%. In the long term, a slight elevation in proteinuria and a small rise in blood pressure accompany unilateral nephrectomy.

Around 35% of potential living donor transplant recipients will be ABO blood group incompatible with their intended donor, which until recently precluded transplantation. However, there are now two potential solutions to this problem. The first is 'paired donation' in which incompatible donor/recipient pairs exchange kidneys between pairs to allow ABO compatible transplantation (Fig. 77.18). Recruitment of more than two pairs to facilitate 'pooled donation' increases the likelihood of matching donors with compatible recipients and, although such schemes pose logistic challenges, they are now operating successfully in several countries. An alternative approach is to transiently deplete the recipient of ABO antibodies by passing their blood through special absorption columns, along with administration of pre-transplant immunosuppressive agents. This approach has been successful in Korea and Scandinavia and more recently elsewhere but graft survival is probably worse than for paired donation. Both paired donation and antibody depletion strategies are also potentially applicable to recipients in which HLA antibodies preclude transplantation.

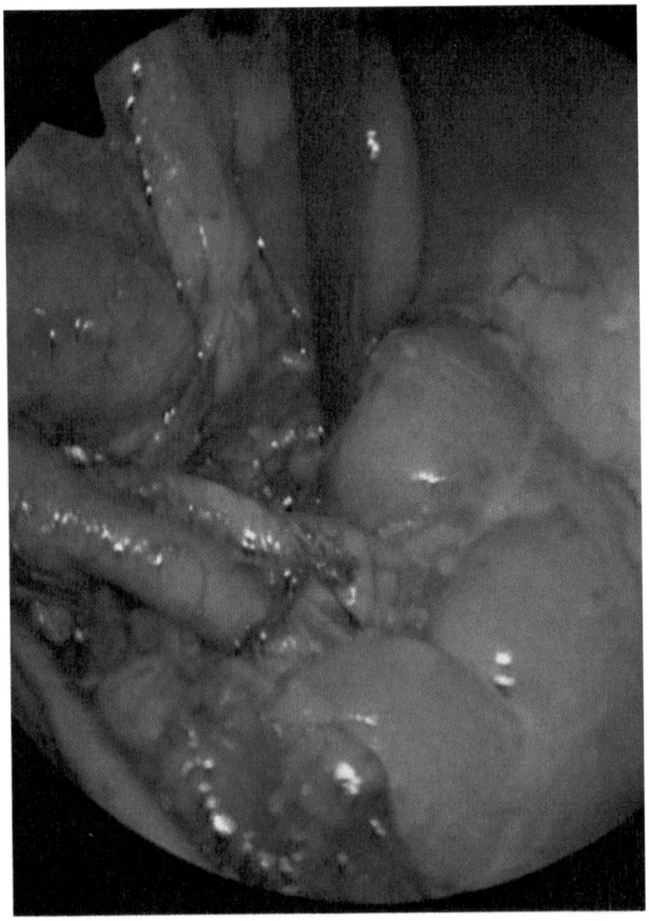

Living liver donors

Living donor liver transplantation is now undertaken in a number of centres worldwide and is relatively common in some countries where deceased donation is not practised for cultural or religious reasons. The concept was first pioneered to allow children to receive the left lobe or lateral segment from an adult donor. In countries where transplantation from a heart-beating cadaveric donor is undertaken, living donor liver transplantation in children has to a large extent been superseded by the techniques of liver reduction or liver splitting. Split-liver transplantation, first performed by Pichlmayr in 1988, allows the liver from a deceased

Figure 77.16 Laparoscopic living donor nephrectomy. The left kidney has been mobilised on its vascular pedicle ready for staple transection of the renal vessels and removal via a small midline incision.

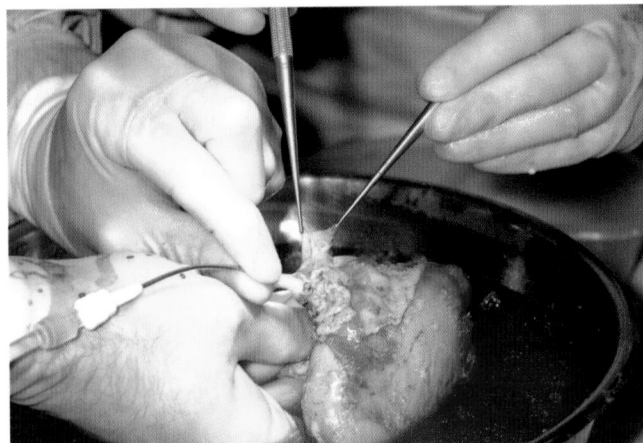

Figure 77.17 After removal from the donor the kidney is flushed with chilled organ preservation solution and, if necessary, stored briefly on ice until transplanted into the recipient.

Rudolph Pichlmayr, **1932–1997, Surgeon of Hannover, Germany.**

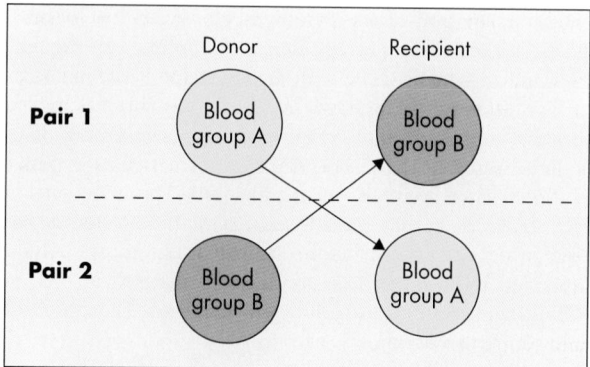

Figure 77.18 Paired living donor kidney transplantation. Paired donation allows patients with willing but blood-group-incompatible donors to be transplanted by pairing them with other incompatible donor–recipient pairs. In the example shown the two willing donors are incompatible with their intended recipients (blood groups A to B and B to A), but by paired donation each recipient can receive an ABO-compatible kidney transplant (blood groups A to A and B to B).

donor to be split in two. The right lobe is used for an adult and the left lobe is usually used for a child, although occasionally a split liver has been used for two adults (Fig. 77.19). In adult-to-adult living donor liver transplantation, the right lobe of the liver is transplanted. The donor procedure has a reported mortality rate of around 0.2% and one of the complications is bile leak.

Living donors: other organs

Occasionally, living donors have provided segments of pancreas, small bowel and lung for transplantation, but this is more controversial. In North America, living donor combined kidney and segmental pancreas transplantation has been undertaken to treat insulin-dependent diabetics with end-stage renal disease. In occasional patients, living donor small bowel transplantation has been performed using a small bowel graft, which comprises a length of around 1.5 m of ileum. Finally, a small number of living donor segmental lung transplants have been performed. To

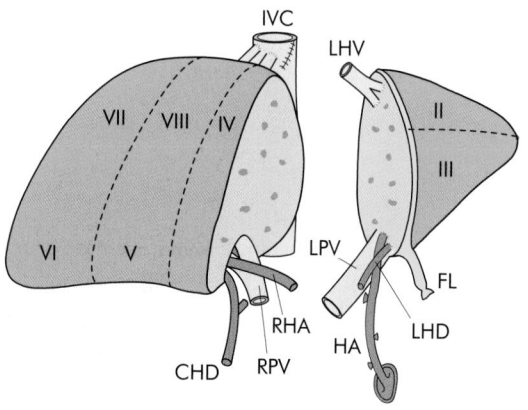

Figure 77.19 An adult liver may be split (according to Couinard's segments) so that the left lateral segment (segments II and III) can be transplanted into a child and the right lobe (together with segment IV) can be transplanted into an adult. CHD, common hepatic duct; FL, falciform ligament; HA, hepatic artery (on aortic patch); IVC, inferior vena cava; LHD, left hepatic duct; LHV, left hepatic vein; LPV, left portal vein; RHA, right hepatic artery; RPV, right portal vein.

provide sufficient pulmonary tissue without compromising the donor it is necessary to use segments from two different donors for each recipient. The ethical issues raised by living donation for extrarenal organs are understandably complex.

Resumption of function following organ transplantation

It is crucial that following heart, lung or liver transplantation the transplanted organ resumes satisfactory function immediately. If primary non-function occurs, the only option is rapid re-transplantation. After kidney, pancreas or small bowel transplantation, immediate graft function is desirable but not vital. The factors that determine the functional integrity of a transplanted organ are shown in Summary box 77.8.

> **Summary box 77.8**
>
> **Factors determining organ function after transplantation**
>
> *Donor characteristics*
> - Extremes of age
> - Presence of pre-existing disease in the transplanted organ
> - Haemodynamic and metabolic instability
>
> *Procurement-related factors*
> - Warm ischaemic time
> - Type of preservation solution
> - Cold ischaemic time
>
> *Recipient-related factors*
> - Technical factors relating to implantation
> - Haemodynamic and metabolic stability
> - Immunological factors
> - Presence of drugs that impair transplant function

KIDNEY TRANSPLANTATION

Patient selection

Renal transplantation is the preferred treatment for many patients with end-stage renal disease because it provides a better quality of life than dialysis. Transplantation releases patients from the dietary and fluid restrictions of dialysis and the physical constraints imposed by the need to dialyse. Transplantation is also more cost-effective and probably improves survival.

In the UK, around 80–100 people per million of the population develop end-stage renal disease and the incidence increases with age. The causes of end-stage renal disease are numerous and include:

- glomerulonephritis;
- diabetic nephropathy;
- hypertensive nephrosclerosis;
- renal vascular disease;
- polycystic disease;
- pyelonephritis;
- obstructive uropathy;
- systemic lupus erythematosus;
- analgesic nephropathy;
- metabolic disease (oxalosis, amyloid).

Frequently, the primary cause of end-stage renal disease is uncertain. For renal transplantation, as for other types of organ transplantation, careful patient selection is essential. Before acceptance as a suitable candidate on the waiting list, all patients should be formally assessed by a transplant surgeon and nephrologist. A significant number are likely to be considered unsuitable because of major comorbidity, especially cardiovascular disease. In the UK, around 30–40% of the dialysis population are on the waiting list for renal transplantation.

The nature of the primary renal disease does not generally affect the decision to proceed to transplantation. Some of the glomerulonephritides [notably immunoglobulin (Ig)A and focal segmental glomerulosclerosis] may subsequently affect a transplanted kidney, but this only occasionally results in failure of the graft in the first 5 years. In the case of primary oxalosis, combined kidney and hepatic transplantation is usually undertaken to eliminate the metabolic defect and thereby prevent early graft failure from the formation of further oxalate stones.

The age of patients with end-stage renal failure accepted for dialysis has gradually risen over the last two decades, and in the UK the mean age of patients starting dialysis is around 70 years. There is no absolute upper age limit to transplantation but, inevitably, older patients (over the age of 65 years) are less likely to be considered because of major comorbidity.

A careful assessment of comorbid disease that might significantly reduce the chances of a successful outcome after transplantation is essential (Summary box 77.9).

Summary box 77.9

Evaluation of potential recipients for organ transplantation

- Evaluation undertaken by appropriate multidisciplinary team including a surgeon and physician
- Determine presence of comorbidity
- Exclude malignancy and systemic sepsis
- Evaluate against organ-specific criteria for transplantation
- Determine probable ability to cope psychologically with transplant and comply with immunosuppression
- Evaluate need for any preparative surgery required to facilitate transplantation
- Optimise recipient condition prior to transplantation

Rigorous evaluation of the cardiovascular system is particularly important. Cardiovascular disease is very common in the dialysis population, especially those with diabetes, and is the major cause of death after transplantation. Before listing patients for transplantation it is important to ensure that their urinary tract is functional and that there is no need for corrective urological surgery. Only when there is intractable renal sepsis or very large polycystic kidneys that intrude into both iliac fossae is native nephrectomy required before transplantation. Finally, the prospective transplant recipient must be deemed able to cope psychologically with transplantation and likely to comply with immunosuppressive therapy.

Immunosuppressive therapy increases the risk of infection and malignancy after transplantation. Consequently, pre-existing malignancy is an absolute contraindication and, even after curative treatment, transplantation should not usually be considered for at least 3 years. Similarly, the presence of active infection is an absolute contraindication.

Technique of renal transplantation

The transplant kidney is placed in the iliac fossa in the retroperitoneal position leaving the native kidneys *in situ*. Using a retroperitoneal approach the donor renal vein is anastomosed end-to-side to the external iliac vein. The donor renal artery on a Carrel patch of donor aorta is anastomosed end-to-side to the external iliac artery (Fig. 77.20a). If the donor renal artery lacks an aortic patch, as in the case of a living donor transplant, it may be preferable to anastomose the donor artery end-to-end to the recipient internal iliac artery (Fig. 77.20 b).

Following completion of the venous and arterial anastomoses, the vascular clamps are removed and the kidney is allowed to reperfuse with blood. The ureter, which is kept reasonably short to avoid the risk of distal ischaemia, is then anastomosed to the bladder (Fig. 77.21). This is most often achieved by direct implantation of the ureter into the dome of the bladder with a mucosa-to-mucosa anastomosis followed by closure of the muscular wall of the bladder over the ureter to create a short tunnel, the Lich–Gregoir technique. A double-J ureteric stent is left *in situ* to reduce the risk of urine leak or early obstruction and removed

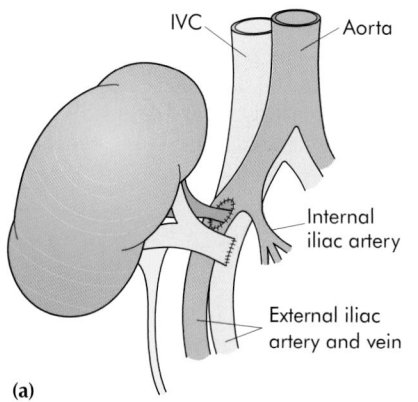

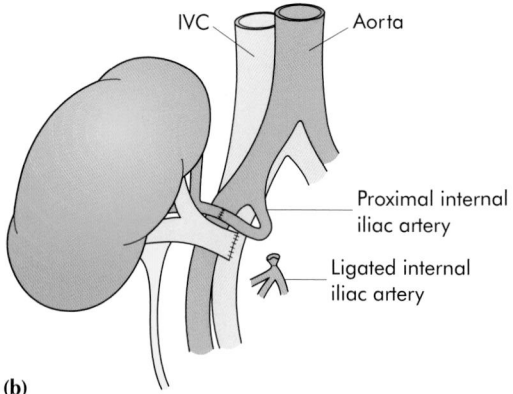

Figure 77.20 Implantation of a renal allograft. (a) The renal artery on a Carrel patch is anastomosed to the external iliac artery. (b) The renal artery is anastomosed end-to-end to the internal iliac artery. IVC, inferior vena cava.

Robert Lich, Jr., **a Urologist of Louisville, KY, USA.**
Willy Gregoir, **Chef du Clinique Urologique, Brussels, Belgium from 1962–1987.**

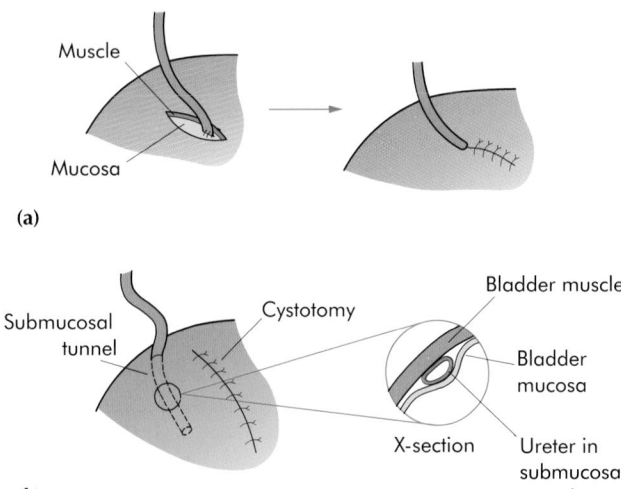

Figure 77.21 Ureteric implantation. (a) Lich–Gregoir technique. (b) Leadbetter–Politano technique.

after several weeks during cystoscopy. If the donor ureter is too short to reach the bladder the native ureter can be divided and the distal segment anastomosed to the ureter or renal pelvis of the donor kidney. The proximal segment of the native ureter can usually be ligated and the native kidney left *in situ* without causing a problem. Before closing the transplant wound it is very important to ensure that the kidney is lying in a satisfactory position without kinking or torsion of the renal vessels.

Technical complications

Vascular complications

The incidence of vascular complications after renal transplantation is low. Renal artery thrombosis occurs in approximately 1% of cases. Renal vein thrombosis is more common (up to 5% of cases) and, although sometimes caused by technical error, the aetiology is often uncertain. It presents during the first week after transplantation with sudden pain and swelling at the site of the graft. The diagnosis is confirmed by Doppler ultrasonography. Urgent surgical exploration is indicated and, in most cases, transplant nephrectomy is required. The incidence of renal vein thrombosis can be minimised by giving low-dose heparin or aspirin prophylaxis. Renal artery stenosis usually presents late (often years) after transplantation with increasing hypertension and decreasing renal function. It may occur in up to 10% of grafts and is diagnosed by angiography. Renal artery stenosis is best treated by angioplasty but, if unsuccessful or not technically possible, the condition can be treated by open surgery and vascular reconstruction.

Urological complications

Urological complications occur in around 5% of patients in the early post-transplant period, but their incidence can be reduced markedly by leaving a temporary ureteric stent *in situ*. Urinary leaks result from technical errors at the ureteric anastomosis or because of ureteric ischaemia. They present with discomfort and

Guy W. Leadbetter, a Urologist of Cambridge, VT, USA.
Victor A. Politano, a Urologist who was at The Massachusetts General Hospital, Boston, MA, and is now at the University of Florida, FL, USA.

leakage of urine from the wound and usually require surgical intervention and reimplantation of the ureter into the bladder or anastomosis of the transplant ureter to the ipsilateral native ureter. Obstruction of the transplant ureter may occur early or late. Causes of obstruction include technical error, external pressure from a haematoma or lymphocele and ischaemic stricture. Ureteric obstruction presents with painless deterioration of graft function and is confirmed by demonstrating hydronephrosis and ureteric dilatation on ultrasound examination. Initial treatment is by percutaneous antegrade nephrostomy and sometimes insertion of a stent. Some ureteric strictures may be amenable to treatment by balloon dilatation but most are best treated by surgical intervention, reimplanting the donor ureter into the bladder or anastomosing it to the native ureter.

Lymphocele

Peri-transplant lymphoceles are usually asymptomatic but occasionally they become large enough to cause ureteric obstruction or oedema of the ipsilateral leg. Initial treatment is usually by ultrasound-guided percutaneous drainage. In the case of large or recurrent lymphoceles, the repeated instillation of povidone-iodine into the lymphocele cavity by a percutaneous drain may lead to resolution. Surgical intervention may be needed to drain a persistent lymphocele into the peritoneal cavity, and this can often be achieved by an ultrasound-guided laparoscopic approach.

Investigation of graft dysfunction

Graft dysfunction during the early postoperative period is a common problem (Summary box 77.10).

Summary box 77.10

Causes of allograft dysfunction

Early
- Primary non-function (irreversible ischaemic damage)
- Delayed function (reversible ischaemic injury)
- Hyperacute and acute rejection
- Arterial or venous thrombosis of the graft vessels
- Drug toxicity (e.g. calcineurin toxicity)
- Infection (e.g. CMV disease in the graft)
- Mechanical obstruction (ureter/common bile duct)

Late
- Chronic rejection
- Arterial stenosis
- Recurrence of original disease in the graft (glomerulonephritis, hepatitis C)
- Mechanical obstruction (ureter, common bile duct)

Delayed graft function (defined as the need for dialysis post-transplantation) as a result of acute tubular necrosis occurs in up to 30% of heart-beating deceased donors and up to 50% of NHBD kidney transplants, but is uncommon (< 5%) following living donor transplantation. Often, recipients produce significant volumes of urine from their native kidneys, making the diagnosis of delayed function more difficult. The incidence of delayed function can be minimised by optimising donor management before kidney procurement and reducing the cold ischaemia time by avoiding unnecessary delay before implantation. As a first step in the management of early graft dysfunction, the urinary catheter should be irrigated in case it is occluded by a blood clot.

Hypovolaemia, if present, should be corrected with the aid of central venous pressure (CVP) monitoring. A Doppler ultrasound examination of the graft is the single most important investigation as it allows exclusion of vascular thrombosis and urinary obstruction as causes of graft dysfunction. Renal radionucleotide scanning provides information on renal perfusion and excretion and may be helpful. If graft dysfunction is still present after several days, it is usual to perform an ultrasound-guided needle biopsy of the kidney to ensure that graft rejection is not present and to repeat the investigation every week until graft function occurs. To avoid the risk of nephrotoxicity, calcineurin blockers are often withheld or given in reduced doses until graft function is established. If calcineurin blockers are not withheld it is important to monitor their blood levels carefully to avoid nephrotoxicity. Acute tubular necrosis usually resolves within the first 4 weeks of transplantation but a small number of grafts (< 5%) suffer primary non-function (i.e. never function).

Allograft dysfunction developing late (> 1 month after transplant) may be a result of:

- acute/chronic rejection;
- drug toxicity;
- ureteric obstruction (lymphocele/ureteric stricture);
- recurrent disease;
- urinary tract infection.

Blood levels of ciclosporin or tacrolimus are assessed to ensure that they are not elevated, and ultrasound examination of the graft is performed to determine whether ureteric obstruction is present. If obstruction is detected, it is further investigated by percutaneous antegrade pyelography and treated as above. If there is uncertainty about the cause of graft dysfunction, transplant biopsy should be performed to establish if allograft rejection is present.

Outcome after transplantation

The results of organ transplantation are generally defined in terms of patient and graft survival (Summary box 77.11).

Summary box 77.11

Outcome after transplantation

- **Transplantation improves the quality and duration of life in most recipients**
- **Transplant outcome has improved progressively over the last two decades and continues to improve**
- **Improved outcome is due to better immunosuppression, organ preservation, chemoprophylaxis and technical advances**
- **Graft survival after kidney, liver and heart transplantation is around 90% at 1 year and 80% at 5 years**
- **The results of lung and small bowel transplantation are less impressive**
- **Chronic rejection is the most common cause of graft failure after all types of solid-organ transplant**
- **Recurrence of the original disease necessitating transplantation may also lead to graft failure**
- **Death from cardiovascular disease with a functioning transplant is relatively common**
- **Up-to-date transplant outcomes for different organs can be found in the online national and international transplant databases (see end of chapter for website addresses)**

Patient survival after deceased donor renal transplantation is > 90% at 1 year and > 80% at 5 years. Graft survival is around 90% at 1 year and 75% at 5 years. Graft survival after a second transplant is only marginally worse than after a first graft. After living-related kidney transplantation, overall graft survival is around 95% at 1 year and 85% at 5 years. Graft survival after transplantation can also be expressed in terms of the half-life of the graft. The half-life of grafts obtained from living donors is longer than that of cadaveric grafts:

- deceased donor grafts: 13 years;
- living unrelated grafts: 14 years;
- living haploidentical grafts: 15 years;
- living identical sibling grafts: 27 years.

If a kidney transplant fails late after transplantation the graft can often be left *in situ*, but transplant nephrectomy may be indicated if the graft is causing symptoms. The operation is undertaken via the original wound, but the kidney is dissected free from the renal capsule and delivered into the wound. The renal vessels are then ligated and divided, leaving behind the original vascular anastomosis.

In addition to graft survival it is important to consider the extent to which transplantation improves the physical and mental well-being of the patient and allows him or her to lead a satisfactory social life. In the case of the kidney, as in other types of solid organ transplant, successful transplantation undoubtedly leads to a substantial improvement in quality of life. However, although some recipients return to a normal or near-normal life, others fare less well and, for the group overall, the quality of life after transplantation falls short of that seen in normal healthy individuals. Renal transplantation is best regarded, therefore, as an effective form of therapy rather than a complete cure.

PANCREAS TRANSPLANTATION

Successful pancreas transplantation restores the normal control of glucose metabolism and obviates the need for insulin therapy in patients with diabetes mellitus. Improved control of blood glucose levels undoubtedly reduces the progression of secondary complications such as retinopathy, peripheral vascular disease and nephropathy. However, in considering the indications for pancreas transplantation, these advantages have to be weighed carefully against the risks of both the transplant procedure itself and the immunosuppressive therapy. For most patients with diabetes these risks are such that the operation can be justified only when kidney transplantation for diabetic nephropathy is also being undertaken. The only additional risks of pancreas transplantation in such patients relate to the transplant operation itself. In the USA, around one-half of all diabetic patients undergoing kidney transplantation also receive a pancreas transplant. In most cases, the kidney and pancreas are obtained from the same donor, so-called simultaneous pancreas and kidney transplantation (SPKT). Pancreas transplantation is sometimes performed in patients who have already undergone successful kidney transplantation; this is called pancreas after kidney transplantation (PAKT). Occasionally, pancreas transplantation alone (PTA) can be justified to treat life-threatening diabetic complications such as hypoglycaemic unawareness.

Careful patient selection is essential to avoid excessive mortality and morbidity. The procedure is usually reserved for those patients with type I diabetes who are relatively young (under the age of 55 years) and who do not have advanced coronary artery disease or peripheral vascular disease. Investigation of the heart's response to stress, either using echocardiography or nuclear medicine imaging, is mandatory.

Surgical technique

Most centres now perform transplantation of the whole pancreas together with a segment of duodenum, essentially as pioneered by Lillehei in 1966. Segmental pancreas transplantation is still performed occasionally. SPKT is usually performed through a midline incision (Fig. 77.22). The pancreas graft is placed intraperitoneally in the pelvis, usually on the right, and the kidney graft is placed on the left. The donor vessels of the pancreas graft are anastomosed to the recipient iliac vessels and the exocrine secretions are most commonly dealt with by anastomosing the graft duodenum to the small bowel (enteric drainage), often via a Roux-en-Y loop. The duodenum may also sometimes be anastomosed to the bladder (urinary drainage). The pancreas graft functions immediately after revascularisation, although supplementary insulin may be required for a few days. Technical complications usually occur early and include vascular thrombosis of the graft (5%) and anastomotic leaks. Wound infection occurs in up to 10% of cases and intra-abdominal infection is relatively common. The specific complications of enteric drainage include intra-abdominal sepsis and adhesive small-intestinal obstruction. Bladder drainage of the exocrine pancreas may result in the following complications:

- bladder/duodenal anastomotic leaks;
- cystitis (because of the effect of pancreatic enzymes);
- urethritis/urethral stricture;
- reflux pancreatitis;
- urinary tract infection;
- haematuria;
- metabolic acidosis (caused by loss of bicarbonate in the urine).

Urinary drainage of the pancreas has the advantage that urinary amylase levels can be used to monitor graft rejection. However, urinary complications are common after bladder drainage and in around 20% of cases they are severe enough to require conversion to enteric drainage. Most centres now prefer primary enteric drainage after SPKT.

Acute rejection after SPKT is relatively common (10–20% of cases) and, if detected early, responds to steroids. Because it usually involves both the kidney and pancreas grafts, serum creatinine can be used as a surrogate marker for pancreas graft rejection. Serum lipase and amylase levels are useful indicators of pancreas graft inflammation, of which acute rejection is one cause. Urinary drainage has the advantage after PTA and PAKT of allowing pancreas graft rejection to be monitored by serial measurements of urinary amylase. A fall in urinary amylase is indicative of acute rejection. Elevation of the blood glucose level is a late feature of acute rejection and often indicates the process is beyond reversal.

Results of pancreas transplantation

The principal aim of pancreas transplantation is to prolong life in diabetic patients who otherwise have high mortality rates at 10 years after receiving a kidney transplant alone. It also provides freedom from insulin treatment and improves quality of life.

The results of pancreas transplantation have improved significantly over the last decade. After SPKT, the 1-year patient survival rate is > 95% and the 1-year graft survival rates for pancreas and kidney grafts are 85% and 95% respectively. Most deaths are due to cardiovascular complications or overwhelming infection. Patient and kidney graft survival after SPKT in patients with diabetic nephropathy is at least as good as after kidney transplant alone in this group. The results of PTA are not as good as after SPKT (1-year pancreas graft survival 70%) because acute rejection is more difficult to monitor in the absence of a kidney allograft.

Transplantation of isolated pancreatic islets

Treatment of diabetes by transplantation of isolated islets of Langerhans is a more attractive concept than vascularised pancreas transplantation because major surgery and the potential complications of transplanting exocrine pancreas are avoided. Pancreatic islets for transplantation are obtained by mechanically disrupting the pancreas after injection of collagenase into the pancreatic duct. The islets are then purified from the dispersed tissue by density-gradient centrifugation and can be delivered into the recipient liver (the preferred site for transplantation) by injection into the portal vein. Until recently, human islet transplantation had been performed intermittently and with very disappointing results. Although some degree of islet cell function often occurred initially, this was rarely sustained. However, in 2000, Shapiro and colleagues in Edmonton, Canada, reported success with islet transplantation in seven patients with type I diabetes. Sequential islet transplantation from two or three donor

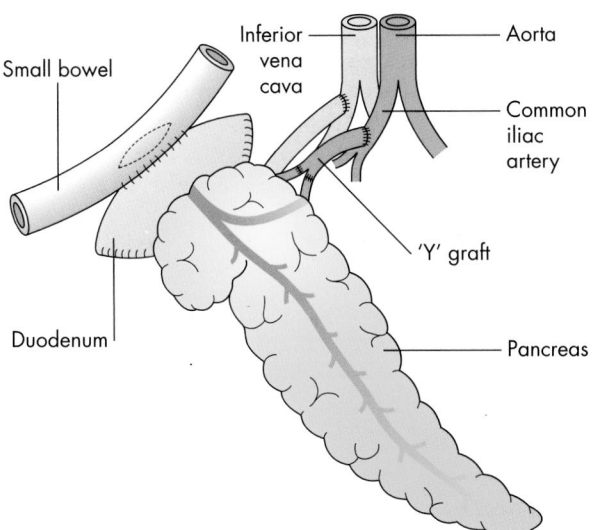

Figure 77.22 Pancreas transplant operation with enteric drainage of the exocrine secretion via a duodenoenterostomy. A 'Y' graft using the donor iliac artery is usually used to reconstruct the divided splenic and superior mesenteric arteries of the graft prior to implantation.

Richard Lillehei, **Surgeon, The University of Minnestoa, Minneapolis, MI, USA.**
Cesar Roux, **1857–1934, Professor of Surgery and Gynaecology, Lausanne, Switzerland, described this method of forming a jejunal conduit in 1908.**

Paul Langerhans, **1847–1888, Professor of Pathological Anatomy, Freiburg, Germany.**
Andrew Mark James Shapiro, **Chairman of Clinical Research in Transplantation, CIHR/Wyeth Canada, Edmonton, Alberta, Canada.**

CHAPTER 77 | TRANSPLANTATION

pancreas glands was required to produce insulin independence and, although the long-term success was less than initially hoped for, some patients remained free from exogenous insulin.

As an alternative to preventing islet cell rejection through immunosuppressive therapy, attempts have been made to protect isolated islet cells from rejection by encapsulating them inside semi-permeable membranes. The protective membranes are designed with a pore size that allows insulin to pass through but prevents antibodies and leucocytes from reaching the islets, thereby avoiding the need for immunosuppressive therapy. A major attraction of this approach is that islets isolated from animals can be used and bioartificial pancreas grafts containing xenogeneic islets are currently under evaluation.

LIVER TRANSPLANTATION

Starzl first attempted liver transplantation in 1963 and, by 1967, had achieved prolonged survival rates. The first liver transplant performed outside the USA was performed in Cambridge in 1968 by Calne. Throughout the 1970s, liver transplantation remained hazardous and frequently failed. However, since then, the results have progressively improved as a result of better patient selection, improved immunosuppression and chemoprophylaxis, better organ preservation, refinements in the operative technique, and advances in per- and postoperative management. Liver transplantation is now a routine operation in specialist centres.

Indications and patient selection

The indications for liver transplantation fall into four groups:

- cirrhosis;
- acute fulminant liver failure;
- metabolic liver disease;
- primary hepatic malignancy.

The most common indication for transplantation is chronic liver failure. In adults the most common causes are alcoholic liver disease, viral liver disease (hepatitis C in Europe and the USA and hepatitis B in some other countries), primary biliary cirrhosis and sclerosing cholangitis. In children, who account for around 10–15% of all liver transplants, biliary atresia is the most common indication. Acute fulminant liver failure requiring transplantation on an urgent basis accounts for approximately 10% of activity and is usually viral or drug induced (e.g. paracetamol overdose in the UK). There are a variety of metabolic diseases for which transplantation offers the prospect of cure. These include Wilson's disease, oxalosis and alpha-1-antitrypsin deficiency. Primary hepatic malignancy is more common in patients with cirrhosis, especially virally induced disease, and may be best treated by transplantation because tumour resection may leave insufficient functional liver tissue behind. Cholangiocarcinoma has a high recurrence rate and is seldom an indication for transplantation.

Technique of liver transplantation

A transverse abdominal incision with a midline extension is made and the diseased liver is mobilised (Fig. 77.23). Because of portal hypertension, the recipient hepatectomy is often the most difficult

Thomas Earl Starzl, **Professor of Surgery, Pittsburgh, PA, USA.**
Samuel Alexander Kinnier Wilson, **1878–1936, Professor of Neurology, King's College Hospital, London, England, described this condition in 1912.**

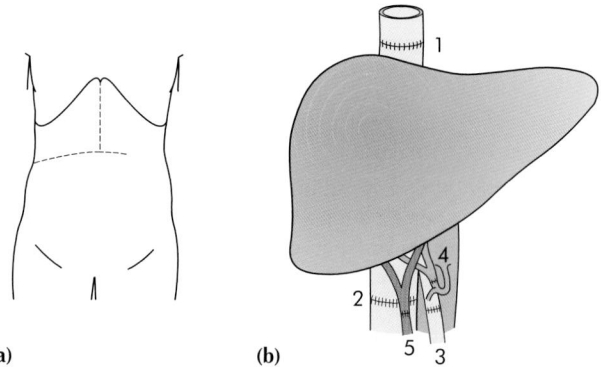

Figure 77.23 (a) Incision used for liver transplantation. (b) Completed implantation. The anastomoses, in order of performance, are: (1) suprahepatic vena cava; (2) infrahepatic vena cava; (3) portal vein; (4) hepatic artery; (5) bile duct.

part of the operation, especially if there has been previous surgery. The common bile duct is divided, as is the hepatic artery. The inferior vena cava is clamped and divided above and below the liver, and the portal vein is clamped and divided, allowing the recipient liver to be removed. Occlusion of the vena cava and portal vein results in a reduction in cardiac output and may necessitate the use of veno-venous bypass. The bypass circuit delivers blood from the portal vein and inferior vena cava back to the heart via a cannula inserted into the axillary vein or the internal jugular veins. After placing the donor liver in position, the supra- and infrahepatic caval anastomoses are performed. The portal vein and the hepatic arterial anastomoses are then completed and the graft is reperfused. Finally, biliary drainage is re-established, usually by a duct-to-duct anastomosis (without the use of a T-tube). It may be necessary, for example in recipients with biliary atresia or sclerosing cholangitis, to reconstruct the biliary drainage by a bile duct to Roux loop anastomosis. An alternative 'piggyback' technique of liver transplantation is sometimes preferred in which the diseased native liver is dissected from the intact inferior vena cava and the suprahepatic vena cava of the donor is anastomosed end-to-side to the anterior wall of the recipient vena cava.

Many patients undergoing liver transplantation are extremely ill and the surgery involved can be very demanding. Optimal perioperative management is crucial for success and presents a major challenge. Blood loss during and after the transplant procedure can be very considerable and management of coagulopathy is particularly important. Coagulation is assessed repeatedly throughout the transplant period and corrected appropriately with fresh frozen plasma, cryoprecipitate and platelets as necessary.

Technical complications

Haemorrhage

Meticulous haemostasis during the transplant operation is essential. It may be necessary, occasionally, to pack the peri-transplant area for 2–3 days to achieve adequate haemostasis when there is diffuse oozing despite correction of coagulopathy. Evacuation of extensive perihepatic haematoma may be required to avoid secondary infection.

Vascular complications

Hepatic artery thrombosis may occur spontaneously or as a result of acute rejection and is more common in children. It may present as a rise in serum transaminase levels, unexplained fever or bile leak. Doppler ultrasonography or angiography is used to confirm the diagnosis and urgent re-transplantation is usually required. Portal vein thrombosis presents more insidiously and does not usually require re-transplantation.

Biliary complications

Biliary leaks are now relatively uncommon and biliary stenosis is the more common problem. It usually occurs late and is managed by endoscopic dilatation and stenting; less often it is managed by surgical correction.

Paediatric liver transplantation

Until recently, the major factor limiting paediatric liver transplantation was the lack of donor livers of suitable size. However, as noted earlier, the development of techniques for using adult livers that have been reduced in size by cut-down techniques has greatly alleviated the problem. For small children the lateral segment of the left lobe is often used but the entire left lobe or the right lobe may also be used.

Outcome after liver transplantation

The outcome after liver transplantation depends on the underlying disease; the best results are seen in patients with chronic liver disease (Fig. 77.24). Patients undergoing transplantation as a result of acute liver failure have a higher mortality rate in the early post-transplant period because of multi-organ failure, but those who recover have very good long-term liver allograft survival. Conversely, patients transplanted for tumour have a very good early outcome but ultimately fare less well because of recurrence. Patients receiving a liver transplantation following hepatitis B or C infection may develop graft failure as a result of recurrent viral disease but the availability of improved anti-viral therapy has helped reduce this problem.

SMALL BOWEL TRANSPLANTATION

Progress in small bowel transplantation has lagged behind that of other types of solid organ transplantation but it is now a well-established therapy for highly selected recipients. Intestinal transplants stimulate a particularly strong graft rejection response, probably because the small intestine contains large amounts of lymphoid tissue. Moreover, ischaemia and rejection increase intestinal permeability and allow translocation of bacteria from the lumen of the bowel. Added to this, the operation is often complex and is made technically difficult because of repeated previous abdominal surgery. Consequently, graft rejection and infection remain major problems and the results obtained are inferior to those obtained after other types of organ transplantation. Small bowel transplantation is a treatment option for patients with intestinal failure as defined by the loss of intestinal function to the extent that long-term parenteral nutrition is required. Intestinal failure may result from short bowel syndrome after resection of the intestine or from intestinal dysfunction. Indications for transplant include the following:

- intestinal atresia;
- necrotising enterocolitis;
- volvulus;
- disorders of motility;
- mesenteric infarction;
- Crohn's disease;
- trauma;
- desmoid tumours.

Because of the substantial risks associated with small bowel transplantation, the procedure should be considered only for those patients in whom long-term total parenteral nutrition (TPN) has failed, usually because venous access has become impracticable or because of frequent life-threatening line sepsis. The need for small bowel transplantation is estimated at around 0.5–1.0 patient per million of the population and around 50% of cases are children.

Small bowel transplantation may be carried out as an isolated procedure, performed together with a liver transplant or undertaken as a component of a multivisceral transplant. When possible, isolated small bowel transplantation is undertaken because patient survival is higher.

A small bowel transplant from a deceased donor comprises the entire small bowel, but it is no longer considered advisable to include the ascending colon in the graft. The superior mesenteric artery of the graft (with an aortic patch) is anastomosed to the recipient aorta, and the superior mesenteric vein is anastomosed to the inferior vena cava or to the side of the portal vein. The proximal end of the small bowel graft is anastomosed to the

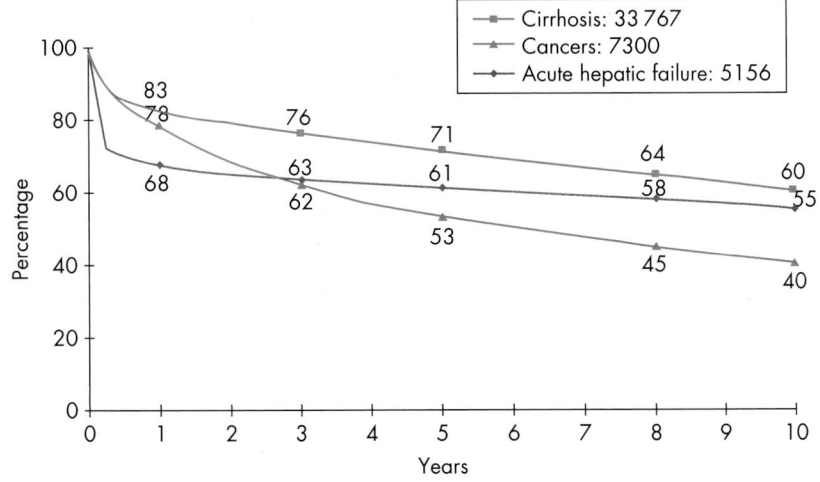

Figure 77.24 Outcome after liver transplantation according to the initial liver disease. Patients transplanted for acute liver disease have a higher early mortality but good long-term outcome. Patients transplanted because of liver tumour have a good initial outcome but survival continues to decline progressively (data obtained from the European Liver Transplant Registry, 2007).

recipient jejunum or duodenum. The distal end of the graft is anastomosed to the side of the colon (with a loop ileostomy) or is fashioned as an end-ileostomy. A gastrostomy tube (to overcome delayed gastric emptying) and a feeding jejunostomy tube are inserted.

About one-half of all patients who require small bowel transplantation have cholestatic liver disease secondary to TPN and require combined liver and small bowel transplantation. Cholestatic liver disease due to TPN is especially common in children. When combined liver and small bowel transplantation is carried out, the two grafts are transplanted *en bloc*. The donor aorta is fashioned into a conduit including the superior mesenteric and coeliac arteries and anastomosed to the recipient aorta. The portal vein anastomosis is as for isolated liver transplantation.

Multivisceral or 'cluster' transplants may be necessary in the case of large desmoid tumours when excision of both the small bowel and adjacent organs is required, when there has been extensive thrombosis of the splanchnic vessels and for generalised disorders of gastrointestinal motility.

The 1-year graft survival rate after small bowel transplantation is about 65% for both isolated small bowel transplantation and for combined liver and small bowel transplantation. After 3 years, the graft survival rate is around 45%. As already noted, however, patient survival is better after isolated small bowel transplantation than after combined liver and small bowel transplantation, when loss of the graft usually equates with death of the recipient. Most of the mortality after small bowel transplantation is due to sepsis and multi-organ failure. The risk of infection after small bowel transplantation is heightened by the additional requirements for immunosuppression to control graft rejection. This accounts for the relatively high incidence of lymphoproliferative disease (around 10%) observed in patients who have undergone small bowel transplantation. Because of the large amount of donor lymphoid tissue transplanted, GVHD may be an added complication. However, despite the hazards, small bowel transplantation offers patients with intestinal failure a chance to lead an active life, free from the constraints of long-term nutritional support.

THORACIC ORGAN TRANSPLANTATION

Heart transplantation

Barnard performed the first human heart transplant in Cape Town, South Africa, in 1967. The operation was based on the experimental work of Lower and Shumway at Stanford, and Shumway subsequently went on to pioneer successful cardiac transplantation in the clinic. Heart transplantation is now considered an effective treatment for selected patients with end-stage cardiac failure. The most common indications are ischaemic heart disease and idiopathic cardiomyopathy, but other indications include valvular heart disease, myocarditis and congenital heart disease.

Transplantation is considered only in patients with end-stage heart disease that has failed to respond to all other conventional

Christiaan Neethling Barnard, **1922–2001, Professor of Cardiac Surgery, The University of Cape Town, Cape Town, The Republic of South Africa.**
Richard Rowland Lower, **Contemporary, Thoracic Surgeon, Richmond, VA, USA.**
Norman Edward Shumway, **1923–2006, Cardiothoracic Surgeon, Stanford University School of Medicine, Palo Alto, CA, USA.**

therapy and when predicted survival without transplantation is only 6–12 months. Transplantation is usually limited to patients under the age of 65 years who do not have irreversible damage to other organ systems. The preoperative assessment is rigorous and measurement of pulmonary vascular resistance is mandatory because, when it is raised, perioperative mortality is high.

Technique of heart transplantation

A median sternotomy is performed and the patient is given systemic heparin, placed on cardiopulmonary bypass and cooled to 29°C. After cross-clamping the aorta, the recipient heart is excised at the mid-atrial level. The donor heart is then prepared and the left atrium is opened by making incisions (Fig. 77.25) in the posterior wall between the orifices of the pulmonary veins to create an atrial cuff. The left and then right atrial anastomoses are performed and the pulmonary and aortic arterial anastomoses are then completed (Fig. 77.26). The patient is then rewarmed and weaned from cardiopulmonary bypass. Occasionally, heterotopic cardiac transplantation is undertaken, when the donor heart is placed adjacent to and augments the recipient's own heart.

Heart–lung, single-lung and double-lung transplantation

Pulmonary transplantation became a clinical reality when Reitz performed the first successful combined heart–lung transplant in 1981. Combined heart–lung transplantation is still sometimes performed, usually in patients with pulmonary vascular disease in

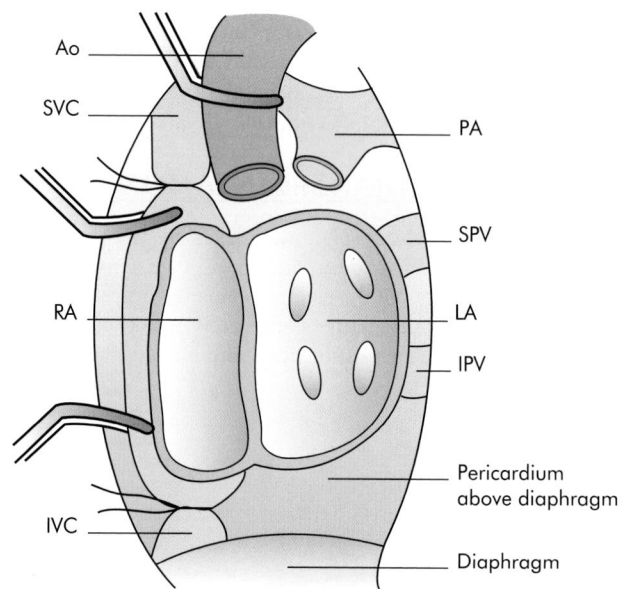

Figure 77.25 Recipient cardiectomy. After median sternotomy, the recipient is placed on cardiopulmonary bypass. Venous cannulae for bypass are sited in the superior vena cava (SVC) and inferior vena cava (IVC) via punctures in the right atrium (RA), and oxygenated blood is returned via a cannula in the ascending aorta (Ao). The diseased recipient heart is excised, leaving behind cuffs of right and left atria. IPV/SPV, inferior/superior pulmonary veins; LA, left atrium; PA, pulmonary artery (courtesy of J. Dunning).

Bruce Arnold Reitz, **Thoracic Surgeon, Stanford University School of Medicine, Palo Alto, CA, USA.**

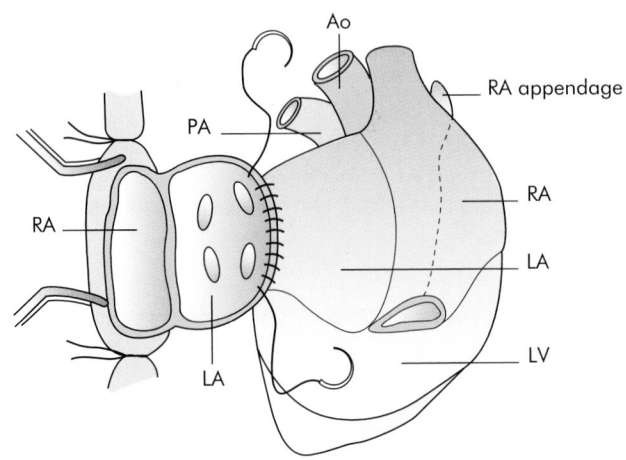

Figure 77.26 Implantation of the donor heart. The donor left atrium is opened by an incision connecting the four pulmonary veins, excising the central portion. The left atrial anastomosis is performed, starting at the lateral wall of the donor and continuing inferiorly and superiorly, concluding with the inter-atrial septum. The right atrial anastomosis is performed, matching the recipient atrium by an incision towards the donor right atrial appendage (dotted line), which avoids the sinus node at the cavoatrial junction. Finally, the pulmonary artery and aortic anastomosis are completed. Abbreviations as for Fig. 77.25 (courtesy of J. Dunning).

whom there is cardiac dysfunction because of congenital (e.g. Eisenmenger's syndrome, in which the left-to-right shunt is reversed because of pulmonary hypertension) or acquired cardiac dysfunction. For most patients with end-stage pulmonary disease, however, single- or double-lung transplantation has now replaced heart–lung transplantation. Lung transplantation is more economical in terms of organ use although, if heart–lung transplantation is undertaken for isolated respiratory disease, the healthy native heart can be used for transplantation, the so called 'domino procedure'. Heart–lung transplantation is performed through a median sternotomy, taking particular care to avoid injury to the phrenic, vagus and recurrent laryngeal nerves during excision of the recipient heart and lungs. The recipient right atrium and aorta are divided as for orthotopic cardiac transplantation and the donor heart–lung block readied for implantation, incising the right atrium from the divided inferior vena cava. An end-to-end tracheal anastomosis is performed and the right atrial and aortic anastomoses are performed as for cardiac transplantation.

Single- and double-lung transplantation are effective therapies for selected patients with end-stage chronic lung disease, in whom declining lung function limits life expectancy despite optimal medical therapy. Common indications are pulmonary fibrosis, pulmonary hypertension, emphysema and cystic fibrosis. Single-lung transplantation can be performed for pulmonary fibrosis. Single-lung transplantation is performed through a posterolateral thoracotomy and double-lung transplantation through a bilateral thoracotomy or median sternotomy. During lung transplantation, the donor pulmonary veins on a left atrial cuff are anastomosed to the recipient left atrium. Next, the bronchial anastomosis and the pulmonary arterial anastomosis are completed. Cardiopulmonary bypass is usually required if pulmonary hypertension is

present. Dehiscence of the airway anastomosis used to be common after heart–lung and lung transplantation, but improvements in organ preservation and surgical technique have dramatically reduced the incidence of this often fatal complication to < 5%. Late airway stenosis at the bronchial anastomosis because of ischaemia occurs in around 10% of bronchial anastomoses and is treated by dilatation.

Outcome after thoracic organ transplantation

The 1- and 5-year graft survival rates after heart transplantation are around 85% and 70% respectively. The results after heart–lung and lung transplantation are less good, with 1-year graft survival rates of around 75% and 5-year survival rates of around 40%.

FUTURE PROSPECTS

The two major problems in organ transplantation are:

- chronic graft rejection and the side-effects of non-specific immunosuppression;
- the shortage of organs for transplantation.

New immunosuppressive agents that have fewer or different agent-specific side-effects from existing therapies are likely to enter clinical practice and there is continuing research into the development of non-invasive biomarkers (in urine or blood) that will allow early diagnosis of graft rejection. A longstanding goal in organ transplantation has been the development of strategies for inducing specific immunological tolerance. Transplantation tolerance would eliminate the need for long-term non-specific immunosuppressive agents, leaving the immune system intact for defence against infection. It has long been possible to induce transplant tolerance in experimental animals with a variety of preconditioning regimens that often involve pretreatment schedules using donor bone marrow cells or donor antigen. So far, however, there is no clinically applicable strategy for inducing transplant tolerance.

The demand for human organs for transplantation is so great that deceased donors cannot ever satisfy it. Many consider that the solution is to perfect xenotransplantation, and there is general agreement that the pig is the most suitable source of xenogeneic organs. However, all humans have pre-formed antibodies directed against carbohydrate antigens expressed by pig organs and these cause hyperacute rejection. The dominant carbohydrate antigen responsible is gal-1,3-αgal. Progress has been made towards circumventing hyperacute xenograft rejection and pigs that have been genetically engineered not to express the gal-1,3-αgal antigen have been produced. However, organs from genetically modified pigs are still rejected within a few weeks by primates, despite the use of potent immunosuppressive agents. In addition to the complex immunological problems posed by xenotransplantation there is a risk that pig organs may transmit infectious agents, and there is particular concern about the risks posed by porcine endogenous retrovirus (PERV). Lastly, there are unanswered questions regarding the extent to which pig organs are able to fulfil the physiological demands required of them after transplantation into a human.

Finally, looking to the future, there is optimism that human pluripotent stem cells may ultimately provide a source of tissue transplants for treating a wide range of diseases. Attempts are now under way to define the cell signals needed to guide human

CHAPTER 77 | TRANSPLANTATION

embryonic and adult stem cells to differentiate *in vitro* into functional tissue of the desired cell type. These include insulin-producing cells, cardiac myocytes and neuronal tissue. Although cell transplantation is the initial goal, by combining the developments in stem cell medicine with those taking place in tissue engineering and biomaterials it may one day be possible to engineer more complex vascularised grafts for transplantation (Summary box 77.12).

Summary box 77.12

Future developments in transplantation

- Novel immunosuppressive agents
- Development of non-invasive biomarkers for monitoring rejection
- Strategies for inducing donor-specific immunological tolerance
- Xenotransplantation
- Stem cell medicine and tissue engineering

FURTHER READING

Busuttil, R.M. and Klintmalm, G.B. (eds) (2005) *Transplantation of the Liver*, 2nd edn. W.B. Saunders, Philadelphia, PA, USA.

Collins, G.M., Dubernard, J.M., Land, W. and Persijn, G.G. (eds) (1997) *Procurement, Preservation and Allocation of Vascularised Organs*. Kluwer Academic Publishers, Dordrecht, Netherlands.

---

in vitro **is Latin for 'in the glass'.**

Danovitch, G.M. (ed.) (2004) *Handbook of Kidney Transplantation.* Lippincott Williams & Wilkins, Philadelphia, PA, USA.

Forsythe, J.L.R. (ed.) (2005) *Transplantation – a Companion to Specialist Surgical Practice*, 3rd edn. W.B. Saunders, London.

Morris, P.J. (ed.) (2001) *Kidney Transplantation: Principles and Practices*, 5th edn. W.B. Saunders, Philadelphia, PA, USA.

Schofield, P.M. and Corris, P.A. (1998) *Management of Heart and Lung Transplantation Patients*. W.B. Saunders, Philadelphia, PA.

WEBSITE ADDRESSES FOR SELECTED NATIONAL AND INTERNATIONAL TRANSPLANT DATABASES

Collaborative Transplant Study (Europe): www.ctstransplant.org
European Liver Transplant Registry: www.eltr.org
Scandiatransplant: www.scandiatransplant.org
UK Transplant: www.uktransplant.org.uk
United Network for Organ Sharing (USA): www.unos.org

WEBSITE ADDRESSES FOR USEFUL CLINICAL GUIDELINES IN ORGAN TRANSPLANTATION

UK guidelines on CMV in transplantation: www.bts.org.uk
UK guidelines for living donor kidney transplantation: www.bts.org.uk
UK guidelines relating to solid organ transplantation from NHBD. www.bts.org.uk

Common instruments on the general tray

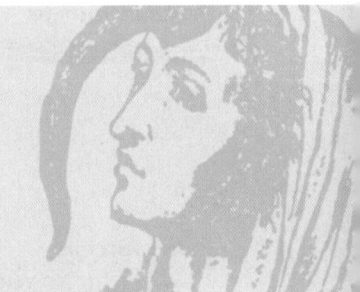

This is a list of common instruments on the general tray with some information how they are used and about the people associated with them.

Langenbeck retractor

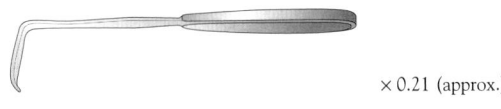

× 0.21 (approx.)

This small general purpose retractor is useful for holding open wounds, such as in an open appendicectomy. They are often used in pairs (one in each of the assistant's hands). They stay in position best if the handles are lifted slightly so that the tips lock in under the fascia. Bernhard Rudolf Konrad von Langenbeck (1810–1887) was Professor of Surgery successively at Keil and Berlin, Germany. He performed the first internal fixation of a femoral neck fracture in 1850.

Morris retractor

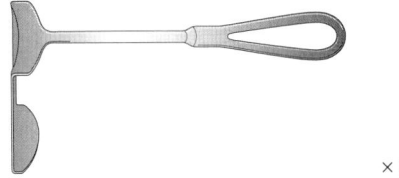

× 0.20 (approx.)

This is a big retractor which is useful for giving maximum exposure in large incisions such as those used in the abdomen. It can be used to improve visibility off to one side of an incision (by pulling firmly in that direction) so is valuable during the initial phase of a laparotomy. Sir Henry Morris (1844–1926) was a surgeon at the Middlesex Hospital, London, UK.

Deaver retractor

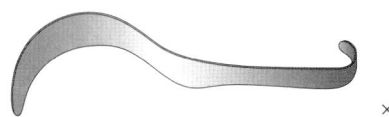

× 0.15 (approx.)

This retractor is specifically designed for holding the liver up out of the way during a cholecystectomy. It needs to be used carefully to avoid damaging the liver. Some surgeons protect the liver with an abdominal pack before placing the blade on top. John Blair Deaver (1855–1931) was Professor of Surgery at the University of Pennsylvania Medical School, Philadelphia, USA. He also described a paramedian incision for appendicectomy.

McIndoe scissors

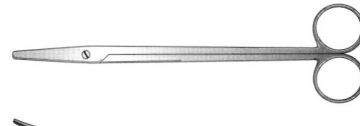

× 0.42 (approx.)

Scissors are used by surgeons to perform dissection respecting anatomical planes. The closed blades are inserted into a fascial plane, and then gently opened. The tissue to be divided can then be seen clearly and divided without risk of damage to vital structures. Sir Archibald Hector McIndoe (1900–1960) was a plastic surgeon at St Bartholomew's Hospital, London, and the Queen Victoria Hospital, East Grinstead, UK. He was born in New Zealand (cousin of Harold Gillies) and became a consultant plastic surgeon to the RAF during WW2. He supervised the rehabilitation of badly disfigured airmen who later formed the Guinea Pig Club.

DeBakey forceps

× 0.21 (approx.)

These forceps allow the surgeon to grasp tissues firmly while minimising damage to the tissue held in the jaws of the forceps. They are useful for holding vessel walls in vascular surgery. Michael Ellis DeBakey (born 1908) was Professor of Surgery at Baylor University College of Medicine, Houston, USA. He was the first to successfully implant an artificial heart, and he also performed the first successful carotid endarterectomy.

Gillies forceps

× 0.29 (approx.)

These forceps have teeth and are ideal for holding tough tissues such as skin. Sir Harold Gillies (1882–1960) was a plastic surgeon at St Bartholomew's Hospital, London, UK. He was born in New Zealand (cousin of Archibald McIndoe) and became one of the founders of British plastic surgery. He originated the tubed pedicle flap.

Adson forceps

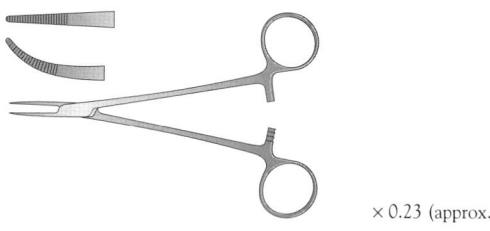

These forceps are non-toothed, and so are ideal for holding delicate tissues such as bowel. Alfred Washington Adson (1887–1951) was Professor of Neurosurgery at the Mayo Clinic, Rochester, USA. He was one of the first to use sympathectomy for the treatment of hypertension, and cervical sympathectomy for Raynaud's syndrome.

× 0.23 (approx.)

Allis forceps

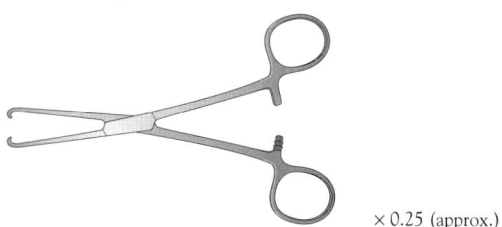

These forceps are used to hold soft tissues for a long period while minimising tissue damage. Using the ratchet they can be locked on to tissue such as bowel and can be used to provide gentle traction. Oscar Huntington Allis (1836–1921) was a surgeon at the Presbyterian Hospital, Philadelphia, USA.

× 0.25 (approx.)

Spencer Wells forceps

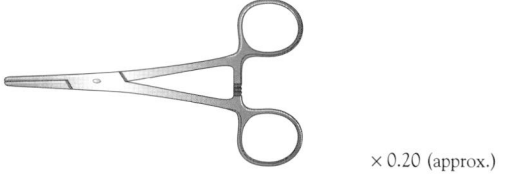

These were one of the first ratchet forceps ever designed and are still very useful. They are often used in pairs for clamping an artery before dividing it. The cut ends of the artery are then tied off, and the forceps removed (carefully!). Sir Thomas Spencer Wells (1818–1897) was a surgeon at the Samaritan Free Hospital for Women and Children, London, UK. He was one of the earliest surgeons to make use of anaesthetics in operation.

× 0.20 (approx.)

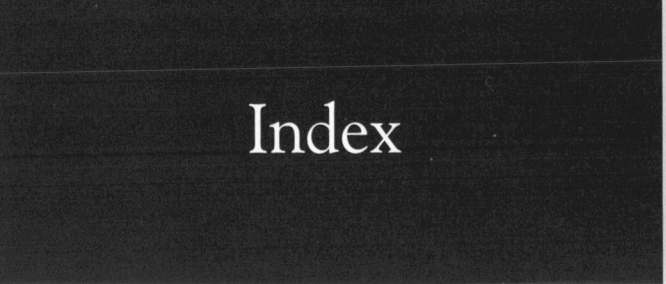

Index

Page references followed by f indicate figures: those followed by t indicate tables and those followed by b indicate boxed material. To save space in the index, the following abbreviations have been used:

CABG – coronary artery bypass grafting
CT – computerised tomography
ERCP – endoscopic retrograde cholangiopancreatography
GORD – gastro-oesophageal reflux disease
MRI-magnetic resonance imaging

Key to letters following page numbers: b, box; f, figure; t, table

To save space in the index, some terms have been abbreviated; see p. 1433

Key to letters following page numbers: b, box; f, figure; t, table

To save space in the index, some terms have been abbreviated; see p. 1433

Key to letters following page numbers: b, box; f, figure; t, table

To save space in the index, some terms have been abbreviated; see p. 1433

INDEX

Key to letters following page numbers: b, box; f, figure; t, table

To save space in the index, some terms have been abbreviated; see p. 1433

INDEX

To save space in the index, some terms have been abbreviated; see p. 1433

Key to letters following page numbers: b, box; f, figure; t, table

INDEX

Key to letters following page numbers: b, box; f, figure; t, table

INDEX

To save space in the index, some terms have been abbreviated; see p. 1433

Key to letters following page numbers: b, box; f, figure; t, table

To save space in the index, some terms have been abbreviated; see p. 1433

INDEX

Key to letters following page numbers: b, box; f, figure; t, table

To save space in the index, some terms have been abbreviated; see p. 1433

INDEX

To save space in the index, some terms have been abbreviated; see p. 1433

Key to letters following page numbers: b, box; f, figure; t, table

To save space in the index, some terms have been abbreviated; see p. 1433

Key to letters following page numbers: b, box; f, figure; t, table

To save space in the index, some terms have been abbreviated; see p. 1433

To save space in the index, some terms have been abbreviated; see p. 1433

Key to letters following page numbers: b, box; f, figure; t, table

To save space in the index, some terms have been abbreviated; see p. 1433

To save space in the index, some terms have been abbreviated; see p. 1433

Key to letters following page numbers: b, box; f, figure; t, table

To save space in the index, some terms have been abbreviated; see p. 1433

To save space in the index, some terms have been abbreviated; see p. 1433

To save space in the index, some terms have been abbreviated; see p. 1433

Key to letters following page numbers: b, box; f, figure; t, table

To save space in the index, some terms have been abbreviated; see p. 1433

Key to letters following page numbers: b, box; f, figure; t, table

To save space in the index, some terms have been abbreviated; see p. 1433

Key to letters following page numbers: b, box; f, figure; t, table

To save space in the index, some terms have been abbreviated; see p. 1433

To save space in the index, some terms have been abbreviated; see p. 1433

Key to letters following page numbers: b, box; f, figure; t, table

To save space in the index, some terms have been abbreviated; see p. 1433

INDEX

Key to letters following page numbers: b, box; f, figure; t, table

To save space in the index, some terms have been abbreviated; see p. 1433

Key to letters following page numbers: b, box; f, figure; t, table

Key to letters following page numbers: b, box; f, figure; t, table

To save space in the index, some terms have been abbreviated; see p. 1433

Key to letters following page numbers: b, box; f, figure; t, table

To save space in the index, some terms have been abbreviated; see p. 1433

Key to letters following page numbers: b, box; f, figure; t, table

Key to letters following page numbers: b, box; f, figure; t, table

To save space in the index, some terms have been abbreviated; see p. 1433

Key to letters following page numbers: b, box; f, figure; t, table

INDEX

To save space in the index, some terms have been abbreviated; see p. 1433

INDEX

To save space in the index, some terms have been abbreviated; see p. 1433

Key to letters following page numbers: b, box; f, figure; t, table

INDEX

To save space in the index, some terms have been abbreviated; see p. 1433

Key to letters following page numbers: b, box; f, figure; t, table

To save space in the index, some terms have been abbreviated; see p. 1433

Key to letters following page numbers: b, box; f, figure; t, table

To save space in the index, some terms have been abbreviated; see p. 1433

INDEX

Key to letters following page numbers: b, box; f, figure; t, table

To save space in the index, some terms have been abbreviated; see p. 1433